COLOR PLATES

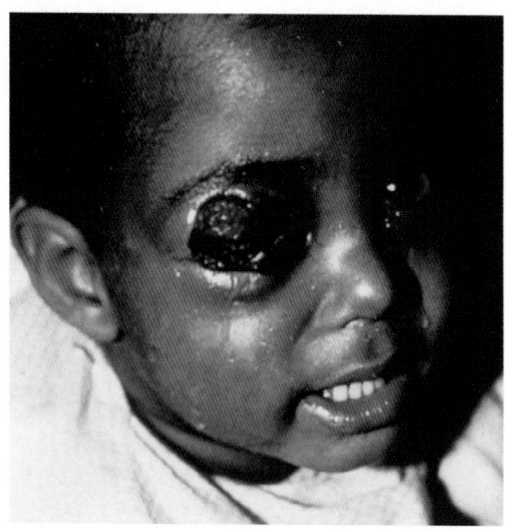

FIGURE 7.2 Cutaneous anthrax on the eyelids of a young child. (Courtesy of Dr. Larry Schwab. From Ostler HB, Maibach HI, Hoke AW, et al. *Diseases of the eye and skin: a color atlas*. Philadelphia: Lippincott Williams Wilkins, 2004, with permission.)

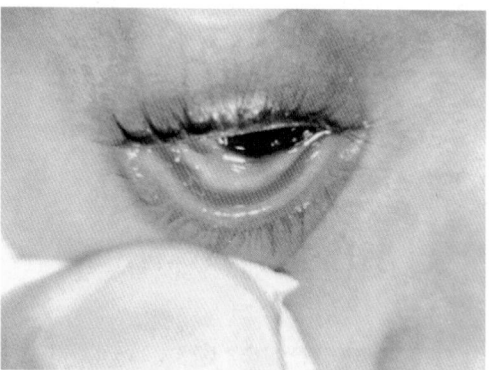

FIGURE 23.1 Pseudomembrane on lower lid palpebral conjunctiva and extending into the inferior fornix in patient with epidemic keratoconjunctivitis (adenovirus).

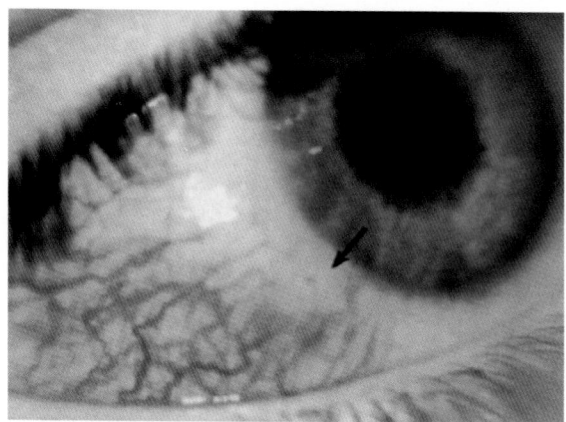

FIGURE 23.5 Red eye caused by chickenpox (varicella) involvement of conjunctiva. Note sectorial injection of conjunctiva. White area *(arrow)* at junction of conjunctiva and cornea is the pox lesion.

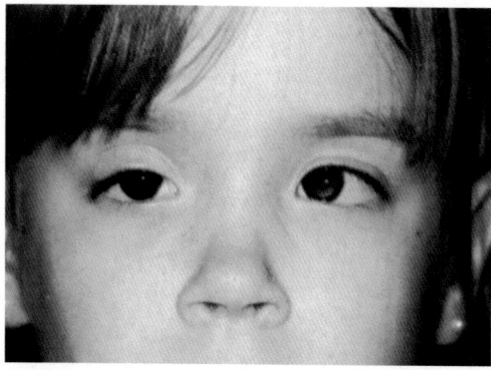

FIGURE 24.7 Left esotropia. Note lateral displacement of Hirschberg light reflex in the left eye. Photograph demonstrates right ptosis. Pupils are pharmacologically dilated. Asymmetry of red reflex is caused by misalignment of the eyes.

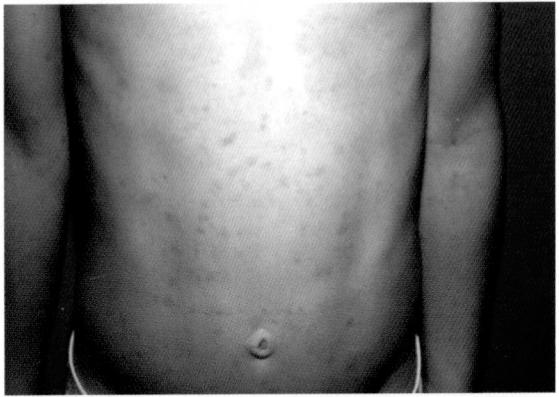

FIGURE 61.2 Pityriasis Rosea. (Courtesy of the Walter W. Tunnessen Pediatric Image Library, which is supported by the Foerderer Foundation.)

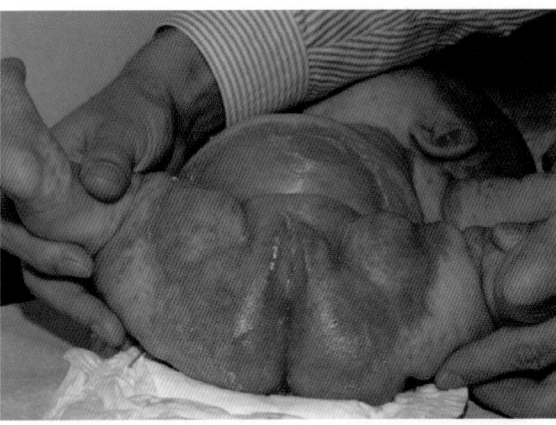

FIGURE 61.3 Candida moniliasis. (Courtesy of the Walter W. Tunnessen Pediatric Image Library, which is supported by the Foerderer Foundation.)

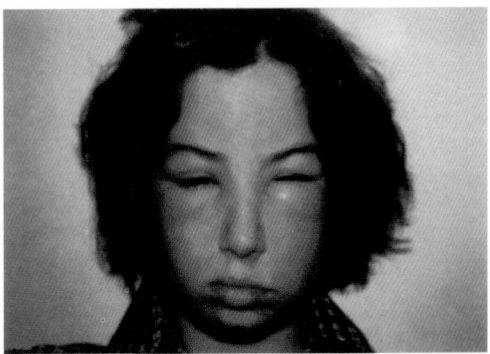

FIGURE 85.12 Facial edema and inflammation in response to exposure to airborne contact allergen (e.g., vaporized oil in smoke of burned poison ivy plants).

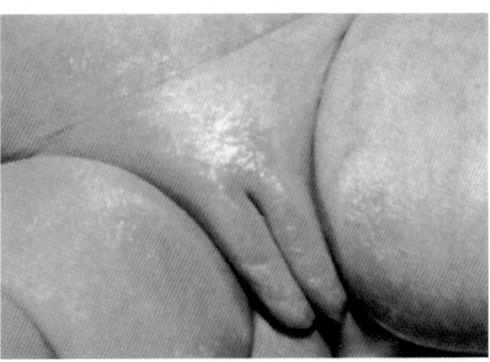

FIGURE 85.15 Infant with occlusion diaper dermatitis.

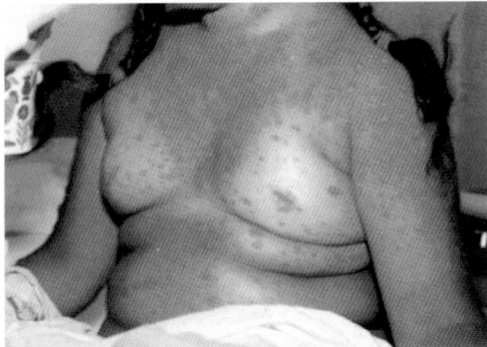

FIGURE 85.19 Same child as seen in Figure 85.18 with Stevens-Johnson syndrome secondary to sulfonamides. Note photo distribution of lesions.

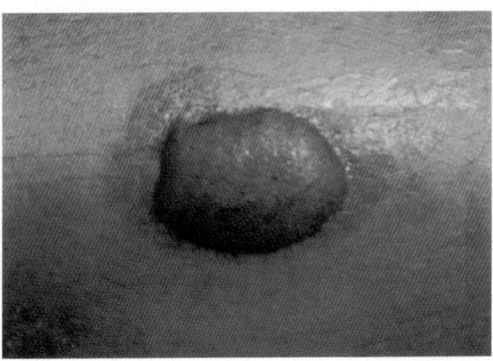

FIGURE 85.21 Hemorrhagic bulla in patient with vasculitis.

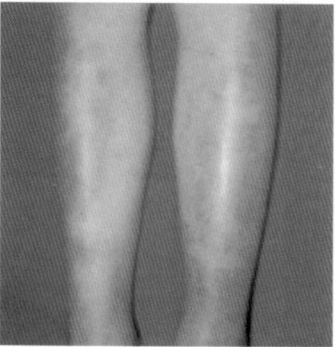

FIGURE 85.22 Extensor surface involved with lesions of erythema nodosum.

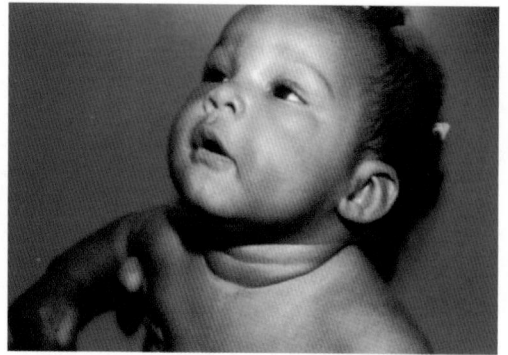

FIGURE 85.41 Infant with popsicle panniculitis of the cheek.

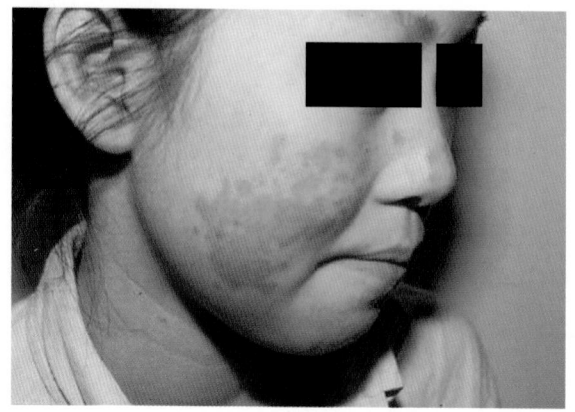

FIGURE 101.6 Adolescent girl with discoid lesions in malar distribution.

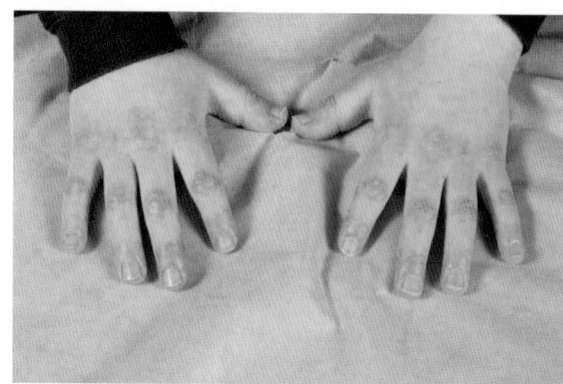

FIGURE 101.9 Gottron papules in juvenile dermatomyositis (JDMS). (Courtesy of Lisa Rider, MD.)

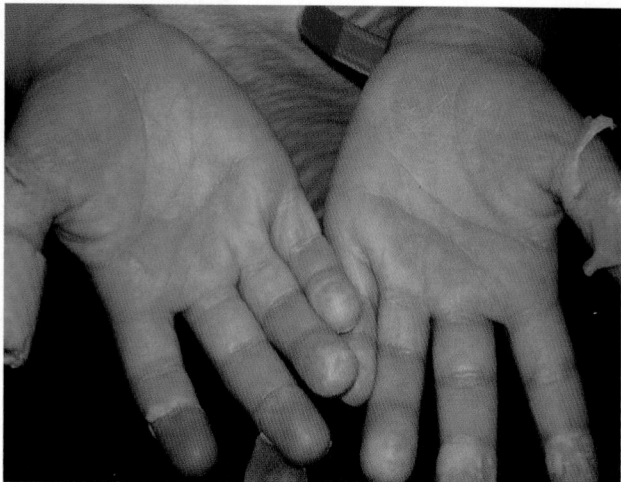

FIGURE 101.13 Periungual desquamation during the convalescent phase of Kawasaki disease.

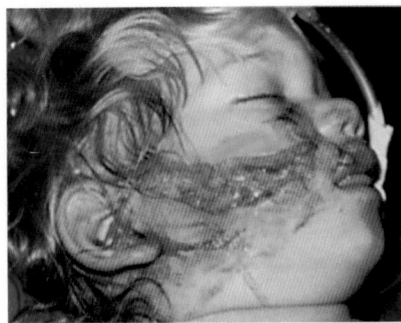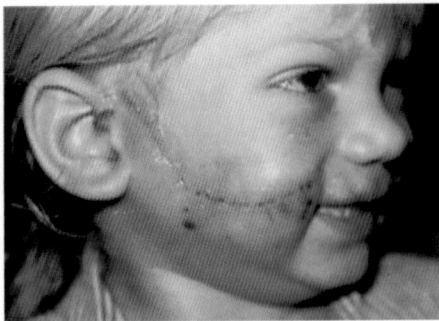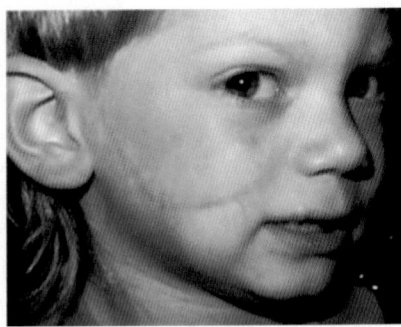

FIGURE 111.6 Photographs of a 3-year-old boy after an attack by a dog. The **top** photograph shows the child before sharp debridement, facial nerve exploration, and layered closure of his complex wound. The **middle** panel is a photograph of the child 1 week after his repair and demonstrates the precise reapproximation of the facial soft tissues. The **bottom** photograph was taken 8 months after the attack and demonstrates a nicely healed facial scar that will continue to fade and soften. (Courtesy of David W. Low, MD.)

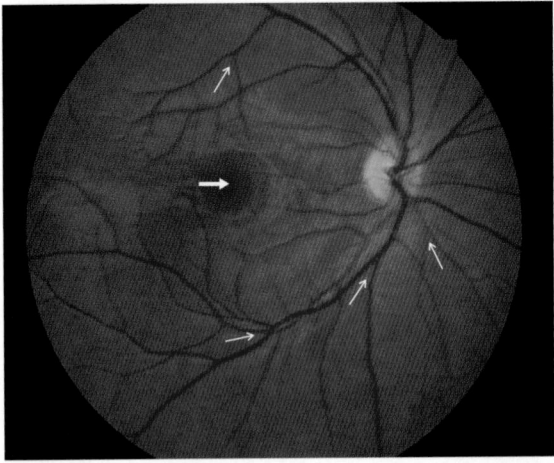

FIGURE 117.2 Normal right retina as viewed by indirect ophthalmoscope. Central dark area *(thick arrow)* represents fovea. Note that the apex of the branch point of the blood vessels *(thin arrows)* always points back toward the direction of the optic nerve head.

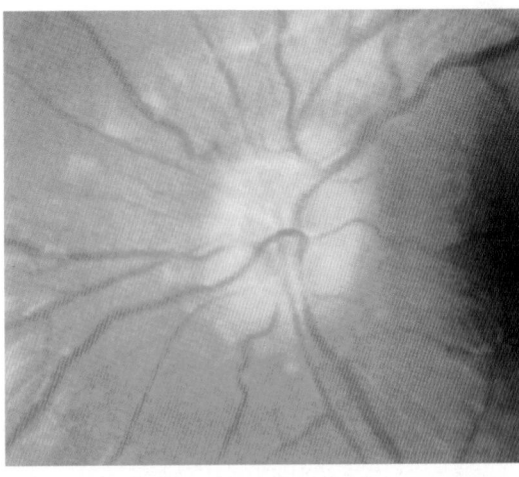

FIGURE 117.3 Papilledema. Note blurred disc margins and loss of view of blood vessels on disc.

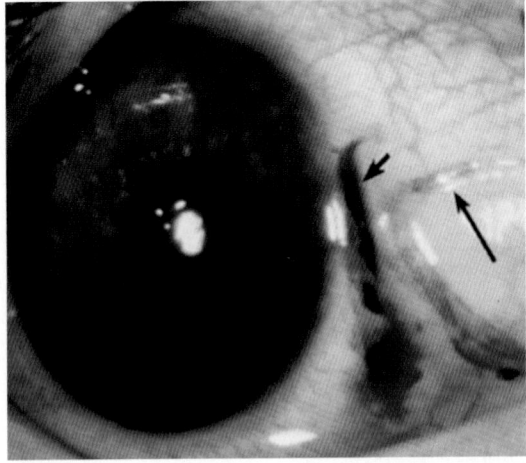

FIGURE 117.7 Ruptured globe. The scleral laceration *(short arrow)* appears as a linear brown line on the white of the eye. The pupil has a teardrop shape, the apex of which points in the direction of the rupture. The *long arrow* points to the upper border of a large conjunctival laceration. Note that the underlying sclera is intact under the conjunctival laceration. There is a diffuse hyphema in the anterior chamber, which partially obscures the pupil.

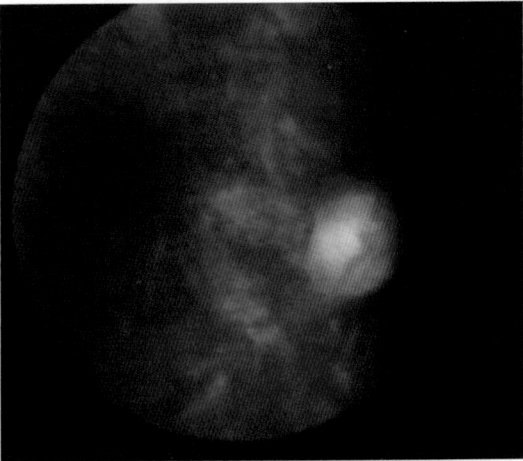

FIGURE 117.14 Retinal hemorrhages in abusive head injury.

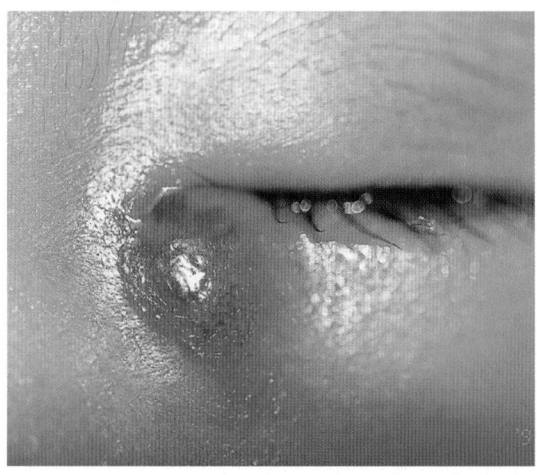

FIGURE 119.5 Dermoid cyst abscess. (From Fleisher GR, Ludwig W, Baskin MN, eds. *Atlas of pediatric emergency medicine*. Philadelphia, PA: Lippincott Williams & Wilkins, 2004. Reprinted with permission.)

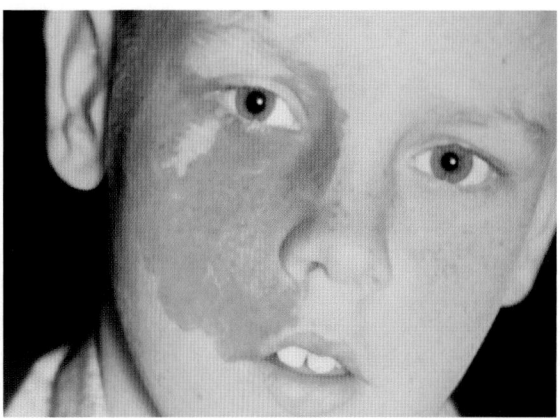

FIGURE 119.15 Facial port-wine stain. (From Weber J, Kelley J. *Health assessment in nursing*, 2nd ed. Philadelphia, PA: Lippincott Williams & Wilkins, 2003.)

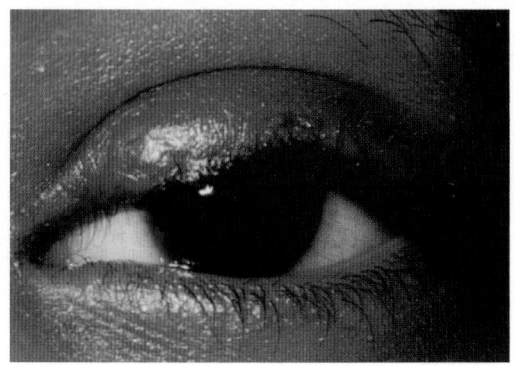

FIGURE 127.4 Acute sty (external hordeolum).

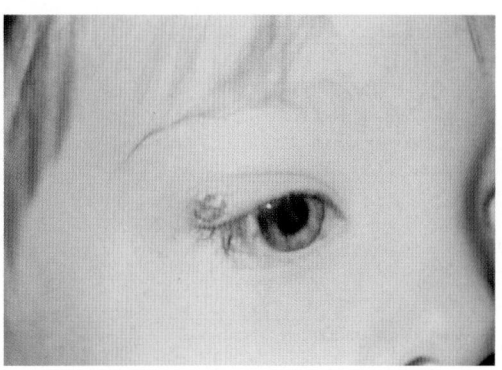

FIGURE 127.5 Chalazion draining spontaneously via skin.

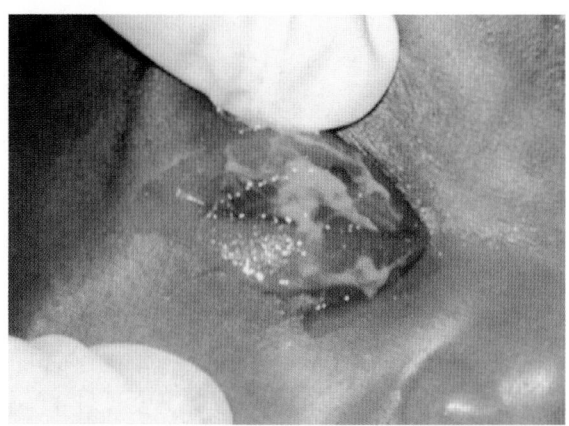

FIGURE 127.7 Neonatal gonorrheal conjunctivitis. Note the dramatic lid swelling and severe purulent discharge.

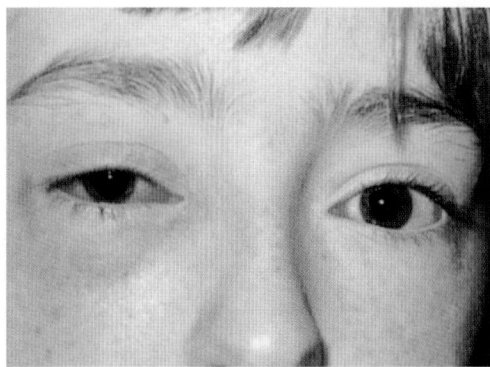

FIGURE 127.8 Patient with right epidemic keratoconjunctivitis infection. Note the lid swelling, red eye, and absence of purulent discharge. Patient also has right preauricular adenopathy (not visible). Note the early injection of left eye, representing sequential involvement.

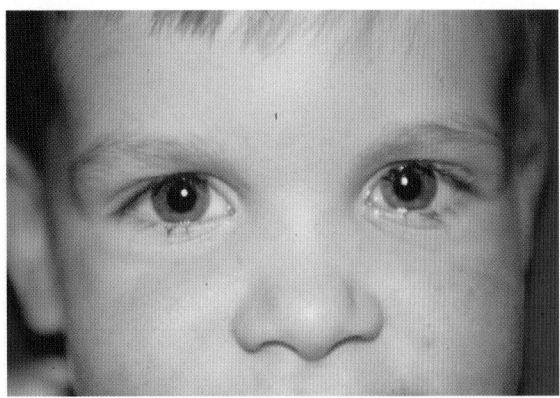

FIGURE 127.10 Left nasolacrimal duct obstruction. Note discharge on medial lower lid and wet lower lid lashes. The conjunctiva is non-inflamed (no "red eye") indicating that the child does not have conjunctivitis.

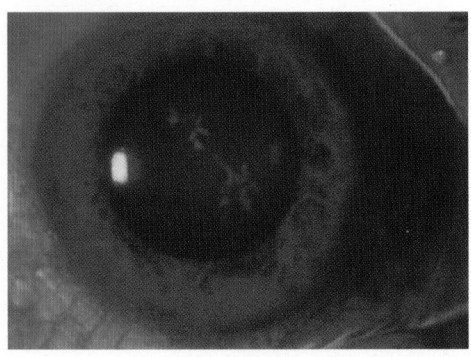

FIGURE 127.11 Fluorescein staining pattern of herpes simplex virus corneal infection. Eye is illuminated with blue light to demonstrate yellow/green branching fluorescein staining pattern of herpetic dendrite.

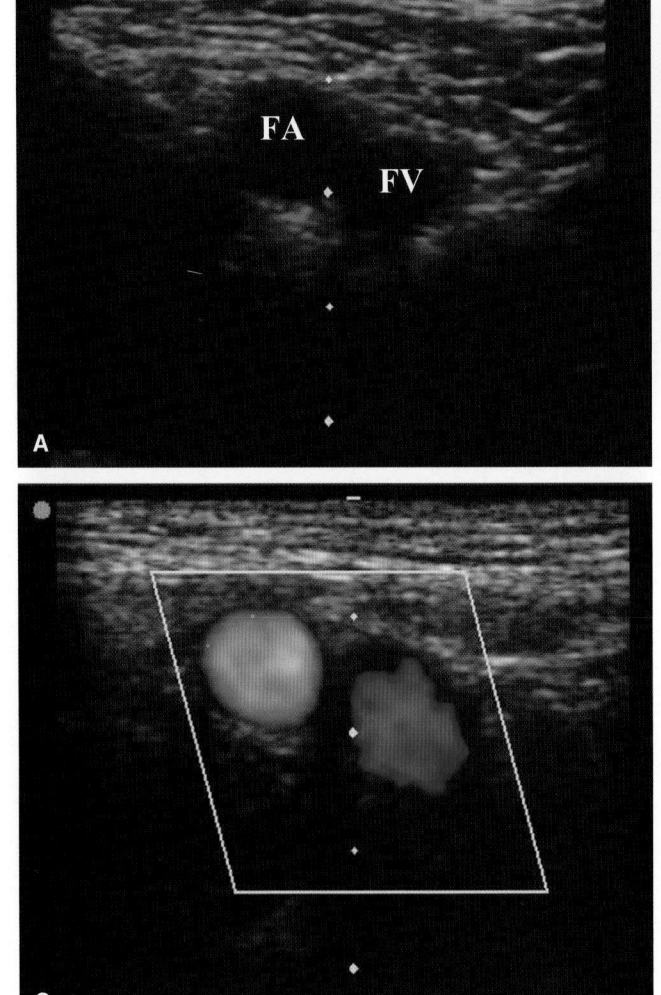

FIGURE 134.20 Femoral vascular anatomy. A: Femoral artery *(FA)* and femoral vein *(FV)*. B: During compression, the vein collapses and is not visible, whereas the artery remains patent and visible by ultrasound. C: The femoral artery will pulsate, whereas the vein will have low constant flow or no flow depending on the sensitivity settings of the color Doppler.

SIXTH EDITION

TEXTBOOK OF PEDIATRIC EMERGENCY MEDICINE

SIXTH EDITION

TEXTBOOK OF PEDIATRIC EMERGENCY MEDICINE

Editors

Gary R. Fleisher, MD
Egan Family Foundation Professor
Department of Pediatrics
Harvard Medical School;
Pediatrician-in-Chief and Chair
Department of Medicine
Children's Hospital of Boston
Boston, Massachusetts

Stephen Ludwig, MD
Professor of Pediatrics and Emergency Medicine
University of Pennsylvania School of Medicine
Senior Advisor for Medical Education
John H. and Hortense Cassel Jensen Chair
Children's Hospital of Philadelphia
Philadelphia, Pennsylvania

Associate Editors

Richard G. Bachur, MD
Associate Professor
Department of Pediatrics
Harvard Medical School
Chief, Division of Emergency Medicine
Children's Hospital Boston
Boston, Massachusetts

Marc H. Gorelick, MD, MSCE
Professor
Departments of Pediatrics and Population Health
Medical College of Wisconsin;
Jon E. Vice Chair in Emergency Medicine
Children's Hospital of Wisconsin
Milwaukee, Wisconsin

Kathy N. Shaw, MD, MSCE
Professor and Associate Chair
Department of Pediatrics
University of Pennsylvania School of Medicine;
Division Chief
Department of Emergency Medicine
The Children's Hospital of Philadelphia
Philadelphia, Pennsylvania

Richard M. Ruddy, MD
Professor of Clinical Pediatrics
Department of Pediatrics
University of Cincinnati College of Medicine;
Director
Division of Emergency Medicine
Cincinnati Children's Hospital Medical Center
Cincinnati, Ohio

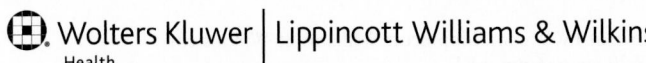

Wolters Kluwer | Lippincott Williams & Wilkins
Health
Philadelphia • Baltimore • New York • London
Buenos Aires • Hong Kong • Sydney • Tokyo

Acquisitions Editor: Frances DeStefano
Product Director: Julia Seto
Production Manager: Bridgett Dougherty
Senior Manufacturing Manager: Benjamin Rivera
Senior Marketing Manager: Angela Panetta
Design Coordinator: Terry Mallon
Production Service: Aptara®, Inc.

Printed in China

Library of Congress Cataloging-in-Publication Data

Textbook of pediatric emergency medicine / editors Gary R. Fleisher,
Stephen Ludwig.—6th ed.
    p. ; cm.
    Includes bibliographical references and index.
    ISBN 978-1-60547-159-4 (alk. paper)
1. Pediatric emergencies. I. Fleisher, Gary R. (Gary Robert), 1951–
II. Ludwig, Stephen, 1945–
    [DNLM: 1. Child. 2. Emergencies. 3. Critical Care. 4. Emergency
Treatment. 5. Infant. WS 205 T355 2010]
    RJ370.T48 2010
    618.92′0025—dc22   2010002547

Care has been taken to confirm the accuracy of the information presented and to describe generally
accepted practices. However, the authors, editors, and publisher are not responsible for errors or omissions or for any consequences from application of the information in this book and make no warranty,
expressed or implied, with respect to the currency, completeness, or accuracy of the contents of the publication. Application of the information in a particular situation remains the professional responsibility
of the practitioner.

The authors, editors, and publisher have exerted every effort to ensure that drug selection and
dosage set forth in this text are in accordance with current recommendations and practice at the time of
publication. However, in view of ongoing research, changes in government regulations, and the constant
flow of information relating to drug therapy and drug reactions, the reader is urged to check the
package insert for each drug for any change in indications and dosage and for added warnings and precautions. This is particularly important when the recommended agent is a new or infrequently employed
drug.

Some drugs and medical devices presented in the publication have Food and Drug Administration
(FDA) clearance for limited use in restricted research settings. It is the responsibility of the health care
provider to ascertain the FDA status of each drug or device planned for use in their clinical practice.

To purchase additional copies of this book, call our customer service department at (800) 638-3030 or
fax orders to (301) 223-2320. International customers should call (301) 223-2300.

Visit Lippincott Williams & Wilkins on the Internet: at LWW.com. Lippincott Williams & Wilkins customer service representatives are available from 8:30 am to 6 pm, EST.

10 9 8 7 6 5 4 3 2 1

■CONTRIBUTING AUTHORS

Michael S.D. Agus, MD
Assistant Professor
Department of Pediatrics
Harvard Medical School;
Director
Medicine Critical Care Program
Department of Medicine
Children's Hospital Boston
Boston, Massachusetts

Evaline A. Alessandrini, MD, MSCE
Professor
Department of Pediatrics
University of Cincinnati College of Medicine;
Director, Quality Scholars Program in Health Care
    Transformation
Divisions of Health Policy & Clinical Effectiveness and
    Emergency Medicine
Cincinnati Children's Hospital Medical Center
Cincinnati, Ohio

Elizabeth R. Alpern, MD, MSCE
Associate Professor
Department of Pediatrics, Division of Emergency Medicine
The University of Pennsylvania School of Medicine;
Director of Research and Attending Physician
Department of Pediatrics, Division of Emergency Medicine
The Children's Hospital of Philadelphia
Philadelphia, Pennsylvania

Angela C. Anderson, MD, FAAP
Associate Professor of Emergency Medicine and Pediatrics
The Warren Alpert School of Medicine at Brown University
Brown University;
Physician, Pediatric Emergency Medicine
Departments of Emergency Medicine and Pediatrics
Rhode Island and Hasbro Children's Hospitals
Providence, Rhode Island

Amy M. Arnett, MD
Assistant Professor
Department of Pediatrics
The Ohio State University College of Medicine;
Attending Physician, Emergency Medicine
Pediatric Medical Director, NCH Critical Care
    Transport Team
Department of Emergency Medicine
Nationwide Children's Hospital
Columbus, Ohio

Paul L. Aronson, MD
Instructor
Department of Pediatrics
The University of Pennsylvania School of Medicine;
Fellow
Division of Emergency Medicine
The Children's Hospital of Philadelphia
Philadelphia, Pennsylvania

Magdy W. Attia, MD
Professor
Department of Pediatrics
Jefferson Medical College
Philadelphia, Pennsylvania;
Fellowship Director, Associate Director
Division of Emergency Medicine
Alfred I. DuPont Hospital for Children
Wilmington, Delaware

Jeffrey R. Avner, MD, FAAP
Professor
Department of Pediatrics
Albert Einstein College of Medicine;
Section Chief
Pediatric Emergency Medicine
Children's Hospital at Montefiore
Bronx, New York

Lynn Babcock Cimpello, MD
Associate Professor of Clinical Pediatrics
Division of Emergency Medicine
University of Cincinnati College of Medicine;
Cincinnati Children's Hospital Medical Center
Cincinnati, Ohio

David Bachman, MD
Department of Emergency Medicine
Central Maine Medical Center
Lewiston, Maine

Richard G. Bachur, MD
Associate Professor
Department of Pediatrics
Harvard Medical School
Chief, Division of Emergency Medicine
Children's Hospital Boston
Boston, Massachusetts

Donald S. Bae, MD
Assistant Professor
Department of Orthopaedic Surgery
Harvard Medical School;
Attending Physician
Department of Orthopaedic Surgery
Children's Hospital Boston
Boston, Massachusetts

M. Douglas Baker, MD
Professor
Department of Pediatrics
UT Southwestern Medical Center
Dallas, Texas

Marc N. Baskin, MD
Assistant Professor
Department of Pediatrics
Harvard Medical School;
Associate Physician in Medicine
Division of Emergency Medicine
Children's Hospital Boston;
Service Chief
Short Stay Unit
Children's Hospital Boston
Boston, Massachusetts

Carl R. Baum, MD
Associate Professor of Pediatrics
Yale University School of Medicine;
Attending Physician
Section of Pediatric Emergency Medicine and Center
    for Children's Environmental Toxicology
Yale-New Haven Children's Hospital
New Haven, Connecticut

Louis M. Bell, MD
Professor
Department of Pediatrics
University of Pennsylvania;
Associate Chair of Clinical Activities
Department of Pediatrics
The Children's Hospital of Philadelphia
Philadelphia, Pennsylvania

Deena Berkowitz, MD, MPH
Assistant Professor
Departments of Pediatrics and Emergency Medicine
The George Washington University School of Medicine
    and Health Sciences;
Attending Physician
Department of Emergency Medicine
Children's National Medical Center
Washington, DC

Amy L. Billett, MD
Associate Professor in Pediatrics
Harvard Medical School;
Director of Safety and Quality
Department of Pediatric Oncology
Dana-Farber Cancer Institute
Boston, Massachusetts

Charles D. Blackwell, MD
Attending Physician
Department of Pediatric Emergency Medicine
Children's Hospitals and Clinics of Minnesota
Minneapolis, Minneapolis

Robert G. Bolte, MD
Professor
Department of Pediatrics
University of Utah School of Medicine;
Associate Director, Trauma Service
Division of Pediatric Emergency Medicine
Primary Children's Medical Center
Salt Lake City, Utah

Alison Brent, MD
Associate Professor
Department of Emergency Medicine
University of Colorado Health and Sciences Center
Aurora, Colorado
The Children's Hospital

Linda L. Brown, MD, MSCE
Assistant Professor of Emergency Medicine
    and Pediatrics
Warren Alpert Medical School of Brown University;
Physician
Pediatric Emergency Medicine
Hasbro Children's Hospital
Providence, Rhode Island

Robyn L. Byer, MD
Instructor of Pediatrics
Department of Pediatrics
Harvard Medical School;
Attending Physician
Division of Emergency Medicine
Children's Hospital Boston
Boston, Massachusetts

James M. Callahan, MD
Associate Professor of Clinical Pediatrics
Department of Pediatrics
University of Pennsylvania School of Medicine;
Director of Medical Education
Division of Emergency Medicine
The Children's Hospital of Philadelphia
Philadelphia, Pennsylvania

Leslie Castelo-Soccio, MD, PhD
Instructor
Department of Dermatology
University of Pennsylvania School of Medicine;
Attending Physician
Section of Pediatric Dermatology
Children's Hospital of Philadelphia
Philadelphia, Pennsylvania

Laura L. Chapman, MD
Assistant Professor
Department of Emergency Medicine
Warren Alpert Medical School of Brown University;
Physician
Department of Pediatric Emergency Medicine
Rhode Island and Hasbro Children's Hospitals
Providence, Rhode Island

Vincent W. Chiang, MD
Associate Professor
Department of Pediatrics
Harvard Medical School;
Chief
Inpatient Services
Department of Medicine
Children's Hospital Boston
Boston, Massachusetts

Maryanne R.K. Chrisant, MD
Division of Gastroenterology
University of Virginia Health System
Charlottesville, Virginia

Thomas H. Chun, MD
Associate Professor
Department of Emergency Medicine and Pediatrics
Brown University;
Attending Physician
Emergency Department
Hasbro Children's Hospital
Providence, Rhode Island

Sarita Chung, MD
Instructor in Pediatrics
Department of Pediatrics
Harvard Medical School;
Assistant in Medicine
Division of Emergency Medicine
Children's Hospital Boston
Boston, Massachusetts

Theodore J. Cieslak, MD
Defense Department Liaison Officer
Centers for Disease Control and Prevention
Atlanta, Georgia

Joy L. Collins, MD, FAAP
Assistant Professor
Department of Surgery
University of Pennsylvania;
Attending Surgeon
Department of General and Thoracic Surgery
The Children's Hospital of Philadelphia
Philadelphia, Pennsylvania

Erika Constantine, MD
Assistant Professor
Department of Emergency Medicine and Pediatrics
Warren Alpert Medical School of Brown University;
Attending Physician
Department of Pediatric Emergency Medicine
Rhode Island and Hasbro Children's Hospitals
Providence, Rhode Island

Jacqueline Bryngil Corboy, MD
Instructor
Department of Pediatrics
Feinberg School of Medicine;
Attending Physician
Department of Pediatrics
Children's Memorial Hospital
Chicago, Illinois

Howard M. Corneli, MD
Professor
Department of Pediatrics
University of Utah School of Medicine;
Staff Physician
Emergency Department
Primary Children's Medical Center
Salt Lake City, Utah

Kathleen M. Cronan, MD
Associate Professor
Department of Pediatrics
Jefferson Medical College
Philadelphia, Pennsylvania;
Attending Physician, Emergency Department
Director of Health Content Integration, Nemours Center for
    Children's Health Media
Nemours A. I duPont Hospital for Children
Wilmington, Delaware

Joanne M. Decker, MD (Deceased)

Carlos A. Delgado, MD, FAAP
Attending Physician, Emergency Department
Department of Pediatric Emergency Medicine
Pediatric Emergency Medicine Associates (PEMA)
Children's Healthcare of Atlanta at Scottish Rite
Atlanta, Georgia

Robert Jay Deutsch, MD, MPH, FAAP
Attending Physician, Pediatric Emergency Medicine
Department of Emergency Medicine
Emergency Medical Associates;
Attending Physician, Pediatric Emergency Medicine
Department of Emergency Medicine
Saint Barnabas Medical Center
Livingston, New Jersey

Cinnamon Dixon, DO
Pediatric Emergency Medicine Fellow
Division of Emergency Medicine
Cincinnati Children's Hospital Medical Center
Cincinnati, Ohio

Henry L. Dorkin, MD
Department of Pediatrics
Harvard Medical School;
Division of Respiratory Diseases
Children's Hospital Boston
Boston, Massachusetts

David E. Drum, MD, PhD
Clinical Associate Professor
Department of Radiology
Harvard Medical School
Boston;
Staff Physician
Department of Nuclear Medicine
VA Boston Health Care
West Roxbury, Massachusetts

Nanette C. Dudley, MD
Professor (Clinical)
Department of Pediatrics
University of Utah School of Medicine;
Attending Physician
Emergency Department
Primary Children's Medical Center
Salt Lake City, Utah

Karen Dull, MD
Instructor
Department of Pediatrics
Harvard Medical School;
Attending Physician
Division of Emergency Medicine
Children's Hospital Boston
Boston, Massachusetts

Dennis R. Durbin, MD, MSCE
Associate Professor
Departments of Pediatrics and Epidemiology
The University of Pennsylvania School of Medicine;
Director
Section of Research;
Attending Physician
Department of Emergency Medicine
The Children's Hospital of Philadelphia
Philadelphia, Pennsylvania

Edward M. Eitzen Jr., MD, MPH
Adjunct Associate Professor
Department of Emergency Medicine, Pediatrics
Uniformed Services University of the Health Sciences
Bethesda, Maryland;
Senior Partner
Biodefense and Public Health Programs
Martin-Blanck and Associates
Falls Church, Virginia

Lisa M. Elden, MD, CM
Associate Otolaryngologist
The Children's Hospital of Philadelphia;
Assistant Professor
Department of Otolaryngology
University of Pennsylvania;
Academic Institution Hospital or Institution
Philadelphia, Pennsylvania

Karan McBride Emerick, MD
Division of Gastroenterology
Connecticut Children's Medical Center
Hartford, Connecticut

Michele Burns Ewald, MD
Assistant Professor
Department of Pediatrics
Harvard Medical School;
Attending Physician and Medical Toxicology
    Fellowship Director
Division of Emergency Medicine
Children's Hospital Boston
Boston, Massachusetts

Joanna R. Fair, MD, PhD
Assistant Professor of Radiology
Department of Radiology
University of New Mexico Health Sciences Center
Albuquerque, New Mexico

Mirna M. Farah, MD
Associate Professor of Pediatrics and Emergency
    Medicine
University of Pennsylvania School of Medicine
Philadelphia, Pennsylvania

Joel A. Fein, MD, MPH
Associate Professor
Department of Pediatrics
The University of Pennsylvania School
    of Medicine;
Attending Physician
Emergency Department
The Children's Hospital of Philadelphia
Philadelphia, Pennsylvania

Gary R. Fleisher, MD
Egan Family Foundation Professor
Department of Pediatrics
Harvard Medical School;
Physician-in-Chief and Chair
Department of Medicine
Children's Hospital Boston
Boston, Massachusetts

Todd A. Florin, MD
Instructor
Department of Pediatrics
University of Pennsylvania School of Medicine;
Fellow
Pediatric Emergency Medicine
Department of Pediatrics
The Children's Hospital of Philadelphia
Philadelphia, Pennsylvania

Janet H. Friday, MD
Clinical Professor
Department of Pediatrics
University of California, San Diego
La Jolla;
Attending Physician
Emergency Department
Rady Children's Hospital San Diego
San Diego, California

Ronald A. Furnival, MD
Professor
Department of Pediatrics and Emergency Medicine
University of Minnesota Medical School;
Medical Director
Department of Pediatric Emergency Medicine
University of Minnesota Amplatz Children's Hospital
Minneapolis, Minneapolis

Carmen Teresa Garcia, MD
Attending Physician
Department of Pediatric Emergency
Jackson Memorial and Holtz Children's Hospitals
Miami, Florida

Andrew L. Garrett, MD, MPH
Associate Research Scientist
Mailman School of Public Health
Columbia University;
Director of Planning and Response
National Center for Disaster Preparedness
Mailman School of Public Health
Columbia University
New York City, New York

Michael H. Gewitz, MD
Professor and Vice Chairman
Department of Pediatrics
New York Medical College;
Physician-in-Chief/Executive Director
Chief, Pediatric Cardiology
Maria Farari Children's Hospital at Westchester
Valhalla, New York

Javier A. Gonzalez Del Rey, MD
Professor of Clinical Pediatrics
Department of Pediatrics
University of Cincinnati College
    of Medicine;
Associate Director
Division of Emergency Medicine;
Director, Pediatric Residency Programs
Department of Pediatrics
Cincinnati Children's Hospital
    Medical Center
Cincinnati, Ohio

Marc H. Gorelick, MD, MSCE
Professor
Departments of Pediatrics and Population Health
Medical College of Wisconsin;
Jon E. Vice Chair in Emergency Medicine
Children's Hospital of Wisconsin
Milwaukee, Wisconsin

Monika Goyal, MD
Department of Pediatric Emergency Medicine
Children's Hospital of Philadelphia
University of Pennsylvania School
    of Medicine
Philadelphia, Pennsylvania

Rose C. Graham, MD, MSCE
Clinical Assistant Professor of Pediatrics
Division of Pediatric Gastroenterology, Hepatology
    and Nutrition
The Children's Hospital of Philadelphia
Philadelphia, Pennsylvania

David S. Greenes, MD
Department of Medicine
Children's Hospital Boston;
Clinical Assistant Professor
Department of Pediatrics
Harvard Medical School
Boston, Massachusetts

Karen D. Gruskin, MD
Assistant Professor
Department of Medicine
Harvard Medical School;
Director of Network Services
Department of Medicine
Children's Hospital Boston
Boston, Massachusetts

Steven D. Handler, MD, MBE
Professor
Otolaryngology: Head and Neck Surgery
University of Pennsylvania School of Medicine;
Associate Director
Otolaryngology
The Children's Hospital of Philadelphia
Philadelphia, Pennsylvania

Marvin B. Harper, MD
Associate Professor
Department of Pediatrics
Harvard Medical School;
Chief Medical Information Officer
Department of Medicine
Children's Hospital Boston
Boston, Massachusetts

Fred M. Henretig, MD
Professor of Pediatrics and Emergency Medicine
University of Pennsylvania School of Medicine;
Director
Section of Clinical Toxicology
The Children's Hospital of Philadelphia
Philadelphia, Pennsylvania

Joeli Hettler, MD
Assistant Professor
Department of Emergency Medicine
Tufts University School of Medicine
Boston, Massachusetts

Dee Hodge III, MD
Associate Professor
Department of Pediatrics
Washington University in St. Louis
Attending Physician
Emergency Services
St. Louis Children's Hospital
St. Louis, Missouri

Paul J. Honig, MD
Professor Emeritus
Department of Pediatrics and Dermatology
University of Pennsylvania School of Medicine;
Attending Physician
Section of Pediatric Dermatology
Children's Hospital of Philadelphia
Philadelphia, Pennsylvania

Cynthia R. Jacobstein, MD, MSE
Clinical Assistant Professor
Department of Pediatrics
The University of Pennsylvania School of Medicine;
Attending Physician
Division of Emergency Medicine
The Children's Hospital of Philadelphia
Philadelphia, Pennsylvania

David M. Jaffe, MD
Dana Brown Professor of Pediatrics
Department of Pediatrics
St. Louis Children's Hospital
Washington University in St. Louis School of Medicine;
Director
Emergency Services
St. Louis Children's Hospital
St. Louis, Missouri

Vaishali Jha, MD
Fellow
Department of Pediatric Emergency Medicine
University of Minnesota;
Fellow
Department of Pediatric Emergency Medicine
Children's Hospital and Clinics of Minnesota
Minneapolis, Minnesota

Mark D. Joffe, MD
Associate Professor
Department of Pediatrics
University of School of Medicine;
Director, Community Pediatric Medicine
Children's Hospital of Philadelphia
Philadelphia, Pennsylvania

Howard A. Kadish, MD, MBA
Professor
Department of Pediatrics
University of Utah;
Medical Director, Rapid Treatment Unit
Department of Pediatrics
Primary Children's Medical Center
Salt Lake City, Utah

Emily R. Katz, MD
Director, Child & Adolescent Psychiatry Consultation
    Liaison Service
Department of Psychiatry
Rhode Island and Hasbro Children's Hospitals
Providence, Rhode Island

Ken Kazahaya, MD, MBA
Associate Professor of Clinical Otorhinolaryngology
Department of Otorhinolaryngology: Head and
    Neck Surgery
The University of Pennsylvania School of Medicine;
Director, Pediatric Skull Base Surgery, and
    Medical Director, Cochlear Implant Program
Division of Pediatric Otolaryngology & Human
    Communication
The Children's Hospital of Philadelphia
Philadelphia, Pennsylvania

Jennifer C. Kesselheim, MD, M.Ed
Instructor
Department of Pediatrics
Harvard Medical School;
Attending Physician
Department of Medicine
Children's Hospital Boston
Boston, Massachusetts

Brent R. King, MD, MMM
Professor and Chairman
Department of Emergency Medicine
The University of Texas Medical School at Houston;
Chief of Service
Emergency Department
Memorial Hermann (TMC) and Lyndon B. Johnson
    General Hospitals
Houston, Texas

Christopher King, MD, FACEP
Associate Professor of Emergency Medicine
    and Pediatrics
Department of Emergency Medicine
University of Pittsburgh School of Medicine;
Attending Physician
Department of Emergency Medicine
Children's Hospital of Pittsburgh of UPMC
Pittsburgh, Pennsylvania

Bruce L. Klein, MD
Associate Professor of Pediatrics and Emergency
    Medicine
The George Washington School of Medicine and Health
    Sciences;
Chief
Division of Transport Medicine
Children's National Medical Center
Washington, DC

Susanne Kost, MD, FAAP, FACEP
Associate Professor of Pediatrics
Thomas Jefferson University Medical College
Philadelphia, Pennsylvania
Attending Physician
Division of Emergency Medicine
Nemours/Alfred I. duPont Hospital for Children
Wilmington, Delaware

Nathan Kuppermann, MD, MPH
Professor
Department of Emergency Medicine and Pediatrics
University of California Davis School of Medicine;
Chair
Department of Emergency Medicine
University of California Davis Medical Center
Sacramento, California

Jane M. Lavelle, MD
Associate Professor
Department of Pediatrics
University of Pennsylvania;
Medical Director
Division of Emergency Medicine
The Children's Hospital of Philadelphia
Philadelphia, Pennsylvania

Eva Leder, MD
Clinical Fellow in Pediatrics
Department of Pediatrics
Harvard Medical School;
Clinical Fellow in Pediatrics
Division of Respiratory Diseases
Children's Hospital Boston
Boston, Massachusetts

Lois K. Lee, MD, MPH
Instructor
Department of Pediatrics
Harvard Medical School;
Associate
Department of Medicine
Children's Hospital Boston
Boston, Massachusetts

Alex V. Levin, MD, MHSc, FRCSC
Professor
Department of Ophthamology
Jefferson Medical College of Thomas Jefferson
    University;
Chief
Pediatric Ophtalmology and Ocular Genetics
Wills Eye Institute
Philadelphia, Pennsylvania

Jason Levy, MD
Instructor in Pediatrics
Department of Pediatrics
Harvard Medical School;
Division of Emergency Medicine
Children's Hospital Boston
Boston, Massachusetts

William J. Lewander, MD
Professor and Associate Chair of Pediatric Emergency
    Medicine
Department of Emergency Medicine and Pediatrics
Warren Alpert Medical School of Brown University;
Medical Director
Hasbro Pediatric Emergency Department
Hasbro Children's Hospital
Providence, Rhode Island

Lisa L. Lewis, MD
Attending Physician
Division of Emergency Medicine
Cincinnati Children's Hospital Medical Center
Cincinnati, Ohio

Chris A. Liacouras, MD
Associate Professor
Department of Pediatrics
The University of Pennsylvania School of Medicine;
Director
Department of Pediatric Endoscopy;
Attending Physician
Department of Gastroenterology and Nutrition
The Children's Hospital of Philadelphia
Philadelphia, Pennsylvania

Erica L. Liebelt, MD, FACMT
Professor
Departments of Pediatrics and Emergency Medicine
University of Alabama at Birmingham School
    of Medicine;
Medical Director of Medication Safety
Departments of Pediatrics and Emergency Medicine
The Children's Hospital of Alabama
Birmingham, Alabama

John M. Loiselle, MD
Associate Professor
Department of Pediatrics
Jefferson Medical College
Philadelphia, Pennsylvania;
Chief
Division of Emergency Medicine
Department of Pediatrics
Alfred I. duPont Hospital for Children
Wilmington, Delaware

Stephen Ludwig, MD
Professor of Pediatrics and Emergency Medicine
University of Pennsylvania School of Medicine
Senior Advisor for Medical Education
John H. and Hortense Cassel Jensen Chair
Children's Hospital of Philadelphia
Philadelphia, Pennsylvania

Dennis P. Lund, MD
Professor of Surgery & Division Chair
Department of Surgery
UW School of Medicine & Public Health;
Surgeon-in-Chief
Department of Surgery
American Family Children's Hospital
Madison, Wisconsin

**James M. Madsen, MD, MPH, FCAP, FACOEM,
    COL, MC-FS**
Adjunct Associate Professor, Preventive Medicine and
    Biometrics
Assistant Professor, Military and Emergency
    Medicine
Assistant Professor, Pathology
Uniformed Services University of the Health Sciences
    (USUHS)
Bethesda, Maryland;
Fellow, Medical Toxicology
Hahnemann University Hospital;
Fellow, Medical Toxicology
Division of Medical Toxicology
Department of Emergency Medicine
Drexel University College of Medicine
Philadelphia, Pennsylvania

Richard Malley, MD
Associate Professor of Pediatrics
Harvard Medical School;
Senior Associate in Medicine
Division of Infectious Diseases
Children's Hospital Boston
Boston, Massachusetts

Kenneth D. Mandl, MD, MPH
Associate Professor
Department of Pediatrics
Harvard Medical School;
Senior Associate Physician in Medicine
Department of Pediatrics
Children's Hospital Boston
Boston, Massachusetts

Shannon F. Manzi, PharmD
Adjunct Associate Professor
School of Pharmacy
Northeastern University;
Team Leader, Emergency Services
Department of Pharmacy
Children's Hospital Boston
Boston, Massachusetts

Constance M. McAneney, MD, MS
Associate Professor
Department of Pediatrics
University of Cincinnati College of Medicine;
Associate Director
Division of Emergency Medicine
Cincinnati Children's Hospital Medical Center
Cincinnati, Ohio

Rakesh D. Mistry, MD, MS
Assistant Professor
Department of Pediatrics
University of Pennsylvania School of Medicine;
Attending Physician
Department of Emergency Medicine
Children's Hospital of Philadelphia
Philadelphia, Pennsylvania

Matthew Mittiga, MD
Assistant Professor of Clinical Pediatrics
Department of Pediatrics
University of Cincinnati College of Medicine;
Attending Physician
Division of Emergency Medicine
Cincinnati Children's Hospital Medical Center
Cincinnati, Ohio

Ameer P. Mody, MD, MPH
Assistant Professor
Department of Emergency Medicine
Division of Pediatric Emergency Medicine
Loma Linda University Medical Center
Loma Linda;
Clinical Director
Department of Pediatric Emergency Medicine
Children's Hospital of Orange Country
Orange, California

Cynthia J. Mollen, MD, MSCE
Assistant Professor
Department of Pediatrics
Division of Emergency Medicine
The University of Pennsylvania;
Attending Physician
Department of Pediatrics
Division of Emergency Medicine
The Children's Hospital of Philadelphia
Philadelphia, Pennsylvania

David P. Mooney, MD
Chief, Trauma Surgery
Children's Hospital Boston;
Assistant Professor of Surgery
Harvard Medical School
Boston, Massachusetts

Fran Nadel, MD, MSCE
Associate Professor
Department of Pediatrics
University of Pennsylvania School of Medicine;
Attending Physician
Division of Emergency Medicine
Children's Hospital of Philadelphia
Philadelphia, Pennsylvania

Joshua Nagler, MD
Assistant Professor
Department of Pediatrics
Harvard Medical School;
Attending Physician
Department of Emergency Medicine
Children's Hospital Boston
Boston, Massachusetts

Michael L. Nance, MD
Associate Professor
Department of Surgery
University of Pennsylvania;
Director, Pediatric Trauma
Department of Surgery
The Children's Hospital of Philadelphia
Philadelphia, Pennsylvania

Howard L. Needleman, DMD
Clinical Professor
Developmental Biology (Pediatric Dentistry)
Harvard School of Dental Medicine;
Senior Associate
Department of Dentistry
Children's Hospital Boston
Boston, Massachusetts

Douglas S. Nelson, MD
Professor
Department of Pediatrics
University of Utah School of Medicine;
Medical Director
Emergency Department
Primary Children's Medical Center
Salt Lake City, Utah

Linda P. Nelson, DMD, MSCD
Assistant Clinical Professor of Pediatric Dentistry
Department of Developmental Biology
Harvard School of Dental Medicine;
Senior Attending Physician
Department of Pediatric Dentistry
Children's Hospital Boston
Boston, Massachusetts

Mark I. Neuman, MD, MPH
Assistant Professor of Pediatrics
Department of Pediatrics
Harvard Medical School;
Attending Physician
Division of Emergency Medicine
Children's Hospital Boston
Boston, Massachusetts

Kevin C. Osterhoudt, MD, MS
Associate Professor
Departments of Pediatrics and Emergency Medicine
The University of Pennsylvania School of Medicine;
Medical Director
The Poison Control Center
The Children's Hospital of Philadelphia
Philadelphia, Pennsylvania

Bonnie L. Padwa, DMD, MD
Associate Professor
Department of Oral and Maxillofacial Surgery
Harvard Medical School;
Oral Surgeon-in-Chief
Department of Plastic and Oral Surgery
Children's Hospital Boston
Boston, Massachusetts

Jan E. Paradise, MD
Department of Pediatrics
Signature Medical Group
Brockton, Massachusetts

Ronald I. Paul, MD
Professor
Department of Pediatrics
University of Louisville;
Chief of Emergency Medicine
Emergency Department
Kosair Children's Hospital
Louisville, Kentucky

Barbara B. Pawel, MD
Clinical Associate Professor
Department of Pediatrics
The University of Pennsylvania School
  of Medicine;
Attending Physician
Division of Emergency Medicine
The Children's Hospital of Philadelphia
Philadelphia, Pennsylvania

Catherine E. Perron, MD
Assistant Clinical Professor
Department of Pediatrics
Harvard Medical School
Boston;
Attending Physician
Division of Emergency Medicine
Children's Hospital Boston
Director of Pediatric Emergency Medicine
South Shore Hospital
Weymouth, Massachusetts

Holly E. Perry, MD
Assistant Professor
Department of Emergency Medicine
Tufts University School of Medicine
Boston, Massachusetts
Attending Physician
Department of Emergency Medicine
Baystate Medical Center
Springfield, Massachusetts

Jill C. Posner, MD, MSCE
Associate Professor of Clinical Pediatrics
Department of Pediatrics
The University of Pennsylvania School of Medicine;
Attending Physician
Emergency Department
The Children's Hospital of Philadelphia
Philadelphia, Pennsylvania

William P. Potsic, MD, MMM
Professor
Department of Otorhinolaryngology, Head and Neck Surgery
University of Pennsylvania School of Medicine;
Senior Surgeon, Division of Otolaryngology
Vice Chairman for Clinical Affairs and Director of
  Ambulatory Surgical Services
Department of Surgery
The Children's Hospital of Philadelphia
Philadelphia, Pennsylvania

Carla Maria Pruden, MD, MPH
Fellow
Division of Emergency Medicine
Cincinnati Children's Hospital Medical Center
Cincinnati, Ohio

Elizabeth B. Rand, MD
Division of Gastroenterology
The Children's Hospital of Philadelphia
Philadelphia, Pennsylvania

Mark G. Roback, MD
Professor of Pediatrics and Emergency Medicine
University of Minnesota Medical School;
Director, Division of Emergency Medicine
Department of Pediatrics
University of Minnesota Amplatz Children's Hospital
Minneapolis, Minnesota

Nancy M. Rodig, MD
Instructor in Pediatrics
Harvard Medical School;
Division of Nephrology
Children's Hospital Boston
Boston, Massachusetts

Henry D. Royal, MD
Professor of Radiology
Department of Nuclear Medicine
Mallinckrodt Institute of Radiology
St. Louis, Missouri

Richard M. Ruddy, MD
Professor of Clinical Pediatrics
Department of Pediatrics
University of Cincinnati College of Medicine;
Director
Division of Emergency Medicine
Cincinnati Children's Hospital Medical Center
Cincinnati, Ohio

Richard A. Saladino, MD
Associate Professor of Pediatrics
Department of Pediatrics
University of Pittsburgh School of Medicine;
Chief
Division of Pediatric Emergency Medicine
Children's Hospital of Pittsburgh
Pittsburgh, Pennsylvania

Stephen Santora, MD
Department of Orthopedic Surgery
University of Utah School of Medicine;
Primary Children's Medical Center
Salt Lake City, Utah

Richard J. Scarfone, MD
Associate Professor
Department of Pediatrics
University of Pennsylvania School of Medicine;
Medical Director, Emergency Preparedness
The Children's Hospital of Philadelphia
Philadelphia, Pennsylvania

Jeff E. Schunk, MD
Professor
Department of Pediatrics
University of Utah School of Medicine;
Department of Pediatrics
Primary Children's Medical Center
Salt Lake City, Utah

Sara A. Schutzman, MD
Assistant Professor
Department of Pediatrics
Harvard medical School;
Associate in Medicine
Department of Medicine
Division of Emergency Medicine
Children's Hospital Boston
Boston, Massachusetts

Jeffrey A. Seiden, MD
Clinical Instructor
Department of Pediatrics
The University of Pennsylvania School of Medicine;
Fellow
Department of Emergency Medicine
The Children's Hospital of Philadelphia
Philadelphia, Pennsylvania

Steven M. Selbst, MD
Professor of Pediatrics
Department of Pediatrics
Jefferson Medical College
Philadelphia, Pennsylvania;
Vice Chair for Education
Attending Physician, Division of Emergency Medicine
Department of Pediatrics
Alfred I. duPont Hospital for Children
Wilmington, Delaware

Sonal N. Shah, MD, MPH
Instructor
Department of Pediatrics
Harvard Medical School;
Attending Physician
Division of Emergency Medicine
Children's Hospital Boston
Boston, Massachusetts

Michael Shannon, MD, MPH
Deceased
Division of Emergency Medicine
Children's Hospital Boston
Boston, Massachusetts

Kathy N. Shaw, MD, MSCE
Professor and Associate Chair
Department of Pediatrics
University of Pennsylvania School of Medicine;
Division Chief
Department of Emergency Medicine
The Children's Hospital of Philadelphia
Philadelphia, Pennsylvania

Stephen Shusterman, DMD
Associate Clinical Professor of Developmental Biology
Department of Pediatric Dentistry
Harvard University School of Dental Medicine;
Dentist-in-Chief, Emeritus
Children's Hospital Boston
Boston, Massachusetts

Colin A. Sieff, MD
Associate Professor
Department of Pediatrics
Harvard Medical School;
Senior Associate in Medicine
Department of Medicine
Children's Hospital Boston
Boston, Massachusetts

Benjamin K. Silverman, MD
Professor, Pediatrics
Department of Pediatric Emergency Medicine
UCLA/Harbor Hospital
UCLA School of Medicine
Torrance, California

Jonathan I. Singer, MD
Professor of Emergency Medicine and Pediatrics
Boonshoft School of Medicine
Wright State University;
Attending Physician
Children's Medical Center
Dayton, Ohio

Howard M. Snyder III, MD
Professor of Surgery in Urology
Department of Urology
University of Pennsylvania
School of Medicine;
Director of Surgical Teaching
Division of Urology
The Children's Hospital of Philadelphia
Philadelphia, Pennsylvania

Philip R. Spandorfer, MD, MSCE
Associate Research Director
Department of Pediatric Emergency Medicine
Children's Healthcare of Atlanta at
    Scottish Rite
Atlanta, Georgia

Anne M. Stack, MD
Assistant Professor of Pediatrics
Harvard Medical School;
Clinical Chief
Division of Emergency Medicine
Children's Hospital Boston
Boston, Massachusetts

Dale W. Steele, MD
Associate Professor
Department of Emergency Medicine and Pediatrics
Warren Alpert Medical School of Brown University;
Attending Physician and Fellowship Director
Department of Pediatric Emergency Medicine
Providence, Rhode Island

Molly (Martha W.) Stevens, MD, MSCE
Assistant Professor
Pediatrics; Section of Emergency Medicine
Medical College of Wisconsin;
Attending Physician
Emergency Medicine and Trauma Center
Children's Hospital of Wisconsin
Milwaukee, Wisconsin

Michelle D. Stevenson, MD, MSE
Assistant Professor of Pediatrics
Department of Pediatrics
University of Louisville School of Medicine;
Research Director
Division of Emergency Medicine
Kosair Children's Hospital
Louisville, Kentucky

Robert P. Sundel, MD
Associate Professor of Pediatrics
Department of Pediatrics
Harvard Medical School;
Director of Rheumatology
Department of Medicine
Division of Immunology (Rheumatology)
Children's Hospital Boston
Boston, Massachusetts

Stephen J. Teach, MD, MPH
Professor
Departments of Pediatrics and Emergency Medicine
George Washington University School of Medicine and
    Health Sciences;
Associate Chief
Division of Emergency Medicine
Children's National Medical Center
Washington, DC

Valerie T. Thompson, MD
Assistant Professor of Pediatrics
University of Miami Miller School of Medicine;
Director
Division of Pediatric Emergency Medicine
Holtz Children's Hospital
Miami, Florida

Susan B. Torrey, MD
Associate Clinical Professor of Pediatrics
Department of Pediatrics
Baylor College of Medicine
Staff Physician
Department of Pediatric Emergency Medicine
Texas Children's Hospital
Houston, Texas

Nicholas Tsarouhas, MD
Associate Professor of Clinical Pediatrics
Department of Pediatrics
University of Pennsylvania School of Medicine;
Associate Medical Director, Emergency Department
Medical Director, Emergency Transport Team
Division of Emergency Medicine
The Children's Hospital of Philadelphia
Philadelphia, Pennsylvania

Daniel S. Tsze, MD, MPH
Assistant Professor
Department of Pediatrics
Columbia University College of Physicians and Surgeons;
Attending Physician
Division of Pediatric Emergency Medicine
Morgan Stanley Children's Hospital of NewYork-
    Presbyterian
New York, New York

Leah Tzimenatos, MD
Assistant Professor Pediatric Emergency
    Medicine
Department of Emergency Medicine
University of California Davis School of Medicine
Sacramento, California

Cheryl Vance, MD
Professor
Department of Emergency Medicine and Pediatrics
University of California Davis School of Medicine;
Chief, Pediatric Emergency Medicine
Department of Emergency Medicine
University of California Davis Medical Center
Sacramento, California

Rebecca L. Vieira, MD
Instructor
Department of Pediatrics
Harvard Medical School;
Assistant in Medicine
Division of Emergency Medicine
Children's Hospital Boston
Boston, Massachusetts

Robert J. Vinci, MD
Professor of Pediatrics
Department of Pediatrics
Boston University School of Medicine;
Vice Chairman
Department of Pediatrics
Boston Medical Center
Boston, Massachusetts

Mark L. Waltzman, MD
Assistant Professor
Department of Pediatrics
Harvard Medical School;
Assistant Medical Director, Division of Emergency
    Medicine
Co-Director, Travel and Geographic Medicine
Department of Medicine and Division of Emergency
    Medicine
Children's Hospital Boston
Boston, Massachusetts

Vincent J. Wang, MD
Associate Professor of Clinical Pediatrics
Department of Pediatrics
Keck School of Medicine of University of Southern
    California;
Associate Division Head
Division of Emergency Medicine
Department of Pediatrics
Childrens Hospital Los Angeles
Los Angeles, California

Debra L. Weiner, MD, PhD
Attending Physician
Department of Emergency Medicine
Children's Hospital Boston;
Assistant Professor of Pediatrics
Harvard Medical School
Boston, Massachusetts

Heidi C. Werner, MD
Pediatric Residency Program
The Children's Hospital of Philadelphia
Philadelphia, Pennsylvania

James F. Wiley II, MD, MPH
Clinical Professor
Departments of Pediatrics and Emergency
    Medicine/Traumatology
University of Connecticut School of Medicine
Farmington;
Attending Physician
Emergency Department
Connecticut Children's Medical Center
Hartford, Connecticut

Michael Witt, MD, MPH
Medical Director
Department of Pediatric Emergency Medicine
Elliot Hospital
Manchester, New Hampshire

Joanne N. Wood, MD, MSHP
Attending Physician
Department of Pediatrics
The Children's Hospital of Philadelphia
Philadelphia, Pennsylvania

Amy L. Woodward, MD, MPH
Assistant Professor
Department of Pediatrics
Indiana University School of Medicine;
Attending Physician in Pediatric Rheumatology
Department of Pediatrics
Riley Hospital for Children
Indianapolis, Indiana

George A. Woodward, MD, MBA
Professor and Chief
Department of Pediatrics and Division of Emergency
    Medicine
University of Washington School of Medicine;
Chief and Medical Director
Emergency Medicine and Transport Medicine
Seattle Children's Hospital
Seattle, Washington

Paul K. Woolf, MD
Professor
Department of Pediatrics
New York Medical College;
Associate Director, Pediatric Cardiology
Department of Pediatrics
Children's Hospital Westchester
Valhalla, New York

**Loren G. Yamamoto, MD, MPH, MBA,
FAAP, FACEP**
Professor of Pediatrics
Department of Pediatrics
John A. Burns School of Medicine
University of Hawaii;
Emergency Medicine Director and Vice Chief of Staff
Kapi'olani Medical Center for Women and Children
Honolulu, Hawaii

Albert C. Yan, MD
Associate Professor
Department of Pediatrics and Dermatology
University of Pennsylvania School of Medicine;
Section Chief
Department of Pediatric Dermatology
The Children's Hospital of Philadelphia
Philadelphia, Pennsylvania

Emily A. Zajano, MD
Teaching Fellow
Department of Pediatrics
Warren Alpert Medical School of Brown University;
Pediatric Emergency Medicine Fellow
Department of Pediatric Emergency Medicine
Rhode Island and Hasbro Children's Hospitals
Providence, Rhode Island

Joseph Zorc, MD, MSCE
Associate Professor
Department of Pediatrics and Emergency Medicine
University of Pennsylvania School of Medicine;
Attending Physician
Emergency Department
The Children's Hospital of Philadelphia
Philadelphia, Pennsylvania

The term "innovation" has found its way into many conversations in recent times. Whether the topic is medical care, medical education, research, or advocacy—innovation is the mantra. As we bring forth the 6th edition of the *Textbook of Pediatric Emergency Medicine*, the term "innovation" is on our minds as well.

Certainly, as we look back, we note the very dramatic innovations that have taken place in our subspecialty. Prior to our first edition in 1983, there was no official subspecialty of pediatric emergency medicine either in pediatrics or in emergency medicine. Current day trainees cannot fathom that historical perspective. Many of the treatments, testing modalities, procedural techniques, technologic aids, and organized approaches to care of the ill or injured child did not exist. For example, there were no dedicated trauma centers and no attention to the elements of the emergency medical services system for children (EMSC). Certainly, there was little in the way of new knowledge being developed through research. Teaching methods were also very primitive and there were no basic training programs like Pediatric Advanced Life Support (PALS), Advanced Pediatric Life Support (APLS), or advanced fellowship training programs. We would like to think that the *Textbook of Pediatric Emergency Medicine* helped to spark the creation of a new subspecialty and stimulated the many, many innovations that have helped children across the United States and around the world. It gives a great sense of pride to think that our textbook has played some small part in the development of the now more than 1,400 board-certified Pediatric Emergency Medicine specialists, of more than 65 fellowship training programs in the United States and Canada, of the PALS and APLS courses, of the PECARN Research Network, and of the many local and regional CME courses that have helped emergency physicians and pediatricians stay abreast of the latest and most efficient therapies.

But while reflecting on the innovations of the past is satisfying, it is not as important as thinking about the innovations of the future. We hope that this 6th edition will continue to stimulate improvement. To do so, we have revised and updated each and every chapter. Suggested readings now come from the current era of publications. We have added to and expanded our table of contents by including chapters on palpitations, cystic fibrosis, travel-related emergencies, and ultrasound. In particular, there is a new chapter on practice pathways; establishing such pathways will be very important to our future, as we focus on quality and safety and gauge practice variations among our various centers. Our chapter authors formerly came from subspecialty perspectives and now they primarily are practicing PEM specialists. Many of our authors have become experts in some subfield of PEM.

In this edition we have enlisted the help of three new associate editors: Richard Bachur, Marc Gorelick, and Kathy Shaw. These individuals symbolize the new era of PEM specialists who are all fellowship trained. They represent a next generation of PEM leaders.

With this edition of the textbook, we are also offering the text on the TPEM website. This will make it possible for the owner of the text to use the book in the traditional way and also to have online access to updated information, journal articles from *Pediatric Emergency Care*, interactive practice pathways, and other helpful features. The TPEM website will transform the book into a living document always capable of growth and development.

Whether the innovation is of the past or of the future, we feel honored to be a part of this great professional movement that has helped so many children and families. Pediatric care in the Emergency Department is now more effective, safer, more pain free, and kinder and more supportive of children and families. No longer is the Emergency Department the "pit" as it was often referred to at many training centers in decades past. Now it is a great place for patient care, teaching, research, and advocacy. Many of our readers tell us—"I keep your book open in the ED." "I like it because it tells me what to do and what not to miss." "I always carry it with me on-call." Indeed, these were our motivation for writing this text in the early 1980's. Beyond all of our innovations, this feedback continues to be our constant and guiding principle.

Gary R. Fleisher, MD
Boston, MA

Stephen Ludwig, MD
Philadelphia, PA

■ ACKNOWLEDGMENTS

As we complete the final pages of the 6th edition of *Textbook of Pediatric Emergency Medicine*, we would like to acknowledge and sincerely thank those around us who have made it all possible.

The writing and editing of this edition, like that of its predecessors, is a process that did not take place in the office between 8 a.m. and 6 p.m. Most of the work transpired during very early morning hours, nights, and weekends. When deadlines drew close, it encroached on vacations and on holidays. The precious commodity of time has been the very time that we have taken from our families. Their commitment to us and to our objectives and aspirations has been tremendous. Their donation of their own time has been magnanimous. Without their love and support our work would not have meaning. It is the treasure of our own families that drives us to help other children and their parents. To Jan and Zella, we give our love and gratitude. To Daniel, Carl, and Madeline Fleisher, to Susannah Ludwig & Mike Poppleton, Elisa Ludwig & Jesse Pires, Aubrey Ludwig and a new generation, Jack Ellis Poppleton, we offer our appreciation for sharing and understanding. Your only payback can come through the health and well-being of strangers of your generation and from those to come.

To our coeditors—our closest colleagues—we extend our greatest respect and thanks. Rich Ruddy has continued to be by our side and has been joined by a great trio of new associate editors. Unfortunately, Fred Henretig and Ben Silverman could not continue with the project as associate editors but we would not be working on the 6th edition without their dedication to the previous five versions. We also miss the contributions and positive support of the late Michael Shannon, MD. For all our closest colleagues, we hope that your level of personal satisfaction fills the void of our inability to say enough about your skills and dedication to the project.

During the years of the six editions, we have had so many associates and coworkers that it is impossible to name them all without forgetting some and thereby inadvertently offending them. They have worked by our side in the emergency department. They have taught with us in lectures, conferences, and workshops. They have served on committees, task forces, and boards. They have written and rewritten chapters based on our whims and notions. They have covered some of our nights and weekends. They have taught us, questioned us, stimulated us, and always supported us. Some remain at our sides at Children's Hospital Boston and The Children's Hospital of Philadelphia. But equally valuable are others who have moved to centers of pediatric emergency care around the United States and around the world. Those who have moved beyond the "nests" are not forgotten. We continue to appreciate and acknowledge all of you, our colleagues, both near and far.

We offer a special note of acknowledgement to our trainees. We appreciate all those we have encountered as medical students, residents, fellows, and continuing medical education students. We thank you all. It is you who have asked the questions. It is you who have longed for the information. You have held out the expectation that we provide the answers in an accurate and available form.

We have also learned from our many thousands of our patients and their parents. They too have kept the bar of expectation high, forcing us to try to meet those expectations.

In each of our offices there has been a coworker of special patience and extraordinary skills. For this edition, Cindy Chow and Carolyn Trojan have gone above and beyond the call. We have not forgotten those who were there for other editions: Rose Beato, Pat Parkinson, and Carmen Christmas. Work without these devoted colleagues would be unimaginable.

To our coworkers at Wolters Kluwer Lippincott Williams & Wilkins, we extend our thanks also. For this edition in particular, we appreciate your insight into the field of Pediatric Emergency Medicine, your consistency, and your dedication to the broad educational enterprise that we have built together over the past 20 years. In particular, we thank Julia Seto, Satvinder Kaur and Fran DeStefano who kept us moving forward.

A final note goes to our teachers, chairmen, and mentors. There are and have been many and we thank you all. To the late Jean Cortner, MD, we offer a special note of thanks. He was there when it all began. He bet on two young faculty members. I hope he knows that his bet has had adequate pay out. And for each of us, there has been a special advocate and advisor in our careers. To the late David Cornfeld and the very active David Nathan, we often think about how you would have done it. We believe that this is the highest compliment that one can offer to a mentor.

Stephen Ludwig, MD
Gary R. Fleisher, MD

■CONTENTS

SECTION I ■ LIFE-THREATENING EMERGENCIES

SECTION II ■ SIGNS AND SYMPTOMS

SECTION III ■ MEDICAL EMERGENCIES

SECTION IV ■ TRAUMA

SECTION V ■ SURGICAL EMERGENCIES

SECTION VI ■ PSYCHOSOCIAL EMERGENCIES

■ LIST OF ALGORITHMS

CHAPTER 1 ■ RESUSCITATION—PEDIATRIC BASIC AND ADVANCED LIFE SUPPORT

STEPHEN LUDWIG, MD, AND JANE M. LAVELLE, MD

The most critical and dramatic of all emergency situations is the application of cardiopulmonary resuscitation (CPR). CPR is a series of interventions aimed at restoring and supporting vital function after apparent death. The urgent and immediate goal of resuscitation is to reestablish substrate delivery to meet the metabolic needs of the myocardium, brain, and other vital organs. The overall goal is to return the child to society without morbidity related either to the underlying disease process or to the resuscitation process.

Instruction in CPR techniques has come from two widely disseminated national courses: pediatric advanced life support (PALS) and advanced pediatric life support (APLS). Both of these courses have been overwhelmingly successful in training health-care providers in the appropriate resuscitative techniques. Both courses stress the early recognition of the child who is in need of resuscitative efforts. But despite these educational efforts, the outcome of resuscitation in situations in which there has been asystolic arrest is still poor, although improving. As in many conditions we manage in pediatric patients, primary prevention, or at least early recognition, is the most successful strategy.

The paradigm for pediatric CPR has been based largely on the adult model. In 2005 the International Liaison Committee on Resuscitation (ILCOR) reviewed the science of resuscitation. There is an orderly progression through the assessment and management of the ABCs—airway, breathing, and circulation. Like its adult counterpart, pediatric CPR is best performed by a well-coordinated team of physicians, nurses, respiratory therapists, and other support personnel. Recent trends have resulted in inclusion of parents in the resuscitation room.

BACKGROUND

Incidence

There are no incidence data for pediatric resuscitations performed annually in the United States. But it is estimated that 16,000 children die annually from out-of-hospital cardiopulmonary arrests. Table 1.1 shows the childhood mortality rates and the leading causes of death in the United States for children for 2007. Table 1.2 shows the leading causes of death in the United States in different age groups and the relative rates per population. Note that there is a relatively higher mortality rate for young children. Note also that, of the causes of death listed in Table 1.1, most are potentially reversible. Trauma is

the leading cause of death in childhood. Table 1.3 details the leading causes of unintentional injury by age group for the years 2000 to 2005. Special techniques of trauma management are presented in Chapters 104 and 105. We believe the techniques of basic and advanced life support, when readily available and skillfully supervised and applied, contribute to the significant reduction in childhood mortality.

Patient Characteristics

Age

In many series of CPR cases, most children were at the younger end of the pediatric age range. In a series published from The Children's Hospital of Philadelphia, the mean age was 1.98 years and the median was 5 months. The age range was between 2 weeks and 16 years (Fig. 1.1). Although pediatric CPR education generally should be tailored to the anatomic and physiologic characteristics of the young child, emergency department (ED) staff must be prepared to cope with the full spectrum of age and size.

Etiology

The most common primary diagnoses of hospitalized pediatric patients requiring resuscitation involve the respiratory system (Table 1.4). Conditions such as pneumonia, bronchiolitis, asthma, aspiration, and respiratory distress syndrome account for the largest group of diagnoses. Cardiac diagnoses and central nervous system (CNS) disorders occur in roughly equal frequency, but half as often as respiratory diagnoses. Common cardiovascular diagnoses include congenital heart disease, septic shock, and severe dehydration. CNS diagnoses include hydrocephalus (ventricular shunt failure), meningitis, seizure, and tumor.

In the ED, the physician is more likely to encounter children whose out-of-hospital cardiac arrest deaths result from trauma (20% to 30% of cases), sudden infant death syndrome (SIDS), or unknown causes. Primary cardiac etiologies are much rarer in the pediatric population. Approximately 10% of out-of-hospital cardiac arrest patients have ventricular tachycardia (VT) or ventricular fibrillation (VF). Children with congenital anomalies, chronic sequelae of prematurity, and birth trauma, and those with chronic relapsing disease are also seen in the ED, as increasing numbers of children have survived the neonatal period, transplantation, complex surgery, and cancer therapy and have been discharged from

TABLE 1.1

DEATHS AND DEATH RATES FOR 2007 AND AGE-ADJUSTED DEATH RATES AND PERCENT CHANGES IN AGE-ADJUSTED RATES FROM 2006–2007 FOR THE 15 LEADING CAUSES OF DEATH: UNITED STATES

Rank[a]	Cause of death (based on the *International Classification of Diseases, Tenth Revision*, 2nd ed., 2004)	Number	Death rate	Age-adjusted death rate (2007)
	All causes	2,424,059	803.7	760.3
1	Diseases of heart (I00–I09, I11, I13, I20–I51)	615,651	204.1	190.7
2	Malignant neoplasms (C00–C97)	560,187	185.7	177.5
3	Cerebrovascular diseases (I60–I69)	133,990	44.4	41.6
4	Chronic lower respiratory diseases (J40–J47)	129,311	42.9	41.2
5	Accidents (unintentional injuries) (V01–X59, Y85–Y86)[b]	117,075	38.8	37.8
6	Alzheimer's disease (G30)	74,944	24.8	22.8
7	Diabetes mellitus (E10–E14)	70,905	23.5	22.4
8	Influenza and pneumonia (J09–J18)[c]	52,847	17.5	16.3
9	Nephritis, nephrotic syndrome and nephrosis (N00–N07, N17–N19, N25–N27)	46,095	15.3	14.4
10	Septicemia (A40–A41)	34,851	11.6	11.0
11	Intentional self-harm (suicide) (U03, X60–X84, Y87.0)[b]	33,185	11.0	10.8
12	Chronic liver disease and cirrhosis (K70, K73–K74)	28,504	9.5	8.9
13	Essential hypertension and hypertensive renal disease (I10, I12, I15)	23,769	7.9	7.3
14	Parkinson's disease (G20–G21)	20,136	6.7	6.4
15	Assault (homicide) (U01–U02, X85–Y09, Y87.1)[b]	17,520	5.8	5.8
	All other causes	465,069	154.2	

[a]Rank based on number of deaths.
[b]For unintentional injuries, suicides, and homicides, preliminary and final date may differ because of the truncated nature of the preliminary file.
[c]New code J09 (Influenza due to identified avian influenza virus) was added to the category in 2007.
Source: Xu J, Kochanek KD, Tejada-Vera B. *Deaths: Preliminary data for 2007.* National vital statistics reports. Vol 58, No. 1. Hyattsville, MD: National Center for Health Statistics, 2009.

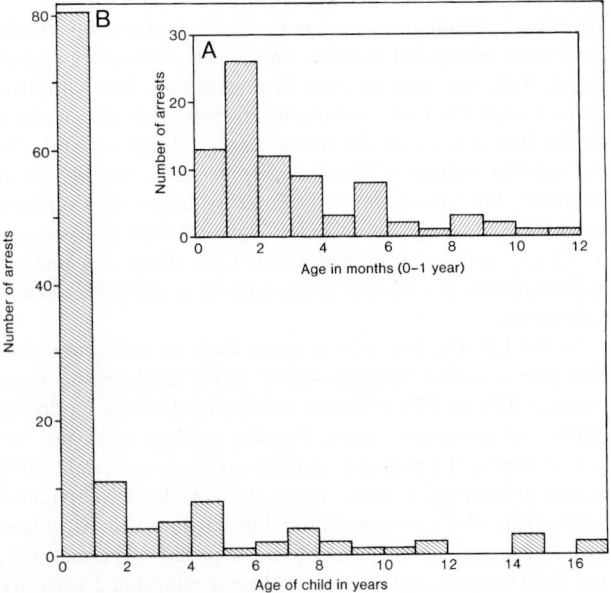

FIGURE 1.1 Histogram showing frequency of cardiac arrest as related to age in months (**A**) and years (**B**) from The Children's Hospital of Philadelphia survey.

the hospital (see Chapter 120). The broad range of diagnoses encountered in our review of resuscitation is noted in Table 1.4. This clearly differs from the adult circumstance of resuscitation, in which case most arrests are related to myocardial infarction secondary to coronary artery disease.

The PALS course teaches that the many etiologies of arrest follow one of two pathways: respiratory distress to respiratory failure to arrest or circulatory compromise to circulatory failure to arrest. In our experience, 80% of children who have arrested have followed the first pathway (Fig. 1.2). Twenty percent of patients follow the circulatory failure pathway to arrest. It is difficult in some cases to determine which mechanism was primary.

Demographics

There are no national demographic studies to identify socioeconomic, ethnic/racial, familial, or community characteristics of the pediatric patient who requires life support intervention. Such studies would be important for developing profiles of the high-risk patient population for subsequent development of surveillance or prevention programs. It is most important to study such factors on a local level, where local solutions may be implemented. Some states have begun child death review efforts that might shed light on prevention strategies.

TABLE 1.2

DEATHS AND DEATH RATES FOR THE 10 LEADING CAUSES OF DEATH IN SPECIFIED AGE GROUPS: UNITED STATES, PRELIMINARY 2007

Rank[a]	Cause of death (based on the *Intentional Classification of Diseases, Tenth Revision, 2nd ed., 2004*) and age	Number	Rate
All age groups[b]			
	All causes	2,424,059	803.7
1	Diseases of heart (I00–I09, I11–I13, I20–I51)	615,651	204.1
2	Malignant neoplasms (C00–C97)	560,187	185.7
3	Cerebrovascular diseases (I60–I69)	133,990	44.4
4	Chronic lower respiratory diseases (J40–J47)	129,311	42.9
5	Accidents (unintentional injuries) (V01–X59, Y85–Y86)	117,075	38.8
	Motor vehicle accidents (V02–V04, V09.0, V09.2, V12–V14, V19.0–V19.2, V19.4–V19.6, V20–V79, V80.3–V80.5, V81.0–V81.1, V82.0–V82.1, V83–V86, V87.0–V87.8, V88.0–V88.8, V89.0–V89.2)	43,098	14.3
	All other accidents (V01, V05–V06, V09.1, V09.3–V09.9, V10–V12, V15–V18, V19.3, V19.8–V19.9, V80.0–V80.2, V80.6–V80.9, V81.2–V81.9, V82.2, V82.9, V87.9, V88.9, V89.1, V89.3, V89.9, V90–V99, W00–X59, Y85–Y86)	73,977	24.5
6	Alzheimer's disease (G30)	74,944	24.8
7	Diabetes mellitus (E10–E14)	70,905	23.5
8	Influenza and pneumonia (J09–J18)[c]	52,847	17.5
9	Nephritis, nephrotic syndrome and nephrosis (N00–N07, N17–N19, N25–N27)	46,095	15.3
10	Septicemia (A40–A41)	34,851	11.6
	All other causes (residual)	588,203	195.0
1–4 years			
	All causes	4,651	28.2
1	Accidents (unintentional injuries) (V01–X59, Y85–Y86)	1,566	9.5
	Motor vehicle accidents (V02–V04, V09.0, V09.2, V12–V14, V19.0–V19.2, V19.4–V19.6, V20–V79, V80.3–V80.5, V81.0–V81.1, V82.0–V82.1, V83–V86, V87.0–V87.8, V88.0–V88.8, V89.0–V89.2)	529	3.2
	All other accidents (V01, V05–V06, V09.1, V09.3–V09.9, V10–V12, V15–V18, V19.3, V19.8–V19.9, V80.0–V80.2, V80.6–V80.9, V81.2–V81.9, V82.2, V82.9, V87.9, V88.9, V89.1, V89.3, V89.9, V90–V99, W00–X59, Y85–Y86)	1,037	6.3
2	Congenital malformations, deformations and chromosomal abnormalities (Q00–Q99)	506	3.1
3	Assault (homicide) (U01–U02, X85–Y09, Y87.1)	365	2.2
4	Malignant neoplasms (C00–C97)	361	2.2
5	Diseases of heart (I00–I09, I11, I13, I20–I51)	163	1.0
6	Influenza and pneumonia (J09–J18)[c]	106	0.6
7	Certain conditions originating in the perinatal period (P00–P96)	77	0.5
8	Septicemia (A40–A41)	74	0.4
9	In situ neoplasms, benign neoplasms and neoplasms of uncertain or unknown behavior (D00–D48)	55	0.3
10	Cerebrovascular diseases (I60–I69)	52	0.3
	All other causes (residual)	1,326	8.1
5–14 years			
	All causes	6,091	15.2
1	Accidents (unintentional injuries) (V01–X59, Y85–Y86)	2,157	5.4
	Motor vehicle accidents (V02–V04, V09.0, V09.2, V12–V14, V19.0–V19.2, V19.4–V19.6, V20–V79, V80.3–V80.5, V81.0–V81.1, V82.0–V82.1, V83–V86, V87.0–V87.8, V88.0–V88.8, V89.0–V89.2)	1,264	3.1
	All other accidents (V01, V05–V06, V09.1, V09.3–V09.9, V10–V12, V15–V18, V19.3, V19.8–V19.9, V80.0–V80.2, V80.6–V80.9, V81.2–V81.9, V82.2, V82.9, V87.9, V88.9, V89.1, V89.3, V89.9, V90–V99, W00–X59, Y85–Y86)	893	2.2
2	Malignant neoplasms (C00–C97)	929	2.3
3	Congenital malformations, deformations and chromosomal abnormalities (Q00–Q99)	356	0.9
4	Assault (homicide) (U01–U02, X85–Y09, Y87.1)	337	0.8
5	Diseases of heart (I00–I09, I11, I13, I20–I51)	209	0.5
6	Intentional self-harm (suicide) (U03, X60–X84, Y87.0)	195	0.5
7	Influenza and pneumonia (J09–J18)[c]	111	0.3
8	Chronic lower respiratory disease (J40–J47)	98	0.2
9	Cerebrovascular diseases (I60–I69)	85	0.2
10	In situ neoplasms, benign neoplasms and neoplasms of uncertain or unknown behavior (D00–D48)	82	0.2
	All other causes (residual)	1,532	3.8

(continued)

TABLE 1.2

DEATHS AND DEATH RATES FOR THE 10 LEADING CAUSES OF DEATH IN SPECIFIED AGE GROUPS: UNITED STATES, PRELIMINARY 2007 (CONTINUED)

Rank[a]	Cause of death (based on the *Intentional Classification of Diseases, Tenth Revision,* 2nd ed., 2004) and age	Number	Rate
	15–24 years		
	All causes	33,788	79.5
1	Accidents (unintentional injuries) (V01–X59,Y85–Y86)	15,356	36.1
	Motor vehicle accidents (V02–V04, V09.0, V09.2, V12–V14, V19.0–V19.2, V19.4–V19.6, V20–V79, V80.3–V80.5, V81.0–V81.1, V82.0–V82.1, V83–V86, V87.0–V87.8, V88.0–V88.8, V89.0–V89.2)	10,507	24.7
	All other accidents (V01, V05–V06, V09.1, V09.3–V09.9, V10–V12, V15–V18, V19.3, V19.8–V19.9, V80.0–V80.2, V80.6–V80.9, V81.2–V81.9, V82.2, V82.9, V87.9, V88.9, V89.1, V89.3, V89.9, V90–V99, W00–X59, Y85–Y86)	4,849	11.4
2	Assault (homicide) (*U01–*U02, X85–Y09, Y87.1)	5,284	12.4
3	Intentional self-harm (suicide) (*U03, X60–X84, Y87.0)	4,030	9.5
4	Malignant neoplasms (C00–C97)	1,609	3.8
5	Diseases of heart (I00–I09, I11, I13, I20–I51)	991	2.3
6	Congenital malformations, deformations and chromosomal abnormalities (Q00–Q99)	373	0.9
7	Cerebrovascular diseases (I60–I69)	197	0.5
8	Pregnancy, childbirth and the puerperlum (O00–O99)	166	0.4
9	Septicemia (A40–A41)	156	0.4
10	Influenza and pneumonia (J09–J18)[c]	154	0.4
	All other causes (residual)	5,472	12.9

Source: Deaths: Preliminary data for 2007. National vital statistics reports. Vol 58, No. 1. Hyattsville, MD: National Center for Health Statistics, 2009.

TABLE 1.3

LEADING CAUSES OF UNINTENTIONAL INJURY DEATH AMONG CHILDREN 0 TO 19 YEARS USING THE MODIFIED MATRIX, BY AGE GROUP, UNITED STATES, 2000–2005

	Age group in years				
Rank	<1 (*n* = 5,883)	1–4 (*n* = 10,203)	5–9 (*n* = 7,144)	10–14 (*n* = 9,088)	15–19 (*n* = 40,734)
1	Suffocation 66%	Drowning 27%	MVT—occupant 22%	MVT—occupant 26%	MVT—occupant 41%
2	MVT—occupant 8%	Pedestrian 15%	MVT—unspecified 15%	MVT—unspecified 15%	MVT—unspecified 28%
3	Drowning 7%	Fires/burns 14%	Pedestrian 14%	Pedestrian 12%	Poisoning 7%
4	MVT—Unspecified 5%	MVT—occupant 13%	Fires/burns 13%	Drowning 10%	MVT—other 6%
5	Other injuries 5%	MVT—unspecified 9%	Drowning 13%	MVT—other 9%	Pedestrian 5%
6	Fires/burns 4%	Suffocation 8%	Other injuries 7%	Other injuries 8%	Drowning 5%
7	Poisoning 2%	Other injuries 8%	MVT—other 6%	Fires/burns 6%	Other injuries 5%
8	Falls 2%	Falls 2%	Pedal cyclist 4%	Pedal cyclist 6%	Falls 1%
9	Pedestrian 1%	Poisoning 2%	Suffocation 4%	Suffocation 4%	Fires/burns 1%
10	MVT—other 0.5%	MVT—other 2%	Falls 1%	Poisoning 2%	Suffocation 1%
11	Pedal cyclist 0.02%	Pedal cyclist 0.3%	Poisoning 1%	Falls 2%	Pedal cyclist 1%

Source: CDC/NCHS National Vital Statistics System.

TABLE 1.4

DIAGNOSES OF CHILDREN REQUIRING LIFE SUPPORT BY BODY SYSTEM

Respiratory	Central Nervous System (CNS)
Pneumonia	Acute hydrocephalus
Aspiration	Head trauma
Asthma	Seizure
Epiglottitis	Tumor
Laryngotracheobronchitis	Meningitis
Respiratory failure/chronic lung disease	Hemorrhage
Bronchiolitis	**Gastrointestinal**
Botulism	Trauma
Primary apnea	Enterocolitis
Bronchopulmonary dysplasia	Bowel perforation
	Bowel obstruction
Cardiovascular	Tracheoesophageal fistula
Congenital heart disease	**Miscellaneous/Multisystem**
Septic shock	Sudden infant death syndrome
Dehydration	Drug ingestion
Pericarditis	Tumors (non-CNS)
Congestive heart failure	Multiple trauma
Myocarditis	

Source: From The Children's Hospital of Philadelphia 1976–1980.

Treatment

Pediatric CPR presents the emergency physician with several complexities and frustrations. The first difficulty often encountered is that the patient may have received only basic life support (BLS) care (see Chapter 6). Although this is changing with enhanced development of emergency medical services for

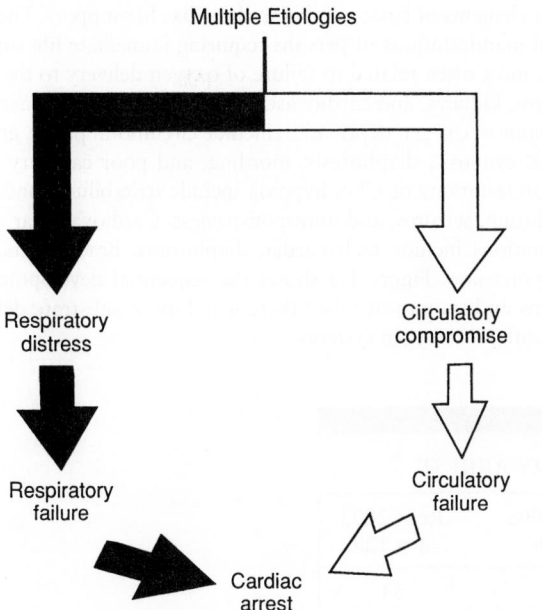

FIGURE 1.2 Pathophysiologic pathways from etiologies to cardiac arrest. (Adapted from PALS, American Heart Association.)

children, pediatric patients are likely to be brought to the ED without the same level of field treatment that adult patients receive routinely. Due to the fact that the overwhelming majority of cardiac/respiratory arrests occur in adults, paramedics may have limited exposure and thus a lower comfort level during pediatric arrest situations. There is controversy about how much prehospital care should be performed in other emergency situations, but cardiac arrest requires an immediate and effective response. Although paramedics are trained and equipped to provide both adult and pediatric life support, they may be forced to initiate pediatric life support at the most basic level. In other areas, paramedics are limited by laws, regulations, or negative attitudes. Absent or inadequate prehospital care leads to longer periods of hypoxia and hypoperfusion, which directly affect prognosis and CNS morbidity (see Chapter 6). Seidel documented the difference in survival rates between traumatized adults and children who require prehospital care, as well as the lack of adequate pediatric equipment in prehospital care systems. Other investigators have documented the deficiencies in emergency care provided in freestanding emergency care centers and in primary care providers' offices. Walsh-Kelly et al. documented this issue in primary care offices in one state.

The wide spectrum of age and diagnoses adds additional complexity. The resuscitation team must provide an array of technical skills, drugs, and equipment. Without delay, the team must have the flexibility to adjust to the correct sizes and drug dosages for children.

Our experience shows that careful management of airway and breathing is extremely important. Because the cause of the arrest is often related to respiratory failure and because the child's myocardium is relatively resilient to hypoxemia, the rapid correction of hypoxemia may be all that is necessary to effect resuscitation.

For those patients who do not respond to airway and breathing management alone, life support will be significantly more difficult. In the ED, the lack of an immediate patient response usually predicts a need for multiple drug interventions.

One of the common frustrations when administering drugs is the establishment of an intravenous (IV) line. This technical skill continues to be the most common obstacle toward achieving successful CPR. However, the use of intraosseous (IO) technique and central line placement has been a great advance in solving the access problem. Thus far, ultrasound guidance of CVP placement has not improved outcomes but this technique may help as PEM physicians become more facile with it.

Arrhythmia management is a relatively infrequent problem in pediatric life support. The absence of atherosclerotic vascular disease makes the child's myocardium less susceptible to arrhythmia. As a result, antiarrhythmic medications and defibrillation are infrequently used. The most common cardiac rhythms to be recognized and managed are sinus bradycardia, pulseless electrical activity (PEA), and asystole. The expectations to this are those children with congenital heart disease (preoperative and postoperative) and those who have sustained direct myocardial trauma (see Chapters 84 and 118). These children may have unusual and difficult arrhythmias that require esoteric management to achieve a successful outcome.

Perhaps the greatest difficulty comes not with specific knowledge or technical skill but with attitude. Many EDs are unaccustomed to resuscitating children and will become immobilized

OUTCOME FOR OUT-OF-HOSPITAL PEDIATRIC CARDIOPULMONARY ARREST

	% of Patients (% Survival)			
	Donoghue 2005	Young 2004	Sirbaugh 1999	Young 1991
Witnessed	30.8 (13.1)	34 (16)		31 (19)
Bystander CPR	30.7 (9.4)	31	26	30 (26)
ROSC	22.8	29	11	
Survival to hospital admission	23.9	25		
Survival to hospital discharge	6.7	8.4	2.4	8.4
Good neurologic outcome	2.2	31	17	

when faced with the task. There is a fear that the child is somehow more fragile. In other circumstances, there is overcompensation to the point that the resuscitation of a child is prolonged beyond an optimal point for either the child or the family.

However, many pediatric emergency physicians are uncomfortable with the adult patient who may be a visitor or employee at the pediatric hospital who is brought to the ED with acute chest pain and possible myocardial infarction. Pediatric emergency physicians are encouraged to take the American Heart Association's Advanced Cardiovascular Life Support (AHA-ACLS) course.

The ED team should review the effectiveness of each individual resuscitation effort and the collective effort of the ED. This audit may be accomplished using one or more of the following approaches: (i) postresuscitation debriefing and conference; (ii) review of the videotape recording of resuscitation; (iii) monthly morbidity mortality conferences; (iv) chart audit; (v) review of resuscitation database (e.g., cross-referencing morbidity and mortality with various shifts, personnel teams, and prehospital treatment); and (vi) performance on practice codes on the use of patient simulation manikin. When the team recognizes that its efficiency and effectiveness are less than ideal (or less than they are with adult patients), specific remedial education should be undertaken.

Prognosis

The outlook for survival after CPR is very variable for pediatric patients. In our experience, if respiratory arrest is recognized rapidly and managed skillfully, immediate survival may be as high as 90%. These figures are based on a hospitalized population of children who require resuscitation within the hospital. The use of rapid response teams have improved these outcomes. For patients arriving to the ED *in extremis*, the outcome is not as good. Although this rate has been substantially improved over the last 10 years presumably due to improve-

ments in physician education, equipment, and techniques, children who arrive in the ED in asystolic arrest still have a poor prognosis. The poorer prognosis for patients in the ED may be attributed to delayed recognition of the arrest and limited prehospital care. Several case series have documented an overall prognosis, as shown in Tables 1.5 and 1.6.

CPR research is extremely difficult to perform. Most of our information is based on retrospective studies such as those reported in Tables 1.5 and 1.6. Patient populations, characteristics, terminology, and methodology vary among studies, making it difficult to compare one investigator's work with another's. Performing a prospective study is challenged by legal and ethical considerations in enlisting patients at a time when "informed consent" is impossible. In 1997, a conference was held and a special report issued to bring uniformity to the terminology of CPR research. This important report may bring more clarity to the CPR research of the future.

CLINICAL MANIFESTATIONS

Infants and children who have experienced disruption of oxygen or glucose delivery to the brain may benefit from the various elements of basic or advanced cardiac life support. The clinical manifestations of persons requiring immediate life support are most often related to failure of oxygen delivery to the skin, brain, kidneys, and cardiovascular system. Cutaneous manifestations of oxygen deprivation include circumoral pallor, grayish hue, cyanosis, diaphoresis, mottling, and poor capillary refill. Manifestations of CNS hypoxia include irritability, confusion, delirium, seizures, and unresponsiveness. Cardiovascular manifestations include tachycardia, diaphoresis, bradycardia, and hypotension. Figure 1.3 shows the sequential development of signs and symptoms when there is failure of substrate delivery to different oxygen systems.

OUTCOME FOR IN-HOSPITAL PEDIATRIC CARDIOPULMONARY ARREST

	Meaney 2006 $n = 464$	Nadkarni 2006 $n = 880$	Reiss 2002 $n = 129$
ROSC	50	52	64
Survival to hospital discharge	23	27	16
Good neurologic outcome	64 (67/105)	65 (154/236)	90 (19/21)

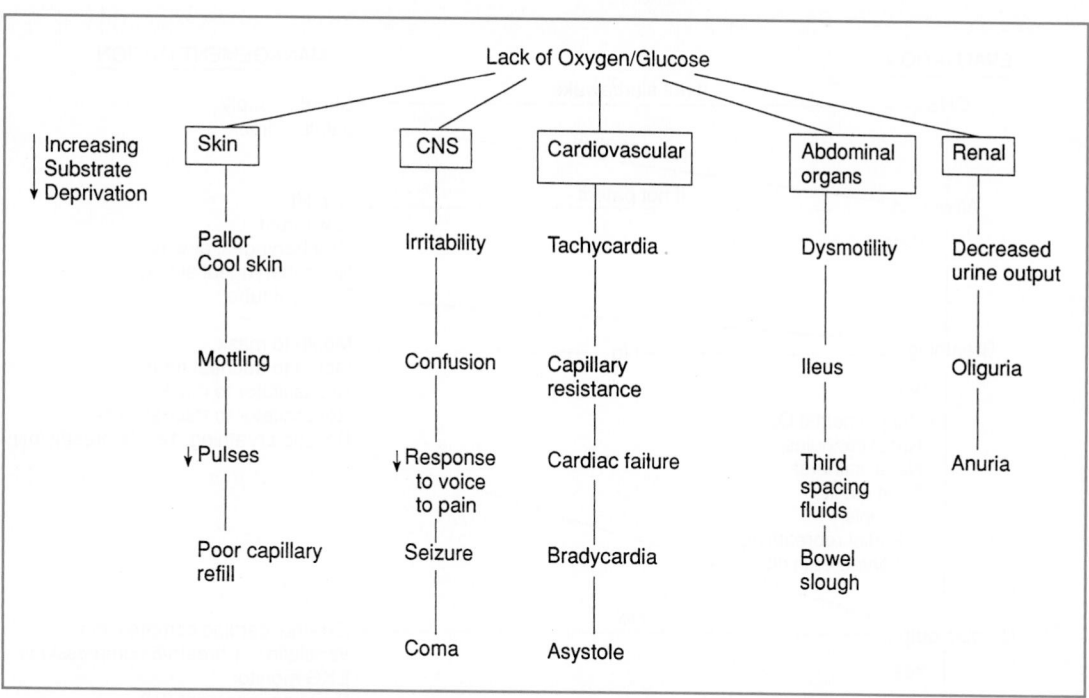

FIGURE 1.3 Signs and symptoms of lack of substrate delivery to vital organ systems. CNS, central nervous system.

Glucose is the second essential substrate necessary for maintenance of CNS integrity. Severe hypoglycemia may be just as devastating as severe hypoxemia. Clinical manifestations are often similar to hypoxemia, including seizures and coma. In addition, the effect of hypoglycemia on the cardiovascular system may lead to a secondary failure of oxygen delivery because of hypotension and related hypoperfusion.

A patient who has experienced a failure of substrate delivery to the central circulation must be resuscitated or supported until more specific diagnosis and management can be determined. It is also essential to identify patients who are *at risk* for failure of substrate delivery. This can be accomplished by a physical examination with emphasis on evaluation for airway patency, gas exchange, and cardiovascular integrity. In detecting those at risk, pulse oximetry, if available, may be useful in identifying mild degrees of hemoglobin desaturation. In addition, laboratory tests may be helpful because patients with a low partial pressure of arterial oxygen (PaO_2), pH, glucose, hemoglobin, hemoglobin saturation, or high PaO_2 are at risk. Also, recognition of certain disease entities allows early intervention, careful monitoring, and prevention of cardiovascular collapse. Examples include croup, airway foreign body, meningitis, and increased intracranial pressure (ICP).

MANAGEMENT

Management Sequence

Once it is determined that a child requires life support, a sequence of evaluations and interventions should be accomplished (Fig.

1.4). Initially, CNS integrity must be evaluated: Is the patient alert? Does he or she respond to a shout or painful stimulus? If there is no response, the assumption is that the brain is no longer receiving an adequate amount of oxygen, and the three basic sequences of evaluation and management are initiated.

First, the airway is maneuvered to move the mandibular block of tissue up and off the posterior pharyngeal wall. The physician places his or her cheek next to the mouth and nose while listening and feeling for movement of air. At the same time, the physician is watching the chest for any evidence of chest wall movement. If the patient is moving air independently, the physician simply continues to support the airway and looks to provide a mechanism for delivering supplemental oxygen. If the patient is not breathing spontaneously, the work of breathing must be assumed by the care provider, using an expired air technique when a manual resuscitator is not available. As soon as advanced life support breathing technology is available, it should be used. With the recognition that the airway is open and ventilation is occurring, the third phase of oxygen delivery is evaluated by feeling for arterial pulsations. The physician should palpate the brachial, carotid, or femoral arteries. If palpable pulses are not present after a 15-second evaluation, external cardiac compression (ECC) is initiated to provide a circulation. The adequacy of ECC is initially determined by feeling for pulses. In determining whether the oxygen delivery system has been reestablished, the physician should look for improvement in the level of consciousness, a return to spontaneous breathing, or an inherent cardiac rhythm.

More specific management sequences are offered at the end of this chapter.

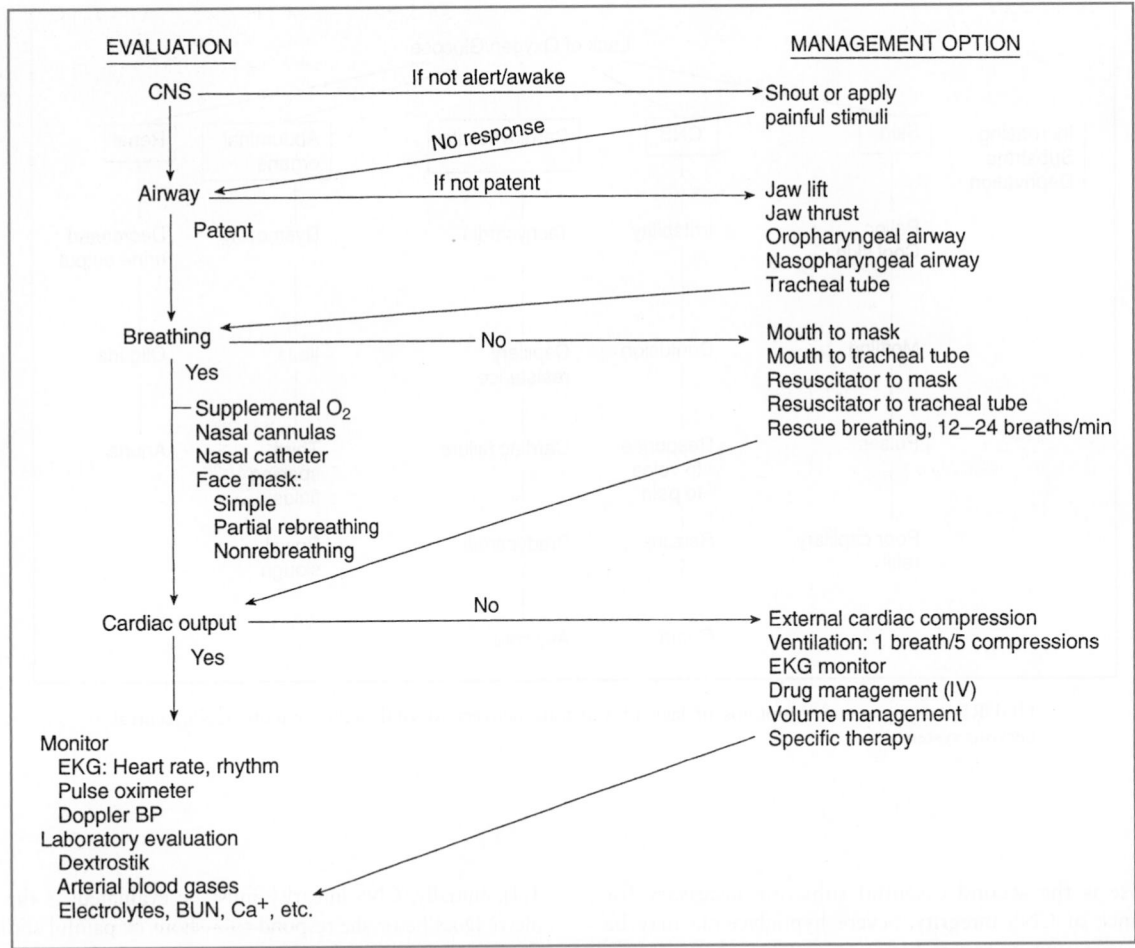

FIGURE 1.4 Management sequence for pediatric life support. CNS, central nervous system; EKG, electrocardiogram; BP, blood pressure; BUN, blood urea nitrogen.

Airway

Evaluation

The first priority in the sequential evaluation and management paradigm of basic and advanced life support is evaluation and treatment of the airway. The physician should look, listen, and feel for evidence of gas exchange. The physician should *look* at the chest to see whether there is chest wall or abdominal movement suggestive of breathing effort. The physician should *listen* over the mouth and nose for the sound of air movement. With a stethoscope, the physician should listen over the trachea and the axilla for air entry. The physician should *feel* with his or her cheek for evidence of air movement. If there is evidence of spontaneous breathing and no evidence of gas movement through the central airway, the presumptive diagnosis is that of airway obstruction.

Management

If trauma is suspected, the head and cervical spine must be stabilized during evaluation and management of the airway. Someone must be assigned to hold the head in the midline position while applying gentle cephalad traction. The most effective noninvasive maneuver for clearing an obstructed airway involves tilting the head back slightly and lifting the chin forward by pulling or pushing the mandibular block of tissue forward (Fig. 1.5). The traditional mechanism of gentle flexion of the cervical spine on the thoracic spine may open the airway, but it provides less efficient ventilation and is hazardous if cervical spine trauma has occurred.

Most airway obstruction is related to the mandibular block of tissue falling posteriorly and lying against the posterior wall of the hypopharynx. This can be relieved by physically grasping the mandibular block and pulling it forward so the lower anterior central incisors are anterior to the maxillary central incisors. The same result can be obtained by pushing the mandibular block of tissue forward. The fingers should be placed behind the angle of the jaw and the jaw pushed forward so the lower central incisors are in a plane anterior to the upper central incisors (Fig. 1.5). These noninvasive maneuvers should be attempted before any of the more invasive airway adjuncts are tried. Table 1.7 lists airway equipment and respiratory monitoring equipment that should be available for pediatric life support.

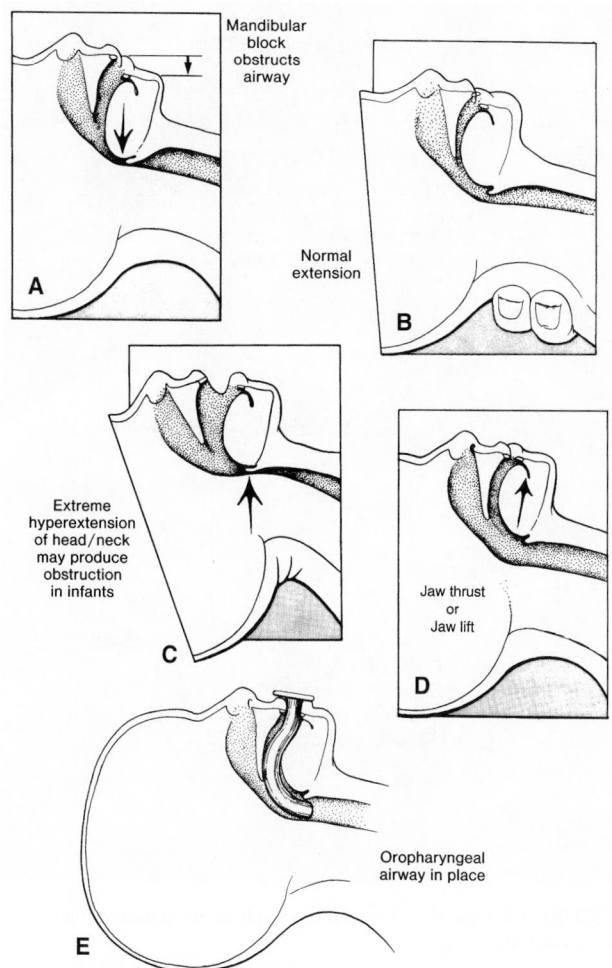

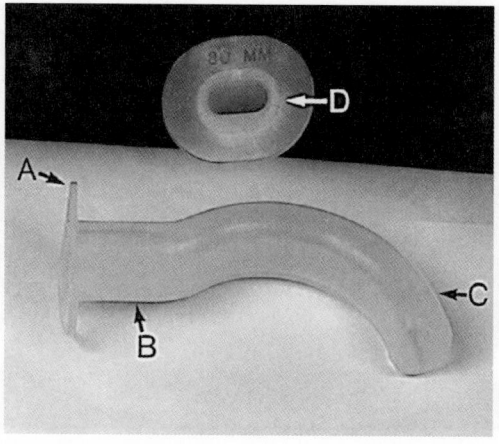

FIGURE 1.6 Oropharyngeal airway: flange (**A**), bite block (**B**), stent (**C**), and gas exchange or suction conduit (**D**).

FIGURE 1.5 **A:** Upper airway obstruction related to hypotonia. **B:** Partial relief of airway obstruction by means of head extension (danger of cervical spine injury in cases of trauma). **C:** Extreme hyperextension causing upper airway obstruction. **D:** Fully open airway through use of jaw thrust or jaw lift. **E:** Oropharyngeal airway stenting mandibular block off of posterior pharyngeal wall.

TABLE 1.7

AIRWAY EQUIPMENT KIT FOR PEDIATRIC
RESUSCITATION

Masks
Laryngoscope handle with laryngoscope blades:
    Miller 0, 1, 2, 3,
    MacIntosh 2, 3, 4
Wis-Hipple 1.5
Oropharyngeal airways: all sizes
Nasopharyngeal airways: French sizes 12, 16, 20, 24, 28
Endotracheal tubes: ID sizes
    Uncuffed: 2.5 to 7.5 mm in 0.5-mm increments
    Cuffed: 5.0 to 10 mm in 0.5-mm increments
    Stylet: infant, adult
Magill forceps: child, adult
Extra batteries and laryngoscope lamps
Suction catheters: French sizes 6, 8, 10, 12, 14
Yankauer suction tip
End-tidal CO_2 monitor, pulse oximeter, CR monitor
Defibrillator, Q-CPR puck, adhesive pads

Artificial Airways

Oropharyngeal Airways. Oropharyngeal airways are used when manual manipulation of the airway cannot maintain airway patency. The purpose of the oropharyngeal airway is to stent or support the mandibular block of tissue off the posterior pharyngeal wall. There are three basic parts to this airway device (Fig. 1.6). The flange is used to prevent the airway from falling back into the mouth. It also serves as a point of fixation for adhesive tape. The bite block portion is designed to prevent approximation of the central incisors. A forceful bite may produce obstruction of an oral tracheal tube. The stent of the oropharyngeal airway is designed specifically to hold the tongue away from the posterior pharyngeal wall. Secondarily, the stent may provide an air channel or suction conduit through the mouth. The proper size oropharyngeal airway can be estimated by placing the airway alongside the face so the bite block portion is parallel to the palate. The tip of the airway should just approximate the angle of the mandible.

The primary use of the airway is in the unconscious patient. The airway should be placed by using a wooden spatula or tongue depressor to press the tongue into the floor of the mouth. The airway is then passed so the stent conforms to the contour of the tongue. If the oropharyngeal airway is not inserted properly, it may push the tongue backward into the posterior pharynx, aggravating or creating upper airway obstruction. If the airway is too long, it may touch the larynx and stimulate vomiting or laryngospasm.

Nasopharyngeal Airways. The nasopharyngeal airways stent the tongue from the posterior pharyngeal wall (Fig. 1.7). It may also be used to facilitate nasotracheal suctioning. The length of the nasopharyngeal airway is estimated by measuring the distance from the nares to the tragus of the ear. The outside diameter of the airway should not be so large that it produces sustained blanching of the skin of the ala nasae. The nasopharyngeal airway is inserted through the nares and passed along the floor of the nostril into the nasopharynx and oropharynx so it rests between the tongue and the posterior pharyngeal wall. Nasopharyngeal airways may lacerate the vascular adenoidal tissue found in the nasopharynx of children. Therefore, adenoidal

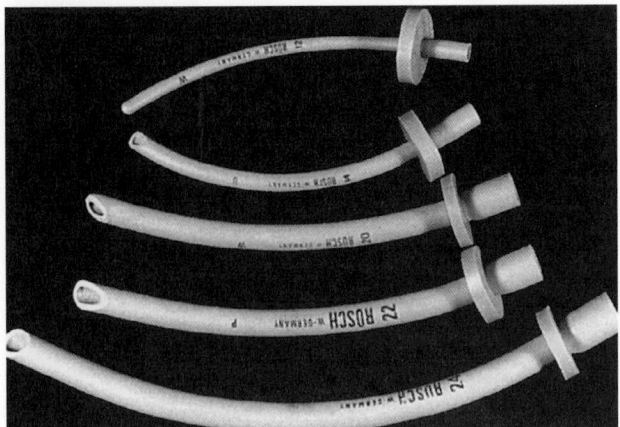

FIGURE 1.7 Nasopharyngeal airways in a variety of sizes.

hypertrophy and bleeding diatheses are relative contraindications to the use of these airways.

Endotracheal Tubes. The endotracheal (ET) tube (Fig. 1.8) supplies a stable alternate airway. ET tubes are used to (i) overcome upper airway obstruction, (ii) isolate the larynx from the pharynx, (iii) allow mechanical aspiration of secretions from the tracheal bronchial tree, and (iv) facilitate mechanical ventilation or end-expiratory pressure. The correct tube size can be approximated by using a simple formula based on the patient's age:

$$\text{Inside diameter (ID) in mm} = \frac{16 + \text{Age in years}}{4}$$

Because this is an estimate, it is prudent to have the next smaller and larger size ET tube available. Estimation of tube size based on the size of the patient's fifth finger is not accurate. Tube size may also need to be modified based on the cause of the arrest (e.g., croup). In the pediatric patient, uncuffed tubes are used and are compatible with positive-pressure ventilation. This is because in children, there is a normal narrowing of the trachea at the level of the cricoid ring (Fig. 1.9). With proper tube selection, this narrowing serves as a functional seal. In the hospital setting either cuffed or uncuffed tubes may be used for airway management. When using a cuffed tube add 0.5 mm to the tube size.

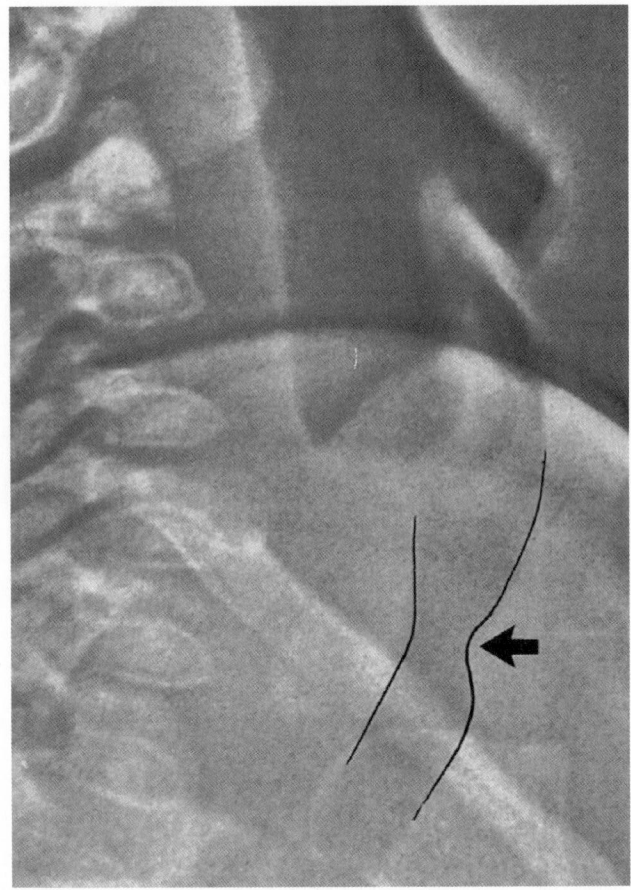

FIGURE 1.9 Lateral neck xeroradiograph showing narrowing at level of cricoid ring.

A variety of ET tubes are available. Tracheal tubes (Fig. 1.8) should be translucent to facilitate inspection of internal debris or occlusion, have a radiopaque tip marker, have the internal diameter noted proximally so it is visible after intubation, have a distal vocal cord marker so when the marker is placed at the level of the vocal cords, the tip of the tube is in a midtracheal position, have centimeter markings along the course of the tube to be used as reference points for detecting tube movement, and meet the American National Standard Institute Z-79 guidelines for tracheal tubes and cuffs. The

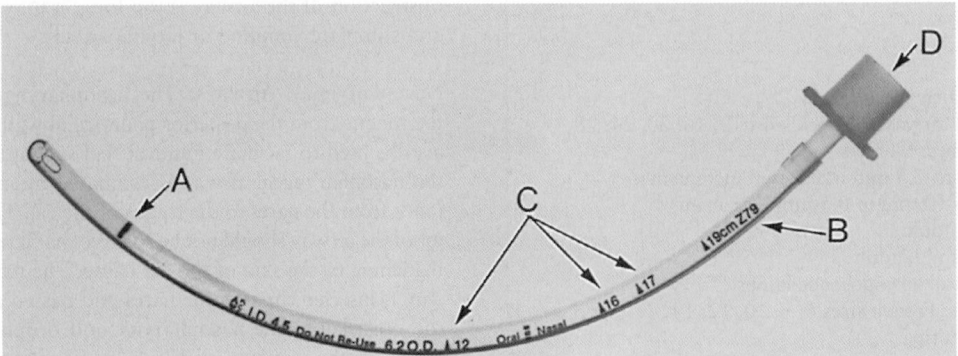

FIGURE 1.8 Oral tracheal tube: vocal cord marker (**A**), manufacturer's indication that tube meets ANSI-Z79 subcommittee standards (**B**), distance in centimeters from tip of tube (**C**), and standard 15-mm connector (**D**).

distance the tube is inserted into the trachea may be calculated by using the formula:

$$\text{Insertion distance (cm mark at teeth)} = \frac{\text{Age in years}}{2} + 12$$

Other Techniques. Alternative airway management systems, including esophageal/tracheal tubes, laryngeal mask airways, and transtracheal ventilation systems, have all been used with adult patients with varying degrees of success. All the methods have been approved by governmental agencies and professional societies, but their use in children has not been well tested or researched. There is more experience with the use of the laryngeal masks in children. This method may be used by experienced providers when ET intubation is not possible (Class 11b).

Laryngoscopy and Intubation (see Chapter 5, Procedure 8 in Chapter 135). Laryngoscopy creates a spatial plane through the mouth to the larynx through which an ET tube can be passed into the trachea. The laryngoscope consists of a blade and a handle. It is used to identify the glottis and to compress the intervening soft-tissue structures into the floor of the mouth. The three components of the laryngoscope blade are the spatula, the tip, and the flange (Fig. 1.10). The spatula may be curved or straight and is used to compress tissue. The tip of the blade is used for positioning the spatula so an optimal compression of the mandibular block or soft tissue can be achieved. The flange keeps the tongue out of the way of the intubating channel. The laryngoscope is introduced into the mouth so the tip of the blade slides down the right side of the tongue. As the tip of the blade follows the tongue posteriorly, it bumps into the anterior pillars of the tonsils. The tip is moved around the pillars of the tonsils until it bumps into the epiglottis. When using a curved spatula, the tip is placed in the vallecula, the space between the tongue and epiglottis. When using a straight spatula, the tip is placed under the epiglottis with the leading edge resting on the aryepiglottic folds. Once the tip is properly placed, the spatula is shifted from the right side of the mouth to the middle of the mouth. This left lateral movement of the spatula allows the flange to push the tongue ahead of it so the tongue eventually occupies the middle third of the mouth. The right one-third of the mouth is then available as a channel through which the tracheal tube can pass. Once the tip of the blade is properly positioned and the flange has moved the tongue into the left corner of the mouth, the full surface of the spatula is used to compress the tongue into the floor of the mouth. With compression of the soft tissue of the mouth, the glottis should be exposed and the tracheal tube can be passed. The tracheal tube should be fitted with a stylet. The purpose of the stylet is to provide some degree of curvature to the tube for those circumstances where a totally straight channel cannot be achieved. The tracheal tube is passed through the glottis so the ring marker near the tip of the tube is aligned with the vocal cords. If the tube selected is the proper size and the ring marker is placed directly at the vocal cords, the tip of the tube should be at a midtracheal position.

Proper positioning of the tube is confirmed most accurately by end-tidal CO_2 monitoring (Fig. 1.11) and by auscultating for breath sounds and observing for symmetric chest movement. The child's small chest wall may transmit sounds widely and thus mislead the physician into thinking the positioning is correct. The physician should listen carefully. He or she should listen over the stomach and both axillas and look for improved color of the patient. If breath sounds are not equal or end-tidal CO_2 monitoring is not available, the tube should be withdrawn slightly and the breath sounds and chest movement reevaluated. When circumstances allow, tube position should be confirmed with an anteroposterior (AP) chest roentgenogram. On the AP film, the tip of the tracheal tube should be at a T2 to T3 vertebral level or directly between the lower edges of the medial aspect of the clavicles (Fig. 1.12).

Loss of an established airway is an unnecessary complication. The tracheal tube should be thoroughly secured with adhesive tape. The skin to which the adhesive tape is affixed should be cleansed, dried, and painted with tincture of benzoin (Fig. 1.11).

The management of airway obstruction is detailed in a separate section at the end of this chapter, and Chapter 5 covers other advanced aspects of airway management.

Breathing

Evaluation

When a clear and stable airway has been established, the patient should be reassessed. The physician should look, listen, and feel for evidence of gas exchange. In infants, adequacy of ventilation is assessed by observing free uniform expansion of the lower chest and upper abdomen. This is in contrast to older children and adolescents in whom one looks for uniform upper chest expansion as a sign of adequate ventilation. Gas exchanges should be confirmed by auscultation and by electronic monitoring of end-tidal CO_2 and pulse oximetry. First, the physician should listen over the trachea to establish quickly that gas exchange is occurring through the central airway. Then, he or she should listen to breath sounds bilaterally to assess for peripheral aeration and symmetric lung expansion.

Management

Spontaneous Ventilation. If the airway has been established and the patient is breathing spontaneously, supplemental oxygen should be administered. Although elimination of carbon dioxide is important, it is not nearly as important as delivery

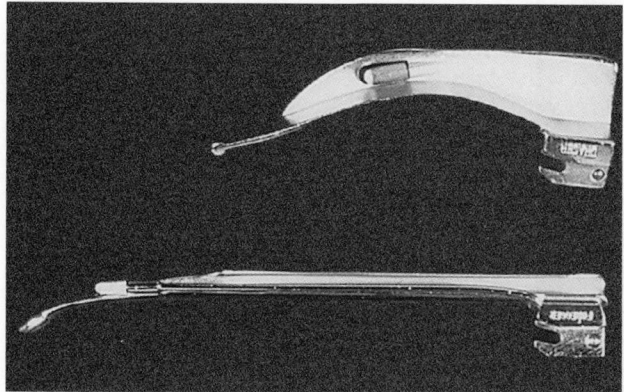

FIGURE 1.10 Laryngoscope blades—straight blade (Miller) and curved (MacIntosh).

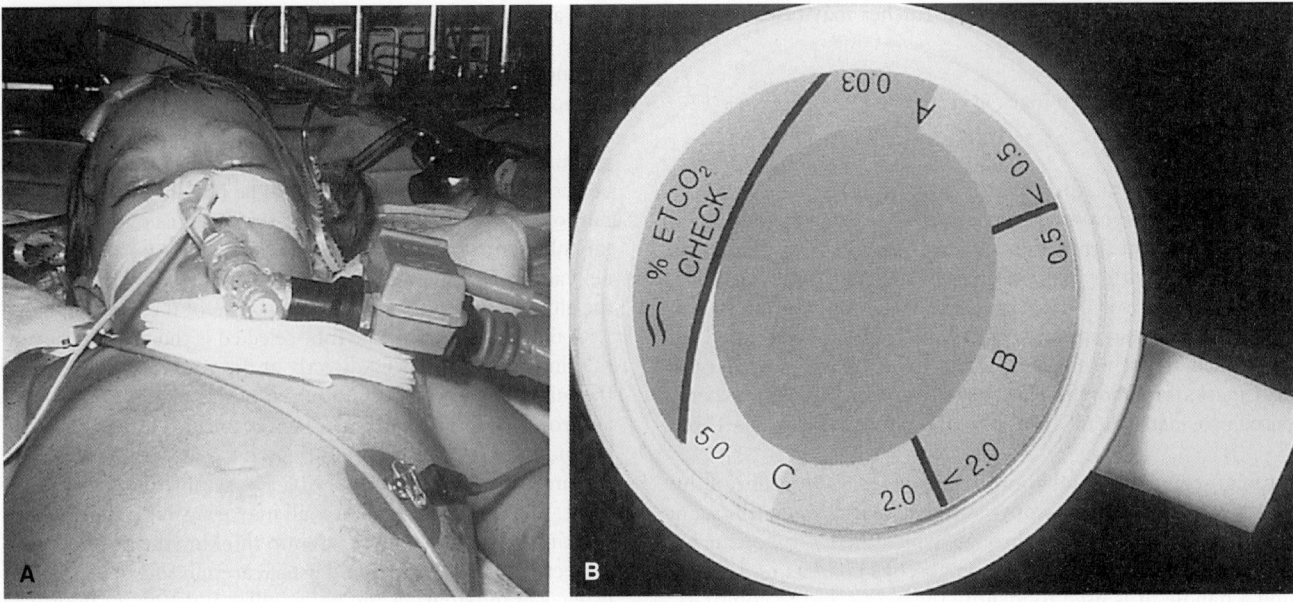

FIGURE 1.11 End-tidal CO_2 monitor. **A:** Inline on patient's endotracheal tube. **B:** Disposable-type monitor.

of oxygen. Children are quite resistant to the effects of severe hypercarbia and respiratory acidosis. However, they do not tolerate even short periods of oxygen deprivation.

Oxygen Delivery Devices. A variety of oxygen delivery devices are available for use in patients who have stable airways without ET tubes.

Nasal cannulas. Nasal cannulas have two hollow plastic prongs that arise from a flexible hollow face piece. Humidified oxygen delivered through the hollow tubing is directed to the nostrils. One hundred percent oxygen is run through a bubbler into the cannula system at a flow of 4 to 6 L per minute. Because of oropharyngeal and nasopharyngeal entrainment of air, the final oxygen delivery is usually 30% to 40%. The advantages of

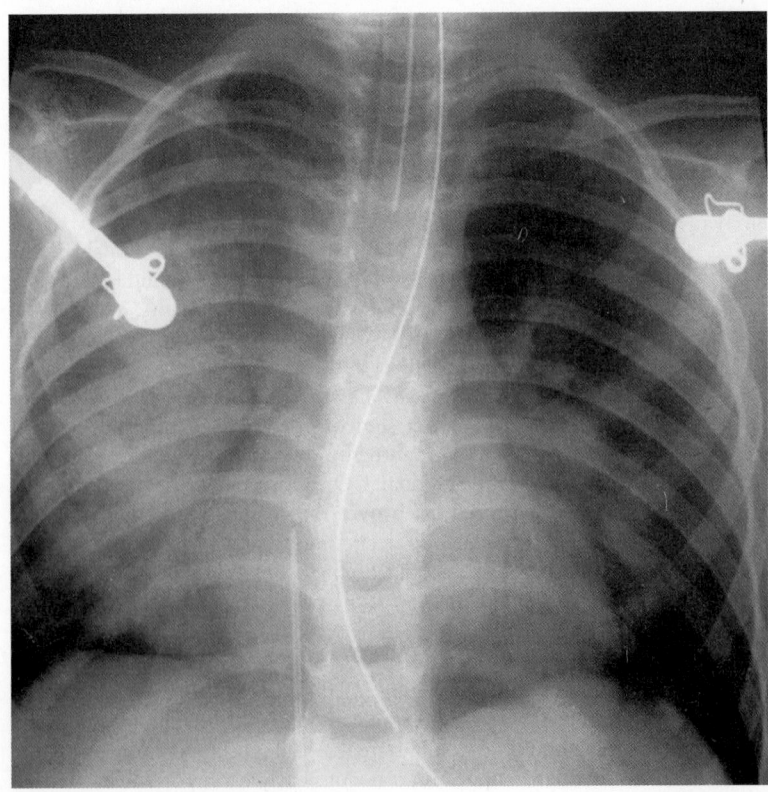

FIGURE 1.12 Chest radiograph showing proper endotracheal tube placement at T2 to T3 vertebral level.

cannulas are that they are easy to apply, lightweight, economical, and disposable. Inefficiency of the bubbler humidifier is compensated for by the fact that the normal humidification and warming systems of the upper airway are not bypassed. The use of this device presumes the patient's oxygen needs can be met with substantially less than 100% oxygen. This method of oxygen delivery is best tolerated by the older child.

Oxygen hoods. Oxygen hoods are clear plastic cylinders with removable lids (Fig. 1.13) or clear, soft, plastic tents just large enough to accommodate the infant's head. They are used for delivery of oxygen to infants and come in a variety of sizes. They usually have a gas inlet system for wide-bore tubing and a port for positioning the cylinder across the neck. Their purpose is to maintain a controlled environment for oxygen, humidity, and temperature. This can be done without producing a tight seal at the neck. Hoods are best used for newborns and infants. One can, without difficulty, deliver oxygen concentrations in the 80% to 90% range simply by increasing the oxygen flow to flood the canister. Another advantage is that the oxygen may be well humidified. Because of their potential for delivering concentrations of oxygen that may be toxic to the eyes or lungs of the infant, it is imperative to monitor both the fraction of inspired oxygen (FiO_2) and the PaO_2.

Oxygen tents. The oxygen tent provides a controlled and stable environment for humidity, temperature, and oxygen. Tents are useful for delivery of oxygen between 21% and 50%. Oxygen concentration may be variable because of a poor seal and frequent entry. Therefore, a tight fit and only necessary entry should be allowed. Tents potentially impede access to the patient, and if mist is used, the patient may be hidden in a cloud, which makes skin color difficult to evaluate.

Oxygen masks. The most often used equipment for the spontaneously breathing patient is the oxygen mask. Several types of oxygen masks can be used to offer the patient a wide range of inspired oxygen concentrations. Masks seem to be better tolerated than nasal cannula by the young child, particularly when the mask is held by a calm parent or by ED personnel. There are several mask types from which to select. As with all equipment, even masks have associated hazards. In patients prone to vomit, the mask can block the flow of vomitus and increase the risk of aspiration. The obtunded patient wearing a mask must always be observed.

SIMPLE MASKS. The simple face mask delivers a moderate concentration of oxygen. These masks are lightweight and inexpensive. They should be clear to allow observation of the child's color. They can be used in a loose-fitting fashion and are relatively comfortable. If the flow of oxygen is inadvertently disrupted, the child can breathe through side ports. A minimal flow of oxygen is necessary to flush potential dead space. This type of oxygen delivery device does not bypass the upper airway mechanisms for warming and humidification of inspired gas. The disadvantages of the simple mask lie in the fact that it is difficult to provide a known and stable FiO_2. The FiO_2 will vary with the inspiratory flow rate of the patient and with the oxygen flow into the system. The actual pharyngeal FiO_2 may be difficult to predict or measure.

PARTIAL REBREATHING MASKS. Partial rebreathing masks allow delivery of a higher oxygen concentration than simple masks do. They are also helpful in conserving oxygen. This system is a combined face mask and reservoir bag. When the flow rate into the bag is greater than the patient's minute ventilation and when the oxygen is adjusted so the bag does not collapse during inhalation, there is negligible CO_2 rebreathing. Partial rebreathing masks are usually used for midrange oxygen delivery. We use one when we are trying to maintain FiO_2 between 35% and 60%.

NONREBREATHING MASKS. Nonrebreathing masks are combined face mask and reservoir bag devices that have nonrebreathing valves incorporated into the face mask. They are useful for giving oxygen concentrations up to 100%.

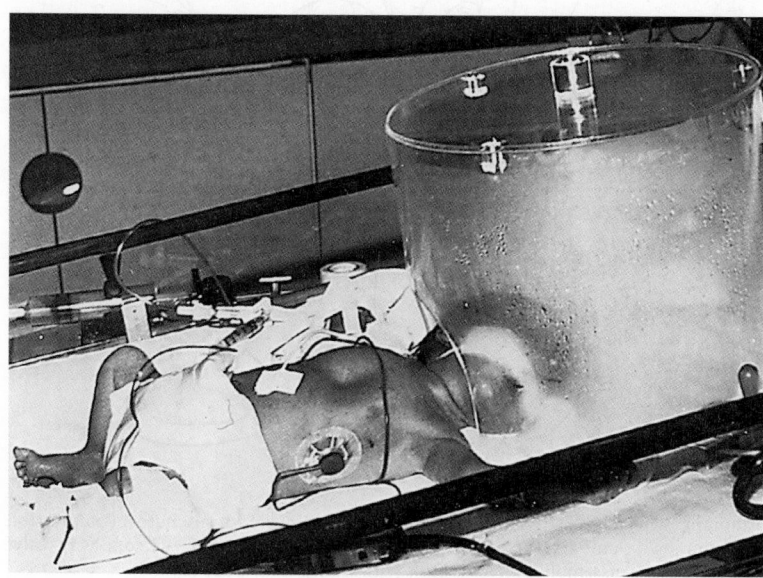

FIGURE 1.13 Infant oxygen hood. Oxygen hoods are clear plastic cylinders with removable lids or clear, soft, plastic tents just large enough to accommodate the infant's head.

Assisted Ventilation. If the airway has been established and the child is not breathing spontaneously or gas exchange is not adequate, artificial ventilation should be started. The recommended rates for rescue breathing in infants and children are 20 to 24 for an infant and 16 to 20 for an older child. Rates may need modification based on the etiology of the child's arrest (e.g., treatment of ICP may require a faster rate).

If adjuncts for mechanical ventilatory support are not available, an expired air technique may be used. Patient size, type of available airway, and trial will determine which type should be used. Because of risk of human immunodeficiency virus (HIV) transmission, mouth-to-mouth resuscitation is no longer recommended. Instead, rescue breathing should be done with a pocket mask that contains an appropriate millipore filter (Fig. 1.14). Placement of the mask over the mouth alone, over the mouth and nose, or over a tracheostomy site depends on the patient and the equipment available (Fig. 1.14). See Chapter 120 for care of the patient with tracheostomy.

Expired Air Techniques

Hand-squeezed, self-inflating resuscitators. Hand-squeezed, self-inflating resuscitators are the most commonly used resus-

citators for infants and children. The elasticity of a self-inflating bag allows the bag to refill independently of gas flow. This feature makes the self-inflating bag easy to use for the inexperienced operator. Many of the self-inflating bags are equipped with a pressure-limiting pop-off valve that is usually preset at 30 to 35 cm H_2O to prevent delivery of high pressures. Self-inflating bags that are not pressure limited should have a manometer in line. For gas to flow, the bag must be squeezed. Thus, for the patient who is breathing spontaneously, the operator must time the bag compressions to the patient's efforts. These resuscitators should be adapted to deliver high concentrations of oxygen. In most cases, this involves using an oxygen reservoir adaptation with the unit (Fig. 1.15). More recent research has shown that even with an attached reservoir, only oxygen concentrations of 60% to 90% were obtainable. Units without oxygen reservoir adaptations often deliver low concentrations of supplemental oxygen and, therefore, should be avoided.

The resuscitator may be used with a mask. When selecting a family of mask sizes, select a mask type that seals a variety of facial contours. Also, the body of the mask should be sufficiently transparent so vomitus can be recognized easily through the mask. Masks with a pneumatic cuff design allow for the easiest and most efficient fit that avoids air leaks around the mask. Resuscitators, masks, and ET tubes should be standardized so any resuscitator can connect with any mask or ET tube. A recent study by Davidovic demonstrated the value of two-person technique.

Anesthesia bags. Anesthesia bags depend on an adequate gas flow to maintain a compressible unit that propels gas toward the patient (Fig. 1.16). An exit port must also be present so the bag does not become a carbon dioxide reservoir. When used

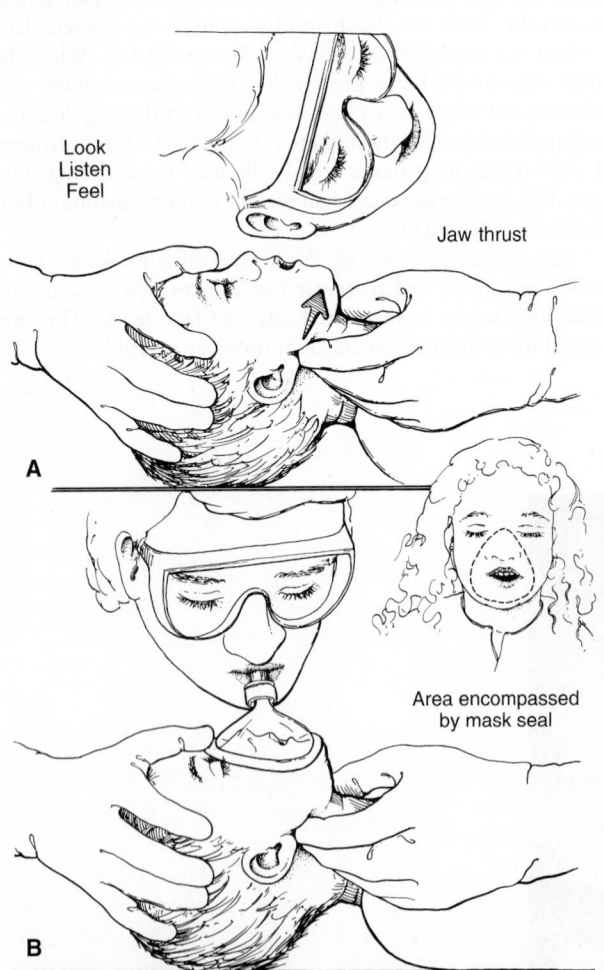

FIGURE 1.14 Basic life support—airway and breathing. **A:** Positioning of head to open airway and evaluation for spontaneous ventilation. **B:** Expired air (mouth-to-mask) ventilation.

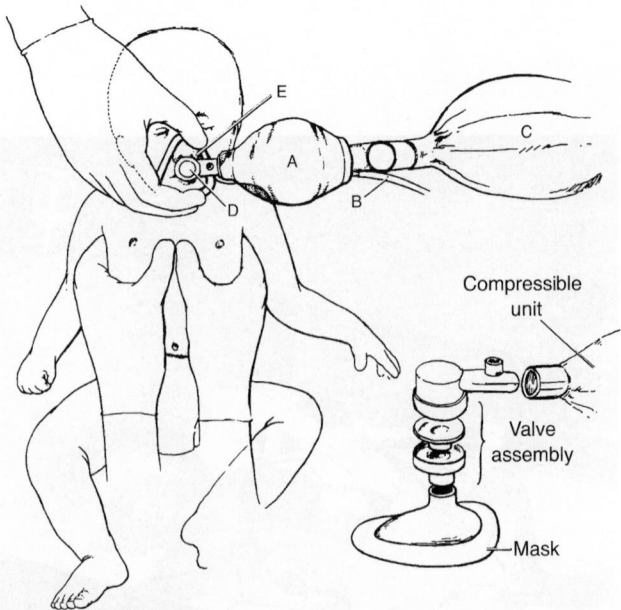

FIGURE 1.15 Self-inflating hand-powered resuscitator: compressible unit (**A**), oxygen source (**B**), oxygen reservoir (**C**), one-way valve assembly (**D**), and mask with transparent body (**E**).

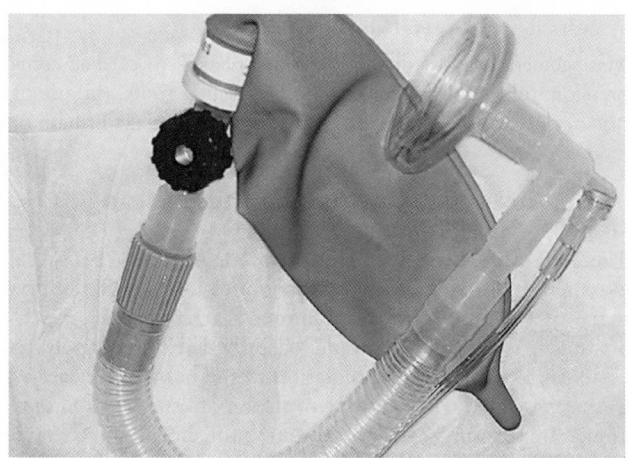

FIGURE 1.16 Family of clear plastic, air-filled collar facial masks.

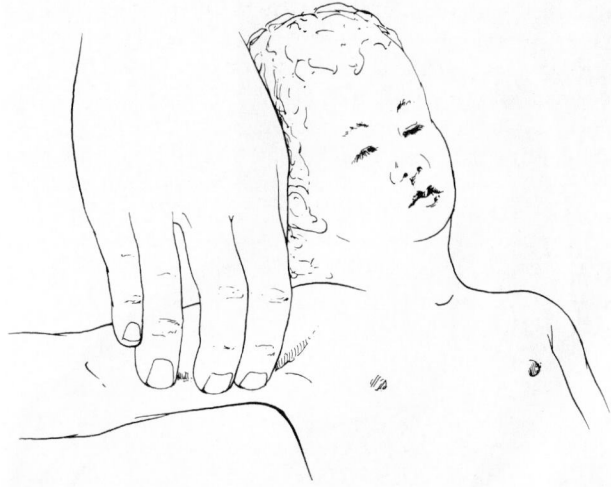

FIGURE 1.18 Palpation of brachial pulse on medial aspect of the upper arm in the subbicep groove.

with an oxygen blender, any desired concentration of oxygen may be provided for the patient because this system directly delivers the gas flowing into it. When used correctly, this device allows 100% oxygen to be delivered as well as maintaining end-expiratory pressure. However, the major disadvantage of this type of bag is that considerable experience is needed to use it effectively, which has prompted some to recommend the use of the self-inflating bag as the primary mode of ventilation. One must be able to accurately judge the rate of gas flow into the bag and the rate of gas escape from the exit port so underfilling or overfilling does not occur. If the bag is removed from a leak-tight patient application, it promptly deflates and one must wait for the reservoir to refill. Overfilling the bag is dangerous because high pressures can be transmitted to the lung and stomach (Fig. 1.17).

Mechanical ventilators. The ED should also be equipped with a mechanical ventilator. If the resuscitation is successful, this is important for maintenance of ventilation while the patient awaits transfer or transport to a critical care unit. A mechanical ventilator is also crucial in the event of multiple arrest victims in order to free personnel for other vital tasks.

Circulation

As with the other components of CPR, the circulation must be first assessed and then managed.

Evaluation

Once the airway has been opened and gas exchange ensured, the physician must evaluate the effectiveness of circulation by (i) observing skin and mucous membrane color, and (ii) palpating a peripheral pulse and checking capillary refill. If the patient's color is ashen or cyanotic, the circulation will need to be treated.

The palpation of a peripheral pulse and assessment of capillary refill is mandatory. Often, ineffective cardiac activity can be palpated over the child's thin chest wall. Thus, the presence of an apical pulse may not be meaningful. The palpation of a strong femoral or brachial pulse (Fig. 1.18) indicates presumptively that the cardiac output is adequate. Capillary refill should be assessed repeatedly (Fig. 1.19).

Most modern defibrillators have a "quick-look" paddle configuration that allows a rapid evaluation of cardiac rhythm to be made by placing the defibrillation paddles on the chest and using them as monitoring electrodes.

The resuscitation team will also find it helpful to have continuous blood pressure monitoring. Blood pressure measurements will help quantify the effectiveness of cardiac function. An ultrasound or portable Doppler device may be necessary to detect systolic pressure at low levels in small infants (Fig. 1.20).

As soon as possible, the team will also require continuous electrocardiogram (EKG) monitoring to assess the development of arrhythmia as the resuscitation proceeds.

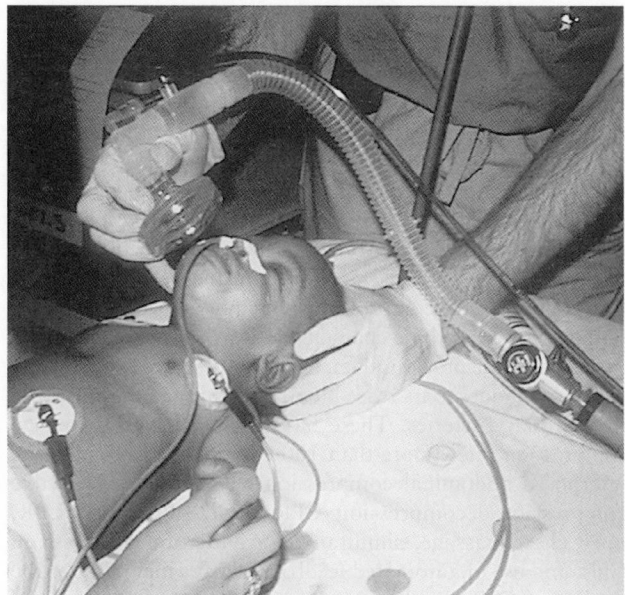

FIGURE 1.17 Anesthesia bag in use.

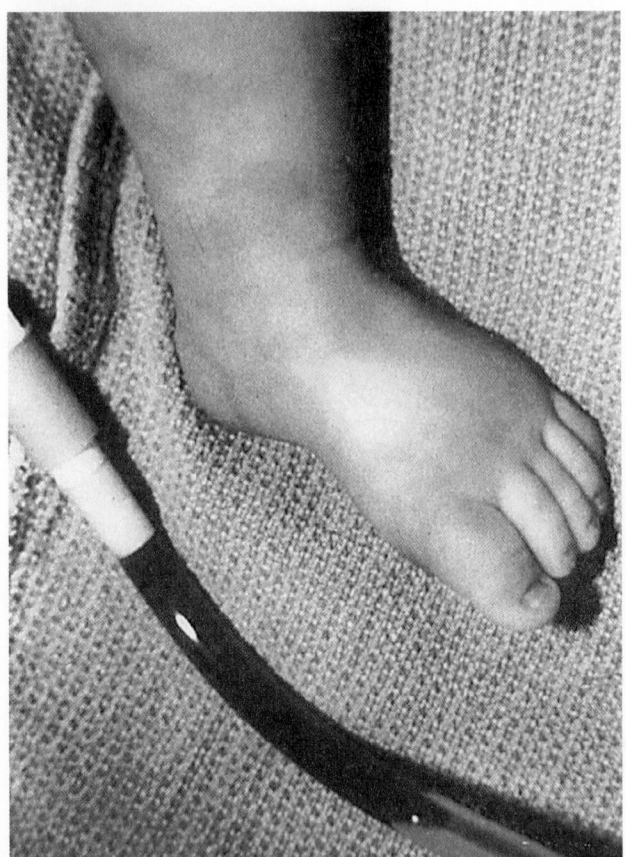

FIGURE 1.19 Delayed capillary refill.

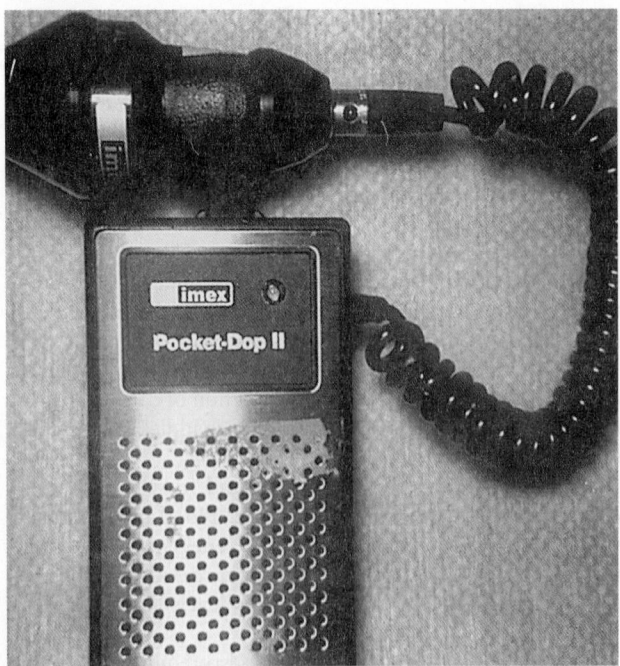

FIGURE 1.20 Portable Doppler device for determining blood pressure during resuscitation.

Management

Management may be divided into five phases: (i) cardiac compression, (ii) establishment of an intravascular route, (iii) use of primary drugs, (iv) use of secondary drugs, and (v) defibrillation.

External Cardiac Compression

The 2005 AHA Guidelines emphasize the importance of well-executed external cardiac chest compressions (CPR) as primary treatment for cardiopulmonary arrest. In the newly arrested patients, CPR should be provided immediately to establish a minimum of circulation to the brain and heart as this is associated with improvements in both survival and outcome. Importantly, several recent published reports have clearly shown that the quality of CPR administered in both out-of-hospital and in-hospital settings does not meet the standards set forth by the AHA.

In the newly arrested child, vigorous, high-quality chest compressions generate approximately one-third of the normal cardiac output. This generates a coronary artery perfusion pressure (CAPP) of approximately 10 mm Hg. This decreases over time as the myocardium becomes damaged by hypoxemia and metabolic derangements. It is estimated that CAPPs of 25 to 30 mm Hg are needed to produce forward flow through the aorta in order to reperfuse the myocardium and "jump start" the heart into a perfusing rhythm to provide sufficient blood flow to all vital organs.

The mechanism by which blood moves during CPR continues to be the subject of investigation. Techniques that augment this forward flow could potentially improve the rates of successful return of spontaneous circulation (ROSC) and neurologic survival. "Direct compression" and "thoracic pump" describe the current mechanisms that explain how blood flows during CPR. In the "direct compression" model, the heart is squeezed between the sternum and the posterior vertebrae. During compression, "systole," blood moves through the AV valves and the aorta. During relaxation, "diastole," blood fills the myocardium in preparation for the next systole. In the "thoracic pump" model, the heart is viewed as a conduit. During compression, venous valves at the thoracic inlet close preventing retrograde flow, the venous side of the circulation is compressed, and blood moves forward through the AV valves and the aorta. During relaxation, negative intrathoracic pressures suck blood into the pulmonary bed and heart in preparation for the next systole. In practice, both methods probably contribute to blood flow. Because of the compliance and elasticity of the chest wall and the intrathoracic structures, direct compression may play a larger role in the pediatric patient. Additionally, chest compressions may provide greater cardiac output because of these characteristics.

Based on the previous data, investigators have explored different techniques to increase blood flow through the aorta and the coronary arteries. These have included high-frequency compression rates (more than 100 compressions per minute), interposed abdominal compression CPR (IAC-CPR), active compression-decompression CPR (ACD-CPR), vest CPR, open chest massage, simultaneous ventilation-compression CPR, and use of automated feedback devices that monitor the quality of CPR. To date, compression rates and automated performance feedback have been the most promising.

Compression rates clearly affect the cardiac output. During CPR, CAPP rises during consecutive chest compressions and falls during pauses in compressions and with positive-pressure ventilation. Compression rates of more than 100 have been shown to improve cardiac output, CAPP, and 24-hour survival when compared with rates less than 80. Although the optimal compression rate remains unknown, compression rate of 100 per minute is now recommended for all ages beyond the neonatal period. There is some evidence in adults that compression-only CPR (no ventilation) produces similar survival rates. Because of the etiology of pediatric arrest, in addition to higher metabolic rate and lower functional residual capacity, this practice is not recommended for children.

The optimal duty cycle also remains unknown. To date, a duty cycle of 50% (compression:relaxation, 1:1) is believed to provide the highest flow rates. Leaning or incomplete decompression of the chest during the relaxation phase occurs commonly and may affect the cardiac output generated by CPR by decreasing venous return.

Other techniques such as IAC-CPR (interposed-abdominal compression CPR) and mechanical devices developed for adults and used in adult resuscitation such as ACD (active compression-decompression), vest CPR, mechanical CPR, simultaneous ventilation-compression CPR, and phased thoracic-abdominal compression-decompression CPR are not recommended for use in pediatric arrest because of lack of experience and data.

Open cardiac massage provides better blood flow to vital organs in animals and in adults when compared with CPR. Because of the compliance of the thoracic structures in children, this technique may not offer any benefit. There is inadequate data to recommend its use in the resuscitation of children regardless of the etiology of the arrest.

It is imperative that the provider assess the efficacy of CPR. Evaluating for the presence of the femoral artery pulse with compressions is helpful. Although this pulse may represent venous rather than arterial pulsations, it still provides important, easily accessible information to the provider. Continuous end-tidal CO_2 monitoring can also serve as a marker of blood flow. Exhaled CO_2 rises as pulmonary blood flow and cardiac output increases. Weil and others have worked on a method of measuring CO_2 by means of a sublingual probe. This technique offers promise for monitoring cardiac output and may be useful as a predictor of terminal hypoperfusion. One of the most innovative additions to CPR has been the development of monitors with accelerometers and force sensors that provide real-time feedback to the provider. A puck is placed on the child's chest and feedback including compression rate and force is displayed on the defibrillator screen. Verbal feedback is also provided. Currently, this technology is available for use in children older than 8 years of age.

Over the past decade there have been several reports that have demonstrated the delivery of suboptimal CPR by practitioners both in the out-of-hospital and in-hospital setting. It is now known that high-quality CPR is linked to both improved rates of ROSC, to survival to hospital admission and perhaps to better neurologic outcome. Wik et al. published a case series of paramedic practice for out-of-hospital cardiac arrest and found that chest compressions were delivered only half of the available time and were compliant with AHA guidelines only 28% of the time. Ashton et al. showed that the rate and depth of compres-

sions decreased significantly after 2 minutes even though rescuers denied feeling fatigue. Kramer-Johansen et al. compared quality of CPR and outcome in out-of-hospital cardiac arrest in adult patients with and without automated real-time verbal and visual feedback provided by a prototype defibrillator. Compression depth, the percentage of compressions with adequate depth, and the compression rate increased when feedback was given. Increased compression depth was associated with increased survival to hospital admission. Abella et al. found that higher compression rates (greater than 80) resulted in higher rates of ROSC. Edelson et al. demonstrated that longer preshock pauses were associated with defibrillation failure. Thus, CPR quality is a critical determinant of survival after CPR. Monitoring and feedback defibrillators can enhance this quality. The AHA 2005 Guidelines recommend the following: Push hard and fast (100 per minute, IIa), ensure full chest recoil (IIb), minimize interruptions in chest compressions, avoid hyperventilation, and change rescuers every 2 minutes in less than 5 seconds. The proper technique for providing CPR is essential and all healthcare emergency medicine should be familiar with this technique. The rescuer should compress the lower half of the sternum, avoiding the xiphoid process, one-third to one-half the depth of the chest. The child should be supine on a firm surface that is wider than the patient's torso and extends from the shoulders to the waist. For infants (younger than 1 year), the Thaler or two thumb-encircling hands technique is the preferred method for health-care providers (Figs. 1.21 and 1.22). The recommended rate of compressions for all ages except neonates is 100 compressions per minute. The compression and relaxation phases of each compression should be equal. Once the airway has been secured, coordination of compressions and rescue breathing is no longer necessary (Table 1.8).

Intravenous Access

The site used for vascular access depends on the patient's condition and the provider's experience. The most common sites used in the ill pediatric patient include peripheral venous access, central venous access via the femoral vein, and IO access.

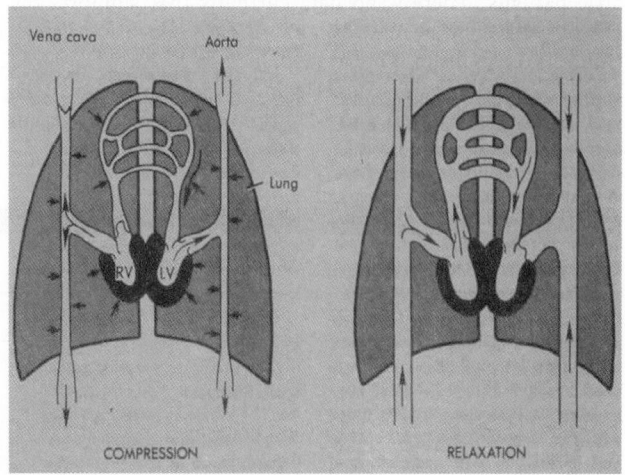

FIGURE 1.21 Movement during external cardiac compression. RV, right ventricle; LV, left ventricle.

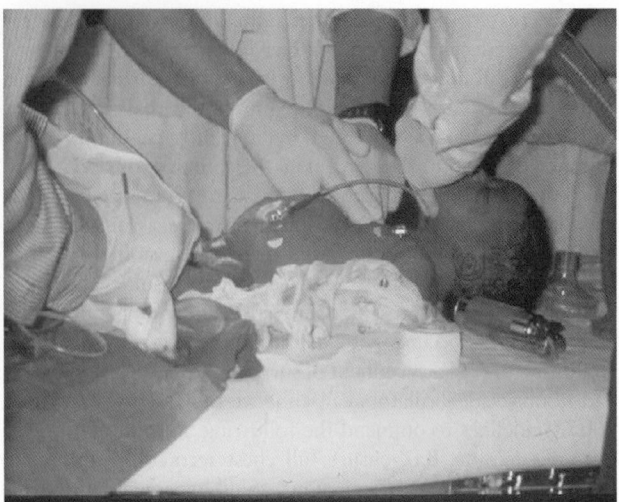

FIGURE 1.22 External cardiac compression.

In the arrested patient, access is challenging and time-consuming. IO access is the first and best choice for this scenario because this procedure is simple and can be accomplished quickly (30 to 60 seconds). This route can be safely used for all drugs and fluids needed during resuscitation. The onset of action of drugs administered via this route is comparable to that of drugs administered into the central circulation. Manual pressure or use of a pressure bag is necessary when giving fluids to restore the vascular volume in order to overcome the resistance of the marrow venous plexus. The preferred site in children is the medial surface of the tibia 1 to 3 cm below the tibial tuberosity (Fig. 1.23). Alternative sites include the anterior surface of the distal femur, the medial malleolus, and the anterior iliac spine. There are several types of rigid, styletted needles commercially available for this procedure in infants and children. There are also some new IO devices available on the market now. The bone injection gun (BIG) is a spring-loaded device that can be used in adolescents/adults and can effectively penetrate the thicker bony cortex. The EZ-IO® (Vidacare, San Antonio, TX) a battery-powered hand-held drill, is available for use in pediatric patients. There is no data currently that supports the use of these new needles over those currently used widely. Contraindications to IO placement include recently fractured bone, osteogenesis imperfecta, and osteopetrosis. Complications are rare and have been reported in less than

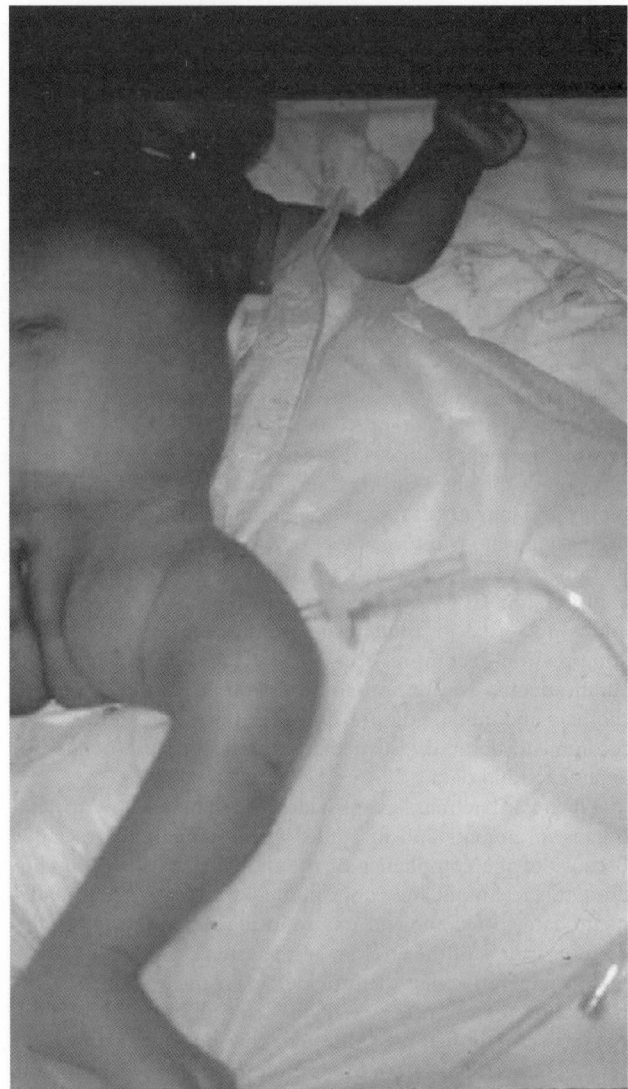

FIGURE 1.23 Intraosseous needle placed in distal femur.

1% of patients. These have included extravasation, epiphyseal injury, fracture, compartment syndrome, fat embolism, and thrombosis (see Section VII for description of procedure). Peripheral venous access provides an adequate route for resuscitation as long as it is achieved quickly. Veins of the hands, forearm, and ankle are most commonly used (see Section VII for

TABLE 1.8

CHEST COMPRESSION PARAMETERS

Age	Depth	Rate	Technique	Landmark
Neonate		90	Thaler, 2 Fingers	Just below the nipple line
	1/3–1/2 chest diameter	100		Between the nipples in the center of the chest
1 yr to puberty	1/3–1/2 chest diameter		1 or 2 Hands	
Adult	1½–2 inches	100	2 Hands	Between the nipples in the center of the chest

Adapted from the American Heart Association 2005 Guidelines for Cardiopulmonary Resuscitation and Emergency Cardiovascular Care.

TABLE 1.9

SAMPLE PROTOCOL FOR INTRAVENOUS ACCESS

1. First 1.5 min
   Peripheral IV catheter, two sites
2. 1.5–5 min
   a. If intubated: give drugs via endotracheal tube (including epinephrine/atropine/lidocaine)
   b. If not intubated: intraosseous—one site
      Continued peripheral IV—one site
3. Longer than 5 min
   a. Femoral vein percutaneous
   b. External/internal jugular percutaneous
   c. Subclavian vein percutaneous
   d. Saphenous vein cutdown

Adapted from Kanter RK, Zimmerman JJ, Strauss RH, et al. Pediatric emergency intravenous access. *Am J Dis Child* 1986;140:144.

description of this procedure). There should be an established protocol for the sequence of IV access steps (Table 1.9).

The femoral vein is the easiest central vein to access in the critically ill child when many interventions are ongoing simultaneously. There are also less complications associated with this route. Central venous access provides a more secure route, allows the capability of monitoring central venous pressure, and allows for blood sampling. In adults, this route has been shown to provide more rapid onset of action and higher peak drug levels that theoretically could affect outcome. This has not been shown to be the case in the pediatric patient. In the child with uncompensated shock or arrest, this type of access may follow IO access through which initial resuscitation can occur rapidly.

The femoral vein lies medial to the femoral artery. If there is no pulse present, the artery can be found by locating the midpoint between the anterior iliac spine and the pubic symphysis. The right femoral vein is easier to access and is less likely to enter the posterior lumbar venous plexus. The

Seldinger technique is preferred for catheter placement. By placing a small towel underneath the child's buttocks and slightly externally rotating the hip, the inguinal area is flattened, making venous entry easier. The needle should enter at a 45-degree angle, approximately one finger breadth below the inguinal ligament. Complications associated with this procedure include thrombosis and suppurative thrombophlebitis. See Procedure Section VII for description of this procedure and see Table 1.10 for catheter sizes.

Drugs of Resuscitation

Estimating Body Weight

Appropriate drug doses, fluid therapy, and equipment size vary depending on the size of the child in need of resuscitation. Recommended drug doses are based on kilograms of body weight. The 50th percentile weight from a standardized growth curve can be used if based on the child's known/estimated age. The "Broselow tape" allows a simple, accurate method of estimating the weight and drug doses based on the measured height. The tape is placed alongside the child in supine position and has appropriate drug dosages and equipment sizes printed on it at intervals (Fig. 1.24). Standard drugs and drug dosages are shown in Table 1.11.

Endotracheal Route of Administration

The pulmonary bed provides a surface for absorption of lipid-soluble drugs and can be used before vascular access is available. Currently, lidocaine, epinephrine, atropine, and naloxone (LEAN) can be used via this route. The optimal drug dosage remains unknown because absorption likely varies widely because of its dependence on pulmonary blood flow. Animal studies have shown that standard doses of epinephrine (0.01 mg per kg) achieve serum levels that are approximately 10% of those achieved by the intravascular route. Thus, the recommended dose of epinephrine to be given via the ET tube is 0.1 mg

TABLE 1.10

CATHETER SIZE AND LENGTH FOR FEMORAL CENTRAL VENOUS ACCESS

Age	Average weight (kg)	Average height (cm)	Average catheter length (cm)
1 mo	4.2	55	15.7
3 mo	5.8	61	17.3
6 mo	7.8	68	19.1
9 mo	9.2	72	20.1
1 yr	10.2	76	21.1
1.5 yr	11.5	83	22.9
2 yr	12.8	88	24.2
4 yr	16.5	103	28.1
6 yr	20.5	116	31.4
8 yr	26	127	34.2
10 yr	31	137	36.8
12 yr	39	149	39.9
14 yr	50	165	44.0
16 yr	62.5	174	46.3

Adapted from Henretig FM, King C, eds. *Textbook of pediatric emergency procedures.* Baltimore: Williams & Wilkins, 1997.

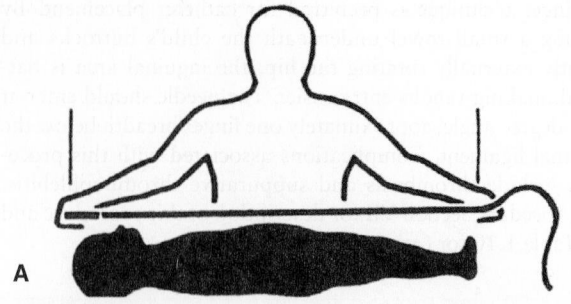

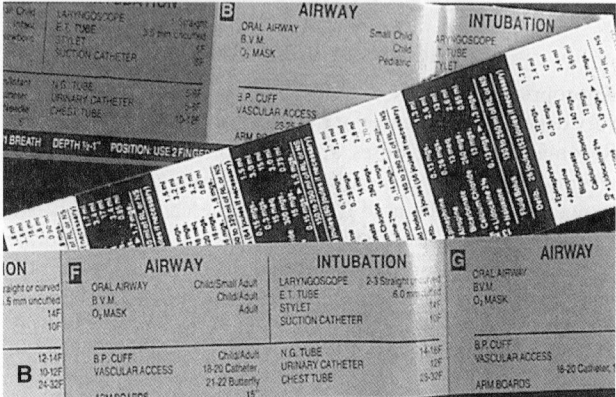

FIGURE 1.24 Broselow tape for determining drug dosage schedule based on patient length. **A:** Placement of tape. **B:** Equipment size and drug dosage schedule printed on tape.

TABLE 1.11

DRUGS AND DOSES OF RESUSCITATION

Drug	Dose (IV/IO)
Adenosine	0.1 mg/kg, max 6 mg Repeat 0.2 mg/kg, max 12 mg
Atropine	0.02 mg/kg, min 0.1 mg ETT: 0.03 mg/kg Maximum single dose 　　Child　　　　0.5 mg 　　Adolescent　　1 mg
Amiodarone	5 mg/kg, repeat to 15 mg/kg, max 300 mg
Calcium chloride (10%)	20 mg/kg or 0.2 mL/kg
Dobutamine	2–20 μg/kg/min infusion
Dopamine	2–20 μg/kg/min infusion
Epinephrine	IV: Use 1:10,000 0.01 mg/kg or 0.1 mL/kg, max 1 mg 0.1–1 μg/kg/min infusion ETT: Use 1:1000 0.1 mg/kg or 0.1 mL/kg, max 10 mg
Glucose 10%	0.5–1 g/kg, 5–10 mL/kg
Lidocaine	1 mg/kg load, max 100 mg 20–50 μg/kg/min ETT: 2–3 mg
Magnesium sulfate	25–50 mg/kg, max 2 g
Naloxone	<5 yr or <20 kg 0.1 mg/kg >5 yr or >20 kg 2 mg IV
Procainamide	15 mg/kg over 30–60 min
Sodium bicarbonate	1 mEq/kg (after adequate ventilation)
Vasopressin	40 IU

IV, intravenous; IO, intraosseous.
Adapted from The American Heart Association 2005 Guidelines for Cardiopulmonary Resuscitation and Emergency Cardiovascular Care.

per kg, 10 times the recommended IV dose. Larger doses of the LEAN drugs are also recommended ranging from 2 – 10x the IV dose. All drugs should be diluted up to 5 mL of saline and given with five manual ventilations to distribute it across the alveolar surface (Table 1.11).

Epinephrine. Epinephrine is the primary drug for pediatric cardiopulmonary arrest because the rhythms most commonly encountered are asystole or bradycardia (Table 1.11). Epinephrine is an endogenous catecholamine with potent alpha- and beta-adrenergic properties. At higher doses, the alpha effects are most prominent and result in intense vasoconstriction. This results in improved aortic diastolic pressure, which is associated with improved outcomes. It is also associated with increased coronary artery and cerebral blood flow. Epinephrine also augments myocardial contraction and increases the intensity of fine ventricular fibrillation that yields higher rates of successful defibrillation.

There has been much debate over the optimal dose of epinephrine. In the original AHA guidelines, the recommended epinephrine dose for adults was 1 mg to be repeated every 3 to 5 minutes. Subsequent to this, in 1986, using an animal model, Brown demonstrated significant increases in blood flow to vital organs with increasing epinephrine doses. At higher doses, however, significant side effects such as hypertension, malignant dysrhythmias, and endocardial ischemia became more prominent.

Multiple studies in both adult and pediatric populations have failed to show improved outcomes with high-dose epinephrine. In fact, a recent prospective study of children with in-hospital cardiac arrest showed that the use of high-dose epinephrine was associated with worse survival. Another study of out-of-hospital arrest in pediatric patients did not show any benefit with high dose over standard dose epinephrine.

After a decade of experience, the new guidelines recommend standard dose epinephrine (0.01 mg per kg) for initial and subsequent IV doses for unresponsive or refractory pediatric asystolic arrest. High-dose epinephrine may be considered for patients with calcium channel blocker toxicity. It is important to be familiar with the two available concentrations for epinephrine dosing to avoid error. Once ROSC has occurred, an infusion of epinephrine can be titrated to achieve the desired effects. Epinephrine should be given in a secure IV or IO to avoid ischemia-associated infiltration. Infusions are best given via a central catheter. It should not be mixed with bicarbonate solutions to prevent drug inactivation. Side effects include hypertension, tachycardia, widened pulse pressure, malignant dysrhythmias, and excessive vasoconstriction.

Vasopressin. In an effort to improve rates of ROSC, investigators have looked at a number of other vasoconstrictors, including vasopressin, norepinephrine, phenylephrine, and endothelin-1. To date, none of these has replaced epinephrine. Vasopressin is an endogenous hormone that is found in high levels in patients undergoing CPR. Levels of this hormone are higher in patients that survive the event. Vasopressin acts at V_1 receptors causing (i) intense vasoconstriction in skeletal muscle, intestine, and skin; (ii) slightly less vasoconstriction in coronary and renal vessels; and (iii) vasodilatation in cerebral vessels.

There have been several adult studies comparing vasopressin and epinephrine. None of these to date have shown clear benefit of using vasopressin over epinephrine. A few pediatric case series have appeared in the literature, these do not provide clear evidence for its use in children (2005 AHA guidelines indeterminate).

Sodium Bicarbonate. Initial AHA guidelines recommended the use of sodium bicarbonate to treat the profound acidosis associated with low or no-flow states. Subsequent to these earlier recommendations, investigations reported potential deleterious effects of its use resulting in a change in the 1992 guidelines, which stated that the use of sodium bicarbonate may be considered in the scenario of prolonged cardiopulmonary arrest. Its use remains controversial in the literature.

Adequate ventilation and restoration of pulmonary blood flow and tissue perfusion is the foundation of acid–base balance during resuscitation. This treats the respiratory component of acidosis. It is known that significant acidosis develops within minutes of cardiopulmonary arrest. Controversy exists regarding the treatment of the metabolic component. During arrest, a substantial gradient exists between central venous pH, arterial pH, and P_{CO_2}. These differences resolve once circulation is restored. Buffering with the administration of sodium bicarbonate occurs via production of CO_2, which must then be removed through ventilation. This results in an increase in intracellular acidosis when pulmonary blood flow is low or absent. Other potential detrimental effects of sodium bicarbonate therapy include hyperosmolarity, hypernatremia, leftward shift of the oxyhemoglobin dissociation curve, increased lactate production, catecholamine inactivation, and reduction of coronary artery perfusion pressure.

Several retrospective studies have failed to demonstrate improved outcomes with the use of sodium bicarbonate. However, retrospective reviews lack accurate down times, initial pH measurements, and presenting rhythms among other important data points. A single, double-blinded, randomized trial of adult out-of-hospital arrest ($n = 502$, asystole, ventricular fibrillation) comparing a mixture of bicarbonate-trometamol-phosphate with normal saline failed to show increased rates of hospital admission or survival to discharge. However, in this study, the mean response time was 5.8 minutes, 48% of cases had bystander CPR, and 44% had VF, all factors suggesting early intervention and effective resuscitation.

Animal studies have shown conflicting results. Some have shown no benefit, whereas others have demonstrated an improved resuscitation success with reduced neurologic deficit. The experimental model used may differ considerably from real clinical scenarios. In most, the arrest was less than or equal to 5 minutes and buffer is administered early in the resuscitation effort.

Current guidelines recommend that the use of sodium bicarbonate may be considered in prolonged pediatric arrest only after adequate ventilation is ensured and epinephrine and chest compressions have been instituted (Class IIa). The initial recommended dose is 1 mEq per kg. Subsequent doses should be determined by measured acidosis, or empiric 0.5 to 1 mEq per kg can be considered after every 10 minutes of persistent arrest. Half-strength (0.5 mEq per mL) solution should be used in neonates. Sodium bicarbonate is also recommended for the treatment of hyperkalemia, hypermagnesemia, tricyclic antidepressant overdose, and sodium channel blocker poisoning.

Atropine. Atropine is a parasympatholytic drug, which has peripheral and central effects. Peripherally, it is vagolytic and accelerates sinus and atrial pacemakers and increases conduction through the AV node. Centrally, it stimulates the medullary vagal nucleus, which causes bradycardia. This effect occurs when the drug is administered in low doses.

Atropine is recommended for the treatment of bradycardia that is known to be vagally mediated (such as bradycardia associated with ET intubation). It may be used in children with symptomatic bradycardia when adequate oxygenation and ventilation is not successful. Practitioners should prepare for transcutaneous pacing. The recommended dose is 0.02 mg per kg, with a minimum dose of 0.1 mg, and a maximum dose of 0.5 mg in a child and 1.0 mg in adolescents. The dose may be repeated every 5 minutes to a maximum of 1 mg in a child and 2 mg in an adolescent.

Glucose. Glucose is a major substrate for both the brain and the myocardium. Because of high metabolic rate and decreased glycogen stores, children have high requirements for glucose. Losek performed a cross-sectional study of 49 consecutive children presenting to a pediatric ED requiring resuscitative interventions for altered mental status, seizures, respiratory and cardiac failure, and cardiopulmonary arrest. Eighteen percent of these patients were hypoglycemic. Current data remains controversial as to whether or not hyperglycemia affects neurologic outcome. Therefore, it is currently recommended that glucose be monitored in the post-arrested patient. Hypoglycemia should be treated (Class IIb). Continuous infusions are most physiologic. The recommended dose is 0.5 to 1 g per kg, which can be given as 5 to 10 mL per kg of D_{10}. It may also be important to treat significant hyperglycemia.

Adenosine. Adenosine is a short-acting purine nucleoside that slows conduction through the AV node and blocks reentry circuits by direct action on AV nodal adenosine receptors. It depresses the automaticity of primary pacemaker cells. It is metabolized by adenosine deaminase, which is present on the surface of red blood cells, and thus has an extremely short half-life. It has proven to be very effective in the treatment of supraventricular tachycardia (SVT) in children. It is the treatment of choice for stable and unstable SVT (Class IIa). The recommended dose is 0.1 mg per kg, with a maximum of 6 mg. A second dose of 0.2 mg per kg, with a maximum of 12 mg may be given. Adenosine must be administered via rapid IV bolus during continuous EKG monitoring. A two-syringe method with stopcock is recommended; one syringe contains the drug, and the second contains a 5-mL saline flush. Its effects are seen within 15 to 30 seconds. Transient side effects include facial flushing, chest pain, anxiety, and dyspnea. However, because of its extremely short half-life, these effects disappear within 10 to 20 seconds. Other more serious side effects include bronchospasm or apnea, accelerated ventricular rhythm, wide complex tachycardia, and brief asystole. These have been reported rarely, probably because of the short half-life of the drug. However, they emphasize the need for appropriate equipment and personnel to be available during administration of this medication.

Amiodarone. Amiodarone is a class III antiarrhythmic. Potassium channels are blocked, which prolongs phase 3 of the cardiac action potential and thus prolongs the refractory period. This is the principal effect of the drug. Amiodarone also has properties of sodium channel and beta-adrenoreceptor blockade. Amiodarone is used for the treatment of adult patients with shock refractory VT and VF/VT. The trial amiodarone versus lidocaine in prehospital VF (ALIVE) was a prospective, double-blinded, randomized, controlled trial of amiodarone versus lidocaine in 347 patients with out-of-hospital cardiac arrest resulting from refractory VF. Survival to hospital admission was 22.8% in the amiodarone group versus 12% in the lidocaine group. There was no difference between the groups in survival to hospital discharge. The widespread use of amiodarone in adults is supported by research; however, experience with its use in pediatric patients has demonstrated its effectiveness. Current guidelines recommend a loading dose of 5 mg per kg with a maximum of 15 mg per kg per day. Avoid use with class I antiarrhythmics (lidocaine, procainamide) because all these medications prolong the QT interval. It is metabolized by the liver, is highly protein bound, and is rapidly distributed and highly lipophilic. The main adverse effects include bradycardia, tachydysrhythmias, and hypotension. In the scenario of VF or pulseless VT, it should be administered as a rapid bolus; otherwise, it is given as an infusion over 20 to 60 minutes (Class IIb). The concentration should not exceed 2 mg per mL to avoid local phlebitis. No light protection is required after the drug has been reconstituted.

Lidocaine. Lidocaine is a class I antiarrhythmic and functions as a sodium-channel blocker, reducing the slope of phase 4 repolarization of the myocyte-decreasing automaticity. More recent experience has called its role in resuscitation into question. There is little evidence that lidocaine is superior to other drugs or to placebo when treating adults in the out-of-hospital setting. In fact, a recent, randomized, prospective study of adults with out-of-hospital VF compared the use of lidocaine to epinephrine after defibrillation. There was no difference in survival to hospital admission or discharge between the two groups. As discussed earlier, the ALIVE trial showed higher rates of survival to both hospitalization and discharge in adults treated with amiodarone versus lidocaine for the treatment of shock-resistant VF. The Amiodarone in Out-of-Hospital Resuscitation of Refractory Sustained Ventricular Tachycardia (ARREST) trial also suggested that amiodarone is superior to lidocaine for shock-resistant out-of-hospital VF. Thus, evidence is mounting that supports the use of amiodarone over lidocaine for resuscitation. Current recommendations state that lidocaine may be used for shock-resistant VF or pulseless VT in children. A loading dose of 1 mg per kg is given intravenously, followed by an infusion of 20 to 50 mcg per kg per minute. Side effects include myocardial depression, CNS depression, seizures, and muscle twitching.

Calcium. Calcium has an important role in vascular smooth muscle excitation–contraction coupling. Calcium enhances systolic function and systemic vascular resistance via vascular smooth muscle contraction. Calcium administration does not improve outcome in patients with out-of-hospital asystolic arrest. It has also been demonstrated that increases in intracellular calcium contribute to cell death due to reperfusion injury.

The 2005 AHA Guidelines do not recommend the routine administration of calcium in children with asystolic arrest. A recent review of pediatric patients from the National Registry of Cardiopulmonary Resuscitation revealed that calcium was used in 45% of cases. Importantly, use of calcium was associated with decreased survival to discharge. Calcium treatment is indicated for children with documented hypocalcemia, hypermagnesemia, hyperkalemia, and calcium channel overdose. Calcium should be monitored and hypocalcemia treated in ill children, particularly those with sepsis.

The most favorable dosing for calcium remains unclear. Calcium chloride 10% (100 mg per mL, 27.2 mg per mL of elemental calcium) seems to offer the best bioavailability. The current recommended dose is 5 to 7 mg per kg of elemental calcium. Therefore, 0.2 mL per kg of calcium chloride (20 mg calcium chloride/kg) can be given slow IV push during arrest or more slowly, over 5 to 10 minutes, in more stable patients. The recommended dose for calcium gluconate 10% (100 mg per mL, 9 mg per mL of elemental calcium) is 60 to 100 mg per kg or 0.6 to 1 mL per kg.

Magnesium. Magnesium inhibits calcium channels, decreasing intracellular calcium resulting in smooth muscle relaxation. Severe magnesium deficiency is associated with arrhythmias, sudden death, and congestive heart failure. Available information does not reveal any effect on outcomes for patients receiving magnesium during resuscitation. Magnesium has been shown to be effective in children with severe asthma who have persistent respiratory distress despite aggressive beta-agonist therapy. Current guidelines recommend the use of magnesium sulfate for documented hypomagnesemia, torsades de pointe, and severe asthma. A dose of 25 to 50 mg per kg (maximum of 2 g) is given intravenously over 10 to 20 minutes.

Fluid Resuscitation

Restoration of the circulating intravascular volume is an important element of successful resuscitation. Crystalloids in 20 mL per kg aliquots remain the mainstay of acute volume resuscitation. Dextrose solutions should not be used in the initial phases of fluid resuscitation.

Hypertonic saline causes an osmotic shift of fluid from the intracellular and interstitial spaces to the extracellular compartment, providing rapid volume expansion with less interstitial edema. In addition, less volume is required, which can be given over a shorter period of time. Hypertonic solutions are also believed to reduce ICP by establishing an osmotic gradient across the blood–brain barrier that draws water from the brain into the vascular space. Conversely, potential ill effects include continued hemorrhage from injured blood vessels, and increased ICP due to leakage of sodium through a disrupted blood–brain barrier. Currently, there is not enough data to support the use of hypertonic crystalloid instead of isotonic crystalloid for the resuscitation of patients.

TABLE 1.12A

PRESENTING RHYTHM IN PEDIATRIC PATIENTS WITH OUT-OF-HOSPITAL
CARDIOPULMONARY ARREST (%)

	n	Asystole	VT/VF	PEA
Young 1999	548	67	9	24
Sirbaugh 1999	300	83	4	12
Diechmann 1995	65	83	9	8
Young 2004	3,097	75	10	
Donoghue 2005	2,734	78	8	13
Gerein 2006	503	77	4	16

Serum albumin concentration has been shown to be inversely related to mortality risk. Thus, its use in the resuscitation of ill patients has been explored. It is 30 times more expensive than crystalloid solutions and has limited availability. Systematic reviews have failed to show benefit its administration; in fact, its use may be associated with an increased risk of death. Albumin is believed to have some anticoagulant properties and may leak across the capillary wall promoting edema. The ongoing, prospective x trial saline vs. albumin fluid evaluation (SAFE) aims to answer this question.

Defibrillation and Cardioversion

The true prevalence of VT and VF in children with cardiopulmonary arrest is not known. In published reports the incidence varies from 9% to 10% in pediatric out-of-hospital arrest (Table 1.12A–B). The incidence of an initial rhythm of VT/VF amongst pediatric inpatient arrest is also approximately 10%. An additional 10% to 15% will develop VT/VF as a subsequent rhythm. Although the need for defibrillation is relatively uncommon, it should always be considered, particularly in older children, children with a history of congenital heart disease or dysrhythmias, or children who experience a witnessed sudden arrest.

Defibrillation is the asynchronous delivery of a shock to the myocardium in an attempt to produce simultaneous depolarization of a critical mass of myocardial cells to allow spontaneous repolarization and the resumption of a perfusing cardiac rhythm. Defibrillators can deliver monophasic or biphasic wave forms. Biphasic wave forms allow for successful defibrillation at a lower energy of 150 J. Biphasic defibrillators have largely replaced monophasic defibrillators. Standard adult paddles are 8 to 13 cm in diameter. Pediatric paddles 4.5 cm in diameter are available with most defibrillators. The correct paddle size is that which makes complete uniform contact with the chest wall. The large paddle can usually be used for infants older than 1 year of age and/or weighing more than 10 kg if placed on front and back. Larger paddle surfaces result in decreased intrathoracic impedance, which optimizes the energy reaching the myocardium. Electrode paste should be used to decrease impedance and prevent injury to the skin. Saline soaked pads should never be used because they can create a bridge between the two electrodes. Paddles should be applied with pressure on the anterior chest wall at the upper right side of the chest below the clavicle and to the left of the nipple in the anterior axillary line directly over the heart, never touching each other. Now most defibrillators have disposable adhesive pads that allow rhythm recognition through which a shock can be delivered. These can be applied to the chest, or anteriorly and posteriorly if appropriate, of the arrested child immediately at the beginning of the resuscitation and can aid in preventing delays in rhythm checks and treatment. The initial dose for defibrillation is 2 J per kg, increased to 4 J per kg if the first attempt is unsuccessful. Automated external defibrillators (AEDs) automatically interpret the cardiac rhythm and, if VF is present, advise the operator to deliver a charge. They are small, easy to use, and have batteries that last for 5 years. For patients with VF, early rapid defibrillation is the treatment of choice. AEDs have been proven to be highly sensitive and specific when used on adults, and there is good evidence that its use in the out-of-hospital setting has resulted in a dramatic improvement in survival of adults with VF. Cecchin et al. studied 696 rhythm strips from children younger than 12 years of age to test the accuracy of AEDs. There was 100% sensitivity for nonshockable rhythms, and the sensitivity for

TABLE 1.12B

PRESENTING RHYTHM IN PEDIATRIC PATIENTS WITH IN-HOSPITAL
CARDIOPULMONARY ARREST (%)

	Asystole	VT/VF	PEA
Reiss[a] 2002	55	1	11
Nadkarni 2006	40	14	24

[a]Children with heart disease not in the study population

VF was 96%. Since the 2005 guidelines, new information has shown that AEDs can be used to deliver shocks safely in children older than 1 year of age (Class IIb). Data is lacking to make a recommendation for or against its use in children younger than 1 year of age. Available AEDs deliver a standard adult charge between 150 and 200 J. More recently, an attenuating pediatric electrode system has become available that decreases the charge delivered to 50 J.

Synchronous cardioversion is the delivery of a charge that is timed with the patient's R wave. This reduces the risk of inducing VF by avoiding delivery of the charge during the T wave. This is indicated for treatment of rhythms in which the patient still has a pulse but has evidence of compromised perfusion, such as VT and SVT. The initial charge for synchronized cardioversion is 0.5 to 1 J per kg. This dose can be doubled to 2 J per kg if the tachydysrhythmia persists. Sedation and analgesia should be considered during this procedure.

Special Scenarios

The chain of survival includes rapid access to emergency medical services, rapid CPR, rapid defibrillation when indicated, and rapid advanced care. Once in the ED, the process of resuscitation is best accomplished with an effective leader that organizes and directs a skilled team. The American College of Surgeons divides the resuscitation into the primary and secondary surveys. During the primary survey, the life-threatening condition is identified and appropriate interventions are undertaken. These include the so-called ABCDEs of resuscitation, which includes attention to A, airway/breathing/cervical spine; B, breathing; C, circulation; D, disability, dextrose, decontamination; and E, exposure and environment. This phase of resuscitation should be completed within the first 5 to 10 minutes of arrival. Monitors (cardiorespiratory, pulse oximeter, end-tidal CO_2, blood pressure cuff) should be placed, IV access should be obtained, and a Foley catheter placed, if necessary. The secondary survey is a head-to-toe examination to determine the etiology of the illness. During this portion of the resuscitation, diagnostic studies are done, consultants are called, and arrangements for definitive care are completed. The ABCs should be reassessed frequently throughout the resuscitation.

Teamwork in Resuscitation. The new PALS and ACLS curricula have incorporated curricula on leadership, role clarity, and communication. Effective leaders and team members must have cognitive skill (fund of knowledge), technical and procedural skills, and behavioral skills. Recent information reveals lack of effective teamwork skills and their negative impact on resuscitation outcomes. Effective education includes challenging active exercises, such as high-fidelity simulation. Video-recording of resuscitation provides another venue for reviewing errors and providing constructive feedback on team management skills.

Specific Resuscitation Scenarios

In the 2005 AHA resuscitation guidelines, an international expert panel updated guidelines for pediatric prearrest/arrest scenarios. Figures 1.25 to 1.28 summarize these guidelines along with the following commentary. It is important to remember that no algorithm can cover every clinical situation; the treating team of health-care professionals must consider the many etiologies of arrest and modify therapies accordingly. Early recognition and intervention of/for respiratory and circulatory failure, vascular access, and frequent reassessment are the foundation of successful resuscitation efforts for all scenarios encountered in the pediatric ED.

Asystole/Bradycardia

The algorithms for the treatment of asystole and bradycardia adapted from the expert consensus statement are outlined in Figures 1.25 and 1.26. These are the most common prearrest/arrest scenarios encountered in the pediatric ED. As stated earlier, impending or existing respiratory failure is the most common etiology. As always, early recognition and intervention to support the respiratory system and other vital functions reduces morbidity and may be lifesaving. Other etiologies of bradycardia include heart block, heart transplant, increased ICP, hypoglycemia, hypercalcemia, drug effect, increased parasympathetic tone, and hypothermia. The first step in the treatment of children with bradycardia is airway management. Remember that increase in heart rate is the primary mechanism by which children increase their stroke volume, bradycardia readily leads to hypotension. Chest compressions should begin when perfusion is inadequate. Assess the rhythm on the cardiac monitor. If the bradycardia is believed to be due to increased vagal tone or heart block, atropine is an appropriate intervention. For most situations, epinephrine is the drug of choice. In children with heart block, cardiac pacing may be necessary.

In the pulseless child, it is important to identify the rhythm on the monitor so the correct intervention can be instituted. Asystole, PEA, pulseless VT, or VF are all possibilities, although in pediatric cardiopulmonary arrest, asystole predominates. In a witnessed, sudden arrest, primary cardiac etiologies should be considered. For asystole and PEA, SDE is the drug of choice. Always consider treatment of reversible causes such as hypovolemia, hypothermia, electrolyte abnormalities, poisonings, tension pneumothorax, and cardiac tamponade.

Tachydysrhythmias

The differential diagnosis of tachycardias includes sinus tachycardia (ST), SVT, and VT. Narrow complex morphology and beat-to-beat variability are usually present in children with ST. Rates rarely exceed 220 beats per minute (bpm) in infants and 180 bpm in children. Common causes of ST include hypoxemia, hypovolemia, hyperthermia, metabolic abnormalities, and pain/anxiety. Therapy is directed at treating the underlying cause.

SVT can be distinguished from ST by its lack of beat-to-beat variability and rate (most often greater than 220 bpm in infants and greater than 180 bpm in children). In children, aberrant conduction yielding a wide complex rhythm occurs less than 10% of the time. SVT is most commonly caused by accessory reentry pathways. The algorithm for the treatment of tachydysrhythmias appears in Figure 1.27. Patients with stable SVT have adequate oxygenation and perfusion; those with unstable SVT have inadequate perfusion and thus require rapid intervention. Chemical or electrical conversion can be used for the treatment of unstable SVT. Because of the efficacy and safety of adenosine in the treatment of SVTs, most practitioners have adopted this as first-line treatment when vascular or IO access is available. It is optimal to obtain a 12-lead EKG prior to and during treatment to aid in the diagnosis. Resuscitation equipment and drugs should be close at hand. If the patient fails to convert to sinus

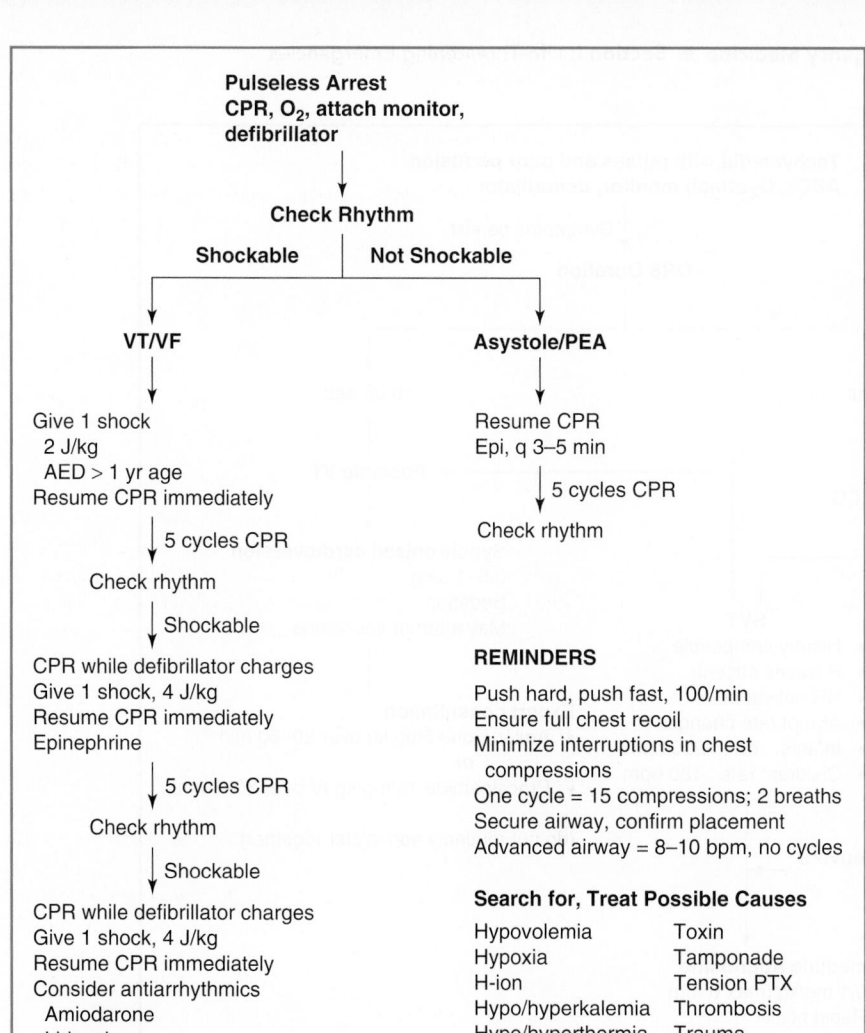

Pulseless Arrest
CPR, O₂, attach monitor, defibrillator

Check Rhythm

Shockable | Not Shockable

VT/VF

Give 1 shock
2 J/kg
AED > 1 yr age
Resume CPR immediately

5 cycles CPR

Check rhythm

Shockable

CPR while defibrillator charges
Give 1 shock, 4 J/kg
Resume CPR immediately
Epinephrine

5 cycles CPR

Check rhythm

Shockable

CPR while defibrillator charges
Give 1 shock, 4 J/kg
Resume CPR immediately
Consider antiarrhythmics
  Amiodarone
  Lidocaine
  Magnesium

Asystole/PEA

Resume CPR
Epi, q 3–5 min

5 cycles CPR

Check rhythm

REMINDERS

Push hard, push fast, 100/min
Ensure full chest recoil
Minimize interruptions in chest
  compressions
One cycle = 15 compressions; 2 breaths
Secure airway, confirm placement
Advanced airway = 8–10 bpm, no cycles

Search for, Treat Possible Causes

Hypovolemia | Toxin
Hypoxia | Tamponade
H-ion | Tension PTX
Hypo/hyperkalemia | Thrombosis
Hypo/hyperthermia | Trauma

FIGURE 1.25 Management approach to pulseless arrest. ABCDE: A, airway/breathing/cervical spine; B, breathing; C, circulation; D, disability, dextrose, decontamination; E, exposure and environment; CPR, cardiopulmonary resuscitation; IO, intraosseous; IV, intravenous; PEA, pulseless electrical activity; PTX, tension pneumothorax; VF, ventricular fibrillation; VT, ventricular tachycardia. (Adapted from American Heart Association Guidelines 2005 for Cardiopulmonary Resuscitation and Emergency Cardiovascular Care [Supplement]. *Circulation* 2005;112.)

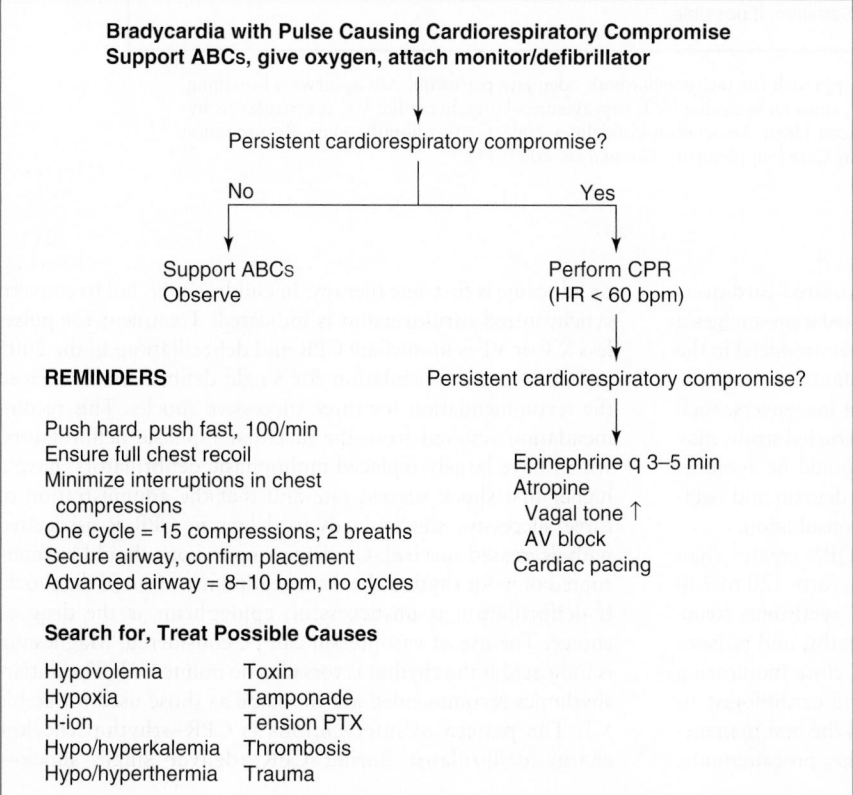

Bradycardia with Pulse Causing Cardiorespiratory Compromise
Support ABCs, give oxygen, attach monitor/defibrillator

Persistent cardiorespiratory compromise?

No | Yes

Support ABCs
Observe

Perform CPR
(HR < 60 bpm)

Persistent cardiorespiratory compromise?

Epinephrine q 3–5 min
Atropine
  Vagal tone ↑
  AV block
Cardiac pacing

REMINDERS

Push hard, push fast, 100/min
Ensure full chest recoil
Minimize interruptions in chest
  compressions
One cycle = 15 compressions; 2 breaths
Secure airway, confirm placement
Advanced airway = 8–10 bpm, no cycles

Search for, Treat Possible Causes

Hypovolemia | Toxin
Hypoxia | Tamponade
H-ion | Tension PTX
Hypo/hyperkalemia | Thrombosis
Hypo/hyperthermia | Trauma

FIGURE 1.26 Management approach for bradycardia. CPR, cardiopulmonary resuscitation. (Adapted from American Heart Association Guidelines 2005 for Cardiopulmonary Resuscitation and Emergency Cardiovascular Care [Supplement]. *Circulation* 2005; 112.)

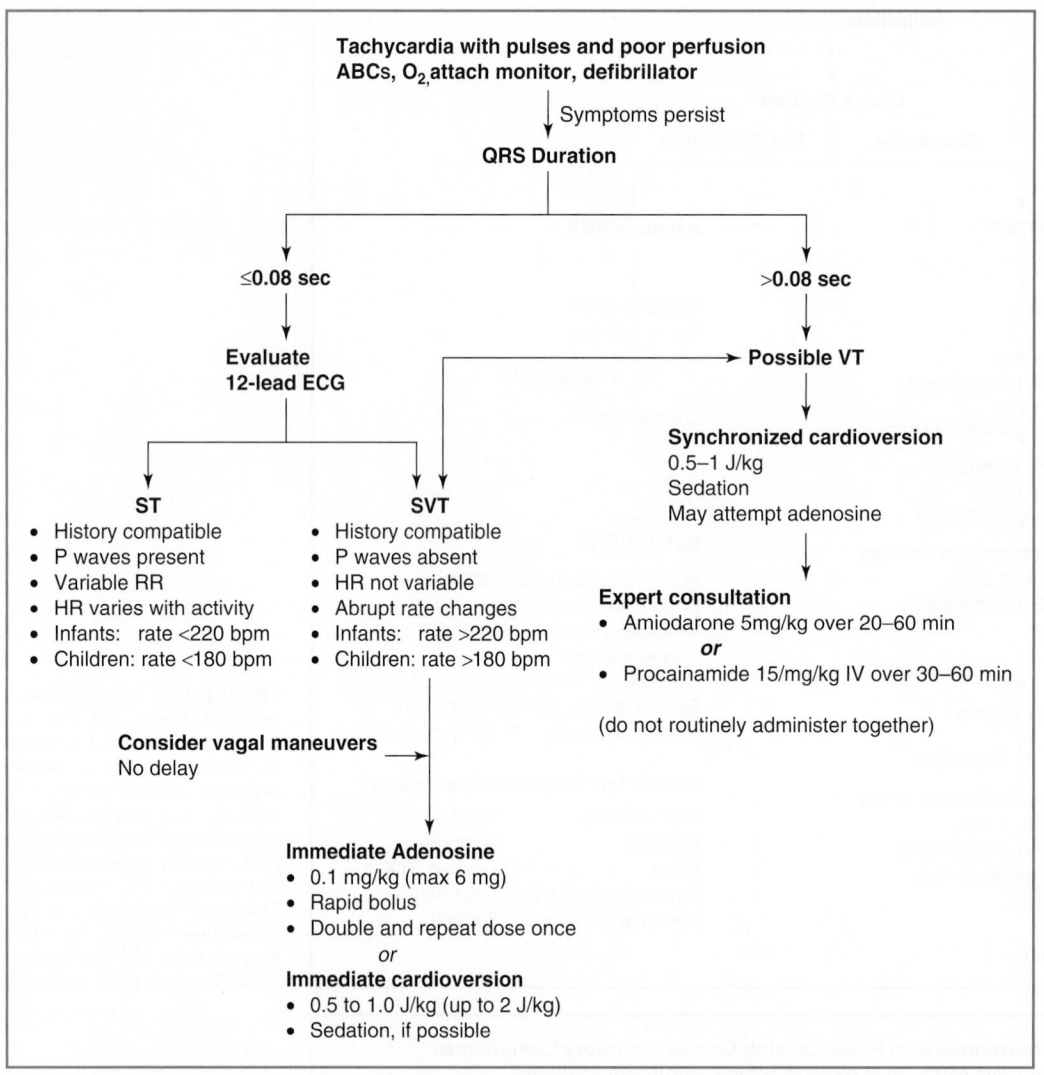

FIGURE 1.27 Management approach for tachycardia with adequate perfusion. ABCs, airway, breathing, circulation HR, heart rate; ST, sinus tachycardia; SVT, supraventricular tachycardia; VT, ventricular tachycardia. (Adapted from American Heart Association Guidelines 2005 for Cardiopulmonary Resuscitation and Emergency Cardiovascular Care [Supplement]. *Circulation* 2005; 112.)

rhythm after two doses of adenosine, synchronized cardioversion (0.5 J per kg) is recommended. Use of sedation analgesia should be considered. Vagal maneuvers were reintroduced in the 2000 AHA guidelines for stable SVT. In infants, ice may be applied to the face; in older children, Valsalva maneuvers, such as knee to chest or forceful blowing on an obstructed straw, may be attempted. Ocular and carotid pressure should be avoided. Use of other therapies such as procainamide, digoxin and beta-blockers may be considered after cardiology consultation.

VT is characterized by wide complex (QRS greater than 0.08 seconds) and typically has a rate ranging form 120 to 200 bpm. Etiologies of VT include prolonged QT syndrome, structural heart disease, myocarditis, cardiomyopathy, and poisonings. In children presenting with stable VT, close monitoring and immediate consultation with a pediatric cardiologist to determine etiology and definitive treatment is the best management. Chemical conversion using amiodarone, procainamide,

or lidocaine is first-line therapy. In children who fail to convert, synchronized cardioversion is indicated. Treatment for pulseless VT or VF is immediate CPR and defibrillation. In the 2005 guidelines, recommendation for single defibrillation replaced the recommendation for three successive shocks. This recommendation resulted from the fact that biphasic defibrillators, which have largely replaced monophasic defibrillators, have a higher first shock success rate and that the administration of three successive shocks leads to delays in CPR is associated with decreased survival. Cardiac compressions should be interrupted only for rhythm checks and administration of the shock. If defibrillation is unsuccessful, epinephrine is the drug of choice. The use of vasopressin can be considered. Magnesium is indicated if the rhythm is torsades de pointes VT. The antiarrhythmics recommended are the same as those used for stable VT. The pattern of interventions is CPR→rhythm check→ charge defibrillator during CPR→deliver single shock→

immediate CPR→brief rhythm check →resume CPR as drug is prepared and administered. Interruptions in CPR should be held to very brief periods to check the rhythm and to administer shocks. The resuscitation team should anticipate the need for the next interventions.

Extracorporeal Cardiopulmonary Resuscitation

There is now some information regarding the use of extracorporeal CPR (E-CPR) to treat refractory cardiac arrest in children presenting to an ED setting. Currently, it is an option available in large, tertiary care Children's Hospitals. The majority of the literature to date comes from the treatment of inpatients with primary cardiac disease. Use of E-CPR for these patients following a witnessed arrest seems to increase the chance for favorable outcome. The 2005 Guidelines state "Consider extracorporeal CPR for in-hospital cardiac arrest refractory to initial resuscitation attempts if the condition leading to cardiac arrest is reversible or amenable to heart transplantation, if excellent conventional CPR has been performed after no more than several minutes of no-flow cardiac arrest, and if the institution is able to rapidly perform extra-

corporeal membrane oxygenation (ECMO) (Class IIb). MacLaren et al. published a retrospective case series of children with septic shock who were treated with ECMO. Forty percent of the 45 cases received CPR prior to cannulation and 47% of the 45 cases survived to hospital discharge. Posner et al. presented case reports of two children treated with E-CPR in the ED, one patient with prolonged QT survived neurologically intact. Use of E-CPR can be considered for children with refractory arrest who have had a short downtime and have received high-quality CPR when the resources and personnel are available.

STABILIZATION AND TRANSPORT

Once resuscitation efforts have achieved cardiorespiratory stability, the patient should be transported to an inpatient special care unit for the critically ill. This transport may require a move of several hundred yards or several hundred miles to an appropriate pediatric hospital. In either circumstance, the patient should be transported with advanced support technology in place and qualified personnel in appropriate numbers in attendance, with options for further interventions immediately available. Medications for resuscitation, sedation, and muscle relaxation should also be available (Fig. 1.28).

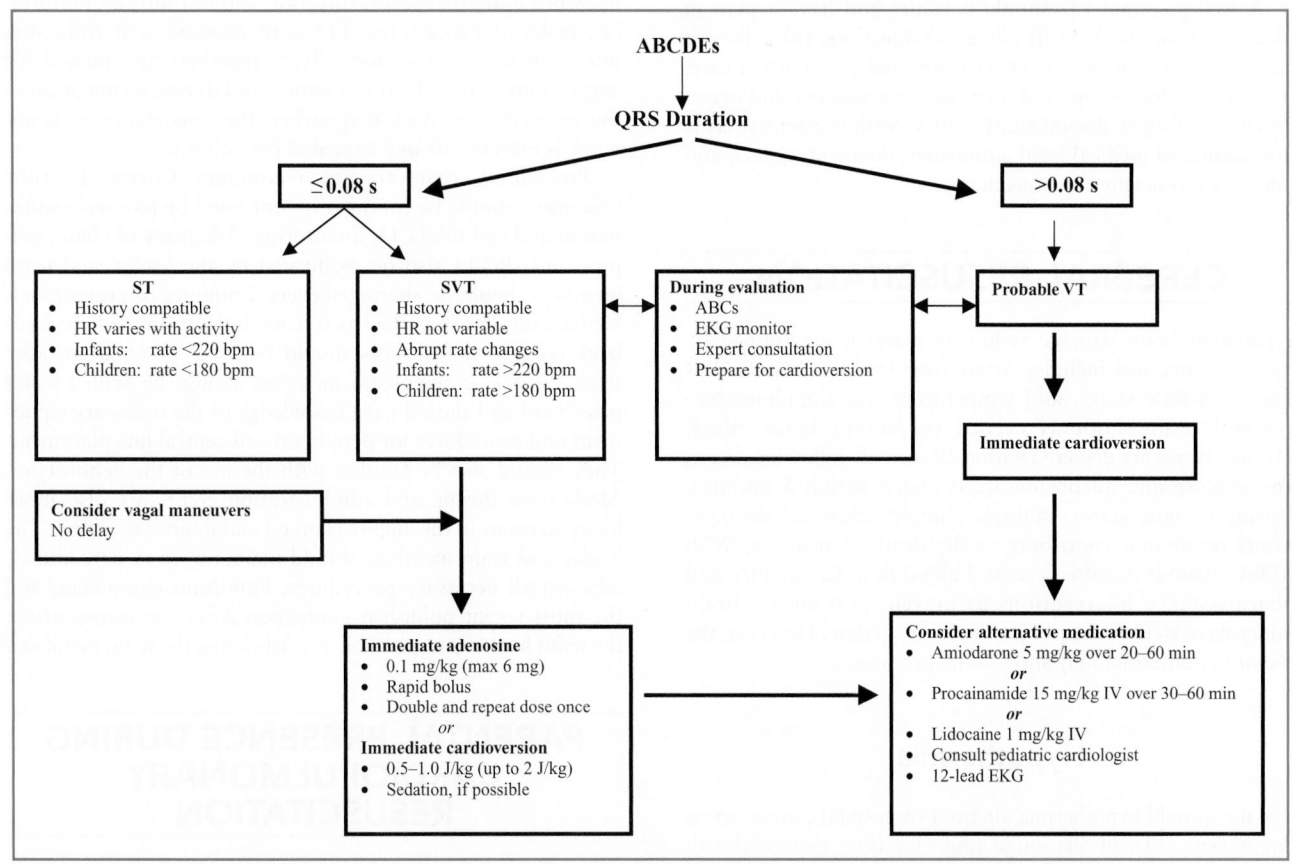

FIGURE 1.28 Management approach to tachycardia with poor perfusion. ABCs, airway, breathing, circulation; ABCDE, A, airway/breathing/cervical spine; B, breathing; C, circulation; D, disability, dextrose, decontamination; E, exposure and environment; bpm, beats per minute; EKG, electrocardiogram; HR, heart rate; IV, intravenous; ST, sinus tachycardia; SVT, supraventricular tachycardia; VT, ventricular tachycardia. (Adapted from American Heart Association Guidelines 2000 for cardiopulmonary resuscitation and emergency cardiovascular care [Supplement]. *Circulation* 2000;102(8) and American Academy of Pediatrics/American Heart Association. *PALS provider manual.* 2002.)

DISCONTINUATION OF LIFE SUPPORT

If well-executed resuscitative measures fail to achieve ROSC, resuscitative efforts should be discontinued. There is now good evidence that if cardiac muscle remains unresponsive to aggressive airway intervention, cardiac massage, and two doses of epinephrine, there is no chance for a successful resuscitation. Thus, a brief, well-executed resuscitation is indicated for the child who arrives to the ED with cardiopulmonary arrest. This includes definitive airway management; vigorous, monitored chest compressions; IO access; and one to two doses of epinephrine. During this time, the leader of the resuscitation can review the history and complete the primary and secondary survey. Prolonged resuscitation efforts past 20 minutes, without ROSC, are usually futile unless other treatable problems exist such as hypothermia, drug overdose, or VT/VF. Ultimately, the diagnosis of death and subsequent discontinuation of resuscitative efforts is a judgment that is made by the team leader. A decision not to begin resuscitation is generally not made in the ED unless there is a written do not resuscitate (DNR) document provided by the child's parent or guardian. Baren and Mahon have written about other end-of-life issues in the pediatric ED.

A well-prepared ED should consider and have a plan in place for issues such as (i) advanced directives, (ii) palliative care issues, (iii) bereavement measures and postmortem care, (iv) survivor follow-up, and (v) request for autopsy and organ donations. Proper documentation of a death is essential, as is notification of medical legal authorities, donor programs, and referring physicians and consultants.

CEREBRAL RESUSCITATION

Permanent brain damage following arrest is determined by many factors and includes arrest time (no-flow state), CPR time (low-flow state), and temperature. Cardiopulmonary–cerebral resuscitation is needed to prevent brain injury. Oxygen stores are depleted within 20 seconds following arrest, and glucose and adenosine are depleted within 5 minutes. During no-flow states, multiple complex chemical derangements occur that contribute to the death of neurons. With ROSC, there is impaired cerebral blood flow. Circulatory and pharmacologic interventions to prevent post-anoxic brain injury have yielded disappointing results to date. However, the use of hypothermia may show some promise.

Hypothermia

The use of mild hypothermia after out-of-hospital cardiac arrest due to ventricular fibrillation in adults has been associated with improved neurologic outcome and is generally tolerated without significant complication. The Hypothermia after Cardiac Arrest Study Group reported on 275 adult patients resuscitated from out-of-hospital VF cardiac arrest, who were randomized to either mild hypothermia (32°C to 24°C) for 24 hours or standard normothermic postresuscitation management. Favorable neuro-

logic outcome at 6 months was seen in 55% of the patients in the hypothermia group versus 39% in the normothermic group, $p < 0.009$. Death occurred less frequently in the hypothermia group, 41% versus 55%, $p < 0.02$. A second study by Bernard et al. produced similar results. Seventy-seven patients were randomized to hypothermia versus normothermia; 49% of those treated with hypothermia versus 26% with normothermia were discharged with good neurologic function. A recent trial of induced hypothermia for asphyxiated neonates was associated with a significant decrease in outcomes of death or moderate disability at 18 months. A multicenter trial of induced hypothermia following pediatric arrest is now ongoing. Currently, cooling to 32°C to 34°C for 12 to 24 hours may be considered for children who remain comatose post-arrest (Class IIb).

COMMON ERRORS IN RESUSCITATION

Because of the complexity and stress of these situations, many errors are possible. Lack of effective leadership is a common problem, especially in the setting of large, tertiary care, teaching hospitals. Effective leaders assign specific roles and tasks to the members of the resuscitation team. They make clinical decisions and give specific direction without directly performing tasks or procedures. Frequent reassessment following interventions is cornerstone. Team members are queried for suggestions during the resuscitation and during termination of the resuscitation. As stated earlier, the importance of teamwork is essential to well-executed resuscitation.

Procedural errors are not uncommon. Correct ET tube placement should be continually confirmed by physical examination and end-tidal CO_2 monitoring. Adequacy of chest compressions should also be monitored by the leader, and team members should be alternated every 2 minutes to prevent ineffective compressions due to rescuer fatigue. Immediate feedback compression devices should be used for children older than 8 years of age. Team members should be skilled in IO placement and should have knowledge of the necessary equipment and procedures for peripheral and central line placement. They should also be familiar with the use of the defibrillator. Medication dosing and administration errors are also more likely to occur in this highly charged and intense situation. The leader and team members should maintain up-to-date knowledge on all necessary procedures, important equipment, and the most recent published guidelines. After the resuscitation, the team leader is responsible for debriefing the team members.

PARENTAL PRESENCE DURING CARDIOPULMONARY RESUSCITATION

Parental presence in the resuscitation room is becoming routine practice. A recent study by Dingeman et al. documented that 87% of families wanted this choice, 86% believed it was their right, and 94% said that they would choose it again. There remains a high variation of practice, 22% to 93% honor the families' request. Parents want to be with their child during what may be the last moments of life. They also want to be certain that they and the ED staff have done all that is possible. Thus, in many centers, it is now recommended that parents be asked if they want to be in the resuscitation area. If they assent, they should be accompanied by a nurse or social worker who can serve as a support person and an interpreter. The decision to allow or not allow family presence is one that must be made by each ED, and there must be staff education, preparation, and quality assessment for this practice to be effective in easing the pain of the worst tragedy a human being can face—the loss of their child.

ETHICAL ISSUES IN PEDIATRIC CARDIOPULMONARY RESUSCITATION

Fearon, in a more recent publication, discussed many unique ethical challenges faced by the emergency physician. In providing CPR, emotions are often highly charged and, at times, a dirth of data is provided on which to base the immediate decisions that must be made. Fearon raised several important considerations: When are resuscitation attempts futile, and is the ED physician obligated to provide care at the families' insistence? How do family religious beliefs play a role in decision making? What is the role of parental presence? Should procedures be performed on the recently dead? Can resuscitation research be performed without informed consent? Some of these issues have been addressed in policy statements made by professional organizations, but each question needs to be considered in discussions that occur at the local ED level.

SUMMARY

In most circumstances, resuscitation of the pediatric patient can be approached with a sense of optimism for reversing the process that acutely threatens the child's life. Well-organized and well-qualified personnel can affect a high rate of successful resuscitation. However, organization and qualification require advanced planning, training, and preparation. Inherent in this preparation is the development of personnel disciplined to follow the sequence of evaluation and management of the ABCs. In addition, personnel must stay knowledgeable about the science of resuscitation and prevention, new interventions, new equipment, and new procedures to provide the best possible care to children.

Suggested Readings

Abella BS, Alvarado JP, Myklebust H, et al. Quality of cardiopulmonary resuscitation during in-hospital cardiac arrest. *JAMA* 2005;293(3):305–310. Available at: http://jama.ama-assn.org/cgi/content/full/293/3/305

Abella BS, Aufderheide TP, Eigel B, et al. Reducing barriers for implementation of bystander-initiated cardiopulmonary resuscitation: a scientific statement from the American Heart Association for healthcare providers, policymakers, and community leaders regarding the effectiveness of cardiopulmonary resuscitation. *Circulation* 2008;117:704–709. Available at: http://circ.ahajournals.org/cgi/content/full/117/5/704

Alzaga-Fernandez AG, Varon J. Open-chest cardiopulmonary resuscitation: past, present and future. *Resuscitation* 2005;64:149–156.

American Academy of Pediatrics/American Heart Association. *PALS provider manual*. Dallas: AHA publication, 2002:1–434.

American Heart Association Guidelines 2000 for Cardiopulmonary Resuscitation and Emergency Cardiovascular Care [Supplement]. *Circulation* 2000;102(8).

American Heart Association Guidelines 2005 for Cardiopulmonary Resuscitation and Emergency Cardiovascular Care [Supplement]. *Circulation* 2005;112.

American Heart Association. Infant CPR Anytime Personal Learning Program. Available at: http://www.americanheart.org/print_presenter.jhtml?identifier=3045660

Ashton A, McCluskey A, Gwinnutt CL, et al. Effect of rescuer fatigue on performance of continuous external chest compressions over 3 min. *Resuscitation* 2002;55:151–155.

Atkinson E, Mikysa B, Conway JA, et al. Specificity and sensitivity of automated external defibrillator rhythm analysis in infants and children. *Ann Emerg Med* 2003;42:185–196.

Aufderheide TP, Lurie KG. Death by hyperventilation: a common and life-threatening problem during cardiopulmonary resuscitation. *Crit Care Med* 2004;32(9):S345–S351.

Babbs CF, Nadkarni V. Optimizing chest compression to rescue ventilation ratios during one-rescuer CPR by professionals and lay persons: children are not just little adults. *Resuscitation* 2004;61:173–181.

Babbs CF, Sack JB, Kern KB. Interposed abdominal compression as an adjunct to cardiopulmonary resuscitation. *Am Heart J* 1994;127:412–421.

Baren JM, Mahon M. End-of-life issues in the pediatric emergency department. *Clin Pediatr Emerg Med* 2003;4:265–272.

Bar-Joseph G. The use of acid buffers during cardiopulmonary resuscitation: a time to change again? *Curr Opin Crit Care* 1999;5:201–210.

Bartlett RH, Roloff DW, Custer JR, et al. Extracorporeal life support: the University of Michigan experience. *JAMA* 2000;283:904–908.

Berg MD, Nadkarni VM, Berg RA. Cardiopulmonary resuscitation in children. *Curr Opin in Crit Care* 2008;14:254–260.

Bernard S, Gray TW, Buist MD, et al. Treatment of comatose survivors of out-of-hospital cardiac arrest with induced hypothermia. *N Engl J Med* 2002;346:557–563.

Bobrow BJ, Clark LL, Ewy GA, et al. Minimally interrupted cardiac resuscitation by emergency medical services for out-of-hospital cardiac arrest. *JAMA* 2008;299(10):1158–1165.

Bonnin MJ, Pepe PE, Kimball KT, et al. Distinct criteria for termination of resuscitation in the out-of-hospital setting. *JAMA* 2000;284:1438–1441.

Bordley WC, Travers D, Scanlon P, et al. Office preparedness for pediatric emergencies: a randomized, controlled trial of an office-based training program. *Pediatrics* 2003;112:291–295.

Brown K, Bocock J. Update in pediatric resuscitation. *Emerg Med Clin North Am* 2002;20(1):1–17.

Brown J, Kellerman AL. The shocking truth about external defibrillators. *JAMA* 2000;284:1438–1441.

Brown CG, Martin DR, Pepe PE, et al. A comparison of standard-dose and high-dose epinephrine in cardiac arrest outside the hospital. *N Engl J Med* 1992;327:1051–1055.

Bunch TJ, White RD, Gersh BJ, et al. Long-term outcomes of out-of-hospital cardiac arrest after successful early defibrillation. *N Engl J Med* 2003;348:2626–2633.

Bunn F, Roberts I, Tasker R, et al. Hypertonic versus isotonic crystalloid for fluid resuscitation in critically ill patients. *Cochrane Database Syst Rev* 2004; Issue 3. Art. No. CD002045.

Caffrey SL, Willoughby PJ, Pepe PE, et al. Public use of automated external defibrillators. *N Engl J Med* 2002;347:1242–1247.

Carpenter TC, Stenmark KR. High-dose epinephrine is not superior to standard-dose epinephrine in pediatric in-hospital cardiopulmonary arrest. *Pediatrics* 1997;99:403–408.

Cecchin F, Jorgenson DB, Berul CI, et al. Is arrhythmia detection by external automated defibrillators accurate for children?: sensitivity and specificity of an automated external defibrillator algorithm in 696 pediatric arrhythmias. *Circulation* 2001:103;2483–2488.

David JS, Gueugniaud PY, Riou B, et al. Does the prognosis of cardiac arrest differ in trauma patients? *Crit Care Med* 2007;35:2251–2255.

Davidovic L, LaCovey D, Pitetti RD. Comparison of 1- versus 2-person bag-valve-mask techniques for manikin ventilation of infants and children. *Ann Emerg Med* 2005;46:37–42.

Dieckmann RA, Vardis R. High-dose epinephrine in pediatric out-of-hospital cardiopulmonary arrest. *Pediatrics* 1995;95:901–913.

Dingeman RS, Mitchell EA, Meyer EC, et al. Parent presence during complex invasive procedures and cardiopulmonary resuscitation: a systematic review of the literature. *Pediatrics* 2007;120:842–854.

Donoghue AJ, Nadkarni V, Berg RA, et al. Out-of-hospital pediatric cardiac arrest: an epidemiologic review and assessment of current knowledge. *Ann Emerg Med* 2005;46:512–522.

Donoghue AJ, Nadkarni VM, Elliott M, et al. Effect of hospital characteristics on outcomes from pediatric cardiopulmonary resuscitation: a report from the national registry of cardiopulmonary resuscitation. *Pediatrics* 2006;118:995–1001.

Dorian P, Cass D, Schwartz B, et al. Amiodarone as compared with lidocaine for shock-resistant ventricular fibrillation. *N Engl J Med* 2002;346: 884–890.

Dyson E, Smith GB. Common faults in resuscitation equipment—guidelines for checking equipment and drugs used in adult cardiopulmonary resuscitation. *Resuscitation* 2002;55:137–149.

Edelson DP, Abella BS, Kramer-Johansen J, et al. Effects of compression depth and preshock pauses predict defibrillation failure during cardiac arrest. *Resuscitation* 2006;71:137–145.

Eiesenberg MS, Mengert TJ. Primary care: cardiac resuscitation. *N Engl J Med* 2001;344:1304–1313.

Emergency Cardiac Care Committee and Subcommittees, American Heart Association. Guidelines for cardiopulmonary resuscitation and emergency cardiac care. VI. Pediatric advanced life support. *JAMA* 1992;268: 2262–2275.

Ewy GA. Cardiac resuscitation—when is enough enough? *N Engl J Med* 2006;355: 510–512.

Fearon DM. Ethical issues in pediatric resuscitation. In: Cahill JD, ed. *Updates in emergency medicine*. New York: Kluwer Academic/Plenum Publishers, 2003:56–63.

Fiedor ML. Pediatric simulation: a valuable tool for pediatric medical education. *Crit Care Med* 2004;32(2):S72–S74.

Fingerhut LA, Warner M. The ICD-10 injury mortality diagnosis matrix. *Injury Prevention* 2006;12:24–29.

Fiser RT, Morris MC. Extracorporeal cardiopulmonary resuscitation in refractory pediatric cardiac arrest. *Pediatr Clin North Am* 2008;55:929–941.

Froehlich CD, Rigby MR, Rosenberg ES, et al. Ultrasound-guided central venous catheter placement decreases complications and decreased placement attempts compared with the landmark technique in patients in a pediatric intensive care unit. *Crit Care Med* 2009;37:1090–1096.

Frost P, Wise MP. Cardiorespiratory arrests and rapid response teams in pediatrics. *JAMA* 2008;299(12):1423–1424. Available at: http://jama.ama-assn.org/cgi/content/full/299/12/1423-a

Gerein RB, Osmond MH, Stiell IG, et al. What are the etiology and epidemiology of out-of-hospital pediatric cardiopulmonary arrest in Ontario, Canada? *Acad Emerg Med* 2006;13:653–658.

Grenvik A, Schaefer J. From Resusci-Anne to Sim-Man: the evolution of simulators in medicine. *Crit Care Med* 2004;32(2):S56–S57.

Hall WL, Myers JH, Pepe PE, et al. The perspective of paramedics about on-scene termination of resuscitation efforts for pediatric patients. *Resuscitation* 2004;60:175–187.

Hallstrom A, Cobb L, Johnson E, et al. Cardiopulmonary resuscitation by chest compression alone or with mouth-to-mouth ventilation. *N Engl J Med* 2000; 342:1546–1553.

Hallstrom A, Ornato JP, Weisfeldt M, et al. Public-access defibrillation and survival after out-of-hospital cardiac arrest. *N Engl J Med* 2004;351:637–646.

Hazinski MF, Markenson D, Neish S, et al. Response to cardiac arrest and selected life-threatening medical emergencies. *Circulation* 2004;109:278–291.

Holzer M, The Hypothermia After Cardiac Arrest Study Group. Mild therapeutic hypothermia to improve the neurologic outcome after cardiac arrest. *N Engl J Med* 2002;346:549–556. http://jama.ama-assn.org/cgi/content/full/295/22/2646

Huikuri HV, Castellanos A, Myerburg RJ. Sudden death due to cardiac arrhythmias. *N Engl J Med* 2001;345:1473–1482.

Jorgenson D, Morgan C, Snyder D, et al. Energy attenuator for pediatric application of an automated external defibrillator. *Crit Care Med* 2002;30(4S):S145–S148.

Laffey JG, Kavanagh BP. Hypocapnia. *N Engl J Med* 2002;347:43–53.

Lavelle J, Costarino A. Central venous access and central venous pressure monitoring. In: Henretig FM, King C, eds. *Textbook of pediatric emergency procedures*. 2nd ed. Baltimore: Williams and Wilkins, 2008.

Losek J. Hypoglycemia and the ABC's (sugar) of pediatric resuscitation. *Ann Emerg Med* 2000;35:43–46.

Ludwig S, Kettrick RG, Parker M. Pediatric cardiopulmonary resuscitation: a review of 130 cases. *Clin Pediatr* 1984;23:71–76.

MacLaren G, Warwick B, Best D, et al. Extracorporeal membrane oxygenation for refractory septic shock in children: one institution's experience. *Pediatr Crit Care Med* 2007;8:447–451.

Marsch SCU, Tschan F, Semmer N, et al. Performance of first responders in simulated cardiac arrests. *Crit Care Med* 2005;33(5):963–967.

Mayr VD, Wenzel V, Voelckel WG, et al. Developing a vasopressor combination in a pig model of adult asphyxial cardiac arrest. *Circulation* 2001;104: 1651–1656.

McIntyre KM. Vasopressin in asystolic cardiac arrest. *N Engl J Med* 2004; 350:179–181.

McKee MR. Amiodarone—an "old" drug with new recommendations. *Curr Opin Pediatr* 2003;15:193–199.

Meaney PA, Nadkarni VM, Cook EF, et al. Higher survival rates among younger patients after pediatric intensive care unit cardiac arrests. *Pediatrics* 2006;118:2424–2433.

Merchant RM, Soar J, Skrifvars MB, et al. Therapeutic hypothermia utilization among physicians after resuscitation from cardiac arrest. *Crit Care Med* 2006;34:1935–1940.

Morris MC, Nadkarni VM. Pediatric cardiopulmonary-cerebral resuscitation: an overview and future directions. *Crit Care Clin* 2003;19:337–364.

Morris M, Wernovsky G, Helfaer M, et al. Survival outcomes following extracorporeal cardiopulmonary resuscitation from in-hospital pediatric cardiac arrest. *Pediatr Crit Care Med* 2004;5:440–446.

Nadkarni V, Hazinski MF, Zideman D, et al. Paediatric life support: an advisory statement by the Paediatric Life Support Working Group of the International Liaison Committee on Resuscitation. *Resuscitation* 1997;34:115–127.

Nadkarni VM, Larkin GL, Peberdy MA, et al. First documented rhythm and clinical outcome from in-hospital cardiac arrest among children and adults. *JAMA* 2006;295:50–57.

Nolan JP. Post resuscitation care—time for a care bundle? [Editorial]. *Resuscitation* 2008;76:161–162.

Nolan JP, Morley PT, Vanden Hoek TL, Hickey RW. Therapeutic hypothermia after cardiac arrest. An advisory statement by the Advanced Life Support Task Force of the International Liaison Committee on Resuscitation. *Circulation* 2003;108:118–121.

Nowak JE, Brilli RJ. Pediatric rapid response teams: is it time? *JAMA* 2007;298:2311–2312.

Page R, Joglar J, Kowal R, et al. Use of automated defibrillators by a US airline. *N Engl J Med* 2000;343:1210–1215.

PALS provider manual. American Academy of Pediatrics and the American Heart Association, 2002.

Peberdy MA, Ornato JP. Progress in resuscitation: an evolution, not a revolution. *JAMA* 2008;299(10):1188–1190. Available at: http://jama.ama-assn.org/cgi/content/full/299/10/1188

Peberdy MA, Ornato JP, Larkin GL, et al. Survival from in-hospital cardiac arrest during nights and weekends. *JAMA* 2008;299:785–792.

Peddy SB, Hazinski MF, Laussen PC, et al. Cardiopulmonary resuscitation: special considerations for infants and children with cardiac disease. *Cardiol Young* 2007;17(suppl 2):116–126.

Perkins GD, Stephenson BTF, Smith CM, et al. A comparison between over-the-head and standard cardiopulmonary resuscitation. *Resuscitation* 2004;61: 155–161.

Perondi MBM, Reis AG, Paiva EF, et al. A comparison of high-dose and standard-dose epinephrine in children with cardiac arrest. *N Engl J Med* 2004;350:1722–1730.

Posner JC, Osterhoudt, Mollen CJ, et al. Extracorporeal membrane oxygenation as a resuscitative measure in the pediatric emergency department. *Pediatr Emerg Care* 2000;16:413–415.

Prengel AW, Linder KH, Keller A, et al. Cardiovascular function during the post-resuscitation phase after cardiac arrest. *Crit Care Med* 1996;24: 2014–2019.

Reilly PM, Howell DJ. What's the P_{SL} CO_2?—The role of sublingual carbon dioxide measurement in patient care. *AACN News* 2003;20:1–6.

Reis AG, Nadkarni V, Perondi MB, et al. A prospective investigation into the epidemiology of in-hospital pediatric cardiopulmonary resuscitation using the international Utstein reporting style. *Pediatrics* 2002;109:200–209.

Riscii CE, Foster KS, Voorhees WD, et al. Electroventilation in the baboon. *Am J Emerg Med* 1988;6:561–565.

Rudner R, Jalowiecki P, Karpel E, et al. Survival after out-of-hospital cardiac arrest in Katowice (Poland): outcome report according to the "Utstein style". *Resuscitation* 2004;61:315–325.

Safar P, Behringer W, Bottiger B, et al. Cerebral resuscitation potentials for cardiac arrest. *Crit Care Med* 2002;30(4 suppl):S140–S144.

Samson RA, Berg RA, for the American Heart Association and Bingham R, for the European Resuscitation Council. Use of automated external defibrillators for children: an update—an advisory statement from the Pediatric Advanced Life Support Task Force, International Liaison Committee on Resuscitation. *Pediatrics* 2003;112(1):163–168.

Samson RA, Nadkarni VM, Meaney PA, et al. Outcomes of in-hospital ventricular fibrillation in children. *N Engl J Med* 2006;354:22.

Sayre MR, Berg RA, Cave DM, et al. Hands-only (compression-only) cardiopulmonary resuscitation: a call to action for bystander response to adults who experience out-of-hospital sudden cardiac arrest: a science advisory for the public from the American Heart Association Emergency Cardiovascular Care Committee. *Circulation* 2008;117:2162–2167. Available at: http://circ.ahajournals.org/cgi/content/full/117/16/2162

Seidel JS, Hornbein M, Yoshiyama K, et al. Emergency medical services and the pediatric patient: are the needs being met? *Pediatrics* 1984;73:769–772.

Shankaran S, Laptook AR, Ehrenkranz RA, et al. Whole-body hypothermia for neonates with hypoxic-ischemic encephalopathy. *N Engl J Med* 2005;353: 1574–1584.

Sharek PJ, Parast LM, Leong K, et al. Effect of a rapid response team on hospital-wide mortality and code rates outside the ICU in a Children's Hospital. *JAMA* 2007;298(19):2267–2274.

Sirbaugh PE, Pepe PE, Shook JE, et al. A prospective, population-based study of the demographics, epidemiology, management, and outcome of out-of-hospital pediatric cardiopulmonary arrest. *Ann Emerg Med* 1999;33: 174–184.

Srinivasan V, Morris MC, Helfaer MA, et al. Calcium use during in-hospital pediatric cardiopulmonary resuscitation: a report from the National Registry of Cardiopulmonary Resuscitation. *Pediatrics* 2008;121:e1144–e1151.

Stadbauer KH, Wagner-Berger HG, Wenzel V, et al. Survival with full neurologic recovery after prolonged cardiopulmonary resuscitation with a combination of vasopressin and epinephrine in pigs. *Anesth Analg* 2003;96: 1743–1749.

Stevenson AGM, McGowan J, Evans AL, et al. CPR for children: one hand or two? *Resuscitation* 2005;64:205–208.

Stiell IG, Hebert PC, Wells GA, et al. The Ontario trial of active compression-decompression cardiopulmonary resuscitation for in-hospital and prehospital cardiac arrest. *JAMA* 1996;275:1417–1423.

Stiell IG, Wells GA, Field B, et al. Advanced cardiac life support in out-of-hospital cardiac arrest. *N Engl J Med* 2004;351(7):647–656.

Tang W, Weil MH, Schock RB, et al. Phased chest and abdominal compression-decompression: a new option for cardiopulmonary resuscitation. *Circulation* 1997;95:1335–1340.

The Albumin Reviewers (Alderson P, Bunn F, Lefebre C, et al). Human albumin solution for resuscitation and volume expansion in critically ill patients. *Cochrane Database Syst Rev* 2004; Issue 3. Art. No. CD001208.

The Hypothermia after Cardiac Arrest Study Group. Mild therapeutic hypothermia to improve neurologic outcome after cardiac arrest. *N Engl J Med* 2002;346:549–556.

Truog RD, Christ G, Browning DM, et al. Sudden traumatic death in children: "We did everything, but your child didn't survive". *JAMA* 2006;295(22): 2646–2654.

Tsai E. Should family members be present during cardiopulmonary resuscitation? *N Engl J Med* 2002;346:1019–1021.

Valenzuela TD, Roe D, Nichol D, et al. Outcomes of rapid defibrillation by security officers after cardiac arrest in casinos. *N Engl J Med* 2000;343: 1206–1209.

Voelckel WG, Lurie KG, Sweeney M, et al. Effects of active compression-decompression cardiopulmonary resuscitation with the inspiratory threshold valve in a young porcine model of cardiac arrest. *Pediatr Res* 2002;51: 523–527.

Walsh-Kelly CM, Bergholte J, Erschen MJ, et al. Office preparedness for pediatric emergencies: baseline preparedness and the impact of guideline distribution. *Pediatr Emerg Care* 2004;20:289–294.

Wenzel V, Krismer AC, Arntz HR, et al. A comparison of vasopressin and epinephrine for out-of-hospital cardiopulmonary resuscitation. *N Engl J Med* 2004;350:105–113.

Wenzel V, Lindner KH, Augenstein S. Intraosseous vasopressin improves coronary artery perfusion pressure rapidly during cardiopulmonary resuscitation. *Crit Care Med* 1999;27:1565–1569.

Wik L. Rediscovering the importance of chest compressions to improve the outcome from cardiac arrest. *Resuscitation* 2003;58:267–269.

Wik L, Kramer-Johansen J, Myklebust HBE, et al. Quality of cardiopulmonary resuscitation during out-of-hospital cardiac arrest. *JAMA* 2005;293(3):299–304.

Xavier LC, Kern KB. Cardiopulmonary resuscitation guidelines 2000 update: what's happened since? *Curr Opin Crit Care* 2003;9:218–221.

Xu J, Kochanek KD, Tejada-Vera B. *Deaths: Preliminary data for 2007. National Vital Statistics Reports.* Vol 58, No. 1. Hyattsville, MD: National Center for Health Statistics, 2009.

Young KD, Gausche-Hill M, McClung CD, et al. A prospective, population-based study of the epidemiology and outcome of out-of-hospital pediatric cardiopulmonary arrest. *Pediatrics* 2004;114:157–164.

Young KD, Seidel J. Pediatric cardiopulmonary resuscitation: a collective review. *Ann Emerg Med* 1999;33:195–205.

CHAPTER 2 ■ NEONATAL RESUSCITATION

PAUL L. ARONSON, MD, AND EVALINE A. ALESSANDRINI, MD, MSCE

EPIDEMIOLOGY

More than 100 million babies are born each year worldwide, and approximately 4 million are born each year in the United States. Although more American women are seeking prenatal care in the first trimester of their pregnancies and there has been a decline in women who receive late or no prenatal care, the United States has one of the highest infant mortality rates of developed countries: 6.78 per 1,000 live births in 2004. This rate is markedly affected by birth weight. The infant mortality rate in 2004 was 2.26 per 1,000 for infants who weighed 2,500 g or more, 57.64 per 1,000 for infants who weighed less than 2,500 g, and 244.50 per 1,000 for those weighing less than 1,500 g. The infant mortality rate had declined by more than 75% between 1950 and 2004. These declines have been linked to improved access to care, advances in neonatal medicine, and educational campaigns such as the "Back to Sleep" campaign aimed at reducing sudden infant death syndrome. Still, the infant mortality rate has not declined significantly since 2004, and racial and ethnic disparities remain. Infant mortality rates are highest for infants of non-Hispanic black mothers, and lowest for infants of Asian mothers.

Amazingly, nearly 90% of neonates transition from intrauterine to extrauterine life without resuscitative needs. However, the remaining 10% require some assistance, and 1% require extensive resuscitative efforts. Resuscitative needs also vary greatly by birth weight. Approximately 6% of term newborns will require resuscitation at birth, compared with nearly 80% of infants weighing less than 1,500 g. Resuscitation of the newborn in the emergency department (ED) is an uncommon yet critical event that can cause an ED team well versed in other resuscitative scenarios to lose their usual level of confidence in critical situations. The key to a successful newborn resuscitation for the ED team includes preparedness of staff and equipment and anticipation of high-risk births.

EMERGENCY DEPARTMENT PREPAREDNESS

The best place for the birth of a newborn infant is in the delivery suite. However, because of varying circumstances, infants are born at home, in the prehospital setting, and in the ED. Most neonatal resuscitations in the ED occur without prior notice. Any knowledge that can be obtained before the arrival of the laboring mother or recently born infant will aid in the success of the resuscitation. Discussions with local prehospital providers to offer early notification to ED staff regarding anticipated or recent births will aid in more successful new-

born resuscitations. Education of staff, available and functioning equipment, and familiar policies and procedures are critical for preparedness.

Staff

The American Heart Association (AHA) and the American Academy of Pediatrics (AAP) have been leaders in developing guidelines for and offering training in neonatal resuscitation since 1979. Their Pediatric Advanced Life Support course offers didactic and skills teaching for neonatal resuscitation that occurs outside the delivery room. In addition, resuscitation in the delivery room is addressed in depth in the Neonatal Resuscitation Program (NRP). In concert with the goals of the AHA and the AAP, all personnel responsible for care of newborns, including ED staff, should complete courses and maintain their skills in the area of newborn resuscitation. At least one person skilled in newborn resuscitation should attend every birth in a delivery room. Additional trained personnel must be available for high-risk deliveries, such as most of those occurring in the ED or other locations outside the delivery room. Ideally, there should be at least three members on the team that are trained to work together. Identification and training of staff is the first step in preparation for neonatal resuscitation.

Equipment

In addition to a standard obstetric tray, every ED should have a newborn resuscitation kit that is readily accessible, maintained meticulously with other emergency equipment, and rapidly restocked after use. Necessary equipment and medications are listed in Table 2.1. A medication dosing chart by weight and a radiant warmer are invaluable to a neonatal resuscitation.

Policies and Procedures

As soon as the need for neonatal resuscitation becomes evident, a prearranged plan should be activated to organize personnel and assemble equipment. Readily available policies for accessing pediatric and neonatal consultants, as well as neonatal transport teams for transfer to regional centers, are critical. Because neonatal resuscitations in the ED are uncommon, simulations, mock codes, and scavenger hunts for newborn equipment on a routine basis allow staff to remain familiar with their neonatal resuscitation skills and supplies.

TABLE 2.1

NEONATAL RESUSCITATION EQUIPMENT
AND DRUGS

Equipment
Gowns, gloves, and masks for universal precautions
Radiant warmer with temperature probe
Warm towels and blankets
Bulb syringe
Suction equipment with manometer
Suction catheters (5F, 8F, and 10F)
Meconium aspirator
Oxygen with flow meter and tubing
Self-inflating resuscitation bag (500 mL) with oxygen reservoir or anesthesia (flow-inflating) bag with manometer (must be capable of delivering 90–100% oxygen and be no larger than 750 mL)
Face masks (premature, newborn, and infant sizes)
Oral airways (sizes 000, 00, and 0)
Endotracheal tubes (2.5, 3.0, 3.5, and 4.0) and small stylets
Laryngoscope handles and straight blades (nos. 0 and 1)
Extra batteries and laryngoscope bulbs
Laryngeal mask airways
Stethoscope
Tape
Scissors
Sterile umbilical catheterization tray
Umbilical catheters (3.5F and 5F)
Three-way stopcocks
Needles and syringes
Nasogastric feeding tubes (8F and 10F)
Cardiorespiratory monitor
Small electrocardiographic leads
Pulse oximeter with newborn probe
End-tidal CO_2 detector
Chest tubes (8F and 10F)
Magill forceps, small

Drugs
Weight-based resuscitation chart
Epinephrine 1:10,000 (0.1 mg/mL)
Dextrose in water, 10%
Naloxone (1 mg/mL or 0.4 mg/mL)
Sodium bicarbonate 4.2% (0.5 mEq/mL)
Isotonic crystalloid: normal saline, Ringer's lactate

HIGH-RISK BIRTHS

Most births that occur outside the delivery room have high-risk components such as trauma-induced labor and unexpected or teenage pregnancy. There is usually little time to obtain a complete obstetric history, but a brief period of questioning may reveal pertinent information that will affect a successful newborn resuscitation. Particularly important information includes prematurity, multiple gestation, meconium-stained amniotic fluid, and maternal drug use. The team can then anticipate the need for assisted ventilation, simultaneous resuscitations, tracheal suctioning, or pharmacologic interventions. Table 2.2 lists other risk factors associated with the need for neonatal resuscitation. Knowledge of many of these factors will only be available in a more controlled delivery room setting, but familiarity with this high-risk profile will benefit those involved in newborn resuscitation.

PATHOPHYSIOLOGY

Physiology of Intrauterine Development

The lungs develop over the second and third trimesters of pregnancy. Terminal airways develop by approximately 24 weeks' gestation, and the alveoli develop by 30 to 32 weeks. Surfactant is initially produced by about 23 to 24 weeks; however, sufficient amounts for opening the airways are usually not present until 34 weeks' gestation. In utero, the lung is filled with amniotic fluid, which is primarily removed by chest compression during vaginal birth. Preterm infants or those born by cesarean section tend to have more fluid in their lungs. At birth, the key physiologic change is the initiation and maintenance of respiration. Factors such as cold, touch, hypoxia, and hypercarbia help stimulate respiration. However, severe acidosis, prolonged hypoxia, maternal drugs, and moderate hypothermia depress this effort.

The heart and circulatory system begin developing during the third week of gestation. In utero, the circulation is more like a parallel circuit rather than a series circuit because of the foramen ovale and ductus arteriosus that serve as bypasses. After birth, these structures close physiologically. Severe acidosis, hypoxia, hypovolemia, and hypothermia can impair the closure. Anatomic closure of the bypasses may not occur for 2 to 4 weeks. The fetal heart is also sensitive to hypoglycemia because of the neonate's limited energy stores, and myocardial failure can occur if the infant becomes hypoglycemic.

Changes at Birth

The fetus has two large right-to-left shunts: one from the right atrium to the left atrium through the foramen ovale, and the second from the pulmonary artery to the aorta across the ductus arteriosus. The placenta is the gas-exchange organ that provides a low-resistance shunt compared with the high resistance of the fetus' pulmonary circulation. At birth, two major changes occur that eliminate these shunts: The umbilical cord is clamped, and then respirations are initiated. Expansion of the lungs increases the neonate's PaO_2 and pH, which causes pulmonary vasodilation and a fall in pulmonary vascular resistance. The normal heart rate will vary between 100 and 200 beats per minute initially and then stabilize between 120 and 150 beats per minute.

The normal newborn will begin spontaneous respirations within seconds after birth. The normal rate will be between 35 and 60 breaths per minute. The initial breaths taken by the infant must inflate the lungs and effect a change in vascular pressures so that the lung water is absorbed into the pulmonary arterial system and cleared from the lung. This inflation pressure is a powerful mechanism for the release of pulmonary surfactant, which increases compliance of the lung and establishes a functional residual capacity.

The neonate oxidizes free fatty acids released from the brown fat stores for heat production and increases oxygen consumption. The neonate experiences substantial heat loss by all four heat-loss mechanisms, especially if he or she is not dried promptly and thoroughly.

TABLE 2.2

NEONATAL HIGH-RISK PROFILE

Prenatal	Natal	Postnatal
Maternal Older than 35 yr of age Younger than 16 yr of age Diabetes Hypertension Third-trimester bleeding Infection Premature rupture of membranes Drug ingestion or therapy Drug abuse Anemia Rh sensitization Cardiac, liver, or renal disease Toxemia Preeclampsia, eclampsia No prenatal care **Fetal** Fetal distress on monitor Multiple gestation Meconium-stained amniotic fluid Premature labor Postmature labor Intrauterine growth retardation	**Maternal** Hypotension Prolonged labor Placenta previa Abruptio placenta Drugs Cesarean section **Fetal** Abnormal presentation Prolapsed cord Abnormal heart rate Meconium-stained fluid Polyhydramnios or oligohydramnios Forceps delivery Asphyxia	**Fetal** Respiratory distress Asphyxia Hypotension Meconium staining Prematurity Small for dates

Asphyxia

Asphyxia is defined as the failure to provide the cell with oxygen and remove carbon dioxide, resulting in metabolic acidemia. Both ventilation and circulation are essential to avoid asphyxia. Multiple stimuli at birth initiate respirations and alter the prenatal circulation. The actual stimuli for initiating respirations are believed to include a rise in $PaCO_2$, interruption of umbilical circulation, and tactile and temperature stimulation.

Neonatal asphyxia can result from multiple factors, as listed in Table 2.3. The initial response to asphyxia will be

TABLE 2.3

CAUSES OF NEONATAL ASPHYXIA

Maternal	Fetal
Diabetes	Abnormal presentation
Hypertension	Meconium aspiration
Toxemia	Sepsis
Preeclampsia	Hypovolemia
Eclampsia	Prolapsed cord
Exposure to alcohol, magnesium,	Congenital anomalies
β-adrenergic agents, narcotics	
Isoimmunization	
Infection	
Abruptio placenta	
Placenta previa	

hyperpnea for 2 to 3 minutes and sinus tachycardia. If there is no significant increase in PaO_2, respirations will stop for 1 to 1.5 minutes (primary apnea). During primary apnea, stimulation such as drying or slapping of the feet will restart breathing. If the apnea is prolonged, the infant loses muscle tone and becomes mottled, cyanotic, and then bradycardic. The infant may attempt gasping, nonrhythmic respiratory efforts of 6 to 10 times per minute for several minutes, while the heart rate continues to fall. Soon thereafter, the child ceases to gasp (secondary apnea). At this point, stimulation will not cause the infant to resume breathing, but rather ventilatory support must be initiated for the newborn to survive. Brain and other organ damage progresses rapidly beyond this point.

It is important to realize that when one evaluates a neonate in distress or full arrest, the asphyxial event may have begun in utero. It is difficult to document the beginning of the hypoxic period. Indeed, the infant may have passed through both stages of apnea in utero. Thus, there must be aggressive intervention if the infant is to survive. A rule of thumb is that for every minute of secondary apnea, the infant will require 4 minutes of artificial ventilation before rhythmic breathing is reestablished. An apneic infant must be treated as if he or she is in a secondary apneic stage, and resuscitation must begin immediately. If a rapid increase in heart rate does not occur with assisted ventilation, chest compressions and aggressive circulatory support will be required. If hypoxemia remains untreated, there may be further pulmonary vasoconstriction and increased right-to-left shunting through the ductus arteriosus and foramen ovale, as well as a persistence of fetal circulation.

ASSESSMENT OF THE NEWLY BORN

Successful resuscitation of a depressed newborn requires accurate assessment of the infant's respiratory effort, heart rate, color, and tone. In addition, attention to the newborn's temperature must accompany all resuscitative efforts.

Assessment of these critical parameters occurs simultaneously with management of any detected abnormality in a rapid and timely fashion. The evaluation of the clinical manifestations of a depressed newborn should occur along with resuscitative efforts within the first minute after birth. Complete assessment is performed after the infant is dried and placed in a warm environment, the airway is cleared, and stimulation has been provided.

Respiratory Effort

Most newborns will begin to breathe effectively in response to mild stimulation. The infant should be assessed for respiratory rate (between 35 and 60 breaths per minute is normal). Adequacy of respirations is noted by evaluating chest rise, auscultating good air movement, and confirming a heart rate above 100 beats per minute with improving color of the infant. Observation of tachypnea, retractions, or grunting warrants close evaluation and management. A gasping, cyanotic, or unresponsive infant requires immediate respiratory support with oxygenation and ventilation (see "Management" section).

Heart Rate

The newborn's heart rate is an excellent objective measurement of the success of the resuscitation and should be monitored closely with assessment of respiratory effort. The heart rate may be determined in many ways: (i) palpation of the pulse at the base of the umbilical cord, (ii) auscultation of heart tones with a stethoscope, (iii) palpation of the femoral or brachial pulse, and (iv) placement of a cardiac monitor. Auscultation of the apical heart rate is often difficult in a noisy environment, and the electrodes of a cardiac monitor may be difficult to place while vernix covers the newborn's body. The normal infant's heart rate is greater than 100 beats per minute at birth. The average awake infant's heart rate is between 120 and 150 beats per minute shortly after birth. Variations in heart rate commonly occur with hypoxia, hypovolemia, hypothermia, and maternal drug use. Trends in heart rate are followed closely during resuscitation and postresuscitation stabilization. The average mean arterial pressure of term infants in the first 12 hours of life is between 50 and 55 mm Hg.

Color

As respirations begin and pulmonary vascular pressures fall, the newborn rapidly becomes pink. Acrocyanosis, or persistent cyanosis of the distal extremities, may persist for several hours after birth. Acrocyanosis is not a reflection of inadequate oxygenation, but it may indicate hypothermia if persistent. Pallor may be a sign of decreased cardiac output, anemia, hypovolemia, hypothermia, or acidosis. Its cause should be investigated and corrected promptly. Central cyanosis that has not resolved with administration of oxygen and ventilation within the first minute of life must be emergently evaluated for heart disease, sepsis, diaphragmatic hernia, other congenital anomalies, or other causes.

Temperature

Particular attention must be paid to the thermoregulation of all infants, especially those born in a prehospital setting or ED, where the ambient temperature is lower than ideal for a newborn. As the patient is dried and placed under a radiant warmer, the temperature should be monitored via the axillary route using electronic thermometers with a disposable tip. Normal axillary temperatures fall between 36.5°C and 37.4°C. Rectal temperatures are reserved for infants whose core temperature may be in question. Recovery from acidosis is delayed by hypothermia. In addition, hypothermia increases metabolic needs and produces hypoxia, hypercarbia, metabolic acidosis, and hypoglycemia. Thus, efforts to maintain a normal body temperature are crucial to a successful resuscitation.

Apgar Score

The Apgar score is a useful guide to evaluate the newborn at specific intervals after birth. Although the Apgar score has been used as an indicator of responsiveness to resuscitative efforts, the score is not used to determine the need for resuscitation. Five objective signs—heart rate, respirations, muscle tone, reflex irritability, and color—are assessed 1 minute and 5 minutes after birth. Each sign receives a score between 0 and 2, and the points are then totaled for the final score (Table 2.4). If the 5-minute Apgar score is less than 7, additional scores may be obtained every 5 minutes until the infant is 20-minutes old. The score at 5 minutes and beyond is more predictive of survival and neurologic status. Although experienced physicians have developed these guidelines, they have not undergone rigorous clinical trials. Thus, if resuscitative efforts are needed for a newborn infant, they should be started immediately and not be delayed while the Apgar score is obtained.

MANAGEMENT

Initiation and Termination of Resuscitation

When and if to begin resuscitative efforts on a newborn is fraught with emotion and difficult to objectively address. Studies have shown that between 40% and 50% of apparently stillborn term newborns survived. Approximately two-thirds of these infants had a normal neurologic outcome. Current recommendations state that noninitiation of resuscitation is appropriate in some conditions that include gestational age less than 23 weeks, anencephaly, or known trisomy 13. Otherwise, resuscitative efforts should be performed on any term infant. There are multiple ethical issues regarding initiation of resuscitation of the very low-birth-weight infant.

TABLE 2.4

APGAR SCORE

Sign	Score		
	0	1	2
Heart rate	Absent	<100 beats/min	>100 beats/min
Respirations	Absent	Slow, irregular	Good, crying
Muscle tone	Limp	Some flexion	Active motion
Reflex irritability	None	Grimace	Cough, sneeze, cry
Color	Blue or pale	Pink body, blue hands and feet	Completely pink

However, with surfactant therapy and improved management of these infants, outcomes have improved over time and the controversy of resuscitation remains. Current recommendations note that a birth weight less than 400 g may be one criterion to not initiate resuscitation. At the stressful time of an emergency delivery, if there is any question of viability, it is probably best to initiate resuscitative efforts.

A difficult decision is when to stop resuscitation. One predictor is the Apgar score. Survival is extremely unlikely if the 10-minute Apgar score remains 0. In this circumstance, a 10-minute period of resuscitation is usually warranted; but if the Apgar score remains 0 or 1 at that time, resuscitation may be terminated because of extremely poor outcomes. It is imperative to believe that every resuscitative step has been performed correctly and repetitively prior to termination of resuscitation. In addition, emergency staff with neonatal expertise on site should be invited to participate in these resuscitative efforts and decisions to terminate resuscitation.

Initial Management Priorities

Four questions should be asked when an infant is born:

1. Is the infant term?
2. Is the amniotic fluid clear of meconium?
3. Is the baby breathing or crying?
4. Does the baby have good muscle tone?

If the answers to these questions are yes, it is likely that the newborn will do well and require routine care. However, most births occurring outside the delivery suite will have high-risk attributes and require supportive or ongoing newborn care. The initial steps of neonatal resuscitation include positioning and clearing the airway, drying and warming with prevention of heat loss, stimulating, and repositioning. These steps occur within 30 seconds and are followed immediately by an evaluation of respirations, heart rate, and color. When possible, all resuscitation equipment should be ready for use, the radiant warmer on, and a team with preassigned roles assembled. Figure 2.1 is a flow diagram of neonatal resuscitation.

Thermoregulation

The initial step of drying the infant to minimize heat loss is extremely important, and further resuscitation is continued after warming has begun. Premature infants are at greater risk of hypothermia because of their greater body surface area-to-weight ratio, minimal fat stores, and thinner epidermis and dermis. As previously stated, recovery from acidosis is delayed by hypothermia, and hypothermia is a special problem for the infant born outside the hospital. Thus, simply resuscitating the baby in a warm environment, under a prewarmed radiant warmer while drying the amniotic fluid from the infant and removing wet linens from contact with the skin will markedly decrease heat loss. These maneuvers will maximize the infant's chance of recovery. Alternative methods of warming infants, particularly while awaiting a radiant warmer in the case of an unexpected delivery, include warm blankets and towels. Placing the infant naked against the mother's body and covering both mother and infant with blankets may also warm the stable infant. Although preventing heat loss is vital, hyperthermia should be avoided because it is associated with perinatal respiratory depression and hypoxic-ischemic injury may be worsened.

Cerebral hypothermia has been advocated by some as a means to protect asphyxiated infants from further brain injury. A multicenter, randomized controlled trial showed that systemic hypothermia initiated within 6 hours of life reduced death or neurologic disability in infants with moderate or severe hypoxic-ischemic encephalopathy. Another randomized controlled trial showed improved neurodevelopmental outcomes with selective head cooling in asphyxiated infants with less severe encephalopathy. However, there remain insufficient data to recommend the routine use of systemic or selective hypothermia in asphyxiated infants until further clinical trials are undertaken. In the ED, maintenance of a normal body temperature and avoidance of hyperthermia are critical.

Suctioning

Many newborns have excessive secretions, including amniotic fluid, cervical mucus, and meconium, which may obstruct their airways. (Meconium is a special situation discussed in the following section.) These secretions can generally be removed by placing the infant on his or her side and gently suctioning the mouth and then the nose with a bulb syringe. Mechanical suction with an 8F or 10F suction catheter may also be used. To avoid soft-tissue injury, negative pressure from mechanical suctioning should not exceed 100 mm Hg. Deep suctioning of the oropharynx in a newborn is likely to cause vagally mediated bradycardia and/or apnea. Excessive suctioning may also contribute to atelectasis. Most clear fluid is resorbed by the lungs into the arterial system. Consequently, suctioning should be gentle and brief because this is usually adequate to remove secretions.

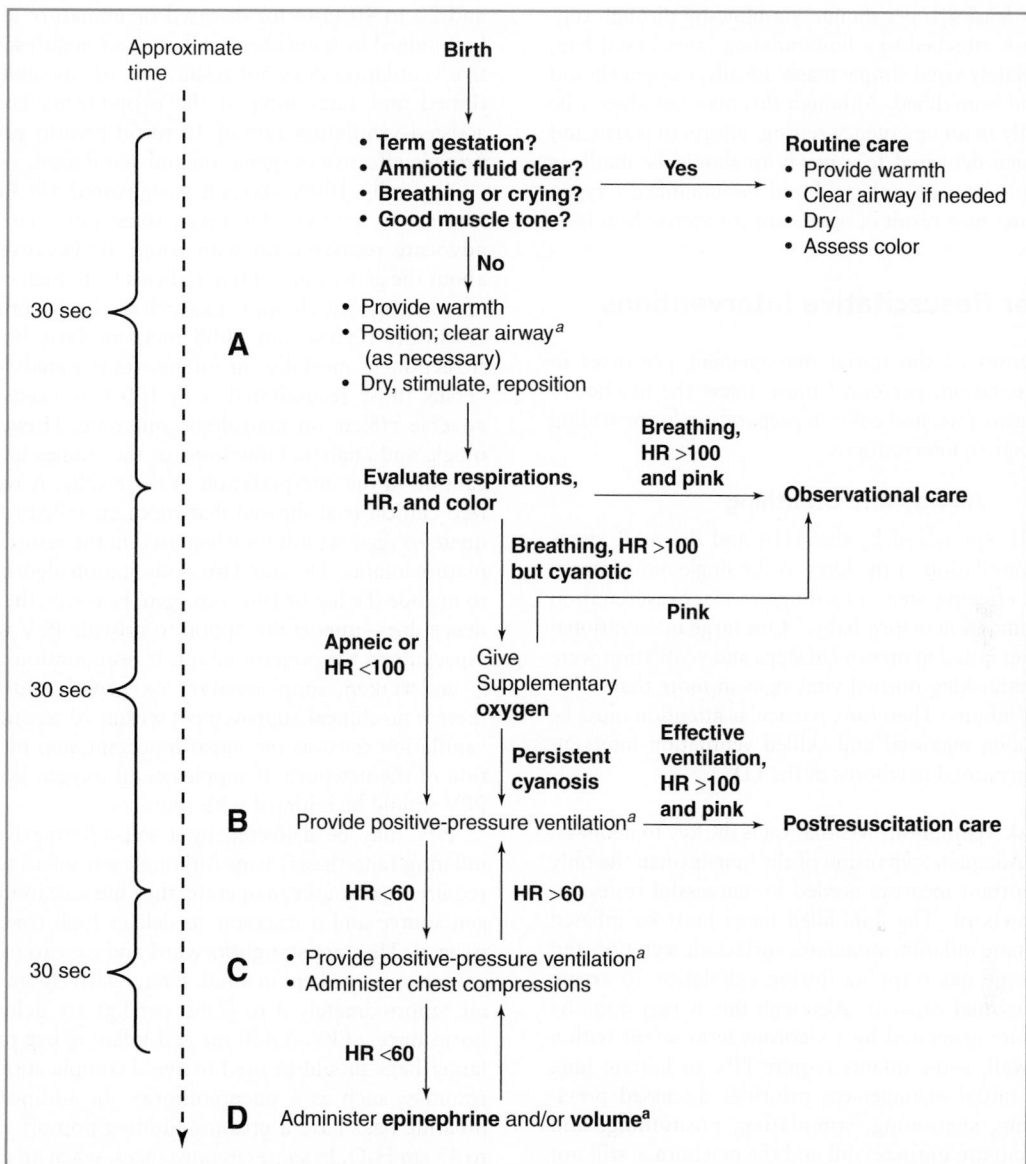

FIGURE 2.1 Overview of neonatal resuscitation. (Adapted from Kattwinkel J, Short J, Boyle D, et al. *Textbook of neonatal resuscitation.* 5th ed. Elk Grove Village, IL: American Academy of Pediatrics and American Heart Association, 2006.)

Stimulation

Most newborns will begin effective breathing during stimulation from routine drying and suctioning. Other methods of safe stimulation include flicking the heels and rubbing the back of the newborn infant. More vigorous methods of stimulation are unnecessary and may be associated with harmful consequences. If after a brief period of stimulation, suctioning, and drying (no more than 30 seconds; Fig. 2.1), effective respirations have not been established, positive-pressure ventilation (PPV) is initiated.

Airway Positioning and Oxygen Administration

Most infants require only warming, drying, stimulation, and suctioning after birth for a smooth transition to their extrauterine environment. If a newborn is exhibiting signs and symp-

toms of airway obstruction after routine suctioning, the airway should be repositioned. Correct positioning, with the neck slightly extended in the "sniffing position," will bring the posterior pharynx, larynx, and trachea inline and facilitate air entry. This maneuver may also be accomplished by placing a towel or blanket beneath the shoulders and upper back of the supine infant. By elevating the shoulders and upper back approximately 1 inch, the airway is again slightly extended into a neutral position, compensating for the infant's relatively large occiput. Avoid flexion or hyperextension of the newborn's neck, which is likely to exacerbate airway obstruction.

An infant who exhibits central cyanosis, yet is making adequate, spontaneous respirations and has a heart rate above 100 beats per minute, needs supplemental oxygen. It is important to deliver as close to 100% oxygen as possible, with a flow rate of at least 5 L per minute via blow-by through tubing, a face mask attached to a flow-inflating (anesthesia) bag, or an appropriately sized simple mask. Ideally, oxygen should be warmed and humidified. Although this may not always be possible initially in an emergency setting, efforts to warm and humidify oxygen delivered to a newborn should be made as soon as possible because unheated and unhumidified oxygen at high flow rates may result in significant convective heat loss.

Further Resuscitative Interventions

Upon completion of the initial management priorities in neonatal resuscitation, personnel must assess the newborn's respirations, heart rate, and color in preparation for providing further resuscitative interventions.

Airway and Breathing

The 2005 NRP, sponsored by the AHA and the AAP, states repeatedly: "Ventilation of the lungs is the single most important and most effective step in cardiopulmonary resuscitation of the compromised newborn baby." One large observational study noted that initial management steps and ventilation were effective in establishing normal vital signs in more than 99% of newly born infants. Therefore, particular attention must be paid to providing maximal and skilled ventilation interventions for compromised newborns in the ED.

Bag-valve-mask Ventilation. Ventilation is the key to neonatal resuscitation. Adequate expansion of the lung is often the only and most important measure needed for successful resuscitation of the newborn. The fluid-filled lungs must be inflated with air. Adequate inflation stimulates surfactant secretion and also allows some gas trapping during exhalation to create a functional residual capacity. Although this is best done by negative pressure generated by a vigorous term infant with a strong chest wall, some infants require PPV to initiate lung expansion. If initial management priorities discussed previously (warming, suctioning, stimulating, positioning, and blow-by oxygen) are unsuccessful and the newborn is still not breathing or is gasping, the heart rate is less than 100 beats per minute, and/or the color remains cyanotic despite 100% oxygen, PPV must be initiated. Indications for PPV are summarized in Table 2.5.

PPV is best achieved with a well-fitted face mask, which covers the infant's nose and mouth but does not place pressure on the eyes. A cushioned rim on the face mask allows the best possible seal. A relatively high inflation pressure, between 25 and 40 cm H_2O, delivered slowly over several seconds is necessary for the infant's first breath. Subsequent ventilations typically require less pressure (15 to 20 cm H_2O for normal lungs

and 20 to 40 H_2O for diseased or immature lungs), and are best judged by good chest wall rise and breath sounds. If effective ventilation does not result, the airway should be repositioned and suctioning of the oropharynx considered. An assisted ventilatory rate of 40 to 60 breaths per minute will provide effective oxygenation and ventilation.

Typically 100% oxygen is delivered via PPV for rapid reversal of hypoxia. However, some physician investigators advocate resuscitation with room air because of concerns about the generation of free radicals from high concentrations of oxygen, which may exacerbate brain injury. A 2005 Cochrane review and 2008 meta-analysis both showed a reduction in mortality in infants resuscitated with room air versus those resuscitated with 100% oxygen, without any adverse effects on neurologic outcome. However, methodologic and analytic limitations of the studies have resulted in caution in the interpretation of the results. A recent randomized clinical trial showed that room air failed to provide adequate oxygen saturation when used in the resuscitation of premature infants. The standard resuscitation algorithm continues to include the use of 100% oxygen; however, the available evidence does support the option to provide PPV with room air, especially in the preterm infant. If resuscitation with room air is undertaken, supplementary oxygen should be utilized if there is no clinical improvement within 90 seconds of birth. As ventilation remains the most important step in the resuscitation of the newborn, if supplemental oxygen is not available, PPV should be initiated with room air.

PPV may be delivered by a self-inflating bag or a flow-inflating (anesthesia) bag. Although self-inflating bags do not require a gas source to operate, they must be used with an oxygen source and a reservoir to deliver high concentrations of oxygen. They are straightforward and easy to use, but several caveats must be kept in mind. First, relatively small volumes of air (approximately 4 to 6 mL per kg) are delivered to newborns during PPV. A 450-mL self-inflating bag rather than the larger bags should be used to avoid complications from barotraumas, such as a pneumothorax. In addition, many self-inflating bags have a pressure-limiting pop-off valve set at 30 to 45 cm H_2O. In some circumstances, when an infant requires higher initial inflation pressures, the bag may not allow the resuscitator to deliver enough pressure to the newborn for an adequate first breath. Unless the valve is occluded, effective inflation may be prevented.

To inflate properly, flow-inflating bags require adequate airflow and a good mask seal. Consequently, the resuscitator must be facile at positioning the airway and mask, controlling the flow valves, and monitoring the manometer, which is needed to monitor peak ventilatory pressures delivered to the infant. Benefits of the flow-inflating bag include the ability to deliver a wide range of peak inspiratory pressures, positive end-expiratory pressure, high concentrations of oxygen compared with the self-inflating bag, and ease of determination whether there is a tight seal. Proper use requires training and practice.

If bag-valve-mask ventilation is required for longer than several minutes, an orogastric tube should be placed to decompress the stomach so further effective ventilation is not inhibited. This tube should be left in place. The infant should be reevaluated after 30 seconds of PPV for spontaneous respirations and heart rate. If the infant has begun breathing and the heart rate is

TABLE 2.5

INDICATIONS FOR POSITIVE-PRESSURE VENTILATION

Apnea or gasping respirations
Heart rate <100 beats/min
Persistent central cyanosis despite administration of 100% oxygen

TABLE 2.6

INDICATIONS FOR ENDOTRACHEAL INTUBATION

Ineffective bag-valve-mask ventilation
Prolonged need for positive-pressure ventilation
Suctioning of meconium in an infant who is not vigorous
When chest compressions are required
Administration of resuscitation medications
Advanced resuscitation situations such as extreme prematurity

above 100 beats per minute, PPV may be slowly discontinued. If respirations are inadequate or the heart rate remains less than 100 beats per minute, assisted ventilation must be continued and endotracheal (ET) intubation must be considered.

Endotracheal Intubation. Most resuscitative efforts succeed with bag-valve-mask ventilation alone. In the event that there is a prolonged need for PPV or mask ventilation has not been effective in restoring vital functions, ET intubation is indicated. Indications for ET intubation are summarized in Table 2.6. Once the decision to intubate the trachea has been made, supplies from the newborn resuscitation tray are organized. Sizes of airway equipment can be determined by birth weight (Table 2.7). ET tube size can also be estimated by gestational age:

$$\text{ET tube size in mm} = \text{Gestational age in weeks}/10$$

Thus, a 35-week premature infant would require a 3.5-mm ET tube.

ET intubation is typically performed via the orotracheal route during direct laryngoscopy with a straight blade. The laryngoscope blade is inserted into the vallecula or onto the epiglottis and reveals the vocal cords during a gentle lifting movement. Laryngoscopy in the newborn is challenging because of the infant's large tongue and secretions, which may obscure airway landmarks. Attempts at ET intubation should be limited to 20 seconds per attempt. If the glottis is not visualized or the tube is not inserted into the trachea within 20 seconds, oxygenate the infant with 100% oxygen provided by bag-valve-mask ventilation, and then try again. Successful ET intubation also requires proper tube positioning. Most neonatal ET tubes have a black vocal cord line near the tip. When this guide is placed at the level of the vocal cords, the tip of the tube is likely to be positioned properly in the trachea. Another estimate for the insertion distance of the ET tube is

$$\text{Total cm at gum line} = 6 + \text{Weight of the infant in kg}$$

Proper positioning of the ET tube must be confirmed by auscultation of equal breath sounds in both axillae; good, symmetric chest wall movement; and improvement of the infant's cardiorespiratory status. Once positioning is clinically verified, the ET tube must be securely taped in place, and positioning may then be confirmed with a radiograph as indicated. End-tidal CO_2 detectors are the recommended means of confirming ET tube placement during newborn resuscitation. It is important to note that they may be associated with false-negative results, particularly in infants with extremely compromised cardiac output. Other issues, such as decreased pulmonary blood flow and small tidal volume, may influence end-tidal CO_2 detection in newborns. If ET tube positioning is uncertain and the end-tidal CO_2 detector does not detect exhaled carbon dioxide, the safest measure is to extubate, provide bag-valve-mask ventilation, and reintubate the trachea. Note that pulse oximetry is not routinely used in newborns after delivery. Some studies have shown that the readings did not correlate with blood gas values. Furthermore, the definition of a "normal" oxygen saturation immediately after birth is unknown, and aggressively attempting to increase the saturation to near 100% may cause oxygen toxicity.

More recently, investigators found laryngeal mask airways (LMAs) successful for ventilating full-term or near-term newborns, particularly in cases of ineffective bag-valve-mask ventilation or failed ET intubation. Although LMAs may be used as a secondary device to ventilate term newborns by healthcare practitioners skilled in their use, data supporting use of LMAs in preterm infants are insufficient to routinely recommend their use in this scenario. Furthermore, LMAs cannot replace ET intubation when meconium suctioning is required.

Circulation

Chest Compressions. Chest compressions are rarely needed during neonatal resuscitation. Most series have demonstrated that less than 0.1% of all births require chest compressions. Bradycardia and asystole in the newborn are virtually always a result of respiratory failure, hypoxemia, and tissue acidosis. Consequently, oxygenation and ventilation are most critical to successful infant resuscitation. Chest compressions should be started whenever the heart rate remains less than 60 beats per minute despite 30 seconds of PPV. Indication for chest compressions, which are always performed simultaneously with PPV with 100% oxygen, are listed in Table 2.8.

Current recommendations state that three chest compressions are followed by a brief pause for one ventilation. Thus, in 1 minute, the newborn should receive 90 chest compressions and 30 ventilations. This technique allows for optimal

TABLE 2.7

SELECTION OF AIRWAY EQUIPMENT BY WEIGHT

Weight (g) or gestational age (wk)	Endotracheal tube size (mm)	Suction catheter (F)	Oral airway	Laryngoscope straight blade
<1,000 or <28	2.5	5, 6	000	0
1,000–2,000 or 28–34	3.0	6, 8	000 or 00	0
2,000–3,000 or 34–38	3.5	8	00 or 0	0, 1
>3,000 or >38	3.5, 4.0	8 or 10	0	1

TABLE 2.8

INDICATION FOR CHEST COMPRESSIONS

Heart rate <60 beats/min despite 30 s of effective positive-
pressure ventilation

lung expansion by not compressing the chest during PPV, and
the most important aspects of reversing neonatal asphyxia,
good oxygenation and ventilation, are maximized.

Two techniques of performing chest compressions in the
neonate or young infant are recommended. The preferred
method involves placing the thumbs on the lower third of the
sternum, encircling the chest and supporting the back with
the fingers (Fig. 2.2). The thumbs should be placed side by
side just below the nipple line. However, if the neonate is
very small or if the resuscitator is large, the thumbs may need
to be superimposed. Pressure must be placed on the sternum
and not the adjacent ribs. In the event that the resuscitator's
hands are too small to encircle the newborn's chest or encircling the chest obstructs other resuscitative efforts such as
umbilical line placement, then the two-finger technique may
be used. This method entails placing the ring and middle fingers on the sternum just below the nipple line for chest compressions.

With either method of chest compression, the resuscitator
should compress the chest approximately one-third of the
anterior-posterior diameter of the chest to generate a palpable
pulse. The compression stroke should also be somewhat
shorter in duration than the relaxation phase for generation of
maximum cardiac output. In addition, the fingers or thumbs
should not be lifted off the chest at any time to save time with
correct finger positioning; maintain control over compression
depth and preserve correct finger positioning to prevent damage to underlying organs.

After approximately 30 seconds of well-coordinated chest
compressions and ventilation, stop chest compressions to check
the spontaneous heart rate by palpating the pulse at the base
of the umbilical cord. Ventilations can be continued while using
this method of pulse check. If auscultating the left chest for
heart rate check, compressions and ventilations will need to be
suspended. If the heart rate is at least 60 beats per minute, compressions can stop, but ventilation should be continued at the
40 to 60 breath per minute rate. If the heart rate remains below
60 beats per minute, compressions must be continued and epinephrine should be given (see below). In addition, resuscitators
must be sure they are providing adequate ventilation with
100% oxygen, resulting in good chest wall movement and
coordinated compressions and ventilations.

Vascular Access. A newborn requires vascular access for
administration of medications or volume expansion.
Bradycardia or asystole unresponsive to effective oxygenation,
ventilation, and chest compressions warrant pharmacologic
therapy. Infants exhibiting signs of poor perfusion, particularly those with risk for hypovolemia, such as fetal hemorrhage or maternal hypotension from placental abruption,
require volume expansion.

Several methods of vascular access may be used in the newborn. The umbilical vein is often considered a preferred site for
vascular access during neonatal resuscitation because it is easily located and cannulated, and medication delivery requires
insertion only to the point at which blood is able to be aspirated (usually 2 to 4 cm). (See Section VII: Umbilical Vein
Catheterization for methods.) A skilled resuscitator may elect
to cannulate the umbilical artery to obtain arterial blood gases
and monitor arterial pressures in critically ill infants; however,
administration of medications is not recommended via this
route. (See Section VII: Umbilical Artery Catheterization.)
Vascular access may also be obtained by placing peripheral
catheters in the extremities or scalp. In a newborn resuscitation

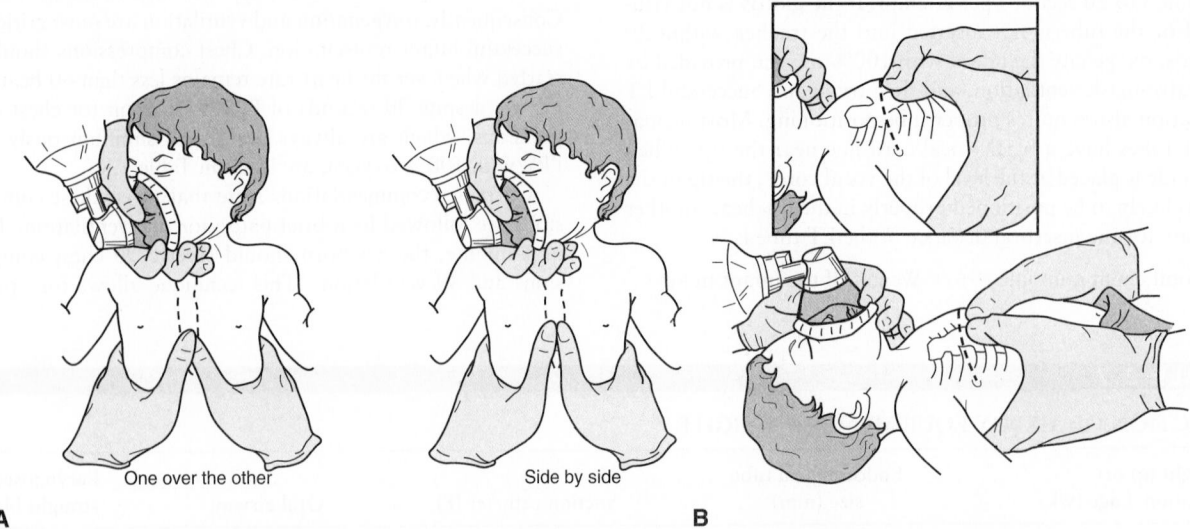

One over the other   Side by side

A   **B**

FIGURE 2.2 **A:** Thumb method of chest compressions. Infant receiving chest compressions with thumb
1 fingerbreadth below the nipple line and hands encircling chest. **B:** Hand position for chest encirclement
technique for external chest compressions in neonates. Thumbs are side by side over the lower third of the
sternum. In the small newborn, thumbs may need to be superimposed *(inset)*. Gloves should be worn during resuscitation.

TABLE 2.9

MEDICATIONS FOR NEONATAL RESUSCITATION

Medication	Concentration	Dosage	Route	Comment
Epinephrine	1:10,000	0.1–0.3 mL/kg	IV, ET, IO	Rapid push, dilute with 2 mL saline via ET tube
Sodium bicarbonate	0.5 mEq/mL (4.2% solution)	1–2 mEq/kg	IV, IO	Slowly over 2 min with effective ventilation
Naloxone	1 mg/mL	0.1 mg/kg	IV, IO	Rapid push
	0.4 mg/mL		IM, SC	Only in well-perfused neonate
Dextrose	10%	2–5 mL/kg	IV, IO	Correction of hypoglycemia

IV, intravenous; ET, endotracheal; IM, intramuscular; SC, subcutaneous.

scenario, peripheral venous access may be difficult. In the event that fluids and medications are required and other methods of vascular access have failed, intraosseous lines may be used (see Section VII: Intraosseous Infusion). Although experience with other infants is extensive in this arena, experience in the neonate is limited. A 20- or 22-gauge spinal needle may replace the 16- or 18-gauge larger intraosseous needles; however, the procedure for line placement in the proximal tibia is the same as for older children (see Appendix 3.8). Recall that premature infants have a small intraosseous space. Finally, the ET tube may be used for administration of epinephrine when vascular access has not yet been established.

Medications and Volume Expanders for Acute Resuscitation
Epinephrine. Although medications are rarely required for neonatal resuscitation, epinephrine is the most commonly indicated medication. Because asystole and bradycardia are usually the result of respiratory failure and tissue acidosis, epinephrine therapy is indicated when the newborn's heart rate remains less than 60 beats per minute, despite 30 seconds of effective ventilation with 100% oxygen and another 30 seconds of coordinated chest compressions and ventilation. Epinephrine works because of its α-adrenergic effects. Swine models have demonstrated that epinephrine induces vasoconstriction secondary to α-receptor agonism in infants, increases the diastolic and mean arterial pressures, and thus increases the perfusion pressure to the coronary arteries, enhancing oxygen delivery to the heart. The β-adrenergic effects of epinephrine that increase myocardial contractility and stimulate spontaneous contractions appear less important.

The dose of epinephrine therapy in neonates is 0.01 to 0.03 mg per kg of a 1:10,000 concentration, or 0.1 to 0.3 mL per kg (Table 2.9). It may be administered via an umbilical venous catheter, a peripheral IV, an intraosseous line, or the ET tube. The dose should be repeated every 3 to 5 minutes as needed throughout the resuscitation. Intravenous epinephrine should be administered as rapidly as possible and followed by a 1-mL normal saline flush. The safety and efficacy of high-dose epinephrine (0.1 to 0.2 mg per kg) has not been studied in neonates. A concern that large doses of epinephrine may lead to prolonged hypertension and subsequent intracranial hemorrhage in neonates has precluded the investigation of changing dosing recommendations. The AHA does recommend giving a higher dose of endotracheally administered epinephrine, between 0.03 and 0.1 mg per kg. However, given

that there are no data from newborn infants to assess the safety of higher doses of intratracheal epinephrine, IV administration remains the preferred route. Given the need to distribute the medication throughout the lungs, ET epinephrine should be followed by 1 to 2 mL of normal saline and several positive-pressure breaths.

Volume expanders. Volume expanders are indicated for the treatment of hypovolemia. Both historical and physical examination findings suggest the need for volume expansion. Historical factors include fetal hemorrhage from an avulsed cord or trauma, or maternal hypotension from placenta previa, placental abruption, or trauma. Umbilical cord prolapse may cause hypovolemia in the newborn. Physical examination findings include pallor that persists despite oxygenation, weak peripheral pulses, persistently high or low heart rate, and a poor response to resuscitation, including effective ventilation.

Volume expanders (Table 2.10) are administered intravenously in 10 mL per kg aliquots and should be given fairly quickly (over 5 to 10 minutes), but not so rapidly as to increase the risk of intracranial hemorrhage from delicate vascular beds. The umbilical vein is the best site for administration of volume expanders, although the intraosseous or peripheral IV route may be used. After each infusion, the infant is reassessed for improvements in perfusion, blood pressure, and oxygenation. Current recommendations are to begin with a crystalloid solution, such as normal saline or Ringer's lactate. Administration of O-negative red blood cells (crossmatched with mother's blood if time allows) may be indicated for large volume blood loss or poor response to crystalloid

TABLE 2.10

VOLUME EXPANDERS FOR NEONATAL RESUSCITATION

Fluid	Dosage (mL/kg)	Route
Normal saline	10	IV
Ringer's lactate	10	IV
Packed red blood cells	10	IV

IV, intravenous.

infusion. Albumin-containing solutions are no longer recommended because of cost, limited availability, risk of infection, and potential increased mortality.

Other Medications

Sodium bicarbonate. There are insufficient data to recommend routine use of bicarbonate therapy in neonatal resuscitation. Bicarbonate therapy may contribute to respiratory acidosis and a worsening intracellular acidosis, which may actually impair myocardial and cerebral function. Thus, its use is discouraged in brief resuscitations. In prolonged resuscitations and after establishment of adequate ventilation, bicarbonate may be given for documented metabolic acidosis or hyperkalemia using arterial blood gases and serum chemistries to guide administration. The dose of sodium bicarbonate is 1 to 2 mEq per kg administered intravenously and slowly over 2 minutes to decrease adverse effects associated with its hypertonicity. For the same reason, only the 0.5 mEq per mL (4.2%) solution should be administered to neonates. If only the 1 mEq per mL solution is available, it should be diluted 1:1 with sterile water before intravenous delivery. Because of its caustic nature, bicarbonate should never be administered via the ET route. Little research data exist to support the choice of other buffers, such as tris(hydroxymethyl)aminomethane (THAM), for documented metabolic acidosis, although many practitioners use this medication to reduce the occurrence of hypernatremia. This controversial area requires rigorous research.

Naloxone hydrochloride. Naloxone is a narcotic antagonist that reverses respiratory depression induced by narcotics. Naloxone is indicated for infants displaying signs of respiratory depression after PPV has restored a normal heart rate and color, and for those infants whose mothers have received narcotics within the 4 hours before delivery. Prompt and effective oxygenation and ventilation must be provided and the infant must have adequate perfusion before the administration of naloxone. The current dosing recommendation for naloxone is 0.1 mg per kg, which is given as 0.1 mL per kg of the 1 mg per mL concentration (Table 2.9). Caution must be used, as there are several concentrations of naloxone available. Naloxone is best administered via the intravenous, intraosseous, or intramuscular routes. ET administration is not recommended because of lack of data. Furthermore, the resuscitator must remember that repetitive doses of naloxone may be required because the duration of action of narcotics may exceed that of naloxone. Finally, do not give naloxone to the newborn of a mother suspected of narcotic addiction because this may precipitate acute narcotic withdrawal and seizures.

Atropine. Atropine is not recommended for acute neonatal resuscitation. Atropine is a parasympatholytic drug that reduces vagal tone and accelerates sinus or atrial pacemakers and atrioventricular conduction. Because vagal stimulation does not cause bradycardia in neonatal resuscitation, atropine is not indicated. Furthermore, many investigators believe that the bradycardic vagally mediated response to hypoxia is a valuable reflex to guide resuscitative efforts and should not be pharmacologically abolished by atropine.

The usual dose of atropine is 0.02 mg per kg with a minimum dose of 0.1 mg and a maximum dose of 2 mg. Because most newborns weigh less than 5 kg, their dose would require

the 0.1 mg minimum. If smaller doses are given, paradoxical bradycardia and slowed atrioventricular conduction will likely occur. In conclusion, the efficacy of atropine in newborn resuscitation is unproven and anecdotal and could have deleterious consequences.

Postresuscitation Stabilization

After appropriate resuscitative efforts, continuous monitoring and anticipation of complications must occur until the patient is safely transported to a neonatal facility. Priority must be given to thermoregulation by providing the infant with a warm environment and repetitively monitoring the temperature. Measures of effective oxygenation and ventilation are assessed. Pulse oximetry and arterial blood gases are performed. ET tubes are securely taped and a chest radiograph is ordered to confirm tube and venous access placement. Vascular access is secured, and correction of metabolic acidosis and hypovolemia is continued. Glucose monitoring and the avoidance of hypoglycemia are also paramount as low blood glucose has been associated with poor neurologic outcome.

If mechanical ventilation is required while waiting transport to the neonatal facility, a pressure ventilator is used. Peak pressures are determined by clinical evaluation of adequate chest wall rise and blood gas analyses. A good starting point for peak pressure is the pressure needed for good chest wall rise and breath sounds during resuscitation as shown on the manometer. In general, this is between 15 and 30 cm H_2O. The physician should try to use the lowest pressure necessary for good clinical and laboratory response. Excessive positive pressure will decrease venous return to the heart, decrease cardiac output, and cause injury to lung tissue.

SPECIAL SITUATIONS

Meconium

Management of meconium-stained amniotic fluid has changed substantially with the most recent recommendation of the NRP. Meconium staining of the amniotic fluid complicates between 10% and 20% of all pregnancies. The risk of meconium-related complications at delivery increases to nearly 30% in infants born after 42 weeks' gestation. Approximately 2% to 5% of infants born with meconium in the amniotic fluid will experience some degree of aspiration syndrome, ranging from mild tachypnea to very severe pneumonitis with persistent pulmonary hypertension (Fig. 2.3). The management of an infant born through meconium differs from that previously discussed for other depressed infants.

When meconium staining is detected during delivery, resuscitative personnel must be prepared in the event that specific interventions are needed (Fig. 2.4). In the event the delivery occurs in the ED or a setting where health-care personnel are present and there is meconium staining of the amniotic fluid, the infant should be immediately transferred to the resuscitation team without intrapartum suctioning of the infant's mouth and nose. This recommendation is a change from previous guidelines after a multicenter randomized trial showed no decrease in the risk of meconium aspiration syndrome

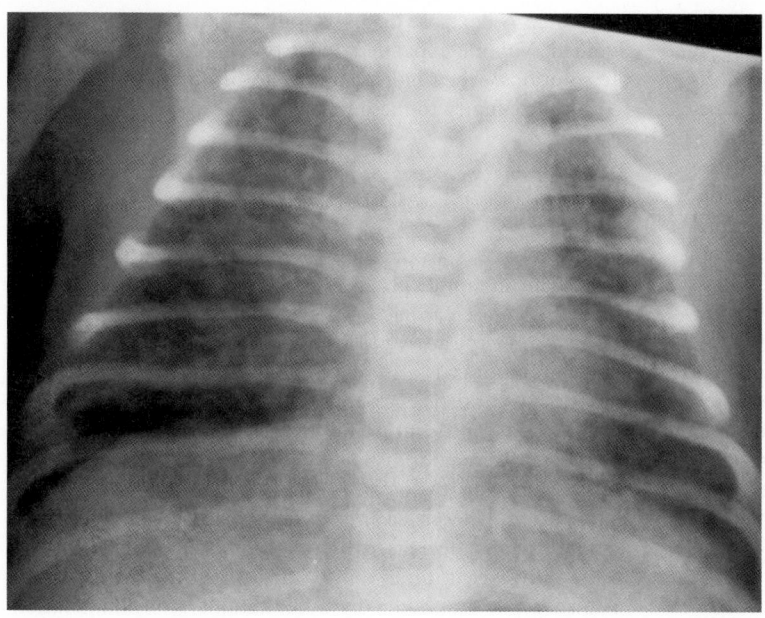

FIGURE 2.3 Meconium aspiration radiograph.

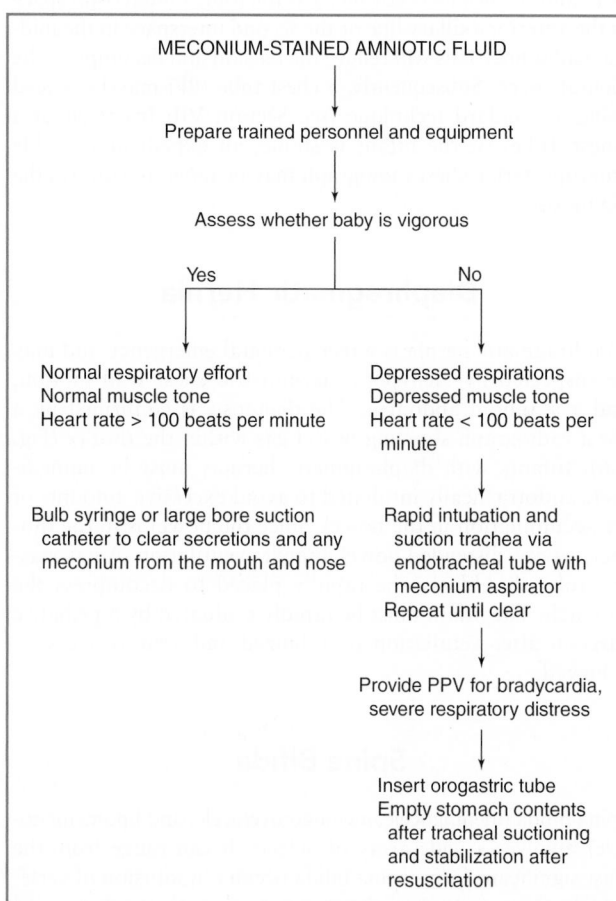

FIGURE 2.4 Management of infant born with meconium-stained amniotic fluid. PPV, positive-pressure ventilation.

when suctioning was performed after delivery of the infant's head but before delivery of the body.

Current guidelines for further management of newborns with meconium in the amniotic fluid are based on the status of the newborn rather than the consistency of the meconium. If meconium is present and the baby is not vigorous—that is, a baby with depressed respirations, depressed muscle tone, or a heart rate less than 100 beats per minute—direct suctioning of the trachea soon after delivery is indicated before many respirations have occurred. After delivery, the infant is placed in a warm environment, and before other usual resuscitative efforts, meconium suctioning is completed. First, the trachea is intubated, and suctioning of the lower airway occurs. Because the ET tube itself is the largest diameter item placed in the trachea, it is the most effective means of suctioning meconium. Thus, a meconium aspirator (Fig. 2.5) directly attached between the ET tube and mechanical suction is the preferred method of removing meconium from the lower airway. Negative pressure is applied by occluding the opening on the side of the aspirator with a finger. Mechanical suctioning should not exceed 100 mm Hg. Repeat intubation and

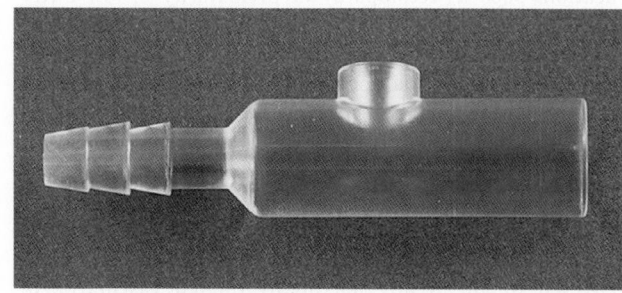

FIGURE 2.5 Meconium aspirator.

suctioning with another ET tube may be required until the aspirated material is clear. After initial tracheal suctioning, it may be necessary to begin PPV if the heart rate or respirations are severely depressed, despite persistent meconium in the airway. Wait until completion of tracheal suctioning and resuscitation to place an orogastric tube to empty meconium from the newborn's stomach, which could potentially be aspirated later.

When meconium is present and the baby is vigorous, defined as a baby with a normal respiratory effort, normal muscle tone, and a heart rate greater than 100 beats per minute, a bulb syringe or large-bore (12F or 14F) suction catheter is used to clear secretions and any meconium from the mouth and nose. Tracheal suctioning should be eliminated in vigorous infants, regardless of the consistency of the meconium. This recommendation is based on several large randomized trials that demonstrated that routine tracheal suctioning did not decrease morbidity or mortality from meconium aspiration syndrome.

Prematurity

Premature infants have an increased likelihood of needing newborn resuscitation. Early involvement of neonatologists and neonatal centers adept in the management of low-birth-weight infants is crucial to improve outcome. Only 15% of hospitals have specialized neonatal units. Hospitals without neonatal units need easily available guidelines and established relationships for accessing neonatal consultation and transport. Several factors have added importance in the resuscitation of the preterm infant. These include greater risk for heat loss, greater mechanical ventilation needs, and greater risk of intraventricular hemorrhage.

Premature infants are at greatest risk for heat loss because of their higher ratio of body surface area to body mass. Premature infants require the strictest attention to maintenance of normal body temperature.

Premature infants are more likely to develop respiratory distress than term infants. As a result, assisted ventilation must be provided effectively but gently. ET intubation is usually necessary for surfactant administration and transport to a neonatal facility. Too much ventilatory pressure may result in barotrauma to the lungs and decreased cardiac output as a result of decreased venous return. Good clinical judgment should be used by watching for adequate chest wall rise and listening for good breath sounds. The physician should use the lowest pressure necessary to achieve a heart rate greater than 100 and good color; inflation pressures can generally be initiated at 20 to 25 cm H_2O and titrated to these clinical endpoints. Hyperoxia may lead to complications such as retinopathy of prematurity in low-birth-weight infants, and so beginning the resuscitation with less than 100% inspired oxygen is a reasonable option. If no improvement in heart rate or color occurs by 90 seconds, the fraction of inspired oxygen should be increased. Once the infant is stabilized after initial resuscitative care, the fraction of inspired oxygen can be decreased while monitoring pulse oximetry.

The germinal matrix of the preterm infant's brain is vulnerable to bleeding. Factors contributing to subsequent intracranial hemorrhage include excessive pressure or osmolality delivered to an already maximally dilated vascular bed. Subsequently, in premature infants, hyperosmolar solutions

such as 25% dextrose or 8.4% sodium bicarbonate should be avoided. Volume expanders, dextrose, and sodium bicarbonate solutions, when indicated, should be administered slowly to minimize injury to these vascular beds.

Pneumothorax

Pneumothorax is a potentially lethal problem in the neonate because it can rapidly progress to a tension pneumothorax and thereby decrease cardiac output. It is often the result of PPV, positive end-expiratory pressure, or resuscitation.

Pneumothorax is also more common in premature infants with surfactant deficiency and in infants with meconium aspiration. Signs and symptoms include grunting respirations; intercostal, sternal, and substernal retractions; elevated respiratory rate; and tachycardia followed by bradycardia and hypotension. The physical examination findings may include asymmetrically decreased breath sounds and distant heart tones. However, it often may not be possible to diagnose or localize a pneumothorax by auscultation. Transillumination by a high-intensity light in a dark room will reveal increased light transmission on the side of the pneumothorax.

If significant respiratory distress is present and pneumothorax is suspected, rapid decompression may be achieved with a large syringe, 20-gauge needle or catheter over needle, and three-way stopcock. The chest is cleansed with antiseptic solution, and the needle is advanced at the fourth intercostal space in the anterior axillary line or the second interspace in the midclavicular line. This will relieve the tension and decompress the pleural space. Subsequently, a chest tube (8F) may be placed using a standard technique (see Section VII: Insertion of a Chest Tube). If the infant is stable, an expedient portable anteroposterior chest radiograph may be taken to confirm the diagnosis.

Diaphragmatic Hernia

Diaphragmatic hernia is a true neonatal emergency and may be suspected by tachypnea, asymmetric chest wall motion, and a scaphoid abdomen. The diagnosis is confirmed by a chest radiograph showing bowel gas within the thorax (Fig. 2.6). Infants with diaphragmatic hernias must be immediately endotracheally intubated to avoid excessive amounts of air accumulation in the bowel. Since the bowel is in the thoracic cavity, distended bowel impedes ventilation. A nasogastric tube should also be rapidly placed to decompress the stomach. The infant must be rapidly evaluated by a pediatric surgeon after ventilation is stabilized and venous access is achieved.

Spina Bifida

Spina bifida (meningocele, meningomyelocele, and lipomeningocele) involves a wide array of defects. It can range from the least significant form (spina bifida occulta, nonfusion of vertebral laminar arches) to the severe form with meninges and neural tissue protruding, with poorly organized cord tissue

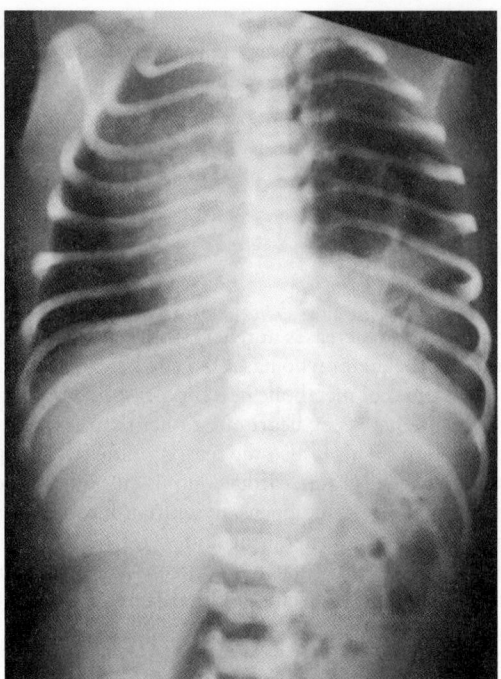

FIGURE 2.6 Left diaphragmatic hernia.

exposed to the surface. Neurologic deficit ranges from none to severe impairment and associated hydrocephalus. The child should receive proper supportive care, oxygen and fluid (as needed), sterile moist dressings to the exposed sac or tissues, and prompt referral to a pediatric neurosurgeon.

Suggested Readings

American Heart Association; American Academy of Pediatrics. 2005 American Heart Association (AHA) guidelines for cardiopulmonary resuscitation (CPR) and emergency cardiovascular care (ECC) of pediatric and neonatal patients: neonatal resuscitation guidelines. *Pediatrics* 2006;117:e1029–1038.

Escrig R, Arruza L, Izquierdo I, et al. Achievement of targeted saturation values in extremely low gestational age neonates resuscitated with low or high oxygen concentrations: a prospective, randomized trial. *Pediatrics* 2008;121: 875–881.

Gluckman PD, Wyatt JS, Azzopardi D, et al. Selective head cooling with mild systemic hypothermia after neonatal encephalopathy: multicentre randomised trial. *Lancet* 2005;365:663–670.

Grein AJ, Weiner GM. Laryngeal mask airway versus bag-mask ventilation or endotracheal intubation for neonatal resuscitation. *Cochrane Database Syst Rev* 2005;2:CD003314.

Halliday HL. Endotracheal intubation at birth for preventing morbidity and mortality in vigorous, meconium-stained infants born at term. *Cochrane Database Syst Rev* 2001;1:CD000500.

Kattwinkel J, Short J, Boyle D, et al. *Textbook of neonatal resuscitation.*, 5th ed. Elk Grove Village, IL: American Academy of Pediatrics and American Heart Association, 2006.

Mathews TJ, MacDorman MF. Infant mortality statistics from the 2004 period linked birth/infant death data set. *Natl Vital Stat Rep* 2007;55:1–32.

Perlman JM, Risser R. Cardiopulmonary resuscitation in the delivery room: associated clinical events. *Arch Pediatr Adolesc Med* 1995;149:20–25.

Salhab WA, Wyckoff MH, Laptook AR, et al. Initial hypoglycemia and neonatal brain injury in term infants with severe fetal acidemia. *Pediatrics* 2004;114:361–366.

Saugstad OD, Ramji S, Soll RF, et al. Resuscitation of newborn infants with 21% or 100% oxygen: an updated systematic review and meta-analysis. *Neonatology* 2008;94:176–182.

Shankaran S, Laptook AR, Ehrenkranz RA, et al. Whole-body hypothermia for neonates with hypoxic-ischemic encephalopathy. *N Engl J Med* 2005;353: 1574–1584.

Tan A, Schulze A, O'Donnell CP, et al. Air versus oxygen for resuscitation of infants at birth. *Cochrane Database Syst Rev* 2005;2:CD002273.

Vain NE, Szyld EG, Prudent LM, et al. Oropharyngeal and nasopharyngeal suctioning of meconium-stained neonates before delivery of their shoulders: multicentre, randomised controlled trial. *Lancet* 2004;364:597–602.

Wang CL, Anderson C, Leone TA, et al. Resuscitation of preterm neonates by using room air or 100% oxygen. *Pediatrics* 2008;121:1083–1089.

CHAPTER 3 ■ SHOCK

LOUIS M. BELL, MD

All physicians who care for ill children will be faced with managing the clinical syndrome of shock. Many common childhood illnesses, such as trauma, gastroenteritis, infection, and accidental drug ingestions, can lead to shock. Ultimately, without timely medical intervention, the child in shock will follow a common pathway to multiorgan system failure and death. Early recognition and appropriate therapy are vital if we hope to reduce the morbidity and mortality associated with this serious syndrome.

The first section of this chapter is devoted to early recognition, which demands a clear understanding of the definition, pathophysiology, and clinical manifestations of shock. Next, the etiologic types of shock, including hypovolemic, cardiogenic, distributive (septic), dissociative, and obstructive shock, are discussed.

Finally, the appropriate therapy and prevention of shock are discussed. Exciting developments are occurring within this area. Advances in molecular biology and immunology have led to a better understanding of the biochemical mediators involved in initiating and maintaining shock. Noninvasive methods for measurement of cardiac output are being developed for use in the emergency department (ED). Treatment modalities that antagonize or prevent the inflammatory cascade that lead to shock, multiorgan dysfunction syndrome (MODS), and death are now being studied. Combined with aggressive supportive and microbial therapies, these experimental immunotherapies may further reduce the morbidity and mortality associated with shock.

DETERMINANTS OF CARDIAC OUTPUT AND THE DEFINITION OF SHOCK

Circulation in the Child

Normal circulatory function is maintained by the complex interplay between the central pump (heart) and blood flow at the regional level, all done with the sole purpose of delivering oxygen and nutrients to the tissues.

The cardiac output is calculated by multiplying the stroke volume (volume of blood ejected by the left ventricle) by the heart rate (ejection cycles per minute). The stroke volume depends on the filling volume of the ventricle (preload), myocardial contractility (Starling's curve), and the resistance against which the heart is pumping blood into the systemic vasculature (afterload).

Heart rate is controlled through the vagus nerve and endogenous catecholamine release. Hypertension and severe hypoxemia can lead to increases in vagal tone and bradycardia. In times of flight, fright, or stress, endogenous cate-cholamine release increases adrenergic tone with an increased heart rate. In the infant who has relatively less myocardial contractility, in times of metabolic need, increase in cardiac output depends on an increasing heart rate rather than on an increase in stroke volume. This is also the reason bradycardia is poorly tolerated in this age group; cardiac output falls quickly because there is little ability to compensate with an increase in stroke volume. Conversely, faster heart rates are best tolerated in infants, in whom ventricular filling time is less critical in contributing to stroke volume and, ultimately, to cardiac output.

Definition of Shock

An understanding of normal physiology allows us to define *shock* as an acute syndrome that occurs because of cardiovascular dysfunction and the inability of the circulatory system to provide adequate oxygen and nutrients to meet the metabolic demands of vital organs. Note that this definition recognizes that shock can and does exist without hypotension, especially in children.

PATHOPHYSIOLOGY

Microcirculatory Dysfunction

The clinical manifestations of shock can be directly related to the abnormalities seen on the tissue, cellular, and biochemical levels. Microcirculatory dysfunction, common to all etiologic types of shock, is characterized by maldistribution of capillary blood flow. Local sympathetic, vasoconstrictor nerve activity and circulatory vasoactive substances (Table 3.1) cause smooth muscle contraction in the precapillary sphincters and arterioles. As shock continues, mechanical obstruction of capillary beds occurs by blockage with cellular debris. Normally, polymorphonuclear leukocytes undergo extensive deformation as they squeeze through the capillaries. Hydrostatic pressure within the capillary makes this possible. However, hydrostatic pressures fall by 30% to 40% during shock states. As a result, capillary beds are blocked and endothelial damage occurs. Subsequent complement activation causes still further aggregation of platelets and granulocytes. During septic shock, exposure to endotoxin directly damages vascular endothelium. Once damaged, endothelial cells can generate procoagulant activity, which may explain the mechanism by which fibrin is deposited in the microcirculation. Superoxide radicals, lysosomal metabolites, and cytokines produced by macrophages and neutrophils for bacterial killing can result in further tissue damage, especially to endothelium, adding to the vicious cycle of damage to the microcirculation.

TABLE 3.1

ENDOGENOUS (HOST-DERIVED) VASOACTIVE MEDIATORS IN SHOCK

Mediator	Stimulus	Major sources	Major actions
Norepinephrine	Hypovolemia Head trauma	Sympathetic nervous system Adrenal medullae	Vasoconstriction β_1, β_2 stimulation
Epinephrine	Hypovolemia Hypercapnea	Adrenal medullae	Vasoconstriction α, β_1 stimulation
Angiotensin II	Hypovolemia	Kidneys, brain, blood	Vasoconstriction
Arachidonic acid metabolites			
Leukotrienes	Tumor necrosis factor Bacterial antigens	Macrophages	Capillary permeability Vasoconstriction, release of lysomal hydrolases
Thromboxane A_2	Hypoxia	Platelets	Vasoconstriction, platelet aggregation
Prostaglandins F_2	Hypoxia	Platelets Vascular smooth muscle	Vasoconstriction

Prostaglandins I_2	Hypoxia	Healthy vascular
		  endothelium
			Vasodilator counterbalances
			  thromboxane A_2

Myocardial depressant factor	Ischemia Tissue damage	Pancreas	Direct negative inotropic effects
Opiates (B-endorphins)	Hypoxia	Pituitary	Decreased myocardial contractility Decreased sympathetic tone hypotension
Inducible nitrous oxide	Inflammatory cytokines	Leukocytes	Vasodilation of vascular smooth muscle

Tissue Ischemia

Tissue ischemia is also basic to all forms of shock. The consequences of poor tissue perfusion sustain the cascade of events that occur during shock. When there is a lack of oxygen, energy production at the cellular level becomes inefficient, producing only 2 moles of adenosine triphosphate (ATP) per mole of glucose instead of the normal 38 moles of ATP produced by aerobic metabolism.

In addition, anaerobic metabolism depletes glycogen stores with an accumulation of lactate and associated acidosis. The decreasing energy and acidosis lead to an efflux of potassium and an influx of sodium and calcium with an obligate influx of water into the cell. Cellular swelling and further cellular dysfunction occur, which is seen clinically as edema.

Release of Biochemical Mediators

Biochemical mediators play an important role in the development and continuation of all types of shock. These vasoactive and inflammatory mediators are endogenous (host-derived) products primarily from cells of nervous system and hematopoietic origin. Although in septic shock these mediators are stimulated after exposure to microbial products (e.g., endotoxin) and play a primary role in initiating shock, in hypovolemic and cardiogenic shock, they are released secondarily in response to ischemic cellular injury as just described.

Vasoactive Mediators

The vasoactive mediators exert their effect primarily by induction of severe vasoconstriction and vasospasm, induction of platelet aggregation and thrombus formation, increased capillary permeability, and redistribution of blood flow away from vital tissues (Table 3.1).

Inflammatory Mediators

In the past, it was believed that invasive microbial agents were directly responsible for the cellular damage and microcirculatory dysfunction seen in septic shock. However, since the mid-1990s, it has become clear that endogenous inflammation mediators are the real culprits in the pathogenesis of septic shock and that lethal tissue injury occurs when production of these mediators escalates out of control. The concept that shock (and particularly septic shock) is an uncontrolled inflammatory response is being challenged as more is discovered about the types of cytokines that are secreted by the immune system. As we know, the CD4 T cells secrete cytokines with inflammatory properties from type 1 helper T cells (TH1s). Cytokines with *anti*inflammatory [type 2 helper T-cell (TH2)] properties, such as interleukin (IL)-4 and IL-10, are also produced. Although the factors that determine whether the T cells have a TH1 or TH2 response is unknown, it is clear that the cascade of events that lead to shock is a complicated interaction between pathogen and host immunity.

ENDOGENOUS (HOST-DERIVED) INFLAMMATORY MEDIATORS IN SHOCK

Mediator	Stimulus	Major sources	Major action
Platelet-activating factor	TNF Bacterial antigens	Platelets Neutrophils	Thrombosis Vascular permeability
Cytokines			
Tumor necrosis factor α (TNF-α)	Bacterial antigens Severe trauma	Macrophages Monocytes	Induces other mediators Adhesion to endothelium Enhanced TNF-x production
Interferon-gamma	Bacterial antigens	T cells	
Interleukin (IL)-1 beta	TNF Bacterial antigens	Mononuclear Phagocytes	Fever Leukocytosis Acute-phase reactants Adhesion to endothelium
IL-6	TNF IL-1	Monocytes Endothelial cells	Fever Leukocytosis Thrombosis
IL-8	Endotoxin TNF	Monocytes Endothelial cells	Neutrophil activation
Complement fragments	TNF Bacterial antigens	Alternate pathway	Chemotactic activity
Toxic oxygen species	TNF Bacterial antigens	Neutrophils	Cellular damage

Septic shock starts with exposure to microbial products. Perhaps the most potent stimulator of the inflammatory cascade is the outer cell membrane of gram-negative bacteria, a lipopolysaccharide (LPS) coat, also called *endotoxin*. Once in the bloodstream, the LPS attaches to a plasma protein called *LPS-binding protein* (LBP). This complex (LPS-LBP) binds to the CD14 receptor on the surface of the monocyte/macrophage, which leads to stimulation of tumor necrosis factor alpha (TNF-α) and IL-1, and ultimately, to the entire cascade of inflammatory mediators.

As a group, these protein mediators are called *cytokines* (Table 3.2). TNF plays a pivotal role in triggering the production of not only other cytokines, but also other inflammatory mediators. TNF is one known endogenous factor that is capable of inducing a broad range of vasoactive and inflammatory mediators. Because of this, treatment of shock with anti-TNF antibodies has been attempted with mixed results (see "Initial Therapy" section). TNF in physiologic amounts has beneficial effects in tissues and promotes wound healing, tissue remodeling, and neovascularization. In pathogenic amounts, TNF and other inflammatory mediators (Table 3.2) cause severe septic shock in animal models and act primarily by inducing fever, increasing the white blood cell counts, inducing production of procoagulant and cell adhesion molecules by endothelial cells, causing aggregates of hematopoietic cells, and increasing vascular permeability.

Nitric Oxide

Although nitric oxide synthases (NOS) are absent in resting cells, it is known that the gene is rapidly expressed in response to stimuli by inflammatory cytokines. For example, after exposure to TNF-α and IL-1, a variety of cells, including macrophages, vascular endothelium, vascular smooth muscle, hepatocytes, and cardiac myocytes, are induced to increase nitric oxide (NO) production. In these pathologic amounts, NO causes vasodilation of vascular smooth muscle, vascular hyporesponsiveness, and hypotension and shock. In physiologic amounts, NO has beneficial effects that make it important in host defense against infection as a neurotransmitter and in cardiovascular homeostasis.

Complement Activation

The complement system is activated by circulating bacteria and bacterial products. The low-molecular-weight peptides that are released as a result induce both vasoactive and inflammatory effects. Vasoactive effects are seen with C3 and C5 fragments, which promote the release of histamine and other vasoactive mediators, which produce increased permeability and vasodilation. Complement fragments also stimulate an inflammatory response by promoting the activation and aggregation of platelets and granulocytes.

Myocardial Depressant Factor

Myocardial depression occurs in all types of shock. More recent investigation suggests that myocardial depression may occur as a result of mediators that act directly on myocardial tissue. Discovered in 1970, a small peptide called *myocardial depressant factor* is produced when the pancreas is ischemic and hypoperfused. Myocardial depressant factor has been shown to have negative inotropic effects in isolated heart muscle and causes constriction of the splanchnic vascular bed. In 1985, Parker, using isolated heart muscle preparation, found altered inotropic responsiveness within 1 to 2 hours of endotoxin treatment, demonstrating *in vitro* what is apparent in patients with shock syndrome. Other pathways have been implicated in myocardial depression including NO-induced cytokine production.

Intrinsic myocardial depression, either primarily as in septic shock or secondarily as in hypovolemic or cardiogenic shock, adds to other circulatory derangements that have been discussed. Understanding this intrinsic or direct cardiac depression is important in designing treatment strategies.

CLINICAL MANIFESTATIONS

Early or Compensated Shock

Regardless of the etiology, shock begins when there is absolute or functional hypovolemia. Absolute hypovolemia exists in cases of severe emesis and diarrhea, trauma with blood loss, peritonitis, and "third spacing" of fluids or increased capillary permeability, as in sepsis. Functional hypovolemia exists when vascular capacity increases, as in septic shock, spinal cord injury, anaphylaxis, and barbiturate overdose.

The signs of early shock include tachycardia, mild tachypnea, slightly delayed capillary refill (more than 2 to 3 seconds), orthostatic changes in blood pressure or pulse, and mild irritability. These earliest symptoms result from an effort to compensate for shock, increase cardiac output, and maintain perfusion of vital organs (brain, heart, kidneys). Unexplained tachycardia without other signs may be one of the earliest signs of shock. Tachycardia occurs to compensate for a diminished

stroke volume (Fig. 3.1). Delayed capillary refill occurs as increases in sympathetic tone by endogenous catecholamines cause peripheral vasoconstriction. In some cases of early septic shock, the skin may be warm and dry without a decrease in capillary refill, reflecting cutaneous vasodilation in a state of increased cardiac output and increased venous capacitance—so-called *warm distributive shock*. As systemic vascular resistance falls, cardiac output must increase to maintain normal arterial pressure. Often, in this form of distributive (septic) shock (i.e., high cardiac output and low systemic vascular resistance), the pulse will be bounding and the pulse pressure widened.

Late or Uncompensated Shock

As shock continues, these early compensatory mechanisms are not enough to meet the metabolic demands of the tissue, and uncompensated shock follows (Fig. 3.1). In uncompensated shock, the effects of cellular ischemia with the associated release of vasoactive and inflammatory mediators begin to affect the microcirculation, and the child shows signs of brain, kidney, and cardiovascular compromise.

Tachycardia and tachypnea continue. Tachypnea becomes more severe because an increasing acidosis elicits a compensatory increase in the minute ventilation, resulting in a fall in Pa_{CO_2} and a compensatory respiratory alkalosis. The skin may be mottled or

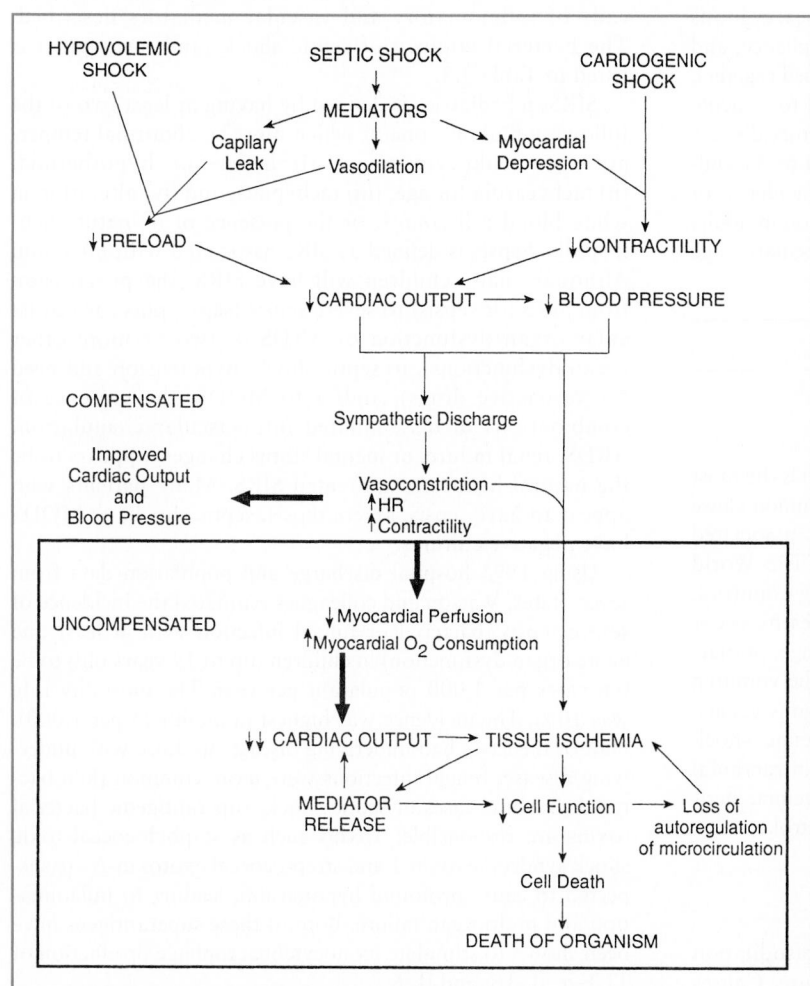

FIGURE 3.1 Sequence of pathophysiologic events in clinical shock states. (From Witte MK, Hill JH, Blumer JL. Shock in the pediatric patient. *Adv Pediatr* 1987;34:139–173, with permission.)

pale and extremities cool as vasoconstriction and diminished blood flow to the skin occur. Capillary refill becomes markedly delayed (more than 4 seconds). Hypotension is noted. Decreased cardiac output and vasoconstriction cause a decrease in renal perfusion, and oliguria is noted. The gastrointestinal tract is also underperfused and may become ischemic. Under these conditions, decreased motility, distension, release of vasoactive and inflammatory mediators, and fluid accumulation may occur. In patients with septic shock, fever (greater than 38.3°C rectally) or hypothermia (less than 35.6°C rectally) may occur.

As perfusion of the brain is compromised, irritability progresses to agitation, confusion, hallucinations, alternating periods of agitation and stupor, and finally coma. The MODS secondary to ongoing shock and exaggerated inflammatory responses is at the end of a continuum that has been termed *systemic inflammatory response syndrome* (SIRS), a syndrome that is meant to describe the nonspecific inflammatory process, which may occur after trauma, infection, burns, pancreatitis, and other diseases. (See "Distributive Shock" section.)

The effects of a dysfunctional microcirculation, tissue ischemia, and release of vasoactive and inflammatory mediators obviously affect all tissues, including the pulmonary tissues and vasculature. Damage to the capillary endothelium in the lung allows fluid to fill the interstitium of the intraalveolar septum. If the shock syndrome progresses, fluid accumulation will eventually lead to fluid leakage into the alveolar spaces, which prevents adequate gas exchange. As the damage to the lungs continues, the child demonstrates dyspnea, tachypnea, cyanosis refractory to oxygen therapy, decreased lung compliance, and diffuse alveolar infiltrates. These signs, when grouped together, represent syndromes of pulmonary injury referred to as acute lung injury (ALI) and the more severe acute respiratory distress syndrome (ARDS). Carcillo found that 11 (32%) of 34 children with septic shock developed ARDS. The incidence of ALI/ARDS is approximately 10 times more common in adults (22 to 86 cases per 100,000 persons) than in the pediatric age group (2 to 8 cases per 100,000 persons per year).

TYPES OF SHOCK

Hypovolemia

Hypovolemia (decreased circulating blood volume) is the most common cause of shock in children. The most common cause of hypovolemic shock occurs from water losses associated with diarrhea and vomiting (see Chapter 18). The World Health Organization estimates that in developing countries, 1.5 to 2.5 million diarrhea-associated infant deaths occur annually among children younger than 5 years of age, primarily because of hypovolemic shock, secondary to the vomiting and diarrhea that occurs with a variety of infectious agents, such as rotaviruses. Other causes of hypovolemic shock include blood losses (trauma, gastrointestinal, intracranial hemorrhage), plasma losses (burns, hypoproteinemia, peritonitis), and water losses (glycosuric diuresis, sunstroke).

Distributive Shock

Distributive shock occurs primarily because of vasodilation and pooling of blood in the peripheral vasculature. Causes

TABLE 3.3

BACTERIAL ETIOLOGY OF INVASIVE DISEASE IN INFANTS AND CHILDREN[a]

Streptococcus pneumoniae
Neisseria meningitides
Group B *Streptococcus*
Listeria monocytogenes
Haemophilus influenzae type b
Gram-negative bacilli[b]
Staphylococcus aureus
Pseudomonas aeruginosa
Salmonella enteritidis
Fungus

[a]Isolated from blood or cerebrospinal fluid.
[b]Includes *Escherichia coli* and *Enterobacter* species.
Based on data from Schuchat A, Robinson K, Wenqer JD, et al. *N Engl J Med* 1997;337:970–976 and Watson RS, Carcillo JA, Linde-Zwirble WT, et al. *Am J Respir Crit Care Med* 2003;167:695–701.

include anaphylaxis, central nervous system (CNS) or spinal injuries, drug ingestions, and most commonly in children, sepsis. The primary derangements in septic shock results from exposure to microbial components (e.g., endotoxin, teichoic acid, viral proteins), which trigger the cascade of inflammatory and vascular mediators described. The bacterial etiology of septic shock (and meningitis) is listed in Table 3.3.

SIRS in pediatrics is defined by having at least two of the following findings, one of which must be abnormal temperature or leukocyte count: (i) hyper- or hypothermia, (ii) tachycardia for age, (iii) tachypnea, and (iv) alteration in white blood cell counts, or the presence of immature neutrophils. Sepsis is defined as SIRS associated with infection. Although many children will have SIRS, the progression from SIRS (or sepsis) to severe sepsis (sepsis plus cardiovascular organ dysfunction *or* ARDS *or* two or more other organ dysfunctions), to septic shock (hypotension and need for vasoactive drugs), and/or to MODS (the presence of combinations of disseminated intravascular coagulation, ARDS, renal failure, or mental status changes) appears to be the natural history of untreated SIRS. Many patients who appear to have sepsis, severe sepsis, septic shock, or MODS have negative cultures.

Using 1995 hospital discharge and population data from seven states, Watson and colleagues estimated the incidence of severe sepsis (bacterial or fungal infection with at least one acute organ dysfunction) in children (up to 19 years old) to be 0.6 cases per 1,000 population per year. The mortality rate was 10%. The incidence was highest in infants (5 per 1,000). Half of the cases had underlying disease. In those with underlying disease, fungal infections were more common than bacterial. In some cases of septic shock, superantigenic bacterial toxins are responsible. Toxins such as staphylococcal toxic shock syndrome toxin-1 and streptococcal exotoxin-A are suspected to cause profound hypotension, leading to inflammation and multiorgan failure. Both of these superantigens have been shown to stimulate monocyte/macrophage production of TNF-α, IL-1β, and IL-6.

Cardiogenic Shock

Cardiogenic shock can usually be distinguished from other forms of shock because of associated signs of congestive heart failure, including rales auscultated throughout the lungs, a gallop cardiac rhythm, enlarged liver, and jugular venous distension.

Regardless of the etiology, cardiogenic shock leads to decreased cardiac output, in most cases as a result of a decrease in myocardial contractility. As we have seen, direct myocardial damage occurs in all types of shock as a late manifestation. Other common etiologies of cardiogenic shock in children include viral myocarditis, arrhythmia, drug ingestions, postoperative complications of cardiac surgery, metabolic derangements (hypoglycemia), and congenital heart disease. Occasionally, congenital heart disease is diagnosed in an infant, usually within the first 3 months of life, when the infant presents to the ED in congestive heart failure and shock. These infants invariably have congenital heart abnormalities, such as truncus arteriosus, transposition of the great vessels, or left hypoplastic heart syndrome, that depend on flow through the ductus arteriosum to maintain adequate oxygen delivery. The closure of the ductus precipitates congestive heart failure and eventually cardiogenic shock.

The management of obstructive shock, which is caused by mechanical obstructions to ventricular outflow and occurs with pericardial tamponade or tension pneumothorax (see Chapter 107 and Section VII), and dissociative shock, which occurs secondary to carbon monoxide poisoning (see Chapter 87) or methemoglobinemia, are discussed elsewhere.

TREATMENT

Initial Therapy

To determine proper therapy, recall the definition and pathophysiology of shock. *Shock* is defined as an acute syndrome that occurs because of cardiovascular dysfunction, as well as the inability of the circulatory system to provide adequate oxygen and nutrients to meet the metabolic demands of vital organs. Therefore, initial therapy in the ED can be applied universally, regardless of the etiology of shock, and is directed to reverse or halt further tissue injury. To underscore this, in 1991, Carcillo compared hemodynamic and oxygen use in children with either cardiogenic shock or septic shock. These data suggested that there was little difference physiologically, and therefore, initial treatment should be similar. Furthermore, the early recognition and aggressive fluid resuscitation and inotropic therapies appear to be vital in improving outcomes. The American College of Critical Care Medicine—Pediatric Advanced Life Support (ACCM-PALS) guidelines for hemodynamic support of newborns and children in septic shock recommends a therapeutic guideline (Fig. 3.2). In community hospitals (prior to transport) a retrospective cohort of 91 infants and children presenting with suspected septic shock were significantly more likely to survive if the guidelines were followed (8% vs. 38% survival). Survival was most dependent on early aggressive fluid resuscitation.

As noted previously, the basic defects are in shock hypovolemia, microcirculatory dysfunction, tissue ischemia, and cardiovascular dysfunction. Each defect becomes more severe the longer the shock state exists, so prompt and aggressive treatment is mandatory. The etiology of shock can be determined as therapy begins.

With this pathophysiology in mind, the first steps of therapy are to (i) establish an adequate airway; (ii) determine whether breathing is adequate; (iii) provide oxygen at 100% FiO$_2$; (iv) establish vascular access and obtain laboratory samples; and (v) provide aggressive fluid resuscitation, beginning with 20 mL per kg of crystalloid 0.9% sodium chloride or Ringer's lactate given intravenously as rapidly as possible (in minutes). Repeat intravenous boluses of 20 mL per kg (up to a total of 60 mL per kg should be done over 10 to 15 minutes. Reassessment after each therapeutic maneuver is vital (Fig. 3.3). After the initial therapy, the following questions should be addressed: (i) Is tracheal intubation needed? (ii) Should additional intravenous therapy be given? If so, blood, crystalloid, or colloid? (iii) Are positive inotropic drugs needed? If so, which one initially? (iv) What is the urine output? (v) What other drugs are needed (antibiotics)? (vi) Is the patient at risk for adrenal insufficiency? (vii) Should arrangements for admission to the ICU be initiated?

Simultaneously, a history should be obtained while the initial treatment is started. If possible, another physician can obtain a history from the caregivers. Questions pertaining to trauma, fever, diarrhea, vomiting, medication, allergies, heart disease, immune competence, and seizures should be addressed. The step-by-step initial approach to pediatric shock is outlined in Figure 3.2.

Decision and Monitoring in the Emergency Department

Oxygenation

Oxygen delivery to the tissues remains our primary focus in children with shock. While the airway and ventilatory effort is assessed, 100% oxygen should be provided via a bag-valve-mask apparatus. Assisted bag-valve-mask may be indicated. If there is any question that the airway is obstructed or that ventilatory effort is inadequate, the insertion of an artificial airway is indicated. We suggest the orotracheal intubation route initially. Measurements of the PaO$_2$ by an arterial blood sample or pulse oximetry should be performed throughout the decision-making process. The goal is to maintain the arterial oxygen tension above 65 mm Hg; therefore, 100% oxygen should be continued until that is achieved. It should be noted that, given a hemoglobin concentration of 10 g per dL and 100% arterial oxygen saturation, a mixed venous oxygen saturation (measured from the superior vena cava) of more than 70% is associated with improved outcome in the first 6 hours of presentation in septic shock (see "Fluid Administration" section).

Vascular Access

Vascular access is vital in treatment. If possible, a large-bore intravenous catheter should be inserted in a peripheral vein. However, in many instances, the peripheral extremities will be

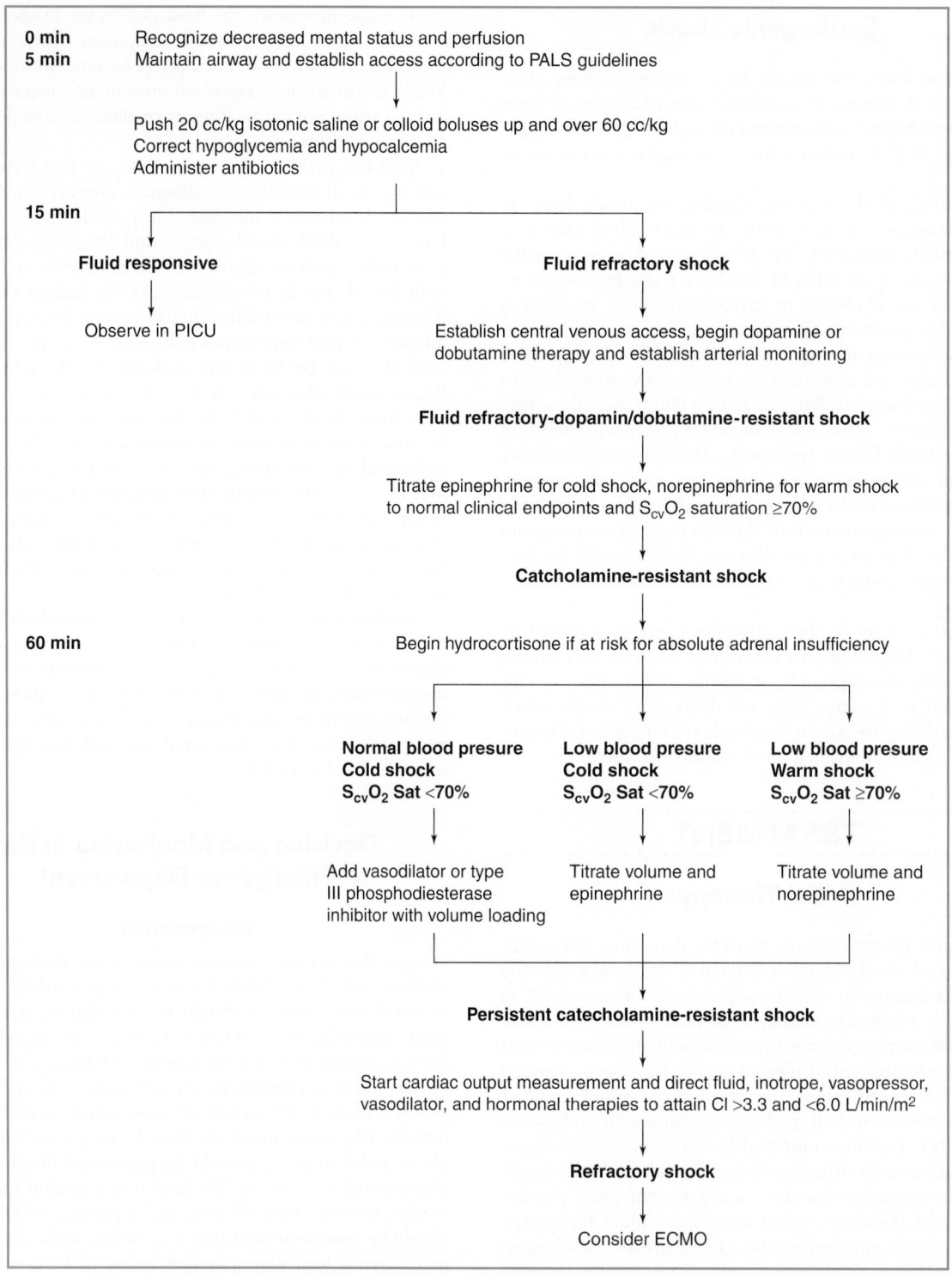

FIGURE 3.2 Approach to pediatric shock. PALS, Pediatric Advanced Life Support; PICU, pediatric intensive care unit; CI, cardiac index; ECMO, extracorporeal membrane oxygenation. (From Dellinger RP, Levy MM, Carlet JM, et al. Surviving sepsis campaign: international guidelines for management of severe sepsis and septic shock: 2008. *Crit Care Med* 2008;36(1):296–327.

cool because of vasoconstriction and no vein is found. Central vein venous placement by the Seldinger technique (see Section VII, Procedure 3.2) is the next step. Use of the femoral vein is preferred in infants and younger children. In older children and adolescents, cannulation of the internal jugular, external

jugular, and subclavian veins can also be considered. If there is any delay in accomplishing prompt placement of a central venous catheter, an intraosseous line should be placed.

In children younger than 5 years of age, needle placement into the marrow space of the medial portion of the proximal

---

Oxygenate/Ventilate
- O_2 by bag-valve-mask
- Intubation (consider early)
- Maintain Pao$_2$ >65

Vascular Access
- Peripheral vein
- Femoral vein
- Internal jugular
- External jugular
- Subclavian vein
- Intraosseous infusion (consider early in those with hypotension)
- Peripheral venous cutdown

Administer Fluids
- Saline 20 mL/kg initially
- Hgb <10g/dL blood; saline
- Hgb >10g/dL saline; 5% albumin

Drug Therapy
- Positive inotropic agents
- Treat acidosis
- Vasodilator agents
- Hypoglycemia
- Hypocalcemia
- Low-dose hydrocortisone for adrenal insufficiency (see text)

Specific Therapy
- Control hemorrhage
- Antibiotics (see text)
- Immunotherapies (see text)

FIGURE 3.3 Management of shock—overview.

tibia, angulated away from the growth plate and 1 to 2 inches below the tibial tuberosity, is indicated (see Section VII, Procedure 3.8). In older children (older than 5 years of age) and adults, needle placement 1 to 2 inches above the medial malleolus is indicated. If central line placement is delayed, intraosseous fluid replacement is an excellent interim step in infants and children who require fluid resuscitation. In 1991, Velasco et al. found this technique to be useful in resuscitation in a hemorrhagic shock model and now it is an accepted method of achieving vascular access if reliable venous access cannot be rapidly attained. Others have commented on the safety and ease of placement. Intravenous fluid, blood products, bicarbonate, and catecholamines are among the therapies successfully given using this technique and are comparable in effect to the central or peripheral intravenous routes.

The last resort in establishing venous access would be for a venous cutdown (see Section VII, Procedure 3.1). Simultaneous with attempts at vascular access, venous blood samples can be obtained for complete blood cell count, platelets, prothrombin and partial thromboplastin times, electrolytes, blood urea nitrogen, creatinine, glucose, and blood culture (if indicated). An arterial blood sample should also be obtained.

Fluid Administration

After venous access is established, 20 mL per kg of 0.9% normal saline or Ringer's lactate is infused as rapidly as possible by push. Then reassessment should occur. The decision to give additional intravenous fluids can be based on arterial pressures, heart rate, and oxygenation. If blood pressure is normal, additional fluids will depend on urine output, heart rate, capillary refill, and mental status. If the child remains hypotensive after the initial fluid challenge, an additional 20 to 40 mL per kg

should be infused and, if possible, titrated against central venous or right atrial pressures because they correlate better with intravascular volume than does systemic arterial pressure. Once in the intensive care setting, placement of a balloon-tipped, flow-directed pulmonary artery catheter or careful monitoring of mixed venous gases and central venous pressures (12 to 15 mm Hg) may be needed to assess more accurately the filling pressures of the heart, especially in children with fluid-refractory and dopamine-resistant shock.

Low cardiac output, rather than low systemic vascular resistance, is associated with increased mortality in children with septic shock. In most cases, careful monitoring of the clinical signs of perfusion, maintenance of perfusion pressures [mean arterial pressure–central venous pressure (CVP)], and maintenance of superior vena cava oxygen saturation at levels of more than 70% will ensure adequate cardiac output, thereby improving survival.

Accurate, noninvasive methods to measure cardiac output in the initial stages of fluid and inotropic support in the ED may be beneficial. One modality currently being evaluated is impedance cardiography. Using this noninvasive technique stroke volume, cardiac output and contractility can be determined. While its use in the pediatric ICU is being evaluated, it may become an important tool in the ED.

If these types of measurements are not possible in the ED or if transfer to the ICU is imminent, changes in vital signs and perfusion can be used to guide fluid management. Although we do not base fluid management on an absolute amount and are guided by the child's clinical condition, some ballpark figures for initial fluid resuscitation can be provided. In 1991, Carcillo et al. studied all children with septic shock who presented to the ED over a 6-year period and who had a pulmonary artery catheter inserted within 6 hours of presentation. Interestingly, fluid resuscitation in excess of 40 mL per kg in the first hour improved survival and was not associated with an increased risk of either cardiogenic pulmonary edema or ARDS, compared with children who received smaller amounts of fluid. Therefore in severe shock, fluid resuscitation, if indicated, up to 60 mL per kg or approximately 50% of the circulation blood volume, may be given within the initial phase of therapy (within the first 15 to 20 minutes). The important point to remember is that, in most cases of shock, not enough fluid is given and the child remains in relative hypovolemic shock. In 2002, Carcillo and Fields recommended that in the absence of rales, gallop rhythm, hepatomegaly or increased work of breathing, fluid can be administered to as much as 200 mL per kg in the first hours directed toward achieving normal perfusion and blood pressure. Monitoring such signs as heart rate, capillary refill, mental status, and urine output (at least 1 mL per kg per hour) is helpful in determining the amount of fluids needed in the initial phases of resuscitation. Monitoring of cardiac output is essential for children with cerebral damage or those in cardiogenic shock, in which case the need for adequate fluid resuscitation must be balanced with concerns over cerebral edema or cardiac disease, respectively.

Choice of Fluids and Blood Products

The initial choice of fluid should be 0.9% saline or Ringer's lactate given as described earlier, beginning with 20 mL per kg over minutes. Packed red blood cells should be given at 10 mL per kg over 1 to 2 hours to maintain a hemoglobin of 10 g per dL.

Children with cyanotic heart disease, or neonates, may require higher hematocrit percentages to ensure adequate tissue delivery.

If the hemoglobin is over 10 g per dL or if blood is not available, 5% albumin in 0.9% sodium chloride can be used in combination with crystalloid fluids. Initially, albumin can be given in 10 mL per kg doses. When colloids (albumin) are used, appropriate intravascular monitoring should be considered when possible to guard against circulatory overload.

Improving Myocardial Function and Circulation

Catecholamines (adrenergic agents) are the drugs of choice for improving myocardial contractility in patients with shock because of their very short half-life (2 to 3 minutes) and potency (Table 3.4). A brief review of adrenergic receptor physiology is important if we are to have a rational approach to their use.

There are at least three broad populations of adrenergic receptors, termed alpha (α), beta (β), and dopaminergic (DA) receptors. Although all have been subdivided further, in general, β_1-receptors mediate inotropic (contractility), chronotropic (rate), and dromotropic (increased conduction velocity) activity. β_2-Receptors mediate vasodilation and bronchial smooth muscle relaxation. α-Receptors mediate arteriole constriction systemically and bronchial muscle constriction. DA receptors, termed DA_1 and DA_2, mediate smooth muscle relaxation and increase renal blood flow and sodium excretion.

Catecholamines may stimulate some adrenergic receptors more strongly than others, providing some rationale for selection. In general, the mechanism of action for most positive inotropic agents seems to be an increased concentration of or sensitivity to intracellular calcium during systole. If the desired effect is not achieved with one agent, combinations of several agents together may be necessary. It is important to note that there may be decreased responsiveness to adrenergic stimulation in patients with congenital heart disease, after heart transplantation, or in those with bronchopulmonary dysplasia.

Currently, dopamine is the first choice to improve cardiac function and improve splanchnic and renal circulation if the patient is relatively stable but remains hypotensive after initial fluid resuscitation. At low dosages (2 μg per kg per minute), dopamine increases renal blood flow up to 50% and sodium excretion up to 100%. Cardiac output is increased with dosages of 5 to 10 μg per kg per minute. At higher dosages (more than 10 μg per kg per minute), x-adrenergic effects predominate, leading to arterial vasoconstriction and an increase in blood pressure. Improvement in perfusion as measured by increased urine output, blood pressure, and warming of the extremities can be seen early. More accurate measurements of cardiac index, arterial mixed venous difference, or left ventricular stroke work can be used to titrate the dosage in the ICU.

In some cases of profound septic shock and hypotension, epinephrine should be considered initially. A low dosage (less than 0.2 μg per kg per minute) of epinephrine stimulates both β_1 cardiac effects and β_2 peripheral vascular effects, which results in an increase in skeletal muscle blood flow and a decrease in diastolic blood pressure. Dosages higher than 0.3 μg per kg per minute are associated with increased α-adrenergic effects and increases in blood pressure. If the child is unresponsive to fluid resuscitation and dopamine, epinephrine may be useful in maintaining blood pressure and cardiac output. Experts recommend the use of low-dose norepinephrine for fluid-refractory, dopamine-resistant hyperdynamic (warm) shock.

Vasodilatory therapy should be considered in patients when epinephrine is being used and there are still signs of shock but with a normal blood pressure. Nutrient flow may be improved, left ventricular stroke work enhanced, and myocardial oxygen consumption decreased by lowering impedance to left ventricular ejections. A short-acting vasodilating drug, such as sodium nitroprusside, beginning with 0.1 μg per kg per minute, is preferred. The infusion can be increased until evidence of decreased peripheral vascular resistance exists or until the generally accepted safe dosage of between 8 and 10 μg per kg per minute is reached. Toxicity results from the accumulation of thiocyanate (cyanide), which should be monitored. The use of this therapy in the ED is rarely needed for the indication of shock, although in cases in which transfer to the ICU is delayed, it may be indicated.

TABLE 3.4

POSITIVE INOTROPIC AGENTS

Agent	Dose range (μg/kg/min)	Mechanism[a]	Considerations
Dopamine	2–20	β_1, β_2, DA stimulation	Increases renal flow 1–2 μg/kg/min, cardiac output 5–10 μg/kg/min
Epinephrine	0.1–1.0	β_1, β_2, α stimulation	Dose over 0.3 μg/kg/min associated or α effects
Dobutamine	2.5–15	β_1, β_2 stimulation	Increase cardiac output with no increase in heart rate, not as effective in those <12 mo (see text)
Milrinone	1–10	Phosphodiesterase F[111] inhibition	Positive inotrope with smooth muscle relaxation
Isoproterenol	0.1–1.0	β_1, β_2 stimulation	Increases myocardial oxygen consumption
Norepinephrine	0.1–1.0	α, β_1 stimulation	Infrequent use due to renal vasoconstriction

[a]Adrenergic receptors: Beta (β_1) receptors mediate inotropic, chronotropic, and dromotropic activity; intestinal relaxation. Beta (β_2) receptors mediate vasodilation and bronchial smooth muscle relaxation. Alpha (α) receptors mediate arteriole constriction systemically; bronchial muscle constriction. Dopaminergic (DA) receptors mediate smooth muscle relaxation, as well as increases in renal blood flow and sodium excretion.

Dobutamine should be considered initially in patients with cardiogenic shock because it is a very selective stimulant of β_1 receptors. In patients with cardiogenic shock (elevated cardiac filling pressures and low cardiac output), it tends to increase cardiac output without increasing the heart rate. Starting dosages should be 2 to 5 μg per kg per minute. If dobutamine fails, epinephrine should be used.

Finally, milrinone represents a class of inotropic agents distinct from the catecholamines. Although the mechanism of action is not fully understood, data favor inhibition of myocardial cyclic adenosine monophosphate phosphodiesterase (c-AMPase). A direct relaxant effect on vascular and vasodilation that results in smooth muscle causes afterload, and preload reduction contributes to the improved hemodynamic state. Milrinone facilitates atrioventricular conduction, relaxes smooth muscle, and dilates coronary arteries. At this time, there is seldom an indication to start this agent in the ED.

Acid–Base Abnormalities

It is clear that unless perfusion and ventilation are adequate, infusion of sodium bicarbonate rarely maintains arterial pH. There is increasing concern that the use of sodium bicarbonate may be detrimental at worst or of no benefit at best. The 2005 American Heart Association guidelines for CPR no longer recommend therapy with buffers during cardiac arrest in adults. The use of sodium bicarbonate to treat metabolic acidosis in children and neonates is also under scrutiny. Some experts have concerns about the effects of bicarbonate with respect to hemodynamics, left ventricular function, intracellular pH, and oxygen delivery and consumption. It seems most prudent that when treating shock in the pediatric patient that the focus be on correcting the underlying cause of acidosis, rather than the use of bicarbonate. Ultimately, improved blood flow will result in a decrease in acid products of anaerobic metabolism and only then will pH concentration remain normal.

Steroids

Bone, in a prospective, randomized, double-blind, placebo-controlled study of adults, concluded that high-dose corticosteroids provided no benefit in the treatment of septic shock. Patients in this study who exhibited serum creatinine levels above 2 mg per dL and who received steroids experienced a significantly higher mortality rate than the placebo group. Furthermore, patients who received high-dose methylprednisolone died as a result of secondary infection more often than their placebo-treated counterparts. Therefore, high-dose corticosteroids are of no therapeutic value in patients with septic shock. More recently, however, there have been several studies in adults with septic shock (most requiring ongoing vasopressor therapy) given physiologic doses of corticosteroids. The results suggested that this supplemental therapy may benefit some patients with vasopressor-dependent septic shock. A multicentered trial in France revealed that adults with catecholamine refractory septic shock who received low-dose hydrocortisone had a reduced risk of death. Currently, hydrocortisone therapy in children is only indicated for catecholamine resistance and suspected or proven adrenal insufficiency (defined as a total cortisol level between 0 and 18 mg per dL). Children at risk for adrenal insufficiency include those with purpura fulminans and associated Waterhouse-Friedrickson syndrome, those who have previously received steroids for

chronic illness, and those with known pituitary or adrenal abnormalities.

Disseminated Intravascular Coagulation

As we have seen, microcirculatory dysfunction, tissue ischemia, and cardiovascular dysfunction, regardless of etiology, leads to shock and consumption of coagulation factors and platelets. This consumption is characterized by thrombocytopenia, an increase in fibrin split products, a decrease in fibrinogen, and abnormally prolonged prothrombin time and partial thromboplastin times (see Chapter 91). Management includes platelet transfusions (if indicated for bleeding or platelet counts less than 50,000 per mm³) with infusion of 0.2 unit per kg. Fresh frozen plasma, 10 mL per kg intravenously, may be given for prolonged prothrombin and partial thromboplastin times.

Antibiotics

Antibiotics are given presumptively in most cases of severe shock when the etiology is unclear. Antibiotics are chosen based on age and suspected bacterial pathogens. If the child is younger than 4 weeks of age and there is no suspicion or evidence of meningitis, ampicillin and gentamicin is one effective combination. From 4 to 12 weeks of age, ampicillin and cefotaxime are favored by many pediatric infectious diseases specialists when meningitis is ruled out.

In some cases, the infant or child is too unstable to tolerate a lumbar puncture. Presumptive antibiotics should not be delayed in these cases. After resuscitation, the lumbar puncture can safely be performed and the cerebrospinal fluid (CSF) profile will still indicate a bacterial etiology. Latex agglutination tests can be obtained on urine plus CSF if the CSF culture and blood culture are negative. Presumptive antibiotics in children with shock and meningitis or when meningitis cannot be ruled out would include vancomycin and ceftriaxone or cefotaxime for the possibility of a strain of *Streptococcus pneumoniae* that is resistant to penicillin or cefalosporins. Vancomycin should be considered in the patient with suspected sepsis in an area that has increased methicillin-resistant *Staphylococcal aureus*. In children with underlying disease that affect the immune system, fungal infections should be considered. Invasive candidiasis would be most likely and amphotericin B or voriconazole would be a reasonable presumptive choice.

An Approach to Pediatric Shock

Considering all of the above, an approach to pediatric shock has been suggested by Carcillo and others (Fig. 3.2). The guideline includes a timeline underscoring the importance of early recognition of shock and prompt fluid resuscitation as the vital first steps in management.

Experimental Therapies

Over the last several years, identification of the mediators of septic shock has led to a better understanding of how these mediators cause and contribute to the pathophysiology of shock. Coincidentally, the use of monoclonal antibody techniques has allowed for the production of large quantities of antibody that are free from human infection and are of known isotype and epitope specificity. This new knowledge has led to the development of a number of investigational therapies aimed at different components of the inflammatory cascade.

TABLE 3.5

EXPERIMENTAL THERAPIES[a] FOR THE TREATMENT
OF SEPTIS SHOCK (SELECTED)

Category	Product and mechanism of action
Antimicrobial	
E5	Murine IgM monoclonal antibody; binds to lipid A of endotoxin
HA-1A	Human IgM monoclonal antibody; binds to lipid A of endotoxin
Soluble CD14	Blocks binding of endotoxin to macrophage
Anti-CD14 antibody	Blocks binding of endotoxin to macrophage
Anticytokine	
Anti-tumor necrosis factor (TNF) antibody	Blocks inflammatory cascade
TNF soluble receptor	Binds TNF, inhibits inflammatory cascade
Interleukin (IL)-1 receptor antagonist	Blocks IL-1 binding
Nitric Oxide (NO) Inhibitors	
L-NMA	L-*arginine* analogs; inhibits NO synthase and decreases NO production, thereby preventing vasodilation
L-NAA	Same as above
Anticoagulation/ Antiinflammatory	
Recombinant human activated protein C	Antithrombotic; antiinflammatory and profibrinolytic activity, modulates and improves microcirculatory dysfunction
Antithrombin III	Glycoprotein; reduces interactions between endothelial cells and neutrophils, decreases cytokine production
Antioxidant	
N-acetylcysteine	Antioxidant; reduces proinflammatory factors, IL-8

[a]The safety and efficacy studies of these agents in humans and animals have been mixed. In some cases, use of these products has resulted in an increased mortality as compared with controls. Further research is needed.

These therapies can be divided into four broad categories (Table 3.5): (i) agents aimed at blocking the effects of circulating microbial products, (ii) agents that block cytokines, (iii) agents that reduce or prevent NO production, and (iv) agents that act as anticoagulants.

Although initially there was much optimism as to whether these products would reduce mortality by blunting the proinflammatory effects of cytokines or the vasodilatory effects of NO or thrombus formation, subsequent animal and human studies have revealed mixed results. In fact, some of these studies have been associated with an increased mortality. One potential useful agent is activated protein C [drotrecogin alfa (activated)] because procoagulation and subsequent thrombus formation are always components of the pathophysiology of shock. Reduced levels of activated protein C, an endogenous protein that promotes fibrinolysis and inhibits thrombosis and inflammation, are associated with an increased risk of death in septic adults. Randomized, double-blind, placebo-controlled trials in adults with sepsis determined that administration of activated protein C was associated with improved survival, with the potential for bleeding during the infusion as a risk. In November 2001, the U.S. Food and Drug Administration approved this agent for use in adults with severe sepsis. In adults, the incidence of serious bleeding was higher in those receiving protein C than the placebo group (3.5% vs. 2.0%) in a 2001 study. Protein C levels in children reach adult values at the age of 3 years. There is interest in studying this therapy in children. In a safety study in 83 children with severe sepsis, serious bleeding was seen in 2.4% to 4.8%. Currently, protein C should be considered for use only in adults with sepsis-induced organ dysfunction with a clinical assessment of high risk of death.

The use of these agents needs further study in children. If proven effective, we can almost certainly expect to use these agents in the ED. Therefore, emergency medicine physicians will need to understand the indications and risks of these agents as new data are made available for review.

Laboratory Indications of Improvement in Shock

The initial phase of treatment for shock is directed to improve oxygen delivery to the tissues by ensuring adequate ventilation, correcting hypovolemia, and improving cardiac function.

The success of the initial resuscitation is usually reflected in signs of improved perfusion (skin, kidneys, brain, heart rate) and indications of normal CVP if invasive monitoring is required. However, other laboratory parameters may be useful, if monitored sequentially, in determining whether the shock syndrome is persisting despite early clinical improvement. Sequential measurements of serum lactate levels, and expired CO_2 gas (end-tidal CO_2) and cardiac output measurement may indicate that continued aggressive resuscitation is needed despite signs of improvement.

In 1983, Vincent et al. found that a 5% reduction in serum lactate in the first hour was a good prognostic sign for patients presenting in circulatory shock. Lactate should fall over time as perfusion and oxygen delivery to the tissue improves. High serum lactate levels (approximately 4 mm per L) or serum lactate levels that continue to rise despite therapy are indications of severe shock. Aggressive therapeutic maneuvers to reverse the shock should be redoubled in this setting.

In addition, end-tidal CO_2 is a noninvasive laboratory value that may indicate continued hypovolemia. In hypovolemia and poor perfusion of the peripheral tissues and pulmonary tissues, CO_2 is not excreted in the lungs. Subsequently, there is a reduction of expired CO_2 gas, which is measured as a decreased end-tidal CO_2. As perfusion improves, end-tidal CO_2 increases. Investigators hope to correlate whether sequential end-tidal CO_2 measurements can be used to titrate the amount of intravenous fluid needed during resuscitation of the patient in shock. These measurements are noninvasive and may be a valuable adjunct in accessing improvements in perfusion in children with severe hypovolemia in the ED.

The feasibility of using a noninvasive technique to determine cardiac output by continuance wave Doppler ultrasound is being studied in ED settings in Australia. This technique was used in 30 children with suspected fluid-resistant septic shock in England as well. Determining the hemodynamic patterns (high cardiac index with low systemic vascular resistance vs. low cardiac index) was helpful in management. This technique may help to direct therapy in the treatment of severe sepsis in the future.

Suggested Readings

Annane D, Sebille V, Charpentier C, et al. Effect of treatment with low doses of hydrocortisone and fludrocortisone on mortality in patients with septic shock. *JAMA* 2002;288:862–871.

Aschner J, Poland RL. Sodium bicarbonate: basically useless therapy. *Pediatrics* 2008;122(4):831–835.

Barton P, Kalil AC, Nadel S, et al. Safety, pharmacokinetics, and pharmacodynamics of Drotrecogin alfa (activated) in children with severe sepsis. *Pediatrics* 2004;113(1):7–17.

Beale RJ, Hollenberg SM, Vincent JL, et al. Vasopressor and inotropic support in septic shock: An evidence-based review. *Crit Care Med* 2004;32(11):S455–S465.

Bernard GR, Vincent JL, Laterre PF, et al. Efficacy and safety of recombinant human activated protein C for severe sepsis. *N Engl J Med* 2001;344(10):699–709.

Bochud PY, Bonten M, Marchetti O, et al. Antimicrobial therapy for patients with severe sepsis and septic shock: an evidence-based review. *Crit Care Med* 2004;32(11):S495–S512.

Bone RC. A critical evaluation of new agents for the treatment of sepsis. *JAMA* 1991;266:1686–1691.

Bone RC, Fisher CJ, Clemmer TP, et al. A controlled clinical trial of high-dose methylprednisolone in the treatment of severe sepsis and septic shock. *N Engl J Med* 1987;317:653–658.

Brierley J, Peters MJ. Distinct hemodynamic patterns of septic shock at presentation to pediatric intensive care. *Pediatrics* 2008;122(4):752–759.

Brilli RJ, Goldstein B. Pediatric sepsis definitions: past, present, and future. *Pediatr Crit Care Med* 2005;6(3):S6–S8.

Burgner D, Rockett K, Kwiatkowski D. Nitric oxide and infectious diseases. *Arch Dis Child* 1999;81:185–188.

Carcillo JA, Davis AL, Zaritsky A. Role of early fluid resuscitation in pediatric septic shock. *JAMA* 1991;266:1242–1245.

Carcillo JA, Fields AI. Clinical practice parameters for hemodynmaic support of pediatric and neonatal patients in septic shock. *Crit Care Med* 2002;30(6):1400–1401.

Dellinger RP, Levy MM, Carlet JM, et al. Surviving sepsis campaign: international guidelines for management of severe sepsis and septic shock: 2008. *Crit Care Med* 2008;36(1):296–327.

Dey I, Sprivulis P. Emergency physicians can reliably assess emergency department patient cardiac output using the USCOM continuous wave Doppler cardiac output monitor. *Emerg Med Australas* 2005;17:193–199.

Falk JL, Rackow EC, Weil MH. End-tidal carbon dioxide concentration during cardiopulmonary resuscitation. *N Engl J Med* 1988;318:607.

Goldstein B, Girior B, Randolph A, et al. International pediatric sepsis consensus conference: definitions for sepsis and organ dysfunction in pediatrics. *Pediatr Crit Care Med* 2005;6(1):2–8.

Han YY, Carcillo JA, Dragotta MA, et al. Early reversal of pediatric-neonatal septic shock by community physician is associated with improved outcome. *Pediatrics* 2003;112(4):793–799.

Hotchkiss RS, Karl IE. The pathophysiology and treatment of sepsis. *N Engl J Med* 2003;248:138–150.

Keh D, Sprung CL. Use of corticosteroid therapy in patients with sepsis and septic shock: an evidence-based review. *Crit Care Med* 2004;32(11):S527–S533.

Landry DW, Oliver JA. The pathogenesis of vasodilatory shock. *N Engl J Med* 2001;345:588–595.

Parker MM, Hazelzet JA, Carcillo JA. Pediatric considerations. *Crit Care Med* 2004;32(11):S591–S594.

Pinsky MR. Antioxidant therapy for severe sepsis: promise and perspective. *Crit Care Med* 2003;31:2697–2698.

Rangel-Frausto MS, Pihhet D, Costigan M, et al. The natural history of the SIRS: a prospective study. *JAMA* 1995;273:117–123.

Rivers E, Nguyen B, Havstad S, et al. Early goal-directed therapy in the treatment of severe sepsis and septic shock. *N Engl J Med* 2001;345(19):1368–1377.

Summers RL, Shoemaker WC, Peacock WF, et al. Bench to bedside: electrophysiologic and clinical principles of noninvasive hemodynamic monitoring using impudence cardiography. *Acad Emerg Med* 2003;10:669–680.

Velasco AL, Delgado-Paredes C, Templeton J, et al. Intraosseous infusion of fluids in the initial management of hypovolemic shock in young subjects. *J Pediatr Surg* 1991;26:4–8.

Vincent JL, Dufaye P, Berre J, et al. Serial lactate determinations during circulatory shock. *Crit Care Med* 1983;11:449–451.

Vincent JL, Gerlach H. Fluid resuscitation in severe sepsis and septic shock: an evidence-based review. *Crit Care Med* 2004;32(11):S451–S454.

Warren BL, Eid A, Singer P, et al. High dose antithrombin III in severe sepsis: a randomized controlled trial. *JAMA* 2001;286:1869–1878.

Watson RS, Carcillo JA, Linde-Zwirble WT, et al. The epidemiology of severe sepsis in children in the United States. *Am J Respir Crit Care Med* 2003;167:695–701.

Ziegler EJ, Fisher CJ, Sprung CL, et al. Treatment of gram-negative bacteremia and septic shock with HA-1A human monoclonal antibody against endotoxin. *N Engl J Med* 1991;324:429–436.

CHAPTER 4 ■ SEDATION AND ANALGESIA

JOEL A. FEIN, MD, MPH, AND STEVEN M. SELBST, MD

The relief of pain and suffering is one of the most common reasons for seeking care in an emergency department (ED). Injuries and painful medical conditions are common among children, and ED physicians are morally obligated to manage pain appropriately. Pain is defined as an unpleasant sensory and emotional experience usually characterized in terms of tissue damage, which is signaled by some form of visible or audible behavior. Acute pain serves a useful function and is necessary for survival; it alerts us to avoid certain painful stimuli, and it warns us that some body tissues may be damaged. However, pain must be relieved as quickly as possible; chronic pain serves no useful function and it has been noted that even acute pain can inhibit healing.

BACKGROUND

Historical Undertreatment of Pain in the Emergency Department

There have been great advances in recognition, assessment, and management of pain in children in recent years. The care of infants and children who undergo painful procedures in the ED has also improved considerably. Unfortunately, pain control is still not always addressed satisfactorily. Some recent studies still show that children, especially children younger than 2 years of age, still often fail to receive analgesia for painful conditions. Pain experienced by children in the ED is often poorly assessed and documented. Inadequate dosing of medications for children upon discharge from the ED is a significant problem. Emergency physicians and pediatricians are equally unlikely to give analgesics to children.

Barriers to Treatment of Pain in Children

Many theories try to explain why pediatric pain is not successfully managed in the ED. Physicians expect babies to cry, so this nonspecific response to pain is often tolerated instead of controlled. Moreover, because young children and infants cannot describe or localize their pain, it is often ignored or presumed not to exist. Adult patients who clearly indicate that they are in pain generally get a direct response from a physician, whereas a young child who is crying or whimpering may not. In addition, some ED physicians avoid giving adequate analgesics to children because they fear it will lead to drug addiction. This is fear unfounded, however, because narcotic addiction is extremely rare when medications are used appropriately to manage acute pain. Hypotension and respiratory depression are other feared consequences of narcotic use with

children, and although these fears may be legitimate, respiratory depression and hypotension are unlikely to occur if proper protocols are adhered to. These unlikely occurrences should be manageable in the ED, and they should not inhibit the attempt to control pain. Furthermore, it is likely that ED physicians are often forced to concentrate on other aspects of resuscitation and care before managing pain. Plans for pain control, therefore, may be forgotten because of other priorities. Some physicians avoid analgesics because they do not want to mask symptoms. Also, in some cases, pain is ignored because it is inconvenient to wait for topical analgesics to take effect. This can delay care, so some physicians may underuse analgesics and convince a young child that a painful procedure or repositioning of an extremity will hurt only for a minute. Brute force (instead of medication) is then used, and more pain is inflicted on an already uncomfortable child.

Pain control may not be properly addressed with children because some physicians are unfamiliar with sedative and analgesic agents for children. In some EDs, these agents are not available. Also, children are often unable to cooperate or provide good verbal descriptions of pain, so it may be difficult to assess or quantify pain or to measure success in treating it. However, great progress has been made lately in the assessment of pain in children. Table 4.1 summarizes some reasons for inadequate pain control with children.

ASSESSMENT OF PAIN IN CHILDREN

The clinical evaluation of pain may be accomplished through physiologic measurements, behavioral assessment, or self-report. Infants and preschool children (younger than 5 years of age) cannot understand the nature of self-report scales, and their assessment, therefore, relies on observer report. *Physiologic* indicators of pain include heart and respiratory rates, blood pressure, and palm sweating. Of interest, but not yet of practical use in the emergency setting, is the correlation between an individual's pain and the acutely measured levels of stress hormones, such as cortisol, catecholamines, and glucagon.

Observational *behavioral pain assessments* can, however, measure behavioral distress experienced by the child. For example, the Behavioral Pain Score categorizes facial expressions (positive, negative, or neutral), crying (laughing, not crying, moaning, sobbing), and movements (playing, not moving, withdrawal, complex agitation). The Children's Hospital of Eastern Ontario Pain Scale is a widely used instrument that measures crying, facial expression, verbal expression, torso position, touch, and leg position. The scale has been found to be valid and reliable for assessing pain in younger children and

POSSIBLE REASONS FOR INADEQUATE PAIN
CONTROL IN EMERGENCY DEPARTMENT

Inability of young children to talk
Misconception that infants cannot feel pain
Misconception that children will not remember pain
Misconception that children will get addicted to narcotics
Fear of respiratory depression and hypotension
Unfamiliarity with analgesics and dosages
Other conditions taking priority

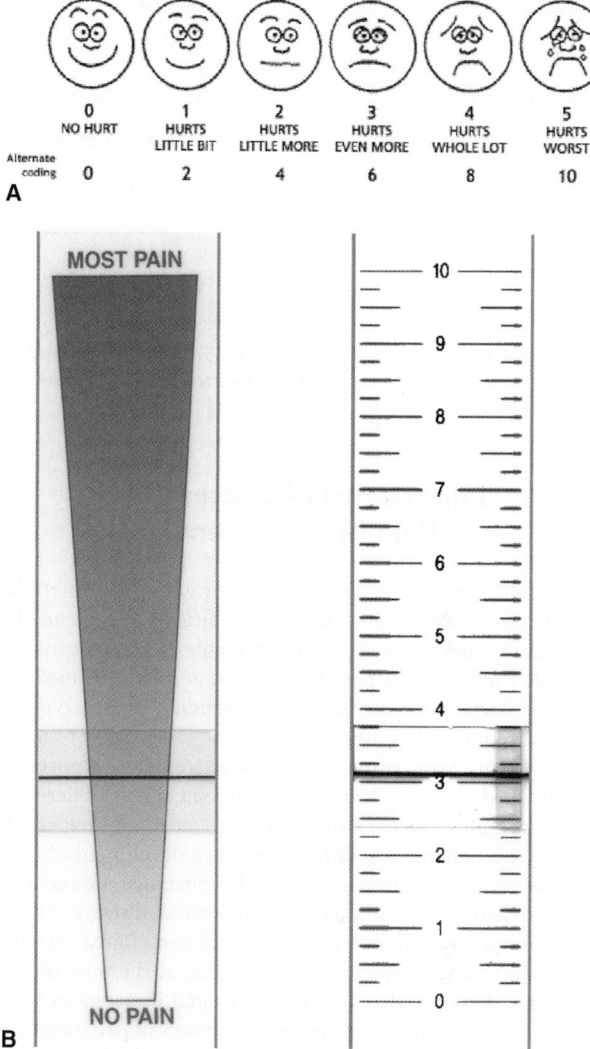

infants. Some observational pain scales use a combination of behavioral and physiologic measurements.

Self-report pain scales are the best indicators of pain and are the gold standard for assessing pain in children. Standard self-report assessment tools, such as visual analog scales (VASs), are more reliable indicators of pain when completed by the patient rather than by observers. Young children (between ages 4 and 7 years) can reliably use picture scales with faces in different phases of happiness and crying. The Wong-Baker FACES Pain Rating Scale (Fig. 4.1A) is one example of this type of ordinal scale.

For older children and adults, a VAS consists of a 10 cm (100 mm) horizontal line with end points marked as "no pain" (0) to "worst possible pain" (10) (Fig. 4.1B). Patients indicate the level of their pain by marking the line. A decrease in the VAS by 10 mm has been noted to correlate with the patients reporting "a little" improvement in their pain. Another study in adults demonstrated that patients who are in more pain to begin with require up to 30 mm decrease before considering their pain "a little better." The VAS has been further enhanced for children by allowing them to use multiple modalities for pain rating. These more versatile instruments allow the child to determine changes in height, thickness, and color as the pain intensity increases, as well as capitalize on the child's ability to discriminate his or her pain using at least one of these dimensions.

Impact of Pain on Children and Families

Emergency physicians must understand that pain is an individual experience and many factors contribute to the degree of pain that a child experiences for any given condition. Children of all ages can experience pain; it is believed that even neonates by 26 weeks' gestation respond to tissue injury with specific behavior and with autonomic, hormonal, and metabolic signs of distress. Newborns feel pain and react to painful stimuli (e.g., circumcision) with wiggling motions and crying. Young children often exaggerate the size and power of needles, while older children may be better able to understand the need for a painful procedure; they are usually less anxious and better able to tolerate the inflicted pain. However, an older child may have a better understanding of the significance of an injury or an illness that could cause depression, anxiety, and more pain. Similarly, parental response (anxiety or reassuring calm) may affect a child's perception of pain. Caregivers can experience elevated heart rate, blood pressure, and anxiety during the child's IV cannulation. Not surprisingly, parental distress-promoting behaviors increase childhood dis-

FIGURE 4.1 **A:** The Wong-Baker FACES Pain Rating Scale. (From Wong DL, Hockenberry-Eaton M, Wilson D, et al. *Wong's essentials of pediatric nursing.* 6th ed. St. Louis: Mosby, 2001:1301. Copyright Mosby, Inc. Reprinted by permission.) **B:** The front and back of a visual analog scale.

tress during IV cannulation. Other psychological factors, such as the child's emotional state, personality traits, gender, or cultural background, may impact his or her anxiety, and this can also alter the degree of pain. Some children seem to have a hypersensitivity to pain, whereas others tolerate it well. Recent work has demonstrated that certain genotypes, such as the CYP2D6 polymorphisms and opioid receptor OPRM1, can mediate the metabolism and efficacy of certain opiate medications. The context of the situation also plays a role; children who are hit during play may not complain of pain, yet may experience pain if the injury was meant as an attack or as punishment. A child's past experience with painful stimuli is also meaningful. One study showed that inadequate analgesia for one painful procedure might diminish the effect of adequate analgesia in subsequent procedures. Of course, the painful stimulus itself is important, and a stimulus that causes a great deal of tissue damage may hurt more than one that causes minor injury. Figure 4.2 summarizes the components of a pediatric patient's pain experience.

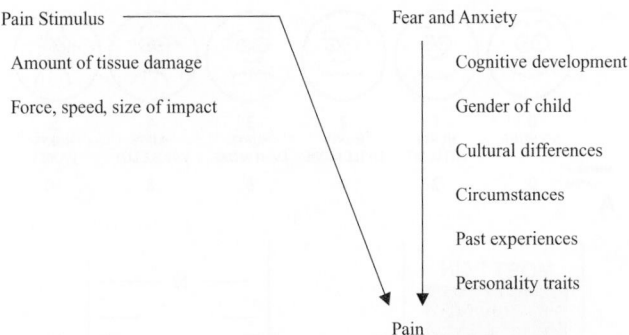

FIGURE 4.2 Components of pain. (Adapted from Schecter NL. Pain and pain control in children. *Curr Probl Pediatr Adolesc Health Care* 1985;15:4–67.)

Importance of Successful Pain Management

Realistically, pain in the pediatric patient who presents to the ED may never be eliminated completely. Efforts must be made, however, to relieve pain as much as possible. Several means are available for managing pain in children, and various medications and techniques can be used, depending on the type of pain that requires treatment.

Successful pain management is extremely important. Uncontrolled pain may lead to hyperalgesia, a state where the painful stimulus causes more pain than normally expected. Infants who undergo a painful experience develop an altered response to future episodes of pain. For instance, infants circumcised without anesthesia show increased distress during routine immunizations at 4 to 6 months of age, compared with those who received topical local anesthetic at the time of circumcision. This has also been demonstrated in neonates who had repeated heel sticks. Furthermore, surveys of patients, parents, and families show that satisfaction with the ED experience is highly dependent on the degree of pain a patient experiences and the efforts made to alleviate the pain. One study demonstrated that more than 75% of caregivers would be willing to pay $15 and more than one third would pay $100 to make an IV cannulation procedure painless. The Joint Commission has specific guidelines stating that patients have the right to pain assessment and treatment. This pain must be frequently reassessed, and the pain must be appropriately addressed with adequate analgesia.

NONPHARMACOLOGIC METHODS FOR PAIN CONTROL

Regardless of the procedure performed or the medications used during procedural sedation and analgesia (PSA), the patient's developmental level and acute level of anxiety will directly impact the success of a procedure and the patient's eventual subjective experience. There are many nonpharmacologic methods used to decrease the child's fear and incorporate the family into the therapeutic objectives. In general, these methods are low cost, consume very little time, and have few, if any, side effects. Thus, nonpharmacologic techniques can be used alone or as "adjuncts" to sedation drug therapy.

Children need gentle reassurance and carefully chosen words to reduce fear and pain. One should keep in mind that young children understand more than they say. Avoid casual teasing, condescension, or talking about the child while excluding him or her. As many choices as possible should be offered, but only if they are real choices. Do not tell a child that something will not hurt unless you are sure that it will not. It is important to be honest with the child about any pain or discomfort that he or she will experience. Once a child is surprised by a painful stimulus, he or she will become more vigilant and less amenable to distraction or relaxation techniques. In general, the time between informing the child about potential discomfort and the actual procedure performance should be brief. Long delays between the explanation and the actual procedure increase anticipatory distress prior to the procedure. One study showed that an empathic (age-appropriate) explanation of an upcoming needle stick reduced crying among patients compared with a group of children who received impersonal instructions. Fassler showed that allowing an older child to read about a procedure and then allowing role-playing and discussion was helpful in reducing pulse rates, as well as other physiologic and behavioral responses to pain. Such explanations and role-playing are time consuming, and it is helpful to enlist the child's parents to assist in these techniques. In some EDs, child life specialists help children with preparation and distraction for procedures, and they help educate the staff (and sometimes even families) about the most appropriate language to use for a specific child.

Most pediatric centers advocate family member presence during painful procedures. Recent research demonstrates that family presence does not increase the pain or distress of the parent or child, nor does it adversely affect the clinicians' abilities to provide safe and effective care. Giving the family the option to remain in the room during procedures and resuscitations increases the family's overall satisfaction with the visit, and should be incorporated into the plans for PSA.

Distraction of a child during a painful procedure may help reduce pain and distress. This includes having the child perform rhythmic breathing or blowing bubbles. A recent meta-analysis showed that music therapy is effective in reducing anxiety and pain for children undergoing procedures. Music can be used as adjunctive therapy in some clinical situations involving pain in the ED. Age-appropriate distraction has been demonstrated to reduce self-reported anxiety and parental perception of pain in children during laceration repair. For younger children, parents can also help with singing and storytelling. Visually intriguing toys, paintings on the walls or ceiling of a procedure room, and music or videotapes may also distract a young child. *Guided imagery*, in which children are coached to imagine a pleasant memory or scenario, may also be helpful. For example, one could ask the child to think of the funniest movie he or she has ever seen and to imagine the pain getting less intense with each laugh. Or, the child could be asked to imagine the pain as a color that is fading away and is painted over with the child's favorite color. *Hypnosis* has been used to treat pain in children for several years, and it has been successful in children as young as 2 years of age. Some physicians believe that the technique better serves children than adults because children have vivid imaginations and can more easily intertwine fantasy and reality. Hypnosis is of proven value for chronic pain syndromes such as migraine headaches or long-term illnesses. Hypnosis has also been recommended for the acute management of burns, fractures, and other injuries; however, its use for painful procedures in a busy ED has not been rigorously evaluated.

Counterstimulation is a technique by which someone repetitively and persistently rubs or touches an area of the body close to the area that is being hurt. This technique is based on the gate theory of pain. Transmission of pain information from dorsal horn cells occurs through a "gate," which opens in response to signals from the affected small fibers. The gate can be "closed" by large neurons that are stimulated by nonpainful touching or pressing of the skin. The theory explains why we rub our elbow when we hit it against something: The rubbing stimulates these large fibers and suppresses the anticipated painful sensation.

Restraint should not be used in lieu of appropriate sedation and analgesics for the pediatric patient. Although proper *restraint* of a child for a painful procedure does not always reduce fear or anxiety, it does allow the physician to perform the task better. This indirectly reduces pain because fewer attempts may be necessary to accomplish the task. One should never attempt a painful procedure on a moving subject! The need for restraint should be explained to the parents, who should not be involved in the actual process. Instead, the child might be wrapped in hospital sheets or papoose boards with Velcro straps, with the parents attempting to calm the child afterward. Experienced clinicians using papoose boards often use sheets between the child and the Velcro straps to avoid skin abrasion by the Velcro itself. The technique should be monitored carefully to avoid the uncommon complications of minor bruising, edema, or transient vascular compromise.

SPECIFIC AGENTS

Analgesics for Mild to Moderate Pain

Conditions such as headache, myalgia, chest pain, pharyngitis, otitis media, arthralgia, sunburn, strains, and sprains often produce mild pain in children. For treatment of less intense pain, aspirin, acetaminophen, ibuprofen (nonnarcotics), and codeine (narcotic) are excellent oral analgesic medications. *Aspirin* is one of the oldest analgesic medications, but it is rarely used now because of the better side effect profile of other analgesics and the perceived risk of Reye's syndrome.

Acetaminophen acts centrally on nonopioid receptors in the brain to inhibit prostaglandin synthetase. Acetaminophen is a good choice for pain associated with minor trauma or otitis media because it is well tolerated and comes in liquid form, making it easy to give to young children. One study showed that 1,000 mg of acetaminophen is equal to 60 mg of codeine for postpartum pain. In addition, acetaminophen does not cause bleeding and is unlikely to cause bronchospasm in asthmatics. It is dosed at 10 to 15 mg per kg per dose every 4 hours and takes effect in 20 to 40 minutes, with a peak effect in 2 hours. Rectal administration produces delayed and variable uptake. Higher doses may be needed, but clearance may be prolonged so the rectal dose interval should be extended to 6 or 8 hours. Single rectal doses of 20 mg per kg produced safe plasma concentrations in preterm neonates. In general, high dosages of acetaminophen are usually well tol-

erated, but therapy in children should not exceed 75 mg per kg day (60 mg per kg per day in infants and newborns). Updated guidelines and product labeling are anticipated from the FDA in the near future, decreasing the total daily dosage that is considered safe. Acetaminophen has no antiinflammatory effects, and therapeutic doses rarely are associated with side effects in children; overdose, however, can cause liver toxicity. Addition of codeine may enhance the analgesic effect in a subset of children.

Nonsteroidal antiinflammatory drugs (NSAIDs) (e.g., ibuprofen) are potent inhibitors of the COX pathway and they prevent the formation of prostaglandin, a known mediator of pain, fever, and inflammation. NSAIDs are excellent choices for treating minor pain, such as headache, dysmenorrhea, or musculoskeletal injuries. Some studies show that NSAIDs provide better analgesia than acetaminophen, and others show no difference. NSAIDs have a longer half-life than acetaminophen. The recommended dosage of ibuprofen is 8 to 10 mg per kg given every 6 hours. The recommended dosage for ibuprofen in older children is 200 to 400 mg per dose given every 6 hours (maximum 40 mg per kg per day) for mild to moderate pain. Ibuprofen is available in liquid form, making it suitable for use in very young children. Ibuprofen and the other NSAIDs, such as naproxen and ketorolac, are nonaddictive and does not cause respiratory or cardiac depression. NSAIDs may cause gastrointestinal bleeding, but this risk is very small. These agents also cause renal and hepatic dysfunction; therefore, they should be used with caution in children with renal or hepatic disease. They may prolong bleeding time, but their effect on platelets (inhibition of aggregation) is reversible. NSAIDs are subject to a ceiling effect, in which a maximum dose is achieved, beyond which there is no additional analgesic effect.

A newer group of NSAIDs, the COX-2 inhibitors, may have fewer side effects than ibuprofen in children. There is concern in adults that COX-2 inhibitors may result in a greater number of cardiac adverse events, but this has not been shown to be true in children without underlying cardiac disease. These agents do not impair platelet function and are less likely to cause gastritis. Currently, these medications are recommended for those who require long-term NSAID administration for chronic pain syndromes. They should be used with caution, as recent evidence links some of these medications with heart disease and stroke in adult patients.

Furthermore, *codeine* is a narcotic analgesic that can be given orally (even to young children) to control minor pain. Codeine usually is given orally because it maintains two-thirds of its effectiveness in oral form compared with parenteral use. It is believed to be more potent than aspirin but less potent than meperidine; thus, it is valuable for moderate pain (dental abscess, severe otitis media, or stomatitis) in some children and has a low addiction potential. Significant effort has been invested in uncovering the pharmacogenetic effects of codeine in children. When given the same dose, some children will have a suboptimal response, others will respond well and still others will have toxic manifestations. The recommended dosage is 0.5 to 1 mg per kg per dose every 4 to 6 hours (maximum 60 mg per dose). Codeine can be ordered as a liquid form for use in young children, and it can be combined with acetaminophen to produce an even greater analgesic effect than when either is used alone. Codeine can cause respiratory depression, but this occurs very rarely. It has little renal or hepatic toxicity and does not alter platelet function, but

TABLE 4.2

ANALGESICS FOR MILD PAIN

Analgesic	Advantages	Disadvantages
Acetaminophen	Well tolerated, safe	Liver toxicity if overdosed
Ibuprofen	Long duration of action	Gastrointestinal irritation
Codeine	Good safety record	Nausea, constipation
Sucrose	Maybe useful for infants for procedural pain. No adverse effects.	Not always affective for babies older than 30 days.

it can cause the same gastrointestinal side effects (e.g., nausea, vomiting, constipation) as noted for other narcotics.

Finally, sucrose has been shown to be safe and effective in managing pain, especially for procedural pain, such as heel sticks and injections, for infants younger than 6 months of age. The effect of sucrose is strongest in the newborn and decreases gradually over the first 6 months of life. It is recommended to use a 25% sucrose solution and administer 2 mL orally by allowing the infant to suck on a pacifier. Alternatively, use a syringe and apply 1 mL orally to each cheek. The sucrose should be administered no more than 2 minutes before beginning the painful procedure.

The benefits of using codeine and the other analgesics described here for mild pain far outweigh the few side effects involved with their use in young children. Table 4.2 summarizes the advantages and disadvantages of these analgesics for treating minor pain in children.

Analgesics for Moderate to Severe Pain

Opioid medications are extremely important for treating patients in the ED with moderate to severe pain (burns, fractures, sickle cell vasoocclusive crises). Most opioids can cause important adverse effects (primarily respiratory depression and hypotension) that are dose related and may be reversed with naloxone if necessary, remembering that with reversal of the narcotic induced side effect will also reverse pain control. For this reason, naloxone may be dosed according to level of reversal needed (e.g., mild respiratory depression can be reversed with 1 – 10 mcg/kg) to preserve some level of pain control. Because of pharmacokinetic differences in young infants that may predispose them to respiratory depression, these drugs should be used with caution and with reduced doses in infants younger than 3 months of age who are not ventilated mechanically. Opioid analgesics can be given by various routes of administration. In general, the intramuscular (IM) route should be avoided because the injection itself is painful, it causes delayed drug absorption, and the dosage of drug given cannot be titrated. The intravenous (IV) route is more advantageous because titration is possible, although some pain is involved in starting the IV line. Subcutaneous administration can also be an option in patients without IV access. Some physicians choose to deliver the opioids with a patient-controlled analgesia device that allows the patient to self-administer the drug at a safe dosage as it is needed. This allows patients to have some control over their own pain while relieving the ED nurse of time needed to administer the drugs.

For severe pain from a significant burn, sickle cell crisis, fracture, or other injury, *morphine* is an excellent choice. The usual dosage of morphine is 0.1 to 0.2 mg per kg per dose, titrated to effect and given intravenously over a few minutes. The maximum dose is generally 10 mg for opioid-naive subjects, and the medication may be repeated every 2 to 4 hours. The higher dosage, and a dosing interval of every 1 to 2 hours, is suggested for those who take narcotics often (e.g., those with sickle cell disease or cancer) because they may have some tolerance to the drug. If needed, a subsequent dose is reduced to 0.05 mg per kg if the patient is moderately sedated. Young infants should receive 0.05 mg per kg every 4 to 8 hours and they should be closely monitored. Morphine can also be given as a continuous infusion at 0.01 mg per kg per hour for infants younger than 6 months of age and 0.025 to 0.04 mg per kg per hour for children older than 12 months of age. It can be titrated, if needed (increase 25% every 3 hours). When given intravenously, its effect is almost immediate, with the peak effect occurring in 20 minutes. Morphine can cause pooling of blood by decreasing peripheral vascular resistance and histamine release, both of, which may result in hypotension. This is more often a concern in the patient with a severe injury who may be hypovolemic or those experiencing histamine release. Certainly, the fluid status of an injured child requires careful attention from the ED staff, but pain control should not be withheld after IV fluids have corrected volume depletion. If the child is awake, alert, and screaming in pain, morphine can be given safely as long as the patient is monitored carefully. If the patient has persistent hypotension, other agents such as fentanyl can be used to control pain.

Meperidine is another opioid agent that can be used to treat moderate to severe pain. It can be given intravenously at a dose of 0.5 to 1 mg per kg, or intramuscularly at a dose of 1 to 1.5 mg per kg given every 3 to 4 hours. The maximum recommended dose for opioid-naive patients is 100 mg. It has no significant advantages over morphine, and there can be problems with its use. For example, it may cause nervousness, tremors, disorientation, and even seizures when used intravenously because of accumulation of its metabolite normeperidine. Meperidine should be used with great caution, if at all, in patients with head trauma or increased intracranial pressure as it has the potential to decrease respirations and increase intracranial pressure. Likewise, it should be used with great caution in infants, as it may decrease respiration. In general, morphine may be a better opioid for severe pain unless a patient indicates that meperidine works best.

Fentanyl is a synthetic opioid that should be given at a dose of 1 to 3 μg per kg per dose intravenously *slowly* over 3 to 5 minutes. It has a rapid onset of action (almost immediately) and a short duration of action (30 to 60 minutes), which makes it useful in the ED. Fentanyl also appears to be effective when used intranasally or via nebulizer. It is an excellent agent for severe pain from fractures. Fentanyl also has several other advantages. It is a relatively safe drug and rarely causes hypotension, making it an excellent choice for injured children in severe pain. Respiratory depression can occur within minutes of fentanyl administration, but this is reported in only 0.7% of adult patients, some of whom were intoxicated with alcohol. There is a greater risk of respiratory depression when coadministered with other sedatives and in infants younger than 3 months of age. Apnea occurs even less often, and this may be related to a rapid rate of infusion of fentanyl rather than the dosage. Although these adverse effects are serious, they can be reversed with naloxone and avoided if the dosage guidelines are followed and the drug is given slowly. Individualized dosing titrated to effect may reduce these side effects. Also, equipment and personnel who can manage an obstructed airway should be nearby when fentanyl is used.

An uncommon event caused by fentanyl is neuromuscular blockade, with severe thoracic and abdominal muscle rigidity. However, this "wooden chest syndrome" has not been reported during procedural sedation in which lower doses are used, and when the drug is administered slowly. Most often, this side effect is reversible with naloxone, but succinylcholine and manual ventilation may be required. Despite the problems already noted, fentanyl remains a valuable analgesic that can be used in the ED when a child has severe pain. Fentanyl has been used for safe repair of complicated facial lacerations that might otherwise have required general anesthesia. It should be noted that fentanyl causes an unusual tendency for children to reach up and scratch their faces. If fentanyl is used for repair of lacerations, restraints may be needed to prevent a child from contaminating a sterile field. Even better, the parent can be assigned to scratch the child's nose if so requested. Fentanyl can also be given in the form of a transmucosal lozenge, but this is contraindicated in patients who are not opioid tolerant and in the management of acute pain.

Ketorolac tromethamine is a parenteral NSAID that has been used to treat moderate to severe pain. IV ketorolac has been found to be as effective as morphine for postoperative pain in children with fewer side effects. Some studies show that ketorolac is comparable to narcotic agents for treatment of musculoskeletal pain, headaches, sickle cell crises, and orthopedic injuries with less sedation and fewer side effects. Other studies show that children with sickle cell disease and fractures do not have a narcotic-sparing effect with ketorolac. It is often the drug of choice for patients with acute renal colic. However, some believe the drug is comparable to oral ibuprofen and there is little advantage of injectable NSAIDs over oral administration. Ketorolac does not cause respiratory depression or nausea or vomiting. Dosing guidelines are not well established, but many pediatric centers use ketorolac with a dose of 0.5 mg per kg intravenously to a maximum of 30 mg IV every 6 hours for a maximum of 5 days.

Other Agents

Hydromorphone (Dilaudid) is a semisynthetic agent used for management of moderate to severe pain for children in the ED, as a substitute for morphine and codeine. This is often given orally, rectally, or parenterally, and the analgesic effects last 4 to 5 hours. It is less sedating than morphine. Serious errors have occurred when hydromorphone dosing is confused with morphine dosing. No more than 0.015 mg/kg (max 4 mg/dose) should be given intravenously for initial dosing. Likewise, oxycodone and hydrocodone are oral analgesics that are more potent than codeine with less associated nausea and vomiting. Oxycodone and hydrocodone are about equal to morphine as analgesics and respiratory depressants. Like codeine, they retain about 60% of their efficacy when given orally. Oxycodone is often combined with nonopioid medications such as aspirin (Percodan), acetaminophen (Percocet, Tylox), or ibuprofen. One recent study found that oxycodone was no more effective than ibuprofen in reducing pain related to orthopedic injuries in children and combining oxycodone with ibuprofen did not add further pain relief. Sustained-release oxycodone should not be used for acute pain management.

Table 4.3 summarizes the advantages and disadvantages of several analgesics used to treat moderate to severe pain.

LOCAL ANESTHETIC AGENTS FOR WOUND REPAIR

Lidocaine

Lidocaine is an excellent local anesthetic that has been used frequently in the ED for wound repair, foreign body removal, insertion of IV infusion lines or lumbar puncture needles, drainage of abscesses, and arterial puncture. Lidocaine is usually administered as a 1% solution (10 mg per mL) at a maximum dosage of 5 mg per kg. A 0.5% solution is used for infiltration when large volumes are needed or in smaller patients when it is desirable to limit the total number of milligrams per kilograms given. When vasoconstriction is desired for suturing, lidocaine can be used in combination with epinephrine, at a

TABLE 4.3

ANALGESICS FOR MODERATE TO SEVERE PAIN

Analgesic	Advantages	Disadvantages
Morphine	Rapid onset, potent analgesia	Respiratory depression, hypotension
Meperidine	Potent analgesia	Respiratory depression, seizures
Fentanyl	Potent analgesia, less hypotension	Respiratory depression, apnea
Ketorolac	Nonnarcotic NSAID	Use for more than 5 days can result in renal damage

dosage of (lidocaine) 7 mg per kg. Slightly lower doses should be used in neonates (4 to 5 mg per kg). Lidocaine should not be combined with epinephrine for use in areas supplied by end arteries, such as the digits, penis, or pinna of the ear. Lidocaine is advantageous because it provides excellent local anesthesia and takes effect quickly (within a few minutes). The effect lasts long enough to complete most procedures (about 1.5 to 2 hours). It is generally a safe drug because few people have a true allergy to it. Serious toxicity, such as seizures and cardiac arrest, can occur, but only when large amounts are injected inadvertently or when the drug is injected directly into a blood vessel.

The major disadvantage of using lidocaine as a local anesthetic is that a painful injection is required for administration. This pain can be reduced, however, if a long, small (27- or 30-gauge) needle is used to produce a "fanning" effect of the anesthetic. To avoid inadvertent injection into a vessel while injecting deep into tissue, a larger needle is needed to aspirate blood. Otherwise, the small needle is recommended, and only a small amount of lidocaine should be injected to avoid tissue distortion. Some physicians recommend using a syringe with a thumb ring during infiltration for better control. It is best to inject lidocaine slowly, perhaps over 30 seconds. This may cause less rapid distension of local tissue and activation of fewer nerve endings. Warming the lidocaine by storing the medication and syringes in fluid warmed to 98.6°F seems to reduce the pain of infiltration. It may also hurt less to inject the lidocaine into the damaged tissue inside the wound instead of into the intact skin. The needle should be pulled out to the tip and the injection given again at 90-degree angles to minimize the number of punctures. Subsequent injections to extend the area of anesthesia should be given through anesthetized tissue when possible. It is helpful to rub the skin near the site of injection first because this reduces pain by stimulating other nerve endings according to the gate theory of pain. Buffered lidocaine, prepared by mixing lidocaine and sodium bicarbonate in a 9:1 ratio, which is more alkaline and subsequently less painful when administered. Buffered lidocaine can be made as needed in the ED or in advance, and it will remain stable for approximately 2 weeks. In all cases, a few minutes should be allowed for the anesthesia to take effect. Table 4.4 summarizes some hints to reduce the pain of lidocaine infiltration.

Other Injectable Local Anesthetics

Bupivacaine 0.25% is similar to lidocaine but may have a longer duration of action and may help reduce pain for 6 hours after a

wound is repaired. To avoid toxicity, inject no more than 2 to 2.5 mg per kg of bupivacaine. Diphenhydramine, 0.5% and 1%, has been used and studied as a local anesthetic in adult patients. However, it seems to cause more pain on infiltration than lidocaine and has resulted in tissue necrosis. Therefore, it is not recommended as an injectable anesthetic. Benzyl alcohol has been shown as a reasonable alternative to lidocaine for subcutaneous anesthesia in the rare patient that has a history of allergy to amide anesthetics. Multidose vials of physiologic saline solution that contain 0.9% benzyl alcohol can be mixed in a 1:100 dilution with epinephrine 1:1,000 strength to create a solution that has comparable effectiveness to 1% lidocaine for laceration repair and IV insertion. Note that the duration of action of benzyl alcohol is shorter than that of lidocaine and may not be as effective for prolonged procedures. Benzyl alcohol should never be used in infants.

Topical Anesthetics for Wound Repair

LET is a solution of 4% lidocaine, 0.1% epinephrine, and 0.5% tetracaine. It can be made in gel form with hydroxyethyl cellulose. LET has been used successfully and safely for repair of uncomplicated facial and scalp lacerations in children. The major advantage to using LET for suturing is that the anesthetic can be applied painlessly, without the use of a needle. This reduces the fear and anxiety involved in wound repair and may help the suturing go more smoothly. Even in the small number of children who have inadequate anesthesia from LET, the application of this topical anesthetic will reduce the pain of subsequent administration of lidocaine by injection. The gel can be applied directly to the wound and allowed to remain for approximately 20 to 30 minutes, the solution can be "painted" onto the wound with a cotton-tipped swab, or a saturated cotton ball can be applied to the wound and held in place manually or with tape. Subsequently, the surrounding skin will be well blanched, indicating adequate local anesthesia. Like lidocaine, LET should not be applied to body parts where vasoconstriction is contraindicated. LET has essentially replaced TAC (tetracaine, adrenaline, cocaine compound) as the preferred topical anesthetic for wound repair because it is much less costly and has reduced toxicity. TAC carries the risk of cocaine toxicity and can lead to seizures and death, especially if used near mucous membranes where rapid absorption can occur. TAC should no longer be used as an anesthetic for wound repair in children.

TOPICAL ANESTHETIC AGENTS FOR IV PLACEMENT AND VENIPUNCTURE

A plethora of products are currently available for topical anesthesia through intact skin and have been found helpful in relieving pain associated with IV catheter placement and venipuncture in children. Studies have shown that decisions about IV line placement can often be made at triage. If preparing for IV line placement, one should prepare multiple sites in case the first attempt is unsuccessful, which occurs between 50% and 75% of the time, depending on whether or not the child is dehydrated. These products are also useful for draining

---

TABLE 4.4

HINTS TO REDUCE PAIN OF LIDOCAINE INFILTRATION

1. Do not allow child to see needles involved in preparing lidocaine.
2. Warm and buffer lidocaine with sodium bicarbonate.
3. Use a long, small needle for infiltration.
4. Rub skin around injection site before infiltration.
5. Infiltrate through devitalized tissue or anesthetized areas.
6. Inject slowly, only what is needed.
7. Wait for anesthetic effect.

an abscess or paronychia, arthrocentesis, lumbar puncture, or access for fully implantable central venous catheters.

All topical anesthetics currently available contain lidocaine either alone or mixed with another anesthetic and have variable mechanisms of delivery and onset times. The delivery mechanism must traverse the stratum corneum, which contains highly ordered lipid bilayers that block the entry or exit of water or water-soluble substances. Products can traverse this barrier using direct injection below the skin, using needle-less injection using pressurized gas by passive diffusion, or by interrupting or bypassing the barrier using heat, ultrasound, or electricity.

Multiple studies have demonstrated that intradermal injection of lidocaine, or saline with benzyl alcohol, can reduce IV insertion pain; although this technique requires an additional needle stick, most patients prefer it to no anesthesia at all. Anesthesia is almost immediate, offering a distinct advantage over other modalities. Newer products using pressurized helium or CO_2 to achieve needle-less subcutaneous infiltration of 1% or 2% powdered lidocaine achieve anesthesia within 1 to 3 minutes. One pediatric study that showed good efficacy did not find that this method caused pain on administration, contrary to the adult studies using the same method. Ethyl chloride vapocoolant spray applied to the puncture site has demonstrated variable effectiveness in multiple studies. Perhaps because the needle stick needs to follow the topical application almost immediately, vapocoolants have been found more effective for IM injection than for IV insertion.

Passive diffusion can be time-consuming, and during the time required for onset of anesthesia, young children may become agitated, perspire, and have difficulty keeping the anesthetic in the correct skin location. The oldest and most studied of these products, topical EMLA cream, is a eutectic mixture of lidocaine and prilocaine. EMLA is applied with an occlusive dressing directly to the skin for 60 minutes before it is effective, so it is not practical for some situations in the ED. A newer topical anesthetic cream, LMX-4, has been shown to be a very effective topical skin anesthetic. This is a topical formulation of 4% lidocaine in a liposomal delivery medium. An occlusive dressing is ideal but not required for application. In contrast to EMLA cream, LMX4 does not contain prilocaine and, therefore, does not increase the risk of methemoglobinemia in neonates. The 20-minute onset of action makes this a better topical anesthetic choice for use in the ED, but still requires some ability to predict who will need these procedures. Although there have been no safety studies in children younger than 2 years of age, there have been no reports of lidocaine toxicity in any age group with this medication.

Heat, ultrasound, laser, and iontophoresis have all been used to disrupt or more effectively bypass the lipid bilayers in the stratum corneum, thereby decreasing the anesthetic onset time for topical agents. Many of these products have proven efficacy and work efficiently; however, most require an additional mechanical apparatus attached to the skin. One more recently tested product is a self-contained topical patch containing lidocaine and prilocaine that generates heat once removed from its airtight pouch, allowing for a 20-minute onset of action. This product offers the advantage of keeping the medication where it is placed, without the potential for leakage; however, it must also be applied well in advance of the procedure, requiring accurate site choice and potentially higher cost for application at more than one site.

NERVE BLOCK

Lidocaine can be used for peripheral nerve block if the physician has appropriate knowledge of anatomy and the nerve supply to the wound is superficial. The skin at the nerve site should be anesthetized, and then lidocaine (5 mg per kg) should be infiltrated more deeply into the nerve in the same manner as the local anesthesia. During this infiltration, the physician should aspirate to ensure a blood vessel has not been penetrated inadvertently.

Some EDs use lidocaine for regional nerve block. The preferred technique for fracture reduction at some institutions is a Bier block or "mini-Bier" block. With this technique, a double pneumatic tourniquet or two blood pressure cuffs are placed above the elbow and IV lines are started in the child's upper extremities. One of these lines is for administration of lidocaine, and the other is reserved for other medications, if needed. Diazepam, midazolam, and thiopental should be available in case seizures result from lidocaine infiltration, and the child should be attached to a cardiac monitor during the procedure. Newer literature suggests the utility of intralipids in local anesthetic overdose or inadvertent IV administration, particularly with bupivacaine. The affected limb is elevated for exsanguination as the upper cuff is inflated to occlude the arterial blood supply. Then lidocaine (without epinephrine) is infused into the affected extremity at a dosage of 3 mg per kg (Bier block) or 1.5 mg per kg (mini-Bier block) (maximum 100 mg). This should be given slowly, and tourniquet pressures must be maintained so the drug does not escape under the tourniquet. Once the injured extremity has local anesthetic in an isolated compartment, the lower cuff, which should be wrapped around an anesthetized area, can be inflated. The upper cuff can be deflated. This lower cuff can be deflated very slowly after the procedure but not less than 15 minutes after the lidocaine infusion was given. The child should be observed in the ED for at least 1 hour. The Bier block has been found to be slightly more effective than the mini-Bier block. There are risks to this procedure, including seizures, coma, confusion, and cardiac arrest, if the child were to unintentionally receive a massive amount of lidocaine rapidly. Three randomly controlled trials involving Bier blocks, found no adverse effects among more than 500 procedures. Still some physicians prefer to perform the Bier block or mini-Bier block in the operating room, where circumstances can be better controlled.

PROCEDURAL SEDATION AND ANALGESIA (PSA)

PSA has replaced *conscious sedation* in the lexicon of emergency medical treatment of ill or injured patients. The American College of Emergency Physicians (ACEP) defines PSA as "techniques of administering sedatives or dissociative agents with or without analgesia to induce a state that allows the patient to tolerate unpleasant procedures while maintaining cardiorespiratory function." This definition eliminates the confusion that results when rendering a patient *less* conscious during "conscious sedation" and allows for the attainment of different levels of sedation depth dependent on the specific patient needs. The Joint Commission accepts the continuum of depth of sedation proposed by the American Society of Anesthesiologists (ASA) in 1999 (Table 4.5).

DEFINITIONS OF FOUR LEVELS OF SEDATION AND ANESTHESIA

Level	Respond purposefully (not reflexively) to	Airway and breathing maintained	Cardiovascular function maintained
Minimal sedation	Verbal commands	Yes	Yes
Moderate sedation/analgesia	Light tactile stimulation	Yes	Yes
Deep sedation/analgesia	Painful stimulation	Potentially not	Yes
Anesthesia	None	No	Potentially not

Adapted from American Academy of Pediatrics, American Academy of Pediatric Dentistry, Coté CJ, et al. Guidelines for monitoring and management of pediatric patients during and after sedation for diagnostic and therapeutic procedures: an update. *Pediatrics* 2006;118:2587–2602.

The regimens used for PSA can provide anxiolysis, sedation, dissociation, analgesia, or any combination of the four. As clinicians involved in this decision, our selection of medication is informed by knowing details about the procedure, the patient, and the particulars about the available medications (Table 4.6). The terminology assigned to a particular episode of PSA is most accurately determined by the intended effects, rather than by the specific medications used. For example, the clinician can decide that a child needs some assistance in keeping still, an increased receptiveness to distraction techniques, or amnesia for the procedure. This child requires anxiolysis rather than sedation, and will receive a relatively smaller dose of a medication that will not require cardiorespiratory monitoring. However, a child who needs to be still during a delicate procedure may require a larger dose of the same medication, after which he or she has some risk of cardiorespiratory compromise that requires more intensive monitoring.

It is best to obtain information about the procedure from the person performing it. It is important to know the length of time that the procedure will take to complete, and the time that the child may need to remain immobile. For example, one may decide to use morphine rather than fentanyl if a procedure is expected to last longer than 10 minutes. It is equally important to know the duration and severity of pain usually involved in this procedure. Some procedures, such as fracture reduction, are only brief but very painful and also require the child to remain immobile during the casting portion of the procedure. The same is true for procedures in which the administration of regional anesthesia is painful, but the remainder of the procedure is not. Finally, one must consider the level of distress that visualization of the procedure may

cause for patient and family members. Agents that provide an amnesic effect may be desirable in the case where a child could be frightened by the sight of blood or other body fluid.

The child's reaction to the procedure can be estimated from his or her current pain rating, developmental level, and initial reaction to health-care providers. Parents are often the best source of information about the child's expected reaction to the procedure. Some parents may know that, despite a pain-free procedural technique using topical anesthetic for a facial laceration, their child will be so fearful of strangers that nonpharmacologic techniques will not suffice. Conversely, a mother may express that her child was calm throughout his or her last laceration repair and believe that she can adequately distract him or her during the procedure.

SEDATION PROTOCOLS

Progression from mild sedation or analgesia to general anesthesia cannot be simply divided into discrete stages. In general, as the dose of analgesic and sedative agents increases, consciousness decreases and the risk of cardiorespiratory depression increases. A child may continue to advance along the sedation continuum until protective airway reflexes are lost and he or she is effectively under general anesthesia. It is not always possible to predict how a child will respond to medications. Although the ED physician may intend to achieve mild sedation, moderate or deep sedation may result. Thus, individuals administering moderate or deep sedation and anesthesia should be qualified (and have appropriate credentials) to manage patients at whatever level of sedation or anesthesia is achieved, either intentionally or unintentionally.

INFORMATION THAT CAN ASSIST CLINICIAN IN DETERMINING TYPE OF AGENT NEEDED FOR PROCEDURAL SEDATION AND ANALGESIA

Procedure	Patient	Agent
Expected pain severity	Current pain rating	Onset
Expected pain duration	Prior experiences	Duration
Required duration of immobility	Developmental age	Desired effects
Distressful or frightening appearance of procedure	Initial reaction to provider	Unwanted effects
	Parental expectation	

Because of the potential for respiratory depression with the sedative and analgesic agents discussed in this chapter, it is imperative that EDs develop protocols for their use. Several organizations, such as the American Academy of Pediatrics (AAP), the ACEP, and the ASA, have prepared guidelines for sedation in children. These protocols differ in certain fine points, but there is general agreement on major issues. The specifics of the ED protocol should be modified at each individual institution.

Evaluation and Preparation of Patient Prior to Sedation

The ASA recommends that clinicians administering sedation/analgesia should be familiar with aspects of the patient's medical history that may relate to the medication about to be given. This includes abnormalities of any major organ system; previous adverse experience with sedation analgesia; drug allergies; current medications; time of last oral intake of solids and liquids; and use of alcohol, tobacco, or drugs of abuse. Patients should have a focused physical examination before sedation is administered. This should include vital signs, auscultation of the heart and lungs, and evaluation of the airway. Conditions that may make endotracheal intubation more difficult (such as short neck, small mandible, large tongue, or trismus) should be noted.

For moderate and deep sedation, the ASA recommends providing patients and parents with information on the risks, benefits, and alternatives to sedation and analgesia before a procedure. The importance of preprocedure fasting is controversial, and it is not known whether preprocedure fasting results in decreased incidence of adverse outcomes. That said, the AAP recommends several dietary precautions before sedation: Infants should not have milk or solids for several hours before elective sedation (not within 4 hours for infants younger than 5 months, 6 hours for those 6 to 36 months, and 8 hours for older children). Intake of clear liquids may continue, but should cease in all cases within 2 hours of the scheduled sedation. ACEP publications have noted that there is insufficient evidence to fully support these time intervals, and offers a "level B recommendation" (moderate clinical certainty) that "procedural sedation may be safely administered to pediatric patients who have had recent oral intake." Those at risk for aspiration of gastric contents (such as those with history of gastroesophageal reflux, extreme obesity, pregnancy, or previous esophageal dysfunction) may benefit from appropriate pharmacological treatment to reduce gastric volume and increase gastric pH. For the emergency patient, sedation should still be preceded by an evaluation of food and fluid intake. It is prudent to assume that patients in the ED have full stomachs when planning the use of sedatives or analgesics. The increased risks of sedation must be weighed against the benefits and the lightest affective sedation used. Some patients may benefit from delaying the procedure or administration of appropriate pharmacological treatment to reduce gastric volume and increase gastric pH. Consider airway protection before emergency sedation.

Personnel

Personnel who are trained in pediatric life support should be available, and at least one additional support personnel should be on hand to monitor the patient. Personnel must understand the pharmacology of the sedatives they use. For deep sedation, the AAP recommends that a third person trained in pediatric resuscitation should be available to assist the patient.

Equipment

For children who are undergoing moderate sedation, emergency equipment should be available for children of all ages and sizes. This should include a suction device and a positive-pressure oxygen delivery system capable of delivering at least 90% FiO_2. In areas where moderate and deep sedation are being administered, endotracheal tubes should also be available. Reversal agents such as naloxone and flumazenil should be immediately available in the ED. Additional equipment recommendations include a nearby defibrillator and medications that might be needed for resuscitation.

Monitoring

A designated person must continuously observe the child's face and chest wall motion. Unless truly unavoidable, equipment and special drapes must not block this observation. Patients should have continuous monitoring of oxygen saturation, respiration, and heart rate with (at least) intermittent monitoring of blood pressure during and after the procedure. Continuous electrocardiographic monitoring has not been proven to affect outcome; however, it is simple, readily available, and should be routine. Monitoring with pulse oximetry is essential because of the proven difficulty in recognizing hypoxemia even by experienced personnel. Measurement of exhaled carbon dioxide ($EtCO_2$) is another modality that has been used extensively in anesthetized patients and has recently been introduced into the emergency medicine arena. Noninvasive capnography by nasal cannula is available for pediatric patients; some units combine this nasal cannula device with an oxygen delivery component as well. The visualization of the "sidestream" $EtCO_2$ waveform over time can offer the clinician insight into the ventilatory status of a nonintubated patient who has normal baseline lung function. Studies have demonstrated that monitoring of $EtCO_2$ provides earlier detection of respiratory depression than traditional monitoring techniques. Although it is not yet clear which patients require $EtCO_2$ monitoring, it would clearly be a helpful adjunct for patients receiving deep sedation, for those whose ventilation cannot be observed while receiving moderate sedation, and for those who are receiving supplemental oxygen empirically thus blunting the already limited ability of the pulse oximeter to detect hypoventilation or apnea.

The bispectral index (BIS) monitor is an electroencephalographic device that is attached to a patient's forehead and has been introduced as a potential marker of a patient's sedation level. The device has been widely used for monitoring patients receiving general anesthesia in the operating room. A patient with a BIS value of 0 has no electrical activity, and a patient with a score of 100 is wide awake. Unfortunately, specific numerical BIS values may not correlate well with other observational measurements of sedation in children undergoing ED procedures, and can be highly variable at lighter levels of sedation. Further research is needed to determine how BIS monitoring can be effectively used in pediatric emergency patients.

If a patient is expected to have deep sedation, it is recommended that an IV line be established before sedation and maintained throughout the procedure and until a patient is no longer at risk for cardiorespiratory depression. If a patient is receiving an IM agent, the clinician should determine the need for an IV based on the risk for cardiovascular compromise or the potential need for rapid sequence intubation.

Vital signs should at least be measured at baseline, after drug administration, after the procedure is completed, during early recovery, and at the completion of recovery. If deep sedation is anticipated or the child has an underlying illness, the frequency of measurement of vital signs should be increased (e.g., to every 5 minutes). Patients are at highest risk for complications from sedation during the 5 to 10 minutes after administration of the medication and during the period immediately after the procedure when stimuli are discontinued. After the procedure, appropriate staff should continue to observe patients who received sedation and continuous pulse oximetry, and monitoring of heart rate should continue until the patient has met discharge criteria. Before discharge, any child who has received moderate or deep sedation should be awake enough to sit and speak without assistance and preferably able to ambulate. Younger children should be able to perform age-appropriate functions. The child should also have adequate hydration status, documentation of stable cardiovascular function, and an adequate airway.

CHOICE OF TECHNIQUES AND MEDICATIONS

Taking the previous information into consideration, clinicians must first decide whether the child requires anxiolysis, sedation, analgesia, or some combination of the three. Patients who undergo nonpainful procedures, such as computed tomography (CT) scans or magnetic resonance imaging (MRI) scans, or those receiving regional analgesia, may be best served by receiving an agent that provides anxiolysis or sedation

alone. The following sections discuss the onset, duration, effects, and potential adverse consequences of these agents.

Anxiolysis and Sedation

Children who are undergoing painless procedures may be too young, anxious, or emotionally labile to remain still enough for the procedure to be successful. Examples include CT scans, echocardiography, and electroencephalography. Benzodiazepines can be used to provide the appropriate level of anxiolysis or sedation. It is important to remember that these agents do not provide any analgesia and should not be used alone for painful procedures. In addition, the sedative/hypnotic agents include chloral hydrate, pentobarbital, etomidate, propofol, and nitrous oxide (N_2O). Barbiturates include pentobarbital, thiopental, and methohexital. The relative advantages and disadvantages of these agents are listed in Table 4.7.

Benzodiazepines can provide anxiolysis, sedation, muscle relaxation, and amnesia during frightening or painful procedures. Benzodiazepines, such as midazolam, depress all levels of the central nervous system by binding to the gamma-aminobutyric acid (GABA) receptor complex and modulating GABA, which is a major inhibitory neurotransmitter in the brain. The dosage, routes, onset, and duration of action of the commonly used benzodiazepines are presented in Table 4.8. Of these, midazolam is considered the most efficacious during PSA, offering the advantage of rapid onset, rapid offset, and relatively wide therapeutic range. It is important to remember that the higher doses used in the transmucosal administration of benzodiazepines render the medication just as potent as if administered intravenously. The other distinct advantage of midazolam is the multiple potential routes of administration. Parenteral administration is the fastest and more reliable method; however, it requires another painful procedure (IV

TABLE 4.7

AGENTS USED FOR SEDATION OF CHILDREN IN EMERGENCY DEPARTMENT

Agent	Advantages	Disadvantages
Benzodiazepines	Multiple routes of administration Short acting Amnestic	Potentiates respiratory depression when used as adjunct
Chloral hydrate	Oral or rectal routes Pure sedative	Slow onset Long duration Paradoxical hyperactivity
Pentobarbital	Pure sedative effects Wide therapeutic range Rapid onset	Cardiorespiratory depression if given rapidly or at high dosage
Thiopental	Very rapid onset and offset	Circulatory depression
Methohexital	Very rapid onset and offset Rectal route possible	Circulatory depression Respiratory depression Twitching
Propofol	Short duration Deep sedation, amnesia	Narrow therapeutic range Respiratory depression
Etomidate	Short duration Deep sedation, amnesia	Myoclonus Possible adrenal suppression

TABLE 4.8

FEATURES OF BENZODIAZEPINES

Drug	Dosage (mg/kg)	Route	Onset (min)	Duration (h)
Midazolam (Versed®)	0.05–0.1	Intravenous (IV)	2–3	1–2
	0.1–0.2	Intramuscular (IM)	10–20	1–2
	0.5	Oral	15–30	1–1.5
	0.3–0.5	Rectal	10–30	1–1.5
	0.2–0.5	Intranasal	10–15	1
Diazepam (Valium®)	0.2 (max 10 mg)	IV, IO	1–3	0.5
	0.5 mg/kg	Rectal	10	1
Lorazepam (Ativan®)	0.05 mg/kg (max 2 mg)	IV, IO, IM	15–30	8–12

placement or IM injection). Children tolerate oral midazolam well; younger children find it less caustic than the intranasal route, and older children find it less intrusive than rectal administration. A recent report noted that midazolam can be given intranasally for anxiolysis for minor procedures in the ED, in a safe and effective manner, using an atomized delivery device. Since benzodiazepines have no analgesic properties, they are often used concomitantly with analgesics during painful procedures. This combination can lead to more side effects, particularly respiratory depression, than use of either drug alone. A reversal agent, flumazenil, can be used in case of severe adverse effects due to benzodiazepine administration. The initial dose of flumazenil is 0.01 mg per kg (maximum dose 0.2 mg) and may be repeated every 1 minute to total maximum dose of 1 mg. The duration of action is less than 60 minutes, so resedation may occur if medium- or long-acting benzodiazepines are used.

Chloral hydrate has no analgesic effects, but at recommended doses produces a light level of sleep and allows airway reflexes to be maintained. Its effects are more reliable in infants and children younger than 3 years old. Chloral hydrate is absorbed rapidly through the oral or rectal mucosa, and is then metabolized by the liver to trichloroethanol, the active ingredient. At doses of 50 to 100 mg per kg, the onset of action of chloral hydrate is between 10 and 15 minutes with the peak effect at about 60 minutes, and its effects last up to 4 to 8 hours. Although the transmucosal route of administration is advantageous, the onset and duration of action of chloral hydrate render it less useful in many emergency situations. Other clinically significant adverse effects seen in the ED are respiratory depression, hypotension, and gastrointestinal distress. Paradoxical excitability can be notable, particularly in children with developmental delay or preexisting emotional problems. The cardiorespiratory effects can be more pronounced in very young infants or those born prematurely, and the dosage, monitoring, and observation periods should be adjusted concomitantly. The recommended dose for neonates is 25 mg per kg per dose for sedation prior to procedures. Repeated doses should be used with great caution as drug metabolites accumulate with repeated use. At some centers, children younger than 1 month of age or premature infants younger than 60 weeks' postgestational age are monitored for 23 hours after chloral hydrate administration. Chloral hydrate should not be used in children with hepatic, renal, or cardiac disease.

The barbiturate medications, pentobarbital, thiopental, and methohexital, depress the reticular activating system via the GABA receptors. Barbiturates have no analgesic properties of their own and may actually increase pain perception, so they are not ideal for painful procedures. Pentobarbital is the most common barbiturate used in the ED. It has the greatest use for nonpainful procedures such as imaging studies. Sedation occurs rapidly after IV administration of 1 mg per kg (infants older than 6 months) to 2 mg per kg (children), and the effect dissipates in 15 to 20 minutes. Repeated doses of 1–2 mg/kg can be administered to a total of 3 mg/kg for infants and 6 mg/kg for children (maximum 100 mg/dose, total max 300 mg). Narcotics can also be combined with pentobarbital, but this may result in prolonged sedation, making the combination less convenient to use in a busy ED. Although used with relative success in adults, IV administration of thiopental or methohexital is not recommended when sedating children, given the severe complications resulting from intraarterial injection or local tissue infiltration. Rectal administration of methohexital offers some advantages, however, and has demonstrated shorter onset and recovery times than chloral hydrate. Rectal methohexital (20 to 30 mg per kg, maximum 500 mg) has a faster onset of action, with effects demonstrated in approximately 15 minutes. Thiopental is generally used rectally for procedural sedation in children. The rectal dose of thiopental is 5 to 10 mg per kg per dose for sedation. The barbiturates can cause respiratory depression and decrease the respiratory response to hypoxemia and can also cause decreased venous return and subsequent hypotension in hypovolemic patients. Thoipental decreases intracranial pressure and may be useful if increased intracranial pressure is a concern.

Propofol is an ultra-short-acting sedative-hypnotic with no analgesic properties. Propofol has gained favor in the ED because it has a rapid onset of action, a rapid offset, and some antiemetic and amnesic properties. However, this potent sedative has a relatively narrow therapeutic range, and the incidence of adverse events such as partial airway obstruction and apnea are slightly higher than other standard regimens. Some experts suggest using $EtCO_2$ monitoring for every propofol sedation; however, it is not yet clear that this alters outcomes in ED patients who are otherwise well monitored using standard clinical examination and monitoring procedures. Transient hypotension is expected with administration of this agent, albeit more common in patients with hypovolemia or fragile cardiovascular status. A number of studies using propofol in pediatric ED patients have indicated excellent efficacy and safety, demonstrating short recovery times and shorter overall ED times. Some have begun using propofol in conjunction with an opiate medication such as fentanyl or alfentanyl; however, this increases the risk of adverse events. Notably, the procedures performed in these studies were limited to brief, intensely painful experiences, which seem to be best suited for this medication regimen. The volume of distribution and elimination of propofol is the same in children as it is in adults, making dosing recommendations similar as well. It is administered slowly as a bolus dose of 1 mg per kg (maximum 40 mg), supplemented by 0.5 mg per kg aliquots every 3 minutes to a maximum of 4.5 mg per kg. A continuous infusion rate of 67 to 100 μg per kg per minute is preferred for procedures of longer duration. Propofol can be mixed with 0.5 mg per kg lidocaine to decrease the pain of injection, or the 0.5 mg per kg of lidocaine can be given IV into a tourniqueted arm prior to propofol administration. If used with alfentanyl, this technique may not be needed, because that drug has also been noted to decrease the incidence of pain at the IV site. Patients who are allergic to eggs or soy should not receive propofol.

Etomidate is an imidazole hypnotic agent that has gained favor as an induction agent for endotracheal intubations. It has a rapid onset of action, short duration, and exhibits less hemodynamic and respiratory effects than other sedative/hypnotic agents. Whereas the dosage used for pediatric intubations is 0.3 mg per kg, the suggested dose for sedation is 0.15 mg per kg.

Etomidate may be useful in certain rapidly performed procedures such as anterior shoulder dislocations; however, a small number of patients experience clinically significant myoclonus. The adrenal suppression ascribed to the use of etomidate is rarely clinically apparent after one dose in the emergency setting.

N_2O is an odorless gas that can be an effective agent for painful procedures (Table 4.9). It has the distinct advantage that it can be delivered painlessly through inhalation. Onset and offset of effects are 4 to 5 minutes. If no effects are noted after 5 minutes of administration, then another agent should be selected. N_2O affects the cerebral cortex, not the brainstem, so circulatory and respiratory depression does not occur and there is little relaxation of skeletal muscle. N_2O provides mainly sedative, dissociative, and amnesic effects. Frequently, the patient remains awake and able to follow instructions during the procedure. Although N_2O exhibits some analgesic effects, not all patients report complete pain relief with N_2O. Studies

have demonstrated marked pain relief in 29% of patients and partial pain relief in 61%. Because of the additional sedative effects of N_2O, it is not recommended for children who are already sedated, unconscious, or intoxicated. Patients who receive this gas describe feeling as if they are floating, drowsy, or euphoric, with some describing heaviness in their extremities. Some patients have experienced vomiting; however, this is less dangerous than other sedation regimens because patients maintain their cough and gag reflexes. Vomiting is more common in patients who report that they are susceptible to motion sickness. Prolonged intermittent dizziness has also been reported after N_2O–oxygen administration. Oversedation can occur, especially in patients who have received other sedating medications. Because N_2O rapidly diffuses into air-filled body cavities, its administration is contraindicated in patients with pneumothorax, bowel obstruction, or head injury. It is also contraindicated in pregnant patients, and pregnant staff members should not administer N_2O.

N_2O is useful for procedures that do not require systemic analgesia, either because the procedure is not very painful or the area cannot easily be anesthetized locally. This includes incision and drainage, paronychia, skin and vaginal foreign-body removal, laceration repair, burn dressing, and zipper entrapment.

Commercially available N_2O devices provide a 50-50 mixture of N_2O–oxygen, and contain a fail-safe system that shuts off the flow of N_2O when oxygen flow stops. Some delivery units require the patient to create a negative pressure of 3 to 5 cm H_2O to open the mask's "demand valve" that delivers the gas. This type of delivery system is best for children 8 years of age and older. A continuous-flow nasal mask can also be used to deliver N_2O and is more acceptable to younger children; some practitioners have developed a continuous-flow face mask that is potentially more reliable in children who typically breathe through their mouths. Each unit is fitted with a scavenger system that is connected to the vacuum system in the patient's room. The equipment is portable, but can cost several thousand dollars and must be inspected daily to ensure safety. In addition, the patient who receives N_2O requires the attention of a staff member who is skilled and experienced in the administration of the agent.

Ketamine

Ketamine hydrochloride is a dissociative anesthetic agent. It causes amnesia and a trancelike state in which the child cannot respond verbally. It also can provide some analgesia at subanesthetic doses. Ketamine is both water and lipid soluble, and therefore, can be used by IV (0.5 to 2 mg per kg) and IM routes (3 to 4 mg per kg) with equal success. The drug has a rapid onset of action (1 minute intravenously, 5 to 10 minutes intramuscularly). A single IV dose lasts about 15 minutes; however, with repeated doses or continuous infusion, its effect can last 1 to 2 hours. Ketamine can also be given orally (10 mg per kg), in which case sedation occurs within 30 to 45 minutes and lasts about 2 hours.

At the dosages used in ED procedures, ketamine does not characteristically depress spontaneous ventilation. It also allows a patient to maintain pharyngeal function and protective airway reflexes. Thus, the risk of airway compromise is less with ketamine than with some other agents. Laryngospasm may occur in less than 2% of patients; neonates and those with active respiratory infections are at higher risk for this compli-

---

TABLE 4.9

NITROUS OXIDE–OXYGEN ANALGESIA

Advantages	Disadvantages
Has rapid onset, short duration of action	Fail-safe system required
Causes sedation, dissociation, and amnesia	Expensive equipment
Is useful when local anesthesia is impractical	Scavenger device needed
May be used for young children	Not all patients benefit
Is safe when mixed with oxygen	More personnel required

cation. Importantly, the vast majority of patients who experience laryngospasm respond well to mask ventilation and do not require endotracheal intubation. The increased salivation caused by ketamine can also contribute to pharyngeal obstruction, but can be effectively prevented by prior administration of atropine (0.01 mg per kg) or glycopyrrolate (0.005 mg per kg). In summary, like any of the other PSA agents, ketamine should be used only by someone who is familiar with the uncommon complications and skilled in airway management.

In approximately 7% to 10% of pediatric patients, ketamine causes unusual, unpleasant sensations and dreams with subsequent flashbacks. Two recent prospective studies that administered midazolam *after* ketamine to pediatric patients found no effect of midazolam on recovery agitation or emergence phenomena. However, because preprocedure anxiety is strongly associated with recovery agitation, further research is needed to determine the effects of a benzodiazepine *before* the ketamine is administered. Regardless of the clinician's choice in this matter, all efforts should be made to control the environment to provide the child with a soothing, relaxing sedation induction. This includes dim lights and a prohibition on noisy movement, especially those that involve the child noticing the instruments to be used in the procedure. It is helpful to have the child choose a "dream" for himself, and ask the parent to help facilitate that dream through music, singing, or storytelling. Because of the potential agitation effects, ketamine is not recommended for use in psychotic or emotionally disturbed patients.

Vomiting can occur in up to 20% of patients who receive ketamine. However, this usually occurs in the recovery phase and may be less likely if midazolam is administered. Ketamine also can elevate blood pressure, intracranial pressure, and pulmonary artery pressure, so patients with head trauma, CNS malformations, and cardiovascular disease should not receive this drug. For many years, ketamine has been associated with increased ICP and avoided in head trauma and status epilepticus. Recent studies have cast doubt on this assumption and further research is needed.

SPECIAL SITUATIONS

The Emotionally Labile Child

There are a number of issues the clinician faces when caring for an injured child who is known to be emotionally labile. This includes children with autism, mental retardation, or an adjustment disorder. It is important to assess the child's expected emotional response in a foreign environment, use the social and emotional support available to the child at the time of the visit, and determine the need for and choice of medications for sedation and analgesia.

The parents' or caregiver's assessment of the child's anticipated emotional response is paramount in defining the best approach for the procedure. Despite an apparent lack of response to usual vocal or calming techniques, many of these children still do well if their caregivers stay near, and if it seems to them that there is less change occurring in their surroundings. These children may be taking medications already, and drug interactions must be considered when choosing a procedural sedative. However, if the child's initial medication has sedative properties (e.g., those found in phenobarbital or benzodiazepines), then simply adding or increasing a dose may be all that is needed.

Studies have demonstrated that, despite the potential for paradoxical reactions in children with emotional disorders, benzodiazepines used in the correct dosage result in better cooperation through procedures. In fact, too little of the medication may simply reduce the patient's inhibitions and worsen the situation. Ketamine, in contrast, is more likely to cause a severe emotional response at any therapeutic dose in emotionally reactive children, and so it is usually avoided in these cases. The route of administration is also an important consideration, in that some children have a strong aversion to manipulation of certain body parts.

Abdominal Pain

Few, if any, over-the-counter medications are efficacious in relieving abdominal pain. Historically, there has been a conflict between the desire to alleviate pain and the concern that analgesics will obscure the ability to accurately diagnose the patient's condition. Recent studies suggest that this concern is unwarranted: Administration of morphine lowered the pain scores of children with abdominal pain but did not alter the location of tenderness, the confidence or diagnostic accuracy of the treating physicians, or the number of children who suffered perforation of the appendix. Dispelling the myth that analgesic medications are forbidden in patients with abdominal pain is an important advance in the consideration of the "ouchless" ED.

COMPLICATIONS AND ERRORS

Most children who receive sedation and analgesia in the ED have a good outcome and benefit from the efforts to reduce pain and anxiety during a procedure. However, administration of sedative and analgesic agents to children in the ED always carries some risk to the patient and potential liability for the provider. There is always a chance for error with such medications. Some errors are fatal; many are preventable. One study showed that up to 17% of pediatric procedural sedations have some type of complication. Most adverse events are respiratory and 1/200 require interventions to maintain a patent airway and to ventilate the patient. One in every 1,500 sedations results in an event that requires unanticipated admission to the hospital. Those providing care to sedated children must take steps in advance of a procedure, and vigilantly monitor the child during a procedure in order to minimize potential adverse outcomes. A recent study showed inadequate and inconsistent monitoring (particularly failure to use or appropriately respond to pulse oximetry) was a major factor contributing to poor outcome in sedated children.

The needs of the provider or the institution must not be placed ahead of the safety or comfort of the patient. A physician should always prepare, and ensure adequate staffing, for a deeper level of sedation than originally planned.

Medication Errors

All ED staff, including physicians, nurses, pharmacists, support staff, and others should take steps to prevent medication errors. Look-alike and sound-alike drugs, sometimes with similar packaging, are contributing factors in some errors. Caution should be used in stocking medications.

Allergic reactions are potential complications with any medications. Preventable errors related to medication allergies may occur when the health-care provider fails to obtain an adequate medical history, fails to read the record, or does not review previously documented allergies.

Some of the more serious medication errors involve a misplaced decimal point, which can result in a tenfold error. It is thus recommended when writing medication orders to place a zero before a decimal point to express a number less than one (e.g., 0.5 mL). However, one should never use a terminal zero (e.g., 5.0) because failure to see the decimal point may result in the patient getting ten times the dose desired. Also, write the word "units" rather than "u," which can be misinterpreted as an extra zero. Many other medication errors are due to incorrect computation. Some of these may be preventable by electronic order technology where only approved drug doses are accepted by the computer. Studies performed on inpatient units have shown that computerized physician order entry systems have reduced medication errors by 55%. More studies in the ED setting need to be conducted to determine if this reduction is comparable.

Institutions are required by the Joint Commission and the Center for Medicaid and Medicare Services (CMS) to establish a list of "high-alert" drugs that would require special or additional checks in their dosing, preparation, and administration. Double check medication dosages before any drugs are given. Research shows that 95% of all mistakes are found when someone checks the work of another. Double checks are more effective when performed independently. It is best to verify a colleague's result without visually examining the calculations that allowed them to arrive at that result. The checker might otherwise be drawn into the calculator's mistake, when he or she is only shown his or her calculations. Tenfold errors are easily missed this way.

Having a satellite pharmacy that serves the ED with unit dosing rather than having nurses prepare medications may be beneficial. It is interesting to note that, in the hospital setting, 39% of errors are detected before reaching the patient. In the ED setting, only 23% of errors are detected before reaching the patient. This may be related to the lack of a pharmacist's involvement in most ED decisions.

Take time to be sure all necessary equipment and medications are in place before giving sedative agents. The SOAPME checklist is familiar to many and reminds the clinician to plan in advance [Suction, Oxygen, Airway (appropriate-sized equipment), Pharmacy (drugs needed), Monitors, Equipment (perhaps a defibrillator)]. The Joint Commission advocates a "time-out" before any medication is given to verify the correct patient, site, and medications. Anticipate complications such as laryngospasm. Have a back-up plan for complications before they arise. The Joint Commission emphasizes the concept of "sedation rescue," which is essential to safe sedation. The ability to rescue a patient after an adverse event is also emphasized by AAP guidelines.

Documentation

Careful documentation of the use of sedatives and analgesics is extremely important. If an inpatient or outpatient record already exists, there is no need to repeat the information previously documented. However, a brief note is recommended to indicate that the chart was reviewed before giving sedative agents. A note indicating the child's pre-sedation status is helpful and there should be a notation that the patient's condition has not changed since arrival or since the last exam in the record.

When using sedatives and analgesics, a well-designed, time-based record is essential. The use of a separate form or checklist is particularly useful as a supplement to the ED note. The checklist may improve efficiency. It may serve to remind the caregiver to ask specific questions or perform a specific part of the physical examination. The record should indicate any history of allergies or adverse drug reactions, as well as medications used prior to sedation. It is wise to place this information near the section for writing the sedation orders so they can be reviewed when medications are ordered.

The physical examination should focus on the airway and cardiovascular system. The patient's weight must be carefully recorded in an obvious location in the record and it is best to record this consistently in kilograms. Dosing errors are the leading category of mishaps involving medications and about 10% of these are related to an incorrect weight (obtained or recorded incorrectly) for the child. It is also helpful to document the child's level of consciousness during the procedure (e.g., how he or she responds to verbal commands or tactile stimulation). Note the patient's level of consciousness again prior to discharge.

Discharge instructions must be reviewed with the child's guardian before the patient is allowed to go home. They may be preprinted and include a reminder to parents that the child should not be involved in activities that require coordination such as bicycle riding or skating for perhaps 24 hours. Adult supervision should be recommended for at least 8 hours. Unsupervised bathing and use of electrical devices or other possibly dangerous items should not be permitted for at least 8 hours.

SUMMARY

It is common to encounter children in pain in the pediatric ED. It is often difficult, but not impossible to avoid inflicting pain on some children in this setting. Management should be accomplished with nonpharmacologic techniques such as hypnosis and distraction, along with various narcotic and nonnarcotic analgesics, local and topical anesthetics, and sedative-hypnotics. Other agents, such as N_2O, ketamine, and propofol, play a more limited role in reducing pain and distress in the pediatric patient. Gentle restraint is needed occasionally and reassurance is of paramount importance.

Suggested Readings

Agrawal D, Manzi SF, Gupta R, et al. Preprocedural fasting state and adverse events in children undergoing procedural sedation and analgesia in a pediatric emergency department. *Ann Emerg Med* 2003;42:636–646.

Alexander J, Manno M. Underuse of analgesia in very young pediatric patients with isolated painful injuries. *Ann Emerg Med* 2003;41:617–622.

Allison KP, Smith G. Burn management in a patient with autism. *Burns* 1998;24:484–486.

American Academy of Pediatrics, American Academy of Pediatric Dentistry, Coté CJ, et al. Guidelines for monitoring and management of pediatric patients during and after sedation for diagnostic and therapeutic procedures: an update. *Pediatrics* 2006;118(6):2587–2602.

American Society of Anesthesiologists Task Force on Sedation and Analgesia by Non-Anesthesiologists. Practice guidelines for sedation and analgesia by non-anesthesiologists. *Anesthesiology* 2002;96:1004–1017.

Annequin D, Carbajal R, Chauvin P, et al. Fixed 50% nitrous oxide oxygen mixture for painful procedures: a French survey. *Pediatrics* 2000;105(4):e47. Available at: http://www.pediatrics.org/cgi/content/full/105/4/e47.

Bartfield JM, Janikas JS, Lee RS. Heart rate response to intravenous catheter placement. *Acad Emerg Med* 2003;10:1005–1008.

Bassett KE, Anderson JL, Pribble CG, et al. Propofol for procedural sedation in children in the emergency department. *Ann Emerg Med* 2003;42: 773–782.

Berde CB, Sethna NF. Analgesics for the treatment of pain in children. *N Engl J Med* 2002;347:1094–1091.

Bijur PE, Silver W, Gallagher EJ. Reliability of the visual analog scale for measurement of acute pain. *Acad Emerg Med* 2001;8:1153–1157.

Bird SB, Dickson EW. Clinically significant changes in pain along the visual analog scale. *Ann Emerg Med* 2001;38:639–643.

Boudreaux ED, Francis JL, Loyacano T. Family presence during invasive procedures and resuscitations in the emergency department: a critical review and suggestions for future research. *Ann Emerg Med* 2002;40:193–205.

Brown JC, Klein EJ, Lewis CW, et al. Emergency department analgesia for fracture pain. *Ann Emerg Med* 2003;42:197–205.

Burton JH, Bock AJ, Strout TD, et al. Etomidate and midazolam for reduction of anterior shoulder dislocation: a randomized controlled trial. *Ann Emerg Med* 2002;40:496–504.

Cravero JP, Bilke GT, Beach M, et al. Incidence and nature of adverse events during pediatric sedation/anesthesia for procedures outside the operating room: report from the pediatric sedation research consortium. *Pediatrics* 2006;118: 1087–1096.

Di Liddo L, D'Angelo A, Nguyen B, et al. Etomidate versus midazolam for procedural sedation in pediatric outpatients: a randomized controlled trial. *Ann Emerg Med* 2006;48:433–440.

Dingeman RS, Mitchell EA, Meyer EC, et al. Parent presence during complex invasive procedures and cardiopulmonary resuscitation: a systematic review of the literature. *Pediatrics* 2007;120:842–854.

Doyle L, Colletti JE. Pediatric procedural sedation and analgesia. *Pediatr Clin North Am.* 2006;53:279–292.

Drendel AL, Brousseau DC, Gorelick MH. Pain assessment for pediatric patients in the emergency department. *Pediatrics* 2006;117:1511–1518.

Eichenfield LF, Funk A, Fallon-Friedlander S, et al. A clinical study to evaluate the efficacy of ELA-Max (4% liposomal lidocaine) as compared with eutectic mixture of local anesthetics cream for pain reduction of venipuncture in children. *Pediatrics* 2002;109:1093–1099.

Fassler D, Wallace N. Children's fear of needles. *Clin Pediatr* 1982;21:59–60.

Fein JA, Boardman CR, Stevenson S, et al. Saline with benzyl alcohol as intradermal anesthesia for intravenous line placement in children. *Pediatr Emerg Care* 1998;14:119–122.

Gill M, Green SM, Krauss B. Can the bispectral index monitor quantify altered level of consciousness in emergency department patients? *Acad Emerg Med* 2003;10:175–179.

Gradin M, Eriksson M, Holmqvist G, et al. Pain reduction at venipuncture in newborns: oral glucose compared with local anesthetic cream. *Pediatrics* 2002;110:1053–1057.

Green SM, Kupperman N, Rothrock SG, et al. Predictors of adverse events with intramuscular ketamine sedation in children. *Ann Emerg Med* 2000;35:35–42.

Green SM, Rothrock SG, Lynch EL, et al. Intramuscular ketamine for pediatric sedation in the emergency department: safety profile in 1,022 cases. *Ann Emerg Med* 1998;31(6):688–697.

Green SM. Fasting is a consideration—not a necessity—for emergency department procedural sedation and analgesia. *Ann Emerg Med* 2003;42(5): 647–650.

Green SM. Research advances in procedural sedation and analgesia. *Ann Emerg Med* 2007;49:31–36.

Hardwick WE, Givens TG, Monroe KW, et al. Effect of ketorolac in pediatric sickle cell vaso-occlusive pain crisis. *Pediatr Emerg Care* 1999;15:179–182.

Havel CJ Jr, Strait RT, Hennes H. A clinical trial of propofol vs. midazolam for procedural sedation in a pediatric emergency department. *Acad Emerg Med* 1999;6:989–997.

Hertzog JH, Dalton HJ, Anderson BD, et al. Prospective evaluation of propofol anesthesia in the pediatric intensive care unit for elective oncology procedures in ambulatory and hospitalized children. *Pediatrics* 2000;106: 742–747.

Joint Commission on Accreditation of Healthcare Organizations. *Comprehensive accreditation manual for hospitals: The official handbook by the JCAHO.* Oakbrook Terrace, IL: Joint Commission on Accreditation of Healthcare Organizations, 2005.

Kelly AM, Powel CV, Williams A. Parent visual analogue scale ratings of children's pain do not reliably reflect pain reported by child. *Pediatr Emerg Care* 2002;18(3):159–162.

Kennedy RM, McAllister JD. Midazolam with ketamine: who benefits? *Ann Emerg Med* 2000;35:297–299.

Kim MK, Strait RT, Sato TT, et al. A randomized clinical trial of analgesia in children with acute abdominal pain. *Acad Emerg Med* 2002;9:281–287.

Klassen JA, Liang Y, Tjosvold L, et al. Music for pain and anxiety in children undergoing medical procedures: a systematic review of randomized controlled trials. *Ambul Pediatr* 2008;8:117–128.

Koller DM, Myers AB, Lorenz D, Godambe SA. Effectiveness of oxycodone, ibuprofen or the combination in the initial management of orthopedic injury-related pain in children. *Pediatr Emerg Care* 2007;23:627–633.

Lane RD, Schunk JE. Atomized intranasal midazolam use for minor procedures in the pediatric emergency department. *Pediatr Emerg Care* 2008;24: 300–303.

Luhmann JD, Kennedy RM, Lang Porter F, et al. A randomized clinical trial of continuous-flow nitrous oxide and midazolam for sedation of young children during laceration repair. *Ann Emerg Med* 2001;37:20–27.

Mace SE, Brown LA, Francis L, et al. Clinical policy: critical issues in the sedation of pediatric patients in the emergency department. *Ann Emerg Med* 2008;51:378–399.

McGrath PJ, Johnson G, Goodman JT, et al. CHEOPS: a behavioral scale for rating postoperative pain in children. In: Fields HL, eds. *Advances in pain research and therapy.* New York: Raven Press, 1985:395–402.

Migita RT, Klein EJ, Garrison MM. Sedation and analgesia for pediatric fracture reduction in the emergency department—A systematic review. *Arch Pediatr Adolesc Med* 2006;160:46–51.

Miner JR, Biros MH, Heegaard W, et al. Bispectral electroencephalographic analysis of patients undergoing procedural sedation in the emergency department. *Acad Emerg Med* 2003;10:638–643.

Pershad J, Kost S. Emergency department based sedation services. *Clin Pediatr Emerg Med* 2007;8:253–261.

Powell CV, Kelly AM, Williams A. Determining the minimum clinically significant difference in visual analog pain score for children. *Ann Emerg Med* 2001;37:28–31.

Priestly S, Kelly AM, Chow L, et al. Application of topical local anesthetic at triage reduces treatment time for children with lacerations: a randomized controlled trial. *Ann Emerg Med* 2003;42:34–40.

Probst BD, Lyons E, Leonard D, et al. Factors affecting emergency department assessment and management of pain in children. *Pediatr Emerg Care* 2005; 21:298–305.

Roback MG, Bajaj L, Wathen JE, et al. Preprocedural fasting and adverse events in procedural sedation and analgesia in a pediatric emergency department: are they related? *Ann Emerg Med* 2004;44:454–459.

Roback MG, Wathen JE, Bajaj L, Bothner JP. Adverse events associated with procedural sedation and analgesia in a pediatric emergency department: a comparison of common parental drugs. *Acad Emerg Med* 2005;12:508–513.

Sacchetti A, Gerardi M. Procedural sedation for patients with special health needs. In: Krauss B, Brustowicz R, eds. *Pediatric procedural sedation and analgesia.* Philadelphia: Lippincott Williams & Wilkins, 1999:189–199.

Selbst SM, Clark M. Analgesic use in the emergency department. *Ann Emerg Med* 1990;19:1010–1013.

Sherwin TS, Green SM, Khan A, et al. Does adjunctive midazolam reduce recovery agitation after ketamine sedation for pediatric procedures? A randomized, double-blind, placebo-controlled trial. *Ann Emerg Med* 2000;35:229–238.

Singer AJ, Gulla J, Thode HC, Jr. Parents and practitioners are poor judges of young children's pain severity. *Acad Emerg Med* 2002;9:609–612.

Singer AJ, Stark MJ. LET versus EMLA for pre-treating lacerations: a randomized trial. *Acad Emerg Med* 2001;8:223–230.

Sinha M, Christopher N, Fenn R, et al. Evaluation of nonpharmacologic methods of pain and anxiety management for laceration repair in the pediatric emergency department. *Pediatrics* 2006;117:1163–1168.

Taddio A, Nulman I, Koren BS, et al. A revised measure of acute pain in infants. *J Pain Symptom Manage* 1995;10:456–463.

Taddio A, Shah V, Gilbert-MacLeod C, et al. Conditioning and hyperalgesia in newborns exposed to repeated heel lances. *JAMA* 2002;288:857–861.

Van Der Walt JH, Moran C. An audit of perioperative management of autistic children. *Paediatr Anaesth* 2001;11:401–408.

Wathen JE, Roback MG, Mackenzie T, et al. Does midazolam alter the clinical effects of intravenous ketamine sedation in children? A double-blind, randomized, controlled, emergency department trial. *Ann Emerg Med* 2000;36: 579–588.

Williams DG, Hatch DJ, Howard RF. Codeine phosphate in paediatric medicine. *Br J Anaesth* 2001;86:413–421.

Yen K, Kim M, Stremski ES, et al. Effect of ethnicity and race on the use of pain medications in children with long bone fractures in the emergency department. *Ann Emerg Med* 2003;42:41–47.

Young KD. Pediatric procedural pain. *Ann Emerg Med* 2005;45:160–171.

Zempsky WT, Cravero JP, Committee on Pediatric Emergency Medicine and Section on Anesthesiology and Pain Medicine, et al. Relief of pain and anxiety in pediatric patients in emergency medical systems. *Pediatrics* 2004;114: 1348–1356.

Zempsky WT, Schecter NL. What's new in the management of pain in children. *Pediatr Rev* 2003;24:337–347.

Zempsky WT. Developing the painless emergency department: a systematic approach to change. *Clin Pediatr Emerg Med* 2000;1:253–259.

CHAPTER 5 ■ EMERGENCY AIRWAY MANAGEMENT—RAPID SEQUENCE INTUBATION

LOREN G. YAMAMOTO, MD, MPH, MBA, FAAP, FACEP

Management of the airway is a critical initial step in the stabilization of patients who present to the emergency department (ED) with a life-threatening emergency. Endotracheal (ET) intubation is often the most reliable means of maintaining airway control. Indications for ET intubation include cardiopulmonary arrest, apnea, respiratory insufficiency, actual or potential airway obstruction, respiratory depression, severe burns, severe multiple trauma, severe head injury, increased intracranial pressure (ICP), a depressed sensorium, and a loss of the normal protective airway reflexes.

Airway management is most optimal when the ED staff is trained to recognize the need for intubation and to accomplish this while minimizing complications. The equipment necessary for ET intubation should be readily available at the bedside for immediate access and use during the management of any critically ill patient in the ED (Table 5.1).

ET intubation can be difficult when seizures, agitation, combativeness, and inadequate muscle relaxation, result in poor airway visualization. Laryngoscopy and intubation potentially result in ICP elevation, pain, bradycardia, and a higher risk of gastric regurgitation and hypoxemia. Patients who arrive in the ED often have not been fasted.

Although intubation can often be accomplished under these circumstances, the conditions are optimized and the adverse effects are minimized when a patient is intubated using rapid sequence intubation (RSI)—a rapid induction of general anesthesia that induces unconsciousness and muscle relaxation. The purpose of RSI is to rapidly render a patient unconscious and paralyzed so that intubation can be facilitated. Emergency intubations performed under a fully relaxed state are usually easier to perform and have fewer adverse effects, such as pain and ICP elevation.

While RSI and rapid sequence induction are both referred to as RSI, the former terminology is more commonly used in emergency medicine, while the latter is used more commonly in anesthesia. This difference is not absolute; however, the purpose of RSI in the ED is most often to emergently intubate a patient, while the purpose of RSI in the operating room is less emergent.

Pharmacologic paralysis makes it impossible to perform a neurologic examination on the patient and eliminates all respiratory effort by the patient. Would it be preferable to sedate a patient without paralysis for intubation because of these considerations? Although this was a common practice in the past, intubation using sedation alone has a higher complication rate than RSI does, making RSI the preferred technique.

RSI is not necessarily indicated in cardiac arrest. In cardiac arrest, for example, intubation without RSI would generally be preferable unless cardiopulmonary resuscitation, brain perfusion, muscle tone, and/or some degree of consciousness were maintained, in which case RSI may be of benefit. Understanding the principles of RSI is the best means of determining when it is indicated.

A typical RSI consists of premedications (most often lidocaine and/or atropine) to block vagal stimulation, a sedative to induce unconsciousness, and a muscle relaxant to induce paralysis. This typical sequence can become rather complicated when more considerations are added. It should be noted that the drugs for pediatric RSI have been recommended in their most basic forms as (i) premedications, (ii) sedative, and (iii) muscle relaxant. This chapter addresses the following controversies surrounding RSI: sedative selection, muscle relaxant selection, priming or defasciculation, and adjunctive medications such as lidocaine and fentanyl.

RAPID SEQUENCE INTUBATION SEDATIVES

The most common sedatives used in RSI include thiopental, ketamine, etomidate, propofol, midazolam (and other benzodiazepines). Narcotic analgesics such as fentanyl can also be used, but this is less common. Each drug has both beneficial and detrimental properties that must be understood to select the best sedative for RSI in the patient at hand. The advantages and disadvantages of each drug are summarized in Table 5.2. The most recent controversies in sedative selection include RSI indications for ketamine, etomidate and propofol.

Thiopental (an ultrashort-acting barbiturate) was initially one of the most commonly used sedatives for RSI. Its advantages are reliability and rapid onset (10 to 20 seconds), short duration, and a cerebral protective effect accomplished by reducing ICP, cerebral metabolism, and cerebral oxygen demand. Its main disadvantages are vasodilation and myocardial depression, which may result in profound hypotension. Thiopental should be avoided or used in lower dosages in hypotensive or hypovolemic patients. These effects can be also minimized by slowing the rate of injection. Thiopental causes respiratory depression and may result in coughing, laryngospasm, and bronchospasm. Thiopental is contraindicated in porphyria and status asthmaticus.

Ketamine produces rapid sedation, amnesia, and analgesia. It is described as a dissociative agent that induces a trancelike state in which the patient is unaware, but not necessarily asleep. In combination with a paralyzing agent as in RSI, this difference is not noticeable. Ketamine results in sympathetic stimulation and an increase in systemic blood pressure (BP); however, reduced doses or avoidance of a sedative are still recommended

TABLE 5.1

EQUIPMENT NEEDED FOR RAPID SEQUENCE
INTUBATION

Pulse oximeter
End-tidal CO_2, monitor or detector
Electrocardiogram monitor
Uncuffed endotracheal tubes, sizes 2.5–6.0
Cuffed endotracheal tubes, sizes 6.0–8.5 (cuffed tubes smaller
    than 6.0 are available)
Endotracheal tube stylets
Laryngoscopes (straight blade sizes 0–3, curved blade sizes 2–4)
Oral airways
Oxygen masks, preferably a nonrebreather
Ventilation masks in all sizes for bag-valve-mask ventilation
Large and small self-inflating ventilation bag with oxygen
    reservoir tail and positive end-expiratory pressure valve
    attachment. Rusch type anesthesia bags can also be used
    but require a pressurized oxygen source and can be more
    difficult to ventilate large patients.
Laryngeal mask airways in all sizes
Oxygen source
Suctioning source
Large-bore stiff suction tips
Flexible suction catheters
Nasogastric tubes
Tracheostomy tubes
Tracheostomy surgical instrument set
12- and 14-gauge needle catheters for needle cricothyrotomy
Preassembled transtracheal ventilation setup

in potentially hypovolemic patients. Adverse effects, which include ICP elevation, intraocular pressure elevation, hallucinations, excessive airway secretions, and laryngospasm, limit its use to ED patients who have hypotension, hypovolemia, or status asthmaticus. Recent studies have been published addressing the use of ketamine in patients with elevated ICP, long thought to be a contraindication. More research is needed to substantiate these findings. Ketamine increases airway secretions, so routine atropine premedication is recommended. Ketamine has a bronchodilating effect, making it useful for RSI of patients with severe bronchospasm that requires intubation. Ketamine is contraindicated in patients with hypertension, head injury, psychiatric problems, glaucoma, or an open globe injury. In some older children the psychological reactions to ketamine have severely limited its use. However, this is rarely a problem when using ketamine for RSI as the effect of the medication will generally dissipate prior to extubation and awakening. These reactions usually disappear upon awakening but can be recurrent. The frequency of psychiatric disturbances with ketamine (sometimes reported to be 5% to 30%) are less common in children. Other reports have shown no significant adverse psychological effects compared with other sedatives. The use of benzodiazepines during ketamine anesthesia have been alleged to reduce the likelihood of adverse psychological effects; however recent studies do not clearly prove this. It is unclear whether benziodiazepine treatment is necessary, but its downside risk is minimal when using during RSI.

Etomidate has more recently been advocated as an RSI sedative. Although most RSI sedatives have advantages in certain clinical situations and disadvantages in others, etomidate has advantages in the broadest range of RSI patients. It shares some advantages of thiopental—rapid and reliable onset of unconsciousness, ICP reduction, and reduction of cerebral metabolic demand. Etomidate has minimal cardiovascular depression compared with thiopental. Etomidate at first glance appears to have superior cerebroprotective properties because it lowers ICP and cerebral metabolism with better preservation of cerebral perfusion pressure compared with thiopental. Etomidate is associated with myoclonus-resembling seizures. The frequency with which this occurs ranges from 10% to 80% in various reports. However, the etiology is not well-defined. Although etomidate has some anticonvulsant properties, it also appears to stimulate

TABLE 5.2

SIGNIFICANT PROPERTIES OF RAPID SEQUENCE INTUBATION SEDATIVES

Drug	Onset	Duration	Cerebroprotective effect	Cardiovascular effect	Bronchial effect	Other disadvantages
Thiopental	Rapid	Brief	Good	Significant depression	Bronchospasm	
Ketamine	Rapid	Brief	Adverse	Stimulatory	Bronchodilatory	Psychic reactions and excessive airway secretions
Etomidate	Rapid	Brief	Good	Neutral	Neutral	Myoclonus, cortisol suppression
Propofol	Rapid	Brief	Good	Significant depression	Neutral	Less experience with agent in emergency department rapid sequence intubation (RSI)
Midazolam	Less rapid	Brief	Modest	Neutral	Neutral	Titration recommended, is not feasible in RSI
Fentanyl	Less rapid	Brief	Modest	Neutral	Neutral	Seizure-like activity and chest wall rigidity

seizures in others. Etomidate suppresses glucocorticoid and mineralocorticoid levels. This effect is clearly clinically significant in long-term administration of etomidate. Single use as in ED RSI results in measurable decreases in corticosteroid levels, and more recent studies have concluded that this is likely to be clinically significant in shock states, especially in septic shock. It is unproven, but it makes logical sense to administer corticosteroids when etomidate is used to offset this problem. Although unproven, etomidate should not be used in patients with partial seizures and adrenal insufficiency. Because of its broad applicability for RSI, some experts have recommended that etomidate be the standard sedative used for RSI. Etomidate clearly has the broadest set of indications in RSI. Sedative selection is a difficult aspect of RSI, and etomidate potentially simplifies this decision. It is important for the clinician to remember that etomidate has no analgesic properties and is extremely short acting (~5 minutes), and plans must be in place for post-intubation sedation and analgesia.

Propofol use in the ED is increasing in frequency. It is largely used by anesthesiologists for short-term sedation and general anesthesia. It can be used as a sedative in RSI, but its degree of experience here is limited and it does not have substantial advantages over other sedatives. Propofol shares many features with thiopental. Propofol decreases ICP and cerebral metabolism. Propofol's onset is rapid and brief, but it can result in significant cardiovascular depression. Although propofol can be used in instances when thiopental could be used, there is more experience with thiopental.

Midazolam (and other benzodiazepines such as diazepam) has a slower onset than thiopental. It is more commonly used for mild or moderate sedation or as an adjunctive agent in general anesthesia. Midazolam is capable of anesthesia induction at higher dosages. Cardiovascular and respiratory depression occur less often than with barbiturates. Lack of recall or anterograde amnesia results from benzodiazepines used for anesthesia. Benzodiazepines should not be used in patients with glaucoma. Midazolam has many properties that suggest its use for RSI in the ED. Many reports in the literature have advocated its use despite the lack of data to document its deep sedation efficacy. The dosing range is suggested at 0.1 to 0.3 mg per kg. The lower dosage is clearly insufficient to reliably induce unconsciousness. Because these drugs also result in amnesia, studies may never be able to retrospectively assess the degree of unconsciousness attained during RSI.

Fentanyl is a short-acting narcotic analgesic that results in rapid analgesia and unconsciousness at higher dosages. Adverse effects associated with fentanyl are less than those of morphine. The doses of narcotics required to produce complete anesthesia are much higher than the doses required for analgesia alone and may vary extensively. Chest wall rigidity may occur with rapid injection of fentanyl, but this is preventable with slow administration and is sometimes reversible with naloxone, although a muscle relaxant may be required to adequately ventilate the patient. Fentanyl use has been associated with seizure-like activity. Fentanyl is used most often in cardiovascular surgery in combination with other anesthetics. Although it has some properties useful for RSI performed in the ED, literature sources to support fentanyl use for RSI in the ED are lacking. Fentanyl should not be used with monoamine oxidase inhibitors.

Although myocardial depression is most pronounced with thiopental, all sedatives cause some degree of cardiovascular depression, especially in hypotensive or hypovolemic patients. Because no sedative is entirely free of cardiovascular depression in the hypovolemic or hypotensive patient, such patients should receive reduced dosages or no sedative at all, depending on their cardiovascular status.

SEDATIVE SELECTION

Sedative selection remains one of the most controversial aspects of RSI. Etomidate appears to have the broadest applicability, but each agent should be well understood so individual practitioners can make the best decisions about which agent would be most optimal in each clinical situation. The clinical situation determines the optimal sedative selection. Table 5.3 summarizes sedative selections in different clinical categories.

The purpose of the sedative is to render the patient unconscious, while the paralyzing agent facilitates intubation. However, at least one study has demonstrated that thiopental and propofol facilitate intubation better than etomidate, ketamine, and benzodiazepines.

Although etomidate and propofol are said to be cerebroprotective, it is difficult to find the original data that compares the cerebroprotective properties of etomidate and propofol compared to thiopental and other barbiturates. Propofol has no significant advantages over thiopental and etomidate for RSI, making it difficult to justify its use here. It is generally agreed that barbiturate coma remains the standard means of cerebroprotection. Etomidate coma has not replaced barbiturate coma in this regard suggesting that etomidate's cerebroprotection has not been demonstrated to be superior to that of barbiturates. Additionally the risk of increased morbidity and mortality from adrenocortical suppression associated with continuous infusion or repeated doses of etomidate makes it unappealing for this use.

Etomidate can potentially be used in most clinical situations, but upon careful consideration, there may be superior alternatives in many situations. Thiopental can be used for all patients except those with hypotension, hypovolemia, status asthmaticus, or porphyria. In patients with suspected head injuries who have severe hypovolemia or hypotension, thiopental should be avoided. Any sedation agent may compromise cardiovascular function in such a state. There is not enough information in the literature to establish a clear consensus about which sedative would be the most optimal in this situation. Etomidate, a low-dose sedative or no sedative would be among the best options.

In potentially hypovolemic patients with suspected head injuries, etomidate, midazolam, or low-dose thiopental may be used in conjunction with volume resuscitation. Midazolam has the major disadvantage of ideally requiring titration, which is not feasible in RSI, making it difficult to justify its selection. Etomidate might be preferred over low-dose thiopental here.

In head injury patients without hypovolemia or hypotension, thiopental or etomidate both have cerebroprotective properties; however, if barbiturate cerebroprotection is superior to etomidate's cerebroprotection, then thiopental should be preferred. While propofol could be used here, it has no properties that make it superior to thiopental or etomidate for RSI. In a patient without head injuries who has hypotension/hypovolemia, ketamine or etomidate may produce the least

TABLE 5.3

RAPID SEQUENCE INTUBATION DRUGS AND DOSES (in mg)

Age	2 mo	6 mo	1 yr	3 yr	5 yr	7 yr	9 yr	11 yr	12 yr	14 yr	16 yr	Adult
Average weight (kg)	5	8	10	15	19	23	29	36	44	50	58	65

1. Preoxygenation: Positive-pressure ventilation with cricoid pressure only if hypoventilating or hypoxic
2. Adjunctive agents

   Atropine (0.01–0.02 mg/kg): Optional in adults not requiring ketamine (1 mg maximum dose)

	2 mo	6 mo	1 yr	3 yr	5 yr	7 yr	9 yr	11 yr	12 yr	14 yr	16 yr	Adult
	0.1	0.15	0.2	0.3	0.3	0.4	0.5	0.5	0.5–1	0.5–1	0.5–1	0.5–1

   Lidocaine (1.5 mg/kg): Use when ICP elevation is suspected (otherwise, it is optional—see text)

	2 mo	6 mo	1 yr	3 yr	5 yr	7 yr	9 yr	11 yr	12 yr	14 yr	16 yr	Adult
	8	12	15	22	28	35	44	54	66	75	90	100

3. Assess ability to establish ventilation if intubation fails; do not proceed if inability to mask ventilate is anticipated
4. Sellick maneuver (cricoid pressure): Do not release until intubation is confirmed
5. Paralyzing agent: Choose one—see text

	2 mo	6 mo	1 yr	3 yr	5 yr	7 yr	9 yr	11 yr	12 yr	14 yr	16 yr	Adult
Rocuronium (0.6–1 mg/kg)	4	6	9	12	15	20	25	30	40	45	50	60
Succinylcholine (1–2 mg/kg)	8	12	15	25	30	40	50	55	60	65	70	80
Vecuronium (0.1–0.2 mg/kg)	0.5	1.5	2	3	4	5	6	7	8	10	11	13

6. Sedation agent: problem specific

   Head injury without hypotension: (i) thiopental, (ii) etomidate
   Head injury with mild hypotension: (i) etomidate, (ii) half dose thiopental
   Hypotension: (i) ketamine, (ii) etomidate. Consider reduced dose or no sedative at all since any sedative can worsen hypotension.
   Status asthmaticus: (i) ketamine, (ii) etomidate
   Status epilepticus: (i) thiopental, (ii) benzodiazepine

	2 mo	6 mo	1 yr	3 yr	5 yr	7 yr	9 yr	11 yr	12 yr	14 yr	16 yr	Adult
Thiopental (3–5 mg/kg)	15–25	24–40	30–50	45–75	60–90	70–115	90–145	110–180	130–200	150–250	170–290	200–325
Etomidate (0.3 mg/kg)	1.5	2.5	3	4.5	6	7	9	10	13	15	17	20
Ketamine (1–2 mg/kg)	5–10	8–16	10–20	15–30	19–38	23–46	30–60	35–70	45–90	50–100	60–100	65–100

7. Intubate

	2 mo	6 mo	1 yr	3 yr	5 yr	7 yr	9 yr	11 yr	12 yr	14 yr	16 yr	Adult
[endotracheal (ET) tube size]	3.5	3.5	4.0	4.5	5.0	5.5	6.0	6.5	7.0	7.0 female, 8.0 male		
ET tube depth at lip (cm)	11	12	13	14	15	16	18	19	20	22	22	22
Laryngoscope blade size	1	1	1	2	2	2	2	2	3	3	3	3–4

8. Optional NG/OG tube (F)

	2 mo	6 mo	1 yr	3 yr	5 yr	7 yr	9 yr	11 yr	12 yr	14 yr	16 yr	Adult
	8	10	10	12	12	12	14	14	16	16	16	16

9. Longer-acting sedation and/or paralysis as needed
10. If reversal of rocuronium is needed (see text)

adverse effects. Atropine should be used with ketamine. No sedative or a low dosage of sedative (ketamine, etomidate, or thiopental) is recommended in severe hypotension/hypovolemia to reduce the likelihood of cardiovascular collapse in patients with maximal endogenous sympathetic stimulation while ensuring that the patient is not aware of being paralyzed. Etomidate's adverse effect of adrenal suppression becomes potentially more important in shock states.

Ketamine or benzodiazepines have been recommended for sedating patients with status asthmaticus who require intubation; however, ketamine is associated with a bronchodilatory effect, whereas benzodiazepines are not. Etomidate can be used here, but ketamine has superior characteristics for severe status asthmaticus.

Both thiopental and benzodiazepines have potent anticonvulsant effects, making these drugs useful for RSI in status epilepticus.

In patients with severe cardiovascular compromise or unconsciousness, a sedative may be considered optional to prevent further cardiovascular compromise.

MUSCLE RELAXANTS

Muscle relaxants result in total muscle paralysis, yet the patient may be fully conscious.

Succinylcholine is a depolarizing muscle relaxant with a rapid onset (30 to 60 seconds) and short duration (3 to 12 minutes). Even though it has been the most common muscle relaxant used in RSI, it has numerous disadvantages. Although not contraindicated in head injuries, it causes elevated ICP. Intraocular and intragastric pressure elevations may occur. Muscle fasciculations that might result in muscle pain, rhabdomyolysis, and myoglobinuria might also occur. These are more severe in muscular patients and can be prevented by a defasciculating dose of rocuronium before succinylcholine (this is not necessary in children younger than 5 years of age). Atropine premedication may prevent the bradycardia and excessive bronchial secretions associated with succinylcholine, although recent data has questioned this effect particularly in older children. Other less preventable adverse effects include negative inotropic and chronotropic effects, an association with malignant hyperthermia, hyperkalemia, hypertension, and arrhythmias. Another caution is the use of succinylcholine in a patient with neuromuscular disease. Succinylcholine is contraindicated in patients with glaucoma, penetrating eye injuries, significant neuromuscular disease, history or family history of malignant hyperthermia, and pseudocholinesterase deficiency. At 3 to 60 days after trauma or burns (in other words, day 3 or later following trauma or burns), succinylcholine results in an increased frequency of the risks described here and should not be used. Patients with severe burns or large crush injuries may already be acutely hyperkalemic; thus, the decision to use succinylcholine should consider this as well.

Of the nondepolarizing muscle relaxants, rocuronium currently has the fastest onset and shortest duration. Vecuronium was commonly used prior to rocuronium's introduction. Both agents have minimal cardiovascular effects. Onset times for rocuronium and high dose vecuronium are 30 to 90 seconds. Standard dose vecuronium (0.1 mg/kg) results in an onset time of 90–120 seconds. Duration for rocuronium is 25 to 60 minutes, wheras vecuronium can persist for up to 2 hours when true RSI doses of 0.3 mg/kg are used. Rocuronium is available in a premixed vial ready to use, and vecuronium comes in a powder that must be reconstituted. This factor gives rocuronium another advantage when the time to intubation may be prolonged because of medication preparation.

Other nondepolarizing muscle relaxants include pancuronium, atracurium, and mivacurium. Pancuronium has a slower onset and more cardiovascular side effects. Atracurium and mivacurium have rapid onset times but are associated with histamine release and cardiovascular side effects. Rocuronium is currently the nondepolarizing muscle relaxant of choice. A newer drug, rapacuronium has a rapid onset time and shorter duration than rocuronium, so its use could increase once experience with it is better described.

MUSCLE RELAXANT SELECTION

In comparing rocuronium and succinylcholine, rocuronium has fewer adverse effects, whereas succinylcholine has a shorter duration. The onset times are similar. Some view rocuronium as preferable because it is safer. The contrary view is that because of succinylcholine's shorter duration (which allows restoration of spontaneous ventilation within 3 to 12 minutes compared with 25 to 60 minutes for rocuronium), succinylcholine is better if intubation fails.

In most patients, neuromuscular blockade facilitates both intubation and bag-mask ventilation. For patients with risk factors that suggest a difficult intubation or will require frequent neurologic checks, succinylcholine may be preferable. For others, rocuronium may be preferable. Whether the shorter duration of succinylcholine justifies its greater risk of adverse effects is essentially a personal judgment that individual clinicians must make.

Rocuronium can be reversed pharmacologically. While edrophonium was commonly recommended, this drug is no longer available. Neostigmine (given with atropine or glycopyrrolate to block muscarinic bradycardia and excessive secretions) can be used; however, this is not clinically routinely useful because reversal cannot be achieved immediately. Reversal must wait for some degree of spontaneous recovery to occur, which occurs later than the duration of succinylcholine. Sugammadex is a new agent reported in trials to rapidly reverse rocuronium and vecuronium in the early stage (known as profound neuromuscular blockade). This might become a routinely available option in the future.

Defasciculation and Priming

Defasciculation refers only to the use of succinylcholine, which might cause fasciculations, muscle pain, rhabdomyolysis, and myoglobinuria. This effect is most pronounced in muscular individuals. Fasciculations might increase muscle tone and increase the risk of gastric regurgitation during RSI. To prevent fasciculations, "defasciculation" is recommended, where one-tenth the paralyzing dose of a nondepolarizing muscle relaxant (e.g., rocuronium 0.1 mg per kg) is administered 1 to 3 minutes before succinylcholine administration. This "defasciculating" dose of rocuronium will prevent fasciculations caused by succinylcholine. Defasciculation is most beneficial in muscular individuals. Defasciculation is not necessary in children 5 years of age or younger. Note that this defasciculating step delays the time to intubation and adds complexity to RSI.

Priming in RSI refers to nondepolarizing muscle relaxants only. Its purpose is to shorten the onset time of nondepolarizing muscle relaxants. A priming dose is one-tenth the paralyzing dose of a nondepolarizing muscle relaxant. Using vecuronium as an example, a priming dose of 0.01 mg per kg is administered. Five minutes should elapse for the "priming" to take effect. The paralyzing dose of 0.1 mg per kg is then administered. The full paralyzing onset time of vecuronium is about 100 seconds without priming, 50 seconds with priming. Unfortunately, priming adds an additional 5-minutes delay to intubation while saving 50 seconds in accelerating the onset of the full dose of vecuronium. Because the onset time of rocuronium is considerably faster, the advantage of priming is minimal. Although some experts still recommend priming, it appears to have little benefit in the ED when immediate intubation is required.

Defasciculation and priming are often confused because they both require one-tenth of the paralyzing dose of a nondepolarizing muscle relaxant. However, the two principles are different, even though they have similar characteristics in that they are optional, they delay the time to intubation, and they add complexity to the drug administrations in RSI. Most ED

RSI protocols have removed defasciculation and priming options from routine use.

ADJUNCTIVE AGENTS

The RSI sequence shown in Table 5.3 considers the use of atropine and lidocaine. Atropine use prior to intubation was considered routine in children to prevent bradycardia, although this has recently been challenged in the literature. Use of atropine is optional in adults, unless ketamine is used as a sedative, in which case, atropine is recommended in some protocols in adults as well. Lidocaine is more controversial. It has been shown to reduce ICP and airway reactivity under certain conditions when given 2 minutes before intubation. If ICP elevation is suspected, a cerebroprotective sedative (thiopental or etomidate) is generally preferred in RSI. Lidocaine is cerebroprotective in isolation, but it is unclear whether lidocaine results in additional benefit when added to a cerebroprotective RSI regimen that includes thiopental or etomidate. Despite this controversy, most practicing academic centers and consensus reports recommend the use of intravenous (IV) lidocaine prior to intubation if ICP elevation is suspected. In addition to IV lidocaine, topical lidocaine has been recommended to blunt the adverse reaction to ET intubation. This adds considerable complexity to the laryngoscopy procedure, especially in patients in whom neck immobilization is critical and/or airway visualization may be less than optimal. The recommendation that lidocaine be used in intubating asthmatics stems from its beneficial effect in attenuating bronchospasm. If one truly believes that lidocaine has such a benefit, then if possible, it should be administered long before the patient requires intubation (i.e., to prevent respiratory failure and the need for intubation), as opposed to administering it during RSI.

Opiate analgesics such as fentanyl and morphine have been advocated as adjunctive agents in RSI to further reduce the adverse effects of intubation. Ketamine has analgesic properties; thus, coadministration of analgesics is unnecessary with ketamine. Sedatives such as benzodiazepines, etomidate, and thiopental have little or no analgesic properties. The coadministration of analgesics has been recommended to address this. When considering that the patient is fully unconscious when reliable sedatives such as etomidate and thiopental are used, the additional benefit of analgesics to reduce the amount of "pain" felt by an unconscious patient becomes small. Narcotic analgesics have adverse reactions, and the additional risk that these pose may not justify their routine use. Benzodiazepines must ideally be titrated to assess the degree of sedation; thus, the degree of sedation with these agents is less reliable in RSI, in which case, coadministration of analgesics may be more beneficial.

If RSI is to accomplish its goal of rapid ET intubation, the addition of adjunctive agents should be critically considered because each additional agent adds time and complexity to RSI. This factor is often not considered when discussing the benefit of an individual adjunctive agent in isolation. Therefore, the RSI protocol described in Table 5.3 includes atropine for pediatric patients and IV lidocaine as an optional adjunctive agent for head trauma. Other adjunctive agents may be considered, but they have not been included in the table.

RAPID SEQUENCE INTUBATION PROTOCOL

After patient assessment, immediate stabilization, and IV/IO access, patients should be assessed for any contraindications to RSI or its agents. The major contraindication to RSI is the likelihood that intubation or ventilation might not be possible, as in cases of limited cervical mobility, a receding mandible, limited jaw opening, major facial or laryngeal trauma, upper airway obstruction, or distorted facial or airway anatomy.

To simplify RSI, a table such as Table 5.3 should be adapted. This table should be taped to the wall in the critical care area of your ED. This table is not a substitute for thoroughly understanding the characteristics of each agent and for the critical thinking necessary to select the agents. The following list explains the protocol shown in Table 5.3:

1. Preoxygenation (by spontaneously inspiring or mask-ventilating 100% oxygen for 2 to 5 minutes) results in an oxygen reserve. Positive-pressure mask ventilation may inflate the stomach and increase the likelihood of gastric regurgitation; thus, this procedure, in conjunction with cricoid pressure (see item 4), should be performed only if needed to oxygenate and ventilate the patient adequately. Hyperoxygenation is impossible in some patients. Pulse oximetry and an electrocardiogram monitor should be considered mandatory for patients undergoing RSI. If a self-inflating bag is used, oxygen is *not* delivered through the mask unless the bag is squeezed. Thus, if the patient is spontaneously breathing, a mask attached to a self-inflating bag should *not* be used; instead, a standard oxygen mask, such as a nonrebreather, should be used.

2. Atropine premedication is routinely administered in children. It prevents bradycardia and reduces oral secretions. This is considered optional for adults unless ketamine is used, in which case atropine is recommended. Lidocaine lowers ICP and suppresses the cough reflex. It may be beneficial to patients with ICP elevations. When used in conjunction with other ICP-lowering agents, however, its additional benefit is unclear. Lidocaine is generally recommended for patients with suspected ICP elevation.

3. Before proceeding, it should be ascertained that a good mask seal and an open airway can be maintained. In most instances, muscle relaxation facilitates mask ventilation and intubation. If an inability to intubate and/or mask ventilate is suspected, RSI should not proceed until additional assistance can be obtained.

4. The Sellick maneuver (application of pressure on the cricoid ring sufficient to occlude the esophageal lumen without compressing the airway lumen or moving the cervical spine) is alleged to reduce the likelihood of passive gastric regurgitation and aspiration and the likelihood of gastric distention resulting from mask ventilation. It should, therefore, be performed prior to positive-pressure mask ventilation, unless this results in gagging. It should be maintained until tracheal intubation is confirmed. Data

supporting the benefit of the Sellick maneuver are weak at best and at least one study has demonstrated that it is performed unreliably by ED staff.

5. After appropriate selection, a muscle relaxant followed by a sedative should be administered in rapid sequence. Administering the muscle relaxant first allows the sedative to be administered gradually while waiting for the full onset of the muscle relaxant. Some experts prefer the reverse sequence. For muscle relaxants, Table 5.3 lists rocuronium and succinylcholine. Optional priming (applies to nondepolarizing agents only) and defasciculation (applies to succinylcholine only) are not included in the sequence described in Table 5.3.

6. Intubation can take place when there is full relaxation of the airway muscles, usually 45 seconds after rocuronium or succinylcholine administration.

7. Once intubation is completed, proper ET tube placement should be confirmed by auscultation, end-tidal CO_2 ($ETCO_2$) detection, and the maintenance of oxygenation monitored by pulse oximetry. A confirmatory radiograph should be obtained.

8. Gastric evacuation can be performed with a nasogastric (NG) or orogastric (OG) tube at this time. Significant gastric distention noted prior to intubation can be deflated by an NG or OG tube prior to intubation if clinically tolerable by the patient.

9. Longer-acting sedatives and nondepolarizing muscle relaxants should be administered to maintain unconsciousness and paralysis as needed.

10. If reversal of rocuronium is necessary, neostigmine together with atropine can be administered to accelerate recovery; however, some degree of spontaneous recovery must be present for reversal to occur.

Nasal Intubation Compared with Oral Intubation in the Trauma Patient

Trauma victims who arrive in the ED have suspected cervical spine (C-spine) injuries in addition to other injuries. When it is not possible to rule out a C-spine injury before RSI, the head and neck should be immobilized during intubation.

Unless contraindicated, emergency intubation of pediatric patients should generally be performed orally. In spontaneously breathing patients, older literature sources have recommended blind nasal tracheal intubation, whereas newer recommendations prefer oral tracheal intubation using RSI. If the need for intubation is emergent, nasal tracheal intubation may not be as reliable as oral tracheal intubation. Nasal tracheal intubation is noxious, and it may cause the conscious patient to gag or become agitated, resulting in more neck movement, an increase in ICP, and possible vomiting. Nasal tracheal intubation is more difficult in children. Epistaxis, sinusitis, and cribriform fracture complications are other concerns with nasal tracheal intubation. Studies have not been able to show that nasal tracheal intubation results in less C-spine movement than oral tracheal intubation.

There is concern that laryngoscopy during oral tracheal intubation may displace a C-spine fracture. When using RSI, however, laryngoscopy manipulation and neck movement are minimized under these more ideal conditions. The concern that the loss of cervical muscle tone on an unstable C-spine will reduce its splinting effect and increase its instability has not been supported by evidence.

In a critical situation, intubation is best carried out by the means with which the clinician is most familiar for the given clinical condition. Oral tracheal intubation using RSI appears to be the best means of securing an airway for most clinicians.

Cervical Spine Immobilization During Endotracheal Intubation

The terms that describe C-spine immobilization are ambiguous. For example, traction has been used synonymously with immobilization, although "traction" generally indicates a pulling action with an undefined degree of force. Manual cervical immobilization implies that hands are somehow used to immobilize the neck. Cervical immobilization implies the use of a stiff collar and other devices to immobilize the neck. Philadelphia collars used with manual stabilization do not provide any additional C-spine stability compared with manual stabilization alone. Axial (inline) traction has been shown to worsen C-spine stability in patients. One preferred method is to remove the anterior portion of the cervical collar with an assistant immobilizing the head and neck after the patient is rendered unconscious and paralyzed. This enables the jaw to open wider, providing better visualization during laryngoscopy without sacrificing cervical immobilization.

Alternative Intubation and Airway Techniques

Because the experience level of most ED physicians is greatest with oral tracheal intubation, it is unwise to deviate from this in managing a critically ill child who requires intubation. Alternative procedures should be reserved for instances in which conventional airway techniques prove unsuccessful.

Flexible fiberoptic scopes, lighted stylets to guide nasal tracheal intubation, retrograde intubations, and surgical airways all require high skill and experience levels to be performed optimally. These procedures have less documented experience in children. Directly visualizing the airway through a fiberoptic scope is appealing; however, it requires extensive practice, and it may be especially difficult in critical intubations or in agitated patients. Intubation aided by bronchoscopy, lighted stylets, and the retrograde wire technique are not recommended in ED RSI because of the lack of spontaneous breathing during RSI and the time required for these procedures.

The Combitube™ (Sheridan Catheter Corporation, Argyle, NY) is a double-lumen airway that is blindly inserted through the mouth. One lumen exits through the distal end of the Combitube. The other lumen exits through multiple side holes proximal to the distal end. An inflatable (distal) balloon separates these two (the distal end hole and the more proximal side holes). Because the Combitube is inserted blindly, it will enter either the trachea or the esophagus. If it enters the trachea, the distal balloon is inflated and the distal end-hole lumen is used to ventilate the patient just as if this were a conventional tracheal tube. If the Combitube enters the esophagus, the inflation of the distal balloon occludes the esophagus and the lumen ending in the more proximal side holes is used to ventilate the patient. The esophageal position of this tube is similar to an esophageal obturator airway. Use of the Combitube requires familiarity with its function and method of insertion. It has been demonstrated to be effective in providing an airway during resuscitation, but failures occur as well. Widespread experience with the Combitube in pediatric patients is lacking as there are no specific pediatric sizes.

The laryngeal mask airway (LMA) is another airway device. LMAs come in several different sizes, and their use in pediatric patients has been demonstrated. Experience with LMAs is growing. The correct insertion and placement position of the LMA is critical. The LMA is inserted blindly, taking about 15 to 20 seconds. LMA insertion methods are best taught using video or hands-on instruction. In-depth understanding of the LMA and previous hands-on experience are required to consider it as an airway management option. The LMA does not prevent aspiration but it may be useful when one is unable to successfully intubate.

Surgical airways, such as tracheostomy or cricothyrotomy, may be considered. Complications, including incorrect tube placement, subcutaneous emphysema, pneumomediastinum, pneumothorax, bleeding, tracheal stenosis, subglottic stenosis,

arterial injury, blood aspiration, and persistent tracheocutaneous fistulae, are more common when the procedure is performed on an emergency basis in children. Cricothyrotomy is faster and easier to perform than tracheostomy and also has a lower complication rate. However, in small children, the cricothyroid membrane is not readily palpable and may be too small for an airway. It is not recommended in children younger than 10 years of age. Electrocautery devices should be avoided during these procedures because the presence of high-flow oxygen can result in spontaneous combustion.

Because surgical airways are difficult to perform in children, needle cricothyrotomy may be beneficial for children who cannot be ventilated by any other route, although the complications are similar to those of surgical airways and the experience level with this procedure in children is minimal as well. An over-the-needle 12- or 14-gauge IV catheter is directed inferiorly through the cricothyroid membrane, the needle is removed, and the catheter is left in place. It is vital to have a ventilation device preassembled and ready to use before such an emergency because ventilation through a transtracheal catheter requires a special setup. Many recommendations for transtracheal ventilation have appeared in the literature. Special transtracheal airway kits are available commercially that are generally superior to using an IV catheter. Two ventilation examples are shown in Figure 5.1. These use a wall outlet or tank oxygen pressure directly into the transtracheal catheter. It is the most optimal means to deliver

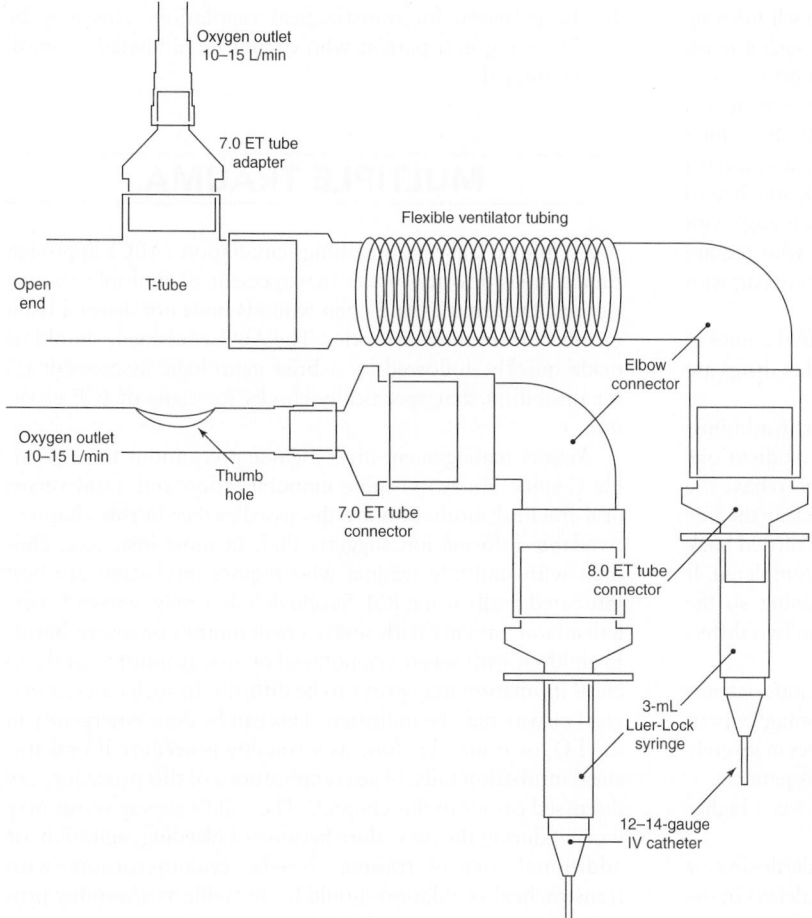

FIGURE 5.1 Transtracheal ventilation setup. (Adapted from Yamamoto LG. Rapid sequence anesthesia induction and advanced airway management in pediatric patients. *Emerg Med Clin North Am* 1991;9: 611–638, copyright by WB Saunders, with permission from author and publisher.)

an adequate tidal volume through the small catheter. By occluding the T tube or the side hole, oxygen is forced through the catheter at high pressure. Chest movement should be used as a visible indicator of adequate ventilation. Exhalation occurs passively through the larynx and not through the catheter. If exhalation is obstructed as well, transtracheal ventilation is contraindicated. The catheter must be held securely because a kink or movement of the catheter would compromise this fragile airway. Another common recommendation is to attach a ventilation bag to the transtracheal catheter through an ET tube connector (about size 3.0). Delivering an adequate tidal volume by aggressively squeezing the bag is possible, but such exaggerated motion may dislodge or kink the catheter.

Transtracheal ventilation is only a temporizing measure, and a more definitive airway should be established as soon as possible. It is important to have ED staff members familiarize themselves with the transtracheal ventilation setup. By attaching a balloon or glove to the transtracheal catheter, air flow can be visualized during practice sessions.

AVOIDING PROBLEMS

Being prepared by becoming aware of the following problems commonly encountered during RSI can greatly improve the success of the procedure.

1. Oxygen delivery devices must be well understood by the staff. New nurses and residents often do not know that oxygen is *not* delivered to the mask attached to a self-inflating bag unless the bag is squeezed. Thus, putting such a mask in front of a patient who is spontaneously breathing will deliver only 21% oxygen (room air), and the patient will fail to hyperoxygenate. For spontaneously breathing patients, oxygen should be delivered using a standard oxygen mask, such as a nonrebreather. A mask attached to a closed-circuit bag (anesthesia-type bag, Rusch bag) with 100% oxygen can also be used. For patients who require positive-pressure mask ventilation, a self-inflating bag with an oxygen reservoir tail is satisfactory.

2. Drug preparation is time consuming. Thiopental comes in kits that require reconstitution before use. Other drugs are less troublesome.

3. Sedatives and muscle relaxants may interact if administered together. The line between the two medications should be cleared. When RSI begins, it is better to have the IV running at a high rate to more effectively clear the line to prevent interaction. The IV rate should be turned back to baseline when RSI drug administration is completed. It may be more optimal to have two IVs running so the drugs can be administered in rapid sequence in two different lines.

4. Paralysis is not a substitute for sedation. Conscious patients remain conscious during paralysis (a frightening experience). It may be safer, however, to avoid sedatives in severely hemodynamically compromised or unconscious patients.

5. Intubation using a sedative without paralysis has a higher complication rate than RSI.

6. Incorrect weight estimates can result in underdosing or overdosing of drugs and can cause significant delays in the onset of RSI.

7. Avoiding unrecognized extubation and esophageal intubation is critical. Frequent clinical reevaluation, $ETCO_2$ monitoring, and pulse oximetry are highly recommended because they often can prevent this serious complication. $ETCO_2$ monitoring (capnometry) is preferable to $ETCO_2$ color detection because it permits quantitative PCO_2 monitoring, which is useful in patients who are difficult to ventilate or in those who require the PCO_2 to be maintained in a strict range. $ETCO_2$ color detectors work only for a short period. After 15 minutes or so, moisture renders them nonfunctional; thus, these should not be used for long transports unless they are frequently replaced.

8. Mainstem bronchial intubation can occur easily in small children who have a small degree of tracheal tube movement.

9. The duration of the sedative is frequently shorter than the duration of the muscle relaxant, potentially resulting in consciousness while paralyzed. Avoid this by maintaining sufficient sedation during the duration of paralysis.

10. RSI protocols should be reviewed with the ED staff at periodic in-services. A common problem occurs when the person who applies the Sellick maneuver releases it prematurely to tend to a seemingly more important task. This person should be dedicated to this maneuver alone and must not release it until intubation is confirmed.

11. Suction devices may malfunction; therefore, there always should be a backup available. Standard Yankauer tips may be clogged by food particles, so newer stiff suction tips with larger openings may be more useful.

12. Be prepared for transtracheal ventilation. This may be lifesaving in a patient who cannot be intubated or mask ventilated.

MULTIPLE TRAUMA

A disciplined airway, breathing, circulation (ABC) approach should take priority in the management of multiple trauma victims. Deformities and open wounds must not distract team members from these priorities. The ABC assessment should be made quickly, followed by a brief neurologic assessment (*D* for disability) that specifically checks for signs of ICP elevation.

Airway management must include precautions for a possible C-spine injury. (C-spine immobilization and nasal versus oral tracheal intubation are discussed earlier in this chapter.) Available information suggests that, in most instances, children with multiple trauma who require intubation are best intubated orally using RSI. Succinylcholine may worsen hyperkalemia in patients with severe crush injuries or severe burns. In children with severe craniofacial or airway injuries, oral tracheal intubation may prove to be difficult. In such cases, a surgical airway may be indicated. This can be done emergently in the ED, or it may be done as a standby procedure if oral tracheal intubation fails. (The complications of this procedure are discussed earlier in this chapter.) The child's airway status may worsen during the procedure because of bleeding, agitation, or additional airway trauma. Needle cricothyrotomy with transtracheal ventilation should be available as a standby procedure if further airway difficulties occur.

Oxygenation may be compromised by pulmonary injuries such as pneumothorax, hemothorax, chest wall injuries, pulmonary contusions, or aspiration. In addition to these, ventilation may be compromised by airway trauma and central nervous system depression. Oxygen administration should be considered routine for all multiple trauma victims. Intubation is indicated in patients who have ventilatory compromise, a potential for airway compromise, moderate or severe shock, and hypoxemia despite supplemental oxygen. Positive-pressure ventilation may worsen a pneumothorax if a chest tube is not in place.

Circulation should be assessed by using multiple clinical parameters. Early mild shock should be treated aggressively to reverse any progression toward late shock and hypotension, which is associated with a poorer outcome. Acute symptoms and signs of early shock are subtle and often underestimated. These signs and symptoms include agitation, restlessness, lethargy, pallor, delayed capillary refill, coolness of the feet, metabolic acidosis, a short perfusion bar/wave on the pulse oximeter, and difficulty in picking up a pulse oximetry signal. Tachycardia and hypotension are indicators of late, severe shock. Paradoxical bradycardia has been noted in shock with hypotension; therefore, the absence of tachycardia cannot be used to rule out shock. Dismissing a low BP as "normal for a child" because of the absence of tachycardia is not valid.

Sedatives and agents used for RSI may have significant adverse effects on BP because of myocardial depression or vasodilation. In hypovolemic or hypotensive children, sedative doses should be reduced or avoided, depending on the clinical situation.

The initial treatment of shock related to hypovolemia consists of frequent clinical reassessment and fluid restoration with volume-expanding crystalloids such as normal saline or lactated Ringer's solution. The usual initial bolus should be 20 mL per kg. This is followed by reassessment of clinical shock parameters. This process should be repeated if evidence of shock persists until fluid volume is restored. Red blood cells should be transfused if excessive hemorrhage is sustained. Large volume fluid resuscitation can result in complications because of hypothermia. When large fluid volumes are anticipated or the patient is very small, crystalloid solutions should be warmed gently and blood products should be infused through a blood warmer.

HEAD TRAUMA

The same priorities should be followed with head trauma as with multiple trauma. Children with head injuries who have depressed sensoriums may be hypoxic, hypovolemic, hypotensive, or acidotic. Although intracranial hemorrhage alone cannot account for significant hypovolemia that results in shock in an older child or adult, this is possible in an infant. Unconscious patients should be intubated using RSI. Patients responsive only to painful stimuli may also need to be intubated. Some patients with lesser degrees of sensorium depression may need intubation using RSI, depending on the degree of head injury and the rate of deterioration. Patients at risk of ICP elevation should be given thiopental or etomidate in addition to lidocaine pretreatment as part of RSI unless hypovolemia or hypotension exist, in which case the dose should be

reduced or eliminated, depending on the clinical circumstances. Thiopental and etomidate lower ICP and cerebral metabolic oxygen demand.

Patients with head injuries may develop posttraumatic seizures related to cerebral contusions, cerebral edema, or intracranial hemorrhage. Under RSI, these seizures are not visible because of pharmacologic paralysis. It is prudent in most instances to give a loading dose of phenytoin (10 to 20 mg per kg) or fosphenytoin (10 to 20 mg PE/kg) after intubation is confirmed to treat prophylactically any undiagnosed posttraumatic seizure focus.

BURNS

Children with severe burns represent a special form of multiple trauma. Burn patients may also sustain blunt trauma, and ABCs are still the priority. Early intubation using RSI is advocated for patients at risk of airway injury because airway edema is expected to worsen rapidly. These cases include children with evidence of soot in sputum or vomitus, burns of the face, singed nasal hairs, lip burns, wheezing, stridor, or severe burns. The possibility of carbon monoxide poisoning should be considered. It may be preferable to avoid succinylcholine in patients with severe burns for fear of worsening hyperkalemia.

Pulmonary compromise may result from smoke inhalation, burn injury, bronchial edema, bronchospasm, blunt trauma, or adult respiratory distress syndrome. Initial chest radiographs may fail to show some of these injuries.

Children with severe burns have significant hypovolemia because of external fluid losses. Lactated Ringer's or normal saline boluses of 20 mL per kg should be used to immediately correct hypovolemia in conjunction with guidelines for fluid replacement based on body surface area (BSA) of the burns.

STATUS EPILEPTICUS

In patients presenting to the ED with prolonged seizures, the standard approach of ABC support and immediate administration of benzodiazepines is generally initiated. Loading with IV phenytoin/fosphenytoin and/or phenobarbital may also be considered if seizures continue. This process of administering anticonvulsants and waiting to assess its effect occurs in 3- to 5-minute cycles. If seizures fail to respond to several doses of anticonvulsants, the child could be continuously seizing for an additional 30 to 60 minutes.

Prolonged seizures result in hypoxia and respiratory acidosis due to poor ventilation. The brain is simultaneously hypermetabolic with greater oxygen demand. The agents used for RSI may effectively reverse this hypermetabolic process. Skeletal muscle activity stops. Oxygenation and ventilation are restored. The brain may still be hypermetabolic because it may still be epileptogenic, but at least hypoxia and acidosis are decreased. Thiopental is cerebroprotective, and both thiopental and benzodiazepines have potent anticonvulsant activity. Simultaneous IV administration of high dosages of benzodiazepines, phenytoin/fosphenytoin, phenobarbital, and/or other newer IV anticonvulsants (valproic acid, levetiracetam) can potently reduce the seizure potential of the brain while maintaining oxygenation and ventilation. The major adverse effect of most anticonvulsants is respiratory depression. Following RSI, this is no longer a concern and maximum doses of anticonvulsants can be administered to provide maximum anticonvulsant activity.

In refractory status epilepticus, the duration of seizures, hypoxia, and acidosis is likely to contribute to cerebral injury. Refractory status epilepticus can be anticipated if the seizures fail to stop after initial IV benzodiazepine doses, at which point the failure of conventional anticonvulsants should be considered high risk and RSI followed by maximum anticonvulsant administration should be considered. Because potentially injurious seizure durations of 40 minutes or more can occur in the management of such patients, it may be prudent to initiate RSI earlier rather than later. The concern that seizures may be protracted yet can no longer be visibly appreciated after RSI should be tempered by the clinical benefits of RSI as described. Electroencephalogram (EEG) monitoring in the ED is often recommended, but it is not feasible in most hospitals, although portable bispectral index monitors (functionally, a portable EEG device) may have some potential to monitor this.

AGITATED PATIENTS WHO REQUIRE PROCEDURES OR TRANSPORT

Agitated or combative patients with head injuries or possible intracranial lesions that require computed tomography scanning cannot be scanned in such a condition. Sedation alone can be considered for such patients. In patients who fail to respond to standard sedation measures or in patients who may benefit from ET intubation, RSI provides an effective means of immediately securing airway control, breathing, and movement so imaging can be completed with minimal trauma to the patient. Patients who require transport to another facility, and who are agitated and difficult to control, may be unmanageable during transport. After the clinical situation has been assessed, RSI may be indicated if its benefits outweigh its risks. Patients are more difficult to monitor during procedures and transports. The immediate detection of unrecognized extubation or hypoxemia is crucial. Portable pulse oximeters and $ETCO_2$ monitors can monitor oxygenation and confirm intubation continuously.

Suggested Readings

Bledsoe GH, Schexnayder SM. Pediatric rapid sequence intubation: a review. *Pediatr Emerg Care* 2004;20(5):339–443.

Bonomo JB, Butler AS, Lindsell CJ, et al. Inadequate provision of postintubation anxiolysis and analgesia in the ED. *Am J Emerg Med* 2008;26(4):469–472.

Butler J, Jackson R. Best evidence topic report. Lignocaine as a pretreatment to rapid sequence intubation in patients with status asthmaticus. *Emerg Med J* 2005;22(10):732.

Cheng CA, Aun CS, Gin T. Comparison of rocuronium and suxamethonium for rapid tracheal intubation in children. *Paediatr Anaesth* 2002;12(2):140–145.

Clark RK, Trethewy CE. Assessment of cricoid pressure application by emergency department staff. *Emerg Med Australas* 2005;17(4):376–381.

Ellis DY, Harris T, Zideman D. Cricoid pressure in emergency department rapid sequence tracheal intubations: a risk-benefit analysis. *Ann Emerg Med* 2007;50(6):653–665.

Fastle RK, Roback MG. Pediatric rapid sequence intubation: incidence of reflex bradycardia and effects of pretreatment with atropine. *Pediatr Emerg Care* 2004;20(10):651–655.

Fengler BT. Should etomidate be used for rapid-sequence intubation induction in critically ill septic patients? *Am J Emerg Med* 2008;26(2):229–232.

Guldner G, Schultz J, Sexton P, et al. Etomidate for rapid-sequence intubation in young children: hemodynamic effects and adverse events. *Acad Emerg Med* 2003;10(2):134–139.

Hildreth AN, Mejia VA, Maxwell RA, et al. Adrenal suppression following a single dose of etomidate for rapid sequence induction: a prospective randomized study. *J Trauma* 2008;65(3):573–579.

Ivy ME, Cohn SM. Addressing the myths of cervical spine injury management. *Am J Emerg Med* 1997;15(6):591–595.

Jones RK, Caldwell JE, Brull SJ, Soto RG. Reversal of profound rocuronium-induced blockade with sugammadex: a randomized comparison with neostigmine. *Anesthesiology* 2008;109(5):816–824.

Oglesby AJ. Should etomidate be the induction agent of choice for rapid sequence intubation in the emergency department? *Emerg Med J* 2004;21(6):655–659.

Perry JJ, Lee JS, Sillberg VA, et al. Rocuronium versus succinylcholine for rapid sequence induction intubation. *Cochrane Database Syst Rev* 2008;16(2):CD002788.

Pühringer FK, Rex C, Sielenkämper AW, et al. Reversal of profound, high-dose rocuronium-induced neuromuscular blockade by sugammadex at two different time points: an international, multicenter, randomized, dose-finding, safety assessor-blinded, phase II trial. *Anesthesiology* 2008;109(2):188–197.

Robinson N, Clancy M. In patients with head injury undergoing rapid sequence intubation, does pretreatment with intravenous lignocaine/lidocaine lead to an improved neurological outcome? A review of the literature. *Emerg Med J* 2001;18(6):453–745.

Sagarin MJ, Chiang V, Sakles JC, et al. National Emergency Airway Registry (NEAR) investigators. Rapid sequence intubation for pediatric emergency airway management. *Pediatr Emerg Care* 2002;18(6):417–423.

Sivilotti ML, Filbin MR, Murray HE, et al. Does the sedative agent facilitate emergency rapid sequence intubation? *Acad Emerg Med* 2003;10(6):612–620.

Turner BK, Wakim JH, Secrest J, et al. Neuroprotective effects of thiopental, propofol, and etomidate. *AANA J* 2005;73(4):297–302.

Zed PJ, Mabasa VH, Slavik RS, et al. Etomidate for rapid sequence intubation in the emergency department: is adrenal suppression a concern? *CJEM* 2006;8(5):347–350.

Zelicof-Paul A, Smith-Lockridge A, Schnadower D, et al. Controversies in rapid sequence intubation in children. *Curr Opin Pediatr* 2005;17(3):355–362.

Zuckerbraun NS, Pitetti RD, Herr SM, et al. Use of etomidate as an induction agent for rapid sequence intubation in a pediatric emergency department. *Acad Emerg Med* 2006;13(6):602–609.

CHAPTER 6 ■ EMERGENCY MEDICAL SERVICES AND TRANSPORT MEDICINE

GEORGE A. WOODWARD, MD, MBA, ANDREW L. GARRETT, MD, MPH, BRENT R. KING, MD, MMM, AND M. DOUGLAS BAKER, MD

OVERVIEW OF EMERGENCY MEDICAL SERVICES

Infants, children, and adolescents are commonly treated by emergency medical services (EMS) systems worldwide. This discipline of medicine is also termed *prehospital care*, and the terms are used interchangeably. In the United States, approximately 5% to 15% of calls for an ambulance will be for a patient younger than 18 years of age. This subgroup of the population usually enjoys relatively good health; however, accidental trauma is the leading cause of death. Similar to older patients, pediatric patients are also susceptible to acute medical illness and exacerbations of chronic conditions such as asthma and diabetes. Infants may also present with complications of congenital cardiac, respiratory, or oncologic disease, or with perinatal complications during and after delivery out of the hospital. Many of these sick or injured children will enter the EMS system for initial evaluation, treatment, and transport to the hospital. Pediatric patients consistently represent a challenge to most EMS systems and providers. They may be too small to fit most of the conventional EMS equipment. They may be one part of a large family unit needing care and they present an emotional challenge to the provider. Despite these difficulties, the goal is to seamlessly integrate the prehospital care of children in the prehospital environment into EMS systems that were originally designed to care for adults.

Summarized by Ludwig and Selbst, EMS for children (EMSC) is a concept for an all-encompassing, multidisciplinary care system that includes parents, primary care providers, prehospital care providers and transport systems, community hospital and tertiary care referral center emergency departments (EDs), and pediatric inpatient units, including critical care facilities. The elements of this system should be linked by effective communication and transportation systems and governed by well-established policies and procedures. The provision of pediatric EMS, although a single link in this chain, is a critical component. EMS providers are continually balancing the need for rapid transport to the hospital with the ability to stabilize the sick or injured child in the field. This must all be done with the patient's best interest in mind, being mindful that prehospital care is only one portion of the patient's medical management.

Until the 1970s, prehospital care was largely the part-time purview of taxi services and mortuary owners. There were no organized EMS systems to speak of, other than basic first aid providers. Changes began to occur when military patient movement systems successfully explored the lifesaving inter-vention of rapid transportation and surgery for injured soldiers. At that time, the success of physician-staffed civilian prehospital systems in Ireland led to the formation of experimental EMS systems in the United States, using specially trained "para-medics" instead of physicians. California, Florida, and Ohio had early EMS systems that proved successful in saving the lives of patients with cardiac emergencies. The *EMS Systems Act* of 1973 led to the establishment of several hundred new EMS regional systems across the United States, albeit without a clear mandate for physician oversight initially. The television show *Emergency!* (NBC 1972–1978) was pivotal in changing the public's perception and expectation of care outside of the hospital, and assisted in rapidly advancing the discipline from its infancy into adolescence.

In just over thirty years, EMS capabilities have grown to provide emergency prehospital access to nearly every American. There are more than 15,000 EMS systems in the United States utilizing approximately 800,000 EMS personnel who respond to an estimated 16 million requests a year. It can be estimated that approximately 800,000 to 1.5 million of these requests are for pediatric patients.

EMS systems exist across a broad range of environments beyond the use of ambulances to transport sick or injured patients to the hospital. In 2005, after Hurricane Katrina impacted the U.S. Gulf Coast, much attention was focused on the role of the EMS system and the challenges that were faced during the surge in demand for services that occurred. This incident in particular emphasized the role that EMS stakeholders must play in disaster preparedness and planning if they are to best serve the public during a crisis. Additionally, EMS professionals are becoming involved in providing care in non-traditional settings such as international humanitarian relief as well as with law enforcement tactical or SWAT teams. As these EMS disciplines continue to grow in complexity and capability, so will the need to oversee the care of children that occurs in these situations.

WHERE HAVE EMS SYSTEMS TRADITIONALLY FALLEN SHORT FOR CHILDREN?

The formalization of pediatric emergency medicine as a specialty helped enable an organized approach to investigating and developing EMS systems for children. The need to improve the capacity of EMS to manage sick and injured pediatric patients initially came from the providers themselves as well as the physicians who received those patients. Shortfalls in provider training, pediatric-specific emergency equipment, established standards of care, and quality pediatric EMS research severely limited the advancement of the specialty.

Epidemiologic studies helped clarify the specific needs of children in the EMS system, and in doing so, identified many of its shortfalls. Tsai and Kallsen found those at the pediatric age extremes to be the principal users of prehospital services—teenagers for trauma and infants and preschoolers for illness (primarily seizures, ingestions, and respiratory diseases). Yamamoto et al. showed that persons with disabilities were also more likely to use an ambulance; however, ambulance personnel felt less prepared to handle those patients. This is an important consideration, as the prevalence of children with special health-care needs (CSHCN) is estimated at 13% to 18%. Baker and Ludwig found that infants with serious illness were more likely to be transported by EMS than were adolescents. The fact that most childhood cardiopulmonary arrests occur in children younger than 4 years of age emphasizes the need of EMS systems to provide age-appropriate equipment and personnel properly trained in pediatric resuscitative care, especially in the youngest age groups.

Institute of Medicine Report Findings and Significance

Recently, the Institute of Medicine (IOM) was commissioned to analyze and report on the capabilities of both prehospital- and hospital-based pediatric emergency care in the United States. They published two documents: *Emergency Care for Children: Growing Pains* and *Emergency Medical Services at the Crossroads* in 2007. While complimentary of the past accomplishments of the EMS system, their findings also highlighted many of the shortfalls that exist around the care of all patients, as well as children, in all of the components of the EMS system, and also suggested a system of interventions to address these issues. These reports highlighted the following:

■ Insufficient coordination of EMS systems and hospitals
■ Disparities in response times to emergency calls, with a focus on the flow of information from 911 operator to dispatcher to responder
■ Uncertainties around the quality of EMS care, with an emphasis on a lack of a way to measure EMS quality overall
■ A "divided" professional identity in EMS—meaning those who work in EMS often feel a lack of support from their partners in the field, typically fire and police services, as well as their hospital-based partners, physicians and nurses
■ A general lack of disaster preparedness considering the role that EMS providers may play in a large incident or terrorist attack
■ An overall lack of evidence exists to inform how EMS is evolving as a professional and medical specialty
■ A significant percentage of EDs that lack all of the recommended equipment to care for a critically injured or sick child
■ Pediatric training for EMSC is underemphasized and in many cases not required to be part of continuing education requirements for EMS personnel

■ Pediatric treatment patterns vary widely between EMS and hospital-based care providers

While critical of the EMS system in many ways, the IOM reports do reflect the "still developing" nature of EMS as a discipline—one which is growing quickly since its birth in the 1970s, and still has a way to go to appreciate exactly what its role is. The onus is on EMS systems themselves to address these challenges as much as possible to ensure that they are providing excellent care to all of their patients, regardless of age.

It is difficult to perform quality clinical research in the EMS system. There are few large-scale, randomized clinical studies that have been undertaken in the pediatric EMS population. Even with well-designed research, it may be difficult to generalize the findings outside the study population and locale due to the high level of variability within EMS systems across the United States. No two systems are designed or operate in exactly the same way with regard to staffing, protocols, oversight, demographics, or training. The paucity of scientific scrutiny of EMS in general highlights the need for future research focusing on both EMS and EMSC. The emergence of EMS fellowships has given academic physicians an opportunity to specialize in EMS, and by doing so, to increase the likelihood of having future leaders in the field who are committed to quality research as an important component of medical oversight. The establishment of a federal EMSC program under the U.S. Department of Health and Human Services, as well as the federally funded EMSC National Resource Center, were important steps to assist EMS academicians in defining a research agenda around EMSC as well as providing avenues for funding these projects. As the discipline evolves, we must resist the temptation to quickly add new technologies, procedures, and protocols to prehospital care without ensuring that these modalities have proven efficacy. There is a real concern that in an effort to aid one patient, others will suffer from unnecessary intervention or inappropriate allocation or utilization of resources.

GOVERNANCE OF EMS SYSTEMS

As mentioned above, there is no nationally standardized definition of what constitutes an EMS system. In all 50 states, EMS legislation exists to provide a statutory basis for individual EMS to exist and operate. In addition to control at the state level, municipal, county, or regional local government may regulate the organization and authorization of services provided by EMS personnel. This patchwork of governance over EMS systems may make it very difficult to speak with a unified voice when it comes to patient care, training, and certification, and makes it difficult for EMS professionals to move between communities, much less across state lines. Although there is a National Registry of Emergency Medical Technicians (NREMTs) that serves as a centralized credentialing group, this organization does not authorize an EMT to practice in a state or region, and there is little consistency around the issue of states granting reciprocity for EMS providers.

After the *Emergency Medical Services Act* of 1973, all states identified lead agencies that coordinate EMS activities within the state. In most states, the lead agency is headed by an EMS director who reports to the state department of health. Often, state-level advisory councils exist to direct and assist in the development of protocols and minimum standards of operation.

States are frequently divided into EMS regions, at which level prehospital care becomes operational, and where local government, hospitals, and ambulance services interact with each other. Regional advisory councils may exist as well. Pediatric clinicians should be encouraged to become involved in these regional committees as advocates of the pediatric needs within their systems.

COMPONENTS OF PREHOSPITAL CARE SYSTEMS

The prehospital component of EMSC is an architecture that involves a variety of personnel and equipment, only some of which is standardized and regulated. To understand the extent of the services provided by prehospital care systems, it is important to understand the training, capabilities, and scope of practice of prehospital personnel and the equipment available to them.

Prehospital Personnel

In the past, prehospital personnel were not always trained to provide the specialty care that their patients required. It was not until 1964 that the first reports of attempts to train fire and police personnel in basic cardiopulmonary resuscitation (CPR) appeared in the literature. Since then, several classifications of prehospital care providers have emerged, each with different levels of training and varying degrees of capabilities. Several categories (and certification levels) of prehospital personnel exist (Table 6.1): first responders (FRs), basic life support (BLS) providers, intermediate life support providers (ILS), and advanced life support (ALS) providers. Some states and regions use their own notations for the skill levels of providers, but their personnel typically fit into one of the categories described here. Training standards and requirements for certification exist for all these groups, established by the U.S. Department of Transportation (DOT) and the National Highway Traffic Safety Administration (NHTSA). These agencies publish national standard curricula (NSC) for each level of provider, and they are periodically reviewed and updated. The NSC is a guideline only—the DOT does not conduct training or issue licenses or certifications to EMTs. There has been an extensive recent effort to create the language to standardize the training of personnel by proscribing a list of "competencies" for each level of provider. Nowhere is this more evident than in the recent publication The National EMS Scope of Practice Model, developed by NHTSA. This document can be accessed at http://www.nhtsa.dot.gov/staticfiles/DOT/NHTSA/Communication%20&%20Consumer%20Information/Articles/Associated%20Files/EMSScope.pdf.

First Responders

The layperson definition of a "first responder" to an emergency is the person who happens on the scene first to provide patient aid. In the context of classification of providers, however, a *first responder* refers to a person who is certified in limited but

TABLE 6.1

NATIONAL HIGHWAY TRAFFIC SAFETY ADMINISTRATION, U.S. DEPARTMENT OF TRANSPORTATION, TRADITIONAL NATIONAL STANDARD CURRICULA SKILLS AND MEDICATIONS FOR PREHOSPITAL PROVIDERS

First Responder
Cardiopulmonary resuscitation
First aid
Basic airway management
Patient assessment
Basic wound care
Childbirth
Safe patient movement
Assisted ventilation (external)
Automated external defibrillator (AED) (elective)

EMT-Basic
All first responder scope, plus:
Vital signs assessment
Oxygen administration
AED
Assist patient with nitroglycerine, inhalation medications (e.g., albuterol)
Epinephrine autoinjector, oral glucose
On-scene triage
Splinting, spinal immobilization, helmet removal
Extrication and transport
Nasogastric tube (elective)
Orotracheal intubation (elective)

EMT-Intermediate
All EMT-Basic scope, plus some or all of the following:
Medical communications
Basic electrocardiogram (EKG)
Dual-lumen airway device or similar
Pulse oximetry
Orotracheal intubation (in some areas)
Naso- and orogastric tube
Basic determination of death
Manual defibrillation and pacing
Needle thoracotomy
Meconium aspiration
Administration of limited medications (in some areas)

EMT-Paramedic[a]
Scope of EMT-Intermediate, plus some or all of the following:
Termination of resuscitation/grief support
Needle or surgical cricothyrotomy (in some areas)
Digital or transilluminated intubation
Nasotracheal intubation
Peak expiratory flow rate (PEFR) testing
12-lead EKG
Rapid-sequence/medication-enhanced intubation (in some areas)
Use of intravenous, intramuscular, and oral medications

[a]The current paramedic National Standard Curricula does not make specific recommendations for an EMT-Paramedic pharmacopoeia.
From National Highway Traffic Safety Administration, U.S. Department of Transportation, National Standard Curricula. Adapted from http://www.nhtsa.dot.gov/.

significant lifesaving capabilities. A certified FR course with a standardized 40-hour curriculum has been developed, and providers can be registered by NREMT. The role of the FR is vital in rural and wilderness areas where extended response times are common, and skills such as hemorrhage control, airway positioning, and early defibrillation can be truly lifesaving. In suburban and urban EMS areas, this level of provider has been phased out in lieu of more highly trained volunteer and professional EMT-Basics (EMT-Bs), -Intermediates (EMT-Is), and -Paramedics (EMT-Ps), but is still prevalent in the police and non-EMS fire services, as well as in some rural areas.

Although the exact capabilities of FRs vary according to local standards, most are trained to help clear an obstructed airway, control blood loss, use an automated external defibrillator (AED), and to administer first aid or CPR while awaiting the arrival of more advanced personnel. Spinal immobilization, oxygen administration, and medication administration are skills typically beyond the capabilities of most FRs. Generally, FRs do not (and should not) provide patient transport in ambulances as the primary caregiver. In the new NHTSA model, this level provider is referred to as an Emergency Medical Responder (EMR).

Basic Life Support Providers—EMT-Basic

The proliferation of many certification levels of EMS providers has led to some confusion with regard to who can do what in the field. *EMT-Bs* are providers who have skills that exceed those of FRs. EMT-Bs are capable of patient assessment, spinal immobilization, noninvasive ventilatory assistance, and defibrillation with AEDs. In some areas, EMT-Bs who are certified in AED use may be classified as *EMT-D* (defibrillation). In the past, EMT-Bs were classified as EMT-A (ambulance) or EMT-NA (non-ambulance) based on their work environment, but this has been discontinued. EMT-Bs are trained to recognize and treat pulselessness, apnea, upper airway obstruction, and extremity deformity, as well as recognize respiratory distress, altered mental status, shock, mechanisms of injury, and obvious death.

EMT-B training typically requires 100 or more hours as well as observation time in an ED. This level is popular with volunteer fire department members and others who provide EMS on a volunteer basis. It is also the standard level of training for private industry EMTs who perform the interfacility and discharge transport of medically stable patients from a hospital, nursing home, or other medical facility. The EMT-B curriculum typically involves one educational module on infants and children, representing a relatively small percentage of the total training exposures. They learn basic resuscitation skills and external airway management as well as some of the nuances of injury that apply to children and infants. In the new NHTSA model, EMT-B's are referred to as simply Emergency Medical Technicians, or EMTs.

Midlevel Providers—EMT-Intermediate

Midlevel classifications developed in response to the specific perceived needs of local jurisdictions, regions, or states. The *EMT-I* provider possesses additional clinical skill beyond that of the EMT-B based on the region they practice, but less than those of a paramedic. This frequently includes the ability to acquire vascular access (including interosseous access) or to perform advanced airway management. Tracheal intubation typically remains an intervention for EMT-Ps, but in some cases EMT-Is are locally authorized to perform this skill. More typically, the mid-level provider's advanced airway management capabilities are limited to a dual-lumen airway device. Most systems will review pediatric skills during the approximately 175- to 225-hour training curriculum, and in the associated internship and clinical preceptorship. The EMT-I invasive airways are typically contraindicated in children and infants due to the size of the device.

The benefits of performing intermediate-level procedures in the field are and have been a topic of much debate. It is a concern that intermediate-level providers may focus their efforts on learning interventions that (independently) may be of diminished value or on skills that may easily deteriorate because of infrequent use. It is important that EMT-Is be expert providers of BLS skills and not overly reliant on rarely performed advanced interventions, especially in children. It is important to consider that, although this level of training may be ideal for someone who is paired with an EMT-P, it is rarely an acceptable alternative to paramedic-level services except when the EMS system would otherwise not be able to operate beyond the BLS level. The benefit of developing and initiating the use of skills that lengthen scene time but do not lead to immediate definitive treatment, such as intravenous (IV) access without the authorization to administer medications, and routine glucometer use without the approval to administer IV dextrose, must be evaluated carefully by each system and its medical director. Overall, the current trend is toward phasing out this level of EMT classification but EMT-Is still play an important role in providing EMS in rural and occasionally suburban settings when paired with an EMT-P. Under the new NHTSA model, this level of provider is classified as an Advanced EMT (AEMT).

Advanced Life Support Providers—EMT-Paramedic

ALS providers are EMT-Ps, or "paramedics." They have 1,000 hours to, in some cases, more than 3,000 hours of training, internship, and clinical hospital time, and they are capable of administering a high level of medical care in the field. Their capabilities include advanced diagnostic skills, recognition and treatment of arrhythmias, and advanced airway management, including endotracheal intubation and in some areas emergent surgical airways and medication-enhanced intubation using sedatives and paralytics. In addition, they can administer lifesaving medications and fluids in the field. Their ability to use diagnostic tools and diagnose suspected cardiac disease, stroke, and trauma in the field can lead to the diversion of eligible patients to medical centers that can provide the most appropriate care. This level of training has become the standard of prehospital care in the United States, but it can be prohibitively expensive for a volunteer service or smaller community to support. Paramedics have formal didactic training in the emergency care of children, which may include the AAP's (American Academy of Pediatrics) Pediatric Education for Prehospital Professionals (PEPP) or AHA's (American Heart Association) Pediatric Advanced Life Support (PALS) courses, but most will admit to being uncomfortable with younger patients due to the lower volume of and limited exposure to pediatric patients and the perceived (or actual) difficulty of performing advanced procedures and assessments in the prehospital environment. In the new NHTSA model, EMT-Paramedics are classified as Paramedics to simplify the concept.

EMS Physicians

In some cases a physician may serve in the role of a field responder. This may be a doctor who is serving as a service's medical director, or it may be as a specialized provider or as an EMS Fellow in a larger system. Physicians may also be a part of law enforcement tactical teams, to immediately provide the highest level of care in situations where there may be a risk of casualties. Although the field is not the typical practice environment for physicians in the United States (it is much more common in other countries), there are distinct advantages to having a physician responder. The first is that they may provide direct medical control to the intermediate and paramedic providers on a scene. Second, they may bring the ability to perform advanced interventions for patients with specialized needs, such as a field amputation of an entrapped extremity. Third, they may play an important role in the management of complex incidents, such as a mass casualty incident. EMS physicians should be specifically oriented and trained before working in this environment—this includes learning how to establish scene safety, proper lifting, emergency vehicle operation, and how to use the communications equipment properly.

Equipment and Modes of Transport

Until the 1970s, ambulances were little more than hearses, sometimes painted white, which were sparsely equipped and minimally attended. In 1969 and 1973, the National Academy of Science and the DOT published documents that generally defined the purpose of an ambulance and its contents. Since then, many states have established much more comprehensive ambulance licensing standards, some of which pertain specifically to pediatric equipment, and there is a list of both adult and pediatric equipment for ambulances published collectively by the American College of Surgeons (ACS), the American College of Emergency Physicians (ACEP), and the National Association of EMS Physicians (NAEMSP), with input from the AAP, which was revised in 2008. This list is commonly used to establish the minimum requirements for EMS programs.

There are typically two classes of ambulances now in service in the United States—each is primarily dedicated either to advanced (EMT-P) or basic (EMT-B) life support service. BLS units are equipped to conform to the previously mentioned list (Table 6.1). Included are ventilation and airway equipment, immobilization devices, bandages, two-way communication equipment, obstetric kits, extrication equipment, and other miscellaneous items.

In 1988, the ACEP published a position paper that detailed the staffing and equipment appropriate for ALS units. In addition to the equipment contained in the BLS list, these ALS units carry intubation and vascular access equipment, a portable monitor-defibrillator, and a variety of ALS medications. They must also carry at least one EMT-P. In some areas, the standard is two. Most states now require that the electrocardiogram (EKG) equipment be 12-lead capable in order to diagnose and potentially reroute a patient with suspected cardiac disease to a center with a cardiac catheterization facility.

AEDs have been approved for use in the pediatric population older than 1 year of age. Special pediatric step-down pads may be used that attenuate the delivered shock, but their use is not mandatory as per AHA recommendations. AEDs with adult and pediatric pads should be carried on all BLS ambulances, and should be optional for ALS ambulances that have other manual defibrillation capabilities. Some newer manual defibrillators have an AED option built in as an additional resource to the EMT.

Pediatric Equipment

Since the mid-1990s, great strides have been made in appropriately equipping BLS and ALS ambulances to safely manage pediatric patients. In 2009, a document outlining collaboratively developed standards regarding equipment needed in ambulances was developed and endorsed by the ACS Committee on Trauma, the AAP, the ACEP, NAEMSP, and the Pediatric Equipment Guidelines Committee–EMSC partnership for Children Stakeholder Group and published in the July 2009 Bulletin of the ACS (available at: www.facs.org/fellows_info/bulletin/2009/ambulance0709.pdf) and as a July 2009 AAP Policy Statement (available at: http://pediatrics.aappublications.org/cgi/reprint/124/1/e166) (Table 6.2). This list includes much of the specialized pediatric equipment that until 2009 had been recommended separately by the EMSC and other organizations. The new document details the minimum recommended equipment to be able to care for either an adult or pediatric patient.

Because of the limited space on an ambulance, most EMS crews will not have all the mechanical or pharmacologic options available in a hospital. Examples are a paramedic crew that carries morphine but not fentanyl for analgesia, or normal saline and not lactated Ringer's solution for fluid resuscitation. An example of a state-approved list of medications for ALS ambulances is provided in Table 6.3. More technically sophisticated equipment and medications can often be added if required, as long as its use is established and monitored by the medical director for the EMS service.

Interfacility Transport

An increasing trend is the use of ALS ambulances and paramedic crews for the interfacility transport of stabilized patients who require admission or treatment at another facility. This is typically done by private ambulance companies that are providing a service to the hospital industry, or by community EMS units in extraordinary circumstances or in remote rural areas. The transport by EMS of hospital-stabilized pediatric patients can be challenging for many reasons. For example, the EMT-P is not traditionally trained in the long-term monitoring of disease processes, continuation or titration of hospital-initiated therapies such as dopamine or insulin infusions, or the mechanics of using a hospital programmed IV pump or central line monitors. For this reason, prior to undertaking this type of transfer, the crew must have additional training that certifies their competency in using the required specialized equipment. There is a subspecialized level of training termed *critical care paramedic*, which emphasizes these issues.

Specialty Teams and Emergency Medical Services

In many geographic areas, the medical needs of the population served require specialty ALS or critical care transport services. Such services can be either air or ground equipment, and may be

TABLE 6.2

EQUIPMENT FOR AMBULANCES

REQUIRED EQUIPMENT: BASIC LIFE SUPPORT (BLS) AMBULANCES

A. Ventilation and Airway Equipment
1. Portable and fixed suction apparatus with a regulator (per federal specifications; see Federal Specification KKK-A-1822F reference)
   - Wide-bore tubing, rigid pharyngeal curved suction tip; tonsillar and flexible suction catheters, 6–16F, are commercially available (have 1 between 6F and 10F and 1 between 12F and 16F)
2. Portable oxygen apparatus capable of metered flow with adequate tubing
3. Portable and fixed oxygen-supply equipment
   - Variable flow regulator
4. Oxygen-administration equipment
   - Adequate length tubing; transparent mask (adult and child sizes), both nonrebreathing and valveless; nasal cannulas (adult, child)
5. Bag-valve mask (manual resuscitator)
   - Hand-operated, self-reexpanding bag; adult (>1000 mL) and child (450–750 mL) sizes, with oxygen reservoir/accumulator; valve (clear, disposable, operable in cold weather); and mask (adult, child, infant, and neonate sizes)
6. Airways
   - Nasopharyngeal (16–34F; adult and child sizes)
   - Oropharyngeal (sizes 0–5; adult, child, and infant sizes)
7. Pulse oximeter with pediatric and adult probes
8. Saline drops and bulb suction for infants

B. Monitoring and Defibrillation
All ambulances should be equipped with an automated external defibrillator (AED) unless staffed by ALS personnel who are carrying a monitor/defibrillator. The AED should have pediatric capabilities, including child-sized pads and cables.

C. Immobilization Devices
1. Cervical collars
   - Rigid for children aged 2 years or older; child and adult sizes (small, medium, large, and other available sizes)
2. Head immobilization device (not sandbags)
   - Firm padding or commercial device
3. Lower extremity (femur) traction devices
   - Lower extremity limb-support slings, padded ankle hitch, padded pelvic support, traction strap (adult and child sizes)
4. Upper and lower extremity immobilization devices
   - Joint-above and joint-below fracture (sizes appropriate for adults and children), rigid support constructed with appropriate material (cardboard, metal, pneumatic, vacuum, wood, or plastic)
5. Impervious backboards (long, short; radiolucent preferred) and extrication device
   - Short (extrication, head-to-pelvis length) and long (transport, head-to-feet length) with at least three appropriate restraint straps (chin strap alone should not be used for head immobilization) and with padding for children and handholds for moving patients

D. Bandages
1. Commercially packaged or sterile burn sheets
2. Triangular bandages
   - Minimum of two safety pins each
3. Dressings
   - Sterile multitrauma dressings (various large and small sizes)
   - ABDs, 10″ × 12″ or larger
   - 4″ × 4″ gauze sponges or suitable size
4. Gauze rolls
   - Various sizes
5. Occlusive dressing or equivalent
   - Sterile, 3″ × 8″ or larger
6. Adhesive tape
   - Various sizes (including 1″ and 2″), hypoallergenic
   - Various sizes (including 1″ and 2″), adhesive
7. Arterial tourniquet (commercial preferred)

E. Communication
Two-way communication device between EMS provider, dispatcher, and medical control

F. Obstetrical Kit (Commercial Package Is Available)
1. Kit (separate sterile kit)
   - Towels, 4″ × 4″ dressing, umbilical tape, sterile scissors or other cutting utensil, bulb suction, clamps for cord, sterile gloves, blanket
2. Thermal absorbent blanket and head cover, aluminum-foil roll, or appropriate heat-reflective material (enough to cover newborn)

G. Miscellaneous
1. Sphygmomanometer (pediatric and adult regular- and large-sized cuffs)
2. Adult stethoscope
3. Length/weight-based tape or appropriate reference material for pediatric equipment sizing and drug dosing based on estimated or known weight
4. Thermometer with low temperature capability
5. Heavy bandage or paramedic scissors for cutting clothing, belts, and boots
6. Cold packs
7. Sterile saline solution for irrigation (1-L bottles or bags)
8. Flashlights (two in number) with extra batteries and bulbs
9. Blankets
10. Sheets (minimum of four), linen or paper, and pillows
11. Towels
12. Triage tags
13. Disposable emesis bags or basins
14. Disposable bedpan
15. Disposable urinal
16. Wheeled cot (conforming to national standard at the time of manufacture)
17. Folding stretcher
18. Stair chair or carry chair
19. Patient care charts/forms
20. Lubricating jelly (water soluble)

H. Infection Control (*Latex-free equipment should be available*)
1. Eye protection (full peripheral glasses or goggles, face shield)
2. Face protection (e.g., surgical masks per applicable local or state guidance)

(continued)

TABLE 6.2

CONTINUED

3. Gloves, nonsterile (must meet 1999 National Fire Protection Association requirements, which can be found at http://www.nfpa.org/)
4. Coveralls or gowns
5. Shoe covers
6. Waterless hand cleanser, commercial antimicrobial (towelette, spray, liquid)
7. Disinfectant solution for cleaning equipment
8. Standard sharps containers, fixed and portable
9. Disposable trash bags for disposing of biohazardous waste
10. Respiratory protection (e.g., N95 or N100 mask—per applicable local or state guidance)

I. **Injury-prevention Equipment**
   1. All individuals in an ambulance need to be restrained (there is currently no national standard for transport of uninjured children; see NHTSA Web site, http://www.nhtsa.gov/ for list of EMS-approved child occupant protection devices)
   2. Protective helmet
   3. Fire extinguisher
   4. Hazardous material reference guide
   5. Traffic-signaling devices (reflective material triangles or other reflective, nonigniting devices)
   6. Reflective safety wear for each crew member (must meet or exceed American National Standards Institute/International Safety Equipment Association performance class II or III if working within the right of way of any federal-aid highway; visit http://www.reflectivevest.com/federalhighwayruling.html for more information)

REQUIRED EQUIPMENT: ADVANCED LIFE SUPPORT (ALS) AMBULANCES

For emergency medical technician-paramedic services, include all of the required equipment listed for the basic-level provider, plus the following additional equipment and supplies. For emergency medical technician–intermediate services (and other nonparamedic advanced levels), include all of the equipment for the basic-level provider and selected equipment and supplies from the following list, on the basis of local need and consideration of prehospital characteristics and budget.

A. **Airway and Ventilation Equipment**
   1. Laryngoscope handle with extra batteries and bulbs
   2. Laryngoscope blades, sizes 0–4, straight (Miller); sizes 2–4, curved, (MacIntosh)
   3. Endotracheal tubes, sizes 2.5–5.5 mm uncuffed and 6–8 mm cuffed (two each), other sizes optional
   4. Meconium aspirator adaptor
   5. 10-mL non–Luer-Lock syringes
   6. Stylettes for endotracheal tubes, adult and pediatric
   7. Magill (Rovenstein) forceps, adult and pediatric
   8. Lubricating jelly (water soluble)
   9. End-tidal CO_2—detection capability
      - Colorimetric (adult and pediatric) or quantitative capnometry

B. **Vascular Access**
   1. Crystalloid solutions, such as Ringer's lactate or normal saline solution (1000-mL bags × 4); fluid must be in bags, not bottles; type of fluid may vary depending on state and local requirements

2. Antiseptic solution (alcohol wipes and povidone-iodine wipes preferred)
3. Intravenous-fluid pole or roof hook
4. Intravenous catheters, 14–24 gauge
5. Intraosseous needles or devices appropriate for children and adults
6. Venous tourniquet, rubber bands
7. Syringes of various sizes, including tuberculin
8. Needles, various sizes (one at least 1½″ for intramuscular injections)
9. Intravenous administration sets (microdrip and macrodrip)
10. Intravenous arm boards, adult and pediatric

C. **Cardiac**
   1. Portable, battery-operated monitor/defibrillator
      - With tape write-out/recorder, defibrillator pads, quick-look paddles or electrode, or hands-free patches, EKG leads, adult and pediatric chest attachment electrodes, adult and pediatric paddles
   2. Transcutaneous cardiac pacemaker, including pediatric pads and cables
      - Either stand-alone unit or integrated into monitor/defibrillator

D. **Other Advanced Equipment**
   1. Nebulizer
   2. Glucometer or blood glucose measuring device
      - With reagent strips
   3. Large-bore needle (should be at least 3.25″ in length for needle chest decompression in large adults)

E. **Medications (Preloaded Syringes When Available)**
   Medications used on advanced-level ambulances should be compatible with current guidelines as published by the American Heart Association's Committee on Emergency Cardiovascular Care, as reflected in the advanced cardiac life support and pediatric advanced life support (PALS) courses, or other such organizations and publications (ACEP, ACS, NAEMSP, and so on). Medications may vary depending on state requirements. Drug dosing in children should use processes that minimize the need for calculations, preferably a length-based system. In general, medications may include:
   - Cardiovascular medication such as 1:10000 epinephrine, atropine, antidysrhythmic agents (e.g., adenosine and amiodarone), calcium-channel blockers, β-blockers, nitroglycerin tablets, aspirin, vasopressor for infusion
   - Cardiopulmonary/respiratory medications such as albuterol (or other inhaled β-agonist) and ipratropium bromide, 1:1000 epinephrine, furosemide
   - 50% dextrose solution (and sterile diluent or 25% dextrose solution for pediatrics)
   - Analgesics, narcotic, and nonnarcotic
   - Antiepileptic medications such as diazepam or midazolam
   - Sodium bicarbonate, magnesium sulfate, glucagon, naloxone hydrochloride, calcium chloride
   - Bacteriostatic water and sodium chloride for injection
   - Additional medications as per local medical director

OPTIONAL BASIC EQUIPMENT
This section is intended to assist EMS providers in choosing equipment that can be used to ensure delivery of quality prehospital care. Use should be based on local resources. The equipment in this section is not mandated or required.

(continued)

TABLE 6.2

EQUIPMENT FOR AMBULANCES (CONTINUED)

A. Optional Equipment

1. Glucometer (per state protocol)
2. Elastic bandages
   - Nonsterile (various sizes)
3. Cellular phone
4. Infant oxygen mask
5. Infant self-inflating resuscitation bag
6. Airways
   - Nasopharyngeal (12F, 14F)
   - Oropharyngeal (size 00)
7. Alternative airway devices [e.g., a rescue airway device such as the esophageal-tracheal double-lumen airway (ETDLA), laryngeal tube, or laryngeal mask airway (LMA)] as approved by local medical direction
8. Alternative airway devices for children (few alternative airway devices that have been approved by the Food and Drug Administration have been studied in children; those that have been studied, such as the LMA, have not been adequately evaluated in the prehospital setting)
9. Neonatal blood pressure cuff
10. Infant blood pressure cuff
11. Pediatric stethoscope
12. Infant cervical immobilization device
13. Pediatric backboard and extremity splints
14. Topical hemostatic agent
15. Appropriate chemical, biological, radiologic, nuclear, explosive personal protective equipment (CBRNE PPE), including respiratory and body protection
16. Applicable chemical antidote autoinjectors (at a minimum for crew members' protection; additional for victim treatment based on local or regional protocol; appropriate for adults and children)

B. Optional Advanced Equipment

1. Respirator
   - Volume-cycled, on/off operation, 100% oxygen, 40–50 psi pressure (child/infant capabilities)
2. Blood-sample tubes, adult and pediatric
3. Automatic blood pressure device
4. Nasogastric tubes, pediatric feeding tube sizes 5F and 8F, sump tube sizes 8F–16F
5. Pediatric laryngoscope handle
6. Size 1 curved (MacIntosh) laryngoscope blade
7. 3.5- to 5.5-mm cuffed endotracheal tubes
8. Needle cricothyrotomy capability and/or cricothyrotomy capability (surgical cricothyrotomy can be performed in older children in whom the cricothyroid membrane is easily palpable, usually by the age of 12 years)

OPTIONAL MEDICATIONS

A. Optional Basic Life Support Medications

1. Albuterol
2. EpiPens
3. Oral glucose
4. Nitroglycerin (sublingual tablet or paste)

B. Optional Advanced Life Support Medications

1. Anxiolytics
2. Intubation adjuncts including neuromuscular blockers

INTERFACILITY TRANSPORT

Additional equipment may be needed by ALS and BLS prehospital care providers who transport patients between facilities. Transfers may be done to a lower or higher level of care, depending on the specific need. Specialty transport teams, including pediatric and neonatal teams, may include other personnel such as respiratory therapists, nurses, and physicians. Training and equipment needs may be different depending on the skills needed during transport of these patients. There are excellent resources available that provide detailed lists of equipment needed for interfacility transfer such as the American Academy of Pediatrics Guidelines for Air and Ground Transport of Neonatal and Pediatric Patients.

APPENDIX: EXTRICATION EQUIPMENT

Adequate extrication equipment must be readily available to the EMS responders but is more often found on heavy rescue vehicles than on the primary responding ambulance. In general, the devices or tools used for extrication fall into several broad categories: disassembly, spreading, cutting, pulling, protective, and patient related. The following is necessary equipment that should be available either on the primary response vehicle or on a heavy rescue vehicle:

Disassembly tools
- Wrenches (adjustable)
- Screwdrivers (flat and Phillips head)
- Pliers
- Bolt cutter
- Tin snips
- Hammer
- Spring-loaded center punch
- Axes (pry, fire)
- Bars (wrecking, crow)
- Ram (4 ton)

Spreading tools
- Hydraulic jack/spreader/cutter combination

Cutting tools
- Saws (hacksaw, fire, windshield, pruning, reciprocating)
- Air-cutting gun kit

Pulling tools/devices
- Ropes/chains
- Come-along
- Hydraulic truck jack
- Air bags

Protective devices
- Reflectors/flares
- Hard hats
- Safety goggles
- Fireproof blanket
- Leather gloves
- Jackets/coats/boots

Patient-related devices
- Stokes basket

Miscellaneous
- Shovel
- Lubricating oil
- Wood/wedges
- Generator
- Floodlights

Local extrication needs may necessitate additional equipment for water, aerial, or mountain rescue.

TABLE 6.3

EXAMPLE OF REQUIRED MEDICATIONS FOR ADVANCED LIFE SUPPORT AMBULANCES

Activated charcoal	EpiPen	Terbutaline
Adenosine	Furosemide	Thiamine
Albuterol	Glucagon	Intravenous (IV) normal saline
Aspirin	Oral glucose	
Atropine	Lidocaine	**Optional**
Atrovent for nebulization	Magnesium sulfate	Amiodarone
Calcium chloride	Midazolam	Cyanide antidote kit
Cetacaine spray or 2% lidocaine jelly	Morphine sulfate	Lorazepam
Dextrose D10, D25, D50	Naloxone	Metoprolol
Diazepam	Nitroglycerin	Mark I kit autoinjectors
Diltiazem HCl	Nitropaste	Nifedipine
Diphenhydramine	Oxygen	Pralidoxime
Dopamine	Saline for flushes	Tetracaine
Epinephrine 1:1,000, 1:10,000	Sodium bicarbonate	D5W or LR IV solutions

From Commonwealth of Massachusetts. *OEMS EMS pre-hospital treatment protocols*. 5th ed. Boston, MA: office of Health & Human Services, 2004, with permission.

EMS or hospital-based. Examples of specialty transport units are those assigned to neonatal or pediatric transport teams, high-risk obstetrics teams, and mobile intensive care units (MICUs). For each of these, specialized equipment and staffing are incorporated beyond the scope of EMS providers (typically for nurses, respiratory therapists, or physicians), although EMTs are frequently used as primary or secondary team members. For more information, see "Pediatric Interfacility Transport" section.

Air Transport

The gradual introduction of air medical transport into civilian prehospital care began in the 1960s. During that time, a National Academy of Sciences Research Council document recommended the initiation of pilot programs to evaluate ground and air ambulance services in sparsely populated areas. Since then, air medical transport has developed into a common part of some EMS systems.

Regardless of their degree of involvement, physicians should be aware of the air medical transport resources and capacities in their region. Two basic types of air transport exist: helicopter and fixed-wing (FW) aircraft. Helicopters [rotor-wing (RW) craft] are common in both rural and urban EMS systems, although they are typically hospital-based and usually carry a nurse, respiratory therapist, or physician as one (or more) of their crew members. The Association of Air Medical Services' Atlas and Database of Air Medical Services (ADAMS) notes that in the United States, as of September 2008, there are 310 Air Medical Services, 699 bases with helicopters (RW), 154 bases with FW aircrafts for a total of 840 RW aircrafts and 292 FW aircrafts. It is estimated that approximately 400,000 patients are transported by helicopter annually, with another 100,000 transported by FW aircraft.

ADAMS also estimate that 95% of those services provide emergency service to medical and trauma scenes. Many services have an EMT-P as a primary crew member. The unique capabilities of rapid, direct scene response give the RW craft a distinct advantage over FW aircraft and ground units in some

cases. Helicopter EMS have allowed for the provision of ALS services to larger rural areas incapable of sustaining independent ALS units and have provided access to tertiary care centers for patients in regions without such centers. In both rural and crowded metro and suburban areas, RW aircraft offer the benefit of time saved in transit—a benefit in cases such as trauma and coronary syndromes. However, such a benefit comes at a high cost. One recent research project has suggested that direct air transport from an accident scene to a trauma center for pediatric patients may not improve survival when compared with local hospital stabilization prior to air transfer. Air medical transport is a specialized service and is typically an adjunct to, and not a substitute for, ground transport, with certain exceptions such as prolonged vehicle extrications or other situations where a patient is entrapped at an emergency scene. The proper provision of air medical services requires specialized equipment, staffing, and medical oversight, both on the ground and in the air. Additionally, the issue of medical helicopter safety was thrust to the forefront in 2008, with an unprecedented series of fatal medical helicopter incidents occurring in that year. The industry is aggressively exploring the issue of safety, and the National Transportation Safety Board (NTSB) has made the issue of medical helicopter safety one of its top ten priorities. It is likely that increased regulation of the industry will be the result along with elimination of some of the latitude that medical helicopters have had in the past with regards to freedom of operations.

MEDICAL OVERSIGHT OF EMERGENCY MEDICAL SERVICES

There are two types of medical oversight—direct (online) and indirect (offline). Both models require initial and ongoing input by physicians, and each model has its own risks and benefits. A physician "with experience and knowledge of EMS" (Emergency Medical Services Systems Act of 1973) is required to be involved in the operations of all ALS (and now most BLS) EMS systems.

Level I—Adult and Pediatric
❏ Adult: SBP < 90 any reading   ❏ Pedi: SBP < 2 × age (yr) + 70 mm Hg
❏ Adult: GCS ≤ 10   ❏ Pedi: GCS ≤ 8
    ❏ Adult: all GSW neck/chest/abd/extrem above elbow or knee
    ❏ Pedi: all GSW
❏ Transfer receiving blood
❏ Penetrating injury with large blood loss at scene, exsanguinating hemorrhage, expanding hematoma
❏ Respiratory compromise
❏ Major impalement
❏ Complete or partial amputation above elbow/knee
❏ Other blunt or penetrating injury to neck, chest, or abdomen
❏ Any patient initially stable that then deteriorates
❏ Emergency department physician discretion: _____
❏ Other:_____

Level II—Adult and Pediatrics
Anatomic:
❏ head❏ face ❏ neck❏ chest ❏ abdomen ❏ extremities ❏ burns
Mechanism:
❏ high-speed MVA ❏ pedestrian ❏ bicycle ❏ falls
Other:
❏ multisystem trauma ❏ hypothermia ❏ drowning with trauma ❏ assault with LOC
❏ helicopter transport ❏ intentional injury ❏ comorbid factors
❏ initially stable/deterioration ❏ emergency department physician discretion
❏ pregnant ❏ age > 55 yr

Level III—Adult and Pediatrics
❏ all intoxicated (EtOH/drug) with evidence of traumatic injury
❏ traumatic event in past 24 hr requiring hospital admission (normal VS, GCS 15, with no other criteria noted)
❏ any pediatric burn >5% and <10% without other involvement of face, genitalia, and/or accompanied by inhalation or other injuries
❏ all falls in children >5 ft, <20 ft

FIGURE 6.1 Sample hospital-based protocol for trauma team activation by EMS report. SBP, systolic blood pressure; GCS, Glasgow Coma Score; GSW, gunshot wound; MVA, Motor vehicle accident; EtOH, ethyl alcohol; LOC, loss of consciousness; VS, vital signs. (From University of Massachusetts, Worcester, MA, with permission.)

Direct Medical Control

Direct medical oversight refers to the real-time provision of supervision or authorization of EMS activities by a physician using radio, phone, or on scene, sometimes referred to as "medical control" or "medical command." This model enables a clinician to direct care by EMS after an assessment is transmitted to them. This may include voice reports and electronic broadcast of data, such as a 12-lead EKG. The benefit of such an arrangement is true customized care, but the drawbacks include additional time spent reporting instead of treating, demand on the base station staff, the potential for technical problems with the communications gear, and the potential supervision of field EMS personnel by base station clinical staff who are not experienced in the EMS setting. Although once a common model, many EMS systems are trending toward using indirect oversight, such as the use of standing order protocols, to reduce some of the quality variability and time requirements associated with direct medical control.

Indirect Medical Control

Indirect medical control includes the medical management of an EMS system through the use of established care guidelines in place before the call for help arrives. The EMS medical director for a service, who is ultimately responsible for every aspect of patient care, authorizes the EMS personnel to utilize standard protocols for the care of patients in order to save time and reduce the variability of orders. In most systems, the option remains for EMS personnel to call in to speak with a clinician for direct medical control if they have questions or if the protocol does not clearly apply. This may also be necessary for certain procedures or medications considered to be higher risk to the patient. In many cases the protocols may be established by the regional or state EMS authority (Fig.6.1).

Figure 6.2 provides an example of a regional protocol for pediatric altered mental status. Note that there are a different set of actions for basic, intermediate, and paramedic providers. This protocol also clearly states when to contact online medical control for additional guidance. This enables the providers in the field to have a preestablished, physician-evaluated course of action for most patient care situations. This has the enormous benefit of saving time in critical situations as well as reducing interoperator variability in patient assessment in the field and medical decision-making at the hospital base station. The EMSC National Resource Center publishes model pediatric protocols that can be a very useful adjunct when designing or reviewing protocols.

THE TIMELINE OF EMS CARE

When an EMS system is activated, this places into motion a chain of events to efficiently deliver the most appropriate personnel to the patient for safe transport to the most appropriate

PARAMEDIC PROCEDURES

1. Ensure scene safety and maintain body substance isolation precautions as appropriate.
2. Maintain open airway and assist ventilations as needed. This may include repositioning of the airway, suctioning, and/or the use of airway adjuncts (NP airway/OP airway) as indicated. Assume spinal injury if associated with trauma and manage accordingly.
3. Administer oxygen using appropriate delivery device, as clinically indicated.
4. ALS STANDING ORDERS
    a. Advanced airway management if indicated
    b. Initiate IV normal saline KVO. If a hypovolemic etiology is suspected, administer fluid bolus at 20 mL/kg.
    c. Cardiac monitoring (12-lead EKG)/dysrhythmia recognition
    d. Treatment for specific etiologies
        i. Known Diabetic
            1. Dextrose 10% 0.5 g/kg IV bolus (neonates)
            2. Dextrose 25% 0.5 g/kg IV bolus (estimated body weight <50 kg)
            3. Dextrose 50% 0.5 g/kg IV bolus (estimated body weight >50 kg)
            4. Glucagon 0.1 mg/kg Push, IO, IM, or SC up to max. of 1 mg
        ii. Coma of Unknown Etiology
            1. Age less than 5 yr:
                a. Naloxone HCL: 0.1 mg/kg to max. dose of 2 mg, IV push, ET, IO, SC, IM
                b. Dextrose as listed previously
            2. Age greater than 5 yr:
                a. Naloxone HCL: 2 mg IV push, ET, IO, IM, SC
                b. Dextrose as listed previously
5. Initiate transport as soon as possible.
6. Contact MEDICAL CONTROL. The following may be ordered:
    a. Glucagon 0.1 mg/kg IV push, IO, IM, SC up to max. of 1 mg
    b. Normal saline fluid bolus 20 mL/kg
    c. Dextrose
        i. Dextrose 10% 0.5 g/kg IV bolus (neonates)
        ii. Dextrose 25% 0.5 g/kg IV bolus (estimated body weight <50 kg)
        iii. Dextrose 50% 0.5 g/kg IV bolus (estimated body weight >50 kg)
    d. Naloxone HCL
        i. If age <5 yr: 0.1 mg/kg to max. dose of 2 mg IV bolus, ET, IM, SC, IO
        ii. If age ≥ 5 yr: 2 mg IV bolus, ET, IM, SC, IO
    e. Additional fluid boluses of 20 mL/kg NS at intervals as needed
    f. If coma caused by specific drug overdose, physician may order:
        i. Atropine 0.02 mg/kg IV bolus or ET (min. dose of 0.1 mg), or IO
            1. NB: If given via ET route, follow with 2 mL sterile saline via ET
        ii. Sodium bicarbonate 1 to 2 mEq/kg as slow IV infusion. CAUTION: Pediatric patients must have adequate ventilatory function prior to the administration of sodium bicarbonate.
    g. Monitor and record vital signs every 5 min at a minimum if unstable, or every 15 min if stable.
    h. Notify receiving hospital.

FIGURE 6.2 Sample EMS protocol for pediatric altered mental status. (From Central Massachusetts EMS Regional Authority, with permission.)

receiving hospital. There are many steps to achieving this ideal goal; the major ones are presented in the following sections.

EMS Activation

It is typically the parent, caregiver, or bystander who recognizes that a child requires emergency medical help, and contacts EMS through the 911 emergency number. With widespread 911 education in place now, from time to time children make the call themselves. Nearly every community has 911 service, with many having Enhanced 911 (E-911) services that provide the dispatcher with the address of the caller. Using a cell phone to contact 911 is increasingly common, and improving technologies (wireless E-911 systems) can allow for the localization of the caller using the global positioning satellite (GPS) technology built into many wireless phones.

Receiving the Call and Dispatching Assistance

In most systems, a trained 911 operator will receive the emergency call and direct the request to the appropriate police, fire, or EMS agency. In many communities, the dispatchers are trained in emergency medical dispatch (EMD) to provide standardized medical advice to the 911 caller through the use of algorithms or protocols. Some dispatchers are trained as EMTs themselves and can assist the caller as needed until help arrives. It should be a goal in every community to have reliable medical advice available for the 911 caller while awaiting EMS response. The dispatchers are also responsible for simultaneously initiating the response of appropriate resources. In a *tiered system*, there is a set of criteria that determine whether an ALS or BLS response is indicated and dispatched, based on the caller's chief complaint.

For example, a call for an isolated minor foot injury would receive a unit with EMT-Bs. In contrast, a call for a seizure would receive a paramedic ambulance. In a *nontiered system*, the highest level of provider is dispatched to all calls for help, typically EMT-Ps. Based on local policies, other resources such as police and fire units may be dispatched along with EMS.

Field Treatment

When EMTs arrive, assessment and treatment is begun using established protocols or online medical control, the patient is rapidly stabilized, and transport to the receiving hospital is begun without delay. In many cases, transport will be initiated immediately and any assessment and procedures will be conducted while en route to the hospital to save time. Based on protocol and/or the online medical control, a decision is made regarding the receiving hospital, or point of entry (POE). The POE selection is based on various factors: patient condition, the capabilities of the receiving hospital, such as a cardiac catheterization team on-call or a pediatric trauma center, and the distance and time to a receiving facility. Many EMS systems are now specifying certain hospitals as approved POE for conditions such as stroke, acute coronary syndrome, or pediatric trauma. This assures that the patient is going to a facility that can best manage their condition.

A challenging situation for EMS providers is when a clinician unknown to the EMS service stops at an emergency scene and wishes to direct the medical care. This is a precarious situation for both the provider and the clinician, since there is no way to verify the qualifications of the bystander. Wherever possible, this situation should be guided by a protocol, and at no time should the clinician be allowed to endanger the patient or the providers. ACEP has produced a policy statement that outlines the issues involved in having a bystander clinician involved in the care of the EMS patient. Because of the liabilities involved in having an unknown bystander take a role in an established system of providing prehospital care, this is a circumstance where online medical control should be contacted to determine the ways in which the bystander may assist. Options may range from providing an extra set of hands to having the clinician assume control for the patient and accompanying them to the ED. It is strongly encouraged that EMS draft an information card or document to give to on-scene providers to explain how this will work for a specific service. This should be written in conjunction with the EMS service's medical director.

Transit to the Hospital

Once the child is en route to the receiving hospital, either medical control or the EMS unit itself should notify the receiving hospital of the transport. Based on the nature of the child's illness or injury, the facility then can begin to assemble personnel and equipment for prompt treatment. This is especially important for hospitals where some resources may not be immediately accessible and, in cases of trauma or serious illness, when a specific resuscitation team can be assembled to meet the EMTs in the treatment room. On arrival, essential information concerning the child's condition and the field treatment is transferred by verbal report to the accepting care team. It is important for ED staff to maintain a good working relationship with their community EMS providers. Taking the time to listen to and acknowledge their report and participation is both a professional courtesy and an important way to get another perspective on the patient's emergency that will be difficult to access once they depart the ED. Each encounter should be considered as a potential learning and teaching experience, and deficits noted as a stepping stone for future improvement. Providing patient follow-up, where allowable, is another way of including the EMTs in the care continuum.

ISSUES AND CONTROVERSIES IN EMS CARE

Lights and Siren Use

One of the most important aspects of the transit to the hospital is patient and provider safety. There are few times when a higher-speed drive with lights and siren (L&S) will be of benefit to a sick or injured child—in fact, this practice may be one of the most dangerous things EMS providers could do for the patient. Clawson published in 2002 that an estimated 15,000 to 25,000 ambulance or rescue vehicle accidents occur per year in the United States while the vehicles are using L&S, with over 100 fatalities. Sixty percent of these accidents are the fault of the emergency vehicle driver. Intersections are the most common site for accidents involving EMS vehicles operating L&S. Interventions in Salt Lake City that reduced the number of emergency vehicles responding to incidents using L&S (in units other than the first responding vehicle) resulted in a nearly 80% reduction in emergency vehicle-related collisions. Although in some communities it is legal for emergency vehicles to exceed the speed limit and pass through red lights, this does not mean that it is safe to do so. A NAEMSP position paper from 1994 recommends that an EMS service develops a policy on L&S use that should be reviewed by the medical director because accidents while running "hot" with L&S are a common cause of litigation. The same should be said for having multiple vehicles respond to an incident using L&S, something that is frequently done but is likely unnecessary. Emergency vehicle accidents are an area of high, and frequently unnecessary, liability in EMS that is borne more out of a tradition of L&S use than a medical necessity for the patient. This is a good example of a nonmedical aspect of an EMS system that does, in fact, directly affect patient care.

Transport Safety

Accidents involving ambulances are becoming tragically common, and when they do occur, the rear compartment of the vehicle is an extremely dangerous place to be. Every patient must be safety restrained in the vehicle with shoulder and body straps, in a position that minimizes further injury and protects the airway; however, this can pose a significant challenge with pediatric patients. Every ambulance should have the capacity to secure a child or infant safely. If the patient is an infant and his or her medical condition permits, the use of an approved child safety seat (CSS) should be encouraged in a forward facing seat without an airbag. Note that these are not available in most ambulances. For those pediatric patients that are to be secured on the ambulance cot, there are techniques that can be

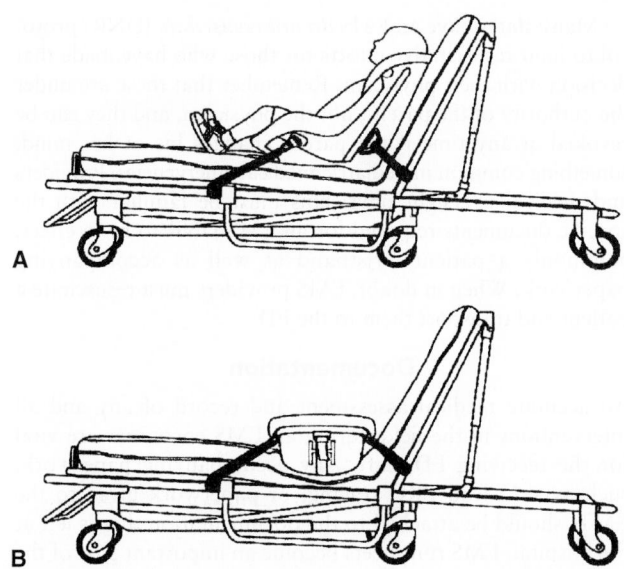

FIGURE 6.3 Diagram of a car seat attached to an ambulance cot. **A:** Recommended method for restraining children up to about 18 kg who can tolerate a semi-upright seated position, showing belt attachment to the cot and routing through the convertible child restraint. **B:** Recommended method for restraining infants who cannot tolerate a semi-upright seated position, showing belt attachment to the cot and routing through the car bed loops. (From Bull MJ, Talty J, et al. Crash protection for children in ambulances, recommendations and procedures. In: 45th annual proceedings of the Association for the Advancement of Automotive Medicine, 2001:353–367. Reprinted with permission from the Association for the Advancement of Automotive Medicine.)

used to make this practice as safe as possible to reduce the chance of another injury if the EMS vehicle is involved in an accident (Fig. 6.3). In many ambulances there is a seat in the rear of the vehicle that can be opened into a CSS that may be appropriate. New products are currently available that can secure a child to the ambulance cot and which have been crash-tested to establish their capabilities, such as a restraint developed by SafeGuard (Westfield, Indiana) (http://www.safeguardseat.com/ems); such a device can be used for children too large to fit in a CSS. Although specialized products do exist to secure a child to an ambulance cot, the EMS provider must take great care to ensure that it is properly attached to the cot, and that the child's head, torso, and pelvis are appropriately secured to prevent injury in an accident. It is important to keep in mind that many of these products may not have established crashworthiness, and the degree of protection they provide is unclear. The NHTSA, the federal entity that oversees EMS in the United States, has convened a work group in 2009 to establish the best practices for safety transporting pediatric patients in EMS and those results are pending. The family's own car seat secured properly in the ambulance may often be the best alternative providing it is medically safe and appropriate for the patient's condition. This also encourages a safe discharge home from the hospital by already have the child's safety seat available in the emergency department. EMS providers and parents must also be restrained in the ambulance whenever possible to prevent a secondary collision with the patient during an accident. Sixty percent of the fatalities in a study of ambulance crashes were EMTs who were unrestrained in the patient compartment. Any monitoring equip-

ment must be secured to the frame of the ambulance because even a low-speed collision can turn loose objects into fatal missiles to a child or the provider. It is an additional recommendation that a child not be transported in an ambulance unless it is medically necessary. Other alternatives, such as a family member or a patrol car with a child seat, should be explored. With almost no exceptions, it is unacceptable to transport a child on the lap of a parent in an ambulance, regardless of how the child is secured to the parent or stretcher.

Medical-Legal Issues

Prehospital care providers and their medical overseers are legally responsible for their actions or lack thereof. *Good Samaritan* laws are variable by state and may not provide any coverage if a provider, from an EMT to a physician, is being paid to be present at the scene of the emergency. It is vital to understand what type of professional liability coverage exists for both EMS providers as well as medical control clinicians.

Prehospital care providers practice in a precarious setting. They commonly attend to children in cramped, poorly lit conditions; encounter crowded, emotional, or even hostile environments; and may lack the appropriate equipment for pediatric patients. Despite these and other obstacles, prehospital care providers often must make important decisions about the management and transport of critically ill children with rapidly changing conditions. Because of inadequate pediatric training or experience, some prehospital care providers might not feel prepared well enough to provide such management. Many lawsuits that involve EMS result from the transport of patients to inappropriate facilities, deviation from standardized protocols, perceived or actual slow response time, or the failure to transport patients when indicated (a "no load"). When in doubt, it is usually safest to transport the patient. Language barriers can be an important factor in accurately assessing a patient and situation, and it is important to address how to approach language incompatibilities ahead of time. There are numerous resources for telephone-based interpreters available (at a cost), but these are difficult to access unless the EMS service already has an existing account with a translation service (such as Language Line®). Using telephone interpreters is cumbersome in the EMS setting due to the need for privacy and mobility, but at times it is the only option. It may also be useful to have printed medical translation cards specific to the demographics of the EMS service area.

EMTs can minimize their risks by attending to the three Ds: details, duties and documentation. When a situation is unclear, prehospital care providers should consult with the online medical control physician.

Details of Standards of Care

All prehospital providers and medical control personnel should provide care that mirrors the standards of practice that apply to their profession. As previously discussed, some areas rely heavily on the use of protocols to standardize prehospital care activities, where others require real-time discussions with an online medical control base station. Whichever model is followed, the onus is on the provider to ensure that the care they are giving is not operator dependent but dictated by the scenario being faced. Standards of care and medical control are established to protect the EMS provider professionally as well as serve the patient. Deviating from one's level of training or from an established and reviewed protocol with or without the involvement of medical control can expose the EMT to unfortunate legal scrutiny in the event of a poor patient outcome.

Attention to the routine details of emergency care and transport is vital, as many complaints and lawsuits are based on minor deviations from the standards of care, which may seem insignificant at the time of an emergency. It is important to look at each EMS run as a part of a whole. There are many routine details of care that are vital but are frequently overlooked on a case by case basis. This mentality should be avoided, as it will likely lead to a problem. Examples include

- improperly restraining adult and pediatric patients
- using excessive speed or failing to yield
- the inappropriate use of lights and siren
- having patients with painful or cardiac complaints ambulate to the ambulance
- improperly extricating patients from motor vehicle accidents
- incomplete spinal immobilization onto a backboard when it is indicated

Duties to Provide Care

All health-care providers must understand their duties to provide care. Questions often arise concerning issues of consent, especially when children are involved. The *doctrine of implied consent* permits the treatment of minors without parental consent when a medical emergency exists. In general, any minor with a condition that threatens "life and limb" is considered an emergency and should be treated and transported. This is typically true even in the difficult situation when a parent refuses EMS for a patient who appears to be emergent. Minor patients cannot refuse treatment and transport in an emergency situation. The same is true when parents are incapable of understanding the risks of refusing care because of cognitive impairment from intoxication or injury. The use of online medical command can help evaluate and resolve a situation where there may be disagreement at the scene regarding the need for transport.

If parents are present and refuse care for their injured or ill child, they should be asked to sign a standard form releasing the EMS system from responsibility. If at all possible, an assessment should be done to determine if there is a medical emergency, and online medical control should be sought if the EMTs are unclear about whether a threat to life or limb exists. The parents must be informed of the risk of not transporting a sick or injured pediatric patient, which typically may include death or permanent disability. Regardless of religious beliefs or parental desires, a child must be treated and transported if there is a life-threatening emergency or if providers suspect child abuse, even if parents refuse. Involve medical control early in these situations, and utilize law enforcement resources as necessary to ensure that the patient receives the necessary emergency stabilization and transport. Remember that all EMTs, regardless of certification level, have a *duty to report* suspected child abuse at all times and in all patients. Even if the ED says that they will report a suspected case later on, it is important to still immediately file a report with the authorities to protect the EMS provider.

Many states have an EMS *do not resuscitate* (DNR) protocol to limit resuscitative efforts for those who have made that decision with their physician. Remember that these are under the authority of the parent, not the physician, and they can be revoked at any time if the parent changes his or her mind, something common in pediatric medical emergencies. Providers and medical oversight physicians must be familiar with the specific documents required for an EMS DNR to be in effect, commonly a patient wristband as well as accompanying paperwork. When in doubt, EMS providers must resuscitate a patient and transport them to the ED.

Documentation

An accurate medical assessment and record of any and all interventions in the field during an EMS encounter are vital for the receiving ED staff. Any accompanying paperwork, such as a 12-lead EKG tracing, or paperwork given to the EMTs should be attached to the documentation that is left at the hospital. EMS run sheets become an important part of the patient's permanent medical record and may play an important role in determining the patient's hospital care. Especially important aspects of documentation are vital signs, medical allergies, initial evaluation and responses to interventions, and any changes en route as well as a record of the mechanism of injury and details that helps put the incident in perspective.

In addition, in our increasingly litigious society, proper documentation of EMS activities is the best defense against potential legal action. Special attention should be given to accurately documenting the patient's condition on arrival, including vital signs, position and restraint during transport, medication and fluid administration, airway status, and other interventions. Of special importance is the documentation of a properly placed, secured, and patent airway if intubation is performed by EMTs. Some departments use a separate intubation checklist with multiple redundant confirmations for this important but inherently risky procedure. It is important to realize that no EMS will have a 100% intubation success rate, but they must have a 100% success rate at airway management including detecting misplaced or displaced tubes.

All EMS documentation should be completed legibly, with errors noted by a single line cross out, initial, and date. The provider's signature must be legible and include a printed name and credentials. The EMS chart is a medical-legal document as well as a simple record of what transpired in the field. The chart must tell the story and relay all the important assessment and treatment data. It should reflect the medical decision-making thought process as well as document any online medical control orders that were acquired. For paramedics, it is essential to have times associated with any medications that were given.

Increasingly, EMS services are utilizing electronic medical records (EMR) or other electronic charting, typically done with tablet-style laptop computers connected wirelessly to the patient-monitoring equipment and to the hospital's centralized information system. This has the potential to improve the accuracy of collecting data associated with patient care, although this information is typically unfiltered and may not accurately reflect the real-time condition of the patient because of problems with the equipment, motion artifact, or other variables in the EMS setting.

TABLE 6.4

EMERGENCY MEDICAL SERVICES–RELATED ORGANIZATIONS AND ONLINE RESOURCES

Organization	Online resource
Air Medical Physician Association	www.ampa.org
American Academy of Pediatrics	www.aap.org
American College of Emergency Physicians	www.acep.org
American Heart Association	www.americanheart.org
American Trauma Society	www.amtrauma.org
Association of Air Medical Services	www.aams.org
Commission on Accreditation of Medical Transport Systems	www.camts.org
EMSC	http://bolivia.hrsa.gov/emsc/
Language Line	www.languageline.com/page/industry_healthcare/
National Association of Emergency Medical Physicians	www.naemsp.org
National Association of Emergency Medical Technicians	www.naemt.org
National Association of State EMS Directors	www.nasemsd.org
National Highway Traffic Safety Institute	www.nhtsa.dot.gov
National Registry of Emergency Medical Technicians	www.nremt.org
Pediatric Advanced Life Support (PALS)	www.americanheart.org/presenter.jhtml?identifier=3012001

EMERGENCY MEDICAL SERVICES FOR CHILDREN—RESOURCES AND LINKS

We recommend that physicians and other advanced health-care providers become involved in the EMSC system in their community, especially those who work in emergency medicine, critical care, pediatrics, surgery, and family medicine. On a local, regional, or state level, physicians can contact the EMSC organization for ways to advocate for pediatric EMS issues. The state Office of EMS or its equivalent can be contacted for a schedule of local community medical services meetings. This is a good way for an interested physician to learn more about the issues facing their EMS providers. There are standardized educational opportunities that can afford the teacher and provider more experience with pediatric EMS, such as the PEPP curriculum through the AAP. More and more EMTs are undertaking the PALS course (AHA) to supplement their pediatric training, and physician educators play an important role in the success of this course.

Many other organizations exist to serve as educational resources and as forums for discussing, teaching, and implementing policies used to promote the specific needs of pediatric EMS. National organizations and their web sites are listed in Table 6.4. EMSC is an example of a national initiative designed to reduce child and youth disability and death due to severe illness and injury. Medical personnel, parents, volunteers, community groups, businesses, national organizations, and foundations contribute to the effort. Examples include the many projects on childhood injury prevention and the previously referred to list of essential pediatric EMS equipment for ambulances.

PEDIATRIC INTERFACILITY TRANSPORT

Pediatric interfacility transport involves patient transfer from one medical location to another. Patient status can vary from relatively stable to critically ill. The disease processes involved are detailed throughout this text and include inpatients with progressive or unresolved problems and the entire spectrum of neonatal illness. Although the ABC (airway, breathing, circulation) approach to care remains the integral focus during interfacility transport, it is essential to understand the disease process and expected progression of the disease during the transport period.

Interfacility transport can originate from or be directed to hospitals, emergency care centers, physician offices, clinics, or other medical care facilities. There may not be a clear distinction between interfacility and prehospital transport in terms of equipment, process, and in some instances, personnel. Many interfacility transport teams routinely transport patients from the prehospital care environment, and EMS may be involved in interfacility transport. The differences between prehospital and interfacility transport teams often revolve around extrication issues, personnel education, and experience.

Although transport teams care for patients with disease processes similar to those seen in ED and critical care units, the delivery of care can differ. The transport environment offers many opportunities for problems if care is not managed appropriately. Although issues of transport team organization can be found in other texts, we briefly review important concepts of interfacility transport here.

Interfacility transport begins with the recognition of a need or a desire for medical care not available at the patient's current location. Reasons for transport can include a requirement for advanced or specialized levels of care or services, a patient's preference for a particular caregiver, the desire to obtain a second opinion, insurance issues, and parent or provider frustrations. However, as outlined in the Consolidated Omnibus Budget Reconciliation Act of 1985 and the federal Emergency Medical Treatment and Active Labor Act (EMTALA) regulations, interfacility transport cannot be used as a method to avoid initial assessment, stabilization, or intervention, especially with regard to a patient's ability to pay.

To prepare for interfacility transport, a transport system must have access to specialized equipment, trained personnel, and appropriate licenses (Tables 6.5A to 6.5D). The transport system

TABLE 6.5A

AN EXAMPLE OF EQUIPMENT AND PHARMACEUTICAL SUPPLIES USEFUL FOR PEDIATRIC CRITICAL CARE
TRANSPORT: CONTENTS OF A "UNIVERSAL" PEDIATRIC CRITICAL CARE TRANSPORT EQUIPMENT BAG[a]

Center Lid Zippered Panel
Heimlich valve (2)
Chest tubes (1 each)
  10F, 12F, 16F
  Stylette (1 each)
    Neonatal and adult
Ventilator circuit
Cricothyroid kits
  3 or 3.5 mm (1)
  4 mm (1)
Pneumothorax kit

Center Panel—Pouch
AAA batteries (2)
AA batteries (4)
C batteries (2)
9-Volt batteries (1)
Electrocardiogram electrodes
  Infant and pediatric
pH paper
Nonsterile gauze
Lancets
Thermometer

Center Panel
Infant/pediatric self-inflating bag
Adult self-inflating bag
Buretrol and secondary
  medication set
Folder with extra paperwork
  Flowsheets
  Consent forms
  Progress note paper
  IV solution recipe list
  STATMed card
  Parent handbook
  i-STAT reference
Salem sump (1 each)
  Sizes: 6, 8, 10, 12, 14, 16, 18
Replogle tube
Infant Oxyhood
Nasal cannula (1 each)
  Infant and pediatric
Assorted respiratory masks
Venturi tube
Green bubble tubing
Face masks (1 each)
  Preemie, infant, toddler
  Child and adult
Suction catheters (3 each)
  6F, 8F, 10F, 12F, 14F
Intraflow transducer

Center Panel—Airway Pouch
Green O_2 suction catheters (2 each)
  10F, 14F
Extra laryngoscope bulbs (large and
  small)
Saline vials for suctioning
Laryngoscope handles (2)
Laryngoscope blades
  Miller: 0, 1, 2, 3
  Wis-Hipple: 1.5
  MacIntosh: 2, 3, 4
Oral airways (1 each)
  Sizes: 4, 5, 6, 7, 8, 9
Magill forceps
Tygon
Benzoin
Yankauer
K-Y Jelly
Humidivent
Tongue blades
5-cc Syringe
Nipples
White tape

Center Panel—IV Kit
NSS flushes (3)
3-cc syringes (3)
5-cc syringes (3)
Saline vials (2)
Heparin flush (3)
Stopcocks (3)
T-connectors (3)
Clear tape
Tourniquet or rubber bands
Blood culture bottle
Bullets (1 each)
  Clear, red, green, purple
Uterine artery/uterine vein (UA/UV)
  catheter (2 each)
  3.5F, 5.0F, 8.0F
Jelco and Flash catheters (3 each)
  18, 20, 22, 24 gauge
Butterflies (2 each)
  19, 23, 25, 27 gauge
Alcohol swabs
Betadine swabs
PRN adapters (3)
Band-Aids
Interosseous needles (1 each)
  16 and 18 gauge
  Arm boards (1 each size)

Right-side Pocket
Goggles
Hot packs (3)
Neonatal pulse oximetry probes (2)
Easy Cap O_2 Sensor

Back Pocket
Mapelson circuit with metal valve
Mapelson circuit with disposable valve
Endotracheal tube (2 each)
  2.5, 3.0, 3.5, 4.0, 4.5, 5.0, 5.5, 6.0, 6.5,
  7.0
Cuffed endotracheal tube (2 each)
  5.0, 6.0, 7.0, 8.0, 9.0
Manometer
Extra bags (0.5 L, 1 L, 2 L)

Left Front Pocket
Nebulizer pouch
  Nebulizer
  Adapter for Mapelson
  Albuterol 5 mg/mL 20-mL bottle
  Albuterol Jets 2.5 mg/5 mL
  Saline vials
  Racemic epinephrine
Lacri-Lube
Penlight
5-in-1 Connector (1)
6-in-1 Connector (1)
O_2 tank key
Nasopharyngeal airways (1 each)
  12, 14, 16, 18, 20, 22, 24, 26, 28, 30
Arterial pressure tubing (3)
Arterial set (1)
Microtubing (3)
Extension tubing (4)
Bifurcated connector (1)
Trifurcated connector (1)

Right Front Pocket
Syringes
  1, 3, 5, 10 cc (5 each)
  20, 30 cc (3 each)
  60 cc (4), 60 cath tip (1)
Assorted needles
Pressure bag

Left-side Pocket
Formulary
DINAMAP cuffs (1 each)
  1, 2, 3, 4, 5
Safe cuffs (1 each)
  Infant, child, small and large adult

[a]Transport teams must be self-sufficient during the transfer process; therefore, care should be taken to ensure adequate and appropriate supplies.
Specifics may vary as per team function and intended patient population.

is responsible for ensuring the safety of the patient, team, and family members during the transport as well as guaranteeing that the patient is cared for in the medically appropriate environment. The transport system should have an identifiable medical director who is responsible for ensuring adequate training and education as well as continuing assessment of the transport per-

sonnel and process. The medical director is the person ultimately responsible for ensuring a safe, reliable transport system.

Significant preparation is required to be an efficient user of transport services. The users of a transport system (the referral hospitals and physicians) must ensure the transport services meet the standards required for the transfer of their patients.

TABLE 6.5B

ADDITIONAL TRANSPORT EQUIPMENT TO BE CONSIDERED WHEN EQUIPPING A PEDIATRIC CRITICAL CARE TRANSPORT TEAM

Cardiorespiratory monitors	Infusion pumps
Noninvasive	Single and/or multichannel
Invasive	Blood sample measuring devices
Ventilators	Point of care testing
Pressure	Glucometer
Volume	Portable suction
Capnography	Portable oxygen
Pulse oximeter	Cellular phone(s)
Defibrillator with pacing capability	

The referral providers must avoid the mind-set of getting the patient out of the initial care environment as quickly as possible without first ensuring transport safety and medical stability.

Transport medicine is an established section within the AAP. Many other groups, such as the Air Medical Physicians Association, are dedicated to ensuring optimal care for transported patients. These organizations offer continuing education and are conduits for information regarding transport medicine. The AAP published the third edition of its "Guidelines for Air and Ground Transport of Neonatal and Pediatric Patients" in 2007. There are several listservs dedicated to pediatric transport. These include the pediatric interhospital transport discussion list (PEDTPT-L@listserv.brown.edu) and the AAP transport section listserv (transmedaap@listserv.aap.org). Subscribe to these lists by contacting listserv@listserv.brown.edu and www.aap.org/sections/transmed/.

Transport Considerations

Familiarity and the ability to understand the transport environment and troubleshoot as necessary is critical for the successful transport of a patient. Therefore, emergently configuring a transport team in response to an acute request for patient transport, unless there has been adequate preparation and training, should be avoided. Logistic issues to consider include ensuring proper equipment and medication supplies; intervening in a potentially cramped, moving environment; safely securing the patient to the stretcher and the stretcher to the transport vehicle; and recognizing and managing the loss of inverter power. In addition, oxygen delivery and suction—as well as the issue of motion sickness—can be difficult for the non–transport-oriented participant. Noise, vibration, and temperature can also be formidable problems for the patient and provider if not anticipated and planned for.

In the transport process, one must be prepared for all types of patients and complications. When the transport team arrives, the patient's status may be significantly different than

TABLE 6.5C

A STANDARD PEDIATRIC/NEONATAL CRITICAL CARE TRANSPORT MEDICATION SUPPLY[a]

Medication	Number	Medication	Number
Albumin 5% 250 mL	1	Procainamide 100 mg/mL 10 mL	1
Albumin 25% 50 mL	1	Propanolol 1 mg/mL 1 mL	2
Ampicillin 1 g	2	Sodium chloride 0.9% 10 mL	4
Amiodarone 50 mg/mL 3 mL	5	Sterile water injection 10 mL	4
Benzocaine spray 20%	1	Terbutaline 1 mg/1 cc 1 mL	10
Cefazolin 1 g	1	Tolazoline 25 mg/mL 4 mL	2
Cefotaxime 2 g	1	Vancomycin 500 mg	2
Dexamethasone 4 mg/mL 30 mL	1	Vasopressin 20 U/mL	5
Digoxin 100 μg/mL 1 mL	4	Verapamil 2.5 mg/mL 2 mL	3
Diphenhydramine 50 mg/mL 1 mL	1		
Furosemide 10 mg/mL 2 mL	4	**IV Solutions**	
Gentamicin 10 mg/mL 2 mL	4	Dextrose 5% 0.2 NS 1,000 mL	1
Glucagon 1 mg	2	Dextrose 10% 1,000 mL	1
Heparin 1,000 U/mL 10 mL	1	Sodium chloride 0.9% 1,000 mL	1
Hydrocortisone 100 mg/2 mL	2	Theophylline 4 mg/cc 50 cc	1
Lidocaine spray 10% 33 g	1		
Magnesium sulfate 4 mEq/mL 2 mL	2	**Additional Medications to Consider**	
Mannitol 25% 50 mL	2	Albuterol-metered inhaler	
Methylprednisolone 125 mg/2 mL	2	Albuterol 5 mg/mL 20 mL	
Methylprednisolone 1,000 mg	1	Albuterol jet 2.5 mg/3 mL	
Neostigmine 0.5 mg/mL 1 mL	2	Insulin 100 U/mL	
Nifedipine capsule 10 mg	3	Lorazepam 2 mg/mL	
Oxymetazoline nasal spray 15 mL	1	Prostaglandin E 0.5 mg/mL	
Phenylephrine 10 mg/mL	1	Racemic epinephrine 2.25%, 15 mL	
Phenytoin 50 mg/mL 5 mL	2	Survanta 8 mL	
Potassium chloride 2 mEq/mL 10 mL	2	Topical thrombin 1,000 U	
		Tromethamine 500 mL	

[a]Care should be taken to ensure all medications are current (not expired).

TABLE 6.5D

A RAPIDLY ACCESSIBLE "STAT" MEDICATION SUPPLY
SHOULD BE INCLUDED

Medication	Number
Adenosine 3 mg/mL 2 mL	5
Albumin 5% 50 mL	2
Amiodarone 50 mg/mL 3 mL	5
Atropine 0.4 mg/mL 1 mL	4
Calcium gluconate 100 mg/mL 10 mL	3
Dextrose 50% 50 mL	1
Dobutamine 12.5 mg/mL 20 mL	1
Dopamine 40 mg/mL 5 mL	3
Epinephrine 1 mg/mL 1 mL	3
Epinephrine 1 mg/mL 30 mL	1
Isoproterenol 0.2 mg/mL 5 mL	2
Lidocaine 20 mg/mL 5 mL	2
Naloxone 1 mg/mL 1 mL	4
Nitroprusside 60 mg/mL	1
Pancuronium 1 mg/mL 10 mL	1
Sodium bicarbonate 44.6 mEq/mL 50 mL	3
Sodium chloride 0.9% 10 mL	2
Sterile water injection 10 mL	3
Succinylcholine 20 mg/mL 10 mL	1
Thiopental syringe 250 mg/10 mL	1
Vecuronium 10 mg	2
Controlled Substances	
Diazepam 5 mg/mL 2 mL	3
Fentanyl 50 μg/mL 5 mL	1
Ketamine 10 mg/mL 20 mL	1
Midazolam 5 mg/mL 2 mL	2
Morphine Tubex 2 mg/mL	5
Phenobarbital 65 mg/mL	3

that initially described. This can be the result of a change in the patient's condition, incomplete assessment by the referring physician or transport team, or inadequate information flow. The ability to correctly assess severity of illness or injury before transport, from both the referring physician and the receiving physician perspectives, helps facilitate appropriate triage, advice and pretransport care of the patient, mode of transport, and personnel configuration decisions. Orr et al. have done considerable work in studying predictive models to help appropriately triage for and critically assess the use of pediatric transport systems. This research suggests several factors are useful in predicting in-hospital mortality. These include blood pressure, respiratory rate, oxygen requirement, and altered mental status. They also found that risk of mortality increased with performance of major interventions, as did the occurrence of unplanned events. Orr et al's 2009 paper "Pediatric specialized transport teams are associated with improved outcomes" clearly demonstrates the positive patient impact of specialty pediatric transport teams. Others have looked at the Shock Index (SI) in an attempt to determine stability and level of illness, while other systems use specific triage tools to determine optimal response required (ALS, level of critical care transport) for each particular patient. Kanter et al. evaluated use of the PRISM score in the pre-ICU populations. Use of electronic adjuncts to care is also increasing. Telemedicine interactions prior to and during transport can potentially improve information flow and accessibility, ultimately improving patient care and safety. The transport team

may also be asked to transfer a different patient if a more critical patient has presented to the same referring institution. Inadequate numbers or types of personnel, equipment, or medications can render the transport team less effective in these situations.

The medical capabilities of the transport systems are important to assess. All transport teams do not have equivalent levels of pediatric skills. Transport services can vary from specialized pediatric teams, such as those supplied by tertiary care pediatric hospitals, to generalized transport services. In addition, some teams have additional capabilities (in addition to specialized personnel support), such as those who perform or transport patients requiring (or receiving) extracorporeal membrane oxygenation (ECMO), inhaled nitric oxide, and high-frequency ventilation or oscillation. Foley et al. presented a review of 100 patients, including 32 children, transported while on ECMO. A generalized transport service accepts all ages and types of patients; unfortunately, there are no universal standards or regulations regarding the level of experience or expertise in pediatrics required to transport pediatric patients. There are, however, accrediting agencies and standards that can be reviewed. The most specific accreditation process for transport systems is through the Commission on Accreditation of Medical Transport Systems (CAMTS). Although this is often a voluntary appraisal of a system, certification has been used as a mandatory review for licensing of some services in specific states. All hospital-based teams must, however, comply with Joint Commission on Accreditation of Healthcare Organizations requirements for patient care and safety. The 2003 National Patient Safety Goals mandate to improve safety of high-alert medications does not exempt transport teams from compliance. The mandate to remove concentrated electrolytes (including, but not limited to, potassium chloride, potassium phosphate, and sodium chloride greater than 0.9%) from patient care units, moving from use of the rule of 6s and standardizing and limiting the number of drug concentrations available in the transport organization, has been a challenge for some systems, but must be accomplished for optimal patient safety. Transport personnel need to potentially predict certain electrolyte needs prior to transport, or ensure availability at the referring facility, if they do not have the availability to carry or prepare specific fluids during the process because of this restriction.

Although pediatric patients can be efficiently and safely transported by different types of transport systems, the referring physician is responsible for assessing each program for medical sophistication and safety. Pediatric diseases and processes are different from those in adults, and one should not assume a general transport service has adequate experience in pediatrics to offer the appropriate or optimal level of care. Although patient transport by a general team may be quickly accomplished, the process may be classified as getting the patient to pediatric care quickly as opposed to rapidly bringing pediatric care to the patient. For many patients, this is an academic distinction. For example, the stable trauma patient, the child with a clearly defined medical process, or the patient needing referral for a nonprogressive, non–life-threatening issue may be adequately transported by a transport team without extensive pediatric experience. It is imperative, however, that general ALS and/or critical care skills be available for most of these transports. Consultation with a pediatric expert should also be included. When the differential diagnosis needs to be explored during the transport process or when the patient's condition is rapidly changing, an experienced pediatric team is usually preferred. In geographic locations where specialized pediatric transport is unavailable, involvement of an appropriately skilled acute care/critical care pediatrician on the referring and/or receiving end is important. When possible, an unstable patient should not be referred from a nonpediatric provider to a pediatric institution via a transport team inexperienced in pediatric disease process and management. Ideally, advanced pediatric care should begin the moment the transport team is contacted. Pediatric medical or surgical advice, as well as adequate instruction before arrival of the transport team, can be stabilizing and potentially lifesaving for that particular patient.

Technical skill capability in general transport teams does not necessarily translate into technical skill competence in the treatment of children. This is perhaps most evident in children needing advanced airway intervention. A child's anterior larynx and the recommendation to avoid nasal intubation in children can preclude successful airway intervention by personnel who are not sufficiently educated or experienced in managing the pediatric airway. This discussion is not meant to cause one to avoid nonpediatric transport services, but only to ensure that the technical skill and competency necessary for adequate assessment and care of the patient during the transport process are optimal and that the cognitive components, if necessary, are augmented by an outside pediatric specialist.

When a decision is made to transport a pediatric patient, there is often a discussion of the appropriate mode of transport. Nonmedical transports include a parent's automobile or a taxicab. Problems with these choices include lack of assurance of direct transport to the receiving facility, inability to ensure patient safety, and the lack of available medical care during the transfer. Even the accompaniment of a physician or nurse does not markedly improve the ability for medical intervention in these nonmedical vehicles. A BLS ambulance offers

direct transportation to the receiving institution, but does not offer much in the way of pediatric expertise or intervention capability. Physician or nurse accompaniment in a BLS ambulance increases potential level of medical care; however, the BLS environment is limited with regard to basic personnel, pediatric equipment, and medications. ALS transport offers more sophisticated resuscitation abilities but may provide variable and inconsistent levels of pediatric experience and/or expertise. Physician accompaniment may increase the level of available medical care within the ALS environment, but that impact may be decreased by the particular service's use of protocols and offline medical direction. Critical care transport services can increase the medical sophistication of ALS providers by ensuring the presence of a critical care transport nurse, but these providers may be lacking significant pediatric training, experience, expertise and/or skills. Pediatric critical care transport systems include critical care participants (nurses and physicians) with significant pediatric experience and expertise.

When transport services are needed, the modes to be considered include ground ambulance, RW aircraft (helicopter), and FW aircraft (jet or prop plane) (Figs. 6.4 to 6.6). Often, the decision is straightforward. For example, the available transport system may be ground only, or inclement weather may prevent air transport. Alternatively, the distance may be so great or traffic issues significant enough that ground ambulance transport is impractical. Several important issues should be considered when mode of transport is discussed. The first is personnel availability. If the transport modes require or offer different personnel configurations, the mode with the most appropriate personnel should be strongly considered. Ideally, a pediatric transport service with the capability for air and ground transport is available so comparative personnel issues are not the major deciding factors. A choice between speed of transport and appropriate medical personnel can be difficult, although they

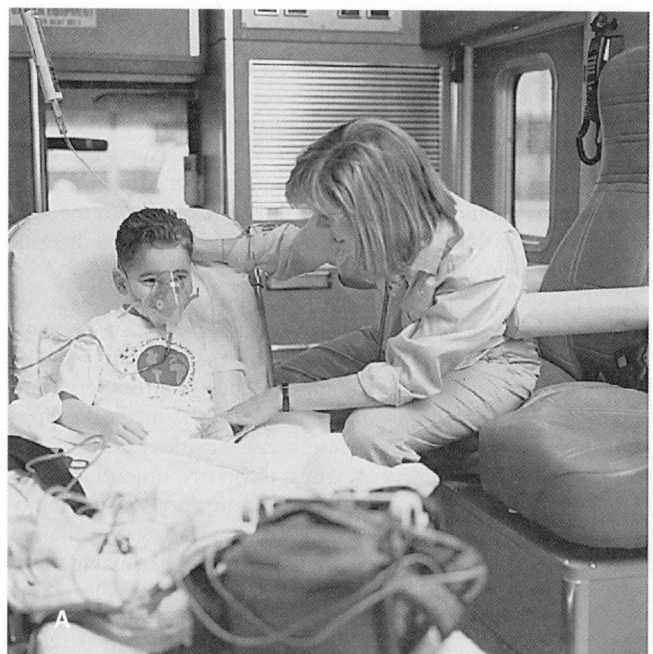
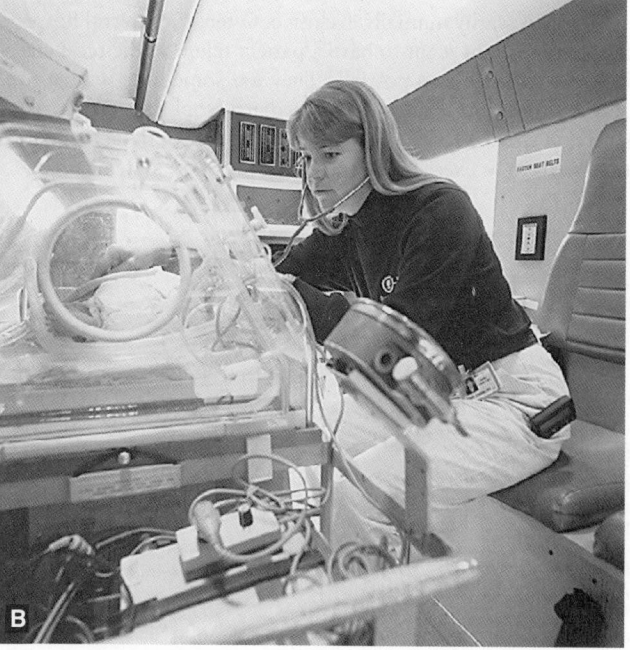

FIGURE 6.4 **A, B:** Pediatric interfacility ambulance environment. Examples of patients being transported within the ambulance environment. Note relative limitations of space and patient access. (Used with permission, © The Children's Hospital of Philadelphia, Philadelphia, PA.)

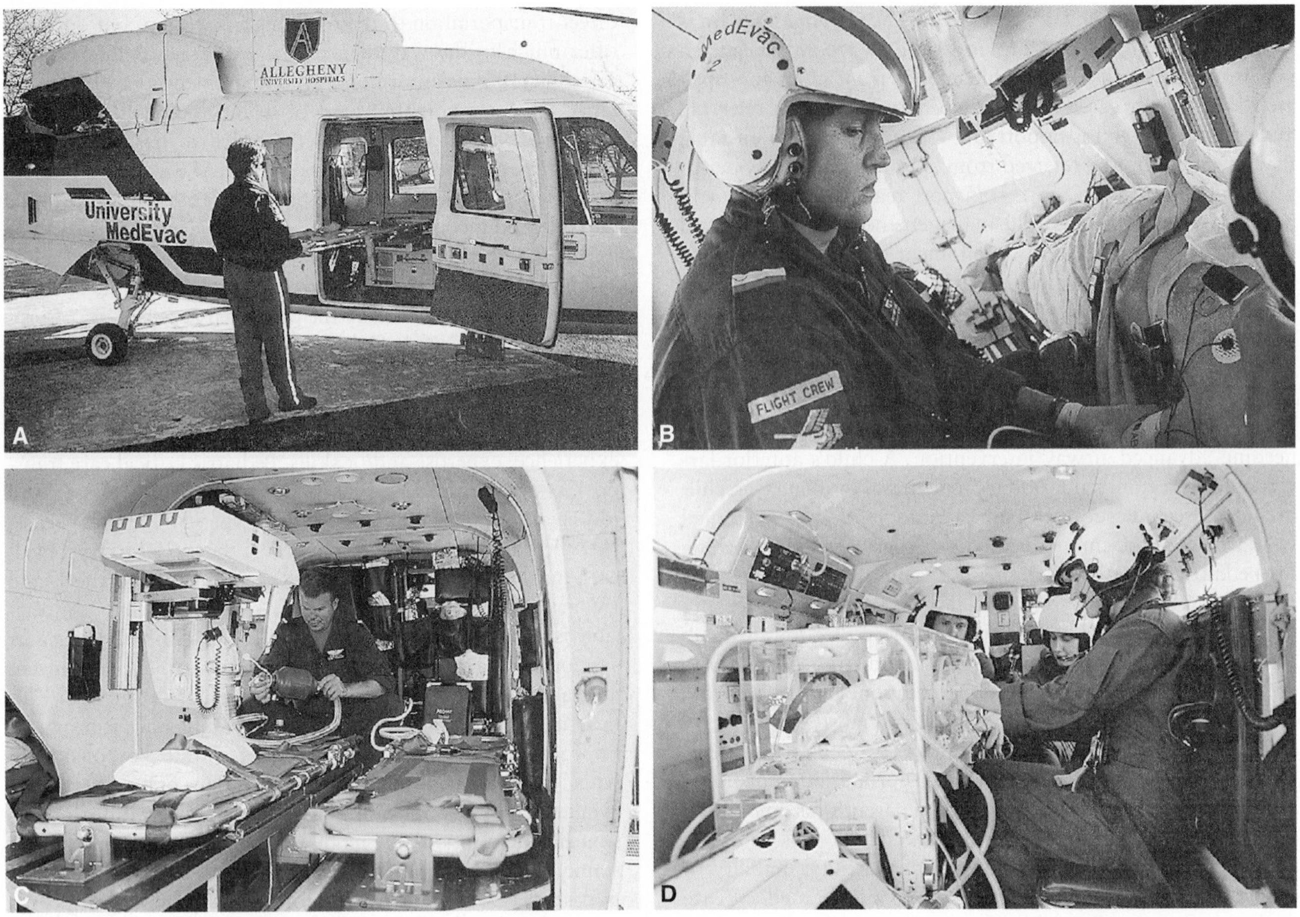

FIGURE 6.5 **A–D:** Air medical transport environment. Examples of design of a medical helicopter ("rotor-wing"). Note relative space and patient access limitations. (A–C: From Hahnemann University Hospital, University MedEvac, Philadelphia, PA, with permission; D: Used with permission, © The Children's Hospital of Philadelphia, Philadelphia, PA.)

are not necessarily mutually exclusive. Often, the referral hospitals or physicians want to have a patient taken to the receiving hospital as quickly as possible. They are sometimes willing to accept a transport team with little pediatric sophistication based solely on speed. Occasionally this may be appropriate, but caution needs to be exercised to ensure the transport system is capable of handling issues that can occur during the transport process. The referral physicians must be proactive in the mode of transport decision. This includes being aware of the transport systems that are available and evaluating those systems before using them. In areas without tertiary care pediatric transport options, local pediatric providers and the receiving pediatric physicians should be available to provide expertise to the general transport services to help bridge the gap between the general (primarily adult) and pediatric providers.

Transport across international borders may also be required. This mode of transport requires significant preplanning. Specific issues to be considered for these patients include, but are not limited to, language issues of providers (and patients), compatibility and redundancy of medical equipment, power sources, medication issues with customs, communications during process, visas, passports, other documentation, and logistics of transport durations. For many international, long-distance transports, air crews are required to "time out," necessitating transport times that may go into days or use of additional personnel for the process. The same concerns, although not as rigid in established requirements, must be afforded to the health-care personnel as well. Options and solutions to some of these issues are available, but must be anticipated prior to need. Several services specialize in international transport and should be consulted for one trying to

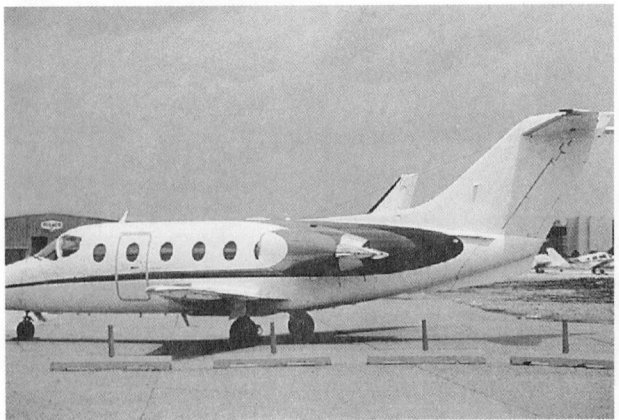

FIGURE 6.6 Fixed-wing transport. Both jet and piston (propeller) aircraft are used. Picture used with permission, Airlift Northwest, Seattle Washington.

determine or arrange optimal international transport options. During international operations, if both custodial parents are not accompanying the patient, it may be necessary to have a certified letter from the parent(s) not present giving the team permission to leave the country.

The disease process must also be considered in mode of transport decisions. The patient with developing petechiae, fever, and hypotension should not be transported several hours by ground if a quicker method of transport is available. Thomas et al. reported an association between helicopter transport and increased survival in blunt trauma patients (adult and pediatric). However, a short air transport for a relatively stable patient may not be an appropriate use of resources or be in the patient's or team's best interest. Eckstein et al. and Arfken et al. suggested that helicopter services may be overused and may not influence outcomes when compared with alternative modes of transport. One must be cognizant of the many issues surrounding the mode of transport choices. These choices should be individualized for each patient. Although appropriate medical care should not be withheld for financial reasons, a cost comparison of air and ground transports is often useful, especially if done before the acute transport. This may be an important factor in the decision process; however, if the referral or receiving physician or hospital is responsible for guaranteeing the cost of the transport. In general, RW (helicopter) transport costs two to three times as much as a ground transport for local transfers. However, the cost may potentially be offset by the savings in time. A helicopter, which can travel directly to and land at the patient's location, is much quicker than an ambulance, which must take a more circuitous route. If the helicopter cannot land directly at the referring or receiving center, however, the time savings by air transport may be less significant. In that situation, in addition to the decreased time savings, the patient may be placed at greater risk with the multiple transfers from referral center to ambulance to helicopter to ambulance to receiving hospital. The riskiest time for the patient is often during transfer from stretcher to stretcher or vehicle to vehicle (Fig. 6.7). These transfers increase the opportunities for dislodgement of endotracheal tubes, central venous catheters, chest tubes, and other lifesaving equipment. Communication center personnel, transport team, members and medical command physicians should all be aware of times, distances, and particular medical and logistical nuances of each referring institution and location.

Personnel Issues

Many types of providers can function effectively as part of a pediatric transport team. Nurses, ARNPs, respiratory therapists, EMTs, paramedics, and physicians serve on various transport teams. The choice of personnel depends on several factors, but the most important are the team's primary mission and the resources available for training and skill maintenance. In general, the personnel chosen for the transport team should have experience in the care of critically ill infants and/or children, and they must be competent in the transport environment. The best bedside clinician may be ineffective if he or she does not know where to find resources in the ambulance or helicopter, or how to turn on the oxygen or suction. The team may also be functionally limited if one of the providers is limited in knowledge or ability to perform specific patient care tasks, such as medication administration and delivery. The

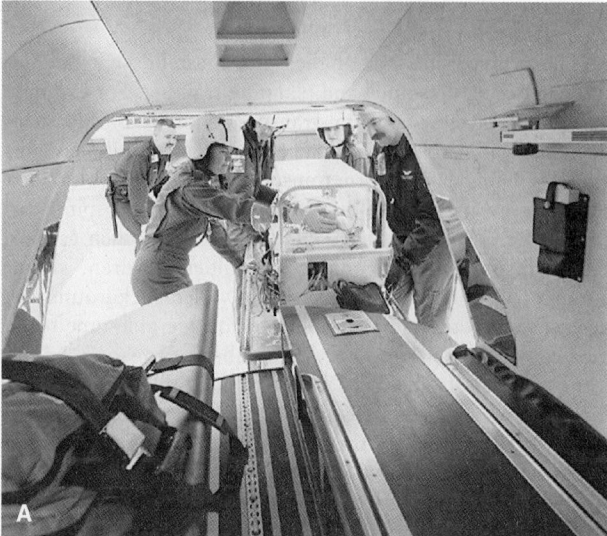

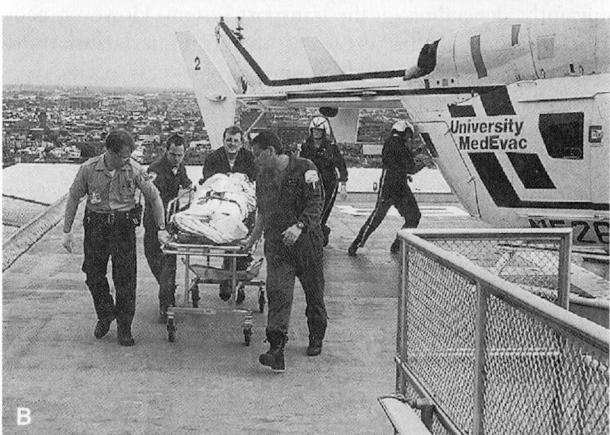

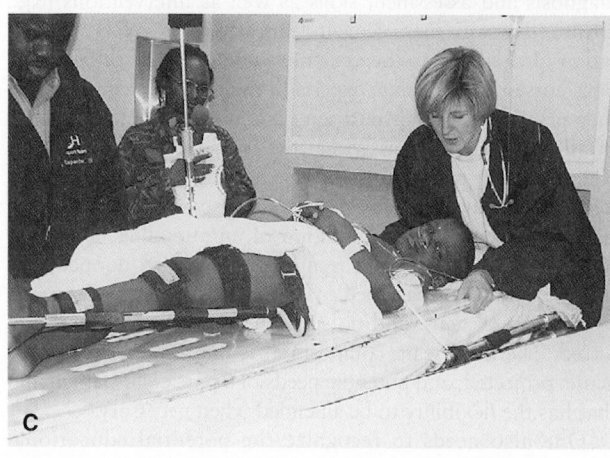

FIGURE 6.7 **A–C:** Transfer of patient during transport process. Patient transfer between vehicles or stretchers can be risky to the patient. Tube, line, oxygen, or medication disconnection or disruption, as well as shifts in immobilization, must be avoided. (**A, C:** Used with permission, © The Children's Hospital of Philadelphia, Philadelphia, PA; **B:** From Hahnemann University Hospital, University MedEvac, Philadelphia, PA, with permission.)

transport environment is not the appropriate place to learn basic pediatric critical care skills.

The primary mission of the team must be kept in mind when selecting personnel and planning training. For example, a team devoted to neonatal transport should consider team members with experience in the care of critically ill neonates, whereas teams that perform transports from nonhospital locations may want to employ personnel with prehospital care experience. Teams that have multiple missions, such as those that transport both neonates and older children, should attempt to recruit team members from varied backgrounds. By necessity, such teams have to devote considerable time to the medical cross-training of staff members. However, having team members from varied backgrounds offers the potential for those members to assist in the training and care delivery processes. Regardless of the medical background of the transport participants, education and experience in the transport environment is imperative.

Transport team capabilities and types of personnel vary significantly, depending on the transport system. However, pediatric critical care transport teams, the ideal interfacility transport configuration for children, often have several specific types of providers. At the heart of most pediatric critical care transport teams are highly trained pediatric critical care transport nurses. These nurses usually have significant critical care or emergency medicine experience before becoming members of the transport service. They have often had their technical and cognitive skills enhanced by formal or informal specialized training, as described here. Such training may allow them to be classified as practitioners with advanced skill certification in certain jurisdictions. Depending on the sophistication of the transport system, training opportunities, skills and assessment, and medical licensure issues, transport nurses often provide advanced management for these children. This can include diagnosis and assessment skills as well as interventions (e.g., advanced airway management, central venous access, resuscitation). In addition to their cognitive and technical skills, transport nurses have become experts in the environment in which they practice. The transport nurse should be intimately aware of all operating systems within the transport environment as well as safety procedures for the patient and the transport team. The medical skills of pediatric transport nurses can often be complemented by the addition of an attending, fellow, or resident physician; ARNP; respiratory therapist; nonpediatric transport nurse; or paramedic. Team compositions vary greatly in different systems, and no single team configuration is preferred. The ideal team composition is one that addresses the acute, projected, and potential needs of a particular patient and that has the flexibility to be amended when necessary.

One also needs to recognize the potential educational value (as compared with service use) of resident trainees during the transport environment. Many pediatric programs include residents and fellows as part of the patient care team, while in some cases, they participate as additional members in primarily an educational role. Durbin et al., as well as Fazio et al., reviewed the use and educational value associated with residents on transport. If residents or fellows are used in more than an educational role, they must bring a skill set to the transport environment that is additive and complementary to the other team members and equals or exceeds that of those who could take their place. If the resident cannot function as a full member of the team, and has replaced

someone who could, reassessment of personnel configurations is indicated.

In addition to the personnel already described, transport teams usually include drivers or pilots who may have no role in patient care or who may assist the other personnel. Communications specialists may be employed as part of the team's call receipt and dispatch process. Finally, all transport teams should have a clearly identified supervisory medical director(s) and appropriate medical command physicians who are involved with every transport.

Other important educational considerations are the resources of both time and money available to devote to training and maintaining competencies for team members. If training time is limited, the transport team must consider hiring staff that is already well trained. For instance, a neonatal team could hire neonatal nurse practitioners. However, such well-trained staff usually demand higher wages, making them potentially more expensive than instituting an ongoing training program. Many teams do not have the opportunity to hire nurse practitioners or other previously trained and highly skilled personnel; therefore, those teams especially need to devote significant time and resources to training team members. The amount of time necessary varies with the team's mission and its customary personnel composition. A team with a well-defined scope of practice, such as neonatal transport, should employ experienced neonatal nurses. In this circumstance, only those additional skills that are new to the team members need to be added, although competency in all expected cognitive and technical skills need to be assured. Likewise, if a team usually includes a physician, the other team members may not need to learn advanced skills such as tracheal intubation. Teams must ensure their members, regardless of background and previous education/experience are competent in all procedural and management skills that may be required during transport. Such extensive training usually includes a didactic component, a skills segment, and rotations through various clinical care areas. If the group is large enough, the didactic component may be a series of lectures. However, this type of experience is difficult to arrange for one or two new team members. Alternatives to formal lectures include video- or audiotaped lectures or a modular self-study curriculum.

Unfortunately, skill acquisition is only the beginning. Rarely used skills are quickly forgotten, so a process for skill maintenance must be established. Furthermore, as in all areas of medical practice, the knowledge base in transport medicine is constantly changing, making continuing education vital. Skill retention and continuing education are best accomplished using a three-part process. The first component is renewal of basic procedural and cognitive skills. Such retraining may include rotations through the operating room to practice airway techniques; dry or animal laboratory experiences for interosseous infusion, cricothyroidotomy, thoracostomy tube placement, and other important but rarely needed procedures; and simulated codes to practice resuscitation.

The second component is formal continuing education through regularly scheduled programs, including lectures, journal clubs, and presentations of particularly unusual or difficult patients. In addition, such forums may be used to learn about new medical equipment, communication devices, and vehicle issues.

The final component of an effective education program is quality improvement. Routine, periodic case reviews should take place by the transport service in conjunction with other medical experts. A formal morbidity and mortality conference may be included as a part of such a program. In addition, topics such as response times and parent satisfaction may be discussed. The focus of these sessions should be on the process of patient transport. Determining and assigning blame for less-than-optimal outcomes is important only when the staff member involved was clearly negligent. It is far more important to focus on ways in which the team's practices may be changed to improve performance and minimize risk of similar events in the future.

Although the team's mission dictates most of the cognitive and technical aspects of training, all teams will need to work together in a cohesive fashion. This might be particularly challenging for transport teams as they practice in a unique and somewhat isolated environment and in a fashion that might be quite different from the traditional medical hierarchy. The interactions and relationships necessary for success in this type of practice may have more in common with other high-performance teams, such as military special forces units and aircraft crews, than with those found in many other healthcare situations. A growing body of evidence from the airline industry, and now from health care, suggests that these team skills can be learned and that, when fully integrated into the culture of the program, serve to improve team performance and decrease medical errors.

Communication

A key component of any transport team is effective communication. Referring physicians must be able to contact the transport service, including the appropriate medical command physicians, quickly and easily, and teams in the field must be able to communicate with the receiving facility and providers. The ability to communicate with a command physician is particularly important for teams using resident physicians or nonphysician practitioners because they may need online medical direction. Ideally, a single point of contact (e.g., a dispatch/communication center) should be established to help ensure centralized access, to help ensure that no calls are missed, and that all communications are properly documented (Fig. 6.8).

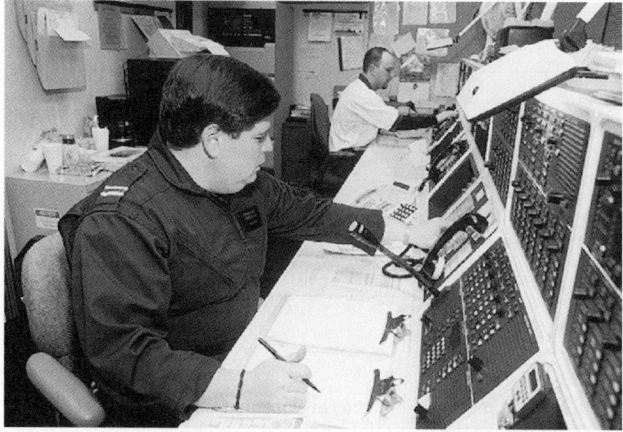

FIGURE 6.8 Transport communication center. A dedicated transport communication center and personnel are invaluable in coordinating all aspects of pediatric transport. The system need not be as elaborate as demonstrated, but should include dedicated phone lines, radio access, personnel notification capability systems, and personnel. (From Hahnemann University Hospital, University MedEvac, Philadelphia, PA, with permission.)

Communication with the transport team begins with an initial call from the referring provider. This initial contact is best managed by the use of a protocol or template, which helps ensure that the necessary patient and logistical information is properly received by the transport team (Fig. 6.9). During the initial call or soon thereafter, the referring provider may request advice regarding the medical management of the patient. Alternatively, such advice may be offered by the receiving physician. For critically ill infants and children, medical advice via telephone may be needed intermittently from the time of initial contact through arrival, evaluation, and departure from the referring facility until arrival at definitive location in the receiving facility. For these reasons, it is preferable to have transport requests initiated and received by senior physicians who can ask for and offer appropriate advice directly. The more people between the source of the information and the final recipient, the greater the potential for significant changes or omissions that may be vital to the patient. We also recommend that transport nurse–to–referral bedside nurse conversation to evaluate the patient from the nursing perspective be an expected part of the transport process. Together, these two avenues of information flow offer the greatest potential for complete awareness of all aspects of the patient's disease process and current medical condition.

After the transport team has arrived at the referring facility and performed a preliminary evaluation of the patient, they often need to communicate with one or more people at the receiving hospital. These calls can involve patient review and logistical issues such as patient disposition, scheduling of studies, and need for consultants. The ability to conference in various participants, such as specialty physicians, charge nurses, and bedside nurses, can greatly impact the information flow, logistics, and potential delivered care of the patient. Such calls are best facilitated by a communication center.

En route to the receiving hospital, it may be necessary for the transport team to contact the medical command physician either for advice or because the patient's medical condition has changed. Reliable communications are especially important at this point in the transport. The team should be equipped with redundant systems to ensure a reliable means of communication is always available. These should include cellular technology, long-range alpha beepers, land radio communications systems and satellite phone where necessary. Newer technologies, including telemedicine and global positioning systems, may improve communication and logistics capabilities. The transport command physician should be immediately accessible to the transport team by telephone or designated beeper.

After arrival at the receiving hospital, the transport team is responsible for ensuring an efficient, informative, and seamless transition of care to the inpatient physician and nursing team. Adequate communication and information flow must take place to fully inform the inpatient team of the patient's disease process and care to date. Complete documentation, written in a clear, concise fashion, is mandatory (Fig. 6.10). Anything less than a complete transfer of information and a seamless transition from referral physician to transport team to receiving physicians is a disservice to the patient and a source of potential liability.

It is important to remember that transport communications have other medical-legal ramifications. The most important of these involves the giving of medical advice and the assumption of legal responsibility for patient management. When giving or

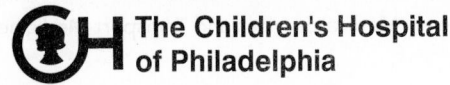

The Children's Hospital
of Philadelphia

NUR-1032
Rev. 01/03

TRANSPORT TEAM
REFERRAL FORM

(PATIENT PLATE IMPRINT)

INITIAL CALL TIME: _____ DATE OF REQUEST: ____ / ____ / ____ DATE OF TRANSPORT: ____ / ____ / ____

NAME: _____ AGE: _____ / D.O.B.: _____

REFERRING HOSPITAL: _____ ACCEPTING HOSPITAL: _____ WEIGHT _____ Kg

REFERRING M.D.: _____ ACCEPTING M.D.: _____ REFERRING PH. #: _____

REFERRING UNIT/LOCATION: _____ ACCEPTING UNIT: _____ ACCEPTING PH. #: _____

HISTORY AND INITIAL ASSESSMENT: **PROVISIONAL DIAGNOSIS:**

_____

_____

_____

_____

_____

ALLERGIES: _____ EXPOSURE TO COMMUNICABLE DISEASE: _____

RESPIRATORY		**CARDIOVASCULAR**	**NEUROLOGIC**	

RESPIRATORY

SUPPLEMENTAL O₂   Y   N

SaO₂: in RA _____ %
            in O₂ _____ %

FiO₂ being delivered by:

Nasal Cannula   face mask

Oxyhood   blowby

INTUBATED   Y   N Size _____

IMV _____   PIP/PEEP _____

TV _____   PS _____

BLOOD GASES

TIME	
SITE	
pH	
pCO₂	
pO₂	
BE	

CARDIOVASCULAR

COLOR:

CAPILLARY REFILL:

URINE OUTPUT:

MURMUR:

NEUROLOGIC

GLASGOW COMA SCALE

Eye Opening	Spontaneous	4
	To Voice	3
	To Pain	2
	None	1
Verbal Response	Oriented	5
	Confused	4
	Inappropriate Words	3
	Incomprehensible Sounds	2
	None	1
Motor Response	Obeys Commands	6
	Localizes (Pain)	5
	Withdraw (Pain)	4
	Flexion (Pain)	3
	Extension (Pain)	2
	None	1
TOTAL		

PUPILS:
Response to light:
EQUAL
UNEQUAL
FIXED

SEIZURES
Y   N
GENERALIZED
FOCAL

VITAL SIGNS

	TIME	TEMP	HR	RR	BP
INITIAL					
@REFERRAL					
@UPDATE					

LAB RESULTS

OTHER LABS:

CULTURES SENT:

CSF:
WBC _____   RBC _____
PROT _____   GLUC _____

X-RAYS/CT:

COMPLETED BY REFERRING HOSPITAL	**RECOMMENDATIONS BY CHOP**

VENDOR:

☐ ETT
☐ ALS
☐ BLS

☐ PCA
☐ Medevac
☐ Stat Medevac
☐ Referral to arrange air
☐ Referral to arrange ground
☐ Other (specify) _____

AUTHORIZATION:

AUTHORIZATION CONTACT NAME: _____

CONTACT PHONE #: _____

AUTHORIZATION #: _____

SIGNATURES:

RN _____   MCP _____

☐ **See updates on back page**

FIGURE 6.9 Transport referral form. A standardized form for recording transport referral information is important. This form should be readily accessible to those who receive the referral. Copies can also be distributed to referral centers to help streamline the process. The forms should, at least, be in duplicate to allow for an official medical record copy (which stays with the command physician during the transport process to document transport progress) and one to accompany the transport team, which eventually resides in the patient's transport record. (Used with permission, © The Children's Hospital of Philadelphia, Philadelphia, PA.)

THE CHILDREN'S HOSPITAL OF PHILADELPHIA
EMERGENCY TRANSPORT RECORD

FIGURE 6.10A Transport record form (flow sheet). The intratransport period must be documented in an efficient fashion. It must document general medical information, as well as progression and response to specific interventions, in a timed, sequential fashion. This should also be, at least, in duplicate to allow for a medical record copy and one that remains with the transport system. (Used with permission, © The Children's Hospital of Philadelphia, Philadelphia, PA.)

THE CHILDREN'S HOSPITAL OF PHILADELPHIA

Calculation of Continuous Drug Infusions
Ordered in Base Concentration (based on weight)

Drug _____

Patient Weight (kg) _____

PATIENT PLATE IMPRINT

Fill in the appropriate horizontal row for the base concentration ordered. Complete correlating solution preparation boxes using the calculation examples on the back of this form. <u>Verify that the continuous infusion drug label matches the calculated information below.</u> Solution preparation boxes should be verified by each new nurse caring for the patient.

____ u/kg/hr to run at 10 mL/hr (Insulin)		A. ____ u/hr	B. ____ u/10ml	C. ____ u/ml	D. ____ u/ ____ ml
____ u/kg/hr to run at 1 mL/hr		E. ____ u/hr		F. ____ u/ml	G. ____ u/ ____ ml
____ u/ kg/min to run at 1 mL/hr	H. ____ u/min	I. ____ u/hr		J. ____ u/ml	K. ____ u/ ____ ml
____ mcg/kg/min to run at 1 mL/hr	L. ____ mcg/min	M. ____ mcg/hr	N. ____ mg/hr	O. ____ mg/ml	P. ____ mg/ ____ ml
____ mcg/kg/hr to run at 1 mL/hr		Q. ____ mcg/hr	R. ____ mg/hr	S. ____ mg/ml	T. ____ mg/ ____ ml
____ mg/kg/hr to run at 1 mL/hr			U. ____ mg/hr	V. ____ mg/ml	W. ____ mg/ ____ ml

Document most recent MD order in the Ordered Dose box. Calculate Rate (ml/hr) using example on the back of this form. <u>This section must be completed at the initiation of the infusion, at the beginning of each shift, with dose change, and when changing the bottle/bag/syringe.</u>

Date/Time Reason	Ordered Dose	X. Rate (ml/hr)	Syringe Exp. date/time	RN Signature

FIGURE 6.10B.1 Drug infusion charts and medication dosage charts based on weight may be useful for the transport team. (Used with permission, © The Children's Hospital of Philadelphia, Philadelphia, PA.)

units/kg/hr to run @ 10 ml/hr (INSULIN ONLY)

Box A Calculate **units/hr:** Base concentration X ___ pt wt = ___ units/hr to run @ 10 ml/hr
e.g.: 0.1 units/kg/hr to run @ 10 ml/hr X 6 kg = 0.6 units/hr to run @ 10 ml/hr

Box B When run at 10 ml/hr, units/hr is the same as **units/10 ml**
Therefore: 0.6 units/hr @ 10 ml/hr is the same as 0.6 units/10 ml

Box C Calculate **units/ml:** units/10 ml ÷ 10 = ___ units/ml
e.g.: 0.6 units/10 ml ÷ 10 = 0.06 units/ml

Box D Calculate **total units in container:** units/ml X ___ container size = ___ total units / ___ container
e.g.: 0.06 units/ml X 100 ml bottle = 6 units/100 ml bottle

units/kg/hr to run @ 1 ml/hr

Box E Calculate **units/hr:** Base concentration X ___ pt wt = ___ units/hr to run @ 1 ml/hr
e.g.: 15 units/kg/hr to run @ 1 ml/hr X 8kg = 120 units/hr to run @ 1 ml/hr

Box F When run at 1 ml/hr, units/hr is the same as **units/ml**
Therefore: 120 units/hr to run @ 1ml/hr to run @ 1 ml/hr is the same as 120 units/ml

Box G Calculate total units in container: units/ml X ___ container size = ___ total units/ ___ container
e.g.: 120 units/ml X 250 ml bottle = 30,000 units/250 ml bottle

units/kg/min to run @ 1 ml/hr

Box H Calculate **units/min:** Base concentration X ___ pt wt = ___ units/min to run @ 1 ml/hr
e.g.: 0.01 units/kg/min to run @ 1ml/hr X 7 kg = 0.07 units/min to run 1ml/hr

Box I Calculate **units/hr:** ___ units/min X 60 min/hr = ___ units/hr
e.g.: 0.07 units/min X 60 min/hr = 4.2 units/hr

Box J When run at 1ml/hr, units/hr is the same as **units/ml**
Therefore: 4.2 units/hr to run @ 1ml/hr to run @ 1 ml/hr is the same as 4.2 units/ml

Box K Calculate **total units in container:** units/ml X ___ container size = ___ total units/ ___ container
e.g.: 4.2 units/ml X 50 ml syringe = 210 units/ 50 ml syringe

mcg/kg/min to run @ 1ml/hr

Box L Calculate **mcg/min:** Base concentration X ___ pt wt = ___ mcg/min to run @ 1 ml/hr
e.g.: 10 mcg/kg/min to run @ 1 ml/hr X 9 kg = 90 mcg/min to run 1 ml/hr

Box M Calculate **mcg/hr:** ___ mcg/min X 60 min/hr = ___ mcg/hr
e.g.: 90 mcg/min X 60 min/hr = 5400 mcg/hr

Box N Calculate **mg/hr:** ___ mcg/hr ÷ 1000 mcg/mg = ___ mg/hr
e.g.: 5400 mcg/hr ÷ 1000 mcg/mg = 5.4 mg/hr

Box O When run at 1ml/hr, mg/hr is the same as **mg/ml**
Therefore: 5.4 mg/hr run @ 1 ml/hr is the same as 5.4 mg/ml

Box P Calculate **total mg in container:** mg/ml X ___ container size = ___ total/ ___ container
e.g.: 5.4 mg/ml X 50mL syringe = 270 units/50 ml syringe

mcg/kg/hr to run @ 1 ml/hr

Box Q Calculate **mcg/hr:** Base concentration X ___ pt wt = ___ mcg/hr to run @ 1 ml/hr
e.g.: 5 mcg/kg/hr to run@1ml/hr X 12 kg = 60 mcg/hr to run 1 ml/hr

Box R Calculate **mg/hr:** ___ mcg/hr ÷ 1000 mcg/mg = ___ mg/hr
e.g.: 60 mcg/hr ÷ 1000 mcg/mg = 0.06 mg/hr

Box S When run at 1 ml/hr, mg/hr is the same as **mg/ml**
Therefore: 0.06 mg/hr run @ 1 ml/hr is the same as 0.06 mg/ 1 ml
Calculate **total mgs in container:** mg/ml X ___ container size = ___ total mg/ ___ container

Box T e.g.: 0.06 mg/ml X 50 ml syringe = **3 mg/50 ml syringe**

mg/kg/hr to run @ 1 ml/hr

Box U Calculate **mg/hr:** Base concentration X ___ pt wt = ___ mg/hr to run @ 1 ml/hr
e.g.: 2 mg/kg/hr to run @ 1ml/hr X 18 kg = 36 mg/hr to run@1ml/hr

Box V When run at 1 ml/hr, mg/hr is the same as **mg/ml**
Therefore: 36 mg/hr to run @ 1 ml/hr is the same as 36 mg/ml

Box W Calculate **total mg in container:** mg/ml X ___ container size = ___ total mg/ ___ container
e.g.: 36 mg/ml X 50 ml syringe = 1800 mg/50 ml syringe

Box X Rate Calculations/Changes:

"Desired Method"
Have
$$\frac{\text{Ordered Dose (units/kg/hr)}}{\text{Base Concentration (units/kg/hr)}} \times \text{Base Conc Rate (ml/hr)} = \text{Ordered Dose Rate}$$

Example 1: Physician order reads: Insulin.... Base concentration 0.1 units/kg/hr equal to 10 ml/hr; Dose: 0.07 units/kg/hr.

$$\frac{0.07 \text{ units/kg/hr}}{0.1 \text{ units/kg/hr}} \times 10 \text{ ml/hr} =$$

$$0.7 \times 10 \text{ ml/hr} = 7 \text{ ml/hr}$$

"Ratio Method"
$$\frac{\text{Base Concentration (units/kg/hr)}}{\text{Base Concentration Rate (ml/hr)}} = \frac{\text{Ordered Dose (units/kg/hr)}}{\text{Ordered Dose Rate (X ml/hr)}}$$

Example 1: Physician order reads: Insulin....Base concentration 0.1 units/kg/hr equal to 10 ml/hr. Dose: 0.07 units/kg/hr.

$$\frac{0.1 \text{ units/kg/hr}}{10 \text{ ml/hr}} = \frac{0.07 \text{ units/kg/hr}}{X \text{ ml/hr}}$$

$$(0.1 \text{ units/kg/hr})(X) = (0.07 \text{ units/kg/hr})(10 \text{ ml/hr})$$

$$0.1 \text{ units/kg/hr } (X) = 0.7 \text{ units/kg/hr}$$

$$\frac{0.1 \text{ units/kg/hr } (X)}{0.1 \text{ units/kg/hr}} = \frac{0.7 \text{ units/kg/hr}}{0.1 \text{ units/kg/hr}}$$

$$X = 7 \text{ ml/hr}$$

FIGURE 6.10B.2 Rate calculation worksheet. (Used with permission, © The Children's Hospital of Philadelphia, Philadelphia, PA.)

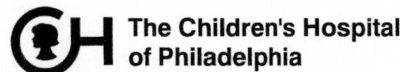

**The Children's Hospital
of Philadelphia**

TRN-004
Rev. 08/02

**AUTHORITY FOR TRANSFER, TREATMENT AND
TRANSPORTATION BY THE EMERGENCY TRANSPORT
TEAM OF THE CHILDREN'S HOSPITAL OF PHILADELPHIA**

(PATIENT PLATE IMPRINT)

I hereby consent to the transfer and transport of _____
Patient's name

from _____ to _____
Referring medical facility   Accepting medical facility or home

I consent to the transfer and transport of the patient to any other hospital or medical facility enroute to the location mentioned above should it become indicated by the Emergency Transport Team of The Children's Hospital of Philadelphia for the patient's safety or well being.

I understand that the condition of the above patient is such that the referring physician recommends transfer of the patient by the Emergency Transport Team of The Children's Hospital of Philadelphia.

I acknowledge there are potential unanticipated risks to the transportation such as possible traffic hazards, adverse weather conditions, vehicle operator errors, failure of medical equipment and the vehicle, and consequences of actions of persons outside of the control of transport personnel, all of which could have an impact on the patient.

I understand that this transport may be accomplished with or without a physician in attendance but under the direction of protocols or telephone triage orders from the Medical Command Physician from The Children's Hospital of Philadelphia.

I also consent to the treatment and care that may be provided to the patient during the transportation. I acknowledge that there may be a delay or interruption of the patient's previous medical treatment during the period of transport. I understand that not all the resources required to fully diagnose and treat the patient are available during transport. These delays, interruptions or lack of resources may increase the severity of the patient's condition and may in rare cases, result in the death of the patient.

I have considered the above risks, and other risks not mentioned by the transport team and the alternatives and benefits of the transfer and transportation, and consent to the transfer and transportation provided by The Children's Hospital of Philadelphia.

I authorize The Children's Hospital of Philadelphia to provide medical information to the patient's family physician(s).
☐ yes   ☐ no

I authorize The Children's Hospital of Philadelphia to provide medical information to the patient's referring physician(s).
☐ yes   ☐ no

I acknowledge that I have read the above authorizations and that no guarantee or assurance has been made to me as to the results that may be obtained. I have read this form and completely understand it.

_____   _____
Printed name of consenting party   relationship to patient

_____   _____
Signature of consenting party   date and time

_____   _____
Signature of The Children's Hospital of Philadelphia employee acting as witness   date and time

FIGURE 6.10C.1 Written consent for transport is mandatory. (Used with permission, © The Children's Hospital of Philadelphia, Philadelphia, PA.)

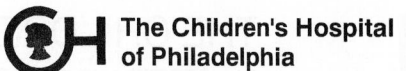

The Children's Hospital of Philadelphia

TRN-004
Rev. 08/02

(PATIENT PLATE IMPRINT)

AUTHORITY FOR TRANSFER, TREATMENT AND TRANSPORTATION BY THE EMERGENCY TRANSPORT TEAM OF THE CHILDREN'S HOSPITAL OF PHILADELPHIA

Oral consent

Consent obtained by: ☐ telephone   ☐ other _____

_____
Consenting party's name and relationship to patient

_____   _____
Signature of person obtaining oral consent   date and time

_____   _____
Signature of witness   date and time

Emergency consent if parent or legal guardian not available

I, _____, as the referring physician

of _____, have personally or through my designees, made
Referring hospital
unsuccessful attempts to locate parents or legal guardians to obtain oral consent to transfer and transport the patient to The Children's Hospital of Philadelphia. After medical examination of the patient, I have determined that the medical benefits of transferring to and transporting by The Children's Hospital of Philadelphia outweigh the increased risks to the patient if any further delay is made in locating parents or legal guardian.
I, acting on the behalf of the patient, consent to the transfer and transport to The Children's Hospital of Philadelphia.

_____
Printed name of attending physician acting as consenting party

_____   _____
Signature of attending physician   date and time

_____   _____
Signature of The Children's Hospital of Philadelphia employee acting as witness   date and time

FIGURE 6.10C.2 Example of emergency and oral consent documentation form. (Used with permission, © The Children's Hospital of Philadelphia, Philadelphia, PA.)

receiving management advice by telephone, both parties should remember that the transport command physician is usually unable to see and are always unable to examine the child in question. Therefore, his or her advice will often be somewhat general. The receiving physician must do his or her best to offer clear and complete information, especially when specific information is requested. Suggestions for care must be clearly and completely communicated. For example, if the transport command physician believes that a fluid bolus is needed, that advice should include type and amount of fluid and speed of infusion to avoid any misinterpretation of advice or an inadvertent mistake in one of those parameters. All advice should be documented in writing and/or by audio recording. The referring physician is under no obligation to accept the advice of the receiving physician, but he or she would be prudent to give it serious consideration. If the referring physician is unable or unwilling to perform suggested interventions because of dis-

agreement, personnel issues, equipment limitations, or other reasons, this should be discussed with the receiving physician. Likewise, results from interventions or marked changes in the patient's condition during the referral process should be communicated to the receiving physician and transport service. Clear, precise, efficient, and honest communication is imperative for the patient to receive the most appropriate care.

Communication with the patient and family is also important during the transport process. Straightforward communications about disease process and expectations can help prepare a family to accept the consequence of the illness or injury. Lack of communication or reluctance to give bad news can cause a family to expect different outcomes than they should and may pave the way for anger and resentment.

Written communication of all data regarding the patient's care is imperative. Patient summaries, copies of all medical paperwork, laboratory values, and radiographs should be

FOUNDED 1855

THE CHILDREN'S HOSPITAL OF PHILADELPHIA

34th STREET AND CIVIC CENTER BOULEVARD • PHILADELPHIA, PA 19104 • (215) 590-1000

Medical Record # _____

DEPARTMENT OF MEDICAL RECORDS

AUTHORIZATION FOR THE RELEASE OF MEDICAL INFORMATION

I hereby consent to and authorize *The Children's Hospital of Philadelphia* to release information from the records of the patient listed below. In addition, if the record contains any of the following information, I consent to and authorize its release by checking the appropriate box:

Drug/Alcohol Treatment: ☐	Psychological Treatment: ☐	HIV Related Treatment: ☐

PATIENT'S NAME: _____

DATE OF BIRTH: _____

RELATIONSHIP:

       Circle one: Son   Daughter   Self   Foster Child   Other: _____

The information is to be released to:

NAME OF PERSON: _____

NAME OF ORGANIZATION: _____

STREET ADDRESS: _____

CITY: _____ STATE: _____ ZIP: _____

Disclosure Parameters:

Reason for release of information: _____

The date, event or condition upon which this authorization will expire, if not earlier revoked: _____

The information to be released and date(s) service:

    ☐ Emergency Department   Date(s): _____

    ☐ Outpatient Department   Department: _____

                               Date(s): _____

    ☐ Inpatient Admission   Date(s): _____

    ☐ Immunization Records   Date(s): _____

    ☐ Other Information: (Explain) _____

This authorization may be revoked at any time except to the extent that *The Children's Hospital of Philadelphia* has already acted in reliance on it.

Signature (if not the patient, I certify I am parent/legal guardian of the patient): _____

Date: _____   Telephone #: _____

The Children's Hospital is an equal opportunity employer and patients are accepted without regard to race, creed, color, handicap, national origin or sex

MR-109

FIGURE 6.10D A written release for medical records will help with transmission of information at time of discharge to referring physicians and the primary care physician. (Used with permission, © The Children's Hospital of Philadelphia, Philadelphia, PA.)

The Children's Hospital *of* **Philadelphia**

34th Street and
Civic Center Boulevard
Philadelphia, Pa. 19104-4399

Emergency Transport Service

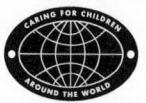

George A. Woodward, M.D.
Medical Director

Kirsten Johnson Moore, R.N., M.S.N.
Nursing Director

Phone 215-590-4988
Fax 215-590-1394
To arrange transport:
800-590-2160

Patient's name _____   **Date** _____

Parent's name _____

Referring facility/address/personnel

_____

_____   **Physician** _____

_____   **Unit Manager** _____

Phone   _____   **Unit Contact** _____

Fax   _____

Beeper   _____

Family physician/pediatrician

_____

_____

_____

_____

Phone   _____

Fax   _____

Beeper   _____

Other (specialist/consultant)   **Other (specialist/consultant)**

_____   _____

_____   _____

_____   _____

Phone   _____   **Phone**   _____

Fax   _____   **Fax**   _____

Beeper   _____   **Beeper**   _____

Laboratory phone number   _____

Radiology phone number   _____

Other phone numbers   _____

<u>**Pre-Transport Checklist**</u>

o **Family notified and consents to transport**

o **Order written for transport**

o **Insurance pre-authorization for admission if necessary**

o **Medical record copied**

o **Transport summary if available**

o **Laboratory data copied**

o **X-rays and radiology reports copied**

FIGURE 6.10E A standardized form can be distributed to referral centers to allow demographic information to be collected prior to the arrival of the transport team. Identification of all principals involved in the patient's care can help future flow of information regarding the patient's diagnosis and outcome. (Used with permission, © The Children's Hospital of Philadelphia, Philadelphia, PA.)

available for the transport team on their arrival at the referring location. A transport referral checklist may be useful to help streamline the process (Fig. 6.11). Adequate preparation of these documents before arrival of the transport team can greatly improve the efficiency of the transport process and the transition of care. Availability of the referring personnel at the time of transport can also make the process more efficient for all concerned. Telephone and fax numbers and the addresses of the referring and primary physicians should be available to the transport team so follow-up information may be easily conveyed. Likewise, the referring and primary physicians should be given contact numbers for the transport team and its medical and administrative directors.

Finally, the family should receive preprinted directions to the receiving facility. Information about the facility, parking, city, local transit, and the visiting policies of the receiving unit should also be provided. Enabling a family member to accompany the transport team has been shown to be important to both the patient and family, while not diminishing the delivered quality of care. Recognition of the family's role in the overall care of the child will pay dividends to the team, patient, and family.

Patient and Team Safety

Safety is a key consideration for the transport team. The team should do everything possible to provide for the safety of all involved in the transport process. This includes more than providing pediatric medical expertise for the patient during the transport. It starts with vehicle selection, driver or pilot capabilities, and ongoing licensure requirements. The transport medical director is responsible for continually assessing the capabilities of the particular modes of transport and the personnel involved with those functions. This goes beyond licensure issues. Active inspections and evaluations, as well as continuous quality improvement (CQI) issues, are important. Unsafe vehicles or personnel must be attended to or removed from service. Safety of the transport personnel must also be a priority. Avoiding the use of RW transport in bad weather is a good example of a safety decision in the transport environment. Improvement in helicopter EMS (HEMS) safety profiles were recognized when pilots were isolated from patient care information. Instead of being informed that a critical child might die without their intervention, pilots now often make "go" or "no go" decisions based solely on weather and equipment issues. If an appropriate "no go" decision is made, this should not be questioned or countermanded by medical or administrative personnel. If a "no go" decision is made based on weather considerations, another mode of transport or other patient care options must be considered. Competition between transport programs or aeromedical providers can be a safety hazard. In their desire to gain a competitive advantage, one or all the programs (or specific personnel) may be willing to bend weather and safety rules. It is the policy of our systems that if one air service has denied a transport for weather-related issues, another air service is not contacted unless it is located in a separate environment that may change the weather issues. There is no excuse for risking or losing the lives of several caregivers for any one particular transport. Unfortunately, the HEMS industry has seen an unprecedented accident and fatal-

ity rate over the past several years. In 2006, the National Transportation Safety Board (NTSB) critical reviewed 55 EMS accidents from January 2002 to January 2005. These included 54 fatalities and 19 serious injuries. They determined that 29 of the 55 fatalities could have been prevented with systematic corrective actions. This review resulted in safety initiative recommendations, which are outlined in the NTSB publication, *Special Investigative Report on Emergency Medical Services Operations*, available at www.ntsb.gov. As per that report and the Blumen's referenced 2002 safety review, the number of HEMS flight hours increased approximately 85% from about 162,000 to 300,000 (1991–2005) and the average accident rate increased during the last 5 years of the report from 3.53 (1992–2001) to 4.56 (1997–2001) per 100,000 flight hours. The following recurring safety issues were noted: (i) less stringent requirements for EMS operations conducted without patients on board; (ii) lack of aviation flight risk-evaluation programs for EMS operations; (iii) lack of consistent, comprehensive flight dispatch procedures for EMS operations; and (iv) no requirements to use technologies such as terrain awareness and warning systems (TAWS) to enhance EMS flight safety. There were two accidents with four fatalitiesin 2006 and two accidents with seven fatalities in 2007. From December 2007 to October 2008, there were nine fatal HEMS accidents with 35 fatalities. The Federal Aviation Administration (FAA) reported that there were 33 EMS helicopters involved in 32 fatal accidents, with 83 related fatalities from 2002 through September 2008, resulting in an annual average of 4.5 fatal accidents and 12 deaths per year. It was noted that 23 of these accidents, and 65 of the fatalities occurred at night. Compared to ground ambulance transport (15 million annual patient exposures), the fatal accident rate is greater for helicopter transport by approximately 13.5 times, and the helicopter fatality rate exceeds that seen with ground ambulances by 34 times. Interventions by the FAA have resulted in safety improvements, including certification of night vision goggles (NVG) for helicopter use. Other recommendations included TAWS, more stringent flight operation requirements, improved preflight risk management and hazard identification, and mitigation programs and formalized dispatch procedures to include up-to-date weather information and assistance in flight risk-assessment decisions.

Although there is not a singular intervention or assessment tool that will guarantee risk-free air transport, accreditation by the CAMTS demonstrates adherence to the safety standards proposed for the air medical transport industry.

STABILIZATION FOR TRANSPORT

The patient care paradigm of most interfacility transport teams stands somewhat in contrast to that of prehospital care systems. EMS providers are usually bringing a patient from an environment without medical care (e.g., home or accident scene) to a hospital. In many of these cases, the patient is better served to have the minimum stabilization necessary at the scene followed by rapid transport to an appropriate hospital, with further intervention being performed en route or on arrival. In contrast, the interfacility transport team is most often taking a patient from a hospital, usually an ED or another monitored setting, to a monitored bed within a higher level or specialty

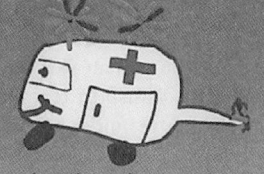

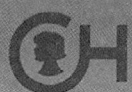

The Children's Hospital *of* Philadelphia
Emergency Transport Team

Emergency Transport Team 800-590-2160 Fax 215-590-4868

Your call will be immediately answered by a transport communication specialist who will record your name, location, phone number, patient's name, age and diagnosis and connect you with the appropriate transport medical command physician

Prior to transport
☐ Obtain parental consent for transport
☐ Notify family that one parent may usually ride in ground ambulance with their child

Please provide the transport team with copies of
☐ Patient's medical record
☐ Transfer summary (if appropriate)
☐ Laboratory values
☐ Radiographic studies
☐ Patient registration information
☐ Names, addresses, phone and fax numbers of physicians involved in the patient's care (private and referring physicians, specialists) to aid in providing follow-up information after arrival at The Children's Hospital of Philadelphia

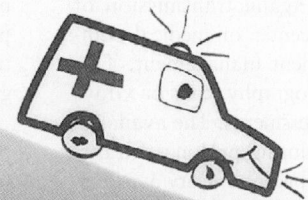

Pediatric and Neonatal Transport
800-590-2160

FIGURE 6.11 Referral checklist. Transport referral checklists can decrease the transition time at the referring hospital by allowing the referral team to anticipate the logistics of the pretransport process and accomplish many tasks prior to the arrival of the transport team. (Used with permission, © The Children's Hospital of Philadelphia, Philadelphia, PA.)

care center. The transport team, therefore, is responsible for maintaining an appropriate advanced level of care between the two centers. Ideally, the transport team should provide the level of care that the patient will have at the receiving facility. At a minimum, the transport team must maintain the patient's present level of care under difficult circumstances. Stabilization before transport is the key to this process.

Initial preparation for transport often begins when the referral caregivers recognize that the patient requires care beyond the capabilities of their center. Appropriate advice and suggestions from transport personnel or the receiving physician may allow much of the necessary stabilization, interventions, and preparation for transport to be accomplished before the team arrives. Telemedicine promises to improve the pre-transport assessment opportunities in the future. Availability of visual and other data to be reviewed by local experts should offer a more individualized, higher level of initial assessment and suggested advice.

When the transport team arrives, they should review the medical history, including all therapeutic maneuvers and interventions performed at the referring hospital. An immediate and thorough physical examination is mandatory. During this pre-transport review process, endotracheal tubes, chest tubes, IV and intraarterial catheters, and other indwelling devices should be checked for proper placement and stabilization. When doubt exists, devices should be replaced or better secured.

After this initial assessment, the transport team, in concert with the medical command physician, should decide which, if any, further medical interventions are required to be initiated and/or continued before leaving the referring center. Such interventions are most appropriate when they may have a direct impact on patient outcome. For example, the child who may have meningitis should definitely receive antibiotics before or during the transport process, but a lumbar puncture may be deferred until he or she arrives at the receiving hospital. The appropriateness of interventions will, to some degree, be dictated by the distance to the receiving hospital. For example, a child with a circumferential burn of an extremity may require a fasciotomy to prevent vascular compromise. If the receiving hospital is 5 minutes away, this might be appropriately deferred. However, if the receiving hospital is 2 hours away, it may be prudent to have the procedure performed before departing from the referring center. Again, transmission of images or materials to the receiving center or medical command physicians can help in the patient management. This could include images of computed tomography scans or x-rays as well as copies of EKGs or other assessments. The availability of point-of-care testing is helpful during prolonged transport processes to assess metabolic or other laboratory markers.

After the patient is optimally prepared for transport, he or she must then be moved from the referral facility's bed to the transport stretcher and then to the vehicle. Such movements represent great risk to the patient. If an IV catheter or an endotracheal tube is going to be displaced, it will likely occur while the patient is being moved. This fact has several implications. First, patients should be subjected to the fewest transfers necessary to get them from the referring hospital to the definitive bed/location they will occupy at the receiving hospital. Movement from the transport stretcher to a holding bed in the ED is often unnecessary and can be avoided with advanced planning. Second, extra vigilance should be used during patient transfer. Personnel should be assigned to secure lines and tubes, and the movement should be coordinated by a team leader. Precautions such as planned, temporary disconnection of the ventilator from the endotracheal tube may need to be considered during these moves. Finally, the patient must be reassessed immediately after each movement. The team must be assured that the airway is stable, immobilization is secure (if appropriate), and that potentially lifesaving tubes, lines, and medications have not become dislodged or disrupted.

Monitoring is imperative during the transport process. Observation and palpation may be hindered by patient position relative to the caregiver within the vehicle. This may be especially evident in a small transport helicopter. Auscultation may also be impaired in a noisy transport environment. The air transport environment, especially in a RW or turbo prop aircraft, may be 50% louder than a comparable ground transport. Therefore, more reliance is placed on sophisticated monitoring tools, including cardiorespiratory, pulse oximetry, capnography, and gas delivery monitors with audible and visual alarms as well as point-of-care laboratory testing.

ALTITUDE PHYSIOLOGY AND THE AIR MEDICAL ENVIRONMENT

When pediatric patients are transported by helicopter or FW aircraft, one must be cognitive of issues regarding altitude physiology. An increase in altitude brings with it a decrease in ambient oxygen as well as the potential for an increase in the size of air spaces. For most patients, however, these should not be major issues. For patients with severe hypoxia at sea level, diving injuries, or large, enclosed pockets of air, however, air transport can be dangerous.

Two gas laws are most important in the transport process. Boyle's law states that with a constant temperature, the volume of a gas varies inversely with the pressure ($P_1V_1 = P_2V_2$) (Fig. 6.12). As altitude increases, barometric pressure decreases; therefore, the volume of the gas increases. Dalton's law (the law of partial pressure) says that the partial pressure of a gas mixture is the sum of all the partial pressures of the gas within the mixture ($PT = P_1 + P_2 + P_3 \ldots$) (Fig. 6.13). For example, the total pressure of air is 1. The partial pressure of nitrogen is 0.78, oxygen is 0.21, and other gases are 0.01. The partial pressure of oxygen will always be 21%. At higher altitudes, air becomes less dense and the partial pressure of oxygen, while still 21%, offers diminished oxygen availability.

These issues can be important during the air medical transport. Entrapped air, if not vented, can be painful (middle ear sinus, teeth, bowel), annoying (flatus, belching), and dangerous (pneumothorax). Use of tight-fitting earplugs in flight can cause an artificial air pocket that may trigger the same problems. More significant air space issues include simple pneumothorax and pneumocephalus, which can become symptomatic at high altitudes. Patients with bowel obstructions may have increased gas volume, leading to vomiting and potential aspiration. Air in military antishock trousers may vary with altitude as will the air in pressure splints and blood pressure cuffs. Air in endotracheal tube cuffs and Foley catheters may also be affected and might need to be adjusted during flight. Patients with an air embolism from a diving injury or other cause are especially prone to gas volume–related issues during air transport.

Altitude (ft)	Barometric Pressure (mm Hg)	Atmospheres	Relative Volume
18,000	380	0.50	2.0
12,000	483	0.64	1.6
8,000	565	0.77	1.33
5,000	632	0.83	1.2
Sea level	760	1.0	1.0

FIGURE 6.12 Boyle's law ($P_1V_1 = P_2V_2$ or $P_1/P_2 = V_1V_2$). As altitude increases, barometric pressure decreases and volume of gas increases. The diagram illustrates enclosed gas expansion at specific altitudes. "Atmospheres" is compared with the amount of pressure exerted by an overlying 1 square inch air column. At sea level, this equals 14.7 pounds per square inch (psi) and one-half that amount (7.35 psi) at 18,000 ft. (From Woodward GA, Vernon DD. Aviation physiology in pediatric transport. In: Jaimovich DG, Vidyasagar D, eds. *Pediatric and neonatal transport medicine.* Philadelphia: Hanley and Belfus, Inc., 1995:40, with permission.)

Hypoxia can also be a major issue. This can usually be overcome with addition of 100% FiO_2—unless the patient is already hypoxic at lower altitudes on 100% oxygen. Positive end-expiratory pressure is usually not effective in augmenting the hypoxemia that occurs secondary to an increase in altitude.

Most air transports, however, do not reach an altitude that will greatly influence the patient's care. Helicopter transport routinely occurs at 1,000 feet or less above ground level, although this can be greatly altered in mountainous regions where traversing high-altitude peaks may be necessary. FW transport aircraft are usually pressurized, meaning that they can simulate the atmospheric pressure of a lower environment. Air pressure in these aircraft is often set at a level of 5,000 to 8,000 feet, which can, however, still lead to a significant increase in gas volume. Opportunities for achieving higher ambient pressure (lower altitude pressure) may be available, depending on the limitations of the particular aircraft. If an aircraft cannot be pressurized to a higher pressure, one can consider flying at a lower altitude. Trade-offs include increased turbulence, speed restrictions, and fuel issues.

Other issues to be considered in air transport include vibration, turbulence, noise, humidity, temperature, air sickness, exhaust fumes, specific aircraft dangers, and gravitational forces. Helipad availability, landing zones, and other issues of aircraft accessibility must also be determined. Although these logistical issues are ultimately the responsibility of the air transport service and are usually predetermined for the interfacility

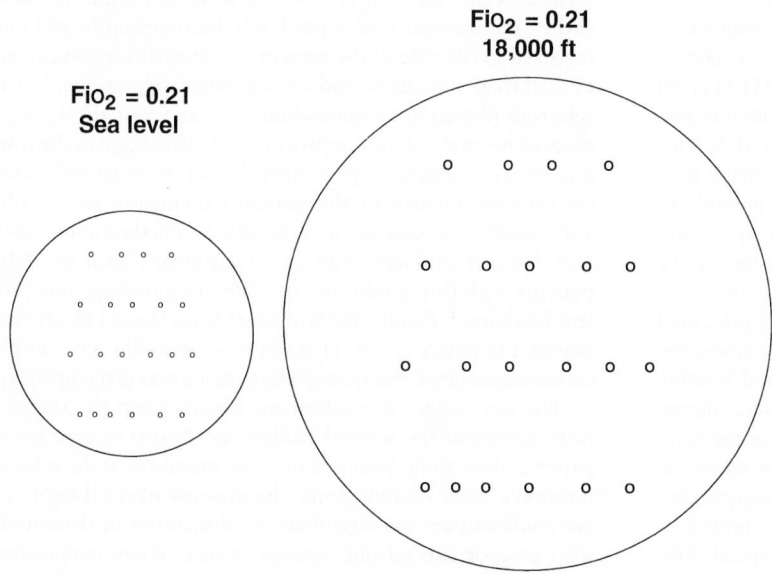

A

FioO$_2$ = 0.21
Sea level

FioO$_2$ = 0.21
18,000 ft

	Altitude (1000 feet)			
	0	**10**	**20**	**30**
Barometric pressure	760	523	349	225
PO_2	160	110	73	47
H_2O vapor pressure	47	47	47	47
"Dry barometric pressure"	713	476	302	178
$PaCO_2$	40	40	40	40
PaO_2				
FiO_2 0.21	100	50	13	0
FiO_2 0.5	307	194	107	45
FiO_2 1.0	663	436	262	138

B

FIGURE 6.13 **A:** Dalton's law (law of partial pressure): ($P_T = P_1 + P_2 + P_3 \ldots$). The total pressure of a gas is the sum of its component gases. The diagram illustrates that the percentages of air components (oxygen illustrated and represents 21% of air) at different altitudes does not change, although air is less dense at a higher altitude. **B:** The effects of altitude and decreased barometric pressure on oxygen availability. (From Woodward GA, Vernon DD. Aviation physiology in pediatric transport. In: Jaimovich DG, Vidyasagar D, eds. *Pediatric and neonatal transport medicine.* Philadelphia: Hanley and Belfus, Inc., 1995:41, with permission.)

transport, any additional information should be offered by the referral center personnel. One must be especially careful around running (hot) aircraft. The helicopter's tail rotor and plane's propellers are often invisible when turning but capable of inflicting severe damage upon those who venture too close. Loose clothing, medical equipment, and stretcher pads can become entangled in a helicopter's rotors, causing severe damage to the vehicle and to the passengers of the transport. In general, no one should approach an aircraft other than crew and specifically trained personnel. Approach to the aircraft should be done under the direction of the flight crew or designated flight safety personnel.

MEDICAL–LEGAL ISSUES

Patient transport is governed by a variety of federal, state, and local statutes. Transport teams and their members may be sued for malpractice under traditional tort law. Therefore, it is important that all members of the transport team understand applicable regulations and avoid unnecessary medical-legal risk. Timely, legible, and complete documentation is imperative. This includes not only the team members on site, but also the communications personnel and the medical team receiving information or giving advice. This documentation should address any decision points and inconsistencies in standard of delivery of care, including responsiveness, mode of transport, personnel notification, preparation for patient's needs, and any delays that may be anticipated or encountered.

Of all regulations, the EMTALA has the greatest impact on the management of patient transport. Woodward's review of legal issues in transport discusses the impact of EMTALA on the interfacility transport populations. Frew and Williams also offer excellent in-depth publications describing EMTALA. This act places clear duties on both the referring and receiving hospitals. The referring clinicians must do everything possible to stabilize the patient's medical condition before transport and may not transfer a patient against his or her will unless the facility cannot provide the appropriate level of care. Furthermore, the referring physician must obtain informed consent for transfer and, as part of this process, must advise the patient or the parents of a minor about the risks and benefits associated with transfer. Under EMTALA rules, these discussions should not include the financial ramifications of the decision. This aspect of the law is particularly important when the patient is being transferred solely because of a managed care contract. It seems only fair that parents know that a refusal of transfer may leave them responsible for a hospital bill. However, under EMTALA rules, such information, however, well-intentioned, may be construed as financial coercion to enable the transfer. Instead, the patient should be told to contact the representatives of his or her insurer or the hospital financial personnel to discuss these issues. The referring team is also responsible for selecting an appropriate means of transport. Obviously, the more critical the need for medical care and expertise, the more sophisticated the transport capabilities need to be. This is an important point for the referral physician to remember. The desire to transfer a child to a more appropriate medical facility as soon as possible is understandable, but if the method chosen places the child in a medical environment that does not offer at least the level of care at the referral cen-

ter, that center and physician will be liable for any untoward effects that can be construed as having occurred because of the choice of transport. Finally, EMTALA requires the receiving hospital to accept the patient in transfer if the appropriate type and level of care are available. The ability of the patient to pay for medical care cannot be considered by either the referring or the receiving facility. In addition to the EMTALA, there are often local regulations that direct transport services. For example, some cities have laws designating certain agencies as official providers of prehospital services. Such laws must be considered when offering transport services. It is important to note, however, that guidelines, such as trauma center transfer protocols, do not negate or supersede EMTALA guidelines. Any law that contradicts or conflicts with EMTALA is considered preempted by EMTALA.

The Health Insurance Portability and Accountability Act (HIPAA) of 1996 also impacts the traditional transport system. Limitations are placed on information dispersion that could be potentially linked to a specific patient. Although this should not impact patient information flow between primary providers or the assessment of services by an established CQI system, the generic follow-up letters that many systems used for feedback and as a marketing tool are no longer permitted. Legal advice should be sought on how to replace this time-honored, but now outdated, method of generic communications.

Traditional tort law also applies to the transport team. Most of these issues are no different than those encountered in other health-care venues. However, one potential source of medical-legal risk is unique to the transport team. As stated earlier, the transport team gradually becomes more and more involved in the care of the patient. At first, this involvement is limited to giving advice and management suggestions. It is the referring physician's responsibility to carry out these suggestions as he or she deems appropriate. At this stage in the transport process, transport personnel should try to gain the clearest possible picture of the patient's condition so the most appropriate suggestions may be given. Furthermore, advice may be best prefaced with general phrases such as "Most patients with this condition" or "We often manage this problem by doing." Finally, the transport team should clearly document any advice given, in writing or by audio recording, in case disagreements regarding what advice was given arise later.

The next stage of involvement occurs when the transport team arrives at the referral facility and begins to care for the patient, often along with one or more members of the referring hospital's staff. At this point, the greatest medical-legal risks are conflicts over management and difficulties in determining who gave or carried out medical orders. When management conflicts arise, the medical command physician should be contacted, and he or she should resolve these conflicts by speaking directly with the referring physician. The medical record should clearly reflect who gave and who carried out each order.

Finally, the transport team assumes total responsibility for the care of the patient when they leave the referral center. The team should be assured that the patient is as stable as possible before leaving. If an unstable patient is transported, the team must document why it was in the patient's best interest to undertake transport at that time.

In some cases, transfer agreements exist between hospitals. Typically, such agreements stipulate that the receiving hospital will accept all transfers from the referring hospital. In the past, transfer agreements served to decrease the time needed to accept the patient by eliminating or shortening the approval process. More recently, transfer agreements have become less important for two reasons. First, the EMTALA places a duty on the receiving hospital to accept the patient as long as there is an appropriate bed location available. Second, for patients who are not critically ill, managed care organizations often stipulate certain facilities. In such cases, the transfer agreement exists between the managed care organization and the receiving hospital. However, the referring hospital must still meet obligations to the patient under the EMTALA.

Finally, if the transport team operates under specific guidelines or protocols, these may become the focus of legal action. Therefore, it is imperative that all guidelines represent the current standard of care. Furthermore, guidelines should be designed to ensure providers do not exceed their scope of practice as defined by state and local regulations. Periodic review of existing protocols and guidelines is warranted. New guidelines should be developed in conjunction with recognized authorities and should be reviewed by risk-management specialists before implementation.

REIMBURSEMENT FOR TRANSPORT SERVICES

As the costs of health care continue to increase, reimbursements to providers and hospitals have largely remained level or decreased. Hospital operating margins have become increasingly narrow, forcing administrators to make difficult programmatic decisions. This situation may increase the need for transport teams to recoup as much of their costs as possible. Unfortunately, in most cases, only services provided by a licensed provider can be billed to third-party payers. In practical terms, this places the burden of documentation and billing upon the shoulders of physicians and licensed nurse practitioners. Teams that do not include these individuals as members will be unable to bill some payers.

There are, in essence, three types of current procedural terminology (CPT) codes that may be used for transport billing:

1. Codes for giving direction or advice to other providers by telephone (e.g., 99373). These codes were originally intended to allow physicians to receive reimbursement for the time spent advising patients by telephone. However, they may also be used when the transport physician is advising personnel at the referring hospital on the management of a patient prior to the arrival of the transport team. The interaction must be documented and, even with documentation, many payers will not reimburse for this service.
2. Codes for directing the transport team by phone or radio (e.g., 99288). This code was originally intended to reimburse physicians for time spent directing the actions of prehospital providers. To be reimbursed, the physician must be in direct communication with the team and must be making the medical decisions. These interactions must also be documented.
3. Codes for the provision of transport services (e.g., 99289, 99291). These codes designate transport services provided by the physician. Currently, codes 99289 and 99290 are intended, respectively, for the initial and subsequent care of

patients younger than 2 years of age, whereas 99291 and 99292 are used for children older than 2 years. Critical care physicians will recognize that codes 99291 and 99292 are the same codes that are used for the critical care services. For billing purposes, transport is considered to be critical care and the same rules apply. First, the billing provider must be physically present during the transport. Second, the patient must meet the definition for critical illness. Third, just as in critical care situations, the provider can only bill for procedures that he or she performs personally or that a resident physician performs under his or her direct supervision. To be billed separately from critical care time, the time spent performing the procedure must be deducted from the overall critical care time. For example, a transport physician attending to a neonate spends a total of 80 minutes directly attending to the patient and reviewing records, but 10 minutes of that time was spent placing a thoracostomy tube. Then the physician is able to bill for 70 minutes of critical care time and for the procedure.

In most cases, services and procedures that are "bundled" under traditional critical care codes are also "bundled" under transport codes.

Suggested Readings

Emergency Medical Services

American College of Emergency Physicians. EMS communication network. *Ann Emerg Med* 2006;47:510.

American College of Surgeons Committee on Trauma, American Academy of Pediatrics, American College of Emergency Physicians, et al. Equipment for ambulances. July 2009. Available at: www.facs.org/fellows_info/bulletin/2009/ambulance0709.pdf, and http://pediatrics.aappublications.org/cgi/reprint/124/1/e166.

Arfken CL, Shapiro MJ, Bessey PQ, Littenberg B. Effectiveness of helicopter versus ground ambulance services for interfacility transport. *J Trauma Injury Infect Crit Care* 1998;45(4):785–790.

Arendts G, Elgafi S. Announcing the emergent patient in the emergency department: a randomised trial. *Emerg Med J* 2006;23:388–390.

Association of Air Medical Services. *Atlas and database of air medical services.* Available at: www.aams.org/GISdatabase.htm

Baker MD, Ludwig S. Pediatric transport and the private practitioner. *Pediatrics* 1991;88:691–695.

Barnes SL, Branson R, Gallo LA, et al. En-route care in the air: snapshot of mechanical ventilation at 37,000 feet. *J Trauma* 2008;64:S129–S134; discussion S134–S135.

Becker LR. Ambulance crashes: protect yourself and your patients. *JEMS* 2003;28:24–26.

Becker LR, Zaloshnja E, Levick N, et al. Relative risk of injury and death in ambulances and other emergency vehicles. *Accid Anal Prev* 2003;35:941–948.

Bell A, Lockey D, Coats T, et al. Physician response unit—a feasibility study of an initiative to enhance the delivery of pre-hospital emergency medical care. *Resuscitation* 2006;69:389–393.

Blumen IJ; UCAN Safety Committee. *A safety review and risk assessment in air medical transport.* Salt Lake City, UT: Air Medical Physician Association; 2002. http://www.flightweb.com/article.php?story=20051122120054921&query=blumen.

Bohm K, Rosenqvist M, Hollenberg J, et al. Dispatcher-assisted telephone-guided cardiopulmonary resuscitation: an underused lifesaving system. *Eur J Emerg Med* 2007;14:256–259.

Brown E, Bleetman A. Ambulance alerting to hospital: the need for clearer guidance. *Emerg Med J* 2006;23:811–814.

Browning Carmo KA, Williams K, West M, et al. A quality audit of the service delivered by the NSW neonatal and paediatric transport service. *J Paediatr Child Health* 2008;44:253–272.

Bull MJ, Weber K, Talty J, et al. Crash protection for children in ambulances. 45th annual proceedings of the Association for the Advancement of Automotive Medicine, 2001;353–367.

Clawson J, Olola C, Heward A, et al. Cardiac arrest predictability in seizure patients based on emergency medical dispatcher identification of previous seizure or epilepsy history. *Resuscitation* 2007;75:298–304.

Clawson JJ. Unnecessary lights and siren use: a public health hazard. *Public Manag* 2002;84(9):12–14.

Committee on Ambulance Equipment and Supplies, National Emergency Medical Services for Children Resource Alliance. Guidelines for pediatric equipment and supplies for basic and advanced life support ambulances. *Ann Emerg Med* 1996;28:699–701.

Crystal R, Bleetman A. Ambulance alerting of paediatric emergencies to a general hospital. *Resuscitation* 2004;63:321–325.

Davis DP, Peay J, Good B, et al. Air medical response to traumatic brain injury: a computer learning algorithm analysis. *J Trauma* 2008;64:889–897.

Deasy C, Ryan D, O'Donnell C, et al. The impact of a pre-hospital medical response unit on patient care and emergency department attendances. *Ir Med J* 2008;101:44–46.

Dissmann PD, Le Clerc S. The experience of Teesside helicopter emergency services: doctors do not prolong prehospital on-scene times. *Emerg Med J* 2007;24:59–62.

Dunford J, Domeier RM, Blackwell T, et al. Performance measurements in emergency medical services. *Prehosp Emerg Care* 2002;6:92–98.

Fakhry SM, Scanlon JM, Robinson L, et al. Prehospital rapid sequence intubation for head trauma: conditions for a successful program. *J Trauma* 2006;60:997–1001.

Fallis WM, Silverthorne D, Franklin J, et al. Client and responder perceptions of a personal emergency response system: lifeline. *Home Health Care Serv Q* 2007;26:1–21.

Forslund K, Kihlgren M, Sorlie V. Experiences of adding nurses to increase medical competence at an emergency medical dispatch centre. *Accid Emerg Nurs* 2006;14:230–236.

Frew SA, Giese K. *Quick risk and compliance answers.* 2nd ed. Racine, WI: Johnson Insurance Services, LLC, 2008.

Garrison HG, Maio RF, Spaite DW, et al. Emergency Medical Services Outcomes Project III (EMSOP III): the role of risk adjustment in out-of-hospital outcomes research. *Ann Emerg Med* 2002;40:79–88.

Gausche M, Lewis RJ, Stratton SJ, et al. Effect of out-of-hospital pediatric endotracheal intubation on survival and neurological outcome: a controlled clinical trial. *JAMA* 2000;283:783–790.

Gausche-Hill M, Barata I, Baren J, et al. The role of the emergency physician in emergency medical services for children. *Ann Emerg Med* 2003;42:206–215.

Gebbie KM, Silber S, McCollum M, et al. Activating physicians within a hospital emergency plan: a concept whose time has come? *Am J Disaster Med* 2007;2:74–80.

Gratton MC, Ellison SR, Hunt J, et al. Prospective determination of medical necessity for ambulance transport by paramedics. *Prehosp Emerg Care* 2003;7:466–469.

Guyette FX, Roth KR, LaCovey DC, et al. Feasibility of laryngeal mask airway use by prehospital personnel in simulated pediatric respiratory arrest. *Prehosp Emerg Care* 2007;11:245–249.

Haines CJ, Lutes RE, Blaser M, et al. Paramedic initiated non-transport of pediatric patients. *Prehosp Emerg Care* 2006;10:213–219.

Hedges JR, Newgard CD, Mullins RJ. Emergency Medical Treatment and Active Labor Act and trauma triage. *Prehosp Emerg Care* 2006;10:332–339.

Hjalte L, Suserud BO, Herlitz J, et al. Why are people without medical needs transported by ambulance? A study of indications for pre-hospital care. *Eur J Emerg Med* 2007;14:151–156.

Houghton RJ, Baber C, McMaster R, et al. Command and control in emergency services operations: a social network analysis. *Ergonomics* 2006;49:1204–1225.

Huddleston KC. Pediatric health policy analysis: the Emergency Medical Services for Children (EMSC) Act and the Wakefield Act, utilizing social construction of target populations. *Pediatr Nurs* 2006;32:167–172.

Jenkin A, Abelson-Mitchell N, Cooper S. Patient handover: time for a change? *Accid Emerg Nurs* 2007;15:141–147.

Jenkinson E, Currie A, Bleetman A. The impact of a new regional air ambulance service on a large general hospital. *Emerg Med J* 2006;23:368–371.

Johnson TD, Lindholm D, Dowd MD. Child and provider restraints in ambulances: knowledge, opinions, and behaviors of emergency medical services providers. *Acad Emerg Med* 2006;13:886–892.

Kannikeswaran N, Mahajan PV, Dunne RB, et al. Epidemiology of pediatric transports and non-transports in an urban emergency medical services system. *Prehosp Emerg Care* 2007;11:403–407.

Kerby JD, MacLennan PA, Burton JN, et al. Agreement between prehospital and emergency department glasgow coma scores. *J Trauma* 2007;63:1026–1031.

Kost S, Cronan K, Gorelick M, et al. Ambulance use by high-acuity patients in a pediatric ED. *Am J Emerg Med* 2000;18(6):679–682.

Levick NR. A crisis in ambulance safety. *Emerg Resp Disaster Manage* 2002;4:20–22.

Lubin JS, Delbridge TR, Cole JS, et al. EMS and emergency department physician triage: injury severity in trauma patients transported by helicopter. *Prehosp Emerg Care* 2005;9:198–202.

Ludwig S, Selbst S. A child-oriented emergency medical services system. *Curr Probl Pediatr* 1990;20:115–158.

Machen I, Dickinson A, Williams J, et al. Nurses and paramedics in partnership: perceptions of a new response to low-priority ambulance calls. *Accid Emerg Nurs* 2007;15:185–192.

Maio RF, Garrison HG, Spaite DW, et al. Emergency Medical Services Outcomes Project IV (EMSOP IV): pain measurement in out-of-hospital outcomes research. *Ann Emerg Med* 2002;40:172–179.

Markenson DS, Domeier RM. National Association of EMS Physicians Pediatric Task Force and Standards and Clinical Practices Committee. The use of automated external defibrillators in children. *Prehosp Emerg Care* 2003;7:258–264.

McLean SA, Maio RF, Domeier RM. The epidemiology of pain in the prehospital setting. *Prehosp Emerg Care* 2002;6:402–405.

Melton JT, Jain S, Kendrick B, et al. Helicopter Emergency Ambulance Service (HEAS) transfer: an analysis of trauma patient case-mix, injury severity and outcome. *Ann R Coll Surg Engl* 2007;89:513–516.

National Association of EMS Physician, National Association of State EMS Directors. Use of warning lights and siren in emergency medical vehicle response and patient transport. *Prehosp Disaster Med* 1994;9:133–136.

Newton A, Ratchford A, Khan I. Incidence of adverse events during prehospital rapid sequence intubation: a review of one year on the London Helicopter Emergency Medical Service. *J Trauma* 2008;64:487–492.

Orr RA, Felmet KA, Han Y, et al. Pediatric specialized transport teams are associated with improved outcomes. *Pediatrics* 2009;124:40–48.

Patterson PD, Baxley EG, Probst JC, et al. Medically unnecessary emergency medical services (EMS) transports among children ages 0 to 17 years. *Matern Child Health J* 2006;10:527–536.

Pitetti R, Glustein JZ, Bhende MS. Prehospital care and outcome of pediatric out-of-hospital cardiac arrest. *Prehosp Emerg Care* 2002;6:283–290.

Pons PT, Haukoos JS, Bludworth W, et al. Paramedic response time: does it affect patient survival? *Acad Emerg Med* 2005;12:594–600.

Price L. Treating the clock and not the patient: ambulance response times and risk. *Qual Saf Health Care* 2006;15:127–130.

Qazi K, Kempf JA, Christopher NC, et al. Paramedic judgment of the need for trauma team activation for pediatric patients. *Acad Emerg Med* 1998;5:1002–1007.

Quan L. Pediatric resuscitation and emergency medical services. *Ann Emerg Med* 1999;33:214–217.

Ringburg AN, Spanjersberg WR, Frankema SP, et al. Helicopter emergency medical services (HEMS): impact on on-scene times. *J Trauma* 2007;63:258–262.

Roudsari BS, Nathens AB, Arreola-Risa C, et al. Emergency Medical Service (EMS) systems in developed and developing countries. *Injury* 2007;38:1001–1013.

Samson RA, Berg RA, Bingham R, et al. Use of automated external defibrillators for children: an update: an advisory statement from the Pediatric Advanced Life Support Task Force, International Liaison Committee on Resuscitation. *Circulation* 2003;107:3250–3255.

Sayre MR, White LJ, Brown LH, et al. The national EMS research agenda executive summary. Emergency Medical Services. *Ann Emerg Med* 2002;40:636–643.

Scribano PV, Baker MD, Holmes J, et al. Utilization of prehospital interventions for the pediatric patient in an urban emergency medical service system [abstract]. *Arch Pediatr Adolesc Med* 1996;150(suppl):36.

Seidel JS, Henderson D, Tittle S, et al. Priorities for research in emergency medical services for children: results of a consensus conference. *Ann Emerg Med* 1999;33:206–210.

Silverman RA, Galea S, Blaney S, et al. The "vertical response time": barriers to ambulance response in an urban area. *Acad Emerg Med* 2007;14:772–778.

Silvestri S, Rothrock SG, Kennedy D, et al. Can paramedics accurately identify patients who do not require emergency department care? *Prehosp Emerg Care* 2002;6:387–390.

Spaite DW, Maio R, Garrison HG, et al. Emergency Medical Services Outcomes Project II (EMSOP II): developing the foundation and conceptual models for out-of-hospital outcomes research. *Ann Emerg Med* 2001;37:657–663.

Svenson JE, Abernathy MK. Ketamine for prehospital use: new look at an old drug. *Am J Emerg Med* 2007;25:977–980.

Talbot R, Bleetman A. Retention of information by emergency department staff at ambulance handover: do standardised approaches work? *Emerg Med J* 2007;24:539–542.

The National Transportation Safety Board Accident Database. Available at: http://www.ntsb.gov/NTSB/Query.asp. Accessed January 13, 2006.

Tsai A, Kallsen G. Epidemiology of pediatric prehospital care. *Ann Emerg Med* 1987;16(3):284–292.

Tung BJ. The pediatric rescue airway. *Air Med J* 2005;24:55–58.

Wagner C, Mazurek P. Current practice in pediatric immobilization–an editorial. *Air Med J* 2006;25:144–148.

Williams DM. 2005 JEMS 200-city survey. A benchmark for the EMS industry. *JEMS* 2006;31:44–61, 100–101.

Wilson P. Fasten their seatbelts: legal restraint of children in car seats and road ambulances. *Paediatr Nurs* 2007;19:14–18.

Wilson GD, Sittig SE, Schears GJ. The laryngeal mask airway at altitude. *J Emerg Med* 2008;34:171–174.

You JS, Park S, Chung SP, et al. The era of audiovisual dispatch using cellular phones with video telephony. *Resuscitation* 2008;76:486–487.

Interfacility Transport

Adams K, Scott R, Perkin RM, et al. Comparison of intubation skills between interfacility transport team members. *Pediatr Emerg Care* 2000;16(1):5–8.

American Academy of Pediatrics, Committee on Pediatric Emergency Medicine, American College of Critical Care Medicine, et al. Consensus report for regionalization of services for critically ill or injured children. *Pediatrics* 2000;105:152–155.

Ammon AA, Fath JJ, Brautigan M, et al. Transferring patients to a pediatric trauma center: the transferring hospital's perspective. *Pediatr Emerg Care* 2000;16(5):332–334.

Aoki BY, McCloskey K. *Evaluation, stabilization, and transport of the critically ill child.* St Louis, MO: Mosby–Year Book, 1992.

Council of the Society of Critical Care Medicine. Consensus report for regionalization of services for critically ill or injured children. *Crit Care Med* 2000; 28:236–239.

Craig SS. Challenges in arranging interhospital transfers from a small regional hospital: an observational study. *Emerg Med Australas* 2005;17:124–131.

Crocker M, Fraser G, Boyd E, et al. The value of interhospital transfer and emergency MRI for suspected cauda equina syndrome: a 2-year retrospective study. *Ann R Coll Surg Engl* 2008;90:513–516.

Davey AL, Macnab AJ, Green G. Changes in pCO_2 during air medical transport of children with closed head injuries. *Air Med J* 2001:20(4):27–30.

Durbin DR, Giardino AP, Costarino AT. Residents on the transport team: balancing service and education. *Arch Pediatr Adolesc Med* 1996;150:529–534.

Eckstein M, Jantos T, Kelly N, et al. Helicopter transport of pediatric trauma patients in an urban emergency medical services system: a critical analysis. *J Trauma* 2002;53(2):340–344.

Fazio RF, Wheeler DS, Poss WB. Resident training in pediatric critical care transport medicine: a survey of pediatric residency programs. *Pediatr Emerg Care* 2000;16:166–169.

Flabouris A, Hart GK, George C. Outcomes of patients admitted to tertiary intensive care units after interhospital transfer: comparison with patients admitted from emergency departments. *Crit Care Resusc* 2008;10:97–105.

Flabouris A, Hart GK, George C. Observational study of patients admitted to intensive care units in Australia and New Zealand after interhospital transfer. *Crit Care Resusc* 2008;10:90–96.

Foley D, Pranikoff T, Younger JG, et al. A review of 100 patients transported on extracorporeal life support. *ASAIO J* 2002;48(6):612–619.

Golestanian E, Scruggs JE, Gangnon RE, et al. Effect of interhospital transfer on resource utilization and outcomes at a tertiary care referral center. *Crit Care Med* 2007;35:1470–1476.

Green A, Showstack J, Rennie D, et al. The relationship of insurance status, hospital ownership, and teaching status with interhospital transfers in California in 2000. *Acad Med* 2005;80:774–779.

Haji-Michael P. Critical care transfers—a danger foreseen is half avoided. *Crit Care* 2005;9:343-344.

Harrison TH, Thomas SH, Wedel SK. Success rates of pediatric intubation by a non-physician staffed critical care transport service. *Pediatr Emerg Care* 2004;20:101–107.

Hill AD, Vingilis E, Martin CM, et al. Interhospital transfer of critically ill patients: Demographic and outcomes comparison with nontransferred intensive care unit patients. *J Crit Care* 2007;22:290–295.

Hinkelbein J, Floss F, Denz C, et al. Accuracy and precision of three different methods to determine Pco2 (Paco2 vs. Petco2 vs. Ptcco2) during interhospital ground transport of critically ill and ventilated adults. *J Trauma* 2008;65:10–18.

Holleran RS, Linsler R. Pediatric transport team: intermountain life flight. *Pediatr Emerg Care* 2006;22:374–378.

Ishimine P, Zorc JJ, Woodward GA. Sometimes it's not so clear: altered mental status and transport. *Pediatr Emerg Care* 2001;17:282–288.

Jaimovich DG, Vidyasagar D, eds. *Handbook of pediatric and neonatal transport medicine.* 2nd ed. Philadelphia: Hanley and Belfus, Inc., 2001.

Kahale J, Osmond MH, Nesbitt L, et al. What are the characteristics and outcomes of nontransported pediatric patients? *Prehosp Emerg Care* 2006;10: 28–34.

Kanter RK, Edge WE, Caldwell CR, et al. Pediatric mortality probability estimated from pre-ICU severity of illness. *Pediatrics* 1997;99:59–63.

Kaszynski SB. EMTALA: duty extends to even non-transferring emergency patients. *J Law Med Ethics* 2001;29:102–103.

King BR, Foster RL, Woodward GA, et al. Procedures performed by pediatric transport nurses: how "advanced" is the practice? *Pediatr Emerg Care* 2001;17(6):410–413.

King BR, Woodward GA. Procedural training for pediatric and neonatal transport nurses: part I—training methods and airway training. *Pediatr Emerg Care* 2001;17:461–464.

King BR, Woodward GA. Pediatric critical care transport—the safety of the journey: a five-year review of vehicular collisions involving pediatric and neonatal transport teams. *Prehosp Emerg Care* 2002;6:449–454.

King BR, Woodward GA. Procedural training for pediatric and neonatal transport nurses: part 2—procedures, skills assessment, and retention. *Pediatr Emerg Care* 2002;18(6):438–441.

Koval KJ, Tingey CW, Spratt KF. Are patients being transferred to level-I trauma centers for reasons other than medical necessity? *J Bone Joint Surg Am* 2006;88:2124–2132.

Larson JT, Dietrich AM, Abdessalam SF, et al. Effective use of the air ambulance for pediatric trauma. *J Trauma* 2004;56:89–93.

Ligtenberg JJ, Arnold LG, Stienstra Y, et al. Quality of interhospital transport of critically ill patients: a prospective audit. *Crit Care* 2005;9:R446–R451.

Lim MT, Ratnavel N. A prospective review of adverse events during interhospital transfers of neonates by a dedicated neonatal transfer service. *Pediatr Crit Care Med* 2008;9:289–293.

Limprayoon K, Sonjaipanich S, Susiva C. Transportation of critically ill patient to pediatric intensive care unit, Siriraj Hospital. *J Med Assoc Thai* 2005;88 (suppl)8:S86–S91.

Macnab AJ, Grant G, Stevens K, et al. Cost: benefit of point-of-care blood gas analysis vs. laboratory measurement during stabilization prior to transport. *Prehospital Disaster Med* 2003;18(1):24–28.

Mainie P, Carmichael A, McCullough S, et al. Endotracheal tube position in neonates requiring emergency interhospital transfer. *Am J Perinatol* 2006;23: 121–124.

Maloney GE Jr, Pakiela JA. Characteristics of patients transported by an aeromedical service for acute toxicologic emergencies: a 5-year experience. *Air Med J* 2008;27:48–50.

Markakis C, Dalezios M, Chatzicostas C, et al. Evaluation of a risk score for interhospital transport of critically ill patients. *Emerg Med J* 2006;23:313–317.

Mazur SM, Pearce A, Alfred S, et al. Use of point-of-care ultrasound by a critical care retrieval team. *Emerg Med Australas* 2007;19:547–552.

McPherson ML, Jefferson LS, Graf JM. A validated pediatric transport survey: how is your team performing? *Air Med J* 2008;27:40–45.

Mitchell AD, Tallon JM, Sealy B. Air versus ground transport of major trauma patients to a tertiary trauma centre: a province-wide comparison using TRISS analysis. *Can J Surg* 2007;50:129–133.

Newgard CD, Hedges JR, Stone JV, et al. Derivation of a clinical decision rule to guide the interhospital transfer of patients with blunt traumatic brain injury. *Emerg Med J* 2005;22:855–860.

Newgard CD, McConnell KJ, Hedges JR, et al. The benefit of higher level of care transfer of injured patients from nontertiary hospital emergency departments. *J Trauma* 2007;63:965–971.

Odetola FO, Shanley TP, Gurney JG, et al. Characteristics and outcomes of interhospital transfers from level II to level I pediatric intensive care units. *Pediatr Crit Care Med* 2006;7:536–540.

Orf J, Thomas SH, Ahmed W, et al. Appropriateness of endotracheal tube size and insertion depth in children undergoing air medical transport. *Pediatr Emerg Care* 2000;16(5):321–327.

Orr RA, Venkataraman ST, McCloskey KA, et al. Measurement of pediatric illness severity using simple pretransport variables. *Prehosp Emerg Care* 2001;5(2):127–133.

Philpot C, Day S, Marcdante K, et al. Pediatric interhospital transport: diagnostic discordance and hospital mortality. *Pediatr Crit Care Med* 2008;9: 15–19.

Reinhart RO. *Basic flight physiology.* 2nd ed. New York: McGraw-Hill, 1996.

Shatney CH, Homan SJ, Sherck JP, et al. The utility of helicopter transport of trauma patients from the injury scene in an urban trauma system. *J Trauma* 2002;53:817–822.

Smith J, Lynch J, Sugrue M, et al. An evaluation of compliance with practice guidelines on interhospital trauma transfer. *Injury* 2005;36:1051–1057.

Southard PA, Hedges JR, Hunter JG, et al. Impact of a transfer center on interhospital referrals and transfers to a tertiary care center. *Acad Emerg Med* 2005;12:653–657.

Stevenson A, Fiddler C, Craig M, et al. Emergency department organization of critical care transfers in the UK. *Emerg Med J* 2005;22:795–798.

Teasdale D, Hamilton C. Baby on the move: issues in neonatal transport. *Paediatr Nurs* 2008;20:20–25.

Thomas SH, Harrison TH, Buras WR, et al. Helicopter transport and blunt trauma mortality: a multicenter trial. *J Trauma* 2002;52(1):136–145.

Thomas AH, Orf J, Peterson C, et al. Frequency and costs of laboratory and radiograph repetition in trauma patients undergoing interfacility transfer. *Am J Emerg Med* 2000;18:156–158.

Trevisanuto D, Doglioni N, Ferrarese P, et al. Neonatal pneumothorax: comparison between neonatal transfers and inborn infants. *J Perinat Med* 2005;33: 449–454.

Trevisanuto D, Verghese C, Doglioni N, et al. Laryngeal mask airway for the interhospital transport of neonates. *Pediatrics* 2005;115:e109-e111.

van Lieshout EJ, de Vos R, Binnekade JM, et al. Decision making in interhospital transport of critically ill patients: national questionnaire survey among critical care physicians. *Intensive Care Med* 2008;34:1269–1273.

van Lieshout EJ, Vroom MV. ICU transport: interhospital transport of critically ill patient with dedicated intensive care ventilator. *Chest* 2005;127:688–689; author reply 689.

Vernon DD, Furnival RA, Hansen KW, et al. Effect of a pediatric trauma response team on emergency department treatment time and mortality of pediatric trauma victims. *Pediatrics* 1999;103:20–24.

Vos G, Engel M, Ramsay G, et al. Point-of-care blood analyzer during the interhospital transport of critically ill children. *Eur J Emerg Med* 2006;13:304–307.

Warren J, Fromm RE Jr, Orr RA, et al. American College of Critical Care Medicine. Guidelines for the inter- and intrahospital transport of critically ill patients. *Crit Care Med* 2004;32:256–262.

Williams A. Diversion: air medical liability issue? *Air Med J* 2001;20:11–12.

Williams A. *Outpatient department EMTALA handbook 2002.* New York: Aspen Law and Business/Aspen Publishers, 2001.

Wong K, Levy RD. Interhospital transfers of patients with surgical emergencies: areas for improvement. *Aust J Rural Health* 2005;13:290–294.

Woodward GA. Transport case 1: a time to fly? A dilemma in pediatric transport. *Pediatr Emerg Care* 1996;12:122–125.

Woodward GA. Pediatric head trauma. *Air Med* 1999;5(6);6–8.

Woodward GA. Legal issues in pediatric interfacility transport. Ethical and legal issues in pediatric emergency medicine. *Clin Pediatr Emerg Med* 2003;4: 256–264.

Woodward GA, editor in chief. *Guidelines for air and ground transport of neonatal and pediatric patients.* 3rd ed. Elk Grove Village, IL: Section on Transport Medicine of American Academy of Pediatrics, 2006.

Woodward GA, Chun T, Miles DK. It's not just a seizure: etiology, management and transport of the seizure patient. *Pediatr Emerg Care* 1999;15:147–155.

Woodward GA, Fein JA. Transport of sedated patients. In: Kraus B, Brustowicz R, eds. *The practice of pediatric sedation and analgesia in the outpatient setting.* Baltimore: Williams & Wilkins, 1999.

Woodward GA, Fleegler EW. Should parents accompany pediatric interfacility ground ambulance transports? The parent's perspective. *Pediatr Emerg Care* 2000;16(6):383–390.

Woodward GA, Fleegler EW. Should parents accompany pediatric interfacility ground ambulance transports? Results of a national survey of pediatric transport team managers. *Pediatr Emerg Care* 2001;17:22–27.

Woodward GA, Insoft RM, Pearson-Shaver AL, et al. The state of pediatric interfacility transport: consensus of the second National Pediatric and Neonatal Interfacility Transport Medicine Leadership Conference. *Pediatr Emerg Care* 2002;18(1):38–43.

Woodward GA, King B. "Interfacility" transport from the home or office. *Pediatr Emerg Care* 1997;13:164–168.

Woodward GA, Levy RJ, Weinzimer SA. Diabetes and transport: a potentially bittersweet combination. *Pediatr Emerg Care* 1998;14:71–76.

Woodward GA, Moore KJ, Needle MN. Oncology and transport: beware the presentation and anticipate the clinical course. *Pediatr Emerg Care* 1996;12:454–459.

Woodward GA, Posner JC, Bolte RG, et al. Just another asthmatic? The many faces of asthma in pediatric transport. *Pediatr Emerg Care* 1998;14:237–245.

Woodward GA, Somogyvari Z. The Hungarian (Budapest) neonatal interfacility transport system: insight into program development and results. *Pediatr Emerg Care* 1997;13:290–293.

Woodward GA, Wernovsky G, Rhodes LA, et al. Sepsis, septic shock, acute abdomen? The ability of cardiac disease to mimic other illness. *Pediatr Emerg Care* 1996;12:317–324.

Yamamoto LG. Wireless teleradiology and fax using cellular phones and note-book PCs for instant access to consultants. *Am J Emerg Med* 1995;13: 184–187.

Yamamoto LG, Inaba AS, DiMauro R. Personal computer teleradiology inter-hospital image transmission to facilitate tertiary pediatric telephone consul-tation and patient transfer: soft-tissue lateral neck and elbow radiographs. *Pediatr Emerg Care* 1994;10:237–277.

Zimmermann M, Bein T, Philipp A, et al. Interhospital transportation of patients with severe lung failure on pumpless extracorporeal lung assist. *Br J Anaesth* 2006;96:63–66.

CHAPTER 7 ■ EMERGENCY DEPARTMENT RECOGNITION AND MANAGEMENT OF VICTIMS OF BIOLOGICAL AND CHEMICAL TERRORISM

RICHARD J. SCARFONE, MD, FRED M. HENRETIG, MD, THEODORE J. CIESLAK, MD, JAMES M. MADSEN, MD, MPH FCAP, FACOEM, COL, MC-FS, AND EDWARD M. EITZEN JR., MD, MPH

BACKGROUND—THE THREAT OF BIOLOGICAL AND CHEMICAL TERRORISM

In the aftermath of the release of the nerve agent sarin in the Tokyo subway system in 1995, another 1995 plot to release chlorine gas in California's Disneyland theme park, the events of September 11, 2001, and the intentional spread of anthrax through the U.S. mail, the potential for emergency care providers being confronted with children who are victims of terrorism is greater than ever. Biological and chemical terrorism, in particular, involve the use of highly virulent or toxic agents with the intent to cause mass casualties, an outcome that could overwhelm regional emergency medical services (EMS) capacity and pose unique medical management challenges. Only through comprehensive community planning, research and development, and medical education can this potential catastrophe be mitigated. This chapter discusses the use of biological and chemical weapons as agents of terror, indicates specific pediatric vulnerabilities, offers initial approaches to syndrome recognition for potential victims of such attacks, and highlights the major biological and chemical agents of concern and their management.

BIOLOGICAL AND CHEMICAL WEAPONS

Microbial pathogens, biologic toxins, and highly toxic chemicals have long been considered for use as military weapons. Currently, considerable concern surrounds their possible use on civilian populations, including children, by terrorist groups. These agents are often included in the category "weapons of mass destruction" but are more properly termed *mass-casualty weapons*, because they do not necessarily destroy infrastructure and because of their potential to cause hundreds to thousands of casualties, especially in scenarios involving a large-scale attack via an aerosol release. However, even smaller-scale, technologically primitive incidents can cause considerable morbidity and wreak havoc on regional medical care systems thereby successfully terrorizing a population. Modern examples of the latter include the intentional spread of salmonella on restaurant salad bars in Oregon in 1984; the Tokyo subway

sarin attack in 1995 in which perpetrators punctured plastic garbage bags, allowing sarin vapor to escape; and the mail-borne anthrax attacks in the fall of 2001.

The medical consequences and epidemiology of a large-scale attack with these agents would mimic more traditional disasters, but with some distinct differences (Table 7.1). A chemical attack may combine elements of traditional mass disasters of high acuity (e.g., earthquake, bomb explosion, airplane crashes) and hazardous materials incidents (e.g., chemical tank car crash, factory explosion). Casualties in these disasters would occur almost immediately and first responders such as paramedics, police, and fire personnel as well as "first receivers" such as emergency department (ED) physicians and nurses may be disproportionately affected.

The details of the Tokyo sarin attack illustrate many of these features. At about 8:00 a.m., five subway cars were attacked simultaneously. By 8:28 a.m., an ambulatory victim arrived to one area ED a short distance from the affected subway stations. At 8:43 a.m., the first ambulance arrived, and the next hour brought an additional 500 patients, including three in cardiopulmonary arrest. Citywide, 5,510 persons sought emergency medical treatment at more than 200 facilities within a few hours of the attack; about 25% required hospitalization. Of note, most of the victims went to hospitals by taxi, bus, or private vehicles, rather than by formal EMS transport, further compounding the initial chaos. Until the identity of the agent was known, significant efforts at patient decontamination were lacking, resulting in several cases (most mild) of secondary exposure to hospital workers from "off-gassing" from casualties.

A covert (unannounced) biological attack, in contrast, would more likely simulate a natural infectious disease outbreak and present as a public health crisis evolving over a longer period of time. Illness onset would be delayed by variable incubation periods with victims typically presenting some time and distance from the point of exposures. The "first responders" for most exposed children would actually be first receivers such as pediatricians and ED physicians. Of note, the mail-borne anthrax cases in the fall of 2001 had elements of both overt (e.g., the letters opened by Senate office workers) and covert (e.g., postal workers unknowingly exposed and then becoming infected) attacks.

In this context, pediatric ED providers should have a grasp of the fundamental principles of epidemiology and be able to apply these principles in working up an unexpected outbreak

TABLE 7.1

CHARACTERISTICS OF CHEMICAL AND BIOLOGICAL ATTACKS

Chemical weapons attack (differences in comparison to "routine" hazardous materials incidents)	Biological weapons attack (differences in comparison to natural infectious disease epidemics)
Intent to cause mass casualties	Intent to cause mass casualties
More toxic substances	More virulent agents
Initial substance identification delayed	Rare, nonendemic diseases, delayed diagnosis
Greater risk to EMS first responders	Greater risk to physicians and other first receivers
Overwhelming numbers of patients	Overwhelming numbers of patients
Many "worried well"	Many "worried well"
Mass hysteria, panic	Mass hysteria, panic
Discovery of chemical dispersal device	Discovery of biological agent dispersal device
	More compressed time frame of outbreak
	Very high infection rates, morbidity, mortality
	More respiratory forms of disease than in natural forms
	Multiple epidemics at once
	Reduced rate of infection in sheltered persons
	Infected, dying animals

EMS, emergency medical services.
Adapted from Henretig FM, Cieslak TJ, Eitzen EM Jr. Biological and chemical terrorism. *J Pediatr* 2002;141: 311–326.

of unusual illness. Attempts should be made to (i) identify who is affected, (ii) determine possible routes of exposure, (iii) describe clinical findings of the disease, (iv) formulate a case definition, (v) quantify the number of cases, and (vi) calculate the attack rate in an attempt to identify the causative organism. The epidemic can then be described in terms of timing, place, routes of exposure, and other clinical characteristics of ill patients. Thus, pediatric ED providers can play a pivotal role on the "front lines" of our nation's public health infrastructure in our defense against both terrorism-induced and naturally occurring diseases. In some systems, real time ED visit data is captured by syndromic surveillance engines, alerting monitoring organizations (i.e. CDC) and thus potentially identifying an epidemic early in the course.

SPECIFIC PEDIATRIC CONCERNS

Several physiologic, developmental, and psychological considerations are unique to the pediatric population in the context of planning for biological and chemical terrorism. In addition, there are specific vulnerabilities within our EMS system as it responds to critically ill children that might well be exacerbated by such an incident. These challenges and some potential remedies are highlighted in Table 7.2.

Pediatricians may experience unique problems in managing childhood victims of biological or chemical terrorism. For example, many of the drugs useful in treating such casualties are unfamiliar to pediatricians or have relative contraindications in childhood. To date, there have been no formal consensus guidelines authored or endorsed by authoritative pediatric societies that specifically address the treatment of pediatric victims. The recommendations offered herein, therefore, represent the authors' best interpretation of current pediatric infectious disease and toxicology experience as extrapolated to this context.

BIOLOGICAL AGENTS

A working group convened by the Centers for Disease Control and Prevention (CDC) has identified anthrax, smallpox, plague, botulinum toxin, tularemia, and the viral hemorrhagic fevers as the biological diseases that would constitute the gravest threats to public health and security; the causative microorganisms are termed Category A agents. We thus limit our focus here to these six agents (Table 7.3). In addition, we add a brief discussion of the phytotoxin (plant toxin) ricin because of its ready availability and ease of production. Treatment protocols for these uncommon conditions are likely to evolve continuously, particularly if future incidents occur, as was the case when the mail-borne anthrax outbreak unfolded. The CDC offers a telephone hotline and a website for up-to-date management advice (Table 7.3).

Of note, the fluoroquinolones and/or tetracyclines are currently considered drugs of choice in the treatment and prophylaxis of anthrax, plague, and tularemia. Although these have been little used by pediatricians in the past, there is now considerable recent experience with the use of these antibiotics for selected serious pediatric infections. Furthermore, the risk of morbidity and mortality from these biological agent-induced diseases far outweighs the putative minor risks (arthropathy with fluoroquinolones, dental staining with tetracyclines) associated with short-term pediatric use of these medications. In fact, ciprofloxacin and doxycycline appear to be relatively free of these adverse effects, and more recently became U.S. Food and Drug Administration approved medications specifically for use in children for the prophylaxis and treatment of anthrax following inhalational exposure (i.e., in the context of terrorism).

Specialized laboratory services would likely be required to rapidly identify these agents or confirm a diagnosis of disease

TABLE 7.2

PEDIATRIC VULNERABILITIES TO BIOLOGICAL AND CHEMICAL TERRORISM

Realm	Potential vulnerability	Potential response
Physiologic	Increased respiratory exposure (higher minute ventilation, live "closer to the ground")	Early warning, sheltering[a] (gas masks for the general population are not advised at present due to risk of poor fit, suffocation)
	Increased dermal exposure (thinner, more permeable skin; larger body surface area/mass ratio)	Protective clothing, earlier decontamination[a]
	Increased risk of dehydration, shock with toxin-induced vomiting, diarrhea (decreased fluid reserves, larger body surface area/mass ratio)	Recognition, aggressive fluid therapy
	Increased risk of hypothermia during decontamination (larger body surface area/mass ratio)	Warm-water decontamination
	More fulminant disease (possible), immunologic immaturity, more permeable blood–brain barrier	Pediatric-specific research for early diagnosis and treatment of biological- and chemical-weapons victims[a]
	Differing disease manifestations	Education
	Relative antibiotic contraindications	Research trials in children
Developmental	Less capacity to escape attack site, take appropriate evasive actions (developmental immaturity, normal dependence on adult caregivers who might be injured or dead) or be reunited with families	Increased public education, especially of parents, teachers, and caregivers
Psychological	Less effective coping skill of children who suffer injury or witness parental, sibling death (psychological immaturity)	Child psychiatry involvement, cognitive therapy, research for preventing pediatric posttraumatic stress disorder[a]
	Greater anxiety over reported incidents, hoaxes, media coverage, etc.	Pediatric counseling of parents and children[b]
EMS	Less capacity to cope with influx of critical pediatric patients, loss of routine hospital transfer protocols, limited ability to expand pediatric hospital bed capacity through NDMS	Community and regional planning with significant pediatric input

EMS, emergency medical services; NDMS, national disaster medical system.
[a]Plausible, but unproven or unstudied, and/or not intuitively obvious.
[b]See Chapters 20, 129, and 131.
Adapted from Henretig FM, Cieslak TJ, Eitzen EM Jr. Biological and chemical terrorism. *J Pediatr* 2002;141:311–326.

---

caused by them. Further, work with most of these agents is very hazardous. As such, a national Laboratory Response Network (LRN) has been established to facilitate the timely detection of bioterrorism-related diseases. This network involves laboratories at local, state, and federal levels. The latter include the CDC in Atlanta, Georgia, and the U.S. Army Medical Research Institute of Infectious Diseases (USAMRIID) at Fort Detrick in Frederick, Maryland. If pediatric emergency care providers suspect such an illness, they should immediately inform their hospital microbiology laboratory and infection control office, as well as the local public health departments, to effect prompt notification and transport of specimens to the appropriate laboratory. In addition, the CDC and USAMRIID may be contacted directly (Table 7.3).

Early Recognition of a Covert Biological Attack

Pediatricians and ED physicians face seriously ill and injured children in their practices every day, but rarely encounter children who are victims of biological agent exposure. Considering three critical epidemiological characteristics of such an attack might enhance early recognition: an *epidemic*

number of patients, a common *exposure* history, and *exotic* disease presentations. A large number of patients, out of proportion to time of year and expected clinical syndromes, might trigger suspicion. Although some variations in the incubation period may occur after a biological agent attack, most persons would initially be exposed at the same time, and thus become ill and present in a relatively compressed time frame. In contrast, most natural epidemics evolve with a gradual rise in disease incidence because persons are progressively exposed to increased numbers of infectious patients, fomites, or vectors that spread the organism.

A history of geographic connection among patients, or some observation of an unusual source of exposure, such as a powder in an envelope, might also sound the alarm. By exotic diseases, it is suggested that many infections caused by biological weapons, particularly with advanced disease, are relatively unusual and unique. Diseases that are rare, not endemic in the area of exposure, or that are normally spread by vectors that are not indigenous to the relevant geographic area would also be suspect, especially if numerous cases developed simultaneously.

Additional clues to a biological agent attack might include especially high infection rates among exposed persons, high rates of patients with atypical pneumonia, particularly high

TABLE 7.3

PRIMARY THREAT BIOLOGICAL AGENTS OF TERRORISM

Syndrome	Clinical presentation	Incubation period	Transmission and precautions	Diagnosis	Treatment	Prophylaxis
Acute respiratory distress with fever	*Inhalational Anthrax*—Abrupt onset of fever, chest pain, respiratory distress; mediastinitis; progression to shock and death within 24–36 h	1–5 days (may be weeks)	Person-to-person transmission: None Standard Precautions	Chest x-ray: widened mediastinum, hemorrhagic pleural effusion Isolation of *B. anthracis* from affected tissue (usually blood, nasal secretions, or pleural fluid)	Ciprofloxacin [a,b] 15 mg/kg q 12 h, or Doxycycline[c] ■ **If >8 yr and >45 kg: give** 200 mg loading dose, then 100 mg q 12 h; ■ **If >8 yr and ≤45 kg: give** 4.4 mg/kg loading dose then 2.2–4.4 mg/kg/day in 2 divided doses; ■ **If ≤8 yr: same as >8 yr and ≤45 kg,** **Therapy if strain is susceptible:** Penicillin G[d] 400,000 units/kg/day in divided doses (if susceptible) Treat for 60 days	Ciprofloxacin 15–20 mg/kg PO q 12 h (not to exceed 1 gm/day), or doxycycline ■ **>8 yr and >45 kg: give** 200 mg loading dose, the 100 mg q 12 h; ■ **>8 yr and ≤45 kg: give** 4.4 mg/kg loading dose then 2.2–4.4 mg/kg/day in 2 divided doses; ■ **≤8 yr: same as >8 yr and ≤45 kg,** **Therapy if strain is susceptible:** Amoxicillin ■ If ≥20 kg: give 500 mg PO q 8 h; or If <20 kg: give 40 mg/kg divided into 3 doses to be taken q 8 h Prophylaxis for 60 days
	Pneumonic Plague—Apparent severe community-acquired pneumonia; hemoptysis, cyanosis, gastrointestinal symptoms, septic shock	2–3 days	Person-to-person transmission: YES Droplet precautions	Gram-negative bacilli/coccobacilli in sputum, blood or lymph node; safety-pin appearance with Wright or Giemsa stain. Confirmation with isolation of *Y. pestis* from blood or sputum	**Preferred Therapy** Gentamicin 2.5 mg/kg IM or IV 3 times daily[e] **Alternative Choices** Doxycycline ≥45 kg give adult dose <45 kg give 2.2 mg/kg IV 2 times daily (Maximum 200 mg daily) Ciprofloxacin 15 mg/kg 2 times daily[f] Chloramphenicol 15 mg/kg IV 4 times daily[g]	Doxycycline[b] If ≥45 kg give adult oral dose If <45 kg give 2.2 mg/kg orally 2 times daily or Ciprofloxacin 20 mg/kg orally 2 times daily[d] Prophylaxis for 10 days
	Ricin (aerosolized)—Acute onset of fever, chest pain, and cough, progressing to respiratory distress and hypoxemia; not improved with antibiotics; death in 36–72 h	Symptomatic within hours	Person-to-person transmission: None Standard precautions	Isolation of toxin from respiratory secretions or serum	Supportive therapy	Supportive therapy

		Incubation	Transmission	Diagnosis	Preferred Therapy	Preferred Choices[b]
	Tularemia (pneumonic)— Abrupt onset fever, fulminant pneumonia	2–10 days	Person to person transmission: None Standard precautions	Chest x-ray: infiltrate, hilar adenopathy, effusion. Small, faintly staining, slow-growing, gram-negative coccobacillus in sputum or blood.	**Preferred Therapy** Gentamicin 2.5 mg/kg IM or IV 3 times daily[e] **Alternative Choices** Doxycycline = 45 kg give adult dose <45 kg give 2.2 mg/kg IV 2 times daily (Maximum 200 mg daily) Ciprofloxacin 15 mg/kg 2 times daily[f] Chloramphenicol 15 mg/kg IV 4 times daily[g]	**Preferred Choices**[b] Doxycycline[b] If ≥45 kg give adult oral dose If <45 kg give 2.2 mg/kg orally 2 times daily or Ciprofloxacin 20 mg/kg orally 2 times daily[d]
Acute rash with fever	*Cutaneous anthrax*— Papule progressing to vesicle, to ulcer, then to depressed black eschar, with marked edema. May not be associated with fever.	1–10 days	Person to person transmission: YES Contact precautions	Isolation of *B. anthracis* from affected tissue	As with inhalation anthrax	Not recommended
	Plague (bubonic)— Tender, enlarged, fluctuant lymph node in the distribution of the infected flea bite; fever and malaise; progresses to DIC, sepsis	4–7 days	Person to person transmission: None Standard Precautions	Confirmation with isolation of *Y. pestis* from blood or bubo aspirate	If signs/symptoms of sepsis, treat as with pneumonic plague	Not recommended
	Smallpox—Macules and papular evolve to pustules and scabs; fever; headache; delirium; rash is synchronous and is more prominent on the extremities	7–17 days	Person to person transmission: YES Airborne precautions	Clinical diagnosis with laboratory confirmation	Supportive therapy	Smallpox vaccine within 96 h of exposure

(continued)

TABLE 7.3

PRIMARY THREAT BIOLOGICAL AGENTS OF TERRORISM (CONTINUED)

Syndrome	Clinical presentation	Incubation period	Transmission and precautions	Diagnosis	Treatment	Prophylaxis
	Viral hemorrhagic fever (e.g. Ebola)—Fever with mucous membrane bleeding, petechiae, thrombocytopenia, hypotension	7–42 days (virus-specific)	Person to person transmission: YES Airborne precautions	Clinical diagnosis with laboratory confirmation	Supportive therapy	Supportive therapy
Neurologic syndromes	*Botulism*—Acute bilateral descending flaccid paralysis beginning with cranial nerve palsies	1–3 days	Person to person transmission: None Standard precautions	Clinical diagnosis with confirmation after toxin isolation	Supportive therapy; an anti-toxin may prevent disease progression	Supportive therapy

[a]Therapy with ciprofloxacin may be initiated either as IV (preferred method) or oral dosage. The pharmacokinetics are such that oral ciprofloxacin is rapidly absorbed in the GI tract with no substantial loss by first-pass metabolism. Maximum serum concentrations are attained 1–2 h after oral dosing.
[b]Ciprofloxacin dose should not exceed 1 g/day in children.
[c]In 1991 the American Academy of Pediatrics amended their recommendation to allow treatment of young children with tetracyclines for serious infections such as Rocky Mountain spotted fever for which doxycycline may be indicated. Doxycycline is preferred for its twice-a-day dosing and low incidence of GI side effects.
[d]If laboratory testing reveals isolate is penicillin-susceptible, therapy should be changed to IV penicillin.
[e]Other fluoroquinolones can be substituted at doses appropriate for age. Ciprofloxacin dosage should not exceed 1 g daily in children.
[f]Concentration should be maintained between 5 and 20 μg/mL. Concentrations greater than 25 μg/mL can cause reversible bone marrow suppression. Children younger than 2 yr should not receive chloramphenicol.
[g]In children, ciprofloxacin does should not exceed 1 g daily, chloramphenicol should not exceed 4 g daily. Children younger than 2 yr should not receive chloramphenicol. In neonates, gentamicin-loading dose of 4 mg/kg should be given initially.
[h]Tetracycline may be substituted for doxycycline.

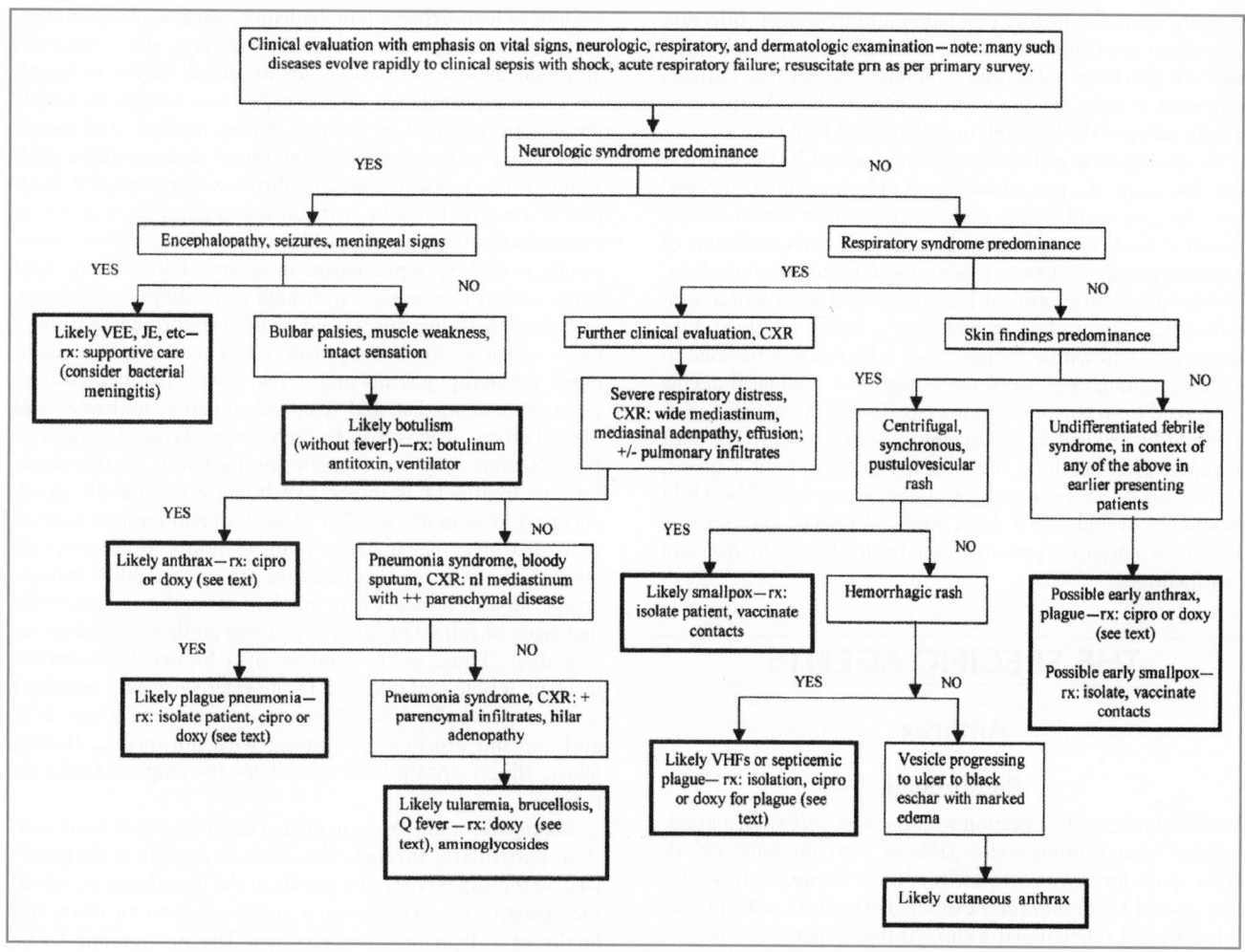

FIGURE 7.1 Approach to the early recognition and diagnosis of an attack with an unknown biological agent. VEE, venezuelan equine encephalitis; JE, Japanese encephalitis; rx, treatment; CXR, chest x-ray; VHF, viral hemorrhagic fever. (From Henretig FM, Cieslak TJ, Kortepeter MG, et al. Medical management of the suspected victim of bioterrorism: an algorithmic approach to the undifferentiated patient. *Emerg Med Clin North Am* 2002;20:351–364, with permission from Elsevier.)

morbidity or mortality, several epidemics at once, attack rates lower in persons sheltered from the suspected route of exposure, presence of infected or dying animals, and the discovery of suspicious actions or potential delivery systems.

Most of the primary biological threat agents can be categorized as causing the subacute onset of effects (e.g., days after exposure) and further divided into predominantly respiratory, neurologic, or dermatologic syndromes. Thus, with a careful medical and epidemiological history, physical examination, and limited, routine laboratory evaluation, an early suspicion of a biological attack might be raised, and initial diagnostic impression considered, as outlined in Figure 7.1. This in turn could trigger appropriate requests for infectious disease consultation and more definitive laboratory testing, as well as early empiric therapy. A similar approach, applied universally with unusual increases in patient volume or illness presentations, might also help practitioners to participate in the early recognition of a new or reemerging natural infectious disease (e.g., West Nile disease or severe acute respiratory syndrome, to name more recent examples). If a pediatrician recognizes, or

even suspects, any such natural or intentional outbreak, immediate reporting to local and regional public health authorities is appropriate, even before a specific diagnosis can be confirmed.

Minimizing Spread of Infection

As soon as ED staff suspect that a patient may be the victim of biological terrorism, appropriate steps must take place to prevent or minimize exposure to limit the spread of disease. The level of ED mitigation and preparedness activities will largely depend on the level of awareness of the disease outbreak. For example, if society were faced with a known release of smallpox by terrorists, EDs would need to take dramatic steps to protect staff and patients. Such steps might include setting up screening stations outside of the hospital, staffed by clinicians wearing gowns, gloves, N-95 respirators, and eye protection. If a child suspected to have smallpox were encountered at the screening station, he or she would need to be covered with a sheet, provided a mask, and escorted directly to a negative-pressure room for further evaluation and treatment. Infection Prevention and Control specialists would need to provide guidance on specimen collection, handling, and testing. Patients suspected to have smallpox would need to be cohorted into specific units of the hospital, or in dedicated facilities.

At the opposite end of the spectrum, would be the inadvertent discovery of a patient suspected to have an infectious disease. Perhaps an ED triage nurse discovers that within a short period of time two separate children arrive with complaints of floppiness and weakness, raising the concern for botulism. Perhaps a pediatric resident becomes concerned about a viral hemorrhagic fever after encountering a highly febrile and ill-appearing child with a purpuric rash who recently traveled to Africa. Although not all of the Category A biological agents are spread from person to person (see Table 7.3), in these cases it would be prudent to assume this mode of spread. The staff member, after washing his hands, should put on a gown, gloves, an N-95 respirator, and eye protection. The child should be covered with a sheet, provided a mask, and escorted directly to a negative-pressure room for further evaluation and treatment.

THE SPECIFIC AGENTS

Anthrax

Background

Anthrax is caused by infection with *Bacillus anthracis*, a gram-positive spore-forming rod capable of surviving long periods in its spore form without nutrients or moisture. Natural disease caused by *B. anthracis* exhibits cutaneous, gastrointestinal (GI), and inhalational forms. Anthrax spores can be formulated in a manner to enhance aerosolization. The resulting small particles may drift long distances with air currents, produce lethal infection when inhaled, and resist environmental degradation, making them a formidable terrorist weapon.

The anthrax attack of 2001 was characterized by 22 confirmed or suspect cases (11 inhalational, 11 cutaneous), with five deaths, resulting from presumed or known exposure to anthrax-contaminated mail. The attack resulted in enormous public anxiety, as well as major demands for medical care and public health resources. Antibiotic prophylaxis was prescribed for more than 30,000 persons, and decontamination of the Hart Senate Office Building alone took months and cost an estimated $23 million. Many bioterrorism defense experts, however, fear an even more widespread aerosol release (e.g., from a small cropduster-type airplane) that could potentially sicken hundreds of thousands.

Inhalational anthrax is the disease form that poses the greatest threat. Following the accidental release of anthrax spores from a Soviet military facility at Sverdlovsk in 1979, 66 of 77 known victims of inhalational anthrax died. In the recent U.S. attack, all five deaths were among the 11 patients with this form of disease.

Pathophysiology/Common Manifestations

Inhalational anthrax results from spore uptake in the alveoli by pulmonary macrophages, followed by bacterial germination and toxin production in the mediastinal lymph nodes,

leading to hemorrhagic lymphadenitis, mediastinitis, and sepsis. Symptoms typically begin 1 to 5 days after exposure, although incubation periods up to several weeks in length have been reported. The disease begins as a nonspecific febrile illness, characterized by fever, headache, myalgia, and cough. The relative lack of eye, nose, and throat findings such as red, watery eyes, rhinorrhea, or sore throat with pharyngeal injection or exudate helps to distinguish this phase from common viral infections, such as those due to rhinovirus. A brief intervening period of improvement sometimes follows, but rapid deterioration then ensues with high fever, dyspnea, cyanosis, and shock marking this second phase. Hemorrhagic meningitis occurs in up to 50% of cases. Chest radiographs or computed tomography scans may reveal a widened mediastinum or prominent mediastinal lymphadenopathy; infiltrates and pleural effusions may also be seen. Gram stains of peripheral blood smears may demonstrate the bacterium at this stage. Prompt treatment is imperative because historically death occurred in as many as 95% of inhalational anthrax cases if such treatment began more than 48 hours after symptom onset. Even with modern intensive care, in the 2001 anthrax attack, all four patients with inhalational anthrax who exhibited signs of fulminant disease prior to antibiotic administration died. Thus, in the context of a known bioterrorism incident, a potential dilemma facing emergency care providers is deciding which patients who may have been exposed to anthrax and are now presenting with nonspecific flulike, febrile illness are optimal candidates for empiric antibiotic therapy.

Cutaneous anthrax occurs when organisms gain entry into skin, particularly through abrasions or cuts. It is characterized by the appearance of a papule at the inoculum site, which then progresses over days to a vesicle, then to an ulcer, and finally to a depressed, black eschar. The surrounding tissue becomes markedly edematous, but not particularly tender, distinguishing this infection from typical cellulitis. It is, however, quite amenable to therapy with a variety of antibiotics, and, with timely institution of treatment, is rarely fatal. In the 2001 outbreak, all 11 patients with cutaneous anthrax survived. The one pediatric victim of the 2001 attack was a 7-month-old boy with cutaneous anthrax on his arm, presumably contracted after a brief visit to a New York City television news studio that had received contaminated mail (a similar lesion is pictured on the face of a child in Fig. 7.2 [see also color plate]). He was suspected initially of having a brown recluse spider bite, and the correct diagnosis was only confirmed after the discovery of anthrax contamination at another television studio. Of note, he also developed evidence of hemolysis, thrombocytopenia, and renal insufficiency, features not usually observed in otherwise uncomplicated cases of cutaneous disease, thus raising the possibility of a particular vulnerability in infancy.

The finding of gram-positive rods in skin biopsy material (in the case of cutaneous disease) or in blood smears, pleural fluid, or spinal fluid should suggest anthrax. Chest radiographs demonstrating a widened mediastinum in the context of fever and constitutional signs should also lead one to consider the diagnosis. Confirmation may be obtained by blood culture. State health laboratories, USAMRIID, and the CDC can also confirm a diagnosis of anthrax by polymerase chain reaction and immunohistochemical assay.

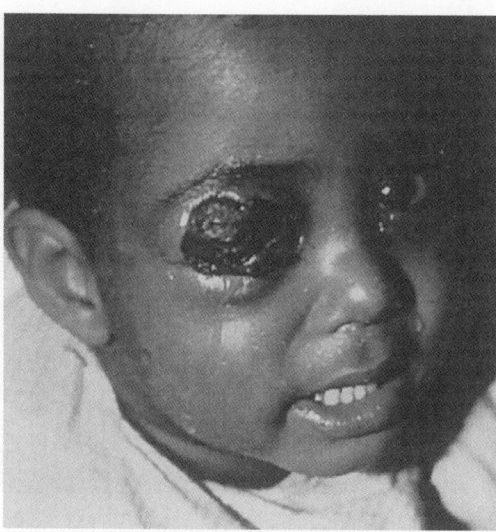

FIGURE 7.2 Cutaneous anthrax on the eyelids of a young child. (Courtesy of Dr. Larry Schwab. From Ostler HB, Maibach HI, Hoke AW, et al. *Diseases of the eye and skin: a color atlas.* Philadelphia: Lippincott Williams Wilkins, 2004, with permission.)

Management

As anthrax has little potential for person-to-person transmission, standard precautions (Table 7.3) are adequate for healthcare workers caring for anthrax victims. Given the usual 1- to 5-day incubation period, decontamination of victims presenting days after exposure is unwarranted. Reaerosolization of organisms from skin or clothing likewise poses little threat under typical circumstances, but bathing and laundry with soap and water would seem prudent soon after direct physical contact with a suspect substance.

Although naturally occurring strains of *B. anthracis* are usually quite sensitive to penicillin G, penicillin-resistant strains of *B. anthracis* are known; thus, many experts consider ciprofloxacin [10 to 15 mg per kg, max 400 mg, IV (intravenous) q12h] or doxycycline (2.2 mg per kg, max 100 mg, IV q12h) as essential components of first-line treatment for victims of intentional anthrax. Infectious Disease and Emergency Preparedness experts can provide advice regarding postexposure prophylaxis. See Table 7.3 for detailed treatment recommendations for children. Newer treatments under development include the use of monoclonal antibodies and anthrax immune globulin; these are not currently available nor have they been tested for use in children.

Plague

Background

Plague, caused by infection with the gram-negative bipolar-staining rod *Yersinia pestis*, is usually transmitted in nature via the bite of fleas. Endemic disease is still seen in areas of the southwestern U.S., South and Southeast Asia, as well as in South America and Africa. Plague has long appeared attractive as an agent of bioterrorism. Testimony to its extreme lethality and infectivity can be obtained by considering that the "Black Death" eliminated one-third of the population of Europe during the Middle Ages.

Pathophysiology

Y. pestis is a facultative intracellular pathogen that is able to survive temporarily within macrophages, thus aiding its dissemination to distant sites following inoculation or inhalation. It is lymphotropic, and significantly tender regional lymphadenopathy (e.g., in the distribution of a flea bite) is often a prominent feature of bubonic plague. Pneumonic plague (along with smallpox) is one of the few bioterrorist threats readily transmissible from person to person via the respiratory route, and coughing patients are often highly contagious. However, because plague, unlike smallpox, is spread by large respiratory droplets, close contact is needed for transmission.

Clinical Manifestations

Bubonic plague is characterized by the classic bubo, a tender, enlarged, fluctuant lymph node in the distribution of the infected flea bite. Fever and malaise are usually present. Bubonic plague may progress to septicemia as bacteria gain access to the circulation; 80% of bubonic plague victims have positive blood cultures. Petechiae, purpura, and overwhelming disseminated intravascular coagulation (DIC) may develop.

Pneumonic plague may arise secondarily after blood-borne seeding of the lungs or may be seen primarily after aerosol exposure. Symptoms include high fever, chills, malaise, fatigue, headache, and cough. Chest radiographs may reveal a patchy or consolidated broncho-pneumonia, and the classic clinical finding is one of blood-streaked sputum; DIC and an overwhelming sepsis may develop as the disease progresses. Meningitis develops in 6% of cases. Untreated pneumonic plague has a mortality rate approaching 100%.

A presumptive diagnosis of plague can be made by observing the classic bipolar-staining "safety pin"–like rods in Gram or Wayson stains of sputum, aspirated lymph node material, or cerebrospinal fluid. Confirmation is obtained via blood, sputum, or aspirate culture. The organism grows on standard blood or MacConkey's agars but is often misidentified by automated systems.

Management

Droplet precautions should be employed in cases of suspected pneumonic plague. Such precautions should be continued in confirmed cases until sputum cultures are negative. Standard precautions are adequate in managing bubonic plague victims. Given the incubation period, decontamination would not be necessary in a clinical setting. A previously licensed plague vaccine is currently out of production. This vaccine was developed to prevent bubonic plague in endemic regions, and animal data suggest that it is unlikely to protect against the pneumonic form of the disease. See Table 7.3 for detailed treatment recommendations for children.

Smallpox

Background

The global eradication of smallpox represents one of the great success stories of public health, with the last endemic case occurring in Somalia in 1977. Since then, research stockpiles of variola virus have been consolidated into two World Health Organization (WHO)—approved stores—at the CDC in Atlanta and at a Russian institute in Koltsovo, near Novosibirsk. This achievement would seem to make terrorist use of this virus impossible; however, several factors give cause for concern. First is the fear that other stockpiles already exist in the hands of belligerent nations unbeknownst to WHO. Second, the entire viral genomic sequence is known and published; therefore, it is likely only a matter of time before technology permits reconstruction of the virus. Finally, although the virulence factors of variola virus are poorly understood, it may be possible for someone to manipulate related orthopoxviruses such as monkeypox to enhance their virulence in humans and create a disease similar to smallpox. In light of these considerations, the CDC in 2003 recommended a strategy of reintroducing vaccination in the United States after a nearly 30-year hiatus, with the initial goal of vaccinating up to 10,000,000 front-line EMS and health-care providers. This program has subsequently proven controversial and has been suspended in light of cardiac toxicities not described previously; probably fewer than 50,000 civilians were vaccinated. The U.S. military, however, has vaccinated several hundred thousand personnel in recent years very successfully and serious adverse events have been rare.

Several factors might make smallpox an attractive weapon to potential belligerents. First, the duration of immunity after vaccination is a matter of some controversy, with some studies suggesting a duration of only 3 to 5 years while other studies suggest the possibility of lifelong immunity. Second, until the recent licensing of a new product (ACAM2000, Acambis Corporation), vaccine had long been out of production, and stockpiles of vaccinia vaccine were dwindling and losing potency; susceptibility to the disease has thus become nearly universal. Also, effective therapy is lacking and health-care providers are unfamiliar with the disease. Finally, the potential for rapid spread potentially permits a terrorist to cause widespread disease and panic with a minimum of infectious material.

Pathophysiology

Although infectivity is highest when the smallpox rash first appears, the disease may be spread by exposed persons about 24 hours before the exanthem appears. During the 7- to 17-day-long incubation period, the virus replicates in upper respiratory tract mucosa, giving rise to a primary viremia. The liver and spleen are then seeded, further amplification of the virus occurs, and a secondary viremia ultimately develops. The skin is seeded with this secondary viremia, and the classic exanthem of smallpox develops.

Clinical Manifestations

Clinical illness begins rather abruptly during the phase of secondary viremia and is characterized by fever, malaise, rigors, vomiting, headache, and backache. The classic exanthem typically begins 2 to 4 days later as macules on the face and extremities. These lesions progress in synchronous fashion to papules, then to pustules, and finally form scabs. As scabs separate, survivors are left with disfiguring depigmented scars. The rash spreads centrally to the trunk but remains more abundant at the periphery. This centrifugal distribution and synchrony distinguish smallpox from the principal differential diagnostic consideration, chickenpox, which has a centripetal distribution of lesions in varying stages of development (Fig. 7.3). An enanthem usually accompanies the characteristic exanthem, and internal organs become viral targets as well.

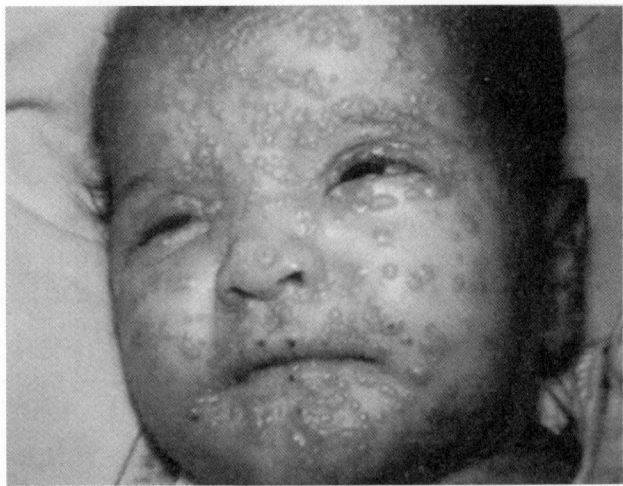

FIGURE 7.3 A child with smallpox. (From Henretig FM, McKee MR. Preparedness for acts of nuclear, biological and chemical terrorism. In: Gausche-Hill M, Fuchs S, Yamamoto L, eds. *APLS: the pediatric emergency medicine resource.* American Academy of Pediatrics and American College of Emergency Physicians. Sudbury, MA: Jones and Bartlett, 2004:568–591, with permission.)

Death occurs in 30% of variola major (the predominant form of smallpox in the past) patients and typically results from hypotension and immune complex–associated toxemia, as well as visceral organ involvement. Eye involvement leads to blindness in a small number of victims. Uncommon variants with lesser (variola minor) or greater (hemorrhagic and flat-type variants) mortality also existed.

Management

The diagnosis of smallpox should be suspected on clinical grounds. Laboratory confirmation (e.g., cultures, electron microscopy, polymerase chain reaction) is probably best effected by emergent notification and specimen of pustule fluid transported to the CDC or local health department.

Based on past experience, vaccination (with vaccinia, an orthopoxvirus closely related to variola) of smallpox-exposed persons within the first 4 days after exposure may prevent the development of overt disease. Although the vaccine has been used safely and successfully in even young infants, it has a relatively high rate of serious complications in certain patients. Notably, fetal vaccinia and resultant fetal demise can occur when pregnant women are vaccinated. Vaccinia gangrenosa, a frequently fatal complication, occurred when immunocompromised persons were inadvertently vaccinated. Eczema vaccinatum may occur in those with preexisting skin conditions and can be serious. Myocarditis and pericarditis may occur. A severe postvaccinial encephalitis was well-known albeit relatively rare during the era of widespread vaccination; because this complication occurs only in primary vaccines, it would disproportionately affect pediatric patients. Autoinoculation can occur when virus from the primary lesion arising at the site of vaccination is transferred by scratching to eye or other areas of the skin. Young children would likely be at greater risk for such inadvertent transmission, although this might be mitigated by the use of folded gauze and a semipermeable adhesive membrane (not a water-tight dressing) to cover vaccination sites. To manage these complications, vaccinia immune globulin (VIG) should be available when undertaking a vaccination campaign. VIG [0.6 mg per kg intramuscularly (IM)] may be given to vaccine recipients who experience severe complications or to significantly immunocompromised individuals exposed to smallpox in whom vaccination would be unsafe. Today, stocks of vaccine and VIG are controlled by the CDC. Even a single case of smallpox occurring anywhere in the world today would represent a grave public health emergency. A suspected case should thus prompt immediate notification and consultation with health authorities. Strict airborne, droplet, and contact precautions should be instituted immediately for victims and should continue until all scabs have separated. Decontamination of symptomatic patients is unnecessary. Contacts must be observed closely for 17 days following their last potential exposure. The development of fever during this period would be cause for isolation. Multiple victims would ideally be managed as a cohort at dedicated sites removed from conventional hospital facilities.

Botulism

Background

Botulism occurs as a result of exposure to one of seven botulinum neurotoxins (A through G). Only types A, B, E, and rarely, F appear to cause human botulism in nature. Botulinum toxin was included in the U.S. biological arsenal in the 1950s and 1960s, and was weaponized by Iraq in the 1980s. The Aum Shinrikyo cult in Japan tried unsuccessfully to disseminate botulinum toxin before deciding to release sarin in the Tokyo subway system.

Pathophysiology

Botulinum toxins are produced by certain strains of *Clostridium botulinum*, a strictly anaerobic spore-forming gram-positive rod commonly found in soil. In addition, a few cases of type F neonatal botulism have been described; in these cases, *Clostridium baratii* was believed to be the source of toxin. Most cases of natural botulism result from ingestion of preformed toxin (food poisoning) or intestinal toxin formation (infant form). Infant botulism has additional unique epidemiologic considerations; more extensive discussion of this form, and of botulism in general, may be found elsewhere in this text (see Chapters 92 and 96). The botulinum neurotoxins are the most toxic substances known to man, with an LD_{50} (for type A toxin) of 0.001 mcg per kg. These toxins function at the peripheral cholinergic presynaptic nerve terminals, principally the neuromuscular junction, by preventing the release of acetylcholine and thereby leading to a generalized flaccid paralysis and autonomic symptoms. In keeping with the fact that toxins are chemical poisons produced by biological organisms, it is important to keep in mind that most cases of terrorist-caused botulism will represent chemical intoxication rather than a disease caused by colonization and infection of tissues by replicating *C. botulinum* organisms.

Clinical Manifestations

Following a latent period ranging from 24 hours to several days, victims begin to experience cranial nerve dysfunction, manifesting as bulbar palsy, ptosis, photophobia, and blurred vision owing to difficulty in accommodation. Symptoms progress to include dysarthria, dysphonia, and dysphagia. Ultimately, a descending, symmetric, flaccid paralysis ensues, although sensorium and sensation are not affected primarily. The mucous membranes are dry; this fact, along with mydriasis, the nature of the paralysis (lack of initial fasciculations), and the latent period, all differentiate botulism from nerve agent intoxication. A solitary case of botulism must also be differentiated from myasthenia gravis, Guillain-Barré syndrome, tick paralysis, and a few other uncommon neurologic disorders. The presence of multiple casualties with similar symptoms should raise the concern for botulism.

Management

Supportive care, with meticulous attention to ventilatory support, remains the mainstay of botulism management. Patients may require such support for several months, making the management of a large-scale botulism outbreak especially problematic in terms of medical resources. Diagnosis of botulism is made through identifying toxin in serum, stool, gastric aspirate, or contaminated food. Infant botulism is best detected through stool culture. These methods may be time consuming. Use of nerve conduction studies may lend support to the clinical diagnosis and antitoxin administration should not wait for final culture results.

A bivalent (types A and B) botulinum antitoxin is licensed and available through the CDC. A separate investigational anti-E preparation is similarly available after consultation with CDC experts. Although administration of antitoxin is unlikely to reverse disease (the antitoxin is most effective when given during the clinically asymptomatic, or latent, period following inhalation of the toxin), it may be useful in preventing progression when administered to exposed persons. The antitoxin is prepared from horse serum and requires that a test dose be administered before therapy; patients reacting to this test dose require desensitization prior to treatment.

In addition, an investigational heptavalent despeciated (Fab2) antitoxin, also produced in horses, is now available in the Strategic National Stockpile through the CDC. Finally, a licensed human botulinum immunoglobulin is available to treat infant botulism (see also Chapters 96 and 102). While the product (BabyBIG) contains antibody against botulinum toxin types A–E, it has only been studied, and is thus only licensed, to treat type A and B intoxication. Botulism is not contagious, and standard precautions are adequate for patient care.

Tularemia

Tularemia is a highly infectious plaguelike disease caused by the gram-negative coccobacillus *Francisella tularensis*. Several clinical forms of naturally occurring tularemia are known, but pneumonic tularemia would presumably be the most likely clinical presentation in the event of an intentional bioaerosol release of *F. tularensis*. The onset of symptoms may be abrupt and include fever, nonproductive cough, substernal tightness, pleuritic chest pain, occasional hemoptysis, chills, headache, malaise, anorexia, and fatigue. Chest radiographs may show infiltrates, hilar adenopathy, pleural effusion, or miliary infiltrates (may mimic tuberculosis).

Tularemia is not contagious, and standard precautions are adequate in patient care. However, processing cultures is a very significant risk to laboratory staff, who thus must be notified of a suspected case. See Table 7.3 for detailed treatment recommendations for children.

Viral Hemorrhagic Fevers

The viral hemorrhagic fevers are a heterogeneous group of illnesses caused by infection with lipid-enveloped RNA viruses belonging to the families *Arenaviridae, Bunyaviridae, Filoviridae,* and *Flaviviridae.* These viruses may cause fulminant illnesses with fever, hypotension, and bleeding diathesis. The capacity for human-to-human transmission and high lethality makes the filoviruses (e.g., Ebola and Marburg viruses) and arenaviruses (e.g., Lassa Fever virus) particularly concerning. Supportive care remains the cornerstone of therapy for most of the viral hemorrhagic fevers. IV ribavirin appears somewhat efficacious in treating disease due to the *Arenaviridae.*

Ricin

The distinction between biological agents, which are living organisms capable of causing infections, and chemical agents, which are nonliving poisons, is obvious. Toxins, such as ricin, however, are chemical poisons produced by biological organisms and are increasingly seen as "midspectrum agents." Although discussed with biological agents, it should be kept in mind that they cause chemical intoxication (poisoning) rather than infections, do not replicate in hosts, and do not produce communicable, or contagious, conditions.

Ricin is a toxin derived from the castor bean, and its production is not technologically challenging. It is quite toxic if ingested, and far more so if injected or inhaled. It is infamous as a homicidal weapon of espionage used by the Bulgarian secret service during the Cold War against defector Georgi Markov. More recently, in February 2004, it was discovered in a U.S. Senate office building, apparently having been delivered through the mail. At least 16 persons required decontamination, although no one became ill. Ricin is an inhibitor of cellular protein synthesis via enzymatic attack on the 28S ribosomal subunit.

The clinical presentation of ricin intoxication depends on the route of exposure. Exposures due to aerosols are dose dependent. Four to 8 hours after inhalation, fever, chest tightness, cough, dyspnea, nausea, and arthralgias can be expected followed within 36 hours by progressive cough, dyspnea, cyanosis, and pulmonary edema resulting in respiratory failure. If ingested, necrosis of the GI epithelium, local hemorrhage, and hepatic, splenic, and renal necrosis can be expected followed by vascular collapse and death. If injected, severe local necrosis of muscle and regional lymph nodes with moderate visceral organ involvement will be seen.

Ricin poisoning is not contagious. Establishing a diagnosis may be challenging. Early post exposure (zero to 24 hours) nasal or throat swabs and respiratory secretions may be submitted for toxin assay for epidemiological purposes, although positive nasal swabs do not prove penetration of toxin to the lungs and negative swabs do not exclude exposure in any given patient. In addition, toxin assays and measurement of antibody response can be performed on serum. Management is primarily supportive, although the U.S. military has found that postexposure prophylaxis with an investigational toxoid is efficacious in animal trials.

Other Agents

Numerous other agents may present bioterrorist threats of varying degrees. In addition to previously discussed incidents, terrorists and belligerents have attempted to use *Salmonella, Shigella,* glanders, cholera, typhus, and probably many other organisms or toxins to induce disease. Many of these agents are discussed adequately elsewhere in this and other texts; a few warrant additional comment here.

Venezuelan equine encephalitis makes an attractive weapon because of its high infectivity; virtually all nonimmunes contracting the virus become symptomatic. In adults, this disease is usually self-limiting, with few patients developing encephalitis. In infants and young children, however, the disease can be severe, with as many as 4% developing overt encephalitis, often leading to permanent sequelae and death. In nature, the disease is transmitted via the bite of Culex mosquitoes. When delivered intentionally via aerosol, access to the olfactory bulbs may produce more rapid and/or more severe neurologic disease. Treatment is supportive.

Staphylococcal enterotoxin B (SEB) is a bacterial toxin that has been weaponized in the past. Although familiar to many clinicians as a common cause of food poisoning, SEB would also be a potent incapacitating toxin if delivered by aerosol. Symptoms produced in this manner would begin 3 to 12 hours after exposure and consist of fever, headache, chills, myalgias, and nonproductive cough. Dyspnea and chest pain accompanies high dosages of inhaled toxin. Nausea, vomiting, and diarrhea may occur as a result of inadvertently swallowed toxin. Treatment is supportive; meticulous attention should be paid to fluid management. Patients may be ill for as long as 2 weeks with aerosol exposure.

Various fungal toxins, such as the trichothecene mycotoxins, have been mentioned in a biowarfare or bioterrorism context. After the Vietnam War, the U.S. government accused the Soviets of using a trichothecene toxin, T-2 (otherwise known as "yellow rain"), against Hmong tribesmen. The Iraqis are known to have weaponized another fungal toxin, aflatoxin, which in addition to acute clinical effects, is a potent hepatic carcinogen. Symptoms produced by various mycotoxins are variable and depend on the route of exposure. The trichothecene mycotoxins are different from virtually all other bioterrorist agents in that they are dermally active. Treatment is supportive.

CHEMICAL AGENTS

Background

Chemical warfare dates back to antiquity, when the Chinese used arsenical smokes in about 1000 BC and Spartan allies used burning sulfur and coal smoke during the Peloponnesian

War. World War I became the venue for the first large-scale use of such agents, particularly the gases chlorine and phosgene and the vesicating agent sulfur mustard, resulting in thousands of casualties. During the Holocaust, the Nazis infamously used the commercially available fumigant Zyklon B to release cyanide, as the genocidal agent in their concentration camps. Furthermore, both Allied and Axis powers also produced and stored enormous amounts of both vesicants and (after the war) nerve agents, leaving a heritage of chemical-weapon stockpiles throughout the world today. Iraq is known to have used chemical agents against Iran and also its own Kurdish population during the Iraq–Iran war in the 1980s. During the 1991 Gulf War, the existence of the Iraqi chemical agent armamentarium was well-known and led to an increased determination to prepare and defend American military forces against such an attack. Finally, religious terrorists used sarin against civilians in a residential neighborhood of Matsumoto, Japan, in June 1994, and again, as previously noted, in the more infamous attack on the Tokyo subways in March 1995.

Most chemical warfare agents are liquids at room temperature, but may exist as aerosols (visible mists or fogs composed of tiny droplets suspended in the atmosphere, or invisible aerosols composed of even smaller particles) after dispersal by munitions. Liquids are also volatile to varying degrees, and thus, may vaporize into a typically invisible gaseous phase, particularly in conditions of high temperature, strong wind, and deposition onto relatively nonporous surfaces. A few agents—for example, chlorine, phosgene, and hydrogen cyanide—exist primarily as gases in typical summertime conditions. Chemical agents may also be characterized by their environmental persistence, which is inversely related to volatility. Persistent agents, such as mustard and the nerve agent VX, pose a greater secondary contamination hazard from exposed terrain or material, or via contact by rescue or health-care workers with a victim's clothing or skin, than do the nonpersistent agents chlorine, phosgene, hydrogen cyanide, and the G nerve agents.

Toxic effects from chemical agents usually follow dermal or inhalational exposure and may present as (i) topical effects to the skin, the eyes, and the respiratory epithelium of the respiratory tract following contact and superficial absorption, (ii) effects on the body as a whole following systemic distribution, and (iii) both local and systemic effects. Although certain chemical agents under the appropriate conditions may be volatile, dermally active, or both, biological agents in general possess neither of these properties. Most of the modern medical literature on the clinical effects of chemical warfare agents focuses on the nerve agents, which are emphasized in this chapter. Clinical syndromes related to vesicants, pulmonary agents, cyanide, and riot-control agents are also briefly summarized (Table 7.4). General principles of supportive care for poisoned patients are detailed in Chapter 102; these principles also apply largely to the general support of chemical warfare agent victims.

Early Recognition of a Covert Chemical Attack with an Unknown Agent

By analogy with the previous parallel discussion regarding early recognition of a biological attack, alert pediatric emergency care providers will again be cognizant of three critical epidemiologic features: an epidemic number of patients, a common exposure history, and exotic disease presentations. In the context of chemical attack, this will manifest as an acute illness onset (within seconds to minutes, or hours in the case of some of the vesicants and pulmonary agents). In the more severe chemical incident scenarios, the recognition that such an attack has occurred will not be subtle; there might be numbers of persons collapsing, or dying, within minutes of exposure. As for the biological agents, it is convenient to categorize chemical weapons as causing predominantly neurologic, respiratory, or dermatologic syndromes that can help the practitioner in distinguishing attacks with nerve agents or cyanide, chlorine or phosgene, or vesicants, respectively (Fig. 7.4). Further input into more definitive diagnosis and management advice may be available from public health authorities or the regional poison control center (1-800-222-1222).

The most critical emergent decision will likely be the distinction of cyanide from nerve agent attack because the immediate antidotal therapies are quite different. As noted previously, in both cases, there may be numbers of victims with sudden collapse, coma, and seizures, with many deaths occurring rapidly. Nerve agent casualties will be more likely to be cyanotic, have miotic pupils with altered vision, have copious oral and nasal secretions, and have findings of acute bronchospasm and bronchorrhea, but clinical differentiation may be difficult in an individual case.

General Management, Decontamination, and Personal Protection Strategies

The general treatment of chemically contaminated victims begins with extrication, triage, emergent resuscitation as needed, and decontamination performed by rescue workers or health-care providers garbed in appropriate personal protective equipment (PPE). Patient decontamination has two important purposes: (i) prevention of secondary exposure of health-care workers and facilities and (ii) prevention or minimization of continuing absorption of agent into the patient. *This latter point is typically underemphasized, but by preventing absorption of a lethal dose of agent, immediate decontamination can be the most important life-saving action available for a chemical casualty.* This process would ideally occur at the scene, and thus ED staff would be spared the considerable challenges posed by the arrival of contaminated patients to their facility. However, as noted previously, in a large-scale terrorist incident, it is far more likely that some victims will self-transport to the ED. In this context, decontamination must take place prior to significantly contaminated patients being allowed into the ED. In brief, airway and cardiopulmonary support, including bag-valve-mask ventilation, possibly endotracheal intubation, and emergent antidotal therapy are provided as necessary, while contaminated clothing is removed as soon as possible. Simple disrobing may remove as much as 90% of the contamination hazard to health-care personnel. This is accompanied or followed immediately by more definitive decontamination as detailed in the following section. ED staff in bulky protective gear may find it difficult to provide significant advanced life support to small children prior to decontamination. In many cases, such support may be limited to manual airway maneuvers, provision of oxygen, bag-valve-mask ventilation, and the

TABLE 7.4A
PRIMARY THREAT CHEMICAL AGENTS OF TERRORISM

Agent	Toxicity	Clinical findings	Onset	Decontamination[a]	Management
Nerve agents: Tabun, sarin, soman, VX	Anticholinesterase: muscarinic, nicotinic, and CNS effects	Vapor: miosis, rhinorrhea, dyspnea Liquid: diaphoresis, vomiting Both: coma, paralysis, seizures, apnea	Seconds: vapor Minutes–hours: liquid	Vapor: fresh air, remove clothes, wash hair Liquid: remove clothes, copious washing skin, hair with soap and water, ocular irrigation, *decontaminate as soon as possible!*	ABCs Optimal therapy for individual, critical patients includes parenteral atropine and pralidoxime as follows: Atropine: 0.05 mg/kg IV[b], IM[c] (min 0.1 mg, max 5 mg), repeat q2–5 min pm for marked secretions, bronchospasm Pralidoxime: 25 mg/kg IV, IM[d] (max 1 g IV, 2 g IM), may repeat within 30–60 min pm, then again q1 h for 1 or 2 doses pm for persistent weakness, high atropine requirement Treatment of mass casualties in the ED or the prehospital setting may be better effected by use of autoinjectors of atropine and pralidoxime (see Table 7.4.b) Diazepam: 0.3 mg/kg (max 10 mg) IV; Lorazepam: 0.1 mg/kg IV, IM (max 4 mg); Midazolam: 0.2 mg/kg (max 10 mg) IM pm seizures, or severe exposure
Vesicants: Mustard	Alkylation and inflammation	Skin: erythema, vesicles Eye: inflammation Respiratory tract: inflammation	Hours (immediate pain with Lewisite)	Skin: soap and water Eyes: water (both: major impact only if done within minutes of exposure)	Symptomatic care (possibly BAL
Lewisite	Arsenic toxicity, including increased vascular permeability				3 mg/kg IM q4–6 h for systemic effects of Lewisite in severe cases)

Agent	Mechanism	Signs/Symptoms	Decontamination	Treatment
Pulmonary agents:				
Chlorine	Liberation of HCl; alkylation	Eyes, nose, throat irritation (especially chlorine) Respiratory: bronchospasm, pulmonary edema (especially phosgene)	Fresh air and water to skin	Symptomatic care
Phosgene	Alkylation (primary effect), liberation of HCl (at higher doses)	Minutes: eyes, nose, throat irritation, bronchospasm; Hours: pulmonary edema		
Cyanide	Cytochrome oxidase inhibition: cellular anoxia, lactic acidosis	Tachypnea, coma, seizures, apnea	Fresh air Skin: soap and water	ABCs, 100% oxygen Na bicarbonate prn metabolic acidosis Choose antidote: Nitrite/Thiosulfate or Hydroxocobalamin (both IV)
Riot Control agents: CS CN (Mace®) Capsaicin (pepper spray)	Nonspecific irritation (most agents); stimulation of release of substance P (pepper spray)	Eye: tearing, pain, blepharospasm Nose and throat irritation Pulmonary failure (rare)	Fresh air Eyes: lavage	Ophthalmics topically, symptomatic care

Na Nitrite

Dose (mL/kg)	Estimated Hgb (g/dL)
0.27	10
0.33	12 (est. for average child)
0.39	14

(max 10 mL)

Na thiosulfate (25%): 1.65 mL/kg (max 50 mL)

Hydroxocobalamin 70 mg/kg (adult dose 5 g) May repeat 35–70 mg/kg (2.5–5 g adults) prn severe toxicity

CNS, central nervous system; ABCs, airway, breathing and circulatory support; min, minimum; max, maximum; prn, as needed; BAL, British Anti-Lewisite; HCl, hydrogen chloride; Hgb, hemoglobin concentration; est, estimated hemoglobin concentration.

[a]Decontamination, especially for patients with significant nerve agent or vesicant exposure, should be performed by health-care providers garbed in adequate personal protective equipment. For ED staff, this consists of nonencapsulated, chemically resistant body suit, boots, and gloves with a full–face air–purifier mask/hood.

[b]Intraosseous route is likely equivalent to intravenous.

[c]Atropine might have some benefit via endotracheal tube inhalation, as might aerosolized ipatropium.

[d]Pralidoxime is reconstituted to 50 mg/mL (1 g in 20 mL water) for IV administration, and the total dose infused over 30 min, or may be given by continuous infusion (loading dose 25 mg/kg over 30 min, then 10 mg/kg/h). For IM use, a higher concentration of 300 mg/mL (1 g added to 3 mL water—by analogy to the U.S. Army's Mark 1 autoinjector concentration) might be utilized to effect a reasonable volume for injection; the contents of an autoinjecter can also be obtained by injection into an empty sterile vial (see text).

TABLE 7.4B

AUTOINJECTOR ADMINISTRATION OF ATROPINE AND PRALIDOXIME FOR MASS CASUALTIES AND/OR PREHOSPITAL SETTINGS

Atropine autoinjector therapy		
Approximate age	Approximate weight (kg)	Autoinjector size (mg)[a]
<6 mo	<7.5	0.25
6 mo–4 yr	7.5–18	0.5
5–10 yr	18–30	1
>10 yr	>30	2 (adult size)

Pralidoxime autoinjector therapy[b]			
Approximate age (yr)	Approximate weight (kg)	Number of autoinjectors	Pralidoxime dose range (mg/kg)
3–7	13–25	1	24–46
8–14	26–50	2	24–46
>14	>51	3	35 or less

[a]Administer one autoinjector.
[b]Pediatric autoinjectors of pralidoxime are not FDA approved or available at this time. Adult-intended autoinjectors (600-mg pralidoxime in 2 mL), while not approved for pediatric use, might be considered as initial treatment in dire (especially prehospital) circumstances, for children with severe, life-threatening nerve agent toxicity who lack intravenous access, and for whom more precise, mg/kg IM dosing (as per Table 7.4A) would be logistically impossible. Suggested dosing guidelines are offered: note potential excess of initial pralidoxime dose for age/weight, although within general guidelines for recommended total over first 60–90 min of therapy of severe exposures.
Adapted from Henretig FM, Cieslak TJ, Eitzen EM Jr. Biological and chemical terrorism. *J Pediatr* 2002;141:311–326.

use of autoinjector-delivered IM antidotes in severe cases of nerve agent toxicity. A partial solution resides in the recent recommendations of the Occupational Safety and Health Administration (OSHA) to establish a hospital decontamination corridor ("warm zone") in which more maneuverable PPE can be used than at the site of exposure (the "hot zone"). Following decontamination in the hospital decontamination corridor, only standard precautions then need to be used in the decontamination zone ("cold zone"), which would begin at or before the entrance to the emergency room unless the emergency room itself becomes contaminated.

Decontamination

Decontamination of casualties contaminated with chemical agents is usually of far greater immediacy than is decontamination of biological agents. The reason is that most biological agents will not penetrate intact skin, whereas chemical agents, particularly liquid nerve agents and vesicants as either liquids or vapors, can be absorbed within only a few minutes. Although the effects of percutaneously absorbed chemical agents may not appear for minutes to hours, tissue damage from vesicants occurs within a few minutes and agent that penetrates the skin is far less amenable to decontamination than is agent that has not yet been absorbed.

Until very recently, providing decontamination to critically ill children in the hospital setting would have constituted a significant challenge for most emergency care providers. Traditionally, hospital EDs had one designated area for a (single!) contaminated patient; often, this facility would go unused for years at a time and ED staff was not frequently drilled in its proper utilization. It is now recognized, however, that a special decontamination treatment area in proximity to the ED (in the OSHA-designated hospital decontamination corridor, or warm zone) would markedly facilitate this process and accred-

itation agencies have mandated that all hospitals provide such decontamination capacity; thus most hospitals have taken steps to create such areas in recent years.

Decontamination capability must be available on a short set-up time basis. Many models have been proposed, but most authorities recommend an outdoor facility with multiple patient stations, arranged so that parallel lines of ambulatory and non-ambulatory patients may be processed simultaneously (Fig. 7.5). An outdoor facility is more capable of handling multiple patients and may make the use of copious water irrigation easier; however, it may be challenging to protect victims from inclement weather in temperate climate zones, an issue especially important in the management of young children. An alternative might be the use of a facility that is enclosed, and adjacent but separate structurally from the main ED, with a separate and high-volume ventilation system vented directly outdoors (Fig. 7.6).

Optimally, the surface would allow drainage, minimizing risk of patients slipping and falling and risk of further exposure to contaminated rinse water. Medical personnel in warm-zone-appropriate PPE (OSHA provides suggested lists) should staff an initial triage station at the entrance to the decontamination structure. Triage at this point facilitates rapid identification of patients requiring immediate antidotal or other life-saving intervention, as well as diversion of nonambulatory patients to the appropriate area with medical assistance. Ideally triage is done by EMT or paramedic level practitioners who are used to rapid field triage. Ambulatory patients are instructed in self-decontamination. Obviously, young children require assistance or may be accompanied by parents if present. An outdoor facility must provide adequate water, some temperature control during environmental extremes, and measures to maintain personal modesty, such as curtains or other barriers separating shower lines for males from lines for females.

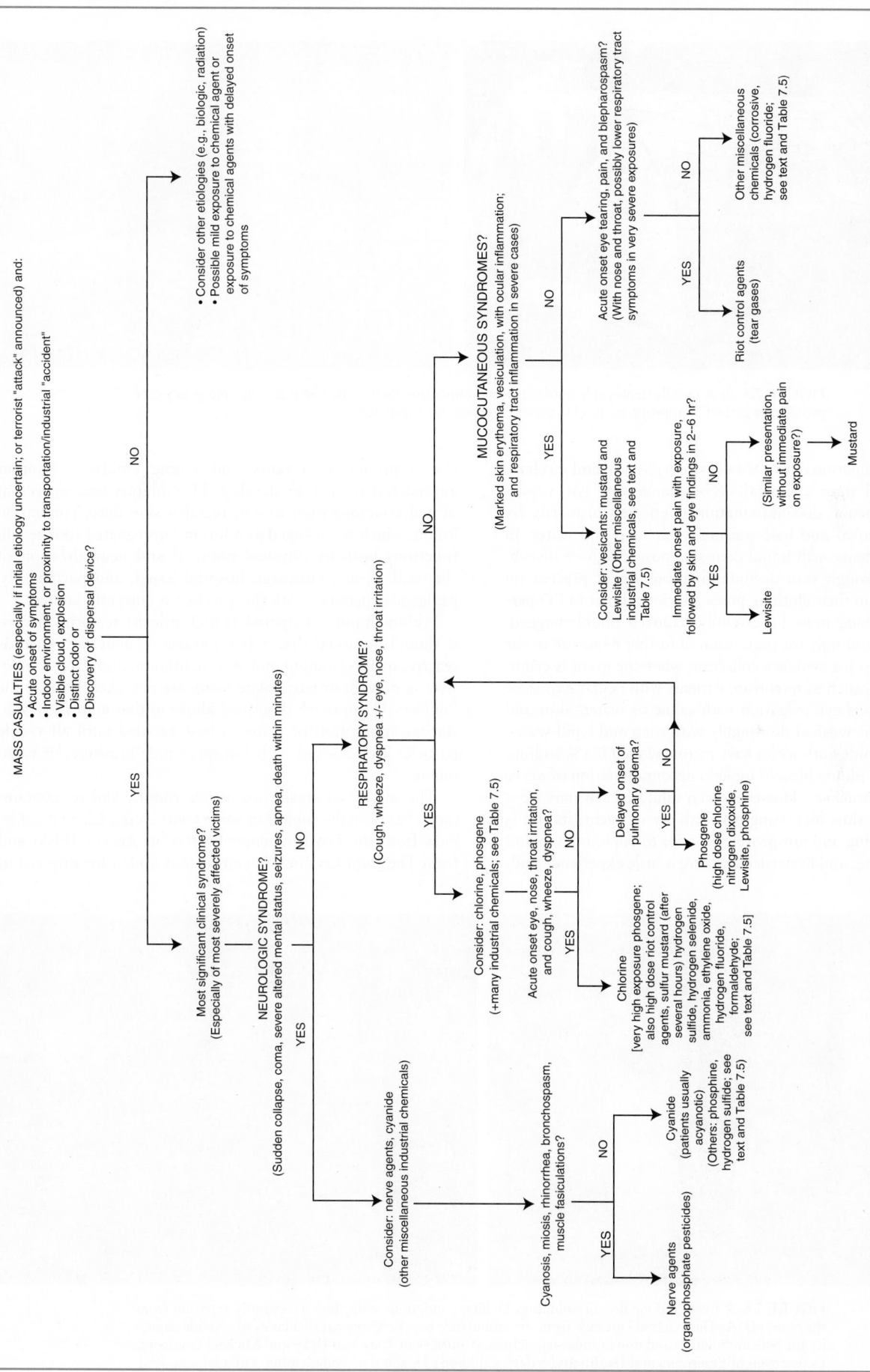

FIGURE 7.4 Approach to the recognition and diagnosis of an attack with an unknown chemical agent.

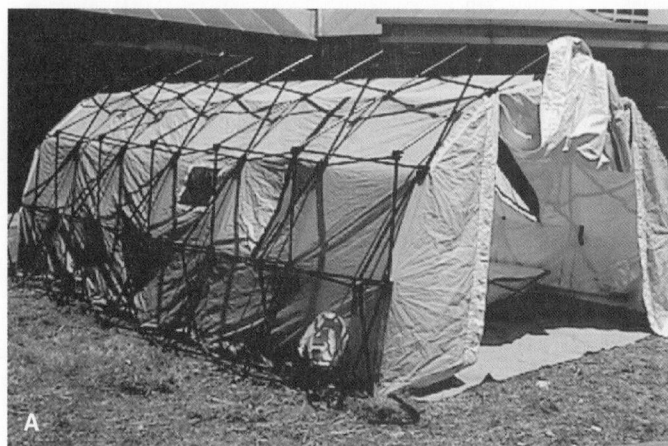
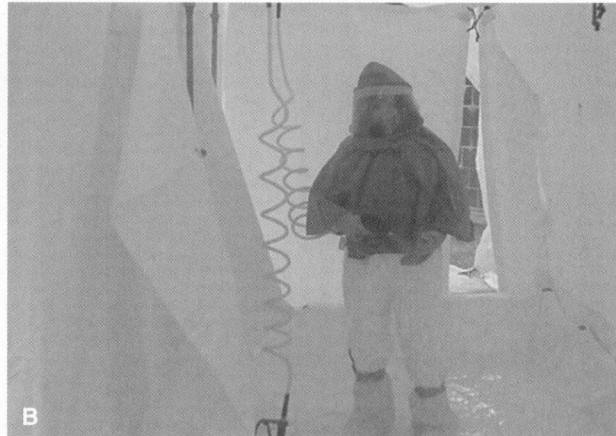

FIGURE 7.5 **A:** A rapidly deployable outdoor decontamination facility. **B:** The pediatric emergency care provider is garbed in appropriate level C personal protective equipment.

Decontamination efforts should stress physical and mechanical removal over chemical decontamination. For vapor-exposed patients, decontamination is effected primarily by clothing removal and hair washing with soap and water. In contrast, patients with liquid dermal exposure require disrobing and thorough skin decontamination. Agent present on their skin or in their clothing poses a serious threat to ED personnel. Clothing must be carefully removed double-bagged, and labeled, not only for prevention of further exposure to the agent but also for evidence collection when the event is criminal in nature, such as terrorism. Patients with ocular exposure require copious eye irrigation with saline or water. Skin and hair should be washed thoroughly with soap and tepid water. Previously, some authorities have recommended 0.5% sodium hypochlorite (dilute bleach) for skin decontamination of nerve agents and vesicants. However, even dilute bleach may be a skin irritant, thus increasing permeability to agent, its use is time consuming and not proven superior to copious soap and water washing, and in particular, there is little experience with

this approach in infants and young children. Another approach that has been developed for military field use is that of a decontamination lotion, reactive skin decontamination lotion, which is packaged as a lotion-impregnated sponge and functions both by physical removal and neutralization of chemical agents. However, hospital-based, and particularly, pediatric experience with this product is currently limited.

Although not anticipated as high-priority terrorist threats, it should be noted that a few hazardous materials, such as reactive metals (sodium, potassium, lithium) and strong corrosives in powder or particulate form, are rare exceptions to the "universal" approach described above in that with these substances application of water is best avoided until all visible particles are removed with forceps, gentle brushing, or vacuuming.

The matter of wash/rinse water runoff, and its containment, has been the subject of some controversy. Current guidelines from the Environmental Protection Agency (EPA) and from The Joint Commission stress that a plan for disposal of

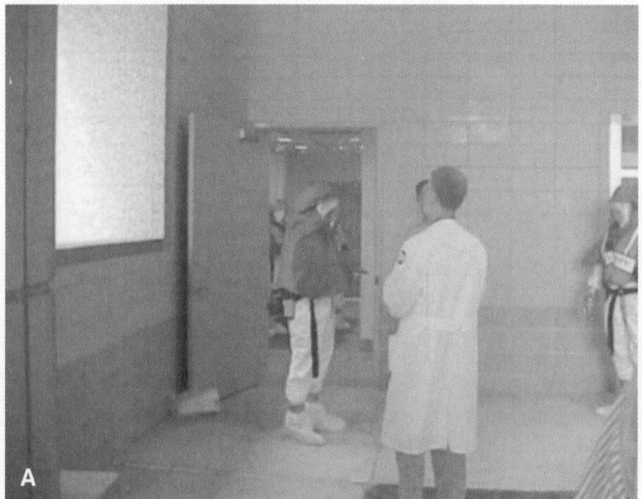
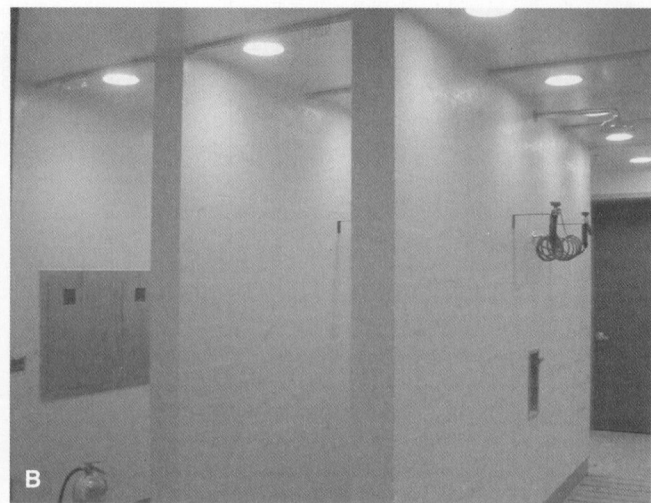

FIGURE 7.6 A fixed, indoor decontamination facility, contiguous with, but structurally separate from the main ED. **A:** The external entrance from the ambulance bay. **B:** Three parallel lanes to provide capacity for both ambulatory and nonambulatory victims. (Courtesy of Tony Van Dyke and Michael Goldberg, Department of Environmental Health and Safety, ■ Children's Hospital of Philadelphia, Philadelphia, PA.)

contaminated waste needs to be put into place by hospitals as part of their preparation for an event. Appropriate PPE for ED staff is an important consideration. The amount of chemical agent believed to contaminate patients who would arrive alive at the ED after a WMD (weapon of mass destruction) attack would consist essentially of that on their skin and clothing, and would thus be of far lower concentration than rescue workers would face at the scene of exposure. Most authorities thus believe that adequate protection in the hospital decontamination corridor (warm zone) would be afforded to ED staff garbed in level C PPE, which consists of a nonencapsulated chemically resistant body suit, gloves, and boots, with a full-face air purifier mask containing a cartridge with both an organic-vapor filter for chemical gases and vapors and a HEPA filter to trap aerosols of biological and chemical agents (Fig. 7.5). Such PPE is much less cumbersome to work in than level A or B outfits (which use self-contained breathing apparatus) and is much less expensive.

Choices regarding specific materials used in level C PPE options are difficult because few such barrier materials have been tested against WMD agents. At least one such material, DuPont's Tyvek F, has been found effective against mustard and organophosphate agents, but given the predicted low concentration and short contact times relevant to the ED decontamination process, less expensive fabrics may be adequate. Again, OSHA provides a list of suggested PPE for use in the warm zone. Biological agents require a considerable degree of energy to reaerosolize from contaminated skin or clothing, and they are not (in contrast to chemical agents) either volatile or (with the exception of trichothecene mycotoxins) dermally active (i.e., they neither cause skin lesions nor penetrate intact skin to cause disease). Thus, surface decontamination of biological agents, although still necessary after gross contamination, is nevertheless considered less critical than decontamination of chemical agents.

Nerve Agents

Nerve agents are organophosphorus esters, and, like the less potent "organophosphate" (OP) insecticides, are potent and essentially irreversible inhibitors of acetylcholinesterase (see Chapter 102). Certain oximes can dissociate bound nerve agents from acetylcholinesterase but only initially; after a variable period (depending on the structure of the nerve agent), a portion of the organophosphate is cleaved (in a process called *aging*) and the resulting nerve agent—cholinesterase complex becomes refractory to oxime action. The "G" (for "German") nerve agents, developed in Germany just before and during World War II, include GA, or tabun; GB, or sarin; and GD, or soman. VX (reportedly "Venom" X) was developed by Great Britain and the United States in the late 1940s and early 1950s. All four nerve agents are liquids at temperate conditions but may be aerosolized by spraying or during an explosive detonation.

The G agents are moderately volatile and relatively nonpersistent; the most volatile, sarin, evaporates at almost exactly the same rate as does water. Although VX is minimally volatile, potentially lasting weeks or longer on contaminated surfaces, at temperatures above 100°F (37.8°C) it can cause significant inhalational toxicity. The time required for these agents to undergo aging varies from a few minutes for soman

to 48 hours for VX. The nerve agent vapors are all heavier than air and would thus affect persons closer to the ground (e.g., those in trenches and basements, and perhaps young children) disproportionately. Although all these agents are hazardous by ingestion, inhalation, and cutaneous absorption, the primary danger from the G agents is inhalation of vapor, whereas VX is primarily a skin contact hazard, except in hot environments or when it is explosively aerosolized.

Toxicology

Nerve agent–induced inhibition of acetylcholinesterase causes the neurotransmitter acetylcholine to accumulate in cholinergic synapses and in neuromuscular and neuroglandular junctions; this excess of acetylcholine initially causes end-organ stimulation that may then lead to end-organ failure. Cholinergic sites are found in the central nervous system (CNS), in the neuromuscular junctions of somatic nerves, and in several autonomic nervous system sites, including parasympathetic nerve endings, some sympathetic nerve endings (e.g., sweat glands), and both parasympathetic and sympathetic ganglia.

The cholinergic syndrome thus produced is classically divided into CNS, nicotinic (neuromuscular junction and sympathetic ganglia), and muscarinic (smooth muscle and exocrine gland) effects.

CNS effects include altered mental status progressing through lethargy to coma, ataxia, convulsions, and respiratory depression (central apnea). Although seizure initiation is initially largely a result of excess cholinergic stimulation of excitatory glutamate receptors, antagonism of inhibitory gamma-aminobutyric acid receptors may also play important roles in seizure propagation. Neuropathological changes observed in animal studies also suggest that prolonged seizure activity further disturbs excitatory amino acid and N-methyl-D-aspartate receptor function, ultimately leading to neuronal calcium influx and neuronal injury.

Nicotinic effects include muscle fasciculations and twitching, and then weakness progressing to flaccid paralysis. Nicotinic effects on sympathetic activity may also result in tachycardia, hypertension, and metabolic aberrations (e.g., hyperglycemia, hypokalemia, metabolic acidosis).

Muscarinic toxicity is manifested by (i) ocular findings (miosis, visual blurring, eye pain, lacrimation); (ii) respiratory findings (watery rhinorrhea, bronchospasm, increased bronchial secretions causing cough, wheezing, dyspnea); (iii) dermal findings (flushing, sweating, cyanosis); (iv) GI findings (salivation, nausea, vomiting, diarrhea progressing to fecal incontinence and abdominal cramps); (v) genitourinary findings (frequency, urgency, incontinence); and (vi) cardiovascular findings (bradycardia, hypotension, atrioventricular block). Because muscarinic effects on the heart are opposed by the cardiovascular effects of nicotinic hyperstimulation at autonomic ganglia, heart rate and blood pressure in nerve agent victims may be either elevated or depressed and are not reliable indicators of the severity of nerve agent intoxication.

Clinical Presentation

The clinical presentation in a given patient depends on dose and route of exposure. For vapor exposures, mild toxicity would be suggested by miosis, rhinorrhea, mild dyspnea, and wheezing—all local effects caused by contact of vapor with epithelial surfaces. As the dose increases, and systemic distribution of the agent occurs, the victim might experience increased respiratory secretions and dyspnea, nausea, vomiting, and muscle weakness. In the Tokyo experience with sarin vapor exposure, miosis (99%), dyspnea (63%), nausea (60%), and headache (74%) were particularly common among moderately symptomatic patients at hospital admission. In severe cases with exposure to high vapor concentrations, rapid onset of paralysis and seizures leading to death from respiratory arrest may occur within minutes. In the Tokyo sarin incident, 3 of 640 patients presented to one ED in cardiopulmonary arrest. One patient was unresponsive to resuscitation, 1 patient experienced severe hypoxic damage and died on hospital day 28, and 1 patient recovered fully.

With vapor inhalation, affected patients do not typically deteriorate once they are removed from the exposure. In contrast, with dermal exposure, symptoms may progress even after the agent is removed from the skin surface. Initial findings after a small dose might include localized sweating, followed by localized fasciculations of underlying muscle. Systemic effects from larger doses of liquid usually begin with GI signs and symptoms, and then progress to generalized fasciculations, muscle weakness, paralysis, convulsions, and death resulting from respiratory failure from CNS depression and respiratory muscle paralysis. Eye findings and obstructive respiratory effects tend to be less prominent in these patients, at least early in the course and with low doses. Because of the time (up to 18 hours for a small drop of VX) needed for liquid nerve agent to penetrate the skin, dermal exposures have a longer latency, and patients may not become symptomatic for several hours after exposure, even after decontamination. However, a pin head–size droplet (10 mg) of VX may cause sudden collapse with paralysis, apnea, and death after a latent interval of only 10 to 30 minutes.

Management

The diagnosis of nerve agent poisoning is primarily by clinical recognition and response to antidotal therapy. Routine toxicological studies do not identify organophosphorous compounds or their metabolites in blood or urine. Measurements of acetylcholinesterase in plasma or in erythrocytes have traditionally been used to confirm OP insecticide poisoning, and the activity of these enzymes is decreased after significant nerve agent toxicity as well. Erythrocyte acetylcholinesterase activity is a more accurate guide to acute toxicity, whereas measurements of plasma cholinesterase (pseudocholinesterase or butylcholinesterase) are more useful for monitoring patient recovery during the weeks after exposure. However, correlation between cholinesterase levels and clinical effects is poor in mild to moderate exposures, and the test is not widely available. Treatment for symptomatic patients is indicated without awaiting cholinesterase levels, but antidotal therapy is not needed for exposed asymptomatic patients, even if cholinesterase levels are depressed. These patients, however, should be carefully observed if there is any possibility of concomitant exposure to liquid nerve agent. The overall treatment approach for these agents focuses on airway and ventilatory support, aggressive use of antidotes, particularly atropine and pralidoxime chloride, prompt control of seizures, and the provision of decontamination as necessary (Table 7.4). Atropine is used for its antimuscarinic effects and pralidoxime serves to reactivate acetylcholinesterase. Atropine treats bronchospasm and increased bronchial secretions, bradycardia, GI effects of

nausea, vomiting, diarrhea, and cramps, and may lessen seizure activity. However, atropine will not improve skeletal muscle paralysis. Pralidoxime (2-PAM) cleaves organophosphate away from the cholinesterase and regenerates the intact enzyme if aging has not yet occurred. This effect is observed most at neuromuscular junctions, with improved muscle strength.

Both atropine and pralidoxime are administered IV in severe cases, although intraosseous access is likely equivalent to IV. However, animal data suggest that hypoxia should be corrected, if possible, prior to IV atropine use, to prevent arrhythmias; otherwise, IM use might be safer initially. Atropine is dosed initially at 0.05 mg per kg, with minimum dose 0.1 mg and maximum 5 mg; pralidoxime is dosed at 25 mg per kg, with maximum doses of 1 g IV or 2 g IM (Table 7.4). Atropine has also been administered by the endotracheal or inhalational route in some contexts, and such use (or that of ipratropium as an aerosol) might also have salutory effects.

Pediatric experience with OP pesticide poisoning suggests that the continuous infusion of pralidoxime may be optimal. However, the IM route is acceptable if IV access is not readily available. This might be quite relevant in a pediatric masscasualty incident. In fact, most U.S. EMS systems now stock military IM autoinjector kits of 2-mg atropine and 600-mg 2-PAM. Pediatric-size autoinjectors of atropine are now available in 0.25-, 0.5- and 1-mg doses. Of note, during the Gulf War, 240 Israeli children, none of whom were exposed to nerve agent, were evaluated for accidental autoinjection of atropine, as reported by Amatai et al. Systemic anticholinergic effects occurred in many of these patients, but seizures, severe dysrhythmias, and deaths were not observed.

Pediatric-size 2-PAM autoinjectors are not currently available in the United States. However, in dire circumstances, even the adult autoinjectors with 0.8-inch needle insertion lengths and 600-mg pralidoxime might find utility in children older than ages 2 to 3 years or who weigh more than 13 kg (suggested guidelines and weight-based dosing for children of all sizes are detailed in Table 7.4A and 7.4B). For infants, one might consider using the adult pralidoxime autoinjector as a convenient source of concentrated (300 mg per mL) pralidoxime solution suitable for IM injection. This can be effected by the discharge of one or several autoinjector's contents into an emptied 10-mL sterile saline vial (Fig. 7.7). The solution may then be withdrawn through a filter needle into one or several syringes suitable for small-volume IM injections, each of which are then capped with new needles appropriate for IM use. Finally, the routine administration of anticonvulsant doses of benzodiazepines is recommended in significant cases, even without observed convulsive activity, because animal studies have indicated some amelioration of subsequent seizures and morphologic brain damage with such use. Potential future advances in nerve agent treatment currently under investigation include the use of more effective bis-quaternary oximes, such as HI-6, fetal bovine serum acetylcholinesterase, scopolamine for anticholinergic effects (potentially better CNS penetration than atropine), and the use of ketamine as an adjunct to treat prolonged nerve agent–induced seizures.

Specific Pediatric Considerations

Little experience is available to comment on differences between pediatric and adult patients in the dose–response

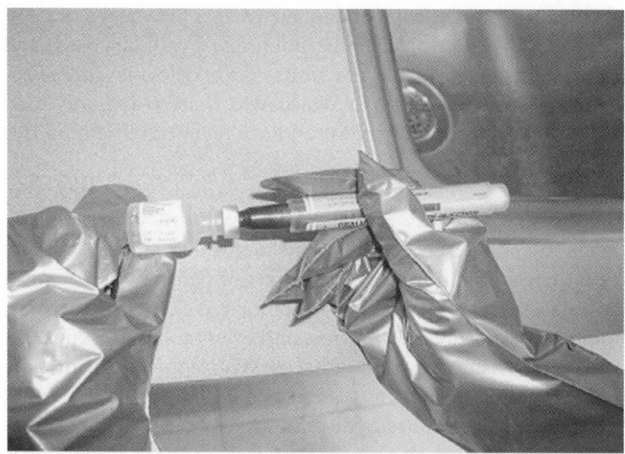

FIGURE 7.7 Autoinjector-packaged proalidoxime can be injected into an empty vial for subsequent reuse in small pediatric patients. (From Henretig FM, Mechem C, Jew R. Potential use of autoinjector-packaged antidotes for treatment of pediatric nerve agent toxicity. *Ann Emerg Med* 2002;40:405–408, with permission.)

curve or the toxic-effect spectrum with exposure to nerve agents, or in response to therapy. The thinner skin of children and greater surface area to mass ratio might make them more susceptible to dermal absorption on a mg per kg basis in comparison to adults. Likewise, the immature blood–brain barrier in infants might increase the relative risk of CNS toxicity. One case series of anticholinesterase pesticide poisoning in children found that depressed sensorium and muscle weakness/flaccidity were more prominent than muscarinic findings. Nevertheless, more than half of these patients did demonstrate miosis (80%), tearing and excess salivation (60%), and GI findings (52%). Also, severe OP pesticide poisoning in children may certainly manifest by dramatic muscarinic findings, including respiratory compromise, in many cases (see Chapter 102). It seems doubtful that the nerve agent toxidrome, and hence the appropriate management approach, would differ significantly in children from that in adults. Nevertheless, the clinician should be prepared for subtle and sometimes significant differences in children from the classic cholinergic toxidrome seen in adults.

Disposition and Prognosis

The disposition of exposed patients depends on severity of symptoms and route of exposure. Most patients presenting after vapor exposure manifest peak toxicity by the time of hospital arrival, and when their symptoms have either resolved or abated to only mild eye findings (miosis from exposure to nerve agent vapor may persist for up to 6 weeks), they may be discharged. After dermal exposure, symptom onset may lag up to 18 hours, even after thorough skin decontamination, and most experts recommend a 24-hour observation period even in initially asymptomatic victims.

The prognosis for apparently full recovery from even severe nerve agent poisoning appears to be good with timely life support interventions and adequate antidotal therapy. Apneic patients have recovered ventilatory function within 3 hours, and once consciousness was regained, muscle weakness and obtundation have resolved over a few days, whereas miosis and subtle mental status effects have persisted for several weeks. Nerve agents, unlike some pesticides, have not been implicated in delayed peripheral neuropathy, although some follow-up studies on survivors of the Tokyo sarin attack suggest a considerable incidence of neurocognitive and affective sequelae.

Vesicants

The major vesicants, or blistering agents, are cellular poisons and include the mustards (sulfur mustard and nitrogen mustards) and Lewisite. The mustards are believed to act primarily as alkylating agents, whereas Lewisite is an organic arsenical believed to affect the thiol groups in critical cellular enzymes. However, because little clinical experience with Lewisite exposure exists, this discussion focuses on mustard.

Mustard exists as an oily, yellow to dark brown liquid with a garlic or mustard odor. It has relatively low volatility and is considered persistent, although at high temperatures its vapor hazard is considerable. Mustard vapor, unlike most other chemical vapors, can penetrate skin and lead to early tissue damage and eventual blistering. This fact is the warrant for the exception of vesicants to the general rule that skin decontamination is not an immediate priority for vapor-exposed chemical casualties. An estimated 80% of mustard casualties during World War I were caused by mustard vapor exposure (although 80% of *fatalities* from chemical warfare agents were caused by pulmonary agents). The lethality of mustard to well-protected troops on the battlefield in World War I was less than 5%, but this agent would be far more deadly against unsuspecting and unprotected civilians; an amount as little as 1 teaspoon may kill a 70-kg adult.

Mustard forms a cyclic ethylsulfonium ion that is a potent alkylating agent causing injury to rapidly reproducing cells (its systemic effects are often described as radiomimetic), and its local effects are most evident on the skin, in the eyes, and in the respiratory tract. With severe exposures, the bone marrow, GI mucosa, and the CNS may also be damaged. Although mustard-induced cell injury begins within the first few minutes after exposure, clinical effects of mustard usually follow a latent period that is inversely related to dose but that is often 4 to 6 hours. Skin lesions after liquid contact begin with erythema, followed by blister formation, or if the dose is large enough, skin sloughing without blister formation (Fig. 7.8). The burns are usually partial thickness (second degree). Blister fluid does not contain active mustard and is not hazardous. Vapor exposure results in later, and usually milder, skin injury.

Ocular lesions from vapor include conjunctival inflammation, corneal damage, and often severe lid edema. Permanent blindness is a rare complication, but many patients presenting for treatment may be functionally blind because the pain and blepharospasm induced by mustard renders them unwilling to open their eyes. Vapor-induced pulmonary effects begin with upper respiratory tract irritation, and may progress through dyspnea and a productive cough to a severe necrotizing tracheobronchitis with pseudomembrane formation. Patients may succumb to secondary bacterial bronchopneumonia. Bone marrow damage may occur in severe cases on about the third to fifth days after exposure, and manifest as progressive pancytopenia. Low leukocyte counts (less than 500 per mm³), or a precipitous decreases in the leukocyte count, portend a

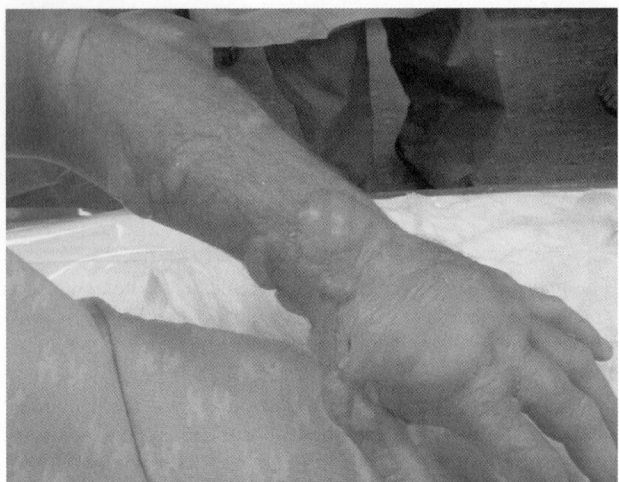

FIGURE 7.8 A patient with mustard-induced skin blisters. (From Greenberg MI. Greenberg's Text-Atlas of Emergency Medicine. Philadelphia: Lippincott Williams & Wilkins, 2005:968.)

serious risk of sepsis and death. An accident involving the explosion of a mustard-containing shell caused a heavy exposure to three children. These patients presented acutely with altered mental status and muscle activity, and two of them died 3 to 4 hours after exposure. A case series of Iranian children and adolescents exposed to mustard during the Iraq–Iran War found that compared with adults, the younger victims exhibited a shorter onset and more severe dermal lesions, attributable to the more delicate skin in this age group.

Because mustard penetrates tissue rapidly and binds to cellular components within the first two to five minutes, the most important early intervention is immediate (i.e., at the scene) decontamination as soon as possible after exposure. Skin and eye decontamination are accomplished similarly as discussed for nerve agents. Additional, or delayed, decontamination at the time of ED arrival may still be of value in preventing continuing absorption and thus systemic distribution in patients and secondary contamination of the patient and health-care workers, although it must again be pointed out that blister fluid from mustard casualties does not pose a contamination threat. No specific antidotes to mustard poisoning are available. Supportive care for skin lesions is analogous to that provided for burn injury, although fluid requirements are usually far less than with comparable body-surface-area thermal burns. Additional treatment of respiratory tract inflammation, ocular injury, and immunosuppression associated with leucopenia may be required (see Chapters 108, 98, 117, and 91, respectively). Research directions in management include the potential salutary effect of granulocyte colony-stimulating factor in the further treatment of mustard-induced leucopenia, and the use of oral *N*-acetylcysteine both as a potential prophylactic agent and for mitigating chronic pulmonary effects.

Pulmonary Agents

Toxic inhalant agents, including chlorine and phosgene, may cause injury in several ways, including simple asphyxia by displacing oxygen, topical damage to airways or alveoli, systemic absorption through the pulmonary capillary bed, and allergic hypersensitivity reactions. Both chlorine and phosgene were used in battle in World War I, are commonly used for industrial purposes today, and are reviewed briefly in this section.

Chlorine is considered a gas with relatively low to intermediate water solubility and chemical reactivity, whereas phosgene is considered to have low solubility and reactivity. Because the initial irritant symptoms of gas exposure tend to correlate directly with water solubility and chemical reactivity, low-dose exposures to chlorine, and even moderate exposures to phosgene, might cause either no symptoms at all or only mild irritation of eyes, nose, and upper airways during exposure. Victims could easily dismiss these effects, thus prolonging exposure and the severity of the ultimate lung injury. Chlorine lung injury is probably mediated by both hydrochloric acid generation in the upper airway and by free oxygen radical cascade at the alveolocapillary membranes in the lower airway.

Phosgene (carbonyl chloride) is also believed to generate hydrochloric acid, contributing particularly to upper airway, nasal, and conjunctival irritation at higher doses (as mentioned, lower but still potentially lethal doses may not give rise to any irritation at all) as well as a carbonyl group that participates in acylation reactions at the pulmonary alveolocapillary membranes; the resulting leaking of fluid across damaged membranes eventually leads, after an asymptomatic period, to pulmonary edema and acute lung injury. Phosgene lung injury may also be mediated in part by an inflammatory reaction associated with leukotriene production.

Chlorine is a dense, acrid yellow-green gas of intermediate solubility and intermediate chemical reactivity that tends to settle close to the ground. Initial effects after mild to moderate exposure include ocular and nasal irritation, followed by cough, and progressing to a choking sensation and substernal chest tightness. Bronchospasm often occurs, especially in patients with a history of reactive airway disease. Pulmonary edema may follow significant exposures within 2 to 4 hours. Severe exposures result in the rapid onset (within 30 to 60 minutes) of pulmonary edema, in addition to the initial irritation.

Mild to moderate exposures to phosgene may be initially asymptomatic, with only the perception of a pleasant odor of newly mown hay. Thus, lung exposure time may be significant before the victim removes himself from the affected area. Pulmonary edema occurs after a considerable delay, typically 4 to 6 hours, but with lower exposures as late as 24 hours after exposure. In these cases, dyspnea precedes objective clinical or radiologic findings. With higher exposures, early lacrimation may be followed by cough and dyspnea, and pulmonary edema, although still delayed, supervenes earlier than with a low-dose exposure. The pulmonary edema may be so severe as to result in hypotension from hypovolemia. The onset of dyspnea within the first 4 hours after exposure to phosgene portends the eventual development of massive pulmonary edema and a grave prognosis.

Management of exposure to pulmonary agents is primarily supportive (see Chapter 98). Decontamination is primarily removal to fresh air. Careful attention to control of pulmonary secretions, bronchospasm, and pulmonary edema, as well as to aggressive treatment of secondary bacterial infection (often occurring 3 to 5 days after exposure) is required. Animal studies suggest a modest benefit of steroid therapy in mitigating lung injury after chlorine inhalation, and thus steroids may be considered for patients with chlorine exposure, especially as an adjunct to bronchodilators in those manifesting bronchospasm and/or a history of asthma. In addition, some symptomatic relief has also been reported for chlorine exposure with nebulized 3.75% sodium bicarbonate therapy, but the impact of this regimen on pulmonary damage is unknown. Animal models have suggested a benefit of antiinflammatory agents, including ibuprofen and *N*-acetylcysteine, to ameliorate phosgene-induced pulmonary edema, as well as the utilization of low tidal volume ventilation (protective ventilation), but these interventions have not yet been reported in clinical trials.

Cyanide

Compounds containing the cyanide ion (CN^-) have a long history as favored agents for homicide and suicide, but their efficacy as chemical warfare agents is somewhat limited by their volatility in open air and, on the battlefield, by their flammability. However, if released nonexplosively in a crowded, closed room, they could have devastating effects. Chemical agents containing cyanide include the liquids hydrocyanic acid (hydrogen cyanide, HCN) and cyanogen chloride (ClCN), both of which rapidly vaporize after release.

ClCN may cause some initial eye, nose, and airway irritation from its chlorine moiety, but its systemic effects are the same as those of HCN and result from toxicity of its cyanide anion. Hydrogen cyanide dissociates only minimally to hydrogen ions and cyanide, but the intact molecule (HCN) appears to act by the same mechanism as the cyanide anion itself.

Toxicology

Some cyanide is normally present in human tissues and several pathways exist for its metabolism. Cyanide reacts reversibly with metals such as ferric ion (Fe^{3+}) and cobalt; in the body, the reaction of hydroxocobalamin with cyanide yields cyanocobalamin, or vitamin B_{12}. Cyanide also reacts with sulfur-containing compounds. Recent evidence also supports a significant interaction of cyanide with endogenous nitric oxide (NO). The enzyme rhodanese detoxifies cyanide by catalyzing its reaction with a sulfur donor to form the relatively nontoxic thiocyanate and sulfite ions, which are then renally excreted. The ability of the body to metabolize small quantities of cyanide, given sufficient time, accounts for the dependence of cyanide toxicity on conditions of concentration and exposure time. The same amount of cyanide that will kill when given over a few minutes may be successfully metabolized by the body if administered over several hours.

Doses of cyanide large enough to overwhelm normal metabolism inhibit electron transport at the cytochrome-aa_3 complex (cytochrome oxidase) of the mitochondrial cytochrome chain. The inactivation of this enzyme site, critical to aerobic adenosine triphosphate production, results in cellular anoxia and a decreased arteriovenous oxygen difference (from inability of cells to use delivered oxygen), metabolic acidosis (from accumulation of hydrogen ions not incorporated with oxygen) and increased lactic acid (from the failure to generate energy aerobically).

Clinical Manifestations

Clinical manifestations of cyanide poisoning relate to cellular anoxia; thus, those organs that are metabolically most active, particularly the brain and heart, are most severely affected. The carotid body chemoreceptors, which receive the highest relative blood flow and oxygen delivery of any tissue in the body, are rapidly stimulated by the presence of high concentrations of cyanide, and mediate a pronounced gasping reflex, which increases rate and depth of respiration. They also indirectly stimulate the adrenal medulla to release epinephrine, with resulting initial tachycardia and hypertension. Thus, high concentrations of cyanide vapor initially produce tachypnea, hyperpnea, and hypertension within 10 to 15 seconds. Anoxic injury to the CNS and myocardium soon follow, with unconsciousness and seizures (30 seconds after exposure), opisthotonus, trismus, decerebrate posturing, bradycardia, arrhythmias, hypotension, and eventually cardiac arrest (as soon as 4 to 8 minutes after exposure).

Exposure to low concentrations of vapor produces nonspecific effects such as headache, light-headedness, nausea, and ataxia. "Classic" signs of cyanide poisoning are said to include severe dyspnea without cyanosis, or even cherry-red skin (because of lack of peripheral oxygen use), and a bitter almond odor to breath and body fluids. However, some cyanide-poisoned patients develop cyanosis, and only about half the population is genetically capable of detecting the cyanide odor. Noteworthy laboratory abnormalities in cyanide poisoning include an abnormally high mixed venous oxygen saturation with resultant decreased arteriovenous oxygen content difference (one of the most useful laboratory indicators of cyanide poisoning), high-anion-gap metabolic acidosis, and increased blood lactate.

Sidell has emphasized that in a chemical attack the observation that people are convulsing or dying within minutes of exposure implies that the weapon is either cyanide or a nerve agent. With high concentrations of cyanide, seizures begin within seconds and death ensues within minutes, often with little cyanosis or other findings. Exposure to lethal concentrations of a nerve-agent liquid or vapor may also lead to sudden collapse with preterminal apnea and convulsions. Cyanosis in such cases tends to be more common than in cyanide casualties. Miosis and increased nasoocular secretions indicate exposure to nerve agent vapor rather than to cyanide but could be absent in a victim exposed only to lower doses of nerve-agent liquid.

Management

Management of cyanide poisoning begins with removal to fresh air. Dermal decontamination is unnecessary if exposure has been only to vapor, but wet clothing should be removed and the underlying skin should be washed with soap and water, or with water alone if liquid on the skin is a possibility. Attention to the basics of intensive supportive care is critical and includes (i) provision of 100% oxygen to all significantly symptomatic patients (regardless of arterial Po_2), (ii) mechanical ventilation as needed, (iii) circulatory support with crystalloid and vasopressors, (iv) correction of metabolic acidosis with IV sodium bicarbonate, and (v) seizure control with benzodiazepine administration. The cyanide-induced inhibition of cellular oxygen use might lead to the expectation that supplemental oxygen would not be of use in cyanide poisoning, but in fact, administration of 100% oxygen has been found to empirically exert a beneficial effect, possibly by directly displacing cyanide from cytochrome oxidase-binding sites.

Symptomatic patients, especially those with severe manifestations, may further benefit from specific antidotal therapy. Currently, two regimens are available in the United States, and many hospitals are now considering the stocking of one system or the other; thus, both are described here in some detail.

The older cyanide antidote approach utilized a two-step process. First, a methemoglobin-forming agent such as amyl nitrite or sodium nitrite is administered. The ferric ion (Fe^{3+}) in methemoglobin has an even higher affinity for cyanide than does cytochrome aa_3. The equilibrium of this reaction causes dissociation of bound cyanide from the cytochrome oxidase and restores aerobic energy production. Nitrites may also have therapeutic efficacy independent of methemoglobin formation, possibly via conversion to NO with subsequent beneficial vasodilatory effects. However, nitrite administration is potentially hazardous because too rapid IV infusion may cause or exacerbate hypotension, and overproduction of methemoglobin may compromise oxygen-carrying capacity. Thus, nitrite is probably not indicated for conscious patients with minimal symptoms and is relatively contraindicated in patients whose cyanide toxicity is complicated by existing impaired oxygen delivery (e.g., smoke inhalation victims from a house fire, with likely concomitant lung injury and carbon monoxide poisoning).

These potential adverse effects of nitrites would obviously be less compelling in the context of a severely intoxicated, prostrate casualty of a terrorist cyanide vapor attack, and careful attention to proper dosing and rate of administration should allow safe use of this antidote. Pediatric nitrite dosing depends on body weight and hemoglobin concentration. The recommended initial pediatric dosage, assuming hemoglobin concentration of 12 g per dL, is 0.33 mL per kg of the standard 3% sodium nitrite solution, given slowly IV over 5 to 10 minutes; the initial adult dosage is 10 mL. Dosing may be adjusted for patients with significant anemia, although this knowledge would rarely be available in the context of emergent treatment of a critically poisoned child. The second step is provision of a sulfur donor, typically sodium thiosulfate, which is used as a substrate by rhodanese for its conversion of cyanide to thiocyanate. Thiosulfate itself is efficacious, relatively benign, and also synergistic with oxygen administration, and thus may be used without nitrites in situations such as smoke inhalation. The initial thiosulfate dose for children is 1.65 mL per kg of the standard 25% solution IV, and the initial adult dose is 50 mL. Second treatments with one half the initial dose of nitrite and thiosulfate may be given 30 minutes after the original dose if needed in severe cases.

The newer antidote available in the United States is hydroxocobalamin. This compound is the hydroxy form of cobalamin, and in the presence of cyanide exchanges its hydroxy group for cyanide, forming cyanocobalamin (vitamin B_{12}), which is subsequently excreted by the kidneys. Its use is not complicated by the potential for nitrite-induced hypotension or methemoglobinemia, and has a low order of toxicity. Thus, hydroxocobalamin may be especially suited for use in the prehospital and ED management of a mass-casualty incident with cyanide. The recommended initial dose is 5 g in adults or 70 mg per kg in children, administered IV over 15 minutes. A second dose (2.5 to 5 g in adults, 35 to 70 mg per kg in children) may be repeated in severely affected patients, with the second infusion rate ranging from 15 minutes to 2 hours based on patient condition. Hypertension is a predictable side effect of hydroxocobalamin administration. The medication is dark red in color, and treatment does result in reddening of skin and mucous membranes and red-colored urine that may last several days. This phenomenon may also skew some common laboratory results that are based on colorimetric tests, such as creatinine, bilirubin, and hepatic transaminases, as well as co-oximetry results. Although no human controlled trials are available to compare hydroxocobalamin to nitrite/thiosulfate-based therapies, many authorities currently feel that hydroxocobalamin's efficacy and safety profile favor it as the cyanide antidote of choice, especially for children in the mass-casualty context.

The combined use of hydroxocobalamin and thiosulfate in severe cases might provide synergistic effects and still avoid the potential hazards of nitrite therapy. Lastly, newer compounds with oral availability are under investigation, and include cobinamide, a cobalamin precursor with high cyanide affinity, and analogs of 3-methylpyruvate, which like thiosulfate enhance conversion of cyanide to thiocyanate.

Because clinical distinction between cyanide and nerve-agent casualties may be difficult, any patient thought to have been exposed either to cyanide or to a nerve agent but who does not respond to antidotal therapy specific for the suspected agent should be given a trial of the antidotes for the other agent.

Riot Control Agents

Riot control agents, also called lacrimators ("tear gas," although they are actually aerosols rather than gases), include several compounds, the most important of which are CS (*o*-chlorobenzylidene malononitrile), CN [1-chloroacetophenone, "Mace" (although Mace is also often used to refer to pepper spray)], and pepper spray (containing capsaicin). CS and CN are solids and are typically dispersed as an aerosol of fine particles. Although the United States does not consider riot control agents to be official chemical warfare weapons, these agents are widely available, cause significant incapacitating effects in closed spaces, and could conceivably be used in a terrorist attack; therefore, they are outlined briefly in this section.

Their mechanism of action after low-level exposure is unclear but, in the case of pepper spray, appears to be related to the release of the pain-modulating neurotransmitter substance P. All these agents can cause (i) transient ocular effects, including burning sensation, tearing, blepharospasm, and photophobia; (ii) irritation of the nose, throat, and upper airway; and (iii) skin burning, erythema, and (at high concentrations and high ambient temperatures and humidity) vesication. A few riot control agents, such as Adamsite (DM), cause pronounced vomiting in addition to delayed-onset irritation of the eyes and the upper airway, and are referred to as vomiting agents. Most victims under usual circumstances of exposure become symptomatic within seconds from the traditional lacrimating agents (irritation after exposure to DM may take up to 20 minutes to develop) but remain so for only 20 to 60 minutes.

However, high concentrations in closed spaces or discharge of agent close to the victim's face have been associated with serious medical complications, including severe ocular toxicity, dermal burns, and pulmonary failure. A few lethal cases have been described in which death was caused by severe tracheobronchitis with pseudomembrane formation and pulmonary edema.

Management includes careful ocular and dermal decontamination. The skin should be washed with soap and water, although this may cause transient increased pain. Hypochlorite solution should not be used because it may exacerbate dermal burns via the creation of toxic by-products. The eyes should be thoroughly lavaged after a single dose of topical anesthetic if necessary. Respiratory complications must be managed supportively, as previously described for mustard and pulmonary agent toxicity. Severe respiratory effects may not manifest for 12 to 24 hours; therefore, patients with dyspnea or any objective findings should probably be observed in the hospital. Severe respiratory complications from exposure to riot control agents have been described in at least two young infants, one of whom was in a house into which CS was sprayed. A canister of pepper spray was accidentally discharged directly into the face of the other infant. Both survived with prolonged care, the latter requiring ventilatory support, including five days of extracorporeal membrane oxygenation. A few cases of children ingesting CS powder are known, which resulted only in transient diarrhea and abdominal cramping.

Miscellaneous Chemicals

The potential of a terrorist attack on industrial sources of dangerous chemicals such as factories, railroad and vehicular tank cars, or storage depots expands the list of potential "chemical weapons" considerably. In addition, the development of potent incapacitating agents, such as fentanyl derivatives, by law enforcement or military agencies for use in combating terrorist incidents, might unfortunately lead to mass casualties requiring medical treatment, as occurred in the October 2002 theater hostage incident in Moscow. Further, the advent of such agents may allow them to fall into terrorist hands for use as an offensive weapon. A full discussion of all such possible chemical injuries and their management is obviously beyond the scope of this discussion. In general, many of the relevant industrial chemicals (e.g., methyl isocyanate, ammonia, nitrogen dioxide, sulfur oxides) might be expected to induce respiratory effects analogous to those of chlorine or phosgene discussed previously; others (e.g., strong acids or alkalies, hydrogen fluoride, formaldehyde, acrolein) could cause dermatologic injury from irritant or caustic properties, as well as more systemic effects in severe exposures (Table 7.5). Fentanyl derivatives can be lethal from suppression of the respiratory center in the medulla of the brain. Some of the principles in managing such toxic injuries are discussed in Chapter 102, and further information is available from standard reference toxicology texts and by consultation with the regional poison control center (1-800-222-1222).

EMERGENCY DEPARTMENT PREPAREDNESS

The ED response to WMD incidents will need to be integrated into the hospital's standing disaster plan. Appropriate protocols for notifying additional personnel, using hospital security for patient direction and diversion at the ED entrance and around the decontamination site, and handling the dissemination of information to the public and news media should be anticipated. Hospital spaces that are not routinely used for patient care, such as cafeterias, may be used as holding areas for large numbers of exposed but minimally symptomatic patients. Routine hospital supplies such as gowns and towels may be depleted rapidly in the face of mass casualties. Demands for hospital beds, and particularly intensive care unit beds, are likely to be overwhelming. Alternative care facilities staffed by outside help may be needed in mass-casualty situations (e.g., warehouses or other such buildings might need to be converted to temporary care sites). Predisaster planning for both "natural" disasters and WMD incidents must take into account such factors. A framework exists for activating medical assistance plans at the federal level through the National Response Framework and the National Disaster Medical System, augmented if necessary by military medical assets from the Department of Defense.

The issue of stocking-specific antidotes, medications, and vaccines in the context of planning for a WMD event involving the potential for mass casualties poses additional challenges. Many hospitals do not routinely stock adequate amounts of such pharmaceuticals for even one critical patient. WMD incident planning should establish some mechanism for local or regional stockpiling of these critical medications and/or a means to rapidly acquire them. Table 7.6 offers an attempt to quantify the amount of antidotal medications that might be needed in one ED for the management of a nerve agent or cyanide attack involving both pediatric and adult victims on a scale of the Tokyo sarin attack. A biological agent attack would place similar enormous demands on the hospital pharmacy for antibiotics, vaccines, antitoxins, and so on. A federal system for stockpiling pharmaceuticals and emergency medical supplies, managed through the CDC, has been created to augment local resources in this critical logistical arena. The first large-scale deployment of this Strategic National Stockpile occurred in the hours following the September 11, 2001 attacks on New York and Washington, DC. However, because prompt treatment is crucial in chemical emergencies, national stockpiles should be viewed as a resupply source and do not obviate the need for each hospital to develop its own stockpile of antidotes that might be needed during the first few hours after such a mass-casualty incident.

Obviously, many unanswered questions remain regarding ED preparedness for a biological- or chemical-agent attack, including (i) optimal decontamination techniques, especially for young children; (ii) optimal PPE for ED staff; (iii) logistics of patient and hospital staff flow, and isolation, in the context of a potentially lethal, contagious disease (e.g., smallpox,

TABLE 7.5

REPRESENTATIVE CLASSES OF INDUSTRIAL CHEMICALS—SUMMARY OF PEDIATRIC
MANAGEMENT CONSIDERATIONS

Agent	Clinical findings	Onset	Decontamination	Management
Strong acids/ bases	Eye—caustic injury Skin—chemical burns GI—chemical burns of mouth, larynx, esophagus, stomach	Rapid	GI: defer, immediate ED referral Ocular, skin: immediate copious water irrigation	Supportive care, early endoscopy for significant ingestion; antibiotics and steroids controversial, should be individualized, consult PCC
Respiratory tract irritants (e.g., ammonia, HCl and HF gases)	ENT and respiratory tract irritation with cough, chest pain, dyspnea, wheeze (possible pulmonary edema in severe cases)	Rapid	Move to fresh air	Supportive respiratory care (consider nebulized calcium gluconate solution for HF, consult PCC)
Fentanyl and other opioids	CNS and respiratory depression, miosis	Rapid	Move to fresh air (for aerosol exposure): consider AC for ingestion, consult PCC	Supportive care, naloxone 0.01–0.1 mg/kg
Cellular asphyxiants: Phosphine, sodium azide	Cough, dyspnea, headache, dizziness, vomiting, tachycardia, hypotension, severe metabolic acidosis, may progress to coma, seizures, death; may have delayed onset pulmonary edema with phosphine	Rapid (except pulmonary edema with phosphine)	Move to fresh air (consider AC for ingested sodium azide—caution with vomitus, which may emit toxic hydrazoic acid fumes: consult PCC)	ABCs, 100% oxygen
Arsine	Severe hemolysis	2–4 h	Move to fresh air	Supportive care, enhance urine flow, consider alkalinization, consult PCC

GI, gastrointestinal; ED, emergency department; PCC, poison control center (1-800-222-1222); HCl, hydrogen chloride; HF, hydrogen fluoride; EENT, eye, ear, nose, and throat; CNS, central nervous system; AC, activated charcoal 1 g/kg p.o. or n.g.; ABCs, airway, breathing and circulatory support.

TABLE 7.6

PHARMACEUTICAL STOCKING ESTIMATES FOR ONE EMERGENCY DEPARTMENT IN A HYPOTHETICAL
CHEMICAL AGENT ATTACK[a]

Agent/antidote	Pediatric dose	Adult dose	Total requirement (for 500 patients)
Nerve Agents			
Atropine	0.02–0.05 mg/kg (minimum dose, 0.1 mg)	2–5 mg	6,875 mg = 17,188 amps (1 mL of 0.4 mg/mL); 859 vials (20 mL of 0.4 mg/mL)
Pralidoxime	25–50 mg/kg	1–2 g	1,875 g = 1,875 vials (1 g each)
Cyanide			
Na nitrite (3%)	0.33 mL/kg (for Hgb 12 g/dL)	10 mL	4575 mL
Na thiosulfate (25%)	1.65 mL/kg	50 mL	25,000 mL = 500 vials (50 mL each)
Hydoxocobalamin	70 mg/kg	5 g	2138 g

Note: Cyanide treatment would require either 375 nitrite/thiosulfate-based or 428 hydroxcobalamin-based cyanide antidote kits.
Na, sodium; Hgb, hemoglobin.
[a]Assumptions: 500 patients to one emergency department (as per one hospital's experience in the Tokyo sarin attack); one-half the patients are children with average weight of 10 kg; if nerve agent attack, severe exposure necessitating maximal doses of atropine and pralidoxime; five atropine doses over 12 h; three pralidoxime doses over 12 h; if cyanide attack, severe exposure necessitating initial full dose of Na nitrite/Na thiosulfate, or hydoxocobal-amin, followed by 50% of initial dose × 1.

plague, viral hemorrhagic fevers); (iv) safety of decontamination water runoff into public drainage systems; (v) the communitywide needs for education and training; and (vi) financial considerations for individual hospital and regional planners. Continued activity on an expert consensus basis, as well as new research, should help to address many of these issues.

CONCLUSION

The prospect of a mass-casualty incident from the terrorist use of biological or chemical agents is unfortunately more likely now than ever before. Although the impact of such an event is almost unimaginable, at the same time, efforts must be made to prepare for the "unthinkable." Such preparedness requires highly coordinated responses involving local and regional EMS systems, HAZMAT (hazardous materials) teams, police and fire departments, hospital EDs, local and federal public health agencies, and military medical specialists. In particular, EDs must consider important issues, including (i) the early recognition, triage, decontamination, treatment, and disposition of multiple casualties of such an attack; (ii) protection of health-care workers and existing patients; and (iii) the integrity of the ED itself to provide ongoing care to later-arriving casualties and to continue to meet normal patient demands. Fortunately, in 2009, our pediatric emergency care providers, academic medical centers, regional health departments, and several federal agencies, including the U.S. Departments of Health and Human Services, Homeland Security, and Defense, are actively engaged in confronting these vital public health and national security challenges.

Suggested Readings

General

American Academy of Pediatrics. Chemical-biological terrorism and its impact on children. *Pediatrics* 2005;118:1267–1278.

Centers for Disease Control and Prevention. Biological and chemical terrorism: strategic plan for preparedness and response. *MMWR Morb Mortal Wkly Rep* 2000;49(RR-4):114.

Eitzen EM Jr. Education is the key to defense against bioterrorism. *Ann Emerg Med* 1999;34:221–223.

Henretig F. Biological and chemical terrorism defense: a view from the "front lines" of public health. *Am J Public Health* 2001;91:718–720.

Henretig FM, Cieslak TJ, Eitzen EM Jr. Biological and chemical terrorism. *J Pediatr* 2002;141:311–326.

Henretig FM, McKee MR. Preparedness for acts of nuclear, biological and chemical terrorism. In: Gausche Hill M, Fuchs S, Yamamoto L, eds. *APLS: the pediatric emergency medicine resource.* American Academy of Pediatrics and American College of Emergency Physicians. Sudbury, MA: Jones and Bartlett, 2004:568–591.

Macintyre AG, Christopher GW, Eitzen E Jr, et al. Weapons of mass destruction events with contaminated casualties: effective planning for health care facilities. *JAMA* 2000;283:242–249.

Scarfone RJ, Alexander S, Coffin SE, et al. Emergency preparedness for pandemic influenza. *Pediatr Emerg Care* 2006;22(9):661–669.

Sidell FR. Nerve agents. In: Sidell FR, Takafuji ET, Franz DR, eds. *Textbook of military medicine. Part 1: medical aspects of chemical and biological warfare.* Washington, DC: Office of the Surgeon General, Walter Reed Army Medical Center, 1997:129–179.

Biological Terrorism

Arnon SS, Schechter R, Inglesby TV, et al. Botulinum toxin as a biological weapon: medical and public health management. *JAMA* 2001;285:1059–1070.

Borio L, Inglesby T, Peters CJ, et al. Hemorrhagic fever viruses as biological weapons: medical and public health management. *JAMA* 2002;287:2391–2405.

Breman JG, Henderson DA. Diagnosis and treatment of smallpox. *N Engl J Med* 2002;346:1300–1308.

Christopher GW, Cieslak TJ, Pavlin JA, et al. Biological warfare: a historical perspective. *JAMA* 1997;278:412–417.

Dennis DT, Inglesby TV, Henderson DA, et al. Tularemia as a biological weapon: medical and public health management. *JAMA* 2001;285:2763–2773.

Fine AM, Wong JB, Fraser HSF, et al. Is it influenza or anthrax? A decision analytic approach to the treatment of patients with influenza-like illness. *Ann Emerg Med* 2004;43:318–328.

Freedman A, Afonja O, Chang MW, et al. Cutaneous anthrax associated with microangiopathic hemolytic anemia and coagulopathy in a 7-month-old infant. *JAMA* 2002;287:869–874.

Henderson DA, Inglesby TV, Bartlett JG, et al. Smallpox as a biological weapon: medical and public health management. *JAMA* 1999;281:2127–2137.

Henretig FM, Cieslak TJ, Kortepeter MG, et al. Medical management of the suspected victim of bioterrorism: an algorithmic approach to the undifferentiated patient. *Emerg Med Clin North Am* 2002;20:351–364.

Inglesby TV, Dennis DT, Henderson DA, et al. Plague as a biological weapon: medical and public health management. *JAMA* 2000;283:2281–2290.

Inglesby TV, O'Toole T, Henderson DA, et al. Anthrax as a biological weapon, 2002: updated recommendations for management. *JAMA* 2002;287:236–2252.

Madsen JM. Toxins as weapons of mass destruction: a comparison and contrast with biological-warfare and chemical-warfare agents. *Clin Lab Med* 2001;21:593–605.

Madsen JM. Military personnel Part II—biologic threats. In: Greenberg M, Hamilton R, Phillips S, McCluskey GJ (eds). *Occupational, Industrial, and Environmental Toxicology*, 2nd edition. Philadelphia: Mosby, 2003, pp. 244-257.

Madsen, JM. Biological warfare and terrorism: toxins and other mid-spectrum Agents. In: Wexler P (editor-in-chief). *Encyclopedia of toxicology.* Vol 1–4. Oxford: Elsevier, 2005:273–279.

Torok TJ, Tauxe RF, Wise RP, et al. A large community outbreak of salmonellosis caused by intentional contamination of restaurant salad bars. *JAMA* 1997;278:389–395.

U.S. Army Medical Research Institute of Infectious Diseases. *Medical management of biological casualties—handbook.* Ft. Detrick, MD: U.S. Army Medical Research Institute of Infectious Diseases, 1998.

White S, Henretig F, Dukes R. Vulnerable populations in the setting of bioterrorism. *Emerg Med Clin North Am* 2002;20:365–392.

Chemical Terrorism

Amitai Y, Almog S, Singer R, et al. Atropine poisoning in children during the Persian Gulf crisis. A national survey in Israel. *JAMA* 1992;268:630–632.

Billmore DF, Vinocur C, Ginda M, et al. Pepper-spray-induced respiratory failure treated with extracorporeal membrane oxygenation. *Pediatrics* 1996;98:961–963.

Brennan RJ, Waeckerle JF, Sharp T, et al. Chemical warfare agents: emergency medical and emergency public health issues. *Ann Emerg Med* 1999;34:191–204.

Burklow TR, Yu CE, Madsen JM. Industrial chemicals: terrorist weapons of opportunity. *Pediatr Ann* 2003;32:230–234.

Davis KG, Aspera G. Exposure to liquid sulfur mustard. *Ann Emerg Med* 2001;37:653–656.

Douidar SM. Nebulized sodium bicarbonate in acute chlorine inhalation. *Pediatr Emerg Care* 1997;13:406–407.

Hall AH, Dart R, Bogdan G. Sodium thiosulfate or hydroxocobalamin for the empiric treatment of cyanide poisoning? *Ann Emerg Med* 2007;49:806–813.

Henretig FM, Mechem C, Jew R. Potential use of autoinjector-packaged antidotes for treatment of pediatric nerve agent toxicity. *Ann Emerg Med* 2002;40:405–408.

Holstege CP, Kirk M, Sidell FR. Chemical warfare: nerve agent poisoning. *Crit Care Clin* 1997;13:923–942.

Kales SN, Christiani DC. Acute chemical emergencies. *N Engl J Med* 2004;350:800–808.

Kerns W II, Beuhler M, Tomaszewski C. Hydroxocobalamin versus thiosulfate for cyanide poisoning. *Ann Emerg Med* 2008;51:338–339.

Kozer E, Mordel A, Bar Haim S, et al. Pediatric poisoning from trimedoxime (TMB4) and atropine automatic injectors. *J Pediatr* 2005;146:41–44.

Lee EC. Clinical manifestations of sarin nerve gas exposure. *JAMA* 2003;290:659–662.

Momeni AZ, Aminjavheri M. Skin manifestations of mustard gas in a group of 14 children and teenagers: a clinical study. *Int J Dermatol* 1994;33:184–187.

Occupational Safety and Health Administration. OSHA best practices for hospital-based first receivers of victims from mass casualty incidents involving the release of hazardous substances. Available at: http://www.osha.gov/dts/osta/bestpractices/html/hospital_firstreceivers.html.

Okumura T, Suzuki K, Fukuda A, et al. The Tokyo subway sarin attack: disaster management. Part 2: hospital response. *Acad Emerg Med* 1998;5: 618–624.

Okumura T, Takasu N, Ishimatsu S, et al. Report on 640 victims of the Tokyo subway sarin attack. *Ann Emerg Med* 1996;28:129–135.

Platoff GE, Baskin SI, Madsen JM. Military personnel Part III—chemical threats. In: Greenberg M, Hamilton R, Phillips S, et al. (eds). *Occupational, industrial, and environmental toxicology*. 2nd ed. Philadelphia: Mosby, 2003:258–273.

Rotenberg JS, Newmark J. Nerve agent attacks on children: diagnosis and management. *Pediatrics* 2003;112:648–658.

Russell D, Blaine PG, Rice P. Clinical management of casualties exposed to lung damaging agents: a critical review. *Emerg Med J* 2006;23:421–424.

Sauer SW, Keim ME. Hydroxocobalamin: improved public health readiness for cyanide disasters. *Ann Emerg Med* 2001;37:635–641.

Scarfone RJ, Henretig FH, Sullivan FJ. Decontamination and the use of personal protective equipment. *Pediatr Emerg Care* 2006;22(6):445–453.

Sofer S, Tal A, Shahak E. Carbamate and organophosphate poisoning in early childhood. *Pediatr Emerg Care* 1989;5:222–225.

U.S. Army Medical Research Institute of Chemical Defense. *Medical management of chemical casualties—handbook*. Aberdeen Proving Grounds, MD: U.S. Army Medical Research Institute of Chemical Defense, 1999.

Vinsel PJ. Treatment of acute chlorine gas inhalation with nebulized sodium bicarbonate. *J Emerg Med* 1990;8:327–329.

Wax PM, Becker CE, Curry SC. Unexpected "gas" casualties in Moscow: a medical toxicology perspective. *Ann Emerg Med* 2003;41:700–705.

CHAPTER 8 ■ ABDOMINAL DISTENSION

JEFFREY R. AVNER, MD, FAAP

Abdominal distension is generally defined as an increase in the breadth of the abdominal cavity. Often, the distension is large and thus easily noticeable to the child or parent. However, subtle increases in abdominal girth may be first appreciated by the child's sensation of abdominal pressure, fullness, or bloating. In general, abdominal distension is often due to an increase in intraabdominal volume by air, fluid, stool, mass, or organomegaly. Nevertheless, care should be taken not to confuse true abdominal distension with certain conditions that cause an *apparent* increase in abdominal girth such as poor posture, the natural exaggerated lordosis of childhood, abdominal wall weakness, obesity, and pulmonary hyperinflation. Examination of the patient in both the supine and upright positions assists the clinician in recognizing these factors before considering diagnoses that truly increase the volume of the abdominal cavity.

Abdominal distension is a nonspecific sign. That is, the causes of abdominal distension are numerous (Table 8.1). Even when the discussion is limited to the more common causes (Table 8.2) or emergent and urgent causes of abdominal distension (Table 8.3), the list is long. When confronted with a patient with abdominal distension, one approach is to divide the causes into the following generic categories: distended bowel, extraluminal gas (e.g., free air), extraluminal fluid, massive hepatomegaly, massive splenomegaly, and other causes. This categorization is more easily described on paper than discerned at the bedside. A large cystic mass can be easily mistaken for ascitic fluid. A Wilms' tumor may feel much like splenomegaly. Another difficulty in the clinical application of this categorization is that many pathologic processes that lead to abdominal distension do so through several of the previously mentioned categories. For example, kwashiorkor causes abdominal distension secondary to hepatosplenomegaly and ascites. For these reasons, the reader is urged to regard this initial categorization, when used at the bedside, as tentative, pending confirmation from plain radiograph, ultrasound, computed tomography (CT), or other imaging studies.

DIFFERENTIAL DIAGNOSIS

Bowel distension occurs secondary to mechanical or functional intestinal obstruction, aerophagia, malabsorption, or obstipation. Mechanical obstruction most commonly occurs in infants secondary to congenital malformations (atresia, volvulus, Hirschsprung's disease), incarcerated hernia, duplication cysts, or intussusception. At any age, a history of previous abdominal surgery usually suggests intraabdominal adhe-sions as the cause of intestinal obstruction. The amount of bowel distension is often related to the level of obstruction. The more distal the obstruction, the more proximal is the bowel distension to the obstruction. After many hours, most of the gas distal to the obstruction is passed, leaving an airless segment distally. Therefore, the lack of air in the rectum and sigmoid colon on a prone cross-table lateral radiograph of the abdomen supports the diagnosis of mechanical obstruction. Functional obstruction, or paralytic ileus, is suggested by tympanitic abdominal distension with the absence of bowel sounds. In general, all parts of the gastrointestinal (GI) tract are dilated, but the colon is usually more distended than the small intestine. Paralytic ileus may occur secondary to numerous causes. Signs such as involuntary guarding and pain with movement suggest peritoneal irritation secondary to infection, pancreatic enzymes, bile, or blood. Fever without peritoneal signs suggests intestinal inflammation, gastroenteritis, systemic infection, or anticholinergic poisoning (see Chapters 92 and 102). Various poisonings (atropinics), toxins (botulism), antimotility drugs (loperamide), and metabolic abnormalities (hypokalemia, hypercalcemia, uremia, acidosis) may also result in an ileus. These will most likely occur in the patient who has no abdominal findings other than tympanitic abdominal distension. In these cases, the abdomen is usually nontender. Toxic megacolon, an extensive dilatation of the colon, is a potentially fatal complication of severe colitis. This condition is usually seen with ulcerative colitis but may accompany Crohn's disease or antibiotic-related pseudomembranous colitis. Children with toxic megacolon have abdominal distension along with diarrhea, pain, fever, dehydration, and possibly sepsis. It is important to note that some conditions such as sepsis and peritonitis may cause a combination of functional and mechanical obstruction. Finally, gastric dilatation may result from several causes, including localized paralytic ileus (due to gastroenteritis or a pulmonic process), aerophagia, and iatrogenic reasons (bag-valve-mask respirations or esophageal intubation). The resulting gastric distension is an extremely important entity that may result in significant respiratory embarrassment secondary to upward pressure on the diaphragm unless decompressed through a nasogastric tube or other means.

Bulky, foul-smelling, or diarrheal stools suggest malabsorption secondary to many causes, which may include formula enteropathies, bacterial overgrowth, parasites, and cystic fibrosis (see Chapters 89 and 92). In lactose intolerance, bacterial metabolism of unabsorbed lactose produces intestinal gas causing abdominal distension, cramping, flatulence, and diarrhea. The severity of the symptoms is related primarily to

TABLE 8.1

DIFFERENTIAL DIAGNOSIS OF ABDOMINAL DISTENSION

Spurious
Poor posture
Obesity
Pulmonary hyperinflation
Lordotic posture of childhood
Abdominal muscle weakness/
  hypotonia

Bowel Distension
Aerophagia
  Postprandial
  Post–positive-pressure ventilation
    with bag-valve-mask device
  Tracheoesophageal fistula
Intestinal obstruction (mechanical)
  Volvulus
  Incarcerated hernia
  Intussusception
  Adhesive bands
  Duplications and other masses
  Meconium ileus
Ileus
  Toxic megacolon
  Infection
    Abscess
    Appendicitis
    Peritonitis
    Botulism
    Gastroenteritis
    Pneumonia
    Sepsis
    Necrotizing enterocolitis
Intraperitoneal blood (trauma,
  ruptured ectopic pregnancy,
  aneurysm)
Electrolyte abnormalities
  Hypokalemia
  Hypercalcemia
Poisoning/medications (e.g.,
  anticholinergic, opiate, loperamide,
  botulism)
Trauma
Shock
Severe pain secondary to
  Biliary colic
  Renal colic
Malabsorption
  Congenital causes
  Bacterial overgrowth
  Parasites
  Formula enteropathy
  Lactose intolerance
  Celiac disease
Obstipation
  Functional
  Hirschsprung's disease
  Hypothyroidism

Free Peritoneal Air
Intestinal perforation
Pneumomediastinum

Extraluminal Fluid
Hypoproteinemia
  Malnutrition
  Nephrotic syndrome
  Renal failure
  Cirrhosis
  Protein-losing enteropathy
  Congenital syphilis and TORCH
    infections
Blood
  Hepatic laceration
  Splenic laceration
Peritoneal inflammation
  Bile peritonitis
  Peritonitis
  Leukemia
  Tuberculosis
  Pancreatitis
Cirrhosis
  Biliary atresia
  Chronic active hepatitis
  Wilson's disease
  α_1-Antitrypsin disease
  Tyrosinemia
  Galactosemia (late)
Portal hypertension
Chylous ascites
Congestive heart failure/pericarditis
Budd-Chiari syndrome

Hepatomegaly
Congestive heart failure/constrictive
pericarditis (chronic)
Budd-Chiari syndrome
Biliary atresia
Inflammation
  Abscess
  AIDS
  Hepatitis
  Tyrosinemia
  Galactosemia
  Wilson's disease
  Congenital syphilis and TORCH
    infections
Neoplastic disease
  Hodgkin's disease
  Neuroblastoma
  Leukemia
  Lymphoma (non-Hodgkin's)
  Hepatoblastoma
Storage disease
Hemolytic anemia
  Sickle cell
  β-Thalassemia
  Malaria
Hepatic laceration (subcapsular
  hematoma)

Splenomegaly
Portal hypertension
Neoplastic disease
  Hodgkin's disease
  Leukemia
  Lymphoma (non-Hodgkin's)
Hemolytic anemia
  Sickle cell
  Spherocytosis
  β-Thalassemia
  Malaria
Inflammation
AIDS
Storage diseases
Hemorrhage
  Trauma (subcapsular hematoma)
Sequestration (sickle cell)

Mass
Cysts
  Choledochal cyst
  Ovarian cyst
  Mesenteric cyst
  Peritoneal cyst
  Omental cyst
  Polycystic kidneys
Obstructive uropathy
Uterine enlargement
  Pregnancy
  Hematocolpos
Neoplastic disease
  Wilms' tumor
  Ovarian tumor
  Teratoma
Inflammatory masses
  Regional enteritis

TABLE 8.2

COMMON CAUSES OF ABDOMINAL DISTENSION[a]

Aerophagia (crying, feeding)
Gastroenteritis
Obstipation
Pregnancy
Traumatic ileus
Intestinal obstruction (mechanical)
Obstructive uropathy (infants)
Pneumonia/sepsis
Peritonitis
Intraabdominal bleeding
Hemolytic disease
Congestive heart failure
Hepatitis

[a]Listed in approximate order of frequency.

the quantity of lactose ingested. Celiac disease may present with prominent abdominal distention, especially in children younger than 2 years, along with nonspecific GI symptoms and poor weight gain. Obstipation is a common cause of abdominal distension. The patient usually has a history of

TABLE 8.3

LIFE-THREATENING CAUSES OF ABDOMINAL DISTENSION

Infectious
Peritonitis
Sepsis/pneumonia
Botulism
Pancreatitis
Congenital syphilis
Hepatitis
Tuberculosis

Congenital
Tyrosinemia
Galactosemia
Hemolytic disease

Traumatic
Intraabdominal bleeding

Neoplastic
Leukemia and other malignancies

Other
Intestinal obstruction (mechanical)
Electrolyte abnormality
Renal failure
Poisoning
Necrotizing enterocolitis
Intestinal perforation
Shock
Budd-Chiari syndrome
Congestive heart failure
Pericarditis
Portal hypertension
AIDS
Toxic megacolon

irregular stooling or chronic constipation. This is often due to a severe functional disturbance, but pathologic processes, including Hirschsprung's disease and other defects in bowel enervation, and hypothyroidism should be excluded.

Extraluminal gas usually causes abdominal distention only when present as free peritoneal air. This may result from intestinal perforation (due to trauma, inflammation, ulcer, foreign-body ingestion, or other causes) or secondary to a pneumomediastinum. It is demonstrated with an upright or cross-table lateral radiograph of the abdomen or on an upright chest radiograph. An ileus generally contributes to the abdominal distension.

Extraluminal fluid in the abdomen may be an effusion, blood, chyle, bile, urine, or pus. The most common reason in pediatrics for the accumulation of fluid in the abdominal cavity is secondary to a low serum albumin. This may be the result of protein loss due to nephrotic syndrome or protein-losing enteropathy, or due to decreased protein synthesis such as that which occurs in cirrhosis and malnutrition. There is usually associated peripheral edema and pleural effusion. Increased venous and lymphatic resistance through the portal and hepatic veins may also cause accumulation of abdominal fluid. Obstruction of blood flow through the liver is suggested by distended abdominal wall veins, a history of hemoptysis, and an enlarged spleen. The obstruction may occur at the prehepatic level (portal venous thrombosis), within the liver parenchyma (end-stage cirrhosis), at the hepatic veins (Budd-Chiari syndrome), or at the intrathoracic level [congestive heart failure (CHF), pericarditis]. Obstruction at the porta hepatis is usually idiopathic, although a history of umbilical venous catheterization or omphalitis in the newborn period should suggest this possibility. Obstruction at this level generally does not cause marked ascites. Although cirrhosis evolves gradually, its clinical presentation may be abrupt. It results from Wilson's disease, α_1-antitrypsin disease, biliary atresia, and other congenital problems, or occasionally, from chronic active hepatitis. Decreased clotting factors would be among the many laboratory findings of cirrhosis. Obstruction of flow at the hepatic veins or above occurs as a result of Budd-Chiari syndrome, CHF, or constrictive pericarditis (see Chapter 82). The liver is engorged, resulting in hepatomegaly and right upper quadrant tenderness in each of these entities. Finally, a diseased peritoneum from infectious, inflammatory, or malignant causes can also cause an intraabdominal effusion.

A history of recent trauma and signs of shock point to intraperitoneal bleeding, usually due to a splenic or hepatic laceration. An ileus secondary to both peritoneal inflammation and shock likely contributes to the abdominal distension. Trauma in the recent past suggests chylous ascites. Finally, a diffusely tender abdomen suggests infectious peritonitis, pancreatitis, or bile peritonitis.

Extreme hepatomegaly that develops acutely occurs secondary to inflammation, congestion due to increased central venous pressure or vascular obstruction, or trauma (see Chapter 89). There will be marked right upper quadrant tenderness and general systemic toxicity. Causes include hepatitis, CHF, constrictive pericarditis, and congenital enzyme deficiencies. Neoplastic disease, especially the proliferative blood cell disorders (leukemia, lymphoma), commonly cause significant hepatomegaly and splenomegaly. Other causes of extreme hepatomegaly include storage diseases and congenital hemolytic anemias. However, the hepatomegaly in these conditions usually develops gradually and is accompanied by many other signs of chronic illness.

Extreme splenomegaly without marked hepatomegaly in the toxic-appearing child suggests intraparenchymal bleeding with an intact capsule, sickle cell sequestration crisis, or malaria (see Chapters 91, 92, and 103). In the nontoxic child, portal hypertension, neoplastic disease, and chronic hemolysis should be suspected. Neoplastic disease often results in a spleen with an irregular surface. Chronic hemolysis secondary to sickle cell disease, β-thalassemia, and hereditary spherocytosis may also result in a very large spleen. In the case of hemoglobin "SS" disease, but not hemoglobin "SC" disease or sickle-thalassemia, splenic enlargement is followed by splenic atrophy beyond 5 years of age. A peripheral blood smear generally identifies this group of causes of massive splenomegaly (see Chapter 91).

Other causes of abdominal distension include cysts, masses, tumors, uterine enlargement, obstructive uropathy, bowel duplication, and inflammation. Cystic lesions include ovarian cysts; mesenteric, omental, or peritoneal cysts; choledochal cysts; and polycystic kidneys. These conditions generally present with a subacute history and physical examination. The exception is torsion of the large ovarian cyst, which produces vomiting and marked abdominal pain. Abdominal ultrasound generally identifies intraabdominal cysts readily. Of course, an abdominal CT scan is also diagnostic but is associated with significant radiation exposure. Renal masses are probably the most common cause of abdominal distension in early infancy. Renal cystic disease is the most common cause of flank mass in the neonate. Hydronephrophesis due to ureteral-pelvic junction obstruction or posterior urethral valves may also cause abdominal distention in the neonate. Over time, bilateral renal obstruction may cause dehydration, renal failure, and shock. Although the diagnosis of obstructive uropathy is supported by an abnormal urinalysis or blood urea nitrogen (BUN):creatinine ratio, these results may be normal. Confirmation of renal anomalies is made by ultrasound. Tumors such as neuroblastoma, Wilms' tumor, an ovarian tumor, and a teratoma generally can be palpated easily as firm, discrete abdominal masses by the time they are causing frank abdominal distension (see Chapter 97). Bowel duplication can be a subtle diagnosis until a complication such as mechanical bowel obstruction or hematochezia develops. A contrast CT scan of the abdomen, however, generally confirms this diagnosis once suspected. Regional enteritis with sufficient inflammatory mass to cause abdominal distension is preceded by a long history of obstructive and malabsorptive symptoms. Acute-phase reactants such as the sedimentation rate are likely to be abnormal in regional enteritis. Finally, a midline pelvic mass should suggest pregnancy or hematocolpos.

EVALUATION AND DECISION

History

The history should attempt first to differentiate acute from chronic symptomatology by focusing on the rate of progression, recent trauma, weight loss, or weight gain. Parents may note early, subtle changes in these symptoms before they

become apparent to the clinician. Next, systemic signs such as fever, anorexia, edema, and lethargy further define the acuteness of the problem and, to some degree, narrow the diagnostic possibilities. One must always be on the alert, however, for an acute complication superimposed on a more subtle chronic condition. Next, symptoms relative to specific organs, including the GI, renal, cardiac, and gynecologic systems, should be pursued. These include questions about nausea, vomiting (bilious or nonbilious), abdominal pain, change in bowel habits, stool history (color, consistency), shortness of breath, cough, hemoptysis, urine output (including strength of stream and any abnormality of urinary color or foamy urine), menstrual history, and sexual activity (asked in a confidential manner). Other important historical information includes stress or anxiety (associated with aerophagia), previous abdominal surgery, and recent medication use (including laxatives and antidiarrheal agents). Finally, a family history of anemia, early infant death among relatives or metabolic disease, a travel history, and a careful newborn history may be revealing.

Physical Examination

After ruling out life-threatening respiratory embarrassment and shock, the physical examination should focus on determining whether the cause of the abdominal distension is related to bowel (air or stool) (Fig. 8.1), free fluid (Fig. 8.2), massive hepatomegaly (Fig. 8.3), massive splenomegaly (Fig. 8.4), inspissated stool, or a discrete mass (Fig. 8.5). A tympanitic abdomen suggests bowel distension (either by a mechanical obstruction or an ileus) or, especially in a toxic-appearing child, free air. A fluid wave or shifting dullness (more reliable in younger children) suggests ascites. Palpable loops of bowel or a palpable descending colon suggests stool. Massive hepatomegaly and splenomegaly generally are defined easily by palpation. However, care should be taken to begin palpation in the pelvic area and advance superiorly so as not to overlook the liver edge. Furthermore, the examiner must be cautious since other masses may mimic hepatomegaly and, in particular, splenomegaly. Thus, it is important to note not only the location of the mass, but also whether it is firm, fixed (suggesting retroperitoneal origin), cystic, smooth, or nodular. Other key physical findings include signs of CHF, abdominal tenderness, peripheral edema, signs of trauma or easy bruising, lymphadenopathy, pallor, and jaundice. A rectal examination for a mass, tenderness, gross (frank blood, currant jelly stool) or occult blood, and the presence or absence of stool is also helpful. More specific findings may be pursued once an initial hypothesis is made based on the algorithms in this chapter.

Laboratory

The initial laboratory evaluation of abdominal distension is determined by the clinical findings and may include complete blood count with smear, erythrocyte sedimentation rate, C-reactive protein, and reticulocyte count; liver function tests, including serum albumin and clotting studies; electrolytes with BUN, creatinine, lipase, and amylase; a urinalysis with reducing substances; and a chest radiograph and a two-view abdomen plain radiograph. The radiographs are helpful in

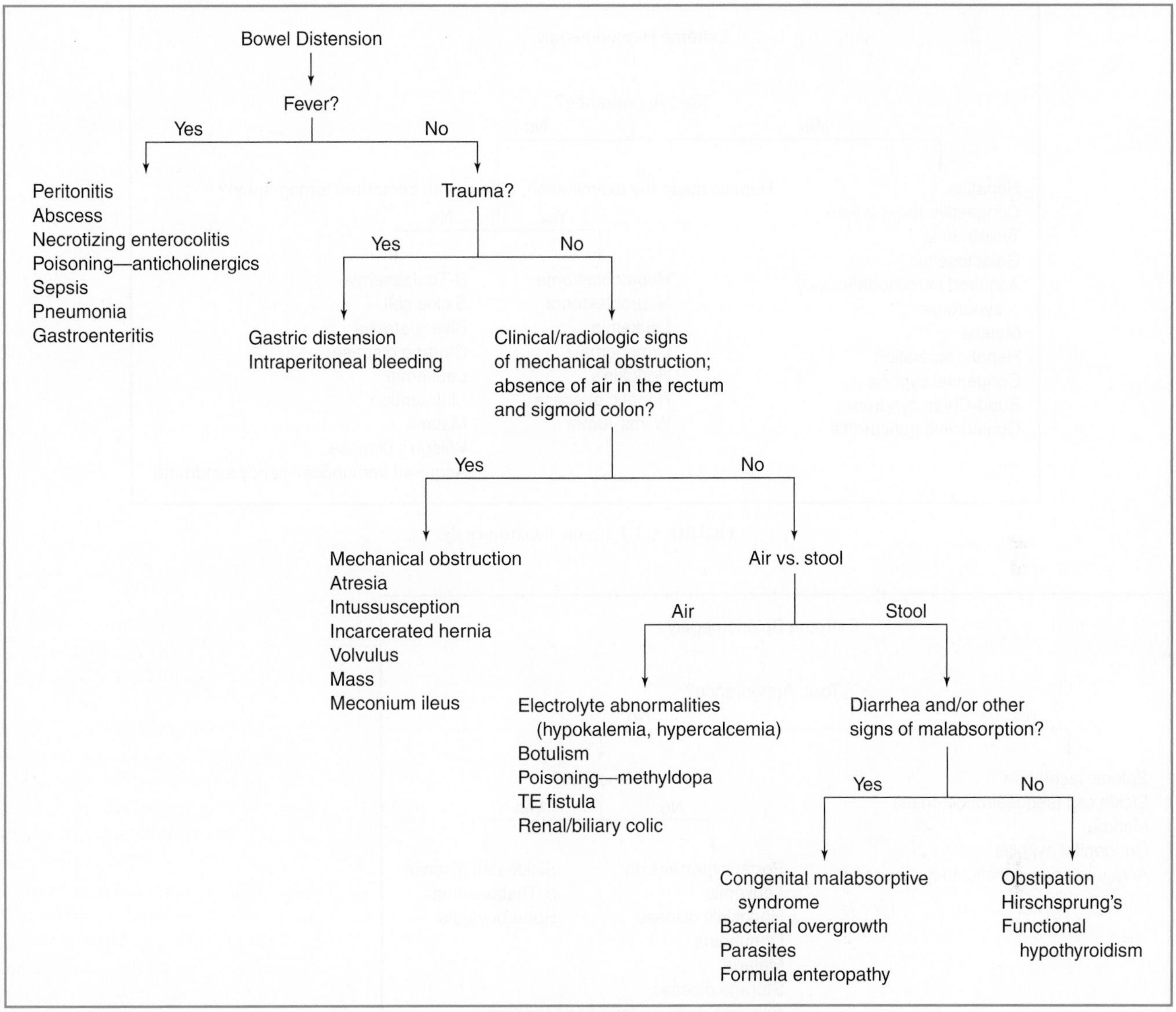

Bowel Distension

↓

Fever?

Yes ← → No

Yes:
Peritonitis
Abscess
Necrotizing enterocolitis
Poisoning—anticholinergics
Sepsis
Pneumonia
Gastroenteritis

No → Trauma?

Yes ← → No

Yes:
Gastric distension
Intraperitoneal bleeding

No: Clinical/radiologic signs of mechanical obstruction; absence of air in the rectum and sigmoid colon?

Yes ← → No

Yes:
Mechanical obstruction
Atresia
Intussusception
Incarcerated hernia
Volvulus
Mass
Meconium ileus

No → Air vs. stool

Air ← → Stool

Air:
Electrolyte abnormalities (hypokalemia, hypercalcemia)
Botulism
Poisoning—methyldopa
TE fistula
Renal/biliary colic

Stool → Diarrhea and/or other signs of malabsorption?

Yes ← → No

Yes:
Congenital malabsorptive syndrome
Bacterial overgrowth
Parasites
Formula enteropathy

No:
Obstipation
Hirschsprung's
Functional hypothyroidism

FIGURE 8.1 Bowel distension (TE, tracheoesophageal).

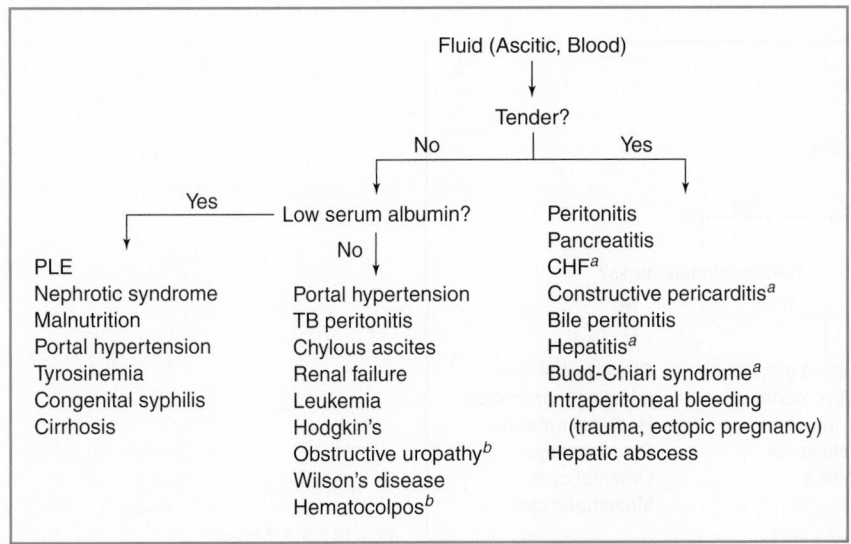

Fluid (Ascitic, Blood)

↓

Tender?

No ← → Yes

No → Low serum albumin?

Yes ← → No

Yes:
PLE
Nephrotic syndrome
Malnutrition
Portal hypertension
Tyrosinemia
Congenital syphilis
Cirrhosis

No:
Portal hypertension
TB peritonitis
Chylous ascites
Renal failure
Leukemia
Hodgkin's
Obstructive uropathy[b]
Wilson's disease
Hematocolpos[b]

Yes:
Peritonitis
Pancreatitis
CHF[a]
Constructive pericarditis[a]
Bile peritonitis
Hepatitis[a]
Budd-Chiari syndrome[a]
Intraperitoneal bleeding (trauma, ectopic pregnancy)
Hepatic abscess

FIGURE 8.2 Fluid (ascitic, blood). PLE, protein-losing enteropathy; TB, tuberculosis; CHF, congestive heart failure. [a]right upper quadrant tenderness; [b]newborn period only or primarily.

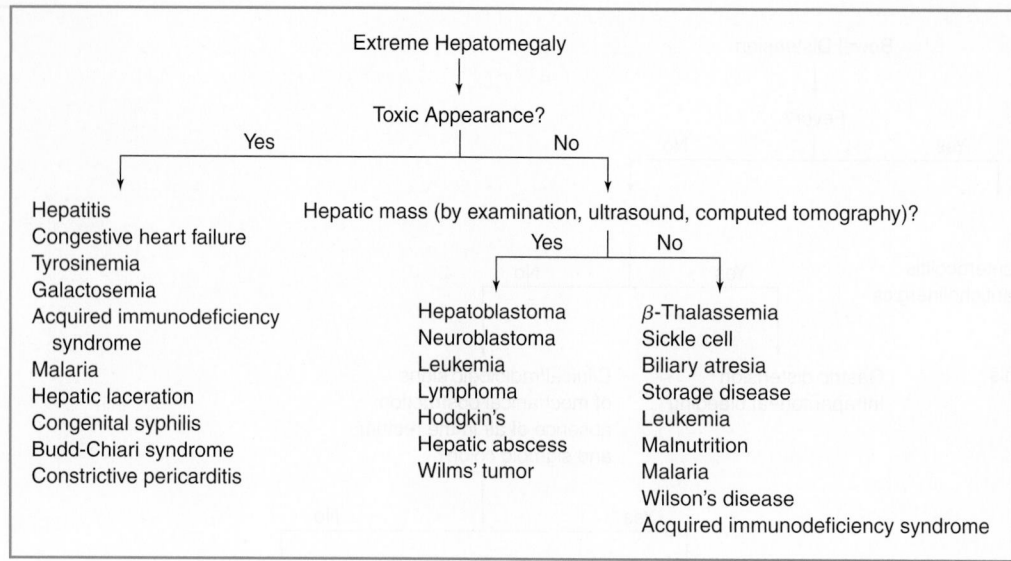

FIGURE 8.3 Extreme hepatomegaly.

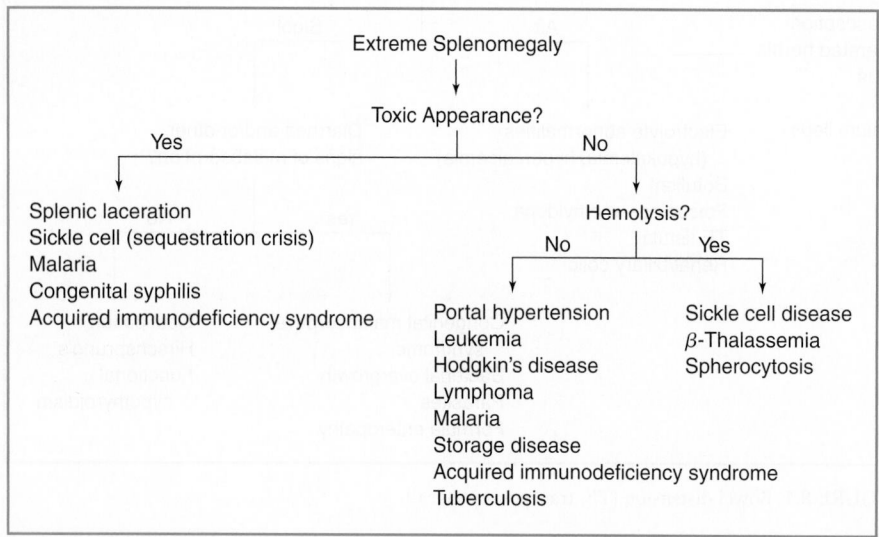

FIGURE 8.4 Extreme splenomegaly.

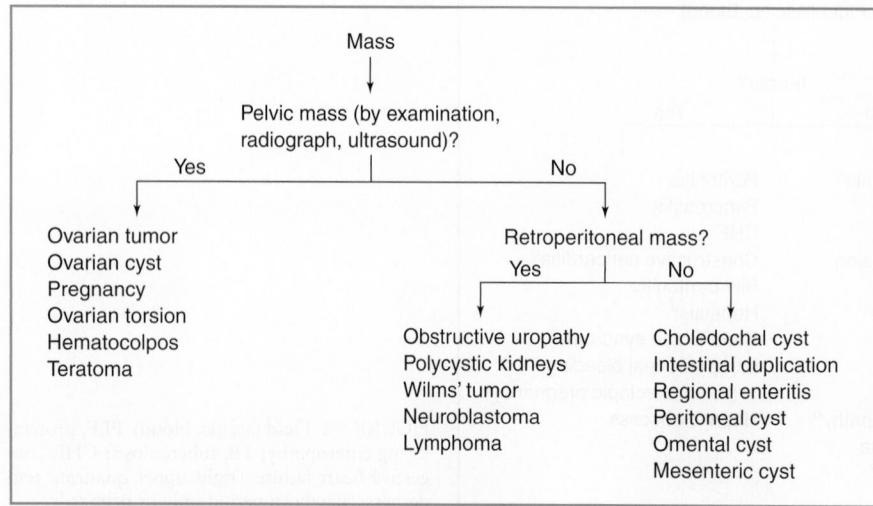

FIGURE 8.5 Mass.

determining the intestinal gas pattern, presence of free intraabdominal air, and presence of intraabdominal calcifications. If intestinal obstruction is suspected, one of the plain radiographs should be a prone cross-table lateral view to determine the presence or absence of air in the rectum and sigmoid colon. The addition of a left lateral decubitus view to the supine radiograph of the abdomen adds to the diagnostic utility if an intussusception is suspected.

Often, after the initial history, physical examination, and laboratory evaluation, further imaging studies will be necessary. Ultrasound is an excellent first step since it is becoming widely available and is portable, has no ionizing radiation, is inexpensive, and can usually determine the presence and characteristics of a mass, organomegaly, and ascites (see Chapter 134). It is also fairly accurate in the diagnosis of GI obstruction, malrotation, and intussusception. Furthermore, physical exam findings (site of maximal tenderness and/or distention) can be correlated with ultrasound findings. An abdominal CT scan is the preferred study in the evaluation of abdominal distention if an ultrasound is inconclusive or unable to be obtained (i.e., obesity). Focused abdominal sonography for trauma (FAST) is a useful screening tool in the initial evaluation of abdominal trauma in pediatrics (see Chapter 107). However, the FAST exam should not be used as the sole diagnostic test to exclude suspected intraabdominal injury; CT scanning has higher sensitivity and specificity in this setting.

Management

Abdominal distension by itself may represent a medical emergency. First, this occurs when the distension is so severe that diaphragmatic excursion is compromised. For example, gastric and bowel distension secondary to aerophagia and ileus posttrauma may significantly impair a child's respiratory status. Massive ascites and free peritoneal air may also compromise respiration. Therefore, the first step in management is to assess and stabilize the child's respiratory status, including the use of positive-pressure ventilation and/or emergent relief of distension, if needed. Passage of a nasogastric or orogastric tube may also result in dramatic improvement in the child's respiratory status.

The second, far less common situation in which abdominal distension may represent an emergent situation in itself is compression of the inferior vena cava (IVC), resulting in a compromised cardiovascular status. For example, occasionally, a child with severe obstipation may present with weak pulses and cool extremities. In this situation, rapid infusion of intravenous fluids, as well as disimpaction, will improve the patient's perfusion status rapidly. Managing the child in the lateral decubitus position may relieve pressure on the IVC. When the airway, breathing, and circulation have been stabilized, the diagnostic evaluation can proceed with laboratory and imaging studies as discussed previously.

Suggested Readings

Belamarich PF. Abdominal distention. In: McInerny TK, Adam HM, Campbell DE, et al., eds. *American academy of pediatrics textbook of pediatric care.* Elk Grove Village, IL: American Academy of Pediatrics, 2009:1369–1376.

Chavhan GB, Masrani S, Thakkar H, et al. Sonography in the diagnosis of pediatric gastrointestinal obstruction. *J Clin Ultrasound* 2004;32(4):190–199.

Heyman MB. Lactose intolerance in infants, children, and adolescents. *Pediatrics* 2006;118(3):1279–1286.

Hill ID. Celiac disease–a never-ending story? *J Pediatr* 2003;143(3):289–291.

Holmes JF, Gladman A, Chang C. Performance of abdominal ultrasonography in pediatric blunt trauma patients: a meta-analysis. *J Pediatr Surg* 2007; 42(9):1588–1594.

Hooker RL, Hernanz-Schulman M, Yu C, et al. Radiographic evaluation of intussusception: utility of left-side-down decubitus view. *Radiology* 2008;248(3):987–994.

Maglinte DD, Heitkamp DE, Howard TJ, et al. Current concepts in imaging of small bowel obstruction. *Radiol Clin North Am* 2003;41(2):263–283.

Rasquin A, Di Lorenzo C, Forbes D, et al. Childhood functional gastrointestinal disorders: child/adolescent. *Gastroenterology* 2006;130(5):1527–1537.

Swischuk LE. The abdomen. In: Swischuk LE, ed. *Emergency imaging of the acutely ill or injured child,* 4th ed. Baltimore: Williams & Wilkins, 2000: 149–289.

SIGNS AND SYMPTOMS

CHAPTER 9 ■ APNEA

SUSAN B. TORREY, MD

Neonates and infants can experience apneic episodes in response to a variety of physiologic and pathophysiologic processes not seen in later life. Differences in maturity of the central nervous system (CNS), respiratory reserve, and susceptibility to infectious agents are among the factors that interact to make the very young patient unique. The causes of apnea in older children are similar to those in adults, although the susceptibility and reserve of the child, again, are different. In this chapter, the neonate and the young infant are emphasized, but for completeness, the older child also is considered.

Apnea is defined as a respiratory pause of greater than 20 seconds, or of any duration if there is associated pallor or cyanosis and/or bradycardia. Apnea must be distinguished from periodic breathing, which is a common respiratory pattern in young infants and is characterized by cycles of short respiratory pause followed by an increase in respiratory rate. Normal newborn infants display respiratory patterns that vary by gender and by conceptual age, as well as by sleep state. Research studies have demonstrated that premature infants typically have more apneic episodes than do term infants. Normal-term infants experience significantly more episodes of nonperiodic apnea during rapid eye movement (REM) sleep than during non-REM sleep, although respiratory failure occurs more often during non-REM sleep. Severe apnea may be accompanied by change in color, muscle tone, or mental status, or by choking. Such an episode is described as an acute life-threatening event (ALTE).

PATHOPHYSIOLOGY

Control of respiration by respiratory centers in the pons and medulla through output to the upper airway and bellows apparatus is modulated by peripheral factors such as hypoxia, hypercarbia, and laryngochemical stimulation. The immature response of the neonate and the young infant to these influences, in comparison to that of the older child, accounts for some of the vulnerability of these small patients. The adult response to hypoxemia is to increase respiratory rate in proportion to the decrease in oxygen partial pressure (PO_2). Tachypnea is maintained for the duration of the hypoxic stimulus. In contrast, the neonate demonstrates a brief increase in respiratory rate followed by depression of respiratory drive and, often, apnea. As an example, during sleep, infants who are mildly hypoxic tend to breathe periodically or develop apneic spells. Furthermore, hypoxemia during sleep may not cause arousal. Hypoxemia also results in less of a response to rising arterial carbon dioxide tension ($PaCO_2$) with further depression of respiratory drive.

Feeding affects ventilation in young infants. Poor coordination of sucking and breathing can result in apnea. Furthermore, infants can develop apnea with hypoxia and bradycardia as the result of exaggerated laryngeal chemical reflexes in response to regurgitation. Mild hypoxia, as can occur in association with feeding or sleep, exacerbates this response.

A number of exogenous factors, including toxins and metabolic derangements, affect respiratory control by causing medullary depression. Clinical experience demonstrates that newborn and very young infants are particularly sensitive to these factors; for example, hypoglycemia can be manifested as apnea in young infants, and anemia is often related to apnea in premature babies. The young infant is susceptible to bellows failure on a purely mechanical basis. The infant's thoracic cage is extremely pliable, which can cause the chest wall to collapse during inspiration. More muscular effort is then required to produce an adequate tidal volume, resulting in increased work of breathing. In addition, the diaphragmatic muscles have limited glycogen stores and tire easily, resulting in greater vulnerability to respiratory failure as a result of respiratory distress.

DIFFERENTIAL DIAGNOSIS

The differential diagnosis of apnea is extensive (Table 9.1). Gastroesophageal reflux is frequently diagnosed in infants with an ALTE, with or without a history of vomiting. Several infectious processes can cause apnea. Meningitis, even in the absence of fever, must be included in the differential diagnosis. Respiratory syncytial virus, the predominant cause of bronchiolitis, may cause apnea in infants who were premature or have preexisting lung disease or congenital heart disease. Pertussis can cause apnea in small infants. Infant botulism is a diagnosis that will hopefully be made before apnea occurs. It must be suspected on the basis of age, symptoms, and clinical findings. Apnea may be the only clinical manifestation of seizure activity. This may be particularly difficult for emergency physicians to identify if they did not witness the episode and neurologic examination may be normal in the postictal period. Apnea may be a symptom of several systemic disease processes, including metabolic abnormalities that result in hypoglycemia, and sepsis. Congenital abnormalities must always be considered in newborns and in young infants. Prolongation of the QT interval can cause a dysrhythmia that is manifested as an ALTE. Finally, there have been well-substantiated reports of ALTE as the result of life-threatening child abuse such as Munchhausen's by proxy or inflicted head injury. Frequently, no cause for the ALTE is identified.

Of great concern to both parents and physician is the risk of sudden infant death syndrome (SIDS) for an infant who has an

TABLE 9.1

DIFFERENTIAL DIAGNOSIS OF APNEA

	Neonate, infant	Older child
Central nervous system	Infection (meningitis, encephalitis) Seizure Prematurity Inflicted head injury Increased intracranial pressure (ICP) Congenital anomaly (e.g., Arnold-Chiari) Breath-holding spell	Infection Toxin Tumor Seizure Increased ICP (trauma, hydrocephalus) Idiopathic hypoventilation ("Ondine's curse")
Upper airway	Laryngospasm (e.g., gastroesophageal reflux) Infection (e.g., croup, pertussis) Congenital anomaly (e.g., Down syndrome)	Obstructive sleep apnea Infection (epiglottitis, croup) Foreign body
Lower airway	Infection (pneumonia, bronchiolitis) Congenital anomaly	Infection Asthma
Other	Infant botulism Hypocalcemia, hypoglycemia Anemia Sepsis Dysrrhythmia	Guillain-Barré syndrome Spinal cord injury Flail chest Dysrrhythmia Ingestion

unexplained ALTE. Multiple studies have identified no causal relationship between ALTE and SIDS. Furthermore, although the rate of SIDS in the United States has dropped dramatically since 1992 when the American Academy of Pediatrics recommended that infants be placed supine or on the side during sleep, there has been no change in the incidence of ALTEs. In addition, the vast majority of SIDS events occur at night, whereas infants typically experience ALTEs during the day.

EVALUATION AND DECISION

Initial Stabilization

The first priority of the emergency physician, after immediate resuscitation of the patient, is to identify life-threatening conditions (Fig. 9.1) such as persistent or recurrent apnea, hypoxia, septic shock, or hypoglycemia. In addition to assessment of the vital signs, including a rectal temperature and blood pressure, the general appearance and mental status should be noted. Regardless of the cause, apnea is life threatening; therefore, a diagnostic investigation, guided by history and physical findings, should be performed to evaluate the child for several common etiologies (Table 9.2). The next phase of evaluation addresses two key questions: (i) Is this episode of clinical significance? (ii) What is the risk of recurrence? Factors to consider include signs of another acute illness, the age of the child, and other possible risk factors for clinically significant or recurrent apnea (Table 9.3).

Has a Significant Apneic Episode Occurred?

The key to answering the two questions is invariably in the history (Table 9.3). A clear initial history from a firsthand observer without the predictable influence of repeated questions is vital. This may not be a simple task, considering the observer's recent stressful experience. The following details should be included: (i) where the event took place; (ii) how long the event lasted; (iii) whether the infant was awake or asleep; (iv) whether there was an associated color change and, if so, to what colors and in what order; (v) description of associated movements, posture, or changes in tone; (vi) what resuscitative efforts were made and the infant's response to them; and (vii) when the infant was last fed. The response to these questions may provide the physician with clues to the diagnosis. As an example, an 8-month-old infant who was interrupted in a favorite activity, began to cry, turned red and blue, and finally had several seconds of tonic-clonic motor activity likely had a breath-holding spell. In contrast, a history of 40 minutes of cyanosis and apnea in a now well-appearing child may be unreliable. Other recent events that should be documented are symptoms of other illnesses, including changes in behavior, activity, and appetite, as well as recent trauma and immunizations.

In many cases, the description of the event may be concerning, although the child appears well. In this situation, hospitalization for further workup, as outlined next, is warranted. A typical case might be the previously well 5-week-old child who was noted by the parents to be apneic during a nap. The infant was described as limp and blue and "looked like he was dead." There was no response to tactile or verbal stimulation

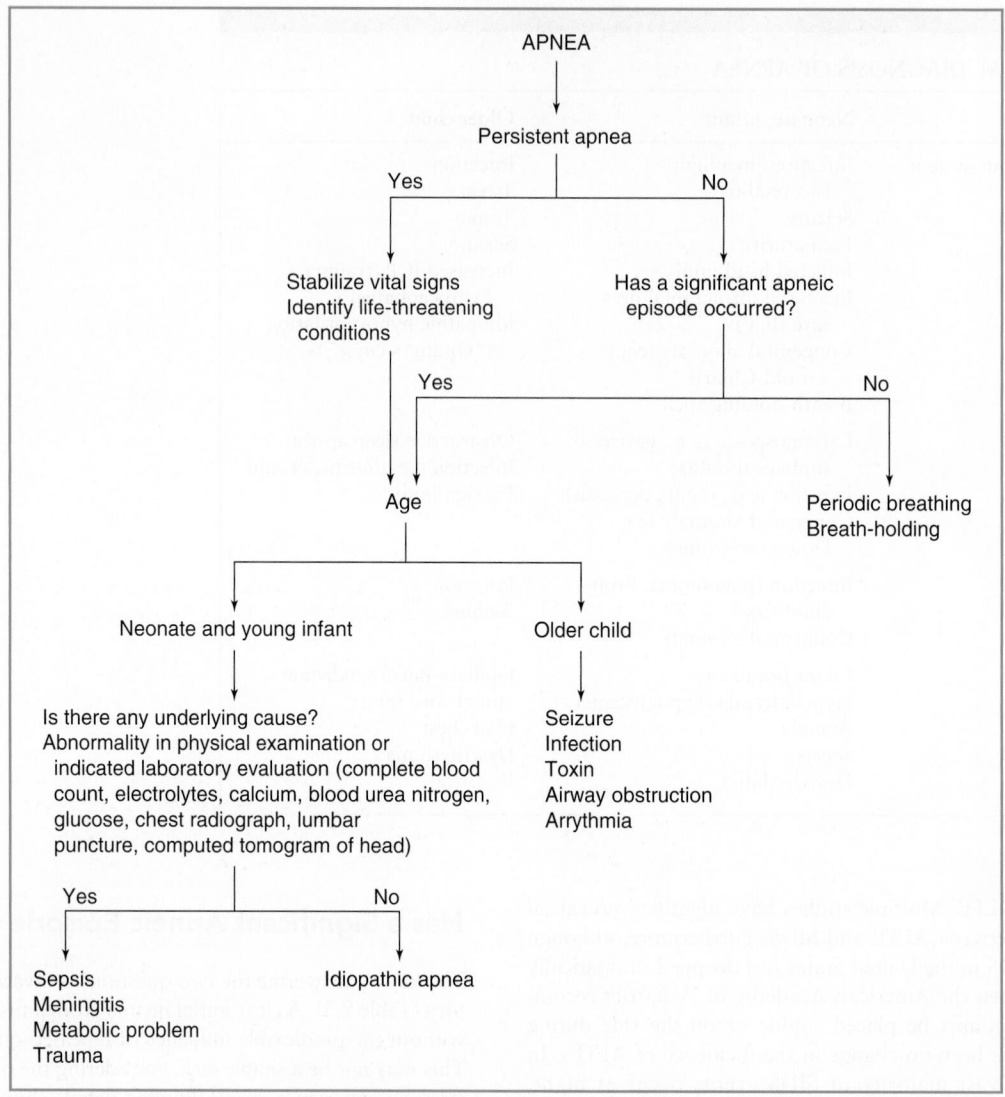

FIGURE 9.1 Approach to the diagnosis and management of apnea.

for 5 to 10 seconds, but after 15 to 20 seconds of mouth-to-mouth breathing, the child coughed, gagged, and began to breathe. His color improved over the next 30 seconds, and the parents rushed him to the emergency department (ED). Although the baby now looks entirely normal, he may be at grave risk for experiencing another ALTE.

The medical history also may provide important information regarding infants at risk for significant or recurrent apnea.

TABLE 9.2

COMMON LIFE-THREATENING CONDITIONS
THAT CAUSE APNEA

Pneumonia
Sepsis/meningitis
Hypoglycemia
Seizures
Intracranial hypertension
Shock
Ingestion (e.g., analgesics, sedatives, muscle relaxants)

The physician should ask specifically about previous similar episodes. Information about perinatal events, including gestational age (birth weight), labor and delivery, maternal health, and nursery course, is helpful. A family history with specific reference to seizures, infant deaths, and serious illnesses in young family members also should be included. Finally, information regarding poisons available in the household may be important in treating an older child.

Is There an Underlying Cause?

A careful physical examination identifies many treatable acute illnesses that can cause apnea. One clue to serious systemic disease is fever or hypothermia. Tachypnea suggests either a respiratory problem or a metabolic problem. Shock may be secondary to sepsis or hypovolemia from occult trauma. Evaluation of the nervous system should include notation of mental status, palpation of the fontanelles, and funduscopic examination. Dysmorphic features might suggest an underlying congenital abnormality; however, an entirely normal physical

TABLE 9.3

HISTORICAL FEATURES OF APNEA

History	Significant apnea
Duration of event	Greater than 20 s or of any duration associated with pallor, cyanosis, and/or bradycardia
Was child asleep or awake?	Either, but apnea during sleep is more worrisome
Color change	Pallor or cyanosis
Associated movements, posture, or change in tone	Seizure activity Hypotonia "He/she looked dead"
Resuscitative efforts and response	Color change or hypotonia requiring cardiopulmonary resuscitation to improve
Interval since last feeding	If shortly after feeding, consider gastroesophageal reflux
Where event occurred	Association with sleep, trauma

examination provides no reassurance that the described event was clinically insignificant and will not recur.

Laboratory evaluation should be guided by the history and physical examination. Tests to consider in the ED include a measurement of blood glucose and serum electrolytes. Any indication that the infant could have a serious infection should be pursued with cultures of blood and urine and by examination of cerebrospinal fluid. Urine and blood for toxicologic analysis should be obtained from patients who may have been exposed to toxic substances or medications. Noninvasive pulse oximetry is adequate to identify hypoxemia, and significant metabolic acidosis will be apparent on determination of serum electrolytes. The arterial or venous blood gas examination does not serve as a screening test for a serious event and should be obtained on the basis of specific indications. Radiologic studies, (such as of the lateral neck, chest, abdomen, or computed tomography of the head) should be performed as indicated by the history and physical examination.

The tasks of the emergency physician faced with a young patient who has had an apneic episode are to identify whether he or she should be hospitalized and to treat underlying conditions. If a careful history and physical examination suggest that a significant apneic episode has not occurred, the diagnosis of periodic breathing or breath-holding can be made, and the patient can be discharged after appropriate counseling of the parents and arrangements for follow-up. The evaluation of a young child with apnea, however, rarely will be so straightforward. If historical information indicates that significant apnea has occurred, the infant is at risk for a recurrence of this life-threatening event. An aggressive search for an underlying cause is necessary and often includes laboratory studies, lumbar puncture, chest radiograph, and electrocardiogram (EKG). Hospital admission should be arranged for observation and further diagnostic evaluation.

A significant apneic episode in the absence of systemic disease leaves the emergency physician in a quandary. There may not be an explanation for the event that satisfies the physician or the anxious parents. Thus, it is judicious to refer the family to an available specialist or center. There is considerable practice variation in the inpatient evaluation and management of an ALTE. The approach that is usually pursued is designed to identify known causes of primary apnea. It generally includes in-hospital observation with monitoring and an evaluation of the CNS with an electroencephalogram, some type of sleep study, a chest radiograph, and an EKG. Respiratory function is evaluated with a pneumogram, and a barium swallow and esophageal pH study might identify gastroesophageal reflux. An ultrasound or CT of the head would be indicated if a central (CNS) cause for apnea, such as inflicted head injury, is suspected. The decision to recommend home cardiorespiratory monitoring is beyond the scope of emergency practice.

In many instances, a thorough history and careful physical examination with appropriate laboratory studies will suggest that a significant apneic event has not occurred and that there is no serious underlying illness. In this situation, the emergency physician should reassure and educate the family before discharging the patient. Good medical practice dictates that the parents also should be given specific instructions regarding indications for another ED visit and a follow-up visit to a primary care provider.

Suggested Readings

Abu-Shaweesh J. Maturation of respiratory reflex responses in the fetus and neonate. *Semin Neonatol* 2004;9:169–180.

Brand D, Altman R, Purtill K, et al. Yield of diagnostic testing in infants who have had an apparent life-threatening event. *Pediatrics* 2005;115:885–893.

Claudius I, Keens T. Do all infants with apparent life-threatening events need to be admitted? *Pediatrics* 2007;119:679–683.

Cote A, Bairam M, Deschenes M, et al. Sudden infant deaths in sitting devices. *Arch Dis Child* 2008;93:384–389.

Esani N, Hodgman J, Ehsani N, et al. Apparent life-threatening events and sudden infant death syndrome. *J Pediatr* 2008;152(3):365–370.

McGovern M, Smith M. Causes of apparent life-threatening events in infants: a systematic review. *Arch Dis Child* 2004;89:1043–1048.

Meehan W, Merschman J, Chiang V. An 18-month-old girl with recurrent apneic spells. *Pediatr Emerg Care* 2008;24:546–549.

Pitetti R, Whitman E, Zaylor A. Accidental and nonaccidental poisonings as a cause of apparent life-threatening events in infants. *Pediatrics* 2008;122: e359–e362.

Tieder J, Cowan C, Garrison M, et al. Variation in inpatient resource utilization and management for apparent life-threatening events. *J Pediatr* 2008;152: 629–635.

Wilwerth B, Harper M, Greenes D. Identifying hospitalized infants who have bronchilolitis and are at high risk for apnea. *Ann Emerg Med* 2006;48:441–447.

CHAPTER 10 ■ ATAXIA

JANET H. FRIDAY, MD

Acute childhood ataxia is an uncommon presenting complaint in the emergency department. *Ataxia* is defined as a disturbance in coordination of movements and may be manifest as an unsteady gait. When it occurs, it is a distressing problem to both parent and clinician. It is important to establish the sign because true ataxia may be difficult to differentiate from clumsiness in toddlers. Parents are generally more sensitive to gait abnormalities in this age group. In older children, ataxia may be confused with weakness or vertigo. Life-threatening causes of pure ataxia are rare in children. After consideration of these, the problem may be approached in a cautious, stepwise fashion.

PATHOPHYSIOLOGY

The cerebellum coordinates complex activities such as walking, talking, and eye movements. Ataxia may be caused by a pathologic condition at either a focal or global level within the cerebellum or by disruptions in the afferent or efferent pathways. Anatomically, the cerebellum is located in the posterior cranial fossa, separated from the cerebrum by the tentorium. The ventral borders of the cerebellum form the roof of the fourth ventricle. Space-occupying lesions such as posterior fossa tumors and cerebellar hemorrhage may impede cerebrospinal fluid (CSF) flow, leading to hydrocephalus and increased intracranial pressure (ICP). Conversely, direct pressure on the cerebellar peduncles may cause ataxia to present.

The cerebellum links with other portions of the central nervous system through the superior, middle, and inferior peduncles via the midbrain, pons, and medulla. Proprioceptive and sensory afferent impulses from muscles, joints, and tendons are carried via inferior peduncles to the cerebellar cortex. Labyrinthine afferent input is also conducted through the inferior peduncles. Connections from frontal motor cortex travel through the middle cerebellar peduncles. The superior peduncles carry efferent output to musculoskeletal tracts from the nuclei of the cerebellum.

The cerebellum is composed of two hemispheres. Because of the decussation patterns, a lesion that affects only one side of the cerebellum will result in movement abnormalities of the ipsilateral side, with distal movements more affected than proximal ones. Midline lesions lead to truncal ataxia, with swaying during standing, sitting, and walking, and/or with titubations (small rhythmic movements) of the head and neck. Finally, the intrinsic function of the cerebellum may be disrupted by toxins and autoimmune and metabolic disorders.

DIFFERENTIAL DIAGNOSIS

Ataxia as a presenting sign invokes a broad differential diagnosis (Table 10.1). Distinguishing among acute, intermittent, and chronic progressive and chronic nonprogressive ataxia may be helpful, although some diagnoses have overlap in their time course at presentation. Fortunately, common causes of pure ataxia (Table 10.2) are not rapidly progressive. Acute cerebellar ataxia or postinfectious cerebellitis is truncal in nature and occurs 8 days to 3 weeks after an infectious illness (see Chapter 92). Children ages 1 to 3 years are most commonly affected. Varicella is the classically identified culprit. Other prodromal infections include mumps, Epstein Barr virus, and mycoplasma. Nystagmus is the most common accompanying symptom. The ataxia is most severe at its onset. Complete recovery usually is noted after several weeks, but has been described as several months. CSF may show mild lymphocytosis and increased protein. Imaging studies are normal. A small percentage of patients may show long-term sequelae such as learning disabilities or coordination problems.

Ingestions of anticonvulsants, alcohol, or sedative-hypnotics generally cause depressed mental status (see Chapter 102) and may have associated ataxia. However, for certain substances (phenytoin, carbamazepine, primidone), ataxia may be the most remarkable feature of intoxication.

When an ataxic patient presents with weakness and areflexia, Guillain-Barré syndrome may be present. If ophthalmoplegia and areflexia are prominent, the Miller-Fisher variant can be suspected. Neuroimaging is normal, and the CSF may show a mild leukocytosis and elevated protein. Tick paralysis may present similarly, with the discovery of an engorged tick (which may be hidden by long hair), as the diagnostic finding.

Ataxia may be an early prominent sign of posterior fossa tumors (especially medulloblastoma) and other conditions associated with increased ICP, including hydrocephalus and supratentorial tumors (see Chapter 97). Labyrinthitis and benign paroxysmal vertigo are rarely seen in young children but are occasionally encountered in adolescents. The sensation of loss of balance classically produces a wide-based gait. Conversion disorder should be suspected in a patient who walks with a narrow gait and has elaborate "near falls."

Life-threatening causes of ataxia (Table 10.3) rarely present as ataxia alone. In a few cases, bacterial meningitis has been reported with ataxia as the first symptom. Viral cerebellitis may occur as a result of enteroviral disease. Neuroblastoma

TABLE 10.1

DIFFERENTIAL DIAGNOSIS

Acute or Recurrent Ataxia
Acute cerebellar ataxia (postinfectious)
Guillain-Barré syndrome
Tick paralysis
Drug intoxication
Labyrinthitis
Vasculitis or Kawasaki disease
Vertebrobasilar occlusion
Meningitis
Viral encephalitis
Intracranial hemorrhage
Postconcussion syndrome
Benign paroxysmal vertigo
Conversion reaction
Multiple sclerosis
Acute demyelinating encephalomyelitis
Migraine
Epilepsy (pseudoataxia)
Transient ischemic attacks
Hartnup disease
Wilson's disease
Episodic ataxia type 1 (paroxysmal ataxia and myokymia)
Episodic ataxia type 2 (acetazolamide-responsive ataxia)
Maple syrup urine disease
Pyruvate decarboxylase deficiency

Chronic or Progressive
Hydrocephalus
Posterior fossa tumors
Cerebellar Hemangioblastoma (von Hippel-Lindau disease)
Chiari I malformation
Vermal aplasia (Dandy-Walker malformation and Joubert's syndrome)
Spinocerebellar degenerations
Basilar impression
Cerebellar hemisphere hypoplasia or agenesis
Abetalipoproteinemia (vitamin E deficiency)
Freidrich's ataxia
Juvenile sulfatide lipodosis
Juvenile GM$_2$ gangliosidosis
Ataxia telangiectasia
Ataxia with oculomotor apraxia
Refsum disease
Familial periodic ataxia
Hartnup disease
Marinesco-Sjögren syndrome

may present with titubations, myoclonic ataxia, and chaotic eye movements. The syndrome is immune mediated. It should be suspected in patients with acute ataxia that waxes and wanes over several days. One should consider vertebrobasilar occlusion in a patient with neck trauma and ataxia, cerebellar

TABLE 10.2

COMMON CAUSES OF ACUTE ATAXIA

Acute cerebellar ataxia
Drug ingestion
Guillain-Barré syndrome

TABLE 10.3

LIFE-THREATENING CAUSES OF ATAXIA

Meningitis
Drug intoxication
Brain tumor
Neuroblastoma
Cerebral vascular accident (stroke)
Intracranial hemorrhage

hemorrhage with ataxia and headache, and vasculitis in a child with features of Kawasaki disease.

Migraine, seizure, transient ischemic attack, and metabolic disease are the most common causes for intermittent ataxia. Chronic progressive ataxias may have a basis in metabolic defects, some of which are treatable. When a progressive ataxia acutely worsens, this may signify severe hydrocephalus or hemorrhage into a posterior fossa tumor. A variety of familial, metabolic, and congenital causes exist for chronic nonprogressive ataxias.

EVALUATION AND DECISION

The approach to the problem should begin with a thorough history and physical examination. The duration and progression of the illness can be established and will help define the ataxia as acute, intermittent, or chronic. Chronic ataxia should be further divided into progressive or nonprogressive. Key historical points to cover include recent illnesses such as varicella or other infectious diseases and access to medications or alcohol (Table 10.4). Family history may be helpful in recurrent or genetic causes.

Physical examination should focus on signs of increased ICP (bulging fontanel, papilledema, bradycardia, hypertension, abnormal respirations), meningeal irritation (nuchal rigidity, Kernig's or Brudzinski's sign), fever, rash, attached tick, and evidence of middle ear disease. A detailed neurologic

TABLE 10.4

DRUGS AND TOXINS THAT MAY CAUSE ATAXIA

Phenytoin
Alcohol
Carbamazepine
Benzodiazepines
Tricyclic antidepressants
Antihistamines
Dextromethorphan
Lead
5-Fluorouracil
Ethylene glycol
Primidone
Phenothiazines
Topiramate
Risperidone
Gabapentin

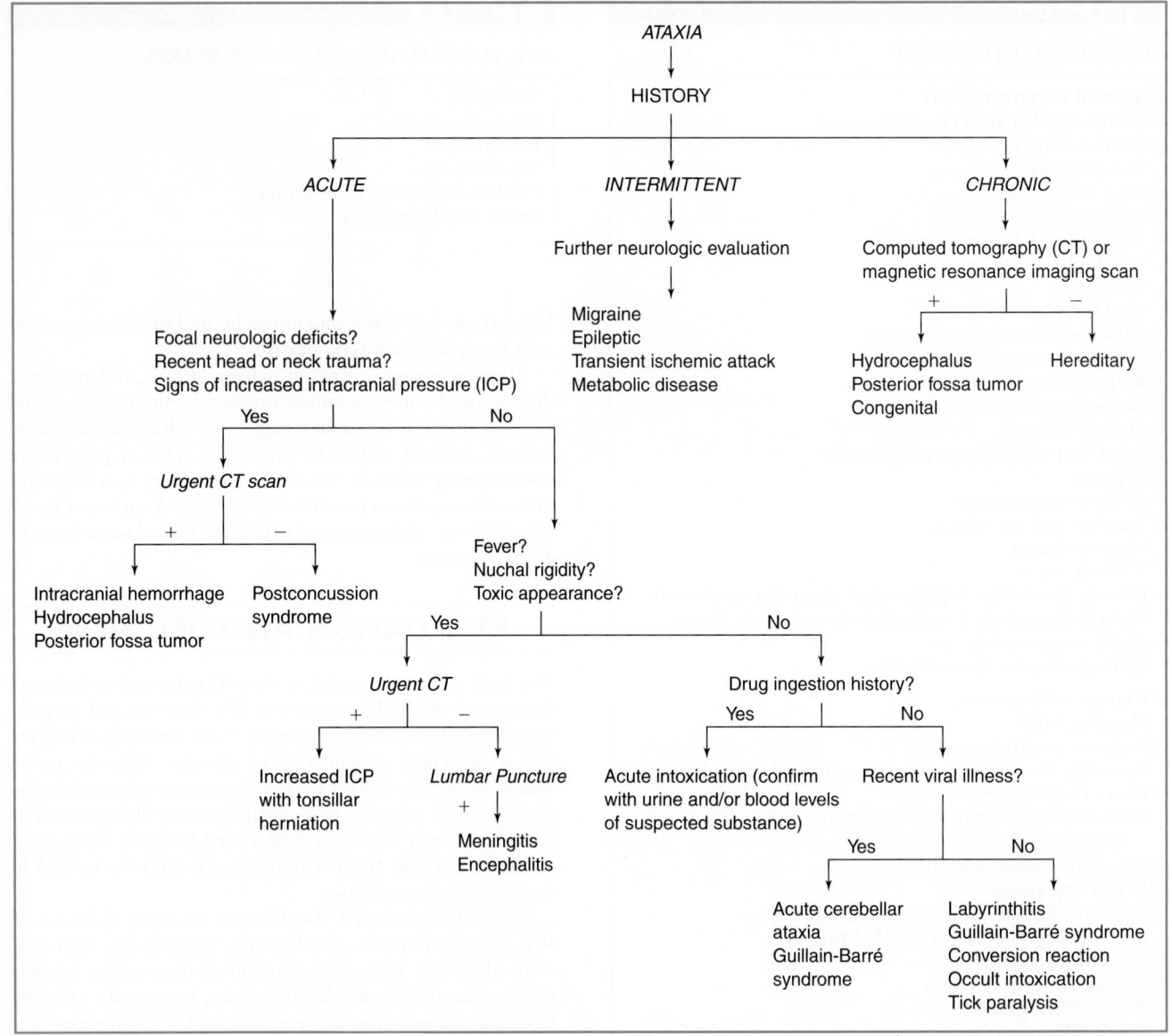

FIGURE 10.1 The diagnostic approach to the child with ataxia.

examination should document general level of consciousness, cranial nerve function, strength, tone, reflexes, sensation, and proprioception. Romberg's test will demonstrate a sensory deficit. Observation of the actual movements will help sharpen the diagnosis because particular syndromes have more truncal versus distal involvement, or unilateral versus bilateral involvement. Specific testing of cerebellar function is impossible in young children. However, a cooperative older child can be asked to perform a finger–nose–finger test, heel–shin test, and rapid alternating movements to further delineate neurologic dysfunction.

The decision to pursue specific laboratory testing is outlined in the algorithm shown in Figure 10.1. Patients with an acute presentation, focal neurologic deficits, recent head trauma, or signs of increased ICP warrant urgent evaluation via cranial computed tomography scan. Evidence of

intracranial hemorrhage, hydrocephalus, or posterior fossa tumor provides an etiology for the ataxia. Neurosurgical involvement should be sought. If the imaging study is normal, the diagnosis may be postconcussion syndrome for patients with head trauma. Consultation with a neurologist may be indicated if physical examination findings other than ataxia persist.

If the patient appears "toxic" with fever or nuchal rigidity, an emergent imaging of the head is indicated because cerebellar tonsil herniation may cause neck stiffness. If imaging results are negative, a lumbar puncture can be performed safely. When bacterial meningitis is strongly suspected, appropriate antibiotics may be administered before the testing is done.

When other causes have been eliminated, it is prudent to suspect drug or alcohol ingestion (Table 10.4). With the exception of benzodiazepines, the routine toxicologic screen of urine will not detect many of these drugs. Thus, specific blood levels are indicated when intoxication is suspected.

Management of ataxia in children is directed at the underlying cause. Fortunately, the most common cause, acute cerebellar ataxia, is a self-limiting illness that resolves completely in most cases. During periods of significant ataxia, head protection may be warranted because of the risk of falling. Also, special caution with sedatives is necessary because their effect may be greatly heightened.

Suggested Readings

Connolly AM, Dodson WE, Prensky AL, et al. Course and outcome of acute cerebellar ataxia. *Ann Neurol* 1994;35:673–679.
Fenichel GM. Ataxia. In: *Clinical pediatric neurology: a signs and symptoms approach*, 5th ed. Philadelphia: Elsevier Saunders, 2005:219–237.
Nussinovitch M, Prais D, Volovitz B, et al. Post-infectious acute cerebellar ataxia in children. *Clin Pediatr* 2003;42:581–584.
Ryan MM, Engle EC. Acute ataxia in childhood. *J Child Neurol* 2003;18: 309–316.

CHAPTER 11 ■ BREAST LESION

RAKESH D. MISTRY, MD, MS

Complaints related to the breast usually involve pain, discharge, and either discrete or diffuse enlargement. Presentation of a breast lesion in a pediatric patient in the emergency setting is uncommon; however, pediatric emergency physicians must be able to distinguish etiologies that require immediate intervention from those that are more appropriately handled by referral to a specialist or close follow-up with a general pediatrician. Fortunately, most breast lesions in children and adolescents are benign and self-limited. However, many patients and their families will benefit from reassurance that neoplastic diseases of the breast are extremely rare in all pediatric age groups. This chapter covers the spectrum of disorders that pediatric emergency physicians are likely to encounter, focuses on the diagnostic approach to breast lesions, and discusses the management of common etiologies.

DIFFERENTIAL DIAGNOSIS

Breast lesions in children can be easily divided into the following categories: infections, benign cysts or masses, malignant masses, abnormal nipple secretions, lesions associated with pregnancy and lactation, and miscellaneous causes, including both anatomic and physiologic entities (Table 11.1). A complete history and physical examination are essential to narrow the differential diagnosis and usually provides sufficient information to guide management. With few exceptions, most breast lesions require little diagnostic testing in the emergency department (ED) and typically can be evaluated using outpatient referral to an appropriate specialist. The commonly encountered disorders (Table 11.2) are almost always benign, but consideration must be given to potentially life-threatening processes (Table 11.3).

Breast Infections

Infection in the breast may take the form of a generalized cellulitis (mastitis) or an abscess. The incidence to breast infection occurs bimodally, with the early peak in the neonatal age group and the later, more common, peak in postpubertal females. Neonatal breast infection (mastitis neonatorum) most frequently presents in the first few weeks of life, commonly resulting from infection of the already enlarged breast bud produced by intrauterine maternal estrogen stimulation. As a result, mastitis neonatorum is more likely to occur in full-term, as opposed to premature infants. In some cases, excessive handling of the hypertrophied tissue by concerned caregivers may facilitate introduction of bacteria.

The most common infecting organism is *Staphylococcus aureus*; however, gram-negative enterics and group B streptococci are frequently isolated. More recent studies have demonstrated an increased incidence of community-associated methicillin-resistant *S. aureus* (CA-MRSA), and the presence of anaerobic bacteria in neonatal, adolescent, and adult breast infections.

The clinical presentation of neonatal breast infection is characterized by local signs of inflammation, such as edema, erythema, and warmth. Fever may be present in just 22% to 38% of cases and, although systemic symptoms are uncommon, the potential exists for seeding and associated invasive infections, including bacteremia, osteomyelitis, and pneumonia. For this reason, a complete evaluation for sepsis should be strongly considered in the presence of neonatal breast mastitis or abscess under the age of 2 months, especially in the setting of ill or toxic appearance. For older, well-appearing neonates, the emergency physician may elect to perform only a blood culture, and culture of purulent discharge, if present. Initial ED therapy consists of empiric broad-spectrum intravenous antibiotic for *S. aureus* (CA-MRSA if indicated by local resistance rates), group B streptococcus, and gram-negative enterics; appropriate choices may include vancomycin (no gram-negative coverage), third-generation cephalosporins, or combination therapy with a beta-lactamase–resistant penicillin and an aminoglycoside. Subsequent antibiotic therapy can be guided by the results of a Gram stain and lesion culture. For cases where a breast abscess has developed, removal of purulent material is indicated. However, great care must be taken to avoid damaging the breast bud; therefore, specialty consultation is recommended, and needle aspiration is preferred to incision and drainage of the abscess.

Breast infection in postpubertal females can be further classified as lactational or nonlactational. Lactational mastitis is discussed later in this chapter. Nonlactational mastitis and, less commonly, breast abscess can develop in the central or peripheral regions of the breast and is usually the result of the introduction of bacteria from the skin into the ductal system. These infections are more likely to occur in women who are overweight, have large breasts, have nipple piercings, or practice poor hygiene. Peripheral mastitis can be associated with diabetes, rheumatoid arthritis, steroid treatment, granulomatous disease, and trauma. Other predisposing factors for mastitis include previous radiation therapy, foreign body, sebaceous cysts, hidradenitis suppurativa, and trauma to the periareolar area. Signs and symptoms of infection include local erythema, warmth, pain, and tenderness, and may also include dimpling of the overlying skin and

TABLE 11.1

BREAST ENLARGEMENT/MASSES

I. Inflammatory Conditions
   A. Cellulitis and Mastitis
   B. Breast Abscess
II. Noninflammatory Conditions
   A. Infancy
      1. Physiologic hypertrophy
      2. Tumor (rare)
   B. Childhood
      1. Premature thelarche
      2. Precocious puberty
      3. Prepubertal gynecomastia (male)
      4. Malignancy (rare)
   C. Adolescence
      1. Male
         a. Postpubertal (physiologic) gynecomastia
         b. Exogenous hormonal stimulation
         c. Endocrinopathy
         d. Nipple cyst
         e. Malignancy (rare)
      2. Female
         a. Isolated, benign cyst
         b. Fibroadenoma
         c. Fibrocystic disease
         d. Juvenile hypertrophy
         e. Hematoma/fat necrosis (posttraumatic)
         f. Papillomatosis
         g. Cystosarcoma phylloides and other cancers (rare)

purulent nipple discharge. Systemic signs, including fever, are less commonly present. Organisms commonly implicated in this age group include both methicillin-sensitive and resistant *S. aureus*, streptococcal species, *Enterococcus*, *Pseudomonas* species, and anaerobic organism such as *Bacteroides* species.

Recommended treatment for mastitis in the postpubertal female includes initiation of antistaphylococcal oral antibiotic therapy and warm compresses. Patients should be instructed to keep the area as clean and dry as possible, to wear a clean cotton bra to help prevent excessive sweating, and to avoid

TABLE 11.2

COMMON BREAST LESIONS

Newborn
Physiologic hypertrophy
Mastitis (mastitis neonatorum)

Prepubertal Child
Premature thelarche (female)

Pubertal/Postpubertal Male
Pubertal gynecomastia

Pubertal/Postpubertal Female
Enlargement/galactorrhea secondary to pregnancy
Mastitis and Breast Abscess
Fibroadenoma
Fibrocystic disease
Benign, isolated cysts

TABLE 11.3

LIFE-THREATENING BREAST LESIONS

Newborn
Mastitis (mastitis neonatorum)

Prepubertal Child
Breast enlargement with precocious puberty (secondary to hormonal secretion by a tumor)

Postpubertal Male
Breast enlargement with abnormal sexual development (secondary to hormonal secretion by a tumor)

Postpubertal Female
Neoplastic mass
Galactorrhea secondary to prolactin-secreting tumor

skin creams or talcum powders. The majority of patients may be managed as outpatients, but require a follow-up appointment in 24 to 48 hours to ensure the infection is improving. For patients with systemic symptoms, those who appear toxic, or demonstrate a lack of response to outpatient antibiotics, hospital admission for intravenous antibiotics is indicated. If a breast abscess is suspected, confirmation via ultrasonography is preferred. Breast abscesses should be drained via needed aspiration by a surgical specialist; incision and drainage are only occasionally necessary.

Benign Cysts and Masses

Enlargement of breast tissue may occur at any age, even in the neonatal period. As previously discussed, the male and female neonatal breast bud is hypertrophied in the first few weeks of life secondary to in utero maternal estrogen stimulation. This is a normal physiologic response and will abate over time; therefore, treatment is not required and caregivers should be instructed to avoid manual stimulation. In preschool age girls, a temporary unilateral or bilateral enlargement of the breast bud may occur. This is typically consistent with isolated premature thelarche in the absence of other manifestations or development of secondary sexual characteristics. If premature thelarche is suspected, reassurance should be provided; the enlargement will most likely spontaneously resolve and can be followed up with the primary care physician. The presence of breast enlargement in young girls in the setting of secondary sexual characteristics (precocious puberty), or in young boys (prepubertal gynecomastia), is atypical, and a specific cause should be aggressively pursued. Careful history and examination focused on the presence of adrenal, ovarian, or hypothalamic pathology, including hormone-secreting tumors and intracranial tumors, are indicated in these cases. Recent medication usage should be reviewed as several medications can cause gynecomastia. Unless an intracranial mass is suspected, most young children can be referred for outpatient workup with an experienced physician or endocrinologist.

Fibroadenomas are the most common benign breast lesion in the pediatric and adolescent age groups, accounting for approximately 75% of breast masses. When present in adolescent girls, these lesions are sometimes called juvenile fibroadenomas.

Fibroadenomas are usually discovered by self-examination and present as solitary, mobile, rubbery, occasionally tender masses with normal overlying skin. Fibroadenomas are more common in African Americans and are more likely to occur in the upper outer quadrants of the breast. These lesions are benign and do not require extensive evaluation. If the emergency physician feels imaging is required, breast ultrasound is most helpful to confirm the diagnosis and exclude more severe pathologies. Of note, mammography is usually not helpful, owing to the increased fibroglandular tissue present in children and adolescents. Fibroadenomas can be observed over time, and reassurance that the malignant potential of a fibroadenoma is very low should be provided. If treatment is required, for example, with giant fibroadenomas (>5 cm), referral to a pediatric surgeon or breast surgeon for excisional biopsy is preferred.

Fibrocystic disease is a benign, progressive process that is generally seen in women during adolescence and young adulthood that may be encountered by emergency physicians. Fibrocystic masses may be solitary or multiple, unilateral or bilateral, feel nodular within the breast tissue, and are most prominent in the upper outer quadrants of the breast. Frequently, presentation is that of cyclically painful masses, with changes in size or nodularity during the course of the menstrual cycle, with the worst degree of pain during the premenstrual phase. Nipple discharge may also be present and is typically nonbloody, green, or brown. Importantly, in the pediatric and adolescent population, these lesions are not considered precancerous. Breast ultrasonography can be used to confirm the diagnosis and surgical intervention is rarely required. Treatment is largely symptomatic with breast support, nonsteroidal analgesics, and avoidance of caffeine. Oral contraceptive agents can reduce symptoms in severe cases for adults, but are not typically prescribed for fibrocystic disease in childhood and adolescent. Follow-up and subsequent evaluation by a primary care physician is recommended; referral to a surgeon for needle aspiration or excisional biopsy is indicated for painful, large, solitary lesions.

Nipple masses represent another group of generally benign breast masses. Benign intraductal papillomatosis is the most common etiology and can be seen in prepubertal or pubertal boys and girls, often coming to attention because of bleeding from the nipple. Occasionally, the lesion may obstruct the nipple and become more painful and possibly infected. In extremely rare instances, a nipple mass can represent an intraductal carcinoma. In these cases, cytologic examination of the bloody nipple discharge can be of diagnostic value. Therefore, expedient referral to a breast surgeon or pediatric surgeon is indicated after detection. In cases of benign nipple masses, careful observation for several weeks by an experienced primary care physician or surgical specialist is indicated. If the nipple mass or bleeding persists, excision is the treatment of choice.

Trauma to the breast can commonly result in the formation of hematomas and fat necrosis, both of which can be palpated as firm, well-circumscribed breast masses. Initially, these lesions may be tender. If left untreated, they may develop into areas of scar tissue that are affixed to the skin. Breast trauma and fat necrosis are relatively common, but the differentiation from other more serious lesions may be difficult, requiring consultation with a surgeon in cases of uncertainty.

Malignant Masses

Cancers of the breast have been reported in young children, but are exceedingly rare, accounting for less than 1% of all breast tumors in adolescence. In both children and adolescents, metastatic disease secondary to rhabdomyosarcoma, Hodgkin's and non-Hodgkin's lymphoma, neuroblastoma, and leukemia are far more common than primary breast malignancies. Adolescent or childhood breast tumors are often classified as secretory carcinomas that behave more benignly than breast cancers in adults. Other histologic classifications of breast malignancies reported in children and adolescents include carcinomas, sarcomas, and cystosarcoma phylloides, which can have both benign and malignant features. Physical examination characteristics suggestive of malignancy include a hard, nontender, solitary mass with ambiguous margins. The mass may be fixed to surrounding tissues, and overlying skin changes such as edema, warmth, skin dimpling, and/or nipple retraction may be present. Other signs include bleeding from the nipple and local lymphadenopathy. The appropriate treatment for suspected malignant lesions is the same as that for a benign mass–prompt referral to a pediatric surgeon or breast surgeon for definitive workup, usually consisting of excisional biopsy. Risk factors for malignant breast masses in the pediatric population include chest irradiation, such as for Hodgkin's disease or radioiodine treatment for thyroid cancer, and a strong familial history of breast malignances, such as patients who are offspring of women with inherited cancer syndromes. Important for detection of potential malignant breast masses is self-examination of the breast; adolescents should be encouraged to routinely perform self-examinations, especially if they are at increased risk of developing breast cancer.

Abnormal Secretions (Nipple Discharge)

There are multiple etiologies of abnormal nipple secretions in children and adolescents. These can be divided according to their potential for surgical management. Nonsurgical causes typically present as nonspontaneous discharges. The most common example is discharge fluid expressed during breast self-examination. The fluid may be milky, multicolored, and sticky and is a normal, physiologic discharge of little concern. When breast infection (mastitis or abscess) is present, a purulent discharge may be expressed or occur spontaneously.

Galactorrhea is the most common spontaneous nipple discharge and usually occurs bilaterally. Pregnancy and lactation are typical causes of galactorrhea; however, in the absence of these conditions, increased prolactin states should be suspected. Structural lesions of the hypothalamus and pituitary (e.g., adenomas) and exogenous medications can cause increased prolactin levels. Drugs implicated in increased prolactin secretion include oral contraceptives, tricyclic antidepressants, phenothiazines, metoclopramide, reserpine, α-methyldopa, and anabolic steroids. As mentioned earlier, in utero estrogen exposure can lead to breast bud hypertrophy in neonates; additionally, this hypertrophy can be accompanied by a colostrum-like material that has been referred to as "witch's milk." This discharge occurs temporarily, until maternal estrogen levels decline, and is not considered pathologic.

Other nonsurgical spontaneous nipple discharges have been described as multicolored, grossly bloody, serous, or clear and watery. Nonbloody discharges are rarely indicative of malignancy. Mammary duct ectasia, traumatic nipple erosions (e.g., "jogger's nipple"), and eczema are among the more common causes of nonbloody discharges. These disorders can be treated with nipple hygiene, warm compresses, and topical antibiotics, if necessary. When nipple discharge is described as serosanguinous or frankly bloody, or when it tests positive for occult blood, the potential for surgical pathology increases, particularly when a mass is palpable below the nipple. However, surgical etiologies are rare, with malignancy only present in 6% of bloody nipple discharges. More common causes include mammary duct ectasia, intraductal papillomas, intraductal cysts, chronic cystic mastitis, and pregnancy. Any pediatric patient with spontaneous nipple discharge not explained by an obvious cause (e.g., jogger's nipples) should be referred to a breast or surgical specialist for close follow-up and further diagnostic and therapeutic evaluation.

Lesions Associated with Pregnancy and Lactation

Significant changes occur in the female breast as a result of pregnancy, most prominently an increase in breast size and weight. Although pregnant patients may have any of the breast lesions seen in nonpregnant patients, they are prone to develop some unique conditions. The most frequent of these is puerperal (lactational) mastitis, which develops in up to one-third of lactating women, usually within the first few weeks postpartum. Lactational mastitis is likely to result from infection with *S. aureus*, with an increasing incidence of CA-MRSA. *Streptococcus* species, gram-negative organisms, mycobacteria, *Candida*, and *Cryptococcus* have all been implicated as causative organisms of lactational mastitis. Breast abscess may also occur secondary to mastitis and frequently requires drainage of purulent material. Treatment of lactational mastitis consists of warm compresses, antistaphylococcal antibiotic therapy, and frequent evacuation of breast milk. Breast engorgement may exacerbate the symptoms of breast infection; therefore, continued feeding or pumping is recommended. The risk of mother-to-infant transmission of infection is rare and breastfeeding can typically continue. In cases where there is substantial pain, or the infant does not like the taste of infected milk, feeding can proceed in the opposite breast. Mastitis within the first 2 weeks postpartum is often a result of cracked nipples, infant attachment difficulties, and anatomic abnormalities (e.g., cleft lip or palate); later onset is usually a result of poor hygiene or inadequate emptying of the breast with subsequent milk stasis, engorgement, and colonization of bacteria within the milk.

Pregnant patients may also have simple milk-filled cysts called galactoceles, which are often tender and located on the periphery of the breast. Ice packs, breast support, and aspiration may be needed to relieve the obstruction of the milk-filled ducts.

Nonlactating pregnant patients may develop bloody discharge from the nipple during the second or third trimester, representing a benign condition from epithelial cell proliferation. If the discharge persists after delivery, a more thorough investigation for alternate etiologies is recommended. Fibroadenomas often increase in size during pregnancy to the point of infracting and may result in significant pain. Excision is often advised for any solitary mass and the patient should be expediently referred to a breast surgeon. The number of cases of breast malignancy diagnosed during pregnancy is very low.

Miscellaneous Breast Lesions

Congenital Lesions

Supernumerary breasts (polymastia) and supernumerary nipples (polythelia) are congenital conditions that are unlikely to present as chief complaints in the ED, but that may be discovered incidentally on examination. The incidence of polymastia is unknown, but it is more common in girls and results from failure of the embryonic mammary ridges to regress. Polymastia is present at birth, often resembling skin tags or nevi, and may not be noticed until the tissue is hormonally influenced during puberty, pregnancy, or lactation. Supernumerary breasts are most commonly found in the axillae but have been reported to occur in several locations. This ectopic tissue may become tender with menses and has been reported to develop the same range of pathology as normal breast tissue, necessitating excision under certain circumstances.

Polythelia is present in 0.6% of Caucasians and 1.5% of African Americans. It is both sporadic and familial. Polythelia is most commonly found on the left, inferior to the normal nipple. In newborns, polythelia may appear as small, wrinkled lesions with or without pigmentation. The significance of polythelia is questionable. One series of patients with polythelia had a 23% incidence of associated unsuspected urologic anomalies. For this reason, patients with polythelia should be referred for at least a primary screening of underlying urologic disease. Other reported associations include pyloric stenosis, hypertension, congenital heart disease, and cardiac conduction defects. Otherwise, this disorder requires no treatment unless the diagnosis is uncertain (e.g., the lesion looks like a possible melanoma) or is perceived as a cosmetic problem.

Premature Thelarche

Premature thelarche refers to isolated breast development without other signs of puberty. Minimum acceptable ages for thelarche are 7 years for Caucasian females and 6 years for African American females. Typically appearing within the first 2 years of life in its most common form, premature thelarche is a benign, transient condition of unknown etiology. Cases of premature thelarche usually present to the ED secondary to concern raised by parents of prepubertal girls, and reassurance is usually all that is required. However, premature thelarche may be the first sign of true precocious puberty or pseudopuberty, or exposure to exogenous estrogens, and careful follow-up with the primary physician is required.

Juvenile Breast Hypertrophy

Juvenile breast hypertrophy is a rare disorder characterized by sudden, rapid, massive breast enlargement at a time of intense endocrine stimulation, usually between 8 and 16 years of age, after onset of menarche. It is believed to result from end-organ hypersensitivity to estrogen. The hypertrophy is usually bilateral and asymmetric and may progress at an alarming rate over 36 months. The differential diagnosis of this lesion includes cystosarcoma phylloides, juvenile fibroadenoma, and precocious puberty; however, true endocrine or neoplastic lesions are uncommon. In some cases, the hypertrophy regresses in 1 to 3 years, but referral to a breast surgeon is always indicated; breast reduction or even total ablation may become necessary. This disorder is often associated with extreme emotional and psychosocial distress for patients and families.

Gynecomastia

Gynecomastia is a term commonly used to describe a broad spectrum of clinical breast lesions in boys, including excess breast tissue, breast enlargement, and masses of tissue below the nipple that are discrete and nonadherent to the chest wall. Some authorities assert that it is almost always unilateral; others claim it is exclusively bilateral. Additionally, gynecomastia has been described as the male equivalent of fibrocystic changes in the female breast. Despite the confusion in the literature, histologically, there is a proliferation of dense periductal connective tissue with hyperplasia of ductal epithelial cells, which is the result of an increased effective estrogen–testosterone ratio in the serum or in the breast tissue. Causes of this relative hormone imbalance include physiologic changes (neonatal, puberty, aging); exogenous medications; tumors of the testes, adrenal glands, and lungs; metabolic conditions (cirrhosis, hyperthyroidism, renal disease); and hypogonadism.

From a clinical perspective, gynecomastia occurs in about 50% of all boys between the ages of 11 and 18 years and typically lasts about 2 years. It can be associated with growth spurts and can also cause a significant degree of pain. The glandular enlargement is about 4 cm and resembles the early stages of female breast budding. More commonly, gynecomastia will present to the emergency physician because of the anxiety in adolescent boys. If the patient with gynecomastia has normal-size genitalia and none of the predisposing conditions listed earlier, reassurance is all that is required. There is often particular concern about gynecomastia in obese boys, since they may appear to have an overabundance of fatty tissue in the breast region. Surrounding fatty tissue may also give the illusion of small genitalia; however, these patients have no higher incidence of gynecomastia than their nonobese counterparts. Rarely, a few conditions can be mistaken for physiologic gynecomastia, such as lipomastia, a round adipose tissue mass, or neoplasm. If there is any concern for these entities or systemic diseases, then the patient should be urgently referred to an endocrinologist. Overall, gynecomastia is best managed by referral to the primary care physician for continued follow-up.

Physiologic Mastalgia

During the first trimester of pregnancy, some teenage girls may complain of breast fullness. Occasionally, nongravid patients may have breast pain for which no underlying cause is grossly apparent or suspected. These patients may have mastalgia that is likely related to the hormonal milieu of the breast throughout the menstrual cycle. Mastalgia is often described as a bilateral, poorly localized, heavy, dull, achy pain that radiates to the axillae. The pain is often worse with activity and relieved with the onset of menses. In general, there are no abnormal physical findings, except tender, nodular breasts. The differential diagnosis includes costochondritis, Tietze's syndrome, cervical root syndromes, old breast trauma that has resulted in fat necrosis or hematoma, lung disease, and gallstones. Once these possibilities can be reasonably ruled out, mastalgia is the likely diagnosis. Most patients will improve with reassurance, analgesics such as nonsteroidal antiinflammatory medications, warm compresses, and breast support. If the pain is refractory to these measures, other suggested therapies include caffeine avoidance, salt restriction, and diuretics. Danazol, a synthetic androgen, is reserved for severe, debilitating pain.

EVALUATION AND DECISION

History and Physical Examination

Initial evaluation of a breast lesion begins with a careful history and physical examination (Table 11.4). The two most common categories of breast lesions presenting in children are infections and structural or mass lesions. When infection is suspected, especially in neonates or infants, particular attention should be given to the presence of systemic symptoms such as fever, chills, malaise, poor appetite, and lethargy. For the evaluation of mass lesions, it is imperative to obtain a detailed menstrual history and a chronology of the development

---

TABLE 11.4

IMPORTANT HISTORICAL AND PHYSICAL EXAMINATION COMPONENTS IN THE EVALUATION OF A BREAST LESION

History
Onset and duration of lesion
Pain
Nipple discharge
Relationship of lesion with menses
Complete menstrual and sexual development history, including sexual activity and previous pregnancies
Family history of breast disease
Diet
Medications
Concomitant medical disorders
Systemic symptoms: fever, weight loss, sweating, headaches, visual changes

Physical Examination
Breasts: symmetry, skin appearance, temperature, areola, nipples, secretions, masses, chest wall, axillae
Lymph nodes
Hair distribution
Genitalia

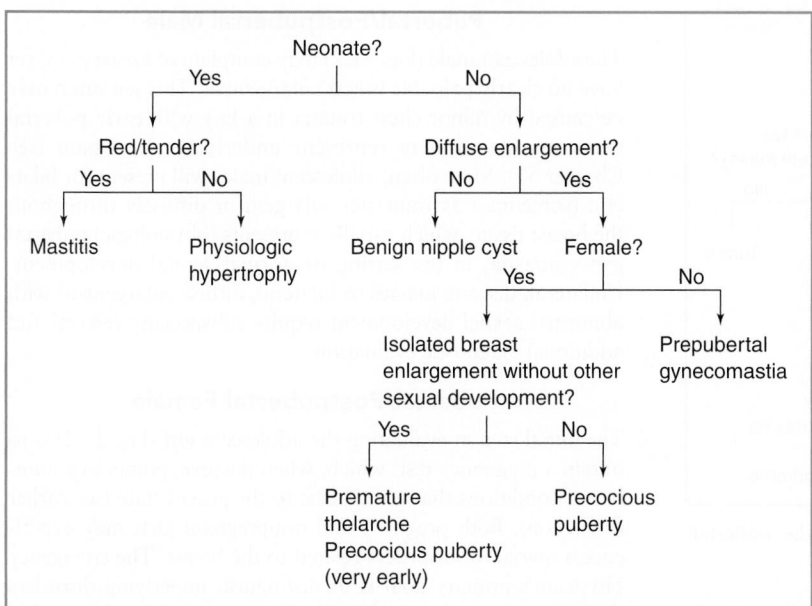

FIGURE 11.1 Approach to breast complaints in the prepubertal child.

of secondary sexual characteristics. Features of intracranial masses, including headaches or visual changes, should be assessed. Pregnant or lactating patients may also present to a pediatric ED. These patients should be queried regarding breastfeeding or breastfeeding attempts, as well as about general symptoms related to changes in the breast tissue. Medications may have an effect on the growth of certain breast lesions and may also affect hormonal pathways, leading to abnormal breast secretions. Therefore, a detailed medication history should be obtained. Few breast disorders may have a familial pattern; however, a careful family history can be helpful.

A comprehensive physical examination should be performed on any pediatric patient who complains of a breast mass or lesion. Premature appearance of secondary sexual characteristics, hirsutism, or abnormal skin coloring may indicate the presence of an endocrinopathy. A detailed evaluation of the breasts and adjacent structures is essential. The chest wall should be inspected for any gross deformities, asymmetry, or skin changes. The physician should have the patient lean forward with hands on hips and again observe for any asymmetry or skin retraction. With the patient supine with arms above the head, the physician should palpate each breast in a series of concentric circles radiating outward from the nipple, looking and feeling for nodules, cysts, masses, or inconsistencies in the breast tissue. Each areola should be gently compressed to assess for masses or nipple discharge. If present, the color, character, and odor of any discharge should be noted. The physician should feel for the presence of any masses or lymphadenopathy in both axillae.

Diagnostic Testing

The majority of patients presenting to the ED will not require intensive laboratory or radiologic testing. All postmenarchal girls should have a pregnancy test performed; breast tenderness and swelling are among the earliest signs of pregnancy. The most helpful test in the emergency setting is breast ultrasonography, which is useful in distinguishing between masses and cystic lesions as well as the presence of abscess with mastitis. Other imaging studies are rarely helpful. Mammography is of little value in children and adolescents, owing to the high proportion of fibroglandular tissue within the breast. Chest radiography is rarely helpful, except when the examiner believes that signs and symptoms from the lungs or chest wall are referred to the breast. If nipple discharge is present, Gram stain, culture, and rarely cytology can be of value. Fine needle aspiration is used in a limited fashion in children and adults, since the majority of lesions are typically benign. Serum endocrinology testing may be indicated for some breast lesions, although these generally take place outside the ED.

Approach

The approach to the patient with complaints related to the breast primarily depends first on whether the patient is prepubertal or pubertal/postpubertal. Among patients who are pubertal/postpubertal, the considerations vary greatly between boys and girls. Finally, unique considerations pertain to the pregnant or lactating girl, as discussed earlier in this chapter.

Prepubertal Child

Among prepubertal children (Fig. 11.1), the most common breast disorders are physiologic hypertrophy in the newborn period and premature thelarche in young girls. When physiologic hypertrophy is noted in newborns, erythema or tenderness should be assessed, and mastitis and potential serious bacterial infection should be considered. Breast development in prepubertal girls, without other signs of puberty, particularly in

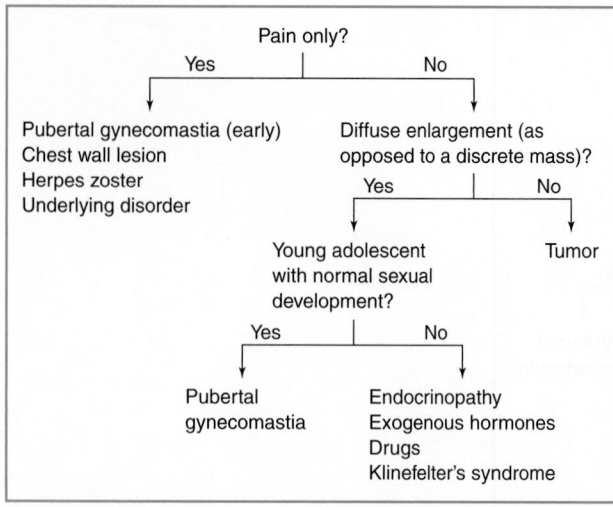

FIGURE 11.2 Approach to breast complaints in the pubertal/postpubertal boy.

those younger than 2 years of age, is likely due to the common and benign condition of premature thelarche. Nevertheless, since this may be the first sign of precocious puberty, urgent follow-up with the primary care physician and/or an endocrinologist for additional testing is recommended. Also among prepubertal children, isolated lesions underneath the nipple may be noted and are usually benign cysts.

Pubertal/Postpubertal Male

The adolescent male (Fig. 11.2) may complain of breast pain, yet have no clearly palpable breast enlargement. This sensation may be caused by minor chest trauma in a boy with early pubertal gynecomastia or may represent underlying chest pain (see Chapter 51). Most often, adolescent males will present for bilateral (sometimes asymmetric) enlargement diffusely throughout the breast tissue, which usually represents (physiologic) pubertal gynecomastia, in the setting of normal sexual development. Unilateral, discrete masses or bilateral, diffuse enlargement with abnormal sexual development require subspecialty referral and additional diagnostic evaluation.

Pubertal/Postpubertal Female

The initial step in evaluating the adolescent girl (Fig. 11.3) is to obtain a pregnancy test, which, when positive, points to a number of conditions that are specific to the gravid state (see earlier discussion). Both pregnant and nonpregnant girls may experience a myriad of disorders related to the breast. The emergency physician's primary goal is to distinguish underlying disorders that are causing chest rather than breast pain (see Chapter 51) and to assess for a few relatively minor problems, including cellulitis, abscess, hematoma, and traumatic erosions. In cases where there is concern for deeper infection or an irregular or large breast mass, breast ultrasonography can be used to rule out severe, life-threatening etiologies. Less severe causes of breast enlargement, masses, and discharge require outpatient follow-up and evaluation by an appropriate specialist.

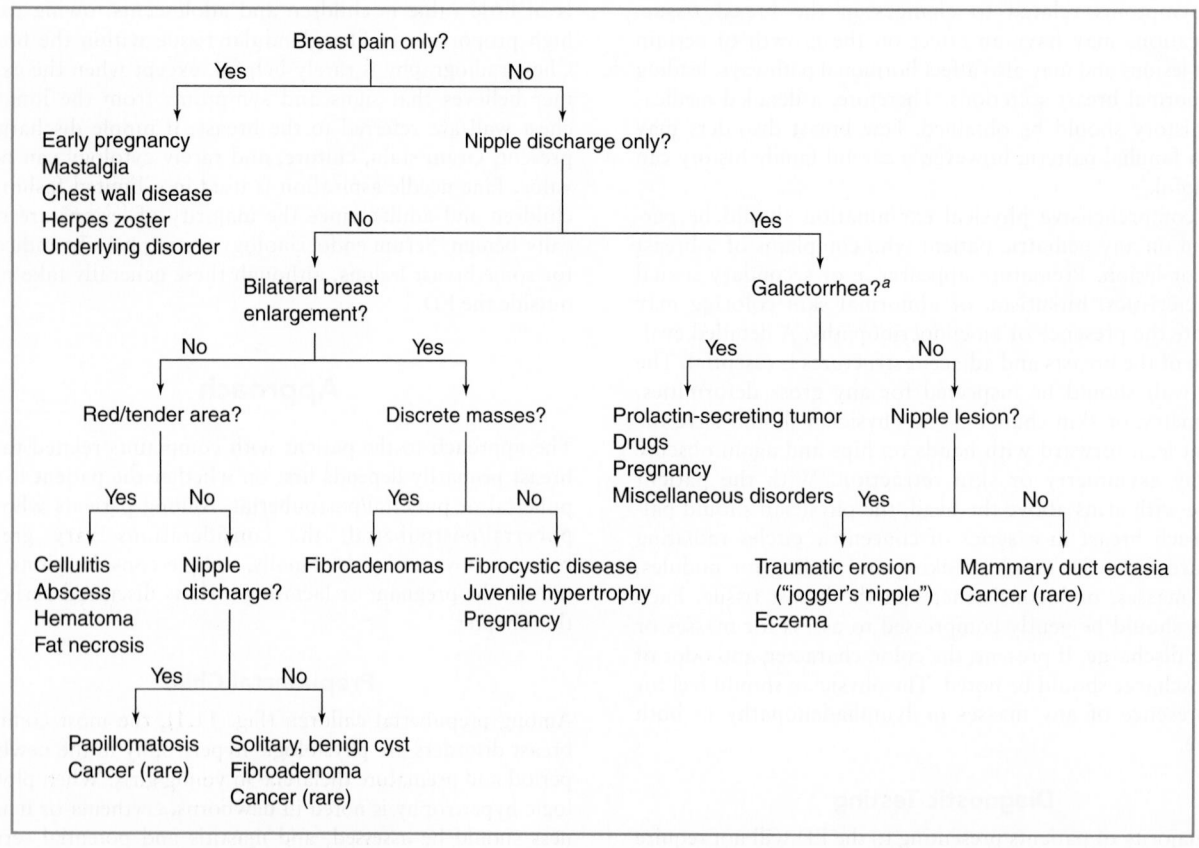

FIGURE 11.3 Approach to breast complaints in the pubertal/postpubertal girl. *a*Galactorrhea refers to milky, as opposed to bloody, serous, or purulent discharge.

ACKNOWLEDGMENT

The author acknowledges Jill M. Baren, MD, for her significant contribution to this chapter.

Suggested Readings

Arca MJ, Caniano DA. Breast disorders in the adolescent patient. *Adolesc Med* 2004;15:473–485.

Brook I. Cutaneous and subcutaneous infections in newborns due to anaerobic bacteria. *J Perinat Med* 2002;30:197–208.

Garcia CJ, Espinoza A, Dinamarca V, et al. Breast US in children and adolescents. *Radiographics* 2000;20:1605–1612.

Hansen N, Morrow M. Breast disease. *Med Clin North Am* 1998;82:203–222.

Lazala C, Saenger P. Pubertal gynecomastia. *J Pediatr Endocr Metab* 2002;15: 553–560.

Merlob P. Congenital malformations and developmental changes of the breast: a neonatological view. *J Pediatr Endocr Metab* 2003;16:471–485.

Michie C, Lockie F, Lynn W. The challenge of mastitis. *Arch Dis Child* 2003;88 (9):818–821.

Neinstein LS. Breast disease in adolescent and young women. *Pediatr Clin North Am* 1999;46(3):607–629.

Scott-Conner CE, Schorr SJ. The diagnosis and management of breast problems during pregnancy and lactation. *Am J Surg* 1995;170:401–405.

Spencer JP. Management of mastitis in breastfeeding women. *Am Fam Physician* 2008;78:727–732.

Stafford I, Hernandez J, Laibl V, et al. Community-acquired methicillin-resistant staphyloccocus aureus among patients with puerperal mastitis requiring hospitalization. *Obstet Gynecol* 2008;112:533–537.

Stricker T, Navrath F, Sennhauser FH. Mastitis in early infancy. *Acta Paediatr* 2005;94:166–169.

Templeman C, Hertweck SP. Breast disorders in the pediatric and adolescent patient. *Obstet Gynecol Clin North Am* 2000;27(1):19–34.

West KW, Rescoria FJ, Scherer LR, et al. Diagnosis and treatment of symptomatic breast masses in the pediatric population. *J Pediatr Surg* 1995;30: 182–187.

CHAPTER 12 ■ COMA AND ALTERED LEVEL OF CONSCIOUSNESS

DOUGLAS S. NELSON, MD

Consciousness refers to the state of being awake and aware of oneself and one's surroundings. It is a basic cerebral function that is not easily compromised; impairment of this faculty may therefore signal the presence of a life-threatening condition. An altered level of consciousness (ALOC) is not in itself a disease. It is a state caused by an underlying disease process, which must be addressed quickly to maximize a patient's chance of recovery. *Coma* refers to a state of complete unawareness and unresponsiveness (e.g., unconsciousness) from which a patient cannot be roused; this represents the most extreme form of ALOC. The term *coma* is often modified with descriptors such as light or deep. Lesser levels of impairment are described using other terms whose meanings may overlap. *Lethargy* refers to depressed consciousness resembling a deep sleep from which a patient can be aroused but into which he or she immediately returns. A patient is said to be stuporous or obtunded when he or she is not totally asleep but demonstrates greatly diminished responses to external stimuli. Because neurologic status may vary dramatically over time, it may be difficult to describe such symptoms using a single descriptor. Recording the comatose patient's specific response (body movement, type of vocalization) to a defined stimulus (e.g., a sternal rub) is usually preferable (Table 12.1).

PATHOPHYSIOLOGY

The state of wakefulness is mediated by neurons of the ascending reticular activating system (ARAS) located in the brainstem and pons. Neural pathways from these locations project throughout the cortex, which is responsible for awareness. If the function of these neurons is compromised or if both cerebral hemispheres are sufficiently affected by disease, an ALOC will result.

Proper function of the ARAS and cerebral hemispheres depends on many factors, including the presence of substrates needed for energy production, adequate blood flow to deliver these substrates, absence of abnormal serum concentrations of metabolic waste products or extraneous toxins, maintenance of body temperature within normal ranges, and the absence of abnormal neuronal excitation or irritation from seizure activity or central nervous system (CNS) infection.

Disorders that produce coma by raising intracranial pressure (ICP) increase the volume of an existing intracerebral component such as brain, blood, or cerebrospinal fluid (CSF). Alternatively, a new component such as a tumor may be introduced. The brain can initially compensate for this altered volume relationship by regulating blood flow and CSF production. When the limits of these compensatory mechanisms are reached, ICP will rise abruptly, decreasing cerebral perfusion pressure (defined as mean arterial pressure minus ICP) and placing the patient at risk for herniation.

Herniation, the displacement of a part of the brain from its usual position into an unfamiliar intracranial compartment, can occur in several locations within the cranium, as shown in Figure 12.1. Central herniation results from an increase in volume and pressure in both cerebral hemispheres, compressing and displacing the midbrain and upper brainstem downward through the tentorium. Cingulate gyrus herniation occurs as a result of unilateral cerebral hemisphere volume increase when the gyrus is displaced laterally underneath the falx, crossing the midline of the cranium. This unilateral volume increase may instead cause uncal herniation because the lower midline portion of a cerebral hemisphere and adjoining hippocampal gyrus are directed downward through the tentorium. Foramen magnum (or tonsillar) herniation is a consequence of increased pressure in the posterior fossa, forcing the cerebellar tonsils through the foramen magnum at the base of the skull.

DIFFERENTIAL DIAGNOSIS

A differential diagnosis for children presenting in or near coma is shown in Table 12.2. Conditions arising from trauma or disease within the CNS are separated from those affecting the brain diffusely due to extracranial problems. The more commonly encountered causes of coma are listed in Table 12.3. These most likely causes of coma should be considered in every patient presenting in this condition. Life-threatening causes of ALOC are listed in Table 12.4 and must be considered in every patient. If present, these disorders require emergent treatment. More than one problem may be present simultaneously; for example, a drowning victim may incur a head injury when falling into a swimming pool, or a deeply postictal patient with known seizure disorder may have ingested a toxin.

Primary Central Nervous System Disorders

Trauma

Coma-producing brain lesions that result from trauma include subdural and epidural hematomas, intraparenchymal and subarachnoid hemorrhage, penetrating injuries, cerebral contusion, diffuse cerebral edema, and concussion (see Chapter 116). Penetrating injuries are rare and of obvious origin. Most

TABLE 12.1

GLASGOW COMA SCALE

Eye Opening	
Spontaneous	4
To speech	3
To pain	2
None	1
Best Motor Response	
Obeys verbal command	6
Localizes to painful stimulus	5
Flexion withdrawal	4
Flexion decorticate	3
Extension decerebrate	2
No response	1
Best Verbal Response[a]	
Oriented, converses	5
Disoriented, converses	4
Inappropriate words	3
Incomprehensible sounds	2
No response	1

[a]Preverbal children should receive full verbal score for crying with stimulation.

cases of pediatric head injury are blunt in nature, involving rapid deceleration against an automobile interior or the ground. Inflicted injury is also common in young children. The site of hemorrhage may be located opposite external signs of trauma due to the rebounding of the brain within the skull after impact (contrecoup injury). Patients may present in a comatose state or may be alert for variable periods after impact. All traumatic lesions of the brain may increase ICP, which is the chief cause of the resulting vomiting, lethargy, and/or coma seen in these patients. Increased ICP reduces cerebral perfusion pressure initially and may eventually result in herniation.

Epidural hematomas are caused by bleeding from cerebral arteries or veins; 85% are associated with an overlying skull fracture. Epidural hematomas may occur after relatively minor trauma; in one series, 24 of 53 children with epidural hematoma had fallen less than 5 feet. The classic location of the injury is the temporal lobe, due to tearing of the middle meningeal artery. Such arterial bleeding produces a faster onset of symptoms such as headache, vomiting, and decreased level of consciousness (LOC) than venous hemorrhage. Approximately 40% of these patients may appear neurologically normal on presentation, during the classically described "lucid interval." On computed tomography (CT) scan, epidural hematomas usually appear sharply localized and are unilateral with a lenticular (lenslike) shape.

Subdural hematomas, produced by tearing of cortical bridging veins between the dura and arachnoid, can occur bilaterally and are five to ten times more common than epidural bleeding. They may occur on a chronic basis in young, abused children and are associated with skull fractures in 30% of cases. When imaged, these lesions are classically crescent shaped. Retinal hemorrhages may be found in 75% of abused patients with subdural hematomas.

Diffuse cerebral edema is more common than focal lesions after brain trauma and is unfortunately less amenable to neurosurgical intervention. Characteristic CT findings of loss of gray–white interface may not be visible for 12 to 24 hours after the trauma was sustained. When radiographic abnormalities appear, they may be similar to those produced by hypoxia. *Concussion* is an inexact term for a transient alteration in normal neurologic function after experiencing head trauma. A postconcussion syndrome may last for hours to days and is characterized by nausea, vomiting, dizziness, headache, and lethargy. Neuroimaging studies are normal, yet patients may be symptomatic enough to require admission for observation and intravenous (IV) hydration.

Seizures

LOC is greatly diminished both during and after periods of seizure activity. Although generalized seizure activity is readily recognizable by the rhythmic motor activity accompanying an ALOC, partial or absence seizure activity may present in a

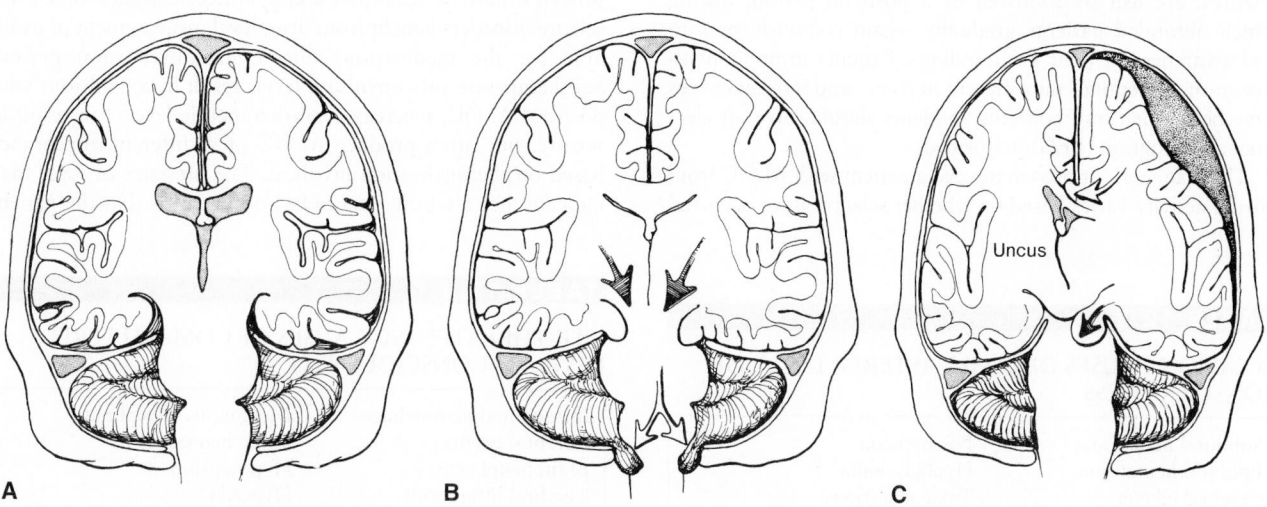

FIGURE 12.1 Intracranial contents. **A:** Normal relationships. **B:** *Dark arrows,* central herniation; *light arrows,* foramen magnum or tonsillar herniation. **C:** *Dark arrow,* uncal herniation; *light arrow,* cingulate gyrus herniation.

TABLE 12.2

ETIOLOGY OF ACUTE-ONSET COMA/ALTERED LEVEL OF CONSCIOUSNESS

I. Conditions Arising from Head Trauma or Primary Central Nervous System Disease
   A. Trauma
      1. Intracranial hematoma (subdural, epidural, intra-parenchymal)
      2. Cerebral contusion
      3. Cerebral edema
      4. Concussion
   B. Seizures
      1. Status epilepticus (convulsive, nonconvulsive)
      2. Postictal state
   C. Infection
      1. Meningitis
      2. Encephalitis
      3. Focal infections (brain abscess, subdural empyema, epidural abscess)
   D. Neoplasms
      1. Tumor (edema, hemorrhage)
   E. Vascular disease
      1. Cerebral infarct (thrombotic, hemorrhagic, embolic)
      2. Central venous thrombosis
      3. Subarachnoid hemorrhage
      4. Vascular malformation/aneurysm
   F. Hydrocephalus
      1. Obstructive (from tumor or other cause)
      2. Cerebrospinal fluid shunt malfunction
II. Conditions Affecting the Brain Diffusely
   A. Vital sign abnormalities
      1. Hypotension, hypertension
      2. Hypothermia, hyperthermia
   B. Hypoxia
      1. Pulmonary disease
      2. Severe anemia

      3. Methemoglobinemia
      4. Carbon monoxide
      5. Posthypoxic encephalopathy
   C. Intoxications
      1. Sedative drugs: antihistamines, barbiturates, benzodiazepines, ethanol, gamma-hydroxybutyrate (GHB) and analogs, narcotics, phenothiazines
      2. Tricyclic antidepressants
      3. Anticonvulsants
      4. Salicylates
   D. Metabolic abnormalities
      1. Hypoglycemia (sepsis, insulin overdose, ethanol intoxication)
      2. Hyperglycemia (diabetic ketoacidosis, hyperglycemic hyperosmolar syndrome)
      3. Metabolic acidosis
      4. Metabolic alkalosis
      5. Hyponatremia, hypernatremia
      6. Hypocalcemia, hypercalcemia
      7. Hypomagnesemia, hypermagnesemia
      8. Hypophosphatemia
      9. Uremia (kidney failure)
      10. Liver failure
      11. Acute toxic encephalopathy (Reye's syndrome)
      12. Inherited metabolic disorders
   E. Other
      1. Intussusception
      2. Hemolytic uremic syndrome
      3. Dehydration
      4. Sepsis
      5. Rheumatologic conditions (SLE, Behçet's)
      6. Psychiatric conditions

more subtle fashion with staring, tremors, eye blinking, rhythmic nodding, or other inappropriate repetitive motor activity. Seizures of all types, except absence and simple partial seizures, are usually followed by a postictal period, during which obtunded patients gradually regain responsiveness to and awareness of their surroundings. Patients in nonconvulsive status epilepticus may present in coma, and if other causes have been ruled out, comatose patients should have an electroencephalogram (EEG) performed.

The diagnostic approach toward a patient with ALOC from seizure activity varies based on whether seizures have occurred

in the past and the progression or resolution of his or her neurologic abnormalities (see Chapter 69). Posttraumatic or new focal seizures are assumed to reflect an intracranial lesion until proven otherwise. Children taking anticonvulsants for known seizure disorders benefit from drug-level measurement (if available for the medication) during an observation period. Subtherapeutic anticonvulsant levels result in convulsions with postictal ALOC, whereas supratherapeutic levels can result in seizure, but often produce ALOC of a different appearance based on the medication involved. The presence of fever may indicate that a febrile seizure has occurred or that the patient

TABLE 12.3

COMMON CAUSES OF COMA/ALTERED LEVEL OF CONSCIOUSNESS

Subdural hematoma	Posthypoxia
Epidural hematoma	Hypoglycemia
Cerebral edema	Toxic ingestions
Postictal state	Meningitis
Hypotension	

TABLE 12.4

LIFE-THREATENING CAUSES OF COMA/ALTERED LEVEL OF CONSCIOUSNESS

Intracranial hemorrhage	Meningitis, encephalitis
Cerebral edema	Toxic ingestions
Brain neoplasms	Hypotension
Cerebral infarctions	Hypoxia
Cerebrospinal fluid shunt malfunction	Sepsis

has contracted a CNS infection such as meningitis or encephalitis (see Chapters 92 and 96). The new onset of afebrile generalized seizures requires a more elaborate evaluation, as detailed in Chapter 69.

Infection

Coma-inducing infections of the CNS may involve large areas of the brain and surrounding structures, as in meningitis or encephalitis, or they may be confined to a smaller region, as in the case of cerebral abscess or empyema (see Chapter 92). Bacterial meningitis remains the most common infection severe enough to produce profoundly diminished LOC. Despite the overall decrease in cases since the introduction of vaccines effective against *Haemophilus influenzae* and *Streptococcus pneumoniae*, infections with the latter organism and *Neisseria meningitidis* still occur and are now the most common etiologic agents after the neonatal period. Meningitis may also be caused by viral (enteroviruses, herpes), fungal (*Candida, Cryptococcus*), mycobacterial (tuberculosis), and parasitic (cysticercosis) organisms. These nonbacterial infections usually have a slower onset of symptoms. The incidence of viral meningitis peaks in late summer, when enterovirus infections are most common.

Encephalitis, or inflammation of brain parenchyma, may also involve the meninges (see Chapter 92). It occurs most commonly as a result of viral infection or immunologic mechanisms. Mumps and measles viruses were common etiologic agents before immunizations against these diseases, and they still occur in unimmunized individuals. Varicella encephalitis occurs 2 to 9 days after the onset of rash. The incidence of arthropod-borne encephalitides varies by geographic location but usually peaks in late summer and early fall. The herpes simplex virus remains the most common devastating cause of encephalitis, causing death or permanent neurologic sequelae in more than 70% of patients. It affects the temporal lobes most severely (outside the neonatal period), leading to seizures and parenchymal swelling, which can cause uncal herniation.

Focal CNS infections include brain abscesses, subdural empyemas, and epidural abscesses (see Chapter 92). Brain abscesses occur most often in patients with chronic sinusitis, chronic ear infection, dental infection, endocarditis, or uncorrected cyanotic congenital heart disease. One-fourth of the cases of brain abscess occur in children younger than 15 years of age, with a peak incidence between 4 and 7 years of age. Subdural empyema also occurs secondary to chronic ear or sinus infection, but it is most commonly seen as a sequela of bacterial meningitis. Cranial epidural abscess is rare, but most cases occur from extension of sinusitis, otitis, orbital cellulitis, or calvarial osteomyelitis.

Neoplasms

Alterations in consciousness as a result of intracranial neoplasms (see Chapter 97) may be caused by seizure, hemorrhage, increases in ICP caused by interruption of CSF flow, or direct invasion of the ARAS by the malignancy (which is unlikely to cause coma of rapid onset). The location of the tumor determines additional symptoms: ataxia and vomiting for infratentorial lesions versus seizures, hemiparesis, and speech or intellectual difficulties resulting from supratentorial neoplasms. Acute hydrocephalus secondary to tumor growth most commonly presents with headache, lethargy, and vomiting.

Vascular

Coma of cerebrovascular origin is caused by interruption of cerebral blood flow (stroke) as a result of hemorrhage, thrombosis, or embolism (see Chapter 96). Hemorrhage is often nontraumatic, stemming from an abnormal vascular structure such as an arteriovenous malformation (AVM), aneurysm, or cavernous hemangioma. Rupture of an AVM is the most common cause of spontaneous intracranial bleeding among pediatric patients. The hemorrhage is arterial in origin and located within the parenchyma, but it can rupture into a ventricle or the subarachnoid space. Aneurysm rupture is less common and is unusual in that repetitive episodes of bleeding may occur ("sentinel bleeds"), with rising morbidity and mortality from each subsequent episode of bleeding. Subarachnoid blood may be present in either case, although more commonly with aneurysm rupture. Cavernous and venous hemangiomas are lower-flow lesions that produce a less acute onset of symptoms.

Stroke may also occur from thrombosis or embolism of a normal vessel. Cerebral infarction caused by occlusion of the anterior, middle, or posterior cerebral artery usually produces focal neurologic deficit, not coma. Acute occlusion of the carotid artery, however, may produce sufficient unilateral hemispheric swelling that herniation and coma may ensue; infarction may also lead to hemorrhage. Central venous thrombosis is most commonly seen with hypercoagulable states or as a sequela of infections of the ear or sinus.

Swelling or hemorrhage from infarcted brain can cause increased ICP, leading to interruption of blood flow to the ARAS and resultant coma. Focal symptoms vary based on the size and location of brain denied adequate blood supply. Vascular accidents in the cerebellum present with combinations of ataxia, vertigo, nausea, occipital headache, and resistance to neck flexion. Coma is an unusual early sign of infarction of cerebral structures but becomes more common as lower anatomic centers are affected. Occlusion of the basilar artery may result in upper brainstem infarction, resulting in rapid onset of coma, as does hemorrhage or infarction of the pons.

Cerebrospinal Fluid Shunt Problems

Children with congenital or acquired hydrocephalus as a result of prematurity, neoplasm, or trauma depend on the continued function of a neurosurgically placed shunt to drain CSF and to prevent rises in ICP (see Chapter 126). The most common shunt type is ventriculoperitoneal (VP), draining CSF from a lateral cerebral ventricle, up through a small hole in the skull, through a valve with an attached reservoir located beneath the scalp and into the peritoneum via tubing placed under the skin of the neck, chest, and abdomen. CSF shunts may malfunction for many reasons, including tubing rupture, valve malfunction, tubing blockage, tubing disconnection, and shunt infection. The risk of failure is greatest during the first 6 months after shunt placement or revision. Coma in children has also been noted after intrathecal baclofen overdose resulting from intrathecal pump misuse, or in the immediate postoperative setting after receipt of an inadvertent intraoperative bolus of baclofen.

Systemic Abnormalities

The second major category of disorders causing coma listed in Table 12.2 arises in organs other than the CNS and affects the brain diffusely. These abnormalities alter neuronal activity by a variety of means, including decreasing metabolic substrates required for normal function (e.g., hypoxia, hypotension, hypoglycemia, other electrolyte abnormalities), altering the rate of intracellular chemical reactions (e.g., hypothermia, hyperthermia), and introducing extraneous toxins into the CNS.

Hypoxia

Oxygen delivery to the brain may be adversely affected by disorders that compromise a patient's airway, breathing, or circulation. Neurons are the cells most sensitive to oxygen deprivation, and they will cease to function within seconds after being deprived of adequate levels of oxygen. Hypoxic coma may result from airway obstruction, pulmonary disease, severe acute anemia, severe methemoglobinemia, carbon monoxide poisoning, or asphyxia (e.g., drowning). Permanent CNS dysfunction results from total anoxia lasting more than 4 to 5 minutes at normal body temperatures; lesser degrees of hypoxia may be tolerated for longer periods. Submersion in cold water may cool the brain sufficiently to exert a neuroprotective effect. It is usually unclear in the emergency department how much permanent neurologic damage has taken place as a result of hypoxia. Hypercarbia may accompany hypoxia and also be responsible for neurologic depression and coma.

Cardiovascular Abnormalities

Hypotension may be the product of numerous causes, including hemorrhage, dehydration, sepsis, arrhythmia, and intoxication. The end result is poor cerebral perfusion, which produces diminished mental status (see Chapter 3). Hypertensive encephalopathy is distinguished by headache, nausea, vomiting, visual disturbance, ALOC, or coma in the presence of a blood pressure greater than the 95th percentile for age and gender (see Chapter 34). The acute onset of severe hypertension may reflect ongoing renal (e.g., unilateral renal artery stenosis, acute glomerulonephritis), endocrine (e.g., pheochromocytoma), or cardiac (e.g., aortic coarctation) pathology, or it may be the result of a toxic ingestion (e.g., cocaine). Cerebral hemorrhage may result. Hypertension or hypotension accompanied by bradycardia may indicate increased ICP.

Disorders of Thermoregulation

Hypothermia or hyperthermia in the pediatric patient is usually caused by prolonged environmental exposure to temperature extremes, such as those found in cold water or in a closed car in sunlight (see Chapter 87). The child who becomes comatose as a result of abnormal core temperature will have multiple organ system abnormalities in addition to CNS dysfunction. Mental impairment is progressive as body temperature is lowered because each fall of 1°C produces a 6% decline in cerebral blood flow. At 29°C to 31°C, confusion or delirium is present, as is muscular rigidity. Patients with core temperatures of 25°C to 29°C are comatose with absent deep tendon reflexes and fixed, dilated pupils. CNS findings in hyperthermia include headache, vomiting, and obtundation, leading to coma and/or seizures, especially above 41°C.

Toxic Ingestions

Pediatric toxic ingestions are often not witnessed, may involve a large dose on a milligram per kilogram basis, may be intentionally inflicted, and are usually complicated by the young patient's inability to provide information on the quantity or identity of the substance ingested (see Chapter 102). Table 12.2 lists many drug classes that cause coma when an overdose is taken. Exogenous toxins may impair neuronal function directly or by causing hypoxia, acidosis, enzyme inhibition, hypoglycemia, or seizures. Overdoses of street drugs, resulting in coma, have been reported in young children coerced into "body packing" drugs in their intestines.

Metabolic Alterations

Abnormal serum concentrations of any substrate or product involved in neuronal metabolism can produce ALOC leading to coma. Hypoglycemia is the most common disorder in this category, especially in infants and young children, whose capacity for hepatic gluconeogenesis is limited. Disorders known to produce hypoglycemia include serious bacterial infections, sepsis, dehydration, and toxic ingestions (especially ethanol, beta blockers, and oral hypoglycemics). Diabetes mellitus, especially of new onset, may present with profoundly depressed consciousness from the combination of hyperosmolarity, dehydration, hypotension, and lactic acidosis and ketoacidosis. Patients under treatment for diabetic ketoacidosis may also develop ALOC due to cerebral edema. Patients with type 2 diabetes may present in a hyperglycemic hyperosmolar nonketotic coma, which can be complicated by malignant hyperthermia.

Metabolic acidosis or alkalosis of sufficient degree produces ALOC. Severe dehydration that leads to significant metabolic acidosis is the most common disorder of this type seen in children. Abnormal concentrations of any serum electrolyte, including sodium, calcium, magnesium, and phosphorus, can also produce altered mental status. The degree of resulting neurologic compromise will be affected by the duration of the problem and concurrent disorders. Severe dehydration alone may also produce profound lethargy in infants and children, even in the absence of significant electrolyte abnormalities.

Other causes of metabolic coma in the pediatric age group include kidney or hepatic failure, both of which may result in progressive apathy, confusion, and lethargy. Urea cycle defects may present with ALOC and hyperammonemia in young infants (see Chapter 94). Acute toxic encephalopathy (Reye's syndrome) is a rare but devastating illness caused by mitochondrial injury of unknown origin that affects all organs of the body, particularly the brain and liver (see Chapter 96). An epidemiologic association exists between the disorder and an antecedent viral illness (including varicella) from which a patient is recovering. Patients with Reye's syndrome typically develop severe vomiting, followed by combative delirium that progresses to coma. Cerebral edema, increased ICP, and central herniation may occur with typically poor outcome.

Miscellaneous Conditions

Other causes of coma or ALOC in children are less easily categorized. Children with intussusception, the most common cause of bowel obstruction in childhood, may have significant apathy and lethargy in addition to vomiting, intermittent abdominal pain, and bloody stools. As a result, they are often treated for dehydration, sepsis, or meningitis before the appropriate diagnosis is discovered. CNS involvement in hemolytic uremic syndrome may produce a comatose state secondary to cerebral infarction, most commonly occurring in the basal ganglia. Breastfed infants of

TABLE 12.5

MNEMONIC FOR CAUSES OF COMA

DPT
Dehydration
Poisoning
Trauma

OPV
Occult trauma
Postictal or postanoxia
Ventriculoperitoneal shunt problem

HIB
Hypoxia or hyperthermia
Intussusception
Brain masses

MMR
Meningitis or encephalitis
Metabolic
Reye's syndrome, other rarities

Modified from Schunk JE. The pediatric patient with altered level of consciousness: remember your "immunizations." *J Emerg Nurs* 1992;18(5):419–421.

vegan mothers have presented in coma, suffering from severe vitamin B$_{12}$ deficiency. Children with adrenoleukodystrophy may present acutely with coma, as can those with rheumatologic diseases such as systemic lupus erythematosus and Beçhet's disease.

Psychiatric disorders may produce a true stuporous state. More commonly, neurologically intact patients attempt to feign unresponsiveness for reasons known only to them, and they may be remarkably successful at remaining immobile despite painful stimuli. The nature of their "impairment" may be discovered by a detailed neurologic examination. Conscious patients will usually avoid hitting their face with a dropped arm, may resist eyelid opening, will raise their heart rate to auditory or painful stimuli, and will have intact deep tendon, oculovestibular, and oculocephalic reflexes.

A useful mnemonic incorporating the common causes of coma in children has been proposed by Schunk and is listed in Table 12.5. It is based on the names of childhood immunizations: DPT (for *d*ehydration, *p*oisoning, *t*rauma), OPV (*o*ccult trauma, *p*ostictal or *p*ostanoxia, *v*entriculoperitoneal shunt problem), HIB (*h*ypoxia or *h*yperthermia, *i*ntussusception, *b*rain masses), and MMR (*m*eningitis or encephalitis, *m*etabolic, *R*eye's syndrome, other *r*arities).

EVALUATION AND DECISION

An approach for the evaluation of pediatric patients presenting with coma is summarized in Figure 12.2. All patients need rapid assessment of their airway, breathing, and circulation, followed by a focused history, physical examination, and consideration of laboratory and imaging studies. This approach is based on the selective use of the following critical clinical and laboratory findings: (i) vital signs; (ii) a history of recent head trauma, seizure activity, or ingestion; (iii) signs of increased ICP or focal neurologic abnormality; (iv) fever; (v) laboratory results; (vi) brain CT scan results; and (vii) CSF analysis. The

evaluation of the comatose patient should follow an orderly series of steps, addressing the more life-threatening problems of hypoxia, hypotension, or increased ICP before investigating less urgent disorders. If one or more of the former are present, immediate resuscitative efforts are begun.

History and Physical Examination

Although open-ended questions have merit in medicine, goal-directed questioning pertaining to suspected diagnoses is required in cases of coma of unknown origin. Specific queries regarding current medications, medications and substances available to ingest, seizures, fever, headache, irritability, vomiting, changes in gait, and behavioral abnormalities should be made. The most important historical finding in a comatose patient is a history of recent head trauma. If no history of head trauma is present, it should continue to be considered as a potential cause of ALOC if a pediatric patient was unsupervised at any time within 24 hours of presentation, if all caregivers are not available, or if the veracity of caregivers seems questionable.

A patient's vital signs will reveal the presence of fever, hypotension, or hypertension. The LOC of a neurologically impaired patient may initially be evaluated using a simple AVPU scale, representing four major levels of alertness: *a*lert, responsive to *v*erbal stimuli, responsive to *p*ainful stimuli, and *u*nresponsive. Elements of a more detailed neurologic evaluation are discussed in the following section.

The patient should be carefully examined for physical findings consistent with head trauma, including retinal hemorrhage, hemotympanum, CSF otorrhea or rhinorrhea, postauricular hematoma (Battle's sign), palpable or visual damage to scalp or skull, and periorbital hematoma ("raccoon eyes"). Child abuse should be suspected if unexplained bruising is present or the stated mechanism of injury is disproportionate to the degree of physical damage present. Other significant physical findings include anisocoria, absent or reduced pupil reactivity, papilledema, and nuchal rigidity. Purpuric or varicelliform rashes may signify the presence of systemic infections with CNS involvement. Incontinence of urine or stool may indicate that an unwitnessed seizure has occurred.

Neurologic Examination and Scoring

The neurologic examination of the comatose patient should include standard tests of eye opening, responsiveness to verbal and tactile stimuli, and deep tendon reflexes as well as the more specialized examinations described in this section. Any focal (unilateral) abnormal finding is always significant because it may indicate a structural CNS lesion. Abnormal findings on neurologic examination reflect the underlying pathologic condition causing coma and may allow localization of a lesion within the brain.

Patients with ALOC benefit from quantification of their impairment using standard measurements. This allows evaluation of patients' changing neurologic status over time and the recording of this information in the medical record. The effect of medical interventions may then be more easily assessed. The use of accepted scoring systems also facilitates communication

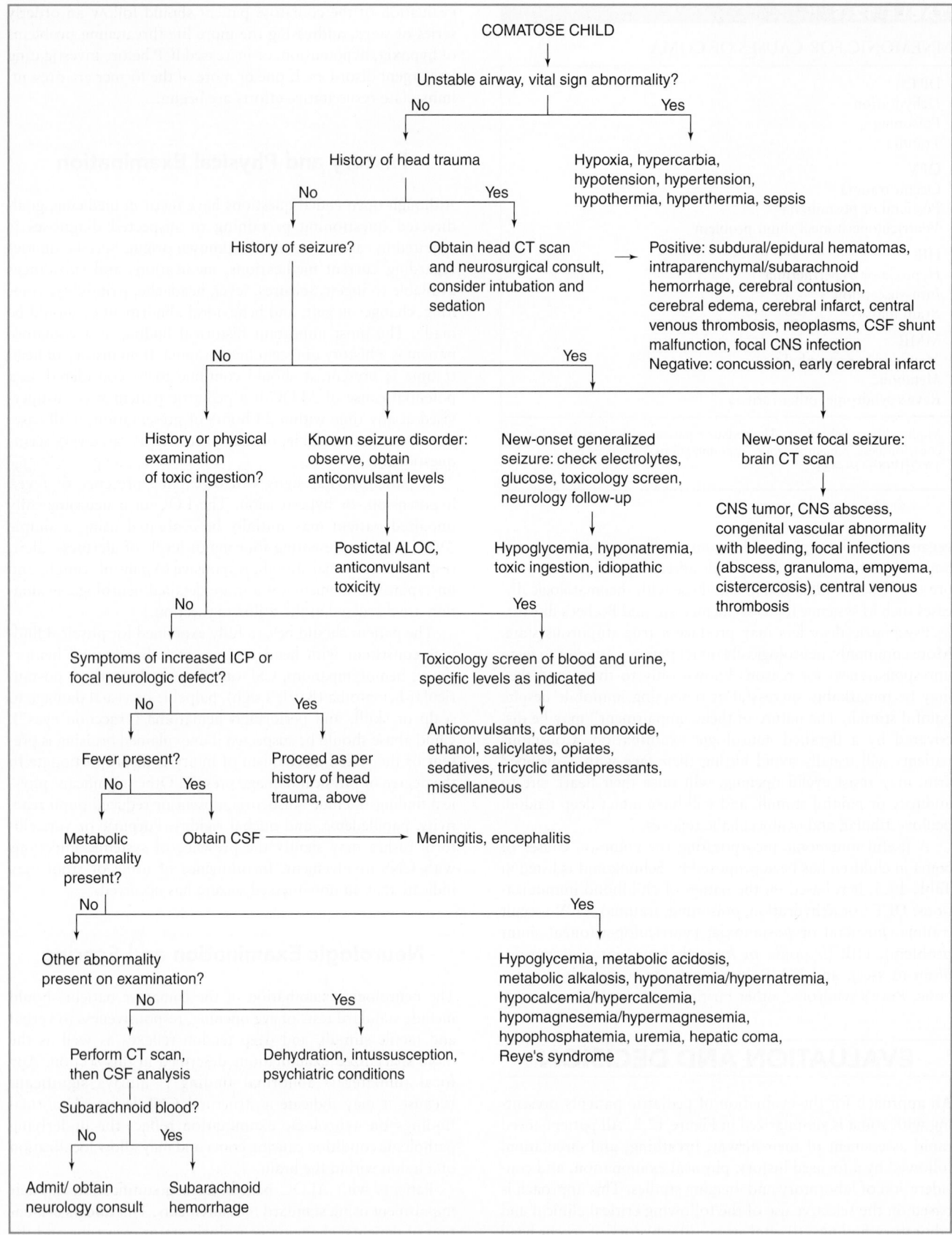

FIGURE 12.2 Evaluation of the comatose child. CT, computed tomography; CSF, cerebrospinal fluid; CNS, central nervous system; ALOC, altered level of consciousness; ICP, intracranial pressure.

with consultants such as neurologists and neurosurgeons. In addition, many outcome measures of neurologically injured patients rely on scales used to assess neurologic function. Although originally developed for trauma, a widely used measurement of consciousness is the Glasgow Coma Scale (GCS) shown in Table 12.1. Patients are graded on three areas of neurologic function: eye opening, motor response, and verbal responsiveness. A GCS score of 3 is the minimum score possible and represents complete unresponsiveness; a GCS score of 15 is assigned to fully alert patients.

Pupillary responses provide the most direct window to the brain of a comatose patient. A unilaterally enlarging pupil (greater than 5 mm) that becomes progressively less reactive to light indicates either progressive displacement of the midbrain or medial temporal lobe, or downward displacement of the upper brainstem. Bilateral enlarged and unreactive ("blown") pupils indicate massive CNS dysfunction and are most commonly seen with posttraumatic increases in ICP. Conditions affecting the brain diffusely usually spare pupillary responses. Exceptions include opiate intoxication, which may cause pinpoint pupils whose constriction is so subtle that it may be detected only with an ophthalmoscope. Intoxication with substances having anticholinergic effects, such as scopolamine, is accompanied by widely dilated pupils that may not react to light.

Other ocular signs noted in patients with depressed LOC are the roving side-to-side conjugate eye movements seen in lighter stages of metabolic coma. Persistent conjugate deviation of the eyes to one side may be caused by focal seizure activity, its resultant postictal state, or focal lesions within the brain. Ongoing seizure activity is usually apparent because of the jerking ocular movements present. Most structural brainstem lesions abolish conjugate eye movements, but it is rare for a metabolic disorder to do so. Oculocephalic reflexes (doll's eye movements) consist of conjugate turning of the eyes in the direction opposite brisk head rotation. They should not be checked in any patient who has suffered a traumatic injury because cervical spine injury may be exacerbated. In the comatose patient, the presence of this reflex implies an intact brainstem and cranial nerves. Deepening ALOC may also be measured by the reduction and loss of spontaneous blinking, then loss of blinking caused by touching the eyelashes, and finally loss of blink with corneal touch. Both eyes should always be tested to detect asymmetry. Neurologically normal patients with 30 degrees of head elevation exhibit an oculovestibular (caloric) response to irrigation of each ear with 10 mL of ice water, consisting of slow conjugate deviation of the eyes toward the irrigated ear with fast beats of nystagmus away from that side. Comatose patients with intact brainstem lose the nystagmic component and have eyes that remain deviated toward the irrigated side for several minutes.

Limb movement and postural changes seen in comatose patients include the bilateral restless movements of the limbs of patients in light coma. Unilateral jerking muscular movements may indicate focal seizure activity or generalized convulsions in a patient with hemiparesis. Decerebrate rigidity refers to stiff extension of limbs with internal rotation of the arms and plantar flexion of the feet. It is not a posture that is held constantly; it usually occurs intermittently in patients with midbrain compression, cerebellar lesions, or metabolic disorders. Decorticate rigidity, when arms are held in flexion and adduction and legs are extended, indicates CNS dysfunc-

tion at a higher anatomic level, usually in cerebral white matter or internal capsule and thalamus. Signs of meningeal irritation include Kernig's sign, resistance to bent knee extension with the hip in 90 degrees flexion, and Brudzinski's sign, involuntary knee and hip flexion with passive neck flexion.

The abnormal breathing pattern most commonly seen in comatose patients is Cheyne-Stokes respirations, where intervals of waxing and waning hyperpnea alternate with short periods of apnea. Other abnormal breathing patterns that occur with brainstem lesions include central neurogenic hyperventilation, which can produce respiratory alkalosis, and apneustic breathing, in which a 2- to 3-second pause occurs during each full inspiration.

Laboratory and Radiologic Studies

Laboratory tests commonly obtained on comatose patients include electrolytes, blood urea nitrogen, creatinine, glucose, blood gas, hemoglobin, hematocrit, osmolality, ammonia, and anticonvulsant levels. Toxicologic screening of both blood and urine should be obtained in patients with ALOC of unknown origin. If bedside glucose determination is available, it should be performed on every patient with nontraumatic ALOC. Comatose patients need IV access, and laboratory tests may often be obtained at the time of IV catheter placement. A noncontrast CT scan of the brain can reveal many of the lesions associated with coma, such as cerebral edema, hydrocephalus, malignancy, hematomas, and abscesses. Infarction and thromboses may require the addition of contrast or the use of magnetic resonance imaging scanning to be fully defined.

Vital Sign Abnormalities

Evaluation and treatment of airway, breathing, and circulatory compromise always take precedence over neurologic problems in the child with ALOC. Airway patency and respiratory effort are both compromised by decreased mental status and may result in hypoxia and/or hypercarbia. The former may be readily measured using pulse oximetry, although values will be inaccurate if a toxic hemoglobinopathy, such as methemoglobinemia or carboxyhemoglobinemia, is present. Hypoxia is usually evident by cyanosis of the lips and nailbeds and pulse oximetry values below 90% (see Chapter 15). Arterial blood gas analysis with co-oximetry is useful to quantify respiratory status and identify altered hemoglobin states. The treatment of hypoxia, regardless of the cause, always begins with supplemental oxygen.

The numerical definition of hypotension varies with age, but pallor and evidence of poor peripheral perfusion, with capillary refill time greater than 4 seconds, is recognizable even before placement of a sphygmomanometer cuff. Immediate administration of IV crystalloid therapy starting with 20 mL per kg of normal saline or lactated Ringer's solution is indicated, followed by additional boluses and vasopressors if needed (see Chapter 3). Efforts should be made during IV placement to draw blood for laboratory tests. Of the empiric antidotal therapies often used in adults, only glucose (0.25 to 0.5 g per kg) is routinely administered to children. An empiric trial of naloxone (0.1 mg per kg, max 2 mg per dose) is sometimes justified, whereas flumazenil and thiamine are given only when specific indications for their use exist (see Chapter 102).

Severe hypertension is less easily discerned on physical examination. If confirmed in more than one extremity, antihypertensives should be administered via the IV route (see Chapters 34 and 100). Mental status should improve after blood pressure is lowered to high normal levels. Patients in hypertensive crises are at risk for hemorrhagic stroke and should be evaluated with a head CT scan if they are neurologically abnormal after blood pressure lowering. Moderate hypertension in the comatose patient with increased ICP may represent a physiologic response to maintain cerebral perfusion pressure (by raising mean arterial pressure), and in this context, should not be treated with antihypertensives.

Hypothermia and hyperthermia are readily recognized once a core (rectal) temperature less than 35°C or greater than 41°C is obtained. The mental status of these patients should begin to improve as body temperature approaches the normal range. A significant percentage of patients with abnormal core temperatures have drowned, fallen through ice, or were engaged in sporting activities in extreme environments. Adolescents with hypothermia may have associated ethanol toxicity. Head trauma, hypoxia, and/or cervical spine injury may be present in these patients.

History of Head Trauma

The patient with deeply depressed consciousness (GCS score less than 9) after head trauma is presumed to have increased ICP until proven otherwise. Rapid sequence intubation with 1 mg per kg of lidocaine added to standard paralytics and sedatives (to blunt rises in ICP caused by laryngeal manipulation) is indicated. Cervical spine injury should be assumed and cervical immobilization maintained at all times. An emergent noncontrast brain CT scan should be obtained and neurosurgery consulted.

History of Seizures

The patient with ALOC in the absence of trauma should be evaluated for recent seizure activity with current postictal state (see Chapters 69 and 96). A history of previous seizures, witnessed convulsive activity, and ALOC consistent with previous postictal periods are valuable clues to this etiology of coma. Ongoing seizure activity may be revealed by the presence of muscular twitching, increased tonicity, nystagmus, or eyelid fluttering. Subtle or completely nonconvulsive forms of status epilepticus may require an EEG to diagnose. The mental status examination of the postictal patient should gradually improve over several hours. Although temporary focal neurologic deficits may follow seizures of any cause, they must be presumed to indicate the presence of focal CNS lesions until proven otherwise.

The evaluation of neurologically depressed patients with seizures varies based on the patient's history, type of seizure, and presence or absence of fever. Patients with a history of seizures should have serum anticonvulsant concentrations measured and be observed until they approach their neurologic baseline. Children who have had a simple febrile seizure (see Chapter 69) should return to their baseline state soon, usually within 1 hour. Those who remain lethargic or irritable past this point (especially after antipyretics have been administered) should be suspected of having meningitis and are candidates for lumbar puncture. Patients with new-onset generalized seizures who do not meet criteria for simple febrile seizures (see Chapters 27, 69, and 96) require more extensive evaluation, which may include measurements of electrolytes (especially sodium, glucose, and calcium), toxicologic screening, examination of CSF, and neurology consultation.

The new onset of focal seizures, with or without the presence of fever, should be evaluated with a head CT scan (using contrast when indicated) to determine the presence of a focal lesion such as a tumor, abscess, or hemorrhage. Only after the results of this study are known should a lumbar puncture be performed. If neuroimaging is unavailable and meningitis or encephalitis is a concern, empiric treatment for bacterial meningitis or herpetic encephalitis may be administered and lumbar puncture deferred (see Chapter 92).

History of Toxic Ingestions

If no history or physical examination findings suggestive of head trauma or seizures are present, a toxic ingestion should be considered, especially in toddlers and adolescents. The availability in the home of any substances capable of depressing CNS function should be thoroughly explored. In general, coma from toxic ingestions is of slower onset than that from trauma and may be preceded by delirium or other abnormal behaviors.

Chapter 102 lists major toxidromes that result from ingestions that produce CNS depression. The pupils of a poisoned comatose patient are a particularly valuable source of information. Miosis occurs with ingestions of narcotics, clonidine, organophosphates, gamma-hydroxybutyrate (GHB), phencyclidine, phenothiazines, and occasionally, barbiturates and ethanol. Mydriasis is produced by ingestions of anticholinergic agents (e.g., atropine, antihistamines, and tricyclic antidepressants) and sympathomimetic compounds (e.g., amphetamines, caffeine, cocaine, LSD, and nicotine). Nystagmus may indicate the ingestion of barbiturates, ketamine, phencyclidine, or phenytoin. Pupillary responses are more likely to be preserved in toxic or metabolic comas. Systemic toxins do not cause unequal pupils; anisocoria in the setting of ALOC should be pursued with neuroimaging.

A toxicologic screen of blood and urine should be considered in all children with coma of unknown origin. Specific assays for other chemicals may be ordered as suspected. A serum acetaminophen level should be ordered in all children with significant ingestions. Table 12.6 lists compounds capable of causing coma that are not typically detected by drug screening; the compounds are grouped by pupillary effects.

The poisoned patient with depressed consciousness should be intubated with a cuffed endotracheal tube for airway protection before decontamination efforts are made. Naloxone may be administered as empiric antidotal therapy for coma-producing toxic ingestions involving unknown medications. Flumazenil should not be given routinely to these patients because seizures may result. Its use is limited to

TABLE 12.6

POISONS UNDETECTED BY DRUG SCREENING
THAT CAUSE COMA

Miosis Present
Bromide
Clonidine
Chloral hydrate
Gamma-hydroxybutyrate (GHB)
Organophosphates
Tetrahydrozoline
Selected opiates (especially synthetic)

Mydriasis Present
Carbon monoxide
Cyanide
Methemoglobinemia
LSD

pure benzodiazepine overdoses in patients with no history of seizures or drug habituation.

Increased Intracranial Pressure or Focal Neurologic Defect

Nontraumatic causes of increased ICP or focal neurologic deficits include neoplasms, CSF shunt malfunction, and hemorrhage secondary to cerebrovascular disease (see Chapters 96 and 126). These patients may present with a history of headache, vomiting, confusion, lethargy, meningismus, focal neurologic dysfunction, seizure activity, or deep coma. Initial physical signs of increased ICP include a bulging fontanelle in infants and sluggishly reactive pupils. More severe and prolonged increases in ICP produce a unilaterally enlarged pupil, other cranial nerve palsies (III, IV, VI), papilledema, and Cushing's triad of hypertension, bradycardia, and periodic breathing. All may signal impending or progressive herniation. From the standpoint of the emergency physician, which type of herniation is present is unimportant; all are life threatening, and the initial treatment is identical for all. Endotracheal intubation using rapid sequence induction (with lidocaine administration and cervical immobilization) is performed to minimize increases in ICP while gaining airway control. Evaluation should parallel that for traumatic head injury, bearing in mind the increased desirability of using IV contrast for CT imaging. Urgent neurosurgical consultation is recommended for all patients in this category regardless of focality of scan findings. Comatose patients with a CSF shunt may need their shunt reservoir or ventricle tapped emergently to treat increased ICP.

Fever

Coma accompanied by fever indicates that CNS infection may be present (see Chapters 27 and 92). Resistance to neck flexion is the most important physical finding in meningitis, the most common infection of this type, although children younger than 2 years of age may lack this finding. Historical data may also include a steadily increasing headache, irritability, vomiting, and worsening oral intake. Kernig's and Brudzinski's signs

may be present. Other useful physical clues to CNS infection are the rashes that accompany meningococcemia, varicella, and Rocky Mountain spotted fever. The historical and physical findings in encephalitis are similar to those in meningitis; meningismus may be absent, however. Seizures are particularly common if herpes simplex is the causative agent.

A history of localized CNS dysfunction or seizures before the onset of febrile coma or the presence of concomitant focal neurologic signs may indicate the presence of a focal cerebral infection such as an abscess, granuloma, or subdural empyema. In addition, either diffuse or focal infections may present with signs of increased ICP secondary to abscess formation, cerebral edema, or blockage of CSF flow. If this is the case, a head CT scan should be obtained before lumbar puncture is performed. A contrast-enhanced study is desirable if concern about focal infection is present. The ill-appearing patient should receive antibiotics before neuroimaging is performed.

CSF analysis remains the key to establishing the diagnosis of CNS infection. Abnormalities of CSF white blood cell count (pleocytosis), glucose, and protein occur in roughly predictable patterns with bacterial or viral meningitis, and pathogens may be visible using Gram and other stains (see Chapter 92). Rapid testing with agglutination studies or polymerase chain reaction tests might also be used to identify pathogens. CSF pleocytosis in encephalitis is variable and, if present, is usually mild (less than 500 cells per mm^3), with normal levels of glucose and protein being common. CSF in herpes simplex encephalitis contains red blood cells in 50% of cases. Bloody or xanthochromic CSF under increased pressure in the absence of signs of infection indicates subarachnoid hemorrhage.

Metabolic Abnormalities

The presence of a metabolic disorder leading to coma is usually apparent once the results of routine laboratory tests are available. These values for glucose, sodium, potassium, bicarbonate, calcium, magnesium, and phosphorus make any deficiency or excess of these serum components readily apparent and treatable. Blood gas analysis for evaluation of acidosis or alkalosis from metabolic or respiratory causes may also be indicated. Decreased LOC caused by diabetic ketoacidosis may initially worsen because of a paradoxical temporary decrease in CSF pH and/or cerebral edema complicating therapy.

Renal and hepatic function should be quantified with analysis of blood urea nitrogen, creatinine, and ammonia. Markedly elevated serum blood urea nitrogen and creatinine, oliguria, hypertension, anemia, acidosis, and hypocalcemia indicate the presence of uremic coma as a result of renal failure. Hyperammonemia with decreased mental status may be caused by hepatic failure, acetaminophen ingestion with resultant hepatotoxicity, valproic acid toxicity, Reye's syndrome, or inborn metabolic errors. The hyperammonemia of Reye's syndrome is accompanied by a history of antecedent viral illness (possibly varicella) resolving within the past week and likely treated with aspirin (see Chapter 96). Unremitting vomiting is soon accompanied by encephalopathy, in the absence of jaundice, scleral icterus, focal neurologic signs, or meningeal irritation. Hyperammonemia without accompanying liver failure in the young infant may indicate the presence of a congenital urea cycle defect.

TABLE 12.7

COMMON ERRORS IN THE EVALUATION AND
MANAGEMENT OF CHILDREN WITH COMA

Assuming no head trauma has taken place if no such history
is given

Neglecting to secure the airway before imaging studies are
performed

Hyperventilating intubated patients to a P_{CO_2} well below
35 mm Hg

Not sedating patients once they are paralyzed and intubated

Believing that a toxic ingestion has not occurred because the
"tox screen" is negative

Coma of Unknown Origin

Patients with coma of unknown origin not falling into any of the
diagnostic categories discussed previously usually benefit from a
noncontrast brain CT scan, CSF analysis, and neurologic consultation, in that order. If meningeal irritation is present without
fever or other signs of infection, a subarachnoid hemorrhage
may be the cause. Common avoidable errors in the evaluation
and management of children with coma are listed in Table 12.7.
Patients presenting in a comatose state usually need admission
for continuing treatment, observation, and specialized care,
except when there is an easily recognized and reversible cause,
such as hypoglycemia in an individual with known diabetes.

Suggested Readings

Adams RD, Victor M, Ropper AH. Coma and related disorders of consciousness. In: Adams RD, Victor M, Ropper AH, eds. *Principles of neurology*, 8th
ed. New York: McGraw-Hill, 2005:302–321.

Anderson KJ, Farmer JP, Brown K. Reversible coma in children after improper
baclofen pump insertion. *Paediatr Anaesth* 2002;12(5):454–460.

Beno S, Calello D, Baluffi A, Henretig FM. Pediatric body packing: drug smuggling reaches a new low. *Pediatr Emerg Care* 2005;21(11):744–746.

Brust JCM. Coma. In: Rowland LP, ed. *Merritt's textbook of neurology*, 11th
ed. Baltimore: Lippincott Williams & Wilkins, 2005:20.

Cochran JB, Walters S, Losek JD. Pediatric hyperglycemic hyperosmolar syndrome: diagnostic difficulties and high mortality rate. *Am J Emerg Med* 2006;
24(3):297–301.

Codazzi D, Sala F, Parini R, Langer M. Coma and respiratory failure in a child
with severe vitamin B(12) deficiency. *Pediatr Crit Care Med* 2005;6(4):
483–485.

Duzova A, Bakkaloglu A. Central nervous system involvement in pediatric
rheumatic diseases: current concepts in treatment. *Curr Pharm Des*
2008;14(13):1295–1301.

Fourtner SH, Weinzimer SA, Levitt Katz LE. Hyperglycemic hyperosmolar nonketotic syndrome in children with type 2 diabetes. *Pediatr Diabetes* 2005;
6(3):129–135.

Kirkham FJ. Non-traumatic coma in children. *Arch Dis Child* 2001;85(4):
303–312.

Ravid S, Diamond AS, Eviatar L. Coma as an acute presentation of
adrenoleukodystrophy. *Pediatr Neurol* 2000;22(3):237–239.

Schunk JE. The pediatric patient with altered level of consciousness: remember
your "immunizations." *J Emerg Nurs* 1992;18(5):419–421.

Shaoul R, Gazit A, Weller B, et al. Neurological manifestations of an acute
abdomen in children. *Pediatr Emerg Care* 2005;21(9):594–597.

Theobald I, Kuwertz-Bröking E, Schiborr M, et al. Central nervous system
involvement in hemolytic uremic syndrome (HUS)—a retrospective analysis
of cerebral CT and MRI studies. *Clin Nephrol* 2001;56(6):S3–S8.

Towne AR, Waterhouse EJ, Boggs JG, et al. Prevalence of nonconvulsive status
epilepticus in comatose patients. *Neurology* 2000;54(2): 340–345.

Wong CP, Forsyth RJ, Kelly TP, et al. Incidence, aetiology, and outcome of nontraumatic coma: a population based study. *Arch Dis Child* 2001;84:
193–199.

CHAPTER 13 ■ CONSTIPATION

ROSE C. GRAHAM, MD, MSCE, AND STEPHEN LUDWIG, MD

Constipation is an important problem in the pediatric emergency department for many reasons. It is one of the most common pediatric complaints, accounting for 3% of primary care visits. There are many causes for constipation (Table 13.1), some rare and some very common (Table 13.2). Occasionally, the presentation of constipation is atypical, with chief complaints that superficially seem unrelated to the gastrointestinal tract (Table 13.3). Although relatively rare, some causes of constipation are potentially life threatening and need to be recognized promptly by the emergency physician (Table 13.4). In addition, constipation may produce symptoms that mimic other serious illnesses such as appendicitis.

DEFINITION

Although constipation most commonly is defined as decreased stool frequency, there is not one simple definition. The stooling pattern of children changes based on age, diet, and other factors. Average stooling frequency in infants is approximately 4 stools per day during the first week of life, decreasing to 1.7 stools per day by 2 years of age, and approaching the adult frequency of 1.2 stools per day by 4 years of age. Nevertheless, normal infants can range from 7 stools per day to 1 stool per week. Older children can defecate every 2 to 3 days and be normal.

It is easier to define constipation as a problem with defecation. This may encompass infrequent stooling, passage of large and/or hard stools associated with pain, incomplete evacuation of rectal contents, involuntary soiling (encopresis), or inability to pass stool at all.

PHYSIOLOGY

The passage of food from mouth to anus is a complex process. The intestine relies on input from intrinsic nerves, extrinsic nerves, and hormones to function properly. Normal defecation involves voluntary and involuntary components. Disruption of any of these can result in constipation.

The colon is specialized to transport fecal material and balance water and electrolytes contained in the feces. When all is functioning well, the fecal bolus arrives in the rectum formed but soft enough for easy passage through the anus.

Normal defecation requires the coordination of the autonomic and somatic nervous systems and normal anatomy of the anorectal region. The internal anal sphincter is a smooth muscle, which is innervated by the autonomic nervous system. It is tonically contracted at baseline. It relaxes in response to the arrival of a fecal bolus in the rectum, allowing stool to descend to the portion of the anus innervated by somatic nerves. At this point, the external anal sphincter, striated muscle under voluntary control, tightens until the appropriate time for fecal passage. Before defecation, squatting straightens the angle between the rectum and the anal canal, allowing easier passage. Voluntary relaxation of the external anal sphincter allows passage of the feces, and increasing intraabdominal pressure via Valsalva aids the process.

EVALUATION AND DECISION

The evaluation of the child presumed to have constipation should begin with a thorough history and physical examination. Special attention should be paid to the age of the patient, duration of symptoms, timing of first meconium passage after birth, changes in frequency and consistency of stool, stool incontinence, pain with defecation, rectal bleeding, presence of abdominal distention and/or palpable feces, and a rectal exam to assess anal position, sphincter tone, widening of the rectal vault, and presence of hard stool.

A complaint of constipation is not sufficient for diagnosis. A decrease in stool frequency or the appearance of straining is often interpreted as constipation. The physician should be aware of the grunting baby syndrome, or infant dyschezia, in which an infant grunts, turns red, strains, and may cry while passing a soft stool. This is the result of poor coordination between Valsalva and relaxation of the voluntary sphincter muscles. Examination reveals the absence of palpable stool in the rectum or abdomen. Complaints of constipation not supported by history or physical examination are called pseudo-constipation (Fig. 13.1).

Acute Constipation

Constipation is not a disease; it is a symptom of a problem. Constipation is acute when it has occurred for less than 1 month's duration. The patient's age and the duration of the constipation are important when determining the cause and significance of the problem.

The infant younger than 1 year of age with true constipation is particularly concerning. Potential causes include serious diseases such as dehydration, malnutrition, and infant botulism. A recent viral illness accompanied by dehydration from excessive water loss through vomiting, diarrhea, fever, and increased respiratory rate can precipitate acute constipation in an infant. Adynamic ileus or decreased intake after gastroenteritis may cause slower transit time through the colon, which can also lead to hard stools. Anal fissures and/or diaper rash

TABLE 13.1

ETIOLOGY OF CONSTIPATION

I. Functional
   A. Fecal retention
   B. Depression
   C. Harsh toilet training
   D. Toilet phobia
   E. Avoidance of school bathrooms
   F. Fecal soiling
   G. Anorexia nervosa
II. Pain on Defecation
   A. Anal fissure
   B. Foreign body
   C. Sexual abuse
   D. Laxative overuse
   E. Proctitis
   F. Rectal prolapse
   G. Rectal polyps
   H. Perianal streptococcal infection
III. Mechanical Obstruction
   A. Hirschsprung's disease
   B. Pelvic mass
   C. Upper bowel obstruction
   D. Rectal stenosis
   E. Anal atresia (newborn)
   F. Meconium ileus (newborn)
   G. Pregnancy
IV. Decreased Sensation/Motility
   A. Drug induced
   B. Viral "ileus"
   C. Neuromuscular disease
      1. Hypotonia
      2. Werdnig-Hoffmann disease
      3. Cerebral palsy
      4. Down syndrome
   D. Metabolic abnormalities
      1. Hypothyroidism
      2. Hyperparathyroidism
      3. Hypercalcemia
      4. Diabetes insipidus
      5. Renal tubular acidosis
      6. Heavy metal poisoning
   E. Infant botulism
   F. Spinal cord tumor
   G. "Prune belly" syndrome
V. Stool Abnormalities
   A. Dietary
   B. Dehydration
   C. Malnutrition
   D. Celiac disease
VI. Pseudoconstipation
   A. Breastfed infant
   B. Normal variation in stool frequency

TABLE 13.2

COMMON CAUSES OF CONSTIPATION

Functional
Anal fissure
Viral illness with ileus
Dietary

TABLE 13.3

SOME ATYPICAL PRESENTATIONS OF CONSTIPATION

Anorexia
Headaches
Lethargy
Limp
Refusal to walk
Seizure-like activity (shaking, staring spells)
Urinary retention
Urinary tract infection

after a bout of diarrhea may precipitate painful defecation, resulting in stool retention. In this case, the infant may assume a retentive posture consisting of extension of the body with contraction of the gluteal and anal muscles.

Excessive intake of cow's milk, inadequate fluid intake, and malnutrition should all be uncovered by a complete dietary history. Recent courses of medication cannot be overlooked because many can cause constipation (Table 13.5). Ingestion of lead is also a potential and serious reason for constipation.

Infantile botulism commonly presents with acute constipation, weak cry, poor feeding, and decreasing muscle tone (see Chapter 96). Acute constipation can also be a symptom of a bowel obstruction, but is normally a less prominent feature than other symptoms (see Chapter 121).

Acute constipation in the child older than 1 year of age occurs for many of the same reasons as in the infant. History may reveal recent viral illness or use of medication, as well as the presence of underlying illness, such as neuromuscular disease. Physical examination suffices to rule out anal malformations and other physical problems that could result in trouble defecating.

Chronic Constipation

Constipation of more than 1 month's duration in an infant, although probably a functional problem, is especially concerning and should prompt consideration of an underlying illness. Spinal muscular atrophy, amyotonia, congenital absence of abdominal muscles, dystonic states, and spinal dysraphism, which cause problems with defecation, can be readily diagnosed with history and physical examination.

TABLE 13.4

LIFE-THREATENING CAUSES OF CONSTIPATION

Acute Constipation
Mechanical obstruction
Dehydration
Infantile botulism

Chronic Constipation
Hirschsprung's disease
Abdominal/pelvic mass
Anorexia nervosa

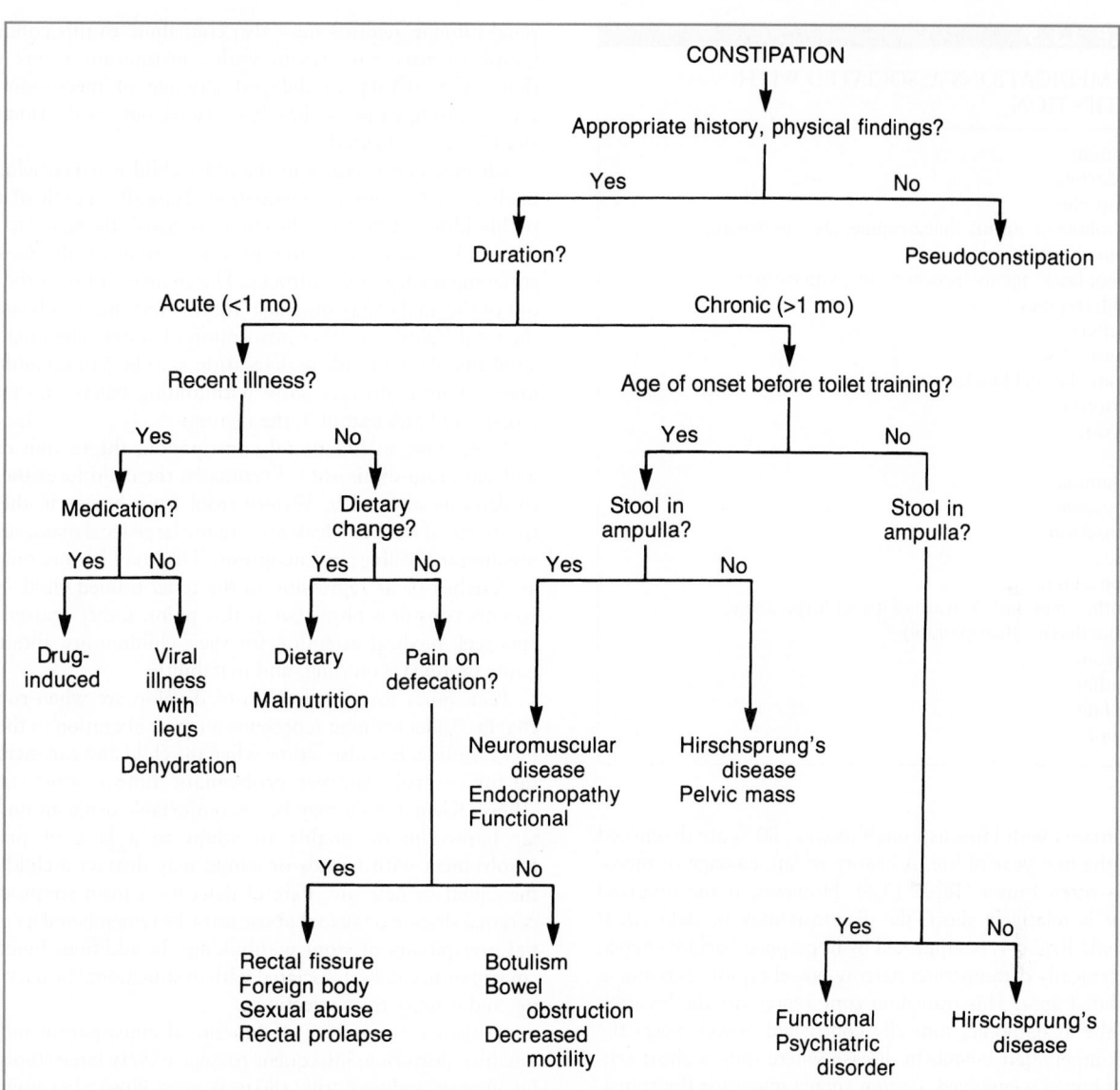

FIGURE 13.1 Approach to constipation.

Anorectal anomalies occur in approximately 1 in 2,500 live births. Anal stenosis causes the passage of ribbonlike stools with intense effort. Diagnosis is made by anal examination, which demonstrates a tight, constricted canal. The condition is treated by repeated anal dilations, sometimes over several months. The anus can be covered by a flap of skin, leaving only a portion open for passage of stool. This "covered anus" may require anoplasty with dilation. Anterior displacement of the anus is believed to cause constipation by creating a pouch at the posterior portion of the distal rectum that catches the stool and allows only overflow to be expelled after great straining. The treatment may be medical or surgical.

Hirschsprung's disease, or congenital intestinal aganglionosis, is rare but must be considered in the constipated infant because it has the potential to cause life-threatening complications. The incidence is 1 in 5,000 live births, with a male:female predominance of 4:1. As a result of failure of migration of ganglion cell precursors along the gastrointestinal tract, there is the absence of ganglion cells in the submucosal and myenteric plexuses of the affected segment. The absence of ganglion cells leaves the affected segment tonically contracted, blocking passage of stool. The segment proximal to the blockage dilates as the buildup of stool progresses. In most cases, the child never feels the urge to defecate because the blockage is proximal to the internal sphincter and anal canal.

In Hirschsprung's disease, abdominal examination often yields a suprapubic mass of stool that may extend throughout the abdomen. Rectal examination reveals a constricted anal canal with the absence of stool in the rectal vault, commonly followed by expulsion of stool when the finger is removed. The combination of palpable abdominal feces and an empty rectal vault is abnormal and must be further investigated.

Megacolon in Hirschsprung's disease can lead to enterocolitis characterized by abdominal distension; explosive stools, which are sometimes bloody; and fever progressing to sepsis and hypovolemic shock. Enterocolitis represents a major cause of mortality in this condition.

SOME MEDICATIONS ASSOCIATED WITH
CONSTIPATION

Aluminum
Amiodarone
Amitriptyline
Anticholinergic agents (benztropine, glycopyrrolate,
  promethazine)
Antineoplastic agents (procarbazine, vincristine)
Benzodiazepines
β-Blockers
Calcium salts
Calcium-channel blockers
Cholestyramine
Diazoxide
Iron
Mesalamine
Omeprazole
Ondansetron
Opioids
Phenobarbital
Phenothiazines and derivatives (prochlorperazine,
  promethazine, haloperidol)
Phenytoin
Ranitidine
Sucralfate
Ursodiol

Of infants with Hirschsprung's disease, 80% are diagnosed within the first year of life. A history of late passage of meconium is often found (Table 13.6). However, if the involved segment is relatively short, the diagnosis may be delayed. If suspected, diagnosis is supported by unprepped barium enema, which typically demonstrates narrow bowel rapidly expanding to a dilated area. This transition zone represents the location where the aganglionic, tonically contracted bowel meets the dilated, innervated bowel. In disease where only a short segment of bowel is involved, barium enema may miss the transition zone and anal manometry aids in diagnosis. Confirmation is achieved by demonstration of aganglionosis on biopsy (see also Chapter 121).

Hypothyroidism in the infant may present with constipation. Water-losing disorders such as diabetes insipidus and

FINDINGS IN HIRSCHSPRUNG'S DISEASE AND
FUNCTIONAL CONSTIPATION

	Hirschsprung's	Functional
Onset in infancy	Common	Rare
Delayed passage of meconium	Common	Rare
Painful defecation	Rare	Common
Stool-withholding behavior	Rare	Common
Soiling	Rare	Common
Stool in rectal vault	Rare	Common
Failure to thrive	Common	Rare

renal tubular acidosis may also contribute to this condition. Cystic fibrosis can present with constipation alone; when there is a history of delayed passage of meconium and Hirschsprung's disease has been ruled out, evaluation by a sweat test is indicated.

Chronic constipation in the older child is overwhelmingly likely to be functional constipation. Typically, a cycle of stool-withholding starts when the child disregards the signal to defecate and strikes a retentive posture—rising on the toes and stiffening the legs and buttocks. This maneuver forces the stool out of the anal canal and back into the rectum, which subjects the fecal bolus to further absorption of water. The longer the stool sits, the more likely defecation is to be painful and traumatic. This reinforces stool-withholding behavior, creating larger and harder stool in the rectum.

Over time, in functional constipation, the rectum dilates and sensation diminishes. Eventually, the child loses the urge to defecate altogether. Watery stool from higher in the gastrointestinal tract can leak around the large fecal mass, causing involuntary soiling, or encopresis. This may be misconstrued as diarrhea or as regression in the toilet-trained child. Many parents consult a physician at this point. Other reasons parents seek medical attention for their children are abdominal pain, anorexia, vomiting, and irritability.

Peak times for constipation to develop are when routines change. Toilet training represents a major alteration in the toddler's routine. It is also a time when the child and caregiver battle for control. Another problematic time is after starting school, when a child may be uncomfortable using an unfamiliar bathroom or unable to adapt to a lack of privacy. Involvement with friends or games may distract a child from the signal to defecate. Painful defecation from streptococcal perianal disease or sexual abuse must be remembered as potential precipitants of stool withholding. In addition, functional constipation can be associated with dysfunctional urinary voiding and urinary tract infections.

A history supportive of functional constipation includes retentive posturing, infrequent passage of very large stools, and involuntary soiling during the peak ages. Physical examination typically reveals palpable stool in the abdomen. The back should be inspected for skin changes over the sacral area, which would suggest spinal dysraphism. Normal deep tendon reflexes and strength in the lower extremities in conjunction with a normal anal-wink reflex virtually excludes neurologic impairment. The anus should be normal in placement and appearance. Rectal examination typically yields a dilated vault filled with stool. Abdominal flat-plate x-ray can be helpful but is not necessary (Fig. 13.2). Failure to thrive is not associated with functional constipation and, if present, should prompt further investigation.

Although functional constipation encompasses most cases of chronic constipation in the child older than 1 year of age, the less common causes must always be considered.

As in the infant, endocrine abnormalities and other disorders can cause and present as constipation. Hypothyroidism is often associated with constipation, as well as with sluggishness, somnolence, hypothermia, weight gain, and peripheral edema. Diabetes mellitus produces increased urinary water loss and, in the long term, intestinal dysmotility, which can lead to constipation. Hyperparathyroidism and hypervitaminosis D, which lead to increased serum calcium, cause

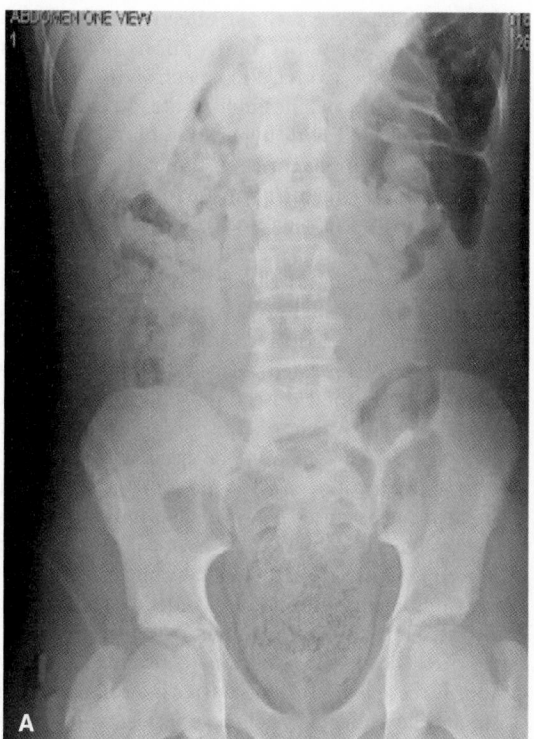 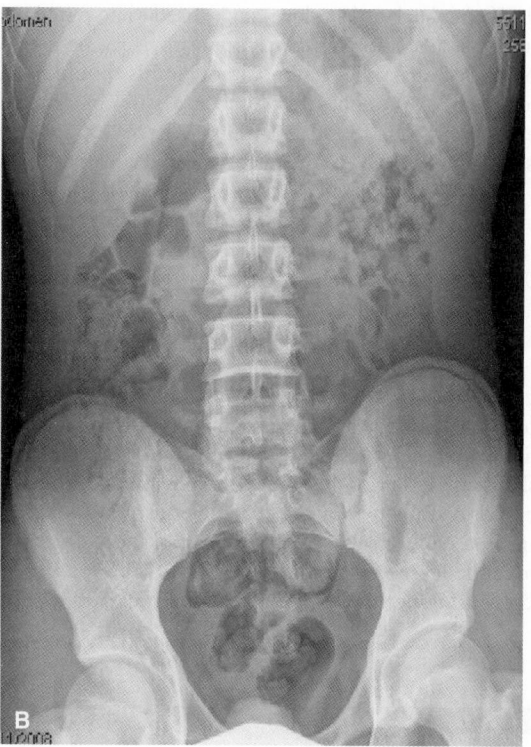

FIGURE 13.2 Both abdominal radiographs demonstrate evidence of constipation with extensive retained fecal material throughout the colon and rectum. The rectum in figure (**A**) is widened and contains a large fecal impaction while that in figure (**B**) is less widened and the stool is less compacted.

constipation through decreased peristalsis. Celiac disease is also recognized as a cause of chronic constipation.

Rarely, an abdominal or pelvic mass may present with chronic constipation. Careful abdominal examination will demonstrate the mass. Rectal masses may present similarly. Follow-up again is emphasized because a mass that does not resolve after clearance of impaction needs further evaluation. Hydrometrocolpos can present with constipation and urinary frequency; therefore, a genital examination is indicated in girls to document a perforated hymen. One must also remember that intrauterine pregnancy is a common cause of pelvic mass and constipation in adolescent girls.

Children with neuromuscular disorders often develop chronic constipation. Myasthenia gravis, the muscular dystrophies, and other dystonic states can predispose children to constipation through a number of mechanisms. A detailed history and physical examination should recognize most neuromuscular problems, allowing symptomatic treatment to be provided.

Psychiatric problems must not be forgotten in the evaluation of constipation. Depression can be associated with constipation secondary to decreased intake, irregular diet, and decreased activity. Many psychotropic drugs can cause constipation. Anorexia nervosa may present with constipation because of decreased intake or metabolic abnormalities, and laxative abuse can cause paradoxical constipation.

TREATMENT

Simple acute constipation in an infant should be treated initially with dietary changes (Table 13.7). Decreasing con-

sumption of cow's milk, possible formula change, and increasing fluid intake when appropriate may be enough to alleviate the symptoms. In addition, supplementing the diet with sorbitol as found in prune, pear, white grape, and apple juice can be helpful to soften the stool and improve stool passage. If dietary measures are not sufficient, lactulose or barley malt soup extract (Maltsupex®) may be useful as osmotic agents. Historically, Karo® corn syrup had been used as an osmotic agent, but its use has fallen out of favor after concerns that the syrup may contain spores of *Clostridium botulinum*. Stool lubricants such as mineral oil should not be used in children younger than 3 years of age and should also be avoided in some older children when aspiration is a risk. Polyethylene glycol solutions such as MiraLax® have gained increased use in the outpatient setting (see discussion below). When perianal irritation or anal fissures are present, local perianal care may decrease the risk of painful defecation, which, in turn, may decrease stool-retentive behavior. Follow-up is the most important aspect of treating simple constipation.

Therapy for acute functional constipation in the child older than 1 year of age should be the same as that for the infant, with dietary changes and stool softeners as mainstays; however, attention should also be paid to psychological factors such as recent stress that may be complicating the situation.

Treatment for chronic constipation in the infant younger than 1 year of age should include ongoing dietary measures including several daily servings of pureed fruits and vegetables, sorbitol-containing juices, and possible formula change. If dietary measures alone are insufficient to control symptoms, a daily stool softener such as lactulose can be used to help maintain soft stool passage and a glycerin suppository can be used on occasion to disimpact the rectum, although this should not be used regularly. Although safety data are still emerging, polyethylene glycol (PEG) 3350 (MiraLax®, GlycoLax®) may also be a safe and effective treatment for chronic constipation in infants. Loening-Baucke and colleagues studied 20 children and Michail and colleagues studied 12 children younger than 1 year of age, who were safely and successfully treated with PEG 3350 used for several months or more. Although more safety data is needed to make specific recommendations, this will likely become one of the therapeutic options for this age range.

Treatment (Table 13.7) for chronic functional constipation in the child older than 1 year of age begins with disimpaction and evacuation of the stool remaining in the colon. This is accomplished with either oral or rectal therapy or a combination of the two. A study by Youssef et al. demonstrated that in fecally impacted children whose palpable stool mass did not extend above the level of the umbilicus, PEG 3350 at a dose of 1 to 1.5 g per kg per day (up to a maximum of 100 g per

day) given for 3 days was an effective method of disimpaction and evacuation. Other oral options include lactulose, sorbitol, senna, bisacodyl, PEG electrolyte solution, magnesium hydroxide, and magnesium citrate. Rectal disimpaction can be accomplished with hypertonic phosphate (Fleet®) enemas or bisocodyl suppositories. A mineral oil enema administered the night before the first phosphate enema may soften existing stool, allowing less painful passage. Phosphate enemas are typically dosed at one adult-sized enema (133 mL) for patients 3 years and older, and one pediatric-sized enema (66 mL) for those 1 to 3 years of age. Phosphate enemas should not be used in children younger than 1 year. The enema may be repeated, spaced 24 hours apart, with a maximum of three total doses. Subsequent doses should only be given if evacuation of the previous dose has occurred. Phosphate enemas should be used with caution in patients with dehydration, prolonged enema retention, or renal impairment because such use has rarely been associated with severe hyperphosphatemia, hypocalcemia, and tetany, and consequent life-threatening complications. Tap water and soapsuds enemas should be avoided because of the possibility of water intoxication. Enemas will disimpact but oral agents are often needed in addition to produce full bowel evacuation. If there is no response after 2 days, more aggressive disimpaction under physician supervision is indicated. Oral phospho-soda preparations should never be used in children and have been removed from the market secondary to serious electrolyte abnormalities.

The long-term maintenance phase of therapy, which is equally as important as the disimpaction and evacuation phase, involves nonstimulant osmotic laxatives, lubricants, fluids, fiber, and behavioral therapy. Laxatives include hyperosmolar agents such as lactulose and PEG 3350. Lubricants such as mineral oil and Kondremul® are helpful to lubricate the intestine for easier passage of stool. These should only be used in children older than 3 years of age and those without a high risk for aspiration. Some have advocated the use of fat-soluble vitamin supplementation when mineral oil products are used, but there is little evidence to suggest this is truly necessary. Increasing fluid and fiber intake is also critical to long-term success in treating constipation. Table 13.8 outlines the recommended daily fiber intake for different ages. Fiber should be increased gradually toward the goal to minimize side effects of flatulence. Regular toileting should be encouraged with positive reinforcement in the school-age child. Toilet training should be discontinued in the training toddler until retentive behaviors have improved. Education of patients and parents about the pathophysiology of constipation, the etiology of encopresis when present, and the expectations of therapy are vital. Close follow-up is a mainstay of treatment. Successful therapy may take months to years to complete.

TABLE 13.7

TREATMENT STEPS FOR FUNCTIONAL CONSTIPATION: "DEFECATE"

D—Disimpact
  oral route: PEG 3350, PEG electrolyte solution,
    magnesium hydroxide, magnesium citrate, lactulose,
    sorbitol, senna, or bisacodyl
  rectal route: hypertonic phosphate enema (Fleet®),
    mineral oil enema, glycerin suppository (infants),
    bisocodyl suppository (children)
E—Evacuate/empty bowel
  PEG 3350 (MiraLax®)
  PEG electrolyte solution (GoLYTELY®)
  lactulose
  senna
  bisocodyl
F—Fluids
  increase fluid intake
  decrease caffeine intake
E—Eat fiber
  foods high in fiber
  fiber supplements such as FiberCon®, Metamucil®,
  Benefiber®, Konsyl®, and high-fiber juices (Optimize™)
    increase nonabsorbable carbohydrates (i.e., sorbitol)
C—Cathartics, softeners, and lubricants
  PEG 3350 (MiraLax)
  lactulose
  barley malt (Maltsupex®)
  lubricants such as mineral oil, Kondremul®, and Milkinol®
A—Album (diary/journal)
  daily record of bowel movements with details
T—Toileting
  set bathroom time after meals
  proper height of toilet with foot support
  reward systems/positive reinforcement
  local perineal care, ointment, sitz baths
E—Education and early follow-up
  critical for success of therapy

TABLE 13.8

RECOMMENDED FIBER DOSE IN GRAMS PER DAY

Toddler	8–10
Preschool	12–14
School-age	14–16
Adult	20–35

Approach to the Patient with Severe Chronic Constipation

Disimpaction and evacuation of stool in the patient with severe chronic constipation or one who has failed simple therapy presents a challenge, particularly in the emergency department setting. A series of phosphate enemas may not be sufficient to disimpact a larger stool mass. Use of PEG with electrolytes solution (GoLYTELY®) as a lavage either orally or via nasogastric tube at a dose of 10 to 25 mL per kg per hour up to 1000 mL per hour until stool is clear may be helpful to treat more severe impactions. This method should be done in the hospital under supervision of a physician with close monitoring of the patient's volume and cardiovascular status and electrolytes. Risks may be higher in patients with complex medical conditions such as cardiac disease. Gastrograffin or N-acetylcysteine enemas may be an additional method of disimpaction, especially in the case of distal intestinal obstructive syndrome as occurs in patients with cystic fibrosis. In cases of very severe fecal impaction, surgical disimpaction may be necessary. The use of milk and molasses enemas in children is falling out of favor in many institutions as a result of safety concerns following several case reports of serious adverse events, including one death, after administration. The other components of constipation therapy apply as already outlined previously and in Table 13.7.

Suggested Readings

Benninga MA, Voskuijl WP, Taminiau JAJM. Childhood constipation: Is there new light in the tunnel? *J Pediatr Gastroenterol Nutr* 2004;39:448–464.

Constipation Guideline Committee of the North American Society for Pediatric Gastroenterology, Hepatology and Nutrition. Evaluation and treatment of constipation in infants and children: recommendations of the North American Society for Pediatric Gastroenterology, Hepatology and Nutrition. *J Pediatr Gastroenterol Nutr* 2006;43:e1–e13.

Loening-Baucke V. Prevalence, symptoms and outcome of constipation in infants and toddlers. *J Pediatr* 2005;146:359–363.

Loening-Baucke V, Krishna R, Pashankar DS. Polyethylene glycol 3350 without electrolytes for the treatment of functional constipation in infants and toddlers. *J Pediatr Gastroenterol Nutr* 2004;39:536–539.

Michail S, Gendy E, Preud'Homme D, et al. Polyethylene glycol for constipation in children younger than eighteen months old. *J Pediatr Gastroenterol Nutr* 2004;39:197–199.

Nurko S, Youssef NN, Sabri M, et al. PEG3350 in the treatment of childhood constipation: a multicenter, double-blinded, placebo-controlled trial. *J Pediatr* 2008;153:254–261.

Pashankar D, Loening-Baucke V, Bishop W. Safety of polyethylene glycol 3350 for the treatment of chronic constipation in children. *Arch Pediatr Adolesc Med* 2003;157:661–664.

Walker M, Warner BW, Brilli RJ, Jacobs BR. Cardiopulmonary compromise associated with milk and molasses enema use in children. *J Pediatr Gastroenterol Nutr* 2003;36:144–148.

Youssef N, Peters JM, Henderson W, et al. Dose response of PEG 3350 for the treatment of childhood fecal impaction. *J Pediatr* 2002;141(3):410–414.

SIGNS AND SYMPTOMS

CHAPTER 14 ■ COUGH

RICHARD G. BACHUR, MD

Cough is a common pediatric complaint with a variety of causes. Although cough is usually a self-limited symptom associated with upper respiratory illnesses, it occasionally indicates a more serious process. Under most circumstances, history and physical examination can accurately determine the cause.

PATHOPHYSIOLOGY

Cough is a reflex designed to clear the airway. Although a cough can be initiated voluntarily, it is usually elicited by stimulation of receptors located throughout the respiratory tract, from the pharynx to the bronchioles. The receptors are triggered by inflammatory, chemical, mechanical, and thermal stimuli. Direct (central) stimulation of a cough center in the brain occurs more rarely. The reflex consists of a forced expiration and sudden opening of the glottis, which rapidly forces air through the airway to expel any mucus or foreign material.

DIFFERENTIAL DIAGNOSIS

The causes of cough differ in the type of stimulus and the site of involvement in the respiratory tract (Table 14.1). The common causes of cough are listed in Table 14.2. Potentially life-threatening causes are listed in Table 14.3.

In distinguishing the etiologies of cough, the clinician must consider features that are atypical for simple upper respiratory infections (URIs) or routine asthma. Although pertussis exists as a URI in the catarrhal phase, infants with paroxysms of coughing, color change, significant posttussive emesis or apneic episodes should be tested and managed as possible pertussis. Similarly, toddlers and young children with new onset wheezing following a choking episode, those infants with wheezing unresponsive to usual therapy, and those with persistent lobar pneumonia should be evaluated for a foreign body. Finally, children who present with cough and associated stridor may have croup, but recurrent stridor, associated dysphagia, or chronic hoarseness must be evaluated for a foreign body, extrinsic compression of the trachea (vascular ring, tumor), or laryngeal pathology (papilloma, hemangioma).

EVALUATION AND DECISION

The history and physical examination are the keys to establishing a diagnosis for cough. The first priority is to recognize and treat any life-threatening conditions. Patients with significant respiratory distress should receive supplemental oxygen and rapid assessment of their airway and breathing (Fig. 14.1).

History

Cough can occur as an acute or chronic symptom, depending on the underlying process. Most common and serious causes of cough have an acute onset (Fig. 14.1). Certain conditions, such as asthma, may present with an acute or a chronic history of cough.

The relationship of the cough to other factors is helpful. Cough in the neonate must raise the possibility of congenital anomalies, gastroesophageal reflux, congestive heart failure, and atypical pneumonia (e.g., *Chlamydia*). If the cough began with other upper respiratory tract symptoms or fever, an infectious cause is likely. A cough that started with a choking episode, especially in an older infant or toddler, suggests a foreign-body aspiration. Cough associated with exercise or cold exposure, even in the absence of wheezing, may be a sign of reactive airway disease. A primarily nocturnal cough often stems from allergy, sinusitis, or reactive airway disease. Systemic complaints should also be considered in patients with a cough: headache, fever, facial pain or pressure (sinusitis), acute dyspnea (asthma, pneumonia, cardiac disease), chest pain (asthma, pleuritis, pneumonia), dysphagia (esophageal or pharyngeal foreign body), dysphonia (laryngeal edema or tracheal mass), or weight loss (malignancy or tuberculosis).

The quality of the cough may also be helpful in localizing the process. A barking, seal-like cough with or without stridor supports the diagnosis of laryngotracheitis. A paroxysmal cough associated with an inspiratory "whoop," cyanosis, or apnea is characteristic of pertussis. Tracheitis gives a deep "brassy" cough, whereas conditions accompanied by wheezing (asthma or bronchiolitis) typically produce a high-pitched "tight" (often termed *bronchospastic*) cough. Determining whether a cough is productive can be difficult in young children who often swallow, rather than expectorate, their sputum. However, many parents can convey whether the cough is "dry" or "wet." Although a productive-sounding cough may be seen with uncomplicated URIs, sinusitis and lower respiratory tract infections are commonly accompanied by a productive cough.

Typically, the onset of cough with rhinorrhea suggests a viral URI. However, if a child with an apparent URI becomes more ill or has persistent symptoms, secondary bacterial infections and pertussis as well as other noninfectious etiologies should be considered.

Physical Examination

Patients with a cough require evaluation of the entire respiratory system. Older patients may be able to initiate a typical cough for assessing the quality, and with younger children,

TABLE 14.1

CAUSES OF COUGH IN CHILDREN

Infection
Upper respiratory infection
Sinusitis
Tonsillitis
Laryngitis
Laryngotracheitis (croup)
Tracheitis/tracheobronchitis
Bronchiolitis
Acute bronchitis
Pneumonia
Pleuritis
Bronchiectasis/pulmonary abscess

Inflammation/Allergy
Allergic rhinitis
Laryngeal edema
Reactive airway disease
Chronic bronchitis
Cystic fibrosis

Mechanical or Chemical Irritation
Foreign-body aspiration
Neck/chest trauma
Chemical fumes
Inhaled particulates
Smoking

Neoplasm
Pharyngeal or nasal polyp
Hemangioma of the larynx or trachea
Papilloma of the laryrnx or trachea
Lymphoma compressing airway
Mediastinal tumors

Congenital Anomalies
Cleft palate
Laryngotracheomalacia
Laryngeal or tracheal webs
Tracheoesophageal fistula
Vascular ring
Pulmonary sequestration

Miscellaneous
Gastroesophageal reflux
Congestive heart failure
Swallowing dysfunction
Granulomatous diseases (e.g., pulmonary tuberculosis)
Psychogenic cough
Foreign body in otic canal
Medications (e.g., angiotensin-converting enzyme inhibitors)

gentle gagging with a tongue depressor can trigger a cough. Usually, the cause of the cough can be localized to the upper or lower respiratory tract by the physical examination. Rhinorrhea, congestion, swollen turbinates, sinus tenderness,

TABLE 14.2

COMMON CAUSES OF COUGH

Upper respiratory infection	Acute bronchitis
Sinusitis	Pneumonia
Laryngotracheitis	Allergic rhinitis
Bronchiolitis	Reactive airway disease

TABLE 14.3

LIFE-THREATENING CAUSES OF COUGH

Reactive airway disease	Laryngeal edema
Croup	Pertussis
Bronchiolitis	Toxic inhalation
Foreign body	Congestive heart failure
Pneumonia	Bacterial tracheitis

and pharyngitis are all signs of upper respiratory tract involvement. Allergic features include boggy nasal mucosa, an allergic nasal crease, and allergic "shiners." An otoscopic exam may reveal a small foreign body (e.g., hair) in the otic canal, which may cause chronic cough. Laryngitis and/or stridor generally imply inflammation or obstruction at the level of the trachea or larynx. Unequal breath sounds, wheezes, ronchi, and rales are signs of lower respiratory tract disease. A careful cardiac evaluation should be performed to detect evidence of congestive heart failure, and any clubbing should be noted, as this finding is suggestive of a chronic, cyanotic condition such as cystic fibrosis. Young infants may have respiratory distress with localized upper airway congestion, but older infants and children usually have lower respiratory tract disease if significantly distressed (except in the obvious case of stridor).

Ancillary Studies

For most children with a cough, the history and physical examination should be sufficient to make a diagnosis. In patients with unexplained cough or significant or persistent pulmonary signs, a chest radiograph is warranted. In children with an uncomplicated exacerbation of their asthma, a radiograph is unnecessary. If a radiolucent foreign body is suspected, inspiratory and expiratory films or decubitus films should be obtained to detect air trapping; in cases where the imaging studies are negative, bronchoscopy may be warranted if the suspicion for aspiration is high, particularly in the case of peanuts (see Chapter 28). Other studies that could be useful in selected patients include sinus films, lateral neck radiographs, barium swallow, and computed tomography of the sinuses, neck, or chest.

In addition, laboratory tests may be necessary for specific diagnoses. Such tests include a complete blood count and differential, blood culture, tuberculin test, nasopharyngeal swab for rapid assays or culture (commonly for pertussis, respiratory syncytial virus, and influenza), Wright stain of nasal secretions (eosinophils with allergic rhinitis, neutrophils with sinusitis), and sputum culture and Gram stain (neutrophils and gram-positive diplococci with pneumococcal pneumonia). Pulmonary function testing can be useful to diagnose or follow obstructive airway disease. In cases of airway masses, airway anomalies, foreign bodies, or atypical pneumonias, bronchoscopy may be necessary.

Approach

The major considerations in evaluating a child with cough include the quality of the cough, associated choking or emesis,

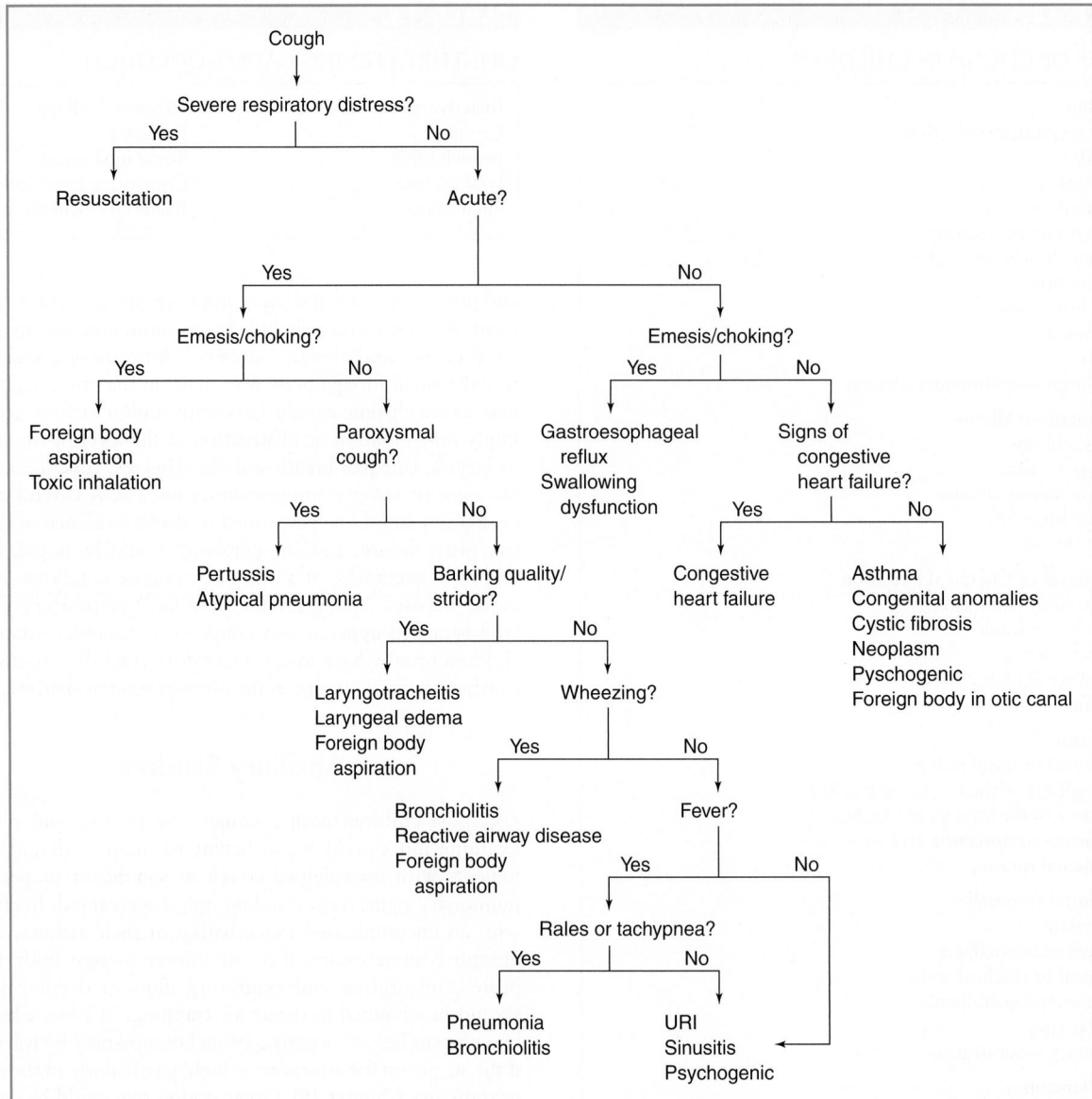

FIGURE 14.1 Approach to the child with cough.

and the findings of lower respiratory tract signs or fever (Fig. 14.1). Any child with respiratory distress needs immediate attention to their oxygenation and ventilation.

Most patients with cough of acute onset will have a simple URI, asthma, bronchiolitis, or pneumonia. A sudden onset with choking or gagging, especially in the preverbal child, is suspicious for a foreign-body aspiration (see Chapter 28). A barky cough, with or without stridor, in a child 3 months to 3 years of age suggests laryngotracheitis. Paroxysms of coughing associated with perioral cyanosis, posttussive emesis, or apnea points to pertussis. Visualizing the posterior pharynx with a tongue blade will often elicit an episode of coughing.

Physical examination should include inspection of the nares, otic canal, and oropharynx and auscultation of the chest. Wheezing indicates bronchiolitis, asthma, or, rarely, foreign-body aspiration. Patients with asthma may complain only of cough and deny any wheezing. Careful auscultation during

forced exhalation may detect wheezing or a prolonged expiratory phase. In an older child, significant lower airway obstruction can be measured with a handheld peak flow meter. Asymmetric, or focal, wheezing is seen with lower airway masses and foreign bodies. Rales, ronchi, and decreased breath sounds are characteristic of lower respiratory tract infection.

The remaining patients with a cough of acute onset will have pneumonia or a URI such as viral nasopharyngitis, sinusitis, pharyngitis, or tracheitis. Although rales, decreased breath sounds, or focal wheezing are signs associated with pneumonia, a small proportion of patients with pneumonia may not have any findings by auscultation. Therefore, in cases of significant cough, especially in very young children and those with high fever or elevated white blood cell counts, a chest radiograph is useful to exclude the diagnosis of pneumonia.

Children with chronic cough are likely to have reactive airway disease, allergic rhinitis, or sinusitis. In young children with failure to thrive or recurrent pulmonary infections, cystic fibrosis (see Chapter 99) should be considered. Chronic cough with a history of recurrent pneumonias or chronic bronchitis can also be suggestive of immunodeficiency or anatomic lesions (see Chapters 98 and 128). Choking with feeding or emesis followed by cough or wheezing in young infants is typical of gastroesophageal reflux. Newborns who exhibit a cough deserve special consideration for airway anomalies, atypical pneumonias, and congestive heart failure (see Chapters 84, 92, 98, and 123). Persistent cough during the day that stops with distraction or sleep is supportive of a psychogenic cause.

TREATMENT

The primary goal should be to treat the underlying process rather than to attempt to suppress the cough. Patients with any distress need supplemental oxygen and immediate assessment of the airway and breathing. Wheezing from asthma is primarily treated with inhaled beta-2 agonists (see Chapter 82). The treatment for bronchiolitis is mainly supportive; a trial of a bronchodilator may be beneficial in a fraction of infants. In children with suspected reactive airway disease based on history alone, a trial of bronchodilator therapy is warranted. Follow-up with the primary care physician is crucial for establishing a treatment plan. Children with suspected foreign bodies or airway masses (intrinsic or extrinsic to the airway) need appropriate intervention for their removal. Croup treatment consists of mist therapy in mild cases, and racemic epinephrine, steroids, and oxygen for more severe episodes. Treatment of pneumonia depends on the age and suspected pathogen. Patients with pertussis require antibiotics for eradication of the organism, and young infants or any child with significant paroxysms need hospitalization.

Antitussive medications have limited value and should not be used routinely in young infants. It is better to give specific therapy (bronchodilators in asthma, antibiotics in sinusitis) and avoid suppressing a cough in conditions with increased sputum production (e.g., asthma, pneumonia). In older children with a nonproductive cough that interrupts sleep, antitussives can be prescribed. Using cool mist humidifiers and elevating the head during sleep can be beneficial for coughs associated with viral URIs.

Suggested Readings

Asilsoy S, Bayram E, Agin H, et al. Evaluation of chronic cough in children. *Chest* 2008;134(6):1122–1128.

Bisgaard H, Szefler S. Prevalence of asthma-like symptoms in young children. *Pediatr Pulmonol* 2007;42(8):723–728.

Callahan CW. Etiology of chronic cough in a population of children referred to a pediatric pulmonologist. *J Am Board Fam Pract* 1996;9(5):324–327.

Chang AB, Glomb WB. Guidelines for evaluating chronic cough in pediatrics: ACCP evidence-based clinical practice guidelines. *Chest* 2006;129 (1 suppl):260S–283S.

de Jongste JC, Shields MD. Cough. 2: chronic cough in children. *Thorax* 2003;58(11):998–1003.

Eigen H. The clinical evaluation of chronic cough. *Pediatr Clin North Am* 1982;29(1):67–78.

Farah MM, Padgett LB, McLario DJ, et al. First-time wheezing in infants during respiratory syncytial virus season: chest radiograph findings. *Pediatr Emerg Care* 2002;18(5):333–336.

Gern JE, Lemanske RF Jr. Infectious triggers of pediatric asthma. *Pediatr Clin North Am* 2003;50(3):555–575, vi.

Gilger MA. Pediatric otolaryngologic manifestations of gastroesophageal reflux disease. *Curr Gastroenterol Rep* 2003;5(3):247–252.

Halstead LA. Role of gastroesophageal reflux in pediatric upper airway disorders. *Otolaryngol Head Neck Surg* 1999;120(2):208–214.

Klig JE. Current challenges in lower respiratory infections in children. *Curr Opin Pediatr* 2004; 16(1):107–112.

Lerou PH. Lower respiratory tract infections in children. *Curr Opin Pediatr* 2001; 13(2):200–206.

Mackey JE, Wojcik S, Long R, et al. Predicting pertussis in a pediatric emergency department population. *Clin Pediatr (Phila)* 2007;46(5):437–440.

McGuirt WF Jr. Gastroesophageal reflux and the upper airway. *Pediatr Clin North Am* 2003; 50(2):487–502.

Murphy CG, van de Pol AC, Harper MB, et al. Clinical predictors of occult pneumonia in the febrile child. *Acad Emerg Med* 2007;14(3):243–249.

Rachelefsky GS, Katz RM, Siegel SC. Chronic sinusitis in the allergic child. *Pediatr Clin North Am* 1988;35(5):1091–1101.

Roback MG, Dreitlein DA. Chest radiograph in the evaluation of first time wheezing episodes: review of current clinical practice and efficacy. *Pediatr Emerg Care* 1998;14(3):181–184.

Vernacchio L, Kelly JP, Kaufman DW, et al. Cough and cold medication use by US children, 1999–2006: results from the slone survey. *Pediatrics* 2008;122(2):e323–e329.

Walsh-Kelly CM, Hennes HM. Do clinical variables predict pathologic radiographs in the first episode of wheezing? *Pediatr Emerg Care* 2002; 18(1):8–11.

Yellon RF, Goldberg H. Update on gastroesophageal reflux disease in pediatric airway disorders. *Am J Med* 2001;111(suppl 8A):78S–84S.

SIGNS AND SYMPTOMS

CHAPTER 15 ■ CYANOSIS

ANNE M. STACK, MD

Cyanosis, a bluish-purple discoloration of the tissues, is a disturbing condition commonly confronted by the pediatric emergency physician. It is most easily appreciated in the lips, nail beds, earlobes, mucous membranes, and locations where the skin is thin and may be enhanced or obscured by lighting conditions and skin pigmentation.

PATHOPHYSIOLOGY

The three factors that ultimately determine the occurrence of cyanosis are the total amount of hemoglobin (Hb) in the blood, the degree of Hb oxygen saturation or qualitative changes in the Hb, and the state of the circulation.

Oxygenated Hb is bright red, and deoxygenated Hb is purple. Cyanosis is evident when the reduced or deoxygenated Hb in the blood exceeds 5 g per 100 mL or when oxygen saturation approaches 85%. When the total amount of Hb in the blood is increased, as in polycythemia, this substantial contribution is evident in the overall appearance of the patient from the increased red blood cell mass, and the patient may appear ruddy. The relative increase in the amount of unsaturated Hb in the polycythemic patient will add a blue hue to the skin. Conversely, when the total amount of Hb is decreased, as in anemia, the patient appears pale, and even if Hb is desaturated, cyanosis may not appear.

The degree of Hb saturation is determined by several factors, including the partial pressure of oxygen (PO_2) in the alveolus, the ability of oxygen (O_2) to diffuse across the alveolar epithelial cell wall into the capillary bed and subsequently into the red cell itself, and the Hb molecule. First, because the PO_2 in the alveolus is determined by a balance between the amount of O_2 added during alveolar ventilation and that removed by blood flow throughout the alveolar capillary bed, if the level of alveolar ventilation falls, so does the PO_2 of alveolar gas, causing a fall in arterial PO_2 and desaturation. Second, the ability of O_2 to diffuse across the alveolar wall into the red cell, or gas–blood barrier, is greatly affected by the circumstances of the barrier itself. According to *Fick's law*, the volume of gas per unit time moving across a tissue sheet is directly proportional to the area of the sheet and the difference in partial pressures between the two sides but inversely proportional to the thickness. Any condition that diminishes surface area or increases the thickness will decrease the amount of O_2 in the blood. Third, the Hb molecule itself has unique properties that affect the amount of oxygen it can carry. Although the complexities of Hb and its ability to carry O_2 are beyond the scope of this chapter, to understand cyanosis it is critical to note that the color of whole blood is in part determined by the state of the Hb molecule. Oxygen binds reversibly to the iron molecule

of the Hb subunit, changing its conformation, and oxygenated Hb is bright red. Consequently, factors that affect O_2 binding to Hb will affect the color of the blood. For example, carbon monoxide competitively binds to the ferrous portion of heme, but at an affinity 200 times more than that of oxygen. The change in conformation of Hb with carbon monoxide occupying all the iron in the heme tetramer gives carboxyhemoglobin a cherry red hue, despite the fact that little oxygen is bound to the Hb molecule. In addition, when heme iron is oxidized to the ferric state (it is normally in the ferrous state, even when bound to O_2), known as methemoglobin, it is also incapable of binding O_2. Therefore, Hb will remain deoxygenated, and methemoglobin itself is a brownish-purple color.

The state of the circulation plays an important role in the presence and degree of cyanosis. If a shunt is present, cyanosis can result. A *shunt* is defined as a mechanism by which blood that has not traveled through the ventilated alveolar capillary bed mixes with arterial blood. Deoxygenated blood mixing with oxygenated blood reduces the arterial PO_2, and if the shunt is large, the reduction in PO_2 can be severe, leading to marked cyanosis. Another contribution from the state of the circulation on presence of cyanosis concerns blood as it travels through a capillary bed. Oxygen is unloaded to the tissues as blood travels through a capillary, with the relative concentration of unsaturated Hb increasing from one end of the capillary bed to the other. Factors that slow blood flow, such as poor perfusion states and cold temperature, favor the unloading of oxygen and thus increase the amount of unsaturated Hb in the tissue capillaries. A third contribution from the circulation concerns the ratio of blood flow to ventilation within the lung. Simply stated, in an upright lung, the apex is ventilated more than the base, and the base is perfused more than the apex. Because most of the blood flow in the lung then comes from the relatively less ventilated areas of the lung, depression of the blood PO_2 is inevitable. In normal healthy subjects, this depression is only a few millimeters of mercury; however, in patients with diseased lungs, the contribution of ventilation/perfusion inequality to lowering of blood PO_2 can be significant.

DIFFERENTIAL DIAGNOSIS

The most common causes of cyanosis are cardiac and respiratory diseases that lead to a decrease in the arterial PO_2, but many other conditions can also cause a patient to appear blue (Tables 15.1 and 15.2). Therefore, consideration of the pathophysiologic framework outlined previously allows an orderly approach to the differential diagnosis of cyanosis. Life-threatening causes of cyanosis are summarized in Table 15.3.

TABLE 15.1

CAUSES OF CYANOSIS

I. Respiratory
  A. Decrease in inspired O_2 concentration
  B. Upper airway
    1. Foreign body
    2. Croup
    3. Epiglottitis
    4. Bacterial tracheitis
    5. Traumatic disruption
    6. Congenital anomalies (e.g., vascular malformation, hypoplastic mandible, laryngotracheomalacia)
  C. Chest wall
    1. External compression
    2. Flail chest
  D. Pleura
    1. Pneumothorax
    2. Hemothorax
    3. Empyema/effusion
    4. Diaphragmatic hernia
  E. Lower airway
    1. Asthma
    2. Bronchiolitis
    3. Cystic fibrosis
    4. Pneumonia
    5. Hyaline membrane disease
    6. Adult respiratory distress syndrome
    7. Bronchopulmonary dysplasia
    8. Foreign body/aspiration
    9. Congenital hypoplasia
II. Vascular
  A. Cardiac
    1. Cyanotic congenital defects
      a. Tetralogy of Fallot
      b. Transposition of the great vessels
      c. Truncus arteriosus
      d. Pulmonary atresia
      e. Severe pulmonary stenosis with patent foramen
      f. Tricuspid atresia
      g. Ebstein's anomaly
      h. Total anomalous pulmonary venous drainage
      i. Atrioventricular canal defect
    2. Congestive cardiac failure
    3. Cardiogenic shock
  B. Pulmonary
    1. Pulmonary edema
    2. Primary pulmonary hypertension of the newborn
    3. Pulmonary hypertension
    4. Pulmonary embolism
    5. Pulmonary hemorrhage
  C. Peripheral
    1. Moderate cold exposure
    2. Shock: septic/cardiogenic
    3. Acrocyanosis of the newborn
III. Neurologic
  A. Drug or toxin-induced respiratory depression (e.g., morphine, barbiturates)
  B. Central nervous system lesions (e.g., intracranial hemorrhage, contusion)
  C. Seizure
  D. Breath holding
  E. Neuromuscular disease (e.g., Guillain-Barré, spinal muscular atrophy)
IV. Hematologic
  A. Polycythemia
  B. Methemoglobinemia
V. Dermatologic
  A. Blue dye
  B. Pigmentary lesions
  C. Tattoos
  D. Amiodarone therapy

SIGNS AND SYMPTOMS

TABLE 15.2

COMMON CAUSES OF CYANOSIS

I. Local cyanosis
  A. Acrocyanosis of the newborn
  B. Moderate cold exposure
II. Generalized cyanosis
  A. Respiratory dysfunction
  B. Congenital heart disease

With regard to the amount of Hb, polycythemia, as in newborns with twin–twin transfusion, infants of diabetic mothers, children with high erythropoietin states, or other conditions associated with increased red cell mass, may give the appearance of cyanosis because of the relative increase in the amount of unsaturated Hb.

The degree of Hb saturation is affected by many factors, which can be grouped conveniently by systems. First is the significant contribution from respiratory conditions. Any circumstance leading to a decrease in the concentration of inspired oxygen, such as a house fire where oxygen is consumed by combustion, confinement to a small unventilated space such as being locked inside a discarded refrigerator, or high altitude, can eventually lead to diminished PO_2 and cyanosis. Likewise, upper airway obstruction, as with a foreign body, croup, epiglottitis, bacterial tracheitis, tracheal/bronchial disruption, or congenital airway abnormalities, quickly leads to decreased alveolar ventilation and hypoxemia. Age, events leading to presentation, and examination features, such as barking cough, can help distinguish these. Cyanosis ensues rapidly when chest wall movement or lung inflation is impeded. This condition is often a result of trauma and includes external chest compression, flail chest, or hemothorax. Tension pneumothorax, whether traumatic or as a result of preexisting lung disease such as asthma or cystic fibrosis, is diagnosed by dyspnea, deviated trachea, and possibly distended neck veins with diminished breath sounds on the affected side. Empyema or pleural effusion caused by infection, malignancy, or large chylothorax may be associated with fever, respiratory distress, dullness to percussion, and an asymmetric examination on auscultation. Importantly, any lung dysfunction that directly affects pulmonary gas exchange can lead to cyanosis. The most common conditions in children are asthma, bronchiolitis, pneumonia, cystic fibrosis, pulmonary edema, and hyaline

TABLE 15.3

LIFE-THREATENING CAUSES OF CYANOSIS

I. Respiratory
  A. Decreased inspired O_2 concentration
  B. Upper airway obstruction/disruption
  C. Chest wall immobility
  D. Tension pneumothorax
  E. Massive hemothorax
  F. Lung disease leading to hypoxemia
II. Vascular
  A. Cardiac
    1. Cyanotic congenital defects
    2. Congestive heart failure
    3. Cardiogenic shock
  B. Pulmonary
    1. Pulmonary edema
    2. Primary pulmonary hypertension of the newborn
    3. Pulmonary embolism
    4. Pulmonary hemorrhage
  C. Peripheral
    1. Septic shock
III. Other
  A. Neurologic conditions leading to hypoxemia
  B. Severe methemoglobinemia

membrane disease. Other causes include bronchopulmonary dysplasia, foreign body or substance aspiration, and congenital pulmonary lesions, to list a few.

Circulatory or vascular conditions leading to diminished arterial PO_2 are also associated with cyanosis. One of the most common causes of cyanosis in children is congenital heart disease. Although most newborns with cyanotic congenital heart disease are discovered while still in the newborn nursery, on occasion, such a newborn will initially present to the emergency department (ED) in the first few days or weeks of life with cyanosis. One condition particularly prone to such late presentation is tetralogy of Fallot, specifically in those infants with concomitant pulmonary atresia who have patent ductus arteriosis–dependent pulmonary blood flow. When the ductus closes, profound cyanosis ensues. Rarely, an infant with mild tetralogy of Fallot (or "pink tet") may present with intermittent cyanosis during a "tet spell," which is a 15- to 30-minute self-limited episode of cyanosis caused by increased right-to-left shunting and decrease in pulmonary blood flow. Diagnosis in the pink tet is facilitated by presence of a loud systolic murmur. The causes of cyanotic congenital heart disease are listed in Table 15.1 (II, A). Although many mixing lesions are correctable, several congenital lesions remain with significant shunting of blood from right to left, and these cyanotic children will inevitably be seen in the ED over the course of their lives. Cyanosis may also be caused by pulmonary congestion from cardiac failure or left-to-right cardiac lesions leading to increased pulmonary blood flow and diminished diffusion of O_2 across the gas–blood barrier. (For a detailed discussion of cardiac disease, see Chapter 84.) Several pulmonary vascular abnormalities can also lead to cyanosis. These include primary pulmonary hypertension of the newborn or pulmonary hypertension from other causes where, because of high pulmonary pressures, blood is shunted away from the lungs and the child becomes hypoxemic. Pulmonary embolism and pulmonary

hemorrhage, although rare in children, also impair lung perfusion and must be considered.

Low perfusion states may lead to local cyanosis, particularly of the hands, feet, and lips. Moderate cold exposure slows transit time for red cells across capillary beds, leading to greater unloading of oxygen to the tissues and local blueness. Patients in septic or cardiogenic shock may have perfusion-related cyanosis with long capillary refill times as a result of vascular collapse of sepsis or pump failure. Poor perfusion can also result from hyperviscous states such as polycythemia or leukemia. Acrocyanosis, or blueness of the hands and feet with preserved pinkness in the mucous membranes and elsewhere, is seen commonly in newborns and is related to variable perfusion in the extremities. It is seen in well-appearing babies and resolves within the first few days of life.

Neurologic conditions can also lead to Hb desaturation and cyanosis. Patients who hypoventilate because of central nervous system (CNS) depression, whether from primary CNS lesions or drugs/toxins that depress the respiratory center, are often centrally cyanotic at presentation to the ED. Episodic blue spells in infants and young children who are otherwise well may be caused by breath holding, especially when associated with a sudden insult such as fright, pain, frustration, or anger. Vigorous crying is believed to cause cerebral ischemia via vasoconstriction from decreased PCO_2, decreased cardiac output from Valsalva maneuver, and hypoxemia from apnea (see Chapter 131). Seizures are often associated with cyanosis from inadequate respiration during the convulsion. A variety of neuromuscular diseases that affect chest wall or diaphragmatic function may ultimately lead to hypoventilation.

With respect to the Hb molecule itself, methemoglobinemia is an unusual but not rare reason for presentation to the pediatric ED. Methemoglobin can be either congenital or acquired. Congenital methemoglobinemia is caused by either Hb variants designated M hemoglobins or deficiency of NADH-dependent methemoglobin reductase. The more commonly acquired form occurs when red blood cells are exposed to oxidant chemicals and drugs. Young infants with gastroenteritis or oxidant toxin exposure are particularly susceptible to the development of methemoglobinemia as a result of immature enzyme systems required to reduce Hb. Symptoms, caused by decreased blood oxygen content and cellular hypoxia, include headache, dizziness, nausea, dyspnea, confusion, seizure, and coma. Even at low levels, skin discoloration is prominent, often with intense or "slate gray" cyanosis from the presence of methemoglobin as perceived through the skin. (For a more detailed discussion of methemoglobinemia, see Chapter 91.)

Other conditions leading to a blue appearance of the skin may be confused with cyanosis. A rare but perplexing presentation is that of the well-appearing child with unusually localized cyanosis, which after some head scratching, turns out to be related to blue dye of clothing. Slate blue discoloration of the face, neck, and arms has been noted in patients on chronic amiodarone therapy. Certain pigmentary lesions such as mongolian spots can be confused with cyanosis, especially when uncharacteristically large or in unusual locations. Adolescents will occasionally "tattoo" areas of the body that may appear as local cyanosis.

EVALUATION AND DECISION

A careful yet rapid history and physical examination are critical to the approach to the cyanotic patient because timely correction may be lifesaving. Many historical features can help narrow the differential diagnosis and lead to prompt evaluation and treatment. The onset and pattern, location, quality, temporal nature, and presence of palliative or provocative features must be explored. Age of the patient with respect to onset of cyanosis, whether at birth, shortly after birth, or acquired later, is critical. In newborns, congenital cardiac and respiratory diseases are the most common causes of cyanosis. Special attention must also be paid to known preexisting heart or lung disease that may predispose to the acute onset of cyanosis. History of exposure to environmental conditions or toxins, such as cold, trauma, clothing dye, smoke inhalation, confinement to an airtight space, drugs, or chemicals, is crucial. Known history or family history of M hemoglobin or deficiency of NADH-dependent methemoglobin reductase may lead directly to the cause of cyanosis. A history of sudden pain or fright with crying or seizure occurrence should be sought.

The physical examination must include a complete general examination, with special attention paid to the vital signs, oxygen saturation, and cardiovascular and pulmonary systems. An immediate and key physical examination feature is the presence or absence of respiratory distress. In general, children with respiratory distress are likely to have *respiratory* dysfunction, and careful examination of the airway, breathing, and circulation should be rapidly initiated. Presence of cough, "sniffing position," stridor, retractions, or fever should be determined. Lung examination may reveal adventitious (e.g., wheezing or rales) or diminished breath sounds. Presence of a cardiac murmur suggests cardiac disease. Careful attention to the peripheral circulation, including pulses, capillary refill, and temperature, is also helpful. A rapid neurologic examination should be performed. Hypoventilation and subsequent hypoxemia can be the result of many conditions affecting the CNS.

Location of cyanosis helps determine its cause. Central cyanosis is noted in the mucous membranes, tongue, trunk, and upper extremities. It is most often the result of decreased arterial PO_2 but can also result from severe methemoglobinemia or polycythemia. If the cyanosis is peripheral only (hands, feet,

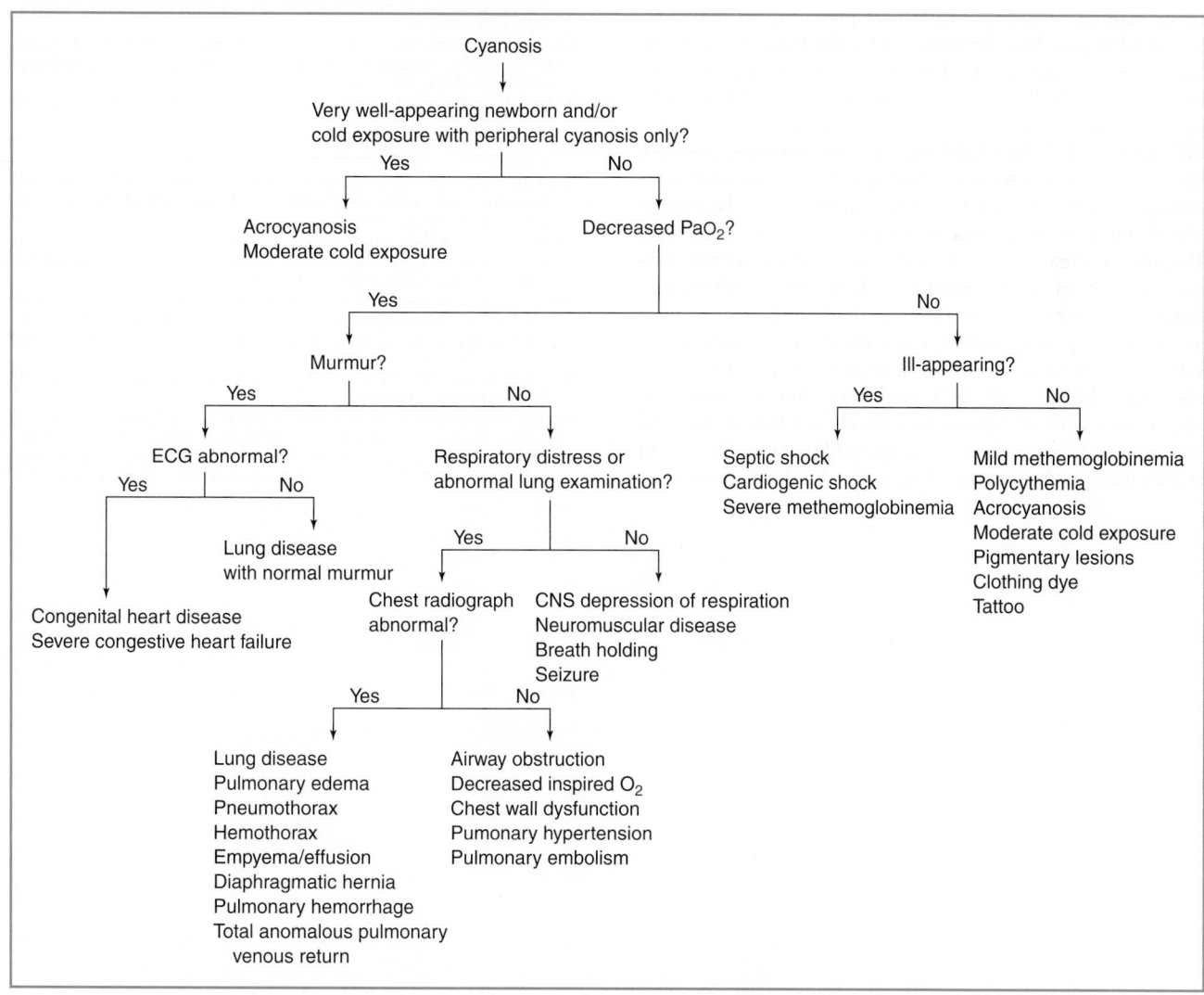

FIGURE 15.1 Laboratory evaluation of cyanosis. EKG, electrocardiogram; CNS, central nervous system.

lips), moderate cold exposure, newborn acrocyanosis, shock states, or mild methemoglobinemia may be the cause. Local blue discoloration of a single extremity corresponds to compromise of distal circulation or autonomic tone as seen in traumatic vascular lesions or reflex sympathetic dystrophy. Cyanosis and swelling of just the head may be seen with superior vena cava syndrome. In addition, a local blue hue to the skin may also be a result of simple phenomena such as pigmentary lesions or blue clothing dye. If blue coloring appears on an alcohol swab wiped across the discolored area of skin, dye is responsible. Differential cyanosis of the lower body versus the upper body may indicate high pulmonary vascular resistance with right-to-left shunting via the ductus arteriosis. Transposition of the great arteries with pulmonary-to-aortic shunt of oxygenated blood through the ductus arteriosis is represented in the rare instance that the upper body is blue and the lower body pink.

The path of the laboratory evaluation depends on the historical features and physical findings established on initial encounter (Fig. 15.1). All patients, except very well-appearing newborns and well-appearing cold-exposed patients with peripheral cyanosis only, require measurement of arterial PO_2. (Oxygen saturation by pulse oximetry may be helpful in determining if hypoxemia is the cause of cyanosis, but it may also be misleading when forms of Hb are present other than oxyhemoglobin and deoxyhemoglobin.) If the PO_2 is normal, the laboratory evaluation is determined by the degree of ill appearance. Well-appearing oxygenated children with cyanosis usually have less urgent conditions, such as polycythemia, mild methemoglobinemia, cold exposure, newborn acrocyanosis, or dermatologic findings. In this case, laboratory evaluation might include a methemoglobin level and complete blood count, or no further investigation may be warranted. Despite a normal PO_2, an ill-appearing cyanotic patient may have a more emergent condition such as severe methemoglobinemia or septic or cardiogenic shock and may require aggressive laboratory investigation, including complete blood cell count, methemoglobin level, blood cultures, and blood chemistry. Blood with high methemoglobin content may appear very dark or "chocolate brown" and fails to turn red on exposure to air, such as in a drop on filter paper. Treatment is then directed at the underlying cause. Methemoglobinemia may improve with intravenous methylene blue. If the PO_2 is decreased, oxygen therapy should be instituted. In general, cyanosis caused by decreased alveolar ventilation or diffusional abnormalities often improves with delivery of 100% O_2. However, hypoxemia caused by decreased pulmonary perfusion or shunt responds little to oxygen therapy. Next, a chest radiograph should be obtained. Abnormalities of the lungs may confirm pulmonary disease as a major contributor to hypoxemia, and changes in the cardiac size or silhouette may suggest cardiac causes. If the chest radiograph is normal, other reasons for diminished arterial PO_2, such as CNS- or chest wall–related respiratory depression, upper airway obstruction, or pulmonary perfusion abnormalities, must be entertained. If a concomitant murmur or other concern for cardiac disease exists, an electrocardiogram (EKG) is essential. Abnormal EKGs suggest cardiac dysfunction, either congenital or acquired (Table 15.1), and the addition of echocardiography will help establish the definitive diagnosis.

Suggested Readings

Barker SJ, Curry J, Redford D, et al. Measurement of carboxyhemoglobin and methemoglobin by pulse oximetry: a human volunteer study. *Anesthesiology* 2006;105(5):892–897.

Bradberry SM. Occupational methaemoglobinaemia. Mechanisms of production, features, diagnosis and management including the use of methylene blue. *Toxicol Rev* 2003;22(1):13–27.

DiMario FJ Jr. Prospective study of children with cyanotic and pallid breath-holding spells. *Pediatrics* 2001;107:265.

Driscoll DJ. Evaluation of the cyanotic newborn. *Pediatr Clin North Am* 1990;37:123.

Grant JB, Saltzman AR. Respiratory functions of the lung. In: Baum GL, Wolinsky E, eds. *Textbook of pulmonary diseases*, 5th ed. Boston: Little, Brown and Company, 1994.

Lundsgaard C, Van Slyke DD. Cyanosis. *Medicine* 1923;2:15.

Martin L, Khalil H. How much reduced hemoglobin is necessary to generate central cyanosis? *Chest* 1990;97:182–185.

Umbreit J. Methemoglobin–it's not just blue: a concise review. *Am J Hematol* 2007;82(2):134–144.VanRoekens CN, Zuckerberg AL. Emergency management of hypercyanotic crises in tetralogy of Fallot. *Ann Emerg Med* 1995;25:256–258.

Watcha M, Connor MT, Hing AV. Pulse oximetry in methemoglobinemia. *Am J Dis Child* 1989;143:845–847.

West JB. Gas transport to the periphery. In: West JB, ed. *Physiological basis of medical practice*, 12th ed. Baltimore: Williams & Wilkins, 1990;538–545.

West JB. Pulmonary gas exchange. In: West JB, ed. *Physiological basis of medical practice*, 12th ed. Baltimore: Williams & Wilkins, 1990;546–559.

CHAPTER 16 ■ CRYING AND COLIC IN EARLY INFANCY

BARBARA B. PAWEL, MD, AND FRED M. HENRETIG, MD

Crying is the means by which an infant may express discomfort, ranging from normal hunger and desire for company to severe, life-threatening illness. Many common minor irritations and illnesses are excluded by careful history and physical examination. Often, however, a normal, thriving baby will develop a chronic pattern of daily paroxysms of irritability and crying known as colic. The attacks usually have their onset in the second to third week of life and may last for several hours, more commonly in the late afternoon or evening. The typical episode is described as paroxysmal crying that develops into a piercing scream, as if the baby were in pain. The child may draw up the legs, the abdomen may appear distended, bowel sounds are increased, and flatus may be passed, leading parents to conclude that their child has abdominal distress. The emergency physician may be confronted with such a patient and the worried, occasionally hostile parents (usually no earlier than midnight). Colic cannot be cured in the emergency department (ED), and only when crying episodes are repeated and stereotypical and other causes of crying are excluded can the diagnosis of colic be considered. Establishing an orderly approach to the infant with unexplained crying is important to rule out the occasional physical illness and to provide preliminary guidance to the family.

PATHOPHYSIOLOGY

Any unpleasant sensation can cause an infant to cry. Pain or an altered threshold for discomfort (irritability) may be caused by diverse physical illnesses. Those most likely to present abruptly in a young infant are listed in Table 16.1. Numerous unproven theories abound about the etiology of colic. Cow's milk allergy, immaturity of the gastrointestinal tract or central nervous system, parental anxiety, maternal smoking during pregnancy, poor feeding technique, and individual temperament characteristics all have been invoked. The search for a specific cause of colic continues. Gastroesophageal reflux has been suggested as a possible etiology of infant colic; however, studies have shown placebos to be equivalent to antireflux medications in reducing colicky crying. Moreover there is poor correlation between irritability/crying and pH probe documented reflux episodes.

Two polypeptides produced in the gastrointestinal tract (motilin and ghrelin) have been found to be elevated in colicky infants and may play a role by affecting gastrointestinal motility.

No single theory (or concomitant therapy) has gained uniform acceptance. Colic may be a syndrome that represents the manifestations of some or all these factors in varying degrees

in a normal population of babies whose tendency to cry varies along a normal distribution. Brazelton's original data on infant crying patterns have been supplemented by larger-scale studies in Canada and England. All studies revealed crying levels to increase from birth to a peak of approximately 3 hours per day at 6 to 8 weeks, followed by a rapid decline.

Early infant crying was also shown to cluster more commonly in afternoon and evening hours. These estimates of crying time over the first 12 weeks of life seem to reflect a certain degree of inconsolable crying behavior that normal infants are destined to exhibit in the first 3 months of life. An encounter with a health-care provider is more likely if the infant is difficult to console or if the crying episode is believed to be associated with pain. Although there are variations in the literature, most agree that a reasonable definition for colic embraces Wessel's criteria: An infant younger than 3 months of age with more than 3 hours of crying per day occurring more than 3 times per week for more than 3 weeks.

EVALUATION AND DECISION

A careful history and physical examination with emphasis on the head, eyes, ears, skin, abdomen, genitalia, and extremities, plus analysis and culture of a urine specimen, will usually enable the physician to diagnose identifiable illnesses or injuries causing severe paroxysms of crying (Table 16.1). Initially, this clinical evaluation must focus on those conditions that are potentially life-threatening: meningitis, child abuse, intussusception, incarcerated hernia, severe intoxication, and metabolic disturbance. Other less critical but more common conditions should be sought next; corneal abrasion or foreign body, otitis media, aerophagia, teething, gastroenteritis, and anal fissure are most commonly seen. As noted in Table 16.1, other diagnoses are encountered occasionally.

The history should include special attention to the onset of crying and any associated events—particularly recent immunization ("screaming spells" lasting up to 24 hours have been described after pertussis vaccine), trauma, fever, or use of medications. Physical examination must be thorough, with the baby completely undressed. Vital signs may reveal fever, suggesting infection (although not always present in young infants with serious infections), or hyperpnea, suggesting metabolic acidosis.

The head should be explored for evidence of trauma and the fontanel should be palpated. Eyes must be examined with fluorescein to look for corneal abrasion, even in infants with no symptoms referable to the eyes. In addition, eversion of the

TABLE 16.1

TABLE 16.1

CONDITIONS ASSOCIATED WITH ABRUPT ONSET OF
INCONSOLABLE CRYING IN YOUNG INFANTS

I. Discomfort Caused by Identifiable Illness
  A. Head and neck
    1. Meningitis[a]
    2. Skull fracture/subdural hematoma[a]
    3. Glaucoma
    4. Foreign body (especially eyelash) in eye[b]
    5. Corneal abrasion[b]
    6. Otitis media[b]
    7. Caffey's disease (infantile cortical hyperostosis)
    8. Child abuse[a]
    9. Prenatal/perinatal cocaine exposure
  B. Gastrointestinal
    1. Excess air (improper feeding/burping technique)
    2. Gastroenteritis[b]
    3. Intussusception[a]
    4. Anal fissure[b]
    5. Cow's milk protein intolerance
    6. Gastroesophageal reflux/esophagitis
  C. Cardiovascular
    1. Congestive heart failure[a]
    2. Supraventricular tachycardia[a]
    3. Coarctation of the aorta[a]
    4. Anomalous origin of left coronary artery from
       pulmonary artery[a]
  D. Genitourinary
    1. Torsion of the testis
    2. Incarcerated hernia[a]
    3. Urinary tract infection
  E. Integumentary
    1. Burn
    2. Strangulated finger, toe, penis (hair tourniquet)
  F. Musculoskeletal
    1. Child abuse[a]
    2. Extremity fracture (following a fall)
  G. Toxic/metabolic
    1. Drugs: antihistamines, atropinics, adrenergics,
       cocaine (including passive inhalation), aspirin[a]
    2. Metabolic acidosis, hypernatremia, hypocalcemia,
       hypoglycemia[a]
    3. Pertussis vaccine reactions
II. Colic—Recurrent Paroxysmal Attacks of Crying[b]

[a] Life-threatening causes.
[b] Common causes.

upper eyelids can exclude a foreign body. Fundoscopy should be attempted (retinal hemorrhages are common signs of abuse, especially in shaken baby syndrome). Careful otoscopy is required to visualize the tympanic membranes. The heart should be evaluated for signs of congestive failure, arrhythmia, or rare ischemia-producing lesions (Table 16.1, I.C). Abdominal and rectal examinations must be performed to look for signs of anal fissure or intussusception. The diaper must be removed, and a careful search should be made for incarcerated hernia, testicular torsion, or strangulation of the penis or clitoris by an encircling hair. Crying may be the primary symptom of an occult urinary infection, so a suitable specimen of urine should be obtained for urinalysis and culture. Careful palpation of all long bones despite the absence of obvious signs of trauma can detect fracture sites that might otherwise have been overlooked. Each finger and toe should be inspected closely to rule out strangulation by hair or thread. Further consideration of laboratory or radiographic evaluation is made in light of the clinical findings. A low threshold for urine toxicology screening is warranted in the persistently irritable baby, given the prevalence of illicit drug use. Infants with unexplained, incessant crying may have a limited physical examination necessitating an extensive evaluation and hospitalization.

Many infants will have a completely negative examination, and the history (or subsequent follow-up) will be suggestive of colic. Over the time in which the crying attacks recur, the infant must demonstrate adequate weight gain (average 5 to 7 oz per week in the first months of life) and absence of physical disorders on several examinations before underlying illnesses can be excluded and colic can be diagnosed confidently (Fig. 16.1). When it becomes clear that a given infant is experiencing colic, the practitioner faces a vexing problem. No dramatic cure is currently available, but the symptoms almost invariably resolve within 3 months of onset. Many studies on the etiology and treatment of colic have methodologic weaknesses, making it difficult for clinicians to use and compare results. In general, no safe and effective medical treatment for colic is available. The efficacy of simethicone is not supported by good quality trials but there have been no reported side effects and it is widely used by physicians who treat colic. Methylscopolamine is neither effective nor safe. Dicyclomine, once believed to be effective, is no longer recommended in infants younger than 6 months because of its dangerous anticholinergic side effects. Elimination of cow's milk protein through formula changes is only useful in the small subset of cases (4%) with cow's milk protein intolerance. Maternal hypoallergenic diets while breast-feeding have yielded mixed results. Herbal tea mixtures appear to reduce crying times, however, there are multiple drawbacks, including compromised nutrition due to the large volume required for symptomatic relief and lack of standardized dosing and strength. In addition, there is a potential for GI or neurotoxicity if certain ingredients with similar names are inadvertently added. A recent study adding a probiotic dietary supplement to breast-fed infants' diets showed decreased crying times in 95% of patients within 28 days. There is not enough support at present to recommend practice changes but further research may be promising. A study by Taubman found that parental counseling (to be more responsive to infant crying with immediate efforts at consoling) was far more effective than dietary manipulation. Interestingly chiropractic manipulation has gained some popularity and although studies have shown no benefit to colicky infants, visits were associated with an overall increase in parent satisfaction. The safest and most effective course of treatment at this time seems to be counseling and empathy. The physician can reassure the parents that their baby is thriving and will outgrow the colic and develop normally.

The emergency physician must be aware of colic as an entity to initiate the evaluation already described, rule out acute treatable illness, and refer the family to a pediatrician for follow-up. Colic is not serious and does not last forever, but it probably will be a nuisance for several weeks to come. The physician should stress to all family members the importance of sharing in the baby's care, so the mother can get

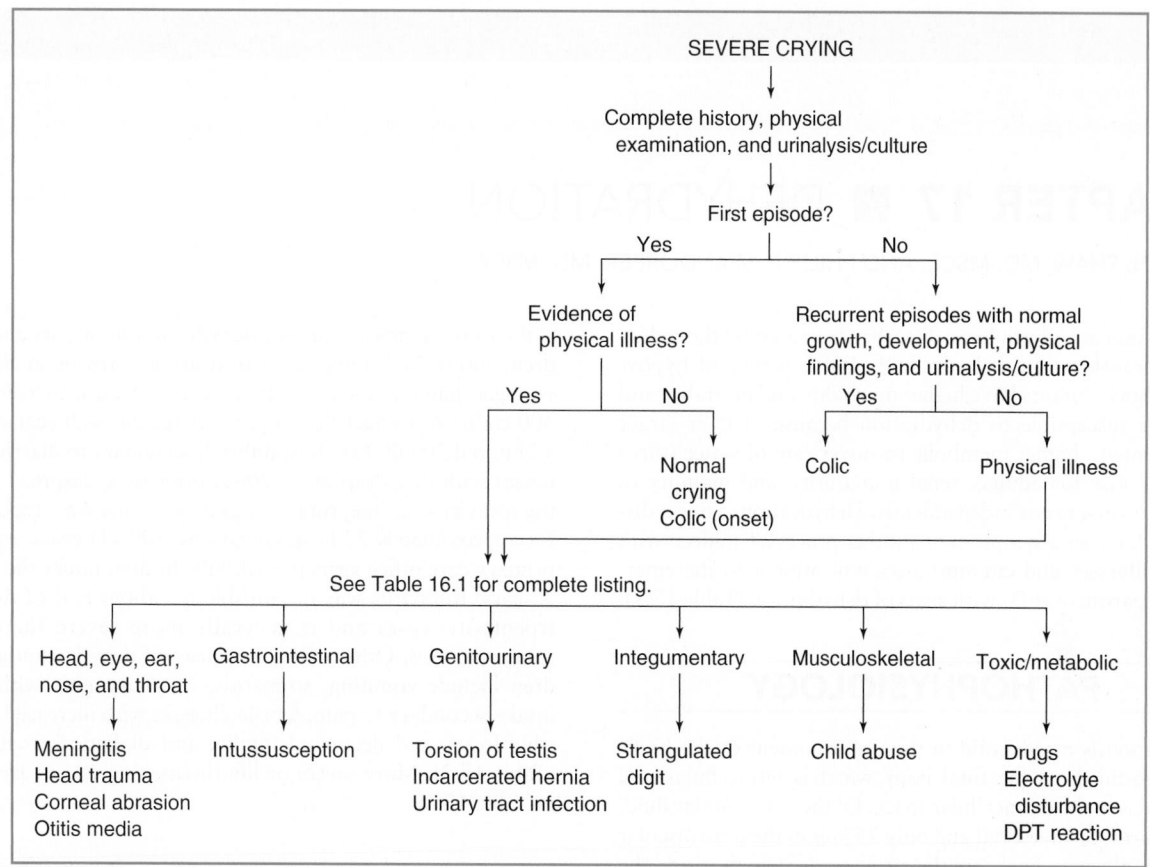

FIGURE 16.1 Approach to abrupt onset of severe crying in infancy. DPT, diphtheria-pertussis-tetanus (vaccine).

some periods of rest and relief from full-time responsibility for the infant. The emergency physician is responsible for investigating the vulnerability of families and children who present with excessive crying. Assessment of the parents' emotional state and the status of available support systems are mandatory. Exhaustion of the parents may be dangerous for the infant, both psychologically and physically. The National Center for Shaken Baby Syndrome acknowledges that excessive crying is a risk factor for abuse. They have launched a prevention campaign, including a website that provides helpful tips for parents on how to safely cope with the frustration and despair often associated with colic. For immediate amelioration of crying at the time of the ED visit, no drug therapy or feeding change is recommended. Rather, most colicky babies derive some temporary relief from rhythmic motion, such as rocking, being carried, or riding in a car, and from continual monotonous sounds, such as those from a washing machine or electric fan. A purposefully chosen circuitous route for the car ride home (one that combines motion and sound) should suffice as therapy for the first visit.

Suggested Readings

Barr RG. Changing our understanding of infant colic. *Arch Pediatr Adolesc Med* 2002;156:1172–1174.

Brazelton TB. Crying in infancy. *Pediatrics* 1962;29:579–588.

Brotherton H, Philip RK. Anomalous left coronary artery from pulmonary artery (ALCAPA) in infants: a 5-year review in a defined birth cohort. *Eur J Pediatr* 2008;167:43–46.

Evanoo G. Infant crying: A clinical conundrum. *J Pediatr Health Care* 2007;21: 333–338.

Fireman L, Serwint J. Colic. *Pediatr Rev* 2006;27:357–358.

Garrison MM, Christakis DA. A systematic review of treatments for infant colic. *Pediatrics* 2000;106:184–190.

Hardoin RA, Henslee JA, Christenson CP, et al. Colic medication and apparent life-threatening events. *Clin Pediatr* 1991;30:281–285.

Herman M, Le A. The crying infant. *Emerg Med Clin North Am* 2007;25: 1137–1159.

Hughes S, Bolton J. Is chiropractic an effective treatment in infantile colic? *Arch Dis Child* 2002;86:382–384.

Lehtonen LA, Rautava PT. Infantile colic: natural history and treatment. *Curr Probl Pediatr* 1996;26:79–85.

National Center on Shaken Baby Syndrome. Crying, a trigger to violence. Available at: http://www.DONTSHAKE.org.

Poole SR. The infant with acute, unexplained, excessive crying. *Pediatrics* 1991; 88(3):450–455.

Reijneveld SA, Brugman E, Hirasing RA. Excessive infant crying: the impact of varying definitions. *Pediatrics* 2001;108:893–897.

Savino F. Focus on infantile colic. *Acta Paediatr* 2007;96:1259–1264.

Savino F, Grassino EC, Guidi C, et al. Ghrelin and motilin concentration in colicky infants. *Acta Paediatr* 2006;95:738–741.

Savino F, Pelle E, Palumeri E, et al. *Lactobacillus reuteri* (American type culture collection strain 55730) versus simethicone in the treatment of infantile colic: A prospective randomized study. *Pediatrics* 2007;119(1):e124–e130.

Sondergaard C, Henriksen TB, Obel C, et al. Smoking during pregnancy and infantile colic. *Pediatrics* 2001;108:342–346.

St James-Roberts I. Persistent infant crying. *Arch Dis Child* 1991;31(3): 653–655.

Taubman B. Parental counseling compared with elimination of cow's milk or soy milk protein for the treatment of infant colic syndrome: a randomized trial. *Pediatrics* 1988;81:756–761.

Wessel MA. Paroxysmal fussing in infancy, sometimes called "colic." *Pediatrics* 1975;14:421–435.

CHAPTER 17 ■ DEHYDRATION

KATHY N. SHAW, MD, MSCE, AND PHILIP R. SPANDORFER, MD, MSCE

Dehydration is a physiologic disturbance caused by the reduction or translocation of body fluids and is a type of hypovolemic shock. Infants have higher morbidity and mortality and are more susceptible to dehydration because of their larger water content, higher metabolic turnover rate of water (three times the rate for adults), renal immaturity, and inability to meet their own needs independently. Dehydration is not a disease itself, rather a symptom of another process. Children with various illnesses and circumstances will present to the emergency department (ED) with signs of dehydration (Table 17.1).

PATHOPHYSIOLOGY

Dehydration is a reduction in the water content of the body. Over two-thirds of the total body water is intracellular and one-third is in the extracellular space. Of the extracellular fluid, three-fourths is interstitial and only 25% is in the intravascular space as plasma. Early in the process of dehydration, the majority of the water loss is from the extracellular compartment, which contains 135 mEq per L of sodium and negligible potassium. However, with time, there is an equilibration from the intracellular compartment to the extracellular compartment, which has 150 mEq per L of potassium and negligible sodium. As the electrolyte composition of extracellular fluid and intracellular fluid vary greatly, an understanding of this process helps the clinician gauge the optimal composition and rate of fluid deficit correction (see Chapter 100).

Dehydration is often categorized by the serum osmolarity and severity (degree of fluid deficit), which is helpful in determining fluid therapy. Based on the initial serum sodium, most children have isonatremic dehydration (also referred to as isotonic dehydration, serum sodium 130 to 150 mEq per L), whereas others have hypernatremic dehydration (hypertonic dehydration, serum sodium greater than 150 mEq per L) or hyponatremic dehydration (hypotonic dehydration, serum sodium less than 130 mEq per L). Severity is judged by the amount of body fluid lost or the percentage of weight loss, and is typically characterized as mild (less than 50 mL per kg, or less than 5% of total body weight), moderate (50 to 100 mL per kg, or 5% to 10% of total body weight), and severe (greater than 100 mL per kg, or greater than 10% of total body weight).

DIFFERENTIAL DIAGNOSIS

Fluid imbalance in dehydration results from (i) decreased intake; (ii) increased output secondary to insensible, renal, or gastrointestinal (GI) losses; or (iii) translocation of fluid such as occurs with major burns or ascites (Table 17.1). Gastroenteritis is the most common cause of dehydration in infants and children, and is the leading cause of death worldwide in children younger than 4 years of age. In the United States, an average of 300 children younger than 5 years of age die each year, and an additional 200,000 are hospitalized, secondary to diarrheal illnesses with dehydration. In 2006, prior to widespread use of the rotavirus vaccine, rotavirus gastroenteritis was responsible for approximately 22 hospitalizations, 300 ED visits, and 300 primary care office visits per 10,000 children under the age of 3 years. Rotavirus was responsible for about half of the gastroenteritis cases and is generally more severe than nonrotavirus cases. Other common causes of dehydration in children include vomiting, stomatitis, or pharyngitis with poor intake secondary to pain, febrile illnesses with increased insensible losses and decreased intake, and diabetic ketoacidosis (Table 17.2). More severe or life-threatening causes are listed in Table 17.3.

EVALUATION AND DECISION

The first step in evaluating a child with dehydration is to assess the severity or degree of dehydration, regardless of the cause (Table 17.4). Most children with clinically significant dehydration will have two of the following four clinical findings: (i) capillary refill greater than 2 seconds, (ii) dry mucous membranes, (iii) no tears, and (iv) ill appearance. Dehydration is a type of hypovolemic shock. Mild, moderate, and severe dehydration correspond to impending, compensated, and uncompensated states of shock, respectively (see Chapter 3). If there is severe dehydration or uncompensated shock, the child must be treated immediately with isotonic fluids to restore intravascular volume, as detailed later in this chapter.

History

A thorough history is needed to assess the child with dehydration to determine the cause and degree of dehydration (Fig. 17.1). Particular attention should be paid to the child's output and intake of fluids and electrolytes. Overt GI losses from diarrhea and vomiting are the most common causes of dehydration in children, therefore, information about the amount and character of these losses is critical in determining a cause (see Chapters 18 and 78). The child may not be drinking because of physical restriction (e.g., dependence on a caregiver, pain, altered consciousness, anorexia). Fever, high ambient temperatures or bundling a baby, sweating, and hyperventilation may cause increased insensible losses. It is important to note whether there is any underlying disease that would contribute

TABLE 17.1

CAUSES OF DEHYDRATION

Decreased Intake
  Physical restriction
    Infant
    Central nervous system depression
  Anorexia
  Voluntary or imposed cessation of drinking
    Pharyngitis, stomatitis
    Respiratory distress
    Child abuse
  Hypothalamic hypodipsia
Increased Output
  Insensible losses
    Fever
    Sweating
    Heat prostration
    High ambient temperature/low humidity
    Hyperventilation
    Cystic fibrosis
    Thyrotoxicosis
  Renal losses
    Osmotic
    Diabetic ketoacidosis
    Acute tubular necrosis
    High protein feeds
    Mannitol usage
  Nonosmotic
    Diabetes insipidus
    Sustained hypokalemia-hypercalcemia
    Sickle cell disease
    Chronic renal disease
    Bartter's syndrome
  Sodium-losing
    Congenital adrenal hypoplasia
    Diuretics
    Sodium-losing nephropathy
    Pseudohypoaldosteronism
  Gastrointestinal losses
    Diarrhea (see Chapter 18)
      Secretory vs. nonsecretory
    Vomiting (see Chapter 78)
      Obstructive vs. nonobstructive
Translocation of Fluids
  Burns
  Ascites (e.g., nephrotic syndrome)
  Intraintestinal
    Paralytic ileus
    Postabdominal surgery

to dehydration (e.g., cystic fibrosis, diabetes, hyperthyroidism, renal disease).

Asking the parents about documented weight loss, amount of urine output, and the presence or absence of tears is helpful in determining the severity of the dehydration. Although

TABLE 17.2

COMMON CAUSES OF DEHYDRATION

Gastroenteritis	Febrile illness
Stomatitis/pharyngitis	Diabetic ketoacidosis

TABLE 17.3

LIFE-THREATENING CAUSES OF DEHYDRATION

Gastroenteritis (especially infants)	Heat prostration
Diabetic ketoacidosis	Gastrointestinal obstruction
Burns over 25% of body surface area	Cystic fibrosis
Thyrotoxicosis	Diabetes insipidus
Congenital adrenal hyperplasia	Child abuse

decreased urine output is an early sign of dehydration, only 20% of patients with the complaint of decreased urine output will be dehydrated. All ingested fluids should be noted because diluted juices or water can be associated with hyponatremic dehydration, whereas excess salt intake or low liquid intake may indicate hypernatremic dehydration. Further, inquiring how the infant formula is prepared may lead to the discovery of electrolyte abnormalities with dehydration if too little or too much water is added.

Physical Examination

Measurement of vital signs is an important and objective part of the evaluation of the child with dehydration (Table 17.4). The first sign of mild dehydration is tachycardia, whereas hypotension is a very late sign of severe dehydration. In mild to moderate dehydration, the respiratory rate is usually normal. As a child becomes more acidotic and fluid is depleted, the respiratory rate increases and the breathing pattern becomes hyperpneic. Unfortunately, vital signs alone are not always reliable. Tachycardia also may be caused by fever, agitation, or pain; respiratory illness affects respiratory rates; and orthostatic signs are difficult to obtain in babies and young children.

Age of the child, nutritional status, and type of dehydration may also affect clinical assessment, which is critical to effective management of the acutely dehydrated child. In general, older children show signs of dehydration sooner than babies do because of their lower levels of extracellular water. Babies with excess subcutaneous fat may look less dehydrated than they really are, whereas severely malnourished babies may appear to be more dehydrated secondary to wasted supporting tissues. Signs of dehydration may be less evident or appear later in hypernatremic dehydration. Excessive irritability with increased muscle tone, and doughy or smooth and velvety skin, often are noted with this type of dehydration. Conversely, signs of dehydration may be more pronounced or appear sooner in hyponatremic dehydration. Keeping these caveats in mind, particular attention should be paid to the overall appearance, mental status, eyes, and skin on physical examination. The mildly dehydrated child usually appears well and may be tired, have decreased tearing and a slightly dry mouth. Dry mucous membranes are an early sign of dehydration, but this finding is affected by rapid breathing and ingestion of fluids. Conversely, the severely dehydrated baby classically appears quite ill with lethargy or irritability, a dry mouth, sunken fontanel, and absent tears. More moderate states of dehydration, however, require more careful evaluation.

TABLE 17.4

CLINICAL ESTIMATION OF DEGREE OF DEHYDRATION[a,b]

Clinical finding	PPV	NPV	Sensitivity (95% CI)	Specificity (95% CI)
Decreased skin elasticity	0.57	0.93	0.35 (0.23–0.49)	0.97 (0.92–0.99)
Capillary refill >2 s	0.57	0.94	0.48 (0.35–0.61)	0.96 (0.90–0.99)
Ill appearance (tired, listless)	0.42	0.95	0.59 (0.46–0.71)	0.91 (0.84–0.95)
Absent tears	0.40	0.96	0.67 (0.53–0.78)	0.89 (0.82–0.94)
Abnormal respirations	0.37	0.94	0.43 (0.30–0.56)	0.86 (0.78–0.91)
Dry mucous membranes	0.29	0.99	0.80 (0.67–0.89)	0.78 (0.70–0.85)
Sunken eyes	0.29	0.95	0.60 (0.47–0.72)	0.84 (0.76–0.90)
Abnormal radial pulse	0.25	0.93	0.43 (0.30–0.56)	0.86 (0.78–0.91)
Tachycardia (>150)	0.20	0.93	0.46 (0.32–0.61)	0.79 (0.72–0.87)
Decreased urine output (parental report)	0.17	0.97	0.85 (0.73–0.93)	0.53 (0.44–0.62)

[a]The 10-point dehydration score listed in descending PPV.
[b]One to two findings indicate mild dehydration <5% total body weight, three to six findings indicate moderate dehydration (5% to 10% total body weight), and seven to ten findings indicate severe dehydration (>10% total body weight).
PPV, positive predictive value; NPV, negative predictive value; CI, confidence interval.
Reproduced by permission of *Pediatrics*, Vol. 99, Page(s) e6, Table 2, Copyright 1997.

The skin is a reliable organ to assess for signs of peripheral perfusion because it is an indicator of the child's systemic vascular resistance and degree of shunting that is occurring to maintain blood pressure. Peripheral and central pulses and skin temperature should be compared. Cool peripheral extremities are an early sign of poor perfusion, whereas weak central pulses are a very late sign. One of the more objective measures of dehydration is assessment of skin perfusion by measuring capillary refill time. Although the child's body temperature does not affect capillary refill time, it may be falsely prolonged when measured on the foot or in a cool room. Thus, the test should be performed on the fingertip or nail bed in a warm room. Light pressure is applied to blanch the fingernail bed, and the time is measured until color returns (Fig. 17.2). Delays of only 2 to 3 seconds indicate moderate dehydration, and a measurement of more than 3 seconds occurs with severe fluid losses. Skin elasticity can be assessed by determining whether there is a delay in return of skin to its original state after it is pinched into folds (tenting). This is a less reliable finding in older children and malnourished babies who have less subcutaneous tissue.

Laboratory

The quantity and quality of urine produced are also important indicators of the cause or degree of dehydration. Progressive decrease in urine output and increase in specific gravity and osmolarity are expected with increasing severity of dehydration when normal renal function is preserved. If the physical examination indicates significant dehydration and there is dilute or copious urine, a renal or adrenal origin is most likely. In addi-tion, polyuria and the presence of glucose or ketones may indicate diabetic ketoacidosis, whereas a history of disorders of the central nervous system (CNS) suggests diabetes insipidus.

In children who are judged to have moderate to severe dehydration that requires intravenous (IV) rehydration, laboratory tests of electrolytes, glucose, blood urea nitrogen, and creatinine are usually obtained to determine osmolarity and renal function. Approximately one-third of moderately to severely dehydrated children will have hypoglycemia less than 60 mg per dL. The acid–base status may be assessed further with an arterial or venous blood gas.

Diagnostic Approach

In approaching the patient with presumed dehydration, the initial assessment serves to determine whether compensated or uncompensated shock is present. If the child appears to be in shock, resuscitation should begin and a number of life-threatening disorders need to be considered, as listed in Table 17.3 and discussed in Chapter 3. Patients with obvious burns or diseases that disrupt the integument in the same way (e.g., scalded skin syndrome) are presumed to have become dehydrated through transudation of fluid through the skin.

If the patient does not have an obvious cutaneous source for dehydration, GI losses provide the most likely explanation. A history of vomiting (see Chapter 78) or diarrhea (see Chapter 18) should be sought. Most children with vomiting or diarrhea have viral gastroenteritis, but many diseases (Tables 18.1 and 78.1) produce these symptoms. Additional history serves to establish the adequacy of oral intake. Several common minor

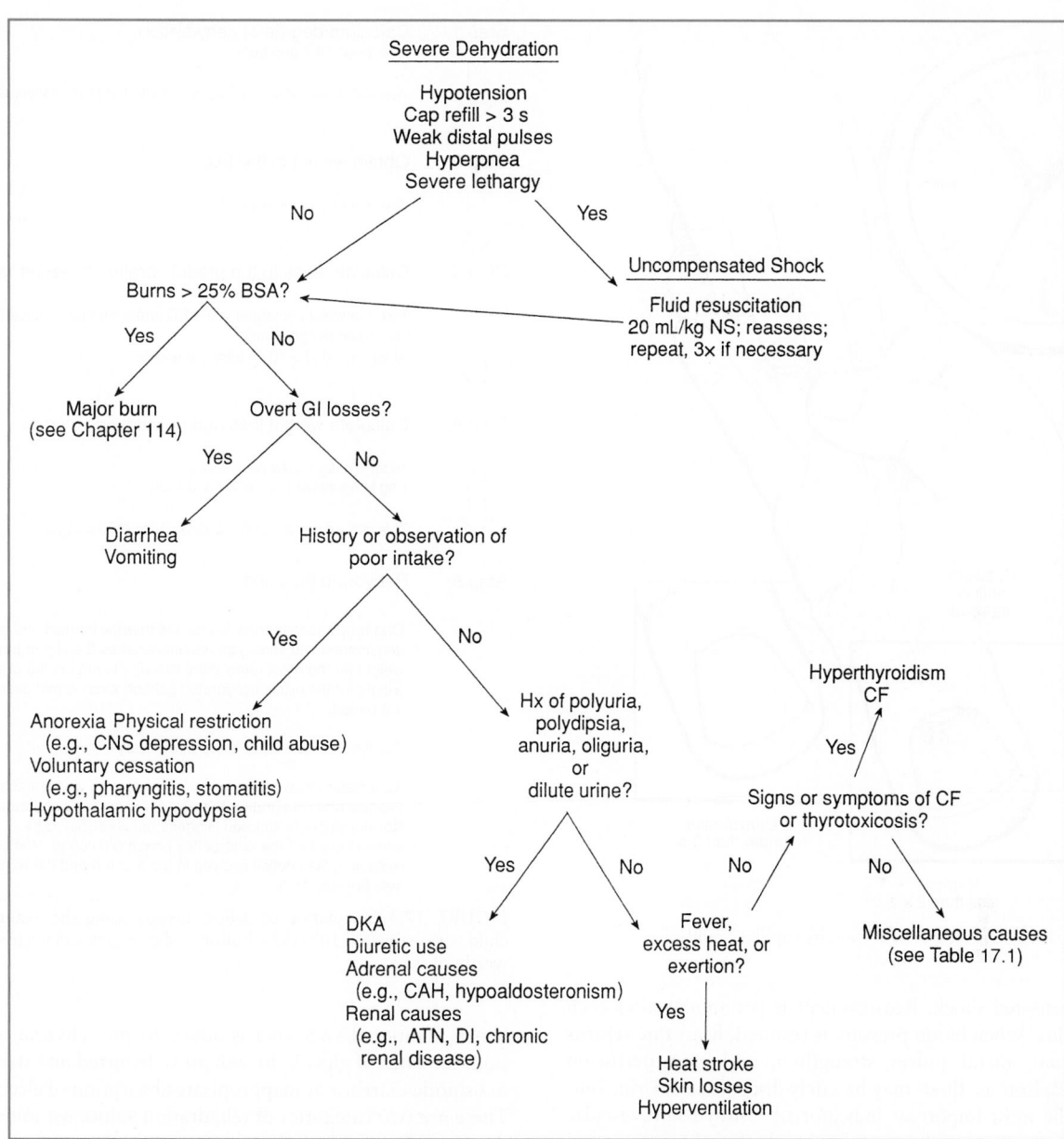

FIGURE 17.1 Suspected dehydration. BSA, body surface area; NS, normal saline; GI, gastrointestinal; CNS, central nervous system; CF, cystic fibrosis; DKA, Diabetic ketoacidosis; Hx, History; CAH, congenital adrenal hyperplasia; ATN, acute tubular necrosis; DI, diabetes insipidus.

infections, such as pharyngitis and stomatitis, as well as more serious disorders of the CNS, cause dehydration as a result of voluntary or involuntary limitation of fluids taken orally.

Next, the history should address the nature and quantity of the urine output. With dehydration, one expects to find oliguria or anuria if normal renal concentrating function remains intact. Severe oliguria or anuria may also, however, be manifest if severe dehydration and shock has led to acute renal failure (see Chapter 100). The unexpected discovery of polyuria points to diabetes mellitus or insipidus, adrenal insufficiency, diuretic use, or renal injury or disease with resultant loss of concentrating ability (Fig 17.1).

By this point, the physician will have established a diagnosis in most patients. In hot weather or when there is prolonged fever, skin losses must be considered. Patients with cystic fibrosis

(see Chapter 99) are prone to dehydration because of a high concentration of sodium in the sweat (the finding of hyponatremic dehydration seemingly unexplained by the estimated fluid loss should suggest this diagnosis). Additional considerations are listed in Table 17.1.

Initial Management

The dehydrated child must be examined immediately for the degree of dehydration or state of hypovolemic shock. If there is severe dehydration or uncompensated shock, the patient is treated acutely with isotonic fluids to restore intravascular volume regardless of serum osmolarity or cause of the dehydration (Fig. 17.3). Normal saline or Ringer's lactate is given via an IV or intraosseous line in 20 mL per kg aliquots over approximately 15 to 30 minutes, or as quickly as possible if there is

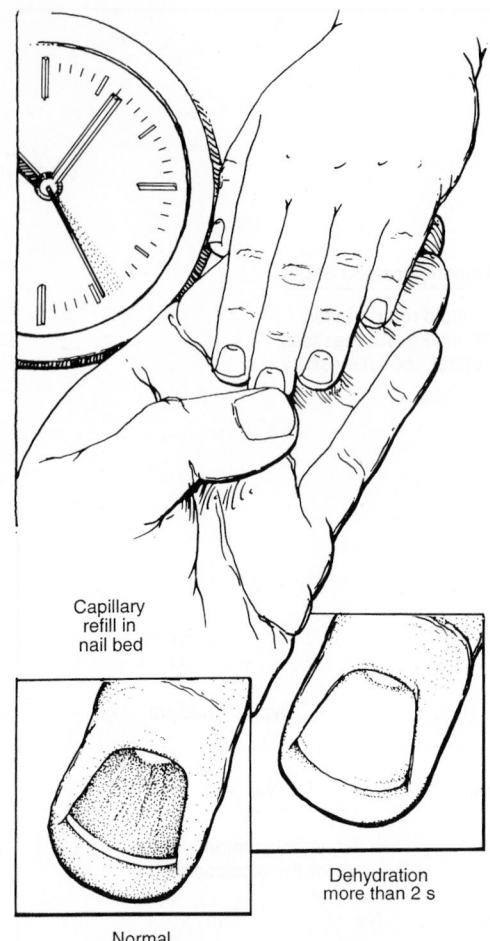

Capillary
refill in
nail bed

Normal
less than 2 s

Dehydration
more than 2 s

FIGURE 17.2 Assessing dehydration by capillary refill.

Step 1:   Calculate degree of dehydration.
          (see Table 18.4 and text)

          Assume a patient is moderately dehydrated (10% dehydration).

Step 2:   Obtain weight in the ED.

          The patient weighs 9 kg.

Step 3:   Calculate back to the predehydration baseline weight.

          Take the weight obtained in the ED and divide by 1 minus the
          proportion dehydration.
          (9 kg)/(1 − 0.1) = 10 kg baseline weight

Step 4:   Calculate weight loss and deficit fluid volume.

          10 kg − 9 kg = 1 kg weight loss
          1 kg is equivalent to 1,000 mL deficit

          This patient has a 1,000 mL fluid deficit (100 cc/kg).

Step 5:   Rehydrate the child.

          Oral rehydration therapy is first-line therapy for mild and moderate
          dehydration and should be administered as 2 cc/kg of baseline
          weight for the moderately dehydrated patient (1 cc/kg of baseline
          weight for the mildly dehydrated patient) every 5 min over a
          4-h period.

          2 cc/kg x 10 kg = 20 cc every 5 min orally

          Administer intravenous fluids for those who were unable to
          tolerate oral rehydration therapy or for severe dehydration.
          Normal saline or lactated Ringer's boluses should be
          administered for the emergency phase (20 cc/kg). Half of the
          remaining fluid deficit is given in the first 8 h and the remainder
          over the next 16 h.

FIGURE 17.3 Calculation of deficit therapy using the example of a child with estimated 10% dehydration and emergency department (ED) weight of 9 kg.

uncompensated shock. Reassessment is paramount after each fluid bolus. When blood pressure is restored, heart rate returns to normal, distal pulses strengthen, and skin perfusion improves, isotonic fluids may be safely discontinued. Urine output is the most important indicator of restored intravascular volume in patients with intact renal and adrenal function, and without diabetes mellitus or insipidus, and should be a minimum of 1 mL per kg per hour. If dextrose is needed initially for low serum glucose, 0.5 to 1 g per kg is given in a single bolus of 10% or 25% dextrose and the serum level is rechecked.

Oral Rehydration Therapy

If the child is determined to be mildly or moderately dehydrated, then oral rehydration therapy (ORT) is the therapeutic option of choice. ORT is the frequent administration of small volumes of an appropriate rehydration solution, typically with an oral syringe. The use of ondansetron, a serotonin $5HT_3$ selective receptor antagonist, has clearly been shown to improve the success of rehydration with ORT (Table 17.5). An appropriate rehydration solution has the correct balance of glucose and sodium, which enables the body to absorb the water passively via the sodium glucose cotransport mechanism in the small intestine. The glucose-to-sodium ratio is an important determinant in the acceptability of these solutions. Optimal solutions have a 1:1 or a 2:1 glucose:sodium ratio.

When additional sweetener is added to the rehydration solution, the ratio of glucose to sodium is distorted and may result in osmotic diarrhea or inappropriate absorption of electrolytes. There are two categories of rehydration solutions: initial rehydration solutions that contain 60 to 90 mEq per L of sodium (e.g., Rehydralyte, World Health Organization oral rehydration solutions) and maintenance solutions that contain 40 to 60 mEq per L of sodium (e.g., Pedialyte). If the etiology of the dehydration is presumed to be due to cholera, then the higher sodium concentration is appropriate because there is a large sodium loss in the diarrhea stools of cholera patients. However, if the etiology of the dehydration is presumed to be viral gastroenteritis, then the lower sodium concentration solutions would be appropriate and are more readily available. Both rehydration and maintenance solutions have approximately 20 mEq per L of potassium and a low glucose concentration of 2% to 2.5%. Soda, juice, popsicles, sports drinks, and soups are inappropriate rehydration solutions in dehydrated infants and children and should be strongly discouraged. These fluids do not have the appropriate glucose-to-sodium ratio and are not absorbed as easily as electrolyte solutions.

The amount of fluid to be administered is dependent on the degree of dehydration. Mild dehydration reflects up to 5% weight loss, so 5% of the child's body weight (50 mL per kg)

TABLE 17.5

ONDANSETRON DOSING FOR GASTROENTERITIS

Patient weight	Dose
<10 kg	1 mg liquid
10–20 kg	2 mg orally disintegrating tablet
>20 mg	4 mg orally disintegrating tablet

should be administered as small-volume frequent feeds. Likewise, moderate dehydration represents up to 10% weight loss, so 10% of the child's weight (100 mL per kg) should be administered. An easy rule of thumb to remember is that a mildly dehydrated patient can receive 1 mL per kg every 5 minutes and a moderately dehydrated patient can receive 2 mL per kg every 5 minutes. As the child tolerates the feeds, the volume can be increased as well as the frequency. The rehydration should be completed over a 4-hour time frame (Fig. 17.3). ORT has been shown to be equivalent to IV fluid therapy in terms of rehydration efficacy. Interestingly enough, it has been shown that it takes less time to institute therapy with ORT (i.e., teach the parents how to administer the fluids) than to start an IV line in a child, and there is less staff time involved in administering care to these patients as well as shorter ED stays. There are a significant number of patients with gastroenteritis that will be unable to perform ORT and will subsequently require alternative methods for rehydration. Nasogastric (NG) tube use is an acceptable alternative as it has been shown to be as effective as IV hydration. They are relatively easy to place and the patient does not need to remain awake while receiving the rehydration solution. A small feeding tube is better tolerated for fluid administration than a larger NG tube. However, they are considered one of the more noxious interventions and practitioners may choose parenteral rehydration over NG.

Parenteral Rehydration

Approximately 20% of patients will be unable to tolerate oral syringe administration of ORT because of persistent vomiting, high stool outputs, or inability to cooperate. If the patient is unable to tolerate ORT or is severely dehydrated, then administration of 20 mL per kg boluses of isotonic saline or lactated Ringer's solution intravenously would be appropriate. The number of boluses required depends on the patient's physiologic response to the fluid that has been administered. Once the initial resuscitation phase is completed, an IV fluid is determined for the maintenance phase (see Chapter 100). The initial fluid often is D51/2NS with 20 mEq per L of potassium chloride. Notable exceptions include major burn patients who continue to require isotonic fluids (see Chapter 108), children with diabetic ketoacidosis who do not require dextrose initially (see Chapter 86), and children with severe electrolyte disturbances, such as may occur with pyloric stenosis or severe hypernatremic dehydration (see Chapter 100). There are recent studies advocating for the use of isotonic fluids for all patients who require maintenance of hydration. The benefit of isotonic solutions (such as normal saline) is to avoid fatal hyponatremia.

The fluid rate is determined by the estimated fluid deficit and ongoing losses (Fig. 17.3). Usually, 50% of the child's fluid deficit is given over the first 8 hours in addition to one-third of the daily maintenance fluid requirements. In hypertonic states, after initial stabilization with isotonic fluids, the replacement solution is given more slowly to allow equilibration across the blood–brain barrier (see Chapter 100).

Parenteral rehydration via an IV catheter has been used extensively. The advantages of IV rehydration are numerous including familiarity with the procedure, widespread acceptance, and direct vascular access to rehydrate a patient. There are disadvantages associated with IV catheter use, primarily difficulty in obtaining access in dehydrated children, particularly those younger than 3 years, pain associated with placement, and the time and resources required for placement. Subcutaneous rehydration was common prior to the widespread use of IV catheters. There is evidence that using human recombinate hyaluronidase (Hylenex®) with a subcutaneous catheter may be an alternative for mild and moderately dehydrated children who have failed ORT. Hyaluronidase temporarily dissolves hyaluronic acid and allows fluid to be administered subcutaneously, which is subsequently absorbed into the vascular system. Advantages of subcutaneous fluid administration include ease of placement and decreased pain with insertion. More research in this new modality is required.

In all types of dehydration and their methods of treatment, the patient must be monitored closely. Physical exam and vital signs should be reassessed continually, urine output monitored closely, ongoing losses quantified and replaced, and therapy individualized.

Suggested Readings

Allen CH, Etzwiller LS, Miller MK, Harb G. Subcutaneous hydration in children using recombinant human hyaluronidase: Safety and ease of use. *Ann Emerg Med* 2008;52(4 suppl):S75–S76.

American Academy of Pediatrics, Provisional Committee on Quality Improvement, Subcommittee on Acute Gastroenteritis. Practice Parameter. The management of acute gastroenteritis in young children. *Pediatrics* 1996;97:424.

Atherly-John YC, Cunningham SJ, Crain EF. A randomized trial of oral vs intravenous rehydration in a pediatric emergency department. *Arch Pediatr Adolesc Med* 2002;156:1240.

Finberg L, Kravath RE, Hellerstein S, eds. *Water and electrolytes in pediatrics: physiology, pathophysiology, and treatment.* 2nd ed. Philadelphia: WB Saunders, 1993.

Fonseca BK, Holdgate A, Craig, JC. Enteral vs. intravenous rehydration therapy for children with gastroenteritis. *Arch Pediatr Adolesc Med* 2004;158: 483–490.

Freedman SB, Adler M, Seshadri R, et al. Oral ondansetron for gastroenteritis in a pediatric emergency department. *N Engl J Med* 2006;354(16):1698–1705.

Gorelick MH, Shaw KN, Murphy KO. Validity and reliability of clinical signs in the diagnosis of dehydration in children. *Pediatrics* 1997;99:1. Available at: http://www.pediatrics.org/cgi/content/full/99/5/e6.

Hartling L, Bellemare S, Wiebe N, et al. Oral versus intravenous rehydration for treating dehydration due to gastroenteritis in children. *Cochrane Database Syst Rev* 2006, Issue 3. Art. No.: CD004390. DOI: 10.1002/14651858. CD004390.pub2.

King CK, Glass R, Bresee JS, et al. Managing acute gastroenteritis among children: oral rehydration, maintenance, and nutritional therapy. *MMWR* 2003;52(RR-16):1–16.

Moritz ML, Ayus, JC. Prevention of hospital-acquired hyponatremia: a case for using isotonic saline. *Pediatrics* 2003;111:227–230.

Spandorfer PR, Alessandrini EA, Joffe M, et al. Oral vs. intravenous rehydration of moderately dehydrated children: a randomized controlled trial. *Pediatrics* 2005;115:295–301.

World Health Organization. *The treatment of diarrhoea. A manual for physicians and other senior health workers.* WHO/CDD/SER/80.2. 4th ed. Geneva: Division of Diarrhoeal and Acute Respiratory Disease Control, World Health Organization, 2005.

SIGNS AND SYMPTOMS

CHAPTER 18 ■ DIARRHEA

GARY R. FLEISHER, MD

Diarrhea refers to a softening in the consistency of the stool with or without an increase in the number of stools. Although the World Health Organization defines diarrhea as the passage of three or more loose or watery stools per day, because of the variability in the frequency and type of stools among children, absolute limits of normalcy are difficult to define. Rather, any deviation from the child's usual pattern should arouse at least a mild concern, regardless of the actual number of stools or their water content. Some infants, particularly those who are breastfed, often have five or six loose stools daily routinely; other healthy infants may produce only one formed stool every other day.

DIFFERENTIAL DIAGNOSIS

Diarrhea, with or without vomiting, often prompts a visit to the emergency department (ED). An estimated 15 to 20 million children younger than 5 years of age have between 20 and 40 million episodes of diarrhea annually in the United States. Approximately 12% of all hospitalizations of children 1 month through 4 years of age include diarrhea as one of the top three discharge diagnoses. Although most bouts of diarrhea seen in the ED in developed countries result from self-limiting infections, diarrhea may be the initial manifestation of a wide spectrum of disorders, as outlined in Table 18.1.

Of the many causes of diarrhea, a few are particularly common: infections with viruses and bacteria, parenteral diarrhea (diarrhea due to a nongastrointestinal infection), and diarrhea induced by antibiotic administration (Table 18.2). The single most common disorder seen in the ED is viral gastroenteritis.

Any cause of diarrhea may produce, on rare occasions in developed countries, a fatality secondary to dehydration or electrolyte disturbance. Several hundred young children die annually in the United States from gastroenteritis; however, most of the disorders, particularly viral gastroenteritis, are mild. The emergency physician must be vigilant in recognizing the few children who have diseases that are likely to be life threatening from among the majority of children who have self-limiting infections. Particularly urgent are intussusception, pseudomembranous colitis, hemolytic uremic syndrome (HUS), and appendicitis (Table 18.3). In addition, children may develop severe dehydration with diarrhea secondary to any pathogen.

Intussusception, although not typified by presentation with diarrhea, is the most common of these serious disorders to have diarrhea as a symptom. Most children with intussusception primarily have severe, episodic abdominal pain, but a few are brought to the hospital with the complaint of bloody diarrhea. Intussusception peaks in frequency between 5 and 10 months of age and tapers off rapidly after 2 years of age, unless there is a predisposing pathologic condition. Although the child may be febrile, the temperature is usually normal. Classically, intussusception causes colicky abdominal pain, vomiting, and an abdominal mass, in addition to a "currant jelly" stool. The finding of a mass in association with colicky abdominal pain, vomiting, and blood in the stool is highly suggestive of intussusception, but a mass actually is palpable in fewer than 20% of cases. Thus, the physician should consider this diagnosis even in the absence of a mass when a child in the first year or two of life has the combination of bloody diarrhea and severe, colicky abdominal pain. In addition, the child who is flaccid or lethargic out of proportion to the degree of dehydration should raise suspicion, as intussusception can evoke "neurologic" signs. Plain films of the abdomen may be diagnostic (intussusceptum seen on the basis of air contrast), suggestive (mechanical obstruction), or nonspecific (normal or ileus); thus, a high index of suspicion mandates either an ultrasound or a contrast enema with air or barium.

HUS, although uncommon, merits consideration in any child with bloody diarrhea because it is a potentially fatal illness. Children are affected most often in the first 3 years of life. Typically, over the course of several days, an initially mild gastroenteritis becomes complicated first by hematochezia and then by pallor (anemia), purpura (thrombocytopenia), and oliguria (acute renal failure). When HUS is suspected, a complete blood count, urinalysis, and coagulation studies should be performed. The peripheral blood smear, in addition to reduced numbers of platelets, shows evidence of intravascular hemolysis, including helmet cells and red blood cell fragments. The urine tests positive for blood (both hemoglobin and red cells).

Another serious disorder that may cause bloody diarrhea is pseudomembranous colitis. This disease results from an overgrowth of toxin-producing clostridial organisms in the bowel and must be considered after a course of antibiotic therapy, which can decimate the normal gut flora. It may occur at any age but is uncommon in early childhood. Although the incidence of pseudomembranous colitis is highest after treatment with clindamycin, a less frequently prescribed antibiotic, any of the antibacterial drugs may be the culprit. In fact, because of its common use, amoxicillin is responsible for most cases of pseudomembranous colitis in childhood, even though the incidence after therapy with this agent is low. Occasional cases occur in children with no recent usage of antibiotics. Clinically, the patient with pseudomembranous colitis usually appears ill with prostration, abdominal distension, and significant amounts of blood in the stool. Stool toxin analysis provides the mainstay of diagnosis.

TABLE 18.1

CAUSES OF DIARRHEA

Infections
Enteral
  Viruses: rotavirus, Calciviruses (Norwalk and sapporo viruses), enteroviruses, adenoviruses, astroviruses
  Bacteria: *Salmonella, Shigella, Yersinia, Campylobacter,* pathogenic *Escherichia coli, Aeromonas hydrophila, Vibrio* spp., *Clostridium difficile,* tuberculosis
  Parasites: *Giardia lamblia, Entamoeba histolytica, Cryptosporidia*
Nongastrointestinal (parenteral diarrhea)

Dietary Disturbances
Overfeeding, food allergy, starvation stools

Anatomic Abnormalities
Intussusception, Hirschsprung's disease, partial obstruction, appendicitis, blind loop syndrome, intestinal lymphangiectasia, short bowel syndrome

Inflammatory Bowel Disease
Ulcerative colitis, Crohn's disease

Malabsorption or Increased Secretion
Cystic fibrosis, celiac disease, disaccharidase deficiency, acrodermatitis enteropathica, secretory neoplasms

Systemic Illnesses
Immunodeficiency
Endocrinopathy: hyperthyroidism, hypoparathyroidism, congenital adrenal hyperplasia

Psychogenic Disturbances (Irritable Bowel Syndrome)

Miscellaneous
Antibiotic-induced diarrhea, secondary lactase deficiency, neonatal drug withdrawal, toxins (e.g., organophosphate ingestion), hemolytic-uremic syndrome

---

Appendicitis manifests primarily with abdominal pain, followed by anorexia, vomiting, or fever. Less commonly, appendicitis may cause diarrhea. The presumed mechanism for the diarrhea is irritation of the colon by the inflamed appendix. In most cases, careful questioning about the nature of the diarrhea will reveal a description of frequent, very low volume stools, with mucus. Particularly in very young children or among patients of any age who have a perforated appendix and a long duration of illness, the diagnosis of appendicitis as the cause of diarrhea may be delayed because the classic con-

TABLE 18.2

COMMON CAUSES OF DIARRHEA

Infections
  Enteral
    Viruses
    Bacteria
  Nongastrointestinal ("parenteral" diarrhea)
Dietary disturbances
Psychogenic disturbances
Miscellaneous
  Antibiotic induced
  Secondary lactase deficiency

TABLE 18.3

LIFE-THREATENING CAUSES OF DIARRHEA

Intussusception
Hemolytic uremic syndrome
Pseudomembranous colitis
Appendicitis
Salmonella gastroenteritis (with bacteremia in the neonate or immunocompromised host)
Hirschsprung's disease (with toxic megacolon)
Inflammatory bowel disease (with toxic megacolon)

---

stellation of findings is often absent. However, the examiner will usually be able to elicit abdominal tenderness greater than would be expected with gastroenteritis.

EVALUATION AND DECISION

The initial evaluation of the child with diarrhea should serve the dual purpose of exploring the possible causes and assessing the degree of illness. Preexisting conditions in the child may account for the diarrhea or predispose him or her to unusual causes; in particular, the emergency physician should search for a history of gastrointestinal surgery or chronic illnesses, such as ulcerative colitis or regional enteritis. Immunodeficiency syndromes, neoplasms, and immunosuppressive therapy all lead to an increased susceptibility to infection. Institutionalized children and those recently returning from underdeveloped countries are more likely to harbor bacterial or parasitic pathogens.

A history of abdominal pain, particularly if severe, raises the index of suspicion for intussusception and appendicitis. Bloody diarrhea points particularly to bacterial enteritis but occasionally occurs with viral infections and may also herald the onset of HUS or pseudomembranous colitis. The combination of episodic abdominal pain and blood in the stool characterizes intussusception. Vomiting in association with diarrhea is very suggestive of viral gastroenteritis, whereas vomiting in isolation (see Chapter 78) is more concerning for intestinal obstruction.

With the initial interview, the physician should attempt to reconstruct historically the child's intake and output during the course of the illness. Detailed questions about the number and size of stools, the frequency of emesis, and the amount of liquid taken orally allow for an estimate of fluid balance. Decreases in the frequency or volume of urination (or the number of diaper changes in the infant) suggest an inadequate output, reflecting the development of dehydration.

The general physical examination can provide clues to an underlying illness in the child who appears malnourished or small for his or her age. The body weight should be measured and compared to a premorbid weight. If fever is present, infectious causes are most likely. The pulse and blood pressure, together with the turgor of the skin and mucous membranes, are useful in assessing the degree of dehydration (Table 18.4), except in the child who has hypernatremia, as relatively normal skin turgor is preserved in this condition even with dehydration. On abdominal examination, the finding of a mass (regional enteritis, intussusception) or evidence of obstruction

TABLE 18.4

CLINICAL FINDINGS IN DEHYDRATION

Degree of dehydration (%)	Skin	Mucosa	Pulse	Blood pressure
0	Good turgor	Moist	Normal	Normal
5	Dry	Dry, no tears	Mildly increased	Orthostatic decrease
10	Tenting present	Very dry	Moderately increased, weak	Mildly decreased
15	Poorly perfused	Parched	Markedly increased, thready	Markedly decreased

is important. A rectal examination should be performed in the child who has chronic diarrhea. With overflow stools secondary to prolonged constipation, the rectal ampulla often contains a large amount of hard stool, but it is usually empty in the patient with Hirschsprung's disease. For selected children, laboratory measurements may assist in the evaluation of dehydration, but they often fall in the normal range despite marked loss of fluids.

A diagnostic approach to the pediatric patient with diarrhea is outlined in Fig. 18.1. The physician should first determine

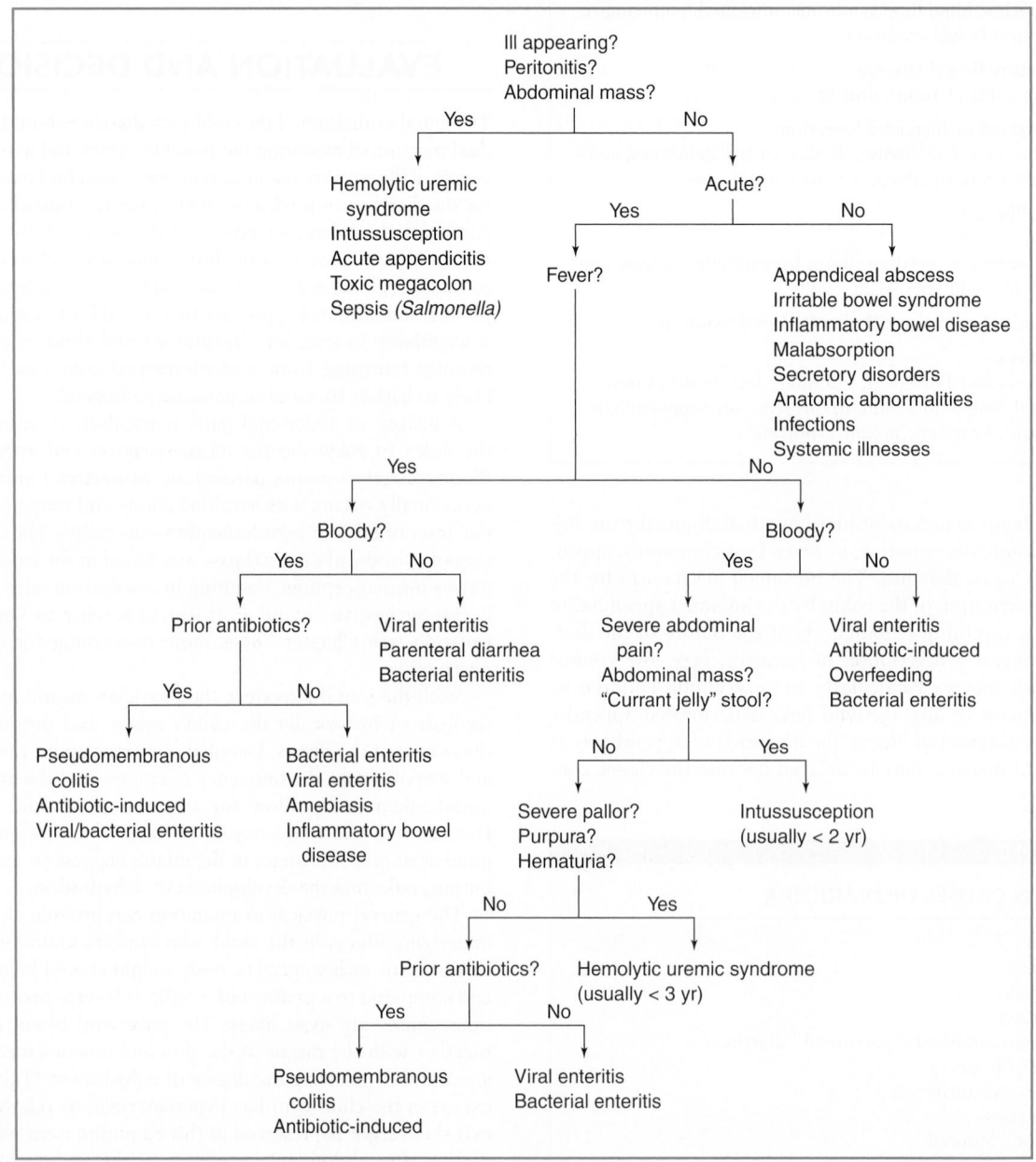

FIGURE 18.1 Diagnostic approach to the immunocompetent child with diarrhea.

whether the child appears seriously ill or has signs of a surgical abdominal process. Once it has been determined that immediate signs of a life-threatening condition are absent, more than any other feature, the duration of diarrhea dictates the initial diagnostic considerations. Children with chronic diarrhea (more than 5 days) are more likely than their counterparts with illnesses of briefer duration to have irritable bowel syndrome, bacterial infections, inflammatory bowel disease, or various malabsorptive disorders. Such conditions, if uncomplicated, do not require a definitive diagnosis emergently, with the possible exception of bacterial enteritis in a febrile or toxic-appearing patient, but rather an evaluation over time.

Acute Diarrhea

With the acute onset of diarrhea, most children have an infectious cause for their disorder and will require at least a brief evaluation in the ED. Fever, the hallmark of infection, serves as the first branch point in the approach to such patients. Although not all children with infectious enteritis have fevers, the finding of an elevated temperature points strongly in this direction. At the same time, the absence of fever, particularly in the presence of bloody stools, should alert the physician to the possibility of one of several serious noninfectious diseases, particularly intussusception and HUS.

The next question is whether hematochezia (bloody stool) is present. Blood is seen in the stool of approximately 10% of children with diarrhea. In most cases, the blood appears in small quantities as drops on the surface of the stool and should not be construed as ominous. A small percentage of children with diarrhea, however, have more profuse rectal bleeding. In these patients, one must exclude life-threatening disorders such as intussusception, HUS, and pseudomembranous colitis.

Febrile children with bloody diarrhea (Fig. 18.1) almost invariably have an infectious enteritis. Pseudomembranous colitis should be considered particularly in patients who have received antibiotic therapy, but this diagnosis usually can be discarded on clinical grounds in the absence of systemic toxicity, abdominal distension, and gross blood in the stools. If pseudomembranous colitis is strongly suspected, admission to the hospital and a full diagnostic evaluation should be considered. Bacterial diarrhea should be sought by culture in febrile children with frankly bloody diarrhea but will be found only in 15% to 20% of cases; viral enteritis is much more common. In the first few months of life, in the infant for whom *Salmonella* gastroenteritis represents a more serious illness, a stool smear for polymorphonuclear leukocytes is useful because the finding of sheets of inflammatory cells strongly points to a bacterial origin. Amebiasis merits consideration only in endemic areas and among travelers. Finally, an occasional child with inflammatory bowel disease may present with an initial episode of acute, bloody diarrhea. In most of these cases, the physician can elicit a preceding history of weight loss or recurrent abdominal pain; in the remainder, the diagnosis emerges only over time, when bloody diarrhea persists in the face of negative cultures.

Most febrile children with nonbloody diarrhea (Fig. 18.1) have viral enteritis. The physician must perform a thorough examination because nonenteric infections, particularly otitis media, may cause "parenteral" diarrhea. For similar reasons,

a urine culture is indicated if any historical factors point to an infection of the urinary tract. Although a small percentage of these patients have a bacterial enteritis, routine cultures of stool are not recommended for nonbloody diarrhea of brief duration in otherwise healthy children. Immunocompromised patients, such as those with acquired immunodeficiency syndrome (HIV/AIDS) (see Chapter 93), require a more thorough evaluation, including bacterial cultures and examination for ova and parasites.

Afebrile children with bloody diarrhea (Fig. 18.1) represent the most worrisome category because most patients with intussusception, HUS, and pseudomembranous colitis have this symptom constellation. In particular, intussusception should be considered carefully in any child younger than 1 year of age with grossly bloody diarrhea that does not appear to have an infectious cause. Although the finding of a mass or a currant jelly stool is pathognomonic, a history of severe, colicky abdominal pain in a lethargic child warrants an abdominal ultrasound or contrast enema. Obvious pallor, purpura, and hematuria point to HUS, an unusual but potentially life-threatening disease. Once again, prior antibiotic therapy raises the possibility of pseudomembranous colitis. The most common diagnosis, infectious enteritis, should be assigned only after exclusion of the more serious disorders by history, physical examination, and occasionally, laboratory or imaging studies.

Afebrile children with nonbloody diarrhea (Fig. 18.1) are usually judged to have viral enteritis. Those who receive antibiotic agents, such as amoxicillin, may be suffering from a drug-related gastrointestinal disturbance (antibiotic-induced diarrhea) but not usually from pseudomembranous colitis. During the first 6 to 12 months of life, overfeeding may manifest as diarrhea. The tip-off to this diagnosis is the history of excessive intake in the overweight child. Bacterial enteritis, although a possibility, does not merit a stool culture in the usual clinical circumstances.

Chronic Diarrhea

Chronic diarrhea precipitates a visit to an ED by a child less often than does acute gastroenteritis. An apparent worsening of a long-standing disease may be a final frustration on the part of the parents, however, particularly on a weekend when the family's usual physician may be unavailable. The evaluation of chronic diarrhea usually requires a period of observation and laboratory evaluation beyond the scope of the ED. In the management of these children, the role of the emergency physician is to identify those few individuals who have urgent conditions and refer the remainder to their regular source of care. Particularly in the infant, consideration must be given to Hirschsprung's disease and to cystic fibrosis. A history of delayed passage of meconium, constipation since birth, and abdominal distension are compatible with Hirschsprung's disease. Malabsorptive stools and respiratory infections suggest cystic fibrosis. Failure to thrive, thrush, and pneumonia occur in association with human immunodeficiency virus (HIV) infection. A stool culture and examination for parasites serve to diagnose the serious infections of the gastrointestinal tract and provide a head start on the evaluation for the physician who subsequently sees the child.

The child who returns to the ED with the persistence of an acute diarrheal illness, presumed to be viral in origin and with no evidence of malnutrition or dehydration, often may be managed without an extensive evaluation. Three causes are common: (i) bacterial infections, (ii) secondary lactase deficiency from mucosal sloughing, and (iii) starvation stools in the child who inadvertently has been continued on a clear liquid diet for several days. A stool culture should be obtained, and testing for clostridial toxin is indicated in the presence of recent or ongoing antibiotic therapy. If the child has remained on a clear liquid diet, gradual refeeding is recommended. Milk and all milk products should be proscribed temporarily when secondary lactase deficiency is suspected.

TREATMENT

The treatments for the myriad causes of diarrhea are covered in the medical and surgical sections of this book; however, the therapy for viral gastroenteritis or parenteral diarrhea merits a brief summary. Although all children with circulatory compromise and many children with moderate to severe dehydration need intravenous fluids, the majority of patients with gastroenteritis can be managed with oral solutions. Most children, even those with vomiting, will tolerate frequent, small feedings, but occasionally delivery of fluids via a nasogastric tube may be helpful.

Optimal oral therapy emphasizes the use of appropriate glucose and electrolyte solutions, as well as the early reintroduction of feeding. The ideal solutions, based on formulas carefully tested by the World Health Organization (WHO), have a carbohydrate:sodium ratio that approaches 1:1. Although some recommend, particularly for young infants, initial rehydration with a solution that contains 75 to 90 mEq/L of sodium (i.e., Rehydralyte®) and subsequent maintenance with a more hypotonic formulation (i.e., Pedialyte®), most clinicians use a single preparation during the course of routine, brief illnesses. Older children with mild gastroenteritis tolerate juices and other commercial products, even though the carbohydrate:sodium ratio deviates from the WHO standard.

In general, antidiarrheal agents are ineffective and have no role in the treatment of infectious gastroenteritis during childhood; agents that decrease intestinal mobility (i.e., Lomotil®) carry an additional risk of toxicity. Preliminary studies that pointed to a decrease in stool output with bismuth subsalicylate (Pepto-Bismol®) have not been replicated to a point where routine utilization can be recommended. When selected bacterial or parasitic pathogens are isolated or strongly suspected, appropriate antimicrobial agents should be prescribed (see Chapter 92).

Suggested Readings

Mauer AM, Dweck HS, Finberg L, et al. American Academy of Pediatrics Committee on Nutrition: use of oral fluid therapy and posttreatment feeding following enteritis in children in a developed country. *Pediatrics* 1985;75:358–361.

Blanton LH, Adams, SM, Beard RS, et al. Molecular and epidemiologic trends of Calciviruses associated with outbreaks of acute gastroenteritis in the United States, 2000–2004. *J Infect Dis* 2006;193:413–426.

Bonadio WA, Hennes HH, Machi J, et al. Efficacy of measuring BUN in assessing children with dehydration due to gastroenteritis. *Ann Emerg Med* 1989;18:755–757.

Centers for Disease Control. Severe Clostridium difficile-associated disease in populations previously at low risk. *MMWR Morb Mortal Wkly Rep* 2005;54:1201–1205.

Brown KH. Dietary management of acute childhood diarrhea: optimal timing of feeding and appropriate use of milk and mixed diets. *Pediatrics* 1991;118(pt 2):S92–S98.

Cohen MB. Etiology and mechanisms of acute infectious diarrhea in infants in the United States. *J Pediatr* 1991;118(pt 2):S34–S39.

Finkelstein JA, Schwartz JS, Torrey S, et al. Common clinical features as predictors of bacterial diarrhea in infants. *Am J Emerg Med* 1989;7:469–473.

Frezen PD. Mortality due to gastroenteritis of unknown etiology in the United States. *J Infect Dis* 2003;187:441–452.

Gerber A, Karch H, Allerberger F, et al. Clinical course and the role of Shiga toxin-producing *Escherichia coli* infection in hemolytic-uremic syndrome in pediatric patients, 1997–2000 in Germany and Austria: a prospective study. *J Infect Dis* 2002;186:493–500.

Glass RI, Lew JF, Gangarosa RE, et al. Estimates of morbidity and mortality rates for diarrheal diseases in American children. *J Pediatr* 1991(pt 2); 118:S27–S33.

Goldman RD, Friedman JN, Parkin PC. Validation of the clinical dehydration scale for children with acute gastroenteritis. *Pediatrics* 2008;122:545–549.

Gorelick MH, Shaw KN, Murphy KO. Validity and reliability of clinical signs in the diagnosis of dehydration in children. *Pediatrics* 1997;99:E6.

Gremse DA. Effectiveness of nasogastric rehydration in hospitalized children with acute diarrhea. *J Pediatr Gastroenterol Nutr* 1995;21:145–148.

Ho MS, Glass RI, Pinsky RF, et al. Diarrheal deaths in American children. Are they preventable? *JAMA* 1988;260:3281–3285.

Horwitz JR, Gursoy M, Jaksic T, et al. Importance of diarrhea as a presenting symptom of appendicitis in very young children. *Am J Surg* 1997;173:80–82.

Huicho L, Sanchez D, Contreras M, et al. Occult blood and fecal leukocytes as screening tests in childhood infectious diarrhea: an old problem revisited. *Pediatr Infect Dis J* 1993;12:474–477.

Koehler KM, Lasky T, Fein SB, et al. Population-based incidence of infection with selected bacterial enteric pathogens in children younger than five years of age, 1996–1998. *Ped Infect Dis J* 2006;25:129–134.

Levy JA, Bachur RG. Intravenous dextrose during outpatient rehydration in pediatric gastroenteritis. *Acad Emerg Med* 2007:14:324–330.

Musher DM, Musher BL. Contagious acute gastrointestinal infections. *N Engl J Med* 2004;351:2417–2427.

Picus D, Shackelford GD. Perforated appendix presenting with severe diarrhea. Findings on barium-enema examination. *Radiology* 1983;149:141–143.

Reid SR, Bonadio WA. Outpatient rapid intravenous rehydration to correct dehydration and resolve vomiting in children with acute gastroenteritis. *Ann Emerg Med* 1996;28:318–323.

Rockx B, De Wit M, Vennema H, Vinjé J, et al. Natural history of *Calicivirus* infection: a prospective cohort study. *Clin Infect Dis* 2002;35:246–253.

Rowe PC, Orrbine E, Lior H, et al. Risk of hemolytic uremic syndrome after sporadic *Escherichia coli* O157:H7 infection: results of a Canadian collaborative study. Investigators of the Canadian Pediatric Kidney Disease Research Center. *J Pediatr* 1998;132:756–782.

Snyder JD. Use and misuse of oral therapy for diarrhea: comparison of U.S. practices with American Academy of Pediatrics recommendations. *Pediatrics* 1991;87:28–33.

Sorrano-Brucker H, Avendano P, O'Ryan M, et al. Bismuth subsalicylate in the treatment of acute diarrhea in children: a clinical study. *Pediatrics* 1991;87:18–27.

Torrey S, Fleisher G, Jaffe D. Incidence of *Salmonella* bacteremia in infants with *Salmonella* gastroenteritis. *J Pediatr* 1986(5 pt 1);108:718–721.

CHAPTER 19 ■ DISTURBED CHILD

LAURA L. CHAPMAN, MD, EMILY R. KATZ, MD, AND THOMAS H. CHUN, MD

This chapter presents an approach for the diagnosis of the acutely disturbed child who manifests agitation and aggression. Additional details of management of the conditions discussed here are found in Chapter 133.

At times, the child's ways of responding to external events and changes in the environment are inadequate. In other situations, a previously supportive environment no longer provides security and protection. As a result, the child may no longer be in control of his or her social and emotional responses. It is usually at this point of crisis that the emergency physician meets the child and his or her caregivers.

The agitated child is typically anxious, upset, and unresponsive to attempts at support. The child may pace back and forth and may threaten staff or family. Speech is often loud and may be abusive. Some children may also be disoriented and out of contact with reality. When agitated, younger children may be out of control, running about the examining room and having severe temper tantrums. They may cry or strike out at the parent or physician. Older children and adolescents may be distraught, sullen, and angry as they meet the examiner. Some children or adolescents, however, may appear to be calm and under control when seen in the emergency department (ED). Information from the parents may reveal significant destructiveness at home before coming to the hospital. In many cases, the improvement in the child's behavior in the ED is a response to the structure provided and the sense that help will be forthcoming.

DIFFERENTIAL DIAGNOSIS

A wide variety of medical and psychiatric conditions can lead to a child's development of significant agitation and aggression. These disorders are listed in Table 19.1 and include severe psychiatric disturbances, life-threatening medical conditions, and minor aberrations in the child's ability to respond to stressful events.

Medical Conditions

Agitation, especially in the presence of disorientation, abnormal vital signs, or decreased level of consciousness, should be considered due to an emergent medical cause until proven otherwise. Clinicians should resist the temptation to immediately ascribe agitation or aggression to psychiatric causes, even in children with a preexisting psychiatric diagnosis. These children remain susceptible to medical illness and are at even higher risk than their peers for engaging in substance use and high-risk behaviors. The first step in evaluating a child with a

chief complaint of sudden personality change or confusion is to rule out any potentially life-threatening medical causes.

The history and physical exam can provide multiple diagnostic clues to help the emergency physician differentiate medical from psychiatric causes (Table 19.2). In general, medical causes of agitation have an acute onset and the patient is likely to be disoriented, particularly with regard to time and place. Recent memory can be impaired. In addition, hallucinations may be visual, tactile, or gustatory, rather than auditory in nature (auditory hallucinations are less common). In contrast, psychiatric causes of agitation and confusion have a gradual onset, often following a prolonged period of progressive social and emotional withdrawal. Hallucinations with psychiatric conditions are most frequently auditory. On physical exam, it is important to review vital signs, complete a full exam including a complete neurologic exam, and to consider medical etiologies if abnormalities are found. Further discussion of the evaluation of the agitated child can be found later in this chapter.

Table 19.3 lists medical conditions that can induce agitation in a child. Most of these diagnoses present acutely. For example, a patient with closed head trauma or a cerebral hemorrhage will present with an acute change in mental status and agitation that worsens over a period of minutes to hours. These patients may also be acutely intoxicated, making the evaluation challenging. Careful assessment of vital signs, and in this case, head imaging and toxicologic screening will lead to the correct diagnosis. Other medical conditions, such as thyroid disease, diabetes mellitus, and electrolyte imbalances, will present subacutely. These disorders are usually preceded by medication changes or by a period of weeks to months of symptoms such as weight change, hair loss, diarrhea or vomiting, or fatigue. A patient with a chronic condition such as heart or renal disease can present with agitation during a period of acute worsening of their chronic illness. It is therefore critically important to obtain an accurate history of current and previous medical problems.

A special consideration in pediatrics, especially in the preverbal, autistic or mentally delayed child, is pain. These children may appear agitated, when in fact they have an acute medical condition or an acute injury. A careful physical exam and a broad diagnostic workup is necessary to fully evaluate these children. Child abuse should always be considered, especially in the autistic or mentally delayed child, as these children have been shown to be at higher risk.

Toxicologic Ingestion or Withdrawal

Acute ingestion of a toxicologic substance, or in the case of a chronic user, withdrawal from a substance, commonly leads to

TABLE 19.1

DIFFERENTIAL DIAGNOSIS OF AGITATION AND AGGRESSION IN CHILDHOOD

Psychosis, caused by
　Medical illness
　Ingestion of toxic substance
　Pervasive developmental disorder (e.g., autism)
　Adult type schizophrenia
　Manic-depressive illness
Depression
Conduct disorder
Adjustment reaction of childhood or adolescence
Attention-deficit disorder
Medical illness in the absence of psychosis (e.g., thyrotoxicosis, temporal lobe epilepsy)
Sensory deficit: blindness, deafness
Severe communication disorder (e.g., childhood aphasia)

TABLE 19.3

MEDICAL CONDITIONS THAT MAY LEAD TO AGITATION AND DELIRIUM

Central Nervous System Lesions
　Tumor
　Brain abscess
　Cerebral hemorrhage
　Meningitis or encephalitis
　Temporal lobe epilepsy
　Closed head trauma
Cerebral Hypoxia
　Pulmonary insufficiency
　Severe anemia
　Cardiac failure
　Carbon monoxide poisoning
Metabolic and Endocrine Disorders
　Electrolyte imbalance
　Hypoglycemia
　Hypocalcemia
　Thyroid disease (hyper- and hypo-)
　Adrenal disease (hyper- and hypo-)
　Uremia
　Hepatic failure
　Diabetes mellitus
　Porphyria
　Reye's syndrome
　Wilson's disease
Collagen-vascular Diseases
　Systemic lupus erythematosus
　Polyarteritis nodosa
Infections
　Malaria
　Typhoid fever
　Subacute bacterial endocarditis
　HIV and complicating infections
　Pain

agitation and may lead to psychosis (Table 19.4). In obtaining a history, a frequent important clue in drug intoxication is the acute onset of disordered thinking in the presence of visual hallucinations. A history of drug abuse and the availability of toxic substances are other important historical clues. Intoxication with alcohol, sedatives, antidepressants, anticholinergic agents, and heavy metals can be life threatening if enough of the agent has been ingested. Withdrawal syndrome in patients habituated to alcohol or sedative-hypnotic agents may likewise result in severe agitation, psychosis, seizure, and death.

Delirium

Delirium can be broadly defined as acute, fluctuating global cerebral dysfunction due to a medical condition. The presentation can be quite variable but the core feature is a disturbance in consciousness with a decreased ability to focus, sustain, or shift attention (Table 19.5). While many delirious patients may be agitated or suffering from hallucinations, others can appear hypoactive, quiet, and withdrawn.

Irritability, mood fluctuation, and anxiety are common findings in pediatric patients suffering from delirium. If delirium is present, priorities should be maintaining the patient's safety while evaluating and treating the underlying cause (Table 19.6).

TABLE 19.2

DIFFERENTIATING FEATURES OF ORGANIC AND PSYCHIATRIC PSYCHOSIS[a]

Evaluation feature	Organic psychosis	Psychiatric psychosis
Onset	Acute	Gradual
Pathologic autonomic signs[b]	May be present	Absent
Vital signs	May be abnormal	Normal
Orientation	Impaired	Intact
Recent memory	Impaired	Intact
Intellectual ability	May be impaired	Intact
Hallucinations	Visual	Auditory

[a]Children with both functional and organic psychoses will have impaired reality testing, inappropriate affect, thought disorder, poor behavior control, and disturbed relating ability.
[b]Increase or decrease in heart rate, respiratory rate, blood pressure, and temperature; miosis or mydriasis; and skin color changes.

TABLE 19.4

EXOGENOUS SUBSTANCES CAUSING AGITATION AFTER INGESTION OF SIGNIFICANT QUANTITY OR OVERDOSE, OR DURING WITHDRAWAL WHEN HABITUATED

Intoxication/Overdose
Alcohol
Marijuana
Cocaine
Opioids (e.g., heroin, methadone)
Amphetamines
Methamphetamines/MDMA(ADHD medications, ecstacy)
Hallucinogens—LSD, peyote, mescaline
Corticosteroids (adverse therapeutic effect)
Phencyclidene (PCP)
Barbiturates
Methaqualone (Quaalude)
Anticholinergic compounds
Antipsychotics (e.g., phenothiazines)
Opioids (e.g., heroin, methadone)

Withdrawal
Alcohol
Barbiturates
Benzodiazepines
Other sedative-hypnotic agents

Psychiatric Conditions

A number of psychiatric conditions can present with agitation or aggression. Agitation or aggressive behavior may be the final common pathway for a number of psychiatric conditions. These conditions are discussed below and in greater detail in Chapter 133.

Psychotic Disorders

Psychosis refers to a mental state in which major disturbances in thinking, relating, and reality testing occur. They

TABLE 19.5

CLINICAL DISTURBANCES OF DELIRIUM

Consciousness	Decreased awareness of the environment
Attention	Impaired ability to focus, sustain, or shift attention
Cognition	Disorientation, disorganization, thought disturbance (e.g., paranoia, confusion, language, or memory deficit)
Perception	Hallucinations (especially tactile and visual), illusions, misperceptions
Sleep	Sleep–wake cycle disturbances, fluctuating symptoms (i.e., "sundowning"—waxing and waning symptoms)
Behavior	Agitation, hyper- or hypoactivity, restlessness
Mood/affect	Anxious, depressed, irritable, labile
Neurologic	Diffuse EEG slowing, myoclonus, asterixis, abnormal tone

TABLE 19.6

"I WATCH DEATH" MNEMONIC FOR DELIRIUM

Infection	Meningoencephalitis, HIV, sepsis, abscess
Withdrawal	Alcohol, barbiturates, benzodiazepines, other sedative hypnotics
Acute Metabolic Disturbance	Acidosis, alkalosis, electrolyte abnormality, hepatic or renal failure
Trauma	Head injuries, heatstroke, postoperative complications, severe burns
CNS Pathology	Increased intracranial pressure (e.g., hydrocephalus), seizures, neoplasms, vasculitis
Hypoxia	Anemia, carbon monoxide poisoning, cardiopulmonary failure, impaired cerebral circulation
Deficiencies	Vitamins B_{12}, B_1 (thiamine), B_3 (niacin), folate
Endocrine Disturbances	Hyper- and hypocortisol states, hyper- and hypoglycemia, myxedema, hyperparathyroidism
Acute Vascular Events	Stroke, arrhythmia, shock, hypertensive encephalopathy
Toxins/Drugs	Illicit drug use, prescription drugs, pesticides, solvents
Heavy Metals	Lead, mercury, manganese

Adapted from Wise MG, Terrell CD. In: Hall JB, Schmidt GA, Wood LD, eds. Delirium in the Intensive Care Unit. Principles of Critical Care. 2nd ed. New York: McGraw-Hill; 1998;969–72

may have hallucinations, delusions (fixed, false beliefs), and/or grossly disorganized behavior and speech. Psychotic patients do not express themselves clearly and have difficulty answering direct questions. They also may be extremely suspicious and hostile. In children, psychosis is less likely to be due to a primary psychotic disorder such as schizophrenia and more likely due to a medical illness or another psychiatric disorder that can present with psychotic symptoms [e.g., severe anxiety, posttraumatic stress disorder (PTSD), depression, or mania].

Primary psychotic disorders include brief psychotic disorder, schizophreniform disorder, schizophrenia, delusional disorder, and schizoaffective disorder. These illnesses share core diagnostic criteria but differ primarily based on duration of symptoms. Brief psychotic disorder requires the presence of psychotic symptoms for greater than 1 day but less than one month. Schizophreniform disorder requires active psychotic symptoms for 1 to 6 months. The diagnosis of schizophrenia is reserved for patients who have demonstrated active, prodromal, and/or residual symptoms lasting greater than 6 months. Delusional disorder is diagnosed in otherwise well-functioning children who have non-bizarre delusions and no hallucinations or disorganization. Schizoaffective disorder is diagnosed when patients have bipolar or major depressive episodes superimposed on symptoms consistent with a diagnosis of schizophrenia.

It is useful to assess the child presenting with psychotic symptoms for their level of premorbid functioning as well as any recent stressors. Primary psychotic disorders can present in children who have been previously well adjusted or may have had mild to moderate emotional problems but have been exposed to acute or chronic unmanageable stressor(s) such as trauma or abuse. For children who present with a prolonged prodromal period of progressive social and emotional withdrawal, an eventual diagnosis of a chronic disorder such as schizophrenia is more likely.

It is important for clinicians to reserve the use of the term schizophrenia for patients meeting full diagnostic criteria, since the prognosis for brief psychotic disorder, schizophreniform disorder, and the other psychiatric disorders that can present with psychosis can often be good. Using the term schizophrenia in the ED setting, before it has been determined that full diagnostic criteria have been met, can be unduly devastating and demoralizing for patients and their families. Liberal use of this term may also lead to insufficient evaluation for alternative and potentially treatable diagnoses.

Depression

The depressed child who presents to the ED may appear sad, hopeless, anxious, anhedonic, or withdrawn. However, some depressed children present with irritability as their main symptom and deny feeling sad. This irritability can, in turn, lead to agitated and aggressive behavior. Thus, the emergency physician should ask about other common symptoms of depression including depressed mood and a disturbance in "SIGECAPS" (Table 19.7), a family history of mood disorders, and any major recent changes in the child's life. While depression and resulting irritability can occur in the absence of any major apparent stressors, common precipitants of depression and a sense of hopelessness may include parental divorce or separation, loss of a parent through death, a recent devaluation of personal abilities through poor academic performance, peer rejection, or the onset of significant physical illness. Once depression is identified, it is extremely important to inquire about the presence and nature of any suicidal ideation.

Manic/Mixed Episodes

While mania is primarily associated with elation or elevated mood, the main symptom, especially in children, can be irri-

TABLE 19.7

"SIGECAPS" MNEMONIC FOR DEPRESSION

Sleep (decreased, increased, or disturbed sleep)
Interests (loss of interests, morbid preoccupations)
Guilt (excessive guilt)
Energy (decreased energy)
Concentration (decreased or problems with concentration)
Appetite (decrease or increase in appetite)
Psychomotor functioning (decreased or problems with functioning)
Suicidal ideation

Adapted from Caplan JP, Stern TA. Mnemonics in a mnutshell: 32 aids to psychiatric diagnosis. Current Psychiatr 2008;7:27.

TABLE 19.8

"DIG FAST" MNEMONIC FOR MANIA

Distractibility (attention too easily drawn to unimportant or irrelevant external stimuli)
Indiscretion (excessive involvement in pleasurable activities that have a high potential for painful consequences such as buying sprees/shoplifting, sexual indiscretions, or driving recklessly)
Grandiosity (excessively inflated self-esteem, feeling invincible, reporting they have or are planning to achieve wildly unrealistic goals)
Flight of ideas (rapidly leaping from one idea to the next or subjective experience that thoughts are racing)
Activity increase (socially, at school, or at home) or psychomotor agitation
Sleep deficit (decreased need for sleep while still feeling rested or energized)
Talkativeness/pressured speech (difficult or impossible to interrupt)

Adapted from Caplan JP, Stern TA. Mnemonics in a mnutshell: 32 aids to psychiatric diagnosis. Current Psychiatr 2008;7:27.

tability. In fact, signs of elation may be completely absent. As with depression, the irritability can be severe and judgment can be so impaired that children can become aggressive and violent. A manic episode is defined as a 7-day period (or shorter if hospitalization is required) of a persistently elevated or irritable mood along with symptoms of distractibility, indiscretions/hypersexuality, grandiosity, flight of ideas, increased goal-directed activity, rapid or pressured speech, and decreased need for sleep (Table 19.8). Some children will have a mixed episode, simultaneously meeting criteria for mania and depression. Irritability, agitation, violent acts, and suicidality are more likely to occur when mixed symptoms are present. Children and adolescents experiencing mixed or manic symptoms may be difficult to engage in an interview. They tend to speak rapidly and have pressured speech, have difficulty staying still, and find it difficult or impossible to concentrate long enough to answer questions. As with all presentations of psychiatric symptoms, a high suspicion for an organic etiology should be maintained, especially if abnormal vital signs, confusion, and/or disorientation exist.

Anxiety

Children with anxiety disorders can become quite agitated and even aggressive in an effort to avoid something they are afraid of. For example, children with separation anxiety may become violent—kicking and punching caregivers, destroying property—in their increasingly desperate attempts to prevent their parents from dropping them off at daycare. Children with obsessive–compulsive disorder (OCD) can become agitated and/or aggressive when they are kept from carrying out a compulsion. Agitation and aggression tend to escalate as the fear of the event or activity draws near and may resolve rather precipitously when the event has passed. For example, the child with a school phobia may become increasingly irritable as the weekend draws to a close. It may worsen to the point of trying to jump out of a moving school bus. However, that same child may then appear perfectly safe and happy within 15 minutes of starting the school day. Typically, children whose anxiety leads to severe irritability or aggression will have a long-standing history of anxiety symptoms, and the patient or their parents are usually able to give a clear history of precipitating events. In the absence of such a history and/or a clear precipitating event, suspicion for an organic contribution should be raised.

Trauma

Children and adolescents who have been victims of past or ongoing physical or sexual abuse or other severe trauma may develop acute agitation brought on by posttraumatic stress disorder. The symptoms of this disorder include fluctuating behavior with episodes of excitement, fearfulness, or irritability; recurrent nightmares or flashbacks; and lack of involvement in usual friendships or activities. Children who experience posttraumatic reactions often avoid or refuse to talk about the trauma, and thus, parents may be confused about the reasons for the child's disturbed behavior. If parents are aware of the traumatic event, they may be upset or feel guilty about its occurrence.

Alternatively, one or more of the child's parents may be the perpetrators of the trauma. Parents and children should thus be asked about trauma separately, as part of the diagnostic assessment. Children who are upset about a previous trauma may be particularly difficult to evaluate. They will appear frightened, may behave erratically, and may be uncomfortable with discussing previous traumatic events. A quiet environment and gentle support from the physician may help these children express their thoughts and fears. Younger children who are frightened and who do not easily separate from their parents should raise the possibility of past or current trauma.

Disruptive Behavior Disorders

Disruptive behavior disorders include attention-deficit/hyperactivity disorder, oppositional defiant disorder, and conduct disorder; these disorders are discussed in greater length in Chapter 133. Children with each of these disorders commonly present with out-of-control, agitated, and/or violent behavior. Acute agitation or aggression that requires an ED visit is likely to result from some consequence of the child's difficulties at school or at home. Usually their presenting symptoms fit into a long-standing pattern of similar behaviors. Children with disruptive behavior disorders are at increased risk for substance abuse and suffering trauma-related injuries. Therefore, any acute change in behaviors, especially if accompanied by any physical symptoms or abnormal vital signs, should raise suspicion of a medical contribution to the patient's presentation.

Adjustment Disorders

Adjustment disorder is characterized by a deterioration of functioning from a previously higher level. The decline in function occurs in the presence of some precipitating event or situation that leads to significant emotional or behavioral distress or a symptomatic response in excess of what would be expected given the specific stressor. At times, the precipitant may be a developmental event, such as enrollment in a new school, increased peer pressure, or the emergence of secondary sexual characteristics during puberty. The precipitant also may be an acute event such as the loss of a parent through death or divorce. Children with adjustment reactions can present with anxiety, depressed mood, and/or behavioral disturbances. Behaviors that may fall under this category include those that violate the rights of others or other major age-appropriate societal norms and rules (truancy, vandalism, fighting, etc.).

The child with an adjustment reaction is oriented and usually can explain his or her problems well, although those who present with behavioral disturbances may be quite angry and difficult to engage. In order for a diagnosis of adjustment disorder to be made, the patient's symptoms must not meet criteria for any other major psychiatric disorder. The agitation and aggression of an adjustment reaction can be as dangerous and require intensive intervention as other psychiatric disorders. As such, patients with adjustment reactions need to be screened for suicidality, homicidality, and safety to return home.

Pervasive Developmental Disorders Including Autism

These disorders are discussed in greater length in Chapter 133. Children with pervasive developmental disorders (PDD) who present with agitation or aggression can pose a significant diagnostic and treatment challenge. The range of causes of such behavior is extremely broad, and the patient's ability to report his or her current symptoms can be severely impaired. Clinicians should pay special attention to questioning caregivers about any recent changes in the patient's life or behaviors, no matter how insignificant they may initially appear. Small changes in the patient's routine or apparently minor medical ailments such as constipation can lead to severe behavioral disturbances including self-injurious behavior. Suspicion for medical causes/contributions to the patient's presentation must be extremely high and consultation with the patient's primary clinicians should be sought whenever available. While interventions for agitated and aggressive behavior will be discussed in detail later in this chapter and in Chapter 133, it should be noted that special care should be taken with PDD spectrum patients. Caregivers should be consulted in order to ascertain what calming/distracting techniques have been useful for the patient in the past, and clinicians should use caution when dosing sedative medications, as patients with PDD spectrum often require smaller doses than other children and are especially sensitive to medication side effects.

EVALUATION AND DECISION

The emergency assessment of the agitated or withdrawn child or adolescent involves three complementary areas. The first area involves determination of whether the problematic behavior is caused by some medical condition or organic state. Potential life-threatening effects of the medical condition must be recognized and treated. Second, the psychiatric manifestations of the presenting condition, whether organic or psychiatric, are assessed. Third, the family system and social support for the child are assessed. Once these three areas have been evaluated, the physician can make an appropriate decision regarding disposition and further treatment.

General Approach/Initial Stabilization

The first priority when approaching an agitated and/or aggressive patient is to ensure the safety of both the patient and the ED staff. Pharmacologic and non-pharmacologic interventions that can be employed are discussed in Chapter 133.

Medical Conditions

First, to determine whether the child's agitation or withdrawal is organically based, the physician should bear in mind the differential diagnosis of these behaviors, which include psychiatric as well as organic origins (Table 19.1). A complete history of the acute events that led up to the ED visit, including any changes in behavior or functioning of the child, should be obtained. The possibility of drug use or ingestions should be explored with the parents and with the child. The child's medical history should be documented carefully, and any previous episodes of the current behavior should be reviewed. In general, organically based problems are acute in onset and result from an ingestion, an injury, or the worsening of a medical condition. The differentiating features of organic psychoses and psychiatric psychoses have already been discussed and are listed in Table 19.2.

The medical evaluation of agitation and withdrawal requires that each child who presents to the ED with these behaviors receive a complete physical examination, including full neurologic evaluation. This makes it possible to detect most significant ongoing organic illnesses and neurologic disease of traumatic, infectious, or structural origin. Mild incoordination, abnormalities of rapid alternating movements, and impaired tandem gait may be present in children with an attention-deficit disorder. In situations in which an acute intoxication is being considered, blood and urine should be obtained and sent for specific drug determination or toxic screening, as appropriate. Additional laboratory studies should be pursued in accordance with the findings of the physical examination and may include a complete blood count, sedimentation rate, urinalysis, electrolytes, blood glucose, calcium, blood urea nitrogen, ammonia, and liver function tests. Thyroid studies are indicated when ongoing thyroid disease is suspected. A computed tomography scan or magnetic resonance imaging examination may be helpful when trauma or a mass lesion is being considered (Table 19.9).

Psychiatric Evaluation

The second major area in the ED approach to an agitated or withdrawn child involves assessment of psychiatric manifestations of the presenting condition. This is achieved through a thorough history of present illness (HPI), mental status examination (MSE), in conjunction with an evaluation of the child's

TABLE 19.9

MEDICAL EVALUATION OF THE AGITATED CHILD

Baseline evaluation
  Physical examination including neurological exam

If intoxication suspected
  Toxicologic screening
  Specific drug testing
  Anion/osmolar gap
  Blood gas

If suggested by history or physical exam
  CBC
  ESR
  Urinalysis
  Electrolytes
  Blood glucose
  BUN
  Ammonia
  LFTs
  Pregnancy test
  Thyroid function tests
  EKG

If trauma or mass lesion suspected
  Head CT or MRI

CBC, complete blood cell count; ESR, erythrocyte sedimentation rate; BUN, blood urea nitrogen; LFTs, liver functions tests; EKG, electrocardiogram; CT, computed tomography; MRI, magnetic resonance imaging.

previous level of adjustment, past psychiatric history, and family psychiatric history. In older children and adolescents, the Folstein "Mini-Mental Status Examination" (MMSE) can be a useful screening tool. In younger children who cannot complete the tasks of the MMSE, bedside observation and questioning of parents (or nursing staff) will be the mainstay of assessment. All patients should be asked whether their thinking is confused, whether they are seeing or hearing any strange things, and about the any homicidal or suicidal ideation. The ED physician can obtain much of the MSE during the history and physical examination. Other areas will require direct questioning of the child by the physician.

The categories of the MSE, as described in Chapter 133, are also summarized here. The child's appearance will have already been noted. Orientation to person, place, time, and situation should be determined. Short- and long-term memory should be tested, as should cognitive functions, which include intelligence, fund of knowledge, and the ability to reason and think (much of this information can be determined from the flow of the interview). The child's behavior should be assessed for activity level and age appropriateness. Particularly important in the emergency assessment of the child are affect and thinking. Affect refers to the predominant feelings displayed by the child. The examiner should observe the nature of the affect (e.g., happy, sad, angry, flat), its degree of appropriateness to the situation, and how it changes as various subjects are discussed. Thinking includes thought processes and thought content. The coherence and goal directedness of verbal communication are assessed, and loose associations and speech that lack internal consistency are noted.

Evaluation of thought content involves identifying the child's major themes and concerns. Preoccupations, such as hallucinations, delusions, and ideas of reference (present in psychosis), or sadness, hopelessness, and feelings of depression (present in depression) should also be sought. The child's strengths can be assessed from spontaneous statements and from forthrightness in answering specific questions. The child's insight into the current problem should be noted, and their capacity to suggest a plan for the present crisis should be evaluated.

Determining the presence or absence of suicidal or homicidal ideation and intent is an essential part of the MSE and provides an opportunity to ask about past attempts. The circumstances and intent of any previous suicidal or homicidal attempts should be explored thoroughly and should include questioning about how the patient feels about the fact that prior attempts have failed. If the patient reports suicidal or homicidal ideation, they should be asked whether they have a plan, if they have the means to carry out that plan, what they think will happen if they carry it out, and what, if anything, has kept them from acting on their plan already. The most effective way of determining such intent is by asking the child directly. Such an approach opens the subject in a way that is often reassuring, thereby enabling the discussion to proceed.

As the MSE is carried out, the physician develops a picture of the child that leads to certain diagnostic possibilities. For example, the psychotic child will have bizarre or inappropriate affect, speech that is not goal directed, and possibly, hallucinations or delusions. Such a child typically relates poorly to the physician, avoiding eye contact, failing to respond to the physician's attempts to empathize, and perhaps, engendering in the physician feelings of confusion and uneasiness. If the psychotic child is oriented with intact memory and cognitive functions, it is likely that the psychosis is psychiatric in origin. If the child's orientation, memory, and cognitive functions are significantly impaired, the psychosis is more likely organic in nature. When the child's thinking is coherent and the affect is not bizarre or inappropriate, it is likely that psychosis is not present.

While interviewing the patient, physicians should pay attention to the feelings they experience when interacting with the child, as this can be a rich source of useful information. For example, an interview with a depressed child will often leave the physician feeling sorry for the patient. The manic patient may leave the physician feeling either stressed or more cheerful and talkative. With disruptive behavior disorders, child's manner of relating may be distant or manipulative. The physician may feel angry at such children. Psychotic children may seem odd or absent and leave the physician feeling disconnected or uneasy. Most importantly, the physician should pay close attention to any threatening feelings, as this may be the first sign that a patient may become violent. While awareness of this emotional response to a patient is not, in and of itself, diagnostic, it can still be clinically useful—especially when the patient or family members are reluctant or unreliable historians, or difficult to engage. Recognition of the feelings engendered by a patient can be useful in helping physicians summon empathy and prevent themselves from acting in a counter-therapeutic or unnecessary manner (i.e., being overly aggressive with physical restraints).

Evaluation of Support Systems

Finally, emergency evaluation includes assessment of the family and social support system. Information about who lives at home with the child, the nature of their relationships with each other, and any recent changes in family composition or in the child's living situation help in understanding the current problem and in determining treatment.

The physician can gain information about the family through observation and direct questioning. Information about family relationships, including the parents' level of concern and their ability to appreciate the child's current situation, is obtained. The parents' description of the child during the history taking offers insight into how the child is perceived in the family. The extent to which the parents try to engage a withdrawn child or to calm and set limits with an agitated child should be noted, as well as the child's response to these efforts.

As the child is questioned by the physician, the parents' responses are also informative. Do the parents answer for the child and interrupt when he or she tries to speak? The parental response suggests the degree to which the child's independent thinking and behavior are encouraged. If the child is not cooperative during the psychiatric or physical examinations, how effective are the parents in telling the child that he or she must cooperate? The parents' success in gaining the child's cooperation during the ED visit may offer a valuable clue about their ability to manage their child effectively at home.

The physician can assess the degree of coping by the family in part by the way in which the family members describe problems. Responses that suggest that the parents are overwhelmed and disorganized should lead the physician to consider psychiatric consultation and possible hospitalization. The openness of the family in discussing recent difficulties also is important. Some families are extremely guarded and deny problems, despite the presence of a major crisis that they are unable to manage. Other families offer a more balanced view of family functioning, instilling greater confidence in the physician. If the child's parents are divorced, assessing the relationship between the parents is important. Arguments and disagreements, as well as the possibility of violence, lead to a lack of safety and security for the child in crisis. The degree of support that a single parent receives from extended family and neighbors is also an important factor in evaluating family support and capacity.

Before discharge, the physician should be confident that the child is safe; otherwise, social work or psychiatric consultation should be obtained.

Disposition

In determining the disposition of a child with a psychiatric problem in the ED (Fig. 19.1), the physician should be guided by the severity of the problem and by the ability of the family to manage the child on an outpatient basis. The physician should inquire about what social supports are available to the parents. If extended family or close friends are available and the parents believe that their participation would be helpful, the physician should encourage the parents to enlist such help. If other agencies are working with the family, their efforts

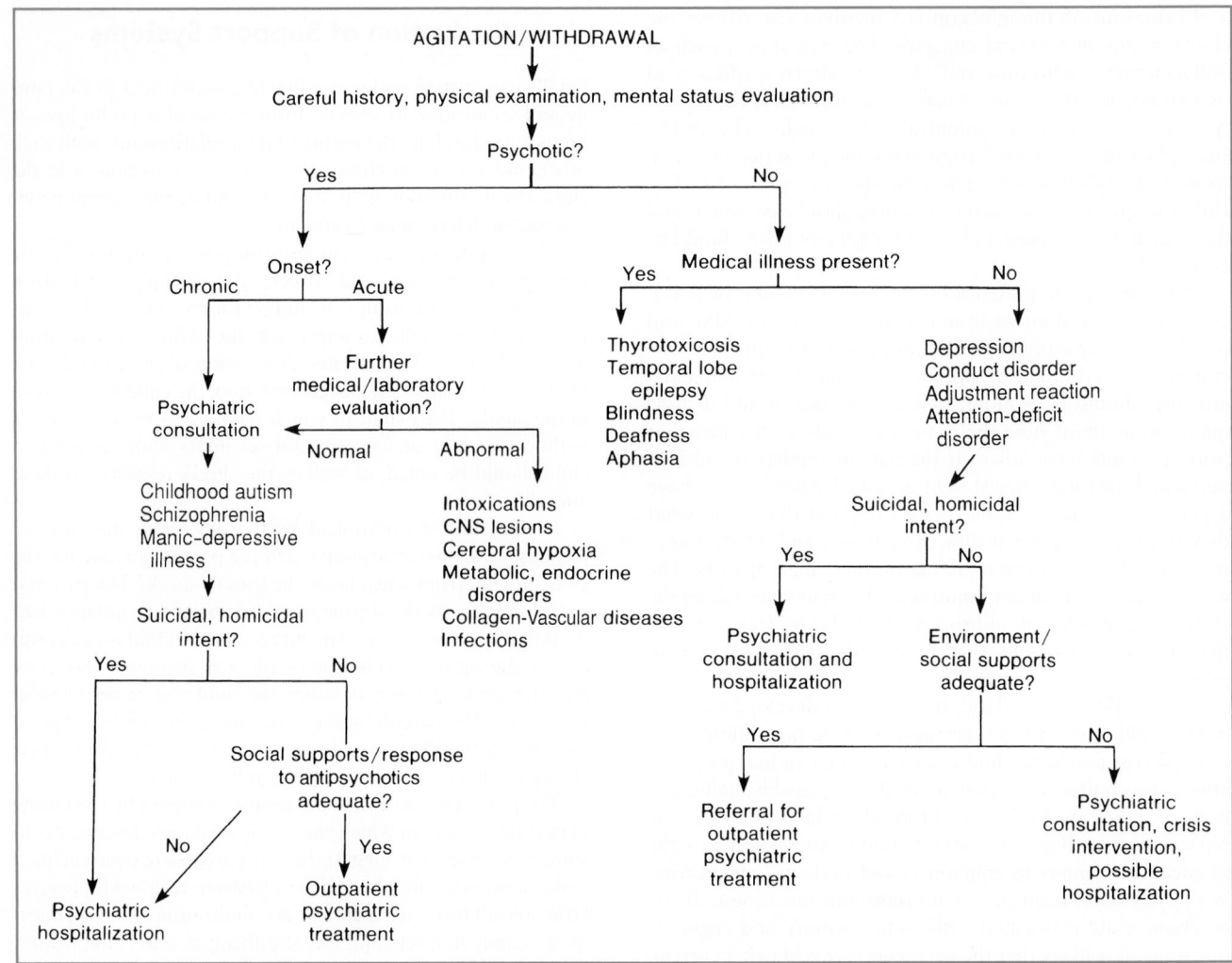

FIGURE 19.1 Approach to the diagnosis and initial disposition of the acutely disturbed child. CNS, central nervous system.

should be coordinated with those of the hospital or mental health facility at which the child receives treatment. Many families express a clear preference about whether their child should be hospitalized. The physician should keep this preference in mind, but should make the decision based on the data about the child's physical and emotional well-being and the assessment of the family support system.

When organic etiologies are suspected or delirium is present, full medical evaluation, observation, and treatment of the underlying condition is required. This is best accomplished through medical hospitalization. Psychiatric consultation is indicated in all cases of psychiatric psychosis, mania, and/or suicidal or homicidal intent. Social work or child protection team consultation is indicated whenever abuse or neglect are suspected.

Psychotic patients who are not suicidal, homicidal, or aggressive and who are able to engage in normal activities of daily living may be referred for ongoing outpatient treatment after a positive response to antipsychotic medication (see Chapter 133).

Patients who have suicidal or homicidal intent are usually hospitalized, as are patients who are unable to maintain their own safety due to mania. Patients with disruptive behavior disorders sometimes require brief inpatient hospitalization when current outpatient and community supports are inadequate to prevent further violence. In the absence of suicidal ideation, homicidal ideation, impaired decision making leading to unsafe behaviors, inability to carry out basic daily functions, or extreme acts of aggression, the ability of the family and social support system to control the child's behavior and prevent further emotional and physical harm should be assessed. If the support system is adequate and timely and appropriate treatment is available, referral to outpatient treatment may be appropriate. When the support system is not adequate and/or appropriate outpatient treatment options are not available, psychiatric hospitalization may be necessary, especially with such behaviors as fire setting, persistent aggressiveness, or failure of prior or current outpatient treatment.

If a child is already in treatment, every effort should be made to contact the child's providers in order to obtain their assessment as to the appropriate disposition and to attempt to arrange for follow-up as close to ED discharge as possible. The physician who discharges a child for outpatient psychiatric treatment should help the family develop short-term measures to manage the child and relieve his or her distress until outpatient psychiatric treatment begins.

Suggested Readings

American Academy of Child and Adolescent Psychiatry. Practice parameters for the assessment and treatment of children and adolescents with schizophrenia. *J Am Acad Child Adolesc Psychiatry* 2001;40(suppl):4S–23S.

Benoit MB. Emergency assessment and suicide assessment in child and adolescent psychiatry. In: Noshpitz JD, ed. *Handbook of child and adolescent psychiatry.* Vol 7. *Advances and new directions.* New York: John Wiley & Sons, 1998:369–379.

Folestein MF, Folstein SE, McHugh PR. A practical method for grading the cognitive state of patients for clinicians. *J Psychiatr Res* 1975;12(3):189–198.

Kahn AU. *Psychiatric emergencies in pediatrics.* Chicago: Year Book Medical Publishers, 1979.

Sadka S. Psychiatric emergencies in children and adolescents. *New Dir Ment Health Serv* 1995 Fall;67:65–74.

Sargent J, Silver M, Hodas G, et al. Crisis intervention in children and adolescents. *Clin Emerg Med* 1984;4:245–262.

Terr LC. Childhood traumas: an outline and overview. *Am J Psychiatry* 1991;148:10–20.

Thomas LE, King RA. Child and adolescent psychiatric emergencies. In: Lewis M, ed. *Child and adolescent psychiatry: a comprehensive textbook.* 3rd ed. Philadelphia: Lippincott Williams & Wilkins, 2002:1104–1110.

Turkel SB, Tavaré CJ. Delirium in children and adolescents. *J Neuropsychiatry Clin Neurosci* 2003;15(4):431–435.

Volkmar FR. Childhood and adolescent psychosis: a review of the past 10 years. *J Am Acad Child Adolesc Psychiatry* 1996;35:843–851.

Wise MG, Brandt G. Delirium. In: Hales RE, Yudofsky SC, eds. *Textbook of neuropsychiatry.* 2nd ed. Washington, DC: American Psychiatric Press, 1992:302.

CHAPTER 20 ■ DIZZINESS

STEPHEN J. TEACH, MD, MPH

Patients may present with "dizziness" as an isolated complaint or as part of a constellation of symptoms related to an underlying illness. True vertigo, the perception that the environment is rotating relative to the patient or that the patient is rotating relative to the environment, arises in the peripheral or central vestibular system. It can be immensely disturbing, even frightening, to patients and their families. Preverbal children, unable to articulate the sensation, may merely be irritable, vomit, and prefer to lie still. Older children and adults may have difficulty describing the sensation.

Unfortunately, most patients who use the term "dizziness" are in fact describing one of numerous nonvertiginous disturbances (pseudovertigo), which may be difficult for the practitioner to distinguish from true vertigo. Light-headedness, presyncope, intoxication, ataxia, visual disturbances, unsteadiness, weakness, stress, anxiety, hyperventilation, depression, and fear can initially all present with a complaint of dizziness.

Therefore, when evaluating a child complaining of dizziness, the practitioner should listen carefully to the details of the history as these may allow him or her to distinguish true vertigo from pseudovertigo. The key element in the history that strongly suggests true vertigo is the subjective sense of rotation. Often, the best response to a chief complaint of being dizzy is to say, "Tell me what you mean by 'dizzy.'" Initially vague complaints often become increasingly concrete, and the underlying diagnosis may become increasingly clear.

PATHOPHYSIOLOGY

True vertigo arises from a disturbance in either the peripheral or central components of the vestibular system. The two peripheral sensory organs of the system (together known as the labyrinth) are the semicircular canals (stimulated by rotary motion of the head) and the vestibule (stimulated by gravity). Both organs lie near the cochlea within the petrous portion of the temporal bone. The proximity of the vestibular and cochlear apparatus explains the frequent association of vertigo with hearing impairment.

Afferent impulses from these organs travel via the vestibular portion of the eighth cranial nerve to the vestibular nuclei in the brainstem and in the cerebellum. Cortical projections terminate in the superior temporal gyrus and the frontal lobe. Efferents from the cerebellum and vestibulospinal tract to the peripheral muscles complete the circuit by which the vestibular system helps maintain balance and position sense. Additional impulses from the vestibular nuclei ascend within the medial longitudinal fasciculus to cranial nerves III, IV, and VI, accounting for the oculovestibular reflexes. Almost all patients complaining of true vertigo should have nystagmus, at least when the vertiginous symptoms are peaking. If not, then a vestibular defect is much less likely. When present with true vertigo, the fast component of the nystagmus is almost always in the same direction as the perceived rotation.

DIFFERENTIAL DIAGNOSIS

As discussed earlier, dizziness is best divided into vertiginous conditions (true vertigo) and nonvertiginous conditions (pseudovertigo). Table 20.1 lists the differential diagnosis of true vertigo and highlights the life-threatening causes. Table 20.2 lists the most common causes of vertigo. Table 20.3 lists numerous nonvertiginous conditions that may initially be described as dizziness. Because the spectrum of nonvertiginous conditions is so broad, the following discussion will concentrate on true vertigo.

Vertigo follows a dysfunction of the vestibular system within the semicircular canals, vestibule, or vestibular nerve (peripheral vertigo), or within the brainstem, cerebellum, or cortex (central vertigo). It can also be divided into conditions in which hearing is impaired (usually peripheral causes) and into conditions in which hearing is spared (usually central causes). Finally, vertigo can be divided into acute (usually infectious, postinfectious, traumatic, or toxic) and chronic-recurrent groups (usually caused by seizures, migraine, or benign paroxysmal vertigo of childhood).

Infections

Both acute and chronic bacterial and viral infections of the middle ear with or without associated mastoiditis may cause both vestibular and auditory impairment (see Chapter 31). Severe, untreated, acute suppurative otitis media with effusion may extend directly into the labyrinth. Even without direct invasion of the pathogens, inflammatory toxins can cause a serous labyrinthitis.

Chronic and recurrent otitis media can produce a cholesteatoma of the tympanic membrane, an abnormal collection of keratin caused by repeated cycles of perforation and healing. Cholesteatomas can erode the temporal bone and the labyrinth, producing a draining fistula from the labyrinth that presents as vertigo, nausea, and hearing impairment. Computed tomography (CT) scans show destruction of the temporal bone.

Viral infections can directly affect the labyrinth or the vestibular nerve; together these conditions are known as *vestibular neuronitis*. Known pathogens include mumps, measles, and the Epstein-Barr virus. Herpes zoster infection of the ear canal and facial palsy (Ramsay Hunt syndrome) may

TABLE 20.1

CAUSES OF VERTIGO IN CHILDREN

Peripheral causes	Central causes
Suppurative or serous labyrinthitis	Tumor[a]
External ear impaction (especially cerumen)	Meningitis[a]
	Encephalitis[a]
Ramsay Hunt syndrome	Increased intracranial pressure[a]
Cholesteatoma	Multiple sclerosis
Perilymphatic fistula	Trauma[a]
Vestibular neuronitis	Seizure (usually complex partial)
Benign paroxysmal vertigo	
Ingestions[a]	Migraine
Temporal bone fracture[a]	Stroke[a]
Posttraumatic vestibular concussion	Motion sickness
Ménière's disease	Paroxysmal torticollis of infancy

[a]Life-threatening causes of vertigo.

also involve the 8th nerve. More commonly, a nonspecific upper respiratory tract infection may precede the illness. Onset is usually acute and can be severe. Nystagmus is usually present. Patients prefer to lie motionless with their eyes closed. Recovery is from 1 to 3 weeks. Early use of prednisone may shorten the course.

Migraine

Vertigo may be a prominent feature of classic migraine or migraine equivalent, in which there is no associated headache (see Chapters 55 and 96). Up to 19% of children with migraine may have vertiginous symptoms during their aura. Basilar migraine presents as a throbbing occipital headache following signs and symptoms of brainstem dysfunction (including vertigo, ataxia, tinnitus, and dysarthria). Vertigo from migraine equivalent (without pain) is typically seen in patients with a family history of migraine headache and is associated with other transient neurologic complaints (e.g., weakness, dysarthria). Symptoms may suggest temporal lobe epilepsy. The latter is distinguished by altered consciousness.

The differential diagnosis of headache and vertigo includes a brainstem or cerebellar mass, hemorrhage, and infarction.

TABLE 20.2

COMMON CAUSES OF VERTIGO

Suppurative or serous labyrinthitis
Benign paroxysmal vertigo
Migraine
Vestibular neuronitis
Ingestions
Seizure
Motion sickness

TABLE 20.3

COMMON CAUSES OF PSEUDOVERTIGO

Depression	Cardiac disease
Anxiety	Anemia
Hyperventilation	Hypoglycemia
Orthostatic hypotension	Pregnancy
Hypertension	Ataxia
Heat stroke	Visual disturbances
Arrhythmia	Psychogenic disturbance

These uncommon disorders are best assessed by magnetic resonance imaging (MRI).

Benign Paroxysmal Vertigo

Considered by many to be a form of migraine, benign paroxysmal vertigo is most common in children between the ages of 1 and 5 years. Patients have recurrent attacks, usually one to four per month, and occasionally in clusters. Onset is sudden—the child often cries out at the start of each episode—and is associated with emesis, pallor, sweating, and nystagmus. Episodes are brief, lasting up to a few minutes, and may be mistaken for seizures. In fact, the electroencephalogram (EEG) is normal. Consciousness and hearing are preserved, and the neurologic examination is otherwise normal. The disorder spontaneously remits after 2 to 3 years.

Ototoxic Drugs

Most agents that disturb vestibular function will also disturb auditory function. Specific agents include aminoglycoside antibiotics, furosemide, ethacrynic acid, streptomycin, minocycline, salicylates, and ethanol. Toxic doses of certain anticonvulsants and neuroleptics can produce measurable disturbances of vestibular function, although associated complaints of vertigo are rare.

Posttraumatic Vertigo

Several mechanisms account for posttraumatic vertigo. The most obvious is fracture through the temporal bone with damage to the labyrinth. Presentation includes vertigo, hearing loss, and hemotympanum. CT scanning of the temporal bone should be obtained when there is hemotympanum or posttraumatic evidence of vestibular dysfunction.

More subtle causes of posttraumatic vertigo include trauma-induced seizures, migraine, or a postconcussive syndrome. The latter disorder (vestibular concussion) typically follows blows to parietooccipital or temporoparietal regions and presents with headache, nausea, vertigo, and nystagmus. Although it generally remits with time, intermittent and recurrent episodes can occur. Hyperextension and flexion ("whiplash") injuries can be associated with vestibular dysfunction, probably caused by basilar artery spasm with subsequent impairment of their labyrinth and cochlear connections. Symptoms may mimic basilar artery migraine.

Seizures

Two types of seizures are associated with vertigo: vestibular seizures (seizures causing vertigo) and vestibulogenic seizures ("reflex" seizures brought on by stimulating the semicircular canals or vestibules by sudden rotation or caloric testing). Vestibular seizures, the more common type, consist of sudden onset of vertigo with or without nausea, emesis, and headache, and are invariably followed by loss or alteration of consciousness. The EEG is abnormal. Anticonvulsants may be of benefit.

Motion Sickness

Motion sickness is precipitated by a mismatch in information provided to the brain by the visual and vestibular systems during unfamiliar rotations and accelerations. The most common situation occurs when a child travels in a car or airplane and is deprived of a visual stimulus that confirms movement. Symptoms include vertigo, nausea, and nystagmus. Attacks can be prevented by allowing patients to watch the environment move in a direction opposite to the direction of body movement. In car travel, encouraging children to "look out the window" is helpful.

Ménière's Disease

Uncommon in children younger than 10 years, Ménière's disease is characterized by episodic attacks of vertigo, hearing loss, tinnitus, nystagmus, and autonomic symptoms of pallor, nausea, and emesis. Between episodes, patients may complain of impaired balance. The underlying cause is believed to be an overaccumulation of endolymph within the labyrinth, which causes a rupture (endolymphatic hydrops). Typical attacks last from 1 to 3 hours and usually begin with tinnitus, a sense of fullness within the ear, and increasing hearing impairment. Attacks are intermittent and unpredictable, often lasting for years and, at times, evolving to permanent hearing loss.

Miscellaneous Causes

Vertigo may occur at any point in the clinical course of multiple sclerosis when the central demyelination interferes with the vestibular nuclei in the brainstem or its efferents or afferents. Diagnosis is confirmed by MRI and lumbar puncture. Paroxysmal torticollis of infancy consists of spells of head tilt associated with nausea, emesis, pallor, agitation, and ataxia. Episodes are brief and self-limited and may recur for months or years. The cause is unclear, although some authors see it as a prelude to later benign paroxysmal vertigo (considered by some to be a migraine variant). Perilymphatic fistula is an abnormal communication between the labyrinth and the middle ear, with leakage of perilymphatic fluid through the defect. It may be congenital or acquired by trauma, infection, or surgery. The diagnosis may be suspected when vertigo is provoked by sneezing or coughing, actions that can increase perilymphatic drainage. Diagnosis is confirmed by middle ear exploration. Finally, vertigo may be associated with diabetes mellitus and chronic renal failure.

EVALUATION AND DECISION

Differentiation of True Vertigo and Pseudovertigo

Evaluation of children complaining of dizziness begins by separating those with true vertigo from those with pseudovertigo (Tables 20.1 and 20.3). True vertigo is always associated with a subjective sense of rotation of the environment relative to the patient or of the patient relative to the environment. All vertigo is made worse by moving the head, and acute attacks are usually accompanied by nystagmus. Pseudovertigo is suggested by complaints involving light-headedness, flushing, weakness, ataxia, unsteadiness, weakness, fatigue, pallor, anxiety, stress, hyperventilation, and fear.

True Vertigo

History and Physical Examination. Once true vertigo (Fig. 20.1) is identified, its severity, time course, and pattern must be established. In general, the most severe attacks of vertigo are due to peripheral causes, whereas central causes tend to be more recurrent, chronic, and progressive. Sudden onset of sustained vertigo suggests central or peripheral trauma, infection, stroke, or ingestion. Recurrent episodic attacks suggest seizures, migraine, or benign paroxysmal vertigo. More persistent episodes suggest brainstem or cerebellar mass lesions.

Recurrent, transient, altered mental status suggests seizure or basilar migraine. Episodes of prior head injury suggest concussion syndromes. Recent upper respiratory tract infections may suggest vestibular neuronitis. History of ototoxic drug or intoxicant use is important, as is a family history of migraine. Age of the patient is especially useful—benign paroxysmal vertigo is unusual after age 5 years, whereas Ménière's disease is unusual before age 10 years. A family history of migraine may be helpful.

The physical examination focuses on the middle ear and on neurologic and vestibular testing. Visualization of the external ear canal may reveal cerumen impaction, foreign body, or zoster lesions (Ramsay Hunt syndrome). Perforation or distortion of the tympanic membrane should be noted. A pneumatic bulb will enable the examiner to see whether abrupt changes in the middle ear pressure trigger an episode of vertigo, a suggestion that a perilymphatic fistula may be present (Hennebert's sign).

The neurologic examination must be complete, focusing closely on the auditory, vestibular, and cerebellar systems. Both vestibular and cerebellar disorders may present with an unsteady gait. In both situations, when there is a unilateral lesion, the child will fall toward the side of the lesion. The two may at times be distinguishable by the nature of the nystagmus (described below). In addition, if cerebellar dysfunction is present, there may be dysmetria and ataxia. All cases of suspected vestibular or cerebellar dysfunction require close follow-up evaluation because of the risk of a posterior fossa mass.

Nystagmus is a highly specific sign for both central and peripheral vertiginous disorders. Nystagmus from a peripheral origin usually occurs without other neurologic signs (except, perhaps, auditory changes and tinnitus). Nystagmus from

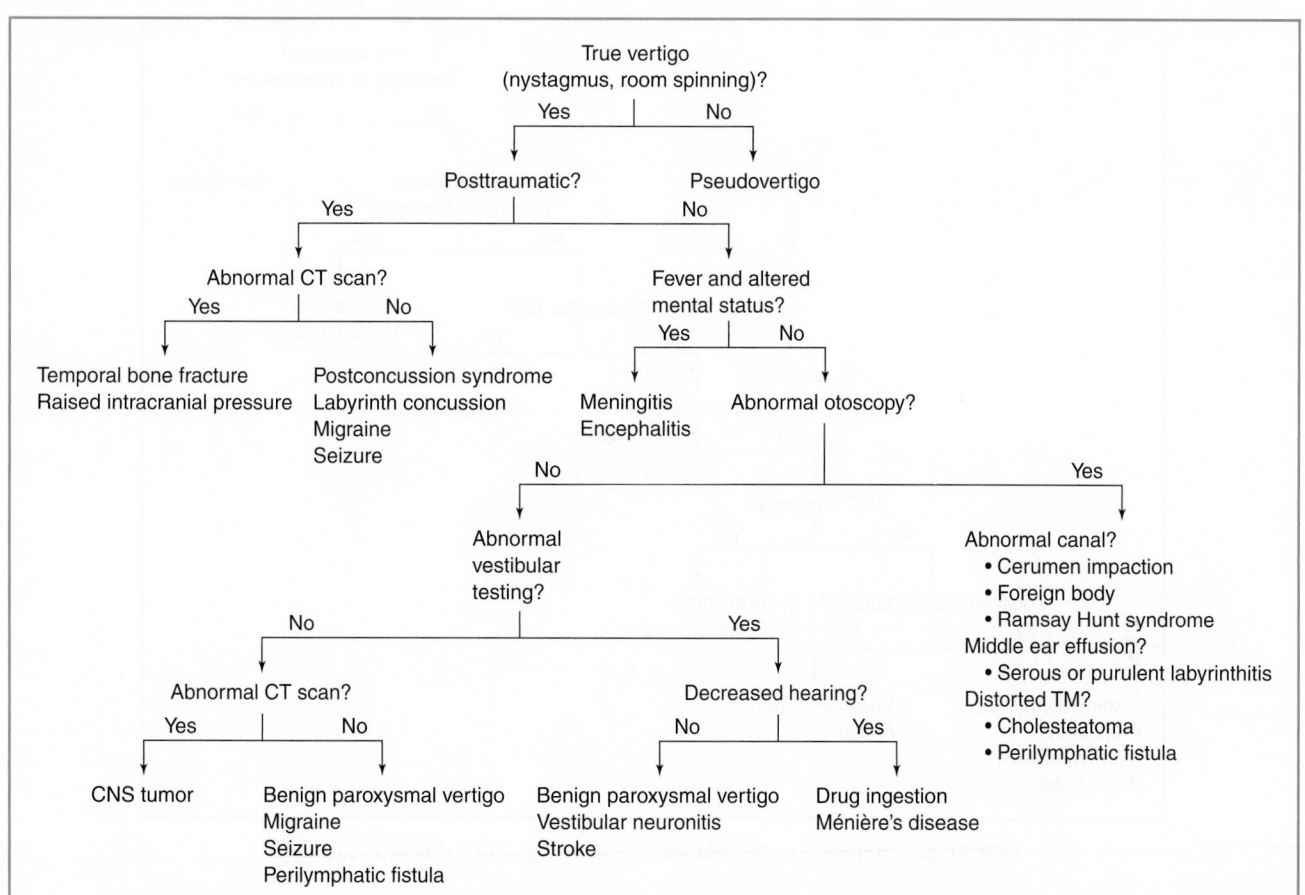

FIGURE 20.1 Approach to the child with true vertigo. CT, computed tomography; TM, tympanic membrane; CNS, central nervous system.

central causes, on the other hand, is usually accompanied by such signs. In addition, a patient complaining of dizziness with vertigo may not have nystagmus at the time that he or she is examined. Tests to elicit positional vertigo and nystagmus can therefore be helpful in identifying and even distinguishing central and peripheral vestibular dysfunction, particularly if the tests elicit or increase the patient's complaint.

Initially, nystagmus should be sought in all positions of gaze and with changes in head position. Peripheral vestibular disorders are characterized by a "jerk" nystagmus with the slow component toward the affected side. Central lesions are characterized by nystagmus with the fast component toward the affected side and reversal of the fast component when changing from right to left lateral gaze. The Nylen-Hallpike test is performed by moving a child rapidly from a sitting to a supine position with the head 45 degrees below the edge of the examining table and turned 45 degrees to one side. Nystagmus and a vertiginous sensation may result as the vestibular system is stressed. Certain features of the nystagmus elicited may be helpful in distinguishing central from peripheral vestibular dysfunction. In central dysfunction, for example, onset of nystagmus is immediate; in peripheral vestibular disorders, it is delayed. Finally, visual fixation tends to dampen peripheral nystagmus while it usually does not affect nystagmus from central causes.

The cold caloric response tests for integrity of the peripheral vestibular system. Slow and careful irrigation of either 100 mL of tap water 7°C below body temperature or 10 mL of ice water into the external ear canal through a soft plastic tube, with the child lying about 60 degrees recumbent, should induce a slow movement of the eyes toward the stimulus and a fast movement away. Instillation of warm water (44°C) will cause an inverse reaction. Vestibular damage will suppress the response on the affected side. Absence of nystagmus indicates absence of peripheral vestibular function. The test is contraindicated if the tympanic membrane is perforated.

Laboratory Data. Laboratory investigations have a limited role in the evaluation of vertigo. Useful initial tests include a complete blood count, a serum glucose, and an electrocardiogram. Together, these may help identify patients with pseudovertiginous conditions caused by anemia, hypoglycemia, and rhythm abnormalities. Further laboratory testing may reveal diabetes or renal failure, both of which have been associated with vertigo. Toxicologic testing including specific anticonvulsant levels and an ethanol level, if indicated, may be helpful. A lumbar puncture is indicated in cases of suspected meningitis or encephalitis.

Radiologic imaging of the central nervous system, preferably by MRI for adequate visualization of the posterior fossa

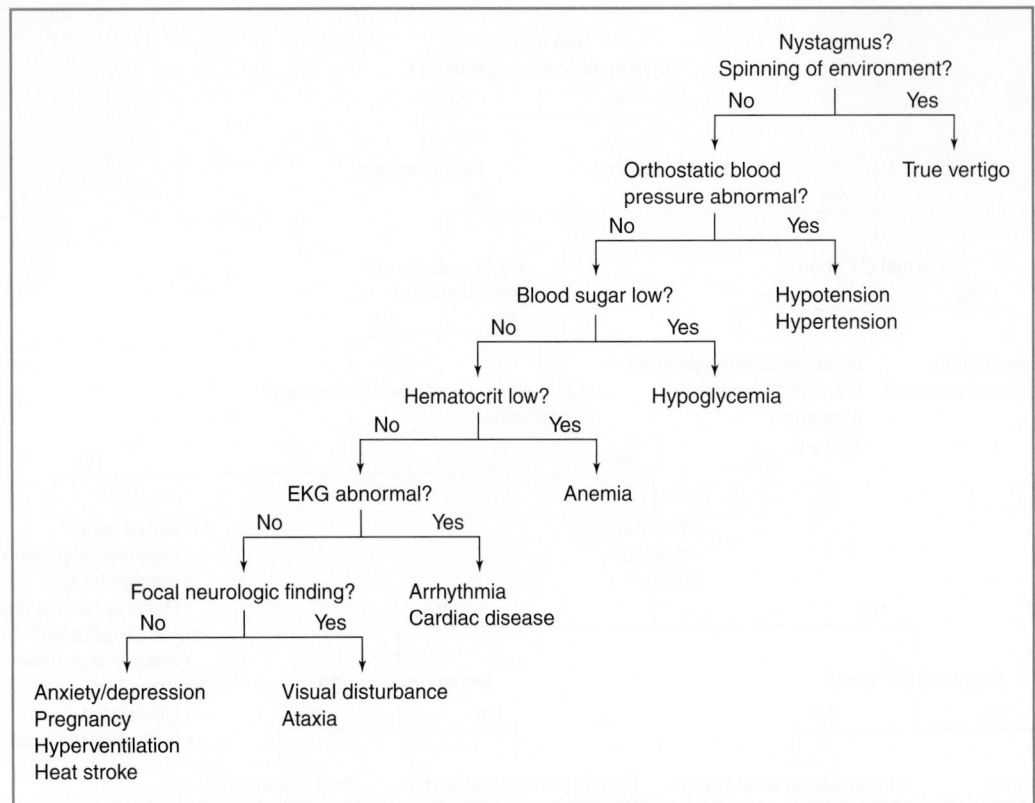

FIGURE 20.2 Approach to the child with pseudovertigo. EKG, electrocardiogram.

and brainstem, is indicated in cases of chronic and recurrent vertigo to exclude mass lesions. Children with vertigo and an underlying bleeding diathesis or a predisposition toward ischemic stroke (i.e., sickle cell disease) may also need an emergent cranial CT or MRI. Posttraumatic vertigo, especially when accompanied by hearing loss or facial nerve paralysis, is best assessed by CT including adequate images of the temporal bone.

Some children with true vertigo will require referral for more extensive testing. An EEG is indicated when vertigo accompanies loss of consciousness or other manifestations of a seizure. Audiometry is indicated when vertigo accompanies otalgia, hearing loss, or tinnitus. Specialized testing for nystagmus, including electronystagmography, which measures eye movements at rest and at extremes of gaze, can separate central from peripheral vestibular disorders. It may be combined with caloric and positional testing.

Management. Specific disorders causing vertigo are treated directly. Suppurative or serous labyrinthitis, for example, is treated with antibiotics. An erosive cholesteatoma may require surgical removal. Anticonvulsants may diminish vestibular and vestibulogenic seizures. Motion sickness may respond to simple behavioral changes (e.g., encouraging children to look out the window). Other causes of vertigo spontaneously remit without therapy and merit only close monitoring. Vestibular neuronitis and benign paroxysmal vertigo are examples.

Subspecialist consultation is indicated in certain situations. Neurosurgical evaluation after trauma may be indicated in cases of suspected basilar skull fracture. Suspected perilymphatic fistula, cholesteatoma, or complicated otitis media may merit otorhinolaryngologic evaluation. Neurologists may be helpful in cases of suspected seizure or migraine.

Children with severe or recurrent attacks of vertigo may require treatment with specific antivertiginous medications. The antihistamines dimenhydrinate (12.5 mg to 25 mg orally every 6 to 8 hours, maximum dose 75 mg per day for ages 2 to 6 years and 25 mg to 50 mg every 6 to 8 hours for ages 6 to 12 years, maximum dose 150 mg per day) and meclizine (12.5 mg to 25 mg orally every 12 hours in children older than 12 years of age) may be helpful. Concomitant use of a benzodiazepine such as diazepam (0.1 to 0.3 mg per kg per day orally divided every 6 to 8 hours, maximum 10 mg per dose) as a sedative may be necessary in severe cases.

Pseudovertigo

Pseudovertigo (Fig. 20.2) refers to a broad array of diagnoses that present with symptoms such as light-headedness, presyncope, intoxication, ataxia, visual disturbances, unsteadiness, stress, anxiety, and fear. Uniformly absent are a sense of rotation and ocular nystagmus. Underlying causes are numerous; several of the most common causes are listed in Table 20.3 (see also discussions of syncope in Chapter 73). Careful consideration of the patient's age, gender, detailed history, and physical examination, together with a limited number of ancillary tests, may help establish the specific diagnosis.

Suggested Readings

Aust G, Novotny M. Ménière's disease and various types of vertigo in children. *Int Tinnitus J* 2005;11:66–68.

Baloh RW. Clinical practice. Vestibular neuritis. *N Engl J Med* 2003;348:1027–1030.

Bower CM, Cotton RT. The spectrum of vertigo in children. *Arch Otolaryngol Head Neck Surg* 1995;121:911–915.

Kitsko DJ, Dohar JE. Inner ear and facial nerve complications of acute otitis media including vertigo. *Curr Allergy Asthma Rep* 2007;7:444–450.

Lewis DW. Pediatric migraine. *Pediatr Rev* 2007;28:43–53.

MacGregor DL. Vertigo. *Peditar Rev* 2002;23:10–16.

Megerian CA, Hadlock TA. Case records of the Massachusetts General Hospital. Weekly clinicopathological exercises. Case 40-2001, an eight-year-old boy with fever, headache, and vertigo two days after aural trauma. *N Engl J Med* 2001;345:1901–1907.

Newman-Toker DE, Hseih YH, Carmargo CA, et al. Spectrum of dizziness visits to US emergency departments. *Mayo Clin Proc* 2008;83:765–775.

Phillips JO, Backous DD. Evaluation of vestibular function in young children. *Otolaryngol Clin North Am* 2002;4:765–790.

Tusa RJ, Saada AA, Niparko JK. Dizziness in childhood. *J Child Neurol* 1994;9:261–274.

Uneri A, Turkdogan D. Evaluation of vestibular functions in children with vertigo attacks. *Arch Dis Child* 2003;88:510–511.

Weber PC, Bluestone CD, Perez B. Outcome of hearing and vertigo after surgery for congenital perilymphatic fistula in children. *Am J Otolaryngol* 2003;24:138–142.

CHAPTER 21 ■ EDEMA

LINDA L. BROWN, MD, MSCE

Edema may be defined as the abnormal swelling of tissues from the accumulation of fluid in the extravascular space. In children presenting for medical care, this fluid may appear as generalized or localized swelling. When significant edema is present, collections of fluid may be visualized as pericardial or pleural effusions or as ascites. When edema is profound and generalized, the patient is described as having anasarca. However, the initial presentation of generalized edema may be subtle. Often the swelling is most prominent in the dependent portions of the extremities or lower back or in distensible tissues such as the eyelids, scrotum, or labia. Obtaining a careful history and completing a physical examination will help to identify these patients and may lead to a definitive diagnosis.

PATHOPHYSIOLOGY

The occurrence of edema in healthy individuals is usually prevented by the balance of oncotic and hydrostatic pressures between the intravascular and interstitial spaces, as well as the normal function of the lymphatic system. Any imbalance in this system may lead to increased interstitial fluid and resultant tissue swelling. Edema may occur as a result of decreased intravascular oncotic pressure, increased venous or lymphatic pressure, or from the loss of normal vascular permeability, as seen with vasculitis from an allergic or hypersensitivity reaction. Tightly controlled serum levels of albumin and sodium maintain normal intravascular oncotic pressure. Hypoalbuminemia may arise from decreased production of proteins caused by hepatic disease, as a result of protein malnutrition or, more commonly from losses of protein through gastrointestinal (GI), renal, or dermal (e.g., burns) conditions. When the albumin level is less than 2.5 g/dL, the oncotic pressure in the vascular space is reduced enough for fluid to move freely into the soft tissues and, if not corrected, generalized edema may result.

When the intravascular albumin and sodium levels are within the normal range and vascular permeability is preserved, the formation of edema requires increased hydrostatic pressures to overcome the oncotic pressure, forcing fluid out of the vascular space. This can occur as a result of hypervolemia from cardiac failure, renal failure, salt retention, estrogen–progesterone excess, or renal tubular insensitivity to the natriuretic and diuretic actions of atrial natriuretic peptide.

In the event of a hypersensitivity reaction, the formation of edema may be rapid, localized, and potentially life threatening. In such patients with a severe allergic reaction associated with anaphylaxis, edema may involve the tissues adjacent to the airway leading to potential airway compromise. More commonly, this allergic reaction is merely uncomfortable with localized swelling of the affected area and occasional pruritis, as seen with insect bites. The onset of symptoms is usually more gradual for causes of generalized edema. In fact, a 10% to 15% weight gain may be accumulated, with symptoms existing for weeks to months, before a patient presents for medical care.

DIFFERENTIAL DIAGNOSIS

A myriad of disease processes can result in either localized or generalized edema (Table 21.1). Localized edema in children is often caused by an allergic reaction, with the most severe reactions resulting from exposure to nuts, shellfish, or hymenoptera venom. Idiopathic nephrotic syndrome, although rare (occurring in just 2 to 3 of every 100,000 children annually), is the most common cause of generalized edema (Table 21.2). Overall, most children who develop edema will have a benign diagnosis and self-limited course. However, potentially life-threatening conditions (Table 21.3) can occur, including severe allergic reactions, soft tissue infections with associated bacteremia (see Chapter 92), deep venous thrombosis, and kidney, liver, or cardiac disease.

EVALUATION AND DECISION

When evaluating the child with edema, it is helpful to classify the swelling as localized or generalized. As with any complaint, it is necessary to perform a complete and thorough history and physical examination. It is important to include information on the location of the edema (facial vs. extremities), and the duration of the symptoms (hours vs. weeks), as well as associated symptoms including fever, shortness of breath, or recent illness. Past medical history, including a dietary history and family history is helpful to identify patients with chronic conditions or inherited disorders such as hereditary angioedema. Current and recent medications or allergies may also help to clarify the diagnosis. Overall, the duration of the symptoms and the patient's age may help to narrow down your differential, as certain disorders will present in the newborn period (congenital lymphedema, Turner's syndrome) while others occur more frequently in school-age children or adolescents (nephrotic syndrome, vasculitis). It is particularly important to inspect for edema around the eyes, scrotum or labia, as well as the distal extremities, as these areas may be the only locations with perceptible swelling.

A urinalysis to rule out proteinuria should be included in the initial evaluation of any patient presenting with generalized edema. It is important to realize that this edema may be the only physical finding of renal disease, the most common cause of hypoalbuminemia. Acquired hypoproteinemia from

TABLE 21.1

CAUSES OF EDEMA

Decreased Oncotic Pressure
Protein loss
    Protein-losing enteropathy
    Nephrotic syndrome
    Cystic fibrosis
Reduced albumin synthesis
    Liver disease
    Malnutrition

Increased Hydrostatic Pressure
Increased blood volume from sodium retention
    Congestive heart failure
    Primary renal sodium retention
        Acute glomerulonephritis
        Henoch-Schönlein purpura
        Premenstrual edema or edema of pregnancy
Venous obstruction
    Constrictive pericarditis
    Acute pulmonary edema
    Portal hypertension
    Budd-Chiari syndrome
    Local venous obstruction
    Thrombophlebitis/deep venous thrombosis
Lymphatic obstruction

Increased Capillary Permeability
Allergic reaction
Angiotensin-converting enzyme inhibitor-induced angioedema
Inflammatory reactions
    Burns
    Cellulitis
Hereditary angioedema
Pit viper envenomations

Other
Edema of the newborn
Hypothyroidism (myxedema)
Lymphedema
Epstein-Barr virus infectious mononucleosis (upper eyelid edema)

hepatic or intestinal disease is unusual but should also be considered, especially after a renal etiology is ruled out. Generalized edema may also be the result of congestive heart failure (CHF). However, these children will usually present with other complaints and physical examination findings, including shortness of breath, gallop, and hepatomegaly.

TABLE 21.2

COMMON CAUSES OF EDEMA

Localized
Allergic reaction
Cellulitis
Trauma
Dependent edema from immobility of extremity

Generalized
Nephrotic Syndrome
Allergic reaction

TABLE 21.3

LIFE-THREATENING CAUSES OF EDEMA

Localized
Allergic reaction with airway involvement
Angiotensin-converting enzyme inhibitor-induced angioedema
Cellulitis
    Group A Streptococcus with varicella
Pit viper envenomations
Thrombophlebitis

Generalized
Cardiac disease
    Congestive heart failure
    Pericardial effusion
Renal disease
    Nephrosis
    Nephritis
Hepatic failure

LOCALIZED EDEMA

Localized edema is a more common presenting complaint in pediatrics than generalized edema (Fig. 21.1). Usually, these areas of localized swelling are caused by minor trauma, infection, or secondary to an allergic reaction. Historical factors and physical examination findings will often lead to a particular diagnosis without the need for further testing. Tenderness to palpation points to trauma or infection, while fever, erythema, and overlying warmth more commonly occur with an infectious cause (Table 21.4). On the face and distal extremities, insect bites may produce swelling and warmth, which can be difficult to distinguish from cellulitis. A therapeutic response to an oral antihistamine or to an intramuscular dose of epinephrine can help to differentiate an allergic reaction from other causes of localized swelling.

Interestingly, localized bilateral upper eyelid edema may be found in patients with Epstein-Barr virus (EBV) infectious mononucleosis. This swelling (Hoagland's sign) may be present in up to 50% of patients, is notable only for the first few days of the illness, and does not lead to any significant discomfort. Although transient, this finding is thought to be very specific for the diagnosis of EBV and may be used to trigger further laboratory evaluation to confirm the diagnosis.

As previously mentioned, when localized edema occurs on the face, it is important that the physician evaluate the child carefully for concurrent airway involvement. When a child presents with severe or recurrent facial edema, especially if there is a family history of a similar problem, the diagnosis of hereditary angioedema (see Chapter 82) should be investigated. Facial edema may also be caused by oral, dental, or sinus infections, including acute sinusitis, orbital cellulitis, or dental abscess. Often these patients will present with a history of dental or facial pain, sinus congestion, erythema, or fever. A history of environmental exposure should lead to the diagnosis of other common causes of localized swelling, including sunburn, frostbite, and plant-induced dermatitis (poison ivy). Although rarely seen, pit viper envenomation may cause rapid onset of painful swelling at the site of injury (see Chapter 83).

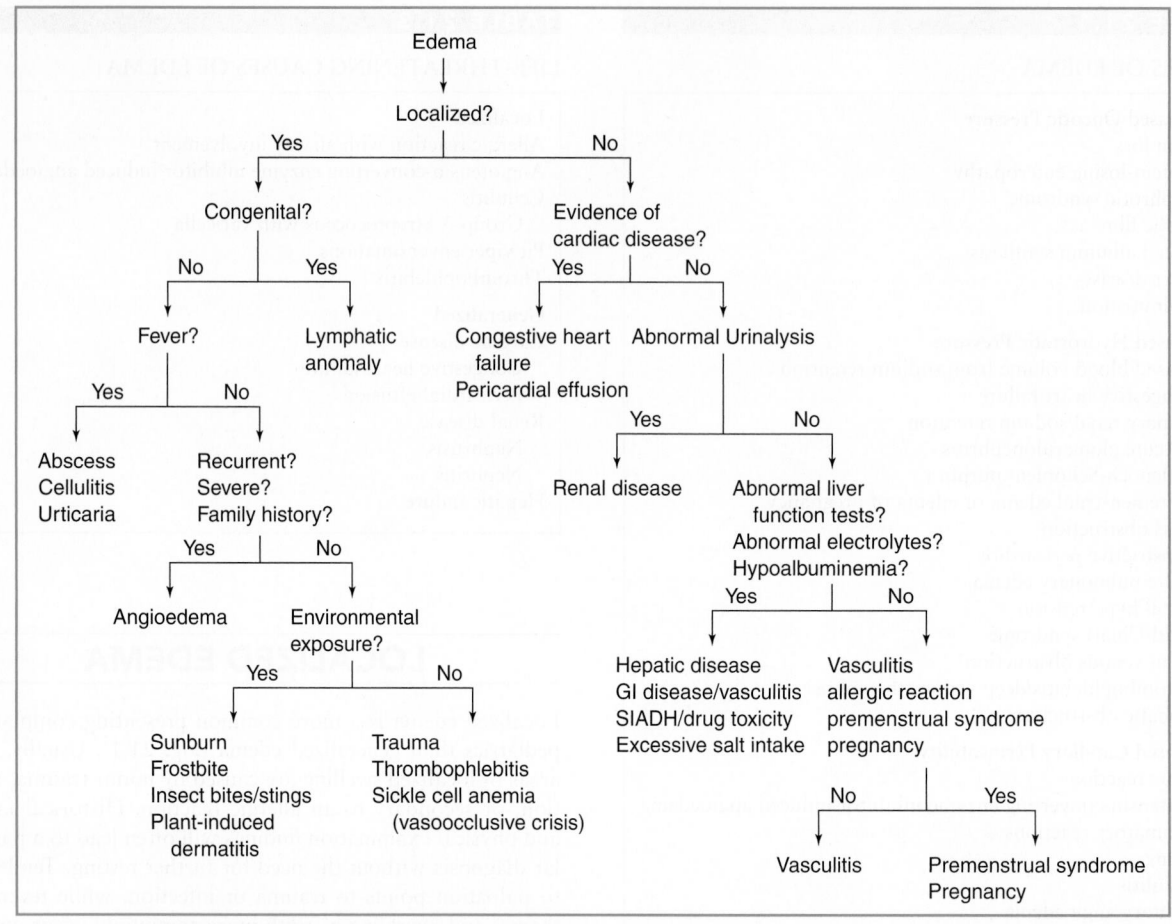

FIGURE 21.1 Edema in children. GI, gastrointestinal; SIADH, syndrome of inappropriate secretion of antidiuretic hormone.

Occasionally, an infant will present with unexplained, localized swelling of an extremity present since birth. In this situation, the possibility of an injury secondary to birth trauma should be explored. Less commonly, congenital lymphedema (Milroy's disease), Turner's syndrome (bilateral leg edema), and Noonan's syndrome (pedal edema) should be considered. Sickle cell anemia may cause swollen and painful digits in young children, referred to as dactylitis (see Chapter 91). Thrombophlebitis or deep venous thrombosis rarely occurs in the prepubertal child but may affect adolescents; inherited hypercoagulable states, weightlifting, and the use of oral contraceptive pills predispose teenagers to this condition. Evaluation of these patients should include an ultrasound of the venous system of the affected limb and a thorough laboratory evaluation. Superior vena cava syndrome may also pre-sent as facial swelling, often with some degree of facial cyanosis or plethora.

GENERALIZED EDEMA

The evaluation of the child presenting with generalized edema must include a complete and thorough cardiovascular examination. Patients with CHF, pericarditis, myocarditis, or cardiomyopathy may present with edema, but these children will usually have additional signs and symptoms. An edematous child presenting with a gallop, tachycardia, tachypnea, inspiratory crackles, or hepatomegaly should be evaluated for cardiac disease (see Chapter 84). For patients with complex heart disease, right-sided failure will lead to generalized edema without

TABLE 21.4

DIFFERENTIATION AMONG THE COMMON CAUSES OF LOCALIZED EDEMA

	Fever	Local tenderness	Local warmth	Lesion/color
Allergic Reaction	No	No	Yes	Erythematous
Trauma	No	Yes	No	Violaceous
Infection	Usually	Yes	Yes	Erythematous or violaceous

the pulmonary findings. In the child with a pericardial effusion, the classic findings of pulsus paradoxus, muffled heart sounds, and jugular venous distension may occur. However, in several studies of patients with cardiac tamponade visible on echocardiography, these findings were absent in 30% to 50% of patients. Evaluation of these children should therefore also include a chest radiograph, which may show an enlarged cardiac silhouette, and an electrocardiogram (EKG). Findings on the EKG will vary greatly with the etiology of the heart failure, including ST-segment elevation and generalized T-wave inversion suggestive of pericarditis or diffusely low voltages suggestive of myocarditis. Ultimately, echocardiography is diagnostic.

Generalized edema, with an otherwise normal exam, occurs most commonly in patients with renal disease, particularly nephrotic syndrome (see Chapter 100). Other forms of renal disease or vasculitis, including glomerulonephritis, hemolytic uremic syndrome, or Henoch-Schönlein purpura (HSP) may also be responsible. In contrast to patients with nephrotic syndrome and edema from low oncotic pressure, edema associated with acute renal failure results from the hypervolemic state. The initial diagnosis of nephrotic syndrome is based on significant proteinuria (3+ or 4+ or >300 mg/dL on a urinalysis). The presence or absence of urine red blood cells, white blood cells, or casts in the urine, along with further laboratory testing including chemistries, albumin and total protein, and complement and triglyceride levels may help to confirm the diagnosis. Various factors, including the presence of hypertension or significant fluid collections in the pleural or peritoneal spaces, must be considered to determine the appropriate initial management of these patients. In the child with HSP, the location of the edema may be helpful. The swelling primarily affects the lower extremities, where the purpuric rash predominates, or is isolated to specific joints when arthritis is present. The purpuric rash, despite normal platelet count and coagulation studies (consistent with a vasculitis), is usually, but not universally, present.

In an edematous patient with a normal cardiac exam and no proteinuria, further evaluation should include a search for hepatic and other GI diseases, as well as other forms of vasculitis. Patients with protein-losing enteropathy, from milk protein allergy, celiac disease, giardiasis, or inflammatory bowel disease, can present with generalized edema with few other physical findings. These patients may have significant protein loss through the GI tract and will often present with hypoalbuminemia. An initial laboratory evaluation, including liver function tests, electrolytes, erythrocyte sedimentation rate, and measurement of total protein and albumin, may reveal abnormalities. However, further evaluation, including more specific

blood, urine, and stool testing, is often required to definitively diagnose the etiology of edema in this subset of patients.

As noted throughout this chapter, generalized edema may be a sign of a serious underlying disease. However, less serious conditions may be causative as well. Certain drugs (oral contraceptive pills, corticosteroids, lithium, nonsteroidal antiinflammatory agents, calcium channel blockers, and others) may cause some people to become edematous. This swelling usually resolves when the medication is discontinued. Cyclical edema related to menstruation occurs frequently in young women. The etiology of this edema is likely hormonally mediated, although the exact mechanisms are unclear. Pregnancy may result in edema as well.

In conclusion, it is important to remember that a complete history and physical examination of the patient with either localized or generalized edema may be enough to arrive at a likely diagnosis. It is of particular importance to focus on the cardiovascular, renal, and GI systems when searching for an etiology for generalized edema. Commonly, patients presenting with symptoms of localized edema will have an allergic, traumatic, or infectious etiology and, with appropriate management, will have resolution of their symptoms without serious sequelae.

Suggested Readings

Baliga R, Lewy JE. Pathogenesis and treatment of edema. *Pediatr Clin North Am* 1987;34:639–648.

Bernardi E, Camporese G, Büller HR, et al. Serial 2-point ultrasonography plus D-dimer vs whole-leg color-coded Doppler ultrasonography for diagnosing suspected symptomatic deep vein thrombosis: a randomized controlled trial. *JAMA* 2008;300:1653–1659.

Charlesworth EN. Urticaria and angioedema: a clinical spectrum. *Ann Allergy Asthma Immunol* 1996;76:484–495.

Fisher DA. Obscure and unusual edema. *Pediatrics* 1966;37:506.

Green ML. Edema. In: *Pediatric diagnosis: interpretation of symptoms and signs in infants, children, and adolescents.* 5th ed. Philadelphia: WB Saunders, 1992:399–403.

Holliday MA, Barratt TM, Avner ED. Edema. In: *Pediatric nephrology*, 3rd ed. Baltimore: Williams & Wilkins, 1994:200–204.

Katz BZ. Epstein-Barr virus infections. In: Long SS, Pickering LK, Prober CG, eds. *Principles and practice of pediatric infectious disease.* 3rd ed. New York: Churchill Livingstone, 2008:1036–1044.

Krishnamurthy A, Naguwa SM, Gershwin ME. Pediatric angioedema. *Clin Rev Allergy Immunol* 2008;34(2):25–259.

Salcedo JR, Thabet MA, Latta K, et al. Nephrosis in childhood. *Nephron* 1995;71:373–385.

Schrier RW. Pathogenesis of sodium and water retention in high-output and low-output cardiac failure, nephrotic syndrome, cirrhosis, and pregnancy. Part I. *N Engl J Med* 1988;319(16):1065–1072.

Schrier RW. Pathogenesis of sodium and water retention in high-output and low-output cardiac failure, nephrotic syndrome, cirrhosis, and pregnancy. Part II. *N Engl J Med* 1988;319(17):1127–1134.

Vogt BA, Avner ED. Pediatric nephrology. In: *Behrman: Nelson textbook of pediatrics.* 17th ed. 2004:1751–1753.

Zuraw, BL. Hereditary Angioedema. *N Engl J Med* 2008;359(10):1027–1036.

CHAPTER 22 ■ EPISTAXIS

FRAN NADEL, MD, MSCE, AND FRED M. HENRETIG, MD

Epistaxis (nosebleeding) is a common symptom in young children and may be alarming to parents who often overestimate the amount of blood loss. It usually is noted first at about age 3 years and increases in frequency with age, until peaking before or in adolescence. An orderly approach to the history and physical examination is necessary to identify the small minority of patients who require emergent hemorrhage control, laboratory investigation, or consultation with an otorhinolaryngologist (ORL) for further management.

PATHOPHYSIOLOGY

Minor trauma, nasal inflammation, desiccation, and congestion, as well as the rich vascular supply of the nose, contribute to the frequency of nosebleeds in otherwise normal children. The nose is a favored site for recurrent minor trauma, especially habitual, often absent-minded, picking. The small vessels that supply the nasal mucous membrane have little structural support because the mucosa is closely applied to the perichondrium and periosteum of the nasal septum and lateral nasal walls. Furthermore, the nasal mucosa is richly supplied with vessels that form plexiform networks. One such anastomosis of common etiologic significance is Kiesselbach's plexus in Little's area of the anterior nasal septum, about 0.5 cm from the tip of the nose (see Fig. 127.4). Any factors that tend to cause congestion of the nasal vessels or drying of the mucosa will enhance the likelihood of epistaxis, resulting from a given degree of trauma.

DIFFERENTIAL DIAGNOSIS

Many types of local and systemic disorders may cause epistaxis (Table 22.1). Local factors predominate in etiologic importance (Table 22.2). In addition to minor accidental trauma and habitual picking, any cause of acute inflammation will predispose the nose to bleeding. Acute upper respiratory infections, whether localized as in colds or secondary to more generalized infections such as measles, infectious mononucleosis, and influenzal illnesses, contribute to the onset of epistaxis. Nasal colonization with *Staphylococcus aureus* may predispose to a more friable mucosa and epistaxis.

Allergic rhinitis may also be a factor. *Rhinitis sicca* refers to a condition that is common in northern latitudes during the winter, in which low ambient humidity, exacerbated by dry hot-air heating systems, leads to desiccation of the nasal mucosa with concurrent tendency to frequent bleeding. Staphylococcal furuncles, foreign bodies, telangiectasias (Osler-Weber-Rendu disease), hemangiomas, or evidence of

other uncommon tumors may be found on inspection. Juvenile nasopharyngeal angiofibroma is usually seen in adolescent boys with nasal obstruction, mucopurulent discharge, and severe epistaxis. These tumors may bulge into the nasal cavity but often require examination of the nasopharynx to be identified. Although benign, they can cause severe problems through local invasion of adjacent structures. A rare childhood malignant tumor, nasopharyngeal lymphoepithelioma, may cause a syndrome of epistaxis, torticollis, trismus, and unilateral cervical lymphadenopathy. Other rare local causes of epistaxis include nasal diphtheria and Wegener's granulomatosis.

Children rarely present with a nosebleed as their only manifestation of a more systemic disease. In children with severe or recurrent nosebleeds, a concerning family history, or constitutional signs and symptoms, the physician should consider a systemic process. von Willebrand's disease and platelet dysfunction are two of the more common systemic diseases that cause recurrent or severe nosebleeds. Other less common systemic factors include hematologic diseases such as leukemia, hemophilia, and clotting disorders associated with severe hepatic dysfunction or uremia. Arterial hypertension rarely is a cause of epistaxis in children. Increased nasal venous pressure secondary to paroxysmal coughing, which can occur in pertussis or cystic fibrosis, occasionally may cause nosebleeds. *Vicarious menstruation* refers to a condition occasionally found in adolescent girls in whom monthly epistaxis related to vascular congestion of the nasal mucosa occurs concordant with menses and is presumably related to cyclic changes in hormone levels. Nosebleeds in infants are rare and one should consider the possibility of child abuse.

EVALUATION AND DECISION

Rarely are nosebleeds in children life threatening or require more than simple measures to gain control of hemorrhage. However, one's evaluation should begin with hemorrhage control and identification of children who are unstable by noting alterations in the patient's general appearance, vital signs, airway, color, and mental status. Perhaps the most crucial step in gaining hemorrhage control is calming the child and family. Success in this effort may be enhanced by having a child sit on a parent's lap while the adult provides pressure to the nose and the child is distracted by a toy or video.

Most childhood nosebleeds are anterior in origin. However, because posterior bleeds may require more extensive therapy, it is important to identify the site of bleeding. In general, posterior sites bleed more profusely, although parents may underestimate the volume because much of the blood is often swallowed. Blood seen in the oropharynx, blood in both nares, difficulty

TABLE 22.1

DIFFERENTIAL DIAGNOSIS OF EPISTAXIS

Local Predisposing Factors
Trauma, direct and picking
Local inflammation
  Acute viral upper respiratory tract infection (common cold)
  Bacterial rhinitis/sinusitis
  Congenital syphilis
    β-Hemolytic streptococcus
  Foreign body
  Acute systemic illnesses accompanied by nasal congestion
    Measles, infectious mononucleosis, acute rheumatic fever
  Allergic rhinitis
  Nasal polyps (cystic fibrosis, allergic, generalized)
  Staphylococcal furuncle
Vascular malformations (telangiectasias as in Osler-
  Weber-Rendu disease, hemangiomas)
Juvenile angiofibroma[a]
Other tumors, granulomatosis (rare)[a]
Rhinitis sicca

Systemic Predisposing Factors
Hematologic diseases[a]
  Platelet disorders
    Quantitative: idiopathic thrombocytopenic purpura,
      leukemia, aplastic anemia
    Qualitative: von Willebrand's disease, Glanzmann's
      disease, uremia
  Hemophilias
    Clotting disorders associated with severe hepatic disease,
      disseminated intravascular coagulation (DIC), vitamin
      K deficiency
    Drugs: aspirin, nonsteroidal antiinflammatory drugs,
      warfarin, valproic acid rodenticide
Vicarious menstruation
Hypertension[a]
  Arterial (unusual cause of epistaxis in children)
  Venous: superior vena cava syndrome or with paroxysmal
    coughing seen in pertussis and cystic fibrosis

[a]Life-threatening condition.

controlling bleeding despite adequate anterior pressure, and a normal anterior exam are more characteristic of a posterior nasal bleed but can be found with an anterior causative site.

After treating any emergent problems, the evaluation of the child with epistaxis begins with a thorough history. Specific features to be sought include frequency of occurrence, difficulty in control (and adequacy of simple at-home first aid), history of trauma, nose picking, frequent upper respiratory infection, allergic and chronic discharge, and obstructive symptoms. Often, asking children which finger they pick their noses with will elicit a more honest answer.

TABLE 22.2

COMMON CAUSES OF EPISTAXIS

Trauma
Foreign body
Allergic rhinitis
Rhinitis sicca
Viral rhinitis

Commonly, parents will note hematemesis or melena, prompting them to seek urgent medical attention. Specific questions regarding evidence for any systemic hemorrhagic disorder or family history of bleeding are asked. In adolescent girls, relation to menses is noted.

Physical examination must include a complete general examination with special attention paid to vital signs, including blood pressure, evidence of hematologic disease (enlarged nodes, organomegaly, petechiae, or pallor), and of course, inspection of the nasal cavity after reasonable efforts to stop the bleeding. When examining a child with a nosebleed, one will need a good light source, suction, and adequate body fluid precautions. Nasal inspection begins with clearing the passages by having the child blow his or her nose or by using gentle suction. On examination, one is looking for the site of bleeding, mucosal color, excoriations, discharge, a foreign body or other mass, and septal hematomas. Using one's thumb, the tip of the nose is pushed upward to allow examination of the vestibule, the anterior portion of the septum, and anterior portion of the inferior turbinate. If the mucosa is too boggy for adequate visualization, a topical vasoconstrictor or decongestant may be beneficial. A more thorough examination requires the use of a nasal speculum. Using one's nondominant hand, the speculum is passed vertically into the nares and opened, allowing examination of the septum, turbinates, and middle meatus. A topical anesthetic and restraints may be necessary for such an examination in young children.

Because most cases of bleeding in children are from the anterior nasal septum, the simplest way to stop the hemorrhage is to apply direct pressure on the bleeding site for 5 to 10 minutes by external compression of the nares between two fingers. In addition, a cotton (dental) roll may be placed under the upper lip to compress the labial artery. Occasionally, the addition of cotton pledgets moistened with a few drops of epinephrine (1:1,000) or application of topical thrombin will help achieve hemostasis. The child should be sitting up, with his or her head tilted slightly forward during these procedures. If an anterior site of bleeding is identified and there is no evidence of a hemorrhagic diathesis— and particularly if bleeding has been recurrent—cautery with a silver nitrate stick may be warranted (see Chapter 135). For management of severe epistaxis not responsive to such measures, nasal packing or surgical ligation of vessels may be necessary (see Chapter 135, Procedure 7.2). The recent advent of expandable nasal tampons has simplified the procedure of anterior nasal packing for the emergency physician, especially in patients who relapse after a successful cautery.

However, nasal tampons pose the risk of toxic shock syndrome, necessitating careful patient instructions and follow-up. For children with nosebleeds from a hemorrhagic diathesis, one must also correct the underlying disorder. No laboratory workup is indicated in children without clinical evidence of severe blood loss in whom systemic factors are not suspected, and for whom an anterior site of bleeding is identified and stopped readily with local pressure. Reassurance and education about appropriate at-home management needs to be provided.

Occasionally, recurrent epistaxis during an acute upper respiratory infection or flare-up of allergic rhinitis may be lessened with use of an antihistamine-decongestant preparation, although care must be taken not to dry the nose excessively, which can cause epistaxis related to dry mucosa. However, potential side effects of these combination products argue against their use in children younger than 6 years. During the winter, especially in the context of forced hot-air heating systems, a cool mist vaporizer may lessen crusting and drying of nasal mucosa with its subsequent predisposition to recurrent bleeding. An emollient, such as petroleum jelly or a topical antibiotic cream, placed in the nostrils twice daily, and saline nasal spray also are useful for maintaining normal moistness of the nasal mucosa. Instructing parents to keep the child's fingernails short is also helpful.

All patients discharged from the emergency department (ED) after evaluation for significant epistaxis should be given specific instructions on nares compression and indications for repeat evaluation. For patients with specific local abnormalities, such as tumors, polyps, or telangiectasias, referral to an ORL is necessary. Such referral might also be considered, even with questionable findings on the ED nasal examination, if bleeding was severe, recurrent, or suspected to be posterior in origin.

Finally, evaluation for hemorrhagic diathesis should be performed in any child with pertinent positive findings on history, family history, or physical examination. This usually would include prothrombin time, partial thromboplastin time, complete blood cell count, and screening study for von Willebrand's disease. Although the yield would be low in the absence of corroborative clinical features, some children with isolated epistaxis that seems particularly severe or frequently recurrent might also deserve such screening. Children with isolated recurrent epistaxis may have mild bleeding abnormalities; however, the diagnosis of these patients may be difficult, requiring more sophisticated laboratory evaluation (e.g., postaspirin bleeding time, factor VIII–related antigen, ristocetin aggregation study) and referral to a hematologist may be helpful. More recently, epistaxis and mild coagulopathy (thrombocytopenia) suggestive

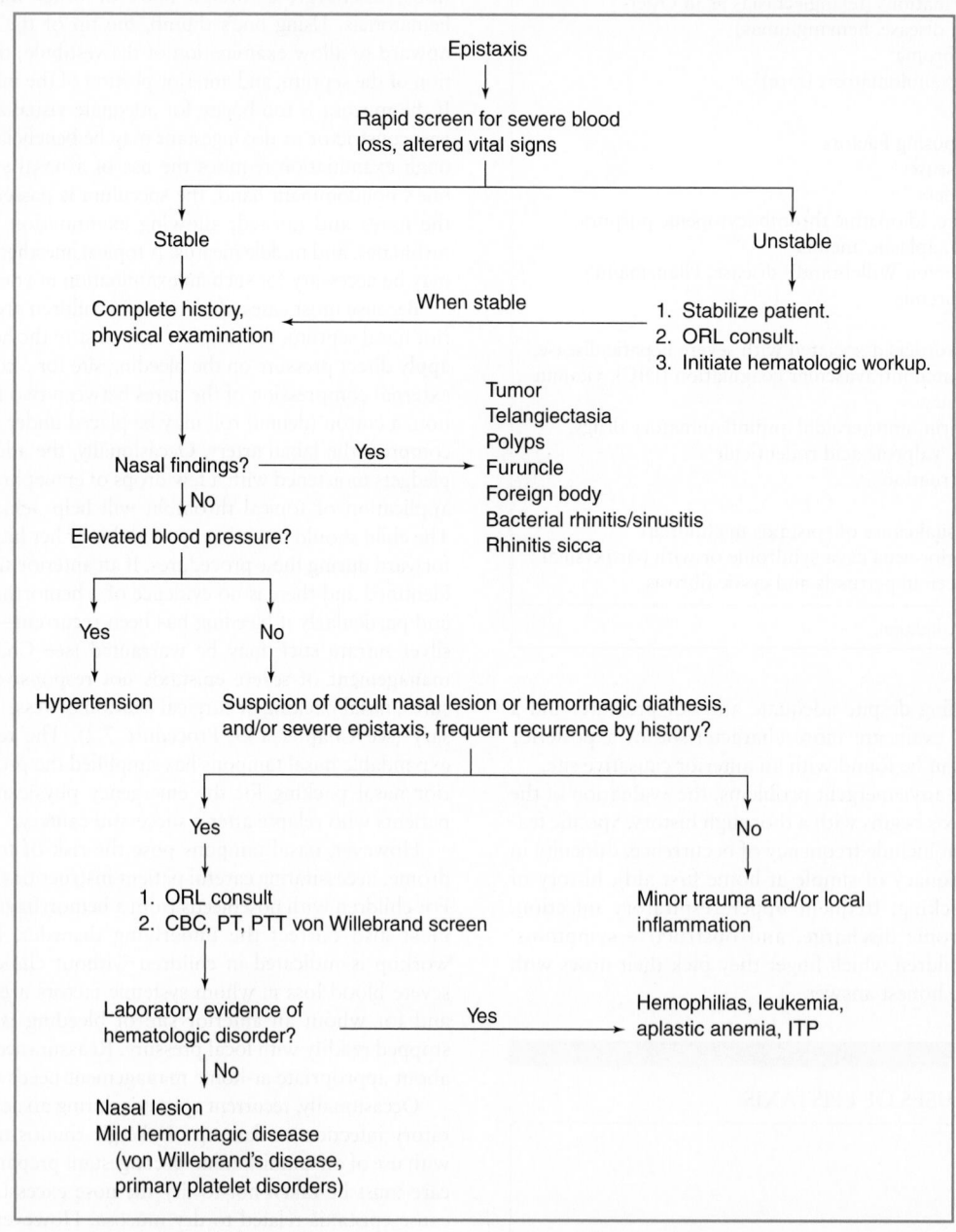

FIGURE 22.1 Approach to diagnosis of epistaxis. ORL, otorhinolaryngologist; CBC, complete blood count; PT, prothrombin time; PTT, partial thromboplastin time; ITP, idiopathic thrombocytopenic purpura.

of acquired von Willebrand's disease has been reported rarely in children receiving chronic valproic acid therapy. These considerations are outlined in the epistaxis algorithm (Fig. 22.1).

Suggested Readings

McIntosh N, Mok JY, Margerison A. Epidemiology of oronasal hemorrhage in the first 2 years of life: implications for child protection. *Pediatrics* 2007;120:1074–1078.

Pallin DJ, Chng YM, McKay MP, et al. Epidemiology of epistaxis in US emergency departments, 1992 to 2001. *Ann Emerg Med* 2005;46:77–81.

Pimpinella PJ. The nasopharyngeal angiofibroma in the adolescent male. *J Pediatr* 1964;64:260–267.

Ritter FN. Vicarious menstruation. In: Strome M, ed. *Differential diagnosis in pediatric otolaryngology.* Boston: Little, Brown and Company, 1975:216.

Sandoval C, Dong S, Visintainer P, et al. Clinical and laboratory features of 178 children with recurrent epistaxis. *J Pediatr Hematol Oncol* 2002;24:47–49.

Schulman I. Clinical conference: the significance of epistaxis in childhood. *Pediatrics* 1959;24:489.

Serdaroglu G, Tutuncuoglu S, Kavakli K, et al. Coagulation abnormalities and acquired von Willebrand's disease type 1 in children receiving valproic acid. *J Child Neurol* 2002;17:41–43.

Whymark AD, Crampsey DP, Fraser L, et al. Childhood epistaxis and nasal colonization with Staphylococcus aureus. *Otolaryngol Head Neck Surg* 2008;138:307–310.

CHAPTER 23 ■ EYE—RED

ALEX V. LEVIN, MD, MHSC, FRCSC

"Red eye" is a generic term that refers to any condition in which the "white of the eye" appears red or pink. A red eye may be caused by local factors, intraocular disease, or systemic problems. Tables 23.1, 23.2, and 23.3 list common and life-threatening causes of red eye. Often, the cause of a red eye can be identified based on the history alone. Discussion here, of chemical conjunctivitis or irritation caused by agents such as smoke or trauma, is limited because the history is almost always known in these situations, making the diagnosis clear. The management of these disorders is discussed in Chapters 117 and 127.

When approaching the problem of "red eye," it is important to determine which tissues are involved. This chapter is confined to disorders in which the conjunctiva, episclera, or sclera are inflamed. Attention must be paid to documenting whether the inflammation is unilateral or bilateral, diffuse or sectorial, and acute or chronic. When bilateral, it is helpful to know whether both eyes were involved simultaneously or sequentially.

PATHOPHYSIOLOGY

With the exception of the cornea, the eye is covered by conjunctiva, a modified mucous membrane covered by nonkeratinized stratified squamous epithelium with goblet cells overlying a substantia propria. The conjunctival epithelium is contiguous with the corneal epithelium. The conjunctiva extends from the surface of the eyeball above and below onto the inner surface of the upper and lower eyelids, creating an upper and lower fornix as it reflects off the eyeball onto the lids (palpebral conjunctiva). These fornices may become repositories for foreign material or exudate. The conjunctiva overlying the sclera (bulbar conjunctiva) may become inflamed without involvement of the palpebral conjunctiva and vice versa. The palpebral conjunctiva contains lymphoid follicular tissues that may become particularly prominent during ages when benign lymphoid hypertrophy (e.g., tonsils, adenopathy) is common. Benign lymphoid hypertrophy appears as small bumps on the palpebral conjunctiva, particularly of the lower lid, best visualized with magnification. A follicular reaction may also occur in some forms of red eye—in particular, viral conjunctivitis. The conjunctiva also covers the caruncle, a small mass of tissue, containing glands, located in the medial corner of the eye at the junction of the upper and lower eyelids.

The sclera (the true "white of the eye") is a largely avascular dense collagenous tissue that provides a tough fibrous outer wall for the eyeball. Four of the six extraocular muscles insert into the anterior sclera, 4 to 8 mm away from the cornea: the superior, medial, inferior, and lateral rectus muscles (see Chapter 24). Although these insertions are not easily visible on the normal eye, inflammation of the muscles makes them apparent. Knowledge of this anatomy may be helpful in the diagnosis of myositis.

The sclera may become inflamed (scleritis). An intermediate layer, the episclera, lies beneath the conjunctiva's substantia propria and another largely avascular fascial layer (Tenon's fascia), where it is firmly attached to the sclera. The episclera and Tenon's fascia do not extend onto the eyelids. The episclera is more vascularized than the sclera and may become inflamed either in a diffuse or localized fashion (diffuse, sectorial, or nodular episcleritis).

The term *conjunctivitis* should be reserved for disorders in which the conjunctiva is inflamed. Inflammation may be caused by direct irritation, infection, inflammation of underlying or contiguous structures (e.g. cornea), immune phenomena, or processes secondary to abnormalities of the lid and lashes. Inflammation within the anterior chamber affecting the iris (iritis) may also result in secondary inflammation of the conjunctiva.

A tear film, which prevents desiccation, is constantly present over the surface of the eye. The tear film is made up of three components: an inner mucinous layer secreted by the goblet cells of the conjunctiva; a middle aqueous layer secreted by the lacrimal glands within the superior temporal anterior orbit and superior conjunctival fornix; and an outer layer secreted by glands in the body of the eyelids, which empty at the eyelid margins (each eyelid contains 20 to 30 glands). A disruption in the function of any three of these anatomic structures may result in an abnormal tear film with secondary desiccation of the ocular surface, resulting in irritation and inflammation (dry eye syndrome).

Innervation of the conjunctiva and cornea comes from the first division of the trigeminal nerve (V1). Abnormalities on the ocular surface may give rise to pain or a foreign-body sensation. The reflex arc that involves the afferent trigeminal nerve and the efferent facial nerve results in a rapid blink, with contraction of the orbicularis oculi muscle, to protect the surface of the eye in response to noxious stimuli. Two other reactions to noxious stimuli may occur: tearing and discharge. Tearing (epiphora) may accompany virtually any conjunctival inflammation or irritation. Tearing may even be a part of some forms of dry eye syndrome, as the lacrimal gland attempts to compensate for ocular surface desiccation due to disruption of the other layers of the tear film. Discharge results either from conjunctival exudation or precipitation of mucus out of the tear film. The latter occurs when the tear film is not flowing smoothly (e.g., nasolacrimal duct obstruction), causing misinterpretation as infection when the problem is actually mechanical.

TABLE 23.1

COMMON CAUSES OF RED EYE[a]

Conjunctivitis
    Infectious: viral (including herpes), bacterial, chlamydial
    Allergic or seasonal
    Chemical (or other physical agents such as smoke)
Systemic disease (Table 23.3)
Trauma
    Corneal or conjunctival abrasion
    Iritis
    Foreign body
Dry eye syndromes
Abnormalities of the lids and/or lashes
    Blepharitis
    Trichiasis due to epiblepharon
    Sty or chalazion (external or internal hordeolum)
    Molloscum of lid margin
    Periorbital or orbital cellulitis
Contact lens–related problems
    Infectious keratitis (corneal ulcer)
    Allergic conjunctivitis
    Corneal abrasion
    Poor fit
    Overwear

[a]Not listed in order of frequency. List not complete.

Although discharge may be a nonspecific finding, the nature of the discharge may be helpful in determining the cause of an infection. Discharge without a red eye is by definition not conjunctivitis. The presence of membranes or pseudomembranes (Fig. 23.1, see also color plate) on the palpebral conjunctiva of an eye with conjunctivitis is also helpful in establishing a cause. For example, pseudomembranes or membranes are more common with adenovirus infection or Stevens-Johnson syndrome. These white or white-yellow plaques are caused by loosely or firmly adherent collections of inflammatory cells, cellular debris, and exudate.

EVALUATION AND DECISION

The approach to the child who presents in the emergency department with a red eye is outlined in the flowchart shown in Figure 23.2.

Any child who wears contact lenses regularly, even if the lens is not in the eye at the time of the examination, should be

TABLE 23.2

LIFE-THREATENING CAUSES OF RED EYE[a]

Systemic disease (Table 23.3)
Child abuse
    Blunt trauma
    Covert instillation of noxious substances [medical child
        abuse (formerly known as Munchausen syndrome by
        proxy)]
Traumatic intracranial arteriovenous fistula (very rare)

[a]List not meant to be complete.

TABLE 23.3

SYSTEMIC CONDITIONS THAT MAY BE ASSOCIATED WITH RED EYE[a]

Collagen vascular disorders
Juvenile rheumatoid arthritis
Infectious diseases
    Varicella, rubeola, otitis media
Kawasaki disease
Inflammatory bowel disease
Cystic fibrosis
Vitamin A deficiency
Cystinosis
Leukemia
Ectodermal dysplasia
Trisomy 21
Cornelia de Lange syndrome
Status post radiation therapy, including ocular field
Bone marrow transplantation
Stevens-Johnson syndrome

[a]Not a complete list: intended to demonstrate multiorgan representation.

referred to an ophthalmologist within 12 hours if he or she has red eye. Red, and often painful, eyes of a person who wears contact lenses may represent potentially blinding corneal infection (corneal ulcer) or the breakdown of the corneal epithelium, which subsequently would predispose the person to corneal infection. Other than removing the contact lens when possible (topical anesthesia may be helpful), further diagnostic or therapeutic interventions by the pediatric emergency physician are not indicated in these patients. It is recommended that empiric antibiotics not be started because the ophthalmologist may want to culture the cornea. Rather, prompt consultation with ophthalmology is essential. The presence of a white spot on the cornea of a contact lens wearer with inflamed conjunctiva is an ominous sign that may represent an ulcer. The absence of such a spot does not rule out corneal ulcer. Other causes of red eye in a contact lens wearer include contact lens solution allergy (which may develop even after years of using the same regimen), overwear, overly tight fit, foreign body, or a damaged contact lens. Examination by an ophthalmologist is perhaps the only way to ensure that a

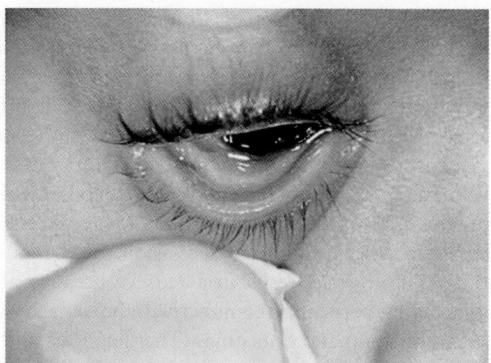

FIGURE 23.1 Pseudomembrane on lower lid palpebral conjunctiva and extending into the inferior fornix in patient with epidemic keratoconjunctivitis (adenovirus).

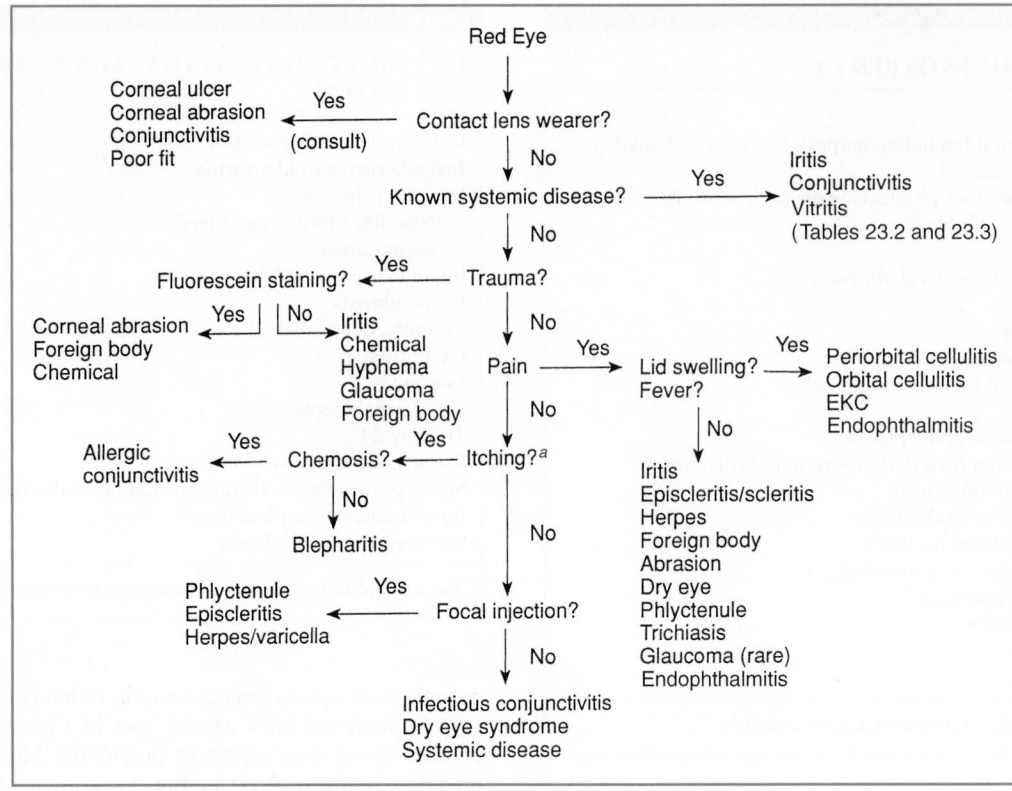

FIGURE 23.2 Diagnostic evaluation of red eye. (EKC = epidemic keratoconjunctivitis)

corneal ulcer is not missed by ascribing the red eye to one of these other etiologies. It is recommended that all contact lens wearers with a red eye be seen an ophthalmologist.

Numerous systemic diseases may be associated with ocular inflammation. A representative sample can be found in Table 23.3. In some systemic diseases, the associated ocular abnormality involves intraocular inflammation (iritis, vitritis), which can then cause secondary conjunctival infection. Patients with these diseases may also have coincidental ocular inflammation unrelated to their underlying conditions. Ophthalmologic consultation may be helpful in making this distinction. For example, in Kawasaki disease, the inflammation of the conjunctiva may be associated with mild iritis. More often, the conjunctiva is inflamed in isolation as part of the systemic mucous membrane involvement. Description of conjunctival inflammation is once again important as the conjunctivitis of Kawasaki disease is usually confined to the bulbar conjunctiva rather than the palpebral, with little, if any, discharge unlike an infective process such as viral conjunctivitis in which the entire conjunctiva is inflamed (Fig. 23.3). Very rarely, head injury may cause the development of an intracranial arteriovenous fistula that may present with proptosis, chemosis, red eye, corkscrew conjunctival blood vessels, and decreased vision.

Traumatic injury may result in a red eye because of other reasons including corneal or conjunctival abrasion, hyphema, iritis, or rarely, traumatic glaucoma. (The diagnosis and treatment of these disorders are summarized in Chapter 117.) If there is no fluorescein staining of the conjunctiva or cornea and there is no obvious evidence of severe intraocular injury (e.g., hyphema, ruptured globe), the examiner may need to consider

the possibility of noxious material coming in contact with the eyeball at the time of trauma. Both acidic and alkaline substances may cause a red eye. (The treatment of these disorders is summarized in Chapter 127.) Likewise, a foreign body may cause ocular pain and inflammation. Foreign bodies often can be difficult to see on brief, superficial examination, especially if the foreign body is smaller than what the naked eye can see. To

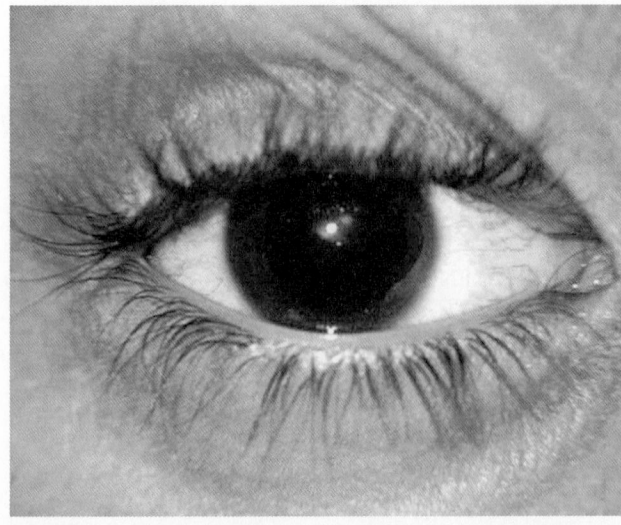

FIGURE 23.3 Bulbar conjunctival injection in patient with Kawasaki disease.

enhance visualization, spin the focusing wheel of a direct ophthalmoscope to the black or green number 10 or more. This will turn the instrument into a self-illuminated hand-held magnifier. All the recesses and redundant folds of the conjunctiva must be inspected. The upper eyelid should be everted (see Chapter 117). The lower eyelid should be pulled down from the globe as the patient looks upward so the inferior fornix can be inspected. The patient should be asked to adduct the affected eye when the lateral canthus (junction of the upper and lower eyelid laterally) is stretched laterally to allow inspection of the lateral fornix. There is no analogous medial fornix.

It is wise to inspect the position of the eyelashes before performing lid eversion and examining the conjunctival fornices. Eyelashes that turn against the ocular surface (trichiasis) may cause a red eye that is accompanied by pain or foreign-body sensation in the absence of lid swelling. Although corneal fluorescein staining may reveal the effect on the corneal epithelium, the condition may be so mild that slit lamp biomicroscopy would be required despite significant symptoms. Trichiasis is particularly common in patients who have had prior injury or surgery to the eyelid and in patients of Asian background. In the latter case, a prominent fold of skin (epiblepharon) may be found medially just below the eyelid margin, causing the lower lid medial eyelashes, and less commonly the upper lid lashes, to rotate toward the eyeball (Fig. 23.4).

In the absence of cornea/conjunctiva abrasion, foreign body, and trichiasis, the painful red eye caused by trauma may have iritis. This may not present for up to 72 hours after the trauma was sustained. Photophobia and vision blurring may also occur. The ipsilateral pupil may be smaller. Occasionally, one will see a cloudy inferior cornea caused by the deposition of inflammatory cells and debris on the inner surface (keratoprecipitates). This finding may be easier to recognize with the direct ophthalmoscope focused as a magnifier (see above). Iritis also may occur in association with systemic disease or as an isolated idiopathic ocular finding. Iritis associated with juvenile idiopathic arthritis (formerly known as juvenile rheumatoid arthritis) is characterized by the distinct absence of signs or symptoms until the disease has progressed significantly, thus underscoring the need for routine screening of these patients. Other systemic causes of iritis include sarcoidosis, tuberculosis, inflammatory bowel disease, collagen vascular disorders, systemic lupus erythematosis, Wegener's, tubular interstitial nephritis uveitis syndrome (TINU), and leukemia. Traumatic iritis and nontraumatic iritis often are indistinguishable except by history. All causes of iritis, regardless of the etiology, require ophthalmologic consultation and follow-up if the diagnosis is not otherwise apparent. The diagnosis of iritis requires slit lamp examination by a skilled observer. Topical steroids should not be prescribed by non-ophthalmologists.

Episcleritis and scleritis may also cause a painful red eye. Although episcleritis is usually an isolated ocular abnormality, scleritis is often associated with an underlying systemic disease, particularly the collagen vascular disorders. Both entities may present with focal or diffuse inflammation. A focal nodular or diffuse elevation may be seen. The eye is often tender, especially with scleritis, where the inflamed area may have a bluish hue. There may also be pain on attempted movement of the eye. Diagnosis and treatment require slit lamp examination and ophthalmologic consultation.

Herpetic corneal infection is another cause of painful red eye. This may be caused by either the simplex or varicella-zoster viruses. Usually, there is no concomitant dermatologic manifestation except in association with chickenpox, when a unilateral or bilateral lesion may be seen on the conjunctiva (usually near or just on the edge of the cornea) with focal injection (Fig. 23.5, see also color plate). Most often, no treatment is required for a conjunctival pox lesion during chickenpox, but herpetic corneal ulcers require urgent treatment to prevent corneal scarring and vision loss. Patients with herpetic corneal ulcers may have a history of prior recurrent painful red eye, although herpes occasionally can be painless because of induced corneal hypoesthesia. Herpes simplex is virtually always unilateral. Fluorescein staining of the cornea may reveal a linear branching pattern referred to as dendrites (Fig. 120.10). If the infected area is located eccentrically on the corneal surface, the injection may be localized to the quadrant of conjunctiva adjacent to the lesion.

If eye pain is relieved by a drop of topical anesthetic (see Chapter 117), the patient most likely has a surface problem (e.g., foreign body, abrasion). If the pain is not relieved and periorbital swelling and fever are present, the red eye may be caused by periorbital or orbital cellulitis. These are emergent

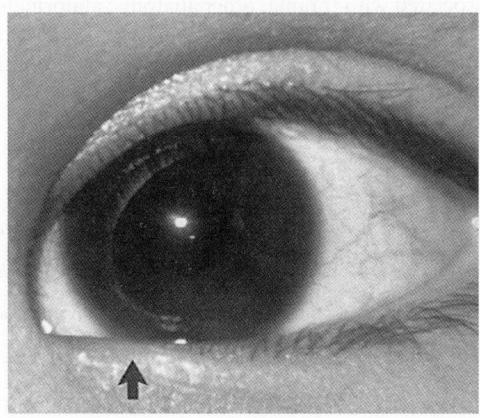

FIGURE 23.4 Epiblepharon. Extra skin fold medially on lower lid *(arrow)* rotates eyelashes back toward eyeball surface.

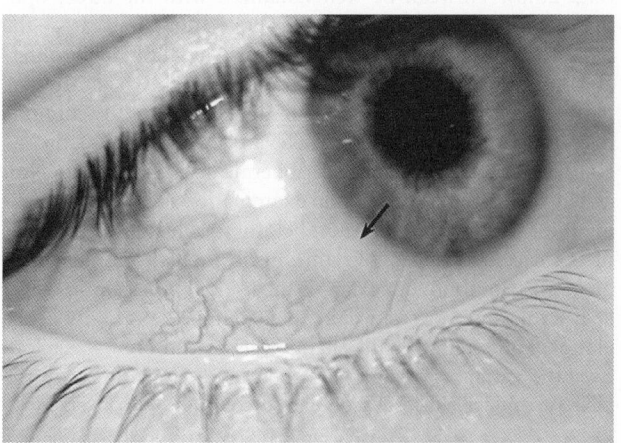

FIGURE 23.5 Red eye caused by chickenpox (varicella) involvement of conjunctiva. Note sectorial injection of conjunctiva. White area *(arrow)* at junction of conjunctiva and cornea is the pox lesion.

conditions, the treatment and diagnosis of which are reviewed in Chapter 127. Eye pain and marked lid swelling also may be associated with epidemic keratoconjunctivitis (EKC) secondary to adenovirus (Fig. 120.8). When questioned further, patients may reveal that they actually have a sandy foreign-body sensation rather than true ocular pain. Pseudomembranes are a fairly diagnostic sign when present (Fig. 23.1). Low-grade fever and tender preauricular adenopathy may also occur, making it difficult to distinguish EKC from periorbital cellulitis. EKC usually affects the eyes consecutively and bilaterally as opposed to the unilateral nature of periorbital cellulitis. There also may be associated prominent photophobia and tearing in adenoviral conjunctivitis, which is not usually seen in cellulitis.

Itching is another important diagnostic symptom. When it is associated with swelling of the conjunctiva, giving it the appearance of a blister-like elevation (chemosis, Fig. 120.9), one should suspect acute allergic conjunctivitis. Unlike chronic, recurrent, seasonal, allergic conjunctivitis, there are usually no associated systemic symptoms. Often, there is no known causative agent, and there may be associated periocular swelling. The condition may be unilateral or bilateral and usually has an acute or hyperacute onset. Photophobia, tearing, and lid swelling may also occur. The emergency physician can prescribe topical antihistamines and/or vasoconstrictors, as well as cool compresses, to relieve the symptoms. Systemic diphenhydramine may also be useful. The etiology is only rarely identified.

Itching may also accompany blepharitis, an idiopathic disorder in which there is suboptimal flow of secretions from the meibomian glands normally present in the eyelids. Because these glands participate in the formation of the lubricating tear film that normally covers the eye, the deficiency of flow may result in an abnormal tear film and rapid corneal desiccation. Symptoms are aggravated by activities associated with prolonged staring and a decreased blink rate (reading, television or computer viewing, and video games) or going outside on windy days. Patients may have photophobia and a sandy foreign-body sensation. To compensate for the tear film deficiency, reflex excess tearing may occur from the lacrimal gland. The most characteristic sign is erythema of the eyelid margins and flaking and crusting at the base of the eyelashes (Fig. 23.6). This can be well visualized with the direct ophthalmoscope as a magnifier (see above). Left untreated, the reduced flow of the meibomian glands may allow for proliferation of the coagulase-negative staphylococci, which are normally present. This overgrowth may lead to an immune response causing an inflamed elevated white spot(s) on the conjunctiva (phlyctenule) or peripheral corneal infiltrates associated with a red eye. Slit lamp examination is helpful in making these diagnoses and is most helpful to rule out the presence of corneal involvement. Erythromycin topical ointment may be useful, but more important is the use of baby shampoo eyelash scrubs once or twice daily to encourage better flow of the glands. Full strength baby shampoo is placed on a washcloth over the caretaker's finger and then used to gently scrub the base of the eyelashes. Accumulated soap is then rinsed away

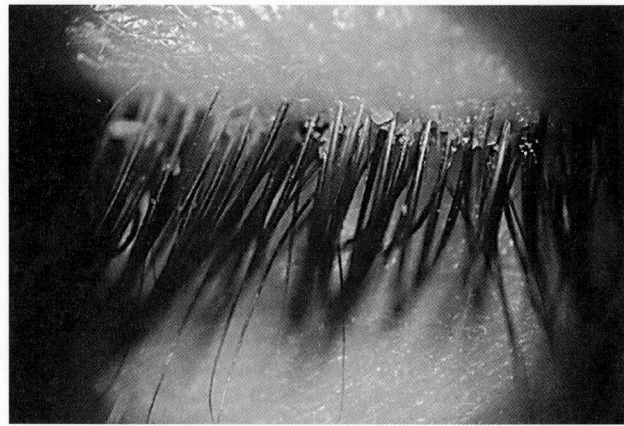

FIGURE 23.6 Blepharitis. Note crusts and flakes at base of eyelashes.

with a washcloth. This should be done once or twice daily and continued for some time even after the symptoms have improved or resolved.

Although itching and pain may be minor symptoms associated with several types of conjunctivitis, it is usually the absence of these symptoms that should lead one to suspect an infectious cause. Conjunctivitis usually causes diffuse inflammation of the conjunctiva, either unilaterally or bilaterally with rare exception (e.g., sectoral herpes keratitis). The differentiation of bacterial, viral, chlamydial, and other types of conjunctivitis is sometimes difficult (see Chapter 127). Purulent discharge is particularly characteristic of bacterial infection.

If the injection is localized, the examiner should consider a specific list of diagnostic possibilities. Herpes keratitis phlyctenule, episcleritis, and scleritis may present with focal involvement, as previously discussed. Localized injection of the conjunctiva may be an indicator of an imbedded foreign body, varicella, or other focal processes that require the attention of an ophthalmologic consultant.

Although much feared, glaucoma in children is very rare. Congenital glaucoma is usually not associated with a red eye or pain. Small children who have glaucoma often have enlarged eyes (buphthalmus) with tearing, photophobia, cloudy cornea and less commonly, heterochromia. Acute acquired glaucoma causes a painful red eye, perhaps associated with corneal clouding and decreased visual acuity. Acquired glaucoma, is most often associated with trauma, other anatomic abnormalities, or iritis that would be apparent on examination. Because it is difficult to determine intraocular pressure in children, ophthalmologic consultation is required in all cases.

Suggested Readings

Fisher MC. Conjunctivitis in children. *Pediatr Clin North Am* 1987;34: 1447–1456.
Greenberg MF, Pollard ZF. The red eye in childhood. *Pediatr Clin North Am* 2003;50:105–124.
Levin AV. Eye emergencies: acute management in the pediatric ambulatory setting. *Pediatr Emerg Care* 1991;7:367–377.
Matoba A. Ocular viral infections. *Pediatr Infect Dis* 1984;3:358–368.

CHAPTER 24 ■ EYE—STRABISMUS

ALEX V. LEVIN, MD, MHSC, FRCSC

Strabismus refers to any misalignment of the eyes such that they are not viewing in the same direction. *Esotropia* refers to eyes that are turned in (cross eyed). *Exotropia* refers to eyes that are turned out (wall eyed). The terms *hypertropia* and *hypotropia* refer to a higher or lower eye, respectively. By convention, vertical misalignment of the eyes is always categorized by the higher eye (e.g., right hypertropia), unless it is known that a specific abnormal process is causing one eye to be held in a lower position (e.g., left hypotropia). (Note: These terms should not be confused with *hyperopia*, the term referring to farsightedness.) Many children with strabismus require a formal evaluation by an ophthalmologist for definitive diagnosis and management, but the emergency physician should attempt to answer two questions: (i) "Is the strabismus an emergency?" and, if so, (ii) "What is the most likely cause?"

PATHOPHYSIOLOGY

Six muscles surround each eyeball (Fig. 24.1). Although several of these muscles may individually move the eye in more than one direction, knowledge of the primary action of these muscles allows for the definition of diagnostic positions of gaze (Table 24.1). This can be helpful in pinpointing specific muscle dysfunction. For example, if a muscle that primarily governs abduction (e.g., lateral rectus) is impaired, the eye is unable to abduct and will usually lie in a position of adduction (esotropia). Likewise, if a muscle that is involved with downgaze (e.g., inferior rectus) is impaired, the eye will have a tendency to remain in relative upgaze (ipsilateral hypertropia).

Although the interactions of the extraocular muscles are complex, the eyeballs should always move symmetrically, both quantitatively and qualitatively, into each direction of gaze. On lateral gaze, the abducting and adducting eye should move far enough so that no sclera is visible laterally or medially, respectively (Fig. 24.2). Both eyes should move symmetrically into upgaze and downgaze such that a straight line, parallel to the horizon, could be drawn between the most superior or inferior part of the iris (Fig. 24.3).

On upgaze, the eyelids should also move up involuntarily. Likewise, on downgaze, the eyelids should move down symmetrically. In the primary position (straight ahead), no sclera should be visible superiorly. The upper eyelid margins should just cross over the iris without crossing over a significant portion of pupil. If one or both lids droop further down, the patient has ptosis. The lower eyelid margin usually crosses within 1 mm above or below the 6 o'clock position of the inferior iris.

Strabismus is categorized into misalignment as a result of impaired muscle function or misalignment in the presence of full normal muscle function. In general, there are only two

emergency reasons why the function of a particular muscle might be impaired: neurogenic palsy or muscle restriction.

Three cranial nerves are responsible for the innervation of the six extraocular muscles (Table 24.1). The sixth cranial nerve innervates the ipsilateral lateral rectus muscle. This nerve exits the ventral pons and then travels on the wall of the middle cranial fossa (clivus), reaching the sphenoid ridge, along which it travels until entering the cavernous sinus. The course of this nerve allows it to be injured by vascular or neoplastic changes in the midbrain, increased intracranial pressure (ICP), large anterior midline craniofacial tumors (e.g., nasopharyngeal carcinoma), otitis media (OM) with involvement of the petrous portion of the sphenoid (Gradenigo syndrome), and any abnormality that involves the cavernous sinus. An abnormality of the sixth cranial nerve will cause a reduction in ipsilateral abduction (Fig. 24.2), and in the straight ahead position, a possible ipsilateral esotropia.

The fourth cranial nerve innervates the superior oblique muscle. It is the only cranial nerve that completely decussates and has a dorsal projection over the midbrain. This position renders the fourth cranial nerve particularly vulnerable to blunt head trauma, one of the most common causes of fourth nerve palsy. The fourth cranial nerve also has a relatively long intracranial course, which makes it particularly susceptible to increased ICP and parenchymal shifts caused by cerebral edema. It also runs through the cavernous sinus. Fourth cranial nerve palsy may be congenital but asymptomatic for several years during childhood until the brain is no longer able to compensate. Acquired or congenital palsy of this cranial nerve causes the eyes to become misaligned vertically (ipsilateral hypertropia). Patients with congenital fourth cranial nerve paresis compensate by tilting their head to the ipsilateral side, which allows for a rebalancing of the eye muscles such that alignment may be achieved. Old photographs may demonstrate this tilt. Facial asymmetry can also be seen after years of this compensatory tilting. Ophthalmic consultation is usually needed to differentiate between congenital and acquired palsy.

The third cranial nerve supplies the remaining four extraocular muscles. It is involved with downgaze, upgaze, and adduction. Parasympathetic innervation to the pupil (see Chapter 25) and innervation to the eyelid muscle (levator palpebrae) are also carried in the third cranial nerve. A complete third cranial nerve palsy results in an eye that is positioned down (from the remaining action of the unaffected superior oblique muscle) and out (from the remaining action of the unaffected lateral rectus muscle) with ipsilateral ptosis and ipsilateral pupillary dilation (Fig. 24.4). Because the third cranial nerve divides into a superior and an inferior division just as it enters the orbit from the cavernous sinus and because the fibers to individual muscles are segregated within

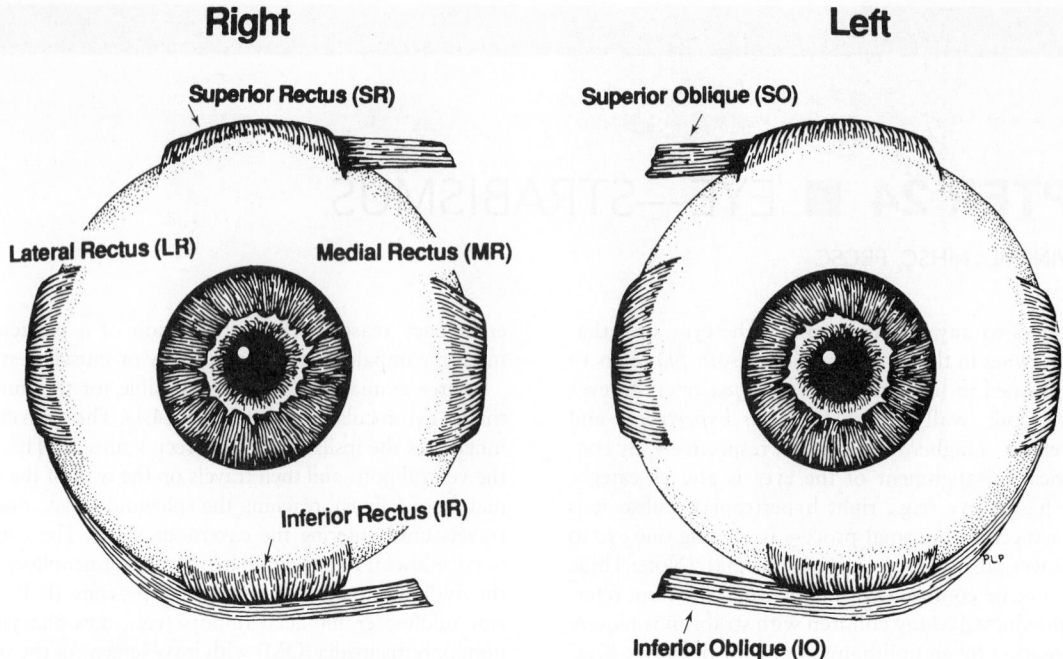

FIGURE 24.1 Normal extraocular muscle anatomy.

the nerve throughout its course, partial third cranial nerve palsies may occur with or without ptosis and/or pupillary dilation. This may leave the patient with complex strabismus, which is best left to the ophthalmologic consultant. (The differential diagnosis of third cranial nerve palsies is summarized in Chapter 25.)

The action of a muscle may also be impaired by restriction. The muscle can become infiltrated with substances that might restrict its action or cause fibrosis. Children with hyperthyroid eye disease (e.g., Graves) can have large, tight eye muscles. An eyeball may also be restricted in its movements by tumors or infection in and around the globe. Orbital tumors, cellulitis, or abscesses that cause restriction may be associated with proptosis or a displacement of the entire eyeball, either vertically or horizontally. After blunt trauma to the eyeball, the globe may be translocated posteriorly, causing an increased intraorbital pressure that may result in a "blowout" fracture of the bony orbital wall. Limitations of movement caused by blowout fractures may not be noticeable until the eye attempts to move. In other words, the eyes may be parallel in the straight ahead position but may be misaligned when they attempt to look in a direction opposite the fracture site. When an orbital wall fracture occurs, the muscle or surrounding tissues that run along that wall may become entrapped within that fracture, tethering the eyeball so the eye cannot look in the direction opposite the fracture. For example, fractures of the orbital floor may entrap the inferior rectus muscle, tethering the eye downward so upgaze is restricted (Fig. 24.5). Sometimes, the eye may also have a limitation of movement in the direction of the fracture. Orbital wall fractures may also be associated with enophthalmos, in which the eye appears to be sunken in the orbit, or proptosis caused by orbital hemorrhage. All patients with orbital fractures must receive a complete ophthalmic examination to rule out accompanying ocular injury. The most common fracture involves the inferior and/or medial walls of the orbit. The lateral wall is rarely fractured. Fracture of the superior wall (orbital roof) is particularly worrisome because it may allow communication between the subfrontal intracranial space and orbit.

TABLE 24.1

EXTRAOCULAR MUSCLES

Muscle[a]	Cranial nerve	Action[b]	Eye position in palsy
Medial rectus	III (inferior division)	Adduction	Exotropia
Inferior rectus	III (inferior division)	Downgaze	Hypertropia
Lateral rectus	VI	Abduction	Esotropia
Superior rectus	III (superior division)	Upgaze	Hypotropia
Superior oblique	IV	Downgaze	Hypertropia
Levator palpebrae[c]	III (superior division)	Eyelid	Ptosis (lid)

[a]Inferior oblique not included for simplicity. Isolated palsy of the inferior oblique is extremely rare.
[b]Action in the horizontal or vertical field only. Cyclorotatory movements not included.
[c]By definition, not truly an extraocular muscle.

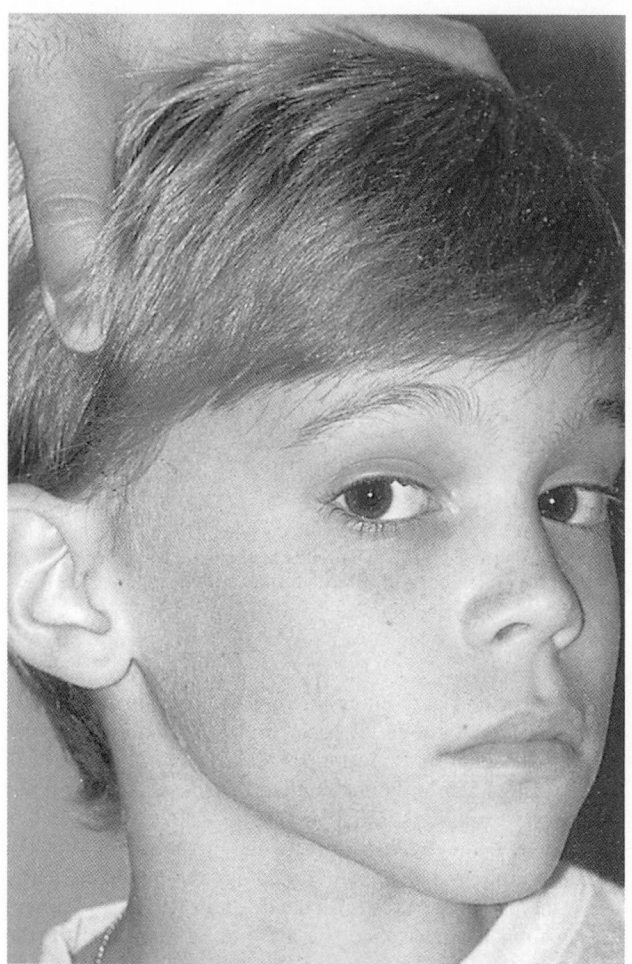

FIGURE 24.2 Patient's head is being rotated passively to patient's left as he looks straight ahead. This causes displacement of eyes into right gaze. Left eye adducts fully, showing no visible sclera medially. Subtle right sixth nerve palsy demonstrated by failure of right eye to abduct fully: sclera is still visible laterally on right eye.

The remaining types of strabismus fall into the category where eye muscle function is unimpaired (nonrestrictive and nonparalytic). These problems are not emergent. The eyes may be misaligned as a result of a failure of the brain to use both eyes simultaneously in a coordinated fashion (idiopathic), a need for glasses or the presence of poor vision in one eye. Uncorrected farsightedness (hyperopia) can result in esotropia (accommodative esotropia), which may have an acute onset, usually between the ages of 2 and 6 years, with the misalignment often worse at near viewing. Uncorrected nearsightedness (myopia) can result in exotropia, especially when the patient views in the far distance. Both types of misalignment may be treated with glasses.

Checking the vision in both eyes (see Chapter 127) is essential in all cases of strabismus with full eye movements to rule out the presence of uncorrected refractive error or a poorly seeing eye. The latter may be due to serious eye problems such as retinoblastoma or cataract.

EVALUATION AND DECISION

The Hirschberg light reflex test can be helpful in determining whether strabismus is present. The physician should shine a penlight or direct ophthalmoscope light at the patient's eyes from 2 to 3 feet while the patient is told to look at the other end of the room. In younger children, the patient may choose to look at the light itself, but all efforts should be made to distract the child with a more distant target. The examiner should observe the white dot light reflex that appears to be located on the cornea, overlying the iris or pupil of each eye. This reflex should be located in a nearly symmetric position in each eye (Fig. 24.6). In the normal state, the light reflex actually falls slightly off-center in the nasal direction in both eyes (Fig. 24.6). If the eyes are misaligned, symmetry would not be preserved (Figs. 24.5 and 24.7, see also color plate).

Two findings are helpful in assessing whether strabismus is emergent: (i) the presence or absence of double vision and

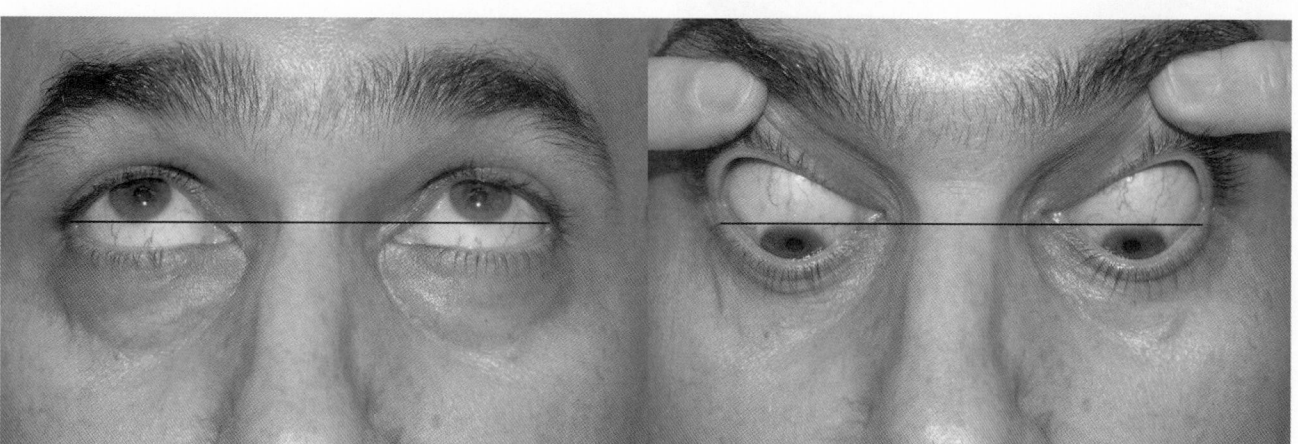

FIGURE 24.3 In normal upgaze, an imaginary line parallel to the horizon can be drawn between the most inferior point of the edge of each iris. In normal downgaze, a similar line can be drawn at the most superior point of the iris.

SIGNS AND SYMPTOMS

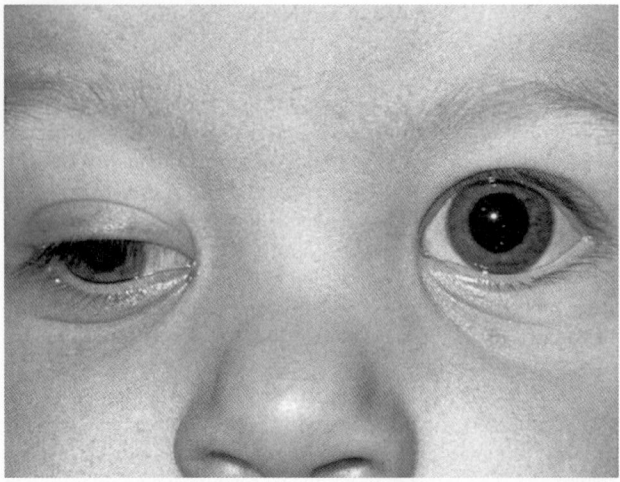

FIGURE 24.4 Right third cranial nerve palsy. When looking straight ahead with left eye, right eye rests in a hypotropic and exotropic position. Note right ptosis. Right pupil is involved (mydriatic), but both pupils were dilated pharmacologically by examiner just before this photograph was taken.

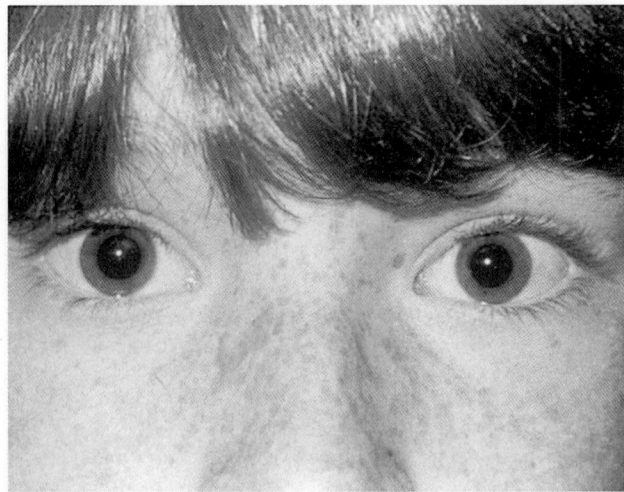

FIGURE 24.6 Normal Hirschberg light reflex test. Light reflexes fall symmetrically in each eye. The reflex in the patient's left eye is a bit nasal to the center, but still within normal limits.

(ii) the status of the eye movements. Although young children may not complain of diplopia, this symptom often indicates an acute or subacute onset of ocular misalignment. Nonemergent childhood strabismus is usually not associated with double vision because the brain becomes adept at suppressing the misaligned nonfixing eye. If a child complains of diplopia, ophthalmologic consultation is appropriate, even if no strabismus appears on examination by the emergency physician.

If the eye movements are completely full and symmetric, one can be virtually certain that the strabismus is not emergent. Problems that cause emergent strabismus do so by impairing the action of one or more muscles. A neurogenic palsy or restrictive phenomenon can not be present if the eye movements are full. If there are any questions about subtle reductions in extraocular movement or if there is prominent nystagmus elicited in one

particular field of gaze (more than the few beats of normal end point nystagmus known as gaze paretic nystagmus), ophthalmologic consultation is most likely appropriate.

Because of fear and noncompliance, some children will not follow the examiner's target that is presented to assess eye movement. If they will not follow the target but look at the examiner only, the examiner should ask the parent to gently move the patient's head to each side and then up and down. The examiner can also do this by putting one hand on the child's head (Fig. 24.2), although this may serve only to heighten the child's anxiety. As the patient continues to look straight ahead when the head is being turned, the eyes are moving passively in reference to the head and orbit. When the head is turned to the left, the eyes move into right gaze to maintain fixation straight ahead (Fig. 24.2). If the head is tilted

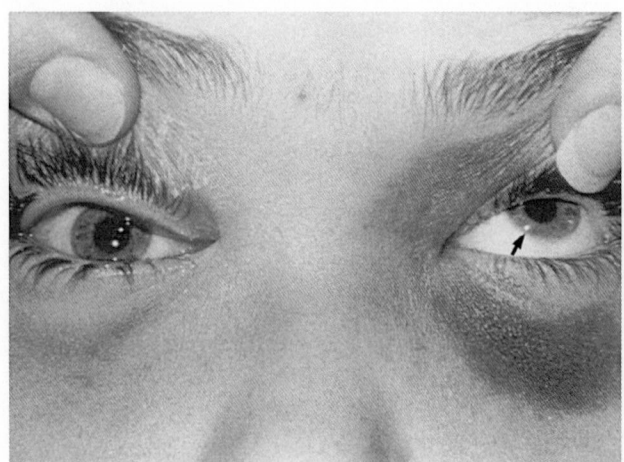

FIGURE 24.5 Patient is looking upward. Right inferior orbital wall blowout fracture causes restriction of upgaze in right eye. Note light reflexes (Hirschberg test). Left reflex (*arrow*) is lower in reference to pupil than right reflex, indicating the presence of a right hypotropia.

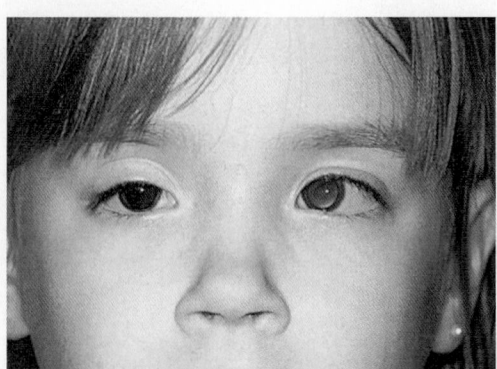

FIGURE 24.7 Left esotropia. Note lateral displacement of Hirschberg light reflex in the left eye. Photograph demonstrates right ptosis. Pupils are pharmacologically dilated. Asymmetry of red reflex is caused by misalignment of the eyes.

up, the eyes are moved into relative downgaze. Essentially, this is the "doll's eye" maneuver used in the assessment of comatose patients. If the eyes move symmetrically and fully on passive movement of the head, this rules out the presence of a neurogenic or restrictive problem with the same accuracy as if the patient had voluntarily followed a target. Although the neuro-ophthalmologic contributions to the assessment of the comatose patient are beyond the scope of this chapter, the presence of a cranial nerve palsy can be ruled out even in the patient who is experiencing an altered mental status related to central nervous system (CNS) disease if the eyes move fully on the doll's eye maneuver as the head is rotated by the examiner.

When an orbital blowout fracture is suspected, confirmation may be obtained by a computed tomography (CT) scan of the orbit. Some controversy exists about the need to perform this test emergently. Some ophthalmologists prefer to image only if the strabismus and diplopia do not spontaneously resolve over 1 to 2 weeks. If there is a concern about intracranial injury or orbital roof fracture as the cause of strabismus, an urgent CT scan of the head is indicated. If there is significant enophthalmos, then early imaging is also recommended. To evaluate the extraocular muscles, it is essential that coronal views be obtained. Contrast enhancement is unnecessary. Plain skull radiographs play virtually no role in the diagnosis and management of orbital fractures.

The causes of pediatric strabismus are summarized in Tables 24.2 through 24.4. The first considerations (Figs. 24.8 and 24.9) are restrictive strabismus and neurogenic palsies. Myasthenia gravis and thyroid ophthalmopathy (hyperthyroidism) can mimic virtually any strabismus with deficiency of extraocular movement and must always be considered in the differential diagnosis in any pattern of ocular misalignment. Myasthenia may cause ptosis, whereas thyroid disease causes retraction of the upper lid. The pupils are not involved in either condition.

TABLE 24.2

DIFFERENTIAL DIAGNOSIS OF STRABISMUS[a]

Neurogenic Palsies
III Cranial nerve palsy (partial or complete)
IV Cranial nerve palsy
VI Cranial nerve palsy
Traumatic extraocular muscle palsy
Myasthenia gravis
Internuclear ophthalmoplegia
Skew deviation

Restrictive Strabismus
Orbital wall fracture
Orbital hemorrhage, tumor, infection, or abscess
Thyroid eye disease
Nonthyroid extraocular muscle infiltration (e.g., metastasis)
Orbital cellulites

Nonneurogenic Nonrestrictive Strabismus
Idiopathic childhood strabismus
Strabismus caused by refractive errors (e.g., accommodative esotropia)
Sensory strabismus (unilateral visual loss)

[a]Not listed in order of frequency.

TABLE 24.3

COMMON CAUSES OF STRABISMUS[a]

Esotropia
Congenital infantile or acquired (with or without farsightedness), nonparalytic, nonrestrictive
Long-standing unilateral visual loss
Medial orbital wall fracture
VI cranial nerve palsy
Orbital mass, hemorrhage, or infection (all uncommon)

Exotropia
Nonparalytic nonrestrictive idiopathic childhood exotropia
Long-standing unilateral visual loss
III cranial nerve palsy
Orbital mass, hemorrhage, or infection (all uncommon)

Hypertropia
Dissociated vertical deviation (a nonparalytic nonrestrictive childhood deviation)
Idiopathic overaction or the inferior oblique muscle (affected eye rises in adduction)
Inferior or superior orbital wall fracture
IV Cranial nerve palsy: congenital or acquired
Orbital mass, hemorrhage, or infection (all uncommon)

Hypotropia
Brown syndrome (tight superior oblique tendon)
Inferior or superior orbital wall fracture
Orbital mass, hemorrhage, or infection (all uncommon)

[a]Not listed in order of frequency.

Esotropia Emergencies

Figure 24.8 summarizes the approach to a patient with esotropia and exotropia. Patients with a restrictive or neurogenic esotropia (deficiency of abduction) may adopt an abnormal head position to place the eyes in the position of best alignment to avoid double vision. By turning the face in the direction of the deficiency (e.g., right face turn for right sixth nerve palsy) when looking straight ahead, the eyes are aligned and appear straight. The patient's head must be held in the straight ahead position to notice that the affected eye is actually crossed.

In the presence of proptosis or a history of eye trauma, one must be concerned that an orbital process is causing the esotropia. Fracture of the medial orbital wall may cause entrapment and restriction of the medial rectus. Fracture of

---

TABLE 24.4

LIFE-THREATENING CAUSES OF STRABISMUS[a]

Intracranial mass	Head trauma
Elevated intracranial pressure	Meningitis
Myasthenia gravis	Neoplastic infiltration of extraocular muscles
Orbital tumor	Superior orbital wall fracture
Orbital cellulitis	Retinoblastoma causing visual loss

[a]Not listed in order of frequency.

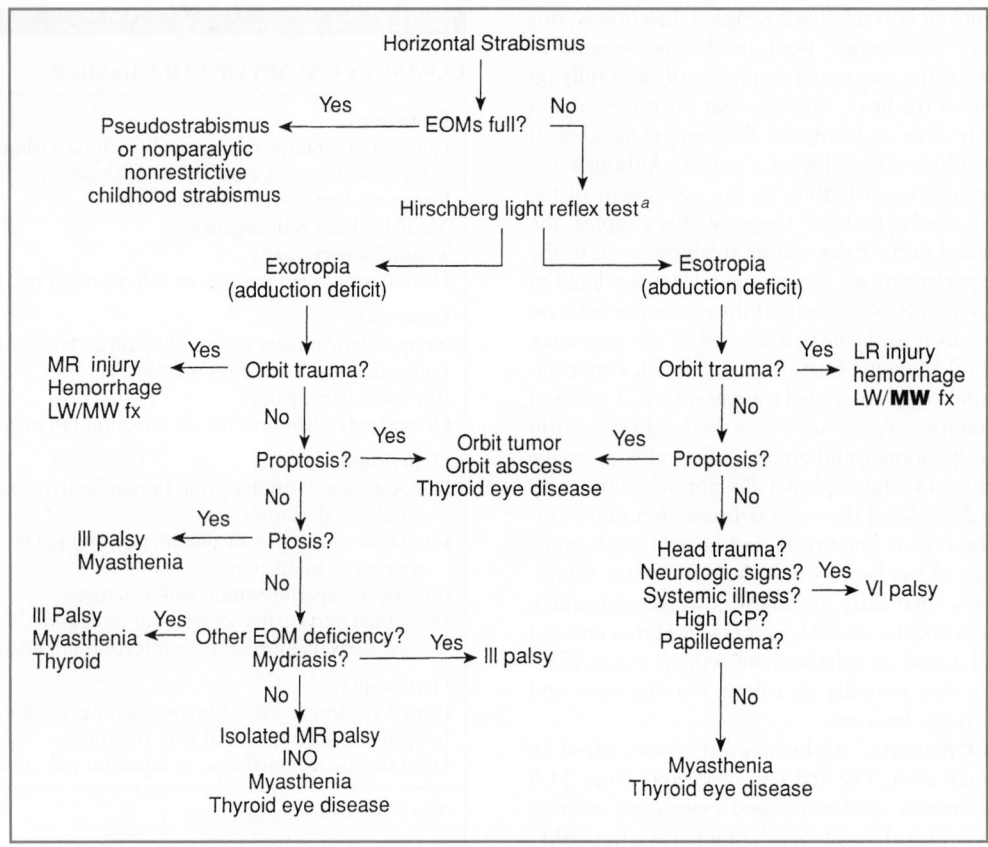

FIGURE 24.8 Evaluation of horizontal strabismus. EOM, extraocular muscle movement; MR, medial rectus; LW, lateral orbital wall; MW, medial orbital wall; fx, fracture; LR, lateral rectus; ICP, intracranial pressure; INO, internuclear ophthalmoplegia; boldface type, most likely fracture. [a]With head held in straight ahead position.

the lateral wall—usually part of a tripod fracture that involves the zygoma and inferior lateral wall—may cause orbital hemorrhage that would displace the eye medially.

Likewise, a lateral orbital tumor or abscess can push the eye toward the nose or restrict abduction. Any infiltrative process that involves the eye muscles may also cause esotropia through restriction. Orbital cellulitis can cause any type of misalignment, including esotropia, with or without abscess formation. A CT scan of the orbit with coronal and axial views is the diagnostic procedure of choice in these situations.

Lateral rectus palsy (sixth cranial nerve palsy) occurs most commonly secondary to head trauma (see Chapter 116) or increased ICP. Other CNS signs, such as papilledema, may be present. Magnetic resonance imaging (MRI) of the brain is the procedure of choice. Sixth cranial nerve palsy can also occur rather precipitously after the placement of ventricular shunts designed to relieve increased ICP even if the palsy was not obvious preoperatively. Sixth cranial nerve palsy may be bilateral, in which case both eyes will be in the crossed position with reduced ability to adduct bilaterally, although possibly asymmetrically.

Exotropia Emergencies

Orbital cellulitis, thyroid eye disease, and orbital tumors may also cause exotropia. Trauma very rarely results in exotropia because lateral wall fractures rarely cause entrapment. Orbital

hemorrhage (with or without medial wall fracture) can have a mass effect, causing the eye to be turned out.

Isolated paresis of the medial rectus muscle, resulting in a deficiency of adduction and a turned out eye, is quite unusual because other muscles are also innervated by the same branch of the third cranial nerve. One should look for accompanying ptosis, pupillary dilation, or deficiencies of upgaze or downgaze to confirm third cranial nerve involvement, even if these findings are subtle.

Unilateral isolated deficiency of adduction may be the result of an intranuclear ophthalmoplegia secondary to a brainstem injury that involves the interconnecting pathways between the third and sixth cranial nerves. Bilateral isolated deficiency of adduction is virtually diagnostic of this condition. MRI of the brainstem should be ordered emergently. The observer should also look for prominent nystagmus on attempted abduction of the contralateral eye.

Hypertropia/Hypotropia Emergencies

Paretic or restrictive vertical eye muscle imbalance must be referred to an ophthalmologist. Figure 24.9 summarizes the approach to the patient with vertical ocular misalignment. To determine whether it is the higher or lower eye that is abnormal, the examiner must have the patient look upward and then downward. If one eye is unable to look downward fully,

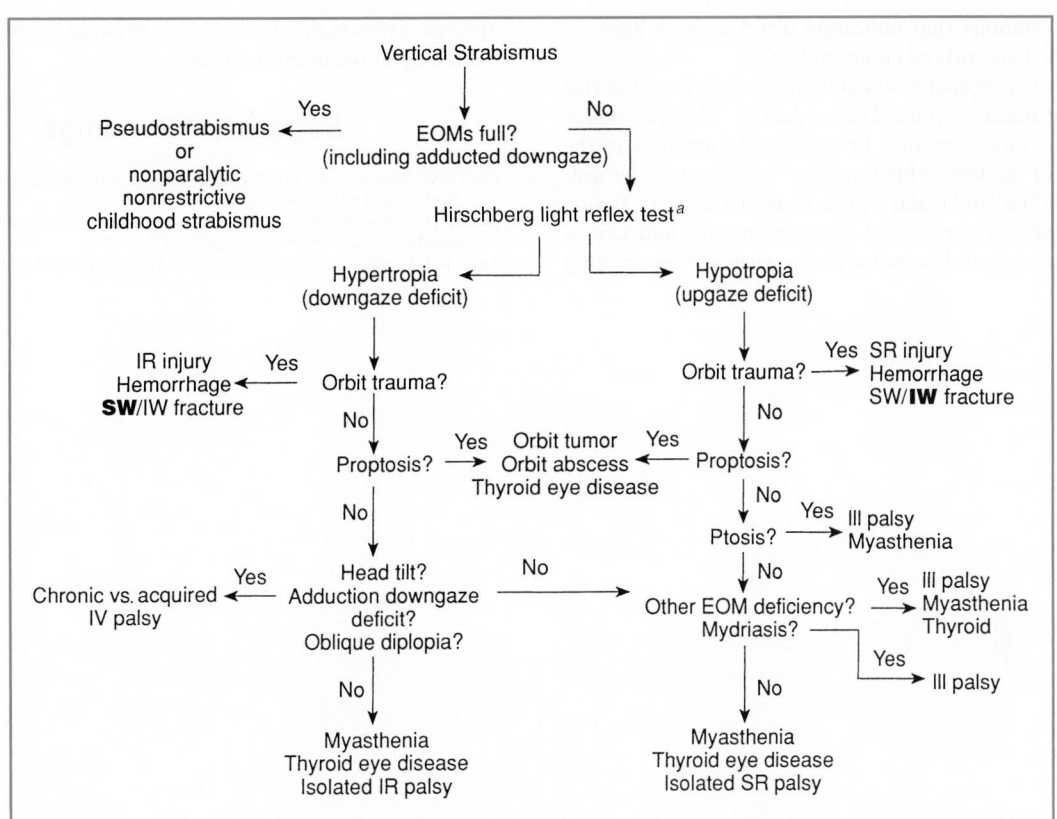

FIGURE 24.9 Evaluation of vertical strabismus. EOM, extraocular muscle movement; IR, inferior rectus; SW, superior orbital wall; IW, inferior orbital wall; SR, superior rectus; **boldface type**, most likely fracture. [a]With head held in straight ahead position.

SIGNS AND SYMPTOMS

the patient has a hypertropia of that eye. If one eye is unable to look upward fully, that eye is hypotropic (Fig. 24.5). Patients may adopt abnormal head positions to compensate for this misalignment. By lifting the chin to look straight ahead, the eyes are placed in relative downgaze, thus indicating that the strabismus is worse when the patient looks up. Likewise, the patient may adopt a chin down position to look straight ahead, indicating that the strabismus is worse in downgaze. A chin up or chin down position does not prove strabismus as there may be other causes (e.g., chin up position as compensation for ptosis, chin up or down position to lessen nystagmus). When a patient has an anomalous head position, it can be useful to examine the patient with the head in the opposite position to better highlight the abnormality for which the spontaneous head position is trying to compensate. For example, if the patient presents with a chin up position, the eyes may appear to be aligned in that position. If the head is moved by the examiner into a chin down position, the vertical misalignment of the eyes will be more apparent. An eye may become hypertropic for several reasons. Any mass underneath the eyeball—for example, an orbital tumor or a mucocele extending upward from the maxillary sinus—may push the eye upward. A tightened superior rectus is unusual but may be seen in thyroid eye disease or after trauma. An inferior orbital wall fracture could injure (weaken) the inferior rectus or cause hemorrhage that would push the eye up into a hypertropic position. A CT scan of the orbit would be the proper diagnostic modality.

Perhaps the most important cause of ipsilateral hypertropia is a lesion that involves the fourth cranial nerve. Although the eye may be able to look straight down fully, there may be a restriction of gaze in the down-and-in position relative to the other eye (which then would be looking down and out). Because of the torsional forces of the superior oblique muscle on the eyeball, the patient may adopt an abnormal head position with a face turn and a head tilt away from the affected eye. One must always consider the possibility that a new fourth nerve palsy actually represents a decompensated congenital abnormality.

Although rare, neurogenic palsies of the inferior oblique or inferior rectus with resultant vertical misalignment may occur. These have been reported after viral illnesses, including varicella. As with exotropia of neurogenic origin, it would be more likely to have other branches of the third cranial nerve involved with other findings. Another type of vertical eye muscle imbalance, skew deviation, can be the presenting sign of a midbrain lesion. Ophthalmologic consultation can be helpful in deciding whether MRI is appropriate.

Hypotropia can be caused by an orbital roof fracture with superior hematoma that pushes the eye down. Alternatively, hypertropia from a deficiency of downgaze due to tethering of the superior rectus muscle in an orbital roof fracture can also occur uncommonly. Orbital roof fracture is an emergent condition. Neuroradiologic evaluation, including coronal views, must be obtained to rule out communication between the orbit and the intracranial cavity. Pulsating proptosis is a particularly ominous sign indicating direct contact between the intracranial and orbital compartments.

Traumatic hypotropia most commonly results from inferior wall blowout fractures (Figs. 24.5 and 24.9). The eye often is enophthalmic, and there may be associated numbness in the distribution of the infraorbital nerve as it innervates the ipsilateral infraorbital and malar region. Orbital lesions, including those that may have extended from the intracranial cavity, may push the eyeball downward and prevent it from looking upward. Thyroid eye disease also can cause hypotropia due to tightening of the inferior rectus.

Suggested Readings

Cibis GW, Waeltermann JM. Rapid strabismus screening for the pediatrician. *Clin Pediatr* 1986;25:304–307.

Dutton JJ, Mason PN, Iliff N, et al. Management of blow-out fractures of the orbital floor. *Surv Ophthalmol* 1991;35:279–298.

Ticho BH. Strabismus. *Pediatr Clin North Am* 2003;50:173–188.

CHAPTER 25 ■ EYE—UNEQUAL PUPILS

ALEX V. LEVIN, MD, MHSC, FRCSC

Abnormalities of the pupils can be helpful diagnostically when assessing central nervous system, autonomic nervous system, orbital, and ocular problems. Pupillary disorders can be divided into two categories: disorders in which the size of one or both pupils is abnormal and disorders in which the shape of one or both pupils are abnormal. The pupil can also be malpositioned (*corectopia*). Congenital or acquired (e.g., after trauma) corectopia generally requires ophthalmology consultation. When the pupils are different in size, the term applied is *anisocoria*. An abnormally dilated pupil is called *mydriasis*. *Miosis* refers to an abnormally constricted pupil. Figure 25.1 represents a flowchart for an approach to anisocoria.

PATHOPHYSIOLOGY

The pupillary dilator muscle receives sympathetic innervation. The pupillary sphincter receives parasympathetic innervation that also supplies the ciliary muscle of the eyeball that governs focusing (accommodation) of the lens.

The first-order sympathetic neurons extend from the hypothalamus through the midbrain, pons, and medulla into the spinal cord, where they synapse with the second-order neurons at the ciliospinal center of Budge-Waller, just before exiting the cord at roots C8–T2.

The cervicothoracic sympathetic trunk then travels over the apex of the lungs to the superior cervical ganglion in the neck, where synapses are made with the third-order neurons. Sympathetic innervation to the face departs from the superior cervical ganglion or at the bifurcation of the common carotid artery. Therefore, complete unilateral anhidrosis in association with unilateral miosis suggests damage to the second-order neurons or superior cervical ganglion. The third-order neurons travel with the internal carotid artery into the cranial vault, where the fibers gain access to the orbit via the nasociliary branch of the first division of the trigeminal nerve. They then travel through the ciliary ganglion in the orbit without synapse. Fibers extend to the iris dilator via the ciliary nerves. Disruption of sympathetic innervation anywhere along its course results in ipsilateral miosis (Horner syndrome) and is often accompanied by mild ptosis, enophthalmos, with or without ipsilateral anhidrosis. The lower lid may be higher than the contralateral side ("upside down ptosis").

Parasympathetic neurons originate in the Edinger-Westphal nuclei, located on the dorsal aspect of the third cranial nerve nucleus in the anterior dorsal mesencephalon at the level of the superior colliculus, ventral to the sylvian aqueduct. These neurons travel with the third cranial nerve, exiting the midbrain on its ventral aspect and passing between the posterior cerebral artery and the superior cerebellar arteries as they arise from the posterior communicating artery in the circle of Willis. The nerve then runs anteriorly and enters the cavernous sinus superiorly and laterally. Just before entering the posterior orbit through the superior orbital fissure, the third cranial nerve splits into a superior and an inferior division. The latter contains the parasympathetic fibers that then pass into the ciliary ganglion, where they synapse. Short ciliary nerves then carry the postsynaptic fibers to the pupillary sphincter muscle and the ciliary muscle (behind the iris). Unilateral mydriasis can be caused by damage to the parasympathetic fibers anywhere along their course. With the exceptions noted next, it is distinctly unusual for the parasympathetic fibers to be damaged without other evidence of third cranial nerve palsy (a deficit in the ability of the eye to adduct, look upward, and/or look downward, and/or ptosis; see Chapter 24).

Local factors can also cause physical changes in the iris or in the surrounding structures that may result in miosis or mydriasis.

EVALUATION AND DECISION

When testing pupillary size, it is essential that the patient be instructed to look at a *distant* target that does not involve reading letters or numbers. This prevents the eyes from needing to accommodate. Because the innervation for accommodation is the same as that for the pupillary sphincter, the accommodating patient also has reflex contraction of the pupils, particularly when focusing at near. Focusing on a near object also stimulates convergence of the eyes toward each other. Crying or forced eyelid closure may also induce miosis.

ANISOCORIA

When evaluating the patient with anisocoria, the emergency physician must answer two critical questions: (i) Which pupil is abnormal, the smaller or the larger? and (ii) Is this abnormality acute or chronic?

To establish which pupil is abnormal, the relative difference in pupillary size should be noted under conditions of bright illumination and dim illumination. Using the largest diameter circle of the direct ophthalmoscope or a bright penlight, both pupils should be illuminated simultaneously in a room with the lights on. The room lights should then be turned off and the handheld light source held tangentially from below or from above so the eyes are illuminated only enough that the examiner can note the pupillary size.

Normally, the pupils constrict equally in response to bright illumination and dilate equally in dim illumination. If the relative

253

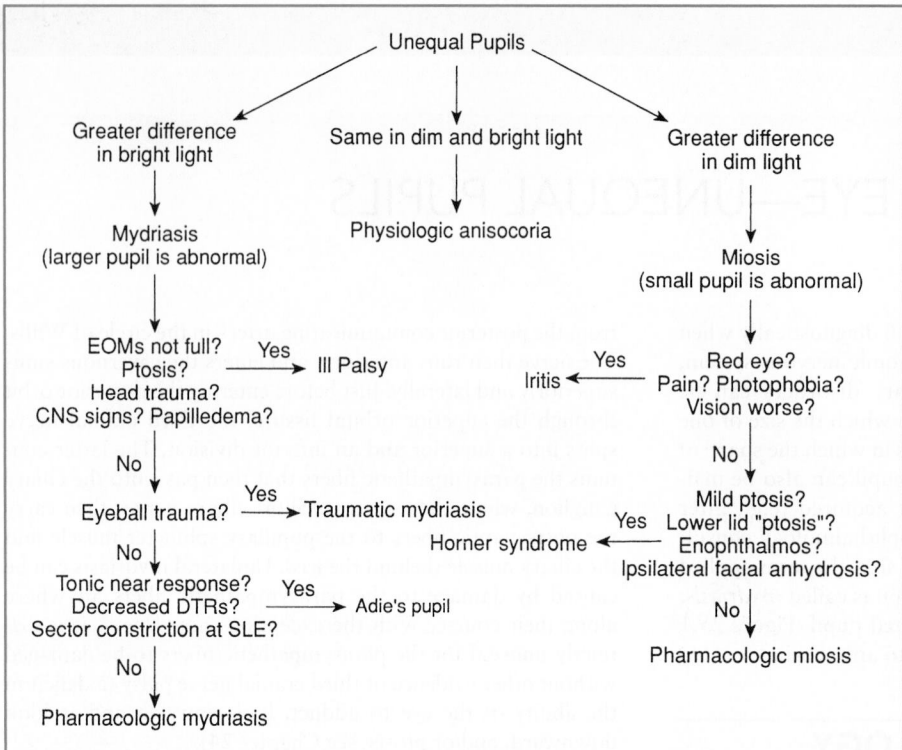

FIGURE 25.1 Unequal pupils. EOM, extraocular muscle movement; CNS, central nervous system; III, third cranial nerve; DTR, deep tendon reflex; SLE, slit lamp examination.

difference in pupillary size increases under bright illumination, the larger pupil is the abnormal pupil: the larger pupil is not constricting normally (Fig. 25.2). If the relative difference in pupillary size increases under dim illumination, the smaller pupil is the abnormal pupil: the smaller pupil is not dilating normally. If the relative difference in pupillary size is the same in both dim and bright illumination, the patient does not have an abnormal pupil (Fig. 25.3). Rather, the patient has physiologic anisocoria. Approximately 20% of people with normal pupils have a difference in the size of their pupils in excess of 0.4 mm.

When trying to establish whether the anisocoria is of relatively recent or acute onset, as opposed to long-standing anisocoria, it is helpful to view old photographs. Sometimes, chronic physiologic anisocoria will not have been noticed previously. The direct ophthalmoscope can be used to provide magnification and illumination of the photograph so the pupils can be viewed. Set the focusing dial on progressively higher black (or green) numbers until adequate magnification has been achieved while viewing through the direct ophthalmoscope. It also is important to note any other symptoms that accompanied the onset of anisocoria (headaches, pain, double vision, or blurred vision). The causes of anisocoria are summarized in Tables 25.1 to 25.3.

MIOSIS

Local Factors

An irritated or inflamed iris sphincter muscle will result in miosis. Iritis, secondary to trauma or other factors, is a common cause (see Chapter 23). The eye is usually injected, and

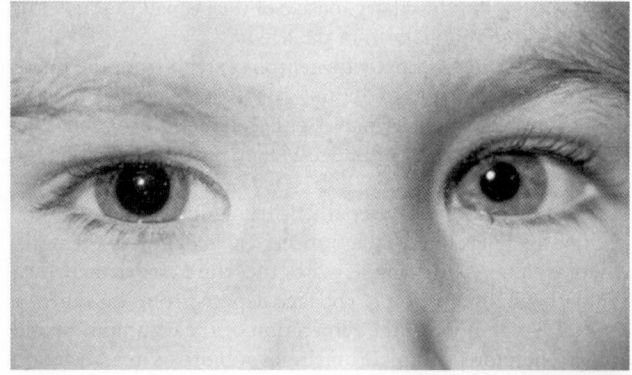

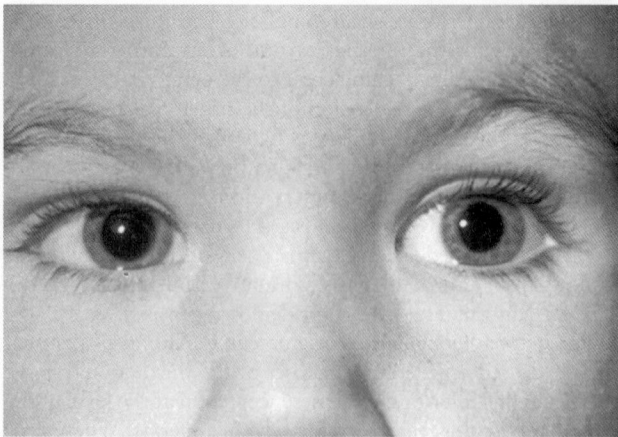

FIGURE 25.2 Patient with right mydriasis. Relative difference between the pupil size is greater in bright illumination (**top**) than in dim illumination (**bottom**).

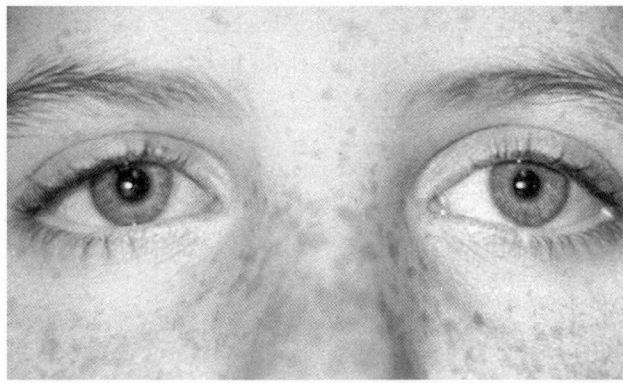

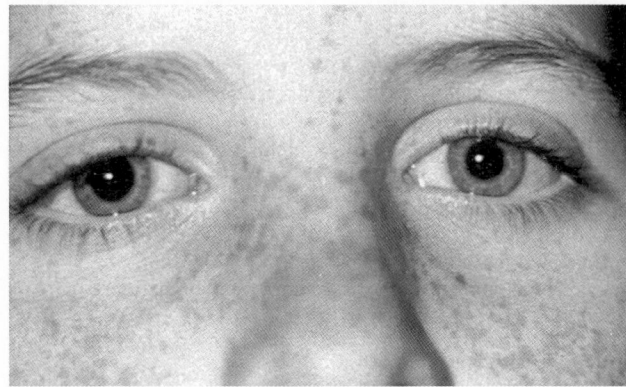

FIGURE 25.3 Physiologic anisocoria. Relative difference in pupil size is the same in bright illumination (**top**) and dim illumination (**bottom**).

there are symptoms of eye pain, photophobia, tearing, with or without decreased vision. Injection may surround the cornea for 360 degrees, creating a ring of erythema ("ciliary blush"). More diffuse injection may also occur. Children with juvenile idiopathic arthritis may not have these classic symptoms associated with their iritis; in fact, they may have no symptoms at all. Traumatic iritis is often not apparent for 12 to 72 hours after eye trauma. Iritis from any cause, especially when long-standing (as is often seen in juvenile idiopathic arthritis with

TABLE 25.1

DIFFERENTIAL DIAGNOSIS OF UNEQUAL PUPILS*a*

Physiologic anisocoria
Pharmacologic (miotics or mydriatics)
Local factors
   Miosis: iritis, surgical trauma
   Mydriasis: trauma
   Abnormal pupil shape from scar formation following prior
     iritis or trauma
Neurologic causes
   Miosis: Horner syndrome
   Mydriasis: third cranial nerve palsy, Adie's pupil
Congenital abnormalities
   Iris coloboma
   Anterior chamber dysgenesis syndromes (e.g., Axenfeld-Rieger)

*a*Not listed in order of frequency.

TABLE 25.2

COMMON CAUSES OF UNEQUAL PUPILS*a*

Physiologic anisocoria
Miosis
   Iritis secondary to trauma, juvenile rheumatoid arthritis,
     or idiopathic
   Abnormal pupil shape from scar formation following prior
     iritis or trauma
   Horner syndrome (Table 25.5)
Mydriasis
   Trauma
   Third cranial nerve palsy
   Adie's pupil
Congenital abnormalities
   Iris coloboma

*a*Not listed in order of frequency.

asymptomatic iritis that escaped recognition), can result in scar tissues between the pupil edge and the lens just behind the pupil (posterior synechia), which prevent pupillary dilation or cause asymmetric irregular dilation of one or both pupils. The diagnosis of iritis is confirmed by slit lamp biomicroscopy. This technique is described in Chapter 117. Ophthalmologic consultation is important for evaluation and treatment.

Other local factors include surgical irritation of the iris and pharmacologically induced unilateral miosis. Mechanical contact with the iris during any intraocular surgical procedure may result in transient postoperative unilateral miosis. Parasympathomimetic or sympatholytic systemic medications and topical drops can also result in transient miosis. A list of commonly used topical miotics is found in Table 25.4. These drops are rarely used in children, with the exception of their occasional bilateral use to treat crossed eyes or unilateral or bilateral use for glaucoma. Systemic drugs from the same categories may result in bilateral miosis. It is helpful to remember that most topical ophthalmic miotics are supplied in bottles that have green caps.

TABLE 25.3

LIFE-THREATENING CAUSES OF UNEQUAL PUPILS*a*

Miosis
Intracranial mass lesion or vascular insult
Spinal cord tumor or compression
Intrathoracic tumor
Aneurysm
Cavernous sinus inflammation, thrombosis, or tumor

Mydriasis
Increased intracranial pressure
Intracranial mass lesion
Aneurysm
Cavernous sinus inflammation, thrombosis, or tumor
Orbital tumor

*a*Not listed in order of frequency.

TABLE 25.4

TOPICAL OPHTHALMIC MIOTICS
(DROPS AND OINTMENTS)

Generic name	Trade names
Cholinergics	
Pilocarpine	Adsorbocarpine, Akarpine, Almocarpine, Isopto Carpine, Miocarpine, Pilagan, Pilocar, Pilocel, Pilogel, Pilomiotin, Piloptic, Ocusert Pilo
Carbachol	Carbacel, Isopto Carbachol
Anticholinesterases	
Physostigmine	Eserine Sulfate, Isopto Eserine
Demecarium	Humorsol
Echothiophate iodide	Echodide, Phospholine Iodide
Isoflurophate (DFP)	Floropyl

Neurologic Factors

Congenital Horner syndrome may result from brachial plexus injury and is often associated with ipsilateral iris hypopigmentation. This sign is not as helpful in the first few months of life when both eyes are normally relatively hypopigmented. More than 50% of children with congenital Horner syndrome have a history of difficult extraction at delivery. Congenital varicella infection may also be a cause.

This testing is best performed by ophthalmologic or neurologic consultants. If the presence of Horner syndrome is questioned, one drop of topical 4% cocaine can be instilled into both eyes. Because cocaine prevents reuptake of norepinephrine at the terminal myoneural junction of the sphincter muscle, pupillary dilation will occur normally. Failure of the miotic pupil to dilate is diagnostic of Horner syndrome. Knowledge of the sympathetic system anatomy can be exploited through the use of other topically applied diagnostic agents to localize the site of the lesion. Table 25.5 summarizes the causes of acquired Horner syndrome in children. All children who have Horner syndrome should receive a complete evaluation unless congenital Horner syndrome is present, based on history, old photographs, and examination.

MYDRIASIS

Local Factors

Both trauma and topical agents can cause unilateral mydriasis. Blunt trauma (and, less commonly, intraocular surgery) can result in a fixed dilated pupil. Traumatic mydriasis usually occurs in a setting in which a clear history of trauma and other intraocular injuries, such as hyphema, are noted. The pupil may be somewhat irregular in shape if the sphincter has irregular tears that appear as V-shaped notches in the pupil margin best seen using the direct ophthalmoscope as a magnifier.

TABLE 25.5

CAUSES OF ACQUIRED HORNER SYNDROME
IN CHILDREN[a]

First-order Neuron
Brainstem glioma or other tumor
Brainstem vascular insult (aneurysm, infarct)
Spinal cord tumor
Syringomyelia
Poliomyelitis
Head or spinal trauma
Postsurgical

Second-order Neuron
Intrathoracic tumor (neuroblastoma, ganglioneuroma, metastatic)
Intrathoracic aneurysm
Cervical tumor or adenitis
Trauma (especially brachial plexus trauma)
Postsurgical

Third-order Neuron
Internal carotid thrombosis or aneurysm
Internal carotid or head trauma
Otitis media
Nasopharyngeal malignancy
Cavernous sinus thrombosis, tumor, or inflammation
Postsurgical

[a]Not listed in order of frequency.

Sometimes, pigment deposition can be seen on the anterior surface of the lens.

Topical parasympatholytics and sympathomimetics can also cause mydriasis. Systemic medications from the same classes can cause bilateral pupillary dilation. A list of topical mydriatics is found in Table 25.6. Most of these drops are supplied in bottles that have red caps. Pharmacologic mydriasis can be diagnosed by the instillation of pilocarpine 1% into both eyes. The pharmacologically dilated pupil will not constrict or will constrict only minimally. Inhaled medications (e.g. ipratropium) can also cause transient mydriasis, often presenting unilaterally.

TABLE 25.6

TOPICAL OPHTHALMIC MYDRIATICS[a]
(DROPS AND OINTMENTS)

Generic name	Trade names
Sympathomimetics	
Phenylephrine	AK-Dilate, Efricel, Mydfrin, Neo-Synephrine, Phenoptic
Cocaine (see text)[b]	
Parasympatholytics	
Atropine	Atropisol, Isopto Atropine, Ocu-Tropine
Cyclopentolate	Ak-Pentolate, Cyclogyl, Pentolair
Homatropine	Homatrocel, Isopto Homatropine
Scopolamine	Isopto Hyoscine, Mydramide
Tropicamide	Mydriacyl, Mydriafair, Tropicacyl

[a]Combination products may also be available.
[b]Diagnostic and anesthetic use only—not prescribed for outpatient use.

Neurologic Factors

When a child with unilateral mydriasis arrives in the emergency department, the initial concern is often cerebral herniation leading to compression and stretching of the third cranial nerve. A rapid neurologic assessment usually is sufficient to diagnose herniation because most patients will have a decreased level of consciousness, focal findings in addition to a dilated pupil, and abnormal vital signs usually with deficiencies of eye movements and/or ptosis (see Chapter 24). Once the physician is certain that increased intracranial pressure (ICP) is not present, a more careful evaluation is appropriate.

Examination by an ophthalmologist is often indicated to help define patterns of extraocular muscle deficit and strabismus, as well as to assess for the possible presence of papilledema. Meningitis and increased ICP have been associated with mydriasis from third cranial nerve involvement without abnormalities of the extraocular muscles. In children, head trauma is the most common cause of acquired third cranial nerve palsy. Other causes are listed in Table 25.7. Neuroradiologic investigation is almost always indicated.

Other problems may mimic the eye muscle imbalance of third nerve palsy. For example, an inferior orbital wall blowout fracture (see Chapter 24) may cause a deficiency in the eye's ability to look up. Trauma may also result in unilateral mydriasis. Together, these findings may mimic a third cranial nerve palsy. This scenario underscores the need for ophthalmologic consultation when pathologic unilateral mydriasis and/or eye muscle deficits are present. Diagnostic clues to the presence of a long-standing third cranial nerve palsy include phenomena associated with aberrant regeneration of the oculomotor nerve. Examples include eyelid elevation when the patient looks down and pupillary constriction when the patient looks upward, downward, or into adduction.

Adie's pupil is most often unilateral. It is caused by parasympathetic denervation at the myoneural junction of the pupillary sphincter muscle. It may be associated with deep tendon hyporeflexia. Also known as tonic pupil, an Adie's pupil constricts slowly to near convergence and then redilates deliberately. Slit lamp examination may reveal serpentine microundulations or asymmetries on constriction to light. Adie's pupil usually has an acute or subacute onset. It has been reported after trauma and

---

TABLE 25.7

CAUSES OF THIRD CRANIAL NERVE PALSY IN CHILDREN[a]

Head trauma
Congenital (isolated or with other cranial nerves involved)
Brain/meningeal tumor
Meningitis/encephalitis
Postviral syndromes
Hydrocephalus
Migraine
Cavernous sinus thrombosis
Aneurysm
Benign idiopathic ("cryptogenic")

[a]Not listed in order of frequency.

---

viral illnesses, including varicella. The denervation is best demonstrated by instillation of weak pilocarpine (0.125% or 0.1%) into both eyes. This concentration is too weak to cause constriction of the normal pupil. The denervated Adie's pupil will become miotic. Acutely, this test may be falsely negative. Perhaps it is best that this test be left to the ophthalmologist so complete ophthalmic examination can be conducted before pharmacologic alterations in pupil size are made.

A common misconception is that poorly seeing eyes have large pupils. Even an eye with very poor vision (light perception) or total blindness may have normal pupil size.

CORECTOPIA AND IRREGULAR PUPILS

Pupils that are located eccentrically rather than centrally are often bilaterally abnormal and represent congenital anomalies. A corectopic pupil can also be due to a progressive change in iris anatomy. Congenital corectopia may be associated with other holes in the iris (polycoria), abnormal iris strands that may be adherent to the cornea, or alterations in iris color. These abnormalities may also be associated with glaucoma and systemic malformations such as dental and umbilical abnormalities (Axenfeld-Rieger spectrum). Progressive changes in pupil location may be because of progressive formation of scar tissue after eye surgery or progressive posterior synechia. After trauma, the presence of corectopia, or a teardrop-shaped pupil, is particularly ominous because this may indicate an underlying associated rupture of the eyeball (see Chapter 117).

The direct ophthalmoscope can be helpful in identifying iris anomalies. The focusing dial should be turned so the iris is in focus (less than 6 in. away from the patient). The dial will be turning in the direction of increasingly higher black (or green) numbers to provide increasing magnification at shorter distances from the eye. The red reflex test (see Chapter 117) can also be helpful when the pupil does not appear as a perfect circle.

Perhaps the most familiar disorder of pupillary shape and/or location is the congenital iris coloboma. This "keyhole" pupil (Fig. 25.4) represents a failure of proper embryologic development of the iris tissue. By itself, iris coloboma is usually asymptomatic and not associated with a functional deficit. Associated colobomatous defects of the retina or optic nerve may exist, and these can result in serious visual compromise. An eye with coloboma may be smaller (microphthalmia).

Occasionally, when dilating drops are instilled initially, the pupil may begin to dilate irregularly and asymmetrically. This is of no concern provided the ultimate shape of the dilated pupil is round. Otherwise, it is wise to seek ophthalmologic consultation in all situations of corectopia or irregular pupillary shape.

UNEQUAL PUPILLARY REACTIVITY

Both pupils should be equally brisk in their constricting reaction to a penlight (or direct ophthalmoscope light). When asymmetry in pupillary reactivity is found, it is always the more sluggish pupil that is abnormal. Often, the more sluggish pupil will be a unilaterally dilated pupil (for which the previous discussion applies). If both pupils are symmetric in their baseline positions, an abnormally sluggish pupil may indicate

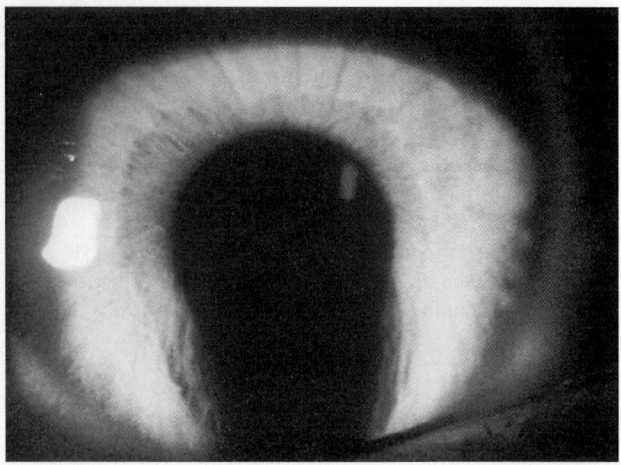

FIGURE 25.4 Iris coloboma creating a "keyhole" pupil. The iris defect is always inferior or inferior-nasal.

the presence of a serious retinal or optic nerve problem that is impairing the ability of the affected eye to perceive the light source equally. Testing visual acuity is essential under these circumstances. A Marcus Gunn pupil [also known as afferent pupillary defect (APD)] occurs when there is unequal perception of light between the two eyes, usually due to a unilateral

or asymmetric optic neuropathy, which could be due to trauma, tumor (e.g., glioma in neurofibromatosis type 1), genetic optic neuropathies (e.g., Leber hereditary optic neuropathy), demyelinating disease, or inflammation of the optic nerve (papillitis). The reader is referred elsewhere (Young and Levin, 1997) for details of the "swinging flashlight test" used to evaluate for a Marcus Gunn pupil.

The pupil should not be pharmacologically manipulated in the ED if there is a concern about a pupil abnormality. Rather, direct referral to an ophthalmologist is appropriate so the pupils may be observed unaltered.

Suggested Readings

Brazis PW. Localization of lesions of the oculomotor nerve: recent concepts. *Mayo Clin Proc* 1991;66:1029–1035.

Brodsky MC, Baker RS, Hamed LM. *Pediatric neuro-ophthalmology.* New York: Springer, 1996.

Hamed LM. Associated neurologic and ophthalmologic findings in congenital oculomotor nerve palsy. *Ophthalmology* 1991;98:708–714.

Jeffery AR, Ellis FJ, Repka MX, et al. Pediatric Horner syndrome. *JAAPOS* 1998;2:159–167.

Miller NR. Solitary oculomotor nerve palsy in childhood. *Am J Ophthalmol* 1977;83:106–111.

Red reflex examination in infants. Section on Ophthalmology. American Academy of Pediatrics. *Pediatrics* 2002;109:980–981.

Thompson HS, Pilley SF. Unequal pupils: a flow chart for sorting out the anisocorias. *Surv Ophthalmol* 1976;21:45–48.

Young TA, Levin AV. The afferent pupillary defect. *Pediatr Emerg Care* 1997;13:61–65.

CHAPTER 26 ■ EYE—VISUAL DISTURBANCES

KAREN DULL, MD

Sudden loss or deterioration of vision (or diplopia) can be caused by numerous diseases and injuries (Tables 26.1 to 26.3). A systematic approach is necessary to reach a correct diagnosis and to minimize the risk of permanent visual impairment. The patient's age, underlying disease conditions, visual history, and history of possible injury must be determined. The extent of the visual impairment, the rapidity of its onset, and the association with other systemic findings are vital pieces of information. It is important to remember that visual acuity improves with age. The normal visual acuity for a toddler is 20/40 and gradually improves to the normal adult acuity of 20/20 by age 5 or 6 years. A careful eye examination, including gross and ophthalmoscopic examination, determination of extraocular movement, and visual acuity, together with the history, leads to correct diagnosis and management of the patient.

Few ocular conditions in the pediatric population are truly emergent (Table 26.4), but many are urgent; most can be treated by the emergency physician or can be referred for appropriate follow-up with an ophthalmologist. Many conditions seen by a pediatric ophthalmologist are not discussed here because they rarely are seen in the emergency department (ED). Such conditions include congenital eye disorders and amblyopia. Likewise, head tilt may represent a visual disturbance and requires a complete ophthalmologic evaluation, although the condition may also be caused by musculoskeletal problems in the neck. Conditions that are more likely to be seen in the ED are emphasized in this chapter.

PATHOPHYSIOLOGY

Vision may be impaired through interference at any point in the visual pathway. Light must reach the eye, pass through the cornea and the anterior chamber, be focused by the lens, pass through the posterior chamber, and reach the retina. The retina must react to the visual stimuli, generate electrical impulses, and transmit these impulses along the optic nerve and eventually to the visual cortex for interpretation. In addition, for binocular vision, the movement of both eyes must be coordinated and smooth. Loss of clarity of the visual media or damage to the conductive tissues anywhere along the visual pathway can lead to decreased vision.

DIFFERENTIAL DIAGNOSIS

Trauma and infections are the two most common causes of acute visual impairment that can interfere with any part of the visual pathway (Tables 26.1 and 26.2). The total spectrum of diseases that cause visual impairment can be understood best if the visual pathway is divided into its parts, and each part is considered sequentially (Table 26.1).

Vision may be limited by periorbital diseases such as periorbital cellulitis, tumor, infection, or allergic swelling of the eyelids. Orbital cellulitis should be considered if decreased vision, proptosis, ophthalmoplegia, or pain with eye movements is present.

Blunt trauma to the eye may cause a blowout fracture of the orbit. The weakest portion of the orbit, the floor, most commonly breaks, and this may entrap the extraocular muscles. Visual impairment may be limited to double vision when looking in a certain direction, particularly upward. Testing the extraocular movements reveals the limitation. Careful inspection of the globe is also necessary.

Diseases of the cornea that cause visual impairment are predominantly infectious or traumatic. Infections of the cornea and conjunctiva can be caused by bacteria, viruses, and fungi (see Chapters 23 and 127). All these diseases may present as a unilateral or bilateral process, usually affecting only the conjunctiva and cornea. Onset is variable but usually occurs over 1 or 2 days, and vision is not greatly impaired. In the newborn period, gonococcal, chlamydial, and herpetic infections must be considered. *Staphylococcus* species are the leading cause of bacterial keratitis. *Pseudomonas* species is the most commonly isolated bacteria in patients who wear contact lenses. In the United States, the most common corneal infection that causes permanent visual impairment is herpes simplex keratoconjunctivitis, whereas trachoma infection is the most common cause worldwide. A careful ophthalmoscopic or slit lamp examination will reveal the characteristic dendritic ulcers of herpes simplex infection after the eye has been stained with fluorescein. Unless this disease is excluded, steroid-containing medications should not be used. Herpes simplex infection may be recurrent, so if a child with a history of previous herpes simplex keratitis complains of a red eye on the previously infected side, recurrent herpes infection must be suspected. With a recent eye injury or foreign-body intrusion, fungal infections are possible.

Traumatic injuries to the cornea include one of the true ophthalmologic emergencies: alkali burns. Alkali burns in general carry a worse prognosis than acid burns. The cause of the chemical injury is usually obvious from the history. Immediate copious irrigation of the eye with normal saline is imperative to prevent permanent visual impairment and to preserve visual acuity. Both ultraviolet and infrared light can cause damage to the cornea, resulting in severe pain and photophobia within 24 hours of exposure. Lacerations with perforation of the cornea usually affect other parts of the eye as well and can lead to significant visual impairment. Careful inspection of the globe with associated lid trauma is mandatory.

TABLE 26.1

CAUSES OF ACUTE VISUAL DISTURBANCES

	Traumatic	Nontraumatic
Periorbital	Eyelid hematoma, edema from trauma	Orbital or periorbital cellulitis, tumor, allergic edema
Cornea and conjunctiva	Chemical burns, thermal burns, ultraviolet or infrared burns, laceration of cornea	Conjunctivitis (bacterial, viral, fungal)
Anterior chamber	Traumatic iritis, hyphema, posttraumatic cataract, dislocation of lens, glaucoma	Acute iritis, glaucoma, uveitis
Posterior chamber	Vitreous hemorrhage	Endophthalmitis
Retina	Severed retinal artery, retinal tears or detachment, commotio retinae	Retinal vein or artery obstruction, spontaneous
Cortex	Head trauma	Optic neuritis, toxins, hysteria, hypoglycemia, leukemia, cerebrovascular accidents, migraine, multiple sclerosis, acute disseminated encephalomyelitis, meningitis, encephalitis, seizure, cerebral venous sinus thrombosis, idiopathic intracranial hypertension
Other	Carotid artery trauma	Poisoning Shunt malfunction Vitamin A deficiencies Measles Neoplasm

The anterior chamber of the eye consists of the aqueous humor, the iris, and the lens. Acute iritis is rare in children, and the cause is often uncertain. There is a sudden onset of pain, redness, and photophobia that usually affects one eye only. The degree of visual impairment varies with the severity of inflammation. Certain diseases, such as juvenile rheumatoid arthritis, have associated iritis. Blunt trauma can also cause iritis, but vision is only slightly impaired unless other structures are involved. Traumatic iritis often presents 24 to 72 hours after the trauma.

Trauma can also cause a hyphema or hemorrhage into the anterior chamber. This can result in little to severe visual impairment in the affected eye, depending on the extent of bleeding and associated trauma. Complications of hyphema include rebleeding, which typically occurs within the first 5 days after injury, and increased intraocular pressure potentially leading to glaucoma. Previously, all patients with hyphema were hospitalized on strict bed rest. However, this was not shown to improve outcome, but close follow up with an opthamologist is recommended. Despite lack of definitive evidence, most ophthalmologists recommend cycloplegic and corticosteroid drops to reduce pain and possibly reduce inflammatory complications. Nonsteriodal antiinflammatory drugs should be avoided. The risk of vision loss is highest in patients with sickle cell disease or trait, greater than 20% of the visual field affected, rebleeding, and residual blood lasting beyond 3 to 4 days duration.

Traumatic injuries can lead to cataract formation, usually within a few days of injury, but onset may be delayed for years. Dislocation of the lens after trauma causes significant visual impairment but can be recognized easily with a careful examination. Glaucoma and a retinal detachment may be late complications of blunt trauma. Pain around the eye, blurred vision, and occasionally, nausea and vomiting in a patient with glaucoma or with a recent eye injury may represent an acute attack of glaucoma. Congenital glaucoma is a major preventable cause of blindness in children; most cases manifest within the first 6 months of life and occasionally present to the ED. Corneal clouding, buphthalmos, or asymmetry in eye size may be the chief complaint. If any one of these is noted as a primary complaint or an incidental finding, immediate referral is required.

TABLE 26.2

COMMON CONDITIONS THAT CAUSE ACUTE VISUAL DISTURBANCES

Trauma
Migraine
Chemical burns
Hyphema
Ruptured globe
Periorbital infection
Conjunctivitis

TABLE 26.3

CAUSES OF ACUTE DIPLOPIA

Blowout fractures
Poisoning
Central nervous system pathology (tumor, bleed, idiopathic intracranial hypertension)
Shunt malfunction
Arnold-Chiari malformation
Myasthenia gravis
Head trauma

TABLE 26.4

EMERGENT CONDITIONS THAT CAUSE VISUAL DISTURBANCES

Alkali or acid burns
Central retinal artery occlusion
Ruptured globe

The uvea consists of the iris, ciliary body, and choroid. One or all portions of the uvea may become inflamed, causing uveitis. Iritis and iridocyclitis may be called anterior uveitis, whereas inflammation of the choroid is often called posterior uveitis. The etiologies may be divided into infectious and noninfectious. Infectious uveitis may be caused by viruses, bacteria, fungi, or helminths. The most common cause of posterior uveitis in children is toxoplasmosis. Noninfectious causes include juvenile rheumatoid arthritis, trauma, ankylosing spondylitis, Behçet's disease, pseudotumor cerebri, peripheral uveitis, sarcoidosis, and sympathetic ophthalmia. Vogt-Koyanagi-Harada syndrome is a panuveitis with meningeal and cutaneous findings. Prompt treatment of this syndrome is necessary for optimal visual outcome.

In addition to blurred vision in one or both eyes, anterior uveitis is also associated with pain in the affected eye, headache, photophobia, and conjunctival injection. On gross examination, the pupil may be constricted and have a ring of redness surrounding the cornea. A slit lamp exam is used to confirm the diagnosis. Anterior uveitis may be confused with conjunctivitis or an acute attack of glaucoma. In posterior uveitis, the pain and photophobia may be less pronounced, but there may be a more pronounced visual impairment.

The posterior chamber is composed of the vitreous humor. The vitreous gel is usually clear, and any diseases that affect the clarity will impair vision. Certain chronic conditions such as uveitis can cause deposits in the vitreous humor, but the visual impairment is very gradual. Infections inside the eye (endophthalmitis) usually result from a penetrating injury, surgery, or an extension of a more superficial infection. Bacterial infections develop more rapidly than do fungal infections. The child will have severe pain in or around the eye and, with bacterial infections especially, may have fever and leukocytosis. The process is usually unilateral, and vision is severely compromised. Purulent exudate is formed in the vitreous humor, and ophthalmoscopic examination may reveal a greenish color with the details of the retina lost. A hypopyon—accumulation of pus in the anterior chamber—is usually present.

Either penetrating or blunt trauma (see Chapter 117) to the eye can lead to vitreous hemorrhage, but this is uncommon in children. Diabetes mellitus, hypertension, sickle cell disease, and leukemia may cause vitreous hemorrhage as well as retinal tears, central retinal vein occlusion, and tumor. There is a sudden loss or deterioration of vision in the affected eye. This may presents as strabismus and nystagmus in younger preverbal patients. Findings on examination depend on the degree of hemorrhage. Blood clots may be visible with the ophthalmoscope, or the fundus reflex may be black, obscuring the retina in more severe cases.

Retinal vein and artery obstruction are also uncommon in pediatric patients. With central retinal artery occlusion, there is a sudden, painless, total loss of vision in one eye. If only a branch is occluded, a field loss will result. Ophthalmoscopic examination reveals the cherry-red spot of the fovea, the optic nerve appears pale white, and the arteries are narrowed significantly. A Marcus Gunn pupil (relative afferent defect) may be present and may be diagnosed by shining a light in one eye, then in the other. When the light is shone in the normal eye, both pupils will constrict. When light is shone in the damaged eye, the pupil will dilate. The retinal artery may be severed by trauma or obstructed by emboli, as in a patient with endocardial thrombi or arterial obstructions in systemic lupus erythematosus (SLE) and in diseases with hypercoagulability, such as sickle cell disease. The arterial spasm associated with migraine may lead to retinal artery obstruction.

As with retinal artery occlusion, retinal vein occlusion causes a painless loss of vision. Visual loss may be severe, with total occlusion of the central retinal vein, or less pronounced, with branch obstruction. Examination of the retina reveals multiple hemorrhages with a blurred, reddened optic disc. The arteries are narrowed, the veins engorged, and patchy white exudates may be evident. These findings will be limited to one area in branch occlusion. Retinal vein obstruction, although rare, may occur with trauma or diseases such as leukemia, cystic fibrosis, or retinal phlebitis.

As mentioned, a tear in the retina may lead to vitreous hemorrhage, causing decreased vision in the affected eye. If the tear is in the macula, the visual loss will be severe. A tear in the retina may not cause immediate visual impairment. Retinal detachment from a retinal tear may be delayed for years. The visual impairment may go unnoticed if the detachment is peripheral. As the detachment progresses or when it involves more central areas, the patient will complain of cloudy vision with lightning flashes (photopsia). This may be followed by a shadow or curtain in the visual field. Visual acuity may remain normal if the macula is not involved. Examination of the eye will reveal a lighter-appearing retina in the area of detachment, and it may have folds. Flashing lights or visual field defects, after trauma, should raise the suspicion of retinal detachment. Retinoschisis, splitting of the layers of the retina, may be seen in shaken baby syndrome.

Commotio retinae, or Berlin's edema, is edema of the retina that may follow blunt ocular trauma by 24 hours. The visual loss is variable, and the retina will appear pale gray because of the edema, but the macula is usually spared.

The optic nerve transmits visual signals to the cortex. Optic neuritis is involvement of the optic nerve by inflammation or demyelination. The process is usually acute and may be unilateral or bilateral. Loss of vision may take from hours to days, and visual impairment ranges from mild loss to complete blindness. Patients often complain of disturbance of color vision. Pain may be absent or present on movement of the eye or palpation of the globe. It is rarely an isolated event in children. Causes include meningitis, viral infections, immunizations, encephalomyelitis, Lyme disease, and demyelinating diseases. Multiple sclerosis uncommonly occurs in childhood, but may present with sudden onset of intermittent episodes of optic neuritis associated with gait disturbances, paresthesisas, and dysesthesias. Pediatric neuromyelitis optica is a demyelinating disease of the central nervous system that is difficult to distinguish from multiple sclerosis. Typically it presents with optic neuritis and transverse myelitis. Visual loss ranges from mild to severe. Similarly, acute disseminated encephalomyelitis may present acutely with hemiplegia, ataxia, cranial nerve palsies, and optic neuritis. It may follow a recent viral infection, and, unlike multiple sclerosis, does not generally reoccur. Exogenous toxins and drugs (e.g., lead poisoning, long-term chloramphenicol treatment) may also cause optic neuritis.

Idiopathic intracranial hypertension (IIH), or pseudotumor cerebri, which is characterized by increased intracranial pressure with normal cerebrospinal fluid content, normal neuroimaging, absence of neurologic signs except cranial nerve VI palsy, and often without discernable cause, can also present with visual loss. Transient visual obscurations due to optic disc edema occur in about three-fourths of IIH patients. The attacks are monocular or binocular. Visual acuity loss and/or visual field defects can be reversed with appropriate therapy.

Pressure on the optic nerve from a neoplastic lesion, such as an optic glioma or craniopharyngioma, may cause visual field loss as an early finding. Optic nerve gliomas can occur anywhere along the optic nerves, chiasm, and optic tract. Optic nerve gliomas are slow growing, and patients present with proptosis, unilateral or bilateral visual loss, strabismus, optic atrophy, or nystagmus. Children with craniopharyngiomas often present with nonspecific complaints of headaches or progressive visual loss of unknown cause. They may also present with endocrine abnormalities related to pituitary dysfunction.

Children with shunts for hydrocephalus may suffer acute visual disturbances—ranging from diplopia to complete blindness during acute shunt failure. Thus, the child with an acute visual disturbance and a shunt must be evaluated for shunt patency, function, and infection. Various toxins are capable of causing impaired vision. The loss may be gradual or sudden, depending on the particular toxin. Toxins usually act on ganglion cells of the retina or on optic nerve fibers, causing contraction of the peripheral field, central visual defect, or a combination. Methyl alcohol, when ingested, may cause bilateral sudden blindness, which may be complete and permanent or may have a more gradual onset. With methyl alcohol ingestion, associated symptoms include nausea, vomiting, abdominal pain, headache, dizziness, delirium, and convulsions. Other toxins include halogenated hydrocarbons, sulfanilamide, quinine, mercury, and quinidine. Large doses of salicylates may cause amblyopia. Digitalis may cause transient amblyopia, visual blurring, or the perception of yellow halos around light (xanthopsia).

Visual impairment may also result from interference with the visual cortex of the brain. Cortical blindness has many causes (Table 26.5). Head trauma (see Chapters 37 and 116) may cause total loss of vision soon after the event. This has been called "footballer's migraine" because of its association with head trauma in soccer. Even trivial head trauma has been known to cause blindness. The apparent hysterical reaction that follows head trauma, especially in young children, may represent complete blindness in a child who is unable to express the problem or is too frightened by the experience. The physical examination may be completely normal. There may be a delay of onset, but the entire course is usually brief, lasting minutes to hours. This form of blindness is often confused with hysterical blindness, the latter being a diagnosis of exclusion. Monocular blindness may be caused by trauma to the carotid artery on the affected side.

Cerebral venous sinus thrombosis may present with headache, diplopia, nausea, vomiting, blurred vision, and

TABLE 26.5

CAUSES OF CORTICAL BLINDNESS

Cardiac arrest
Status epilepticus
Hypoxia
Perinatal asphyxia
Cerebral infarction
Meningitis
Encephalitis
Subacute sclerosing leukoencephalitis
Hypoglycemia
Uremia
Hydrocephalus
Shunt malfunction
Head trauma
Cardiac surgery
Cerebral or vertebral angiography
Drugs (steroids)
Carbon monoxide poisoning
Occipital epilepsy
Postictal states
Hypertensive crisis

photophobia. It may be associated with hypercoagulable states secondary to oral contraceptive usage.

Migraine headaches are a common cause of visual loss in children. Opthalmoplegic migraine, which occurs primarily in children, affects the third cranial nerve causing ptosis, pupillary dilation, exotropia and diplopia, and blurred vision as the headache ends and takes days to weeks to resolve. Basilar migraine are typically occipital, associated with visual disturbances and accompanied by blurred or tunnel vision, dizziness, ataxia, diplopia, and vomiting. Retinal migraine is characterized by sudden loss of vision associated with a headache. Headache and nausea after such an episode are the rule but occasionally may be absent.

Seizures may also present with visual changes, which sometimes manifest as a migraine-like episode. Visual disturbances may also be the only clinical manifestation of childhood occipital epilepsy, but are more commonly associated with more typical seizure activity.

EVALUATION AND DECISION

The absolute ophthalmologic emergencies are alkali burns, a ruptured globe, and retinal artery occlusion. The diagnosis of the first is by history, and therapy must be initiated promptly to minimize the damage to the eye. If there is any doubt about the actual substance to which the eyes have been exposed, treatment for an alkali burn is always prudent. A ruptured globe must be suspected with any possible penetrating injury to the eye. The injury may be subtle, and the vision may be normal. If a possibility of a ruptured globe exists, the eye should be protected and the patient should have immediate evaluation by an ophthalmologist. Retinal artery thrombosis is rare in children, but it should be suspected when there is sudden, unilateral painless loss of vision and a predisposing condition. Predisposing conditions include those associated with

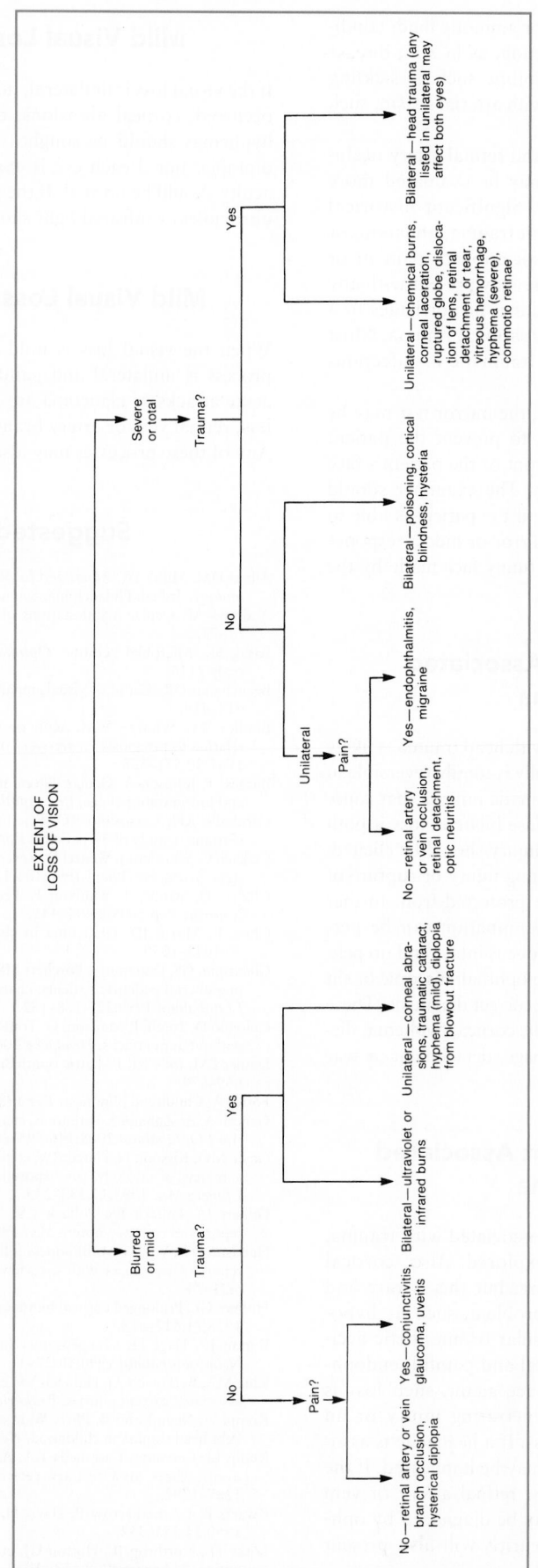

FIGURE 26.1 Diagnostic approach to visual disturbances.

emboli, such as endocardial thrombi or amniotic fluid; conditions with arteritis leading to obstruction, as in SLE; disease states associated with hypercoagulability, such as sickling hemoglobinopathies; and conditions with arterial spasm, such as severe hypertension.

If alkali burns, a ruptured globe, and retinal artery occlusion can be excluded, the patient may be evaluated more carefully before instituting therapy. Significant historical information includes episodes of recent trauma, unilateral or bilateral nature of the loss, and association of pain in or around the eye (Fig. 26.1). Child abuse may present with any of a variety of traumatic injuries. Retinal hemorrhages in a child are almost always caused by intentional trauma. Most children seen in the ED will have a traumatic or infectious process.

If hysterical blindness is suspected, the mirror test may be used. A mirror that is large enough to prevent the patient from looking around it is placed in front of the patient's face and is slowly rocked back and forth. The examiner should observe the patient from above to see if the patient is able to suppress the tendency to follow the mirror or hide a response to another visual stimulus, such as a funny face made by the examiner.

Severe Visual Loss Associated with Trauma

Severe bilateral visual loss associated with head trauma is likely cortical blindness. This condition usually is totally reversible in less than a few hours. Any of the traumatic injuries that cause severe unilateral loss of vision may cause bilateral loss if both eyes are involved. The mechanism of injury should be elicited. If there is any possibility of a penetrating injury or rupture of the globe, the involved eye should be protected from further damage by shielding until careful examination can be performed by a skilled physician. If the globe is intact and no penetration by a foreign body occurred, an ophthalmoscopic or slit lamp examination usually leads to the correct diagnosis. These conditions include chemical burns of the cornea, hyphema, dislocation of the lens, vitreous hemorrhage, detachment or tear of the retina, and commotio retinae.

Severe Visual Loss Not Associated with Trauma

With severe bilateral visual loss not associated with trauma, the possibility of toxins must be explored. Also, cortical blindness may cause a similar picture, but this is rare and generally associated with another problem, such as hypoglycemia, leukemia, and cerebrovascular or anesthetic accidents. If severe visual loss is unilateral and painful, endophthalmitis must be suspected, but once again, such loss is usually the result of a previous penetrating injury or an extension of a local infectious process. If a headache is associated with the visual loss, migraine may be implicated. If the severe loss is unilateral and painless, retinal artery or vein occlusion, or retinal detachment, may be diagnosed by ophthalmoscopic examination. Optic neuritis will also present this way.

Mild Visual Loss with Trauma

If the visual loss is unilateral, not severe, and if trauma recently occurred, corneal abrasions, traumatic cataracts, and small hyphemas should be sought. A blowout fracture may cause diplopia, but if each eye is examined individually, the visual acuity should be normal. If the process is bilateral, exposure to ultraviolet or infrared light should be considered.

Mild Visual Loss without Trauma

When the visual loss is mild and nontraumatic, and if the process is unilateral and painful, conjunctivitis, uveitis, and acute attacks of glaucoma are possible. If the process is painless, retinal vein or artery branch occlusion may be suspected. Any of these processes may also be bilateral.

Suggested Readings

Albert DM, Miller JW. *Albert and Jacobiec's Principles and practice of ophthalmology.* 3rd ed. Philadelphia: Saunders Elsevier, 2008.

Andrews AP. Ocular manifestations of child abuse. *Pa Med* 1996; 99(suppl): 71–75.

Basak SK. Microbial keratitis. *Ophthalmology* 2006;113:2115–2116; author reply 2116.

Beauchamp GR. Cause of visual impairment in children. *Pediatr Ann* 1980;9: 414–418.

Bradley WG, Whitty CWM. Acute optic neuritis: its clinical features and their relation to prognosis for recovery of vision. *J Neurol Neurosurg Psychiatry* 1967;30:531–538.

Burgess P, Johnson A. Ocular defects in infants of extremely low birth weight and low gestational age. *Br J Ophthalmol* 1991;75:84–87.

Caraballo RH, Cersosimo RO, Fejerman N. Childhood occipital epilepsy of Gastaut: a study of 33 patients. *Epilepsia* 2008;49:288–297.

Cedzich C, Schramm J, Wenzel D. Reversible visual loss after shunt malfunction. *Acta Neurochir (Wien)* 1990;105:121–123.

Chabas D, Strober J, Waubant E. Pediatric multiple sclerosis. *Curr Neurol Neurosci Rep* 2008;8:434–441.

Chew E, Morin JD. Glaucoma in children. *Pediatr Clin North Am* 1983; 30:1043–1059.

Cinciripini GS, Donahue S, Borchert MS. Idiopathic intracranial hypertension in prepubertal pediatric patients: characteristics, treatment, and outcome. *Am J Opthalmol* 1999;127:178–182.

Cologno D, Torelli P, Manzoni G. Transient visual disturbances during migraine without aura attacks. *Headache* 2002;42:930–933.

Datner EM, Jolly BT. Pediatric ophthalmology. *Emerg Clin North Am* 1995;13: 669–679.

Foster A. Childhood blindness. *Eye* 1988;2:27–36.

Ganesh A, Al-Zuhaibi S, Pathare A, et al. Orbital infarction in sickle cell disease. *Am J Ophthalmol* 2008;146:595–601.

Gayle MO, Kissoon N, Hered RW, et al. Retinal hemorrhage in the young child: a review of etiology, predisposed conditions, and clinical implications. *J Emerg Med* 1995;13:233–239.

Gilbert JA, Pollack ES, Pollack CV. Vogt-Koyanagi-Harada syndrome: case report and review. *J Emerg Med* 1994;12:615–619.

Harrison DW, Walls RM. Blindness following minor head trauma in children: a report of two cases with a review of the literature. *J Emerg Med* 1990; 6:21–24.

Holmes GL. Prolonged cortical blindness after closed head trauma. *South Med J* 1978;71:612–613.

Kattan JC, Dagi TF. Compensatory head tilt in upbeating nystagmus. *J Clin Neuroophthalmol* 1990;10:27–31.

King MA, Barkovich AJ, Halbach VV, et al. Traumatic monocular blindness and associated carotid injuries. *Pediatrics* 1989;84:128–132.

Kömpf D, Neundorfer B, Ehret W, et al. Transitory impairment of vision after light head trauma in childhood. *Neuropediatrie* 1977;8:354–359.

Kump LI, Cervantes-Castaneda RA, Androudi SN, et al. Analysis of pediatric uveitis cases at a tertiary referral center. *Ophthalmology* 2005;112: 1287–1292.

Kwartz B, Leatherbarrow B, Davis H. Diplopia following head injury. *Injury* 1990;21:351–352.

Lotze TE, Northrop JL, Hutton GJ, et al. Spectrum of pediatric neuromyelitis optica. *Pediatrics* 2008;122:e1039–e147.

Oesterle CS. Exercise induced esotropia. *J Pediatr Ophthalmol Strabismus* 1989;26:150–151.

Recchia FM, Saluja RK, Hammel K, et al. Outpatient management of traumatic microhyphema. *Ophthalmology* 2002;109:1465–1470; discussion 1470–1471.

Salvin JH. Systematic approach to pediatric ocular trauma. *Curr Opin Ophthalmol* 2007;18:366–372.

Spirn MJ, Lynn MJ, Hubbard GB 3rd. Vitreous hemorrhage in children. *Ophthalmology* 2006;113:848–852.

Stretton S, Gopinathan U, Willcox MD. Corneal ulceration in pediatric patients: a brief overview of progress in topical treatment. *Paediatr Drugs* 2002; 4:95–110.

Wagner RS, Aquino M. Pediatric ocular inflammation. *Immunol Allergy Clin North Am* 2008;28:169.

Wall M. Idiopathic intracranial hypertension: mechanisms of visual loss and disease management. *Semin Neurol* 2000:20(1):89–95.

Weaver FA, Wagner WN, Yellin AE, et al. Monocular blindness after penetrating trauma to the carotid artery. *J Vasc Surg* 1989;10:89–92.

Williams JR. Optic neuritis in a child. *Pediatr Emerg Care* 1996;12(3):210–212.

Wong VC. Cortical blindness in children: a study of etiology and prognosis. *Pediatr Neurol* 1990;7:179–185.

Woodward G. Posttraumatic cortical blindness: are we missing the diagnosis in children? *Pediatr Emerg Care* 1990;6:289–292.

Wright KW. *Pediatric opthalmology and strabismus.* St. Louis, MO: Mosby, 1995.

Wright KW. *Pediatric opthalmology for pediatricians.* Baltimore: Williams & Wilkins, 1999.

SIGNS AND SYMPTOMS

CHAPTER 27 ■ FEVER

ELIZABETH R. ALPERN, MD, MSCE, AND FRED M. HENRETIG, MD

Fever, the abnormal elevation of body temperature, has been recognized for centuries by physicians as a sign of disease. Furthermore, the problem of the febrile child is one of the most commonly encountered in clinical pediatrics, accounting for as many as 20% of pediatric emergency department (ED) visits. Despite such considerable clinical experience, only recently has much progress been made in our understanding of the pathogenesis of fever. The problem of appropriate clinical and laboratory evaluation of febrile children, however, remains a major challenge. The approach outlined in this chapter helps the physician treat a febrile child in the ED and proceed systematically with the appropriate diagnostic steps and management. The principal causes of fever in children are listed in Table 27.1.

PATHOPHYSIOLOGY

Fever is a complex process, involving the highly coordinated interplay of autonomic, neuroendocrine, and behavioral responses to a variety of infectious and noninfectious inflammatory challenges. Fever is believed to be an adaptive response that is ubiquitous in animals. Exogenous pyrogens (e.g., toxins, infectious agents, antigen–antibody complexes) from many sources produce fever by inducing the production of proteins, collectively termed endogenous pyrogens, by phagocytic leukocytes. These are now identified as proteins including interleukin-B1, interleukin-6, tumor necrosis factor-α, and several interferons. These proteins enter the circulation after their synthesis and interact with specialized receptor neurons in the organum vasculosum of the preoptic, anterior hypothalamus, one of the "circumventricular organs" of the brain, which is now understood to have no blood–brain barrier and to function as a neurohumoral receptor. Signaling at this site leads to the production of prostaglandins, particularly PGE_2, monoamines, and probably cyclic adenosine monophosphate. PGE_2 is likely the critical mediator of the febrile response and impacts on preoptic neurons to reset the hypothalamic thermostat thereby initiating several responses. The principle effect is on the vasomotor center and results in peripheral vasoconstriction of cutaneous beds with redirection of blood flow to deeper tissues, thus minimizing skin heat loss. In addition, sweating is decreased; vasopressin secretion falls, which results in lowered extracellular fluid volume that requires heating; and behavioral adjustments, such as shivering and seeking a warmer environment, are stimulated. These effects all combine to elevate body temperature. There is some evidence that increased body temperature impairs replication of many microbes and may aid phagocytic bactericidal activity. The febrile response includes further adaptive neuroendocrine effects. Glucose metabolism is curtailed in favor of that based on lipolysis and proteolysis, thus depriving bacteria of their preferred substrate. Fever-induced anorexia further diminishes glucose availability to microbes. Hepatic production of acute-phase reactant proteins may result in binding of divalent cations, which are also growth factors for microorganisms. All these effects combine to further enhance the host's response to microbial invasion. Rarely, fever results from central nervous system (CNS) dysfunction (e.g., hypothalamic tumor, infarction) that alters the thermostatic set point directly, rather than via pyrogen induction. Finally, sometimes hyperpyrexia is not due to altered hypothalmic regulation, but rather to increased heat production (e.g., stimulant drug overdose—see Chapter 102) or exposure to excess environmental heat (heat stroke—see Chapter 87).

It is difficult to pinpoint the lowest temperature elevation considered to be definitely abnormal for all children under all circumstances. Some children normally have rectal temperatures as low as 36.2°C (97°F) or as high as 38°C (100.4°F). Children, like adults, also have diurnal variations in temperature, with the peak usually occurring between 5 p.m. and 7 p.m. This variation is less pronounced in infants. In the 2- to 6-year age range, the temperature may vary by 0.9°C (1.6°F), and in children older than 6 years of age, diurnal variation may span 1.1°C (2°F). Factors such as excessive clothing, physical activity, hot weather, digestion of food, and ovulation can raise temperature in the absence of disease. For the appropriately dressed child who has been at rest 30 minutes, a rectal temperature of 38°C (100.4°F) is defined as fever for this discussion. Using the proper technique to record rectal temperature is important for maximum accuracy. Optimal technique includes appropriate positioning and restraint in infants (prone, supine, or on the side with hips slightly flexed), depth of insertion (about 2 to 3 cm), and time for equilibration (2 to 3 minutes with glass thermometers or several seconds with electronic digital probes). The thermometer should not be placed directly into a fecal mass because the fecal temperature may not have equilibrated with rapid fluctuations in core temperature and thus may be falsely low as temperature rises rapidly. Oral and axillary temperatures are usually about 0.6°C (1°F) and 1.1°C (2°F) lower than rectal temperatures, respectively. More recent attempts to measure temperature with a less invasive technique include temperature-sensitive pacifiers and forehead strips, both of which have been found to be unreliable. However, infrared tympanic membrane thermometry has been more recently adopted in many settings; the tympanic membrane shares vascular supply with the hypothalamus, and it has been shown in adult intensive care settings that there is excellent correlation between core temperature (e.g., pulmonary artery catheter) and tympanic membrane

TABLE 27.1

PRINCIPAL CONDITIONS IN CHILDREN ASSOCIATED WITH FEVER

Infections
  Central nervous system
    Meningitis
    Encephalitis
    Brain abscess
  Ocular
    Periorbital (preseptal) cellulitis
    Orbital cellulitis/abscess
  Airways and upper respiratory tract
    Common cold (upper respiratory infection)
    Pharyngitis/tonsillitis
    Otitis media
    Acute cervical adenitis
    Acute sinusitis
    Peritonsillar, retropharyngeal, lateral pharyngeal wall
      abscess
    Croup
    Epiglottitis
  Oral cavity and salivary glands
    Alveolar abscess
    Viral stomatitis (herpangina, herpetic gingivostomatitis)
    Parotitis (mumps, acute suppurative parotitis)
  Pulmonary
    Bronchiolitis
    Pneumonia
    Bronchitis
    Pulmonary tuberculosis
    Lung abscess
  Cardiac
    Myocarditis
    Endocarditis
    Pericarditis
  Gastrointestinal
    Acute gastroenteritis (viral, salmonella, shigella)
    Appendicitis
    Peritonitis
    Pancreatitis
    Acute mesenteric adenitis
    Hepatitis
    Cholangitis
    Intraabdominal abscesses
  Genitourinary
    Urinary tract infection/pyelonephritis
    Perinephric abscess
    Acute salpingitis, tuboovarian abscess
    Acute prostatitis
    Epididymitis, orchitis
  Musculoskeletal
    Septic arthritis
    Osteomyelitis
    Myositis
  Skin and soft tissue/Lymphoid
    Abscess (methicillin-resistant *Staphylococcus aureus*,
      methicillin-sensitive *S. aureus*, group A *Streptrococcus*)
    Cellulitis
    Necrotizing fasciitis
    Exanthems (systemic infections usually associated with
      prominent rashes)
      Viral: roseola, rubeola, rubella, varicella, hand–foot–
        mouth disease (Coxsackievirus)
      Bacterial toxin: scarlet fever
    Syphilis (secondary)

    Meningococcemia (occasionally other primary septicemia)
    Rocky Mountain spotted fever
    Lymphadenitis
  Systemic infections
    Bacterial sepsis (primary—especially meningococcemia)
    "Occult bacteremia" (especially pneumococcal)
    Viruses (Epstein-Barr, adenovirus)
    Lyme disease
    Rickettsial (Rocky Mountain spotted fever, ehrlichiosis),
      chlamydial, fungal, parasitic, and unusual bacterial
      infections
    Toxic shock syndrome
    Miliary tuberculosis
Vasculitis Syndromes and Hypersensitivity Phenomena
  Acute rheumatic fever
  Juvenile rheumatoid arthritis
  Systemic lupus erythematosus
  Polyarteritis nodosa
  Kawasaki syndrome
  Dermatomyositis/polymyositis
  Mixed connective tissue disease
  Henoch-Schönlein purpura
  Serum sickness
  Stevens-Johnson syndrome
  Drug and immunization reactions
Neoplasms
  Leukemia
  Neuroblastoma
  Lymphoma
  Ewing's sarcoma
Poisonings and Drug Reactions
  Sympathomimetics (e.g., amphetamines, cocaine)
  Anticholinergics (e.g., antihistamines, tricyclic
    antidepressants, atropinic alkaloids)
  Salicylates
  Malignant hyperthermia
  Serotonin syndrome
  Neuroleptic malignant syndrome
  Alcohol/sedative–hypnotic withdrawal
Central Nervous System (CNS) Disorders
  CNS lesions in hypothalamus/brainstem
  Prolonged seizures
  Riley-Day syndrome
Metabolic Diseases
  Thyrotoxic crisis
  Etiocholanolone fever
  Acute intermittent porphyria
Miscellaneous Conditions
  Dehydration
  Intravascular hemolysis
  Hemorrhage into an enclosed space
  Anhydrotic ectodermal dysplasia
  Extreme environmental heat excess
  Hereditary periodic fever syndromes
  PFAPA (periodic fever, aphthous stomatitis, pharyngitis,
    adenitis)
  Cyclic neutropenia
  Sarcoidosis
  Inflammatory bowel disease
  Factitious
  Major trauma (crush injuries)
  Other rare causes

readings. Several studies in children have confirmed the reliability of this technique compared with rectal temperature, although others have questioned the accuracy of tympanic measurements in young infants, especially those younger than 3 months of age. The presence of otitis media (OM) or cerumen does not seem to affect reliability adversely. Temporal artery thermometry has also been recently studied, and though it is more accurate than tympanic thermometry in young children, it has limited sensitivity for detecting temperatures in the fever range. Because even low-grade fever may be clinically significant in young infants and there is at least some doubt about the reliability of axillary, tympanic, or temporal artery measurements in this age group, rectal temperatures should be obtained in this population.

EVALUATION AND DECISION

The importance of fever lies in its role as a sign of disease. The physicians caring for a febrile child should concentrate on discovering the cause of the fever and treating the underlying illness. Any fever may signify serious infection; however, hyperpyrexia, defined as a temperature of 41.1°C (106°F) or higher, is more often associated with diagnoses of pneumonia, bacteremia, or meningitis. As the risk of serious bacterial infection is higher with hyperpyrexia in children, a more thorough assessment for possible bacterial etiology and consideration of empiric antibiotics is indicated. However, the magnitude of reduction of fever in response to antipyretics does not distinguish children with serious bacterial illnesses from those with viral diseases. If no specific treatment for the determined diagnosis is necessary, the physician's goal is then to provide appropriate supportive care and follow-up. Because many parents have "fever phobia," instructions that explain the importance of fever as an indicator of disease, not as an inherently harmful entity, should be given.

A complete *history and physical examination* will provide the most important clues in determining the diagnosis of children with febrile illnesses. The *general impression* obtained in the first few moments of an evaluation is extremely important in the recognition of potentially life-threatening causes of fever (Table 27.2). A great deal of information can be attained by visual assessment of the child while in the arms or lap of the parent. The severity of the illness may become apparent if the child is agitated or uninterested in the surroundings while in this comfortable, safe position. If the child appears nontoxic, observation of the child while the *history* of the present illness and past medical history is being discussed may provide further insight into the diagnosis. Fever has different management implications for distinct subsets of children. Therefore, a clear understanding of the degree, mode of measurement, and duration of fever is especially important in the initial evaluation. The physician should ask questions concerning associated signs and symptoms, medications being given (including antipyretics and antibiotics), presence of ill contacts, travel history, and pet or insect exposures. The medical history should focus on recurrent febrile illnesses and the presence of any diseases or drug regimens that would compromise normal host defenses, such as sickle cell anemia, asplenia (functional, congenital, or surgical), malignancy (noting particularly chemotherapeutic or radiation treatments), human immunodeficiency virus (HIV), renal disease,

TABLE 27.2

LIFE-THREATENING ACUTE FEBRILE ILLNESSES

Infection
  Central nervous system
    Acute bacterial meningitis
    Encephalitis
  Upper Airway
    Acute epiglottitis
    Retropharyngeal abscess
    Laryngeal diphtheria (rare)
    Croup (severe)
  Pulmonary
    Pneumonia (severe)
    Tuberculosis, miliary
  Cardiac
    Myocarditis
    Bacterial endocarditis
    Suppurative pericarditis
  Gastrointestinal
    Acute gastroenteritis (fluid/electrolyte losses)
    Appendicitis
    Peritonitis (other causes)
  Musculoskeletal
    Necrotizing myositis (gas gangrene)/fasciitis
  Systemic
    Meningococcemia
    Other bacterial sepsis
    Rocky Mountain spotted fever
    Toxic shock syndrome

Collagen-vascular
  Acute rheumatic fever
  Kawasaki syndrome
  Stevens-Johnson syndrome

Miscellaneous
  Thyrotoxicosis
  Heat stroke
  Acute poisonings and drug reactions: sympathomimetics, anticholinergics, salicylate, serotonin syndrome, neuroleptic malignant syndrome, malignant hyperthermia, alcohol/sedative-hypnotic withdrawal
  Malignancy

prolonged steroid use, or indwelling catheters or ventriculoperitoneal shunts. Immunization status should also be determined. An understanding of prior evaluation and treatments during this illness may be helpful.

As stated previously, the *physical examination* of the young febrile patient begins during the interview with the caregiver. The physician should note the child's alertness, responsiveness to persons and objects, work of breathing, color, feeding activity, and age-related appropriateness of social interaction and gross motor functions. The *febrile infant who appears irritable and/or lethargic* while being held by a parent before the examination has a high probability of having a serious infection such as meningitis or sepsis. The complaint or observation that a child's crying increases with parental attempts to comfort is critical because "paradoxical irritability" is an important sign of meningitis in infancy.

Other signs of severe or life-threatening infections heralded by fever should be sought early in the examination. CNS infections may be marked by fever with altered sensorium, convulsion, meningismus, or focal neurologic deficits. However, infants younger than 2 years of age with meningitis may not have meningismus, but they may instead have irritability, somnolence, a bulging fontanel, or nonspecific symptoms such as anorexia, lethargy, or vomiting. Severe upper airway infections may present with stridor, excessive drooling, and tripod positioning. A child with pneumonia, pericarditis, endocarditis, or sepsis syndrome may display tachycardia, dyspnea or tachypnea, cyanosis or pallor, poor perfusion or hypotension, as well as altered mental status. Hemorrhagic rashes may signal bacterial or rickettsial infections such as meningococcemia or Rocky Mountain spotted fever.

Although the index of suspicion for serious febrile illness must be high throughout the evaluation of each child, most childhood illnesses with fever are minor and self-limiting. Once the physician has ascertained that the child is not in immediate danger, the examination should focus on sites of common pediatric infections, including the ears, nose, and throat; cervical lymph nodes; respiratory, gastrointestinal, and genitourinary tracts; and skin, joints, and skeletal system (Table 27.3). Evaluation of each child is developed with an understanding of the common infectious entities that affect that child's age group and the presenting signs and symptoms or lack thereof in each infectious entity (see Chapter 92 for a full discussion of infectious diseases).

Many febrile exanthems are characteristic enough to be diagnostic (see Chapters 62–67 and 92). Varicella, rubeola, scarlet fever, and coxsackievirus can all be identified by their pathognomonic rashes. However, if a child with chickenpox presents several days into the illness with a new fever, the possibility of group A β-hemolytic streptococcal or *Staphylococcus aureus* superinfection should be considered. Children with *fever and petechiae* may have invasive meningococcal disease, disseminated streptococcal infection, or Rocky Mountain spotted fever; however, they may simply have a less serious viral infection or streptococcal pharyngitis. Differentiation of these entities is crucial and is based on clinical appearance of the patient and laboratory evaluation. A child with only a few petechiae (especially if only above the nipple line), normal white blood cell (WBC) count, normal platelet count, and well appearance is less likely to have invasive disease. However, any child who appears ill, has distinctly abnormal laboratory results, or has a rapidly progressive petechial rash needs a more complete evaluation for sepsis or meningitis and should receive antibiotics. A patient with fever and diffuse erythroderma should be evaluated carefully for hemodynamic instability or other signs and symptoms of toxic shock syndrome.

On physical examination, acute otitis media is identified by the acute onset of otalgia or fever with changes in the tympanic membranes, such as redness, bulging, decreased mobility, loss of landmarks and light reflex, air–fluid level behind the tympanic membrane, or purulent drainage from a perforation. Careful examination of the head and neck may reveal rhinorrhea and signs of inflammation, suggesting a viral upper respiratory infection (URI). The oropharynx may reveal pharyngitis or stomatitis (see Chapters 48 and 71). Children with a history of a recent respiratory infection may have reactive, tender, swollen cervical lymph nodes; asymmetric enlargement of nodes especially with tenderness and overlying erythema might indicate bacterial adenitis. Croup is readily identified by a barky cough

TABLE 27.3

COMMON CAUSES OF FEVER

Infections
  Central nervous system
    Acute bacterial meningitis
    Viral meningoencephalitis
  Ocular
    Periorbital cellulitis
    Orbital cellulitis
  Upper respiratory tract
    Common cold
    Pharyngitis/tonsillitis
    Cervical adenitis
    Croup
    Acute sinusitis
    Otitis media
  Oral cavity and salivary glands
    Alveolar abscess
    Herpangina
    Herpetic gingivostomatitis
    Mumps (unimmunized child)
  Pulmonary
    Acute tracheobronchitis
    Bronchiolitis
    Pneumonia
  Gastrointestinal
    Acute gastroenteritis
    Appendicitis
  Genitourinary
    Urinary tract infection
    Acute salpingitis
    Tuboovarian abcess
  Musculoskeletal
    Septic arthritis
    Osteomyelitis
  Skin and soft tissue/Lymphoid
    Abscess
    Cellulitis
    Lymphadenitis
    Miscellaneous systemic infections associated with prominent rash (e.g., meningococcemia and Rocky Mountain spotted fever)
    Scarlet fever
    Viral exanthems (especially varicella, measles if unimmunized)
  Systemic
    Primary septicemia—especially meningococcemia
    "Occult" bacteremia
    Viral syndromes
    Vector-borne disease—especially Lyme disease
    Toxic shock syndrome

Miscellaneous
  Drug and vaccine reactions, including serum sickness
  Kawasaki syndrome
  Amphetamine, cocaine, salicylate poisoning

with or without stridor in young children, whereas a distinctive "hot potato voice" with unilateral tonsillar swelling in adolescents indicates a peritonsillar abscess. Wheezing, tachypnea, and fever in infants usually mark bronchiolitis. Pneumonia often presents with cough, fever, tachypnea, auscultatory findings, and hypoxemia. Mild abdominal pain or tenderness, vomiting, and/or diarrhea may suggest viral gastroenteritis or early hepatitis or pancreatitis. More severe findings, particularly the occurrence of peritoneal signs, may indicate appendicitis, intraabdominal abscess, or peritonitis from other causes (see Chapters 49 and 121). However, in children, fever with abdominal pain may also represent lower lobe pneumonia, streptococcal pharyngitis, urinary tract infection (UTI), gastroenteritis, or mesenteric adenitis. Additional findings in UTI may include suprapubic or costovertebral angle tenderness (see discussion below and in Chapter 92). Adolescent girls with pelvic or abdominal pain and fever should be evaluated for pyelonephritis and pelvic inflammatory disease (see Chapter 90). Differentiation of these diverse diagnoses depends on a thorough history, physical examination, and at times, well-directed laboratory evaluation (see Chapter 92).

Continued advancements in *immunizations* have changed the frequency and risk of certain febrile illness in children. The Centers for Disease Control and Prevention report that the *Haemophilus influenzae* type B (Hib) vaccine has drastically changed the risk and causative agents for meningitis in children. There has been a 94% reduction in the incidence of *H. influenzae* meningitis and a shift in the median age of those affected from 15 months to 25 years of age. The current rarity of epiglottitis in children is also due to this decline in *H. influenzae* infections. In addition, a heptavalent pneumococcal conjugate vaccine (PCV) was licensed in 2000. Prior to the availability of this vaccine, 70% of invasive *Streptococcus pneumoniae* infections in children younger than 5 years of age presented as bacteremia without a focus of infection. This vaccine has significantly decreased the risk of invasive pneumococcal diseases in children. However, there has been an overall small, but not inconsequential, increase in invasive bacterial infections in children due to pneumococcal serotypes not contained within the heptavalent vaccine. Recognition of these epidemiologic changes is crucial in evaluating and treating the febrile child. Children between 2 and 18 years of age who have bacterial meningitis will now most likely be infected with *Neisseria meningitides* or nonvaccine serotype *S. pneumoniae*. These findings obviously influence the evaluation and treatment of febrile children with signs of meningitis, as well as those young children without an identified source of infection after thorough historical and physical examination.

Occult bacteremia is the presence of pathogenic bacteria in the blood of a well-appearing febrile child in the absence of an identifiable focus of infection (see Chapter 92). Children with occult bacteremia may develop serious bacterial infections such as septic arthritis, osteomyelitis, meningitis, or sepsis. Children most commonly suspected to be at risk for occult bacteremia are those between the ages of 2 and 36 months with a fever of 39°C (102°F) or higher. Infants younger than 2 months of age are at increased risk for invasive disease and therefore necessitate different evaluation and treatment. The reported incidence of occult bacteremia among highly febrile young children before the initiation of the Hib vaccine program was between 3% and 10%. However, studies in the post-Hib, pre-PCV era showed that the prevalence of occult bacteremia in this group decreased to 1.6%–1.8% and was predominately due to *S. pneumoniae*. As mentioned previously, with the licensure of the PCV, rates of invasive pneumococcal infections including occult bacteremia have decreased. Studies from the post-PCV era indicate the risk of occult bacteremia in immunized children to be less than 1%.

Given these general considerations, an algorithmic *approach to the child with an acute* (less than 5 days) *febrile illness* can be formulated, using the following *key features*: overall degree of *toxicity* and presence of signs or symptoms of life-threatening disease, immunocompromised *host status*, patient's *age, degree of fever*, and presence of *localizing features* on history and physical examination (Fig. 27.1). Laboratory studies are indicated only for selected situations as defined by these clinical features. Most older febrile children do not need routine laboratory testing.

Infants younger than 2 months of age are at increased risk of serious bacterial infections and bacteremia and are more difficult to assess clinically than older children. Thus, for children with fevers of 38°C (100.4°F) or higher who are younger than 2 months of age, many authorities recommend a laboratory investigation for serious infection ("sepsis workup"), including complete blood cell count (CBC), blood culture, urine analysis, urine culture, and lumbar puncture with cerebrospinal fluid (CSF) for cell count, glucose, protein, Gram stain, and culture. Some of these authorities support the same evaluation for infants up to 3 months of age; regardless of the exact age parameter, most clinicians base their approach on one of the several published guidelines for managing febrile infants. Herpes simplex virus polymerase chain reaction (PCR) or culture with presumptive antiviral treatment should be considered in neonates with historical concerns or physical findings of skin, eye, or mouth lesions; respiratory distress; seizures; signs of sepsis; or CSF pleocytosis. Stool for leukocytes and culture should be obtained if diarrhea is present. Respiratory findings are good predictors of clinically significant positive chest radiographs in children younger than 3 months; therefore, chest radiographs may be obtained only when there are clinically evident respiratory signs. Clinical examination alone, without further laboratory evaluation, is generally not considered sensitive enough to identify serious illness in these very young infants. In addition, the peripheral blood WBC count has been shown to be inadequate as an indicator of young febrile infants at risk for meningitis. Biomarkers, including procalcitonin and C-reactive protein, have been recently evaluated as predictors of serious bacterial infection in febrile young infants. Further evaluations of these markers alone and in combination with existing algorithms may provide improved prediction of serious bacterial infection in newborns and young infants. Infants younger than 1 month are usually admitted to the hospital for observation with presumptive antibiotic therapy after full evaluation as noted above in the ED. Many studies (Baker et al., Baskin et al., Dagan et al., Jaskiewicz et al., Garra et al.) found that children between 1 and 2 months of age, who are not pretreated with any antibiotics and who have a pristine physical examination and completely benign laboratory evaluation, may be safely discharged home with careful observation and close follow-up. For such a disposition, parents should be able to watch the infant closely for changes in symptoms, should have ready access to health care, and should be willing to return for evaluation. These studies found that either close observation without antibiotics (e.g., Baker et al.) or after empiric intramuscular ceftriaxone (e.g., Baskin et al.) are safe and effective management strategies in this age group.

Recent work has concentrated on the evaluation of the febrile young infant or child with signs and symptoms suggestive of

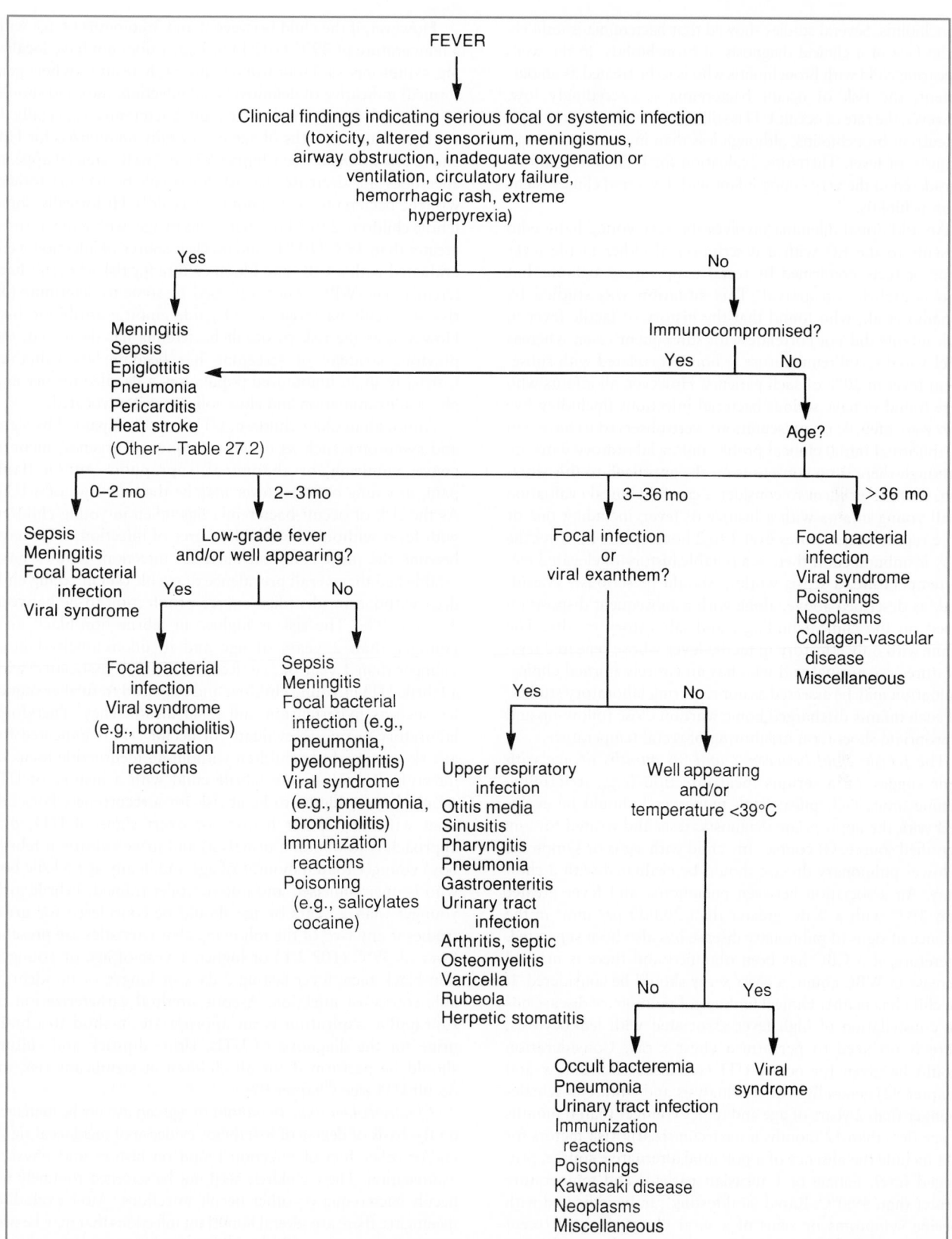

FIGURE 27.1 Approach to the evaluation of the febrile child.

bronchiolitis. Several studies showed that bacteremia is unlikely in the face of a clinical diagnosis of bronchiolitis. In the well-appearing child with bronchiolitis who is to be treated as an outpatient, the risk of occult bacteremia is exceedingly low. However, the rate of occult UTI is still significant in children with concurrent bronchiolitis, although less than in children without a source of fever. Therefore, evaluation for UTI should still be considered in the very young infant with fever and clinical signs of bronchiolitis.

An additional dilemma involves the very young baby who presents to the ED with a description of either tactile fever alone or fever confirmed by rectal temperature at home but who is afebrile on arrival. This situation was studied by Bonadio et al., who found that the history of tactile fever in such infants did not correlate with subsequent fever, whereas an elevated rectal temperature at home correlated with subsequent fever in 20% of such patients. However, all infants who were found to have serious bacterial infections (including five who were afebrile on presentation) were observed to have had an abnormal initial clinical profile and/or laboratory workup. Although there is no consensus on the approach to this situation, it seems prudent to consider a careful clinical evaluation in all young infants with a history of fever, including one or more repeat temperatures over 1 to 2 hours in the ED after the baby is unbundled. If there is a reliable history of elevated rectal temperature, a sepsis workup should be seriously considered, as described above, along with a subsequent disposition based on the clinical findings, and laboratory results. The infant with only a history of tactile fever whose repeated temperatures are normal and who has an entirely normal clinical evaluation may be assessed as not requiring laboratory studies. All such infants discharged home warrant close follow-up and appropriate short-term monitoring of rectal temperature.

The *febrile child between 2 and 36 months of age* with signs suggesting a serious focal infection (e.g., irritability, meningismus, tachypnea, flank tenderness) should be evaluated with the appropriate diagnostic tests and treated for any identified source. Of course, any child with signs or symptoms of lower pulmonary disease should be evaluated with a chest x-ray. An association between pneumonia and fever greater than 39°C with a WBC greater than 20,000 per mm^3 in the absence of signs of pulmonary disease has also been suggested. Therefore, if a CBC has been obtained and there is marked increase in WBC count, a chest x-ray should be considered. If the child has neither clinical findings of pulmonary disease nor the constellation of high fever associated with leukocytosis, there is no need to perform a chest x-ray. Consideration should be given for occult UTI (see discussion below and Chapter 92) generally with a urinalysis and culture in females younger than 2 years of age and males younger than 6 months of age (less than 12 months if uncircumsized). Risk factors for UTI include the absence of a potential alternative source, prolonged fever, female or Caucasian patient, and temperature greater than 39.0°C. Rapid viral testing can be indicated with specific symptoms or signs of a viral illness. Several recent investigations have shown a decreased risk of bacterial infections with positive rapid tests for specific viruses. Despite positive viral tests, children should be evaluated for secondary bacterial infection through careful examination, especially those patients who have an atypical course based on their duration or severity of their symptoms.

However, if the child between 2 and 36 months of age with a temperature of 39°C (102°F) or higher does not have localizing symptoms or laboratory/radiograph results (when performed) indicative of definitive focal infection, the child should be assessed for the risk of occult bacteremia especially if younger than 6 months of age or not fully immunized for Hib and *S. pneumoniae* (see Chapter 92). A "well" clinical appearance does not decrease the risk for occult bacteremia (otherwise the bacteremia would not be "occult"). Historically, some febrile children, 2 to 24 or 36 months of age, with temperatures greater than 39°C (102°F) and no clear source of infection were evaluated with a CBC and blood culture for risk of occult bacteremia. The WBC count was used by some to determine the risk of occult bacteremia and guide empiric antibiotic use. However, as the risk of occult bacteremia has decreased, the previous strategy of screening has become less valuable. Currently, in an immunized population, a detailed history and physical examination and close follow-up is advocated.

Although in older children, UTIs are accompanied by signs and symptoms such as dysuria, frequency, urgency, incontinence, vomiting, or abdominal, suprapubic, and/or flank pain, in young children fever may be the only sign of a UTI. As the risk of occult bacteremia has fallen in young children with fever without identifiable source of infection, UTIs have become the most common bacterial infection. Studies have established the overall prevalence of occult UTI in young children without an identified source of infection to be between 3% and 9%. The risk is highest in febrile non-black girls younger than 2 years of age and in uncircumcised boys younger than 1 year of age. Renal scarring is associated with a febrile UTI in young children and may lead to further sequelae such as hypertension and renal insufficiency. Therefore, laboratory testing to evaluate for occult UTI is indicated for at-risk young febrile children without an identifiable focus of infection. Certainly any febrile child with a history of UTI should be considered to be at risk for a recurrence. For children without a prior history or overt signs of UTI, one approach is to obtain a urinalysis and urine culture in febrile boys younger than 6 months of age and in any age febrile boy who is uncircumcised and not yet toilet trained. Febrile girls younger than 2 years of age should be considered for urine studies if any two of the following characteristics are present: fever of 39°C (102.2°F) or higher, 1 year of age or younger, non-black race, fever lasting 2 days or longer, or no identifiable source of infection. Aseptic urethral catheterization or suprapubic aspiration is an appropriate method to obtain urine for the diagnosis of UTIs. Urine dipstick and culture should be performed for all children at significant risk for occult UTI (see Chapter 92).

Children older than 36 months of age can usually be managed on the basis of degree of irritability, evidence of meningeal signs, and/or other foci of infection found on history and physical examination. These children need not be screened routinely for occult bacteremia or other occult infections. After excluding meningitis, there are several important infections that may be present in ill-appearing, febrile children in this age group, without obvious initial focus. These include meningococcemia, Rocky Mountain spotted fever, and pyelonephritis (see Chapter 92). Early institution of presumptive therapy may be lifesaving in some of these situations, so their possibility must be borne in mind with toxic, febrile children at any age.

Simple febrile seizures occur in 3% to 5% of all children (see Chapter 69). They are defined as generalized tonic-clonic seizures without focal neurologic findings, occurring only once per febrile illness (usually in the first 12 hours of onset of fever) in children 6 months to 5 years of age and lasting less than 15 to 20 minutes in duration. By definition, they are seizures accompanied by fever that occur in children without CNS infection or other underlying cause. The dilemma that faces the emergency physician is to decide whether a febrile seizure is truly such, or if a child presenting with a fever and seizure requires a lumbar puncture to rule out meningitis. Green et al. reviewed 503 cases of meningitis in children 2 to 15 years of age and noted that no cases of bacterial meningitis presented solely as a seizure without any other neurologic signs or symptoms (nuchal rigidity, irritability, prolonged seizure activity, or multiple seizures). Kimia reviewed more than 700 patients with first simple febrile seizure and identified no cases of bacterial meningitis. The decision to perform a lumbar puncture should be determined by the presence of signs or symptoms of meningitis or other CNS infection. As such, any child with irritability, lethargy, abnormal mental status findings after a usual postictal period, or signs of meningitis such as bulging fontanel, should have a lumbar puncture performed. Particular care should be taken in the assessment of children younger than 12 months of age (because of the difficulty in recognizing signs and symptoms of meningitis in very young infants) and in children pretreated with antibiotics (because symptoms of partially treated meningitis may be minimal or absent). Children with atypical or complex febrile seizures should be closely evaluated for CNS infection.

Other causes of acute febrile episodes should be kept in mind, including intoxications, environmental exposure, and immunization reactions. *Toxic exposures*, particularly aspirin, anticholinergics, and sympathomimetics (e.g., amphetamines, cocaine, and methylenedi-oxymethamphetamine or "ecstasy"), may present with severe hyperpyrexia (see Chapter 102). Additional uncommon febrile drug reactions include the *serotonin syndrome* occurring with the combined use of monoamine oxidase inhibitors and analgesic, antitussive, or psychotropic serotonergic medications (e.g., meperidine, dextromethorphan, fluoxetine), and the *neuroleptic malignant syndrome* (see Chapter 102). History of environmental heat exposure preceding severe hyperpyrexia may represent *heat stroke* rather than an infectious cause for the increased temperature (see Chapter 87). Therapeutic exposure to the antiepileptic drug zonisamide can result in oligohydrosis and severe resultant heat stroke. The diphtheria–pertussis–tetanus *immunization* is associated with fever that occurs within 48 hours (occurring less often with diphtheria, tetanus, acellular pertussis vaccine administration), as is the conjugate pneumococcal vaccine administration. Fever, at times accompanied by a faint rash, may occur 7 to 10 days after immunization with the live-attenuated measles vaccine or the measles–mumps–rubella vaccine.

Fevers of unknown origin (FUOs) are defined as daily temperatures of 38.5°C (101.3°F) or higher for at least 2 weeks without discernible cause. Many children evaluated for FUOs actually have consecutive unrelated viral illnesses. Infections commonly causing prolonged fever in children include Epstein-Barr virus infections, osteomyelitis, *Bartonella henselae* infections (cat-scratch disease), UTIs, Lyme disease, and HIV. Although consecutive viral illnesses are the most common etiology for recurrent fevers in a child, occasional cases are due to *periodic fever syndromes* that are marked by recurrence of fever at regular intervals, affecting the child over a period of years. PFAPA (periodic fever, aphthous stomatitis, pharyngitis, and cervical adenitis), familial Mediterranean fever, or cyclic neutropenia are in the differential for the diagnosis of the child with recurrent, intermittent fevers.

Additional noninfectious causes of prolonged fever include neoplasms, collagen vascular diseases, and inflammatory disorders (ulcerative colitis or Crohn's disease).

Symptomatic Treatment

In general, antipyretic therapy should parallel the pathophysiologic basis of the fever. When the fever is caused by altered hypothalamic set point, as in infection, antigen–antibody reactions, and malignancy, attempts to reset the "thermostat" with antipyretic medications are most likely to enhance patient comfort. Antipyretics work via the inhibition of hypothalamic prostaglandin synthesis. If fever is caused by imbalance of heat production and heat loss mechanisms, such as in heat stroke, urgent cooling by physical removal of heat is necessary, such as with ice-water baths, and antipyretics will not help (see Chapter 87). Rarely, a patient with infection will have extreme hyperpyrexia [temperature of 41.1°C (106°F) or higher] and will require urgent temperature reduction with both antipyretics and external cooling. Patients with ongoing febrile seizures also warrant rapid treatment with antipyretics and external cooling, although tepid to cool water sponging is usually sufficient. However, children at risk for recurrent febrile seizures do not, unfortunately, tend to be protected by rapid use of "prophylactic" antipyresis at first sign of fever.

Acetaminophen and ibuprofen are currently the most commonly used pediatric antipyretic medications in the United States (aspirin is no longer recommended for routine antipyretic use in children because of its potential to cause severe gastrointestinal bleeding and its implication as an etiologic risk factor for Reye's syndrome). The current dosage recommendation for acetaminophen is 10 to 15 mg per kg given every 4 to 6 hours, with a maximum of four doses per day, resulting in 40 to 60 mg per kg per day. Several reports and reviews have stressed that, although very rare, repetitive dosing of acetaminophen at the upper limit of, or just slightly above, recommended dosages may result in severe or fatal fulminant hepatic failure. This is particularly the case for children who were fasting (e.g., because of vomiting or diarrhea with febrile illness), younger than age 2 years, treated for several days, or treated with adult-intended preparations.

Ibuprofen is typically dosed at 5 to 10 mg per kg per dose, given every 6 to 8 hours, with a maximum of four doses per day (e.g., 30 to 40 mg per kg per day). Several studies have found that ibuprofen is more effective in reducing fever, especially in single-dose comparisons at 4 and 6 hours after administration, than acetaminophen at commonly used doses of each agent. However, the difference narrows and is, in our view, of little clinical significance for most patients when antipyretic therapy is used repetitively over 12 to 24 hours or more, as typically prescribed for most childhood febrile illnesses (e.g., Hay et al, 2008). Theoretical concern that widespread use of ibuprofen in children might manifest a significantly increased incidence of serious gastrointestinal bleeding, renal failure, or allergic reactions relative to acetaminophen has not been borne out in large, prospective studies (Lesko and Mitchell, 1995). Nevertheless, ibuprofen has been rarely associated with acute renal dysfunction when it was used in children with dehydration. An additional concern with ibuprofen is that its antiinflammatory activity in the treatment of routine febrile illnesses, particularly varicella, might predispose to invasive bacterial, particularly streptococcal, disease. Although not proven to be causally related, it might still be prudent to avoid ibuprofen in such cases of suspected or at-risk streptococcal disease, as well as for children at risk of dehydration. Several studies in the past decade have evaluated the practice of combining or alternating ibuprofen and acetaminophen (Hay et al., Kramer et al, Sarrell et al.). In general, these have found modest increments in antipyretic effect without an increase in observed short-term drug toxicity. However, many commentators (Schmitt, Serwint) have noted that "real-world" safeguards are not equivalent to those enforced in prospective studies, that such complicated regimens pose considerable potential for parental confusion and overdosing, and that they may well add to unreasonable "fever phobia." Thus, our practice is to avoid prescribing such regimens for routine antipyresis, but rather to consider dual therapy in exceptional cases. If instituted, it is prudent to use sub-maximal doses of each agent (acetaminophen 12.5 mg per kg per dose alternating with ibuprofen 5 mg per kg per dose every 4 hours, with a 3 dose per day limit of each) and only with the provision of very detailed instructions and precautions. It is important to remember that many parents greatly fear even moderately high fever in their children and require reassurance that the fever itself, in its usual range of severity, does not cause damage. They need education about appropriate indications for antipyretic treatment, particularly seeking to reduce fever-associated discomfort, rather than a modestly elevated temperature itself. They need further education about appropriate, safe antipyretic dosing regimens, the lack of urgency in treating fever (unless temperature goes above 41.1°C (106°F) or there are prolonged febrile seizures), and most important, the concept that the overall well-being of the child, in context with age, is usually far more important than the temperature per se.

Suggested Readings

Alpern ER, Alessandrini EA, Bell LM, et al. Occult bacteremia from a pediatric emergency department: current prevalence, time to detection, and outcome. *Pediatrics* 2000;106(3):505–511.

Alpern ER, Alessandrini EA, McGowan KL, et al. Serotype prevalence of occult pneumococcal bacteremia. *Pediatrics* 2001;108(2):E23. Available at: http://www.pediatrics.or/cgi/content/full/108/2/e23.

American Academy of Pediatrics, Committee on Drugs. Acetaminophen toxicity in children. *Pediatrics* 2001;108:1020–1024.

American College of Emergency Physicians Clinical Policies Committee, American College of Emergency Physicians Clinical Policies Subcommittee on Pediatric Fever. Clinical policy for children younger than three years presenting to the emergency department with fever. *Ann Emerg Med* 2003; 42(4):530–545.

Bachur R, Harper MB. Reliability of the urinalysis for predicting urinary tract infections in young febrile children. *Arch Pediatr Adolesc Med* 2001; 155(1):60–65.

Bachur RG, Harper MB. Predictive model for serious bacterial infections among infants younger than 3 months of age. *Pediatrics* 2001;108(2):311–316.

Bachur R, Perry H, Harper MB. Occult pneumonias: empiric chest radiographs in febrile children with leukocytosis. *Ann Emerg Med* 1999;33(2):166–173.

Baker MD, Avner JR, Bell LM. Failure of infant observation scales in detecting serious illness in febrile 4- to 8-week-old infants. *Pediatrics* 1990;85(6): 1040–1043.

Baker MD, Bell LM, Avner JR. Outpatient management without antibiotics of fever in selected infants. *N Engl J Med* 1993;329(20):1437–1441.

Baker MD, Fosarelli PD, Carpenter RO. Childhood fever: correlation of diagnosis with temperature response to acetaminophen. *Pediatrics* 1987;80(3): 315–318.

Baskin M, O'Rourke EJ, Fleisher GR. Outpatient treatment of febrile infants 28 to 89 days of age with intramuscular administration of ceftriaxone. *J Pediatr* 1992;120(1):22–27.

Bass JW, Steele RW, Wittler RR, et al. Antimicrobial treatment of occult bacteremia: a multicenter cooperative study. *Pediatr Infect Dis J* 1993;12(6): 466–473.

Benito-Fernandez J, Vazquez-Ronco M, Morteruel-Aizkuren E, et al. Impact of rapid viral testing for influenza A and B viruses on management of febrile infants without signs of focal infection. *Pediatr Infect Dis J* 2006;25: 1153–1157.

Bernard GR, Wheeler AP, Russell JA, et al. The effects of ibuprofen on the physiology and survival of patients with sepsis. The Ibuprofen in Sepsis Study Group. *N Engl J Med* 1997;336:912–918.

Black S, France EK, Isaacman D, et al. Surveillance for invasive pneumococcal disease during 2000–2005 in a population of children who received 7-valent pneumococcal conjugate vaccine. *Pediatr Infect Dis J* 2007;26(9):771–777.

Black S, Shinefield H, Baxter R, et al. Postlicensure surveillance for pneumococcal invasive disease after use of heptavalent pneumococcal conjugate vaccine in Northern California Kaiser Permanente. *Pediatr Infect Dis J* 2004;23:485–489.

Bonadio WA, Hegenbarth M, Zachariason M. Correlating reported fever in young infants with subsequent temperature patterns and rate of serious bacterial infections. *Pediatr Infect Dis J* 1990;9:158–160.

Bonadio WA, Smith DS, Sabnis S. The clinical characteristics and infectious outcomes of febrile infants aged 8 to 12 weeks. *Clin Pediatr* 1994;33(2):95–99.

Bonsu BK, Harper MB. Utility of the peripheral blood white blood cell count for identifying sick young infants who need lumbar puncture. *Ann Emerg Med* 2003;41(2):206–214.

Bramson RT, Meyer TL, Silbiger ML, et al. The futility of the chest radiograph in the febrile infant without respiratory symptoms. *Pediatrics* 1993;92(4):524–526.

Bulloch B, Craig WR, Klassen TP. The use of antibiotics to prevent serious sequelae in children at risk for occult bacteremia: a meta-analysis. *Acad Emerg Med* 1997;4:679–683.

Byer RL, Bachur RG. Clinical deterioration among patients with fever and erythroderma. *Pediatrics* 2006;118(6):2450–2460.

Byington CL, Enriquez FR, Hoff C, et al. Serious bacterial infections in febrile infants 1 to 90 days old with and without viral infections. *Pediatrics* 2004;113(6):1662–1666.

Carstairs K, Tasnen D, Johnson AS, et al. Pneumococcal bacteremia in febrile infants presenting to the emergency department before and after the introduction of the heptavalent pneumococcal vaccine. *Ann Emerg Med* 2007;49:772–777.

Curtis N. Non-steroidal anti-inflammatory drugs may predispose to invasive group A streptococcal infections. *Arch Dis Child* 1996;75:547.

Dagan R, Powell KR, Hall CB, et al. Identification of infants unlikely to have serious bacterial infection although hospitalized for suspected sepsis. *J Pediatr* 1985;107(6):855–860.

Dubos F, Hue, V, Grandbastien B, et al. Bacterial skin infections in children hospitalized with varicella: a possible negative impact of non-steroidal anti-inflammatory drugs? *Acta Derm Venereol* 2008;88:26–30.

Evered LM. Does acetaminophen treat fever in children? *Ann Emerg Med* 2003;41:741–743.

Ferrera PC, Bartfield JM, Snyder HS. Neonatal fever: utility of the Rochester Criteria in determining low risk for serious bacterial infections. *Am J Emerg Med* 1997;15(3):299–302.

Fleisher GR, Rosenberg N, Vinci R, et al. Intramuscular versus oral antibiotic therapy for the prevention of meningitis and other bacterial sequelae in young, febrile children at risk for occult bacteremia. *J Pediatr* 1994;124(4): 504–512.

Garra G, Cunningham SJ, Crain EF. Reappraisal of criteria used to predict serious bacterial illness in febrile infants less than 8 weeks of age. *Acad Emerg Med* 2005;12(10):921–925.

Gorelick MH, Shaw KN. Clinical decision rule to identify febrile young girls at risk for urinary tract infection. *Arch Pediatr Adolesc Med* 2000;154:386–390.

Green SM, Rothrock SG, Clem KJ, et al. Can seizures be the sole manifestation of meningitis in febrile children? *Pediatrics* 1993;92(4):527–534.

Greenes DS, Fleisher GR. Accuracy of a noninvasive temporal artery thermometer for use in infants. *Arch Pediatr Adolesc Med* 2001;155:376–381.

Hasday JD, Fairchild KD, Shanholtz C. The role of fever in the infected host. *Microbes Infect* 2000;15:1891–1904.

Hay AD, Costelloe C, Redmond NM, et al. Paracetamol plus ibuprofen for the treatment of fever in children (PITCH): randomised controlled trial. *BMJ* 2008;337:a1302.

Herz AM, Greenhow TL, Alcantara J, et al. Changing epidemiology of outpatient bacteremia in 3- to 36-month-old children after the introduction of the

CHAPTER 29 ■ GASTROINTESTINAL BLEEDING

STEPHEN J. TEACH, MD, MPH

Gastrointestinal (GI) bleeding is a relatively common problem in pediatrics. Over one 12-month study period at a large urban pediatric emergency department, complaints of rectal bleeding accounted for 0.3% of all visits. Most infants and children who arrive in the ED with what appears to be GI bleeding have an acute, self-limited GI hemorrhage and are hemodynamically stable. In such patients, three important questions must be asked: (i) Is the patient really bleeding? (ii) Is the blood coming from the GI tract? and (iii) Is there more than a trivial amount of blood? Children with only a few drops or flecks of blood in the vomit or stool should not be considered "GI bleeders" if their history and physical examinations are otherwise unremarkable. Caution must be taken, however, as small amounts of blood (whether in emesis or passed per rectum) may be the harbinger of more extensive enteral bleeding.

Likewise, caution must be taken to ensure the passed "blood" actually contains hemoglobin. Many substances ingested by children may simulate fresh or chemically altered blood. Red food coloring (as in some cereals, antibiotic and cough syrups, Jell-O®, and Kool-Aid®), as well as fruit juices and beets, may resemble blood if vomited or passed in the stool. Melena may be confused with dark or black stools due to iron supplementation, dark chocolate, bismuth, spinach, cranberries, blueberries, grapes, or licorice. In these cases, confirmation of the absence of blood with Gastroccult® (vomitus) or Hemoccult® (stool) tests will allay parental anxiety, as well as prevent unnecessary concern and testing. Gastroccult® is a specific and sensitive assay, stable in an acid environment and can detect as little as 300 mcg per dL of hemoglobin.

A careful search for other causes of presumed GI bleeding (recent epistaxis, dental work, menses, hematuria, buttock lesions, and pharyngitis) should be sought. In most cases of upper and lower GI bleeding, the source of the bleeding is inflamed mucosa (infection, allergy, drug induced, stress related, or idiopathic). The emergency physician must be vigilant in differentiating inflammatory conditions that are often self-limited from causes that may require emergent surgical or endoscopic intervention, such as ischemic bowel (intussusception, volvulus), structural abnormalities (Meckel's diverticulum, angiodysplasia), and portal hypertension (esophageal varices). Acute GI bleeding rarely represents a surgical emergency. In the previously noted study, only 4.2% of 95 patients required a blood transfusion or an operative intervention.

INITIAL ASSESSMENT

Because the presentation and differential diagnosis of GI bleeding are broad, a systematic approach to all patients is crucial and includes the following sequential steps:

1. Assessment of the severity of the bleeding and institution of appropriate resuscitative measures if the patient manifests hemorrhagic shock.
2. Establishment of the level of bleeding within the GI tract.
3. Narrowing of the differential diagnosis based on pertinent history, physical examination, and laboratory tests based on knowledge of age-related causes in upper and lower GI bleeding.
4. Evaluation and decision making.

Severity of Bleeding

Estimation of blood loss (a few drops, a spoonful, a cupful, or more) should be obtained initially. This can be extremely difficult and inaccurate. Hemoglobin and hematocrit are also unreliable estimates of acute blood loss because of the time required for hemodilution to occur after an acute hemorrhage. The estimated volume of blood loss should be correlated with the patient's clinical status. The presence of resting tachycardia, pallor, prolonged capillary refill time, and metabolic acidosis point to significant enteral blood loss. An orthostatic decrease in systolic blood pressure of 10 mm Hg or more, or an increase of 20 beats per minute in pulse, suggests a 10% to 20% loss of intravascular volume. Hypotension is a late finding in young children with hemorrhagic shock and demands immediate resuscitative measures.

Establishment of the Level of Bleeding

There are two general categories of GI bleeding: upper and lower. *Upper GI bleeding* refers to bleeding proximal to the ligament of Treitz. *Lower GI bleeding* is distal to the ligament. In most cases, the clinical findings along with nasogastric lavage will delineate the cause of bleeding within the GI tract. *Hematemesis,* defined as the vomiting of blood, can range from fresh and bright red to old and dark (due to the effect of gastric acidity) with the appearance of "coffee grounds." *Hematochezia,* the passage of bright red blood per rectum, suggests lower GI bleeding or upper GI bleeding with a very rapid enteral transit time. *Melena,* the passage of stool that is shiny, black, and sticky as a result of enzymatic or bacterial action on intraluminal blood, reflects bleeding from either the upper GI tract or the proximal small bowel. In general, the darker the blood in the stool, the higher it originates in the GI tract (or, alternatively, the longer it has resided in the GI tract). "Currant jelly" stools indicate vascular congestion and hyperemia of the colon with passage of abundant mucus from the colonic goblet cells, as seen with intussusception.

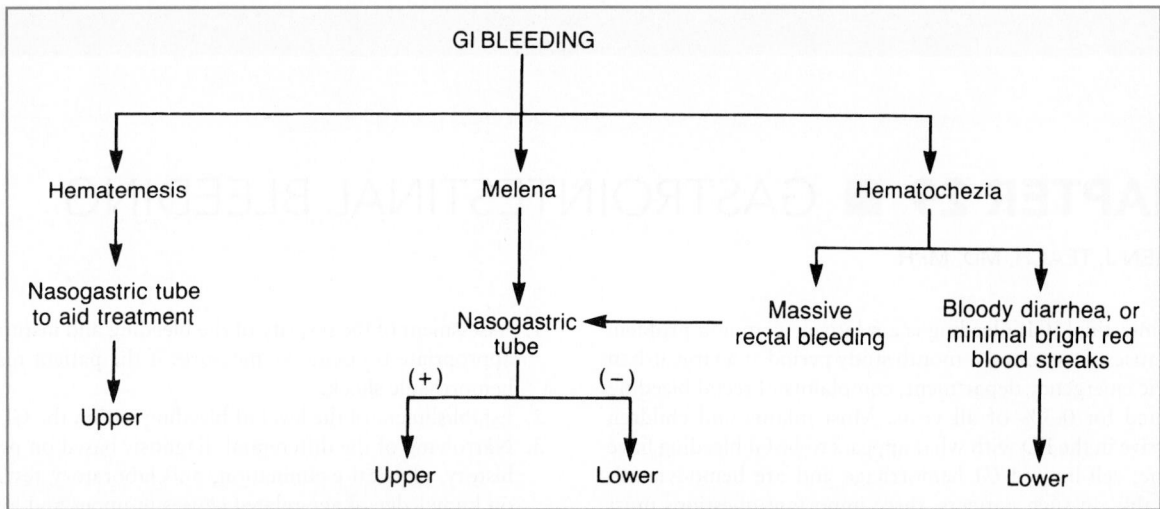

FIGURE 29.1 Establishing level of gastrointestinal (GI) bleeding.

Maroon-colored stools generally occur with a voluminous bleed anywhere proximal to the rectosigmoid area, such as seen with a Meckel's diverticulum.

All patients with a significant bleeding episode should have a nasogastric tube placed for a diagnostic saline lavage (Fig. 29.1). Presence of bilious material indicates an open gastric pylorus. In patients with hematemesis or melena, a positive examination of a nasogastric aspirate confirms an upper source of GI bleeding, whereas a negative result almost always excludes an active upper GI bleed. Occasionally, a postpyloric upper GI lesion, such as a duodenal ulcer, bleeds massively without reflux into the stomach, resulting in a negative aspirate. In such a case, an upper GI endoscopic study may be the best method to detect such a lesion. Patients with significant hematochezia or melena should likewise have a nasogastric tube placed. As noted above, because blood can exert a cathartic action, brisk bleeding from an upper GI lesion may induce rapid transit through the gut, thus preventing blood from becoming melanotic. In patients with hematochezia manifested as bloody diarrhea or minimally blood-streaked stools, a lower GI source should be investigated.

UPPER GASTROINTESTINAL BLEEDING

Differential Diagnosis

As seen in Table 29.1, there is considerable overlap between age groups and causes of upper GI bleeding. Mucosal lesions, including esophagitis, gastritis, peptic ulceration, and Mallory-Weiss tears, are the most common sources of GI bleeding in all age groups (see Table 29.2 and Chapter 89). Of all cases of upper GI bleeding in children, 95% are related to mucosal lesions and esophageal varices. Life-threatening causes of upper GI bleeding are listed in Table 29.3.

Hematemesis in a healthy newborn most likely results from swallowed maternal blood either at delivery or during breast-feeding (i.e., cracked nipples). The Apt test can differentiate neonatal from maternal hemoglobin based on the conversion of oxyhemoglobin to hematin when mixed with alkali. To perform the Apt test, the physician should mix one part bloody stool or vomitus with five parts water, centrifuge at 2,000 rpm

---

TABLE 29.1

ETIOLOGY OF UPPER GASTROINTESTINAL BLEEDING BASED ON AGE[a]

Neonatal period (<4 wk)	Infancy (<2 yr)	Preschool age (2–5 yr)	School age (>5 yr)
Swallowed maternal blood	Gastritis	Epistaxis	Gastritis
Hemorrhagic gastritis	Esophagitis	Gastritis	Mallory-Weiss tear
Peptic ulcer	Mallory-Weiss tear	Esophagitis	Peptic ulcer
Idiopathic	Peptic ulcer	Mallory-Weiss tear	Stress ulcer
Bleeding diathesis	Pyloric stenosis (<2 mo of age)	Toxic ingestion	Toxic ingestion
Esophagitis	Vascular malformation	Peptic ulcer	Esophagitis
Intestinal duplication	Toxic ingestion	Foreign body	Esophageal varices
Vascular malformations	Intestinal duplication	Vascular malformation	Vascular malformation
Pyloric stenosis		Esophageal varices	Hemobilia
		Hemobilia	

[a]In approximate order of frequency of occurrence.

TABLE 29.2

COMMON CAUSES OF UPPER GASTROINTESTINAL BLEEDING BASED ON AGE

Neonatal Period
Swallowed maternal blood

Infancy
Gastritis
Esophagitis
Mallory-Weiss tear

Preschool Age
Epistaxis
Gastritis
Mallory-Weiss tear

School Age
Gastritis
Mallory-Weiss tear
Peptic ulcer

for 2 minutes, and mix the supernatant with 1 mL of 1% sodium hydroxide for every 5 mL of supernatant. Fetal hemoglobin is more resistant to denaturing than adult hemoglobin and remains pink, whereas maternal hemoglobin becomes brown. Obtaining sufficient vomited blood to perform this test may be difficult.

In the breast-fed neonate with new onset of hematemesis and maternal history of cracked nipples, who is well-appearing and with normal examination, another approach is to allow the mother to nurse in the ED. Often, when the infant has been at the breast for a few moments and then is pulled away, an obvious significant degree of bleeding from the mother's nipple is apparent, providing considerable reassurance to both physicians and parents. As an alternative, a breast pump can be used.

Although rare, hemorrhagic disease of the newborn should be considered with prolongation of the prothrombin time. Failure to administer vitamin K in the immediate postpartum period is a critical risk factor for this disorder.

Significant and sometimes massive upper GI hemorrhage in a newborn infant may occur with no demonstrative anatomic lesion or only "hemorrhagic gastritis" at endoscopy. This is usually a single, self-limited event that is benign if treated with appropriate blood replacement and supportive measures. Pyloric stenosis may present with significant hematemesis, often preceded by significant non-bloody emesis.

Critically ill children of any age are at risk for developing stress-related peptic ulcer disease. Such ulcers occur with life-threatening illnesses, including shock, respiratory failure, hypoglycemia, dehydration, burns (Curling's ulcer), intracranial

TABLE 29.3

LIFE-THREATENING CAUSES OF UPPER GASTROINTESTINAL BLEEDING

Ulcer
Esophageal varices
Vascular malformation
Duplication

lesions or trauma (Cushing's ulcer), renal failure, and vasculitis. These ulcers may develop within minutes to hours after the initial insult and primarily result from ischemia. Hematemesis, hematochezia, melena, and/or perforation of a viscus may accompany stress-associated ulcers. Hematemesis secondary to gastroesophageal reflux and esophagitis is uncommon but should be considered in patients who are severely symptomatic with vomiting or aspiration. Hematemesis following the acute onset of vigorous vomiting or retching at any age suggests a Mallory-Weiss tear. These tears occur at the gastroesophageal junction due to a combination of mechanical factors (e.g., retching) and gastric acidity.

Idiopathic peptic ulcer disease is a common cause of GI bleeding in preschool and older children. Most preschool children with idiopathic ulcers develop GI bleeding (hematemesis or melena). Complications, including obstruction and perforation, may occur. Younger children have less characteristic symptoms, often localize abdominal pain poorly, and may have vomiting as a predominant symptom. Older children and adolescents describe epigastric pain in a pattern typical of adults. *Helicobacter pylori* infection has emerged as a leading cause of secondary gastritis, particularly in older children. Similar to adults, pediatric patients with evidence of *H. pylori* infection are treated with triple therapy of amoxicillin, clarithromycin, and a proton pump inhibitor; however, the current recommendations advocate for 10 to 14 days of treatment until the newer short courses (1 to 5 days) being used in adults have been tested in pediatric patients. Preparations of bismuth may be added to the regimen, and metronidazole may be substituted in patients with penicillin allergy. Note that bismuth subsalicylate can turn the stool a darker color, even black.

In older children, the possibility of bleeding esophageal varices must be considered in the differential diagnosis of upper GI bleeding. Although variceal bleeding is rare in infancy, esophageal and gastric varices associated with portal hypertension due to hepatic and vascular disorders are the most common causes of severe upper GI hemorrhage in older children. One-half to two-thirds of these children have an extrahepatic presinusoidal obstruction, often resulting from portal vein thrombosis, as the cause of portal hypertension. Omphalitis with or without a history of umbilical vein cannulation, dehydration, and a number of other factors may contribute. Other children with portal hypertension have hepatic parenchymal disorders such as neonatal hepatitis, congenital hepatic fibrosis, cystic fibrosis, or biliary cirrhosis associated with biliary atresia. Two-thirds of patients with portal hypertension develop bleeding before 5 years of age, and 85% do so by 10 years of age.

Evaluation and Decision: Upper Gastrointestinal Bleeding

History and Physical Examination

Pertinent historical elements to be sought include a history of umbilical catheterization or sepsis in the neonatal period, previous episodes of bleeding from the GI tract or other sites, and past hematologic disorders and liver disease. A family history of peptic ulcer disease can be found in up to 30% of patients with idiopathic ulcers. The presence of prior epigastric pain may suggest more longstanding esophagogastritis or ulcer disease. Ingestions should be sought as a possible cause. These include theophylline, aspirin, iron, nonsteroidal antiinflammatory drugs (NSAIDs), alcohol, and steroids. Massive hemorrhage associated with right upper quadrant pain and jaundice in the post trauma patient indicates bleeding into the biliary tract (hemobilia).

The physical examination should include visualization of the posterior nose and pharynx to eliminate epistaxis as a source of bleeding. Signs of liver disease or portal hypertension may be subtle in children. Icterus, abdominal distension, prominent abdominal venous pattern, hepatosplenomegaly, cutaneous spider nevi, and ascites suggest liver disease and/or portal hypertension with esophageal varices. A rectal examination for the detection of melena, hematochezia, and occult blood is crucial in all cases of GI bleeding.

Laboratory Evaluation

Laboratory tests are not useful for identifying a precise cause of upper GI bleeding. Mucosal lesions are more likely than esophageal varices to be associated with prior occult bleeding. A low mean corpuscular volume and hypochromic, microcytic anemia suggest chronic mucosal bleeding. Initial low white blood cell and platelet counts may be seen in either hypersplenism from portal hypertension or sepsis with associated mucosal ulceration due to stress. Abnormal hepatic studies, including an elevation of serum bilirubin, transaminases, and prothrombin time, and a low serum albumin, are suggestive of esophageal varices. A blood urea nitrogen:creatinine ratio greater than 30 may indicate blood resorption and an upper GI source of bleeding.

Diagnostic Approach

If a significant upper GI bleed has occurred, and once hemodynamic stability is restored, identification of the specific age-related disorder is the next step (Table 29.1 and Fig. 29.2). If the bleeding is mild and self-limited or the gastric aspirate is negative, a minor mucosal lesion is likely. Although mucosal lesions such as esophagitis, gastritis, or peptic ulcer disease can present with severe bleeding, most often bleeding from mucosal lesions is self-limiting and will respond to conservative medical management. In patients with persistent or recurrent hemorrhage, emergent endoscopy may be necessary if the bleeding is considered life threatening (continued transfusion requirement, hemodynamic instability). In a small percentage of patients in whom bleeding is massive, making endoscopic visualization impossible, angiography or radionuclide studies (Technetium-sulfur colloid/Tc-labeled red blood cells) may be indicated. Treatment of specific mucosal conditions and esophageal varices is discussed in Chapter 89.

Eighty percent to 85% of upper GI bleeding stops spontaneously, regardless of the source, before or early in the hospital course. In stable patients who have stopped bleeding, double-contrast barium examination of the upper GI tract and endoscopy provide valuable and often complementary information. In this group of patients, endoscopy need not be performed on an emergent basis and may be done electively in the first 12 to 24 hours after admission. Elective endoscopy should be performed in patients who stop bleeding spontaneously but who have required transfusion and/or have a history of previously unexplained upper GI bleeding episodes.

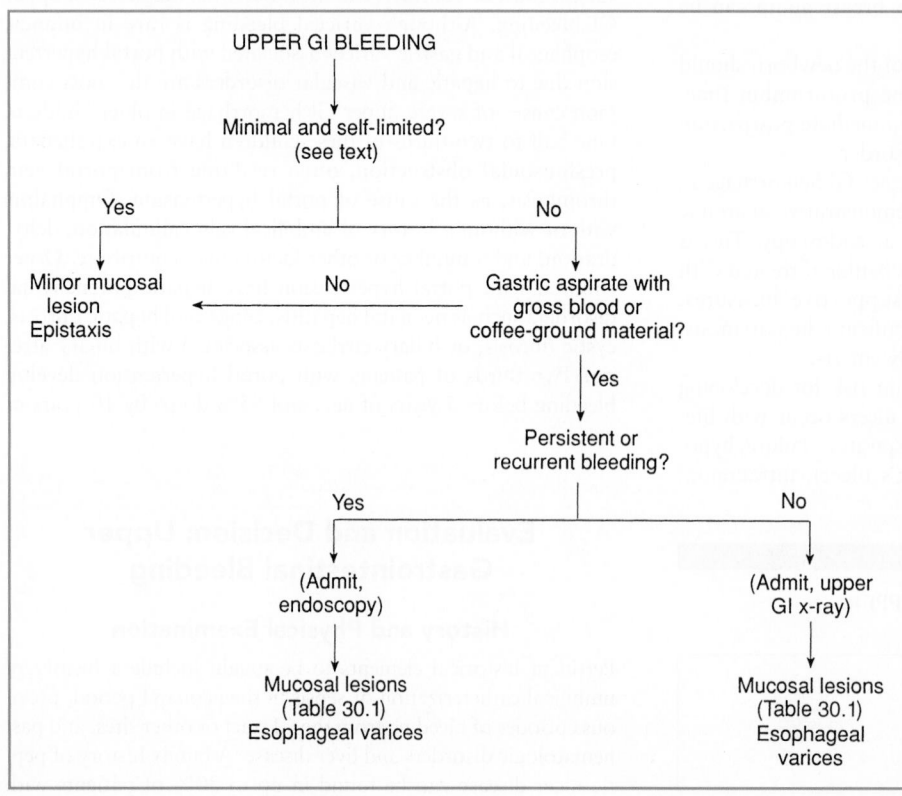

FIGURE 29.2 Diagnostic approach to upper gastrointestinal (GI) bleeding.

TABLE 29.4

ETIOLOGY OF LOWER GASTROINTESTINAL BLEEDING BASED ON AGE[a]

Neonatal period	Infancy (1 mo–2 yr)	Preschool age (2–5 yr)	School age (>5 yr)
Well Infant			
Swallowed maternal blood	Anal fissure	Anal fissure	Infectious colitis
Infectious colitis	Infectious colitis	Infectious colitis	Polyps
Allergic colitis	Allergic colitis	Juvenile polyps	Inflammatory bowel disease
Hemorrhagic disease	Nonspecific colitis	Intussusception	Hemorrhoids
Duplication of bowel	Juvenile polyps	Henoch-Schönlein purpura	Meckel's diverticulum
Meckel's diverticulum	Intussusception	Meckel's diverticulum	Hemolytic uremic syndrome (HUS)
Sick Infant			
Infectious colitis	Meckel's diverticulum	HUS	Pseudomembranous colitis
Midgut volvulus	Duplication	Inflammatory bowel disease	Ischemic colitis
Hirschsprung's disease	HUS	Peptic ulcer	Peptic ulcer
Disseminated coagulopathy	Inflammatory bowel disease	Pseudomembranous enterocolitis	Angiodysplasia
Necrotizing enterocolitis	Pseudomembranous enterocolitis	Ischemic colitis	
Intussusception	Ischemic colitis	Angiodysplasia	
Congestive heart failure	Lymphonodular hyperplasia		

[a]In approximate order of frequency of occurrence.

LOWER GASTROINTESTINAL BLEEDING

Differential Diagnosis

Similar to upper GI bleeding, there is overlap among age groups in the etiology of lower GI bleeding (Table 29.4). The most common disorders by age group are listed in Table 29.5, and the life-threatening causes are listed in Table 29.6. Of note, many cases of lower GI bleeding resolve spontaneously without a specific diagnosis being established.

TABLE 29.5

COMMON CAUSES OF LOWER GASTROINTESTINAL BLEEDING BASED ON AGE

Neonatal Period
Swallowed maternal blood
Infectious colitis
Allergic colitis

Infancy
Anal fissure
Infectious colitis
Allergic colitis

Preschool Age
Anal fissure
Infectious colitis

School Age
Infectious colitis
Intestinal polyp

Neonatal Period (0 to 1 Month)

As is true for upper GI bleeding, a common cause of blood in the stool in well infants is the passage of maternal blood swallowed either at delivery or during breast-feeding from a fissured maternal breast. Although hemorrhagic disease of the newborn is uncommon after prophylactic administration of vitamin K at delivery, maternal drugs that cross the placenta, including aspirin, phenytoin, and phenobarbital, may interfere with clotting factors and cause hemorrhage. Infectious diarrhea can occur in very young infants, and stools may contain blood or mucus. Common bacterial pathogens in this age group include *Campylobacter jejuni* and *Salmonella*.

In ill-appearing neonates with lower GI bleeding, midgut volvulus, necrotizing enterocolitis, and Hirschsprung's disease should be considered (Table 29.4). Malrotation with midgut volvulus is most common during this period. Initially, bilious vomiting, abdominal distension, and pain are present. Melena is seen in 10% to 20% of patients and signifies vascular compromise. Of all cases of necrotizing enterocolitis, 10% occur in term infants. These patients can present with nonspecific signs of sepsis (temperature instability, apnea, and/or bradycardia) and with

TABLE 29.6

LIFE-THREATENING CAUSES OF LOWER GASTROINTESTINAL BLEEDING

Midgut volvulus
Intussusception
Meckel's diverticulum
Hemolytic uremic syndrome
Pseudomembranous colitis
Ischemic colitis
Peptic ulcer

specific GI tract findings, such as abdominal distension, pain, and abdominal wall erythema. GI bleeding can be in the form of occult bleeding or grossly bloody stools. Hirschsprung's disease with enterocolitis may also present with GI bleeding in the neonatal period. Enterocolitis has recently been shown to occur in up to 25% of children with Hirschsprung's disease. The risk of enterocolitis remains high until about 6 months of age. The diagnosis should be considered in any newborn that does not pass meconium in the first 24 to 48 hours of life.

Infancy (1 Month to 2 Years)

In the first 2 years of life, anal fissures are among the most common cause of rectal bleeding and are usually associated with hard stools, constipation, or other trauma. Treatment with stool softeners and sitz baths will often resolve the problem spontaneously in most patients. Milk or soy allergic enterocolitis usually occurs during the first month of life, but it can occur later in infancy and occasionally in older children (depending on when exposure occurs). These infants can present with chronic diarrhea and failure to thrive, with stools containing blood or mucus, or less commonly, with fulminant colitis and shock. Milk-protein allergy responds (often slowly) to a change in formula from cow's milk or soy protein to an elemental formula (Nutramigen®, Alimentum®, Pregestimil®). Breast-fed infants whose mothers drink cow's milk may develop an allergic colitis that responds to removal of cow's milk from the mother's diet. Infectious enterocolitis as a cause of bloody diarrhea is common in all age groups. Bacterial causes (*Salmonella*, *Shigella*, *Campylobacter*, pathogenic *Escherichia coli*, and *Yersinia enterocolitica*) should be identified with stool cultures. In symptomatic infants and children, the presence of leukocytes in a stool smear may aid in preliminary diagnosis. Pseudomembranous colitis should be considered in any infant or child with bloody stools and a history of recent antibiotic therapy. "Nonspecific colitis" has been demonstrated to be a common cause of hematochezia in infants younger than 6 months of age. Although the cause of nonspecific colitis is unknown, it may represent a variation in the colonic response to viral invasion.

Meckel's diverticulum should be suspected in infants or young children who pass bright or dark red blood per rectum. Intermittent painless bleeding or massive GI hemorrhage can occur. Sixty percent of complications from Meckel's diverticulum (hemorrhage and intestinal obstruction) occur in patients younger than 2 years of age.

Idiopathic intussusception may occur in infancy, with 80% occurring before 2 years of age. In children older than 3 years, a lead point (polyp, Meckel's diverticulum, or hypertrophied lymphoid patch) is more often found than in younger children. Paroxysmal pain may be associated with occult blood, hematochezia, or "currant jelly stools" (formed by the combination of fresh blood with mucus elaborated by the colonic wall). Lethargy alone (without pain) has been increasingly recognized as a presenting symptom of intussusception in young children.

Lymphonodular hyperplasia is an uncommon cause of rectal bleeding in this age group and may cause mild, painless hematochezia. The nodular lymphoid response is self-limited and does not require any specific therapy. Intestinal duplications are also an uncommon cause of lower GI bleeding and, when diagnosed, are usually found in children younger than 2 years of age. Duplications can be found anywhere in the GI tract but are most common in the distal ileum. These usually present with obstruction and lower GI bleeding.

Preschool Period (2 to 5 Years)

The two most common conditions to cause bleeding in children 2 to 5 years of age are juvenile polyps and infectious enterocolitis. Most polyps in childhood are inflammatory without significant malignant potential and are often multiple. Between 30% and 40% are palpable on rectal examination. Like a Meckel's diverticulum, polyps may be seen with painless rectal bleeding in this age group. Significant bleeding is unusual. Infectious causes of colitis are similar to those discussed in younger age groups. Hematochezia is often a manifestation of systemic disease in infancy and throughout childhood. Hemolytic uremic syndrome (HUS) is the most prevalent of these conditions reported in infants and children up to 3 years of age. Bloody diarrhea due to *E. coli* O157:H7 may precede the development of renal and hematologic abnormalities in HUS. GI manifestations of Henoch-Schönlein purpura (HSP) occur in 50% of patients and include colicky abdominal pain, melena, and bloody diarrhea. These symptoms precede the characteristic rash in 20% of patients. GI complications among patients with HSP include hemorrhage (5%), intussusception (3%), and rarely, intestinal perforation.

Angiodysplasia is a rare cause of GI bleeding but can be associated with massive hemorrhage. Vascular lesions of the GI tract probably have a congenital basis. Several recognized syndromes, including Rendu-Osler-Weber syndrome and Turner's syndrome, may be associated with intestinal telangiectasia.

School Age through Adolescence Period

For the most part, the diagnostic considerations relevant to the preschool child apply to school-age and adolescent children with the addition of inflammatory bowel disease, which is rare before the age of 10 years. Rectal bleeding is a common presentation of both ulcerative colitis and Crohn's disease. Massive lower GI bleeding occurs in 2% to 5% of children with Crohn's disease. Toxic megacolon is a life-threatening presentation of both ulcerative colitis and Crohn's disease.

Evaluation and Decision: Lower Gastrointestinal Bleeding

History and Physical Examination

Symptoms of an acute abdominal process with bowel obstruction, including abdominal pain, distension, and vomiting, should be elicited. A history of bloody diarrhea may indicate infectious or allergic colitis, intussusception, or HUS. Extraintestinal manifestations of inflammatory bowel disease, including weight loss, anorexia, and arthralgias, may be predominant symptoms in school-age children. The dietary history may suggest features of milk or soy protein intolerance. Firm stool streaked with red blood characterizes anal fissures or lower colonic polyps. A detailed family history (bleeding diathesis, familial polyposis) and drug history (NSAIDs, salicylates, iron) or antibiotics (pseudomembranous colitis) are important in patients with lower GI bleeding. A history of constipation in a young infant with acute onset of bloody diarrhea suggests enterocolitis associated with Hirschsprung's disease.

Physical examination to detect abdominal obstruction (abdominal tenderness, distension, palpable mass, peritoneal signs, hyperactive (early) or hypoactive (late) bowel sounds) is the most urgent task of the evaluating physician. Careful separation of the buttocks with eversion of the anal mucosa may reveal a fissure. Prominent or multiple perianal skin tags may raise suspicion of Crohn's disease. Rectal polyps may be palpable on rectal examination. Cutaneous lesions may provide important diagnostic clues in patients with GI bleeding. Eczema may be associated with milk allergy, whereas erythema nodosum is the most common skin manifestation of inflammatory bowel disease. Mucocutaneous pigmentation (Peutz-Jegher syndrome) and cutaneous or subcutaneous tumors (Gardner's syndrome) indicate intestinal polyposis.

Diagnostic Approach

Rectal bleeding presents in all pediatric age groups (Table 29.4 and Fig. 29.3). The causes of lower GI bleeding vary significantly with age, and are often transient and benign. Occasionally, lower GI bleeding reflects a life-threatening pathologic condition, and establishment of a specific diagnosis becomes urgent.

The priority of the emergency physician in evaluating the patient with lower GI bleeding is to identify lower tract bleeding associated with intestinal obstruction and with other causes of large volume bleeding such as a Meckel's diverticulum. Intussusception and a late presentation of midgut volvulus secondary to malrotation are the major types of intestinal obstruction associated with lower GI hemorrhage. All causes of abdominal obstruction (e.g., adhesions, incarcerated hernia, and appendicitis) eventually result in bleeding if diagnosis is delayed and vascular compromise occurs.

Severe lower GI bleeding leading to hemodynamic instability or requiring transfusion is rare in pediatrics, and gastric lavage is essential in these cases to rule out a possible upper GI tract source. Meckel's diverticulum is the most common cause of severe lower GI bleeding in all age groups. Following Meckel's diverticulum, Crohn's disease and arteriovenous malformation are prominent causes of massive lower GI bleeding in adolescents.

The urgency and extent of evaluation of patients with lower GI bleeding will depend on the amount of bleeding, the patient's age, and associated physical findings. In a healthy infant with a few streaks of blood in the stool and a normal examination, a limited evaluation and observation are reasonable. If more significant hematochezia is found and if a nasogastric aspirate is negative, then significant pathology must be sought. Flat and upright abdominal radiographs should be performed if an obstructive process (e.g., intussusception, volvulus) is suspected by history or physical examination. The absence of radiographic findings should not, however, deter the physician from pursuing further diagnostic evaluation. An upper GI examination can often define the level of small-bowel obstruction. Ultrasound has been increasingly used to identify etiologies of obstruction. An air or barium enema examination may be diagnostic and therapeutic in children with intussusception.

If obstruction is not considered likely, the decision to perform contrast enema examination or colonoscopy will depend on the diagnosis suspected. Air-contrast barium enema can also be extremely valuable in the detection of polyps or inflammatory bowel disease. Indications for colonoscopy include severe bleeding, moderate but persistent bleeding with a negative double-contrast barium enema, or a lesion of unknown nature seen on barium enema. If undefined bleeding persists, radionuclide studies or angiography should be considered. A technetium scan may detect ectopic gastric mucosa as seen in Meckel's diverticulum, whereas angiography will help identify

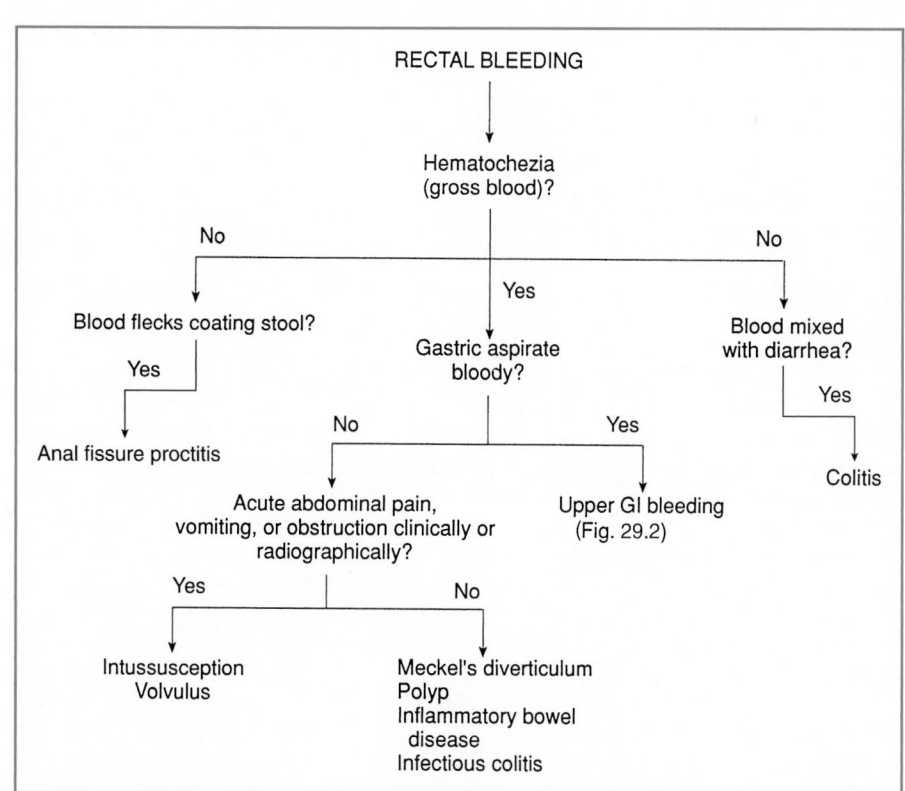

FIGURE 29.3 Diagnostic approach to lower gastrointestinal (GI) bleeding.

bleeding vascular malformations in the GI tract. Ongoing, undiagnosed GI hemorrhage accounts for fewer than 10% of cases in infants and children. Exploratory laparotomy may be necessary and lifesaving in these circumstances.

SUMMARY

Management of acute GI bleeding often requires a team approach, including the emergency physician, surgeon, and gastroenterologist. The foremost goals of ED evaluation of patients with GI bleeding are establishment of hemodynamic stability and determination of level of bleeding. Patients with nontrivial upper GI bleeding should generally be admitted for observation and further evaluation. If an acute abdominal process is suspected, surgical consultation and diagnostic workup should be instituted. If rectal bleeding is mild and self-limited and the history and physical are unremarkable, further investigation with the primary care provider or a gastroenterologist is recommended.

Suggested Readings

Applegate KE. Intussusception in children: imaging choices. *Semin Roentgenol* 2008;43:15–21.

Arvola T, Ruuska T, Keränen J, et al. Rectal bleeding in infancy: clinical, allegological, and microbiological examinations. *Pediatrics* 2006;117:e760–e768.

Boyle JT. Gastrointestinal bleeding in infants and children. *Pediatr Rev* 2008;29:39–52.

Chelimsky G, Czinn S. Peptic ulcer disease in children. *Pediatr Rev* 2001;22:349–355.

Crill CM, Hak EB. Upper gastrointestinal tract bleeding in critically ill pediatric patients. *Pharmacotherapy* 1999;19:162–180.

Czinn SJ. Helicobacter pylori infection: detection, investigation, and management. *J Pediatr* 2005;146:S21–S26.

Fishman SJ, Burrows PE, Leichtner AM, et al. Gastrointestinal manifestations of vascular anomalies in childhood: varied etiologies require multiple therapeutic modalities. *J Pediatr Surg* 1998;33:1163.

Fox VL. Gastrointestinal bleeding in infancy and childhood. *Gastroenterol Clin North Am* 2000;29:37–66.

Leung A, Wong A. Lower gastrointestinal bleeding in children. *Pediatr Emerg Care* 2002;18(4):319–323.

Racadio JM, Agha AK, Johnson ND, et al. Imaging and radiological interventional techniques for gastrointestinal bleeding in children. *Semin Pediatr Surg* 1999;8:181–192.

Teach SJ, Fleisher GR. Rectal bleeding in the pediatric emergency department. *Ann Emerg Med* 1994;23:1252–1258.

CHAPTER 30 ■ GROIN MASSES

DEENA BERKOWITZ, MD, MPH, AND BRUCE L. KLEIN, MD

Children occasionally present to the emergency department (ED) with an inguinal mass. It may be noticed during a diaper change, or the older child may bring it to the parent's attention; sometimes an adolescent arrives alone seeking help. There are many different causes, ranging from inconsequential to serious (Table 30.1). One generally can ascertain the correct diagnosis based on the age and gender of the child, the location of the mass, how painful it is, how rapidly it has evolved, and whether there are any associated symptoms or signs (Fig. 30.1). Lymph node enlargement and retractile, undescended, ectopic, and traumatically dislocated testes are discussed in this section. Hernia and hydrocele (as well as scrotal masses) are addressed in Chapters 57 and 121.

DIFFERENTIAL DIAGNOSIS

Lymphadenopathy and Lymphadenitis

There are two groups of inguinal nodes: superficial and deep. The superficial ones can be subdivided into a horizontal group that runs parallel to the inguinal ligament and a vertical group located lateral to it. The horizontal group drains lymph from (i) the skin of the lower abdominal wall, perineum, and gluteal region; (ii) the skin of the penis and scrotum; (iii) the mucosa of the vagina; and (iv) the lower anal canal. The vertical group drains lymph from (i) the gluteal region, (ii) the penis and deep structures of the scrotum, (iii) the anterior and lateral areas of the thigh and leg, and (iv) the middle and medial portions of the foot. The deep inguinal nodes, which lie beneath the fascia lata medial to the femoral vein, drain (i) all the superficial nodes, (ii) the clitoris or glans of the penis, (iii) the medial areas of the thigh and leg, and (iv) the lateral portion of the foot.

A healthy child can have a few small nodes normally. Normal inguinal nodes are less than 1.5 cm long, and they tend to be oval, firm, slightly moveable, and nontender. If the nodes are enlarged (especially unilaterally) or tender, erythematous, or suppurating, further evaluation is necessary (see Chapter 43).

Inguinal adenopathy—nodes that are enlarged but nontender—is often part of a more generalized lymphadenopathy. The list of causes of generalized lymphadenopathy is extensive and includes collagen vascular diseases (e.g., juvenile rheumatoid arthritis, serum sickness), immunologic disorders (e.g., chronic granulomatous disease), metabolic diseases (e.g., Gaucher's disease, Niemann-Pick disease), and certain hemolytic anemias. Inguinal nodes may be enlarged because of malignancy (e.g., acute lymphocytic leukemia), but this is rarely the sole presentation of a malignant tumor. Of note, some local tumors, such as testicular tumors, metastasize to the inguinal nodes. Although many infections, particularly viral ones (e.g., human immunodeficiency virus, Epstein-Barr virus), produce inguinal adenopathy, these also usually cause generalized lymphadenopathy as well as hepatosplenomegaly and other abnormalities.

Inflammation or infection of the gluteal region, perineum, genitalia, or ipsilateral lower extremity is the most common cause of isolated inguinal adenopathy or adenitis. These areas must be examined carefully. Chronic eczema, tinea cruris, or an innocuous inflammation (e.g., an insect bite, diaper rash) may produce lymphadenopathy. In such cases, treatment of the underlying condition suffices. If lymphadenitis—enlargement with tenderness, erythema, or suppuration—is detected, the node itself is probably infected. Group A β-hemolytic streptococcus, *Staphylococcus aureus*, or an enteric organism is the usual pathogen, depending on the site of the primary infection. A Gram stain and culture from the primary site or node aspirate helps identify the organism. Most children can be treated as outpatients with oral antibiotics (e.g., clindamycin or trimethoprim–sulfamethoxazole where MRSA is prevalent). Children with severe symptoms should be admitted and treated with intravenous antibiotics. Abscesses caused by these pathogens should be aspirated or incised and drained, unless they are already draining spontaneously (see Chapter 92).

Venereal diseases can result in inguinal adenopathy or adenitis in adolescents. Herpes simplex is a common cause of genital ulcerations and bilaterally enlarged, painful lymph nodes. Occasionally, enlarged lymph glands may precede the appearance of vesicles. Oral acyclovir initiated within the first six days of primary disease shortens the duration of symptoms and viral shedding by 3 to 5 days, but is somewhat less effective in recurrences. Topical acyclovir is not recommended. Symptomatic treatment of primary herpetic lesions does not affect the subsequent frequency or severity of recurrence.

The chancre of primary syphilis is painless and has a raised, indurated border and a clean surface. Bilateral (70%) or unilateral, nontender inguinal adenopathy is common. A positive rapid plasma reagin confirms the diagnosis, but this test is nonreactive in up to 30% of patients with primary syphilis. Recommended treatment for primary syphilis in adolescents is benzathine penicillin G, 2.4 million units, intramuscularly.

Chancroid is more common in developing countries than in the United States. It is caused by *Haemophilus ducreyi*, which is hard to isolate and requires selective media. Unlike syphilis, the chancroid ulcer is painful and nonindurated, and has serpiginous borders and a friable base covered with a gray or dirty yellow exudate. About one-half of patients develop painful adenitis, usually unilaterally. The node or nodes often suppurate and drain spontaneously, or require

TABLE 30.1

CAUSES OF INGUINAL MASSES

Painful
Torsion of an undescended testicle[a]
Trauma (e.g., dislocated testicle)[a]
Incarceration or strangulation of an indirect inguinal hernia[a]
Lymphadenitis

Usually or Comparatively Painless
Hernia
Hydrocele
Lymphadenopathy
Retractile or undescended testicle

[a]Urgent or emergent condition.

needle aspiration or surgical incision. Recommended treatments for adolescents include azithromycin, 1 g, orally or ceftriaxone, 250 mg, intramuscularly.

Lymphogranuloma venereum, which occurs mostly in tropical and subtropical countries, is caused by *Chlamydia trachomatis*. The genital papule, vesicle, or ulcer is often missed because it is painless, inconspicuous, and transitory. One or more unilaterally enlarged, moderately tender, fluctuant nodes are characteristic. If left untreated, these nodes can drain and form fistulae. Three weeks of treatment with doxycycline or erythromycin is necessary, or longer until lesions have resolved.

Granuloma inguinale is caused by the gram-negative bacillus *Calymmatobacterium granulomatis*. Granuloma inguinale is rare in the United States but if untreated results in extensive subcutaneous granulomas (pseudobuboes), which mimic inguinal adenopathy. The initial, small red nodule or vesicle progresses to a painless red mass of granulomatous tissue, which ulcerates and coalesces. Both tetracycline and trimethoprim–sulfamethoxazole are reported to be effective.

An enlarged, tender inguinal node can be caused by plague, brucellosis, tularemia, or cat-scratch disease if the portal of entry for the infective organism is the lower extremity. *Yersinia pestis*, which causes plague, is typically transmitted by flea bites and is (extremely) rare in the United States; however, pneumonic plague has become of heightened concern in more recent years as a potential agent of bioterrorism (see Chapter 7). The buboes are firm and extremely tender. The overlying skin is often warm and edematous. Mortality can be as high as 80%. Streptomycin or gentamicin is the drug of choice for children in most cases.

Inguinal lymphadenopathy can be seen in ulcero-glandular tularemia when it is caused by an infected tick bite on the lower extremity. Like plague, pneumonic tularemia is considered a possible bioterrorism threat (see Chapter 7). Enlarged, tender, regional lymph nodes precede the appearance of a small papule (at the portal of entry) that later ulcerates. Streptomycin, gentamicin, or amikacin is recommended for children.

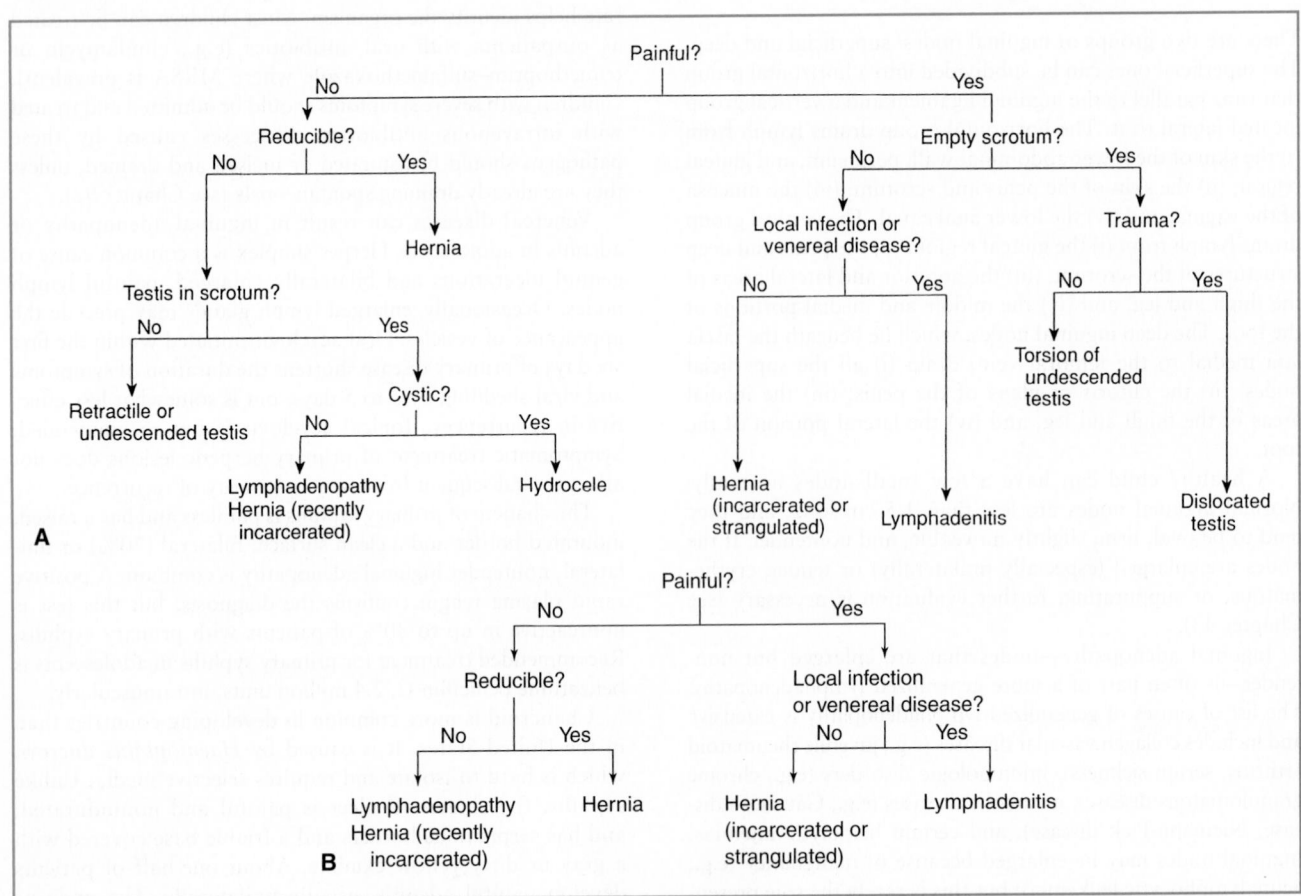

FIGURE 30.1 **A:** Groin masses in boys. **B:** Groin masses in girls.

Infection with *Bartonella henselae* (cat-scratch disease) results in regional lymphadenopathy that is usually red, indurated, and warm. Painful suppurative nodes can be treated with needle aspiration for relief of symptoms; incision and drainage should be avoided and surgical excision is unnecessary. Usually, the lymphadenopathy resolves spontaneously within 2 to 4 months. Antibiotic treatment for immunocompetent children with mild disease is of uncertain value (see Chapter 43).

Filariasis, which is found in the tropics, can produce adenopathy or adenitis associated with lower-extremity lymphedema and scrotal pathology. Diethylcarbamazine citrate (DEC) is the drug of choice for lymphatic filariasis.

Retractile, Undescended, Ectopic, and Traumatically Dislocated Testes

If the inguinal mass is firm, oval, and nontender and is associated with an empty scrotum, it probably is a retractile or undescended testis. A retractile testis, in contrast to a truly undescended one, is pulled into its abnormally high position by a hyperactive cremasteric reflex and can be "milked" back into the scrotum by the examiner. When the testicle is retractile, the scrotum appears fully developed. Although it may retract again, it will ultimately assume a normal position; therefore, no treatment is needed (see Chapter 124).

An undescended testicle occurs in 2% to 4% of term boys. As expected, its incidence correlates inversely with gestational age. For example, cryptorchidism is about ten times more common in boys born at 30 weeks' gestation, and practically all premature boys who weigh less than 900 g at birth are cryptorchid. The incidence falls to about 0.8% by 1 year of age. Because this is similar to the incidence in adult men, it seems that spontaneous descent rarely occurs after 6 months to 1 year of age. The testis can lodge anywhere along its natural line of descent—for example, intraabdominally, in the inguinal canal, or just outside the external inguinal ring. (An intraabdominal testicle is not palpable, and the scrotum appears underdeveloped.) Cryptorchidism is right-sided in about 50% of patients, left-sided in 20%, and bilateral in 30%. There is a right-sided predominance possibly because the right testicle descends later than the left one during embryologic development. Bilateral cryptorchidism occurs more often in premature boys and in conjunction with some anatomic, enzymatic, and chromosomal disorders that are diagnosed in the delivery suite or shortly thereafter. There is an increased incidence of cryptorchidism among family members.

The testis can also be located ectopically—for example, in a superficial pouch near the external ring or, less commonly, in the suprapubic, perineal, or femoral areas. It is important to note that an ectopic testis will never descend into the scrotum spontaneously.

If cryptorchidism is left untreated, various complications, including testicular hypotrophy, infertility, malignancy, injury related to trauma, torsion, and development of an inguinal hernia, can ensue. Regarding infertility, germ cell depletion increases after 15 months of age; other degenerative changes, such as Leydig cell atrophy, smaller seminiferous tubules, and peritubular fibrosis, also develop over time. These histological abnormalities are worse in testicles located more proximally.

Interestingly, sperm counts are diminished in the normally descended testis, too, although not as markedly. The incidence of malignancy is increased four- to sevenfold compared with men who have normally descended testes. The malignancy is usually a seminoma or a nonseminomatous germ cell tumor, presenting later in life. If an undescended testicle is located in the inguinal region, it is more likely to be injured from trauma. Also, torsion occurs more often in cryptorchid testes. Finally, approximately 90% of undescended testicles are associated with a patent processus vaginalis, increasing the possibility that a hernia will develop.

Early referral to a urologist is warranted. Nowadays, laparoscopy is the preferred way to locate an impalpable testis. Although ultrasound, computed tomography scan, or magnetic resonance imaging scan sometimes yield positive findings, there are high false-negative rates with these studies. In no instance should a negative imaging study be interpreted as meaning the testis is not present. Orchiopexy (laparoscopic and/or surgical) is generally performed around 1 year of age, although many urologists recommend earlier treatment. During orchiopexy, the testis, spermatic cord, and vascular structures are mobilized and brought down into the scrotum, where the testis is either pexed or placed into a dartos pouch; in addition, the processus vaginalis is ligated if it is patent. (In some cases of cryptorchidism, the testis cannot be found during exploration or appears maldeveloped.) Although it was hoped that earlier orchiopexy would decrease the incidence of malignancy, this remains controversial. Because the testis can be palpated more easily when it is in the scrotal sac, orchiopexy should facilitate earlier diagnosis of a malignancy; however, this too has never been established. In certain cases, early orchiopexy may improve the chances for fertility.

Hormonal therapy (e.g., human chorionic gonadotropin) to promote testicular descent may benefit a few select cases. However, studies from the United States have demonstrated that it is not very effective, especially when retractile testes are excluded. (In fact, many pediatric urologists use it mainly to differentiate retractile from undescended testes.) Some clinicians report that it works better in infants than older boys. It is ineffective if the testis is located ectopically.

Finally, a traumatically dislocated testicle may be discovered in the groin. Testicular dislocation occurs primarily in the older adolescent and young adult but is rare even then. It usually follows major trauma—for example, a deceleration straddle injury in a motorcyclist. Often an associated injury, such as a pelvis or femur fracture, is found. Despite swelling, ecchymosis, and tenderness, the scrotum feels empty. As mentioned, sometimes the testis is palpated in an abnormal location, most often in the groin in the superficial pouch anterior to the external oblique aponeurosis. Occasionally, the testis can be manually reduced, but if this is unsuccessful, surgery is necessary (see Chapter 112).

EVALUATION AND DECISION

In evaluating a groin mass, one must consider the gender of the child, presence or absence of pain, location of the testis (in boys), response to attempted reduction, history of trauma, and findings of local infection.

Boys

In boys (Fig. 30.1A), pain often heralds a potentially emergent condition, including torsion of an undescended testis, an incarcerated or strangulated hernia, or a significant injury. One begins the evaluation by carefully palpating the scrotum. An empty scrotum points to a dislocated testis after trauma or spontaneous torsion of an undescended testis. In a boy with bilaterally descended testes, an isolated, painful groin mass may be an incarcerated or strangulated inguinal hernia. The finding of penile lesions, such as those of herpes or syphilis, or cutaneous inflammatory lesions, such as insect bites, eczema, or infected lacerations on the legs or lower abdomen, identifies the source of inguinal lymphadenitis.

Painless groin masses in boys are usually not urgent. If the mass is reducible, it is an inguinal hernia, which can be repaired electively. The absence of a testis in the scrotum on the side of the mass suggests a retractile or undescended testis. A retractile testis is more likely in the boy presenting with new-onset swelling; the diagnosis can be confirmed in most cases by "milking" the testis into the scrotum. When both testes are descended, a painless mass is likely to be either a hydrocele or an enlarged lymph node. One must keep in mind that a recently incarcerated hernia may be painless and is easily confused with a solitary, enlarged lymph node.

Girls

As for boys, one should first ascertain the presence or absence of pain. The highest priority in girls with painful masses (Fig. 30.1B) is to identify an incarcerated or strangulated hernia. Local lesions or signs of inflammation point to lymphadenitis.

Although hernias occur less often in girls than boys, they are still relatively common. The ability to reduce the mass with gentle pressure confirms this diagnosis. When a painless mass is irreducible, a recently incarcerated hernia (particularly involving an ovary) or an enlarged lymph node is the most likely cause.

Suggested Readings

Lymphadenopathy and Lymphadenitis

Hammerschlag MR, Rawstron SA. Sexually transmitted infections. In: Jenson H, Baltimore RS, eds. *Pediatric infectious diseases: principles and practice.* Philadelphia: WB Saunders, 2002:1009.

Kelly CS, Kelly RE. Lymphadenopathy in children. *Pediatr Clin North Am* 1998;45:875.

Pickering L, ed. *Red book: 2006 report of the Committee on Infectious Diseases.* 27th ed. Elk Grove Village, IL: American Academy of Pediatrics, 2006.

Tunnessen WW Jr. Lymphadenopathy. In: Roberts KR, ed. *Signs and symptoms in pediatrics.* Philadelphia: JB Lippincott, 1999:63.

Twist CJ, Link MP. Assessment of lymphadenopathy in children. *Pediatr Clin North Am* 2002;49:1009.

Retractile, Undescended, and Ectopic Testicle

Action Committee for Determining Timing of Elective Surgery on the Genitalia of Male Children. Timing of elective surgery on the genitalia of male children with particular reference to the risks, benefits, and psychological effects of surgery and anesthesia. *Pediatrics* 1996;97:590.

Esposito C, Caldamone AC, Settimi A, et al. Management of boys with nonpalpable undescended testis. *Nat Clin Pract Urol* 2008; 5:252–260. Available at http://www.nature.com/clinicalpractice/uro.

Ferrer FA, McKenna PH. Current approaches to the undescended testicle. *Contemp Pediatr* 2000;1:106.

Haynes JH. Inguinal and scrotal disorders. *Surg Clin North Am* 2006;86:371.

Husmann DA. Cryptorchidism. In: Belman B, King L, Kramer S, eds. *Clinical pediatric urology.* London: Martin Dunitz, 2002:1125.

Hutson JM, Clarke MC. Current management of the undescended testicle. *Semin Pediatr Surg* 2007;16:64.

Jordan GH. Laparoscopic management of the undescended testicle. *Urol Clin North Am* 2001;28:23.

Kolon TF. *Cryptorchidism eMedicine Journal* 2002. Available at: http://emedicine.medscape.com/article/438378-overview.

LeungAK, RobsonWL. Current status of cryptorchidism. *Adv Pediatr* 2004;51: 351.

Neely EK, Rosenfeld RG. The undescended testicle: when and how to intervene. *Contemp Pediatr* 1990;7:21.

Petterson A, Richiardi L, et al. Age at surgery for undescended testis and risk of testicular cancer. *N Engl J Med* 2008;356:18.

Rajfer J, Handelsman DJ, Swerdloff RS, et al. Hormonal therapy of cryptorchidism. *N Engl J Med* 1986;314:466.

Rozanski TA, Bloom DA. The undescended testis: theory and management. *Urol Clin North Am* 1995;22:107.

Scrotal Trauma

Chang KJ, Sheu JW, Chang TH, et al. Traumatic dislocation of the testes. *Am J Emerg Med* 2003;21:247.

CHAPTER 31 ■ HEARING LOSS

ROBERT J. VINCI, MD

Normal hearing is crucial for the proper development of speech and language, especially during early childhood development. Persistent hearing loss will distort a child's perception of expressive speech and language and may compromise the ability to attain normal language. Failure to recognize hearing impairment may lead to cognitive impairment and may negatively impact school performance, socialization, and emotional development. Acute hearing loss is of two main types: conductive and sensorineural. Several serious—even life-threatening—disorders can accompany acute hearing loss. Therefore, prompt clinical evaluation is mandated when hearing loss is suspected.

Hearing loss can occur as an isolated symptom or in association with auditory or central nervous system (CNS) dysfunction. The differential diagnosis of hearing loss includes congenital and acquired causes. It may be produced by the abnormal transmission of sound waves to the inner ear (conductive hearing loss) or by the defective processing of sound waves (sensorineural hearing loss) in the inner ear (Table 31.1). In young children, the possibility of acute hearing loss may be suspected by parents when the child does not respond to noise or to simple commands. Abnormal or delayed language development may be a sign of a more chronic process. Older children and adolescents may complain directly of hearing difficulty.

PATHOPHYSIOLOGY

An intricate series of properly aligned anatomic and physiologic connections is responsible for the precise functioning of the auditory system. The auricle or outer ear is designed to receive sensory transmission or "sound waves" from the child's environment. A patent external ear canal is required for the passage of sound waves to the tympanic membrane.

When sound reaches the tympanic membrane, vibrations of the membrane are transmitted and produce movement of the ossicles located within the middle ear. The vibrations of the ossicles produce fluid waves of the inner ear fluid within the cochlea. Here the specialized receptors in the form of hair cells in the spiral organ of Corti convert this mechanical energy to nerve impulses that are transmitted by the cochlear (acoustic) nerve, the auditory portion of the eighth cranial nerve to the brain. These nerve impulses are integrated by the brain and transformed into what we now perceive as sound. It is important to note that, anatomically, the acoustic apparatus is closely related to the vestibular system, which is concerned with the proprioceptive senses of posture and equilibrium. The three semicircular canals of the vestibular system are connected to the cochlear system; therefore, abnormalities

in the inner ear may cause both auditory and vestibular symptoms.

DIFFERENTIAL DIAGNOSIS

Conductive Hearing Loss

In children, conductive hearing loss occurs when there is a decrease in the transmission of sound waves from the external environment to the cochlea or inner ear. Commonly, middle ear effusion (acute or chronic), impacted cerumen, foreign body of the external ear canal, infections of the external ear canal (otitis externa), and fixation or disruption of the middle ear ossicles may produce conductive hearing loss (Table 31.1). In children with chronic recurrent/otitis media (OM), a cholesteatoma—an epidermal inclusion cyst of the middle ear—may develop and cause a slowly progressive conductive hearing loss. Acute head injury, especially in association with a basilar skull fracture, may produce a conductive hearing loss secondary to hemotympanum, rupture of the tympanic membrane, or disruption of the inner ear ossicles. Especially in young children, perforation of the tympanic membrane can occur from self-inflicted injury from a cleaning device such as a cotton swab. Rarely, the conductive hearing loss may be secondary to malformations of the external or middle ears, such as malformations of the auricle, absence of the external ear canal, or atresia of the ossicular chain.

Congenital Sensorineural Hearing Loss

Approximately 1 of every 750 infants is born with congenital hearing loss. Diagnostic possibilities include genetic disorders, chromosomal abnormalities, metabolic and storage diseases, and abnormal development of the auditory apparatus (Table 31.1). Congenital hearing loss secondary to aplasia of the inner ear (Michel's aplasia) and abnormal cochlear development (Mondini's aplasia), or absence of parts of the cochlear apparatus (Scheibe's aplasia, Alexander's aplasia), are reported in children. Sensorineural hearing loss has been described in more than 70 syndromes, including Waardenburg syndrome (facial dysmorphism, white forelock), Jervell and Lange-Nielsen syndrome (prolonged Q-T syndrome), Usher's syndrome (retinitis pigmentosa and sensorineural hearing loss), and Alport's syndrome (nephritis, optic abnormalities, and hearing loss). The chromosomal disorders caused by trisomies (especially trisomies 13 to 15, 18, and 21) are associated with defects in hearing. Many of these patients are diagnosed because of anatomic features associated with each of these disorders,

TABLE 31.1

DIFFERENTIAL DIAGNOSIS OF HEARING LOSS

I. Conductive Hearing Loss
  A. Middle ear effusion
    1. Acute or chronic
  B. Impacted cerumen
  C. Foreign body of external ear canal
  D. Otitis Externa
  E. Ossicle dysfunction (fixation)
  F. Cholesteatoma
  G. Acute trauma
    1. Hemotympanum
    2. Rupture of the tympanic membrane
    3. Disruption of the inner ear ossicles
  H. Malformation of the auricle or external ear canal
  I. Atresia of the ossicle chain
II. Sensorineural Hearing Loss
  A. Congenital or neonatal
    1. Anatomic abnormalities
      a. Aplasia of the inner ear (Michel's aplasia)
      b. Abnormal cochlear development
        i. Mondini's aplasia
        ii. Scheibe's aplasia
        iii. Alexander's aplasia
    2. Syndromes (more than 70 described with hearing loss)
      a. Waardenburg syndrome
      b. Jervell and Lange-Nielsen syndrome (prolonged Q-T syndrome)
      c. Usher's syndrome
      d. Alport's syndrome
    3. Chromosomal abnormalities
      a. Trisomy 13–15
      b. Trisomy 18
      c. Trisomy 21
    4. Infections
      a. TORCH
      b. Congenital syphilis
    5. Metabolic
      a. Hypothyroidism
      b. Storage disorders
    6. Neonatal
      a. Birth asphyxia
      b. Kernicterus
      c. Use of ototoxic drugs
      d. Extreme prematurity
  B. Acquired
    1. Infection
      a. Bacterial meningitis
      b. Viral labyrinthitis
      c. Acute otitis media
    2. Vascular insufficiency
      a. Sickle cell disease
      b. Diabetes mellitus
      c. Polycythemia
    3. Anatomic defect
      a. Perilymphatic fistula
    4. Trauma
      a. Temporal bone fracture
      b. Noise-induced injury
      c. Barotrauma
      d. Lightning
    5. Tumor
      a. Acoustic neuroma
      b. CNS tumors
      c. Leukemic infiltrates
      d. Neurofibromatosis
    6. Autoimmune disease
    7. Functional hearing loss
    8. Miscellaneous
      a. Kawasaki disease
      b. Hypothyroidism
      c. Hypoparathyroidism
      d. Ototoxic drugs (e.g., gentamicin)
    9. Idiopathic

TORCH, toxoplasmosis, other (infections), rubella, cytomegalovirus (infection), and herpes (simplex); CNS, central nervous system.

although the hearing loss that occurs may be present at birth or develop over time. Overall, one-third of patients with congenital hearing loss have associated clinical symptoms of a known syndrome. The remaining two-thirds of patients are classified as having nonsyndromic hearing loss. More recent advances in genetic testing have begun to elucidate gene abnormalities in patients with nonsyndromic hearing loss.

Acquired Sensorineural Hearing Loss

Although acquired sensorineural hearing loss occurs less commonly than congenital hearing loss, the absence of associated symptoms may make it a more difficult diagnosis. An array of clinical problems can produce sensorineural hearing loss during childhood.

Acute Infection

Hearing loss secondary to bacterial meningitis is the most common cause of acquired sensorineural hearing loss. Reported in 15% to 20% of patients with meningitis, the hearing loss is usually profound and often bilateral. The hearing loss associated with meningitis is organism specific and most commonly associated with *Streptococcus pneumoniae* (31%), but was also associated with infections caused by *Haemophilus influenzae* (9% to 18%) and *Neisseria meningitides* (10%), and can develop despite appropriate antimicrobial therapy. Since the mid-1990s, vaccine programs that have led to a decrease in the incidence of *H. influenza* and *S. pneumoniae* infections have been instrumental in decreasing the occurrence of this complication. For patients with acute bacterial meningitis, adjunctive therapy with dexamethasone may decrease the inflammation in the subarachnoid space and lessens neurologic sequelae such as hearing loss. To be most effective, the dexamethasone therapy should be given to the patient before or with the initial administration of antibiotics. All children who have had bacterial meningitis should have a complete hearing evaluation as part of their follow-up from their acute hospitalization.

Congenital infection caused by cytomegalovirus (CMV) is the most common intrauterine infection that produces sensorineural hearing loss. Congenital infection from rubella, syphilis, toxoplasmosis, and perinatally acquired herpes simplex infections are also associated with acquired sensorineural hearing loss. The hearing loss associated with these infections may occur in infants with no other manifestations of congenital infection and may not develop until early childhood. Thus, many experts advocate for universal newborn hearing screening and regular monitoring of children with known congenital infections or high-risk infants such as neonatal intensive care unit graduates.

Viral infections of the labyrinth (also called viral cochleitis) secondary to mumps, parainfluenzae, adenovirus, herpes simplex, CMV, and rubeola have been described and confirmed by serologic studies. Labyrinthitis usually has symptoms related to inflammation of the inner ear and involvement of the vestibular apparatus, and patients may complain of vomiting, tinnitus, and vertigo.

Vascular Insufficiency

Sudden hearing loss secondary to vascular insufficiency has been described in the pediatric patient. Vascular insufficiency may compromise blood flow to the cochlea, producing a hypoxic insult to the sensitive nerve cells in the organ of Corti. Once injured, these nerve cells may not regenerate and profound sensorineural hearing loss can develop. In children, sickle cell disease, long-standing diabetes mellitus, and hyperviscosity states associated with polycythemia can compromise cochlear blood flow and produce sudden hearing loss.

Perilymphatic Fistula

Anatomic defects in the bony or membranous enclosure that normally surrounds the perilymphatic space can produce a perilymphatic fistula. These defects may produce an anomalous communication between the middle and inner ear compartment and should be considered in the differential diagnosis of the pediatric patient with acute sensorineural hearing loss. A perilymphatic fistula can occur at any age. The sudden ingress of air into the inner ear is believed to produce the symptom complex of hearing loss, tinnitus, vertigo, dizziness, and nystagmus. Antecedent trauma usually underlies the development of a fistula. This is especially true in any patient who has a recent history of vigorous exercise or changes in barometric pressure associated with airplane travel or scuba diving. Although unilateral hearing loss is most common, bilateral hearing deficits have been described. Occasionally, a perilymphatic fistula will develop in a child with previously abnormal hearing. Therefore, this diagnosis needs to be considered in any patient who has sudden onset of hearing loss, fluctuation in hearing, or complaints of progressive hearing loss, regardless of baseline hearing function. Patients with a perilymphatic fistula generally have a normal otoscopic examination. If a tympanogram is performed, middle ear effusion is usually absent. Emergent referral to an otolaryngologist is warranted because surgery may be required for closure of the anatomic defect.

Head Trauma

Both the vestibular and cochlear nerves can be injured with fractures of the temporal bone. Assessment of audiologic function should be considered in any child with major head trauma; computed tomography (CT) scan may be required to diagnose these injuries.

Acoustic Trauma

Immediate, severe, and permanent hearing loss can follow even a short period of exposure to sound greater than 140 dB. Exposure to sounds in the 80- to 100-dB range can produce hearing loss with chronic exposure and is most commonly diagnosed in adolescents. Rock concerts, stereo headphones, machinery, and explosive devices are capable of producing sound at the intensity required to produce this condition.

Chronic/Recurrent Otitis Media

A history of chronic/recurrent OM may predispose patients to the development of sensorineural hearing loss. This hearing loss is believed to be related to inflammatory changes in the inner ear produced by the diapedesis of toxins through the round window membrane. Such involvement of the inner ear has been confirmed pathologically by the presence of labyrinthitis in patients with acute OM. Because middle ear effusions produce a conductive hearing loss, the clinician must be aware of the possibility of OM producing a mixed picture.

Functional Hearing Loss

Functional hearing loss may occur in patients who have a psychological component to their presentation. Most commonly occurring during adolescence, functional hearing loss should be considered in patients who present with other manifestations of psychiatric illness. Often, these patients will have a normal physical examination and inconsistent findings with bedside hearing tests. Formal audiologic testing will be normal in these patients and mental health referral is indicated to elucidate the cause of this apparent hearing loss.

Miscellaneous

Acoustic neuroma, CNS tumors, and leukemic infiltrates are also associated with sensorineural hearing loss. Other considerations in pediatric patients include Kawasaki disease, hypothyroidism, lightning injury, hyperlipidemia, and hyperbilirubinemia, or the use of ototoxic drugs in the neonatal period. Finally, some children will have no demonstrable cause for their hearing loss.

EVALUATION AND DECISION

Any complaint of hearing loss requires prompt evaluation. Common causes of acute hearing loss are listed in Table 31.2. Life-threatening causes of acute hearing loss are rare in pediatric patients (Table 31.3). The initial step in evaluation is to confirm the presence of acute hearing loss (Fig. 31.1). Although sophisticated hearing tests are best performed by an audiologist, the emergency physician should attempt bedside testing of gross hearing function. In young children, behavioral responses to loud stimuli can be assessed. Without attracting visual attention, an auditory stimulus (e.g., vigorous hand clapping or ringing a bell) can be presented to the child. Eye blinking or turning toward the stimulus represents a positive response and suggests some degree of intact hearing. In older children or adolescents, hearing can be assessed by asking the patient if he or she hears a low-intensity sound such as a soft whisper or fingers rubbing together. Because hearing dysfunction can be subtle and can occur over the entire range of auditory frequencies, these bedside tests may underestimate the degree of hearing impairment. Therefore, an abnormal test should be considered a confirmation of hearing impairment; a

TABLE 31.2

COMMON CAUSES OF ACUTE HEARING LOSS

Conductive hearing loss	Sensorineural hearing loss
Middle ear effusion	TORCH infections
Impacted cerumen	Birth asphyxia
Foreign body of external ear canal	Viral labyrinthitis
	Bacterial meningitis
	Perilymphatic fistula
	Trauma
	Acoustic neuroma

TORCH, toxoplasmosis, other (infections), rubella, cytomegalovirus (infection), and herpes (simplex).

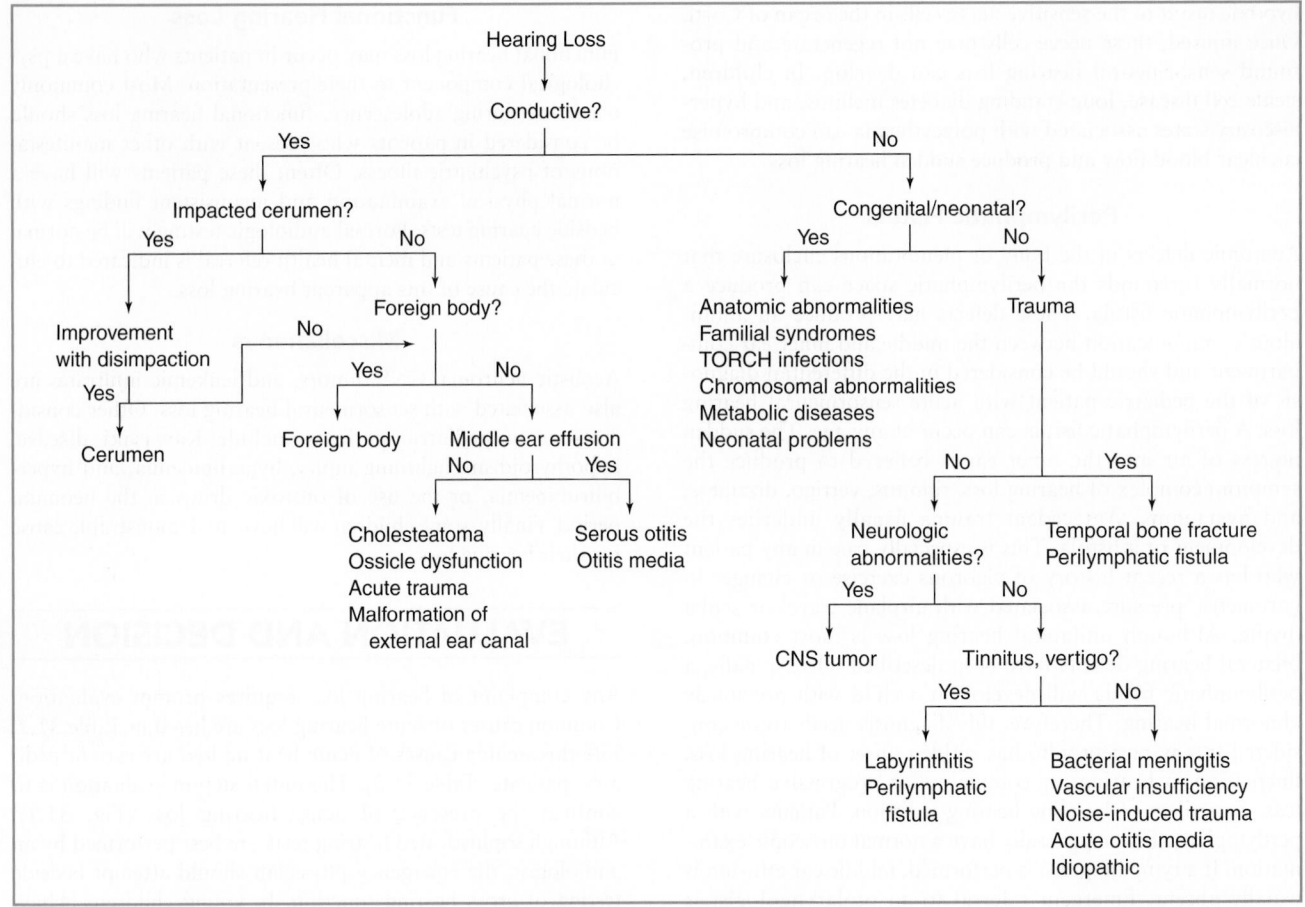

FIGURE 31.1 Evaluation of hearing loss.

negative test needs to be interpreted in the context of the chief complaint of the patient. If the history remains strongly suggestive of hearing loss, the physician should assume some degree of hearing loss despite the results of bedside testing and formal audiology follow-up is required.

Critical elements of the medical history should include the onset of the hearing loss and the duration of symptoms. Family history of hearing loss may suggest the diagnosis of a genetic disorder with delayed presentation of hearing loss. A history of birth asphyxia, prematurity, hyperbilirubinemia, or maternal infection points to a neonatal cause. A more recent history of head trauma or barotrauma (e.g., scuba diving) may suggest the diagnosis of perilymphatic fistula. Fever and otalgia suggest a diagnosis of acute OM. Associated neurologic symptoms such as tinnitus, vertigo, and dizziness suggest inner ear disease or CNS involvement. Headache can be a marker for tumor of the CNS or extension of middle ear infection (Fig. 31.1).

TABLE 31.3

LIFE-THREATENING CAUSES OF ACUTE HEARING LOSS

Acute head injury
Brain tumor
Leukemic infiltrate
Vascular insufficiency

On physical examination, the presence of fever may suggest an infection such as OM or viral labyrinthitis. A detailed otoscopic examination to detect the presence of a middle ear effusion, impacted cerumen or evidence of an external ear infection, perforated tympanic membrane, foreign body, or other abnormality of the tympanic membrane is a priority. Tympanometry can be used to supplement the physical examination, especially if the otoscopic examination suggests the presence of middle ear disease. Because of the intricate relationship between the cranial nerves, a careful neurologic examination is required. Within the petrous bone, the cochlear nerve is closely related to the seventh cranial nerve and the vestibular branch of the eighth cranial nerve. An ipsilateral facial nerve palsy in a patient with hearing impairment suggests an intracranial process. Vestibular function should be tested looking for the presence of nystagmus at rest and with directed gaze. Patients with vestibular dysfunction often fall to one side with Romberg testing or have difficulty with rapid alternating movements or finger-to-nose testing.

Once hearing loss is established, the next step in the emergency department (ED) is to differentiate conductive from sensorineural hearing loss with the use of tuning fork tests (Fig. 31.1). Conductive hearing loss can be confirmed by the Weber test. In the Weber test, a vibrating, 512-Hz tuning fork is placed in the midline of the patient's forehead. Patients with hearing loss will report that the vibrations of the tuning fork lateralize to the side with the conductive hearing loss (vibrations are felt better in the bad ear) or away from the side with the sensorineural hearing loss (vibrations are felt better in the good ear). For the Rinne test, the vibrating tuning fork is placed against the mastoid process. When the patient signals that the vibration has ceased, the tuning fork is placed adjacent to that ear to determine whether the patient can hear the sound of the still-vibrating tuning fork. Patients with conductive hearing loss will not be able to hear the tuning fork. This is a negative Rinne test (bone conduction greater than air conduction). Sensorineural hearing loss shows up as a positive Rinne test (air conduction greater than bone conduction). Finally, a test by confrontation is performed by placing a tuning fork at a point equidistant from both ears. Regardless of the type of hearing loss, the patient will report the sound to be higher on the side with normal hearing.

Laboratory evaluation is seldom necessary in the ED; when needed, it should focus on a diagnosis that may be contemplated after obtaining a detailed history and physical examination. Complete blood cell (CBC) count and peripheral blood smear, renal function tests, serologic tests for syphilis, TORCH titers, and bacteriologic cultures should be performed only if the history and physical suggest an associated diagnosis. Thyroid function tests, lipid profile, and serum calcium levels should be individualized in the context of clinical findings. Referral for genetic testing may be indicated for children with congenital sensorineural hearing loss.

In children with the clinical suspicion of intracranial pathology, a radiologic evaluation assists in the diagnosis. Patients with known or suspected congenital malformation of the middle and inner ears should be evaluated with a CT scan because bony detail is essential for diagnosis. Inner ear abnormalities have been demonstrated in 8% to 20% of patients with sensorineural hearing loss. A CT scan should also be performed in patients with suspected fracture of the temporal bone. Magnetic resonance imaging is indicated for the accurate diagnosis of an acoustic neuroma or for any patient with suspected retrocochlear pathology. With the addition of paramagnetic contrast, high-resolution scanning, and thin-section techniques, excellent detail of the internal auditory canal can be achieved.

Most children with decreased hearing in the ED have a conductive hearing loss. If impacted cerumen is seen on examination, it must be removed because it may be the cause of the decreased hearing and prevents further otoscopic evaluation. Children whose hearing improves after disimpaction and who have a normal otoscopic examination need no further treatment. Patients without impacted cerumen and those who fail to improve after removal of cerumen may have a foreign body in the ear canal. Only large objects that completely obstruct the external auditory canal should impair hearing; thus, this diagnosis is easily established during otoscopic examination. Foreign bodies may be removed either by grasping the object with alligator forceps or by placing a right angle instrument behind the object and then gently withdrawing the instrument and pulling the foreign body with it. Care must be taken to avoid irrigation of an ear canal if the foreign material consists of vegetable matter that could expand from the irrigation. Finally, irrigation is contraindicated with known or suspected perforations of the tympanic membrane.

The next step in the evaluation is a careful examination of the tympanic membrane, including pneumatic otoscopy. Many patients will show evidence of a middle ear effusion, the most common cause of hearing loss seen in the ED. Rarely, a cholesteatoma may be seen through the translucent tympanic membrane. Sensorineural hearing loss is seen less often in the ED. Most children with sensorineural hearing loss have congenital problems that are diagnosed during the course of routine care, although occasional cases will be brought to the attention of the emergency physician. Among the acquired causes, those that must be diagnosed urgently include CNS tumors, vascular accidents, and perilymphatic fistula. In cases of acquired sensorineural hearing loss, a history of trauma should be sought. Direct blows to the head may cause temporal bone fractures or a perilymphatic fistula, and sudden changes in pressure may injure the cochlea. If there is no preceding trauma, a careful neurologic examination should be performed, looking for evidence of CNS tumors. A CT scan is indicated if these lesions are suspected. The most common cause of acquired sensorineural hearing loss seen in children in the ED without a history of trauma is viral labyrinthitis. These patients usually have associated tinnitus, vertigo, and vomiting but no focal neurologic abnormalities. Most of the remaining causes of hearing loss are idiopathic. Vascular insufficiency merits consideration in children with sickle cell anemia, diabetes mellitus, and collagen vascular disease. If the cause of the hearing loss remains uncertain, otolaryngologic consult and evaluation should be considered.

Suggested Readings

Brookhouser PE. Sensorineural hearing loss in children. *Pediatr Clin North Am* 1996;43:1195–1216.

Dennis JM, Neely JG. Basic hearing tests. *Otolaryngol Clin North Am* 1991; 24:253–276.

Mafong DD, Shin EJ, Lalwani AK. Use of laboratory evaluation and radiologic imaging in the diagnostic evaluation of children with sensorineural hearing loss. *Laryngoscope* 2002;112:1

McIntyre PB, Berkey CS, King SM, et al. Dexamethasone as adjunctive therapy in bacterial meningitis: a meta-analysis of randomized clinical trials since 1988. *JAMA* 1997;278:925–931.

Pappas DG, Simpson LC, Godwin GH. Perilymphatic fistula in children with preexisting sensorineural hearing loss. *Laryngoscope* 1988;98:507–510.

Roisen NJ. Etiology of hearing loss in children. *Pediatr Clin North Am* 1999; 46:49–64.

St Martin MB, Hirsch BE. Imaging of Hearing Loss. *Otolayrngol Clin North Am* 2008;41:157–178.

Thompson DC, McPhillips H, Davis RL, et al. Universal newborn hearing screening: summary of the evidence. *JAMA* 2001;286(16):2000–2010.

Tomaski GM, Grundfast KM. A stepwise approach to the diagnosis and treatment of hereditary hearing loss. *Pediatr Clin North Am* 1999;46:35–48.

Van de Beek D, De Gans J, McIntyre P, et al. Corticosteroids in acute bacterial meningitis. *Cochrane Database Syst Rev* 2003, Issue 3. Art. No.: CD004305.

Yoshinago-Itano C, Sedey AL, Coulter DA, et al. Language of early and later identified children with hearing loss. *Pediatrics* 1998;102:1161.

SIGNS AND SYMPTOMS

CHAPTER 32 ■ PATIENTS WITH HEART MURMURS

BENJAMIN K. SILVERMAN, MD

A cardiac murmur is a noise created by the turbulence of blood flow, under varying pressures, through chambers and vessels and across valves that are of unequal sizes and shapes. The murmur itself is not an abnormality. Most murmurs, in fact, are sounds created by normal turbulence and, therefore, are best referred to as "normal" or "flow" rather than the less appropriate adjectives, "innocent" or "functional" (Table 32.1). Some loud murmurs are created by clinically inconsequential defects (e.g., small ventricular septal defects), whereas other, barely discernible, murmurs may be associated with far more serious defects or illnesses, such as acute myocarditis (which has a murmur only in rare patients with severe dilatation causing valvular insufficiency) or transposition of the great vessels. A host of cardiac and several extracardiac conditions can be associated with heart murmurs (Table 32.2).

In a "first encounter" examination of a child, the emergency physician will often hear a murmur and then must determine how to fit this finding into the sometimes complicated evaluation of the patient's current illness. Is the murmur an incidental finding of no relevance? Is it suggestive of heart disease? If so, are there cardiac-related symptoms? Is it related to life-threatening illness, not necessarily of cardiac origin?

Certain priorities prevail that should precede the further definition of the murmur per se. It is not important to pinpoint a primary cardiac lesion immediately, but it is essential to determine whether the patient is in cardiac decompensation, whether life is at risk, and whether there is an incipient need for evaluation by a cardiologist or cardiac surgeon.

The ultimate goal of this chapter is to provide criteria for determining whether a patient's murmur is associated with life-threatening illness of cardiac or extracardiac origin, and whether the patient needs cardiac consultation now, or eventually, or not at all.

DIFFERENTIAL DIAGNOSIS

History

Unless the patient is in extremis, a careful, focused history is always the starting place. For the patient in whom a murmur is heard, in addition to usual history related to the present complaint, relevant questions might include the following:

- If the patient is an infant, were ultrasound aberrations found during pregnancy?
- Has the murmur been known to have been present? If so, since when? Has it been evaluated at any previous examination? If so, what were the findings and conclusion? Has there been cardiac surgery?
- Was there an antecedent illness before discovery of the murmur? Sore throat? Viral infection? Apparent respiratory infection?
- Are there or have there been associated signs or symptoms? Feeding problems? Weight gain or loss? Difficult breathing? Cyanosis? Edema? Hypertension? Chest pain? Joint symptoms? Congenital defects?
- Does the child tire easily (during feedings in infants)? How far can he or she walk? Does the child squat after walking? Climb stairs? Have cyanotic "spells"?

Examination

The examination should consist of as complete a physical as possible under the prevailing circumstances.

Murmur Characteristics

Most physicians cannot dissect a murmur in intricate detail with the precision of a cardiologist. Therefore, although the characteristics are briefly defined here, the subsequent course of this chapter makes only minimal use of them. More detailed descriptions of murmur characteristics are given in the references at the end of this chapter.

- *Timing and duration:* Is the murmur systolic (between the first and second heart sounds) or diastolic (between the second and first sounds)? Early, mid, late, or throughout systole (holosystolic)? Beginning in systole and persisting into diastole (continuous)?
- *Intensity (loudness):* Usually graded from barely discernible (grade I) to accompanied by a palpable thrill (grade IV) to audible without making contact with the chest (grade VI).
- *Shape:* Terms such as *diamond-shaped*, *plateau*, *crescendo*, and *decrescendo* are more easily understood when learned in conjunction with a phonocardiogram; interpreting them by ear requires training and persistent practice.
- *Quality: Musical, blowing, rumbling, wood-sawing, harsh, vibratory, twang, soft, rough, grating,* and *click* are among the subjective terms used.
- *Frequency (pitch):* Described qualitatively as low, medium, or high.
- *Location and transmission:* Location is the point of maximum intensity (upper, lower, or mid left or right sternal margin; apex; midclavicular or axillary line; at which rib interspace?). Transmission refers to the areas of maximal spread of the sound (to the back, to the neck, axilla, throughout entire precordium).

TABLE 32.1

CHARACTERISTICS USUALLY ASSOCIATED WITH A "NORMAL" MURMUR

Timing: midsystole
Intensity: grades I through III
Location of maximal intensity: midsternal border
Radiation: possibly faintly to the precordium and neck, but rarely the back
Quality: "twangy" or "vibratory"
Heart sounds: readily definable, including splitting of S_2

Precordial Examination

The remainder of the precordial examination should be completed; inspect for left- or right-sided chest bulge, palpate for thrills and clicks and points of maximal impulse, and listen carefully for the heart sounds and adventitial sounds. The physician must interpret the first and second sound for intensity and splitting. The third and fourth sounds, opening snaps, clicks, rubs, and some unusual rhythms may be confused for murmurs at times and should be kept in mind as possible confounding factors.

Associated Signs and Symptoms

Vital Signs. Normal ranges of vital signs for age are listed in Appendix D at the end of this book.

■ *Heart rate and rhythm:* Check the heart rate, and listen and palpate for rhythm disturbances (see Chapters 74 and 84). The normally rapid rate of the infant makes evaluation of the murmur even more difficult. Palpate the brachial and femoral artery pulsations.

■ *Blood pressure:* Ascertain that a proper-size cuff is used. Lower-extremity pressures are normally measured 10 to 40 mm Hg higher than upper pressures.

■ *Respirations:* Count the rate and observe for retraction, asymmetry, and hypoexpansion.

■ *Body temperature:* Infants with heart murmurs are subject, of course, to the multiple causes of elevated body temperature as any other child. Particularly, though, infective endocarditis must be thought of in any child with heart disease and fever. Children with acute episodes of acquired entities, such as rheumatic fever and myocarditis, will probably be febrile. Hypothermia may be associated with cardiac shock.

SIGNS AND SYMPTOMS

TABLE 32.2

CONDITIONS THAT MAY BE ASSOCIATED WITH PRESENCE OF A CARDIAC MURMUR[a]

I. Infancy
  A. Cardiac
    1. Noncyanotic
      a. Normal murmur ("innocent" murmur)
      b. Congenital defects
        (1) Patent ductus arteriosus
        (2) Atrial septal defect
        (3) Ventricular septal defect
        (4) Aortic stenosis
        (5) Coarctation of aorta
        (6) Pulmonary stenosis
        (7) Partial anomalous pulmonary venous drainage
      c. Myocarditis
      d. Primary myocardial disease
    2. Cyanotic
      a. Congenital defects
        (1) Tetralogy of Fallot
        (2) Transposition of the great vessels
        (3) Truncus arteriosus
        (4) Pulmonary atresia
        (5) Severe pulmonary stenosis with patent foramen
        (6) Tricuspid atresia
        (7) Ebstein's anomaly
        (8) Total anomalous pulmonary venous drainage
        (9) Atrioventricular canal defect
        (10) Hypoplastic left heart
        (11) Primary Pulmonary Hypertension
    3. Congestive cardiac failure
      a. Secondary to any of the previous, as well as noncardiac causes listed as follows
  B. Extracardiac
    1. Severe anemia
    2. Arteriovenous malformation
    3. Pulmonary insufficiency (including infection, hypoperfusion, pulmonary arterial hypertension)
    4. Hyperpyrexia
II. Older Child
  A. Cardiac
    1. Normal murmur
    2. Congenital defect (same list as for infancy—both cyanotic and noncyanotic)
    3. Mitral valve prolapse
    4. Myocarditis (viral, collagen, toxic, endocrine, genetic)
    5. Acute rheumatic fever
    6. Healed rheumatic carditis
    7. Subacute bacterial endocarditis
    8. Congestive cardiac failure (associated with any of previous or following noncardiac diseases)
  B. Extracardiac
    1. Severe anemia
    2. Arteriovenous malformation
    3. Pulmonary insufficiency (with incidental murmur)
    4. Thyrotoxicosis
    5. Hyperpyrexia

[a]It should be kept in mind that *any* pediatric problem may be coincidentally associated with the presence of a normal cardiac murmur or with one of the other conditions in this table. The algorithms and chapter text are constructed to help sort out the significance of the murmur in the context of patient management.

Pulse Oximetry. Pulse oximetry is used to evaluate the presence and degree of oxygen desaturation and is sometimes referred to as "the fifth vital sign."

Color. Central cyanosis (see Chapters 15 and 98) is diffuse and is best differentiated from peripheral cyanosis by involvement of the tongue. Central cyanosis due to cardiac lesion may be differentiated from cyanosis due to pulmonary disease by the hyperoxia test—exposing the child to 100% oxygen while monitoring with pulse oximetry. Those with pulmonary disease may improve their oximetry reading while those with cardiac lesions probably will not. If accompanied by clubbing of the distal fingers in the older child, cyanosis is probably chronic and persistent. Severe pallor related to marked anemia may be associated with high-output cardiac failure.

Signs Associated with Cardiac Failure. Additional signs that may be associated with cardiac failure are listed as follows (also see Chapter 84):

- *Edema:* More likely to be dependent and pitting in cardiac disease. In the preambulant child, dependent edema may be appreciated best along the back, rather than the lower extremities, and also may be prominent in the periorbital area.
- *Neck veins:* Check for distended jugular veins in the neck of the patient who is lying flat or propped at a 45-degree angle.
- *Respiratory effort:* Look for tachypnea, grunting, difficult breathing (particularly subcostal retractions), and for the patient more comfortable when resting in an upright position. Listen to the lung fields for crackles and wheeze, usually symmetric in a patient in cardiac failure.
- *Organ enlargement:* Palpate for a soft, engorged liver (particularly the left lobe, which becomes palpable early in right-sided congestive heart failure). Check for splenomegaly.

Remaining Examination. Also look for the following signs:

- *Skin:* Look for non-blanching petechiae on the surface of the skin, in the conjunctivae, and under the fingernails. Also search for erythema marginatum and subcutaneous nodules. Look for thoracotomy scars.
- *Joints:* Check for tenderness, redness, heat, and swelling (see Chapter 56).
- *Neurologic:* Examine for cranial nerve malfunction? Paresis? Papilledema?
- *Nutritional evaluation:* Are the child's height and weight within a reasonable percentile compatible with the parents'? Is the weight percentile significantly less or greater than that for height?

Ancillary Diagnostic Aids

None of the following need to be used routinely, but most should be obtainable and interpretable for the emergency department (ED) setting. They should be ordered selectively if clinical assessment of the child does not allow a satisfactory conclusion regarding the significance of the murmur.

Electrocardiography. A full 14-lead electrocardiogram (EKG), using age- and size-appropriate electrodes, should be readily obtainable for screening and evaluation purposes. The emergency physician should have a working knowledge of the criteria for determining normality, which will vary with the age group of the child (see Chapter 84 and Appendix D). A lead II rhythm strip can be used for monitoring the patient in distress or with possible abnormal rhythm.

Echocardiography. Echocardiography allows definitive diagnosis for many congenital cardiac lesions, determination of the severity of cardiac failure, differentiation of myocarditis from pericardial effusion, evaluation of intrathoracic pressure phenomena (tamponade, effusion, tumors), and discovery of coronary artery malpositions or coronary dilatation, as in Kawasaki Disease.

Echocardiography has replaced cardiac catheterization in preoperative diagnosis of most, but not all, lesions. Because it is somewhat expensive and is so technician dependent, the procedure is of optimal value in conjunction with cardiology consultation. The cardiologist can guide the technician as to optimal methodology.

Procedures such as angiocardiography, electrophysiologic mapping, and cardiac flow determinations, although they may prove essential for eventual diagnosis, require cardiac consultation and should not be part of the evaluation in the ED.

Chest Radiograph. Films should be taken in both posteroanterior (PA) and lateral views. The physician should look for gross cardiac enlargement in the PA views, which may be determined in older children by a transverse diameter greater than 50% of the width of the thoracic cage. In infants, the diameter normally may be considerably wider than that ratio. Thymic shadows, scoliosis, rib abnormalities, and less than full inspiration may be confounding factors. The lung fields should be evaluated for infiltrates and for increased or diminished pulmonary vascular flow. Rib notching may be present secondary to long-standing coarctation of the aorta.

Blood Studies. Screening tests that might be of ancillary value under specific circumstances include a complete blood cell count, sedimentation rate and/or C-reactive protein, arterial blood gas measurements, co-oximetry, blood culture, antistreptolysin titer, sickle cell screening, troponin, and brain natriuretic protein (bnp) and anti-nuclear antibody.

EVALUATION AND DECISION

Neonates and older infants usually have differing clinical presentations than older children. Therefore, for the purposes of our first encounter evaluation, we divide murmur patients by two age groups: from birth to 3 years of age (Figs. 32.1A and 32.1B) and older than 3 years of age (Figs. 32.2A to 32.2C). Table 32.2 lists conditions that may be associated with cardiac murmurs.

Infants Younger Than 3 Years of Age with Cardiac Murmur

Neonates or infants younger than 3 years of age in whom a murmur is heard require extremely careful assessment. The

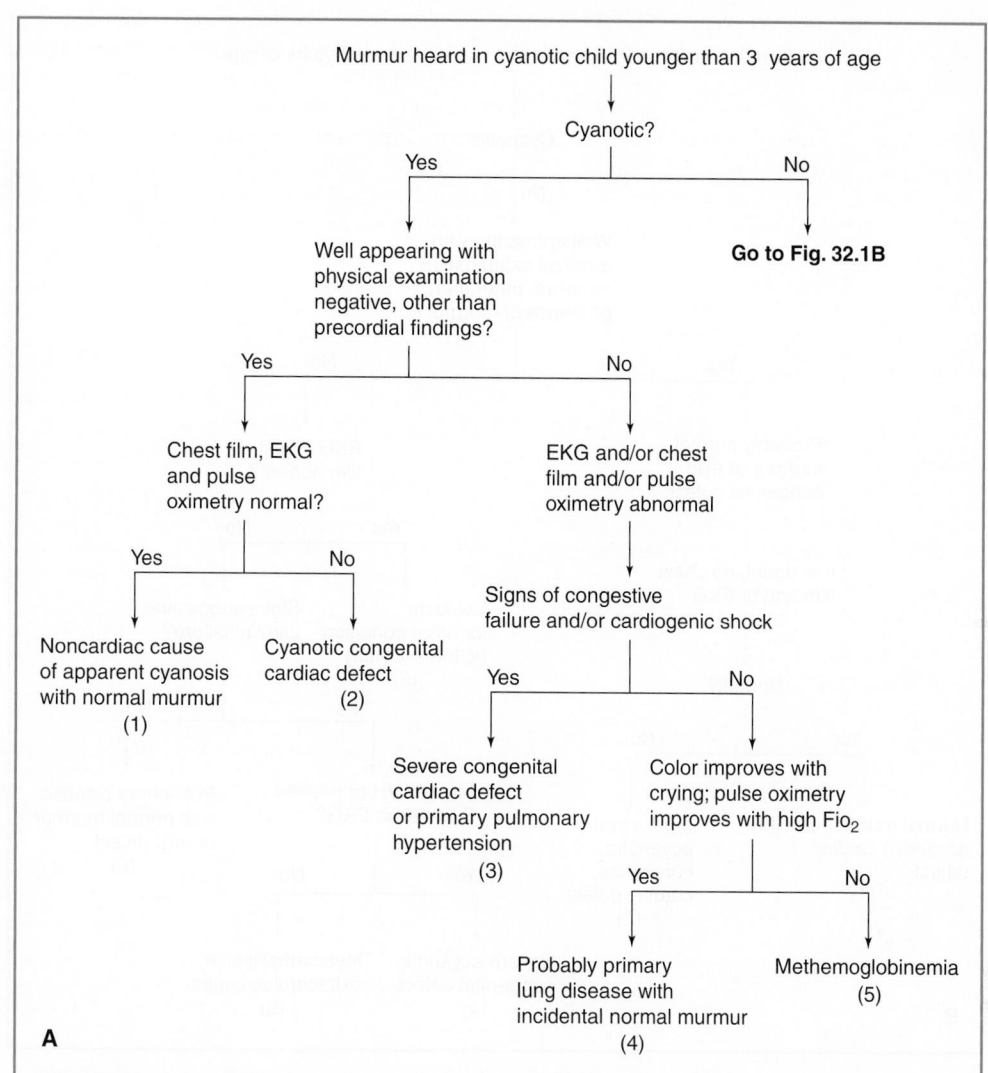

FIGURE 32.1A Assessment of a cyanotic infant younger than 3 years of age in whom a murmur is heard. (Numbers in parentheses refer to specific citations in text.) EKG, electrocardiogram.

lead point in the evaluation is the presence or absence of cyanosis, preferably confirmed by pulse oximetry.

Infants Younger Than 3 Years of Age Who Are Cyanotic

Any baby who has a murmur and appears cyanotic (Fig. 32.1A) should have a thorough physical examination, as well as a pulse oximetry determination, an EKG, chest film, and possibly arterial gases and echocardiography.

If the physical examination is normal, except for the cyanosis and the murmur, and the EKG, film, and pulse oximetry are normal, the infant probably has a normal murmur and a noncardiac cause of only apparent cyanosis (peripheral acrocyanosis, polycythemia, methemoglobinemia) [Fig. 32.1A (1)]. If still in doubt, echocardiography may be supportive.

A cyanotic infant who appears well, but who has an abnormal EKG and chest film and has diminished arterial saturation by oximetry or blood gas evaluation, probably has cyanotic heart disease; however, he or she is not likely to get into early trouble [Fig. 32.1A (2)]. This could include tetralogy of Fallot, transposition of the great vessels with single ventricle, truncus arteriosus, Ebstein's anomaly, tricuspid atresia with patent foramen ovale, anomalous pulmonary venous drainage, or moderately severe pulmonary stenosis with right-to-left shunting through an atrial or ventricular septal defect or a patent ductus. These babies should be referred for early echocardiogram and discussed with a cardiologist. Neonates should be admitted for evaluation and possible treatment in the hospital, but well-appearing children more than 4 weeks old should have early cardiac consultation but do not necessarily need to be admitted.

If the cyanotic infant appears acutely ill, a chest radiograph and/or the EKG will likely be abnormal. If the findings

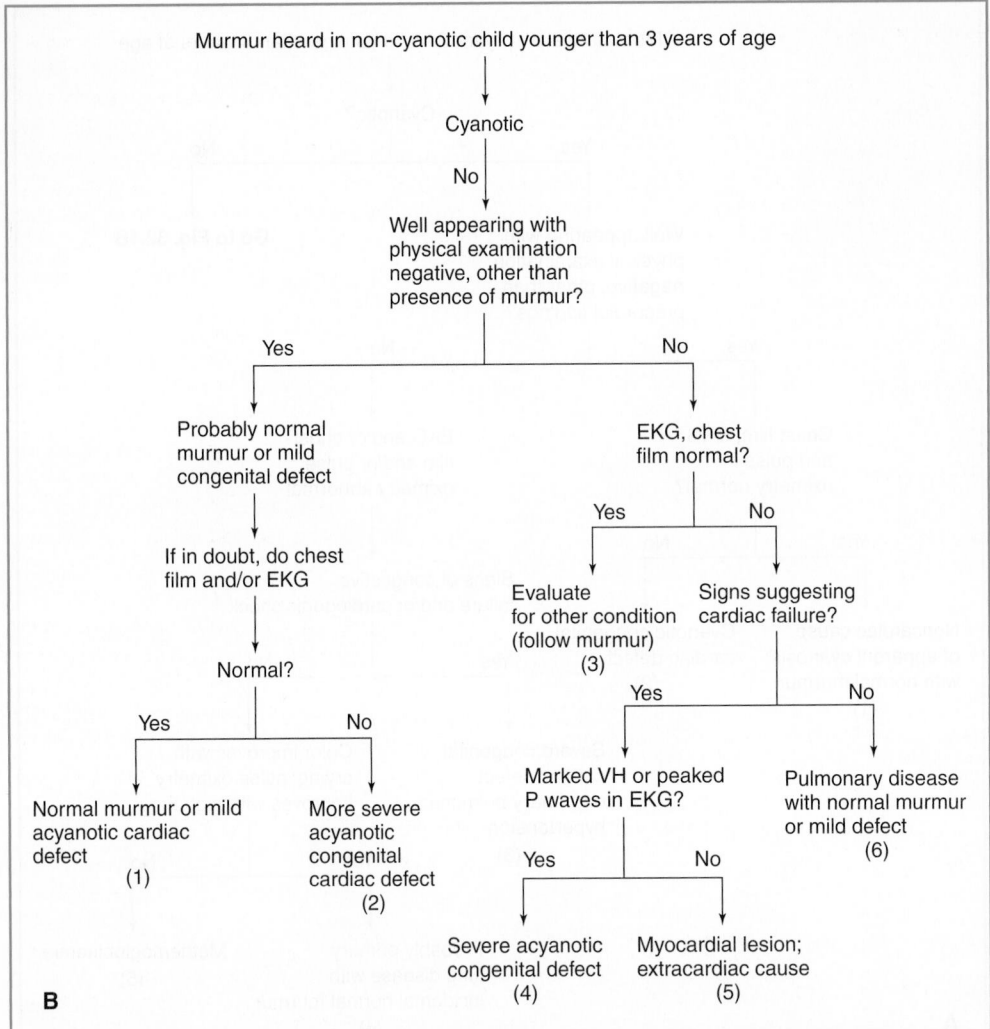

FIGURE 32.1B Assessment of a noncyanotic infant younger than 3 years of age in whom a murmur is heard. (Numbers in parentheses refer to specific citations in text.) EKG, electrocardiogram; VH, ventricular hypertrophy.

on examination suggest congestive heart failure (CHF) and/or cardiogenic shock, the baby probably has severe cyanotic congenital heart disease or an extremely severe acyanotic defect with the cyanosis related to poor perfusion and failure [Fig. 32.1A (3)].

Defects in the neonate could include hypoplastic left heart, extreme aortic or pulmonary stenosis, severe coarctation of the aorta, pulmonary atresia with intact ventricular septum, and tricuspid atresia with closed foramen (Table 32.3). Survival of patients with these severe lesions is dependent on maintaining patency of the ductus arteriosus. Early infusion therapy with prostaglandin E1 (Alprostadil) under carefully controlled monitoring should be considered (see Chapter 84). Interventional cardiac catheterization by experienced cardiologists provides an alternative approach to abetting right-to-left flow.

In the sick cyanotic neonate with respiratory distress, the possibility of primary pulmonary hypertension also should be considered. This might be defined by differential cyanosis—less in the upper body than in the lower. Urgent admission to a neonatal unit, for possible treatment with either inhaled NO or extracorporeal membrane oxygenation (ECMO), is essential [Fig. 32.1A (3)].

In the somewhat older infant, other considerations include Ebstein's anomaly, large arteriovenous malformation, atrioventricular canal defect, large ventricular septal defect, and total anomalous pulmonary venous drainage. These babies should be admitted to the hospital or transferred to a center for diagnostic cardiac workup and therapy.

TABLE 32.3

LIFE-THREATENING CARDIAC LESIONS IN THE LLL AND/OR DEEPLY CYANOTIC NEONATE

Hypoplastic left heart
Extreme coarctation of the aorta
Critical aortic stenosis
Critical pulmonary stenosis
Pulmonary atresia with intact ventricular septum
Tricuspid atresia with closed foramen

For the deeply cyanotic and/or ill-appearing neonate, emergency cardiac consultation should be requested and consideration given to immediate infusion therapy with prostaglandin E1 to ensure patency of the ductus arteriosus.

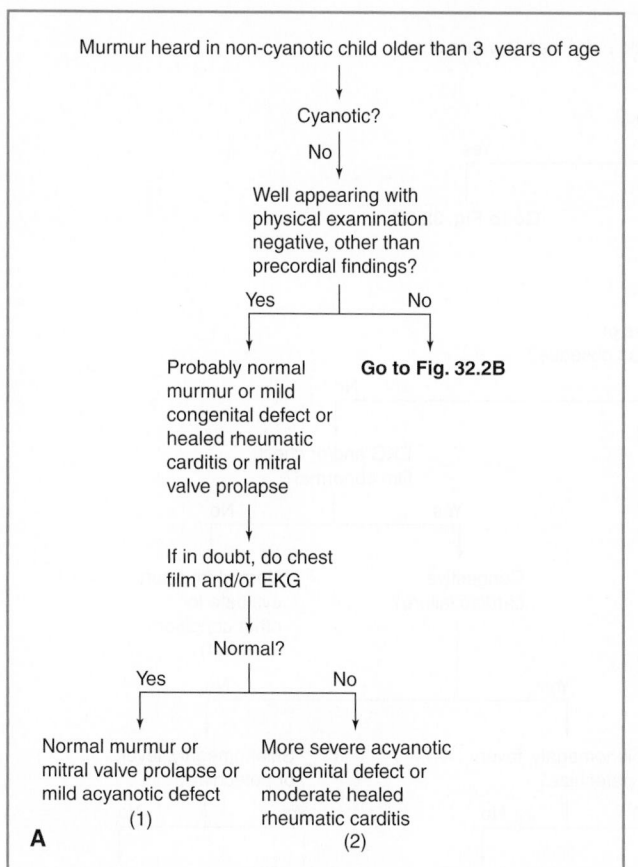

Murmur heard in non-cyanotic child older than 3 years of age

Cyanotic?

No

Well appearing with physical examination negative, other than precordial findings?

Yes / No

Probably normal murmur or mild congenital defect or healed rheumatic carditis or mitral valve prolapse

Go to Fig. 32.2B

If in doubt, do chest film and/or EKG

Normal?

Yes / No

Normal murmur or mitral valve prolapse or mild acyanotic defect
(1)

More severe acyanotic congenital defect or moderate healed rheumatic carditis
(2)

A

FIGURE 32.2A Assessment of a noncyanotic, well-appearing child 3 years of age and older in whom a murmur is heard. (Numbers in parentheses refer to specific citations in text.) EKG, electrocardiogram.

If the evaluation of the sick cyanotic baby does not suggest CHF or shock and the saturation improves somewhat with crying and in oxygen, the baby probably has primary lung disease caused by infection, hypoperfusion, or pulmonary arteriolar hypertension [Fig. 32.1A (4)]. These babies should be admitted for further evaluation and therapy and the murmur followed closely during therapy. If the saturation by oximetry of an infant without cardiac disease does not improve with oxygen, the patient may have methemoglobinemia [Fig. 32.1A (5)], either on a congenital basis or secondary to gastroenteritis. Co-oximetry studies of blood gases should be performed (see Chapter 87).

Infants Younger Than 3 Years of Age Who Are Not Cyanotic

Infants younger than 3 years who are not cyanotic (Fig. 32.1B) should be evaluated carefully, looking for the abnormalities as outlined previously under the "Examination" section.

If the baby has a negative physical examination, except for the murmur, and appears well [Fig. 32.1B (1)], the murmur may represent a congenital cardiac defect that is physiologically insignificant at the time (small patent ductus, atrial or ventricular septal defect, mild aortic or pulmonary stenosis, partial anomalous pulmonary venous drainage) or a normal murmur.

These children can be followed by the primary care physician or referred to a cardiologist. If doubt exists about the infant's status because of the intensity or transmission of the murmur, an EKG and chest film, and possibly echocardiography, should be ordered; if normal, they confirm the previous impression. Peripheral pulmonary stenosis, related to angulation of the distal pulmonary arteries, is a common cause of normal murmurs in neonates; this murmur transmits well to the back, may be quite loud, but in time, will not be discernible.

If the EKG suggests abnormal atrial or ventricular hypertrophy and the chest film shows cardiac enlargement or abnormal pulmonary vasculature, a more significant degree of the same acyanotic defects, or possibly an acyanotic (or "silent") Tetralogy of Fallot, is likely. Nonemergent referral to a cardiologist is warranted [Fig. 32.1B (2)].

If the acyanotic baby with a murmur appears ill, an EKG and a chest film are obtained. If these are normal, the murmur is most likely inconsequential, and the baby should be evaluated for an underlying medical or surgical illness related to the presenting complaints at this visit [Fig. 32.1B (3)]. It is important to think also of noncardiac conditions causing high flow, such as severe anemia or hyperpyrexia, as causes of the murmur.

If the infant has signs suggesting cardiac failure, EKG findings of marked ventricular hypertrophy, and/or abnormally shaped P waves, it might be indicative of a severe acyanotic congenital cardiac defect (large ventricular septal defect, large patent ductus, severe aortic or pulmonary stenosis) [Fig. 32.1B (4)]. Urgent cardiac consultation should be obtained. In the neonate, consideration should be given to indomethacin or an accepted alternative therapy for closure of the ductus arteriosus to lessen the left-to-right shunting.

A baby in failure with only T-wave and/or ST-segment changes on EKG may have viral myocarditis, primary myocardial disease, anomalous origin of the left coronary artery, or an extracardiac problem that causes high cardiac output (severe anemia, large arteriovenous malformation). Some of these babies, although not cyanotic on the basis of their underlying lesion, may show a degree of diminished saturation on pulse oximetry because of the hypoperfusion related to cardiac failure. All such babies need admission or transfer to a tertiary pediatric center for emergency evaluation and treatment [Fig. 32.1B (5)].

If the chest film and/or EKG is not normal and the baby appears ill but does not have signs that suggest CHF, a primary pulmonary disease should be considered, with the murmur being either a normal one or representing a milder acyanotic defect [Fig. 32.1B (6)]. Admission for further evaluation and therapy is appropriate.

Children 3 Years and Older with Cardiac Murmur

The assessment and disposition of an older child in whom a murmur is discovered is somewhat less of a challenge to the emergency physician. The child is more cooperative and generally more interactive than the infant, and as a result, the sometimes subtle evaluation of the child's state of well-being is less uncertain. The heart rate normally is slower, allowing easier dissection of the murmur.

By the time children who live in geographic areas in which modern medical care is available reach 3 years of age, most

SIGNS AND SYMPTOMS

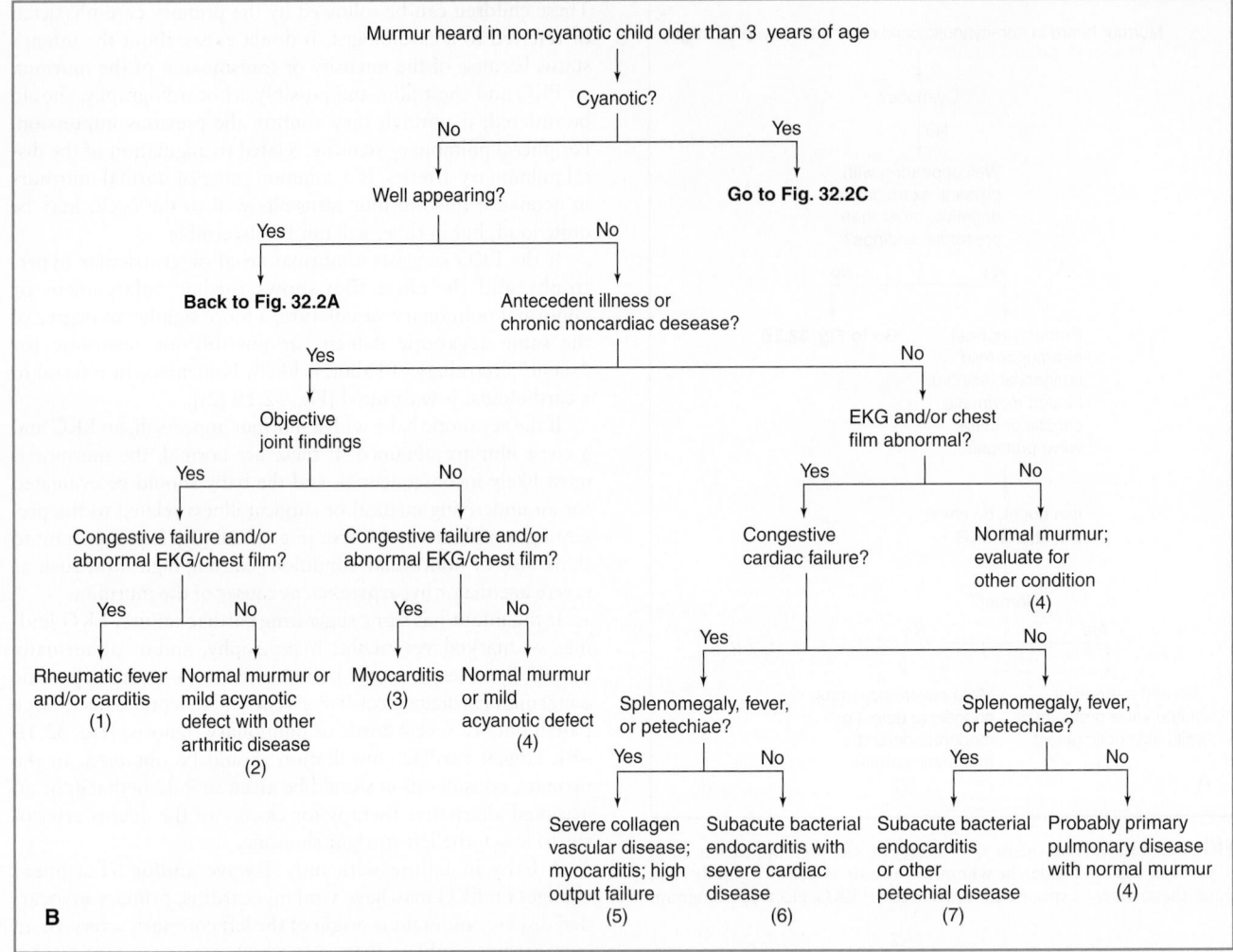

FIGURE 32.2B Assessment of a noncyanotic, sick child 3 years or older in whom a murmur is heard.
(Numbers in parentheses refer to specific citations in text.) EKG, electrocardiogram.

congenital lesions have been discovered and many have been surgically repaired. Acquired cardiac and noncardiac illnesses, therefore, play a more prominent role in assessment. Still, some congenital lesions have gone unrecognized, some do not require surgery, and others that require surgery have not had access because of inadequate insurance or other economic or social reasons.

Normal murmurs are by far the most common ones discovered at a first encounter with an older child. Table 32.1 describes the characteristics generally associated with a normal murmur. If the examining physician is satisfied that the murmur is a normal one and the child has no other symptoms referable to the cardiovascular system, cardiac consultation and further workup is not necessary or advisable. Still, it is often difficult to distinguish a normal murmur from the murmur of relatively benign intracardiac lesions as small atrial or ventricular defects or mild aortic or pulmonic stenosis. The management guidelines outlined in this chapter obviate the need for the emergency physician to be concerned about such a differential. For the purposes of the ED evalua-

tion, it is important to determine only whether the patient is in difficulty or needs further early evaluation. In these age groups also, the presence or absence of cyanosis is a significant finding.

Children 3 Years of Age and Older Who Are Not Cyanotic

The acyanotic child with a murmur who seems essentially well [Fig. 32.2A (1)] and has a negative physical examination other than the precordial finding most likely has a normal murmur but may have a mild acyanotic congenital defect, a healed rheumatic carditis, or a mitral valve prolapse. The femoral artery pulsations should always be palpated for the possibility of coarctation of the distal aorta. In mitral valve prolapse, a midsystolic "click" is a more constant finding than the murmur that follows the click. These children should be followed by the primary care physician. If in doubt because of the intensity or transmission of the murmur, an EKG and chest film, and possibly echocardiography, should be ordered. If these are

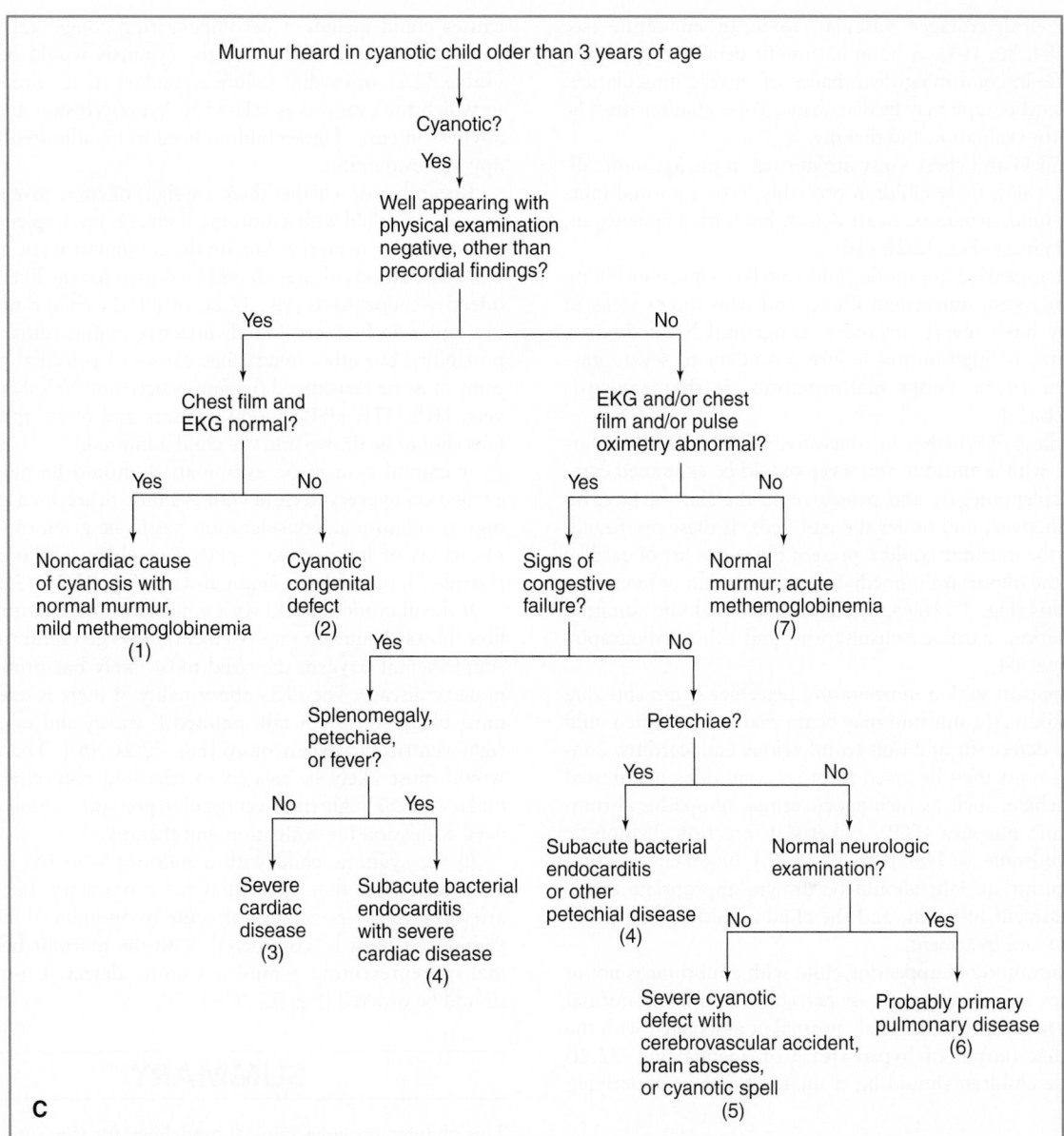

FIGURE 32.2C Assessment of a cyanotic child 3 years of age or older. (Numbers in parentheses refer to specific citations in text.) EKG, electrocardiogram.

normal, one has further assurance that primary care follow-up is all that is necessary. If these are abnormal, there is concern about the possibility of a more severe acyanotic defect or moderately severe healed rheumatic carditis [Fig. 32.2A (2)]. Referral should be made to a cardiologist on a nonemergency basis for further differentiation.

In evaluating the acyanotic child who appears acutely ill and has a murmur [Fig. 32.2B (1)], a careful history should be taken regarding prior or recent antecedent illness, including a significant sore throat or "viral" illness. If there is such a history, the possibility of swollen, red, and tender joints should be sought. If these are present, the child is febrile, and an EKG is abnormal, the child should be hospitalized to be evaluated for the possibility of acute rheumatic fever (see Chapter 84). In

contrast, the acyanotic ill child with objective joint findings but a normal EKG is more likely to have a normal murmur with a concurrent arthritic-like illness, such as septic or reactive arthritis, juvenile rheumatoid arthritis, or Henoch-Schönlein purpura (HSP) [Fig. 32.2B (2)]. These children need diagnostic evaluation of their acute illness and follow-up of the murmur.

The ill-appearing acyanotic child who has a murmur and a history of known chronic or recent antecedent illness, but has no objective joint findings, should have an EKG, a chest film, and echocardiography. If the EKG shows ST-segment and T-wave abnormality and if the heart is enlarged, the patient probably has myocarditis or pericarditis, with the murmur resulting from turbulence created by ventricular dilation or compression and atrioventricular valve insufficiency [Fig. 32.2B (3)]. The cause could be viral, collagen vascular, toxic, or endocrine (see Chapters 84, 86, 101). A brain natriuretic peptide (bnp) might be of value in confirming disturbance of cardiac musculature. The echocardiograph may be diagnostic. These children must be admitted for evaluation and therapy.

If the EKG and chest x-ray are normal in the acyanotic ill-appearing child, these children probably have a normal murmur, or a mild, acyanotic heart defect, but with a concurrent, unrelated illness [Fig. 32.2B (4)].

The ill-appearing acyanotic child who has a murmur but no chronic or recent antecedent illness and who shows signs of CHF may have severe acyanotic congenital heart disease, myocarditis, or high-output failure secondary to severe anemia, large arteriovenous malformation, or thyrotoxicosis [Fig. 32.2B (5)].

Regardless of whether in congestive failure, the ill-appearing infant with a murmur and fever should be examined carefully for splenomegaly and petechiae on the skin surface, on the conjunctivae, and under the nail beds. If these are found, although the murmur could represent the entire list of cardiac diseases, the important immediate concern is that of infectious endocarditis [Fig. 32.2B (5, 6)]. The child should be admitted for evaluation, cardiac consultation, and echocardiography (see Chapter 84).

If the patient with a murmur and petechiae is not showing signs of failure, the murmur may be normal or represent a mild acyanotic defect. In addition to infectious endocarditis, consideration must then be given to other conditions manifested with petechiae, such as meningococcemia, idiopathic thrombocytopenic purpura (ITP), rickettsial infection, hemolytic uremic syndrome, or HSP [Fig. 32.2B (7)]. Blood cultures and other appropriate labs should be drawn, appropriate emergency treatment initiated, and the child admitted for further evaluation and treatment.

If the acyanotic ill-appearing child with a murmur is not in failure, has no splenomegaly or petechiae, and has a normal EKG, the murmur is most likely normal or associated with the high cardiac output of hyperpyrexia or anemia [Fig. 32.2B (4)]. These children should be evaluated for their underlying condition.

Children 3 Years and Older Who Are Cyanotic

As with infants, cyanotic older children (Fig. 32.2C) with murmurs should have an EKG, chest film, pulse oximetry, and possibly an arterial blood gas after a careful history and complete physical examination. If these are normal, except for the cyanosis and murmur, the child probably has a noncardiac cause of the cyanosis (polycythemia, methemoglobinemia) [Fig. 32.2C (1)]. The murmur may be normal or associated with a coincidental acyanotic congenital defect. The primary condition should be investigated. If uncertainty exists about a noncardiac etiology once the studies are obtained, an echocardiogram should her performed.

The cyanotic child who is well appearing but has abnormal EKG, chest film, echocardiography, and pulse oximetry has cyanotic heart disease that possibly could be improved surgically [Fig. 32.2C (2)]. The child should be referred to a cardiologist on a nonemergent basis for further evaluation, including echocardiography.

If the cyanotic child appears acutely ill and has signs of CHF, severe cardiac disease is present [Fig. 32.2C (3)]. The

causes could include a decompensating congenital cyanotic cardiac defect, in which case the cyanosis would be intense (Table 32.2), or cardiac failure secondary to acquired disease, in which the cyanosis is related to hypoperfusion and is usually less intense. These children need to be admitted for therapy and evaluation.

Regardless of whether there are signs of congestive failure in the cyanotic child with a murmur, if there is fever, splenomegaly, and/or petechiae on the skin, on the conjunctivae, or under the nail beds, blood cultures should be drawn for the likelihood of infective endocarditis [Fig. 32.2C (4)]. If the child is not in failure and petechiae are found, infective endocarditis is still a possibility, but other noncardiac causes of petechial presentations must be considered (meningococcemia, Valsalva maneuvers, HUS, ITP, HSP). Blood cultures and other appropriate labs should be drawn and the child admitted.

A careful neurologic examination should be part of the evaluation of every ill child with cyanotic heart disease. If findings are abnormal, consideration has to be given to the complications of hypoxemic "spells," cerebrovascular accident ("stroke"), or, if febrile, brain abscess [Fig. 32.2C (5)].

If the ill cyanotic child with a murmur and abnormal chest film shows significant improvement of oxygen saturation with supplemental oxygen, the child most likely has primary pulmonary disease. The EKG abnormality, if there is one, would most likely consist of tall, pointed P waves and evidence of right ventricular hypertrophy [Fig. 32.2C (6)]. The murmur would most likely be related to tricuspid regurgitation secondary to the high right ventricular pressure. These children need admission for evaluation and therapy.

In the cyanotic child with a murmur who has a normal EKG and chest film, abnormal pulse oximetry, but normal arterial PO_2, the possibility of acute toxin-induced methemoglobinemia must be considered, with the murmur being normal or representing a mild acyanotic defect. Co-oximetry should be ordered [Fig. 32.2C (1, 7)].

SUMMARY

This chapter provides clinical guidelines for the initial assessment and disposition of infants and children in whom a murmur is discovered during a first visit. Although diagnostic pathways have been suggested, it has also been shown that definitive diagnosis of the underlying cardiac defect is not the primary aim of ED evaluation; careful assessment of the patient and safe disposition are required at first encounter. The emphasis, in other words, is on the patient and less so on the murmur.

Suggested Readings

Athreya B, Silverman BK. *Pediatric physical diagnosis*. East Norwalk, CT: Appleton-Century-Crofts, 1985.

Barrett MJ, Lacey CS, Sekara AE, et al. Mastering cardiac murmurs: the power of repetition. *Chest* 2004;126:470–475.

Fuerst RS. Use of pulse oximetry. In: King C, Henretig FM, eds. *Textbook of pediatric emergency procedures*. 2nd ed. Philadelphia: Wolters Kluwer 2008:749–754.

Gersony WM. Major advances in pediatric cardiology in the 20th century. *J Pediatr* 2001;139(2):328–333.

Goldmuntz E. The epidemiology and genetics of congenital heart disease. *Clin Perinatol* 2001;28:1–10.

Hoffmann JIE. Cardiology. In: Rudolph CD, Hoffmann JIE, Rudolph AM, eds. *Pediatrics*. 21st ed. New York: McGraw-Hill, 2003:1780–1842.

SIGNS AND SYMPTOMS

TABLE 34.3

COMMON CAUSES OF HYPERTENSION

Age group	Cause
Newborn infants	Renal artery thrombosis, renal artery stenosis, congenital renal malformations, coarctation of the aorta, bronchopulmonary dysplasia
Infancy–6 yr	Renal parenchymal diseases,[a] coarctation of the aorta, renal artery stenosis
6–10 yr	Renal parenchymal diseases, renal artery stenosis, essential hypertension (including obesity)
Adolescence	Essential hypertension (including obesity), renal parenchymal diseases

[a]Includes renal structural and inflammatory lesions and tumors.
Adapted from the Task Force on Blood Pressure Control in Children. Report of the second task force on blood pressure control in children—1987. *Pediatrics* 1987;79:1–25.

for hypertension and eliciting signs and symptoms of end-organ damage resulting from the hypertensive process. In the absence of any concerning findings in the history or physical examination, the child with mild or moderate hypertension should be referred for follow-up with his or her primary care physician. Although it is appropriate to initiate the process of patient education in the ED regarding weight loss, dietary salt reduction, and exercise, a definitive diagnosis of hypertension should not be offered until the child has had repeated measurements of his or her blood pressure on several occasions.

The workup of a child with severe hypertension requires careful evaluation for the presence of clinical findings that may represent either the primary cause of the elevated blood pressure or the secondary systemic effects of hypertension. Relevant history includes frequent urinary tract infections, unexplained fevers, hematuria, dysuria, frequency, and edema—all suggestive of possible renal disease. A history of umbilical artery catheterization as a neonate may indicate the risk of renal artery stenosis or thrombosis. Ingestion of prescription, over-the-counter, or illicit drugs, or rapid withdrawal of some blood pressure medications used for chronic hypertension, may support the diagnosis of drug-induced hypertension. Alternatively, a history of sweating, flushing, palpitations, fever, and weight loss may indicate a pheochromocytoma.

Physical examination should concentrate on identifying potentially involved organ systems, paying particular attention to cardiovascular, renal, and central nervous systems. The cardiac examination should inspect for the evidence of congestive heart failure (CHF) and pulmonary edema. Absent or decreased femoral pulses are suggestive of aortic coarctation. Abdominal examination may reveal the presence of a bruit or renal mass such as Wilms' tumor, implicating a renovascular cause for the hypertension. Peripheral edema may suggest volume overload from renal failure. Neurologic evaluation should include observation for sensorimotor symmetry and appropriate cerebellar function. Funduscopic examination for hypertensive changes such as hemorrhages, infarcts, and disc

edema should be conducted, in addition to testing the pupillary light reflex and visual acuity.

Initial investigations for severe hypertension in the ED should be limited to the most basic of tests. Blood studies including a complete blood cell count, electrolytes, blood urea nitrogen, serum creatinine, and urinalysis are usually warranted. In addition, a urine culture should be obtained in all girls and in boys with known renal pathologic conditions. A chest radiograph and an echocardiogram may help evaluate the extent damage from hypertension and may help detect the presence of CHF. If there are concerning findings on the initial cardiovascular examination, an echocardiogram may also be warranted. Although several additional studies exist for the evaluation of hypertension, these are rarely part of the routine ED assessment.

When the cause of hypertension is not readily apparent, a systematic approach to evaluation is indicated (Fig. 34.1). Because underlying renal disease is among the more common causes of hypertension in children, assessing for renal pathology based on historical elements, physical examination, and an initial urinalysis is often a good starting point. If this assessment is unrevealing, attention should be directed to the cardiovascular system, as coarctation of the aorta is most likely to manifest in a toddler or an older child with previously undiagnosed hypertension. When a careful evaluation of the renal and cardiovascular systems is not revealing, a detailed neurologic assessment is in order because any condition accompanied by increased intracranial pressure may elevate the systemic blood pressure. The history and signs of head trauma are usually obvious but may be occult when injuries in young children are not witnessed or are intentionally inflicted. Specific questioning about the ingestion of illicit drugs or other medications and a toxicologic screen are an appropriate next step if renal, cardiovascular, and neurologic causes are ruled out. Finally, although the endocrine disorders are relatively rare, a careful history and directed physical examination may identify temperature sensitivity, a goiter or abdominal striae suggestive of hyperthyroidism, or Cushing's syndrome. Intermittent headaches and flushing occur with pheochromocytoma, and elevated circulating catecholamines are responsible for hypertension seen in neuroblastoma. A negative evaluation for an underlying cause of hypertension in the ED is compatible with, but not sufficient for, the diagnosis of essential hypertension. Follow-up is always indicated.

MANAGEMENT (SEE CHAPTER 100)

There is little consistency in the literature as to when treatment of hypertension should be initiated, particularly in the ED setting. Acuteness of the rise in blood pressure levels, the presence of symptoms, preexisting medical problems, and the extent of end-organ damage are all factors to be considered (Fig. 34.2). According to the Fourth Report, immediate evaluation and treatment should be undertaken for patients with symptomatic stage 2 hypertension. However, some authors suggest that severe hypertension, even if asymptomatic, warrants acute treatment. In the end, the decision to treat a patient acutely in the ED setting will be based on a blood

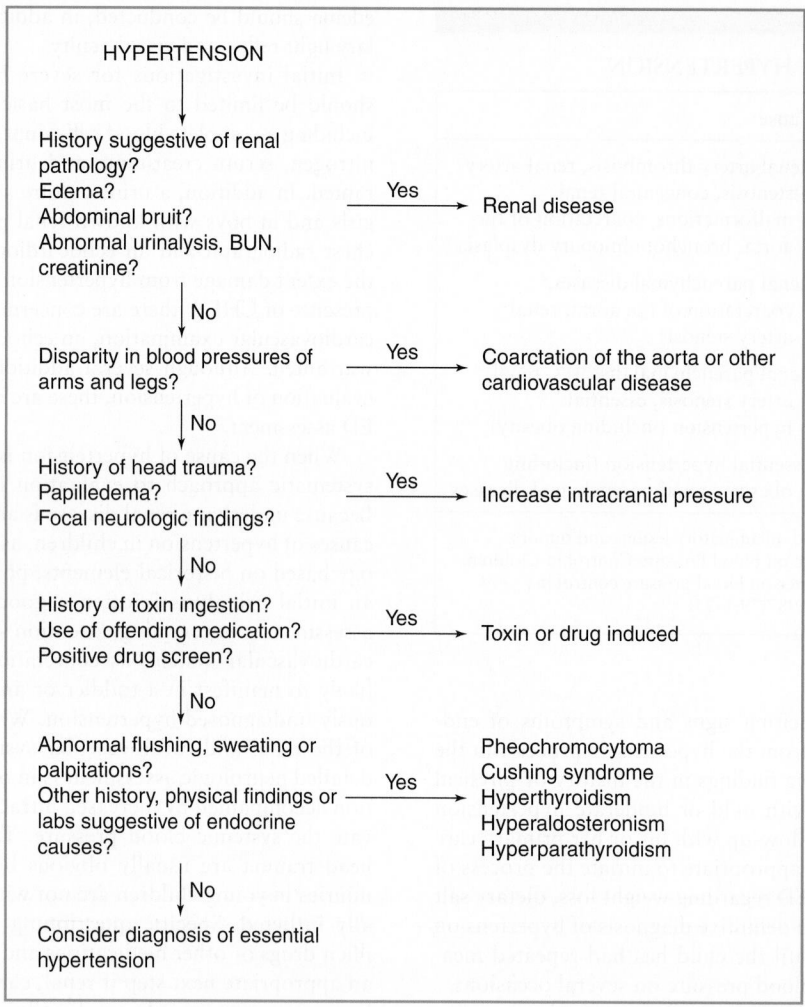

FIGURE 34.1 Diagnostic approach to the most common causes of acute, persistent hypertension in a previously healthy child. CHF, congestive heart failure.

pressure measurement that the clinician feels is imminently dangerous to the patient.

For children with severe hypertension, treatment must be rapid and, at the same time, cautious. There is a compelling reason for a conservative approach. Under normal conditions, autoregulation maintains a constant cerebral perfusion pressure, dilating cerebral vasculature when blood pressure falls and constricting cerebral vasculature when blood pressure level rises. Particularly in chronic hypertension, the range of pressures over which autoregulation occurs shifts upward to protect the brain from excessive perfusion. As such, cerebral vasculature may no longer be able to maintain perfusion pressure at lower ranges of blood pressure values. Too rapid a decrease in blood pressure levels can result in dangerous underperfusion and cerebral ischemia. Although there is no consensus on how slowly blood pressure levels should be lowered, a good rule of thumb is to reduce blood pressure levels by no more than 25% in the first 6 to 8 hours. Thereafter, the goal of therapy should be to normalize the blood pressure levels over a period of 3 to 4 days.

In addition to treating the elevation in blood pressure levels, the child with complications of hypertension may also require treatment of the specific complications. Careful attention should be paid to managing the child's airway, breathing, and circulation. The child with seizures or CHF often requires the standard treatment of these problems in addition to antihypertensive therapy. However, when other complications are believed to be secondary to severe hypertension, treatment of the hypertension should take precedence.

SPECIFIC THERAPY

For the treatment of hypertensive emergencies, it is recommended that an intravenous antihypertensive formulation be used because of its more predictable pharmacokinetic profile and ease of titration. Hypertensive urgencies may be managed using either intravenous or oral antihypertensive agents.

The choice of drugs (Table 34.4) depends on the severity of the patient's hypertension, the patient's current medications,

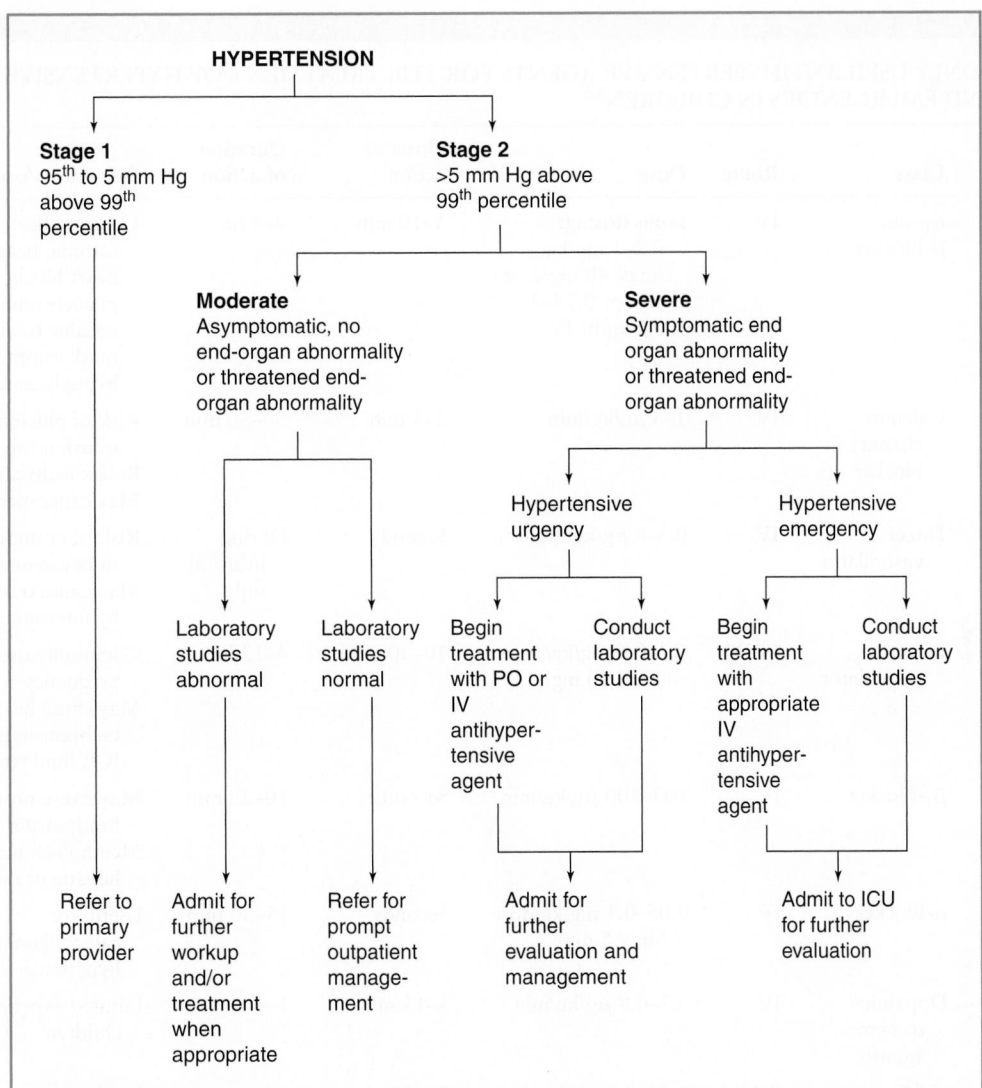

HYPERTENSION

Stage 1
95th to 5 mm Hg
above 99th
percentile

Stage 2
>5 mm Hg above
99th percentile

Moderate
Asymptomatic, no
end-organ abnormality
or threatened end-
organ abnormality

Severe
Symptomatic end
organ abnormality
or threatened end-
organ abnormality

Hypertensive
urgency

Hypertensive
emergency

Laboratory
studies
abnormal

Laboratory
studies
normal

Begin
treatment
with PO or
IV
antihyper-
tensive
agent

Conduct
laboratory
studies

Begin
treatment
with
appropriate
IV
antihyper-
tensive
agent

Conduct
laboratory
studies

Refer to
primary
provider

Admit for
further
workup
and/or
treatment
when
appropriate

Refer for
prompt
outpatient
manage-
ment

Admit for
further
evaluation and
management

Admit to ICU
for further
evaluation

FIGURE 34.2 Approach to the initial emergency department triage and stabilization of the persistently hypertensive child. ICU, intensive care unit.

SIGNS AND SYMPTOMS

underlying medical conditions, the suspected cause of the hypertension, and the organs involved. Ideal medications for the treatment of hypertensive emergencies have a rapid onset of action and short half-life, allowing for the easy titration necessary for controlled blood pressure reduction. It is difficult to recommend one particular type of antihypertensive agent over another, as the choice of agent is so often multifactorial. However, the most commonly used agents for hypertensive emergencies include nicardipine, labetalol, and sodium nitroprusside. Hypertension caused by a catecholamine-secreting tumor (pheochromocytoma) might best be controlled with an α-blocking agent such as phentolamine. Elevated blood pressure levels secondary to high renin states may respond best to an angiotensin-converting enzyme inhibitor such as enalaprilat. However, if hypertension is associated with an intracerebral bleed, medications that cause an increase in cerebral blood flow, such as nicardipine and hydralazine, are best avoided.

Intravenous Antihypertensive Medications

Labetalol

Labetalol is a combined α_1- and β-adrenergic blocking agent. As such, it has the ability to reduce peripheral vascular resistance with little to no effect on heart rate or cardiac output. It has a rapid onset of action (usually 5 to 10 minutes) and a plasma half-life of 3 to 5 hours when given intravenously. Because of its duration of action, labetalol can be more difficult to titrate to effect than other agents and therefore is not routinely used as a continuous infusion.

Dosing recommendations for labetalol use in hypertensive emergencies vary widely. The drug may be administered by intermittent bolus dosing, or by a bolus dose followed by a continuous infusion (See Table 34.4). Recommendations for bolus dosing are 0.2 to 1 mg per kg and for infusion 0.25 to

TABLE 34.4

MOST COMMONLY USED ANTIHYPERTENSIVE AGENTS FOR THE TREATMENT OF HYPERTENSIVE URGENCIES AND EMERGENCIES IN CHILDREN[a,b]

Drug	Class	Route	Dose	Onset of action	Duration of action	Side effects/comments[c]
Labetalol	α_1- and β-Blocker	IV	Bolus dosing: 0.2–1 mg/kg (max 40 mg/dose) Infusion: 0.25–3 mg/kg/hr IV	5–10 min	2–4 hr	Contraindicated in asthma, heart failure, heart block, pheochromocytoma, cocaine toxicity; may mask symptoms of hypoglycemia
Nicardipine	Calcium channel blocker	IV	1–3 μg/kg/min	2–5 min	30–60 min	Risk of phlebitis at infusion site Reflex tachycardia May cause increased ICP
Sodium nitroprusside[d]	Direct vasodilator	IV	0.3–8 μg/kg/min	Seconds	During infusion only	Risk of cyanide/thiocyanate toxicity May cause transient hypotension
Hydralazine[d]	Direct vasodilator	IV/IM	0.2–0.6 mg/kg/dose (max 20 mg)	10–30 min	4–12 hr	Commonly used in pregnancy May cause headaches, tachycardia, increased ICP, fluid retention
Esmolol	β_1-Blocker	IV	100–500 μg/kg/min	Seconds	10–20 min	May cause profound bradycardia Metabolism independent of hepatic or renal processes
Phentolamine[d]	α-Blocker	IV	0.05–0.1 mg/kg/dose (max 5 mg)	Seconds	15–30 min	Useful for catecholamine-induced hypertensive crisis
Fenoldopam[d]	Dopamine receptor agonist	IV	0.2–0.8 μg/kg/min	5–15 min	1–4 hr	Limited experience in children
Nifedipine	Calcium channel blocker	PO	0.25–0.5 mg/kg/dose (max 10 mg)	20–30 min	6 hr	Precipitous decrease in MAP associated with doses > 0.25 mg/kg/dose Difficult to administer in exact doses May cause dizziness, flushing, rebound hypertension
Isradipine	Calcium channel blocker	PO	0.05–0.1 mg/kg/dose (max 5 mg)	30 min–2 hr	12 hr	Limited experience with pediatric use
Clonidine[d]	α_2-Receptor agonist	PO	0.05–0.1 mg/dose, may be repeated up to 0.8 mg of total dose	15–30 min	6–8 hr	Dry mouth, drowsiness
Minoxidil[d]	Direct vasodilator	PO	0.1–0.2 mg/kg/dose (max 10 mg)	Within 1 hr	8–12 hr	Potent vasodilator Hirsutism, fluid retention, primarily seen with long-term use

IV, intravenous; ICP, intracranial pressure; IM, intramuscular; PO, by mouth; MAP, mean arterial pressure.
[a]Because several of these medications have not been extensively tested in children, existing pharmacokinetic data are frequently based on studies in adults.
[b]Dosing recommendations vary by source.
[c]See additional comments and cautions in text.
[d]Indicates drugs with Food and Drug Administration–approved pediatric labeling for use in hypertension.

3 mg per kg per hour. Because of its more potent β-blocking effects, it should be used neither in patients with asthma, heart block, or CHF nor for the treatment of hypertension in patients with pheochromocytoma or sympathomimetic drug overdose (e.g., cocaine; see Chapter 102), due to its potential to cause unopposed alpha effects.

Nicardipine

Nicardipine is a dihydropyridine calcium channel blocker that prevents vascular smooth muscle contraction by blocking the movement of calcium across the cell. This results in a reduction in peripheral vascular resistance without compromising cardiac output. Its onset of action within 1 to 2 minutes of administration and short elimination half-life make it relatively easy to titrate. Nicardipine is the preferred agent for the treatment of hypertensive emergencies at many institutions because of its safety profile, ability to produce a relatively rapid effect, and low risk for causing hypotension. Recommended dosing is 1 to 3 μg per kg per minute by continuous infusion. Excessive reductions in blood pressure levels, though uncommon, can be reversed by the administration of calcium. Because it elevates intracranial pressure, nicardipine should be avoided in patients with increased intracranial pressure. Reflex tachycardia that is usually not clinically significant and phlebitis at the site of administration are known adverse effects of the drug.

Sodium Nitroprusside

Nitroprusside is a powerful vasodilator, affecting both arteriolar and venous smooth muscle cells. Its onset of action is almost immediate, and its duration of action is extremely short, allowing for easy titration of the drug to the desired blood pressure level. Because of its venous dilatory effects, nitroprusside reduces preload and often improves cardiac output if CHF is present. It may also increase intracerebral pressure, though some note that a rise in cerebral blood flow is offset by a concomitant drop in systemic pressure. Nitroprusside is metabolized to thiocyanate, and cyanide is an intermediary in its metabolism. Consequently, cyanide and thiocyanate toxicity must be considered a risk of its use, particularly for infusions lasting more than 24 to 48 hours. Such toxicity is also compounded by liver or renal impairment, as both organ systems are involved in the metabolism of sodium nitroprusside. In cases of renal or liver impairment, and for infusions lasting more than 24 hours, thiocyanate levels should be monitored daily. Because of this toxicity and its propensity to cause more episodes of transient hypotension than other agents, some institutions use only sodium nitroprusside as a second-line agent.

Nitroprusside is given as an intravenous infusion, starting at a dosage of 0.3 to 0.5 μg per kg per minute and increasing as needed to 8 μg per kg per minute. The patient should be kept in the recumbent position because of the frequency of orthostatic hypotension. The degree of drop in blood pressure levels is dose related; thus, the infusion should be started at the low end of the dosage range and titrated to achieve the desired blood pressure levels. The average dosage required for the control of hypertension is approximately 3 μg per kg per minute. Because nitroprus-

side has an extremely short half-life, blood pressure returns to pretreatment levels within 1 to 10 minutes of the cessation of the infusion.

Hydralazine

Hydralazine is an arteriolar vasodilator that can be given intravenously, intramuscularly, and orally, but onset of action is faster, in the order of 10 to 30 minutes, when administered intravenously. Its relative safety and efficacy, combined with extensive clinical experience, make it among the most commonly used agents for hypertension associated with pregnancy. Known side effects include reflex tachycardia, fluid retention, facial flushing, and increased intracranial pressure. These adverse effects and the availability of more potent, faster acting agents have largely replaced its use in the ED setting for nonpregnant patients. Hydralazine is given at a dose of 0.2 to 0.6 mg per kg intravenously or intramuscularly, or at a dose of 0.25 mg per kg orally to a maximum of 25 mg.

Esmolol

Esmolol is a selective β_1-blocker that has traditionally been used for the treatment of early postoperative hypertension following repair of congenital heart disease. Primary effects are at the level of the heart and kidneys. It has an onset of action of approximately 60 seconds and a duration of action of 10 to 20 minutes. It is usually administered by continuous infusion after an initial bolus dose. A single pediatric trial found esmolol to be effective for use after coarctation of the aorta repair by administering an initial bolus of 125 to 500 μg per kg followed by an infusion of 125 to 500 μg per kg per minute. Metabolism is independent of both hepatic and renal processes, making a good choice for use in patients with multiorgan failure. Although reported use in hypertensive children outside of the postoperative setting is limited, the drug certainly has potential for use in the ED setting.

Phentolamine

Phentolamine is an α-adrenergic receptor antagonist that is particularly useful in the treatment of hypertension associated with catecholamine-induced hypertensive crises, as seen with pheochromocytoma or sympathomimetic toxicity. Effectiveness has not been shown to be consistent for other types of hypertensive crises. Dosing recommendations vary widely. Some recommend 0.05 to 0.1 mg per kg per dose intravenously to a maximum of 5 mg, and others recommend a pediatric dose of 1 mg administered intravenously or intramuscularly, repeated as needed to achieve appropriate blood pressure control.

Enalaprilat

Enalaprilat is an angiotensin-converting enzyme inhibitor that can be useful in high renin states. It is contraindicated for use in patients with bilateral renal artery stenosis. Because of the high incidence of renovascular disease in the pediatric population, and limited pediatric experience with its use, caution must be exercised before using this agent for the treatment of severe hypertension in the ED. It should be administered at a dose of 0.05 to 0.1 mg per kg intravenously up to a maximum of 1.25 mg.

Oral Antihypertensive Medications

Nifedipine

Short-acting nifedipine is a calcium channel blocker that works by decreasing peripheral vascular resistance. Its use in children remains controversial, owing to the serious hypotensive side effects of the drug experienced in adults. However, similar exaggerated effects have not been clearly demonstrated in children.

Although traditionally administered sublingually, more recent reports suggest more predictable absorption when the capsule is bitten and swallowed. Nifedipine is administered at a dose of 0.25 to 0.5 mg per kg up to a maximum of 10 mg. Onset of action is within 20 to 30 minutes; duration of action is approximately 6 hours. Precipitous decreases in mean arterial pressure (>25%) have been associated with doses exceeding 0.25 mg per kg. There are also isolated case reports of rebound hypertension causing adverse neurologic events after the use of short-acting nifedipine in children with hypertensive encephalopathy. Because of the difficulties in titrating to effect and its slower onset of action, the use of nifedipine should be limited to hypertensive urgencies only. Facial flushing and increased cerebral blood flow are other side effects of nifedipine administration.

Isradipine

A second-generation dihydropyridine calcium channel blocker, isradipine has received more recent attention for use in children with severe hypertension. Onset of action is usually 30 minutes to 2 hours, with a half-life of 3 to 8 hours. It has selective action on vascular smooth muscle, which allows it to be used in children with compromised myocardial function. At present, only anecdotal experience with its use for severe elevations in blood pressure levels in children exists. Dosing ranges from 0.05 to 0.1 mg per kg per dose to a maximum of 5 mg, given 2 to 4 times daily.

Clonidine

Clonidine is an α_2-adrenergic agonist that works by reducing cerebral sympathetic output. Its onset of action is 15 to 30 minutes following administration. It is recommended by some for the management of hypertensive urgencies, although most studies have evaluated its use as a treatment of chronic primary hypertension. The drug has been approved by the Food and Drug Administration for use in children older than 12 years. Side effects include somnolence and dry mouth.

Minoxidil

Minoxidil is a direct vasodilator that exerts its effect on the potassium channels of smooth muscle cells causing hyperpolarization and eventual relaxation of arterioles. Venous vessels are not affected. This has been shown to be effective particularly in children with chronic hypertension experiencing acute elevations. It is recommended for occasional use in hypertensive urgencies.

Newer Agents

Fenoldopam

Fenoldopam is a selective dopamine agonist causing vasodilation of the renal, coronary, cerebral, and splanchnic vasculature, resulting in a decrease in mean arterial pressure. The use of fenoldopam in pediatric patients has increased in recent years. Case reports have demonstrated success with its use for controlled hypotension during spinal instrumentation and in the intensive care setting when conventional therapy was unsuccessful. More recently, a clinical dose-ranging study of the use of fenoldopam in children showed that although fenoldopam resulted in a decrease in blood pressure levels, this decrease was less than that observed in adults.

In adults, peak effects of fenoldopam have been observed in 5 to 15 minutes, with steady-state serum levels achieved in 30 to 60 minutes. Infusion rates of 0.2 to 0.8 μg per kg per minute are recommended for use in children. Side effects include reflex tachycardia, increased intracranial pressure, and increased intraocular pressure. Although pediatric experience with fenoldopam is limited, it appears to be a reasonable alternative to other more conventional therapies.

Clevidipine

Clevidipine is a recently developed, ultra-short-acting dihydropyridine calcium channel antagonist with high specificity for vascular smooth muscle. Its half-life is only a few minutes, making it relatively easy to titrate when administered as a continuous infusion. Its decreased tendency to cause tachycardia when compared with sodium nitroprusside and more rapid offset of action when compared with nicardipine make it a strong contender for the management of severe elevations in blood pressure levels in the ED. Clevidipine has not yet been approved for use in pediatric patients and no dosing recommendations in children exist as of yet, although pediatric trials are expected to begin in the next few years.

SUMMARY

It is not unusual that a child presenting to the ED will have an elevation in blood pressure levels. In many such cases, the blood pressure level will normalize with rest or acclimation to the environment. Occasionally, however, the elevation in blood pressure levels will be sustained. In children with asymptomatic mild hypertension and no target organ involvement, the emergency physician must ensure adequate follow-up. Moderate or severe hypertension that affects or threatens to affect end organs, in contrast, requires evaluation and initiation of treatment in the ED (Fig. 34.2). In severe or life-threatening cases, blood pressure reduction will often need to be instituted before the cause of the hypertension is known.

Suggested Readings

Adamson PC, Rhodes LA, Saul JP, et al. The pharmacokinetics of esmolol in pediatric subjects with supraventricular arrhythmias. *Pediatr Cardiol* 2006; 27(4):420–427.

Dittrich S, Germanakis J, Dittrich H, et al. Comparison of sodium nitroprusside versus esmolol for the treatment of hypertension following repair of coarctation of the aorta. *Interact Cardiovasc Thorac Surg* 2003;2(2):111–115.

Flynn JT. Pediatric hypertension: recent trends and accomplishments, future challenges. *Am J Hypertens* 2008;21(6):605–612.

Flynn JT, Tullus K. Severe hypertension in children and adolescents: pathophysiology and treatment. *Pediatr Nephrol* 2009 Jun;24(6):1101-12. Epub 2008 Oct 7.

Hammer GB, Verghese ST, Drover DR, et al. Pharmacokinetics and pharmacodynamics of fenoldopam mesylate for blood pressure control in pediatric patients. *BMC Anesthesiol* 2008;8:6.

Heilpern K. Pathophysiology of hypertension. *Ann Emerg Med* 2008;51(3)(suppl):S5–S6.

Lustik SJ, Papadakos PJ, Jackman KV, et al. Nicardipine versus nitroprusside for deliberate hypotension during idiopathic scoliosis repair. *J Clin Anesth* 2004;16(1):25–33.

National High Blood Pressure Education Program Working Group on High Blood Pressure in Children and Adolescents. The fourth report on the diagnosis, evaluation, and treatment of high blood pressure in children and adolescents. *Pediatrics* 2004;114(2)(suppl):555–576.

Patel HP, Mitsnefes M. Advances in the pathogenesis and management of hypertensive crisis. *Curr Opin Pediatr* 2005;17(2):210–214.

Porto I. Hypertensive emergencies in children. *J Pediatr Health Care* 2000;14(6):312–317.

Sahney S. A review of calcium channel antagonists in the treatment of pediatric hypertension. *Pediatr Drugs* 2006;8(6):357–373.

Tabbutt S, Nicolson SC, Adamson PC, et al. The safety, efficacy, and pharmacokinetics of esmolol for blood pressure control immediately after repair of coarctation of the aorta in infants and children: a multicenter, double-blind, randomized trial. *J Thorac Cardiovasc Surg* 2008;136(2):321–328.

Tenney F, Sakarcan A. Nicardipine is a safe and effective agent in pediatric hypertensive emergencies. *Am J Kidney Dis* 2000;35(5):E20.

Tobias JD. Fenoldopam for controlled hypotension during spinal fusion in children and adolescents. *Paediatr Anaesth* 2000;10(3):261–266.

Yiu V, Orrbine E, Rosychuk RJ, et al. The safety and use of short-acting nifedipine in hospitalized hypertensive children. *Pediatr Nephrol* 2004;19(6):644–650.

SIGNS AND SYMPTOMS

CHAPTER 35 ■ IMMOBILE ARM

SARA A. SCHUTZMAN, MD

An infant or child brought for the evaluation of an "immobile arm" is not moving the limb because of pain or weakness. The evaluation is often a challenge because most of these children are preverbal; therefore, the history is second or third hand if available at all, patients are unable to report symptoms or pain location, and the physical examination is often difficult because of children's fear of strangers. These children can be considered as having an upper-extremity equivalent of "limp." By using historical information, physical findings, selective radiologic studies, and laboratory tests, children with this complaint can be diagnosed and managed.

DIFFERENTIAL DIAGNOSIS

Table 35.1 lists most conditions that cause decreased use of the arm. Trauma is by far the most common cause of decreased arm movement in children (Table 35.2). Any injury from the clavicle to the fingertips can cause arm pain in children and can lead to diminished use of the limb. These injuries range from a serious (fracture or dislocation with neurovascular compromise; Table 35.3) to a simple contusion. Most young children with diminished arm use will have a radial head subluxation ("nursemaid's elbow"), fracture, or soft-tissue injury. Although one can often elicit a history of trauma, the diagnosis must be considered even in its absence because of unwitnessed events in preverbal children or, less commonly, intentional injuries inflicted by caregivers who are not forthcoming. With musculoskeletal injuries, the child may have an obvious abnormality, such as a deformity or contusion, or more subtle findings of localized tenderness or decreased arm movement. Children with hemophilia may have hemarthrosis or hematoma with minimal trauma. Radiographs are useful for demonstrating most fractures or dislocations but may appear normal with Salter-Harris type I fractures and nursemaid's elbow, as well as with contusions and other minor soft-tissue injuries (see also Chapter 114).

Although much less common than trauma, infection may also cause decreased use of an arm. There may be a history of fever, and onset of arm disuse is often less abrupt than with trauma. The infection can be located at any point from the shoulder to finger and may be superficial (e.g., cellulitis, paronychia) or deep. Arthritis and osteomyelitis frequently have associated localized swelling, warmth, and tenderness; infected joints usually have limited, painful range of motion. With more severe infections, the child may be febrile and appear ill (especially if bacteremic). Laboratory findings may include elevated white blood cell count, elevated sedimentation rate (ESR), or elevated C-reactive protein (CRP) level, and blood culture results may yield the offending agent. Acutely,

radiographs often are nondiagnostic; if arthritis or osteomyelitis is suspected, ultrasound, bone scintigraphy, or magnetic resonance imaging (MRI) should be considered (depending on the clinical scenario), with arthrocentesis or subperiosteal/bone aspiration as indicated (see Chapters 92 and 125). Congenital syphilis, although unusual, may present as pseudoparalysis in infants due to metaphysitis, periostitis, osteochondritis, or pathologic fracture, with bony changes evident on the radiograph.

Other inflammatory causes of arm pain include noninfectious arthritis and myositis. In addition to a swollen, tender joint, children with arthritis caused by postinfectious, Lyme, and rheumatologic diseases may have multiple joint involvement, rash, fever, adenopathy, heart murmur, hematuria, or bloody stools. If the examination suggests an inflammatory arthritis but cannot exclude a septic process, then arthrocentesis is necessary for definitive diagnosis.

Tumors are a rare cause of diminished arm use. The tumors can be benign or malignant and of bone, cartilage, or muscle, or they may represent neoplastic infiltration of bone marrow (e.g., leukemia, neuroblastoma). Tumors are usually less acute in onset; cardinal symptoms may include pain and, perhaps, increasing mass or joint swelling, although the lesions may be asymptomatic. Occasionally, tumors lead to a pathologic fracture. Systemic complaints, including fever, malaise, and weight loss, may be present. Physical examination may reveal localized tenderness, joint swelling, or a mass of the soft tissue or bone. With leukemia or neuroblastoma, fever, abdominal mass, hepatosplenomegaly, or pathologic adenopathy may also be found. Plain radiographs are of obvious importance; lesion location and radiologic appearance (density and peripheral margin) can be diagnostically significant. Complete blood cell count (CBC) and ESR are helpful in screening for possible infection or bone marrow neoplasm (see Chapter 97).

Children with neurologic abnormalities will have diminished use of an arm because of weakness, with or without pain. An isolated monoplegia may be caused by a radiculopathy, plexopathy, or neuropathy that results from compression, inflammation, or injury. Trauma, particularly traction on the arm, is a common mechanism that leads to neurologic abnormalities (e.g., brachial plexus injury from birth); however, nontraumatic conditions may have an abrupt onset with no apparent antecedent illness. The child will have diminished arm movement, weakness, and may even experience pain; unlike the previously discussed causes of arm disuse, however, the pain (if present) is usually not reproducible with palpation and is not accompanied by swelling or redness. Reflexes may be diminished or absent. It is important to identify any associated neurologic abnormalities because facial or leg weakness may be subtle but would point to a lesion in the central nervous system.

TABLE 35.1

DIFFERENTIAL DIAGNOSIS OF THE IMMOBILE ARM

Trauma
Fracture
Dislocation/subluxation
Hemarthrosis (hemophilia)
Soft-tissue injury
Nerve injury
Splinter/hair tourniquet

Infection
Septic arthritis
Osteomyelitis
Soft-tissue infection
  Cellulitis
  Abscess
  Lymphangitis
  Paronychia/felon/tenosynovitis
Congenital syphilis

Tumor
Primary musculoskeletal
  Bone
  Cartilage
  Soft tissue
Bone marrow infiltration
  Leukemia
  Neuroblastoma
  Lymphoma

Inflammation
Arthritis
  Juvenile rheumatoid arthritis
  Other collagen vascular
  Postinfectious
  Lyme
Myositis

Infarction
Hemoglobinopathy
  Hand-foot syndrome
  Acute pain crisis
  Avascular necrosis
Avascular necrosis

Neurologic
Radiculopathy
Plexopathy
Neuropathy
Injury
  Traction
  Pressure
  Laceration

Miscellaneous
Reflex sympathetic dystrophy

Children with hemoglobinopathies (most commonly sickle cell disease) may present with decreased arm use because of vasoocclusive crisis, causing ischemia or infarction of bone marrow with acute bone pain. Long bones are commonly affected; however, young children frequently have involvement of the small bones of the hands and feet (dactylitis). Usually, no precipitating events are identified. The child experiences pain with localized tenderness and swelling of the involved areas; there may be associated warmth and erythema. Acutely,

TABLE 35.2

COMMON CAUSES OF DIMINISHED ARM USE

Newborns/infants
  Clavicle fracture
  Brachial plexus injury
  Septic arthritis/osteomyelitis

Infants/preschool-aged children
  Nursemaid's elbow
  Fracture
  Soft-tissue injury

there are no bony abnormalities on radiographs. Because the "hand-foot syndrome" may be the first clinical manifestation of sickle cell disease, all children at risk for sickle cell disease with limb pain or swelling (or fever) must be screened for hemoglobinopathy if not tested previously. It is also particularly important to consider septic arthritis and osteomyelitis in children with sickle cell disease, as they are susceptible to infection, and the clinical findings may overlap with bone infarction, particularly if fever and leukocytosis are present (see Chapter 91).

Several other much less common processes can cause decreased upper-limb use. These include avascular necrosis of the humeral head or capitellum in otherwise healthy children and reflex sympathetic dystrophy.

EVALUATION AND DECISION

The evaluation of the child who has diminished arm movement consists of a complete history and a thorough physical examination, with radiologic studies and laboratory tests when indicated. On the basis of these findings, appropriate management can be undertaken.

A history of any trauma should be ascertained. Details of the event may provide clues to the type of injury incurred; a fall onto an outstretched hand may cause a wrist, forearm, or elbow injury, whereas a sudden arm pull by a caregiver can cause dislocation or subluxation of the radial head ("nursemaid's elbow"). Of note is that some children with radial head subluxation may have a mechanism of injury other than a pull. If an immediate causative traumatic event is not elicited, the duration, course, and pattern of diminished arm use should be clarified. Fever, malaise, rash, or weight loss may give clues to a systemic illness. If the patient is an infant, it should be determined whether the arm disuse was from birth: a difficult delivery may lead to clavicular fractures or brachial plexus injuries. It should be remembered that infants do not always mount a

TABLE 35.3

LIFE- AND LIMB-THREATENING CAUSES OF DIMINISHED ARM USE

Septic arthritis/osteomyelitis
Leukemia/other malignancy
Fracture with neurovascular compromise

febrile response to infection and may have only nonspecific symptoms of diminished feeding, increased sleeping, lethargy, or irritability. General medical history should include any history of inflammatory process, hemophilia, or sickle cell disease.

After a careful history, a physical examination should be performed. Fever should be noted and may be indicative of infection or, less likely, inflammatory or neoplastic process. Observation and inspection, sometimes from a distance of several paces, can provide information that might otherwise be unobtainable because many children cry when approached or touched by a stranger. The position of the arm should be noted. A child with nursemaid's elbow often holds the arm pronated and slightly flexed with obvious diminished movement, although often without apparent discomfort; a child with neurologic abnormality may hold the arm limply at the side of the body. Close inspection for areas of deformity, redness, swelling, or bruising should be done. Observation of the child's reach and grasp for an interesting object can provide information about the active range of motion and neurologic function. The clinician should palpate from clavicle to fingertips to identify areas of warmth, swelling, or tenderness (often best accom-

plished in the younger child while he or she is being distracted). Joints should be assessed for warmth, swelling, tenderness, and range of motion; however, if a history of trauma is present, manipulation can be deferred until an acute fracture has been excluded. Neurovascular integrity of the arm should be assessed carefully. A thorough general examination for rash, other joint abnormalities, hepatosplenomegaly, adenopathy, abnormal mass, and neurologic status should be performed, particularly for children without an obvious injury.

Plain radiographs are one of the most useful studies for evaluating children with diminished arm use. They may reveal a fracture or dislocation, joint effusion, or lytic bone lesion. If a discrete area of tenderness is identified, radiographs of that location, including the joint above and below, should be obtained. If the focus of pain is not apparent, it may be necessary to obtain radiographs of the entire limb from clavicle and shoulder to fingers.

A CBC may help in the diagnosis of infection, inflammation, malignancy, or hemoglobinopathy. Although nonspecific, an ESR or CRP levels may be useful in differentiating inflammatory or infectious processes from other causes.

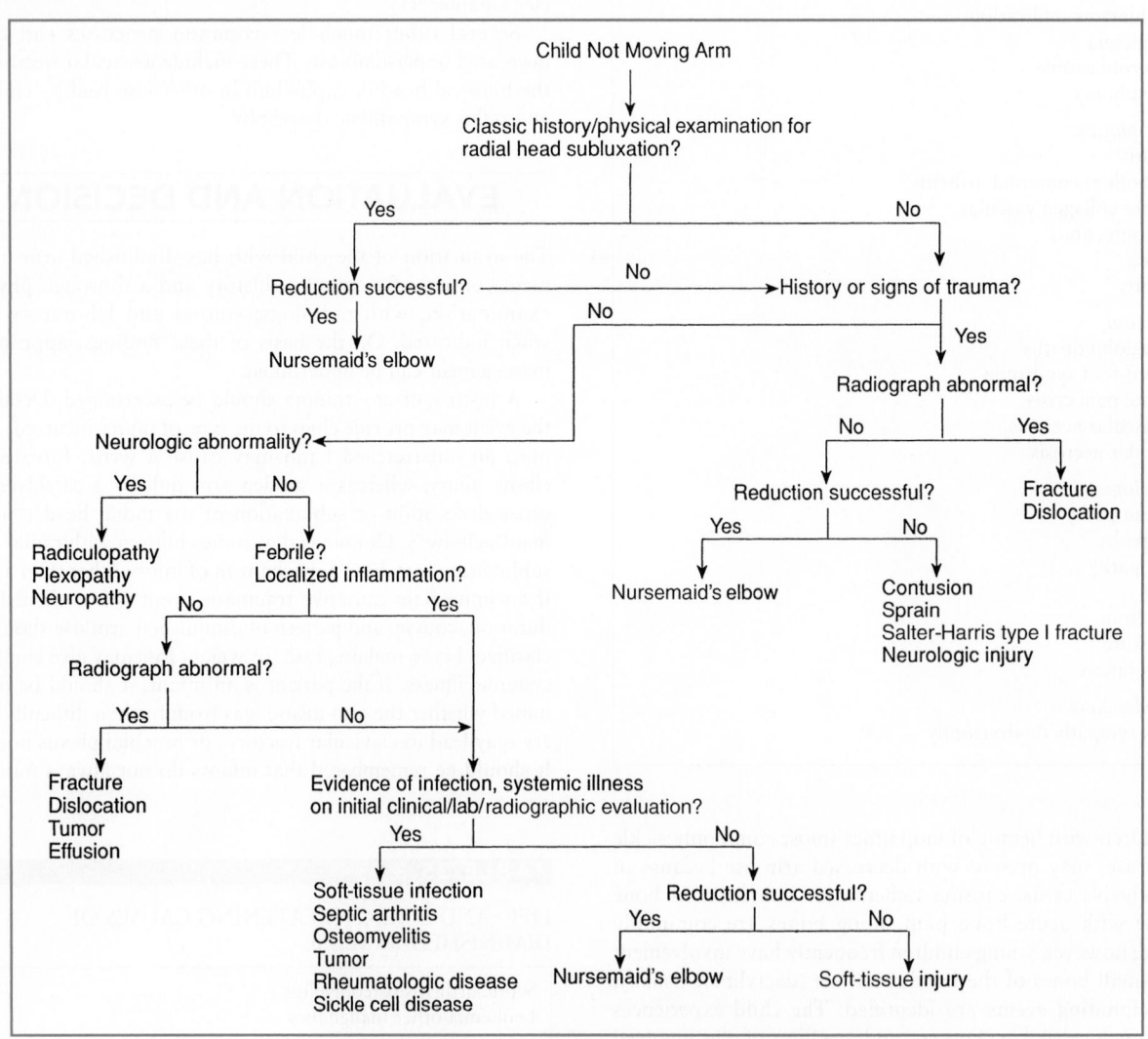

FIGURE 35.1 Approach to the child with diminished arm use.

Other tests helpful in selected cases include blood culture (if an infectious process is suspected), hemoglobin electrophoresis (if sickle cell disease is a possibility), bone scan, or MRI (for osteomyelitis, septic arthritis, aseptic necrosis). Arthrocentesis is imperative if septic arthritis is a possibility, and if osteomyelitis is suspected, evaluation and treatment should proceed urgently.

When a child is brought for the evaluation of diminished arm use, the physician should first determine whether this resulted from a specific traumatic event (Fig. 35.1). If the history is classic for radial head subluxation, the patient is holding the arm pronated and slightly flexed, and there is no localized tenderness or swelling, then the physician may attempt reduction. If the child does not regain full use of the arm quickly, as in all other cases of trauma, radiographs should be obtained. In many cases, the radiographic studies provide the diagnosis (e.g., fracture, dislocation). Normal radiographs in the setting of acute trauma usually imply soft-tissue injury and the patient should be treated symptomatically with close follow-up, provided that neurovascular integrity is established. If radiographs appear normal but the child has reproducible tenderness localized to the epiphyseal plate, then the patient should be presumptively treated for a Salter-Harris type I fracture. Occasionally, a child with a nursemaid's elbow may have an atypical history (e.g., "fell onto arm"); if radiographs exclude a fracture but the patient is holding the arm in a characteristic position, an attempt at reduction should be performed.

Children with neurologic abnormalities should be evaluated urgently to localize the site and cause of the impairment; the appropriate subspecialist (neurologist, neurosurgeon) should be involved.

If the child has no clear history of trauma but is afebrile with no obvious localized findings of infection, the limb should be evaluated radiographically. Abnormalities revealed might include fracture, dislocation, tumor, or effusion. If radiographs are normal in these children, one could consider obtaining a CBC count, ESR, CRP, and blood culture tests, or hemoglobin electrophoresis to evaluate for occult infectious or inflammatory processes.

Children who are febrile, have signs of localized inflammation (e.g., warm, swollen joint), or have evidence of systemic illness should have a CBC and ESR, CRP, and blood culture tests in addition to radiographs. On the basis of specific findings, further evaluation might include arthrocentesis, bone scan, MRI, or rheumatologic tests. When the initial history, physical examination, laboratory tests, and radiographs localize with the site and etiology of the pathology, the physician can begin specific management.

Some children with no history of trauma in whom a thorough initial evaluation is unrevealing will have a nursemaid's elbow. Therefore, an attempt at reduction is warranted in selected cases. Children with persistently diminished arm movement who are afebrile and nontoxic, with no localized findings, normal neurovascular function, and normal laboratory tests, likely have an occult soft-tissue injury and can be managed as outpatients. A few of these children may have indolent pathologic processes or occult fractures; therefore, close follow-up must be ensured. These patients should be reevaluated every few days until normal arm use is regained or until evidence of a pathologic process develops. If arm disuse persists, a more extensive evaluation to diagnose or exclude occult fracture, infection, tumor, or inflammatory process is in order.

Suggested Readings

Carson S, Woolridge DP, Colletti J, et al. Pediatric upper extremity injuries. *Pediatr Clin North Am* 2006;53:41–67.

Cassidy JT, Petty RE, Laxer RM, et al. *Textbook of pediatric rheumatology,* 5th ed. Philadelphia, PA: Elsevier Saunders, 2005.

Fenichel GM. *Clinical pediatric neurology: a signs and symptoms approach,* 5th ed. Philadelphia, PA: Elsevier Saunders, 2005.

Kothari NA, Delchovitz DJ, Meyer JS. Imaging of musculoskeletal infections. *Radiol Clin North Am* 2001;39(4):653–671.

Macias CG, Bothner J, Wiebe R. A comparison of supination/flexion to hyperpronation in the reduction of radial head subluxation. *Pediatrics* 1998;102:e10.

Macias CG, Wiebe R, Bothner J. History and radiographic findings associated with clinically suspected radial head subluxations. *Pediatr Emerg Care* 2000;16:22–25.

Schutzman SA, Teach S. Upper-extremity impairment in young children. *Ann Emerg Med* 1995;26:474–479.

SIGNS AND SYMPTOMS

CHAPTER 36 ■ INJURY—ANKLE

ANGELA C. ANDERSON, MD, FAAP

Approximately 26% of sports-related injuries in school-aged children involve the ankle. Young children with ankle injuries may complain of pain anywhere from their mid-calf to their toes because it is often difficult for children to localize pain. Conversely, pathology in the lower leg and foot can cause referred pain to the ankle.

The ankle joint is composed of three bones: the tibia, the fibula, and the talus. The bony prominence of the distal fibula constitutes the lateral malleolus, whereas the prominence of the distal tibia forms the medial malleolus. The physes are located one to two fingerbreadths above the distal ends of the tibia and the fibula.

The ankle ligaments are attached to the physes. The distal fibular physis is the most commonly injured growth plate in the lower extremities. It is second only to the distal radius in the incidence of physeal injuries.

Growth plates and bones are weaker than ligaments. Consequently, ankle trauma in preadolescent children is much more likely to cause fractures of the physis and the adjacent epiphysis and/or metaphysis than do ligamentous injuries or sprains.

DIFFERENTIAL DIAGNOSIS

A number of traumatic injuries may cause ankle pain (Table 36.1). Although trauma is the most common cause of ankle pain in children, infectious, rheumatologic, inflammatory, neoplastic, and hematologic abnormalities also should be considered (Table 36.2) because trauma may occasionally merely exacerbate pain in children with underlying conditions. Again, keep in mind that a complaint of ankle pain may result from a lesion anywhere between the knee and the toe, particularly in preverbal children. The most common injuries vary according to age (Table 36.3).

Ankle Fractures

Fractures of the ankle account for 5.5% of all fractures in pediatrics. The system used to classify ankle fractures in children differs from the one used in adults because of the presence of growth plates and the possible implications of physeal injuries. The Salter-Harris classification is most commonly applied, as described in Chapter 114.

Inversion ankle injuries in preadolescents most commonly cause a Salter-Harris type I fracture of the distal fibula (Fig. 36.1). Clinically, the patient presents with swelling about the lateral malleolus and tenderness at the distal fibular physis. Fractures confined to the physes may not be visible on radiographs. Consequently, routine radiographs may appear normal despite the presence of a fracture.

In severe inversion injuries, the distal fibular fracture described previously may be accompanied by a fracture of the medial malleolus (Fig. 36.2). This medial malleolus fracture is usually a Salter-Harris type III or IV fracture of the distal tibia. These patients will have tenderness at the medial malleolus and the distal fibular physis.

Fractures resulting from eversion of the ankle are usually a combination of a Salter-Harris type II 2 fracture of the lateral tibia and a transverse fracture of the fibula (Fig. 36.3). The fibular fracture is relatively high (4 to 7 cm above the fibular physis). Therefore, it is important to examine the full length of the fibula in patients with ankle injuries.

Direct axial compression of the ankle is uncommon but can cause a Salter-Harris type V injury to the distal tibia.

External rotation injuries are responsible for lesions known as transitional fractures. Transitional fractures occur during adolescence when closure of the growth plates is beginning. Closure of the distal tibial physis starts at the center of the bone and then spreads medially, posteriorly, and finally laterally. The distal tibial physis closes before the distal fibular physis.

As skeletal maturity (and physeal closure) progresses, the relative strengths of various parts of the tibia change. As a result, the same mechanism of injury may cause very different fracture patterns, depending on the age of the patient. The juvenile Tillaux fracture and the triplane fractures are examples of transitional fractures.

In the juvenile Tillaux fracture, a fragment of bone is torn off the lateral border of the tibia by the anterior tibiofibular ligament (Fig. 36.4). It is a Salter-Harris type III injury of the distal tibia. This fracture is seen almost exclusively in patients between the ages of 12 and 14 years. This is because the closure of the medial aspect of the distal tibial physis begins around 12 to 14 years of age, whereas the lateral aspect remains open and therefore less stable for approximately another 18 months. The greater the skeletal maturity of the patient, the more lateral the epiphyseal fracture line occurs.

Diagnosis of these fractures may be difficult because routine radiographs may not show the fracture line well. If displacement is minimal, the only radiographic sign may be a slight widening of the lateral tibial physis or a faint vertical fracture line through the epiphysis on anteroposterior (AP) or oblique views. In some cases, the only finding may be local tenderness in the area of the lateral tibial physis. Multiple oblique views, computed tomography (CT), or tomography may be needed to adequately delineate the extent of the fracture.

Growth arrest and angular deformity are rare because these fractures occur at the time of physeal closure. However, ankle

TABLE 36.1

DIFFERENTIAL DIAGNOSIS OF TRAUMATIC INJURIES THAT CAUSE ANKLE PAIN

Leg
Tibial fractures (toddler's fracture)
Fibular fractures
Contusions
Compartment syndrome of the calf

Ankle
Fractures
    Distal tibial
    Distal fibular
    Physeal
Sprains
Contusions
Osteochondritis dissecans
Hemarthrosis

Foot
Fractures
    Talar
    Navicular
    Fifth metatarsal (Jones fracture)
    Calcaneal
Sprains
Contusions

TABLE 36.2

DIFFERENTIAL DIAGNOSIS OF ANKLE PAIN

Trauma
    Fractures
    Sprains
    Contusions
    Osteochondritis dissecans
    Hemarthrosis

Inflammatory
    Tendonitis
    Synovitis
    Periostitis
    Sever's disease (calcaneal apophysitis)

Infectious
    Osteomyelitis
    Soft-tissue abscess
    Septic joint
    Brodie's abscess (subacute osteomyelitis of the distal tibia)

Rheumatologic
    Juvenile rheumatoid arthritis
    Rheumatic fever
    Reiter's syndrome

Hematologic
    Sickle cell disease (pain crisis)
    Hemophilia (hemarthrosis)

Osteochondroses (avascular necrosis)
    Kohler's disease (navicular)
    Freiberg's disease (second metatarsal)

Tumors
    Ewing's sarcoma
    Osteoid osteoma

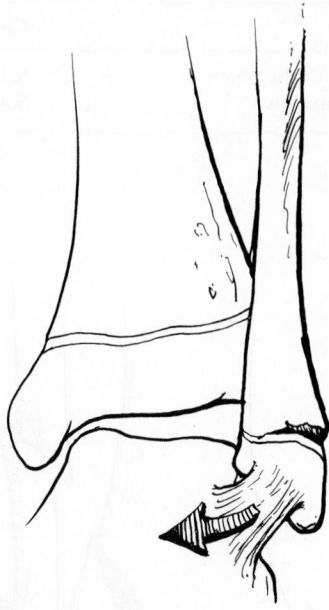

FIGURE 36.1 Inversion injury.

joint arthritis may complicate the long-term outcome if the diagnosis is missed or if reduction is inadequate.

Triplanar fractures are characterized by a fracture line that runs in three planes: coronal, sagittal, and transverse. They are a combination of a juvenile Tillaux fracture and a Salter-Harris type II fracture of the distal tibia. Two types of triplane fractures have been described. The first is a three-fragment fracture (Fig. 36.5). The first fragment is the same as the one found in the juvenile Tillaux fracture—a fragment of the epiphysis torn off the anterolateral quadrant of the tibia. The

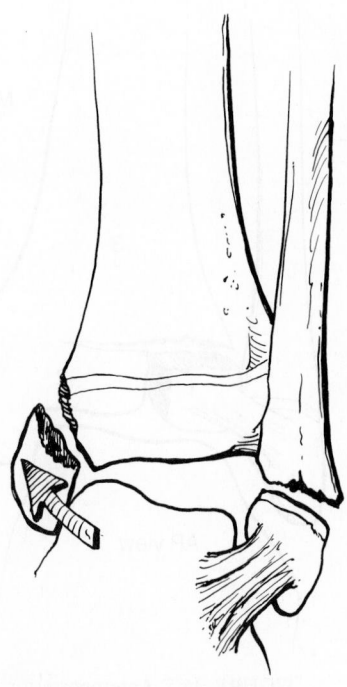

FIGURE 36.2 Severe inversion injury.

TABLE 36.3

COMMON INJURIES ASSOCIATED WITH ANKLE PAIN ACCORDING TO AGE

Toddler	Child	Adolescent
Spiral fracture of the tibia	Salter-Harris type I fracture of the distal fibula	Ankle sprain
Soft-tissue contusion	Soft-tissue contusion	Soft-tissue contusion

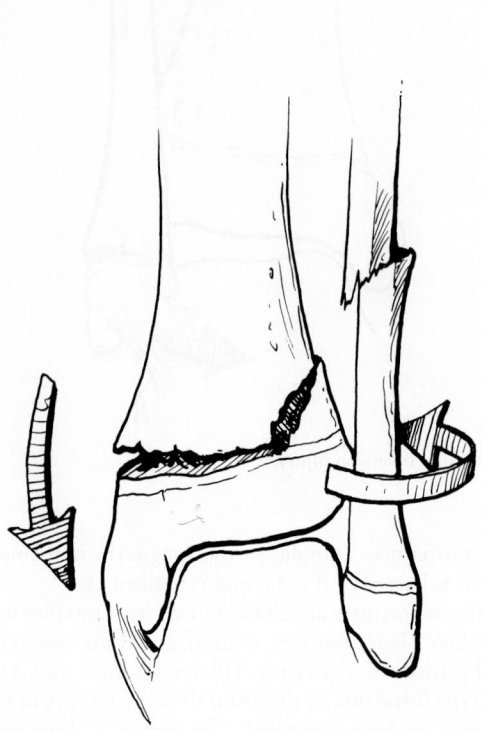

FIGURE 36.3 Eversion injury.

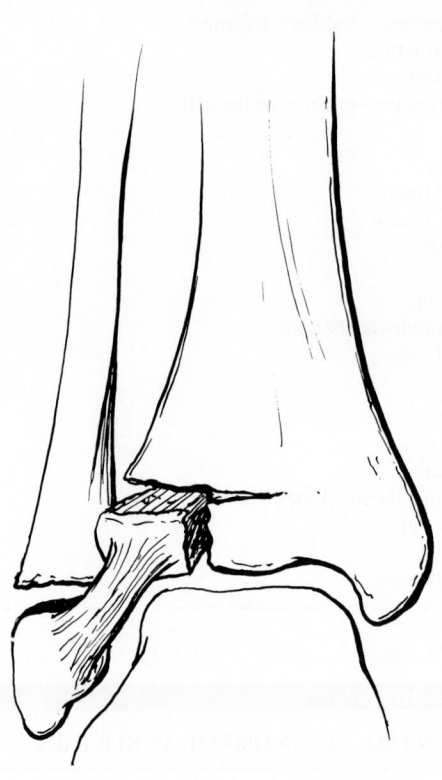

FIGURE 36.4 Juvenile Tillaux fracture or Salter-Harris type III fracture of the distal tibial physis; the medial part of the tibial physis is fused.

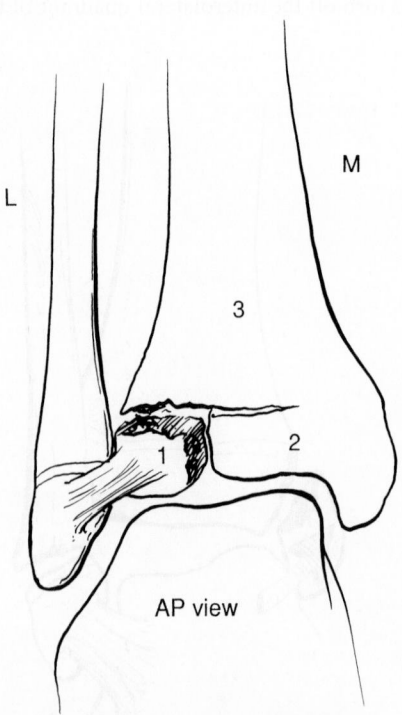

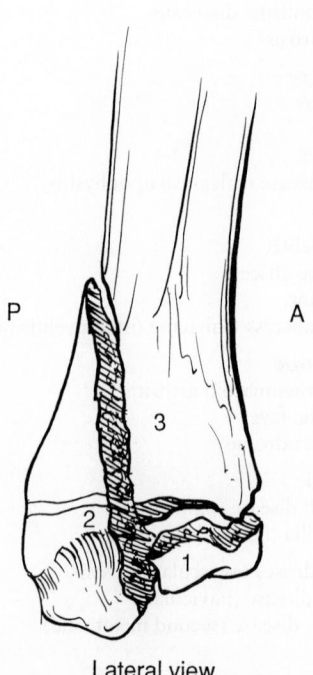

FIGURE 36.5 Anteroposterior and lateral views of three-fragment triplanar fracture. L, lateral; M, medial; P, posterior; A, anterior.

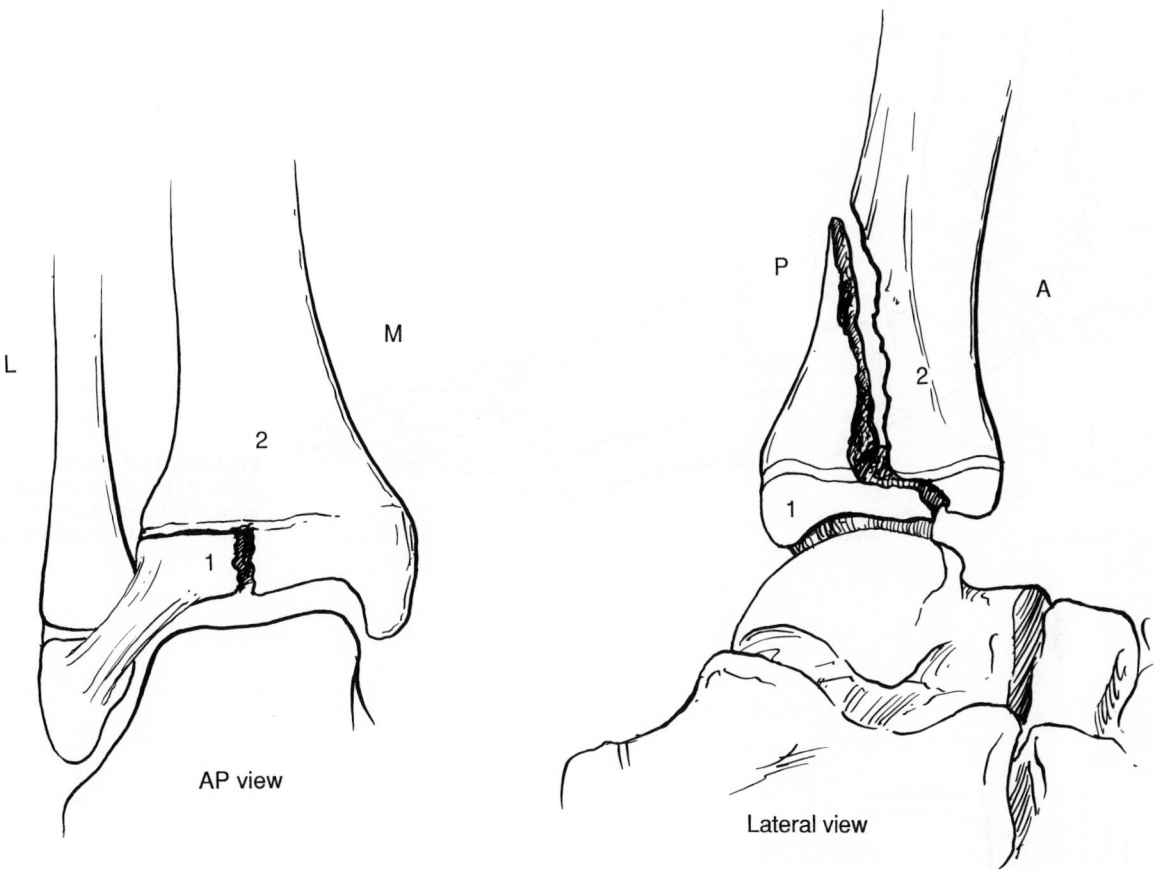

FIGURE 36.6 Anteroposterior and lateral views of two-fragment triplanar fracture. L, lateral; M, medial; P, posterior; A, anterior.

second fragment is the remaining medial part of the epiphysis, which is attached to a posterior spike of the metaphyseal bone. The third fragment is the tibial shaft.

A two-fragment fracture has also been described. The first fragment is again the lateral tibial epiphysis, but it is attached to a posterior spike of the metaphyseal bone. The second fragment is the remaining medial epiphysis and is attached to the tibial shaft (Fig. 36.6).

On a radiograph, triplanar fractures have the appearance of a Salter-Harris type III fracture on the AP view and a Salter-Harris type II fracture on the lateral view. If only the AP view is obtained, it may be difficult to distinguish these fractures from the juvenile Tillaux fracture. The key to diagnosis is the posterior metaphyseal spike seen on the lateral film.

Ankle Sprains

Ankle sprains in children or preadolescents are less common than fractures because the ligaments in this age group are much stronger than growth plates or even bone. If a ligamentous injury occurs in a child with an open growth plate, an associated avulsion fracture is almost always present. However, once skeletal maturity is reached, ankle sprains become the most common of sports injuries.

Inversion injuries cause 85% of ankle sprains. The most commonly injured structures are the lateral ligaments. Three lateral ligaments support the ankle joint: the anterior talofibular (ATFL), the calcaneofibular (CFL), and the posterior talofibular (PTFL) (Fig. 36.7). The ATFL is the weakest and most commonly injured of the three. The CFL is intermediate in strength and is rarely injured without an associated tear of the ATFL. The PTFL is the strongest and least injured of the lateral ligaments. Because its fibers run horizontally, only extreme dorsiflexion will stress this ligament. The peroneus brevis tendon also traverses the lateral aspect of the ankle joint and can be injured by inversion stress. It inserts at the base of the fifth metatarsal.

Eversion injuries account for 15% of ankle sprains. The deltoid ligament, which supports the medial aspect of the ankle, is most commonly affected by this mechanism (Fig. 36.8). It is composed of deep and superficial fibers. Eversion may also cause disruption of the tibiofibular syndesmosis, which connects the distal tibia and the fibula.

Classification of Ankle Sprains

There are many systems of classification for ankle sprains. Table 36.4 provides guidelines that can be used in grading injuries to the lateral ligaments.

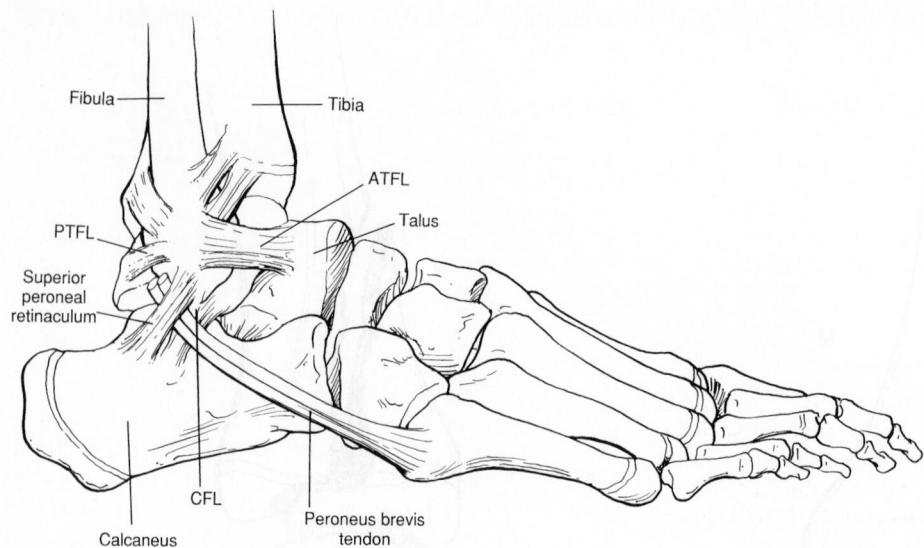

FIGURE 36.7 Lateral view of the ankle. ATFL, anterior talofibular ligament; PTFL, posterior talofibular ligament; CFL, calcaneofibular ligament.

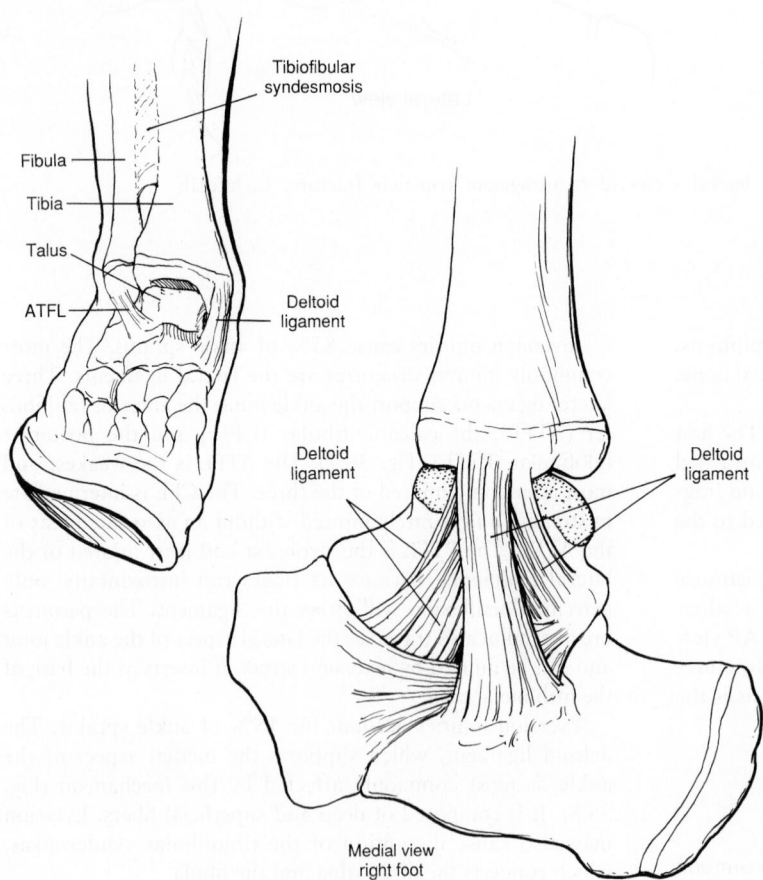

FIGURE 36.8 Ankle eversion injury. ATFL, anterior talofibular ligament.

TABLE 36.4

CLASSIFICATION OF ANKLE SPRAINS

	Grade I: Mild sprain	Grade II: Moderate sprain	Grade III: Severe sprain
Ligament injury	Minor	Near complete tear	Complete rupture
Swelling	Mild	Moderate	Severe
Tenderness	Mild, local	Moderate, diffuse	Marked
Functional loss	Minimal	Ambulates with difficulty	Inability to bear weight

Injuries Associated with Ankle Sprains

Approximately 7% of ankle sprains are accompanied by osteochondral fractures of the talus. The medial dome is more commonly fractured than the lateral dome. Avulsions of the peroneus brevis tendon from the base of the fifth metatarsal have been observed in up to 14% of patients with ankle ligament ruptures. If this injury occurs in children younger than 15 years, the avulsed fragment is usually an apophysis and is considered a Salter-Harris type I injury. In older patients, the displaced portion represents a bony fragment and is known as a Jones fracture.

EVALUATION AND DECISION

History

Trying to obtain a reliable history in ankle injuries can be very unsatisfying. It is a rare occasion when the patient says: "I sustained an inversion injury while playing basketball!" More commonly, the description is: "I twisted it and it hurts." Nevertheless, the mechanism of injury, if obtainable, can provide a clue to the diagnosis. Other questions include the following: (i) When did the injury occur? (ii) Did swelling occur immediately or gradually? (iii) Is there a history of any previous injury to that limb? and (iv) Does the patient have a history of any other medical problems—osseous, neurologic, or muscular disease?

A history of fever, rash, or other joint involvement, in combination with a history of minimal or no trauma, suggests nontraumatic diagnoses such as septic joint, arthritis, or collagen-vascular disease.

Physical Examination

General Inspection

Look for obvious deformities, open wounds, loss of anatomic landmarks, local swelling, and ecchymosis. If an obvious deformity is present, keep manipulation of the extremity to a minimum and assess neurovascular status promptly. Any break in the skin may communicate with the joint space or constitute an open fracture. The need for antibiotic coverage must be evaluated immediately.

Neurovascular Evaluation

Palpate the dorsalis pedis and posterior tibial arteries. Note skin temperature, color, and capillary refill. The absence of pulses or the presence of pallor requires immediate attention. A Doppler device may help identify pulses.

Vascular compromise is usually caused by a posterior dislocation. Traction reduction of the deformity should be attempted as rapidly as is feasible by performing the following steps: (i) sedate the patient; (ii) apply longitudinal traction to the foot; (iii) if relocation is not accomplished in step ii, apply longitudinal traction and pull the foot in a posterior to anterior direction; and (iv) immobilize the ankle and obtain radiographs. If the vascular status has not been compromised, continue with the examination and evaluate the nerves that cross the ankle. Test soft touch and pain sensation of the foot.

Bony Palpation

Trace all three bones of the ankle joint (the tibia, the fibula, and the talus), searching for areas of point tenderness. It is very important to palpate the distal tibial and fibular physes because fractures in these areas may not be evident on radiographs. Any tenderness found along a physis should be considered a Salter-Harris type I fracture at the least, even if radiographic studies are negative. Also keep in mind that the only clue to a juvenile Tillaux fracture may be tenderness at the lateral tibial physis. Remember to palpate the fibula proximal to the ankle joint. External rotation and triplanar injuries may be associated with high fibular fractures.

Finally, examine the foot. This should include palpation of the dome of the talus. This is performed most easily with the foot in plantar flexion. Palpate the base of the fifth metatarsal. Tenderness here suggests an avulsion of the peroneus brevis tendon.

Once one area of point tenderness is found, continue to examine the entire joint. A single injury may cause many abnormalities.

Ligament Palpation

Palpate for tenderness along all three lateral ligaments, remembering that each one arises from the distal fibula. The ATFL can be further tested by inverting and plantar flexing the foot. This will increase pain if injury to this ligament is present. More than 4 cm of swelling in an area of lateral ligament tenderness is highly suggestive of significant ligament injury.

Examine the superficial fibers of deltoid ligament on the medial aspect of the joint. The deep fibers are intraarticular and nonpalpable; therefore, rupture may be present without much medial tenderness. Isolated injuries to the deltoid ligament are rare because of the great strength of this ligament. If the deltoid ligament has been damaged, the tibiofibular syndesmosis is usually disrupted along with it.

Injuries to the tibiofibular syndesmosis may be explored by (i) squeezing the midshafts of the tibia and the fibula together, (ii) dorsiflexing and then externally rotating the foot while holding the tibia and the fibula stable, or (iii) forcefully dorsiflexing the ankle with the patient supine. Exacerbation of pain with these maneuvers suggests syndesmotic disruption.

Stability Testing

An attempt should be made to assess the stability of the ankle joint. However, stability testing in the immediate postinjury period may be limited significantly by pain, swelling, and/or muscle spasm. Several maneuvers are useful, but they are generally not performed if an ankle fracture is present.

■ *Anterior Drawer Test*—The anterior talofibular ligament is the only structure that prevents forward subluxation of the talus. The anterior drawer test is performed to assess the anterior stability of the ankle joint and the integrity of the ATFL (Fig. 36.9). The test result is positive if the foot can be pulled forward by more than 4 mm or if there is a significant difference in the degree of anterior movement in the injured ankle compared with the normal ankle.

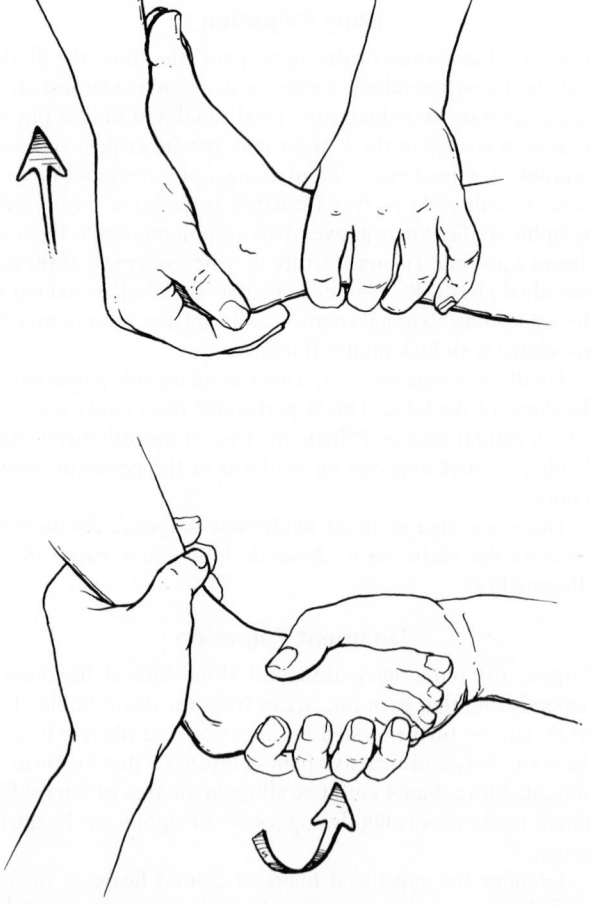

FIGURE 36.9 (**Top**) The anterior drawer test is performed by placing the patient's heel in the palm of the examiner's hand with the ankle at a 90-degree angle to the long axis of the leg. The examiner gently, but firmly, moves the heel and foot forward *(arrow)*. (**Bottom**) In the talar tilt maneuver, the heel is firmly adducted *(arrow)* and assessed for increased laxity or instability compared with the noninjured side.

■ *Talar Tilt Test*—This test is used to examine the lateral stability of the ankle joint. It is performed by firmly adducting the heel, looking for increased laxity compared with the noninjured joint (Fig. 36.9). Both the anterior talofibular and calcaneofibular ligaments must be torn to cause gross lateral ankle instability.

Radiographic Imaging

The Ottawa ankle rules (OARs) were developed to help clinically predict radiographically evident ankle fractures in adults. OARs maintain that ankle radiographs are required only if the patient has pain near the malleoli and one or both of the following: (i) inability to bear weight immediately following the injury and in the emergency department (four steps) and (ii) bone tenderness at the posterior edge or tip of either malleolus. These rules were 100% sensitive in detecting clinically significant fractures in patients older than 18 years; application of these rules allowed for a 28% reduction in the number of radiographs ordered. A more recent study suggests that OARs were 100% sensitive in detecting ankle fractures 3 mm or more in width in children older than 2 years; however, patients with Salter-Harris type I fractures were not included as positive outcomes. One study that investigated OARs in children and included Salter-Harris type I fractures as abnormal determined that OARs had a sensitivity of only 80% if applied to children younger than 15 years. All studies utter warnings regarding the use of OARs to predict ankle fractures in very young children.

Radiographic evaluation of the ankle should include at least three views: AP, lateral, and mortise. If tenderness of the proximal fibula is noted, full-length views of the fibula are essential. Tenderness at the base of the fifth metatarsal mandates visualization of this area on the lateral film. If radiographic findings are questionable, consider obtaining comparison views of the noninjured ankle. The practice of *routinely* obtaining comparison views has not been studied and it is unknown if doing so would change clinical practice or patient outcome.

Note areas of soft-tissue swelling. This may be the only clue to a Salter-Harris type I fracture of the distal fibula. Stress radiographs to evaluate growth plate injuries are rarely necessary and may cause further damage. The value of stress radiographs to assess ligament damage is also questionable. Severe pain and muscle spasms frequently prohibit stress maneuvers. Arthrography may be more helpful but is seldom indicated in the acute care setting. This method uses the location of extravasated contrast material in the ankle joint to identify ligamentous ruptures.

CT scan of the ankle is often necessary to fully evaluate triplane fractures. Magnetic resonance imaging (MRI) may be useful in evaluating patients in whom one has a high clinical suspicion of injury despite normal radiographs. MRI may also delineate suspected tendon and ligament injuries in selected circumstances.

Approach

The approach (Fig. 36.10) to the evaluation and diagnosis of traumatic ankle injuries relies primarily on physical findings

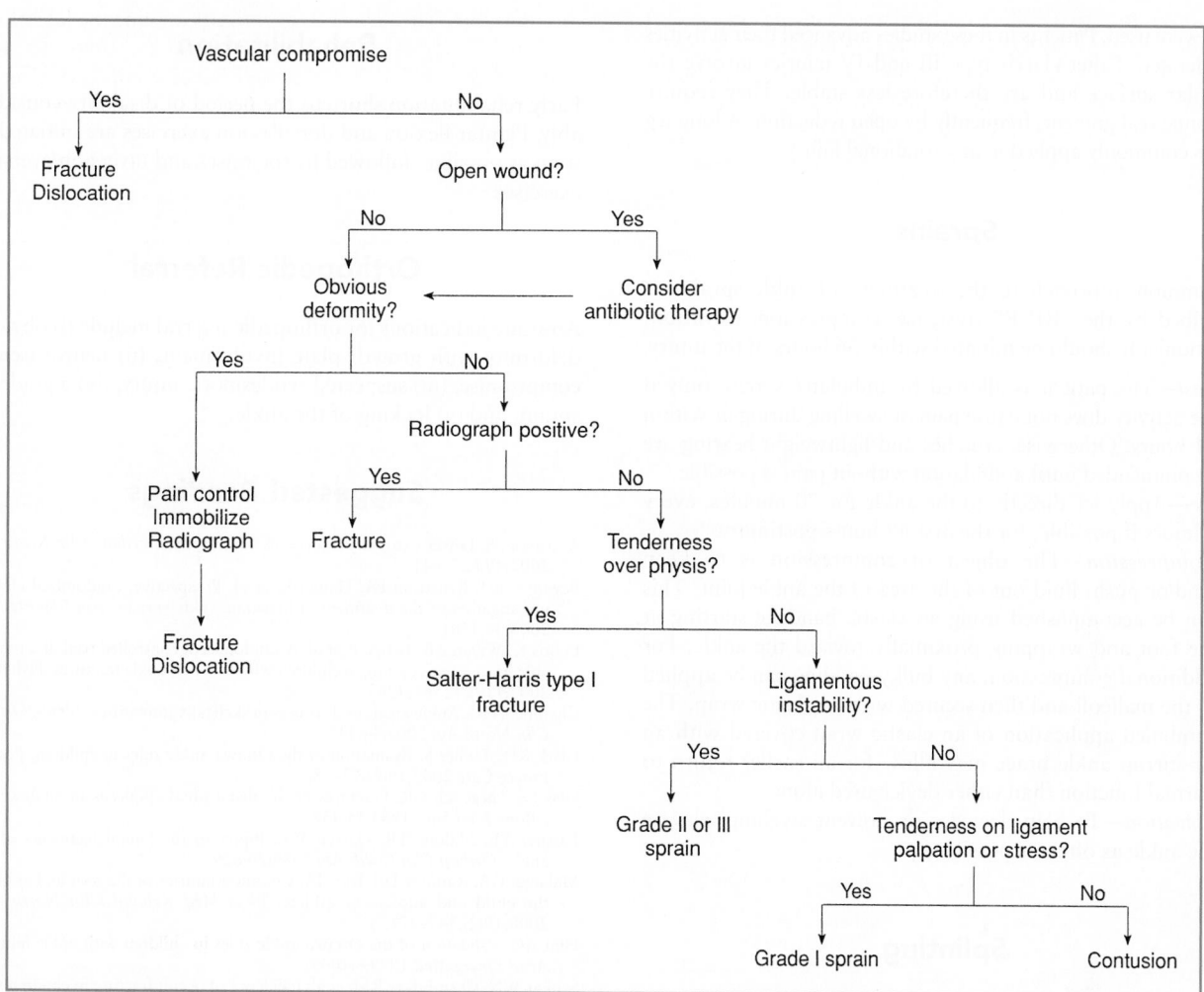

FIGURE 36.10 Evaluation and diagnosis of traumatic ankle injuries.

and the results of radiographic evaluation. Initially, pulses and sensation are assessed. Loss of pulses and/or sensation suggests a fracture/dislocation and the need for a rapid reduction; when available without delay, orthopedic consultation is advisable. After immobilization to prevent further compromise and the provision of analgesia, a radiograph should be obtained immediately. If neurovascular status is adequate and the general inspection reveals no obvious abnormalities, proceed with the rest of the physical examination as described previously.

Next, examine the area for open wounds. If present, fashion a sterile saline dressing and immobilize the extremity before obtaining a radiograph. Consider in addition the administration of intravenous antibiotic therapy and tetanus prophylaxis.

If radiographic studies indicate a fracture or dislocation, provide treatment of the specific injury (see Chapter 114). Administer analgesia as needed.

If no fracture is evident on the radiograph, but tenderness is elicited over a physis, the diagnosis of a Salter-Harris I injury can be made and appropriate immobilization is performed (see Chapter 114). One study demonstrated that approximately 18% of children with tenderness at the distal fibular physis and normal radiographs will develop new periosteal bone forma-

tion, thus implying the presence of an occult fracture. A negative radiographic result in the absence of bony tenderness suggests the diagnosis of contusion or ligamentous injury. The diagnosis of a grade II or III sprain is rendered to the patient with joint instability. If the ankle is stable, but pain is elicited with ligamentous stress or palpation, a grade I sprain is diagnosed.

TREATMENT

Fractures

Fracture reduction is usually accomplished by reversing the mechanism of injury. Closed reduction and a short leg cast are usually adequate for Salter-Harris type I and II fractures of the distal tibia and the fibula (see Chapter 114). Some displacement can be accepted in younger patients because of their ability to remodel. Two studies have suggested that children with nondisplaced Salter-Harris type I fractures my benefit from even more conservative therapy; those treated with crutches, a 5-day period of non–weight bearing, and the use of a removable ankle brace (e.g., an air-stirrup ankle brace or an elastic bandage) were able to return to normal activity sooner than those in whom short leg casts were used. Patients in these studies advanced their activities as tolerated. Salter-Harris type III and IV injuries involve the articular surface and are therefore less stable. They require anatomic realignment, frequently by open reduction. A long leg cast is commonly applied in any rotational injury.

Sprains

A common approach to the treatment of ankle sprains is described by the "RICE" (rest, ice, compression, elevation) mnemonic. It should be initiated within 36 hours of the injury.

- *Rest*—The patient is allowed to ambulate/exercise only if the activity does not cause pain or swelling during or within 24 hours. Otherwise, crutches and lightweight bearing are recommended until ambulation without pain is possible.
- *Ice*—Apply ice directly to the ankle for 20 minutes, every 2 hours if possible, for the first 48 hours postinjury.
- *Compression*—The object of compression is to keep (and/or push) fluid out of the area of the ankle joint. This can be accomplished using an elastic bandage starting at the foot and wrapping proximally toward the ankle. For additional compression, any bulky padding can be applied to the malleoli and then secured with an elastic wrap. The combined application of an elastic wrap covered with an air-stirrup ankle brace may allow for an earlier return to normal function than either device used alone.
- *Elevation*—To help decrease or prevent swelling, elevate the ankle as often as possible.

Splinting

If swelling or pain is severe, apply a stirrup and/or posterior splint to the ankle (see Procedures 12.14a–c). Air splints can also be used; they allow dorsiflexion and plantar flexion while maintaining medial and lateral stability.

Rehabilitation

Early rehabilitation shortens the period of disability considerably. Plantar flexion and dorsiflexion exercises are initiated as soon as possible, followed by toe raises and inversion/eversion exercises.

Orthopedic Referral

Absolute indications for orthopedic referral include (i) obvious deformity with growth plate involvement, (ii) neurovascular compromise, (iii) suspected syndesmotic injury, (iv) a grade III sprain, and (v) locking of the ankle.

Suggested Readings

Anderson, S. Lower extremity injuries in youth sports. *Pediatr Clin North Am* 2002;49:627–641.

Beynnon BD, Renström PA, Haugh L, et al. Prospective, randomized clinical investigation of the treatment of first-time ankle sprains. *Am J Sports Med* 2006;34;1401.

Boutis K, Willan AR, Babyn P, et al. A randomized, controlled trial of a removable brace versus casting in children with low-risk ankle fractures. *Pediatrics* 2007;119;e1256–e1263.

Chambers HG. Ankle and foot disorders in skeletally immature athletes. *Orthop Clin North Am* 2003;34:445.

Clark KD, Tanner S. Evaluation of the Ottawa ankle rules in children. *Pediatr Emerg Care* 2003;19(2):73–78.

Dias LS, Giegerich CR. Fractures of the distal tibial epiphysis in adolescence. *J Bone Joint Surg* 1983;65:438.

Lassiter TE, Malone TR, Garrett WE. Injury to the lateral ligaments of the ankle. *Orthop Clin North Am* 1989;20:629.

Malanga GA, Ramirez Del Toro JA. Common injuries of the foot and ankle in the child and adolescent athlete. *Phys Med Rehabil Clin North Am*. 2008;19(2):347–371, ix.

Plint AC. Validation of the Ottawa ankle rules in children with ankle injuries. *Acad Emerg Med* 1999;6:1005.

Sankar WN, Chen J, Kay RM, et al. Incidence of occult fracture in children with acute ankle injuries. *J Pediatr Orthop* 2008;28:500–501.

Stefanich R, Lozman J. The juvenile fracture of Tillaux. *Clin Orthop Relat Res* 1986;210:219.

Volger HW. Unusual juvenile ankle fracture: explanation and surgical repair. *J Foot Surg* 1990;29:516.

CHAPTER 37 ■ INJURY—HEAD

SARA A. SCHUTZMAN, MD

PEDIATRIC HEAD TRAUMA

Head injuries in children are common, accounting for more than 600,000 emergency department (ED) visits per year in the United States. Although the majority of these injuries are minor, head trauma causes significant pediatric morbidity and mortality. Trauma is the leading cause of death in children older than 1 year, and traumatic brain injury is the leading cause of death and disability caused by trauma in children, resulting in approximately 3,000 deaths annually.

The most common mechanism of injury for pediatric head trauma is falls, followed by motor vehicle and pedestrian accidents and bicycle injuries; the majority of fatal injuries occur secondary to motor vehicle-related accidents. The mechanism of head injury varies with age; younger children are more likely to suffer falls or abuse, whereas older children are often injured in sporting or motor vehicle accidents (in addition to falls).

Many of the serious neurologic complications of head injury are evident soon after the traumatic event; however, some life-threatening injuries can appear initially as minor head trauma. To manage head injuries best, the physician must approach the child in a systematic manner to address all injuries (global resuscitation is the first priority of cerebral resuscitation), identify and treat any neurologic complications, and prevent ongoing cerebral insult.

PATHOPHYSIOLOGY

Neurologic injury following head trauma is related to the unique physiology and pathophysiology of the brain and the intracranial environment. The brain is a semisolid structure bathed in cerebrospinal fluid (CSF) and covered by the fine inner pia-arachnoid membrane and the outer thick fibrous layer of dura, all of which are encased in the skull, which is covered by the five-layered structure of the scalp. After infancy (when the skull sutures fuse), the cranial vault becomes a stiff and poorly compliant structure housing the brain. Because the intracranial volume is relatively fixed, any change in the volume of one of the intracranial components (blood, brain, and CSF) must occur at the expense of the others; if the other components do not decrease proportionally, intracranial pressure (ICP) will increase.

Brain injury occurs in two phases: primary and secondary. The primary injury is the mechanical damage sustained at the time of trauma and can be caused by direct impact of the brain against the internal calvarial structures, by bone or foreign bodies projected into the brain, and by shear forces delivered to the white matter tracts. Secondary brain injury is further neuronal damage sustained after the traumatic event to cells not initially injured. This results from numerous causes, including hypoxia, hypoperfusion, and metabolic derangements, and may also result from sequelae of the primary injury (e.g., cerebral edema, expanding intracranial mass) or be caused by extracranial injuries (e.g., hypotension from excessive blood loss, hypoxia from pulmonary contusion). The clinician's goal is to identify and treat any complications of primary brain injury in order to limit further neuronal damage by secondary brain injury.

One of the most common causes of secondary brain injury is cerebral ischemia resulting from impaired perfusion. Cerebral perfusion pressure is the difference between the mean arterial pressure of blood flowing to the brain and the ICP. In the healthy child, blood flow to the brain is maintained at a constant rate over a wide range of systemic blood pressures by means of autoregulatory changes in the cerebrovascular resistance so that the brain does not suffer ischemia or excessive blood flow during periods of relative hypo- or hypertension, respectively. With severe injuries, this autoregulatory control may be lost and the cerebral blood flow can become directly dependent on the cerebral perfusion pressure; with low mean arterial pressure or increased ICP, there will be inadequate blood flow and cerebral ischemia results. In addition to potential for causing decreased cerebral perfusion, increased ICP, if left unchecked, can lead to brain herniation and compression. This may be caused by a number of posttraumatic conditions, including cerebral edema and expanding intracranial mass.

Clinical symptoms of increased ICP or herniation include headache, vomiting, irritability, lethargy, visual disturbance, gait abnormalities, and weakness. Signs include depressed level of consciousness, abnormal vital signs (bradycardia, hypertension, respiratory irregularity), cranial nerve palsies, hemiparesis, and decerebrate posturing. The classic findings in transtentorial herniation are headache, decreasing level of consciousness followed by ipsilateral pupillary dilatation (cranial nerve III palsy), and contralateral hemiparesis or posturing. If the process continues unchecked, dilatation of the opposite pupil, alteration in respirations, and ultimately, bradycardia and arrest ensue. For a more detailed description of the anatomy, pathophysiology, and treatment of specific head injuries, please see Chapter 105.

DIFFERENTIAL DIAGNOSIS

Head trauma may cause injuries of the scalp, skull, and intracranial contents. Although each is discussed here separately, the clinician must remember that these injuries may occur alone or in combination, and all potential injuries must be considered when dealing with one.

Scalp

The scalp consists of five layers of soft tissue that cover the skull; contusions and lacerations of this structure are common results of head trauma. The outermost layers of the scalp are skin and the subcutaneous tissue; edema and hemorrhage here may produce a mobile swelling. The third layer, the galea aponeurotica, is a strong membranous sheet that connects the frontal and occipital bellies of the occipitofrontalis muscle. The remaining two layers deep to the galea are the loose areolar tissue and pericranium. Subgaleal hematomas may result from more forceful blows as vessels in the fourth layer bleed and dissect the galea from the periostium, or they may be signs of an underlying skull fracture. In subperiostial hematomas, or cephalohematomas, the swelling is localized to the underlying cranial bone and most frequently occurs with birth trauma. Scalp lacerations may occur with or without underlying contusions or fractures and they often require suturing. Given the high vascularity of the scalp, these injuries can result in significant blood loss if not recognized and treated appropriately.

Skull

Skull fractures occurring in the calvarium, or bony skullcap, include frontal, parietal, temporal, and occipital fractures and may be linear, diastatic, depressed, comminuted, or compound. Fractures in the base of the skull are termed *basilar*. Most simple fractures require no intervention but are important in that they are a marker of significant impact to the head and are associated with up to a 20-fold increased risk of intracranial injury (ICI).

Linear fractures account for 75% to 90% of skull fractures in children and often manifest with localized swelling and tenderness. Diastatic fractures are traumatic separations of cranial bones at a suture site or fractures that are widely split. A depressed skull fracture is present when the inner table of the skull is displaced by more than the thickness of the entire bone. These may be palpable and are diagnosed with tangential skull radiographs (SRs) or computed tomography (CT) scans. Compound fractures are those that communicate with lacerations.

Basilar skull fractures may be difficult to detect on routine SR or CT; however, their location produces clinical signs that lead to the diagnosis. Fractures of the petrous portion of the temporal bone may cause hemotympanum, hemorrhagic or CSF otorrhea, or Battle's sign (bleeding into mastoid air cells with postauricular swelling and ecchymosis). Fracture of the anterior skull base may cause a dural laceration with subsequent drainage of CSF into paranasal sinuses and rhinorrhea. Anterior venous sinus drainage may cause blood leakage into the periorbital tissues (raccoon's eyes). Given the location of basilar skull fractures, associated cranial nerve palsies may occur. There is a high incidence of associated ICI in children with basilar skull fracture, even in those with a Glasgow Coma Scale (GCS) score of 15 and normal neurologic examination results.

Intracranial Injury

Insults to intracranial contents include functional derangements without demonstrable lesions on CT scan (concussion,

posttraumatic seizures), hemorrhage [cerebral contusion, epidural hematoma (EDH), subdural hematoma, subarachnoid hemorrhage, and intracerebral hemorrhage], and acute brain swelling. Rarely, penetrating brain injuries occur in children. ICIs may also be classified as focal (e.g., contusions, hematomas, lacerations) or diffuse (e.g., diffuse axonal injury, diffuse brain swelling). Focal injuries are usually apparent on the initial CT scan, even if clinically asymptomatic. Diffuse injuries, in contrast, may not demonstrate striking abnormalities on early CT imaging, even if the patient manifests significant alteration in neurologic function.

Concussion

Concussion is the most minor brain injury and is characterized by posttraumatic alteration in mental status that may or may not involve loss of consciousness (LOC). No consistent associated pathologic lesion in the brain has been identified. The child may have a depressed level of consciousness, pallor, vomiting, amnesia, and confusion; however, the clinical picture usually normalizes within several hours without specific therapy.

Posttraumatic Seizure

Posttraumatic seizures can be divided temporally into immediate, early, and late, and they occur in 5% to 10% of children hospitalized for head trauma.

Immediate seizures occur within seconds of the trauma and may represent traumatic depolarization of the cortex. They usually are generalized and rarely recur.

Early seizures occur within 1 week of the trauma (the majority within 24 hours). Skull fractures, intracranial hemorrhage, and focal signs are associated with increased risk of early posttraumatic seizures; therefore, an early seizure should prompt investigation of these possibilities.

Late seizures occur more than 1 week after the traumatic event and may be attributed to scarring associated with local vascular compromise, distortion, and mechanical irritation of the brain. These seizures are more likely to occur in children with severe head injuries, dural lacerations, and intracranial hemorrhages. A substantial number of patients will have subsequent seizures.

Cerebral Contusion

Cerebral contusion is a bruising or crushing of brain and often results from blunt head trauma. The site of contusion may be a "coup" lesion, with the injured cerebral cortex directly beneath the site of impact (with or without skull fracture), or a "contrecoup" lesion, with damage opposite the site of impact; the contusion is demonstrable by CT scan. Children with cerebral contusion may have had LOC (not imperative), may show a depressed level of consciousness or symptoms of vomiting or headache, and may have focal neurologic signs or seizures.

Epidural Hematoma

Epidural hematoma (EDH) is a collection of blood between the skull and the dura. An overlying fracture is present in 60% to 80% of cases, and, depending on the location and vascular structure involved, the hemorrhage may be of arterial or venous origin; injury to the middle meningeal artery is frequently responsible for temporal EDH. The classic pattern of a "lucid interval" between initial LOC and subsequent neurologic deterioration occurs only in a minority of children with EDH; furthermore, patients may occasionally develop EDH after relatively "minor" trauma with no history of LOC. Although many children present with marked lethargy, focal neurologic signs, or a clinical pattern consistent with temporal lobe herniation as the hematoma expands, some children may be alert with a nonfocal neurologic examination and may have symptoms only of headache or persistent vomiting; nevertheless, rapid deterioration can ensue.

Subdural Hematoma

Subdural hematomas (SDHs) occur as a result of bleeding between the dura and the arachnoid membranes covering the brain parenchyma. They may result from direct trauma or from shaking injuries and are due to tearing of the cortical bridging veins or due to bleeding from the cortex itself. SDHs may be bilateral, and frequently, there is an associated underlying brain injury. Skull fractures occur in only a minority of cases. Children with SDHs often have seizures, may present with evidence of acutely elevated ICP, or may have more non-specific signs of vomiting, irritability, or low-grade fever. Physical examination often reveals an irritable or lethargic child, with a bulging fontanel in infants, who may or may not have neurologic abnormalities. CT scan commonly demonstrates crescent-shaped subdural collections.

Intracerebral Hematoma

Posttraumatic intracerebral hematomas are unusual in children. Blood within the parenchyma is usually the result of severe focal injury or penetrating trauma, usually manifests with severe neurologic compromise, and often portends a poor prognosis.

Subarachnoid Hemorrhage

Subarachnoid hemorrhage may occur following head trauma (including shaking injuries in infants) and may cause headache, neck stiffness, and lethargy in the child.

Diffuse Axonal Injury

Diffuse axonal injury is characterized by injury to the white matter tracts of the brain and is one of the most common causes of prolonged posttraumatic coma in children. The initial CT scan may be normal or may demonstrate multiple petechial hemorrhages in the deep white matter and central structures. The degree of microscopic injury is usually greater than that seen on diagnostic imaging, accounting for clinical symptoms that may be disproportionate to CT scan findings.

Diffuse Brain Swelling

Diffuse brain swelling occurs frequently in children with severe head trauma. It appears to be a reactive phenomenon that occurs within hours of the traumatic event and is likely a final common manifestation of brain injury caused by a variety of pathophysiologic processes. The major effect of this swelling is potential for significant elevation of ICP. These children have a depressed level of consciousness and may have focal neurologic signs or symptoms of herniation.

Penetrating Injuries

Penetrating head injuries are uncommon in children and may be caused by bullets, teeth (e.g., dog bites), or other objects (e.g., dart, pencil, pellet) penetrating the skull. These injuries have obvious potential for extensive damage to the brain and intracranial vessels.

EVALUATION AND DECISION

The clinical spectrum of head injury in children varies from a small contusion of the scalp with no neurologic sequelae to severe ICI that causes death. The general approach is essentially the same as with any child who presents with trauma, paying particular attention to potential CNS damage. Following the ABCs (airway, breathing, and circulation) of resuscitation, the physician must systematically evaluate and stabilize the child with head trauma. The goals of management are to identify complications of the head trauma and to prevent secondary brain injury. Because some complications of head trauma may not manifest immediately, the assessment period includes the initial evaluation in the ED and a more extended observation period, either in the hospital or as an outpatient, as clinically indicated. Specific therapy will vary based on specific diagnosis in each case and may include supportive care and possible neurosurgical intervention. Although complications are more common in children with severe head injury, they also occur in children with apparently minor head trauma; thus, all patients merit some degree of scrutiny.

The immediate management of the child varies with the degree of compromise. A brief initial assessment is performed to determine immediate stability. In the older child, verbal response to a question often establishes the adequacy of the airway, ventilation, and cognitive function. If the child is unconscious or has unstable vital signs, immediate resuscitation is initiated to ensure a patent airway (with cervical spine immobilization), effective ventilation, and adequate tissue perfusion (see Chapter 1); efforts to decrease possible increased ICP may be indicated, depending on the degree of neurologic compromise (see Chapter 105). The child with airway and hemodynamic stability and with only mild to moderate depression of mental status can undergo a more timely evaluation to identify subtle or occult abnormalities.

CLINICAL ASSESSMENT

History

The history should be obtained from the patient (if age and level of consciousness permit) and from any witnesses to determine the nature and severity of the impact and the prehospital course. Specifics of the traumatic event should include how, when, and where the trauma occurred, as well as details such as height of a fall, type of impact surface, and type and velocity of striking objects. Occurrence of LOC as well as duration should be determined. If the event was unwitnessed and the patient is amnestic, the clinician should assume that LOC occurred. Occurrence of seizure activity (including details of time of onset posttrauma, duration, and focality) and the child's level of alertness since the injury should be noted, as well as presence of vomiting, irritability, ataxia, and abnormal behavior—all signs of possible brain injury. Vomiting after a head injury is not uncommon;

however, persistence for more than several hours may signal intracranial abnormalities. If the child is verbal, he or she should be questioned about the presence of headache or neck pain, amnesia, weakness, visual disturbances, or paresthesias. In many cases, elicited symptoms may be the only evidence of underlying CNS injury. In infants, symptoms of ICI may be subtle or absent; therefore, the clinician should pay particular attention to any alteration in behavior in this age group. Progression or resolution of any symptoms, neurologic signs, and level of consciousness since the traumatic episode must be defined clearly. One should also inquire about previous medical history and factors predisposing to head trauma (e.g., seizure disorder, gait disturbance, bleeding diathesis, alcohol abuse, or illicit drug use). When there are discrepancies in the history, when the history does not fit the physical findings, or when there is a skull fracture or ICI in a young child without a history of significant trauma, one should suspect nonaccidental injury.

Physical Examination

After a primary survey with appropriate resuscitation, a thorough physical examination should be performed, with special emphasis on the vital signs, head and neck, and neurologic examination. Bradycardia may be a sign of increased ICP; it is of particular concern when associated with hypertension, abnormal breathing pattern, depressed level of consciousness, or neurologic abnormality. Bradycardia may also be seen with spinal cord injuries caused by unopposed parasympathetic tone; in this case, it is often associated with hypotension, flaccidity, a sensory level, and absent deep tendon reflexes. Tachycardia may reflect hypovolemia (especially if associated with hypotension), hypoxia, or anxiety. Isolated head injuries rarely cause hypovolemia (except in infants with large subgaleal or intracranial hematomas); therefore, hypotension should alert the clinician to a possible extracranial or spinal cord injury.

The head should be inspected and palpated carefully for scalp swelling, lacerations, irregularities of the underlying bony structure, and fontanel fullness (in infants). Signs of basilar skull fracture (periorbital or postauricular hemorrhage in the absence of direct trauma, hemotympanum, CSF otorrhea, or rhinorrhea) and retinal abnormalities (hemorrhage or papilledema) should be noted. All children with depressed mental status or neck pain should have cervical spine immobilization maintained at least until its integrity has been confirmed radiographically; one should note cervical abrasions, deformity, or tenderness—findings that may indicate underlying cervical spine injuries.

Neurologic examination encompasses assessment of the child's mental status, as well as cranial nerve, motor, sensory, cerebellar, and reflex functions. Serial examinations are important in the child with head trauma to document improvement or deterioration. The GCS is a convenient way to quantify the level of consciousness and monitor neurologic progression. The GCS rates patient performance in three areas: eye opening, verbal ability, and motor ability. It also assesses the level of alertness, mentation, and major CNS pathways (Table 37.1); an individual's score may range from a low of 3 to a

TABLE 37.1

GLASGOW COMA SCALE SCORE

Activity	Best response	Score
Eye opening	Spontaneous	4
	To verbal stimuli	3
	To pain	2
	None	1
Verbal	Oriented	5
	Confused	4
	Inappropriate words	3
	Nonspecific sounds	2
	None	1
Motor	Normal spontaneous movements	6
	Localizes pain	5
	Withdraws to pain	4
	Abnormal flexion (decorticate rigidity)	3
	Abnormal extension (decerebrate rigidity)	2
	None	1

high of 15. The score has been modified for more age-appropriate behaviors in infants (Table 37.2). Although ICIs are more common in a child with a low GCS score, even a child with a GCS score of 15 may harbor potentially life-threatening complications of head trauma (e.g., EDH), especially if neurologic abnormalities are present. Further evaluation of mental status includes assessing orientation and memory. Subtle signs (irritability and high-pitched cry) may be indicative of underlying abnormalities in infants.

TABLE 37.2

MODIFIED COMA SCALE FOR INFANTS

Activity	Best response	Score
Eye opening	Spontaneous	4
	To speech	3
	To pain	2
	None	1
Verbal	Coos, babbles	5
	Irritable, cries	4
	Cries to pain	3
	Moans to pain	2
	None	1
Motor	Normal spontaneous movements	6
	Withdraws to touch	5
	Withdraws to pain	4
	Abnormal flexion (decorticate rigidity)	3
	Abnormal extension (decerebrate rigidity)	2
	None	1

Cranial nerve function is assessed by checking for facial symmetry, corneal reflexes, presence of a gag reflex, full extraocular movements, pupillary size, and pupillary reactivity. In the comatose patient or in the child with possible neck injury who is uncooperative, lateral gaze may be tested by caloric stimulation of the vestibular apparatus (but not the "doll's eye" maneuver) once tympanic membrane integrity has been established.

Examination of the motor system to evaluate both CNS and spinal cord function varies with age and level of consciousness. The alert patient should have individual muscle groups tested and gait evaluated. The child with a depressed level of consciousness may have motor responses elicited by noxious stimuli (e.g., sternal rub, nail bed pressure). Deep tendon reflexes and Babinski response should also be evaluated. Obviously, a complete physical examination with attention to possible thoracic, abdominal, pelvic, and extremity injuries should be performed.

Radiographic Investigation

Complications of head trauma may be identified with radiographic studies, which include plain radiographs of the skull and cervical spine and CT scan of the head; specific studies are indicated based on the child's history and physical findings. Although MRI is an additional imaging modality for the cranial contents, limited availability and prolonged study time limit its utility for evaluation of acute trauma at this time. All children with significant head trauma should be evaluated for associated cervical spine injuries. This evaluation will be clinical, with or without radiographic studies, based on the specific circumstances (see Chapter 106).

CT provides excellent images of the intracranial contents, and therefore, is the diagnostic modality of choice when intracranial pathology is suspected. CT imaging, however, has disadvantages, including exposure to ionizing radiation and the possible requirement for pharmacologic sedation, especially in younger patients. Ideally, CT imaging should be used selectively for patients at higher risk for ICI, limiting potentially unnecessary studies for those who are at low risk. Identifying clinical predictors for traumatic brain injury that have both high sensitivity and specificity, however, has been a challenging, and thus far, incompletely accomplished task.

Clear risk factors for possible ICI, for which CT imaging should be obtained, include history of penetrating trauma, altered level of consciousness, focal neurologic abnormalities, and signs of skull fracture. Other factors concerning for possible ICI include seizure, persistent vomiting, progressive or severe headache, loss of consciousness (particularly if more than brief or associated with other symptoms), and a predisposing condition for ICIs (e.g., coagulopathy). Mechanisms of injury that are either very significant or high-impact focal force (e.g., golf club to temporal area) are also more concerning for possible complications. Additional indicators for possible ICI in children younger than 2 years include bulging fontanel, irritability/behavioral change, and suspicion of abuse.

Children younger than 24 months are more challenging to assess because they cannot report symptoms, have a limited behavioral repertoire, are at higher risk for abuse, and are

TABLE 37.3
RISK FACTORS FOR ICI IN CHILDREN YOUNGER THAN 2 YEARS

High risk
Depressed mental status
Focal neurologic examination
Signs of skull fracture
Seizure
Irritability
Bulging fontanel
Persistent/progressive vomiting
Loss of consciousness >1 min
Suspicion of abuse
Underlying condition predisposing to ICI

Intermediate risk
Few episodes vomiting
Brief LOC
History of lethargy/irritability, now resolved (more concerning if behavioral change was prolonged)
Caretakers concerned about child's current behavior
Nonacute skull fracture
Higher force mechanism/fall onto harder surface
Hematoma, particularly if larger, nonfrontal in location, or in younger child
Unwitnessed trauma with possibility of significant mechanism
Vague or no history of trauma, but child with signs or symptoms of head trauma

Low risk
Low energy mechanism
No signs or symptoms
More than 2 h since injury
Older age more reassuring

ICI, intracranial injury; LOC, loss of consciousness.

often minimally symptomatic with ICI (up to one-half of infants with ICI have no symptoms of brain injury). Most of those with ICI and no symptoms, however, have an associated skull fracture, which is typically associated with overlying scalp swelling. Swelling more concerning for underlying fracture is that in younger infants, larger in size, and in nonfrontal location. Published guidelines have divided children younger than 2 years into those at high, intermediate, and low risk for ICI (Table 37.3). Those at high risk should have CT imaging, those at low risk require no imaging, and those at intermediate risk should have imaging or observation, based on the clinical scenario, need for sedation, availability of CT or radiographs, and expertise in image interpretation. The younger the age, the more difficult to assess and the higher the incidence of ICIs (and particularly of occult or asymptomatic ICIs); although this is a continuum, the clinician should have a very low threshold for obtaining a CT scan for infants younger than 3 months with trauma, unless trivial, even without symptomatology. In all cases, the patient's condition must be stabilized before transfer to the neuroradiologic suite; the patient should be monitored appropriately and accompanied by a health-care professional with medication and equipment necessary for resuscitation.

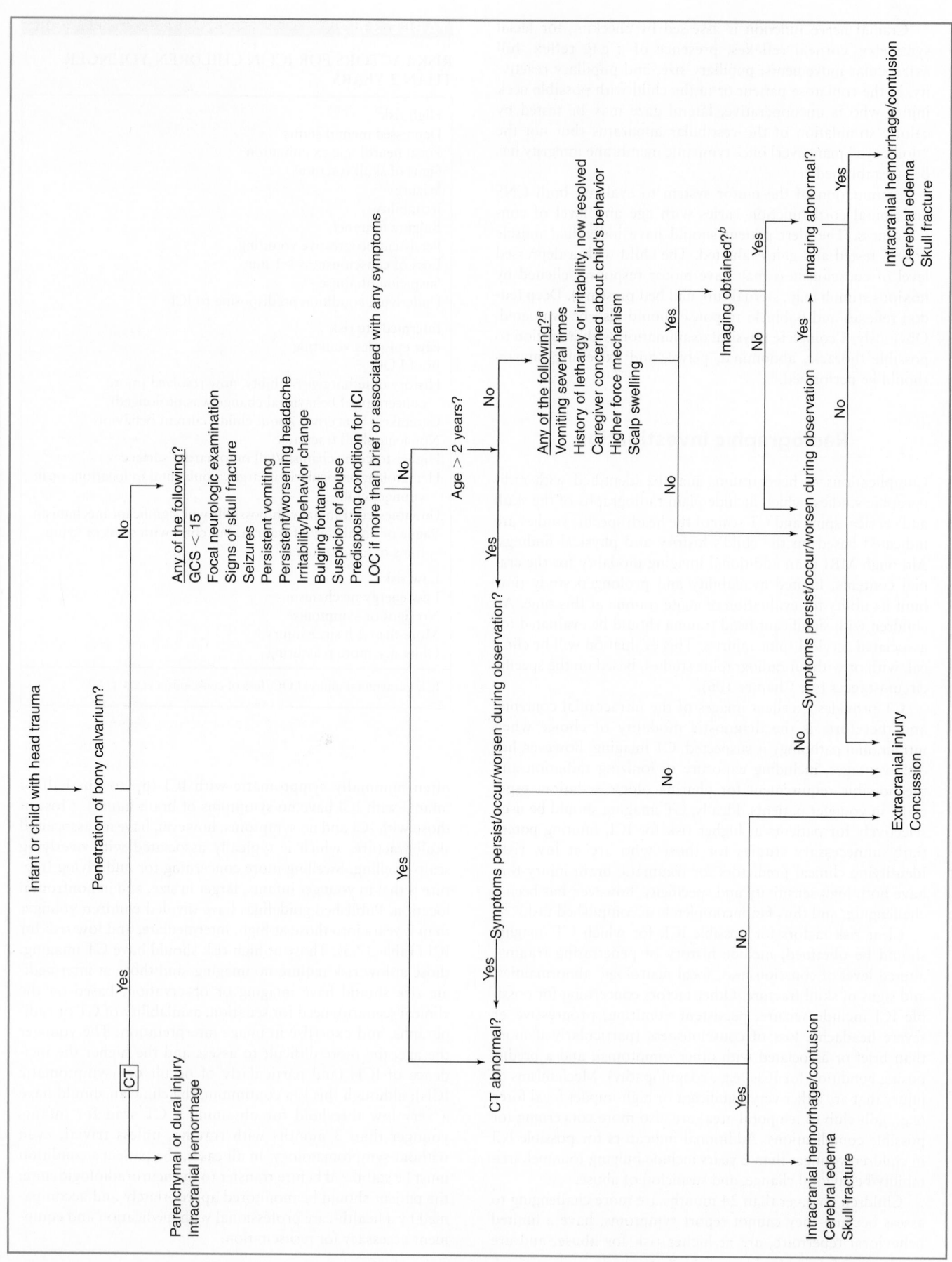

Infant or child with head trauma

Penetration of bony calvarium?

Yes — CT — Parenchymal or dural injury
Intracranial hemorrhage

No

Any of the following?
GCS < 15
Focal neurologic examination
Signs of skull fracture
Seizures
Persistent vomiting
Persistent/worsening headache
Irritability/behavior change
Bulging fontanel
Suspicion of abuse
Predisposing condition for ICI
LOC if more than brief or associated with any symptoms

No

Age > 2 years?

Yes — Symptoms persist/occur/worsen during observation?

Yes — CT abnormal?

Yes — Intracranial hemorrhage/contusion
Cerebral edema
Skull fracture

No — Extracranial injury
Concussion

No

Any of the following?[a]
Vomiting several times
History of lethargy or irritability, now resolved
Caregiver concerned about child's behavior
Higher force mechanism
Scalp swelling

Yes — Imaging obtained?[b]

Yes — Imaging abnormal?

Yes — Intracranial hemorrhage/contusion
Cerebral edema
Skull fracture

No

No — Symptoms persist/occur/worsen during observation — Yes

No — Extracranial injury
Concussion

Symptoms persist/occur/worsen during observation?

No — Extracranial injury
Concussion

Over the years, one of the most controversial issues in the management of head trauma has been use of SRs. Since SRs give no direct information about ICI, their use has appropriately dwindled. However, SRs are useful for demonstrating skull fractures (one of the best predictors for ICI in infants and young children) and have the advantages of delivering lower doses of ionizing radiation, being more universally available, less costly, and not requiring sedation. Certainly, any child for whom there is significant concern for ICI should undergo CT imaging; however, there may still be a very small role for SRs in certain select circumstances when immediate CT is not warranted, yet significant chance of fracture exists to justify the test. Data suggest that a substantial number of children younger than 12 to 24 months with ICI are minimally symptomatic, but most of these asymptomatic children have an associated skull fracture. One possible approach to imaging would be to use SRs as a screening tool in infants and young children with scalp findings (but not an obvious fracture) who do not have other features concerning for ICI. Scalp findings more highly associated with fracture in young children include hematomas that are larger in size, nonfrontal in location, and found in younger infants and children. Those with fractures identified on SRs would need to have CT scans performed because they are at increased risk for associated ICI. Other indications for SRs would include a question of depressed fracture or penetrating trauma, possibility of a foreign body, and as part of a skeletal survey. When considering the use of SRs, the clinician should take into account the experience of the physician/radiologist interpreting the radiographs; SRs of young children can be very challenging to interpret, and the utility of the study depends on an accurate reading.

Approach

The goals of management are to define specific anatomic lesions (e.g., skull fracture and ICI) and to prevent secondary brain injury, while limiting unnecessary cranial irradiation. Pediatricians and emergency physicians will be the initial clinicians to evaluate and manage most children with head trauma. Neurosurgical consultation should be considered for all children with penetrating trauma, abnormal mental status or neurologic examination, skull fractures, and intracranial complications. The urgency of neurosurgical involvement varies with the acuity of the patient's clinical condition.

One approach (Fig. 37.1) to diagnosing complications of head trauma involves determining whether a penetrating injury has occurred. If so, brain or vascular injury is likely and emergent CT scanning and neurosurgical consultation are mandated in addition to stabilization.

If the head injury has resulted from blunt trauma, it must be determined whether an ICI is likely. Suggestive historical features and physical findings include a GCS score less than 15, focal neurologic abnormality, signs of a skull fracture, history of seizure, persistent vomiting, persistent/progressive or severe headache, or underlying condition that predisposes to ICI (e.g., coagulopathy). An additional factor may be LOC, especially if longer than momentary or associated with other complaints. In infants, irritability, significant behavior change, bulging fontanel, and suspicion of abuse are also concerning for possible ICI. If any of these findings are present, in addition to supportive therapy, CT scan and possible neurosurgical consultation are indicated. Abnormalities on CT might include intracranial hemorrhage or contusion, diffuse cerebral swelling, or skull fracture; if the CT scan is normal, then concussion or extracranial injury has likely occurred.

If these findings are not present, then the child will be alert with a nonfocal neurologic examination. The drowsy child who quickly became alert, the one with a history of momentary LOC who is alert with a nonfocal examination, the patient with mild headache or one to two episodes of vomiting, may show no evidence of intracranial complications, yet the child may have had more than a trivial head injury. In the event these patients do not undergo a CT scan, they should be observed in the ED for at least 4 to 6 hours after the injury for signs and symptoms of complications. These would include neurologic abnormalities, mental status depression, persistent vomiting, or increasingly severe headache. A CT scan should be obtained if these signs or symptoms develop. As previously stated, discrete abnormalities may be identified on CT scan, but if the scan is normal, then the child has suffered a concussion or extracranial injury.

For children younger than 2 years, presence of vomiting several times, history of lethargy or irritability reported that has since resolved, caregiver's concern about the child's behavior, a higher force mechanism, and presence of a scalp swelling indicate that more than a trivial injury may have occurred and either imaging or observation for symptoms is indicated. The incidence of complications (fracture and/or ICI) is higher with hematomas that are larger, nonfrontal in location, and present in younger patients. CT is the appropriate imaging modality for any child with symptoms. SRs may be an alternative for the asymptomatic infant with isolated scalp swelling. Decision for CT versus SR imaging for the asymptomatic infant with scalp swelling should be based on the clinical scenario, availability for CT/SR, need for sedation, and expertise in image interpretation. If SRs demonstrate a fracture, then CT scan is indicated to evaluate for ICI. If imaging is not performed, then the child should be observed for a period of time in the ED for onset of symptoms. These would include neurologic abnormalities, lethargy/depressed mental status, persistent vomiting, and

FIGURE 37.1 Approach to the child with head trauma. CT, computed tomography; GCS, Glasgow Coma Scale; ICI, intracranial injury; LOC, loss of consciousness. [a]Children in this group who have had more than trivial head trauma and who should have imaging or observation, as appropriate; the decision will be based on the specific clinical scenario. Patients who are younger, those with a history of more intense/prolonged symptoms, and those with swelling that is larger in size or nonfrontal in location are at greater risk for complications. [b]CT is the appropriate modality for symptomatic patients; skull radiographs may be considered as an alternative to CT for asymptomatic patients with hematoma. The decision for CT/skull radiographs should be based on clinical scenario, availability of CT, need for sedation, expertise in imaging interpretation; if skull radiograph demonstrates fracture, CT is indicated to evaluate for ICI.

CRITERIA FOR DISCHARGE WITH HOME
OBSERVATION

Traumatic force not life threatening
Glasgow Coma Scale score of 15
Nonfocal neurologic examination
No significant symptoms
No history of prolonged loss of consciousness (or normal CT if it did occur)
No intracranial abnormalities on CT (if obtained)
Reliable caregivers who are able to return, if necessary
No suspicion of abuse or neglect
CT, computed tomography.

irritability. A CT scan should be obtained if signs or symptoms develop. As previously stated, discrete abnormalities may be identified on CT scan, but if imaging is normal, then the child has likely suffered a concussion or extracranial injury.

The remaining children who sustained impact of minimal force, had no LOC, and are alert and asymptomatic with normal examinations likely have only minor head trauma with or without extracranial injuries, including contusions and lacerations. Home observation is appropriate management for the majority of these patients. Rarely, intracranial complications develop in these children, causing symptoms hours after the traumatic event; therefore, the caregiver should be given a printed list of signs and symptoms indicative of increased ICP with instructions to check the child at regular intervals and to return to the ED if symptoms occur. Postconcussive counseling (especially with regard to return to sports), when indicated, should also be given. The care-

givers must be reliable and able to return with the child if necessary, and there must be no suspicion of abuse or neglect—otherwise admission for observation in the hospital should be considered (Table 37.4).

Suggested Readings

Atibaki SM, Stiell IG, Bazarian JJ, et al. A clinical decision rule for cranial computed tomography in minor pediatric head trauma. *Arch Pediatr Adoles Med* 2008;162:430–445.

Brenner D, Elliston CD, Hall EJ, Berdon WE. Estimated risks of radiation-induced fatal cancer from pediatric CT. *AJR Am J Roentgenol* 2001;176(2):289–296.

Brody AS, Guillerman RP. Radiation risk from diagnostic imaging. *Pediatr Ann* 2002;31:643–647.

Committee on Quality Improvement, American Academy of Pediatrics. The management of minor closed head injury in children. *Pediatrics* 1999;104: 1407–1415.

Dunning J, Daly JP, Lomas JP, et al. Derivation of the children's head injury algorithm for the prediction of important clinic events decision rule for head injury in children. *Arch Dis Child* 2006;91:885–891.

Greenes DS, Schutzman SA. Clinical significance of scalp abnormalities in head-injured infants. *Pediatr Emerg Care* 2001;17:88–92.

McCrory P, Johnston K, Meeuwisse W, et al. Summary and agreement statement of the Second International Conference on Concussion in Sports, Prague 2004. *Phys Sports Med* 2005;33(4):29–40.

Oman JA, Cooper RJ, Holmes J, et al. Performance of a decision rule to predict need for computed tomography among children with blunt head trauma. *Pediatrics* 2006;117:e238–e246.

Quayle KS, Jaffe DM, Kuppermann N, et al. Diagnostic testing for acute head injury in children: when are head computed tomography and skull radiographs indicated? *Pediatrics* 1997;99:1–8.

Palchak MJ, Holmes JF, Vance CW, et al. A decision rule for identifying children at low risk for brain injuries after blunt head trauma. *Ann Emerg Med* 2003; 42:492–506.

Schutzman SA, Barnes P, Duhaime AC, et al. Evaluation and management of children younger than two years of age with apparently minor head trauma: proposed guidelines. *Pediatrics* 2001;107(5):983–993.

Schutzman SA, Greenes DS. Pediatric minor head trauma. *Ann Emerg Med* 2001;37:65–74.

Schnadower D, Vazques H, Lee J, Dayan P, Roskind CG. Controversies in the evaluation and management of minor blunt head trauma in children. *Curr Opin Pediatr* 2007;19:258–264.

CHAPTER 38 ■ INJURY—KNEE

MARC N. BASKIN, MD

Acute pain or injury to the knee is a common complaint in the emergency department (ED). Many injuries are minor and require only limited therapy; others, however, require consultation with an orthopedist, either in the ED or as outpatients after pain and inflammation subside. The emergency physician can provide appropriate therapy or determine the need for consultation, based on a comprehensive history, physical examination, and an appropriate radiographic evaluation.

DIFFERENTIAL DIAGNOSIS

The differential diagnosis of acute and chronic knee injuries is summarized in Table 38.1. The pertinent anatomy is illustrated in Figures 38.1 and 38.2.

Acute Injuries

Fractures

Fractures of the distal femoral epiphysis are classified by the Salter-Harris pattern (see Chapter 114) and by the displacement of the epiphysis (usually lateral or medial). The injury usually follows significant trauma (e.g., being struck by a car and the knee hyperextended or being hit during contact sports from the lateral side with the foot fixed by cleats). The patient has severe pain, refuses to bear weight, and has extensive soft-tissue swelling and possibly deformity. Distal neurovascular status should be assessed because compromise of the popliteal artery occurs in 1% of cases and peroneal nerve injury occurs in 3% of cases. Radiographs are usually diagnostic but may be normal if the injury is a nondisplaced Salter-Harris type I fracture. Stress views should be considered in this situation if the physis is tender or a large effusion is present.

Fractures of the proximal tibial epiphysis are rarer than those of the distal femoral epiphysis but are more likely to involve vascular compromise because of the proximity of the popliteal artery to the posterior aspect of the tibial epiphysis. The patient has severe pain, limited range of motion (ROM), and commonly, a hemarthrosis. If displaced, the knee will be deformed. Distal neurovascular status should be assessed. Usually, radiographs are diagnostic but may be normal if the injury is a nondisplaced Salter-Harris type I fracture. Lateral and anteroposterior (AP) stress views may be necessary.

Acute traumatic avulsion of the tibial tuberosity is caused by acute stress on the knee's extensor mechanism. The quadriceps muscle group extends the knee by way of the patellar ligament. The patellar ligament inserts on the tibial tuberosity and may avulse it during sudden acceleration (e.g., beginning a jump) or deceleration (e.g., landing after a jump). The patient

will have tenderness and swelling over the tibial tubercle and is unable to extend the knee fully. The patella may be displaced superiorly. A lateral radiograph is diagnostic.

Fractures of the patella are rare in children younger than 6 years because the child's patella is surrounded by cartilage, protecting it from direct trauma. Avulsion fractures can occur. A medial avulsion fracture suggests that the mechanism was a patellar dislocation that spontaneously reduced. The patient's knee will be swollen, the patella tender. A radiograph is diagnostic although a bipartite patella may be confused with an acute fracture. The curved radiolucent line associated with a bipartite patella is usually in the superior lateral quadrant, a rare area for a fracture, and should not be associated with the soft-tissue swelling and effusion seen with a fracture.

Osteochondral fractures are fractures of articular cartilage and underlying bone not associated with ligamentous attachments. These fractures often involve the femoral condyles or the patella. Occasionally, a patient sustains a direct blow to the knee, but, more commonly, the knee is injured during a twisting injury or the patella is dislocated. The patient has severe pain, has immediate swelling, and holds the knee partially flexed. Knee radiographs need to include an intercondylar view because the fragment may be in the intercondylar notch. Osteochondral fractures can be missed because only the small ossified portion of the osteochondral fragment is radiopaque. Magnetic resonance imaging may be necessary.

Analogous to an adolescent who ruptures the anterior cruciate ligament (ACL), patients 6 to 16 years old may sustain avulsion fractures of the tibial spine at the point where the ACL inserts. The tibial spine is incompletely ossified and may avulse before the ligament ruptures. The patient may have a hemarthrosis and will be unable to bear weight. If the patient tolerates an examination, the Lachman test (Fig. 38.3) may be positive because the injury is similar mechanically to an ACL tear. AP, lateral, and intercondylar or tunnel-view radiographs will show the avulsed fragment. The visible ossified fragment may be small because the tibial spine is mostly radiolucent cartilage.

Dislocations

In a child, the knee joint itself rarely dislocates; usually, the distal femoral or proximal tibial epiphysis separates first. Dislocation occurs more frequently when the growth plates have closed and usually with trauma that involves significant force, such as a motor vehicle crash or contact sports. The knee appears obviously deformed with the tibia or femoral condyles abnormally prominent in an anterior or posterior dislocation, respectively. Disruption of the popliteal artery may occur with the dislocation, and the resulting hypoperfusion may be limb threatening. Posterior tibial and dorsalis pedis

TABLE 38.1

DIFFERENTIAL DIAGNOSIS OF THE INJURED KNEE

Acute injuries
  Fractures
    Distal femoral epiphysis[a]
    Proximal tibial epiphysis[a]
    Tibial tubercle avulsion
    Patella
    Tibial spine avulsion
    Osteochondral fractures
  Soft-tissue injuries
    Collateral ligament sprain or rupture
    Anterior cruciate ligament sprain or rupture
    Posterior cruciate ligament sprain or rupture
    Meniscal tears
    Quadriceps tendon rupture
    Patellar tendon rupture
    Hamstring strain[b]
  Posttraumatic infections
    Septic arthritis[a]
    Osteomyelitis[a]
    Cellulitis
    Septic prepatellar bursitis
  Dislocations and subluxations
    Patellar[b]
    Knee joint[a]

Subacute injuries
  Osgood-Schlatter's disease[b]
  Patellofemoral pain syndrome[b]
  Patellar tendon tendinitis (jumper's knee)
  Prepatellar bursitis
  Osteochondritis dissecans
  Baker's cyst
  Iliotibial band friction syndrome

Other
  Pathologic fractures[a]
  Hip disease
    Slipped capital femoral epiphysis
    Aseptic necrosis of the femoral head

[a]Life- or limb-threatening causes of the injured knee.
[b]Common causes of the injured knee.

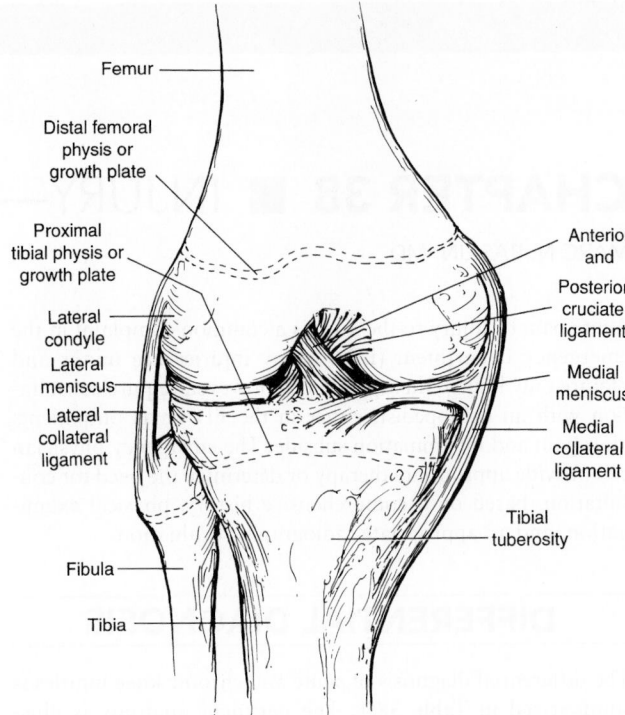

FIGURE 38.1 Anatomy of the knee—anterior view (patella removed).

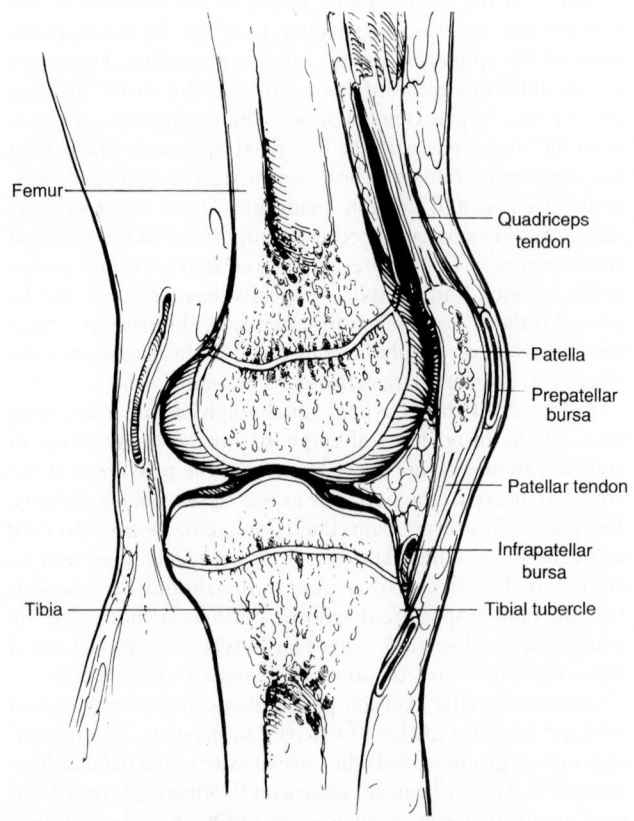

FIGURE 38.2 Anatomy of the knee—sagittal section.

pulses and peroneal nerve function (sensation between the great and second toe and ankle dorsiflexion) must be documented. Radiographs will confirm the diagnosis.

Patellar dislocation occurs as the quadriceps muscles pull along the patellar tendon to extend the knee. If the vastus medialis fibers do not keep the patella in the intercondylar groove, the patella may dislocate laterally. This often recurrent injury rarely occurs from direct force but happens more often during dancing or gymnastics. The patient may feel a ripping or popping sensation. The patient complains of intense pain and holds the knee flexed. The patella is displaced laterally, and the diagnosis is usually made based on history and examination. The dislocation may be reduced before radiographs are taken. Radiographs should be obtained to rule out an associated avulsion fracture of the patella.

If the history is consistent with dislocation but the patient is no longer in pain and has a normal examination results, he or

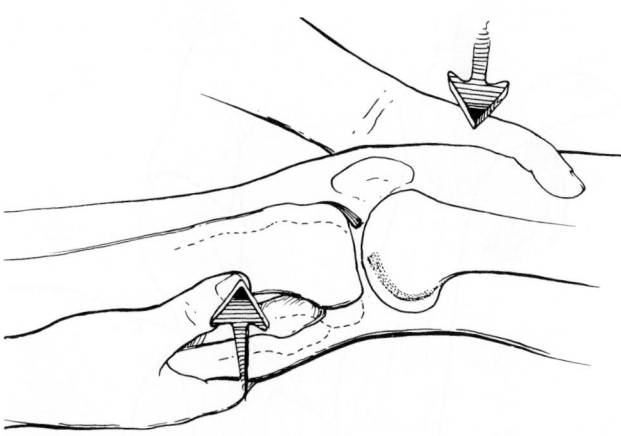

FIGURE 38.3 Testing for anterior cruciate ligament injury with the Lachman test. Flex the knee 20 to 30 degrees, support the thigh with one hand, and grasp the calf with the other hand. Move the tibia forward on the femur. Observe the tibial tubercle for movement and feel for excessive forward movement of the tibia in relation to the femur.

she may have subluxated the patella. A high-riding or laterally displaced patella may be observed. The quadriceps or Q angle formed by a line drawn from the anterior-superior iliac spine to the midpatella and one drawn from the midpatella to the tibial tubercle can be measured. When the angle is above 20 degrees, the extensor mechanism may sublux the patella laterally. The patellar apprehension test is performed by gently attempting to move the patella laterally. If the patient becomes apprehensive or grabs the examiner's hand, this suggests that he or she has subluxated the patella. Radiographs should be obtained to look for an associated osteochondral fracture.

Soft-Tissue Injuries

Medial collateral ligament (MCL) or lateral collateral ligament (LCL) injuries are rare when the epiphysis is open because the involved ligaments are stronger than the growth plate. The LCL inserts on the fibular head proximal to the physis, and the MCL inserts on the tibia distal to the physis. In older patients, the MCL may be damaged by a blow to the lateral side of the knee during contact sports or stress during a skiing accident, when the athlete "catches an edge" and falls forward with the leg rotated externally. Severe collateral ligament injury may be associated with ACL or meniscal damage. On examination, the knee may be swollen only minimally but will be tender over the involved ligament. The knee should then be tested for lateral laxity in full extension (associated with more severe injuries) and in 30 degrees of flexion (associated with less severe injuries), as shown in Figure 38.4. Orthopedic referral may be indicated if the examination reveals lateral or medial laxity.

ACL injuries occur in many scenarios, but usually involve rotational forces on a fixed foot. The patient often reports the sensation of a "pop." The joint usually swells rapidly as a result of hemarthrosis and has a marked decrease in ROM. The Lachman test (Fig. 38.3) is sensitive (0.7 to 0.9) in detecting ACL injuries but may be falsely negative soon after the injury, when the knee is swollen and painful. Examining the uninjured knee can be helpful for comparison. Arthroscopy or magnetic resonance imaging is often needed for definitive diagnosis. ACL

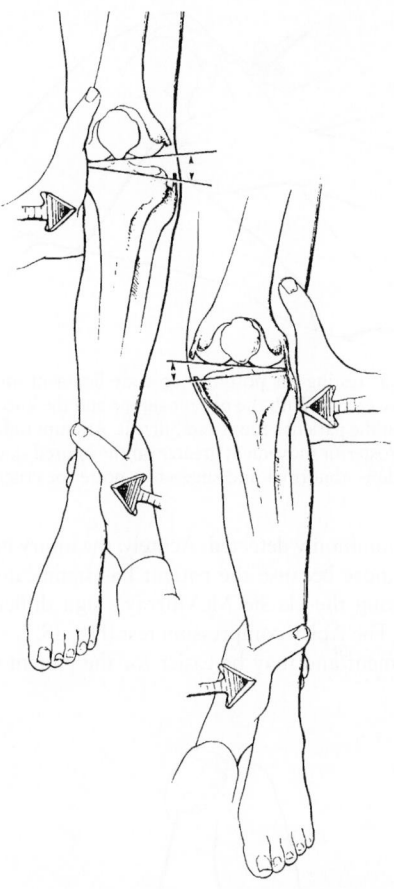

FIGURE 38.4 Testing for collateral ligament injury. Test the knee in full extension and in 30 degrees of flexion. To test for medial collateral ligament injury, hold and apply force to the medial side of the ankle with one hand and apply pressure over the fibular head with the other hand. To test for lateral collateral ligament injury, hold and apply force to the lateral side of the ankle with one hand and apply pressure just below the medial side of the knee with the other hand. If the knee "opens up" laterally or medially more than the uninjured knee, the collateral ligament is injured.

injuries are rare before adolescence because in a child, the ACL's insertion point, the tibial spine, is incompletely ossified. Therefore, the same force that would produce an ACL injury in an adolescent will cause an avulsion fracture of the tibial spine in a child. Radiographs may detect an epiphyseal fracture, tibial spine fracture, or an avulsed bone fragment due to an MCL or LCL injury.

Posterior cruciate ligament injuries are extremely rare and usually result from direct force on the tibial tubercle, pushing the tibia posteriorly on the femur. The posterior drawer sign will be present in most cases (Fig. 38.5).

The menisci are tough fibrocartilage pads that help distribute the body's weight over the femoral and tibial condyles. They can be injured when the knee is twisted during weight bearing. The patient, usually older than 12 years, may report a popping sensation and the feeling of the knee "giving out." More chronically, the patient may report that the knee suddenly refuses to extend fully, "locking up," and then suddenly "unlocking." Joint-line tenderness is frequently present (sensitivity 0.7 to 0.8, specificity 0.2) but must be differentiated from the tenderness associated with collateral ligament injuries. An

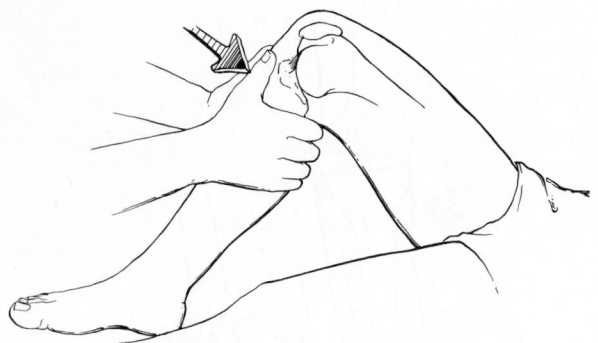

FIGURE 38.5 Testing for posterior cruciate ligament injury with the posterior drawer test. With the patient supine and the knee flexed to 90 degrees, sit on the patient's foot to stabilize it. Attempt to force the tibia posteriorly. Posterior movement greater on the injured side than on the uninjured side is abnormal and suggests a posterior cruciate ligament injury.

effusion is commonly detected. Acutely, the injury may be difficult to diagnose because the patient has significantly reduced ROM, making the classic McMurray's sign difficult to elicit (Fig. 38.6). The Apley compression test (Fig. 38.7) requires less knee movement and may be easier for the patient to tolerate.

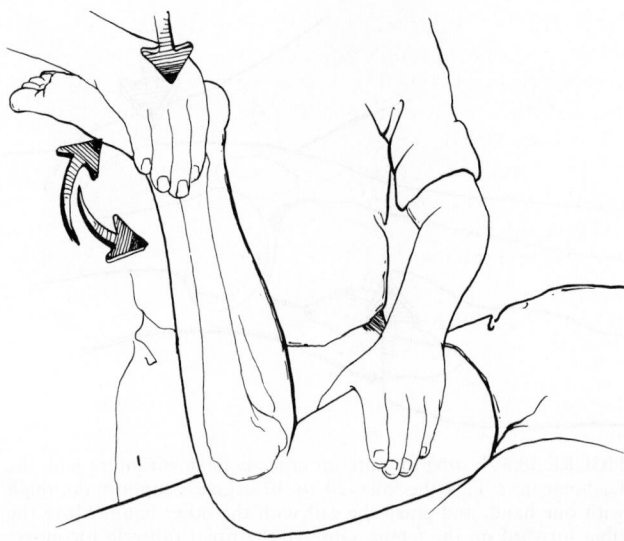

FIGURE 38.7 Testing for meniscal injury with the Apley compression test. With the patient prone and the knee flexed to 90 degrees, apply pressure to the heel while the tibia is rotated. If this produces pain that resolves when the tibia is distracted from the femur while rotated, a meniscal injury should be suspected.

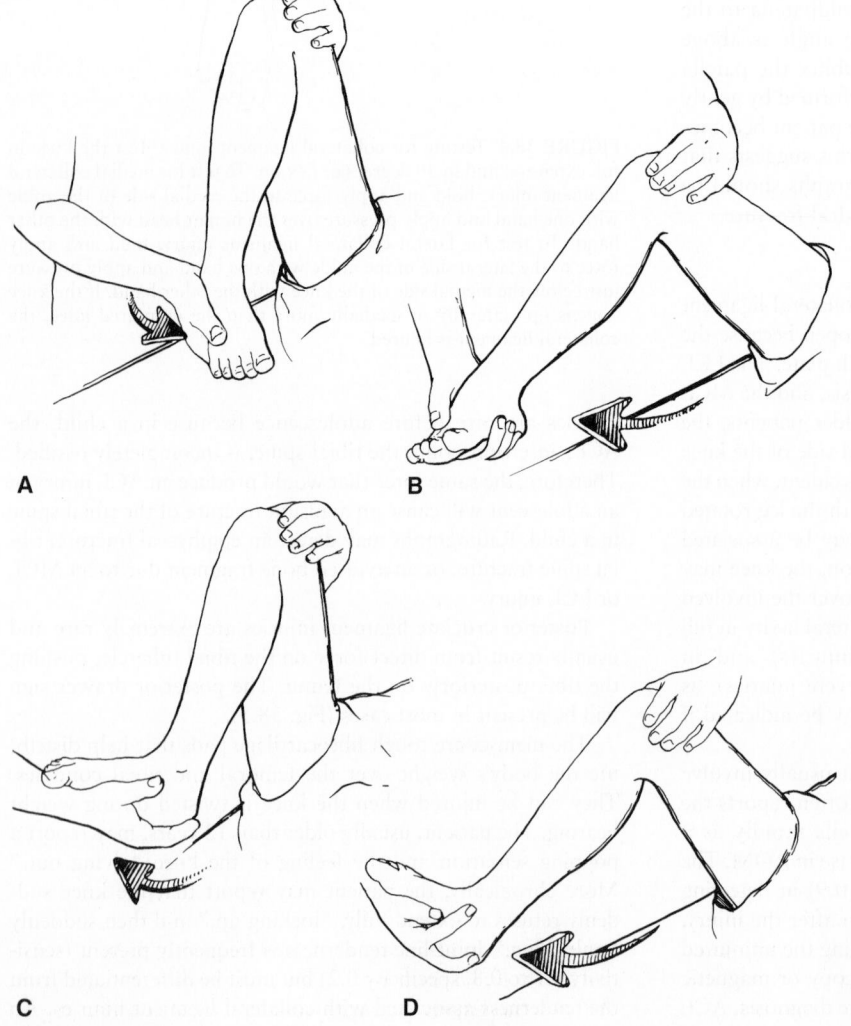

FIGURE 38.6 A–D: Testing for meniscal injury with the McMurray test. Grasp the patient's foot with one hand and place the other hand over the joint lines, push on the lateral side to apply a valgus force. Fully flex and extend the knee while alternately internally and externally rotating the tibia. The injured meniscus may be felt as a click or snapping sensation as the knee is manipulated.

Radiographs are generally obtained to evaluate for other causes of the pain. A subluxating patella, ACL injury, or osteochondral fracture may also cause a popping sensation, and the patellofemoral pain syndrome (PFPS) may be associated with "giving way" of the knee.

The quadriceps or patellar tendon can rupture acutely, especially in an older athlete who jumps or falls a great distance. The patient will not be able to actively extend the knee, the area over the rupture may be tender, and the patella may be positioned abnormally. A hemarthrosis may be present, and radiographs may show the abnormally positioned patella.

The three hamstring muscles (semitendinosus, semimembranosus, and biceps femoris) flex the knee and may be strained in young athletes. The semitendinosus and semimembranosus run along the medial popliteal space, and the biceps femoris tendon runs laterally. The patient may describe an acute pain or even a pop in the back of the thigh or may present subacutely with posterior thigh and popliteal knee pain when the hamstrings are strained by repetitive use. Palpation of the tendons is painful.

Posttraumatic Infection

Although not considered injuries, acute infections may present after a vague history of trauma. Physical findings of acute infection are present. The most common disorders are septic arthritis, osteomyelitis, cellulitis, and septic prepatellar bursitis.

Subacute Injuries

Many subacute knee problems manifest acutely in the ED. Osgood-Schlatter's disease of the tibial tubercle may lead to similar symptoms as a traumatic avulsion of the tubercle; however, with Osgood-Schlatter's disease, the symptoms have been noted for days or weeks. The symptoms of Osgood-Schlatter's disease are exacerbated by squatting or jumping, but they do not cause the same disability as an acute avulsion. The disease is usually seen in patients between 11 and 15 years of age. It may be caused by recurrent contractions of the patellar tendon during knee extension, traumatizing the tendon's insertion on the tibial tubercle during the child's growth spurt. The patients have localized tenderness and occasional swelling over the tibial tubercle. The patient will refuse to extend the knee against force (e.g., perform a deep-knee bend) and have difficulty going up or down stairs, although they may have a normal gait on a level surface. To eliminate the possibility of a neoplasm, the physician should always obtain radiographs. In Osgood-Schlatter's disease, the radiographs will either be normal or show irregularity of the tubercle.

PFPS or chondromalacia patella may be caused by misalignment of the extensor mechanism of the knee. The patella transmits the force of the quadriceps muscles to the patellar tendon to extend the knee. The vastus lateralis, vastus intermedius, and rectus femoris pull the patella slightly laterally and need to be balanced perfectly by the vastus medialis to keep the patella tracking across the articular cartilage correctly. Some of these patients have chondromalacia patella, with softening of the cartilage. The patient with PFPS has patellar pain with running and especially while going down inclines or stairs. The patient may also have the sensation of the knee giving out when descending, although an actual fall does not usually occur. The patient may describe pain when sitting for a prolonged time with the knee flexed at 90 degrees (e.g., in class). The pain disappears once the patient is ambulatory. On examination, the patient may have the medially displaced patella, an increased Q angle, tenderness of the articular surface of the patella, and a positive patellar stress test. This test is performed with the patient in the supine position with the knee fully extended. The patient is asked to relax the quadriceps so that the physician can move the patella. With the patella pulled inferiorly, the physician should gently press down on it and ask the patient to tighten the quadriceps. (A younger patient should be asked to "push the knee into the examination table.") This will move the patella superiorly as the physician continues to press down. A patient with PFPS will have acute pain with this maneuver. Radiographs are normal.

Patellar tendon tendinitis, or "jumper's knee," occurs in patients during their growth spurt, especially those involved in jumping (knee extension) sports. The knee is tender on the inferior pole of the patella and the adjacent patellar tendon, but not on the tibial tubercle; radiographs are generally normal.

Prepatellar bursitis occurs after acute or chronic trauma to this bursa, which overlies the patella. The patient will have swelling over the anterior aspect of the knee, especially over the patella. A septic bursitis may need to be ruled out by needle aspiration.

Osteochondritis dissecans is the separation of a small portion of the femoral condyle with the overlying cartilage. The patient is usually an adolescent with a 1- to 4-week history of nonspecific knee pain. The physical examination may be normal, or the femoral condyle may be tender with the knee flexed. Because AP and lateral radiographs may not show the lesion, a tunnel or intercondylar view should be obtained.

Iliotibial band syndrome usually occurs in older runners who complain of pain over the lateral femoral condyle. The iliotibial band moves in an anterior or posterior direction across the lateral femoral condyle as the knee flexes and extends. This repetitive movement may cause the pain. When examined, the patient is tender over the lateral femoral epicondyle, palpable 2 cm above the joint line. Radiographs are normal.

The Baker's cyst is a herniation of the synovium of the knee joint or a separate synovial cyst located in the popliteal fossa. The patient complains of popliteal pain and swelling only if the cyst enlarges. The sac can be palpated in the posterior medial aspect of the popliteal space and may be transilluminated. For the most part, radiographs will be normal or show soft-tissue swelling.

In any patient with knee pain, with or without a history of trauma and benign (e.g., osteochondroma and nonossifying fibroma) and malignant tumors (e.g., osteosarcoma or Ewing's sarcoma), the various causes of monoarticular arthritis (see Chapter 56) and hip disease that may present with knee pain (e.g., slipped capital femoral epiphysis or aseptic necrosis of the femoral head) must be considered.

EVALUATION AND DECISION

Four points are critical in the patient's history: (i) the activity and forces that led to the injury (e.g., direction of the force, whether the foot was fixed); (ii) the initial location of the pain; (iii) any sensations or noises (e.g., "locking," "pops," or "tears"); and (iv) the timing of any swelling.

The possibility of abuse in young children must always be considered, especially if the injury is unexplained, the history is implausible, or the delay in seeking of medical care was unreasonable.

Most severe injuries (e.g., ACL, collateral ligament, or meniscal injuries) occur when the patient is involved in high-velocity weight-bearing activities, especially running and making sharp cuts or being subjected to direct valgus or varus stress.

Lower-velocity injuries usually result in only patellar dislocation or subluxation. Direct trauma to the front of the knee may cause posterior cruciate ligament injuries or patellar fractures, whereas lateral to medial (valgus) forces may cause collateral or cruciate ligament damage or fractures. Distinct popping noises or tearing sensations are reported in ACL injuries and patellar subluxation. Locking of the knee often may be reported in meniscal injuries but not immediately after the injury. Although the knee may "hurt all over" when seen in the ED, the patient may be able to localize the initial pain. Meniscal or collateral ligament injuries cause pain on the lateral or medial aspect of the knee, whereas ACL injuries hurt just inferior to the patella, and Osgood-Schlatter's disease is painful a few centimeters inferior to the patella over the tibial tubercle. Swelling within 2 hours strongly suggests hemarthrosis and an associated ACL injury, meniscal injury, or osteochondral fracture. Swelling after 4 to 12 hours is more likely to be an isolated effusion without an associated fracture or ligamentous injury.

In subacute injuries, ask about hip or groin pain because the hip and knee share sensory nerves. Legg-Calve-Perthes disease or a slipped capital femoral epiphysis may cause anterior thigh or knee pain. Inquire about changes in physical activities or footwear. Patellar pain and the sensation of the knee giving way without actually falling when going down stairs or inclines suggest PFPS (i.e., chondromalacia patella). Exacerbation doing deep-knee bends suggests Osgood-Schlatter's disease or patellar tendonitis.

Examination of the patient should include walking and standing to check for medially deviated "squinting" patellae. Inspect and palpate the knee in two positions, sitting relaxed with the knees at 90 degrees and supine. When sitting, the knees are inspected for swelling, bony changes (e.g., swelling and tenderness over the tibial tubercle in Osgood-Schlatter's disease), joint-line tenderness (meniscal injuries), and quadriceps atrophy.

With the patient supine, repeat inspection and palpation over the joint line, collateral ligaments, patella, proximal fibula, tibial tuberosity, and popliteal space. If the knee appears swollen, check for an effusion. Normally, synovial fluid coats the patellar surface but does not separate the patella and femur. When fluid separates the two bones, a sharp pat on the patella results in the sensation of a tap as the two bones meet. If the joint contains a large amount of fluid, the patella will not touch the femur but will feel as if it is sitting on a cushion. Document the ROM of the knee.

The physician should test for collateral and cruciate ligament damage, meniscal injuries, patellar subluxation, and PFPS, using the appropriate maneuvers (Table 38.2).

Distal pulses, the posterior tibial, and the dorsalis pedis should be palpated, and the peroneal nerve function should be

TABLE 38.2

SUMMARY OF DIAGNOSTIC MANEUVERS FOR THE INJURED KNEE

Maneuver	Diagnosis
Collateral laxity test (Fig. 38.4)	Collateral ligament injury
Lachman test (Fig. 38.3)	Anterior cruciate ligament injury
Posterior drawer test (Fig. 38.5)	Posterior cruciate ligament injury
McMurray test (Fig. 38.6)	Meniscal injury
Apley compression test (Fig. 38.7)	Meniscal injury
Patellar apprehension test	Patellar subluxation
Patellar stress test	Patellofemoral pain syndrome

assessed. The deep peroneal nerve enervates the ankle dorsiflexors. The extensor hallucis longus can be tested by opposing dorsiflexion of the great toe. The deep peroneal nerve supplies sensation to the web space between the great and second toes.

Patients with knee symptoms should have a careful hip examination because patients with aseptic necrosis of the femoral head or a slipped capital femoral epiphysis may present with anterior thigh or knee pain.

All patients with acute knee injuries should have AP and lateral radiographs, and if indicated, a patellar (or skyline view) radiograph should be taken. If the injury is more chronic, an intercondylar or tunnel view should also be taken to evaluate for osteochondritis dissecans.

The Ottawa Knee Rules have demonstrated 100% sensitivity for knee fractures in large, prospective, multicentered adult trials. Studies in children are more limited but they also demonstrated a sensitivity of 100% (95% confidence interval = 95% to 100%) in a study involving 750 children of whom 70 had fractures. According to the OKR, radiographs are required of children only if the patient has any of the following finding: (i) isolated tenderness of the patella, (ii) tenderness of the head of the fibula, (iii) inability to flex to 90 degrees, (iv) inability to bear weight both immediately and in the ED (4 steps) regardless of limping.

Figure 38.8 summarizes an approach to the child with an acutely injured knee. If the initial evaluation suggests vascular compromise, traction and reduction of the knee should be attempted and an emergency orthopedics consultation should be obtained. If the patella is obviously dislocated, it may be reduced before obtaining radiographs. Postreduction radiographs and a careful examination for physeal tenderness then can exclude the diagnosis of a fracture. If the patient's knee is too painful or swollen to allow a complete examination, or if the patient has a hemarthrosis, ligament or meniscal damage should be suspected. The patient should be instructed to use cruches and remain completely non–weight bearing until medical or surgical follow-up or until the patient improves.

If the patient tolerates an examination, a series of maneuvers may suggest collateral ligament injury, cruciate ligament

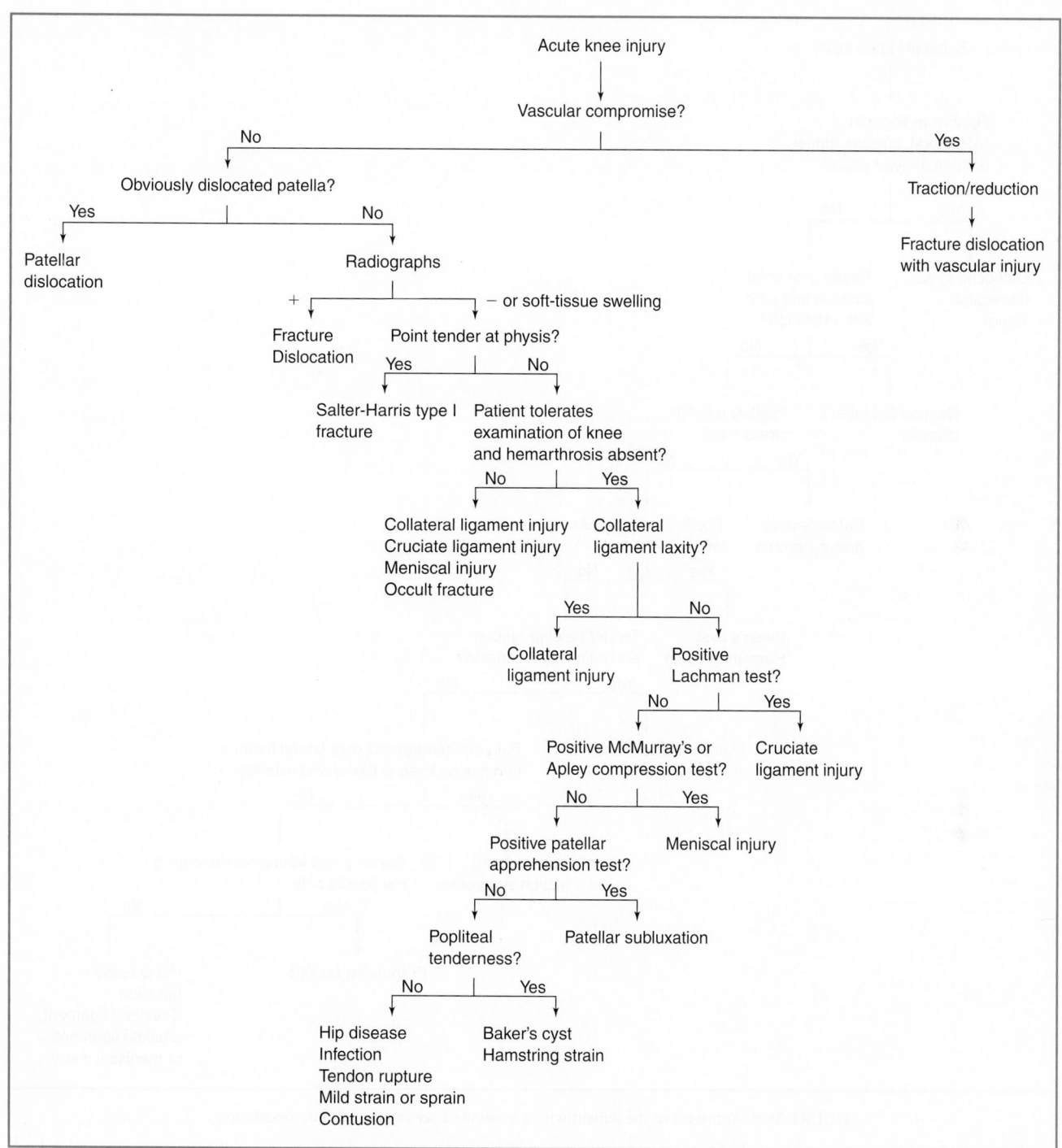

FIGURE 38.8 Approach to the patient with an acute knee injury.

injury, meniscal injury, or patellar subluxation as the diagnosis. (Table 38.2 summarizes the diagnostic maneuvers for the knee.) Next, an assessment for popliteal tenderness, to exclude a Baker's cyst or hamstring strain, is performed. Finally, if no signs of infection or hip disease exist, the patient may have a tendon rupture, mild ligament sprain, or bone contusion.

Often, a patient may come to the ED with a history of trauma and knee pain that has been present for more than 1 or 2 days (Fig. 38.9). In addition to the standard AP, lateral, and patellar views, a tunnel or intercondylar view should be taken to exclude a fracture, tumor, and osteochondritis dissecans. If the initial knee and hip examinations do not suggest a diagnosis and no signs of infection exist, the diagnostic maneuvers in Table 38.2 should be completed. The patient may have an old collateral ligament, cruciate ligament, or meniscal injury and may require an orthopedic referral.

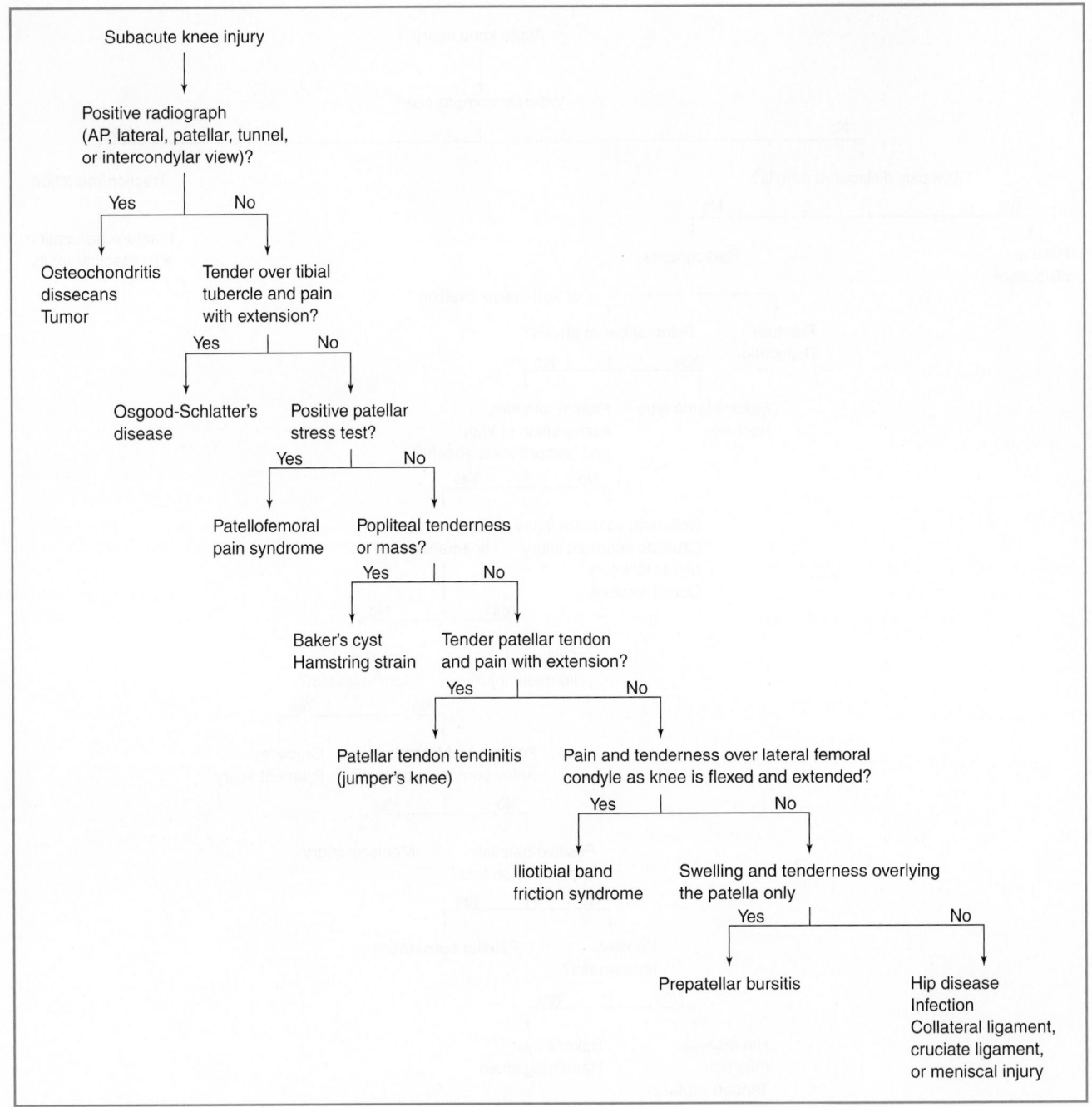

FIGURE 38.9 Approach to the patient with a subacute knee injury. AP, anteroposterior.

Suggested Readings

Beaty JH, Kasser JR, eds. *Rockwood and Wilkins' fractures in children*, 6th ed. Philadelphia, PA: Lippincott Williams & Wilkins, 2006.

Bulloch B, Neto G, Plint A, et al. Validation of the Ottawa Knee Rules in children: a multicenter trial. *Ann Emerg Med* 2003;42:48–55.

Micheli LJ, Kocher MS, eds. *The pediatric and adolescent knee*. Philadelphia, PA: Saunders Elsevier, 2006.

Micheli LJ, Purcell L, eds. *The adolescent athelete: a practical approach*. New York, NY: Springer Verlag, 2007.

Solomon DH, Simel DL, Bates DW, et al. Does this patient have a torn meniscus or ligament of the knee? Value of the physical examination. *JAMA* 2001;286:1610–1620.

CHAPTER 39 ■ INJURY—SHOULDER

MARC N. BASKIN, MD

This chapter focuses on the diagnosis of the child with an acutely injured shoulder. For the preverbal child with a possible shoulder injury presenting with an immobile arm, see Chapter 35. Children have different etiologies for their shoulder injuries than do adults because of their open growth plates, and young patients may be more difficult to examine because of anxiety and limited verbal skills. Figure 39.1 shows the important bony anatomy.

DIFFERENTIAL DIAGNOSIS

The differential diagnosis depends primarily on exactly where the patient has pain and the type of trauma. In this chapter, injuries are described anatomically, from the sternoclavicular joint to the humeral shaft (Tables 39.1 and 39.2).

Physeal (growth plate) fractures of the medial clavicle can be caused by direct trauma to the medial clavicle or by indirect trauma that forces the shoulder medially and separates the growth plate. This injury mimics the sternoclavicular dislocations seen in skeletally mature patients. In patients younger than 22 to 25 years, injury to the sternoclavicular joint causes physeal fractures because the epiphysis of the medial clavicle begins to ossify between 13 and 19 years of age and fuses between 22 and 25 years of age. Once fused, a similar injury will cause sternoclavicular joint dislocations. Most separations are anterior, and the patient has swelling and tenderness over the sternoclavicular joint. Anteroposterior (AP) and superiorly projected lordotic radiographs comparing both clavicles may not visualize the lesion. Computed tomography (CT) is usually necessary to delineate the lesion. If the dislocation is posterior, the aorta or trachea may be injured. The child may remain asymptomatic or may complain of dysphagia or difficulty breathing. If the growth plate and ligaments are not disrupted by the injury, a simple sprain has occurred.

The clavicle is a commonly fractured bone in children, most often in the middle or lateral third of the bone. The clavicle is subject to any medially directed force on the upper limb (e.g., a fall on an outstretched hand) but is commonly fractured by a direct blow. Although subclavian vessels and the brachial plexus are just beneath the clavicle, they are rarely injured because the subclavius muscle is interposed between the bone and vessels, and the thick periosteum of the clavicle rarely splinters. A neonate's birthing injury or an infant's greenstick fracture of the clavicle may go unnoticed until the focal swelling of the developing callus is noted. In the older child, the arm droops down and forward and the head may be tilted toward the affected side because of sternocleidomastoid muscle spasm. Localized swelling, tenderness, and crepitations may be noted. A radiograph will confirm the diagnosis. Rarely,

a radiograph obtained because of clavicular trauma will show a congenital pseudarthrosis or false joint of the clavicle.

Osteolysis of the distal clavicle with resorption of the bone may develop after minor injuries to the clavicle. Patients experience chronic pain and mild swelling 2 to 3 weeks after the initial injury. Radiographs are diagnostic.

Acromioclavicular (AC) joint injuries usually cause physeal fractures of the distal clavicle in patients younger than 14 years. Older children may sprain the AC joint (shoulder separations). Either injury is most often caused by a direct blow to the shoulder. The child will have pain with any motion of the shoulder and tenderness over the AC joint. Grade I and II injuries are nondisplaced. Grade III and IV injuries are displaced 25% to 100%, and Grade V injuries are more than 100% displaced. Bilateral "stress view" radiographs of the AC joint may be obtained to compare the separation on the normal and affected sides. Cosmetic deformities and degenerative changes of the distal clavicle may complicate these injuries, even with appropriate therapy.

Scapula fractures are rare in pediatrics and usually occur only after major direct trauma, such as a motor vehicle accident or a fall from a height. The child will have tenderness over the scapula. The patient often sustains other more life-threatening injuries (e.g., head injuries, rib fractures, or pneumothoraces).

Shoulder or glenohumeral joint dislocations are rare in children younger than 12 years. These injuries become common in adolescence as the skeleton matures. The glenohumeral joint is shallow, allowing a wide range of motion but increasing the risk of dislocation. The patient is injured when an already abducted and externally rotated arm is forcibly extended posteriorly (e.g., blocking in football or missing a slam dunk and striking the rim during basketball). This action leverages the humeral head out of the glenoid fossa. The trauma can damage the axillary nerve or fracture the humeral head. More than 95% of all dislocations are anterior, and less than 5% are posterior. The patient will be in severe pain, supporting the affected arm internally rotated and slightly abducted (i.e., the patient cannot bring the elbow to his or her side). The shoulder contour is sharp, unlike the smooth contour of the opposite shoulder, and the acromion is prominent (Fig. 39.2). Sensation over the lateral deltoid muscle (axillary nerve distribution), lateral proximal forearm (musculocutaneous nerve distribution), and distal pulses should be documented. Radiographs should always be obtained because a humeral head or even a clavicular fracture may mimic a shoulder dislocation. An AP, transscapular lateral (Neer's), and an axillary view will show the position of the dislocation and the presence of any fractures.

If the patient has a history consistent with dislocation but has more range of motion than expected and the radiograph is

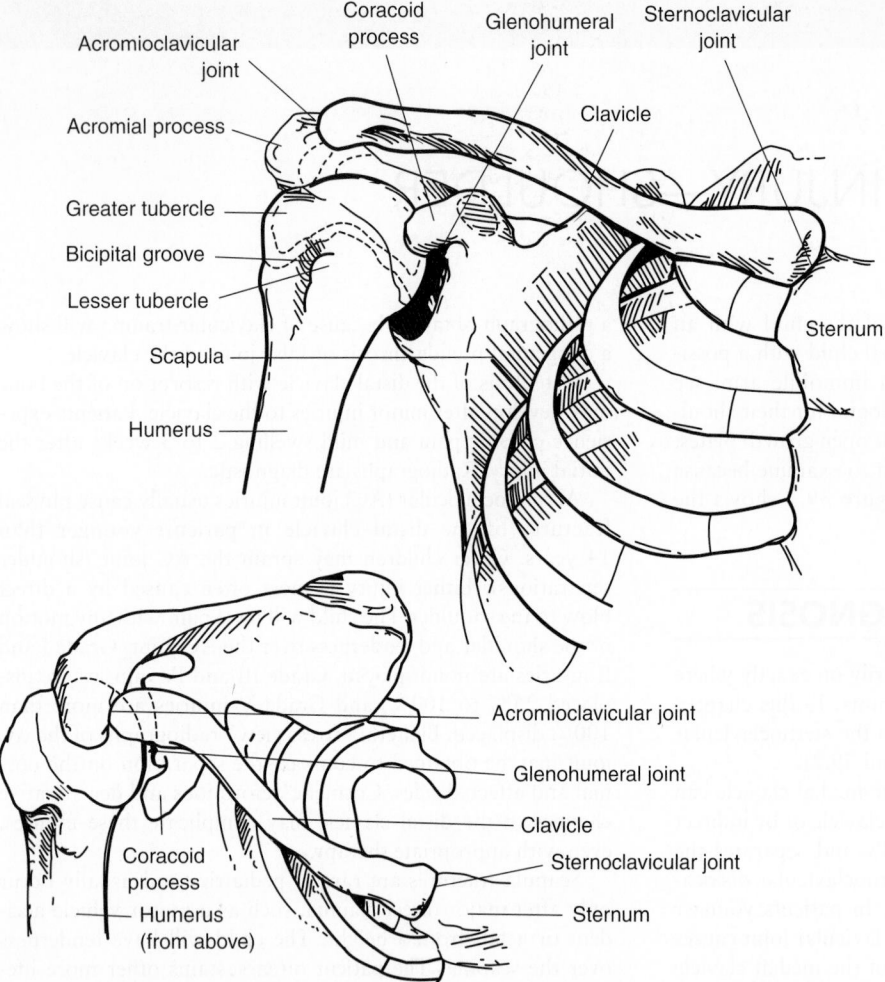

FIGURE 39.1 Anatomy of the shoulder.

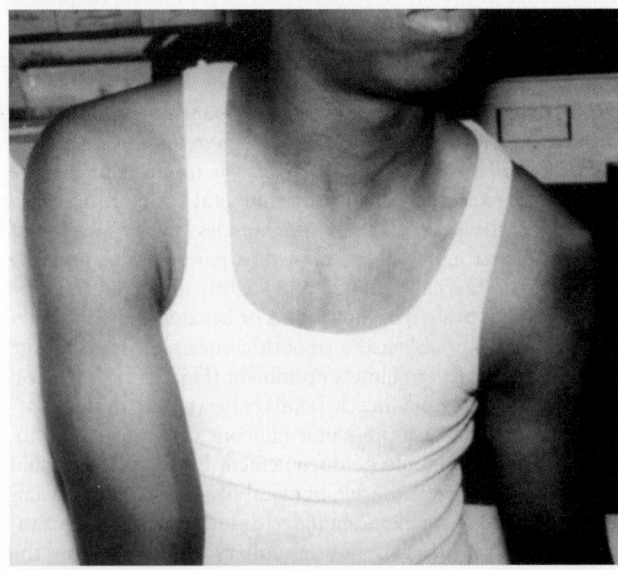

FIGURE 39.2 An older adolescent patient with left anterior gleno-humeral joint dislocation. Notice the sharp contour of the shoulder, the fullness below the glenoid fossa, and the prominent acromion.

normal, the patient may have spontaneously reduced a dislo-cated shoulder or subluxated the glenohumeral joint and only sprained the ligaments overlying the glenoid fossa. An appre-hension test may confirm the diagnosis (Fig. 39.3).

Actual tears of the rotator cuff are uncommon before 21 years of age. However, if the rotator cuff muscles are dam-aged or weak, the humeral head is displaced upward during overhead motion and may impinge the tendon of the supraspinatus muscle as it runs below the acromion. Impinge-ment symptoms usually occur with repetitive overhead motions (e.g., throwing a ball). The pain is poorly localized or most notable over the deltoid area. Pain with passive full forward flexion may be suggestive. The Hawkins' test (Fig. 39.4) and Yocum's test may elicit pain suggestive of rotator cuff injury. For the Yocum's test, have the patient place the hand of the painful side on the opposite shoulder. The examiner should then raise the elbow without raising the affected shoulder. Pain during this maneuver is suggestive of rotator cuff injury. Of the rotator cuff muscles, the most commonly weakened is the supraspina-tus. This can be tested by putting the arm in about 90 degrees of abduction and 30 degrees of forward flexion with the shoul-der internally rotated, that is, thumbs down or "empty the

TABLE 39.1

DIFFERENTIAL DIAGNOSIS OF THE INJURED SHOULDER

Sternoclavicular joint
  Dislocation[a]
  Sprain
Clavicle
  Physeal fracture/separation of medial clavicle
  Fracture
  Contusion (shoulder pointer)
  Osteolysis
Acromioclavicular joint dislocation or sprain (shoulder
  separation)
Scapula fracture
Glenohumeral joint
  Dislocation (shoulder dislocation)
  Subluxation
  Labral tears
Rotator cuff tendonopathy with impingement symptoms
  Rotator cuff tear
Humerus
  Fracture of proximal humeral physis
  Stress fracture of proximal humeral physis (Little League
  shoulder)
  Fracture of shaft
Biceps tendon tendonitis
Pathologic fracture[a]
Referred pain (from)
  Myocardium[a]
  Diaphragm[a]
  Neck
Thoracic outlet syndrome[a]
Brachial plexus injury "pinched nerve" or "stinger"

[a]Potentially life-threatening conditions.

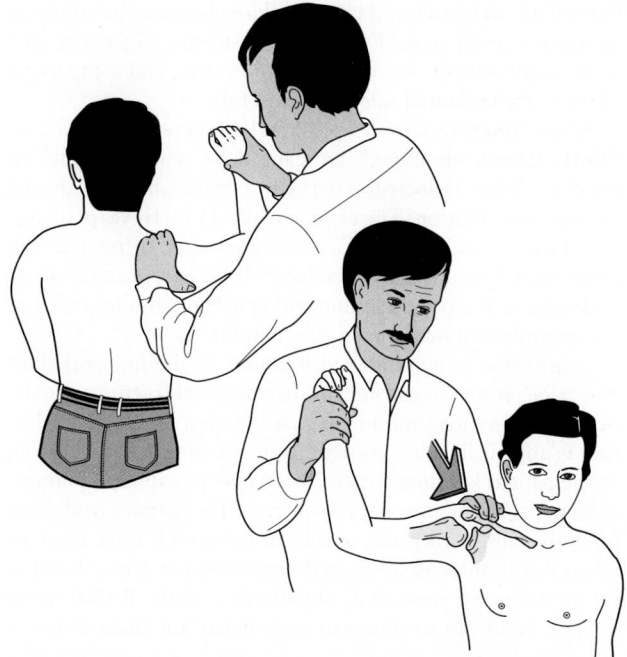

FIGURE 39.3 The apprehension test to evaluate for shoulder subluxation. The patient's shoulder should be abducted passively and rotated externally. If this elicits apprehension or pain, the test is positive. If not, the examiner then should apply anteriorly directed pressure to the posterior aspect of the humeral head. If this elicits pain, then the test also is positive and the patient's shoulder may have subluxed or the patient may have instability of the glenohumeral joint.

can" position. Push down on the arm as the patient resists. Pain without weakness is consistent with rotator cuff injury. Pain with significant weakness suggests possible tendon tear. Plain radiographs are usually normal, and a magnetic resonance imaging may be necessary.

Fracture separations of the proximal humeral epiphysis occur until the patient's epiphysis closes because the ligamentous attachments are stronger than the growth plate. The epiphysis closes between 16 and 18 years of age in males and about 1 year earlier in females. The injury occurs because of direct or indirect trauma, such as an attempt to break a fall with a hand. The patient usually has mild swelling and local tenderness. AP and lateral radiographs confirm the diagnosis, although they are

TABLE 39.2

COMMON CAUSES OF THE INJURED SHOULDER

Clavicle fracture
Glenohumeral joint
  Dislocation (shoulder dislocation)
  Subluxation
Humerus
  Fracture of proximal humeral physis

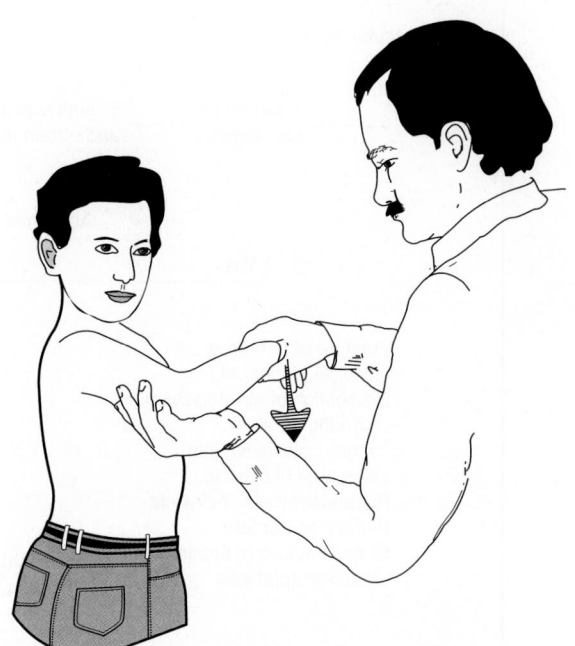

FIGURE 39.4 The Hawkins' test to evaluate for impingement of the supraspinatus tendon. The patient's arm should be held in internal rotation and 90 degrees of forward flexion. Internally rotatate the shoulder further by gently pushing the forearm downward while supporting the elbow. This brings the humeral head up against the acromion. Pain especially localized below the acromion suggests impingement.

less reliable in infants and young children because the epiphysis is mainly cartilaginous. Even in older patients, slight widening of the epiphysis may be difficult to appreciate, and comparison views of the uninjured side may be useful.

Stress fractures of the proximal humeral epiphysis, or "Little League shoulder," are caused by repetitive internal rotation of an abducted, externally rotated shoulder during the throwing motion. The child, usually 11 to 16 years of age, has diffuse shoulder pain that worsens after throwing. The proximal humerus may be tender and radiographs may show widening of the proximal humeral epiphysis. Radiographs of the contralateral humerus may be helpful.

Transverse or comminuted fractures of the humeral shaft may occur from direct trauma, whereas spiral fractures usually occur from indirect trauma (e.g., a fall on a hand). If the history is implausible, inconsistent from one caregiver to another, or the patient is younger than 2 years, the possibility of nonaccidental trauma must be considered. The patient will have obvious pain, tenderness, and local deformity. Care must be taken not to miss an associated neurovascular injury because the radial nerve runs along the humeral shaft. Radial nerve damage results in weakness of wrist extension and anesthesia of the skin between the first and second metacarpals. Radiographs help rule out a pathologic fracture (e.g., through a unicameral bone cyst or tumor).

In older patients, shoulder pain may be due to tendonitis of the tendon of the long head of the biceps. This tendon is palpable as it runs through the bicipital groove just anterior and medial to the greater humeral tuberosity. The patient often has chronic pain and tenderness over the bicipital groove.

A painful shoulder or fracture that follows minimal trauma may be caused by a benign or malignant tumor or by nonneoplastic bone lesions. Osteochondromas (exostoses) are outgrowths of benign cartilage from the bone adjacent to the epiphysis and present with a mass adjacent to a joint. The nonossifying fibromas (called "fibrous cortical defects" if smaller than 0.5 cm) are common asymptomatic lesions that may lead to pathologic fractures.

The malignant chondroblastoma is a rare tumor, but its most common location is the proximal humerus. The patient often has joint pain from an effusion associated with this tumor. Osteogenic sarcomas and Ewing's sarcoma are more common but involve the humerus in only 10% of cases.

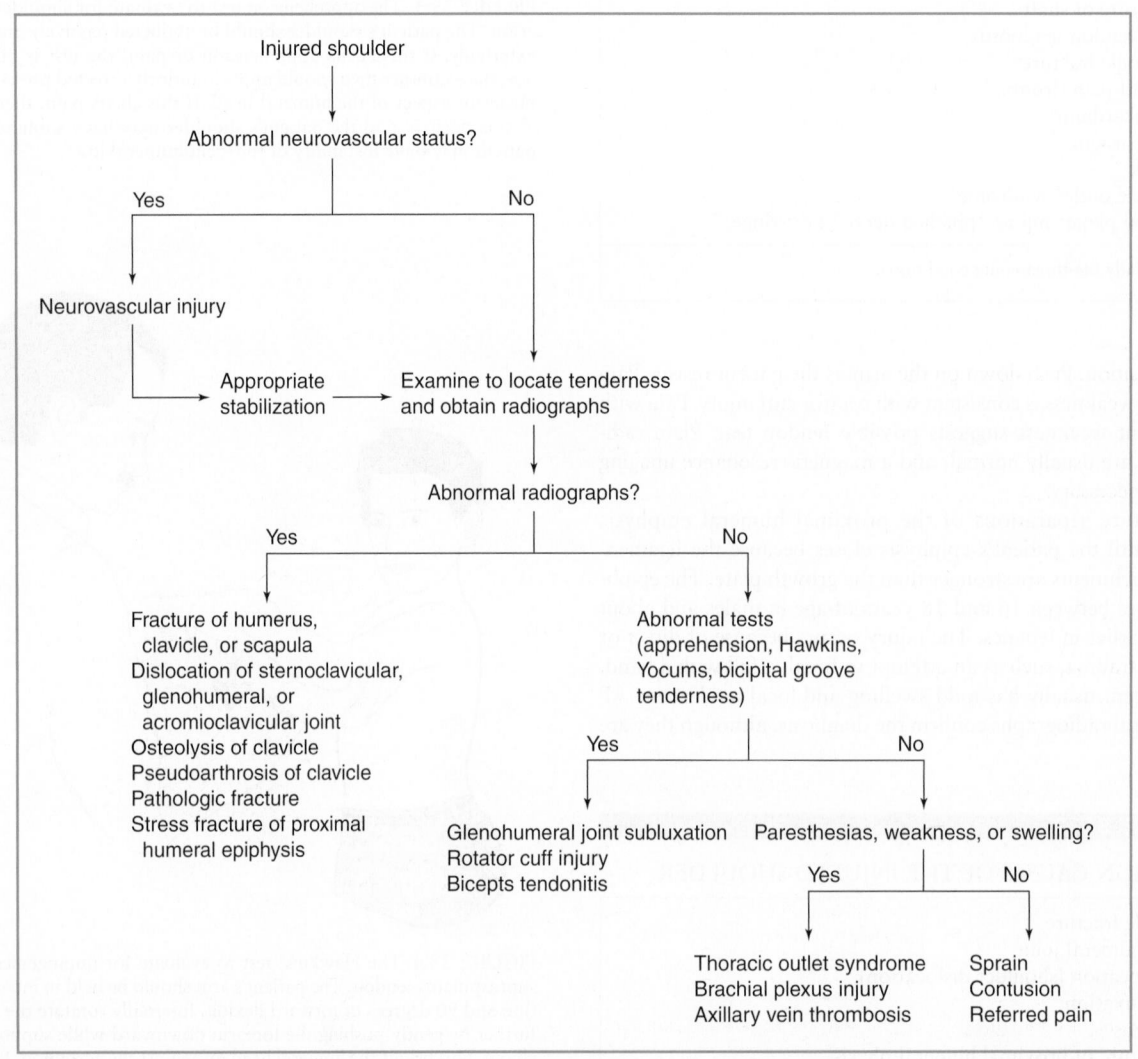

FIGURE 39.5 Approach to the patient with an injured shoulder.

Unicameral and aneurysmal bone cysts are asymptomatic until the bone fractures, but they are not neoplastic lesions. Unicameral or "simple bone" cysts are benign fluid-filled cavities most commonly localized to the proximal humerus.

Shoulder pain may also be referred from the neck (e.g., cervical disc herniation), myocardium, or diaphragm (e.g., a splenic hematoma) after trauma to those areas.

Thoracic outlet syndrome, with compression of the lower roots of the brachial plexus (C8 to T1) may present as shoulder pain. The numbness and paresthesias most commonly follow the dermatome of the ulnar nerve. The symptoms may be induced (Roo's test) by having the patient rapidly open and close their hands for 3 minutes with the arm abducted 90 degrees and the shoulder externally rotated. The test is considered positive if it induces the patient's pain and paresthesias. A chest radiograph may demonstrate a cervical rib. Thoracic outlet symptoms may also be caused by axillary vein thrombosis, most commonly in a pitcher. The patient may have nonspecific arm pain and swelling but may also have dyspnea and chest pain if the thrombus is embolizing. Swelling and discoloration due to venous congestion may be present. Ultrasonography is diagnostic.

Acute brachial plexus injuries ("pinched nerves" or "stingers") are common in high-impact sports. Most commonly, the shoulder is forcefully depressed and the head and neck tilted to the opposite side, stretching the brachial plexus. The patient has immediate arm weakness or paralysis and paresthesias or numbness along a cervical dermatome, most commonly C5 and C6. Less commonly, C8 to T1 can be injured when the arm is forcefully abducted, for example, falling and grabbing a tree branch. The symptoms may resolve prior to the emergency department evaluation. Cervical spine injuries must be excluded.

EVALUATION AND DECISION

Initially, the patient's neurovascular status is assessed and fracture stabilization provided, if necessary (Fig. 39.5).

For an isolated shoulder injury, ask the patient to localize the pain as specifically as possible and determine the mechanism of injury. Determine whether the trauma was direct or indirect and ascertain what position the shoulder was in when the injury occurred. If the pain is chronic, determine the position or motion that most exacerbates the pain (e.g., throwing a ball). Ask the patient about any distal paresthesias, associated pain, and trauma (e.g., neck, chest, abdomen). Always consider the possibility of abuse in young children, especially if the injury is unexplained, the history is implausible, or inconsistent between caregivers, or the seeking of medical care was delayed unreasonably.

Observe the patient without clothes over the shoulder for positioning of the arm, swelling, deformity, or any asymmetry. Ask the patient to point with one finger to the most painful area. This observation period before the formal physical examination is especially important in a young, anxious child and helps prioritize the rest of the evaluation.

If the child seems anxious, examine the uninjured side first. Carefully palpate the entire shoulder from sternoclavicular joint to the shaft of the humerus. Swelling and tenderness at the sternoclavicular joint suggests a physeal separation or dislocation at this site. The clavicle is covered only by a thin platysma muscle, and a fracture is easily seen and palpated. Just lateral to the

clavicle is the AC joint. Elevation of the clavicle above the acromion or tenderness of the articulation suggests AC joint dislocation (shoulder separation) or sprain. Just in front of the greater tuberosity of the humerus is the tendon of the long head of the biceps within the bicipital groove. Pressure may produce exquisite tenderness in this area, so palpation should be gentle; if uncertainty about a finding of tenderness exists, a comparison with the examination of the uninjured side is helpful. Finally, the proximal humeral shaft and the scapula are palpated.

During the neurologic evaluation, it is important to test sensation over the deltoid muscle (to assess axillary nerve damage after shoulder dislocation) and over the lateral proximal forearm (to assess musculocutaneous nerve damage).

Next, examine the patient's active and passive range of motion (Fig. 39.6), checking for abduction, adduction, forward flexion, backward extension, internal rotation, and external rotation. Internal and external rotation can be observed easily in a child by asking the patient to touch behind the neck (external rotation) and lower back to the inferior tip of the opposite scapula (internal rotation).

Once the pain has been localized, appropriate radiographs should be obtained. When indicated, additional specific tests may be performed: the apprehension test for shoulder subluxation and laxity (Fig. 39.3), Hawkins' (Fig. 39.4) and Yocum's tests for rotator cuff injury, and Roo's test for thoracic outlet syndrome.

If the patient has nonspecific pain with numbness, paresthesias, weakness, or diffuse swelling, a brachial plexus injury or thoracic outlet syndrome should be considered.

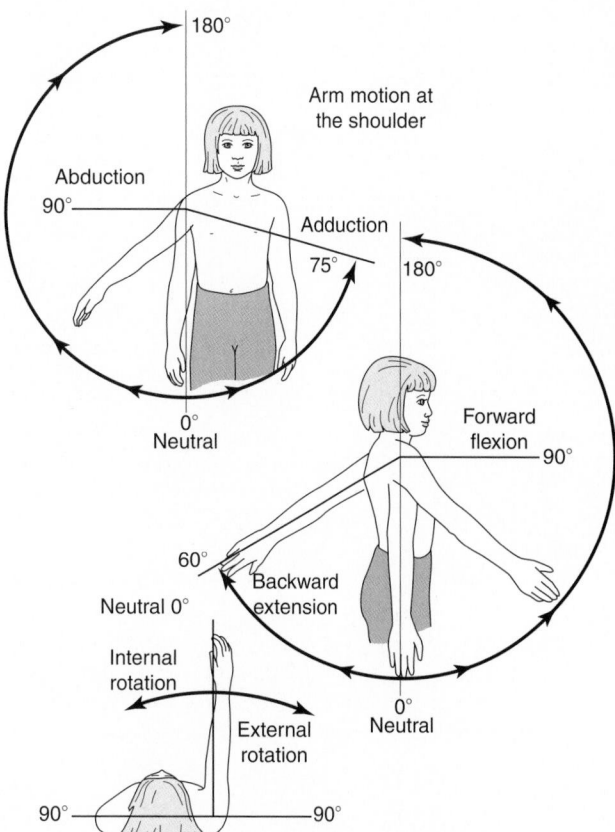

FIGURE 39.6 Range of motion of the shoulder joint.

Patients with normal radiographs and negative maneuvers are most likely to have sprains or contusions, but occasionally, they may be experiencing referred pain.

Suggested Readings

Beaty JH, Kasser JR, eds. *Rockwood and Wilkins' fractures in children*, 5th ed. Philadelphia, PA: Lippincott Williams & Wilkins, 2001.

Chen FS, Diaz VA, Loebenberg M, et al. Shoulder and elbow injuries in the skeletally immature athlete. *J Am Acad Orthop Surg* 2005;13(3):172–185.

Griffin LY, ed. *Essentials of musculoskeletal care*, 3rd ed. Rosemont, IL: American Academy of Orthopaedic Surgeons, 2005.

Hoppenfeld S. *Physical examination of the spine and extremities*. Norwalk, CT: Appleton-Century-Crofts, 1976.

Irvin R, Iversen D, Roy S. Sports medicine: prevention, assessment, management, and rehabilitation. Boston, MA: Allyn & Bacon, 1998.

Micheli LJ, Purcell L, eds. *The adolescent athlete: a practical approach*. New York, NY: Springer, 2007.

CHAPTER 40 ■ JAUNDICE—UNCONJUGATED HYPERBILIRUBINEMIA

KENNETH D. MANDL, MD, MPH

Jaundice—a yellowish discoloration of the skin, tissues, and bodily fluids—indicates an increased production or impaired excretion of bilirubin, leading to hyperbilirubinemia. Both physiologic and pathologic etiologies may give rise to unconjugated (or indirect) hyperbilirubinemia. To distinguish between them, the clinician must consider the patient's age, the rate of increase and peak level of serum bilirubin, and the historical features of the case. Prompt evaluation and therapy for unconjugated hyperbilirubinemia are particularly important for infants younger than 1 week. If bilirubin levels rise too high, these young infants risk developing neurodevelopmental deficits and kernicterus.

PATHOPHYSIOLOGY

Bilirubin is formed from the degradation of hemoglobin and other heme-containing proteins. Heme protoporphyrin becomes oxidized, producing biliverdin, which is then reduced to form bilirubin. In the blood, bilirubin is bound to albumin. The liver uptakes bilirubin for conjugation by a glucuronyl transferase and then excretes the conjugated form into bile. The net balance of its entry into and removal from the circulation determines serum bilirubin concentration. In the newborn infant, multiple factors contribute to hyperbilirubinemia, including increased red blood cell (RBC) volume and decreased red blood cell survival, as well as impaired plasma binding, liver uptake, conjugation, and excretion of bilirubin.

Older children and adults normally have serum bilirubin concentrations below 1 mg per dL and appear jaundiced when the bilirubin level rises above 2 mg per dL. Newborn infants become visibly jaundiced when their serum bilirubin concentration is above 5 mg per dL. In conjugated, or direct, hyperbilirubinemia, the conjugated (or direct reacting) portion of the serum bilirubin exceeds 2.0 mg per dL and is more than 15% to 30% of the total. Otherwise, the hyperbilirubinemia is unconjugated, or indirect (see Chapter 41).

In neonates, severe hyperbilirubinemia (levels greater than 25 to 30 mg per dL), especially when present with hemolysis or other significant illness, may be associated with neurotoxicity, encephalopathy, or kernicterus. Kernicterus is a rare but devastating neurologic disorder, with characteristic yellow staining in the basal ganglia and other brain regions. Kernicterus is found almost exclusively in breastfed infants. Of note, one more recent report found that, in a large, managed care organization, serum bilirubin levels over 30 mg per dL occurred in about 1 per 10,000 neonates and were generally not accompanied by acute neurotoxicity or chronic neurological sequelae.

DIFFERENTIAL DIAGNOSIS

The most common causes of unconjugated hyperbilirubinemia for patients beyond the neonatal period are hemolytic processes resulting in overproduction of bilirubin (Table 40.1). Extravascular blood in a concealed hemorrhage may be metabolized into supraphysiologic concentrations of bilirubin. Enzyme deficiencies and other conditions that impair the hepatic uptake or conjugation of bilirubin can cause jaundice. Upper gastrointestinal (GI) obstruction generally causes conjugated hyperbilirubinemia but may occasionally be associated with an unconjugated hyperbilirubinemia. Jaundice may be associated with dehydration due to inadequate fluid intake—generally in breastfed infants during the first week of life. After the first week of life, jaundice may be associated with the components of the breast milk itself.

Excess Bilirubin Production

The numerous causes of hemolysis may be classified as intravascular or extravascular. Intravascular hemolysis may be further divided into intracorpuscular and extracorpuscular defects (Table 40.1). Inborn errors of metabolism, such as glucose-6-phosphate dehydrogenase (G6PD) deficiency, may result in destruction of RBCs. This disorder is common in African American and Asian children as well as in those of Mediterranean origin. Patients with G6PD deficiency who are exposed to oxidant stress (e.g., fava beans, sulfa drugs) may have acute rapid hemolysis. Neonates with G6PD deficiency have an increased risk of jaundice that is only partially attributable to hemolysis.

Hemoglobinopathies, including sickle cell disease, can result in hemolysis, as can the impairments in hemoglobin chain synthesis that occur in the thalassemias. Defects in the RBC membrane found in hereditary spherocytosis and hereditary elliptocytosis increase the fragility of the corpuscles. Extracorpuscular causes of RBC destruction include the autoimmune, microangiopathic, and drug-induced hemolytic anemias.

Hematomas, pulmonary hemorrhages, and other collections of extravasated blood undergo hemolysis and, if sufficiently large, can elevate serum levels of unconjugated bilirubin. Rarely, hemophilia in young infants can present as jaundice. Various hypersplenic states, including splenic sequestration crisis in sickle cell disease, may result in anemia with accompanying hemolysis and hyperbilirubinemia.

TABLE 40.1

CAUSES OF PRIMARILY UNCONJUGATED
HYPERBILIRUBINEMIA

Excess bilirubin production
Intravascular hemolysis
  Intracorpuscular
    Glucose-6-phosphate dehydrogenase deficiency
    Sickle cell disease
    Thalassemia
    Hereditary spherocytosis, hereditary elliptocytosis
  Extracorpuscular
    Autoimmune hemolytic anemia
    Microangiopathic hemolytic anemia
    Drug-induced hemolytic anemia
Extravascular hemolysis
  Concealed hematomas
  Hypersplenism

Infection
Bacterial sepsis
Malaria (causes hemolysis)
Urinary tract infection

Inherited disorders of bilirubin metabolism
Gilbert's syndrome
Crigler-Najjar syndrome type II

Neonatal only
Physiologic hyperbilirubinemia
Nonphysiologic hyperbilirubinemia
Breast-feeding–associated jaundice in the setting of dehydration
Breastmilk jaundice (after 1 wk of life)
Hemolysis
  Intravascular
    Maternal-fetal blood group incompatibility (ABO, Rh, other)
    Polycythemia
  Extravascular
    Cephalohematoma
    Neonatal intracranial hemorrhage
    Swallowed blood during birth
Upper gastrointestinal obstruction
  Pyloric stenosis
  Meconium ileus
  Hirschsprung's disease
  Duodenal atresia
Endocrine
  Congenital hypothyroidism
  Infant of a diabetic mother
Inherited disorders of bilirubin metabolism
  Crigler-Najjar syndrome type I
  Galactosemia (early)
  Lucey-Driscoll syndrome

Infection

Jaundice may be evident in cases of serious infection. Bacterial endotoxins reduce bile flow and can cause hyperbilirubinemia. The neonate with jaundice, as well as poor feeding, lethargy, or fever, should be evaluated for sepsis and urinary tract infection. Sepsis is exceedingly rare among well-appearing jaundiced neonates who have no additional signs or symptoms, occurring at a rate considerably below 1%. However, young infants, particularly those older than 8 days with the new onset of jaundice, have an elevated risk of urinary tract infection. Malaria,

caused by *Plasmodium* species, is endemic in tropical regions; in patients with malaria, a high degree of parasitemia may result in massive hemolysis presenting with jaundice.

Inherited Disorders of Bilirubin Metabolism

Gilbert's syndrome is a common cause of mild, intermittent, unconjugated hyperbilirubinemia that occurs in as much as 6% of the population. Patients with Gilbert's syndrome have a partial deficiency of glucuronyl transferase. They generally do not present until late childhood or early adolescence, when they may develop nonspecific abdominal pain, nausea, and mild jaundice during an intercurrent illness. Other liver function studies (including hepatic enzymes and measures of liver function including coagulation studies and ammonia level) are normal and there is no evidence of hemolysis or hepatosplenomegaly. The serum bilirubin rarely exceeds 5 mg per dL.

Crigler-Najjar syndrome is characterized by the absence or deficiency of the enzyme bilirubin glucuronyl transferase. Type I, the more severe form, manifests soon after birth and is associated with high morbidity and mortality. Type II, the milder form, caused by an incomplete enzyme deficiency, typically presents in infancy or later in childhood but has been reported to first appear as late as adolescence. The type II form is generally treatable with phototherapy or phenobarbital.

Special Considerations in the Neonate

Physiologic Neonatal Hyperbilirubinemia. Circulating indirect bilirubin is normally conjugated by the liver to direct bilirubin, which is water soluble and excreted with bile acids. Newborns are deficient in the enzyme responsible for this conjugation, and most newborns develop a mild hyperbilirubinemia with approximately 60% manifesting clinical signs of physiologic jaundice. Physiologic jaundice peaks between 3 and 5 days of life in the term infant and requires no treatment. Because at high levels bilirubin may be associated with neurotoxic effects, careful attention should be paid to distinguishing physiologic from nonphysiologic jaundice.

Nonphysiologic Neonatal Hyperbilirubinemia. One percent to 2% of newborns require readmission within the first week of life, and up to 85% of these readmissions are for nonphysiologic neonatal hyperbilirubinemia. Jaundice in the term newborn is nonphysiologic if it is conjugated or appears within the first 24 hours of life. Other indications that jaundice may not be physiologic are a peak serum total bilirubin concentration of 17 mg per dL or higher in the breastfed infant and 15 mg per dL or higher in the formula-fed infant. Also, infants with a persistence of jaundice beyond the first week of life, or whose serum bilirubin level increases more than 5 mg per dL per day, should be followed closely for nonphysiologic jaundice. Risk factors for nonphysiologic neonatal hyperbilirubinemia include the history of a sibling with hyperbilirubinemia, breast-feeding, lower gestational age, maternal diabetes, bruising (from birth trauma), and Asian race. Dehydrated neonates may develop unconjugated hyperbilirubinemia.

Breast-feeding and Jaundice. Breastfed newborns develop a greater degree of hyperbilirubinemia more often than do formula-fed newborns. During the first week of life, breastfed infants are at risk of inadequate intake of fluid and if dehydrated, may develop breast-feeding–associated jaundice. Breast milk jaundice, on the other hand, occurs in 1% of newborns, is associated with the breast milk itself and may be hormonally mediated or related to intestinal excretion and resorption of bile.

Hemolysis. Birth trauma, when associated with a cephalohematoma, extensive bruising, or swallowed maternal blood, can result in hyperbilirubinemia. Intracranial, pulmonary, or other concealed hemorrhage can also lead to extravascular hemolysis. Similarly, polycythemia, caused by delayed clamping of the cord or maternal-fetal or fetal-fetal transfusion (in multiple gestations), increases the RBC mass and causes jaundice in neonates.

Maternal-fetal blood group incompatibility is critical to recognize early. When maternal antibodies are produced against fetal red blood cell antigens, the neonate can develop a Coombs' positive isoimmune hemolytic anemia that incurs a higher risk of kernicterus than the risk in infants with nonhemolytic causes of jaundice. Fetal Rh and A and B blood group antigens are most commonly etiologic in the hemolysis syndrome, although dozens of antigens have been implicated. Rh-negative mothers may become sensitized to an Rh-positive fetus during pregnancy and mount an antibody response to a fetus during a subsequent pregnancy. Administration of Rho (D) immune globulin (RhoGAM) to Rh-negative mothers who have not yet developed anti-Rh antibodies can prevent Rh isoimmunization. ABO hemolytic disease of the newborn generally occurs in infants with A or B blood groups whose mothers have type O blood group. Maternal anti-A and anti-B antibodies are produced and can result in hemolysis with a positive direct Coombs' test.

Upper Gastrointestinal Obstruction. Pyloric stenosis, meconium ileus, Hirschsprung's disease, duodenal atresia, and other causes of upper GI obstruction may present with jaundice and clinical signs of obstruction. In neonates, obstruction can increase enterohepatic circulation or decrease the enzyme activity responsible for bilirubin uptake, resulting in unconjugated hyperbilirubinemia. In contrast, older children and adults with upper GI obstruction and jaundice generally have a conjugated hyperbilirubinemia.

Endocrine Disorders. Unconjugated hyperbilirubinemia may be the presenting sign of congenital hypothyroidism, preceding other manifestations by several weeks. The mechanism probably relates to reduced bile flow. Other signs that may be present include persistent poor feeding, prolonged jaundice, constipation, and hypotonia. Infants of diabetic mothers are also at increased risk of jaundice, with as many as 19% developing nonphysiologic hyperbilirubinemia.

Inherited Disorders of Bilirubin Metabolism. Very high, rapidly rising levels of bilirubin not responsive to phototherapy raise the concern for Crigler-Najjar syndrome type I or Lucey-Driscoll syndrome. Lucey-Driscoll syndrome is probably caused by an inhibition of glucuronyl transferase. Infants with galactosemia may exhibit an unconjugated hyperbilirubinemia during the first week of life. Older infants with galactosemia tend to have a conjugated hyperbilirubinemia. Infants with galactosemia usually also present with vomiting, failure to thrive, poor feeding, abdominal distension, and hypoglycemia.

TABLE 40.2

COMMON CAUSES OF PRIMARILY UNCONJUGATED HYPERBILIRUBINEMIA

Excess bilirubin production
Glucose-6-phosphate dehydrogenase deficiency
Sickle cell disease

Infection
Malaria (causes hemolysis)

Inherited disorders of bilirubin metabolism
Gilbert's syndrome

Neonatal only
Physiologic hyperbilirubinemia
Nonphysiologic hyperbilirubinemia
Breast-feeding–related jaundice
Overproduction of bilirubin
  Hemolysis
    Maternal-fetal blood group incompatibility (ABO, Rh, other)
    Cephalohematoma

EVALUATION AND DECISION

An approach to the patient with unconjugated hyperbilirubinemia is outlined in Figure 40.1. Hemolysis and Gilbert's syndrome are the most common causes of jaundice in the patient beyond the neonatal period (Table 40.2). During the neonatal period, physiologic jaundice and breast-feeding–related jaundice are the most likely causes. The differential diagnosis is broad, and evaluation should always begin with a detailed history and physical examination.

History

A general clinical history may help guide the workup. An infant who has been lethargic or apneic or a child who has been ill and febrile may require evaluation for serious bacterial infections (Table 40.3). A neonate with persistent or bilious emesis may have an upper GI obstruction.

The clinician should ascertain whether there are factors predisposing a patient to jaundice. One such factor is a family history of jaundice or anemia or a racial or ethnic origin associated with hemolytic anemias. African American race and Mediterranean ancestry are associated with G6PD deficiency. Additional causes of jaundice run in families or have racial predisposition. African American patients are much more likely to have sickle cell disease. Mediterranean and Asian children have higher incidence of thalassemia. East Asian neonates are more likely to develop nonphysiologic hyperbilirubinemia.

A history of drug ingestion may lead to the diagnosis of drug-induced hemolysis. Dietary history may identify an agent such as the fava bean that induces hemolysis in patients with G6PD deficiency. Residence in or travel to sub-Saharan Africa, Southeast Asia, or parts of Central and South America carries a risk of exposure to malaria.

Special Historical Considerations in the Neonate

For the newborn, timing of the onset of jaundice is critical. Most jaundice appearing before the first 24 hours of life is pathologic. Maternal blood type and Rho (D) immune globulin

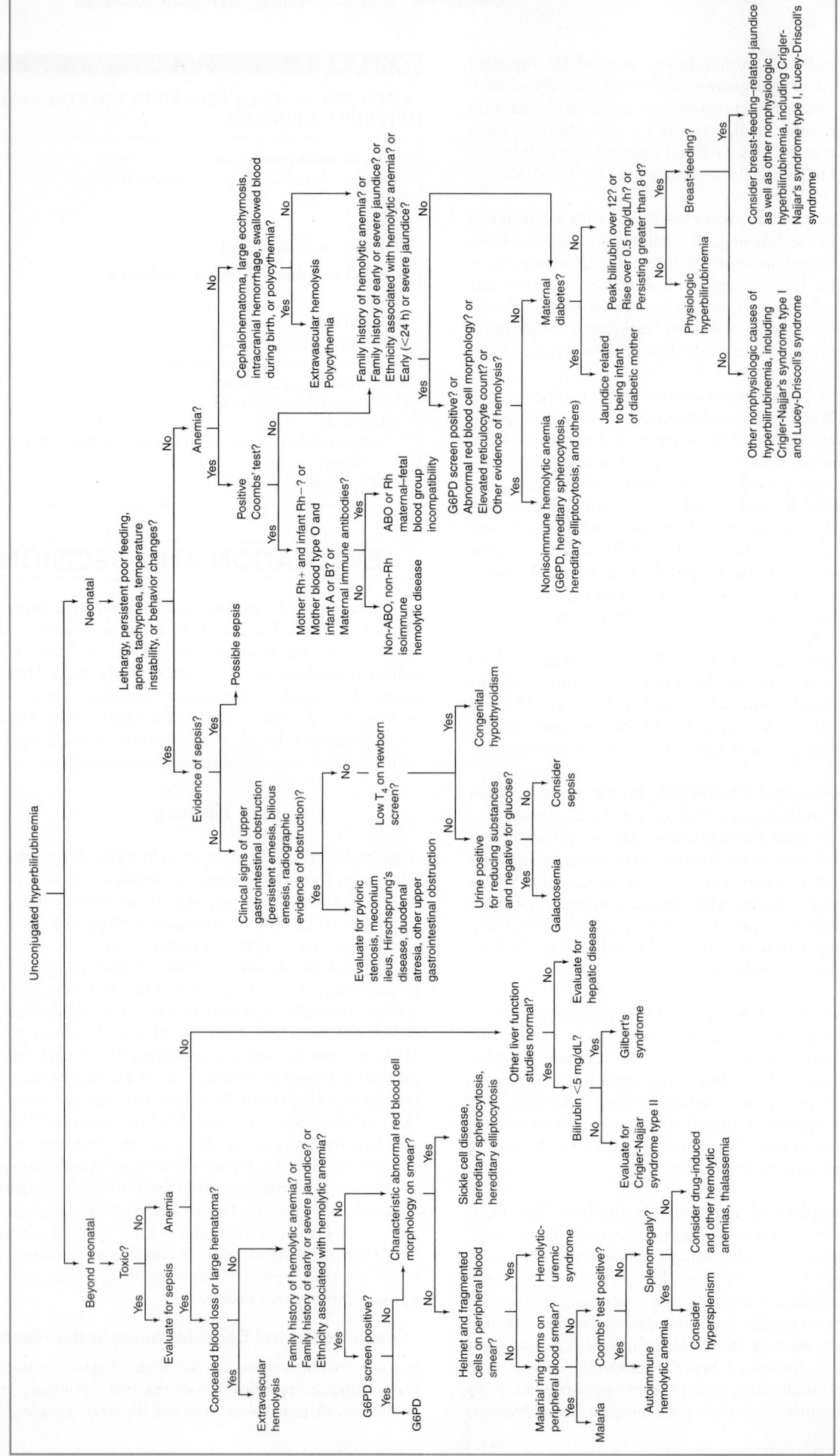

FIGURE 40.1 Evaluation of the pediatric patient with unconjugated hyperbilirubinemia. G6PD, glucose-6-phosphate dehydrogenase.

TABLE 40.3

LIFE-THREATENING CAUSES OF PRIMARILY UNCONJUGATED HYPERBILIRUBINEMIA

Acute hemolysis

Infection
Bacterial sepsis
Malaria (causes hemolysis)

Neonatal only
Nonphysiologic hyperbilirubinemia
Hemolysis
    Maternal-fetal blood group incompatibility (Rh, ABO, other)
    Polycythemia
Upper gastrointestinal obstruction
Endocrine
    Congenital hypothyroidism
Inherited disorders of bilirubin metabolism
    Crigler-Najjar syndrome type I
    Galactosemia (early)
    Lucey-Driscoll syndrome

status should be ascertained to establish risk factors for isoimmune hemolytic anemia. Previous bilirubin levels and the results of Coombs' test should be reviewed. Feeding practices influence development of jaundice; a breastfed infant is at risk for breast-feeding–related jaundice, including jaundice resulting primarily from dehydration. Knowledge of weight gain or loss may help judge hydration status.

Physical Examination

The general appearance of the patient will help guide the clinician as to the likelihood of a serious underlying condition such as bacterial sepsis. In the neonate, poor feeding, lethargy, apnea, tachypnea, and temperature instability may accompany serious infections.

The sclera and skin should be examined closely under adequate light. In a patient with dark skin, palms and soles may be less pigmented and easier to assess for jaundice. Gentle pressure with one finger to blanch the skin facilitates inspection of skin color. In neonates, jaundice progresses in a cephalocaudad direction. Newborns with jaundice below the knees and on the palms have the highest levels of serum bilirubin. Pallor may indicate anemia from hemolysis or bleeding.

Presence of a cephalohematoma or large areas of ecchymosis may suggest extravascular hemolysis as the cause of hyperbilirubinemia. Hepatomegaly may indicate underlying liver dysfunction. Splenomegaly can indicate a hypersplenic state such as splenic sequestration in sickle cell disease. Splenomegaly may also be present in lupus, which is associated with an autoimmune hemolysis. In a neonate with jaundice and vomiting, an abdominal mass suggests upper GI obstruction.

Laboratory Testing

The serum bilirubin level should always be measured as visual inspection alone can be unreliable as a screen for significant neonatal hyperbilirubinemia. Transcutaneous measurements of bilirubin are correlated with serum bilirubin. However, transcutaneous measurements can be inaccurate and thus are best used as a screen with a low threshold to follow up with a serum measurement. Jaundiced patients beyond the neonatal period should be evaluated for anemia with a complete blood cell count and reticulocyte count. Those with evidence of anemia and/or hemolysis should have a peripheral blood smear examined microscopically. Characteristic abnormal morphology, such as sickle cells, spherocytes, or elliptocytes, may be identified. Helmet and fragmented cells are diagnostic of a microangiopathic hemolytic anemia, such as that occurring in hemolytic-uremic syndrome. Malarial ring forms may be apparent. Nucleated RBCs and Howell-Jolly bodies indicate a sustained hemolysis. Patients with anemia or hemolysis should also have a Coombs' test performed to look for evidence of autoimmune hemolysis. Testing for G6PD should be performed if the patient has risk factors or a consistent clinical presentation. Hemoglobin electrophoresis may be used to diagnose hemoglobinopathies, such as sickle cell disease and thalassemia. If hepatomegaly is present or if there is no evidence of anemia, liver function studies should be performed. Patients with no laboratory abnormalities other than serum unconjugated bilirubin below 5 mg per dL have Gilbert's syndrome, a benign condition.

Special Laboratory Considerations in the Neonate

In neonates, it may be important to determine the rate of rise of serum bilirubin with serial measurements. The clinician must know whether a newborn has a setup for maternal-fetal isoimmune anemia.

Therefore, either the mother's blood and Rh type and antibody status should be obtained or the infant's blood type should be determined and Coombs' test performed. A neonate with probable physiologic jaundice does not need to undergo an anemia or hemolysis workup if he or she has no family history of hemolytic disease, no maternal-fetal blood group incompatibility, and no physical stigmata of anemia.

If clinical signs of obstruction are present, the patient should undergo appropriate laboratory testing such as abdominal radiographs, ultrasound, or upper GI series with contrast. The neonate with fever or ill appearance should be evaluated for serious bacterial infection, with peripheral white blood cell count, urine analysis, and cerebrospinal fluid analysis, as well as blood, urine, and cerebrospinal fluid cultures. Results of the newborn screen for congenital hypothyroidism may be available. The newborn with symptoms of congenital hypothyroidism needs to have a determination of T_4 level. A newborn with poor feeding, vomiting, or failure to gain weight should be evaluated for galactosemia. If the newborn with galactosemia has already started feeds, the urine will contain reducing substances (Clinitest positive) but no glucose.

Approach

Beyond the Neonatal Period

In all children with jaundice, a total bilirubin level with fractionation and complete blood cell count should be performed. If a patient appears acutely ill, the physician should proceed with the appropriate evaluation and treatment for sepsis. Among well-appearing patients, the hematocrit determines the likely diagnostic possibilities and appropriate studies.

Anemia. Anemic children are suspect for having hemolytic processes, including autoimmune hemolytic anemia, hemoglobinopathies (e.g., thalassemia or sickle cell anemia), enzyme deficiencies (e.g., G6PD), red blood cell membrane defects (e.g., spherocytosis), hypersplenism, drug reactions, hemolytic-uremic syndrome, and malaria. Extravascular hemolysis and resultant jaundice occur occasionally in children with concealed blood loss or large hematomas. A family history of hemolytic anemia and severe jaundice, particularly among children of Mediterranean descent, suggests G6PD deficiency, whereas abnormal RBC morphology points to sickle cell anemia, hereditary spherocytosis, or heredity elliptocytosis. Additional clues on the peripheral smear include helmet and fragmented cells in hemolytic-uremic syndrome and ring forms in malaria.

A positive Coombs' test is seen with autoimmune hemolytic anemia. In patients with splenomegaly, hemolysis may lead to jaundice. Finally, drug reactions and unusual hemolytic anemias should be considered.

Normal Hematocrit. When unconjugated hyperbilirubinemia occurs without anemia, abnormal liver function studies (transaminases, prothrombin time, and partial thromboplastin time) differentiate hepatic disease from inherited disorders of bilirubin metabolism. Among these latter disorders, only Gilbert's syndrome, which produces a mild elevation in the serum bilirubin level, is at all common.

Neonatal Period

An ill appearance and/or fever suggest sepsis. Other disorders likely to cause lethargy include bowel obstruction, hypothy-roidism, and inborn errors of metabolism, such as galac-tosemia. Among well-appearing neonates, the presence of anemia is important in the differential diagnosis.

Anemia. The foremost consideration in the infant with indirect hyperbilirubinemia and anemia is isoimmune hemolytic disease, caused by blood group incompatibility, because this disorder may lead to kernicterus. The diagnosis can be established by determining the blood group and Rh status of the maternal-infant dyad in combination with a Coombs' test in the infant. Other disorders that produce jaundice include enzymatic and structural disorders of the red blood cell (e.g., G6PD, hereditary spherocytosis) and the poorly understood occurrence of jaundice in infants of diabetic mothers.

Normal Hematocrit. In the absence of anemia, extravascular hemolysis is a common cause of jaundice in the newborn, with the breakdown of hemoglobin occurring in a cephalohematoma, in large ecchymosis, or from swallowed blood. In addition, polycythemic infants are prone to jaundice. Also, hemolysis of even small amounts of hemoglobin may markedly elevate the serum bilirubin level in the infant with an immature liver. Thus, the same disorders that are diagnosed in anemic infants may occur in the jaundiced neonate with a normal hematocrit.

Most infants with indirect hyperbilirubinemia will have a negative evaluation for the disorders previously listed. If the bilirubin level is below 12 mg per dL, rises slowly, and resolves before 8 days of age, one can diagnose physiologic hyperbilirubinemia without further laboratory studies. When these conditions are not met, the most likely cause for the jaundice is the

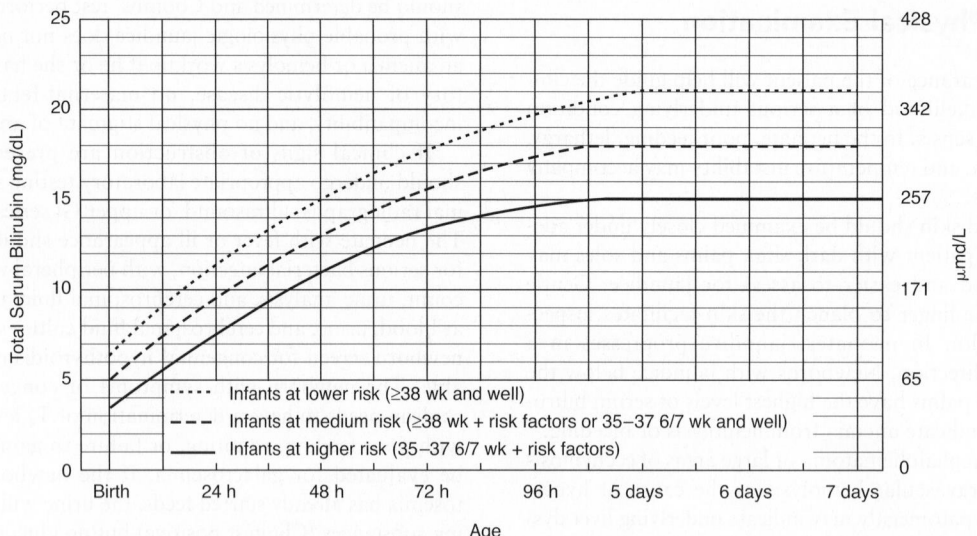

- Use total bilirubin. Do not subtract direct reacting or conjugated bilirubin.
- Risk factors = Isoimmune hemolytic disease. G6PD deficiency, asphyxia, significant lethargy, temperature instability, sepsis, acidosis, or albumin < 3.0 g/dL (if measured)
- For well infants 35−37 6/7 wk can adjust TSB levels for intervention around the medium risk line. It is an option to intervene at lower TSB levels for infants closer to 35 wk and at higher TSB levels for those closer to 37 6/7 wk.
- It is an option to provide conventional phototherapy in hospital or at home at TSB levels 2−3 mg/dL (35−50 mgd/L) below those shown but home phototherapy should not be used in any infant with risk factors.

FIGURE 40.2 Guidelines for phototherapy in hospitalized infants of 35 or more weeks' gestation. The guidelines refer to the use of intensive phototherapy, which should be used when the TSB exceeds the line indicated for each category. Consultation with neonatology and/or hematology is recommended. TSB, total serum bilirubin measured in mg/dL. (From American Academy of Pediatrics Subcommittee on Hyperbilirubinemia. Management of hyperbilirubinemia in the newborn infant 35 or more weeks of gestation. *Pediatrics* 2004;114(1):297–316. Reprinted by permission).

hormonal impairment of bilirubin conjugation. Other possibilities, either alone or in combination with breast milk jaundice, include Crigler-Najjar and Lucey-Driscoll syndromes.

MANAGEMENT

For patients beyond the neonatal period, the management of hyperbilirubinemia is primarily directed at identification and treatment of the underlying cause. In some cases of severe hyperbilirubinemia, such as those caused by Crigler-Najjar syndrome type II, phototherapy or phenobarbital may be indicated. In contrast, newborns with jaundice require careful monitoring and, sometimes, specific therapies for hyperbilirubinemia because the neonatal central nervous system is susceptible to the toxic effects of bilirubin. The emergency physician may initiate the management of term newborn infants with jaundice and arrange hospitalization or subsequent follow-up after discharge. Infants discharged home from their birth hospitalization on the first or second day of life are at increased risk of readmission for hyperbilirubinemia. The management of premature infants with hyperbilirubinemia is highly specialized and not discussed here.

The goal of neonatal hyperbilirubinemia management is to prevent neurotoxicity, encephalopathy, and kernicterus. The jaundiced newborn needs to be kept well hydrated, and enteral feeding should be encouraged to promote bilirubin excretion. When bilirubin levels rise significantly, phototherapy and exchange transfusion may be indicated.

Phototherapy can be initiated with either an overhead bank of lights or a fiberoptic light source in a blanket. Phototherapy primarily promotes (i) photoisomerization of unconjugated bilirubin to a less toxic isomer, which is excreted in the bile and (ii) structural isomerization of bilirubin to lumirubin, which is excreted in the bile and urine.

Indications for phototherapy and exchange transfusion vary according to the age of neonate (see also Chapter 95 for further discussion). For the term neonate who develops jaundice and has no evidence of hemolysis, indications for phototherapy and exchange transfusion as recommended by the American Academy of Pediatrics in 2004 are shown in Figures 40.2 and 40.3. For the ease of understanding, these are summarized by age at 24-hour intervals in Table 40.4, although the action values by age in hours as depicted in the nomograms are the more definitive authority. When there is evidence of isoimmune

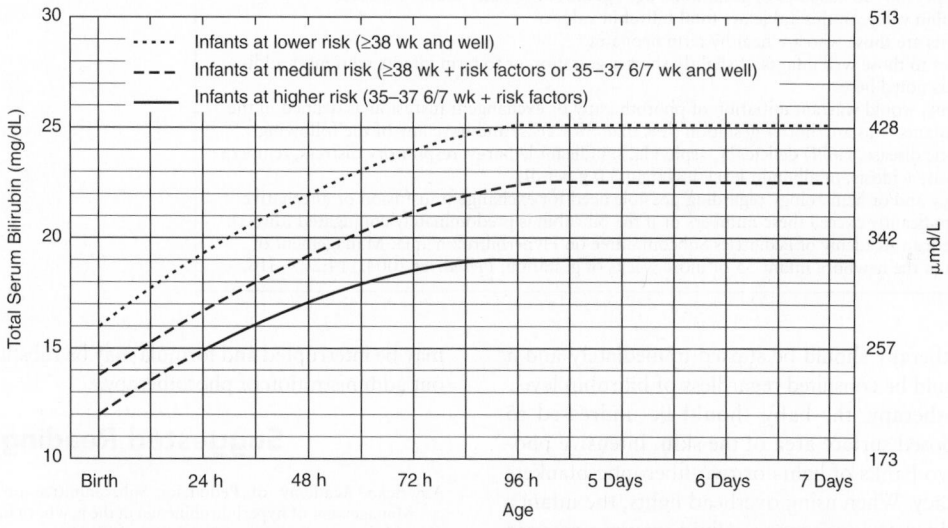

- The dashed lines for the first 24 h indicate uncertainty due to a wide range of clinical circumstances and a range of responses to phototherapy.
- Immediate exchange transfusion is recommended if infant shows signs of acute bilirubin encephalopathy (hypertonia, arching, retrocollis, opisthotonos, fever, high pitched cry) or if TSB is ≥5 mg/dL (85 µmol/L) above these lines.
- Risk factors—isoimmune hemolytic disease, (G6PD) deficiency, asphyxia, significant lethargy, temperature instability, sepsis, acidosis.
- Measure serum albumin and calculate B/A ratio (see legend).
- Use total bilirubin. Do not subtract direct reacting or conjugated bilirubin
- If infant is well and 35–37 6/7 wk (median risk) can individualize TSB levels for exchange based on actual gestational age.

FIGURE 40.3 Guidelines for exchange transfusion in infants 35 or more weeks' gestation. During birth hospitalization, exchange transfusion is recommended if the TSB rises to these levels despite intensive phototherapy. For readmitted infants, if the TSB level is above the exchange level, repeat TSB measurement every 2 to 3 hours and consider exchange if the TSB remains above the levels indicated after intensive phototherapy for 6 hours. Measurement of serum albumin allows calculation of a bilirubin/albumin (B/A) ratio, which may be used together but not in lieu of the TSB level as an additional factor in determining the need for exchange transfusion. The following risk catagories and B/A ratios (TSB mg per dL per Alb g per dL) would suggest consideration of exchange transfusion: infants older than 38 weeks (8.0); infants 35 to 37 6/7 weeks and well or older than 38 weeks with risk factors as noted above (7.2); infants 35 to 37 6/7 weeks and risk factors (6.8). Consultation with neonatology and/or hematology is recommended. TSB, total serum bilirubin measured in mg per dL. (From American Academy of Pediatrics Subcommittee on Hyperbilirubinemia. Management of hyperbilirubinemia in the newborn infant 35 or more weeks of gestation. *Pediatrics* 2004;114(1):297–316. Reprinted by permission.)

TABLE 40.4

MANAGEMENT OF HYPERBILIRUBINEMIA IN THE INFANT 35 WEEKS'
OR MORE GESTATION

Risk category (wks' gestation)	Age (h)	Phototherapy (TSB mg/dL)	Exchange transfusion (TSB mg/dL)
Low risk ≥38 and well	24	12	19
	48	15	22
	72	17.5	24
	96	20	25
	120	21	25
Medium risk 35–37 6/7 and well ≥38 and risk factors	24	10	16.5
	48	13	19
	72	15	21
	96	17	22.5
	120	18	22.5
High risk 35–37 6/7 and risk factors	24	8	15
	48	11	17
	72	13	18.5
	96	14.5	19
	120	15	19

TSB, total serum bilirubin measured in mg/dL.
These guidelines apply only to neonates of gestational age equal to or greater than 35 weeks.
Note that the bilirubin values in this Table are **total bilirubin** values.
The low-risk patients are those who are healthy term neonates.
Medium-risk applies to those well infants of slightly shorter gestation or to term infants who meet additional risk criteria as noted here.
The high-risk patients would warrant initiation of phototherapy or exchange transfusion as defined in the table and include infants who are shorter gestation (less than 38 weeks) and have any of the following: isoimmune hemolytic disease, G6PD deficiency, asphyxia, significant lethargy, respiratory distress, temperature instability, sepsis, acidosis, or albumin level less than 3.0 g per dL.
Consult neonatology and/or hematology regarding possible need for exchange transfusion or alternative therapy if levels significantly exceed these numbers or if the bilirubin is predominantly conjugated (direct).
Adapted from American Academy of Pediatrics Subcommittee on Hyperbilirubinemia. Management of hyperbilirubinemia in the newborn infant 35 or more weeks of gestation. *Pediatrics* 2004;114:297–316.

hemolysis, phototherapy should be started immediately and a neonatologist should be consulted regardless of bilirubin level.

During phototherapy, the baby should be undressed to maximize the exposed surface area of the skin. Intensive phototherapy with two banks of lights or two fiberoptic blankets will improve efficacy. When using overhead lights, the infant's eyes must be shielded and maintenance fluid requirements are increased. Phototherapy is relatively contraindicated in patients with conjugated hyperbilirubinemia because it can cause the "bronze baby syndrome."

When bilirubin levels are toxic, exchange transfusion may be necessary. Exchange transfusion is most commonly indicated in infants with hemolytic disease. Generally, fresh, irradiated, reconstituted whole blood is pushed in through an umbilical vein catheter while blood is pulled out through an umbilical artery catheter. Careful monitoring is necessary. Complications include electrolyte and acid-base disturbances, hemolysis, and infection.

For jaundiced, breastfed infants, the interruption or discontinuation of breast-feeding should be discouraged. Any of several management strategies, however, are accepted, such as following: (i) the infant may be observed while normal breast-feeding continues; (ii) if bilirubin levels are high (Table 40.4), the infant may continue to breast-feed while receiving phototherapy; (iii) breast-feeding may be supplemented with or without administration of phototherapy; and (iv) breast-feeding

may be interrupted and formula may be substituted with or without administration of phototherapy.

Suggested Readings

American Academy of Pediatrics Subcommittee on Hyperbilirubinemia. Management of hyperbilirubinemia in the newborn infant 35 or more weeks of gestation. *Pediatrics* 2004;114(1):297–316.

Garcia FJ, Nager AL. Jaundice as an early diagnostic sign of urinary tract infection in infancy. *Pediatrics* 2002;109(5):846–851.

Ip S, Chung M, Kulig J, et al. An evidence-based review of important issues concerning neonatal hyperbilirubinemia. *Pediatrics* 2004;114(1):e130–e153.

Kuzniewicz MW, Escobar GJ, Wi S, et al. Risk factors for severe hyperbilirubinemia among infants with borderline bilirubin levels: a nested case-control study. *J Pediatr* 2008;153(2):234–240.

Maisels MJ. What's in a name? Physiologic and pathologic jaundice: the conundrum of defining normal bilirubin levels in the newborn. *Pediatrics* 2006;118(2):805–807.

Maisels MJ, McDonagh AF. Phototherapy for neonatal jaundice. *N Engl J Med* 2008;358(9):920–928.

Nathan DG, Orkin SH. *Nathan and Oski's hematology of infancy and childhood*, 7th ed. Philadelphia, PA: WB Saunders, 2009.

Newman TB, Liljestrand P, Escobar GJ. Infants with bilirubin levels of 30 mg/dL or more in a large managed care organization. *Pediatrics* 2003;111(6, pt 1):1303–1311.

Riskin A, Tamir A, Kugelman A, et al. Is visual assessment of jaundice reliable as a screening tool to detect significant neonatal hyperbilirubinemia? *J Pediatr* 2008;152(6):782–787, 787.e1–e2.

Thayyil S, Marriott L. Can transcutaneous bilirubinometry reduce the need for serum bilirubin estimations in term and near term infants? *Arch Dis Child* 2005;90(12):1311–1312.

Watchko JF. Vigintiphobia revisited. *Pediatrics* 2005;115(6):1747–1753.

Watchko JF, Oski FA. Bilirubin 20 mg/dL = vigintiphobia. *Pediatrics* 1983;71:660–663.

CHAPTER 41 ■ JAUNDICE—CONJUGATED HYPERBILIRUBINEMIA

JONATHAN I. SINGER, MD

The presence of jaundice in a child can be a useful indicator of occult pathology. The finding of icterus should set in motion a careful diagnostic search to elucidate the cause. The ultimate goal, to identify precisely the cause of the clinical syndrome, may rest in some cases with the longitudinal caregiver. In all cases, however, the emergency physician at first visit must separate patients whose admission can be temporized from those who require urgent intervention and/or immediate hospitalization.

PATHOPHYSIOLOGY

Unconjugated bilirubin is largely a product of converted heme from senescent red blood cells. Unconjugated bilirubin is transported from extrahepatic reticuloendothelial cells to the liver, bound to albumin. Albumin is detached as the bilirubin gains entry into the hepatocyte. In the liver cell, bilirubin is conjugated with glucuronide by the action of uridine diphosphate glucuronyl transferase. The soluble conjugated digluronide then is secreted across the canalicular membrane into the bile. In the intestine, as a result of the activity of bacterial flora, bilirubin is converted to urobilinogen. A portion of urobilinogen is reabsorbed into the portal circulation and is taken up by the liver cells, only to be reexcreted into the bile. A small percentage of urobilinogen escapes into the systemic circulation and is excreted in the urine. The unabsorbed urobilinogen is excreted in the stool as fecal urobilinogen.

In hepatocellular disease, the damaged liver may be unable to excrete the conjugated bilirubin produced in normal amounts. Or, in the absence of hepatic damage, regurgitation into the plasma of conjugated bilirubin may result from functional cholestasis, disruption of the hepatic architecture, or extrahepatic biliary obstruction. In most instances of jaundice primarily related to hepatic disease, the plasma exhibits elevated concentrations of unconjugated and conjugated bilirubin. Overt mechanical obstruction of bile excretion leads to raised plasma levels of conjugated bilirubin, and only as secondary liver damage occurs do unconjugated bilirubin levels rise.

DIFFERENTIAL DIAGNOSIS

Conjugated hyperbilirubinemia is defined by a conjugated bilirubin level higher than 1 mg per dL if the total bilirubin is less than 5 mg per dL or the conjugated bilirubin level represents more than 20% of the total bilirubin if the total bilirubin is higher than 5 mg per dL. Conjugated hyperbilirubinemia, indicating cholestasis, is considered pathological. Cholestatic jaundice may be congenital or acquired. The differential diagnosis includes a variety of structural defects, infections, hepatotoxins, inborn errors of metabolism, and familial syndromes (Table 41.1).

Although only a few diseases commonly cause conjugated hyperbilirubinemia (Table 41.2), all are serious. In addition, several less common conditions are important considerations because they are life threatening (Table 41.3).

EVALUATION AND DECISION

It is convenient to divide the approach to patients with conjugated hyperbilirubinemia by age, focusing first on those younger than 8 weeks old and then on those who are older (Fig. 41.1). A majority of children who eventually develop life-threatening or chronic liver disease initially present in the first 2 months of life. Early physician recognition may lead to successful treatment and a more favorable prognosis.

Infants Younger than 8 Weeks

In the perinatal period, infants develop conjugated hyperbilirubinemia in response to a variety of conditions that may not be encountered in older patients. The increased sensitivity to insult is a result of different patterns of hepatic enzyme activity and liver immaturity with regard to bile formation. Many systemic or hepatic insults may produce perinatal cholestasis (Table 41.1). However, a small number of disorders account for the overwhelming majority of perinatal cholestasis. They include idiopathic neonatal hepatitis, biliary atresia, α_1-antitrypsin deficiency, cystic fibrosis, tyrosinemia, galactosemia, choledochal cyst, and perinatal infections. These disorders can be separated by the tempo of the presentation and the appearance of the infant.

The tempo of cholestasis is most abrupt with the infections acquired in utero and during the birthing process. Infected patients are more likely to present shortly after birth. Those who have congenital infections will have a low birth weight. They present with cholestatic jaundice, irritability, jitteriness, and/or seizures. On examination, microcephaly, hepatomegaly, splenomegaly, and petechiae may be seen with the perinatal TORCHS complex. These include perinatal infections from toxoplasmosis, other infections, rubella, cytomegalovirus (CMV), herpes simplex, and syphilis. Jaundice may be one of the first signs of bacteremia without apparent focus of infection or bacterial sepsis in the first few days of life. Hyperbilirubinemia may

TABLE 41.1

CAUSES OF CONJUGATED HYPERBILIRUBINEMIA IN INFANTS AND CHILDREN

First 8 wk of life
Hepatic disorders
  Biliary atresia
  Intrahepatic biliary hypoplasia
  Idiopathic neonatal cholestasis or neonatal hepatitis syndrome
  Ischemic hepatitis
Perinatal infections
  Toxoplasmosis
  Rubella
  Cytomegalovirus
  Varicella zoster
  Herpes simplex
  Coxsackievirus
  Human immunodeficiency virus
  Bacterial sepsis
  Listeriosis
  Syphilis
  Babesiosis
  Urinary tract infection
Metabolic disorder
  Galactosemia
  Galactokinase deficiency
  Hereditary fructose intolerance
  Hereditary tyrosinemia
  α_1-Antitrypsin deficiency
  Cystic fibrosis
  Hypothyroidism
  Hypopituitarism
Biliary tree disorders
  Spontaneous perforation of the bile duct
  Choledochal disorders
  Gallstones or biliary sludge

Childhood
Hepatic disorders
  Hepatotoxins (drugs, chemicals)
  Byler disease
  Dubin-Johnson syndrome
  Rotor syndrome
Infections
  Viral hepatitides (A through E)
  Epstein-Barr virus, Coxsackievirus, echovirus
  Liver abscess (usually anicteric)
  Myocarditis
  Urinary tract infection
  Suppurative cholangitis
  Peritonitis
  Pneumonia
Metabolic disorders
  Wolman disease
  Zellweger syndrome
  Glycogen storage (III, IV)
  Wilson's disease
Biliary tree disorders
  Choledocholithiasis
  Cholangitis
  Cholecystitis
  Choledochal cyst
  Pancreatic disease
Miscellaneous
  Abdominal crisis, sickle hemoglobinopathy
  Hepatorenal syndrome
  Kawasaki disease

TABLE 41.2

COMMON CAUSES OF CONJUGATED HYPERBILIRUBINEMIA

Infancy
  Idiopathic neonatal cholestasis
  Biliary atresia
  Perinatal infections (TORCHS)
  Sepsis/urinary tract infection
Childhood
  Viral hepatitis
  Hepatotoxins

TORCHS, toxoplasmosis, other (infections), rubella, cytomegalovirus, herpes (simplex), and syphilis.

occur antecedent to blood cultures becoming positive and may precede findings of anorexia, vomiting, abdominal distension, fever, hepatomegaly, or alterations in respiratory pattern or sensorium. The precise mechanism of jaundice that complicates bacteremia and sepsis is not completely understood. Jaundice may also be an early diagnostic sign of urinary tract infection in the neonatal period. An increase in the conjugated bilirubin fraction may be seen in patients who have afebrile, otherwise asymptomatic urinary tract infection.

The tempo of icterus is subacute with the other common causes of conjugated hyperbilirubinemia. The metabolic and hepatic disorders have variable symptoms at onset. However, the manifestations are far less acute than those seen in the infectious states. Infants with galactosemia, tyrosinemia, and fructose intolerance may appear ill in the emergency department due to metabolic derangement or secondary infection. However, they have had an antecedent history of failure to thrive, developmental delay, and inconstant jaundice. Unexplained fatality in the sibship or unexplained pulmonary, gastrointestinal, neurologic, or psychiatric disturbance in other family members may provoke diagnostic consideration (see Chapter 94).

The tempo of hepatic and biliary tree disorders is chronic. Those with biliary atresia have intermittent, mild conjugated hyperbilirubinemia during the first 6 to 8 weeks of life. They feed well and thrive. Their stools may be intermittently pigmented early on and become permanently without pigment only after 4 to 6 weeks. They have a benign appearance and

TABLE 41.3

LIFE-THREATENING CAUSES OF CONJUGATED HYPERBILIRUBINEMIA

Fulminant hepatic failure
Septicemia
Intraabdominal sepsis
  Pyogenic liver abscess
  Suppurative cholangitis
  Peritonitis
Abdominal crisis, sickle hemoglobinopathy
Hepatorenal syndrome

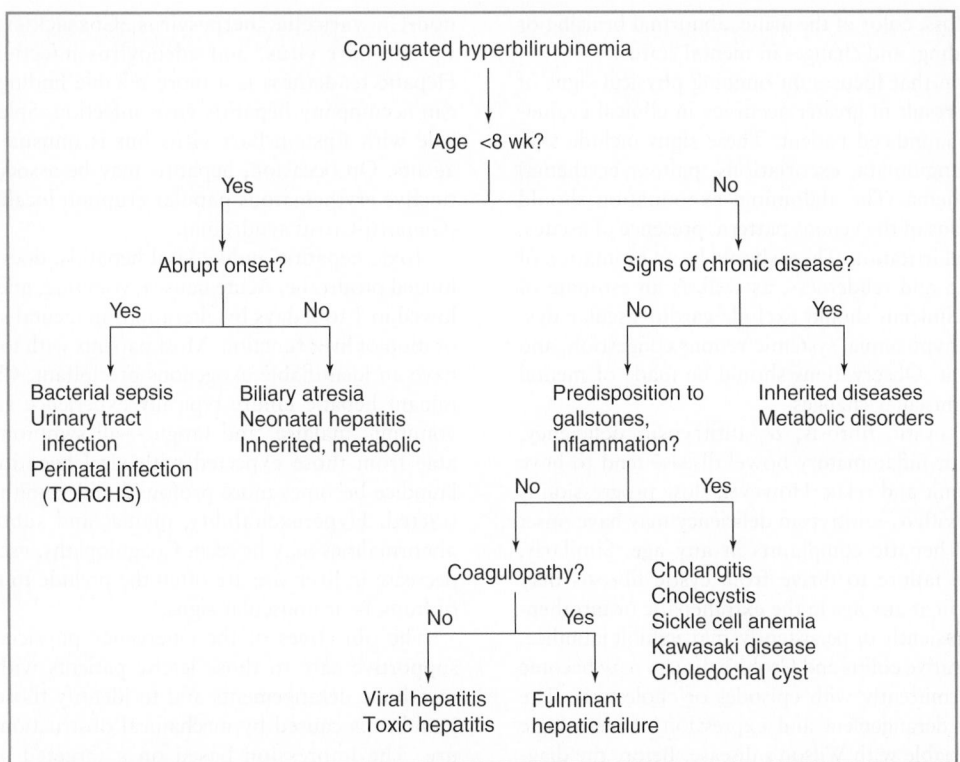

FIGURE 41.1 Approach to the patient with congenital hyperbilirubinemia. TORCHS, toxoplasmosis, other (infections), rubella, cytomegalovirus, herpes (simplex), and syphilis.

SIGNS AND SYMPTOMS

with the exception of jaundice and hepatomegaly seem otherwise well. Those patients without a precise anatomic, genetic, or infectious cause of cholestasis are considered to have idiopathic neonatal cholestasis or neonatal hepatitis syndrome. They have onset of their jaundice from 1 to 30 days, with a mean of 7 days. Initially, their stool color is normal, but the stools may become acholic after several weeks. The presence of acholic stools may make it difficult to differentiate between obstructive jaundice causing hepatocellular disease and that caused by obstruction of the biliary tree.

The priorities for the emergency physician are to diagnose medically treatable infections, identify metabolic disorders for which effective therapy is available, and detect extrahepatic obstructive lesions that are amenable to surgical correction. The evaluation begins with cultures of cerebrospinal fluid, blood, urine, and stool. Infants should also have complete blood cell and platelet counts, coagulation studies, hepatic enzymes (aspartate aminotransferase, alanine aminotransferase, and gamma-glutamyl transpeptidase), ammonia, albumin, total protein, alkaline phosphatase, electrolytes, blood urea nitrogen, creatinine, and blood sugar tests. Urine should be obtained for urinalysis and tested for reducing substances. A right upper quadrant ultrasound should be performed in order to identify anatomic abnormalities such as a choledochal cyst. If cystic fibrosis is suspected, schedule the patient for a sweat chloride iontophoresis or testing for common genetic variants in the cystic fibrosis transmembrane conductance regulator gene. Additional studies of blood and urine that they may find useful include α_1-antitrypsin, TORCHS and hepatitis B virus serology, serum amino acids, thyroid function tests,

red blood cell galactose 1-phosphate uridyltransferase activity, and urine examination for cytomegalovirus.

Inpatient observation is appropriate in this age group because the diagnosis can rarely be established in the emergency department. Empiric therapy for sepsis or urinary infection is often warranted, pending culture results.

Children Older than 8 Weeks

In the evaluation of conjugated hyperbilirubinemia beyond infancy, it is necessary to know if there has been exposure to contagion or a potential for sexual or vertical transmission of infections such as hepatitis or human immunodeficiency virus. Other risk factors for hepatitis (e.g., needle sticks, hemodialysis, transplant, transfusion of blood products, or factor use) need to be evaluated. The physician should pursue possible exposure to industrial toxins or foods previously implicated in hepatic injury (e.g., carbon tetrachloride, yellow phosphorus, tannic acid, alcohol, mushrooms of the *Amanita* species). The emergency physician must inquire about use of acetaminophen, salicylates, nonsteroidal anti-inflammatory drugs, iron salts, erythromycin estolate, ceftriaxone, rifampin, nitrofurantoin, oxacillin, tetracycline, trimethoprim-sulfamethoxazole, ketoconazole, diphenylhydantoin, isoniazid, and chlorpromazine. The presence of prior episodes of jaundice, acholic stools, and/or abdominal pain may suggest an underlying disorder, predisposing the patient to obstruction of the biliary tree. Other historical points include the presence of fever, arthralgia, arthritis, conjunctivitis, rash, pruritus, vomiting, diarrhea, weight loss, color of the urine, abnormal bruising or spontaneous bleeding, and changes in mental status.

An examination that focuses on ongoing physical signs of liver disease may result in greater accuracy in clinical evaluation of the older jaundiced patient. These signs include skin changes (spider angiomata, excoriations, palmar erythema) and peripheral edema. The abdominal examination should include observations of the venous pattern, presence of ascites, mass, or peritoneal irritation. There should be an estimation of liver size, contour, and tenderness, as well as an estimate of spleen size. The clinician should exclude cardiovascular dysfunctions such as hypoxemia, systemic venous congestion, and low cardiac output. Observations should be made of mental status and neuromuscular changes.

Patients with cystic fibrosis, α_1-antitrypsin deficiency, Wilson's disease, or inflammatory bowel disease tend to have symptoms that remit and relax. However, slow progression is the rule. Patients with α_1-antitrypsin deficiency may have onset of respiratory or hepatic complaints at any age. Similarly, infants who have failure to thrive from cystic fibrosis may develop obstruction at any age in the extrahepatic or intrahepatic ducts and, transiently or persistently, may exhibit jaundice. Patients with ulcerative colitis and Crohn's disease may become symptomatic intermittently with episodes of cholestasis. The degree of hepatic derangement and expression of neurologic abnormality is variable with Wilson's disease. Before the diagnosis is entertained, patients typically exhibit dysarthria, tremors, rigidity, or psychic disturbances. Rarely, younger patients without prodromal events have acute jaundice and hepatomegaly and progress to hepatic failure.

Biliary calculi and acute inflammation of the gallbladder are uncommon causes of conjugated hyperbilirubinemia in the pediatric population (Chapter 89). However, a subset of patients is predisposed to these complications. Cholelithiasis may complicate any of the hemolytic anemias, particularly in patients with sickle hemoglobinopathies. These patients have increased incidence of both liver and gallbladder disease. Liver or gallbladder dysfunction accounts for jaundice when more than 10% of an elevated bilirubin in a patient with sickle cell disease is conjugated. Cholecystitis may accompany a variety of acute focal infections, such as pneumonia or peritonitis, and may occur in the course of bacterial sepsis. In this event, shock and hyperpyrexia may divert the clinician from the deranged biliary system. In less severe cases, fever, nausea, vomiting, abdominal distension, and right upper quadrant pain are prominent features of cholecystitis. Right upper quadrant abdominal mass, pain, and jaundice constitute the classic triad in the diagnosis of choledochal cyst. The clinical recognition may be delayed until there is a complication, such as cholangitis. An acute, painful right upper quadrant mass associated with jaundice may also occur in the course of acute hydrops of the gallbladder from Kawasaki disease or systemic streptococcal infection.

In the previously healthy child, the most common cause of conjugated hyperbilirubinemia is acute hepatitis (Chapter 92). The illness may be abrupt in onset, with fever, urticaria, and arthralgia as primary manifestations. More often, the illness is insidious. Viral hepatitis is characterized by low-grade fever and gastrointestinal complaints such as anorexia, malaise, nausea, vomiting, and abdominal pain before the jaundice. Liver enlargement with hepatitis (A, B, C, and non-A, non-B,

non-C), varicella, herpesvirus, Coxsackievirus, echovirus, Epstein-Barr virus, and adenovirus infection is inconstant. Hepatic tenderness is a more reliable finding. Rarely, ascites can accompany hepatitis virus infection. Splenomegaly is the rule with Epstein-Barr virus but is unusual with the other agents. On occasion, hepatitis may be associated with a distinctive erythematous papular eruption localized to the limbs (Gianotti-Crosti syndrome).

Toxic hepatitis, unlike viral hepatitis, does not have a prolonged prodrome. Acute nausea, vomiting, and malaise are followed in 1 to 2 days by alterations in mental status and deterioration of liver function. Most patients with toxic hepatitis will have an identifiable exogenous precipitant. Children with fulminant hepatic failure typically experience anorexia, nausea, vomiting, malaise, and fatigue—all symptoms indistinguishable from those expected with viral hepatitis. The patient's jaundice becomes more profound and vomiting becomes protracted. Hyperexcitability, mania, and subtle psychomotor abnormalities may be seen. Coagulopathy, ascites, and sudden decrease in liver size are often the prelude to the development of frank neuromuscular signs.

The objectives of the emergency physician are to render supportive care to those icteric patients with infectious and metabolic derangements and to identify those cases in which jaundice is caused by mechanical obstruction or hepatic failure. The impression based on a targeted history, physical examination, and clinical algorithms can be bolstered with the following laboratory examinations: complete blood cell count, platelet count, coagulation profile, prothrombin time, total and direct bilirubin, hepatic enzymes, alkaline phosphatase, electrolytes, blood urea nitrogen, and creatinine. Urinalysis, culture, and toxicologic screen should be considered. Chest and abdominal radiographs are indicated when there are pulmonary parenchymal complaints or significant abdominal findings. Other laboratory tests that are often available immediately and that may provide useful information in specific circumstances are serum ammonia, albumin, total protein, lipid profile, pH, and carbon dioxide. If available, abdominal sonography or computed tomography may be helpful occasionally. In no circumstance will results of several important blood and urine tests be of immediate use. Such studies, which are appropriate, include antinuclear antibody, α fetoprotein, and serum for bile acids, ceruloplasmin, protein electrophoretic pattern, polymerase chain reaction assays or serologic evidence of recent infection (e.g., Epstein-Barr virus, mycoplasmal or hepatitis profiles). Urinary analysis includes assessment of organic acids and copper. These investigations may be helpful, however, to the longitudinal caregiver who must maintain a vigilant watch over the jaundiced patient.

Children older than 8 weeks with conjugated hyperbilirubinemia should be admitted to the hospital at the time of their presentation in all cases in which life-threatening conditions may exist (Table 41.3). Inpatient treatment is also suggested when intravenous fluids are necessary to treat symptomatic hypoglycemia or electrolyte imbalance and when operative intervention may prove necessary. Icteric patients who have been diagnosed previously with confidence and who have exacerbation of their symptoms may require admission to reappraise their status. The physician may also be influenced to admit the patient when social factors or geographic barriers inhibit consistent observations. Admission is also indicated for patients who require further diagnostic intervention, such as hepatobiliary scintigraphy, endoscopic retrograde cholangiopancreatography, or liver biopsy to arrive at a definitive diagnosis.

Suggested Readings

Crain EF, Gershel JC. Urinary tract infections in febrile infants younger than 8 weeks of age. *Pediatrics* 1990;86:363–367.

Emerick KM, Whitington PF. Neonatal liver disease. *Pediatr Ann* 2006;35: 280–286.

Garcia FJ, Nager AL. Jaundice as an early diagnostic sign of urinary tract infection in infancy. *Pediatrics* 2002;109:846–851.

Jacquemin E, Lykavieris P, Chaoui N, et al. Transient neonatal cholestasis: origin and outcome. *J Pediatr* 1998;133:563–567.

Moyer V, Freese DK, Whitington PF, et al. Guideline for the evaluation of cholestatic jaundice in infants: recommendations of the North American Society for Pediatric Gastroenterology, Hepatology and Nutrition. *J Pediatr Gastroenterol Nutr* 2004;39:115–128.

Suchy FJ. Approach to the infant with cholestasis. In: Suchy FJ, Balistreri WF, Sokol RJ, eds. *Liver disease in children*, 3rd ed. New York, NY: Cambridge University Press, 2007:187–194.

CHAPTER 42 ■ LIMP

SUSANNE KOST, MD, FAAP, FACEP

Limping is a common complaint in the pediatric acute care setting. A *limp* is defined as an alteration in the normal walking pattern for the child's age. The average child begins to walk between 12 and 18 months of age with a broad-based gait, gradually maturing into a normal (adult) gait pattern by the age of 3 years. Normal walking involves a complex integration of the nervous and musculoskeletal systems, yet it should appear smooth and effortless. A normal gait cycle can be divided into two phases: stance and swing. The stance phase, the time from the heel striking the ground to the toe leaving the ground, encompasses about 60% of the gait cycle. The swing phase involves a sequence of hip then knee flexion, followed by foot dorsiflexion and knee extension as the heel strikes the ground to begin the next cycle.

The causes of limping are numerous, ranging from trivial to life threatening, but most children who limp do so as a result of pain, weakness, or deformity. Pain results in an antalgic gait pattern with a shortened stance phase. The most common causes of a painful limp are trauma and infection. Neuromuscular disease may cause either spasticity (e.g., toe-walking) or weakness, which results in a steppage gait to compensate for weak ankle dorsiflexion. Ataxia may be interpreted by parents as a limp. The Trendelenburg gait, characterized by a pelvic tilt away from the affected hip, is common in congenital or acquired hip disorders. A vaulting gait may be seen in children with limb-length discrepancy or abnormal knee mobility. A stooped, shuffling gait is common in patients with pelvic or lower abdominal pain.

The evaluation of a child with a limp demands a thorough history and physical examination, using an age-based approach. Toddlers generally provide the greatest diagnostic challenge because a history of trauma may be unclear and the ability to describe or localize pain may be lacking. In all age groups, a detailed history of the circumstances surrounding the limp should be obtained, with focus on the issues of trauma, pain, and associated fever or systemic illness. The physical examination must be complete because limping may originate from abnormalities in any portion of the lower extremity, nervous system, abdomen, or genitourinary tract. The location of the pain may not represent the source of the pathology, for example, hip pain may be referred to the knee area. Laboratory and imaging studies should be tailored to the findings in the history and physical examination, keeping in mind an appropriate age-based differential diagnosis.

DIFFERENTIAL DIAGNOSIS

The extensive differential diagnosis of the child with a limp may be approached from several angles: disease category, location of pathology, or age of the child. Table 42.1 presents the differential diagnosis by disease category; Table 42.2 organizes the differential diagnosis by age and the location of pathology. The most common causes of limp are outlined in Table 42.3, and potentially life- or limb-threatening conditions are listed in Table 42.4. This section reviews the differential diagnosis within the framework of an algorithmic approach (Fig. 42.1).

The most common cause of limping in all ages is trauma, either acute or repetitive microtrauma (stress fractures). Older children who limp as a result of trauma can generally describe the mechanism of injury and localize pain well. The toddler and preschool age groups, with their limited verbal ability and cooperation skills, often provide a diagnostic challenge. A common type of injury in this population (often not witnessed) is the aptly named "toddler's fracture," a nondisplaced spiral fracture of the tibial shaft that occurs as a result of torsion of the foot relative to the tibia. Occult fractures of the bones in the foot also occur in young children. Initial plain radiographic findings may be subtle, or at times nonexistent, but will become apparent in 1 to 2 weeks. The advent of digital radiography has led to improved accuracy in the diagnosis of toddler's fracture. Bone scans will identify these lesions sooner. Another fracture often lacking initial radiographic confirmation is a Salter-Harris type I fracture, which presents as tenderness over a physis after trauma to a joint area. Stress fractures may also lack overt radiographic findings. Common sites for overuse injury include the tibial tubercle (Osgood-Schlatter's disease), the anterior tibia (shin splints), and the calcaneus at the insertion of the Achilles tendon (Sever's disease). More information on the subject of fractures is found in Chapter 114.

Trauma may also induce limping as a result of soft-tissue injury. Although young children are more likely to sustain fractures than sprains and strains, the latter can occur. Joint swelling and pain out of proportion to the history of injury raises the possibility of a hemarthrosis as the initial presentation of a bleeding disorder (see Chapter 91). Severe soft-tissue pain and swelling in the setting of a contusion or crush injury suggests compartment syndrome. With compartment syndrome, pain is exacerbated by passive extension of the affected part; pallor and pulselessness are late findings. Severe pain of an entire limb out of proportion to the history of injury suggests complex regional pain syndrome, formerly known as *reflex sympathetic dystrophy*. This entity is most common in young adolescent girls. It may be accompanied by mottling and coolness of the extremity, presumably as a result of abnormalities in the peripheral sympathetic nervous system.

A limp that is accompanied by a history of fever or recent systemic illness is likely to be infectious or inflammatory in origin. However, the absence of fever does not preclude the possibility of a bacterial bone or joint infection, and many infections

TABLE 42.1

DIFFERENTIAL DIAGNOSIS OF LIMP BY
DISEASE CATEGORY

Trauma or overuse
Fracture
Stress fracture
Soft-tissue injury
Spondylolisthesis
Herniated nucleus pulposus

Infectious
Septic arthritis
Osteomyelitis
Lyme arthritis
Discitis
Pelvic inflammatory disease

Inflammatory
Transient synovitis
Reactive arthritis
Rheumatic disease
Appendicitis

Developmental or acquired
Developmental dysplasia of
the hip
Blount's disease
Limb-length discrepancy
Torsional deformities
Avascular necrosis
Slipped capital femoral
epiphysis
Testicular torsion

Congenital
Vertical talus
Tarsal coalition
Other congenital limb
abnormalities
Spinal dysraphism
Inguinal hernia

Neurologic
Muscular dystrophy
Peripheral neuropathy
Complex regional pain
syndrome

Neoplasia
Benign bone tumors
Malignant bone tumors
Leukemia
Intraabdominal tumors
Sacral tumors
Spinal cord tumors

Metabolic
Rickets
Hyperparathyroidism

Hematologic
Sickle cell disease
Hemophilia

bone. A reactive joint effusion may be present. Occasionally, osteomyelitis and septic arthritis will coexist. More detailed discussions of both septic joint and osteomyelitis are found in Chapters 92 and 125.

Rheumatic conditions that may result in limp are numerous; many are accompanied by systemic symptoms and characteristic skin rashes. Examples include Lyme disease, Henoch-Schönlein purpura, erythema multiforme, acute rheumatic fever, juvenile rheumatoid arthritis, and systemic lupus erythematosus. Occasionally, limping from arthralgia will precede the development of the arthritis and systemic involvement. An approach to the child with joint pain is found in Chapter 56, and a detailed discussion of arthritis is found in Chapter 101.

In the absence of obvious trauma, fever, or systemic symptoms, the next step in the approach to the differential diagnosis of a limp is to determine the focality of the findings and the degree of pain. Localized pain suggests repetitive microtrauma, bone tumor, or an acquired skeletal deformity. Repetitive microtrauma may be responsible for avascular necrosis of the foot bones in two locations: the tarsal navicular bone (Kohler's disease) in younger children and the metatarsal heads (Freiberg's disease) in adolescents. Both benign and malignant bone tumors may present with a painful limp. Benign lesions include bone cysts (unicameral or aneurysmal), fibrous dysplasia, and eosinophilic granulomas. Osteoid osteoma, caused by a painful nidus of vascular osteoid tissue, is another benign lesion unique to young people. The most common malignant pediatric bone tumors are osteogenic sarcoma and Ewing's sarcoma. Bone tumor pain may be acute or chronic, with acute pain usually related to a pathologic fracture. Examples of acquired skeletal abnormalities causing painful limp include tarsal coalition and osteochondritis dissecans. Tarsal coalition occurs as a result of gradual calcification of a congenital cartilaginous bar between tarsal bones; it presents most commonly as a painful flatfoot in school-age children. Osteochondritis dissecans is related to separation of articular cartilage from underlying bone; it most commonly affects the knees of adolescent boys.

Localized findings without pain suggest congenital or slowly developing acquired limb abnormalities. Three disorders of the hip fit into this category, each of which is characteristic of a specific age group. Developmental dysplasia of the hip includes a spectrum of abnormalities, ranging from mild dysplasia to frank dislocation. Most affected children with access to primary care are diagnosed with abnormal hip abduction on routine examination in infancy. Occasionally, the diagnosis will be missed, and the child then presents at the onset of walking with a painless short-leg limp, or waddling gait if bilateral, with weakness of the abductor musculature. Legg-Calvé-Perthes disease, an avascular necrosis of the capital femoral epiphysis, presents in young school-age children as an insidious limp with mild, activity-related pain. Slipped capital femoral epiphysis (SCFE) presents in young, typically obese, adolescents with an externally rotated limp. The amount of pain experienced is related to the rate of displacement of the epiphysis, ranging from none to severe. Legg-Calvé-Perthes disease and SCFE are more common in boys. Other acquired skeletal deformities that may cause painless limp include limb-length inequality, Blount's disease (with marked bowing of the proximal tibias), and torsional deformities. Baker's cyst of the

are preceded by a history of minor trauma. Septic arthritis is the most serious infectious cause of joint pain and limp. It is more common in younger children and typically presents with a warm, swollen joint (although swelling in the hip is very difficult to detect clinically). Exquisite pain with attempts to flex or extend the joint is characteristic of septic arthritis, and the degree of pain with motion serves as a helpful clinical sign in distinguishing bacterial joint infection from inflammatory conditions. A common diagnostic challenge is differentiating septic arthritis from transient (or toxic) synovitis in a young child with fever, limp, and pain localized to the hip. Transient synovitis, a postinfectious reactive arthritis, generally follows a milder course. It is usually preceded by a recent viral respiratory or gastrointestinal illness. Acute-phase reactants may be elevated in both conditions, although usually less so in synovitis. A unilateral joint effusion, which is better visualized with ultrasound than plain films, may be present in both. Bilateral effusions are more suggestive of an inflammatory synovitis. Doppler ultrasonography may reveal hyperemia of the femoral head in a septic hip, where increased flow would not be expected in synovitis. Orthopedic consultation for joint aspiration may be required for a definitive diagnosis because a septic hip is a surgical emergency requiring open drainage. Osteomyelitis is another potentially serious infectious cause of limp, although the presentation is typically more chronic than that of a septic joint. Osteomyelitis, which is also more common in younger children, presents with pain and occasionally warmth and swelling, usually over the metaphysis of a long

TABLE 42.2

DIFFERENTIAL DIAGNOSIS OF LIMP BY AGE AND LOCATION OF PATHOLOGY

	Long bone	Skin/soft tissue	Any joint	Hip	Knee	Ankle/foot	Spine
Toddler	Fracture Toddler's Salter type I Periostitis Osteomyelitis Vasoocclusive crisis Congenital Anomaly	Contusion Strain Foreign body Immunization Infection	Septic arthritis Reactive arthritis Rheumatic disease Systemic JRA Hemarthrosis	Transient synovitis DDH	Occult trauma Blount's disease Referred hip pain	Poor shoe fit Occult trauma Vertical talus Kohler's disease	Dysraphism Infection Tumor
School age	Fracture Salter type I Discrepant limb length Osteomyelitis Tumor Vasoocclusive Crisis	Contusion Strain Myositis Growing pains Infection	Sprain Reactive arthritis Rheumatic disease EM, HSP, ARF Septic arthritis Lyme arthritis	Transient synovitis AVN	Baker's cyst Referred hip pain	Poor shoe fit Salter type I fracture Tarsal coalition Kohler's disease	Dysraphism Infection Tumor
Adolescent	Fracture Tumor Osteomyelitis	Contusion Strain Tendonitis CRPS	Sprain Reactive arthritis Rheumatic disease IBD, SLE Septic arthritis Gonococcal Lyme arthritis	SCFE	Osgood-Schlatter's disease Osteochondritis dissecans Chondromalacia Baker's cyst Referred hip pain	Poor shoe fit Salter type I fracture Bunion Freiberg's disease Sever's disease	Scoliosis Spondylolisthesis Herniated disc Infection Tumor

JRA, juvenile rheumatoid arthritis; DDH, developmental dysplasia of the hip; EM, erythema multiforme; HSP, Henoch-Schönlein purpura; ARF, acute rheumatic fever; AVN, avascular necrosis; CRPS, complex regional pain syndrome; IBD, inflammatory bowel disease; SLE, systemic lupus erythematosus; SCFE, slipped capital femoral epiphysis.

TABLE 42.3

COMMON CAUSES OF LIMP

Trauma	**Rheumatic disease**
Fracture	
Soft-tissue injury	**Other hip disorders**
Overuse injuries	Developmental dysplasia
	Legg-Calvé-Perthes disease
Transient synovitis	Slipped capital femoral epiphysis
Infection	
Septic arthritis	
Osteomyelitis	

TABLE 42.4

LIFE- OR LIMB-THREATENING CAUSES OF LIMP

Septic arthritis
Osteomyelitis
Tumor
Developmental dysplasia of the hip
Slipped capital femoral epiphysis
Epidural abscess
Appendicitis

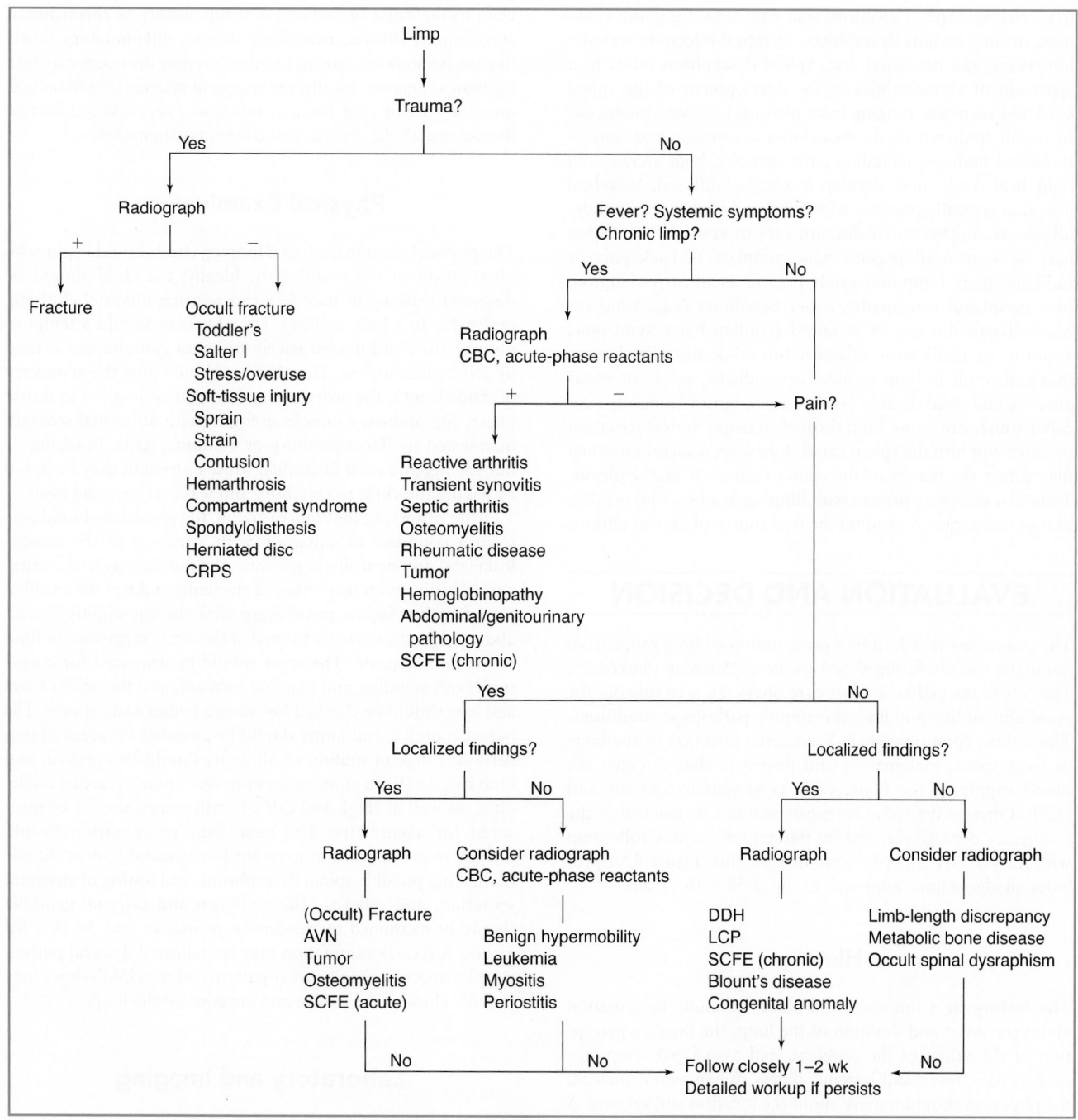

FIGURE 42.1 Algorithmic approach to the child with a limp. CRPS, complex regional pain syndrome; CBC, complete blood cell count; SCFE, slipped capital femoral epiphysis; AVN, avascular necrosis; DDH, developmental dysplasia of the hip; LCP, Legg-Calvé-Perthes disease.

popliteal tendon may cause limping with minimal local discomfort.

Limping in the absence of localized limb findings suggests a systemic (or nonlimb) source such as the spine or the abdomen. A painful limp without localization or with migratory bone pain suggests a hematologic or oncologic cause, such as sickle cell disease or leukemia. Limping with bilateral leg pain localized to the muscles, especially the calves, suggests myositis. Benign acute childhood myositis is common during influenza epidemics. Recurrent diffuse aches after periods of vigorous activity, usually worse at night, suggest benign hypermobility syndrome or "growing pains." A painless, poorly localized limp may occur with metabolic bone disease (e.g., rickets). Spinal problems that can cause leg pain, weakness, or limp include dysraphism, vertebral infection, spondylolisthesis, and herniated disc. Spinal dysraphism refers to a spectrum of abnormalities in the development of the spinal cord and vertebrae ranging from obvious (myelomeningocele) to occult (tethered cord). Associated neurologic and musculoskeletal findings, including pain, atrophy, high arches, and tight heel cords, may develop in early childhood. Vertebral infection typically presents with fever and back pain. Spondylolisthesis and herniated disc are rare in young children but may be seen in adolescents who complain of back pain or radicular pain. Limp may rarely present as an early symptom of a peripheral neuropathy, either hereditary (e.g., Charcot-Marie-Tooth disease) or acquired (Guillan-Barre syndrome, vitamin- or medication-related). Intraabdominal pathology that can result in limp includes appendicitis, pelvic or psoas abscess, and renal disease. Solid tumors, most commonly neuroblastoma, can cause limp through retroperitoneal irritation or extension into the spinal canal. Likewise, a sacral teratoma may affect the nerves of the cauda equina or sacral plexus. Testicular pain may present with limping in a boy who is reluctant or embarrassed to admit the true source of his discomfort.

EVALUATION AND DECISION

The conditions that lead to a presentation of limp range from mundane (poorly fitting shoes) to life threatening (leukemia). The role of the pediatric acute care physician is to rule out the possibility of life- and limb-threatening pathologic conditions. The serious conditions include bacterial infection of the bone or joint space, malignancy, and disorders that threaten the blood supply to the bone, such as avascular necrosis and SCFE. Often, a definitive diagnosis will not be reached in the emergency department, and the patient will require follow-up with the primary care physician or specialist. Figure 42.1 provides an algorithmic approach to the child with a limp.

History

The history in a limping child should include information about the onset and duration of the limp, the family's perception of the origin of the problem, and associated symptoms such as pain, fever, and systemic illness. When pain is present, the physician should inquire about the location and severity. A history of trauma should be addressed, keeping in mind the inherent difficulty in obtaining an accurate trauma history in

very young children. Conversely, obvious trauma in the absence of a consistent history raises the question of inflicted injury. In more chronic presentations, any cyclical or recurrent patterns should be noted. Stiffness and limp primarily in the morning suggest rheumatic disease, whereas evening symptoms suggest weakness or overuse injury. A history of joint or limb swelling should be investigated, with attention to the degree of swelling and any migratory or recurrent patterns.

The medical history should include birth and developmental history. Breech position is associated with developmental dysplasia of the hip, and mild cerebral palsy may present in childhood with abnormal gait. History of viral infections, streptococcal pharyngitis, medication use, and immunizations may provide clues to the cause of limping. A family history of rheumatic or autoimmune disease, neurologic disease, inflammatory bowel disease, hemoglobinopathy, or other bleeding disorders may help facilitate diagnosis. Finally, the review of systems should include questions about past trauma, infections, neoplasia, endocrine disease, metabolic disease, and congenital anomalies.

Physical Examination

The physical examination in a limping child should begin with observation of the child's gait. Ideally, the child should be observed walking in bare feet and wearing minimal clothing, preferably in a long hallway. The physician should attempt to observe the child unobtrusively to avoid gait changes caused by self-consciousness. The observer should note the symmetry of stride length, the proportion of the gait cycle spent in stance phase, hip abductor muscle strength (with abnormal strength manifested by Trendelenburg or waddling gait), in-toeing or out-toeing, and joint flexibility. Muscle strength may be tested by asking the child to run, hop, and walk on toes and heels.

After observing the child in action, the physician should perform a complete examination with attention to the musculoskeletal and neurologic systems. The musculoskeletal examination begins with inspection of the limbs and feet for swelling or deformity. Supine positioning with the leg slightly flexed, abducted, and externally rotated at the hip is suggestive of fluid in the joint capsule. The spine should be inspected for curvature, both standing and bending forward, and the soles of feet and toes should be checked for foreign bodies and calluses. The bones, muscles, and joints should be palpated for areas of tenderness; range of motion of all joints should be checked; and limb lengths (from anterior superior iliac spine to medial malleolus), as well as thigh and calf circumferences, should be measured for asymmetry. The neurologic examination should include inspection of the spine for lumbosacral hair or dimple (indicating possible spinal dysraphism), and testing of strength, sensation, and reflexes. The abdomen and external genitalia should be examined for tenderness or masses and the skin for rashes. A rectal examination may be indicated if sacral pathology is suspected. Finally, wear patterns on the child's shoes may provide clues to the nature and duration of the limp.

Laboratory and Imaging

Plain radiographs remain a mainstay of the workup of a limping child. They provide an excellent means of screening for fracture, effusion, lytic lesions, periosteal reaction, and avascular necrosis. In a child with an obvious focus of pain, the radiographs may be obtained with views specific to that area, noting that children with knee pain may have hip pathology. The need for comparative views (of the normal extremity) depends on the experience of the physician interpreting the films. Some radiographic findings can be subtle, and comparison with the opposite side may be helpful. In a young child or a child lacking obvious focus for the limp, anteroposterior and lateral views of both lower extremities (including the feet) should be ordered as an initial screen. In toddlers lacking a focus of pain and in older children in whom hip pathology is suspected, anteroposterior and frog-leg lateral views of the pelvis are required. The frog-leg lateral view, obtained with the hips abducted and externally rotated, allows excellent visualization of the femoral heads. These radiographs should always include both hips to enable comparison of the femoral heads and width of the joint spaces. Radiographs of the spine are necessary if the child has neurologic signs or symptoms.

In children whose limp is associated with fever or systemic illness, laboratory studies, including a complete blood cell count, C-reactive protein level, and an erythrocyte sedimentation rate, are indicated. An elevated C-reactive protein level is a better independent predictor of disease than is an elevated erythrocyte sedimentation rate, and a C-reactive protein level of more than 2.0 mg per dL (20 mg per L) is strongly suggestive of bacterial infection. These studies serve as screens for infection, inflammation, malignancy, and hemoglobinopathy. Laboratory studies are also indicated in the absence of fever if the child has been limping for several days without evidence of trauma on plain films. Children with evidence of infection or inflammation with a joint effusion may require arthrocentesis for definitive diagnosis. In areas of endemic Lyme disease, a Lyme titer is a reasonable initial screening test in a patient with arthritis. A creatine phosphokinase level may be helpful if muscle inflammation is suspected.

When the initial history, physical examination, imaging, and laboratory evaluation indicate the cause of the limp, specific treatment can be initiated. Abnormalities in the initial workup without a definitive diagnosis should prompt further imaging or laboratory studies. Bone scintigraphy is more sensitive than plain radiographs for occult fracture, infection, avascular necrosis, and tumor; however, it is not specific for a given pathologic process. Computed tomography is an excellent imaging modality for cortical bone; it serves as a useful diagnostic adjunct in certain fractures, bony coalitions, and bone tumors. Ultrasound is the preferred modality for diagnosing hip effusions; it is also useful for guiding needle aspirations of the hip joint. Magnetic resonance imaging is useful in imaging the spinal cord, avascular necrosis, and bone marrow disease. Magnetic resonance imaging is becoming increasingly useful in the evaluation of infectious and oncologic musculoskeletal abnormalities as well, as an adjunct to bone scintigraphy or in place of it when the site of pathology is well localized.

If the initial workup in a limping child is completely normal, including screening radiographs and laboratory studies, the child may be followed closely as an outpatient. The child should be examined every few days until improvement is noted or a cause is determined. If the limp persists beyond 1 to 2 weeks without a diagnosis, further workup or consultation with a specialist is indicated.

Suggested Readings

Caird MS, Flynn JM, Leung YL, et al. Factors distinguishing septic arthritis from transient synovitis of the hip in children: a prospective study. *J Bone Joint Surg Am* 2006;8(6):1251–1257.

Clark MC. Approach to the child with a limp. *UpToDate* 2008;16.3.

Delaney RA, Lenahan B, O'Sullivan L, et al. The limping child: an algorithm to outrule musculoskeletal sepsis. *Ir J Med Sci* 2007;176:181–187.

Do TT. Transient synovitis as a cause of painful limps in children. *Curr Opin Pediatr* 2000;12:48–51.

Fahr MJ, James LP, Beck JR, et al. Digital radiography in the diagnosis of toddler's fracture. *South Med J* 2003;96:234–239.

Fernandez M, Carrol CL, Baker CJ. Discitis and vertebral osteomyelitis in children: an 18-year review. *Pediatrics* 2000;105:1299–1304.

Fischer SU, Beattie TF. The limping child: epidemiology, assessment, and outcome. *J Bone Joint Surg Br* 1999;81:1029–1034.

Halsey MF, Finzel KC, Carrion WV, et al. Toddler's fracture: presumptive diagnosis and treatment. *J Pediatr Orthop* 2001;21:152–156.

Leet AI, Skaggs DL. Evaluation of the acutely limping child. *Am Fam Physician* 2000;61:1011–1018.

Levine MJ, McGuire KJ, McGowan KL, et al. Assessment of test characteristics of C-reactive protein for septic arthritis in children. *J Pediatr Orthop* 2003;23:373–377.

Myers MT, Thompson GH. Imaging the child with a limp. *Pediatr Clin North Am* 1997;44:637–658.

Shavit I, Eidelman M, Galbraith R. Sonography of the hip-joint by the emergency physician: its role in the evaluation of children presenting with acute limp. *Pediatr Emerg Care* 2006;22:570–573.

SIGNS AND SYMPTOMS

CHAPTER 43 ■ LYMPHADENOPATHY

RICHARD MALLEY, MD

Lymphadenopathy is defined as swelling of the lymph nodes. Swollen lymph nodes are a common presenting sign in children, mainly because children have more pronounced lymphoid responses to inflammation than adults do, and they also have relatively more lymphoid tissue. Because the differential diagnosis of lymphadenopathy is extensive, it is helpful to distinguish localized from generalized lymphadenopathy. *Localized* or *regional adenopathy* generally occurs in response to a focal infectious process, although rarely other causes may need to be considered. Because a large number of organisms can cause localized adenopathy, it is often helpful to differentiate between acute and subacute/chronic regional adenopathy. *Generalized lymphadenopathy* is defined as enlargement of more than two noncontiguous lymph node regions. The most common causes of generalized adenopathy are systemic infections (bacterial or viral), autoimmune diseases, and neoplastic processes.

DIFFERENTIAL DIAGNOSIS

Acute Regional Adenopathy

The clinician caring for a child with acute regional adenopathy will benefit from knowledge of the anatomic distribution of nodes in the area and their drainage areas, as described in Table 43.1. The location of lymphadenopathy is often suggestive of a possible cause. For instance, in the head and neck region, swollen nodes are often a response to focal infectious processes occurring in areas that drain in the region of the nodes. Occipital nodes most commonly enlarge in response to bacterial or fungal scalp infections or chronic inflammation, such as occurs in seborrheic dermatitis. Because preauricular nodes drain the conjunctiva and lateral eyelids, these often enlarge in viral conjunctivitis. Epidemic keratoconjunctivitis caused by adenoviruses often presents with an enlarged preauricular node. The combination of conjunctivitis and ipsilateral preauricular adenopathy is called oculoglandular syndrome, or Parinaud's syndrome. Another infection that can present as Parinaud's syndrome is chlamydial conjunctivitis, also called neonatal-inclusion conjunctivitis. Chlamydial conjunctivitis, which generally presents within 5 to 7 days after birth, is diagnosed by the finding of intracytoplasmic inclusion bodies in conjunctival scrapings or, more commonly, by detection of the pathogen by immunofluorescent staining of ocular secretions. Parinaud's syndrome is also occasionally seen in cat-scratch disease, tularemia, and listeriosis. Similarly, the presence of submaxillary and submental nodes indicates the possibility of an infectious process in the oral cavity. Therefore, the physician should perform a careful oral and dental examination in these cases. Dental abscesses or gingival infections may be responsible for lymphadenopathy in these regions.

The differential diagnosis of cervical adenopathy is more extensive, mainly because the anatomy of the region is more complex. As can be seen in Table 43.1, nodes in the cervical region can be divided into three areas: the superior deep nodes below the angle of the mandible, the superficial cervical nodes found anteriorly and posteriorly along the sternocleidomastoid muscle, and the inferior deep nodes at the base of the neck. Enlargement of superior deep or superficial nodes raises the possibility of a lingual, external ear, or parotid gland process. In contrast, the inferior deep nodes have a much wider drainage area, including the head and neck, upper extremities, and the thoracic and abdominal regions. Swelling of these nodes, in particular, scalene and supraclavicular nodes, can be the first sign of occult thoracic or abdominal pathology, such as malignancy. Therefore, nodes found in these regions must be investigated carefully, with thorough physical examinations and, if necessary, radiographic examinations.

By far, the most common cause of acute cervical adenopathy is a viral upper respiratory tract infection. In these cases, lymph nodes are generally symmetrically enlarged and are soft and minimally tender, if at all. The reactive adenopathy may persist for 2 to 3 weeks beyond the resolution of the viral illness, but there should be no progression in the size or extent of the adenopathy. Bacterial cervical adenitis is also a common cause of cervical lymphadenopathy in children, particularly in preschool-age children. It is usually caused by group A β-hemolytic *Streptococcus* or *Staphylococcus aureus* (including methicillin-resistant *S. aureus*), although anaerobes (routinely penicillin-sensitive) may also be involved, particularly in oral infections. A history of a sore throat may be present in a minority of patients. Bacterial adenitis is most often unilateral and presents with firm, tender, and warm lymph nodes. In addition to the cervical area, other common sites of involvement include submaxillary, inguinal, and axillary nodes. If left untreated, these nodes may become erythematous and eventually fluctuant. Drainage of the nodes is sometimes required, even in appropriately treated cases (see Chapter 92).

Epstein-Barr virus (EBV), the agent of infectious mononucleosis, commonly causes posterior cervical lymphadenopathy in older children and adolescents. EBV infections do not always cause generalized adenopathy. The classic presentation of a child with EBV includes malaise, fever, an exudative tonsillopharyngitis, and hepatosplenomegaly. Facial edema may accompany significant EBV adenopathy, presumably reflecting obstructed lymph drainage. Younger children and infants with EBV infection may present less typically with fever alone or with symptoms suggestive of a mild upper respiratory infection. The diagnosis is made most easily with the detection of a

TABLE 43.1

REGIONAL ADENOPATHY

Site	Drainage area	Common causes	Less common causes
Occipital	Posterior scalp/neck	Tinea, seborrhea, pediculosis	Rubella
Preauricular	Conjunctiva	Viral conjunctivitis	Parinaud's syndrome of cat-scratch disease
	Lateral eyelids	*Chlamydia* conjunctivitis	Trachoma
	Temporal skin		Tularemia
Submaxillary /submental	Lip, gums, teeth, buccal mucosa	Chronically cracked lips, dental caries/infection, herpetic gingivostomatitis	
Cervical		**Acute common**	**Acute less common**
Superior (deep)	Tongue	Viral upper respiratory infection	Kawasaki syndrome
Superficial	External ear	Bacterial infection head/neck	
Anterior	Parotid gland	Primary bacterial adenitis	
Posterior		Epstein-Barr virus	
Inferior (deep)	Entire head/neck	**Chronic common**	**Chronic less common**
Scalene	Larynx, trachea	Cat-scratch disease	Anaerobic infection
Supraclavicular	Thyroid gland	Atypical mycobacterium	Epstein-Barr virus
	Arms/superficial thorax	Mycobacterium tuberculosis	Cytomegalovirus
	Lungs/mediastinum		Toxoplasmosis
	Abdomen		Tularemia
			Histoplasmosis
			Leptospirosis
			Brucellosis
			Sarcoid
			Sinus histiocytosis
			Hodgkin's disease
			Non-Hodgkin's lymphoma
			Lymphosarcoma
			Rhabdomyosarcoma
Axillary	Upper extremity	Upper-extremity inflammation	Rheumatologic disease hand/wrist
	Chest wall	Cat-scratch disease	Rat-bite fever
	Upper lateral abdominal wall		Toxoplasmosis
	Breast		
Epitrochlear	Ulnar side hand/forearm	Chronically inflamed hand	Secondary syphilis
		Local infection	Rheumatologic disease hand/wrist
			Tularemia
			Cat-scratch disease
Inguinal	Scrotum/penis	Lower-extremity inflammation	Chancroid
	Vulva/vaginal mucosa	Genital herpes	Lymphogranuloma venereum
	Skin/lower abdomen	Primary syphilis	
	Perineum/gluteal region		
	Lower anal canal		
	Lower extremities		
Iliac	Lower extremities	Lower-extremity inflammation	
	Abdominal viscera	Trauma	
	Urinary tract	Appendicitis	
		Urinary tract infection	
Popliteal	Knee joint	Severe local infection	
	Skin of lower leg/foot		

positive heterophile-agglutinating antibody (e.g., Monospot), although it is important to remember that this test may be falsely negative in children younger than 7 years.

A rarer, but very important, cause of acute cervical lymphadenopathy is Kawasaki disease, a systemic febrile syndrome of as yet undefined cause (see Chapter 101). Kawasaki disease, also called *mucocutaneous lymph node syndrome*, occurs most often in children younger than 4 years and is rare after 8 years of age. It is important to diagnose Kawasaki disease early because prompt treatment with intravenous gamma globulin can prevent coronary artery aneurysms, the most serious complication of this illness. The cervical lymphadenopathy in Kawasaki disease, seen in approximately 50% to 70% of patients, occurs during the early phase of the illness and may be unilateral or bilateral. The nodes are firm and mildly tender and should be at least 1.5 cm in diameter. The presence of a large node in the cervical area, in association with fever of more than 5 days' duration, bilateral conjunctival injection with limbal sparing, mucous membrane involvement, peripheral edema or erythema, and a polymorphous truncal rash, should alert the physician to the possibility of this disorder.

Axillary adenopathy is commonly present with any infection or inflammation of the upper extremities. Most commonly, injuries to the hand, such as occur after falling or with puncture wounds or bites, may present with concomitant axillary adenopathy. Similarly, epitrochlear nodes, which are not normally palpable in children, may become inflamed after infections of the third, fourth, or fifth finger; medial portion of the hand; or ulnar portion of the forearm. Most commonly, these infections are caused by pyogenic bacteria (e.g., *S. pyogenes, S. aureus*), but depending on the inciting event, other pathogens may be responsible (e.g., *S. moniliformis* and *Spirillum minus* in rat-bite fever).

Inguinal adenopathy most often results from lower-extremity infection, although sexually transmitted diseases may also be responsible. For example, acute genital infection with herpes simplex virus-2 often presents with tender inguinal adenopathy, occasionally as the only sign. Similarly, chancroid, lymphogranuloma venereum, and syphilis may present with inguinal nodal swelling and tenderness. The presence of genital lesions, which may be either painful (as in herpes simplex virus or chancroid) or painless (as in syphilis), offers clues to these diagnoses. Therefore, careful history-taking and physical examination are necessary to exclude these possibilities. Enlarged iliac nodes are palpable deeply over the inguinal ligament and become inflamed with lower-extremity infection, urinary tract infection, abdominal trauma, and appendicitis. Of note, iliac adenitis, which can present with fever, limp, and inability to fully extend the leg, may mimic the signs and symptoms of septic hip arthritis. Unlike in hip disease, however, hip motion is not limited on examination. Iliac adenitis may also be confused with appendicitis, but the pain initially occurs in the thigh and hip rather than in the periumbilical region or right lower quadrant.

Chronic Regional Adenopathy

Numerous agents can cause chronic regional lymphadenopathy. Organisms such as *Bartonella henselae* (the etiologic agent of cat-scratch disease), mycobacteria, and atypical mycobacteria are most commonly responsible for chronic adenopathy. Cat-scratch disease is a relatively common cause of chronic axillary or cervical adenopathy (see Chapter 92). Cat-scratch disease is characterized by a history of exposure to kittens (although other animals have also been implicated) and the development of a primary lesion at the site of a scratch. The primary lesion is 2 to 5 mm in size and is typically papular initially, and it may then progress to a pustule. About 2 weeks later, lymphadenopathy develops proximal to the site of the lesion. Typically, the nodes are enlarged but may or may not be inflamed. Lymphangitis does not occur in cat-scratch disease. Fever is present in only about 30% of patients. Other symptoms, such as seizures, may occur but are rare.

Although histopathology may be helpful in diagnosing cat-scratch disease, the most reliable diagnostic method is serology.

Tuberculous cervical lymphadenitis, otherwise known as *scrofula*, most commonly involves the posterior cervical nodes. Scrofula has become less common in the United States, although more recent epidemiologic studies in this country have suggested that the incidence of tuberculosis is rising. A history of exposure to an individual with active tuberculosis is often elicited, and several family members may have positive results on skin tests. Pulmonary and other systemic symptoms, such as fever, fatigue, and weight loss, are often present. The affected nodes are typically bilateral, fixed, and matted. Fluctuance is a late and rare finding in tuberculous adenitis. The diagnosis of tuberculous cervical lymphadenitis is made by a combination of skin testing, chest radiographs, and if possible, culture data from the involved node.

In contrast, atypical mycobacterial adenitis usually involves children younger than 5 years and is generally unilateral. The node is rarely larger than 3 cm. Overlying skin may turn a deep purple and gradually thins, developing a parchment-paper appearance. Fluctuance and ulceration occur commonly. Infected patients generally appear well, with a notable absence of any systemic symptoms. Chest radiographs are normal. A clear history of exposure to atypical mycobacteria (e.g., acquiring the infection via a fish tank) is the exception rather than the rule. Formal diagnosis is made by culture of the infected node, although the clinical appearance of the lesion and careful physical examination will often lead the clinician to the correct diagnosis. Treatment generally involves excision of the node, although, more recently, reports of treatment with newer macrolides suggest a possible role for antimicrobial therapy of these infections.

Other less common causes of chronic adenopathy deserve mention. A prolonged heterophile-negative adenopathy unresponsive to a trial of antibiotics should raise suspicion for one of these possibilities. Cytomegalovirus infection, which is characterized by cervical adenopathy, pharyngitis, and atypical lymphocytosis, may cause prolonged adenopathy in younger children. Toxoplasmosis typically presents as a single, nontender posterior cervical node. Brucellosis, associated generally with axillary and cervical lymphadenopathy, and tularemia with cervical adenopathy, are rare infectious causes of chronic adenopathy in children.

Noninfectious etiologies may also cause chronic regional adenopathy. Various malignancies, such as Hodgkin's disease, lymphosarcoma, neuroblastoma, and rhabdomyosarcoma, may all present with chronic cervical lymphadenopathy (see Chapter 97). For example, Hodgkin's disease usually presents as a slowly growing, painless firm node in the upper third of the neck. Lymphosarcoma also presents as a firm painless node, but it occurs in children younger than those with Hodgkin's and more commonly involves extranodal sites such as the tonsils. Rhabdomyosarcoma, the most common solid tumor of the head and neck in children, often involves the nasopharynx, middle ear, mastoid, or orbit, but it can also occur as a painless mass anywhere in the head and neck.

In African American children, sarcoidosis must be entertained in a child with bilateral chronic cervical adenopathy. Scalene nodes are involved in more than 80% of cases. An abnormal chest film, with hilar adenopathy and peribronchial fibrosis, suggests sarcoidosis. Sinus histiocytosis, a benign form of histiocytosis, can present as a large painless cervical adenopathy. The clinical presentation often includes fever, anemia, leukocytosis, and elevated erythrocyte sedimentation rate. Although the initial clinical presentation may be confused with lymphoma, the disease usually has a benign course, with resolution over a prolonged period.

Generalized Lymphadenopathy

Various systemic illnesses are associated with generalized lymphadenopathy (Table 43.2). The most common causes of generalized lymphadenopathy include bacterial or viral illnesses that disseminate systemically. As an example, the high incidence of vomiting and abdominal pain in streptococcal pharyngitis has been attributed to abdominal node inflammation and swelling, suggesting a more systemic pattern of adenopathy in streptococcal disease. Rarer bacterial causes of generalized lymphadenopathy include bacterial illnesses such as brucellosis and leptospirosis, diagnoses that may be suggested by occupational or dietary history. Common viral causes of generalized adenopathy include EBV or cytomegalovirus mononucleosis, rubella, and measles in parts of the world where the disease is endemic. Another cause of generalized adenopathy includes human immunodeficiency virus (HIV) infection. HIV infection in children can present with persistent generalized adenopathy, hepatosplenomegaly, and failure to thrive. Generalized lymphadenopathy may occasionally be the only presenting symptom in a child with vertical HIV infection.

Noninfectious systemic disease may also present with generalized adenopathy. Approximately 70% of patients with systemic lupus erythematosus or juvenile idiopathic arthritis manifest generalized adenopathy during the acute phase of illness (see Chapter 101). The lymphadenopathy of serum sickness often occurs in the presence of the exanthem but may be seen without rash. The lymphadenopathy of autoimmune hemolytic anemia coincides with each episode of hemolysis.

Neoplastic disease that causes generalized adenopathy may be primary to the lymph node as in Hodgkin's and non-Hodgkin's lymphomas, or it may be metastatic to the node with invasion of the node by extrinsic malignant cells as in leukemia or neuroblastoma (see Chapter 97). Hodgkin's disease, as discussed previously under "Regional Adenopathy", usually manifests as cervical adenopathy. In contrast, non-Hodgkin's lymphoma may present with rapidly enlarging, diffuse adenopathy, often accompanied by abdominal pain, vomiting, and diarrhea secondary to abdominal node involvement. Another neoplastic condition that can present with generalized adenopathy is leukemia. Approximately 70% of patients with acute lymphocytic leukemia and 30% of patients with acute myelogenous leukemia have generalized adenopathy (see Chapter 97). These children usually appear ill, having other systemic signs—hepatosplenomegaly, anemia, and thrombocytopenia with petechiae, purpura, and hemorrhage.

Histiocytosis presents as a spectrum of disease, ranging from a benign, isolated eosinophilic granuloma found in a long bone of an older child to the malignant multiorgan histiocytic infiltration found in infants with Letterer-Siwe disease (see Chapter 97). Lymphadenopathy often occurs in histiocytosis and can be an isolated finding; however, it usually occurs in association with other manifestations of disease.

Rarer causes of systemic adenopathy include lipid storage diseases (Gaucher's and Niemann-Pick's diseases), which can cause diffuse adenopathy, and are almost always associated

TABLE 43.2

GENERALIZED ADENOPATHY

Systemic infection
 Bacterial
  Bacteremia
  Scarlet fever
  Subacute bacterial endocarditis
  Syphilis
  Tuberculosis
  Brucellosis
 Viral
  Varicella
  Rubella
  Rubeola
  Epstein-Barr virus
  Cytomegalovirus
  Human immunodeficiency virus
 Fungal
  Histoplasmosis
  Coccidioidomycosis
 Parasitic
  Toxoplasmosis
  Malaria

Autoimmune disease
 Juvenile idiopathic arthritis
 Systemic lupus erythematosus
 Serum sickness
 Autoimmune hemolytic anemia

Primary lymphoid neoplasm
 Hodgkin's disease
 Non-Hodgkin's lymphoma

Metastatic neoplasm
 Acute lymphocytic leukemia
 Acute myelogenous leukemia
 Neuroblastoma

Histiocytosis
 Letterer-Siwe disease
 Histiocytic medullary reticulosis

Storage disease
 Gaucher's disease
 Niemann-Pick's disease

Drugs
 Aromatic antiepileptics: phenytoin, phenobarbital, carbamazepine, primidone
 Other antiepileptic agents: lamotrigine, valproic acid, ethosuximide
 Antibiotics: isoniazid, dapsone, sulfonamides, minocycline
 Others
  Allopurinol
  Diltiazem
  Zalcitabine

Miscellaneous
 Hyperthyroidism

with hepatosplenomegaly. Bone marrow biopsy, showing lipid-laden histiocytes, is diagnostic.

Certain drugs can be associated with generalized adenopathy. Drug-induced hypersensitivity syndrome deserves particular attention because it has been associated with rather severe presentations, some of which have been fatal. This syndrome is generally, but not always, associated with aromatic anticonvulsants such as phenytoin, phenobarbital, and carbamazepine, but newer antiepileptic and other drugs have also been reported to cause this syndrome (Table 43.2). The aromatic antiepileptic agents have a common benzene ring that is metabolized to arene oxides. It is postulated that anticonvulsant hypersensitivity syndrome occurs in patients who may have a defect in the epoxide hydrolase enzymatic pathway, which normally degrades the toxic arene oxide metabolites formed during oxidation of the antiepileptics. It is important to remember that a patient with a history of a hypersensitivity reaction to one anticonvulsant drug may be at high risk for an even more severe reaction if exposed to another anticonvulsant drug. Although this syndrome can occasionally present with lymphadenopathy alone (which may not even be generalized), the characteristic features generally progress to include fever, rash, and organ involvement (e.g., liver, bone marrow, kidney, and lungs). Beyond cessation of the drug and provision of supportive care, the optimal therapy for this condition is not established at this time, although some have proposed the use of systemic corticosteroids and/or intravenous immune globulin.

Finally, hyperthyroidism can be associated with a nonspecific lymph node hyperplasia, but one should see other signs and symptoms of the illness, such as tachycardia, hypertension, diaphoresis, weight loss, goiter, lid lag, and hyperreflexia, on physical examination.

Life-Threatening Lymphadenopathy

Several disorders associated with lymphadenopathy, primarily but not exclusively oncologic, can be life threatening (Table 43.3). The superior vena cava (SVC) syndrome is an example of life-threatening adenopathy. The SVC is a thin-walled vessel with low intravascular pressure that is approximated tightly to the right mainstem bronchus and completely encircled by the lymph nodes that drain the thoracic cavity. SVC syndrome is obstruction of the SVC, usually caused by massive adenopathy, and manifests as dilated chest wall and neck veins, facial edema, and plethora. Drowsiness or stupor, called "wet brain" syndrome, may also be seen. Superior mediastinal syndrome is a variant of the SVC syndrome, with additional respiratory symptoms caused by trachea or bronchus compression. In contrast with patients with SVC syndrome, those with superior mediastinal syndrome present in respiratory distress with coughing and wheezing.

TABLE 43.3

LIFE-THREATENING CONDITIONS ASSOCIATED WITH LYMPHADENOPATHY

Superior vena cava syndrome	Acute myelogenous leukemia
Hodgkin's disease	Neuroblastoma
Non-Hodgkin's lymphoma	Letterer-Siwe disease
Neuroblastoma	Coronary artery aneurysm
Bone marrow failure/ multiorgan infiltration	Kawasaki disease
Acute lymphocytic leukemia	Drug-induced hypersensitivity syndrome

Almost all patients with SVC or superior mediastinal syndrome have a malignant etiology (see Chapter 97). In children, Hodgkin's and non-Hodgkin's lymphomas are the most common causes, followed by metastatic neuroblastoma. Emergency physicians who treat patients with SVC syndrome must be careful to administer all intravenous therapy in the lower extremities. Poor circulation in the upper extremities and torso because of SVC obstruction results in poor drug distribution and places the patient with SVC syndrome at increased risk of thrombus formation.

EVALUATION AND DECISION

The clinician who evaluates lymphadenopathy is faced with an extensive differential diagnosis. A meticulous history and physical examination can help focus the evaluation of the patient. Historical data that need to be obtained include the time of onset, the rate of growth, and the duration of symptoms. Lymphadenopathy of more than 3 weeks' duration is considered chronic. The presence and duration of fever, history of rash or pruritus, cough, weight loss, anorexia, and nausea are important systemic symptoms. Recent illnesses must be considered, particularly because lymphadenopathy may persist for 2 to 3 weeks after the resolution of common viral illnesses. Certain medications, most notably the aromatic anticonvulsants and other drugs listed in Table 43.2, can cause generalized lymphadenopathy and must be kept in mind because of the potential severity of hypersensitivity reactions. In addition, the presence of certain risk factors, such as young cats in the home (cat-scratch disease) or other animals (e.g., dogs, rabbits, rats), exposure to patients with active tuberculosis, consumption of unpasteurized milk, or exposure to fish tanks (atypical mycobacteria), among others, needs to be ascertained. Finally, the clinician must ask whether any prior treatment, such as antibiotic therapy or attempted aspiration with cultures, has been initiated. For example, children with atypical mycobacterial adenitis may present to the emergency department after a prolonged course of antistaphylococcal antibiotic therapy failed to reduce the size of the node. Knowledge of the response to specific antimicrobial therapy can often guide the physician to exclude certain diagnoses.

The physical examination should include a careful determination of the size of the enlarged nodes and documentation of the number of nodes involved to provide an adequate baseline for follow-up. In general, lymph nodes larger than 1 cm are significant in any location. The presence of erythema, warmth, and tenderness often indicates an acute pyogenic bacterial process. In most disease processes that cause lymphadenopathy in children, the nodes will be firm, rubbery, and mobile. Lymph nodes fixed to underlying tissues or located in deeper fascial planes are rare in children, but when present, they should prompt the physician to consider early surgical evaluation. Finally, because several systemic diseases manifest a specific pattern of adenopathy, examination of all lymph node regions must be performed. Likewise, hepatosplenomegaly, rash, and other signs of systemic involvement must be sought.

The approach to the patient with lymphadenopathy focuses initially on the history and examination findings as noted, with emphasis on the distribution of enlarged nodes: regional or generalized (Fig. 43.1). Regional lymphadenopathy should be categorized as acute or subacute/chronic.

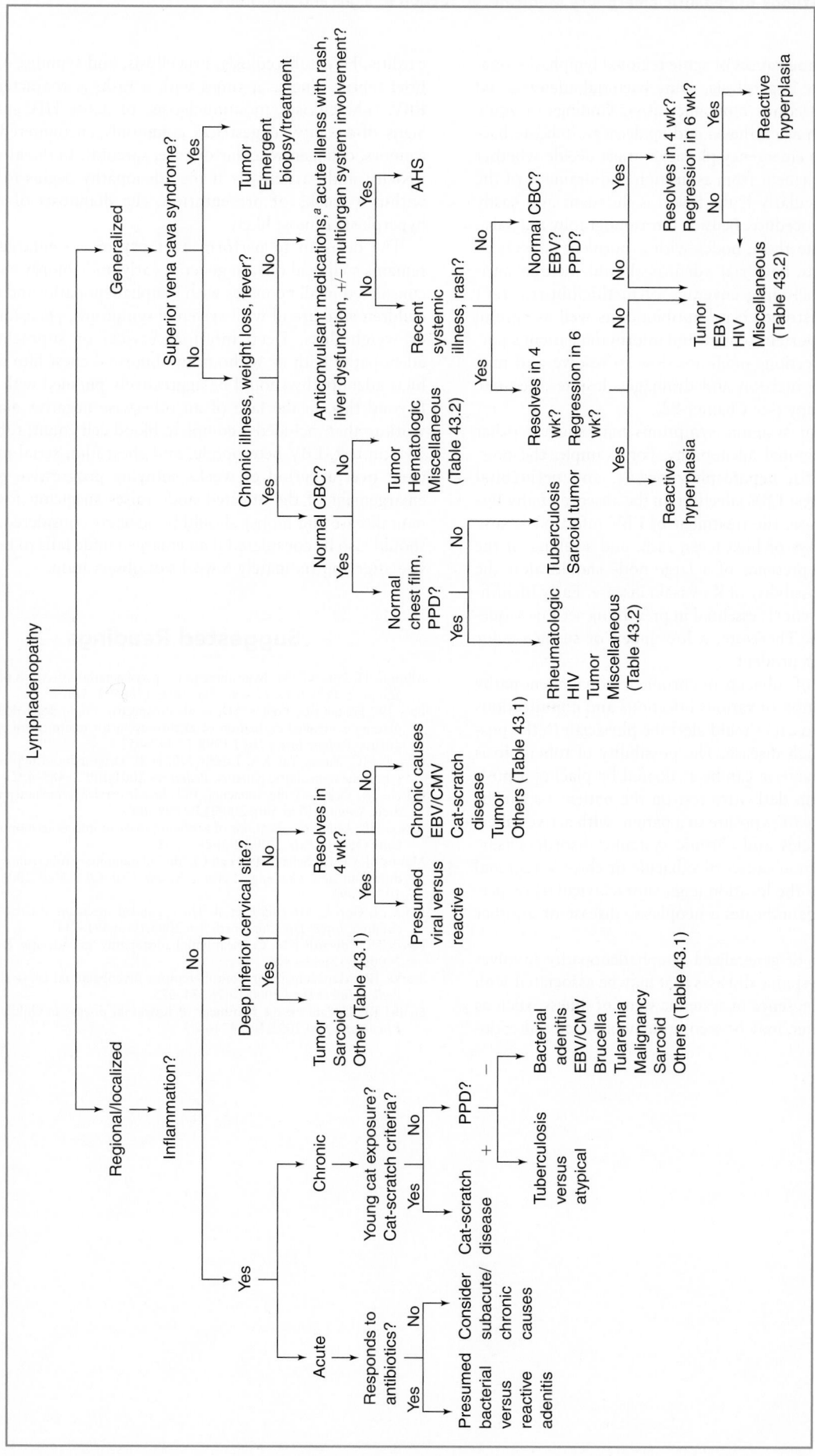

FIGURE 43.1 The diagnostic approach to the child with lymphadenopathy. [a]Rarely, other drugs may cause AHS (Table 43.2). PPD, purified protein derivative; EBV, Epstein-Barr virus; CMV, cytomegalovirus; CBC, complete blood cell count; HIV, human immunodeficiency virus; AHS, anticonvulsant hypersensitivity syndrome.

The most common causes of acute regional lymphadenopathy include reactive hyperplasia, acute bacterial adenitis, and EBV infection (infectious mononucleosis). Findings of acute inflammation, such as erythema and tenderness, indicate bacterial adenitis. The emergency physician must decide whether the patient would benefit from aspiration and drainage of the lymph node, particularly if the lesion is fluctuant and easily amenable to the procedure. Bedside ultrasonography may also help to differentiate those nodes with a purulent collection. Treatment of acute bacterial adenitis should include antistaphylococcal (including coverage of methicillin-resistant *S aureus*) and antistreptococcal antibiotics as well as careful follow-up. It is important to note and inform the patient's parents that these infections often are slow to resolve and may eventually require incision and drainage, despite adequate antimicrobial therapy (see Chapter 92).

The presence of systemic symptoms may suggest other causes of acute regional adenopathy. For example, the presence of pharyngitis, hepatosplenomegaly, and periorbital edema should suggest EBV infection. In the absence of any respiratory compromise, the treatment of EBV infection is supportive. Several days of high fever, rash, and swelling of the extremities in the presence of a large node should alert the physician to the possibility of Kawasaki disease. Early identification of these patients is essential in preventing serious sequelae of this disease. Therefore, a low index of suspicion for Kawasaki disease is prudent.

The evaluation of subacute or chronic regional adenopathy includes consideration of various infectious and noninfectious causes. Exposure to cats should alert the physician to the possibility of cat-scratch disease. The possibility of tuberculosis or atypical mycobacteria can be evaluated by placing a positive purified protein derivative test on the patient or can be elicited by a history of exposure to a patient with active tuberculosis. Malignancies and chronic systemic disorders (sarcoid) are less common causes of subacute or chronic regional adenopathy. Either the location (e.g., supraclavicular) or persistence of the node indicates a neoplastic disease or another serious process.

The evaluation of generalized lymphadenopathy involves consideration of systemic diseases that may be associated with adenopathy. The presence of systemic signs of illness, such as weight loss and fever, may be seen in subacute bacterial endocarditis, HIV, tuberculosis, brucellosis, and syphilis. A recent, brief febrile illness, at times with a rash, is characteristic of EBV, tuberculosis, mononucleosis, or acute HIV infection. Signs of toxicity suggest less commonly encountered causes (tumors, collagen vascular disease, sarcoid). In the absence of toxicity, and particularly if the adenopathy begins to resolve within 4 weeks of presentation, the diagnosis of reactive hyperplasia is most likely.

The decision to perform a biopsy on an enlarged node remains a clinical one. In general, early node biopsy should be considered in all neonates with lymphadenopathy and in older children who are ill with systemic symptoms, persistent fever, or weight loss. Deep inferior cervical or supraclavicular adenopathy with or without an abnormal chest film showing hilar adenopathy should be aggressively pursued with biopsy. Beyond this, in the face of an otherwise negative diagnostic workup that included a complete blood cell count, tuberculosis skin test, EBV heterophile, and chest film, serial measurement over a period of weeks showing progressive or rapid enlargement of the affected node raises suspicion for malignant disease and biopsy should be strongly considered. Biopsy should also be considered if an enlarged node fails to regress in size after approximately 6 weeks of observation.

Suggested Readings

Albright JT, Pranski SM. Nontuberculous mycobacterial infections of the head and neck. *Pediatr Clin North Am* 2003;50(2):503–514.

Bass JW, Freitas BC, Freitas AD, et al. Prospective randomized double blind placebo-controlled evaluation of azithromycin for treatment of cat-scratch disease. *Pediatr Infect Dis J* 1998;17:447–452.

Carroll MC, Yueng-Yue KA, Esterly NB, et al. Drug-induced hypersensitivity syndrome in pediatric patients. *Pediatrics* 2001;108(2):485–492.

Gosche JR, Vick L. Acute, subacute, and chronic cervical lymphadenitis in children. *Semin Pediatr Surg* 2006;15(2):99–106.

Jenson HB. Acute complications of Epstein-Barr virus infectious mononucleosis. *Curr Opin Pediatr* 2000;12(3):263–268.

Marais BJ, Gie RP, Schaaf HS, et al. Childhood pulmonary tuberculosis: old wisdom and new challenges. *Am J Respir Crit Care Med* 2006;173(10):1078–1090.

Massei F, Gori L, Macchia P, et al. The expanded spectrum of bartonellosis in children. *Infect Dis Clin North Am* 2005;19(3):691–711.

Peters TR, Edwards KM. Cervical lymphadenopathy and adenitis. *Pediatr Rev* 2000;21(12):399–405.

Starke JR. Management of nontuberculous mycobacterial cervical adenitis. *Pediatr Infect Dis J* 2000;19(7):674–675.

Sundel RP. Update on the treatment of Kawasaki disease in childhood. *Curr Rheumatol Rep* 2002;4(6):474–482.

CHAPTER 44 ■ NECK MASS

CARLA MARIA PRUDEN, MD, MPH, AND CONSTANCE M. MCANENEY, MD, MS

Neck masses are common in children, and the diagnosis encompasses a multitude of disorders. By definition, neck masses include any visible swelling that disturbs the normal contour of the neck between the shoulder and the angle of the jaw. The patient's age and the location of the neck mass are important in determining the differential diagnosis. In the pediatric population, the four basic classifications of neck lesions are inflammatory, congenital, traumatic, and neoplastic. Inflammatory masses are the most common and usually represent structures normally present, such as lymph nodes, that are undergoing changes from infectious causes. By far, the most common causes of neck masses in children are reactive adenopathy and adenitis. Congenital anatomic defects of the neck are often unapparent or minimally recognizable at birth, but they develop into significant cystic masses over time. Included in this category are cystic hygromas, branchial cleft cysts, hemangiomas, thyroglossal duct cysts, and dermoids. Traumatic neck masses are usually caused by hematoma surrounding vital structures and may lead to significant distress. Malignant lesions of the head and neck must be ruled out, but fortunately, they are fairly uncommon and are often caused by cancer of the lymphatic system. Therefore, an organized thorough history and examination of the head and neck, as well as a working understanding of the embryology of the neck, is important to assist in an appropriate workup to facilitate diagnosis and treatment.

True medical emergencies arise if neck masses compromise adjacent vital structures, including the airway, carotid and jugular blood vessels, and cervical spinal cord. In rare cases, the principal threat to life is from systemic toxicity. Infection that leads to septicemia, or the effects of excess hormone secretion in thyroid storm, can lead to uncompensated shock. Most large neck masses do not encroach on vital structures because their growth points outward. Embarrassment about personal appearance or a concern of malignancy may be factors, however, in the initiation of the emergency department (ED) visit.

This chapter first emphasizes recognition of masses that represent true emergencies (Table 44.1). Then, the approach to nonemergent but commonly seen lesions is described (Table 44.2). Table 44.3 lists causes of neck masses of children by origin.

EVALUATION AND DECISION

The initial history and physical examination should screen rapidly for airway or vascular compromise with consideration of integrity of the cervical spine. The presence of stridor, hoarseness, dysphagia, and drooling indicates respiratory compromise. The quality of breathing, level of consciousness, and integrity of the cervical spine should also be assessed. Appropriate resuscitative measures should be taken if respira-

tory or vascular compromise is evident. The cervical spine should be immobilized if there is history of trauma or if the initial evaluation leads to suspicion. Table 44.1 lists disorders that constitute true emergencies because of local pressure on vital structures or because of systemic toxicity.

Child with Neck Mass and Respiratory Distress or Systemic Toxicity

Trauma from vehicular collisions, falls from heights, or sports injuries may cause bleeding or hematoma formation near vital structures such as the carotid artery or trachea. If the trauma involves the cervical spine, a hematoma may occur over fractured vertebrae. Even mild injuries may lead to severe hemorrhage and compression of vital structures of the neck in children who have clotting factor disorders (i.e., hemophilia) or platelet disorders (i.e., idiopathic thrombocytopenic purpura). Symptomatic arteriovenous fistulas may appear weeks after neck trauma. The emergency physician should be wary of severe trauma or ecchymoses with an "insignificant history" and should consider possible child abuse or an acquired bleeding problem. The progression of a pneumomediastinum to pneumothorax can be rapid although very uncommon and requires close observation of the tachypneic child with a "crepitant" neck mass. Acutely, this may be caused by trauma to the chest and rib cage or by severe airway obstruction caused by asthma or a foreign body. In children with obstructive lung diseases, such as asthma and cystic fibrosis, high transpulmonary pressure generated in these diseases forces air through small alveolar leaks into the mediastinum or pleural space. This may produce a pneumomediastinum that dissects into the neck. Anaphylactic reaction with neck swelling may precipitate an acute emergency if the swelling compromises the airway. Severe, local reactions to bee stings or to other sensitizing allergens may cause enough tissue edema to obstruct the trachea.

Infections associated with life-threatening processes include retropharyngeal, lateral pharyngeal, and peritonsillar abscesses. Lemierre's syndrome, an uncommon parapharyngeal infection involving thrombophlebitis of the internal jugular vein with metastatic pulmonary abscesses, may manifest as respiratory distress and systemic toxicity in the adolescent with a history of pharyngitis. Rarely, epiglottitis may present with associated cervical adenitis or the appearance of submandibular mass from ballooning of the hypopharynx. These patients may have cervical adenitis and concomitant dysphagia, drooling, and stridor. Occasionally, branchial cleft cysts or cystic hygromas can become infected and progress to abscess formation or rarely to mediastinitis. Laryngoceles may become acutely infected and obstruct airflow. Massive tonsillar hypertrophy with infectious

TABLE 44.1

LIFE-THREATENING CAUSES OF NECK MASS

Hematoma secondary to trauma
   Cervical spine injury
   Vascular compromise or acute bleeding
   Late arteriovenous fistula
Subcutaneous emphysema with associated airway or
   pulmonary injury
Local hypersensitivity reaction (sting/bite) with airway edema
Airway compromise with epiglottitis, tonsillar abscess, or
   infection of floor of mouth or retropharyngeal space (with
   adenopathy)
Bacteremia/sepsis associated with local infection of a cyst
   (cystic hygroma, thyroglossal, or branchial cleft cyst)
Non-Hodgkin's lymphoma with mediastinal mass and airway
   compromise
Thyroid storm
Mucocutaneous lymph node syndrome with coronary
   vasculitis
Tumor—leukemia, lymphoma, rhabdomyosarcoma,
   histiocytosis X
Lemierre's syndrome

mononucleosis can manifest with upper airway obstruction. Dental infection that spreads to the floor of the mouth (Ludwig's angina) and neck may cause neck masses and airway compression. More recently, children with human immunodeficiency virus (HIV) infection (see Chapter 93) are reported to have parotitis or generalized lymphadenopathy, particularly visible in the neck as a presenting complaint. Children may have hyperthyroid symptoms when a neck mass represents thyromegaly. Similarly, patients with the mucocutaneous lymph node syndrome (Kawasaki disease) often have cervical lymphadenopathy and, on rare occasions, have active life-threatening vasculitis of the coronary vessels.

Neck tumors in children may become large enough to encroach on vital structures. Lymphoma, an uncommon but important cause of neck mass, is suggested especially by painless enlargement (often of supraclavicular nodes) that occurs over several weeks in the older school-age child. When mediastinal nodes are involved, the patient may rapidly develop a blockage of the intrathoracic trachea that is accentuated on lying down. These children may be fine when sitting, but when supine, the anterior mediastinal masses compress the trachea, causing the airway to collapse. Cystic hygromas and hemangiomas occasionally enlarge sufficiently enough to interfere with feeding or to obstruct the airway. Other tumors, such as rhabdomyosarcoma, leukemia, neuroblastoma, and histiocy-

TABLE 44.2

COMMON CAUSES OF NECK MASS

Lymphadenopathy secondary to viral or bacterial infection
Cervical adenitis (bacterial)
Hematoma
Benign tumors—lipoma, keloid
Congenital cyst (squamous epithelial cysts)

TABLE 44.3

DIFFERENTIAL DIAGNOSIS OF NECK MASS BY ETIOLOGY

Congenital
   Squamous epithelial cyst (congenital or posttraumatic)
   Pilomatrixoma (Malherbe's calcifying epithelioma)
   Hemangioma and cystic hygroma (lymphangioma)
   Branchial cleft cyst
   Thyroglossal duct cyst
   Laryngocele
   Dermoid cyst
   Cervical rib

Inflammatory
   Infection
      Cervical adenitis—streptococcal, staphylococcal, fungal,
         mycobacterial, cat-scratch disease, tularemia
      Adenopathy—secondary to local head and neck infection
      Secondary to systemic "infection"—infectious
         mononucleosis, cytomegalovirus, toxoplasmosis, others
      Retropharyngeal abscess
      Focal myositis—inflammatory muscular pseudotumor
      Lemierre's syndrome
      "Antigen" mediated
      Local hypersensitivity reaction (sting/bite)
      Serum sickness, autoimmune disease
      Pseudolymphoma (secondary to phenytoin)
      Kawasaki disease
      Sarcoidosis
      Caffey-Silverman syndrome

Trauma
   Hematoma
   Sternocleidomastoid tumor of infancy (fibromatosis colli)
   Subcutaneous emphysema
   Acute bleeding
   Arteriovenous fistula
   Foreign body
   Cervical spine fracture

Neoplasms
   Benign
      Epidermoid
      Lipoma, fibroma, neurofibroma
      Keloid
      Goiter (with or without thyroid hormone disturbance)
      Osteochondroma
      Teratoma (may be malignant)
      "Normal" anatomy or variant
   Malignant
      Lymphoma—Hodgkin's disease, non-Hodgkin's
         lymphoma
      Leukemia
      Other—rhabdomyosarcoma, neuroblastoma,
         histiocytosis X, nasopharyngeal squamous cell
         carcinoma, thyroid, or salivary gland tumor

tosis X, are life threatening because of local invasion and metabolic and hematologic effects.

Child with Neck Mass and No Distress

Most children in the ED with a neck mass are not in distress; the leading diagnoses are reactive adenopathy or acute lymphadenitis from viral or bacterial infection. A common concern, however, is deciding which neck mass bears the diagnosis of malignancy and requires biopsy or further evaluation.

History

A careful evaluation of history, establishing the duration of signs and symptoms, as well as ascertaining the involvement of other organ systems (fatigue, weight loss, night sweats, adenopathy elsewhere), often suggests the diagnosis. Presence of sore throat, fever, neck pain, difficulty breathing, or "noisy breathing" (stridor, wheezing) should be elicited. Location of the mass, size and shape of the mass, duration of symptoms, and a history of injury are important. The patient's age at discovery of the lesion should be noted because those found early in infancy increase the risk of a cyst of congenital origin. Birth trauma, with bleeding into the sternocleidomastoid muscle, may cause torticollis, which presents at several weeks of age with a neck mass. It is important to note that not all congenital lesions present at birth or in the first months of life. They are brought to medical attention with acute infection or inflammation, sometimes as a recurrent unilateral neck mass in young infants. Changes in the size of the mass with time or with a child's growth, and whether there has been a change in the character of the lesion, should be noted. Presence of a dimple or sinuses, history of drainage, and other symptoms of infection may assist in making the diagnosis. History of exposure to an infectious agent, including streptococcal pharyngitis, infectious mononucleosis, or recent upper respiratory illness, should be sought. Questions regarding exposure to animal bites or scratches are important. Systemic symptoms that suggest serum sickness (fever, malaise, rash, arthralgias, nephritis) or pseudolymphoma ought to prompt an exposure history for medications (e.g., antibiotics and anticonvulsants, respectively). Figure 44.1 describes a pathway to facilitate some of the differential diagnoses by category.

Physical Examination

After assessment for critical illness is performed, the clinician should perform a thorough examination on a child with a neck mass. It is often valuable to examine the patient thoroughly and then come to examine the area of the head and neck last. Palpation of the mass, noting its location, size, shape, relationship, attachment to normal structures in the neck, and overlying skin changes, should be completed. Figure 44.2 diagrams the locations of many of the causes of neck mass. It is important to ascertain whether crepitation, a thrill, or a bruit is present and the degree to which an inflammatory mass is fluctuant. The surrounding area should be palpated for additional lesions (10% to 20% of branchial lesions are bilateral) and to evaluate normal structures of the neck such as the thyroid gland, sternocleidomastoid muscles, trachea, and cervical spine. The ability of the patient to flex and extend the neck should be ascertained. Inspection of the oral cavity should be performed, noting oral mucosa, dentition, and the orifices such as Stensen's duct (parotid gland) and other glands. The presence of movement of the mass with swallowing or with protrusion of the tongue is important. The examination of the head should be meticulous, including the scalp, ears, sinuses, and nasopharynx.

During auscultation of the chest, special attention should be paid to inspiration because extrathoracic airway obstruction from the trachea or upper airway may produce only faint stridor. Respiratory distress or wheezing that worsens in the supine position may be an early sign of an anterior mediastinal mass. The physical examination should be completed, looking for signs of systemic illness as a cause for the neck mass. The general appearance and color of the child is important, as is the presence of hepatosplenomegaly or an abdominal mass, indicating a high suspicion for a malignancy. Signs of thyroid hormone excess (tachycardia, bounding pulses, systolic hypertension, exophthalmos) or deficiency may be associated with a goiter. Rashes, generalized lymphadenopathy, and fever may indicate an inflammatory or oncologic process. Failure to thrive or weight loss may be found with a number of causes of infection or oncologic illness, including HIV disease, histiocytosis X, mycobacterium infections, and others. Finally, a close examination of the skin, not only observing the overlying skin but also noting any animal scratches or bites of the face and extremities, is imperative.

Details of chronicity, size, and progression and evidence of inflammation help distinguish between infection and neoplasm. Characteristics that some authors have found associated with malignancy include masses that are firm and larger than 3 cm in diameter, nonpainful, progressively enlarging, ulcerating, deep to fascia or fixed to tissue, or discovered in a newborn. These criteria are sensitive but not specific for cancer. Even with these characteristics, most lesions are benign congenital cysts or inflammatory masses. The duration the "node" is present is not discriminating in that, often, inflammatory nodes that are biopsied have been present for more than 2 to 3 months.

DIFFERENTIAL DIAGNOSIS

Congenital Masses

Thyroglossal duct cysts are the most common congenital cyst of the neck. They develop along the line of descent of the thyroid gland in the neck anywhere from the base of the tongue to the sternal notch in the *anterior triangle*. This will occur if the embryologic thyroglossal duct fails to obliterate before the formation of the hyoid bone. Sixty-five percent of these are found to be infrahyoid. Thyroglossal duct cysts are usually midline, adjacent to the hyoid bone, and more than half are diagnosed in children before 10 years of age. Occurrence usually is noticed after an upper respiratory infection or an episode of hemorrhage. Thyroglossal duct cysts are soft, nontender, smooth, and may move cranially when the child swallows or protrudes the tongue. If infected, they may be warm, erythematous, and drain externally. If drainage occurs by way of the foramen cecum, there may be an associated foul taste in the mouth. Antibiotics (for mouth and skin flora), warm compresses, and incision and drainage (if indicated) should be initiated for signs of infection. Complete excision is the treatment of choice after complete resolution of infection.

Cystic hygromas are cystic lymphatic malformations occurring in the *posterior triangle* of the neck. Most are identified at birth, but some may be recognized after injury or upper respiratory infection when "herniation" has occurred after crying,

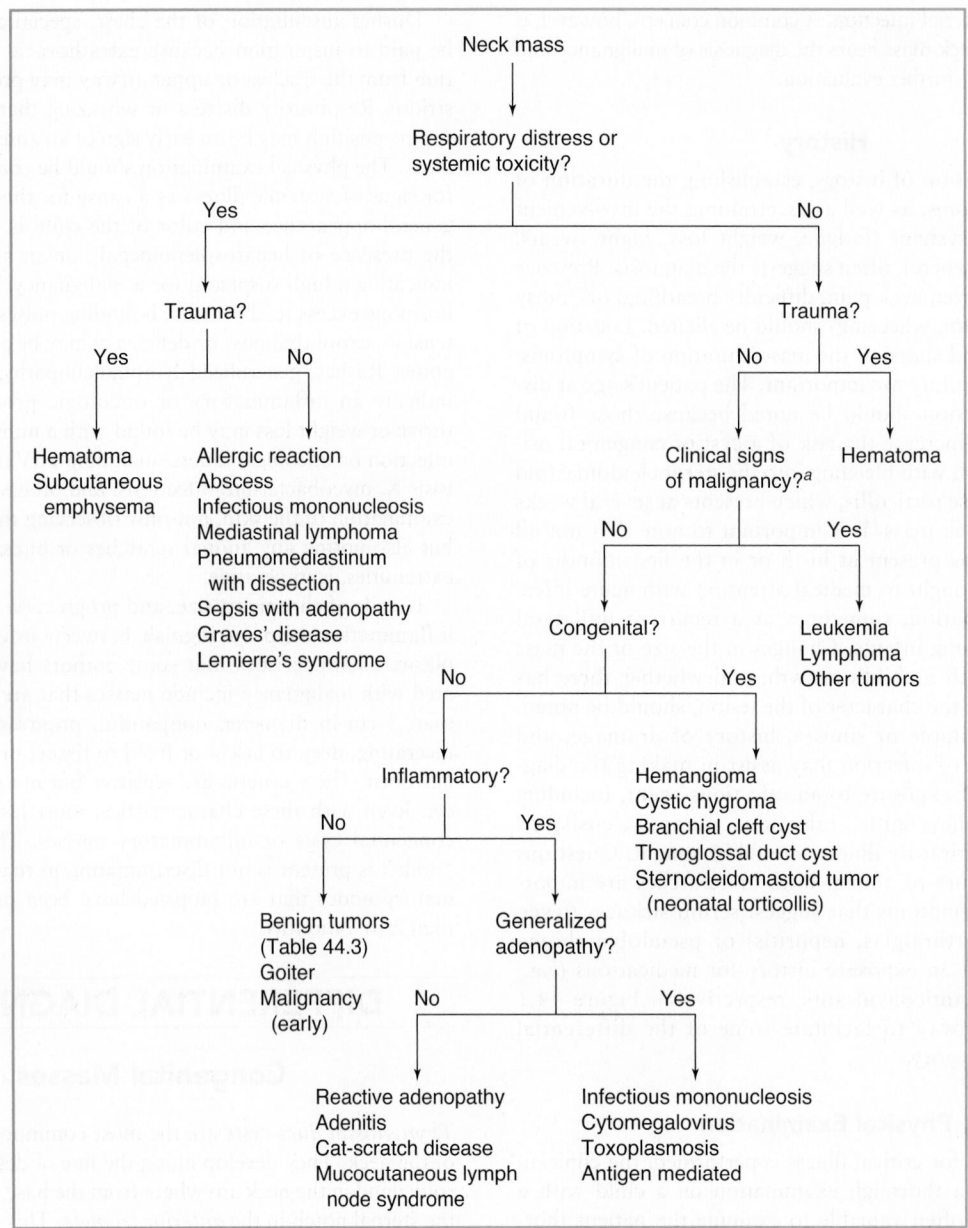

FIGURE 44.1 Evaluation of the child with a neck mass. [a]Malignancy: nontender, >3 cm diameter (and firm), enlarging mass of several weeks' duration, ulceration, location deep to superficial fascia or fixed to tissue, supraclavicular mass, systemic lymphadenopathy and bruising, superior vena cava syndrome.

coughing, or other forceful Valsalva maneuvers. Ninety percent present before the age of 2 years. Cystic hygromas appear discrete, soft, mobile, nontender, and vary greatly in size. Extension to the mediastinum can cause chylothorax or chylo-mediastinum, and rarely, airway compromise can occur; thus, chest radiograph is recommended. Infection is uncommon, but signs of it would be as expected. Ultrasonography is useful in establishing whether the mass is cystic. Computed tomography (CT) imaging or magnetic resonance imaging can determine the extent and involvement of surrounding structures. Spontaneous regression is rare; therefore, complete excision is the treatment of choice.

Branchial cleft anomalies are lesions most commonly occurring from defects in the development of the second branchial arch, giving rise to firm masses along the anterior border of the sternocleidomastoid muscle near the angle of the mandible in the *posterior triangle of the neck*. Branchial cleft sinuses are painless and present with drainage at the junction of the middle and lower thirds of the sternocleidomastoid muscle. Cysts that are usually fluctuant, mobile, and nontender may occur if the sinus tract becomes blocked. If the cyst becomes infected, it can be painful and warm. Probing or injecting the tract may lead to infection. Incision and drainage of a branchial lesion should be avoided because it may result in fistula formation. Ultrasonography may be useful in identifying a thin-walled, anechoic, fluid-filled cyst. Treatment with antibiotics with complete resolution of infection is necessary if the sinus or cyst is infected. Excision of the entire tract and cyst is important to prevent recurrence.

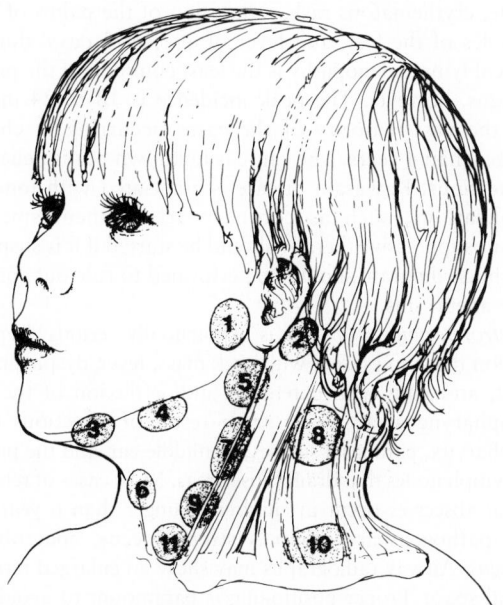

FIGURE 44.2 Differential diagnosis of neck mass by location. *Area 1. Parotid:* Cystic hygroma, hemangioma, lymphadenitis, parotitis, Sjogren's and Caffey-Silverman syndrome, lymphoma. *Area 2. Postauricular:* Lymphadenitis, branchial cleft cyst (1st), squamous epithelial cyst. *Area 3. Submental:* Lymphadenitis, cystic hygroma, sialadenitis, tumor, cystic fibrosis. *Area 4. Submandibular:* Lymphadenitis, cystic hygroma, sialadenitis, tumor, cystic fibrosis. *Area 5. Jugulodigastric:* Lymphadenitis, squamous epithelial cyst, branchial cleft cyst (1st), parotid tumor, *normal*—transverse process C2, styloid process. *Area 6. Midline neck:* Lymphadenitis, thyroglossal duct cyst, dermoid, laryngocele, *normal*—hyoid, thyroid. *Area 7. Sternocleidomastoid (anterior):* Lymphadenitis, branchial cleft cyst (2nd, 3rd), pilomatrixoma, rare tumors. *Area 8. Spinal accessory:* Lymphadenitis, lymphoma, metastasis (from nasopharynx). *Area 9. Paratracheal:* Thyroid, parathyroid, esophageal diverticulum. *Area 10. Supraclavicular:* Cystic hygroma, lipoma, lymphoma, metastasis, *normal*—fat pad, pneumatocele of upper lobe. *Area 11. Suprasternal:* Thyroid, lipoma, dermoid, thymus, mediastinal mass. From May M. Neck masses in children: diagnosis and treatment. *Clin Pediatr* 1976;5:17. Reprinted by permission.

Hemangiomas, which include capillary hemangiomas, strawberry hemangiomas, and capillary-cavernous hemangiomas, are common head and neck lesions identified in infancy and are usually noticed within the first year of life. They are three times more common in female child than in male child. Hemangiomas are soft, mobile, nontender, and bluish or reddish with increased warmth. After compressing the mass, they may refill. A thrill or bruit may be present. They tend to grow larger in the first year of life and then involute over the next several years. Rare complications include thrombocytopenia from platelet consumption, disseminated intravascular coagulation, hemorrhage, airway obstruction, congestive heart failure, ulceration, infection, and necrosis. If located in the beard distribution, these may be associated with glottic and subglottic hemangiomas, increasing the risk for airway compromise. Treatment for most hemangiomas is conservative and nonoperative because the issues are almost solely cosmetic and short term. Other treatments (corticosteroids, laser treatment, resection) are reserved for rapidly growing lesions that are impairing vision and hearing, or which are life threatening.

Neonatal torticollis, also known as *fibromatosis colli*, results from sternocleidomastoid fibrosis and shortening of the muscle. Presenting symptoms of torticollis occur in the first 3 weeks of life, with the infant holding his/her face and chin away from the affected side and the head tilted toward the fibrous mass. The mass is firm and seems attached to the muscle. Physical therapy, including massage, range-of-motion exercises, stretching exercises, and positional changes, is the preferred treatment. Facial and cranial asymmetry can develop without intervention. Surgical intervention is rarely needed.

Inflammatory Masses

Cervical lymphadenopathy is the most common reason for neck masses in children. Up to 90% of children between the ages of 4 and 8 years can have cervical adenopathy without obvious associated infection or systemic illness. Lymphadenopathy in newborns and young infants is rare and warrants investigation. Anterior cervical nodes drain the oropharynx and become enlarged with upper respiratory, oral, and pharyngeal infections. Posterior cervical lymph nodes drain the scalp and nasopharynx and become enlarged with inflammation or infection in these areas. Supraclavicular lymphadenopathy is considered pathologic and should be biopsied. Etiology for cervical adenopathy includes bacterial or viral infection [including rhinovirus, parainfluenza virus, respiratory syncytial virus, cytomegalovirus, and Epstein-Barr virus (EBV)] from local, regional, or systemic illness. With treatment of the underlying infection, cervical lymphadenopathy should resolve.

Cervical lymphadenitis occurs when acute infection is present within the lymph node (see Chapter 93). Bacteria are the most common causes and include methicillin-resistant *Staphylococcus aureus* and group A β-hemolytic streptococci, although those caused by *Haemophilus influenzae*, anaerobic bacteria, and virus have also been noted. Common presentation is usually one or more cervical lymph nodes that become acutely enlarged, tender, warm, and erythematous after an upper respiratory illness, pharyngitis, tonsillitis, or otitis media. Systemic symptoms of fever and malaise may be present. Treatment includes antibiotics and warm compresses. If the patient appears toxic, admission and treatment with intravenous (IV) antibiotics are appropriate. Without antibiotic treatment, enlargement with the development of fluctuation and regional cellulitis may progress. Most cases of acute cervical lymphadenitis resolve with oral β-lactamase–resistant antibiotics. If the patient fails to improve on this treatment, further diagnostic investigation is necessary, which may include serology, ultrasound, fine needle aspiration, and incision and drainage. Purulent fluid should be sent for Gram stain and aerobic and anaerobic cultures, with antibiotic management based on results.

Cat-scratch disease is another common cause of lymph node enlargement in children. Typically, regional lymph nodes enlarge 2 to 4 weeks after a cat scratch (usually a kitten). The lymphadenopathy can be cervical if the head or neck has been scratched (33% to 50%). Fever and malaise may have been present initially (30%), and usually, a single node is involved. The area around the lymph node is warm, tender, indurated, and erythematous. *Bartonella henselae* is the organism most likely responsible. Indirect immunofluorescent antibody assay for detection of serum antibodies to antigens of *Bartonella* organisms is useful in diagnosis. The indirect immunofluorescent antibody test is available in commercial laboratories, state public health department laboratories, and the Centers for Disease Control and Prevention. Polymerase chain reaction assays are available in some commercial and research laboratories. Warthin-Starry silver stain of the lymph node or inoculation site will identify the organism but is not specific. Management is symptomatic with resolution in 2 to 4 months. Needle aspiration provides relief to those with tender, suppurative nodes and aids in diagnosis. Surgical excision is unnecessary and can lead to formation of a draining sinus. Antibiotics should be considered for acutely ill patients with systemic symptoms (hepatic or splenic involvement, endocarditis), the immunocompromised patient and patients with painful adenitis. Oral azithromycin, erythromycin, rifampin, trimethoprim-sulfamethoxazole, and ciprofloxacin have been shown to be effective. Parenteral gentamicin is also effective and is suggested for those patients with endocarditis.

Mycobacterial infection of the cervical lymph nodes is most often caused by the atypical strains of *Mycobacterium avium-intracellulare* and *M. scrofulaceum.* The enlarged lymph nodes are generally submandibular in location and red, rubbery, and minimally tender to palpation. If systemic manifestations are present, an immune deficiency should be considered. In contrast, clinical systemic signs of tuberculosis accompany cervical lymphadenopathy caused by *M. tuberculosis.* The supraclavicular lymph nodes are commonly involved. Children with suspected mycobacterium infection should have a purified protein derivative tuberculin skin test and chest radiograph performed. The purified protein derivative tuberculin test may be negative in atypical mycobacterium infections. An excisional biopsy may need to be performed to differentiate between tuberculous and nontuberculous mycobacteria as the offending organism. Treatment for atypical mycobacterial cervical lymphadenitis is complete surgical excision. Treatment with clarithromycin with ethambutol or rifampin may be indicated in children with recurrent disease or incomplete excision. Incision and drainage result in a draining sinus. Treatment for *M. tuberculosis* lymphadenitis is the same as for pulmonary tuberculosis–6 to 9 months of antituberculosis chemotherapy.

Cervical lymphadenitis can be the result of viral infections (rhinovirus, parainfluenza virus, respiratory syncytial virus, cytomegalovirus, and EBV), most commonly mononucleosis. Classically, the patient has diffuse lymphadenopathy with prominent posterior cervical lymphadenopathy and large, hypertrophied tonsils. *EBV* is the most common cause of mononucleosis. Systemic symptoms of fever, headache, malaise, and the presence of hepatosplenomegaly are common. Exudative pharyngitis may be present, and the throat should be cultured for group A β-hemolytic streptococci. If bacterial pharyngitis is present, the child should be treated with antibiotics. Generally, treatment for mononucleosis is supportive. Corticosteroids (prednisolone/prednisone at 1 mg per kg per day) have been found useful in reducing tonsillar inflammation in patients with airway compromise.

Kawasaki disease (mucocutaneous lymph node syndrome; see Chapter 101) is associated with a single enlarged cervical lymph node (>1.5 cm diameter), nonexudative conjunctival injection, erythematous mouth, cracked lips, strawberry tongue, erythematous rash, induration of the palms of hands and soles of the feet, and fever of at least 3 days' duration. Cervical lymphadenopathy is the least common of the presenting signs, however. The peak incidence is 18 to 24 months, with the vast majority of the cases occurring in children younger than 4 years. The cause is unknown but is believed to be infectious. Kawasaki disease is associated with long-term complications, such as coronary artery aneurysm; thus, immunosuppressive therapy should be started if it is suspected. An echocardiogram should be performed to rule out coronary artery aneurysms.

Retropharyngeal abscess is a potentially serious deep neck infection that can present with neck mass, fever, dysphagia, sore throat, and pain with extension and/or flexion of the neck. Retropharyngeal abscesses are a result of infections of the nasopharynx, paranasal sinuses, or middle ear, and the paramedian lymph nodes that drain those areas. Most cases of retropharyngeal abscesses occur in children younger than 6 years. The usual pathogens are group A streptococcus, anaerobes, or *S. aureus.* Airway radiographs may show an enlarged retropharyngeal space. Proper positioning is paramount to avoid false-positive radiographs seen with wider prevertebral soft tissue in nonextension films. CT scan of the neck is more accurate in determining the presence of retropharyngeal abscess. Treatment includes monitoring for signs of airway compromise and IV antibiotic treatment using clindamycin, ampicillin/sulbactam, or cefazolin. Most children will need drainage, but IV antibiotics and observation may be sufficient for those determined to have retropharyngeal cellulitis.

Lemierre's syndrome is an infection of the parapharyngeal space with septic thrombophlebitis of the internal jugular vein, leading to septic embolization to the lungs and/or central nervous system. It is seen as a complication of inadequately treated tonsillitis but can also be seen with neck abscesses. It is generally seen in adolescents and adults. Sore throat, fever, fullness to one side of the neck, neck pain, trismus, dysphagia, dyspnea, and toxic appearance can be the presenting clinical signs and symptoms. The predominant pathogen is a gram-negative bacillus *Fusobacterium necrophorum.* Treatment consists of either penicillin in combination with a β-lactamase inhibitor or a β-lactamase–resistant antibiotic in combination with a drug that is highly effective against anaerobes (clindamycin or metronidazole) for at least 6 weeks. Anticoagulation is still controversial.

Neoplasms

Fortunately, neoplasms of the head and neck in children are less commonly seen than infection or congenital lesions. It is estimated that 80% to 90% of neck masses in children are benign. Presentation is usually a painless, firm, fixed cervical mass. Systemic symptoms may not be present. Differentiating between a benign and malignant lesion can be difficult. Findings that would prompt further workup to rule out malignancy include supraclavicular lymphadenopathy, a node larger than 2 cm in diameter, enlargement of a node for more than 2 weeks, no decrease in size of a lymph node after 4 to 6 weeks, lack of inflammation, firm or rubbery consistency, ulceration, failure to respond to antibiotics, and systemic symptoms. Neoplastic etiologies for neck mass in children include

Hodgkin's and non-Hodgkin's lymphoma, rhabdomyosarcoma, neuroblastoma, thyroid carcinoma, nasopharyngeal carcinoma, and teratomas. As described in the section on evaluation, duration and characteristics of the neck mass will lead to increased likelihood of cancer. If a malignancy is suspected, a complete blood cell count, chest radiograph, and selective CT or magnetic resonance imaging should be obtained. Treatment is individualized according to specific tumor and extent of disease (see Chapter 97).

LABORATORY TESTING

The clinical impression should be used to ascertain the need for laboratory studies or radiologic imaging. Many of the common conditions are inflammatory or acute infections, and no studies need to be performed. Oxygenation may be determined by pulse oximetry. In processes for which the risk of critical airway obstruction is impending, the utility of the arterial blood gas adds little initially, and the stress may lead to worsening of the obstruction. A complete white blood cell count and differential are most helpful when an oncologic cause or mononucleosis is suspected. When bleeding from trivial trauma is being considered as a cause of neck mass, the platelet count, prothrombin time, and partial thromboplastin time should be obtained. Consider also a bleeding time when a coagulopathy is in the differential. Serum thyroid hormone and thyroid-stimulating hormone levels may be warranted for suspected thyroid masses. Throat culture for streptococcal disease (or a rapid strep screen) should be obtained when pharyngitis is found. A heterophile antibody assay or, especially in the younger child, EBV-specific serologic tests should be performed to confirm infectious mononucleosis.

Cervical spine radiographs need to be obtained for trauma patients when instability or fracture of the cervical spine is suspected. For most patients with a neck mass and concern for deeper-tissue involvement, the imaging study of choice will be CT. Facial or mandibular films may be necessary to evaluate for some lower-face trauma or oral infections. Soft-tissue lateral neck films may be helpful to evaluate for intraoral, retropharyngeal, or airway infectious problems. In the child with respiratory distress, a chest radiograph is necessary to view the mediastinum, pleura, and lung for infection, tumor, pneumothorax, or pneumomediastinum. Ultrasound may be useful in defining the mass; a cystic mass with linear septations is characteristic of a cystic hygroma. Other masses (lymphadenopathy, thyroglossal duct) and fibromatosis colli (congenital torticollis) have fairly definitive patterns. Ultrasound may also help identify adenitis with abscess formation requiring drainage. Although not specific, the finding of calcification within a mass may suggest a teratoma or neuroblastoma.

In studies in which biopsies of neck masses were obtained, several authors have found preoperative diagnoses to be correct as infrequently as 60% of the time. Biopsy of the lesion is required when the suspicion is high for malignancy. As in adults, fine needle aspiration in children is becoming more popular at some centers because it offers high sensitivity and specificity for tumors. This may reduce the need for open biopsies as often as 75% of the time by identifying inflammatory or self-limiting processes.

THERAPY

In the ED, the clinical evaluation most often reveals adenopathy that requires no acute therapy or adenitis that necessitates a course of systemic oral antibiotics and local care. Important to the approach to adenitis is the follow-up in several days to monitor clinical response and need for aspiration and drainage. When the mass is suspicious for tumor or congenital cyst, surgical consultation for biopsy or excision is indicated. Hospitalization and institution of definitive therapy are indicated for the patients with neck masses who present with systemic toxicity, airway compromise, or severe local disease.

Suggested Readings

Aciero SP, Waldhausen JHT. Congenital cervical cysts, sinuses and fistulas. *Otolaryngol Clin North Am* 2007;40:161–176.

Ajulo P, Qayyum A, Brewis C, et al. Lemierre's syndrome: the link between a simple sore throat, sore neck and pleuritic chest pain. *Ann R Coll Surg Engl* 2005;87:303–305.

Al-Dajani N, Wootton SH. Cervical lymphadenitis, suppurative parotitis, thyroiditis, and infected cysts. *Infect Dis Clin North Am* 2007;21(2):523–541.

Anne S, Teot LA, Mandell DL. Fine needle aspiration biopsy: role in diagnosis of pediatric head and neck masses. *Int J Pediatr Otorhinolaryngol* 2008;72:1547–1553.

Brown RL, Azizkhan RG. Pediatric head and neck lesions. *Pediatr Clin North Am* 1998;45:889–905.

Craig FW, Shunk JE. Retropharyngeal abscess in children: clinical perspective, utility of imaging, and current management. *Pediatrics* 2003;111:1394–1398.

Dulin MF, Kennard TP, Leach L, et al. Management of cervical lymphadenitis in children. *Am Fam Physician* 2008;78(9):1097–1098.

Green M. The neck and lymphadenopathy. In: *Pediatric diagnosis*, 6th ed. Philadelphia, PA: Elsevier, 1998;61–65:398–403.

Long SS, Pickering LK, Prober CG. *Principles and practice of pediatric infectious diseases*, 2nd ed. New York, NY: Churchill Livingstone, 2003.

Malik A, Odita J, Rodriguez J, Hardjasudarma M. Pediatric neck masses: a pictorial review for practicing radiologists. *Curr Probl Diagn Radiol* 2002;31:146–157.

Tracy TF, Muratore CS. Management of common head and neck masses. *Semin Pediatr Surg* 2006;16:3–13.

Turkington JRA, Paterson A, Sweeney LE, et al. Neck masses in children. *Brit J Radiol* 2005;78:75–85.

Vieira F, Allen SM, Stocks RM, et al. Deep neck infection. *Otolaryngol Clin North Am* 2008;41:459–483.

CHAPTER 45 ■ NECK STIFFNESS

LEAH TZIMENATOS, MD, CHERYL VANCE, MD, AND NATHAN KUPPERMANN, MD, MPH

Neck stiffness is an important chief complaint in children evaluated in the emergency department. Commonly, neck stiffness is accompanied by neck pain. Certain clinical conditions, however, may lead a child to hold the neck in an abnormal posture without neck pain. The underlying causes of neck stiffness or malposition in children range from relatively benign (e.g., muscle strain, cervical adenitis) to life threatening (e.g., meningitis, fracture, or subluxation of the cervical spine).

Torticollis (meaning "twisted neck" from the Latin roots *tortus* and *collum*) is a subset of neck stiffness. With torticollis, the child holds the head tilted to one side and the chin rotated in the opposite direction, reflecting unilateral neck muscle contraction. This may result from various pathologic processes and may or may not be associated with neck pain. Torticollis is often congenital and muscular in origin; however, it can also be associated with acquired processes such as trauma, infectious or inflammatory illnesses, central nervous system neoplasms, drug reactions, and a variety of different syndromes.

This chapter reviews the differential diagnosis of neck stiffness including torticollis, both with and without neck pain, in children. The proposed algorithm at the end of the chapter helps distinguish potentially life-threatening causes from benign causes of neck stiffness, while providing a broad differential diagnosis for this important clinical finding.

DIFFERENTIAL DIAGNOSIS

Most patients presenting with neck stiffness are well appearing with benign, frequently self-limited conditions; however, the differential diagnosis of neck stiffness is broad and includes many potentially life-threatening causes. These various diagnoses must be considered and, when appropriate, excluded depending on the patient's clinical presentation and history. A history of trauma, signs or symptoms of an infectious or inflammatory process, or any evidence of spinal cord involvement may be helpful in identifying a number of specific diagnoses.

Table 45.1 lists most causes of neck stiffness in children, Table 45.2 lists the common causes, and Table 45.3 lists the life-threatening causes. The following descriptions categorize the causes of neck stiffness in children by underlying mechanism and severity.

Neck Stiffness Associated with Trauma

Potentially Life-threatening Causes

Trauma to the neck is a common cause of neck pain and stiffness in children (see Chapter 115). Fortunately, serious injuries

to the cervical spine (fractures, subluxations, and spinal cord injuries) are uncommon, especially in children younger than 8 years. Because of a higher fulcrum of the cervical spine and relative weakness of the neck muscles compared to adults, these injuries generally occur in the upper cervical spine in younger children, as opposed to the lower cervical spine in adolescents and adults. Neck injuries in children most commonly result from high kinetic energy mechanisms, such as motor vehicle-related collisions, sports injuries, and falls.

Fractures of the Cervical Spine. Fractures of the cervical spine in children are very uncommon, occurring in 1% to 3% of hospitalized pediatric trauma patients. Although some children with fractures of the cervical spine are unresponsive at the time of evaluation, most are alert and verbal, limit their neck movement secondary to pain, and have no demonstrable neurological deficit. At the minimum, the cervical spine should be immobilized and multiple-view radiographs of the cervical spine should be obtained on any child with an altered level of consciousness, pain or stiffness of the neck, any neurological deficits, or distracting painful injuries after blunt trauma. Radiographs should also be obtained in those who are unable to perceive pain (as a result of alcohol or drugs) or describe their symptoms. A large prospective study of blunt trauma victims identified five criteria (posterior midline cervical tenderness, altered alertness, distracting injury, intoxication, and focal neurological signs) that correctly identified all children with cervical spine injuries; however, there were few children younger than 9 years and none younger than 2 years with cervical spine injury in this study. A multicenter attempt to retrospectively validate this decision rule among a different cohort of children (including those younger than 2 years) demonstrated a lower sensitivity, suggesting the need for refinement of these criteria before use in pediatric patients.

Subluxation of the Cervical Spine. Traumatic subluxations of the cervical spine are more common than fractures and may occasionally result from minor trauma (e.g., falls from low heights) but more commonly result from more severe trauma (see Chapter 115). The most commonly occurring of these is rotary (or "rotatory") atlantoaxial subluxation, which generally does not compromise the spinal canal because the transverse ligament of the atlas remains intact. Rotary subluxation typically causes neck pain and torticollis. Sternocleidomastoid (SCM) spasm and neck tenderness are localized to the same side as the head rotation (as the SCM attempts to "reduce" the deformity) in contrast to muscular (inflammatory and congenital) torticollis, in which the spastic, tender SCM muscle is opposite to the direction of head rotation. In addition, in rotary subluxation, there is palpable deviation of the spinous

TABLE 45.1

CAUSES OF NECK STIFFNESS OR MALPOSITION

Trauma
Fracture of the cervical spine
Subluxation of the cervical spine
Epidural hematoma of the cervical spine
Subarachnoid hemorrhage
Muscular contusions/spasm of the neck
Clavicular fracture

Infectious/inflammatory conditions
Bacterial meningitis
Retropharyngeal abscess
Infections of the spine (osteomyelitis, tuberculosis, epidural
   abscesses, discitis)
Minor irritation, malposition, and muscle spasm
Rotary atlantoaxial subluxation as a result of local
   inflammation and/or otolaryngologic procedures
   (Grisel's syndrome)
Primary or reactive cervical lymphadenitis/lymphadenopathy
Intervertebral disc calcification
Collagen vascular diseases (juvenile rheumatoid arthritis,
   ankylosing spondylitis, psoriatic arthritis, and other
   spondyloarthropathies)
Upper lobe pneumonia
Acute suppurative thyroiditis
Otitis media and mastoiditis
Viral myositis
Pharyngotonsillitis
Upper respiratory tract infection

Tumors, vascular lesions of the central nervous system, and
   other space-occupying lesions
Brain tumor
Spinal cord tumor
Subarachnoid hemorrhage (aneurysm rupture)
Other tumors of the head and neck (rhabdomyosarcoma,
   Ewing's sarcoma, lymphoma, nasopharyngeal carcinoma,
   orbital tumor, acoustic neuroma, osteoblastoma, and
   metastatic tumors)
Other space-occupying lesions of the head and neck
   (Arnold-Chiari malformation)
Other space-occupying lesions of the spinal cord (neurenteric
   cyst, arteriovenous malformation, syringomyelia)

Congenital conditions
Congenital muscular torticollis
Skeletal malformations (Klippel-Feil syndrome, Sprengel's
   deformity, hemiatlas, basilar impression, occipitocervical
   synostosis)
Atlantoaxial instability secondary to congenital conditions
   (Down syndrome, Marfan syndrome, Klippel-Feil syn-
   drome, os odontoideum, Morquio syndrome)

Miscellaneous
Ophthalmologic, neurological, and/or vestibular causes
   (strabismus, cranial nerve palsies, extraocular muscle
   palsies, refractive errors, migraine headache, myasthenia
   gravis, Guillain-Barré syndrome, pseudotumor cerebri)
Benign paroxysmal torticollis of infancy
Sandifer syndrome
Spontaneous pneumomediastinum
Spasmus nutans
Dystonic reaction
Psychogenic

TABLE 45.2

COMMON CAUSES OF NECK STIFFNESS OR MALPOSITION

Trauma
Minor trauma (cervical muscular contusions, strains,
   and spasm)
Clavicular fracture
Traumatic rotary atlantoaxial subluxation

Infectious/inflammatory conditions
Minor irritation, malposition, and muscle spasm
Cervical lymphadenitis
Pharyngotonsillitis and other upper respiratory tract
   infections
Viral myositis/myalgias
Bacterial meningitis
Infectious rotary atlantoaxial subluxation (Grisel's syndrome)

Congenital conditions
Congenital muscular torticollis

Miscellaneous
Dystonic reaction

process of C2 in the same direction as the head rotation. In
contrast, during normal neck rotation beyond 20 degrees, the
spinous process of C2 deviates to the contralateral side. With
rotary atlantoaxial subluxation, an anteroposterior open-
mouth radiograph typically shows the rotation of C1 on C2,
with the odontoid in an eccentric position relative to C1.
However, definitive diagnosis is made by dynamic computed
tomography (CT) scans of the neck showing a fixed rotation
between C1 and C2 that fails to resolve with attempts to

TABLE 45.3

LIFE-THREATENING CAUSES OF NECK STIFFNESS OR MALPOSITION

Trauma
Injuries to the cervical spine (fracture, subluxation,
   epidural hematoma)
Subarachnoid hemorrhage

Infection
Bacterial meningitis
Retropharyngeal abscess
Infections of the spine (osteomyelitis, epidural abscesses,
   discitis)
Atlantoaxial subluxation with anterior displacement of the
   atlas as a result of local inflammation

Tumors, vascular lesions of the central nervous system, and
   other space-occupying lesions
Brain tumor
Spinal cord tumor
Subarachnoid hemorrhage (aneurysm rupture)
Other tumors and space-occupying lesions of the head, neck,
   and spinal cord

Congenital conditions
Atlantoaxial instability secondary to congenital conditions

correct the torticollis. Neurological deficits are rare in patients with traumatic rotary subluxation. Most patients can be treated with a cervical collar and antiinflammatory medications. Traction and immobilization, and rarely surgery, are necessary for more severe and/or long-standing rotary subluxation or if reduction is not achieved by conservative measures. Early diagnosis and treatment are important.

Atlantoaxial subluxation with compromise of the spinal canal results when there is ligamentous laxity or rupture with resultant anterior movement of the atlas on the axis. Children with underlying conditions including Down syndrome and Marfan syndrome are more susceptible to this due to laxity of the transverse ligament of the atlas. Radiographic findings may include a widened predental space and prevertebral soft-tissue swelling. Treatment involves immobilization and cervical traction.

Epidural Hematomas of the Cervical Spine. Epidural hematomas of the cervical spine are uncommon but may occur even after apparently minor trauma. These may compress the spinal cord, leading to progressive neurological symptoms and signs as well as neck stiffness or pain. Magnetic resonance imaging (MRI) of the spinal cord clearly demonstrates this injury. Emergent neurosurgical consultation and surgical decompression are indicated.

Subarachnoid Hemorrhage. Subarachnoid hemorrhage after trauma may lead to neck stiffness but is accompanied by headache and/or other physical findings of head trauma. Rarely, subarachnoid hemorrhage may be due to nontraumatic causes such as aneurysm rupture.

Generally Non–life-threatening Causes

Traumatic Muscular Contusions of the Neck. Blunt trauma to the neck may result in neck pain as a result of muscular contusion and/or spasm. This is a diagnosis of exclusion, however, and should not be entertained until a detailed physical (including neurological) examination and radiographs of the cervical spine exclude the possibility of a more serious injury. Treatment includes a soft cervical collar and analgesic medication.

Clavicular Fracture. Fracture of the clavicle in children is common and may cause torticollis because of SCM muscle spasm. However, the diagnosis of clavicle fracture is usually clear because pain, tenderness, and swelling are noted over the fracture site. The acute symptoms associated with clavicle fractures may, on occasion, however, mask an associated rotary atlantoaxial subluxation. Clinicians caring for children should be aware of this association.

Neck Stiffness Associated with Infectious/Inflammatory Conditions

Potentially Life-threatening Causes

Bacterial Meningitis. Bacterial meningitis has become a rare childhood disease in the United States; however, it is still the most important infectious cause of neck stiffness. In the post–HiB and PCV7 vaccine era, the most common bacterial pathogens causing meningitis after infancy are *Streptococcus pneumoniae* (including non-vaccine type strains) and *Neisseria meningitidis*. Children with meningitis typically have findings of neck stiffness on physical examination, although this may not be apparent in young infants and in those children who lack an inflammatory response (i.e., meningococcal meningitis). In a study of 326 children presenting to an emergency department in the Netherlands between 1988 and 1998 with signs of fever and meningeal irritation, 30% had bacterial meningitis and 13% had viral or aseptic meningitis. Torticollis has also been reported in patients with bacterial meningitis, although far less commonly than meningismus.

Retropharyngeal Abscess. There are several other important infectious processes for which neck stiffness and fever usually are the presenting signs. Retropharyngeal abscess is an infection that occupies the potential space between the posterior pharyngeal wall and the anterior border of the cervical vertebrae. Most commonly caused by group A streptococcus, oral anaerobic organisms (*Bacteroides*), and *Staphylococcus aureus*, these infections cause clinical toxicity, drooling, and stridor. Neck pain and/or stiffness are presenting clinical findings in approximately two-thirds of children with these infections. Limitation of neck extension and torticollis are particularly common. Lateral radiographs of the neck can be helpful in making the diagnosis and will reveal soft-tissue swelling anterior to the upper cervical vertebral bodies. These films are often limited, however, due to inadequate neck extension or failure to obtain the image during inspiration. CT imaging with intravenous contrast is currently the imaging modality of choice.

Infections of the Spine. Infectious processes involving the spine (osteomyelitis, epidural abscess, discitis) in children can involve the cervical region, although they occur most commonly in the thoracic and lumbar areas. Localized pain, fever, and elevation of inflammatory markers including erythrocyte sedimentation rate (ESR) and C-reactive protein generally accompany these infections.

Vertebral osteomyelitis occurring in the cervical spine may lead to neck stiffness. Vertebral osteomyelitis is usually bacterial in origin (most commonly caused by *S. aureus*) but may be caused by mycobacteria (tuberculous or nontuberculous) as well. If the cervical spine is involved, radiographs of this area may reveal destruction of the vertebral body, local soft-tissue swelling, or narrowing of the disc space. Technetium bone scanning or MRI will frequently reveal abnormalities of the spine before bony destruction is visible on plain radiography.

Although uncommon, spinal epidural abscesses are associated with significant morbidity and mortality. Epidural abscesses may occur in the cervical spine, although lower spine involvement is much more common. When these abscesses occur in the cervical region, severe neurological deficits may occur, and emergent neurosurgical referral is essential.

Discitis is uncommon in children and usually affects the thoracic or lumbar spine; however, cases of cervical discitis have been reported. This disease is generally seen in children younger than 3 years and is often caused by infection with *S. aureus*, although bacterial cultures are commonly negative, and the cause has been debated. When evaluating for this condition, technetium bone scanning or MRI may be necessary if conventional radiography is nondiagnostic.

Generally Non–life-threatening Causes

Torticollis Due to Minor Irritation, Malposition, and Muscle Spasm. Most well-appearing children with sudden onset of mild torticollis without a history of trauma, fever, or neurological abnormalities do not have serious underlying pathology as a cause of their symptoms. Commonly, the patient awakens with mild neck pain, stiffness, and malposition. On evaluation, there is no history of trauma, fever, preceding illness, pharyngotonsillitis or any additional physical examination abnormality. The examination reveals a well-appearing child with mild torticollis, whose limitation of motion is primarily when he or she attempts correction of the malposition. Such muscular torticollis may be due to SCM spasm from awkward sleeping position or other mild irritation. In cases with this type of benign presentation, history, and examination, nothing more than careful clinical assessment, analgesic/antiinflammatory medication, consideration of soft cervical collar, and close follow-up may be necessary.

Atlantoaxial Subluxation as a Result of Local Inflammation and/or Otolaryngologic Procedures (Grisel's Syndrome). Rotary atlantoaxial subluxation rarely may occur as a result of inflammatory processes in the head and neck region (e.g., rheumatoid arthritis, systemic lupus erythematosus, tonsillitis, pharyngitis, otitis media, retropharyngeal abscess) or after otolaryngologic procedures (e.g., tonsillectomy, adenoidectomy). This condition, also called *Grisel's syndrome*, is believed to occur as a result of ligamentous laxity after an infectious or inflammatory process. The subluxation may or may not be associated with displacement of the atlas, depending on the degree of involvement of the transverse ligament of the atlas. Most children with Grisel's syndrome have torticollis and neck pain, often localized to the ipsilateral SCM muscle. Fever and dysphagia are also common. The child's head is tilted to one side and rotated to the side opposite of the facet dislocation. As with rotary atlantoaxial subluxation from traumatic causes, radiographs may demonstrate abnormality, but dynamic CT scan is diagnostic (see previous discussion). In the uncommon likelihood of severe disease (and certainly in the rare likelihood of spinal cord compression), neurosurgical consultation should be obtained because cervical traction and immobilization are needed. Most commonly, the condition is mild and there is no anterior displacement of the axis. If mild, the condition usually responds to analgesic medication, physical therapy, and a soft cervical collar. In addition to treating the subluxation, antibiotics to treat an underlying bacterial infection, if present, are needed.

Cervical Lymphadenitis. Cervical lymphadenitis, either acute or chronic, is a common cause of neck pain and stiffness. The child with this condition typically has tender swelling over the lateral aspect of the neck, with or without fever. Most cases of cervical lymphadenitis are caused by *S. aureus* or group A streptococcus; however, other bacteria, mycobacteria, and other infectious conditions may be involved (including *Bartonella henselae*, the cause of cat-scratch disease). A purified protein derivative skin test to screen for tuberculosis if any risk factors are present and empirical antibiotics to treat the most common bacterial pathogens are usually sufficient therapy. Cervical adenitis may also occur in response to an infection in a juxtaposing site (i.e., site of lymphatic drainage to the cervical nodes), such as the scalp.

Intervertebral Disc Calcification. Intervertebral disc calcification (IDC) in children is an uncommon, generally self-limited condition in which the nucleus pulposus of one or more intervertebral discs calcifies. Both the underlying cause of the condition and the cause of acute symptoms are unknown. Children typically present with 24 to 48 hours of neck pain associated with neck stiffness or torticollis; fever is often present as well. The ESR is usually elevated in IDC, and leukocytosis occurs in one-third of patients. Radiographs of the spine usually show the disc calcification, and CT scans help localize the calcification within the nucleus pulposus. The calcification resorbs spontaneously, and the disease is generally benign and self-limited, although disc protrusion and cord compression may uncommonly occur. However, one must distinguish infections of the spine and meningitis (see previous discussions) from IDC.

Collagen Vascular Disease. Collagen vascular disease (see Chapter 101) in children may involve the cervical spine and lead to neck stiffness and/or pain. Children with juvenile rheumatoid arthritis may have either insidious or acute onset of symptoms, which commonly include neck stiffness. Although isolated cervical disease is unusual, neck stiffness or torticollis may be the presenting sign of juvenile rheumatoid arthritis. Cervical involvement in ankylosing spondylitis is a late finding as it is in other spondyloarthropathies. Girls with psoriatic arthritis, however, may have cervical involvement preceding sacroiliac and lumbar involvement.

Other Infectious/Inflammatory Conditions. Pharyngotonsillitis, upper respiratory tract infections, otitis media, and mastoiditis may be associated with neck pain. Torticollis may occasionally be seen as these conditions may be accompanied by Grisel's syndrome as well. It is important to remember that if the neck pain is posterior in location and accompanied by fever, a lumbar puncture should be strongly considered to exclude the possibility of meningitis. Similarly, the diagnosis of viral myositis involving the neck can be made only after excluding the possibility of meningitis in a child with neck pain and fever. Upper lobe pneumonia may cause pain referred to the neck with or without associated stiffness. Although rare, acute suppurative thyroiditis is another infectious cause of neck pain and stiffness and is associated with fever and a palpable neck mass (i.e., swelling of the thyroid).

Neck Stiffness Associated with Tumors, Vascular Lesions of the Central Nervous System or Other Space-occupying Lesions

Potentially Life-threatening Causes

Space-occupying lesions of the brain and spinal cord may lead to neck stiffness, malposition, and/or pain. Even if the histology of these lesions is benign, they are potentially life threatening because of the complications of intracranial pressure elevation and the potential for brain and spinal cord compression. Ruptured aneurysms may cause subarachnoid hemorrhage with associated neck stiffness.

Brain Tumors. Children with tumors of the posterior fossa, the most common location for pediatric brain tumors, may present with head tilt, neck stiffness, or torticollis. Posterior fossa tumors may cause any of a number of other symptoms and signs (e.g., vomiting, headache, ataxia, disturbances in vision including diplopia, papilledema, cranial nerve deficits, corticospinal or corticobulbar signs). Head tilt may result from attempts to compensate for diplopia. However, neck stiffness is believed to result from irritation of the accessory nerve by the cerebellar tonsils trapped in the occipital foramen or by tonsillar herniation.

Spinal Cord Tumors. Tumors of the spinal cord are uncommon in children and account for a small fraction of all central nervous system tumors in childhood. The most common spinal cord tumor is an astrocytoma. Typically, spinal cord tumors cause pain at the site of the tumor and neurological defects (sensory and motor defects, impaired bowel and bladder function), but symptoms may be very slow to develop, often leading to delays in diagnosis. Spinal cord tumors may also cause torticollis. Patients with these tumors may also hold their heads in a forward flexed position (hanging head sign). An MRI of the a spine should be obtained on any child with symptoms and signs suggestive of a spinal cord tumor, and emergency neurosurgical consultation should be obtained.

Vascular Anomalies. Congenital berry aneurysms and acquired cerebral aneurysms may rupture spontaneously and result in life-threatening subarachnoid hemorrhage. This can present with abrupt onset of severe headache, meningismus, nausea and vomiting, photophobia, and possibly fever, thus mimicking meningitis.

Other Space-occupying Lesions of the Head and Neck. Head and neck tumors are uncommon in children, and diagnosis requires a high index of suspicion. Presenting signs and symptoms may include neck pain, stiffness, and/or torticollis. Rhabdomyosarcomas, Ewing's sarcomas, and lymphomas account for most of the tumors of the neck but other tumors occurring in this region include nasopharyngeal carcinoma, orbital tumors, acoustic neuromas, osteoblastomas, and metastatic tumors. Arnold-Chiari malformations of the brain may also cause neck pain and stiffness.

Other Space-occupying Lesions of the Spinal Cord. Other uncommon space-occupying lesions of the cervical spine such as neurenteric cysts, arteriovenous malformations, spontaneous spinal epidural hematomas, and syringomyelia may also cause neck pain and stiffness, generally accompanied by neurological findings. Early diagnosis by MRI is essential.

Generally Non–life-threatening Causes

Benign Tumors of the Head and Neck. Osteoid osteoma is a benign bone tumor that typically affects older children and adolescents. Pain is the typical presenting symptom, often worse at night. If the osteoma is in the cervical spine, neck pain and/or stiffness result. Plain radiography is usually diagnostic

(showing a well-demarcated radiolucent lesion surrounded by sclerotic bone). Treatment may be conservative medical management, radiofrequency ablation, or surgical. Eosinophilic granulomas and bone cysts are other benign (and rare) lesions of the spine that may cause neck pain and stiffness.

Congenital Causes of Neck Stiffness

Neck stiffness and/or torticollis from congenital abnormalities are usually not life threatening. These congenital causes are usually muscular or skeletal in origin.

Congenital Muscular Torticollis

Congenital muscular torticollis is the most common cause of torticollis in infancy. The etiology of this condition is unclear but is believed to be related to birth trauma, causing an injury to the SCM muscle with hematoma formation, followed by fibrous contracture of the muscle. Other theories include those suggesting intrauterine malposition, infection, neurogenic causes, and intrauterine compartment syndrome of the SCM muscle. On examination, a palpable mass can often be detected in the inferior aspect of the SCM. The mass is generally not present at birth but appears in the neonatal period. The head is held in the characteristic position, with the patient's chin pointing away from the affected, contracted SCM muscle. Craniofacial asymmetry is commonly found to some degree in these patients, typically with contralateral flattening of the occiput and ipsilateral depression of the malar prominence. Radiographs of the cervical spine may be necessary to exclude other causes of torticollis. Treatment is conservative with active positioning and manual stretching of the involved muscle. If the deformity persists after 6 to 12 months, surgical release of the SCM is required (approximately 5% of cases).

Skeletal Malformations

Klippel-Feil syndrome is characterized by congenital fusion of a variable number of cervical vertebrae, which may result in atlantoaxial instability. The cause of this syndrome is unknown. It is often associated with many other bony abnormalities, and significant scoliosis develops in more than 50% of affected children. Limitation in range of motion of the neck is the most common physical sign. In addition to limited neck motion, the classic triad also includes a low hairline and a short neck; this triad, however, is seen in fewer than half of patients.

Sprengel's deformity is characterized by congenital failure of the scapula to descend to its correct position. The scapula rests in a high position relative to the neck and thorax. In its most severe form, the scapula may be connected by bone to the cervical spine and limit neck movement.

Hemiatlas is a malformation of the first cervical vertebra, which may cause severe, progressive torticollis. In time, the deformity becomes fixed; therefore, posterior fusion is recommended.

Basilar impression is a condition resulting from anomalies at the base of the skull and vertebrae, which lead to a short neck, headache, neck pain, and cranial nerve palsies due to compression of the cranial nerves. Many congenital conditions, including Klippel-Feil syndrome, achondroplasia, and neurofibromatosis, may cause basilar impression. Commonly associated with basilar impression is occipitocervical synostosis, a condition in which fibrous or bony connections between the base of the skull and the atlas cause neck pain, torticollis, high scapula, and several neurological symptoms.

Atlantoaxial Instability

Several congenital conditions may be associated with atlantoaxial instability and may predispose the patient to cervical subluxation. In addition to Down, Marfan, and Klippel-Feil syndromes, these include other skeletal dysplasias and os odontoideum (aplasia or hypoplasia of the odontoid). Children with these conditions should be screened for atlantoaxial instability. Morquio syndrome is a mucopolysaccharidosis resulting in flattening of the vertebrae and multiple skeletal dysplasias. In this syndrome, the odontoid process of the axis is underdeveloped and may lead to atlantoaxial subluxation.

Miscellaneous Causes of Neck Stiffness

Head tilt, neck stiffness, and/or torticollis have been reported in several other conditions, some of which are life threatening and others generally benign.

Ophthalmologic, Neurological, and/or Vestibular Causes

Head tilt or neck malposition may result from abnormalities of vision (strabismus, cranial nerve palsies, extraocular muscle palsies, refractive errors) or the vestibular apparatus. The child attempts to correct for the disturbance through changes in neck position. Careful ophthalmologic and neurological examinations of the child with head tilt are necessary to exclude these possibilities. Torticollis has also been reported in patients with migraine headaches.

Myasthenia Gravis

Patients with myasthenia gravis may develop torticollis, although ptosis, impairment of extraocular muscular movement, and other cranial nerve palsies are generally earlier signs.

Guillain-Barré Syndrome

Neck stiffness has been reported in children with Guillain-Barré syndrome. Neck stiffness in this condition, however, is seen in association with the generalized motor weakness and areflexia.

Pseudotumor Cerebri

Stiff neck and torticollis have also been reported in children with pseudotumor cerebri. In fact, these neck symptoms may be the presenting signs of the condition. Of course, the more usual clinical presentation of pseudotumor is characterized by headache, vomiting, and papilledema. Lumbar puncture and removal of cerebrospinal fluid may quickly resolve the cervical symptoms and signs. This association serves as a reminder to the clinician to inspect the optic discs of children with neck stiffness and/or torticollis.

Benign Paroxysmal Torticollis of Infancy

Benign paroxysmal torticollis of infancy presents as recurrent episodes of head tilt sometimes accompanied by pallor, agitation, and vomiting. Typical onset is between 2 and 8 months of age, and the condition tends to remit by 2 to 3 years. Episodes subside spontaneously within a few hours or days. The etiology is unknown, and there is no effective treatment

Sandifer Syndrome

Sandifer syndrome is the constellation of torticollis, gastroesophageal reflux, and hiatal hernia. Children with this syndrome may have recurrent vomiting and failure to thrive.

Spontaneous Pneumomediastinum

Spontaneous pneumomediastinum may present with neck pain and torticollis. A history of severe coughing and/or retching is usually elicited. Crepitus is generally palpated along the neck.

Spasmus Nutans

Spasmus nutans is an acquired condition of childhood, characterized by nystagmus, head nodding, and torticollis. Children with these findings typically become symptomatic in the first 2 years of life. The condition is generally benign and self-limited. However, some children with the symptoms of spasmus nutans have underlying brain tumors. Therefore, imaging of the brain is necessary to exclude this possibility.

Dystonic Reaction

Certain drugs can cause acute dystonic reactions with torticollis. These include many antipsychotic and antiemetic agents (most commonly haloperidol, prochlorperazine, and metoclopramide), as well as some benzodiazepines, antihistamines, and other agents. Treatment with 1 to 2 mg per kg of diphenhydramine may be diagnostic and therapeutic.

Psychogenic

Hysterical patients may present with torticollis. This diagnosis can be made only after excluding other more serious causes.

EVALUATION AND DECISION

The evaluation of, and treatment plan for, neck stiffness is best organized around several important historical/clinical questions and physical examination findings: (i) Is there evidence of spinal cord involvement? (ii) Is there a history of trauma? (iii) Is there evidence of an infectious or inflammatory process (e.g., history or presence of fever)? (iv) Is a cervical mass present? (v) Are the symptoms acute or chronic?

The approach to the child with a stiff or malpositioned neck should focus initially on whether there is spinal cord involvement, as detailed in Fig. 45.1. The studies included in the figure represent potential diagnostic modalities to be considered for a child with those signs/symptoms; however, these studies are not required. Decisions regarding specific diagnostic modalities will depend on each patient's individual presentation, history, and examination.

For any child with neck stiffness or pain, a history of weakness or paresthesias of the extremities or of functional abnormalities of the bowel or bladder should be sought. In addition,

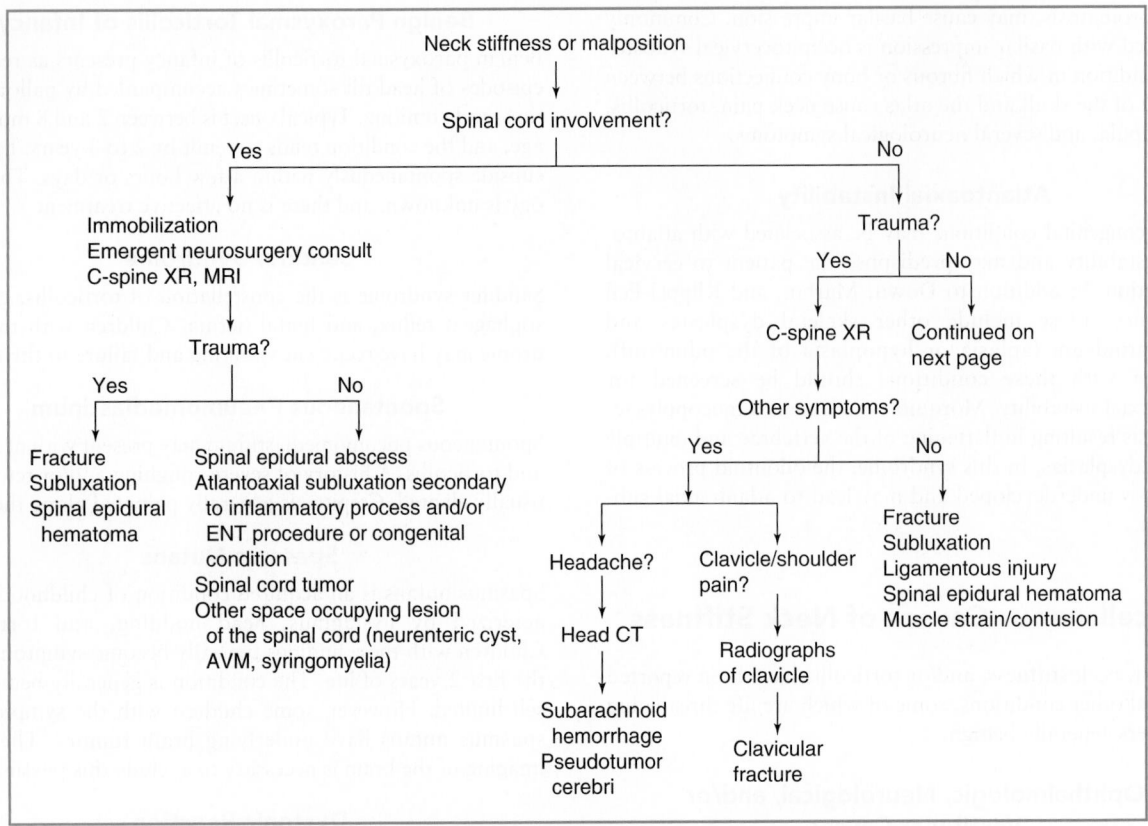

FIGURE 45.1 Approach to the child with stiff or malpositioned neck. Diagnostic studies included in this approach are intended to be *considerations* that may assist with making a diagnosis depending on the specific clinical scenario. C-spine XR, cervical spine radiograph; MRI, magnetic resonance imaging; ENT, ear, nose, and throat; AVM, arteriovenous malformation; CT, computed tomography; CBC, complete blood count; ESR, erythrocyte sedimentation rate; CRP, C-reactive protein; PPD, purified protein derivative; TB, tuberculosis; SCM, sternocleidomastoid; CXR, chest radiograph. (*continued*)

a complete ophthalmologic and neurological examination should be performed, with the latter focusing on spinal cord function. Included in this examination should be an assessment of muscle strength, sensation, deep tendon reflexes, the Babinski reflex, and anal tone. Extra vigilance must be used if the patient is too young or incapacitated to provide an accurate history.

If *spinal cord involvement* is detected, immobilization, neurosurgical consultation, and imaging of the cervical spine (radiographs and MRI of the cervical spine) are necessary. Conditions causing cervical spinal cord compromise may rapidly lead to permanent disability or death if not immediately addressed. If secondary to trauma, one should suspect cervical spine fracture, subluxation, or spinal epidural hematoma. In the setting of fever, a spinal epidural abscess should be considered. Atlantoaxial subluxation with instability secondary to otolaryngologic diseases or procedures should be considered in children with spinal cord involvement and consistent histories. Finally, spinal cord tumors and other space-occupying lesions should be considered if the development of symptoms is gradual and not associated with trauma or fever.

The next issue to be considered is whether the neck stiffness is the result of an *acute traumatic event*. If acute trauma is the

cause of the neck stiffness, the cervical spine should be properly immobilized (see Chapter 115) and multiple radiographic views of the cervical spine obtained. Fractures and subluxations/dislocations will generally be identified on plain radiography of the cervical spine. Other modalities (e.g., flexion-extension views, CT, MRI) may be useful to detect ligamentous injury, rotary subluxation, or spinal epidural hematomas. Cervical muscle strain and/or contusion are diagnoses of exclusion in the setting of trauma, and neck stiffness after the possibility of more serious conditions is excluded. If other symptoms in addition to the neck stiffness are present, appropriate studies should be obtained. For example, the patient with neck stiffness and headache may have a subarachnoid hemorrhage for which a head CT scan would be indicated. The patient with clavicle fracture may have spasm of the SCM muscle and torticollis. However, tenderness is noted over the injured clavicle, and radiographs will confirm the diagnosis. On occasion, rotary atlantoaxial subluxation may be associated with clavicle fracture.

Fever in the setting of neck stiffness suggests the presence of an infectious, inflammatory, or neoplastic process. The presence of meningitis must be excluded either clinically or with a lumbar puncture (see Chapter 92). On examination, the finding of meningismus should be sought. A lumbar puncture

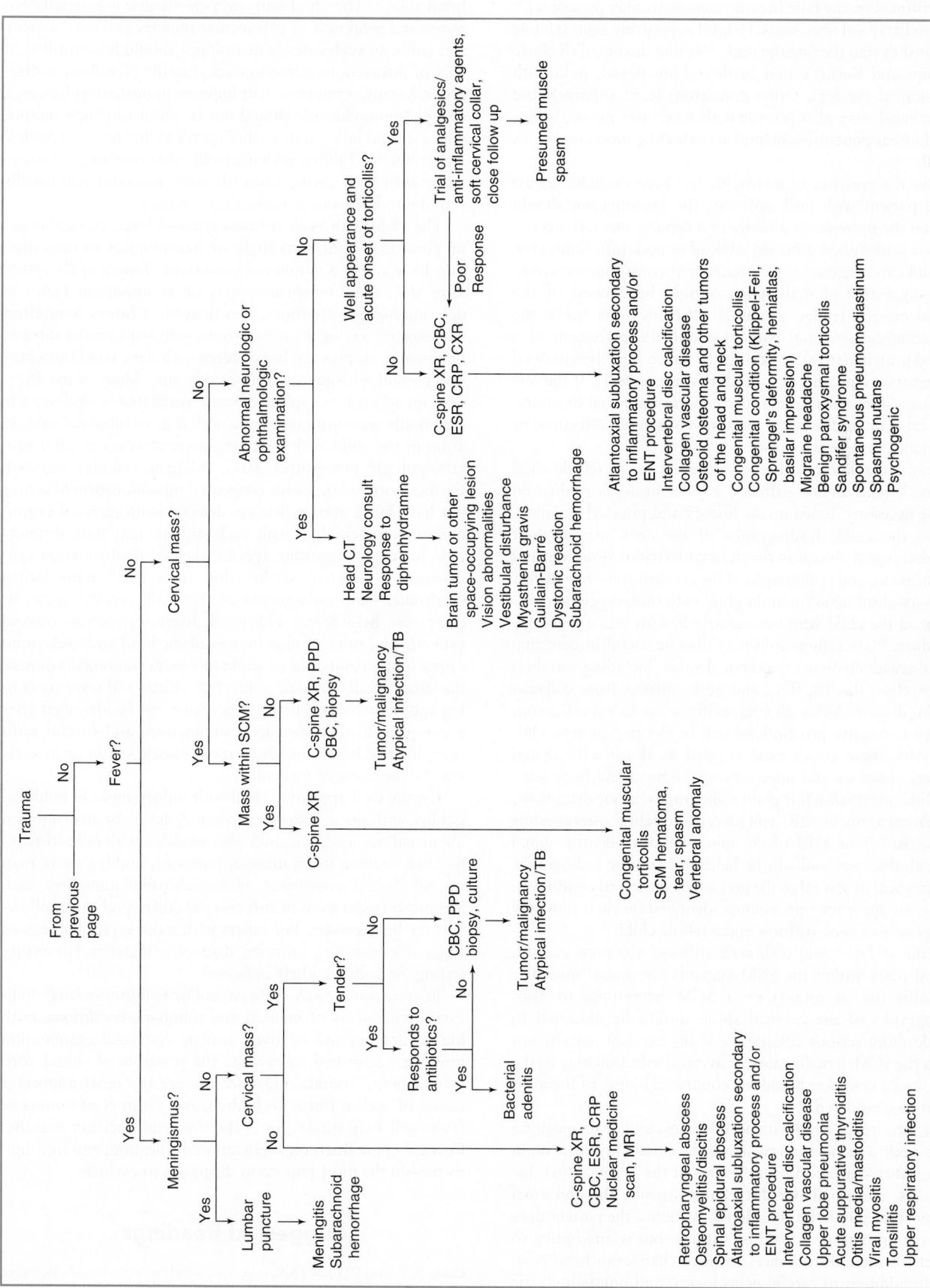

FIGURE 45.1 (*Continued*)

should be seriously considered in the presence of fever and neck stiffness of any type because meningitis may present with fever and atypical neck signs. Helpful supporting signs include Brudzinski's sign (flexing the neck, eliciting flexion of the knee and hip) and Kernig's sign (with the hip flexed, pain with extension of the leg). Other conditions (e.g., subarachnoid hemorrhage) may also present with fever and meningismus, and a lumbar puncture is helpful in evaluating these conditions as well.

After the presence of meningitis has been excluded in the febrile patient with neck stiffness, the examination should focus on the *presence or absence of a cervical mass*. If a cervical mass is identified, a history of head or neck infections, contact with cats suggestive of *Bartonella*, or constitutional symptoms suggestive of malignancy should be elicited. If the cervical mass is tender, a trial of antibiotics directed at the most common bacterial pathogens and the placement of a purified protein derivative skin test to screen for tuberculosis if risk factors are present may be all that is necessary. If the cervical mass does not respond to an appropriate trial of antibiotics, cat-scratch disease, atypical mycobacterial infection, or malignancy may be the cause.

If no palpable cervical mass is present in the febrile child with neck pain and/or stiffness, a more in-depth evaluation may be necessary, based on the history and physical examination of the child. Radiographs of the neck may suggest retropharyngeal abscess in the child with stridor, drooling, and neck stiffness, and radiographs of the cervical spine may detect atlantoaxial subluxation in the child with otolaryngologic disease or in the child who has recently had an otolaryngologic procedure. Plain radiographs may also be useful in detecting other diseases involving the cervical spine, including vertebral osteomyelitis, discitis, IDC, and neck stiffness from collagen vascular disease. Although nonspecific, white blood cell count, ESR, or C-reactive protein level will be elevated in most children with these conditions, as well as those with spinal epidural abscesses and infections of the head and neck (e.g., tonsillitis, mastoiditis). If plain radiography is not diagnostic, technetium scans or MRI will identify vertebral osteomyelitis or discitis. CT or MRI of the spine will also identify spinal epidural abscesses and can be helpful if routine radiographs are equivocal in several of the previously described conditions. Finally, an upper lobe pneumonia identified on chest film may be the cause of neck stiffness in the febrile child.

In the *afebrile* child with neck stiffness, the presence of a cervical mass within the SCM suggests congenital muscular torticollis (in an infant) or a SCM hematoma or tear. Radiographs of the cervical spine should be obtained to exclude more serious conditions. If the cervical mass is not within the SCM, a malignancy or atypical infection may be the cause, and a complete blood cell count and biopsy of the mass should be considered.

For the afebrile child with neck stiffness and/or malposition of the neck and no cervical mass, the possibility of a brain tumor, other space-occupying lesions of the brain, visual disturbances, and vestibular disturbance causing the abnormal neck posture should be considered. At times, the patient does not have primary neck pain or stiffness but is attempting to correct for these disturbances through changes in head position. In addition to careful neurological and ophthalmologic examinations, a head CT scan is necessary to exclude the pos-

sibility of a space-occupying lesion of the brain, including a brain tumor. The child with myasthenia gravis generally has ptosis and weakness of extraocular muscles and may develop torticollis. In such cases, a neurologist should be consulted. A trial of intravenous edrophonium chloride (Tensilon) is diagnostic because symptoms will improve immediately; however, edrophonium chloride should not be given to young infants, who are especially prone to this agent's ability to cause cardiac arrhythmias. Children with torticollis after receiving neuroleptic or antiemetic medications (dystonic reaction) will usually respond to intravenous diphenhydramine.

The child with neck stiffness without fever, cervical mass, or abnormal ophthalmologic or neurological examination may have any of a number of conditions. *Timing of the symptoms (i.e., acute or chronic)* may be an important factor in determining the appropriate evaluation. Chronic symptoms may suggest a congenital syndrome, collagen vascular disease, or a neoplastic process, but children with these conditions may also present with acute onset of symptoms. Many of the disorders mentioned as typically being associated with fever are commonly seen without fever as well (e.g. atlantoaxial subluxation in the child with otolaryngologic diseases or after otolaryngologic procedures, IDC, collagen vascular disease). Furthermore, infants with congenital muscular torticollis may not have SCM masses that are detectable on physical examination. Some children with neck stiffness may have dysmorphic features, suggesting specific skeletal malformation syndromes or cervical subluxation in a child with Down syndrome. Plain radiographs of the head, cervical spine, or chest may help detect additional diagnoses such as osteoid osteoma and other benign tumors of the head and neck or an upper lobe pneumonia or spontaneous pneumomediastinum, the latter usually in association with a history of severe coughing and/or retching. Finally, if no cause can be identified after a complete history, detailed examination, and careful radiographic and laboratory evaluation, muscle spasm or hysteria may be the cause of torticollis.

For the well-appearing child with sudden onset of mild torticollis without a history of trauma, fever, or neurological abnormalities (e.g., the child who awakens with mild torticollis after sleeping in an unusual position), nothing more than careful clinical assessment, analgesic/anti-inflammatory medication, consideration of soft cervical collar, and close follow-up may be necessary. For others with more severe findings or suggestive histories, however, diagnostic imaging, laboratory testing, or both are likely indicated.

In conclusion, neck stiffness and/or malposition may indicate a wide array of medical and traumatic conditions, both life-threatening and relatively benign. A careful examination must be performed to exclude the presence of spinal cord involvement. Trauma and infection are the most important causes of neck stiffness in children, and a history of trauma or fever will help guide the evaluation and decision making. Cervical spine fracture, subluxation/dislocation, and meningitis remain the most important diagnoses to exclude.

Suggested Readings

Cheng JCY, Tang SP, Chen TMK, et al. The clinical presentation and outcome of treatment of congenital muscular torticollis in infants—a study of 1,086 cases. *J Pediatr Surg* 2000;35:1091–1096.

Chi H, Lee YJ, Chiu NC, et al. Acute suppurative thyroiditis in children. *Pediatr Infect Dis J* 2002;21:384–387.

Cornejo VJF, Martinez-Lage JF, Piqueras C, et al. Inflammatory atlanto-axial subluxation (Grisel's syndrome) in children: clinical diagnosis and management. *Child Nerv Syst* 2003;19:342–347.

Craig FW, Schunk JE. Retropharyngeal abscess in children: clinical presentation, utility of imaging, and current management. *Pediatrics* 2003;111: 1394–1398.

Cirak B, Ziegfeld S, Knight VM, et al. Spinal injuries in children. *J Pediatr Surg* 2004;39:607–612.

Dai LY, Ye H, Qian QR. The natural history of cervical disc calcification in children. *J Bone Joint Surg Am* 2004;86:1467–1472.

Fernandez M, Carrol CL, Baker CJ. Discitis and vertebral osteomyelitis in children: an 18-year review. *Pediatrics* 2000;105:1299–1304.

Gupta AK, Roy DR, Conlan ES, et al. Torticollis secondary to posterior fossa tumors. *J Pediatr Orthop* 1996;16:505–507.

Leonard J, Kuppermann N, Olsen C, et al. Sensitivity of the NEXUS C-spine criteria within the PECARN C-spine injury (CSI) cohort. *Acad Emerg Med* 2008;15:S6.

Nigrovic LE, Kuppermann N, Malley R, et al. Children with bacterial meningitis presenting to the emergency department during the pneumococcal conjugate vaccine era. *Acad Emerg Med* 2008;15:522–528.

Oostenbrink R, Moons KG, Theunissen CC, et al. Signs of meningeal irritation at the emergency department: how often bacterial meningitis? *Pediatr Emerg Care* 2001;17:161–164.

Subach BR, McLaughlin MR, Albright AL, et al. Current management of pediatric atlantoaxial rotatory subluxation. *Spine* 1998;23:2174–2179.

Viccellio P, Simon H, Pressman BD, et al. A prospective multicenter study of cervical spine injury in children. *Pediatrics* 2001;108:e20.

Vitale MG, Goss JM, Matsumoto H, et al. Epidemiology of pediatric spinal cord injury in the United States years 1997 and 2000. *J Pediatr Orthop* 2006;26: 745–749.

CHAPTER 46 ■ ODOR—UNUSUAL

ALISON BRENT, MD

The human nose is able to discriminate approximately 4,000 odors! Occasionally, parents bring an infant or child to the emergency department (ED) complaining of an unusual smell. Adolescents are more likely to note a new or unusual odor themselves and present to the ED with specific complaints.

Unfortunately, olfaction is a sense that most medical professionals are not trained to use, quantify, or describe. Before the development of sophisticated laboratory tests, clinicians relied heavily on the sense of smell. Even today, early diagnostic clues that can lead the clinician to a more selective workup, rapid diagnosis, and prompt therapeutic intervention may be obtained. In some situations, a prompt diagnosis can be lifesaving or can improve the quality of life.

PATHOPHYSIOLOGY

The olfactory area extends from the roof of the nasal cavity approximately 10 mm down the septum and superior turbinates bilaterally. The exact mechanism of stimulation of the olfactory receptors is unknown. Smell is more acute in the darkness and is believed to be linked to blood cortisol levels.

The unique odor emitted by a person is produced by a combination of body secretions and excretions, particularly those from the oropharynx and nasopharynx and the respiratory tract, plus aromas from the skin and cutaneous lesions, urine, feces, and flatus. The most significant components of odor in healthy humans are the apocrine glands. These secretions are initially odorless, but bacterial breakdown that results in fatty acid production can cause an offensive odor. Body odor is altered by hygiene, metabolism, toxins, infections, and systemic diseases.

When a child is unable to detect odor, anosmia should be considered. When a child complains of strange odors, especially if no one else is able to identify them, temporal lobe epilepsy should be contemplated.

DIFFERENTIAL DIAGNOSIS

A number of conditions, including metabolic disorders, dermatologic conditions, intoxications, infections, foreign bodies, various abnormalities of the body orifices, and a variety of systemic diseases, may result in an abnormal body odor (Table 46.1).

Metabolic Disorders

The most common metabolic disorder that has a characteristic odor is diabetic ketoacidosis (Table 46.2). The characteristic breath odor is caused by acetone and is described as sweet or fruity. It is important to note that any condition that results in a marked metabolic acidosis and ketosis will result in the characteristic sweet or fruity breath.

Inborn errors of metabolism that result in altered body, breath, or skin odors are unusual individually, but as a composite, they reflect a significant percentage of life-threatening illnesses of infancy (see Chapter 94). Although definitive diagnosis depends on specific identification of serum and urine amino and organic acid levels, many such conditions are associated with a positive ferric chloride test, which when performed in the ED can yield presumptive diagnosis.

Phenylketonuria is a disorder of amino acid metabolism associated with a deficiency of phenylalanine dehydroxylase and dihydropteridine reductase, which forces use of minor metabolic pathways of phenylalanine, resulting in the buildup of phenylacetic acid. It is the buildup of phenylacetic acid in the sweat and urine that causes a musty, mousy, horsey, wolflike, or barny odor. Clinical features of untreated phenylketonuria include white-blond hair, blue eyes, fair complexion, eczema, microcephaly, hypertonicity, increased risk for pyloric stenosis, seizures, and progressive mental deterioration. Although neonatal screening detects most of these cases, the observation of a characteristic odor in an infant should prompt appropriate laboratory studies, which may include a ferric chloride test in the ED. Prompt diagnosis and dietary restriction of phenylalanine promote a normal outcome.

Maple syrup urine disease is caused by a metabolic defect in the decarboxylation of the ketoacids of the branch-chain amino acids (leucine, isoleucine, and valine), which results in their accumulation in the blood. It is apparently a metabolite of isoleucine in the urine that results in the characteristic odor of maple syrup, caramelized sugar, or boiled Chinese herbal medicine. Children with this disorder can have variable clinical manifestations, ranging from decreased appetite, vomiting, and ataxia to progressive acidosis, seizures, coma, and death. Prompt diagnosis and limitation of dietary branched-chain amino acids promotes normal development.

Oasthouse urine disease, or methionine malabsorption syndrome, is caused by defective transport of methionine and, to a lesser extent, leucine, isoleucine, valine, tyrosine, and phenylalanine by the intestines and kidneys. The unabsorbed methionine in the gut is broken down by colonic bacteria to α-hydroxybutyric acid, which causes the characteristic odor described as yeast, celery, malt, or a brewery. Clinical presentation includes fair hair and skin, hyperpnea, extensor spasms, fever, edema, and mental retardation. Successful treatment consists of a methionine-restricted diet.

The odor of sweaty feet syndrome, or isovaleric acidemia, is caused by a defect in the catabolism of leucine. The characteristic

TABLE 46.1

CLINICAL SOURCE AND CAUSE OF UNUSUAL ODORS

Urine		Body	
Metabolic diseases	**Metabolic disease odors**	**Toxins**	**Toxin odors**
Phenylketonuria	Mousy, musty, horsey, wolflike, barny	Nitrites, lacquer, ethanol, isopropyl alcohol, chloroform	Sweet, fruity
Maple syrup urine disease (branched-chain ketonuria)	Maple syrup, caramel, boiled Chinese herbal medicine	Paraldehyde, chloral hydrate	Pears
Oasthouse urine disease (methionine malabsorption)	Yeast, celery, malt, brewery	Cyanide	Bitter almonds, peach pits
Odor of sweaty feet syndrome (isovaleric acidemia)	Sweaty feet or socks, ripe cheese	Cicutoxin	Carrots
Odor of cat's urine syndrome (biotin-responsive multiple carboxylase deficiency)	Tomcat urine	Disulfiram, mercaptan, hydrogen sulfide	Rotten eggs
Fish odor syndrome (trimethylaminuria)	Dead fish	Zinc phosphide	Musty, fish, raw liver
Odor of rancid butter syndrome (tyrosinemia)	Fishy, musty, rotten cabbage	Arsenic, phosphorous, dimethyl sulfoxide, thallium, tellurium, parathion, malathion, selenium	Garlic
		Camphor, naphthalene, p-dichlorobenzene	Mothballs
Toxins	**Toxin odors**	Vacor	Peanuts
Turpentine	Violets	O-Chlorobenzylidene, malonitrile	Pepper
Infectious diseases	**Infectious disease odors**	Ethchlorvynol	Aromatic, vinyl-like
Urinary tract infection	Ammonia	Nitrobenzene	Shoe polish
Foreign body	**Foreign body odors**	Methyl salicylate	Oil of wintergreen
Urethral foreign body	Foul, putrid	Alcoholic beverages	Alcoholic beverages
		Metabolic diseases	**Metabolic disease odors**
		Phenylketonuria	Mousy, musty, horsey, wolflike, barny
		Odor of sweaty feet syndrome (isovaleric acidemia)	Cheesy, sweaty socks
		Infectious diseases	**Infectious disease odors**
		Typhoid fever	Freshly baked bread
		Yellow fever	Butcher shop
		Smallpox	Menagerie
		Scrofula	Stale beer
		Diphtheria	Sweet
		Rubella	Freshly plucked feathers
		Miliary fever	Rotten straw
		Omphalitis	Foul
		Miscellaneous diseases	**Miscellaneous disease odors**
		Scurvy	Putrid
		Gout	Fetid
		Pellagra	Sour or musty butter
		Psychiatric diseases	**Psychiatric disease odors**
		Schizophrenia	Pungent, heavy
		Antibiotics	**Antibiotic odors**
		Cephalosporin	Musty
		Penicillin	Ammonia
		Skin diseases	**Skin disease odors**
		Hidradenitis	Pungent
		Darier's disease (keratosisfollicularis)	Burned tissue
		Bromhidrosis	Pungent
		Ichthyosis, ulcers, necrosis, pemphigus	Foul, unpleasant
		Burns	Charred flesh

(continued)

TABLE 46.1

CLINICAL SOURCE AND CAUSE OF UNUSUAL ODORS (CONTINUED)

Breath		Body fluids	
Toxins	**Toxin odors**	**Sputum**	**Sputum**
Amphetamines	Bad breath	*Infectious diseases*	*Infectious disease odors*
Cyanide	Bitter almonds	Bronchitis, empyema, abscess	Foul, putrid
Arsenic, phosphorus,	Garlic	**Vomitus**	**Vomitus**
tellurium, parathion,		*Infectious diseases*	*Infectious disease odors*
malathion		Peritonitis	Feculent
Iodine	Metallic	*Systemic diseases*	*Systemic disease odors*
Chloroform, lacquer, salicylate	Fruity, ripe apples	Gastrointestinal obstruction	Feculent
Chloral hydrate, paraldehyde	Pears	*Toxins*	*Toxin odors*
Methyl salicylate	Oil of wintergreen	Arsenic, phosphorus	Garlic
Ethchlorvynol	Aromatic, vinyl-like	Turpentine	Violets
Camphor naphthalene,	Mothballs	**Stool**	**Stool**
p-dichlorobenzene		*Infectious diseases*	*Infectious disease odors*
Hydrogen sulfide	Rotten eggs	Shigella, salmonella	Rank
		Steatorrhea	Foul
Infectious diseases	**Infectious disease odors**	*Systemic diseases*	*Systemic disease odors*
Pharyngitis, tonsillitis, acute	Foul, putrid	Malabsorption, cystic fibrosis,	Foul, vile
ulcerative gingivitis		celiac disease, chronic disease	
(Vincent's angina, trench		*Toxins*	*Toxin odors*
mouth), lung abscess,		Arsenic	Garlic
halitosis, dental abscess		**General**	**General**
Diphtheria	Sweet grapes	*Foreign body*	*Foreign body odors*
		Rectal foreign body	Foul, putrid
Metabolic diseases	**Metabolic disease odors**	**Pus**	**Pus**
DKA or any other condition	Fruity or sweet	*Infectious diseases*	*Infectious disease odors*
that causes ketosis		Gas gangrene	Sweet, rotten apples
Odor of sweaty feet syndrome	Sweaty feet or socks, ripe	Foreign body	Fetid, putrid
(isovaleric acidemia)	cheese	Proteophylic bacteria	Feculent, ripe cheese
		Clostridium gas gangrene	Rotten apples
Systemic diseases	**Systemic disease odors**	*Proteus*	Mousy
Uremia	Fishy, ammonia	Proteolytic bacteria	Overripe cheese
Hepatic failure	Musty fish, raw liver,	**Vaginal discharge**	**Vaginal**
	clover, feculent	*Infectious diseases*	*Infectious disease odors*
Gastrointestinal obstructions	Foul, feculent	Vaginitis, foreign body	Fishy, foul
		Systemic diseases	*Systemic disease odors*
Foreign body	**Foreign body odors**	Malignancy	Fetid
Nasal foreign body	Foul, putrid	*Foreign body*	*Foreign body odors*
		Vaginal foreign body	Foul, putrid
		Ear discharge	**Ear discharge**
		Metabolic diseases	*Metabolic disease odors*
		Maple syrup urine disease	Maple syrup, caramel, boiled
			Chinese herbal medicine
		Infectious diseases	*Infectious disease odors*
		Pseudomonas	Foul
		Foreign body	*Foreign body odors*
		Otic foreign body	Foul, putrid

odor described as sweaty feet or socks or ripe cheese comes from the buildup of isovaleric acid. Clinically, children experience vomiting, dehydration, acidosis, and slowly progressive mental deterioration. Treatment consists of restriction of leucine in the diet.

In the odor of cat's urine syndrome, the enzymatic defects are in the biotin-dependent enzymes β-methylcrotonyl-CoA carboxylase, pyruvate carboxylase, and propionyl-CoA car-

boxylase. The cause of the distinctive aroma of cat urine is unknown. Clinically, children have failure to thrive, ketoacidosis, and neurologic symptoms similar to Werdnig-Hoffmann's disease. Treatment consists of a low-leucine diet and the addition of biotin.

Fish odor syndrome, trimethylaminuria, results from an unidentified defect that possibly relates to choline metabolism. The dead fish odor in the urine results from buildup of

TABLE 46.2

METABOLIC DISEASE ASSOCIATED WITH UNUSUAL ODORS

Disease	Odor	Odor source	Enzyme defect	Clinical features	Treatment	Rapid emergency department diagnosis
Diabetic ketoacidosis	Sweet or fruity	Breath	Lack of insulin or insulin activity	Polyuria, polydipsia, polyphagia, weight loss, coma, acidosis	Insulin administration	1 mL urine + 10% ferric chloride—red-brown color
Phenylketonuria	Musty, mousy, horsey, wolflike, barny	Urine and body	Phenylalanine hydroxylase	Progressive mental retardation, eczema, decreased pigmentation, seizures, spasticity, white-blond hair, blue eyes, pyloric stenosis, microcephaly	Diet low in phenylalanine	1 mL urine + 10% ferric chloride—green color
Maple syrup urine disease (branched-chain ketonuria)	Maple syrup, caramel, boiled Chinese herbal medicine	Urine	Branched-chain ketoacid decarboxylase	Marked acidosis, seizures, vomiting, ataxia, decreased appetite, coma leading to death in first year or two of life or mental subnormality without acidosis or intermittent acidosis without mental retardation	Diet low in branched-chain amino acid; protein restriction and/or thiamine in large doses	1 mL urine + 10% ferric chloride—blue, yellow, or blue-green color
Oasthouse urine disease (methionine malabsorption)	Yeast, celery, malt, brewery	Urine	Defective transport of methionine, branched-chain amino acids, tyrosine, and phenylalanine	Mental retardation, spasticity, hyperpnea, fever, edema, fair hair and skin0	Restrict methionine in diet	1 mL urine + 10% ferric chloride—purpleor red-brown color
Odor of sweaty feet syndrome (isovaleric acidemia)	Sweaty feet or socks, ripe cheese	Urine, body, breath, all body fluids	Isovaleryl-CoA dehydrogenase	Recurrent bouts of acidosis, vomiting, dehydration, coma, aversion to protein foods, lethargy, hypotension	Restrict leucine in diet	N/A
Odor of cat's urine syndrome (biotin-responsive multiple carboxylase deficiency)	Tomcat urine	Urine	β-Methylcrotonyl-CoA carboxylase, pyruvate carboxylase, propionyl-CoA carboxylase	Neurologic disorder resembling Werdnig-Hoffmann's disease, ketoacidosis, failure to thrive	Leucine restriction? Biotin administration	N/A
Fish odor syndrome (trimethylaminuria)	Dead fish	Urine	Unknown defect in choline metabolism	Stigmata of Turner syndrome, neutropenia, recurrent infections, anemia, splenomegaly	Unknown	N/A
Odor of rancid butter syndrome (tyrosinosis)	Rancid butter, rotten cabbage, fishy, musty	Urine	Unknown	Poor feeding, irritability, progressive neurologic deterioration, seizures, hepatic dysfunction, death	Response to decreased phenylalanine and tyrosine intake?	1 mL urine + 10% ferric chloride—transient blue-green color

N/A, not applicable.

SIGNS AND SYMPTOMS

trimethylamine. Clinical presentation includes stigmata of Turner syndrome, normal complement of chromosomes, neutropenia, recurrent pulmonary infections, and abnormal platelet function.

The odor of rancid butter syndrome, tyrosinosis, results from an unidentified defect in metabolism. It is hypothesized that a buildup of α-ketogammame-thiolbutyric acid in the urine results in the characteristic smell of rancid butter. Clinical presentation includes poor feeding, irritability, seizures, coma, progressive neurologic deterioration, and early death secondary to infection and liver failure. In some cases, restriction of dietary phenylalanine and tyrosine has been helpful.

Dermatological Conditions

Many dermatologic diseases (Table 46.1) are associated with specific odors. Any cause of hyperhidrosis results in an offensive body odor. Hidradenitis has a characteristic pungent odor, whereas Darier's disease is noted to have a pervasive aroma of burned tissue. An abscess or cellulitis is identified by the characteristic odors of the responsible microorganisms.

In burn patients, there is the typical odor of charred flesh, which when infected with *Pseudomonas aeruginosa*, takes on a characteristic sweet, grapelike odor.

Toxicologic Considerations

Recognition of a characteristic odor is vital for rapid, accurate diagnosis and treatment of some potentially lethal ingestions before laboratory identification (Table 46.1) (see Chapter 102).

Penicillins give off an ammoniacal scent, whereas cephalosporins are noted to have a musty odor. Topical benzoyl peroxide, applied in large quantities, emits a pungent, pervasive aroma.

A strong garlic odor is typical of arsenic, arsine gas, phosphorus, tellurium, parathion, malathion, selenium, dimethyl sulfoxide, and thallium. The odor of bitter almonds or peach pits is indicative of cyanide poisoning, in which the degree of excretion of the odor parallels toxicity (although the ability to detect this odor is genetically determined and may only be present in up to 40% of persons).

Diagnostic odors are found in several sedative-hypnotic medications that primarily have central nervous system manifestations. Ethchlorvynol (Placidyl) is a volatile agent that has an aromatic plastic or vinyl-like breath odor. Ingestion results in coma, hypothermia, respiratory depression, hypotension, and bradycardia. An overdose of chloral hydrate can result in central nervous system depression ranging from slurred speech, ataxia, and incoordination to deep coma, gastritis, and cardiac arrhythmias. It may be seen in children or as an intentional overdose in adults, and it imparts a fruity, pearlike scent. Disulfiram (Antabuse) gives the breath a rotten egg odor because of the sulfide metabolites. The pleasant smell of oil of wintergreen indicates methyl salicylate poisoning.

Infectious Diseases

Many microorganisms produce characteristic odors that suggest the diagnosis of their respective infectious diseases by olfaction alone (Table 46.1) (see also Chapter 92). Omphalitis in the newborn can be life threatening. It presents with a foul or putrid odor associated with a draining, erythematous umbilical area. Less common infections that have been historically associated with characteristic odors include typhoid's aroma of freshly baked bread, yellow fever's butcher shop smell, smallpox's menagerie odor, scrofula's odor of stale beer, diphtheria's sweet smell, and rubella's scent of freshly plucked feathers.

Foreign Bodies

Foreign bodies are capable of producing a foul odor that results from secondary bacterial colonization or infection. Foreign body odors can be localized to a particular orifice, or they may pervade a patient's clothing, body, and surrounding environment. Foul-smelling, fetid, or feculent odors indicate anaerobic infections, whereas a sickly sweet odor is associated with *Escherichia coli,* and *Clostridia* is associated with a mousy odor.

Orifice Odors

Specific orifice odors can be diagnostic of infectious disease processes.

Oropharynx

A healthy mouth does not give off an offensive odor. Halitosis, or bad breath, is the result of a release of volatile sulfur compounds formed when the oral flora metabolizes amino acids from compounds in the saliva that adhere to the tongue, teeth, and gums. Halitosis is increased in states of diminished solid and liquid intake. Tonsillitis (see Chapters 71 and 92) has an offensive odor, and group A β-hemolytic streptococcus gives off a characteristic "strep breath" smell. Dental abscesses (see Chapter 122) and acute ulcerative gingivitis (Vincent's angina or trench mouth) are associated with a penetrating, offensive odor. The oropharynx is also the portal of exit for deeper infections. Lung abscesses, empyema, bronchitis, and bronchiectasis result in foul breath and sputum. Nasal foreign bodies in toddlers are usually associated with an odor identified by parents as bad breath.

Nose

Nasal drainage can be clear and odorless or mucopurulent and odiferous. Nasal drainage and bleeding can reflect local infections, foreign bodies, irritations of the nasal passage, and sinus drainage.

Ear

Sterile inner ear fluid is odorless but gives off a rank smell when infected. Acute otitis externa is usually associated with a mucoid drainage, whereas chronic otitis externa produces a purulent, discolored drainage with a foul odor, usually secondary to *Pseudomonas aeruginosa* or *Staphylococcus aureus*.

Genitalia

Vaginal secretions are combinations of vulvar secretions from sebaceous, sweat, Bartholin's and Skene's glands, transudate through the vaginal wall, exfoliated cells, cervical mucus, endometrial and oviductal fluids, plus vaginal microorganisms and menstrual blood. These secretions are hormonally mediated and vary with the menstrual cycle. Odors are exacerbated by the presence of retained foreign bodies, including tampons and diaphragms.

Bacterial vaginosis (nonspecific vaginitis, *Gardnerella* vaginitis, *Corynebacterium* vaginitis, *Haemophilus* vaginitis, nonspecific vaginosis, and anaerobic vaginosis) is caused by an increase in anaerobic bacteria and a decrease in lactobacilli (see Chapter 90). The anaerobic bacteria act synergistically with *Gardnerella vaginosa*, to produce enzymes and aminopeptidases that degrade protein, and decarboxylases that convert amino acids and other compounds to amines. The amines produce the characteristic "fishy" odor, which is best detected by alkalinization by using 10% potassium hydroxide placed directly on a vaginal swab and smelling immediately. This odor also can be indicative of sexual abuse in children. Vaginal infection with *Trichomonas* often is associated with a fishy odor, whereas *Candida* vaginitis is notably free of odor (see Chapter 94).

A male counterpart, balanoposthitis, is associated with a urethral discharge that produces a fishy odor when alkalinized because of the same process and organisms as occur in bacterial vaginosis.

Urethral Meatus

A urinary tract infection caused by urea-splitting bacteria will emit an ammoniacal odor.

Rectum

Stool odors vary with diet, medications, and microbiologic flora. Various malabsorptive syndromes, such as sprue, cystic fibrosis (see Chapter 99), and Whipple's disease, are associated with foul-smelling stool. The presence of blood in the stool has a distinctive, pungent odor, as does pus. *Shigella* and *Salmonella* (see Chapter 92) have distinctive rank odors.

Systemic Diseases

Several nutritional syndromes (Table 46.1), such as pellagra's stench of sour or musty butter and the putrid or fetid smell of scurvy and gout, have unique odors. Schizophrenia has a characteristic body odor described as heavy, unpleasant, and pungent. The odor-producing substance is *trans*-3-methyl-2-hexanoic acid, which is produced in the sweat. Uremic breath is produced by secondary and tertiary amines, dimethylamines, and trimethylamines that produce a fishy odor. Malignancy—especially when associated with an expanding external mass, bleeding, and necrosis—gives off a trenchant odor because of tissue and cellular breakdown plus gas formation. Hepatic failure gives an odor of "fetor hepaticus" (described as musty, rotten eggs, or garlic) and is noted in the breath or urine. In Crohn's disease (see Chapter 89), the development of gastric fistulae is often heralded by a feculent odor.

A physiologic odor that often heralds the onset of puberty is that emanating from the underarms. This is usually the earliest sign of puberty and precedes all other physical changes. Age of onset is around 6 to 8 years and reflects the onset of adrenarche. Dehydroepiandrosterone sulfate is the androgen believed to be responsible for the pungent aroma of underarm body odor and can be measured for confirmation. Although the adrenal and hypothalamic-pituitary-gonadal axes are separate systems involved with the onset of puberty, they often become active nearly simultaneously.

EVALUATION AND DECISION

The evaluation of a child who presents to the ED should incorporate all the senses, including smell (Fig. 46.1). Both presence and absence of odors can be diagnostic. Each person has a unique odor, ranging from pleasant to offensive. Using the sense of smell should be done in stages; an initial evaluation of the prevailing odor of the examination room, followed by attention to overall body odor and identification of odors from individual orifices and body fluids. Body fluids such as ocular, ear, nasal, sinus tract, or umbilical drainage; vomitus; sputum; genital discharge; stool; ulcers; and superinfection of the dermis have unique identifiable odors.

Good or poor hygiene is readily detected in a closed examination room. When an unusual odor is detected, the history should include information about medications (topical, oral, or rectal), onset and duration of odor, methods used to alter odor, unusual drainage from body orifices, suspicion of foreign body, fever, and other pertinent symptoms.

In the evaluation of the significance of odors, attention must be paid to the child's age and developmental level. At birth, infant odors are a conglomeration of their own and their mother's physical environment. After birth, a well-cared-for, healthy infant should have a very pleasing aroma and odorless breath. Offensive body odor in a newborn suggests an inborn error of metabolism, a localized infection such as omphalitis, or neglect. During infancy, inborn errors of metabolism are relatively common (Table 46.3) and are potentially life-threatening causes of unusual odor (Table 46.4). Infection localized to the umbilicus, omphalitis, produces a foul odor and is easily diagnosed on the basis of erythema, induration, and discharge. Other sources found in older children (foreign bodies, ingestions, and pharyngitis) are unusual in the infant.

In an older child, the physician should determine a child's history and whether clinical signs of chronic systemic diseases, such as diabetes, liver failure, or uremia, are present. The child with ketoacidosis usually appears dehydrated and manifests deep, rapid (Kussmaul) respirations; the breath may smell of ketones. Uremia develops in patients with renal failure who may have short stature, edema, hypertension, and a characteristic fishy odor of their breath. With liver failure, the patient may have jaundice, ascites, lethargy, or mental status changes, as well as breath and urine that takes on the odor of rotten eggs or garlic.

Body odors change with puberty through hormonally induced metabolic changes. The most significant change is the development of axillary odor related to apocrine secretions that are retained or spread by axillary hair. Normal quantities of sweat have a barely perceptible odor, whereas increasing quantities of sweat production cause increasingly noticeable and offensive odor.

Early on, the physician should determine the potential risk of ingestion of a toxic substance. In the adolescent, the risk of a significant ingestion increases and can be life threatening (Table 46.4). Next, the physician should ascertain whether the odor emanates from a particular body orifice such as the ear,

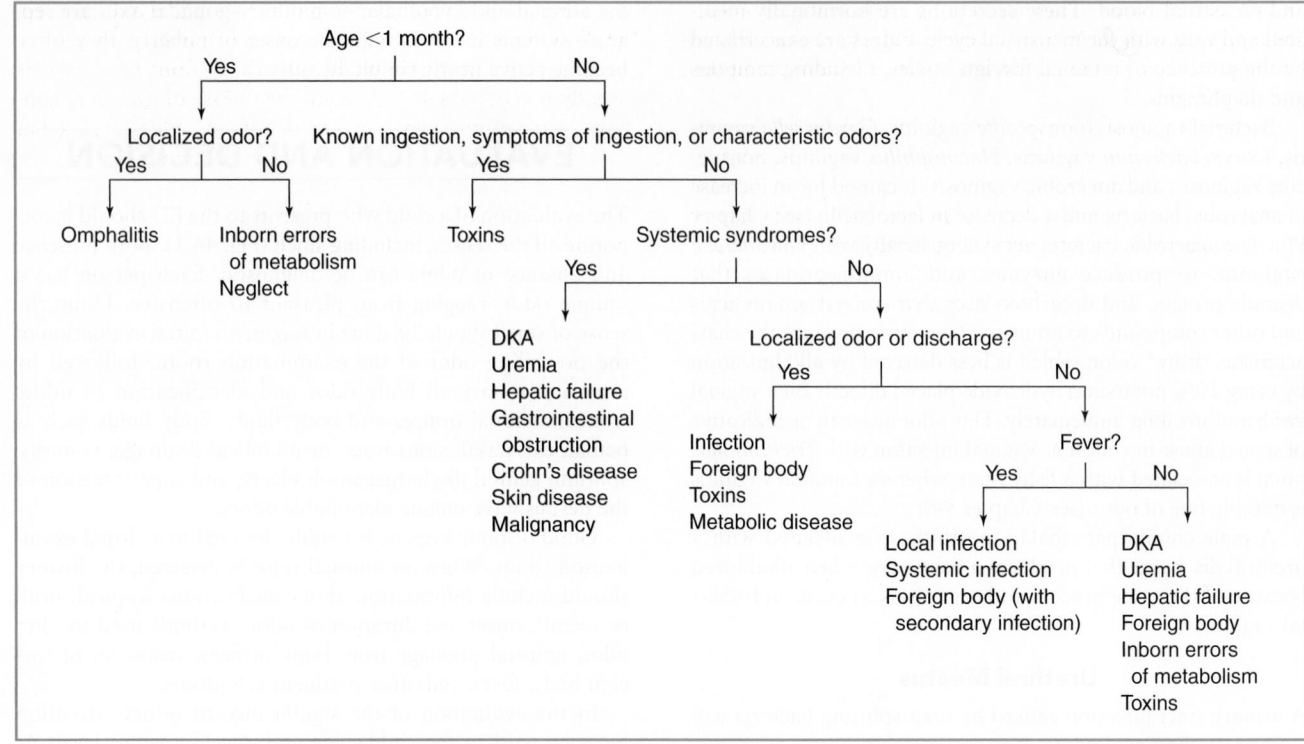

FIGURE 46.1 Evaluation and decision for unusual odors. DKA, diabetic ketoacidosis.

nose, pharynx, vagina, urethra, or rectum. Nasal foreign bodies are particularly common in children between the ages of 1 and 5 years. They may remain hidden for weeks, long beyond the child's memory of placing the object, and eventually, they produce a secondary infection that leads to a foul discharge. In some cases of foreign body, the odor may be so strong that it appears to be generalized. Thus, a careful examination of the

various orifices, with particular attention to the nares, is always advisable. The presence or absence of fever is another crucial variable in the evaluation of odor. Fever suggests an infectious cause, either systemic or localized. Pharyngitis and tonsillitis characteristically cause foul odor to the breath, much like a lung abscess. Occasionally, parents state that their child smells as if he or she had a "strep throat." Although

TABLE 46.3

COMMON CAUSES OF UNUSUAL ODORS

Infants
Inborn errors of metabolism
Omphalitis
Neglect

Toddlers
Foreign bodies
  Otic
  Nasal
  Vaginal
  Urethral
  Rectal
Localized infections
  Stomatitis

Adolescents
Localized infections
  Pharyngitis
  Tonsillitis
  Vaginitis
Toxins
Alcoholic beverages
Puberty

TABLE 46.4

LIFE-THREATENING CAUSES OF UNUSUAL ODOR

Metabolic disease
Inborn errors of metabolism
Diabetic ketoacidosis

Infectious diseases
Omphalitis
Diphtheria
Lung abscess

Toxins
Arsenic
Cyanide
Isopropyl alcohol
Methyl salicylate
Vacor

Systemic disease
Uremia
Liver failure
Gastrointestinal obstruction
Peritonitis

foreign bodies occasionally produce obstruction and a secondary infection of severity sufficient enough to evoke a febrile response, in most cases, the inflammation is localized and the child is afebrile.

In the absence of a known history or obvious findings of chronic systemic disease, a visible foreign body, known ingestion, or fever, the clinician should perform a careful physical examination and a urinalysis. Diabetic ketoacidosis always causes glucosuria and ketonuria, but hepatic or renal failure may be less obvious. In addition, inborn errors of metabolism may first manifest well beyond the newborn period. Foreign bodies may defy routine attempts at visualization and, based on a high index of suspicion, require endoscopy or imaging procedures. Therefore, persistence or an unusual odor or concern for chronic toxicity merits further laboratory evaluation.

In cases in which an explanation of the odor is not uncovered, a follow-up evaluation in 2 to 3 days is prudent.

In patients who have died in the ED, a faint fecal odor is usually noted, possibly related to the release of intestinal contents to the atmosphere. Unique identifiable odors detected at the time of death or autopsy can direct laboratory evaluation toward possible causes of death.

Suggested Readings

Chiang WK. Otolaryngologic principles. In: Goldfrank LR, Flomenbaum NE, Lewin NA, et al, eds. *Toxicologic emergencies*, 8th ed. Stanford, CT: Appleton & Lange, 2006:339–351.

Rezvani I, An approach to inborn errors of metabolism. In: Kliegman RM, Behrman RE, Jenson HB, Stanton BMD, eds. *Textbook of pediatrics*, 18th ed. Philadelphia, PA: WB Saunders, 2007:527–567.

SIGNS AND SYMPTOMS

CHAPTER 47 ■ OLIGOMENORRHEA

JAN E. PARADISE, MD

In this chapter, possible causes of oligomenorrhea and secondary amenorrhea are reviewed. *Oligomenorrhea* means infrequent menstruation and can be defined for the pediatric emergency physician as an interval of more than 6 weeks between two menstrual periods. If menstrual cycles do not resume within 3 to 6 months, the term *secondary amenorrhea* is applied. Some patients with anovulatory menstrual cycles have oligomenorrhea punctuated by episodes of excessive bleeding. An approach to the evaluation of abnormal vaginal bleeding is presented in Chapter 76.

Oligomenorrhea should be distinguished from hypomenorrhea, a nonpathologic pattern of light but regular menstrual periods. This chapter does not include a consideration of primary amenorrhea—that is, failure to menstruate by a specified age, often 16 years. However, some of the disorders discussed here can produce primary rather than secondary amenorrhea as part of an overall delay in pubertal development.

The differential diagnosis of oligomenorrhea is given in Table 47.1.

EVALUATION AND DECISION

Diagnosis of Pregnancy

"Is she pregnant?" is always the first question to answer in evaluating an adolescent with one or several missed menstrual periods (Fig. 47.1). If the patient is not pregnant, her evaluation can proceed at a more deliberate pace. If she is pregnant, however, prompt diagnosis and referral are important for the teenager who intends to seek a therapeutic abortion, as well as for the one who plans to continue her pregnancy. Early and regular prenatal care is associated with reduced morbidity and mortality among pregnant teenagers and their offspring. Early diagnosis also affords the pregnant adolescent more time to decide on and to arrange for a therapeutic abortion if that is her choice. As of 2009, before a minor can have an abortion, 35 states require consent by or notification of a parent (both parents in Minnesota, Mississippi, and North Dakota) or a hearing by a judge, and 25 states require counseling followed by a 24-hour waiting period. The time needed to comply with these requirements can push the procedure into the second trimester, resulting in higher morbidity and higher cost.

Early pregnancy is not always easy to recognize. Symptoms of fatigue, nausea, vomiting (not necessarily in the morning), urinary frequency, and breast growth or tenderness are common but by no means universal or specific. On pelvic examination, the first indications of pregnancy are softening of the

lower uterine segment (Hegar's sign) and of the cervix (Goodell's sign) at 4 to 6 weeks after the last menstrual period. By 6 weeks' gestation, the uterus changes from pear-shaped to globular and by about 8 weeks, the vagina and cervix acquire a bluish hue (Chadwick's sign). These changes occur in ectopic as well as in intrauterine pregnancies. A serviceable rule is that the pregnant uterus grows to about the size of a tennis ball at 8 weeks after the last menstrual period, becomes baseball-sized at 10 weeks, and softball-sized at 12 weeks. When the uterus is retroflexed, its size is more difficult to assess and rectovaginal palpation should be done. After 12 weeks, the uterine fundus is palpable above the symphysis pubis on abdominal examination. Fetal movement can be discerned after about 16 weeks. The fundus reaches the level of the umbilicus at 20 weeks' gestation.

Some patients may report the result of a home pregnancy test. However, because of variability in patients' timing of ovulation and of blastocyst implantation, and because of variability in the test's sensitivity for detecting urinary human chorionic gonadotropin (hCG), home pregnancy test kits commonly give falsely negative results. False-positive results can also occur. Accordingly, the emergency physician should not rely on the reported result of a home pregnancy test to make or to exclude the diagnosis of pregnancy.

Qualitative urine and serum pregnancy tests performed in medical settings generally detect the β-subunit of hCG (β-hCG) at levels above 25 mIU per mL. Quantitative serum tests for β-hCG generally have a sensitivity of around 5 mIU per mL. These sensitivities will permit the detection of a normal pregnancy within about 10 days after conception and, in most but not all cases, by the time an expected menstrual period is missed. Ectopic pregnancies often produce abnormally low levels of β-hCG. The emergency physician should know the detection level of the quantitative and qualitative β-hCG tests used by his or her laboratory.

If a patient with one or several missed menstrual periods also complains of abdominal pain or abnormal vaginal bleeding, the diagnosis of *ectopic pregnancy* must be entertained. (The diagnosis of ectopic pregnancy is discussed at greater length in Chapter 76.) Ectopic pregnancies are less common among adolescents than among older women. Although more than half of women with ectopic pregnancy have no risk factors, prior chlamydial and gonococcal cervicitis and prior pelvic inflammatory disease all increase the likelihood that a subsequent pregnancy will be ectopic.

Pseudocyesis is a rare cause of amenorrhea in women who believe they are pregnant and who exhibit many presumptive symptoms and signs of pregnancy, including nausea, vomiting, hyperpigmented areolae, galactorrhea, and abdominal

TABLE 47.1

DIFFERENTIAL DIAGNOSIS OF OLIGOMENORRHEA ORGANIZED BY PATHOPHYSIOLOGY OF DISORDER OR CONDITION

I. *Hypothalamic-pituitary axis disorders*
   A. Disorders of weight and/or energy expenditure
      1. Anorexia nervosa
      2. Strenuous exercise
      3. Marked thinness or weight loss
      4. Chronic illness
   B. Delayed maturation
   C. Psychological stress
   D. Central nervous system tumors
   E. Pseudocyesis
II. *Ovarian disorders*
   A. Ovarian failure
      1. Gonadal dysgenesis
      2. Alkylating antineoplastic agents
      3. Pelvic irradiation
      4. Autoimmune disease
   B. Hormone-secreting tumors

III. *Uterine disorders*
   A. Endometrial destruction
      1. Surgical
      2. Tuberculosis
IV. *Hyperprolactinemia*
   A. Lactation
   B. Drugs (see Table 47.3)
   C. Pituitary adenoma
   D. Hypothyroidism
V. *Hyperandrogenism*
   A. Polycystic ovary syndrome
   B. Adrenal disease
VI. *Miscellaneous conditions*
   A. Pregnancy
   B. Hormonal contraception
   C. Hypothyroidism or hyperthyroidism

SIGNS AND SYMPTOMS

distension. The diagnosis is made when a patient who insists that she is pregnant nevertheless has no true uterine enlargement, no demonstrable fetal parts or heart sounds, and a negative pregnancy test result. Psychiatric consultation should be obtained for such patients.

Evaluation of Nonpregnant Patients

If the physician can answer "no" to our original question—"Is she pregnant?"—the evaluation of an adolescent with

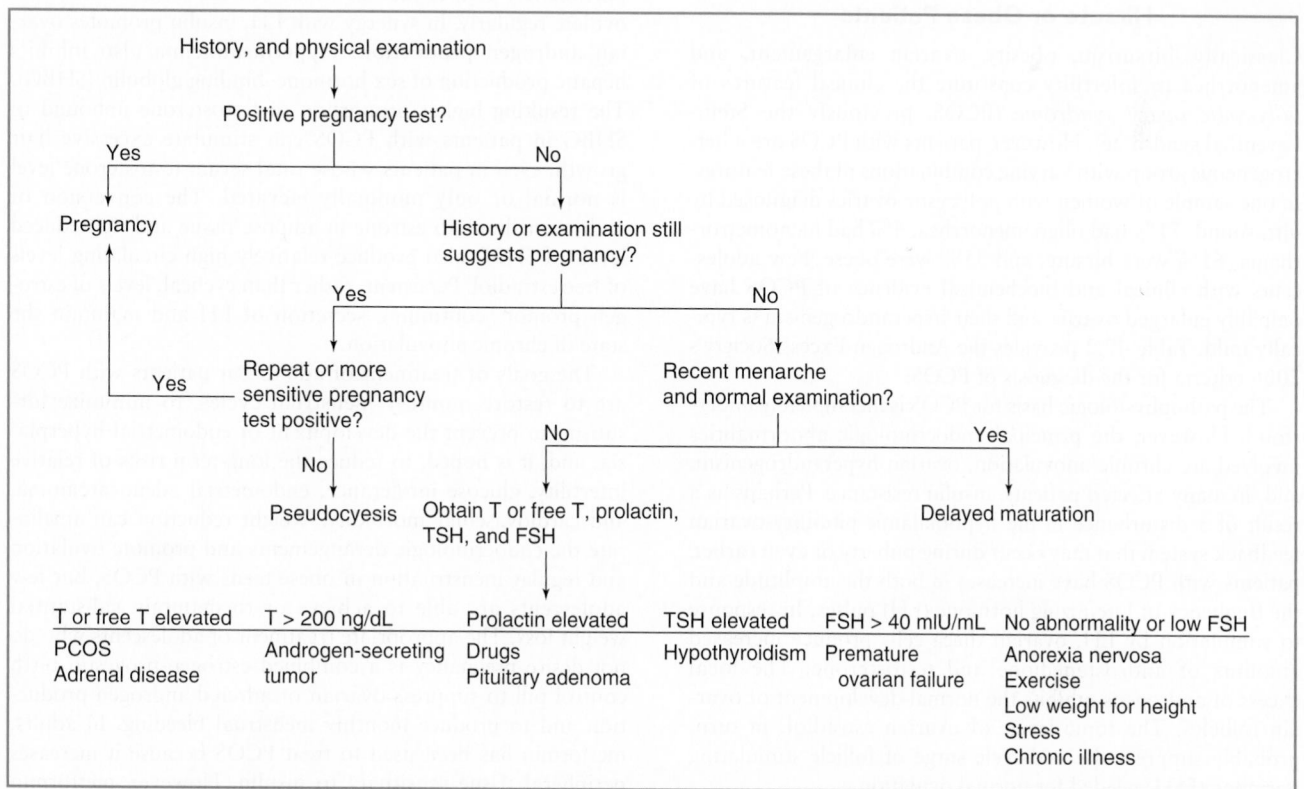

FIGURE 47.1 Strategy for initial diagnostic evaluation of the patient with oligomenorrhea. T, testosterone; TSH, thyroid-stimulating hormone; FSH, follicle-stimulating hormone; PCOS, polycystic ovary syndrome.

oligomenorrhea can proceed at a deliberate pace (Fig. 47.1). During the first 2 years after menarche, it is not unusual for girls to have an occasional menstrual cycle that lasts less than 25 days or more than 40 days. As a rule, if an adolescent complains of only one or two prolonged menstrual cycles, is fewer than 2 years past menarche, and is not sexually active, further investigation in the emergency department (ED) is not warranted. However, the ED physician should be aware that, among adolescents who report oligomenorrhea at baseline (defined as an average cycle length of 42 to 180 days), the prognosis for developing regular cycles is guarded. After 3 years of follow-up, more than half will continue to have abnormally long cycles.

Adolescents with oligomenorrhea that has persisted for longer than 2 years after menarche or that involves three or more cycles longer than 42 days during the past year are candidates for further diagnostic evaluation, although ordinarily this ought to be accomplished in an outpatient setting rather than in an ED. In the interview, historical details about the patient's menstrual pattern, growth, endocrine and central nervous systems, psychological status, and medications should be sought specifically. On physical examination, the patient's height and weight, skin, breasts, and pelvis should be checked. Because galactorrhea is not always spontaneous, the examiner should try to express fluid manually from the patient's breasts. The completed examination will separate the majority of patients who have no notable abnormalities from a minority with the important findings of hirsutism, obesity, galactorrhea, and marked thinness.

Hirsute or Obese Patients

Classically, hirsutism, obesity, ovarian enlargement, and amenorrhea or infertility constitute the clinical features of *polycystic ovary syndrome* (PCOS, previously the Stein-Leventhal syndrome). However, patients with PCOS are a heterogeneous group with varying combinations of these features. In one sample of women with polycystic ovaries diagnosed by ultrasound, 71% had oligoamenorrhea, 4% had menometrorrhagia, 61% were hirsute, and 35% were obese. Few adolescents with clinical and biochemical evidence of PCOS have palpably enlarged ovaries and their hyperandrogenism is typically mild. Table 47.2 provides the Androgen Excess Society's 2006 criteria for the diagnosis of PCOS.

The pathophysiologic basis for PCOS is incompletely understood. However, the principal endocrinologic abnormalities involved are chronic anovulation, ovarian hyperandrogenism, and, in many affected patients, insulin resistance. Perhaps as a result of a disturbance in the hypothalamic-pituitary-ovarian feedback system that may occur during puberty or even earlier, patients with PCOS have increases in both the amplitude and the frequency of luteinizing hormone (LH) pulses. In response to stimulation by LH, ovarian theca cells produce increased amounts of androstenedione and testosterone. The local excess of androgens inhibits the normal development of ovarian follicles. The tonic levels of ovarian estradiol, in turn, probably suppress the mid-cycle surge of follicle-stimulating hormone (FSH) needed for normal ovulation.

A substantial number of patients with PCOS have insulin resistance, and the proportion of women who do have it increases with age. This is independent of obesity: the insulin resistance in both lean and obese women with PCOS is dispro-

TABLE 47.2

ANDROGEN EXCESS SOCIETY CRITERIA FOR THE DIAGNOSIS OF POLYCYSTIC OVARY SYNDROME (2006)

Diagnostic criteria	Comment
1. Hirsutism and/or hyperandrogenemia	Hirsutism present in about 60% of patients; elevated free or total testosterone or DHEAS in 60%–80% of patients
2. Oligoanovulation and/or polycystic ovaries	Oligoamenorrhea present in 70%–100% of patients; ovarian morphology (by transvaginal ultrasound) not required for diagnosis
3. Other potential disorders excluded	Especially nonclassic congenital adrenal hyperplasia and androgen-secreting tumors

DHEAS, dehydroepiandrosterone sulfate.
Adapted from Azziz R, Carmina E, Dewailly D, et al. Position Statement: criteria for defining polycystic ovary syndrome as a predominantly hyperandrogenic syndrome: an Androgen Excess Society guideline. *J Clin Endocrinol Metab* 2006;91:4237–4245.

portionately greater than in women of the same habitus who ovulate regularly. In synergy with LH, insulin promotes ovarian androgen production. Hyperinsulinemia also inhibits hepatic production of sex hormone–binding globulin (SHBG). The resulting higher proportion of testosterone unbound to SHBG in patients with PCOS can stimulate excessive hair growth, even in patients whose total serum testosterone level is normal or only minimally elevated. The conversion of androstenedione to estrone in adipose tissue and the reduced levels of SHBG also produce relatively high circulating levels of free estradiol. Persistent, rather than cyclical, levels of estrogen promote continuing secretion of LH and maintain the state of chronic anovulation.

The goals of treatment of adolescent patients with PCOS are to restore monthly menstrual cycles, to minimize hirsutism, to prevent the development of endometrial hyperplasia, and, it is hoped, to reduce the long-term risks of relative infertility, glucose intolerance, endometrial adenocarcinoma, and cardiovascular morbidity. Weight reduction can ameliorate the endocrinologic derangements and promote ovulation and regular menstruation in obese teens with PCOS, but few adolescents are able to achieve or to maintain substantial weight loss. The appropriate treatment of adolescents who do not desire pregnancy is a combined estrogen-progestin birth control pill to suppress ovarian or adrenal androgen production and to produce monthly menstrual bleeding. In adults, metformin has been used to treat PCOS because it increases peripheral tissue sensitivity to insulin. However, metformin often restores fertility (increasing the risk of unwanted pregnancy in adolescents). Studies to date of metformin use in adolescents have been limited by small numbers of subjects, lack of control groups, and short follow-up intervals.

Nonclassic *congenital adrenal hyperplasia* is a rare cause of oligomenorrhea associated with hyperandrogenism. It is usually indistinguishable clinically from PCOS and can be excluded by a normal 17-hydroxyprogesterone level in the morning during the follicular phase of the menstrual cycle. Other rare causes of oligomenorrhea, including *Cushing's disease* and *ovarian and adrenal tumors*, should be suspected in patients with hirsutism accompanied by signs of glucocorticoid excess, or with rapidly developing, more severe virilization (male-pattern baldness, deepening of the voice, clitoromegaly), and in those with testosterone levels above 200 ng per dL.

Galactorrhea

Hyperprolactinemia occurs in approximately 25% of adult women with secondary amenorrhea but is a much less common cause of oligomenorrhea in adolescents. Nevertheless, the possibility of hyperprolactinemia must be considered in all adolescents with oligomenorrhea because only 40% to 50% of hyperprolactinemic patients have spontaneous or expressible galactorrhea. The constellation of oligomenorrhea, galactorrhea, and hyperprolactinemia can be produced by many drugs (Table 47.3), especially antipsychotic agents; by the discontinuation of birth control pills; rarely by cutaneous or neurogenic stimulation of the breasts; and by excessive secretion of prolactin itself (e.g., primary hypothyroidism, pituitary adenoma). Drugs produce hyperprolactinemia by blocking pituitary dopamine receptors or interfering in other ways with dopaminergic or serotoninergic central nervous system pathways. Rarely, in hypothyroid patients, hypothalamic thyroid-releasing hormone acts as a prolactin-releasing factor, resulting in galactorrhea. Breastfeeding is an obvious physiologic cause of prolactin secretion and oligomenorrhea. The occasional patient with galactorrhea but with a normal prolactin level should be reevaluated periodically in an effort to identify a treatable cause of the problem.

Thin Patients

In patients who have eating disorders or malnutrition, and in those who participate in sports that emphasize thinness, recent research indicates that *caloric intake insufficient to meet energy expenditures* or an "energy drain" is probably the cause of oligomenorrhea. Leptin levels fluctuate in relation to body fat stores, are positively correlated with body mass index, and are lowered during fasting. The normal diurnal pattern of leptin concentration is absent in amenorrheic women. Hypothalamic neurons involved in controlling the gonadotropin-releasing hormone pulse generator have leptin receptors. Levels of the hormone ghrelin are elevated in amenorrheic women with either anorexia nervosa or high levels of exercise. Thus, leptin and possibly ghrelin appear to serve as signals to the hypothalamic-pituitary system concerning overall energy balance.

Accordingly, in assessing the nonpregnant adolescent with oligomenorrhea whose body mass index is low, one should inquire routinely about recent weight loss, chronic illness or other causes of negative energy balance, behavior characteristic of anorexia nervosa (Table 47.4), a restrictive eating pattern, and *strenuous exercise* (especially sports that put a premium on low body weight such as long-distance running, dance, and gymnastics). Many amenorrheic women who are athletes restrict their food intake; amenorrhea, eating disorders, and osteoporosis together are termed "the female athletic triad."

All Other Patients

Among adolescents who do not have hirsutism, obesity, galactorrhea, obesity, or excessive thinness, suppression of the hypothalamic-pituitary axis is the most common cause of oligomenorrhea that occurs more or persists for at least 2 years after menarche. Although oligomenorrhea in otherwise normal-appearing adolescents has historically been ascribed to psychosocial stressors (family disruption, moving, depression), many patients with apparently psychogenic menstrual irregularity prove on careful evaluation to have disordered eating patterns or nutritional deficits.

TABLE 47.3

PARTIAL LIST OF DRUGS THAT CAN CAUSE HYPERPROLACTINEMIA AND/OR GALACTORRHEA

1. *Antipsychotic and antidepressant agents*
   Phenothiazines [e.g., chlorpromazine (Thorazine), clomipramine (Anafranil), fluphenazine (Prolixin), prochlorperazine (Compazine), thioridazine (Mellaril)]
   Haloperidol (Haldol)
   Pimozide (Orap)
   Risperidone (Risperdal)
   Thiothixene (Navane)
2. *Drugs used to treat gastrointestinal disorders*
   Cimetidine (Tagamet)
   Metoclopramide (Reglan)
3. *Antihypertensive Agents*
   Methyldopa (Aldomet)
   Reserpine (Hydromox, Serpasil, others)
   Verapamil (Calan, Isoptin)
4. *Opiates*
   Codeine
   Morphine

TABLE 47.4

DSM-IV-TR CRITERIA FOR THE DIAGNOSIS OF ANOREXIA NERVOSA

1. Refusal to maintain body weight at or above a minimally normal weight for age and height (i.e., weight loss or failure to gain weight leading to body weight <85% of that expected for age and height).
2. Intense fear of gaining weight or becoming fat, even though underweight.
3. Disturbed experience of one's body weight or shape, undue influence of weight or shape on self-evaluation, or denial of the seriousness of the current low body weight.
4. In postmenarcheal females, amenorrhea (i.e., absence of at least three or more consecutive anticipated cycles). Menstruation induced by hormonal treatment is excluded.

Adapted from American Psychiatric Association. *Diagnostic and Statistical Manual of Mental Disorders, Fourth Edition, Text Revision.* Washington, DC: American Psychiatric Association, 2000.

Other diagnostic possibilities for oligomenorrheic patients with no abnormal physical findings include a wide variety of conditions. About half of women using contraceptive *medroxyprogesterone* injections for 12 months have amenorrhea; after 2 years of use, the proportion with amenorrhea is 68%. Amenorrhea also occurs in about 2% of menstrual cycles among patients taking *birth control pills* that contain 50 μg or less of estrogen. However, amenorrhea persisting 12 months after the last injection of medroxyprogesterone or 6 months after birth control pills have been stopped should be evaluated in the standard fashion.

Hypothyroidism and *hyperthyroidism* can both produce menstrual irregularities. Although hypothyroidism has classically been associated with metrorrhagia, recent data indicate that oligomenorrhea is more common than metrorrhagia among women with hypothyroidism.

Many patients with hyperprolactinemia and oligomenorrhea do not have concomitant galactorrhea that would otherwise prompt a medical investigation. Similarly, although hirsutism and obesity are classic features of PCOS, many adolescent patients with oligomenorrhea and the endocrinologic abnormalities of PCOS lack one or both of these signs. A history of hot flashes, antineoplastic chemotherapy, pelvic irradiation, or autoimmune disease suggests the diagnosis of *premature ovarian failure*. *Endometrial destruction* that results from overly vigorous curettage or pelvic tuberculosis is an exceedingly rare cause of oligomenorrhea.

Approach to Diagnosis

Patients with oligomenorrhea but few other symptoms or signs of disease require laboratory evaluation to differentiate among the many potential causes of oligomenorrhea after pregnancy has been excluded. Figure 47.1 outlines a strategy for initial diagnostic evaluation. Determinations of serum levels of FSH, testosterone (T), and/or free testosterone (free T), prolactin, and thyroid-stimulating hormone (TSH) are needed either to corroborate the suspected diagnosis or to categorize the patient whose history and physical examination have provided few diagnostic clues. Other laboratory tests should be performed as warranted by the clinical situation. The finding of a mildly elevated total or free T level constitutes strong evidence for a diagnosis of PCOS. A testosterone level of more than 200 ng per dL suggests an ovarian or adrenal tumor. An elevated prolactin level indicates a pituitary microadenoma in patients who are not taking any of the drugs known to cause hyperprolactinemia and galactorrhea (Table 47.3). An elevated TSH level points to hypothyroidism either as the cause of oligomenorrhea or as a concomitant condition. FSH values of more than 40 mIU per mL confirm ovarian failure as the source of difficulty. If the laboratory evaluation discloses no abnormalities or only a low FSH level, the patient probably has one of the many conditions that cause hypothalamic-pituitary suppression. For definitive diagnosis, which may require additional laboratory testing, and for ongoing clinical management, all patients with oligomenorrhea should be referred to their primary care providers.

The administration of exogenous progestin is often advocated as an in vivo test of ovarian and endometrial function for oligomenorrheic patients. If the hypothalamic-pituitary axis is producing some gonadotropin, the ovaries are responding with some estradiol production, and the uterine endometrium is growing appropriately, then the addition of exogenous progestin (medroxyprogesterone acetate 10 mg per day for 7 days) will be followed by at least scanty menstrual bleeding within 7 days after the treatment is completed. This "withdrawal" flow, if it appears, provides the patient and her physician with tangible evidence of the basic integrity of these organs and indicates that anovulation is the source of the amenorrhea. For diagnosis in adolescents, however, laboratory investigation is much preferable to progestin administration. Nearly all nonpregnant adolescents with oligomenorrhea do have anovulation and will have a withdrawal bleed. Interposing this step merely postpones the laboratory evaluation that the clinician must still conduct to arrive at a diagnosis and to select an appropriate treatment.

Suggested Readings

Bastian LA, Piscitelli JT. Is this patient pregnant? Can you reliably rule in or rule out early pregnancy by clinical examination? *JAMA* 1997;278: 586–591.

Cannavo S, Venturino M, Curto L, et al. Clinical presentation and outcome of pituitary adenomas in teenagers. *Clin Endocrinol* 2003;58:519–527.

Cohen LE. Cancer treatment and the ovary: the effects of chemotherapy and radiation. *Ann N Y Acad Sci* 2008;1135:123–125.

Cole LA, Khanlian SA, Sutton JM, et al. Accuracy of home pregnancy tests at the time of missed menses. *Am J Obstet Gynecol* 2004;190:100–105.

Escobar-Morreale HF, Sanchon R, San Millan JL. A prospective study of the prevalence of nonclassical congenital adrenal hyperplasia among women presenting with hyperandrogenic symptoms and signs. *J Clin Endocrinol Metab* 2008;93:527–533.

Guttmacher Institute. *State policies in brief: Parental involvement in minors' abortions,* and *Counseling and waiting periods for abortion.* New York, NY: Guttmacher Institute, 2009. http://www.guttmacher.org/statecenter/spibs/. Accessed October 13, 2009.

Haddad PM, Wieck A. Antipsychotic-induced hyperprolactinaemia: mechanisms, clinical features and management. *Drugs* 2004;64:2291–2314.

Hillard PJA. Menstruation in adolescents: what's normal, what's not. *Ann N Y Acad Sci* 2008;1135:29–35.

O'Brien RF, Emans SJ. Polycystic ovary syndrome in adolescents. *J Pediatr Adolesc Gynecol* 2008;21:119–128.

Paradise JE. Evaluation of oligomenorrhea in adolescence. *UpToDate* Version 17.2. http://www.uptodate.com. Accessed October 13, 2009.

Pfeifer SM, Dayal M. Treatment of the adolescent patient with polycystic ovary syndrome. *Obstet Gynecol Clin North Am* 2003;30:337–352.

Redmond GP. Thyroid dysfunction and women's reproductive health. *Thyroid* 2004;14(suppl):S5–S15.

Stafford DEJ. Altered hypothalamic-pituitary-ovarian axis function in young female athletes. *Treat Endocrinol* 2005;4:147–154.

Trivax B, Azziz R. Diagnosis of polycystic ovary syndrome. *Clin Obstet Gynecol* 2007;50:168–177.

van Hooff MHA, Voorhorst FJ, Kaptein MBH, et al. Predictive value of menstrual cycle pattern, body mass index, hormone levels and polycystic ovaries at age 15 years for oligo-amenorrhoea at age 18 years. *Hum Reprod* 2004;19: 383–392.

Waggoner W, Boots LR, Azziz R. Total testosterone and DHEAS levels as predictors of androgen-secreting neoplasms: a populational study. *Gynecol Endocrinol* 1999;13:394–400.

Warren MP, Perlroth ME. The effects of intense exercise on the female reproductive system. *J Endocrinol* 2001;170:3–11.

CHAPTER 48 ■ ORAL LESIONS

MARK G. ROBACK, MD

Children of all ages, from birth forward, experience oral lesions, which may represent a wide range of illnesses. Oral lesions may be associated with benign conditions that completely resolve without intervention or may be representative of life-threatening diseases. The differential diagnosis includes a large number of localized congenital and acquired causes; however, lesions associated with systemic disease must also be considered (Fig. 48.1 and Table 48.1). Most often, patients with isolated complaints (e.g., a mouth sore or mass, drooling, pain, fever) represent common, self-limited conditions (Table 48.2). However, a complete history and physical examination is essential for all patients with oral lesions to rule out systemic and potentially life-threatening diseases (Table 48.3) that may present initially with only isolated mouth findings.

PATHOPHYSIOLOGY

Oral lesions may result from localized or systemic pathophysiologic processes. Localized causes include congenital masses and cysts, infectious diseases, and oral tumors. Systemic illnesses with prominent oral involvement include a number of infectious and other inflammatory or toxin-mediated conditions. Given the broad spectrum of illnesses presenting with oral lesions, it is convenient to discuss individual causes under specific headings within the differential diagnosis. Several conditions with typical oral lesions exist that do not comfortably fit under any of these headings and are discussed in the section on miscellaneous oral lesions.

DIFFERENTIAL DIAGNOSIS

Congenital Oral Lesions

Most oral lesions present at birth or early infancy represent benign findings. Patients are largely asymptomatic, and the lesions resolve spontaneously.

Epstein's pearls occur in more than 60% of newborns as small, white milia in the midline of the hard palate. These epithelial inclusion cysts are often found in clusters and resolve over the first few months of life. Epithelial pearls are similar to Epstein's pearls and appear as shiny, small, white, self-limited lesions that occur on the gums.

Bohn's nodules are also self-limited cysts that appear on the mandibular or maxillary dental ridges. Dental lamina cysts occur on the alveolar ridge of newborns and represent trapped remnants of the dental lamina.

Natal teeth are the premature eruption of primary teeth and are found at birth (natal) or within the first month of life (neonatal). These teeth are either supernumerary or true deciduous teeth and are usually found in the lower incisor region. Natal teeth may lead to ulcerations of the underside of the tongue, called Riga-Fede disease.

Patients with ankyloglossia may be referred to as "tongue tied" because of congenital shortening of the lingual frenum, which limits their ability to fully extend the tongue. Surgical correction is considered for patients when speech is affected.

Epulis is a congenital, fibrous, sarcomatous tumor that arises from the periosteum of the mandible or maxilla. The mass is firm and pedunculated and may regress spontaneously. Excision is required if the epulis interferes with feeding or breathing, or for cosmetic reasons.

Lymphangioma is a benign congenital tumor of lymphatic vessels appearing on the tongue, lips, or buccal mucosa at birth or in early infancy. Hemangiomas are benign vascular malformations present at birth that may become more apparent as the patient grows. Oral hemangiomas are typically accompanied by vascular lesions elsewhere in the body, especially on the skin.

Infectious Oral Lesions

Infectious oral lesions are typically manifestations of viral infections but may be caused by bacterial or fungal infections as well (see Chapter 92).

Candidiasis, or thrush, is white plaque on the buccal mucosa, gingivae, and palate that will not "rub off" with a tongue blade. Caused by *Candida albicans*, thrush is common in neonates and infants. When thrush occurs after infancy, the immune status of the patient must be considered. Oral candidiasis most commonly occurs in patients infected with human immunodeficiency virus (HIV).

The typical lesions of herpes simplex virus (HSV) are groups of vesicles on an erythematous base that may become unroofed and appear as erosions in and around the mouth. Infections may be primary or recurrent. Herpes gingivostomatitis, most commonly caused by HSV type 1 (HSV-1), represents primary infection that typically occurs in young children and infants. These patients have pain, fever, and drooling. Herpes labialis manifests as recurrent painful lesions that occur on the lips, most often the lower lip. Herpes labialis, or "cold sores," may be accompanied by an acute febrile illness, extensive sun exposure, or stress.

Hand-foot-mouth disease is characterized by discrete shallow erosions in the mouth, especially on the soft palate, accompanied by erythematous papulovesicular lesions on the hands and feet. High fever may be associated with this enteroviral,

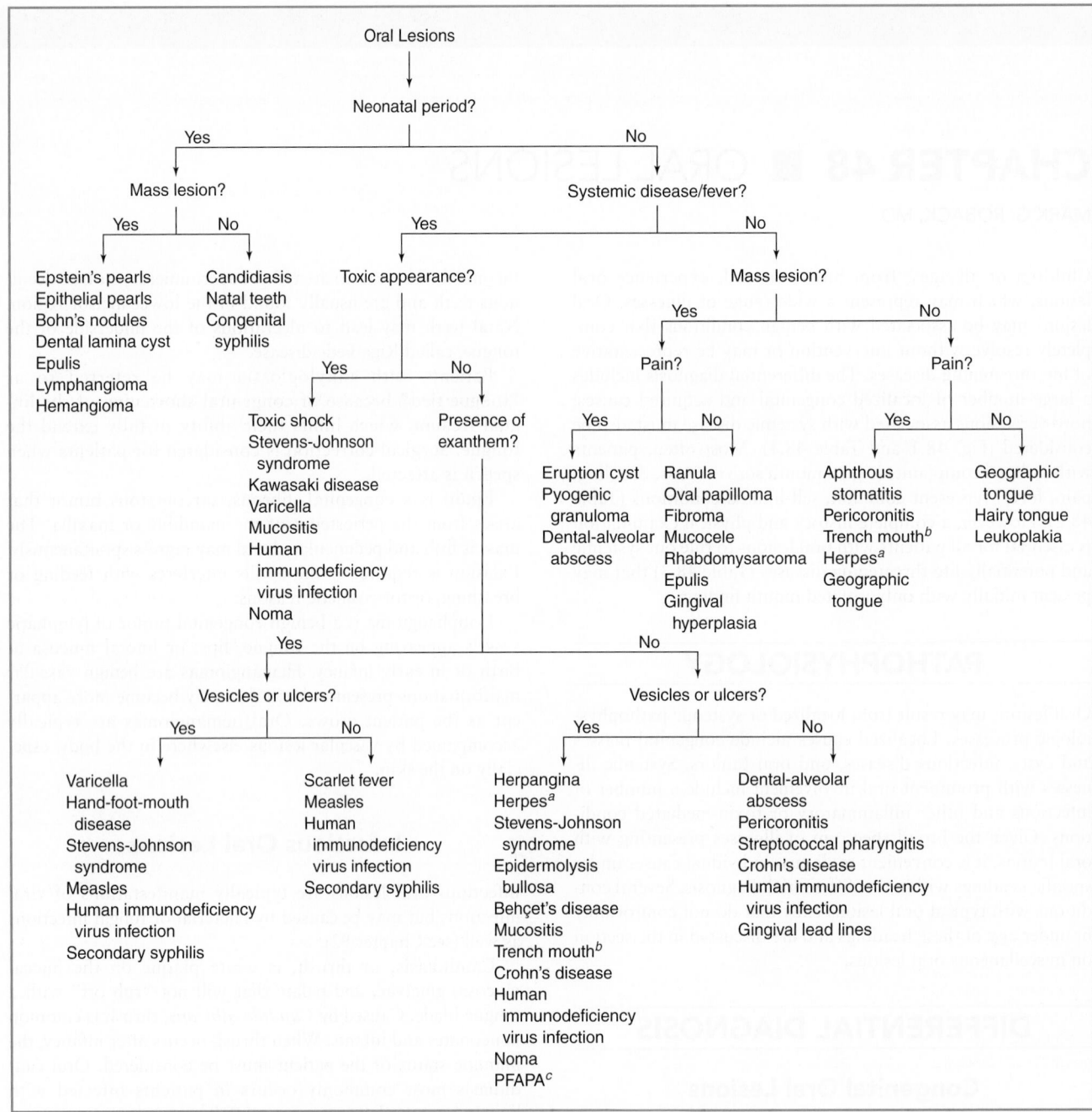

FIGURE 48.1 Oral lesions. [a]Herpes gingivostomatitis or labialis. [b]Trench mouth, acute necrotizing ulcerative gingivitis. [c]PFAPA, *p*eriodic *f*ever, *a*phthous stomatitis, *p*haryngitis, and cervical *a*denitis syndrome.

typically coxsackievirus, mediated disease that is self-limited in nature. Supportive treatment, specifically antipyretics/analgesics and adequate oral hydration, is usually sufficient therapy.

Herpangina is also a group A coxsackievirus infection that is characterized by vesicles or ulcers on the pharynx of patients with fever, muscle aches, and malaise. Similar to hand-foot-mouth disease, the treatment of herpangina is largely supportive in nature.

The characteristic "strawberry tongue" seen in streptococcal scarlet fever is the result of hypertrophic red papillae on a thick white coat. Palatal petechiae are often present, as is the typical "sandpaper" papular rash on an erythematous base that blanches on palpation, involving the trunk and back. Streptococcal pharyngitis without exanthem often presents with strawberry tongue and palatal petechiae.

Koplik's spots—pinpoint white macules on markedly erythematous mucous membranes—occur during the prodrome

TABLE 48.1

DIFFERENTIAL DIAGNOSIS OF ORAL LESIONS

Congenital oral lesions
Epstein's pearls
Epithelial pearls
Bohn's nodules
Dental lamina cysts
Natal teeth
Ankyloglossia
Epulis (gum boil)
Lymphangioma
Hemangioma

Infectious oral lesions
Candidiasis
Herpes simplex
    Gingivostomatitis—primary
    Labialis—recurrent (cold sores)
Hand-foot-mouth disease
Herpangina
Scarlet fever
Streptococcal pharyngitis
Measles
Varicella
Human immunodeficiency virus infection
Dental-alveolar abscess
Pericoronitis
Acute necrotizing ulcerative gingivitis (trench mouth)
Noma
Syphilis
    Acquired (secondary)
    Congenital
Hairy tongue

Tumorous oral lesions
Eruption cyst
Oral papilloma
Fibroma
Mucocele
Ranula
Pyogenic granuloma
Rhabdomyosarcoma

Oral lesions associated with systemic disease
Stevens-Johnson syndrome
Toxic shock syndrome
Mucositis
Kawasaki disease
Crohn's disease
Behçet's syndrome
Epidermolysis bullosa
Gingival lead lines

Miscellaneous oral lesions
Aphthous stomatitis
Geographic tongue
Gingival hyperplasia
Leukoplakia

PFAPA, periodic fever, aphthous stomatitis, pharyngitis, and cervical adenitis.

TABLE 48.2

COMMON CAUSES OF ORAL LESIONS

Candidiasis
Aphthous stomatitis
Herpes simplex
    Gingivostomatitis—primary
    Labialis—recurrent
Hand-foot-mouth disease
Herpangina

of measles, which includes cough, coryza, conjunctivitis, and fever. By the time the characteristic rash occurs, Koplik's spots have typically resolved.

Varicella lesions occurring in the mouth result in painful vesicles, which may become unroofed, on an erythematous base. Patients may be reluctant to swallow because of pain. Unless secondary bacterial infection occurs, these lesions are self-limited.

Oral lesions will be the initial presenting sign in approximately half of children with perinatally acquired HIV infection. Oral candidiasis, parotid enlargement, herpes simplex, hairy leukoplakia, aphthous ulcers, and necrotizing ulcerative gingivitis occur commonly in children infected with HIV. Blue, purple, or red macules, papules, or nodules on the palate suggest oral Kaposi's sarcoma, whereas diffuse swelling, discrete nodules, or ulcers of any oral mucosal surface may indicate non–Hodgkin's lymphoma. The prevalence of oral lesions appears to decrease with highly active antiviral therapy and increase in children with low CD4 percentage and may signal advancing disease.

The pain, erythema, and swelling of the gingiva seen with dental-alveolar abscesses may be associated with fever and loosening or extrusion of the associated tooth. Significant lymphadenopathy and facial cellulitis may develop. Causative organisms are streptococci and anaerobes. Antibiotic therapy with penicillin is secondary in importance to drainage of the abscess.

Pericoronitis is the local infection of the gingiva surrounding an erupting tooth. Although penicillin therapy may be required, good oral hygiene is essential. Lymphadenopathy and facial swelling may accompany pericoronitis.

Acute necrotizing ulcerative gingivitis (ANUG), also called trench mouth or Vincent's angina, is a spirochetal infection of the gingiva that occurs in adolescents. Patients report tender, bleeding gums and breath that has a fetid odor. Gums are hyperemic and appear "punched out" secondary

TABLE 48.3

LIFE-THREATENING CAUSES OF ORAL LESIONS

Stevens-Johnson syndrome
Kawasaki disease
Toxic shock syndrome
Human immunodeficiency virus infection
Noma

to tissue loss between the teeth. Treatment involves attention to oral hygiene, mouth rinses with a dilute hydrogen peroxide solution, oral penicillin, and debridement of necrotic tissue.

Noma, or cancrum oris, is a potentially fatal, gangrenous anaerobic infection of the oral cavity that may rapidly spread outward to involve large areas of the face. It typically begins as an oral mucosal ulcer or as ANUG, particularly after a bout of measles or other intercurrent illness in malnourished or immunocompromised patients. Currently, it is being recognized increasingly in HIV-infected and/or otherwise malnourished children in sub-Saharan Africa.

Although infection is present at birth, the oral lesions of congenital syphilis may not become obvious until several months of age. Erythematous papules are seen in the mouth and other mucocutaneous sites. *Hutchinson's teeth*, peg-shaped, superior, central incisors, are not present until later in life. The secondary stage of acquired syphilis is characterized by patches of ulcers or raised lesions in the mouth and is seen in association with generalized rash, fever, malaise, and adenopathy.

Patients receiving long-term antibiotic therapy may develop elongation of filiform papillae of the dorsum of the tongue and a "hairy" appearance from fungal overgrowth called hairy tongue. Hairy leukoplakia of the lateral aspects of the tongue is found in HIV-infected patients in association with intraepithelial proliferation of Epstein-Barr virus infection.

Tumorous Oral Lesions

The vast majority of tumorous oral lesions in children are self-limited and benign in nature. Congenital oral tumors such as hemangioma, lymphangioma, and epulis have been considered previously.

Eruption cysts are associated with the eruption of teeth, appear on the alveolar ridge, and may contain blood.

Oral papillomas are fingerlike extensions from the epithelium of the tongue, gums, lips, or buccal mucosa. They are typically benign, although a small percentage of papillomas may become malignant.

A fibroma is a benign, smooth mass with a sessile base that frequently develops secondary to soft-tissue injury from minor trauma. The tongue, lips, buccal mucosa, and palate are common sites for the development of fibromas.

Mucoceles are soft, well-demarcated masses that arise secondary to obstruction of salivary glands. Patients are generally otherwise asymptomatic; however, excision or marsupialization is typically required.

Ranula is a retention cyst or mucocele of the submaxillary or sublingual duct. Ranulas are typically seen on the underside of the tongue or on either side of the frenulum on the floor of the mouth. Initial management of pediatric oral cavity ranulas consists of observation for spontaneous resolution. If the lesion does not resolve or recurs repeatedly, surgical treatment is recommended.

Pyogenic granuloma represents granulation tissue that develops in response to an irritant such as a trauma or a foreign body. Most commonly found on the gingiva, pyogenic granulomas are also found on the tongue, lips, and buccal mucosa. Treatment involves incision and drainage. Recurrence is common, especially when a foreign body is present.

Although 35% to 40% of cases will present in the head and neck region, rhabdomyosarcoma is a rare malignant tumor of the oral cavity. These lesions are ulcerative in nature, characterized by rapid growth, and may present with bleeding. Associated signs and symptoms are usually attributed to the mass lesion or obstructive sequelae. Other malignant oral tumors such as fibrosarcoma, carcinoma of the parotid, and osteosarcoma occur but are even more rare than rhabdomyosarcoma.

Oral Lesions Associated with Systemic Disease

Stevens-Johnson syndrome, a severe form of erythema multiforme, consists of an inflammatory process that typically involves mucous membranes in addition to the skin. Oral lesions are erythematous plaques on the mucosa of the oral cavity and lips that develop into vesicles or bullae and may become hemorrhagic. This potentially life-threatening disorder is believed to be secondary to a drug reaction or to follow infections.

Toxic shock syndrome may manifest erythema of the oropharynx and a strawberry tongue in patients with a diffuse erythematous macular exanthem, hyperemic mucous membranes, fever, and signs of shock. This toxin-mediated disease is caused by *Staphylococcus aureus* and may be associated with tampon use or nasal carriage of this organism. Toxin-mediated disease associated with streptococci also presents with diffuse erythema of the skin and oropharynx and may progress to septic shock.

Mucositis presents as ulcers, exudate, and pseudomembranes on the gingivae and buccal mucosa of patients, with neutropenia often secondary to chemotherapy. Lesions are extremely painful, and the breath becomes fetid.

Kawasaki disease is a potentially life-threatening disorder that typically presents with an array of findings, including prolonged fever, rash, lymphadenopathy, nonpurulent conjunctivitis, and edema of the hands and feet. Oral changes of Kawasaki disease include red, dry, cracked lips, erythematous oropharynx, and strawberry tongue. Therapy is directed toward the prevention of coronary aneurysm development.

The inflammatory lesions of Crohn's disease may occur in any portion of the gastrointestinal tract. Oral lesions, seen most often in adolescents and young adults, consist of ulcers, polypoid papulous hyperplastic mucosa, and edema found on the lips, gingiva, vestibular sulci, and buccal mucosa. Immunosuppressive therapy with steroids and azathioprine has yielded mixed results.

Chronic, recurrent ulcers surrounded by erythema and gray exudate are found anywhere in the oral cavity in patients with Behçet's syndrome. Similar lesions occur on the skin, and the genitourinary tract may also be involved. Behçet's syndrome is rare, affecting older children and adolescents, usually boys.

More than 15 types of hereditary epidermolysis bullosa have been described. This rare, vesiculobullous condition affects mucous membranes and teeth, as well as the skin. Scarring may lead to restriction of mouth opening.

Bluish purple "lead lines" on the gingivae have been described, primarily in adults, with chronic lead toxicity and poor oral hygiene.

Miscellaneous Oral Lesions

Aphthous stomatitis is the ulceration of the oral epidermis of unknown cause. These recurrent lesions typically present as 5- to 10-mm ulcerations with a rim of erythema on the buccal mucosa, lips, and lateral aspect of the tongue. The lesions are painful, but patients do not experience fever. The lesions resolve spontaneously after 7 to 10 days.

Less commonly, aphthous stomatitis also occurs with a constellation of symptoms seen in the syndrome of PFAPA (*periodic fever, aphthous stomatitis, pharyngitis, and cervical adenitis*). Children, usually between 2 and 6 years of age, experience the acute onset of periodic fever with temperature more than 39°C, which usually lasts 4 or 5 days in association with aphthous stomatitis, pharyngitis, and cervical adenitis. The fevers and associated symptoms recur every 2 to 8 weeks. Although the episodes resolve spontaneously, the use of glucocorticoids has been reported to be effective in arresting the symptoms of PFAPA. Affected children grow normally without associated disease or long-term sequelae. Tonsillectomy has been reported to prevent recurrence. There is no known etiology of PFAPA.

Geographic tongue represents a benign inflammatory disorder that results in migratory smooth annular patches on the tongue. Although typically asymptomatic, patients may complain of pain. Geographic tongue is typically seen in children younger than 4 years. No treatment is required.

Gingival hyperplasia seen in patients receiving long-term anticonvulsant therapy with phenytoin is irreversible. However, gingival overgrowth that occurs in association with the medications cyclosporine and nifedipine is reversible with discontinuation of the drugs. Poor dental hygiene appears to play a role in the cause. The gingivae undergo fibrous enlargement but are not inflamed or painful. Gingival fibromatosis is an inherited form of gingival hyperplasia.

Leukoplakia of the oral mucosa develops secondary to long-term smokeless tobacco use. These painless, leathery, white patches or plaques occur in areas of greatest tobacco exposure, typically on the mucosa of the buccal sulcus. Significant exposure to tobacco may result in dysplasia or carcinoma.

EVALUATION AND DECISION

When evaluating patients with complaints of oral lesions, it is important to consider a myriad of associated signs and symptoms while taking a complete history and performing the physical examination. The patient's age, general health and appearance, presence of an exanthem or fever, and whether the lesions are painful must be considered. Once the lesions are identified, they should be further characterized by color, type,

and location and considered in the context of any additional physical findings.

Neonates with oral lesions can be divided into two groups on the basis of the morphology of the lesions. Discrete masses usually represent congenital disorders, most of which are self-limited. Candidiasis, which involves the oral cavity more diffusely, is also common.

Among older children, toxic-appearing patients require immediate evaluation for potentially life-threatening disease. Patients with conditions listed in Table 48.3 have associated findings such as diffuse cutaneous rash, hyperemia of other mucous membranes, or poor perfusion indicative of shock. However, Stevens-Johnson syndrome may cause isolated oral lesions initially and then rapidly progress to systemic involvement.

Once life-threatening causes have been considered, careful history and physical examination may lead to the diagnosis of other systemic diseases. Weight loss, abdominal pain, and diarrhea with or without blood loss suggest Crohn's disease, whereas genital ulceration in an adolescent boy points to Behçet's syndrome or secondary syphilis.

The presence of rash and fever makes disorders of infectious etiology more likely. Measles, varicella, scarlet fever, and hand-foot-mouth disease are generally diagnosed by history and physical examination alone. Laboratory evaluation might include a throat culture for streptococci and serologic testing for measles or HIV when these infections are suspected.

Infectious causes of oral lesions without exanthem may display obvious findings such as cachexia and alopecia in the neutropenic patient with mucositis, or they may be relatively localized to the oropharynx as in herpangina, herpes gingivostomatitis or labialis, and dental infections, which may or may not cause fever and lymphadenopathy.

Oral lesions without overt signs of systemic disease are mostly congenital or tumorous in nature. Lesions found in the newborn and during infancy are largely self-limited and most will resolve spontaneously. A few, including lymphangioma, hemangioma, and congenital epulis, may require intervention.

Children and adolescents experience an array of oral lesions not associated with obvious signs of systemic disease that are typically further delineated by considering the type of lesion (i.e., mass, vesicle, ulcer) and whether they are painful. Most of these processes require little or no therapy. Rhabdomyosarcoma is an obvious exception to this observation.

Suggested Readings

Bentley JM, Barankin B, Guenther LC. A review of common pediatric lip lesions: herpes simplex/recurrent herpes labialis, impetigo, mucoceles, and hemangiomas. *Clin Pediatr* 2003;42:475–482.

Berthold P. Noma: a forgotten disease. *Dent Clin North Am* 2003;47:559–574.

Casiglia JW, Woo SB. Oral manifestations of HIV infection. *Clin Dermatol* 2000;18:541–551.

Delaney JE, Keels MA. Pediatric oral pathology. Soft tissue and periodontal conditions. *Pediatr Clin North Am* 2000;47:1125–1147.

de Ru MH, Sukhai RN. Stevens-Johnson Syndrome. *Eur J Pediatr* 2007;166: 1303–1304.

Esmeili T, Lozada-Nur F, Epstein J. Common benign oral soft tissue masses. *Dent Clin North Am* 2005;49:223–240.

Feder HM. Periodic fever, aphthous stomatitis, pharyngitis, adenitis: a clinical review of a new syndrome. *Curr Opin Pediatr* 2000;12:253–256.

Licameli G, Jeffrey J, Luz Jennifer, et al. Effect of adenotonsillectomy in PFAPA syndrome. *Arch Otolaryngol Head Neck Surg* 2008;134:136–140.

Lopez R, Fernandez O, Jara G, et al. Epidemiology of necrotizing ulcerative gingival lesions in adolescents. *J Periodontal Res* 2002;37:439–444.

Okunseri C, Badner V, Wiznia A, et al. Prevalence of oral lesions and percent CD4⁺ T-lymphocytes in HIV-infected children on antiretroviral therapy. *AIDS Patient Care STDS* 2003;17:5–11.

Pandit RT, Park AH. Management of pediatric ranula. *Otolaryngol Head Neck Surg* 2002;127:115–118.

Patel NJ, Sciubba J. Oral lesions in young children. *Pediatr Clin North Am* 2003;50:469–486.

Pittock S, Drumm B, Fleming P, et al. The oral cavity in Crohn's disease. *J Pediatr* 2001;138:767–771.

Tröbs RB, Mader E, Friedrich T, et al. Oral tumors and tumor-like lesions in infants and children. *Pediatr Surg Int* 2003;19:639–645.

Witman PM, Rogers RS. Pediatric oral medicine. *Dermatol Clin* 2003;21:157–170.

tomography (CT) scan should be obtained to evaluate for solid organ injury. Lacerations of the liver and spleen are the most common intraabdominal injuries seen in children. Bedside ultrasound [*focused assessment with sonography in trauma* (FAST)] may be used to evaluate for hemoperitoneum. The sensitivity of ultrasound for the detection of solid organ injury is low, and a significant proportion of children with liver and splenic lacerations have minimal intraabdominal fluid.

Considerations Among Children with Abdominal Distension or Prior Abdominal Surgery

A child who has had prior abdominal surgery and who presents with abdominal pain and vomiting should have abdominal radiographs, including flat and upright views, obtained to evaluate for obstruction. Bowel obstruction is most likely the result of adhesions in this population. Ileus, manifesting clinically with distension and absent bowel sounds, often accompanies surgical conditions, such as volvulus and intussusception, but may also be observed among children with sepsis, infectious enterocolitis, or pneumonia. Obstruction may present with isolated vomiting. A low-grade fever suggests an inflammatory process, including peritonitis.

A patient with episodic colicky pain with interposed quiet intervals, even in the absence of a "currant jelly" stool, makes one suspicious of intussusception or midgut volvulus. With intussusception, on plain radiographs, a paucity of bowel gas may be appreciated in the right lower abdomen and a mass may be visualized in the right mid to upper abdomen. The absence of these findings does not exclude the possibility of intussusception and, thus, in a patient with concerning history or physical examination findings, an ultrasound or contrast enema should be obtained. Although ultrasound has very good sensitivity in the diagnosis of intussusception, the test characteristics of the examination are operator dependant. A contrast enema can be used both to confirm the diagnosis and for therapeutic reduction.

An incarcerated hernia is a common cause of bowel obstruction in infants and young children. Inguinal hernias may incidentally incarcerate during acute illnesses in young, crying infants and may be a cause of abdominal obstruction. Signs of partial or complete obstruction with peritonitis indicate a perforated viscus from intussusception, volvulus, or, occasionally, appendicitis or Hirschsprung's disease. An upper GI radiographic series should be performed if malrotation is suspected.

Abdominal Pain Associated with Peritoneal Signs

Rebound tenderness (including tenderness to percussion) or guarding suggests peritoneal inflammation. Children with peritonitis will often avoid motion and keep their hips flexed to relieve tension on the abdominal musculature. The abdomen may be distended, with decreased or absent bowel sounds. In neonates and young infants, abdominal tenderness, which is associated with peritoneal findings or abdominal distension with or without emesis, should raise suspicion for

necrotizing enterocolitis. Systemic signs such as temperature instability, apnea, and lethargy may be present. The presentation of a child with appendicitis may vary widely, and the clinical signs and symptoms depend upon the stage of disease. Early in the course of illness children will most often complain of diffuse, nonspecific, periumbilical abdominal pain, nausea, and anorexia. As disease progresses, vomiting, fever, and migration of pain to the right lower abdomen are common findings. Ultrasound can be used to confirm the diagnosis of appendicitis, but the diagnosis cannot be excluded if the appendix is not well visualized. CT imaging has excellent test characteristics in the diagnosis of appendicitis; however, the risk of radiation must be considered. Decision rules such as the Pediatric Appendicitis Score, which utilize various historical factors, physical examination findings, and laboratory results such as peripheral white blood cell count, may be used to assess the need for imaging and/or hospitalization.

Peritonitis in a child with nephrotic syndrome may be due to spontaneous bacterial peritonitis. Pain localized to the epigastrium can be due to gastritis; however, the presence of peritonitis should raise suspicion for a perforated ulcer. Cholecystitis and pancreatitis may also produce peritonitis, with abdominal pain localized to the epigastrium or right upper abdomen. A child with Meckel's diverticulum will usually present with painless rectal bleeding; however, abdominal pain may occur because of mucosal ulceration from ectopic gastric mucosa.

Extraabdominal Conditions Associated with Acute Abdominal Pain

A thorough physical examination is required to exclude extraabdominal conditions that can be associated with abdominal pain. On auscultation of the chest, localized, decreased, or tubular breath sounds or adventitious sounds (i.e., crackles) suggest pneumonia, not an uncommon cause of abdominal pain in the febrile infant. Children with "occult pneumonia" may have a normal respiratory rate and no detectable auscultatory findings on physical examination. Urinary symptoms may occur with pyelonephritis, and polydipsia with polyuria may herald the onset of diabetes mellitus with abdominal pain from ketoacidosis.

In males, a complete genitourinary examination should be performed, as testicular torsion and an incarcerated inguinal hernia will often produce pain referred to the abdomen. Infectious mononucleosis and streptococcal pharyngitis may be associated with diffuse abdominal pain. The presence of tachycardia, a friction rub or gallop, or hepatosplenomegaly may suggest a cardiac etiology such as pericarditis or myocarditis. The diagnosis of Henoch-Schönlein purpura can be made if abdominal pain is associated with arthritis, along with a classic petechial or purpural rash of the lower extremities.

Palpable Mass

A palpable mass on the left side of the abdomen may be appreciated in a child with constipation. The diagnosis of constipation should be made on clinical grounds, and radiography should be reserved for children in whom there is concern for obstruction or if the diagnosis is in doubt. A detailed history should include questions regarding the frequency of bowel movements, associated straining, and whether the stool is hard. In suspected constipation, a rectal examination may be helpful to confirm the presence of stool in the rectal vault. A sausage-shaped mass in the right mid-abdomen is sometimes appreciated in children with intussusception. Less commonly, an abdominal abscess or neoplasm (commonly of renal origin) may be palpated.

Focal Tenderness

A child with a history of periumbilical pain that radiates to the right lower abdomen, fever, and vomiting should have high suspicion for the diagnosis of appendicitis. Typically, the child with appendicitis will have focal tenderness in the right lower quadrant; however, diffuse tenderness with involuntary guarding may be seen later in the course. In younger children, it is critical to assess for an atypical presentation of appendicitis. The diagnosis of ovarian torsion should be considered in females with acute onset of lower abdominal pain and vomiting. Epigastric tenderness may be observed in children with gastritis or pancreatitis. Right upper quadrant tenderness may be appreciated among children with hepatitis or cholecystitis. Jaundice or scleral icterus may be present. Pain or limitation of inspiration during palpation of the right upper quadrant (Murphy's sign) may be elicited in patients with acute cholecystitis. Focal tenderness in the flank region suggests pyelonephritis or urolithiasis.

Colicky Pain

Intussusception should be considered in a child with colicky abdominal pain, particularly if younger than 2 years. On examination, a sausage-shaped mass may be palpated in the right upper abdomen with ileocolic intussusception. Usually a "lead" point for an intussusception is seen in older children (e.g., mesenteric adenitis, lymphoma, polyp, cystic fibrosis, anaphylactoid purpura). Abdominal radiographs may be useful in confirming obstruction or the presence of a mass; a contrast enema is indicated urgently if there is a high suspicion for intussusception. In low or moderate probability settings, an ultrasound may yield preliminary findings that rule out the need for a therapeutic study for intussusception. Flank tenderness and/or gross or microscopic hematuria may suggest urolithiasis. Gastroenteritis and constipation can be associated with colicky abdominal pain, but these diagnoses should be made after more serious conditions have been excluded.

Fever

Although most children with appendicitis will have peritoneal signs or focal tenderness, this diagnosis must be considered in any child with fever and abdominal pain. Children with gastroenteritis may have crampy abdominal pain and diarrhea. Although viral pathogens such as rotavirus or adenovirus commonly cause gastroenteritis, the presence of fever, bloody stool, or severe abdominal pain may point to a bacterial etiology. A thorough physical examination should be performed to assess for extraabdominal conditions such as pharyngitis, UTI, and pneumonia. Other conditions associated with abdominal pain and fever are shown in Fig. 49.1

Chronic or Recurrent Pattern

Chronic abdominal pain may occur as a result of many of the conditions listed in Table 49.1. When abdominal pain is recurrent or chronic in infants younger than 3 months and is not accompanied by other findings or symptoms, the physician often makes a diagnosis of "colic" (see Chapter 16) or, based on history, of gastroesophageal reflux. However, several causes of recurrent abdominal pain in infants must be considered. These include recurrent intussusception; malrotation with intermittent volvulus; milk allergy syndrome; and various malabsorptive diseases such as cystic fibrosis, celiac disease, and lactase deficiency.

Abdominal pain and pallor can occur rarely in neoplasia, as with bleeding into an abdominal Wilms' tumor, hepatoma, or neuroblastoma. The presence of pallor and pain also raises the possibility of sickling hemoglobinopathies, with the development of a vasoocclusive crisis, a splenic sequestration, or even an aplastic crisis. Jaundice may be observed in the child with hemolysis or with hepatitis. At times, an intraabdominal vasculitis that causes pain may precede the rash of Henoch-Schönlein purpura or be a prominent finding with Kawasaki disease.

Chronic abdominal pain in the adolescents may be due to inflammatory bowel disease. In these children, inflammatory markers such as erythrocyte sedimentation rate and C-reactive protein levels are commonly elevated. In postpubertal females, dysmenorrhea, endometriosis, chronic PID, chronic UTI, or gallbladder disease can be associated with chronic or recurrent abdominal pain. It is particularly difficult to establish the cause of chronic pain when dealing with adolescents on an episodic basis, making appropriate referral essential.

Functional abdominal pain may be considered only after exclusion of other conditions. Patients will most often have a long-standing history of episodes of abdominal pain and will have no or minimal tenderness on abdominal examination. The presence of focal tenderness, rebound, guarding, or fever should prompt consideration of alternative diagnoses. The emergency physician's task is to allay any fears of serious organic disease during the acute episode. Because the long-term solution to a functional complaint is generally not in the realm of the ED, the physician should explain all the organic illnesses that the pain is *not* believed to be, and suggest a nonorganic cause of the pain. The emergency physician should provide an avenue for continued supportive follow-up through referral to the primary physician.

Additional Considerations in the Postpubertal Female with Acute Abdominal Pain

Among postpubertal females, pregnancy and complications of pregnancy must be considered (Fig. 49.2). A menstrual history and ascertainment of sexual activity are essential, and a urine β-hCG sample should be obtained in all females in whom pregnancy is a possibility.

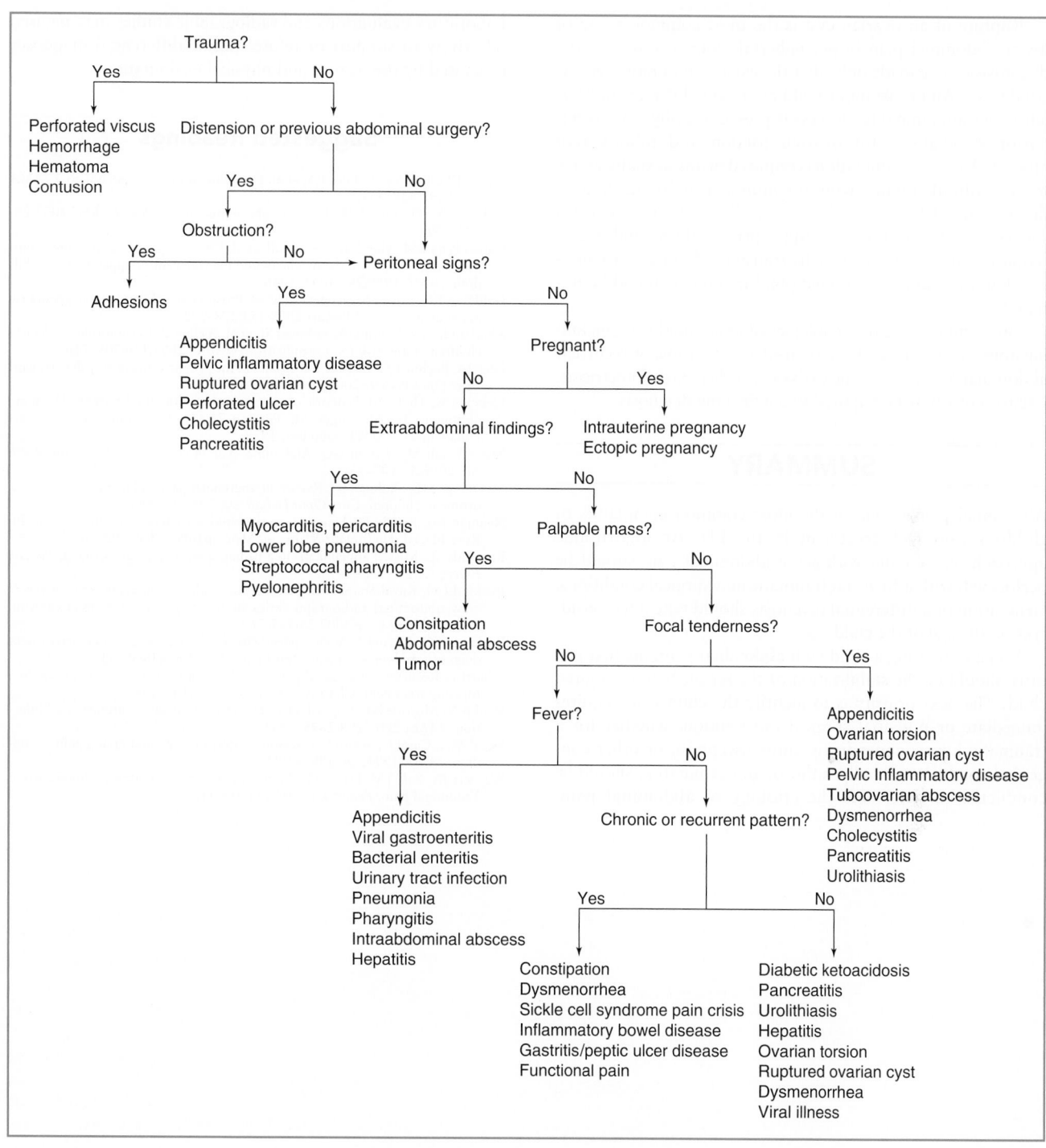

FIGURE 49.2 Acute abdominal pain (postmenarchal female).

The diagnosis of ectopic pregnancy must be considered among women with lower abdominal pain occurring within the first trimester of pregnancy (see Chapter 90). Vaginal bleeding occurs in most patients with ectopic pregnancy but is not always present. A transvaginal or transabdominal ultrasound should be obtained. The diagnosis of ectopic pregnancy is not usually confirmed by ultrasound; however, the presence of an intrauterine gestational sac is reassuring and argues against the diagnosis of ectopic pregnancy. A quantitative serum β-hCG sample should be obtained; it may need to be repeated within 48 to 72 hours if the diagnosis remains uncertain. In addition, RhoD immune globulin (RhoGAM) should be administered to Rh-negative women. Although the diagnosis of ectopic pregnancy should be considered in all pregnant women, crampy lower abdominal pain is commonly reported among women with intrauterine pregnancy.

Rupture of an ovarian cyst is the most common cause of lower abdominal pain in postpubertal women; however, the diagnosis can be made only after the exclusion of more serious conditions. An ultrasound should be obtained if focal right or left lower abdominal tenderness is present on physical examination to evaluate for ovarian torsion and tuboovarian abscess. A pelvic examination is required in any sexually active female with abdominal pain in whom a sexually transmitted disease cannot be excluded. Cervical discharge or tenderness suggests the diagnosis of PID. Appropriate cultures and microscopic examinations for sexually transmitted diseases are indicated and presumptive antimicrobial treatment should be initiated.

Other, nongynecologic etiologies of abdominal pain, including appendicitis, must also be considered. Chronic or recurrent abdominal pain may be due to dysmenorrhea or endometriosis. Laparoscopy may be required to confirm the diagnosis.

SUMMARY

Abdominal pain is one of the most common complaints of children who seek treatment in the ED. An algorithmic approach to the child with acute abdominal pain should be performed, with a focus on traumatic and surgical conditions. Generation of a differential diagnosis should take into consideration the age of the child.

When evaluating a child with abdominal pain, the first priority should be the stabilization of the seriously ill or injured child. The next priority is to identify the child who requires immediate or potential surgical intervention, whether for a traumatic injury, appendicitis, intussusception, or other congenital conditions. Finally, a thorough examination should be conducted to determine the etiology of abdominal pain.

Laboratory evaluations and radiographic studies may be used selectively to support or refute specific differential diagnoses generated by the history and physical examination.

Suggested Readings

Bundy DG, Byerley JS, Liles EA, et al. Does this child have appendicitis? *JAMA* 2007;298:438–451.

Collins BS, Thomas DW. Chronic abdominal pain. *Pediatr Rev* 2007;28: 323–331.

Garcia Peña BM, Mandl KD, Kraus SJ, et al. Ultrasonography and limited computed tomography in the diagnosis and management of appendicitis in children. *JAMA* 1999;282:1041–1046.

Goldman RD, Carter S, Stephens D, et al. Prospective validation of the pediatric appendicitis score. *J Pediatr* 2008;153:278–282.

Kharbanda AB, Taylor GA, Fishman SJ, et al. A clinical decision rule to identify children at low risk for appendicitis. *Pediatrics* 2005;116:709–716.

Levy JA, Bachur RG. Bedside ultrasound in the pediatric emergency department. *Curr Opin Pediatr* 2008;20:235–242.

Liebman W, Thaler M. Pediatric considerations of abdominal pain and the acute abdomen. In: Sleisenger M, Fortran J, eds. *Gastrointestinal disease.* Philadelphia, PA: WB Saunders, 1978.

McCollough M, Sharieff GQ. Abdominal pain in children. *Pediatr Clin North Am* 2006;53:107–137.

McOmber ME, Shulman RJ. Recurrent abdominal pain and irritable bowel syndrome in children. *Curr Opin Pediatr* 2007;19:581–585.

Neuman MI, Ruddy R. Approach to the child with acute abdominal pain. In: Rose BD, ed. *UpToDate.* Waltham, MA: UpToDate Inc, 2007.

Reynolds SL. Missed appendicitis in a pediatric emergency department. *Pediatr Emerg Care* 1993;9:1–13.

Roskind CG, Ruzal-Shapiro CB, Dowd EK, et al. Test characteristics of the 3-view abdominal radiograph series in the diagnosis of intussusception. *Pediatr Emerg Care* 2007;23:785–789.

Rothrock SG, Pagane J. Acute appendicitis in children: emergency department diagnosis and management. *Ann Emerg Med* 2000;36:39–51.

Scharff L. Recurrent abdominal pain in children: a review of psychological factors and treatment. *Clin Psychol Rev* 1997;17:145–166.

Shaikh N, Morone NE, Lopez J, et al. Does this child have a urinary tract infection? *JAMA* 2007;298:2895–2904.

Siegel MN, Carel C, Surrot S. Ultrasonography of acute abdominal pain in children. *JAMA* 1991;266:1987–1989.

Weydert JA, Ball TM, Davis MF. Systematic review of treatments for recurrent abdominal pain. *Pediatrics* 2003;111:e1–e11.

CHAPTER 50 ■ PAIN—BACK

HOWARD M. CORNELI, MD

Back pain has been found to be more common in children than was once thought, but few children see a physician for this complaint. Although back pain is seen less frequently in children than in adults, it is also more likely to signify pathology, especially before adolescence. The evaluation of back pain may be difficult because young children have less ability to describe their pain and even to localize it. Children are subject to conditions causing back pain that are seldom seen in adults, and the common adult causes are uncommon in children. Physicians usually do not see large numbers of children with back pain. Their evaluation, if sometimes challenging, is often important.

DIFFERENTIAL DIAGNOSIS

The causes of back pain are ubiquitous, but this does not mean that children with back pain cannot be diagnosed or that the evaluation is typically difficult or unrevealing. The more likely childhood causes can be divided into a few categories (Tables 50.1 and 50.2).

A history of trauma is important in evaluating back pain but may be misleading in young children whose frequent minor injuries may be seen by the parents as the trigger for a problem that is, in fact, nontraumatic. On the other hand, adolescents with overuse injuries may or may not identify trauma. High-force trauma (e.g., in a car crash) can cause severe back injuries, and careful evaluation for back pain and tenderness is critical in multiple trauma patients, who may have many more obvious injuries. Spinal trauma is covered in Chapter 116, and cervical spine injuries are covered in Chapter 115.

Less severe trauma is common in childhood. Typical falls can produce vertebral compression fractures, which are more common in children. Radicular pain may develop and may occasionally be severe. Contusion is common if bruising and tenderness accompany a history of a direct blow to the back. If this is not over the kidney or spine, simple contusion may be an appropriate diagnosis. Pain after lifting, work, or sports is also common. Although the signs of muscular back strain and lumbar disc herniation are similar to those seen in adults, these conditions occur less commonly in children. Spondylolysis, in contrast, is more common in young people, especially among adolescent athletes. This is a stress fracture or discontinuity of the pars interarticularis. When the vertebra slips forward on the one beneath, the resulting condition is called spondylolisthesis. Either condition can cause back pain, most often in the lower lumbar area or at the L5 to S1 level. These lesions often present during the adolescent growth spurt. The condition is believed to be associated with overuse, especially hyperflexion. Spondylolysis often presents with subacute or recurring pain, but pain may develop acutely in some cases. Lumbar flexion and extension may be limited and, especially in extension, painful. Another condition linked to overuse, Scheuermann's disease, is seen in adolescents as anterior wedging of several vertebrae, especially in the thoracic spine. This condition is painful in about half of those affected. Although disc herniation is much less common in childhood, it does develop in adolescents, especially with activities such as weight lifting. These activities can also cause posterior avulsion fractures of the vertebral apophysis, which displace into the spinal canal producing symptoms similar to disc herniation.

Rare but dangerous causes of back pain deserve special vigilance in children (Table 50.3). A spinal epidural hematoma may follow a fall or blow, sometimes presenting some days later, or it may arise spontaneously, especially in patients with bleeding disorders or those who are receiving anticoagulant therapy. Back pain may only briefly precede symptoms of spinal cord compression. Spinal epidural abscess can present with back pain, low-grade fever, and signs of spinal cord compression. Percussion usually elicits spinal tenderness. Transverse myelitis may be postinfectious, and back pain may precede weakness by as much as 1 to 2 days. These rare but severe conditions underscore the need for a careful neurologic examination in children with back pain. Appreciation of the signs of spinal cord compromise should lead to emergent imaging and neurosurgical consultation.

The infectious causes of back pain are many, yet infection in the back itself can be difficult to diagnose. The symptoms and signs of infection, as well as laboratory markers of inflammation, may be absent. Vertebral osteomyelitis and discitis may present with subtle symptoms in young children, in whom these are the most commonly seen symptoms. Parents may only note refusal to stand or sit. Back pain is often not obvious, and limp may point away from the back. It is advisable to palpate and percuss the back in any child with limp or apparent leg pain. Iliac osteomyelitis and sacroiliac joint infection are seen at times in childhood. Osteomyelitis of the ribs is rare.

Paraspinal or psoas abscess, and pyomyositis in the paraspinal or pelvic muscles, may present as back pain, which may sometimes be severe. Rare spinal infections include spinal tuberculosis (Pott's disease) and brucellosis, in which small vertebral abscesses may accompany lymphadenopathy and hepatosplenomegaly.

Common childhood infections associated with back pain include, of course, urinary tract infection (UTI), which may cause flank pain with or without upper tract involvement, and pneumonia or pleurisy, which present with back pain in some cases. Myalgias and generalized backache may be seen in influenza, mononucleosis, streptococcal pharyngitis, and other

TABLE 50.1

CAUSES OF BACK PAIN

I. *Traumatic, posttraumatic, or injury-related*
  A. Compression fracture
  B. Spondylolysis
  C. Spondylolisthesis
  D. Disk herniation (uncommon in childhood)
  E. Muscle or ligament injury (less common in childhood)
  F. Spinal epidural hematoma (traumatic or spontaneous)
II. *Nontraumatic*
  A. Infectious
    1. Spinal
      a. Discitis
      b. Vertebral osteomyelitis
      c. Spinal epidural abscess
      d. Tuberculosis (Pott's disease)
      e. Brucellosis
    2. Extraspinal
      a. Iliac osteomyelitis/sacroiliac joint infection
      b. Paraspinal/retroperitoneal abscess
      c. Urinary tract infection
      d. Pneumonia or pleurisy
      e. Meningitis
      f. Myalgias
      g. Pyomyositis
    3. Postinfectious—transverse myelitis
  B. Collagen vascular disease
    1. Ankylosing spondylitis
    2. Other spondylitis (regional enteritis etc.)
    3. Juvenile idiopathic arthritis
  C. Other causes
    1. Scheuermann's disease
    2. Sickle cell disease, other hemoglobinopathies
    3. Calcification of intervertebral disc
    4. Cord lesions (diastematomyelia, arteriovenous malformation)
    5. Muscular dystrophies
    6. Aortic dissection (hypertension, Marfan's syndrome)
    7. Developmental anomalies of the spine
  D. Neoplastic
    1. Spinal tumors
      a. Benign
        1. Osteoid osteoma
        2. Eosinophilic granuloma
        3. Osteoblastoma, benign
        4. Aneurysmal bone cyst
        5. Neurenteric cyst
      b. Malignant
        1. Ewing sarcoma
        2. Osteogenic sarcoma
    2. Spinal cord tumors (may cause spinal cord dysfunction)
      a. Gliomas, neurofibromas
      b. Teratomas, lipomas
    3. Extraspinal/paraspinal tumors
      a. Neuroblastoma
      b. Wilms' tumor
    4. Metastatic brain tumor
    5. Leukemia/lymphoma
III. *Referred*
  A. Pancreatitis/gallbladder pain/constipation
  B. Appendicitis
  C. Hematocolpos
  D. Renal colic
IV. *Psychogenic*

TABLE 50.2

COMMON IMPORTANT CAUSES OF BACK
PAIN IN CHILDREN

I. Traumatic
  A. Compression fracture
  B. Spondylolysis/spondylolisthesis
II. Infectious
  A. Discitis
  B. Vertebral osteomyelitis
  C. Urinary tract infection
  D. Pneumonia
III. Neoplastic
  A. Malignant tumors
  B. Benign tumors

generalized infections. Parents occasionally identify meningitis primarily as back pain, especially in an infant; the parent may note that it hurts the child to move the back. Because infections in young children sometimes lack the more obvious symptoms seen in older patients, associated back pain may be more prominent. The young child with a UTI often shows no urinary symptoms as such. Pneumonia may be clinically occult, with little cough and few findings on auscultation.

Abdominal conditions that may present with back pain or flank tenderness include pancreatitis, in which a steady, penetrating pain radiates prominently to the back; gallbladder disease, in which pain may radiate to the back; and appendicitis, especially in a retrocecal location. Ovarian pain, as with torsion or pelvic inflammatory disease, may at times radiate to the back, and intestinal pain, particularly that because of constipation, sometimes manifests as back pain. Kidney stones in children will usually cause typical renal colic and hematuria on urinalysis, but atypical cases with infection or obstruction may present a diagnostic challenge.

Collagen vascular diseases that cause back pain include ankylosing spondylitis and juvenile idiopathic (rheumatoid) arthritis with sacroiliitis. Both of these conditions more often affect boys older than 8 years. The back is notably stiff to flexion, especially in the lumbar region. Spondylitis may also be seen in association with reactive arthritis, regional enteritis, ulcerative colitis, and psoriasis.

TABLE 50.3

SERIOUS CAUSES OF BACK PAIN IN CHILDREN

I. Traumatic
  A. Spondylolisthesis
  B. Spinal epidural hematoma
II. Infectious
  A. Discitis
  B. Vertebral osteomyelitis
  C. Meningitis
  D. Transverse myelitis
  E. Spinal epidural abscess
III. Neoplastic
  A. Malignant tumors
  B. Benign tumors
  C. Leukemia/lymphoma

A host of neoplastic causes, both benign and malignant, may present with back pain (Table 50.1). These are not so rare that they can be ignored in an evaluation of back pain. Leukemia, and especially lymphoma, may present as back pain. Ewing sarcoma may mimic infection, with fever, leukocytosis, and rarefaction of bone on radiographs.

Sickle cell disease and other hemoglobinopathies may cause back pain. Children with sickle cell disease experience vasoocclusive crises in the spine and may be prone to vertebral osteomyelitis. Osteoporosis and osteopenia due to many causes, including chronic bed rest, paraplegia, and osteogenesis imperfecta, will make compression fractures possible after minor or minimal trauma. Dissecting aortic aneurysm has been reported rarely in children, usually with hypertension or with Marfan's syndrome and other connective tissue disorders.

Table 50.1 lists other miscellaneous causes of back pain. Several diagnoses for childhood back pain should be made cautiously or avoided altogether. Growing pains do not affect the back. Idiopathic scoliosis demonstrates back pain only in the most severe cases. Muscle strain is less common in children, especially before adolescence, and this diagnosis should be made only after other causes are excluded. An objective link between back pain and heavy school bags has not been demonstrated, although some children who perceive their loads as heavy may complain of pain. Chronic low back pain has been shown to have emotional and perceptual components in children, but psychogenic pain is less common in children than in adults and acute pain seldom merits this diagnosis. A psychological component may, of course, be suggested by chronic pain undiagnosed after thorough evaluation, a cheerful affect when describing symptoms, disproportional school absence, or unusual family dynamics. Even if suspicion of psychogenic pain exists, a careful initial investigation should be undertaken to exclude organic causes.

EVALUATION AND DECISION

Particular signs and symptoms may be suggestive. Pain at the end of the day, or worsened by exercise, is more likely to be musculoskeletal. Pain with prolonged standing or sitting may be due to vertebral causes, and pain with cough or sneeze can suggest disc disease or related lesions. Pain on arising may signify collagen vascular disease. Night pain may suggest tumor, and if relieved by nonsteroidal antiinflammatory drugs, suggest osteoid osteoma or osteoblastoma. Pain and tenderness over the spine are often skeletal, but such findings off the midline may be more likely muscular. Limp with back pain is worrisome. Relief with traction (as when a parent lifts the child under the arms) can suggest disc or vertebral pain, as in discitis, as can increased pain on spinal flexion or compression (e.g., during diaper changes).

Constitutional symptoms such as fever, diminished appetite, and weight loss suggest serious disease. Pain causing new or progressive kyphosis, scoliosis, or gait disturbance is almost always due to pathology. Sciatica, especially in the adolescent athlete or laborer, may signify disc herniation. Although chronic occasional pain that does not limit activity may turn out to be functional, pain that endures or recurs is often concerning, and worsening pain should be worrisome. Finally, be aware that parents may sometimes feel an infant or a toddler has back pain when adjoining areas are the true source (as in abdominal pain, hip pain, limb pain, or neck pain).

Age may be suggestive of cause. Discitis and osteomyelitis are most common in preschool children. Children older than 10 to 12 years are more prone to overuse injuries, such as spondylolysis.

Fever is likely, of course, to signify infection, but it can also be seen with neoplastic and collagen vascular diseases. Even more important, children with musculoskeletal infections can be afebrile at presentation in a significant proportion of cases.

The most important task in children with back pain is to rule out any sign of neurologic involvement (Fig. 50.1). Conditions that affect the spinal cord are seen often enough in children and their gravity should be borne in mind throughout the evaluation. The history should be reviewed for limb weakness or disuse or for a change in function of the bowel or bladder. Any suspicion of spinal cord involvement warrants prompt neurosurgical consultation.

Certain injury histories suggest specific diagnoses. Axial loading of the spine, as when a child lands in a seated position after a fall, is often associated with compression fractures of the vertebrae. The history of position in falls and collisions, however, is unreliable, and compression fracture is common in children who believe they landed supine.

A history should be sought of sports, lifting, or work-related exposures to back stress. Gymnasts, dancers, weight lifters, football players, and participants in similar sports often hyperextend their back. Unfortunately, not all children who develop stress injuries are engaged in easily identified activities. As excessive competition in sports is introduced to younger children, sports injuries may be seen earlier and more commonly in childhood. Concern also exists that trends to obesity and a sedentary lifestyle may increase back complaints in children.

A history may reveal an underlying disease, chronic inactivity (in the bedridden child), or drug therapy that may cause osteoporosis, which increases the risk of fracture. A review of systems, social history, and family history may reveal helpful clues. Change in posture or gait is important, as is any history of overuse. Headache might be worrisome, and weakness, numbness, or paresthesias would be critical. Family history may be positive in ankylosing spondylitis and related conditions. A family history of back pain can also be revealing in cases of functional pain. School performance and school absence can be relevant, as may social and family stress.

Chronic back pain may be seen in collagen vascular conditions, Scheuermann's disease, or a developmental defect in the spine, but tumors may also progress slowly with chronic back pain being the only noted symptom. On the other hand, the acute onset of pain or neurologic symptoms can be the first signs of a chronic (but expanding) mass lesion.

Physical examination must document spinal cord function in any child with back pain. This includes the evaluation of muscle bulk, tone, and strength; sensitivity to light pinprick as well as light touch; the deep tendon reflexes and Babinski reflex; and anal tone, the anal contracture reflex, and, in boys, the cremasteric reflex. If any neurologic compromise is suspected, additional sensory examination of proprioception, heat, and cold is warranted.

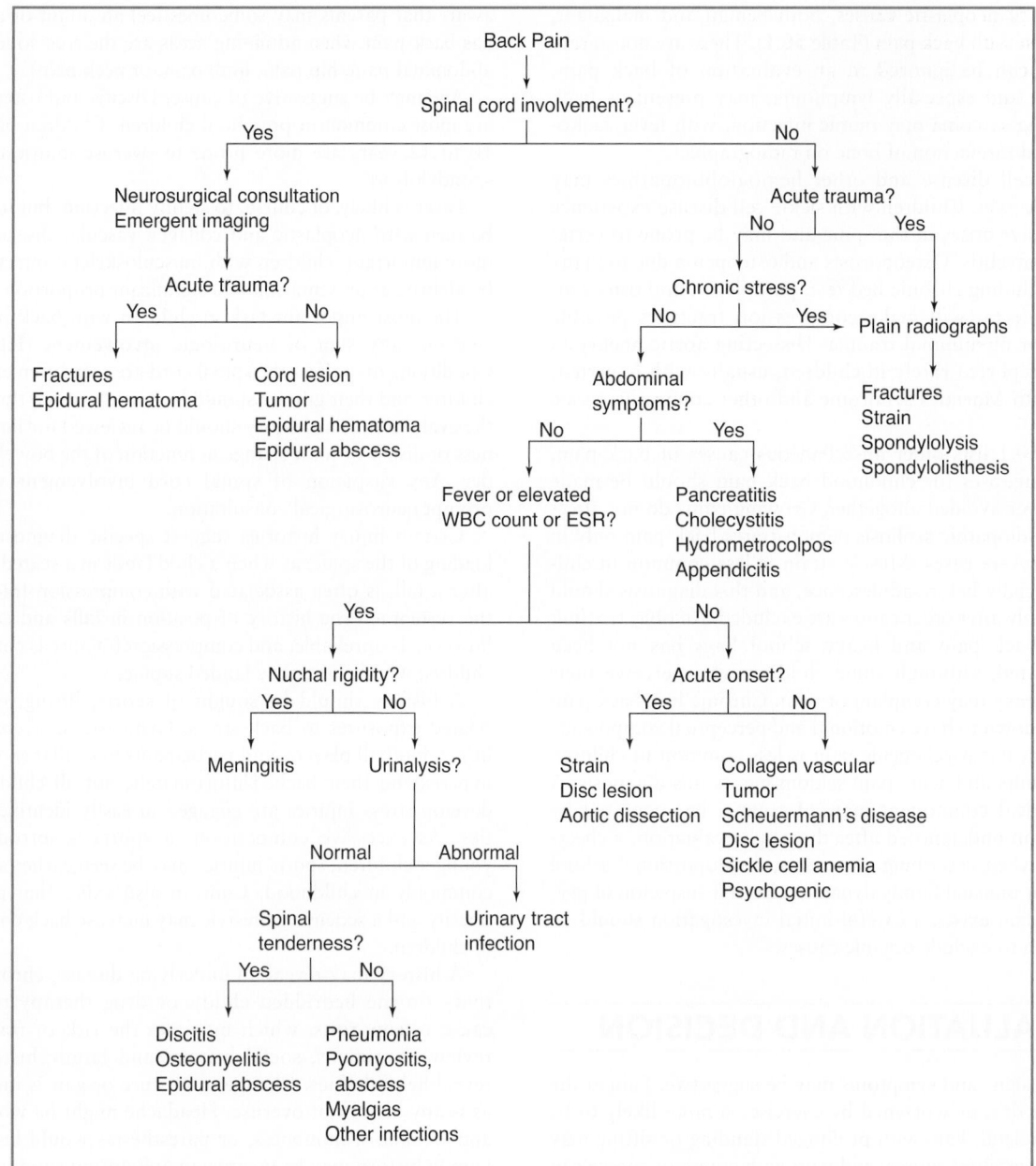

FIGURE 50.1 Approach to the diagnosis of back pain. WBC, white blood cell; ESR, erythrocyte sedimentation rate.

The physical examination should start with the appearance of the spine: unusual kyphosis, lordosis, or scoliosis should be noted. Excessive lumbar lordosis is associated with spondylolysis, spondylolisthesis, disc herniation, and muscular or ligamentous back pain. Pelvic tilt on single-leg standing suggests hip abductor dysfunction. After careful inspection of gait and posture, the examination should move on to palpation and percussion of the spine, flank, and ribs, sacroiliac and paraspinal regions; rotation of each hip; straight-leg raising and evaluation of hamstring tightness; and spinal mobility in rotation, flexion, and extension. Pain on flexion is more common with anterior lesions and pain on extension or hyperextension with posterior lesions. The examiner can provoke extension pain by providing slight resistance as the patient stands from toe touching, and hyperextension may be increased by gentle downward pressure on the shoulders as the patient slumps the shoulders back and the abdomen forward; this maneuver, repeated as the patient stands on one leg and then the other, is especially useful to detect spondylolysis. Spondylolysis should not produce spine tenderness or gait changes but spondylolisthesis may. Chest and abdominal examinations should also be performed, as should rectal and genital inspection. (Hydrometrocolpos has been reported as a cause of back pain, even in premenarchal girls.)

The cause of back pain may remain obscure even after a thorough history and physical examination. In children, it is often appropriate to seek consultation with a radiologist.

Imaging is more often revealing in children than in adults but still must be used selectively; ordering radiographs in all cases of back pain will have a low yield.

Midline pain, tenderness, or pain with motion should lead to radiographic studies, particularly after childhood trauma or falls. Exacerbation by activity, and persistence or progression of pain, also usually warrants imaging. Plain radiographs are almost always obtained first. Plain images are often sufficient to reveal compression fracture, bony tumor, Scheuermann's disease, and spondylolisthesis and may be revealing in spondylolysis and ongoing cases of discitis or osteomyelitis. Oblique views, although helpful when spondylolysis is suspected, may not be as sensitive as single photon emission computed tomography (SPECT). Bone scan has a clear role in finding discitis and vertebral osteomyelitis, and SPECT may enhance accuracy here as well.

Magnetic resonance imaging (MRI) is increasingly used in the evaluation of back pain. Besides other advantages, it defines almost all spine lesions. Note, though, that its most typical indication in adults, disc disease, is uncommon in children. The issues of both expense and sedation should limit its too-ready use. MRI is clearly indicated, however, if spinal cord pathology is suspected and is often useful when other imaging techniques prove inconclusive.

Computed tomography (CT) remains a useful method for emergent evaluation of trauma, in cases of avulsion fracture, or when lesions outside the spine, including kidney stones, are suspected. CT is limited, however, in its ability to delineate densities within the spinal canal and to study the alignment of structures in the vertical axis. MRI overcomes these limitations and provides highly detailed longitudinal images of the spine, the canal, the cord, and other tissues.

Plain chest radiography is indicated if pneumonia is considered. Radiolabeled white blood cell scans may detect soft-tissue infection or abscess. Ultrasound may outline ovarian lesions and abdominal tumors such as neuroblastoma.

Laboratory investigations may not be helpful in traumatic back pain and should be directed by the presentation otherwise. Urinalysis and urine culture will commonly be undertaken. A complete blood count (CBC), C-reactive protein, and sedimentation rate may help if infectious or inflammatory disease is suspected. Blood cultures sometimes give positive results in osteomyelitis and discitis. If a neoplasm is considered, obtaining a CBC, acute-phase reactants, uric acid, and lactate dehydrogenase levels may be helpful, along with urine catecholamine measurement if a neuroblastoma is possible. Sickle cell preparations or hemoglobin electrophoresis may be indicated. Pancreatic enzymes and biliary studies may rule out related pathology. Other evaluations may be used selectively.

The treatment of the varying causes of back pain is discussed in specific sections of this book. Negative results after appropriate diagnostic evaluation may warrant a trial of empiric therapy with nonsteroidal antiinflammatory medication, but close follow-up should be arranged.

In summary, because back pain is less common in children than in adults, and because it more often implies significant pathology, it deserves and must receive a careful evaluation.

Suggested Readings

Davis PJ, Williams HJ. The investigation and management of back pain in children. *Arch Dis Child Educ Pract Ed* 2008;93:73–83.

Herman MJ, Pizzutillo PD, Cavalier R. Spondylolysis and spondylolisthesis in the child and adolescent athlete. *Orthop Clin North Am* 2003;34(3):461–467, vii.

Jones GT, Macfarlane GJ. Epidemiology of low back pain in children and adolescents. *Arch Dis Child* 2005;90:312–316.

Kim HJ, Green DW. Adolescent back pain. *Curr Opin Pediatr* 2008;20:37–45.

Sassmannshausen G, Smith BG. Back pain in the young athlete. *Clin Sports Med* 2002;21:121–132.

SIGNS AND SYMPTOMS

CHAPTER 51 ■ PAIN—CHEST

ROBYN L. BYER, MD

The complaint of chest pain rarely represents a life-threatening emergency in children, in contrast to the same complaint in adults. Although heart disease is an uncommon source of chest pain in children, the fear of a cardiac origin for the pain may evoke anxiety in the child or in the parents. There are a wide variety of etiologies for chest pain including diseases of the respiratory, cardiac, gastrointestinal (GI), neurologic, psychiatric, and musculoskeletal systems; however, it is most commonly due to idiopathic noncardiac origins. Chest pain accounts for approximately 0.6% of all pediatric emergency department (ED) visits and affects boys and girls equally. Clinicians need to take a careful approach to the patient even in the pediatric setting. This chapter first briefly reviews the pathophysiology of chest pain, then outlines the differential diagnosis in children, and finally presents the evaluation, as appropriate in the ED.

PATHOPHYSIOLOGY

To understand the possible origins of chest pain or discomfort, it is important to review how this sensation is transmitted. Musculoskeletal pain is produced by irritation of these tissues and is transmitted through the sensory nerves. The stimulus is carried through the nerves in the dermatomal or intercostal distribution to the dorsal root ganglia, up the spinal afferents and into the central nervous system. This local, peripheral, sharp pain can also be produced by primary dorsal root irritation in the spine. Because of overlap of nerve distribution, pain may be sensed in locations distal to the irritation. For example, the third and fourth cervical nerves evoke pain as far caudally as the nipple line of the chest.

Tracheobronchial pain is transmitted by vagal afferents in the large bronchi and trachea to fibers in the cervical spinal column. Dull, aching, or sharp pain is felt in the anterior chest or neck. The irritation or sensation of cough is transmitted in a similar fashion. Pleural pain arises in the pain-sensitive parietal pleura and then travels through the intercostal nerves in the chest wall, giving rise to sharp, well-localized pain. The visceral pleura is insensitive to pain. The intercostal or phrenic nerves transmit diaphragmatic pain. Peripheral diaphragmatic irritation may cause local chest wall pain because of the intercostal innervation. Central diaphragmatic stimulation travels by the phrenic nerve, with the pain referred to the shoulder of the affected side.

The esophagus appears to be more pain-sensitive in its proximal portion. Pain is transmitted by afferents to corresponding spinal segments, with resultant anterior chest or neck pain. The pericardium is innervated by portions of the phrenic, vagal, and recurrent laryngeal nerves, as well as by the esophageal plexus. This appears to give rise to various sensations, including chest or abdominal pain, dull pressure, and even referred angina-like pain.

Other mediastinal structures, such as the aorta, have pain fibers in the adventitia of the vessel wall. They transmit pain through the thoracic sympathetic chain to the spinal dorsal roots, giving rise to sharp, and variably localized chest pain. Cardiac pain is likely transmitted by a number of routes, including the thoracic sympathetic chain and the cardiac nerves through the cervical and stellate ganglia. It has been proposed that pain arises from abnormal ventricular wall movement and stimulation of the pericardial pain fibers. These routes account for the sensation of cardiac chest pain as pressure or crushing pain substernally or as sharp pain in the shoulder, neck, or arm.

DIFFERENTIAL DIAGNOSIS

A differential diagnosis of chest pain in children is included in Table 51.1. In the case of trauma, cardiac or pulmonary compromise may arise from direct injury to the heart, great vessels, or lung (see Chapter 118). Most chest pain in the nontraumatized child is caused by acute respiratory disease, musculoskeletal injury, anxiety, or inflammation (Table 51.2). Often, the physician does not make a causative diagnosis of the chest pain and calls it nonspecific or idiopathic in origin. Occasionally, this idiopathic chest pain may be unrecognized organic disease, such as gastroesophageal reflux disease. Chest pain in children usually occurs without associated cardiorespiratory signs or symptoms, often as an acute or chronic problem. By the time of the ED visit, frequently, the pain has resolved. Although much less frequent, chest pain in association with cardiorespiratory distress demands immediate attention. Table 51.3 lists the life-threatening causes of chest pain by disease and mechanisms for decompensation. Chest pain in the dyspneic or cyanotic patient most often stems from a respiratory problem, such as pneumonia, asthma, pleurisy, or pneumothorax. Rarely does severe chest pain in an acutely ill child result from myocardial infarction (MI) due to aberrant coronary vessels, cocaine abuse, Kawasaki disease, hyperlipidemia, or other underlying cardiac diseases (aortic stenosis, an acute arrhythmia, or pericardial disease). Every individual evaluation must be started, however, with a broad differential diagnosis in mind to ensure proper diagnosis and management of the child with chest pain.

A cardiac cause for chest pain has been reported in up to 6% of pediatric patients, but this includes both those presenting to an emergency department and those evaluated in a cardiology clinic; the incidence in ED patients is likely to be lower.

TABLE 51.3

CAUSES OF CHEST PAIN

I. **Musculoskeletal/Neural**
  A. Muscle
     Trauma—contusions, lacerations, strain
     Infection—myositis
  B. Breast
     Physiologic (fullness during menses or pregnancy)
     Mastitis
     Fibrocystic disease
     Tumor (adenoma, other)
     Gynecomastia
  C. Bone
     Trauma—contusions, rib fractures
     Osteitis, osteomyelitis
     Costochondritis, Tietze syndrome
     Tumor
     Slipping rib syndrome
  D. Intercostal nerve
     Neuritis—zoster, trauma
     Toxin
  E. Dorsal root
     Trauma
     Radiculitis—viral, postviral
     Spinal disease—scoliosis
II. **Tracheobronchial (Proximal Bronchi)**
  A. Foreign body
  B. Infection
     Tracheitis
     Bronchitis
     Cystic fibrosis
  C. Asthma
III. **Pulmonary/Pleural/Diaphram**
  A. Trauma—penetrating and blunt
  B. Pleurisy/pleurodynia—viral, mycobacterial
  C. Pneumonia
  D. Cystic fibrosis
  E. Pneumothorax, hemothorax, chylothorax
  F. Empyema

G. Pneumomediastinum
H. Malignancy/mediastinal mass
I. Postpericardiotomy syndrome
J. Pulmonary embolus/infarction
K. Vasoocclusive crisis (sickle cell disease)
L. Tumor
M. Subphrenic abscess/hepatic abscess
N. Fitz-Hugh-Curtis syndrome
IV. **Gastrointestinal**
  A. Esophageal
     Foreign body
     Caustic ingestion
     Gastroesophageal reflux/esophagitis
     Esophageal spasms
     Infection—*Candida*
     Esophageal rupture/tear
  B. Hiatal hernia
  C. Gastritis/peptic ulcer disease
  D. Cholecystitis
  E. Pancreatitis
V. **Cardiac (angina, pericardial, aortic)**
  A. Angina—coronary insufficiency,[a] anomalous vessels, pulmonary hypertension
  B. Hypertrophic cardiomyopathy
  C. Aortic stenosis, pulmonary stenosis
  D. Asymmetric septal hypertrophy
  E. Pericardial defects and effusions, pericarditis
  F. Acute arrhythmias[a]
  G. Myocarditis[a]
  H. Aortic aneurysm—idiopathic, syphilitic, Marfan's syndrome
  I. Mitral valve prolapse
VI. **Central**
  A. Psychiatric—anxiety, hyperventilation, conversion reaction, depression, phobia
  B. Idiopathic—Texidor's twinge (precordial catch)
  C. Other—visceral pain–associated disability syndrome

[a]Associated drug induced (especially cocaine).

Major categories include arrhythmias, anatomic lesions, and acquired disorders. Myocardial ischemia is rare in pediatrics but can present with typical unrelenting substernal crushing chest pain with or without radiation to neck or arm, diaphoresis, nausea, dyspnea, and syncope. Patients are usually in distress and have physical examination abnormalities, including

TABLE 51.2

COMMON CAUSES OF CHEST PAIN

Functional (anxiety/psychosomatic)
Musculoskeletal contusion/strain
Costochondritis/myositis
Cough or respiratory infections (bronchitis, pneumonia, pleurisy, upper respiratory infections)
Asthma
Gastroesophageal reflux
Idiopathic

pallor, diaphoresis, a gallop rhythm, a heart murmur, and decreased peripheral perfusion. Myocardial ischemia/infarction can occur as a result of a thrombosed coronary artery aneurysm. These aneurysms, which occur as a sequelae from Kawasaki disease, have both insufficient laminar flow and areas of stenosis that become obstructed via thrombosis, leading to decreased myocardial perfusion. Case reports of myocardial ischemia without risk factors in adolescents have been attributed to vasospasm. Cocaine exposure can result in palpitations and coronary vasospasm, leading to ischemia, MI, arrhythmias, or cardiomyopathy. Patients with cocaine toxicity are often anxious with confusion or combativeness and have significant tachycardia and hypertension. Other toxins have cardiac effects. The herbal medications aconite, ephedra, and licorice have also been implicated as the cause of chest pain, congestive heart failure, arrhythmias, and MIs.

Anomalous coronary arteries that originate from the opposite sinus and traverse between the great vessels usually presents with sudden death but can also cause chest pain with intense

TABLE 51.3

LIFE-THREATENING CAUSES OF CHEST PAIN

Category	Disease/injury	Decompensation
Traumatic	Rib fracture	Tension pneumothorax or shock from hemothorax
	Cardiac contusion	Arrhythmia or myocardial infarction
	Laceration—heart or great vessel	Shock
	Contusion—great vessels	Dissecting aneurysm/shock
	Pulmonary contusion	Adult respiratory distress syndrome
Cardiac	Congenital heart disease	Arrhythmia, shock, pulmonary hypertension
	Myocardial infarction (anomalous coronary artery, Kawasaki disease, cocaine toxicity)	Arrhythmia, cardiogenic shock
	Myocarditis	Arrhythmia, cardiogenic shock
	Pericarditis	Tamponade
	Rheumatic heart disease	Arrhythmia, congestive heart failure
	Aortic aneurysm	Rupture-shock, dissection
	Obstructive cardiac disease	Acute hypertension
Pulmonary	Pneumothorax (asthma, cystic fibrosis, spontaneous)	Tension pneumothorax, pulmonary hypertension, shock
	Hemothorax	Shock, hypoxemia
	Pulmonary infection or empyema	Pulmonary hypertension, sepsis
	Aspiration—foreign body	Acute airway obstruction, progressive pulmonary hypertension
	Acute asthma	Tension pneumothorax, pulmonary hypertension
	Pulmonary embolus	Pulmonary infarction, hypertension, cardiovascular collapse
	Pulmonary venoocclusive disease	Pulmonary hypertension
	Tumor (chest wall, chest, or mediastinum)	Airway compromise, progression of tumor
Miscellaneous	Drug ingestion/overdose (especially cocaine)	Arrhythmia, cardiomyopathy, shock
	Sickle cell crisis	Pulmonary infarction or hypertension
	Cholecystitis	Sepsis, peritonitis

exercise. Pain is thought to be related to inadequate coronary perfusion via either compression of the great vessels, relative ostial stenosis, or both. The history is the key to this significant disease as the physical examination findings are usually normal.

Hypertrophic cardiomyopathy is the most common cardiac cause of sudden death, which is likely due to ventricular dysrhythmias, yet chest pain is not a common feature. This disease follows an autosomal dominant pattern of inheritance; however, spontaneous mutations may occur. Patients often have a systolic murmur that becomes more intense with standing or a Valsalva maneuver. Chest pain can also occur with severe obstruction from aortic stenosis, which is likely to be discovered by the pathological murmur on physical examination. The patient with chest pain that has onset with or worsening with exertion should be evaluated for these conditions.

Arrhythmias are not uncommon in children and usually present with chest pain and palpitations. Symptoms of heart pounding may occur with instantaneous initiation and termination whereas other children have been reported to abruptly stop an activity. Most are benign, such as premature atrial and ventricular contractions; however, children may present with signs of shock, congestive heart failure, or syncope secondary to supraventricular or ventricular tachycardia. Physical examination is often normal in the absence of active arrhythmias, but long-term effects can lead to cardiomyopathy. Dilated cardiomyopathy presents with chest discomfort, fatigue, exercise intolerance, palpitations, and physical examination findings, such as a gallop rhythm and a murmur secondary to mitral valve insufficiency.

Inflammatory conditions such as pericarditis and myocarditis can present with chest pain and systemic symptoms. Pericardial disease includes pericarditis, pericardial effusions, and cardiac tamponade. Pericarditis often presents with fever, a stabbing chest pain that improves with sitting up and leaning forward, respiratory distress, a friction rub, and distant heart sounds. Pericarditis and pericardial effusions can restrict outflow, leading to neck vein distension and, in severe cases of tamponade, pulsus paradoxus (see Chapter 84). The presentation of myocarditis can be subtler with mild chest pain and fatigue for several days, followed by the development of fever, dyspnea, and worsening chest pain. The examination often shows tachycardia (or bradycardia when severe), orthostatic changes not improved by fluid resuscitation, pulsus paradoxus, and a gallop rhythm. Both pericarditis and myocarditis are usually associated with a preceding viral illness. Endocarditis is most often seen in children with a history of congenital heart disease but can present in those with no known predisposing condition. Patients are often ill-appearing with a history of prolonged fever and may have signs of embolization. Other illnesses that can present with carditis include rheumatic heart disease and Kawasaki disease.

Chest pain associated with mitral valve prolapse is controversial. Studies have shown that mitral valve prolapse is not more common in those with chest pain than in the general population, and other etiologies of the chest pain (i.e., esophagitis) may exist in a patient with this condition. However, chest pain in patients with mitral valve prolapse may be secondary to papillary muscle or left ventricular endocardial ischemia. A midsystolic click and late systolic murmur should be found on physical examination. Pain secondary to mitral valve prolapse should be considered only when no other etiology is found.

Patients with connective tissue disorders, such as Marfan syndrome, have the potential to develop aortic dilation, aortic dissection, and rupture. Symptoms of aortic dissection/rupture include generalized distress with unrelenting severe chest pain, decreased cardiac output, dyspnea, and, often, abdominal pain.

Children who present with chest pain days to months after cardiac surgery should be evaluated for signs of pericardial effusion known as *postpericardiotomy syndrome*. Patients with pulmonary hypertension may present with exercise intolerance, palpitations, and syncope. The resultant right ventricular dilatation may be found on physical examination as a narrowed second heart sound, hepatomegaly, and cyanosis if an atrial septal defect or ventricular septal defect is present. Eisenmenger syndrome is severe pulmonary hypertension from an uncorrected congenital heart disease, leading to cyanosis from right to left shunting of blood. Isolated anatomic abnormalities such as atrial septal defects have been known to present with chest pain and may or may not display the classic findings of a hyperactive precordium, widely split fixed second heart sounds, and both systolic and diastolic murmurs.

Unrecognized disease rarely causes isolated chest pain in a child who otherwise appears well, but the physician should consider drug exposure (e.g., cocaine; methamphetamine; nicotine; β-agonist abuse; the triptans; combination cold medications containing chlorpheniramine, dextromethorphan, and phenylpropanolamine; the herbal medications mentioned previously). Although cardiac conditions are infrequent, attention should be paid to diagnosing the rare patient with hypertrophic cardiomyopathy, angina, or early pericardial or myocardial inflammation (see Chapter 84).

Pulmonary diseases are common and account for approximately 12% to 21% of chest pain cases. A first episode of reactive airway disease should be suspected when an associated night cough, history of wheezing, or family history of atopy is present. There is a high incidence of exercise-induced asthma, which often presents with chest tightness, shortness of breath, and wheezing with exercise. These historical features are important, as the physical examination may be completely normal during the ED visit. Infectious diseases of the respiratory tract are associated with fever, malaise, cough, and coryza and may involve several family members simultaneously. Patients with pneumonia (see Chapter 92) often present with tachypnea and hypoxia in addition to fever and cough. Spontaneous (nontraumatic) pneumomediastinum and pneumothorax may occur in patients with reactive airway disease, cystic fibrosis, or as a result of barotrauma (i.e., Valsalva maneuver, forceful vomiting, or coughing). The pain of a pneumothorax is often unrelenting and pleuritic in nature. If the pneumothorax is moderate or large, patients present with significant respiratory distress and decreased breath sounds on the affected side. Spontaneous (nontraumatic) pneumomediastinum is most often reported in male adolescents without underlying lung disease and in those with asthma. It appears to occur with any activity that involves straining against a closed glottis. This is thought to cause a rise in intraalveolar pressure and subsequently a rupture of the alveoli releasing air into the

interstitial space. Air then dissects along fascial planes of the hilum into the mediastinum and neck. Those with spontaneous pneumomediastinum present with substernal chest pain that frequently radiates to the neck and is worse with deep inspiration and position changes, subcutaneous crepitus, Hamman's sign (crunching heart sounds), dysphagia, and dysphonia. This diagnosis must be distinguished from pneumothorax, pericarditis, and esophageal perforation.

Pleural effusions can cause chest pain associated with decreased breath sounds and dullness to percussion on physical examination. Pleurodynia, often secondary to coxsackievirus B infection, causes sharp chest pain, fever, and a friction rub. Aspiration of a foreign body into the trachea or esophagus may occur without such history in a toddler or even in an older child, and approximately 50% of these children may complain of chest pain. Foreign bodies lodged in the airway often present with chest pain, cough, decreased breath sounds, and unilateral wheezing. However, auscultatory findings may be unimpressive despite a positive history.

Although pulmonary embolisms (see Chapter 98) are rare in children, they can present with pleuritic chest pain, cough, hypoxia, hemoptysis, dyspnea, respiratory distress, and the sense of impending doom. Usually, this condition is associated with risk factors such as obesity, oral contraceptive use, pregnancy, collagen vascular disease, nephrotic syndrome, cigarette smoking, recent surgery, immobility, trauma (particularly spinal injury), a positive family history, a hypercoagulable condition (known or unknown), or prior cardiorespiratory problems. Finally, children with sickle cell disease can develop a vasoocclusive crises resulting in acute chest syndrome.

GI diseases account for approximately 4% to 7% of pediatric patients with chest pain. Diseases include gastroesophageal reflux, esophagitis, gastritis, ulcer disease, and, rarely, esophageal rupture or spasm. History is important regarding symptom relationship to meals and body position. Pain of gastroesophageal reflux is typically described as burning, worse in the recumbent position, related to eating, and improved with antacid or H_2 antagonist therapy. The physical examination finding is usually normal or positive for epigastric tenderness. Foreign bodies in the GI tract can cause chest pain, drooling, dysphagia, and odynophagia. The history often uncovers this diagnosis, and radiography may be helpful. Spontaneous esophageal perforation (Boerhaave syndrome) is secondary to transmitted increased pressure against a closed glottis most often seen with vomiting and also with straining, coughing, defecation, seizure, childbirth, or forceful nose blowing. Presentation includes symptoms of chest pain, crepitus, pneumomediastinum, and hematemesis to hemorrhage and shock. Mackler triad includes vomiting, chest pain, and subcutaneous emphysema. There are case reports of adolescents diagnosed with diffuse esophageal spasm via motility testing after persistent chest pain. Intraabdominal processes such as cholecystitis can present with postprandial pain and pain in the right upper quadrant.

Musculoskeletal causes of chest pain are common accounting for 15% to 31% of cases and are typically overuse injuries (muscle strain and inflamed tissue). Chest pain often occurs after physical activity and is reproducible by palpation and contraction of the muscle group on physical examination. Direct trauma may produce a contusion or rib fracture. Costochondritis is an inflammatory condition of the costochondral junctions, which may be preceded by a respiratory illness, and characteristically, has reproducible pain on examination. The pain is described as sharp and exaggerated by physical activity or deep inspiration. Tietze syndrome is a benign inflammatory condition of unknown cause, which results in isolated swelling of a costochondral junction. The inflamed area appears as a mass on the chest wall and results in chest pain that typically radiates to the shoulder or arm. This syndrome usually occurs in adults but has been reported in children and infants. When evaluating a chest wall mass, the differential diagnosis should include osteomyelitis and tumors.

Slipping rib syndrome is a pain syndrome caused by hypermobility of the anterior aspect of the 8th to 10th ribs, which do not directly attach to the sternum but instead are held together by fibrous tissue. It is thought that weakening of the fibrous tissue in the area allows the ribs to rub against the other, irritating the intercostal nerve and referring pain to the chest wall and abdomen. Patients describe a popping or clicking sensation followed by pain, which lasts several minutes. Pain is reproduced by hooking the lower ribs with the hand and pulling anteriorly.

A large group of children with chest pain will have no evidence of organic disease and no history of underlying cardiorespiratory disease or trauma. They may have a family history of chest pain and are able to identify a stressful situation that has precipitated the episode. Such children have psychogenic chest pain and represent approximately 5% to 17% of pediatric chest pain cases. Complaints of chest pain and other somatic aches often are chronic, and other symptoms of psychiatric illness or hyperventilation may be present. Nonorganic chest pain may appear to cause respiratory distress in the hyperventilating teenager, but close examination should distinguish this syndrome from serious problems (see Chapter 131).

Idiopathic etiology is the most common diagnosis of chest pain in pediatrics, representing 23% to 45% of cases. The term is used to describe chest pain when no organic etiology and no psychological factors are present to explain the pain. It is typically described as occasional short episodes of sharp chest pain with or without exercise and no other associated symptoms. Physical examination is completely normal and pain is not reproducible. Precordial catch syndrome, or "Texidor's twinge," is a relatively frequent cause of chest pain in healthy teenagers and young adults. It typically presents with an acute, sharp, well-localized pain (often in the left substernal region) that has a "split second" onset, is of short duration, worsened by deep inspiration, and usually occurs at rest or related to exercise. It is often relieved by position change (sitting up straight), which suggests that posture or ligamentous stretching of the supporting ligaments of the heart may have a role but the true etiology is unknown. The physical examination is normal without reproducible pain.

Other causes of chest pain include male adolescents with gynecomastia and female patients with fibrocystic breast disease. Rarely, chest pain, pressure, or shortness of breath, worse on supine position, will be associated with the presentation of a mediastinal mass.

EVALUATION AND DECISION

Child with Thoracic Trauma

The first step in evaluation of the child with chest pain is to perform a thorough history and physical examination. If the history is positive for a traumatic injury or if there is any evidence of trauma to the chest (see Chapter 118), the patient requires rapid evaluation and may need immediate resuscitation as well (Fig. 51.1A). Correction of cardiac or respiratory insufficiency may diagnose and treat the cause of chest pain.

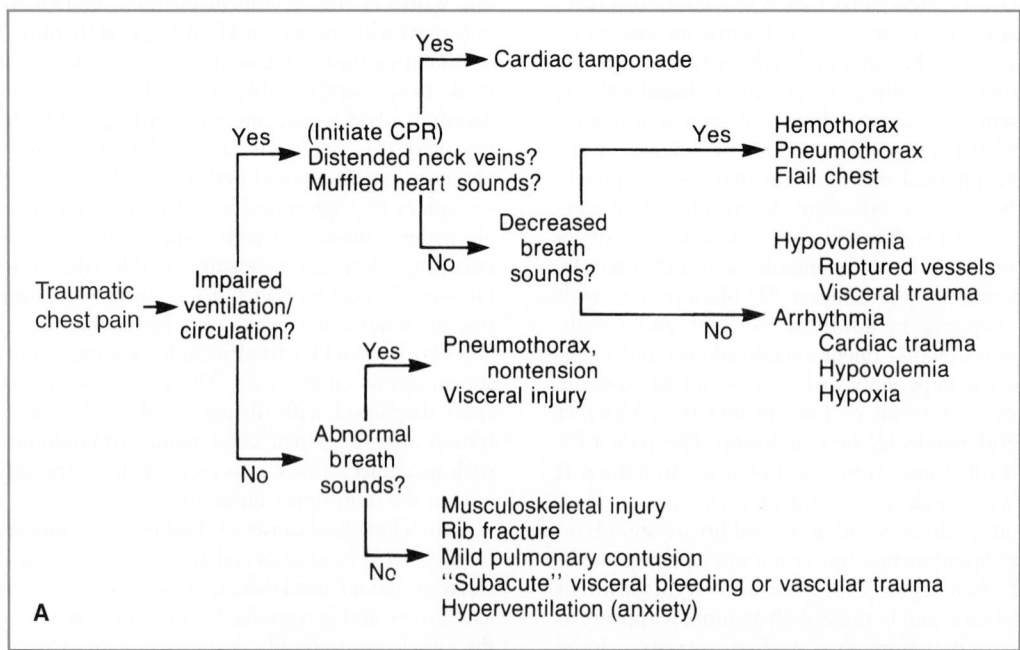

FIGURE 51.1 **A.** Diagnostic approach to traumatic chest pain. CPR, cardiopulmonary resuscitation. (*continued*)

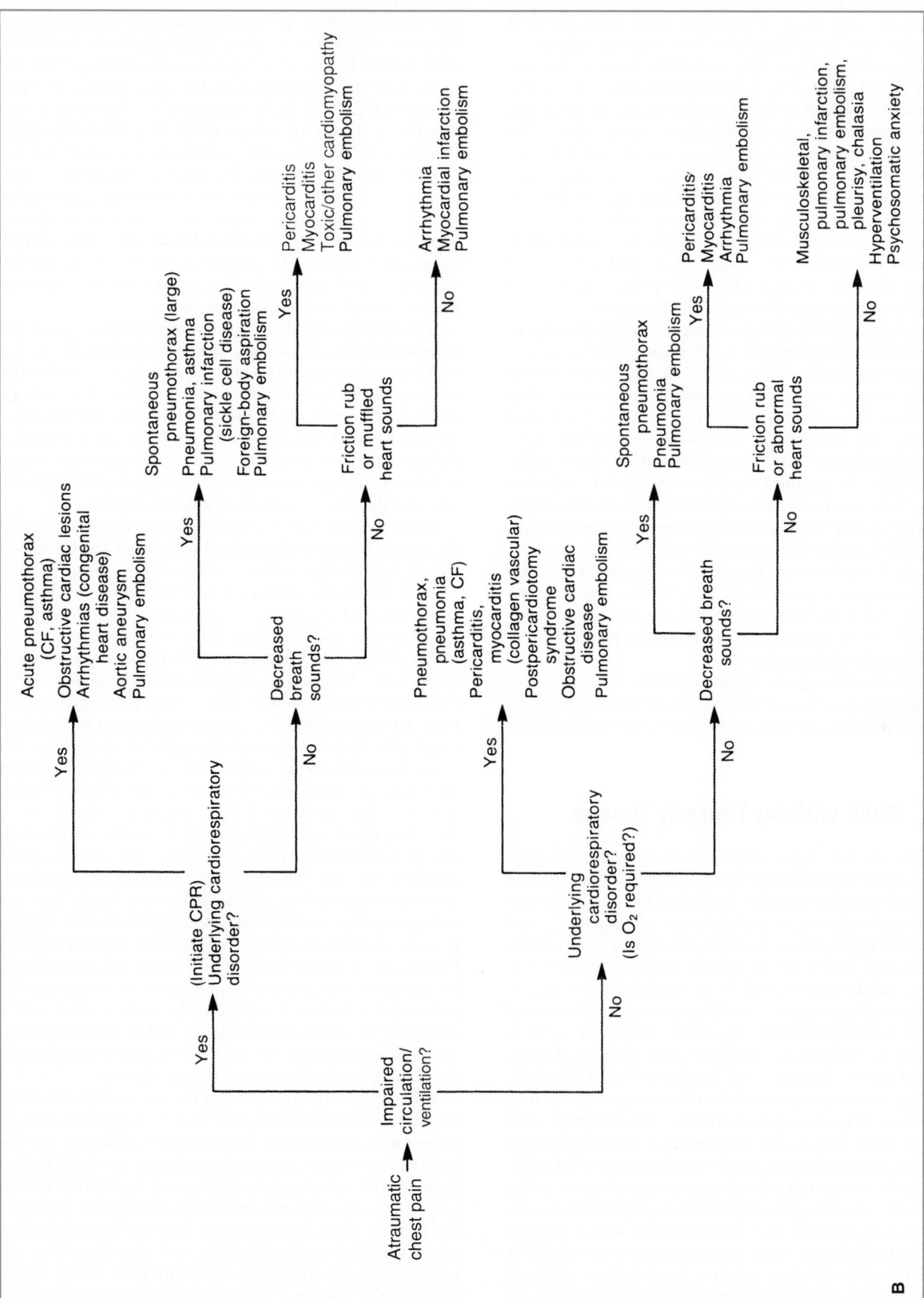

FIGURE 51.1 (*Continued*) **B**. Diagnostic approach to atraumatic chest pain. CPR, cardiopulmonary resuscitation; CF, cystic fibrosis.

Adequacy and symmetry of ventilation should be assessed to distinguish acute respiratory failure from hemothorax or pneumothorax. In children with chest trauma, tachycardia with hypotension is generally caused by hypovolemia secondary to a hemothorax, hemopneumothorax, or vascular injury. Reduced cardiac output and perfusion, however, may also be secondary to a rhythm disturbance (from a myocardial contusion or tension pneumothorax) or cardiac tamponade (which causes muffling of the heart sounds and pulsus paradoxus). A discrepancy of the pulse or blood pressure between the extremities points to aortic diseases, such as traumatic avulsion or aneurysm. Ruptured esophagus and tracheobronchial disruption may result from rapid deceleration injuries and may present with chest pain, subcutaneous emphysema, respiratory distress, and hypotension.

Many children with thoracic injuries but no respiratory distress also complain of chest pain. Although a careful examination is mandatory in an effort to exclude significant intrathoracic trauma, the cause of the pain usually resides in the chest wall: contusions of the soft tissues or rib fractures. A history of significant trauma even in the absence of cardiovascular abnormality dictates that radiographs and an electrocardiogram (EKG) be obtained. Injury to the heart, including myocardial contusions and acute rupture of cardiac structures, can occur during rapid deceleration and compression type injuries. Pulmonary injuries include contusions, pneumothoraces, and hemothoraces. These injuries may present with subtle physical examination findings. Patients have presented with chest pain following blunt trauma that was subsequently complicated by the development of posttraumatic ventricular septal defect and pseudoaneurysm.

Finally, the clinician should consider child abuse if rib fractures are seen in a young infant. In older children, a predisposing cause for fracture (i.e., bone cyst or tumor) should be sought.

Child without Thoracic Trauma

As above, the first step in evaluation of the child with chest pain is to perform a thorough history and physical examination assessing for cardiorespiratory instability (Fig. 51.1B). A thorough history including a complete review of symptoms, social history, and family history should be obtained. The description of chest pain should include quality, intensity, location, frequency, and duration as well as its relationship to exercise, food intake, position, or trauma. Chest pain relieved by leaning forward is consistent with pericarditis, while that which is worsened by reclining may represent gastroesophageal reflux or hiatal hernia. The review of symptoms should be broad, including systemic symptoms such as fever, fatigue, weight loss, diaphoresis, or intolerance to exercise; cardiac symptoms such as palpitations, heart racing, dizziness, or syncope; pulmonary symptoms such as dyspnea, cough, or wheezing; and GI symptoms such as vomiting, dysphagia, abnormal taste in the mouth, or abdominal pain. In general, chest pain that is acute in onset; is described as crushing sternal pain with or without radiation to left arm or neck; awakens a patient at night; or is associated with exertion, syncope, fever, fatigue, dyspnea, decreased exercise tolerance, or palpitations is concerning and demands a more extensive evaluation.

Next, the physician should inquire about a history suggestive of prior cardiorespiratory disease, such as asthma, cystic fibrosis, congenital or structural heart conditions, as well as a past medical history of collagen vascular disease, connective tissue disorders, hyperlipidemia, Kawasaki disease, or a prolonged febrile illness. It also is important to determine if there is a family history of sudden death, hypercholesterolemia, hypercoagulability disorders, or early cardiovascular disease.

Children with respiratory illnesses, such as asthma or cystic fibrosis are at risk for pneumothorax, acute respiratory failure from mucous plugging or pneumonitis, and acute pulmonary hypertension. In the child with a history of cardiac arrhythmias (see Chapter 84), congenital heart disease, cardiac surgery, or pericardial effusions, chest pain may signal an exacerbation of the underlying problem.

The social history should include recent stressors, and cigarette or drug use, including prescription medications such as oral contraceptives, stimulants such as cocaine, and herbal medications. In addition, it may be helpful to determine the patient's perception of the pain and how it is affecting his or her life. Research has shown that approximately one-third of children with chest pain have missed school secondary to their symptoms and approximately half of children with chest pain associate this pain as a problem with their heart.

In the absence of prior cardiopulmonary disease or trauma, the approach must be directed toward unmasking evidence for any of the serious cardiorespiratory illnesses listed in Table 51.3. A thorough examination usually uncovers evidence of the cardiac and respiratory causes of chest pain. The clinician must carefully assess the vital signs, looking for fever, tachycardia, bradycardia, tachypnea, bradypnea, hypertension, hypotension, and hypoxia. The patient may be well-appearing with no apparent distress or ill-appearing with significant distress. Concerning signs of the general appearance include cough, drooling, retractions, lethargy, pallor, or cyanosis. The physical examination in asthma shows a prolonged expiratory phase of respiration, variable degrees of chest hyperinflation, and wheezing accentuated by a forced expiratory effort. However, auscultatory findings, such as crackles or wheezing, may be minimal when obstructive pulmonary disease is moderately severe, and a history of foreign body aspiration should also be sought with new-onset wheezing. Fever, hypoxia, tachypnea, decreased breath sounds, and/or crackles suggests pneumonia, whereas dullness to percussion suggests effusion. Unilaterally absent or decreased breath sounds is concerning for pneumothorax, pneumonia, foreign body aspiration, or a pulmonary embolism. Crepitus of the neck or chest wall is indicative of pneumomediastinum and/or pneumothorax. Tracheal deviation may be seen in severe cases of tension pneumothorax where patients are in obvious distress.

If breath sounds are equal, yet there is an abnormal heart sound, a cardiac etiology is most likely. Pericardial disease can present with a friction rub, distant heart sounds, neck vein distension, hypotension, impaired circulation, pain with leaning forward, and pulsus paradoxus. Signs of myocarditis include persistent tachycardia and orthostasis, bradycardia, and a gallop rhythm. Physical examination findings such as dyspnea, crackles, wheezes, gallop rhythms, neck vein distension, and peripheral edema are seen in those with heart failure or cardiomyopathy. There is a wide range of clinical presentations of children with arrhythmias: They may be stable with irregular heart rates and rhythm, or they can present in cardiovascular shock. Signs of MI include rate and rhythm disturbances, pallor, dyspnea, and diaphoresis, as well as signs of heart failure.

Patients with a pulmonary embolism may present with a variety of physical findings, depending on the degree of arterial obstruction and, thus, hemodynamic compromise (see Chapter 98). Findings may include tachypnea, tachycardia, decreased breath sounds, crackles, fever, a friction rub, an accentuated S2, unexplained cyanosis, pleural friction rub, and/or cardiovascular collapse.

In addition to the usual cardiac and pulmonary examination, one should search for "trigger points," where palpation of the chest wall reproduces the pain, suggesting musculoskeletal inflammation. Reproduction of the pain by a "hooking maneuver" performed over the lower anterior ribs implicates the "slipping rib syndrome." Pain following a dermatome unilaterally suggests intercostal neuritis; children with zoster (shingles) may have pain preceding the development of rash.

When focal, peripheral pain is found without a "trigger point," the physician should consider pain referred from areas of sensory nerve overlap. For instance, relationship of the pain to eating or swallowing suggests esophageal disease, and often, the physical examination may appear normal.

Extrathoracic abnormalities, such as a rash or arthritis, may provide clues to collagen disorders (see Chapter 101) or other systemic illness. Marfan syndrome should be suspected in the tall, thin patient whose upper-extremity span exceeds his or her height and with hyperextensible fingers.

During the examination, it is useful to relate normal findings to the child and family because this reassurance often serves as the major "treatment" of self-limited or functional problems. Some families and patients are simply looking for reassurance that the chest pain is not cardiac in origin. Concerning physical examination findings such as fever, persistent tachycardia, persistent hypertension, hypotension, pathological murmurs, a gallop rhythm, abnormal pulses, abnormal perfusion, hypoxia, and syncope warrant further investigation.

Laboratory studies may be indicated to help confirm a diagnosis and may relieve the anxiety of the child or family; such investigations should be directed toward causes suspected based on the initial evaluation rather than considered as "screening" tests. Pulse oximetry is a quick and inexpensive test that is helpful in determining the severity of any suspected pulmonary disease. Chest radiographs may reveal findings consistent with asthma, pneumonitis, pleurisy, spontaneous pneumothorax, or mass. Foreign bodies ingested and lodged in the esophagus can be visualized if radiopaque (e.g., coins). In the cervical esophagus, they will lie flat and be fully visible in the posteroanterior view of the chest. Airway foreign-body aspiration most frequently manifests, however, by hyperinflation or atelectasis on radiographs because most tracheobronchial foreign bodies are not radiopaque. Inspiratory and expiratory films or decubitus chest radiographs may demonstrate focal hyperinflation (i.e., the lobe with an obstructed bronchus remains inflated in expiration or when placed on the dependent side on a decubitus film). The wide mediastinum from an aortic aneurysm, abnormal cardiac silhouette related to a pericardial effusion or cardiomegaly, rib fractures or bone changes of metabolic bone derangements, and cysts all pro-

duce characteristic radiographic changes. A calcified ring may be visualized in approximately one-third of patients with a history of Kawasaki disease. The presence of atelectasis may suggest mucous plugging or may be subtle evidence of pulmonary infarction from an embolus or a vasoocclusive crisis of sickle cell disease. If found, the presence of a wedge-shaped pulmonary infiltrate with an ipsilateral elevated hemidiaphragm is suggestive of a pulmonary embolism.

An EKG should be performed if cardiac disease is suspected. For example, one would have an elevated level of suspicion for cardiac disease if the physical examination findings are suggestive of myocarditis or pericarditis or if the chest pain is thought to be anginal or exertional, or associated with syncope, dizziness, and/or palpitations. The EKG will be normal in almost all children with chest pain in which the physical examination is unremarkable. It may show signs of cardiac strain or ischemia with valvular heart disease, diseases of outflow obstruction, or ischemia. Acute cocaine exposure may present with classic signs of myocardial ischemia or myocardiopathy. A decreased QRS wave voltage and electrical alternans suggest the presence of a pericardial effusion in the child with muffled heart sounds. Decreased voltages, ST elevations, and T-wave abnormalities may also be seen in diseases such as myocarditis and pericarditis. Heart block and arrhythmias, such as atrial fibrillation and supraventricular tachycardia, can occur secondary to anatomic, ischemic, inflammatory, and drug-induced conditions. These electrical disturbances may be identified by careful evaluation of a rhythm strip. Finally, the S_1-Q_3-T_3 pattern may be seen on EKG evaluation in those with a pulmonary embolism.

Studies other than chest radiographs and EKGs are rarely necessary. An elevated leukocyte count with a shift to the left may point toward infection as the cause of pain. Examination of a peripheral smear and a hemoglobin electrophoresis are indicated in the child suspected of having sickle cell disease as the cause of chest pain. In children with sickle cell disease, a complete blood cell count, reticulocyte count, and blood culture are indicated to assist in ascertaining acute chest syndrome or pneumonia, as well as the presence of acute anemia and its cause. If an intraabdominal source for chest pain from diaphragmatic irritation is under consideration, further testing is appropriate. Serum amylase and lipase levels may be obtained in the workup of pancreatitis. The evaluation of a possible right-sided subdiaphragmatic abscess would include liver function tests and further delineation by ultrasound or computed tomography scan. Esophageal causes of chest pain may often be diagnosed clinically in the ED with a trial of antacid therapy followed by H_2-m receptor antagonist or proton pump inhibitors. To confirm the findings of a hiatal hernia, esophagitis, or a radiolucent foreign body, a barium study or endoscopy may be required. Findings of low PaO_2, EKG abnormalities, and a positive D-dimer are suggestive of pulmonary embolism. This suspected diagnosis requires the performance of a helical computed tomography scan for confirmation. The clinician may consider peak expiratory flow testing and/or therapeutic trial of bronchodilators when asthma is suspected as the cause of chest pain. Only rarely will it become necessary to obtain cardiac-specific creatine phosphokinase fractions and troponin for the evaluation of a possible MI. Toxicologic screens may be useful if the patient is considered at risk of drug abuse, particularly cocaine, or if the diagnosis remains unclear. Consultation with a pediatric cardiologist may be necessary if the chest pain is concerning for a cardiac condition.

Not infrequently, a chest radiograph and an EKG are helpful in allaying parental fears of cardiac disease. However, the clinician should be aware that, in some cases, where a cardiac or respiratory condition is not suspected, ordering unnecessary tests may actually increase a patient's or parent's concern that true pathology exists. Definitive ongoing management requires referral to a primary care physician.

SUMMARY

Chest pain in children is a relatively infrequent sign of serious disease but often has great importance to the patient or family. Most cases can be diagnosed by the emergency physician from the history and physical examination alone, although, at times, a chest x-ray or an EKG is helpful. The physician should always consider drug-induced chest pain (especially associated with cocaine) and other life-threatening conditions. Patients with a history of exercise-induced chest pain and/or syncope, medical history of underlying cardiopulmonary condition, suspected Kawasaki disease, history of drug use, oral contraceptive and cigarette use, and older children with family history of early coronary artery disease or hypercholesterolemia appear to be at higher risk of cardiovascular disease. Psychogenic chest pain is a common occurrence and may be chronic or related to an acute stressful event. The possibility of cardiac disease needs to be addressed directly by the examining physician to alleviate fully the patient's (or family's) anxiety. The most common causes of organic chest pain are musculoskeletal (traumatic or inflammatory) and infectious disorders, usually self-limited or easily treated diseases. Occasionally, serious abdominal, pulmonary, or cardiac problems require immediate attention.

Suggested Readings

Berezin S, Medow MS, Glassman MS, et al. Chest pain of gastrointestinal origin. *Arch Dis Child* 1998;63:1457–1460.
Burns JC, Shike H, Gordon JB, et al. Sequelae of Kawasaki disease in adolescents and young adults. *J Am Coll Cardiol* 1996;28:253–257.
Cava JR, Sayger PL. Chest pain in children and adolescents. *Pediatr Clin North Am* 2004;51:1553–1568.
Chalumeau M, Le Clainche L, Sayeg N, et al. Spontaneous pneumomediastinum in children. *PediatrPulmonol* 2001;31:67–75.
Christensen DD, Vincent RN, Campbell RM. Presentation of atrial septal defect in the pediatric population. *Pediatr Cardiol* 2005;26:812–814.
Dekel B, Paret G, Szeinberg A, et al. Spontaneous pneumomediastinum in children: clinical and natural history. *Eur J Pediatr* 1996;155:695–697.
Ernst E. Cardiovascular adverse effects of herbal medicines: a systematic review of the recent literature. *Can J Cardiol* 2003;19:818–827.
Frommelt PC, Frommelt MA, Tweddell JS, et al. Prospective echocardiographic diagnosis and surgical repair of anomalous origin of a coronary artery from the opposite sinus with an interarterial course. *J Am Coll Cardiol* 2003;42:148–154.
Gitter MJ, Goldsmith SR, Dunbar DN, et al. Cocaine and chest pain: clinical features and outcome of patients hospitalized to rule out myocardial infarction. *Ann Intern Med* 1991;115:277–282.
Glassman MS, Medow MS, Berezin S, et al. Spectrum of esophageal disorders in children with chest pain. *Dig Dis Sci* 1992;37(5):663–666.
Hayes D Jr. Chest pain. *Clin Pediatr* 2007;46(8):746–747.
Hoerbelt R, Keunecke L, Grimm H, et al. The value of a noninvasive diagnostic approach to mediastinal masses. *Ann Thorac Surg* 2003;75:1086–1090.
Horton L, Mosee S, Brenner J. Use of the electrocardiogram in a pediatric emergency department. *Arch Pediatr Adolesc Med* 1994;148:184–188.
Hyman PE, Bursch B, Sood M, et al. Visceral pain-associated disability syndrome: a descriptive analysis. *J Pediatr Gastroenterol Nutr* 2002;35:663–668.
Kocis KC. Chest pain in pediatrics. *Pediatr Clin North Am* 1999;46(2):189–203.
Kundra M, Yousaf S, Maqbool S, et al. Boerhaave syndrome—unusual cause of chest pain. *Pediatr Emerg Care* 2007;23(7):489–491.
Massin MM, Bourguignont A, Coremans C, et al. Chest pain in pediatric patients presenting to an emergency department or to a cardiac clinic. *Clin Pediatr* 2004;43:231–238.
Milov DE, Cynamon HA, Andres JM. Chest pain and dysphagia in adolescents caused by diffuse esophageal spasm. *J Pediatr Gastroenterol Nutr* 1989;9:450–453.
Mukamel M, Kornreich L, Horev G, et al. Tietze's syndrome in children and infants. *J Pediatr* 1997;131(5):774–775.
Rowe BH, Dulberg CS, Peterson RG, et al. Characteristics of children presenting with chest pain to a pediatric emergency department. *Can Med Assoc J* 1990;143(5):388–394.
Sabri MR, Ghavanini AA, Haghighat M, et al. Chest pain in children and adolescents: epigastric tenderness as a guide to reduce unnecessary work-up. *Pediatr Cardiol* 2003;24(1):3–5.
Selbst SM. Chest pain in children. *Pediatr Rev* 1997;18(5):169–173.
Selbst SM, Ruddy RM, Clark BJ, et al. Pediatric chest pain: a prospective study. *Pediatrics* 1988;82:319–323.
Taubman B, Vetter VL. Slipping rib syndrome as a cause of chest pain in children. *Clin Pediatr* 1996;35:403–405.
Tomita M, Suzuki N, Igarachi H, et al. Evidence against strong correlation between chest symptoms and ischemic coronary changes after subcutaneous sumatriptan injection. *Intern Med* 2002;41:622–625.
Yildirim A, Karakurt C, Karademir S, et al. Chest pain in children. *Int Pediatr* 2004;19(3):175–179.
Zavarus-Angelidou KA, Weinhouse E, Nelson DB. Review of 180 episodes of chest pain in 134 children. *Pediatr Emerg Care* 1992;8:189–193.

CHAPTER 52 ■ PAIN—DYSPHAGIA

RONALD A. FURNIVAL, MD, VAISHALI JHA, MD, AND GEORGE A. WOODWARD, MD, MBA

The primary function of swallowing is the ingestion, preparation, and transport of nutrients to the digestive tract. Secondary functions of swallowing are the control of secretions, clearance of respiratory contaminants, protection of the upper airway, and equalization of pressure across the tympanic membrane through the eustachian tube. Dysphagia is defined as any difficulty or abnormality of swallowing. Dysphagia is not a specific disease entity but is a symptom of other, often clinically occult, conditions and may be life-threatening if respiration or nutrition is compromised. Odynophagia (pain on swallowing) or sialorrhea (drooling) may also be present in the dysphagic pediatric patient. Globus pharyngeus refers to the feeling of a lump in the throat. This chapter briefly presents the normal anatomy and physiology of swallowing, the differential diagnosis of disturbances of this process, and the evaluation and treatment of the pediatric patient with dysphagia.

PATHOPHYSIOLOGY

Swallowing begins in utero as early as the 10th to 14th week of gestation, playing an important role in gastrointestinal development and regulation of amniotic fluid volume. By the 34th week of gestation, this complex process, involving 26 muscles, 6 cranial nerves (V, VII, IX, X, XI, and XII), and cervical nerves C1 to C3, is functional, although incompletely coordinated with breathing. In the first few days after birth, each infant develops an individual pattern of sucking, swallowing, and breathing, usually with a 1:1 or 1:2 ratio of breaths per suckle, to prevent aspiration of material into the larynx. This stage of suckling, or suckle feeding, is primarily under medullary control, with minimal input from the cerebral cortex. A transitional period begins at 6 months of age, as the cortex gradually exerts more control over the preesophageal phase of swallowing, allowing for the introduction of solid foods. The preesophageal region depends on normal sensorimotor function of cranial nerves V, VII, IX, and XII, which innervate voluntary skeletal muscles of the face, tongue, and neck, as well as the involuntary muscles of the posterior pharynx. Swallowing in the esophageal region remains an autonomic process, with vagal sensorimotor control coordinating peristalsis of the upper striated and lower smooth muscle of the esophagus. By 3 years of age, the swallowing pattern is mature, although the pediatric patient, unlike the adult, may regress to a less mature stage if normal swallowing is disrupted.

To facilitate suckle feeding and breathing, the infant oropharynx is anatomically different from the adult, with a relatively larger tongue, smaller oral cavity, and more anterior and superior epiglottis and larynx. As the face and mandible grow, the oropharynx enlarges, creating more room for the eventual voluntary use of the tongue and dentition, and the larynx descends, eventually allowing for mouth breathing. Although breathing continues to cease during swallows, the older child depends less on close coordination between eating and breathing.

A normal swallow, using the suckling infant as an example, begins with rhythmic movement of the lips, tongue, and mandible. These parts function as a unit, creating negative intraoral pressure, while also compressing the nipple. The milk expressed from each suckle is stored in the posterior oral cavity until a larger fluid bolus is formed. As the tongue delivers the bolus to the pharynx, the nasopharynx is closed off by the posterior tongue and by elevation of the soft palate. The larynx elevates to a position under the tongue, closing the airway, as the epiglottis inclines to direct the bolus posterior. A pharyngeal wave of contraction sweeps the bolus toward the upper esophagus, where the cricopharyngeal sphincter relaxes, allowing passage into the esophagus. As the esophagus begins peristaltic contractions and the bolus moves past a relaxed lower esophageal sphincter into the stomach, the airway reopens, the cricopharyngeal sphincter constricts to close the upper esophagus, and respirations resume. Dysphagia can result from disruption of normal mechanisms at any stage of the swallowing process.

DIFFERENTIAL DIAGNOSIS

Acute dysphagia is one of the urgent symptoms needing immediate evaluation. While this may be an acute symptom in a healthy child, it may be a new or recurrent symptom in the increasing number of children surviving with chronic conditions. The differential diagnosis for dysphagia is extensive and is commonly divided into preesophageal or esophageal disorders (Table 52.1). Preesophageal causes of dysphagia are further subdivided into anatomic categories, including nasopharyngeal, oropharyngeal, laryngeal, and generalized problems. Infectious and inflammatory disorders of either anatomic region may disrupt swallowing, whereas neuromuscular problems tend to be predominantly preesophageal, given the autonomic function of the esophagus. However, the esophagus can be affected by motility disorders intrinsic to smooth muscle. Finally, the differential diagnosis includes several systemic conditions that may affect the normal swallowing process. In a large case series, Hartnick et al., described 568 pediatric patients who underwent fiberoptic evaluation of swallowing function and their underlying diagnoses. This group included 36% with structural abnormalities of the aerodigestive tract or

TABLE 52.1

DIFFERENTIAL DIAGNOSIS OF DYSPHAGIA

Preesophageal (Nasopharynx, Oropharynx, Larynx)
Mechanical/Anatomic
  General
  Congenital syndromes
    Pierre-Robin
    Treacher-Collins
    Crouzon's
    Goldenhar's
    Cornelia de Lange
  Cysts (tongue, larynx, epiglottis)
  Tumors (neuroblastoma)
  Lymphangioma
  Foreign-body aspiration
  Traumatic (external, endotracheal intubation, endoscopy)
Nasopharyngeal
  Choanal stenosis/atresia
  Nasal septum deflections
Oropharyngeal
  Cleft palate/lip
  Submucosal cleft
  Macroglossia
    Down syndrome (trisomy 21)
    Beckwith-Wiedemann syndrome
  Micrognathia
  Lip/teeth defects
  Tongue/sublingual masses
    Hemangioma
    Lymphangioma
    Lingual thyroid
    Thyroglossal duct cyst
    Branchial cleft cyst
  Hypopharyngeal stenosis
  Temporomandibular joint ankylosis
  Pharyngeal diverticula (congenital/traumatic)
  Adenoidal/tonsillar hypertrophy
Laryngeal
  Tracheostomy
  Tracheoesophageal fistula
  Cervical vertebral osteophytes
  Airway obstruction
  Laryngomalacia
Inflammatory/Infectious
  General
  Anaphylaxis
  Tetanus
  Rabies
  Botulism (especially infant botulism)
  Poliomyelitis
  Angioneurotic edema
  Sydenham's chorea
  Juvenile rheumatoid arthritis
  Stevens-Johnson syndrome
Nasopharyngeal
  Nasal septal abscess
  Sinusitis
Oropharyngeal
  Stomatitis (infectious, allergic)
  Pharyngitis/tonsillitis/uvulitis
  Retropharyngeal abscess

  Peritonsillar abscess
  Cervical adenitis
Laryngeal
  Epiglottitis
  Diphtheria
  Thyroiditis
Neuromuscular
  Prematurity
  Hypoxic injury
  Head trauma
  Neurologic impairment
  Cerebral palsy
  Developmental delay
  Meningitis
  Cerebral abscess
  Cerebral cortical atrophy/hypoplasia/agenesis
  Arnold-Chiari malformation
  Cerebrovascular disease
Cranial nerve palsies (V, VII, IX–XII)
  Palatal paralysis
  Laryngeal paralysis
Spinal cord impairment
  Syringomyelia
  Cricopharyngeal incoordination/spasm
Moebius syndrome
Myotonic muscular dystrophy
Guillain-Barré syndrome
Werdnig-Hoffman
Myasthenia gravis
Myotonic dystrophy
Dermatomyositis
Miscellaneous
  Ingestions (neuroleptic-induced dystonic reaction)
  Familial dysautonomia (Riley-Day syndrome)
  Prader-Willi syndrome
  Cerebrohepatorenal syndrome
  Vitamin deficiencies (pellagra, scurvy)
  Acrodynia
  Infantile Gaucher's disease
  Psychiatric
  Globus hystericus ("lump" in throat sensation)
  Pseudodysphagia
  Conversion reaction
  Hyperphagia
  Munchausen by proxy
Respiratory distress
Esophageal Causes of Dysphagia
Mechanical/Anatomic
  Tracheoesophageal fistula
  Esophageal atresia/stenosis
  Esophageal diverticula/duplication
  Esophageal strictures
    Congenital (webs, fibromuscular, tracheobronchial remnants)
    Acquired (corrosive ingestion, esophagitis, postoperative)

  Foreign-body ingestion
  Thermal injury (burn from hot food/drink)
  Esophageal tumors (hamartomas, leiomyoma, rhabdomyoma)
  Esophageal polyps
  External esophageal compression
  Cardiovascular anomalies (aberrant right subclavian artery, vascular rings, double aortic arch)
  Mediastinal tumors/infiltrations
  Atopic thyroid
  Diaphragmatic hernias
  Paraesophageal hernia
  Hiatal hernia
Altered esophageal motility
  Achalasia
  Gastroesophageal reflux
  Esophageal spasm
Inflammatory/Infectious
  Eosinophilic esophagitis
  Infectious esophagitis
  Candida albicans
  Herpes simplex
  Cytomegalovirus
  Human immunodeficiency virus
Reflux esophagitis
Allergic esophagitis
Radiation injury
Mediastinitis
Esophageal perforation
Crohn's disease
Chagas' disease (*Trypanosoma cruzi*, a South American parasite)
Miscellaneous
  Connective tissue disease
    Scleroderma
    Systemic lupus erythematosus
    Polymyositis
    Dermatomyositis
    Sjögren's syndrome
    Behçet's disease
Hyperkalemia, hypermagnesemia
Muscular hypertrophy of esophagus
Central nervous system tumors
Demyelinating diseases
Epidermolysis bullosa congenita
Lesch-Nyhan syndrome
Wilson's disease
Dyskeratosis congenita
Opitz-Frias syndrome
Lipidosis
Myxedema
Thyrotoxicosis
Alcoholism
Diabetes
Amyloidosis
Posttruncal vagotomy, antireflux surgery
Subcutaneous emphysema

TABLE 52.2

COMMON CAUSES OF DYSPHAGIA

Newborn/Infant
Prematurity
Tracheoesophageal fistula
Choanal stenosis/atresia
Birth trauma
Congenital abnormalities
Gastroesophageal reflux
Respiratory illness
Neurologic/neuromuscular disease
Infectious (botulism, candidiasis, herpetic esophagitis)
Inflammatory

Child
Foreign-body aspiration/ingestion
Caustic ingestion
Infectious
Ingestions (neuroleptic-induced dystonic reaction)
Neurologic impairment (cerebral palsy, mental retardation, head trauma)
Inflammatory

TABLE 52.3

LIFE-THREATENING CAUSES OF DYSPHAGIA

Foreign-body aspiration/ingestion
Anaphylaxis
Tracheoesophageal fistula
Upper airway obstruction
Traumatic esophageal perforation
Epiglottitis
Retropharyngeal abscess
Botulism
Tetanus
Polio
Diphtheria
Central nervous system infection/abscess
Stevens-Johnson syndrome
Corrosive ingestion
Laryngeal paralysis

airway, 26% with neurologic diagnoses, 12% with gastrointestinal disorders, 8% with genetic syndromes, 5% with prematurity, 3% with cardiovascular anomalies, and 2% with metabolic issues presenting with dysphagia.

In the adult patient, dysphagia most commonly results from a variety of neuromuscular disorders, whereas the pediatric patient more often has swallowing difficulty from congenital, infectious, inflammatory, or obstructive causes (Table 52.2). In the newborn or infant, swallowing may be disturbed as a result of prematurity, often associated with respiratory and neurologic disabilities. Gastroesophageal reflux is common in infants, although in a small percentage of patients, it may persist into childhood with reflux esophagitis. Eosinophilic esophagitis has recently been identified as an important cause of dysphagia, particularly in adolescents and young adults with environmental allergies, atopy, and food allergies. Ingestion or aspiration of a foreign body must always be considered in the toddler who has either the acute or chronic onset of dysphagia. Swallowing dysfunction is a common complication following pediatric head injury. In a review of 1,145 pediatric head injury patients, Morgan et al., found that 68% of those with severe injury and 15% of those suffering moderate injury subsequently had dysphagia requiring intervention. Postoperative dysphagia is also common after laryngotracheal reconstruction surgery or cardiovascular surgery. In a review of 2,255 children who had cardiovascular surgery, Jaquiss et al., found that 1.7% had vocal cord dysfunction associated with significant feeding problems and required prolonged gastrostomy feeding. These patients are predisposed to aspiration due to impaired airway protection.

Life-threatening causes of dysphagia may involve airway compromise, serious local or systemic infection, and inflammatory disease (Table 52.3). The newborn may have a congenital anatomic abnormality, such as tracheoesophageal fistula, with aspiration of swallowed fluid into the lungs, or may have traumatic injury to the upper airway and esophagus from iatrogenic instrumentation in the delivery room. The older child may have a foreign body in the airway or esophagus, with the possibility of complete airway obstruction (see Chapter 5). Anaphylaxis or other allergic and infectious processes may present with dysphagia and can threaten airway integrity. These include epiglottitis, retropharyngeal abscess, Stevens-Johnson syndrome, and central nervous system infections.

EVALUATION AND DECISION

The evaluation of dysphagia in the pediatric patient begins with a detailed history, including pregnancy and delivery, family history, feeding history, growth and development, and a history of other illness (Table 52.4). An accurate and complete history should suggest the diagnosis in approximately 80% of patients. Prenatal polyhydramnios, maternal infection, maternal drug or medication use, bleeding disorders, thyroid dysfunction, toxemia, or irradiation may lead to or indicate swallowing problems in the newborn or infant. Association between decreased rate of fetal suckling and digestive tract obstruction or neurologic damage is well known. Maternal myasthenia gravis may also cause temporary feeding problems in the newborn.

A history of traumatic delivery may result in neurologic injury or laryngeal paralysis. Newborn intubation may be associated with trauma to the trachea, larynx, or esophagus, as well as hypoxic brain injury. A history of prematurity, developmental delay, failure to thrive, hypotonia, or associated congenital abnormalities may indicate a neuromuscular cause for dysphagia. The feeding history should include acute or chronic onset of symptoms, age at onset, weight loss, failure to thrive, and type and amount of food the child eats. Presence of fever, pain, respiratory symptoms, facial color, stridor, liquid or solid food intolerance, vomiting, regurgitation, drooling, voice change, position during feeding, and the timing of symptoms in relation to feedings should also be documented. For example, the infant with an upper airway obstruction may become fatigued or begin coughing and choking shortly after beginning to eat. Choking during feeding in an infant may be due to an underlying anatomic abnormality of the trachea, esophagus or larynx. Congenital vascular lesions causing extrinsic compression of the esophagus may remain silent until

TABLE 52.4

IMPORTANT HISTORICAL FEATURES
FOR DYSPHAGIA

General
Age of onset
Acute/gradual onset
Weight gain
Growth and development
Constant, progressive, or intermittent
Pain (location/quality)
Fever
Ingestion history (neuroleptics, foreign bodies, or caustics)
Difficulty chewing
Difficulty swallowing
Change in voice quality
Altered swallowing sensation (lump, sticking, or foreign body)
Drooling/salivation
Solid/liquid intolerance
Cough/choking while feeding
Respiratory symptoms after feeding (stridor, wheezing, or apnea)
Vomiting (gastric contents) vs. regurgitation (food without
    gastric contents, esophageal disorders)
Nasopharyngeal regurgitation
Gastroesophageal reflux
Peptic ulcer disease
Tobacco or alcohol usage
Recent esophageal or airway instrumentation
Arthritis, degenerative joint disease
Antibiotic use
Chemotherapy
Underlying illness, immunodeficiency

Newborn/Infant
Prematurity
Pregnancy history
    Infections
    Medications (especially antihypertensives)
    Bleeding
    Toxemia
    Thyroid dysfunction
    Polyhydramnios
    Fetal irradiation
    Food allergy
Birth history
    Birth trauma
    Hypoxia
    Endotracheal intubation or resuscitation
Cough/gag/cyanosis/fatigue/stridor/irritability with feeding
Feeding times greater than 30 min
Respiratory distress associated with feeding
Vomiting or regurgitation
Level of alertness
Weight gain or failure to thrive
Nasal regurgitation
Refusal to eat age-appropriate foods
Recurrent pneumonias
Family history of neuromuscular disease

the introduction of solid food, or may rarely manifest as dysphagia later in adulthood. Gastroesophageal reflux in infants may manifest as vomiting shortly after feeding or with a history of nighttime cough or emesis. Intrinsic lesions, from inflammation, tumor, or foreign body, may create problems with solid food but cause no difficulty with liquids. Infants with previously unrecognized neuromuscular disorders commonly present initially with dysphagia, particularly for liquids; drooling; prolonged feeding time; weak suckle; or nasal reflux of swallowed material. A history of fever may indicate aspiration pneumonia or other infectious or inflammatory causes of dysphagia. Determining whether symptoms are progressive or intermittent/nonprogressive can also be helpful.

The child with dysphagia should undergo a thorough general physical examination, initially focusing on the patient's cardiopulmonary status. Evidence of respiratory distress or cardiovascular compromise should be treated promptly in the appropriate manner, as outlined elsewhere in this text (see Chapters 1, 2, and 5). Assurance of a secure and stable airway should precede attempts to examine the oropharynx or to remove a foreign body (see Chapter 28).

In the stable dysphagic patient, evaluation of head size and shape, facial structure, mandibular development, tongue disproportion, and ear configuration may provide evidence of an underlying congenital abnormality, such as Pierre-Robin, Treacher-Collins, Crouzon's, and Goldenhar's syndromes. Evaluation of nasal airway patency in the infant can be determined by gently passing an 8F catheter through the nares into the stomach. If the catheter fails to pass easily, choanal stenosis, atresia, or esophageal obstruction must be considered. Inspection of the oral cavity, pharynx, and neck may reveal a cyst, mass, localized infection, or inflammatory cause for dysphagia. Cervical auscultation over the thyroid cartilage during feeding may note evidence of aspiration if upper airway breath sounds are abnormal or if the timing of breathing and swallowing is uncoordinated. The pulmonary examination may also detect signs of aspiration or respiratory compromise, including elevated respiratory rate, increased respiratory effort, stridor, stertor, rales, rhonchi, wheezing, or change in voice quality. Neurologic examination may reveal an altered level of arousal from an underlying brain injury or depressed sensorium from drugs or infection that may limit effective swallowing. Examination of the cranial nerves, particularly V, VII, IX, X, and XII, may reveal abnormalities from traumatic or surgical injury, tumor, or congenital disorder. Evaluation of muscle tone, strength, and reflexes in consideration of other neuromuscular causes of dysphagia completes the general physical examination.

Provided oral intake is not contraindicated by an expected procedure or intervention, observation of a typical feeding, given by a parent or primary caregiver, may help elucidate the cause of dysphagia. The manner of presentation of food to the patient, the consistency and amount given, patient position, duration of feeding, regurgitation (oral or nasal), agitation or behavior change, or the development of respiratory symptoms may further guide the diagnostic evaluation. Patients with upper airway obstruction may have an exacerbation of symptoms when attempting to drink. Patients with lesions such as tracheoesophageal fistula, vascular rings, or esophageal obstruction may begin coughing and choking soon after drinking without any initial difficulty. However, esophageal disorders such as extrinsic compression, strictures, tumors, or altered motility commonly are clinically silent and typically require use of radiographic or direct visual techniques for diagnosis.

Evaluation of the stable dysphagic patient may proceed on the basis of age and acute versus chronic onset of symptom development (Fig. 52.1). The neonate and young infant will require evaluation techniques and consideration of the age-related differential diagnoses outlined in Table 52.2, whereas the older child with an acute onset of dysphagia generally requires a more urgent approach. Witnessed or suspected foreign bodies, either ingested or aspirated, should be investigated with plain radiographs (or contrast studies if a radiolucent object is considered) and, if identified, emergently removed (see Chapter 28). A history of neck trauma or caustic ingestion should lead to the suspicion of aerodigestive tract abnormalities. These patients may present dramatically with neck pain, drooling, and evidence of facial or other trauma, but they may also have a subacute presentation (see Chapters 102, 110, and 115). Presence of fever or signs of systemic illness may result

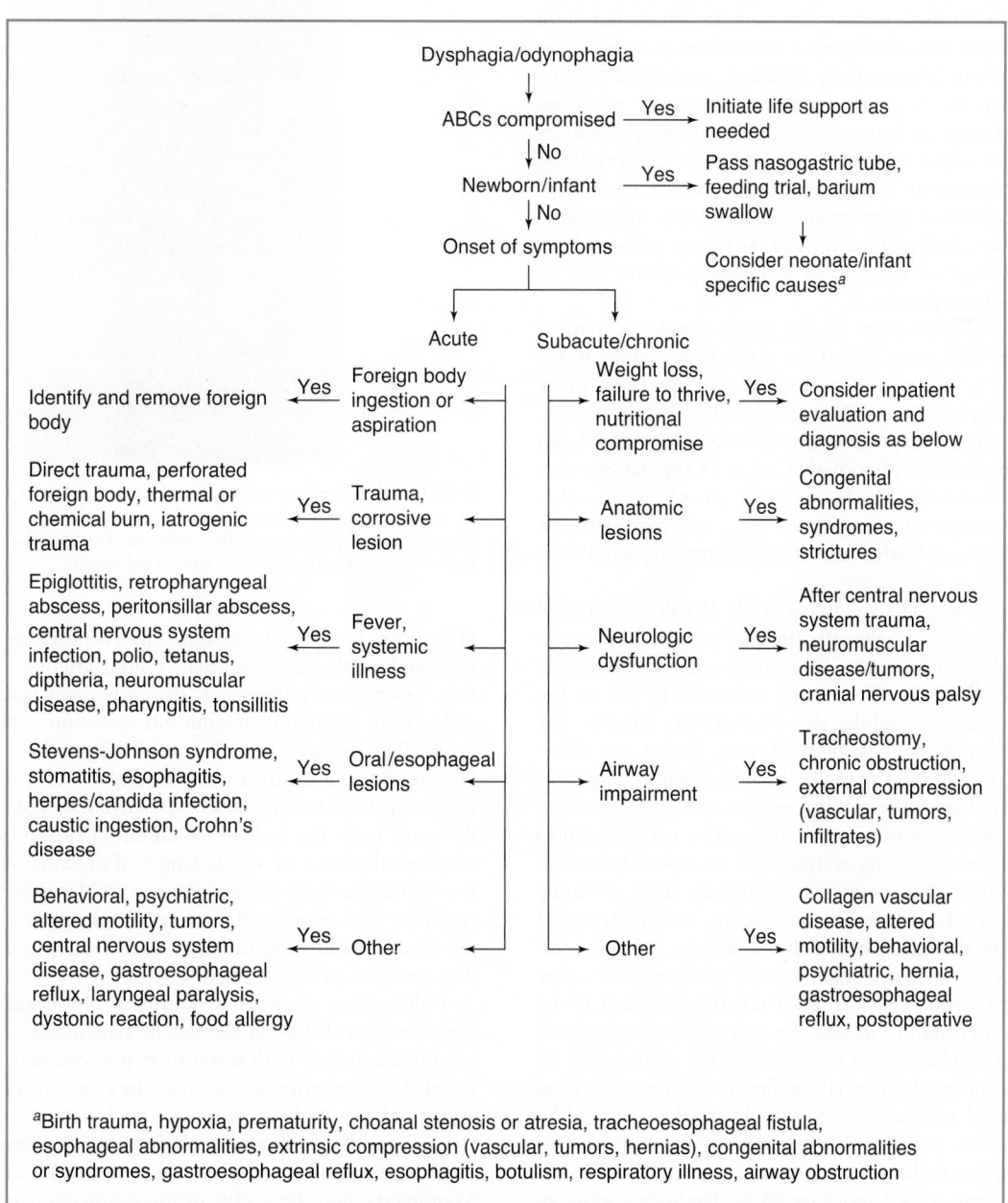

SIGNS AND SYMPTOMS

^{a}Birth trauma, hypoxia, prematurity, choanal stenosis or atresia, tracheoesophageal fistula, esophageal abnormalities, extrinsic compression (vascular, tumors, hernias), congenital abnormalities or syndromes, gastroesophageal reflux, esophagitis, botulism, respiratory illness, airway obstruction

FIGURE 52.1 Evaluation scheme for the child with dysphagia or odynophagia. *Radiographic and assessment options:* neck, chest, abdomen, inspiratory/expiratory films, lateral decubitus films, fluoroscopy (including videofluoroscopy), contrast studies, ultrasonography, echocardiography, angiography, computed tomography, magnetic resonance imaging, esophageal manometry, laryngopharyngeal sensory testing, electromyography, endoscopy. *Laboratory options:* complete blood cell count, blood gas, cultures, toxin identifications, nutritional and electrolyte profile. *Consultant options:* pediatrics, general surgery, otolaryngology, gastroenterology, neurology, infectious disease, cardiology, pulmonology, rheumatology, oncology, nutrition, speech therapy, speech-language pathologist, occupational therapy. ABCs, airway, breathing, circulation.

from potentially life-threatening infectious or inflammatory conditions (Table 52.3). Less severe problems (gingivostomatis or thrush) may present with mouth lesions and can be managed on an outpatient basis after careful assessment of hydration status. Severe problems, including Stevens-Johnson syndrome, herpetic esophagitis, and diphtheria, may be discovered on a detailed examination and may require inpatient management.

Patients with a nonacute history of swallowing difficulty can be evaluated and treated as shown in Figure 52.1. The initial emphasis with these patients lies more in determination of nutritional status and development issues than in acute emergency department intervention, although prolonged feeding difficulty can develop into a life-threatening problem. Evaluation of these patients often involves a multidisciplinary approach. The child with obvious anatomic abnormalities, neurologic impairment, specific syndromes, or a tracheostomy may need referral to appropriate subspecialists after initial evaluation. The child without obvious anatomic or neurologic abnormality who has weight loss or failure to thrive may be evaluated as an outpatient.

Radiographic evaluation of the stable dysphagic patient usually begins with an examination of the airway and soft tissues of the neck, looking for evidence of a foreign body, mass, airway impingement, or other abnormality. A chest radiograph may suggest aspiration pneumonia, congenital heart disease, or mediastinal abnormality or, as in the patient with achalasia, demonstrate fluid levels within an enlarged esophagus. Helical computed tomography scan, echocardiography, or angiography may further identify problems suspected from initial studies.

A videofluoroscopic swallowing study [VFSS or modified barium swallow (BS)] is currently the gold standard for evaluating preesophageal disorders. The patient is fed a typical solid or liquid diet (mixed with contrast material) by his or her parent or caregiver, while the radiologist records the preesophageal and esophageal swallowing phases on videotape. With a swallowing specialist present, such as a speech-language pathologist, the feeding presentation and position, consistency, amount, and type of foods can be varied, both to diagnose problems resulting in dysphagia or aspiration and to evaluate possible therapeutic interventions. This dynamic study may reveal evidence of aspiration, nasopharyngeal reflux, motility disorders, obstructions, masses, cricopharyngeal dysfunction, fistulas, inflammatory processes, or other causes of dysphagia. VFSS differs from the standard BS or upper gastrointestinal (UGI) series in that it does not use pure contrast, but instead uses food mixed with contrast in an attempt to simulate the normal feeding pattern as closely as possible. Several studies suggest multiple swallows should be observed because patients with pathology may not demonstrate those abnormalities on the first few swallows. VFSS is less effective than a UGI series or BS at diagnosing gastroesophageal reflux or lower esophageal, gastric outlet, and small bowel abnormalities (Fig. 52.2), but it is superior in identifying preesophageal causes of dysphagia.

Fiberoptic endoscopic evaluation of swallowing (FEES) is a newly described diagnostic and clinical tool for the pediatric dysphagia patient. With a nasopharyngeal approach under local anesthesia, FEES allows direct visualization of the swallowing process with the ability to document aspiration and functional

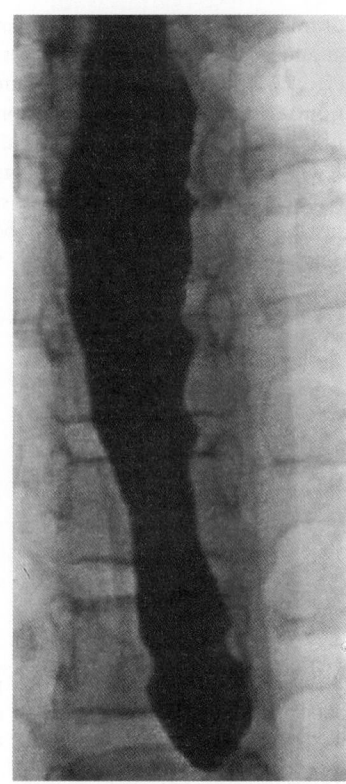

FIGURE 52.2 Upper gastrointestinal series (UGI) of a 14-year-old girl presenting with dysphagia. The UGI demonstrates a significantly dilated upper esophagus, with a functional spasmodic obstruction of the lower esophagus, characteristic of achalasia.

pharyngeal or upper esophageal disorders. FEES may also be indicated for the suspected mass lesion, stricture, caustic ingestion, inflammatory lesion, or foreign body. Advantages of this endoscopic evaluation include no radiation exposure, ready availability, the use of regular positioning and diet (i.e., breast-feeding) without contrast material, and the ability to test sensation in the larynx and pharynx. Disadvantages of FEES primarily result from the lack of visualization of the oral or lower esophageal phases of swallowing and potential intolerance of the endoscope in an awake infant or child. FEES has been successfully used to initially screen dysphagia patients and to reevaluate swallowing function after feeding interventions to diet, position, presentation, and so on.

Other tests, such as a complete blood cell count and appropriate cultures in the febrile patient, or arterial blood gas for the patient with respiratory distress, may also be indicated. Cervical ultrasonography has been used to identify abnormalities with the tissues and function of the palate, tongue, and floor of the mouth; however, it is less useful than contrast studies for assessing airway problems and aspiration. Manometry may be useful in the dysphagic patient with an esophageal motility disorder, but it is better tolerated and more typically used in adults. Esophageal pH testing or radionuclide scintigraphy (milk scans) may document previously unsuspected gastroesophageal reflux. Bronchoscopy with bronchoalveolar lavage is occasionally used to assess recurrent small-volume aspiration. If lavage contains a high percentage of lipid-laden macrophages, aspiration is more likely. However, this technique has low sensitivity and specificity for aspiration. Additional neurologic testing may include studies of brainstem-evoked responses, peripheral nerve conduction, or electromyography. More recent functional magnetic resonance mapping of the swallowing centers in the brain promises improved insight into dysphagia from a central etiology.

Treatment of dysphagia is dictated by the underlying diagnosis. Disorders with the potential to become life-threatening should be treated in the hospital under the care of appropriate specialists. Chronic dysphagia with actual or potential aspiration should be identified. If nutrition has been severely compromised from chronic dysphagia, one should consider nasogastric, nasojejunal, or gastrostomy tube feedings. Many pediatric facilities have developed multidisciplinary feeding/swallowing teams to provide subspecialty expertise, while maintaining continuity and coordination of patient care. Such pediatric teams may include developmental or general pediatricians, speech-language pathologists, pulmonologists, otolaryngologists, gastroenterologists, neurologists, nutritionists, psychologists, occupational or physical therapists, and social service workers. If such a specialty service is not available, involvement of appropriate individual specialists for the management of the patient with dysphagia is imperative as mentioned in Figure 52.1. However, therapy for many disorders can be initiated on an outpatient basis. Gastroesophageal reflux and resultant esophagitis can often be successfully managed with small-volume thickened feeds, positioning, and elevation of the head of the bed. Medical therapy consists of liquid antacids, metoclopramide (should not be used long term due to risk of permanent dystonias), H_2-blockers, or proton pump inhibitors. Children who have failed reflux therapy may be candidates for an evaluation for eosinophilic esophagitis. Treatment of eosinophilic esophagitis includes topical or oral steroids along with proton pump inhibitors. Mycostatin will be helpful in candidal esophagitis, whereas herpetic esophagitis often is self-limiting.

Pediatric dysphagia is an uncommon complaint in the pediatric emergency department but may be the presenting symptom for a wide variety of underlying clinical problems. The history and physical examination first must focus on potentially life-threatening causes and will often lead to a specific diagnosis. Causes of dysphagia not identified from the initial evaluation may require radiographic or subspecialty referral for further diagnostic and therapeutic management.

Suggested Readings

Arvedson JC. Management of pediatric dysphagia. *Otolaryngol Clin North Am* 1998;31(3):453–476.

Bell HR, Alper BS. Assessment and intervention for dysphagia in infants and children: beyond the neonatal intensive care unit. *Semin Speech Lang* 2007;28(3):213–222.

Boesch RP, Daines C, Willging JP, et al. Advances in the diagnosis and management of chronic pulmonary aspiration in children. *Eur Respir J* 2006; 28(4):847–861.

Derkay CS, Schechter GL. Anatomy and physiology of pediatric swallowing disorders. *Otolaryngol Clin North Am* 1998;31(3):397–404.

Farrell TM, Richardson WS, Halkar R, et al. Nissen fundoplication improves gastric motility in patients with delayed gastric emptying. *Surg Endosc* 2001;15(3):271–274.

Furuta GT, Liacouras CA, Collins MH, et al. Eosinophilic esophagitis in children and adults: a systematic review and consensus recommendations for diagnosis and treatment. *Gastroenterology* 2007;133(4):1342–1363.

Garg BP. Dysphagia in children: an overview. *Semin Pediatr Neurol* 2003; 10(4):252–254.

Hartnick CJ, Hartley BE, Miller C, et al. Pediatric fiberoptic endoscopic evaluation of swallowing. *Ann Otol Rhinol Laryngol* 2000;109(11):996–999.

Homer EM. An interdisciplinary team approach to providing dysphagia treatment in the schools. *Semin Speech Lang* 2003;24(3):215–234.

Hurwitz M, Bahar RJ, Ament ME, et al. Evaluation of the use of botulinum toxin in children with achalasia. *J Pediatr Gastroenterol Nutr* 2000; 30(5):509–514.

Hussain SZ, Di Lorenzo C. Motility disorders: diagnosis and treatment for the pediatric patient. *Pediatr Clin North Am* 2002;49(1):27–51.

Karnak I, Senocak ME, Tanyel FC, et al. Achalasia in childhood: surgical treatment and outcome. *Eur J Pediatr Surg* 2001;11(4):223–229.

Kelchner LN, Miller CK. Current research in voice and swallowing outcomes following pediatric airway reconstruction. *Curr Opin Otolaryngol Head Neck Surg* 2008;16(3):221–225.

Lefton-Greif MA, Arvedson JC. Pediatric feeding and swallowing disorders: state of health, population trends, and application of the international classification of functioning, disability, and health. *Semin Speech Lang* 2007;28(3):161–165.

Lefton-Greif MA, Arvedson JC. Schoolchildren with dysphagia associated with medically complex conditions. *Lang Speech Hear Serv Sch* 2008;39(2): 237–248.

Liacouras CA, Spergel JM, Ruchelli E, et al. Eosinophilic esophagitis: a 10-year experience in 381 children. *Clin Gastroenterol Hepatol* 2005;3(12):1198–1206.

Mason SJ, Harris G, Blissett J. Tube feeding in infancy: implications for the development of normal eating and drinking skills. *Dysphagia* 2005;20(1):46–61.

Miller CK, Willging JP. Advances in the evaluation and management of pediatric dysphagia. *Curr Opin Otolaryngol Head Neck Surg* 2003;11(6):442–446.

Miller CK, Willging JP. The implications of upper-airway obstruction on successful infant feeding. *Semin Speech Lang* 2007;28(3):190–203.

Morgan A, Ward E, Murdoch B, et al. Acute characteristics of pediatric dysphagia subsequent to traumatic brain injury: videofluoroscopic assessment. *J Head Trauma Rehabil* 2002;17(3):220–241.

Rosen R, Fritz J, Nurko A, et al. Lipid-laden macrophage index is not an indicator of gastroesophageal reflux-related respiratory disease in children. *Pediatrics* 2008;121(4):e879–e884.

Sachdeva R, Hussain E, Moss MM, et al. Vocal cord dysfunction and feeding difficulties after pediatric cardiovascular surgery. *J Pediatr* 2007;151(3): 312–315, 315 e311–312.

Udall JN Jr. Infant feeding: initiation, problems, approaches. *Curr Probl Pediatr Adolesc Health Care* 2007;37(10):374–399.

SIGNS AND SYMPTOMS

CHAPTER 53 ■ PAIN—DYSURIA

JACQUELINE BRYNGIL CORBOY, MD

Many conditions of the genitourinary tract produce symptoms of pain or burning associated with urination, or *dysuria*. The sensation is produced by the muscular contraction of the bladder and the peristaltic activity of the urethra, both of which stimulate the pain fibers in the edematous and inflamed mucosa. Young children may complain of painful urination when they are instead experiencing related symptoms, such as pruritus. When a child is too young to verbalize his or her symptoms, parents may interpret various nonspecific statements or behaviors by their child as indicative of painful urination.

Dysuria is a commonly reported symptom associated with a number of infectious and noninfectious causes (Table 53.1), but it usually stems from one of several common disorders of childhood and adolescence (Table 53.2). Most children with dysuria as a chief complaint will have primary disorders of the genitourinary tract, and although patients with urethritis secondary to systemic illnesses may have dysuria as one of their many symptoms, it is only occasionally the principal reason for a visit to an emergency department (ED).

Most diseases causing dysuria are self-limited or easily treated; however, the rarely seen systemic causes of urethritis or the spread of some bacterial pathogens beyond the genitourinary tract may be life-threatening (Table 53.3)

DIFFERENTIAL DIAGNOSIS

Systemic Conditions

Stevens-Johnson syndrome is a severe manifestation of erythema multiforme, which may affect the mucous membranes throughout the body, producing conjunctivitis, oral ulceration, and urethritis. The rash that occurs in most patients often has the appearance of target lesions. Although usually self-limited, in some cases, pulmonary involvement leads to death (see Chapter 85).

Skin conditions such as psoriasis, epidermolysis bullosa, and lichen sclerosis et atrophicus can involve the anogenital region, often producing pruritis, pain, and dysuria.

Reiter's syndrome, in the family of juvenile spondyloarthropathies, is characterized by conjunctivitis, arthritis, and urethritis. Rarely diagnosed, it is more common in the male population. Crohn's disease can have genitourinary complications in up to 30% of patients and may present as dysuria, often in the setting of a urinary tract infection, and may be complicated by fistula formation.

Also rare, Behçet's syndrome is another multisystem disease characterized by recurrent oral ulcerations, ocular panuveitis, vasculitis and, less commonly, genital ulcerations that may produce dysuria.

Localized Conditions

Infectious Causes

Infections of the genitourinary tract are the predominant cause of dysuria. In nonsexually active children and adolescents, pyelonephritis is the most serious of these disorders. It usually manifests with fever, often above 39°C (102.2°F), and flank pain or tenderness (older children and adolescents). Patients with cystitis, or lower urinary tract infection (UTI), often present with suprapubic pain or tenderness but may or may not have fever, which, if present, is usually low grade.

Urethritis is a more localized infection that often produces a discharge. Bulbar urethritis is a urologic problem affecting male adolescents, which presents with dysuria and microscopic hematuria, presumably of viral origin. Also in adolescents, *Neisseria gonorrhoeae* and *Chlamydia trachomatis* are the most common bacterial pathogens responsible for urethritis. Asymptomatic infections with these pathogens may lead to the development of pelvic inflammatory disease, which can have serious consequences if left untreated. Non–gonococcal urethritis secondary to *Mycoplasma hominis* and *Ureaplasma urealyticum* infection has been described in male adolescents and to a lesser extent in female adolescents. When herpes simplex causes urethritis, vesicles are usually apparent on examination. Younger children may develop a nonspecific bacterial urethritis with involvement of the glans penis (balanitis) or both the glans and the prepuce (balanoposthitis). In the setting of an urban ED, infectious urethritis and/or cervicitis may be the source of isolated dysuria in up to 30% of adolescent girls, and often goes undiagnosed if urine is sent solely for urinalysis and culture. The development of nucleic acid amplification tests (NAATs), which use ligase chain reaction (LCR) or polymerase chain reaction (PCR) technologies, allows first-catch urine (*not* clean-catch) to be tested for the presence of *C. trachomatis* and *N. gonorrhea* in a noninvasive manner. Where available, these can provide an accurate screening tool for the testing of sexually transmitted diseases (STDs) without performing a cervical or male urethral swab culture. An alternative method of sample collection for NAAT in the female patient is that of the self-collected vaginal swab, which has been shown to be accurate when compared with provider-obtained cervical specimens as well.

Candidal and streptococcal vulvitis and vulvovaginitis, or diaper dermatitis in the non–toilet-trained toddler, may present with a chief complaint of dysuria. Physical examination usually reveals erythema, a cheeselike or mucoid discharge, and, in the case of *C. albicans*, erythematous "satellite" lesions (Chapters 90, 92).

TABLE 53.1

CAUSES OF DYSURIA

I. Systemic Conditions
   A. Stevens-Johnson syndrome
   B. Dermatologic disease (psoriasis, epidermolysis
      bullosa, lichen sclerosis)
   C. Crohn's disease
   D. Reiter's syndrome
   E. Behçet's syndrome
II. Localized Conditions
   A. Infection
      1. Pyelonephritis
      2. Cystitis
         a. Viral (adenovirus)
         b. Bacterial (*Escherichia coli* and other organisms)
      3. Urethritis/balanitis
         a. *Neisseria gonorrhoeae*
         b. *Chlamydia* species
         c. Herpes simplex
         d. *Mycoplasma* and *Ureaplasma*
      4. Vaginosis
         a. Group A streptococcus
         b. *C. albicans*
   B. Chemical irritation
      1. Detergents
      2. Fabric softeners
      3. Perfumed soaps
      4. Bubble baths (unconfirmed)
      5. Medication
   C. Trauma
      1. Local injury
      2. Masturbation
   D. Miscellaneous
      1. Hypercalciuria/uricosuria/urinary stones
      2. Labial adhesions
      3. Urethral stricture
      4. Dysfunctional voiding
      5. Psychogenic dysuria
III. Complaints Misinterpreted As Dysuria
   A. Pinworms
   B. Sexual abuse

Noninfectious Conditions

In young children, certain drugs taken systemically and topical exposures to a variety of chemicals have been reported to irritate the urethral mucosa; however, these findings have not been well documented. Potential local irritants include detergents, fabric softeners, perfumed soaps, and possibly bubble baths. These patients may have either no physical findings or only mild erythema, but they do not have discharge.

Minor injury is another relatively common cause of urethral irritation. In older children and adolescents, normal self-exploratory sexual play, masturbation, voluntary sexual activity, or sexual abuse may be the source of the trauma. As for patients with chemical urethritis, the examination is generally unremarkable.

Urinary stones in children develop in the setting of anatomic abnormalities and/or recurrent infection, and their passage may be associated with complaint of dysuria along with flank pain and hematuria. Children with idiopathic hypercalciuria and idiopathic hyperuricosuria, rare conditions that predispose these patients to produce renal calculi, may complain of dysuria even in the absence of an observable stone (Chapter 100).

Foreign bodies inserted into the urethra should always be considered in the young child. While not common, they can present with urinary symptoms months or years after their original insertion and often require surgical removal.

Urethral strictures, both congenital and acquired, may present with signs of obstruction such as urinary retention, as well as dysuria.

Labial adhesions occur relatively often in young girls. Although they are most often asymptomatic, micro tears may cause dysuria on occasion.

Dysfunctional voiding is a condition that may mimic UTI or urethritis and is responsible for approximately 40% of childhood visits to an urologist. This syndrome is multifactorial in origin and may be initially precipitated by a history of UTI. Behavioral modification or use of anticholinergic medications may be necessary to resolve this condition.

Throughout childhood and into adolescence, a complaint of dysuria may be psychogenic in origin, occurring in the absence of inflammation in the genitourinary tract.

Complaints Misinterpreted As Dysuria

Enterobius vermicularis (pinworms) normally infests the perianal area but occasionally spreads to the vagina in young girls. The pruritus that accompanies this infestation may be expressed as dysuria.

Young children who have experienced sexual abuse may present to the ED with a complaint of dysuria because they experience pain in their genital area or may exhibit behaviors that are interpreted by adult observers as indicative of genital pain.

TABLE 53.2

DIFFERENTIAL DIAGNOSIS OF COMMON CAUSES FOR DYSURIA

Disorder	Cause	Age	Fever	Tenderness
Pyelonephritis	*E. coli*/other bacteria	All	Common, ≥38.5°C	Flank
Cystitis	Viruses/*E. coli*/other bacteria	All	Occasional, ≤38.5°C	Suprapubic
Infectious urethritis	*N. gonorrhoeae*/*C. trachomatis*/*Mycoplasma*/*Ureaplasma*	Adolescents	None	Prostatic/pelvic (occasional)
Vaginitis/dermatitis	*C. albicans*/Group A streptococci	All	None	Local or none
Chemical/traumatic urethritis	Physical insult	Children	None	None

TABLE 53.3

LIFE-THREATENING CAUSES OF DYSURIA

Stevens-Johnson syndrome
Gonococcal urethritis/vaginitis (when complicated by pelvic
    inflammatory disease or systemic spread)

EVALUATION AND DECISION

The approach to the child with dysuria must be broad, and
history will help determine the direction of the workup. A
thorough investigation of possible causes should be conducted, including questions about trauma (both accidental
and nonaccidental), exposure to chemicals such as detergents,
fabric softeners, perfumed soaps, bubble baths, and medications that have been reported to irritate the mucosal lining of
the urethra or bladder. A negative history for injury may not
be accurate, however, because most traumas are not recalled
by young patients or, in the case of masturbation or abuse,
may be denied. The detection of STDs, a common cause of

dysuria in adolescents, may in turn be facilitated by obtaining
a history about the nature and extent of sexual activity or
hampered due to denial by the patient for fear of parental
consequences (Fig. 53.1).

The most important tasks for the emergency physician are
to recognize the rare but serious systemic syndromes and to
diagnose or exclude infections. When dysuria is associated
with a constellation of other symptoms, systemic conditions
must be ruled out. For example, if the patient also complains
of joint pains and conjunctivitis, Reiter's syndrome should be
considered. In a female patient with dysuria and abdominal
pain, pelvic inflammatory disease must be excluded.

Historical findings may be further supported by physical
examination, and special attention should be directed to the
abdomen and genitourinary tract. Careful palpation for the
presence of masses in the abdomen or suprapubic region
should be performed. The presence of discharge, rashes, and
other lesions may identify the source of the problem right
away, negating the need for extensive workup. In both pubertal and prepubertal patients, the finding of vesicles suggests an
infection caused by herpes simplex. Ulcerations without vesicles, however, may be indicative of systemic disorders such as
Behçet's or Stevens-Johnson syndrome. Labial adhesions are

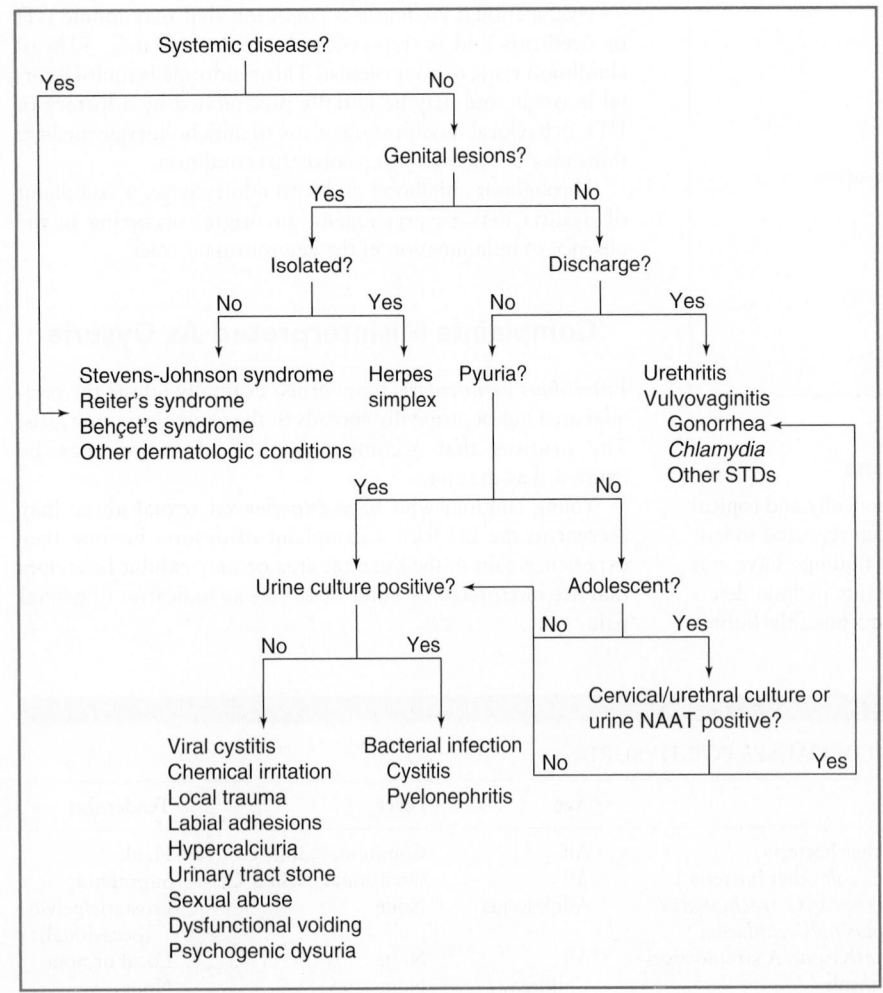

FIGURE 53.1 Approach to the diagnosis of
dysuria. STDs, sexually transmitted diseases;
NAAT, nucleic acid amplification test.

easily recognized on inspection in young girls. A urethral or vaginal discharge suggests an infection of the genitalia: urethritis in the boy and urethritis or vulvovaginitis in the girl. *N. gonorrhoeae* is an organism that commonly causes disease in this area. A Gram stain can be a helpful adjunct in determining the nature of the discharge. In prepubertal girls or boys of any age, the finding of gram-negative intracellular diplococci points to the diagnosis of gonorrhea. However, because nonpathogenic organisms that colonize the vagina after puberty have the same appearance as *N. gonorrhoeae* on Gram stain, this method is an unreliable tool in teenage girls. Urine NAATs, which use LCR or PCR technologies, allow urine to be tested for the presence of *C. trachomatis* and *N. gonorrhea*. These tests, however, are more expensive than traditional swabs but, where available, they can provide a reasonably accurate screening tool for the testing of STDs without performing a cervical or male urethral swab culture. A urethral or vaginal culture should also be obtained on all positive samples for confirmation and susceptibility testing. Postpubertal patients may be treated in the ED, but treatment in young children should await the results of cultures because of medical-legal implications.

If no discharge is seen, the physician should obtain a urinalysis and urine culture. Urinalysis and culture should be performed on specimens obtained by catheter or suprapubic aspiration on female children younger than 2 years and male children younger than 6 months. Clean-catch specimens may be analyzed outside those age groups. A positive result on testing by dipstick (leukocyte esterase and/or nitrites, with the former being more sensitive and the latter more specific) or the finding of pyuria on microscopic analysis increases the likelihood of bacterial infection (urethritis, cystitis, or pyelonephritis) but does not prove the diagnosis and must be confirmed by culture. Inflammatory conditions, such as chemical urethritis, and nonbacterial infections may also evoke a leukocyte response. Thus, the physician may choose to allow the results of cultures to guide the management of children with pyuria, rather than immediately beginning antibiotic therapy, unless clinical suspicion of infection is very high (e.g., prior history of UTI, or presence of fever and flank pain suggesting pyelonephritis).

In the young child with dysuria in the absence of pyuria, local trauma and chemical irritation are the most likely causes for the pain. Because a few children with UTIs do not have either a positive result on testing by dipstick or pyuria, most physicians obtain a urine sample for culture, particularly from febrile patients. However, some experts would argue that the likelihood of infection is low enough in the absence of positive indicators on urine analysis that no further testing is needed. Adolescents require either urine or swab cultures of the genital tract to diagnose mild gonococcal or chlamydial infections.

When no other cause for dysuria is found in a prepubertal girl who has adhesions of her labia minora, these adhesions may be responsible for the painful urination. Most girls with labial adhesions, however, are asymptomatic. Thus, infection or another cause for dysuria should be excluded in girls with this finding.

A few patients with a normal examination and negative cultures may complain persistently of dysuria. In this setting, dysfunctional voiding and idiopathic hypercalciuria represent potential diagnoses. If suspected, the diagnosis of hypercalciuria/uricosuria can be confirmed by measurement of calcium excretion in the urine. Another possible explanation in a female is that the patient is experiencing vaginal pruritus secondary to pinworms. Confirmation of this diagnosis requires either identification of the larvae or ova, or a response to a trial of mebendazole.

Last, the physician should give consideration to both sexual abuse and psychogenic dysuria. In most of these cases, further evaluation outside of the ED will be needed.

SYMPTOMATIC MANAGEMENT

When a specific diagnosis has not been established and the physician is awaiting the results of cultures, therapy directed at the symptom of dysuria can provide some relief. Generally, dilute urine causes less irritation than concentrated urine, so a generous fluid intake should be recommended. Warm water sitz baths may be helpful in the child with urethritis or vulvovaginitis. For the child older than 6 years, phenazopyridine (Pyridium®) at a dosage of 12mg/kg/day divided into three doses (daily maximum 600 mg/day), administered for up to two days, may be helpful as a urinary tract anesthetic.

Suggested Readings

Bachur R, Harper MB. Reliability of the urinalysis for predicting urinary tract infections in young febrile children. *Arch Pediatr Adolesc Med* 2001;155(1):60–65.

Baraff LJ. Management of infants and young children with fever without source. *Pediatr Ann* 2008;37(10):673–679.

Benz MR, Stehr M, Kammer B, et al. Foreign body in the bladder mimicking nephritis. *Pediatr Nephrol* 2007;22(3):467–470.

Berwald N, Cheng S, Augenbraun M, et al. Self-administered vaginal swabs are a feasible alternative to physician-assisted cervical swabs for sexually transmitted infection screening in the emergency department. *Acad Emerg Med* 2009;16(4):360–363.

Best D, Ford C, Miller WC. Prevalence of *Chlamydia trachomatis* and *Neisseria gonorrhoeae* infection in pediatric private practice. *Pediatrics* 2001;108(6):E103.

Bremnor JD, Sadovsky R. Evaluation of dysuria in adults. *Pediatrics* 2002;65(8):1589–1596.

Chon CH, Lai FC, Shortliffe LMD. Pediatric urinary tract infections. *Pediatr Clin North Am* 2001;48(6):1441–1459.

DeLago C, Deblinger E, Schroeder C, et al. Girls who disclose sexual abuse: urogenital symptoms and signs after genital contact. *Pediatrics* 2008;122(2):e281–e286.

Eberz B, Berghold A, Regauer S. High prevalence of concomitant anogenital lichen sclerosis and extragenital psoriasis in adult women. *Obstet Gynecol* 2008;111(5):1143–1147.

Etoubleau C, Reveret M, Brouet D, et al. Moving from bag to catheter for urine collection in non-toilet-trained children suspected of having urinary tract infection: a paired comparison of urine cultures. *J Pediatr* 2009;154(6):803–806.

Fang J, Husman C, DeSilva L, et al. Evaluation of self-collected vaginal swab, first void urine, and endocervical swab specimens for the detection of *Chlamydia trachomatis* and *Neisseria gonrrhoeae* in adolescent females. *J Pediatr Adolesc Gynecol* 2008;21(6):355–360.

Farhat W, McLorie G. Urethral syndromes in children. *Pediatr Rev* 2001;22(1):17–21.

Gorelick MH, Shaw KN. Screening tests for urinary tract infection in children: a meta-analysis. *Pediatrics* 1999;104(5):e54.

Halachmi S, Toubi A, Meretyk S. Inflammation of the testis and epididymis in an otherwise healthy child: is it a true bacterial urinary tract infection? *J Pediatr Urol* 2006;2(4):386–389.

Johnson RE, Newhall WJ, Papp JR, et al. Screening tests to detect *Chlamydia trachomatis* and *Neisseria gonorrhoeae* infections—2002. *MMWR Recomm Rep* 2002;51(RR-15):1–38.

La Manna A, Polito C, Marte A, et al. Hyperuricosuria in children: clinical presentation and natural history. *Pediatrics* 2001;107(1):86–90.

Omar HA. Management of labial adhesions in prepubertal girls. *J Pediatr Adolesc Gynecol* 2000;13(4):183–185.

Parekh DJ, Pope JC, Adams MC, et al. The role of hypercalciuria in a subgroup of dysfunctional voiding syndromes of childhood. *J Urol* 2000;164(3, pt 2):1008–1010.

Poindexter G, Morrell DS. Anogenital pruritus: lichen sclerosus in children. *Pediatr Ann* 2007;36(12):785–791.

Ruffolo C, Angriman I, Scarpa M, et al. Urologic complications in Crohn's disease: suspicion criteria. *Hepatogastroenterology* 2006;53(69): 357–360.

Schlager TA. Urinary tract infections in infants and children. *Infect Dis Clin North Am* 2003;17(2):353–365.

Shaw KN, McGowan KL, Schwartz JS. Screening for urinary tract infection in infants in the emergency department: which test is best? *Pediatrics* 1998;101:E6.

Spitzer RF, Kives S, Caccia N, et al. Retrospective review of unintentional female genital trauma at a pediatric referral center. *Pediatr Emer Care* 2008;24(12): 831–835.

Srinivasin A, Palmer LS. Genitourinary complications of epidermolysis bullosa. *Urology* 2007;70(1):179.e585–e586.

Srivastava T, Schwaderer A. Diagnosis and management of hypercalciuria in children. *Curr Opin Pediatr* 2009;21(2):214–219.

Yazici H. Behçet's syndrome: where do we stand? *Am J Med* 2002;112(1):75–76.

CHAPTER 54 ■ PAIN—EARACHE

AMY M. ARNETT, MD

Ear pain or otalgia is a common symptom of many different conditions in or around the ear (Tables 54.1 to 54.3). Preverbal children may present with fussiness, crying, or waking intermittently at night. Children may have difficulty differentiating tinnitus from ear pain. Ear pain may be primary/otogenic or referred/nonotogenic in origin. A complete history and physical examination is necessary, focusing not only on the ear but also on adjacent areas and those regions innervated by nerves that also innervate the ear. Areas that might be a source of referred pain include the oral cavity, larynx, pharynx, and cervical spine; rarely, referred pain may be from a site below the clavicles. Patients with accompanying central nervous system symptoms, vertigo, or cranial nerve deficits need more extensive evaluation.

DIFFERENTIAL DIAGNOSIS

Otogenic Causes

Trauma is usually evident by physical examination. Hematomas of the pinna or auricle resulting from blunt trauma may occur over the cartilaginous portion or upper half of the ear between the perichondrium and the underlying cartilage. The hematoma may appear as a boggy, purple swelling. Sterile aspiration and a molded pressure dressing are necessary to avoid pressure necrosis of the underlying cartilage and a resulting distorted "boxer's" or "cauliflower" ear.

Body piercing has increased significantly in more recent years, with earlobes and ear cartilage being the most frequent sites. Common complications include infection, allergic reaction, keloid formation, and traumatic tearing. Another complication of piercing is an embedded earring, which often requires local anesthesia and removal. Superimposed infection is the most common complication of ear piercing with local symptoms, including redness, swelling, warmth, pain, and drainage. Earlobe infection is most commonly secondary to *Staphylococcus aureus* and responds well to local treatment and topical or oral antistaphylococcal antibiotics. Complications of ear piercing that involve auricular cartilage such as the helix include chondritis, perichondritis, or perichondrial auricular abscess from *Pseudomonas aeruginosa*. These patients may also present with systemic symptoms, including fever, chills, or nausea. Presentation may be 3 to 4 weeks after piercing and may require incision and drainage, debridement, and fluoroquinolone antibiotics to treat *Staphylococcus* and *Pseudomonas* and *Streptococcus pyogenes*. Nickel earrings may cause earlobe dermatitis. These earrings should be replaced with gold or stainless steel earrings, and topical corticosteroids should be applied as an antiinflammatory agent. Insect or spider bites may cause a local allergic reaction or secondary cellulitis of the ear. Swelling and erythema may occur with either; so, signs of infection such as pain, fever, and tenderness may help determine treatment by antihistamine versus antibiotic. Keloid formation may be pruritic or painful. These patients may be referred for definitive treatment. Tearing of the ear from a piercing may be repaired as any laceration; consider a location involving cartilage may require a layered repair by a facial trauma specialist.

Preauricular pits are asymptomatic until they become infected. Physical examination reveals a warm, erythematous, tender area anterior to the tragus. Treatment includes oral antibiotics to cover skin flora, occasional incision and drainage, and referral for eventual resection.

Frostbite of the auricle is painful. The ear usually appears pallid secondary to vasoconstriction. With thawing, it becomes hyperemic and edematous, and vesicles may appear. It is treated by rapid rewarming with application of moist gauze or cloths soaked in 40°C (104°F) water and continued through reperfusion pain. There is some literature to support aspiration of clear blisters, but hemorrhagic vesicles should be left intact. Consult your burn specialist for their current recommendations. Analgesics should be given for pain control. No debridement of damaged tissue is performed until full demarcation of tissue loss is determined, usually weeks later.

Furunculosis is a gram-positive, usually staphylococcal infection of a hair follicle at the external auditory meatus that causes marked pain and occasional otorrhea. This generally occurs in the cartilaginous portion of the canal and may cause cervical adenopathy. Treatment consists of warm compresses to encourage spontaneous drainage. Topical or oral antistaphylococcal antibiotics are rarely indicated. If spontaneous drainage does not occur, incision and drainage may be necessary. Coalescence of furuncles produces a carbuncle or abscess, which often requires drainage. In the era of colonization with methicillin-resistant *Staphylococcus aureus* (MRSA), culture and antibiotic coverage should be considered.

Herpes zoster oticus is a painful viral infection characterized by vesicles on the auricle, the external auditory meatus, and occasionally, the tympanic membrane (TM). It is caused by a residual *Varicella zoster* viral infection of the seventh and eighth cranial nerves. Complications include facial paralysis as in Ramsay Hunt syndrome, hearing loss, and vertigo. Other cranial nerves may be affected. Although this normally presents in adults, it may occur at any age. Patients in the early stages may be treated with an antiviral agent and/or systemic steroids; otherwise, treatment is mainly symptomatic.

Otitis externa (OE) usually presents in warm, humid weather. Because swimming can predispose the canal to this condition, it is often called "swimmer's ear." The initial presenting symptom may be pruritus. Scratching the canal may

TABLE 54.1

CAUSES OF EARACHE

Otogenic
External
  Trauma
  Ear piercing—infection/dermatoses
  Preauricular pit infection
  Frostbite
  Furunculosis
  Herpes zoster oticus (Ramsay Hunt syndrome)
  Insect/spider bites
Canal
  Otitis externa—swimmer's ear
  Otomycosis
  Foreign body (FB)
  Dermatoses—seborrhea or psoriasis
  Contact dermatitis
  Impacted cerumen
  Trauma
Tympanic Membrane/Middle Ear
  Acute otitis media
  Otitis media with effusion/serous otitis media
  Traumatic perforation
  Myringitis
  Hemotympanum
  Aerotitis or acute barotitis
  Cholesteatoma
Inner Ear/Periauricular Structures
  Labyrinthitis
  Subperiosteal abscess/acute mastoid osteitis
  Intracranial infections
  Facial nerve palsy
	Nonotogenic—Referred Pain
	Trigeminal Nerve (V)
	  Oral cavity: stomatitis, gingivitis, trauma
	  Dental: impacted teeth, trauma, caries, abscess
	  Temporomandibular joint dysfunction
	  Sinusitis
	  Mastoiditis
	  Parotitis
	Facial Nerve (VII)
	  Bell's palsy
	  Herpes zoster infection—Ramsay Hunt syndrome
	Glossopharyngeal Nerve (IX)
	  Oropharynx: tonsillitis, posttonsillectomy, retropharyngeal abscess
	  Nasopharynx
	Vagus Nerve (X)
	  Larynx: trauma, FB
	  Esophagus: FB, burn
	C2/C3
	  Lymphadenitis
	  Branchial cleft cysts
	  Cervical spine: trauma, infection
	Psychogenic
	Drug Ingestions (Causing Tinnitus)
	  Quinine, quinidine, ethacrynic acid, salicylates, nicotine, aminoglycosides

damage the skin and predispose the area to secondary bacterial infection. Ear pain, itching, and discharge are the primary complaints. Examination reveals pain with movement of the auricle or tragus, an erythematous canal with edema, and sometimes foul-smelling, yellow, brown, white, or gray discharge. *P. aeruginosa* and *S. aureus* are the most common causative organisms. Treatment includes cleaning and acidifying the ear canal, controlling pain, and possible antibiotic coverage. An otic suspension combining an acidic medium with an antiinflammatory and/or antibiotic is the usual treatment. Topical polymyxin/neomycin, ciprofloxacin, and ofloxacin all provide good bacterial coverage for *P. aeruginosa* and *S. aureus*. The fluoroquinolones are less ototoxic if middle ear entry is a concern. A wick may be inserted into the canal if it is too edematous to allow the drops to enter. If there is any

accompanying cellulitis, oral antibiotics may be added. Ear plugs for swimmers and acidifying drops after swimming are good preventive measures. Typical pain may be treated with ibuprofen or acetaminophen but may require oral narcotics.

A serious complication of OE is malignant or necrotizing external otitis, which is a fulminant bacterial OE, usually with *P. aeruginosa*. This may extend beyond the limits of the external auditory canal, producing cellulitis, chondritis, osteitis, osteomyelitis, facial nerve paralysis, or septic thromboembolism. These patients require further radiographic evaluation for bony or sinus involvement, otorhinolaryngology (ORL)

TABLE 54.2

COMMON CAUSES OF EARACHE

Otogenic	Nonotogenic
Acute otitis media	Dental caries or abscess
Otitis externa	Pharyngitis
Foreign body	Sinusitis
	Cervical adenopathy

TABLE 54.3

SERIOUS CAUSES OF EARACHE

Hemotympanum secondary to basilar skull fracture
Local spread of acute otitis media to:
  Mastoid cavity—subperiosteal abscess with acute mastoid osteitis
  Vascular structures—lateral sinus thrombosis
  Intracranial region—meningitis, extradural abscess, subdural empyema, focal encephalitis, brain abscess
  Temporal bone—facial nerve paralysis
  Inner ear—labyrinthitis
Ingestions

consultation, and probable admission for combination intravenous antibiotics.

Impacted cerumen in the canal is a common cause of ear pain or discomfort. Normally, asymptomatic cerumen accumulation need not be removed; however, earwax removal is often necessary to complete an ear examination. Careful immobilization is essential. Removal under direct visualization through an otoscope is ideal. An ear curette or small cotton swab may be used. Removal of hard cerumen adherent to the canal may cause bleeding. The wax may be softened with a ceruminolytic agent, such as mineral oil, hydrogen peroxide, or docusate sodium, and then irrigated with warm water. A plastic syringe attached to the plastic tubing end cut from a butterfly needle may be used. A water jet device may also be used, but it must be set on low pressure to prevent damage to the TM. A perforated TM is a contraindication to ceruminolytics or irrigation. An antibiotic/antiinflammatory otic suspension is sometimes recommended as prophylaxis to prevent OE after canal irritation or irrigation.

Foreign bodies (FBs) may be painless, or they can cause trauma or an inflammatory reaction that may elicit pain. Physical examination visually confirms an FB. Successful extraction is dependent on good immobilization, visualization, and availability of equipment. Removal is accomplished by instrumentation with an ear curette or alligator forceps, irrigation with warm water, or suctioning depending on the type of FB. Inflamed canals may be treated with topical antibiotic/hydrocortisone otic drops. Long-standing or hazardous FBs such as button batteries can cause erosion and may require further evaluation and treatment after removal. Referral to ORL should be arranged if FB removal is unsuccessful.

Otomycosis is a fungal infection of the external canal. It may be acute or chronic, primary or secondary to bacterial infection and prolonged use of antibiotic drops. *Aspergillus niger* and *Candida* are the most common causative pathogens. The primary complaint may be pruritus. On physical examination, the canal is erythematous and edematous with grayish, whitish, or blackish debris that resembles dirty cotton. Treatment consists of cleaning and acidifying the ear canal with drops. Topical or systemic antifungals such as nystatin or clotrimazole may be necessary.

Dermatoses of the ear can also cause ear discomfort. Seborrheic dermatitis and psoriasis can affect the external auditory canal and produce scaling or drainage. The primary complaint may be itching. Usually, other areas are also affected, including the retroauricular region and scalp. Removal of crusts can be helpful. Treatment consists of topical corticosteroids.

Contact dermatitis may occur from topical medicines and should be considered in patients with persistent edema and erythema of the canal and auricle, despite appropriate OE treatment. Treatment of the contact dermatitis includes removing the causative agent, cleaning the ear, and applying acidic solutions or topical steroids to decrease the inflammation.

Acute otitis media (AOM) is the most common illness resulting in office visits to physicians who care for children (see Chapter 92). Ear pain is the most reliable symptom on presentation for AOM. In 2000, a review of office visits in the United States showed that approximately 16 million were related to AOM, resulting in 13 million prescriptions. Children in the first 2 years of life have more infections due to eustachian tube dys-

function with its more horizontal position and shorter length as compared with that of the adult; immature or impaired immunity; and increased frequency of upper respiratory infections with day care center exposure. History often includes recent viral upper respiratory infection, followed by deep-seated otalgia, fever, and decreased hearing in older patients.

In 2004, the American Academy of Pediatrics (AAP) and the American Academy of Family Physicians (AAFP) published Clinical Practice Guidelines for AOM. The definition of AOM includes acute onset of symptoms within 48 hours, presence of middle ear effusion, and signs of middle ear inflammation. Physical examination parameters used to evaluate the TM for AOM are position/bulging, color/translucency, and mobility. AOM may show a hyperemic, opaque, bulging TM with poor mobility and serous fluid or yellow pus filling the middle ear space. The auricle is usually normal. A conductive hearing loss may result from accumulation of fluid in the middle ear and impairment of the drum motion. Treatment options vary depending on the severity of infection, with a severe infection defined as the patient having a fever [temperature, more than 39°C (102.2°F)] and severe pain with AOM.

The pathogenesis of AOM often involves coinfection with viral and bacterial pathogens. The three major bacterial pathogens are *Streptococcus pneumoniae* (pneumococcus), nontypeable *Haemophilus influenzae*, and *Moraxella catarrhalis*. *Streptococcus pyogenes*, *S. aureus*, *Mycoplasma pneumoniae*, and gram-negative enteric bacilli are sometimes the causes. Children now receive routine heptavalent pneumococcal conjugate vaccine (PCV7) that should reduce pneumococcal otitis media. Amoxicillin (80 to 90 mg per kg per day divided in two doses) remains the first-line drug for nonsevere episodes of AOM because of its antibacterial coverage, safety, low cost, good taste, and narrow microbiologic spectrum (see Chapter 92). Amoxicillin-clavulanate (90 mg amoxicillin per kg per day divided in two doses), with better coverage for β-lactamase–producing bacteria should be considered as first-line treatment for patients with severe AOM, child care exposure, treatment with amoxicillin for less than 30 days prior, or age less than 2 years. Treatment is usually for 10 days, although shorter courses of 5 to 7 days may be considered in the patient at least 6 years old with uncomplicated disease. If symptoms do not improve in 48 to 72 hours, the patient should be examined and considered for second-line therapy to cover resistant strains of *Haemophilus*, *Moraxella*, or pneumococcus. Those antibiotics include amoxicillin-clavulanate for patients on amoxicillin, or intramuscular ceftriaxone for 3 days for patients on amoxicillin-clavulanate. Other oral cephalosporins or azithromycin may be considered, especially for penicillin-allergic patients. Although AOM has not always been well defined in previous studies, up to 80% of patients diagnosed with AOM improved within 72 hours without treatment. Therefore observation therapy or watchful waiting is now a consideration for treatment. The AAP guidelines suggest considering this for uncertain diagnosis of AOM in children older than 6 months and for routine AOM in children older than 24 months. Subsequent studies support delay in antibiotic treatment only in children older than 2 years. Children aged 2 to 12 years are treated for 48 to 72 hours with pain management; antibiotics are started only if symptoms persist or worsen. Many children have sterile effusions, which are presumed to be viral or unresolved effusions from previously treated infections and are not acutely infected. Pain may be treated with oral analgesics, such as acetaminophen and ibuprofen, or topical anesthetic drops for temporary relief if there is no perforation. Oral decongestants, antihistamines, and intranasal decongestants have not proven to be effective. For those AOM patients with tympanic perforation and purulent drainage, a topical antibiotic drop such as ofloxacin otic or antibiotic/hydrocortisone otic suspension is sometimes given to treat the inflammatory reaction in the ear canal. Perforated TMs usually heal spontaneously, but they may lead to more chronic unhealed perforations, cholesteatoma, or tympanosclerosis. Children with significant recurrent infections may require further evaluation for immunologic problems and/or an ORL consultation for tympanostomy tube placement.

For a child with tympanostomy tubes, discharge from the ear canal is the most common symptom of a middle ear infection. Although most otorrhea is secondary to a viral illness, for persistent drainage, an ototopical therapy such as fluoroquinolone drops for 3 to 5 days is recommended as the first-line treatment. These patients may also be treated initially with oral pain medication.

Although rare, dangerous complications of AOM include local spread to the mastoid cavity, soft-tissue and vascular structures of the neck, intracranial region and temporal bone, or inner ear. On examination for subperiosteal abscess with acute mastoid osteitis, the pinna may be displaced inferiorly and anteriorly, with obliteration of the postauricular crease as a result of swelling. The eardrum may appear gray, not bulging or perforated. This most commonly occurs in infants due to immature immune systems. Treatment includes intravenous antimicrobials such as vancomycin and ceftriaxone, or ampicillin/sulbactam, and in some cases, surgical drainage.

Facial or abducens nerve paralysis is rarely associated with AOM and is treated with antibiotics and possible surgical nerve decompression. The middle ear and mastoid air cells are adjacent to the posterior and middle cranial fossa and sigmoid venous sinus of the brain. Local infection may spread to these adjacent structures leading to intracranial complications that are rare in developed countries, such as meningitis, extradural abscess, subdural empyema, focal encephalitis, brain abscess, lateral sinus thrombosis, and otitic hydrocephalus. All patients with facial or abducens nerve palsy, vertigo, or central nervous system signs require further radiographic evaluation, such as a computed tomography (CT) scan.

Otitis media with effusion (OME) or serous otitis media is defined as inflammation of the middle ear in which a collection of mucoid or serous liquid is present in the middle ear space without signs or symptoms of acute infection. Approximately 2.2 million cases are diagnosed annually, representing 25% to 35% of all otitis cases. The fluid may occur spontaneously due to eustachian tube dysfunction or as an inflammatory response after AOM. In 2004, the AAP published their Clinical Practice Guideline for OME, developed in conjunction with the AAFP and American Academy of Otolaryngology-Head and Neck Surgery. Although most effusions resolve spontaneously, the length of time for resolution is variable, and there is significant concern regarding conductive hearing loss during early speech and language development. Physical examination should include pneumatic otoscopy to test TM mobility. Tympanometry or acoustic reflectometry may be used to confirm an effusion. For healthy children with no craniofacial or neurologic abnormalities or sensory deficits, the effusion may be managed with

observation for up to 3 months, with the more complicated patients receiving closer follow-up. Bacterial pathogens are identified in many children having tympanostomy tube placement for OME; however, studies have shown that antibiotics provide only temporary resolution of fluid and are not routinely recommended. Steroids, antihistamines, and decongestants are not recommended. Chronic effusions may require tympanostomy tube placement for drainage by ORL.

TM perforation may be caused by pressure from fluid behind the membrane or by external trauma. Trauma often occurs with compressive injuries such as a slap with an open hand or injuries from instruments such as cotton-tipped applicators being placed into the ear canal. Pain may be severe immediately after the injury, but it becomes duller with time. Most perforations heal spontaneously. If prophylactic antibiotic eardrops are considered, avoid ototoxic agents. Oral antibiotics are reserved for injuries from contaminated objects or those in a location believed to be infectious. If the perforation involves more than 20% of the drum, a referral for possible repair is needed. Acute hearing loss, facial paralysis, and severe vertigo associated with the perforation require ORL evaluation because of possible ossicle damage or direct injury to the facial nerve or labyrinth.

Bullous myringitis is a painful, usually viral, but possibly bacterial or mycoplasma infection of the TM, characterized by serous or hemorrhagic vesicles or bullae. The course is usually self-limited with treatment consisting of analgesics.

Hemotympanum secondary to a basilar skull fracture may be a serious finding on examination of the ear. The TM may appear dark red or purple secondary to the blood behind it. These patients may have other findings consistent with basilar skull fractures such as Battle's sign—ecchymoses behind the ear, raccoon eyes—periorbital ecchymoses, or cerebrospinal fluid drainage from the nose or ears. The most common complications include facial nerve paralysis, hearing loss, and vertigo. A CT scan is indicated to determine the extent of the injuries. If no significant intracranial injury is found, usually no acute treatment is needed. Antibiotic prophylaxis to prevent meningitis is not routinely recommended.

Aerotitis, or acute barotitis, is a special type of AOM, caused by middle ear barotrauma. A sudden change in altitude in an airplane or the pressure exerted during deep-sea diving can cause eustachian tube closure and produce a severe and painful pressure change in the middle ear with extravasation of blood into the middle ear space. The drum may appear edematous, bloody, or blue because of bleeding behind it. The patient has severe pain and hearing loss. Physical examination reveals a hemorrhagic TM and tenderness over the eustachian tubes. The process is self-limited, lasting 2 to 3 days and resolving spontaneously. Treatment consists of analgesics for pain and decongestants to encourage opening of the eustachian tube. Myringotomy is performed only for severe pain or persistent fluid. Vertigo or sensorineural hearing loss requires ORL referral.

Cholesteatomas may be visualized in the middle ear. These cyst-like structures, which consist of epithelial cells and cholesterol, may be congenital or acquired, often secondary to previous perforation with residual TM epithelial cells in the middle ear. Enzymes formed within the sac may cause erosion of adjacent bones. Although rare, abnormal growths in the canal or middle ear must be evaluated for possible neoplasm and should be referred for evaluation by ORL.

Nonotogenic Causes

Inflammation, infection, neoplasm, or trauma along the course of any nerves innervating the auricle or the external auditory canal, including cranial nerves V, VII, IX, and X and cervical nerves C2 and C3, can produce pain that the patient may interpret as originating from the region of the ear. Therefore, a full head and neck examination, as well as radiographic examinations may be necessary to disclose the cause of ear pain if the ear examination results are normal.

The trigeminal nerve (V) supplies some of the most common areas of referred ear pain, including those of dental origin, such as erupting teeth or abscesses and oral mucosal ulcerations from aphthous ulcers or viral stomatitis. Sinusitis, sialadenitis, or lymphadenitis in these regions may also cause pain. Early mumps may present as ear pain before obvious parotid swelling.

Facial nerve (VII) pain may be a precursor of Bell's palsy or herpes zoster oticus.

The glossopharyngeal nerve (IX) supplies the oropharynx, nasopharynx, and posterior third of the tongue. Inflammation of these areas from pharyngitis or tonsillitis is another common cause of referred earache. Peritonsillar abscess or cellulitis may produce unilateral pain. Earache may also occur after adenotonsillectomy. Nasopharyngeal or oropharyngeal tumors, such as lymphoma or rhabdomyosarcoma, although rare in children, may be associated with ear pain.

The vagus nerve (X) supplies the base of the tongue, larynx, and trachea. Inflammatory or mass lesions in these areas may refer pain to the ear.

Cervical nerves C2 and C3 supply the mastoid and posterior pinna; therefore, ear pain may result from cervical spine injuries, arthritis, or disc disease, as well as any generalized neck disorder.

When otologic examination is normal and no pathology is found in the distribution of the cranial or cervical nerves, the pain may be psychogenic, especially in a person with anxiety or depression. Also, children may not be able to describe tinnitus and refer to it as pain. Certain drug ingestions, such as quinine, quinidine, salicylates, nicotine, ethacrynic acid, and aminoglycosides, are possible causes.

EVALUATION AND DECISION

A history is always important in determining the cause of pain or discomfort and should include questions about other ear symptoms, including tinnitus, hearing loss, vertigo, drainage, and itching, as well as systemic symptoms, such as fussiness, crying when lying down, upper respiratory infection, fever, and alteration in oral intake. Children may have difficulty describing pain. Parents may attribute pulling on ears or fussiness to ear pain. Studies disagree on the relevance of ear pulling; it may not be significant when presenting alone but may be with other signs or symptoms. Preverbal children being evaluated for suspected ear pain need careful evaluation for other causes of their fussiness.

Physical examination should always be complete, especially in children who are not old enough to verbalize that their fussiness is ear pain. Most children do not like to be immobilized for evaluation of the ears and throat; so, otoscopy and visualization of the pharynx should be the last part of the examination. Initial examination of the ear includes gross examination of the auricle, otoscopy of the external auditory canal and TM, and then pneumatic otoscopy to examine the middle ear. Important aids to the examination include positioning of the child and removal of cerumen. The child may be positioned on the parent's lap or shoulder or placed supine on the examination table. Cerumen removal may be accomplished with the use of a small, cotton-tipped applicator, wire loop, or plastic cerumen curette; application of ceruminolytics; irrigation with warm water; or suctioning (see Chapter 135).

Particularly important components of the examination include the external ear, the auditory canal, the TM, the surrounding structures of the head and neck, and the neurologic evaluation (Fig. 54.1).

EXTERNAL EAR EXAMINATION

External problems are usually obvious on initial examination. Trauma, erythema, or vesicles on the auricle may be easily seen. Palpation of the area around the ear may reveal swelling or tenderness either from nodes, mastoiditis, parotitis, or preauricular pit infection.

Abnormal Otoscopy

Otogenic causes are usually diagnosed by visualization with otoscopy (Fig. 92.7). Inflammation in the canal or middle ear, FBs, abnormal lesions, perforations, or cholesteatomas may be seen. Evaluation of the TM for signs of infection includes describing position, color/translucency, and mobility. Despite teaching that redness of the TM is not helpful since it may occur with increased blood flow from fever or crying, recent studies show that distinct erythema of the TM is a predictor of AOM. Mobility is evaluated by applying pressure to the rubber bulb attached to the otoscope with a good seal in the canal and looking for inward movement with positive pressure and outward movement with negative pressure. Purulent discharge in the canal may be wicked out with cotton to better visualize the TM for possible perforation or FBs. Any patient with accompanying vertigo, facial nerve palsy, hemotympanum, or central nervous system symptoms requires further evaluation with a CT scan.

Normal Otoscopy

A normal otoscopic evaluation should prompt a search for referred pain. Evaluation of the cervical spine, oropharynx, and neck should reveal possible sources of inflammation from shared sensory nerves. Radiographs to evaluate dental sources are usually not required emergently. A history of possible drug ingestions should be obtained. If there is a clinical suspicion of disease in the nasopharynx or larynx, an examination with a nasopharyngoscope may be needed. A patient with a completely normal examination and no other accompanying complaints

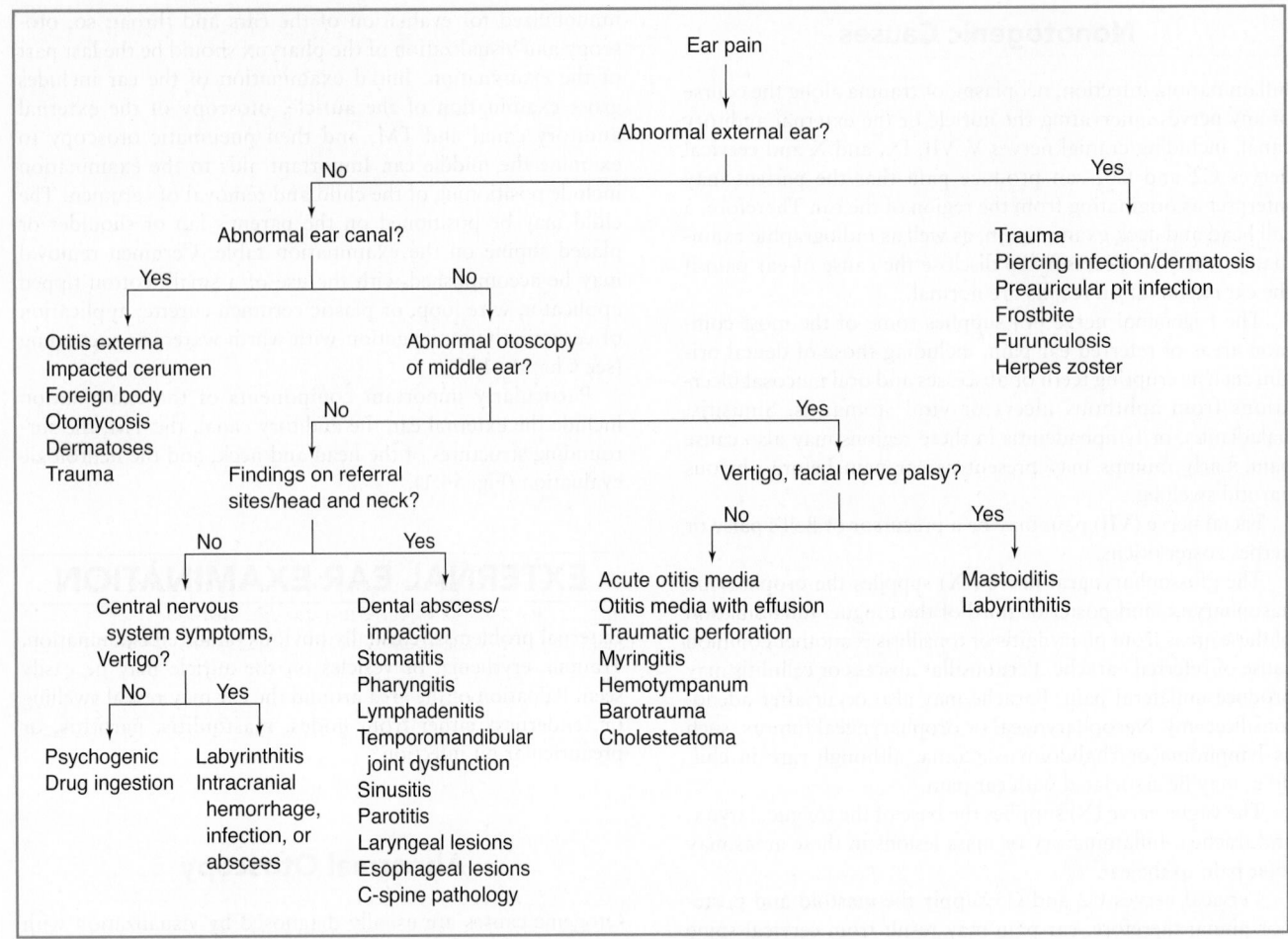

FIGURE 54.1 Approach to the diagnosis of earache. C-spine, cervical spine.

should be referred back to his or her physician for follow-up before a psychogenic cause is given.

Suggested Readings

American Academy of Family Physicians, American Academy of Otolaryngology-Head and Neck Surgery, and American Academy of Pediatrics Subcommittee on Otitis Media With Effusion. Otitis media with effusion. *Pediatrics* 2004;113:1412–1429.

American Academy of Pediatrics Subcommittee on Management of Acute Otitis Media. Diagnosis and management of acute otitis media. *Pediatrics* 2004; 113:1451–1465.

Chan LS, Takata GS, Shekelle P, et al. Evidence assessment of management of acute otitis media, II: research gaps and priorities for future research. *Pediatrics* 2001;108:248–254.

McCormick DP, Chonmaitree T, Pittman C, et al. Nonsevere acute otitis media: a clinical trial comparing outcomes of watchful waiting vs immediate antibiotic treatment. *Pediatrics* 2005;115:1455–1465.

Powers JH. Diagnosis and treatment of acute otitis media: evaluating the evidence. *Infect Dis Clin North Am* 2007;21:409–426.

Rothman R, Owens T, Simel DL. Does this child have acute otitis media? *JAMA* 2003;290:1633–1640.

Rovers MM, Glasziou P, Appelman CL, et al. Antibiotics for acute otitis media: a meta-analysis with individual patient data. *Lancet* 2006;368:1429–1435.

Sarrell EM, Cohen HA, Kahan E. Naturopathic treatment for ear pain in children. *Pediatrics* 2003;111:e574–e579.

Spiro DM, Tay KY, Arnold DH, et al. Wait-and-see prescription for the treatment of acute otitis media: a randomized controlled trial. *JAMA* 2006; 296:1235–1241.

Stirn A. Body piercing: medical consequences and psychological motivations. *Lancet* 2003;361:1205–1215.

CHAPTER 55 ■ HEADACHE

CHRISTOPHER KING, MD, FACEP

Headache is a common complaint of pediatric patients in the emergency department (ED). It is estimated that by the age of 15 years, up to 75% of children have experienced headaches, although most are cared for at home. Parents may seek medical care if the child has a new-onset headache that is particularly painful and does not respond to nonprescription medications, if the child complains of progressively more severe headaches, or if the child has headaches that are recurrent over days, weeks, or months. Children with known migraine headaches are normally seen by a physician only when their standard medication regimen is not effective. Headache as an isolated complaint is a relatively unusual presentation in pediatric patients; it is more often one of a number of symptoms, such as fever, lethargy, sore throat, neck pain, and vomiting.

Like other challenging presentations, headache is seen with regularity and is almost always benign, but in a small subset of patients, it can portend a potentially life-threatening illness. Just as it can be difficult to identify the one child with appendicitis from a succession of patients with viral gastroenteritis, so too the clinician's skill can be tested in distinguishing which child among the many with headache has a serious underlying process. Therefore, the primary responsibility of the emergency physician is to make this important discrimination between "bad" headaches and benign headaches.

Fortunately, this can almost always be done successfully after a thorough history and physical examination, and when necessary, laboratory and radiographic tests. One notable exception to this rule, however, is brain tumor. Although most serious illnesses that cause headache (e.g., meningitis, encephalitis, ruptured vascular anomaly) will be readily classified in the "bad" category, the presence of a brain tumor may not be. The history can be subtle, and the examination is commonly unrevealing, often leading to a delay in diagnosis. Therefore, characteristics of headaches caused by a brain tumor are described in detail in this chapter. Above all, the key to proper management of such patients is ensuring appropriate follow-up care.

PATHOPHYSIOLOGY

For a headache to occur, there must obviously be some noxious stimulus that affects one or more pain-sensitive structures. Injury to an area that is insensitive to pain, as occurs with most types of nonhemorrhagic stroke, may cause significant morbidity but will not manifest as headache. It is therefore useful to consider the sensory innervation of the head and neck. All extracranial structures are sensitive to pain. Thus, processes that affect the sinuses, oropharynx, scalp, neck musculature, and so on often cause patients to complain of headache. In contrast, certain intracranial structures are sensi-

tive to pain and others are not. For example, the brain, ependymal lining, choroid plexus, and much of the dura and pia-arachnoid over the hemispheres are insensitive to pain. Pathologic processes affecting these areas can cause headache, but only by impinging on adjacent pain-sensitive structures. The most pain-sensitive intracranial structures are the proximal portions of the large cerebral arteries at the base of the brain, the venous sinuses, and the large cerebral veins.

Various physiologic mechanisms come into play in causing headache. Painful stimuli can be broadly categorized as resulting from vascular effects, muscle contraction, inflammation, and traction/compression (Table 55.1). Examples of each of these types of headache etiology are described in the following discussion of differential diagnosis. It should be noted that visual problems are an unlikely cause of significant headaches in children. A child with persistent headaches that have previously been attributed to "eye strain" may, therefore, deserve a more careful evaluation.

Attempting to predict the neuroanatomic location of a pathologic process using only the site of headache described by a child is unreliable. In part, this is attributable to the unpredictable displacement of structures caused by a mass lesion. In addition, the extremely complex relationships of the various nerves involved in pain sensation of the head and neck lead to unexpected patterns of referred pain. Thus, a posterior fossa lesion can cause frontal or orbital pain, and supratentorial lesions may result in pain localized to the occiput or the back of the neck.

DIFFERENTIAL DIAGNOSIS

A comprehensive discussion of the various causes of headache in pediatric patients is beyond the scope of this chapter. The conditions described here are those most likely to be seen in acute- and emergency-care settings (Table 55.2) and those with the greatest potential for imminent morbidity or mortality (Table 55.3).

Vascular

Headaches associated with vascular changes are believed to be caused primarily by vasodilation, although the exact mechanism has yet to be fully described. One common example of this type of headache is migraine. Migraine headaches are typically chronic and remitting, with a characteristic pattern that is easily described by the patient or parents (see Chapter 96). Often, a strong family history of migraines is present. For the emergency physician, the main issue with migraine patients is

TABLE 55.1

PATHOPHYSIOLOGIC CLASSIFICATION OF HEADACHES

I. Vascular
   A. Febrile illness
   B. Migraine
   C. Systemic hypertension
   D. Hypoxia
   E. Caffeine withdrawal
II. Muscle Contraction (Tension)
III. Inflammation
   A. Intracranial infections
      1. Meningitis
      2. Encephalitis
      3. Brain abscess
   B. Pharyngitis
   C. Dental infections
   D. Sinus infections
   E. Retroorbital cellulitis/abscess
IV. Traction/Compression
   A. Brain tumor
   B. Intracranial hemorrhage
   C. Increased intracranial pressure
      1. Cerebral edema
      2. Hydrocephalus
      3. Idiopathic intracranial hypertension (pseudotumor cerebri)
   D. Brain abscess
   E. Lumbar puncture
   F. Arterial dissection
V. Others
   A. Posttraumatic/postconcussive
   B. Psychogenic

generally pain control, because the diagnosis is already known. However, a significant change in the quality, severity, or timing of headaches in these patients may represent a separate and potentially more serious problem. In such cases, the clinician should not be dissuaded by the existing diagnosis from pursuing an appropriate workup as indicated.

Headaches accompanying fever are also believed to be mediated by vascular effects. Because fever is such a common

TABLE 55.2

COMMON CAUSES OF HEADACHE

Vascular
Febrile illness
Migraine

Inflammatory
Pharyngitis
Sinus infections
Dental infections

Muscle Contraction
Tension

Others
Psychogenic
Posttraumatic/postconcussive

TABLE 55.3

LIFE-THREATENING CAUSES OF HEADACHE

Vascular
Hypertension
Hypoxia

Inflammatory
Meningitis
Encephalitis

Traction/Compression
Brain tumor
Intracranial hemorrhage
Hydrocephalus
Cerebral edema
Brain abscess
Arterial dissection

symptom, this is probably the most common cause of headaches in pediatric patients seen in the ED. Hypertension is another possible cause of vascular headaches in children. Hypertension causes not only global changes in cerebral vasculature, but also possibly a component of increased intracranial pressure (ICP) that leads to headache.

Finally, hypoxia is a potent stimulus for cerebral vasodilation and can produce headaches on that basis. Therefore, children who experience a hypoxic insult (e.g., carbon monoxide poisoning) or those with disease states that predispose to hypoxia (e.g., cystic fibrosis, cyanotic heart disease) may present with headaches resulting from an acute process or an exacerbation of an underlying illness.

Muscle Contraction

Headaches can be caused by contraction of the scalp or neck muscles. This is the classic "tension" headache that so often plagues adults. These headaches usually occur when a patient has experienced prolonged periods of mental or emotional stress. This leads to recurrent episodes of muscle tension and/or spasm, which cause muscle soreness. The patient can often localize a specific site where the pain is felt, and the involved muscles may be tender to palpation. Although muscle contraction is an unlikely cause of headache in younger children, the stress of life during adolescence will often produce this type of headache. Onset is typically at the end of the day. A headache that is present on arising in the morning or that awakens a patient from sleep would be an unusual manifestation of muscle contraction.

Inflammation

A wide variety of inflammatory conditions can result in headache, ranging from benign to potentially life-threatening entities. Children with bacterial meningitis or encephalitis may present with headache, although this is usually only one of a constellation of symptoms, such as fever, lethargy, neck pain, confusion, or coma. Headache is unlikely to be the sole complaint in these patients. However, an older child or adolescent

emergent basis (many EDs have a dedicated scanner). Scanning time is also much shorter for CT, and the potentially unstable patient can be more easily observed. These characteristics make CT the test of choice to evaluate patients at risk for problems such as intracranial hemorrhage, cerebral edema, and herniation syndrome. CT is especially useful for patients with head trauma. However, CT does not offer the quality of image resolution provided by MRI. Smaller lesions, particularly those of the posterior fossa and brainstem, are more reliably detected by MRI. This is true even when the CT scan is performed using contrast material. Consequently, MRI is superior for children suspected of having a brain tumor who have a normal neurologic examination and no signs of elevated ICP. If these patients have a normal head CT scan in the ED, they will likely also require an outpatient MRI. Such duplication of testing is costly and usually unwarranted. While the use of MRI in the acute management of stroke has lead to a substantial increase in overall scanning capacity, limited availability continues to be the main drawback of MRI. Nonemergent MRI scans are often difficult to obtain from the ED even in large institutions. As discussed in the following, the emergency physician must take these and other factors into account in determining which, if any, imaging modality is indicated for a child with headaches.

Treatment and Disposition

Patients with headaches caused by a potentially life-threatening process (e.g., meningitis, encephalitis, ruptured vascular anomaly) require specific treatment approaches discussed elsewhere in this textbook. A patient with pseudotumor cerebri requires drainage of CSF to reduce the ICP, which, in turn, often relieves the headache pain. Children with headaches that are presumptively diagnosed as benign can almost always be successfully treated with acetaminophen or ibuprofen. The various options available for treating pediatric migraine patients are described in Chapter 96.

Although most children complaining of headache can be safely discharged from the ED with an appropriate follow-up plan, some will require admission to the hospital for further evaluation and treatment. For example, a child with headaches who is found to be significantly hypertensive must be admitted both for management of the blood pressure and investigation of the underlying cause. Any patient with pseudotumor cerebri who also has decreased visual acuity requires emergent evaluation by an ophthalmologist and possibly a surgical procedure to relieve the pressure on the optic nerve. Patients with migraine who have intractable headache pain may also warrant admission to receive a more effective analgesic regimen. The child with a ventricular shunt who has severe headaches will usually require a shunt series, a CT scan of the head, and neurosurgical evaluation to assess the need for possible shunt revision. If neurosurgical consultation is not immediately available, the patient should be transported to an appropriate receiving facility.

A potentially confusing issue that the emergency physician will inevitably face is how to properly manage a child who is suspected of having a brain tumor. Should all these patients have a brain imaging study in the ED? As discussed previously, the resolution of even a contrast-enhanced head CT scan is inferior to MRI for detecting certain types of tumors. Also, a small but finite risk is associated with the administration of contrast material. However, obtaining a nonemergent MRI from the ED may not be an available option. What then is the appropriate diagnostic approach?

In general, a child with headaches who is suspected of having a brain tumor should undergo a head CT scan in the ED if there are any signs or symptoms of elevated ICP. These include an altered mental status, visual changes, persistent vomiting, papilledema, and focal neurologic deficits. Because mass lesions that cause elevated ICP are usually larger and more easily detectable, the reduction in image resolution with CT is less likely to result in missing an abnormality in such cases. Of note, if the CT scan is normal in a child with headache and new focal deficits on neurologic examination, it may be necessary to obtain an emergent MRI to exclude the diagnosis of stroke (e.g., arterial dissection), although this may simply represent the first presentation of a complex migraine syndrome.

However, what about the child with a suspicious history (e.g., increasing frequency or duration of pain, headaches that awaken the child from sleep or occur every morning) who has a normal neurologic examination and no signs of elevated ICP? In most cases, if MRI is not available for a nonemergent scan from the ED, such patients can be safely discharged with an outpatient MRI scheduled within 24 to 48 hours. A delay in diagnosis of 1 or 2 days is usually acceptable if this allows the appropriate diagnostic study to be performed. Obviously, parents must be clearly instructed that any sign of deterioration, such as mental status changes or persistent vomiting, requires that the child be immediately returned to the ED for a reevaluation.

Suggested Readings

Brna PM, Dooley JM. Headaches in the pediatric population. *Semin Pediatr Neurol* 2006;13(4):222–230.

Burton LJ, Quinn B, Pratt-Cheney JL, et al. Headache etiology in a pediatric emergency department. *Pediatr Emerg Care* 1997;13:1–4.

de Ribaupierre S, Rilliet B, Cotting J, et al. A 10-year experience in paediatric spontaneous cerebral hemorrhage: which children with headache need more than a clinical examination? *Swiss Med Wkly* 2008;138:59–69.

Hershey AD. Pediatric headache. *Pediatr Ann* 2005;34:426–429.

Honig PJ, Charney EB. Children with brain tumor headaches: distinguishing features. *Am J Dis Child* 1982;136:121–141.

Kan G, Nagelberg J, Maytal J. Headaches in pediatric emergency department: etiology, imaging and treatment. *Headache* 2000;40:25–29.

Lewis DW, Qureshi F. Acute headache in children and adolescents presenting to emergency department. *Headache* 2000;40:200–203.

Masi G, Favilla L, Millepiedi S, et al. Somatic symptoms in children and adolescents referred for emotional and behavioral disorders. *Psychiatry* 2000;63:140–149.

Mercille G, Ospina LH. Pediatric idiopathic intracranial hypertension: a review. *Pediatr Rev* 2007;28(11):e77–e86.

Metsähonkala L, Anttila P, Sillanpää M. Tension-type headache in children. *Cephalalgia* 1999;19(suppl 25):56.

Newton RW. Childhood headache. *Arch Dis Child Educ Pract Ed* 2008;93:105–111.

Pavlakis SG, Frank Y, Chusid R. Hypertensive encephalopathy, reversible occipitoparietal encephalopathy, or reversible posterior leukoencephalopathy: three names for an old syndrome. *J Child Neurol* 1999;14:277–281.

Reulecke BC, Erker CG, Fiedler BJ, et al. Brain tumors in children: initial symptoms and their influence on the time span between symptom onset and diagnosis. *J Child Neurol* 2008;23:178–83.

Rubin DH, Suecoff SA, Knupp KG. Headaches in children. *Pediatr Ann* 2006;35(5):345–53.

The Childhood Brain Tumor Consortium. The epidemiology of headache among children with brain tumor. Headache in children with brain tumors. *J Neurooncol* 1991;10:31–46.

Walker DM, Teach SJ. Emergency department treatment of primary headaches in children and adolescents. *Curr Opin Pediatr* 2008;20:248–54.

Wilne SH, Ferris RC, Nathwani A, et al. The presenting features of brain tumours: a review of 200 cases. *Arch Dis Child* 2006;91(6):502–6.

CHAPTER 56 ■ PAIN—JOINTS

RICHARD J. SCARFONE, MD

Arthritis and arthralgia are common reasons for children to seek care in the emergency department (ED). Arthritis is joint inflammation marked by swelling, warmth, and limitation of motion, whereas arthralgia is simply joint pain without signs of inflammation. Establishing a diagnosis for the child with joint pain is challenging because the differential diagnosis is lengthy (Table 56.1), clinical and laboratory findings are rarely specific for a particular disease, and disease patterns for many of the etiologies are often highly variable among different patients. Among the most common causes of joint pain in children are infections, trauma, and postinfectious conditions (Table 56.2), whereas those most likely to be life-threatening are due to systemic disease and malignancy (Table 56.3). This chapter serves as a guide to an approach to the child with arthritis or arthralgia, with an emphasis on historical points and physical examination findings that can serve to narrow the diagnostic possibilities.

DIFFERENTIAL DIAGNOSIS

The possible causes of joint complaints in children are extensive (Table 56.1). The initial differential diagnosis usually focuses on the most common etiologies (Table 56.2). Children from 6 to 24 months of age have the highest incidence of nongonococcal bacterial (septic) arthritis, and boys are affected twice as often as girls. Septic arthritis results primarily from the hematogenous dissemination of an organism into the joint or the bony metaphysis. The diagnosis of septic arthritis of the hip should not be delayed because pressure in the joint space will compromise the vascular supply to the femoral head, leading to necrosis (see Chapter 92).

Osteomyelitis involving the distal end of long bones may manifest as arthralgia with or without objective signs of joint inflammation. Children with sickle cell anemia and type 1 diabetes mellitus are at higher risk for osteomyelitis. Onset of symptoms is typically more indolent compared to that in septic arthritis.

In the first 10 days of illness, children with Kawasaki disease may have arthritis or arthralgia, often involving smaller joints in the hand. Beyond that time, involvement of larger joints of the lower extremities is more common. If an arthrocentesis is performed, the synovial fluid analysis resembles that seen with septic arthritis with 100,000 to 300,000 white blood cells (WBCs) per cubic millimeter (mm^3). However, synovial fluid Gram stain and cultures will be negative among children with Kawasaki disease (see Chapter 101).

In the absence of a clear history of a tick bite, Lyme disease may be a challenging diagnosis to establish because only about 40% to 70% of children have the characteristic erythema migrans rash, constitutional symptoms may be mild, and serologic tests will be normal in the early stages of disease.

Transient (also called toxic) synovitis is a poorly understood inflammation of the hip joint, afflicting children 3 to 6 years of age. The diagnosis is typically made on clinical grounds, and this self-limited disease does not result in joint destruction. When the hip is involved, the challenge for clinicians is to distinguish transient synovitis from septic arthritis.

Reactive, or postinfectious, arthritis is probably more common than septic arthritis. Arthritis following various enteric infections is not rare in children, and joint complaints after parvovirus B19 infection are seen among adolescents. *Chlamydia trachomatis* infection of the genitourinary tract should be considered in any sexually active adolescent with new-onset arthritis. With postinfectious arthritis, antimicrobial treatment does not modify the disease course.

Traumatic injuries to a joint may cause periarticular swelling or an effusion indicative of a hemarthrosis. In addition, ligamentous or tendon injuries will result in joint pain and impaired range of motion. Serum sickness and Henoch-Schonlein purpura are marked by characteristic rashes.

EVALUATION AND DECISION

Figure 56.1 depicts an algorithm for the diagnostic approach to the child with joint pain. The evaluation should include inquiries about the specific joint(s) involved, symptom duration, and history of trauma, fever, rash, tick bites, sexual risk factors, intravenous drug use, and recent illnesses. The child's past medical and family histories should be reviewed. A family history of systemic lupus erythematosus (SLE), inflammatory bowel disease, or rheumatoid arthritis increases the child's risk for these diseases.

A comprehensive physical examination should be performed with particular attention paid to a search for rashes, heart murmurs, and abdominal abnormalities. Assessment of the affected joint(s) should determine if it is warm, swollen, or tender as well as its range of motion.

A complete blood cell (CBC) count and differential, C-reactive protein, and erythrocyte sedimentation rate (ESR) are indicated for the febrile child with signs of joint inflammation, especially in the absence of trauma. Additional laboratory studies, such as an antistreptolysin-O titer or antinuclear antibody (ANA) test, should be guided by the history and physical examination. Radiographs of the affected joint are particularly useful in the setting of trauma or acute monoarthritis without an obvious cause, although ultrasound is more sensitive than plain radiographs in detecting an effusion. The Ottawa knee rules can be used to guide the decision to obtain radiographs

TABLE 56.1

JOINT PAIN—DIFFERENTIAL DIAGNOSIS

Infection
Septic arthritis (bacterial)
  Staphylococcus aureus
  Streptococcus pneumoniae
  Haemophilus influenza
  Group B streptococci
  Escherichia coli
Gonococcal
Other infectious arthritis
  Viral
  Mycobacterial
  Fungal
Osteomyelitis

Postinfectious
Viral: hepatitis B, parvovirus, Epstein-Barr virus,
  cytomegalovirus, varicella-zoster, herpesvirus 6,
  enterovirus, adenovirus
Bacterial: acute rheumatic fever, Lyme disease, chlamydia
  (Reiter's syndrome), mycloplasma, shigella, campylobacter

Trauma/Overuse
Contusion
Hemarthrosis
Fracture
Inflicted injury
Ligamentous sprain
Bursitis
Tendonitis
Slipped capital femoral epiphysis
Legg-Calvé-Perthes disease
Osteochondritis dissecans
Chondromalacia patellae
Osgood-Schlatter disease

Immune-mediated/Vasculitic
Juvenile idiopathic arthritis
Serum sickness
Kawasaki disease
Inflammatory bowel disease
Systemic lupus erythematosus
Henoch-Schönlein purpura

Other
Transient synovitis of the hip
Malignancy
  Leukemia
  Neuroblastoma
  Bone tumor
  Hemophilia

TABLE 56.2

COMMON CAUSES OF JOINT PAIN

Septic arthritis (bacterial)
Osteomyelitis
Kawasaki disease
Lyme disease
Transient synovitis of the hip
Postinfectious (reactive)
Traumatic
Serum sickness
Henoch-Schönlein purpura

TABLE 56.3

LIFE-THREATENING CAUSES OF JOINT PAIN

Acute rheumatic fever
Kawasaki disease
Malignancy
  Leukemia
  Neuroblastoma
  Bone tumor

of the knee following injury. In a recent study, the rules were found to be 100% sensitive in detecting fractures while eliminating the need for about one-third of the radiographs. Most febrile children with monoarthritis and joint effusions will need an arthrocentesis to assist in determining the etiology. Magnetic resonance imaging is most useful to detect subtle fractures not visualized on plain films and to help establish a diagnosis of osteomyelitis.

A key initial point in the history is whether trauma preceded the pain. It is easy to be led astray by parents trying to recall what traumatic event could have led to the child's symptoms. The clinician should be mindful that if the mechanism was not severe enough to prevent the child from continuing an activity, it is unlikely to be the cause of a significantly swollen and painful joint. However, if there was a definite traumatic event preceding the onset of symptoms, particularly in the absence of fever, one can proceed with that aspect of the algorithm.

A radiograph will detect fractures or a slipped capital femoral epiphysis (SCFE). Classically, a SCFE occurs in the obese adolescent boy with hip or knee pain (see Chapters 114 and 125), although it should be considered in any child 8 to 14 years of age with hip or knee pain. Importantly, only about half of children will report preceding trauma and there may be bilateral disease in about one third of children. Plain radiographs (including the frog-leg view of the hip) showing a widened epiphysis and caudal displacement of the femoral head establish the diagnosis.

Metaphyseal corner fractures resulting in joint pain are highly suggestive of inflicted injury. These typically occur in children age 3 years or less and there may not be a clear history of trauma. These fractures result from traction or torsion forces such as occurs when the arms or legs are pulled or swung violently.

Radiographs may also aid in determining whether swelling is caused by a joint effusion or is simply soft-tissue swelling outside the joint space, a distinction that is often difficult to make on physical examination alone. In the setting of acute trauma and in the absence of fever, an effusion is indicative of a hemarthrosis and is rarely a diagnostic or therapeutic indication for performing an arthrocentesis. Such a patient will typically experience only temporary relief from the aspiration of fluid, followed by a reaccumulation of blood. Clinicians must have a high index of suspicion for hemarthrosis in the child with hemophilia or other clotting disorder who presents with joint swelling, even without a clear history of trauma.

In the absence of an effusion, inquiries about the duration of symptoms should be made. Children with conditions such as bursitis, tendonitis, and Osgood-Schlatter disease typically have chronic, low-grade pain and may inadvertently come to

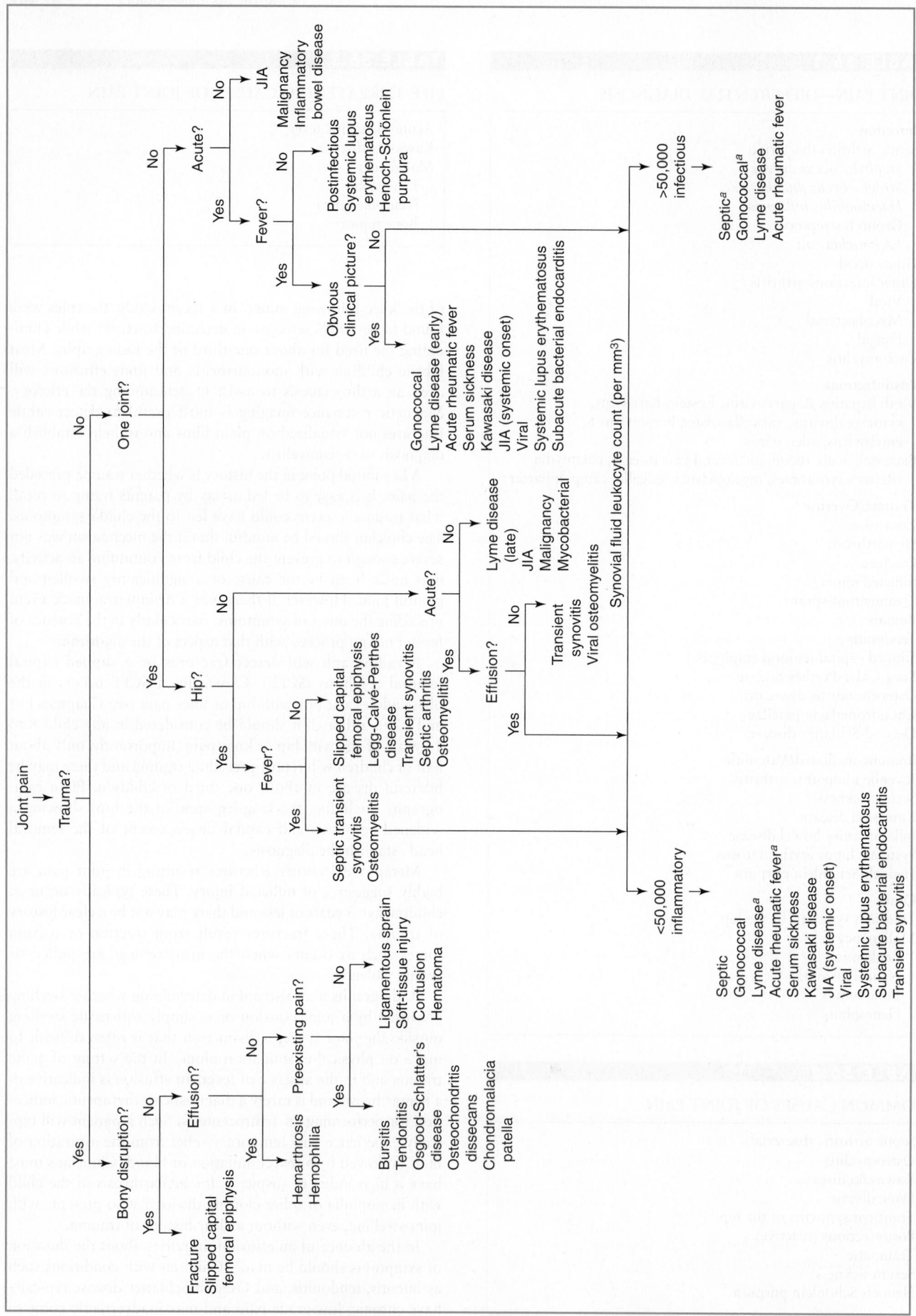

FIGURE 56.1 A diagnostic approach to joint pain. JIA, juvenile idiopathic arthritis. [a]Most likely leukocyte count.

medical attention after minor trauma. New-onset periarticular swelling and pain immediately after acute trauma suggests ligamentous or other soft-tissue injury.

In the absence of trauma, monoarthritis of the hip may represent a true orthopedic emergency. Septic hips require operative drainage to prevent osteonecrosis and the most important prognostic factor is the length of delay between the onset of infection and the institution of therapy. Unlike most other causes of fever and arthritis, septic arthritis involves only a single joint in more than 90% of affected children; 80% of these are hip, knee, or ankle infections. The absence of fever does not preclude the diagnosis; just 60% to 70% of children with septic arthritis are febrile at presentation. A child with septic arthritis of the hip will typically maintain external rotation of the hip, resist even the slightest range of motion and be unable to ambulate. In fact, if the child allows full range of motion, the diagnosis is highly unlikely. Neonates, on the other hand, will often present with thigh swelling, pseudoparalysis, and external rotation at the hip.

A child with acute onset of monoarthritis of the hip or any other large joint, marked by an effusion and severely restricted range of motion, with or without fever, needs an arthrocentesis. The study may be performed with ultrasound guidance and the synovial fluid should be analyzed for cell count and differential, glucose and protein, Gram stain, and culture. *Staphylococcus aureus* is the most common infecting agent for older children, whereas group B *Streptococcus* and gram-negative enteric organisms must also be considered in neonates. In recent years, clinicians are encountering a greater prevalence of community-associated methicillin-resistant *Staphylococcus aureus* as a causative agent. In two large series, about half of the children with septic arthritis of the hip had negative synovial fluid cultures. In these cases, children with synovial fluid WBC counts greater than 50,000 per mm^3 and positive blood cultures were presumed to have septic arthritis and managed accordingly.

In contrast to septic arthritis, children with transient synovitis of the hip usually appear well, may be afebrile or have only mildly elevated temperatures, often are able to bear weight but have a limp, and allow almost complete range of motion of the affected joint. A prospective study of over 150 children presenting with an irritable hip found that just 2% of children had septic arthritis if all of these four risk factors were absent: fever > 38.5°C, refusal to bear weight, ESR > 40 mm per hour, and WBC > 12,000 cells per mm^3.

Often, based on clinical findings, a physician can make a diagnosis of transient synovitis without the need for laboratory testing or arthrocentesis. In more equivocal cases, inflammatory markers may be helpful. The absence of all four factors listed above has a very high negative predictive value in excluding septic arthritis. The presence of one or more risk factors, especially in an ill-appearing child, justifies further diagnostic work-up, including an arthrocentesis.

Inflammatory markers are usually elevated in patients with osteomyelitis, as well. In contrast to those with septic arthritis, children with osteomyelitis have a more subacute onset of pain, are less likely to be febrile, will have greater range of motion at the joint, and may not have signs of joint inflammation.

Legg-Calvé-Perthes disease, a condition of uncertain cause, occurs overwhelmingly in boys, with an onset between 4 and

TABLE 56.4

DISTINGUISHING CLINICAL FEATURES OF ETIOLOGIES OF POLYARTHRITIS

Disease	Clinical characteristics
Gonococcal	Adolescent, tenosynovitis, rash
Lyme	Tick bite, erythema migrans, endemic region, seasonality
Acute rheumatic fever	Recent streptococcal infection, extreme migratory pain, carditis
Serum sickness	Urticaria, angioedema
Kawasaki disease	Prolonged fever, rash, conjunctivitis, mouth changes
Subacute bacterial endocarditis	Congenital heart disease, fever, new murmur, splinter hemorrhages
Systemic lupus erythematosus	African-American female, skin, renal disease
Henoch-Schönlein purpura	Purpura below the waist, nephritis, abdominal pain, scrotal swelling
Inflammatory bowel disease	Abdominal pain, diarrhea, weight loss, anemia

8 years of age. The pain, which may be localized to the hip or referred to the thigh or knee, is insidious in onset. The aseptic necrosis of the femoral head will be manifest on plain radiographs as a small, osteopenic femoral head with a widened joint space, although films obtained early in the clinical course may be normal.

Historical and physical examination findings help narrow the choices among the many causes of polyarthritis (Tables 56.4 and 56.5). The ill-appearing adolescent with migratory arthritis, tenosynovitis involving the extensor tendons of the wrist or ankle, and scattered crops of vesiculopustules on an erythematous base should be strongly suspected for gonococcal arthritis. This occurs three to five times more often in girls, often during

TABLE 56.5

FEVER AND JOINT PAIN

Usually Febrile at Presentation
Septic arthritis (bacterial)
Osteomyelitis
Gonococcal
Acute rheumatic fever
Juvenile idiopathic arthritis (systemic onset subcategory)
Subacute bacterial endocarditis
Serum sickness
Kawasaki disease

May or May Not Be Febrile at Presentation
Leukemia
Mycobacterial
Postinfectious (reactive)
Lyme disease
Systemic lupus erythematosus
Inflammatory bowel disease

menstruation. Of note, few patients report lower abdominal pain or vaginal discharge concurrently, and cultures of blood and synovial fluid are typically negative. The highest yield for establishing the diagnosis is by Gram stain of the skin lesions showing gram-negative intracellular diplococci or by recovering the organism from the cervix, rectum, or throat. Joint involvement with Lyme disease has two distinct patterns. In early disseminated disease when erythema migrans is the principal clinical sign, the child may develop episodic migratory polyarthritis, affecting mainly large joints. However, more typically at this stage, the child has arthralgia without signs of joint inflammation. Weeks to months (mean 4 to 6 weeks) after the tick bite, half of untreated children develop an intermittent monoarthritis, usually of the knee. The joint is significantly swollen but only mildly painful, and patients are usually afebrile at this stage and without a history of trauma. Extremely painful, migratory joint inflammation involving multiple joints in a child with recent evidence of a group A streptococcal infection should raise the concern for acute rheumatic fever. Evidence of carditis, erythema marginatum, subcutaneous nodules, or a positive serology for antistreptococcal antibodies supports the diagnosis. The presence of diffuse urticaria and angioedema accompanying arthralgia or arthritis, especially 3 to 10 days after initiation of an antibiotic, helps distinguish serum sickness from other causes of polyarthritis and fever. Kawasaki disease is characterized by high and persistent fever, conjunctival injection without exudate, mouth and lip swelling and cracking, swelling and erythema of the hands and feet, a nonspecific rash, and lymphadenopathy. About 30% of patients will also develop arthritis or arthralgia, with about one-third of these having onset in the first 10 days of illness. Both small interphalangeal joints and large weight-bearing joints may be involved. Daily temperature spikes exceeding 40°C, especially if accompanied by a transient pink rash, suggest systemic-onset juvenile rheumatoid arthritis (JRA), one of the categories of juvenile idiopathic arthritis (JIA). A common viral-related arthritis is that caused by hepatitis B infection. The arthritis precedes the symptoms of hepatitis and resolves when the jaundice appears. Parvovirus B19 is the causative agent of erythema infectiosum; about 5% of affected children will complain of transient, bilateral joint inflammation. Joint manifestations due to this virus can also occur in the absence of a rash causing a sudden onset of symmetric, self-limited polyarthritis, particularly in the hands. With subacute bacterial endocarditis, musculoskeletal symptoms are variable, ranging from asymptomatic joint effusions to frank arthritis of up to three joints. Preexisting congenital heart disease, a prolonged fever, a new murmur, and splinter hemorrhages may all be clues to the diagnosis of this rare entity in children.

A joint aspiration is rarely necessary to establish a diagnosis for a child with polyarthritis and fever. If an arthrocentesis is obtained, typically the synovial fluid will be sterile and the leukocyte count will characterize the process as inflammatory, although some disease processes may yield counts that could be consistent with either inflammatory or infectious causes (Fig. 56.1).

Postinfectious arthritis is one of the more common causes of acute polyarthritis without fever. One to 2 weeks after an illness (especially *Chlamydia trachomatis*, *Shigella*, or *Salmonella*) or urogenital infection (Reiter's syndrome), a child may develop an asymmetric joint inflammation predominantly involving large joints of the lower extremities. The severity of the antecedent illness has little correlation with the arthritis, and the intensity of synovitis and fever is mild or absent at this stage. As with many of the diseases discussed to this point, SLE has a variable clinical presentation with regard to musculoskeletal involvement. In fact, no two patients have an identical pattern of immune complex formation or clinical disease expression. A symmetric polyarthritis involving peripheral joints of the hands or feet may be seen. However, small effusions of the knee are also common with active disease, and the arthritis may also be intermittent or migratory. Patients with this type of arthritis are usually afebrile, yet high fever may be a prominent finding. Further, although arthritis is one of several diagnostic criteria, it is uncommon for patients with SLE to present with isolated arthritis. Arthritis of the small joints, a positive test for ANA, and abnormalities of the skin, kidneys, or central nervous system should raise the clinician's suspicion for SLE.

Henoch-Schönlein purpura (HSP) is rarely a diagnostic challenge, thanks to the presence of petechiae and purpura in the characteristic below-the-waist distribution. Affected children may also have polyarthritis or arthralgia, colicky abdominal pain, and nephritis. As with the rash, periarticular swelling usually involves joints below the waist.

Chronic arthritis is less common than acute arthritis in children younger than age 16 years, with an incidence of 20 to 150 cases per 100,000. JIA is a newer term used to classify chronic childhood arthritis. It encompasses all of the diseases referred to as JRA, as well as other causes of idiopathic arthritis. Subclassifications of disease are based on the patient's age at onset of symptoms, duration and pattern of arthritis, and presence or absence of systemic signs such as fever or rash. This term describes children younger than age 16 years with joint inflammation for at least 6 weeks, in whom other causes have been eliminated. That they appear at several points in the diagnostic algorithm reflects their diversity. Tests for rheumatoid factor or ANA may assist in establishing a specific diagnosis. These are difficult diagnoses for ED physicians to establish based on a single patient encounter; children with chronic arthritis should be referred to a rheumatologist.

In the absence of fever, chronic pain of one or more joints may also indicate malignancy. Specifically, leukemia or neuroblastoma can both present with true joint swelling, as can bony tumors. Pallor, adenopathy, weight loss, and other constitutional complaints, as well as anemia or cytopenias, would support this diagnosis.

A large joint oligoarthritis occurs as an extraintestinal complication of inflammatory bowel disease in about one-third of children, usually during times of active disease. Clues to the diagnosis include abdominal pain, hematochezia, anemia, and weight loss.

In summary, this review of joint pain in children should serve as a guide to the diagnostic evaluation. The clinician must choose from many different causes, each with variable and nonspecific characteristics. In addition, laboratory studies are rarely specific for a particular disease. However, by asking the appropriate questions, performing a careful physical examination, selectively obtaining adjunct studies, and developing pattern recognition skills, the clinician can follow the correct diagnostic path.

Suggested Readings

Bulloch B, Neto G, Plint A, et al. Validation of the Ottawa knee rule in children: a multicenter study. *Ann Emerg Med* 2003;42:48–55.

Caird MS, Flynn JM, Leung YL, et al. Factors distinguishing septic arthritis from transient synovitis of the hip in children. A prospective study. *J Bone Joint Surg Am* 2006;88:1251–1257.

Gough-Palmer A, McHugh K. Investigating hip pain in a well child. *BMJ* 2007; 334:1216.

Herring JA, Kim HT, Browne R. Legg-Calve-Perthes disease. Part II: Prospective multicenter study of the effect of treatment on outcome. *J Bone Joint Surg Am* 2004;86-A:2121.

Jones OY, Spencer CH, Bowyer SL, et al. A multicenter case-control study on predictive factors distinguishing childhood leukemia from juvenile rheumatoid arthritis. *Pediatrics* 2006;117:e840.

Kocher MS, Bishop JA, Weed B, et al. Delay in diagnosis of slipped capital femoral epiphysis. *Pediatrics* 2004;113:e322.

Kocher MS, Mandiga R, Zurakowski D, et al. Validation of a clinical prediction rule for the difference between septic arthritis and transient synovitis of the hip in children. *J Bone Joint Surg Am* 2004;86:1629–1635.

Kocher MS, Zurakowski D, Kasser JR. Differentiating between septic arthritis and transient synovitis of the hip in children: an evidence-based clinical prediction algorithm. *J Bone Joint Surg Am* 1999;81-A:1662–1670.

Lehman TJA. Classification of juvenile rheumatoid arthritis. In: Rose BD, ed.Waltham, MA: UpToDate, 2009. http://www.uptodate.com/online/content/topic.do?topicKey=gen_pedi/21233&selectedTitle=1~60&source=search_result. Accessed 10/28/2009.

Nigrovic PA. Overview of hip pain in childhood. In: Rose BD, ed. Waltham, MA: UpToDate, 2009 http://www.uptodate.com/online/content/topic.do?topicKey=gen_pedi/21233&selectedTitle=1~60&source=search_result. Accessed 10/28/2009.

Uziel Y, Butbul-Aviel Y, Barash J, et al. Recurrent transient synovitis of the hip in childhood. Longterm outcome among 39 patients. *J Rheumatol* 2006; 33:810.

Wilking AP. An approach to the child with joint pain. In: Rose BD, ed. Waltham, MA: UpToDate, 2009. http://www.uptodate.com/online/content/topic.do?topicKey=pedirheu/12386&selectedTitle=2~150&source=search_result. Accessed 10/28/2009.

CHAPTER 57 ■ PAIN—SCROTAL

CATHERINE E. PERRON, MD

Acute scrotal swelling or pain in a child should be considered a potential surgical emergency. Although some causes of acute scrotal swelling may be benign and require no more than observation and reassurance to the patient and parent, other causes may lead to the rapid loss of a testis if diagnosis and treatment are delayed. The patient with such a complaint should be evaluated promptly. Many diagnoses in cases of scrotal pain are most reliably made clinically, differentiating by age, historical features relating to the evolution of pain and associated symptoms, and physical examination findings.

PATHOPHYSIOLOGY

The anatomic structures contained in the scrotum include the testes; the epididymis; appendages of the testis; and the nerve, vascular, and lymphatic structures that constitute the spermatic cord and traverse the inguinal canal into the scrotum (Fig. 57.1). The anatomy of the testicle, its related structures, and the layers of tissue that surround each testicle in the scrotum may each relate to the pathology seen in this area. The descent of the testis, at approximately 32 to 40 weeks' gestation, through the inguinal canal from the abdomen to its eventual position in the scrotum, also contributes to the risk of pathology in the scrotum and associated groin area. The testis descends within the process vaginalis, which is an out-pouching of the peritoneal cavity. After the descent of the testis, the abdominal portion of the process vaginalis closes and the remaining portion, called the *tunica vaginalis,* is a potential space that encompasses the anterior two-thirds of the testicle. Within this space, fluids of various etiologies can collect. Pathophysiologic causes of acute conditions of the scrotum include ischemia, inflammation, trauma, and tumor. Since these processes often alter blood flow to structures within the scrotum, appropriate imaging modalities, when correlated with clinical history and examination, are often useful in coming to the correct diagnosis.

DIFFERENTIAL DIAGNOSIS

Table 57.1 lists the principal causes of acute scrotal swelling, and Table 57.2 provides the most common diagnoses by age.

Causes of Painful Scrotal Swelling

Torsion of the Testis

Testicular torsion is the most significant condition causing acute scrotal pain and represents a true surgical emergency. As a common cause of acute, painful scrotal swelling in children, testicular torsion accounts for approximately 30% of cases of acute scrotal pain. Testicular torsion is more common in the newborn period and during the early stages of puberty. Approximately two-thirds of the cases of intravaginal torsion occur in children between the ages of 12 and 18 years, overlapping the peak incidence of appendage torsion (see also Chapter 124).

Torsion results from an inadequate fixation of the testis to the intrascrotal subcutaneous tissue (Fig. 57.2), resulting in the so-called "bell-clapper" deformity. The testis, which hangs more freely within the tunica vaginalis in this deformity, may rotate, producing torsion of the spermatic cord, venous engorgement of the testis, and subsequent arterial infarction (Fig. 57.3).

The sudden onset of severe scrotal pain and tenderness, often with radiation to the abdomen, and associated nausea and vomiting is typical. Often, these episodes have their onset in the early morning. At other times, they may be associated with sports activity or mild testicular trauma that may be perceived by the patient as the cause of the pain. A history of trauma is often misleading in patients with testicular torsion. The patient may recall prior episodes of similar pain that resolved spontaneously, suggesting intermittent torsion and spontaneous detorsion.

With torsion of the testis, typically the testis is acutely swollen and diffusely tender and usually lies higher ("horizontal or transverse lie") in the scrotum than the contralateral testis. Since the pain may be referred to the abdomen, it is essential that the genitalia are examined carefully in every child who complains of abdominal pain. There may be overlying erythema of the skin of the scrotum. The cremasteric reflex (retraction of the testis with stroking of the inner thigh) is usually absent with testicular torsion but may be present in early or incomplete torsion. The cremasteric reflex may be absent in infants younger than 30 months. Urinalysis is usually negative.

Time is important in establishing the diagnosis of torsion of the testis. If a testis has been twisted sufficiently to fully obstruct its blood supply for more than 6 to 12 hours, surgical detorsion is unlikely to salvage the gonad. It is impossible to determine clinically, however, whether the torsion has been partial or total. Therefore, it is an oversimplification to assume that if symptoms have been present for more than 6 to 12 hours, an irreversible situation has developed that would preclude any attempt at testicular salvage. The duration of symptoms does not always determine functional recoverability.

Although the diagnosis continues to be established most reliably by a skilled examiner familiar with acute scrotal lesions in children, diagnostic imaging studies may be valuable, particularly in cases where the diagnosis is uncertain.

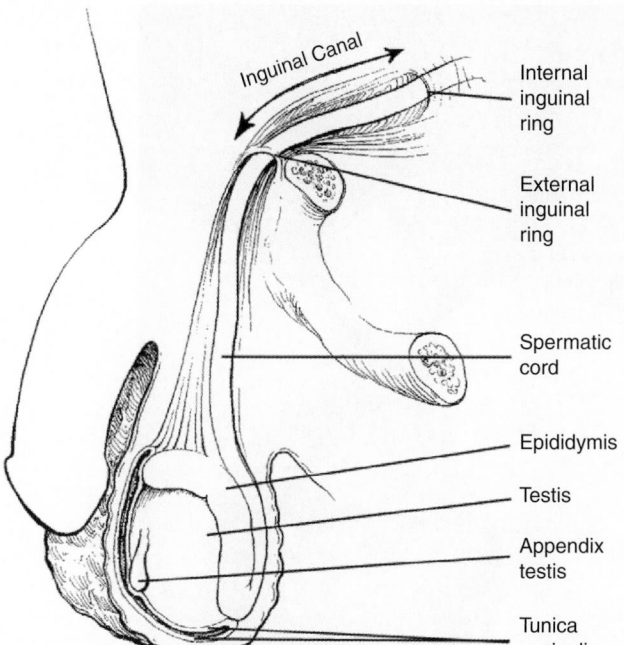

FIGURE 57.1 Anatomy of the scrotal contents.

Color Doppler sonography or nuclear testicular scanning reveals decreased or absent arterial blood flow within the affected testicle when compared with the other. It must be stressed that, if the history and physical examination strongly suggest testicular torsion or if any appreciable time would be lost in arranging for these studies, the preferred course is to proceed with surgical exploration or an attempt at manual detorsion (Fig. 57.4) if surgical intervention is not readily available.

SIGNS AND SYMPTOMS

TABLE 57.1

CAUSES OF ACUTE SCROTAL SWELLING

Painful Scrotal Swelling
Torsion of testis
Torsion of appendage of testis
Trauma—hematocele, hematoma, epididymitis, testicular
  rupture
Epididymitis
Orchitis
Hernia—incarcerated
Tumor[a]—acute hemorrhage

Painless Scrotal Swelling
Hydrocele
Hernia
Varicocele
Spermatocele
Idiopathic scrotal edema
Henoch-Schönlein purpura[a]
Kawasaki disease[a]
Testis tumor[a]
Antenatal torsion of the testis

[a]Life-threatening causes.

TABLE 57.2

COMMON CAUSES OF ACUTE SCROTAL SWELLING

Infancy
Hydrocele
Hernia

Childhood
Hernia
Torsion of the appendix testes
Torsion of the testes
Trauma

Adolescence
Epididymitis
Torsion of the appendix testes
Torsion of the testes
Trauma

Color Doppler flow ultrasound can assess anatomy and blood flow (Fig. 57.5). Swelling and fluid collections can be localized by ultrasound, which can be particularly helpful in trauma. Ultrasound has become the standard of imaging for the acute scrotum as it is now more widely available and has anatomic detail and time advantages over the testicular nuclear perfusion scans. Limitations associated with Doppler sonography must also be recognized, particularly related to small, lower flow prepubertal testes and the operator-dependent nature of this test. False-negative ultrasounds may occur from spontaneous detorsion or in cases of late torsion in which a severe degree of overlying scrotal edema may be associated with sufficient, increased vascularity to obscure the underlying ischemic testis. The testicular nuclear perfusion scan with technetium-99 pertechnetate is less time efficient but another possible imaging modality that also has limitations. Technetium is injected and the scrotum scanned. Impeded blood flow to the torsed testicle results in a cold spot. The presence of a hydrocele, abscess, hematoma, or scrotal hernia may result in

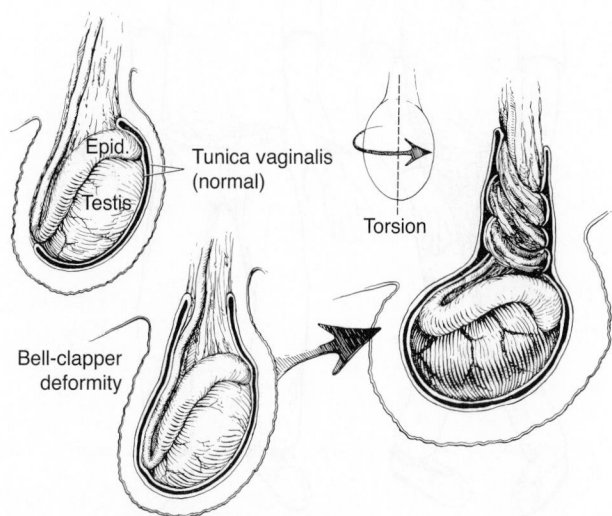

FIGURE 57.2 Torsion testis. Abnormality of testicular fixation—bell-clapper deformity—permits torsion of spermatic vessels with subsequent infarction of the gonad. Epid., epididymis.

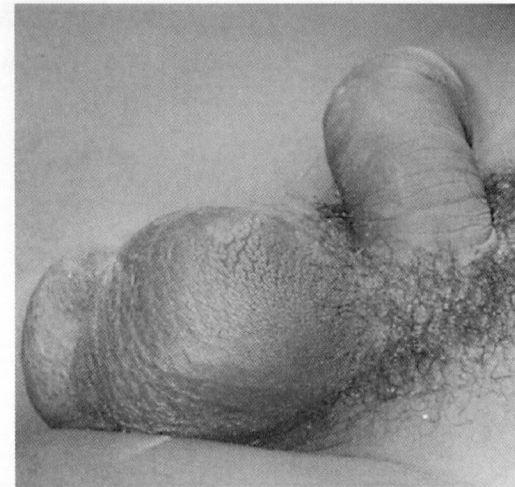

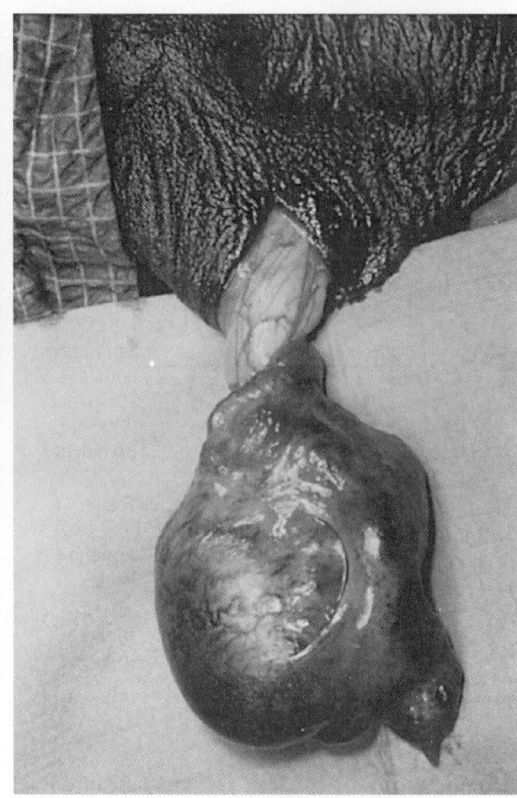

FIGURE 57.3 Torsion of testis. **A:** Swollen, diffusely tender testis high in the scrotum (from twisting of cord structures). **B:** Surgically exposed testis showing torsion of cord structures. Testis was infarcted and was removed.

decreased counts on that side of the scrotum and may be confused with torsion of the testis. False-negative scans may occur for similar reasons as ultrasound related to edema and increased vascularity of late torsion obscuring an ischemic testis. Another pitfall encountered with use of both sonography and nuclear scan is incomplete or intermittent torsion in which the study may indicate normal, increased, or decreased flow, depending on timing.

The therapy for testicular torsion is surgical exploration, detorsion, and fixation of both the torsed and contralateral testis. A nonviable testis requires orchiectomy and fixation of the contralateral testis. If a child is seen within a few hours of the onset of his torsion, before severe scrotal swelling has ensued, it may be possible to accomplish detorsion of the

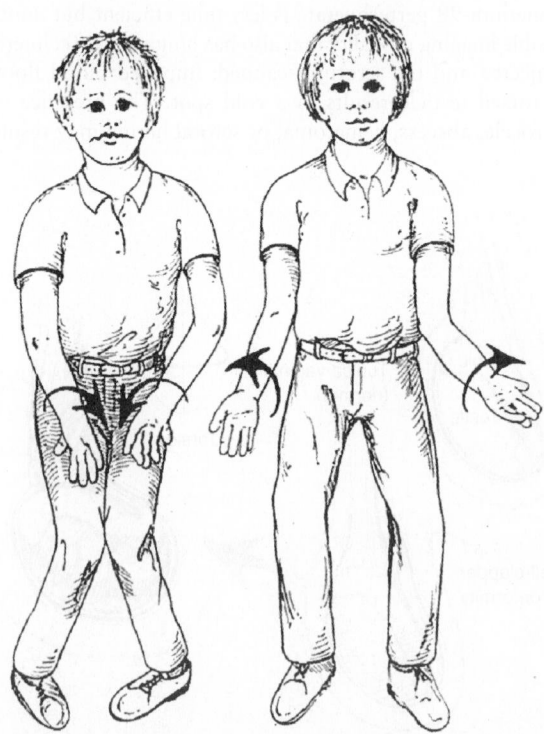

FIGURE 57.4 Torsion of testis. Because torsion typically occurs in a medial direction, manual detorsion should be attempted initially by rotating the testis outward toward the thigh.

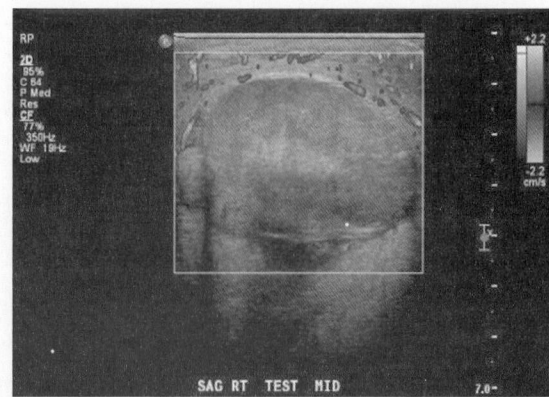

FIGURE 57.5 Torsion of testis (several days old). Ultrasound reveals enlarged testicle and Doppler flow demonstrates no flow to necrotic testis.

spermatic cord manually and thus restore blood supply to the testis. Ideally, this is undertaken by a physician experienced with the technique. The Doppler ultrasound stethoscope provides a noninvasive evaluation of testicular blood flow and is a useful adjunct in manual detorsion of the testis. Initial examination reveals decreased arterial flow to the affected testis, compared with the contralateral one. Intravenous fentanyl (1 to 3 μg per kg) or morphine (0.1 mg per kg) is administered just before attempting detorsion. Because torsion typically (in two-thirds of cases) occurs in a medial direction, detorsion should initially be carried out by rotating the testis outward toward the thigh (Fig. 57.4). Relief of pain and reposition of the testis in a lower position in the scrotum suggests a successful outcome. This can be confirmed with the Doppler stethoscope or color Doppler ultrasound by noting a return of normal arterial pulsations to the testis. Although successful completion of manual detorsion may avoid the necessity of an emergency anesthetic for surgical reduction, it does not remove the necessity for surgical fixation of the testis to prevent the recurrence of this condition. An orchiopexy of the affected testis, as well as of the contralateral one, which is malfixed in more than 50% of cases, is recommended during the same procedure.

Torsion of Testicular Appendage

Several vestigial embryologic remnants are commonly attached to the testis or epididymis that may twist around their base, producing venous engorgement, enlargement, and subsequent infarction. Appendage torsion is most common in boys of ages 7 to 12 years but can occur at any age. Scrotal pain is the usual presenting feature, although the pain is typically less severe and more indolent in onset than the pain associated with testicular torsion. Although there may be associated nausea, vomiting, and diaphoresis, these symptoms are less common than with torsion of the testis (see Chapter 124).

If the child is seen early after the onset of pain, scrotal tenderness and swelling may be localized to the area of the twisted appendage, typically on the superior lateral aspect of the testis. It may be possible to hold the testis gently and have the patient point to the specific point of pain. If this site is indicated to be the upper pole of the testis with the remainder of the testis being nontender, the diagnosis of torsion of a testicular appendage is likely. Although the classic "blue dot" sign of an infarcted appendage may be visible, it often cannot be seen because of overlying edema. In some cases evaluated later in the clinical course, the degree of scrotal tenderness and edema increases to the point at which differentiation from torsion of the testis becomes difficult. In early and late presentations, the cremasteric reflex should be intact. Color Doppler sonography or nuclear scanning demonstrates normal or increased flow to the affected testicle or epididymis compared with the opposite side, representing the inflammation that occurs with torsion of the appendage. Occasionally, surgical exploration may be required to be certain that a torsion of the testis is not present.

If the examiner is confident in the diagnosis of torsion of an appendix testis, surgical exploration is not needed. The child should be sent home with analgesic/antiinflammatory medications, support to the scrotum, and instructions to rest quietly. The pain usually resolves in 2 to 12 days, but in most cases, pain should improve somewhat within a few days. The patient should be reevaluated clinically within 48 hours. In most cases, the child's pain will have lessened, and nothing further is indicated. Occasionally, however, a child will seem to have a disproportionate degree of discomfort from the torsion of these tiny appendages. For these children, removal of the appendage may shorten their morbidity. Contralateral scrotal exploration for this condition is not indicated.

Trauma/Hematocele

In children, most trauma to the scrotum results from a direct blow to the perineum or a straddle injury that forcefully compresses the testicle against the pubic bone. Penetrating injuries are less common, and the small size and greater mobility of the prepubertal testis make testicular injuries rare in this group.

Scrotal trauma includes a spectrum of injuries that ranges from minimal scrotal swelling to rupture of the testis with a tense, blood-filled scrotum (Fig. 57.6A). Urgent surgical

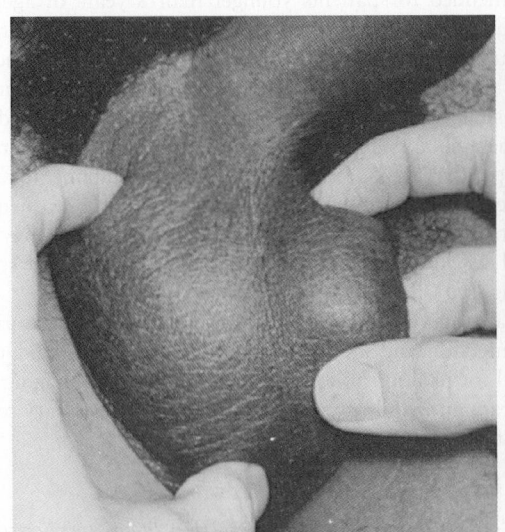
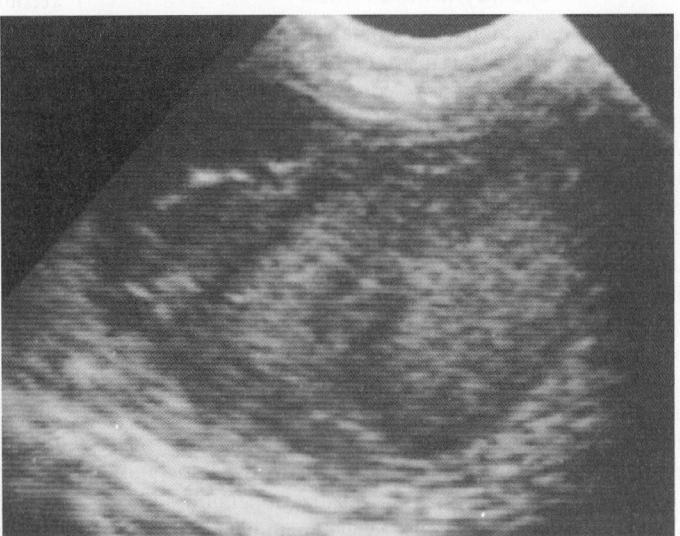

A **B**

FIGURE 57.6 Rupture of testis. **A:** Testicular swelling and tenderness following kick to scrotum. **B:** Ultrasound examination of testis—central linear sonolucent area reflects site of testicular rupture. Surgical repair resulted in a well-preserved gonad.

evaluation should be undertaken, unless the testis clearly can be felt to be normal and without significant tenderness. Often scrotal ultrasound examination is useful (Fig. 57.6B). When any question of testicular rupture remains, surgical exploration is indicated. This approach is based on two facts: (i) a ruptured testis has the best salvage rate when surgically repaired and (ii) testicular torsion may present with a spurious history of trauma (see Chapter 112).

A hematocele, or blood within the tunica vaginalis, may represent severe testicular injury. An obvious ecchymosis of the scrotal wall in the setting of trauma suggests a hematocele. Sonography can identify the fluid collection within the tunica because blood is more echogenic than hydrocele fluid. Scrotal exploration is indicated if testicular rupture is present, or in cases of large hematoceles, which heal more readily after surgical drainage.

Scrotal trauma can also result in an intratesticular hematoma or laceration of the tunica albuginea. Ultrasound can assist in determining the location of blood. Any question or indication of testicular laceration requires surgical exploration and drainage of the hematoma with repair of the laceration. If the tunica albuginea can be determined to be intact, no surgical intervention is necessary.

Traumatic epididymitis is local inflammation, resulting from blunt trauma to the scrotum, which usually occurs within a few days. Typically, short-lived acute pain associated with trauma is followed by a pain-free period after which pain returns. On examination, scrotal erythema, edema, and tenderness of the epididymis may be found. In this noninfectious variety of epididymitis, the urinalysis is negative. Sonography is helpful to rule out any more severe injury and will demonstrate hyperemia associated with the inflammation. Treatment is supportive.

If a scrotal laceration is present, it is essential that the testis and spermatic cord be evaluated for possible injury. This may require an examination under general anesthesia or an inguinal cord block with more severe injuries. For simple scrotal lacerations, careful hemostasis and closure of the laceration with chromic catgut is sufficient.

Epididymitis/Orchitis

Epididymitis is an infection or inflammation of the epididymis, which is most commonly seen in adolescents and adults. In sexually active adolescents, it is commonly associated with *Chlamydia trachomatis*; *Neisseria gonorrhea*, *Escherichia coli*, *Mycobacterium*, and viruses also contribute to cases. In HIV-infected males, *Mycobacterium*, cytomegalovirus, and *Cryptococcus* should also be considered. Epididymitis is seen less frequently in prepubertal boys, in whom it is often associated with a urinary tract infection caused by structural abnormalities of the urinary tract.

The onset of swelling and tenderness is typically more gradual than with torsion of the testis or a testicular appendage. Associated symptoms of urinary frequency, dysuria, penile discharge, or fever may be present. Early on, the epididymis may be selectively enlarged and tender, readily distinguished from the testis. With time, inflammation spreads to the testis and surrounding scrotal wall, making localization impossible. Although elevation of the scrotum relieves pain in epididymoorchitis (Prehn's sign) but causes increased pain in torsion in adults, this finding has not been found to be reliable in children. The cremasteric reflex should be preserved.

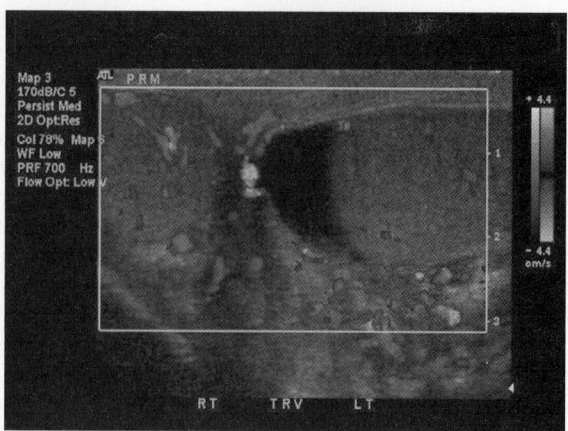

FIGURE 57.7 Epididymitis. Ultrasound image of enlarged epididymis seen on left side of image, testis on right. Color Doppler flow ultrasound reveals increased blood flow to inflamed epididymis.

Although white cells in the urinary sediment are seen more often in epididymitis than in torsion, they are not consistently present. A urinalysis and culture of the urine should always be obtained. The Centers for Disease Control and Prevention recommends a Gram stain and culture of urethral discharge or intraurethral swab, or nucleic acid amplification tests for *N. gonorrhea* and *C. trachomatis* and a urinalysis and culture. Color Doppler sonography typically demonstrates an increase in size and blood flow to the affected testis and epididymis (Fig. 57.7). Nuclear scan shows increased activity in the affected testis. Initial treatment for epididymitis includes antibiotics, analgesics, scrotal support, elevation, and bed rest. In sexually active adolescent males, in whom the most likely cause is chlamydia and gonorrhea, ceftriaxone (250 mg IM in single dose) plus doxycycline (100 mg PO twice a day for 10 days) is recommended. Patients allergic to cephalosporins and/or tetracyclines, or in whom enteric organisms are suspected, can be treated with ofloxacin (300 mg PO twice a day for 10 days) or levofloxacin (500 mg PO once a day for 10 days). Of note, doxycycline is not recommended for patients younger than 8 years of age, and fluoroquinolones are approved for use in patients younger than 18 years of age only for complicated urinary tract infection, unless no other alternatives exist. In prepubertal boys, bacteria responsible for urinary tract infections should be considered. Treatment choices that cover coliforms and attain adequate levels in epididymal tissue include trimethoprim-sulfamethoxazole, cephalexin, or tetracycline. The patient should be warned that this process is frustratingly slow to resolve and that he may have several weeks of gradually subsiding discomfort and scrotal swelling (see Chapter 124).

At any age when epididymitis is associated with a urinary tract infection and in all prepubertal boys with epididymitis, referral for urologic follow-up and urinary tract imaging with sonogram and voiding cystourethrogram are necessary to rule out a structural problem.

Orchitis

Orchitis is an inflammation or infection of the testis resulting from the extension of epididymitis, rarely as hematogenous spread of a systemic bacterial infection, or following certain viral infections, including mumps. Other viruses implicated include adenovirus, Epstein-Barr virus, coxsackievirus, and echoviruses. Although rare before puberty, orchitis occurs in about 18% of postpubertal boys with mumps parotitis. In 70% of cases, it is unilateral. It results in testicular atrophy, but not necessarily sterility, in 50% of affected testes. Fortunately, it is much less common since the advent of vaccine against mumps. The onset of mumps orchitis occurs from 4 to 6 days after parotitis manifests. Although rare, orchitis has been reported in the absence of parotitis. Adrenocorticotropic hormone and corticosteroids in adults may produce some degree of local relief of symptoms, but the course of mumps orchitis is not altered.

Causes of Painless Scrotal Swelling

Hydrocele

An accumulation of fluid within the tunica vaginalis that surrounds the testis—a hydrocele—may be seen with torsion of the testis or an appendage, epididymitis, trauma, or tumor. In these cases, examination of the underlying testis is abnormal. If the testis can be felt to be normal and the hydrocele is not associated with any abnormality of the overlying scrotal soft tissues, it is much more likely to be a simple hydrocele. In the infant, this is the result of fluid being left in place after the processus vaginalis has closed. When the size of the hydrocele has no history of waxing or waning, it is considered a noncommunicating, simple hydrocele, and it may simply be observed. Usually, the fluid will be reabsorbed in the first 12 to 18 months of life.

If the hydrocele has a clear-cut history of changing in size (often with crying or exertion), particularly if it is associated with thickening of the cord structures as they are felt against the pubic tubercle (the silk-glove sign), then the processus vaginalis is patent and the diagnosis is that of a communicating hydrocele (Fig. 57.8). Here the patent processus vaginalis

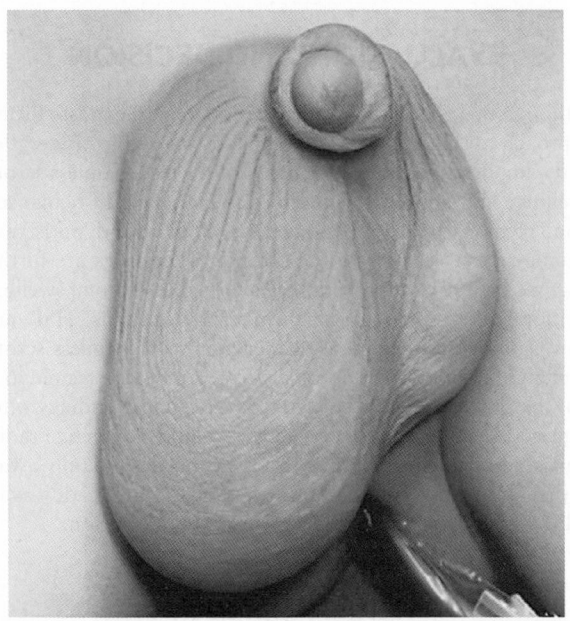

FIGURE 57.8 Hydrocele. Waxing and waning of size indicates a communicating hydrocele with a patent processus vaginalis, requiring surgical correction.

does not generally close spontaneously and may enlarge to permit the development of hernia. Surgical exploration and high ligation of the processus vaginalis with a wide opening of the tunica vaginalis to complete the decompression of the hydrocele is appropriate treatment. Because a scrotal hernia may be confused with a hydrocele, aspiration should never be carried out in children, except by an experienced urologist.

Occasionally, a hydrocele of the cord presents as a scrotal swelling just above the testis. Differentiation from an incarcerated hernia may be difficult and occasionally may require surgical exploration. Ultrasound may also be helpful in determining the nature of the swelling. Surgical treatment like that for a hydrocele of the testis is appropriate.

Hernia

Although most inguinal hernias present in children with a mass in the groin, occasionally the hernia may extend and present as a scrotal swelling. An incarcerated hernia may produce pain in some patients. The diagnosis and treatment of inguinal hernias are discussed in Chapter 121.

Varicocele

A usually painless scrotal swelling, called a *varicocele,* is caused by a collection of abnormally enlarged spermatic cord veins and is most commonly found on routine examination of asymptomatic boys ages 10 to 15 years. Most varicoceles occur on the left, representing spermatic vein incompetence caused by the left spermatic vein draining into the renal vein at a sharp angle, whereas the right spermatic vein drains into the inferior vena cava.

On occasion, a varicocele can present with mild pain or discomfort. The hemiscrotum appears full but does not have overlying skin changes. The testis and epididymis should be palpated to be normal. A mass of varicose veins described as "a bag of worms" can be appreciated above the testicle. Standing examination often reveals the varicocele, which is more prominent when standing. Doppler ultrasound is diagnostic, demonstrating both normal flow to the testis and the collection of tortuous veins. Most varicoceles can be managed conservatively under observation by a urologist. Some large varicoceles may require internal spermatic vein ligation or testicular vein embolization and may have some impact on testicular size and fertility. Most varicoceles are asymptomatic and benign. Inferior vena cava obstruction should be considered when the patient is prepubertal or if the varicocele is acute in onset, right sided, or remains unchanged in the supine position. Patients determined to have a varicocele, especially when they present with discomfort, should be referred for urologic follow-up.

Spermatocele

Located above and posterior to the testicle in postpubertal boys, spermatoceles are sperm-containing cysts of the rete testes, ductuli efferentes, or epididymis. Multiple or bilateral spermatoceles may occur. On examination a small, nontender mass that transilluminates may be appreciated distinct from and posterior to the testicle. These masses must be differentiated from a hydrocele or tumor. Sonography may confirm the location distinct from the testis and help distinguish a spermatocele from tumor. Referral to an urologist is indicated for the excision of large uncomfortable spermatoceles or for aspiration to differentiate a hydrocele from a spermatocele. Otherwise, no specific treatment is needed (see Chapter 124).

Idiopathic Scrotal Edema

Idiopathic scrotal edema is a rare entity that represents only 2% to 5% of acute scrotal swellings in otherwise normal children. Typically, a prepubertal child presents with the rapid onset of painless but notable edema of the scrotal wall that may be bilateral and may extend up onto the abdominal wall. The skin of the scrotum may be erythematous. The child is usually afebrile, and urinalysis is negative. Through the edematous scrotum, the testes can be felt to be normal in size and nontender. This edema of the scrotal wall is of unknown origin, although it is believed to represent a form of angioneurotic edema. Insect bites, allergic reactions, cellulitis, and contact dermatitis can also be contributors to localized scrotal swelling. No specific therapy for idiopathic scrotal edema has been demonstrated to be effective. Bed rest and scrotal elevation may help. Children spontaneously begin to improve within 48 hours, regardless of treatment. Cellulitis, allergic reactions, and contact dermatitis should be appropriately treated. Occasionally, scrotal edema is seen secondary to diseases that cause generalized edema and/or ascites, such as nephrosis and cirrhosis.

Henoch-Schönlein Purpura

Occasionally, a child may be seen with a petechial rash on the scrotum as the initial presentation of this systemic vasculitic syndrome, characterized by nonthrombocytopenic purpura, arthralgia, renal disease, abdominal pain, and gastrointestinal bleeding. More typically, the rash begins on the lower extremities or buttocks and later may involve the scrotum. If the associated swelling is not great, the cord structures and testes can be felt to be uninvolved and normal. In other cases with severe swelling, surgical exploration may be necessary to rule out testicular torsion, which rarely has been noted to coexist. When skin lesions are present, the diagnosis of Henoch-Schönlein purpura (HSP) must be suspected. Occasionally, the acute scrotum is the dominant presenting symptom. Ultrasound may help rule out testicular torsion in these instances. A more detailed discussion of the management of this disease can be found elsewhere in this text (see Chapters 65 and 85).

Kawasaki Disease

Another vasculitis that can produce scrotal swelling and mild pain is Kawasaki disease, which has characteristic features, including fever, adenopathy, rash, conjunctivitis, and irritability. Although discussed in detail elsewhere (see Chapter 101), it is important to note the association of scrotal swelling with this systemic disease to avoid unnecessary surgical explorations or delay in diagnosis of the underlying vasculitis.

Testis Tumor

Testicular or paratesticular tumors are rare in young children. However, in young males of ages 15 to 35 years, it is the most common solid tumor and represents 20% of cancers diagnosed in males. Testicular cancer usually presents as painless, unilateral, and firm to hard scrotal swellings. They may be discovered by the patient or physician on physical examination. Some patients report an achy feeling, and in rapid-growing tumors

associated with hemorrhage or infarction, acute scrotal pain may be reported. Leukemic infiltration of the testis may present bilaterally. The mass does not transilluminate, but an associated reactive hydrocele may do so. In children younger than 2 years of age, the tumor usually is a yolk sac carcinoma, or teratoma. After puberty, germinal cell tumors, as found in the adult population, are seen. Evaluation of a solid testicular mass involves an initial testicular ultrasound examination usually followed by surgical exploration through a groin incision to permit control of the spermatic vessels and a possible radical inguinal orchiectomy.

Antenatal Torsion Testis (Newborn)

A newborn boy may present with a painless, smooth, testicular enlargement that does not transilluminate and is usually dark in color. There should be no or minimal edema of the overlying scrotum. This presentation, in approximately 70% of newborn cases of torsion, usually represents prenatal, extravaginal torsion of the testis (twisting of the entire testis, spermatic cord, and tunica vaginalis), and most commonly occurs during the late period of embryonic development, as the testis descends into the scrotum. At this time, the testicular tunics are not yet attached to the scrotal tissue, and torsion of the entire testis with its tunics can occur. Because fixation of these tissues occurs during the first and second weeks of life, postnatal torsion of a previously normal testis in the neonatal period also occurs, but less frequently (30%). Even though the conventional course of action has been surgical exploration, salvage of the testis believed to have torsed in the prenatal period has been rare; therefore, management remains controversial. It has been argued that the contralateral testis may be malfixed and at risk for subsequent torsion, and therefore, should undergo surgical fixation. Torsion has been reported rarely, however, and current practice is simply to observe these children. After 4 to 6 months, the torsed testis has usually been reabsorbed. Exploration is indicated in the case of rare, bilateral torsion or in newborn boys with suspected postnatal torsion to attempt salvage.

EVALUATION AND DECISION

Although this chapter is entitled scrotal pain, the most efficient approach to the differential diagnosis is through consideration of the important entities causing painful versus painless scrotal swelling. This approach is outlined in Fig. 57.9. Testicular torsion, torsion of an appendage, orchitis, epididymitis, and trauma-related injuries to the scrotum or testicles are further discussed as the common etiologies for painful scrotal swelling. Hemorrhage into a tumor, incarcerated hernias, HSP, and Kawasaki disease may cause either painful or painless scrotal swelling. No one aspect of the history or physical examination may be diagnostic, but collectively the clinical findings often suggest a diagnosis. More recently available adjunctive radiologic studies may be helpful when the clinicians are fully aware of their capabilities and limitations, and they are readily available so as not to delay necessary surgical intervention.

Initial Approach

As a first step in the evaluation of the child with a complaint of scrotal swelling or pain, the physician should determine

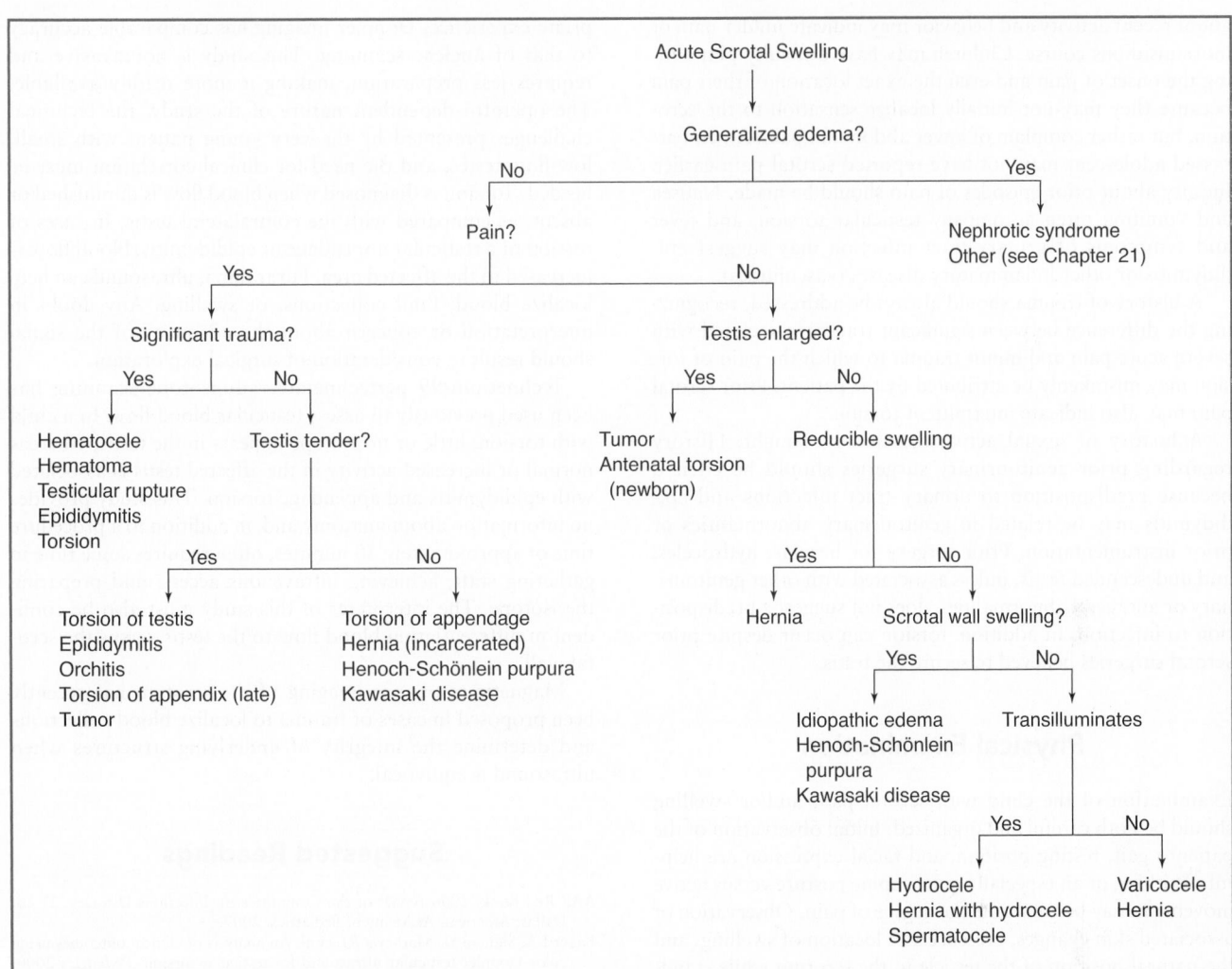

FIGURE 57.9 Diagnostic approach to acute scrotal swelling.

whether the child is suffering from a generalized edematous state, such as the nephrotic syndrome. When the problem is localized to the scrotum, patients can be divided into those who have a painless swelling and those who are experiencing pain.

In the immediate neonatal period, antenatal torsion may cause painless scrotal enlargement. In infancy, the most common causes of painless scrotal swelling (Table 57.2) are hernias and hydroceles; a hernia is often reducible. Beyond infancy, the physician must consider hernia, tumor, spermatocele, and varicocele when evaluating painless scrotal swelling determined to be within the scrotum. Kawasaki disease, HSP, and idiopathic scrotal edema involve the scrotal sac and cause swelling that is either painless or mildly painful.

Painful swelling may follow a well-documented injury, in which case the likely diagnoses are hematocele, hematoma, testicular rupture, and traumatic epididymitis. The physician should bear in mind that boys with testicular torsion often give a history of having had an incidental minor injury. Nontraumatic scrotal pain raises the suspicion of a testicular torsion, if the testis is tender. Unless the diagnosis of a systemic disorder (HSP, Kawasaki disease) is obvious, another structure such as an appendage is reliably determined to be the source of pain within the scrotum, the patient is an adolescent with the classic signs of epididymitis, or an incarcerated hernia is reduced, imaging via Doppler ultrasound or nuclear scan is usually indicated. All patients in whom torsion is suspected, after an initial evaluation by the emergency physician, require a surgical consultation.

History

The age of the child should be considered in evaluating scrotal pain and/or swelling, but overlaps in characteristic age at presentation exist. Testicular torsion occurs in the newborn or early pubertal age range. Torsion of an appendage of the testis, HSP, idiopathic scrotal edema, and Kawasaki disease commonly occur in the prepubertal age group. Epididymitis is more common in adolescents but may occur in prepubertal boys.

Historical features regarding swelling, pain, and associated symptoms should be considered. A history of change in testicular or scrotal size should be determined. If there is pain associated with scrotal swelling, the examiner should determine its onset and severity. Pain is abrupt in onset and severe in testicular torsion, whereas the pain of appendage torsion and epididymitis may be less severe and more gradual. Questions about recent activity and behavior may indicate milder pain or more insidious course. Children may have difficulty pinpointing the onset of pain and even the exact location of their pain because they may not initially localize sensation to the scrotum, but rather complain of lower abdominal pain. An embarrassed adolescent may not have reported scrotal pain earlier. Inquiry about prior episodes of pain should be made. Nausea and vomiting often accompany testicular torsion, and fever and symptoms of urinary tract infection may suggest epididymitis or other inflammatory diseases (vasculitides).

A history of trauma should always be addressed, recognizing the difference between significant trauma associated with severe acute pain and minor trauma to which the pain of torsion may mistakenly be attributed by the patient. Prior scrotal pain may also indicate intermittent torsion.

A history of sexual activity should be sought. History regarding prior genitourinary surgeries should be elicited because predisposition to urinary tract infections and epididymitis may be related to genitourinary abnormalities or prior instrumentation. Prior surgery for hernias, hydroceles, and undescended testis, unless associated with other genitourinary or anorectal abnormalities, does not suggest a predisposition to infection. In addition, torsion can occur despite prior scrotal surgeries believed to secure the testis.

Physical Examination

Examination of the child with scrotal pain and/or swelling should be both careful and organized. Initial observation of the patient's gait, resting position, and facial expression are helpful. Writhing or an especially quiet supine posture versus active movement may best indicate the degree of pain. Observation of associated skin changes, presence and location of swelling, and the natural position of the testicle in the scrotum while standing should then be appreciated. The cremasteric reflex elicited by stroking the upper inner thigh should cause the testicle to elevate when intact. Next, the lower abdomen, inguinal canal, and cord should be palpated. Finally, the scrotum and its contents should be sequentially palpated. Asking the patient to localize his pain with one finger at this time may be especially helpful. The unaffected hemiscrotum should always be palpated first. Knowledge of the location and specific attempt at palpation of the appendix testis and epididymis is beneficial before palpation of the testis itself (Fig. 57.2). Use of a cotton-tipped swab to discretely localize tenderness in these areas may be helpful, and also less threatening to the anxious, uncomfortable patient. Appreciation of swelling, tenderness, and consistency should be noted for all intrascrotal structures. Transillumination may be helpful in some cases (Fig. 57.9).

Imaging Modalities

Color Doppler imaging with pulsed Doppler allows both visualization of scrotal anatomy and intratesticular arterial blood vessel flow determination and comparison. This study can differentiate scrotal wall from testicular blood flow. With appro-priate experience, Doppler imaging has comparable accuracy to that of nuclear scanning. This study is noninvasive and requires less preparation, making it more readily available. The operator-dependent nature of the study, the technical challenges presented by the very young patient with small, low-flow testes, and the need for clinical correlation must be heeded. Torsion is diagnosed when blood flow is diminished or absent, as compared with the contralateral testis. In cases of torsion of a testicular appendage or epididymitis, blood flow is increased to the affected area. For trauma, ultrasound can help localize blood, fluid collections, or swelling. Any doubt in interpretation or concern about the adequacy of the signal should result in consideration of surgical exploration.

Technetium-99 pertechnetate radioisotope scanning has been used previously to assess testicular blood flow. In a child with torsion, little or no isotope appears in the testis, whereas normal or increased activity in the affected testis is associated with epididymitis and appendage torsion. This study provides no information about anatomy and, in addition to a procedure time of approximately 30 minutes, often requires some time in gathering staff, achieving intravenous access, and preparing the isotope. The interpreter of this study must also be confident in differentiating blood flow to the testis versus the scrotal wall.

Magnetic resonance imaging of the scrotum has recently been proposed in cases of trauma to localize blood collections and determine the integrity of underlying structures when ultrasound is equivocal.

Suggested Readings

AAP Red Book. 2006 report of the Committee on Infectious Diseases. 27 ed. Dallas: American Academy of Pediatrics, 2007.

Baker LA, Sigman D, Mathews RI, et al. An analysis of clinical outcomes using color Doppler testicular ultrasound for testicular torsion. *Pediatrics* 2000; 105:604–607.

Buckley JC, McAninch JW. Diagnosis and management of testicular ruptures. *Urol Clin North Am* 2006;33:111–116.

Center for Disease Control and Prevention. Sexually transmitted disease treatment guidelines 2006. *MMWR* 2006;55(RR11):1–94.

Garel L, Dubois J, Azzie G, et al. Preoperative manual detorsion of the spermatic cord with Doppler ultrasound monitoring in patients with intra-vaginal acute testicular torsion. *Pediatr Radiol* 2000;30:41.

Haecker FM, Hauri-Hohl A, von Schweinitz D. Acute epididymitis in children: a 4-year retrospective study. *Eur J Pediatr Surg* 2005;15:180–186.

Jefferson RH, Pérez LM, Joseph DB. Critical analysis of the clinical presentation of acute scrotum: a 9-year experience at a single institution. *J Urol* 1997: 158(3);1198–1200.

Kim SH, Park S, Choi SH, et al. The efficacy of magnetic resonance for the diagnosis of testicular rupture: a prospective preliminary study. *J Trauma* 2009; 66:239–242.

Klin B, Zlotkevich L, Horne T, et al. Epididymitis in childhood: a clinical retrospective study over 5 years. *Isr Med Assoc J* 2001;3:833–835.

Kravchick S, Cytron S, Leibovici O, et al. Color Doppler sonography: its real role in the evaluation of children with highly suspected testicular torsion. *Eur Radiol* 2001;11(6):1000–1005.

Leslie JA, Cain MP. Pediatric urologic emergencies and urgencies. *Pediatr Clin North Am* 2006;53:513–527.

Nussbaum Blask AR, Bulas D, Shalaby-Rana E, et al. Color Doppler sonography and scintigraphy of the testis: prospective, comparative analysis in children with acute scrotal pain. *Pediatr Emerg Care* 2002:18(2):67–71.

Preston MA, Carnat T, Flood T, et al. Conservative management of adolescent varicoceles: a retrospective review. *Urology* 2008;72:77–80.

Richman MN, Bukowski TP. Pediatric epididymitis: pathophysiology, diagnosis and management. *Infect Urol* 2001;14:31–39.

Somekh E, Gorenstein A, Serouf F. Acute epididymitis in boys: evidence of a post-infectious etiology. *J Urol* 2004;171:391–394.

CHAPTER 58 ■ PALLOR

SONAL N. SHAH, MD, MPH

Pallor, or the absence of skin coloration, is a relatively common problem in childhood. Throughout the world, the presence of pallor is often used as a screening tool to identify illness. The development of pallor can be acute and associated with a life-threatening illness, or it can be chronic and subtle, occasionally first noted by someone who sees the child infrequently. The onset of pallor can provoke anxiety for parents who are familiar with descriptions of the presentation of leukemia in childhood. In some instances, only reassurance may be needed, as in the case of a light-complexioned or fair-skinned, nonanemic child. Even if there is a hematologic cause for the pallor, it is often a temporary condition readily amenable to therapy. However, pallor can portend a severe disease, and especially when acute in onset, can herald a true pediatric emergency for which rapid diagnosis and treatment are essential.

The degree of pallor depends on the concentration of hemoglobin in the blood and the distribution of blood in the blood vessels of the skin. Any condition that decreases the concentration of hemoglobin or alters the distribution of blood away from the body's surface may present as pallor. Clinically, pallor caused by anemia can usually be appreciated when the hemoglobin concentration is below 8 to 9 grams per deciliter, although the complexion of the child and the rapidity of onset may influence this value. The hematologic causes for pallor in children are discussed later, and further details regarding their management may be found in Chapter 91. Nonhematologic causes of pallor are outlined briefly in Table 58.1.

DIFFERENTIAL DIAGNOSIS

The differential diagnosis of the major hematologic causes of pallor in children is outlined in Table 58.2. The concentration of hemoglobin in the blood can be lowered by three basic mechanisms: decreased erythrocyte or hemoglobin production, increased erythrocyte destruction, and blood loss. The most common causes of pallor and anemia seen in the emergency department (ED) are iron deficiency and blood loss (Table 58.3), but several less common diseases remain important considerations.

Decreased Production of Hemoglobin and Red Cells

Nutritional Anemias

Nutritional iron deficiency is the most common cause of decreased hemoglobin production in children. A peak in the prevalence of iron deficiency anemia occurs between 12 and 24 months of age, when dietary iron content is often insuffi-cient to meet the demands of a rapidly increasing red cell mass. Premature infants are more susceptible to developing iron deficiency anemia because iron stores at birth are less than those found in term infants, whereas the growth (and therefore, expansion of the red cell mass) of the premature infant is often faster than that of term infants. The early exhaustion of iron stores in premature babies may result in pallor by 6 months of age, whereas in normal infants, signs of iron deficiency anemia are uncommon before 10 to 12 months of age.

A thorough history and physical examination will provide important clues in the diagnosis of iron deficiency anemia. History suggestive of a lack of iron in the diet may be readily apparent or may be recognized only after careful questioning, particularly regarding the daily consumption of cow's milk. The infant with severe iron deficiency is usually irritable and very pale. A compensatory increase in cardiac output is seen, which, when coupled with conditions that increase systemic demands on the heart (such as fever), may provoke the development of congestive heart failure (see Chapter 82).

Serum hemoglobin concentration may be as low as 2 grams per deciliter in severe iron deficiency anemia. Red blood cells are markedly microcytic and hypochromic. Variation in red cell size and shape is usually present, and elongated, pencil-like cells are particularly common. Although the percentage of reticulocytes may be elevated moderately, the absolute reticulocyte count is low.

As the diagnosis of iron deficiency as the cause for an anemia can often be made on the basis of the history alone, treatment is usually instituted before confirmatory laboratory studies are available. Free erythrocyte protoporphyrin, the protein species to which iron is chelated to form mature hemoglobin, is increased in iron deficiency anemia and readily assayed. Thus, this test is particularly useful in the evaluation of the severely anemic child. Measurements of serum iron and ferritin levels have too long of a turnaround time to be of much value in the emergency management of anemia, but are valuable confirmatory tests.

Other nutritional anemias, such as vitamin B_{12} or folic acid deficiency, are uncommon in children in the United States. When present, these anemias are likely associated with particular conditions such as a grossly altered diet, extended hyperalimentation, intestinal resection, or chronic diarrhea. Affected infants usually present with failure to thrive and developmental delay. Older patients more commonly exhibit weight loss, constipation, and weakness. The diagnosis of vitamin B_{12} or folic acid deficiency may be suggested by the finding of anemia with megaloblastic features. Megaloblastic anemia is characterized by normochromic, macrocytic red blood cells, hypersegmented neutrophils, and an elevated serum level of lactic dehydrogenase. Unusual inborn alterations of B_{12} and

TABLE 58.1

PALLOR WITHOUT ANEMIA

Physiologic ("fair-skinned")
Shock: septic, hypovolemic, neurogenic, cardiogenic, anaphylactoid
Hypoglycemia and other metabolic derangements
Respiratory distress
Skin edema
Pheochromocytoma

folic acid absorption and metabolism may cause symptoms similar to those of the nutritional megaloblastic anemias. Megaloblastic anemia is rarely severe enough to be life-threatening. The diagnosis is confirmed by the finding of low serum levels of folic acid or vitamin B_{12} and the response to folic acid or vitamin B_{12} replacement therapy.

Hypoplastic and Aplastic Anemia

Pallor is usually the first sign of aplastic or hypoplastic anemia. These anemias may be congenital or acquired. Congenital aplastic anemias are most commonly part of larger syndromes, with the two major syndromes recognized being Diamond-Blackfan and Fanconi's anemia.

Diamond-Blackfan syndrome is a congenital hypoplastic anemia commonly detected in the first few months of life. The anemia can be severe at the time of diagnosis. The red cells are normocytic or macrocytic. The reticulocyte count is character-

TABLE 58.3

RELATIVELY COMMON CAUSES OF PALLOR OR ANEMIA

Decreased Erythrocyte or Hemoglobin Production
Iron deficiency
Transient erythroblastopenia of childhood

Increased Erythrocyte Destruction
Sickle cell syndromes
Autoimmune hemolytic anemia
G6PD deficiency

Blood Loss

G6PD, glucose-6-phosphate dehydrogenase.

istically low with a leucopenia noted in approximately 10% of affected patients. Thrombocytopenia occurs only rarely. Associated congenital anomalies include microcephaly, cleft palate, web neck, and thumb irregularites. The diagnosis is made by examination of a bone marrow aspirate evidencing markedly reduced or absent erythrocyte precursors with normal marrow cellularity.

Fanconi's anemia is an autosomal recessive condition that results in progressive bone marrow failure generally after age 3 or 4 years. Fanconi's anemia is characterized by a normochromic or macrocytic anemia as well as reductions in both white cell and platelet counts, in contradistinction to Diamond-Blackfan syndrome. Other phenotypic abnormalities

TABLE 58.2

PALLOR WITH ANEMIA

I. Decreased Erythrocyte or Hemoglobin Production
  A. Nutritional deficiencies
    1. Iron deficiency
    2. Folic acid and vitamin B_{12} deficiency or associated metabolic abnormalities
  B. Aplastic or hypoplastic anemias
    1. Diamond-Blackfan anemia
    2. Fanconi's anemia
    3. Aplastic anemia[a]
    4. Transient erythroblastopenia of childhood
    5. Malignancy: leukemia, lymphoma, neuroblastoma[a]
  C. Abnormal heme and hemoglobin synthesis
    1. Anemia of chronic disease
    2. Lead poisoning[a]
    3. Sideroblastic anemias
    4. Thalassemias
II. Increased Erythrocyte Destruction
  A. Erythrocyte membrane defects: hereditary spherocytosis, elliptocytosis, stomatocytosis, pyknocytosis, paroxysmal nocturnal hemoglobinuria
  B. Erythrocyte enzyme defects
    1. Defects of hexose monophosphate shunt: G6PD deficiency most common
    2. Defects of Embden-Meyerhof pathway: pyruvate kinase deficiency most common

  C. Hemoglobinopathies
    1. Sickle cell syndromes[a]
    2. Unstable hemoglobins
  D. Immune hemolytic anemia
    1. Autoimmune hemolytic anemia[a]
    2. Isoimmune hemolytic anemia[a]
    3. Infection
      a. Viral: mononucleosis, influenzas, coxsackievirus, measles, varicella, cytomegalovirus
      b. Bacterial: *Escherichia coli, Pneumococcus, Streptococcus,* typhoid fever, *Mycoplasma*
    4. Drugs: antibiotics
    5. Inflammatory and collagen vascular disease
    6. Malignancy[a]
  E. Microangiopathic anemias
    1. Disseminated intravascular coagulation[a]
    2. Hemolytic uremic syndrome[a]
    3. Cavernous hemangioma
III. Blood Loss
  A. Severe trauma[a]
  B. Anatomic lesions
    1. Meckel's diverticulum
    2. Peptic ulcer
    3. Idiopathic pulmonary hemosiderosis[a]

G6PD, glucose-6-phosphate dehydrogenase.
[a]Conditions that are known to present with acute, life-threatening anemia or are associated with other serious abnormalities.

associated with Fanconi's anemia include hyperpigmentation or hypopigmentation, microcephaly, strabismus, small stature, mental retardation, and anomalies of the thumbs and radii. The diagnosis may be made in the proper clinical context by the presence of increased chromosomal breakage in lymphocytes cultured in the presence of DNA cross-linking agents.

Acquired aplastic anemia can also present with severe pallor in children. The anemia is usually associated with granulocytopenia and thrombocytopenia. Acquired aplastic anemia is often idiopathic but has been associated with exposure to certain drugs and chemicals (e.g., chloramphenicol, felbamate, lindane, gold, benzene, pesticides), radiation, and viral infections (especially hepatitis). The diagnosis is made by an examination of the bone marrow.

Transient erythroblastopenia of childhood (TEC) is a condition that is often associated with a recent viral illness and is characterized by moderate to severe anemia caused by diminished red cell production. The age at presentation can vary from infancy to 10 years, with a median of 18 to 26 months. The mean corpuscular volume (MCV) is usually normal at the time of diagnosis. The reticulocyte count is decreased, and a Coombs test is negative. The anemia of TEC may be associated with a normal or moderately decreased white cell count and a normal platelet count. Bone marrow examination shows an initial reduction or absence of erythrocytic precursors followed by erythroid hyperplasia during recovery. Transient erythroblastopenia that occurs in the first 6 months of life may be difficult to distinguish from Diamond-Blackfan anemia. Spontaneous recovery ultimately confirms the diagnosis of TEC.

Hypoplastic anemia can be the presenting symptom of childhood malignancies. The pallor can be severe, and although all three cell lines of the bone marrow are usually affected, anemia may be the only notable hematologic abnormality. The diagnosis can be suspected from the presence of other symptoms or findings, such as lymphadenopathy, bruising, limb pain, gum bleeding, or an abdominal mass.

Red cell aplasia may develop in patients with underlying hemolytic anemias such as hereditary spherocytosis or sickle cell (SC) disease, usually in association with parvovirus B19 infection. Decreased red cell production in the face of ongoing hemolysis causes an exacerbation of the anemia. The elevated reticulocyte count usually seen in hereditary hemolytic anemias falls to inappropriately low levels, often less than 1%. Although platelets and white cells are generally unaffected, they may be mildly decreased. Red cell transfusions are appropriate if the anemia is associated with cardiovascular compromise or if continuing reticulocytopenia indicates that the anemia is likely to become severe before the usual spontaneous recovery after 3 to 7 days. Patients with decreased erythrocyte production from a condition such as iron deficiency anemia or human immunodeficiency virus (HIV) infection may also experience a transient aplastic crisis from parvovirus B19 infection. Hematologically normal children with underlying (though sometimes unrecognized) immunologic disorders may also develop parvovirus-induced anemia as a result of prolonged viremia.

Disorders of Heme and Globin Production

Pallor may be the presenting sign of nonnutritional disorders of hemoglobin synthesis, including the sideroblastic anemias and thalassemia syndromes. These disorders are characterized by a microcytic, hypochromic anemia. Sideroblastic anemia may be inherited (sex linked) or acquired such as in cases of alcohol, chloramphenicol, or isoniazid exposure, copper deficiency, and zinc toxicity. Although the etiology can be diverse, the inciting factors share a final common pathway, which is a defect in the synthesis of heme in the red cell precursor. As a result, iron use within the developing red cell is abnormal, accounting for the presence of diagnostic ringed sideroblasts in the bone marrow. The serum iron and ferritin levels are often markedly elevated.

In the thalassemias, production of the globin portion of the hemoglobin molecule is impaired because of genetic defects in heme chain synthesis. The anemia is hypochromic and microcytic with an elevated reticulocyte count. Cooley's anemia (β-thalassemia major) presents with severe pallor usually between 6 and 12 months of age, as fetal hemoglobin levels decline and the normal rise in adult hemoglobin (HbA) levels is compromised by a reduced or absent β-globin production. The anemia is the result of a unique combination of decreased hemoglobin synthesis and, as a result of imbalanced α and β globin chain production, accelerated red cell destruction. Consequently, erythropoietic hyperplasia of the bone marrow and extramedullary hematopoiesis occur. In severe β-thalassemia major, extramedullary hematopoiesis within craniofacial bones leads to a spectrum of characteristic facial features including prominence of frontal and parietal bones, depression of the nasal bridge, and protrusion of the upper teeth, resulting in so-called "chipmunk facies." Bone marrow hyperplasia results in thinning of the cortex, widening of the medullary spaces, and osteoporosis. There is delayed skeletal maturation. This constellation of characteristic facies, bony abnormalities, presence of hepatosplenomegaly and characteristic red cell morphology, including marked variation in red cell shape, usually makes this diagnosis readily apparent. Although β-thalassemia is often associated with Mediterranean ancestry, this disease and other thalassemias (e.g., E-β thalassemia, HbH disease) are also seen commonly in children of Southeast Asian, Indian, Pakistani, Arab, and Chinese ethnicity.

Lead poisoning affects heme synthesis, but significant anemia is unusual unless blood lead levels are markedly elevated. Iron deficiency is common in children with increased lead levels and usually accounts for the microcytic anemia found in these patients. If a concomitant hematologic disorder cannot be found in the anemic patient with plumbism, particular care should be given to the possibility of severe lead intoxication.

Systemic Disease

Numerous disorders that are not primarily hematologic may be associated with pallor and anemia due to decreased production of hemoglobin or red cells. Occasionally, pallor is the only presenting finding of a serious systemic disorder. Chronic inflammatory diseases, such as juvenile idiopathic arthritis (JIA) and ulcerative colitis, are often accompanied by a normocytic or microcytic anemia related to impaired iron utilization by hematopoetic cells. The serum iron is reduced; however, low iron-binding capacity distinguishes this anemia of chronic inflammation from the anemia of iron deficiency. Similar clinical and laboratory findings may be associated with chronic infections such as HIV and subacute bacterial endocarditis. Other diseases in which anemia may be a prominent component include chronic renal disease, hyperthyroidism, and hypothyroidism. The anemia in these disorders is not severe enough to be considered a hematologic emergency unless complicated by other hematologic abnormalities. However, anemia may be the first clue to an underlying disease in which early treatment may improve the outcome substantially.

Increased Red Cell Destruction

The numerous conditions associated with shortened red cell survival can be congenital, as in the case of the hemoglobinopathies and membrane and enzyme defects. Acquired causes of shortened red cell survival include autoimmune hemolytic anemia, drug-associated hemolytic anemias, disseminated intravascular coagulation (DIC), and hemolytic–uremic syndrome (HUS). The hemoglobin levels in these disorders can be normal, slightly depressed, or so low as to be life-threatening. The steady state hemoglobin concentration is determined by a balance between the severity of the defect and the bone marrow's ability to respond to the presence of a shortened red cell survival. Compensation is achieved by an increase in erythrocyte production as is evident from the elevated reticulocyte count that is usually found in these conditions.

When the child with increased red cell destruction cannot compensate and make more red blood cells, this may result in a severe, life-threatening exacerbation of the underlying anemia (e.g., as is the case with acquired red cell aplasia from parvovirus B12 as discussed above). An aplastic crisis should be suspected in a patient with a known hemolytic anemia who develops increasing pallor and anemia associated with a reticulocyte count depressed in relation to its normally elevated baseline. The differential diagnosis of these underlying hemolytic conditions that result in red cell destruction is presented below.

Membrane Disorders

The degree of pallor associated with anemia caused by erythrocyte membrane abnormalities depends on the hemoglobin level. Hereditary spherocytosis, the most common of the membrane disorders, is usually characterized by well-compensated chronic hemolysis, which becomes clinically apparent only when the hemolysis is exacerbated by intercurrent infection. In rare instances, patients with hereditary spherocytosis may develop significant anemia, jaundice, and pallor in the newborn period. Moderate or severe anemia is less common in the other membrane disorders, such as hereditary elliptocytosis and hereditary stomatocytosis. The anemia of the erythrocyte membrane disorders is accompanied by reticulocytosis. A direct antiglobulin (Coombs) test will be negative. Red cell morphology usually permits the diagnosis to be made from the peripheral smear. Because these disorders are often inherited in an autosomal dominant fashion, a family history of anemia, splenomegaly, splenectomy, or cholecystectomy may be helpful. However, a particularly severe form of spherocytosis occurs as an autosomal recessive disorder, and even some children with more typical disease lack an informative family history. Consequently, the diagnosis should not be dismissed in the absence of other affected family members.

Infantile pyknocytosis is a hemolytic anemia seen during the first few months of life and is characterized by distorted and contracted erythrocytes and burr cells. The disorder may be associated with pallor and hyperbilirubinemia. Spontaneous recovery usually occurs by 6 months of age.

Enzyme Disorders

Erythrocyte enzymatic defects, such as pyruvate kinase deficiency and certain variants of glucose-6-phosphate dehydrogenase (G6PD) deficiency, may be associated with pallor due to increased red blood cell destruction. G6PD deficiency is the most common human enzyme defect, with predominance in people of Middle Eastern, South Asian, and African descent. This regional distribution is likely explained by the protection G6PD deficiency confers against malaria. In G6PD deficiency, pallor may be accentuated by acute hemolytic crises after exposure to oxidant stress (e.g., naphthalene-containing mothballs, antimalarials, sulfonamides, aspirin, methylene blue, or acidosis). Although alterations in red cell morphology are sometimes found in these enzyme disorders, assays of specific enzymes or substrates are required for definitive diagnosis.

Hemoglobinopathies

Pallor may result from the low hemoglobin level found in patients with sickle cell anemia and related hemoglobinopathies. Acute accentuation of pallor can result from an aplastic crisis, a complication of hemolytic disorders that is particularly common in sickle cell anemia. During an aplastic crisis, the normally elevated reticulocyte count may fall to zero, and the hemoglobin level may fall as low as 1 to 2 grams per deciliter, resulting in severe pallor and signs of high-output cardiac failure.

The sequestration crisis of sickle cell anemia (HbSS) and related hemoglobin disorders (SC disease, S-β^0 thalassemia, S-β^+ thalassemia) is a true hematologic emergency. The presence of increased pallor and acute enlargement of the spleen in a patient with a sickling disorder should prompt immediate investigation of possible sequestration crisis. The condition results from pooling of red cells and plasma in the spleen resulting in sudden and severe anemia with associated hypovolemia. Emergent intervention is warranted as untreated cases may rapidly lead to death. Although this complication rarely occurs in children with homozygous sickle cell disease or S-β^0 thalassemia after the age of 5 years, sequestration crises may occur much later in children with sickling disorders such as SC disease or S-β^+ thalassemia, in which early splenic infarction is less common.

Immune Hemolytic Anemia

Pallor caused by autoimmune hemolytic anemia is usually acute in onset and may be associated with severe anemia. Symptoms include jaundice, dark urine, splenomegaly, and cardiovascular derangement. The presence of only moderate anemia (6 to 8 grams per deciliter) at diagnosis should not detract from consideration of this disease as a hematologic emergency because brisk hemolysis may result in a sudden, additional fall in hemoglobin level. Autoimmune hemolytic anemia is usually, but not always, characterized by a positive direct antiglobulin (Coombs) test and an increased reticulocyte count. Spherocytes are commonly seen in the peripheral smear. Other causes of immune hemolytic anemia include infections, drug exposure, inflammatory diseases, and malignancies.

Microangiopathic Anemia

Alterations in the normal laminar flow of blood through the vascular system may cause increased red cell destruction. In DIC, abnormal fibrin deposition within small blood vessels results in mechanical injury to the erythrocytes. Thrombocytopenia and clotting abnormalities, which often herald the onset of DIC, may also contribute to the anemia via blood loss. The main diagnostic findings are red cell fragments in the peripheral blood smear, platelet and clotting abnormalities typical of a consumptive coagulopathy (see Chapter 91), and the clinical features of an underlying entity such as septic shock or extensive trauma, with which DIC is associated.

The increased red cell destruction in HUS and thrombotic thrombocytopenic purpura (TTP) is also caused by intravascular fibrin deposition. Thrombocytopenia and uremia may lower the hemoglobin concentration even further via blood loss, impaired red cell production, shortened red cell survival, and increased plasma volume. In some instances, anemia may be severe despite only mild uremia and absent thrombocytopenia, leaving doubt about the correct diagnosis. In more typical cases, however, the diagnosis is readily apparent from the findings of oliguria, central nervous system abnormalities, increased blood urea nitrogen, thrombocytopenia, and abnormalities of red cell morphology on peripheral blood smear, including fragments and helmet cells.

Another form of microangiopathic anemia involves the proliferation of blood vessels within a cavernous hemangioma that may trap red cells or initiate a localized consumptive coagulopathy, causing erythrocyte destruction. Anemia in these cases is rarely severe unless the thrombocytopenia, which is more typical of the disorder, causes chronic blood loss.

Blood Loss

Although sudden, massive hemorrhage is usually accompanied by signs of hypovolemic shock, the repeated loss of smaller amounts of blood may be associated with few findings other than pallor. The finding of iron deficiency anemia despite normal dietary iron intake or iron supplementation may be a clue to the presence of chronic blood loss from the gastrointestinal (GI) tract or within the lungs.

EVALUATION AND DECISION

The initial assessment of the child with pallor should include an immediate determination of the degree of illness. Rapid treatment may be imperative for the severely ill child. In the presence of hypovolemic shock, immediate support of vascular volume is required. When high-output cardiac failure from severe anemia occurs, transfusion with small aliquots of packed red cells is necessary. Only after these initial therapeutic efforts have been completed can a thorough evaluation of the anemia proceed.

If the child with pallor is not acutely ill, a deliberate search for the cause of pallor should be undertaken (Fig. 58.1). This may be accomplished by obtaining a thorough yet focused history, performing a detailed physical examination, and ordering appropriate laboratory investigations. The history should focus on several major components. First, particular attention should be paid to the time of onset of pallor. The slow development of pallor suggests diminished red cell production, as is found in bone marrow aplasia or iron deficiency. However, the acute onset of pallor is consistent with the brisk hemolysis of autoimmune hemolytic anemia or the splenic sequestration of sickle cell disease.

After establishing the time course of the anemia, the history can be directed toward more narrow categories of anemia or specific diseases. A detailed dietary history, with particular attention to milk intake, is important in young children with suspected iron deficiency as excessive consumption of cow's milk often results in iron deficiency. Vitamin B_{12} deficiency may accompany strict vegetarian diets from which meat and egg products are excluded and may occur in breast-fed infants of vegetarian mothers or mothers with pernicious anemia. Nutritional folic acid deficiency is rare and can usually be readily deduced from the presence of severe dietary alterations and evidence of other vitamin deficiencies.

The family history helps in the diagnosis of hemoglobinopathies and inherited disorders of red cell membranes and enzymes. Because results of previous hemoglobin testing may have been explained inadequately or recalled inaccurately, a negative family history or newborn screening for hemoglobinopathies should not preclude evaluation of the patient's hemoglobin phenotype if a sickling disorder is suspected. The presence of a microcytic anemia unresponsive to iron in the parents suggests a thalassemic disorder. A history of splenomegaly, splenectomy, or cholecystectomy in family members may help identify a hemolytic disorder such as hereditary spherocytosis or pyruvate kinase deficiency.

Finally, a well-directed review of systems is essential in looking for systemic disorders such as chronic renal disease, hypothyroidism, or JIA. Pallor may be the presenting complaint in these and other disorders.

In the examination of the anemic patient, pulse and blood pressure (BP) should be measured to be sure hypovolemic shock and high-output cardiac failure are neither present nor imminent. If anemia or volume loss is mild, tachycardia may be present with a preserved BP. A systolic flow murmur is often heard if the hemoglobin level is below 8 grams per deciliter. In the severely anemic patient, pallor of the skin and mucous membranes is usually readily apparent. When anemia is less severe or when the skin color is dark, pallor may be appreciated only in the nail beds, palmar surfaces and palpebral conjunctivae. Lymphadenopathy and splenomegaly may suggest a malignancy or an infectious disease such as mononucleosis. When splenomegaly occurs without lymphadenopathy, however, attention is drawn to hemolytic disorders such as hereditary spherocytosis and autoimmune hemolytic anemia or hemoglobinopathies (e.g., sickling disorders or thalassemia major). Scleral icterus may also be present in these disorders of shortened red cell survival. The finding of an unusually large and firm spleen in the absence of increasing scleral icterus suggests that red cells are being sequestered (e.g., splenic sequestration crisis of sickle cell disease, hypersplenism).

The skin in a patient with pallor should be examined for evidence of underlying disorders. The presence of hemangiomas might suggest microangiopathic anemia. If increased bruising or bleeding accompanies pallor, multiple blood elements are probably affected. The circulation time of platelets is short in comparison with that of red cells. Therefore, clinical findings of thrombocytopenia are often present by the time pallor develops in patients with acquired aplastic anemia, Fanconi's anemia, and acute leukemia. Clinical evidence of thrombocytopenia may also suggest microangiopathic anemia as described earlier. Careful auscultation of the abdomen and head may detect unseen hemangiomas. Sources of internal or external blood

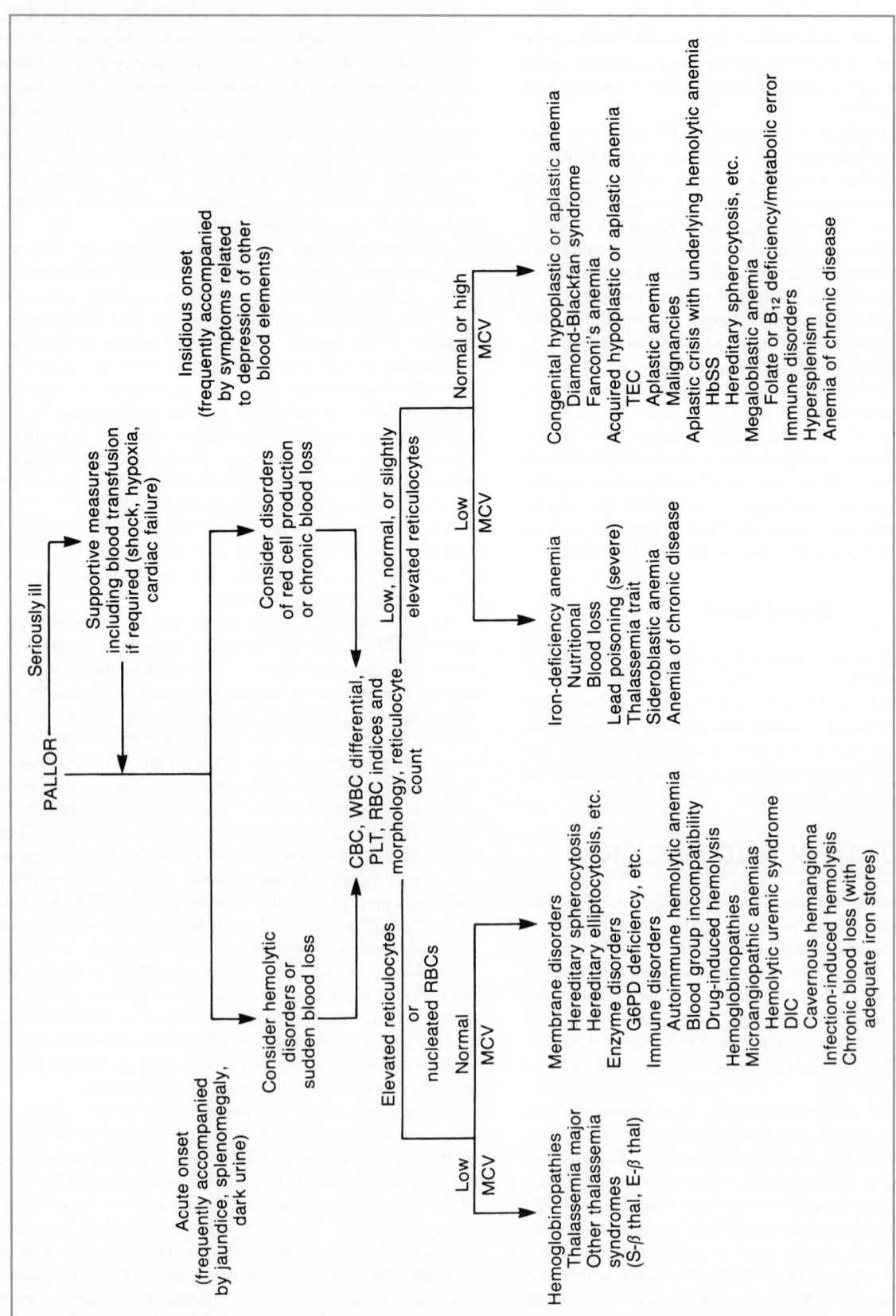

FIGURE 58.1 The diagnostic approach to pallor. CBC, complete blood cell; WBC, white blood cell; PLT, platelet; RBC, red blood cell; MCV, mean corpuscular volume; G6PD, glucose-6-phosphate dehydrogenase; DIC, disseminated intravascular coagulation; TEC, transient erythroblastopenia of childhood; HbSS, sickle cell anemia.

loss should be carefully sought. Chronic GI bleeding may escape detection until iron deficiency anemia develops. Similarly, small pulmonary hemorrhages associated with idiopathic pulmonary hemosiderosis are often mistaken for other pulmonic processes until several recurrences of iron deficiency anemia suggest a hidden site of blood loss. Bony abnormalities associated with red cell disorders include frontal bossing from compensatory expansion of the bone marrow in hemolytic diseases and radial and thumb anomalies found in some patients with Fanconi's anemia.

Numerous classifications of anemia have been used to assist the physician in the laboratory investigation of pallor. Historically, the reticulocyte count and the MCV have been helpful measurements in categorizing causes of anemia. The reticulocyte count can be performed rapidly and, as shown in Fig. 58.1, distinguishes anemias caused by impaired red cell production (e.g., iron deficiency, hypoplastic anemia) from those caused by shortened red cell survival (e.g., hemoglobinopathies, membrane disorders). The MCV provides a quick, accurate, and readily available method of distinguishing the microcytic anemias (iron deficiency, thalassemia syndromes) from the normocytic (membrane disorders, enzyme deficiencies, autoimmune hemolytic anemia, most hemoglobinopathies) or macrocytic (bone marrow/stem cell failure, disorders of B$_{12}$ and folic acid absorption or metabolism) anemias.

The reticulocyte count and MCV should be interpreted with caution. As shown in Fig. 58.1, disorders of shortened red cell survival are not always characterized by an increased reticulocyte count. For example, reticulocytopenia may occur in autoimmune hemolytic anemia, despite active hemolysis and increased erythropoiesis in the bone marrow. Chronic hemolytic disorders, such as sickle cell anemia or hereditary spherocytosis, may first be detected during an aplastic crisis when the reticulocyte count is low. Unless the underlying disorder is recognized, the physician may be misled by this finding. Furthermore, because the reticulocyte count is expressed as a percentage of total red cells, it must be indexed for the degree of anemia. The easiest way to calculate the reticulocyte index is to multiply the reticulocyte count by the reported hemoglobin or hematocrit [HCT pt (patient)] divided by normal hemoglobin or hematocrit [HCT nl (normal)]:

$$\text{Reticulocyte index} = \text{Reticulocyte count} \times \frac{\text{HCT (pt)}}{\text{HCT (nl)}}$$

For example, a reticulocyte count of 5% in a child with severe iron deficiency anemia and a hematocrit of 6% is not elevated when corrected for the degree of anemia ($5\% \times 6\%/33\% = 0.9\%$). The normal reticulocyte index is between 1.0 and 2.0.

The MCV varies with age, necessitating the use of age-adjusted normal values (Table 58.4). In addition, the measured MCV represents an average value. If microcytic and macrocytic red cells are present in the peripheral blood as, for example, in a patient with combined iron deficiency and B$_{12}$ deficiency, the MCV may remain normal. Therefore, the peripheral smear should be examined carefully to determine whether the MCV reflects a single population of red cells of uniform size, or two or more populations of distinctly different size. The red cell distribution width is elevated in the presence of increased variation in red cell size.

As shown in Fig. 58.1, the reticulocyte count and MCV help in the initial classification of anemia but leave the physi-

TABLE 58.4

AGE-RELATED VALUES FOR MEAN CORPUSCULAR VOLUME

Age (yr)	MCV (fL)	
	Median	Lower limit[a]
0.5–2	77	70
2–5	79	73
5–9	81	75
9–12	83	76
12–14:		
Female	85	77
Male	84	76
14–18:		
Female	87	78
Male	86	77

fL, femtoliters.
[a]Third percentile.

cian with broad categories of disease, rather than specific diagnoses. In many instances, the history and physical examination, when coupled with these laboratory measurements, permit identification of a particular disorder. Additional laboratory studies and careful examination of the peripheral smear may be required, however, and can be performed readily when the patient is in the ED. The application of these procedures to diseases that are commonly encountered or that are associated with unusually severe anemia is discussed next.

Increased Reticulocytes and Low Mean Corpuscular Volume

The thalassemia syndromes associated with moderate or severe anemia can be recognized by the distinctive abnormalities of red cell morphology. In Cooley's anemia (β-thalassemia major), the red cells are generally small but vary markedly in size and shape. Many cells appear to contain little or no hemoglobin; the central pallor of the red cell by light microscopy extends to the cell membrane. Nucleated red cells, basophilic stippling, and polychromasia reflect active erythropoiesis. The parents of an affected child usually have a low MCV characteristic of thalassemia trait.

Children with HbS-β-thalassemia often have microcytic red cells, although the alterations of red cell morphology are not as dramatic as in Cooley's anemia. Sickled forms are often but not always present. Target cells are common. The solubility tests are positive because of the presence of HbS. Hemoglobin electrophoresis reveals HbS (single sickle allele) and reduced (less than 50%) or absent HbA (normal adult hemoglobin).

Increased Reticulocytes and Normal Mean Corpuscular Volume

Most membrane disorders can be readily identified by the characteristic changes in red cell shape that lend their names to the diseases (e.g., spherocytosis, elliptocytosis, stomatocytosis).

When the diagnosis of a membrane disorder is uncertain, examination of the parents' peripheral smears may be helpful because, in many cases, the inheritance pattern is autosomal dominant.

Abnormalities of red cell morphology are less striking in erythrocyte enzymatic defects. Blister cells and cells with asymmetric distribution of hemoglobin may be found, however, during episodes of active hemolysis in G6PD deficiency. If transfusion is necessary, a pretransfusion sample should be saved for assay of specific enzymes.

The reticulocyte count is usually markedly elevated in autoimmune hemolytic anemia but may be normal or only slightly elevated during the first days of the disease. In rare instances, reticulocytopenia persists. Spherocytes are usually present on the peripheral smear. Clumping of red cells from agglutination may be seen. This agglutination sometimes causes a falsely elevated MCV because the electronic counter measures the volume of red cell couplets or triplets. The direct antiglobulin test is positive in 90% of cases. Patients with a negative direct antiglobulin test present a challenging diagnostic problem because the initial findings may be similar to those in hereditary spherocytosis.

The recognition of homozygous sickle cell disease (HbSS) is usually accomplished by the finding of sickled red cells on the peripheral smear. Rarely, however, such cells are absent, even during an acute illness. Target cells are commonly found in sickle cell disease but are more prominent in HbSC. Solubility tests are positive. Hemoglobin electrophoresis reveals the presence of the abnormal hemoglobin(s) and the absence of HbA. This confirmatory test takes less than 30 minutes to complete and should be performed when important therapeutic decisions depend on the result.

Red cell fragments are found in those diseases characterized by microangiopathic anemia. In HUS or TTP, thrombocytopenia is present, renal or neurologic function is usually impaired, and thrombotic complications may be present. The platelet count is also low in DIC, and clotting studies are abnormal. If intravascular hemolysis is severe, as in anemia associated with certain artificial cardiac valves, hemosiderin may be detected in the urinary sediment.

Low, Normal, or Slightly Elevated Reticulocytes and Low Mean Corpuscular Volume

In severe iron deficiency anemia, red cells are markedly microcytic and hypochromic and show substantial variation in size and shape. Elongated red cells (pencil forms) are common. Platelet count is often increased but may occasionally be decreased. As discussed previously, the erythrocyte protoporphyrin concentration is usually increased in iron deficiency, although values are lower than those found in severe lead poisoning.

Anemia is uncommon in lead poisoning but, when present, resembles the anemia of iron deficiency in its red cell morphology. Basophilic stippling is found in a small percentage of cases. The erythrocyte protoporphyrin is markedly elevated, and the rapid measurement of this compound helps the physician in the ED to distinguish severe lead poisoning, which

requires hospitalization and intensive chelation, from iron deficiency, which usually can be treated on an outpatient basis.

Low, Normal, or Slightly Elevated Reticulocytes and Normal or Elevated Mean Corpuscular Volume

With the exception of mild macrocytosis, red cell morphology is usually normal in childhood disorders of bone marrow or stem cell failure. Thrombocytopenia and neutropenia are present in aplastic anemia and Fanconi's anemia. Although the platelet count and white count occasionally may be low in patients with Diamond-Blackfan syndrome, the red cells are most severely affected. Erythropoiesis is most severely affected in TEC and acquired pure red cell aplasia, although neutropenia may accompany the former disorder.

The clinical features at the onset of acute leukemia may closely resemble those of aplastic anemia. The presence of blast cells in the peripheral smear may indicate a diagnosis of leukemia, but examination of a bone marrow aspirate is required to distinguish these disorders definitively as well as to characterize the type of leukemia. This procedure is rarely performed in the ED. Therapy, such as corticosteroids, which might interfere with the interpretation of the bone marrow aspirate, should be withheld until a definitive diagnosis has been made.

As discussed, children with hemolytic disorders may escape detection until pallor is noted during an aplastic crisis when the reticulocyte count is similar to that found in primary disorders of red cell production. An underlying hemolytic disease such as sickle cell anemia or hereditary spherocytosis can usually be recognized during an aplastic crisis, however, by finding characteristic red cells on the peripheral smear. In the autosomal dominant disorders of the red cell membrane, the presence of abnormal erythrocytes in the peripheral blood of one of the parents may support the diagnosis. Solubility tests for HbS or hemoglobin electrophoresis should be performed to detect sickling disorders.

The MCV is usually increased in megaloblastic anemias unless other nutritional disorders are present. Hypersegmentation of the polymorphonuclear leukocytes is characteristic. In severe or long-standing megaloblastic anemia, neutropenia and thrombocytopenia may also be found. In such cases, the findings in the peripheral blood may be similar to those of aplastic anemia or even acute leukemia; examination of the bone marrow and measurement of specific nutrients (B$_{12}$, folic acid) are necessary to distinguish these disorders.

Suggested Readings

Bizzarro M., Colson E., Ehrenkranz R. Differential diagnosis and management of anemia in the newborn. *Pediatr Clin North Am* 2004;51:1087–1107.

Chalco JP, Huicho L, Alamo C, et al. Accuracy of clinical pallor in the diagnosis of anaemia in children: a meta-analysis. *BMC Pediatr* 2005;5:46.

D'Andrea AD, Dahl N, Guinan EC, et al. Marrow failure. *Hematology (Am Soc Hematol Educ Program)* 2002;1:58–72.

Kazal LA Prevention of iron deficiency in infants and toddlers. *Am Fam Physician* 2002;66(7):1217–1224.

Orkin SH, Ginsburg D, et al., eds. *Hematology of infancy and childhood.* 6th ed. Philadelphia: WB Saunders, 2003:409–418.

Oski FA, Brugnara C., Nathan DG. A diagnostic approach to the anemic patient. In: Nathan DG, Servey JT, Reamy BV, Hodge J. Clinical presentations of parvovirus B19 infection. *Am Fam Physician* 2007;75(3):373–376.

CHAPTER 59 ■ PALPITATIONS

JAMES F. WILEY II, MD, MPH

Palpitations represent a disagreeable perception of the heartbeat by the patient. Descriptions commonly given include "pounding," "fluttering," "jumping in the chest," or a sensation of the heart "stopping." In adults, palpitations frequently arise from serious underlying cardiac pathology. In children, most etiologies are benign. Pediatric patients demonstrate a high degree of variation in their sensitivity to changes in the heart rate (HR) or rhythm. A patient who actually has trivial cardiac events may express severe symptoms while children with a significant arrhythmia may remain asymptomatic. The challenge to the emergency physician is to determine which complaint can be managed in the emergency department (ED) and which merits further consideration by a cardiologist.

PATHOPHYSIOLOGY

The heart is innervated by the vagus nerve (cranial nerve X) and the sympathetic ganglion. Cardiovascular reflexes (e.g., vasovagal bradycardia) are transmitted by the vagus nerve. Pain sensation (e.g., related to myocardial ischemia) travels through afferent fibers associated with the sympathetic ganglia. In most patients, the sensation of the heartbeat is not felt. Children with documented arrhythmias, such as supraventricular tachycardia (SVT) and stable ventricular tachycardia, may not complain of any symptoms. Even patients with heart murmurs audible to the unassisted ear can learn to ignore this obvious cue.

Patients with palpitations often relate an indirect perception of increased force of cardiac contraction, tachycardia, or irregular heartbeat. Increased force of the contraction is often detected when the patient is supine. At times, it may be described as a rushing or pounding in the ears, particularly when the ear is pressed against a pillow. Caffeine or alcohol consumption, illicit drug use, exercise, and emotional arousal can produce this sensation of a large ventricular stroke volume.

Patients with premature contractions and a compensatory pause may describe the feeling that their hearts "flip-flop" or "stop." Many patients with premature atrial or ventricular contractions notice the subsequent beat after the initial "short" beat because of the increased stroke volume ejected. Other patients may complain of a choking or full sensation in the neck. Jugular venous pulsation associated with right atrial contraction against a closed tricuspid valve (atrioventricular (AV) block with or without atrial tachycardia) can present in this way.

True cardiac arrhythmias arise from various mechanisms that are discussed in Chapter 84.

DIFFERENTIAL DIAGNOSIS

Many conditions may produce palpitations (Table 59.1). Most children with palpitations do not have significant cardiac pathology (Table 59.2). However, many life-threatening conditions can come to medical attention because of abnormal cardiac sensation (Table 59.3). Wolff-Parkinson-White (WPW) syndrome and the prolonged QT syndrome are two potentially lethal diseases that may be diagnosed on a resting electrocardiogram (EKG). A patient with palpitations during exercise should also raise concern for hypertrophic cardiomyopathy, SVT, ventricular tachycardia, or myocardial ischemia. In addition, palpitations in children with known congenital heart disease are frequently caused by a serious cardiac arrhythmia.

Diagnosis of noncardiac causes of life-threatening palpitations, including hypoxemia, hypoglycemia, hyperkalemia, and hypocalcemia, can be made by characteristic EKG changes, serum electrolyte determinations, rapid bedside glucose, and oxygen saturation measurements.

Hyperdynamic Cardiac Activity

Increased HR and contractility are physiologic responses to catecholamine release, like that which may occur with exercise, emotional arousal, hypoglycemia, and pheochromocytoma. Similarly, increased cardiac work accompanies conditions that increase the basal metabolic rate such as fever, anemia, and hyperthyroidism. Sympathomimetic and anticholinergic drugs are among a group of commonly available substances that directly modulate the autonomic nervous system, causing tachycardia, hyperdynamic cardiac activity, and palpitations (Table 59.4).

Postural orthostatic tachycardia syndrome (POTS) describes a form of orthostatic intolerance characterized by tachycardia (more than 30 beats per minute over baseline or more than 120 beats per minute in adults) typically without hypotension upon standing. POTS is commonly seen in teenage girls and manifests as palpitations, dizziness, and tremulousness. The diagnosis may be made when no other serious cause for symptoms is found and the patient has replication of symptoms with head-up tilt table testing. Volume repletion, increased salt diet, and/or fludrocortisone may attenuate symptoms in affected patients.

Sinus Bradycardia

Low basal metabolic rate associated with hypothyroidism may present with a slow HR and sinus rhythm. Similarly, in the

TABLE 59.1

DIFFERENTIAL DIAGNOSIS OF PALPITATIONS

Hyperdynamic Cardiac Activity
Exercise
Anxiety/hyperventilation syndrome
Emotional/sexual arousal
Fever
Anemia
Drug-induced (Table 59.4)
Hypoglycemia
Hyperthyroidism
Pheochromocytoma
Postural orthostatic tachycardia syndrome

Sinus Bradycardia
Sleep
Drug-induced (Table 59.4)
Hypothyroidism
Advanced physical training (e.g., marathon runners)

True Cardiac Arrhythmias
Tachyarrhythmias
    Supraventricular tachycardia
        Drug-induced (Table 59.4)
        Wolff-Parkinson-White syndrome
    Congenital heart disease (e.g., Ebstein's anomaly)
    Postoperative cardiac repair (especially Fontan, Mustard,
        and Senning procedures)
    Ventricular tachycardia
    Drug-induced (Table 59.4)
    Prolonged QT syndrome
    Myocarditis
    Acute rheumatic fever
    Mitral valve prolapse
    Hypertrophic cardiomyopathy
    Myocardial ischemia/hypoxemia
    Hyperkalemia
    Hypocalcemia
    Postoperative cardiac repair (especially tetralogy of Fallot
        repair)
Irregular rhythm or bradyarrhythmia
    Sinus arrhythmia/respiratory variation
    Premature atrial contractions
    Premature ventricular contractions
    Complete heart block
    Sick sinus syndrome
    Postoperative cardiac repair (especially ventriculoseptal
        defect, atrioventricular canal repairs)

TABLE 59.2

COMMON CAUSES OF PALPITATIONS

Exercise
Anxiety/hyperventilation syndrome
Emotional arousal
Drug-induced (e.g., caffeine, over-the-counter
    sympathomimetic agents)
Supraventricular tachycardia
Mitral valve prolapse
Postural orthostatic tachycardia syndrome
Premature atrial or ventricular contractions

TABLE 59.3

LIFE-THREATENING CAUSES OF PALPITATIONS

Cardiac
Wolff-Parkinson-White syndrome
Prolonged QT syndrome
Hypertrophic cardiomyopathy
Congenital heart disease/postoperative cardiac repair
Myocarditis/acute rheumatic fever
Mitral valve prolapse
Sick sinus syndrome
Complete heart block
Myocardial ischemia

Noncardiac
Hypoxemia
Hypoglycemia
Hyperkalemia
Hypocalcemia
Pheochromocytoma
Poisoning (see Table 59.4)

absence of significant sympathetic nervous system input, the
HR may be slow. This state may be responsible for the sinus
bradycardia associated with sleep or with ingestion of drugs
such as clonidine, sedative-hypnotics, or narcotics. Advanced
physical training results in a highly efficient heart with high
ventricular ejection fraction and sinus bradycardia.

True Cardiac Arrhythmias

SVT represents the most common tachyarrhythmia of childhood (see Chapter 84). Possible underlying causes include
drug exposure, congenital heart disease, and WPW syndrome.
Sympathomimetics in cough and cold preparations are the
most common drugs to incite SVT in children. As of 2008, the
U. S. Food and Drug Administration recommends that over-
the-counter cough and cold preparations not be used in children younger than 2 years. Also, palpitations with cardiac
arrhythmias have occurred following ingestion of sympathomimetic additives to unregulated dietary supplements, such
as ephedra (and its congeners, often advertised as "ephedra-
free" products) and high caffeine energy drinks. Cardiac
lesions associated with SVT include Ebstein's anomaly,
repaired dextrotransposition of the great arteries, and single
ventricle lesions status post-Fontan operation. Up to 75% of
patients with WPW syndrome have a shortened P-R interval or
delta wave on resting EKG (see Chapter 84). However,
approximately 50% of children with SVT have no physical
findings and no EKG abnormalities between episodes. In these
patients, descriptions of abrupt onset and rapid termination of
palpitations ("like a light switch") can often be elicited.

Infection, especially viral myocarditis and acute rheumatic
fever, constitutes one of the most common causes of acquired
ventricular tachycardia in children with normal cardiac
anatomy. Similarly, ingestion of drugs that block fast sodium
channels and/or potassium channels (e.g., tricyclic antidepressants, phenothiazines, and antiarrhythmic agents) is a preventable cause of torsades de pointes (polymorphic ventricular
tachycardia) and unstable ventricular tachycardia in the otherwise normal child (Table 59.4). Palpitations associated with

TABLE 59.4

DRUGS THAT CAUSE PALPITATIONS/ARRHYTHMIAS

Sinus or Supraventricular Tachycardia
Ephedrine, pseudoephedrine
Herbal stimulants
Ephedra
Khat (*Catha edulis* leaves, popular in Africa and the
　　Middle East)
Amphetamines
Cocaine
Albuterol, metaproterenol
Antihistamines
Phenothiazines
Antidepressants
Tobacco
Caffeine, theophylline

Ventricular Tachycardia or Torsades de Pointes
Tricyclic antidepressants
Phenothiazines
Antiarrhythmic agents (e.g., quinidine, procainamide,
　　mexiletine, flecainide, encainide)
Chloral hydrate
Chloroquine
Organophosphate pesticides
Chlorinated hydrocarbons
Digoxin
Caffeine, theophylline
Amphetamines
Cocaine
Arsenic

Bradycardia
β-Adrenergic blockers
Calcium channel blockers
Digoxin
Clonidine
Sedative/hypnotic agents
Narcotics
Organophosphate pesticides

exercise may be caused by ventricular tachyarrhythmias that occur in conjunction with hypertrophic cardiomyopathy or myocardial ischemia (usually secondary to congenital anomalies of the coronary arteries). Patients with the prolonged QT syndrome have a genetically determined predisposition to fatal ventricular arrhythmias that can be detected by calculation of the corrected QT interval on a resting 12-lead EKG (see Chapter 84). Patients who have undergone ventriculotomy for tetralogy of Fallot comprise another group who are at high risk for ventricular arrhythmias as a result of the postoperative development of scarring in the right ventricular outflow tract. Finally, electrolyte disturbances, particularly hyperkalemia, hypocalcemia, and hypomagnesemia, may be causative in a child with palpitations and ventricular tachycardia (see Chapter 100).

Premature atrial contractions produce the most common arrhythmia of childhood, with 50% of normal children experiencing at least one premature atrial contraction per day. Premature ventricular contractions (PVCs) also account for many reports of irregular heartbeat. Although this arrhythmia can herald serious underlying pathology, patients with an unremarkable history, normal physical examination, and unifocal PVCs that disappear with exercise do not require further evaluation. Patients with significant sinus or AV node dysfunction as a cause of an irregular or slow heartbeat often have a history of syncope or seizure, slow HR (25 to 50 beats per minute) on examination, a pulmonic flow murmur, or signs of congestive heart failure. Patients who have undergone intraatrial repairs (d-transposition of the great arteries and atrial septal defect) are at highest risk for these potentially life-threatening arrhythmias.

EVALUATION AND DECISION

The ill-appearing child with palpitations requires rapid assessment for the presence of hypoxemia, shock, hypoglycemia, or an existing life-threatening arrhythmia. Further evaluation should include measurement of hemoglobin, serum glucose (Dextrostick), serum electrolytes, calcium, and pulse oximetry or arterial blood gas. The presence of heart disease should be assessed by a 12-lead EKG and rhythm strip, followed by continuous monitoring, frequent vital signs, and chest radiograph (Fig. 59.1). Specific arrhythmias should be treated as outlined in Chapter 84.

The asymptomatic child with palpitations by history may also have an intermittent or continuing arrhythmia. Continuous cardiac monitoring and a resting 12-lead EKG performed while the patient is in the ED increase the likelihood that this abnormality will be detected. Patients with repeated episodes of palpitations may benefit from 24-hour ambulatory (Holter) or longer-term event monitoring, and warrant referral to a pediatric cardiologist. Any patient with a history of syncope, congenital heart disease, or particularly, postoperative or exercise-induced palpitations is at greater risk for having a true cardiac arrhythmia as the cause of his or her symptoms. Similarly, the presence of a short P-R interval with the typical delta wave morphology of WPW syndrome or a prolonged corrected Q-T interval (see Chapter 84) indicates the need for evaluation and consultation by a pediatric cardiologist.

The presence or recent history of fever or an upper respiratory infection should prompt the emergency physician to look for signs and symptoms of myocarditis or acute rheumatic fever. Myocarditis describes inflammation of the muscle wall of the heart. Multiple organisms can cause this pathology, with the most common identified agent being coxsackie virus. Clinical features of this disease are fever, tachycardia out of proportion to activity or degree of fever, pallor, cyanosis, respiratory distress secondary to pulmonary edema, muffled heart sounds with gallop, and hepatomegaly caused by passive congestion of the liver. The EKG findings are nonspecific and include low-voltage QRS complexes (less than 5 mm total amplitude in limb leads), "pseudoinfarction" pattern with deep Q waves and poor R-wave progression in the precordial leads, AV conduction disturbances that range from P-R prolongation to complete AV dissociation, and tachyarrhythmias such as ventricular tachycardia and SVT. A child with palpitations and clinical findings suggestive of myocarditis requires emergent supportive care (see Chapter 3), echocardiography, and admission to a unit capable of intensive monitoring and rapid treatment of cardiac arrhythmias and hemodynamic instability.

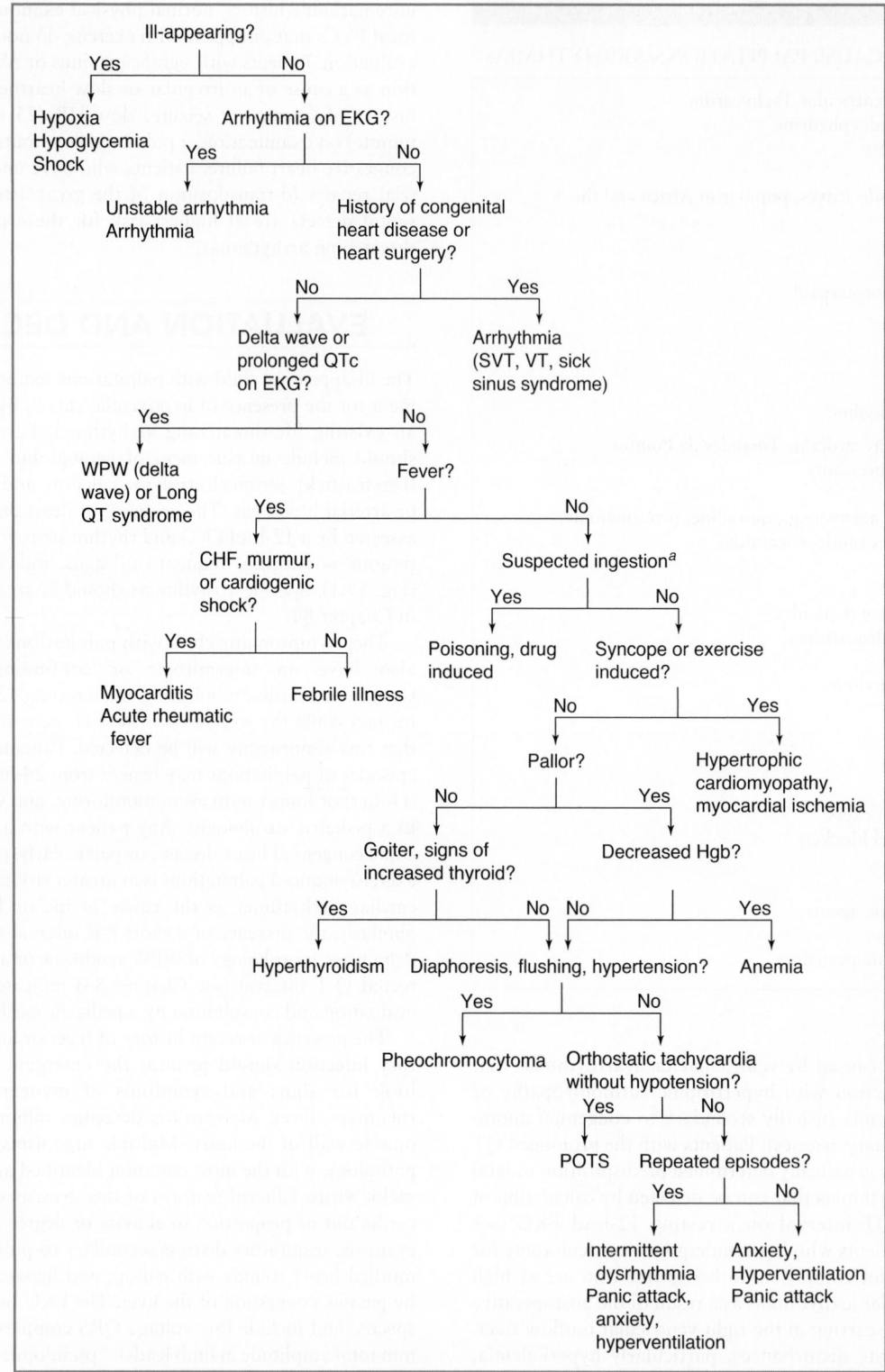

FIGURE 59.1 A diagnostic approach to palpitations. EKG, electrocardiogram; SVT, supraventricular tachycardia; VT, ventricular tachycardia; WPW, Wolff-Parkinson-White; CHF, congestive heart failure; Hgb, hemoglobin; POTS, postural orthostatic tachycardia syndrome. [a]Especially caffeine, diet supplements, herbal preparations, sympathomimetic medications, cocaine, or amphetamines.

Acute rheumatic fever follows pharyngeal streptococcal infection and is an inflammatory disease that targets the heart, vessels, joints, skin, and central nervous system (CNS). Diagnosis and management of acute rheumatic fever are discussed separately (see Chapter 84).

A detailed history of recent medications or precipitating events may reveal the cause of palpitations in some patients. Ingestion of highly caffeinated beverages (including soft drinks and energy drinks), cough and cold preparations, herbal preparations, dietary supplements, "health" drinks with herbal additives, illicit drugs, and a smoking history should be ascertained. The patient's emotional state before the onset of palpitations should be discussed to determine the likelihood of anxiety or emotional arousal as the cause of symptoms (see Chapter 131). The presence of diaphoresis, hypertension, and headache should encourage the assessment for pheochromocytoma, whereas widened pulse pressure and thyroid enlargement suggest hyperthyroidism (see Chapter 86). Anemia may be the cause of symptoms in a patient with pallor (see Chapter 91).

In some patients, an exact cause of palpitations cannot be determined at the time of ED evaluation. Patients with a single episode should have close follow-up arranged with their primary care physicians and should be instructed to return for further evaluation if symptoms recur. Patients with multiple episodes of palpitations deserve further evaluation and consultation with a pediatric cardiologist.

Suggested Readings

Alexander ME, Berul CI. Ventricular arrhythmias: when to worry. *Pediatr Cardiol* 2000;21(6):532–541.

Batra AS, Hohn AR. Consultation with the specialist: palpitations, syncope, and sudden cardiac death in children: who's at risk? *Pediatr Rev* 2003;24(8):269–275.

Bohn D, Benson L. Diagnosis and management of pediatric myocarditis. *Paediatr Drugs* 2002;4:171–181.

Doniger SJ, Sharieff GQ. Pediatric dysrhythmias. *Pediatr Clin North Am* 2006;53:85–105.

Ginsburg GS, Riddle MA, Davies M. Somatic symptoms in children and adolescents with anxiety disorders. *J Am Acad Child Adolesc Psychiatry* 2006;45: 1179–1187.

Haller CA, Benowitz NL. Adverse cardiovascular and central nervous system events associated with dietary supplements containing ephedra alkaloids. *N Engl J Med* 2000;343:1833–1838.

Kaltman J, Shah M. Evaluation of the child with an arrhythmia. *Pediatr Clin North Am* 2004;51:1537–1551.

Maron BJ, Shirani J, Poliac LC, et al. Sudden death in young competitive athletes. Clinical, demographic, and pathological profiles. *JAMA* 1996;276(3):199–204.

Moss AJ. Long QT syndrome. *JAMA* 2003;289:2041–2044.

Olson KR. Emergency evaluation and treatment. In: Olson KR, ed. *Poisoning and drug overdose*, 2nd ed. New York: Lange Medical Books/McGraw-Hill Companies, 2004:11–15.

Saisch SG, Wessely S, Gardner WN. Patients with acute hyperventilation presenting to an inner-city emergency department. *Chest* 1996; 110:952–957.

Sandroni P, Opfer-Gehrking TL, McPhee BR, et al. Postural tachycardia syndrome: clinical features and follow-up study. *Mayo Clin Proc* 1999;74:1106–1110.

Weber BE, Kapoor WN. Evaluation and outcomes of patients with palpitations. *Am J Med* 1996;100:138–148.

Wisten A, Messner T. Symptoms preceding sudden cardiac death in the young are common but often misinterpreted. *Scand Cardiovasc J* 2005;39:143–149.

Woods WA, McCulloch MA. Cardiovascular emergencies in the pediatric patient. *Emerg Med Clin North Am* 2005;23:1233–1249.

SIGNS AND SYMPTOMS

CHAPTER 60 ■ POLYDIPSIA

RONALD I. PAUL, MD

Polydipsia, or excessive thirst, is an uncommon complaint in children. Although fluid consumption varies greatly among individuals, pathologic conditions exist when excessive drinking of fluids interferes with daily life or is accompanied by bizarre behavior, such as drinking from a toilet bowl. Polydipsia is routinely accompanied by urinary frequency (see Chapter 75). Other accompanying symptoms depend on the underlying cause.

PATHOPHYSIOLOGY

The sensation of thirst and subsequent fluid intake is influenced by complex mechanisms that involve the hypothalamus, extracranial thirst receptors, and kidneys. As water is lost from the body, thirst centers in the hypothalamus are stimulated by an increase in serum osmolality. In response to signals from the hypothalamus, the pituitary gland releases an antidiuretic hormone, vasopressin, which causes reabsorption of water in the collecting ducts of the kidney. In addition to physiologic controls of thirst, cortical involvement and social conditioning also play a role and may be responsible for the wide variability in fluid consumption.

DIFFERENTIAL DIAGNOSIS

Diabetes mellitus (DM) is the single most common cause of polydipsia (Table 60.1). Additional prominent symptoms of DM include weight loss and polyuria. Other common causes of polydipsia include sickle cell anemia and diabetes insipidus (DI) (Table 60.2). In sickle cell anemia, chronic sickling of cells in the medulla of the kidney results in a limited ability to concentrate urine and mild polydipsia. In DI, a wide variety of lesions in the hypothalamus and neurohypophysis result in a deficiency of antidiuretic hormone. Inherited forms of nephrogenic DI may be autosomal dominant, autosomal recessive, or X-linked recessive. In instances in which the cause of DI cannot be readily determined, patients are diagnosed as idiopathic. These patients need frequent reevaluations because many are later diagnosed with intracranial tumors.

Less common metabolic and endocrine causes of polydipsia include electrolyte imbalances, catecholamine excess, and cystinosis. Primary renal causes of hyposthenuria include interstitial nephritis, renal tubular acidosis, medullary cystic disease (nephrophthisis), and obstructive uropathy. In nephrogenic DI, the renal tubule is unresponsive to antidiuretic hormone. Patients with nephrogenic DI usually have onset of symptoms in infancy and present with recurrent episodes of dehydration, fever, failure to thrive, and psychomotor retarda-

tion. Pharmacologic causes of polyuria and polydipsia include methylxanthines and diuretics. In addition, chronic lithium therapy may result in nephrogenic DI.

Primary polydipsia is diagnosed when the ingestion of water is in excess of that needed to maintain water balance. It can be caused by an inappropriate psychological thirst drive (psychogenic polydipsia or compulsive water drinking) or by hypothalamic damage that alters thirst but not antidiuretic hormone release (neurogenic polydipsia).

Most children with polydipsia have serious but nonacute problems. Potential life-threatening conditions may develop in certain circumstances (Table 60.3). Patients with DI or nephrogenic DI may develop severe dehydration if water is withheld for prolonged periods. Conversely, urgent management of hypernatremia is usually unnecessary if patients are able to drink and may be harmful if it is of chronic duration. Diabetic ketoacidosis may be an initial presentation of patients with DM, and can result in extreme electrolyte and acid–base imbalances. Patients with primary polydipsia who overload their kidneys' ability to excrete free water may present with hyponatremic seizures. Many of the brain lesions that cause DI can become life-threatening. Patients with severe brain injury often develop DI toward the end of life.

EVALUATION AND DECISION

When evaluating a child with polydipsia, the physician should seek information from the parent regarding the quantity of fluid taken each day and whether the child has used any unusual methods to satiate thirst. A history of nocturnal polydipsia and polyuria is helpful because most children with psychogenic polydipsia do not wake in the middle of the night for fluids. A medical history should include questions on growth and development, as well as past episodes of severe dehydration. Inquiries should be made about known causes of polydipsia such as sickle cell disease, DM, chronic kidney disorders, head trauma, and medications (Fig. 60.1). The physical examination should include a careful evaluation for known systemic and intracranial causes of DI.

If the history and physical examination are not revealing, a urinalysis should be obtained. In almost all cases of polydipsia, the urine-specific gravity will be low (less than 1.010). A specific gravity greater than 1.020 should represent appropriate thirst. If the urinalysis is abnormal, DM, sickle cell disease or trait, or an intrinsic renal disorder should be suspected. If the urinalysis is normal, electrolytes, calcium, and renal function tests may reveal conditions associated with electrolyte imbalances. Patients with DI or nephrogenic DI may have hypernatremia if they are examined when dehydrated. A

TABLE 60.1

CAUSES OF POLYDIPSIA

Diabetes mellitus
    Electrolyte imbalances
    Hypercalcemia
    Hypokalemia

Bartter's syndrome
    Catecholamine excess
    Pheochromocytoma
    Neuroblastoma
    Ganglioneuroma

Cystinosis

Diabetes insipidus (antidiuretic hormone deficient)
    Craniopharyngioma
    Pituitary adenoma
    Histiocytosis
    Head trauma
    Sarcoidosis
    Leukemia
    Infection

    Aneurysm
    Intraventricular hemorrhage
    Hereditary

Drugs
    Methylxanthines
    Diuretics
    Lithium

Renal causes
    Renal tubular acidosis
    Nephrogenic diabetes insipidus
    Sickle cell trait
    Sickle cell diseases
    Interstitial nephritis
    Obstructive uropathy

Primary polydipsia
    Psychogenic polydipsia
    Neurogenic polydipsia

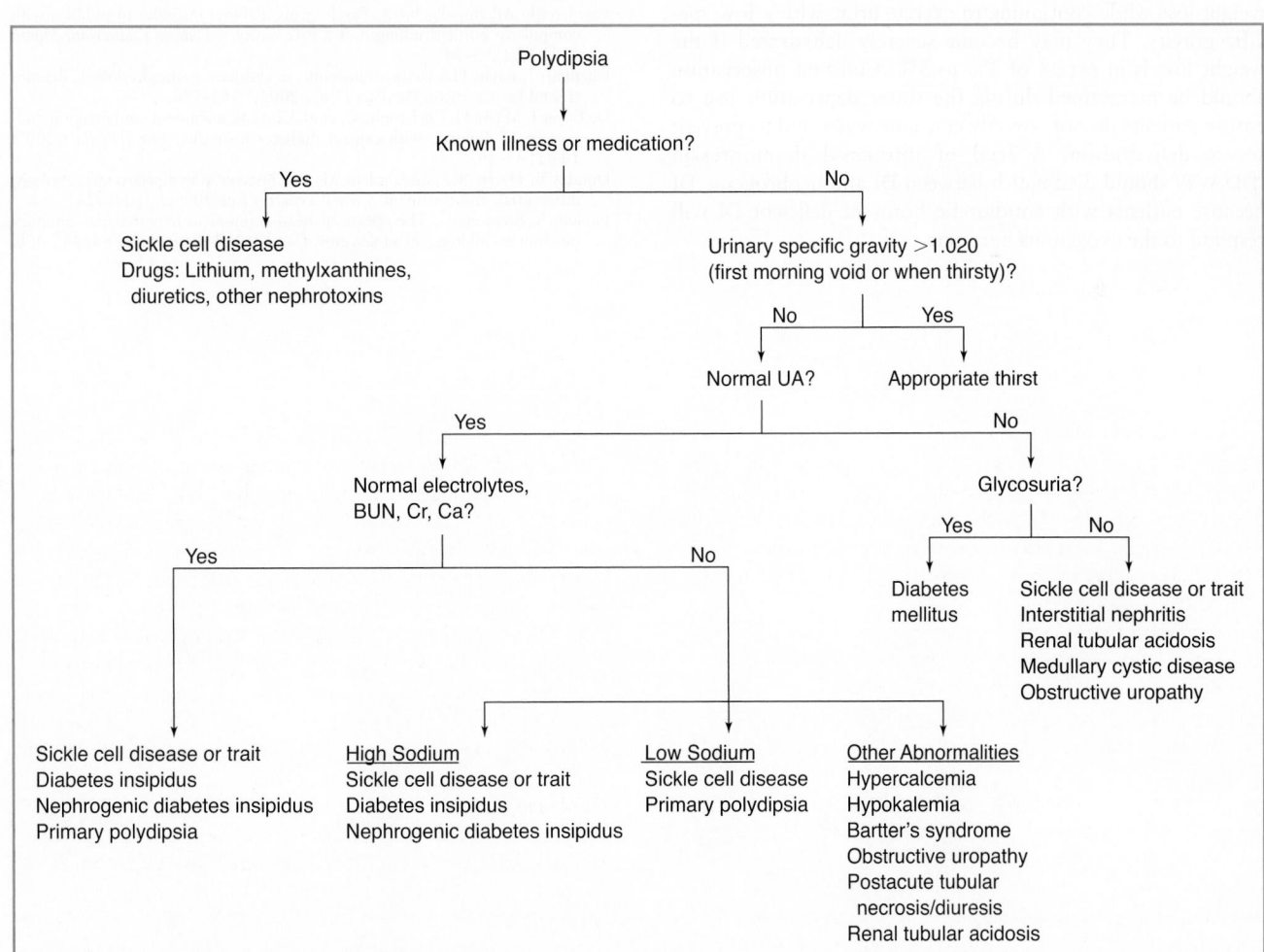

FIGURE 60.1 Diagnostic approach to a child with polydipsia. UA, urinalysis; BUN, blood urea nitrogen; Cr, creatinine; Ca, calcium.

TABLE 60.2

COMMON CAUSES OF POLYDIPSIA

Diabetes mellitus
Sickle cell anemia
Diabetes insipidus (antidiuretic hormone deficient)

TABLE 60.3

LIFE-THREATENING CAUSES OF POLYDIPSIA

Diabetes insipidus (antidiuretic hormone deficient)
Nephrogenic diabetes insipidus
Diabetes mellitus
Primary polydipsia

hemoglobin electrophoresis may be needed to determine whether the patient has sickle cell disease or trait. However, patients with sickle cell disease usually have the diagnosis confirmed before the development of tubular dysfunction and polydipsia. Computed tomography and magnetic resonance imaging scans may be necessary to diagnose intracranial abnormalities.

Patients suspected of having primary polydipsia, DI, and nephrogenic DI require further testing that can be dangerous. These tests should be performed in controlled settings and are usually inappropriate in the emergency department.

Patients with primary polydipsia should respond to a water deprivation test by increasing their urine gravity and osmolality. Patients with DI and nephrogenic DI should have rapid weight loss while continuing to excrete urine with a low specific gravity. They may become severely dehydrated if the weight loss is in excess of 3% to 5%. Constant observation should be maintained during the water deprivation test to ensure patients do not covertly consume water and to prevent severe dehydration. A trial of intranasal desmopressin (DDAVP) should distinguish between DI and nephrogenic DI because patients with antidiuretic hormone-deficient DI will respond to the exogenous hormone.

Unfortunately, even these tests are fraught with some inaccuracies. Patients with primary polydipsia who have chronic overhydration and diminished capacity to concentrate urine may have a blunted response to water deprivation. In addition, patients with DI and nephrogenic DI may produce a hypertonic urine if the glomerular filtration rate is decreased as severe dehydration ensues. Radioimmunoassay for antidiuretic hormone can be helpful in confusing cases.

Suggested Readings

Bichet DG. Nephrogenic diabetes insipidus. *Adv Chronic Kidney Dis* 2006; 13(2):96–104.

Cermeroglu AP, Buyukgebiz A. Psychogenic diabetes insipidus in toddlers with compulsive bottle-drinking: not a rare entity. *J Pediatr Endocrinol Metab* 2002;15(1):93–94.

Chetham T, Baylis PH. Diabetes insipidus in children: pathophysiology, diagnosis and management. *Paediatr Drugs* 2002;4:785–796.

De Buyst J, Massa G, Christophe C, et al. Clinical, hormonal, and imaging findings in 27 children with central diabetes insipidus. *Eur J Pediatr* 2007; 166(1):43–49.

Dundas B, Harris M, Narasimhan M. Psychogenic polydipsia reiew: etiology, differential, and treatment. *Curr Psychiatry Rep* 2007;9(3):236–241.

Einaudi S, Bondone C. The effects of head trauma on hypothalamic-pituitary function in children and adolescents. *Curr Opin Pediatr* 2007;19(4):465–470.

CHAPTER 61 ■ RASH—ECZEMATOUS

TODD A. FLORIN, MD, AND JAMES M. CALLAHAN, MD

Pediatricians often use the terms *eczema* and *atopic dermatitis* interchangeably. However, *eczema* is often used more generally to describe a complex of signs and symptoms, including erythema, edema, vesiculation, scaling, and pruritus. This use of the term is more appropriate because many disease processes and exposures may cause eczematous rashes (see Chapter 85). The distinct forms of eczema are labeled by cause, pattern, or associated conditions such as atopy. Acute eczema consists of erythema, edema, exudation, clustered papulovesicles, scaling, and crusting. Chronic eczema is characterized by lichenification, changes in skin pigmentation, and excoriation. Diagnosis of the underlying cause of the eczematous eruption relies on historical and dermatologic features, as histology is typically not specific.

DIFFERENTIAL DIAGNOSIS

Atopic Dermatitis

Atopic dermatitis (see Chapter 85) is by far the most common cause of an eczematous rash in children (Tables 61.1 and 61.2). It is a chronic or relapsing condition characterized by pruritic eczematous eruptions and occurs in 10% to 20% of all children. There is often a personal or family history of allergic rhinitis, hay fever, or asthma. Most patients have the onset of symptoms before age 6 months, with up to 90% developing symptoms by 5 years of age. Dry conditions or frequent bathing often lead to exacerbations. Stress, sweating, and exposure to environmental allergens may also precipitate flares. Infants and young children may experience worsening symptoms with exposure to certain foods.

Diagnosis is not based on any single defining criteria, but rather has its basis in essential, important, and associated features. Several groups have developed diagnostic criteria, including a United Kingdom Working Party (Table 61.3A) and the American Academy of Dermatology (Table 61.3B). The broad differential diagnosis requires the exclusion of other skin conditions that present in a similar fashion such as seborrheic dermatitis, scabies, contact dermatitis, impetigo, psoriasis, nutritional deficiencies (i.e., zinc), immune deficiencies, and cutaneous lymphoma.

With acute flares, lesions are poorly demarcated, erythematous, scaly, and often weepy and crusted. Chronic lesions are thickened, hyperpigmented, and often excoriated. Distribution varies by age. Infants have lesions on the cheeks, trunk, diaper area, and extensor surfaces. Children show involvement of the feet and flexor areas, such as the antecubital and popliteal fossae and the neck. In adolescents and adults, flexor areas, hands, and feet are usually involved. Xerosis (dry skin),

ichthyosis vulgaris (inherited fishlike scaling), keratosis pilaris (chicken-skin appearance caused by cornified plugs in the upper hair follicles), infraorbital eyelid folds (Dennie-Morgan sign), hyperlinear palms, pityriasis alba (scaly hypopigmented patches), and follicular accentuation may be seen. The pruritus of atopic dermatitis often results in a cycle of excoriation, potentially resulting in microbial colonization and secondary infection. Superimposed bacterial (*Staphylococcus aureus* or group A streptococcus), fungal, and viral infections (eczema herpeticum caused by herpes simplex virus) are common.

Particularly severe or persistent symptoms should prompt consideration of an underlying systemic disorder associated with eczematous eruptions.

Contact Dermatitis

Contact dermatitis (see Chapter 85) is an inflammatory reaction of the skin caused by an allergic stimulus or primary irritant. Acute eruptions have intense pruritus, severe erythema, edema, vesicles, and erosions with serous discharge and crusting. A sharp demarcation between involved and unaffected skin usually exists. Subacute reactions have mild erythema, dry scale, less vesiculation, and mild thickening of the skin. Chronic exposures may result in lichenification, fissures, scales, excoriations, and hyperpigmentation. Vesicles are rare.

Allergic Contact Dermatitis

Allergic contact dermatitis is caused by a classic delayed T-cell–mediated hypersensitivity reaction (type IV). Repeated exposure causes an allergic sensitization. The eruption is delayed after the initial exposure for up to 7 to 10 days. Repeated exposures can cause the rapid appearance of an acute dermatitis (within 12 hours). Rhus dermatitis, caused by an oleoresin in the sap of poison ivy, poison oak, or poison sumac plants, is the most common cause of allergic contact dermatitis in the United States. Delayed exposure may occur because of contact with objects that have had contact with the plants. Typical presentation includes pruritus and erythema followed by development of papules, vesicles and bullae, usually in a streak-like arrangement. Burning of plants leads to aerosolization of the allergen, and may cause a widespread and severe outbreak on exposed skin surfaces. Other plants, flowers, pollens (especially ragweed), clothing, shoes, metals (e.g., nickel in jewelry), cosmetics, adhesive tape, and latex-containing products can also cause an allergic contact dermatitis. Nickel dermatitis occurs on earlobes as a result of nickel-containing earrings and on the abdomen due to pant buttons. Shoe dermatitis, the only form of allergic dermatitis to affect the soles (in contrast to irritant dermatitis, which does affect palms and soles),

TABLE 61.1

DIFFERENTIAL DIAGNOSIS OF ECZEMATOUS RASH

Allergy	**Infectious**
Atopic dermatitis	Seborrheic dermatitis
Allergic contact dermatitis	Dermatophyte infection
Autoeczematization	Scabies
Drug reaction	Molluscum contagiosum
	Pityriasis rosea
Exogenous	Candida
Irritant contact dermatitis	Eczema herpeticum
Lichen simplex chronicus	Human immunodeficiency
Nummular eczema	virus
Asteatotic eczema	
Dyshidrotic eczema	**Oncologic**
(pompholyx)	Histiocytosis
Intertrigo	(Letterer-Siwe)
Frictional lichenoid	Cutaneous T-cell
dermatitis	lymphoma
Photoallergic reaction	Leukemia and lymphoma
Immunologic	**Nutritional**
Wiskott-Aldrich syndrome	Acrodermatitis
Hyperimmunoglobulin E	enteropathica
syndrome	
Omenn's syndrome	**Other**
Severe combined	Psoriasis
immunodeficiency	Exfoliative dermatitis[a] (see
Graft-versus-host disease	Table 61.6)
Agammaglobulinemia	Netherton's syndrome
Immune dysregulation,	
polyendocrinopathy,	
enteropathy, X-linked	
(IPEX)	

[a]Potentially acute life-threatening condition

usually occurs on the dorsal surfaces on the feet, sparing interdigital spaces, in a symmetric manner.

Allergic contact dermatitis is rare in infants because of their impaired ability to react to allergens. By age 3 to 8 years, children react to allergens in a fashion similar to adults. The distribution, shape, and pattern of the rash, and exposure history, may elucidate the cause. Airborne processes (e.g., smoke-containing rhus oleoresin) cause a problem on exposed surfaces, including eyelids, whereas a photoallergic contact dermatitis involves sun-exposed areas [e.g., rash resulting from use of a sunscreen that contains paraaminobenzoic acid (PABA)].

Irritant Contact Dermatitis

A primary irritant dermatitis is a nonallergic reaction of the skin caused by a single exposure or a series of brief contacts with an irritating substance. Strong soaps and detergents, citrus juices, saliva, urine, stool contents, fiberglass particles or

TABLE 61.2

COMMON CAUSES OF ECZEMATOUS RASH

Atopic dermatitis	Dermatophyte infections
Contact dermatitis	Scabies
Allergic	Molluscum contagiosum
Irritant	Pityriasis rosea

TABLE 61.3A

U.K. WORKING PARTY DIAGNOSTIC CRITERIA FOR ATOPIC DERMATITIS

The diagnosis of atopic dermatitis is established when a history of an itchy skin condition exists and at least three of the following criteria are met:

■ History of involvement of the skin creases such as folds of elbows, behind the knees, front of ankles, or around the neck (including cheeks in children younger than 10 years of age)

■ A personal history of asthma or hay fever (or family history of atopic disease in children younger than 4 years of age)

■ A history of general dry skin in the last year

■ Visible flexural eczema (or eczema of the cheeks/forehead and outer limbs in children younger than 4 years of age)

■ Onset before the age of 2 years (not used if the child is younger than 4 years of age)

Source: From Williams HC, Burney PGJ, Pemborke AC, et al. The UK Working Party's diagnostic criteria for atopic dermatitis. III. Independent hospital evaluation. *Br J Dermatol* 1994;131:406–416.

other abrasive materials, and bubble baths are common causes in children. Perioral irritant contact dermatitis occurs as a result of excessive drooling or lip licking, typically presenting as a sharply demarcated rash around the mouth. Juvenile plantar dermatosis is a form of irritant contact dermatitis resulting from alternating excessive hydration and rapid moisture loss of the feet. This presents with extensive skin fissuring and glazed appearance of the planter surface of the foot, largely in prepubertal children who wear occlusive footwear. It may be treated with emollients. Frictional lichenoid dermatitis is likely

TABLE 61.3B

AMERICAN ACADEMY OF DERMATOLOGY CONSENSUS CONFERENCE FEATURES OF ATOPIC DERMATITIS

Essential Features (must be present)
Pruritus
Eczematous skin changes with chronic or recurring history, typical morphology, and distribution
■ Face, neck, extensor involvement in infants and children
■ Flexural lesions in any age group
■ Sparing of groin and axillary regions

Important Features (seen in most cases, support the diagnosis)
Early age at diagnosis
Personal or family history of atopy

Associated Features
Atypical vascular responses (e.g., facial pallor, white dermographism, delayed blanch response)
Keratosis pilaris/hyperlinear palms/ichthyosis
Ocular/periorbital changes
Other regional findings (e.g., perioral changes/periauricular lesions)
Perifollicular accentuation/lichenification/prurigo lesions

Source: From Eichenfield LF, Hanifin JM, Luger TA, et al. Consensus conference on pediatric atopic dermatitis. *J Am Acad Dermatol* 2003;49(6):1088–1095.

to recur. Cutaneous nodules and purpura are suggestive. Hepatosplenomegaly, lymphadenopathy, anemia, thrombocytopenia, and osseous lesions are associated findings.

EVALUATION AND DECISION

The most important points in reaching an accurate diagnosis of an eczematous rash include the distribution of the lesions, the duration of the disease, and the patient's age (see Fig. 61.6A).

Generalized

If a patient presents with a generalized eczematous process, red and scaly from head to toe, this suggests exfoliative dermatitis or erythroderma (Figs. 61.5 and 61.6B). This unusual condition is not a specific diagnosis but instead has multiple causes. It can be a manifestation of an underlying dermatologic process, an infection, a drug reaction, or a systemic illness. Skin biopsy is often necessary for diagnosis. In infancy, an immune dysfunction should be considered, especially if the patient has diarrhea, recurrent infections, or failure to thrive.

Acute Onset or Chronic Problem

The next step in determining a diagnosis is deciding if the rash is of acute onset or has been present for a period of time (Fig. 61.6A). Although not all conditions can be classified exclusively in this way (e.g., atopic dermatitis is a chronic disease but it is often characterized by acute symptomatic flares), this is a useful construct in reaching a diagnosis. Infectious causes mostly present acutely. Eczematous rashes due to systemic diseases are often chronic.

Extensive But Not Generalized

Eruptions that may be extensive but with some areas of non-involved skin include atopic dermatitis, seborrheic dermatitis, scabies, autoeczematization reactions, pityriasis rosea, or contact dermatitis (Fig. 61.6A). A family or personal history of atopy, a history of flares and remittance, extreme pruritus, and a distribution compatible with the patient's age suggest atopic dermatitis. No specific laboratory tests aid in diagnosis. Seborrheic dermatitis is seen only in infancy and after puberty. Features that help distinguish seborrhea from atopic dermatitis in infancy include minimal pruritus; salmon-colored, greasy plaques; and predominant involvement of the scalp and intertriginous regions. Scabies may be distinguished from atopic dermatitis by a history of acute onset, contacts with recent onset of a pruritic eruption, and polymorphous appearance. Occasionally, children with scabies have a chronic rash that has been diagnosed as atopic dermatitis, without a history of rash in contacts. One should always be suspicious of scabies, especially if a child aged 3 years or older presents with the recent onset of an eczematous, pruritic rash. Id reactions can be extensive. A history of an initial contact dermatitis or scaly scalp (tinea capitis) followed by a widespread eczematous rash suggests an autoeczematization reaction. Id reactions tend to be worse in areas near the initial rash. An allergic or irritant contact dermatitis could be extensive, depending on the exposure. Eruptions that are unusually severe, persistent, recalcitrant to treatment, or associated with systemic signs should prompt consideration of an underlying systemic illness. With these processes, the skin findings may be extensive such as that seen with Hyper-IgE syndrome or immune dysregulation, polyendocrinopathy, enteropathy, X-linked (IPEX) or more localized (e.g., the diaper and postauricular areas in children with Langerhans cell histiocytosis).

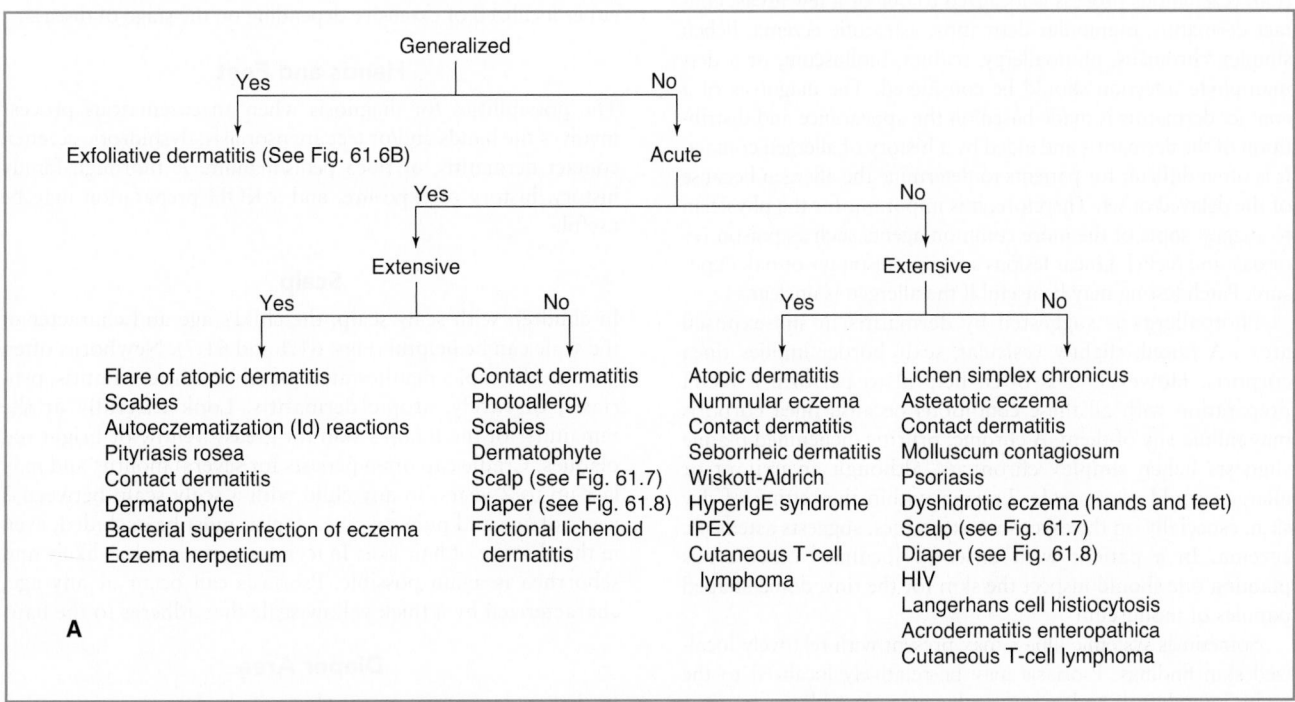

FIGURE 61.6 **A:** Diagnostic approach to the child with an eczematous process. (*continued*)

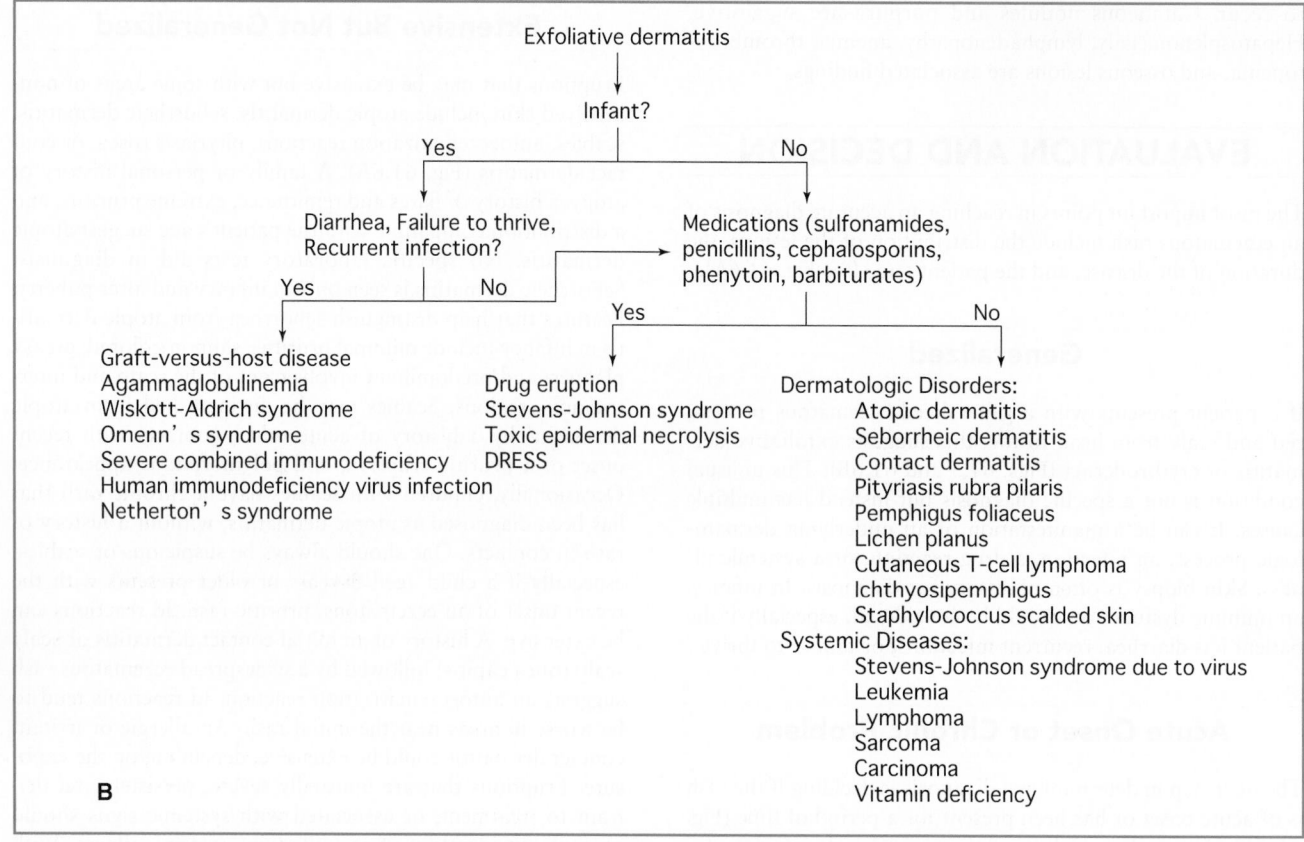

Exfoliative dermatitis

Infant?

Yes / No

Yes: Diarrhea, Failure to thrive, Recurrent infection?

Yes / No

No: Medications (sulfonamides, penicillins, cephalosporins, phenytoin, barbiturates)

Yes / No

Graft-versus-host disease
Agammaglobulinemia
Wiskott-Aldrich syndrome
Omenn' s syndrome
Severe combined immunodeficiency
Human immunodeficiency virus infection
Netherton' s syndrome

Drug eruption
Stevens-Johnson syndrome
Toxic epidermal necrolysis
DRESS

Dermatologic Disorders:
  Atopic dermatitis
  Seborrheic dermatitis
  Contact dermatitis
  Pityriasis rubra pilaris
  Pemphigus foliaceus
  Lichen planus
  Cutaneous T-cell lymphoma
  Ichthyosipemphigus
  Staphylococcus scalded skin
Systemic Diseases:
  Stevens-Johnson syndrome due to virus
  Leukemia
  Lymphoma
  Sarcoma
  Carcinoma
  Vitamin deficiency

B

FIGURE 61.6 (*Continued*) **B:** Diagnostic approach to the child with an exfoliative dermatitis.

Localized

If an eczematous process is localized to one or a few areas, contact dermatitis, nummular dermatitis, asteatotic eczema, lichen simplex chronicus, photoallergy, scabies, molluscum, or a dermatophyte infection should be considered. The diagnosis of a contact dermatitis is made based on the appearance and distribution of the dermatitis and aided by a history of allergen contact. It is often difficult for patients to determine the allergen because of the delayed onset. Therefore, it is important for the physician to suggest some of the more common agents such as poison ivy or oak and nickel. Linear lesions suggest poison ivy or oak exposure. Patch testing may be useful if the allergen is unclear.

Photoallergy is suggested by dermatitis in sun-exposed areas. A raised, slightly vesicular, scaly border implies tinea corporis. However, it is often helpful to perform a KOH preparation with all these conditions because tinea corporis may mimic any of them. A chronic, pruritic, lichenified plaque suggests lichen simplex chronicus, although an irritant or allergen could play a role. Eczema within the setting of dry skin, especially on the extensor extremities, suggests asteatotic eczema. In a patient with onset of localized eczematous plaques, one should inspect the skin for the tiny, dome-shaped papules of molluscum.

Sometimes systemic illness may present with relatively localized skin findings. Psoriasis may be relatively localized to the scalp, intergluteal, and postauricular areas in addition to areas that are prone to epidermal injury such as extensor surfaces of the hand and elbows. Associated findings such as nail dystrophy

and bright red plaques with a silvery scale suggest this diagnosis. HIV infection may be manifested by a seborrheic-like dermatitis. Cutaneous T-cell lymphoma is very rare in children but may be either localized or extensive depending on the stage of disease.

Hands and Feet

The possibilities for diagnosis when an eczematous process involves the hands and/or feet are psoriasis, dyshidrotic eczema, contact dermatitis, or tinea pedis/manum. A thorough family history, history of exposure, and a KOH preparation may be useful.

Scalp

In children with scaly scalp, the child's age and character of the scale can be helpful (Figs. 61.1 and 61.7). Newborns often have cradle cap, a manifestation of seborrheic dermatitis, psoriasis, or rarely, atopic dermatitis. Look carefully at the remainder of the infant's skin for greasy yellow or bright red plaques. Cradle cap often persists for several months and may last up to 2 years. In any child with a scaly scalp between 2 years of age and puberty, tinea capitis must be excluded, even in the absence of hair loss. In teenagers, tinea is less likely and seborrhea is again possible. Psoriasis can occur at any age, characterized by a thick yellow scale that adheres to the hair.

Diaper Area

In diaper dermatitis, morphology of the lesions is important (Figs. 61.3 and 61.8). A bright red, well-demarcated plaque with scale could be psoriasis, candida, or acrodermatitis

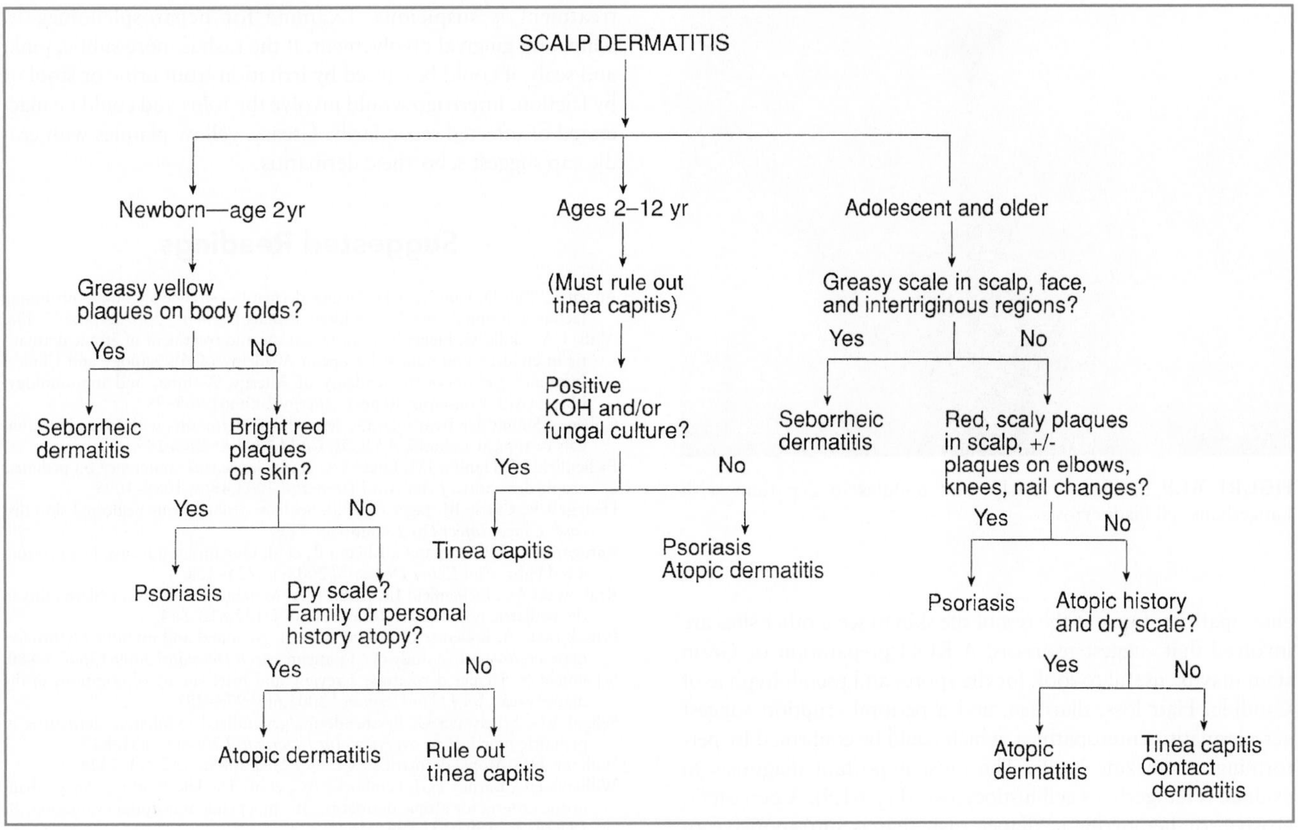

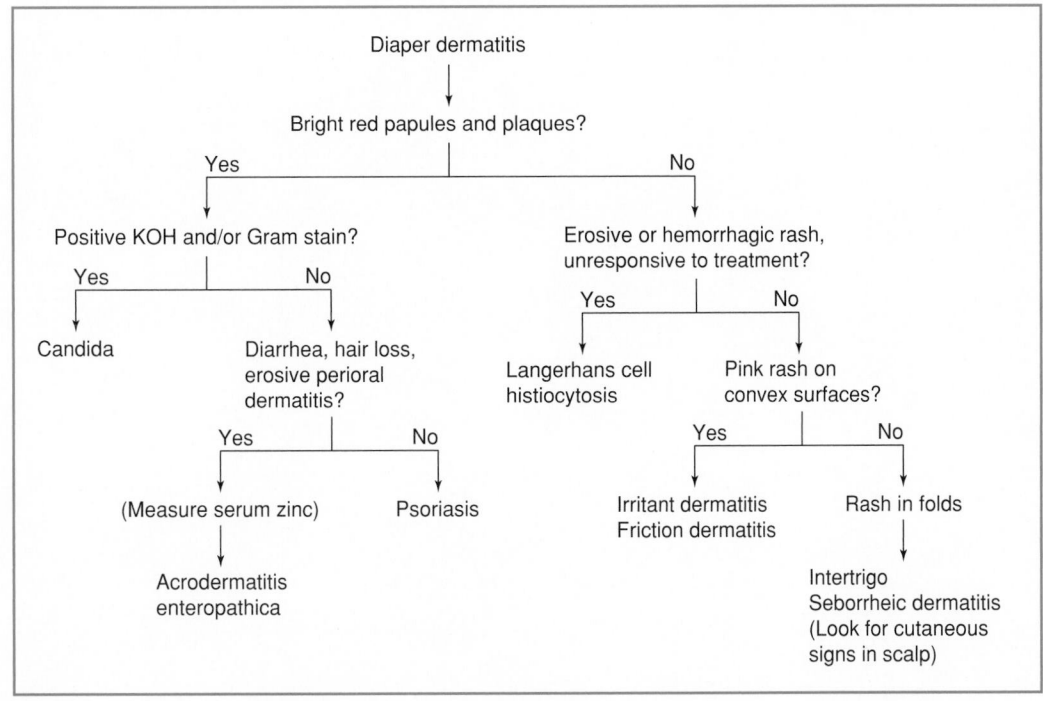

FIGURE 61.7 Diagnostic approach to the child with a scaly scalp.

FIGURE 61.8 Diagnostic approach to diaper dermatitis.

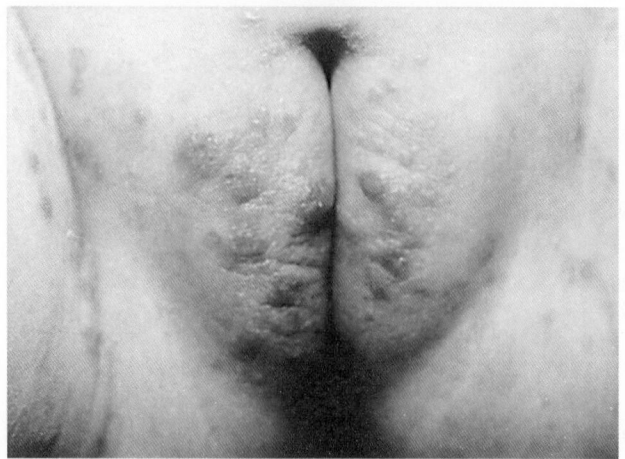

FIGURE 61.9 Persistent vesicles and nodules in a patient with Langerhans cell histiocytosis.

enteropathica. Look at the rest of the skin to see if other sites are involved that suggest psoriasis. A KOH preparation or Gram stain may be useful to look for the spores and pseudohyphae of Candida. Hair loss, diarrhea, and a perioral eruption suggest acrodermatitis enteropathica, which could be confirmed by performing serum zinc levels. The most important diagnosis to exclude is Langerhans cell histiocytosis (Fig. 61.9). A persistent, erosive, or hemorrhagic diaper rash that is unresponsive to treatment is suspicious. Examine for hepatosplenomegaly, scalp, and gingival involvement. If the rash is more subtle, pink, and scaly, it could be caused by irritation from urine or stool or by friction. Intertrigo would involve the folds and could be macerated or infected secondarily. Greasy, yellow plaques with cradle cap suggest seborrheic dermatitis.

Suggested Readings

Adalat S, Wall D, Goodyear H. Diaper dermatitis—frequency and contributing factors in hospital attending children. *Pediatr Dermatol* 2007;24(5):483–488.

Akdis CA, Akdis M, Bieber T, et al. Diagnosis and treatment of atopic dermatitis in children and adults: European Academy of Allergology and Clinical Immunology/American Academy of Allergy, Asthma, and Immunology/PRACTALL Consensus Report. *Allergy* 2006;61:969–987.

Cohen S. Should we treat infantile seborrhoeic dermatitis with topical antifungals or topical steroids? *Arch Dis Child* 2004;89:288–289.

Eichenfield LF, Hanifin JM, Luger TA, et al. Consensus conference on pediatric atopic dermatitis. *J Am Acad Dermatol* 2003;49(6):1088–1095.

Hengge UR, Currie BJ, Jager G, et al. Scabies: a ubiquitous neglected skin disease. *Lancet Infect Dis* 2006;6:769–779.

Katugampola RP, Morgan G, Khetan R, et al. Omenn's syndrome: lessons from a red baby. *Clin Exper Dermatol* 2008;33:425–428.

Krakowski AC, Eichenfield LF, Dohil MA. Management of atopic dermatitis in the pediatric population. *Pediatrics* 2008;122:812–824

Pruszkowski A, Bodemer C, Fraitag S, et al. Neonatal and infantile erythrodermas: a retrospective study of 51 patients. *Arch Dermatol* 2000;136:875–880.

Scheinfeld N. Diaper dermatitis: a review and brief survey of eruptions in the diaper area. *Am J Clin Dermatol* 2005;6(5):273–281.

Sehgal VN, Srivastava G. Erythroderma/generalized exfoliative dermatitis in pediatric practice: an overview. *Int J Dermatol* 2006;45:831–839.

Williams HC. Atopic dermatitis. *N Engl J Med* 2005;352:2314–2324.

Williams HC, Burney PGJ, Pemborke AC, et al. The UK Working Party's diagnostic criteria for atopic dermatitis. III. Independent hospital evaluation. *Br J Dermatol* 1994;131:406–416.

CHAPTER 62 ■ RASH—MACULOPAPULAR

KAREN D. GRUSKIN, MD

Maculopapular rashes are common in pediatric practice, and children often present to the emergency department (ED) for their evaluation and treatment.

Before beginning a discussion of specific causes of maculopapular rashes, it is important to define the clinical characteristics of these types of rashes. A *papule* is a small, solid, mostly elevated lesion that is usually less than 1 cm in diameter. *Macules* are circumscribed flat lesions that differ from surrounding skin because of their color. Both papules and macules may have any size, shape, or color. Commonly, a rash may have papular and macular components, which leads to the term *maculopapular rash*.

The causes of maculopapular rashes are diverse (Table 62.1) and range from benign to life-threatening (Table 62.2). Common causes include viral exanthems, contact dermatitis, insect bites, and scabies (Table 62.3). The diagnostic approach to these disorders is based on the presence or absence of fever, characteristic clinical appearance, location, and chronicity (Fig. 62.1). Some of these conditions have very characteristic clinical appearances (Table 62.4); however, manifestations of these illnesses can be sufficiently variable that a proportion of the cases are difficult to diagnose.

DIFFERENTIAL DIAGNOSIS

Presence of Fever

The potentially life-threatening maculopapular rashes (Table 62.2) are all acute illnesses most commonly associated with fever and significant systemic symptoms. Hence, most patients with these illnesses will appear toxic. Erythema multiforme (EM) and rubeola have recognizable clinical appearances, whereas Kawasaki disease (KWD), Rocky Mountain spotted fever (RMSF), and dengue fever require a high level of clinical suspicion. Other, less severe, febrile illnesses associated with maculopapular rashes are listed in Fig. 62.1.

Potentially Life-threatening Illnesses

Erythema Multiforme

EM is believed to result from an immune-mediated acute hypersensitivity reaction to exposure to a sensitizing antigen (see Chapter 85). Common offenders include drugs, especially trimethoprim-sulfamethoxazole, cefaclor, and phenytoin (more recently, lamotrigine and abacavir have also been implicated); foods, especially nuts and shellfish; and infections by any number of viral, bacterial, protozoal, or fungal organisms.

Herpetic and *Mycoplasma pneumoniae* infections rank among the most common infectious causes.

The rash of EM is characterized by diffuse erythematous macules with central clearing, often called a *target* or *iris lesion*. Lesions may also include erythematous papules, macules, urticarial raised lesions, vesicles, and/or bullae. The distribution is most commonly symmetric and may be noted anywhere on the body with a predilection for the hands and feet, including palms and soles. Lesions may appear in isolation or as a more confluent rash. In the past, patients were classified as having EM minor or EM major/Stevens-Johnson syndrome (SJS). Current theory proposes that EM, SJS, and toxic epidermal necrolysis (TEN) represent a continuum of disease with increasing skin involvement, morbidity, and mortality. EM is primarily a benign, self-limited process whereas TEN is associated with a high fatality rate. EM minor is characterized by cutaneous involvement alone or mucosal involvement that is limited to one surface (usually the mouth) and minimal systemic symptoms. SJS is characterized by extensive skin and mucosal involvement associated with significant systemic symptoms, including fever, chills, and malaise. Skin involvement can progress to sloughing with significant extravascular fluid losses. The term *TEN* is used in cases of severe skin sloughing. Conjunctivitis and keratitis are common features and can lead to permanent corneal scarring. Pulmonary, cardiac, and renal involvement may occur especially in severe cases.

Treatment is predominantly supportive (see Chapter 85). Due to extensive epidermal sloughing, patients with severe SJS or TEN behave similarly to burn patients, and transfer to a pediatric burn unit should be considered. Potentially inciting drugs should be immediately discontinued. For mild cases with pruritus, antihistamines may provide some relief. Oral topical applications of 1:1 mixtures of diphenhydramine and Maalox may provide pain relief from oral lesions. In severe cases, patients require aggressive fluid support and narcotic pain relief. Systemic steroids and intravenous immunoglobulin therapy (IVIG) are of unproven benefit. In fact, some reports suggest a possible increase in morbidity with steroid therapy. Conversely, other data indicate that IVIG may be of benefit in severe cases; however, more studies are required to prove efficacy. Patients with ocular involvement should undergo ophthalmologic evaluation.

Kawasaki Disease

KWD is a well-described illness of unknown cause assumed to be infectious in origin because of its epidemiologic and clinical presentation. However, no infectious agent has been identified and new research suggests that instead an infectious agent initiates an immune cascade that causes the symptoms of KWD

TABLE 62.1

MACULOPAPULAR RASH: ETIOLOGIC CLASSIFICATION

Infectious	*Fungal*
Viral	Pityriasis versicolor
Roseola infantum	*Other Infections*
Rubeola	Rocky Mountain spotted
Rubella	fever
Erythema infectiosum	Ehrlichiosis
(fifth disease)	Mycoplasma (15% of
Varicella (early manifestations	cases)
before bullae)	*Etiology Uncertain But*
Epstein-Barr virus (10–15%	*Thought to Be Viral*
of cases have macular or	Pityriasis rosea
maculopapular rash)	Kawasaki disease
Molluscum contagiosum	Papular acrodermatitis
(papules)	**Noninfectious**
Dengue	*Bites and Infestations*
"Nonspecific" viral	Insect bites
Enterovirus	Scabies
Echovirus	*Miscellaneous*
Coxsackievirus	Drug reaction
Adenovirus	Allergic contact dermatitis
Bacterial	Irritant contact dermatitis
Scarlet fever	Papular urticaria
Syphilis	Erythema multiforme
Disseminated gonorrhea	Guttate psoriasis
	Pityriasis lichenoides
	Lichen nitidus

TABLE 62.2

POTENTIALLY LIFE-THREATENING ILLNESSES ASSOCIATED WITH MACULOPAPULAR RASH

Rocky Mountain spotted fever
Kawasaki disease
Erythema multiforme
Dengue fever
Rubeola
Ehrlichiosis

TABLE 62.3

COMMON DISORDERS ASSOCIATED WITH MACULOPAPULAR RASH

Generalized Rash
Nonspecific viral disease
Enteroviruses
Adenoviruses
Roseola infantum
Erythema infectiosum (fifth disease)
Hand-foot-mouth disease
Scarlet fever
Pityriasis rosea

Localized Rash
Contact dermatitis
Irritant dermatitis
Scabies

sterile pyuria, hepatic dysfunction, arthritis, aseptic meningitis, pericardial effusion, hydrops of the gallbladder, and myocarditis. No laboratory studies are included among the diagnostic criteria; however, certain findings may support the diagnosis. Systemic inflammation causes elevated erythrocyte sedimentation rates and C-reactive protein. Leukocytosis is common with a left shift followed in the second week by marked elevation of platelets (greater than 750,000 per mm³). Other abnormal laboratory results may include a normocytic, normochromic anemia; sterile "mononuclear" pyuria (requires microscopic urine examination as dipstick for leukocyte esterase will be negative); elevation of transaminases; cerebrospinal fluid mononuclear pleocytosis without hypoglycorrhachia or protein elevation; and, hyponatremia (serum sodium lesser than 135 mEq per L) that is associated with an increased risk of coronary artery aneurysms.

The acute phase is usually self-limited but requires accurate diagnosis to prevent the development of coronary artery aneurysms that occur in approximately 20% of cases without therapy. There is an increasing recognition of incomplete disease seen in patients with fever and fewer than four of the previously listed clinical features. Because of the potential for development of coronary artery aneurysms, index of suspicion must remain high and children with possible incomplete disease should be considered candidates for therapy. Atypical disease is more common in children younger than 6 to 12 months of age. A small percentage of those patients who develop aneurysms progress to heart failure, valvular regurgitation, or myocardial infarction, which may prove fatal.

Consultation with a specialist with KWD expertise, usually a pediatric cardiologist or rheumatologist, is recommended prior to initiating therapy. Therapy consists of antiinflammatory agents, specifically high-dose intravenous immunoglobulin (IVIG) and aspirin. Therapy is most often protective against aneurysm development if started during the first 10 days of symptoms. Sadly, there are an increasing number of affected children exhibiting resistance to IVIG therapy who require a second dose for persistent fever and a smaller subset who will not respond to additional doses (for details, see Chapter 101).

(see Chapter 101). Most common in children younger than 5 years, the diagnosis is based on an unremitting fever of at least 5 days' duration and four of the five following features: (i) rash; (ii) nonexudative bulbar conjunctivitis with limbal sparing; (iii) red cracked lips, strawberry tongue, and erythematous oropharynx; (iv) erythema, swelling, and/or induration of peripheral extremities; and (v) a solitary unilateral cervical lymph node of greater than 1.5-cm diameter.

The most commonly associated rash is a generalized pruritic urticaria-like exanthem with raised erythematous plaques; however, the rash may also present with an erythematous maculopapular, morbilliform, scarlatiniform, or erythema marginatum-like pattern. The exanthem may be fleeting or persist for 2 to 3 days. During the later stages of the acute phase, periungual desquamation and peeling of the palms, soles, or perineal area develop. Other complications include

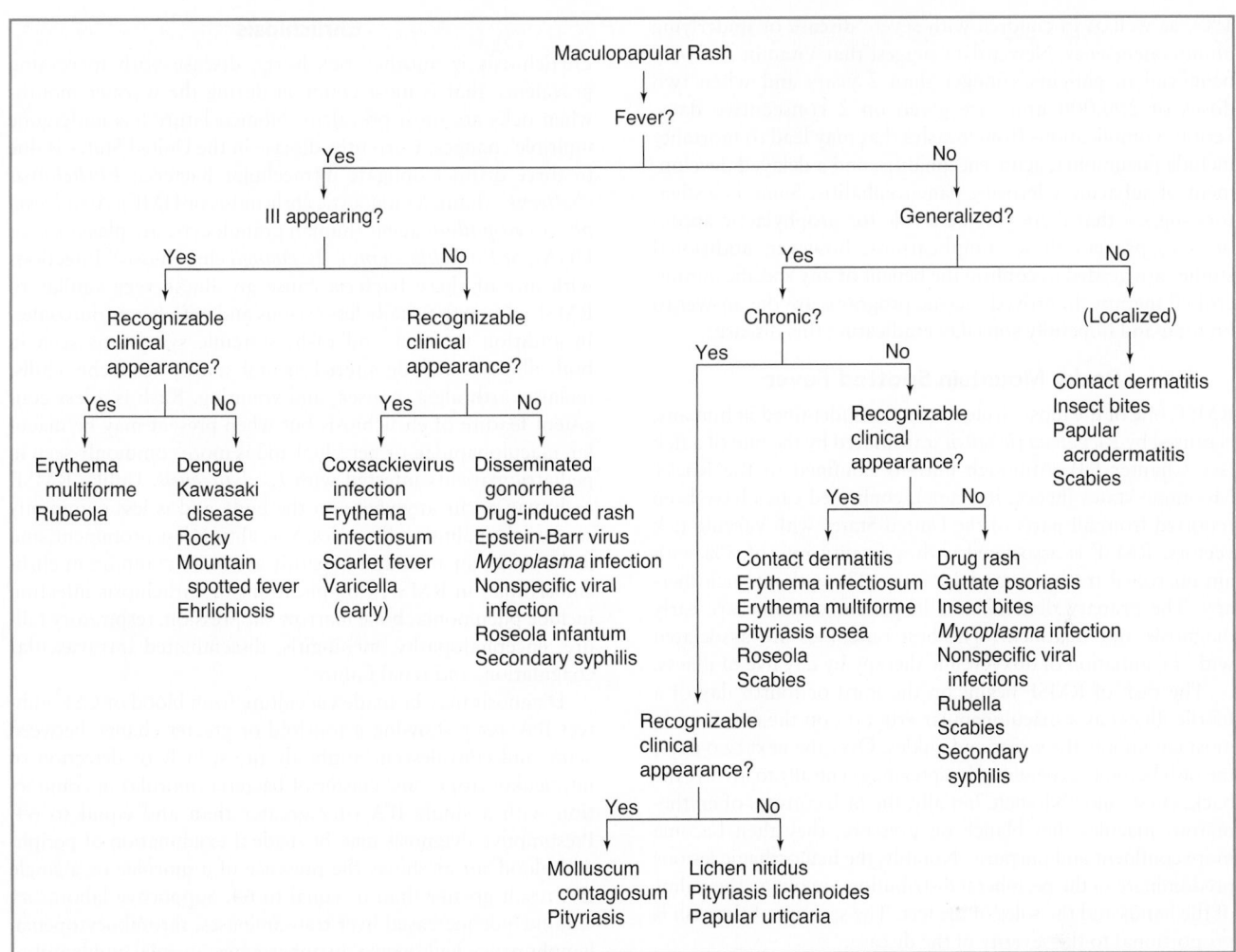

FIGURE 62.1 Diagnostic approach to maculopapular rash.

Measles (Rubeola)

Measles was one of the most common viral exanthems before the advent of the measles vaccine (see Chapter 92). The illness is transmitted by direct contact with droplets from a person infected with the causative RNA-containing paramyxovirus. The incubation period is 10 to 14 days. In its classic form, measles has a highly characteristic natural history. Two to

TABLE 62.4

MACULOPAPULAR RASHES THAT OFTEN HAVE
CHARACTERISTIC CLINICAL APPEARANCES

Rubeola
Erythema infectiosum (fifth disease)
Hand-foot-mouth disease (coxsackievirus A 16)
Molluscum contagiosum
Scarlet fever
Pityriasis versicolor
Pityriasis rosea
Roseola infantum
Insect bites
Erythema multiforme

3 days after the onset of the prodromal symptoms of cough, coryza, conjunctivitis and fever, Koplik spots occur in the mouth, followed 12 to 24 hours later by the cutaneous exanthem. Most typically, Koplik spots appear as pinpoint white lesions on a red base on the buccal mucosa adjacent to the molars; however, they may be seen on any of the mucosal surfaces of the oral cavity except the tongue.

The measles exanthem begins on the head as reddish maculopapules and spreads caudally during the next 4 to 5 days. Within 1 to 2 days of its appearance, the discrete maculopapular lesions coalesce to produce the confluent phase of the rash. Hence, within 2 to 3 days of onset, the rash on the face becomes confluent, whereas the rash on the lower extremities still consists of individual maculopapules. Modified measles occurs in children who have received serum immunoglobulin after exposure to measles. Measles may still occur, but the incubation period may be delayed up to 21 days. The symptoms, although following the usual progression, will be milder. A faint rash and mild febrile illness may occur 7 to 10 days after immunization with the live attenuated measles vaccine.

Diagnosis may be confirmed by testing for measles IgM antibody. No specific therapy exists; however, vitamin A supplementation has been recommended in geographic areas with a high deficiency rate or high measles fatality rate (greater than

1%), as well as in children with severe disease or underlying immunodeficiency. Newer data suggest that Vitamin A is only beneficial in patients younger than 2 years and when two doses of 200,000 units are given on 2 consecutive days. Serious complications from measles that may lead to mortality include pneumonia, acute encephalitis, and a delayed development of subacute sclerosing panencephalitis. Some investigators suggest that there may be a role for prophylactic antibiotics to prevent these complications; however, additional studies are needed to confirm the benefit of any specific antimicrobial therapy. Improved vaccine programs are the answer to limiting and hopefully someday eradicating this disease.

Rocky Mountain Spotted Fever

RMSF, one of the most virulent infections identified in humans, is caused by *Rickettsia rickettsii* transmitted by the bite of a tick (see Chapter 84). Although initially confined to the Rocky Mountain states (hence, its name), confirmed cases have been reported from all parts of the United States with varying tick vectors. RMSF is associated with a fatality rate of 5% with antimicrobial treatment and 13% to 40% without such therapy. The primary determinants in patient outcome are early diagnosis and treatment. The best outcomes are associated with the initiation of doxycycline therapy by day five of illness.

The rash of RMSF begins on the third or fourth day of a febrile illness as a maculopapular eruption on the extremities, most commonly the wrists and ankles. Over the next two days, the rash becomes generalized by spreading centrally to involve the back, chest, and abdomen. Initially, the rash consists of erythematous macules that blanch on pressure; they then become more confluent and purpuric. Notably, the hemorrhagic lesions predominate in the peripheral distribution, involving the palms of the hands and the soles of the feet. The severity of the rash is proportional to the severity of the disease.

All patients with RMSF have some degree of vasculitis that is the basis for many of the associated systemic symptoms. An overall toxic appearance is common. Systemic signs and symptoms include fever, headache, myalgia, conjunctivitis, vomiting, seizures, myocarditis, heart failure, shock; periorbital, facial, or peripheral edema; and disseminated intravascular coagulation or purpura fulminans.

Most commonly, the diagnosis is based on clinical presentation with a history of potential tick exposure. The causative organism is not routinely cultured because of the danger to laboratory personnel. Diagnosis is best made by a serologic test such as indirect immunofluorescence antibody (IFA) assay. Antibodies can be detected 7 to 10 days after onset of illness. Some reference laboratories are now offering polymerase chain reaction (PCR) testing. Thrombocytopenia, hyponatremia and increased aminotransferases usually develop as the disease process progresses but antibiotics should hopefully have been started prior to the development of these findings.

Doxycycline is the drug of choice for therapy in patients of all ages, despite its risk for potentially staining developing teeth at a dose of 4 mg per kg per day in two divided doses (maximum of 100-mg b.i.d.), intravenously or orally. Chloramphenicol is a less optimal alternative and is not effective against ehrlichiosis, which is a common "look-alike" to RMSF. Therapy is continued until the patient is afebrile for at least 2 to 3 days, which usually equals about 7 to 10 days of antibiotic therapy.

Ehrlichiosis

Ehrlichiosis is another tick-borne disease with increasing prevalence that is most common during the warmer months when ticks are most prevalent. Nomenclature has undergone multiple changes. Currently, disease in the United States is due to three distinct obligate intracellular bacteria: *Ehrlichiosis chaffeensis* (human monocytic ehrlichiosis or HME); *Anaplasma phagocytophilum* agent (human granulocytic anaplasmosis or HGA); or *Ehrlichia ewingii* (*E. ewingii* ehrlichiosis). Infections with any of these bacteria cause an illness very similar to RMSF, although usually less serious and with better outcomes. In addition to fever and rash, systemic symptoms seen in both illnesses include altered mental status, headache, chills, malaise, arthralgia, nausea, and vomiting. Rash is a less consistent feature of ehrlichiosis but when present may be macular, maculopapular, or petechial and is more commonly seen in pediatric patients infected with *E. chaffeensis*. Unlike RMSF, rash may occur anywhere on the body and is less commonly seen on the palms and/or soles. Vasculitis is less prominent, and leukopenia, anemia, and hepatitis are more common in ehrlichiosis than in RMSF. Complications of ehrlichiosis infection include pneumonia, bone marrow suppression, respiratory failure, encephalopathy, meningitis, disseminated intravascular coagulation, and renal failure.

Diagnosis may be made via culture from blood or CSF, indirect IFA assay showing a fourfold or greater change between acute and convalescent antibody titers, PCR or detection of intraleukocytoplasmic cluster of bacteria (morula) in conjunction with a single IFA titer greater than and equal to 64. Presumptive diagnosis may be made if examination of peripheral blood smear shows the presence of a morulae or a single IFA result greater than or equal to 64. Supportive laboratory data include increased liver transaminases, thrombocytopenia, lymphopenia, leukopenia, hyponatremia, anemia, and lymphocytic CSF pleocytosis with increased protein concentration.

As for RMSF, doxycycline is the drug of choice for therapy in patients of all ages and at the same dose (see above). Therapy is continued until the patient is afebrile for at least 2 to 3 days and for a minimum total course of 5 to 10 days. Clinical improvement is usually apparent within 3 days, and if not, an alternative diagnosis should be sought. Disease may be more severe or even fatal in untreated patients. Early initiation of therapy minimizes morbidity and mortality.

Dengue Fever

Dengue fever is caused by four dengue viruses transmitted by Aedes mosquitos and is seen in tropical and subtropical areas of almost all continents (including areas of Puerto Rico and the Caribbean basin). The incidence of severe dengue is increasing and may be related to global warming. Many cases are asymptomatic. In symptomatic cases, initial constitutional symptoms include sudden onset of high fever, severe headache, myalgia, arthralgia, and abdominal pain. During the course of fever that lasts 2 to 7 days, back and leg pain may be severe, hence, the disease's nickname "breakbone" fever. The development of a hemorrhagic vasculitis, most common in patients younger than 15 years, leads to the more concerning subtype called dengue hemorrhagic fever. The term dengue shock syndrome is used in even more severe cases when increased vascular permeability leads to shock. Encephalopathy, hepatitis, myocardiopathy, intestinal bleeding, and pneumonia are other complications.

Two distinct rashes may be seen, which coincide with the disease's biphasic fever pattern. The first rash is a generalized, transient, macular rash that blanches under pressure and is seen within the first 24 to 48 hours of the onset of systemic symptoms. The second rash coincides with or occurs 1 to 2 days after defervescence and is a generalized morbilliform or maculopapular rash, sparing the palms and soles.

Diagnosis is based on clinical suspicion and potential exposure based on the virus's geographic distribution. Serologic testing is available as is viral isolation and measurement of serum immunoglobulin antibodies in paired serum specimens obtained 4 weeks apart. Treatment is supportive, and may require aggressive fluid management and pain control. Since a pulse pressure less than or equal to 10 mm Hg has been associated with a worse prognosis, normal saline should be bolused with intensive monitoring to keep the pulse pressure greater than or equal to 30 mm Hg. There are some data from the adult literature suggesting intravenous immunoglobulin and/or plasma exchange may be of benefit is severe cases.

Causes of Other Maculopapular Rashes Associated with Fever

Among non–life-threatening illnesses associated with fever and maculopapular rash are coxsackievirus infections, erythema infectiosum, scarlet fever, and early varicella. Harder to diagnose are rashes associated with Epstein-Barr virus, *Mycoplasma* infections, roseola infantum, disseminated gonorrhea, secondary syphilis, nonspecific viral eruptions, and drug-induced rash. The latter two diagnoses are particularly important to consider in sexually active or potentially abused children.

Coxsackievirus Infections

Coxsackievirus infections of groups A and B (multiple types) can all cause maculopapular exanthems. The classic exanthem of coxsackievirus A16 infection, also appropriately called *hand-foot-mouth disease*, is common and easily recognized. Infections may occur in epidemics, most commonly in the late summer or early fall. Multiple infected members within a household are common.

Coxsackievirus A16 infection begins with a prodrome of low-grade fever, anorexia, mouth pain, and malaise, followed within 1 to 2 days by an oral enanthem and then shortly thereafter by a maculopapular exanthem. The oral lesions begin as small red macules, most often located on the palate, uvula, and anterior tonsillar pillar, which evolve into small vesicles that ulcerate and heal over a 1- to 6-day period. The exanthem begins as maculopapular lesions that develop into small crescent or football-shaped vesicles on an erythematous base. These vesicles, which may be pruritic or mildly tender, are usually located on the dorsal and lateral aspects of fingers, hands, and feet but may develop on the buttocks, arms, legs, and face. The lesions either reabsorb over 2 to 7 days or ulcerate and scab.

The other types of coxsackievirus all cause similar or even indistinguishable exanthems, which may more commonly involve the face, trunk, and proximal extremities. Often, children with these exanthems will be diagnosed with nonspecific

viral infections. Other symptoms attributed to coxsackievirus infection include aseptic meningitis and less commonly myopericarditis, encephalitis, or paralysis. Severe and/or persistent infections may be seen in immunocompromised hosts.

Diagnosis is usually made clinically, although the virus can be easily cultured. PCR assays are available for CSF specimens. The virus is commonly shed for weeks. Coxsackievirus infections are usually self-limiting, so no specific treatment is necessary. IVIG with high antibody titer or pleconaril (a new antiviral drug currently under clinical investigation and available for compassionate use only) may be considered for immunocompromised patients or in life-threatening neonatal infections.

Erythema Infectiosum (Fifth Disease)

Erythema infectiosum is a benign disease caused by parvovirus B19, the same virus that can causes aplastic crises in patients with sickle cell anemia. For the normal, nongravid host, fifth disease is usually of no consequence, with the only systemic symptom being fever in 15% to 30% of cases. On the face is a characteristic, intensely erythematous, "slapped cheek" rash often with a relative circumoral pallor. In addition, a symmetric maculopapular, lacelike rash is seen on the arms and then trunk, buttocks, and thighs, which may be pruritic. In its acute phase, the rash usually lasts only for a few days but can wax and wane in intensity with environmental changes (e.g., exposure to heat or sunlight) for weeks and sometimes months. In a small subset of patients, parovirus B19 causes the atypical papular purpuric gloves and socks syndrome (PPGSS) with a typically painful purpuric exanthem limited to the hands and feet. Immunocompromised children or those with hemolytic anemias can develop red cell aplasia and symptoms associated with a chronic anemia.

Diagnosis is usually made on a clinical basis alone but may be confirmed in an immunocompetent host by measuring parovirus B19–specific IgM antibody. PCR is the best modality for diagnosis in an immunocompromised host. No specific therapy is necessary in immunocompetent hosts. For a chronic infection in an immunodeficient patient, IVIG therapy should be considered. Because parvovirus is associated with fetal anemia, congestive heart failure and hydrops-exposed pregnant women should be referred to their physicians to discuss possible parvovirus antibody testing.

Scarlet Fever

Scarlet fever is caused by phage-infected group A streptococcus that makes an erythrogenic toxin. This disease is still seen with regularity but does not appear to be any more serious than group A streptococcal infection without rash. Scarlet fever is most commonly associated with streptococcal pharyngitis but may occur in association with pyoderma or an infected wound.

The diagnosis of scarlet fever can be made clinically in a child with signs and symptoms of pharyngitis who has a fine, raised, generalized maculopapular rash. The skin has a coarse or sandpapery feel on palpation. Typically, there is sparing of the circumoral area, leading to circumoral pallor. There is usually a bright erythema of the tongue and hypertrophy of the papillae, leading to the term *strawberry tongue*. Pastia's lines, bright red, orange, or even hemorrhagic lines, can occasionally be seen in the axillae or antecubital fossa. The rash generally lasts 3 to 5 days, followed by brownish discoloration and peeling of the skin as small flakes to entire casts of the digits. A rapid streptococcal test or throat culture should be sent to confirm infection. Various antibiotic regimens provide effective treatment (see Chapter 84).

Varicella (Chickenpox)

Although varicella is an easily recognizable vesiculobullous eruption, on occasion, the earliest phase can be confusing. The initial skin manifestations of varicella virus infection are small, red macules. Some of the lesions remain as macules, but most progress to papules and then the characteristic umbilicated, tear-shaped vesicles. The earliest lesions appear on the chest and spread centrifugally, but there are many exceptions to the pattern of spread. Occasionally, a child with mild chickenpox may have only a few scattered macules with only one or two progressing to the more typical vesicular lesions. Of children receiving varicella vaccine, 7% to 8% may develop a mild maculopapular or varicelliform rash within 1 month of vaccination (see Chapter 84).

Epstein-Barr Virus

Between 5% and 15% of patients with Epstein-Barr viral infection, otherwise known as infectious mononucleosis, will have an erythematous maculopapular eruption. Infection in young children is usually asympomatic or so mild that diagnosis is not sought. Older patients between 15 and 25 years of age are more likely to present for evaluation. In addition, 50% to 100% of patients with infectious mononucleosis develop a maculopapular rash after receiving concurrent ampicillin or amoxicillin-containing antibiotics—most commonly for an incorrectly diagnosed streptococcal pharyngitis.

The illness begins insidiously with headache, malaise, and fever, followed by sore throat, membranous tonsillitis, and lymphadenopathy. Splenomegaly is common. The exanthem occurs within 4 to 6 days as a macular or maculopapular morbilliform eruption most prominent on the trunk and proximal extremities. An enanthem consisting of discrete petechiae at the junction of the hard and soft palate occurs in approximately 25% of patients. A small subset of patients develop more serious disease often involving the central nervous system.

Diagnosis is often presumed clinically but may be supported by an absolute increase in atypical lymphocytes, a positive heterophile antibody (monospot) test (obtained after the first week of symptoms) or confirmed by serology. The heterophile antibody test is less sensitive in children younger than 4 years of age. The illness is most commonly self-limited, requiring no therapy, but due to the frequency of associated splenomegaly, affected children should not be allowed to participate in contact sports until fully recovered and the spleen is no longer palpable. Amoxicillin should be avoided for any concurrent infections. Corticosteroids may be considered for patients with particularly severe tonsillitis (see Chapter 84).

Mycoplasma Infections

Infections with *Mycoplasma* pneumoniae may cause maculopapular rashes in up to 15% of cases. The classic clinical presentation is of a child with malaise, low-grade fever, and prominent cough. The cough is initially nonproductive but may become productive, particularly in older children, and may persist for 3 to 4 weeks. Physical examination may show bilateral rales. Roentgenographic examination of the chest, if abnormal, most commonly shows diffuse nonspecific infiltrates.

Diagnosis can be suggested by serum cold hemagglutinins, which are present in more than 50% of cases by the beginning of the second week. If further confirmatory studies are needed, acute and convalescent serum sera should be assayed for specific mycoplasmal antibodies by complement fixation or immunofluorescence. Erythromycin, clarithromycin, or azithromycin is the treatment of choice (see Chapter 84).

Roseola Infantum

Roseola infantum, also called *exanthem subitum* or *sixth disease*, is attributed to primary infection with human herpes virus (HHV)-6. The illness is characterized by the onset of a maculopapular rash that appears following a 3- to 4-day febrile illness. The fever is characteristically high. The rash is widely disseminated, appearing as discrete, small, pinkish macules that rarely coalesce, beginning on the trunk and then extending peripherally. The rash may last for hours to days. The occurrence of the rash within 24 hours of defervescence rather than the morphologic appearance of the rash leads to the correct diagnosis. The rash can appear very similar to that seen in measles, but the child with roseola appears well and no longer febrile. Diagnosis is made clinically and care is supportive.

Disseminated Neisseria Gonorrhea

Disseminated *Neisseria gonorrhoeae* should be considered in sexually active or potentially abused children, especially if associated with a history of vaginal or penile discharge. A distinct minority of patients develop disseminated gonorrhea infection through hematogenous spread. Disseminated gonorrhea may cause a range of cutaneous lesions, including small erythematous papules, petechiae, or vesicle-pustules on a hemorrhagic base. These cutaneous lesions usually develop on the trunk but may occur anywhere on the extremities.

An etiologic diagnosis can be established by demonstration of the organism on Gram stain of the skin lesion, positive blood culture, or positive culture of oral or genital sites. Based on resistance patterns, recommended current therapy is ceftriaxone 50 mg per kg per day (maximum 1 g per day) until clinical improvement is seen, at which point it can be changed to an oral antibiotic, such as cefixime, ciprofloxacin, ofloxacin, or levofloxacin, for a total of a 7-day course. Quinolones should not be used for infections in men who have intercourse with men or in those with a history of recent foreign travel or partners' travel, or infections acquired in other areas with increased resistance. Concomitant sexually transmitted diseases should be sought and treated empirically (see Chapters 84 and 94).

Secondary Syphilis

One needs a high level of suspicion when viewing rashes in sexually active (or potentially abused) children to make the diagnosis of secondary syphilis, caused by the spirochete *Treponema pallidum*. Manifestations of secondary syphilis usually occur 6 to 8 weeks after the appearance of the primary lesion, which may have gone unnoticed. The exanthem extends rapidly and is usually pronounced, lasting for only hours or persisting for several months.

The rash of secondary syphilis is characterized by a generalized cutaneous eruption, usually composed of brownish, dull-red macules or papules that range in size from a few millimeters to 1 cm in diameter. They are generally discrete and symmetrically distributed, particularly over the trunk, where they follow the lines of cleavage in a pattern similar to pityriasis rosea. Papular lesions on the palms and soles, as well as the presence of systemic symptoms, such as general malaise, fever, headaches, sore throat, rhinorrhea, lacrimation, and generalized lymphadenopathy, help differentiate secondary syphilis.

Acquired syphilis is sexually contracted from direct contact with ulcerative lesions of the skin or mucous membranes of an infected individual. Diagnosis may be presumed after a positive nontreponemal test, such as the VDRL slide test, rapid plasma reagin test, or the automated reagin test. Diagnosis should be confirmed by a treponemal test, such as the fluorescent treponemal antibody absorption test, the microhemagglutination test for *Treponema palladium*, or the *T. palladium* immobilization test. Definitive diagnosis may also be made by identifying spirochetes by microscopic dark-field examination or direct fluorescent antibody tests of lesion exudate or tissue. Penicillin is the treatment of choice unless contraindicated, in which case tetracycline, doxycycline, ceftriaxone, or erythromycin may be substituted. Length of therapy should be based on duration and stage of infection. Concomitant sexually transmitted diseases should be sought and treated empirically. HIV testing is recommended for patients with secondary syphilis (see Chapters 84 and 94).

Nonspecific Viral Exanthems

Many times, a specific diagnosis cannot be made even after considering such factors as exposure history, history of preceding illness, description of eruption, time and site of onset, character of initial lesion, progression, distribution patterns, and occurrence of mucosal lesions. This should not be surprising, given the large number of viruses that can be associated with macular or maculopapular eruptions. In particular, enteroviruses and adenoviruses can cause a macular or maculopapular eruption. In fact, enterovirus 71 is now known to be the cause of a subset of cases of hand-foot-mouth disease. There is little to distinguish the rash caused by one of these viruses from that of another, based on the location and morphology, with the exception of those viral infections previously discussed. One usually arrives at the diagnosis of nonspecific viral exanthem in a child in whom other diagnoses have been excluded and who may have signs of associated illness or systemic features such as fever. If specific diagnosis is required, it can be determined by viral isolation and/or a rise in diagnostic titer.

Drug-Induced Rash

Multiple drugs can cause maculopapular rashes in susceptible patients. Most commonly, these rashes have an abrupt onset, are generalized, and may be accompanied by systemic signs such as fever, arthralgia, lymphadenopathy, and hepatomegaly. It is often difficult to distinguish drug eruptions from viral exanthems. This is especially true when an emergency physician is faced with a child who recently was started on one or several medications, often including antibiotics, who now presents with the emergence of a new rash associated with or following a viral-type illness.

The diagnosis of drug eruption depends on a carefully obtained history, including the duration and frequency of all medications taken by the child during the week preceding the onset of the rash. The presence of eosinophilia suggests, but does not confirm, the diagnosis. Often, the final diagnosis is left to the intuition of the physician. In the case of a severe eruption, the potentially offending drug should be discontinued. In milder cases, which more closely resemble nonspecific viral exanthems, a physician may opt to continue therapy as long as the rash does not worsen, with the distinct exception of lamotrigine and abacivir. Regardless of the extent of the rash, both drugs should be discontinued, not reintroduced, and immediately referred to the appropriate specialist for management. The disadvantage of simply discontinuing any other potentially offending drug is that the patient is often labeled as "allergic" to the drug for life. In addition, reactions may be caused by preservatives or dyes in a drug preparation and not by the drug itself.

Illnesses Associated with Maculopapular Rashes without Fever

Maculopapular rashes associated with nonfebrile illnesses tend to be benign. Erythema infectiosum, EM, *Mycoplasma* infections, roseola infantum, secondary syphilis, and nonspecific viral exanthems, which in mild cases may not be associated with fever, have been previously discussed. In approaching the acute afebrile disorders associated with maculopapular rash, it is useful to distinguish between those that cause generalized eruptions and those that cause localized ones. Disorders not usually associated with fever but that cause generalized eruptions include rubella, guttate psoriasis, and pityriasis rosea. Conditions that cause mostly local eruptions include papular acrodermatitis (Gianotti-Crosti syndrome), contact dermatitis, insect bites, and scabies. The chronic duration of some maculopapular rashes not associated with fever helps to lead to the correct diagnosis; examples include lichen nitidus, molluscum contagiosum, papular urticaria, pityriasis lichenoides (Mucha-Habermann disease), and pityriasis versicolor. Molluscum contagiosum, pityriasis rosea, pityriasis versicolor, and forms of contact dermatitis also present with clinically recognizable rashes.

Generalized Eruptions Without Fever

Guttate Psoriasis

About one-third of psoriasis cases begin in the first two decades of life among individuals with a genetic predisposition. The guttate form commonly occurs in younger age groups. The rash is characterized by multiple small discrete round or oval macules or papules (up to 1 cm in diameter) with a loosely adherent scale. The lesions develop predominantly on the trunk, but the face and scalp may be involved. The distal extremities, palms, and soles are usually spared. The lesions of guttate psoriasis are less hyperkeratotic as other types of chronic psoriatic plaques and may respond better to standard psoriasis therapy.

Pityriasis Rosea

Pityriasis rosea is a benign, self-limited condition that most commonly affects older children and adolescents, although it can occur at younger ages. The cause is unknown but is likely to be viral (see Chapter 99).

Pityriasis rosea follows a characteristic clinical course. The initial lesion, the herald patch, is an oval-shaped plaque that occurs in about 80% of cases. The center of the lesion is flat, whereas the borders are raised, red, and scaly. The herald patch can occur anywhere on the body but is most commonly seen on the trunk, neck, or proximal extremities. The herald patch is often mistaken for tinea corporis. One to 2 weeks later, a more generalized, sometimes pruritic, rash erupts. The rash is most dense on the trunk, neck, and proximal limbs. The face and distal extremities are relatively spared but may be involved in younger children. Individual lesions are erythematous papulosquamous ovals that often resemble smaller versions of the herald patch. The long axes of the ovals tend to orient along the lines of cleavage, creating a characteristic "Christmas tree" distribution along the patient's posterior trunk. Atypical distributions (predominantly peripheral) and other individual lesions (papules, vesicles, pustules, urticarial, or purpuric lesions) can occur.

Rubella

Rubella is rarely seen in the postvaccine era in the United States. In a classic case of rubella, the rash, similar to measles, begins on the head and spreads caudally. The progression occurs over 2 to 3 days, and typically, the rash is entirely gone by the fourth day. The rash always remains macular and never becomes confluent, which is an important distinguishing characteristic. One-third of all rubella virus infections are clinically silent (i.e., they have no exanthem). The rash of rubella may show extensive variation in location, progression, and duration, at times disappearing within 12 hours or being localized to one part of an extremity without any progression.

Unlike measles, in which systemic toxicity and fever are the rule, fever is uncommon. Associated symptoms and complaints in rubella include joint pain and adenopathy (most commonly suboccipital, postauricular, and cervical). Arthralgia that occurs with a viral exanthem is highly characteristic for rubella. Diagnosis is based on clinical presentation, and treatment is supportive.

Localized Eruptions without Fever

Contact dermatitis, insect bites, papular acrodermatitis, and scabies usually present in a localized distribution; however, all may appear as a more generalized eruption in extensive cases.

Contact Dermatitis

Contact dermatitis may be caused either by a primary exposure to an irritant or by an acquired delayed hypersensitivity response to a sensitizing substance (see Chapter 99). In the former case, it is termed an *irritant contact dermatitis*, whereas the latter is referred to as a true *allergic contact dermatitis*. Although distinct in etiology, both rashes usually are localized and assume the pattern of an irritating or a sensitizing agent. A sharp demarcation commonly exists between the involved and uninvolved skin areas. Affected skin is erythematous with variable numbers and combinations of macules, papules, vesicles, and/or bullae.

Irritant dermatitis arises from direct contact with agents such as detergents, soaps, acids, alkalis, or rough sheets/clothes. This disorder often is seen in infancy when the skin is relatively thin and susceptible to mechanical or chemical irritation. Allergic contact dermatitis, exemplified by rhus dermatitis (e.g., poison

ivy, poison oak) or nickel dermatitis (jewelry, wristwatches), is more common in older children after exposure to the offending agents.

Diagnosis depends on obtaining a thorough history of exposure and the presence of a characteristic localized pattern of rash. Treatment for both types of these dermatitides includes eliminating exposure to offending irritants, providing topical or systemic antipruritic agents, and for more severe cases, providing topical or systemic steroids (see Chapter 99).

Insect Bites

Virtually all children experience insect bites. Mosquitoes, fleas, and bedbugs are the most common offenders. Diagnosis depends on the season, the climate, exposure to animals, and distribution and appearance of the lesions. In temperate climates, mosquito bites occur exclusively in the warmer months of the year, whereas flea and bedbugs afflict patients year-round. Often, a series of bites occurs in groups, causing a maculopapular appearance. Local reactions can be extensive and take several days to resolve. Care is aimed at minimizing discomfort with topical or systemic antihistamines and/or topical steroids.

Papular Acrodermatitis (Gianotti-Crosti Syndrome)

Papular acrodermatitis is an eruption of unclear cause that has been associated with hepatitis B, EBV, and other viral infections in young children. In the pediatric population, 85% are younger than 3 years. The eruption may follow a low-grade fever or mild upper respiratory symptoms.

The eruption consists of flesh-colored papules that occur anywhere on the body but often concentrate on the extensor surfaces of the arms, legs, and buttock. Lesions are particularly prominent over the elbows and knees. The rash usually lasts 2 to 8 weeks and then disappears. No treatment is needed for the cutaneous eruption; however, a subset of patients with cutaneous lesions develops generalized lymphadenopathy and hepatosplenomegaly. These children should be evaluated for hepatitis and follow-up in 2 weeks is recommended for patients with only cutaneous involvement to exclude hepatitis (see Chapter 93).

Scabies

Scabies is a contagious infestation of the *Sarcoptes scabiei* female mite that selects a favorable body site, burrows beneath the stratum corneum, and deposits eggs along the way. In older children and adults, the usual sites of infestation include the anterior axillary lines, the areolae, the lower part of the abdomen, buttocks, genitals, wrists, interdigital webs, and ankles. In young children, the lesions are usually more diffuse and may also occur on the palms, soles, scalp, and neck (see Chapter 99).

The pathognomonic primary lesion may be visible as a linear, gray-brown, threadlike burrow a few millimeters in length, with a central black dot (the mite). More frequently, the lesions appear as erythematous papules that may be excoriated and possibly secondarily infected because of intense pruritus. On occasion, generalized urticarial or "id" reactions develop.

Diagnosis is usually based on clinical suspicion, although definitive confirmation can be made by identifying the adult mite on microscopic examination of a scraping of suspicious burrows. The treatment of choice in children over 2 months of age is the topical application of permethrin 5% cream, which may be repeated in 2 weeks, if necessary. Pruritus often persists for several weeks after the mites have been eradicated. It is advisable to treat close family members or personal contacts with or without evidence of infestation. Because mites are unable to survive away from their human hosts or at high temperatures, clothing, bedding, and stuffed animals should be laundered in hot water (greater than 50°C, or 120°F) or stored away for several days in plastic bags. Antihistamines provide symptomatic relief for itching that often continues for several weeks despite of successful treatment. Treatment options for nonresponders to permethrin include crotamiton 10%, ivermectin and lindane; however, these therapies are not universally approved for scabies and need to be used with caution.

Chronic Eruptions without Fever

Chronic eruptions are defined as those that are usually present for a minimum of 2 weeks.

Lichen Nitidus

Lichen nitidus is a relatively rare, benign skin disorder that occurs predominatly in preschool and school-age children. It is believed to perhaps be a variant of lichen planus. The eruption consists of groups of tiny, shiny, flesh-colored papules. The lesions commonly occur in lines of local trauma (Kobner's phenomenon) and are most often seen on the trunk, abdomen, forearm, and genitalia. There is no known effective treatment, and the eruption can last for years.

Molluscum Contagiosum

Molluscum contagiosum is caused by a viral infection and consists of discrete flesh-colored papules, usually 2 to 3 mm in diameter, with umbilicated centers (see Chapter 99). Axillary lines of the trunk, abdomen, genital region, inner aspect of the thighs, and the face are the most common sites of presentation, although any hair-free surface may be involved. Usually, a child will have approximately ten scattered lesions; however, on occasion, some may have many more. The lesions tend to persist anywhere from 2 weeks to 1.5 years and may be spread by autoinoculation. Spread can occur between individuals involved in contact sports. The lesions are asymptomatic, with the exception of a minority of patients who develop an inflammatory reaction. When deemed necessary, treatment involves techniques such as liquid nitrogen, curettage, or topical cantharidin or imiquimod (see Chapter 99).

Papular Urticaria

Papular urticaria, a benign condition seen most commonly in young children, is manifested by a chronic or recurrent papular eruption caused by a sensitivity reaction to insect bites. The lesions are usually papules with a central punctum that may rest on an urticarial base. The lesions are most commonly seen in the warm months, when exposure to insects is most intense. Diagnosis is usually made clinically. Treatment is aimed at minimizing exposure to insect bites and providing therapy with simple sedation, topical calamine, or topical corticosteroid to minimize pruritus (see Chapter 99).

Pityriasis Lichenoides (Mucha-Habermann Disease)

Pityriasis lichenoides, or Mucha-Habermann disease, is a relatively rare disorder of unknown cause that can appear in childhood and young adulthood. There are two forms: acute and chronic. The acute disease is characterized by a macular, papular, or papulovesicular rash that is often distributed most heavily on the trunk and upper arms. The lesions occur in successive crops rapidly evolving into vesicular, necrotic, and even purpuric lesions, which may leave pocklike scars. Resolution occurs spontaneously but may take several weeks to months and recurrences may occur. Parents may describe these recurrences as "he keeps getting the chickenpox." The more chronic form may evolve from the acute form or may arise de novo and often lasts for several years. There is no established therapy.

Pityriasis Versicolor

Pityriasis Versicolor (formly Tinea versicolor) is a superficial skin disease caused by the fungus *Pityrosporum orbiculare*, formerly called *Malassezia furfur* (see Chapter 99). Although adolescents and young adults are most commonly affected, the disorder can occur at any age. The distribution of scaly macular lesions is patchy and occurs most commonly over the upper trunk and proximal arms. Occasionally, the face and other areas of the body can become involved. In summer, affected areas are relatively hypopigmented compared to the surrounding unaffected skin because the organism blocks tanning. In winter, the affected areas appear darker than the unaffected skin because the fungus causes mild erythema. This phenomenon of variable coloration of the affected skin gives the disease its name.

The diagnosis is often made by recognition of the characteristic rash. Wood's light examination in a darkened room produces a reddish-brown fluorescence. Microscopic examination of scrapings will demonstrate characteristic hyphae and spores in grapelike clusters ("spaghetti and meatballs" appearance). Initial treatment usually consists of selenium sulfide shampoos weekly for 3 weeks and then monthly for 3 months. Oral antifungal therapy is another option but has not been approved for this usage. Infection may recur and repigmentation may take several months.

EVALUATION AND DECISION

In approaching a child with a maculopapular exanthem, the initial steps are to take a history and to fully examine all cutaneous surfaces. The most important historical features include the duration of the rash (acute or chronic), initial distribution, extent of spread (generalized or localized), ill contacts (including sexual partners of adolescent patients), and any associated systemic symptoms, including fever. The physical examination should include a careful systematic inspection of all mucocutaneous surfaces, with special attention paid to involvement of the oropharynx, palms and soles, extensor or flexor surfaces, scalp, and trunk.

For patients who do not appear ill, certain exanthems will have distinctive patterns that will immediately strike the examiner and make the diagnosis readily apparent. EM, rubella, coxsackievirus infections, erythema infectiosum, scarlet fever, varicella, molluscum contagiosum, pityriasis versicolor, pityriasis rosea, and roseola all have recognizable clinical appearances. Many of these illnesses have characteristic distributions or associated signs and symptoms that aid in their diagnoses. If the pattern of the rash does not evoke immediate recognition from the examiner, a more methodical approach is indicated, as outlined in Fig. 62.1.

For patients with maculopapular rash who appear particularly ill, the potential diagnoses of rubeola (measles), EM, KWD, RMSF, ehrlichiosis, and dengue fever should spring to mind.

Acutely Ill-appearing Patients

Rubeola and EM both have characteristic rashes that are often associated with oral involvement. Patients with rubeola may have a history of an ill contact and several days of cough, coryza, conjunctivitis, and escalating fever. EM may present with a history of the recent introduction of a medication. KWD should be considered in children who have been febrile for more than 5 days and who have or have had conjunctivitis, red lips/strawberry tongue, a solitary enlarged cervical lymph node, and a rash. Clues to the possibility of RMSF, ehrlichiosis, or dengue fever may be obtained from a travel history or known cases within the geographic location. Patients with RMSF may have history of tick bite, and the hemorrhagic rash characteristically remains more peripherally distributed involving the palms and soles. Often confused with RMSF is ehrlichiosis, which may also present with history of tick bite and is clinically similar to RMSF but is associated with fewer vasculitic-type symptoms. Dengue fever should be considered in patients with a biphasic fever pattern and musculoskeletal pain.

Other Generalized Febrile Eruptions

An acute, generalized febrile maculopapular exanthem is usually the result of a nonspecific viral or streptococcal (scarlet fever) infection. The disorders that are seen in acutely ill-appearing patients, discussed previously, may present as milder versions and should be considered as possible causes in less acutely ill febrile children with generalized eruptions. Other viral and bacterial infections may require a higher index of suspicion and confirmatory studies.

Nonspecific viral exanthems most characteristically consist of multiple, closely spaced small papules. The finding of pharyngitis, a strawberry tongue, or intensely erythematous lines in the antecubital fossae points to scarlet fever; however, a throat culture or rapid screening test for streptococcal infection should still be obtained.

Coxsackievirus infections, erythema infectiosum, and early varicella should be able to be diagnosed based on their clinical appearance. It should be remembered that the eruption of varicella is initially maculopapular; however, close inspection usually reveals a few vesicles by the time the child is brought to medical attention.

The final considerations in febrile patients with generalized maculopapular rash are Epstein-Barr virus infections (infectious mononucleosis), *Mycoplasma* infections, roseola infantum, disseminated gonorrhea, and secondary syphilis. The exanthem of infectious mononucleosis should be suspected in the child or, more commonly, in the adolescent who has strep-

tococcal negative pharyngitis and/or history of taking ampicillin or a closely related antibiotic. For children with nonspecific viral symptoms with prominent cough, *Mycoplasma* infection may be the diagnosis. Roseola infantum should be considered in the child who develops maculopapular rash after fever has defervesced. Finally, disseminated gonorrhea and secondary syphilis should be considered in sexually active adolescents and appropriate tests should be sent for confirmation.

Generalized Afebrile Eruptions

Although nonspecific viral illnesses that cause rash are more often than not associated with fever, a minority of children with viral exanthems remain afebrile. Often, no specific diagnosis is possible. Again, the appearance of a diffuse rash in an infant or toddler immediately after the defervescence of a high fever indicates the clinical diagnosis of roseola. Similarly, pronounced posterior occipital lymphadenopathy in an unvaccinated child suggests rubella. If a child is taking any medications, drug rash must be considered. Because a drug reaction is difficult to exclude initially, consideration for discontinuing medications is warranted in severe cases. Also common, pityriasis rosea is distinguished by its characteristic predominantly truncal distribution along the skin folds. Rarely does guttate psoriasis present acutely with a diffuse maculopapular eruption.

Localized Eruptions

The most common causes for acute, localized maculopapular eruptions are contact dermatitis and insect bites. Contact dermatitis may be caused by irritation or allergy. History may be helpful in establishing a diagnosis, as in the case of a child who returns from camp with an allergic dermatitis on the arms and legs (rhus dermatitis or poison ivy) or a teenager who gets an irritant dermatitis of the wrist after wearing a new watch. Irritant reactions are usually exclusively maculopapular, whereas allergic eruptions may become vesicular or eczematous and may also have a characteristic linear appearance. The papules of insect bites are usually isolated lesions, as opposed to the confluent rash seen in contact dermatitis. In temperate climates, insect bites occur most commonly in the summer, but the possibility of bedbugs or fleas should not be overlooked during the colder months. Scabies is a relatively common and potentially difficult diagnosis. Linear lesions and involvement of the web spaces are characteristic; however, often a diagnostic scraping or presumptive therapy is indicated. Gianotti-Crosti syndrome is a rare disorder that produces primarily an eruption limited to the distal extremities. Any of the causes of localized eruptions may appear more generalized in extensive or severe cases.

Chronic Eruptions

Chronic maculopapular eruptions are usually, and more appropriately, seen by physicians in settings other than the ED. However, parents may become acutely concerned about a real or perceived change in a chronic eruption; thus, the emergency physician should be familiar with the more common disorders.

The most commonly seen of the chronic maculopapular eruptions are papular urticaria, molluscum contagiosum, and pityriasis versicolor. Papular urticaria is most common in warm weather but may occur at any time of the year; the characteristic lesions have an urticarial wheal around a central papule. The papules of molluscum contagiosum have an easily recognizable umbilicated central core. Pityriasis versicolor consists of hypopigmented and hyperpigmented areas, predominantly on the trunk. This diagnosis can be confirmed by microscopy or culture. Although uncommon, secondary syphilis needs to be considered in any sexually active patient and a serologic test performed as indicated.

Suggested Readings

Baumer JH, Love SJL, Gupta A, et al. Salicylate for the treatment of Kawasaki disease in children. *Cochrane Database Syst Rev* 2006, Issue 4. Art. No.: CD004175. DOI: 10.1002/14651858.CD004175.pub2.

Buckingham SC. Rocky Mountain spotted fever: a review for the pediatrician. *Pediatr Ann* 2002;31(3):163–168.

Centers for Disease Control and Prevention. Sexually transmitted diseases treatment guidelines 2006. *MMWR* 55(No. RR-11):1–94.

Forman R, Koren G, Shear NH. Erythema multiforme, Stevens-Johnson syndrome and toxic epidermal necrolysis in children: a review of 10 years' experience. *Drug Saf* 2002;25(13):965–972.

Genzi J, Miron D, Spiegel R, et al. Kawasaki disease in very young infants: high prevalence of atypical presentation and coronary arteritis. *Clin Pediatr* 2003;42(3):263–267.

Homan RC, Paddock CD, Curns AT, et al. Analysis of risk factors for fatal Rocky Mountain spotted fever: evidence for superiority of tetracyclines for therapy. *J Infect Dis* 2001;184(11):1437–1444.

Huiming Y, Chaomin W. Meng M. Vitamin A for treating measles in children. Cocharane Database Syst Rev 2005, Issue 4. Art. No.: CD001479. DOI: 10.1002/14651858.CD001479.pub3.

Kabra SK, Lodha R, Hilton DJ. Antibiotic for preventing complications in children with measles. *Cochrane Database Syst Rev* 2008, Issue 3. Art. No.: CD001477. DOI: 10.1002./14651858.cd001477.pub3.

Kahwaji IY, Connuck DM, Tafari N, et al. A national survey on the pediatric cardiologist's clinical approach for patients with Kawasaki disease. *Pediatr Cardiol* 2002;23(6):639–646.

Meissner HC, Leung DYM. Kawasaki syndrome: where are the answers? *Pediatrics* 2003;112(3):672–676.

Oates-Whitehead RM, Baumer JH, Haines L, et al. Intravenous immunoglobulin for the treatment of Kawasaki disease in children. *Cochrane Database Syst Rev* 2003, Issue 4. Art. No.: CD004000. DOI: 10.1002/14651858. CD004000.

Orenstein, WA. The role of measles elimination in development of a National Immunization Program. *Pediatr Infect Dis J* 2006;25(12):1093–1101.

Paller AS, Mancini AJ. *Hurwitz clinical pediatric dermatology: a textbook of skin disorders of childhood and adolescence.* 3rd ed. Philadelphia: WB Saunders, 2005.

Pickering LK, Baker CJ, Long SS, et al., eds. *Red Book: 2006 Report of the Committee on Infectious Disease.* 27th ed. Elk Grove Village, IL: American Academy of Pediatrics, 2006.

Prendiville J. Stevens-Johnson syndrome and toxic epidermal necrolysis. *Adv Dermatol* 2002;18:151–173.

Schutze GE, et al. and the Tick-borne Infections in Children Study (TICS) Group. Human monocytic ehrlichiosis in children. *Pediatr Infect Dis J* 2007;26:475–479.

Sexton DJ, Kaye KS. Rocky Mountain spotted fever. *Med Clin North Am* 2002;86(2):351–360.

Shann F. Severe dengue: coming soon to a pediatric intensive care unit near you? *Pediatr Crit Care Med* 2005:6 (4):490–492.

Singh-Behl D, La Rosa SP, Tomecki KJ. Tick-borne infections. *Dermatol Clin* 2003;21(2):237–244.

Tremoulet B, Best S, Song S, et al. Burns. Resistance to intravenous immunoglobulin in children with Kawasaki disease. *J Pediatr* 2008;153(1):117–121.

SIGNS AND SYMPTOMS

CHAPTER 63 ■ RASH—PAPULAR LESIONS

PAUL J. HONIG, MD, LESLIE CASTELO-SOCCIO, MD, PHD, AND ALBERT C. YAN, MD

Physicians are often confronted by parents who are concerned about "bumps" on their child's skin surface. Most parents will be comforted by a physician's reassurance and recommendations for treatment. Obviously, therapeutic interventions cannot be made until a definitive diagnosis is made. The following algorithm is used to help practitioners diagnose varying papular lesions (Fig. 63.1 and Table 63.1).

PAPULES WITH A CHARACTERISTIC CLINICAL APPEARANCE

Many conditions can be diagnosed on sight. The experienced eye can easily distinguish milia from molluscum contagiosum (MC) and warts from the uncommon xanthoma. Papules caused by bites are localized to exposed surfaces (face and extremities), are often clustered into crops of three or four lesions (the so-called "breakfast, lunch, and dinner" pattern), and classically demonstrate small central puncta. Several clues make the process of separating these entities from one another easier (see "Papules with a Noncharacteristic Clinical Appearance" section).

The distinction between flat warts and xanthomas is more subtle. At times, it is impossible to tell the difference. Because warts are caused by the human papillomavirus, a scratch through any of the lesions may inoculate the virus along the scratch line. This produces flat-topped papules in a linear distribution (a quasi-Koebner's phenomenon—i.e., appearance of the primary eruption located elsewhere on the body at sites of trauma). Therefore, linearly arranged yellow, tan, or flesh-colored flat-topped papules should arouse suspicion of the presence of flat warts, especially if the lesions are distributed on the face, backs of the hands, and knees—favored sites for flat warts. Xanthomas are unusual during childhood. When present, however, they usually are associated with elevations of serum lipids, which gives these lesions their often yellowish hue, especially when diascopy is applied; this can be accomplished by applying a glass slide to a lesion, which may accentuate the yellow color of the lesion. A lipid profile can be helpful in distinguishing these two flat-topped papules from one another. If all else fails, the help of a dermatologist experienced in caring for children can be sought. This is true for any of the entities discussed in this chapter. Skin biopsy is a valuable tool available to the dermatologist and may be required to differentiate many of the entities discussed here.

Milia

Milia are 1- to 2-mm firm, white papules. They are produced by retention of keratinous and sebaceous material in follicular openings. Newborns often have milia on their face. Fortunately, they frequently disappear by the age of 1 month. Milia can also arise from skin trauma, and can be seen in scars after burns and in healed wounds in patients with epidermolysis bullosa. Persistent milia may be a manifestation of the oral-facial-digital syndrome, hereditary hypotrichosis (Marie-Unna type), and certain rare ectodermal dysplasias (Basan's syndrome). Because lesions that are not associated with syndromes disappear spontaneously, no therapy is indicated.

Molluscum Contagiosum

For additional information about MC, see Figure 85.42.

Warts

For additional information about warts, see Chapter 85.

Xanthomas

Papules, plaques, nodules, and tumors that contain lipid are called *xanthomas*. These lesions can appear on any skin surface and are often associated with disturbances of lipoprotein metabolism (Table 63.2).

The most interesting, but the most rare, of hyperlipidemias that arise in the pediatric (infancy to adolescence) age group are the Fredericksen type I hyperlipidemias. This is caused by lipoprotein lipase or apolipoprotein II deficiency or by the presence of inhibitors of lipoprotein lipase. Fifty percent of patients present with episodic abdominal pain that may be acute at times. Malaise, anorexia, fever, and leukocytosis may be present. The cause of the pain is unclear; however, pancreatitis and splenic infarcts have been hypothesized. Eruptive xanthomas occur in more than 50% of the patients. These are 1- to 4-mm yellow/orange papules that appear in crops on the face, extremities, and buttocks. Their sudden appearance causes significant concern. Hepatosplenomegaly is also commonly present, as are lipemia retinalis and creamy plasma. Patients are found to have increased chylomicrons, slightly elevated cholesterol, and significantly elevated triglycerides. With age, patients develop elevated, very low density lipoproteins. Secondary diseases include pancreatitis and diabetes. Dietary modification is the most effective treatment for this disease.

The homozygous form of type IIa hyperlipidemia is seen in children. An elevated low-density lipoprotein, significantly elevated cholesterol, and mildly elevated triglycerides characterize this disorder. Tendinous and tuberous xanthomas and xanthelasmas are seen clinically. The plane xanthomas (xanthelasmas)

TABLE 63.1

PAPULAR LESIONS

Granuloma annulare (common)
Insect bites (common)
Juvenile xanthogranuloma
Lichen nitidus
Mastocytomas, urticaria pigmentosa
Milia (common)
Molluscum contagiosum (common)
Pyogenic granuloma (common)
Spitz nevus
Warts (common)
Xanthomas

may be misinterpreted as flat warts when seen in skin areas away from the eyelids. Secondary disorders include hypothyroidism and nephrotic syndrome. Patients die of atherosclerotic coronary artery disease in their twenties and thirties. Low-density lipoprotein apheresis, liver transplantation, and lipid altering medications are among the current therapies available for this disorder.

Insect Bites

For additional information about insect bites, see Chapter 85.

PAPULES WITH A NONCHARACTERISTIC CLINICAL APPEARANCE

When the diagnosis is not obvious, the algorithm presented in Figure 63.1 can be used.

Presence of White or Translucent Core

Milia and MC have white cores. Sidelighting and a magnifying glass may be needed to see the core within the central portion of the papule in MC. Therefore, it is essential to sidelight all papules about which one is not sure. The obvious white core in milia fills the entire papule rather than a small central portion of the papule (as in MC). The other differentiating point is that milia are hard and beady white; MC are more fleshy. As MC lesions age and desiccate, the central core often retracts resulting in a central umbilication.

Absence of White or Translucent Core

Rapid Growth of Hemangioma-like Lesions

Hemangiomas generally present within the first month of life. Two lesions that may mimic hemangiomas generally manifest after this period. These lesions are the pyogenic granuloma and Spitz nevus. They are differentiated by the fact that the Spitz nevus has a red, smooth, dome-shaped surface, as opposed to the

SIGNS AND SYMPTOMS

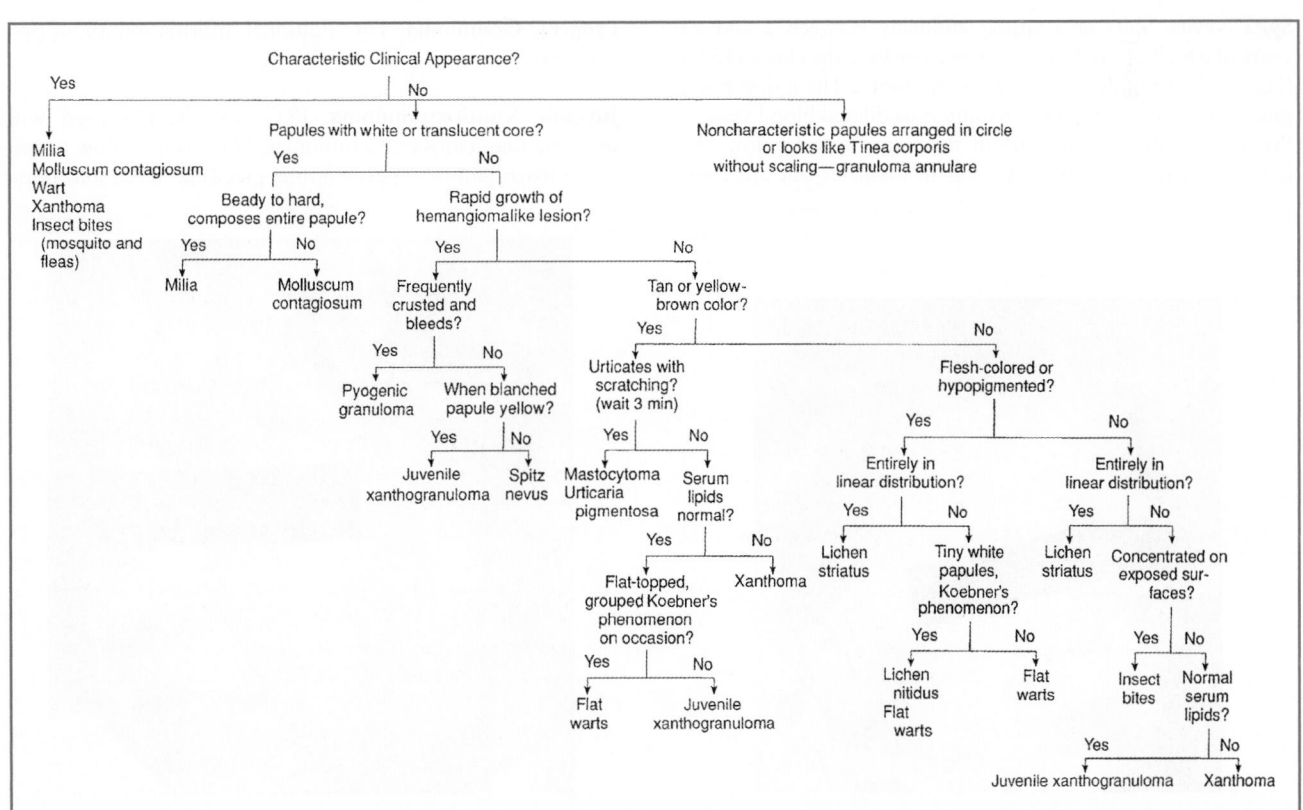

FIGURE 63.1 Approach to the diagnosis of papular lesions.

TABLE 63.2

HYPERLIPIDEMIAS

Type	Age of onset	Clinical presentation	Inheritance
I	Early childhood	Eruptive xanthomas Abdominal pain Hepatosplenomegaly Creamy plasma	AR
IIa	Early childhood	Tendinous xanthomas Xanthelasmas Tuberous xanthomas Corneal arcus	AD
IIb	Early childhood	Same as IIa	AD
III	Adulthood	Palmar xanthomas Tendinous xanthomas Associated diseases: thyroid, renal, liver, diabetes	AR
IV	Adulthood	Obesity and insulin resistance Tuberous xanthomas Eruptive xanthomas	AD
V	Adulthood	Same as IV	AR

AR, autosomal recessive; AD, autosomal dominant.

crusted granular surface of a pyogenic granuloma. The last differentiating point is the common occurrence of bleeding of pyogenic granulomas following minor trauma. Juvenile xanthogranulomas (JXGs) are typically yellow but can be red and appear suddenly. These are firm rather than spongy (like a hemangioma). The characteristic underlying color can often be elicited by using diascopy to blanch the lesion to reveal the yellow color.

Spitz Nevus. Spitz nevi appear suddenly between 2 and 13 years of age. Preferred sites of growth include the cheek (15%) (Fig. 63.2), shoulder, and upper extremities. The lesion has a pink to red surface because of numerous dilated blood vessels. Pressure produces blanching of this pink to red color. The lesions can reach a size of 1.5 cm in diameter but are com-

pletely benign. Pigmented Spitz nevi, another variant of Spitz nevi, often appear black in the skin rather than pink-red, and their appearance is often worrisome for malignant melanoma. Because the histologic appearance of these lesions can be confused easily with a malignant melanoma, an experienced histopathologist should interpret the findings. Most clinicians still recommend that Spitz nevi be removed surgically.

Pyogenic Granuloma. For additional information about pyogenic granulomas, see Figure 99.38.

Juvenile Xanthogranuloma. JXGs can be confused with urticaria pigmentosa or xanthomas. Numerous yellow or reddish-brown papules appear on the face (Fig. 63.3) and upper

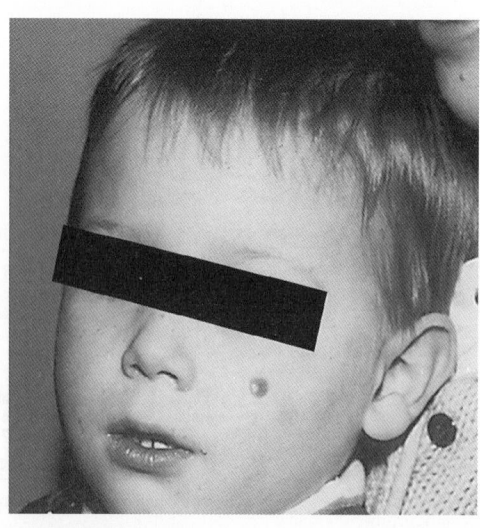

FIGURE 63.2 Red papule that appeared 2 months ago and grew rapidly to this size (Spitz nevus).

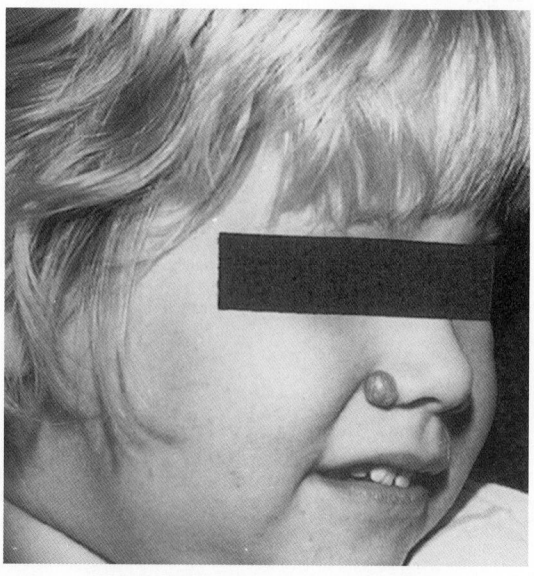

FIGURE 63.3 Blanching erythematous papule on the ala nasi of this child. Biopsy showed this lesion to be a juvenile xanthogranuloma.

trunk in the first year of life. The number of lesions may increase until the child is 18 months to 2 years of age. Serum lipid levels are normal, and the Darier's sign (urtication after scratching—see "Mastocytoma, Urticaria Pigmentosa" section) is negative. The lesions often disappear spontaneously after 2 years of age; therefore, intervention is generally unnecessary. When JXGs are multiple, particularly on the head and neck, evaluation of the eyes for intraocular JXGs is recommended because of their potential for visual impairment. The presence of JXGs in a young child with neurofibromatosis (type 1) has been a marker associated with an increased risk of juvenile myelomonocytic leukemia.

No Hemangioma-like Lesion: Yellow, Tan, or Brown Papule

The yellow, tan, and brown papules include the lesions seen in urticaria pigmentosa (a single, large lesion is called a *mastocytoma*), flat warts, xanthomas, insect bites, and JXGs.

A first step to differentiate the various papules from one another is to scratch them. If hiving of a scratched lesion (Darier's sign) occurs within a short period of time (3 to 5 minutes), the lesion must contain mast cells (i.e., a mastocytoma or urticaria pigmentosa). Make sure to scratch normal skin to rule out the presence of dermographism. The latter condition will produce a false-positive Darier's sign. When no urtication occurs, blood should be drawn to check lipid levels. If lipid levels are normal, the next step is to differentiate two of the entities (i.e., flat warts and JXGs). Flat warts tend to be grouped, are flat topped, and can be autoinoculated in scratch lines (pseudo-Koebner's phenomenon). Lesions characteristic for JXGs are not flat topped, tend to be singular in number (or when multiple are scattered about), and do not demonstrate the Koebner's phenomenon (recapitulation of the eruption in traumatized areas). JXG lesions may also look like xanthomas. Unlike xanthomas, however, abnormal lipid levels do not occur with JXGs.

Mastocytoma, Urticaria Pigmentosa

Parents who bring children with mastocytomas or lesions of urticaria pigmentosa to the physician generally describe a single yellow–tan–brown lesion that was present at or soon after birth (mastocytoma) or multiple pigmented papules that erupt during the first year of life (urticaria pigmentosa). One important clue is a history of these lesions becoming red (Fig. 63.4), hivelike, or blistered. The lesions may ooze and form crusts much like impetigo; however, they do not respond to antibacterial preparations.

Physical examination of the lesion provides the next clue. The surface has a peau d'orange appearance at times. Some papules are often yellow and are easily mistaken for xanthomas. When they are tan to brown, they are believed to be raised moles. The clincher is finding a positive Darier's sign (histamine-induced erythema, swelling, and urtication secondary to scratching and subsequent degranulation of mast cells).

Table 63.3 lists medications and physical stimuli that cause mast cell degranulation and histamine and/or prostaglandin D_2 release. These agents should be avoided.

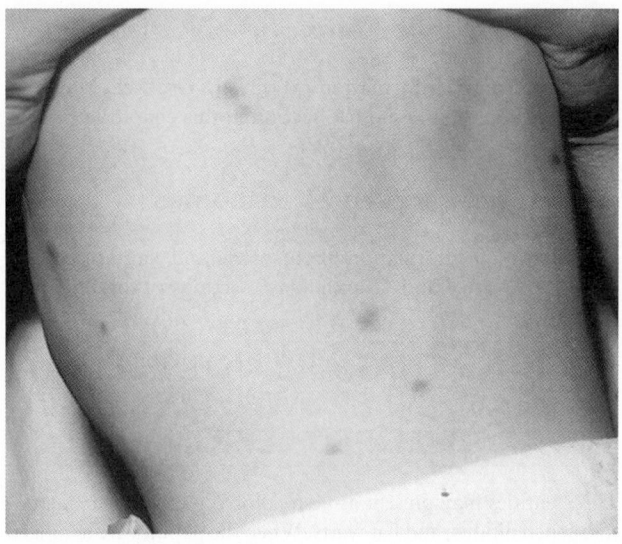

FIGURE 63.4 Erythematous papules representative of urticaria pigmentosa. They will urticate with scratching (Darier's sign).

When large amounts of these mediators are released, generalized flushing, persistent diarrhea, or hypotension may ensue. Children with these symptoms require therapy directed against histamine and prostaglandin D_2. The H_1-receptor antagonists (chlorpheniramine, hydroxyzine, or diphenhydramine) and H_2-receptor antagonists (cimetidine, ranitidine, or famotidine) or occasionally combined H_1- and H_2-receptor antagonists (cyproheptadine or doxepin) may be required. In addition, nonsteroidal antiinflammatory drugs such as indomethacin or ibuprofen may be required to inhibit prostaglandin biosynthesis. Children who suffer from persistent histamine-induced diarrhea may benefit from the addition of oral cromolyn sodium. An epinephrine pen should be provided for patients with systemic disease or extensive symptoms.

Fortunately, with aging, the skin is no longer reactive, and most of the lesions disappear completely.

TABLE 63.3

MEDICATIONS AND PHYSICAL STIMULI TO BE AVOIDED IN PATIENTS WITH URTICARIA PIGMENTOSA

Medications	Physical stimuli
Alcohol	Rubbing of the skin
Aspirin	Extremes of water
Codeine	temperature
Decamethonium	
Dextran	
D-tubocurarine	
Gallamine	
Morphine	
Opiates	
Polymyxin B	
Procaine	
Quinine	
Radiographic dyes	
Scopolamine	

SIGNS AND SYMPTOMS

Juvenile Xanthogranulomas

For additional information about JXGs, see previous "Juvenile Xanthogranuloma" section in this chapter.

Warts and Xanthomas

For additional information about warts and xanthomas, see previous "Warts" and "Xanthomas" sections of this chapter.

LESIONS THAT ARE NOT YELLOW, TAN, OR BROWN: FLESH-COLORED LESIONS

Three entities may present as flesh-colored papules: lichen striatus, lichen nitidus, and flat warts. When the papules are arranged linearly, streaming down an extremity or across the face or neck, lichen striatus should be considered. If the papules are not arranged linearly but are tiny pinpoint, flesh-colored papules, lichen nitidus should be considered, especially if a Koebner's phenomenon is present. Flat warts may be flesh colored.

Lichen Striatus

Lichen striatus is an asymptomatic eruption of unknown cause. The flat-topped papules are arranged linearly and may be confluent. Lesions may occur in a wide band but remain characteristically linear or more accurately curvilinear patterns corresponding to lines of Blaschko. The lesions are flesh colored to erythematous in Caucasians and hypopigmented in African Americans. The eruption follows the long axis of an extremity (Fig. 63.5) or may involve any other part of the skin surface (especially the face). Because the eruption resolves spontaneously within 2 years, no treatment is necessary.

Lichen Nitidus

Lichen nitidus is characterized by tiny, pinpoint, flat-topped, flesh-colored papules (Fig. 63.6). The papules are often grouped and are found in scratch lines (i.e., the Koebner's phenomenon). Although any skin surface may be involved, the trunk and genitalia are common sites. The lesions are often asymptomatic but may occasionally itch. The lesions persist for variable periods and generally do not respond to therapy.

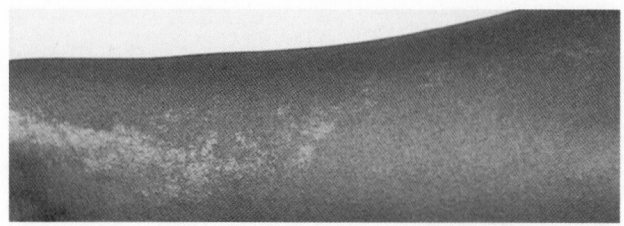

FIGURE 63.5 Hypopigmented papules running linearly along the long axis of the arm in a child with lichen striatus.

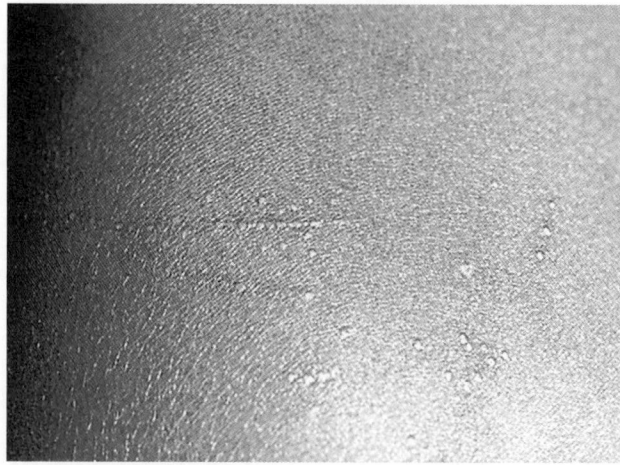

FIGURE 63.6 Tiny flesh-colored to hypopigmented papules in a child with lichen nitidus. Note that the papules are arranged linearly (Koebner's phenomenon).

Flat Warts

See section about flat warts in Chapter 85.

NON–FLESH-COLORED LESIONS

Lichen striatus can be composed of hypopigmented or erythematous papules arranged linearly. Red papules not arranged linearly and concentrated on exposed surfaces usually indicate the presence of insect bites. JXGs can be yellow or reddish-brown. They can be hypopigmented and brown-orange in African-American children. Xanthomas may be yellow or yellow-red. As discussed previously, the serum lipid levels are normal in patients with JXG and elevated in children with xanthomas.

NONCHARACTERISTIC PAPULES

Papules Arranged in Circles—Looks Like Tinea Corporis without Any Scaling

Granuloma Annulare

Granuloma annulare is believed to be an idiosyncratic response to trauma. The location of the changes (i.e., the shins, forearms, back of hands, ankles, and dorsum of the feet) seems to confirm this hypothesis. This skin change may begin as a flesh-colored or violaceous papule that clears centrally as the margins advance, or it may appear as a group of papules arranged in a ringlike configuration (Fig. 63.7). The central portion of the lesion is dusky or hyperpigmented. The key point on physical examination is the lack of scaling. This physical finding distinguishes granuloma annulare from tinea corporis and cannot be stressed enough. The border is firm on palpation, unlike tinea corporis. The rings can be 5 cm in diameter or larger.

A potassium hydroxide test would be definitive in ruling out tinea corporis. It would be difficult to obtain scales from a granuloma annulare lesion using this procedure. It is important

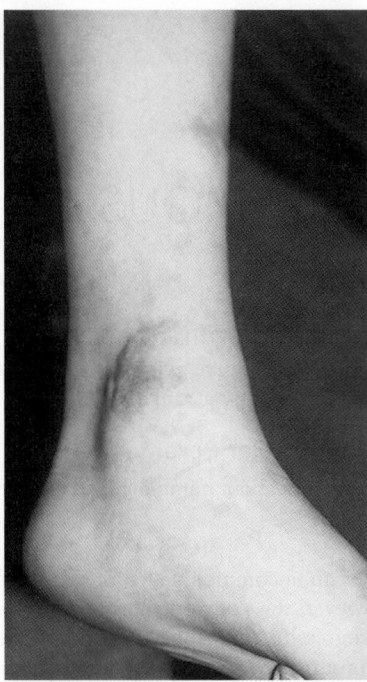

FIGURE 63.7 Note erythematous to violaceous papules arranged in a circle in this child with granuloma annulare.

to diagnose this entity correctly because one can reassure parents that three-fourths of lesions clear spontaneously within a 2-year period. Recurrences are common until children outgrow this tendency. Too often, treatment for tinea corporis is instituted unnecessarily for what is really granuloma annulare.

If this algorithm has not helped in making a diagnosis, a consultant should be called. Many entities can be difficult to differentiate. A dermatologist can often resolve the matter, however, with a skin biopsy sent for histologic review.

Suggested Readings

Briley LD, Phillips CM. Cutaneous mastocytosis: a review focusing on the pediatric population. *Clin Pediatr (Phila)* 2008;47:757–761.

Brown J, Janniger CK, Schwartz RA, Silverberg NB. Childhood molluscum contagiosum. *Int J Dermatol* 2006;45:93–99.

Bunimovich O, Grassi M, Baer MR. Systemic mastocytosis: classification, pathogenesis, diagnosis and treatment. *Cutis* 2009;83:29–36.

Chang MW. Update on juvenile xanthogranuloma: unusual cutaneous and systemic variants. *Semin Cutan Med Surg* 1999;18:195–205.

Dillman AM, Miller RC, Hansen RC. Multiple pyogenic granulomata in childhood. *Pediatr Dermatol* 1991;8:28.

Feoli-Fonseca JC, Levy E, Godard M, et al. Familial lipoprotein lipase deficiency in infancy: clinical, biochemical and molecular study. *J Pediatr* 1998;133:417–423.

Gelbard SN, Tripp JM, Marghoob AA, et al. Management of Spitz nevi: a survey of dermatologists in the United States. *J Am Acad Dermatol* 2002;47:224–230.

Groff KL, Nascimento AG. Subcutaneous granuloma annulare in childhood: clinicopathologic features in 34 cases. *Pediatrics* 2001;107:E42.

Grosshans EM. Acquired blaschkolinear dermatoses. *Am J Med Genet* 1999;85:334–337.

Hanson SG, Levy ML. Granuloma annulare. *Pediatrics* 1999;103:195–196.

Heide R, Tank B, Oranje AP. Mastocytosis in childhood. *Pediatr Dermatol* 2002;19:375–381.

Hernandez-Martin A, Baselga E, Drolet BA, et al. Juvenile xanthogranuloma. *J Am Acad Dermatol* 1997;36:355.

Lin RL, Janniger CK. Pyogenic granuloma. *Cutis* 2004;74:229–233.

Maher-Wiese VL, Marmer EL, Grant-Kels JM. Xanthomas and the inherited hyperlipoproteinemias in children and adolescents. *Pediatr Dermatol* 1991;7:166.

Rohrs HJ, Schatz D, Winter WE, et al. Pediatric lipid disorders in clinical practice. Emedicine Pediatrics [overview]. Available at: http://emedicine.medscape.com/article/901837. Updated April 23, 2008.

Sandwich JT, Davis LS. Granuloma annulare of the eyelid: a case report and review of the literature. *Pediatr Dermatol* 1999;16:375–376.

Shin HT, Harris MB, Orlow SJ. Juvenile myelomonocytic leukemia with features of hemaphagocytic lymphohistiocytosis presenting in association with neurofibromatosis and juvenile xanthogranulomas. *J Pediatr Hematol Oncol* 2004;261:591–593.

Smith KJ, Skelton H. Molluscum contagiosum: recent advances in pathogenic mechanisms and new therapies. *Am J Clin Dermatol* 2002;3:535–545.

Sugandhan S, Khandpur S, Sharma K. Familial chlyomicronemia syndrome. *Pediatr Dermatol* 2007;24:323–325.

Tilly JJ, Drolet BA, Esterly NB. Lichenoid eruptions in children. *J Am Acad Dermatol* 2004;51:606–624.

Wells RS, Smith MA. The natural history of granuloma annulare. *Br J Dermatol* 1963;75:199.

SIGNS AND SYMPTOMS

CHAPTER 64 ■ RASH—PAPULOSQUAMOUS LESIONS

PAUL J. HONIG, MD, LESLIE CASTELO-SOCCIO, MD, PHD, AND ALBERT C. YAN, MD

PAPULOSQUAMOUS ERUPTIONS

Of skin conditions seen in a pediatric dermatology clinic, 10% are papulosquamous (i.e., have a papular and scaling component). The algorithm contained in this chapter should be used as a guide to differentiate these disorders (Table 64.1 and Fig. 64.1). Each key point that distinguishes one disease from another is discussed here.

Presence or Absence of Pruritus

The initial symptom that should be considered is pruritus. Pruritus is absent in the six conditions listed in Table 64.2. Palmar involvement is prominent in secondary syphilis and papulosquamous drug eruptions but is rare in pityriasis rosea. A positive rapid plasma reagin (RPR) test helps differentiate syphilis from pityriasis rosea and a drug eruption. Pityriasis rosea begins with a herald patch, followed by a truncal eruption in a "Christmas or fir tree" distribution. Finally, the Koebner's phenomenon separates lichen nitidus from other entities.

Conditions That Lack Pruritus

Drug Eruption—Papulosquamous

The diagnosis of a drug eruption is based on the history of current or recent intake of a medication and the disappearance of the eruption after discontinuation of the medication. Drug eruptions may manifest in a form that mimics lichen planus, pityriasis rosea, pityriasis rubra pilaris (PRP), psoriasis, seborrheic dermatitis, and syphilis (Table 64.3). The cutaneous manifestations of a drug eruption that resemble one of the previously described disorders, however, will be atypical (e.g., lack of a herald patch and typical truncal distribution in a pityriasis rosea look-alike drug eruption or lack of a violaceous color and feathery white buccal changes in a lichenoid drug eruption). Remember that drug eruptions may or may not itch and may or may not have palmar and plantar involvement.

Lichen Nitidus

Lichen nitidus is a common disorder of children, seen especially in African Americans. There is a 4:1 male:female predominance. Lichen nitidus involves the abdomen, genitalia (shaft and glans), and extremities with tiny, pinpoint, sharply demarcated, flat-topped, flesh-colored papules. Often, these lesions are closely grouped and are linear. Linear grouping of lesions is caused by the Koebner's phenomenon (Table 64.4; appearance of the primary lesion at sites of trauma), which

often occurs in lichen nitidus (Fig. 64.2). The lesions generally are nonpruritic. The course is variable, and the cause is unknown. Therapy is not warranted.

Nummular Eczema (Xerosis)

For more information about nummular eczema, see Chapter 85.

Parapsoriasis

Parapsoriasis is an uncommon pediatric skin condition. When it occurs, however, the course is chronic and, on rare occasions, may progress to cutaneous lymphoma. The appearance of this eruption is easily mistaken for nummular eczema, psoriasis, tinea corporis, or a lichenoid change. Small oval scaling, erythematous (Fig. 64.3) to yellow-brown macules are concentrated on the trunk. The skin lesions are asymptomatic, and the patient feels healthy.

Treatment is unnecessary because the disease is asymptomatic. Topical steroids may be helpful but may not entirely clear the skin changes. The eruption clears spontaneously after varying periods.

Pityriasis Rosea

For more information about pityriasis rosea, see Chapter 85.

Secondary Syphilis

The secondary phase of syphilis is a great mimicker. Therefore, one must suspect this condition to make the correct diagnosis. The eruption may be localized to the trunk, palms, and soles, as well as to any other skin surface. Other clues should be sought by history and physical examination (a primary chancre, condyloma lata, or white mucous patches on the tongue, buccal, and labial surfaces). Generalized lymphadenopathy is usually present. It may be difficult to differentiate secondary syphilis and pityriasis rosea; however, Table 85.11 (see Chapter 85) may be helpful in separating the two entities clinically.

A positive RPR or fluorescent treponemal antibody makes the diagnosis. Remember, a false-negative RPR can occur with antibody excess (the prozone phenomenon). Therefore, dilution of the specimen by the laboratory should be requested if the presence of syphilis is highly suspected. This simple maneuver will result in a positive test for the presence of syphilis.

Color of the Skin Eruption and Pruritus

The eye can discern subtle differences in color. A pruritic papulosquamous eruption that does not look erythematous should suggest one of four disorders. First, a violaceous (bluish-red) or purple appearance generally indicates lichen planus or a lichenoid drug eruption. However, tones of yellow or salmon

TABLE 64.1

PAPULOSQUAMOUS SKIN DISORDERS

Acrodermatitis enteropathica[a]	Pityriasis rosea (common)
Drug eruption, papulosquamous (common)[a]	Pityriasis rubra pilaris
Lichen nitidus	Psoriasis (common)
Lichen planus	Reiter's syndrome
Nummular eczema (common)	Seborrheic dermatitis
Parapsoriasis	Syphilis, secondary (common)

[a]Potentially life-threatening

TABLE 64.2

NONPRURITIC PAPULOSQUAMOUS SKIN DISORDERS

Drug-eruption—papulosquamous	Parapsoriasis
Lichen nitidus	Pityriasis rosea
Nummular eczema	Secondary syphilis

Violaceous or Yellow- or Salmon-colored (Orange-red) Eruptions or Flesh-colored (Nonerythematous) Eruptions

Lichen Planus

Lichen planus is seen occasionally in pediatric patients as a chronic, pruritic, reddish-blue (violaceous) to purplish eruption. Two percent to 3% of cases occur in patients younger than 20 years of age.

The eruption generally involves the flexors of the wrist, forearms, and legs, especially the dorsum of the foot and ankles. The highly pruritic lesions appear as small, violaceous, shiny, flat-topped, polygonal papules (Fig. 64.4). These qualities may be recalled with the alliterative mnemonic of the five

(orange-red) suggest the presence of seborrheic dermatitis or an unusual disorder called PRP. The latter two diseases can be differentiated by looking for yellow thickening of the palms and soles (i.e., in PRP) or knowing that seborrheic dermatitis classically occurs before 12 months of age or after puberty. Lichen nitidus is obvious when tiny, discrete, flesh-colored papules (white papules in African Americans) are found, with some arranged linearly (Koebner's phenomenon).

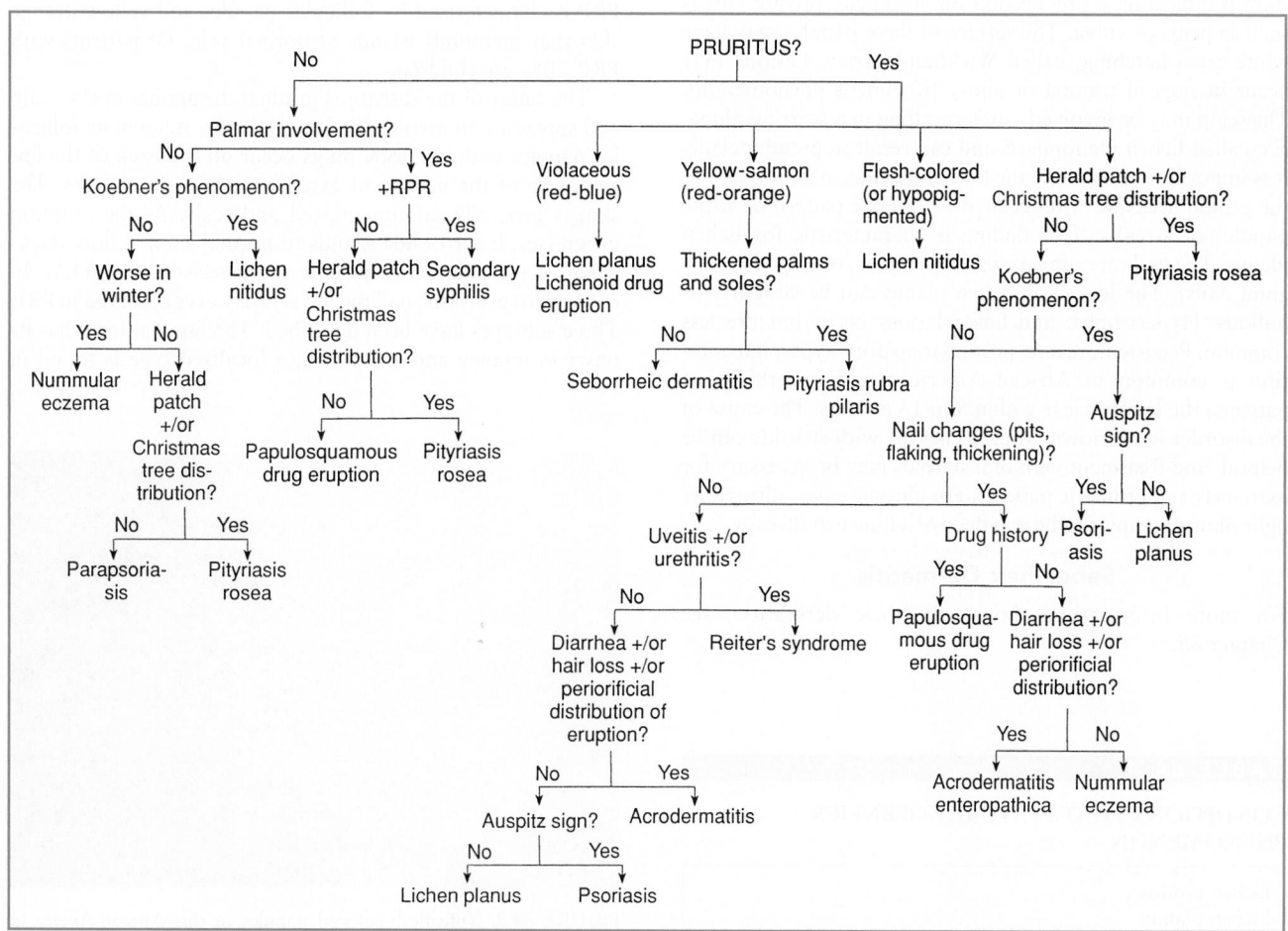

FIGURE 64.1 Algorithm to distinguish papulosquamous lesions. RPR, rapid plasma reagin test.

TABLE 64.3

DRUG ERUPTIONS THAT MAY MIMIC OR INDUCE VARIOUS PAPULOSQUAMOUS LESIONS

Lichen Planus		Pityriasis Rosea
Antimalarial agents	Isoniazid	Barbiturates
β-Blockers	Naproxen	β-Blockers
Captopril	D-penicillamine	Captopril
Carbamazepine	Phenytoin	Gold
Chloral hydrate	Spironolactone	Griseofulvin
Diazoxide	Tetracyclines	Ketotifen
Furosemide		Metronidazole
Gold		Penicillin
Griseofulvin		Tripelennamine
Hydrochlorothiazide		
		Psoriasis
Pityriasis Rubra Pilaris		Antimalarials
β-Blockers		β-Blockers
		Lithium
Seborrheic Dermatitis		? Nonsteroidal antiinflammatory drugs
Contraceptives with progesterone		
(derived from 19-nortestosterone)		
Testosterone		
Syphilis		
Any drug		

ps: pruritic, purplish, planar, polygonal papules. Some add a sixth p indicating a predilection for so-called "private" areas such as penis or vulva. The surface of these papules may have white cross-hatching, called Wickham's striae. Lesions may occur in sites of trauma or injury (Koebner's phenomenon). The scalp may be involved, often resulting in a scarring alopecia, called lichen planopilaris and can result in pseudopelade. It is important to examine the buccal mucous membranes and the genital areas for a reticulated or lacelike pattern of white papules or streaks. This finding is characteristic for lichen planus. The nails are often pitted, dystrophic, or ridged (pterygium nails). The lesions in lichen planus can be vesicular or bullous. Hypertrophic and linear lesions occur but are less common. Persistent, severe, postinflammatory hyperpigmentation is common in African Americans. In two-thirds of patients, the lesions clear within 8 to 15 months. The cause of the disorder is unknown. Topical therapy with steroids can be helpful, and treatment with oral steroids may be necessary for extremely symptomatic patients. For chronic cases, ultraviolet light phototherapy can be an effective adjunct to therapy.

Seborrheic Dermatitis

For more information about seborrheic dermatitis, see Chapter 85.

TABLE 64.4

CONDITIONS THAT FEATURE KOEBNER'S PHENOMENON

Lichen nitidus
Lichen planus
Psoriasis

Pityriasis Rubra Pilaris

PRP is characterized by follicular papules and yellow-orange skin that surrounds islands of normal skin. Of patients with PRP, 30% are children.

The onset of the disease is gradual, beginning in the scalp and spreading to involve the face and ears. Acuminate follicular papules with keratotic plugs occur on the back of the fingers, side of the neck, and extensors of the extremities. The skin is generally salmon-colored and scaly. As the eruption progresses, it surrounds islands of normal skin. Yellow thickening of the palms and soles is characteristic (Fig. 64.5). In contrast to psoriasis, nail pitting is rarely ever observed in PRP. Three subtypes have been described: The familial form has its onset in infancy and childhood, a localized type is found in

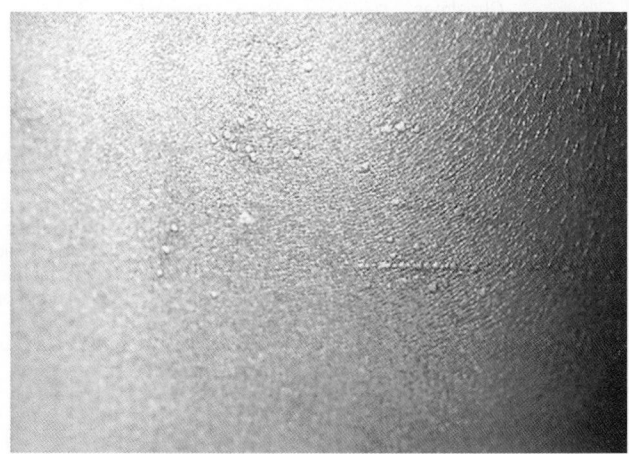

FIGURE 64.2 Note flesh-colored papules in this African-American patient with lichen nitidus. The Koebner's phenomenon also is seen (papules arranged linearly in a scratch).

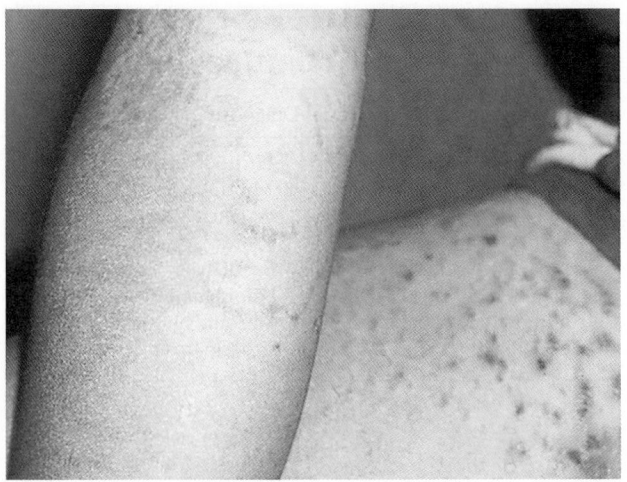

FIGURE 64.3 Red, scaling lesions on arm of child with parapsoriasis.

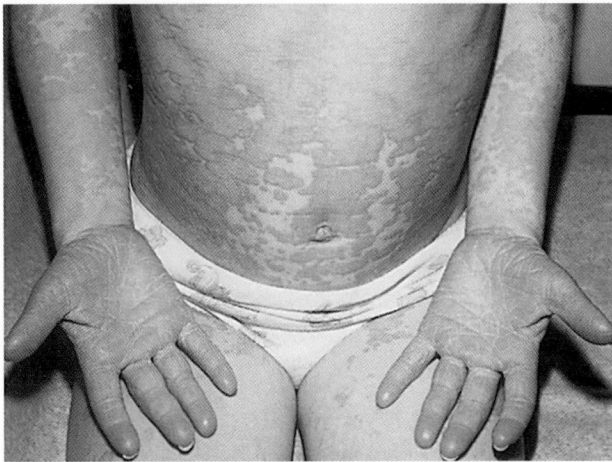

FIGURE 64.5 Hyperkeratosis of palms and islands of normal skin seen in this child with pityriasis rubra pilaris.

60% of cases, and the acquired form occurs in persons older than 15 years. The cause of this disease is unknown, although it is a disorder of keratinization. The condition responds to vitamin A and its derivatives.

Differentiating the Pruritic, Red Papulosquamous Lesions

Pityriasis rosea also should be included in this part of the algorithm. Because the rash of pityriasis rosea may or may not itch, the first differentiating point is to inquire about a history of a herald patch and look for the characteristic Christmas tree distribution (along lines of skin cleavage known as Langer's lines). If one or both is present, a diagnosis of pityriasis rosea is made. If not, one must look for the Koebner's phenomenon. The Koebner's phenomenon is defined as the appearance of the existing rash in areas of traumatized skin (e.g., in scratches,

abrasions, blistered sunburns). This phenomenon is discussed further in the "Psoriasis" section of this chapter.

Another clue to the presence of psoriasis is the finding of abnormal nails (e.g., nail pits, flaking, thickened nails). Reactive arthritis (formerly known as Reiter's syndrome) and acrodermatitis enteropathica may also manifest nail abnormalities. These entities can be differentiated from one another by a history or finding of uveitis and/or urethritis (reactive arthritis) or diarrhea and/or hair loss (acrodermatitis enteropathica).

Psoriasis

Psoriasis is a chronic papulosquamous disease that makes up 4% of all skin disorders encountered in children. The female:male ratio is 2:1. There is a predisposition for involvement of the scalp, perineum (particularly in infants), and the extensor surfaces of the body, particularly the elbows and knees.

One-third of adults with psoriasis experience onset of disease in childhood or adolescence. Psoriasis occurs in 12% of children before the age of 10 years. The major human leukocyte histocompatibility antigens (HLAs) are important genetic markers of psoriasis. Of these, HLA-B13, HLA-BW17 and HLA-CW6 are associated with early onset of disease. The HLA-B13 and HLA-CW6 antigens are associated with a history of antecedent streptococcal infections. The HLA-BW17 antigen is more commonly identified with extensive skin involvement and a strong familial history.

Psoriasis occurs in three forms during childhood: guttate, erythrodermic, and pustular. Any or all of these types may develop with silvery scales into the chronic, plaque-type psoriasis (Fig. 64.6). When a scale is removed, pinpoint areas of bleeding occur on the surface (Auspitz sign). Guttate psoriasis is the most common form, occurring in childhood. Guttate or droplike erythematous papules are scattered over the body. The characteristic silvery scale is only minimally expressed, and the lesions may appear quite red. This form is often preceded by a streptococcal infection. Infants often have involvement in the diaper area as well. Erythrodermic psoriasis is less common and more severe. Onset may be abrupt or gradual, with a diffuse erythema and severe desquamation. In the

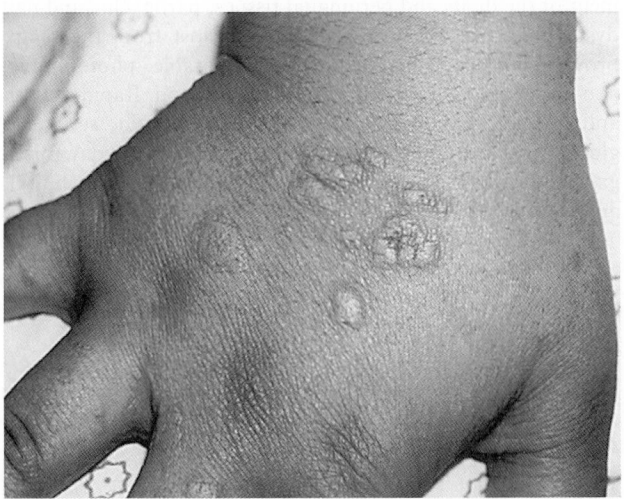

FIGURE 64.4 Note child with red-blue color of flat-topped papules representative of lichen planus.

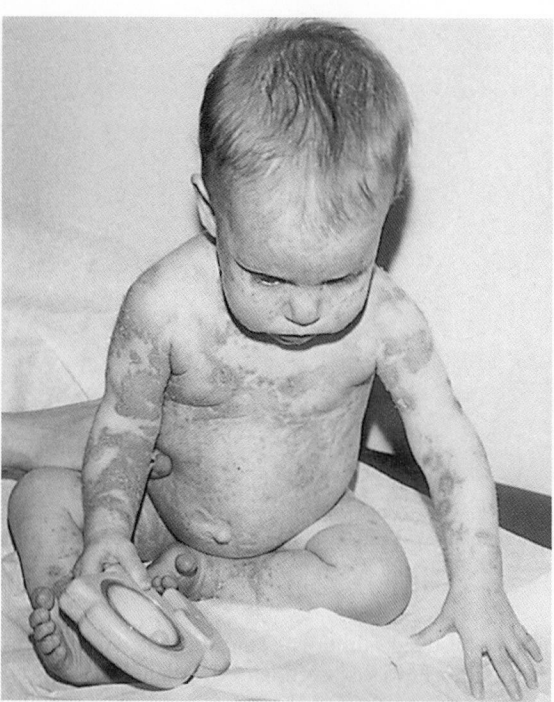

FIGURE 64.6 Plaque-type psoriasis in this infant. Note scaling in scalp.

growing child, there may be associated failure to thrive. Pustular psoriasis is rare and the least commonly occurring form of psoriasis seen in children and may begin in intertriginous areas. Various size sterile and superficial pustules develop on an erythrodermic background. Avoidance of systemic steroids may be prudent in patients with psoriasis because withdrawal of systemic steroids can precipitate pustular flares of the disease.

Characteristically small, pitted lesions are seen on the nails in 25% to 50% of patients in all forms of the condition. Eighty percent of children have scalp involvement, especially at the hair margins. A small number of patients develop arthritis between 9 and 12 years of age; some develop it before the onset of the skin eruption. The distal interphalangeal joints of the hands and feet are involved most often. Therapy with topical agents, including steroids, tar derivatives, vitamin A (tazarotene) and D (calcipotriene) derivatives, emollients, and ultraviolet light, help slow the turnover rate of the epidermis. For severe cases, patients may be treated with systemic immunomodulating agents, including methotrexate, cyclosporine, acitretin, and recently approved biological modifiers that address specific targets in T-cell physiology.

Reactive Arthritis

The skin changes seen in reactive arthritis look much like those in psoriasis. A symmetric arthritis of major joints, uveitis, and urethritis complete the syndrome. Although most cases occur in young adult men, on occasion, the syndrome will be seen in adolescents. Only ten cases have been reported in children younger than 12 years of age. Ninety percent of patients are HLA-B27 positive. A postinfectious cause has been hypothesized.

The palms and soles are the major sites of involvement. Yellow, scaly, hyperkeratotic lesions appear on an erythema-

TABLE 64.5
ACRODERMATITIS ENTEROPATHICA

Differential Diagnosis	
Mucocutaneous candidiasis	Histiocytosis X
Biotin deficiency	Multiple carboxylase deficiency
Cystic fibrosis	Psoriasis
Essential fatty acid deficiency	Seborrheic dermatitis
Glucagonoma syndrome	Anorexia nervosa
Ornithine transcarbamylase deficiency	Chronic bullous dermatosis of childhood

tous base in those locations. The skin lesions may begin as macules, vesicles, or pustules. The palmar plantar changes have been called *keratoderma blennorrhagicum*. The scalp and penis also are characteristically involved with psoriasiform lesions. Erythema and superficial ulcerations may be present in the mouth. Abnormalities of the nails (e.g., dystrophy, onycholysis) are common. (See the "Reactive Arthritis" section for therapy recommendations.)

Acrodermatitis Enteropathica

Acrodermatitis enteropathica is characterized by skin rash, diarrhea, and alopecia. The condition is caused by zinc deficiency, with plasma zinc levels less than 50 *mc*g per dL. This may result from low zinc intake, increased zinc losses from malabsorption, and an autosomal recessive genetic defect in the ability to absorb zinc via zinc transporters in the gastrointestinal tract. The disease generally begins around 9 months of age (1 week to 20 months). Rarely, older children develop this condition as a result of inflammatory bowel disease, cystic fibrosis, inborn errors of metabolism, and anorexia nervosa.

The infant usually presents with a psoriasiform diaper eruption, followed by similar involvement of periorificial (eyes, ears, nose, and mouth) and acral skin. The skin is often eroded and crusted but involved areas often are sharply demarcated. These changes may be confused with a severe candida infection (Table 64.5) or impetigo. Because of involvement of the digits and periungual tissues, paronychia and nail dystrophies are often present. Hair is lost from the scalp, brows, and lashes. The children are irritable, photophobic, and apathetic. Growth retardation is common. Rapid growth and correction of zinc deficiency occurs with zinc sulfate or gluconate 0.5 to 1 mg per kg of elemental zinc per day (often given in divided doses to improve gastrointestinal tolerability), and the dose titrated depending on the response to therapy.

If this algorithm does not lead to a clear diagnosis, many of the entities can be clarified with a skin biopsy or referral to a dermatologist.

Suggested Readings

Acrodermatitis Enteropathica

Maverakis E, Lynch PJ, Fazel N. Acrodermatitis enteropathica. *Dermatol Online J* 2008; 13:11.
Nakano A, Nakano H, Nomura K, et al. Novel SLC39A4 mutations in acrodermatitis enteropathica. *J Invest Dermatol* 2003;120:963–966.

Quirk CM, Seykora J, Wingate BJ, et al. Acrodermatitis enteropathica associated with anorexia nervosa. *JAMA* 2002;288:2655–2656.

Wang F, Kim BE, Dufner J, et al. Acrodermatitis enteropathica mutations affect transport activity, localization, and zinc responsive trafficking of mouse ZIP4 zinc transporter. *Hum Mol Genet* 2004;13:563–371.

Lichen Nitidus

Hassanen A, Nouv-Eldin O, Arun J. Generalized lichen nitidus. *Pediatr Dermatol* 2005;22:158–160.

Tilly JJ, Drolet BA, Esterly NB. Lichenoid eruptions in children. *J Am Acad Dermatol* 2004;51:606–624.

Parapsoriasis

Lam J, Pope E. Pediatric pityriasis lichenoides and cutaneous T cell lymphoma. *Curr Opin Pediatr* 2007;19:441–445.

Sehgeal V, Srivastava G, Aggarwal AK. Parapsoriasis: a complex issue. *Skinmed* 2008;6:280–286.

Pityriasis Rosea

Gonzalez LM, Allen R, Janniger CK, et al. Pityriasis Rosea: an important papulosquamous disorder. *Int J Dermatol* 2005;44:57–64.

Sharma PK, Yadav TP, Gautam RK, et al. Erythromycin in pityriasis rosea: a double-blind, placebo-controlled clinical trial. *J Am Acad Dermatol* 2000;42:241–244.

Pityriasis Rubra Pilaris

Allison DS, El-Azhary RA, Calobrisi SD, et al. Pityriasis rubra pilaris in children. *J Am Acad Dermatol* 2002;47:386–389.

Sehgal VN, Srivasta G. Juvenile pityriasis rubra pilaris. *Int J Dermatol* 2006;45:438–446.

Yang CC, Shih IH, Lin WL, et al. Juvenile pityriasis rubra pilaris: report of 28 cases in Taiwan. *J Am Acad Dermatol* 2008;59:943–948.

Psoriasis

Benoit S, Hamm H. Childhood psoriasis. *Clin Dermatol* 2007;25:555–562.

Janniger CK, Schwartz RA, Musumeci ML, et al. Infantile psoriasis. *Cutis* 2005;76:173–177.

Morris A, Rogers M, Fischer G, et al. Childhood psoriasis: a clinical review of 1262 cases. *Pediatr Dermatol* 2001;18:188–198.

Rogers M. Childhood psoriasis. *Curr Opin Pediatr* 2002;14(4):404–409.

Sukhatme SV, Gottlieb AB. Pediatric psoriasis: updates in biologic therapies. *Dermatol Ther* 2009;22:34–39.

Reactive Arthritis (Reiter's Syndrome)

Kim PS, Klausmeier TL, Orr DP. Reactive arthritis: a review. *J Adolesc Health* 2009;44:309–315.

Manimegalai N, Rajamurugan PS, Rajendran CP, et al. Childhood reactive arthritis. *J Clin Rheumatol* 2008;14:292–293.

Moorthy LN, Gaur S, Peterson MG, et al. Poststreptococcal reactive arthritis in children: a retrospective study. *Clin Pediatr (Phila)* 2009;48:174–182.

Wu IB, Schwartz RA. Reiter's syndrome: the classic triad and more. *J Am Acad Dermatol* 2008;59:113–121.

Syphilis

Workowski KA, Levine WC. *Sexually transmitted diseases treatment guidelines.* Atlanta: U.S. Department of Health and Human Services, 2002.

SIGNS AND SYMPTOMS

CHAPTER 65 ■ RASH—PETECHIAE AND PURPURA

REBECCA L. VIEIRA, MD

Petechiae and purpura refer to blood within the skin or mucosal membranes. Because of their common underlying pathophysiology and overlapping differential diagnoses, petechiae and purpura are often considered together. Purpura, from the Latin *purpura*, meaning "purple" describes lesions between 0.3 and 1 cm in size. Lesions less than 0.3 cm are referred to as petechiae and are usually bright red. The term ecchymoses includes lesions greater than 1 cm. Petechial, purpuric and ecchymotic lesions do not blanch, a characteristic that distinguishes them from vascular dilation and vascular anomalies. Parents and patients often describe petechiae and purpura simply as "rash." However, the finding of petechiae, purpura, or unexplained ecchymoses by a physician should raise concern, as they may be the presenting signs of many diseases, some benign and others life-threatening, some treated easily and others requiring complex therapy.

Patients presenting critically ill with petechiae or purpura will obviously require immediate evaluation and intervention. However, even in well-appearing children these findings could be the first signs of potentially life-threatening conditions. The etiology of petechiae and purpura should be established as rapidly as possible, as in many conditions early treatment will lead to a more favorable outcome. An understanding of the pathophysiology, a careful history and physical examination, and an appropriate laboratory evaluation will often help establish the diagnosis. This chapter presents the initial assessment and differential diagnosis of children with petechiae, purpura, and ecchymoses. The management of emergency situations associated with these symptoms is discussed in Chapter 91.

PATHOPHYSIOLOGY

Normal hemostatis involves complex interactions between the vasculature, platelets, and soluble clotting factors. Defects or deficiencies in any of these components can lead to abnormal bleeding resulting in petechiae, purpura, and ecchymoses. Normally, when a blood vessel is injured, vasoconstriction and retraction occur immediately and decrease blood flow to the affected area. Facilitated by von Willebrand factor, platelets adhere to the subendothelium of the damaged wall and, in response to the exposed subendothelial collagen, release adenosine diphosphate. This reaction causes platelet aggregation at the site of the injury and the formation of a platelet plug that is responsible for primary hemostasis. Acquired and congenital conditions that disrupt normal collagen synthesis or decrease vascular integrity affect this early stage of hemostatis. Alternatively, a decrease in the number of circulating platelets or an alteration in platelet metabolism and aggrega-

tion can also prevent normal primary hemostasis and can result in pathologic bleeding.

Normally, primary hemostasis is followed by the formation of a fibrin clot (secondary hemostasis) through the activation of the coagulation cascade. There are two main pathways of the coagulation cascade (Fig. 65.1). The intrinsic pathway is activated by the exposed collagen of a damaged vessel. This initiates a sequence of enzymatic reactions, beginning with the binding of factor XII to the exposed subendothelium. The extrinsic pathway is activated by tissue thromboplastin. Both pathways ultimately trigger the common pathway, resulting in the formation of a fibrin clot at the site of the injury. Factors XII, XI, IX, and VIII are involved exclusively in the intrinsic pathway, whereas factor VII is involved solely in the extrinsic pathway. Factors X, V, II (prothrombin), and I (fibrinogen) contribute to both pathways. As is the case with primary hemostasis, alterations in secondary hemostasis may result from intrinsic abnormalities of the clotting factors or from abnormalities related to systemic diseases.

Disruption of any aspect of normal hemostasis may result in abnormal bleeding leading to petechiae, purpura or ecchymoses. A basic understanding of normal hemostasis enables the physician to categorize petechial and purpuric disorders into the following categories: loss of vascular integrity, platelet disorders, and coagulation deficiencies. In general, patients with vasculitic disorders present with palpable purpura, patients with platelet disorders present with petechiae and abnormal mucosal bleeding, and patients with coagulation disorders are prone to ecchymoses and hemarthrosis.

DIFFERENTIAL DIAGNOSIS

Petechiae and purpura may result from loss of vascular integrity, thrombocytopenia, disorders of platelet function, or deficiencies of clotting factors. The most common causes of petechiae and purpura include trauma, infections, Henoch-Schönlein purpura (HSP), and idiopathic (or immune) thrombocytopenic purpura (ITP) (Table 65.1). Infections can affect normal hemostasis at many different stages in the process and are thus discussed separately.

Infection

Petechiae and purpura can be the initial manifestation of numerous infectious processes. Infection can disrupt normal hemostasis by several mechanisms. Even minor infections can cause significant thrombocytopenia from decreased platelet production or antiplatelet antibody formation, while severe

TABLE 65.4

COMPARISON OF LABORATORY VALUES IN DISSEMINATED INTRAVASCULAR COAGULATION, LIVER DISEASE, AND VITAMIN K DEFICIENCY

	PT	PTT	Fibrinogen	FSP	Platelet count	Factor V	Factor VII	Factor VIII
DIC	↑	↑	↓	↑	↓	↓	↓	↓
Vitamin K deficiency	↑	↑	N	N	N	N	↓	N
Liver disease	↑	↑	N to ↓	N to ↑	N to ↓	↓	↓	N to ↑

PT, prothrombin time; PTT, partial thromboplastin time; FSP, fibrin split products; DIC, disseminated intravascular coagulation; ↑, increased or prolonged; ↓, decreased; N, normal.

Synthesis of coagulation factors occurs in the liver, with the exception of von Willebrand factor. Thus, congenital and acquired hepatocellular disorders can result in decreased factor production and coagulopathy. Vitamin K is necessary for the activation of coagulation factors VII, IX, X, and prothrombin, and thus plays a vital role in secondary hemostasis. Coagulopathies caused by severe hepatocellular disease or vitamin K deficiency can present with some of the same clinical and laboratory findings as DIC. A comparison of the laboratory values in these three disorders is shown in Table 65.4.

Hemorrhagic disease of the newborn, with clinical manifestations that range from purpura to intracranial hemorrhage, may occur in infants who do not receive prophylactic vitamin K at birth. This may be the case with babies who are born at home or who have unexpected complications during delivery. Vitamin K deficiency in newborns can result from inadequate stores of vitamin K due to maternal deficiency or exclusive breastfeeding. In older children, vitamin K deficiency may occur with malabsorption or chronic diarrhea. Purpura caused by warfarin (Coumadin) therapy or ingestion can resemble vitamin K deficiency clinically.

Circulating anticoagulants in children are associated with viral infections, malignancies, and collagen vascular disorders. They are usually characterized by a prolonged PTT that fails to correct with the addition of normal plasma. Because most acquired inhibitors in children, particularly lupus anticoagulants, are not associated with increased bleeding, the identification of an inhibitor in a patient with purpura should not preclude an investigation of other coagulation abnormalities.

Numerous coagulation abnormalities have been demonstrated in vitro in patients with renal disease and uremia. However, bleeding is most commonly related to altered platelet function rather than to defects in the fluid phase of coagulation. Abnormalities that resemble those found in DIC have been associated with cyanotic congenital heart disease, and the severity of the coagulopathy is generally related to the degree of polycythemia.

EVALUATION AND DECISION

Patients with petechiae, purpura, and unexplained ecchymoses require timely and thorough evaluation. The diagnostic approach is outlined in Figure 65.2. The initial approach should be dictated by the general appearance of the child and the presenting vital signs. It goes without saying that a well-appearing child with normal vital signs can be approached with less urgency than a febrile, lethargic child or a child with signs of impending respiratory or cardiovascular failure.

The evaluation of critically ill children with petechiae and purpura should occur after restoring and maintaining adequate ventilation and perfusion, administering early antibiotics, if indicated, and identifying and controlling life-threatening hemorrhage, often with the administration of blood products. The most important early studies include CBC, PT, PTT, blood cultures, and typing and cross-matching of blood.

In the well-appearing child, the evaluation of petechiae and purpura can proceed in an orderly fashion. The recent and past medical history should be reviewed carefully with the parents and child. The presence or history of fever should raise the suspicion for an infectious process. Acute onset of petechiae or purpura after a recent viral illness or immunization is consistent with an acquired disorder such as ITP or a circulating anticoagulant. Recurrent petechiae and purpura since infancy, however, suggests an inherited abnormality of platelets or clotting factors. Specific inquiries about past surgeries, dental extractions, or significant trauma should be made because the absence of bleeding under these conditions would be unusual in most inherited disorders of even moderate severity. When previous bleeding has occurred, the site of bleeding may be helpful in establishing the alteration in the hemostatic mechanisms. Hemarthroses, a common problem in severe hemophilia, are rarely associated with platelet abnormalities. Conversely, petechiae and subconjunctival hemorrhages are commonly found in children with platelet disorders but occur rarely in hemophilia. The parents of a child with petechiae or purpura should be questioned closely regarding the recent use of any medications, including over-the-counter drugs and home remedies.

The family history should be reviewed for bleeding disorders. A positive family history in male relatives on the maternal side suggests factor VIII or factor IX deficiency. A history of bleeding or bruising in numerous family members of both sexes suggests a condition with dominant inheritance such as von Willebrand disease. As noted earlier, however, a negative family history does not preclude the diagnosis of von Willebrand disease or hemophilia.

A careful review of systems should also be obtained to evaluate for underlying conditions such as uremia, hepatic disease, congenital heart disease, or malabsorption that might be associated with a coagulopathy.

During the physical exam, particular attention should be paid to the skin, and all areas of the skin and mucus

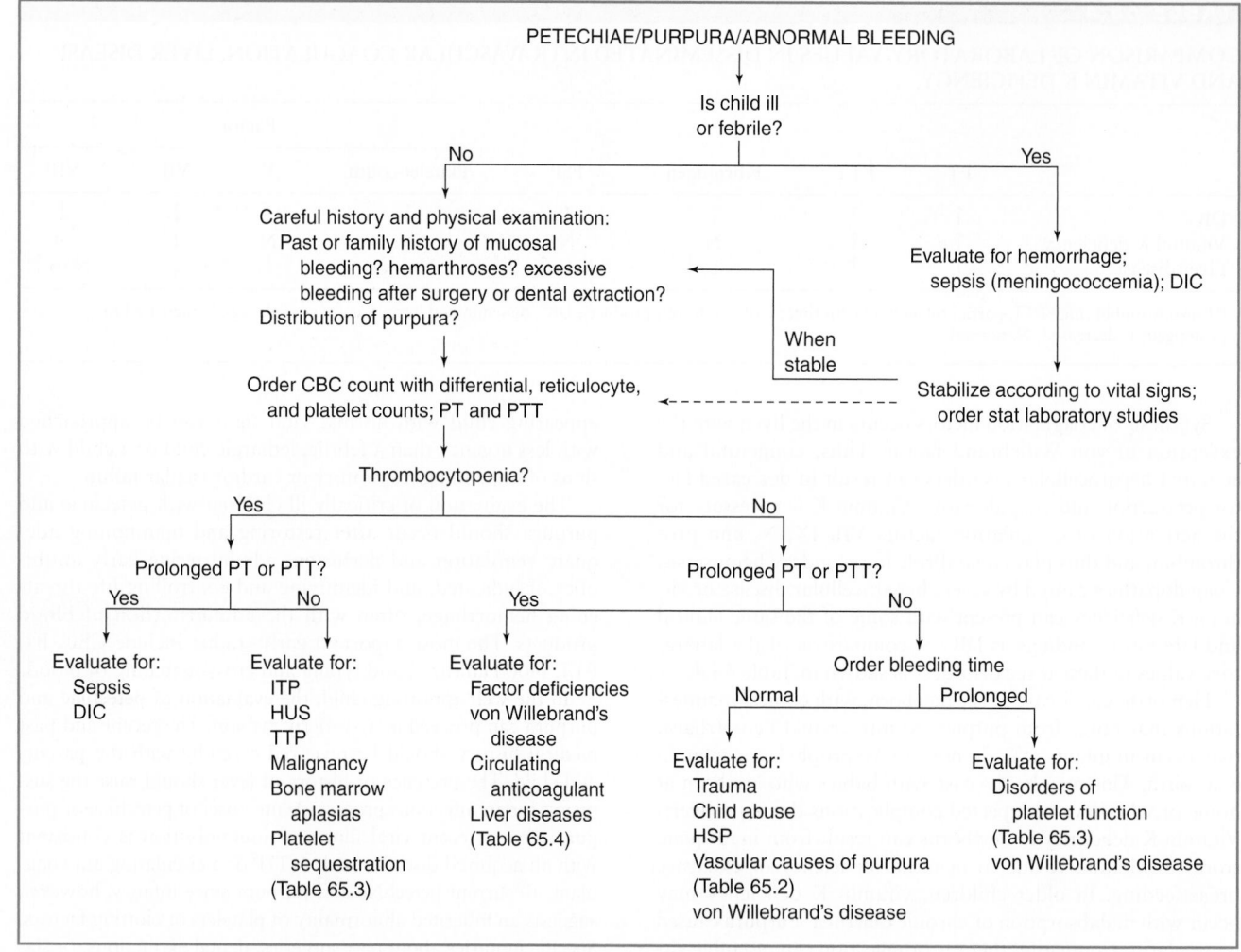

FIGURE 65.2 The approach to the child with petechiae, purpura, or abnormal bleeding. CBC, complete blood cell; PT, prothrombin time; PTT, partial thromboplastin time; DIC, disseminated intravascular coagulation; ITP, idiopathic (immune) thrombocytopenic purpura; HUS, hemolytic uremic syndrome; TTP, thrombotic thrombocytopenic purpura; HSP, Henoch-Schönlein purpura.

membranes should be examined. The distribution of purpura should be noted. Purpura on the lower extremities and buttocks or dependent regions suggests HSP, while purpuric lesions on the palms and soles are often seen with rickettsial infections. When the purpuric or ecchymotic lesion has an unusual shape, such as a folded cord or belt, child abuse should be suspected. A careful neurologic exam is important when there is suspicion of head trauma in the face of a coagulopathy. The eyes should be examined for the presence of conjunctival, scleral, or retinal hemorrhage. Additionally, the presence of lymphadenopathy or hepatosplenomegaly should be evaluated. Lymphadenopathy may be present in certain malignancies (leukemias) or viral infections (infectious mononucleosis, CMV) that can present with petechiae and purpura. Hepatomegaly may signal an underlying hepatic disorder that can cause a coagulopathy. Splenomegaly can be seen in infectious mononucleosis, leukemia, hepatic disease, and the glycogen storage diseases. Inflammation or synovial thickening of the large joints is consistent with the hemarthroses seen in hemophilia.

The laboratory approach to patients with petechiae and purpura is also influenced by the initial presentation and history. All patients who presents with petechiae, purpura, and unexplained bruising should have a complete blood cell count with a differential and platelet count, a PT, and a PTT. In most hospitals, these tests can be performed quickly so therapy can be chosen or modified on the basis of the results. A decreased hematocrit or hemoglobin concentration may indicate past or present blood loss, red blood cell destruction, or bone marrow failure. The WBC count can provide information suggestive of sepsis or leukemia. Atypical lymphocytes are seen with many viral infections, especially mononucleosis.

Causes of abnormal screening coagulation studies (platelet count, PT, PTT, bleeding time) are outlined in Table 65.5. Depending on the results of these initial tests and the clinical impression derived from the history and physical examination, a more sophisticated laboratory evaluation can be undertaken. If emergency therapy is required before the cause of abnormal bleeding is known, pretreatment plasma should be saved for later investigation of disorders such as von Willebrand disease

TABLE 65.5

TESTS COMMONLY USED IN THE INITIAL
EVALUATION OF PETECHIAE, PURPURA OR
SUSPECTED BLEEDING DISORDERS

Platelet Count (normal 150,000–500,000/mm^3)
  Decreased: increased platelet destruction, decreased platelet
  production, platelet sequestration, some platelet function
  disorders (Table 65.3)
Prothrombin Time (normal range may vary between
  laboratories)
  Prolonged: disseminated intravascular coagulation; vitamin
  K deficiency; warfarin ingestion; deficiencies of factors II,
  V, VII, X; abnormalities of fibrinogen; liver disease; renal
  disease; congenital heart disease
Activated Partial Thromboplastin Time (normal range may
  vary between laboratories)
  Prolonged: disseminated intravascular coagulation; von
  Willebrand disease; deficiencies of factors II, V, VIII, IX,
  X, XI, XII; abnormalities of fibrinogen; vitamin K defi-
  ciency; heparin therapy or sample contamination; liver
  disease; congenital heart disease
Fibrinogen (normal >150 mg/100 mL)
  Decreased: disseminated intravascular coagulation, liver
  disease, L-asparaginase therapy, dysfibrinogenemia,
  afibrinogenemia
Fibrin Split Products (normal <1:20)
  Increased: disseminated intravascular coagulation, liver
  disease
Bleeding Time (modified Ivy) (normal <8 min, 30 s)
  Prolonged: idiopathic thrombocytopenic purpura (early)
  and other thrombocytopenias, von Willebrand disease,
  platelet function disorders

or other inherited factor deficiencies. Other laboratory studies
that may be performed include an antinuclear antibody titer as
a screening test for collagen vascular disorders and a reticulocyte count and direct antiglobulin (Coombs) test to detect
immune hemolytic anemia.

The emergency management of children with petechiae and
purpura is discussed in detail in Chapter 91. However, the
general principles are straightforward. When petechiae and
purpura is associated with a serious underlying disorder such
as meningococcemia, treatment of that disorder is usually the
first priority. Treatment of the coagulopathy is based on the
degree and site of bleeding and the actual hemostatic defects.
In primary disorders of hemostasis, appropriate replacement
therapy is used when the specific alteration is known. When
the disease has not been fully defined, broad treatment with
one or more blood products may be required while further laboratory studies are performed.

Suggested Readings

Allen GA, Glader B. Approach to the bleeding child. *Pediatr Clin North Am*
  2002;49:1239–1256.
Bolton-Maggs PH, Pasi KJ. Haemophilias A and B. *Lancet* 2003;361:1801–1809.
Cines DB, Blanchette VS. Immune thrombocytopenic purpura. *N Engl J Med*
  2002;346:995–1008.
Kaplan RN, Bussel JB. Differential diagnosis and management of thrombocy-
  topenia in childhood. *Pediatr Clin North Am* 2004;51:1109–1140.
Leung AK, Chan KW. Evaluating the child with purpura. *Am Fam Physician*
  2001;64:419–428.
Lusher J. Clinical and laboratory approach to the patient with bleeding. In:
  Nathan DG, Orkin SH, Ginsburg D, et al., eds. *Hematology of infancy and
  childhood.* 6th ed. Philadelphia: WB Saunders, 1998:1515–1526.
Robertson J, Lillicrap D, James PD. Von Willebrand disease. *Pediatr Clin North
  Am* 2008;55:377–392.

CHAPTER 66 ■ RASH—URTICARIA

WILLIAM J. LEWANDER, MD, AND EMILY A. ZAJANO, MD

Urticaria is a common cutaneous vascular reaction experienced by nearly 20% of the population at some time during their lives. The etiology remains unknown in the majority of cases. Urticaria is usually acute and transient, but is classified as chronic if it persists for longer than 6 weeks. Although chronic urticaria is sometimes associated with physical agents or systemic illnesses [i.e., viral hepatitis, juvenile rheumatoid arthritis, systemic lupus erythematosus (SLE), lymphoma], the etiology remains unknown in more than 75% of cases.

Urticarial lesions appear as erythematous papules or wheals from edema in the upper dermis with a surrounding flare of erythema caused by vasodilation. They are pruritic, multiple, and of varying size and shape. Individual lesions are transient, usually lasting 12 to 24 hours or less. They often appear suddenly, resolve almost completely, and may reappear. The cutaneous distribution varies, but lesions secondary to physical agents are generally concentrated in areas of direct stimulation (i.e., dermographism).

Urticaria may be accompanied by angioedema and is associated with systemic symptoms from direct visceral involvement or from symptoms secondary to the release of circulating chemical mediators. Lesions of angioedema are often nonpruritic and involve deeper dermal and subcutaneous tissues with swelling that may involve the lips and eyelids. The respiratory, cardiovascular, and gastrointestinal systems may be involved, resulting in a potential life-threatening reaction. Signs and symptoms may include hoarseness, stridor, shortness of breath, wheezing, and general respiratory distress (from laryngospasm and bronchospasm), as well as hypotension, nausea, vomiting, diarrhea, and abdominal pain.

PATHOPHYSIOLOGY

Urticaria is characterized by superficial dermal edema, vasodilation and transudation of fluid and red blood cells, dilated lymphatics, and a mononuclear perivascular infiltrate. Angioedema occurs when these changes involve the deeper portion of the dermis and subcutaneous tissue. Urticaria and angioedema may occur independently or in association. Angioedema is mediated through mast-cell degranulation or via kinin-mediated pathway. Urticaria can be seen in conjunction with angioedema when it occurs via mast-cell degranulation. The release of histamine and various other vasoactive and chemotactic substances from mast cells and basophils appears to play a central role in the pathogenesis.

Acute urticaria is often triggered by infections, medications, and food reactions. Papular urticaria is a form of acute urticaria from hypersensitivity to insect bites. Chronic urticaria can be associated with autoimmune processes, but is more commonly idiopathic. Autoimmune urticaria is mediated by antibodies directed against either the IgE high-affinity receptor or the IgE molecule directly.

DIFFERENTIAL DIAGNOSIS

As shown in Table 66.1, urticaria may be classified on the basis of the mechanism responsible for its formation or, if unknown, as idiopathic.

Multiple factors—both immunologic and nonimmunologic—are capable of initiating the release of these mediators that result in the histopathologic findings described. The type I hypersensitivity reaction that involves the interaction of an antigen with a mast cell– or basophil-bound IgE with release of histamine represents the most common immunologic mechanism. However, type III (immune complex) reactions can also stimulate mediator release through activation of the complement system. Examples include urticaria seen in association with viral hepatitis, infectious mononucleosis, serum sickness, SLE, and some reactions to blood products. Nonimmunologic causes of urticaria include direct mast cell–releasing agents (i.e., opiates, radio contrast media) and agents that presumably alter arachidonic acid metabolism (i.e., aspirin, nonsteroidal antiinflammatory agents, azo dyes). Angiotensin-converting enzyme inhibitors are believed to enhance bradykinin synthesis.

Genetic factors are important in several relatively rare causes of urticaria and angioedema, including hereditary angioedema, familial cold, and localized heat urticaria. The most common etiologies of urticaria are listed in Table 66.2. Although idiopathic urticaria is the most common form, it is a diagnosis reached mainly by exclusion.

EVALUATION AND DECISION

Urticaria is diagnosed by its characteristic appearance and is only rarely confused with erythema multiforme, certain vasculitides (i.e., Henoch-Schönlein purpura), urticaria pigmentosa, or infectious exanthems.

Following clinical recognition, the patient should be evaluated for the presence of an associated systemic reaction that involves cardiopulmonary compromise (outlined in Fig. 66.1). Any form of urticaria that involves the airway or cardiovascular system is potentially life-threatening. Following any needed stabilization of cardiopulmonary compromise, evaluation for a specific etiology should begin with a thorough history and physical examination. Although the cause often remains unknown, Tables 66.1 and 66.2 outline the general classifications and most common identifiable causes of urticaria. In the

TABLE 66.1

CLASSIFICATION OF URTICARIA/ANGIOEDEMA

Immunologic
IgE dependent
    Specific antigen sensitivity
    Physical: dermographism, cold, cholinergic, heat, solar
    Contact
Complement mediated
    Serum sickness
    Reaction to blood products
    Hereditary angioedema
    Systemic lupus erythematosus

Nonimmunologic
Direct mast cell–releasing agents
    Opiates
    Radiocontrast media
Agents that alter arachidonic acid metabolism
    Aspirin and nonsteroidal antiinflammatory agents
    Azo dyes and benzoate preservatives
    Angiotensin-converting enzyme inhibitors

Idiopathic

Adapted from Soter NA. Acute and chronic urticaria and angioedema. *J Am Acad Dermatol* 1991;25:146–154.

context of acute onset, the patient and family must be questioned about specific precipitants, including drugs, foods, and hymenoptera stings. Febrile patients must be examined for clinical findings suggestive of viral and streptococcal infection, mononucleosis, and hepatitis. Latex allergy is uncommon in the general population, but health care workers and children with spina bifida appear to be at high risk for latex allergy. These patients may experience urticaria, conjunctivitis, bronchospasm, and anaphylaxis following contact with or inhalation of latex antigens. Laboratory tests

TABLE 66.2

COMMON CAUSES OF URTICARIA/ANGIOEDEMA[a]

Foods	Insect Bites
Peanuts	Hymenoptera venom
Eggs	**Infections**
Chocolate	Hepatitis
Shellfish	Streptococcus
Milk	Infectious mononucleosis
Strawberries	Mycoplasma
Food dyes and	Parasitic infection
preservatives	Upper respiratory
Drugs	infection
Penicillin	**Physical Agents**
Opiates	Cold
Radiocontrast media	Heat
Aspirin and nonsteroidal	Dermographism
antiinflammatories	Latex
Angiotensin-converting	
enzyme inhibitors	

[a]Essentially all may be life-threatening if accompanied by systemic reaction (see text).

are generally not helpful or necessary in the evaluation of acute urticaria.

Patients with chronic urticaria must be questioned about exposure to parasites, hepatitis, or a family history of urticaria and must be examined for findings suggestive of collagen–vascular disease or thyroid disease. Laboratory tests that may be useful in the evaluation of chronic urticaria include complete blood cell count with differential, erythrocyte sedimentation rate, urinalysis, monospot, antinuclear factor, liver function tests, and thyroid studies. Decreased levels of C_1 esterase inhibitor are found in hereditary angioedema. Stool for ova and parasites should be sent if there is eosinophilia present or if symptoms are consistent with parasitic infection. Provocative tests may be tried cautiously if certain physical urticarias are suspected.

If the etiology of chronic urticaria cannot be determined or if a severe systemic reaction occurs, then referral to an allergist should be considered after initial treatment is instituted.

MANAGEMENT

The initial management of urticaria follows assessment of the patient for a systemic reaction (e.g., anaphylaxis) with cardiopulmonary compromise (i.e., stridor, wheezing, hypotension; see Chapter 82). If cardiopulmonary compromise is present, airway, breathing, and circulation should be stabilized. Medications that may be used include oxygen, epinephrine (1:1,000) (0.01 mg per kg intramuscularly, maximum dose 0.5 mg, may be repeated every 15 minutes), diphenhydramine 1 mg per kg intravenously/intramuscularly, and volume resuscitation followed by vasopressors (i.e., continuous infusion epinephrine) if there is no response. Systemic corticosteroids (i.e., methylprednisolone 1 to 2 mg per kg) are slow to work but may block or reduce late-phase reactions. H_2-blockers may also play a role.

Although any precipitating factor may result in urticaria accompanied by a systemic reaction, cold, cholinergic and solar urticaria, and hereditary angioedema have been associated with severe attacks. Mortality from hereditary angioedema has been reported to be as high as 30% and generally results from airway obstruction. Danazol®, an attenuated androgen, is the preferred long-term prophylactic treatment. Acute attacks often require careful airway management, infusions of fresh frozen plasma, or concentrates of partly purified C_1 esterase inhibitor, and supportive care.

The general management of the more common presentation of urticaria without systemic involvement consists of removing or avoiding the inciting agent (if it can be identified) and providing symptomatic relief with antihistamines of the H1 class. The two most commonly used oral medications are hydroxyzine (Atarax® or Vistaril®, 2 mg per kg per day) and diphenhydramine (Benadryl®, 5 mg per kg per day) each in three to four divided daily doses for at least 3 to 5 days. Second-generation H1 antagonists can also be used, with the benefit of decreased CNS side effects due to decreased penetration of the blood–brain barrier. Cetirizine (Zyrtec®, dosing is age dependent) and loratadine (Claritin®) are a second-generation H1 antagonist used commonly in pediatric chronic urticaria. Cyproheptadine (Periactin®, 0.5 mg per kg per day

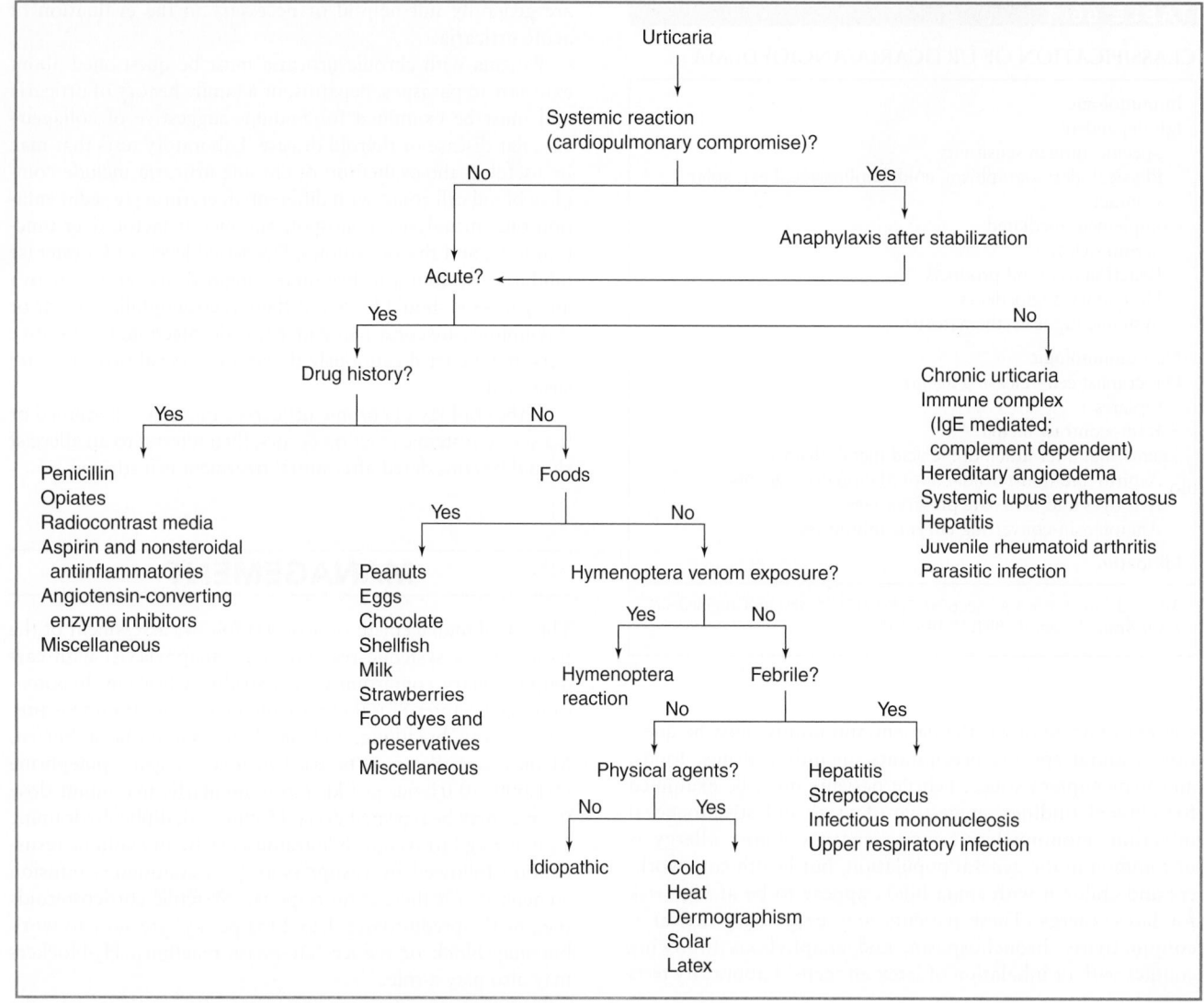

FIGURE 66.1 Algorithm for the evaluation of urticaria.

in three to four divided doses) has also been found to be effective. If there is severe pruritus, a rapidly progressing urticarial rash, or angioedema, then more rapid relief may be achieved with epinephrine (1:1,000) 0.01 mg per kg intramuscularly (maximum dose 0.5 mg) and diphenhydramine, 1 mg per kg IM. Systemic corticosteroids are inconsistent in their benefit, but they may suppress the appearance of new urticarial lesions and are indicated primarily in severe, inadequately controlled cases in which an infectious origin has been excluded.

Recurrent or persistent urticaria sometimes responds to cimetidine (Tagamet®, 20 to 30 mg per kg per day) in four divided oral doses, or cetirizine (Zyrtec®), dose dependent upon age. Cimetidine has numerous clinically important drug-drug interactions and caution should be used when adding cimetidine to an existing drug regimen.). Following or concurrently with treatment, an effort should be made to determine the etiology (Tables 66.1 and 66.2) so that the patient can avoid the precipitating agent.

Suggested Readings

Bailey E, Shaker M. An update on childhood urticaria and angioedema. *Curr Opin Pediatr* 2008;20(4):425–430.

Cicardi M, Agostoni A. Hereditary angioedema [Editorial; comment]. *N Engl J Med* 1996;334(25):1666–1667.

Cribier B. Urticaria and hepatitis. *Clin Rev Allergy Immunol* 2006;30:25–29.

Dreskin S, Andrews K. The thyroid and urticaria. *Curr Opin Allergy Clin Immunol* 2005;5:408–412.

Faurschou A, Wulf HC. Synergistic effect of broad-spectrum sunscreens and antihistamines in the control of idiopathic solar urticaria. *Arch Dermatol* 2008;144(6):765–9.

Gavignet B, Piarroux R, et al. Cutaneous manifestations of human toxocariasis. *J Am Acad Dermatol* 2008;59(6):1031–1042.

Horowitz R, Reynolds S. New oral antihistamines in pediatrics. *Pediatr Emerg Care* 2004;20(2):143–146.

Krishnamurthy A, Naguwa S, Gershwin M. Pediatric Angioedema. *Clin Rev Allergy Immunol* 2008;34:250–259.

Landwehr LP, Boguniewicz M. Current perspectives on latex allergy. *J Pediatr* 1996;128:305–312.

Najib U, Sheikh J. The spectrum of chronic urticaria. *Allergy Asthma Proc* 2009;30:1–10.

Schad C, Skoner D. Antihistamines in the pediatric population: achieving optimal outcomes when treating seasonal allergic rhinitis and chronic urticaria. *Allergy Asthma Proc* 2008;29:7–13.

CHAPTER 67 ■ RASH—VESICOBULLOUS

PAUL J. HONIG, MD, LESLIE CASTELO-SOCCIO, MD, PHD, AND ALBERT C. YAN, MD

Basic to all vesicobullous (blistering) disorders is the disruption of cellular attachments. Blister formation, therefore, follows intracellular degeneration, intercellular edema (spongiosis), or damage to the anchoring structures associated with the basement membrane (hemidesmosomes, basal lamina, anchoring fibrils). The location of these changes, as seen in Table 67.1, can help the physician ascertain a specific diagnosis. When histologic information is not readily available or nondefinitive, however, the historical and clinical features of the case must be relied on.

Such an approach is outlined in Figure 67.1. The key features used in this algorithm to distinguish the various entities are a characteristic clinical appearance, chronicity and/or presence at birth, associated fever or systemic illness, distribution of lesions, and the child's age. The diagnosis of vesicobullous lesions in children younger than 1 month of age is not discussed in this chapter. Figure 67.1 also outlines the frequency and potential severity of these diseases.

CHARACTERISTIC CLINICAL APPEARANCE

Many times, the appearance of a rash is so characteristic that a diagnosis becomes obvious. Such is the case with the conditions listed in Table 67.2.

Linear or geometric areas of vesiculation are the best clues to the presence of allergic contact dermatitis (see Chapter 99). The shape of the dermatitis provides the information that helps identify the offending agent. A history of playing in a shrubbed area, camping, hiking, or being near burning leaves is helpful. Because children brush against poison ivy leaves, vesicles often are in a line and on exposed surfaces (e.g., the face, extremities). A round group of vesicles on the back of the wrist would point to contact sensitivity to nickel contained in the metal case of a wristwatch.

Dermatomal distribution of vesicles or bullae usually indicates the presence of herpes zoster. On rare occasions, in infants, the same dermatomal appearance may represent zosteriform herpes simplex infections. A positive Tzanck smear indicates the presence of the herpes virus. Viral cultures, rapid slide tests using monoclonal antibodies, or more and more commonly, polymerase chain reaction tests are utilized to differentiate herpes simplex from herpes zoster.

Target or iris lesions are pathognomonic of erythema multiforme. The lesion has a dusky center that may blister and has successive bright red bordering rings. At times, a doughnut-shaped blister occurs. This contrasts with annular urticaria where incompletely round (arcuate or polycyclic) wheals are observed and individual lesions typically resolve within less than 24 hours.

Pigmented lesions that blister after stroking or trauma (Darier's sign) indicate the release of histamine from a mast cell collection. This collection may be isolated (mastocytoma of the wrist) or generalized (urticaria pigmentosa). Blistering of such lesions generally occurs only until 2 years of age. After this time, only urtication occurs.

A delicate "tear drop" vesicle is characteristic of varicella (chickenpox). Lesions usually begin on the upper trunk and neck. A progression through papules, vesicles, and crusts occurs rapidly (6 to 24 hours). All stages are present in an area at any given time. Mucous membranes are involved. Fever and malaise are usually present but are variable. Variola (smallpox) may initially resemble varicella. However, following the initial enanthem, the rash begins on the face and spreads to arms and then legs and trunk. In contrast to the lesions of varicella, variola lesions are monomorphic because they progress from macules to papules and pustules, with all the lesions in the same stage of evolution. The pustules are classically umbilicated.

DURATION

If there is no characteristic clinical appearance, the duration of the rash must be considered. If it has been present for 4 weeks or more, it should be considered chronic. Rashes that come and go but take not more than 4 weeks to disappear completely are not considered chronic.

Chronic Rash (Duration 4 Weeks or More)

If the blistering disease has been present since birth (congenital), consider the diagnoses listed in Table 67.3.

Epidermolysis Bullosa Syndromes

Blisters usually occur in areas predisposed to trauma or friction (Fig. 67.2). See Table 67.4 for differentiation of the various types.

Urticaria Pigmentosa

Mast cell disease (mastocytoma or urticaria pigmentosa) may cause blistering until 2 years of age. The pigmented solitary lesion most often occurs on the arm near the wrist (Fig. 67.3). Lesions may be generalized. When a pigmented lesion feels infiltrated, the physician should think of this cause. Gentle mechanical irritation of such lesions causes urtication or blistering (Darier's sign).

TABLE 67.1

PATHOLOGIC DIAGNOSIS OF VESICOBULLOUS ERUPTIONS

Type of blister	Site of formation	Disease
Subcorneal blister	Subcorneal	Impetigo Staphylococcal scalded skin syndrome
Blister from intracellular degeneration	Upper epidermis	Bullous congenital ichthyosiform erythroderma Epidermolysis bullosa of hands and feet Friction blisters
Spongiotic blister	Intraepidermal	Incontinentia pigmenti
Viral blister	Intraepidermal	Variola Herpes simplex Varicella-herpes zoster
Blister from degeneration of basal cell	Subepidermal	Epidermolysis bullosa simplex Lichen planus Lupus erythematosus
Blister from degeneration of basement zone	Subepidermal	Epidermolysis bullosa, dystrophic type Urticaria pigmentosa Bullous pemphigoid Dermatitis herpetiformis Erythema multiforme, dermal type Drug-induced toxic epidermal necrolysis

Epidermolytic Hyperkeratosis (Congenital Bullous Ichthyosiform Erythroderma)

Epidermolytic hyperkeratosis, an autosomal-dominant trait, is categorized under the ichthyotic syndromes. Children with this problem have recurrent bullous lesions during infancy and childhood. The skin has a background of erythema and scaling, and peels. The flexures are always affected with thickening of the skin (hyperkeratosis), as are the palms and soles; findings that develop in response to chronic trauma; erosions; and healing.

Incontinentia Pigmenti

Incontinentia pigmenti, a rare condition, occurs almost exclusively in females. Inflammatory vesicles and bullae erupt in crops in a linear or curvilinear distribution (especially on the extremities) for the first several weeks to months of life (Fig. 67.4). These affected areas then go on to a warty stage. Finally, swirl-like pigmentation occurs but not necessarily in the areas previously involved with warty or blistering lesions. During the vesicobullous stage, a high degree of peripheral eosinophilia occurs (18% to 50%). Because of the multisystem organ involvement often seen in incontinentia pigmenti, children with this condition should seek consultation with dermatologists or geneticists, who can help determine what other system evaluations may be necessary (such as neurology, ophthalmology, dentistry or oral-maxillofacial surgery, or immunology).

If the blistering is noncongenital, chronic bullous dermatosis of childhood (Fig. 67.5), dermatitis herpetiformis, and bullous pemphigoid should be considered. These conditions can be differentiated as outlined in Table 67.5.

Child Who Is Ill

When the blistering lesions occur acutely, it must be determined whether the child is febrile or ill. Conditions that cause such systemic findings with associated blisters include those listed in Table 67.6.

Varicella (Chickenpox)

For more information about varicella, see the discussion under "Characteristic clinical appearance."

Variola (Smallpox)

Although international efforts have been successful at eradicating smallpox, more recent geopolitical events have raised the spectre of bioterrorism and the potential for smallpox to be employed as a biological weapon. For more information about smallpox, see the section immediately preceding and Chapter 7.

Hand-foot-mouth Disease

Caused by coxsackievirus A16 and enterovirus 71, hand-foot-mouth disease is fairly characteristic. Vesicles are present on the palms, on the soles, and in the mouth. Other parts of the body may be involved. Fever, malaise, and abdominal pain may be present. Other coxsackie strains such as A5 and A10 less commonly cause hand foot and mouth disease.

Viral (Nonspecific) and Other Causes

Vesicles have been described in association with other coxsackievirus types (A4, A5, B1, B4), echovirus, reovirus, and *Mycoplasma pneumoniae* infections. These children are usually ill.

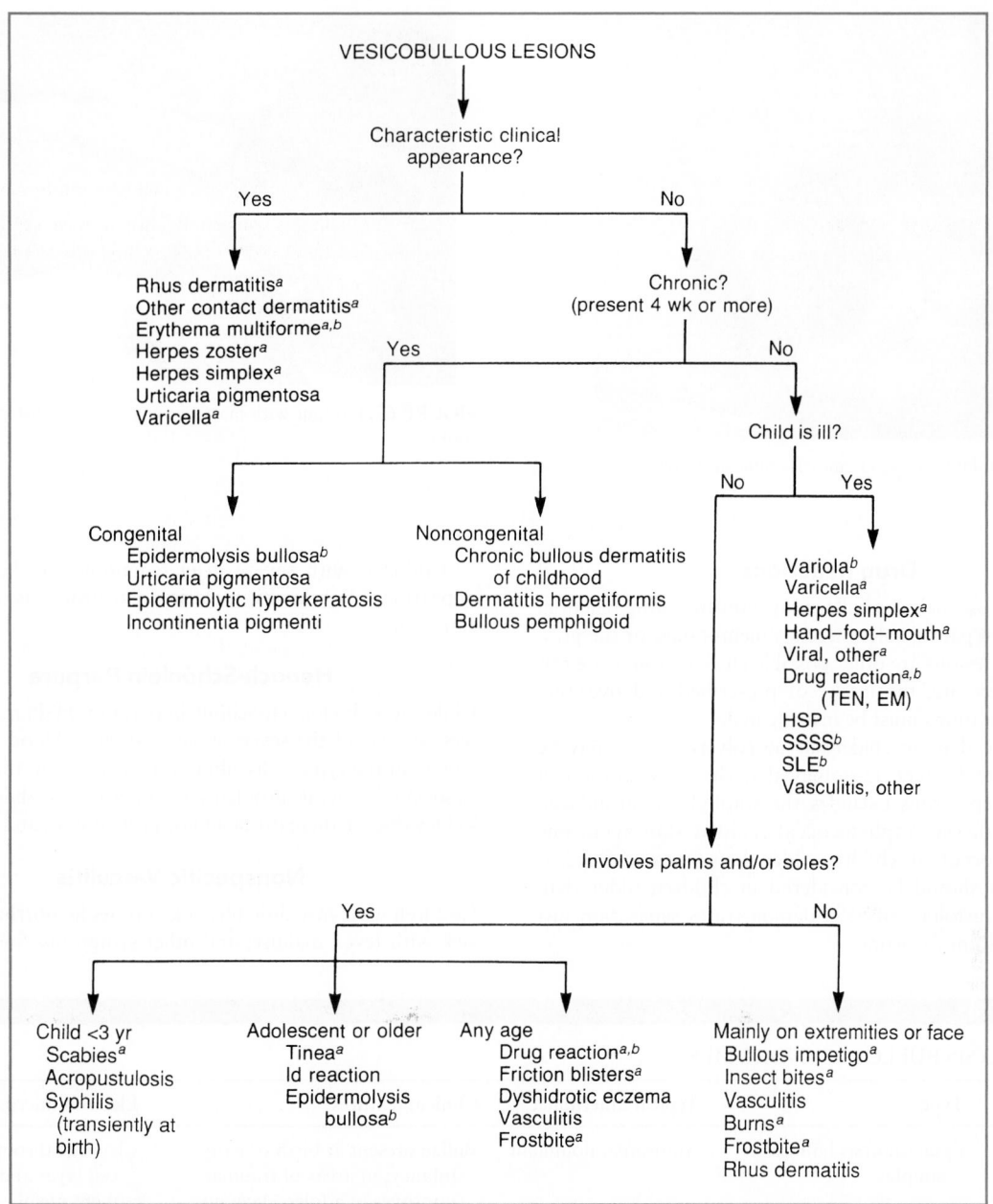

FIGURE 67.1 The diagnostic approach to the child with vesicobullous lesions. TEN, toxic epidermal necrolysis; EM, erythema multiforme; HSP, Henoch-Schönlein purpura; SSSS, staphylococcal scalded skin syndrome; SLE, systemic lupus erythematosus. [a]Common. [b]Potentially life threatening.

TABLE 67.2

VESICOBULLOUS RASHES WITH CHARACTERISTIC CLINICAL APPEARANCE

Rhus dermatitis	Urticaria pigmentosa
Other contact dermatitides	Herpes simplex
Erythema multiforme	Varicella
Herpes zoster	

TABLE 67.3

CONGENITAL BLISTERING DISEASES

Epidermolysis bullosa	Epidermolytic hyperkeratosis
Urticaria pigmentosa	Incontinentia pigmenti

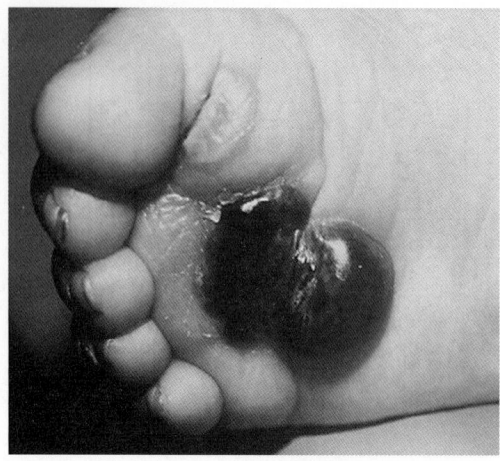

FIGURE 67.2 Infant with epidermolysis bullosa simplex.

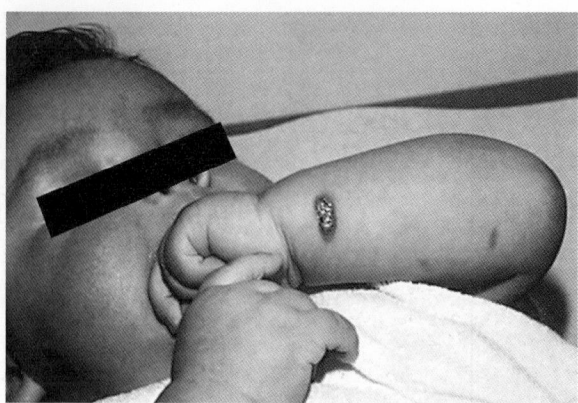

FIGURE 67.3 Infant with mastocytoma that has blistered because of trauma.

Drug Reactions

The presence of vesicles or bullae may indicate a drug reaction. Involvement of palms, soles, mucous membranes, or the presence of target lesions are other possible clues that indicate this problem. Therefore, the intake of prescribed and over-the-counter preparations must be investigated.

Drug-induced toxic epidermal necrolysis (TEN) may be associated with blisters. Histology that shows separation of dermis from epidermis excludes the staphylococcal-induced problem. Also, the staphylococcal scalded skin syndrome (SSSS) rarely occurs in children older than 6 years of age. A drug reaction should be considered in children older than 6 years. The histology of SSSS demonstrates separation just below the stratum corneum.

Children with severe drug reactions may be very toxic appearing. High fevers, malaise, joint problems, and the like can occur.

Henoch-Schönlein Purpura

Children with Henoch-Schönlein purpura (HSP) may have blisters because of the severe inflammation of blood vessels (vasculitis) in the typical distribution that occurs in this condition. Associated systemic problems include arthritis, abdominal pain, kidney disease (hematuria and/or proteinuria), and seizures.

Nonspecific Vasculitis

Children with vasculitic blisters, at times hemorrhagic, may be sick with fever, malaise, and other symptoms. Some go on to

TABLE 67.4

EPIDERMOLYSIS BULLOSA SYNDROMES

	Type	Typical inheritance	Clinical features	Electron microscope
Nonscarring	Epidermolysis bullosa simplex	Autosomal dominant	Bullae present at birth or early infancy; in areas of trauma; improves in adolescence; no mucous membrane involvement; nail involvement (20%)	Cleavage through basal cell layer above basement membrane
	Recurrent bullous eruption of hands and feet (Weber-Cockayne disease)	Autosomal dominant	May present in first 2 years of life but usually not before adolescence or early adulthood	Epidermal cleavage may be anywhere from suprabasal to lower granular cell layer
	Junctional epidermolysis bullosa (Herlitz disease)	Autosomal recessive	Usually at birth; spontaneous bullae and large areas of erosion	Cleavage at junction of dermis and epidermis (above basement membrane)
Scarring	Dominant dystrophic epidermolysis bullosa (dominant dermolytic bullous dermatosis)	Autosomal dominant	Early infancy and later; little or no involvement of hair and teeth; mucous membrane lesions and nail dystrophy	Dermal–epidermal separation beneath basement membrane
	Recessive dystrophic epidermolysis bullosa (recessive dermolytic bullous dermatosis)	Autosomal recessive	Present at birth; widespread scarring and deformity; severe involvement of mucous membranes and nails	Separation at dermal–epidermal junction (beneath basal lamina)

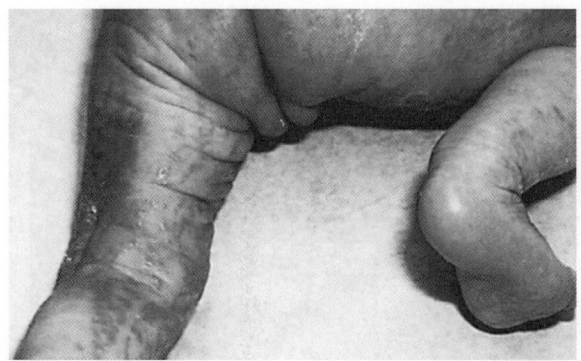

FIGURE 67.4 Linear arrangement of lesions (blisters in some cases) in a child with incontinentia pigmenti.

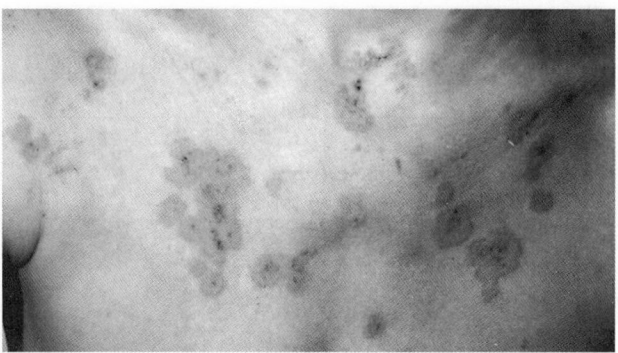

FIGURE 67.5 Chest of patient with chronic bullous dermatosis of childhood. Notice the resemblance to erythema multiforme.

well-defined collagen vascular disease, whereas others smolder, with no diagnosis ever being made.

Herpes Simplex

Primary infection with this virus may cause fever and regional lymphadenopathy. The first encounter for young children is usually herpetic gingivostomatitis. Vesicles involve the lips and the rest of the mouth. These children are often uncomfortable and commonly refuse to eat or drink.

Herpes progenitalis may produce fever and local lymphadenopathy as well. Characteristic clusters of vesicles occur on an erythematous base.

Often, erosions or ulcerations evolve on the vulva or penis. Diagnosis can be confirmed by a Tzanck smear that shows aggregates of multinucleated giant cells (see Chapter 99), a rapid slide test (immune-specific immunofluorescent antibody placed on cells scraped from the blister base), viral culture, or polymerase chain reaction.

Systemic Lupus Erythematosus

Although not characteristic, bullous lesions can occur in systemic lupus erythematosus (SLE). Multisystem involvement

suggests the diagnosis. Laboratory confirmation, which may include a skin biopsy and lupus band test, in conjunction with the complete clinical picture, is necessary for diagnosis.

Palm and Sole Involvement

If the child is not ill, the physician should search for blisters on the palms and soles. The child's age helps differentiate some disorders (Table 67.7).

CHILD YOUNGER THAN 3 YEARS

Scabies

Infants and very young children can have vesicobullous lesions on the palms (Fig. 67.6), soles, head, and face. It is important to not be misled by this distribution and appearance. Generally, the mother or father or other close family contact is also infested and exhibits the typical appearance of this disorder.

TABLE 67.5

NONCONGENITAL CHRONIC BLISTERING DISEASE

	Bullous disease of childhood	Bullous pemphigoid	Dermatitis herpetiformis
Type of lesions	Large, tense, clear bullae; annular plaques with active vesicular borders	Large, tense bullae	Grouped papulovesicles, bullae, or urticarial lesions
Distribution	Scalp, lower trunk, genitals, buttocks, inner thighs	Trunk and flexor surfaces of extremities	Back, buttocks, scalp, extensor surface of extremities, often symmetric
Pruritus	None to severe	Mild	Intense
Mucous membrane involvement	Usually not	Yes	No
Duration	Months to years	Months to years	Months to years
Immunofluorescence	+ or − Linear IgA basement membrane (+ circulating IgA)	+ Linear IgG on basement membrane (+ circulating IgG)	+ Granular IgA at tips of dermal papilla of uninvolved perilesional skin
Treatment	Corticosteroids and dapsone	Corticosteroids	Sulfapyridine or dapsone

TABLE 67.6

BLISTERING DISEASES ASSOCIATED WITH FEVER
AND/OR SYSTEMIC ILLNESS

Chickenpox
Hand-foot-mouth disease
Viral (nonspecific) + other
Drug reaction (toxic epidermal necrolysis, erythema
   multiforme)
Henoch-Schönlein purpura
Nonspecific vasculitis
Herpes simplex
Staphylococcal scalded skin syndrome
Systemic lupus
Atypical measles

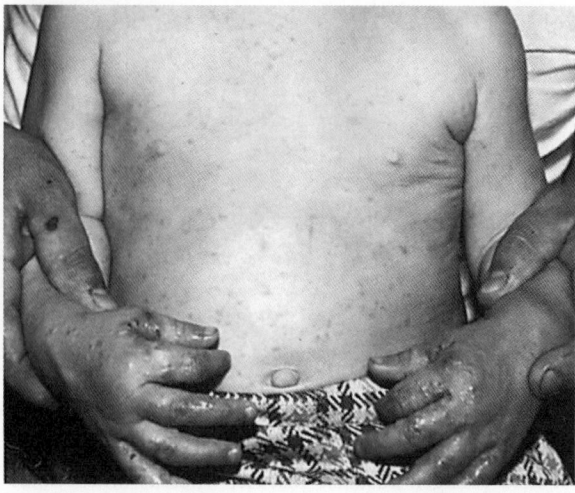

FIGURE 67.6 Blisters on hands of child infested with scabies.

Acropustulosis of Infancy

The appearance of pruritic vesicopustules between 2 and
10 months of age on the palms and soles (Fig. 67.7), typically
in African-American children, suggests acropustulosis of
infancy. Vesicles often involve the lateral aspects of the fingers,
palms, and soles. This condition was commonly diagnosed as
dyshidrotic eczema in the past. Some speculate a relationship
with antecedent scabies infestation in a subset of patients and
may refer to this phenomenon as postscabetic pustulosis in this
setting. Cyclic eruptions occur every 2 to 3 weeks, lasting 7 to
10 days. Spontaneous disappearance occurs at 2 to 3 years of
age. Treatment with topical steroids may moderate some of
the pruritus.

Syphilis

Congenital syphilis may produce transient blisters on the
palms and soles immediately after birth. "Snuffles," rhagades,
condyloma lata, and violaceous to reddish-brown macules on
the palms and soles may be observed. Hepatosplenomegaly is
often present. Osteochondritis is an early and common sign.

TABLE 67.7

ACUTE VESICOBULLOUS DISEASES INVOLVING
PALMS AND SOLES

Child <3 Years Old
Scabies
Acropustulosis of infancy
Syphilis (transiently at birth)

Adolescent or Older
Tinea pedis or manus
"Id" reaction
Epidermolysis bullosa of hands and feet

Any Age
Drug reaction
Friction blisters or burns
Dyshidrotic eczema
Vasculitis (e.g., Henoch-Schönlein purpura)
Frostbite

Severe tenderness of a limb may cause pseudoparalysis of
Parrot. The dilutional serologic test for syphilis is always positive in children with clinical manifestations.

ADOLESCENT OR OLDER

Tinea Pedis or Manus

Certain organisms that cause tinea pedis or manus (e.g.,
Trichophyton mentagrophytes) induce a severe inflammatory
reaction on the hands and feet. Vesicobullous lesions erupt on
the palms, instep, or medial aspect of the foot. A potassium
hydroxide (KOH) preparation or dermatophyte screen (fungal
culture) confirms the presence of hyphae in either location.

"Id" Reaction

If an adolescent's palms have blisters, the physician should
look at the feet. Patients with tinea pedis may have allergic

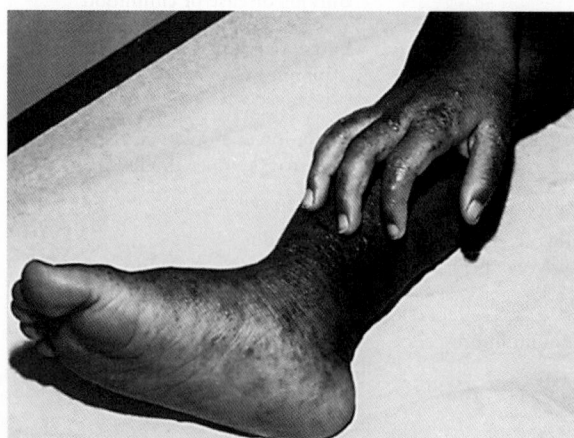

FIGURE 67.7 Note vesicles and pustules on child with acropustulosis
of infancy.

reactions to dissemination of antigen typified by blistering on uninvolved areas, characteristically on the palms. Because this represents a reaction to antigen and not to the intact organism, KOH preparation of the lesions on the palms will be negative for fungus.

Epidermolysis Bullosa of the Hands and Feet

For more information, see "Epidermolysis Bullosa Syndromes" section in this chapter (Table 67.4).

ANY AGE

Drug Reaction

For more information about drug reactions, see "Child Who Is Ill" section in this chapter.

Friction Blisters or Burns

Blistering on the palms and soles appears after trauma to the skin. The trauma is often related to a new activity (e.g., golfing, rowing, football) or to new, possibly poorly fitted, shoes.

Occasionally, accidental burns or burns secondary to child abuse are seen. Abused children may have had cigarette burns or have had their feet dipped in scalding water.

Dyshidrotic Eczema (Pompholyx)

A recurrent rash with episodes of vesicles that involve the palms, soles, and lateral aspects of the fingers is called dyshidrotic eczema. On occasion, large bullae occur. The problem is generally bilateral. Often, there is a personal or family history of atopy. A KOH preparation or fungal culture of scrapings from the palms or soles is generally negative.

Vasculitis

Vasculitis, also called HSP, may involve the palms and/or soles. See "Child Who Is Ill" section in this chapter for more information.

Frostbite (Pernio)

Fingers, toes, feet, nose, cheeks, and ears are affected by extreme cold. After exposed areas are damaged by the cold temperature, symptoms occur on rewarming. Erythema, swelling, and burning pain occur at first, followed by vesicles and bullae [at times hemorrhagic (Fig. 67.8)] within 24 to 48 hours.

Extremities

If there is no involvement or minimal involvement of the palms and soles and the rash is concentrated on the extremities,

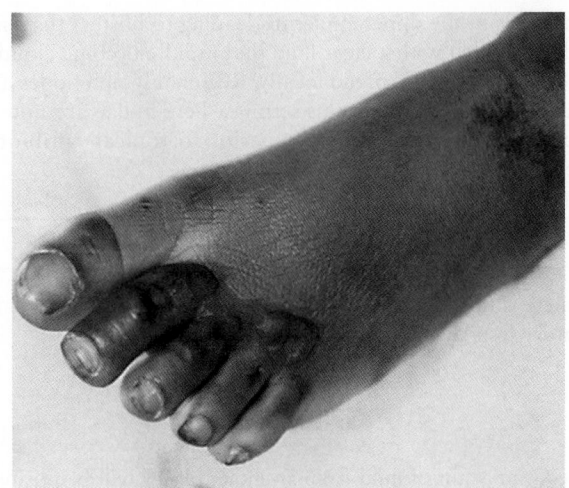

FIGURE 67.8 Frostbite. Child played in the snow for a prolonged period on a cold day wearing sneakers.

insect bites, vasculitis, burns, frostbite, and bullous impetigo should be considered.

INSECT BITES

Insects generally bite exposed skin surfaces. Therefore, heaviest involvement occurs on the head, face, and extremities. Mosquito bites occur in the warm weather months, whereas flea bites occur throughout the entire year. Historical information includes contact with pets, camping trips taken, and involvement in outdoor activities. When blisters are present, the more characteristic urticarial papules are usually present in other locations. If not, confusion with bullous impetigo is easily ruled out with a Gram stain or bacterial culture. In the case of bullous insect bites, these would be negative for bacteria.

VASCULITIS

Concentration of hemorrhagic bullae on the extremities and buttocks indicates HSP. The lower extremities are the area most often involved because of settling of immune complexes and cryoglobulins in that location.

BURNS

Exposed areas are commonly involved. Children accidentally rub against hot objects, causing burns and blistering. In cases of child abuse, children are burned intentionally with cigarettes (often mistaken for lesions of impetigo) or other heated objects. At times, children are submerged in scalding water. Usually, both lower extremities are involved.

BULLOUS IMPETIGO

In bullous impetigo, *Staphylococcus aureus* is usually present in pure culture. The bullae are caused by elaboration of a bacterial toxin that acts as a protease to cleave cell adhesion molecules in the upper epidermis leading to blisters that initially are filled with a clear fluid that rapidly become cloudy. The lesions tend to spread locally. Regional lymph nodes are usually not enlarged. In this setting where bullae are noted, oral antibiotics may prove superior to topical antibiotic therapy.

LABORATORY EVALUATION

If there is no clear idea about what caused the blister, the laboratory tests described next can be helpful.

Gram Stain

The Gram stain of fluid from an intact blister will be positive in impetigo and in a secondarily infected lesion. It will be negative, however, in all other conditions.

Tzanck Smear

Multinucleated giant cells will be present on a Tzanck smear (Fig. 99.7) of material scraped from the base of an intact, freshly opened vesicle caused by herpes simplex, herpes zoster, and varicella.

Rapid Slide Test for Direct Immunofluorescence

Fluorescent-tagged monoclonal antibody is applied to cells scraped from the blister base and can differentiate herpes simplex virus (HSV)-1, HSV-2, or varicella-zoster virus. Results can be available in 1 to 2 hours.

Bacterial or Viral Cultures

Occasionally, cultures help confirm an etiologic diagnosis when Gram stain, Tzanck smears, and direct immunofluorescence (DIF) are negative or indeterminate.

Polymerase Chain Reaction

An alternative or adjunct to traditional culture techniques, polymerase chain reaction techniques, allows for amplification of DNA or RNA present within a specimen and rapid identification of the etiologic pathogen. The technique is useful even when the pathogen present is no longer viable.

Skin Biopsy

For perplexing cases undiagnosed by clinical and/or simple laboratory evaluation, dermatologic consultation and skin biopsy are required.

On histologic examination, many characteristic changes can be found that lead to a definitive diagnosis (Table 67.1). Lichen planus, SLE, TEN, SSSS, and vasculitis are some of the diseases that can be identified by histologic studies.

If the picture on histology is compatible with erythema multiforme, DIF should be considered. DIF will be negative in erythema multiforme but will be positive in bullous pemphigoid [linear immunoglobulin G (IgG) on basement membrane], dermatitis herpetiformis [granular immunoglobin A (IgA) at tips of dermal papillae of uninvolved perilesional skin], and chronic bullous disease of childhood (CBDC) (linear IgA on basement membrane). DIF can be negative in CBDC.

Indirect immunofluorescence can be performed to test for circulating antibodies. Circulating IgG is found in bullous pemphigoid; circulating IgA is found in CBDC.

Suggested Readings

Carr DR, Houshmand E, Heffernan MP. Approach to the acute, generalized, blistering patient. *Semin Cutan Med Surg* 2007;26:139–146.

Centers for Disease Control. *Emergency preparedness and response—smallpox.* Available at: http://www.bt.cdc.gov/agent/smallpox/index.asp.

Fine JD, Eady RA, Bauer EA, et al. Revised classification system for inherited epidermolysis bullosa: report of the second international consensus meeting on diagnosis and classification of epidermolysis bullosa. *J Am Acad Dermatol* 2008;58:931–950.

Frieden IJ. The dermatologist in the newborn nursery: approach to the neonate with blisters, pustules, erosions, and ulcerations. *Curr Probl Dermatol* 1992;4:123.

Kalil C, Fachinello FZ, Cignachi S, et al. Bullous dermatoses in childhood: part I. *Skinmed* 2007;6:73–78.

Kalil C, Fachinello FZ, Cignachi S, et al. Bullous dermatoses in childhood: part II. *Skinmed* 2007;6:128–134.

Kim S, Dedeoglu F. Update on pediatric vasculitis. *Curr Opin Pediatr* 2005;17:695–702.

O'Neil KM. Progress in pediatric vasculitis. *Curr Opin Rheumatol* 2009;21(5): 538–546.

Orion E, Marcos B, Davidovici B, et al. Itch and scratch: scabies and pediculosis. *Clin Dermatol* 2006;24:168–175.

Steen CJ, Carbonaro PA, Schwartz RA. Arthropods in dermatology. *J Am Acad Dermatol* 2004;50:819–842.

Strong M, Johnstone PW. Interventions for treating scabies. *Cochrane Database Syst Review* 2007, Issue 18. Art. No.:CD000320.

Wagner A. Distinguishing vesicular and pustular disorders in the neonate. *Curr Opin Pediatr* 1997;9:396–405.

Wolf R, Orion E, Marcos B, et al. Life threatening acute adverse cutaneous reactions. *Clin Dermatol* 2005;23:171–181.

CHAPTER 68 ■ RESPIRATORY DISTRESS

DEBRA L. WEINER, MD, PHD

Respiratory distress is one of the most common chief complaints of children seeking medical care. It accounts for nearly 10% of all pediatric emergency department visits and 20% of visits of children younger than 2 years. Twenty percent of patients admitted to the hospital and 30% of those admitted to intensive care units are admitted for respiratory distress. Primary respiratory processes account for approximately 5% of deaths in children younger than 15 years and 20% in infants. In addition, respiratory distress contributes substantially to deaths in patients with other primary processes. Respiratory arrest is one of the five leading causes of death in pediatric patients, along with congenital anomalies, trauma, neoplasm, and cardiac disease. Respiratory distress results from interruption of the respiratory or ventilatory pathway. The cause of respiratory distress may be within the respiratory system or within organ systems that control or impact respiration. Respiratory failure is caused by an inability to meet metabolic demands for oxygen (O_2) or by inadequate carbon dioxide (CO_2) elimination. Young children are at particular risk of respiratory distress because of their respiratory anatomy and physiology. Rapid evaluation and aggressive treatment of respiratory distress, as well as anticipation and prevention of impending respiratory distress and failure, are essential to optimize outcome. Respiratory distress is usually reversible, but failure to treat the condition may result in cardiac arrest with long-term neurologic sequelae or death.

PATHOPHYSIOLOGY

Respiration is a complex multisystem process. The primary goals of respiration are to meet metabolic demands for O_2 and to eliminate CO_2. Secondary functions include acid-base buffering, host defense, and hormonal regulation. The upper airway or conducting zone, which includes the nose, nasopharynx, oropharynx, larynx, trachea, major bronchi, and terminal bronchioles, serves as a conduit for air movement. The lower airway, or respiratory zone, consists of the acini and interstitium. Each acinus originates from a terminal bronchiole and includes respiratory bronchioles, alveolar ducts, sacs, and alveoli. The interstitium, which consists of the alveolar walls and interstitial septa, is the fibrous structural framework of the lower airway. Exchange of O_2 and CO_2 between the lungs and the blood occurs at the alveolocapillary membrane and depends on adequate and appropriately matched ventilation and perfusion.

Control of respiration is mediated by central and peripheral neural mechanisms. Respiration is an intrinsic brainstem function of the respiratory centers of the medulla. The dorsal respiratory group produces rhythmic inspiration, whereas the ventral respiratory group controls expiration. Respiration is modulated by impulses within the brain and among the brain, respiratory system, blood, cerebrospinal fluid, and peripheral tissues. In the pons, the apneustic center increases the duration and depth of inspiration, whereas the pneumotaxic center shortens the duration and depth of respiration. Central chemoreceptors in the medulla respond to changes in the pH of cerebrospinal fluid. Peripheral chemoreceptors in the carotid and aortic bodies respond to changes in O_2, CO_2, and pH in arterial blood. In the airways, lungs, and chest wall, stretch, juxtacapillary, and irritant reflex mechanoreceptors respond to lung volume, changes in pulmonary microvasculature, chest wall muscle activity, and environmental irritants. Respiration is further influenced by the cerebellum, which alters respiration with postural change; by the hypothalamus, which controls respiration on a moment-to-moment basis; by the limbic system, which modulates respiration in response to emotion; and by the motor cerebral cortex, which controls volitional respiratory activity, including hyperventilation and hypoventilation and speech. Afferent information is transmitted to the brain primarily by the vagus [cranial nerve (CN) X] from the aortic body and mechanoreceptors, the glossopharyngeal (CN IX) from the carotid body, and the spinal motor neurons from muscle proprioceptors. Efferent impulses are transmitted from the brain via the vagus and spinal nerves to the larynx, trachea, bronchi, bronchioles, and acini; the glossopharyngeal to the pharynx; the hypoglossal (CN XII) to the tongue; and the spinal accessory (CN XI) to accessory muscles.

Impulses are also transmitted via spinal motor neurons in the anterior spinal horn to the cervical nerves (C2 to C4), the phrenic nerve (C3 to C5), and the intercostal nerves (T1 to T12), which innervate accessory muscles, the respiratory diaphragm, and intercostal muscles, respectively. The muscles and bones of the chest wall provide structural support and, along with the muscles of the abdomen, impact lung excursion and thus movement of air in and out of the lung. Cardiovascular and lymphatic drainage maintain the fluid balance of the lung and thus impact gas exchange.

Respiratory distress results from dysfunction or disruption of the respiratory/ventilatory pathway and/or systems that control or modulate respiration.

Respiratory failure is the inability to meet the metabolic demand for O_2 (hypoxia) or the inability to eliminate CO_2 (hypercapnia). Criteria for defining respiratory failure vary widely; one set of criteria is presented in Table 68.1. Hypoxia can be categorized on the basis of mechanism. Hypoxic or arterial hypoxemia is the most common type of hypoxemia. It results from an inability to deliver adequate O_2 to the blood.

TABLE 68.1

CRITERIA FOR RESPIRATORY FAILURE[a]

Clinical	Laboratory
Tachypnea, bradypnea, apnea, irregular respirations	$PaO_2 < 60$ mmHg in 60% O_2[b]
Pulsus paradoxus > 30 mmHg	$PaCO_2 > 60$ mmHg and rising
Decreased or absent breath sounds	pH < 7.3
Stridor, wheeze, grunting	Vital capacity < 15 mL/kg
Severe retractions and use of accessory muscles	Maximum inspiratory pressure ±25 cm H_2O
Cyanosis in 40% O_2[b]	
Depressed or heightened level of consciousness, decreased response to pain	
Weak to absent cough or gag reflex	
Poor muscle tone	

[a]Respiratory failure is likely if two clinical findings and one laboratory finding exist.
[b]Excluding cyanotic heart disease.
[c]Without underlying pulmonary disease.

Most often, this type of hypoxia results from hypoventilation secondary to airway obstruction, central respiratory depression or impairment, neuromuscular or skeletal insufficiency, or restricted lung expansion. Other causes of hypoxemic hypoxia include low atmospheric PO_2 (e.g., high altitude), diffusion impairment (e.g., pulmonary edema, pulmonary fibrosis, acute respiratory distress syndrome, O_2 toxicity), anatomic or physiologic shunt (e.g., atelectasis, pneumonia, abnormal pulmonary blood flow), or increased metabolic demand (e.g., exercise, systemic illness). Anemic hypoxia is the result of the blood's inability to deliver adequate O_2 to tissues as a result of decreased hemoglobin oxygen-carrying capacity. It is caused by inadequate red blood cell number (decreased production, increased destruction, loss), low erythrocyte hemoglobin concentration (anemia), abnormal hemoglobin, carboxyhemoglobin, or methemoglobin. Hypokinetic, ischemic, or stagnant hypoxia also results in an inability of the blood to transport O_2 to the tissues. This type of hypoxia is caused by decreased blood flow to a localized area secondary to compromised cardiac output (e.g., cardiac failure), poor tissue perfusion (e.g., shock), sludging (e.g., polycythemia), or obstructed flow (e.g., vascular obstruction). Histotoxic hypoxia results from inability to metabolize O_2 at the tissue level as a result of inactivation of metabolic enzymes by a chemical such as cyanide. Hypercapnia is caused by inadequate alveolar ventilation [e.g., central nervous system (CNS) depression, spinal cord injury, neuromuscular disease, diaphragmatic dysfunction], ventilation-perfusion imbalance with relative hypoventilation (e.g., restrictive airway disease, pulmonary embolism), or increased CO_2 production (e.g., metabolic/endocrine disturbance). Hypercapnia often contributes to respiratory failure as a result of hypoxemia and is less commonly the primary cause.

Infants are at an increased risk of respiratory distress compared with children and adults because of anatomic and physiologic differences (Table 68.2). These differences result in greater risk of airway obstruction, less efficient respiratory effort, limited respiratory reserve, and dysfunction of CNS respiratory control.

DIFFERENTIAL DIAGNOSIS

Establishing a diagnosis for respiratory distress in part depends on localizing the source of the distress to a particular organ system. Respiratory distress may result directly from a disturbance of the upper or lower respiratory system. It may also be caused by inability of the CNS or peripheral nervous system to interpret or process respiratory requirements, or of the musculoskeletal system to perform the work of breathing. Alternatively, disease or dysfunction of other organ systems may indirectly result in respiratory disturbance by compromising respiratory system function or by stimulating compensatory respiratory mechanisms (Tables 68.3 to 68.5). Treatment of the underlying cause is essential for definitive treatment of the respiratory distress.

Respiratory System

Conditions may be congenital or acquired. They may be caused by upper or lower airway obstruction or by disorders of the parenchyma or interstitium. Upper airway obstruction is common in infants and young children in part because of their airway anatomy and physiology (see Chapter 72). Manifestations of upper airway obstruction include nasal flaring, stertor or snoring, gurgling, drooling, dysphagia, aphonia, hoarseness, stridor, retractions, and paradoxical chest/abdominal wall movement. In neonates, the common causes include nasal obstruction, congenital upper airway anomalies (particularly laryngotracheomalacia), and congenital or postintubation subglottic stenosis. Common causes for acquired upper airway obstruction in infants and children include adenotonsillar hypertrophy, peritonsillar abscess, croup, foreign body, retropharyngeal abscess, tracheitis, and airway edema from trauma, thermal or chemical burn, or allergic reaction. *Epiglottitis*, although less common, is one of the most life-threatening causes of respiratory distress and is a true emergency. The incidence of epiglottitis has declined significantly since routine immunization against *Haemophilus influenzae* B, the pathogen that once caused at

TABLE 68.2

ANATOMIC/PHYSIOLOGIC DIFFERENCES IN INFANT/CHILD AND ADULT AIRWAYS

Difference	Consequence
Nose: infants <4 mo obligate nose breathers	Nasal congestion may result in significant respiratory distress
Larynx: higher (C3–C4 vs. C6), funnel shaped, narrowest at cricoid ring, softer, more elastic	More difficult to intubate
	Collapses more easily, particularly with fixed obstruction (i.e., Bernoulli's principle—as the velocity of flow through a collapsible tube increases, the pressure that holds the tube open decreases)
Trachea: one-third diameter of adult at birth, shorter	Poiseuille's law—resistance varies inversely with fourth power of the radius; 1-mm thickening decreases cross-sectional diameter by 20% in adult and by 80% in child
	More difficult to intubate/maintain proper depth
Alveoli: elastic fibers less well developed	Alveoli collapse more easily, results in ventilation-perfusion mismatch
Lungs: lower functional residual capacity	Reserve small, therefore limited protection when ventilation is interrupted, PaO_2 decreases more rapidly
Respiratory control apparatus: immature—reflexes that inhibit respiration, particularly Hering-Breuer reflex, which responds to stretch of lung, are very strong; central nervous system processing of information markedly affected by sleep state, cold, drugs, other metabolic derangements	Apnea or inability to respond appropriately to mechanical respiratory obstruction or increased metabolic demand
Chest wall: more compliant; intercostal muscles immature; ribs more horizontal; diaphragm flatter, fatigues; during rapid eye movement sleep, intercostal muscle movements become uncoordinated	Accessory muscle retractions
	Diaphragm does more work but is less effective

least 75% of cases. Epiglottitis should be suspected in children who have abrupt onset of fever, dysphagia, drooling, muffled voice, labored respirations, and stridor. Children appear toxic and anxious and assume a sniffing position with protruding jaw and extended neck. These children are at risk of abrupt onset of respiratory arrest from obstruction. *Peritonsillar and retropharyngeal abscess* may present with symptoms similar to epiglottitis but have more gradual onset. *Croup* or laryngotracheobronchitis is the most common cause of upper airway obstruction in children 3 months to 3 years of age. Croup causes subglottic narrowing and is characterized by a barky cough, inspiratory stridor, and hoarseness that are worse at night. Viral croup, most often caused by parainfluenza virus, has an insidious onset following several days of upper respiratory infection symptoms with normal temperature or low-grade elevation. Spasmodic or allergic croup has acute onset, usually with wakening during the night, in a child who was well before going to sleep. Children with recurrent or prolonged croup may have an underlying fixed or functional airway abnormality, most commonly subglottic stenosis or hemangioma. Children with chronic stridor, particularly those younger than 2 years, are also likely to have an underlying congenital anomaly. *Tracheitis*, a bacterial infection of the trachea, usually due to *Staphylococcus* or *Streptococcus*, may occur as a primary infection with abrupt onset, high fever similar to epiglottitis or more commonly as a secondary infection in a child with a croup-like illness and is suggested by worsening clinical course. In patients with respiratory failure due to upper airway infection, tracheitis is now more likely to be the etiology than epiglottitis or croup.

Foreign-body aspiration, which has a peak age of occurrence of 1 to 5 years, may cause obstruction of the upper or lower airway and is a leading cause of accidental death in toddlers. A history of abrupt onset of choking or gagging is suggestive. Drooling, dysphagia, and stridor suggest an upper airway foreign body, whereas unilateral wheeze, particularly first-time wheeze with acute onset, suggests lower airway position. Presentation, particularly with lower airway foreign body, may be delayed by days to weeks from time of aspiration.

Other common causes of lower airway obstruction involve inflammation and bronchospasm and include asthma, allergy, and bronchiolitis. Wheeze, most often diffuse, is usually a predominant feature of these conditions (see Chapter 80). *Asthma* may be triggered by infection, exercise, environmental irritants, stress, and/or gastroesophageal reflux. Allergy, usually accompanied by coryza, congestion, mucosal edema, and/or rash, may be in response to environmental exposures, food, or medications. *Bronchiolitis*, most often caused not only by respiratory syncytial virus but also by parainfluenza, influenza, adenovirus, metapneumovirus, and less commonly other viruses, presents with wheeze in children younger than 2 years. These conditions cause airway obstruction by decreasing airway lumen secondary to bronchospasm, edema, or thickening of the wall of the lumen. Lower airway obstruction is also caused by include filling of the airway lumen by excessive secretions (e.g., from inflammation, infection, toxin such as organophosphate) or aspirated fluids and decrease in lumen diameter due to loss of radial traction of the airway wall, as with emphysema and masses.

TABLE 68.3

CAUSES OF RESPIRATORY DISTRESS

Respiratory system
Upper airway obstruction
  Nasopharynx (craniofacial anomalies, choanal atresia, adenotonsillar hypertrophy, nasal congestion, foreign body, trauma, mass)
  Oropharynx (macroglossia, micrognathia, midface hypoplasia, tonsillitis, peritonsillar abscess, Ludwig's angina, trauma)
  Larynx (laryngomalacia, hemangioma, papilloma, webs, cysts, laryngoceles, laryngotracheal cleft, subglottic stenosis, croup, epiglottitis, retropharyngeal abscess, tracheitis, anaphylaxis, angioneurotic edema, thermal or chemical burn, foreign body, vocal cord paralysis, trauma)
  Trachea (tracheomalacia, stenosis, tracheoesophageal fistula, foreign body)
  Bronchi (bronchomalacia, stenosis, bronchogenic cyst, bronchitis, foreign body)
Lower airway obstruction/acinar/interstitial disease
  Bronchioles (asthma, bronchiolitis, allergy, angioneurotic edema, bronchiectasis)
  Acini/interstitium
  Disorders of lung maturity (transient tachypnea of newborn, respiratory distress syndrome, bronchopulmonary dysplasia, persistent fetal circulation, Wilson-Mikity syndrome)
  Congenital malformation (congenital emphysema, cystic adenomatoid malformation, sequestration, pulmonary agenesis/aplasia/hypoplasia, pulmonary cyst)
  Aspiration (meconium, foreign body, near drowning, gastroesophageal reflux, vomiting)
  Infection (pneumonia; bacterial, atypical bacteria, viral, chlamydial, pertussis, fungal, pneumocystis)
  Pulmonary collapse, fluid, mass (atelectasis, edema, hemorrhage, embolism, mass)
  Environmental/trauma (high-altitude pulmonary edema, thermal or chemical burn, smoke, carbon monoxide, hydrocarbon, drug-induced pulmonary fibrosis, bronchopulmonary traumatic disruption, pulmonary contusion)

Central nervous system
Structural abnormality (agenesis, hydrocephalus, mass, arteriovascular malformation)
Dysfunction/immaturity (apnea, hyperventilation/hypoventilation)
Infection (meningitis, encephalitis, abscess)
Inherited degenerative disease
Intoxication (alcohol, barbiturates, benzodiazepines, opiates)
Seizure
Trauma (birth asphyxia, hemorrhage)
Spinal cord (congenital anomaly, tetanus, trauma)
Anterior horn (poliomyelitis, transverse myelitis, spinal muscular atrophy)

Peripheral nervous system
Peripheral motor nerve (phrenic nerve injury, Guillain-Barré syndrome, multiple sclerosis, tick paralysis, heavy metal or organophosphate toxicity, porphyria)
Neuromuscular junction (myasthenia gravis, botulism, snake bite, organophosphate toxicity, antibiotics)
Muscle (muscular/myotonic dystrophies, IEM, carnitine deficiency, polymyositis/dermatomyositis, fatigue)

Chest wall/intrathoracic
Air leak (pneumothorax, tension pneumothorax, pneumomediastinum, pneumopericardium)
Space-occupying (esophageal foreign body, pleural effusion, empyema, chylothorax, hemothorax, anomalies great vessels, diaphragmatic hernia, cyst, mass)
Boney and/or muscular deformity or dysfunction (congenital bone/muscle absence, spine deformity, pectus excavatum/carinatum, diaphragmatic hernia, contusion, rib fractures/flail chest, burn)

Cardiovascular
Congenital (structural defect, arrhythmia)
Acquired (myocarditis, myocardial ischemia or infarction, pericardial effusion, pericardial tamponade, aortic dissection or rupture, mass, coronary artery dilation/aneurysm, congestive heart failure)

Gastrointestinal
Distension/pain (necrotizing enterocolitis, mass, obstruction, perforation, laceration, hematoma, contusion, appendicitis, infection, inflammation, ascites)

Metabolic/endocrine
Acidosis (exercise, fever, hypothermia, dehydration, sepsis, shock, IEM, liver disease, renal disease, diabetic ketoacidosis, salicylates)

Hyperammonemia (IEM, liver failure)
Serum chemistry disturbance (hyperkalemia/hypokalemia, hypercalcemia/hypocalcemia, hypophosphatemia, hypermagnesemia/hypomagnesemia)
Respiratory chain disturbance (cyanide)
Endocrine (hyperglycemia/hypoglycemia, hyperthyroidism/hypothyroidism, hyperparathyroidism, adrenal hyperplasia)

Hematologic
Anemia, abnormal hemoglobin (inadequate erythrocyte numbers, decreased production, loss, hemoglobinopathy, methemoglobin, carboxyhemoglobin)
Polycythemia

IEM, inborn error of metabolism.

TABLE 68.4

MOST COMMON CAUSES OF RESPIRATORY DISTRESS

Neonates	Infants/children
Nasal obstruction	Peritonsillar abscess
Congenital airway anomalies	Croup
Transient tachypnea	Tracheitis
Respiratory distress syndrome	Foreign body
Meconium aspiration	Bronchiolitis
Pneumonia	Asthma
Sepsis	Allergy
Congenital heart disease	Pneumonia
	Fever
	Sepsis
	Gastroenteritis/dehydration

Disorders of the alveoli and interstitium involve pus or fluid collection, collapse, and structural or functional abnormality. Alveolar and interstitial disease is characterized by tachypnea, cough, grunting, crackles, rhonchi, wheeze, and decreased and/or asymmetric breath sounds with or without fever. In neonates, transient tachypnea of the newborn and meconium aspiration are common causes. *Pneumonia* is one of the most common causes of lower airway disease in neonates, infants, and children. Findings are more likely to be localized in the setting of bacterial pneumonia, whereas patients with viral and atypical pneumonias, such as *Mycoplasma* infection, *Chlamydia* infection, and pertussis, tend to have diffuse peribronchial, interstitial processes. Severe acute respiratory syndrome (SARS), first seen in November 2002, is a form of atypical pneumonia caused by a coronavirus (SARS-CoV). The most common symptoms of SARS are fever, chills, malaise, myalgias, cough, tachypnea, dyspnea, and hypoxia. Chest x-ray (CXR) films reveal focal infiltrates with progression to general patchy, interstitial infiltrates similar to pneumonia or respiratory distress syndrome. Less commonly, aspiration, hemorrhage, and pulmonary edema cause fluid collection in the acini and interstitium. Atelectasis, or airway collapse, resulting from loss of air from the pulmonary parenchyma, often occurs secondary to other processes, including pneumonia, particularly viral; bronchospasm; and inadequate lung expansion, most often resulting from pain, neuromuscular disease, or inactivity. Structural and/or functional abnormalities include bronchopulmonary dysplasia, hyaline membrane disease or respiratory distress syndrome, bronchiectasis (most commonly seen in cystic fibrosis), congenital or acquired emphysema, and pulmonary fibrosis (usually from radiation and chemotherapy).

Several biological and chemical agents that are potential weapons of terrorism or warfare produce respiratory distress as their most predominant effect. These include the biological

TABLE 68.5

MOST COMMON ACUTE LIFE-THREATENING
CAUSES OF RESPIRATORY DISTRESS

Foreign body	Pericardial tamponade
Tension pneumothorax	Epiglottitis

agents inhalational anthrax, pneumonic plague, pneumonic tularemia, melioidosis, and the toxins *Staphylococcus* enterotoxin B and ricin, and the chemical agents chlorine and phosgene (see Chapter 7). Respiratory findings include cyanosis, chest pain, cough, hemoptysis, dyspnea, tachypnea, stridor, rales, and/or wheeze. CXR films may reveal infiltrates, pulmonary edema, pleural effusions, widened mediastinum, abscesses, and/or granulomas.

Nervous System

CNS disturbances may result in hypoventilation or hyperventilation, loss of protective airway reflexes, or airway obstruction from loss of pharyngeal tone. These conditions include CNS malformation, immaturity, infection, degenerative disease, seizures, mass, trauma, and intoxication. Focal neurologic deficits, visual disturbances, pupillary abnormalities, papilledema, abnormal muscle tone, and altered level of consciousness suggest CNS processes. Spinal cord trauma and anterior horn cell disease cause bulbar and respiratory muscle dysfunction, which results in airway obstruction and/or hypoventilation. Peripheral neuromuscular (i.e., peripheral nerve, neuromuscular junction, muscle) disorders result in muscle weakness or paralysis. Physical findings that suggest significant chest wall weakness may include hypotonia, hyporeflexia, muscle weakness, weak cry, hoarse voice, cough, gag, shallow or irregular respiratory pattern, and inability to lift the head or extremities (see Chapter 83).

Chest Wall/Thoracic Cavity

Musculoskeletal deformity or disease involving the support structures of the chest may severely restrict lung expansion, limiting normal ventilatory efforts or attempts at compensatory ventilation for respiratory dysfunction and other systemic disturbances.

Intrathoracic conditions that may produce respiratory distress include air leak and space-occupying lesions, including fluid collections and masses. Air leak is most commonly caused by pneumothorax or tension pneumothorax, which may be traumatic or spontaneous. Pneumothorax occurs when air enters the pleural space either by chest wall penetration (open pneumothorax) or by rupture of lung through the visceral pleura (closed pneumothorax) and causes collapse of the lung. With tension pneumothorax, air is able to enter but not egress. Pneumothorax, in addition to nonspecific signs of respiratory distress, is suggested by chest wall hyperexpansion, decreased or absent breath sounds, and hyperresonance on the side of the air leak. Rarely, a patient will have bilateral pneumothoraces. With tension pneumothorax, there is also jugular venous distension (JVD) and deviation of the trachea and mediastinum away from the air leak. Tension pneumothorax decreases venous return and thus cardiac output. It is therefore life threatening and must be relieved immediately by thoracentesis. The most commonly occurring space-occupying lesion is pleural effusion. Pleural effusion, which may be caused by infection, inflammation, ischemia, trauma, malignancy, major organ failure, drug hypersensitivity, or venous or lymphatic obstruction, is suggested on physical examination by decreased breath sounds and a pleural rub. Mass lesions include congenital or traumatic diaphragmatic hernia, esophageal anomalies, benign or neoplastic masses, and vascular malformations (see Chapter 95).

Cardiovascular

Congenital and acquired heart disease may result in respiratory distress from decreased cardiac output, reduced O_2 saturation, and/or congestive heart failure. Compromised cardiac output, most commonly caused by congenital structural heart defects, cardiac arrhythmias, myocarditis, pericardial effusion, pericardial tamponade, or hypotension, may result in insufficient tissue O_2 delivery to meet metabolic demands. *Pericardial tamponade* causes decreased cardiac output as a result of compromised cardiac filling. Classic physical examination findings of arterial hypotension, JVD, and distant heart sounds, referred to as Beck's triad, are seen in fewer than one-third of patients. Pericardial tamponade may be caused by trauma, infection, inflammation, malignancy, or cardiac surgery. Acute tamponade may be immediately life threatening and must be relieved expeditiously by pericardiocentesis. Cardiac anomalies with right-to-left shunting of deoxygenated blood result in reduced O_2 saturation of blood entering the systemic circulation, hence causing hypoxia with cyanosis. Cardiac defects causing left-to-right shunting result in pulmonary overcirculation, pulmonary venous congestion, and pulmonary edema that directly compromises pulmonary function. In children, congenital heart defects are the most common cause of *congestive heart failure* (CHF). Other cardiac causes of CHF include valvular heart disease, myocardial dysfunction, arrhythmias, ischemia, and infarction. Metabolic disturbances, sepsis, fluid overload, and severe anemia may also result in CHF. Pulmonary manifestations of CHF include tachypnea, increased work of breathing, dyspnea on exertion, orthopnea, cough, wheeze, and bibasilar rales. Other manifestations include poor feeding, failure to thrive, fatigue, tiring with feeds, diaphoresis, edema, tachycardia, weak thready pulses, JVD, displaced point of maximum impulse, cardiac murmur, gallop, rub, cardiomegaly, and hepatosplenomegaly. Vascular causes of respiratory distress include pulmonary embolism, pulmonary hypertension, and pulmonary arteriovenous fistula (see Chapter 82).

Gastrointestinal

Abdominal obstruction, perforation of hollow viscous, laceration of solid organs, hematoma, contusion, appendicitis, infection, inflammation, ascites, or mass may result in impaired diaphragmatic excursion secondary to abdominal distension and/or pain. Prolonged shallow respiration may result in pulmonary hypoventilation. Gastroesophageal reflux or vomiting, particularly in children unable to protect their airway, may result in pulmonary aspiration (see Chapter 93).

Metabolic and Endocrine Disturbances

Metabolic disturbances often manifest as compensatory alterations in respiratory status. Metabolic acidosis results in rapid, deep breathing. Hyperammonemia directly stimulates the respiratory center to produce tachypnea, which results in primary respiratory alkalosis with secondary metabolic acidosis. Metabolic disruption of O_2 metabolism is another cause for respiratory distress. Endocrine disturbances that cause alterations in metabolic rate or chemical imbalances also result in respiratory distress (see Chapters 97 and 98).

Hematologic

Inadequate concentrations of hemoglobin or hemoglobin with decreased oxygen-carrying capacity result in deficient O_2 delivery to tissues. Polycythemia results in sludging of blood and therefore compromised O_2 delivery (see Chapter 87).

EVALUATION AND DECISION

Triage and Stabilization

Every child with significant respiratory distress must be considered to be at potential risk of respiratory collapse. Airway patency, breathing, and circulation should be rapidly assessed and, if compromised, should be established and optimized immediately (Table 68.6). For the child in respiratory arrest, cardiac arrest, if not already present, is imminent.

Cardiorespiratory status should be continuously monitored. A health care provider skilled in airway management and resuscitation should remain with the patient at all times. Evaluation that is stepwise and focused is critical for determining the source and severity of respiratory distress. Anticipation and rapid aggressive management are essential for optimizing outcome. In the child who is alert and otherwise healthy, the position that he or she has naturally assumed is likely to be the one that minimizes respiratory distress and thus should be maintained. A child with significant respiratory distress should be allowed to remain with the parents and should not be agitated. Anxiety increases minute ventilation and adds significantly to the child's O_2 consumption. Any patient believed to have ventilatory compromise should be treated immediately with humidified O_2 at the highest concentration available. Supplemental O_2 provides a small but often crucial margin of safety in ensuring adequate cerebral and myocardial oxygenation. In patients with decreased sensorium or neuromuscular disease, a position to optimize airway patency must be established. Airway devices or assisted ventilation may be necessary. For management of cardiorespiratory arrest, resuscitation efforts must be initiated immediately, as detailed in Chapters 1, 2, and 5.

History

A detailed history usually provides important clues to the cause of respiratory distress, but in a critically ill child, comprehensive detail should not be obtained at the expense of patient care. A brief history can be obtained while emergent treatment is initiated. Details can follow once the child is stabilized. Information obtained by history should include a description of respiratory and other symptoms, onset and duration of symptoms, possible precipitating factors including ill contacts, environmental exposures and recent travel, therapeutic interventions, history of previous similar symptoms, underlying medical conditions,

TABLE 68.6

LIFE-SAVING MANEUVERS TO RELIEVE RESPIRATORY DISTRESS

Maneuvers	Indications	Comments
Heimlich maneuver (abdominal thrusts) for age ≥ 1 yr	Relieve upper airway obstruction caused by foreign body	Contraindicated if conscious patient able to phonate
Back/chest blows for age < 1 yr Manual foreign-body extraction		Remove visible foreign body in the oropharynx, blind sweep contraindicated
Head tilt/chin lift, jaw thrust	Relieve oropharyngeal obstruction	Head tilt/chin lift contraindicated if neck trauma
Nasopharyngeal airway	Relieve nasopharyngeal obstruction	Conscious or unconscious patient Contraindicated if bleeding diathesis, cerebrospinal fluid leak, nasal deformity
Oropharyngeal airway	Relieve obstruction by the tongue	Unconscious patient
Suction	Remove excess secretions, mucous plug	Nose, mouth, and, if intubated, trachea
Bag-valve-mask ventilation	Provide mechanical ventilation, deliver high-concentration oxygen	Self-inflating or anesthesia bag
Endotracheal intubation/assisted ventilation	Control ventilation for depressed central nervous system	Relatively contraindicated if severe midface trauma
	Absent pharyngeal reflexes	If epiglottitis, consider intubation in operating room
	Mechanical support for weak chest wall Artificial airway for obstructed airway Supplemental oxygen for damaged alveoli Control intracranial pressure by hyperventilation Provide tracheopulmonary toilet Provide positive end-expiratory pressure to increase lung volume	Avoid intubation in severe asthma if possible
Needle cricothyroidotomy	Emergent artificial airway required to sustain life, upper airway obstruction cannot otherwise be relieved, tracheostomy cannot be immediately performed	Temporizing measure, tracheostomy to follow immediately
Tracheostomy	Emergent artificial airway required to sustain life, upper airway obstruction cannot be relieved by endotracheal intubation	Should be performed in operating room by experienced physician
Thoracentesis	Evacuation pneumothorax, tension pneumothorax, hemothorax, drainage pleural effusion, empyema	Chest tube placement to follow immediately or performed instead
Thoracostomy	Evacuate, prevent reaccumulation pneumothorax, tension pneumothorax, hemothorax, effusion, empyema	Thoracentesis first if chest tube cannot be placed immediately in life-threatening situation
Pericardiocentesis	Relieve tamponade: effusion, hemopericardium, pneumopericardium	Improve cardiac output
Bronchoscopy	Foreign-body removal	Do not agitate the child before the procedure Esophagoscopy for esophageal foreign body

SIGNS AND SYMPTOMS

particularly those that predispose to respiratory compromise, medications, allergies, and immunizations.

Physical Examination

The physical examination should assess the degree of respiratory distress and should identify the site and likely cause of respiratory distress (Figs. 68.1A and 68.1B). Continuous cardiopulmonary monitoring and frequent assessment are important because respiratory status can change instantaneously. General appearance, level of consciousness, vital signs, respiratory rate, respiratory effort, and adequacy of oxygenation and ventilation give immediate information regarding the severity of respiratory distress and possible sites. Heightened level of consciousness, manifesting as restlessness, anxiety, or combativeness, is more likely an early sign of hypoxia, whereas diminished level of consciousness, manifesting as somnolence,

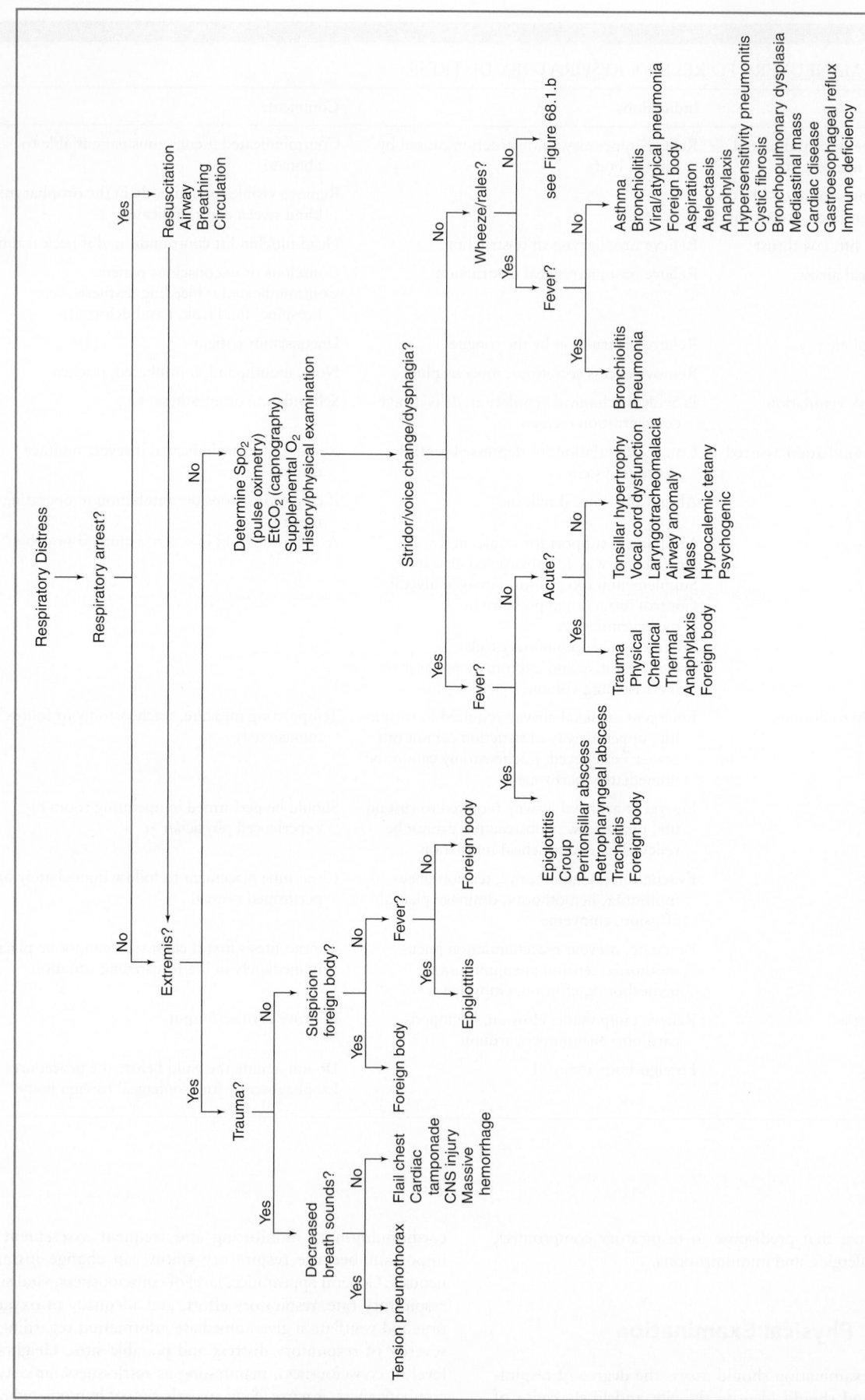

FIGURE 68.1 A: Approach to the child with respiratory distress. (*continued*)

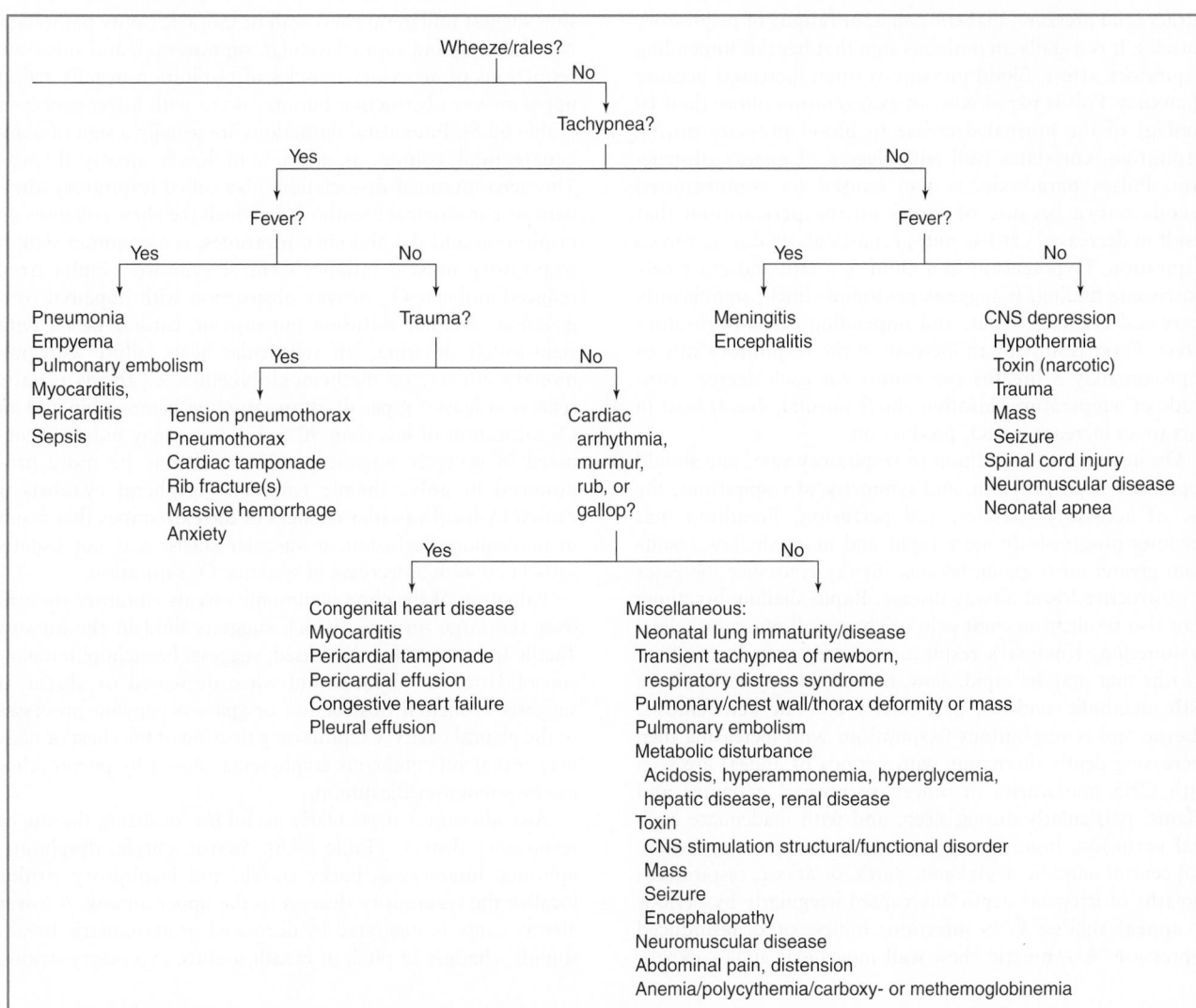

FIGURE 68.1 (*Continued*) **B:** Approach to the child with respiratory distress. SpO₂, percentage oxygen saturation; O₂, oxygen; EtCO₂, end tidal carbon dioxide; CNS, central nervous system.

lethargy, stupor, obtundation, or coma, tends to result from hypercarbia or severe hypoxia. The child's posture may suggest the site of the disturbance. Children with upper airway obstruction tend to assume a sniffing position, an upright sitting posture with neck slightly flexed and head extended. For lower airway obstruction, a tripod position, in which the child is sitting up and leaning forward, may be preferred.

TABLE 68.7

NORMAL RESPIRATORY RATES

Age group	Respiratory rate (breaths/min)
Neonates	35–50
Older infants/toddlers	30–40
Elementary school-aged children	20–30
Older children/adolescents	12–20

Vital sign abnormalities provide important clues about the severity of illness and adequacy of compensatory mechanisms. To maintain cardiac output (CO), children are more dependent on increasing heart rate (HR) than on stroke volume (SV) (CO = HR × SV). Tachycardia is one of the early signs of respiratory compromise and is expected because of increased sympathetic tone due to respiratory distress. Bradycardia in a hypoxic child is a late and ominous sign that often signals impending cardiac arrest. Cardiac arrhythmias that compromise cardiac output may result in respiratory distress. Respiratory rate in children varies with age (Table 68.7). Tachypnea is a compensatory mechanism for hypoxia, hypercapnia, and acidosis, and it also occurs with pain, anxiety, and exercise. Although not specific for respiratory distress, tachypnea is one of the findings most consistently present with respiratory distress and is particularly pronounced with lower airway processes. Tachypnea may be the only manifestation of lower respiratory infection in children younger than 6 months. Bradypnea, or decreased respiratory rate, may reflect central respiratory depression, increased intracranial pressure, diabetic coma, or fatigue of respiratory muscles. It is usually an ominous sign that heralds impending respiratory arrest. Blood pressure is often increased because of anxiety. Pulsus paradoxus, an exaggeration (more than 10 mmHg) of the normal decrease in blood pressure during inspiration, correlates well with degree of airway obstruction. Pulses paradoxus is also caused by compromised venous return because of forces on the pericardium that result in decreased cardiac output, particularly during forced inspiration. Hypotension in a child is a late and extremely worrisome finding. It suggests profound shock, significantly decreased cardiac output, and impending cardiorespiratory arrest. Fever results in an increase in the respiratory rate of approximately 3 breaths per minute for each degree centigrade of temperature elevation above normal, due at least in part to an increase in CO_2 production.

On inspection, in addition to respiratory rate, one should appreciate depth, rhythm, and symmetry of respirations; the use of accessory muscles; and perfusion. Breathing that becomes progressively more rapid and more shallow results from greater air trapping because airway resistance increases in obstructive lower airway disease. Rapid shallow breathing may also result from chest pain or chest wall musculoskeletal dysfunction. Kussmal's respirations (deep, regular, sighing breaths that may be rapid, slow, or normal in rate) are seen with metabolic acidosis, particularly diabetic ketoacidosis. Cheyne-Stokes respirations (respirations with increasing then decreasing depth alternating with periods of apnea) are seen with CNS immaturity in otherwise normal neonates and infants, particularly during sleep, and with inadequate cerebral perfusion, brain injury, increased intracranial pressure, and central narcotic depression. Biot's, or ataxic, respirations (breaths of irregular depth interrupted irregularly by periods of apnea) suggest CNS infection, injury, or drug-induced depression. Asymmetric chest wall movement and/or expansion suggest unilateral chest wall or thoracic cavity pathology. Nasal flaring and supraclavicular, suprasternal, and subcostal retractions of accessory muscles of respiration usually reflect upper airway obstruction but may occur with lower processes (Table 68.8). Intercostal retractions are usually a sign of inadequate tidal volume as a result of lower airway disease. Thoracoabdominal dissociation, also called respiratory alternans or paradoxical breathing, in which the chest collapses on inspiration and the abdomen protrudes, is a common sign of respiratory muscle fatigue. Central cyanosis results from reduced ambient O_2, airway obstruction with impaired oxygenation, alveolar diffusion impairment, cardiac defect with right-to-left shunting, left ventricular heart failure with pulmonary edema, or methemoglobinemia. Cyanosis usually reflects at least 5 g per dL of unsaturated hemoglobin and an O_2 saturation of less than 90%. Cyanosis may not be recognized in severely anemic patients and may be more pronounced in polycythemic patients. Peripheral cyanosis is caused by local vascular changes of the extremities that result in inadequate perfusion or vascular stasis; it is not usually associated with a decrease in systemic O_2 saturation.

Palpation of the chest commonly reveals vibratory rhonchi over the large airways, which suggests fluid in the airway. Tactile fremitus, when increased, suggests bronchopulmonary consolidation or abscess, and when decreased or absent, it suggests bronchial obstruction or space-occupying processes of the pleural cavity. Crepitus on palpation of the chest or neck may reveal subcutaneous emphysema caused by pneumothorax or pneumomediastinum.

Auscultation is particularly useful for localizing the site of respiratory distress (Table 68.8). Stertor, gurgle, dysphonia, aphonia, hoarseness, barky cough, and inspiratory stridor localize the respiratory distress to the upper airway. A lower airway cause is suggested by decreased or asymmetric breath sounds, changes in pitch of breath sounds, expiratory stridor,

---

TABLE 68.8

LOCALIZATION OF RESPIRATORY DISTRESS BY PHYSICAL EXAMINATION FINDINGS

Flaring: reflexive opening of nares during inspiration with upper airway obstruction
Retractions: inward collapse of chest wall as a result of high negative intrathoracic pressure from increased respiratory effort; supraclavicular, suprasternal, and subcostal retractions reflect upper airway obstruction, intercostal retractions reflect lower airway obstruction or disease
Stertor: snoring with nasal congestion, adenotonsillar hypertrophy, neuromuscular weakness
Gurgle: inspiratory and expiratory bubbling sounds caused by secretions oropharynx, trachea, large bronchi
Aphonia/dysphonia: vocal cord obstruction, dysfunction
Hoarseness: laryngeal obstruction, dysfunction
Barky cough: subglottic, tracheal obstruction
Stridor: abnormal turbulence over airway obstruction; (i) inspiratory: quiet, high pitched from glottic, subglottic region; (ii) expiratory: loud, harsh from carina or below; and (iii) biphasic: loud, harsh from trachea
Grunt: expiration against a closed glottis to maintain expiratory lung volume with lower airway, gastrointestinal process
Wheeze: continuous, musical; (i) obstructed bronchi, bronchioles—polyphonic (variable, pitched, regional differences) expiratory as in asthma; (ii) obstructed central airway—monophonic (low pitched, same in all lung fields) expiratory ± inspiratory as with tracheal foreign body, tracheomalacia
Crackles (rales): discontinuous, usually high-pitched, inspiratory; moist, from thin secretions in (i) bronchi, bronchioles (medium rales), or (ii) alveoli (fine rales)
Rhonchi (coarse rales): discontinuous, usually low-pitched, inspiratory; moist or dry, from exudate, edema, inflammation in larger bronchi
Pleural friction rub: loud, low-pitched, inspiratory ± expiratory, due to pleural inflammation
Bronchophony, egophony, whispered pectoriloquy: alterations in voice sounds as a result of lobar pneumonia, pleural effusion

grunting, and/or adventitial sounds, including crackles, rhonchi, wheeze, rub, bronchophony, egophony, and whispered pectoriloquy. The ratio of inspiratory to expiratory phase of respiration, normally 1:1, is often useful in distinguishing an upper from lower respiratory tract cause of respiratory distress. Respiratory distress from upper airway disease usually results from difficulty of inward air movement. The inspiratory phase is often increased relative to the expiratory phase to between 1:1 and 2:1. Lower airway processes often impede outward air movement and may result in a prolonged expiratory phase with ratios of 1:3 to 1:4. Absence or disappearance of wheeze in a child with continued or worsening respiratory distress may represent severe obstruction and should not be considered reassuring but rather may herald impending respiratory arrest.

Percussion of the chest may reveal either hyperresonance, suggesting air trapping, or dullness, suggesting an area of consolidation, a mass in the lung or pleural space, or pleural fluid. Air trapping is further suggested by depressed position of the diaphragm. Diaphragmatic excursion can be accessed by measuring the difference between the level of dullness on percussion during full inspiration and full expiration. Poor diaphragmatic excursion may reflect diaphragmatic dysfunction.

The remainder of the physical examination should concentrate on the nervous, cardiac, gastrointestinal, renal, skin, metabolic/endocrine, and hematologic systems and may reveal pathology of these organ systems that localizes the underlying source of respiratory distress.

Approach

The approach to the child with respiratory distress (Figs. 68.1A and 68.1B) begins with the assessment of airway patency, oxygenation and ventilation, and, as required, appropriate resuscitation as per Pediatric Advanced Life Support guidelines. Patients in extremis (Fig. 68.1A) most commonly due to airway obstruction, tension pneumothorax, flail chest, or cardiac tamponade require immediate treatment of these conditions. History and physical examination to determine etiology, most commonly foreign body, infection, anaphylaxis, or injury and to guide further evaluation and management should be obtained while providing emergent treatment.

For patients with mild to moderate respiratory distress, allow patients to assume and maintain a position that maximizes their respiratory function. Every effort should be made to avoid agitating the child as this may result in critical airway compromise and increased metabolic demand for O_2. The initial focus of the examination should be on the respiratory and cardiac systems. Assessment begins with the observation of patient position, general appearance, work of breathing, and respiratory sounds that can be appreciated without a stethoscope and is followed by auscultation to assess abnormal cardiopulmonary sounds, oxygenation, and ventilation. The remainder of the examination is performed when the child is sufficiently stable to tolerate the examination.

Nearly all patients with respiratory distress should have their oxygenation level tested by pulse oximetry. Arterial blood gas or capnography, which measures end-tidal carbon dioxide (EtCO$_2$) and CO_2 waveform, and chest radiograph are the tests most likely to be helpful in the determination of respiratory failure and impending failure, particularly because of lower airway processes, and may provide insights into its cause. Measurement of EtCO$_2$ and CO_2 waveform is indicated in all intubated patients to access and monitor endotracheal tube placement and ventilation and is recommended in spontaneously breathing patients to diagnosis upper or lower airway obstruction.

Stridor, altered phonation, and/or dysphagia suggest partial airway obstruction. Children with abnormal auscultatory findings (i.e., wheeze, rales, rhonchi, and/or asymmetric breath sounds) and fever are likely to have pneumonia or bronchiolitis, whereas asthma, bronchiolitis, and foreign-body aspiration are common in afebrile patients.

Patients can be further categorized on the basis of tachypnea (Fig. 68.1B). Children with rapid respirations and fever may have pneumonia, even in the absence of rales; empyema, pulmonary embolism, and encephalitis are also important considerations. Tachypnea without fever points to trauma, cardiac disease, metabolic disturbances, toxic ingestions or exposures, and miscellaneous disorders. Biological and chemical warfare agents may produce tachypnea with or without fever. The identity of the agent is suggested by characteristic onset, progression, and multisystem constellation of symptoms.

Febrile children without tachypnea may have apnea or bradypnea as late manifestations of CNS infection. In afebrile patients, considerations include the myriad causes of CNS depression, spinal cord injury, neuromuscular disease, and neonatal apnea. Diagnostic tests should be used selectively to rule out diagnoses suggested by history and physical examination (Table 68.9).

Treatment

Regardless of the cause of respiratory distress, aggressive treatment must be initiated immediately to rapidly restore oxygenation and ventilation. Airway patency, if inadequate, must be established. In the patient with decreased sensorium, positioning of the airway by chin lift (contraindicated if neck injury is suspected) or jaw thrust may relieve soft-tissue obstruction of the airway. The oral cavity should be cleared of secretions, vomitus, blood, and visible foreign matter. The unconscious patient may benefit from the placement of an oropharyngeal airway or endotracheal intubation. In the alert patient with suspected soft-tissue obstruction of the airway, a nasopharyngeal airway may improve airway patency. Placement of a nasogastric tube to decompress a distended abdomen often improves respiratory effort by allowing full expansion of the lungs. The child in whom airway patency cannot be maintained or adequate ventilation and oxygenation cannot be established likely requires endotracheal intubation.

Indications for intubation directly related to respiratory distress include respiratory failure or impending failure, apnea, airway obstruction, inability to handle secretions, and risk of aspiration.

TABLE 68.9

DIAGNOSTIC STUDIES FOR EVALUATION OF RESPIRATORY DISTRESS

Test	Indications	Comments
Pulse oximetry	Respiratory distress, failure	Measures oxygen saturation Relative contraindication if agitation will worsen distress Not reliable if severe anemia No information about ventilation
Capnography	Respiratory distress, failure Confirm, monitor endotracheal tube placement, ventilatory failure Diagnose, differentiate upper, lower airway obstruction, monitor therapeutic interventions	Measures end-tidal CO_2 ($EtCO_2$), CO_2 waveform Can be used in intubated or nonintubated patients Approximates ABG $PaCO_2$ if cardiovascular status intact; $EtCO_2$ values 2–5 mmHg $<$ $PaCO_2$ Characteristic waveforms for apnea, hypoventilation, obstruction
ABG	Respiratory distress, failure, acidosis, carboxyhemoglobin, methemoglobin	Information about ventilation Most useful for lower airway process Relative contraindication if agitation will worsen distress ABG changes occur late and may not be seen until arrest (A-a) O_2 gradient increase suggests ventilation-perfusion mismatch
CBC count, blood cx, + CSF analysis, cx, mono spot/EBV titer	Infection, allergy	Relative contraindication if agitation or positioning for lumbar puncture will worsen distress
Electrolytes, BUN, CR, glucose, Ca, PO_4, Mg, LFTs, ammonia, TFTs	Metabolic/endocrine disease, metabolic disturbance	Calculate anion gap
PT/PTT	Bleeding/clotting disorder, pulmonary embolism	May be normal
Toxicologic screen blood, urine	Ingestion/intoxication	Central nervous system depressants, neuromuscular blockade, electron transport chain poisons
Nasal, ocular, rectal swab: DFA, PCR, cx	Bronchiolitis, *Chlamydia* infection, pertussis, viral pneumonia	Neonates, infants
Sputum: stains, cx	Bacterial, TB, pneumocystis, fungal	Adolescents
TB skin test	TB	
Radiograph		
Lateral neck radiograph	Tracheitis, abscess, foreign body	Not necessary for the diagnosis of croup Relative contraindication unstable airway Consider portable if unstable
Chest radiograph (AP/lateral)	Lower respiratory disease, foreign body, barotrauma, effusion, mass, chest wall trauma/deformity, cardiac process	
Forced expiratory or bilateral decubitus	Foreign body	Air trapping behind object
	Distinguish effusion from infiltrate	Effusion layers
Unilateral decubitus	Abdominal mass, obstruction, perforation	
AP supine/prone, upright/cross-table lateral		
Fluoroscopy	Upper airway obstruction; structural or functional anatomic, foreign body, paralysis vocal cords, diaphragm	
Laryngoscopy/bronchoscopy	Upper or lower airway obstruction; structural or functional, foreign body	Esophagoscopy for esophageal processes

(continued)

TABLE 68.9

CONTINUED

Test	Indications	Comments
Head CT scan	Central mass, hydrocephalus	
Chest CT scan	Congenital anomaly, mass—tumor, abscess, diaphragmatic hernia	
Abdomen CT scan	Obstruction, mass, appendicitis	
Chest and cardiac US	Pleural or pericardial effusion, tamponade	
Electrocardiogram	Cardiac anomaly, failure, pericarditis	
Thoracentesis, pericardiocentesis cytology, biochemical, cx	Infection, inflammation, oncologic process chest, heart, lymphatics	Also therapeutic Consider ultrasound guidance
Ventilation-perfusion scan	Pulmonary embolism	
Barium swallow	Tracheoesophageal fistula, vascular ring, reflux	
Pulmonary function tests	Central or peripheral nervous system depression of chest wall function, respiratory system disease	Measures lung volume, flow, compliance
Electromyography	Central respiratory drive depressed, neuromuscular disease	Measures muscle activity generated by neural outflow from respiratory centers
Angiography	Vascular anomaly	

ABG, arterial blood gas; CBC count, complete blood cell count; cx, culture; CSF, cerebrospinal fluid; EBV, Epstein-Barr virus; BUN, blood urea nitrogen; CR, creatinine; Ca, calcium; PO_4, phosphate; Mg, magnesium; LFTs, liver function tests; TFTs, thyroid function tests; PT, prothrombin time; PTT, partial thromboplastin time; IFA, immunofluorescence assay; TB, tuberculosis; AP, anteroposterior; CT, computed tomography.

SIGNS AND SYMPTOMS

SUMMARY

Respiratory distress is one of the most common chief complaints of children seeking medical care. The causes of respiratory distress are numerous and varied. History and physical examination provide important clues that allow rapid localization of the site of impairment. The underlying cause must be identified and may be within the respiratory system or organ systems that control or impact respiration. Any disorder that causes respiratory distress may be life threatening. Airway and ventilatory problems not only must be recognized but also must be anticipated and addressed aggressively. The underlying cause must also be treated. Patients must be monitored continuously and reassessed frequently. Airway, breathing, and circulation must be established and maintained. Diagnostic evaluation of body fluids, radiologic studies, direct visualization, and specialized tests of organ function must be performed prudently so that respiratory status is not further compromised.

Suggested Readings

American Academy of Pediatrics Subcommittee on Diagnosis and Management of Bronchiolitis. Diagnosis and management of bronchiolitis. *Pediatrics* 2006;118:1774–1793.

Bernstein T, Brilli R, Jacobs B. Is bacterial tracheitis changing? A 14-month experience in a pediatric intensive care unit. *Clin Infect Dis* 1998;27:458–462.

Bjornson CL, Johnson DW. Croup. *Lancet* 2008;371:329–339.

Canducci F, Debiaggi M, Sampaolo M, et al. Two-year prospective study of single infections and co-infections by respiratory syncytial virus and viruses identified recently in infants with acute respiratory disease. *J Med Virol* 2008;80(4):716–723.

Cherry JD. Clinical practice. Croup. *N Engl J Med* 2008;358:384–391.

Custer JR. Croup and related disorders. *Pediatr Rev* 1993;14:19–29.

Darville T, Yamauchi T. Respiratory syncytial virus. *Pediatr Rev* 1998;19:55–61.

Fireman P. The wheezing infant. *Pediatr Rev* 1986;7:247–254.

Flori HR Glidden DV, Rutherford GW, et al. Pediatric acute lung injury: prospective evaluation of risk factors associated with mortality. *Am J Respir Crit Care Med* 2005;171:995–1001.

Gaston B. Pneumonia. *Pediatr Rev* 2002;23:132–140.

Henretig FM, Cieslak TJ, Kortepeter MG, et al. Medical management of the suspected victim of bioterrorism: an algorithmic approach to the undifferentiated patient. *Emerg Med Clin North Am* 2002;20:351–364.

Hopkins A, Lahiri T, Salerno R, et al. Changing epidemiology of life-threatening upper airway infections: the emergence of bacterial tracheitis. *Pediatrics* 2006;118:1418–1421.

Kahn JS. Human metapneumovirus: a newly emerging respiratory pathogen. *Curr Opin Infect Dis* 2003;16:255–258.

Kahn JS. Newly discovered respiratory viruses: significance and implications. *Curr Opin Pharmacol* 2007;7(5):478–483.

King C, Henretig FM, King BR, et al, eds. *Textbook of pediatric emergency procedures*, 2nd ed. Baltimore, MD: Williams & Wilkins, 2007:85–251, 383–409, 823–901.

Klassen TP. Recent advances in the treatment of bronchiolitis and laryngitis. *Pediatr Clin North Am* 1997;44:249–261.

Kopelman AE, Mathew OP. Common respiratory disorders of the newborn. *Pediatr Rev* 1995;16:209–217.

Kravitz RM. Congenital malformations of the lung. *Pediatr Clin North Am* 1994;41:453–472.

Larson GL. Asthma in children. *N Engl J Med* 1992;326:1540–1545.

Loughlin GM, Moscona A. The cell biology of acute childhood respiratory disease: therapeutic implications. *Pediatr Clin North Am* 2006;53:929–959.

Malhotra A, Krilov LR. Viral croup. *Pediatr Rev* 2001;22:5–11.

Mancuso RF. Stridor in neonates. *Pediatr Clin North Am* 1996;43:1339–1356.

Margolis P, Gadomski, A. The rational clinical examination. Does this infant have pneumonia? *JAMA* 1998;279:308.

McIntosh K. Community-acquired pneumonia in children. *N Engl J Med* 2002;346(6):429–437.

Patt HA, Feigin RD. Diagnosis and management of suspected cases of bioterrorism: a pediatric prospective. *Pediatrics* 2002;109:685–692.

Rafei K, Lichenstein R. Airway infectious disease emergencies. *Pediatr Clin North Am* 2006;53:215–242.

Rotta AT, Wiryanwan B. Respiratory emergencies in children. *Respir Care* 2003;48:248–258.

Shah S, Sharieff GQ. Pediatric respiratory infections. *Emerg Med Clin North Am* 2007;25:961–979.

Stroud RH, Friedman NR. An update on inflammatory disorders of the pediatric airway: epiglottitis, croup and tracheitis. *Am J Otolaryngol* 2001;22:268–275.

CHAPTER 69 ■ SEIZURES

VINCENT W. CHIANG, MD

Seizures are the most common neurologic disorder in childhood and among the more common symptoms that lead to an emergency department (ED) visit. Studies have shown that 4% to 6% of all children will have at least one seizure in the first 16 years of life. These can range from a self-limited, nonrecurring episode to a prolonged, life-threatening event. The pediatric emergency physician must have a fundamental knowledge of all aspects of seizure management, including initial stabilization, determination of cause (differential diagnosis), appropriate definitive treatment, and patient disposition.

BACKGROUND

A *seizure* is defined as a transient, involuntary alteration of consciousness, behavior, motor activity, sensation, and/or autonomic function caused by an excessive rate and hypersynchrony of discharges from a group of cerebral neurons. A *convulsion* is a seizure with prominent alterations of motor activity. *Epilepsy*, or seizure disorder, is a condition of susceptibility to recurrent seizures.

Seizures may be generalized or partial. Generalized seizures reflect involvement of both cerebral hemispheres. These may be convulsive or nonconvulsive. Consciousness may be impaired and this impairment may be the initial manifestation. Motor involvement is bilateral. Types of generalized seizures include absence (petit mal), myoclonic, tonic, clonic, atonic, and tonic-clonic (grand mal) seizures.

Partial (focal, local) seizures reflect initial involvement limited to one cerebral hemisphere. Partial seizures are further classified on the basis of whether consciousness is impaired. When consciousness is not impaired, the seizure is classified as a simple partial seizure. Simple partial seizures may have motor, somatosensory/sensory, autonomic, or psychic symptoms. When consciousness is impaired, the seizure is classified as a complex partial seizure. Both simple and complex partial seizures may evolve into generalized seizures (e.g., Jacksonian march).

Status epilepticus is the condition of prolonged seizure activity (more than 5 minutes) or persistent, repetitive seizure activity without recovery of consciousness in between episodes.

A postictal (decreased responsiveness) period usually follows the seizure. During this time, the patient may be confused, lethargic, fatigued, or irritable; also, headache, vomiting, and muscle soreness may occur. In general, the length of the postictal period is proportional to the length of the seizure. For brief seizures, there may be few or no postictal symptoms. Transient focal deficits (e.g., Todd's paralysis) may occur during the postictal period, but one must first rule out a focal central nervous system (CNS) deficit.

PATHOPHYSIOLOGY

The underlying abnormality in all seizures is the hypersynchrony of neuronal discharges. Cerebral manifestations include increased blood flow, increased oxygen and glucose consumption, and increased carbon dioxide and lactic acid production. If a patient can maintain appropriate oxygenation and ventilation, the increase in cerebral blood flow is usually sufficient to meet the initial increased metabolic requirements of the brain. Brief seizures rarely produce any lasting effects. However, prolonged seizures may result in permanent neuronal injury.

Systemic alterations may occur with seizures and result from a massive sympathetic discharge, leading to tachycardia, hypertension, and hyperglycemia. Failure of adequate ventilation, especially in patients in whom consciousness is impaired, can lead to hypoxia, hypercarbia, and respiratory acidosis. Patients with impaired consciousness may be unable to protect their airway and are at risk for aspiration. Prolonged skeletal muscle activity can lead to lactic acidosis, rhabdomyolysis, hyperkalemia, hyperthermia, and hypoglycemia.

DIFFERENTIAL DIAGNOSIS

It is important to remember that a seizure does not constitute a diagnosis but is merely a symptom of an underlying pathologic process that requires a thorough investigation (Table 69.1). Often, no underlying condition is "identified," and the diagnosis of idiopathic epilepsy is made. However, it is important not to exclude potentially treatable causes prematurely. For instance, seizures that result from metabolic derangements (e.g., hyponatremia, hypoglycemia) are often refractory to anticonvulsant therapy until the abnormality is corrected. Furthermore, every effort should be made to rule out a potentially life-threatening cause of seizures (e.g., intracranial injury or hemorrhage, meningitis, ingestions) before a less serious diagnosis is accepted.

Although the diagnosis of a seizure is often made in the ED on the basis of the clinical history, other childhood paroxysmal events are often mistaken for seizure activity (Table 69.2). Occasionally, these events are referred to as an apparent life-threatening event (ALTE). An ALTE is not a diagnosis per se but rather any episode that frightens an infant's caregiver (see Chapter 10). Typically, these events involve apnea, color change (cyanosis, erythema, or pallor), marked change in muscle tone (limpness), or choking and gagging. Although a seizure itself may be the cause of an ALTE, the differential diagnosis (as for seizures themselves) of an ALTE is quite broad. Every attempt should be made to differentiate these events from seizures to ensure appropriate diagnosis, correct

TABLE 69.1

ETIOLOGY OF SEIZURES[a]

Infectious	Metabolic
Brain abscess	Hepatic failure
Encephalitis	Hypercarbia
Febrile (nonspecific)	Hyperosmolarity
Meningitis	Hypocalcemia
Parasites (central nervous system)	Hypoglycemia
Syphilis	Hypomagnesemia
Idiopathic	Hyponatremia
Withdrawals	Hypoxia
Alcohol	Inborn errors of metabolism
Anticonvulsants	Pyridoxine deficiency
Hypnotics	Uremia
Toxicologic	Vascular
Anticonvulsant	Cerebrovascular accident
Camphor	Hypertensive encephalopathy
Carbon monoxide	Oncologic
Cocaine	Primary brain tumor
Heavy metals (lead)	Metastatic disease
Hypoglycemic agents	Endocrine
Isoniazid	Addison's disease
Lithium	Hyperthyroidism
Methylxanthines	Hypothyroidism
Pesticides (organophosphates)	Obstetric
Phencyclidine	Eclampsia
Sympathomimetics	Traumatic
Tricyclic antidepressants	Cerebral contusion
Topical anesthetics	Diffuse axonal injury
Degenerative cerebral disease	Intracranial hemorrhage
Hypoxic ischemic injury	Congenital anomalies

[a]Bold type denotes most common causes. Given their nature, virtually all these etiologies are potentially life threatening, except perhaps simple febrile seizures.

TABLE 69.2

DIFFERENTIAL DIAGNOSIS OF PAROXYSMAL EVENTS

Seizure disorders	Movement disorders
Pseudoseizures	Paroxysmal choreoathetosis
Head trauma	Tic disorders
Loss of consciousness	Shudder attacks
Posttraumatic seizures	Benign myoclonus
Syncope	Psychiatric disorders
Hypovolemia	Daydreaming
Hypoxia	Attention-deficit hyperactivity disorder
Reduced cardiac output	Panic attacks
Sleep disorders	Gastrointestinal disorder
Nightmares	Sandifer syndrome (gastroesophageal reflux)
Night terrors	Abdominal migraines
Narcolepsy	Cyclic vomiting
Sleep-apnea hypersomnia	Breath-holding spells
Somnambulism	Pallid, cyanotic
Atypical migraines	Apparent life-threatening event

SIGNS AND SYMPTOMS

period, and patients often possess a clear mental status after the event. Pseudoseizures also rarely occur during sleep. The diagnosis can often be made upon history and physical examination alone but may also require long-term video and electroencephalographic (EEG) monitoring to confirm the diagnosis. Further complicating the issue is that pseudoseizures are most likely to occur in patients with an underlying seizure disorder.

Breath-holding spells are common, affecting 4% to 5% of all children (see Chapter 131). They typically present between the ages of 6 and 18 months and disappear by 5 years of age. The two types of breath-holding spells—cyanotic and pallid—have common features, including a period of apnea and an alteration in the state of consciousness. Usually, some initiating event (e.g., pain, fear, agitation) triggers the episode. The diagnosis is based on the clinical findings, and the prognosis is excellent.

A variety of movement disorders can mimic seizures. Paroxysmal choreoathetosis is often associated with a positive family history for seizures and exacerbated by intentional movement. Tic disorders can be manifested by twitching, blinking, head shaking, or other repetitive motions. These are usually suppressible and are not associated with any loss of consciousness. Shudder attacks are whole-body tremors similar to essential tremor in adults. Benign myoclonus of infancy can look like infantile spasms but is associated with a completely normal EEG.

Sleep disorders, such as somnambulism, night terrors (preschool-aged children), and narcolepsy (typically in adolescents) can often be diagnosed on the basis of the history alone (see Chapter 131). Infants with gastroesophageal reflux may exhibit torticollis or dystonic posturing (Sandifer syndrome). Atypical migraines and pseudoseizures are often diagnosed after other causes are excluded.

INITIAL STABILIZATION

The first priority in the seizing patient is to address airway, breathing, and circulation (the ABCs; see Chapter 1). An adequate airway is necessary to allow for effective ventilation and

treatment, and accurate prognosis. Each episode or "spell" should be evaluated by examining the preceding events, the episode itself, and the nature and duration of the postictal impairment. Obviously, a thorough physical examination needs to be performed. If any of these features seem atypical, an alternative diagnosis should be considered.

Syncope, or the transient loss of consciousness that results from inadequate cerebral perfusion or substrate delivery, is the most common alternative diagnosis given to patients who present for the evaluation of a seizure episode (see Chapter 73). Further complicating matters is the fact that a small percentage of patients with syncope exhibit some sort of convulsive movement. Although vasovagal episodes or orthostatic hypotension is the most common causes for syncope, it is important to evaluate these patients for potential underlying cardiac disease.

Pseudoseizures are a movement disorder that resemble seizure activity but have no corresponding abnormal brain electrical activity. The movements can be quite startling, are typically bizarre and thrashing, and are often associated with a great deal of vocalization. There is usually no biting, incontinence, or injury associated with pseudoseizures. There is also rarely a postictal oxygenation. Patients with impaired consciousness as part of their seizure are at risk for obstruction (the tongue, oral secretions, emesis), aspiration (loss of protective reflexes), and hypoventilation. Simple maneuvers such as the jaw thrust or suctioning of the oropharynx may improve the compromised airflow. The use of adjunctive airways (oral or nasopharyngeal) may also help maintain an adequate airway. In patients who are actively seizing, it may be difficult to insert these adjuncts and may cause injury if the intervention is forced. Furthermore, in patients for whom trauma is a possibility, these maneuvers must be undertaken with cervical spine (C-spine) immobilization. In patients in whom the airway remains unstable despite these actions, endotracheal intubation is warranted. When it is necessary to use a muscle relaxant to intubate a seizing patient, one should use the shortest acting agent possible. The presence of motor activity may be the only clinical manifestation of seizure, and a long-acting muscle relaxant will mask the ongoing seizure activity.

The patient's circulatory status must also be closely monitored. Seizures generally cause a massive sympathetic discharge that results in hypertension and tachycardia. Continuous cardiac monitoring and intravenous (IV) access should be obtained. Blood samples, including rapid blood glucose testing, should be acquired at this time in an attempt to establish a diagnosis. Peripheral IV access, which is often difficult in the pediatric age group, may be nearly impossible in the actively seizing patient. Intraosseous and/or central venous access may be required in the patient with prolonged seizures.

Once the respiratory and circulatory functions have been assessed and maintained, efforts should be directed at making a diagnosis and stopping any ongoing seizure activity. As long as adequate ventilation and oxygenation are maintained, long-term sequelae are unlikely to result from a transient seizure. The initial increase in cerebral blood flow compensates for any increase in brain metabolic requirements. Consensus management suggests the initiation of anticonvulsant treatment of anyone who has been seizing for more than 10 minutes. This likely represents all patients who are brought to the ED actively seizing.

EVALUATION AND DECISION

History

As a result of the numerous potential causes of seizures, as well as the large number of events that can be mistaken for a seizure, a focused history is important. The parent or caregiver needs to carefully describe the episode and the preceding events. Was there a warning (aura) that the patient was about to have an event? Was there a loss of consciousness, tongue biting, or incontinence? Did the event involve the entire body or only a portion? How long did the event last? How did the patient act after the event was over?

In addition to the episode itself, the preceding events are also crucial. Was there a history of trauma, toxin exposure or ingestion, fever, or other systemic signs of illness (e.g., headache, ataxia, vomiting, diarrhea)? Does the child have an underlying seizure disorder, history of seizures, or other neurologic problems? Is the child taking any anticonvulsants? If yes, was there a recent change in dose, or were any new medications started or old medications stopped? Is there a chance that the

patient could have a subtherapeutic level? Other questions that should be asked include if there was any other significant medical history (including abnormal developmental history), any significant surgical history (including the placement of a ventricular shunt), family history of seizures, other medication use, and travel history to an endemic region (neurocysticercosis is one of the leading worldwide causes of seizures)?

Physical Examination

With the history, a directed physical examination is performed to look for a possible cause of the seizure. Vital signs, including temperature, need to be obtained. An elevated temperature points to a potential infectious cause. The entire body needs to be examined for the evidence of trauma, either as a preceding cause or as a result of falling during the seizure episode. The skin should be examined for rashes or other congenital skin lesions. Dysmorphic features may be associated with other congenital CNS anomalies. Stigmata of underlying hepatic, renal, or endocrinologic disorders should also be noted.

The head should be carefully examined for swelling, deformity, or other signs of trauma. The presence of a ventricular shunt should be noted. The pupils are studied for shape, size, reactivity, and equality. The fundi are examined for the presence of retinal hemorrhages or papilledema. The tympanic membranes are examined for the presence of hemotympanum or for a source of potential infection. The mouth should be examined for the evidence of tongue biting.

The neck is assessed for meningeal irritation. If there is a history or other physical signs of trauma, neck immobilization should be maintained until the C-spine can be "cleared." Examination of the chest, lungs, and abdomen is performed in the usual fashion. The extremities are examined for the evidence of trauma, especially as the result of falling during a seizure.

The neurologic examination may be limited by either ongoing seizure activity or a postictal state and may consist solely of the pupillary examination and an assessment of any asymmetric movements (focality). Any abnormal posturing (decerebrate or decorticate) should be noted and dealt with immediately.

If there is a question of a possible ingestion, the examination is also directed at uncovering a potential toxicologic syndrome (toxidrome) that may suggest a specific class of drugs or toxins that are responsible for the seizure (see Chapter 88). Important variables include temperature, heart rate, blood pressure, pupil size, sweating, flushing, and cyanosis.

As the patient recovers from the seizure episode, periodic reassessment is needed to assess for any underlying neurologic abnormalities.

Diagnostic Approach

Once it has been determined that a seizure may have taken place, the initial diagnostic evaluation (Fig. 69.1) starts with the history and physical examination. Laboratory, radiologic, and other neurodiagnostic testings (e.g., EEG) are other tools that can be a part of the seizure evaluation.

Patients with obvious trauma who are seizing should be treated per advanced trauma life support (ATLS) guidelines (see Chapter 103), with close attention to possible intracranial injury (see Chapter 105).

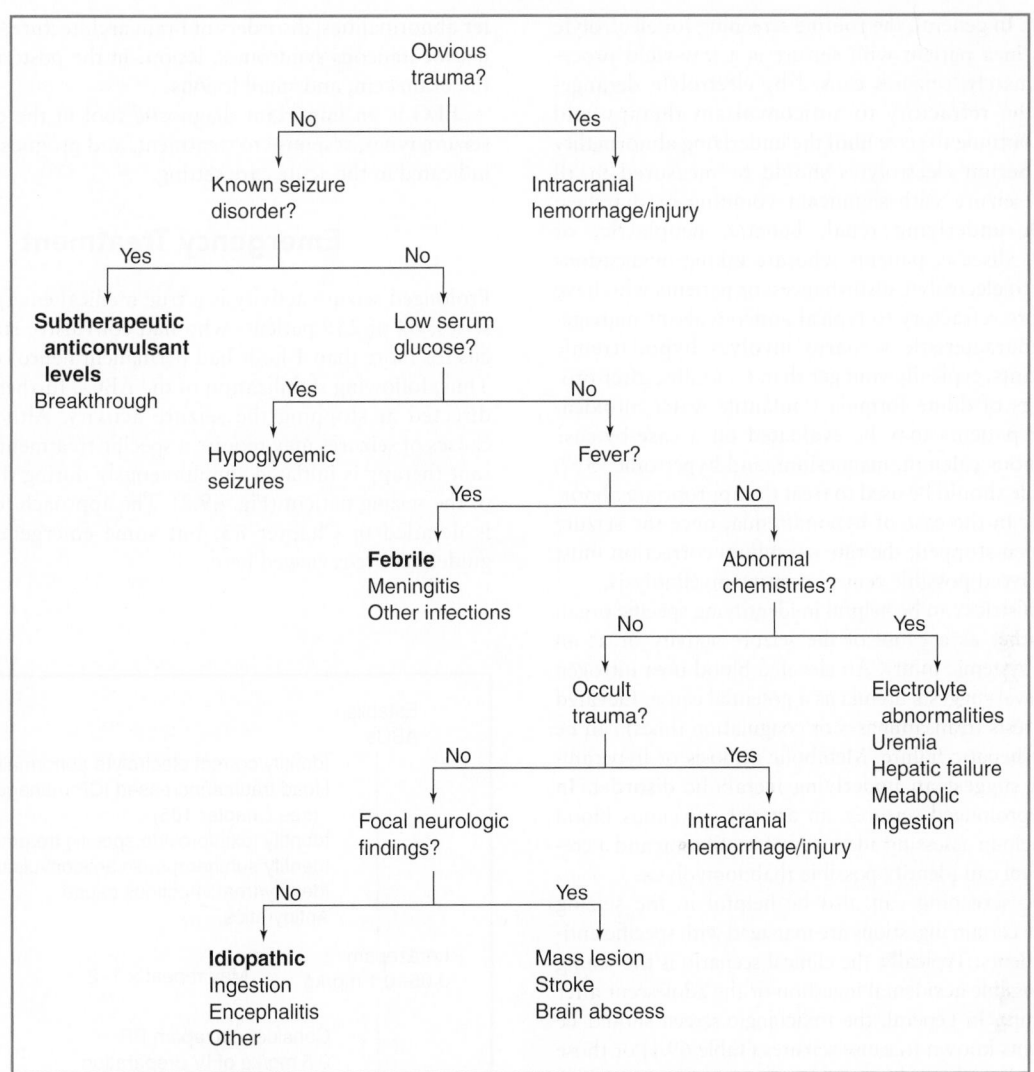

FIGURE 69.1 Diagnostic approach to seizures. The most common causes are in bold type.

Often, patients with a known seizure disorder will present to the ED actively seizing. Patients known or suspected to be taking anticonvulsants should have drug levels evaluated. A subtherapeutic anticonvulsant level is among the most common reasons for patients to present with seizures.

Many different laboratory tests may reveal a cause for a seizure and, as a result, suggest a potential treatment. A rapid glucose reagent strip test should be performed with the initial blood sample. Hypoglycemia is a common problem that can often precipitate seizure activity. If hypoglycemia is documented or a rapid assessment is not available, treatment with 0.25 to 1 g per kg of dextrose is indicated.

A *febrile seizure* is defined as a seizure caused by a fever, but this is a diagnosis of exclusion. Other infectious etiologies that present with a fever and can be the direct cause of a seizure (e.g., meningitis) must first be ruled out (see Chapters 28 and 84). Furthermore, infections not involving the CNS may still be the cause of the seizure through the elaboration of fever. Presence of fever or an elevated white blood cell (WBC) count should direct one to look for a potential infectious cause. Blood cultures should be drawn with the initial samples from

patients at risk for bacteremia in an effort to identify a specific pathogen. Urinalysis and chest radiographs can also be used to confirm a source of infection.

A lumbar puncture (LP) with analysis of the cerebrospinal fluid (CSF) is the only way to make the diagnosis of meningitis and should be performed when meningitis is being considered. An elevated CSF protein and CSF WBC count and a low CSF glucose level are all suggestive of CNS infection. CSF cultures, Gram stain, latex studies, and polymerase chain reaction may identify a specific agent. Ideally, CSF cultures should be obtained before antibiotic therapy is initiated. However, in the critically ill or unstable patient, antibiotics should not be withheld until an LP is performed. Furthermore, in cases in which a potential metabolic disease is being considered, CSF lactate, pyruvate, or amino acid level determinations can be used to diagnose a specific disorder. In these cases, it is often helpful to collect an extra tube of CSF to be frozen and used for later analysis. In any patient with suspected elevated intracranial pressure (ICP), an LP should not be performed until head imaging can be done.

Electrolyte abnormalities may also cause seizures, with hyponatremia, hypocalcemia, and hypomagnesemia being most common. In general, the routine screening for electrolyte abnormalities in a patient with seizure is a low-yield procedure. Unfortunately, seizures caused by electrolyte derangements are often refractory to anticonvulsant therapy and patients will continue to seize until the underlying abnormality is corrected. Serum electrolytes should be measured in all patients with seizure with significant vomiting or diarrhea; patients with underlying renal, hepatic, neoplastic, or endocrinologic disease; patients who are taking medications that may lead to electrolyte disturbances; or patients who have seizures that are refractory to typical anticonvulsant management. One characteristic scenario involves hyponatremic seizures in infants, typically younger than 6 months, after prolonged feedings of dilute formula ("infantile water intoxication"). Other patients may be evaluated on a case-by-case basis. Intravenous calcium, magnesium, and hypertonic (3%) sodium chloride should be used to treat the appropriate abnormal condition. In the case of hyponatremia, once the seizure activity has been stopped, the rate of sodium correction must be titrated to avoid possible central pontine myelinolysis.

Other chemistries can be helpful in identifying specific organ dysfunction either as a cause of the seizure activity or as an assessment of systemic injury. An elevated blood urea nitrogen or creatinine level suggests uremia as a potential cause. Elevated liver function tests (transaminases or coagulation times) can be a reflection of hepatic failure. Metabolic acidosis or hyperammonemia can suggest an underlying metabolic disorder. In patients with prolonged seizures, an arterial or venous blood gas level can help in assessing adequacy of ventilation and a creatine kinase level can identify possible rhabdomyolysis.

Toxicologic screening can also be helpful in the seizing patient because certain ingestions are managed with specific antidotes or treatments. Typically, the clinical scenario is the young child with a possible accidental ingestion or the adolescent after a suicide attempt. In general, the toxicologic screen should be directed at agents known to cause seizures (Table 69.1) or those suggested by a clinical toxidrome.

Radiologic imaging of the patient with seizure generally consists of either a computed tomography (CT) scan or a magnetic resonance imaging (MRI) study in the acute care setting. The following situations should be considered emergent: (i) a patient who has signs or symptoms of elevated ICP, (ii) a patient who has a focal seizure or a persistent focal neurologic deficit, (iii) a patient who has seizures in the setting of head trauma, (iv) a patient who has persistent seizure activity, or (v) a patient who appears ill. Until C-spine injury is ruled out, it is important to maintain C-spine immobilization when head trauma is a concern. Patients with transient generalized seizures in whom a cause of the seizure activity is identified probably do not require any further head imaging studies. Patients with transient generalized seizures in whom no cause is identified and who appear clinically well can have their head imaging performed on a nonemergent basis.

In the past, because of easier availability and lack of a need for sedation for most patients, CT scans were most often the study of choice in the ED for a patient who presented with a seizure. However, given the recent heightened awareness of the risks of ionizing radiation associated with CT scans, patients who do not require emergent imaging may have an MRI study instead. An MRI study also has several other advantages over a CT scan. MRI is better at identifying underlying white mat-

ter abnormalities, disorders of brain architecture, lesions in the neurocutaneous syndromes, lesions in the posterior fossa and the brainstem, and small lesions.

EEG is an important diagnostic tool in the evaluation of seizure types, response to treatment, and prognosis. It is rarely indicated in the acute care setting.

Emergency Treatment

Prolonged seizure activity is a true medical emergency. In one series, 88 of 239 patients who had convulsive status epilepticus for more than 1 hour had permanent neurologic sequelae. Thus, following stabilization of the ABCs, further treatment is directed at stopping the seizure activity. Although certain causes of seizures may require a specific treatment, anticonvulsant therapy is initiated simultaneously during the evaluation of the seizing patient (Fig. 69.2). The approach to this subject is detailed in Chapter 83, but some emergency treatment guidelines are reviewed here.

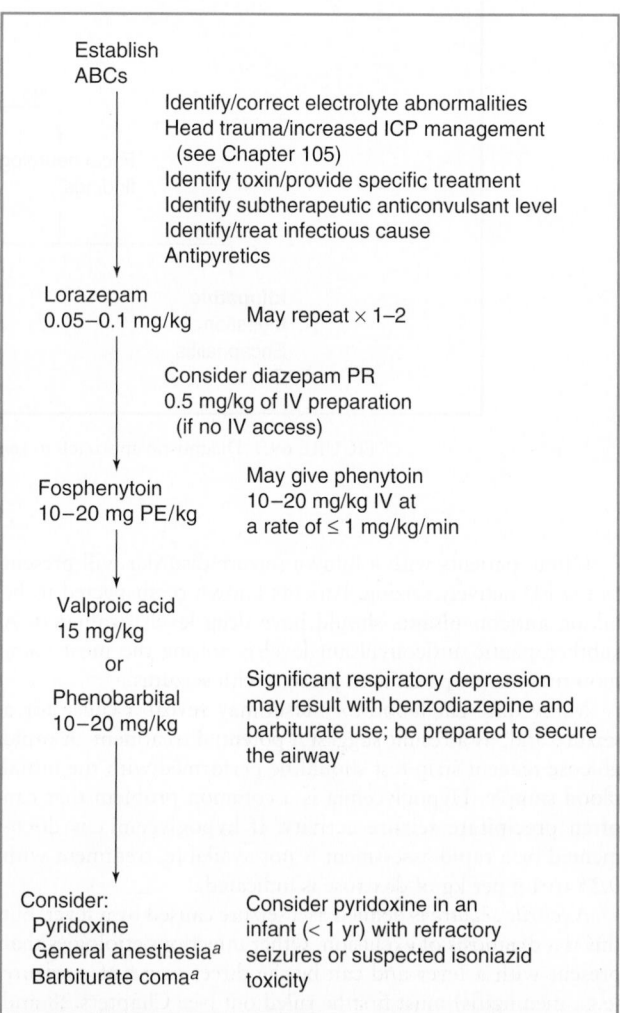

FIGURE 69.2 Management of status epilepticus. [a]Electroencephalogram monitoring and ICU setting required. ABCs, airway, breathing, circulation; ICP, intracranial pressure; PR, per rectum; IV, intravenous; PE, phenytoin equivalent; ICU, intensive care unit.

The benzodiazepines are the initial drug of choice for the treatment of seizures. Lorazepam (Ativan) has a rapid onset of action (less than 5 minutes) and can be given intravenously or intramuscularly. The dose is 0.05 to 0.1 mg per kg, with a maximal dose of 4 mg and can be given over 1 to 2 minutes. Its anticonvulsant effects can last for several hours. It may be repeated at 10- to 15-minute intervals, but its effectiveness decreases with successive doses. The major side effects are respiratory depression and sedation (dose dependent), especially when combined with phenobarbital.

Diazepam (Valium) had been the standard initial treatment of seizures for many years before the development of the newer benzodiazepines. Diazepam is similar to lorazepam, but because of its increased lipid solubility, it has a much shorter half-life. Diazepam has an advantage in that it can be given rectally, which is useful when a patient does not have IV access. More recently, a rectal gel has been introduced in fixed doses of 5, 7.5, 10, 12.5, 15, 17.5, or 20 mg. The IV preparation of the drug may be used alternatively. Recommended rectal dosing for children up to 5 years of age is 0.5 mg per kg.

Phenytoin (Dilantin) is a second-line agent for the treatment of seizures. The dose is 10 to 20 mg per kg as an initial load. It has several limitations as compared with the benzodiazepines. First, peak CNS concentrations may not be reached until 10 to 30 minutes after its infusion is completed and, thus, it is much slower in onset. Furthermore, it must be administered slowly (no faster than 1 mg per kg per minute) because of concerns of cardiac conduction disturbances, which further lengthens its onset of action. It cannot be given in dextrose-containing solutions.

As a result of the limitations in the administration of phenytoin, fosphenytoin (Cerebyx) was created. It is a prodrug whose active metabolite is phenytoin. The drug is dosed as phenytoin equivalents (PE), and the loading dose is 10 to 20 mg PE per kg. The advantages are that it can be given much more rapidly (up to 150 mg PE per minute) and that it may be given in either normal saline or a 5% dextrose-containing solution or intramuscularly.

Phenobarbital (Luminal) is another second-line agent for the treatment of seizures. The loading dose is 10 to 20 mg per kg. Its advantage over phenytoin is that it can be given much more rapidly (100 mg per minute). However, it has an extremely long half-life (up to 120 hours) and a pronounced sedating effect. Furthermore, it can cause significant respiratory depression, especially when given after a benzodiazepine. One must be prepared to intubate a patient who has received both a benzodiazepine and a barbiturate for the treatment of seizures. It is important to remember that if a patient needs to be intubated, a muscle relaxant can mask the motor manifestation of seizure activity. With the introduction of fosphenytoin, phenobarbital should now be considered a third-line agent.

Valproic acid (Depokene) is a commonly used antiepileptic agent and the IV preparation had been used in the past to rapidly attain therapeutic levels. Recently, there have been a few case series demonstrating its effectiveness in treating seizures in children who have been refractory to the first-line agents. As such, many now consider it a third-line agent for the treatment of status epilepticus. It is given intravenously at a dose of 15 mg per kg. It is generally well tolerated and is less sedating than the barbiturates.

Pyridoxine deficiency is an uncommon cause of seizures in newborns. One should consider its use in patients younger than 1 year whose seizure activity is refractory to the other therapies (100 mg). It is also used in the treatment of isoniazid overdose (usual initial dose 70 mg per kg).

If all the described therapies fail, patients may require general anesthesia to abort the seizures. A variety of agents, such as inhalational anesthetics (e.g., halothane, isoflurane) or large doses of short-acting barbiturates (e.g., pentobarbital) or benzodiazepines (e.g., continuous infusion midazolam), can be used. The patient needs both to be intubated (if not already done) and to have continuous EEG monitoring in an intensive care unit. The level of anesthesia should be sufficient to maintain either a flat-line or burst-suppression pattern on the EEG. The anesthesia can be then withdrawn slowly to see if any electrical seizure activity persists.

SPECIAL CONSIDERATIONS

Febrile Seizures

Febrile seizures are the most common convulsive disorder in young children, occurring in 2% to 5% of the population (see Chapter 83). A consensus statement by the National Institutes of Health defines a febrile seizure as a seizure occurring between 6 months and 5 years of age that is associated with a fever [temperature higher than 38°C (100.4°F)] but without the evidence of intracranial infection or other defined cause or neurologic disease.

Febrile seizures can be of any type, but most commonly, they are generalized tonic-clonic seizures. They are usually self-limited and last for only a few minutes. Febrile seizures are classified as simple febrile seizures, which last less than 15 minutes, are generalized, and occur only once during a 24-hour period. In contrast, complex febrile seizures are prolonged, recur within 24 hours, and have a focal onset. Simple febrile seizures (85%) are much more common. There is a family history of febrile seizures in an immediate family member in 25% to 40% of cases. Viral infections are frequently associated with febrile seizures, and more recent studies have shown human herpesvirus as a commonly identified agent.

After the first febrile seizure, approximately 33% of patients will have at least one recurrence and about 9% will have three or more episodes. The younger the patient is at first presentation, the greater the likelihood of recurrence. In addition, recurrences are more likely to recur in patients with lower temperatures on presentation of their first seizure (lower than 40°C) and shorter duration of fever before the seizure (less than 24 hours) and in patients with a family history of febrile seizures. Most recurrences (75%) will also happen within 1 year. The exact risk of developing epilepsy after a febrile seizure is unknown, but most studies indicate that it is less than 5%. Risk factors for developing epilepsy after a febrile seizure include abnormal development before the episode, a family history of afebrile seizures, and a complex first febrile seizure.

The treatment of a patient who presents with a febrile seizure is nearly identical to that for other seizure types. The primary goal is the establishment of a clear airway; secondary efforts are then directed at the termination of the seizure and concurrent lowering of body temperature. However, because

SIGNS AND SYMPTOMS

most febrile seizures are brief in duration, the typical patient who presents for the evaluation of a febrile seizure is no longer seizing upon arrival to the ED. In those instances, if the history is consistent with a simple febrile seizure, the patient has no stigmata of a CNS infection, and the patient's neurologic examination is completely "normal" (the patient may be postictal or slightly hyperreflexive), further evaluation for the cause of the seizure is unnecessary. As such, routine laboratory studies are not recommended for the patient with a simple febrile seizure. Furthermore, routine neuroimaging or EEG screening is also not recommended for the patient with a first-time simple febrile seizure. However, the evaluation should focus on the possible cause of the fever.

It is important to note that typical signs of meningitis may be absent in patients younger than 12 to 18 months. Furthermore, seizure may be the first presentation of meningitis. Thus, one should strongly consider an LP in all patients younger than 12 months who present with a simple febrile seizure, and one should maintain a low threshold to perform one in patients 12 to 18 months of age. LP is recommended in patients younger than 18 months with a complex febrile seizure or a concerning physical or neurologic evaluation, including irritability, lethargy, or poor feeding.

Patients who have a simple febrile seizure may be safely discharged to home. Parents should be reassured that febrile seizures are common and that most patients have no further episodes. They need to be cautioned that a recurrence may happen and should be given simple instructions on what to do should another seizure occur. Furthermore, parents should understand that patients with recurrent febrile seizures may still contract meningitis and may require clinical evaluation for this possibility. They can also be instructed on the proper use of antipyretics, even though studies have failed to demonstrate that this is effective in reducing the recurrence rate. Finally, any identified source of the fever should be properly treated.

Suggested Readings

Freedman SB, Powell ED. Pediatric seizures and their management in the emergency department. *Clin Pediatr Emerg Med* 2003;4(3):195–206.

Hanhan UA, Fiallos MR, Orlowski JP. Status epilepticus. *Pediatr Clin North Am* 2001;48(3):683–694.

Reuter D, Brownstein D. Common emergent pediatric neurologic problems. *Emerg Med Clin North Am* 2002;20(1):155–176.

Riviello JJ Jr, Holmes GL. The treatment of status epilepticus. *Semin Pediatr Neurol* 2004;11:129–38.

Sharma S, Riviello JJ Jr, Harper MB, et al. The role of emergent neuroimaging in children with new-onset afebrile seizures. *Pediatrics* 2003;111(1):1–5.

Uberall MA, Trollmann R, Wunsiedler U, et al. Intravenous valproate in pediatric epilepsy patients with refractory status epilepticus. *Neurology* 2000;54(11):2188–2189.

Warden CR, Zibulewsky J, Mace S, et al. Evaluation and management of febrile seizures in the out-of-hospital and emergency department settings. *Ann Emerg Med* 2003;41(2):215–222.

CHAPTER 70 ■ THE SEPTIC-APPEARING INFANT

STEVEN M. SELBST, MD

A young infant may be brought to the emergency department (ED) because he or she "just doesn't look right" to the parents. Even inexperienced parents whose first baby is just a few weeks old may notice when their child is unusually sleepy, fussy, or not drinking as well as usual. To the physician in the ED, such an infant may appear quite ill with pallor, cyanosis, or ashen color. There may be notable irritability or lethargy, and fever may or may not be present. The infant may be found to have tachypnea, tachycardia, or both. Hypotension or other signs of poor perfusion may also be apparent.

Generally, an ill-appearing infant, such as the one described, will be immediately considered to have sepsis and will be managed reflexively. Although this may be the correct approach in most cases, the physician should remember that several other conditions could produce a septic-appearing infant.

This chapter establishes a differential diagnosis for infants in the first 2 months of life who appear quite ill. An approach to the evaluation and management of such an infant is discussed.

DIFFERENTIAL DIAGNOSIS

Numerous disorders (Table 70.1) may cause an infant to appear septic. The most common of these disorders (Table 70.2) includes certain bacterial infections and viral syndromes. The remaining disorders, although uncommon, demand diagnostic consideration because they are potentially life threatening, yet treatable.

Sepsis

Sepsis (see Chapter 91) should always be considered when the emergency physician is confronted with an ill-appearing infant. The signs and symptoms of sepsis may be subtle. The history may vary, and some infants may seem to be ill for several days whereas others deteriorate rapidly. Likewise, any one or combination of symptoms, such as lethargy, irritability, diarrhea, vomiting, anorexia, or fever, may be a manifestation of sepsis. Fever is generally an unreliable finding in the septic infant; most septic infants younger than 2 months will be hypothermic instead. On physical examination, a septic infant may be pale, ashen, or even cyanotic. The skin is often cool and may be mottled because of poor perfusion. The infant may seem lethargic, obtunded, or irritable. There is often marked tachycardia, with the heart rate approaching 200 beats per minute, and tachypnea may be noted (respiratory rate more than 50 breaths per minute). If disseminated intravascular coagulopathy (DIC) has developed, there may be scattered petechiae or purpura may be evident. If meningitis is also present, a bulging or tense fontanel may be found. Likewise, if the infection has localized elsewhere, there may be otitis media, abdominal rigidity, joint swelling, or tenderness in one extremity or possibly chest findings such as rales. Finally, if the disease process has progressed, the infant may develop shock and may be hypotensive.

The laboratory is often helpful in suggesting a diagnosis of sepsis; however, definitive cultures require time for processing. A complete blood cell (CBC) count may reveal a leukocytosis or left shift. In addition, a coagulation profile may show evidence of DIC, and blood chemistries may reveal hypoglycemia or metabolic acidosis. If localized infection is suspected, aspiration and Gram stain of urine, joint fluid, spinal fluid, or pus from the middle ear may reveal the offending organism. Similarly, a chest radiograph may show a lobar infiltrate if pneumonia is present. A Gram stain of a petechial scraping may also reveal the responsible organism.

Viral Infections

Overwhelming viral infections may mimic sepsis in the young infant. About 25% of infants younger than 1 month with *enteroviral infections* develop a sepsis-like illness. Respiratory distress and hemorrhagic manifestations, including gastrointestinal bleeding and bleeding into the skin, are commonly seen. Seizures often occur, as well as icterus, splenomegaly, congestive heart failure, and abdominal distension. Mortality from enteroviral infections is high among neonates. This infection is indistinguishable from bacterial sepsis, except that bacterial cultures will give negative results, whereas viral isolates from stool and cerebrospinal fluid (CSF), or enterovirus polymerase chain reaction (PCR) of the CSF, may confirm the offending enterovirus.

Epidemics of *respiratory syncytial virus* (RSV) occur in the wintertime, and babies younger than 2 months may present with apnea or respiratory distress with cyanosis. Those born prematurely or with previous respiratory or cardiac disorders are especially susceptible to apnea. These infants often appear septic, but knowledge of illness in the community and a predominance of wheezing on chest examination may lead to the suspicion of RSV bronchiolitis. Still, some infants develop wheezing later in the course and, thus, the initial diagnosis is difficult. A rapid nasal wash test for RSV, if available, will be quickly diagnostic. Culture for RSV requires several days. A CBC count may show a lymphocytosis, but because of stress, a left shift can also be found. Chest radiographs may show diffuse patchy infiltrates and, possibly, lobar atelectasis.

Another viral infection to consider is *herpes simplex*, which usually causes systemic symptoms and encephalitis at 7 to 21 days of life. Neonates present with fever, coma, apnea, fulminant

TABLE 70.1

DIFFERENTIAL DIAGNOSIS OF THE
SEPTIC-APPEARING INFANT

Infectious diseases
Bacterial sepsis
Meningitis
Urinary tract infection
Viral infections—enterovirus, respiratory syncytial virus,
   herpes simplex
Pertussis
Congenital syphilis

Cardiac disease
Congenital heart disease
Supraventricular tachycardia
Myocardial infarction
Pericarditis
Myocarditis
Kawasaki disease

Endocrine disorders
Congenital adrenal hyperplasia

Metabolic disorders
Hyponatremia, hypernatremia
Cystic fibrosis
Inborn errors of metabolism, galactosemia
Hypoglycemia
Drugs/toxins—aspirin, carbon monoxide

Renal disorders
Posterior urethral valves

Hematologic disorders
Severe anemia
Methemoglobinemia

Gastrointestinal disorders
Gastroenteritis with dehydration
Pyloric stenosis
Intussusception
Necrotizing enterocolitis
Appendicitis
Volvulus

Neurologic disease
Infant botulism
Shunt obstruction, infection
Child abuse—intracranial hemorrhage

TABLE 70.2

MOST COMMON DISORDERS THAT MIMIC SEPSIS

Urinary tract infection	Congestive heart failure
Viremia	Gastroenteritis with dehydration

lobe. The diagnosis is confirmed by culture of a skin vesicle, mouth, nasopharynx, eyes, urine, blood, CSF, stool, or rectum.

Pertussis is another infection to consider when evaluating a very ill infant. Apnea, seizures, and death have been reported in this age group. Parents may report respiratory distress, cough, poor feeding, and vomiting (often posttussive). History of exposure to pertussis may be lacking because the infant usually acquires the disease from older children or adults who have only symptoms of a common upper respiratory infection. Physical examination will distinguish the infection from sepsis if the infant has a paroxysmal cough. The characteristic inspiratory "whoop" after a coughing paroxysm (a hallmark in older patients) is uncommon in very young infants. Auscultation of the chest is usually normal; tachypnea and cyanosis may be present. Initial laboratory studies may not identify the condition. The CBC count in young infants may fail to show a marked lymphocytosis as expected in older patients with pertussis. Likewise, the chest radiograph may not show the typical "shaggy right heart border." Atelectasis or pneumonia may be present. Nasopharyngeal culture for *Bordetella pertussis* is confirmatory. PCR technique can reliably identify the condition from nasopharyngeal specimens.

Infants with *congenital syphilis* may present in the first 4 weeks of life with extreme irritability, pallor, jaundice, hepatosplenomegaly, and edema. They may have pneumonia and often have painful limbs. Snuffles and skin lesions are common. Although these infants may appear to be ill on arrival in the ED, their histories reveal that they also have been chronically ill. Certainly, if a history of maternal infection is obtained, the diagnosis should be considered. Laboratory tests will be helpful in that radiographs of the infant's long bones may reveal diffuse periostitis of several bones. A serologic test is needed to confirm the diagnosis.

Cardiac Diseases

In addition to infections, cardiac disease should be considered with a very ill infant. An infant with underlying *congenital heart disease* (CHD), such as ventriculoseptal defect, valvular insufficiency, valvular stenosis, hypoplastic left heart syndrome (HLHS), or coarctation of the aorta, may present with shock or congestive heart failure and clinical findings similar to those of an infant with sepsis. There may be tachycardia and tachypnea, as well as pallor, duskiness, or mottling of the skin. Cyanosis is not always present. There may also be sweating or decreased pulses, and hypotension caused by poor perfusion. However, a careful history and physical examination may help the physician differentiate CHD with heart failure from sepsis. For instance, a chronic history of poor growth and poor feeding may suggest heart disease. Also, the presence of a cardiac murmur may suggest a structural lesion. Moreover, a gallop rhythm, hepatomegaly, neck vein distension, and

hepatitis, pneumonitis, coagulopathy, and seizures, which are often difficult to control. History of maternal genital herpes should lead to suspicion of systemic herpes infection in the neonate. In most cases, however, the mother is completely asymptomatic. Ocular findings such as conjunctivitis or keratitis may be noted, as well as focal neurologic findings. If vesicular lesions are present on the skin, this infection should be strongly considered. However, they are present in only one-third to one-half of patients. Rapid diagnostic tests are available. PCR is a sensitive method to detect the virus from CSF in infants suspected of herpes encephalitis. Direct fluorescent antibody staining of vesicle scrapings is specific but less sensitive than culture. A Tzanck preparation has low sensitivity and is not recommended as a rapid diagnostic test. An electroencephalogram (EEG) or computed tomography (CT) scan may also be helpful and may reveal abnormalities of the temporal peripheral edema may lead one to consider primary cardiac pathology. Intercostal retractions and rales, rhonchi, or wheezing are nonspecific findings and may be present on chest examination in either heart failure or pneumonia. An infant with HLHS or coarctation of the aorta may present with shock toward the end of the first week of life as the patent ductus arteriosus (PDA) closes. In a young baby, difference between upper- and lower-extremity blood pressures suggests coarctation of the aorta. If cardiac output is inadequate, however, pulse differences may not be detected. Normal femoral pulses do not exclude a coarctation because the widely patent ductus arteriosis provides flow to the descending aorta.

Laboratory evaluation is essential in establishing cardiac disease as the cause of an infant's moribund condition. A chest radiograph often shows cardiac enlargement and may show pulmonary vascular engorgement or interstitial pulmonary edema rather than lobar infiltrates (as in pneumonia). The electrocardiogram (EKG) may be helpful in revealing certain congenital heart lesions. For instance, in HLHS, the EKG invariably shows right-axis deviation, with right atrial and ventricular enlargement. The EKG is often a nonspecific indicator of cardiac decompensation; however, an echocardiogram is more helpful. Finally, a complete blood count may be helpful in that the absence of leukocytosis and left shift may make sepsis a less likely consideration. Rarely, an infant with anomalous or obstructed coronary arteries will develop myocardial infarction and appear to be septic initially. Such young infants may have dyspnea, cyanosis, vomiting, pallor, and other signs of heart failure; however, these infants usually have cardiomegaly on chest radiograph. This will prompt the physician to perform an EKG, which usually shows T-wave inversion and deep Q waves in leads I and AVL. Echocardiogram and cardiac catheterization with contrast are needed to confirm the diagnosis.

In addition to CHD, certain *arrhythmias* may cause an infant to appear ill. For instance, a young baby with *supraventricular tachycardia* (SVT) often presents with findings similar to those of a septic infant. This arrhythmia may be idiopathic (50%), associated with CHD (20%), or related to drugs, fever, or infection (20%). Often young infants with SVT go unrecognized at home for 2 days or more because, initially, they have only poor feeding, fussiness, and some rapid breathing. As this condition goes untreated, however, the infants will develop congestive heart failure and may present with all the signs of sepsis, including shock. Because fever can be a precipitating cause of the arrhythmia, the condition is obviously confused with sepsis. However, a careful physical examination will make the diagnosis of SVT obvious. Particularly, the cardiac examination will reveal such extreme tachycardia in the infant that the heart rate cannot even be counted. It is usual for the heart rate to exceed 250 to 300 beats per minute in such infants. With this information, laboratory aids can confirm the diagnosis. An EKG will show regular atrial and ventricular beats with 1:1 conduction, although P waves appear different than sinus P waves and may be difficult to see at all. They are often buried in the T waves. Moreover, a chest radiograph may show cardiomegaly and pulmonary congestion.

Additional cardiac pathologies to consider include *myocarditis* and *pericarditis*. Pericarditis may be caused by bacterial organisms such as *Staphylococcus aureus*; myocarditis usually results from viral infections such as coxsackievirus B. In infants, these often are fulminant infections and the baby

with such a condition will appear critically ill, with fever and grunting respirations. A complete physical examination may help the physician distinguish these conditions from sepsis in that signs of heart failure may be seen and unexplained tachycardia is often present. Also, pericarditis may produce neck vein distension and distant heart sounds if a significant pericardial effusion exists. In addition, a friction rub may be present. Laboratory tests may be helpful in that a chest radiograph will show cardiomegaly and a suggestion of effusion if pericarditis is present. The EKG will show generalized T-wave inversion and low-voltage QRS complexes, especially if pericardial fluid is present. Also, ST-T-wave abnormalities may be seen. The echocardiogram will confirm the presence or absence of a pericardial effusion and poor ventricular function in the case of viral myocarditis. The CBC count will not distinguish these infections from sepsis because leukocytosis is common and a left shift may be present.

Kawasaki disease with associated coronary artery aneurysms is very rare in young infants and is associated with a poor prognosis. A baby with Kawasaki disease may present with cyanosis and shock. Usually, history reveals prolonged and unexplained fever, rash, and mucous membrane inflammation. The physical examination may distinguish this illness from sepsis if there is a diffuse, raised, erythematous rash or cracked red lips, swollen hands and feet, conjunctivitis, and cervical lymphadenopathy. However, these classic features, found in older infants and children, may be absent in young babies. Neonates with Kawasaki disease often have an atypical presentation. Routine laboratory studies may not differentiate this condition from sepsis either. A CBC count may reveal leukocytosis and/or thrombocytosis. CSF usually shows a pleocytosis, with a lymphocytic predominance. Sterile pyuria is sometimes noted. In some cases, findings consistent with myocardial ischemia or an arrhythmia may be noted on EKG. Normal findings or nonspecific abnormalities are more common. Coronary artery aneurysms may be discovered with an echocardiogram, making the diagnosis highly likely.

Endocrine Disorders

Certain endocrine disorders can also mimic sepsis. For instance, infants with *congenital adrenal hyperplasia* (CAH) may present in the first few days or weeks of life with a history of vomiting, lethargy, or irritability. On arrival, signs of marked dehydration may be present, with tachycardia and possibly hypothermia. The recent history may be revealing in that such infants may have been poor feeders since birth and the symptoms may be progressive over a few days. The physical examination can be extremely helpful in establishing the diagnosis in females if ambiguous genitalia are noted. The laboratory evaluation is also helpful in that the presence of marked hyponatremia with severe hyperkalemia should make CAH a likely diagnosis. Other nonspecific laboratory findings in this disorder include hypoglycemia, metabolic acidosis, and peaked T waves or arrhythmias on EKG. Specifically, the finding of elevated 17-hydroxyprogesterone and renin with decreased aldosterone and cortisol in the serum confirms the diagnosis of CAH. Treatment with hydrocortisone 100 mg/m^2 (or 2 mg/kg) intravenously should be initiated as soon as the diagnosis is suspected.

Metabolic Disorders

Various metabolic disorders can also look like sepsis and should be considered in the differential diagnosis. Prolonged diarrhea or vomiting can produce *dehydration, electrolyte disturbances,* and *acid-base abnormalities* such that an infant will appear quite ill. For instance, young infants with diarrhea may develop marked hyponatremia caused by iatrogenic water intoxication. This is seen when well-meaning parents give excess free water to a young infant or improperly mix concentrated formula, leading to a rapid drop in serum sodium. Such infants may appear extremely lethargic, with slow respirations, hypothermia, and, possibly, seizures that are difficult to control. Likewise, dehydrated infants with *hypernatremia* may be lethargic or irritable, with muscle weakness, seizures, or coma. Infants with persistent vomiting may have hypochloremic alkalosis with hypokalemia, and they may appear weak or have cardiac dysfunction (see Chapters 17 and 78).

A special cause of hyponatremic dehydration to consider is *cystic fibrosis* (see Chapter 99). The history in these cases may not be helpful initially, except that the infant usually gets very ill in hot weather. The mother may report poor intake, poor growth, and increased lethargy. Only with specific questioning might the mother report that the baby's skin tastes "salty" or that the baby had meconium plug syndrome (transient form of distal colonic obstruction secondary to inspissated meconium) as a newborn or prolonged neonatal jaundice. In some cases, pulmonary symptoms such as cough, tachypnea, or pneumonia may have been treated earlier in life. On examination, the dehydrated baby looks much like any other septic infant. However, laboratory tests that show profound hypoelectrolytemia, especially when not accounted for by gastrointestinal losses, should suggest cystic fibrosis. A sweat test or DNA analysis will help confirm the diagnosis.

In addition, rare inborn errors of metabolism such as *inherited urea cycle disorders* may produce vomiting in young infants, who will then present with lethargy, seizures, or coma resulting from metabolic acidosis, hyperammonemia, or hypoglycemia (see Chapter 94). Galactosemia is an important metabolic problem that can cause a young infant to appear septic. Galactosemia is caused by a genetic defect in the metabolism of galactose. Neonates with this enzyme deficiency, who are exposed to galactose, present with vomiting, acidosis, failure to thrive, and jaundice. Some may have hypoglycemia and many will have liver dysfunction with a significant coagulopathy. Many develop urinary tract infections or sepsis due to gram-negative organisms. Inquiry about neonatal screening for galactosemia is important. When considering these conditions, it is essential to evaluate the CBC count, electrolytes, bicarbonate, blood glucose, liver function (including coagulation studies), and, possibly, plasma ammonia levels in young infants with significant symptoms of gastroenteritis, lethargy, or irritability. A urinalysis including ketones is helpful. Collect extra plasma (2 mL) and urine (5 mL) for additional testing. Consider sending a follow-up blood filter paper specimen to the newborn screening laboratory. A rapid bedside test for blood sugar level is recommended for immediate recognition of hypoglycemia. *Hypoglycemia* also can be secondary to sepsis, certain drugs, or alcohol intoxication

Another metabolic problem to consider is that of *toxins* (see Chapter 94). Obviously, young infants are incapable of accidental ingestions, but well-meaning parents may rarely cause salicylism in their attempts to aggressively treat fever with aspirin (despite current Reye's syndrome warnings). Affected infants can then present with vomiting, hyperpnea, hyperpyrexia, or convulsions and coma. In such cases, the history of medication given is crucial because the physical examination will not distinguish this ill baby from the infant with sepsis. The laboratory evaluation may lead to the suspicion of some metabolic problem because abnormalities of sodium, blood sugar, or acid-base balance are often found. Moreover, hypokalemia can be seen in salicylism, as well as abnormal liver function or renal function studies. An elevated salicylate level in the serum confirms the diagnosis of aspirin poisoning, but in chronic poisoning, the aspirin level may be relatively low despite a fatal course.

Carbon monoxide poisoning may present as an unknown intoxication when families are unaware of a defective heating system in the home. The young baby may have a history of sluggishness, poor feeding, and vomiting. A more careful history generally reveals that other family members are also ill with headache, syncope, or flulike symptoms. Their symptoms may improve after leaving the home environment. The classic "cherry red" skin color may be lacking, and physical examination may reveal only lethargy. Elevation of the carboxyhemoglobin level is diagnostic.

Renal Disorders

A young infant may also appear extremely ill because of renal failure or dysplasia. Such renal failure could be caused by *posterior urethral valves* that cause bladder outlet obstruction, especially in males. About one-third of these cases are diagnosed by 1 week of age, but more than half go undetected for the first few months of life. The parents may give a history of vomiting or poor appetite, or they may say that the baby has not grown well or that the infant's abdomen appears swollen. On physical examination, hypertension or an abdominal mass (hydronephrosis) may be detected, as well as urinary ascites. Laboratory tests will elucidate the diagnosis even more. Suprapubic ultrasound may demonstrate the dilated posterior urethra and bladder, strongly suggesting posterior urethral valves. A voiding cystourethrogram should be obtained; this will show a dilated posterior urethra, hypertrophy of the bladder neck, and trabeculated bladder. The serum creatinine and blood urea nitrogen levels may be markedly elevated. Urosepsis is a possible complication of posterior urethral valves.

Hematologic Disorders

It is also important to consider hematologic disorders when confronted with a critically ill infant. Any infant with severe *anemia* caused by aplastic disease, hemolytic process, or blood loss can look quite ill (see Chapters 33 and 91). In addition to anemia, disorders of hemoglobin such as *methemoglobinemia* can cause an infant to appear toxic. Although the chronic forms are uncommon inherited disorders of hemoglobin structure or enzyme deficiency, transient methemoglobinemia in infants is occasionally caused by environmental toxicity from oxidizing agents such as nitrates found in some specimens of well water or oxidant drugs (e.g., topical benzocaine in teething gels). This intoxication presents in very young infants with cyanosis, poor feeding, failure to thrive, vomiting, diarrhea, and then lethargy. In other patients, the oxidant stress is less obvious. Methemoglobinemia has been described in infants with gastroenteritis and metabolic acidosis. Often, the associated diarrhea is severe, and it has been believed that the infectious agent that causes the diarrhea or the secondary metabolic acidosis may produce an oxidant stress that leads to methemoglobin formation. On examination, such infants have been described as toxic and lethargic, with hypothermia, tachycardia, tachypnea, and hypotension. They often appear mottled, cyanotic, or ashen. One key to the diagnosis of methemoglobinemia is that oxygen administration does not affect the cyanosis, yet no cardiac problem exists. Also, laboratory tests show a profound acidosis (pH 6.9 to 7.2), yet the PaO$_2$ is normal despite the cyanosis. Leukocytosis and thrombocytosis are present. The blood itself may appear chocolate brown (most easily noted when a drop of blood on filter paper is waved in the air and compared with a normal control), and methemoglobin levels will be elevated up to 65% (normal 0% to 2%). Hemoglobin electrophoresis will be normal (except in rare cases of hemoglobin M), as is the glucose-6-phosphate dehydrogenase assay in most cases. Prerenal azotemia may be noted. With appropriate treatment, the methemoglobin level returns to normal. However, death can occur from methemoglobinemia in infants if not treated promptly.

Gastrointestinal Disorders

Gastrointestinal disorders can cause an infant to appear acutely ill. *Gastroenteritis*, even without electrolyte disturbances, can lead to profound dehydration. In a very young infant with little reserve, this can quickly lead to lethargy and even shock. Bacterial infections such as *Salmonella* may cause sepsis in a young infant, and viral agents may mimic this. A history of bloody diarrhea may suggest this diagnosis. Stool cultures will diagnose bacterial infections, but a few days are needed for isolation. Viral isolation takes even longer. In the ED, a stool smear may reveal polymorphonuclear leukocytes, suggesting bacterial infection. A CBC count with many band forms and a white blood cell (WBC) count in the normal range suggest *Shigella*. Laboratory tests are otherwise not helpful. Fluid resuscitation may improve the infant's appearance and make dehydration the likely diagnosis. However, sepsis often cannot be ruled out in the ED, regardless of laboratory studies and initial therapy.

Also, *pyloric stenosis* causes severe vomiting in the young infant. This is most often seen in male infants 3 to 6 weeks old. An infant with pyloric stenosis may present to the ED with significant dehydration and may be lethargic. Usually, no fever is present. A careful history reveals that vomiting is the predominant feature of the illness, and there may be a positive family history for pyloric stenosis. The physical examination may reveal an abdominal mass, or "olive," in less than half of the cases, which would strengthen the diagnosis of pyloric stenosis. Rarely, a peristaltic wave can be noted to pass over the epigastric area. Electrolytes typically show hypochloremia and hypokalemia, and alkalosis is prominent. Plain radiographs of the abdomen, a barium study, or ultrasound of the upper gastrointestinal tract may be needed to confirm the diagnosis.

Another gastrointestinal disorder to consider is *intussusception*. Although this rarely occurs in infants younger than 5 months, it has been noted in some infants 2 to 3 months old. These infants may present with vomiting, fever, or signs of abdominal pain (e.g., legs drawn up, irritability). The infant may appear to have spasms of pain during which he or she is fretful. This can be followed by apathy and listlessness. Diarrhea may be seen, and if the typical currant jelly stool is noted, the diagnosis of intussusception should be strongly suspected. This is considered a late finding in this condition. On physical examination, an abdominal mass may be palpated or bloody stool found on rectal examination. The laboratory may show nonspecific abnormalities such as leukocytosis and possibly anemia on the CBC count. However, a plain radiograph of the abdomen will likely show the evidence of small bowel obstruction in advanced cases that mimic sepsis and an air-contrast enema will show a filling defect usually near the ileocecal valve. A history of colicky behavior and the physical findings point to a gastrointestinal lesion rather than to sepsis.

Several other unusual but important gastrointestinal disorders have to be considered in infants. *Necrotizing enterocolitis* (NEC) occurs in premature infants in the first few weeks of life and can also occur in term infants, usually within the first 10 days of life. A history of an anoxic episode at birth or other neonatal stresses may suggest NEC. These infants are quite ill, with lethargy, irritability, anorexia, distended abdomen, and bloody stools. Radiographs of the abdomen may be helpful and usually show pneumatosis cystoides intestinalis caused by gas in the intestinal wall. Neonatal *appendicitis* is a rare event, but several cases have been reported to closely mimic sepsis. The mortality for this disorder is close to 80%, and perforation obviously worsens the prognosis. Thus, rapid diagnosis is essential. The most common presenting signs include irritability, vomiting, and abdominal distension on examination. There may also be hypothermia, ashen color, and shock as the condition progresses, as well as edema of the abdominal wall, localized to the right flank, and, possibly, erythema of the skin in that area. The WBC count may be elevated, with a left shift, and there may be a metabolic acidosis, as well as DIC. Abdominal radiographs may show a paucity of gas in the right lower quadrant, evidence of free peritoneal fluid, or a right abdominal wall thickened by edema.

Another gastrointestinal emergency to consider includes *volvulus* secondary to malrotation. About half of infants with this condition present in the first month of life. Neonates with this condition appear very ill and present with bilious vomiting and possibly bloody stools. Physical examination may reveal abdominal distention, signs of peritonitis as intestinal ischemia progresses, and shock. A plain radiograph of the abdomen may give abnormal finding; however, a limited upper gastrointestinal contrast study (designed to visualize the duodenum and proximal jejunum) is imperative for diagnosis. Finally, consider rare diagnoses such as perforation caused by *trauma* from enemas or thermometers, and *Hirschsprung's enterocolitis*.

Neurologic Diseases

Neurologic problems should be considered in the evaluation of a critically ill infant. For instance, an unusual process that produces a sepsis-like picture is *infant botulism*. This illness is produced by neurotoxins elaborated by *Clostridium botulinum*. An infant with botulism is often lethargic at presentation to the ED, with a weak cry and, possibly, signs of dehydration. These infants are usually afebrile. A thorough history may help distinguish botulism from sepsis. If constipation has preceded the acute illness, botulism should be seriously considered. The disease is also associated with the ingestion of honey, breast-feeding, a recent change in feeding practices, a rural environment, or nearby construction. The parents may note a more gradual progression with this illness. On physical examination, infants with botulism are notably hypotonic and hyporeflexic and may have increased secretions caused by bulbar muscle weakness. Infants with botulism differ from those with sepsis because they are generally well perfused with normal cardiovascular parameters. Also, the presence of a facial droop, ophthalmoplegia, and decreased gag reflex are consistent with botulism, whereas they remain unusual findings with a septic infant. The diagnosis of infant botulism is usually made by clinical findings; however, laboratory evaluation (cultures) should rule out bacterial illness. Moreover, abnormal (decreased) pulmonary function tests, such as the measurement of maximal inspiratory force and vital capacity, lend supportive evidence to the diagnosis of botulism. Finally, specific tests will confirm the diagnosis of botulism. A stool specimen to identify toxins of *C. botulinum* may be diagnostic but requires considerable time for identification. However, electromyography will show decreased muscle action potential with the "staircase" phenomenon in this disease. The WBC count is normal in infants with botulism.

A young baby with a ventriculoperitoneal shunt in place because of hydrocephalus can develop serious complications that cause the baby to appear extremely ill. *Shunt infection* could present with fever and irritability in a young infant. Abdominal pain or tenderness may be found on examination, as well as erythema or pus around the shunt itself. The definitive diagnosis is made by shunt aspiration under sterile conditions, but other causes of fever, such as meningitis, should be ruled out first. *Shunt obstruction* may result in increased intracranial pressure that causes a young infant to present with a history of lethargy or poor feeding. On examination, the baby may have bradycardia, apnea, coma, opisthotonic posturing, bulging fontanel, or cranial nerve VI palsy. The shunt may be found to pump poorly. Laboratory tests such as radiographic evaluation of the shunt may be helpful if it shows a disconnection. Otherwise, a CT scan will demonstrate ventricle size and indicate the adequacy of shunt function.

Child Abuse

Intracranial hemorrhage that results from child abuse (see Chapter xxx) must be considered in the very ill infant. It must be emphasized that the absence of bruises on an infant does not rule out child abuse. Vigorous shaking of an infant, followed by throwing the baby against a soft surface such as a mattress or sofa, can produce subdural or subarachnoid hemorrhages. The history may or may not be helpful in establishing a diagnosis. The parents may note that the child seemed to be in respiratory distress at home; only a few may admit to shaking the infant. Reports that the infant was well and is now suddenly in critical condition should raise suspicion of abuse. On examination, the infant may appear gravely ill with apnea,

bradycardia, hypothermia, bradypnea, and possibly, seizures. However, a careful physical examination may suggest abuse rather than sepsis. For instance, bruises may be present elsewhere on the body. More often, no external evidence of trauma is present. Respiratory distress without stridor or lower airway sounds may be apparent, leading to the consideration of a central nervous system cause. The head circumference is often at the 90th percentile, and the fontanel may be full or bulging. Retinal hemorrhages are often found, strongly suggesting trauma or intracranial hemorrhage rather than meningitis. Some neurologic signs may be confused with meningitis, such as nuchal rigidity, irritability or coma, seizures, or posturing. The laboratory is helpful in confirming suspicions of intracranial bleeding. Although the CBC count often shows a leukocytosis and thus is confusing, the spinal fluid from a shaken baby is usually bloody and fails to clear as the fluid is collected. A noncontrast CT scan or magnetic resonance imaging (MRI) usually demonstrates a small posterior, interhemispheric subdural hematoma. Such shaken babies have a high incidence of serious morbidity and mortality.

EVALUATION AND DECISION

Any infant who is critically ill in the first few months of life should initially be presumed to have sepsis. Because such illness is a life-threatening situation that may respond to early treatment, it is imperative to stabilize the child rapidly (Fig. 70.1). After airway, breathing, and circulation have been restored, vascular access should be obtained. Unless another diagnosis is immediately obvious, it is best to give intravenous antibiotics while pursuing alternative diagnoses. If time permits, cultures should be sent to the laboratory before giving antibiotics. Use of prostaglandins should be considered if cardiogenic shock due to PDA closure is suspected.

A complete history should be obtained. It is important to learn of any previous medical problems such as known heart disease or failure to thrive. The time of onset of symptoms, exposure to infection, medications given at home, and specific symptoms noted by the parents must be determined. Next, careful physical examination must be performed because specific findings may lead to a diagnosis other than sepsis (Table 70.3). After the physical examination, a complete laboratory evaluation should be performed. A rapid test for blood sugar level should be obtained promptly as hypoglycemia may be life threatening. All sick infants should have blood culture and urine culture specimens obtained by a urethral catheter or suprapubic bladder tap. A lumbar puncture should also be performed unless physical findings point strongly to a diagnosis other than sepsis or the infant is too ill to tolerate the procedure. A chest radiograph is also essential to look for pulmonary infection and to evaluate the heart size. A CBC count should be obtained; leukocytosis will add support to a suspicion of sepsis but also may be found in various other disorders including viral infections, myocarditis, pericarditis, intracranial bleeds, NEC, appendicitis, intussusception, and methemoglobinemia. Because metabolic problems (disturbances in acid-base balance, electrolytes, blood sugar) can result from sepsis or be the primary problem that mimics sepsis, all sick infants should have chemistries to evaluate serum sodium, potassium, chloride, glucose, and bicarbonate levels.

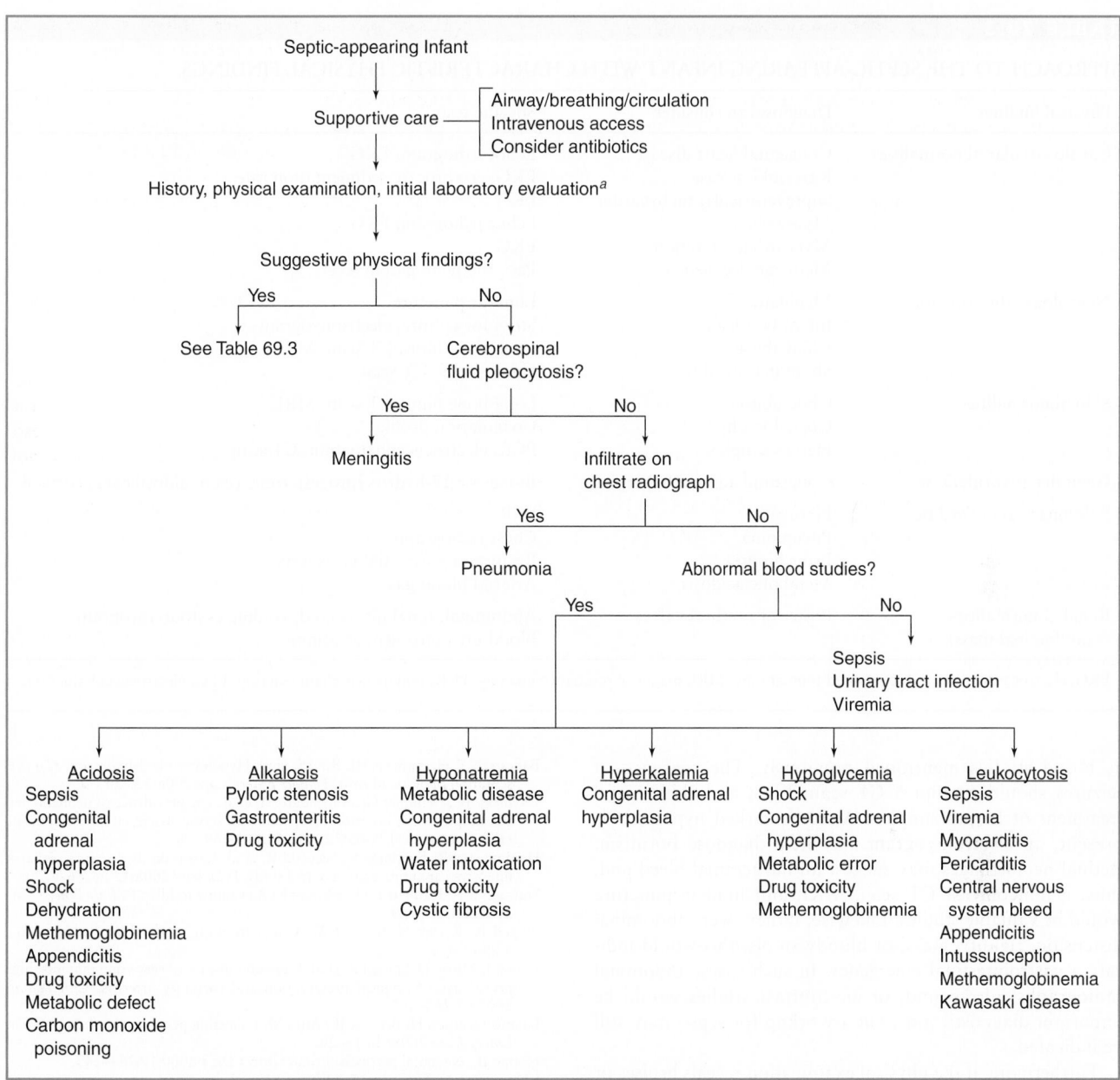

FIGURE 70.1 Initial approach to the septic-appearing child. [a]Initial laboratory evaluation: culture of blood, urine, usually cerebrospinal fluid, chest radiograph, complete blood cell count, urinalysis, electrolytes, glucose, bicarbonate, and maybe arterial blood gas.

If hyponatremia is found, water intoxication, aspirin toxicity, cystic fibrosis, and CAH should be considered. If there is also a marked hyperkalemia, CAH is most likely. If there is hypochloremic alkalosis or alkalosis alone, then pyloric stenosis, aspirin toxicity, or gastroenteritis should be considered. If there is hypoglycemia, it should be considered secondary to poor glucose reserves in an ill infant or related to drug (aspirin) toxicity, inborn errors of metabolism, CAH, or methemoglobinemia. If the serum bicarbonate level is low, this should be confirmed with an arterial blood gas level. Then, if acidosis is present, poor perfusion caused by shock should be considered, as well as dehydration, drug toxicity, methemoglobinemia, appendicitis, CAH, and inborn errors of metabolism, as primary problems.

Finally, if laboratory tests are not revealing for a specific disorder or the patient does not improve quickly as an inpatient receiving antibiotics, stool and CSF isolates for viruses should be considered.

If the physical examination suggests a specific problem, it may be necessary to obtain additional laboratory tests (Table 70.3). For instance, if the examination reveals pallor, cyanosis, or cardiac abnormality (muffled heart sounds, murmur, unexplained tachycardia, or arrhythmia), the physician should consider various cardiac disorders and, possibly, methemoglobinemia. An EKG, arterial blood to measure PaO_2, and possibly an echocardiogram should then be obtained. If there are unusual neurologic findings, such as a bulging fontanel, a lumbar puncture should be performed to rule out meningitis, as well

TABLE 70.3

APPROACH TO THE SEPTIC-APPEARING INFANT WITH CHARACTERISTIC PHYSICAL FINDINGS

Physical findings	Diagnoses to consider	Specific tests
Cardiovascular abnormalities	Congenital heart disease	Echocardiogram, EKG
	Kawasaki disease	EKG, erythrocyte sedimentation rate
	Supraventricular tachycardia	EKG
	Myocarditis	Echocardiogram, EKG
	Myocardial infarction	EKG
	Methemoglobinemia	PaO_2 methemoglobin level
Neurologic abnormalities	Meningitis	Lumbar puncture
	Infant botulism	Stool for culture, electromyogram
	Child abuse	Long bone films, CT scan, MRI
	Shunt malfunction	Shunt series, CT scan
Skin abnormalities	Child abuse	Long bone films, CT scan, MRI
	Coagulopathy	Coagulation profile
	Herpes simplex	PCR, electroencephalogram, CT scan
Genitalia abnormalities	Congenital adrenal hyperplasia	Blood for 17-hydroxyprogesterone, renin, aldosterone, cortisol
Pulmonary abnormalities	Pertussis	PCR
	Pneumonia	Chest radiograph
	Bronchiolitis	Respiratory syncytial virus tests
	Metabolic acidosis	Arterial blood gas
Renal abnormalities (abdominal mass)	Posterior urethral valves	Abdominal, renal ultrasound, voiding cystourethrogram
		Blood urea nitrogen, creatinine

EKG, electrocardiogram; CT, computed tomography; MRI, magnetic resonance imaging; PCR, polymerase chain reaction; EEG, electroencephalogram.

as blood studies mentioned previously. The presence of seizures should prompt a CT scan, EEG, and culture and treatment of herpes simplex. Also, if marked hypotonia is present, an electromyogram may help diagnose botulism. Retinal hemorrhages may suggest an intracranial bleed and, thus, a noncontrast CT scan, MRI, and lumbar puncture would be valuable studies. Likewise, if there were abdominal distension, rigidity, mass, or bloody stools, this would indicate a gastrointestinal emergency. In such cases, abdominal radiographs, ultrasound, or air-contrast studies would be important diagnostic aids, but a workup for sepsis may still be indicated.

Furthermore, if the physical examination reveals bruises or purpura, further evaluation for child abuse, coagulopathy, and sepsis should be considered. In addition, long bone radiographs, coagulation profile (including platelet count), and Gram stain of the purpura may then be desirable. If vesicular lesions are seen on the skin, a PCR and culture for herpes should be obtained. If ambiguous genitalia are noted, blood should be drawn for 17-hydroxyprogesterone, renin, aldosterone, and cortisol levels to rule out CAH (see Chapter xx). Finally, if wheezing is detected on chest examination, a nasopharyngeal swab should be sent for rapid detection of RSV or for the culture of RSV.

Suggested Readings

Bachur RG, Harper MB. Predictive model for serious bacterial infections among infants younger than 3 months of age. *Pediatrics* 2001;108:311–316.

Ballestero Y, Hernandez MI, Rojo P, et al. Hyponatremic dehydration as a presentation of cystic fibrosis. *Pediatr Emerg Care* 2006;23:725–727.

Caviness AC, Demmier GJ, Almendarez Y, et al. The prevalence of neonatal herpes simplex virus infection compared with serious bacterial illness in hospitalized neonates. *J Pediatr* 2008;153:164–169.

Dominguez SR, Friedman K, Seewald R, et al. Kawasaki disease in a pediatric intensive care unit: a case-control study. *Pediatrics* 2008;122:e786–e790.

Durracq MA, Daubert P, Osterhoudt K. A cyanotic toddler. *Pediatr Emerg Care* 2007;23:195–199.

Floyed R, Kerley N, Steele RW. A neonate with sepsis. *Clin Pediatr* 2003; 42:467–470.

Genizi J, Miron D, Spiegel R, et al. Kawasaki disease in very young infants: high prevalence of atypical presentation and coronary arteritis. *Clin Pediatr* 2003;42:263–267.

Guinto-Ocampo H, Bennett JE, Attia M. Predicting pertussis in infants. *Pediatr Emerg Care* 2008; 24:16–20.

Hoppe JE. Neonatal pertussis. *Pediatr Infect Dis J* 2000;19:244–247.

Khetsuriani N, LaMonte A, Oberste S, et al. Neonatal enterovirus infections reported to the national entervirus surveillance system in the United States, 1983–2003. *Pediatr Infect Dis J* 2006;889–893.

Kohl S. The diagnosis and treatment of neonatal herpes simplex virus infection. *Pediatr Ann* 2002;31:726–732.

Korson MS. Advances in newborn screening for metabolic disorders: what the pediatrician needs to know. *Pediatr Ann* 2000;29:294–301.

Levi D, Alejos J. Diagnosis and treatment of pediatric viral myocarditis. *Curr Opin Cardiol* 2001;16(2):77–83.

Long SS. Infant botulism and treatment with BIG-IV. *Pediatr Infect Dis J* 2007;26:261–262.

Risko W. Infant botulism. *Pediatr Rev* 2006;27:36–37.

Sard B, Tunnessen WW. Little boy blue: a cyanotic 3 week old. *Contemp Pediatr* 2001;18:25–33.

Titus MO, Wright SW. Prevalence of serious bacterial infections in febrile infants with respiratory syncytial virus infection. *Pediatrics* 2003;112:282–284.

Underwood K, Rubin S, Deakers T, et al. Infant botulism: a 30 year experience spanning the introduction of botulism immune globulin intravenous in the intensive care unit at Childrens Hospital Los Angeles. *Pediatrics* 2007;120: e1380–e1385.

Weber MA, Ashworth MT, Malone M, et al. Clinicopathological features of paediatric deaths due to myocarditis: an autopsy series. *Arch Dis Child* 2008;93:594–598.

CHAPTER 71 ■ SORE THROAT

GARY R. FLEISHER, MD

Sore throat refers to any painful sensation localized to the pharynx or the surrounding areas. Because children, particularly those of preschool age, cannot define their symptoms as precisely as adults, the physician who evaluates a child with a sore throat must first define the exact nature of the complaint. Occasionally, young patients with dysphagia (see Chapter 52), which results from disease in the area of the esophagus or with difficulty swallowing because of a neuromuscular disorder, will verbalize these feelings as a sore throat. Careful questioning usually suffices to distinguish between these complaints.

Although a sore throat is less likely to portend a life-threatening disorder than dysphagia or the inability to swallow, this complaint should not be dismissed without a thorough evaluation. Most children with sore throats have self-limiting or easily treated pharyngeal infections, but a few have serious disorders such as retropharyngeal or lateral pharyngeal abscesses. Even if the reason for the complaint of sore throat is believed to be an infectious pharyngitis, several different organisms may be responsible. Symptomatic therapy, antibiotics, antiinflammatory drugs, or surgical intervention may be appropriate at times. Most children experience no adverse consequences from misdiagnosis and inappropriate therapy, but a few may develop local extension of infection or sepsis, chronically debilitating illnesses such as rheumatic fever, or life-threatening airway obstruction.

DIFFERENTIAL DIAGNOSIS

Infectious Pharyngitis

Infection is the most common cause of sore throat and is usually caused by respiratory viruses including adenoviruses, coxsackievirus A (various serotypes), or parainfluenza virus (see Chapter 92; Tables 71.1 to 71.3). Several of the respiratory viruses produce easily identifiable syndromes, including hand-foot-mouth disease (coxsackievirus) and pharyngoconjunctival fever (adenovirus). These viral infections are closely followed in frequency by bacterial infections caused by group A streptococci (*Streptococcus pyogenes*). In the winter months during streptococcal outbreaks, as many as 30% to 50% of episodes of pharyngitis may be caused by *S. pyogenes* in school-aged children. The only other common infectious agent in pharyngitis is the Epstein-Barr virus, which causes infectious mononucleosis. Although infectious mononucleosis is not often seen in children younger than 5 years (Fig. 71.1), it cannot be considered rare even during these early years of life. More commonly, however, it affects the adolescent. An additional consideration in adolescents with an infectious

mononucleosis-like syndrome is human immunodeficiency virus (HIV), which does not commonly cause significant pharyngeal inflammation.

Other organisms produce pharyngitis only rarely; these include *Neisseria gonorrhoeae*, *Corynebacterium diphtheriae*, *Francisella tularensis*, and other bacteria. *N. gonorrhoeae* may cause inflammation and exudate but more often remains quiescent, being diagnosed only by culture. Diphtheria is a life-threatening but seldom encountered cause of infectious pharyngitis, characterized by a thick membrane and marked cervical adenopathy. Oropharyngeal tularemia is rare and should be entertained only in endemic areas among children who have an exudative pharyngitis that cannot be categorized by standard diagnostic testing and/or persists despite antibiotic therapy. Although unusual, mixed anaerobic infections should be considered in the ill-appearing adolescent with a severe pharyngitis because these organisms occasionally lead to sepsis (Lemierre's disease). Other pathogens—group C and G streptococci, *Arcanobacterium haemolyticum*, *Mycoplasma pneumoniae*, and *Chlamydia pneumoniae*—have been implicated as agents of pharyngitis in adults, but in childhood, their roles remain unproved and their frequency is unknown. Of these, *A. haemolyticum* is the most frequent, having been isolated from 0.5% to 2.0% of adolescents with pharyngitis, often in association with a maculopapular rash.

Irritative Pharyngitis/Foreign Body

Drying of the pharynx may irritate the mucosa, leading to a complaint of sore throat. This condition occurs most commonly during the winter months, particularly after a night's sleep in a house with forced hot-air heating. Occasionally, a foreign object such as a fishbone may become embedded in the pharynx.

Herpetic Stomatitis

Stomatitis caused by herpes simplex virus is usually confined to the anterior buccal mucosa but may extend to the anterior tonsillar pillars occasionally and involve the upper esophagitis in immunocompetent patients on rare occasions. Particularly, in these more extensive cases, the child may complain of a sore throat.

Peritonsillar Abscess

A peritonsillar abscess may complicate a previously diagnosed infectious pharyngitis or may be the initial source of a child's

TABLE 71.1

DIFFERENTIAL DIAGNOSIS OF SORE THROAT IN THE
IMMUNOCOMPETENT HOST

Infectious pharyngitis
   Respiratory viruses
   Group A streptococci
   Epstein-Barr virus (infectious mononucleosis)
   Human immunodeficiency virus
   Neisseria gonorrhoeae
   Anaerobic bacteria
   Group C and G streptococci
   Arcanobacterium haemolyticum
   Mycoplasma pneumoniae (unconfirmed)
   Chlamydia pneumoniae (unconfirmed)
   Francisella tularensis
   Corynebacterium diphtheriae (diphtheria)

Other causes
   Herpetic stomatitis
   Irritative pharyngitis
   Foreign body
   Peritonsillar abscess
   Retropharyngeal and lateral pharyngeal abscesses
   Epiglottitis
   Kawasaki disease
   Stevens-Johnson syndrome
   Chemical exposure
   Psychogenic pain
   Referred pain

discomfort. This disease is most common in older children and
adolescents. The diagnosis is evident from visual inspection,
augmented occasionally by careful palpation. These abscesses
produce a bulge in the posterior aspect of the soft palate, deviate the uvula to the contralateral side of the pharynx, and have
a fluctuant quality on palpation.

Retropharyngeal and Lateral Pharyngeal Abscesses

Retropharyngeal abscess is an uncommon cause of sore throat,
usually occurring in children younger than 4 years. Although
most children with this disorder appear toxic and have respiratory distress, a few complain of sore throat and dysphagia
without other manifestations early in the course. Occasional
infants and young children may also manifest torticollis. A
soft-tissue radiographic examination of the lateral neck
demonstrates the lesion readily in most cases, whereas direct
visualization is often impossible. Unfortunately, even limited

TABLE 71.2

COMMON CAUSES OF SORE THROAT

Infectious pharyngitis
   Respiratory viruses
   Group A streptococci
   Epstein-Barr virus

Irritative pharyngitis
   Forced hot air heating

TABLE 71.3

LIFE-THREATENING CAUSES OF SORE THROAT

Retropharyngeal and lateral pharyngeal abscesses
Epiglottitis
Tonsillar hypertrophy (severe) with infectious mononucleosis
Diphtheria
Peritonsillar abscess
Lemierre's syndrome

flexion of the neck during the radiograph may cause a buckling of the retropharyngeal tissues that resembles a purulent
collection. The physician must insist on a radiograph with the
neck fully extended before hazarding an interpretation. If the
diagnosis remains uncertain despite adequate radiographs, a
computed tomography (CT) scan should be obtained.

Lateral pharyngeal abscesses manifest in a fashion similar
to retropharyngeal infections but occur less often. High fever
is a common symptom, and both trismus and swelling below
the mandible may be seen. To confirm the diagnosis, a CT scan
is appropriate.

Epiglottitis

The incidence of epiglottitis, a well-appreciated cause of life-
threatening upper airway infection, has declined significantly
since the introduction of vaccination against *Haemophilus
influenzae* type b. This disease manifests with a toxic appearance, high fever, stridor, and drooling. In every reported series
of cases, sore throat appears on the list of symptoms. Although
rarely this may be the primary complaint in a child, other more
striking findings almost always predominate. Epiglottitis

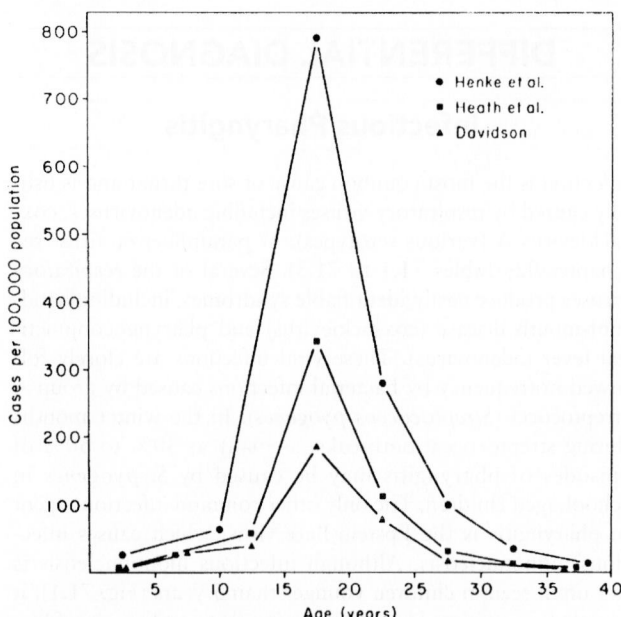

FIGURE 71.1 Incidence by age of infectious mononucleosis in three
large studies.

should be excluded easily as a diagnosis in the patient with a sore throat who is without stridor and appears relatively well.

Kawasaki Disease

Kawasaki disease is characterized by high fever along with at least four of the five following findings: (i) conjunctivitis, (ii) mucositis, (iii) peripheral erythema and/or edema, (iv) truncal rash, and (v) cervical adenopathy (see Chapter 101). The mucositis most commonly involves the lips, but occasionally pharyngitis may be a prominent feature. Other systemic inflammatory conditions (Behçet's syndrome) may involve the pharynx as well.

Stevens-Johnson Syndrome

Stevens-Johnson syndrome, a disease of unknown etiology but presumed to be immune mediated, is characterized by vesicular and ulcerative lesions of the mucosa, including the pharynx, the genitalia, and the conjunctivae. In addition, children with this condition may have a diffuse rash, often characterized by target lesions or vesicles and bullae. Usually self-limited, an occasional case may lead to dehydration or progress to involve the pulmonary system.

Chemical Exposure

Certain ingestions, such as paraquat and various alkalis, may produce a chemical injury to the mucosa of the pharynx (see Chapter 102). Usually, these findings occur in the setting of a known ingestion and are accompanied by lesions of the oral mucosa.

Referred Pain

Occasionally, pain from the inflammation of extrapharyngeal structures is described as arising in the pharynx. Examples include dental abscesses, cervical adenitis, and, occasionally, otitis media.

Psychogenic Pharyngitis

Some children who complain of a sore throat have no organic explanation for their complaint after a thorough history and physical examination and a throat culture. In these cases, the physician should consider the possibility of anxiety, at times associated with frequent or difficult (globus hystericus) swallowing.

Pharyngitis in the Immunosuppressed Host

Immunosuppressed hosts may develop pharyngitis from any of the previously discussed causes. In addition, these patients exhibit a particular susceptibility to infections with fungal organisms such as *Candida albicans*.

EVALUATION AND DECISION

The history and physical examination should focus on findings seen with systemic illnesses causing pharyngitis and the appearance of the oral cavity. A medical history of an immunosuppressive disorder or missed immunizations raises the specter of unusual infections. A sudden onset is most characteristic of epiglottitis.

Fever, either historical or measured, points to an infection or, less commonly, Kawasaki disease. Toxicity and/or respiratory distress occur with infections leading to respiratory obstruction, such as peritonsillar, retropharyngeal, and lateral pharyngeal abscesses; epiglottitis; diphtheria; and infectious mononucleosis with severe tonsillar hypertrophy. Conjunctivitis suggests pharyngoconjunctival fever (adenovirus), Kawasaki disease, or Stevens-Johnson syndrome; generalized adenopathy occurs with infectious mononucleosis and HIV; and a rash is seen with scarlet fever (group A streptococci), Kawasaki disease, infectious mononucleosis, particularly after the administration of amoxicillin, and rarely with A. *hemolyticum* in adolescents.

The tendency of most clinicians is to assume that one of the common organisms is the cause of pharyngitis in the child with a sore throat. Before settling on infectious pharyngitis, however, the emergency physician should first at least briefly consider several more serious disorders (Fig. 71.2). Conditions

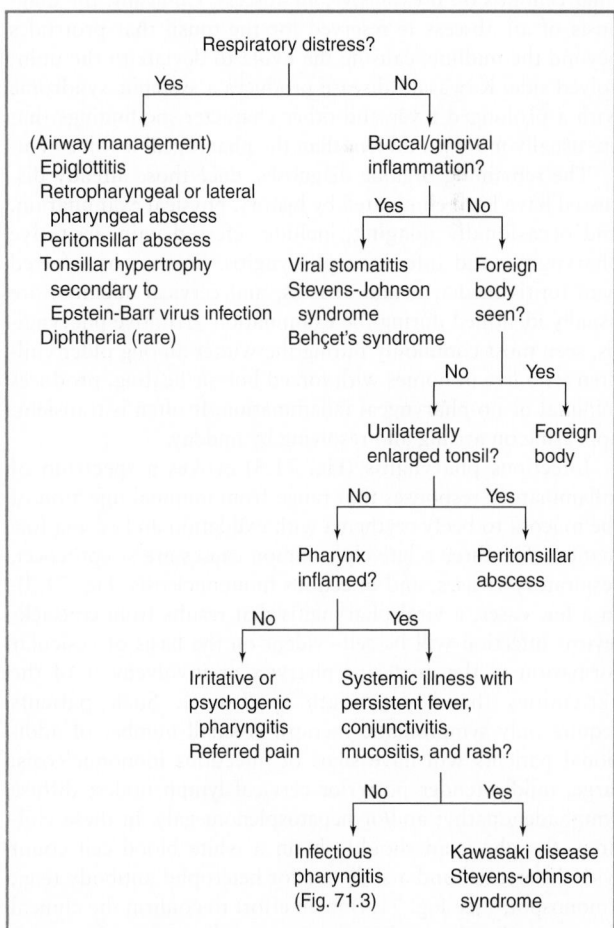

FIGURE 71.2 Diagnostic approach to the child with sore throat.

SIGNS AND SYMPTOMS

that have immediate life-threatening potential include epiglottitis, retropharyngeal and lateral pharyngeal abscesses, peritonsillar abscess, severe tonsillar hypertrophy (usually as an exaggerated manifestation of infectious mononucleosis), and diphtheria. Generally, stridor and signs of respiratory distress accompany the complaint of sore throat in epiglottitis and retropharyngeal abscess. Drooling and voice changes are common in children with these two conditions, as well as in patients with peritonsillar abscess and severe infectious tonsillar hypertrophy. In cases of epiglottitis or retropharyngeal abscess that are not clinically obvious, a lateral neck radiograph, obtained under appropriate supervision, is confirmatory. Peritonsillar abscess and tonsillar hypertrophy are diagnosed by visual examination of the pharynx. Diphtheria is rarely a consideration except in unimmunized children, particularly those from underdeveloped nations.

The next phase of the evaluation of the child with a complaint of sore throat hinges on a careful physical examination, particularly of the pharynx (Fig. 71.2). The appearance of vesicles on the buccal mucosa anterior to the tonsillar pillars points to a herpetic stomatitis or noninfectious syndromes such as Behçet's or Stevens-Johnson syndrome (erythema multiforme). Uncommonly, a small, pointed foreign body, most commonly a fishbone, becomes lodged in the mucosal folds of the tonsils or pharynx; usually, the history suggests the diagnosis, but an unanticipated sighting may occur in the younger child. Significant asymmetry of the tonsils indicates a peritonsillar cellulitis or, if extensive, an abscess. Clinically, the diagnosis of an abscess is reserved for the tonsil that protrudes beyond the midline, causing the uvula to deviate to the uninvolved side. Kawasaki disease produces a systemic syndrome with a prolonged fever and other characteristic findings that are usually more prominent than the pharyngeal involvement.

The remaining organic diagnoses, once those already discussed have been eliminated by history, physical examination, and occasionally imaging, include referred pain, irritative pharyngitis, and infectious pharyngitis. Sources of referred pain (otitis media, dental abscess, and cervical adenitis) are usually identified during the examination. Irritative pharyngitis, seen most commonly during the winter among older children who live in homes with forced hot-air heating, produces minimal or no pharyngeal inflammation. It often is transient, appearing on arising and resolving by midday.

Infectious pharyngitis (Fig. 71.3) evokes a spectrum of inflammatory responses that range from minimal injection of the mucosa to beefy erythema with exudation and edema formation. The three relatively common causes are streptococci, respiratory viruses, and infectious mononucleosis (Fig. 71.3). In a few cases, a viral pharyngitis that results from coxsackievirus infection will be self-evident on the basis of vesicular formation in the posterior pharynx or involvement of the extremities (hand-foot-mouth syndrome). Such patients require only symptomatic therapy. A small number of additional patients will have signs of infectious mononucleosis: large, mildly tender posterior cervical lymph nodes; diffuse lymphadenopathy; and/or hepatosplenomegaly. In these children, the physician should obtain a white blood cell count with differential and a slide test for heterophil antibody (e.g., "monospot," see Fig. 71.4) in an effort to confirm the clinical diagnosis, thereby guiding therapy and discussion of prognosis. Some children, especially those younger than 5 years, will

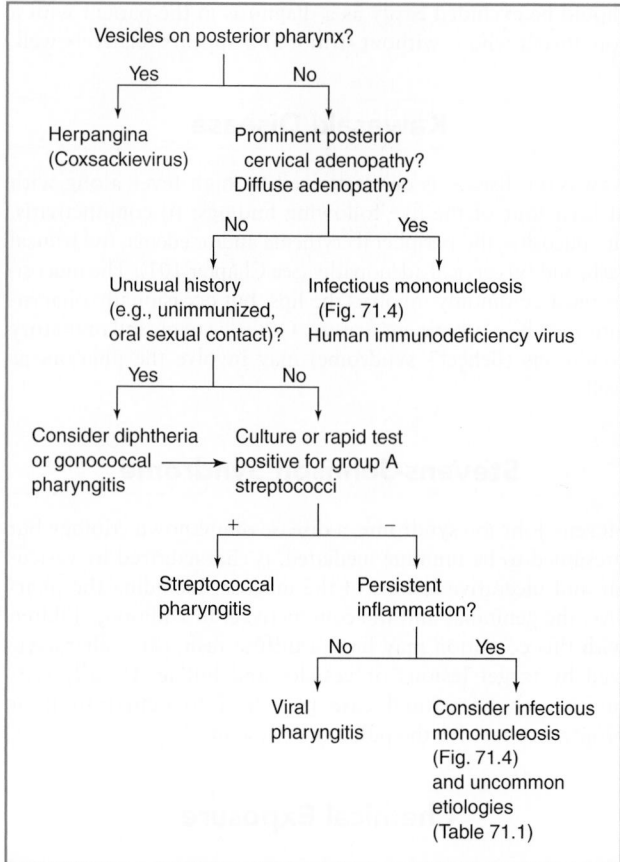

FIGURE 71.3 Diagnostic approach to infectious pharyngitis in the immunocompetent child.

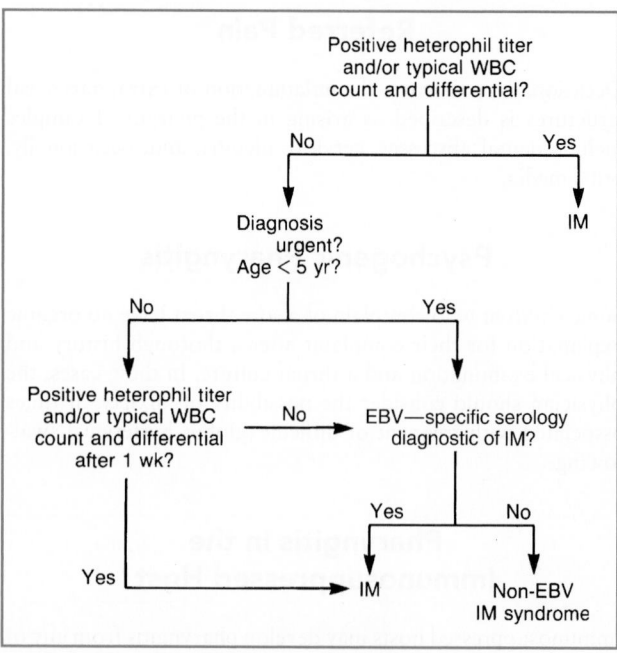

FIGURE 71.4 Diagnostic approach when findings are clinically suggestive for mononucleosis. WBC, white blood cell; IM, infectious mononucleosis; EBV, Epstein-Barr virus.

not have the characteristic lymphocytosis or heterophil antibody response and will require repeated testing or specific serologic assays for antibodies to Epstein-Barr virus. In the rare child with an unusual history, the physician must pursue diagnoses such as gonococcal pharyngitis (sexual abuse, oral sex) or diphtheria (immigration from an underdeveloped nation, lack of immunization).

Ultimately, most children will have a mildly to moderately inflamed pharynx but no specific etiologic diagnosis based solely on the history and physical examination. Although certain symptoms and signs favor streptococcal infection, none is conclusive. Thus, obtaining a rapid test (latex agglutination or optical immunoassay) for group A streptococci, followed by a culture, if negative, is prudent. Rapid tests are most helpful when a positive result is obtained because specificity of the tests is high; however, a negative test result does not exclude streptococcal infection reliably, although some authorities would be satisfied with a negative optical immunoassay alone. With the more recent reported rise in the incidence of rheumatic fever, the accurate diagnosis of streptococcal pharyngitis assumes increasing importance. Generally, symptomatic therapy suffices in the patient with a negative rapid test, although the physician may elect to initiate therapy, usually with a penicillin (penicillin V or amoxicillin) but occasionally with a cephalosporin or macrolide, while awaiting the results of the throat culture in selected cases with highly suggestive clinical features.

Suggested Readings

Bisno AL, Gerber MA, Gwalteny JM, et al. Diagnosis and management of streptococcal pharyngitis: a practice guideline. *Clin Infect Dis* 1997;25:574–583.

Breese BB. A simple scorecard for the tentative diagnosis of streptococcal pharyngitis. *Am J Dis Child* 1977;131:514.

Casey JR, Pichichero ME. Metaanalysis of short course antibiotic treatment for group A streptococcal tonsillopharyngitis. *Pediatr Infect Dis J* 2005;24:909–917.

Craig FW, Schunk JE. Retropharyngeal abscess in children: clinical presentation, utility of imaging, and current management. *Pediatrics* 2003;111:1394–1398.

Davidson RJ. A survey of infectious mononucleosis in the North-East Regional Hospital Board area of Scotland, 1960-9. *J Hyg* (Lond) 1970;68(3):393–400.

El-Daher NT, Hijazi SS, Rawasdeh NM, et al. Immediate vs. delayed treatment of group A beta-hemolytic streptococcal pharyngitis with penicillin V. *Pediatr Infect Dis J* 1991;10:126.

Fleisher GR, Lennette ET, Henle G, et al. Incidence of heterophil antibody responses in children with infectious mononucleosis. *J Pediatr* 1979;94:723.

Gieseker KE, MacKenzie T, Roe MH, et al. Comparison of two rapid *Streptococcus pyogenes* diagnostic tests with a rigorous culture standard. *Pediatr Infect Dis J* 2002;21:922–927.

Gieseker KE, Roe MH, MacKenzie T, et al. Evaluating the American Academy of Pediatrics diagnostic standard for *Streptococcus pyogenes* pharyngitis: backup culture versus repeat rapid antigen testing. *Pediatrics* 2003;111:e666–e670.

Goldenberg NA, Knapp-Clevenger R, Hayes T, et al. Lemierre's and Lemierre's-like syndromes in children: survival and thromboembolic outcomes. *Pediatrics* 2005;116:e543–e548.

Heath CW, Brodsky AC, Potolsky AI. Infectious mononucleosis in a general population. *Am J Epidemiol* 1972;96(2):87–93.

Henke CD, Kurland LT, Elveback LR. Infectious mononucleosis in Rochester, Minnesota 1950 through 1969. *Am J Epidemiol* 1973;98(6):483–90.

Kaltwasser G, Diego J, Welby-Sellenriek PL, et al. Polymerase chain reaction for *Streptococcus pyogenes* used to evaluate optical immunoassay for the detection of group A streptococci in children with pharyngitis. *Pediatr Infect Dis J* 1997;16:748–753.

Komaroff AL, Aronson MD, Pass TM, et al. Serologic evidence of chlamydial and mycoplasmal pharyngitis in adults. *Science* 1983;222:927.

Lieu TA, Fleisher GR, Schwartz JS. Clinical evaluation of a latex agglutination test for streptococcal pharyngitis: performance and impact on treatment rates. *Pediatr Infect Dis J* 1988;7:847.

Lieu TA, Fleisher GR, Schwartz JS. Cost-effectiveness of rapid latex agglutination testing and throat culture for streptococcal pharyngitis. *Pediatrics* 1990;85:246.

MacKenzie A, Fuite LA, King J, et al. Incidence and pathogenicity of *Arcanobacterium haemolyticum* during a 2-year study in Ottawa. *Clin Infect Dis* 1995;21:177–181.

Niland ML, Bonsu BK, Nuss KE, et al. A pilot study of 1 versus 3 days of dexamethasone as add-on therapy in children with streptococcal pharyngitis. *Pediatr Infect Dis J* 2006;25:477–481.

Wald ER, Green MD, Schwartz B, et al. A streptococcal scorecard revisited. *Pediatr Emerg Care* 1998;14:109–111.

Webb KH. Does culture confirmation of high-sensitivity rapid streptococcal tests make sense? *Pediatrics* 1998;101:E2.

Weisner PJ, Tronca E, Bonin P, et al. Clinical spectrum of pharyngeal gonococcal infection. *N Engl J Med* 1973;288:181.

SIGNS AND SYMPTOMS

CHAPTER 72 ■ STRIDOR

HOLLY E. PERRY, MD

Stridor, although a relatively common occurrence, can be frightening to both children and parents. The presence of stridor necessitates a complete and careful evaluation to determine the cause of this worrisome and occasionally life-threatening symptom. This chapter presents the causes of stridor and provides the emergency practitioner with guidelines for initial evaluation and management.

PATHOPHYSIOLOGY

Stridor is an externally audible sound associated with respiration. It is produced by turbulent airflow through large airways. It occurs when a normal respiratory volume of air moves through narrowed airways, which results in the normal laminar flow becoming turbulent. Stridor thus signifies partial airway obstruction.

The level of obstruction can be inferred from several characteristics of stridor: associated phase of respiration, pitch, and length of respiratory phase. Inspiratory stridor occurs with obstruction of the extrathoracic trachea, biphasic stridor when both extrathoracic and intrathoracic tracheas are involved, and expiratory stridor when only the intrathoracic trachea is involved. The pitch of the stridor also helps determine the location of the obstruction. Laryngeal and subglottic obstructions are associated with high-pitched stridor. In contrast, obstruction of the nares and nasopharynx results in lower pitched snoring or snorting sounds also called stertor. Because the passage of saliva and the flow of air are impeded in pharyngeal obstruction, these patients often have a gurgling quality of breathing. Finally, the relative length of inspiratory and expiratory phases may be helpful. Laryngeal obstruction results in an increased inspiratory phase, whereas expiration tends to be prolonged in bronchial obstruction. Both inspiratory and expiratory phases are increased in patients with tracheal obstruction.

DIFFERENTIAL DIAGNOSIS

Stridor may occur in a wide variety of disease processes affecting the large airways from the level of the nares to the bronchi but most often arises with disorders of the larynx and trachea (Table 72.1). For the purposes of differential diagnosis, it is helpful to categorize the common causes of stridor as chronic or acute in onset and to further divide acute onset into febrile and afebrile causes (Table 72.2). Life-threatening causes of stridor must be considered early during the evaluation process (Table 72.3).

Stridor with Acute Onset in the Febrile Child

Laryngotracheitis (croup) is by far the most common cause of stridor in the febrile child. Other diagnoses that should be considered include bacterial tracheitis (see Chapter 92), epiglottitis, retropharyngeal abscess, and laryngeal diphtheria in the unimmunized child. Although less common than croup, these diseases have a greater potential for life-threatening airway compromise.

Croup typically affects children between 7 and 36 months of age but is seen throughout childhood. The illness begins with upper respiratory tract symptoms and fever, usually ranging from 38°C to 39°C (100.4°F to 102.2°F). Within 12 to 48 hours, a barky, "seal-like" cough and inspiratory stridor are noted. Supraclavicular and subcostal retractions may be present. Symptoms are aggravated by crying and ameliorated by nebulized epinephrine. Most children appear only mildly or moderately ill.

Bacterial tracheitis presents in a variety of ways but may closely resemble croup. However, affected patients generally appear toxic, tend to be older, and do not respond as well to nebulized epinephrine. Dysphagia is common, and drooling may be present. The verbal child may complain of anterior neck pain or a painful cough.

Epiglottitis is an infection of the supraglottic structures. It may be divided into disease caused by *Haemophilus influenzae* or that caused by a number of other pathogens including *Staphylococcus aureus*, *Streptococcus pneumoniae*, and β-hemolytic streptococci. The incidence of epiglottis due to *H. influenzae* has plummeted to as low 0.02 per 100,000 in Western countries, following the introduction of the conjugate vaccine. Patients with *H. influenzae* epiglottitis typically are febrile, drooling, and appear toxic. Respiratory distress and a tripod stance (upright position, neck extended, and mouth open) are characteristic symptoms. Sudden airway compromise may occur and is frequently precipitated by the manipulation of the oropharynx.

In contrast, epiglottitis caused by pathogens other than *H. influenzae* has a slower onset, is much more common in adults, and is almost universally associated with difficulty swallowing or sore throat. Importantly, the risk of airway compromise is less than with epiglottitis caused by *H. influenzae*. However, any child with epiglottitis should be managed as if he or she has disease caused by *H. influenzae* and should have the airway inspected under controlled conditions.

A retropharyngeal abscess is another possible cause of stridor, although respiratory distress does not dominate the clinical presentation. More commonly, patients have fever, limitation of neck movement, agitation, or lethargy.

TABLE 72.1

CAUSES OF STRIDOR BY ANATOMIC LOCATION

Nose and pharynx
Congenital anomalies
  Lingual thyroid
  Choanal atresia
  Craniofacial anomalies (Apert's and Down's syndromes;
    Pierre Robin sequence)
  Cysts (dermoid, thyroglossal)
  Macroglossia (Beckwith's syndrome)
  Encephalocele
Inflammatory
  Abscess (parapharyngeal, retropharyngeal, peritonsillar)
  Allergic polyps
  Adenotonsillar enlargement (acute infection, infectious
    mononucleosis)
Neoplasm (benign, malignant)
Adenotonsillar hyperplasia
Foreign body
Neurologic syndromes with poor tongue/pharyngeal
  muscle tone

Larynx
Congenital anomalies
  Laryngomalacia
  Web, cyst, laryngocele
  Cartilage dystrophy
  Subglottic stenosis
  Cleft larynx
Inflammatory
  Croup
  Epiglottitis
  Tracheitis
  Angioneurotic edema
  Miscellaneous: tuberculosis, fungal infection, diphtheria,
    sarcoidosis
Vocal cord paralysis (multiple causes)
Neoplasm
  Subglottic hemangioma
  Laryngeal papilloma
  Cystic hygroma (neck)
  Malignant (e.g., rhabdomyosarcoma)
Laryngospasm (hypocalcemic tetany)

Trachea and bronchi
Congenital
  Vascular anomalies
  Webs, cysts
  Tracheal stenosis
  Tracheoesophageal fistula
Neoplasm
  Tracheal
  Compression by adjacent structure (thyroid, thymus,
    esophagus)
Foreign body (tracheal or esophageal)

Physical examination may reveal midline fullness of the oropharynx.

Stridor with Acute Onset in the Afebrile Child

A foreign body in either the trachea or the esophagus may produce stridor. There may be a history of choking on food or a

TABLE 72.2

COMMON CAUSES OF STRIDOR

Acute, febrile
Croup
Tracheitis
Epiglottitis
Retropharyngeal abscess

Acute, afebrile
Foreign body
Caustic or thermal injury to airway
Spasmodic croup
Angioneurotic edema

Chronic
Laryngomalacia
Vascular anomalies
Adenotonsillar hyperplasia

small object. Physical examination varies, depending on the location of the foreign body.

Both ingestion and inhalation of caustic or thermally damaging substances may result in injury to the airway or hypopharynx. Symptoms of airway compromise may be delayed for as long as 6 hours. Blind finger sweeps have also been reported rarely to result in stridor. Other causes to consider include spasmodic croup, angioneurotic edema, and trauma (see Chapter 112).

Chronic Stridor

The differential diagnosis is determined by the age at onset. Stridor noted shortly after birth is most likely caused by a structural defect. This type of stridor tends to slowly worsen and is severe only when the infant is stressed, such as during crying. Laryngomalacia is the most common cause of congenital stridor accounting for up to 75% of chronic stridor in children younger than 1 year. Stridor associated with laryngomalacia is positional and is worsened by placing the infant in the supine position. It frequently disappears when the child cries. Other congenital causes of stridor include laryngeal webs, laryngeal diverticula, vocal cord paralysis, sub-

TABLE 72.3

LIFE-THREATENING CAUSES OF STRIDOR

Usually febrile
Epiglottitis
Retropharyngeal abscess
Tracheitis

Usually afebrile
Foreign body
Angioneurotic edema
Neck trauma
Neoplasm (compressing trachea)
Thermal or caustic injury

glottic stenosis, tracheomalacia, and vascular anomalies such as a double aortic arch or a vascular sling. Stridor in infants has also been reported to be associated with gastroesophageal reflux.

Stridor in older children may be caused by papillomas or neoplastic processes. Patients with papillomas generally present between 2 and 4 years of age with complaints of hoarseness and stridor. Neoplastic processes causing tracheal compression can also lead to stridor in the older child.

Psychogenic stridor, also called functional stridor, is an uncommon cause of stridor in the older child. Cases have been reported in adolescents, with the youngest age being 10 years. Adolescent girls are diagnosed three times more often with this condition than are adolescent boys. More than 50% of patients meet diagnostic criteria for a psychiatric disorder. Characteristically, stridor improves when the patient is unaware that he or she is being observed, and it may clear with cough. The diagnosis can only be confirmed by direct laryngoscopy in the symptomatic patient when the vocal cords are noted to be adducted during inspiration.

EVALUATION AND DECISION

The first priority is to ensure that the airway is adequate by assessing the level of consciousness, color, perfusion, air entry, breath sounds, and work of breathing, including respiratory rate, nasal flaring, and retractions. Resuscitative measures should be instituted as necessary (see Chapter 5). The child

may then be evaluated systematically. In the child with acute onset of stridor, history should focus on associated symptoms such as fever, duration of illness, drooling, rhinorrhea, and history of choking (Fig. 72.1). Immunization status should be verified, particularly *H. influenzae* vaccination. In the case of a child with chronic stridor, important historical points include age at onset and progression of stridor, as well as ameliorating and aggravating factors.

Physical examination should include careful inspection of the nares and oropharynx, with particular attention to increased secretions, drooling, visible mass, and abnormal phonation. Quality of the voice or cry should be noted as normal, hoarse (croup, vocal cord paralysis, papilloma), weak (neuromuscular disorder), or aphonic (laryngeal obstruction by a foreign body). Regional findings such as adenopathy, neck masses, meningismus, trauma, or bruising should also be sought. Position of comfort should be noted. Children with airway obstruction at the level of the larynx and above usually hyperextend the neck and lean forward ("sniffing" position) in an effort to straighten their upper airway and maximize air entry. This posture does not help relieve more distal obstruction. Finally, response to therapies, such as nebulized racemic epinephrine, should be noted.

Emergency management of the child with stridor depends on its severity and its likely cause. Oxygen, nebulized epinephrine, corticosteroids, laryngoscopy, intubation, and even emergency cricothyroidotomy or tracheostomy all have specific roles in the emergency department (ED) management of stridor, depending on its cause (see Chapters 110 and 123).

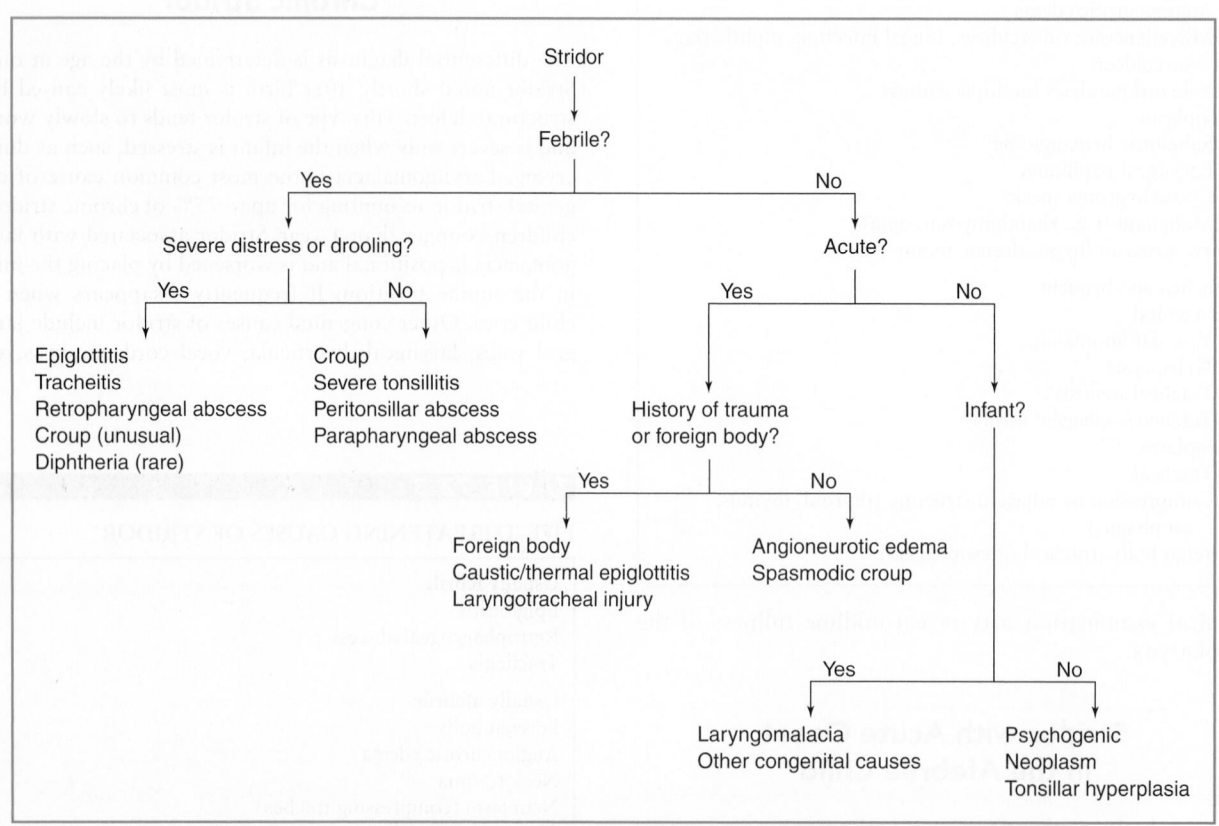

FIGURE 72.1 Diagnostic approach to stridor.

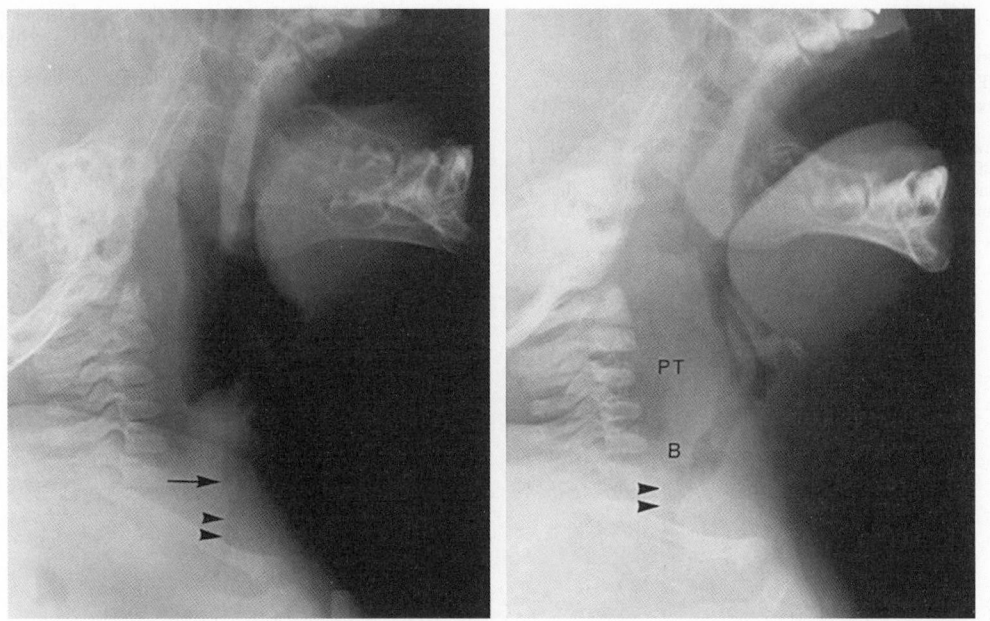

FIGURE 72.2 Inspiratory (**A**) and expiratory (**B**) lateral neck radiographs of a child with upper airway obstruction secondary to a granuloma *(arrow)* in the upper trachea. Note ballooning of the pharynx during inspiration (**A**) and narrowing of the trachea *(arrowheads)* below the level of obstruction. On expiration (**B**), note the normal pharyngeal lumen and dilation *(arrowheads)* of the trachea distal to the obstruction. The "bunching up" of the pharyngeal tissues *(PT)* and the buckling of the trachea *(B)* are normal findings on expiratory films.

Febrile Child

In the febrile child with stridor, the onset is generally acute and the most common cause is croup. Other diagnostic possibilities that should be considered include bacterial tracheitis, epiglottitis, and retropharyngeal abscess. The child whose clinical picture is consistent with mild to moderate croup needs no further evaluation. Although, history and physical examination are the most important diagnostic tools, anteroposterior and lateral neck radiographs may add some useful information and should be considered for the ill-appearing child or one who does not respond as anticipated to treatment. If epiglottitis is strongly suspected, a lateral neck radiograph should be obtained in the ED or the child should be taken to the operating room to have direct visualization of the epiglottis under controlled conditions.

Airway radiographs must be interpreted with care because they are affected by positioning, crying, swallowing, and the phase of respiration. To properly interpret the prevertebral space, the lateral neck radiograph must be taken with the patient's head extended and during inspiration. Normal tracheal buckling, which is seen during expiration in a young child, may be misinterpreted as tracheal mass lesion or deviation from an extrinsic mass (Fig. 72.2). Abnormal findings on a lateral neck radiograph include swollen epiglottis or aryepiglottic folds (epiglottitis), irregular tracheal borders or stranding across the trachea (tracheitis), and increased prevertebral width (retropharyngeal abscess). In children, the prevertebral space should be less than 75% the width of the body of C4 (cervical vertebra).

Radiographic findings consistent with croup are a narrowed subglottic area on anteroposterior view (the "steeple sign") and ballooning of the hypopharynx, best appreciated on the lateral view.

Afebrile Child

In the afebrile child with acute onset of stridor, the duration of stridor, the likelihood of foreign-body aspiration, and the child's age are all key elements to consider. Emergent otolaryngologic or surgical consultation should be obtained in a child with an evidence of airway obstruction if either aspirated foreign body or trauma is a likely cause of stridor. Angioneurotic edema, an autosomal-dominant trait, is characterized by rapid onset of swelling without discoloration, urticaria, or pain. Symptoms may occur in affected patients as young as 2 years of age but usually are not severe until adolescence; they may be precipitated by trauma, emotional stress, or menses. Determination of the C_1-esterase inhibitor level should be considered if angioneurotic edema is suspected.

A child with chronic stridor generally does not require an extensive evaluation in the ED unless significant respiratory distress is present. The infant with chronic stridor who is otherwise well should be referred back to the private pediatrician or to an otolaryngologist. Once a neoplastic cause is deemed unlikely, the older child with chronic stridor should be referred to otolaryngology for evaluation, including direct visualization of the vocal cords.

Suggested Readings

Craig FW, Schunk JE. Retropharyngeal abscess in children: clinical presentation, utility of imaging, and current management. *Pediatrics* 2003;111: 1394–1398.

Derkay CS, Wiatrak B. Recurrent respiratory papillomatosis: a review. *Laryngoscope* 2006;118:1236–1247.

Guldfred L-A, Lyhne D, Becker BC. Acute epiglottitis: epidemiology, clinical presentation, management and outcome. *J Laryngol Otol* 2008;122: 818–823.

Hopkins A, Lahiri T, Salerno R, et al. Changing epidemiology of life-threatening upper airway infections: the reemergence of bacterial tracheitis. *Pediatrics* 2006;118:1418–1421.

Kavanagh KR, Batti JS. Traumatic epiglottitis after foreign body ingestion. *Int J Pediatr Otorhinolaryngol* 2008;72:901–903.

Kuppersmith R, Rosen DS, Wiatrak BJ. Functional stridor in adolescents. *J Adolesc Health* 1993;14:166–171.

Walner DL, Ouanounou S, Donnelly LF, et al. Utility of radiographs in the evaluation of pediatric upper airway obstruction. *Ann Otol Rhinol Larynol* 1999;108:378–383.

Zoumalan R, Maddalozzo J, Holinger LD. Etiology of stridor in infants. *Ann Otol Rhinol Larynol* 2007;116:329–334.

CHAPTER 73 ■ SYNCOPE

CARLOS A. DELGADO, MD, FAAP

From the Greek *synkoptein*, meaning "to cut short," syncope is defined as the temporary loss of consciousness and postural tone, resulting from an abrupt, transient, and diffuse reversible disturbance of cerebral function. Often, the terms *fainting* or *blackout* spells are used. Pathophysiologically, syncope can be explained as a sudden reduction in delivery of substrates such as O_2 or glucose to the brain. Most transient altered consciousness events in children include seizures, syncopes, or hysteric episodes ("fits, faints, or fakes"), and the approach to diagnosis of syncope is to exclude the other two.

Syncope during childhood is generally a benign, brief, isolated event, followed by a complete recovery without sequelae, although in few instances, it can represent potentially life-threatening causes. A thorough, detailed history and physical examination, with attention to clues provided by the premonitory signs and symptoms, are usually sufficient to provide the cause of syncope in most cases. All syncopal events associated with exercise or exertion must be considered dangerous. An overall incidence in the pediatric population of 0.1% to 0.5% has been reported. Syncope occurs predominantly in teenagers, with a peak incidence occurring between 15 and 19 years of age. Females were evaluated more commonly than males. It is estimated that at least 50% of all individuals will have a least one syncopal episode during their adolescence. Syncopal events account for 1% to 3% of all emergency department visits, and, in this setting, the patient has usually regained consciousness by the time of initial assessment by a physician.

DIFFERENTIAL DIAGNOSIS

Pathophysiologically, all causes of transient and abrupt onset of alterations of consciousness can be best categorized into three broad groups (Table 73.1): (i) true syncope reflecting any mechanism that causes a transient decrease in substrate delivery to the brain (e.g., O_2, glucose, blood); (ii) all seizures; and (iii) hysterical pseudoloss of consciousness. Most children and adolescents who faint have orthostatic syncope, vasovagal episodes, or breath-holding spells (Table 73.2). This is in marked contrast to adults, who often have cardiovascular disease. Studies report additional diagnoses in "fainting" children including migraines (11%), seizures (8%), and cardiac causes (6%).

The goal in evaluating syncopal episodes must be to accurately identify the occasional warning signs of serious pathology from the common benign events. The causes of true syncope may be classified into three etiologic categories: *autonomic* (vasovagal), *cardiovascular*, and *metabolic*. Table 73.3 provides a list of the major causes of syncope and conditions that mimic it.

Vasovagal Syncope

Vasovagal syncope is also called neurocardiogenic syncope, vasodepressor syncope, or fainting spell. It is by far the most common cause of fainting in children and adolescents and accounts for more than 50% of cases of childhood syncope.

The pathophysiologic mechanism of vasovagal syncope is similar to an exaggerated Bezold-Jarisch reflex. This reflex is responsible for maintaining blood pressure during orthostatic stress. In patients prone to syncope, the cascade of events begins with a decrease in systemic venous return and, therefore, decreased preload after prolonged upright posture. Enhanced or compensatory sympathetic activity causes an elevation of circulating catecholamines (particularly epinephrine), which increase left ventricular contractility in a relatively empty ventricle. In response, a negative feedback loop via vagal afferents results in sympathetic withdrawal (*hypotensive vasodepressor response*) and augmented vagal tone (*the bradycardic cardioinhibitory response*). The factors that trigger this abnormal response are still unclear. It is probable that a combination of abnormal catecholamine response to orthostatic or other stress, exaggerated ventricular contraction, diminished ventricular volume from venous pooling in the upright position, and enhanced sensitivity of ventricular mechanoreceptors are all involved in the clinical predisposition to recurrent vasovagal syncope.

Most episodes occur while the patient is standing or during a rapid change from a supine or sitting position to standing. Syncope represents a cascade of signs and symptoms that begin with a brief prodrome or presyncopal phase. This progresses to a brief and sudden stage of unconsciousness that typically lasts 1 to 2 minutes and ends with arousal to a previous level of consciousness within a short period.

A syncopal episode may be triggered by a wide array of emotional events such as pain, fear, and anxiety that increase circulatory catecholamines in response to a real or perceived threat. The prodromal symptoms may include light-headedness, dizziness, nausea, shortness of breath, diaphoresis, pallor, and visual changes. Physical conditions such as anemia, dehydration, exertion, hunger, pregnancy, and/or concurrent illness can predispose to a syncopal event. Other factors include confinement to enclosed or poorly ventilated spaces and environmental heat. The patient may remain nauseated, pale, and diaphoretic for several hours after the syncopal episode.

A full syncope can be avoided if the patient recognizes the prodromal symptoms and assumes a supine or Trendelenburg position. Prognostically, vasovagal syncope is considered a benign illness. A prophylactic approach is taken to prevent symptoms of presyncope or near-syncope. Patient education

TABLE 73.1

PATHOPHYSIOLOGIC CLASSIFICATION
OF TRANSIENT, PAROXYSMAL,
ALTERED CONSCIOUSNESS

1. Transient decrease in substrate delivery to the brain:
   syncope
2. Seizures
3. Hysterical pseudoloss of consciousness

must be geared toward rapid symptom recognition, allowing the patient to assume a recumbent position and abort a potential syncopal event. Other preventative measures may include avoiding dehydration and using salt-enriched diets during athletic activity or environmental stress.

Several other related forms of autonomic syncope are orthostatic hypotensive syncope and situational syncope related to micturition, defecation, coughing, and swallowing. Orthostatic hypotensive syncope is associated with an excessive and prolonged fall in blood pressure level on assuming the erect posture from a recumbent position. An unusual and uncommon condition, micturition syncope, follows rapid bladder decompression, in which reduced cardiac return is associated with both postural effects and splanchnic vascular stasis. Hair-pulling syncope has been described in girls. Underlying medical conditions such as anemia or pregnancy may exacerbate the tendency toward any of these vasovagal events.

Another common, usually benign, pediatric variant of vasovagal syncope is that of breath-holding spells, which occur in two forms (see Chapter 131). *Pallid* breath-holding spells result from vagally mediated cardiac inhibition. *Cyanotic* breath-holding spells involve interplay between hyperventilation, Valsalva maneuver, expiratory apnea, and intrinsic pulmonary mechanisms. In pallid breath-holding spells, an inconsequential injury induced by a sudden emotional stimulus such as pain, fright, or anger provokes one or two short cries, followed by pallor and sudden loss of consciousness. In cyanotic breath holding spells, the event occurs as a reflexive response a stressor and is characterized by an initial shrill cry; forced expiration and apnea ensues and progresses to cyanosis and brief loss of consciousness. These spells typically occur in children between 6 months and 5 years of age.

Cardiac Syncope

Syncope caused by significant cardiac or vascular pathology occurs far less often than autonomic syncope. It is suspected when fainting occurs in any of the following situations: a patient with known heart disease, sudden fainting, fainting during exercise, incontinence during fainting, injury during

TABLE 73.2

COMMON CAUSES OF SYNCOPE

Vasovagal	Hyperventilation
Orthostatic	Breath-holding

TABLE 73.3

CLASSIFICATION OF SYNCOPAL EPISODES

I. Syncope
  A. Autonomic
    1. Vasovagal syndrome
    2. Excessive vagal tone—athletes
    3. Volume depletion (orthostatic)—hemorrhage or anemia, dehydration, diuretic abuse
    4. Reflex
      a. Breath-holding spells
      b. Situational—cough, micturition
    5. Pregnancy
  B. Cardiovascular
    1. Structural heart disease
      a. Tetralogy of Fallot
      b. Hypertrophic cardiomyopathy
      c. Valvular aortic stenosis
      d. Primary pulmonary hypertension
      e. Eisenmenger's syndrome
      f. Atrial myxoma
      g. Dilated cardiomyopathy
      h. Pericarditis with tamponade
    2. Tachyarrhythmias
      a. Long QT syndromes
        (1) Congenital
        (2) Acquired, including drug/toxin induced (antiarrhythmics, arsenic, tricyclic antidepressants, phenothiazines, antihistaminics, cisapride)
      b. Supraventricular tachycardia—idiopathic, Wolff-Parkinson-White syndrome, many drugs and toxins (Chapter 74, Table 74.4)
      c. Ventricular tachycardia
    3. Bradyarrhythmias
      a. Atrioventricular block
      b. Sinus node disease
    4. Vascular
      a. Vertebrobasilar insufficiency
  C. Metabolic
    1. Transient hypoglycemia, hypoxia, hyperammonemia, carbon monoxide poisoning
II. Conditions that mimic syncope
  A. Psychological
    1. Hysteric faints
    2. Malingering
    3. Hyperventilation
    4. Panic disorder
    5. Munchausen syndrome by proxy
  B. Neurologic
    1. Seizures
    2. Migraines

the event, family history of sudden cardiac death, and/or an abnormal heart rhythm on the electrocardiogram (EKG) at presentation. It does not follow the stimuli typical of vasovagal syncope. Hypercyanotic spells, usually associated with tetralogy of Fallot, can occur with any heart defect associated with intracardiac right-to-left shunting. An increase in obstruction to pulmonary blood flow or a fall in systemic vascular resistance can precipitate such a spell. The most common arrhythmia causing syncope with an apparently structurally normal heart is supraventricular tachycardia (SVT), especially in the context of Wolff-Parkinson-White (WPW) syndrome. Arrhythmias occur more often in structurally abnormal hearts. Many drugs and toxins may also induce arrhythmias (Chapter 74, Table 74.4).

Prolonged QT syndrome is estimated to be present in 1 of every 5,000 individuals, and approximately one-third of those newly diagnosed have been previously asymptomatic. It is estimated that long QT syndrome may be responsible for as many as 3,000 otherwise unexplained deaths in children and young adults each year in the United States. The diagnosis is made by documenting the prolongation of the corrected QT interval (QTc; by more than 0.45 seconds) by Bazett's formula. The prolongation of QTc results from an extended refractory period of the ventricular myocardium, which places it at risk for "torsade de pointes," a malignant form of ventricular tachycardia (VT; see Chapter 84). This form of VT will impede adequate blood flow to the brain, causing sudden loss of consciousness. Prolonged QT syndrome can be congenital or acquired. Syncope occurs secondary to paroxysmal episodes of rapid VT. Of the congenital forms, the rare Jervell and Lange-Nielsen syndrome is associated with autosomal-recessive deafness. The Romano-Ward syndrome is now being recognized with increasing frequency and is associated with an autosomal-dominant trait in families with normal hearing. More recent work has identified the genetic basis of the congenital forms of long QT syndrome and relates them to at least a dozen distinct heritable arrhythmia syndromes, several disease-susceptibility autosomal-dominant genes, and hundreds of implicated mutations coding for abnormal myocardial K^+ and Na^+ ion channels and, in some cases, inner ear endolymph proteins. The altered ion channel function produces a prolongation of the action potential and cardiac repolarization and propensity to torsade de pointes VT. Long QT syndromes often present as syncope on exercise or exertion and can also masquerade as a seizure. In acquired forms, QTc will be prolonged as a result of electrolyte abnormalities (hypokalemia, hypocalcemia), increased intracranial pressure, or medication use or overdose. Drug exposure may be intentional or accidental. A thorough history should include the types of medications available in the home, possible environmental exposures such as carbon monoxide poisoning, and illicit drug use. Numerous medications including some antibiotics, antiarrhythmics, antihistamines, and psychotropics may prolong QTc. In addition, other drugs such as erythromycin, trimethoprim-sulfamethoxazole, and ketoconazole may prolong QTc themselves or, if taken concomitantly with some of the former classes of medications, may inhibit hepatic metabolism of the latter and thus exacerbate QTc prolongation (Chapter 82, Table 82.17).

Episodic, complete heart block accompanied by syncope may occur in children and adolescents with baseline abnormalities of cardiac conduction. Children who have undergone surgical repair of ventricular defects, such as in tetralogy of Fallot, are also at risk.

Hypertrophic cardiomyopathy (IHSS), is associated with recurrent syncope and is a disease that presents with a thickened left ventricular myocardium, resulting in subaortic stenosis that causes obstruction to ventricular outflow. Patients with severe aortic valvular stenosis present with the classic triad of syncopal episodes, anginal chest pain, and dyspnea on exertion.

Noncardiac Syncope and Disorders that Mimic Syncope

Metabolic causes of syncope include hypoglycemia, which is often associated with pallor, dizziness, and diaphoresis and is unrelated to position. Seizures may occur and unconsciousness may be prolonged, and patients will often require the administration of glucose for recovery. Hypoglycemia may be a component of other childhood disorders that include diabetes mellitus, ketotic hypoglycemia, hepatic enzyme deficiencies, and drug or toxin ingestion, especially ethanol and oral hypoglycemics. Other metabolic causes of syncope include hypoxia alone or in association with mild to moderate carbon monoxide poisoning, which is notorious for producing syncope. Recovery occurs when the child is removed from the offending environment. Hyperammonemia may rarely cause syncope by direct cytotoxic central nervous system effect.

Hyperventilation, associated with high anxiety and emotional events during which the patient will complain of shortness of breath, tachypnea, chest pain, paresthesias, and lightheadedness, may result in syncope. This results from cerebral vasoconstriction in response to self-induced hypocapnia.

Loss of consciousness often occurs with generalized seizures, which may be difficult to distinguish from vasovagal syncope if the event was not witnessed. Seizures are likely to be preceded by an aura, followed by a prolonged postictal state. Both neonatal and complex partial seizures may be subtle and particularly difficult to differentiate from syncope (Table 73.4; see Chapter 69).

Basilar artery migraine may cause syncope. It is usually preceded by an aura, followed by severe occipital headache. It should be considered in patients with syncope and paroxysmal headaches, especially with family history of migraine. Narcolepsy should be considered in the differential diagnosis in adolescents. These episodes characterized by irresistible sleep attacks may last seconds to minutes. In the severe form of cataplexy, the patient experiences sudden loss of muscle tone brought about by intense emotion or physical activity.

Syncope-like events caused by hysteria are common in the adolescent patient. Characteristic features of the clinical event are helpful in differentiating hysteria from organic causes of true syncope. Hysterical "syncope" may be associated with hyperventilation, usually occurs in the presence of an audience, and lacks true loss of consciousness. No overt or objective prodromal symptoms such as hypotension or bradycardia are recognized. It may occur when the patient is in the supine position, which is virtually unreported with vasovagal syncope. There may be a peculiar fluttering of the eyes behind half-closed eyelids. The patient usually describes the event in a calm and indifferent manner and vividly recalls the event, suggesting a lack of complete loss of consciousness. The association of the onset of hysterical syncope and sexual molestation or sexual abuse has also been observed. The presence of a psychiatric disorder is associated with an increased incidence of recurrent events. These patients tend to be anxious and more prone to panic disorders and avoidance-oriented coping strategies.

TABLE 73.4

DIFFERENTIATING SYNCOPE FROM OTHER "SPELLS"

	Syncope, vasovagal	Metabolic (e.g., hypoxia, hypoglycemia)	Seizure	Breath-holding
Period of unconsciousness	Usually seconds	Variable	Minutes or longer	Seconds
Prodrome	Fright, pain, "feels faint"	Confusion, altered mental status, ↑ heart rate, diaphoresis	Occasional aura	Pain, fright → vigorous → cry apnea → LOC
Incontinence	Absent	Absent	May be present	Absent
Confusion on awakening	Absent or mild	Mild	Marked	Absent
Tonic-clonic movements	Occasionally present, if LOC is prolonged	May occur	Commonly present	Rare, may see 1–2 beats
Electroencephalogram	Normal	Normal	Often abnormal	Normal

LOC, loss of consciousness.

Drug or toxin exposure may be accidental or intentional and, in addition to precipitating arrhythmias as previously noted, may occasionally cause an acute, transient loss of consciousness or gradual altered mental status changes leading to syncope rather than the typical prolonged alterations in consciousness. Such an effect may be more characteristic of carbon monoxide poisoning or volatile inhalant abuse (e.g., see Chapter 88). Antihypertensives, β-blockers, diuretics, antiarrhythmics, and drugs that decrease cardiac output such as barbiturates, tricyclic antidepressants, and phenothiazines may cause syncope. Substances of abuse such as alcohol, sedative-hypnotics, and opiates can cause alterations in consciousness that mimic syncope but are usually more prolonged. Anaphylactic reactions characterized by hypotension, pallor, asthenia, nausea, vomiting, and profuse sweating may also mimic syncope.

EVALUATION AND DECISION

In the era of rising health care costs and cost containment, one must be mindful of the utility and expense of diagnostic studies used to evaluate syncope. Extensive and expensive testing is usually unnecessary. A thorough history and physical examination will often suggest the diagnosis. One should pay attention to the airway, respiratory effort, and hemodynamic stability. Vital signs including orthostatic blood pressure and pulse oximetry measurements must be documented and reviewed. In most cases, a complementary EKG screen is useful to rule out symptomatic arrhythmias or long QT syndrome. This approach, emphasizing evaluation of the clinical features of the syncopal episode, supplemented by EKG, is outlined in Fig. 73.1.

The primary goal in evaluating a syncopal child or adolescent is to identify conditions that are associated with a risk of serious injury or are life threatening. Table 73.5 highlights clinical features of syncope that suggest such conditions and thus indicate hospitalization.

A thorough history is the most important part of the evaluation. Parents and relatives often contribute important information to the cause of the syncopal event. A prodromal sign or symptom precedes a typical vasovagal spell. Most occur while standing. Stressful situations, emotional upset, and mild physical trauma can trigger such an event.

Syncope occurring during intense physical activity may identify those patients who have potentially fatal conditions. These patients' symptoms may also suggest vagal tone and/or volume depletion caused by dehydration and heat stress. A detailed evaluation should be considered for patients who have syncope during exercise or have a family history of sudden death, myocardial disease, or arrhythmias. A history of palpitations before syncope should alert the physician to the possibility of tachyarrhythmias. Palpitations are also reported in hyperventilation episodes. History is sought regarding medication use, recent food intake, and intercurrent illnesses for consideration of additional causes of nonvasovagal syncope. A medical history or family history of cardiac or neurodevelopmental disorders is important to elicit possible cardiac or neurologic causes of syncope. If there are no suggestive historical features of either vasovagal or the more worrisome causes of syncope, it may be prudent to cautiously consider some psychological assessment questions, particularly in well-appearing adolescents.

TABLE 73.5

CLINICAL FEATURES OF SYNCOPE REQUIRING HOSPITALIZATION

Presence of cardiovascular disease or abnormal cardiovascular examination—congestive heart failure, arrhythmias
Abnormal electrocardiogram—prolonged QT interval, tachyarrhythmias, atrioventricular or severe bundle branch blocks
Chest pain with syncope
Cyanotic spells
Apnea or bradycardic spells requiring vigorous stimulation
Abnormal neurologic findings—focal signs, status epilepticus, signs of meningeal irritation
Acute toxic ingestions
Orthostatic hypotension resistant to fluid therapy

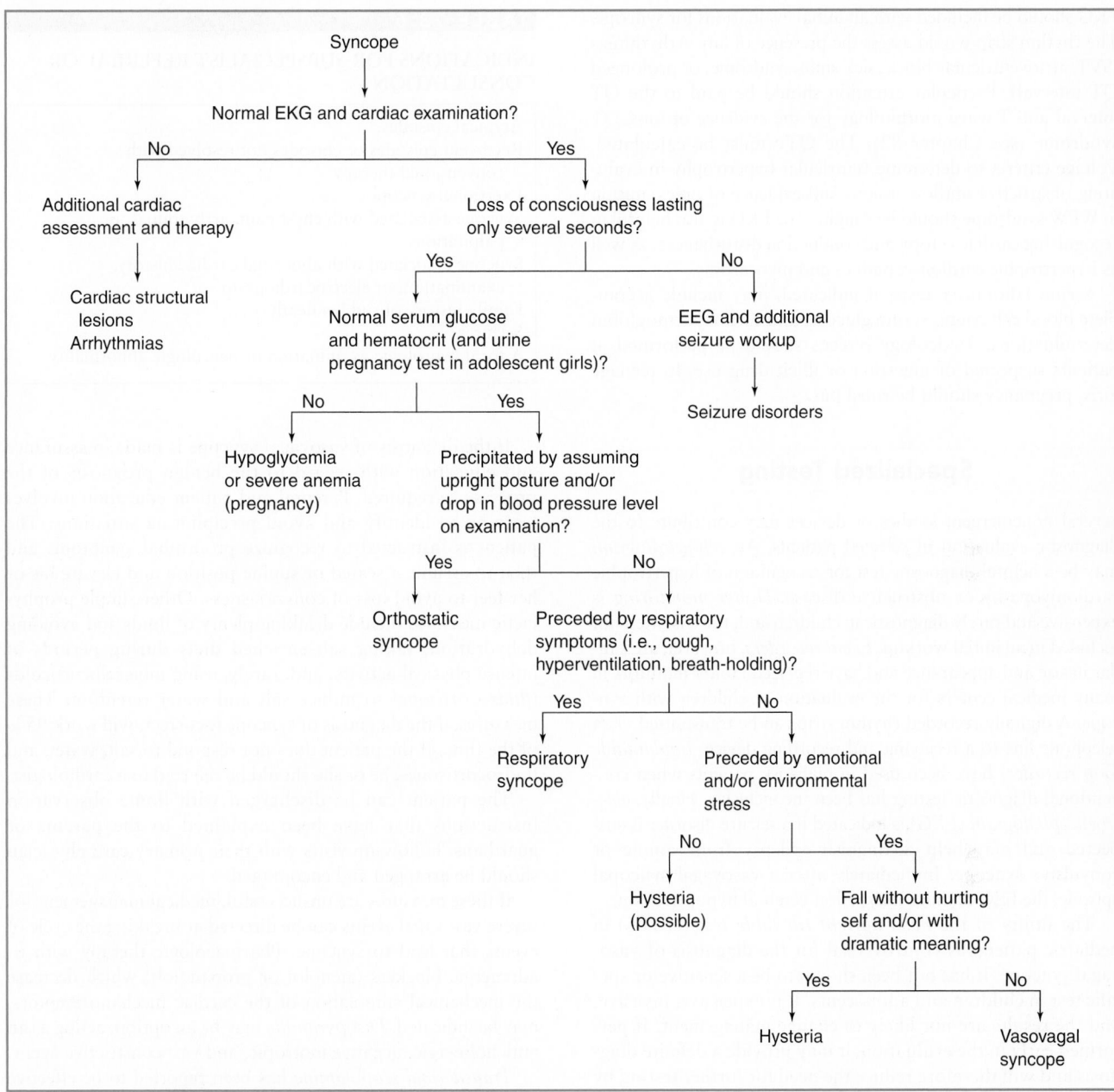

FIGURE 73.1 The diagnostic approach to syncope. EKG, electrocardiogram; EEG, electroencephalogram.

On physical examination, heart rate and blood pressure should be measured first while the patient is supine and then standing. In orthostatic hypotension caused by autonomic dysfunction, dehydration, or blood loss, the patient will have an abnormal decrease in systolic blood pressure (more than 20 mmHg) or an abnormal increase in heart rate with this change in posture. The presence of orthostatic vital signs is confirmatory, but even if normal, the vital signs should not trump the history and clinical findings. Palpation of an abnormal apical impulse or peripheral pulses may suggest a structural heart disease. On auscultation, a loud systolic ejection murmur in the midsternum and upper sternum is present in severe aortic stenosis or IHSS. In addition, the diastolic murmur of a rare left atrial myxoma may be heard. A fourth heart sound may be present in

hypertrophic cardiomyopathy. The general physical examination should include a careful neurologic examination, auscultation for cervical and carotid bruits, an assessment of hydration status, and consideration of the presence of any toxidrome.

Routine Laboratory Testing

The emergency physician must assess the cardiac status of all children who present with a history of a syncopal episode. While in the emergency department, the patient should be placed on a continuous cardiac monitor for the evaluation of heart rate, rhythm, and conduction intervals, unless an obvious noncardiac cause is revealed by the clinical examination. An

EKG should be included with all initial evaluations for syncope. The rhythm strip would assess the presence of any arrhythmias (SVT, atrioventricular block, sick sinus syndrome, or prolonged QT interval). Particular attention should be paid to the QT interval and T-wave morphology for the evidence of long QT syndrome (see Chapter 82). The QTc must be calculated. Voltage criteria to determine ventricular hypertrophy in evaluating obstructive outflow lesions and evidence of preexcitation in WPW syndrome should be sought. The EKG is also helpful in recognizing cardiac ectopy and conduction disturbances, as well as hypertrophic cardiomyopathies and myocarditis.

Serum laboratory tests, if indicated, may include a complete blood cell count, serum glucose, and carboxyhemoglobin determinations. Toxicology screens should be performed in patients suspected of ingestion or illicit drug use. In teenage girls, pregnancy should be ruled out.

Specialized Testing

Several nonemergent studies or devices may contribute to the diagnostic evaluation in selected patients. An *echocardiogram* may be a helpful diagnostic test for recognition of hypertrophic cardiomyopathy or obstructive disease. *Holter monitoring* is expensive and rarely diagnostic in children and, thus, is often not included in an initial workup. *Event recorders*, however, are similar in size and appearance and have replaced Holter monitors in many medical centers for the evaluation of children with syncope. A digitally recorded rhythm strip can be transmitted via a telephone line to a receiving and recording device. *Implantable loop recorders* have been used in high-risk patients when conventional diagnostic testing has been inconclusive. Finally, *electroencephalogram (EEG)* is indicated if a seizure disorder is suspected and may help distinguish epilepsy from simple or convulsive syncope. Immediately after a vasovagal syncopal episode, the EEG findings may reflect cerebral hypoperfusion.

The utility of the *head-upright tilt table test* (HUTT) in pediatric patients is controversial for the diagnosis of vasovagal syncope. It has not been shown to be a sensitive or specific test in children and adolescents. It is expensive, invasive, and the results are not likely to change management. If performed early in the evaluation, it may provide a definite diagnosis and will therefore reduce the need for further testing by demonstrating the physiologic response leading to syncope. It has emerged as a laboratory method for provoking episodes of neurally mediated (vasodepressor) syncope in susceptible individuals. Children, usually pubertal girls with a positive response to HUTT, often have had syncope in special circumstances (e.g., prolonged standing, anxiety, and fright) and experienced a prodrome such as pallor, lightheadedness, and nausea. Children with recurrent unexplained syncope may be referred to appropriate specialists (e.g., a neurologist or an otorhinolaryngologist) for such testing.

THERAPY

Any therapeutic approach to the child with syncope should be individualized on the basis of several issues including the likely pathologic process, frequency and nature of symptoms, likelihood of recurrence, and risk of adverse outcomes.

TABLE 73.6

INDICATIONS FOR SUBSPECIALIST REFERRAL OR CONSULTATION

Atypical episodes
Recurrent episodes or episodes not resolved with
  conventional therapy
Exertional syncope
Syncope associated with chest pain, arrhythmias, or
  palpitations
Syncope associated with abnormal cardiac history,
  examination, or electrocardiogram
Family history of sudden death
Seizures
A focal neurologic examination or neurologic abnormality

If the diagnosis of vasovagal syncope is made, reassurance and education with regard to the benign prognosis of the process are required. Parental and patient education involves learning to identify and avoid precipitating situations. The patient is instructed to recognize prodromal symptoms and then to assume a seated or supine position and elevate his or her feet to avoid loss of consciousness. Other simple prophylactic measures include drinking plenty of fluids and avoiding dehydration, taking salt-enriched diets during periods of intense physical activity, and, rarely, using mineralocorticoids (*fludrocortisone*) to induce salt and water retention. These measures, if the diagnosis of syncope is correct, will work 95% of the time. If the patient does not respond to salt, water, and fludrocortisones, he or she should be referred to a cardiologist.

The patient can be discharged with home observation instructions that have been explained to the parents or guardians. Follow-up visits with their primary care physician should be arranged and encouraged.

If these measures are unsuccessful, medical management for severe vasovagal events can be directed at breaking the cycle of events that lead to syncope. Pharmacologic therapy with β-adrenergic blockers (atenolol or propanolol), which decrease the mechanical stimulation of the cardiac mechanoreceptors, may be indicated. *Disopyramide* may be an option, acting as an anticholinergic, negative inotropic, and vasoconstrictive agent.

Transdermal scopolamine has been reported to be effective presumably by reducing the vagal tone associated with these episodes. More recently, *sertraline* has been shown to be successful in decreasing the frequency of syncope. Midodrine, a peripheral α-stimulating agent, is also effective in adult patients with recurrent neurocardiogenic syncope refractory to other forms of therapy. Pacemaker implantation or implantable cardioverter-defibrillators for vasovagal syncope are reserved for the rare refractory case that has failed aggressive pharmacologic measures.

Table 73.6 offers guidelines regarding which patients require referral to pediatric subspecialists, such as a cardiologist or neurologist.

Suggested Readings

Ackerman MJ. Cardiac causes of sudden unexpected death in children and their relationship to seizures and syncope: genetic testing for cardiac electropathies. *Semin Pediatr Neurol* 2008;12(1):52–58.

Brignole M, Alboni P, Benditt DG, et al. Guidelines on management (diagnosis and treatment) of syncope—update 2004: the Task Force on Syncope, European Society of Cardiology. *Eur Heart J* 2004;25(22):2054–2072.

Cohen GA, Lewis DA, Berger S. Reproducibility of head-up tilt-table testing in pediatric patients with neurocardiogenic syncope. *Pediatr Cardiol* 2005; 26:772–774.

Dovgalyuk J, Holstege C, Mattu A, et al. The electrocardiogram in the patient with syncope. *Am J Emerg Med* 2007;25(6):688–701.

Friedman MJ, Mull CC, Sharieff GQ, et al. Prolonged QT syndrome in children: an uncommon but potentially fatal entity. *J Emerg Med* 2003;24(2):173–179.

Goldenberg I, Moss AJ, Peterson DR, et al. Risk factors for aborted cardiac arrest and sudden cardiac death in children with the congenital long-QT syndrome. *Circulation* 2008;117(17):2184–2191.

Kouakam C, Lacroix D, Klug D, et al. Prevalence and prognostic significance of psychiatric disorders in patients evaluated for recurrent unexplained syncope. *Am J Cardiol* 2002;89(5):530–535.

Mathias CJ, Deguchi K, Schatz I. Observations on recurrent syncope and pre-syncope in 641 patients. *Lancet* 2001;357(9253):348–353.

McLeod KA. Syncope in childhood. *Arch Dis Child* 2003;88:350–353.

Stephenson JBP. Clinical diagnosis of syncopes (including so-called breath-holding spells) without electroencephalography or ocular compression. *J Child Neurol* 2007;22(4):502–508.

Millichap JG. Classification, diagnosis, and treatment of syncope. *AAP Grand Rounds* 2003;10(1):2–3.

Roden D. Clinical practice. Long-QT syndrome. *N Engl J Med* 2008;358(2): 169–176.

Steinberg LA, Knilans TK. Syncope in children: diagnostic tests have a high cost and low yield. *J Pediatr* 2005;146(3):355–358.

Strieper MJ, Auld DO, Hulse JE, et al. Evaluation of recurrent pediatric syncope: role of tilt table testing. *Pediatrics* 1994;93(4):660–662.

CHAPTER 74 ■ TACHYCARDIA

JAMES F. WILEY II, MD, MPH

Fast heart rate or tachycardia is a common sign in children receiving emergency care. It may be noticed on initial evaluation by the emergency provider or may be raised as a concern by the caregiver who notes a rapid heart rate while holding the child or observes rapid jugular venous pulsations, increased apical heart rate, or pulse rate. The definition of tachycardia varies by age [callout to the table of normal vital signs in Appendix C, "Resting Heart Rate"]. In infants and young children, the higher resting heart rate, relative to older children adolescents and adults, reflects higher tissue oxygen utilization and metabolic rate. In most instances, the underlying cause for tachycardia in children is benign. However, children with a life-threatening etiology for their tachycardia require prompt recognition and treatment.

PATHOPHYSIOLOGY

Cardiac muscle has intrinsic automaticity that allows it to beat without any external stimulus. Under normal circumstances, the heartbeat is initiated by an electrical impulse in the sinoatrial (SA) node and travels through the atria to the atrioventricular (AV) node. From there, the electrical impulse is propagated in a coordinated fashion via the His-Purkinje conduction system to the ventricles.

Resting heart rate typically reflects a balance of input from the vagus nerve (cranial nerve X) and the thoracic sympathetic ganglion (levels T1 to T4). Vagal stimulation results in slowing of the heart rate mediated by cholinergic receptors and has a greater impact on resting heart rate than on the sympathetic nervous system. Thus, medications with anticholinergic receptor effects (e.g., antihistamines, atropine) may cause tachycardia. Sympathetic stimulation results in increased heart rate and force of contraction primarily through the β_1-adrenergic receptors. These receptors may also be stimulated by circulating endogenous substances (e.g., epinephrine, increased carbon dioxide tension, hypoxemia) and by exogenous agents (e.g., sympathomimetic drugs).

Life-threatening cardiac tachyarrhythmias [e.g., supraventricular tachycardia (SVT), ventricular tachycardia] arise from various mechanisms that disrupt normal electrical conduction in the heart. The pathophysiology of these arrhythmias is discussed separately (see Chapter 84).

DIFFERENTIAL DIAGNOSIS

Many conditions may produce tachycardia (Table 74.1). Most tachycardic children exhibit sinus tachycardia without significant cardiac pathology (Table 74.2). However, life-threatening

conditions frequently come to medical attention because of fast heart rate and may reflect cardiac and noncardiac origins (Table 74.3).

Sinus Tachycardia

Fever, pain, and emotional arousal (e.g., crying, anxiety) are the most frequent causes of sinus tachycardia in children. Sympathetic stimulation from other conditions such as hypoxemia, hypoglycemia, hypercarbia, anemia, and excess circulating catecholamines (e.g., hyperthyroidism, pheochromocytoma) also increase SA node firing rate (see Table 74.2). In addition, exogenous sympathomimetic or anticholinergic substances may cause sinus tachycardia. Over-the-counter medications that contain antihistamines or pseudoephedrine, "energy" drinks and diet pills that have high concentrations of caffeine, and commonly abused drugs (cocaine, amphetamines) are frequently implicated (see Table 59.4).

Shock is a life-threatening cause of sinus tachycardia that requires rapid recognition and reversal to prevent permanent organ damage or death (see Chapter 3). Circulatory shock may result from intravascular volume loss, inadequate cardiac contractility, a marked drop in systemic vascular resistance, or a combination of these mechanisms. Physical findings help differentiate the different forms of shock (hypovolemic, cardiogenic, septic, and distributive) and identify the underlying cause (Fig. 74.1).

Life-threatening Tachyarrhythmias

SVT represents the most common tachyarrhythmia of childhood (see Chapter 84). The typical heart rate in infants with SVT exceeds 220 beats per minute, whereas older children usually have a heart rate in excess of 180 beats per minute. Infants and children with SVT demonstrate a spectrum of physical signs including no symptoms, palpitations, chest pain, tachypnea (often with feeding in infants), diaphoresis, and severe cardiogenic shock.

The most common form of SVT involves an accessory AV pathway. Additional etiologies include drug exposure, congenital heart disease, and Wolff-Parkinson-White syndrome. Sympathomimetics in cough and cold preparations are the most common drugs to incite SVT in children. As of 2008, the US Food and Drug Administration recommends that over-the-counter cough and cold preparations should not be used in children younger than 2 years. Unregulated dietary supplements such as ephedra (and its congeners, often advertised as "ephedra-free" products) and high-caffeine energy drinks also

TABLE 74.1

DIFFERENTIAL DIAGNOSIS OF TACHYCARDIA

Sinus tachycardia
Fever
Crying
Pain
Hypoglycemia
Hypoxemia
Hypercarbia
Shock
Anemia
Poisoning (see Table 59.4)
Sepsis
Anaphylaxis
Hyperthyroidism
Pheochromocytoma
Drug induced (e.g., antihistamines, caffeine, dietary
    supplements)
Anxiety

Life-threatening cardiac tachyarrhythmias
Supraventricular tachycardia
Atrial flutter
Ventricular tachycardia (monomorphic and polymorphic/
    torsades de pointes)

Other cardiac causes
Myocarditis
Acute rheumatic fever
Kawasaki disease
Pericardial effusion with tamponade

TABLE 74.3

LIFE-THREATENING CAUSES OF TACHYCARDIA

Sinus tachycardia
Anaphylaxis
Hypoxia
Hypoglycemia
Sepsis
Shock
Pheochromocytoma
Poisoning (see Table 59.4)

Cardiac
Supraventricular tachycardia
Ventricular tachyarrhythmias
Atrial flutter

Other cardiac causes
Myocarditis
Pericardial effusion with tamponade

have the potential to precipitate SVT. Cardiac lesions associated with SVT include Ebstein's anomaly, repaired dextro-transposition of the great arteries, and single-ventricle lesions status post-Fontan operation.

Ventricular tachycardia (monomorphic or polymorphic/torsades de pointes) and atrial flutter rarely occur in children (see Chapter 84). Congenital heart disease, electrolyte disturbance (especially hyperkalemia, hypocalcemia, and hypomagnesemia), genetic predisposition (long QT syndromes), or poisoning accounts for most cases of ventricular tachycardia in children. Atrial flutter usually arises from an intraatrial reentry circuit. Most children with atrial flutter have congenital heart disease. Although rare, atrial flutter carries a significant risk of sudden death if not controlled by medications or surgical intervention.

TABLE 74.2

COMMON CAUSES OF TACHYCARDIA

Fever
Pain
Crying
Anxiety
Anemia
Drug induced (e.g., caffeine, herbal medications, dietary
    supplements, illicit drugs)
Hypovolemic shock

Other Cardiac Causes

Cardiac inflammation associated with viral myocarditis, acute rheumatic fever, or Kawasaki syndrome frequently presents with sinus tachycardia (see Chapter 84). Patients with these conditions, especially myocarditis, are also at risk for life-threatening arrhythmias, myocardial ischemia, congestive heart failure, and/or cardiogenic shock. For patients with pericardial effusion, sinus tachycardia is a physiologic response to impaired cardiac outflow in order to maintain cardiac output (see Chapter 84). Pericardial effusion with tamponade may complicate pericarditis, blunt chest trauma, or recent cardiac surgery and results in decreased cardiac output with significant impairment of systemic circulation. In this setting, pericardiocentesis or surgical pericardiotomy is life saving [see Chapter 135, Fig. 9.1, Illustrated techniques of pediatric emergency procedures].

EVALUATION AND DECISION

The child with tachycardia requires rapid assessment for the presence of hypoxia, hypoglycemia, an existing life-threatening arrhythmia, or shock (see Fig. 74.2). Respiratory distress with cyanosis or low pulse oximetry (less than 90%) demands immediate provision of supplemental oxygen and further management of airway and breathing (see Chapter 5). Hypoglycemia typically presents with altered mental status, diaphoresis, and/or hypertension and can be confirmed by measuring rapid blood glucose level. If an arrhythmia is suggested by an extremely rapid heart rate or a concerning tracing on the bedside cardiac monitor, a 12-lead electrocardiogram (EKG) and rhythm strip is necessary to confirm this impression and to guide further treatment (see Chapter 84). Children with congenital heart disease or a family history of sudden death are at increased risk for a life-threatening tachyarrhythmia. Consultation with a pediatric cardiologist and emergent echocardiography are warranted. In patients with shock, additional history and physical findings help guide the clinician

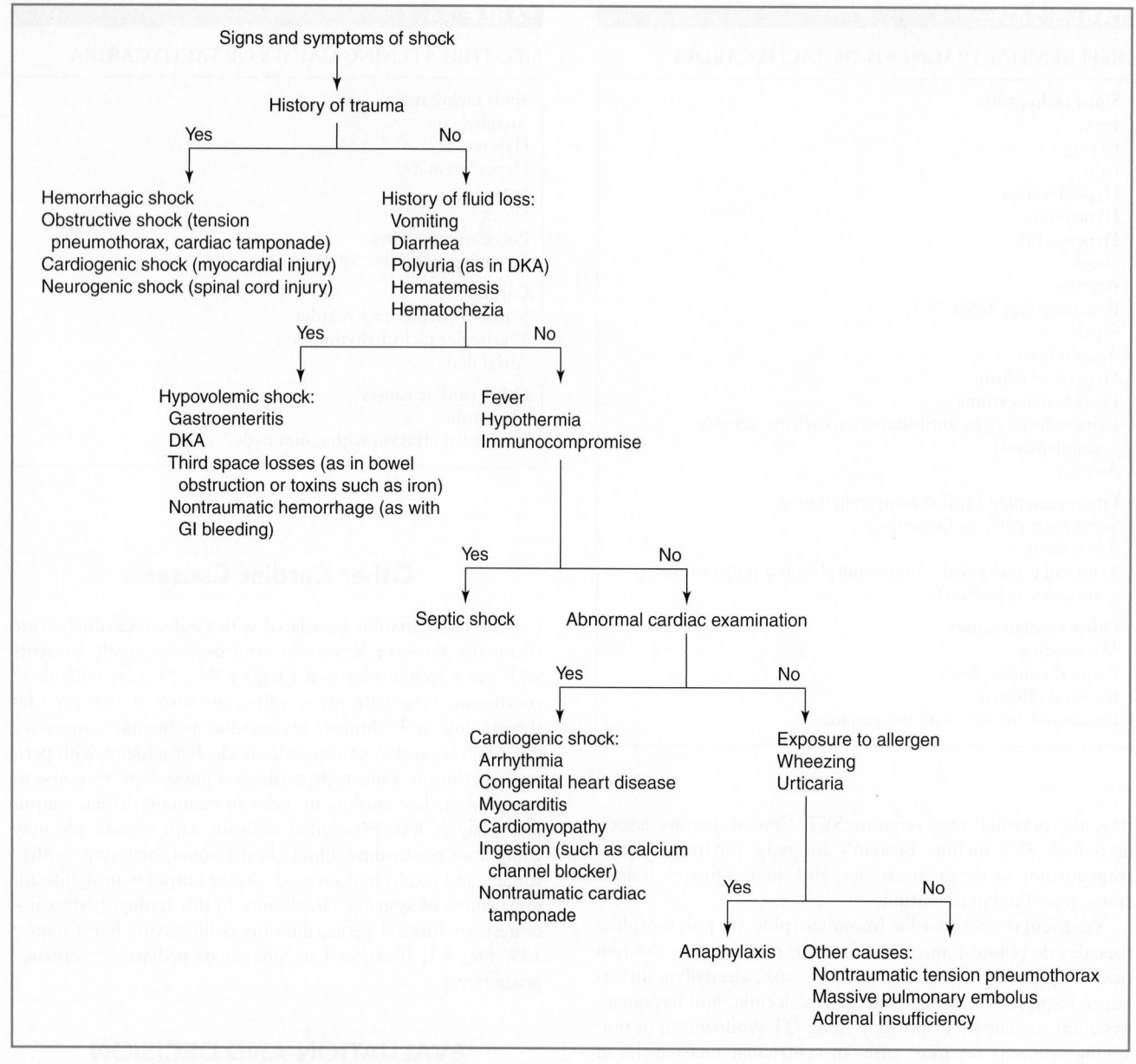

FIGURE 74.1 Approach to the classification of undifferentiated shock in children. DKA, diabetic ketoacidosis; GI, gastrointestinal. (Reproduced with permission from Waltzman, M. Initial evaluation of shock in children. In: UpToDate, Basow, DS (Ed), UpToDate, Waltham, MA, 2009.)

(see Fig. 74.1). Although the etiology may not be initially apparent, rapid treatment is imperative (see Fig. 3.3).

Children with fever and sinus tachycardia typically have a self-limited febrile illness. However, fever is also present in patients with cardiac pathology, including myocarditis, pericardial effusion, Kawasaki syndrome, and acute rheumatic fever, as well as in rare patients with thyroid storm. Myocarditis describes inflammation of the muscle wall of the heart. Multiple organisms can cause this pathology, with the most common identified agent being coxsackievirus. Clinical features of this disease are fever, tachycardia out of proportion to the activity or degree of fever, pallor, cyanosis, respiratory distress secondary to pulmonary edema, muffled heart sounds with gallop, and hepatomegaly caused by passive congestion of the liver (see Chapter 59). A child with tachycardia and clinical findings suggestive of myocarditis requires

emergent supportive care (see Chapter 3), echocardiography, and admission to a unit capable of intensive monitoring and rapid treatment of cardiac arrhythmias and hemodynamic instability.

Pericardial effusion may occur after blunt chest trauma, viral infection, or as a component of inflammatory diseases such as systemic lupus erythematosus. Small effusions may be detected as a friction rub. Large effusions often cause cardiogenic shock and may lead to muffling of heart sounds and EKG changes, such as low-voltage or T-wave flattening with "strain" pattern in leads V1 through V6, but are nonspecific. Pericardial effusions are best identified using ultrasound. Patients with evidence of significant circulatory impairment should undergo a pericardial drainage procedure (e.g., placement of a pericardial catheter percutaneously under ultrasound guidance, pericardial window procedure).

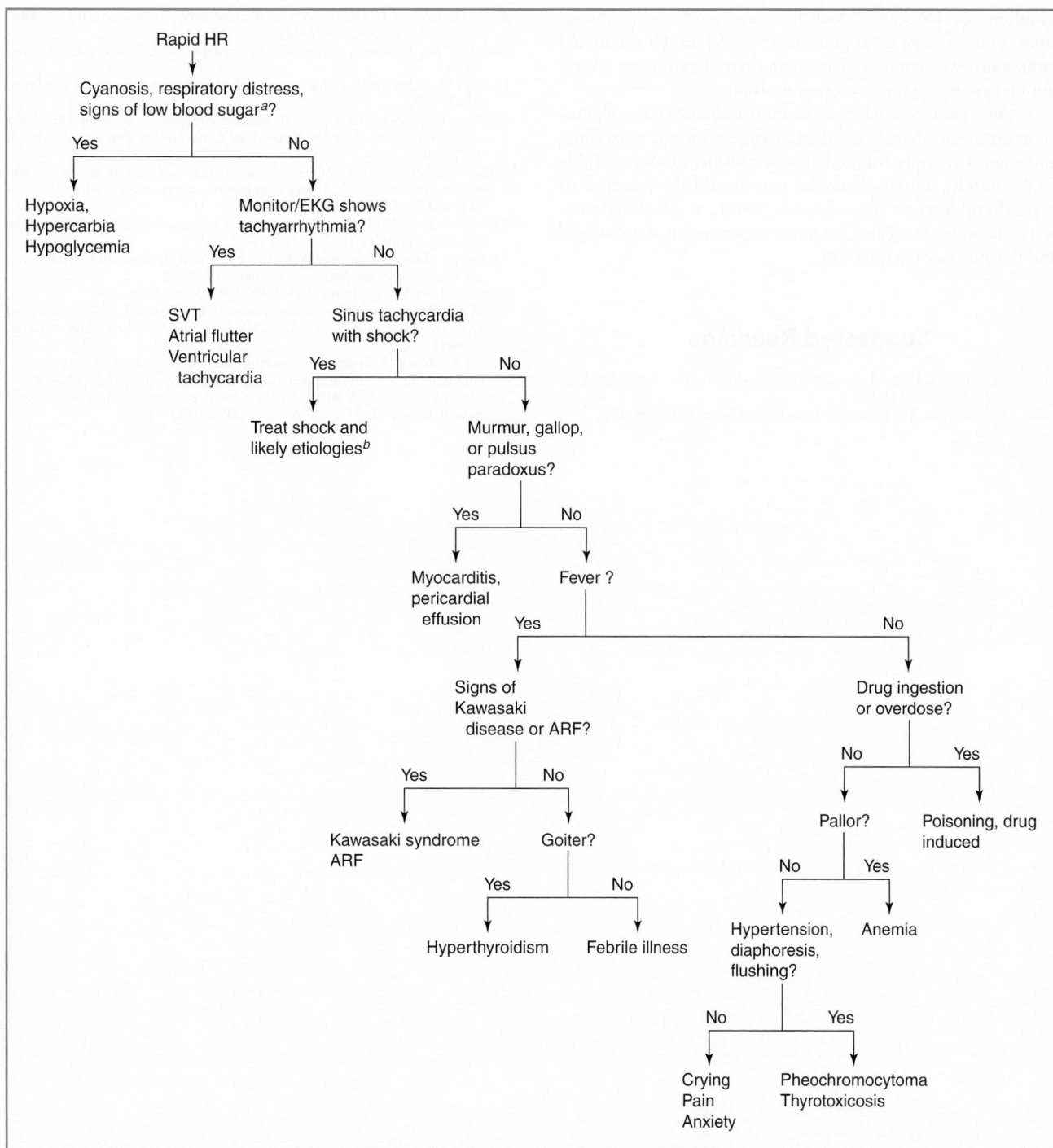

FIGURE 74.2 A diagnostic approach to tachycardia. HR, heart rate; SVT, supraventricular tachycardia; EKG, electrocardiogram; ARF, acute rheumatic fever. *a*Altered mental status, diaphoresis, hypertension. *b*See Fig. 74.1.

Acute rheumatic fever follows pharyngeal streptococcal infection and is an inflammatory disease that targets the heart, vessels, joints, skin, and central nervous system (CNS). Diagnosis and management of acute rheumatic fever are discussed separately (see Chapter 84). Clinical criteria for Kawasaki disease consist of prolonged high fever, conjunctivitis with perilimbic sparing, strawberry tongue, painful swelling of the hands and feet, rash, and lymphadenopathy. Early recognition and treatment of Kawasaki disease with

intravenous γ-globulin is necessary to prevent the development of coronary artery aneurysms with potential for myocardial ischemia (see Chapter 101).

Patients with thyroid storm may have marked sinus tachycardia, fever, goiter, and CNS stimulation (agitation, delirium, psychosis, seizures) accompanied by congestive heart failure (see Chapter 86). Trauma, thyroid infection, thyroid surgery, and acute iodine load are frequent precipitants. Rapid recognition and institution of therapy to treat adrenergic symptoms (β-adrenergic blockers), block hormone synthesis (methima-zole), prevent peripheral conversion of T4 to T3 (iodinated radiocontrast agents), and prevent thyroid hormone release (iodine) are necessary to prevent mortality.

Crying, pain, or anxiety is the most frequent cause of sinus tachycardia in afebrile children. Drug ingestion, poisoning, and anemia are important additional considerations (see Table 59.4). Rarely, sinus tachycardia may herald the presence of hyperthyroidism or pheochromocytoma, a catecholamine-secreting tumor that causes extreme hypertension, diaphoresis, and flushing (see Chapter 86).

Suggested Readings

Alexander ME, Berul CI. Ventricular arrhythmias: when to worry. *Pediatr Cardiol* 2000;21(6):532–541.

Baker AL, Newburger JW. Kawasaki disease. *Circulation* 2008;118:e110.

Bohn D, Benson L. Diagnosis and management of pediatric myocarditis. *Paediatr Drugs* 2002;4:171–181.

Demmler GJ. Infectious pericarditis in children. *Pediatr Infect Dis J* 2006; 25:165.

Doniger SJ, Sharieff GQ. Pediatric dysrhythmias. *Pediatr Clin North Am* 2006; 53:85–105.

Ginsburg GS, Riddle MA, Davies M. Somatic symptoms in children and adoles-cents with anxiety disorders. *J Am Acad Child Adolesc Psychiatry* 2006;45: 1179–1187.

Haller CA, Benowitz NL. Adverse cardiovascular and central nervous system events associated with dietary supplements containing ephedra alkaloids. *N Engl J Med* 2000;343:1833–1838.

Kaltman J, Shah M. Evaluation of the child with an arrhythmia. *Pediatr Clin North Am* 2004;51:1537–1551.

Mazor S, Mazor R. Approach to the child with tachycardia. *UpToDate*. www.uptodate.com. Accessed December 19, 2008.

Moss AJ. Long QT syndrome. *JAMA* 2003;289:2041–2044.

Olson KR. Emergency evaluation and treatment. In: Olson KR, ed. *Poisoning and Drug Overdose*, 2nd ed. New York, NY: Lange Medical Books/McGraw-Hill, 2004:11–15.

Wisten A, Messner T. Symptoms preceding sudden cardiac death in the young are common but often misinterpreted. *Scand Cardiovasc J* 2005;39:143–149.

Woods WA, McCulloch MA. Cardiovascular emergencies in the pediatric patient. *Emerg Med Clin North Am* 2005;23:1233–1249.

CHAPTER 75 ■ URINARY FREQUENCY IN CHILDHOOD

ROBERT G. BOLTE, MD

Urinary frequency is a symptom of several commonly encountered, clinical pediatric problems such as urinary tract infection (UTI), urethritis, vulvovaginitis, diabetes mellitus (DM), drug side effect (with caffeine, theophylline, and diuretics), or psychogenic stress. Moreover, urinary frequency may suggest underlying disease processes with life-threatening potential such as diabetic ketoacidosis, diabetes insipidus (DI), or congenital adrenal hyperplasia that require emergent diagnosis and management. Therefore, an organized approach in the emergency department (ED) evaluation of this symptom is important for any clinician providing acute care to children.

Urinary frequency (pollakiuria) is defined as an increase in the number of voids per day. It is a symptom distinct from polyuria (excretion of excessive amounts of urine). Although the two symptoms can be related, most children who present to the ED with frequency have a normal daily urine output, although the individual voids are frequent and small. Frequency is also distinct from *enuresis*, which is defined as inappropriate urination at an age when bladder control should be achieved.

PATHOPHYSIOLOGY

More than 90% of newborns void during the first day of life. Infants void between 6 and 30 times each day. Over the next 2 years, the number of voidings per day decreases by about half, whereas the volume of urine produced increases fourfold. Children between 3 and 5 years of ages average 8 to 14 voids per day. By 5 years of age, the number of voids decreases to 6 to 12 times per day. Adolescents average 4 to 6 voids per day. In the school-aged population, urinary frequency is usually defined as voiding more often than every 2 hours.

Normal bladder mucosa is both pressure sensitive and pain sensitive. An uncomfortable sensation is produced when urine volume approaches the age-dependent capacity of the bladder. Voiding is initiated by relaxation of the striated muscles of the urinary sphincter. There is an associated contraction of the smooth muscle of the bladder, resulting in bladder emptying. This mechanism is mediated by sacral nerves II to IV. Uncontrolled, "uninhibited" bladder contractions are the normal mechanism for infant and toddler voiding. Uninhibited (parasympathetic-mediated) bladder contractions do not normally occur after toilet training. By 5 years of age, 90% of children have achieved direct voluntary mastery of the voiding reflex and exhibit the adult pattern of urinary control.

Urinary frequency may be caused by reduced bladder capacity, polyuria, or psychological stress. The urinary volume per voiding will be low if frequency is related to reduced bladder capacity or psychological stress. Moreover, there will not be associated polydipsia. If frequency is secondary to polyuria, the urine volume per voiding will be normal or high, and there usually is associated polydipsia (see Chapter 60).

A reduced bladder capacity may also be secondary to inflammation of the bladder, changes in the bladder wall induced by distal obstruction, or extrinsic masses pressing on the bladder. When the bladder is inflamed, its pain/pressure sensitivity threshold is markedly decreased, so less stimuli are necessary to initiate the urge to void.

Distal infravesical obstruction leads to bladder muscle hypertrophy because of the increased effort needed to empty the bladder. This hypertrophied muscle has a higher resting tone, so smaller than normal urine volumes are necessary to initiate the desire to void. A decrease in the size and force of the urinary stream and/or straining to urinate may be noted. Eventually, the bladder muscle fatigues and cannot empty the bladder effectively. This decompensated bladder has an increased residual urine volume with a resultant decrease in the functional bladder capacity. This large, hypotonic bladder contracts poorly, resulting in small, frequent voids.

Extrinsic extravesical masses that impinge on the bladder may cause frequency by mechanically interfering with normal bladder expansion. Extrinsic masses may also stimulate frequent voiding by causing an irritable focus in the bladder wall.

Normal pediatric values for urine output are useful in determining the presence of polyuria. The traditional definition of polyuria is a urinary output of more than 900 mL per m^2 per day. An infant/toddler up to 2 years of age rarely exceeds 500 mL per day. Children 3 to 5 years of age void up to 700 mL per day. Children 5 to 8 years of age have an approximate maximum volume of 1,000 mL per day. Children 8 to 14 years of age void up to 1,400 mL per day. When polyuria is the cause of urinary frequency, the urine volume per void generally is more than 2 mL per kg.

Polyuria with dilute urine is classically associated with a decreased production of antidiuretic hormone or with impaired renal responsiveness to circulating antidiuretic hormone. Polyuria with dilute urine can also be seen when the stimulus for antidiuretic hormone release is absent (e.g., chronic water overloading). In all these situations, the specific gravity of urine seldom is greater than 1.005 and urine osmolality rarely exceeds 200 mOsm per kg. This contrasts with a normal urinary concentrating ability, which is confirmed by a specific gravity of greater than 1.020.

Polyuria with isotonic or slightly hypertonic urine occurs with an osmotic or solute diuresis. Unlike a water diuresis, there are increases in both urine flow rate and solute excretion. The urine osmolality is never lower than 300 mOsm per kg. However, the specific gravity of urine is variable, ranging from 1.010 when the solute is primarily electrolytes and urea (e.g., renal failure, administration of diuretics) to as high as 1.045 when the solute mass is large (e.g., DM, intravenous contrast agents).

Psychogenic/emotional stress may also induce urinary frequency. Cystometric studies have documented significant anxiety-related increases in intravesical pressure, usually accompanied by a desire to void.

DIFFERENTIAL DIAGNOSIS

A differential diagnosis of urinary frequency is outlined in Table 75.1. In-depth discussions of many of these subjects can be found in other chapters of this textbook (in particular, see Chapters 27, 34, 53, 60, 86, 92, 100, 124). The following discussion highlights selected topics in the differential diagnosis.

Frequency is often associated with UTIs; therefore, this diagnosis must always receive significant consideration in the differential, particularly in the febrile Caucasian female patient younger than 2 years (see Chapters 27 and 92). Accurate diagnosis of pediatric UTI is important to ensure both appropriate initial treatment and follow-up evaluation.

The term *urethral syndrome* refers to an entity that can be seen in female adolescents, characterized by acute onset of frequency and dysuria with "insignificant" bacterial counts (less than 10^5 per mL). Pyuria is generally, but not absolutely, present. Vaginitis is a common cause of the urethral syndrome. *Chlamydia trachomatis* is also a relatively common etiology. The urethral syndrome can also occasionally be associated with *Neisseria gonorrhoeae*. There is evidence to support the causal relationship of low-level bacteriuria and symptomatic disease. Therefore, in the context of the urethral syndrome, after all other causes have been excluded, "significant" bacteriuria may be considered as 10^2 *Enterobacteriaceae* or more per mL.

Irritative vulvovaginitis (e.g., secondary to poor hygiene or bubble baths) is a relatively common cause of frequency, usually associated with dysuria but not with pyuria. Frequency may be secondary to urethral trauma secondary to straddle injuries, catheterization, masturbation, or sexual abuse. Pinworms (*Enterobius vermicularis*) may occasionally cause frequency in young females. Children with pinworm infestation may or may not present with perineal itching. Pyuria and dysuria are usually absent.

Frequency may be a presenting symptom of a pelvic mass pressing on the bladder, such as appendicitis, appendiceal abscess, or ovarian torsion. There is obvious potential for significant morbidity. Associated abdominal pain, by history and examination, should be present. Pyuria, microscopic hematuria, and proteinuria (but generally not bacteriuria) may also be present.

Frequency may be secondary to a partial distal urethral obstruction. The urinary stream in the male infant or child who presents with posterior urethral valves is usually nonforceful and nonsustained. Straining to urinate may also be noted. A lower abdominal mass (enlarged bladder) may be palpable.

A neurogenic bladder associated with a spinal cord lesion (e.g., tethered cord) may present with urinary frequency. There

TABLE 75.1

DIFFERENTIAL DIAGNOSIS OF URINARY FREQUENCY

Bladder/urethra
Urinary tract infection (bacterial)[a]
Cystitis (viral)[a]
Cystitis (chemical)
   Methicillin
   Cyclophosphamide (Cytoxan)
Urethritis
   Vulvovaginitis/balanitis (infectious, irritative/abusive, or foreign body)[a]
   Meatal ulcerations/local trauma[a]
   Urethral (frequency-dysuria) syndrome[a]
   Pinworms (*Enterobius vermicularis*)
   Urethral foreign body
Appendicitis or ovarian torsion (pelvic/abscess)[b]
Posterior urethral valves[b]
Neurogenic bladder (spinal cord lesion/injury)[b]
Constipation[a]
Pregnancy[a,b]
Uninhibited (unstable) bladder[a]
Mental retardation/behavioral disorders
Ectopic ureter

Renal
Osmotic diuresis
   Diabetes mellitus[a,b]
   Excess solute intake (inappropriately concentrated formula)[b]
   Intravenous contrast agent
Intrinsic renal parenchymal disease[b]
Sickle cell anemia or trait[a]
Hypercalciuria[a]
Urinary calculi
Congenital adrenal hyperplasia (salt-losing form)[b]
Hypercalcemia
Chronic hypokalemia
Diabetes insipidus (nephrogenic)[b]
Diabetes insipidus (central)[b]
   Head injury
   Brain tumors (e.g., craniopharyngioma, optic nerve glioma)
   Septooptic dysplasia
Drugs[a]
   Caffeine (colas, coffee)
   Theophylline
   Ethanol
   Lithium
   Diuretics
   Vitamin D

Psychogenic/stress
Extraordinary urinary frequency syndrome[a]
Water intoxication[b]
   Psychogenic water drinking
   Munchausen syndrome by proxy

[a]Relatively common causes of frequency.
[b]Emergent/life-threatening causes of frequency.

may be associated lumbosacral abnormalities (hairy patches, cutaneous dimples or tracts, lipoma, or bony irregularities). Decreased anal tone, as well as lower-extremity weakness or reflex abnormalities, may be noted. An enlarged bladder may be palpable.

It is well recognized that in children with urinary tract dysfunction, an association with constipation is often present. Large fecal masses may restrict maximal bladder capacity or directly produce symptoms of frequency by stimulating uninhibited bladder contractions. Resolution of the fecal accumulation decreases frequency symptoms.

Pregnancy should always be considered as a cause of frequent urination in the adolescent female. A lower abdominal mass may be palpable. To state the obvious, adolescent sexual histories are notoriously unreliable.

Uninhibited bladder contractions ("unstable bladder" syndrome) occur involuntarily in children who have failed to gain complete voluntary control over the voiding reflex. This appears to represent a delay in nervous system maturation. A child who attempts to maintain continence must constrict the voluntary urinary sphincter tightly. If the sphincter is relatively weak, urinary frequency associated with urgency and enuresis may result. Females may exhibit the so-called "curtsey" sign, so named because the child squats and attempts to prevent leakage by compressing the perineum with the heel of one foot. This maneuver will usually prevent major incontinence but generally small amounts of urine leakage occur. A history of recurrent UTIs is associated with the presence of this maneuver. If performed, a screening ultrasound examination would reveal normal (minimal) residual urine volumes. With maturity, spontaneous resolution of uninhibited contractions occurs in most cases. In children with significant mental retardation or behavioral disorders, the infantile pattern of spontaneous bladder contraction may persist. Unstable bladder syndrome may also develop in otherwise normal children who have undergone normal toilet training. If symptoms are persistent, a trial of extended-release oxybutynin, behavioral therapy, and/or biofeedback techniques after urologic consultation may be warranted.

Anatomic anomalies of the urogenital tract may result in a chronic leakage of urine. Ectopic ureter would be an example of such an anatomic defect.

Uncontrolled DM is a potentially life-threatening condition that can present with frequent urination. Polyuria results from a glucose-induced osmotic diuresis. At initial presentation, polydipsia, polyphagia, Kussmaul respirations, lethargy, and/or weight loss may also be noted.

In chronic renal failure and in certain diseases of the renal parenchyma (e.g., renal tubular acidosis, Fanconi's syndrome, and Bartter's syndrome), the renal tubules lose their ability to concentrate urine. This leads to polyuria and frequency with large volumes of relatively dilute urine. A concentration defect may also occur with sickle cell disease or trait and may be evident as early as 6 months of age.

Hypercalciuria has been reported as a significant noninfectious cause of the "frequency-dysuria syndrome" in pediatric patients. Onset of symptoms generally ranges from 2 to 14 years of age. Occasionally, hypercalciuria can present in early infancy, where irritability is a hallmark symptom. Symptoms often spontaneously resolve within 2 months. There may be a positive family history of calcium urolithiasis. Dysuria may or may not be present. Hematuria (generally microscopic) and/or crystalluria are often seen. However, the urinalysis may be normal. If the diagnosis is suspected and symptoms persist, studies of urinary calcium excretion and urologic consultation should be considered. A spot urinary calcium-creatinine ratio of 0.2 or more denotes hypercalciuria. Voiding dysfunction in the majority of patients with hypercalciuria responds to behavioral therapy and anticholinergics, with only a small minority of patients requiring treatment with thiazides.

The salt-losing form of congenital adrenal hyperplasia is a life threatening, although a relatively rare, cause of frequency. Excessive urinary excretion of sodium leads to severe water loss and marked dehydration with associated hyperkalemia and hyponatremia. However, at initial presentation (usually in the first 2 months of life), urinary frequency as a symptom is generally not appreciated. Female infants may exhibit virilization of the external genitalia. Male infants may demonstrate increased pigmentation of the external genitalia and/or a relatively enlarged phallus.

Diabetes insipidus is an uncommon, although life-threatening, cause of frequency in the ED. It is clinically characterized by polyuria (with resultant frequency) and polydipsia. It is caused by an inability of the kidneys to concentrate urine. This is related to a deficiency in the hypothalamic production of antidiuretic hormone (central DI) or a renal unresponsiveness to antidiuretic hormone (nephrogenic DI). Some causes of central DI (e.g., septooptic dysplasia) present in the neonatal period. However, most causes of central DI are acquired (e.g., head injury, brain tumors) and therefore can present at any age. The most common type of nephrogenic DI in childhood is the X-linked recessive type, which presents in males during early infancy. If fluids are not accessible or if the thirst sensation is impaired, hypernatremic dehydration develops. If DI is suspected, oral fluids should not be limited. The child should be admitted to the hospital for evaluation and treatment under strict medical supervision.

Drugs are a relatively common cause of frequency in childhood. Methylxanthines (caffeine, theophylline) and ethanol inhibit the production of antidiuretic hormone. Lithium, chronic hypokalemia, hypercalcemia, and vitamin D are also associated with urinary frequency, interfering with renal responsiveness to antidiuretic hormone. Diuretic agents may cause urinary frequency. These agents represent only a few of the many drugs that can cause urinary frequency as a side effect. Therefore, a detailed pharmacology history should be obtained in the child who presents with urinary frequency.

Frequency may result from polyuria secondary to water intoxication. Absence of nocturia and enuresis in the presence of polyuria would suggest an excessive fluid intake. The serum sodium and osmolality would generally be decreased. Psychogenic water drinking is an extremely unusual diagnosis in young children but may present in adolescence. Water intoxication secondary to Munchausen syndrome by proxy, an unusual presentation of abuse in the younger child, is also a consideration.

The "extraordinary urinary frequency syndrome" probably represents a relatively common cause of urinary frequency in pediatric primary care settings. Average age of onset is about 6 years (with a range of about 2 to 11 years). Daytime frequency occurs as often as every 5 minutes. Dysuria is not present. Nocturia is present in about half the cases but usually occurs only about one to two times per night. Polydipsia and polyuria are absent. The physical examination is normal. The urinalysis and serum electrolytes are also normal. If the diagnosis of "extraordinary urinary frequency syndrome" is likely, reassurance and follow-up are indicated. Initial radiologic

SIGNS AND SYMPTOMS

evaluation and pharmacologic therapy are generally unnecessary. Left untreated, frequent voiding often resolves spontaneously within about 2 months, although in some children, the duration of symptoms can be markedly longer. The etiology is unclear but often has a psychogenic component, with an apparent "trigger" (school problems, parental death, sibling illness, etc.) identifiable in about 40% of cases. Parekh et al. reported a 21% rate of hypercalciuria (positive spot urinary calcium-creatinine ratio) in their series of 38 pediatric patients with this syndrome. More extensive urologic and possibly psychological evaluation is warranted if isolated urinary frequency persists for more than 2 months. After consultation, a trial of extended-release oxybutynin, behavior modification, and/or biofeedback techniques are therapeutic considerations.

As an isolated symptom, frequency would be an atypical presentation of pediatric sexual abuse. However, urinary frequency may be seen in association with pertinent history or physical findings (e.g., vulvovaginal venereal infection or genital trauma), which would be suggestive of sexual abuse.

EVALUATION AND DECISION

The primary role of the emergency physician in evaluating the child with urinary frequency is to exclude significant underlying pathology that may result in morbidity and to identify treatable conditions. When confronted with a child whose chief complaint is frequent urination, it should initially be determined whether the criteria for true urinary frequency have been met (see the "Pathophysiology" section above for age-related normal values). Additional history should then focus on symptoms related to the infection of the urinary tract. Are associated symptoms of dysuria, fever, or flank pain also present? Is there a history of UTIs? Questions specifically related to DM should also be included (polyuria, polydipsia, polyphagia, weight loss, family history). The presence or absence of nocturia and enuresis are also important historical points. The urine volume per voiding should be determined (large vs. small). Generally, the presence of polyuria (copious volumes of dilute urine) is obvious from the history. The onset and duration of the symptoms and the quality of the urinary stream should be documented.

In addition, other historical features may be pertinent. For example, are there symptoms to suggest central DI (polydipsia, nocturia, central nervous system abnormalities)? Is there a history of poor growth, suggesting renal disease? Is there a family history of sickle cell disease or trait? Is the child taking any medication or drug (including caffeinated beverages) associated with frequency? Is there a history of chronic constipation, vulvovaginal infection/trauma, or pruritis ani? Are there

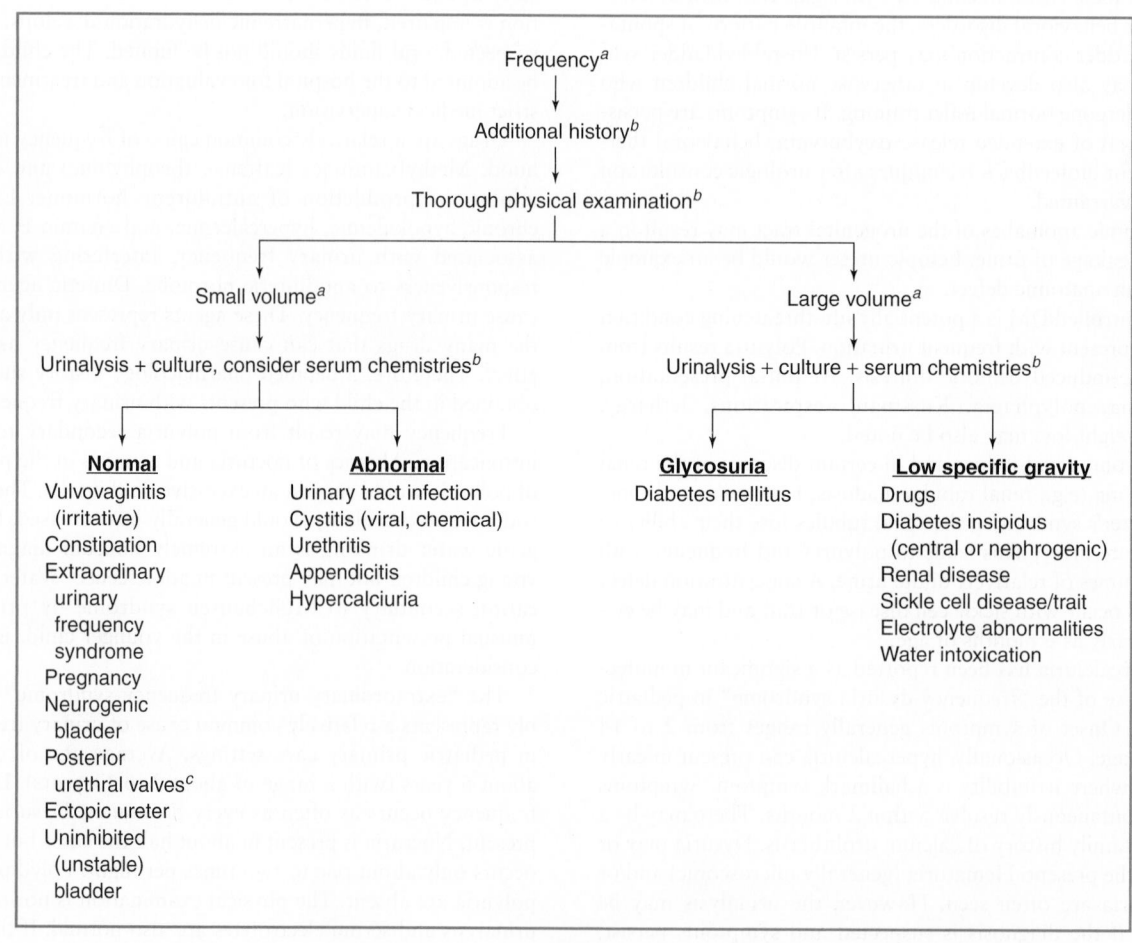

FIGURE 75.1 Evaluation of urinary frequency. *a*Refer to the "Pathophysiology" section for age-related normal values. *b*Refer to the "Evaluation and Decision" section. *c*Renal function tests may be abnormal.

symptoms of abdominal pain, suggesting the possibility of acute appendicitis or appendiceal abscess? In young male patients, what is the quality of the urinary stream? In an adolescent female patient, when was her last menstrual period? Is there a family history of urolithiasis or renal disease?

A complete physical examination should be performed, including an accurate blood pressure measurement. The child's growth parameters should be plotted, and the blood pressure should be compared with age-specific normal values to screen for hypertension (see Chapter 34). The abdomen should be palpated carefully for the presence of abdominal masses and/or tenderness. Percussion of the flanks should be performed. The lumbosacral area should be examined closely for anomalies (hairy patches, dimples, tracts, etc.). Special attention should be focused on the function of sacral nerves II to IV (anal wink and sphincter tone). Unless the diagnosis is readily apparent, a rectal examination should be performed, noting tone, tenderness, masses, and the quality and quantity of stool in the rectal vault. The external genitalia should always be thoroughly examined, meticulously searching for signs of infection, trauma, or anatomic abnormalities. Signs of virilization (in the female) or hyperpigmentation (in the male) should be evaluated. A thorough neurologic examination with careful attention to the retinal fundi and visual fields is warranted.

The laboratory evaluation is fairly straightforward. A urinalysis (including specific gravity) and urine culture should be performed in all cases. Caution should be exercised in interpreting pyuria and/or bacteriuria from a "bag" or "midstream" urine specimens in the infant or toddler. If a UTI is a significant differential consideration, then a catheterized specimen should be the standard in all children still wearing diapers. If a UTI is confirmed, additional elective radiologic evaluation should be considered. Glycosuria obviously suggests the diagnosis of DM.

If the diagnosis is not apparent at this point, serum chemistries (including electrolytes, glucose, blood urea nitrogen, creatinine, and calcium) should be obtained. A sickle cell preparation should also be considered in the African-American child, and a pregnancy test should be performed in the adolescent female patient. This workup is generally sufficient for those children who do not have both daytime and nighttime symptoms or anatomic and/or neurologic abnormalities.

In the child with progressive or worrisome urologic symptoms or signs (e.g., nocturia, persistent dysuria, poor urinary stream, straining to urinate, growth failure, hypertension, fixed low urinary specific gravity), urologic and/or nephrologic consultations are recommended. Additional studies may include a screening ultrasonogram of the urinary tract and abdomen, a voiding cystourethrogram, urinary calcium studies, and possible urodynamic investigation. If the presence of polyuria is in doubt, a 24-hour urine collection may be necessary to establish the diagnosis. If a neurogenic bladder (related to a spinal cord lesion such as a tethered cord) or a brain tumor is suspected, emergent radiologic evaluation with neurosurgical consultation is indicated.

A simplified schematic approach to the evaluation of the child with urinary frequency is outlined in Fig. 75.1.

Suggested Readings

Asnes RS, Mones RL. Pollakiuria. *Pediatrics* 1973;52:615–617.

Corigliano T, Renella R, Robbiani A, et al. Isolated extraordinary daytime urinary frequency of childhood: a case series of 26 children in Switzerland. *Acta Pediatr* 2007;96:1347–1349.

Glazier DB, Anken MK, Ferlise V, et al. Utility of biofeedback for the daytime syndrome of urinary frequency and urgency of childhood. *Urology* 2001;57:791–794.

Hellerstein S, Linebarger JS. Voiding dysfunction in pediatric patients. *Clin Pediatr* 2003;42:43–49.

Loening-Baucke V. Urinary incontinence and urinary tract infection and their resolution with treatment of chronic constipation of childhood. *Pediatrics* 1997;100:228–232.

Parekh DJ, Pope JC, Adams MC, et al. The role of hypercalciuria in a subgroup of dysfunctional voiding syndromes of childhood. *J Urol* 2000;164:1008–1010.

Reinberg Y, Crocker J, Wolpert J, et al. Therapeutic efficacy of extended release oxybutynin chloride, and immediate release and long acting tolterodine tartrate in children with diurnal urinary incontinence. *J Urol* 2003;169:317–319.

Shaikh N, Morone NE, Bost JE, et al. Prevalence of urinary tract infection in childhood: a meta-analysis. *Pediatr Infect Dis J* 2008;27:302–308.

Wiener JS, Scales MT, Hampton J, et al. Long-term efficacy of simple behavioral therapy for daytime wetting in children. *J Urol* 2000;164:786–790.

Youdim K, Kogan BA. Preliminary study of the safety and efficacy of extended-release oxybutynin in children. *Urolology* 2002;59:428–432.

Zorc JJ, Levine DA, Platt SL, et al. Clinical and demographic factors associated with urinary tract infection in young febrile infants. *Pediatrics* 2005;116:664–668.

Zoubek, J, Bloom DA, Sedman AB. Extraordinary urinary frequency. *Pediatrics* 1990;85:1112–1114.

SIGNS AND SYMPTOMS

CHAPTER 76 ■ VAGINAL BLEEDING

JAN E. PARADISE, MD

Vaginal bleeding can be either a normal event or a sign of disease and, when pathologic, can indicate variously a local genital tract disorder, systemic endocrinologic or hematologic disease, or a complication of pregnancy. During childhood, vaginal bleeding is abnormal after the first week or so of life and before menarche. After menarche, abnormal vaginal bleeding must be differentiated from menstruation and, in turn, menstrual bleeding must be categorized as either normal or excessive. *Menstruation* is defined as the spontaneous, periodic shedding of endometrial tissue and blood.

Menstrual patterns during the first 2 years after menarche vary, but it is possible to set outside limits. Ninety-five percent of young adolescents' menstrual periods are between 2 and 8 days long. A duration of 10 days or more is abnormal. An occasional interval of less than 21 days from the first day of one menstrual period to the first day of the next is normal for teenagers, but several short cycles in a row are abnormal. Whether the quantity of a patient's menstrual bleeding is normal can be difficult to determine historically. However, it is uncommon for adolescents to soak more than six to eight perineal pads or tampons a day. Normal menstrual bleeding never produces an acute fall in hemoglobin or hematocrit. Because the relative prevalence of disorders that produce vaginal bleeding correlates more closely with patients' hormonal status than with their chronologic age, the diagnostic approach outlined in this chapter is presented in two sections divided according to patients' menarcheal status (Table 76.1).

VAGINAL BLEEDING BEFORE NORMAL MENARCHE (FIG. 76.1)

Evaluation and Decision

During the patient's general physical examination, the emergency physician should be particularly alert for signs of hormonal stimulation (i.e., breast development, pubic hair growth, a dull pink vaginal mucosa, or physiologic leukorrhea). For the initial examination of the genitalia, an infant or a child should be placed in a frog-leg position either on the parent's lap or on the examining table (Fig. 90.2A). The physician then separates and applies gentle outward traction to the child's labia majora, inspecting the introitus for a bleeding site. A vaginal speculum should not be used. If the vulva is normal, the child should next be placed in the knee-chest position for examination of her vagina (Fig. 90.2B). In this position, the girl is encouraged to relax her abdominal muscles while the examiner gently separates her labia and buttocks. As air enters the vaginal vault, it falls open. The physician can then use an otoscope light to look for a bleeding site or a foreign body. If no bleeding site or foreign body is seen, the child is returned to the supine position and a vaginal specimen for culture is obtained, using either a soft plastic medicine dropper or a cotton-tipped swab moistened with nonbacteriostatic saline solution. Finally, if the interior of the vagina could not be seen well but the examiner suspects a foreign body or trauma, vaginal examination under sedation or general anesthesia should be considered.

Vulvar Bleeding

The vulva consists of several structures: the labia majora, the labia minora, the clitoris, and the vaginal introitus. A premenarcheal girl with the complaint of vaginal bleeding whose vulva looks abnormal may have a vaginal disorder, a vulvar disorder, or both.

Trauma to the vulva often produces lacerations, ecchymoses, or both. Even a minor vulvar injury should alert the emergency physician to the possibility of concurrent, potentially serious vaginal or rectal injuries. Vulvar lacerations do not usually bleed excessively, but hematomas can extend widely through the tissue planes, forming large, painful masses that occasionally produce enough pressure to cause necrosis of the overlying vulvar skin. Because minor periurethral injuries can produce urethral spasm that leads to acute urinary retention, the injured child's ability to void should be checked. The possibility of sexual assault must be considered in the management of every child with a genital injury.

Urethral prolapse (see Chapter 90) is probably the most common cause of apparent vaginal bleeding during childhood. Some patients with urethral prolapse complain of dysuria or urinary frequency, but most have bleeding as their only symptom. A prolapse is diagnosed by its characteristic doughnut shape (Fig. 90.5). The ring of protruding urethral mucosa above the introitus is swollen and dark red with a central dimple that indicates the meatus. When the child is supine, the prolapse is often large enough to cover the vaginal introitus and appears to protrude from the vagina. Bleeding comes from the ischemic mucosa. Urethral prolapse is sometimes mistaken for a malignant tumor, which is a rare cause of vaginal bleeding. If the diagnosis is in doubt, one may safely catheterize the bladder through the prolapse to obtain urine. Some patients with small prolapses whose urethral tissue is still pink will improve with the use of sitz baths alone for several days. However, if the prolapsed tissue looks dark or necrotic at the time of the patient's examination, or if sitz baths are not effective, elective surgical excision of the prolapsed tissue will be needed within a few days after diagnosis.

TABLE 76.1

DIFFERENTIAL DIAGNOSIS OF VAGINAL BLEEDING

I. At any time
  A. Trauma
  B. Tumor
II. Before normal menarche
  A. Hormonal
    1. Neonatal bleeding
    2. Exogenous estrogen
    3. Precocious puberty
  B. Nonhormonal
    1. Urethral prolapse
    2. Genital warts
    3. Lichen sclerosus
    4. Infectious vaginitis
    5. Foreign body
III. After menarche
  A. Bleeding diathesis
  B. Pelvic infection
  C. Endocrinologic problem
    1. Midcycle spotting
    2. Dysfunctional uterine bleeding
      a. Hormonal contraception
      b. Axis immaturity
      c. Polycystic ovary syndrome
      d. Hypothyroidism
      e. Ovarian cyst
  D. Ectopic pregnancy
  E. Spontaneous abortion
  F. Placenta previa
  G. Abruptio placentae

Genital warts, like a urethral prolapse, can be recognized by inspection (Fig. 90.12) and can produce bleeding when they are located on the mucosal surface of the introitus or just inside the hymenal ring. Because the presence of such warts in a child indicates that sexual contact may have occurred, the child should be screened for other sexually transmitted infec-

tions and consideration should be given to reporting the case to the state child protective services agency (see Chapter 132). Topical podophyllin can produce systemic toxicity if a large amount is absorbed. Accordingly, to select an appropriate treatment for bleeding genital warts, a gynecologist or other knowledgeable clinician should be consulted.

Vulvar inflammation can be seen in some patients with vaginal bleeding resulting from bacterial or fungal vulvovaginitis (see also Chapter 77). Infections caused by *Shigella* species, group A hemolytic streptococci, *Neisseria gonorrhoeae*, and *Candida albicans* produce vaginal bleeding or bloody discharge in varying proportions of cases. A few children with rectal *Enterobius vermicularis* (pinworm) infestations scratch so vigorously that they excoriate the perineal area and cause bleeding. Pinworm ova can often be discovered by low-power microscopic examination of perianal material that is collected with clear cellophane tape and then attached to a glass slide.

Although bleeding per se is not common, ecchymoses, fissures, and telangiectasias are frequent clinical manifestations of lichen sclerosus (Fig. 76.2), an uncommon, chronic, idiopathic skin disorder that most often affects the vulva. In this condition, white, flat-topped papules gradually coalesce to form atrophic plaques that involve the vulvar and perianal skin in a symmetric hourglass pattern. Topical treatment with ultrapotent steroids or an immunomodulator is helpful in most cases.

VAGINAL BLEEDING WITHOUT SIGNS OF HORMONAL STIMULATION

Trauma, infection, and foreign bodies are the most common causes of vaginal bleeding during childhood. Vaginal bleeding after trauma indicates a potential emergency. A penetrating narrow object can damage the rectum, bladder, or abdominal viscera without producing much external evidence of injury. Because vaginal lacerations do not always produce a great deal

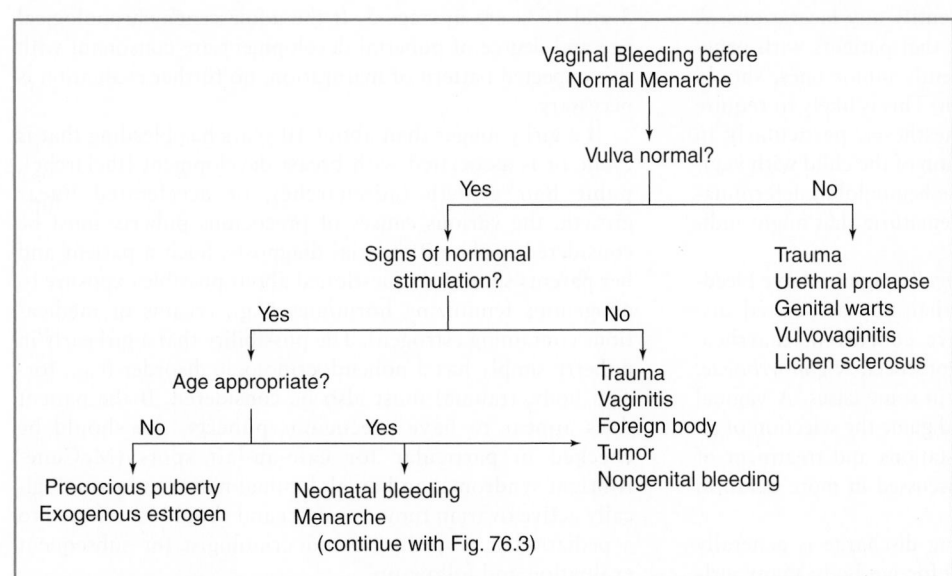

FIGURE 76.1 Diagnostic approach to vaginal bleeding before normal menarche.

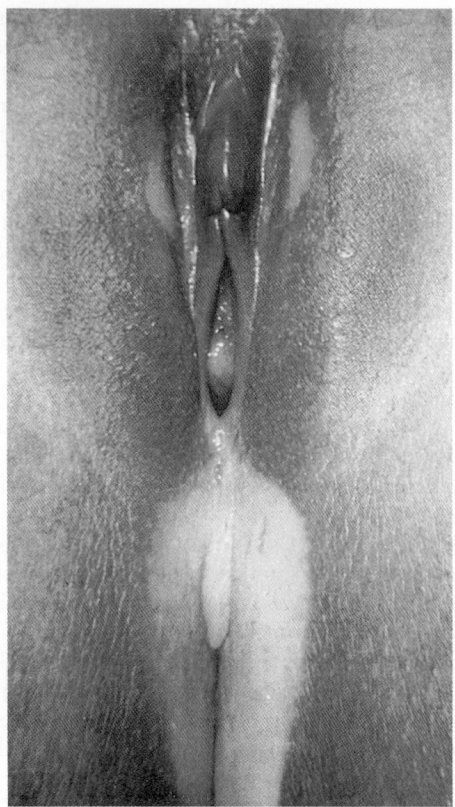

FIGURE 76.2 Figure-of-eight pattern of vulvar and perianal hypopigmentation in a 10-year-old girl with lichen sclerosus.

of bleeding or pain, the emergency physician cannot rely on the severity of the patient's symptoms to indicate the extent of the injury. When a child sustains a genital injury, the physician must consider the possibility that it was inflicted during a sexual assault.

If the clinician knows or suspects that trauma has occurred, the girl's abdomen should be evaluated carefully. Lower quadrant tenderness may provide a clue to intraabdominal injury. The vulva is inspected for bruises, and a rectal examination is performed to identify any lacerations. A general principle of management is that patients with penetrating genital injuries, even apparently minor ones, should undergo careful vaginal examination. This is likely to require procedural sedation or general anesthesia, particularly in young children. Laboratory evaluation of the child with vaginal trauma should include a baseline hemoglobin determination and a urinalysis to screen for hematuria that might indicate urethral or bladder injury.

About half of all patients with *Shigella* vaginitis have bleeding that may be more noticeable than any associated discharge. Most patients do not have concurrent diarrhea. Vaginal infections with group A streptococci, *N gonorrhoeae*, and *C albicans* also cause bleeding in some cases. A vaginal culture will provide the diagnosis and guide the selection of an appropriate antibiotic. The manifestations and treatment of vaginal infections in children are discussed in more detail in Chapters 77 and 90.

Although a chronic, foul-smelling discharge is generally considered the hallmark of a vaginal foreign body, many girls have intermittent scanty vaginal bleeding alone or with an unimpressive discharge. Direct inspection of the vaginal vault using the knee-chest position (Fig. 90.2B) usually allows the examiner to find a foreign body easily. If a foreign body is strongly suspected but cannot be seen using the knee-chest position, the patient should receive a rectal examination and either gentle vaginal lavage (using saline solution, a 50-mL syringe with the plunger discarded, a red rubber catheter, and gravity) or an examination under procedural sedation or anesthesia. Because the most common foreign body—toilet paper—is not radiopaque, pelvic roentgenography is not often likely to be helpful and should be avoided.

Occasionally, a prepubertal patient with a history of bleeding has no abnormalities and no bleeding at the time of the examination. This history should not be dismissed lightly because most parents are good observers, but the patient's urine and stool should also be checked for blood. Vaginal foreign body, genital trauma, and inapparent hormonal stimulation (see the following text) are also in the differential diagnosis.

VAGINAL BLEEDING WITH SIGNS OF HORMONAL STIMULATION

During the first 2 to 3 weeks of life and late in puberty, hormonal fluctuations produce physiologic endometrial bleeding. Before female infants are born, high levels of placental estrogen stimulate growth of both the uterine endometrium and the breast tissue. As this hormonal support wanes after birth, some infants have an endometrial slough that results in a few days of light vaginal bleeding. The bleeding will stop spontaneously and requires no treatment except reassurance for the parents.

Occasionally, an adolescent girl is brought to the emergency department (ED) by her parents to confirm their belief that she is having her first menstrual period. About 65% of girls are in sexual maturity stage 4 (Tanner stage 4) for breast development when menarche occurs (Table 76.2). Of the remaining girls, about 25% are in breast development stage 3 and 10% are in stage 5. If the adolescent's chronological age and degree of pubertal development are consonant with this expected pattern of maturation, no further evaluation is necessary.

If a girl younger than about 10 years has bleeding that is cyclic or is associated with breast development (thelarche), pubic hair growth (adrenarche), or accelerated linear growth, the various causes of precocious puberty must be considered in the differential diagnosis. Such a patient and her parents should be questioned about possible exposure to exogenous feminizing hormones (e.g., creams or medications containing estrogen). The possibility that a girl early in puberty simply has a nonendocrinologic disorder (e.g., foreign body, trauma) must also be considered. If the patient does appear to have precocious puberty, she should be checked in particular for café-au-lait spots (McCune-Albright syndrome) and an abdominal mass (endocrinologically active ovarian tumor or cyst) and should be referred to a pediatrician or pediatric endocrinologist for subsequent evaluation and follow-up.

TABLE 76.2

MEDIAN AGE AT ENTRY TO EACH STAGE OF BREAST DEVELOPMENT DURING PUBERTY IN US GIRLS, BY ETHNICITY[a]

Sexual maturity stage	Description of stage	Median age at entry to pubertal stage (yr)		
		Non-Hispanic blacks (n = 788)	Mexican-Americans (n = 763)	Non-Hispanic whites (n = 594)
2	Breast buds; areolar elevation	9.5	9.8	10.4
3	More growth; no separation of contours	10.8	11.4	11.8
4	Areola projects beyond breast contour	12.2	13.1	13.3
5	Mature breast	13.9	14.7	15.5

[a]Data from US Third National Health and Nutrition Examination Survey, 1988–1994.
Adapted from Sun SS, Schubert CM, Chumlea WC, et al. National estimates of the timing of sexual maturation and racial differences among US children. *Pediatrics* 2002;110:911–919.

ABNORMAL BLEEDING AFTER MENARCHE

Evaluation and Decision

For postmenarcheal adolescents, the first discrimination the emergency physician must make is between those patients whose menstrual bleeding is heavier, more prolonged, or more frequent than they would like but is nevertheless normal, and those patients whose bleeding falls outside the limits presented at the beginning of this chapter. After that, patients with abnormal bleeding will be divided for evaluation and management into two groups: patients who are pregnant and those who are not. For all patients, historical points will include the adolescent's age at menarche, her usual menstrual pattern, and the date of onset of her most recent normal menstrual period. Because anovulatory bleeding is nearly always painless, the presence of dysmenorrhea argues against a diagnosis of anovulatory dysfunctional uterine bleeding (DUB). Other pertinent historical details include the presence or absence of trauma, fainting or dizziness, fever, easy bruising, and excessive bleeding at other sites. While the patient is alone, and after assuring her of confidentiality, the patient should be asked whether she has experienced sexual intercourse. Sexually experienced patients should be asked whether they have ever had a sexually transmitted infection or been pregnant. Current and recent methods of contraception should also be ascertained.

The patient's pulse and blood pressure are noted and checked for orthostatic change. After a routine general examination, a complete pelvic examination is performed for patients who are either not pregnant or within the first trimester of pregnancy. A speculum examination is not necessary for virginal adolescent patients who have not been injured, but a bimanual examination should generally be carried out because teenagers are not always candid about their sexual activity. If it is more comfortable, bimanual rectoabdominal palpation with the patient in the lithotomy position can be substituted, or the examiner can place one finger intravaginally instead of two.

A urine pregnancy test should be obtained early in the evaluation of most postmenarcheal adolescents presenting to the ED because of vaginal bleeding. For the occasional parent who finds it difficult to understand the rationale for this test for his or her daughter, it may be helpful to point out that the medical consequences of failing to diagnose pregnancy can be substantial. A pregnancy test should be obtained even if the patient with an episode of abnormal bleeding says she has had regular menstrual periods, because about 25% of patients with ectopic pregnancies do not report having missed a menstrual period.

BLEEDING IN THE PREGNANT PATIENT (FIG. 76.3)

Bleeding During Late Pregnancy

If the patient is 20 weeks pregnant or more by history or abdominal examination, potential causes of bleeding that must be identified urgently are placenta previa, premature separation of the placenta (abruptio placentae), and a bloody show during labor. Placenta previa occurs in about 1 of 200 pregnancies and abruption in about 1 in 100. However, the risk of both of these pregnancy complications is lower in adolescents than in older women. An obstetrician should be consulted at the earliest opportunity regarding further ED management of the pregnant patient with second- or third-trimester bleeding.

Because digital vaginal examination of a patient with placenta previa can provoke uncontrollable hemorrhage, the emergency care of a patient with vaginal bleeding after the 20th week of pregnancy starts with the management of potential hypovolemic shock (see Chapter 3) rather than with an examination to determine the anatomic site of bleeding. Thus, the patient's vital signs are recorded, the fetal heart rate is monitored, and a large-bore intravenous catheter is inserted. The patient with an apparently normal initial blood pressure is followed carefully nonetheless because her baseline pressure during pregnancy may have been elevated. Initial laboratory evaluation should include determinations of the blood type and antibody screen, hematocrit, platelet count, fibrinogen level, and coagulation studies to screen for disseminated intravascular coagulation, which may be present in moderate and severe abruption. If the patient continues to bleed while in

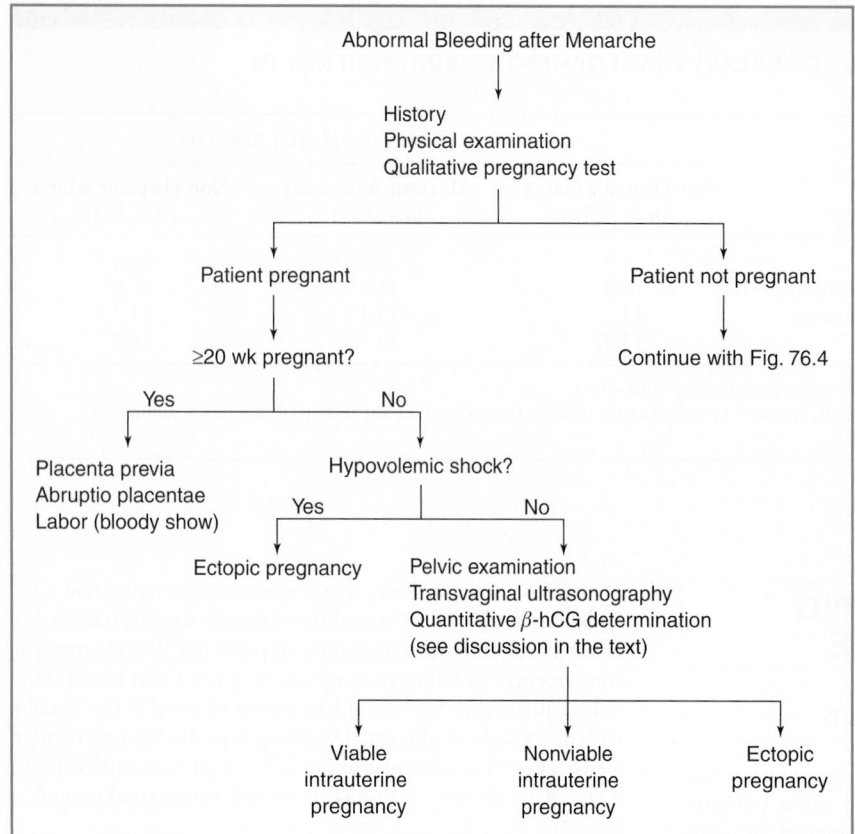

FIGURE 76.3 Diagnostic approach to abnormal uterine bleeding after menarche—pregnant patients. β-hCG, β-human chorionic gonadotropin.

the ED, volume replacement is initiated. If the patient is stable and the fetus is in no distress, the goal of subsequent investigation is to determine the location of the placenta and to identify the cause of the bleeding if it is not placenta previa.

Bleeding during Early Pregnancy

Although the ED physician should be able to recognize and begin managing complications of early pregnancy, an obstetrician should be consulted about any pregnant adolescent who has vaginal bleeding.

Bleeding with Shock

If the patient with vaginal bleeding is in the first or second trimester of pregnancy and has shock or early signs of cardiovascular instability (pallor, perspiration, vomiting), ruptured ectopic pregnancy must be ruled out. In this case, the treatment of shock and diagnostic measures should be undertaken simultaneously. Pelvic examination is performed and obstetric consultation should be obtained rapidly. Emergency laparoscopy or laparotomy may be necessary for critically ill patients. If the patient is relatively stable, transabdominal or transvaginal ultrasonography may help to clarify the diagnosis.

Bleeding without Shock

Among adults in the first trimester of pregnancy presenting to an ED with abdominal pain or vaginal bleeding, approxi-

mately 60% have normal pregnancies, 30% have nonviable intrauterine pregnancies, and 10% have ectopic pregnancies. Corresponding data for adolescents are not known, but the risk of ectopic pregnancy is lower among adolescents than among older women. Apart from older age, the factors that convey the highest risk for ectopic pregnancy (e.g., prior tubal surgery, previous ectopic pregnancy) are rare in adolescents. But, in any case, most patients with ectopic pregnancy do not have any of these risk factors.

The standard terminology for spontaneous abortion includes threatened, incomplete, and complete abortions. Three less common but more complex manifestations of abortion deserve special consideration by the ED physician. *Septic abortion* is diagnosed if signs of infection, usually fever, disproportionately severe pelvic pain, and leukocytosis, are present during a spontaneous or induced abortion. After an induced abortion, persistent or heavy bleeding can indicate *retained products of conception* that will require removal. In a *missed abortion*, the embryo is not expelled from the uterus within 4 weeks of its death. Dark bleeding is often seen. The patient's symptoms of pregnancy may have regressed, the uterus is smaller than it should be according to her menstrual history, and disseminated intravascular coagulation can occur.

In a pregnant patient with abdominal pain or vaginal bleeding in the first trimester, symptoms that favor an intrauterine pregnancy (either normal or abnormal) include mild pain, pain located in the midline, and uterine size greater than 8 weeks. Sharp pain, lateralized pain, and pain of moderate to severe intensity favor ectopic pregnancy. On examination, the diagnosis of incomplete miscarriage is straightforward if the internal cervical os is open or tissue fragments are visible. Examination findings that favor ectopic pregnancy include cervical motion tenderness, lateral pelvic tenderness, and signs of peritoneal irritation. The amount of bleeding and the presence of an adnexal mass on examination are nondiagnostic. If products of conception are not visible, then no constellation of symptoms and signs can accurately distinguish intrauterine from ectopic pregnancy, and diagnostic testing will be crucial.

To identify the cause of bleeding in a pregnant adolescent, a quantitative β-human chorionic gonadotropin (β-hCG) level and findings on transvaginal ultrasonography must be correlated. A single β-hCG level can establish the diagnosis of pregnancy but not its location. Transvaginal ultrasonography can establish that a pregnancy is intrauterine but does not always predict its viability. Clinical assessment of the patient relies on the observation that a normal intrauterine pregnancy should be visible on transabdominal ultrasound when the β-hCG level reaches about 6,000 mIU per mL at the sixth or seventh gestational week (4 to 5 weeks after conception) and should be visible on transvaginal ultrasound when the level reaches between 1,000 to 2,000 mIU per mL at approximately the fifth week of gestation (3 weeks after conception). This so-called "discriminatory threshold" will vary to some extent with operator skill and ultrasound sensitivity. In addition, it should be remembered that β-hCG levels for any given gestational age are higher in twin pregnancies.

Failure to visualize a gestational sac on transvaginal ultrasound in a patient whose β-hCG level exceeds 3,000 mIU per mL strongly suggests a nonviable pregnancy but does not identify its location. Among patients with vaginal bleeding, no intrauterine gestational sac on transvaginal sonography, and a β-hCG level of 2,000 mIU per mL or higher, about 40% will miscarry, about 55% have ectopic pregnancies, and only about 5% have normal intrauterine pregnancies. Because vaginal bleeding is uncommon very early in the course of normal pregnancy, and because ectopic pregnancies produce lower than normal amounts of β-hCG, the likelihood of ectopic pregnancy is increased in symptomatic patients whose β-hCG levels are less than 1,500 mIU per mL.

Sonographic signs suggestive of ectopic pregnancy include a solid or complex adnexal mass, a pelvic mass, particulate fluid in the fallopian tube, an endometrial pseudogestational sac, and cul-de-sac fluid that is either moderate to large in volume or echogenic.

An obstetrician should direct the management of pregnant patients with vaginal bleeding and indeterminate results on transvaginal ultrasonography. Ordinarily, the patient will require either admission to the hospital or close outpatient follow-up. The obstetrician will evaluate serial quantitations of β-hCG. In a normal pregnancy, between days 5 and 42 after conception and above an initial level of 100 mIU per mL, the β-hCG level doubles approximately every 2 days. A decline in β-hCG levels on serial measurement or an increase of less than 66% in 48 hours suggests a nonviable fetus but cannot differentiate intrauterine from extrauterine pregnancy.

Serum progesterone measurement can predict a pregnancy's outcome. Approximately 90% of patients with vaginal bleeding whose progesterone concentrations are higher than 20 ng per mL have normal pregnancies. At a progesterone level below 5 ng per mL, only about 0.16% of pregnancies will be viable. However, because a progesterone level cannot indicate whether a nonviable pregnancy is intrauterine or ectopic, many experts feel that, for ED management, it does not add appreciably to the information afforded by transvaginal ultrasound combined with a β-hCG level.

BLEEDING IN THE NONPREGNANT ADOLESCENT PATIENT (FIG. 76.4)

Vaginal or Cervical Bleeding

On pelvic examination, only a few patients will prove to have vaginal or cervical bleeding. Patients with bleeding from significant vulvar, vaginal, or cervical lacerations should be referred to a gynecologist. The evaluation and management of victims of sexual assault are discussed in detail in Chapters 90 and 132. Hymenal tears produced by coitus rarely require treatment beyond reassurance for the patient. Bleeding genital warts should not be treated with topical podophyllin because toxic amounts of the resin can be absorbed systemically (see Chapter 90). Malignant genital tract tumors are a rare cause of vaginal bleeding during adolescence.

Patients are unlikely to be aware of cervical friability or bleeding caused by infection. On examination, however, punctate cervical hemorrhages (a strawberry cervix) can be seen in about 3% of women with trichomonal vaginitis. Cervical bleeding after swabbing and mucopurulent discharge are common manifestations of cervicitis caused by *Chlamydia trachomatis* and *Neisseria gonorrhea*. Cervical lesions resulting from herpes simplex virus infection may also cause a small amount of bleeding.

Undiagnosed Uterine Bleeding

Most adolescents with vaginal bleeding are not pregnant, and their bleeding is uterine in origin. For these patients, the history, physical examination, and selected laboratory investigations will lead the emergency physician to consider as more or less likely each of three main categories of disease: hematologic problems, pelvic infection, and endocrinologic problems.

The patient should receive a complete blood cell count to screen for anemia and thrombocytopenia. The most common hematologic cause of excessive menstrual bleeding is thrombocytopenia (caused by, for example, idiopathic thrombocytopenic purpura, hematologic malignancy, or chemotherapeutic agents). Clotting factor disorders produce menometrorrhagia much less frequently than does thrombocytopenia, but von Willebrand's disease should be considered in the differential diagnosis.

If the nonpregnant patient with abnormal uterine bleeding also has pelvic pain or tenderness, then pelvic inflammatory disease is a likely possibility. Abnormal bleeding occurs in nearly one-third of patients with pelvic inflammatory disease, generally as a result of endometritis. Pelvic inflammatory disease is discussed in detail in Chapter 90. Every sexually active patient with abnormal vaginal bleeding should be screened for *N. gonorrhoeae* and *C. trachomatis* genital tract infections.

Endocrinologic phenomena—whether physiologic, pharmacologic, or pathologic—are the most common causes of abnormal uterine bleeding in nonpregnant adolescents. During physiologically normal menstrual cycles, the occasional adolescent has spotty bleeding for 24 hours or less in association with the

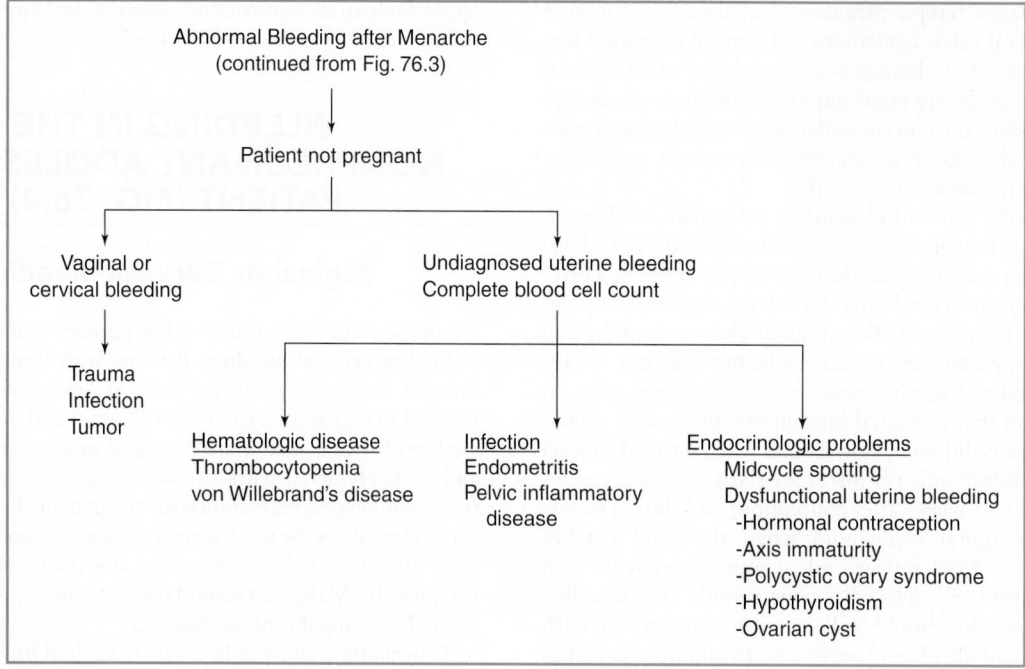

FIGURE 76.4 Diagnostic approach to abnormal uterine bleeding after menarche—nonpregnant patients.

transient decline in estrogen level that occurs at midcycle. The unilateral pain of mittelschmerz can accompany this brief bleeding episode.

Hormonal contraception is a common, pharmacologic cause of irregular menstrual bleeding. Of women who use birth control pills containing 35 μg or less of estrogen, 5% to 10% will have breakthrough intermenstrual spotting or bleeding, especially during the first 3 months of contraceptive pill use. Breakthrough bleeding is also a common side effect of progestin-only contraceptive pills, injectable medroxyprogesterone, and long-acting progestin implants. Many patients using birth control pills experience estrogen withdrawal bleeding if they forget to take one or several pills.

Abnormal uterine bleeding unassociated with either pregnancy or hormonal contraception nearly always indicates lack of regular ovulation and is commonly termed DUB. In adolescents with DUB, the most common underlying causes of anovulation are functional immaturity of the hypothalamic-pituitary-ovarian axis and polycystic ovary syndrome (see Chapter 47). Hypothyroidism should be considered if the patient has other symptoms or signs of thyroid dysfunction. A functioning ovarian cyst is a less common cause of DUB but should be considered especially in the teenager with abnormal uterine bleeding and an adnexal mass or tenderness. The management of DUB is detailed in Chapter 90.

Suggested Readings

General

Boyle C, McCann J, Miyamoto S, et al. Comparison of examination methods used in the evaluation of prepubertal and pubertal female genitalia: a descriptive study. *Child Abuse Neglect* 2008;32:229–243.

Vaginal Bleeding During Childhood

Hill NCW, Oppenheimer LW, Morton KE. The aetiology of vaginal bleeding in children: a 20-year review. *Br J Obstet Gynaecol* 1989;96:467–470.
Lacy J, Brennand E, Ornstei M, et al. Vaginal laceration from a high-pressure water jet in a prepubescent girl. *Pediatr Emerg Care* 2007;23:112–114.
Paradise JE, Willis ED. Probability of vaginal foreign body in girls with genital complaints. *Am J Dis Child* 1985;139:472–476.
Poindexter G, Morrell DS. Anogenital pruritus: lichen sclerosus in children. *Pediatr Ann* 2007;36:785–791.
Scheidler MG, Shultz BL, Schall L, et al. Mechanisms of blunt perineal injury in female pediatric patients. *J Pediatr Surg* 2000;35:1317–1319.
Sugar NF, Feldman KW. Perineal impalements in children: distinguishing accident from abuse. *Pediatr Emerg Care* 2007;23:605–616.
Valerie E, Gilchrist F, Frischer J, et al. Diagnosis and treatment of urethral prolapse in children. *Urology* 1999;54:1082–1084.

Vaginal Bleeding During Pregnancy

Barnhart KT, Casanova B, Sammel MD, et al. Prediction of location of a symptomatic early gestation based solely on clinical presentation. *Obstet Gynecol* 2008; 112:1319–1326.
Dart R, Ramanujam P, Dart L. Progesterone as a predictor of ectopic pregnancy when the ultrasound is indeterminate. *Am J Emerg Med* 2002;20:575–579.
Dart RG, Kaplan B, Varaklis K. Predictive value of history and physical examination in patients with suspected ectopic pregnancy. *Ann Emerg Med* 1999;33:283–290.
Kohn MA, Kerr K, Malkevich D, et al. Beta-chorionic gonadotropin levels and the likelihood of ectopic pregnancy in emergency department patients with abdominal pain or vaginal bleeding. *Acad Emerg Med* 2003;10:119–126.
Sinha P, Kuruba N. Ante-partum haemorrhage: an update. *J Obstet Gynecol* 2008;28:377–381.
Tulandi T. Clinical manifestations, diagnosis, and management of ectopic pregnancy. *UpToDate* Online Version 16.3. http://www.utdol.com/online/content/author.do?topicKey=gen_gyne/8302. Accessed December 12, 2008.

Vaginal Bleeding in the Nonpregnant Adolescent

Hillard PJA. Menstruation in adolescents: what's normal, what's not. *Ann N Y Acad Sci* 2008;1135:29–35.
James A, Matchar DB, Myers ER. Testing for von Willebrand disease in women with menorrhagia: a systematic review. *Am Coll Obstet Gynecol* 2004; 104:381–388.
Strickland JL, Wall JW. Abnormal uterine bleeding in adolescents. *Obstet Gynecol Clin North Am* 2003;30:321–335.

CHAPTER 78 ■ VOMITING

MOLLY (MARTHA W.) STEVENS, MD, MSCE, AND FRED M. HENRETIG, MD

Vomiting is defined as the forceful, coordinated act of expelling gastric contents through the mouth. Vomiting may be caused by a number of problems in diverse organ systems. Although it often represents a transient response to a self-limited infectious, chemical, or psychological insult, it also may portend serious infections, metabolic disturbances, or diseases in gastrointestinal (GI), neurologic, or other major organ systems. Thus, an orderly approach to diagnosis is crucial.

Vomiting is a highly complex act, involving coordinated closure of gastric pylorus and glottis; relaxation of stomach, cardioesophageal junction, and esophagus; and vigorous diaphragmatic and abdominal wall muscular contraction. A series of interconnected coordinating centers in the medulla have been identified, with varying responsiveness to afferent signals from diverse areas of the body, including nocireceptors, chemoreceptors, and mechanoreceptors in the pelvic and abdominal viscera and peritoneum, genitourinary system, pharynx, labyrinth, and heart. The chemoreceptor trigger zone in the floor of the fourth ventricle contains chemoreceptors that monitor both blood and cerebrospinal fluid and is probably the key center initiating the emetic response to drugs (especially cytotoxic chemotherapeutic agents) and metabolic aberrations. More recent therapeutic advances arise from an evolving understanding of neurotransmitter activity in the central nervous system (CNS), GI tract, and other sites. Serotonin (5-hydroxytryptamine) receptors are prevalent in the CNS and gut and participate in the induction of emesis. Use of serotonin receptor antagonists (such as ondansetron and granisetron) has proven to be successful in decreasing or preventing emesis associated with many chemotherapeutic and radiotherapeutic cancer treatments, in emetogenic poisonings, and most recently, in children with viral gastroenteritis.

A related complaint, also often heard in the emergency department (ED), is that of young infants who "spit up." This refers to the nonforceful reflux of milk into the mouth, which often accompanies eructation. Such nonforceful regurgitation of gastric or esophageal contents is most often physiologic and of little consequence, although it occasionally represents a significant disturbance in esophageal function.

It is convenient to attempt to organize the many diverse causes of regurgitation and vomiting into age-related categories (Table 78.1). Although overlap is considerable, the most common and serious entities tend to fall into such groupings.

EVALUATION AND DECISION

General Approach

A brief perusal of the long list of causes for vomiting in Table 78.1 serves to emphasize the need for an orderly approach to

the differential diagnosis of this symptom. The approach advocated here focuses on three key clinical features: child's *age*, evidence of *obstruction*, and signs or symptoms of *extraabdominal organ system disease*. Other important points to consider include *appearance* of the vomitus, *overall degree of illness* (including the presence and severity of dehydration or electrolyte imbalance), and *associated GI symptoms*.

History

The history should focus on the key elements already listed. The patient's age is often critical because certain important entities (especially those that cause intestinal obstruction) are seen exclusively in neonates, older infants, or children beyond the first year of life. Evidence of obstruction, including symptoms of abdominal pain, obstipation, nausea, and increasing abdominal girth, is sought in addition to vomiting. Other associated GI symptoms may include diarrhea, anorexia, flatulence, and frequent eructation with reflux. The suspicion of significant extraabdominal organ system disease is raised by neurologic symptoms such as severe headache, stiff neck, blurred vision or diplopia, clumsiness, personality or school performance change, or persistent lethargy or irritability; by genitourinary symptoms such as flank pain, dysuria, urgency and frequency, or amenorrhea; by common infectious complaints such as fever, sore throat, or rash; or by respiratory complaints such as cough, increased work of breathing, or chest pain (Tables 78.2 and 78.3).

The appearance of the vomitus (by history and inspection when a specimen is available) is often helpful in establishing the site of pathology. Undigested food or milk should suggest reflux from the esophagus or stomach caused by lesions such as esophageal atresia (in the neonate), gastroesophageal (GE) reflux, or pyloric stenosis. Bilious vomitus suggests obstruction distal to the ampulla of Vater, although it occasionally is seen with prolonged vomiting of any cause when the pylorus is relaxed. Fecal material in the vomitus is seen with obstruction of the lower bowel. Hematemesis usually reflects a bleeding site in the upper GI tract; its evaluation is detailed in Chapter 29.

Physical Examination

The physical examination is directed first toward evaluating the overall degree of toxicity. Does the baby look septic? Is there the inconsolable irritability of meningitis? Are there signs of life-threatening dehydration or concern for symptomatic hypoglycemia? Does the child exhibit the bent-over posture, apprehensive look, and pained avoidance of unnecessary

TABLE 78.1

VOMITING AND REGURGITATION: PRINCIPAL CAUSES BY USUAL AGE OF ONSET AND ETIOLOGY

Newborn (Birth to 2 wk)
Normal variations
Gastroesophageal reflux (± hiatal hernia)
Esophageal stenosis, atresia
Infantile achalasia
Obstructive intestinal anomalies
  Intestinal stenosis, atresia
  Malrotation of bowel (± midgut volvulus)
  Meconium ileus (cystic fibrosis)
  Meconium plug
  Hirschsprung's disease
  Imperforate anus
  Enteric duplications
Other gastrointestinal causes
  Necrotizing enterocolitis
  Cow's milk allergy
  Lactobezoar
  Gastrointestinal perforation with secondary peritonitis
Neurologic
  Subdural hematoma
  Hydrocephalus
  Cerebral edema
  Kernicterus
Renal
  Obstructive uropathy
  Renal insufficiency
Infectious
  Meningitis
  Sepsis
Metabolic
  Inborn errors of urea cycle; amino acid, organic acid, and carbohydrate metabolism (phenylketonuria, galactosemia)
  Congenital adrenal hyperplasia

Older Infant (2 wk to 12 mo)
Normal variations
Gastroesophageal reflux
Acquired esophageal disorders (corrosive esophagitis ± stricture, foreign bodies, retroesophageal abscess)
Rumination
Gastrointestinal obstruction
  Bezoars, foreign bodies
  Pyloric stenosis
  Malrotation (with or without volvulus)
  Enteric duplications
  Meckel's diverticulum (complications of)

Intussusception
Ascariasis
Incarcerated hernia
Hirschsprung's disease
Other gastrointestinal causes
  Gastroenteritis
  Celiac disease
  Peritonitis
  Paralytic ileus
Neurologic
  Brain tumors
  Other intracranial mass lesions
  Cerebral edema
  Hydrocephalus
Renal
  Obstructive uropathy
  Renal insufficiency
Infectious
  Meningitis
  Sepsis
  Urinary tract infection
  Otitis media
  Pertussis
  Hepatitis
Metabolic
  Metabolic acidosis (inborn errors of amino acid and organic acid metabolism, renal tubular acidosis)
  Galactosemia
  Fructose intolerance
  Adrenal insufficiency
Drug overdose
  Aspirin
  Theophylline
  Digoxin
Respiratory (posttussive)
  Reactive airways disease
  Respiratory infection
  Foreign body (FB)

Older Child (Older than 12 mo)
Gastrointestinal obstruction
  Acquired esophageal strictures
  Foreign bodies, bezoars
  Peptic ulcer disease
  Posttraumatic intramural hematoma
  Malrotation (with or without volvulus)
  Meckel's diverticulum (complications of)
  Meconium ileus equivalent (cystic fibrosis)
  Ascariasis
  Incarcerated hernia

Adhesions (postsurgical, peritonitis)
Intussusception
Hirschsprung's disease
Superior mesenteric artery syndrome
Other gastrointestinal causes
  Gastroenteritis, gastritis, duodenitis
  Gastroesophageal reflux
  Appendicitis
  Peptic ulcer disease
  Pancreatitis
  Peritonitis
  Paralytic ileus
  Crohn's disease
Neurologic
  Brain tumors
  Other intracranial mass lesions
  Cerebral edema
  Migraine
  Motion sickness
  Postconcussion syndrome
  Seizures
Renal
  Obstructive uropathy
  Renal insufficiency/renal tubular acidosis
Infectious
  Meningitis
  Urinary tract infection
  Hepatitis
  Upper respiratory infection (postnasal mucous drip)
Metabolic
  Diabetic ketoacidosis
  Reye's syndrome
  Adrenal insufficiency
  Inborn error of metabolism (urea cycle or fatty acid oxidation defect; acute, intermittent porphyria)
Toxins and drugs
  Aspirin
  Ipecac
  Theophylline
  Digoxin
  Iron
  Lead (chronic)
Respiratory (posttussive)
  Asthma exacerbation
  Infectious respiratory disease
  FB
Other
  Pregnancy
  Psychogenic
  Cyclic vomiting

movement typical of peritoneal irritation in appendicitis? Next, attention is aimed at the abdomen. Are there signs of obstruction such as ill-defined tenderness, distension, high-pitched bowel sounds (or absent sounds in ileus), or visible peristalsis? A complete physical examination must include a search for signs of neurologic, infectious, toxic/metabolic, and

genitourinary causes, as well as an evaluation of hydration status (see Chapter 17).

The diverse nature of causes for vomiting makes a "routine" laboratory or radiologic screen impossible. The history and physical examination must guide the approach in individual patients. Some well-defined clinical pictures demand urgent

TABLE 78.2

LIFE-THREATENING CAUSES OF VOMITING

Newborn (Birth to 2 wk)
Anatomic anomalies—esophageal stenosis/atresia; intestinal obstructions (Table 78.1), especially malrotation and volvulus; Hirschsprung's disease
Other gastrointestinal (GI) causes
Necrotizing enterocolitis
Peritonitis
Neurologic—kernicterus, mass lesions, hydrocephalus
Renal—obstructive anomalies, uremia
Infectious—sepsis, meningitis
Metabolism—inborn errors, especially congenital adrenal hyperplasia

Older Infant (2 wk to 12 mo)
Gastroesophageal reflux, severe
Esophageal disorders
Rumination
Intestinal obstruction (Table 78.1), especially pyloric stenosis, intussusception, incarcerated hernia, malrotation with volvulus
Other GI causes, especially gastroenteritis (with dehydration)
Neurologic—mass lesions, hydrocephalus
Renal—obstruction, uremia
Infectious—sepsis, meningitis, pertusis
Metabolic—inborn errors
Drugs—aspirin, theophylline, digoxin

Older Child (Older than 12 mo)
GI obstruction, especially intussusception (Table 78.1)
Other GI causes, especially appendicitis, peptic ulcer disease
Neurologic—mass lesions
Renal—uremia
Infectious—meningitis, sepsis
Metabolic—diabetic ketoacidosis, Reye's syndrome, adrenal insufficiency, inborn errors of metabolism
Toxins, drugs—aspirin, ipecac, theophylline, digoxin, iron, lead

TABLE 78.3

COMMON CAUSES OF VOMITING

Newborn (Birth to 2 wk)
Normal variations ("spitting up")
Gastroesophageal reflux
Gastrointestinal (GI) obstruction—congenital anomalies
Necrotizing enterocolitis (premature birth)
Infectious—meningitis, sepsis

Older Infant (2 wk to 12 mo)
Normal variations
Gastroesophageal reflux
Gastrointestinal (GI) obstruction—especially pyloric stenosis, intussusception, incarcerated hernia
Gastroenteritis
Infectious—sepsis, meningitis, urinary tract infection, otitis media
Posttussive—reactive airways disease, respiratory infection, foreign body
Drug overdose—aspirin, theophylline

Older Child (Older than 12 mo)
GI obstruction—incarcerated hernia, intussusception
Other GI causes—gastroenteritis, gastroesophageal reflux, appendicitis
Infectious—meningitis, urinary tract infection
Posttussive—asthma, infection, foreign body
Metabolic—diabetic ketoacidosis
Toxins/drugs—aspirin, theophylline, iron, lead
Pregnancy

SIGNS AND SYMPTOMS

age-related basis. An algorithm for such an approach that uses the key clinical features previously outlined is illustrated in Figure 78.1.

Neonates

A careful history should focus on the perinatal events, onset and duration of vomiting, nature of the vomitus, associated GI symptoms, and the presence of symptoms referable to other organ systems. Newborn babies with the onset of vomiting in the first days of life should always be suspect for one of the common *congenital GI anomalies* that cause obstruction, such as esophageal or intestinal atresia or web, malrotation, meconium ileus, or Hirschsprung's disease. If the vomiting is bilious, bright yellow, or green, an urgent surgical consultation is required. In most cases, a serious and possibly life-threatening mechanical obstruction may be the cause of bilious vomiting. All patients in whom the possibility of GI obstruction is entertained must have immediate flat and upright abdominal films. Other clinical features, such as toxicity, dehydration, and lethargy, usually attest to the length of time of the obstruction and its severity. Except for the later presentations of malrotation, most neonates with a congenital basis for their bowel obstruction will present during their initial nursery stay. Therefore, it is uncommon to see such babies for the first time in the ED. Neonates or infants with malrotation and volvulus may present with abdominal pain (crying, drawing up their knees, poor feeding), with evidence of obstruction (bilious emesis), or an acute abdomen (abdominal distension or rigidity). The diagnosis of malrotation is confirmed by the abnormal

radiologic workup. For example, abdominal pain and bilious vomiting in a child requires supine and upright plain films, as well as a limited upper GI series for evaluation of congenital obstructive anomalies such as malrotation, or a child with paroxysms of colicky abdominal pain and grossly bloody stools requires immediate flat and upright abdominal films, and usually a contrast (air or barium) enema for the likely diagnosis and reduction of intussusception. Other situations require no imaging studies (e.g., a typical case of viral gastroenteritis or a classic history for pyloric stenosis with definite palpation of the pyloric tumor). In many cases, body fluid cultures or serum chemical analyses are essential for making a diagnosis (e.g., meningitis, aspirin toxicity, Reye's syndrome, pregnancy) or for guiding management (e.g., degree of metabolic derangement in pyloric stenosis, diabetic ketoacidosis). For most straightforward, common illnesses (e.g., gastroenteritis, cold with posttussive emesis), laboratory investigation is unwarranted.

APPROACH TO CHILDREN BY AGE GROUPS

With these introductory concepts in mind, we can approach the differential diagnosis of the principal causes of vomiting on an

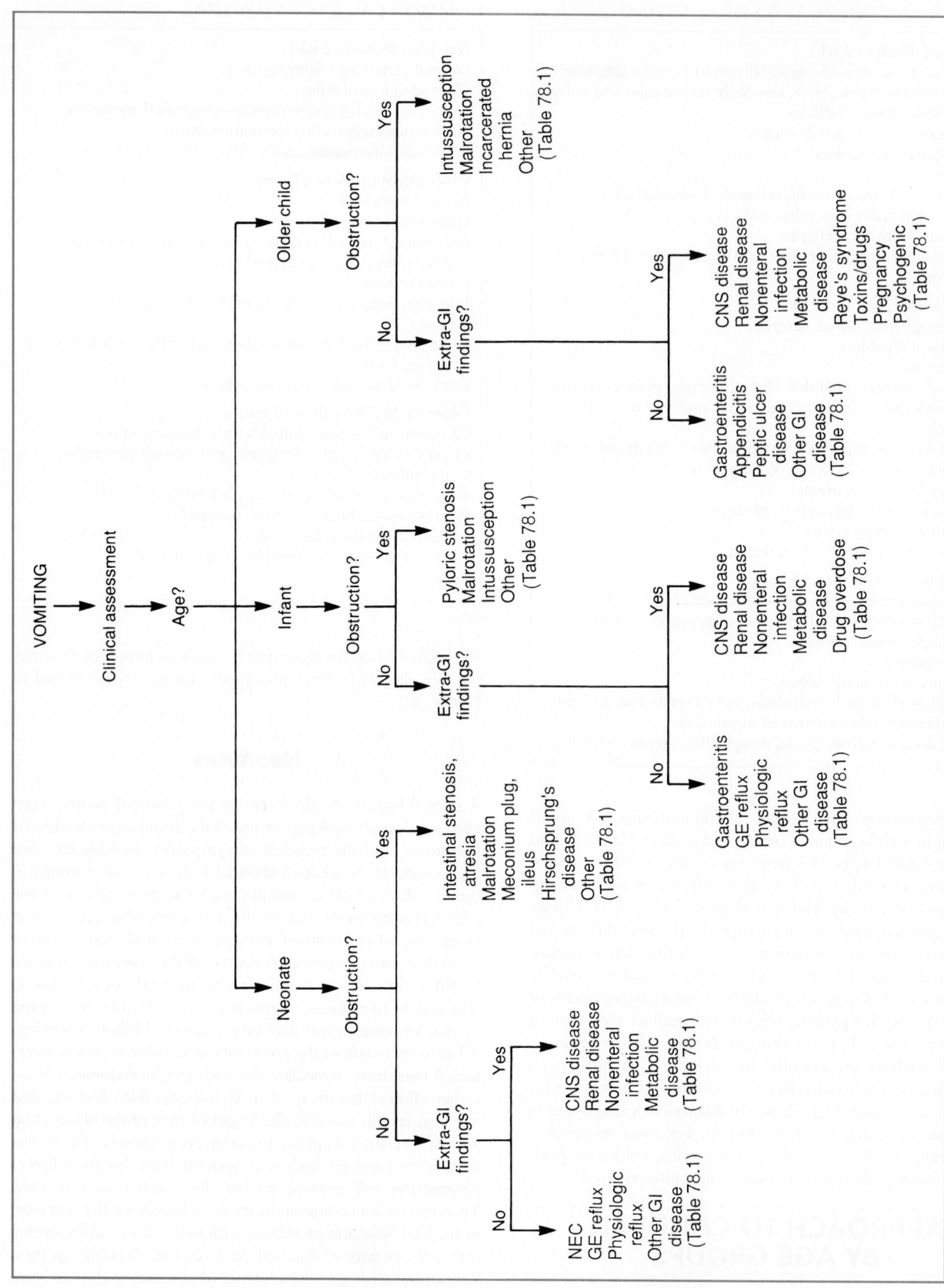

FIGURE 78.1 Differential diagnosis of vomiting. GI, gastrointestinal; NEC, necrotizing enterocolitis; GE, gastroesophageal; CNS, central nervous system.

radiographic location of the duodenal–jejunal junction (upper GI series) and/or the cecum (contrast enema).

Other serious causes of neonatal vomiting that may present to the ED include *infection*, such as meningitis, sepsis, pyelonephritis, or necrotizing enterocolitis (it should be noted that such serious infections are often not accompanied by fever in the neonate); *increased intracranial pressure* (ICP) related to cerebral edema, subdural hematoma, or hydrocephalus; *metabolic acidosis* or *hyperammonemia* caused by the rare inborn errors of amino acid and organic acid metabolism; and *renal insufficiency* or *obstruction*. Such infants usually appear ill, with associated lethargy and irritability; sometimes fever, a full fontanel, a diminished urinary stream, an abdominal mass, or respiratory signs will suggest the correct cause. Obviously, any ill neonate with vomiting, even in the absence of obstruction, also requires hospitalization and prompt evaluation for sepsis and neurologic, renal, and metabolic disease.

Commonly, however, a young infant in the first 2 to 4 weeks of life who appears entirely well is brought to the ED with the complaint of persistent vomiting. The birth history and perinatal course are unremarkable. The baby has gained weight appropriately (usually 5 to 7 oz per week after the first week of life), is vigorous, and has an entirely normal physical examination. Usually, a close description of the "vomiting" (or even better, a trial feeding in the ED) reveals the problem to be *physiologic regurgitation* or *reflux*; so-called spitting up. This is a common (nearly 20% of infants reflux) and insignificant problem, probably representing some normal variation in the developmental maturation of the lower esophageal sphincter (LES). These infants do not exhibit forceful abdominal contractions but rather reflux milk effortlessly into their mouths, which dribbles out, usually when prone, and often with a burp. The degree of reflux may be increased by improper feeding techniques, such as failure to burp the baby, using nipples with holes that are too small, bottle propping, or overfeeding. Observation of a feeding trial and emphasis on good technique suffices for initial management of such babies. Like all newborns, they should be referred for ongoing pediatric care. Most babies outgrow such regurgitation by 6 to 9 months of age, and 95% have resolution of symptoms by 12 months.

Other infants who regurgitate easily may not be managed so easily. Their course may have more significant symptoms of pain, arching, and high volume and frequency of regurgitation, or it may be complicated by distal esophagitis or gastritis, failure to thrive, esophageal–peptic strictures, pulmonary disease, or rarely, apnea or near sudden infant death syndrome, or SIDS, event. Such infants are diagnosed as having *gastroesophageal reflux disease* (GERD), a more severe or pathologic degree of LES dysfunction that is much less common (1:500). Several imaging and physiologic studies may be used to confirm the diagnosis and to correlate a patient's signs and symptoms with episodes of reflux. A 24-hour intraesophageal pH probe is the most sensitive diagnostic test for GE reflux. Based on the patient's history, evaluation of delayed gastric emptying can be done by GE scintiscan, or by an upper GI series to rule out an anatomic cause for the delay. Endoscopy is used to assess suspected complications (esophagitis or stricture); esophageal manometry is primarily a research tool in this disease. Infants with GE reflux should be followed closely by a pediatrician. In uncomplicated GE reflux, reassurance, postural management, and dietary measures are usually adequate. For more severe symptoms or with complications, additional medical management includes the use of histamine H_2 antagonists (ranitidine or famotidine) or gastric acid secretion inhibition with a proton pump inhibitor (omeprazole or lansoprazole). The use of prokinetic drugs has become limited, due to the recall of cisapride for pediatric use (due to the risk of severe cardiac arrhythmias) and the adverse effects of the alternatives, metoclopramide and erythromycin (pyloric stenosis) (dystonic reactions and agitation). GERD that is resistant to vigorous medical therapy (continues to cause serious complications) may be considered for surgical fundoplication (see Chapters 89 and 121).

Older Infant

Infants who present with vomiting after the first few weeks of life may still have intestinal obstruction, but the underlying causes are somewhat different than in the neonate. The important lesions responsible for mechanical obstructions in this age group include congenital hypertrophic pyloric stenosis (HPS), malrotation, intussusception, incarcerated hernia, enteric duplications, and complications of Meckel's diverticulum. Occasionally, other anomalies that might be expected to present in the neonate, such as Hirschsprung's disease, will appear only after several weeks or months of life. In all cases, these conditions have physical findings suggestive of intestinal obstruction and are often specific for the level of obstruction. Having a high index of suspicion for both common and uncommon forms of intestinal obstruction is important to making a timely diagnosis.

The typical infant with *pyloric stenosis* (see Chapter 121) typically appears in the ED at 3 to 6 weeks of age (95% present by 3 months; rarely after 20 weeks) with a chief compliant of projectile vomiting during or shortly after a feeding. The vomiting in pyloric stenosis is typically crescendo in nature, with increasing frequency and severity over days to weeks. In contrast, vomiting caused by GE reflux tends to be relatively consistent over time; in malrotation, vomiting is sudden in onset and can be episodic. The vomitus is nonbilious, reflecting obstruction at the pylorus, and usually voluminous, nearly the entire content of the feeding. The infant may become constipated if vomiting has been of sufficient duration. On examination, an olive-size mass may be palpated (most easily after vomiting has occurred) in the right upper quadrant to the right of the midline and just above the umbilicus. Peristaltic waves may be visualized, moving from left upper to right upper quadrants, again indicating obstruction at the pylorus. Unless the infant is significantly dehydrated, the child is usually vigorous and active, although irritable because of hunger. These infants often develop hypochloremic, hypokalemic metabolic alkalosis, which should be corrected before surgery (see Chapter 100).

The diagnosis of pyloric stenosis is clinical, based on the classic history of projectile, nonbilious emesis, and examination with hyperperistalsis and palpation of a pyloric mass or "olive." Imaging studies [ultrasound (US) or upper GI series] are not necessary if the history and examination are conclusive. In more recent years, however, earlier presentations have resulted in a greater number of infants evaluated before the development of the diagnostic clinical hallmarks, and consequently, an increased reliance on imaging studies to confirm the diagnosis. Early diagnosis has been beneficial with a decrease in the proportion of patients with alkalosis, shortened hospital stay, and decreased morbidity. US has become the diagnostic modality of choice with characteristic findings in HPS of a thickened pyloric wall (greater than 3 mm) with a lengthened canal (greater than 15 mm). However, some centers have found upper GI series to be more cost-effective because of greater operator experience with the procedure, and therefore, fewer repeat studies, as well as the ability to provide information on other origins of nonbilious vomiting. Endoscopy has more recently been recommended as an adjunct test for complicated cases in which clinical examination, US, and/or upper GI series were inconclusive. Surgical pylorotomy, the standard treatment for HPS, is scheduled as soon as dehydration and metabolic derangements (if present) have been corrected. Medical management with intravenous or oral atropine has been successful in a more recent reinvestigation. Still, a larger, well-controlled trial and cost analysis would be necessary before its use is recommended in place of surgical correction.

Between 2 months and about 5 to 6 years of age, the most common cause of obstruction is *intussusception* (see Chapter 121). Most children develop this disorder between 3 months and 2 years of age; the average was 16 months old in a more recent large series. Early symptoms usually include paroxysms of colicky abdominal pain and vomiting, suggesting a GI illness. Initially, the infant may appear relatively well between attacks, but some children will fall asleep or seem prostrate at these times. Stools may be initially normal, then become positive for occult blood. Within 6 to 12 hours of onset, dark maroon blood may be passed per rectum; this blood is often mixed with mucus earning the descriptive label of "current jelly" stool. However, some infants with intussusception may present primarily with lethargy and decreased responsiveness, without striking GI symptoms (so-called neurologic or painless intussusception). Examination of the abdomen usually reveals a somewhat tender, sausage-shaped mass on the right side. The mass may be more easily appreciated by bimanual rectal and abdominal examination, and a test for occult blood may be positive in the absence of gross blood.

Recommendations for the diagnosis and treatment of suspected intussusception include supine and right-side up decubitus radiographs (decubitus to look for abnormal air-fluid levels, free air, or mass at the hepatic flexure region; supine for signs of obstruction such as dilated bowel loops, paucity of gas, or mass effect). US can also be used if experienced personnel are available. Reduction is attempted by contrast (air or liquid) enema if perforation (free air on radiograph or peritonitis) or shock is not evident. More recent success rates for reduction in pediatric centers using air- or liquid-contrast enemas have improved to the range of 80% to 90%, with some centers reporting their increased success with repeated attempts after short intervals (45 to 60 minutes). Open reduction with laparotomy is reserved for patients with perforation or shock at initial diagnosis or when enema reduction is unsuccessful.

Other important causes of obstruction in the older infant include incarcerated inguinal hernia, volvulus, Hirschsprung's disease, or complications related to Meckel's diverticulum. The presence of an incarcerated hernia will be apparent on examination. Volvulus of the bowel is virtually always associated with bilious vomiting. A good clue to the diagnosis of Hirschsprung's disease is asking, "Has your child ever had a normal (unstimulated) bowel movement?" (see Chapters 13 and 121). The obstructive complications of Meckel's diverticu-

lum include intussusception and volvulus and have similar presentations of these types of obstruction related to other causes.

The principal nonobstructive causes of vomiting in the older infant include GI, neurologic, renal, infectious, and metabolic disorders. Nonobstructive GI disturbances are probably the most common cause for vomiting in this age group. *Viral gastroenteritis*, although usually appearing predominantly as diarrhea associated with vomiting, often begins with a prodromal phase of vomiting alone (see Chapter 92). Physical findings are usually limited to ill-defined and inconsistent abdominal pain and signs of a variable degree of dehydration. Vomiting in older infants is also caused at times by persistent GE reflux, as well as by abdominal disorders uncommon in infancy, such as peptic ulcer disease or appendicitis. Occasionally, vomiting is seen in paralytic ileus related to infection (pneumonia, peritonitis) or electrolyte disorders.

Neurologic causes of vomiting in infancy also include *mass lesions* such as tumor, abscess, and intracranial hematoma (see Chapter 96), as well as *meningitis* and *encephalitis*. There may be evidence of increased ICP: increasing head circumference, bulging fontanel, and split sutures (papilledema is rarely noted during infancy). However, some brainstem tumors cause protracted vomiting by direct effect on the vomiting center without an accompanying increased ICP. Again, it is to be emphasized that meningismus is rarely seen with meningitis in infancy and that signs of increased ICP occur late (see Chapter 92). Early findings include fever, vomiting, lethargy, and irritability, especially the paradoxic irritability of increased crying with parental fondling.

Infections outside the GI and neurologic systems may cause vomiting in infants and, occasionally, in older children. Some of the more important infections are *otitis media* (OM), *urinary tract infection* (UTI), *respiratory infections*, and *viral hepatitis*. Positive physical findings on otoscopic examination are seen in OM, along with mild irritability, and often, fever (see Chapter 92). UTIs may be surprisingly devoid of localizing signs and symptoms in preschool children (see Chapter 124); nonspecific GI complaints, including vomiting and abdominal pain, fever, irritability, and anorexia, may be the only presenting symptoms. Urinalysis and culture provide the specific diagnosis. Vomiting also is a common event after the paroxysms of coughing seen in infants with pertussis (see Chapter 92). It is a common symptom in the prodromal phase of infectious hepatitis, usually preceding the onset of jaundice (see Chapter 89). Abnormal liver function tests substantiate this latter diagnosis.

Renal and *metabolic disorders* also cause vomiting in the older infant. Renal failure, renal tubular acidosis, or rarely, diabetic ketoacidosis may be seen in this age group. Hypoadrenalism, hepatic failure, Reye's syndrome, and inborn errors of metabolism such as galactosemia and fructose intolerance also may present in infancy and may have vomiting as a prominent symptom in an ill-appearing infant.

Occasionally, parental overzealous use of over-the-counter or prescribed drugs in infants will lead to *intoxication*. Drugs that often produce vomiting in excessive doses include aspirin, theophylline, and digoxin; all these intoxications are easily verified by associated signs and symptoms and specific drug levels. The problem of accidental ingestion is discussed later.

An additional rare cause of regurgitation or vomiting in infants, with onset usually at 6 to 12 months of age, is *rumination* (see Chapter 131). This severe psychiatric disorder of infancy, related to abnormal maternal–infant relationship, may progress to severe failure to thrive and to death. These infants seem to self-induce the reflux, often by gagging themselves, and often appear to partially rechew and reswallow their vomitus.

Older Child

Many of the causes of intestinal obstruction and other important GI diseases described in neonates and older infants, such as volvulus associated with malrotation, Hirschsprung's disease, a meconium ileus "equivalent" in the child with cystic fibrosis, and an incarcerated hernia, may occasionally first appear in the older child. Older children with malrotation and/or volvulus will often have a previous episodic history of vomiting or intermittent colicky abdominal pain. In addition, older children are often subjected to blunt abdominal trauma; persistent vomiting after such injury may reflect obstruction related to a duodenal intramural hematoma or ileus secondary to pancreatitis. Older children with a prior history of intraabdominal surgery may present with obstruction from adhesions as a late complication. Gastroenteritis, as in infants, continues to be the most common cause of vomiting in the older child seen in the ED. Two entities that usually occur in older children, appendicitis and peptic ulcers, are discussed here, although they occur rarely in infancy as well.

Appendicitis (see Chapter 121) in a preadolescent child classically begins with periumbilical, crampy abdominal pain and anorexia, often followed by vomiting. Then the pain shifts to the right lower quadrant and fever may develop. Younger children may deviate from this pattern by exhibiting less specific symptoms early in their illness and a more rapid progression to perforation and generalized peritonitis. As peritoneal irritation becomes well established, the child attempts to minimize any motion to the abdomen. Physical examination usually reveals localized involuntary right lower quadrant guarding and tenderness that, when mild, may be easier to elicit by asking the child to cough or to hop on one foot. In addition, there may be rebound and referred rebound tenderness along with a tender fullness high on the right during rectal examination. Atypical positions of the appendix (e.g., retrocecal, retroileal, pelvic) will be reflected in atypical areas of maximal tenderness, as well as in confusing symptoms such as diarrhea or dysuria (caused by appendiceal inflammation adjacent to colon or ureter/bladder). Pertinent laboratory findings often include leukocytosis with a left shift in the differential count, but a normal white blood cell count in an afebrile patient does not rule out appendicitis. The urinalysis is usually normal. Occasionally, in an atypical patient, abdominal radiographs may be helpful in showing a right lower quadrant fecalith, localized obstruction, a mass effect with a paucity of gas or isolated air–fluid levels in the right lower quadrant, or lumbar spine scoliosis. Appendicitis is a clinical diagnosis, but when the differential diagnosis is difficult or in early or equivocal cases (approximately one-third of patients with appendicitis have been reported to have atypical clinical findings), imaging studies can be helpful. US and computed tomography (CT) have become the modalities of choice in most centers for children in whom clinical diagnosis is not straightforward, but there is a great amount of variability in their utilization. The advantages of US include lower cost, absence of ionizing radi-

ation, and the ability to assess vascularity. It can be particularly helpful in distinguishing tuboovarian pathology or renal pathology from appendicitis. CT scan has become the imaging study of choice in adults; more recent studies show excellent sensitivity of right lower quadrant CT with rectal contrast. In children, findings of higher diagnostic accuracy with CT than US probably reflect less operator dependency. In the case of appendicitis with complications such as perforation or abscess, CT has been noted to offer better delineation of disease extent.

Vomiting as a symptom of *peptic ulcer disease* in children is usually seen in association with abdominal pain (see Chapter 93). In young children, the pain is often nonspecific and not easily related to meals. In adolescents, the pattern becomes more classically related to food or antacids, and may cause nighttime awakening and weight loss. There may be hematemesis and/or melena. The abdominal examination may be normal or reveal mild to moderate epigastric tenderness. A strong clinical suspicion of peptic ulcer disease should be confirmed with an upper GI series or endoscopy. Other inflammatory lesions of the upper GI tract (gastritis, duodenitis, and Crohn's disease) can also cause persistent vomiting.

Genitourinary causes of vomiting in the older child include UTI and obstructive urologic disease. An important additional concern in adolescent girls is early *pregnancy* (see Chapter 48). It is common for such patients to visit the ED with the chief complaint of persistent vomiting (not necessarily only in the morning) for several weeks, and often sexual activity and/or amenorrhea is initially denied. Physical findings at this stage of pregnancy may be subtle. Thus, prolonged vomiting in a postmenarchal girl should be pursued with the appropriate urine or serum gonadotropin assays (see Chapters 47 and 90).

The important extra-GI infectious diseases of the older child that cause vomiting have been discussed for the most part under the neonatal and infantile headings of this chapter. Serious infections localize symptoms more readily in this older age group. Meningitis is usually accompanied by meningismus after the age of 2 years. Lower urinary infections tend to present with dysuria, frequency, and urgency as children approach school age, and pyelonephritis with fever and lower back pain or tenderness. The toddler or school-age child also may vomit with pharyngeal irritation (pharyngitis, postnasal mucous drip) or have posttussive emesis with persistent or severe cough caused by asthma, respiratory infection, or respiratory foreign body.

Neurologic disease that causes vomiting in the older child again represents (primarily) with lesions that cause increased ICP or direct irritation of the medullary vomiting center; they usually lead to papilledema and/or abnormal neurologic findings on examination. One important exception is childhood *migraine* (see Chapter 96). Preadolescent children do not usually present with the classic migraine picture with aura, hemicranial headache, and scotomas. More often, they complain of rare but severe, poorly localized headaches accompanied by nausea and vomiting and followed by sleep. The physical examination between attacks is usually normal. Another common but minor form of vomiting on a neurologic basis (caused by labyrinthine stimulation) would be the propensity to motion sickness.

Metabolic aberrations, including hepatic, renal, and adrenal failure, may cause vomiting in the older child (as well as during infancy). *Ketoacidosis* presenting for the first time in an as yet undiagnosed diabetic occurs more commonly in older children, especially at school entrance age and later as adolescence begins (see Chapter 86). Vomiting may be the chief complaint of such children, although careful questioning usually uncovers a preceding 3- to 4-week history of polyuria, polyphagia, polydipsia, and at times, weight loss. A fruity breath odor, dehydration, hyperpnea, and varying degrees of altered sensorium are typically present, and a urinalysis and serum glucose determination confirm the diagnosis of diabetic ketoacidosis.

The other important, but now increasingly rare, cause of vomiting is *Reye's syndrome* (see Chapter 89). It is characterized by an acute metabolic encephalopathy and liver disease that presents, typically after a preceding viral illness, with severe recurrent vomiting progressing to varying stages of encephalopathy. Abnormal laboratory data in Reye's syndrome include elevated serum transaminase and ammonia, prolonged prothrombin time, and often, hypoglycemia; bilirubin is usually normal. It has been emphasized that the differential in cases meeting the criteria for Reye's syndrome include Reye's-like syndromes: inherited metabolic disorders and viral and toxic diseases. Because of the substantial morbidity and mortality of Reye's syndrome in the past, the recommendations for the substitution of acetaminophen for aspirin for antipyresis in childhood viral illnesses will most likely continue in the United States until the debate over the association of aspirin in the etiology of these syndromes is settled.

In the discussion regarding older infants, mention was made of occasional inadvertent drug overdose by parents, causing intoxication-related vomiting. In children 1 to 4 years of age, *accidental ingestion* is a common problem. Acute poisonings that cause vomiting as a prominent symptom include aspirin, theophylline, digoxin, and iron sulfate (see Chapter 102). Chronic *lead poisoning* also occurs in this pica-prone age group. Early symptoms of lead intoxication are vomiting, colicky abdominal pain, anorexia, constipation, and irritability. Tragically, many such youngsters have been diagnosed as having nonspecific gastroenteritis syndromes initially, only to return days to weeks later with frank encephalopathy, and ultimately, severe neurologic sequelae. The history of pica and lead paint exposure (peeling paint chips, especially in homes dating back to the 1940s and 1950s) should be sought in every toddler with persistent vomiting. The diagnosis of plumbism can be confirmed with elevated blood levels of lead and erythrocyte protoporphyrins (see Chapter 102).

Cyclic vomiting syndrome is described in a consensus statement as a disorder with recurrent, time-limited episodes of vomiting. It is a diagnosis of exclusion, characterized by an absence of positive laboratory, radiographic, and endoscopic testing. It is often managed by a pediatric gastroenterologist after a prolonged course of primary care and ER visits for disabling nausea and dehydration. The etiology and pathogenesis are unknown, but links with pediatric migraines have been made and postulated mechanisms include episodic dysautonomia, mitochondrial DNA mutations, and/or a heightened hypothalamic stress response.

Finally, the school-age child or adolescent may vomit on a *psychological* basis. Acutely, brief episodes of vomiting may occur with any emotionally disturbing event. Children with school phobia or other significant psychiatric problems may vomit persistently. Adolescents are at risk for self-induced vomiting in the context of the anorexia nervosa and bulimia syndromes (see Chapters 130 and 133). Before the physician attributes the vomiting to a psychological cause, however, a careful history, general examination, and complete neurologic examination are necessary to minimize the likelihood of missing any organic origin. An assessment of disturbed family dynamics, history of emotional disorders, or evidence of depression and/or anxiety during the ED interview may corroborate the suspicion of vomiting on a psychological basis and may warrant a psychiatric referral.

Suggested Readings

General

Boyle JT. *Pediatric gastrointestinal disease.* In: Walker WA, ed. *Pathophysiology, diagnosis, management.* 4th ed. Hamilton, Ontario, Canada: BC Decker, 2004.

D'Agoustino J. Common abdominal emergencies in children [review]. *Emerg Med Clin North Am* 2002;20(1):139–153.

Endo T, Minami M, Ogama T, et al. Neurochemistry and neuropharmacology of emesis–the role of serotonin [review]. *Toxicology* 2000;153(1–3):189–201.

Hasler WL. Serotonin receptor physiology: relation to emesis. *Dig Dis Sci* 1999;44(suppl 8):108S–113S.

McCollough M, Sharieff GQ. Abdominal pain in children [review]. *Pediatr Clin North Am* 2006;53(1):107–137.

Roy CC, Silverman A, Cozzetto FJ. *Pediatric clinical gastroenterology.* 4th ed. St. Louis, MO: Mosby, 1994.

Malrotation

Strousse PJ. Malrotation [review]. *Semin Roentgenol* 2008;43(1):7–14.

Gastroesophageal Reflux Disease

Cadranel S. Medical and surgical therapies for GERD. *J Pediatr Gastroenterol Nutr* 2001;32(suppl 1):S19–S20.

Colleti RB, DiLorenzo C. Overview of pediatric gastroesophageal reflux disease and proton pump inhibitor therapy. *J Pediatr Gastoenterol Nutr* 2003;37 (suppl 1):S7–S11.

Guimaraev EV, Marguel C, Camargos PA. Treatment of gastroesophageal reflux disease [review]. *J Pediatr* 2006;82(5 suppl):S133–S145.

Micheal S. Gastroesophageal reflux [review]. *Pediatr Rev* 2007;28(3):101–110.

Vandenplas Y, Salvatore S, Vieira MC, et al. Will esophageal impedance replace pH monitoring? [review]. *Pediatrics* 2007;119(1):118–122.

Pyloric Stenosis

Hernan Z, Schulman M. Infantile hypertrophic pyloric stenosis [review]. *Radiology* 2003;227(2):319–31.

Letton RW Jr. Pyloric Stenosis [review]. *Pediatr Ann* 2001;30(12):745–750.

MacMahon B. The continuing enigma of pyloric stenosis of infancy; a review. *Epidemiology* 2006;17(2):195–201.

Intussusception

Applegate KE. Intussusception in children: imaging choices. *Semin Roentgenol* 2008;43(1):15–21.

Ein SH, Alton D, Palder SB, et al. Intussusception in the 1990s: has 25 years made a difference? *Pediatr Surg Int* 1997;12:374–376.

Ko HS, Schenk JP, Tröger J, et al. Current radiological management of intussusception in children [review]. *Eur Radiol* 2007;17(9):2411–2421.

Appendicitis

Bundy DG, Byerley JS, Liles EA, et al. Does this child have appendicitis? *JAMA* 2007;298(4):438–451.

Hale DA, Molloy M, Pearl RH, et al. Appendectomy: a contemporary appraisal [review]. *Ann Surg* 1997;225(3):252–261.

Klein MD. Clinical approach to a child with abdominal pain who might have appendicitis [review]. *Pediatr Radiol* 2007;37(1):11–14.

Sivit CJ, Siegel MJ, Applegate KE, et al. When appendicitis is suspected in children [review]. *Radiographics* 2001;21(1):247–262.

Imaging

Gupta H, Dupuy DE. Advances in imaging of the acute abdomen [review]. *Surg Clin North Am* 1997;77(6):1245–1263.

Strousse PS. Sonographic evaluation of the child with lower abdominal or pelvic pain [review]. *Radiol Clin North Am* 2006;44(6):911–23.

Vasavada P. Ultrasound evaluation of acute abdominal emergencies in infants and children [review]. *Radiol Clin North Am* 2004;42(2):445–56.

Reye's Syndrome

Casteels-Van Daele M, Van Geet C, Wouters K, et al. Reye syndrome revisited: a descriptive term covering a group of heterogeneous disorders. *Eur J Pediatr* 2000;159(9):641–648.

Schror K. Aspirin and Reye syndrome: a review of the evidence. *Paediatr Drug* 2007;9(3):195–206.

Gastroenteritis and Ondansetron

Alhashimi D, Alhashimi H, Fedorowicz Z. Antiemetics for reducing vomiting related to acute gastroenteritis in children and adolescents. *Cochrane Database Syst Rev* 2006, Issue 3. Art. No. CD005506. DOI: 10.1002/14651858.CD005506.pub4.

Cubeddu LX, Trujillo LM, Talmecin I, et al. Antiemetic activity of ondansetron in acute gastroenteritis. *Aliment Pharmacol Ther* 1997;11:185–191.

DeCamp LR, Byerley JS, Doshi N, et al. Use of antiemetic agents in acute gastroenteritis: a systematic review and meta-analysis. *Arch Pediatr Adolesc Med* 2008;162(9):858–865.

Freedman SB, Adler M, Seshadri R, et al. Oral ondansetron for gastroenteritis in a pediatric emergency department. *N Engl J Med* 2006;354(16):1698–1705.

Reeves JJ, Shannon MW, Fleisher GR. Ondansetron decreases vomiting associated with acute gastroenteritis: a randomized, controlled trial. *Pediatrics* 2002;109(4):e62. Available at: www.pediatrics.org/cgi/content/full/109/4/e62.

SIGNS AND SYMPTOMS

CHAPTER 79 ■ WEAKNESS

NICHOLAS TSAROUHAS, MD, AND JOANNE M. DECKER,[†] MD

Weakness is defined as an inability to generate normal voluntary force in a muscle or normal voluntary torque about a joint. Although often associated, *hypotonia* is not always synonymous with weakness. Neurologists define hypotonia as decreased resistance to "passive" motion. Not all hypotonic patients are weak; for example, a patient with Down Syndrome may have normal strength (i.e., not weak), yet have decreased tone on physical examination.

PATHOPHYSIOLOGY

Weakness is a reflection of a disease process that may involve any component of the motor neuron unit. These diseases are classically categorized as upper or lower motor unit disorders (Table 79.1). Upper motor neuron disease affects structures extending from the motor strip of the cerebral cortex, through the corticospinal tracts of the spinal cord, to (but not including) the anterior horn cell. Although upper motor neuron disease is generally characterized by increased deep tendon reflexes (DTRs) and spasticity, early in the clinical course there may be flaccid paralysis. Lower motor neuron disease may involve the anterior horn cell, the peripheral nerves, the *neuromuscular junction* (NMJ), or the muscle fibers. In general, it is associated with hyporeflexia, fasciculations, muscle atrophy, weakness, and hypotonia.

DIFFERENTIAL DIAGNOSIS

The *cerebral cortex* can be damaged by *cerebrovascular accidents* (CVAs), which include *cerebral infarctions* and *hemorrhages*. CVAs, while rare (2.1 to 13.1 per 100,000 children per year), cause some of the most catastrophic cases of weakness (Table 79.2). These children usually present with sudden weakness that is most commonly unilateral or asymmetric.

Cerebral hemorrhage is usually due to a *ruptured arteriovenous malformation* (AVM) but may also be caused by a *ruptured aneurysm*. Most AVMs are asymptomatic until rupture, but some children do complain of periodic "migraine-like" headaches. *Brain tumor hemorrhage* may also present acutely as weakness, severe headache, and vomiting.

Cerebral infarctions usually occur in the setting of predisposing factors, which include sickle cell disease, homocystinuria, and hypercoagulable states from antithrombin III, protein C and S deficiencies, and factor V Leiden mutations. Other more common hypercoagulable states include pregnancy, malignancy, infections, or severe dehydration. Substance abuse with

cocaine or amphetamines has also been associated with cerebral infarction. *Embolic* causes should be considered in patients with congenital heart disease, mitral valve prolapse, or a history of rheumatic fever.

Transient ischemic attacks (TIAs) often present with resolving weakness. TIAs are defined as transient neurologic deficits referable to a cerebral artery territory in a child whose MRI shows no acute ischemia, but whose history/work-up suggests cerebrovascular disease. Transient focal deficits are common after the cessation of a seizure. This *Todd's postictal paralysis* almost always resolves within minutes to hours after a seizure has ended. It is most important to ensure an intracranial hemorrhage or other mass lesion is not the cause of the focal weakness, however. A head computed tomography (CT) scan is indicated in cases of prolonged postictal paralysis, especially if the mental status remains impaired, or if other focal deficits persist.

Traumatic injuries may seriously damage or compress the spinal cord. *Spinal cord concussion* is defined as a transitory disturbance in spinal cord function secondary to a direct blow to the back. Symptoms may include flaccid paraplegia or quadriplegia, a sensory level at the site of injury, loss of tendon reflexes, and urinary retention. Recovery usually begins within a few hours and is usually complete within a week. *Spinal epidural hematoma* may cause spinal cord compression as the hematoma expands. Emergent magnetic resonance imaging (MRI) scanning is indicated when an epidural hematoma is suspected. Other traumatic injuries include vertebral body compression fractures, dislocations, and spinal cord transections.

Another serious cause of spinal cord compression is *epidural abscess*, which is usually caused by hematogenous spread of bacteria, most commonly *Staphylococcus aureus*, or by direct spread from an adjacent carbuncle or vertebral osteomyelitis. Patients commonly present with fever and back pain, but also headache, vomiting, stiff neck, and bowel and bladder dysfunction. Point tenderness may be elicited over the affected area. The diagnosis is confirmed by MRI, which helps also to distinguish the abscess from a *vertebral discitis*. Similarly, spinal cord tumors are another important cause of spinal cord compression.

Transverse myelitis is an acute demyelinating disorder of the spinal cord. It is frequently attributed to a preceding viral infection, but also may be immune mediated. It presents as an acute episode of fever and back pain at the level of cord involvement. Leg paresthesias and weakness evolve rapidly over the course of 2 days. Asymmetric leg weakness is common. Tendon reflexes may be increased or reduced. Bowel and bladder continence are often lost. The level of myelitis is usually thoracic and is demarcated by a sensory loss. MRI of the spine is required to exclude cord compression.

[†]Deceased.

TABLE 79.1

DIFFERENTIAL DIAGNOSIS OF WEAKNESS

Upper motor unit disorders	Lower motor unit disorders
Cerebral Cortex	**Anterior Horn Cell**
Cerebrovascular infarction	Poliomyelitis
Cerebrovascular hemorrhage	Postasthmatic amyotrophy
■ Ruptured arteriovenous malformation	Spinal muscular atrophy
■ Ruptured aneurysm	Amyotrophic lateral sclerosis
Brain tumor hemorrhage	
Cerebral embolism	**Peripheral Nerve**
Transient ischemic attack	Guillain-Barré syndrome
Todd's postictal paralysis	Erb's/Klumpke's palsy
Amyotrophic lateral sclerosis	Heavy metal poisoning
	Pharmacologic medicines
Spinal Cord	Marine toxins
Trauma	Acute intermittent porphyria
■ Cord concussion	
■ Epidural hematoma	**Neuromuscular Junction**
■ Fracture	Botulism
■ Dislocation	Myasthenia gravis
■ Transection	Tick paralysis
Epidural abscess	Organophosphates
Diskitis	Neuromuscular blockers
Spinal cord tumor	
Transverse myelitis	**Muscle**
Anatomic	Muscular dystrophy
■ Atlantoaxial dislocations	Myotonic dystrophy
■ Chiari malformations	Dermatomyositis
■ Tethered spinal cord	Infectious
Amyotrophic lateral sclerosis	■ Pyomyositis
	■ Viral myositis
Miscellaneous disorders	■ Trichinosis
Benign congenital hypotonia	Metabolic abnormalities
Alternating hemiplegia	Periodic paralysis
Acute hemiplegic migraine	Rhabdomyolysis/myoglobinuria
Critical illness neuromuscular disease	Inborn errors of metabolism
Conversion disorder/malingering	Endocrine disorders
	Steroid myopathy

SIGNS AND SYMPTOMS

Anatomic anomalies of the spine and spinal cord associated with weakness also include the *atlantoaxial dislocations* associated with Klippel-Feil and Down Syndrome. Patients with *Chiari malformations/myelomeningoceles* also have weakness (as well as other deficits). In the growing child, a *tethered spinal cord* may cause weakness and neurologic deficits as the tether causes the spinal cord to stretch. Clumsiness may be the presenting symptom of leg weakness. Bladder control problems are also common.

TABLE 79.2

LIFE-THREATENING CAUSES OF WEAKNESS

Cerebrovascular accident
Brain tumor hemorrhage
Epidural hemorrhage/abscess
Heavy metal/organophosphate poisoning
Myoglobinuria/rhabdomyolysis
Guillain-Barré syndrome
Myasthenia gravis
Botulism
Tick paralysis

Juvenile amyotrophic lateral sclerosis (ALS) is a rare hereditary disorder involving upper and lower motor neurons. Similar to "adult" ALS, or Lou Gehrig's disease, it causes spasticity and muscular atrophy. The course is progressive and is ultimately fatal.

Anterior horn cell disease affects the most proximal component of the lower motor neuron unit. Because these diseases affect the motor neurons, sensory function is normal. Reflexes are generally lost early in the course of the disease. Ultimately, muscle atrophy and fasciculations develop. Cranial nerve nuclei are often affected as well.

Poliomyelitis is the classic example of an anterior horn cell disease. Poliovirus is a neurotropic inhabitant of the intestinal tract that produces paralytic diseases by destroying the motor neurons of the brainstem and spinal cord. Initial symptoms include fever, sore throat, and malaise. There appears to be a transient improvement, then fever recurs, with headache, vomiting, and meningeal signs. Extremity and back pain often lead to weakness and paralysis. Usually the weakness is asymmetric, with one limb most affected. Bulbar involvement may lead to compromise of respiratory, autonomic, and circulatory centers of the brainstem, as well as weakness of the muscles of respiration and swallowing.

Fortunately, widespread immunization has virtually eradicated polio from the United States.

A peculiar entity that mimics poliomyelitis is idiopathic *postasthmatic amyotrophy*, or Hopkins syndrome. It presents as a sudden onset of weakness, generally 1 to 2 weeks after an acute asthma attack. Like polio, prognosis is poor, with all patients left with some degree of permanent paralysis.

The three pediatric types of *spinal muscular atrophy* (SMA) comprise a group of autosomal recessive genetic disorders in which the anterior horn cells in the spinal cord and motor nuclei of the brainstem are progressively lost. There is widespread muscle denervation and atrophy. The weakness in SMA may present from birth to adulthood. The weakness is usually a symmetric, progressive, proximal weakness. Cardiac and smooth muscle is usually spared. Bulbar involvement becomes evident as the disease progresses. Late in the course, atrophy and fasciculations of the tongue are seen. DTRs are reduced or absent. There is no sensory loss, intellectual retardation, or sphincter disturbance.

Spinal muscular atrophy I (acute infantile SMA, or Werdnig-Hoffman disease) is the most severe form of SMA. The weakness and severe generalized hypotonia begin before 6 months of age. These patients can never sit alone. Death often occurs by 4 years of age, usually from overwhelming pneumonia. *Spinal muscular atrophy II* (chronic infantile SMA) usually has its onset of weakness between 6 and 18 months. These patients can sit alone, but can never walk. In this "intermediate" SMA, survival to adulthood is expected. *Spinal muscular atrophy III* (mild juvenile SMA, or Kugelberg-Welander disease) usually presents with weakness after 18 months. Many present in late childhood or adolescence. This is the mildest form of the SMAs, as these patients can walk without support.

Neuropathies (primary disorders of the axon or its myelin sheath) usually present as progressive symmetric distal weakness. Weakness and sensory loss may move in a "glove and stocking" fashion. Tendon reflexes are usually lost early. Dysesthesias ("pins and needles" or burning sensations) usually occur in acquired conditions.

Guillain-Barré syndrome (GBS; acute inflammatory demyelinating polyradiculoneuropathy) is the classic acquired immunologic neuropathic disorder. It is the most common cause of acute motor paralysis in children. GBS occurs when activated immune mechanisms, induced by an antecedent viral infection, trigger inflammation and demyelination (see Chapter 96). Many viruses have been implicated including adenovirus, Epstein-Barr virus, cytomegalovirus, human immunodeficiency virus, varicella-zoster virus, measles virus, Rubulavirus (mumps), and vaccinia virus. *Mycoplasma pneumoniae* and *Campylobacter jejuni* infections, as well as some vaccines (i.e. swine flu 1976), have also been implicated.

The most common complaint is weakness, but patients also present with leg and back pain, and in younger children, an abnormal gait. The weakness is usually symmetric and may be ascending or descending. There is often a sensory loss, as well as loss of position and vibratory sense. DTRs are diminished or absent in the weak muscles. Bowel and bladder incontinence, autonomic dysfunction (hypotension), and cardiac dysrhythmias also occur.

Respiratory paralysis occurs in 20% to 30%. Cranial nerve involvement is seen in 30% to 40% of patients, usually manifested by facial weakness or ocular paresis. The Miller Fisher variant of GBS includes the triad of ataxia, areflexia, and ophthalmoplegia. Symptoms of GBS may progress for days to weeks.

Required clinical criteria for diagnosis include a progressive motor weakness of more than one limb and areflexia. Examination of the cerebrospinal fluid demonstrates an elevated protein without pleocytosis (albuminocytologic dissociation). Important diseases to consider in the differential diagnosis include acute cerebellar ataxia, transverse myelitis, toxic neuropathy, tick paralysis, botulism, myasthenia gravis (MG), and acute viral myositis. A chronic form of GBS, chronic inflammatory demyelinating polyradiculoneuropathy, also exists.

Birth trauma may produce traction injuries to the nerve roots causing a restricted pattern of focal weakness. *Erb's palsy*, a proximal (C5/C6) brachial plexus palsy, is the most common brachial plexus injury. These infants assume the "waiter's tip" posture: arm adducted, humerus internally rotated, elbow extended, forearm pronated, wrist flexed. A *Klumpke's palsy*, an injury to the lower trunk (C8/T1) of the plexus, is much rarer. Flaccid weakness of the arms and legs may result from excessive traction on the spinal cord during a difficult delivery.

Heavy metals, such as lead, mercury, arsenic, and thallium, are known neuropathic toxins. Lead, in particular, may cause a distal motor weakness with foot and wrist drop. Drug-induced neuropathies occur with drugs of abuse, as well as pharmacologic medicines. Several antimicrobials (isoniazid, nitrofurantoin, and zidovudine), as well as antineoplastics (vincristine, vinblastine, cytosine arabinoside, and cisplatin), are known to cause paresthesias and muscle weakness. The seas also harbor deadly neurotoxins. Ciguatera and paralytic shellfish poisoning are caused when toxin-elaborating dinoflagellates are ingested by fish or shellfish, which are then eaten by unsuspecting humans. Cone snail stings, blue-ringed octopus bites, sea snake bites, and puffer fish ingestion may also result in life-threatening paralysis.

Acute intermittent porphyria is an autosomal dominant inborn error of metabolism that usually presents after puberty with severe abdominal pain and is accompanied by central and peripheral neuropathies. Motor weakness is more common than sensory symptoms, and the proximal muscles are more affected than the distal musculature. Autonomic dysfunction and mental status changes also occur. Many medications, such as griseofulvin, barbiturates, sulfonamides, and estrogens, are known to trigger attacks. Alcohol has also been implicated in initiating these attacks.

Diseases of the NMJ can be recognized by their cranial nerve abnormalities and autonomic dysfunction. Importantly, sensory function is unaffected. In botulism, *Clostridium botulinum*, a gram-positive anaerobe, produces several potent neurotoxins that prevent presynaptic release of acetylcholine at the NMJ, resulting in descending flaccid paralysis. Preformed toxin may be ingested from improperly home-canned foods or any incompletely cooked food. Botulinum spores are also found in the soils of some areas of the United States, particularly in eastern Pennsylvania and California. There are three distinct clinical presentations of natural disease: infant botulism, classic botulism, and wound botulism (see Chapter 96). In addition, the potential use of botulinum toxin as a weapon of bioterrorism has been described (see Chapter 7).

In *infant botulism*, the bacterial spores are ingested, and then they germinate and colonize in the intestinal tract, leading to in vivo toxin production. Infant botulism has been linked to

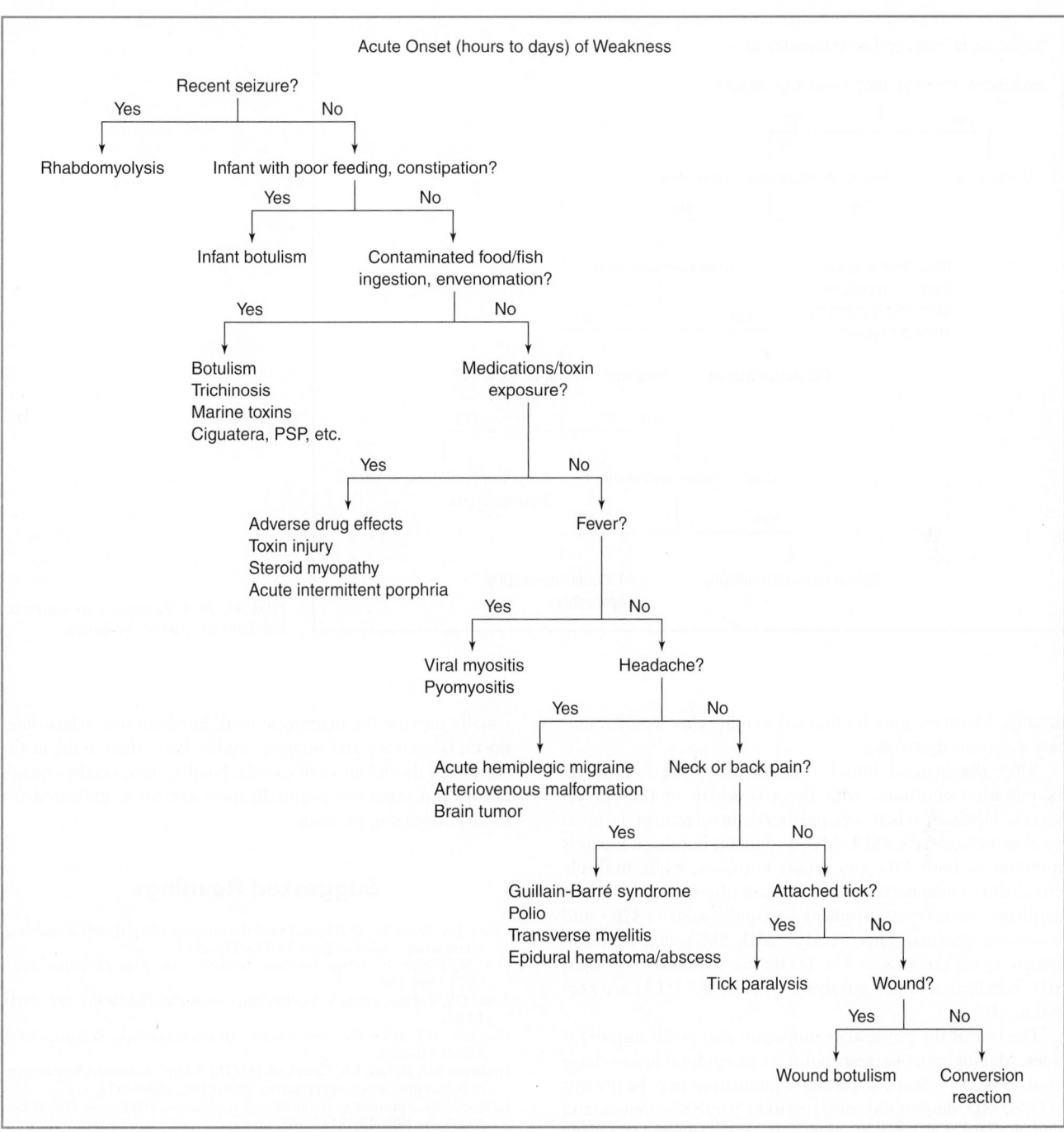

FIGURE 79.3 Approach to acute onset of weakness. PSP; paralytic shellfish poisoning.

TABLE 79.6

GRADING SCALE OF MUSCLE WEAKNESS

0	No movement
1	Trace movement
2	Movement in a horizontal plane but not against gravity
3	Movement against gravity but not against resistance
4	Weak strength against resistance
5	Full strength against resistance

be valuable for identifying patients with bulbar muscle compromise and for monitoring these children during times of decompensation.

Inspection of the muscles should be carried out for the atrophy and fasciculations common in lower motor neuron diseases, such as SMA. Hypertrophy and large "doughy" muscles suggest the muscular dystrophies. Muscle tenderness suggests inflammation or infection, such as would be found with a bacterial pyomyositis or a viral myositis. Focal tenderness of the back may be a clue to an epidural abscess or transverse

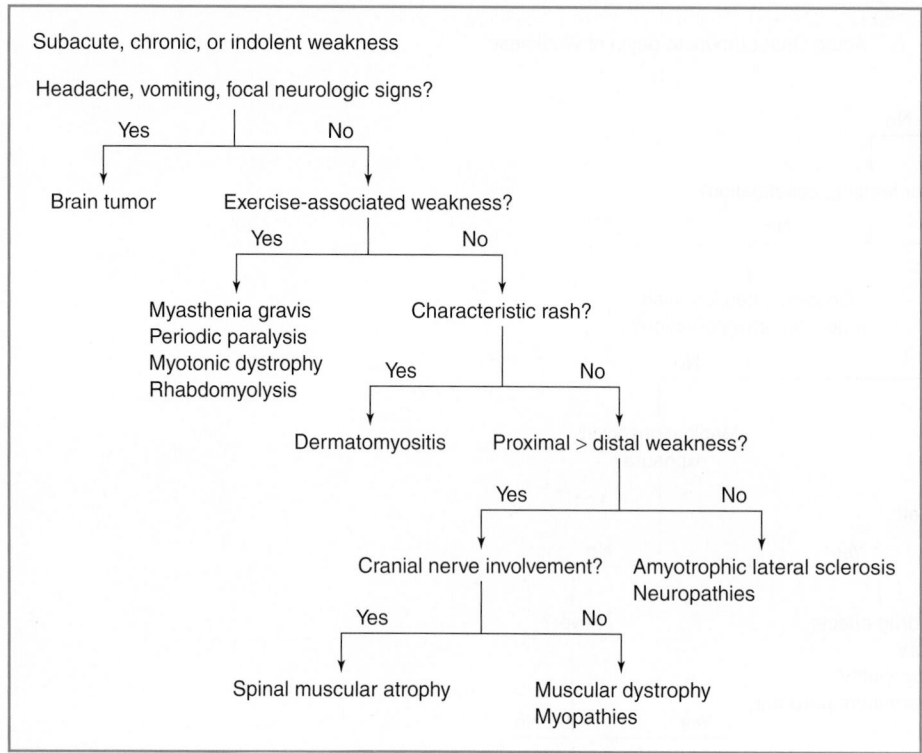

FIGURE 79.4 Approach to subacute, indolent, or chronic weakness.

myelitis. Myotonic muscles that fail to fully relax would implicate myotonic dystrophy.

After the general muscle examination, the neurologic examination continues with the assessment of the cranial nerves. Diseases where cranial nerve involvement is most notable include GBS, SMA, MG, and infant botulism. Ptosis is common to both MG and infant botulism, while multiple prominent cranial nerve palsies are most often seen with infant botulism. Sensory involvement is usually seen in GBS and transverse myelitis, whereas MG, MD, SMA, and botulism usually spare the senses. The DTRs are diminished in GBS, MD, botulism, and tick paralysis, whereas the DTRs are normal in MG.

The rest of the physical examination also yields important clues. Meningismus suggests polio, or an epidural hemorrhage or abscess. An abnormal cardiac examination may be present in GBS, MD, dermatomyositis, periodic paralysis, uremia, and acid maltase deficiency (Pompe's disease). The characteristic heliotrope rash is the hallmark of dermatomyositis. Finally, when the examination is illogical or does not correspond to anatomic or physiologic principles, one should consider a conversion disorder or malingering.

In conclusion, weakness can be a vexing presenting complaint. The differential diagnosis is extensive and the disease processes complex. Although Figure 79.1 outlines a diagnostic approach, as always in emergency medicine, therapeutics should precede diagnostics when the patient is in existing or impending crisis. Patients with acute neurologic, respiratory, or circulatory compromise should have meticulous attention paid to their stabilization first. Trauma patients require adequate cervical spine immobilization to prevent further injury. Once the patient is stable, a careful history and physical will usually narrow the diagnostic field. Furthermore, select diagnostic laboratory and imaging studies may often assist in the search for the definitive diagnosis. Finally, subspecialty consultation and inpatient hospitalization are often indicated for these challenging patients.

Suggested Readings

Chung BH, Wong VC, Ip P. Spinal muscular atrophy: survival pattern and functional status. *Pediatrics* 2004;114(5):e548–e553.

Cox N, Hinkle R. Infant botulism [review]. *Am Fam Physician* 2002; 65(7):1388–1392.

Evans OB, Vedanarayanan V. Guillain-Barré syndrome. *Pediatr Rev* 1997;18(1): 10–16.

Francisco AM, Arnon SS. Clinical mimics of infant botulism. *Pediatrics* 2007; 119(4):826–828.

Hudspeth MP, Holden KR, Crawford TO. The "slurp" test: bedside evaluation of bulbar muscle fatigue. *Pediatrics* 2006;118(2):e530–e533.

Jacobson RD. Approach to the child with weakness or clumsiness. *Pediatr Clin North Am* 1998;45(1):145–168.

LoVecchio F, Jacobson S. Approach to generalized weakness and peripheral neuromuscular disease. *Emerg Med Clin North Am* 1997;15(3):605–623.

Mannix R, Tan ML, Wright R, et al. Acute pediatric rhabdomyolysis: causes and rates of renal failure. *Pediatrics* 2006;118(5):2119–2125.

Mitchell WG, Tseng-Ong L. Catastrophic presentation of infant botulism may obscure or delay diagnosis. *Pediatrics* 2005;116(3):e436–e438.

Patt HA, Feigin RD. Diagnosis and management of suspected cases of bioterrorism: a pediatric perspective [review]. *Pediatrics* 2002;109(4):685–692.

Sander HW, Hedley-White ET. A nine-year-old girl with progressive weakness and areflexia. *N Engl J Med* 2003;348(8):735–743.

Sanger TD, Chen D, Delgado MR, et al. Taskforce on Childhood Motor Disorders. Definition and classification of negative motor signs in childhood. *Pediatrics* 2006;118(5):2159–2167.

Shellhaas RA, Smith SE, O'Tool E, et al. Mimics of childhood stroke: characteristics of a prospective cohort. *Pediatrics* 2006;118(2):704–709.

Stathopulu E, Baildam E. Gower's sign in children with juvenile idiopathic arthritis. *Rheumatology* 2003;42(8):1002–1003.

Tabarki B, Coffiniéres A, Van Den Bergh P, et al. Critical illness neuromuscular disease: clinical, electrophysiological, and prognostic aspects. *Arch Dis Child.* 2002;86(2):103–107.

CHAPTER 80 ■ WHEEZING

VINCENT J. WANG, MD

Wheezes are whistling or musical adventitial sounds that are the hallmark of lower airway constriction and/or obstruction. Whereas rales or crackles are discontinuous or intermittent popping noises, wheezes are continuous sounds most frequently heard during expiration. The most common diseases causing wheezing in children are bronchiolitis and asthma, but the differential diagnosis is broad, and the causes are often multifactorial. An episode of wheezing may occur at least once in 20% of infants younger than 1 year of age, and in almost 50% of children younger than 6 years of age, but less than 15% of children will develop asthma. This chapter presents an organized approach to the diagnosis of conditions associated with wheezing in children beyond the newborn period.

PATHOPHYSIOLOGY

Obstruction to air flow is the common denominator in all conditions that produce wheezing. Wheezing usually results from obstruction of the intrathoracic lower airways (bronchioles) and less commonly by narrowing of the trachea or bronchi. Obstruction of the lower airway passages may be anatomic or physiologic and is the result of extrinsic airway compression or intrinsic airway narrowing. Intrinsic airway narrowing may be caused by bronchial or bronchiolar constriction, inflammation, and/or intraluminal airway blockage. It may also be caused by a combination of these factors simultaneously, as in asthma. When wheezing is audible during the inspiration and expiration phases of respiration, wheezing is more likely to be caused by extrinsic airway compression. In contrast, when wheezing is predominantly expiratory, intrinsic airway narrowing is more likely to be the cause. Table 80.1 provides a pathophysiologic classification of conditions that cause wheezing in children. Some of the diagnoses overlap, however.

DIFFERENTIAL DIAGNOSIS

Table 80.2 lists the life-threatening causes of wheezing, and Table 80.3 outlines the relative prevalence of conditions that may present acutely with wheezing, divided into age groups.

Common Conditions

Bronchiolitis is an acute viral infection of the lower respiratory tract caused predominantly by respiratory syncytial virus (RSV). Other causes include human metapneumovirus, parainfluenza virus, adenovirus, influenza virus, coronavirus, and rhinovirus. Occurring primarily in epidemics between November and March, bronchiolitis primarily affects infants 2 to 12 months of age but may occur in children as old as 2 to 3 years of age. Older children and adults usually have minor upper respiratory symptoms, but may also present with wheezing. Proliferation of cells and submucosal edema lead to obstruction of the bronchioles. Rhinorrhea and a low-grade fever typically accompany a prominent staccato-like cough and a variable degree of respiratory distress. The concurrence of respiratory symptoms in other family members is common. Degree of severity is multifactorial, with factors such as maternal smoking, prematurity, congenital heart disease, reactive airway disease, and others contributing to the individual patient's response to the viral infection.

Asthma is a chronic inflammatory disorder of the airways, characterized clinically by *recurrent* exacerbations involving symptoms of coughing and/or wheezing. Acute asthma attacks are usually triggered by respiratory infections, allergens, and irritants such as cigarette smoke or particulate air pollution. Patients with asthma have a higher incidence of associated atopic diseases, which include allergic rhinitis, conjunctivitis, and atopic dermatitis. Immediate family members are also more likely to be affected by asthma and atopic disease. Although many hesitate to make the diagnosis of asthma in a child younger than 2 years of age, many asthmatics had had their first episode of wheezing before this age. However, 60% of those that wheeze before 3 years of age will not wheeze by school age. In addition, it is unknown if bronchiolitis predisposes patients to develop asthma, or if the response to bronchiolitis is different for a patient who is allergy prone. Also, bronchiolitis may occur in patients who have asthma.

Less Common Conditions

Other infectious causes of wheezing include viral or bacterial pneumonia. Most cases are preceded by several days of upper respiratory tract symptoms and fever. Physical examination will usually reveal tachypnea, retractions, rales, and/or wheezes. Auscultatory findings are often localized rather than diffuse. The most common causes of pneumonia are viral, with RSV being most common, followed by human metapneumovirus, parainfluenza virus, influenza virus, and adenoviruses. Bacterial causes include *Streptococcus pneumoniae*, *Mycoplasma pneumoniae*, *Chlamydia pneumoniae*, group A *Streptococcus*, and *Staphylococcus aureus*. *S. pneumoniae* has been the most common bacterial agent, but the incidence has decreased since the widespread utilization of the conjugate pneumococcal vaccine.

TABLE 80.1

CAUSES OF WHEEZING IN CHILDHOOD

Extrinsic airway compression		**Intrinsic airway narrowing**	
Congenital structural anomalies	*Bronchial constriction*	*Inflammation*	*Intraluminal airway blockage*
Cystic malformations of the lung	Asthma	Asthma	Asthma
Vascular ring/sling	Anaphylaxis	Smoke inhalation/air pollution	Bronchiolitis
Cardiovascular enlargement	Allergic reaction	TEF	Pneumonia
	BPD/CLD	Tracheostomies	Pulmonary aspiration
Mediastinal and thoracic masses	α_1-Antitrypsin deficiency	Pneumonitis	Parasitic infections
Teratoma, lymphoma, thymoma,	Tracheobronchomalacia	GE reflux	Polyps/granulomas
thyroid carcinoma,	Bronchial or lung cyst	Swallowing disorders	Airway hemangioma
neuroblastoma,	Congenital lobar emphysema		Bronchiolitis obliterans
ganglioneuroma,	Cystic adenomatoid		Pulmonary hemorrhage
pheochromocytoma	malformation		Hemosiderosis
Mediastinal lymphadenopathy	Bronchiectasis		Bronchitis
Tuberculosis			Histoplasmosis
Sarcoidosis			

Miscellaneous Causes
Laryngeal cleft (chronic aspiration)
Pulmonary edema (congenital heart disease, congenital heart failure, hypoalbuminemia, nephrotic syndrome, pneumonia, acute
   respiratory distress syndrome, inhaled toxic agents, sepsis, drowing/near-drowning, uremia, lymphatic insufficiency, pancreatitis,
   pulmonary embolism)
Immunodeficiency (severe combined immune deficiency, combined IgA and IgG2 deficiency, B-cell deficiency)
Cystic fibrosis
Immotile cilia syndrome
Psychogenic wheezing

BPD, bronchopulmonary dysplasia; CLD, chronic lung disease; TEF, tracheoesophageal fistula; GE, gastroesophageal.

Pulmonary aspiration is a less common cause of wheezing that occurs in several fairly characteristic clinical circumstances. In otherwise healthy children, the abrupt onset of respiratory distress, associated with an episode of coughing, choking, or gagging, suggests the pulmonary aspiration of a foreign object (see Chapter 28). Foreign-body aspiration is typically seen in toddlers, although older infants may aspirate solid food particles or small objects placed within their reach. Rarely, an older child may also aspirate food particles or other objects. The aspiration of a small object or food substance may not be witnessed, and thus, may go unrecognized for weeks or months until persistent lower respiratory symptoms trigger a search for an underlying cause. In these circumstances, persistent cough, wheezing, and sometimes recurrent fever is associated with an area of consolidation and/or collapse on radiograph. These symptoms fail to resolve despite seemingly appropriate medical therapy for presumed asthma and/or pneumonia.

Recurrent aspiration of food or gastric contents is usually seen in infants younger than 1 year of age, or in older patients with severe developmental delay or neuromuscular disease. Disordered swallowing and esophageal motility, and gastroesophageal (GE) reflux, typically contribute in varying

degrees to the recurrent aspiration that occurs in these patients. Repeated aspiration is also seen in children with tracheostomies and in children with structural anomalies of the tracheolaryngeal complex or an H-type tracheoesophageal fistula. Patients with chronic recurrent aspiration may develop wheezing and respiratory distress in the absence of a well-defined episode of choking or severe coughing because many such patients have depressed cough reflexes or experience "microaspiration." Fever often accompanies pulmonary aspiration, reflecting associated chemical inflammation or infection of the tracheobronchial tree.

Wheezing attributable to an allergic reaction or anaphylaxis (rare) is also of sudden onset and may be accompanied by one or more other clinical findings that include urticaria, angioedema, stridor, and hypotension. When wheezing is the only finding, an allergic reaction or anaphylaxis may be suspected when the onset of respiratory difficulty is associated with Hymenoptera envenomation, medication, food ingestion, or another allergic precipitant. This type of wheezing typically responds promptly to epinephrine administration and/or to bronchodilator therapy.

Transient wheezing may also occur with smoking and air pollutant exposures. Adult patients who smoke cigarettes may present with wheezing. In extension, adolescents who smoke may also wheeze. Wheezing and bronchiolitis have also been associated with passive smoke exposure, and has been shown to increase with increased maternal smoking. Air pollution containing particulate matter less than or equal to 10 microns in diameter, nitrogen dioxide, nitrogen oxide, and carbon monoxide have been associated with wheezing, as well as exacerbation of other causes of wheezing.

Infants and young children with a history of prematurity, assisted ventilatory support, oxygen dependence, and chronic

TABLE 80.2

LIFE-THREATENING CAUSES OF WHEEZING

Asthma	Mediastinal tumor
Bronchiolitis	Congestive heart failure
Foreign-body aspiration	Chemical pneumonitis
Pulmonary hemorrhage	Anaphylaxis

TABLE 80.3

CLINICAL CLASSIFICATION OF WHEEZING: AGE AT DIAGNOSIS AND DISEASE PREVALENCE

Disease prevalence	<1 yr	1–3 yr	>3 yr
Common	Bronchiolitis	Bronchiolitis Asthma	Asthma
Less Common	Pulmonary aspiration GE reflux Swallowing disorders BPD/chronic lung disease Pneumonia	Pulmonary (FB) aspiration Allergic reaction Pneumonia Chronic lung disease	Pneumonia Allergic reaction Chronic lung disease Smoking/Air pollution
Rare	Congenital heart disease Immunodeficiency Cystic malformations of lung Immotile cilia syndrome TEF Cystic fibrosis Tracheobronchomalacia Vascular rings/slings Congenital lobar emphysema	Anaphylaxis Immunodeficiency Mediastinal lymphadenopathy Congenital heart disease Cystic fibrosis Sarcoidosis Parasitic infections Bronchiectasis Pulmonary edema GE Reflux	Anaphylaxis Immunodeficiency Mediastinal lymphadenopathy Bronchitis α_1-Antitrypsin deficiency Cystic fibrosis Parasitic infections Sarcoidosis Psychogenic wheezing Histoplasmosis Bronchiectasis Pulmonary aspiration Tuberculosis Allergic bronchopulmonary Aspergillosis Carcinoid syndrome Pulmonary edema

BPD, bronchopulmonary dysplasia; FB, foreign body; TEF, tracheoesophageal fistula.

SIGNS AND SYMPTOMS

radiographic changes for a variety of conditions occurring in the newborn period may have wheezing caused by bronchopulmonary dysplasia (BPD). Patients without a history of prematurity may also have chronic lung disease (CLD). CLD is the common term referring to infants and children who develop chronic respiratory problems beginning in the neonatal period. This condition is the childhood equivalent of chronic obstructive pulmonary disease and represents a pathophysiologic continuum that includes varying degrees of structural damage and airway inflammation. Although gradual improvement in lung function occurs during infancy and early childhood, bronchial hyperactivity and recurrent episodes of wheezing may persist until later in childhood. Other coexisting problems associated with prematurity such as brain damage, tracheostomy dependence, and GE reflux may complicate the respiratory pathophysiology in patients with BPD or CLD.

Even though the diagnosis of bronchitis is more commonly associated with adult patients, children may develop a nonspecific bronchial inflammation associated with various viral agents. The pathophysiology is similar to bronchiolitis and may be preceded by upper respiratory symptoms. Cough is usually prominent and may be followed by wheezing.

Rare Conditions

Cardiovascular abnormalities are one of many uncommon causes of wheezing in children. Small airway edema in the setting of congestive heart failure or airway impingement by enlarged cardiovascular structures are the usual pathophysiologic mechanism. Most cardiac conditions are associated with other abnormal physical findings, including cyanosis, murmurs, abnormal pulses, poor perfusion, or signs consistent with congestive heart failure. A congenital vascular ring or sling may cause wheezing secondary to extrinsic airway compression. Abnormal cardiac physical findings are generally absent in patients with a vascular ring/sling, although concomitant esophageal compression may result in dysphagia. A right-sided aortic arch is associated with this anomaly.

In addition to respiratory tract involvement, patients with cystic fibrosis (see Chapter 99) will often exhibit steatorrhea and failure to thrive because of pancreatic insufficiency and malabsorption. Cystic fibrosis may be included on the state's newborn screening examination, but testing is not universal, and the screening test does not have 100% sensitivity. Similar to the respiratory tract presentation of cystic fibrosis, patients with the immotile cilia syndrome also develop repeated sinusitis and otitis media, often in association with situs inversus viscerum and bronchiectasis (Kartagener's syndrome).

Wheezing may result from pulmonary edema, which may be caused by congenital heart disease and congestive heart failure. However, pulmonary edema may also be caused by other disease processes, such as pneumonia, acute respiratory distress syndrome, and hypoalbuminemic states, such as nephrotic syndrome and liver failure. Hydrocarbon aspiration, leading to a chemical pneumonitis, may also cause pulmonary edema.

Children with various defects in host defense mechanisms often present with recurrent wheezing and bacterial pulmonary infections. Children with cell-mediated or humoral immune deficiency syndromes can have opportunistic infections or repeated extrapulmonary infections, including meningitis, otitis media, otitis externa, furunculosis, and mucocutaneous candidiasis.

Other uncommon causes of wheezing include extrinsic tracheobronchial compression by an enlarged lymph node or tumor (see Chapter 97). Mediastinal or hilar lymph node enlargement may be the result of leukemia, lymphoma, histoplasmosis, sarcoidosis, or a mycobacterial or fungal infection. Mediastinal tumors that are most likely to produce pulmonary symptomatology include neuroblastoma, pheochromocytoma, ganglioneuroma, thymoma, teratoma, or thyroid carcinoma. The oncologic causes may also metastasize to the lungs and cause extrinsic compression of the airways.

Congenital structural anomalies of the respiratory tract, including bronchogenic cysts, cystic malformations of the lung, congenital lobar emphysema, intrinsic stenosis, and webs, are among the rarest causes of wheezing in children. Respiratory symptoms typically begin in the neonatal period or early infancy. The predominant clinical features will be determined by the site of abnormality within the tracheobronchial tree. Stridor and a croupy cough are typical of laryngotracheal constriction, whereas wheezing and recurrent pneumonia are more characteristic of bronchial narrowing. Respiratory findings generally worsen with intercurrent respiratory infection and may accentuate with crying and activity. Some diagnoses are discovered only with persistence of symptoms, necessitating radiographic evaluation.

Bronchiectasis is the common end result of various causes leading to this irreversible bronchial dilatation. The most common cause is cystic fibrosis, but bronchiectasis may also be caused by immotile cilia syndrome, immune deficiency syndromes, congenital causes, and infection (measles, pertussis, and tuberculosis). Cough is prominent, accompanied by purulent sputum production.

Occasionally, an adolescent patient may present with moderate to severe respiratory distress that is unresponsive to beta agonist therapy. Consideration should be given to precipitating factors and the diagnosis of psychogenic wheezing. These patients may generate wheezing noises in their larynx.

Other rare conditions are listed in Table 80.3.

EVALUATION AND DECISION

History

Thorough history-taking is the key to arriving at an accurate diagnosis in a child with wheezing. In particular, consideration of the age at onset, course and pattern of illness, and associated clinical features provide a useful framework for approaching a differential diagnosis (Figs. 80.1 and 80.2).

In patients with respiratory distress, a focused history pertaining to life-threatening causes of wheezing (Table 80.2) may be necessary based on an abbreviated version of the aforementioned figures. Such a battery of questions may resemble the following: (i) How acutely did the symptoms present? (ii) Has this occurred before? (iii) Does anyone in the family have asthma? (iv) Are there concurrent upper respiratory symptoms? (v) Was the patient choking or did he or she become cyanotic? (vi) Is there any history of cardiac disease or failure

TABLE 80.4

MAJOR CAUSES OF WHEEZING WITH ASSOCIATED CLINICAL FEATURES

Causes	Associated clinical features
Bronchiolitis	Age <3 yr. Upper respiratory symptoms November through March occurrence Concurrent upper respiratory symptoms in close contacts
Asthma	Recurrent episodes Family history of asthma History of atopy Upper respiratory symptoms Environmental trigger (weather change, etc.)
Pneumonia	Upper respiratory symptoms Fever Unilateral wheezing/rales/decreased breath sounds
Foreign-body aspiration	Age >6 mo Choking episode associated with onset of symptoms Abrupt onset or prolonged symptoms despite appropriate therapy Unilateral wheezing or decreased breath sounds Developmental delay, mental retardation History of tracheal surgery/tracheostomy Swallowing disorder, gastroesophageal reflux
Anaphylaxis	Sudden onset Accompanying urticaria, angioedema, stridor, or hypotension New exposure or Hymenoptera envenomation
Congestive heart failure/cardiac disease	History of failure to thrive Heart murmur, hepatomegaly, poor perfusion Cardiomegaly
Cystic fibrosis	History of failure to thrive Recurrent respiratory tract infections Steatorrhea

Adapted from Martinati LC, Boner AL. Clinical diagnosis of wheezing in early childhood. *Allergy* 1995;50:701–710.

to thrive? Table 80.4 reviews salient features of common disorders that cause wheezing.

The onset of wheezing in the neonatal period is associated with congenital structural airway anomalies, although a history of prematurity, mechanical ventilation, and oxygen dependence is more suggestive of BPD or CLD. The *first episode* of wheezing in an otherwise healthy infant in association with cold symptoms indicates bronchiolitis, especially if the episode occurs between November and March. Recurrent episodes of wheezing precipitated by colds and a variety of other triggers are the hallmark of asthma. However, recurrent

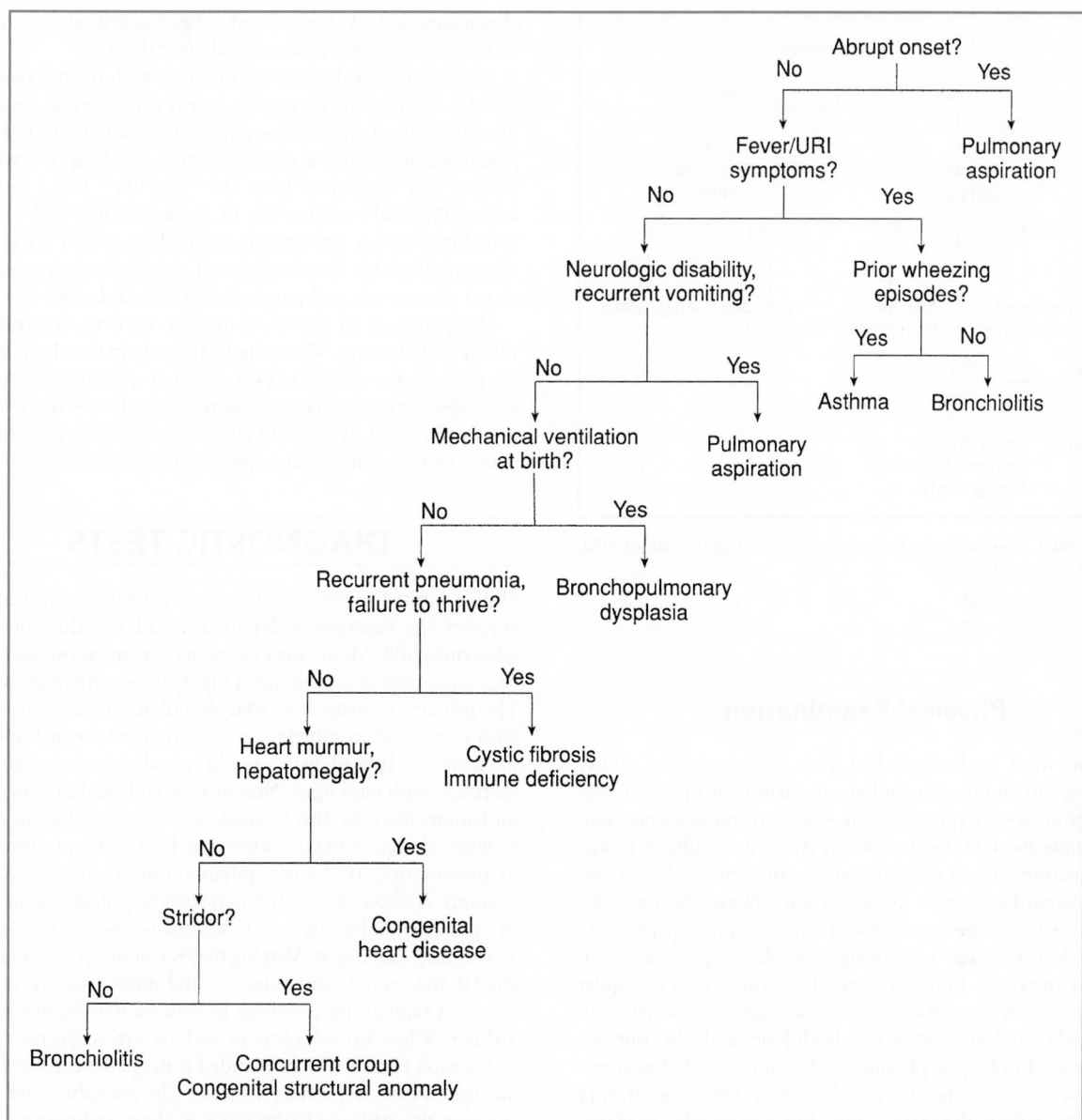

FIGURE 80.1 Approach to wheezing in children younger than 1 year. URI, upper respiratory infection.

wheezing beginning in infancy, or "difficult to control asthma" at any age, should lead to a consideration of cystic fibrosis, GE reflux, recurrent pulmonary aspiration, a retained airway foreign body, immune deficiency, and other diagnoses. Persistent wheezing at any age suggests mechanical airway obstruction from a variety of causes, including congenital airway narrowing, pulmonary foreign body, and compression by a mediastinal tumor. The sudden onset of wheezing is characteristic of pulmonary aspiration, an allergic reaction, or anaphylaxis.

As indicated previously, the diagnosis of a chronic wheezing disorder, such as asthma, relies on the identification of recurrent episodes of obstructive lower airway disease. Subtle manifestations of asthma are often misinterpreted as episodes of bronchitis, pneumonia, or bronchiolitis. Accordingly, it is often useful to ask if the child has ever had any of these or

other "breathing problems," or has ever been treated with a "breathing medicine." In a large longitudinal study from Tucson, major risk factors for asthma included eczema or a parental history of asthma, and minor risk factors included wheezing between viral illnesses, nonviral rhinitis, and eosinophilia.

Cough as a salient feature in patients with obstructive lower airway disease cannot be overemphasized (see Chapter 14). In fact, in many patients with asthma, recurrent cough may be the predominant presenting clinical feature and wheezing may be absent despite careful lung auscultation because it is characteristic of cough variant asthma. Further inquiry might reveal that a patient usually experiences severe or persistent bouts of coughing in association with colds or that coughing is the cause of recurrent nighttime awakening.

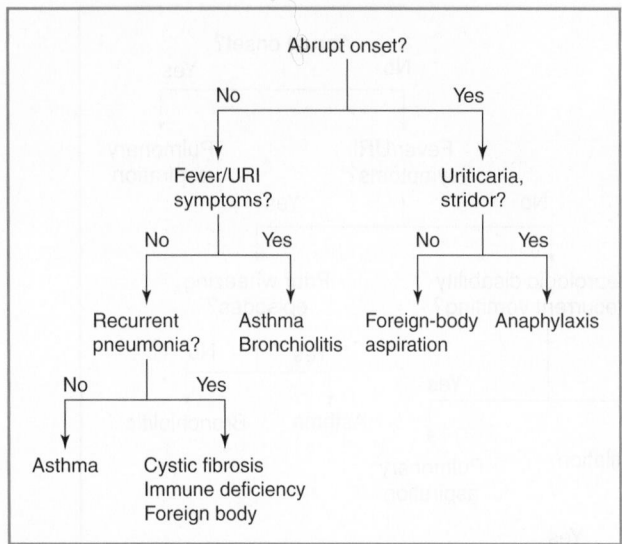

FIGURE 80.2 Approach to wheezing in children 1 year or older. URI, upper respiratory infection.

Physical Examination

Wheezing must be distinguished from other causes of "noisy breathing" in children, including the stridor of upper airway obstruction (see Chapter 72), the stertor of nasal congestion, and audible rhonchi. Because of the dynamic flexibility of airway structures, these clinical features of airway obstruction vary in accordance with the respiratory phase. Accordingly, upper airway collapse and stridor are worse on inspiration, whereas lower airway narrowing and wheezing are accentuated on expiration. Moreover, sounds originating in the upper airway passages (e.g., stridor, stertor) are transmitted with uniform quality and intensity across both lung fields. In contrast, wheezes tend to be polyphonic in pitch and distributed somewhat unevenly in intensity and location. This auscultatory asymmetry reflects the variation in airway narrowing that typically occurs from one lung segment to another. Conversely, wheezes consistently limited to a single lung field suggest a localized obstructive process, such as a foreign body, pneumonia, or an extrinsic mass lesion.

The intensity of wheezes and their pitch and duration are a function of the degree of airway narrowing and the velocity of airflow at the site(s) of obstruction. In patients with minimal airway obstruction, wheezing may be difficult to detect. When such instances are suspected, forced exhalation may reveal low-pitched wheezes limited to the end of expiration. Subtle wheezes can be accentuated further by combining forced exhalation with simultaneous manual compression applied by the examiner in the anteroposterior dimension of the chest (so-called "squeezing the wheeze").

As airway narrowing and minute ventilation increase, wheezes become louder and higher pitched. However, as airway obstruction becomes progressively more severe, airflow and wheezes will diminish proportionately. A "quiet chest" in the face of significant respiratory distress may indicate respiratory failure. Conversely, in patients with reversible bron-chospasm, air exchange and wheezes are often noted to increase in response to bronchodilator therapy.

The clinical evaluation of a patient with obstructive lower airway disease will invariably reveal a prominent cough. To the experienced clinician or parent, this cough will usually be perceived as having a characteristic whistling or "wheezy" quality that is distinct from the "seal-like" barky cough of croup. Physical examination of the wheezing child may also reveal inspiratory and expiratory crackles, which are far more often attributable to subsegmental atelectasis than to an associated pneumonia and parenchymal consolidation.

Auscultation of the neck may be used to determine the source of wheezing. Wheezing heard only in the chest, and not the neck, is more likely to be associated with intrathoracic airway obstruction, whereas wheezing heard over the neck, but not in the chest, is more likely associated with upper airway causes of wheezing, such as psychogenic wheezing.

DIAGNOSTIC TESTS

Only a limited number of diagnostic modalities are needed to support the emergency department (ED) evaluation of the wheezing child. Many other necessary investigations can be performed as part of a subsequent inpatient or outpatient workup. The primary measurement that should accompany any patient with respiratory complaints is pulse oximetry, which measures oxygenation. Indeed, many would consider this a standard measurement with vital signs. Noninvasive end-tidal carbon dioxide measurements may also be made to assess ventilation. A chest radiograph may assist in identifying disease complications such as pneumonia, atelectasis, pneumothorax, or pneumomediastinum. A chest radiograph may also help diagnose heart disease, mediastinal masses, and radiopaque foreign bodies of the airway and esophagus. Varying degrees of hyperaeration, bronchiolar thickening, and subsegmental atelectasis are the most common radiographic findings in patients with bronchiolitis or asthma. When bronchiolitis or asthma are suspected, a chest radiograph can usually be avoided if the patient is afebrile and has little to no respiratory distress. The available data do not support the utility of obtaining a chest radiograph for all patients with their first episode of wheezing.

When bronchiolitis is a suspected cause of wheezing, no further diagnostic testing is required. But in cases of uncertainty, it may be helpful to identify RSV in nasopharyngeal secretions by performing a rapid immunoassay while the patient is in the ED. The diagnosis of asthma can be supported by demonstrating improvement in clinical response or peak flow measurements after bronchodilator treatment. Other patients with asthma may benefit from formal pulmonary function evaluation or bronchial challenge testing performed at a later time.

Patients suspected of having aspirated oropharyngeal or gastric contents should have plain radiographs taken of the chest. Nonspecific findings consistent with lower airway obstruction generally precede the appearance of infiltrates. Patients believed to have recurring episodes of pulmonary aspiration subsequently should have further testing to identify swallowing dysfunction, GE reflux, or actual tracheobronchial soiling. Such inpatient or outpatient tests might include a barium esophagram, esophageal pH monitoring, esophageal endoscopy and biopsy, or radionuclide scintigraphy. Fiberoptic bronchoscopy may be required to diagnose patients with a tracheoesophageal fistula.

An immediate and aggressive workup is always justified in patients suspected of having an airway foreign body (see Chapter 28) on the basis of acute and sudden symptomatology. In this setting, chest radiographs are usually normal, although occasionally they can demonstrate a radiopaque object, the faint outline of a radiolucent foreign body, segmental atelectasis, or a focal area of hyperinflation. Patients with a persistent lower airway foreign body are more likely to show focal collapse and consolidation that is evident on standard chest roentgenograms. Bilateral decubitus views, inspiratory and expiratory radiographs, or airway fluoroscopy may be used to provide additional diagnostic information. Bronchoscopy is the procedure of choice both from a diagnostic and therapeutic perspective when a foreign body is strongly suspected.

The diagnosis of BPD or CLD is established on the basis of chronic respiratory symptoms superimposed on a background of neonatal lung disease. Nevertheless, a chest radiograph characteristically shows hyperexpansion and streaky or patchy infiltrates, punctuated by areas of alternating local hyperaeration and atelectasis. Comparison to previous radiographs is often helpful in distinguishing chronic changes from acute processes.

Newborn screening could identify most children with cystic fibrosis, but screening is dependent on the state standards. Nevertheless, infants with recurrent wheezing and those with failure to thrive associated with chronic diarrhea should be referred for sweat chloride or DNA testing.

A patient suspected of having congenital or acquired heart disease should have an electrocardiogram and a chest radiograph performed in the ED. Definitive diagnosis generally requires echocardiography. A barium swallow, computed tomography scan, or magnetic resonance imaging are usually sufficient to diagnose the presence of a vascular ring or sling, although angiography or magnetic resonance angiography may be necessary for exact anatomic definition.

APPROACH

The evaluation of a wheezing child begins with an immediate assessment of the degree of respiratory distress and consideration of the need for general supportive measures. Patients with suspected respiratory failure should be managed aggressively, as outlined in Chapters 1, 5, and 68. Clinical features suggestive of impending respiratory failure include severe respiratory distress, agitation or lethargy, dusky mucous membranes, signs of autonomic excess (tachycardia, diaphoresis, peripheral vasoconstriction), poor air movement on lung auscultation, pulse oximetry reading of less than 90%, and elevated noninvasive end-tidal carbon dioxide measurements. Blood gas analysis will also aid in the determination of respiratory failure, although this may not be necessary.

Supplemental oxygen should be offered promptly to any patient with respiratory distress and adjusted to maintain a pulse oximeter reading of 93% or greater. Higher altitude medical centers may accept lower pulse oximetry readings. In otherwise healthy children with no feeding difficulty or respiratory distress, recent American Academy of Pediatrics recommendations suggest that a pulse oximeter reading of 90% or

greater is acceptable for patients with bronchiolitis. Patients suspected of having reversible bronchospasm should be given a bronchodilator such as albuterol by inhalation, while further evaluation and management are proceeding according to the priorities established earlier in this chapter.

Expeditious management is essential in patients with poor baseline pulmonary function because they can develop respiratory failure quickly. Such patients include children with significant BPD/CLD and advanced cases of progressive chronic lung disorders such as cystic fibrosis. Moreover, careful titration of inspired oxygen concentration is important in patients with chronic respiratory insufficiency to avoid respiratory drive suppression.

CHILDREN YOUNGER THAN 1 YEAR OLD

An algorithm for elucidating the cause of wheezing in the child younger than 1 year old is presented in Fig. 80.1. It is important to note that some diagnoses more commonly presenting after age 1 year may present before 1 year as well. The abrupt onset of wheezing, often immediately preceded by an episode of choking, gagging, or vomiting, is highly suggestive of pulmonary aspiration of a foreign body. If subacute in presentation, accompanying fever or upper respiratory symptoms may point to bronchiolitis or asthma, which may be preceded by these symptoms. Most young infants who present with a first episode of wheezing have bronchiolitis. A similar complex of physical findings in an older infant with a history of bronchiolitis or wheezing and clear improvement after bronchodilator administration is characteristic of asthma.

The remaining disorders are often found in infants who have overt evidence of chronic or severe underlying illness and who typically present with recurrent or persistent episodes of wheezing and respiratory distress. Pulmonary aspiration of gastric contents may occur in young infants and in children with neurologic disability, as well as the occasional otherwise healthy child or adolescent. A report of mechanical ventilation at birth and/or a prolonged neonatal intensive care unit admission may be a clue to BPD or CLD. Recurrent pneumonia, failure to thrive, and steatorrhea are characteristic of infants with cystic fibrosis, whereas pneumonia in association with repeated extrapulmonary infection is suggestive of an immune deficiency. A heart murmur and other clinical findings consistent with congestive heart failure are indicative of congenital heart disease and pulmonary edema. Wheezing accompanied by stridor commonly indicates the coexistence of viral croup but may reflect intrinsic congenital airway narrowing, such as tracheobronchomalacia or extrinsic compression by a mediastinal structure. In the absence of any of the clinical clues listed, the first episode of wheezing in an otherwise healthy child, especially when it occurs during the winter months, is most likely to represent bronchiolitis.

CHILD 1 YEAR OR OLDER

After 1 year of age, congenital diagnoses in children become less prominent, and the evaluation may be thought of similarly with some differences, as noted in Table 80.3. As with the first age group, it is important to note that overlap occurs with each of these age groups. After age 3, symptoms are most likely attributable to asthma, but rare conditions occur in all age groups. Figure 80.2 outlines an algorithmic approach to the more common causes of wheezing in the child who is older than 1 year. The sudden onset of respiratory distress and wheezing associated with an episode of choking and coughing is likely to indicate foreign-body aspiration, particularly in a toddler who has been eating or playing with a small object. An abrupt onset of wheezing may also accompany stridor, urticaria, and hypotension in the older child with an allergic or anaphylactic reaction. When symptoms present subacutely, associated cough and rhinorrhea suggest the diagnosis of bronchiolitis in the toddler 1 to 3 years of age, but most recurrent episodes of wheezing represent asthma. Typically, asthma exacerbations are precipitated by a concurrent upper respiratory infection, weather change, or allergic trigger, and the patient may show responsiveness to bronchodilator administration. Less commonly, recurrent episodes may represent an exacerbation of CLD, whereas nonrecurrent episodes may be caused by pneumonia or bronchitis.

Wheezing and recurrent pneumonia in multiple pulmonary segments are characteristic of patients with defects in host defense mechanisms, such as cystic fibrosis, an immune deficiency syndrome, or the immotile cilia syndrome. Children in this age group who present with these disorders usually have a history of lower respiratory illness that began in infancy, as well as other signs and symptoms suggestive of chronic disease. Repeated pneumonia in the same pulmonary segment in an otherwise healthy child that begins in late infancy or in early childhood is likely to represent a previously unrecognized bronchial foreign body. In the absence of any of the clinical clues previously listed, the first episode of wheezing in an otherwise healthy child is likely to represent asthma.

It is imperative that *all* patients with wheezing receive outpatient follow-up with their primary care provider or, in some instances, with a specialist. With few exceptions, follow-up evaluation should take place within a day to a week of the ED visit.

Suggested Reading

American Academy of Pediatrics, Subcommittee on Diagnosis and Management of Bronchiolitis. Diagnosis and management of bronchiolitis. *Pediatrics* 2006;118(4):1774–1793.

Chernick V, Boat TF, Wilmott RW, et al. eds. *Kendig's disorders of the respiratory tract in children.* 7th ed. Philadelphia: Saunders, 2006.

Edwards DK. The child who wheezes. In: Hilton SW, Edwards DK, eds. *Practical pediatric radiology.* 3rd ed. Philadelphia: Saunders, 2006.

Fakhoury K. Wheezing illnesses other than asthma in children. In: UptoDate, Redding G, ed. UptoDate, Waltham, MA, 2009.

Krauss B, Silvestri S, Falk J. Capnography. In: UpToDate, Rose, BD (Ed), UpToDate, Waltham, MA, 2008.

Martinati LC, Boner AL. Clinical diagnosis of wheezing in early childhood. *Allergy* 1995;50:701–710.

Martinez FD, Wright AL, Taussig LM, et al. Asthma and wheezing in the first six years of life: relation with lung function, total serum IgE levels and skin test reactivity to allergens. *N Engl J Med* 1995;332:133–138.

Taussig LM, Wright AL, Holberg CJ, et al. Tucson children's respiratory study: 1980 to present. *J Allergy Clin Immunol* 2003;111(4):661–675.

WD. Wheezing. http://www.wrongdiagnosis.com/sym/wheezing.htm

Weinberger M, Abu-Hasan M. Pseudo-asthma: when cough, wheezing, and dyspnea are not asthma. *Pediatrics* 2007;120(4):855–864.

CHAPTER 81 ■ WEIGHT LOSS

CYNTHIA R. JACOBSTEIN, MD, MSE

Weight loss occasionally prompts a visit to the emergency department (ED). More commonly, it is an important physical examination finding in a patient presenting with another complaint. Acute weight loss is most commonly caused by a negative fluid balance occurring in the face of illness and can be life threatening. These problems have special importance to the emergency physician. Chronic weight loss may result from a number of medical and nonmedical causes leading to inadequate nutrition. Any complaint of weight loss, or documented weight loss, is a significant finding that demands careful evaluation and follow-up.

PATHOPHYSIOLOGY

The health of infants and children depends on a balanced intake of fluid and nutrients that serve as building blocks for new tissue. The major determinants of body weight are water and the organic fuels, carbohydrates, protein, and fat. Weight loss occurs when the daily energy balance becomes negative for one of these determinants (Fig. 81.1). Overall, during childhood, the major cause of weight loss is protein-energy intake inadequate to meet the energy demands of cell metabolism and tissue synthesis. Causes include decreased energy intake, normal energy intake with increased metabolic requirement, and normal energy intake in the face of malabsorption or impaired use. During acute illness, fluid loss in excess of intake, in the presence of protein-energy malnutrition, is the most common cause. Water losses occur primarily not only through the gastrointestinal (GI) tract but also through the urine and skin. Fever, infection, trauma, and thermal injury all cause a dramatic increase in metabolism that is rarely balanced with intake. During chronic illness, a cyclic pattern of adequate intake alternating with starvation results in gradual weight loss over time.

DIFFERENTIAL DIAGNOSIS

The differential diagnosis of weight loss is extensive and can be thought of as broad mechanistic categories including inadequate fluid and/or energy intake, decreased absorption, excessive wastage, and increased catabolism or abnormal energy use (Table 81.1). Multiple mechanisms may come into play for a given case of weight loss. The single most common cause of acute weight loss in all age groups is dehydration that occurs in conjunction with an acute infectious illness. In infants and toddlers with chronic weight loss or lack of appropriate weight gain, failure to thrive (FTT), or undernutrition, is usually identified in the first 3 years of life. This is a complex disorder resulting from physical and/or psychosocial problems. In older patients with chronic weight loss, an underlying medical or psychiatric illness is more likely than in infants (Table 81.2). In some instances, the exact diagnosis is not made at the time of the ED visit, but a workup may be initiated and an appropriate referral should be made.

A few life-threatening diseases associated with weight loss must be separated out from conditions that carry no immediate risk (Table 81.3). Severe dehydration in the presence of gastroenteritis or other acute illness may be catastrophic in any age group (see Chapter 17). In young infants, several disease states need to be considered. The salt-losing form of congenital adrenal hyperplasia (CAH) presents with anorexia, vomiting, dehydration, and progressive weight loss. In female infants, virilization of the external genitalia provides a clue to the diagnosis; however, this is lacking in male infants. The characteristic electrolyte abnormality of hyponatremia and hyperkalemia, and the rapidity of onset of the patient's illness, supports the diagnosis of CAH (see Chapter 86). Inborn errors of metabolism cause a wide variety of symptoms, but poor feeding, anorexia, vomiting, weight loss, and lethargy are typically present (see Chapter 94). Those presenting in the first weeks of life are severe and fatal if the correct diagnosis is not made. These disorders may masquerade as (or be complicated by) sepsis, hypoglycemia, hypocalcemia, or GI obstruction, but an inborn error must always be considered in neonates presenting with weight loss. Clinical deterioration in a previously normal baby, history of fetal death, or consanguinity increases suspicion. Infants and young children with congenital immune deficiency syndromes have a significant component of weight loss and wasting, in addition to repeated infections, seborrheic dermatitis, alopecia, chronic diarrhea, and hyperplastic joints. Infants with acquired immunodeficiency syndrome often lose weight before diagnosis. Both groups of children with immunodeficiency are at risk for life-threatening infections. Congenital heart diseases and pulmonary diseases are also associated with poor growth and may require short-term intervention.

In older children, a few diseases associated with weight loss are acutely life threatening and include adrenal crisis, diabetes mellitus with ketoacidosis, severe dehydration, and eating disorders. Older children and adolescents with Addison's disease have gradual onset of fatigue and weakness, anorexia, weight loss, and low blood pressure. If the diagnosis is not made, adrenal crisis may supervene, leading to circulatory failure, which may be rapidly fatal. Evidence of hyperpigmentation (particularly around the genitalia, nipples, axilla, and umbilicus) provides a clue to the diagnosis. Ketoacidosis is the initial manifestation in many children with diabetes; these children often give a history of weight loss in the presence of polyphagia, polydipsia, and polyuria. Eating disorders may lead to electrolyte abnormalities and concomitant dysrhythmias.

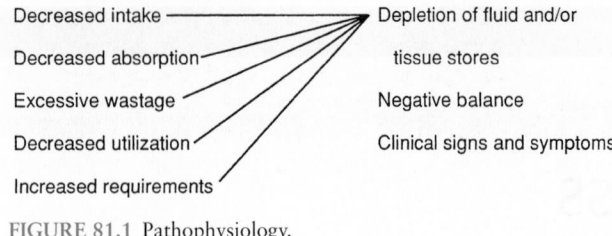

FIGURE 81.1 Pathophysiology.

EVALUATION AND DECISION

General Approach

A thorough history and physical examination are key components in the evaluation of the patient with weight loss. Consideration of the child's age and the severity and duration of the weight loss, along with the presence of other systemic symptoms and specific physical examination findings, help narrow the extensive differential diagnosis. Many diagnoses are exclusive to specific age groups. For the emergency physician, severity is an important consideration because sudden losses are more suggestive of life-threatening disorders that require prompt recognition and treatment.

Acute weight loss (occurring in less than 2 weeks) is most often caused by anorexia, poor fluid and energy intake, increased losses, and increased metabolic need in association with an intercurrent illness. Weight loss is a sensitive indicator for dehydration and commonly occurs in the presence of any significant febrile illness. In this setting, the history includes an estimation of intake, losses, and increased need for fluid and energy intake. The types of losses pinpoint the location of GI pathology. The presence of other symptoms consistent with an acute infectious process substantiates the cause. Circulatory compromise suggests severe depletion (see Chapters 3 and 17) or adrenal crisis (see Chapter 86).

Chronic weight loss (occurring over more than 2 weeks) results from a combination of factors including anorexia, poor utilization or malabsorption, and increased requirements, as well as health consequences imposed by the underlying disease state. When considering the cause of chronic weight loss, broad categories exist, including loss (i) secondary to a medical cause (underlying infection, absorptive defect, inflammatory, or neoplastic disease); (ii) related to a psychosocial or psychiatric cause; or (iii) resulting as a consequence of both

TABLE 81.1

DIFFERENTIAL DIAGNOSIS OF WEIGHT LOSS

Decreased intake	
Anorexia of acute or chronic disease	Major affective disorders
Diencephalic tumor	Anorexia nervosa
Neuromuscular disease	Mental retardation
Congenital syndromes	Failure to thrive
Hypopituitarism	Superior mesenteric artery syndrome
Dieting	Diabetes insipidus
Drug use	Iron deficiency
Gastroesophageal reflux	Plumbism
Constipation	

Decreased absorption	
Pancreatic insufficiency	Enterokinase deficiency
Cystic fibrosis	Amino acid transport defect
Shwachman syndrome	Abetalipoproteinemia
Bile salt deficiency	Hypobetalipoproteinemia
Mucosal abnormalities	Lymphangiectasia
Lactose intolerance	Acute infectious gastroenteritis
Celiac disease	Parasite gastroenteritis
Liver disease	Familial chloride diarrhea
Postinfectious malabsorption	Milk allergy
Inflammatory bowel disease	

Excessive wastage	
Gastroenteritis	Pyloric stenosis
Gastroesophageal reflux/ vomiting/rumination	Secretory diarrhea
Short bowel syndrome	
Hernia/vomiting	
Bulimia	

Increased requirements/Abnormal use	
Chronic infection (e.g., tuberculosis, urinary tract infection)	Inborn errors of metabolism
HIV infection	Addison's disease
Congenital immune deficiencies	Congenital adrenal hyperplasia
Collagen-vascular disease	Hyperthyroidism
Congenital/acquired heart disease	Diabetes mellitus
Chronic pulmonary disease	Hyperthermia
Neoplasm	
Renal insufficiency	
Renal alkalosis/acidosis	
Bartter's syndrome	

TABLE 81.2

COMMON CAUSES OF WEIGHT LOSS

	Infants	Older children/adolescents
Acute	Gastroenteritis	Gastroenteritis
	Acute infectious illness	Acute infectious illness
	Pyloric stenosis	
	Gastroesophageal reflux	
Chronic	Failure to thrive	Inflammatory bowel disease
		Eating disorders
		Affective disorders

TABLE 81.3

POTENTIAL LIFE-THREATENING CAUSES
OF WEIGHT LOSS

Infants	Older children/adolescents
Gastroenteritis, secondary dehydration	Gastroenteritis, secondary dehydration
Inborn errors of metabolism	Diabetes mellitus
Congenital adrenal hyperplasia	Addison's disease
Congenital immune deficiencies	Eating disorder
Acquired immunodeficiency syndrome	
Congenital heart disease	
Pyloric stenosis	

problems. Once again, the importance of a thorough history and physical examination cannot be overemphasized. A complete review of systems, in search of fever, night sweats, arthritis, abdominal pain, and/or diarrhea, dermatitis, and other constitutional symptoms, helps the physician reach the diagnosis. A detailed dietary and feeding history (including frequency, types, and amounts of foods ingested) is invaluable. The attitude of the child and family toward food and eating habits should be explored. An estimation of energy intake is attempted from a record of intake the day preceding the interview. Formula preparation and juice consumption are important historical pieces for babies. Gross overestimation of intake often indicates a psychosocial cause for the poor growth because of an inexperienced parent, poor parent-child interaction, and/or multiple caregivers. A search for a cause of family stress or dysfunction, economic problems, and available resources is essential. The presence or absence of symptoms of depression (poor school performance, disturbed sleep, loss of appetite, and apathy) is also important.

A complete and careful physical examination with attention to vital signs, state of hydration, and findings suggestive of specific disease states (e.g., pallor, jaundice, murmur, and/or cyanosis, clubbing, lymphadenopathy, dermatitis, hyperpigmentation, abdominal mass and/or tenderness, oral ulcers, anal skin tags, arthritis, neurologic abnormalities) provides useful clues. Nutritional inspection includes an evaluation of body fat, muscle mass, hair, skin, and nails. Physical signs associated with specific vitamin deficiencies are nonspecific and occur late in the course of malnutrition. Dysmorphic features should be noted and a thorough neurologic examination should be performed. Infants should be observed nursing or being bottle-fed, with attention to any gagging, choking, reflux, or respiratory distress.

Measurements of weight, recumbent length in babies younger than 2 years, standing height in children older than 2 years, and head circumferences in those younger than 3 years are necessary components of the physical examination. Normal growth is present when sequential measurements consistently lie within the 5th to 95th percentiles on standard growth charts from the National Center for Health Statistics (NCHS). Revisions of the 1977 NCHS growth charts were published in 2000 by the Centers for Disease Control and Prevention (CDC) and are available at the CDC Web site. Values on standard growth curves for children 0 to 36 months old are obtained from recumbent length measurement, as standing height measurements may be as much as 2 cm shorter. Use of growth charts to evaluate the child's weight and height relative to each other and previous values is important. In infants and toddlers with proportionately low measurements of all parameters, head circumference, weight, and height, congenital defects ranging from metabolic/genetic disorders to prenatal or perinatal asphyxia represent the differential diagnosis. This group of children may never achieve normal growth, even in the face of nutritional interventions. Infants/toddlers with normal head circumference and mild or proportionate weight reduction to height include those with constitutional growth delay, genetic dwarfism, or endocrine disorders. The final category represents the majority of infants and toddlers. Children in this group have normal head circumference and low weight out of proportion to height. Inadequate nutrition is the cause. Anthropometric measurements may be helpful in sorting out adequacy of growth of children consistently less than 5% after the ED evaluation. Looking at growth parameters over time is extremely helpful, although usually unavailable in the ED; a consistent fall in a downward direction requires a diligent search for an underlying chronic illness.

The severity of malnutrition can be defined further by using the actual weight expressed as a percentage of the ideal weight for the patient's actual height. Mild protein-energy malnutrition exists when the actual weight is 80% to 90% of the ideal body weight for actual height, moderate when this is 70% to 80%, and categorized as severe when this is 60% to 70%. The degree of malnutrition is important when considering the refeeding regimen and decision making regarding the patient's disposition.

Growth curves have been created for special groups of children who exhibit different growth patterns than does the general population. The growth of premature infants can be evaluated on the basis of their corrected age or on special growth curves. The premature infant normally attains "catch-up" growth during the first 2 years of life (after which normal growth curves can be used). Another standard growth curve has been created for the evaluation of growth during the adolescent age that includes the patient's sexual maturity rating. These graphs account for the variability in the timing of the adolescent growth spurt, and deviation from the standard growth curves should be interpreted with caution.

No routine screening panel of laboratory tests is indicated in patients with undernutrition. Rather, they should be performed as indicated by the history and physical examination. Considerations include complete blood cell count, sedimentation rate, C-reactive protein, iron profile, blood lead, electrolytes, blood glucose, blood urea nitrogen, and creatinine, liver function tests, serum protein profile, urinalysis with urine culture, stool examination, and toxicology screen (Table 81.4).

Infants

Infants should regain their birth weight by 10 to 14 days of age. Average daily weight gain in the first 3 months of life is 25 to 30 g. This decreases to 20 g in the third to sixth months and to 12 g in the second half of the first year. When evaluating the

TABLE 81.4

POSSIBLE LABORATORY TESTS

Primary	Secondary
Complete blood cell count	Bone age
Iron profile	Thyroid function tests
Serum glucose, electrolytes	Immunologic studies
Blood urea nitrogen, creatinine	Chromosomes
Serum proteins	Urine for ketones/reducing substances
Urinalysis, urine culture	Plasma ammonia
Stool hemoccult, clinitest	Plasma lactate
Calcium, phosphate	Serum/urine amino acids
Liver function tests	Urine organic acids
Sedimentation rate, C-reactive protein	Electroencephalogram/head imaging
Chest radiograph	Sweat test
Electrocardiogram	Lactose breath test
Purified protein derivative	Stool for trypsin
Toxicology screen	Stool for fat
	Vitamin B_{12}
	Upper gastrointestinal radiographic study/colonoscopy
	Blood lead level
	Cortisol

infant with weight loss or inadequate weight gain, the physician should include in the history perinatal events and the onset and character of the symptoms. The presence of vomiting and acute weight loss in an otherwise well baby with a good appetite suggests gastroesophageal reflux or pyloric stenosis (Fig. 81.2). Poor sucking or swallowing and delayed development indicate neurologic or neuromuscular disease. Vomiting and anorexia, altered mental status, seizures, and characteristic body fluid odors (see Chapters 46 and 94) point to metabolic disease. Renal insufficiency or tubular disease or liver disease also may cause anorexia and vomiting and, thus, poor growth. Frequent infections, dermatitis, and diarrhea

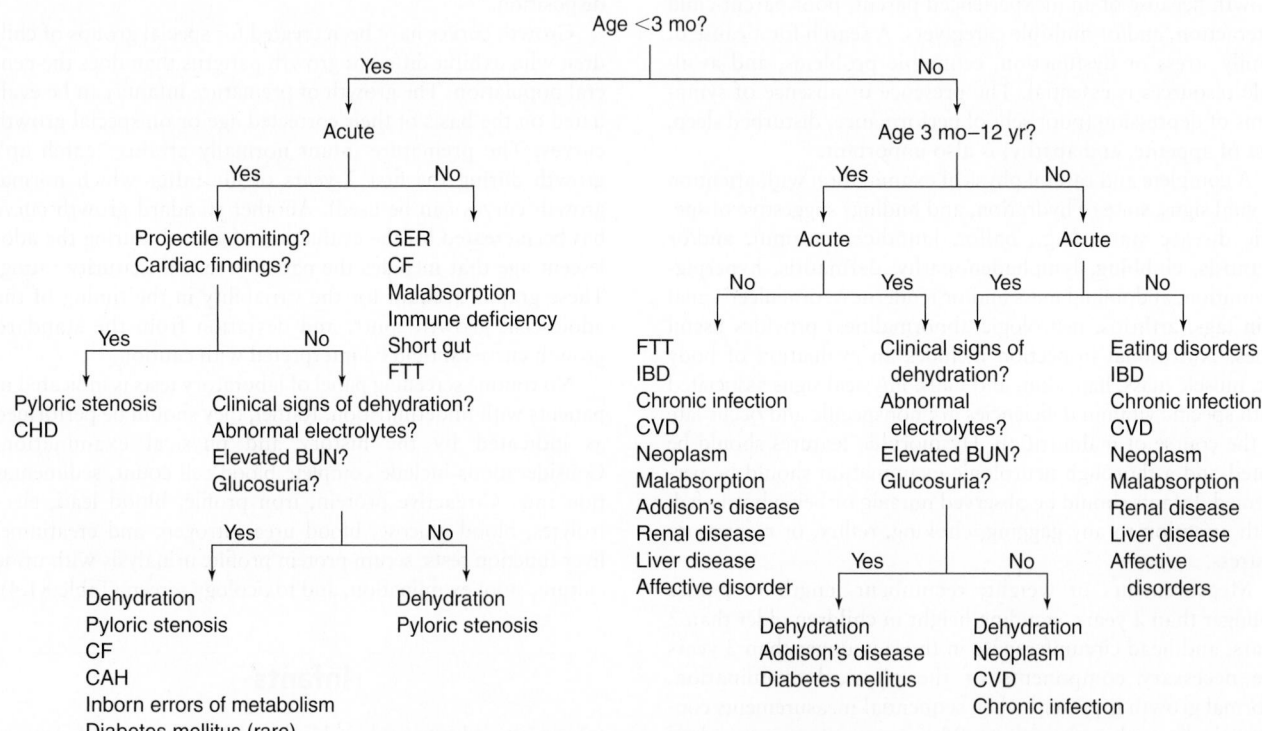

FIGURE 81.2 An approach to the evaluation of weight loss. GER, gastroesophageal reflux; CF, cystic fibrosis; FTT, failure to thrive; IBD, inflammatory bowel disease; CHD, congenital heart disease; CVD, collagen vascular disease; BUN, blood urea nitrogen; CAH, congenital adrenal hyperplasia.

are associated with immune deficiency syndromes. The infant who tires or becomes diaphoretic with feedings may have congenital heart or pulmonary disease. The presence of malodorous, loose stools suggests primary malabsorption or cystic fibrosis. Blood-streaked, water-loss stools may be related to milk protein allergy or infectious (especially bacterial) enteritis.

The physical examination includes measurement of length, weight, and head circumference as described previously. When all three parameters give abnormal measurements, a neurologic, genetic, or metabolic cause is suspect. When length and weight are subnormal but proportional, skeletal dysplasias, endocrinopathies, or constitutional short stature is likely. When only weight is below normal value, an acute illness, dehydration, or deprivation is probably the culprit; the infant should be evaluated for signs of dehydration, cardiac or pulmonary disease, and neurologic abnormalities. As noted previously, observation of a feeding infant may offer some relevant clues. The evaluation of an infant with suspected FTT as a result of child abuse is discussed in Chapter 132.

Older Children

A similar approach to weight loss is used for children beyond infancy (Fig. 81.2). Average weight gain from the age of 2 years until puberty is 2 to 3 kg per year and average growth is 5 to 8 cm per year. A careful history, physical examination, and growth assessment identify the child with growth failure that requires further investigation. Two of the more common causes of chronic weight loss in this age group are diabetes mellitus and inflammatory bowel disease (IBD). For diabetes mellitus, important points include a history of increased appetite, polyuria, and polydipsia. With regard to IBD, colicky abdominal pain, diarrhea, and other symptoms such as arthritis or rash are pertinent. However, weight loss may be the sole manifestation. In this age group, mental health disorders are also an important consideration. The incidence of diagnosed depression in children continues to increase because of both improved recognition and a rising incidence in our society.

Adolescents

Growth failure in adolescents may be the harbinger of chronic illness. The history and physical examination again help uncover the pathology. Consideration of underlying inflammatory, chronic infections, or neoplastic disease is important (Fig. 81.2).

Eating disorders often emerge during adolescence. As in FTT, the diagnosis is made with a careful dietary history and physical examination. These patients exhibit an intense fear of fatness, a relentless pursuit for thinness, a preoccupation with food, and a distorted body image. In cases complicated by severe malnutrition, metabolic derangements, dehydration, or acute psychosis, patients with eating disorders are cared for initially in the hospital. Additional considerations for weight loss in the adolescent include the occurrence of fad dieting and drug use (e.g., stimulants).

Laboratory Tests

The potential list of tests to aid in the evaluation of weight loss is extensive (Table 81.4). Specific diagnostic testing should be performed on a case-by-case basis using a thorough history and physical examination to guide the evaluation. A complete blood cell count serves many purposes and may uncover macrocytosis caused by hypothyroidism or malabsorption of folate or vitamin B_{12}; microcytosis caused by iron deficiency, chronic blood loss, or chronic infection; polycythemia related to chronic heart or lung disease; neutropenia indicative of Shwachman syndrome; elevated neutrophil count secondary to infection; abnormal cell counts or morphologies caused by underlying neoplasm; or thrombocytosis caused by chronic infection or underlying malignancy. Electrolytes may confirm the presence of significant dehydration, and hyponatremia in the presence of hyperkalemia suggests the diagnosis of adrenal insufficiency. Alterations in serum proteins may reflect aberrant absorption, decreased synthesis, or chronic infection. The urinalysis evaluates tubular function and may reveal glucosuria or disaccharide intolerance or galactosemia, as well as infection and renal tubular acidosis. The stool should be checked for the presence of blood, infectious agents, and reducing substances. With the results from this battery of tests, in conjunction with the physical examination and history, a diagnosis or appropriate referral can be made.

SUMMARY

Weight loss is a complaint that requires careful evaluation. With an acute episode of weight loss, many patients seen in the ED will have fluid loss and mild protein-energy malnutrition related to an intercurrent illness with anorexia, increased metabolic need, or increased losses. Most of these children will return to baseline spontaneously when their illness resolves. Chronic weight loss or growth failure is indicative of less common diseases and those for which the differential diagnosis is extensive. In small children, the most common cause is psychosocial growth failure. In older children and adolescents, an organic cause becomes more likely.

Disposition

As always, the general appearance of the infant or child determines the timing and the scope of the evaluation. Hospitalization is indicated in any child who is suspected to have sustained trauma or been abused and may be indicated in those with physical findings consistent with severe malnutrition, hypothermia, bradycardia, or hypotension. Children with mild to moderate protein-energy malnutrition can be referred back to their pediatrician for outpatient management. Nutrition is a central component of well-being in the growing child, and malnutrition carries significant morbidity and mortality. Thus, persons who care for children need to have a sense of normal growth and must develop an approach for the evaluation and treatment of growth failure.

Suggested Readings

Balint JP. Physical findings in nutritional deficiencies. *Pediatr Clin North Am* 1998;45:245–260.

Boswinkel J, Mamula P. Failure to thrive. *Pediatr Case Rev* 2003;3(1):20–29.

Centers for Disease Control and Prevention. CDC growth charts, 2000 version. www.cdc.gov/growthcharts/. Accessed May 30, 2000.

Gahagan S. Failure to thrive: a consequence of undernutrition. *Pediatr Rev* 2006;27:e1–e11.

Judge BS, Eisenga BH. Disorders of fuel metabolism: medical complications associated with starvation, eating disorders, dietary fads, and supplements. *Emerg Med Clin North Am* 2005;23:789–813.

Keane V, Feigelman S. Failure to thrive and malnutrition. In: Kleigman RM, Greenbaum LA, Lye PS, eds. *Practical strategies in pediatric diagnosis and therapy*, 2nd ed. Philadelphia, PA: Elsevier Saunders, 2004:233–247.

Kleinman RE, ed. *Pediatric nutrition handbook*, 6th ed. Elk Grove Village, IL: American Academy of Pediatrics, 2009.

Shah MD. Failure to thrive in children. *J Clin Gastroenterol* 2002;35(5): 371–374.

Sigman GS. Eating disorders in children and adolescents. *Pediatr Clin North Am* 2003;50:1139–1177.

Tunnessen WW, ed. Weight loss. In: *Signs and symptoms in pediatrics*, 3rd ed. Philadelphia, PA: Lippincott Williams & Wilkins, 1999:36–40.

CHAPTER 82 ■ ASTHMA AND ALLERGIC EMERGENCIES

MICHELLE D. STEVENSON, MD, MSE, AND RICHARD M. RUDDY, MD

ASTHMA

Background

Asthma is the most common chronic disease of childhood, affecting approximately 9% of children in the United States. Male, African American, and Puerto Rican children are more likely to experience asthma. Many children, particularly those who are economically disadvantaged, are treated in the emergency department (ED) only during acute exacerbations and receive little or no other ongoing, consistent care. This places the additional burden on the emergency physician both for facilitating appropriate follow-up care and for managing acute exacerbations.

National data demonstrate a significant increase in the annual rate of outpatient visits for asthma since the year 2000, whereas ED visits made by children have appeared to plateau around 750,000 annual visits. In the United States alone, asthma results in an estimated 12 to 14 million school absences per year and was responsible for 186 deaths in children in the year 2004. The reason for sustained high levels of morbidity due to childhood asthma is a subject of active investigation and has not been fully elucidated. However, socioeconomic factors appear to play a major role. Risk factors for life-threatening asthma have been identified and are listed in Table 82.1. Unfortunately, despite these alarming statistics, patients, parents, and physicians often grossly underestimate the life-threatening potential of asthma.

The approach to the assessment and management of acute asthma presented in this chapter is in general agreement with the *Expert Panel Report 3: Guidelines for the Diagnosis and Management of Asthma* developed by the National Asthma Education and Prevention Program (NAEPP), which became available in prepublication form in 2007. This chapter presents an approach based on current knowledge and provides a set of guidelines that can be adapted to meet the needs of the individual patient or ED setting. Areas of controversy and new therapies are also reviewed.

Pathophysiology

Asthma has been increasingly recognized as a multifactorial inflammatory disorder with several phenotypes. Genetic predisposition, environmental exposure, and allergic sensitization play a strong role in the predisposition to wheeze, particularly in children. Therapy must ideally reverse the airway narrowing and block or modify the impact of the cellular role of mast cells, eosinophils, macrophages, neutrophils, T lymphocytes, and epithelial cells.

The two most important components that impact bronchospasm in asthma occur through immunoglobulin E (IgE)-mediated mast cell degranulation and the recruitment of other cellular components that contribute to chronic inflammation and subsequent airway remodeling. Clinically, this separates the immediate reduction in pulmonary function due to antigen stimulation in the first hours from a later reduction beginning at 4 to 12 hours associated with cellular recruitment. Key to this late-phase response is the attraction and impact of inflammatory cells, with TH_2 lymphocytes contributing greatly. The release of leukotrienes, cytokines [particularly interleukin (IL)-4, IL-5, and IL-13], and other mediators drives this process. Neutrophils play a key role in the pathogenesis of severe asthma exacerbations for reasons that are not understood.

In patients with hyperreactive airways, it is clear that viral infection, including respiratory syncytial virus (RSV) and rhinovirus, increase the responsiveness of the airways and bronchial inflammation, probably by cytokine-triggered upregulation. Further defining the contribution of allergic sensitization, the importance of TH_2 cytokine imbalance, and the role of eosinophilic infiltration is an area of ongoing research. Numerous inflammatory mediators are important in the pathogenesis of asthma and may vary across individual patients.

Regardless, the physiologic consequences of asthma are progressive air trapping with dead space ventilation, increased airway resistance, and mismatching of alveolar ventilation and perfusion. As the acute episode progresses, there is further decrease in forced vital capacity, forced expiratory volume at 1 second (FEV_1), and peak expiratory flow rate (PEFR). Each breath is initiated at higher lung volumes that lie on the steep, stiff portion of the compliance curve. At this point, high-pressure changes are required to achieve acceptable tidal volumes. Arterial oxygen saturation decreases with ventilation-perfusion abnormalities. Hypoxemia may cause pulmonary artery hypertension and hyperventilation. Hyperventilation occurs early in the course of acute asthma, out of proportion to any respiratory or metabolic demands. If the acute asthmatic process continues unchecked, minute ventilation cannot be maintained and $PaCO_2$ ultimately rises as the child becomes fatigued.

Metabolic changes also occur with acute asthma. The increased work of breathing increases oxygen and energy consumption, leading to a metabolic acidosis. Compensation for

TABLE 82.1

RISK FACTORS FOR LIFE-THREATENING ASTHMA

Asthma history
  Previous severe exacerbation (e.g., intubation or ICU admission for asthma)
  Two or more hospital admissions for asthma in the past year
  Three or more ED visits in the past year
  Hospitalization or ED visit for asthma within the past month
  Using >2 cannisters of short-acting β_2-agonist per month
  Difficulty perceiving asthma symptoms or severity of exacerbations
  Other risk factors: lack of a written asthma action plan, sensitivity to *Alternaria*

Social history
  Low socioeconomic status/inner-city residence
  Illicit drug abuse
  Major psychological and/or psychosocial problems

Comorbidities
  Cardiovascular disease
  Other chronic lung disease
  Chronic psychiatric disease

ED, emergency department.
Adapted from Expert Panel Report 3 of the National Heart, Lung, and Blood Institute; National Institutes of Health, U.S. Department of Health and Human Services 2007.

this acidosis may not be possible because of already maximal respiratory effort. As respiratory muscles fatigue, respiratory acidosis develops. Combined respiratory and metabolic acidosis set the stage for respiratory failure.

Although the pathophysiology of acute asthma in children and adults is similar, young children are particularly susceptible to status asthmaticus. In children younger than 5 years, peripheral airway resistance is substantially higher than in adults. A small degree of narrowing of peripheral airways results in disproportionate increases in resistance to airflow. Respiratory reserve in children is limited and increases with age as the size of the conducting airways grow larger. Part of this is related to the respiratory surface area being much smaller in children younger than 5 years than in adults. Another age-related mechanical factor, decreased elastic recoil, contributes to earlier small airway closure during normal tidal breathing in young children. This leads to airway collapse and atelectasis during asthma exacerbations or respiratory infection. The horizontal insertion of the diaphragm in infancy makes diaphragmatic recruitment during airway obstruction less efficient. In infants and young children, the contribution of bronchial smooth-muscle constriction to airway obstruction may be less important than that by edema, mucous plugging, and atelectasis.

Triggers

Triggers for acute asthma attacks may be nonspecific and include acute viral infection, allergy, weather change, cigarette smoke or other inhaled irritants, exercise, and cold air. Low-level infections in the upper airways such as sinusitis and otitis media (OM) have been implicated in exacerbations of previ-

ously stable asthma in children. Rhinovirus infections play a significant role in acute exacerbations in children. Allergic reactions not only trigger acute episodes of asthma but can also induce a state of bronchial lability. Allergy may promote acute attacks through immediate mediator release and by chronic airway obstruction through the late-phase inflammatory response. Drug sensitivity, particularly to aspirin products, may induce hyperreactive airways. However, exposure to ibuprofen in patients who are not allergic to aspirin or nonsteroidal antiinflammatory drugs (NSAIDs) does not appear to worsen asthma morbidity and may actually reduce outpatient visits.

Clinical Manifestations

In children with known asthma and an obvious exacerbation, clinical evaluation and initial treatment should begin almost simultaneously. However, for the purposes of clarity, these phases of management are considered in sequence.

The evaluation of the child with wheezing begins with a rapid cardiopulmonary assessment to determine the severity of the episode. This includes the child's general appearance, paying particular attention to the degree of respiratory distress, color, and mental status. Simultaneously, oxygen is administered if there is respiratory distress or oxygen saturation is less than 90% to 92%. If indicated, immediate resuscitative and therapeutic efforts are initiated, as described in the next section. After a baseline evaluation, the child should be reassessed frequently or, when severe, continuously.

In addition to the history and physical examination, other selected studies may be useful in the assessment of acute asthma. Pulse oximetry is valuable in all children with respiratory distress and PEFR can be useful in those older than 6 years, particularly if they have previously performed it. Arterial blood gases (ABGs), chest radiographs, and laboratory blood tests should be used only selectively. Each aspect of the assessment is discussed in more detail later in this chapter. A general guide to several parameters useful for estimating the severity of the episode can be found in Table 82.2.

History

The history should include the duration of the current episode and rapidity of onset, the parent's and/or patient's subjective assessment of severity, other associated symptoms, and the suspected trigger. The child's current medications should be determined, including details of when the medications were started, the dosage, the route, the timing of the last dose, and a history of missed doses from nonadherence or emesis. A history of medications, particularly oral or inhaled steroids in the past 6 months, should be elicited. A recent significant escalation in symptoms and rescue medication use is also worrisome and is a risk factor for near-fatal asthma. In accordance with new guidelines, an estimate of the underlying chronic severity of asthma, level of asthma control, impact of symptoms on quality of life, and risk for a life-threatening episode should be made after the initiation of appropriate therapy. Details about past episodes, such as frequency of ED visits, hospital admissions, intensive care unit (ICU) admissions, and episodes of respiratory failure that required

TABLE 82.2

ESTIMATION OF SEVERITY OF ACUTE ASTHMA EXACERBATION[a]

Sign/symptom	Mild	Moderate	Severe[b]
Respiratory rate[c]	Normal to 30% increase	30%–50% increase	>50% increase
Alertness	Normal or agitated	Normal or agitated	Agitated
Dyspnea	Absent or with exertion/ activity; speech normal	Moderate; speaks in phrases; difficulty feeding	Severe; single words or short phrases; refuses feeding
Accessory muscle use	None to mild intercostal retractions	Moderate intercostal with suprasternal retractions; use of sternocleidomastoid muscles; chest hyperinflation	Severe intercostal and tracheosternal retractions; nasal flaring; chest hyperinflation
Color	Normal	Pale	Possibly cyanotic
Wheeze	Often end expiratory only	Throughout expiration	Throughout inhalation and exhalation, or decreased breath sounds
Oxygen saturation (in room air)	>95%	90%–95%	<90%
Peak expiratory flow rate[c] (% predicted or personal best)	≥70%	40%–69%	<40%
$PaCO_2$	<42 mm Hg	<42 mm Hg	≥42 mm Hg

[a]Within each category, the presence of several parameters, but not necessarily all, indicates general classification of exacerbation. Many of these parameters have not been systematically studied, so they serve only as general guides.
[b]Signs of impending respiratory arrest include the following: drowsy/depressed level of consciousness, paradoxical thoracoabdominal movements, bradycardia, quite chest, or less than 25% PEFR (if obtained).

[c]Normal rates of breathing in awake children		Normal pulse rates in children	
Age	Normal rate (per min)	Age	Normal rate (per min)
<2 mo	<60	2–12 mo	<160
2–12 mo	<50	1–2 yr	<120
1–5 yr	<40	2–8 yr	<110
6–8 yr	<30		

[c]For children 5 years or older who are not experiencing a life-threatening condition.
Adapted from Expert Panel Report of the National Heart, Lung, and Blood Institute, National Institute of Heath, U.S. Department of Health and Human Services 2007.

mechanical ventilation, should be addressed. It must be recognized that even children with intermittent or previously mild asthma may experience a severe exacerbation. Current hydration status should be evaluated with questions regarding recent fluid intake, emesis, and urine output. For children with their first episodes of wheezing, for those with mild histories and usually serious flares, or for those in an episode with focal findings without a trigger, the possibility of a foreign-body aspiration or another cause of wheezing should be explored (Table 82.3). Anaphylaxis due to a food allergy must also be considered early in the differential diagnosis of a child with acute, sudden-onset wheezing.

A personal or family history of atopic disease, including eczema and allergic rhinitis, is suggestive of asthma. The NAEPP Expert Panel Report 3 (EPR3) and others have emphasized the importance of recognition of asthma in early life, particularly in young infants with other atopic conditions, recurrent wheezing, affected sleep, or wheezing without upper respiratory symptoms. Appropriate recognition of the inflammatory process in these infants in partnership with their primary care physician is an essential component of quality asthma care. Finally, the family's ability to cope with the child's disease at home should be assessed in preparation for making a disposition decision.

Physical Examination

As noted previously, the physical examination begins immediately, with an overall assessment of the child's degree of respiratory distress. Severe retractions, accessory muscle use, nasal flaring, cyanosis, decreased muscle tone, and altered mental status are indicative of impending or existing respiratory failure and require immediate intervention. The respiratory rate and heart rate should be noted and compared to age-appropriate standards (Table 82.2).

The remainder of the respiratory examination includes auscultation for decreased breath sounds, wheezing, rhonchi, and crackles. Crackles can occur and are most often caused by focal areas of atelectasis. Any asymmetry in the pulmonary findings should be noted. Children with a severe exacerbation or marked chest pain should undergo palpation of their chest wall, neck, and axillae to examine for the presence of subcutaneous air suggesting pneumomediastinum.

There are several clinical asthma assessment scores in the literature. One such score, the Pediatric Asthma Severity

TABLE 82.3

DIFFERENTIAL DIAGNOSIS FOR WHEEZING

Congenital	Cystic fibrosis
	Lobar emphysema
	Tracheobronchomalacia/laryngomalacia
	Tracheal stenosis
	Bronchial stenosis
	Diaphragmatic hernia
	Tracheoesophageal fistula
	Alpha-1 antitrypsin deficiency
	Vascular ring
Infections	Bronchiolitis
	Pneumonia (viral and bacterial)
	Pertussis
Allergic	Asthma
	Anaphylaxis
	Allergic pulmonary aspergillosis
Acquired/Other	Foreign-body aspiration
	Bronchopulmonary dysplasia
	Bronchiectasis
	Mediastinal bronchial compression
	Recurrent aspiration
	Vocal cord dysfunction
Cardiac	Congestive heart failure
	Pulmonary edema
	Cor triatriatum

Score, has recently been validated in the pediatric, acute care clinical setting and is responsive to changes in patient status during treatment.

Peak Expiratory Flow Rate

PEFR can serve as a simple, quantitative, reproducible, and inexpensive measure of airway obstruction in children with mild to moderate distress. It is recommended by the NAEPP to monitor PEFR in children during an acute asthma flare that is not life threatening. Its utility is limited, however, by the inability of children younger than 5 to 7 years to perform the maneuver reliably. In addition, PEFR is effort dependent and measures predominantly large airway disease.

More recent data from a pediatric ED setting indicate that many children are cooperative to testing with peak flow meters, despite marked underutilization at home. Key components to proper peak flow meter use include use while standing, zeroing the meter, the presence of a good seal from the mouth on the device, and both a good effort and inspiration.

Normal PEFR varies on the basis of the child's sex and height and on some characteristics unique to each peak flow meter model. Knowledge of the child's personal best PEFR can be helpful in the ED. Repeating PEFR 30 to 60 minutes after treatment can assist in determination of the effectiveness of therapy. A flow rate of more than 70% is considered mild, 40 to 69% moderate, and less than 40% severe. The degree of improvement after bronchodilator therapy is more useful than the initial value before therapy. Patients with PEFRs less than 60% of predicted after ED therapy are more likely to relapse after outpatient therapy.

Oxygen Saturation and Arterial Blood Gases

Although ABGs have a role in the evaluation of a severe exacerbation, they have several disadvantages, particularly in children. They can be technically difficult to obtain, are painful, and provide less reliable results in the crying child. Pulse oximetry, however, offers a noninvasive, continuous, and generally valid measure of arterial hemoglobin oxygen saturation (SaO_2). In addition, pulse oximetry provides data regarding the need and adequacy of supplemental oxygen, response to therapy, and appropriate disposition. It should be measured initially in all children with acute asthma in the ED when available. It is one of the few objective measures in young children who are unable to perform PEFRs reliably. Pulse oximetry values of 97% or more on room air, in conjunction with spirometric evidence, may be helpful in identifying adolescent patients with dyspnea due to vocal cord dysfunction. Supplemental oxygen should be provided to maintain an SaO_2 level of more than 90% (some experts recommend at least 93% in young infants), and if hypoxia persists after ED treatment, hospital admission should be considered. For children with mild degrees of hypoxia, studies have shown that initial SaO_2 alone does not predict the need for hospitalization accurately for the individual patient. As a rule, however, children with lower oxygen saturations are more likely to require frequent bronchodilator therapy and hospitalization or to experience relapse. In any case, confirmation of adequate oxygenation is reassuring and obviates the need for ABGs, except in critical cases.

ABGs provide an objective measure of ventilation and oxygenation. In the ED, it should be considered in the evaluation of any child in whom impending or existing respiratory failure is suspected clinically, although it should never delay the initiation of therapy. ABGs must be interpreted in conjunction with the clinical picture. The trend of the PaO_2 and $PaCO_2$ is more important than the initial value. Mild hypoxia and hypocapnia are expected early in the course of acute asthma. As obstruction progresses and fatigue develops in the child, hypoxia becomes more severe and the $PaCO_2$ rises to "normal" or above "normal" range, resulting in a mixed metabolic and respiratory acidosis. It should be emphasized that a "normal" $PaCO_2$ of 40 mm Hg in a child with tachypnea or significant respiratory distress may be a sign of impending respiratory failure and requires aggressive management and close monitoring. Despite the usefulness of the blood gas as an adjunctive measure, the decision to intubate remains clinically based.

Other Studies

The role of chest radiographs in the ED management of acute asthma is limited. Typical findings on routine films such as hyperinflation, atelectasis, and peribronchial thickening do not correlate with severity and rarely alter management. Patients for whom a chest radiograph may alter clinical management include those with persistence of focal findings after bronchodilator therapy, markedly reduced oxygen saturation after therapy, or clinical suspicion of a complication or cause for wheezing other than asthma. These factors also apply to the decision to obtain a chest radiograph in children who present with wheezing for the first time.

Serum potassium measurement should be considered in children at risk for hypokalemia secondary to receiving frequent or prolonged continuous β_2-agonist therapy. A complete blood cell (CBC) count is generally not useful and, if drawn after adrenergic therapy, often reveals a leukocytosis with neutrophil predominance that should not be misinterpreted as secondary to bacterial infection.

Differential Diagnosis

Wheezing (see Chapter 80) is a continuous, high-pitched, musical, auscultatory finding generally most prominent on expiration; it is caused by the obstruction of intrathoracic airways. It must be distinguished from stridor, a harsh, high-pitched, audible sound most prominent on inspiration. Stridor (see Chapter 72) is associated with diseases that cause upper airway obstruction, such as croup and epiglottitis, as discussed in Chapter 92. Croup typically involves the upper airway but not infrequently may present with evidence of both upper and lower airway obstruction.

Some children present with chronic cough (see Chapter 14) as the only symptom of hyperreactive airways or "cough variant asthma." Typically, the cough is worse at night and the child is asymptomatic during the day. Many of these children have a family history of atopic disease or will have reduced peak flows. There are also children whose acute exacerbations are characterized by severe coughing without obvious wheezing. In the ED, the most practical approach may be a trial of bronchodilators that can be therapeutic and diagnostic. It is important to understand that most patients with persistent cough after an upper respiratory tract infection do not respond to inhaled β-agonist therapy. Pertussis should be considered in the differential diagnosis of children with paroxysms of cough.

Although wheezing is most commonly associated with asthma, other explanations should be considered (Table 82.3). Several entities that may cause wheezing can be differentiated from asthma through a careful history, physical examination, and attention to the patient's response to therapy. The two most common problems other than asthma that bring children to the ED with wheezing are bronchiolitis and viral pneumonia. Much less frequent is a foreign-body aspiration.

Bronchiolitis (see Chapter 92) is an acute infection of the small airways most commonly caused not only by the RSV but also by parainfluenza, adenovirus, metapneumovirus, and influenza. Outbreaks usually occur during the winter and peak from January through March. Bronchiolitis generally affects children younger than 1 year most severely and manifests with a history of an upper airway infection, followed by fever, feeding difficulty, progressive wheezing, respiratory distress, and, occasionally, apnea. Some infants, particularly those with chronic lung disease, respond to bronchodilators.

Foreign-body aspiration is seen most commonly in children 6 months to 5 years of age (see Chapter 28). Although the presentation is usually subtler, classically, patients have a history of sudden onset of choking, coughing, or wheezing when eating or playing with a small object. The examination may reveal asymmetric breath sounds or wheezing associated with varying levels of respiratory distress. These children may have some,

although generally incomplete, response to bronchodilators. The chest radiograph is often normal, but in some cases, it may demonstrate differential hyperinflation on inspiratory/expiratory or bilateral decubitus views, focal atelectasis, or, occasionally, a radiopaque foreign body.

Complications

Throughout the ED stay, the potential for complications of acute asthma should be kept in mind. These may be a consequence of the disease itself, the therapy, or both. It is also important to recognize that depression and anxiety are significantly associated with asthma in adolescents, which can lead to impairment in quality of life. Furthermore, epidemiologic studies have shown that asthma, as a chronic condition, is a risk factor for invasive pneumococcal disease.

The most common acute pulmonary complication is atelectasis secondary to mucous plugging. Air leaks that lead to a pneumomediastinum and/or a pneumothorax are potentially life threatening. Children who require positive pressure ventilation of any kind are at particular risk for air leak complications. A pneumothorax should be suspected in any child with a sudden deterioration associated with chest pain, asymmetry of breath sounds, or a shift of the trachea.

Cardiac arrhythmias are associated with adrenergic agents and theophylline. Although theophylline is not recommended for acute asthma, it is still used in chronic asthma control. This drug combination, particularly in association with hypoxemia and acidosis, increases the risk of arrhythmias.

Frequent β_2-agonist therapy can cause hypokalemia and lactic acidosis, although these are rarely clinically significant. The syndrome of inappropriate antidiuretic hormone secretion (SIADH), which may result in symptomatic hyponatremia, is also a potential, although rare, complication of acute asthma.

Management

Initial Approach

The primary goals in the acute management phase of an asthma exacerbation are to correct hypoxemia and to rapidly reverse airflow obstruction. Supplemental oxygen, repetitive β_2-agonists, and the early addition of systemic corticosteroids achieve these goals. Patients should be monitored closely and evaluated serially to determine their response to therapy, to identify those who require more aggressive therapy, and to make a final disposition. For children who are discharged, the emergency physician should prescribe an intensified regimen for a minimum of 3 to 5 days and should recommend that follow-up be kept within a month to monitor outcome and for long term management issues to be addressed.

This section of the chapter presents a stepwise approach to the ED management of acute asthma in children. This approach is generally consistent with the NAEPP EPR3 recommendations and is summarized in algorithm form in Fig. 82.1. Specific dosage recommendations are shown in Table 82.4.

Clinical practice guidelines are increasingly used for commonly encountered ED diagnoses such as asthma. Investigators

MEDICAL EMERGENCIES

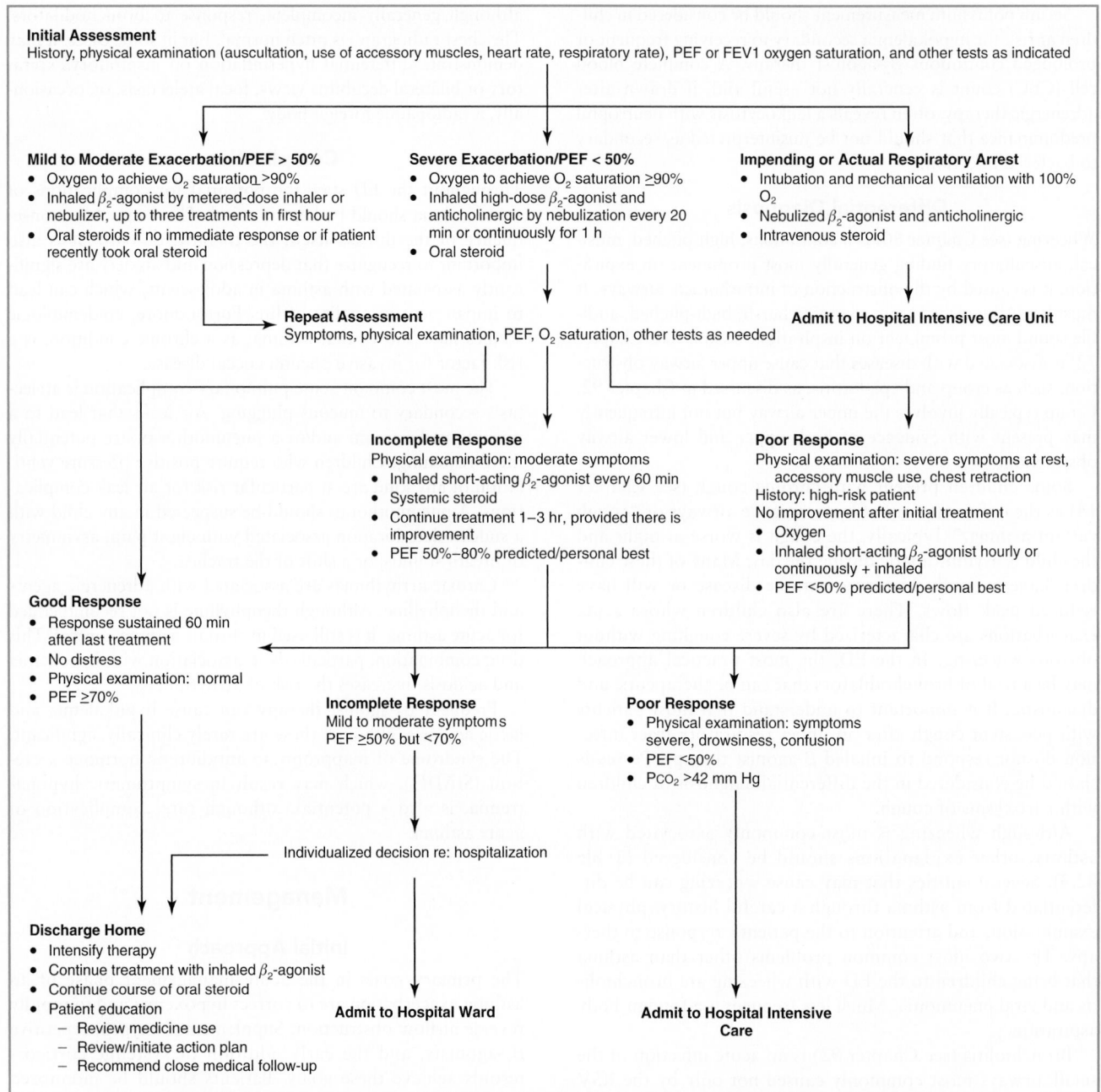

Initial Assessment
History, physical examination (auscultation, use of accessory muscles, heart rate, respiratory rate), PEF or FEV1 oxygen saturation, and other tests as indicated

Mild to Moderate Exacerbation/PEF > 50%
- Oxygen to achieve O_2 saturation >90%
- Inhaled β_2-agonist by metered-dose inhaler or nebulizer, up to three treatments in first hour
- Oral steroids if no immediate response or if patient recently took oral steroid

Severe Exacerbation/PEF < 50%
- Oxygen to achieve O_2 saturation ≥90%
- Inhaled high-dose β_2-agonist and anticholinergic by nebulization every 20 min or continuously for 1 h
- Oral steroid

Impending or Actual Respiratory Arrest
- Intubation and mechanical ventilation with 100% O_2
- Nebulized β_2-agonist and anticholinergic
- Intravenous steroid

Repeat Assessment
Symptoms, physical examination, PEF, O_2 saturation, other tests as needed

Admit to Hospital Intensive Care Unit

Incomplete Response
Physical examination: moderate symptoms
- Inhaled short-acting β_2-agonist every 60 min
- Systemic steroid
- Continue treatment 1–3 hr, provided there is improvement
- PEF 50%–80% predicted/personal best

Poor Response
Physical examination: severe symptoms at rest, accessory muscle use, chest retraction
History: high-risk patient
No improvement after initial treatment
- Oxygen
- Inhaled short-acting β_2-agonist hourly or continuously + inhaled
- PEF <50% predicted/personal best

Good Response
- Response sustained 60 min after last treatment
- No distress
- Physical examination: normal
- PEF ≥70%

Incomplete Response
Mild to moderate symptoms
PEF ≥50% but <70%

Poor Response
- Physical examination: symptoms severe, drowsiness, confusion
- PEF <50%
- P_{CO_2} >42 mm Hg

Individualized decision re: hospitalization

Discharge Home
- Intensify therapy
- Continue treatment with inhaled β_2-agonist
- Continue course of oral steroid
- Patient education
  - Review medicine use
  - Review/initiate action plan
  - Recommend close medical follow-up

Admit to Hospital Ward

Admit to Hospital Intensive Care

FIGURE 82.1 Approach to acute asthma in children. PEF, peak expiratory flow; FEV1, forced expiratory volume in 1 second. Adapted from National Asthma Education and Prevention Program. *Expert Panel Report 3: Guidelines for the Diagnosis and Management of asthma.* U.S. Department of Health and Human Services Publication, Bethesda, MD: National Institutes of Health, National Heart, Lung, and Blood Institute, August 2007.

have shown that these guidelines, when implemented in a pediatric emergency medicine setting, can be useful in implementing and monitoring adherence to important published recommendations. A sample initial order set that may be used for a majority of children with non–life-threatening asthma is given in Fig. 82.2.

Oxygen

All children with acute asthma can be assumed to be hypoxemic unless oxygen saturation is measured immediately and

indicates otherwise. In addition, β_2-adrenergic therapy may exacerbate hypoxemia transiently by increasing blood flow to poorly ventilated areas of the lung, thereby increasing ventilation-perfusion mismatch. Hence, unless SaO_2 is more than 90%, humidified oxygen should be administered immediately. Oxygen is most effectively delivered by mask or nasal cannula. It should be delivered at a flow rate sufficient to maintain SaO_2 levels of more than 90% (93% in infants). In contrast to adults, oxygen-induced suppression of respiratory drive is rare in asthmatic children. It is always recommended to administer

TABLE 82.4

EMERGENCY DEPARTMENT ACUTE ASTHMA THERAPY

Therapy	Dose	Maximum	Comments
Oxygen	Maintain SaO_2 > 90% (>93% in infants)		
Adrenergic agents			
Albuterol (0.5%) nebulizer solution	Intermittent: 0.15 mg/kg q15–20 min in 2 mL NS × 3 and then 0.15–0.3 mg/kg q1–4 h	5 mg/dose	
	Continuous: 0.5 mg/kg/h 2.5 mg minimum	15 mg/h	
Albuterol MDI	4–8 puffs every 20 min × 3 and then every 1–4 h as needed		Use valved holding chamber for all ages Face mask in children <4 yr
Levalbuterol nebulizer solution (0.63 mg/3 mL, 1.25 mg/3 mL)	Intermittent: 0.075 mg/kg (minimum 1.25 mg) q20 min × 3 and then 0.075–0.15 mg/kg q1–4 h	2.5–5 mg	Use one-half the dose of racemic albuterol
	Continuous: 0.25 mg/kg/h	5–7.5 mg/h	
Subcutaneous			
Epinephrine 1:1,000	0.01 mg/kg sq q15–20 min	0.3–0.5 mg	See the text for indications
Terbutaline (0.1%)	0.01 mg/kg sq q15–20 min	0.25 mg	See the text for indications
Intravenous			
Terbutaline (0.1%)	Loading dose: 10 μg/kg over 10 min; initial maintenance: 0.4 μg/kg/min		Titrate up by 0.2 μg/kg/min Usual effective range: 3–6 μg/kg/min
Anticholinergics			
Ipratropium bromide			
Nebulizer solution (0.25 mg/mL)	0.25 mg every 20 min × 3[a] (child) 0.5 mg every 20 min × 3[a] (adult)	0.5 mg	May mix with same nebulizer as albuterol in moderate to severe exacerbations; should be added to β_2-agonist
Metered-dose inhaler (18 μg/puff)	4–8 puffs every 20 min × 3 doses	8 puffs	
Corticosteroids			
Methylprednisolone	1 mg/kg IV bolus	60 mg	
Prednisone	1 mg/kg po	60 mg	
Dexamethasone	0.6 mg/kg po or IM	16 mg	

NS, normal saline; sq, subcutaneous; IV, intravenous; po, orally; IM, intramuscular.
[a]May give with second and third albuterol.

nebulized β_2-adrenergic therapy in children in the ED, with pressurized oxygen.

β_2-Agonists

Repetitive, inhaled β_2-agonists are the mainstay of initial bronchodilator therapy in children. They work by relaxing bronchial smooth muscle directly and may also modulate mediator release from mast cells and basophils. Inhalation therapy has been shown to be as effective as a subcutaneous injection for mild to moderate obstruction and is associated with fewer systemic adverse effects. The highly β_2-selective agent albuterol demonstrates strong potency, good duration of action, and little cardiotoxicity. Frequent (every 15 to 30 minutes) doses of nebulized albuterol appear to be effective in

reversing airway obstruction. Although the ideal dose of albuterol (0.5%) has not been determined, the NAEPP EPR3 guidelines recommend 0.15 mg per kg (0.03 mL per kg) per dose, with a minimum dose of 2.5 mg. From a practical standpoint, patients older than 1 year who weigh less than 30 kg should be given 2.5 mg (0.5 mL) and those who weigh more than 30 kg should be given 5 mg (1 mL), or 0.5 mg per kg per hour via continuous nebulization.

Systematic review has concluded that an albuterol metered-dose inhaler (MDI) and chamber are at least as effective as nebulized treatments of children of all ages and more effective in certain subgroups (younger than 5 years with a moderate to severe exacerbation). It is important to administer four to eight puffs with a valved holding chamber during each treatment

MEDICAL EMERGENCIES

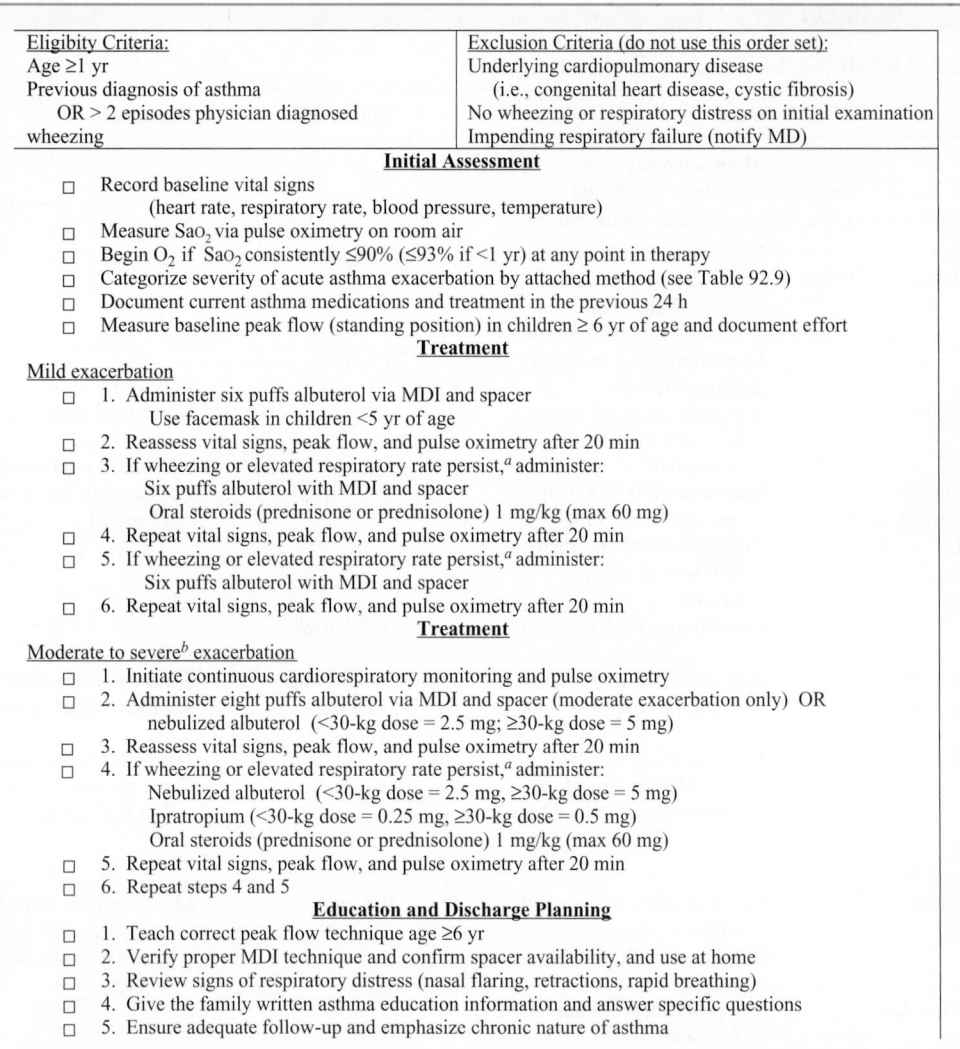

Eligibity Criteria:	Exclusion Criteria (do not use this order set):
Age ≥1 yr	Underlying cardiopulmonary disease
Previous diagnosis of asthma	(i.e., congenital heart disease, cystic fibrosis)
OR > 2 episodes physician diagnosed	No wheezing or respiratory distress on initial examination
wheezing	Impending respiratory failure (notify MD)

Initial Assessment

☐ Record baseline vital signs
     (heart rate, respiratory rate, blood pressure, temperature)
☐ Measure Sao_2 via pulse oximetry on room air
☐ Begin O_2 if Sao_2 consistently ≤90% (≤93% if <1 yr) at any point in therapy
☐ Categorize severity of acute asthma exacerbation by attached method (see Table 92.9)
☐ Document current asthma medications and treatment in the previous 24 h
☐ Measure baseline peak flow (standing position) in children ≥ 6 yr of age and document effort

Treatment

Mild exacerbation

☐ 1. Administer six puffs albuterol via MDI and spacer
     Use facemask in children <5 yr of age
☐ 2. Reassess vital signs, peak flow, and pulse oximetry after 20 min
☐ 3. If wheezing or elevated respiratory rate persist,[a] administer:
     Six puffs albuterol with MDI and spacer
     Oral steroids (prednisone or prednisolone) 1 mg/kg (max 60 mg)
☐ 4. Repeat vital signs, peak flow, and pulse oximetry after 20 min
☐ 5. If wheezing or elevated respiratory rate persist,[a] administer:
     Six puffs albuterol with MDI and spacer
☐ 6. Repeat vital signs, peak flow, and pulse oximetry after 20 min

Treatment

Moderate to severe[b] exacerbation

☐ 1. Initiate continuous cardiorespiratory monitoring and pulse oximetry
☐ 2. Administer eight puffs albuterol via MDI and spacer (moderate exacerbation only) OR
     nebulized albuterol (<30-kg dose = 2.5 mg; ≥30-kg dose = 5 mg)
☐ 3. Reassess vital signs, peak flow, and pulse oximetry after 20 min
☐ 4. If wheezing or elevated respiratory rate persist,[a] administer:
     Nebulized albuterol (<30-kg dose = 2.5 mg, ≥30-kg dose = 5 mg)
     Ipratropium (<30-kg dose = 0.25 mg, ≥30-kg dose = 0.5 mg)
     Oral steroids (prednisone or prednisolone) 1 mg/kg (max 60 mg)
☐ 5. Repeat vital signs, peak flow, and pulse oximetry after 20 min
☐ 6. Repeat steps 4 and 5

Education and Discharge Planning

☐ 1. Teach correct peak flow technique age ≥6 yr
☐ 2. Verify proper MDI technique and confirm spacer availability, and use at home
☐ 3. Review signs of respiratory distress (nasal flaring, retractions, rapid breathing)
☐ 4. Give the family written asthma education information and answer specific questions
☐ 5. Ensure adequate follow-up and emphasize chronic nature of asthma

FIGURE 82.2 Pediatric acute asthma exacerbation initial order set. MDI, metered-dose inhaler. [a]A respiratory score system may be used for decision making. [b]For severe exacerbations, physicians should strongly consider magnesium sulfate (50 mg per kg over 20 minutes IV) and may consider alternative therapies such as continuous albuterol.

and use the appropriate size face mask in younger children (younger than 4 years).

Levalbuterol is available as a nebulized preparation consisting of only the active R-isomer instead of the 1:1 ratio of R- and S-stereoisomers found in racemic β_2-agonists, at significant increased expense. It has been shown to be safe and well tolerated, with minimally fewer side effects, in asthmatic children older than 2 years with stable chronic disease. Data from pediatric ED settings fail to show consistent benefits with levalbuterol when compared with racemic albuterol. Routine preferential use cannot be made without further evidence, including cost analyses. In the meantime, levalbuterol remains an option for children with underlying medical problems, such as congenital heart disease, who may benefit from fewer β_2-agonist effects.

Subcutaneous injection of epinephrine or terbutaline remains an acceptable alternative in settings in which nebulized therapy is unavailable. It may also be indicated as initial therapy for children with severe obstruction, hypoventilation, or apnea in whom the delivery of nebulized medication to the airways is believed to be inadequate. Under these circumstances, the injection can be given simultaneously with the initial aerosol and is recommended to be given intramuscularly.

Corticosteroids

The recognition that inflammation is central to the pathogenesis of acute asthma means that corticosteroids have assumed an increasingly important role in the acute and chronic management of asthma. Early treatment of asthma exacerbations with steroids has been shown to prevent progression of airway obstruction, to decrease the need for emergency treatment and hospitalization, and to reduce morbidity. Steroids are believed to potentiate the effect of β_2-adrenergic agents within hours, in part, through alteration of cell membrane receptors and down-regulation of inflammatory mediator generation. They also appear to decrease small airway inflammation and edema within 24 hours. Steroid therapy may be particularly beneficial for infants in whom the primary pathophysiology is small airway edema and whose response to bronchodilators may be limited.

Because there is a time lag between the administration of steroids and the onset of clinical effect, the first dose is administered as soon as possible. As a rule, almost all children who have had a significant exacerbation ultimately receive steroids. An exception is made for children with mild symptoms who require either no inhaled treatments or, at worst, one treatment that immediately produces adequate resolution in the setting of minimal therapy prior to the arrival in the ED. Exposure to chickenpox in the unvaccinated, susceptible host represents one of the rare instances in which steroids may need to be avoided acutely.

Depending on the level of distress and the child's ability to tolerate oral medications, the dose of corticosteroid is given either intravenously (methylprednisolone 1 mg per kg or equivalent; maximum 60 to 80 mg) or by mouth (prednisone or prednisolone 1 mg per kg; maximum 60 to 80 mg). Guideline 3 reduced the dosage recommended to 1 mg per kg per day in one to two divided doses. Efficacy appears similar in either form.

Dexamethasone has been studied fairly extensively in the treatment of acute asthma in children. A dose of 0.6 mg per kg (maximum 16 mg) of oral dexamethasone for 2 days, started in the ED, is at least as efficacious as a traditional 5-day course of oral steroids. This option is particularly useful in settings of nonadherence or for children prone to emesis.

The data surrounding the use of inhaled corticosteroids in addition to, or in place of, the short course of systemic steroids for the management of acute asthma exacerbations in children are inconsistent. Meta-analyses examining these issues in adults and older children show conflicting results, in part, due to variations across studies in the types of steroids and outcome measures used. Despite the need for further analysis in the acute setting, inhaled steroids are now clearly recognized by the NAEPP as the first-line drug in the chronic management of all classes of persistent asthma in adults and children. Doubling the dose of the patient's usual inhaled corticosteroid is no longer recommended by the NAEPP as a method of treating even minor acute asthma exacerbations, unless there is significant intolerance to oral steroids and the exacerbation is mild. In that case, careful titration of a higher dose of inhaled corticosteroid may be considered.

Anticholinergics

Ipratropium bromide (Atrovent®) is a quaternary ammonium derivative of atropine that limits systemic absorption and decreases its side effects. Ipratropium appears to act synergistically with albuterol, adding additional bronchodilation for patients with moderate to severe airflow obstruction, and may be mixed with albuterol for delivery. Recommendations vary, but the NAEPP EPR3 guidelines suggest 0.25 mg for children (0.5 mg in adolescents and adults) every 20 to 30 minutes, combined with the first three albuterol treatment protocols.

An acceptable alternative is to administer two doses of ipratropium with the second and third albuterol treatment protocols after the assessment of response to the initial albuterol treatment protocol has demonstrated that the exacerbation is moderate to severe. Systematic review has confirmed the utility of multiple doses of ipratropium in severe acute exacerbations in children, with one admission prevented for every 12 children treated with ipratropium [number needed to treat (NNT = 12)].

Intravenous Magnesium Sulfate

Magnesium sulfate acts as a smooth-muscle relaxant to improve bronchodilation. In children with severe acute asthma, it may reduce hospitalizations and improve peak expiratory flow. Its use should be considered especially in children with a severe exacerbation with a poor response to other therapies. Both individual studies in children and a meta-analysis in adults have shown that magnesium sulfate, when given at a dosage of 25 to 75 mg per kg (maximum 2 g), improves outcome in the more severe subgroup. A significant emphasis should be placed on infusion time of 20 minutes, which is shorter than when used for other conditions. Vital signs including blood pressure should be monitored, although most studies report few systemic side effects.

Other Asthma Drugs

Heliox. Heliox is a mixture of helium and oxygen. The gas mixture has a lower density than oxygen and therefore theoretically reduces turbulent flow and airway resistance. This effect reduces work of breathing, which may, in turn, limit or delay respiratory muscle fatigue and allow more time for standard therapeutic agents to take effect. The lower gas density may also improve ventilation to alveoli, with longer time constants resulting in better matching of ventilation and perfusion and more effective delivery of aerosolized medications. Heliox must contain a high concentration of helium (60% to 80%) and it requires a tight-fitting mask, which may limit its acceptance in young children. No adverse effects of heliox have been reported.

Hypoxia can require titration of the heliox-oxygen mixture in the severely hypoxic patient. A systematic review on this agent in adults and children with moderate to severe exacerbations of asthma did not show significant benefits for many outcomes. Improvement in pulmonary function was demonstrated in the most severe subgroups. Consequently, current guidelines recommend considering a trial of heliox-driven albuterol nebulization for severe exacerbations that are unresponsive to therapy or for life-threatening episodes.

Leukotriene Modifiers. Two drugs in this category, zafirlukast and montelukast, have been approved for preventive therapy in chronic asthma in children. Both inhibit bronchoconstriction through antagonism to leukotriene receptors. Zafirlukast (for children 7 years or older) and montelukast (for children 2 years or older) are listed by the NAEPP as an alternative, but not preferred, treatment to inhaled corticosteroids for long-term control of mild persistent asthma or in combination therapy in moderate persistent asthma. There is insufficient evidence to support leukotriene modifiers in the acute management of asthma in children. Recent data suggest that montelukast reduces the risk of worsening asthma symptoms and unscheduled physician visits when added to usual therapy during the dreaded annual September spike in asthma exacerbations.

Omalizumab. Omalizumab is a monoclonal antibody with affinity for IgE at the binding site of the IgE receptor. It can therefore competitively bind free IgE and reduce inflammatory stimulation through IgE receptors. Omalizumab has been studied as a controller medication for moderate to severe persistent asthma in adults and children. Its role in an acute asthma exacerbation has not yet been examined.

Therapies to Avoid in Acute Asthma. Although theophylline has been added as an option in combination therapy for chronic asthma in some children, it currently has no role in the management of acute asthma and NAEPP EPR3 guidelines no longer recommend theophylline for hospitalized patients. Some children with acute asthma will be dehydrated and should receive fluid therapy to return them to a normovolemic state, but aggressive hydration offers no particular advantage. In addition, SIADH is a potential complication. Antibiotics are indicated only for specific bacterial infections such as sinusitis or OM and should be withheld for routine exacerbations of asthma.

Approach to the Child with Respiratory Failure. There is no universally accepted approach to the child with severe asthma who presents with respiratory failure or deteriorates in the ED despite the therapy already outlined. The options include continuous nebulized albuterol, intravenous (IV) β_2-agonist therapy, IV steroids and magnesium sulfate, heliox, and noninvasive and/or mechanical ventilation. The choice of therapy should be guided by the child's mental status, response to therapy, ability to sustain the increased work of breathing, degree of hypoxia, and trend in $PaCO_2$, as well as the physician's familiarity and comfort with the various treatment options. In all cases, these patients require continuous monitoring and constant involvement of clinical personnel. Arrangements should be made for admission to an ICU setting.

The use of continuous nebulized therapy is well established and is equally efficacious to intermittent albuterol in the adult ED setting. Continuous terbutaline and albuterol have been demonstrated to reverse respiratory failure and to eliminate the need for mechanical ventilation. Albuterol is administered as a 0.5 mg per kg per hour (maximum 15 mg per hour) dose.

IV β_2-agonist therapy is an option for children who fail continuous nebulized therapy. In the United States, terbutaline is administered as a 10 μg per kg loading dose over 10 minutes, followed by an initial infusion of 0.4 μg per kg per minute. The infusion is titrated up to effect in increments of 0.2 μg per kg per minute while the child is monitored for unacceptable tachycardia. The usual effective range is 3 to 6 μg per kg per minute. Although not available in the United States, albuterol is the favored IV agent in Canada and Europe.

If the child continues to deteriorate, intubation and mechanical ventilation should be considered. Noninvasive positive pressure ventilation in acute asthma has been studied in adults and children, but its use is controversial and also associated with barotrauma. Because of the difficulty of mechanical ventilation by endotracheal (ET) tube, centers may try it for short, well-monitored intervals while acute therapy is efficiently administered. There is no single ideal approach to the intubation of children with acute asthma, although some general recommendations can be made. The airway should be managed assuming a full stomach, as discussed in Chapter 5. Many authorities consider ketamine (1 to 2 mg per kg IV) to be the induction agent of choice because of its bronchodilating effects. Agents that may increase bronchospasm through histamine release, such as meperidine, morphine, D-tubocurare, and

atracurium, are best avoided. After intubation, all β_2-agonist, anticholinergic, and antiinflammatory drug therapies should continue.

Volume-controlled ventilation is preferred using larger than average tidal volumes (10 to 20 mL per kg), normal respiratory rates for age, and high flow rates to ensure long expiratory times. To achieve these goals, inspiratory pressures must often exceed 50 to 60 cm H_2O. In an effort to minimize barotrauma, incomplete correction of the respiratory acidosis or "controlled hypoventilation" ($PaCO_2$ more than 50 mm Hg) should be the target with a much higher $PaCO_2$ necessary in selected cases. In addition, sedatives and neuromuscular relaxants are generally necessary. Surveillance for barotrauma is critical.

Disposition

After 2 to 4 hours of frequent bronchodilator treatments and the initiation of corticosteroid therapy, as well as potentially IV magnesium sulfate, the limit of routine ED management has been reached and a disposition decision should be made based in part on reliable home resources and follow-up. Continued management of the patient in an "observation unit" or "clinical decision unit" for up to 24 hours may avoid the need for hospital admission.

Criteria for the disposition of acutely ill asthmatic children after ED management are difficult to specifically define. Scoring systems that use various assessment tools are still being developed. As a guideline, however, admission should be considered for children who meet any of the following criteria:

1. Persistent respiratory distress
2. SaO_2 of 91% or less in room air
3. PEFR less than 50% of predicted levels after therapy (or less than 70% with other factors)
4. Inability to tolerate oral medications or fluids (i.e., vomiting)
5. Previous emergency treatment in last 24 hours
6. Underlying high-risk factors: congenital heart disease, bronchopulmonary dysplasia, cystic fibrosis, and neuromuscular disease
7. Evidence of air leak

Other factors that should be considered in conjunction with these criteria include access to emergency care and medical advice, family reliability, sophistication of available home therapy, and severity of past exacerbations.

Children who also meet the criteria listed in Table 82.5 should be admitted to an ICU setting.

TABLE 82.5

CRITERIA FOR INTENSIVE CARE UNIT ADMISSION

Severe respiratory distress
Severity in severe range[a]
$PaO_2 < 60$ mm Hg or $SaO_2 < 90\%$ in 40% O_2
$PaCO_2 > 42$ mm Hg
Significant complications
Pneumothorax
Arrhythmia
Theophylline toxicity

[a]See Table 82.2.

Discharge Management

Children who have an adequate clinical response to ED therapy may be discharged to home. Ideally, they should be observed for 30 to 60 minutes after their last treatment to ensure they do not relapse immediately, except in those who had complete resolution with one treatment. Many discharged children will experience persistent mild to moderate symptoms and considerable acute disability. It is important to understand that the basic pathophysiology, which consists of small airway obstruction, inflammation, and altered lung mechanics, is not immediately reversed in the ED and additional therapy will be required.

Education should be patient and family focused, with emphasis on inhaler technique, the discharge plan and asthma action plan, telephone access to their primary care physician for asthma problems the next 3 to 5 days, and the importance of an asthma-related follow-up appointment in 1 to 4 weeks. An effort should also be made to remove triggers, if possible. Short-course, high-dose oral steroids (i.e., prednisone, 1 mg per kg per day in single or divided dosing up to 60 to 80 mg per day for 3 to 7 days) should be prescribed and administered for essentially all children who present to the ED with a significant exacerbation. The first dose should be given in the ED as previously outlined. Children who experience frequent acute exacerbations, persistent nocturnal symptoms, or multiple absences from school also clearly benefit from the addition of an inhaled corticosteroid to their regular regimen. Inhaled corticosteroid initiation should be strongly considered upon discharge from the ED for these children. Those currently taking an inhaled corticosteroid should be instructed to continue it during the acute exacerbation.

For children who experience their first episode of wheezing or who are not receiving long-term therapy, an albuterol MDI with age-appropriate spacer is generally well tolerated in the subacute phase following the acute episodes. Children younger than 4 years should use either an MDI with a valved holding chamber and face mask or albuterol with a nebulizer. The use of a valved holding chamber device in all ages improves the delivery of medications in MDIs. Partnership with the patient's primary care physician or asthma specialist in this management is recommended. Table 82.6 lists outpatient treatment options.

ANAPHYLAXIS

Background

Anaphylaxis is a potentially life-threatening manifestation of immediate hypersensitivity. The severity of these reactions varies from mild urticaria to shock and death. Anaphylaxis most commonly involves the pulmonary, circulatory, cutaneous, gastrointestinal (GI), and central neurologic systems.

The classic anaphylactic response is an IgE-mediated reaction that occurs after reexposure to an antigen to which the patient has previously been sensitized. The term *anaphylactoid reaction* is sometimes used to refer to a clinically similar syndrome that is not IgE mediated and does not necessarily require previous exposure to the inciting agent. It has become a common practice to use *anaphylaxis* to describe the clinical syndrome, regardless of the responsible mechanism. The annual incidence rate for anaphylaxis in adults and children is estimated to be 49.8 per 100,000 person-years and appears to be on the rise.

Any route of exposure, including parenteral, oral, or inhalation, has been associated with anaphylaxis. Food allergens represent the most common inciting agents in the United States in many studies of adults and children and most often occur outside medical facilities. Other common triggers include hymenoptera stings, drugs, immunotherapy, radiocontrast media, and blood products (Table 82.7). Interestingly, anaphylaxis to immunizations is a relatively rare event, more recently estimated to be 1.5 events per 1 million administrations. The causative agent for anaphylaxis goes undetected in a significant proportion of cases. IgE-mediated anaphylaxis to the latex present in gloves, Foley catheters, and ET tubes was first recognized in the late 1970s. Patients who undergo multiple procedures such as those with myelomeningocele and genitourinary dysplasias, as well as health care workers, appear to be at greatest risk of anaphylaxis to latex-containing products.

Certain conditions are known to increase the risk of fatal anaphylaxis. Peanut, cashew, and other tree nut triggers, especially when consumed outside the home environment, represent an important risk factor. Adolescents appear to be at the greatest risk for death, possibly due to risk-taking behavior. Asthma is also a worrisome historical feature in patients presenting with anaphylaxis, as is a delay in epinephrine administration. Most patients with a fatal reaction to a food have a history of an allergy to the specific food allergen trigger, but the severity of the prior reactions was quite different.

Pathophysiology

Currently, there are three well-established mechanisms that lead to anaphylaxis after exposure to a foreign substance. The first is the classic IgE-mediated reaction. The IgE antibodies form when a person is exposed to the foreign antigen (either in its native state or as a hapten attached to a carrier protein) for the first time. IgE binds to high-affinity receptors on mast cells and basophils. On reexposure, the antigen induces bridging of IgE molecules, leading to degranulation of these cells and to the release of various preformed and rapidly generated mediators. Immune complexes or other agents capable of activating the complement cascade induce the second mechanism. This results in the formation of anaphylatoxins such as C3a and C5a, which directly trigger the release of mediators from mast cells and basophils. The third mechanism involves the ability of certain agents to stimulate the release of mediators directly by an unknown mechanism that does not involve IgE or complement. Agents capable of direct stimulation include hyperosmolar solutions such as mannitol and radiocontrast media.

The sudden release of numerous mediators from mast cells and, perhaps, from basophils is presumed to be responsible for the pathophysiologic features of anaphylaxis (bronchospasm, increased vascular permeability, and altered systemic and pulmonary vascular smooth-muscle tone). The most notable of these mediators is histamine, but others that have been implicated include prostaglandin D2, leukotrienes, platelet-activating factor (PAF), tryptase, chymase, heparin, and chondroitin

TABLE 82.6

OUTPATIENT ASTHMA THERAPY

Medication	Dose	Maximum	Comments
Quick-relief β_2-agonists			
Metered-dose inhaler albuterol	2 puffs q4–6h (routine)	q4h	Use valved holding chamber for all patients, face mask <4 yr
	4–8 puffs q4–6h (exacerbation)		May double dose during exacerbations
			Encourage to consult physician if more frequent use required
Nebulized albuterol	0.05–0.1 mg/kg q4–6h in 2-mL NS	5.0 mg	1.25 mg minimum
			May mix with cromolyn solutions
			May double dose for exacerbations
Long-acting β_2-agonists			Should not be used for symptom relief or for exacerbations
Salmeterol DPI	1 blister q12h (age ≥4 yr)		
Formoterol DPI	1 capsule aerosolized q12h (age ≥5 yr)		
Corticosteroids			
Oral			
Prednisone	1 mg/kg/day × 3–10 day	60 mg/day	May require taper if >7–10 day
Prednisolone			
Inhaled			
Beclomethasone	First-line therapy for persistent asthma		Monitor growth in children
Budesonide			Use valved holding chamber to limit local adverse effects
Flunisolide	Doses vary greatly, depending on severity of chronic asthma		
Fluticasone			
Triamcinolone			
	Consult with primary care physician or asthma specialist		
Cromolyn sodium			
Metered-dose inhaler	2 puffs q6h		
nebulized	20 mg q6h		Age ≥2 yr
Leukotriene modifiers			
Zafirlukast	10 mg bid		Age 5–11 yr
10- or 20-mg tab	20 mg bid		Age ≥12 yr
Zileuton	600 mg 4 times a day		Age ≥12 yr
300- or 600-mg tab			Monitor LFTs
Montelukast	4 mg QHS		Age 12–23 mo (granules)
			Age 2–5 yr (chewable)
4-mg granules; 4- and 5-mg chewable	5 mg QHS		Age 6–14 yr
10-mg tab	10 mg QHS		Age ≥15 yr
Other controller medications			
Theophylline—variety of preparations	Beginning dose 10 mg/kg/day	16 mg/kg/day	Titrate to serum concentration of 5–15 μg/mL with monitoring; many possible drug interactions
Omalizumab (Xolair)	150 mg q2–4 wk	375 mg	Age ≥12 yr
Anti-IgE	Dose dependent on serum IgE		Moderate to severe allergic asthma

NS, normal saline; bid, twice a day; QHS, at bedtime; LFT, liver function tests.

sulfate. Recently, serum PAF, a proinflammatory phospholipid, has been shown to be elevated in patients with anaphylaxis. The activity of PAF acetylhydrolase, which degrades PAF, is inversely correlated with anaphylaxis severity.

Other causes of apparent anaphylaxis for which no clear mechanism has been identified exist. These include reactions after the ingestion of aspirin and other NSAIDs and exercise-induced anaphylaxis in which vigorous exercise, often preceded by a meal or an allergenic food, is the trigger.

Clinical Manifestations

The time between exposure to the inciting agent and onset of symptoms can vary from minutes to hours, although epidemiologic data suggest that the mean latency period in children is 15 to 30 minutes. This interval depends on the sensitivity of the patient and the route, quantity, and rate of administration of the antigen. In approximately 6% of hospitalized children with anaphylaxis in one series, a biphasic reaction occurs in

TABLE 82.7

COMMON CAUSES OF ANAPHYLAXIS

Insect venom
Hymenoptera
Fire ants

Drugs
Antibiotics—penicillin, cephalosporins, sulfonamides
Anesthesia related drugs—lidocaine, neuromuscular blocking
    agents
Aspirin
Radiocontrast media

Foods
Peanuts
Cashews
Other tree nuts
Milk
Seafood—shellfish
Grains
Fruit

Blood products

Immunotherapy
Allergen extracts

Other
Latex
Idiopathic

TABLE 82.8

URTICARIA: CLASSIFICATION

Dermatographism
Physical urticaria
    Cold
    Cholinergic
    Pressure
    Solar
Familial urticaria
    Hereditary angioedema
    Familial cold urticaria
Urticaria secondary to common agents
Urticaria secondary to serum sickness

which symptoms may recur up to 30 hours after the initial reaction. In this series, delayed initial administration of epinephrine was associated with a biphasic reaction.

The signs and symptoms of anaphylaxis vary in both the spectrum and severity of involvement. Reactions may be limited to the skin, as in a mild urticarial reaction, or catastrophically involve multiple systems, leading to shock and death.

Skin manifestations usually emerge first but may be absent. Findings include pruritus, flushing, erythema, urticaria, and, in more severe cases, angioedema. A more detailed discussion of urticaria is found at the end of this section (see also Chapter 66). Mucous membrane involvement may appear as pruritus and congestion of the eyes, nose, and mouth. Swelling of the lips or tongue can potentially impair swallowing and ventilation.

An immediate life-threatening feature of anaphylaxis is upper airway obstruction that results from edema of the larynx, epiglottis, and other surrounding structures. Airway involvement may manifest either as subtle discomfort of the throat or as obvious stridor and respiratory distress. Anaphylaxis can also cause lower airway disease secondary to bronchospasm. This leads to findings similar to acute asthma, such as a sense of chest tightness, cough, dyspnea, wheezing, and retractions.

Another potential life-threatening feature of anaphylaxis is cardiovascular collapse and hypotensive shock. Although the mechanisms are not fully understood, these cardiopulmonary manifestations are believed to result from profound vasodilation, increased vascular permeability, capillary leak, and intravascular volume depletion, as well as a possible direct toxic effect of circulating mediators. Arrhythmias and electrocardiographic evidence of myocardial ischemia may also be seen.

Central nervous system (CNS) involvement can include dizziness, syncope, seizures, and an altered level of consciousness.

These may occur either as a result of hypoperfusion or, possibly, as a direct toxic effect of mediator release.

GI symptoms are relatively common and include nausea, vomiting, diarrhea, and crampy abdominal pain.

Urticaria is a common manifestation of immediate hypersensitivity reactions and a number of other disease processes (Table 82.8). In the patient with acute urticaria from an IgE-mediated process, the urticaria may be localized to the area of exposure, such as the site of a sting. In addition to the localized urticaria, there may be a systemic reaction. Urticaria may be associated with angioedema—swelling of the lower dermis and subcutaneous tissues. The angioedema associated with urticaria is pruritic. Angioedema without pruritus is usually secondary to processes other than immediate hypersensitivity.

Urticaria can be separated into acute and chronic varieties. Most immediate hypersensitivity reactions are associated with an acute reaction, but chronic, recurrent urticaria can be mediated by recurrent exposure to an unknown antigen. In determining the cause of an urticarial reaction, the classification shown in Table 82.8 is important because management may vary.

The physical urticarial reactions may be life threatening, and they should be included in the differential diagnosis of anaphylaxis. Cold urticaria is an acute reaction to cold temperatures, with hives at the site of exposure. Generalized cold exposure, such as immersion in a cold pool, can precipitate an anaphylactic reaction (30%) with hypotension and shock. Therefore, an epinephrine autoinjector should be provided to these patients. The cold urticarias are often acquired and may follow viral infections. There is a familial form of cold urticaria that is rare and associated with a delayed onset, leukocytosis, and pain that distinguishes it from acquired cold urticaria. Cholinergic urticaria is characterized by punctate hives surrounded by an erythematous flare. Exercise, anxiety, shivers, and environmental temperature change can precipitate the reaction. It has been associated with exercise-induced anaphylaxis and often causes systemic manifestations (e.g., abdominal pain, headaches). Solar urticaria is a reaction to light, often sunlight, with the development of pruritus, erythema, and edema. Solar urticaria can be a manifestation of porphyria. Pressure urticaria is associated with hives that develop at the site of significant prolonged pressure in areas of the body. It is often associated with tight clothing.

MEDICAL EMERGENCIES

Management

Initial Assessment

Immediate resuscitative efforts must be initiated for the child who manifests the full-blown anaphylaxis syndrome or any of the independent life-threatening manifestations such as upper airway obstruction or shock. All patients who complain of an "allergic reaction" should be evaluated promptly to determine the extent of involvement, signs of progression, and the need for intervention.

History

The history should be directed toward determining the nature and severity of the reaction, the rapidity with which symptoms evolved, and the evidence of ongoing progression. Change in voice, difficulty in swallowing, dyspnea, and a sense of impending doom are characteristic of potentially serious anaphylaxis.

Attempts should also be made to determine the offending agent. This may be obvious as in a reaction to a bee sting. The history should focus on the 1- to 2-hour period before the onset of symptoms. The association of anaphylactic reactions to food is often confusing. Although patients often identify a particular food as the cause, a more detailed history may implicate something else in the meal. For example, it is common to associate reactions with chocolate whereas the nuts in many chocolate preparations generally are the offending agents.

Factors that may place the child at increased risk for a severe reaction should also be ascertained. These include a personal history of asthma or atopic disease or a previous allergic reaction.

A rapid cardiopulmonary assessment should precede any detailed physical examination to quickly determine whether any evidence of upper airway obstruction, bronchospasm, or shock exists. Once these issues have been identified and treatment has been initiated, a more detailed assessment should be performed to evaluate the patient for less serious cutaneous and GI manifestations.

Management of a life-threatening anaphylactic reaction requires simultaneous evaluation and management of the airway, breathing, and circulation, as well as the immediate administration of epinephrine as illustrated in Fig. 82.3 and

discussed in a sequence in the following section. Delay in the administration of epinephrine increases the risk of adverse outcomes.

Maintenance of the Airway and Oxygenation

The physician should administer 100% oxygen, with bag-valve-mask ventilation, when indicated, to assist ventilation. If there is complete airway obstruction, preparation for immediate ET intubation should parallel the rapid intramuscular administration of epinephrine, which can mitigate or ease the airway management. If intubation is unsuccessful, cricothyrotomy offers a lifesaving alternative.

Epinephrine, the first-line drug for anaphylaxis, should be administered as soon as possible. The threshold for the administration of epinephrine varies somewhat across the literature, but there is no absolute contraindication for its use in anaphylaxis. Epinephrine is clearly indicated when symptoms from more than one organ system are present. It is also recommended promptly for any patient who experiences an isolated cutaneous reaction (urticaria, flushing), who has risk factors for fatal anaphylaxis, or who has a history of a near-fatal episode. The recommendation to administer it sooner, rather than later, in the course of anaphylaxis, comes from the increased likelihood of a fatal reaction among patients who receive delayed administration of epinephrine.

As an α-adrenergic agonist, epinephrine promotes vasoconstriction, which increases blood pressure and decreases capillary leakage. As a β-adrenergic agonist, it relaxes bronchial smooth muscle, increases cardiac rate and contractility, and inhibits further mediator release. Epinephrine should be administered via intramuscular injection to the thigh as a 1:1,000 solution, at a dose of 0.01 mg per kg (maximum 0.5 mL). This dose may be repeated every 5 to 15 minutes for persistent or recurrent symptoms. It has been shown in children that absorption is more rapid and peak plasma levels are higher when intramuscular epinephrine is used than that absorbed via the subcutaneous route.

If the patient is hypotensive or hypoperfused, or if the initial intramuscular dose is ineffective, the epinephrine should be administered intravenously or through an intraosseous needle as a 1:10,000 solution, at a dose of 0.01 mg per kg (maximum 0.1 mL per kg) *over 1 to 2 minutes*. In severe cases, this may need to be followed by a continuous epinephrine infusion of 0.1 μg per kg per minute, which can be titrated to effect up to a maximum dose of 1 μg per kg per minute. Inhaled epinephrine does not achieve adequate plasma levels and should not be substituted for the intramuscular dose during initial therapy for anaphylaxis.

Bronchospasm should be treated aggressively with supplemental oxygen, inhaled β_2-agonists such as albuterol or epinephrine, and corticosteroids, as outlined in the previous section on asthma.

Maintenance of the Circulation

Hypotensive patients should be placed in the Trendelenburg position, and a rapid bolus of 20 mL per kg of a crystalloid solution of normal saline or lactated Ringer's solution should be administered and repeated as necessary. Because plasma volume may fall precipitously by 20% to 40%, large amounts of fluid may be necessary. If hypotension persists after epinephrine administration, normal saline bolus, and positioning,

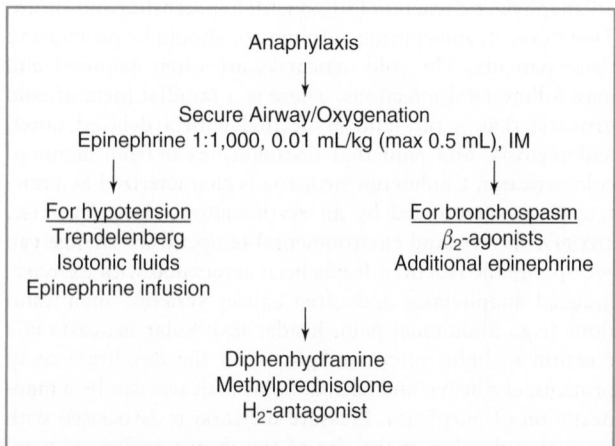

Anaphylaxis
↓
Secure Airway/Oxygenation
Epinephrine 1:1,000, 0.01 mL/kg (max 0.5 mL), IM
↓

For hypotension
Trendelenberg
Isotonic fluids
Epinephrine infusion

For bronchospasm
β_2-agonists
Additional epinephrine

↓
Diphenhydramine
Methylprednisolone
H_2-antagonist

FIGURE 82.3 Management of anaphylaxis. IM, intramuscular.

a continuous infusion of epinephrine should be started as previously described.

Other Therapy

The H$_1$-receptor antihistamines such as diphenhydramine (1 to 1.25 mg per kg intramuscularly or intravenously; maximum 50 mg) are indicated in histamine-mediated allergic reactions. In more stable patients, some authors prefer the oral route of administration. The H$_1$-receptor antihistamines work synergistically with the epinephrine therapy.

Corticosteroids do not take effect during the initial resuscitative phase of anaphylaxis. Their role in preventing biphasic reactions is unclear, but corticosteroids are frequently recommended because of known efficacy for other allergic diseases. They can be administered as methylprednisolone 1 to 2 mg per kg IV (maximum 125 mg) or, for mild symptoms, prednisone 0.5 to 1 mg per kg by mouth (maximum 60 to 80 mg). Children who have received steroids within the last several months or those experiencing severe reactions should receive IV corticosteroids. Stress-dose hydrocortisone should be considered for those with life-threatening anaphylaxis.

Data in adults confirm the additional therapeutic effect of H$_2$-blocking antihistamines such as cimetidine (5 mg per kg; maximum 300 mg) or ranitidine (1 to 2 mg per kg; maximum 50 mg) in addition to H$_1$-blocking antihistamines in acute allergic syndromes. These agents may work synergistically with the H$_1$-blocking antihistamines and are recommended in severe or refractory anaphylaxis.

On occasion, in severe reactions from injection, a venous tourniquet above the injection site of the offending agent and local infiltration of epinephrine 1:1,000 (0.005 mL per kg) and/or the application of ice may decrease further absorption.

Management of Limited Reactions

Most children with allergic reactions present with involvement limited to a diffuse, pruritic rash; localized swelling; or benign involvement of the mucous membranes. Appropriate management of these children varies according to the specific presentation. Options include subcutaneous epinephrine (e.g., for evolving urticaria), oral antihistamines, and corticosteroids.

Diphenhydramine (5 mg per kg per day divided every 4 to 6 hours, with a maximum of 300 mg per 24 hours) and hydroxyzine (2 mg per kg per day divided every 4 to 6 hours, with a maximum of 200 mg per day) are the antihistamines most commonly prescribed for urticaria. In the case of cold urticaria, cyproheptadine (0.25 to 0.5 mg per kg per day divided every 12 hours, with a maximum of 32 mg per day) is the drug of choice whereas hydroxyzine is preferred for cholinergic urticaria or most other chronic urticaria.

Disposition

The recommended period of observation after anaphylaxis should be individualized and based upon severity, risk factors, and access to care. An observation period of 4 to 6 hours may be appropriate for patients with mild to moderate episodes that resolve promptly with therapy. Patients with severe reactions that involve upper airway obstruction or shock generally should be monitored for a minimum of 8 to 24 hours. The incidence of biphasic reactions varies across the literature but approaches 20% in some studies. Children with a history of asthma appear to be at increased risk for delayed, biphasic, and severe reactions and may also require prolonged monitoring. In addition, a longer period of observation may be indicated for patients in whom the allergen could continue to be absorbed, those with a slower onset of symptoms, or those with a history of biphasic reactions.

Patients with less severe manifestations can be discharged home on a course of antihistamines and, in selected cases, corticosteroids. As a rule, therapy initiated in the ED should be continued for a minimum of 48 hours. Follow-up with the child's primary care physician is also advised and referral to an allergist will be indicated in cases of severe disease.

Strategies to avoid exposure to the offending agent should be discussed. All children with a history of significant anaphylaxis, especially those with asthma or a reaction to peanuts or tree nuts, should be instructed to carry a preloaded syringe of epinephrine to be used in emergencies. The chosen dose should be nearest to 0.01 mg per kg per dose [EpiPen (0.3 mg) or EpiPen Jr. (0.15 mg)] and may be rounded up for patients at higher risk of a severe reaction, as outlined previously. In children weighing less than 10 kg, dosing may be more appropriately achieved via syringe administration of a predetermined dose of 1:1,000 epinephrine at 0.01 mg per kg per dose. It has been shown that practical demonstrations at the time of prescription of an epinephrine autoinjector dramatically increase the likelihood of effective administration.

Following an episode of anaphylaxis, approximately 30% of children have a second episode within 7 years. Children with atopic dermatitis, a documented sensitivity to food allergens, or a history of urticaria/angioedema appear to be at increased risk for recurrence.

ANGIOEDEMA WITHOUT URTICARIA

Background

Angioedema without urticaria or other signs of anaphylaxis can be classified as hereditary, acquired, idiopathic, or exposure related (drug, food, bite, or environmental allergen). It results in nonpitting edema of the subcutaneous tissues and is usually bradykinin and complement mediated. Acquired angioedema due to malignancy or autoimmune disease is rare in childhood. Idiopathic angioedema that is chronic is also uncommon in children, but thyroid dysfunction must be considered. A significant percentage of cases with an identifiable causative factor (such as a nonsteroidal antiinflammatory agent or food) will respond to the removal of the offending agent. Many exposure-related and idiopathic cases are presumably histamine mediated (despite lack of urticaria) and will respond to corticosteroids and antihistamines. A detailed review of potential exposures and comprehensive family history are important to guide therapy. Because of the high morbidity and mortality associated with hereditary angioedema, the rest of this section is devoted to its recognition and management.

Hereditary Angioedema

Pathophysiology. Hereditary angioedema is caused by a deficiency of C_1-inhibitor function. It is a rare episodic disorder and can be the result of either low levels of the protein (type I) or poor functionality (type II), causing recurrent episodes of vascular permeability. Because of the autosomal-dominant inheritance pattern, many children with the disorder have a positive family history. However, 20% to 25% of cases are due to spontaneous mutations. School age (8 to 12 years) is the mean age of onset. Patients may present with subcutaneous angioedema (involving circumscribed areas of edema of the skin, most commonly the extremities, without erythema or pruritis), abdominal attacks (severe pain, distention, and vomiting), or laryngeal edema (life-threatening hoarseness, stridor, and voice changes).

Triggers. Episodes of angioedema may be triggered by direct mechanical friction or trauma. Affected children should therefore avoid contact sports. Exposures that result from viral infections should be limited as much as possible (such as early daycare). Puberty often worsens acute episode frequency and duration. Stress, dental manipulation, estrogens, and angiotensin-converting enzyme inhibitors can also serve as the inciting agents of edema.

Clinical Course. Diagnosis of hereditary angioedema early in life is critical but often delayed. A complete history and physical, with special attention to the airway, posterior pharynx, and abdomen, should be performed. Occasionally, abdominal ultrasonography is useful in discriminating angioedema from a surgical process, shows hyperemia of the bowel wall, and often reveals ascites. Patients may report a prodrome of paresthesias at the location where edema will arise, with the self-limited episodes lasting from 2 to 4 days.

The diagnosis is suspected from C4 levels that are usually low because of increased conversion of C4 to C1, while C3 is normal. Functional and antigenic C_1-inhibitor levels should be determined but may be falsely low in infants younger than 2 years.

Management. Supportive care with airway management and monitoring, fluid resuscitation, and pain control represents the mainstay of management. Intubation should be strongly considered in the presence of an inability to swallow, voice changes, or dyspnea. Because of the potential for landmark distortion and an acute increase in edema, direct laryngoscopy is best performed in a controlled setting where a definitive surgical airway can be achieved when required. Unfortunately, corticosteroids and antihistamines are usually ineffective in the management of hereditary angioedema. Epinephrine (nebulized or intramuscular) is also likely to be ineffective but may transiently improve symptoms.

Human C_1-inhibitor concentrate was recently licensed in the United States for routine prophylaxis in adolescents and adults and is widely used in other countries for acute attacks. Efficacy studies of C_1 inhibitor for acute episodes and recombinant product development are underway in the United States. Otherwise, treatment options are limited in children. Currently available in Europe and Canada, C_1-inhibitor concentrate can be administered immediately (10 to 20 units per kg up to 1,000 units) parenterally to children presenting with laryngeal edema or symptoms of an acute abdominal process. This treatment generally begins to alleviate symptoms within 30 to 60 minutes. Repetitive doses are sometimes required. Hospitalization is often necessary in the course of severe laryngeal or abdominal attacks. Currently, in the United States where C_1 inhibitor is not available, fresh frozen plasma (10 mL per kg) may be considered for acute management with consultation with an allergist because its use in hereditary angioedema is controversial. Drugs for long-term prophylaxis (attenuated androgens) are available but not generally used in children. Antifibrinolytics (such as ϵ-aminocaproic acid) are sometimes used for prophylaxis in children, but reports of efficacy in acute therapy remain anecdotal.

SERUM SICKNESS

Background

Serum sickness is an immune complex–mediated disease. It was first described in 1905 in patients who had received heterologous antisera, which, at that time, was used routinely to treat various infectious diseases. Today, the most common cause of serum sickness is exposure to medication, usually described as a serum sickness–like reaction.

The clinical syndromes secondary to an immediate hypersensitivity reaction may appear similar to serum sickness. In the former, IgE is primarily responsible, whereas IgG or IgM immune complexes classically mediate the latter. In many cases, however, elements of both processes are involved. The clinical syndrome of a serum sickness–like reaction that is not mediated by immune complexes has been reported. These reactions are referred to as serum sickness–like reactions. Serum sickness–like reactions appear to be responsible for the relatively common reactions seen in association with cefaclor and many other drugs.

Currently, the medications implicated most frequently in serum sickness or serum sickness–like reactions include the penicillins, sulfonamides, cephalosporins, streptomycin, hydantoins, griseofulvin, bupropion, fluoxetine, and thiouracil. Because these drugs are all low-molecular-weight substances, they cannot act as antigens directly but must bind to proteins, usually through their metabolites. This makes it difficult to substantiate sensitization.

The use of therapeutic agents obtained from heterologous serum has decreased dramatically. These preparations are currently found in antithymocyte globulins used to prevent organ transplant rejection and in antitoxins for the management of clostridial infections, diphtheria, tetanus, and specific arachnid, snake, and scorpion envenomations. Chimeric human-murine monoclonal antibodies such as infliximab (used to treat psoriasis and inflammatory bowel disease) can also induce serum sickness.

Less commonly, exposures to various chemical, infectious agents, or autologous antigens result in a serum sickness–like illness.

Pathophysiology

In the classical serum sickness model, an animal is injected with foreign serum protein. The animal develops the symptoms characteristic of serum sickness 7 to 10 days later. During the initial period after the injection of the foreign protein, there is a period of antigen excess. Antibodies develop approximately 6 to 10 days after the initial antigen injection and then antibody-antigen complexes are formed.

These immune complexes deposit in the tissues and may also activate complement. After this period of immune complex formation, there is a period of antibody excess during which antigen disappears from the system. Symptoms develop when soluble immune complexes are being cleared by the body. These immune complexes can activate the classical complement pathway. The classical pathway of activation begins with the formation of the C1q antibody complex, which activates a C_1 esterase that cleaves the fourth and second complement components (C4 and C2). The C4 and C2 that have been activated can then cleave C3. It is the cleavage of C3 and generation of its active components that allow for the activation of the late-acting complement components (C5 to C9). Because the immune complex activation involves the classical components, C4, C2, and C3, their serum concentration decreases. The complement activation generates the anaphylatoxins C3a and C5a, which then increase vascular permeability, release histamine, and produce bronchospasm. They activate many other cells in the inflammatory process and lead to inflammation around deposits of complexes in various tissues.

Clearance of immune complexes depends on their size and the effectiveness of the reticuloendothelial system. The most vulnerable organs to injury include kidneys and the vascular system.

It has also been shown in experimental animals that immune complex deposition can be enhanced by concomitant activation of an immediate hypersensitivity reaction. The IgE-mediated mast cell degranulation increases vascular permeability, which, in turn, enhances immune complex deposition.

Clinical Manifestations

The severity of serum sickness and the specific clinical manifestations vary widely. The reaction is characterized by fever, malaise, and a rash that is most commonly urticarial but may also appear as maculopapular or vasculitic eruption. Other manifestations include arthralgias or arthritis, lymphadenopathy, angioedema, and nephritis. Other less common problems include abdominal pain, carditis, anemia, and neuritis. Serum sickness is usually self-limited and typically resolves within 1 to 2 weeks with or without therapy.

Characteristically, the onset of symptoms occurs 7 to 14 days after the primary exposure. If there has been prior sensitization, however, reexposure can result in onset of a few days.

History

The history should be directed toward identifying the offending agent and determining the extent and severity of the symptoms. The physician should review possible exposures up to 14 days before symptoms to ascertain a possible cause for the process. Because a secondary exposure can produce a more rapid onset of symptoms (1 to 4 days), inquiries about this interval and about previous exposures may also be revealing.

In addition, the history should elicit information about the extent of systemic illness and the involvement of specific organ systems. It is important to determine the time course and nature of the rash; the degree of joint pain, swelling, or warmth; and evidence of renal involvement such as hematuria, edema, and reduced urine output. In light of the potential for involvement of other organ systems, a complete review of systems is indicated.

Physical Examination

The physical examination serves to determine the severity and extent of involvement of the reaction. A general inspection will help ascertain how ill and uncomfortable the child is. Examination of the skin may reveal a maculopapular eruption, urticaria, or palpable purpura of a cutaneous vasculitis. Painful angioedema is commonly present. Generalized lymphadenopathy often occurs. In more severe reactions, the joints show erythema, warmth, and effusion. Wheezes may be appreciated on auscultation of the lungs, and a pericardial friction rub may be audible if pericarditis is present. The liver and the spleen often enlarge. Rarely, neurologic deficits occur secondary to a vasculitis of the CNS. In serum sickness–like reactions, symptoms are generally limited to fever, pruritis, urticaria/rash, and arthralgias.

Laboratory Findings

The selection of laboratory studies should be determined by the severity of the reaction, the evidence of specific organ system involvement, and the degree of diagnostic uncertainty. For most patients, a urinalysis to look for the evidence of renal involvement is all that is required. A list of other studies that may be indicated for individual patients with immune complex–mediated disease is outlined in Table 82.9.

TABLE 82.9

POSSIBLE LABORATORY EVALUATION OF SERUM SICKNESS[a]

Blood tests
Erythrocyte sedimentation rate
Complete blood cell count with differential
CH50, C3, C4
Blood urea nitrogen, creatinine
Antinuclear antibody
Rheumatoid factor
Hepatic enzymes
Hepatitis B screen
Heterophile antibody
Immune complex assay

Other laboratory tests
Urinalysis
Electrocardiogram
Stool hematest
Computed tomography scan

[a]Laboratory evaluation should be tailored for each individual patient as noted in the text.

The erythrocyte sedimentation rate may be elevated. Both CBC and differential counts may reveal leukopenia or leukocytosis. The C3, C4, and CH5O may decrease because of complement activation. Any of the tests for circulating immune complexes (e.g., cryoglobulins) may be elevated. Stool testing for blood should be considered for patients with abdominal pain or other symptoms involving the GI tract. If carditis is suspected, a screening electrocardiogram and chest radiographs should be obtained; an echocardiogram may also be considered. Severe headache or focal neurologic deficits are indications for neuroimaging, usually a computed tomography scan. Serum sickness–like reactions will not be accompanied by hypocomplementemia or renal dysfunction.

Management

The treatment of serum sickness is based on the extent and severity of the disease. Keeping in mind that the reaction is usually self-limited, the goal is to provide symptomatic relief and to monitor for complications. If possible, the offending antigen should be eliminated.

Pharmacologic management usually involves one or more of the following: antihistamines, NSAIDs, and corticosteroids. Pruritus, rash, and angioedema can be managed with an antihistamine such as hydroxyzine (2 mg per kg per 24 hours divided every 6 to 8 hours, with a maximum of 200 mg per 24 hours). Although experience in the treatment of serum sickness is limited, the use of second-generation, nonsedating antihistamines may also be considered (Table 82.10). Urticarial lesions and angioedema that evolves rapidly may respond acutely to subcutaneous epinephrine (1:1,000, 0.01 mL per kg subcutaneously, with a maximum 0.30 mL). Mild joint involvement and/or fever often improve with the use of an NSAID such as ibuprofen (30 to 50 mg per kg per 24 hours divided every 6 to 8 hours up to a maximum 2.4 g per 24 hours). In more severe disease or after failure to respond to these measures, a burst of corti-

TABLE 82.10

EMERGENCY DEPARTMENT MANAGEMENT OF ALLERGIC RHINITIS

Medication	Dose	Comments
Antihistamines		
Loratadine		Available over the counter
10-mg tab or 10-mg/10-mL syrup	5 mg daily	Age 2–5 yr
	10 mg daily	Age ≥6 yr
Loratadine D		Available over the counter
12 h (loratadine 5 mg/pseudoephedrine 120 mg)	1 tab bid	Age ≥12 yr
24 h (loratadine 10 mg/pseudoephedrine 240 mg)	1 tab daily	Age ≥12 yr
Clarinex® (desloratadine)		
5-mg tab or 0.5-mg/mL syrup	1 mg daily	Age 6–11 mo
	1.25 mg daily	Age 12 mo–5 yr
	2.5 mg daily	Age 6–11 yr
	5 mg daily	Age ≥12 yr
Clarinex® D (desloratadine)		
12 h (desloratadine 2.5 mg/pseudoephedrine 120 mg)	1 tab bid	Age ≥12 yr
24 h (desloratadine 5 mg/pseudoephedrine 240 mg)	1 tab daily	Age ≥12 yr
Allegra® (fexofenadine)	30 mg bid	Age 6–11 yr
30-mg tabs, 60-mg tabs/caps, 180-mg tabs	60 mg bid	Age ≥12 yr
	180 mg	Age ≥12 yr
Allegra D® (fexofenadine 60 mg/pseudoephedrine 120 mg)	1 tab po bid	Age ≥12 yr
Zyrtec® (cetirizine)		Available over the counter
5-mg tabs, 10-mg tabs	2.5 mg daily	Age 6–11 mo
5 mg/5-mL syrup	2.5 mg daily or 2.5 mg bid	Age 1–5 yr
	5–10 mg daily	Age 6–11 and ≥12 yr
Zyrtec D® (cetirizine 5 mg/pseudoephedrine 120 mg)	1 tab bid	Age ≥12 yr
Xyzal® (levocetirizine)		
5-mg tabs, 5 mg/5 mL	2.5 mg daily	Age 6–11 yr
	5 mg daily	Age ≥12 yr
Decongestants		
Oral		
Pseudoephedrine	4 mg/kg/day q6–8 h	Maximum: 180 mg/day
Topical		
Oxymetazoline	Age >6: 0.05%	Limit use to <5 days to avoid
	2–3 drops each nostril bid	rebound congestion

bid, twice a day; po, orally.

costeroids may be prescribed at a dose of 1 to 2 mg per kg per day of prednisone for 7 to 10 days, followed by a taper for 2 weeks (maximum 60 to 80 mg per day). In life-threatening serum sickness with significant circulating immune complexes, plasmapheresis may play a role, but this procedure has not been used extensively for the treatment of this disease. Most children with serum sickness can be managed as outpatients, with close follow-up by their primary care physicians. Children with more severe involvement may benefit from hospitalization.

ALLERGIC RHINITIS

Background

Allergic rhinitis is the most common manifestation of atopic disease. Peak incidence occurs in the pediatric age group, affecting up to 30% of children and adolescents. Although not a life-threatening problem, allergic rhinitis can have a significant, often underestimated, negative impact on the quality of life of affected children. Severe nasal symptoms have been directly linked to poor school performance. Annual direct and indirect costs are estimated to be $2 billion to $5 billion in the United States alone. The morbidity of allergic rhinitis results from the direct manifestations of the disease and from associated complications such as sinusitis, acute asthma, sleep disturbances, dysosmia, and the consequences of chronic mouth breathing.

Pathophysiology

Allergic rhinitis is caused by an IgE-mediated hypersensitivity response of the nasal mucosa to foreign allergens. Following sensitization to a foreign antigen, reexposure triggers an immediate hypersensitivity reaction. This early response is characterized by the activation of mast cells and the release of preformed mediators of inflammation such as histamine and chemotactic factors and newly formed mediators such as prostaglandins and leukotrienes. These mediators cause vasodilation, mucosal edema, mucus secretion, stimulation of itch receptors, and reduction in the threshold for sneezing.

Many children experience a late-phase allergic response that consists of spontaneous release of inflammatory mediators 3 to 12 hours after exposure. There also is a "priming effect" that leads to increased responsiveness to small antigen loads and hyperresponsiveness to environmental irritants.

Historically, allergic rhinitis has been categorized as seasonal or perennial. *Seasonal* allergic rhinitis is most commonly caused by exposure to tree pollens (early spring), grass pollens (late spring and early summer), and ragweed or other weed pollens (late summer and fall). Allergens responsible for *perennial* allergic rhinitis include animal dander, house dust mites, and mold spores. Updated duration-based terminology established by the World Health Organization includes *intermittent* and *persistent* allergic rhinitis. These terms were chosen because not all patient with sensitivity to typical perennial allergens exhibit constant symptoms and because year-round pollens may be found in many parts of the world. It is important to recognize that food allergens to do not typically cause isolated allergic rhinitis.

Clinical Manifestations

The classic symptoms of allergic rhinitis include nasal congestion, paroxysmal sneezing, pruritus of the nose and eyes, and watery, profuse rhinorrhea. Other complaints may include noisy breathing, snoring, repeated throat clearing or cough, itching of the palate and throat, "popping" of the ears, and ocular complaints such as redness, itching, and tearing.

The physical examination is variable but may reveal the "gaping" look of a mouth breather, dark discoloration of skin on the infraorbital ridge caused by venous congestion (allergic shiners), and a transverse external nasal wrinkle secondary to chronic rubbing of the nose (allergic salute). Intranasal findings are variable. The mucosa is often edematous and may appear pale or violaceous. The nasal secretions may be clear, mucoid, or opaque.

Management

There are several approaches to the management of allergic rhinitis. These include the identification and avoidance of environmental allergens and irritants, oral antihistamine drugs, topical decongestants, topical antiinflammatory agents (cromolyn and/or corticosteroids), and immunotherapy.

Recognizing that long-term therapy must be highly individualized, the emergency physician will generally limit interventions to those that safely provide rapid, symptomatic relief and then refer the child to the primary care physician for long-term therapy. Data in adults suggest that adequate treatment of allergic rhinitis in asthmatic patients can significantly reduce health care utilization due to bronchospasm. In this important subgroup, parents should be reminded during the ED visit to seek appropriate chronic management of allergic rhinitis.

Topical corticosteroids have been considered as first-line therapy for chronic allergic rhinitis and may require as long as 2 weeks to achieve maximal relief. Rapid relief can generally be achieved by prescribing an antihistamine in combination with a decongestant (Table 82.10). First-generation antihistamines (such as chlorpheniramine, brompheniramine) are no longer recommended as first-line therapy because of the availability of many inexpensive second-generation antihistamines with a better side effect profile. Antihistamines acutely reduce the rhinorrhea, pruritus, and sneezing associated with allergic rhinitis. A trial of loratadine or cetirizine, now both available without a prescription, is an attractive option for many patients. Recent evidence also indicates that topical therapy with nasal corticosteroids has greater efficacy with an NNT of 4.4 than with an NNT of 15.4 for nonsedating histamines. Topical decongestants such as oxymetazoline hydrochloride present another alternative but should be prescribed for only brief periods (less than 5 days) to avoid tachyphylaxis. Other nonpharmacologic measures such as saline nasal rinses may provide some symptomatic relief.

MEDICAL EMERGENCIES

TABLE 82.11

TOPICAL TREATMENT FOR ALLERGIC RHINITIS

Trade name	Generic name	Dosage	Age
Corticosteroids			
Beconase AQ®	Beclomethasone (aqueous: 42 μg/spray)	1–2 sprays each nostril bid	≥6 yr
Rhinocort AQ®	Budesonide (32 μg/actuation)	1–2 sprays each nostril daily	6–11 yr
		2–4 sprays each nostril daily	≥12 yr
Flonase®	Fluticasone (50 μg/spray)	1–2 sprays each nostril daily	≥4 yr
Nasacort AQ®	Triamcinolone (55 μg/spray)	1 spray each nostril daily	2–5 yr
		1–2 spray each nostril daily	6–11 yr
		2 sprays each nostril daily	≥12 yr
Nasarel®	Flunisolide (29 μg/spray)	2 sprays each nostril bid	6–14 yr
		2 sprays each nostril bid-tid	≥15 yr
Nasonex®	Mometasone furoate (50 μg/spray)	1 spray each nostril daily	2–11 yr
		2 sprays each nostril daily	≥12 yr
Others			
Cromolyn Sodium (available over the counter)	5.2 mg/spray (mast-cell stabilizer)	1 spray each nostril q4–8 h	≥2 yr
Astelin®	Azelastine (137 μg/spray) (antihistamine)	1 spray each nostril bid	5–11 yr
		1–2 sprays each nostril bid	≥12 yr
Ipratropium bromide	0.03%, 21 μg/spray	2 sprays bid-tid	≥6 yr
Singulair®	Montelukast (leukotriene antagonist)	4-mg granules	6–23 mo
4 mg granules		4-mg (chewable) po QHS	2–5 yr
4- and 5-mg chewable		5-mg po QHS	6–14 yr
10-mg tab		10-mg po QHS	≥15 yr

bid, twice a day; tid, twice a day; po, orally; QHS, at bedtime.

Although there is little evidence to support allergen avoidance for indoor allergens, it is logical to limit exposures when possible in patients with significant allergic rhinoconjunctivitis, especially during pollen seasons.

The first-line approach for patients who require long-term therapy is topical cromolyn and/or corticosteroids (Table 82.11) with or without a second-generation oral antihistamine. For completeness, other categories of treatment are also listed in Table 82.11. Children with significant ocular symptoms may also benefit from local ophthalmic treatment (Table 82.12). Immunotherapy and omalizumab are important chronic therapies in development.

TABLE 82.12

OPHTHALMIC DROPS

Trade name	Generic name	Category	Dosage	Age (yr)
Naphcon-A®	Naphazoline and pheniramine	Antihistamine—decongestant	1–2 gtt 4 times/day	≥6
Optivar®	Azelastine hydrochloride	Antihistamine	1 gtt bid	≥3
Alomide®	Lodoxamide tromethamine	Mast-cell stabilizer	1–2 gtt 4 times/day	≥2
Patanol®	Olopatadine	Mast-cell stabilizer and antihistamine	1–2 gtt bid	≥3
Acular®	Ketotifen	Nonsteroidal antiinflammatory drug	1 gtt 4 times/day	≥3
Alamast®	Pemirolast	Mast-cell stabilizer	1–2 gtt 4 times/day	≥3

bid, twice a day; gtt, drops.

ACKNOWLEDGMENT

The discharge instructions for asthma found in Fig. 82.2 were kindly provided by Dr. Stephanie Kennebeck.

Suggested Readings

Asthma

Akinbami L. The state of childhood asthma, United States, 1980–2005. *Adv Data* 2006(381):1–24.

Appel D, Karpel JP, Sherman M. Epinephrine improves expiratory flow rates in patients with asthma who do not respond to inhaled metaproterenol sulfate. *J Allergy Clin Immunol* 1989;84(1):90–98.

Asmus MJ, Hendeles L. Levalbuterol nebulizer solution: is it worth five times the cost of albuterol? *Pharmacotherapy* 2000;20(2):123–129.

Barnett PL, Caputo GL, Baskin M, et al. Intravenous versus oral corticosteroids in the management of acute asthma in children. *Ann Emerg Med* 1997;29(2):212–217.

Benatar SR. Fatal asthma. *N Engl J Med* 1986;314(7):423–429.

Bender BG. Depression symptoms and substance abuse in adolescents with asthma. *Ann Allergy Asthma Immunol* 2007;99(4):319–324.

Bloom B, Dey AN, Freeman G. Summary health statistics for U.S. children: National Health Interview Survey, 2005. *Vital Health Stat 10* 2006(231):1–84.

Borish L, Culp JA. Asthma: a syndrome composed of heterogeneous diseases. *Ann Allergy Asthma Immunol* 2008;101(1):1–8; quiz 8–11, 50.

Boychuk RB, Yamamoto LG, DeMesa CJ, et al. Correlation of initial emergency department pulse oximetry values in asthma severity classes (steps) with the risk of hospitalization. *Am J Emerg Med* 2006;24(1):48–52.

Burkhart PV, Rayens MK, Revelette WR, et al. Improved health outcomes with peak flow monitoring for children with asthma. *J Asthma* 2007;44(2):137–142.

Carl JC, Myers TR, Kirchner HL, et al. Comparison of racemic albuterol and levalbuterol for treatment of acute asthma. *J Pediatr* 2003;143(6):731–736.

Carroll CL, Schramm CM. Noninvasive positive pressure ventilation for the treatment of status asthmaticus in children. *Ann Allergy Asthma Immunol* 2006;96(3):454–459.

Carroll CL, Schramm CM, Zucker AR. Severe exacerbations in children with mild asthma: characterizing a pediatric phenotype. *J Asthma* 2008;45(6):513–517.

Carroll CL, Sekaran AK, Lerer TJ, et al. A modified pulmonary index score with predictive value for pediatric asthma exacerbations. *Ann Allergy Asthma Immunol* 2005;94(3):355–359.

Castro-Rodriguez JA, Rodrigo GJ. Beta-agonists through metered-dose inhaler with valved holding chamber versus nebulizer for acute exacerbation of wheezing or asthma in children under 5 years of age: a systematic review with meta-analysis. *J Pediatr* 2004;145(2):172–177.

Cates CJ, Crilly JA, Rowe BH. Holding chambers (spacers) versus nebulisers for beta-agonist treatment of acute asthma. *Cochrane Database Syst Rev* 2006(2):CD000052.

Ciarallo L, Brousseau D, Reinert S. Higher-dose intravenous magnesium therapy for children with moderate to severe acute asthma. *Arch Pediatr Adolesc Med* 2000;154(10):979–983.

Edmonds ML, Camargo CA Jr, Pollack CV Jr, et al. Early use of inhaled corticosteroids in the emergency department treatment of acute asthma. *Cochrane Database Syst Rev* 2003(3):CD002308.

Expert Panel Report 3: guidelines for the diagnosis and management of asthma. National Institutes of Health; National Heart Lung and Blood Institute. Bethesda, MD: United States Department of Health and Human Services, 2007:1–417.

Fuglsang G, Pedersen S, Borgstrom L. Dose-response relationships of intravenously administered terbutaline in children with asthma. *J Pediatr* 1989;114(2):315–320.

Gorelick MH, Stevens MW, Schultz T, et al. Difficulty in obtaining peak expiratory flow measurements in children with acute asthma. *Pediatr Emerg Care* 2004;20(1):22–26.

Gorelick MH, Stevens MW, Schultz TR, et al. Performance of a novel clinical score, the Pediatric Asthma Severity Score (PASS), in the evaluation of acute asthma. *Acad Emerg Med* 2004;11(1):10–18.

Hederos CA, Janson S, Andersson H, et al. Chest X-ray investigation in newly discovered asthma. *Pediatr Allergy Immunol* 2004;15(2):163–165.

Holgate ST. Pathogenesis of asthma. *Clin Exp Allergy* 2008;38(6):872–897.

Johnston NW, Mandhane PJ, Dai J, et al. Attenuation of the September epidemic of asthma exacerbations in children: a randomized, controlled trial of montelukast added to usual therapy. *Pediatrics* 2007;120(3):e702–e712.

Kayani S, Shannon DC. Adverse behavioral effects of treatment for acute exacerbation of asthma in children: a comparison of two doses of oral steroids. *Chest* 2002;122(2):624–628.

Keahey L, Bulloch B, Becker AB, et al. Initial oxygen saturation as a predictor of admission in children presenting to the emergency department with acute asthma. *Ann Emerg Med* 2002;40(3):300–307.

Kim IK, Phrampus E, Venkataraman S, et al. Helium/oxygen-driven albuterol nebulization in the treatment of children with moderate to severe asthma exacerbations: a randomized, controlled trial. *Pediatrics* 2005;116(5):1127–1133.

Lesko SM, Louik C, Vezina RM, et al. Asthma morbidity after the short-term use of ibuprofen in children. *Pediatrics* 2002;109(2):E20.

Mannix R, Bachur R. Status asthmaticus in children. *Curr Opin Pediatr* 2007;19(3):281–287.

Martinon-Torres F, Rodriguez-Nunez A, Martinon-Sanchez JM. Nasal continuous positive airway pressure with heliox versus air oxygen in infants with acute bronchiolitis: a crossover study. *Pediatrics* 2008;121(5):e1190–e1195.

Mehta SV, Parkin PC, Stephens D, et al. Oxygen saturation as a predictor of prolonged, frequent bronchodilator therapy in children with acute asthma. *J Pediatr* 2004;145(5):641–645.

Mitchell I, Tough SC, Semple LK, et al. Near-fatal asthma: a population-based study of risk factors. *Chest* 2002;121(5):1407–1413.

Mitra A, Bassler D, Goodman K, et al. Intravenous aminophylline for acute severe asthma in children over two years receiving inhaled bronchodilators. *Cochrane Database Syst Rev* 2005(2):CD001276.

Nolan PK, Chrysler M, Phillips G, et al. Pulse oximetry coupled with spirometry in the emergency department helps differentiate an asthma exacerbation from possible vocal cord dysfunction. *Pediatr Pulmonol* 2007;42(7):605–609.

Qureshi F, Zaritsky A, Poirier MP. Comparative efficacy of oral dexamethasone versus oral prednisone in acute pediatric asthma. *J Pediatr* 2001;139(1):20–26.

Qureshi F, Zaritsky A, Welch C, et al. Clinical efficacy of racemic albuterol versus levalbuterol for the treatment of acute pediatric asthma. *Ann Emerg Med* 2005;46(1):29–36.

Richardson LP, Lozano P, Russo J, et al. Asthma symptom burden: relationship to asthma severity and anxiety and depression symptoms. *Pediatrics* 2006;118(3):1042–1051.

Rodrigo G, Pollack C, Rodrigo C, et al. Heliox for nonintubated acute asthma patients [update of *Cochrane Database Syst Rev* 2003;(4):CD002884; PMID: 14583955]. *Cochrane Database Syst Rev* 2006(4):CD002884.

Rodrigo GJ, Castro-Rodriguez JA. Anticholinergics in the treatment of children and adults with acute asthma: a systematic review with meta-analysis [comment]. *Thorax* 2005;60(9):740–746. Erratum in *Thorax* 2006;61(3):274.

Rodrigo GJ, Rodrigo C. Continuous vs intermittent beta-agonists in the treatment of acute adult asthma: a systematic review with meta-analysis. *Chest* 2002;122(1):160–165.

Rodrigo GJ, Rodrigo GJ. Rapid effects of inhaled corticosteroids in acute asthma: an evidence-based evaluation [comment]. *Chest* 2006;130(5):1301–1311.

Scarfone RJ, Capraro GA, Zorc JJ, et al. Demonstrated use of metered-dose inhalers and peak flow meters by children and adolescents with acute asthma exacerbations. *Arch Pediatr Adolesc Med* 2002;156(4):378–383.

Schuh S, Dick PT, Stephens D, et al. High-dose inhaled fluticasone does not replace oral prednisolone in children with mild to moderate acute asthma. *Pediatrics* 2006;118(2):644–650.

Stanley RM, Teach SJ, Mann NC, et al. Variation in ancillary testing among pediatric asthma patients seen in emergency departments. *Acad Emerg Med* 2007;14(6):532–538.

Stevens MM, Scribano PV, Gorelick MH. Screening for poor short-term outcome in acute pediatric asthma. *Ann Allergy Asthma Immunol* 2007;98(5):432–439.

Swischuk LE. Asthma attack: is a chest X-ray necessary? *Pediatr Emerg Care* 2005;21(7):468–470.

Wolf FM, Guevara JP, Grum CM, et al. Educational interventions for asthma in children. *Cochrane Database Syst Rev* 2003(1):CD000326.

Anaphylaxis

Alangari AA, Twarog FJ, Shih MC, et al. Clinical features and anaphylaxis in children with cold urticaria. *Pediatrics* 2004;113(4):e313–e317.

Arkwright PD, Farragher AJ. Factors determining the ability of parents to effectively administer intramuscular adrenaline to food allergic children. *Pediatr Allergy Immunol* 2006;17(3):227–229.

Bansal PJ, Marsh R, Patel B, et al. Recognition, evaluation, and treatment of anaphylaxis in the child care setting. *Ann Allergy Asthma Immunol* 2005;94(1):55–59.

Bochner BS, Lichtenstein LM. Anaphylaxis. *N Engl J Med 20* 1991;324(25):1785–1790.

Bohlke K, Davis RL, Marcy SM, et al. Risk of anaphylaxis after vaccination of children and adolescents. *Pediatrics* 2003;112(4):815–820.

Cianferoni A, Novembre E, Pucci N, et al. Anaphylaxis: a 7-year follow-up survey of 46 children. *Ann Allergy Asthma Immunol* 2004;92(4):464–468.

Davoren M, Peake J. Cashew nut allergy is associated with a high risk of anaphylaxis. *Arch Dis Child* 2005;90(10):1084–1085.

Decker WW, Campbell RL, Manivannan V, et al. The etiology and incidence of anaphylaxis in Rochester, Minnesota: a report from the Rochester Epidemiology Project. *J Allergy Clin Immunol* 2008;122(6):1161–1165.

Ellis AK, Day JH. Incidence and characteristics of biphasic anaphylaxis: a prospective evaluation of 103 patients. *Ann Allergy Asthma Immunol* 2007; 98(1):64–69.

Kemp SF. The post-anaphylaxis dilemma: how long is long enough to observe a patient after resolution of symptoms? *Curr Allergy Asthma Rep* 2008;8(1): 45–48.

Kemp SF, Lockey RF, Simons FE. Epinephrine: the drug of choice for anaphylaxis. A statement of the World Allergy Organization. *Allergy* 2008;63(8): 1061–1070.

Lane RD, Bolte RG. Pediatric anaphylaxis. *Pediatr Emerg Care* 2007;23(1): 49–56; quiz 57–60.

Lee JM, Greenes DS. Biphasic anaphylactic reactions in pediatrics. *Pediatrics* 2000;106(4):762–766.

Lin RY, Curry A, Pesola GR, et al. Improved outcomes in patients with acute allergic syndromes who are treated with combined H1 and H2 antagonists. *Ann Emerg Med* 2000;36(5):462–468.

Sampson HA. Anaphylaxis and emergency treatment. *Pediatrics* 2003;111(6, pt 3):1601–1608.

Sampson HA, Mendelson L, Rosen JP. Fatal and near-fatal anaphylactic reactions to food in children and adolescents. *N Engl J Med* 1992;327(6):380–384.

Sampson HA, Munoz-Furlong A, Bock SA, et al. Symposium on the definition and management of anaphylaxis: summary report. *J Allergy Clin Immunol* 2005;115(3):584–591.

Sampson HA, Munoz-Furlong A, Campbell RL, et al. Second symposium on the definition and management of anaphylaxis: summary report–Second National Institute of Allergy and Infectious Disease/Food Allergy and Anaphylaxis Network symposium. *J Allergy Clin Immunol* 2006;117(2): 391–397.

Shah E, Pongracic J. Food-induced anaphylaxis: who, what, why, and where? *Pediatr Ann* 2008;37(8):536–541.

Simons FE, Roberts JR, Gu X, et al. Epinephrine absorption in children with a history of anaphylaxis. *J Allergy Clin Immunol* 1998;101(1, pt 1):33–37.

Vadas P, Gold M, Perelman B, et al. Platelet-activating factor, PAF acetylhydrolase, and severe anaphylaxis. *N Engl J Med* 2008;358(1):28–35.

Wiener ES, Bajaj L. Diagnosis and emergent management of anaphylaxis in children. *Adv Pediatr* 2005;52:195–206.

Angioedema

Farkas H, Varga L, Szeplaki G, et al. Management of hereditary angioedema in pediatric patients. *Pediatrics* 2007;120(3):e713–e722.

O'Bier A, Muniz AE, Foster RL. Hereditary angioedema presenting as epiglottitis. *Pediatr Emerg Care* 2005;21(1):27–30.

Shah UK, Jacobs IN. Pediatric angioedema: ten years' experience. *Arch Otolaryngol Head Neck Surg* 1999;125(7):791–795.

Zingale LC, Beltrami L, Zanichelli A, et al. Angioedema without urticaria: a large clinical survey. *Can Med Assoc J* 2006;175(9):1065–1070.

Zuraw BL. Clinical practice. Hereditary angioedema. *N Engl J Med* 2008; 359(10):1027–1036.

Serum Sickness

Cochrane CG, Koffler D. Immune complex disease in experimental animals and man. *Adv Immunol* 1973;16:185–264.

Colombel JF, Loftus EV Jr, Tremaine WJ, et al. The safety profile of infliximab in patients with Crohn's disease: the Mayo Clinic experience in 500 patients. *Gastroenterology* 2004;126(1):19–31.

Colton RL, Amir J, Mimouni M, et al. Serum sickness-like reaction associated with griseofulvin. *Ann Pharmacother* 2004;38(4):609–611.

Dart RC, McNally J. Efficacy, safety, and use of snake antivenoms in the United States. *Ann Emerg Med* 2001;37(2):181–188.

Krishnan RS, Hsu S. Serum sickness due to infliximab in a patient with psoriasis. *J Drugs Dermatol* 2004;3(3):305–308.

Lawley TJ, Bielory L, Gascon P, et al. A prospective clinical and immunologic analysis of patients with serum sickness. *N Engl J Med* 1984;311(22): 1407–1413.

LoVecchio F, McBride C. Scorpion envenomations in young children in central Arizona. *J Toxicol Clin Toxicol*. 2003;41(7):937–940.

Lundquist AL, Chari RS, Wood JH, et al. Serum sickness following rabbit antithymocyte-globulin induction in a liver transplant recipient: case report and literature review. *Liver Transpl* 2007;13(5):647–650.

Proctor L, Renzulli B, Warren S, et al. Transfusion Medicine Illustrated. Monoclonal antibody-stimulated serum sickness. *Transfusion* 2004;44(7):955.

Segal AR, Doherty KM, Leggott J, et al. Cutaneous reactions to drugs in children. *Pediatrics* 2007;120(4):e1082–e1096.

Tamburro JE, Esterly NB. Hypersensitivity syndromes. *Adolesc Med* 2001;12(2):vii, 323–341.

Wiggins RC, Cochrane CG. Immune-complex-mediated biologic effects. *N Engl J Med* 1981;304(9):518–520.

Yerushalmi J, Zvulunov A, Halevy S. Serum sickness-like reactions. *Cutis* 2002;69(5):395–397.

Allergic Rhinitis

Al Sayyad JJ, Fedorowicz Z, Alhashimi D, et al. Topical nasal steroids for intermittent and persistent allergic rhinitis in children. *Cochrane Database Syst Rev* 2007(1):CD003163.

Blaiss MS. Pediatric allergic rhinitis: physical and mental complications. *Allergy Asthma Proc* 2008;29(1):1–6.

Bousquet J, Khaltaev N, Cruz AA, et al. Allergic Rhinitis and its Impact on Asthma (ARIA) 2008 update (in collaboration with the World Health Organization, GA(2)LEN and AllerGen). *Allergy* 2008;63(suppl 86):8–160.

Chervinsky P, Casale T, Townley R, et al. Omalizumab, an anti-IgE antibody, in the treatment of adults and adolescents with perennial allergic rhinitis. *Ann Allergy Asthma Immunol* 2003;91(2):160–167.

Fuhlbrigge AL, Adams RJ. The effect of treatment of allergic rhinitis on asthma morbidity, including emergency department visits. *Curr Opin Allergy Clin Immunol* 2003;3(1):29–32.

Garavello W, Di Berardino F, Romagnoli M, et al. Nasal rinsing with hypertonic solution: an adjunctive treatment for pediatric seasonal allergic rhinoconjunctivitis. *Int Arch Allergy Immunol* 2005;137(4):310–314.

Harvey R, Hannan SA, Badia L, et al. Nasal saline irrigations for the symptoms of chronic rhinosinusitis [comment]. *Cochrane Database Syst Rev*. 2007(3):CD006394.

Reed SD, Lee TA, McCrory DC. The economic burden of allergic rhinitis: a critical evaluation of the literature. *Pharmacoeconomics* 2004;22(6):345–361.

Sundberg R, Toren K, Hoglund D, et al. Nasal symptoms are associated with school performance in adolescents. *J Adolesc Health* 2007;40(6):581–583.

CHAPTER 83 ■ BITES AND STINGS

DEE HODGE III, MD

This chapter is oriented to the clinical diagnosis and management of injuries that result from bites and stings, especially as they relate to children. Although the largest proportion of the morbidity and mortality from these injuries occurs in the pediatric age group, little attention has been focused in the pediatric literature on the specifics of treatment.

An overall assessment should include vital signs, location and size of fang or sting marks, pain, swelling, color of surrounding skin, and any systemic symptoms. General care should include relief of pain and itching, tetanus prophylaxis, antibiotics if needed, and emotional support. Animals must be identified as venomous or not. Venomous animals are those that inject their toxin into other animals to produce a harmful effect. Poisonous creatures are those whose tissues are toxic, either in whole or in part. This chapter deals with venomous bites and stings and with wounds inflicted by nonvenomous animals. In evaluating any potential venomous bite or sting, the physician must distinguish between the asymptomatic and the symptomatic bite or sting. Clinical observation may be the only means of distinguishing between the two.

Only those venomous animals found within the continental United States and Canada are discussed here. Only marine life that exists within the tidal zone or is commonly washed ashore is considered. This chapter covers marine invertebrates and vertebrates, terrestrial invertebrates, venomous reptiles, and common mammalian bites.

MARINE INVERTEBRATES

Phylum Coelenterata (Cnidaria)

The phylum is divided into three large classes: the Hydrozoa (hydras, Portuguese man-of-war), Scyphozoa (true jellyfish), and Anthozoa (soft corals, stone corals, anemones).

The phylum includes some of the most beautiful and deadly marine creatures. All members of the phylum have specialized organelles called nematocysts, which are used for entangling, penetrating, anchoring, and poisoning prey (Fig. 83.1). When the tentacles touch an object, the nematocysts fire, releasing toxin-coated, barbed threads. Firing of the nematocysts is not fully understood; the process may be protein- or cation-mediated. The nematocysts of most species cannot penetrate human skin. However, those that do may cause severe pain, serious illness, or even death. The severity of envenomation is related to the degree of toxicity of the venom, number of nematocysts discharged, and general condition of the victim. Stings from sessile forms are generally not as severe as stings from free-floating forms. The various toxins have been named and described but have not been completely biochemically

characterized at the biochemical level. Venom varies from species to species. Jellyfish venoms affect autonomic nervous systems via several mechanisms. Paralysis and central nervous system effects appear to be related primarily to toxic proteins and peptides. Burning pain and urticaria are secondary to the release of various mediators of inflammation, including serotonin, histamine, or histamine-releasing agents in the venom.

Class Hydrozoa

Feathered hydroid (*Pennaria tiarelia*) is found from Maine to Florida and along the Texas coast just below the low-tide line. It is attached to solid objects, including pilings and floats. The mild sting that occurs with handling may be treated with local care.

Portuguese man-of-war (*Physalia physalis*)—commonly considered a jellyfish—is in reality a hydrozoan colony. The float can be up to 30 cm in length. The tentacles hang from the float, may reach a length of more than 75 feet, and contain about 750,000 nematocysts each. This pelagic animal is often driven ashore by storms along the Atlantic coast. Releasing one of the most powerful marine toxins, the nematocysts of the Portuguese man-of-war may discharge even when it is dead and washed up on the beach. Because of the length and transparency of the tentacles in the water, swimmers are often stung without seeing the animal. The toxin contains polypeptides and degradative enzymes. Local effects include pain and irritation. Systemic reactions include headache, myalgias, fever, abdominal rigidity, arthralgias, nausea and vomiting, pallor, respiratory distress, hemolysis, renal failure, and coma. Death may occur if the area stung is extensive in relation to the size of the victim. Treatment is discussed in the next section.

Class Scyphozoa

The common purple jellyfish (*Pelagia noctiluca*) is only mildly toxic. Local skin irritation is the major clinical manifestation.

Sea nettle (*Chrysaora guinguecinda*) is a common jellyfish found along the Atlantic coast. Clinical manifestations are the same as those for purple jellyfish.

Lion's mane (*Cyanea capillata*) is a highly toxic creature that received considerable publicity as the instrument of death in the Sherlock Holmes classic Adventure of the Lion's Mane. The animal reaches a width of 244 cm, with tentacles as long as 61 cm. The shaggy clusters of the golden yellow tentacles that hang from the medusa resemble the mane of a lion. The animal is found along both coasts. Contact with the tentacles produces severe burning. Prolonged exposure causes muscle cramps and respiratory failure.

Treatment of hydrozoan and scyphozoan stings is based on the same general principles. It is directed at three objectives: relieving pain, alleviating effects of venom, and controlling shock. The most important step is to remove the tentacles; as

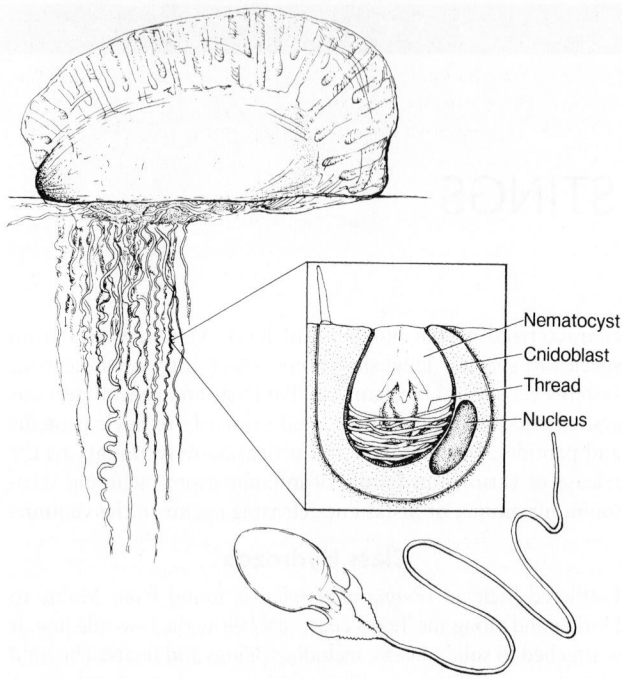

FIGURE 83.1 Marine invertebrate causing human sting.

long as the tentacle adheres to the skin, the nematocysts continue to discharge. The unexploded nematocysts are inactivated with topical application for 30 minutes with vinegar (3% acetic acid), a slurry of baking soda, or meat tenderizer (papain). Papain should not be left on for more than 15 minutes. Vinegar is generally the best disarming agent; however, for Portuguese man-of-war, vinegar has been shown to be ineffective and may activate the nematocysts. The area should be washed with seawater or normal saline. Any adherent tentacles should be carefully removed with instruments or a gloved hand, and the wound area should be immobilized. There is no antivenin available for *Physalia* or the scyphozoans, with the exception of the sea wasp, *Chironex fleckeri*, of Australia. General supportive measures for systemic reactions include oral antihistamines, oral corticosteroids, and codeine or meperidine for pain. Cardiac and respiratory support may be required. Muscle spasms have been treated with 10% solution of calcium gluconate 0.1 mL per kg (10 mg per kg) given intravenously, although the efficacy is controversial. Local dermatitis should be treated with a topical corticosteroid cream.

Class Anthozoa

The anemones found within U.S. tidal zones are only mildly toxic at worst. Coral cuts and stings can be a problem for swimmers off the Florida coast. The stinging ability of stony corals is not well defined but is considered to be of minor significance. Coral cuts, however, are important. The severity of coral cuts stems from a combination of factors, including laceration of tissue, nematocyst venom, foreign debris in the wound, and secondary bacterial infection. The clinical picture is one of stinging sensation followed by wheal formation and itching. If the wound is untreated, an ulcer with an erythematous base may form within a few days. Cellulitis, lymphangitis, fever, and malaise commonly occur.

Treatment consists of cleaning the wound and irrigation with copious amounts of saline. Removal of foreign particles must be accomplished, and debridement may be necessary. The sea provides an excellent inoculum for wound infections. Marine bacteria are generally heterotrophic, motile, and facultatively anaerobic, gram-negative rods. Organisms include *Vibrio* species, *Erysipelothrix rhusiopathiae*, and *Mycobacterium marinum*. Wounds should be left open. Broad-spectrum antibiotic therapy, particularly tetracycline, at a dosage of 40 mg per kg per day in four divided doses, has been advocated but should not be used routinely in children younger than 8 years. For children younger than 8 years, cephalexin (50 mg per kg per day in four divided doses) or trimethoprim-sulfamethoxazole (10 mg TMP per kg per day divided in two doses) should be used.

Phylum Echinodermata

Phylum Echinodermata includes starfish, sea urchins, and sea cucumbers. Of the three classes, only the Echinoedae—sea urchins—have clinical relevance for American children. The long-spined urchins (e.g., Diadema) are dangerous to handle. They do not appear to possess venom as do some of the tropical urchins, but the spines, composed of calcium carbonate, easily pierce the skin and lodge deep in the flesh. The spines may break off readily into the wound and can penetrate wet suits and sneakers. Most injuries occur during wading in shallow water. Clinically, penetration is accompanied by intense pain followed by redness, swelling, and aching. Complications include tattooing of the skin, joint arthritis, secondary infection, and granuloma formation.

In treatment, all spines should be removed as completely as possible. If spines break off in the wound, debridement should be performed with local anesthetic under aseptic conditions, but any spines not reachable will be absorbed in time. Soaking the wound in warm water may be helpful for pain. Systemic antistaphylococcal antibiotics should be used if infection develops.

MARINE VERTEBRATES

Stingrays

Background

Stingrays are the single most important group of venomous fishes, accounting for an estimated 1,000 attacks per year in North America. Stingrays are bottom feeders that have a habit of burying themselves in sand or mud of bays, shoal lagoons, and river mouths. The animals are found along the Atlantic, Pacific, and Gulf coasts and range from several inches in diameter to more than 14 feet in length. Six different species are represented in North American waters. Envenomations usually occur when an unsuspecting swimmer steps on the back of the animal and causes it to hurl its barbed tail upward into the victim as a reflex defense response. Most injuries are confined to the lower extremities, although wounds to the chest and abdomen have been reported.

The venom apparatus consists of a serrated, retropointed, dentinal caudal spine located on the dorsum of the tail. Spines vary in length, depending on the size of the ray, but may reach a length of 122 cm in some species. The spine is encased in an integumentary sheath that contains specialized secretory cells that hold the venom. When the stingray's barb strikes the victim, it easily penetrates the skin, rupturing the integumentary sheath over the spine and causing the venom to pass along the ventrolateral grooves of the barb, into the wound. Laceration of the victim's tissues when the spine is withdrawn facilitates the absorption and distribution of the toxin. The venom is a heat-labile toxin that has been shown to contain at least 15 fractions, including serotonin, 5-nucleotidase, and phosphodiesterase. The toxin depresses medullary respiratory centers, interferes with the cardiac conduction system, and produces severe local pain.

Clinical Manifestations

Because the barb is retropointed, the wound it produces is a combination of puncture and laceration. Wounds may vary in length from 3.5 to 15 cm. The sting is followed immediately by pain, which spreads from the site of injury during the next 30 minutes and usually reaches its greatest intensity within 90 minutes. Pain and edema are most often localized to the area of injury; however, syncope, weakness, nausea, and anxiety are common complaints attributed to both the effects of the venom and the vagal response to the pain. Among other generalized symptoms are vomiting, diarrhea, sweating, and muscle fasciculations of the affected extremity. Generalized cramps, paresthesias, hypotension, arrhythmias, and death may occur. The wound often has a jagged edge that bleeds profusely, and the wound edges may be discolored. Discoloration may extend several centimeters from the wound within hours after injury and may subsequently necrose if untreated. Often, parts of the stingray's integumentary sheath contaminate the wound.

Management

Treatment is aimed at (i) preventing complications evoked by the venom, (ii) alleviating the pain, and (iii) preventing secondary infection. At the scene, the wound should be irrigated with cold saltwater. Flushing can help remove much of the venom. Bleeding should be controlled with direct pressure. On the patient's arrival in the emergency department (ED), shock, if present, should be treated with intravenous (IV) fluids. An attempt should be made to remove any remnants of the integumentary sheath if it can be seen in the wound. The extremity should be placed in hot water [40°C to 45°C (104°F to 113°F)] for 30 to 90 minutes. After soaking, the wound should be reexplored. Further debridement can then be accomplished, and the wound can be closed. Pain relief is best achieved with morphine 0.1 mg per kg IV, intramuscular (IM), or subcutaneous (SC). Tetanus prophylaxis should always be considered, but antibiotics are reserved for wounds that become secondarily infected.

Sharks

Background

Fear of sharks is as old as human history. Sensational media reports of shark attacks—and several popular movies—have asked whether it is safe to go into the water. The answer may be no but not because of sharks. The chance of being assaulted by a shark along the North American coast is roughly 1 in

5 million. Because of the large number of sporting activities that take place in the ocean environment, however, clinicians who practice in coastal areas may be called on to manage a victim of these primitive creatures.

In U.S. waters, most attacks are by the gray reef, great white, blue, and mako sharks. Factors that increase a risk of attack include swimming near sewer outlets, time of the day (late afternoon and early evening), murky warm water, increased commotion, deep channels, and bright objects. Attacks of surfers along the northern California coast were believed to be caused by sharks mistaking surfboard shapes in the water for elephant seals, part of the shark's usual diet.

Clinical Manifestations

Attack victims usually do not see the shark before it strikes. Occasionally, the attack is preceded by one or more "bumps," during which the victim may sustain extensive abrasions from the rough denticles of the shark's skin. Two types of bite wounds are described: tangential injury and a definitive bite. Tangential injury is caused by the slashing movement of the open mouth as the shark makes a close pass. Severe lacerations, incised wounds, and loss of tissue are seen. Definitive bite wounds vary according to the part of the body seized by the shark. Lacerations, loss of soft tissue, amputations, and comminuted fractures are recorded. Most injuries involve only one or two bites and are confined to the extremities.

Management

Hypovolemic shock is the immediate threat to life in shark attacks. Bleeding should be controlled at the scene with direct compression, and intravascular volume should be replaced with crystalloid until blood products are available. The victim should be kept warm and given oxygen when being transported to an ED. Wounds should not be explored in the field.

Tetanus toxoid and tetanus immune globulin therapies should be considered, and prophylactic antibiotics with a third-generation cephalosporin or trimethoprim-sulfamethoxazole are suggested.

Scorpaenidae

Background

The 80 species found in the Scorpaenidae family include the zebra fish, scorpion fish proper, and stonefish. In California, the sculpin is commonly involved. Scorpaenidae are generally found in shallow water, around reefs, kelp beds, or coral. All members of the family are nonmigratory, slow swimming, and often buried in sand. The venom apparatus consists of a number of dorsal, anal, and pelvic spines covered by integumentary sheaths containing venom glands that lie within anterolateral grooves. The venoms are unstable, heat-labile compounds. Most often envenomation occurs when the fish are handled during fishing excursions.

Clinical Manifestations

The clinical signs and symptoms are essentially the same, varying among the species only in degree. Severe pain at the site of the wound is the first and primary clinical sign for all species. The wound and surrounding area becomes ischemic and then cyanotic. Paresthesia and paralysis of the extremity may occur.

Other clinical signs include nausea, vomiting, hypotension, tachypnea proceeding to apnea, and myocardial ischemia with electrocardiographic changes.

Management

Treatment involves irrigating the wound with sterile saline. The injured extremity is then immersed in very hot water [40°C to 45°C (104°F to 113°F)] for 30 to 60 minutes or until the agonizing pain is completely relieved. Pain relief is best achieved with morphine 0.1 mg per kg IV, IM, or SC. The patient should be monitored carefully for cardiotoxic effects and respiratory depression. Antivenin is available only for the stings of the stonefish of Australia.

Catfish

Background

The catfish is a popular food and sport fish found in many lakes and rivers throughout the United States. The venom apparatus consists of a number of spines located in the dorsal and pectoral fins. The integumentary sheaths covering the spines contain venom glands. The venoms are unstable, heat-labile compounds. Most often, envenomation occurs when the fish are handled during fishing excursions. A combination of injuries is seen: wounds secondary to puncture and laceration, foreign-body reaction, and the effects of venom.

Clinical Manifestations

The spines inflict a puncture wound or laceration. The spines may become imbedded in the flesh of the victim, causing soft-tissue swelling, which may become infected or lead to a foreign-body reaction. The venom produces a local inflammatory response—local intense pain, edema, hemorrhage, and tissue necrosis.

Management

Treatment involves irrigating the wound with sterile saline. The injured extremity is then immersed in hot water [40°C to 45°C (104°F to 113°F)] for 30 to 60 minutes or until pain is relieved. Pain relief is best achieved with morphine 0.1 mg per kg IV, IM, or SC. The wound should be explored to locate any retained spines. Adequate debridement is essential. Systemic antibiotics to cover gram-negative organisms are recommended. Wounds may be closed by using a delayed primary closure.

TERRESTRIAL INVERTEBRATES

Phylum Arthropoda

The arthropods make up the largest phylum in the animal kingdom. All arthropods have an exoskeleton with jointed appendages. The phylum is divided into two subphyla: the Chelicerata, which includes scorpions, spiders, ticks, and mites, and the Mandibulata, which includes insects.

Scorpions

Background. Of 650 known scorpion species (class Arachnida), only a limited number are dangerous to humans. In the southwest United States, *Centruroides sculpturatus* is the potentially lethal inhabitant. Although *C. sculpturatus* and *Centruroides exilicauda* (Fig. 83.2) have been considered separate species in the past, more recent taxonomic classification treats the two as one species. The animal has two pinching claws anteriorly and a tail or pseudoabdomen that ends in a telson (Fig. 83.2). The telson houses a pair of poison glands and a stinger. Normally, scorpions grasp their prey with pincers and then sting the victims by arching their tails over their heads. The animals are nocturnal; during the day, they seek shelter under stones and debris. They often crawl into sleeping bags and unoccupied clothing. In one report, 80% of stings occurred in children younger than 10 years.

Clinical Manifestations. The scorpion's poison gland produces a neurotoxin and a local cytotoxin. The general neurotoxicity is excitatory, affecting the autonomic and skeletal neuromuscular system. Common symptoms include local pain, restlessness, hyperactivity, roving eye movements, and respiratory distress. Other associated signs may include convulsions, drooling,

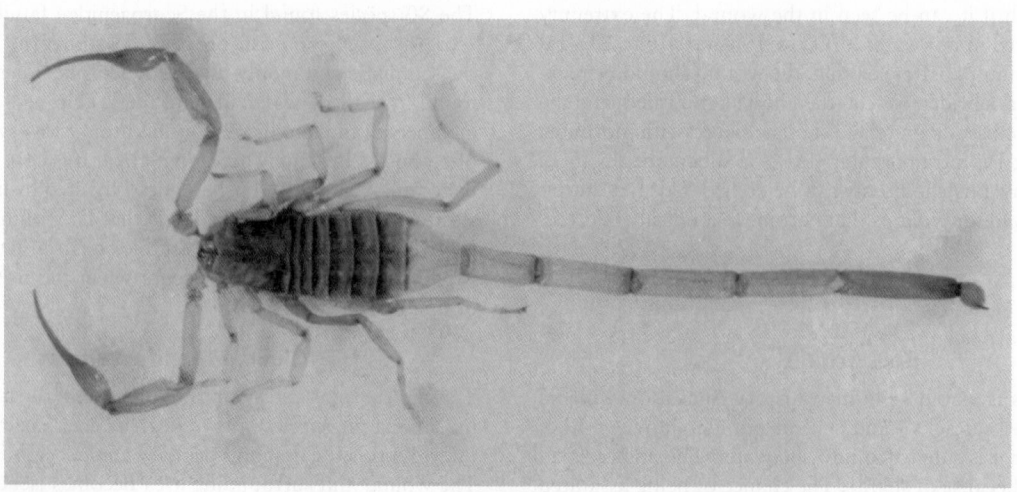

FIGURE 83.2 *Centruroides exilcauda* (sculpturatus). (Courtesy of F. E. Russell.)

wheezing, hyperthermia, cyanosis, gastrointestinal hemorrhage, and respiratory failure. Death may result from respiratory paralysis, pulmonary edema, or shock. The diagnosis may be difficult because history of a sting may not be forthcoming. There is no laboratory test for confirmation of envenomation.

Management. Numerous treatment modalities have been used in addition to general supportive care. Cryotherapy of the site of sting has been advocated to reduce swelling and local induration. An antivenin had been developed and used in Arizona; however, the production ended in 2001. Since the last vials expired, an increase in intensive care unit (ICU) admissions has been reported. Calcium gluconate [0.1 mL per kg (10 mg per kg) of the 10% solution] has been given intravenously to reduce muscular contractions and associated pain, but benefit has not been proved. Sedative-anticonvulsants, in particular, phenobarbital (5 to 10 mg per kg) or benzodiazepines (midazolam 0.05 to 0.1 mg per kg) intravenously are used to treat persistent hyperactivity, convulsions, and/or agitation. A continuous infusion of midazolam may optimize treatment in extreme cases (start at 0.1 mg per kg per hour and titrate to relief of symptoms). Corticosteroids and antihistamines have little, if any, proven benefit.

Spiders

More than 100,000 species of spiders (class Arachnida) are known to exist. All are carnivorous and have fangs and venom by which they immobilize and kill their prey. The risk of serious bites is small, except in a few species. Most spiders are shy and retiring creatures that will not bite people unless provoked. In most species, the fangs are too short and fragile to penetrate human skin, and the venom is mild, however, two species in the United States are capable of producing more severe reactions.

Loxoscelism (Bite of the Brown Recluse Spider). Three species of Loxosceles have caused envenomation, primarily in the southern and midwestern states, but can be found throughout the continental United States. These small spiders (1 to 1.5 cm in length) are characterized by a brown violin-shaped mark on the dorsum of the cephalothorax. They are found outdoors but will establish nests indoors, especially in closets. As its name implies, the most common species, *Loxosceles reclusa*, is shy and will only attack when provoked. The venom is cytotoxic and also contains a factor similar to hyaluronidase.

Clinical manifestations. Clinically, the bite is usually innocuous. Because the bite is initially unnoticed, there is sometimes a

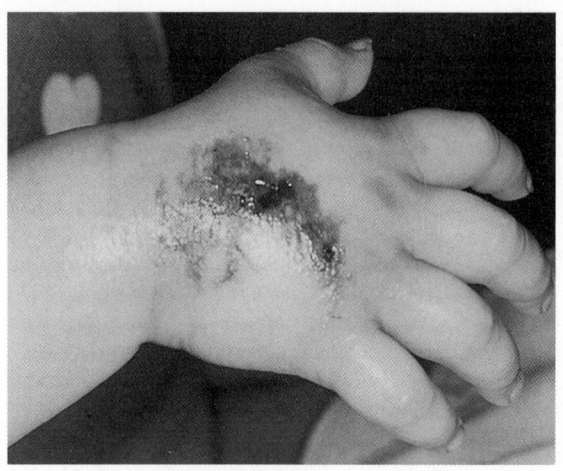

FIGURE 83.3 Spider bite necrotizing.

delay in seeking medical attention. The spectrum of reaction ranges from minor local reaction to severe necrotic arachnidism (Fig. 83.3). The local reaction is characterized by mild to moderate pain 2 to 8 hours after the bite. At the site of the bite, erythema develops with a central blister or pustule. Within 24 hours, subcutaneous discoloration appears and spreads over the next 3 to 4 days, reaching a size of 10 to 15 cm. At this time, the pustule drains, producing an ulcerated "crater." The local reaction varies with the amount of venom injected. Scar formation is rare if there is no evidence clinically of necrosis within 72 hours of the bite. Systemic reaction is most commonly noted in small children. Symptoms are noted 24 to 48 hours after the bite and include fever, chills, malaise, weakness, nausea, vomiting, joint pain, morbilliform eruption with petechiae, intravascular hemolysis, hematuria, and renal failure.

Management. Because of the delay in initial diagnosis, treatment varies with the clinical stage of the bite. There is no specific serologic, biochemical, or histologic test to diagnose envenomation accurately. The range of the brown recluse spider is limited. Many of the presumed bites outside the endemic range are caused by other spiders (Table 83.1) and by other conditions. Pediatric conditions that have been misdiagnosed as brown recluse bites include infections with staphylococci or streptococci, herpes simplex, herpes zoster, erythema multiforme, Lyme disease, fungal infection, pyoderma gangrenosum, chemical burn, poison ivy/oak, and localized vasculitis. Unless all or part of the spider is brought for identification, definitive diagnosis cannot be made. Table 83.1 lists the

TABLE 83.1

SPIDERS KNOWN TO CAUSE NECROTIC LESIONS

Genus name	Common name	Geographic distribution
Argiope	Golden orb weaver	Throughout North America (individual species more restrictive)
Chiracanthium	Running spider	Throughout United States
Loxosceles	Brown recluse	Kansas and Missouri to Texas West to California
Lycosa	Wolf spider	Throughout United States
Phidippus	Black jumping spider	Atlantic Coast to Rocky Mountains

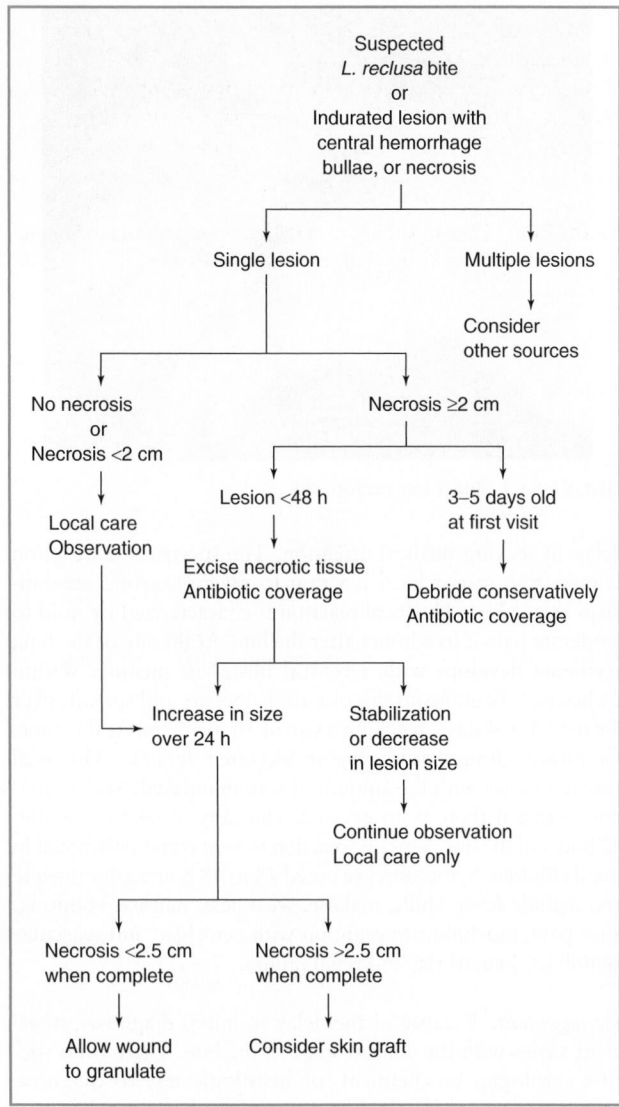

FIGURE 83.4 Management of suspected brown recluse spider bite.

spiders found in the United States, known to cause necrotic lesions. An algorithm for management of suspected bites is shown in Fig. 83.4. One recent series of adult patients suggests that serious complications are rare. Most victims will heal with supportive care. Large-dose steroids have been advocated in the past; however, studies have found no significant alteration of necrosis from the venom by steroids or heparin. Once large areas of necrosis have become demarcated, surgical excision and skin grafting are required, although the need for grafting is rare. Animal studies do not support the use of dapsone, hyperbaric oxygen, or the two in combination in the treatment of these envenomations. However, current recommendations are to limit the use of dapsone to adults with proven brown recluse bites. Dapsone should not be used in children due to the risk of methemoglobinemia. Antivenom is not yet commercially available. For systemic manifestations, vigorous supportive care is needed. Most deaths occur secondary to hemolysis and respiratory failure. A complete blood cell count (CBC) and platelet count for evidence of hemolysis

is needed, as well as monitoring of hemoglobin, urine sediment, blood urea nitrogen (BUN), and creatinine levels for evidence of hemolysis and renal failure.

Latrodectism (Bite of the Black Widow Spider). The bite of *Latrodectus mactans* is the leading cause of death from spider bites in the United States. The animal is shiny black, with a brilliant red hourglass marking on the abdomen. The marking is found on the mature female and may be present on the male. The male is not a threat because it is only one-fourth the size of the female, meaning its fangs are unable to penetrate human skin. The webs are usually found in corners or out-of-the-way places. The female is not aggressive unless guarding her egg sac or provoked. The venom, a complex protein that includes a neurotoxin, stimulates myoneural junctions, nerves, and nerve endings.

Clinical manifestations. Reaction is generalized pain and rigidity of muscles 1 to 8 hours after the bite. No local symptoms are associated with the bite itself. The pain is felt in the abdomen, flanks, thighs, and chest and is described as cramping. Nausea and vomiting are often reported in children. Respiratory distress can occur. Chills, urinary retention, and priapism have been reported. There is a 4% to 5% mortality rate, with death resulting from cardiovascular collapse. The mortality rate in young children may be as high as 50%.

Management. Because of the size, color, and distinctive markings of this spider, bites are seldom mistaken if the child is old enough to describe the spider. A child who has severe pain and muscle rigidity after a spider bite should be considered a Latrodectus bite victim. A clinical grading scale has been developed by Clark (Table 83.2). Treatment with Latrodectus antivenin (Lyovac, Merck, Sharp & Dohme) should be instituted as soon as a bite is confirmed in children who weigh less than 40 kg; the usual dose is 2.5 mL (one vial). Antivenin should be administered by following the package insert and after skin testing to determine the risk of hypersensitivity to horse serum. For children who weigh more than 40 kg, it is not as urgent to institute antivenin treatment, but indications for its use include patients who are younger than 16 years, who have respiratory difficulty, or who have significant hypertension

TABLE 83.2

GRADING SCALE FOR *LATRODECTUS* ENVENOMATION

Grade	Symptoms
1	Asymptomatic Local pain at bite site Normal vital signs
2	Muscular pain—localized Diaphoresis—localized Normal vital signs
3	Muscular pain—generalized Abnormal vital signs Nausea, vomiting Headaches Diaphoresis

(grades II and III). Antivenin is usually effective within 30 minutes and may be repeated once within 2 hours if symptoms return. Serum sickness is a possible side effect. Because the dosage is low, however, serum sickness is uncommon, with a rate lower than those reported for other types of antivenom. Calcium gluconate 10% solution was given in the past to control leg and abdominal cramps. Recent series found calcium gluconate effective in only 4% of cases. Methocarbamol (Robaxin) appears to be even less efficacious than calcium gluconate. Muscle relaxants such as diazepam have also been advocated, but they are variably effective and the effects are short lived. Analgesia may be achieved with morphine or meperidine.

Tarantulas and Others

Tarantulas, although fearsome in size and appearance, do not bite unless provoked. The venom is mild, and envenomation is not a problem. The wolf spider (*Lycosa* species) and the jumping spider (*Phidippus* species) have also been implicated in bites. Like the tarantula, they have mild venom that causes only local reactions. Bites from all three of these spiders should be treated with local wound care.

Tick Paralysis

Ticks are responsible for transmitting a variety of infectious agents, including spirochetes, viruses, rickettsiae, bacteria, and protozoa. Examples of tick-borne illness, which are discussed in Chapter 92, include Rocky Mountain spotted fever, Lyme disease, tularemia, ehrlichiosis, babesiosis, relapsing fever, and Colorado tick fever. Tick paralysis is associated with the bite of the wood tick, *Dermacentor andersonii*; the dog tick, *D. variabilii*; and the deer tick, *Ixodes scapularii*. The gravid engorged tick releases a neurotoxin that can produce cerebellar dysfunction or an ascending weakness. The mechanism of action of the toxin is not well understood.

Clinical Manifestations. Following tick attachment, there is a latent period of 4 to 7 days, followed by symptoms of restlessness, irritability, and ascending flaccid paralysis. Respiratory paralysis and death may follow if the tick is not detected. Laboratory data, including cerebrospinal fluid, are usually normal, but lymphocytic pleocytosis has been reported.

Management. Management is based on general supportive care and a diligent search for the tick. Ticks should be removed using blunt forceps or tweezers. The tick should be grasped as close to the skin surface as possible and pulled upward with a steady even pressure. A twisting or jerking motion may cause the mouthparts to break off. Do not squeeze or crush the body of the tick because this may introduce infective agents. After the tick is removed, the bite site should be cleaned. Once the tick is removed, the paralysis is reversible without apparent sequelae.

Centipedes and Millipedes

Centipedes (class Myriapode order Chilopoda) are venomous, biting with jaws that act like stinging pincers. Bites can be extremely painful; however, the toxin is relatively innocuous, causing only local reaction. Treatment consists of injection of local anesthetic at the wound site and local wound care.

American millipedes (order Diplopoda) are generally harmless.

Insects

The insects (class Insecta) constitute the largest number of animal species. Hymenoptera is the most important order of the class and includes bees, wasps, hornets, yellow jackets, and ants (Fig. 83.5). Because of differences in venom composition and rate of systemic reactions, ants are covered separately in this chapter. Hymenoptera are responsible for 50% of human deaths from venomous bites and stings. A variety of toxic reactions are seen but the most common is allergic.

Bee, Hornet, Yellow Jacket, Wasp

Clinical manifestations. Clinically, the stings of bees and wasps differ because the barbed stinger of the bee remains in the victim's skin, whereas the wasp may sting multiple times. Reactions may vary. The venoms of the bee, hornet, yellow jacket, and wasp contain protein antigens that can elicit an immunoglobulin E antibody response in those who are stung. In addition, venoms contain various biogenic amines, phospholipase, phosphatase, and hyaluronidase. Because of the similarity of the venoms, cross-reactivity can occur. Local reaction to a sting results in pain, erythema, and swelling. Systemic allergic reactions may be grouped by severity. Group I consist of urticaria, generalized erythema, malaise. Group II includes angioedema or two or more of the following: chest or throat tightness, nausea, vomiting, and dizziness. Group III consists dyspnea, wheezing or stridor and two or more of the following: dysphagia, dysarthria, hoarseness, weakness, confusion, feeling of impending disaster. Group IV consists of life-threatening systemic reactions, including hypotension, and shock. Anaphylactic reactions secondary to insect stings occur in 0.5% to 5% of the population.

Management. Because the barbed honeybee stinger with venom sac is avulsed and often remains in the victim's skin, it must be removed if seen. In the past, texts suggested that removal was best accomplished by scraping the stinger and that squeezing or pulling should be avoided. A more recent study compared the effects of delays in removing stings with the effects of different methods of removal. The findings showed that the method of removal is irrelevant (scraping vs. pulling) but that delays in removal are likely to increase the dose of venom received. Stings do not need to be dried with baking soda.

Treatment of stings is based on the severity of the allergic reaction. Local reactions can be treated with cold compresses at the site of sting. Group I reactions are treated with diphenhydramine hydrochloride 4 to 5 mg per kg per day (maximum 200 mg) orally in four divided doses for several days. Group II and Group III reactions are treated with epinephrine 1:1,000 solution 0.01 mL per kg (maximum 0.3 mL) injected intramuscularly followed by diphenhydramine orally. In addition, H_2-blockers may provide additional benefit. Ranitidine (4 to 5 mg per kg per day PO divided q12h) or (2 to 4 mg per kg per day IV divided q6–8h) or famotidine (1 to 2 mg per kg per day PO divided q12h) can be used. Oral steroids (prednisone/prednisolone 2 mg per kg per day) are recommended. These children should be observed in the hospital for 24 hours. Group IV reactions may require intubation if upper airway obstruction is present. Wheezing refractory to epinephrine may be treated with an aminophylline bolus of 6 mg per kg over 20 minutes, followed by a 1.1 mg per kg per hour infusion if needed. Hypotension should be treated with a fluid bolus of saline or

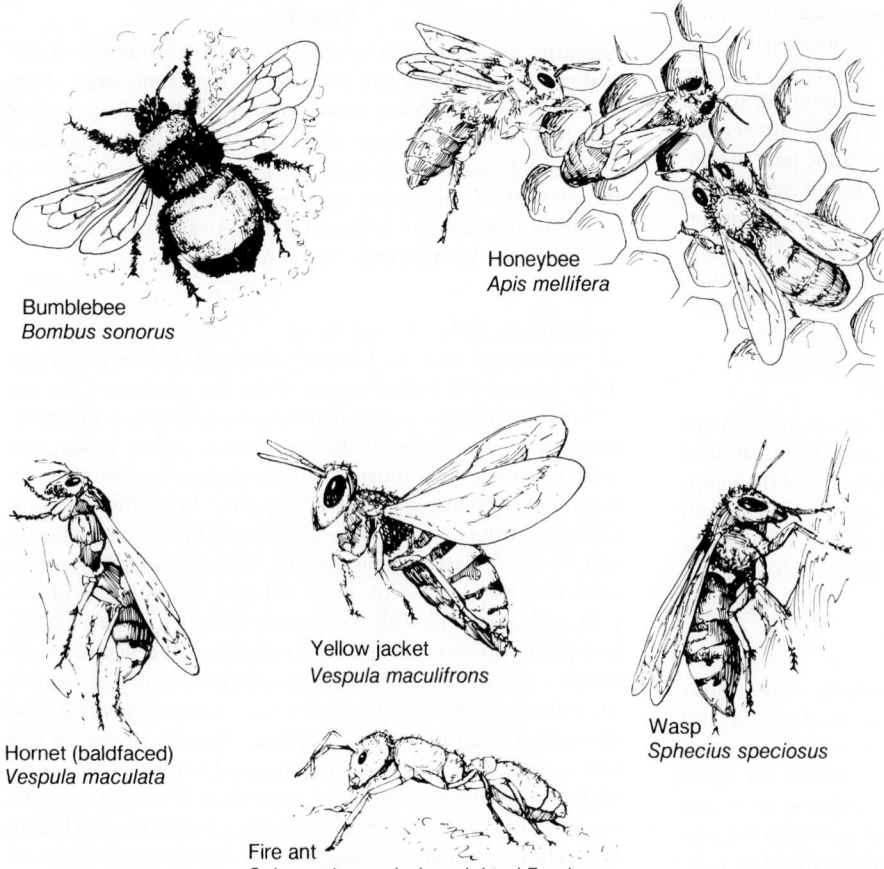

Bumblebee
Bombus sonorus

Honeybee
Apis mellifera

Hornet (baldfaced)
Vespula maculata

Yellow jacket
Vespula maculifrons

Fire ant
Solenopsis saevissima richteri Forel

Wasp
Sphecius speciosus

FIGURE 83.5 Hymenoptera capable of causing allergic reactions.

lactated Ringer's solution 10 to 20 mL per kg given over 20 to 30 minutes. IV epinephrine (1:10,000) should be considered if hypotension fails to respond to IM epinephrine and fluid bolus. Hydrocortisone (2 mg per kg) may be given intravenously for 4 days. All children in this group should be admitted to an ICU. Children who have had a group II, III, or IV reaction should be followed by an allergist for hyposensitization. Parents of these children should keep an insect sting emergency kit. The EpiPen and EpiPen Jr are spring-loaded autoinjectors triggered by placing pressure on the thigh with the instrument. The pens inject 0.3 or 0.15 mg (EpiPen and EpiPen Jr, respectively) of epinephrine. The pens are used as first aid in the field by the parent or guardian and are not meant to substitute for prompt definitive treatment at a medical facility. Parents should receive information regarding the use of epinephrine autoinjectors and avoidance of situations and behaviors that would attract stinging insects.

Fire Ants

Clinical manifestations. An increasing number of bites and envenomations in the South and increasingly northward has been accounted for by fire ants (*Solenopsis richteri* and *Solenopsis invicta*). The venom differs from the other Hymenoptera in that it is an alkaloid with a direct toxic effect on mast cell membranes. There is no cross-reactivity with other members of the order.

The fire ant bites with well-developed jaws and then uses its head as a pivot to inflict multiple stings. The clinical picture of the fire ant sting is one of immediate wheal and flare at the site. The local reaction varies from 1 to 2 mm, up to 10 cm,

depending on the amount of venom injected. Within 4 hours, a superficial vesicle appears. After 8 to 10 hours, the fluid in the vesicle changes from clear to cloudy (pustule), and the vesicle becomes umbilicated. After 24 hours, the lesion is surrounded by a painful erythematous area that persists for 3 to 10 days. Edema, induration, and pruritus at the site occur in up to 50% of patients. Occasionally, systemic reactions occur as with other Hymenoptera.

Management. Treatment of fire ant stings is symptomatic. Local care, such as ice applied to the reactive area, and frequent cleansing of the lesions to prevent secondary infection are all that is usually required. Topical steroids, antibacterial medications, and antihistamines do not appear to be efficacious in prevention of pustule formation. Antihistamines are useful for pruritus. Systemic reactions are rare and should be treated similarly to other Hymenoptera reactions.

TERRESTRIAL VERTEBRATES

Venomous Reptiles

Background

God said to the serpent, "Be accursed beyond all cattle, all wild beasts. You shall crawl on your belly and eat dust every day of your life. I will make you enemies of each other: you and the woman, your offspring and her offspring."

—Genesis 3:14

Throughout recorded history, serpents and their encounters with humans have evoked strong emotions, folklore, and medicinal practices. Research during the past several decades has lessened the mystique surrounding the venomous substances secreted by 15% of the U.S.'s 120 snake species. The more recent emphasis on antivenin therapy and expedient supportive medical care has dramatically reduced mortality and morbidity from poisonous snakebites.

In the United States, an estimated 8,000 people are bitten annually by poisonous snakes. Predictably, the pediatric population, especially males, ages 5 to 19 years, accounts for a disproportionately large number of these victims. The highest incidence occurs in the Southeast and Southwest, between April and October, although venomous snakebites occur at least sporadically in most states. More recent data show 25% of bites are in patients younger than 17 years. Only 10 to 15 deaths are reported per year, but the morbidity in limb dysfunction and other complications, although unknown, is undoubtedly much higher. With appropriate therapy, most long-term morbidity can be prevented.

The poisonous snakes indigenous to the United States are members of the Crotalidae (pit viper) or Elapidae families (Table 83.3). The rattlesnake, water moccasin, and copperhead are pit vipers and are responsible for 99% of venomous snakebites. The coral snake is the only member of the Elapidae family in this country and, along with imported exotic snakes, accounts for the remaining 1% of serious snakebites.

The pit vipers have several characteristic features that distinguish them from nonvenomous snakes (Fig. 83.6): (i) two pits containing heat-sensitive organs that assist these poor-visioned reptiles to localize their prey are located, one on each side of the head, between the eye and nostril; (ii) the pupils are elliptical and vertically oriented in contrast to the usually round pupil of a harmless snake; (iii) two curved fangs or hollow maxillary teeth that are 5 to 20 mm long and, in larger snakes, may be spaced as wide as 3 cm, are folded posteriorly against the palate and advance forward when the pit viper strikes; (iv) the head is relatively more triangular than that of most nonvenomous snakes; and (v) the scutes, or scales, on the ventral portion caudad to the anal plate continue in a single row, whereas nonpoisonous snakes have a cleft, or double row.

The rattlesnake (*Crotalus*) is distributed widely throughout most of the United States and is the culprit in approximately 60% of all pit viper attacks. Several species are notably more menacing and toxic to humans. The large and gold diamondbacks (*Crotalus adamanteus* and *Crotalua atrox*) often stand their ground when approached by humans and inflict most lethal snakebites in North America. Other rattlesnakes that commonly cause the more severe bites include the timber (*Crotalus horridus*), prairie, and pacific (*Crotalus viridus*) rattlesnakes. Several other *Crotalus* species are implicated in less severe human envenomation.

Rattlesnakes vary considerably in size and color, even among species. The eastern diamondback, which inhabits the

TABLE 83.3

POISONOUS SNAKES INDIGENOUS TO THE UNITED STATES

Family	Genus	Species	Common name
Crotalidae			Pit vipers
	Crotalus		Rattlesnakes
		C. adamanteus	Eastern diamondback
		C. atrox	Western diamondback
		C. horridus	Timber rattlesnake
		C. viridus	Western rattlesnake
		C.v. viridis	Prairie rattlesnake
		C.v. helleri	Southern Pacific rattlesnake
		C.v. oreganus	Northern Pacific rattlesnake
		C.v. abussus	Grand Canyon rattlesnake
		C.v. lutosus	Great Basin rattlesnake
		C. cerastes	Sidewinder
		C. ruber	Red diamond rattlesnake
		C. mitchelli	Speckled rattlesnake
		C. lepidus	Rock rattlesnake
		C. tiaris	Tiger rattlesnake
		C. willardi	Ridge-nosed rattlesnake
		C. scutulatus	Mojave rattlesnake
		C. molossus	Black-tailed rattlesnake
		C. pricei	Twin-spotted rattlesnake
	Sistrurus		
		S. catenatus	Massasauga rattlesnake
		S. miliarius	Pygmy rattlesnake
	Agkistrodon		
		A. piscivorus	Water moccasin
		A. contortrix	Copperhead
Elapidae		*Microides euryxanthus*	Sonovan (Arizona) coral snake
		Micrurus fulvius	Eastern coral snake

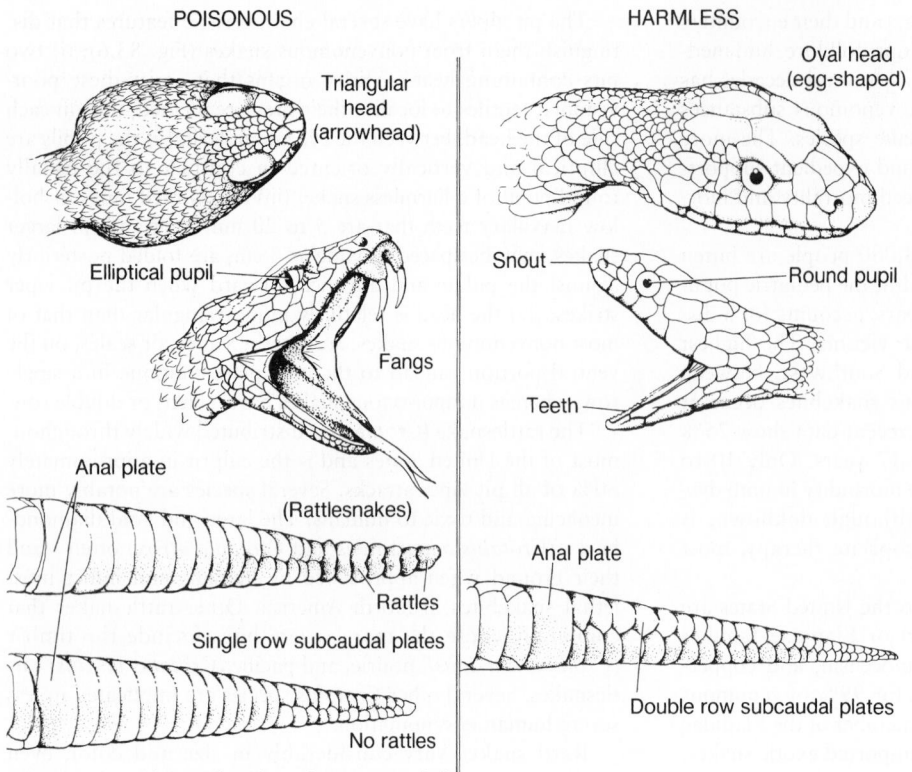

FIGURE 83.6 Comparison of poisonous and nonpoisonous snakes.

coastal Southeast, may be as large as 2 m long and 7 kg in weight; it usually has a brightly outlined symmetric diamond pattern. The timber rattler found in the Northeast and Southeast westward to Texas may be only 1 m long and have nearly black scales (especially in colder climates). Emergency physicians must become familiar with the particular species in their areas.

The pygmy rattler and massasauga are considered rattlesnakes because, in common with *Crotalus* species, they possess a "rattler" on their tail. However, these two relatively small snakes are members of the genus *Sistrorus*, and their bites are not as toxic as those of true rattlesnakes.

The copperhead (*Agkistrodon contortrix*) is a common poisonous snake that lives in the Southeast and much of the Northeast, extending westward as far as Texas and Nebraska. This snake accounts for approximately 30% of venomous snakebites but, luckily, is seldom a serious threat to life or limb. *A. contortrix* is usually 0.6 to 1 m in length and has a light pink to red-brown body, with darker brown crossbands shaped like hourglasses. The head has a coppery tinge.

The water moccasin, also known as the cottonmouth (*A. piscivorus*), is a semiaquatic pit viper indigenous to the Southeast, including the Gulf States and the Mississippi Valley as far north as southern Illinois. These are larger and more belligerent snakes, often traveling with their heads in an aggressive 45-degree angle from the horizontal plane. Their body is olive brown to black, with darker markings on the sides that often fade over the dorsum. The ventral surface is lighter in color. The oral mucosa is distinctively white, hence the name cottonmouth. Like the copperhead, bites from this species are, in general, less serious than those of the *Crotalus* species.

The relatively passive coral snake is responsible for only 10 to 15 snakebite cases per year in this country. As a member of the Elapidae family, it does not share the pit viper's distinctive physical characteristics (i.e., it has round pupils, a blunt head, and ventral caudal scutes, and lacks pits). Unlike the nonpoisonous snakes, the coral snake has two small maxillary fangs.

The snout of the coral snake is always black and is followed by a yellow ring and subsequent black band. Red and black bands then alternate down the approximately 2-feet length of the coral snake, with narrow yellow rings bordering the red band (Fig. 83.7). The nonvenomous king snake is often confused with the coral; it has red bands directly bordered by black bands. The yellow rings in this snake are within the black bands. The adage about coral snakes holds true:

> Red on yellow, kill a fellow.
> Red on black, venom lack.

There are two species of coral snakes: the eastern (*Micrurus fulvius*) and the Arizonan (*Micruroides euryxanthus*). *M. fulvius* is responsible for most human envenomations and is found in most states east of the Mississippi, with the exception of the Northeast. *M. euryxanthus* is indigenous only to Arizona and New Mexico.

Pathophysiology

Snakebite envenomation is a complex poisoning because of the assorted deleterious effects of venoms, as well as the multiple human and snake variables that influence venom toxicity. Venoms are mixtures of potent enzymes, primarily proteinases, and low-molecular-weight peptides that possess extensive pathophysiologic properties. A crotalid venom often has a

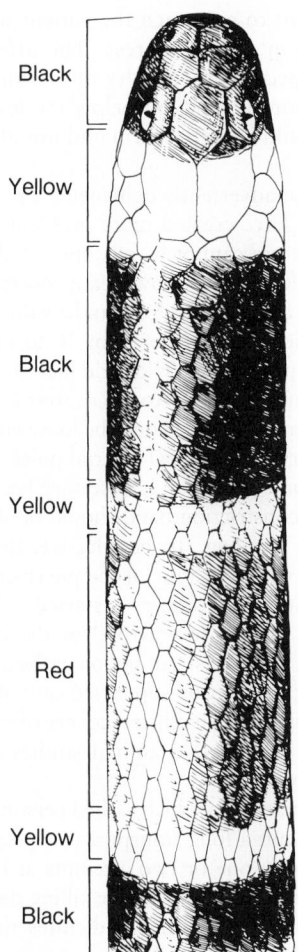

Black

Yellow

Black

Yellow

Red

Yellow

Black

FIGURE 83.7 Coral snake.

combination of necrotizing, hemotoxic, neurotoxic, nephrotoxic, and/or cardiotoxic substances. The neurotoxins comprise a large fraction of the venom of the Mojave rattlesnake. These toxins are related to phospholipase A and bind the nicotinic acetylcholine receptors and thus prevent the depolarizing action of acetylcholine. Proteolytic enzymes aided by hyaluronidase cause much of the local tissue destruction. Many venoms induce increased endothelial permeability and venous pooling, creating intravascular depletion. A transient hemoconcentration may be present during this plasma "leak." Hemotoxic effects induce hemolysis, fibrinogen proteolysis, and thrombocytopenia, which, along with activation of plasminogen, can lead to a bleeding diathesis in severe envenomation. Respiratory failure may occur secondary to pulmonary edema or a shock state.

The ultimate toxicity of the snakebite also depends on human and snake variables. Human factors include the victim's size and general health and wound characteristics that affect venom absorption. A small child is more susceptible to a given volume of venom than a larger person. (Unfortunately, young children are commonly bitten more than once.) Fang penetration of a vessel or subfascial compartment ensures a more rapid absorption and serious systemic effects. Likewise, a bite on the head, neck, or trunk (3% of snakebites) hastens systemic absorption. Approximately one-third of snakebites involve the upper extremity and cause a higher long-term functional morbidity than do lower-extremity wounds.

Snake variables include the snake's size, the amount of venom injected, and the potency of the particular species' venom. Venom secretion is under voluntary muscular control; any condition that facilitates it (e.g., long, healthy fangs or full stores of venom) adds to the toxicity of the bite. An angered and hungry rattlesnake unloads more venom than a recently satiated and surprised rattlesnake.

Clinical Manifestations

Pit Viper. Local pain after a *Crotalus* envenomation is typically intense, and a sensation of burning occurs within a couple of minutes. The pain is greater with ensuing edema and presumably increases with larger inocula of venom. Victims of a significant rattlesnake bite often complain within minutes of a perioral numbness, extending to the scalp and periphery. This paresthesia may be accompanied by a metallic taste in the mouth.

These patients also may have nausea, vomiting, weakness, chills, sweating, syncope, and other more ominous symptoms of systemic venom absorption. A copperhead or pygmy rattlesnake envenomation produces less local symptoms, and systemic consequences are often minimal or nonexistent unless a small child, multiple bites, or larger than average snake is involved. The water moccasin's effects are more variable.

There is a relative lack of serious pain or swelling with the Mojave rattler bite, although, as in other *Crotalus* bites, the patient may complain of paresthesia in the affected extremity. Within several hours, these patients may develop neuromuscular symptoms such as diplopia, difficulty in swallowing, lethargy, nausea, and progressive weakness from the large portion of neurotoxin in this species.

The wound should be inspected for fang punctures, and if two are present, the distance between them should be noted. An interfang distance of less than 8 mm suggests a small snake; 8 to 12 mm, a medium snake; and more than 12 mm, a larger snake. Fang wounds by small snakes such as the pygmy rattler may be extremely subtle; in larger crotalid snakebites, the fang marks may be hidden within hemorrhagic blebs and edema. Occasionally, only one puncture or two scratches will be present, but both wounds may be potentially venomous. However, not all crotalid bites are envenomated; 10% to 20% of known rattlesnake strikes do not inject venom. Other causes of puncture wounds must also be kept in mind—notably rodent bites and thorn wounds. Nonpoisonous snakes sometimes leave an imprint of their two rows of teeth, but the wounds should lack fang puncture marks.

Pit viper envenomations are characterized by intense pain, erythema, and edema at the wound site within 5 to 10 minutes. There may be bloody serosanguinous fluid dripping from the fang punctures. Progressive swelling proportional to the inoculum of venom develops over the next 8 hours and may continue to some degree for an additional 24 hours. Rarely, the venom is deposited predominantly in a muscle compartment, resulting in a deceptively minimal amount of edema. The Mojave rattlesnake bite provides another example of a seemingly innocuous local wound in the setting of a potentially serious envenomation. In a severe diamondback rattlesnake bite, an entire extremity may be swollen within 1 hour.

MEDICAL EMERGENCIES

TABLE 83.4

LOCAL SIGNS OF PIT VIPER ENVENOMATION

Pain	Ecchymosis
Edema	Vesicles
Erythema	Hemorrhagic blebs

Local ecchymoses and vesicles usually appear within the first few hours, and hemorrhagic blebs are often present by 24 hours. Lymphadenitis and lymph node enlargement may also become apparent.

Without appropriate therapy, these local manifestations progress to necrosis and may extend throughout the bitten extremity, effectively maiming the victim. Also, as in any animal wound, secondary infection is a risk; the snake's oral flora includes gram-negative bacteria. Table 83.4 summarizes local characteristics of pit viper bites.

The dramatic signs of crotalid envenomation are derived primarily from the victim's hypovolemic state, hemorrhagic tendencies, and neuromuscular dysfunction. Table 83.5 outlines the more notable physical signs.

Coral Snake. Coral snakes leave unimpressive local signs but can neurologically cripple their prey. The bite may have one or two punctures, at most 7 to 8 mm apart, as well as other small teeth marks. There is usually only mild pain and little, if any, swelling. Local wound and, eventually, extremity paresthesia and weakness may be reported. Over several hours, generalized malaise and nausea, fasciculations, and weakness develop insidiously. The patient may complain of diplopia and have difficulty talking or swallowing. Physical examination reveals bulbar dysfunction and generalized weakness. Respiratory failure may ensue.

Management

Pit Viper. As in all medical emergencies, the airway, breathing, and circulation of the patient must be addressed before attending to the snakebite (Fig. 83.8). The first priority of prehospital care of the snakebite victim is rapid transport to a medical facility. Time is of the essence, and all activities in the field must be tempered by this fact.

TABLE 83.5

SYSTEMIC SIGNS OF CROTALID (PIT VIPER) ENVENOMATION

General
  Anxiety, diaphoresis, pallor, unresponsiveness
Cardiovascular
  Tachycardia, decreased capillary perfusion, hypotension, shock
Pulmonary
  Pulmonary edema, respiratory failure
Renal
  Oliguria, hemoglobinuria, hematuria
Neuromuscular
  Fasciculations, weakness, paralysis, convulsions
Hematologic
  Bleeding diathesis

It is important to approach the patient with reassurance and to place him or her at rest. The affected extremity should be stripped of any jewelry or clothing and immobilized in a position of function below the level of the heart. The patient should be kept warm and not allowed anything by mouth.

Tourniquets, inadvertently tightened for prolonged full vascular occlusion, have created more problems than they have solved and therefore cannot be recommended for prehospital care. In experienced hands, however, a constriction band that obstructs lymph and venous flow can be valuable when a long transport is anticipated (longer than 30 to 60 minutes). The band should be at least 2 cm wide and placed 5 to 10 cm proximal to the wound (proximal to the nearest joint if the wound is nearby). The constriction should be loose enough to admit a finger and preserve good distal arterial pulses. Vigilant observation for adequate perfusion is necessary because of progressive edema; the constriction band should be shifted to remain proximal to the swelling. To be effective, the band must be applied initially within 1 hour of the pit viper bite. It may be removed when antivenin therapy is started.

Incision and suction (extractors) of the pit viper wound while advocated in the past can no longer be advised. The usefulness of extractors can be supported only if applied within minutes of the bite and even then recovery of venom is variable in a laboratory setting. No animal studies have shown an increase in survival.

In the rare situation in which skilled personnel and supplies are at the scene and a long transport is expected, it would be reasonable to allow one or two attempts at IV access. Many authorities also suggest capturing or killing the snake for later verification, but again, prudence dictates that time not be wasted in this adventure and that an inexperienced person not risk the bite of an agitated snake. If the snake arrives in the ED, treat it with respect—more than one person has been bitten by a "dead" snake, and decapitated snakes can bite reflexively for up to 1 hour.

A CBC, coagulation studies, platelet count, urinalysis, and blood crossmatching should be obtained on all patients with suspected venomous snakebite, as blood may be difficult to crossmatch after massive hemolysis. In moderate or severe poisoning, analyses of serum electrolytes, BUN, creatinine, fibrinogen, and arterial blood gas levels are also indicated. Hemolysis, anemia, thrombocytopenia, hypofibrinogenemia, prolonged bleeding times, and metabolic acidosis all may be seen in severe poisoning. Repeat the laboratory studies every 6 hours to ensure no significant changes occur.

Therapy will be based on the clinician's overall grading of venom toxicity. Local and systemic manifestations, as well as laboratory findings, weigh heavily in this judgment. The clinical pattern may change dramatically as the venom's effects unfold; thus, frequent reassessment is crucial. The physician should measure and record the circumference of the injured extremity at the leading point of edema and 10 cm proximal to this level every 30 minutes for 6 hours, then at least every 4 hours for a total of 24 hours. Table 83.6 is derived from a grading system suggested by the Scientific Review Subcommittee of the American Association of Poison Control Centers.

If the history and physical examination on arrival in the ED are consistent with a venomous snakebite, immediate laboratory

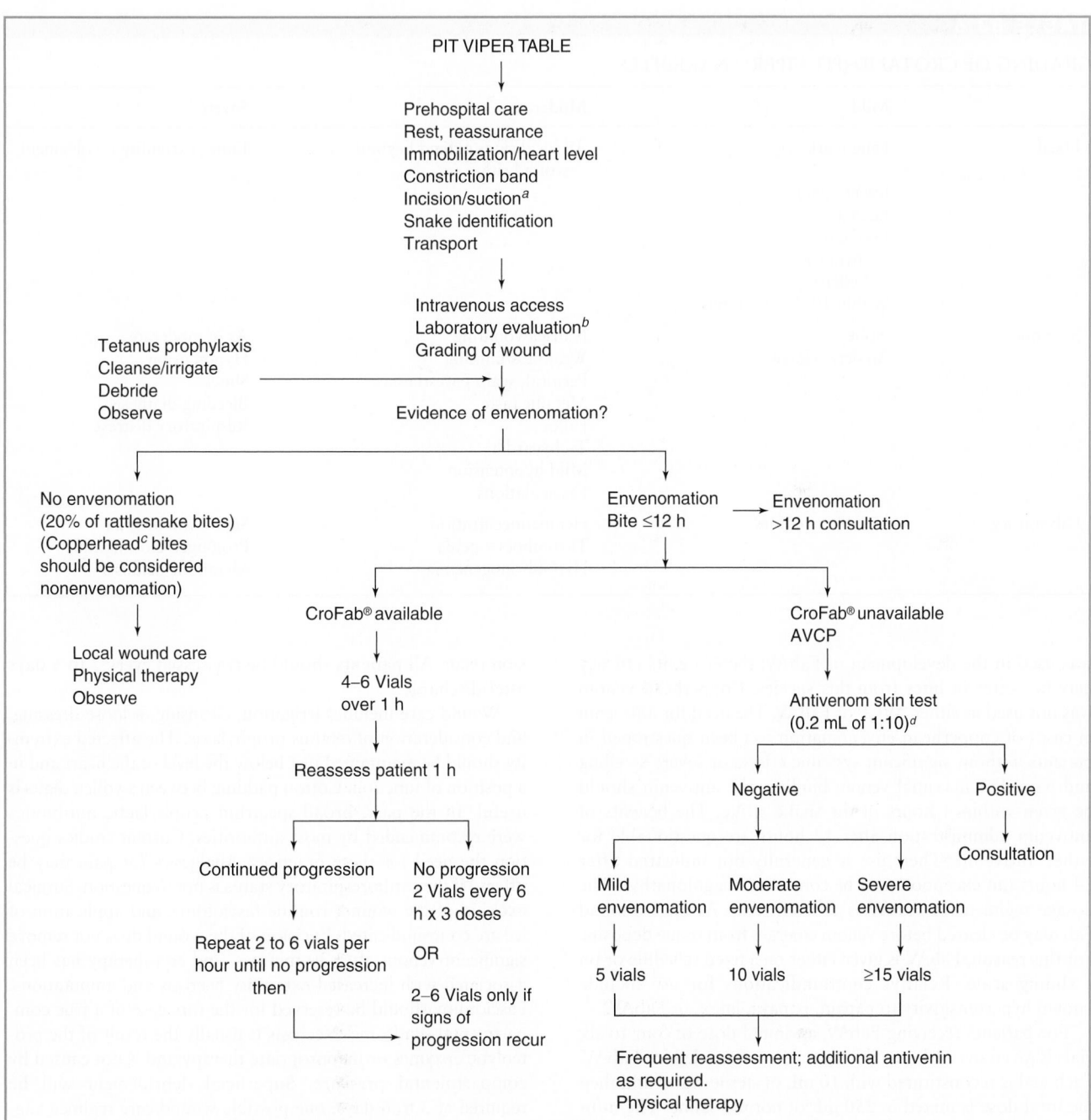

FIGURE 83.8 Management of pit viper bite. [a]Perform within 5 to 10 minutes of bite; continue suction for 30 to 60 minutes. [b]Complete blood cell count, platelet count, prothrombin time, partial thromboplastin time, urinalysis, type and hold; in moderate or severe cases, add fibrinogen, arterial blood gases, electrolytes, blood urea nitrogen, and creatinine. [c]Seldom need antivenin; exceptions with large snakes and small children. d1:100 dilution if allergy history; saline control; resuscitation medications at hand; antivenin seldom indicated if greater than 12 to 24 hours since bite.

evaluation and IV access are indicated. Aggressive supportive medical care must be available if signs of major system dysfunction are present. Any prehospital care (e.g., extremity immobilization) should be rechecked. If an occluding tourniquet is inappropriately present, the physician should place a more proximal constriction band and then cautiously remove the tourniquet, being prepared to respond therapeutically to a systemic release of venom.

The older antivenom (Crotalidae) polyvalent (AVCP; Wyeth-Ayerst Pharmaceuticals) is no longer available and was derived from horse serum and was highly antigenic. The newer antivenom was licensed in 2000 and is a polyclonal, polyvalent Fab affinity purified (FabAV; CroFab® Prothenics, Inc.) product derived from sheep. It has less adverse reactions than seen with AVCP. The antivenom is effective for rattlesnake and water moccasin envenomations. Mojave rattlesnake venom

TABLE 83.6

GRADING OF CROTALID (PIT VIPER) SNAKEBITES

	Mild	Moderate	Severe
Local	Fang mark Intense pain Edema Erythema Ecchymosis ± Vesicles Within 10–15 cm of bite	All local signs extend beyond wound site	Entire extremity involvement
Systemic	None Anxiety related	Nausea/vomiting Weakness/fainting Perioral, scalp paresthesias Metallic taste Pallor Tachycardia Mild hypotension Fasciculations	As in moderate Hypotension Shock Bleeding diathesis Respiratory distress
Laboratory	No abnormalities	Hemoconcentration Thrombocytopenia Hypofibrinogenemia	Significant anemia Prolonged clotting time Metabolic acidosis

was used in the development of FabAV; therefore, its efficacy may be better in bites from this species. Copperhead venom was not used in either AVCP or FabAV. The need for antivenin in cases of copperhead envenomation has been questioned in patients without significant systemic effects or severe swelling and pain. For maximal venom binding, the antivenin should be given within 4 hours of the snake strike. The benefits of antivenin administration after 12 hours are questionable for either antivenin. Their use is generally not indicated after 24 hours (an exception may be continued coagulopathy). The dosage regimen for FabAV is different than AVCP. Unbound Fab may be cleared before venom emerges from tissue deposits. For this reason, FabAV is given either on a fixed schedule or on a sliding scale. Relative contraindications for use include known hypersensitivity to papain, papaya, latex, or FabAV.

For patients receiving FabAV, an initial dose of four to six vials is given over 1 hour. Skin testing is not needed for FabAV. Each vial is reconstituted with 10 mL of sterile water and then the total dose is mixed in 250 mL of normal saline. The infusion should be started slowly, at a rate of 25 to 50 mL per hour for 10 minutes, while observing for allergic reaction. The rate should be increased so the 250 mL is given over 1 hour. If mild allergic manifestations develop, the infusion should be stopped and diphenhydramine (1 to 2 mg per kg IV) given. Once the allergic symptoms have resolved, a minimum of 5 minutes should pass, then the infusion should be restarted at a slower rate. Reactions have been associated with faster infusion rates. Initial dosage from FabAV (CroFab) is given irrespective of degree of envenomation. Subsequent doses are based on signs of progression. The patient should be reassessed after the initial dose. If there is progression of envenomation, then the initial dose should be repeated. If there is no progression, two different schedules are suggested. One choice is to give two vials every 6 hours for three doses. The other regimen is to give two to six vials only if signs of envenomation progres-

sion recur. All patients should be reassessed every 2 to 5 days after discharge.

Wound care includes irrigation, cleansing, a loose dressing, and consideration of tetanus prophylaxis. The affected extremity should be maintained just below the level of the heart and in a position of function. Cotton padding between swollen digits is useful. In the past, broad-spectrum prophylactic antibiotics were recommended by most authorities. Current studies question the need for these practices. Analgesics for pain may be offered if the cardiorespiratory status is not in question. Surgical excision of the wound, routine fasciotomy, and application of ice are contraindicated. Excision of the wound does not remove significant venom after 30 minutes, and cryotherapy has been associated with increased extremity necrosis and amputations. Fasciotomy should be reserved for the rare case of a true compartmental syndrome. Necrosis is usually the result of the proteolytic enzymes or inappropriate therapy and is not caused by compartmental pressure. Superficial debridement will be required at 3 to 6 days; one possible wound care regimen suggested at this stage includes local oxygen, aluminum acetate (1:20 solution) soaks, and triple dye. Physical therapy is beneficial during the healing phase.

The major thrust of supportive care is correction of the intravascular depletion that results from increased venous capacitance, interstitial third spacing, and hemorrhagic losses. Moderate or severe envenomation mandates two IV lines for separate but simultaneous antivenin therapy and volume replacement. Shock usually develops between 6 and 24 hours after the snakebite but may present within the first hour in severe envenomation. Signs of hypovolemia (e.g., decreased capillary perfusion, oliguria, tachycardia, anemia, hypotension) deserve aggressive therapy. Central vascular monitoring and accurate urine output measurements are desirable for optimal therapy. Normal saline or lactated Ringer's solution (20 mL per kg over 1 hour), followed by fresh whole blood or other blood components, often corrects the hypovolemia (see Chapter 3). Vasopressors are usually needed only transiently in the more severe cases. A bleeding diathesis is best managed with fresh whole blood, or blood component therapy, primarily packed cells (10 mL per kg), and fresh-frozen plasma (10 mL per kg). With life-threatening bleeding, platelets (0.2 units per kg) and a more concentrated fibrinogen source (cryoprecipitate—dose one bag per 5 kg body weight) should also be considered. Abnormal clotting parameters, including fibrinogen and platelet and blood counts, should be reevaluated every 4 to 6 hours. Respiratory support is also commonly required when shock has developed. Renal failure is another potential problem in this setting.

The rate of serum sickness with FabAV (CroFab) is much lower than that seen with AVPC. Signs of serum sickness include rashes, arthralgias, edema, malaise, lymphadenopathy, fever, and/or gastrointestinal symptoms that evolve over several days. Prednisone (2 mg per kg per day, maximum 80 mg) until symptoms abate (and then a tapering schedule) has been used with success in most cases. Diphenhydramine (5 mg per kg per day in four divided doses, max 50 mg per dose) is often given as an adjunct.

Coral Snake. When coral snake wounds are present or the history or specimen is consistent with an Eastern coral snakebite, antivenin for *Micrurus fulvius* (Wyeth) is administered before development of further symptoms. The antivenin's access is restricted in the United States (contact http://www.Wyeth.com for information). This is also an equine serum and requires preliminary skin testing (see package insert). The initial recommended dosage is three to five vials by IV; an additional three to five vials may be given as needed for signs of venom toxicity. There is no antivenin available for the Arizona coral snake (*Micruroides euryxanthus*). Supportive care should provide a satisfactory outcome in these cases. Constriction bands, suction and drainage, and other local measures do not retard coral snake venom absorption, and hence, are not indicated.

Exotic Snakes. The clinician confronted with an exotic snakebite or a clinician inexperienced in snakebites should consult a local medical herpetologist, poison control center, or the American Association of Zoologic Parks and Aquariums and the American Association of Poison Control Centers. These centers keep an up-to-date database of exotic antivenoms. Access to this information is available at 800-222-1222. Report all illegally possessed reptiles to the police or to the appropriate fish and game agency.

Mammalian Bites

Background

Children suffer the majority of casualties in this country's growing epidemic of mammalian bites. The overall morbidity of mammalian bites is staggering in terms of infectious complications, cosmesis, disability, psychological trauma, and medical expenses. At least 1 to 2 million people are bitten each year, and about 1% of ED visits are prompted by bite wounds.

Dog bites account for the overwhelming majority (80% to 90%) of these injuries and thus have been the subject of numerous investigations. An estimated 4.5 million dog bites occur in the United States annually, with approximately 885,000 people seeking medical care. The most common dog attack involves a 5- to 14-year-old boy close to home and a large-breed or mixed-breed canine. The dog's owner can be identified 85% to 90% of the time; in fact, in 15% to 30% of cases, the dog belongs to the victim's family. Usually, the dog has never previously bitten anyone and often has been provoked, although most often unintentionally. However, animal jealousy has been implicated in unprovoked biting of infants. A seldom realized mortality of approximately 10 fatal cases occur each year in the United States, primarily in young children and infants.

The remainder of the mammalian bites is perpetrated by cats (5% to 10%), rodents (2% to 3%), and other wild or domesticated animals. Another mammalian species, *Homo sapiens*, inflicts approximately 2% to 3% of the bite wounds that present to medical attention. Human bites share with cat wounds a notoriously high infectious complication rate.

Pathophysiology

Anatomic wound characteristics and the microbiologic inoculum of the offending species determines the pathologic consequences of the bite. For example, many dog bites are localized crush injuries with a substantial amount of infection-prone devitalized tissue—a result of the enormous pressures dogs generate in their bites. Forces of 200 to 400 pounds per square inch, sufficient to perforate sheet metal, have been documented in dogs. Overall, however, only 5% to 10% of dog bites become infected, probably because the resulting lacerations and abrasions are so accessible to good wound hygiene. The typical feline bite, however, is a deep puncture wound and is difficult to irrigate or cleanse, thus subjecting it to a high infection rate (up to 50% in some series). The penetration of tendons, vessels, facial compartments, and bones also has a high infectious risk with increased morbidity. The hand offers all these anatomic components in a relatively small cross-sectional area; therefore, it is potentially prone to serious infections regardless of the biting species. Injuries to deeper structures, including major vasculature, the brain, peritoneum, abdominal organs, and airways, have also been sporadically reported.

Scores of aerobic and anaerobic bacteria indigenous to mammalian oral flora are inoculated into the wound during biting. Cultures of fresh wounds before clinical infection reflect the variety of these contaminants but are not predictive of the causative organism in later infections. The most commonly isolated bacteria in infected cat and dog bite wounds are *Staphylococcus aureus* and *Pasteurella* species, a gram-negative rod. In one series, *P. multocida* and *P. canis* were found in 50% and 80% of infected dog and cat wounds, respectively. Other series have isolated *P. multocida* in only 10% to 20% of infected dog wounds and incriminated other more common bacteria: streptococci, coagulase-negative staphylococci, *S. aureus*, and enteric bacteria. Some unusual isolates in clinical infection have included *Capnocytophaga canimorsus* (DF-2) and *Weeksella zoohelcum* (IIj). Two hundred cases of sepsis following dog bites have been associated with *C. canimorsus*. At least 25% of all infected mammalian bites yield mixed cultures of aerobes and often anaerobes, if carefully sought. Anaerobic bacteria are usually recovered (not alone but only in mixed cultures with aerobes).

Human bite infections are mixed bacterial infections, with *Streptococcus viridans* or *S. aureus* being the predominant organism. Anaerobic bacteria, especially *Bacteroides* and *Peptostreptococcus* species, are commonly cultured. The more serious morbidity in infected human bites of the hand has been correlated with *S. aureus* isolation and, more recently, with *Eikenella corrodens*, a facultative anaerobe.

Finally, the multiple systemic diseases that may be transmitted by mammalian bites need to be considered.

Clinical Manifestations

Mammalian bite wounds cause a spectrum of tissue injuries from trivial to life-threatening. Scratches, abrasions, contusions, punctures, lacerations, and their complications are commonly seen in the ED. The complications usually involve secondary infections or damage to structures that underlie the bite.

Although dog bites are insignificant lesions in at least half of the cases that come to medical attention, 5% to 10% warrant suturing and 2% require hospital admission. Approximately 33% of dog bites involve the upper extremity, presumably while the victim is fending off the attack. Another 33% of wounds are located on the lower extremities and 20% on the head and neck area. The remainder of bites involves multiple areas. Other than bites on the hand, the rate of secondary infection in dog bites given good local care approximates that of nonbite wounds.

Predictably, young children suffer more serious canine injuries. The dog strikes the head and neck in 60% to 70% of victims younger than 5 years and in 50% of those younger than 10 years. These wounds most often involve the lips, nose, and cheek areas, and on rare occasions, they penetrate the skull, with resulting depressed skull fractures and intracranial lesions. It has been estimated that each year 44,000 children suffer facial dog bite wounds, one-third of them requiring complex repair. The uncommon life-threatening injuries occur almost exclusively in young children and include major vascular injury, visceral penetration, and chest trauma. The deaths are usually secondary to acute hemorrhagic shock.

Cat bites are located in the infection-prone upper extremities in two-thirds of cases and are usually puncture wounds rather than lacerations or contusions. Infections that complicate these wounds result from the same organisms isolated in dog bites, but a higher incidence of *P. multocida* is found. *P. multocida* infections characteristically present within 12 to 24 hours of the injury and rapidly display erythema, significant swelling, and intense pain. These infections often respond slowly to adequate drainage and antibiotic therapy. Local infections from other organisms usually present 24 to 72 hours after the bite in a less fulminant manner. Viridans streptococcal infections are occasional exceptions to this generalization and may resemble a *P. multocida* clinical course.

Cat scratches are most commonly located on the victim's upper extremities or periorbital region and are more likely to develop secondary bacterial infection than scratches from the other common domesticated species. Corneal abrasions are also occasionally associated with the periorbital wounds. Cat-scratch disease, an uncommon complication of these injuries, is characterized by a papule at the scratch site and a subsequent regional lymphadenitis. The primary lesion is typically a crusted, erythematous papule, 2 to 6 mm in diameter that develops 3 to 10 days after the scratch. A tender regional lymphadenopathy occurs 2 weeks after the primary lesion.

Malaise and fever are associated symptoms in approximately 25% of patients. Unusual manifestations of this disease include encephalopathy, exanthem, atypical pneumonia, and parotid swelling. The disease is self-limiting, with resolution of the symptoms within 2 to 3 months. *Bartonella henselae* is the causative organism. An indirect fluorescent antibody test to Bartonella is useful in the diagnosis and is available through the Centers for Disease Control and Prevention. Polymerase chain reaction assays are available in some commercial labs.

Human bites in older children and adolescents are most commonly incurred when a clenched fist strikes the teeth of an adversary. The wound typically overlies the metacarpal-phalangeal joint, and on relaxation of the fist, the bacterial inoculum penetrates more deeply into the relatively avascular fascial layers. Hand infections, regardless of infection site, usually present with mild swelling over the dorsum of the hand 1 to 2 days after injury. Infected hand bites may be superficial and localized to the wound, but if there is pain with active or passive finger motion, a more serious deep compartmental infection or tendonitis should be suspected. Osteomyelitis occasionally occurs in hand infections. In younger children, human bites are more often on the face or trunk than on the hands. Often, a playmate inflicts the wound, but child abuse must always be considered. Systemic diseases that may be spread by human bites include hepatitis B and syphilis.

Rodent bites usually occur in disadvantaged socioeconomic groups or among laboratory workers and have a relatively low incidence of secondary infection (10%). Ratbite fever is a rare disease that may present after a 1- to 3-week incubation period with chills, fever, malaise, headache, and a maculopapular or petechial rash. There are two forms: Haverhill fever (*Streptobacillus moniliformis*) and Sodoku (*Spirullum minus*), both of which are responsive to IV penicillin.

Another uncommon bacterium for which lagomorphs, particularly rabbits, are hosts is *Francisella tularensis*. Tularemia is usually spread to humans by rabbit bites, although contact with or ingestion of contaminated animals or insect vectors is sufficient for transmission. Ulceroglandular tularemia is the most common form of the disease, and gentamicin, ciprofloxacin, or doxycycline is the agent of first choice in its treatment. Streptomycin may be used but is no longer readily available in the United States.

Serious infections from multiple bacteria, including osteomyelitis, sepsis, endocarditis, and meningitis, have been reported as complications of mammalian bite wounds, as well as the more esoteric diseases already mentioned. The risk of rabies or tetanus always must be considered in animal bites.

Management

Meticulous and prompt local care of the bite wound is the most important factor in satisfactory healing and prevention of infection. In more extensive wounds, local anesthesia is achieved before wound hygiene. Then, the skin surrounding the wound should be cleaned with a soft sponge, and 1% providone iodine solution can remove obvious contaminants. The wound itself should be forcefully irrigated with a minimum of 200 mL normal saline. A 19-gauge needle or catheter attached to a 30-mL syringe will supply sufficient pressure for wound decontamination and will decrease the infection rate by 20-fold. Stronger irrigant antiseptics—povidone iodine scrub preparation, 20% hexachlorophene, alcohols, or hydrogen peroxide—may damage wound surfaces and delay healing. Soaking in various preparations has not proved helpful in reducing infections.

Most open lacerations from mammalian bites can be sutured if local care is effected within several hours of the injury and good surgical technique is used. Facial wounds often mandate primary closure for cosmetic reasons and, overall, are low infection risks because of the good vascular supply. In fact, one study demonstrated a lower infection rate in sutured dog bite wounds than in those left open. Other more recent studies support the low infection rate in selected sutured bite wounds. The exceptions to suturing are minor hand wounds and other high-risk bites. In large hand wounds, hemorrhage should be carefully controlled. We suggest closing the subcutaneous dead space in these wounds with a minimal amount of absorbable suture material. Cutaneous sutures can be placed after 3 to 5 days if there is no evidence of infection.

Extremities with extensive wounds should be immobilized in a position of function and kept elevated as much as possible. This is especially true of hand wounds, which should have bulky mitten dressings and be supported by an arm sling. All significant wounds should be rechecked in follow-up in 24 to 48 hours.

The following wounds may be considered at high risk for infection: puncture wounds, minor hand or foot wounds, wounds given initial care after 12 hours, cat or human bites, and wounds in immunosuppressed patients. As a rule, these wounds should not be sutured. The use of prophylactic antibiotics is controversial. Suggested indications for antibiotics include the following:

- Human and cat bites through dermis
- Bites closed prematurely
- Bites more than 8 hours old with significant crush injury or edema
- Potential damage to bones, joints, or tendons
- Bites to hands and feet
- Patients with increased risk of infection
- Signs of infection within 24 hours

No single antibiotic is ideal for all the most common organisms involved in infected mammalian bite wounds. Amoxicillin-clavulanic acid (Augmentin) comes close. It is effective in *P. multocida*, Streptococcus, and anaerobe control, as well as in providing methicillin-susceptible staphylococcus aureus (MSSA) coverage. Combination therapy with phenoxymethyl penicillin (penicillin VK) and cephalexin or dicloxacillin has been suggested by some authorities. For high-risk wounds, we recommend amoxicillin-clavulanic acid (30 to 50 mg per kg per day) alone for initial therapy. An extended-spectrum cephalosporin or trimethoprim-sulfamethoxazole PLUS clindamycin is an alternative for the penicillin-allergic patient. The initial dose of antibiotic should be given in the ED and continued for the next 3 to 5 days. It must be emphasized that local care ultimately prevents infection more effectively than any prophylactic antibiotics. Studies indicate that prophylactic oral antibiotics for low-risk dog bite wounds are not indicated because the differences in the rate of infection are not significant and the cost-benefit ratio is not worth the risk of allergic reaction.

Any bite wound with signs of infection deserves aggressive drainage and debridement, as well as antibiotic therapy, after aerobic and anaerobic cultures are obtained. Moderate to severe hand infections or other wounds that involve deep structures usually require debridement and exploration under general anesthesia. Culture swabs should sample the depth of the wound; or, in cases of cellulitis, the specimen can be collected by needle aspiration of the leading edge of erythema. While awaiting cultures, a Gram stain is often helpful in differentiating the probability of staphylococci or streptococci from *P. multocida*.

Parenteral antibiotics and admission to the hospital are indicated if the child has systemic symptoms or has wounds with potential functional or cosmetic morbidity. The choice of parenteral antibiotics should be governed by the same factors considered in selection of prophylactic antibiotics and then modified by culture results.

Tetanus immunization status should be checked in every injury that violates the epidermis, regardless of the cause. Recommendations for tetanus immunoglobulin and immunization are noted elsewhere (Chapter 92).

Concern for rabies is the factor that prompts many patients to seek medical care. Although the incidence of rabies in the United States (one to five cases per year) is extremely low, the physician must always assess the possibility of rabies exposure and promptly initiate prophylaxis when indicated. Dogs and cats account for only 5% of animal rabies in the United States. The history should include the apparent health of the animal and any provocation for attack. Wild carnivores and bats should generally be regarded as rabid; rodents (rats, squirrels) and lagomorphs (rabbits) can usually be considered no risk. Exposure to bats by a sleeping or very young child even without bite or scratch should warrant serious consideration of prophylaxis. Rabies prophylaxis is not indicated in bites by a healthy dog or cat with a known owner, assuming the animal's health does not deteriorate over the following 10 to 14 days. Bites by strays and other domesticated mammals should be considered individually and with consultation of the local health department. Scratches, abrasions, and animal saliva contact with the victim's mucous membranes are capable of rabies spread.

If postexposure antirabies immunization is indicated both passive antibody (RIG, rabies immune globulin, human) and vaccine (HDCV, human diploid cell rabies vaccine) should be given. Immunization with RIG is administered only once, in a dose of 20 IU per kg. Half the dose, or as much as possible, is infiltrated locally around the wound and the remainder is given intramuscularly. The HDCV immunization should be administered intramuscularly in the opposite deltoid (vastus lateralis in infants) from RIG on days 0, 3, 7, 14, and 28 for a total of five doses, each 1.0 mL.

Suggested Readings

General

Auerbach PS. Marine envenomation. *N Engl J Med* 1991;325:486–493.

Halstead BW. *Poisonous and venomous marine animals of the world*. Princeton, NJ: Darwin Press, 1978.

Halstead BW, Vinci JM. Venomous fish stings. *Clin Dermatol* 1991;5:29–35.

Hillman JV. Marine animal exposures in Florida. *J Fla Med Assoc* 1996; 83(3):187–191.

McGoldrick J, Marx JA. Marine envenomations, I: vertebrates. *J Emerg Med* 1991;9:497–502.

McGoldrick J, Marx JA. Marine envenomations, II: invertebrates. *J Emerg Med* 1992;10:71–77.

MEDICAL EMERGENCIES

Singletary EM, Rochman AS, Bodmer JCA, Holstege CP. Envenomations. *Med Clin North Am* 2005;89:1195–1224.

Coelenterata

Armoni M, Ohali M, Hay E, Bibi H. Severe dyspnea due to jellyfish envenomation. *Pediatr Emerg Care* 2003;19:84–86

Bailey PM, Little M, Jelinek GA, et al. Jellyfish envenoming syndromes: unknown toxic mechanisms and unproven therapies. *Med J Aust* 2003; 178:34–37.

Burnett JW, Weinrich D, Williamson JA, et al. Autonomic neurotoxicity of jellyfish and marine animal venoms. *Clin Auton Res* 1998;8:125–130.

Freudenthal AR, Joseph PR. Sunbathers' eruption. *N Engl J Med* 1993;329: 542–544.

Koffman MB. Portuguese man-o'-war envenomation. *Pediatr Emerg Care* 1992;8:27–28.

Mianzan JW, Fenner PJ, Cornelius PFS, et al. Vinegar as a disarming agent to prevent further discharge of the nematocysts of the stinging hydromedusa Olindias sambaquiensis. *Cutis* 2001;68:45–48.

Thomas CS, Scott SA, Galanis DJ, et al. Box jellyfish (Carybdea alata) in Waikiki: the analgesic effect of sting-aid, Adolph's Meat Tenderizer and fresh water on their stings: a double-blinded, randomized, placebo-controlled clinical trial. *Hawaii Med J* 2001;60:205–210.

Echinodermata

Burnett JW, Burnett MG. Sea urchins. *Cutis* 1999;64:21–22.

Stingrays

Bitseff EL, Garoni WJ, Hardison CD, et al. The management of stingray injuries of the extremities. *South Med J* 1970;63:417–418.

Evans RJ, Davies RS. Stingray injury. *J Accid Emerg Med* 1996;13:224–225.

Fenner PJ, Williamson JA, Skinner RA. Fatal and non-fatal stingray envenomation. *Med J Aust* 1989;151(11/12):621–625.

Forrester MB. Pattern of stingray injuries reported to Texas poison centers from 1198 to 2004. *Hum Exp Toxicol* 2005;24:639–642.

Meyer PK. Stingray injuries. *Wilderness Environ Med* 1997;8:24–28.

Sharks

Auerbach PS. Hazardous marine animals. *Emerg Med Clin North Am* 1984;2: 531–544.

Baldridge HD, Williams J. Shark attack: feeding or fighting? *Mil Med* 1969;134: 130–133.

White JAM. Shark attack in Natal. *Injury* 1976;6:191–194.

Scorpaenidae

Bonnet MS. The toxicology of Trachinus vipera: the lesser weeverfish. *Br Homeopath J* 2000;89:84–88.

Kizer KW, McKinney HE, Auerbach PS. Scorpaenidae envenomation: a five-year poison center experience. *JAMA* 1985;253:807–810.

Catfish

Baack BR, Kucan JO, Zook EG, et al. Hand infections secondary to catfish spines: case reports and literature review. *J Trauma* 1991;31:1432–1436.

Zeman MG. Catfish stings: report of three cases. *Ann Emerg Med* 1989;18: 211–213.

Arthropoda

Bentur Y, Taitelman U, Aloufy A. Evaluation of scorpion stings: the poison center perspective. *Vet Human Toxicol* 2003;45(2):108–111.

Berg RA, Tarantino MD. Envenomation by the scorpion Centruroides exilicauda (C. sculpturatus): severe and unusual manifestations. *Pediatrics* 1991;87:930–933.

Brown SGA, Blackman KE, Stenlake V, et al. Insect sting anaphylaxis; prospective evaluation of treatment with intravenous adrenaline and volume resuscitation. *Emerg Med J* 2004;21:149–154.

Clark RF. The safety and efficacy of antivenin Latrodectus mactans. *Clin Toxicol* 2001;39:125–127.

Clark RF, Wethern-Kestner S, Vance MV, et al. Clinical presentation and treatment of black widow spider envenomation: a review of 163 cases. *Ann Emerg Med* 1992;21:782–787.

DeShazo RD, Butcher BT, Banks WA. Reactions to the stings of the imported fire ant. *N Engl J Med* 1990;323:462–466.

Felz MW, Smith CD, Swift TR. A six year-old girl with tick paralysis. *N Engl J Med* 2000;342:90–94.

Freeman TM. Hypersensitivity to hymenoptera stings. *N Engl J Med* 2004; 351;1978–1984.

Gendron BP. Loxosceles reclusa envenomation. *Am J Emerg Med* 1990;8:51–54.

Gibly R, Williams M, Frank W, et al. Continuous intravenous midazolam infusion for Centruroides exilicauda scorpion envenomation. *Ann Emerg Med* 1999;34(5):620–625.

Ginsburg CM. Fire ant envenomation in children. *Pediatrics* 1984;73:689–692.

Gorman RJ, Snead OC. Tick paralysis in three children. *Clin Pediatr* 1978; 17:249–251.

Hobbs GP, Anderson AR, Green TJ, et al. Comparison of hyperbaric oxygen and dapsone on therapy for Loxosceles envenomation. *Acad Emerg Med* 1996;3:758–761.

Iserson KV. Methemoglobin from dapsone therapy for suspected brown spider bite. *J Emerg Med* 1985;3:285–288.

Jerrard DA. ED management of insect stings. *Am J Emerg Med* 1996;14: 429–433.

Key GF. A comparison of calcium gluconate and methocarbamol (Robaxin) in the treatment of latrodectism (black widow spider envenomation). *Am J Trop Med Hyg* 1981;30:273–276.

LoVecchio F, McBride C. Scorpion envenomations in young children in Central Arizona. *J Toxicol Clin Toxicol* 2003;41:937–940.

Milne M, Milne L. Audubon Society field guide to North American insects and spiders. New York, NY: Knopf, 1980.

Moffitt JE, Golden DBK, Reisman RE, et al. Stinging insect hypersensitivity: a practice parameter update. *J Allergy Clin Immunol* 2004;114:869–886.

Osterhoudt KC, Zaoutis T, Zorc JJ. Lyme disease masquerading as brown recluse spider bite. *Ann Emerg Med* 2002;39(5):558–561.

Phillips S, Kohn M, Baker D, et al. Therapy of brown spider envenomation: a controlled trial of hyperbaric oxygen, dapsone and cyproheptadine. *Ann Emerg Med* 1995;25:363–368.

Rees R, Campbell D, Rieger E, et al. The diagnosis and treatment of brown recluse spider bites. *Ann Emerg Med* 1991;16:945–949.

Reeves JA, Allison EJ Jr, Goodman PE. Black widow spider bite in a child. *Am J Emerg Med* 1996;14:469–471.

Sams HH, Hearth SB, Long LL, et al. Nineteen documented cases of Loxosceles reclusa envenomation. *J Am Acad Dermatol* 2001;44(4):603–608.

Saucier JR. Arachnid envenomation. *Emerg Med Clin North Am* 2004;22: 405–422.

Sicherer SH, Simons ER; Section on Allergy & Immunology. Self-injectable epinephrine for first-aid management of anaphylaxis. *Pediatrics* 2007;119: 638–646.

Sofer S. Scorpion envenomation. *Intensive Care Med* 1995;21:626–628.

Vetter RS, Bush SP. Reports of presumptive brown recluse spider bites reinforce improbable diagnosis in regions of North America where the spider is not endemic. *Clin Infect Dis* 2002;35:442–445.

Visscher PK, Veller RS, Camazine S. Removing bee stings. *Lancet* 1996;348: 301–302.

Volcheck GW. Hymenoptera (Apid and Vespid) allergy: update in diagnosis and management. *Curr Allergy Asthma Rep* 2002;2:46–50.

Woestman R, Perkin R, Van Stralen D. The black widow: is she deadly to children? *Pediatr Emerg Care* 1996;12:360–364.

Wright SW, Wrenn KD, Murray L, et al. Clinical presentation and outcome of brown recluse spider bite. *Ann Emerg Med* 1997;30(1):28–32.

Venomous Reptiles

Alberts MB, Shalit M, LoGalbo F. Suction for venomous snakebite: a study of "mock venom" extraction in a human model. *Ann Emerg Med* 2004; 43:181–186.

Behm MO, Kearns GL, Offerman S, et al. Crotaline FAB antivenom for treatment of children with rattlesnake envenomation. *Pediatrics* 2003;112: 1458–1459.

Bond GR. Controversies in the treatment of pediatric victims of Crotalidae snake envenomation. *Clin Pediatr Emerg Med* 2001;2:192–202.

Burgess JL, Dart RC, Egen NB, et al. Effects of constriction bands on rattlesnake venom absorption: a pharmacokinetic study. *Ann Emerg Med* 1992;21: 1086–1093.

Clark RF, McKinney PE, Chase PB, et al. Immediate and delayed allergic reactions to Crotalidae polyvalent immune Fab (Ovine) antivenom. *Ann Emerg Med* 2002;39(6):671–676.

Dart RC, McNally J. Efficacy, safety, and use of snake antivenoms in the United States. *Ann Emerg Med* 2001;37:181–188.

Gold BS, Dart RC, Barish RA. Bites of venomous snakes. *N Engl J Med* 2002;347(5):347–356.

Holstege CP, Wu J, Baer AB. Immediate hypersensitivity reaction associated with the rapid infusion of Crotalidae polyvalent immune Fab (Ovine). *Ann Emerg Med* 2002;39(6):677–679.

Lavonas EJ, Gerardo CJ, O'Malley G, et al. Initial experience with Crotalidae polyvalent immune Fab (ovine) antivenom in the treatment of copperhead snakebite. *Ann Emerg Med* 2004;43:200–206.

Lawrence WT, Giannopoulos A, Hansen A. Pit viper bites: rational management in locales in which copperheads and cottonmouths predominate. *Ann Plastic Surg* 1996;36:276–285.

McKinney PE. Out-of-hospital and interhospital management of crotaline snakebite. *Ann Emerg Med* 2001;37:168–174.

Offerman SR, Bush SP, Moynihan JA, et al. Crotaline Fab antivenom for the treatment of children with rattlesnake envenomation. *Pediatrics* 2002;110:968–971.

Pizon AF, Riley BD, LoVecchio F, et al. Safety and efficacy of Crotalidae polyvalent immune Fab in pediatric crotaline envenomations. *Acad Emerg Med* 2007;14:373–376.

Schmidt JM. Antivenom therapy for snake bites in children: is there evidence? *Curr Opin Pediatr* 2005;17:234–238.

Shaw BA, Hosalkar HS. Rattlesnake bites in children: antivenin treatment and surgical indications. *J Bone Joint Surg* 2002;84:1624–1629.

Spiller HA, Bosse GM. Prospective study of morbidity associated with snake bite envenomation. *Clin Toxicol* 2003;41:125–130.

Trinh HH, Hack JB. Use of CroFab antivenin in the management of a very young pediatric copperhead envenomation. *J Emerg Med* 2005;29:159–162.

Mammalian Bites

Aghababian RV, Conte JE Jr. Mammalian bite wounds. *Ann Emerg Med* 1980;9:79.

Baker MD, Moore SE. Human bites in children. *Am J Dis Child* 1991;141:1285–1291.

Ball V, Younggren BN. Emergency management of difficult wounds: part I. *Emerg Med Clin North Am* 2007;25:101–121.

Blanton JD, Krebs JW, Hanlon CA, et al. Rabies surveillance in the United States during 2005. *J Am Vet Med Assoc* 2006;229:1897–1911.

Brogan TV, Bratton SL, Dowd MD, et al. Severe dog bites in children. *Pediatrics* 1995;96:947–950.

Callaham M. Prophylactic antibiotics in dog bite wounds: nipping at the heels of progress. *Ann Emerg Med* 1994;23:577–579.

Centers for Disease Control and Prevention. Dog bite related fatalities—U.S. 1995–1996. *MMWR Morb Mortal Wkly Rep* 1997;46:463–467.

Centers for Disease Control and Prevention. Rabies prevention. *MMWR Morb Mortal Wkly Rep* 1999;48:RR1.

Centers for Disease Control and Prevention. Nonfatal dog bite-related injuries treated in hospital emergency departments—United States 2001. *MMWR Morb Mortal Wkly Rep* 2003;52(26):605–610.

Chen E, Hornig S, Shepherd SM, et al. Primary closure of mammalian bites. *Acad Emerg Med* 2000;7(2):157–161.

Cummings P. Antibiotics to prevent infections in patients with dog bite wounds: a meta-analysis of randomized trials. *Ann Emerg Med* 1994;23:535–540.

Dire DJ, Hogan DE, Riggs MW. A prospective evaluation of risk factors for infections from dog-bite wounds. *Acad Emerg Med* 1994;1(3):258–266.

Lindsey D, Christopher M, Hollenbach J, et al. Natural course of the human bite wound: incidence of infection and complications in 434 bites and 803 lacerations in the same group of patients. *J Trauma* 1991;27:45.

Moran GJ, Talan DA, Mower W, et al. Appropriateness of rabies postexposure prophylaxis treatment for animal exposures. *JAMA* 2000;284(8):1001–1007.

Morgan M, Palmer J. Dog bites. *BMJ* 2007;334:413–417.

Rupprecht CE, Gibbons CE. Prophylaxis against rabies. *N Engl J Med* 2004;351:2626–2635.

Schmidt JM. Antivenom therapy for snake bites in children: is there evidence? *Curr Opin Pediatr* 2005;17:234–238.

Talan DA, Citron DM, Abrahamian FM, et al. Bacteriologic analysis of infected dog and cat bites. *N Engl J Med* 1999;340(2):85–92.

Wear DJ, Margileth AM, Hadfield TL, et al. Cat scratch disease: a bacterial infection. *Science* 1983;221:1403–1405.

CHAPTER 84 ■ CARDIAC EMERGENCIES

MICHAEL H. GEWITZ, MD, AND PAUL K. WOOLF, MD

Cardiac problems in infancy and childhood are not rare, are frequently complex, and always have important implications for the general health of the child. This chapter provides information regarding the evaluation and management of the more common emergencies that arise from the presence of cardiovascular disease in childhood. For the health-care professional not well-versed in childhood cardiac disease, a brief overview is provided as background for the specific problems discussed in detail.

OVERVIEW

As with other pediatric disorders, cardiac diseases in childhood can be congenital or acquired. Major and minor structural diseases of the heart for the most part result from derangements of embryologic development and thus are present in some form at birth. The clinical manifestations of such problems may be delayed, however, for days, months, or even years. In contrast, many other disorders of cardiac physiology result from problems superimposed on inherently normal cardiac structures. These problems are frequently acute in their development when a relatively sudden change from normal cardiac physiology occurs, leading quickly to the development of symptoms. It should be remembered, however, that acquired cardiac diseases can also be associated with prolonged latent periods. For example, the most prevalent form of acquired heart disease in the United States, coronary artery disease, has its beginnings in childhood in numerous instances, although its appearance as a clinical entity occurs much later. Examples of forms of congenital and acquired pediatric cardiac problems are reviewed in Table 84.1.

The incidence rate of congenital heart disease (CHD) has been fairly constant over the past few decades and is estimated to be approximately 7–8 to 10 cases per 1,000 live births (0.7% to 0.8%). This includes all forms of defects and all ranges of severity but does not include the most common isolated congenital cardiac lesion, bicuspid aortic valve, which occurs in an additional 1% or more of people. The prevalence figures for CHD are continually increasing. It has recently been estimated, in fact, that there are now more adults alive with CHD than there are infants. This "adult CHD" population will continue to increase, of course, as more and better treatment modalities become available to correct and/or palliate even the most severe forms of defects. Many of these patients are beginning to have offspring of their own. Studies have also found the incidence of congenital cardiac problems in children of parents with CHD to range from 5% to 15%. (The disorders seen as part of the spectrum of CHD are extremely variable; comprehensive texts are available for more detailed reviews.)

Age at presentation can vary significantly, depending on the type of congenital cardiac lesion and its impact on cardiac performance. Severe obstruction to pulmonary or systemic flows may be masked in the first few days of life by persistence of a patent ductus arteriosus, whereas the presence of an important ventricular septal defect (VSD) may not become clinically evident until 4 to 6 weeks of age. This wide disparity in age at presentation is related to the physiologic interactions of the systemic and pulmonary vasculature, as well as to the anatomic specifics of any particular lesion. Table 84.2 presents examples of typical presenting ages for the more common forms of CHD. Although it is not important for the emergency practitioner to be versed specifically in all possible defects, knowledge of anatomic and physiologic possibilities is important so the practitioner's awareness of potential problems can lead to appropriate triage and initiation of care. One useful approach is to categorize lesions by the presence or absence of arterial desaturation; thus, there are cyanotic and acyanotic forms of CHD. Table 84.3 reviews some of the congenital lesions that segregate into these two groups.

Even without recalling specific lesions, however, only a few key principles of cyanosis must be understood (Table 84.4) to be able to consider the possibilities when faced with a particular patient. For example, a patient with anemia may have cyanotic CHD, yet not be visibly desaturated, or a patient may have a significant level of pulmonary valve stenosis with significant obstruction to pulmonary blood flow but not appear cyanotic. Conversely, a patient may not have a loud cardiac murmur or any murmur at all and still have a serious cyanotic cardiac lesion (see Chapter 33).

In diagnosing children with possible CHD, therefore, it is not usually necessary to remember long lists of complex lesions. An appreciation of what is anatomically possible and what is physiologically rational, however, usually leads to the ability to discern what is clinically likely in any particular situation.

The next sections deal with specific examples of the melding of these anatomic and physiologic concerns in emergency situations that involve cardiovascular diseases in children.

CONGESTIVE HEART FAILURE

Background

Heart failure is frequently described as a syndrome in which the heart cannot maintain a level of tissue perfusion adequate to meet metabolic needs. During childhood, these needs also include growth and development. This section offers an outline of the primary etiologic and physiologic factors that underlie the clinical presentation of the child in congestive heart failure (CHF).

TABLE 84.1

EXAMPLES OF ACQUIRED AND CONGENITAL FORMS OF PEDIATRIC HEART DISEASE

Forms of pediatric heart disease examples	
Congenital	
Disorders of septal or valvar development	Pulmonary, aortic valve stenosis
	Mitral or tricuspid atresia
	Ventricular septal defect
	Atrial septal defect
Disorders of venous or arterial connection	Transposition of the great vessels
	Anomalies of pulmonary venous return
Disorders of conduction system development	Congenital AV block
	Persistent bypass tract syndromes (preexcitation)
Acquired	
Disorders of cardiac muscular function	Cardiomyopathy associated with cancer therapies
	Acute myocarditis
	Acute pericarditis
Disorders of valvar function	Acute rheumatic fever
	Bacterial endocarditis
Disorders of cardiac rhythm	Drug-induced arrhythmias
	Postsurgical heart block

AV, atrioventricular.

TABLE 84.2

AGE OF PRESENTATION OF CONGENITAL HEART DISEASE[a]

First 2 wk
Left ventricular outflow obstruction
    Coarctation of aorta
    Severe aortic stenosis
    Left heart hypoplasia
Cyanotic lesions
    Transposition of great vessels
    Total anomalous pulmonary venous return
    Atrioventricular (AV) canal malformations
    Truncus arteriosus

First month
Coarctation of aorta
Ventricular septal defect (VSD)
Patent ductus arteriosus (PDA)
Truncus arteriosus
Complex lesions with multiple anomalies (e.g., double-outlet
    right ventricle)

6 Wk to 6 mo
VSD
AV canal malformations
Coronary artery anomalies
Truncus arteriosus

Over 6 mo
VSD
Atrial septal defect
Isolated valvar lesions (e.g., pulmonic stenosis, mitral
    insufficiency)
Small PDA
Partial anomalous pulmonary venous return
Coarctation of aorta

[a]There is considerable overlap regarding any particular lesion and the specific clinical setting. This list is representative and illustrative, not all inclusive.

Etiologic Considerations

Although the primary cause of CHF in infants and children is CHD, a panoply of conditions can be associated with the presentation of CHF in the presence of normal underlying cardiac structure. Table 84.5 lists the more common clinical entities associated with CHF, including primary cardiac disease and conditions in which the heart is affected secondarily. In general, the principal physiologic problems that lead to impaired myocardial performance include (i) excessive pressure loads, such as left heart obstructions; (ii) excessive volume loads, such as with large left-to-right shunts, valvar regurgitation, or severe anemia; (iii) primary inotropic depression, such as with myocarditis, endocrinologic disorders, or coronary perfusion irregularities; and (iv) rhythm abnormalities, such as supraventricular tachycardia (SVT) or severe forms of heart block.

The history is critical in determining the cause of CHF and should not be glossed over in the rush to treat. Knowledge of preexisting cardiac disease is obviously important. A history of known hematologic disorders such as thalassemia or sickle cell anemia should also be sought. Because heart failure can develop as a consequence of pressure overload of the right heart secondary to pulmonary vasoconstriction and hypoxia, a history of respiratory tract difficulties or breathing pattern irregularities should also be reviewed carefully. Knowledge of other systemic conditions is likewise crucial. For example, several studies have indicated that human immunodeficiency virus (HIV) infection can seriously affect cardiac performance seriously on either an acute and chronic basis. Late stages of HIV infection are often complicated by cardiomyopathy and CHF. Careful clinical assessment for signs of cardiac involvement should be part of the evaluation of children with HIV who present with hypotension or who have respiratory problems not responsive to direct pulmonary management. As another example, a history for Kawasaki disease should be sought in patients who present with new-onset CHF that

TABLE 84.3

EXEMPLITIVE CONGENITAL HEART LESIONS

Acyanotic lesions	Cyanotic lesions
Secundum atrial septal defect	Tetralogy of Fallot
Ventricular septal defect	D-transposition of the great vessels
Patent ductus arteriosus	Tricuspid atresia variants
Aortic stenosis/regurgitation	Total anomalous pulmonary venous return
Coarctation of the aorta	Truncus arteriosus
Pulmonic stenosis—valvar	Pulmonary atrioventricular fistula
Peripheral pulmonary stenosis	Complete atrioventricular canal defect
Mitral stenosis/regurgitation	Ebstein's anomaly of the tricuspid valve
Partial anomalous pulmonary venous return	Pulmonary atresia with septal defect
Congenitally corrected transposition of the great vessels	Single ventricle states

appears to be related to inflammatory myocardial disease, even if other classic signs are not overtly present.

In the presence of appropriate physical findings and historical information, the diagnosis of CHF is usually evident in the older child. The principal problem of diagnosis centers on the infant, in whom differentiation between CHF and primary respiratory tract disease can be difficult. Auscultation of cardiac murmurs is helpful, of course, but such murmurs may not always be audible, particularly in severe failure with low output. Parenchymal lung disease may result in systemic desaturation to the same degree as CHF with associated pulmonary congestion and ventilation–perfusion imbalance. Palpation of the liver edge below the costal margin in an infant may be related to hyperexpansion of the lungs and not to systemic venous congestion. Conversely, respiratory tract signs such as wheezing and retractions may be part of the clinical picture of heart failure in the absence of primary lung disease. The chest radiograph often fails to distinguish clearly between cardiac and pulmonary disease because pulmonary markings often mimic infiltrative patterns. Evidence of cardiac enlargement on the radiograph is a useful differential point, although the enlarged thymus of the infant may make interpretation difficult. Other noninvasive methods, such as echocardiography, also can help to establish the diagnosis of cardiac disease.

TABLE 84.4

USEFUL RULES OF CYANOTIC CONGENITAL HEART DISEASE

In the presence of normal hemoglobin moieties and normal cardiac output, right-to-left shunting must be present to produce cyanosis. This can be intrapulmonary, intracardiac, or both.

Obstruction to pulmonary blood flow alone does not produce cyanosis.

A critical mass of reduced hemoglobin must be present to allow visual estimation of cyanosis.

Right-to-left shunts are not usually associated with heart murmurs.

The presence of visible cyanosis depends on the interrelationship of pulmonary and systemic blood flows and hemoglobin concentration.

Pathophysiology

There are four primary determinants of normal cardiac function, each of which may relate to the development of heart failure. The first is *preload*, the volume at end diastole that must be ejected by the left ventricle. This is a close reflection of the intravascular volume status of the child in general, which directly affects cardiac performance through the Frank–Starling relationship. The second, *afterload*, is the opposing force to ventricular ejection and relates to the tension that must be developed by the myocardium to eject a given preload. The third determinant, *contractility*, can be viewed as an intrinsic property of cardiac muscle that permits alterations in cardiac shape necessary for ejection and is determined by fundamental properties of cardiac ultrastructure. The fourth determinant, *heart rate* (HR), is related to intrinsic electrophysiologic capabilities of the specialized cardiac conduction system and to supervening neurologic input. It is directly related to cardiac output (CO) through the classic relationship:

$$CO = HR \times SV \text{ (stroke volume)}$$

Compensatory Responses

To understand the basis for the clinical findings commonly associated with CHF, the physician must consider the physiologic responses to inadequate cardiac function. These include mechanical effects, such as ventricular hypertrophy and ventricular dilatation; neurohumoral effects, principally those that involve the adrenergic nervous system; biochemical effects at the cardiac cellular level that alter myocardial energy metabolism and the excitation–contraction coupling process; and hematologic effects that involve oxygen transport. In addition, pulmonary responses, including increased respiratory frequency and altered respiratory patterns, also comprise an important part of the clinical picture of CHF.

Clinical Manifestations

The clinical manifestations of CHF are directly related to the following compensatory mechanisms:

1. Cardiac enlargement is usually the result of ventricular dilation. Although it may often be possible to detect cardiac

TABLE 84.5

ETIOLOGIC CONSIDERATIONS FOR CONGESTIVE HEART FAILURE

Congenital heart disease	Acquired heart disease	Endocrine/metabolic	Other

Pressure overload
Left ventricular outflow
  obstruction (e.g., aortic
  stenosis, severe coarctation)
	Myocarditis
	Viral infections
	Kawasaki disease
	Collagen-vascular disease
	Cardiomyopathy
		Electrolyte disturbances
		Hypoglycemia
		Hypothyroidism
		Calcium or magnesium
		  disorders
			Ingestions/toxins
			Cardiac toxins (e.g., digitalis)
			Arrhythmogenics
			  (e.g., tricyclic
			  antidepressants)

Left ventricular inflow
  obstruction
  (e.g., cortriatriatum)
	Chronic anemia
	  (e.g., thalassemia major)
	
	Nutritional disorders
		Lipid disorders
		
		Carnitine deficiency
		Carbolic acid disorders
			Chemotherapy agents
			  (e.g., adriamycin)

Volume overload
Left-to-right shunts
  (e.g., ventricular septal
  defect)
	AIDS
	Pericardial disease
	Rheumatic heart disease
		Fatty acid disorders
		Storage Diseases
		Mitochondrial disorders
		Barth syndrome	

Anomalous pulmonary
  venous return
	Cor pulmonale
	Acute (e.g., upper airway
	  obstruction)		

Valvar regurgitation (e.g., aortic insufficiency) Arteriovenous fistulae *Other structural disease* Anomalous coronary artery Traumatic injury *Rhythm disturbance* Supraventricular tachycardia Complete heart block *Postoperative heart disease* Malfunctioning prosthetic valve	Cystic fibrosis Neuropathies *Endocarditis*		

enlargement by displacement of the cardiac impulse, the chest radiograph remains the most readily available method for assessing ventricular dilation (Figs. 84.1 and 84.2). Care must be taken to distinguish the normal cardiothymic silhouette from true cardiomegaly in an infant (Fig. 84.2). The other finding related to mechanical compensatory responses is ven-tricular hypertrophy, which is distinguishable on the electro-cardiogram (EKG; Fig. 84.3). As a compensatory mechanism, hypertrophy occurs before dilatation in pressure overload sit-uations, whereas dilatation may occur first in volume over-load of the heart. In general, cardiac size can be a reliable guide to the overall fluid volume status of the infant or child.

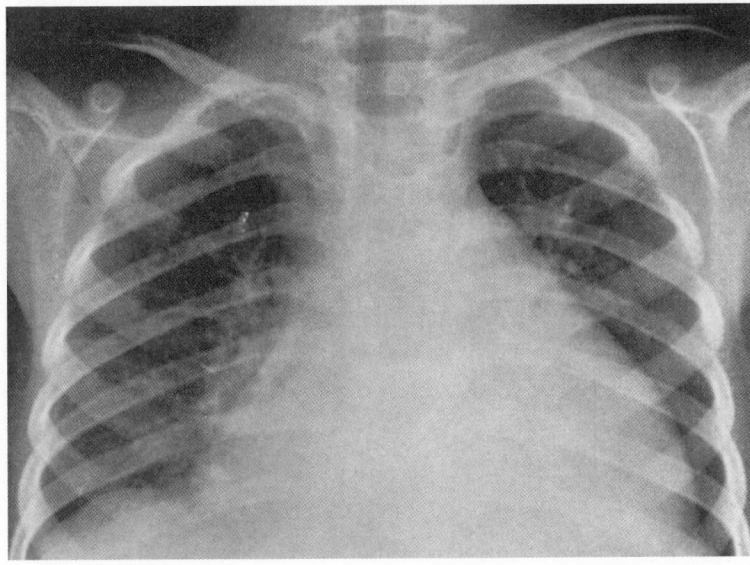

FIGURE 84.1 Chest radiograph of older child with con-gestive heart failure. Note cardiac enlargement and evi-dence of pulmonary venous congestion.

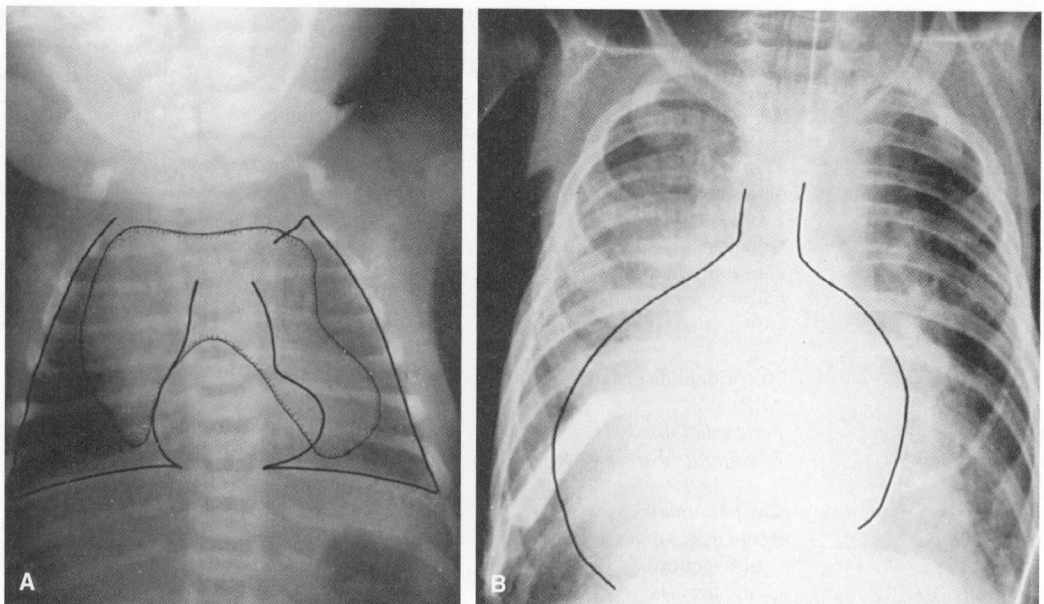

FIGURE 84.2 **A:** Normal cardiothymic shadow. Thymus is demarcated by speckled line and overlies a portion of the heart shadow. **B:** True cardiomegaly in an infant associated with pulmonary edema. Entire area enclosed in outline is cardiac shadow.

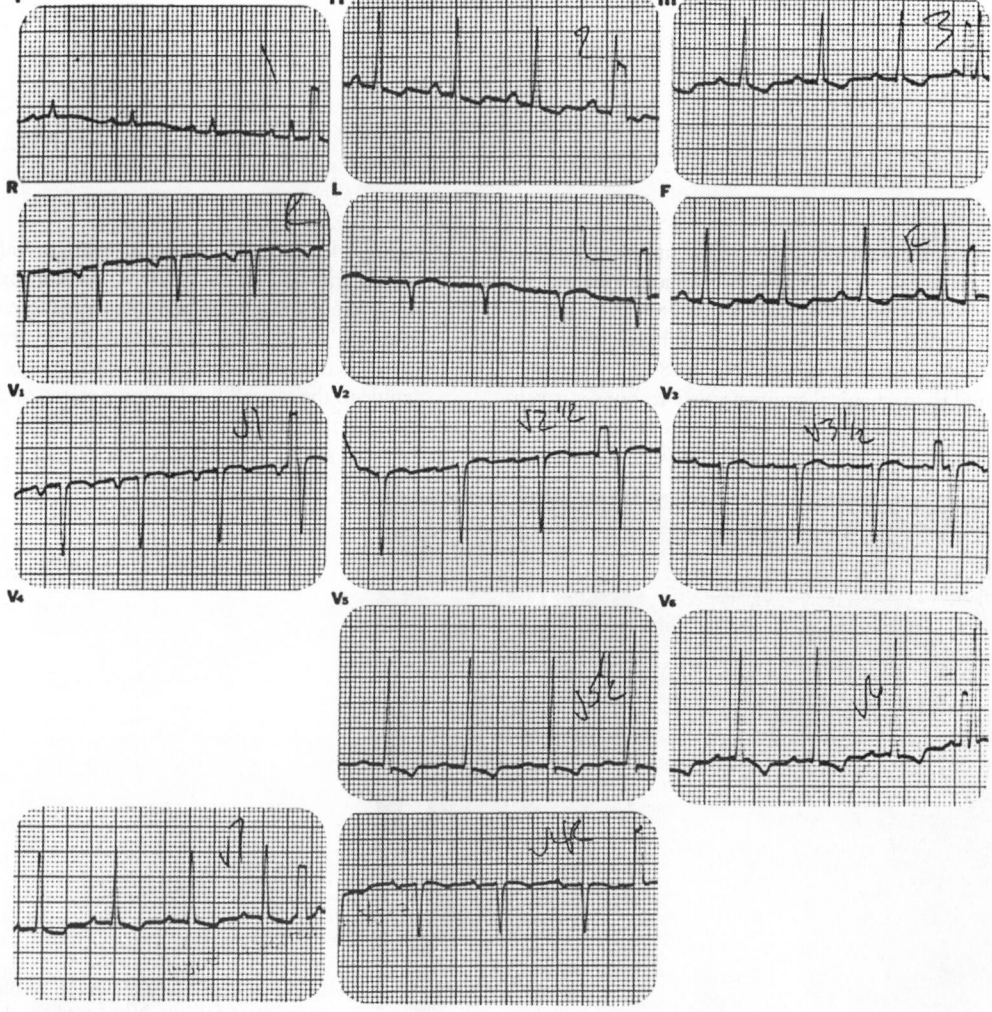

FIGURE 84.3 Electrocardiogram demonstrating left ventricular hypertrophy. Note increased R-wave voltage in left precordial leads and abnormal T-wave changes.

2. Tachycardia is easily detected clinically and, if necessary, confirmed by EKG. A rate of more than 160 beats per minute (bpm) in an infant or 100 bpm in the older child may be a signal for the increased adrenergic tone and catecholamine release associated with the neurohumoral response to diminished CO.

3. Abnormalities of cardiac auscultation are also commonly present. The protodiastolic gallop, or third heart sound (S_3), is a sign of decreased ventricular compliance and increased resistance to filling. Less often, the fourth heart sound, or atrial gallop (S_4), can be heard in children. It should be noted that these auscultatory events can sometimes be normal findings in childhood, and thus, the entire clinical picture must be evaluated before defining their significance in any particular situation.

4. Respiratory responses, notably tachypnea, are usually present as part of the total picture of CHF. Often, rales, rhonchi, and wheezing may be heard and should not be confused as signs of pulmonary parenchymal disease exclusive of heart failure. In contrast, it is not unusual, particularly in infants, for rales to be absent despite the presence of tachypnea or wheezing because considerable alveolar fluid accumulation is necessary for the development of rales. Thus, the presence of rales usually implies severe failure in an infant, whereas pulmonary interstitial fluid collection, which occurs at an earlier stage, may be represented by tachypnea and wheezing alone. In older children, dyspnea with activity and orthopnea may also be present. A chronic cough also may be a sign of pulmonary congestion developing from CHF. Associated with these findings are chest retractions that reflect the large negative intrathoracic pressures needed to ventilate stiff, fluid-filled lungs.

5. Growth failure and undernutrition may be important clinical correlates of chronic CHF. These reflect not only diminished cellular substrate availability as a result of inadequate tissue perfusion, but also increased caloric expenditure associated with heightened oxygen consumption and increased work of breathing. Feeding difficulties, which may be associated with the respiratory patterns previously noted, aggravate caloric balance even further.

6. Cool, moist extremities and a generalized pallor may also be present as a result of peripheral vasoconstriction secondary to catecholamine release and the need to maintain blood pressure (BP) in the face of reduced CO.

7. Central and peripheral fluid accumulation with elevated systemic venous pressure also accompanies CHF, reflecting impaired cardiac emptying as well as impaired sodium and protein balance. Hepatomegaly, jugular venous distention, and peripheral edema represent the clinical manifestations of this aspect of the problem. Peripheral edema, however, is an unusual finding in young infants. Pulsus alternans, a beat-to-beat variability in the strength of the pulse, is also a clinical sign of cardiac mechanical decompensation.

The child with overt CHF who is seen in the emergency department (ED) may present with nearly all the aforementioned signs and symptoms. If the child is severely ill, then pallor will be evident, tachypnea prominent, and intercostal retractions visible. The liver is enlarged and palpable well below the right costal margin; a spleen tip may also be palpable. The pulses are weak and thready, and the skin may be moist and cool to the touch. Auscultation of the chest reveals rales, rhonchi, and sometimes, wheezes. Tachycardia is present, and auscultation of the heart sounds frequently elicits a gallop rhythm. Murmurs may be strikingly absent unless preexisting heart disease is present. A child with this spectrum of findings requires urgent attention. Acute heart failure in a child usually implies an unstable situation with possible rapid deterioration.

Laboratory Findings

Usually, the clinical diagnosis of CHF can be made without extensive radiographs or laboratory tests. However, certain objective changes may corroborate the clinical findings:

1. As noted, a chest radiograph shows an increased cardiothoracic ratio and pulmonary congestion. Kerley B lines or platelike atelectasis at the lung bases, which reflect dilated pulmonary lymphatics, may be present. Pleural effusions are common.

2. The EKG is a nonspecific indicator of cardiac decompensation. The precordial voltages decrease in certain conditions associated with CHF, such as myocarditis, but may be normal or increased in other situations. The EKG can be also helpful for establishing the cause of the CHF, such as cardiac arrhythmia or myocardial ischemia.

3. Echocardiography is useful in evaluating the child with CHF. The differentiation of an enlarged cardiac silhouette secondary to impaired cardiac performance with ventricular chamber enlargement, rather than pericardial fluid accumulation, is best made by ultrasound examination. In addition, functional indices are obtained as an objective measure of cardiac performance and response to therapy. The underlying cardiac structures can also be evaluated for the presence of anatomic lesions.

4. Blood gas abnormalities may be present. Prolonged tissue hypoperfusion can result in metabolic acidosis of a significant degree, and the pulmonary abnormalities already noted may result in hypoxia.

5. Other abnormalities that may be present include electrolyte changes (hyponatremia and hypochloremia) and a reduction in hematocrit, based on dilutional factors. The erythrocyte sedimentation rate (ESR) is usually lowered in active CHF. In addition, in infants with CHF, serum glucose and calcium should be monitored because deficiencies in either may be responsible in large measure for the impaired cardiac function. In situations of suspected perfusion abnormalities or inflammatory myocardial diseases, cardiac enzymes—troponin, in particular—may be elevated.

Management

For the patient who requires emergency treatment of CHF, initial medical therapy includes several therapeutic measures as outlined in Table 84.6. First, supplemental oxygen should be given through a humidified system. In young children, a tight-fitting mask or nasal cannula may not be effective because too much energy is expended fighting such apparatuses. Second, elevation of head and shoulders is helpful in the face of pulmonary edema, with maintenance of the lower extremities in a dependent position to increase peripheral pooling, and thus, diminish pulmonary blood volume. A "cardiac chair" or appropriate modification of an infant seat establishes this posture in the small baby.

MEDICAL EMERGENCIES

TABLE 84.6

EMERGENCY MANAGEMENT OF CONGESTIVE
HEART FAILURE

History and physical examination to define etiology, if
  possible
Elevate head and chest
Ensure adequacy of ventilation
Administer oxygen
Initiate cardiorespiratory monitoring, including frequent
  blood pressure measurement
Achieve venous access and obtain laboratory studies (e.g.,
  complete blood cell count, electrolytes)
Arterial blood gas determination
Achieve rhythm control
Treat pulmonary edema (e.g., diuretics, morphine sulfate)
Provide inotropic support (digitalis or catecholamines)
Consider afterload reduction

Third, morphine sulfate (0.05 to 0.1 mg per kg subcutaneously) can be helpful in the face of agitation and air hunger associated with pulmonary edema. Fourth, positive-pressure respiration by endotracheal intubation is sometimes indicated for severe situations, particularly if arterial blood gas analysis shows respiratory decompensation ($PaCO_2 > 50$ mm Hg). In infants, the use of controlled mechanical ventilation to improve respiratory status greatly enhances survival. Fifth, bicarbonate therapy is sometimes indicated to correct metabolic acidosis that arises from diminished tissue perfusion. Administration of sodium bicarbonate during respiratory decompensation, however, is hazardous since further $PaCO_2$ elevation can occur. In addition, bicarbonate given by rapid infusion can promote cerebral edema and rapidly affect serum osmolarity with deleterious effects. Also, an excessive sodium load can result from injudicious use of bicarbonate. Thus, only for severe acidosis (pH less than 7.2) should bicar-

bonate be considered, and even then, only if respiratory function is satisfactory (see Chapter 95). Sixth, an intravenous (IV) infusion should be started to aid in the administration of drugs and the strict monitoring and administration of fluids.

Blood products in the form of packed cells should be administered if the child is severely anemic. Antibiotics should be reserved for unequivocal evidence of infection or for situations in which circumstantial evidence is strongly suggestive and appropriate cultures have been drawn. The use of corticosteroids may be indicated at times, particularly for heart failure precipitated by rheumatic heart disease. However, decisions of this type should be made with cardiac consultation. Treatment of arrhythmias that result in CHF is discussed subsequently under the "Cardiac Arrhythmias" section.

Although newer pharmacologic agents regularly become available, mainstays of the medical management of acute CHF are still digitalis, or other well-tested inotropic agents, to improve contractility, and diuretics to manipulate ventricular preload and intrapulmonary fluid. Pharmacologic adjustments of afterload have also become important for both acute and chronic CHF treatment. Regardless of the specific therapy, frequent reexamination and reevaluation are mandatory.

Digitalis

The classic drugs for improving the inotropic condition of the heart, unless the CO is severely compromised and the child is acutely ill, are the digitalis glycosides. Modern molecular investigations have helped shape improve our understanding of the mechanisms of action of these agents and how to adjust their administration in specific clinical situations. Although the use of digitalis in infants was reported nearly 60 years ago, until relatively recently dosing regimens have been strictly empiric in their derivations. The use of a radioimmunoassay to determine serum digitalis levels helped define a dosing format. As noted in Table 84.7, a principal clinical value of digitalis pharmacokinetic studies has been to verify that the same unit

TABLE 84.7

DIGITALIZATION WITH DIGOXIN

	I. Usual Doses (IM or oral)	
	Weight (g)	**Dose (TDD)**[a]
Premature infants	500–1,000	20 μg or 0.02 mg/kg
	1,000–1,500	20–30 μg/kg or 0.02–0.03 mg/kg
	1,500–2,000	30 μg/kg or 0.03 mg/kg
	2,000–2,500	30–40 μg/kg or 0.03–0.04 mg/kg
Term neonate		30–40 μg/kg or 0.10–0.04 mg/kg
1 mo–12 yr		40–60 μg/kg or 0.04–0.06 mg/kg
		(Maximum TDD: 1.5 mg)
	II. Alterations in Usual Doses	

Lower if renal function is impaired
Lower in presence of poor myocardial function (cardiomyopathy, myocarditis)
Lower in presence of metabolic imbalance (electrolyte abnormalities, hypoxia, acidosis)
Intravenous/intramuscular dose is 75% of oral dose

[a]TDD, total digitalizing doses. Digitalizing regimen usually given as initial dose: one-half of TDD; second dose: one-fourth of TDD, at 8–12 h; third dose: final one-fourth TDD at 8–12 h after second dose. Maintenance is then started as one-eighth TDD every 12 h. (*Note:* Parenteral preparation contains 100 μg/mL and oral, 50 μg/mL.)

dose per kg of body weight is not necessarily best for children of all ages and that premature infants, in particular, require close adjustment of dose, based on body weight.

The mechanism by which digitalis improves cardiac performance centers on the regulation of the ionic movements that are part of the contractile process. In particular, inhibition of adenosine triphosphatase by digitalis interferes with the sodium and potassium channel mechanism, allowing intracellular accumulation of sodium, and consequently, increasing the level of available calcium for contraction. The associated effect of intracellular potassium depletion may be related to the development of toxicity from digitalis preparations.

The result of digitalis administration for CHF is an increase in the force of cardiac contraction, and thus, an improvement in emptying of the ventricle. Intracardiac filling pressures are reduced, CO rises, cardiac size decreases, and HR slows. Eventually, use of the compensatory mechanisms to maintain CO is mitigated.

Several important points must be remembered when prescribing digitalis glycosides, regardless of the specific one selected or the route of administration. Diligent care must be used in relaying the prescribing information to avoid errors that may have fatal consequences. Calculations of the total digitalizing dose must be double checked and clearly recorded. The microgram dosage should be unequivocally clear, and the corresponding volume to be administered should also be written down. If possible, the prescription should be checked by other medical personnel. Decimal errors are inexcusable but all too common.

The route of administration also has a significant bearing on the dosage prescribed. Parenteral digoxin preparations contain 100 μg per mL, and oral preparations contain 50 μg per mL. In the emergency setting, parenteral administration is often the preferred route. If given IV, the calculated oral dose is reduced by 25%, and the child should be monitored for sudden changes in HR or rhythm. Tissue perfusion levels should be assessed as satisfactory before intramuscular (IM) administration is contemplated because poor absorption from an IM dose (which can be painful) may undercut the therapeutic response.

Digoxin is administered at the dosages described in Table 84.7 (maximum 1.5 mg). The total digitalizing dose is given over 24 hours (one-half initially, then one-fourth in 8 to 12 hours and one-fourth in another 8 to 12 hours). The daily maintenance dosage is one-fourth of the total digitalizing dose divided into twice daily doses for younger children, once daily for older children and adults.

Poisoning from digitalis ingestion may be the precipitating cause for emergency evaluation and for the development of CHF. Various systemic manifestations may be associated with overdosage, including nausea, vomiting, weakness, and worsening of preexisting heart failure. The EKG manifestations of digitalis excess are reviewed subsequently under the "Irregular Heart Rates" section. Care should be taken to clarify the EKG distinctions between "digitalis toxicity" and the more benign "digitalis effect." In general, it is safest to assume the appearance of a new major conduction disturbance in a child who takes a digitalis preparation is related to the drug.

Treatment of digitalis toxicity involves cessation of the drug. Potassium supplementation may be helpful, specifically when potassium depletion has occurred because of dietary factors or diuretic therapy. Potassium should not be given to a patient with digitalis-related atrioventricular (AV) block (see "Cardiac Arrhythmias" section). Diphenylhydantoin (i.e., phenytoin/fosphenytoin) is particularly useful in disorders of impulse formation related to digitalis therapy [e.g., premature ventricular contractions (PVCs)]. In instances of severe heart block, pacing may be required. The presence of digitalis is not an absolute contraindication for cardioversion, and in certain instances, cardioversion may be required to convert even a digitalis-induced rhythm disturbance.

The availability of digoxin antibodies is an important adjunct in the treatment of *digoxin toxicity*.

"Digibind" and other such drugs use the Fab fragment of antibody to digoxin to lower serum concentrations rapidly. Although it is usually necessary to combine vigorous antiarrhythmic therapy (see next section) with digoxin antibody treatment, this form of therapy can provide dramatic improvement in as little as 30 minutes. It must be cautioned, however, that Fab treatment in patients receiving chronic digoxin therapy for CHF may exacerbate CO problems by essentially "withdrawing" the drug. Dosage of Fab is generally equimolar to the estimated amount of digoxin in a patient's body. The onset of action is relatively rapid, as noted and complete reversal of toxicity can occur in 3 to 4 hours. However, close supervision of the patient is needed because with the administration of digoxin antibody, rapid occurrence of hypokalemia can occur. In patients with atrial fibrillation, a rapid ventricular response may occur to exacerbate problems, and occasionally a patient may experience hypersensitivity if sheep protein allergy is present. The elimination of digoxin antibody fragments may take up to several days or longer, especially if renal insufficiency is present, and may interfere with subsequent serum digoxin levels done by radioimmunoassay. Thus, other techniques for assessment of digoxin levels may be needed to follow-up patients at risk.

To use digoxin antibodies, it is assumed that the digoxin total body load (TBL) is proportional to the nanogram per milliliter digoxin level and that each vial of digoxin-immune Fab contains 38 to 40 mg, which neutralizes 0.4 to 0.6 mg digoxin. Thus, the TBL equals serum digoxin (ng per mL) multiplied by the volume of distribution (5.6) multiplied by weight in kg divided by 1,000. The number of vials to be used equals TBL divided by 0.5. For a digoxin level of 5, therefore, in a 20-kg child, approximately 1.1 vials are needed. The TBL may also be assumed to equal 0.8 $\times$ mg of digoxin ingested, if that value is known.

Other Inotropic Agents

In situations of severely compromised CO, isoproterenol or dopamine, both β-receptor agonists, have been used successfully in infants and children. Dobutamine, an analog of dopamine, has also been found to be useful in such circumstances, particularly when impaired myocardial perfusion is part of the underlying problem.

Isoproterenol (Isuprel) has vigorous inotropic effects and marked chronotropic effects. As noted under "Cardiac Arrhythmias," for CHF with persistent bradycardia, isoproterenol is still an important choice. Cardiac rhythm effects may limit the use of isoproterenol, however, because induction of tachyarrhythmias is a consequence of its administration. In addition, hypotension may occur. The starting dose is 0.1 μg per kg per minute by continuous infusion (Table 84.12).

Dopamine has achieved a wide degree of popularity because of its ability, at low doses ("dopaminergic effects"), to augment renal blood flow directly, in addition to improving CO. Furthermore, the chronotropic activity of the drug is somewhat lower than isoproterenol, and there is less of a tendency to produce hypotension. Several studies have established the efficacy and safety of dopamine in infants and children. The drug is available in 5-mL ampules that contain 200 mg of dopamine and is usually diluted in 100 to 250 mL of a neutral or acidic solution (usually 5% to 10% dextrose or saline). Dopamine must not be administered through the same IV solution as sodium bicarbonate because alkali will deactivate the drug. Initial doses in pediatrics range from 2 to 5 μg per kg per minute given by continuous infusion. For severe systemic hypotension, 5 to 10 μg per kg per minute may be used as the starting dose. The response should be relatively prompt, with an increase in HR and BP followed by improvement in urine output. Increasing the infusion rate may be necessary, but at higher doses (5 μg per kg per minute) the beneficial effects of dopamine on renal blood flow are mitigated, and at >20 μg per kg per minute, adrenergic effects predominate and renal blood flow may be reduced. Adverse effects from dopamine include nausea and vomiting, as well as changes in cardiac rhythm, particularly in patients with preexisting arrhythmias and especially at higher infusion ranges (greater than 10 μg per kg per minute). Dopamine may also elevate pulmonary vascular resistance and should be used with caution, if at all, in patients with pulmonary vascular obstructive disease. Monoamine oxidase inhibitors may potentiate the effect of agents such as dopamine.

Dobutamine has achieved widespread popularity for use in the cardiac population because of the relatively rapid response after initiation of infusion and because of the achievement of favorable hemodynamic effects with less myocardial oxygen debt burden than occurs with dopamine. Less chronotropic and arrhythmogenic effects appear to result from dobutamine, and it may have a more direct effect on enhancement of coronary flow. Therefore, dobutamine may have particular efficacy when impaired myocardial perfusion is suspected, as in heart failure from inflammatory myocardial disease or abnormalities that involve the coronary arteries. Dobutamine is administered in similar fashion to dopamine with initial doses that range from 2.5 to 5.0 μg per kg per minute. Higher doses may be used, but complicating adrenergic effects, in particular, potentiation of rhythm disorders, begin to predominate when high doses (15 to 20 μg per kg per minute) are used. As with dopamine, dobutamine can be used in concert with other agents, such as afterload reduction drugs (see below).

These agents should be administered under close supervision, optimally with monitoring of arterial pressure, central venous and/or pulmonary wedge pressure, HR, and urinary output.

Concern remains about the efficacy of dobutamine in the young infant (younger than 1 year of age). In such infants, dobutamine may improve CO but not result in BP elevation. Thus, in severe hypotension in the young infant associated with septic shock, for instance, dobutamine may be more appropriate as an adjunct, and not as a primary inotrope.

Diuretics

Alterations in renal perfusion and salt and water balance are well-known correlates of CHF. Reduced renal blood flow can result in increased circulation volume and increased sodium and water reabsorption (through associated secondary hyper-

aldosteronism). Thus, diuretics play a critical role in the management of the child with CHF.

The so-called "loop diuretics" are used most commonly for the acute treatment of CHF. Furosemide (Lasix®) is the most popular of these agents. Through effects on sodium and chloride transport in the loop of Henle, urinary concentrating capability is diminished and diuresis is achieved. An initial dose of 1 mg per kg IV (max 40 mg/dose) usually results in adequate urine flow within 1 to 2 hours of administration. If 3 to 5 mL per kg per hour urine flow is not achieved, a subsequent dose of furosemide in increments of 1 mg per kg can be given and repeated at hourly intervals to a maximum of 3 to 5 mg per kg. Of note, repeat doses of ethacrynic acid (another loop diuretic) are not advised. Close observation for changes in serum electrolytes, especially potassium, is important, particularly because IV digitalis may be given concurrently.

Thiazide diuretics are less commonly used to treat acute CHF and are now generally reserved for more chronic situations (as oral agents). Nevertheless, agents such as hydrochlorothiazide or chlorothiazide, working at the tubular level, produce good diuretic effects.

Other classes of diuretics may be particularly useful in refractory conditions or in cases in which traditional diuretics are already in use. Of these agents, metalozone (Zaroxolyn®) has been administered most often. It is for oral use; thus, onset of action is delayed. Particularly intense potassium depletion can result from metalozone, and patients who take this drug should be evaluated for potassium loss when they present in the ED.

Spironolactone is an adjunctive form of diuretic therapy. It is not a first-line drug because its diuretic effect may not occur for 2 to 3 days. Aldosterone antagonism makes it suitable for use as an additional agent when potassium loss is a problem, and it may also be useful to directly potentiate myocardial metabolic changes favoring enhanced cardiac contractility.

With the proper use of inotropes and diuretic therapy, improvement can be achieved in most children with CHF. Failure to improve an exacerbation of CHF in children already on these medications requires scrutiny for any of the following: (i) persistent arrhythmia; (ii) untreated or unrecognized infection; (iii) anemia, especially in the infant with CHF; (iv) inadequate or excessive digitalis dose, particularly in the patient with inflammatory myocardial disease; or (v) electrolyte disturbance, such as hypokalemia, which may be worsened with diuretics. If these entities can be ruled out, then more intensive treatment is indicated to improve CO in the face of declining cardiovascular status.

Other Noncatecholamine Agents

Other pharmacologic tools available to treat acute CHF are the bipyridine derivatives amrinone and milrinone. These drugs have the combined effects of inotropic support and peripheral vasodilatation. They are known to be inhibitors of myocardial cyclic adenosine monophosphate (cAMP) phosphodiesterase activity, thereby enhancing intracellular levels of myocardial cAMP. There is also a direct vascular smooth muscle relaxant action. In an ideal sense, this class of therapeutic agents represent a major therapeutic breakthrough because the inotropic effects of these drugs may be additive to other agents, especially to digitalis. Pediatric experience has documented the profound vasodilatory effects of these drugs and the need for careful invasive monitoring when they are used. Adequate filling volumes must be maintained to ensure adequate systemic perfusion. Occasionally, hypersensitivity reactions have occurred with amrinone. Fever and thrombocytopenia are also known side effects, and potassium levels should be followed closely, especially if diuretics are also used. Milrinone may cause less platelet suppression and has become more widely used than amrinone. Chemical interaction with glucose (dextrose) solutions can occur, so these drugs should not be diluted using these fluids. In the patient with CHF in whom standard digoxin and/or catecholamine therapy does not provide improved peripheral perfusion status, use of this class of drugs is standard therapy. Infusion rates for milrinone range from 0.5 to 1.0 μg per kg per minute with a bolus dosage to start therapy of 50 μg per kg given initially over 10 minutes.

Vasodilators

The management of CHF also includes manipulation of loading conditions, following the physiologic principles defined earlier in this chapter. Both afterload and preload interventions can be useful. Agents with effects on cardiac loading have been shown to be efficacious in adults with a variety of chronic forms of cardiac dysfunction and are also appropriate for infants and children with heart failure unresponsive to more conventional treatment regimens. In heart failure, with reduced CO, systemic vascular resistance is often elevated by compensatory mechanisms used to maintain BP. Preload reserve is used through cardiac dilation to increase stroke volume, but this is accomplished at the expense of a decreased ability of the myocardium to shorten as needed to overcome the increase in afterload. Thus, there is a "mismatch" of afterload and preload reserve in heart failure. Vasodilators that work primarily on arteriolar smooth muscle cause afterload reduction, whereas drugs that affect venodilation work on preload by lowering cardiac filling volumes. Some of these agents have mixed effects (Table 84.8). In the vasodilator group, the nitrates, particularly nitroprusside, have been most actively used in the acute care setting. Sodium nitroprusside has both arteriolar and venous actions, a prompt onset of action, and usually a short duration of effect. In the patient with impaired renal function, however, caution must be exercised in its use because the by-product,

thiocyanate, can accumulate with neurologic, endocrinologic, and other toxicity. Other drugs used include α-receptor blockers and angiotensin-converting enzyme inhibitors, although these are more commonly used in the long-term care setting via the oral route. Calcium channel blockers also induce vasodilation and appear to be most useful for diastolic dysfunction conditions. These situations involve heart failure developing in the face of myocardial hypertrophy and/or normal end-systolic volume, such as in hypertrophic cardiomyopathy (HCM). The negative inotropic effects of these agents require their use only with careful cardiac monitoring. A thorough history for the chronic use of these drugs is essential in patients who may present with an exacerbation of heart failure because continuation of such therapy in the acute care setting may be required. Afterload reduction therapy, when used intravenously, usually requires extensive monitoring because failure to maintain adequate cardiac filling can have serious negative results. Emergency use of afterload reduction should be limited to those well-versed in cardiopulmonary physiology, and maintenance of such treatment is best carried out in an intensive care environment.

NEWBORN WITH CHF-ASSOCIATED OBSTRUCTED SYSTEMIC OR PULMONARY BLOOD FLOW

Background

For the baby with cyanotic CHD or with obstruction to systemic blood flow, emergency intervention is crucial, indeed life sparing, and must usually be delivered before permanent long-term therapy can be undertaken. The emergency physician must be able to recognize when such a life-threatening circumstance is present and must be able to initiate therapy even before a precise diagnosis can be accomplished. Although this is most often a problem for the neonatologist or other physician caring for an infant during the first few days of life, these

MEDICAL EMERGENCIES

TABLE 84.8

AFTERLOAD REDUCING AGENTS USED IN CONGESTIVE HEART FAILURE

Agent	Class	Action	Dosage
Nitroprusside	Nitrate	Mixed[a] dilator	1–10 μg/kg/min IV (max 12–15 μg/kg/min)
Nitroglycerin	Nitrate	Venodilator	2–10 μg/kg/min
Hydralazine[a]	Smooth muscle inhibitor	Arteriolar dilator	0.1–0.5 mg/kg/dose every 6 h or 0.2–3 mg/kg single bolus IV
Prazosin	Alpha blockade	Mixed dilator	0.01–0.05 mg/kg/dose by mouth every 8–12 h
Captopril	ACE inhibitor	Mixed	0.1–2.0 mg/kg/dose by mouth every 6 h
Enalapril	ACE inhibitor	Mixed	8 or 12 h (max 6 mg/kg/day)[b]
Diltiazem	Ca^{2+} channel blocker	Arteriolar dilator	0.2–0.5 mg/kg/dose by mouth or sublingual every 8 h
Nifedipine	Ca^{2+} channel blocker arteriolar		0.25–1 mg/kg

ACE, angiotensin-converting enzyme; Mixed, both arterial and venous vasoactivity.
[a]Precise mechanism not identified; may inhibit calcium activity.
[b]Intravenous enalapril is available for an every 8-h regimen (enalaprilat), 0.01–0.05 mg/kg/dose, max enalapril 40 mg/day.

babies are also brought to the ED after having been at home. Still others may need the help of emergency medical personnel as they are transported to cardiac centers for definitive care. Therapy in these critical infants depends on the manipulation of the ductus arteriosus.

Pathophysiology

In fetal life, the ductus arteriosus is the principal conduit allowing the preponderance of right ventricular output to bypass the nonventilating fetal lungs (Fig. 84.4). This pathway thus allows for fetal circulatory viability even in the face of extreme disorders of functional cardiac development (Figs. 84.5 and 84.6). In the case of impaired systemic blood flow, the fetus and later the neonate survives because the ductus allows right ventricular output to reach the systemic circulation. This right-to-left shunt mitigates the effects of even complete aortic and/or mitral atresia. In situations of obstructed pulmonary blood flow, the ductus serves as a conduit for systemic (left ventricular) output to reach the pulmonary circulation. This left-to-right shunt becomes crucial once the newborn becomes dependent on his or her own pulmonary

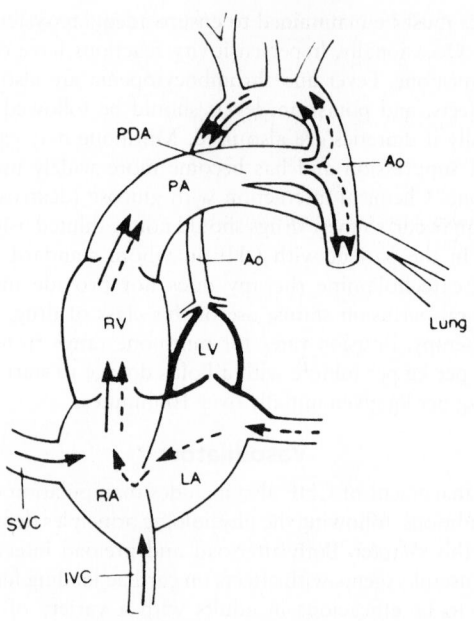

FIGURE 84.5 Aortic and mitral atresia (hypoplastic left heart syndrome in fetus with altered circulatory heart syndrome) in fetus with altered circulatory physiology at ductus and atrial levels. Ao, aorta; IVC, inferior vena cava; LA, left atrium; LV, left ventricle; PA, pulmonary artery; PDA, patent ductus arteriosus; RA, right atrium; RV, right ventricle; SVC, superior vena cava. (Reprinted from Gewitz M. Cardiac disease. In: Polin R, Yoder M, Berg F, eds. *Workbook in practical neonatology.* 2nd ed. Philadelphia: WB Saunders, 1993:267, with permission.)

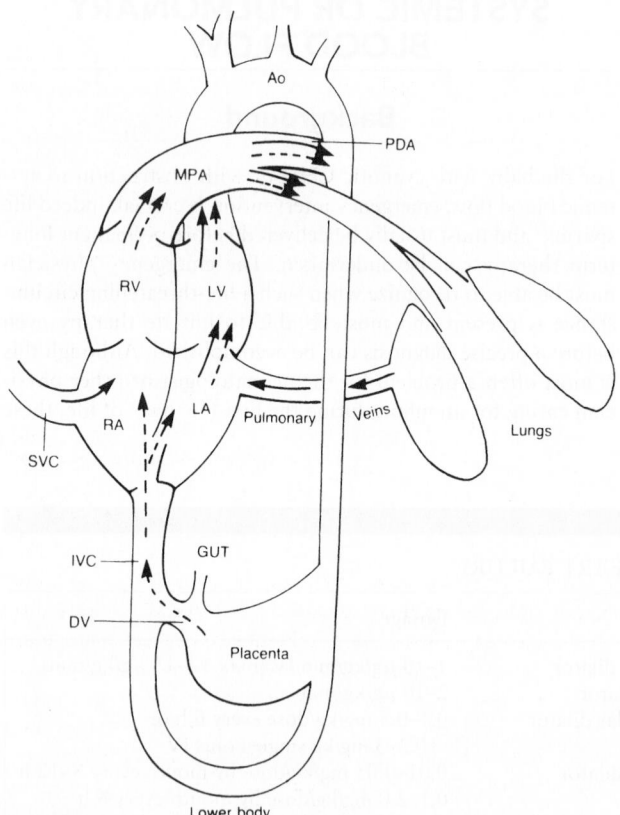

FIGURE 84.4 Normal fetal circulatory pathway including patency of foramen ovale and ductus arteriosus. Ao, aorta; DV, ductus venosus; IVC, inferior vena cava; LA, left atrium; LV, left ventricle; MPA, main pulmonary artery; PDA, patent ductus arteriosus; RA, right atrium; RV, right ventricle; SVC, superior vena cava. (Reprinted from Gewitz M. Cardiac disease. In: Polin R, Yoder M, Berg F, eds. *Workbook in practical neonatology.* 2nd ed. Philadelphia: WB Saunders, 1993:253, with permission.)

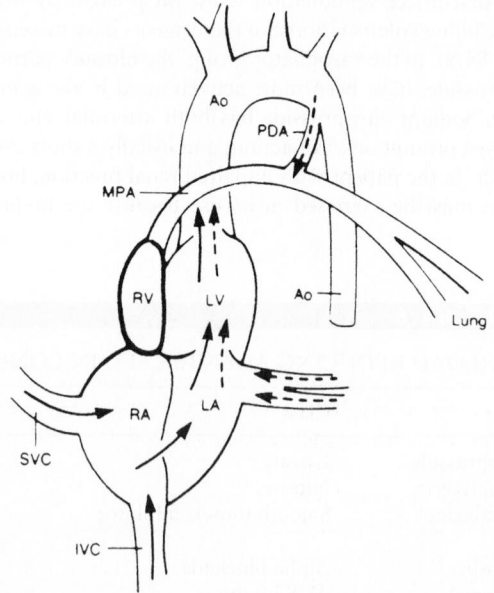

FIGURE 84.6 Pulmonary–tricuspid atresia (right-sided heart hypoplasia) with intact septum in fetus. Altered circulatory physiology at ductus level with enhanced flow at atrial level. Ao, aorta; IVC, inferior vena cava; LA, left atrium; LV, left ventricle; MPA, main pulmonary artery; PDA, patent ductus arteriosus; RA, right atrium; RV, right ventricle; SVC, superior vena cava. (Reprinted from Gewitz M. Cardiac disease. In: Polin R, Yoder M, Berg F, eds. *Workbook in practical neonatology.* 2nd ed. Philadelphia: WB Saunders, 1993:268, with permission.)

TABLE 84.9

DUCTAL-DEPENDENT CARDIAC LESIONS

Ductal-dependent Pulmonary Blood Flow Pulmonary atresia with intact ventricular septum Tricuspid atresia Critical pulmonary stenosis **Ductal-dependent Systemic Blood Flow** Coarctation of the aorta Aortic arch interruption Hypoplastic left heart syndrome (aortic atresia)

Adapted from Gewitz MG. Cardiac disease. In: Polin R, Yoder M, Burg F, eds. *Workbook in practical neonatology.* 2nd ed. Philadelphia: WB Saunders, 1993.

circulation for oxygenation after delivery. Typical conditions that are "ductal dependent" are listed in Table 84.9.

Clinical Manifestations

Any newborn with sudden onset of either collapsed systemic circulation or intense cyanosis should be considered at risk for the presence of a ductal-dependent state. In these babies, closure of the ductus unmasks the underlying circulatory insufficiency, resulting in the clinical picture of severe hypoxemia, shock, or both. These infants may be as old as 1 or 2 weeks, although usually this catastrophe becomes apparent within the first days of life. However, there are times when the process of ductal closure leading to the presentation can be delayed even longer than 2 weeks.

The mechanisms responsible for ductus closure have been defined. Although a prolonged discussion is not relevant in this context, it is important for the emergency physician to understand that these factors center on the balance of dilator and constrictor hormones, namely prostaglandins, and that manipulation of this hormonal system can yield prompt and substantial results. Of course, treatment of heart failure and impaired oxygenation involve more than just ductus manipulation, as outlined elsewhere in this chapter.

Management

Based on the previously described principles, prostaglandin E_1 (PGE$_1$, alprostadil) has become the standard medical intervention used in this urgent situation. PGE$_1$ provides relatively rapid stabilization until more permanent measures can be undertaken. There are few, if any, concerns that would contraindicate the use of PGE$_1$ when any of the conditions noted previously are suspected. Dosage is by infusion at 0.05 to 0.10 μg per kg per minute, after an initial bolus of 0.10 μg per kg. The specific site of infusion is not critical as long as patency of access can be continuously verified. Side effects can be important and, unless prepared for, these can be life-threatening. These include bradycardia, apnea, hypotension, and seizures. Rash and hyperthermia can also develop. Therefore, when PGE$_1$ therapy is initiated, the ability to support respiration and BP should be secured. Intubation may be required and should always be considered if a prolonged transport is planned. It has become evident over the past 25 years that manipulation of the ductus by PGE$_1$ administration has been one of the most important advances in the early treatment of even the most severe forms of CHD.

CARDIAC ARRHYTHMIAS

General Considerations

Background

Disturbances in cardiac rhythm are relatively common in infants, children, and adolescents. An apparent increase in the incidence of cardiac arrhythmias in children can be explained by the extensive use of EKG monitoring equipment in children's hospitals, advances in cardiac surgery that have resulted in the survival of children with complex CHD, new techniques to investigate rhythm disturbances, and an increased awareness on the part of pediatricians and pediatric cardiologists of the manifestations of abnormal cardiac rhythms in children.

Pathophysiology

The electrical impulse that initiates and coordinates the mechanical activity of the heart is propagated in an orderly manner through the normal heart. This electrical activity is initiated in the sinoatrial (sinus) node located at the junction of the superior vena cava and right atrium (Fig. 84.7). Activity then spreads through the atria to the AV node located in the lower part of the right atrium near the coronary sinus and just above the septal leaflet of the tricuspid valve. The impulse continues to the bundle of His, which then divides into the right and left bundle branches in the ventricle. The bundle branches then divide into the Purkinje fibers of the ventricular myocardium, and the entire ventricle is thus depolarized.

Arrhythmias in children are caused by disturbances in impulse formation, conduction, or both. These may occur in association with structural or functional cardiac disease, a systemic disease process that affects cardiac conduction, or because of an isolated, primary cardiac electrophysiologic abnormality. Some types of CHD have a relatively high incidence of associated cardiac arrhythmias. These include corrected transposition of the great vessels, Ebstein's anomaly of the tricuspid valve, mitral valve prolapse, congenital mitral stenosis, and the asplenia-polysplenia syndromes. Postsurgical arrhythmias are commonly seen in children after the Fontan procedure and after repair of tetralogy of Fallot, endocardial cushion defects, large atrial septal defects, or total anomalous pulmonary venous return. Acquired heart diseases that may be associated with rhythm disturbances include hypertrophic and dilated cardiomyopathies (including myocarditis), arrhythmogenic right ventricular dysplasia, bacterial endocarditis, rheumatic heart disease, Kawasaki disease, and cardiac tumors.

Other systemic diseases or abnormalities associated with cardiac arrhythmias include electrolyte disturbances, neuromuscular disorders (muscular dystrophy, Friedreich's ataxia), endocrine disorders (hyperthyroidism or hypothyroidism), inherited disorders of metabolism (glycogen storage disease, Pompe's disease), mitochondrial disorders (acyl Co-A dehydrogenase deficiency, Kearns-Sayre syndrome), collagen diseases (systemic lupus erythematosus), pulmonary diseases (bronchopulmonary dysplasia, cystic fibrosis), hematologic disorders (hemochromatosis, anemia, thalassemia major), neoplasms, renal diseases (uremia), infectious diseases, and central nervous system (CNS) diseases (increased intracranial pressure, encephalitides). Drugs and toxic substances (digitalis, general

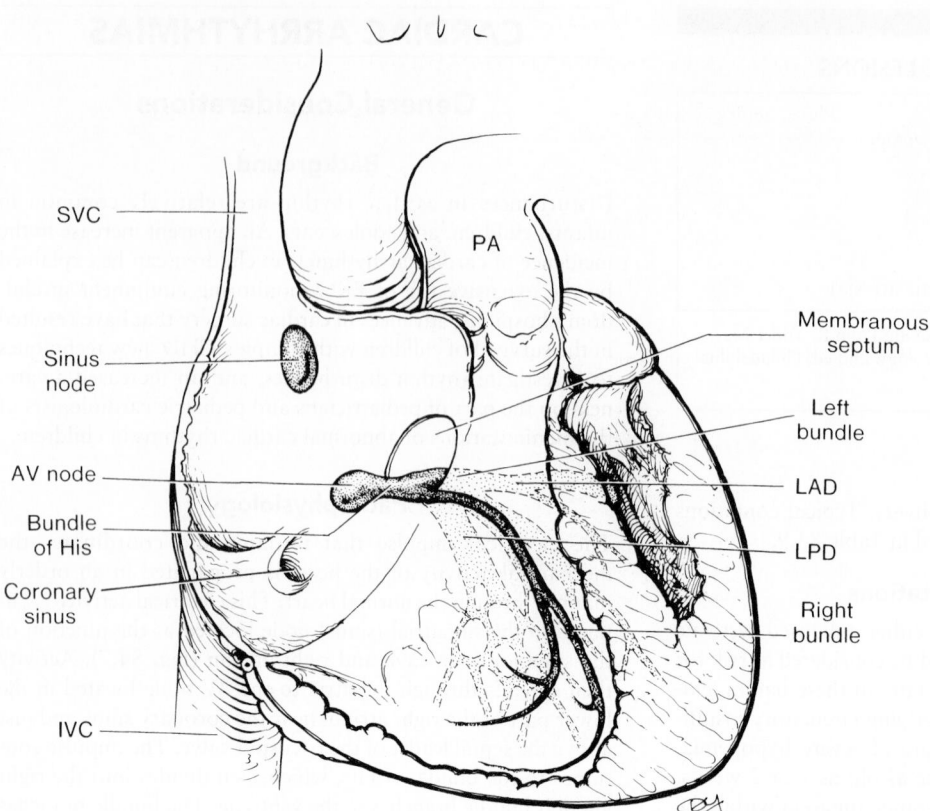

FIGURE 84.7 Schematic representation of the intracardiac conduction system. AV, atrioventricular; IVC, inferior vena cava; LAD, left anterior division; LPD, left posterior division; PA, pulmonary artery; SVC, superior vena cava.

anesthesia, theophylline, sympathomimetic drugs, epinephrine, antihistamines, tricyclic antidepressants) can also lead to abnormalities of cardiac rhythm.

Children may also have AV block, prolonged QT interval, dual AV nodal pathways, or accessory AV pathways [including Wolff-Parkinson-White (WPW) syndrome] in the absence of other systemic or cardiac disease. These represent isolated, primary congenital or acquired cardiac electrophysiologic abnormalities.

Clinical Manifestations

Many children are not aware of or are unable to express awareness of an abnormal cardiac rhythm. Thus, the physician must suspect the diagnosis from the secondary manifestations. Arrhythmias may surface in the following ways:

1. No symptoms. Physical examination reveals an abnormal or irregular HR.
2. Symptoms or signs of CHF (see previous section), shock, or sudden death
3. Symptoms related to decreased cerebral blood flow (syncope, dizziness, irritability, and inappropriate behavior)
4. Symptoms related to decreased coronary blood flow (anginal chest pain)
5. Perception of the rhythm disturbance by the child (palpitations, chest pain, skipped beats)

Management

Management of the child with a cardiac arrhythmia requires recognition of the manifestations of these disorders, diagnosis of the type of rhythm disturbance, understanding of the mecha-

nism of the abnormality, knowledge of appropriate therapy (physiologic, pharmacologic, or electrical), judgment about the appropriate timing and urgency of therapy, and understanding of potential side effects of the therapy. Once an abnormality in cardiac rhythm is suspected or found, the precise diagnosis must be made to institute appropriate treatment. This depends on accurate interpretation of the EKG. The EKG used to evaluate cardiac arrhythmias should include a long rhythm strip in addition to a complete 12- or 15-lead EKG. Lead II is often used for the rhythm strip, but a V_1 lead or another lead in which P waves are prominent may be more helpful. The rhythm on the EKG should be evaluated for rate, regularity, origin of the impulse and mechanism, or origin of any abnormality.

Cardiac arrhythmias become emergencies when they produce or have the potential to produce hemodynamic alterations that result in a decreased CO. Most infants and children who have hemodynamically significant arrhythmias will require cardiac consultation and admission to the hospital for treatment and observation, continuous EKG monitoring (telemetry or bedside with arrhythmia analysis is preferred). Table 84.10 represents an overview of the emergent management of arrhythmias. Children with intermittent palpitations and no signs or symptoms of hemodynamic impairment may be evaluated as outpatients, using ambulatory electrocardiography, transtelephonic event monitoring, or exercise stress testing as deemed appropriate.

The cardiac arrhythmias discussed in this section are classified according to their presentation to the physician: slow HRs, rapid HRs, and irregular HRs. Slow HRs that are most commonly seen in the ED include complete (or third-degree)

TABLE 84.10

EMERGENT MANAGEMENT OF DYSRHYTHMIAS IN CHILDREN (WITH INADEQUATE PERFUSION[a])

Dysrhythmia	Pharmacologic therapies	Definitive electrophysiologic
Slow heart rate		
Complete heart block	Epinephrine (E) bolus of 0.01 mg/kg IV of 1:10,000 dilution, followed by infusion of 0.1–2.0 μg/kg/min	Pacemaker
Sinus bradycardia, sick sinus syndrome	Atropine (At) 0.02–0.04 mg/kg IV (0.1 mg/ min)–(2 mg max)	
Rapid heart rate		
Supraventricular tachycardia	Adenosine (when perfusion deemed sufficient) Initial 0.1 mg/kg (max 6 mg/dose), subsequent 0.2–0.3 mg/kg (max 12 mg/dose) Amiodarone (Amio) 5 mg/kg IV over 20–60 min (max 300 mg/dose) Procainamide (Proc) 5 mg/kg (max 100 mg/dose over 5–10 min, can repeat q 5–10 min) max load 15 mg/kg total (500 mg), digoxin (Dig) (Table 84.7)	Cardioversion, 0.25–2 J/kg, doubling wattage until 10 or successful
Junctional tachycardia	Amiodarone 5 mg/kg IV over 20–60 min (max 300 mg/dose) (Dig) (Proc)	
Ventricular tachycardia	Amiodarone 5 mg/kg IV over 2060 min (max 300 mg/dose) Lidocaine 1 mg/kg	Cardioversion 24 J/kg
Ventricular fibrillation	Defibrillation 2 J/kg	Lidocaine 1 mg/kg and defibrillation 4–10 J/kg
Irregular heart rate		
Premature ventricular contractions	Lidocaine 1 mg/kg	(Amio) (Proc)
Second-degree heart block	(I), (E), (At)	Pacemaker

IV, intravenous.
[a]See text for more complete discussion.

heart block and the sick sinus syndrome with resultant bradycardia of a sinus, junctional or ventricular origin. Rapid HRs include SVT, atrial flutter or fibrillation, and ventricular tachycardia (VT). Irregular rhythms are usually caused by premature ventricular or atrial contractions, sinus arrhythmia, atrial fibrillation, and second-degree heart block.

To determine whether any HR is abnormally fast or slow, one must know the normal range of rates for children of various ages. Results of 24-hour continuous EKG monitoring studies have defined the normal ranges. Table 84.11 illustrates ranges of rates accepted as normal.

TABLE 84.11

NORMAL HEART RATE RANGES

Age	Heart rate (bpm)
Newborn	80–180
1 wk–3 mo	80–180
3 mo–2 yr	80–160
2 yr–10 yr	65–130
10 yr–adult	55–90

Slow Heart Rates

Congenital Complete Heart Block

Complete (third-degree) AV heart block is the most common cause of symptomatic bradycardia in infants and children. Complete heart block, which may be congenital or acquired, results from a complete failure of conduction from atria to ventricles. The atrial rate is always faster than the ventricular rate, which is usually 40 to 80 bpm. A typical EKG is shown in Figure 84.8.

Congenital Heart Block

Congenital complete heart block (CCHB) is due to an abnormality in the region of the AV node (aplasia, hypoplasia, inflammation, or fibrosis) and may be an isolated finding or associated with either specific types of congenital heart defects [corrected or L-transposition of the great arteries, left atrial isomerism/polysplenia syndromes (heterotaxy)], or maternal collagen disease associated with the presence of anti-Ro (SS-A) and anti-La (SS-B). CCHB is being diagnosed more often in utero with the use of fetal monitoring and fetal echocardiography, but it still may not be recognized until weeks or months after birth.

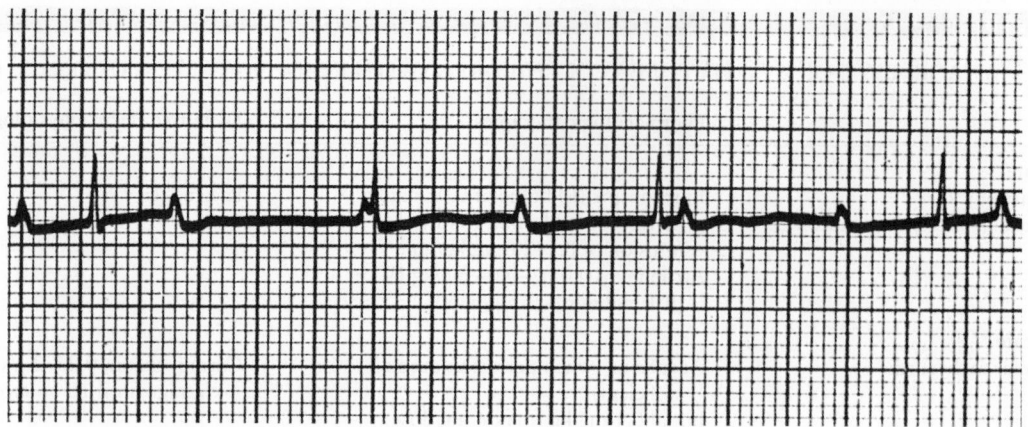

FIGURE 84.8 Example of complete heart block. Note absence of any regular PR interval. Ventricular rate 62 bpm, atrial rate approximately 95 to 115 bpm.

All infants with CCHB have bradycardia. Although some remain asymptomatic, others develop CHF and, occasionally, cardiovascular collapse and sudden death. An EKG will differentiate sinus bradycardia from complete heart block. Sinus bradycardia should respond to the usual resuscitative measures: ventilation and oxygenation, treatment of acidosis, and catecholamine support of HR and BP. The infant with CCHB who has severe CHF or who is in shock will require insertion of a pacemaker, but may also require intubation for adequate ventilation, oxygenation, and treatment of acidosis. If no improvement is obtained with these measures, then infusion of epinephrine may increase the HR slightly, allowing time for the placement of a temporary pacemaker (Table 84.12). A hydropic infant may also require a diuretic such as furosemide (1 mg per kg, IV). Distressed infants with CCHB generally have HRs less than 50 bpm. If an infant is distressed with a rate greater than 50 bpm, one should suspect significant CHD or some other associated problem such as infection or sepsis in addition to CCHB.

The infant in extremis from a slow HR may require immediate temporary pacing in the ED. This may be accomplished by the transcutaneous, transthoracic, or transvenous route.

The transcutaneous route was first introduced by Zoll in 1952. This technique involves the use of pacing electrodes placed on the anterior and posterior chest attached to an external current source. This technique may be used successfully in critical situations to increase the HR; however, the pacing electrodes should be replaced as soon as possible with another type of pacemaker because third-degree burns have been noted under the pacing electrodes after short periods in infants. Special wires available for transthoracic pacing can be placed by the subxiphoid route in infants and children. The procedure uses techniques similar to those used for pericardiocentesis. A pacing wire is inserted through a needle that is subsequently removed once the wire is inside the heart. This type of pacing should be replaced by a transvenous pacemaker once the patient is stable. If time allows, placement of a temporary transvenous pacemaker either through the umbilical vein or femoral vein (see Procedures in Chapter 135) under direct fluoroscopic observation in a cardiac catheterization laboratory is preferred. Temporary transvenous pacing is reserved for infants with signs of CHF, most commonly seen with HRs under 50 bpm or with slightly higher rates in association with a structural CHD. However, an infant with an HR of 45 bpm should not be paced solely on the basis of HR but should be observed for signs of CHF such as tachypnea, poor feeding, or hepatomegaly. The width of the QRS on the EKG does not always correlate with the need for a pacemaker, although wider QRS rhythms frequently are associated with lower escape rates. Only a small percentage of infants with CCHB block require emergency pacing at birth. Many of these infants will not need pacemakers until they are older.

The older child with CCHB may also present with symptoms associated with CHF. More commonly, dizziness, presyncope, syncope, exercise limitation, or fatigue is the presenting complaint in the older child. At times, the appearance of a ventricular arrhythmia may be the presenting sign of difficulty in these patients. Indications for and timing of implantation of a permanent pacemaker in children with CCHB are based on the appearance of these symptoms or signs, or specific electrocardiographic findings such as an excessively slow ventricular rate, ventricular ectopy, or prolonged pauses (greater than 3 seconds).

TABLE 84.12

EVALUATION OF SICK SINUS SYNDROME

Test	Expected normal response
Atropine (0.02–0.04 mg/kg; max: 2 mg)	HR > 90 bpm >25–50% increase in HR
Isoproterenol (0.1–2 μg/min)	>25% increase in HR
Exercise	95% of expected normal rate
Electrophysiology study	Normal CSNRT (<550 ms) Normal SACT (45–105 ms)
24-Hour ambulatory monitor	Normal low rate for age Pauses <3 s

CSRNT, corrected sinus node recovery time; SACT, sinoatrial conduction time; HR, heart rate.

Acquired Nonsurgical Heart Block

Acquired nonsurgical heart block may be idiopathic or associated with congenital heart defects, infectious or inflammatory processes (such as viral or Lyme myocarditis, endocarditis, or rheumatic fever), muscle diseases, cardiac tumors, or cardiac sclerosis. The emergency treatment for congenital or acquired nonsurgical heart block is similar. Pharmacologic therapy may be tried if adequate ventilation, oxygenation, and treatment of acidosis do not produce a normalization of the CO as reflected by the BP and peripheral perfusion. The initial drug to be used should be epinephrine (Table 84.12) because it is most effective in increasing the HR. Adequate intravascular volume should be maintained during epinephrine infusion because its vasodilatory effect may result in lowered BP. If CO is inadequate despite pharmacologic measures, temporary ventricular pacing is indicated.

In this setting, a single typical Stokes-Adams or syncopal attack not related to neurologic disease is considered an indication for pacemaker insertion because these attacks may be fatal. Temporary transvenous pacing may be required during the acute phase of an infectious process, but because resolution of complete heart block may occur in some inflammatory processes (e.g., myocarditis), permanent pacing may not be needed. Persistence of nonsurgical heart block (duration depending on the etiology) does warrant permanent pacemaker insertion. The temporary pacemaker should be left in place during induction of anesthesia for the permanent pacemaker implantation because serious arrhythmias have been noted to occur if adequate CO is not maintained by pacing.

Postsurgical Complete Heart Block

Postsurgical heart block is less common today than in the early days of surgery for CHDs, with a current incidence of less than 1%. Improved knowledge of the location of the conduction system, as well as the implementation of intraoperative mapping techniques, has helped to decrease this serious postsurgical complication. Postsurgical complete heart block generally presents immediately after surgery but it may occur many years after surgery. When it occurs, it may be transient or permanent. All patients with postsurgical complete heart block occurring more than 1 week after surgery should have implantation of permanent pacemakers, due to the unreliability of the escape rhythm. Emergency treatment of symptomatic, late-onset postsurgical complete heart block includes pharmacologic chronotropic agents and temporary pacing until a permanent pacemaker can be placed (as previously).

Sinus Bradycardia

Sinus bradycardia is an HR below the normal range for age (Table 84.11). An EKG is necessary to rule out second-degree or complete heart block; P waves with a normal PR interval must precede each QRS complex in sinus bradycardia. Sinus bradycardia is commonly associated with sinus arrhythmia. It often occurs in the athletic child or in the adolescent as a normal variant, especially during sleep. Other causes of sinus bradycardia include hypothermia; hypothyroidism; significant weight loss (malnutrition or anorexia nervosa); CNS disease, including increased intracranial pressure; and drugs such as morphine, propranolol, or digoxin. Therapy of the underlying disorder is indicated, but in symptomatic patients atropine may be useful as a temporizing measure (Table 84.12). Epinephrine may also be given in this emergency setting (Table 84.12).

Sick Sinus Syndrome

Sick sinus syndrome is a condition in which sinus node function is intrinsically abnormal and may present with a sinus bradycardia or a slow junctional rhythm, often in association with alternating episodes of tachycardia. Syncopal episodes may occur. This abnormal cardiac rhythm may be seen in children who have undergone atrial surgery for closure of an atrial septal defect, particularly of the sinus venosus type, the Mustard procedure for correction of D-transposition of the great arteries, Fontan repair for single ventricle complexes, or in association with a viral myocarditis or as a primary cardiac electrophysiologic abnormality. Table 84.12 outlines the evaluation of the child with a suspected sick sinus syndrome. Evaluation will generally be performed by a pediatric cardiologist.

The urgency of the clinical picture determines the treatment of the child with sick sinus syndrome. The asymptomatic patient with a slow HR can be referred for consultation with a cardiologist. The child with CHF or inadequate perfusion from bradycardia or tachycardia requires therapy directed at the specific arrhythmia and admission to the hospital. Epinephrine infusion (Table 84.12) may increase the HR temporarily in a child with bradycardia but, in this situation, may also precipitate tachyarrhythmias. Epinephrine, therefore, should be administered cautiously under continuous monitoring. Symptomatic slow rhythms may require temporary or permanent cardiac pacing.

Pacemakers

Pacemakers are used frequently in infants and children for the treatment of congenital or acquired (usually postsurgical) complete heart block or sick sinus syndrome. In addition, some patients with tachyarrhythmias or with the long QT syndrome are being treated with pacemakers. Therefore, it has become important for the emergency physician to recognize the normal and abnormal function of a pacemaker.

Pacemaker functions may be complex. They may sense or pace one, two, or three chambers. Pacemakers can be programmed to respond to external factors such as motion or minute ventilation or to synchronize with ventricular and atrial contractions. The universal "letter code" for description of a pacemaker includes three or more letters. The first letter indicates chamber paced (v, ventricle; a, atrium; d, dual; or both), the second letter indicates chamber sensed, and the third letter indicates the mode (I, inhibited; T, triggered; D, dual or both). Additional letters indicate more complex functions, such as rate responsiveness. The goal of current pacing practice is to give the patient a range of HR that can physiologically adapt to activity or other increased metabolic requirements. Rate-responsive and dual-chamber pacemakers (DDD, DDDR) that pace or sense in both the atrium and the ventricle are commonly used in children old enough to have two endocardial wires placed, although synchronized atrial sensing–ventricular pacing can also be accomplished with a single endocardial lead (VDD). Motion-sensing, rate-responsive pacers (VVIR, AAIR) are less useful in young infants than in older children. Rarely, the simple "back-up" modes of VVI or AAI may still be encountered.

Accurate evaluation of pacemaker function in the ED requires knowledge of the specific pacemaker mode. Examples of normal function, failure to capture, and failure to sense are shown in Figure 84.9. When a pacemaker malfunction is suspected, the specific problem should be identified if possible. Each pacemaker manufacturer has a computerized, telemetry-based programmer that enables the practitioner to identify and, if possible, fix the pacemaker malfunction by reprogramming. An EKG lead that shows the largest possible pacemaker stimulus artifact should be chosen with multiple leads providing more information. A pacemaker stimulus that falls outside the cardiac refractory period and fails to result in a ventricular depolarization indicates a failure of capture. In currently available pacemakers, the output of the pacemaker may be reprogrammed externally, often resulting in normal capture. As the battery generator is depleted, the rate on most pacemakers decreases to a predetermined end-of-battery life indicator, which reveals impending battery failure.

An abnormally long pause or an earlier-than-expected paced complex indicates a sensing failure, either inappropriate sensing of another electrical signal (e.g., T-wave sensing instead of QRS) or failure to sense the QRS. Sensing errors can be identified and external reprogramming accomplished.

Any patient with evidence of pacemaker malfunction should be admitted to the hospital if the problem cannot be resolved in the ED. A chest radiograph should be obtained to look for wire fractures or lead displacement. A consultation with a pediatric cardiologist and/or the pacemaker manufacturer's technical staff is generally required to troubleshoot and correct pacemaker problems. The patient with pacemaker malfunction who has symptomatic bradycardia should be managed with the regimens previously discussed (Table 84.12).

The procedure for inserting a temporary pacemaker is described in Section VII.

Fast Heart Rates

Supraventricular Tachycardia

Background. SVT, previously called paroxysmal atrial tachycardia, is the most common significant arrhythmia seen in pediatric practice. SVT describes a group of arrhythmias with similar EKG features but different mechanisms.

A typical EKG seen in a pediatric patient with SVT is shown in Figure 84.10. Note the very rapid rate and the narrow QRS complex. The P waves are different from the usual sinus P wave but may be obscured by the ST segment and not be visible at all. The rate of tachycardia in young infants ranges from 220 to 320 bpm. Older children have tachycardia rates that range from 150 to 250 bpm. SVT with "aberrant conduction" has an EKG with a wide QRS complex and may resemble VT.

Pathophysiology

These mechanisms of SVT have been clarified by the use of intracardiac electrophysiology studies. The majority of instances of SVT in children have been shown to involve reentry circuits utilizing either dual (fast and slow) AV nodal pathways or accessory AV connections (either concealed or manifest as WPW syndrome). Less commonly, enhanced automaticity of sinus nodal, atrial, or AV nodal region fibers may be responsible. More than 90% of infants with SVT have an accessory AV pathway. Older children and adolescents are more likely to have dual AV nodal pathways. Underlying electrophysiologic substrates for SVT may be isolated or seen in conjunction with CHD (approximately 23%, including Ebstein's anomaly or corrected transposition).

Reentrant SVT in the setting of AV accessory pathways is analogous to AV nodal reentrant SVT with the bypass tract functioning like a β pathway (fast conduction, long refractory period) and the AV nodal–His–Purkinje system functioning

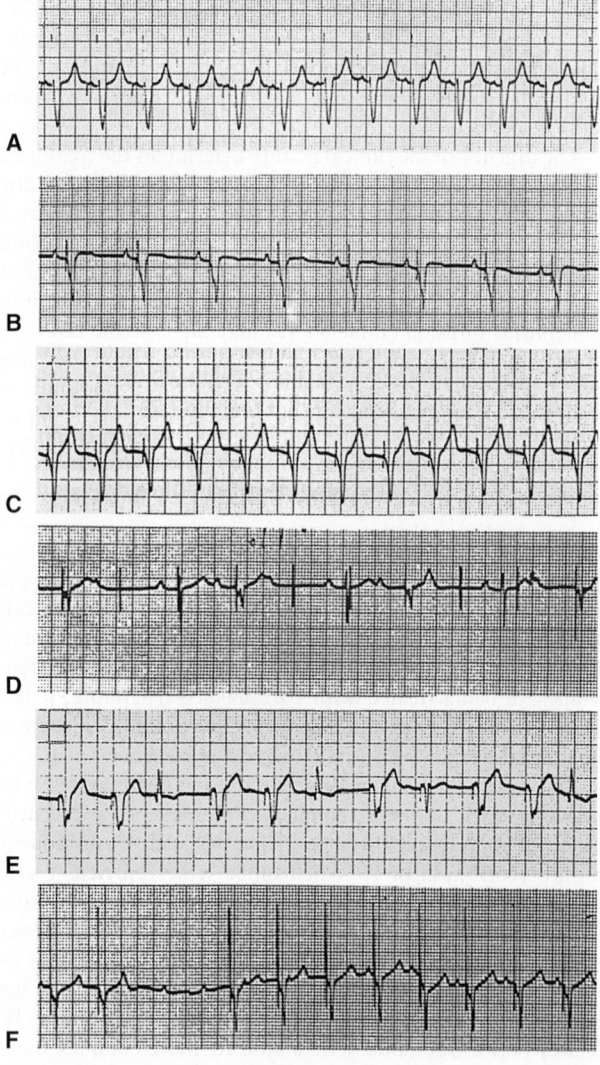

FIGURE 84.9 **A:** Electrocardiogram (EKG) showing pacemaker that paces atrium and, after 150 msec, paces ventricle. Note pacemaker stimulus artifact before the P wave and the QRS complex. **B:** EKG showing pacemaker that senses atrium and paces ventricle after a 150-msec delay. Note that pacemaker stimulus artifact only precedes the QRS complex. **C:** EKG showing ventricular pacing at 100 bpm with normal capture. Note pacemaker stimulus artifact preceding the QRS. **D:** EKG showing ventricular pacing at 85 bpm with intermittent failure of capture. Note several pacemaker stimulus artifacts are not followed by a QRS complex, indicating failure of capture. **E:** EKG showing ventricular pacing at 90 bpm and normal sensing of patient's intrinsic rhythm. **F:** EKG showing ventricular pacing at 100 bpm, as well as inappropriate sensing and failure to stimulate the heart secondary to wire fracture.

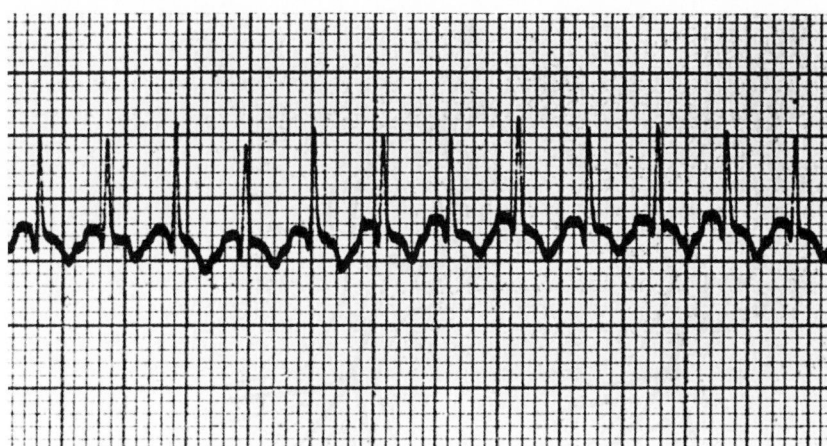

FIGURE 84.10 Supraventricular tachycardia, rate 300 bpm.

like an α pathway (slow conduction, short refractory period). Episodes of SVT are usually initiated by a premature atrial depolarization that blocks antegrade conduction in the accessory pathway and travels to the ventricles over the normal AV conducting system. The impulse, on reaching the ventricular insertion of the bypass tract, can travel retrograde up the bypass tract to the atrium reenter the AV node to start a "circus movement" or reentrant type of tachycardia.

AV accessory tracts may be either manifest on an EKG as WPW syndrome or concealed. In WPW, the pathway conducts antegrade (from atrium to ventricle) during sinus rhythm, resulting in WPW complexes, which consist of a short PR interval and a widened QRS complex with a slurred upstroke (delta wave). These complexes are generally not seen during the tachycardia, but only after conversion to normal sinus rhythm as shown in Figure 84.12. The short PR interval and delta wave characteristic of the WPW syndrome are produced by conduction over the accessory pathway, which has different electrophysiologic properties from the normal AV conduction system. The ventricular complex is a fusion beat with a variable contribution from conduction through the accessory pathway and the AV node. The greater the contribution is from the accessory pathway, the larger the delta wave and more bizarre the QRS. A concealed bypass tract indicates that the bypass tract is used only as the retrograde limb of the reentrant circuit during SVT but is not used for antegrade conduction during normal resting rhythm. Thus, the resting EKG appears normal.

Most commonly, antegrade conduction during AV reentrant SVT occurs through the AV node and the QRS complexes will be normal on the EKG. In patients with WPW, the reentrant circuit may be reversed, with the bypass tract forming the antegrade limb. In these cases, the QRS complexes will be wide and bizarre, and the arrhythmia may stimulate VT. In addition, because the ventricle must be depolarized prior to retrograde conduction up the bypass tract, atrial activation must always follow ventricular activation; therefore, the P wave follows inscription of the QRS complex. The PR interval is usually less than 50% of the R-R interval. In AV nodal reentrant SVT, the P wave may or may not be visible but, if visible, is generally closely related to the preceding QRS complex. The rate of SVT appears to reflect the conduction properties of the AV node and bypass tract when involved. Patients whose AV nodes or bypass tracts conduct slowly have slower rates during SVT. Conduction properties of the various substrates, and consequently, SVT rates can be affected by sympathetic or parasympathetic tone, as well as drugs.

The identification of the mechanism of the tachycardia in SVT is helpful from a therapeutic point of view so a medication known to act specifically on the AV node, the accessory pathway, or the atrial tissue may be chosen.

The infant with SVT is most commonly younger than 4 months of age and is more likely to be male (male:female ratio is 3:2). Episodes may appear to be precipitated by infection, fever, or drug exposure (most commonly, cold medications or bronchodilators containing sympathomimetic amines). Underlying electrophysiologic substrates for SVT may be isolated or seen in conjunction with CHD (approximately 23%, including Ebstein's anomaly or corrected transposition). Accessory AV tracts may be manifest on routine EKG (WPW syndrome: 22%) or concealed. More than 90% of infants with SVT have an accessory AV pathway. Older children and adolescents are more likely to have dual AV nodal pathways. Those previously classified as idiopathic are generally considered to have concealed accessory pathways or other reentrant circuits.

Electrophysiologic catheterization techniques have provided much information about the mechanisms of SVT. SVT in children is most commonly due to a reentrant mechanism; either within the AV node or using an AV bypass tract (either concealed or manifest as WPW). Less commonly, enhanced automaticity of sinus nodal, atrial, or AV nodal region fibers may be responsible for SVT.

An understanding of the concept of reentry is important for understanding the therapeutic approach to SVT. Figure 84.11 illustrates the application of this concept to human SVT in the case of dual AV nodal pathways. By convention, the dual pathways have been labeled alpha (α) and beta (β). The α pathway is slower conducting but has a shorter refractory period than the faster-conducting β pathway. During sinus rhythm, the atrial impulse traverses the faster-conducting β pathway to produce a single QRS complex. The impulse travels simultaneously down the α (slow) pathway, reaching the His bundle shortly after it has been depolarized and rendered refractory by the impulse that was conducted down the β pathway. In response to an atrial premature depolarization, the impulse is blocked in the β pathway as a result of its longer refractory period and proceeds slowly down the α pathway. If conduction

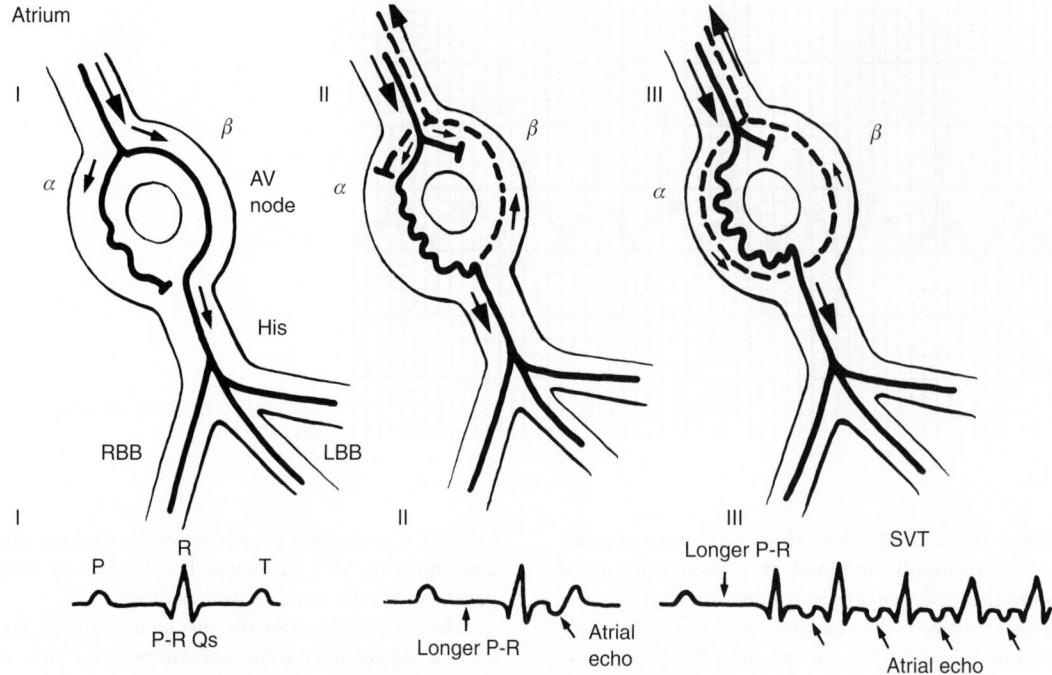

FIGURE 84.11 Schematic representation of conduction pathway and corresponding electrocardiogram in the development of atrioventricular (AV) nodal reentry. See text for full discussion. LBB, left bundle branch; RBB, right bundle branch; SVT, supraventricular tachycardia.

down the α pathway is slow enough to allow the previously refractory β pathway time to recover, a single atrial echo results. An earlier atrial premature depolarization (Fig. 84.11) also blocks in the β pathway, conducts slowly down the α pathway, and arrives later to conduct retrograde through the β pathway back to the α pathway with antegrade conduction producing a sustained AV nodal reentrant tachycardia.

If conduction delay and refractoriness in both pathways are appropriate, a continuously circulating wave front of electrical activity ensues, resulting in a reentrant tachycardia. Additional substrates for reentrant SVT can be found in the sinus node, atrium, and a variety of AV accessory pathways. Reentrant SVT in the setting of AV accessory pathways is analogous to AV nodal reentrant SVT with the bypass tract functioning like a β pathway (fast conduction, long refractory period) and the AV nodal–His-Purkinje system functioning like an α pathway (slow conduction, short refractory period). Episodes of SVT are usually initiated by a premature atrial depolarization that blocks antegrade conduction in the accessory pathway and travels to the ventricles over the normal AV conducting system. The impulse, on reaching the ventricular insertion of the bypass tract, can travel retrograde up the bypass tract to the atrium and reenter the AV node to start a "circus movement" or reentrant type of tachycardia.

AV accessory tracts may be either manifest on an EKG as WPW syndrome or concealed. In WPW, the pathway conducts antegrade (from atrium to ventricle) during sinus rhythm, resulting in WPW complexes, which consist of a short PR interval and a widened QRS complex with a slurred upstroke (delta wave). These complexes are generally not seen during the tachycardia, but only after conversion to normal sinus rhythm as shown in Figure 84.12. The WPW complex repre-sents the presence of a bypass tract connecting atria and ven-tricles. The short PR interval and delta wave characteristic of the WPW syndrome are produced by conduction over the accessory pathway, which has different electrophysiologic properties from the normal AV conduction system. The ven-tricular complex is a fusion beat with a variable contribution from conduction through the accessory pathway and the AV node. The greater the contribution is from the accessory path-way, the larger is the delta wave and more bizarre the QRS. A concealed bypass tract indicates that the bypass tract is used only as the retrograde limb of the reentrant circuit during SVT but is not used for antegrade conduction during normal resting rhythm. Thus, the resting EKG appears normal.

Most commonly, antegrade conduction during AV reen-trant SVT occurs through the AV node and the QRS com-plexes will be normal on the EKG. In patients with WPW, the reentrant circuit may be reversed, with the bypass tract form-ing the antegrade limb. In these cases, the QRS complexes will be wide and bizarre, and the arrhythmia may simulate VT. In addition, because the ventricle must be depolarized prior to retrograde conduction up the bypass tract, atrial activation must always follow ventricular activation; therefore, the P wave follows inscription of the QRS complex. The PR interval is usually less than 50% of the R-R interval. In AV nodal reen-trant SVT, the P wave may or may not be visible but, if visible, is generally closely related to the preceding QRS complex. The rate of SVT appears to reflect the conduction properties of the AV node and bypass tract when involved. Patients whose AV nodes or bypass tracts conduct slowly have slower rates dur-ing SVT. Conduction properties of the various substrates, and consequently, SVT rates can be affected by sympathetic or parasympathetic tone, as well as drugs. Additional substrates

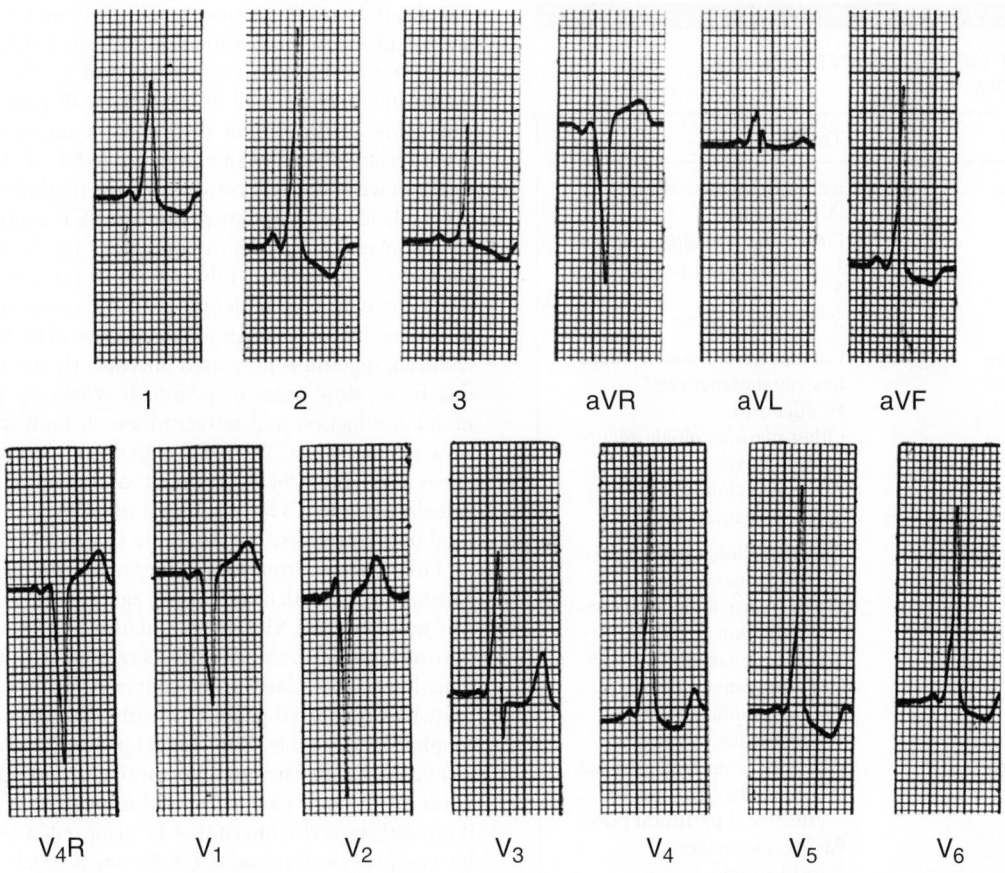

FIGURE 84.12 Electrocardiogram in Wolff-Parkinson-White (WPW) syndrome. Note wide QRS, presence of delta wave (slurred upstroke of R), and short PR interval.

for reentrant SVT can be found in the sinus node, atrium, and a variety of accessory pathways.

The identification of the mechanism of the tachycardia in SVT is helpful from a therapeutic point of view so a medication known to act specifically on the AV node, the accessory pathway, or the atrial tissue may be chosen.

Clinical Manifestations. SVT may occur at any age. Some patients may have only asymptomatic tachycardia. The presence of symptoms or signs of hemodynamic impairment will depend on the rate of duration of the SVT, as well as the presence or absence of preexisting CHD or myocardial dysfunction. The infant with SVT may present with only a fast rate, or with signs of CHF (poor feeding, irritability, respiratory distress) or in shock. The infant may be acidotic with a clinical appearance resembling the septic infant. The older child may complain of palpitations, dizziness, chest pain, respiratory distress, or present with syncope. Because of presenting symptoms, the older child is less likely to be quite as ill when first seen as the infant or young child. The older child with a CHD or primary myocardial disease is more likely to present with signs of CHF. In a patient without CHD or preexisting myocardial dysfunction, CHF usually appears only after 24 hours of SVT.

Episodes of SVT may have no specific inciting factor or may appear to be precipitated by infection, fever, or drug exposure (most commonly, cold medications or bronchodila-tors containing sympathomimetic amines). However, when the patient is first seen in the ED, the precise onset of the SVT is rarely certain and the presence of associated heart defects or dysfunction is unknown. Therefore, all patients must be treated with some degree of urgency.

Management. Treatment of SVT is determined by the clinical condition of the patient and the presumed mechanism. Thus, a different mode of treatment is chosen for the patient with tachycardia in shock than for the asymptomatic patient who has only a fast HR (Table 84.13).

Any patient with SVT who presents with shock or severe hemodynamic compromise should be cardioverted. Synchronized direct current (DC) cardioversion at a dosage of 0.25 to 0.5 J per kg should be used and doubled until effective or until a dosage of 2 J per kg is reached. Underlying acidosis may need to be corrected and adequate ventilation and oxygenation provided because cardioversion may not be successful in the presence of hypoxia or acid–base imbalance. If ventricular fibrillation should occur, defibrillation will generally convert the patient to normal sinus rhythm. The patient may need a sedative or short-acting anesthetic, and preparations should be made for airway support and ventilation if needed. The presence of digoxin in a patient should not prevent the use of cardioversion when needed. A digoxin-related ventricular arrhythmia may be treated with lidocaine.

TABLE 84.13

TREATMENT OF SUPRAVENTRICULAR
TACHYCARDIA

Clinical status	Treatment
Asymptomatic	Ice, vagal maneuvers IV adenosine Other pharmacologic agents 1. IV verapamil (>1 yr old) 2. IV digoxin 3. IV amiodarone
Mild congestive heart failure	Cardioversion, synchronized Ice, vagal maneuvers IV adenosine Other pharmacologic agents 1. IV digoxin 2. IV amiodarone 3. IV procainamide
Moderate congestive heart failure	Cardioversion, synchronized IV adenosine Other pharmacologic agents 1. IV digoxin 2. IV amiodarone 3. IV procainamide Pacing (esophageal or intracardiac)

Severe congestive
heart failure
	Cardioversion, synchronized
	IV adenosine (may not be
	    effective if perfusion poor)
	Pacing, esophageal or
	    intracardiac
	Other pharmacologic agents
	1. IV digoxin
	2. IV amiodarone
	3. IV procainamide

IV, intravenous.

Children who have only moderate, mild, or no hemodynamic impairment can be treated successfully with vagal maneuvers or adenosine. Because the majority of SVT in children is caused by either AV nodal or AV reentry, an intervention that interrupts the reentrant circuit in the AV node will interrupt the tachycardia. There are several effective methods of interfering with AV nodal conduction. In older children and adolescent patients, carotid sinus pressure or the Valsalva maneuver can frequently terminate the tachycardia by increasing vagal tone, thus slowing conduction and prolonging refractoriness within the AV node. In infants and young children, however, these maneuvers are technically difficult and usually ineffective. In this age group, ice water or ice bags applied to the face in the perinasal area for 5 to 10 seconds can be effective in eliciting the diving reflex and stopping the SVT. This technique should be reserved for children who are monitored, with particular caution used in applying these techniques in young infants, because marked sinus slowing may occur.

The pharmacologic agent of choice for the rapid conversion of SVT is IV adenosine, an endogenous purine that breaks the reentry circuit by slowing or blocking conduction in the AV node. When pushed rapidly into as central a vein as possible, it has a rapid onset of action (usually within 10 seconds) and a short half-life with occasional side effects (wheezing, hypotension) lasting less than a minute and rarely being serious. Adenosine may be used in moderately ill patients but should not delay cardioversion in severely compromised patients. Appropriate doses are shown in Table 84.14. The majority of children with SVT will convert to sinus rhythm with adenosine.

If adenosine is not successful, or SVT continues to return after conversion to sinus rhythm, other agents that may be useful and are reviewed in Table 84.14. IV procainamide or amiodarone may be used under the guidance of a cardiologist to terminate reentrant SVT. Although effective in terminating SVT in children, digoxin is now used infrequently for acute treatment due to its slow onset of action. It works by prolonging AV nodal conduction and refractoriness in both the fast (β) and slow (α) pathways. The usual digitalizing dose appropriate for age is used (Table 84.7). As noted earlier, the IV dose should be calculated to be 75% of the oral dose. IV verapamil is rarely used in recent years. The doses are shown in Table 84.14.

Other nonpharmacologic measures can be used as well. Raising the BP with α-adrenergic agents such as phenylephrine can terminate the SVT by stimulating the vagus through the baroreceptor reflexes; SVT that is refractory to the usual pharmacologic agents can also be converted by a pediatric cardiologist by rapid atrial pacing, via either a transvenous or transesophageal electrode. Rapid atrial pacing (faster than the SVT rate) captures the atrium, interrupting the reentrant cycle, and upon cessation of pacing, normal sinus rhythm resumes. Even if normal sinus rhythm cannot be achieved, a slower ventricular rate may be obtained if 2:1 AV nodal block is produced by rapid atrial pacing.

As soon as the patient converts from SVT, an EKG in sinus rhythm should be obtained looking for the presence of WPW syndrome. There is a small but real risk of sudden death in children with WPW, and the presence of WPW on the EKG in sinus rhythm significantly affects chronic therapy. Most pediatric cardiologists will initiate chronic therapy in infants with a prolonged episode of SVT with therapy aimed at preventing recurrences during the first year of life. Chronic maintenance therapy in infants is usually instituted in the hospital on continuous EKG monitoring to observe for adverse side effects of the antiarrhythmic agent. Studies have shown that 20% to 30% of infants will have recurrences on medication. By 1 year of age, many infants will no longer have episodes, allowing for discontinuation of the medication. Persistence of either episodes of SVT or WPW on EKG after 1 year will generally warrant continued therapy. Chronic maintenance therapy in older children with PSVT may be indicated in those with frequent, symptomatic or prolonged episodes that do not convert to sinus rhythm spontaneously and those seen in the setting of WPW. Chronic maintenance therapy may be instituted in older children as outpatients, but the presence of WPW may be an indication for admission.

In the absence of WPW, digoxin is generally the treatment of choice for chronic therapy for prevention of SVT. Digoxin should not be used in the presence of WPW syndrome because of its propensity to shorten the accessory pathway refractory period and promote rapid conduction of supraventricular impulses to the ventricle in atrial fibrillation. Unless one knows from intracardiac electrophysiology study that the accessory pathway refractory period is relatively long and is unaffected by the digoxin, it should not be used primarily in patients with

TABLE 84.14

ANTIARRHYTHMIC AGENTS

Drug	Intravenous	Oral	Desired level
For Supraventricular Tachycardia			
Adenosine	100–400 μg/kg. Initial 100 μg/kg IV Increase by 100 μg/kg every 2 min to 400 μg/kg or 12 mg maximal dose		
Procainamide	5–15 mg/kg over 30–60 min load Infusion 20–80 μg/kg/min	15–50 mg/kg/day divided q3–6h	PA 4–10 μg/kg PA plus NAPA 10–30 μg/mL
Propranolol		0.5–1 mg/kg/dose q6h	50–100 ng/mL
Esmolol	500 μg/kg/dose over 1 min followed by 50 μg/kg/min over 4 min: repeat in 5 min with 500 μg/kg/min over 1 min, 100 μg/kg/min over 4 min	50–200 μg/kg/min	
Verapamil	0.1 mg/kg/dose (max 5 mg/dose)	4–8 mg/kg/day	NA
Not ≤1 yr	Repeat in 30 min if needed. Second dose 0.1–0.3 mg/kg/dose (max 10 mg/dose)		
Digoxin	See Table 84.7	See Table 84.7	0.5–2.0 ng/mL
For Ventricular Tachycardia			
Amiodarone	Amiodarone 5 mg/kg IV over 20–60 min (max 300 mg/dose)	5–10 mg/kg/day	
Procainamide	As above	As above	As above
Lidocaine	1–2 mg/kg/dose Infusion: 20–50 μg/kg/min		1–5 μg/mL
Magnesium sulfate (for torsades)	25–50 mg/kg/dose over 10–20 min (max 2 g/dose)		Mg^{++} 3–4 mg/dL

PA, procainamide; NAPA, N-acetylprocainamide; NA, not available for routine clinical use.

WPW. In patients with WPW, β-blockers including propranolol and atenolol can be very effective in preventing SVT by slowing AV nodal conduction and prolonging refractoriness while having no significant effects on the accessory pathway.

In the absence of WPW, β-blockers, class IA or IC agents such as procainamide or flecainide are also very effective in preventing SVT, by slowing conduction and prolonging refractoriness in the accessory pathway, interrupting the retrograde limb of the reentrant circuit. Verapamil can be effective for chronic therapy, but, like digoxin, may accelerate conduction in AV tracts. Amiodarone can be useful alone or in combination for prevention of SVT due to any mechanism. Older children or infants, who are difficult to control with multiple recurrences, must be managed individually and may require a combination of medications.

Radiofrequency ablation is highly successful in eliminating the substrates for SVT and can be performed safely after 2 years of age. The optimal timing for radiofrequency ablation is individualized on the basis of severity and frequency of episodes, response to therapy, underlying mechanism, and the preference of the patient and family.

Children with SVT should not be treated for upper respiratory tract infections with sympathomimetic amines. Instead, if needed, pure antihistamines, such as those listed in Table 84.15 should be used.

Atrial Flutter and Atrial Fibrillation

Atrial flutter and fibrillation occur uncommonly in children. Atrial flutter consists of rapid, regular atrial excitation at rates of 280 to 480 bpm (Fig. 84.13). The ventricular response depends on AV nodal conduction that may allow 1:1, 2:1, 3:1, or 4:1 conduction. The typical EKG reveals saw-toothed flutter waves best seen in leads 2 and V_1. Atrial flutter is most commonly seen in children with postoperative CHD, especially after the Fontan procedure for single ventricle complexes or the Mustard repair for D-transposition of the great arteries. It may also be encountered in children as an isolated primary electrophysiologic abnormality.

TABLE 84.15

PREFERABLE AGENTS FOR TREATMENT OF UPPER RESPIRATORY INFECTION IN CHILDREN WITH SVT

Chlorpheniramine maleate (Chlor-Trimeton®—Schering) (Teldin®—SKF)
Brompheniramine maleate (Dimetane®—Robbins)
Promethazine HCl (Phenergan®—Wyeth); need a prescription
Diphenhydramine (Benadryl®—Park Davis)
Loratadine (Claritin®—Schering)
Cetirizine HCl (Zyrtec®—Pfizer)
Fexofenadine (Allegra®—Hoechst)
For coughs:
　Robitussin®
　Robitussin DM®
　Robitussin with codeine; need a prescription
　Phenergan with codeine; need a prescription
　Terpin hydrate with codeine—need a prescription

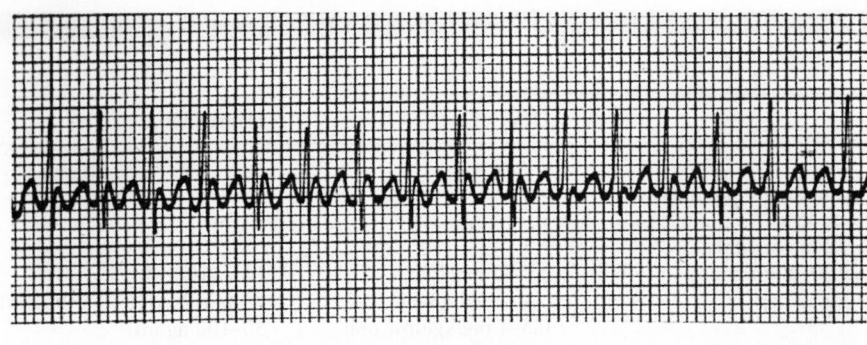

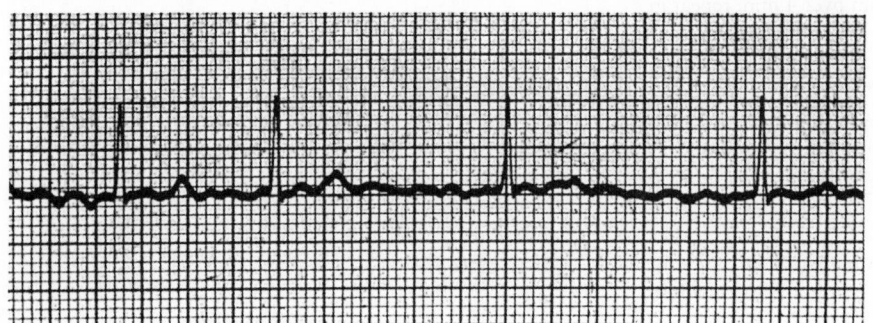

FIGURE 84.13 **A:** Atrial flutter. Sawtooth baseline is apparent. Regular QRS with ventricular rate of 250. **B:** Atrial fibrillation. Irregularly irregular QRS with course erratic baseline undulations representing fibrillatory waves.

Atrial fibrillation consists of totally disorganized rapid atrial activity (at a rate of 400 to 700 bpm) with a variable ventricular rate secondary to varying AV block. Atrial fibrillation is seen most commonly in adolescents with long-standing rheumatic or congenital mitral disease or in patients with hyperthyroidism.

Children with atrial fibrillation or flutter are treated very differently from children with reentrant SVT. Therapy is aimed at either conversion to sinus rhythm or reducing the ventricular rate by increasing AV block, as well as preventing embolization of an atrial thrombus when present. Severe cardiac compromise is an indication for immediate cardioversion. In the presence of normal LV function, a β-blocker (esmolol) or calcium channel blocker (diltiazem, verapamil) can be used to reduce the ventricular rate. In the presence of mild or moderate heart failure, IV digoxin or amiodarone should be used. As with SVT, neither digoxin nor verapamil should be used in patients with WPW. For conversion to sinus rhythm, IV ibutilide, procainamide, amiodarone, flecainide, propafenone, dofetilide, or digoxin may be effective. If atrial flutter or fibrillation has been going on for more than 48 hours, the possible presence of an atrial thrombus should be considered and evaluated by transesophageal echocardiography. In chronic atrial flutter or fibrillation with a possible atrial thrombus, anticoagulation should be instituted prior to either electrical or pharmacologic conversion to sinus rhythm. Since the AV node is not involved in a reentry circuit, adenosine will not convert to sinus rhythm, but will transiently increase AV block, helping to diagnose the exact tachyarrhythmia. In the child who is stable and who has a normal BP and adequate perfusion, the physician can wait for a response to pharmacologic conversion, but failure to achieve a normal rhythm after 24 to 48 hours may call for cardioversion. Therapeutic drug levels for these agents, which should be obtained in a steady state of drug administration, are listed in Table 84.14.

Automatic Atrial Tachycardia

Automatic atrial tachycardia secondary to enhanced automaticity of the sinus node or other atrial tissue can be an isolated electrophysiologic abnormality or seen in association with congenital or acquired heart disease (myocarditis). Adenosine is ineffective, so therapy with β-blockers, calcium channel blockers, amiodarone, procainamide, or digoxin may be used intravenously for acute control, with subsequent chronic oral therapy. Chronic drugs may also include β-blockers, flecainide, and sotalol.

Junctional Tachycardia

Junctional tachycardias most commonly occur after cardiac surgery and may be difficult to control. IV amiodarone and IV procainamide (Table 84.14) have been reported to be effective, as has hypothermia. Electrical cardioversion is ineffective.

Ventricular Tachycardia

VT is encountered much less frequently than SVT in children. VT is a tachycardia with wide QRS complexes and, when P waves are seen, the presence of AV dissociation. It has also been defined as three or more consecutive PVCs (Fig. 84.14). The HR is usually 150 to 200 bpm but may be slower or more rapid.

Clinical Manifestations. Patients may present with asymptomatic tachycardia, but there may be complaints of palpitations, and since the contractions may be hemodynamically inefficient, there may be dizziness, syncope, CHF, or cardiovascular collapse with sudden death. Causes of VT include electrolyte imbalance, metabolic disturbances, prolonged QT syndrome, Brugada syndrome, catecholaminergic polymorphic VT,

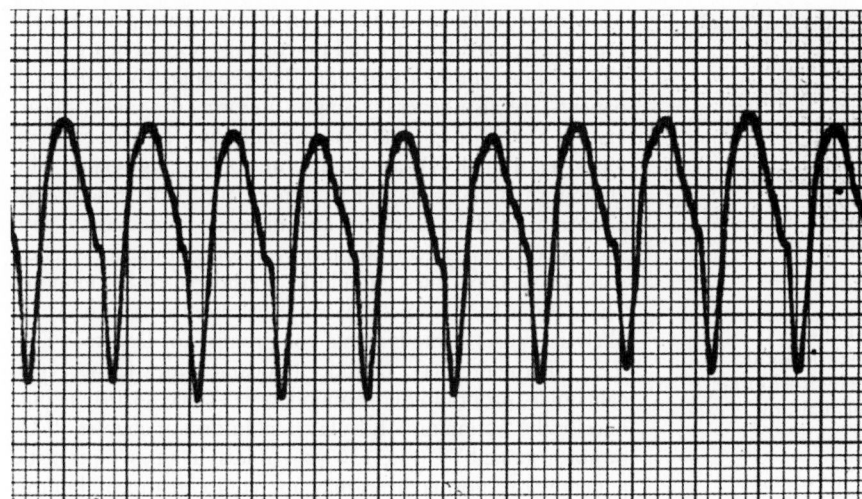

FIGURE 84.14 Ventricular tachycardia. Wide QRS with rate of approximately 250 bpm; sinusoidal pattern.

arrhythmogenic right ventricular dysplasia, drug toxins, congenital or acquired cardiac disease, cardiac tumors or other isolated primary electrophysiologic abnormalities. Specific genetic abnormalities coding for a variety of cardiac membrane channel abnormalities for ventricular arrhythmias have now been identified. Since many of the channelopathies are genetic, a family history of ventricular arrhythmia, unexpected sudden death or syncope in young relatives should be sought. Any family history of hearing deficit should also be noted.

Management. As with SVT patients, the urgency of treatment depends on the clinical status. In cases of shock, impending cardiac decompensation, or cardiac failure, synchronized DC cardioversion at 2 to 4 J per kg up to 10 J per kg should be used. In children with identifiable extra cardiac causes of VT, the underlying disturbance can be treated. Generally, sustained rapid VT requires treatment. Hospital admission and urgent pediatric cardiology consultation are indicated. Patients with CHD and VT often have some degree of hemodynamic compromise and do not tolerate the VT well, requiring urgent therapy. All patients with CHD and sustained VT over 150 bpm require therapy because sudden death occurs in up to 30% of patients with CHD who have VT. Patients with CHD and slower VT or nonsustained VT may also require treatment if hemodynamic instability exists. There is still controversy over whether asymptomatic patients with normal hearts and idiopathic slow VT should be treated with antiarrhythmic agents. The patient should not be made more toxic by the therapy than by the arrhythmia.

Effective emergency pharmacologic therapy includes IV amiodarone, lidocaine, and procainamide (Table 84.14). IV amiodarone is infused at 5 mg per kg over the first hour followed by an infusion of 5 to 10 μg per kg per min. IV lidocaine can be given as a bolus of 1 to 2 mg per kg, followed by a continuous infusion of lidocaine at 20 to 50 μg per kg per minute may be required. IV infusion of IV procainamide at 15 mg per kg given over 30 to 60 minutes, followed by a 20 to 80 μg per kg per minute IV infusion. Rapid ventricular pacing may be used for overdrive suppression for conversion to normal rhythm if pharmacologic therapy fails or is contraindicated.

After conversion to sinus rhythm, the child who has presented with VT, especially of the polymorphic or torsades de pointes type, should have a full EKG with corrected QT intervals carefully measured. There are several special treatment issues pertaining to VT in children with long QT syndrome. Sudden death occurs in 73% of patients with VT who are not treated, secondary to tachyarrhythmias (torsades de pointes) of the type that often degenerates to ventricular fibrillation. In addition, temporary atrial or ventricular pacing at a rate 10% to 20% faster than the underlying sinus rate may be needed to control the arrhythmia, especially in patients with underlying bradycardia, a common association. IV propranolol, phenytoin, and magnesium have been used successfully in these patients. Because class I agents prolong the QT interval in normal patients, they should be avoided in patients with these long QT intervals. A number of medications may prolong the QT interval and produce VT (Table 84.16). Temporary pacing and removal of the offending agent are effective therapies. For management of acquired long QT with ventricular arrhythmias, especially if bradycardia is a prominent factor, an isoproterenol infusion may be therapeutic.

Chronic treatment for VT may include propranolol, atenolol, nadolol, mexiletine, amiodarone, procainamide, sotalol, or propafenone. Those with Purkinje cell tumors, reentry circuits within the ventricle, or ectopic foci may be amenable to catheter radiofrequency ablation in selected cases. An automatic cardioverter-defibrillator may need to be implanted.

Ventricular Fibrillation

Ventricular fibrillation consists of chaotic irregular ventricular contractions with cessation of circulation. Electrical defibrillation with correction of precipitating factors (acidosis, electrolyte imbalance, hypoxia) may result in conversion to normal sinus rhythm. The treatment of cardiac arrest is discussed in Chapter 1. After epinephrine in the resuscitation protocol, the only other drug of proven benefit is IV amiodarone.

Irregular Heart Rates

Premature Ventricular Depolarizations

Background. The primary irregular rhythm that may require attention is the premature ventricular depolarization (PVD).

TABLE 84.16

PHARMACOLOGIC AGENTS THAT PROLONG
QT INTERVAL

Antiarrhythmic Agents	Psychotropic Drugs
Quinidine	Tricyclic antidepressant
Procainamide	amitriptyline
Flecainide	Phenothiazines
Encainide	Haloperidol
Disopyramide	Risperidone
Amiodarone	Pimozide
Sotalol	Lithium carbonate
	Sertraline hydrochloride
Antihistamines	Nefazodone hydrochloride
Terfenadine	Fluvoxamine maleate
Astemizole	
Diphenhydramine	**Cisapride**
Antibiotics/Antifungal Agents	**Probucol**
Erythromycin	*Anthracyclines*
Trimethoprim	*Organophosphates*
Sulfamethoxazole	
Pentamidine	**Epinephrine**
Ketoconazole	
Fluconazole	**Diuretics**
Itraconazole	Potassium loss
Clarithromycin	
Azithromycin	

PVDs are seen as premature, wide, bizarre-shaped QRS complexes. Generally, the T wave is opposite in direction to the main deflection of the QRS. A compensatory pause usually follows the premature beat, and P waves may reveal AV dissociation or retrograde conduction or may be absent. When a rhythmic pattern of PVDs is established, the designation of bigeminy, trigeminy, or quadrigeminy is made, depending on whether that beat followed every second, third, or fourth sinus beat. VT consists of three PVCs or more that last for 10 seconds or less.

Pathophysiology. PVCs often occur without identifiable cause in children and are often considered benign. PVCs are also seen in children with CHD (unoperated or operated) and CHF, viral myocarditis, Lyme myocarditis, cardiac membrane channelopathies resulting in long QT syndrome, cardiomyopathies, cardiac tumors, hemochromatosis, or electrolyte imbalance. They are also seen in association with various forms of drug administration, including general anesthesia, digoxin, sympathomimetic amines, and phenothiazines. PVCs may be precursors of VT or fibrillation.

Clinical Manifestations. Children who present with PVDs are frequently asymptomatic and unaware of their arrhythmia, especially if they are younger than 5 years of age. If the PVC is appreciated, the child may complain of a "skipped" or "hard" beat, a fluttering or pounding in the chest. If the PVDs are frequent and/or associated with heart disease (congenital or acquired), the child may note dizziness or other symptoms of hemodynamic compromise. Frequent PVCs in the presence of preexistent compromised cardiac function may worsen the CO and produce signs and symptoms of CHF.

Management. Isolated PVDs in an asymptomatic patient in the presence of a structurally and functionally normal heart generally do not require treatment. These benign PVDs in such patients are also generally single, uniform (the same appearance in a given lead), and decrease in frequency with exercise. However, if the PVDs are multiform; coupled; associated with an abnormal underlying EKG, abnormal cardiac structure, or abnormal cardiac function; and increase in frequency with exercise or associated with prior symptoms of dizziness, chest pain, or syncope, these should be considered to be ominous. These PVDs may require treatment because they cause (or are likely to cause) hemodynamic compromise, or lead to VT or VF. Treatment may include lidocaine, mexiletine, procainamide, propranolol, or amiodarone (Table 84.14), as outlined in the section on VT. Isolated multiform or coupled PVDs or nonsustained VT (rate 150 bpm or less) in an asymptomatic patient with a normal heart may not require treatment, but this decision must be individualized after consultation with a cardiologist. Rarely is emergency treatment of this type of patient required. Investigations that use 24-hour continuous EKG monitors, transtelephonic event monitoring exercise stress testing, echocardiography, and/or electrophysiologic catheterization studies may be used to determine the appropriate management. Restriction of caffeine and other stimulants should be recommended in all patients with ventricular arrhythmias.

Benign Atrial Arrhythmias

Premature atrial contractions (PADs) are premature P waves, usually followed by a normal-appearing QRS complex. Alternatively, depending on the electrical phase of the heart at the time of the PAD, the impulse may block in the AV node (resulting in no QRS), or be aberrantly conducted through one of the bundle branches (resulting in a wide QRS). PADs generally do not cause symptoms other than palpitations and do not require treatment. Transtelephonic event or continuous 24-hour ambulatory monitoring may be warranted if symptoms suggest the associated occurrence of SVT. Elimination of caffeine or other stimulants such as pseudoephedrine, or other sympathomimetics may decrease the frequency of PADs. Unless the PADs are demonstrated to initiate episodes of SVT, no treatment is indicated.

Variations of normal rhythms commonly seen in children and that do not require treatment include sinus arrhythmia and wandering atrial pacemaker, as long as rates remain in the normal ranges.

First- and Second-degree Heart Block

First-degree heart block reflects slowed conduction from the sinus node to the ventricle (usually in the AV node) and is manifest by a prolonged PR interval. It is seen with digoxin and other antiarrhythmic drugs; certain types of CHD (primum and secundum atrial septal defects); and inflammatory diseases such as rheumatic, viral, or Lyme myocarditis.

Second-degree heart block results in the failure of some impulses to traverse the AV node. Type 1 second-degree AV block (Wenckebach) is manifest as progressive prolongation of the PR interval, culminating in a dropped QRS. Other forms of second-degree heart block include high-grade 2:1, 3:1, and 4:1 block. Type 2 second-degree AV block is manifest as intermittent failure of a QRS to follow a P, without prior PR interval prolongation.

Management. Children with first- and second-degree heart block are generally asymptomatic and do not require cardiac therapy. Type 2 second-degree AV block may reflect an abnormality of the AV node and lead to syncope, requiring pacing. If a manifestation of digitalis toxicity, adjustment of the digitalis dose may be required. If manifestation of myocarditis or endocarditis, treatment of the primary problem is indicated.

Arrhythmias Associated with Electrolyte Abnormalities

Alterations in electrolyte concentrations may influence cardiac rate, rhythm, and automaticity, and may lead to arrhythmias. Potassium and calcium abnormalities are the most common electrolyte alterations that produce arrhythmias, but abnormalities in magnesium and acid–base balance are also important. Commonly, a combination of ionic alterations is responsible for arrhythmias. Any patient with significant arrhythmias should be evaluated for an electrolyte disturbance. The EKG changes may be characteristic and lead to suspicion of a specific electrolyte abnormality. Normal EKG intervals (PR, QRS, QTc) are listed in Table 84.17.

Hyperkalemia. Hyperkalemia is common in hospitalized children and produces recognizable EKG alterations. Peaked T waves are seen at a serum concentration of 5 to 6 mEq per L, and the QRS widens with a concentration exceeding 6 mEq per L. The QT interval increases with the increasing QRS duration. As P-wave amplitude decreases, P-wave duration increases, and the PR interval increases above 7 mEq per L. Above 8 to 9 mEq per L, P waves disappear, the ventricular rate becomes irregular, and severe bradycardia with sinus arrest, block, or idioventricular rhythms occur, often with a sinusoidal wave pattern. Ventricular fibrillation or asystole occurs at serum concentrations greater than 12 to 14 mEq per L. Low serum calcium enhances the myocardial toxicity of hyperkalemia. Likewise, acidosis potentiates hyperkalemia by producing potassium ion efflux from cells.

Hypokalemia. Serum potassium concentrations of less than 2.7 mEq per L generally produce typical EKG changes in ventricular repolarization. These changes may include U-wave amplitude greater than 1 mm, seen best in leads V_2 and V_3, and ST-segment depression greater than 0.5 mm. The QT interval lengthens and the T wave flattens with progressive hypokalemia. The PR interval may be prolonged, and intraventricular conduction may be delayed with widening of the QRS complex. With substantial hypokalemia, P-wave and QRS amplitude may increase. Other arrhythmias that have been associated with hypokalemia include ectopic atrial and ventricular complexes, ectopic atrial tachycardia with block, AV dissociation, second-degree AV block, ventricular bigeminy, VT, and ventricular fibrillation.

Patients on digoxin who become hypokalemic are especially susceptible to arrhythmias because of the synergistic effects of digoxin and hypokalemia on automaticity and conduction.

Hypocalcemia. Hypocalcemia produces characteristic EKG changes that consist of QT interval prolongation secondary to ST-segment prolongation (Fig. 84.15), and occasionally, reversal of the T wave. The EKG changes correlate with ionized calcium because the degree of QT prolongation is generally proportional to the degree of hypocalcemia. Abnormal rhythms, although uncommon, have been reported and include SVT, 2:1 AV block, complete heart block, and torsades de pointes VT. The effects of calcium and potassium on myocardial cells are antagonistic.

Hypercalcemia. Hypercalcemia, with levels above 12 mg per dL, produces a shortened QT interval (Fig. 84.13), a shortened ST segment, and normal or prominent U waves. Severe hypercalcemia causes PR interval prolongation, QRS prolongation, and occasionally, second- and third-degree heart block. Elevated serum calcium decreases the effect of hyperkalemia and potentiates digoxin toxicity. Thus, calcium should be administered cautiously to patients taking digoxin, and the HR should be monitored.

MEDICAL EMERGENCIES

TABLE 84.17

PR INTERVAL AND QRS DURATION RELATED TO RATE AND AGE (AND UPPER LIMITS OF NORMAL)

PR								
Rate	0–1 mo	1–6 mo	6 mo–1 yr	1–3 yr	3–8 yr	8–12 yr	12–16 yr	Adult
<60						0.16 (0.18)	0.16 (0.19)	0.17 (0.21)
60–80					0.15 (0.17)	0.15 (0.17)	0.15 (0.18)	0.16 (0.21)
80–100	0.10 (0.12)				0.14 (0.16)	0.15 (0.16)	0.15 (0.17)	0.15 (0.20)
100–120	0.10 (0.12)			(0.15)	0.13 (0.16)	0.14 (0.15)	0.15 (0.16)	0.15 (0.19)
120–140	0.10 (0.11)	0.11 (0.14)	0.11 (0.14)	0.12 (0.14)	0.13 (0.15)	0.14 (0.15)		0.15 (0.18)
140–160	0.09 (0.11)	0.10 (0.13)	0.11 (0.13)	0.11 (0.14)	0.12 (0.14)			(0.17)
160–180	0.10 (0.11)	0.10 (0.12)	0.10 (0.12)	0.10 (0.12)				
>180	0.09	0.09 (0.11)	0.10 (0.11)					

QPR								
Rate	0–6 mo	1–6 mo	6 mo–1 yr	1–3 yr	3–8 yr	8–12 yr	12–16 yr	Adult
Seconds	0.05 (0.065)	0.05 (0.07)	0.05 (0.06)	0.06 (0.07)	0.07 (0.08)	0.07 (0.09)	0.07 (0.10)	0.08 (0.10)

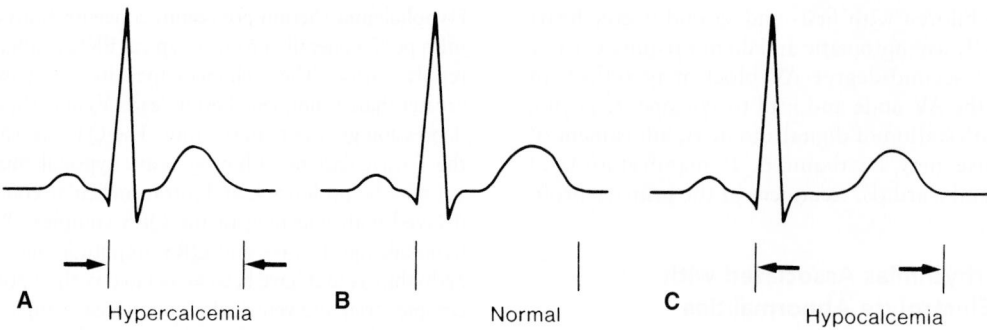

FIGURE 84.15 Electrolyte effects on EKG QT interval. Note prolongation with hypocalcemia, shortening with hypercalcemia.

Hypomagnesemia. Low magnesium levels are often associated with hypokalemia and hypocalcemia. The EKG abnormalities seen may be those associated with any or all these aberrations and include prolongation of the corrected QT interval. Ectopic beats and T-wave changes are commonly noted. Torsades de pointes VT and ventricular fibrillation have been reported.

Hypermagnesemia. Hypermagnesemia of 3 to 5 mEq per L or higher may be associated with a delay in AV and intraventricular conduction. Treatment of these electrolyte abnormalities is discussed in Chapter 100.

Sudden Cardiac Death

Sudden death is a rare occurrence in children, with an overall estimated incidence of 1 in 20,000 to 50,000 per year. In apparently normal children, however, the incidence is estimated to be 1 to 1.5 per 100,000 per year. It is felt that 5% of all deaths in children are due to sudden cardiac death (SCD). Mechanisms of SCD include arrhythmia, ischemia, heart failure, and pulmonary hypertensive crisis. SCD can occur in the setting of a variety of heart diseases (Table 84.18). Of the etiologies of SCD listed, HCM deserves special comment.

Over the 50 years since the landmark pathologic report issued in 1958, the importance of this disease entity (HCM) has become better recognized not only as a cause of sudden death but also as an important cause of ongoing morbidity and clinical concern. The problem includes the spectrum of illnesses

TABLE 84.18

ETIOLOGIES OF SUDDEN CARDIAC DEATH

Hypertrophic cardiomyopathy
Dilated cardiomyopathy
  (including myocarditis)
Coronary artery anomaly
  (left coronary artery from right sinus of Valsalva, ALCAPA)
Repaired congenital heart disease
Aortic dissection
Arrhythmogenic right ventricular dysplasia
Cardiac channelopathies
  (long QT, Brugada, catecholaminergic polymorphic
    ventricular tachycardia)
Wolff-Parkinson-White syndrome

previously classified as IHSS (idiopathic hypertrophic subaortic stenosis), HOCM (hypertrophic obstructive cardiomyopathy), and MSS (muscular subaortic stenosis). The prevalence of HCM is estimated to be 0.2% of the general population. Recently developed fetal information has indicated that asymmetric hypertrophy of the ventricular septum may actually be a component of normal cardiac development whose persistence and further exacerbation after birth underlies a distinct genetically driven pathophysiology. Most commonly, the disease becomes manifest in the adolescent and young adult, and it is known to often progress rapidly during puberty. HCM involves not only myocardial maldevelopment with asymmetric hypertrophy of segments of the heart muscle, most notably but not exclusively the septum, but also distinct mitral valve abnormalities as well. There is now well-delineated, definitively diagnostic genetic analysis possible. Reliable direct DNA sequencing is available to diagnose the typical HCM-causing mutations and to stratify risk.

The clinical findings are quite variable. If left ventricular outflow obstruction is part of the picture, a systolic murmur of varying intensity along the left sternal border is usually present. If the patient is able to change position, or is cooperative, the murmur may be accentuated when changing from supine to upright or with the Valsalva maneuver. Often an S_3 or S_4 can be heard. The arterial pulse palpation can also provide a clue to diagnosis with a "bisferiens" contour. The EKG is abnormal in nearly all patients and often appears quite bizarre. Left ventricular hypertrophy, distinct ST-T changes marked by prominent T inversion patterns, and prominent Q waves, especially in the inferior and midprecordial leads, are characteristic. The echocardiogram, of course, is readily diagnostic and should be obtained, along with cardiac consultation, in any patient with suspected HCM. This is particularly true in the ED setting since management decisions during and after resuscitation and for stabilization of the patient are impacted by the diagnosis. For example, vigorous use of diuretics should be avoided in the patient with HCM and LV outflow obstruction as high preload levels may be required to maintain systemic output. Similarly, catecholamine support for post resuscitation hypotension in HCM must be used with extreme caution, if at all.

Children presenting after resuscitation from a near sudden death episode should have a careful history, including ascertainment of the existence of previous symptoms of cardiac disease (e.g., exertional chest pain, shortness of breath, or syncope), the existence of previous cardiac disease and of a family

TABLE 84.19

CAUSES OF DISEASES OF THE PERICARDIUM

Infectious	Noninfectious, inflammatory	Traumatic	Oncologic	Chronic
Bacterial	Acute rheumatic fever	Postpericardiotomy syndrome	Leukemia	Constrictive pericarditis
Viral	Systemic lupus erythematosus	Chest wall injury	Lymphoma	Subacute effusive pericarditis
Fungal	Uremia	Foreign bodies with cardiac contact	Pericardial cyst	Blood dyscrasias
Parasitic	Radiation		Cardiac rhabdosarcoma	
Tuberculous	Juvenile rheumatoid arthritis Drugs (e.g., Minoxidil)			

history of unexpected sudden death or significant arrhythmia in a young person. A detailed physical exam is also required, regardless of the specific neurologic status. An EKG should be done and assessed for long QT, WPW, or other findings of underlying rhythm or conduction tissue abnormality. The presence of ischemic ST or T-wave abnormalities or electrocardiographic evidence of myocardial infarction should suggest the presence of a rare coronary artery malformation (such as anomalous origin of the left coronary artery from the pulmonary artery or a coronary artery cursing between the aorta and pulmonary artery leading to compression with exercise). An echocardiogram should be performed in order to diagnose structural or functional abnormalities. Consideration should be given to more extensive monitoring, exercise stress testing, cardiac catheterization with coronary angiography, intracardiac electrophysiologic studies or genetic testing for channelopathies when appropriate. Insertion of an AICD for secondary prevention of SCD must be considered as part of the comprehensive cardiac assessment.

PERICARDIAL DISEASE

Background

Few medical situations exist in which a simple, quickly performed medical procedure can result in immediate, lifesaving results. Among these is pericardiocentesis for cardiac tamponade. The technical aspects of pericardiocentesis are discussed elsewhere (see Procedures in Section VII). This section addresses etiologic concerns, clinical findings, and other initial management measures that must be taken to satisfactorily evaluate and treat the child with pericardial disease.

Three forms of illness can affect the pericardium. *Pericarditis*, not always a true medical emergency, is a nonspecific term that denotes inflammatory disease. *Pericardial effusion*, a condition that requires close evaluation but does not necessarily require emergency treatment, implies fluid accumulation within the pericardial space. *Cardiac tamponade*, a true medical emergency that requires immediate attention, connotes a situation in which impairment of ventricular filling has resulted from pericardial fluid accumulation or from constriction of the heart by an abnormally thickened pericardium, resulting in impairment of CO.

Table 84.19 reviews some of the principal causes of pericarditis in childhood. When considering the cause of pericardial disease and its clinical correlates, it is important to remember that the pericardium is in continuity with the surrounding intrathoracic structures. Thus, conditions that affect the pleura, the mediastinal structures, or the diaphragm may affect the pericardium as well.

Infectious diseases remain the most likely cause of pericarditis in childhood. Although a viral etiology frequently is presumed to be causative, in only about 20% to 30% of the time is an actual viral pathogen confirmed. Coxsackie (group B) and enteric cytopathogenic human orphan (ECHO) viruses are paramount, but other agents, including rubella, Epstein-Barr virus, adenovirus, influenza virus, and mumps virus, have all been associated with pericardial inflammation and pericardial effusion. Rarely do viral diseases result in cardiac tamponade.

Purulent pericarditis is often a medical emergency, however, because of associated cardiac tamponade and because of important sequelae that may be mitigated by early effective treatment. Although it is a disease seen at all pediatric ages, approximately 30% of the cases involve children younger than the age of 6 years. *Staphylococcus aureus*, *Haemophilus influenzae*, *Neisseria meningitides*, *Streptococcus pneumoniae*, and other streptococci are the principal bacterial agents responsible for childhood pyogenic pericarditis, although other pathogens have been recovered occasionally. Since *H. influenzae* immunization began, this pathogen is much less frequently seen. Other organisms may also cause pericardial infection and chief among these is *Mycobacterium tuberculosis*. In patients from underdeveloped countries, in fact, *M. tuberculosis* may be equally as common as *S. aureus* as a cause of pericardial infection and must not be overlooked in that population. Associated infections, such as respiratory tract disease, osteomyelitis, or pyogenic arthritis, may be present and may be clinically helpful at indicating the specific organism involved. For example, reviews have noted that many cases of staphylococcal pericarditis were associated with infections distant to the pericardium, such as osteomyelitis, whereas most cases of *H. influenzae pericarditis* were associated with respiratory tract infection. Meningococcemia is associated with pericardial involvement in about 5% of cases.

In childhood, noninfectious pericardial disease can also be significant. The postpericardiotomy syndrome is nearly always associated with pericardial inflammation and must be thought of in the postoperative cardiac patient who develops a pericardial effusion, fever, leukocytosis, and a high ESR after the first week and until several weeks after surgery. This syndrome may occur in as many as 10% to 15% of children who undergo open heart surgery, particularly older children and adolescents. Other important causes of pericardial inflammation include collagen vascular and rheumatic diseases and oncologic diseases, especially mediastinal lymphoma. Kawasaki disease can also be associated with pericardial effusion.

Pathophysiology

As noted earlier, pericardial inflammation is not usually life-threatening. Of concern for the physician who evaluates a child in an emergency situation are the hemodynamic sequelae of either fluid accumulation in the pericardial space or scarring and thickening of the pericardium, leading to restriction of cardiac filling. Usually, a small amount of intrapericardial fluid (less than 30 to 50 mL) exists in an equilibrium state between secretion into the pericardial space and reabsorption. With a sudden accumulation of fluid or with a more gradual increase of large amounts of fluid within the pericardial sac, interference with ventricular filling occurs, leading to decreased stroke volume and to falling BP. Cardiac filling may be compromised through several interrelated mechanisms, including an increased ventricular end-diastolic pressure, a decreased gradient for venous return, premature AV valve closure, and shortened diastolic time. The clinical manifestation of these physiologic aberrations, known as *cardiac tamponade*, is directly related to the severity of these abnormalities and to compensatory mechanisms evoked to overcome them.

Clinical Manifestations

A history of onset of respiratory difficulties after resolution of an upper respiratory illness may indicate pericardial disease in some instances. Chest pain, usually a benign symptom in childhood, is common with pericardial inflammation. This pain varies, depending on position.

Occasionally, abdominal pain may be the presenting symptom. The child with significant pericardial effusion may show clinical signs similar to several of those noted in the preceding section on CHF. Tachypnea, secondary to raised pulmonary venous pressures and decreased pulmonary compliance, is usually present. This may be associated with intercostal retractions. Reduced cardiac output may result in peripheral vasoconstriction, manifested by cool extremities, pallor, or decreased systemic BP. Elevated systemic venous pressures cause neck vein distention, hepatomegaly, and on occasion in more of a chronic picture, protein loss through either the gastrointestinal tract or the urine. Tachycardia is a universal finding and is representative of an effective compensatory mechanism, but only up to a point. This compensation is limited because diastolic filling times are further shortened by the increased HR.

The cardiac auscultatory findings directly relate to the degree of pericardial fluid accumulation. A friction rub (the scratching harsh sound that can be heard throughout the cardiac cycle) is often not audible in the presence of significant amounts of intrapericardial fluid and may become apparent only after pericardiocentesis. The heart sounds are usually distant or muffled, and the apical impulse is weak. In general, the presence of a quiet precordium in the face of the previously noted respiratory and circulatory changes should alert the examiner to the possibility of pericardial disease with effusion.

The sine qua non of cardiac tamponade is pulsus paradoxus. The finding of a paradoxical pulse greater than 20 mm Hg is unequivocal evidence of circulatory compromise. In addition, most clinicians assume as little as 10 mm Hg is suggestive of hemodynamic impairment.

The physiologic mechanisms that underlie pulsus paradoxus can be viewed as exaggerated examples of the integrated functioning of the cardiopulmonary unit. Normally, a small fall (less than 10 mm Hg) in systolic BP is noted with inspiration as a result of several factors. As negative intrathoracic pressure is generated by the inspiratory effort, the gradient for systemic venous return increases, favoring right-sided heart filling. At the same time, diaphragmatic descent exerts a traction effect on the heart, limiting filling and ejection. In addition, there may be some decrease in pulmonary venous return because the gradient from pulmonary veins to left atrium is probably reduced. Thus, left-sided heart output and systemic BP are reduced. The pericardium itself is an additional variable factor. In general, because it envelops the heart, the pericardium tends to retard expansion of ventricular volume, normally only to a limited degree. Thus, in normal respiration, the pericardium exerts an additional volume-reducing effect on the left ventricle. In pericardial disease states, as the pericardium itself becomes more rigid or as fluid in the pericardial space increases and intrapericardial pressure rises, the restriction to left ventricular output becomes greater and the consequent decline in systemic BP becomes steeper.

The best method of detecting pulsus paradoxus is to measure BP first in the usual way at expiration and then to inflate the cuff a second time to a few millimeters of mercury above the systolic BP and allow the cuff to deflate slowly. As the pressure falls, the Korotkoff sounds disappear with each inspiration. At the point at which they cease to disappear, becoming equal to that auscultated during expiration, the measured BP is recorded. The difference between the initial maximum systolic BP and the final measurement is the pulsus paradoxus.

It should be noted that pulsus paradoxus is not a finding unique to cardiac tamponade. It is a common finding in respiratory tract disease (asthma) and also may be present in CHF without pericardial effusion or in conditions with acute volume loss or circulating volume insufficiency.

Laboratory Findings

Laboratory findings vary according to the underlying causes of pericardial disease. Although cardiac tamponade is a clinical diagnosis, certain laboratory tools can be extremely helpful in clarifying the situation.

The EKG shows diminished precordial voltage in most instances of significant intrapericardial fluid accumulation (Fig. 84.16). With pericarditis, an associated current of injury pattern that reflects myocardial involvement, seen as elevations in the ST segments, may also be present. Diffuse T-wave inversions are also common. The heart size is increased on chest radiograph (Fig. 84.17) with pericardial effusion but can be entirely normal

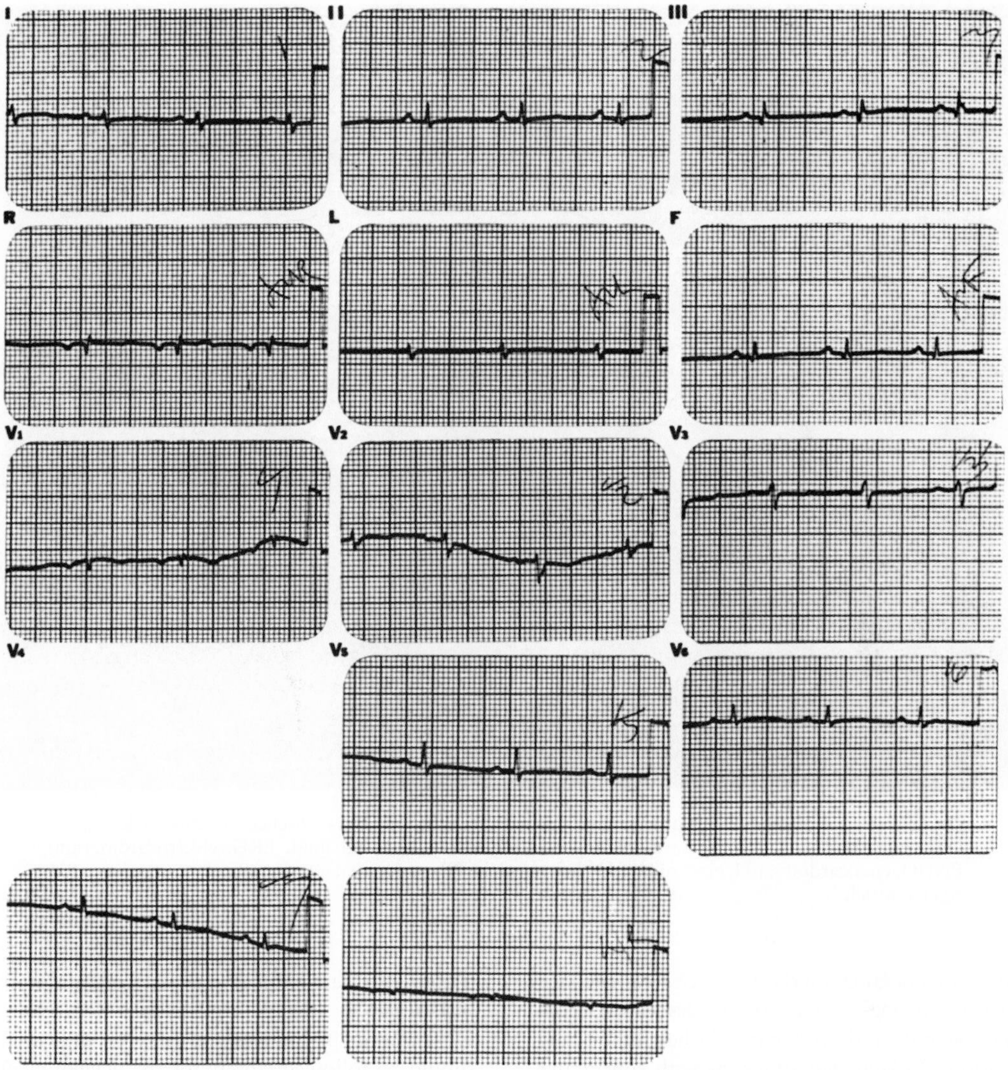

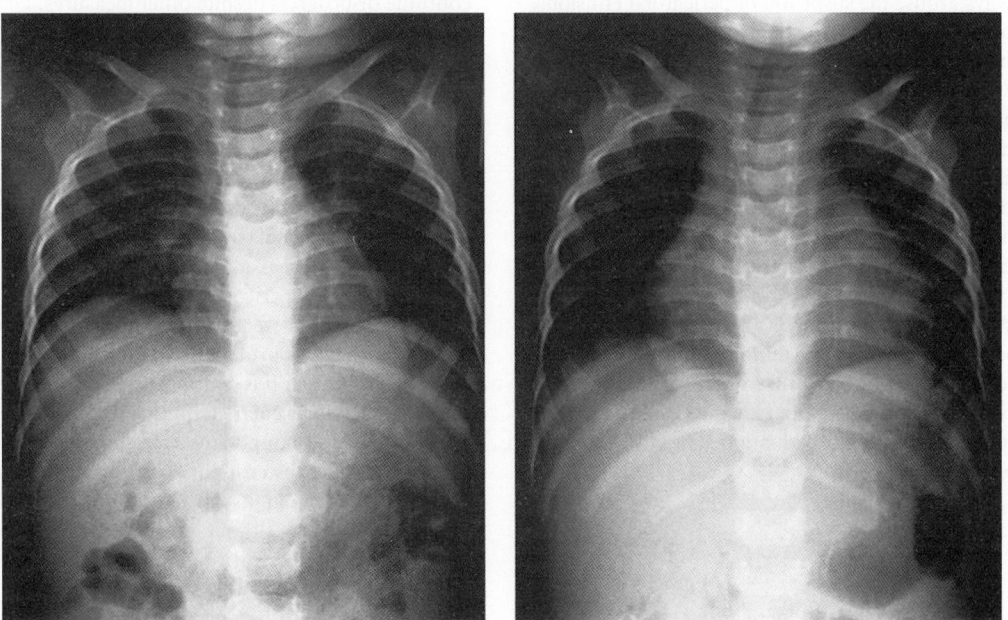

FIGURE 84.16 Electrocardiogram in pericardial effusion. Generalized low voltage present. ST-T wave flattening is present.

FIGURE 84.17 Radiographs from an infant 4 days before and at the time of the diagnosis of purulent pericarditis. Note the increasing heart size and the "water-bottle" silhouette.

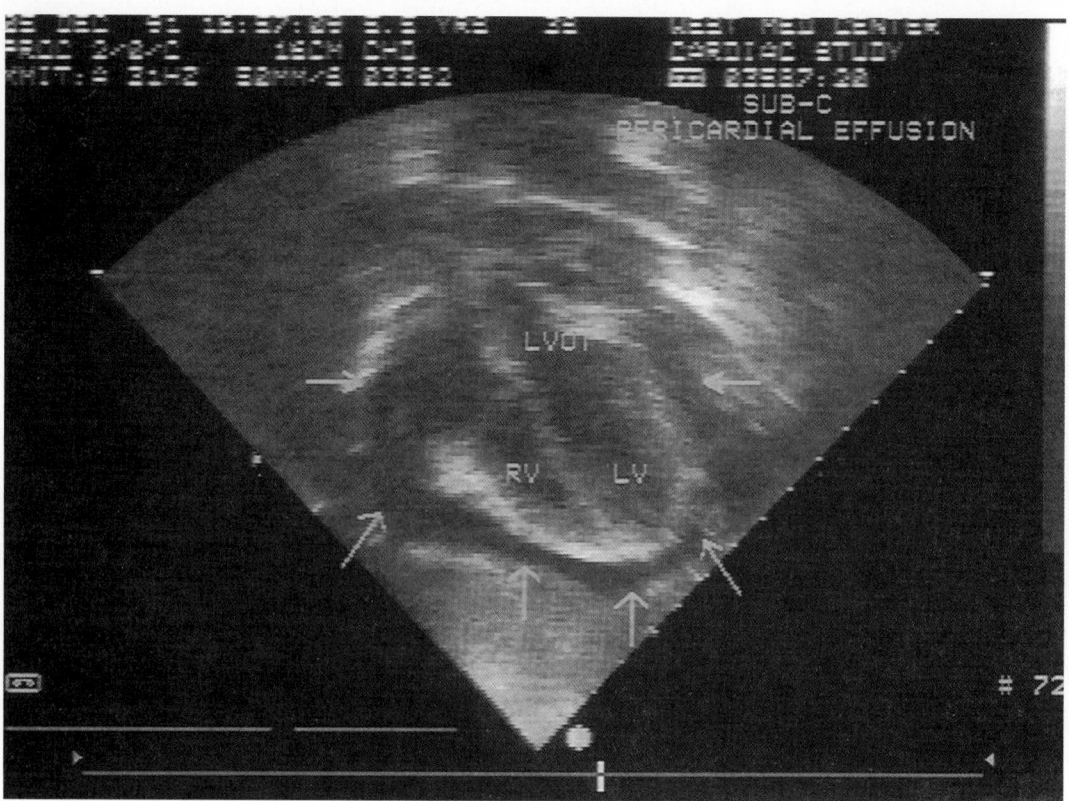

FIGURE 84.18 M-mode echocardiogram in pericardial effusion. Note absence of echoes (clear area) between epicardium and pericardium, representing intrapericardial fluid. EKG, electrocardiogram; ENDO, endocardium; EPI, epicardium; LV, left ventricle; PE, pericardial effusion; PERI, pericardium; RV, right ventricle.

if the amount of intrapericardial fluid is not excessive. The lung fields may be clear, but one should look for associated bronchopneumonia or pleural effusions that may be helpful for diagnostic considerations. In some situations, as with constrictive pericarditis, the heart size may be relatively small. If the patient has had previous chest radiographs, a sudden increase in heart size should always arouse the suspicion of pericardial effusion.

Echocardiography is the diagnostic procedure of choice for determining the presence and amount of intrapericardial fluid. An echo-free space between the epicardium and the pericardium can be readily identified (Fig. 84.18), with a negligible incidence of false-positive diagnoses in experienced hands. Quantitation is not precise, but evidence of anterior and posterior fluid accumulation suggests a large collection. Two-dimensional real-time echocardiographic studies are preferred. In addition, serial evaluation of the pericardial space is easily accomplished with echocardiography and is helpful for observing the effects of treatment and for evaluating indications for further therapeutic maneuvers after initial drainage measures.

As with the evaluation of any other potentially life-threatening infection, when infectious pericardial disease is suspected, a complete bacteriologic evaluation should be initiated before antibiotic therapy is begun.

Management

For pericarditis without evidence of pericardial effusion, emergency invasive treatment is usually not indicated. Symptomatic therapy for pain should be prescribed, and nonsteroidal anti-inflammatory drugs are useful. Bed rest is advisable. Observation in the hospital may be indicated. The patient should be followed closely for the development of complications such as myocarditis, pericardial effusion, or cardiac tamponade. Steroids usually are not indicated unless signs continue or progress despite other measures. Diagnostic evaluation to identify the cause should be initiated.

For newly diagnosed pericardial effusion, when more than mild, a definitive approach is needed. Careful evaluation of vital signs and frequent attention to development of pulsus paradoxus are mandatory. Cardiology consultation should be obtained, and the patient is usually admitted for evaluation. Diagnostic pericardiocentesis often is needed in the de novo presentation, particularly without evidence of other forms of systemic disease; it is almost always required with the suspicion of a purulent pericardial process. Antibiotic therapy alone is not adequate for treatment of purulent pericarditis. Usually, in the presence of purulent pericarditis, an open drainage procedure is indicated. It is contingent on the emergency physician to ensure cardiovascular stability in the presence of pericardial effusion because tamponade can develop rapidly once maximum pericardial distensibility has been reached (Table 84.20).

The management of cardiac tamponade requires intense medical vigilance. Although it may be possible in relatively mild or highly selected situations to manage the effusion conservatively, it is generally necessary to remove the fluid. A full discussion of the techniques used for pericardiocentesis in the emergency situation is available in Section VII of this book.

TABLE 84.20

PURULENT PERICARDITIS: IMMEDIATE MANAGEMENT

1. Ensure adequacy of ventilation and cardiac output
2. Administer oxygen
3. Initiate cardiorespiratory monitoring
4. Obtain laboratory studies (simultaneously with step 5)
   Complete blood cell count, platelet count, electrolytes, blood urea nitrogen, creatinine, glucose, arterial blood gas, blood culture, chest radiograph, electrocardiography, echocardiography
5. Achieve venous access
6. Pericardiocentesis (see Section VII)
   Send specimen for laboratory studies: cultures, CIE, viral titers, antinuclear antibody, Gram stain, cytology, cell count and differential, chemical profile
7. Administer antibiotics[a]
   Oxacillin (150–200 mg/kg/day) or nafcillin or methicillin and chloramphenicol (100 mg/kg/day) or third-generation cephalosporin
   Aminoglycoside (immunocompromised patient)
   Most centers also prefer vancomycin until cultures and sensitivities reported in view of methicillin-resistant staphylococci (MRSA)

CIE, counter immune electrophoresis.
[a]Select antimicrobials to cover *S. aureus*.

This can be a lifesaving technique and, when done successfully, shows clearly the fruitful outcome of appropriate, decisive evaluation and treatment procedures.

INFECTIVE ENDOCARDITIS

Background

One of the persistently complex problems of pediatric cardiovascular medicine has been the evaluation and management of the child with infective endocarditis. Although long-term treatment issues are generally not within the province of emergency medical care, it is critically important for the emergency physician to be aware of the clinical context in which bacterial endocarditis is a consideration. It is also incumbent on the emergency physician to initiate therapy in certain instances, and it is always crucial to avoid unnecessary clouding of the diagnosis.

Etiologic Factors and Prophylaxis Considerations

The clinical picture of infective endocarditis has been evolving steadily during the past 10 to 20 years. Although the most common pediatric setting for this problem is the child with preexisting CHD, variability exists in terms of the types of associated lesions (Fig. 84.19), and it is of concern that a substantial proportion of cases develop in children with no history of cardiac abnormality. These children may be among the most ill, presenting with their illness as part of an acute bacterial endocarditis picture.

Certain physiologic conditions appear to be consistently most important in the development of IE. Diseases characterized by a highly turbulent stream of blood and/or a high velocity of flow are most prone to this complication. Such lesions include VSD, aortic valve stenosis, and mitral valve regurgitation. Children with palliative systemic-to-pulmonary shunts are also in this category. In contrast, secundum atrial septal defect is a lesion with a negligible risk for endocarditis because the shunt flow is of low velocity. It is presumed that in "high velocity–narrow orifice" conditions, damage to cardiac surfaces occurs, resulting in a nidus for platelet deposition and vegetation formation.

While these physiologic factors appear to predispose a child to the development of endocarditis, recent reviews and published guidelines have indicated changed perspectives with regard to iatrogenic influences for IE development. Direct, unequivocal evidence has never been demonstrated to substantiate the belief that dental and medical procedures *per se* are causally related to the development of endocarditis. Dental procedures even without periodontal disease can yield bacteremia of course. Invasive diagnostic medical procedures can

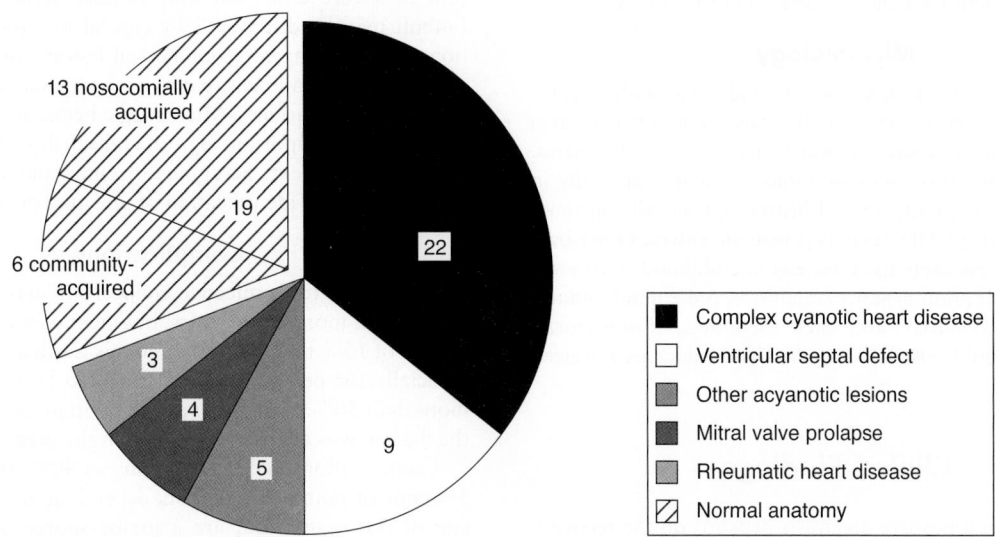

FIGURE 84.19 Distribution of underlying cardiovascular findings in endocarditis in a series of 62 children. (Reprinted from Saiman L, Prince A, Gersony WM. Pediatric endocarditis in the modern era. *J Pediatr* 1993;122:847–853, with permission.)

MEDICAL EMERGENCIES

TABLE 84.21

TRANSIENT BACTEREMIA AND VARIOUS
PROCEDURES OR CONDITIONS

Procedures	Bacteremia (%)
Tooth extractions (no gingivitis)	34
Tooth extractions (gingivitis)	74–75
Endodontic procedures	4
Chewing mint candy	20
Brushing teeth	40
Oral irrigation device	27–50
Massage of infected tonsil	23
Urethral surgery	57
Massage of infected prostate	67
Barium enema	11
Bronchoscopy	15
Sigmoidoscopy	5–10

Modified from Kaye D, ed. *Prophylaxis of endocarditis.* Baltimore:
University Park Press, 1976:245–265, with permission.

TABLE 84.22

CARDIAC CONDITIONS ASSOCIATED WITH HIGH
RISK OF ADVERSE OUTCOME FROM ENDOCARDITIS

Prosthetic cardiac valve
Previous Infective Endocarditis
Congenital heart disease (CHD)[a]
   Unrepaired cyanotic CHD, including palliative shunts and
     conduits
   Completely repaired congenital heart defect with prosthetic
     material or device, whether placed by surgery or by
     catheter intervention, during the first 6 months after the
     procedure[b]
   Repaired CHD with residual defects at the site or adjacent
     to the site of a prosthetic
   Patch or prosthetic device (which inhibit endothelialization)
Cardiac transplantation recipients who develop cardiac valvu-
   lopathy

[a]Except for the conditions listed above, antibiotic prophylaxis is no
longer recommended for any other form of CHD.
[b]Prophylaxis is recommended because endothelialization of prosthetic
material occurs within 6 months after the procedure.
Adapted from Wilson W, Taubert K, Gewitz M, et al. Infective endocarditis. In: Allen H, Shaddy R, Driscoll D, et al., eds. *Moss and
Adams' heart disease in infants, children, and adolescents, including the
fetus and young adult.* 7th ed. Lippincott, Williams & Wilkins, 2008.

as well. Unfortunately, many ordinary daily events are also
associated with at least transient bacteremia (Table 84.21). It
is small wonder, in fact, that more cases of endocarditis are not
evident if bacteremia of oral cavity origin, for instance, were a
singular factor. Conversely, invasive procedures specifically
involving the heart, such as cardiac catheterization, in patients
with even the highest risk, are rarely associated with endocarditis development. Therefore, current recommendations
emanating from scientific bodies worldwide have questioned
the long-held dictum that use of prophylactic antibiotics to
prevent IE after dental or medical procedures is a useful practice in which potential harm outweighs potential risk. Given
this concern, for example, a recent review by The Committee
on Rheumatic Fever, Endocarditis and Kawasaki Disease of
the American Heart Association suggested that prophylactic
antibiotics be considered only for those conditions likely to
predispose to the most serious adverse sequelae *from* endocarditis (Table 84.22). In these selected circumstances, specific
antibiotic regimens have been suggested (Table 84.23).

Microbiology

Causative organisms include bacteria and fungi with streptococci species in general remain the most common causative
agents, with viridans streptococci being the typical isolates.
Staphylococci are also common etiologic agents, especially in
children with structurally normal hearts or, ironically, in those
with postoperative CHD, such as prosthetic valves. Other bacteria are much less likely to be present in childhood endocarditis. These include gram-negative organisms, present in immunocompromised children and sick neonates, *Enterococci*,
Pneumococci, and *Hemophilus* species. These data are reviewed
in Table 84.24.

Clinical Findings

Confirmation of a positive diagnosis depends on the recovery
of organisms obtained by blood culture. To arrive at that
point, however, a high degree of suspicion must be maintained.

Often, early signs and symptoms can be subtle and persist for
considerable time before the diagnosis is made. With viridans
streptococcal endocarditis, this is a common situation. As a
rule, lengthy persistence of fever in any child with CHD should
alert the clinician to consider the possibility of endocarditis.

In the clinical context of CHD, certain conditions should
prompt a careful evaluation for the presence of endocarditis.
These include (i) unexplained fever or a protracted febrile
course in a presumed "viral" syndrome, (ii) pneumonia, (iii) the
development of a new neurologic deficit, (iv) the onset of hematuria, and (v) signs of systemic or cutaneous embolization.

The classic findings of fever, a change in the cardiac examination, splenomegaly, and evidence of emboli are usually present in severe cases but may require serial examinations.
Emboli may be discovered by careful funduscopic examination, by observing for conjunctival lesions, or by meticulous
scrutiny of the nail beds, palms of the hands, soles of the feet,
and other skin surfaces. Microscopic hematuria should be recognized as an important sign of endocarditis in the appropriate clinical context. Scrapings of cutaneous emboli may be
helpful for rapid identification of infecting organisms.

Complications

The mortality from infective endocarditis has decreased considerably in more recent years, but most series still cite a fatality rate of 15% to 20%. Although this is still a high percentage,
especially for pediatric illness, it should be remembered that
more than 50% mortality was the norm in the 1950s and that
the disease was nearly always fatal in the preantibiotic era.

Complications occur in as many as 40% to 60% of cases.
Systemic or pulmonary emboli, depending on the intracardiac
site of the vegetation, are a major source of concern and
require prompt initiation of treatment. Major neurologic
sequelae can arise from focal embolization to the CNS; thus,

TABLE 84.23

ENDOCARDITIS PROPHYLAXIS REGIMENS

Situation	Agent	Regimen
For Dental, Oral, Respiratory Tract, or Esophageal Procedures		
Standard general prophylaxis	Amoxicillin	50 mg/kg po 1 h preprocedure (max 2 g)
Unable to take oral medications	Ampicillin	50 mg/kg IV or IM within 30 min of procedure (max 2 g)
	Or	
	Cefazolin	50 mg/kg IM or IV (max 600 mg)
	Or	
	Ceftriaxone	
Allergic to penicillin	Clindamycin	20 mg/kg po 1 h preprocedure (max 600 mg)
	Or	
	Cephalexin	50 mg/kg po 1 h preprocedure (max 2 g)
	Or	
	Azithromycin or clarithromycin	15 mg/kg po 1 h preprocedure (max 500 mg)
Allergic to penicillin and unable to take oral medication	Clindamycin	20 mg/kg IV within 30 min of procedure (max 600 mg)
	Or	
	Cefazolin	25 mg/kg IV or IM within 30 min of procedure (max 1 g)

Second dose of vancomycin or gentamicin not recommended. Cephalosporins not usable in patients with immediate-type hypertensivity reactions to penicillins.
Adapted from Taubert K, Gewitz M. Infective endocarditis. In: Allen H, Shaddy R, Driscoll D, et al., eds. *Moss and Adams' heart disease in infants, children, and adolescents, including the fetus and young adult.* 7th ed. Lippincott, Williams & Wilkins, 2008.

the presentation of a new neurologic deficit in a child with heart disease can be another clinical clue to the diagnosis of endocarditis. Myocarditis, myocardial abscesses, valvar obstructions associated with large vegetations, and ruptured sinus of Valsalva are other important complications that can be manifested by the appearance of new-onset CHF.

Acute bacterial endocarditis, or the development of an acute situation such as new aortic insufficiency, should be considered a true medical emergency. Often, early reparative surgery is required to save the child's life in this situation. These children are critically ill, and CHF is a grave sign in the context of suspected endocarditis. Characteristic heart murmurs may be absent in this setting; their absence should not be taken as a cause for optimism. Other indications for surgery

include the development of a new cardiac arrhythmia (heart block), continued embolization, and continued positive blood cultures after initiation of appropriate therapy. Hemodynamic changes can transpire quickly, demanding frequent examinations even while the child awaits hospital admission or transfer from the ED.

Management

Treatment of infective endocarditis should be started as early as possible after appropriate evaluation is completed. Blood cultures must be drawn regardless of the presence or absence of classic clinical findings. To facilitate the diagnosis, the

TABLE 84.24

PRINCIPAL PATHOGENIC BACTERIAL AGENTS IN ENDOCARDITIS

	Series		
Organism	Johnson et al. (N = 149)	Martin et al. (N = 76)	Stockheim et al. (N = 11)
Viridans group streptococci	43	38	32
Staphylococcus aureus	33	32	27
Coagulase-negative staphylococci	2	4	12
Streptococcus pneumoniae	3	4	7
HACEK	NA	5	4
Enterococcus species	NA	7	4
Culture negative	6	7	5

Values indicate percentage of patients in the series.
Reprinted from Ferrieri P, Gewitz M, Gerber M, et al. Unique features of infective endocarditis in childhood. *Circulation* 2002;105:2115–2127, with permission.

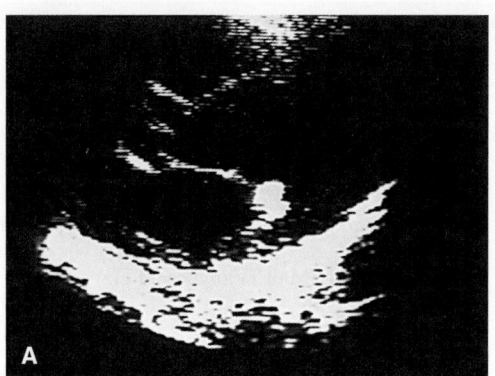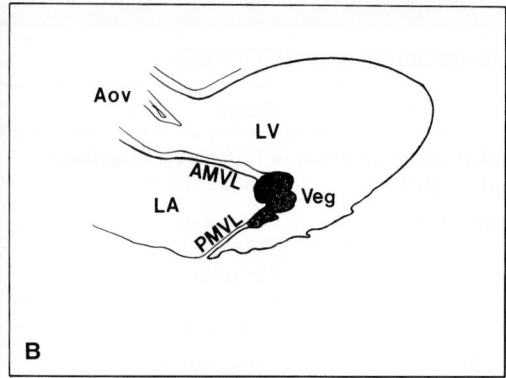

FIGURE 84.20 A: Long-axis parasternal two-dimensional echocardiogram in patient with mitral valve pneumococcal endocarditis. **B:** Schematic view of (**A**). AMVL, anterior mitral valve leaflet; Aov, aortic valve; LA, left atrium; LV, left ventricle; PMVL, posterior mitral valve leaflet; Veg, vegetation.

physician, particularly one who evaluates a child with heart disease with unexplained fever, must obtain blood for appropriate cultures at an early stage. In most cases of endocarditis, the causative organism will be recovered from the initial two blood cultures. Particular emphasis should be placed on avoiding contamination of the sample site. Growth of spurious organisms can be misleading and dangerously time-consuming because bacteria on the skin can be implicated in endocarditis. It is not mandatory to obtain cultures at the time of fever spikes because bacteremia is fairly constant in the untreated patient. Early consultation should be sought from a cardiologist, since specialized procedures such as echocardiography may help pinpoint the diagnosis rapidly, even in relatively difficult situations (Fig. 84.20).

In every instance, the diagnosis of infectious endocarditis implies long-term antibiotic therapy; thus, most management issues arise after the patient has left the emergency area. In general, antibiotic therapy should be instituted as soon as the diagnosis is made. If the patient is critically ill, it may be necessary to initiate therapy even before the results have returned. Certainly, stabilization of the patient with heart failure, initiation of the diagnostic workup, and mobilization of the relevant medical personnel are the responsibilities of the emergency physician in dealing with the child with suspected endocarditis. If the situation requires the initiation of therapy without definition of the microbial agent, many experts recommend the combination of an aminoglycoside, such as gentamicin (5 to 7.5 mg per kg per day), and a penicillinase-resistant penicillin, such as oxacillin (150 mg per kg per day). Others advocate the use of ampicillin (200 mg per kg per day) and gentamicin for the initial therapy in this particular situation plus vancomycin in areas where methacillin-resistant staphylococci are of concern. Cephalosporins such as cefuroxime may also play a role in this context.

It is important to remember that the child with heart disease who presents with a routine febrile illness does not always immediately require antibiotics. Unnecessarily hasty administration of antibiotics when not clearly indicated can be harmful because obfuscation of the ultimate diagnosis may result in damaging delay in the initiation of effective therapy. If systemic antibiotics are contemplated for specific indications, in most cases a blood count and a blood culture should be drawn *before* antibiotic therapy begins. In particular, these

measures should be taken for the child with heart disease and a major infection, such as pneumonia or cellulitis, even if no clinical evidence of endocarditis is immediately apparent. It is not mandatory to admit the child with heart disease and an intercurrent febrile illness to the hospital on every occasion, and the previously noted laboratory studies may be helpful in making such a decision. Clinical judgment remains the best immediate guide for hospitalization. Although a high degree of suspicion for the possibility of endocarditis is mandatory, the emergency physician should resist the temptation to administer antibiotics indiscriminately to the child with heart disease.

HYPOXEMIC ATTACKS

Background

Children with CHD in which pulmonary blood flow is reduced, such as tetralogy of Fallot, may experience periodic episodes of intense hypoxemia. Emergency attention is usually sought for these episodes at the nearest medical location. Therefore, the emergency physician who cares for children should have a good understanding of the associated physiologic and management principles.

Pathophysiology

The reasons for the acute nature of these episodes have never been precisely defined. Initial thoughts that "cyanotic spells" were caused by spasmodic contraction of the portion of right ventricular outflow tract known as the "infundibulum" cannot provide the entire explanation because children with pulmonary atresia in whom no subpulmonic infundibulum has developed can also experience hypercyanotic attacks. Additional theoretical concerns have focused on (i) sudden changes in systemic vascular resistance and in venous return to the heart, which consequently affect the intracardiac right-to-left shunt; (ii) alterations in sensitivity of the respiratory center; (iii) significant changes in HR; or (iv) some combination of these factors. A classic schematic cycle of postulated mechanisms is noted in Fig. 84.21.

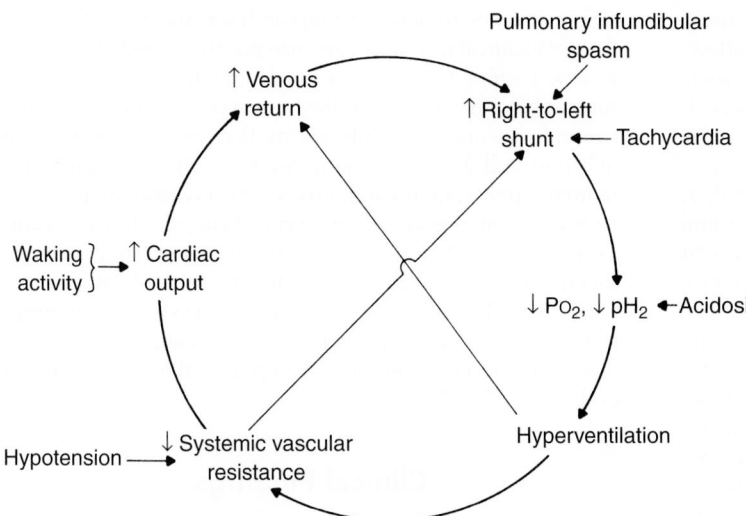

FIGURE 84.21 Schema of interrelated events in the genesis of hypoxemic spells. See text for discussion. (Reprinted from Anthony CL, Arnon RG, Fitch CW, eds. *Pediatric cardiology*. Medical Outline Series. Garden City, NY: Medical Examination Publishing, 1979:193, with permission.)

Any number of precipitant events related to these physiologic factors can be associated with the development of cyanotic spells. Often, they are morning events, noted shortly after awakening. This may be related to the sudden changes in CO that occur after arousal from a long sleep. Other likely times for the appearance of hypercyanosis include periods of dehydration, during invasive medical procedures, or in the face of other significant stresses. The incidence of cyanotic spells is much lower now than in the past because many patients with cyanotic lesions undergo early palliative surgical correction.

Clinical Findings

The diagnosis of a hypoxemic spell usually is self-evident. Aside from the obvious cyanosis and the history of heart disease, there also may be a preceding history of squatting with exertion or of other positional vagaries that parents may recall. It is not necessary for the child to have been overtly cyanotic before the onset of a spell because such episodes can occur in children with little or no preexisting visible cyanosis. During a spell, the child may be irritable and crying or may conversely may be lethargic or even unconscious. Hyperpnea is a feature of the syndrome and should be distinguished from tachypnea or other abnormal respiratory patterns that may signal other medical problems associated with heart disease. During a spell, there may be a notable absence or lessening of a previously heard heart murmur because pulmonary blood flow through the stenotic right ventricular outflow tract is reduced considerably. Laboratory investigations, such as arterial blood gas analysis, ordinarily should be avoided in the initial evaluation. If the attack is prolonged and associated with deepening sensorium changes, assessment of acid–base balance and ventilatory status may then be indicated. Monitoring with peripheral oxygen saturation meters may be helpful to chart responses to therapy.

Management

The child with hypoxemic spells requires immediate attention. Appropriate positioning, oxygen, and administration of morphine are the standard initial therapeutic measures, and these usually result in prompt abatement of the attack (Table 84.25).

Traditionally, subcutaneous morphine has been used in the treatment of cyanotic spells. Relatively large doses are given (0.1 to 0.2 mg per kg), although the precise mechanism of action is not known. Morphine probably does not act to inhibit catecholamine action at the cardiac level but may abort the cycle of hyperpnea and vasomotor changes by depressing the respiratory center. A theoretical negative effect of morphine is its tendency to lower systemic vascular resistance.

Oxygen should be administered because PaO_2 levels may be low and some benefit in terms of oxygen saturation may be obtained from even relatively small increments in dissolved oxygen. In the face of significant reduction of pulmonary blood flow, however, as occurs with a "spell," oxygen may not have a dramatic effect.

The child should be placed in a knee–chest position and calmed, if possible. If the attack persists, additional therapeutic steps are needed. Sodium bicarbonate may be indicated; the dosage depends on arterial pH. High dose IV propranolol has also been recognized as efficacious in this situation, and a dose

TABLE 84.25

ACUTE MANAGEMENT OF HYPOXEMIC SPELLS

Knee–chest position
Oxygen administration
Evaluate and treat cardiac arrhythmia
Morphine sulfate (subcutaneous; 0.1–0.2 mg/kg)
Propranolol IV (0.2 mg/kg over 5 min)
IV fluids
Vasoconstrictors
  Phenylephrine 10–20 μg/kg bolus,
  IM *or* subcutaneous; 0.1–0.5 μg/kg/min infusion IV titrated to HR or BP limits. Higher doses may occasionally be needed.
  Methoxamine 0.10 mg/kg IV
  Bicarbonate (2–3 mEq/kg IV; ensure adequate ventilation)

IV, intravenous; IM, intramuscular.

MEDICAL EMERGENCIES

of 0.2 mg per kg IV over 4 to 5 minutes may yield relatively prompt improvement. Whether propranolol primarily affects the infundibular contraction, the hyperpneic ventilatory response, systemic vasomotor tone, or all these is unclear. It should be remembered that propranolol may exacerbate bronchospasm if the patient has a coincident history of asthma.

IV fluids should be administered during the severe spell, at least in maintenance doses, because pulmonary blood flow and right ventricular output depend on volume. Functionally, right ventricular outflow obstruction may be heightened in the face of depleted intravascular volume.

Vasopressors are used as alternates or adjuncts in treating hypoxemic spells. Phenylephrine can be given as a dilute IV solution of 10 mg per 100 mL and infused at 2 to 10 μg per kg per minute. HR should be monitored and frequent BP assessment carried out if this type of agent is used. Methoxamine (10 mg per 100 mL) or metaraminol (50 mg per 100 mL) may also be used. By increasing systemic vascular resistance, these drugs reduce intracardiac right-to-left shunting favorably and thus improve systemic oxygenation. Digitalis, epinephrine, or norepinephrine, however, should not be used in this setting.

If any underlying condition exists, such as a cardiac rhythm disturbance, prompt correction according to the principles noted under the "Cardiac Arrhythmias" section may alleviate hypoxemic attacks quickly. Cardiac consultation is advisable as soon as feasible to make extended management decisions, even if the spell has abated with the measures already mentioned. In most situations, if the spell has required more than oxygen and positional adjustment to relieve, hospitalization is indicated. Usually, even though relieved with therapy, spells indicate that appropriate surgery for the cardiac defect is required in the near term.

ACUTE RHEUMATIC FEVER

Background

Although the large numbers of patients with rheumatic fever seen in the past in the United States have dissipated because of improved diagnosis and treatment of streptococcal infections, the disease still occurs and has had occasional resurgence in some areas of the United States. Also, rheumatic fever remains one of the most frequent causes of cardiovascular morbidity in children from other countries. The most common age of attack is 5 to 15 years, and winter and spring seasonal peaks are still typical.

Pathophysiology

It has been established clearly that group A beta-hemolytic streptococcal infection is a necessary precedent for the development of rheumatic fever. In particular, a history of infection by this organism of the upper respiratory tract should be sought in any suspected case. The precise mechanistic relationship between antecedent streptococcal infection and rheumatic fever remains ill-defined. Several serologic types of group A streptococci can be associated with acute rheumatic fever so the antigenic factors involved are common to various strains of the organism. The particular host factors that determine

who succumbs to acute rheumatic fever and who does not, despite identical infections, are also poorly defined. A clear-cut genetic pattern has never been identified, although familial susceptibility has been identified for over a century. The more common theoretic considerations that relate streptococcal infection and acute rheumatic fever are (i) an immunologic (autoimmune) response that involves host reaction to infection with a rheumatogenic streptococcus being the heart, specifically, endocardial tissue; (ii) a persistence of organism, despite therapy, with localization to cardiac tissue; and (iii) a direct reaction to the organism, such as cardiotoxicity from streptolysin O produced by the organism. Thus far, no evidence of direct cardiac infection has developed, making experimental evaluation difficult.

Clinical Findings

The diagnosis of rheumatic fever requires a high index of suspicion. The time-honored classic Jones criteria (Table 84.26), if unequivocally present, usually establish the diagnosis, but the situation may not be always so clear-cut.

A complete, careful physical examination is the mandatory first procedure. Special attention should be given to eliciting joint pathology and cutaneous findings, the presence of which may facilitate the diagnosis in difficult cases. The major Jones criteria are derived through clinical examination that usually needs to be repeated at frequent intervals. Of the major criteria, carditis can be over diagnosed easily. Misinterpretation of normal ("innocent") murmurs, whose auscultation is heightened in the presence of fever or other causes of increased CO, can lead to over diagnosis. The presence of an

---

TABLE 84.26

RHEUMATIC FEVER MANIFESTATIONS (CLASSIC)

Major
Carditis
Arthritis
Subcutaneous nodules
Erythema marginatum
Chorea

Minor
Clinical findings
  Arthralgia
  Fever
Laboratory findings
  Elevated acute phase reactants
    Erythrocyte sedimentation rate
    C-reactive protein
  Prolonged PR interval
  Supporting evidence of antecedent group A streptococcal
    infections
      Positive throat culture of rapid streptococcal antibody
        titer
      Elevated or rising streptococcal antibody titer

Adapted from Jones TD. The diagnosis of rheumatic fever. *JAMA* 1944; 126:481, as modified in Dajani A, Ayoub E, Bierman FZ, et al. Guidelines for the diagnosis of rheumatic fever. *JAMA* 1992;268: 2069–2073.

apical systolic murmur (characteristic of mitral insufficiency) or a basal diastolic decrescendo murmur (typical of aortic insufficiency) can be important signs of carditis. The presence of a pericardial effusion, CHF, or pericarditis also strongly suggests the carditis, even in the absence of valvar murmurs. Care must be taken to exclude other causes for cardiac findings, such as deteriorating CHD, which may result in cardiac decompensation not related to a rheumatic process. If possible, the examining physician should attempt to document a change in previous clinical findings in children with preexisting heart disease (or previous rheumatic fever episodes). Although regurgitant lesions such as aortic or mitral insufficiency are common components of the acute manifestations of rheumatic fever, stenotic lesions such as aortic or mitral stenosis are usually not seen with a first attack of acute rheumatic fever.

Polyarthritis is the most frequently found major criterion. It should be remembered that this is true joint inflammation, not arthralgia. Tenderness, motion restriction, heat, redness, and swelling are the typical signs. In contrast to other forms of collagen disease, joint involvement in rheumatic fever is usually migratory and multiple and tends to localize to the larger joints of the extremities. It may be necessary to avoid rapid use of antiinflammatory agents in patients with suspected acute rheumatic fever to clarify the diagnosis of migratory polyarthritis.

The cutaneous criteria are erythema marginatum and subcutaneous nodules. These findings are not as frequent as arthritis and carditis and are rarely present as the only major criteria. Nodules usually occur in situations of recurrent rheumatic fever or chronicity. They are found over extensor surfaces of joints such as elbows or knees, are firm and decidedly nontender, and are movable on palpation. Erythema marginatum characteristically appears on the trunk and proximal extremities and is an extremely evanescent finding. The application of heat may accentuate its appearance. This rash is notable for its fine, lacy appearance with central blanching and a serpiginous pattern. It is not pruritic and is usually easily distinguished from drug rashes or other viral exanthems.

Chorea is the fifth of the major criteria defined by Jones. It is a relatively rare finding limited to children older than the age of 3 years and most often occurs some time after the initial streptococcal infection, making accurate diagnosis difficult. Chorea is typified by involuntary purposeless movement of the extremities and facial grimacing. Notable emotional lability is also a part of the picture. The ED diagnosis of acute rheumatic fever rarely depends on chorea as the principal manifestation. The physician should be aware, however, of the possibility of the diagnosis in a child who presents with this finding and should arrange for appropriate further evaluation of the cause of the chorea.

The "minor criteria" defined by Jones are nonspecific indices of inflammatory disease and, frequently, are sources of overdiagnosis of acute rheumatic fever. The fever associated with acute rheumatic fever is notable for its lack of associated chills or rigor. It is typically low grade, and fevers of greater than 40°C (104°F) or a history of a febrile seizure should point to other illnesses. The wildly fluctuating fever of juvenile rheumatoid arthritis ("quotidian" pattern) is usually not a part of the rheumatic fever picture. Elevation

of the ESR or C-reactive protein should be present in acute rheumatic fever, but severe CHF may lower the ESR. A prolonged PR interval is not only a frequent occurrence in acute rheumatic fever, but is also an extremely nonspecific finding. It does not necessarily correlate with the presence of organic murmurs and can be found in other inflammatory cardiac diseases or as a result of certain drugs. Overemphasis of the significance of PR prolongation is a frequent cause of improper diagnosis.

The most recent modification of the Jones criteria includes evidence of recent streptococcal infection. Culture documentation, or confirmation with the rapid antigen detection test (RADT) can be diagnostic, but specificity of RADT can be low. Serologic evidence may be the most rewarding and diagnostic data. The antistreptolysin O (ASO) is still a commonly used single serologic test and is well standardized. Levels above 250 Todd units in older children and above 333 in younger children are present in active rheumatic fever. As many as 20% of otherwise normal children can have elevated ASO titers and, depending on the time course of the illness, other antibody determinations may be required.

The differential diagnosis of acute rheumatic fever includes many diseases that fall under the classification of "collagen-vascular," as well as other types of diseases. The Jones criteria themselves can include a spectrum of illnesses such as juvenile rheumatoid arthritis, serum sickness, systemic lupus, and even bacterial endocarditis or septic arthritis. Viral processes, such as myocarditis or pericarditis, must also be excluded, as well as unusual intracardiac lesions such as left atrial myxoma.

Careful application of the Jones criteria plus documentation of a streptococcal infection of recent onset should enable the physician to diagnose acute rheumatic fever most, but not all, of the time. Caution must be exercised in arriving at the diagnosis because initiation of therapy may suppress findings critical to the diagnosis. Thus, decisions to treat must be tempered with the understanding that it is vital to collect as much definition of the disease process as possible.

As noted earlier, acute phase reactants such as the ESR and C-reactive protein are elevated in acute rheumatic fever. A complete blood cell count should be drawn to screen for anemia or an elevated white blood cell count. Leukocytosis is not only a manifestation of infection, but may also be considered an "acute phase reactant." Throat cultures (at least two) should be obtained before penicillin therapy is started. In addition, the streptococcal serological screen previously described should be obtained. Blood cultures are frequently drawn, with appropriate concern, to rule out subacute bacterial endocarditis, a problem that can present in an identical fashion to acute rheumatic fever.

A chest x-ray to assess heart size can be helpful for gauging the severity of carditis, as well as for objective verification of its presence. An EKG should be taken to ensure that a rapid pulse rate is the result of sinus tachycardia and to enable measurement of PR interval. If pericardial disease or intracardiac myxoma needs to be ruled out, an echocardiogram can provide highly sensitive information. These latter procedures are usually completed, of course, after cardiac consultation has been requested. The appropriate laboratory procedures to help rule out other forms of collagen-vascular disease are described in Chapter 101.

Echocardiography has been advocated as a method in itself useful to establish the presence of carditis for some experts but such standards have not as yet been universally accepted. Readers should watch the literature for changes in this regards.

Management

Acute rheumatic fever requires admission to the hospital and chronic management. That is, a prolonged treatment course is indicated once the diagnosis is made. Most considerations in caring for a child with acute rheumatic fever are not made in the ED. It should be restated that a rush to treat with antiinflammatory drugs (aspirin or steroids) in a poorly documented case may obscure the ultimate diagnosis and may delay further therapy, thereby compromising more than helping the patient.

Principles of management include (i) treatment of the active streptococcal infection, (ii) rest, (iii) antiinflammatory agents, and (iv) treatment of chorea. All patients with acute rheumatic fever should receive a course of penicillin to eradicate any streptococci. IM benzathine penicillin in appropriate dosage for age and weight (see Chapter 81) is preferable. Reduced activity may be helpful while there is evidence of active inflammation. Antiinflammatory drugs (salicylates or steroids) may be indicated, but the tendency to begin such therapy before confirmation of the diagnosis, as outlined already, should be resisted. If arthritis without carditis is present, aspirin usually is sufficient (see Chapter 101). Treatment of carditis may include steroids, but that decision should be made only after the child is hospitalized and a cardiologist has been consulted. Treatment of chorea is also a long-term management issue, with agents such as diazepam or haloperidol favored. Recent evidence suggests a role for steroids in the treatment of chorea and for the presence of carditis.

Occasionally, the child with acute rheumatic fever may present with significant cardiac compromise that involves CHF associated with a large degree of valvar regurgitation or pericardial effusion that results in cardiac tamponade. Initially, heart failure or tamponade should be managed as outlined in the previous sections, and then consideration should be given to the rheumatic process.

A most important aspect of management of the patient with rheumatic fever is prevention of recurrent attacks. It has been documented clearly that penicillin can be effective in this setting, with minimal patient risk. The most reliable prophylaxis is the IM route, with injections of 600,000 units for children 27 kg or less and 1.2 million units for larger patients of benzathine penicillin G every 28 days being the preferred treatment. Oral penicillin (200,000 units twice daily 250 mg) is an alternative prophylactic regimen. Sulfonamides (Sulfadiazine) may be used in patients allergic to penicillin. Recommended dosages for the sulfonamides are 0.5 to 1.0 g daily, again depending on weight. Recent recommendations suggest continuing antibiotics for a minimum of 5 years or until 21 years of age (whichever is longer) after the initial diagnosis if there is no carditis. If there is persistent valvular disease, prophylaxis should continue until age 40, or in some cases be lifelong. Increasing age may lessen susceptibility to streptococcal disease, but reliable evidence is lacking to substantiate this impression conclusively. The physician who evaluates a child with known rheumatic heart disease for any reason should review the prophylaxis status of the child at every occasion.

Suggested Readings

General

Allen HD, Driscoll DJ, Shaddy RE, et al., eds. *Moss and Adams' heart disease in infants, children, and adolescents.* 7th ed. Philadelphia: Lippincott, Williams & Wilkins, 2008.

Driscoll DJ. *Fundamentals of pediatric cardiology.* Philadelphia: Lippincott, Williams & Wilkins, 2006.

Keane JF, Lock JE, Fyler DC, eds. *Nadas' pediatric cardiology.* 2nd ed. Philadelphia: WB Saunders, 2006.

Shaddy RE, Wernovsky G, eds. *Pediatric heart failure.* New York: Marcel-Decker, 2005.

Rudolph AM. *Congenital diseases of the heart: clinical and physiological considerations.* Wiley-Blackwell, 2009.

Congestive Heart Failure

Booker PD, Evans C, Franks R. Comparison of the hemodynamic effects of dopamine and dobutamine in young children undergoing cardiac surgery. *Br J Anaesth* 1995;74:419–423.

Friedman WF. The intrinsic physiologic properties of the developing heart. In: Friedman WF, Lesch M, Sonnenblock EH, eds. *Neonatal heart disease.* New York: Grune & Stratton, 1973:21.

Gewitz MH, Woolf PK, Frishman WH. Pediatric cardiovascular pharmacology. In: Frishman WH, Sonnenblik EH, Sisca DA, eds. *Cardiovascular pharmaco-therapeutics.* 2nd ed. New York: McGraw-Hill, 2003.

Ross J Jr. Afterload mismatch and preload reserve: a conceptual framework for the analysis of ventricular function. *Prog Cardiovasc Dis* 1976;18:255–264.

Rudolph AM. Cardiac failure in children: a hemodynamic overview. In: Braunwald E, ed. *The myocardium—failure and infarction.* New York: HP Publishing, 1974:102.

Schrier RW, Abraham WT. Hormones and hemodynamics in heart failure. *N Engl J Med* 1999;341:577–585.

Shaddy RE, Curtin LE, Sower B, et al. The pediatric randomized carvedilol trial in children with chronic heart failure: rationale and design. *Am Heart J* 2002;144:383–389.

Weller RJ, Weinbtraub R, Addonizio LJ, et al. Outcome of idiopathic restrictive cardiomyopathy in children. *Am J Cardiol* 2002;90:501–506.

Shaddy RE, Tani L. Chronic congestive heart failure. In: Allen HD, Driscoll DJ, Shaddy RE, et al., eds: *Moss and Adams' heart disease in infants, children, and adolescents.* 7th ed. Philadelphia: Lippincott, Williams and Wilkins, 2008.

Cardiac Arrhythmias

Alexander ME, Berul CI. Ventricular arrhythmias: when to worry. *Pediatr Cardiol* 2000;21:532–541.

Applegate TE. Atrial arrhythmias. *Prim Care* 2000;27:677–708.

Atkins DL, Dorian P, Gonzalez ER, et al. Treatment of tachyarrhythmias. *Ann Emerg Med* 2001;37:591.

Doniger SJ, Sharieff GQ. Pediatric dysrhythmias. *Pediatr Clin North Am* 2006;53:85–105.

Kannakeril PJ, Fish FA. Disorders of cardiac rhythm and conduction. In: Allen HD, Drixcoll DJ, Shaddy RE, et al.,eds. *Moss and Adams' heart disease in infants, children and adolescents: including the fetus and young adult.* 7th ed.. Philadelphia: Lippincott, Williams & Wilkins, 2008, 293–342.

Park MK, Guntheroth WG. *How to read pediatric ECGs.* Chicago: Year Book, 1981.

Walsh EP, Saul JP, Triedman JK, eds. *Cardiac arrhythmias in children and young adults with congenital heart disease.* Philadelphia: Lippincott, Williams & Wilkins, 2001.

Sudden Cardiac Death

Attari M and Dhala A. Role of invasive testing in risk stratification of sudden cardiac death in children and young adults: an electrophysiologic perspective. *Pediatr Clin North Am* 2004;51:1355–1378.

Choi GR, Porter JP, Ackerman MJ. Sudden cardiac death and channelopathies: a review of implantable defibrillator therapy. *Pediatr Clin North Am* 2004;51:1289–1303.

Maron BJ. Hypertrophic cardiomyopathy in childhood. *Pediatr Clin North Am* 2004;51:1305–1346.

Seidman JG, Seidman CE. The genetic basis for cardiomyopathy: from mutation identification to mechanistic paradigms. *Cell* 2001;104:557–567.

Maron BJ. Hypertrophic cardiomyopathy: a systemic review. *JAMA* 2002;287: 1308.

Pericardial Disease

Altman CA. Pericarditis and pericardial diseases. In: Garson AJ, Bricker JT, Fisher DJ, et al. *The science and practice of pediatric cardiology.* 2nd ed. Baltimore: Williams & Wilkins, 1998.

Engle MA, Zabriskie FB, Senterfit LB, et al. Post-pericardiotomy syndrome: a new look at an old condition: modern concepts. *Cardiovasc Dis* 1975;44:59.

Lange RA, Hillis LD. Clinical practice. Acute pericarditis. *N Engl J Med* 2004;351:2195–2202.

Spodick DH. Acute cardiac tamponade. *N Engl J Med* 2003;349:684–690.

Rhenban KS. Pericarditis. *Curr Treat Options Cardiovasc Med* 2005;7:419–427.

Infectious Endocarditis

Baddour LM, Wilson WR, Bayer AS, et al. Infective endocarditis: diagnosis, antimicrobial therapy, and management of complications. *Circulation* 2005;112:2373.

Ferreiri P, Gewitz MH, Gerber MH, et al. Unique features of infective endocarditis in childhood. *Circulation* 2002;105:2115–2126.

Oliver R, Roberts GJ, Hooper L. Penicillins for the prophylaxis of bacterial endocarditis in dentistry. Cochrane Database Syst Rev 2004;(2): CD003813.

Wilson WR, Taubert KA, Gewitz MH, et al. Prevention of infective endocarditis. Guidelines from the American Heart Association: a guideline from the American Heart Association Rheumatic Fever, Endocarditis, and Kawasaki Disease Committee, Council on Cardiovascular Disease in the Young, and the Council on Clinical Cardiology, Council on Cardiovascular Surgery and Anesthesia, and the Quality of Care and Outcomes Research Interdisciplinary Working Group. *Circulation* 2007;116:1736–1754.

Hypoxemic Attacks

Honey M, Chamberlain DA, Howeard J. The effective beta-sympathetic blockage on arterial saturation in Fallot's tetralogy. *Circulation* 1978;30:501.

Morgan BC, Guntheroth WG, Bloom RS, et al. A clinical profile of paroxysmal hyperpnea in cyanotic congenital heart disease. *Circulation* 1965;31:66–69.

Nudel DB, Berman MA, Talner NS. Effects of acutely increasing systemic vascular resistance on oxygen tension in tetralogy of Fallot. *Pediatrics* 1976;58: 248–251.

Acute Rheumatic Fever

Gerber M, Baltimore RS, Eaton CB, et al. Prevention of rheumatic fever and diagnosis and treatment of acute streptococcal pharyngitis: scientific statement from the American Heart Association Rheumatic Fever, Endocarditis, and Kawasaki Disease Committee of the Council on Cardiovascular Disease in the Young, the Interdisciplinary Council on Functional Genomics and Translational Biology, and the Interdisciplinary Council on Quality of Care and Outcomes Research: endorsed by the American Academy of Pediatrics. *Circulation* 2009;119:1541–1551.

Dajani AS, Ayoub E, Bierman FZ, et al. Guidelines for the diagnosis of rheumatic fever. Jones Criteria, updated 1992. Special Writing Group of the Committee on Rheumatic Fever, Endocarditis, and Kawasaki Disease of the Council on Cardiovascular Disease in the Young of the American Heart Association. *JAMA* 1992;268:2069–2079.

Ferreiri P, Jones Criteria Working Group. Proceedings of the Jones Criteria Workshop. *Circulation* 2002;106:2521–2523.

Bryant PA, Robins-Browne R, Carapetis J, et al. Some of the people, some of the time-susceptibility to acute rheumatic fever. *Circulation* 2009;119:742–753.

Miyake C, Gauvreau K, Tani L, et al. Characteristics of children discharged from hospitals in the United States in 2000 with the diagnosis of acute rheumatic fever. *Pediatrics* 2007;120:503–508.

Tani LY, Veasey LG, Minich LA. Rheumatic fever in children younger than 5 years: is the presentation different? *Pediatrics* 2003;112:1065–1068.

MEDICAL EMERGENCIES

CHAPTER 85 ■ DERMATOLOGIC URGENCIES AND EMERGENCIES

PAUL J. HONIG, MD, LESLIE CASTELO-SOCCIO, MD, PHD, AND ALBERT C. YAN, MD

ATOPIC DERMATITIS

Background

The definition of atopic dermatitis has at times been confusing. Many alternative terms are used to describe skin inflammation (dermatitis) that is chronic and relapsing.

Although the eruption may have a variable appearance (erythema, edema, papules, vesicles, serous discharge, and crusting), its constant feature is unrelenting pruritus. The eruption often has a characteristic distribution, depending on age (Fig. 85.1), and often occurs in allergic (atopic) individuals or those with a family history of allergies (e.g., hay fever, asthma, allergic rhinitis, food allergies, eosinophilic gastroenteritis). Although many theories relating to cause exist (e.g., genetic, physiologic, pharmacologic, immunologic), the data are conflicting.

More recent epidemiologic studies indicate that atopic dermatitis affects approximately 15% to 23% of children, beginning at 1 to 2 months of age. Of children who acquire atopic dermatitis, 60% will do so by the end of their first year of life, 90% by 5 years, 95% by 10 years, and 99% between 10 and 20 years of age. The course of an individual case is difficult to predict, but only 30% of those who develop the problem during the first year continue to have the disease during childhood. Of all children who have mild to moderate atopic dermatitis during childhood, 90% will be clear by the time they reach adolescence. For those children suffering from severe atopic dermatitis, only 15% will clear by adolescence.

Pathophysiology

No single theory explains the initiation and progression of atopic dermatitis. Some evidence suggests that a combination of factors, including altered physiologic, pharmacologic, and immunologic mechanisms, is involved in the exaggerated reactivity of the skin.

Various studies have found that patients with atopic dermatitis have altered epidermal barrier function. This is likely related to mutation or downregulation of genes involved in the cornified envelope. Patients with atopic dermatitis have had mutations identified in the filaggrin and collagen XXIX genes, both of which encode for proteins involved in forming the skin's outer protective layer. These changes result in increased transepidermal water loss, decreased quantities of sebaceous gland–derived lipids at the skin surface, and increased transcu-

taneous exposure to allergens. Patients also have an increased sweating response to Mecholyl®. If this drug is injected into the skin of an individual with atopic dermatitis, it causes blanching rather than the usual erythema. Simple scratching of the skin in an atopic will induce white dermatographism. Finally, the β-adrenergic blockade theory hypothesizes that reduced function of the β-adrenergic system leads to decreased production of cyclic adenosine monophosphate (cAMP). This reaction results in an increased release of pharmacologic mediators, such as histamines, producing pruritus and inflammation of the skin.

Atopic dermatitis patients have immune system dysregulation, which includes altered T-cell (Th1/Th2) function, increased production of immunoglobulin E (IgE) by B cells, elevated prostaglandin E_2, abnormal lymphokine secretion profiles, abnormalities of Langerhans cells, deficiencies in the production of endogenous antimicrobial peptides, and defects in response to staphylococcal superantigens. The way in which these changes interact to produce atopic eczema is still not definitive, but the picture is becoming clearer. Production of Th2-related proinflammatory cytokines, such as interleukin (IL)-4, IL-5, IL-13, IgE, and TNF-α, as well as cAMP phosphodiesterase, is abnormally increased. These responses lower cAMP, producing increased release of histamine, prostaglandin E_2, and other cytokines. This leads to decreases in cell-mediated interferon-γ responses and further increases in IL-4 and IL-5 responses. The resulting inflammatory mediators that arise from these complex interactions trigger the itch–scratch cycle.

Clinical Manifestations

The patient's age often determines the distribution and appearance of the skin lesions. During infancy, the itch–scratch cycle, which usually begins at 2 to 3 months of age, produces the erythematous, exudative lesions that appear on the cheeks and extensor surfaces. At times, the process becomes generalized. At about the age of 2 years, more characteristic flexural involvement occurs. Also indicative of atopic dermatitis are (i) varying sized patches of hypopigmentation, especially prominent on the cheeks (pityriasis alba; Fig. 85.2); (ii) patchy or diffuse, fine papules (follicular accentuation; Fig. 85.3); (iii) scaling in the scalp with or without hair loss; and (iv) hyperlinear palms and soles (Fig. 85.4), which may show desquamation. Involvement of the feet in such a manner occasionally leads to the misdiagnosis of tinea pedis, which occurs less often in the pediatric population before adolescence. During adolescence, the distribution remains the same; however, a greater incidence of involvement of the face, neck,

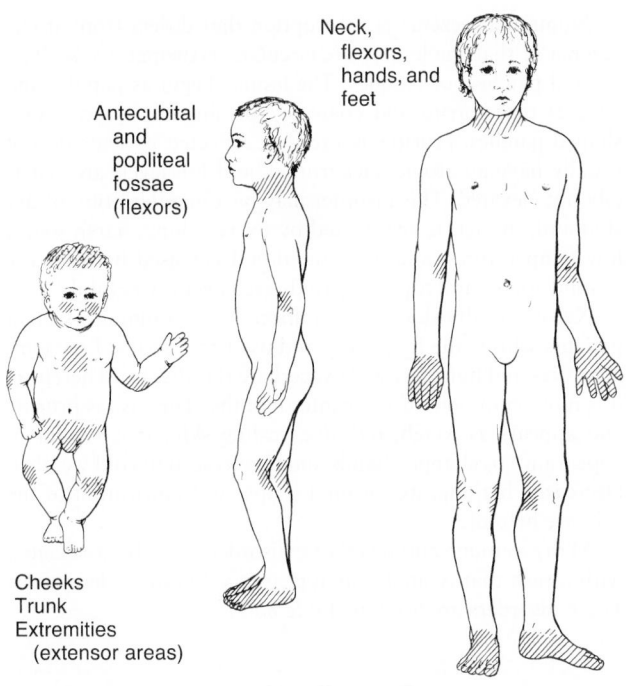

FIGURE 85.1 Distribution of atopic eczema at various ages.

Neck,
flexors,
hands, and
feet

Antecubital
and
popliteal
fossae
(flexors)

Cheeks
Trunk
Extremities
(extensor areas)

posterior auricular areas, and the hands and feet occurs. The major physical findings of chronicity, hyperpigmentation, and lichenification are often present (Fig. 85.5). Characteristically, infants and children with atopic dermatitis show sparing of the nose and perinasal areas when the face is involved.

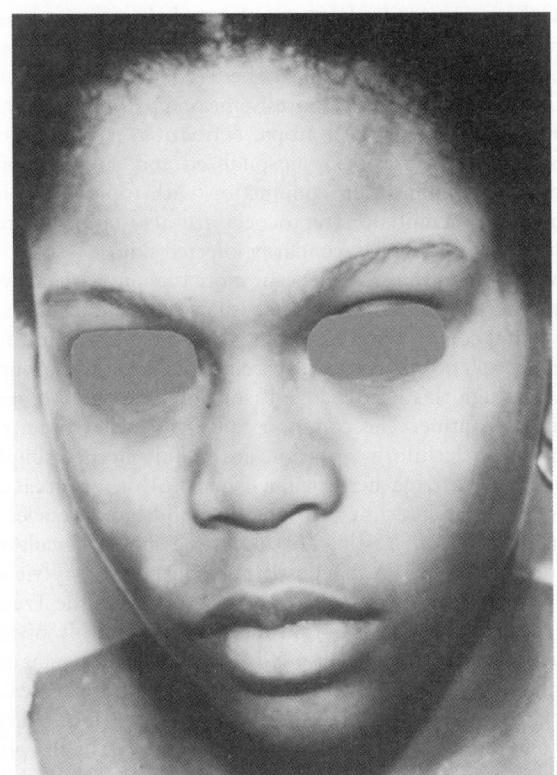

FIGURE 85.2 Postinflammatory hypopigmentation occurring in a child with atopic dermatitis (pityriasis alba).

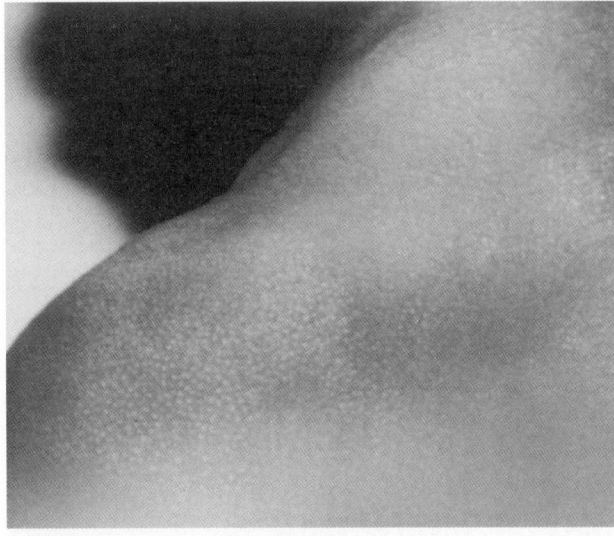

FIGURE 85.3 Follicular accentuation in a patient with atopic eczema.

The diagnosis of atopic dermatitis is based on the presence of pruritus, typical morphology and distribution, as well as a tendency toward chronically relapsing dermatitis. Other possible features are listed in Table 85.1. Unfortunately, laboratory tests are not helpful in the diagnosis of this disorder. Although eosinophilia and elevated serum IgE levels are present, they are not specific for this condition.

Differential Diagnosis

Atopic and seborrheic dermatitis may be difficult to differentiate when first appearing in a 1- to 2-month-old infant. Both conditions may cause scaling in the scalp or diaper dermatitis. Clues pointing to seborrheic dermatitis include involvement of the flexural and intertriginous areas in the infant; a salmon-colored eruption with greasy, yellow scaling; and the lack of

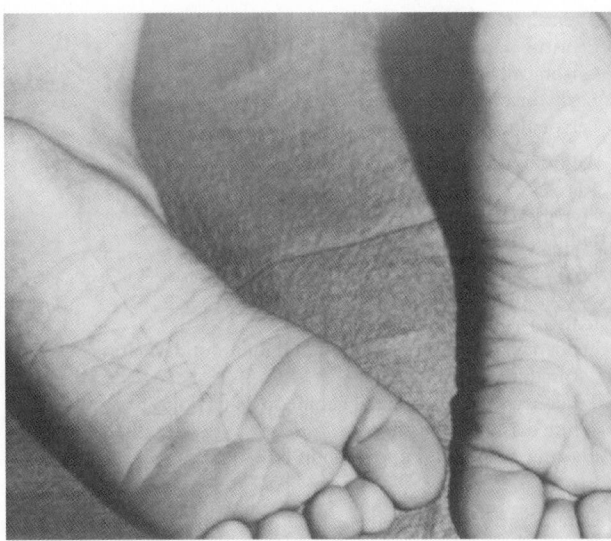

FIGURE 85.4 A patient with atopic eczema who has hyperlinearity of the soles.

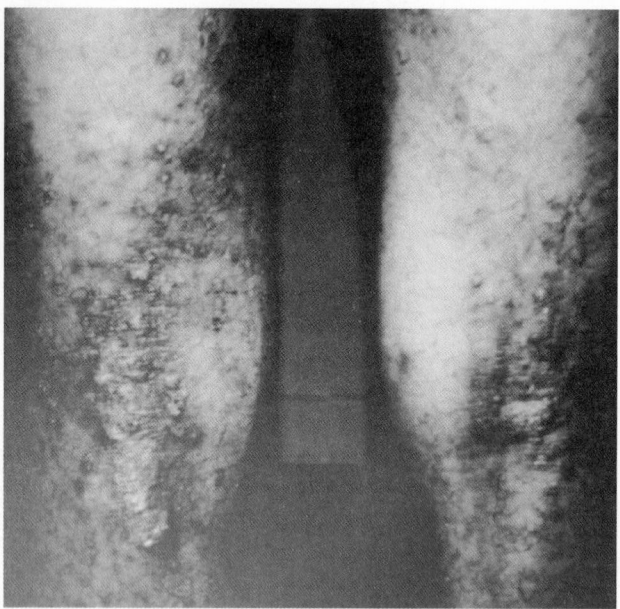

FIGURE 85.5 Chronic changes of hyperpigmentation and lichenification often seen in atopic eczema.

pruritus. Therapeutic clues include a rapid response to antiseborrheic shampoos (such as selenium sulfide) and steroids in seborrheic scaling of the scalp. Atopic dermatitis, in contrast, is often worsened with antiseborrheic shampoos and responds slowly to topical steroids. Infants with seborrheic dermatitis often manifest mild itching if present at all, while pruritus is universally seen in children with atopic dermatitis. Finally, infants with seborrheic dermatitis often show perinasal involvement while those with atopic dermatitis show characteristic sparing of this area.

TABLE 85.1

DIAGNOSTIC FEATURES OF ATOPIC DERMATITIS

Major
Typical morphology and distribution
Pruritus
Chronically relapsing course
Early onset of dermatitis (<2 yr of age)
Personal or family history of atopic disease

Additional Features
Xerosis
Hyperlinear palms and soles
Follicular accentuation
Pityriasis alba
Scaling of the scalp
Ichthyosis
Tendency toward nonspecific hand and foot dermatitis
   (pseudotinea pedis)
Tendency toward repeated cutaneous infections
White dermographism
Elevated serum immunoglobulin E

Minor
Cataracts
Keratoconus
Dennie-Morgan (infraorbital) fold

Nummular eczema is an eruption that differs from atopic eczema in that the lesions are circular, erythematous, scaling, crusted patches, or plaques. The lesions begin as papules and vesicles that spread and coalesce, forming the typical coin-shaped patches. Pruritus is variable. Affected patients do not usually have an atopic background, and IgE levels are generally not elevated. This disorder may be a manifestation of dry skin and, in fact, is aggravated by overwashing, harsh soaps, low temperatures, and low humidity. Decreased bathing, use of mild soaps, and topical steroids are generally helpful.

Xerosis, or dry skin, is a condition that is commonly seen in patients who bathe frequently and use harsh soaps. Low temperatures and humidity will exacerbate this disease. Therefore, it is more common during winter months. The rash is pruritic and appears as rough, red, dry, scaling skin. It is similar in appearance to chapped hands and cheeks seen in cold weather. Decreased bathing, use of mild soaps, and lubrication of the skin are helpful.

Many immune and metabolic disorders are also associated with a rash that is similar in appearance to atopic dermatitis. These disorders are listed in Table 85.2.

Complications

Infection of the existing dermatosis is the principal complication in atopic dermatitis and may in part be explained by a variety of factors: impaired skin integrity exposes epitopes such as fibronectin that allow pathogens an opportunity to bind the skin more effectively and the elaboration of cytokines suppresses normal production of endogenous antimicrobial peptides.

Colonization and infection with *Staphylococcus aureus* is common among atopic children and may account for flare-ups or failure to respond to therapy. There is increasing prevalence of infection with methicillin-resistant *Staphylococcus aureus* (MRSA) in patients with atopic dermatitis, particularly in those who were previously hospitalized and/or used topical calcineurin inhibitors in conjunction with topical steroids. Group A β-hemolytic streptococci are also cultured from many individuals with secondarily infected skin.

Viral skin infections also occur more often in patients with atopic dermatitis. Eczema vaccinatum, once a dreaded and often fatal complication of vaccina (smallpox) immunization, rarely occurs now that routine vaccination has been discontinued although this may change if smallpox vaccination again becomes routine. The common causes for what is termed Kaposi's varicelliform eruption are mainly herpes simplex virus (HSV; eczema herpeticum; Fig. 85.6) or, on occasion, coxsackievirus infection. Groups of umbilicated vesicles or areas of increased crusting and ulceration should be cultured for herpes simplex. A diagnostic procedure that may yield a quick answer to the presence of herpes simplex is the Tzanck test (Fig. 85.7). Material from the base of a freshly opened vesicle is scraped for a Giemsa stain. Multinucleated giant cells and balloon cells indicate the presence of herpes simplex. A much more sensitive and specific test is the rapid direct immunofluorescent test described in Chapter 67 or the polymerase chain reaction systems, which are now more readily available in hospital laboratories. This virus can also cause localized flare-ups of eczema without dissemination. Leyden

TABLE 85.2

IMMUNE AND METABOLIC DISORDERS CAUSING RASH THAT RESEMBLES ATOPIC DERMATITIS

Metabolic disorders	Immunologic disorders
Phenylketonuria	Ataxia-telangiectasia
Acrodermatitis enteropathica	Langerhans cell histiocytosis
Histidinemia	Wiskott-Aldrich syndrome
Gluten-sensitive enteropathy	X-linked agammaglobulinemia
Hartnup disease	Hyperimmunoglobulin E syndrome
Hurler's syndrome	Selective immunoglobulin A deficiency
	Severe combined immunodeficiency

described culture-proven recurrent local attacks of HSV appearing as discrete punched-out ulcerations. As a result, children with atopic dermatitis who develop eczema herpeticum have an increased risk of localized reactivation of HSV, and some of these children may require a period of supervised antiviral prophylaxis on an outpatient basis. Varicella virus lesions also tend to concentrate in areas of inflamed skin as a result of leakage of virions through dilated vessels. The viruses that cause molluscum contagiosum and warts also infect individuals with atopic dermatitis more often than the average patient (Fig. 85.8).

Management (Table 85.3)

Skin tests and hyposensitization are of little value and are rarely indicated. Dietary restrictions may be helpful in certain patients but are difficult to maintain. The four main objectives in the treatment of uncomplicated atopic dermatitis are (i) reduction of pruritus, (ii) reduction of inflammation, (iii) protection of the skin from unknown irritants, and (iv) removal of known irritants and allergens. Reduction of pruritus can be accomplished in numerous ways. The most important of these

methods is limitation of bathing (at times, to only once per week) and the use of a mild soap or synthetic detergent (syndet) cleanser (e.g., Dove®, Oil of Olay®, Tone®, Caress®) Amend the position of registered trade marks. Lubrication of the skin with petrolatum, Aquaphor® ointment, Nivea® cream, Eucerin® cream, or Moisturel® (which contains no lanolin or perfumes) ameliorates dryness, which may be a factor in producing pruritus. Antihistamines can be helpful, although during infancy, the necessity for soporific doses results in their being less therapeutic and infants may experience paradoxical agitation rather than sleepiness. Old standbys include diphenhydramine hydrochloride (5 mg per kg per day in three to four divided doses) and hydroxyzine (2 mg/kg/day in three to four divided doses). Topical diphenhydramine or doxepin is not recommended due to the likelihood of systemic absorption from the skin. Oral agents such as cetirizine, levocetirizine, fexofenadine, loratadine, and desloratadine are also available but because they are less sedating, they may provide less optimal control of pruritus.

Control of inflammation is accomplished with the use of topical steroids (Table 85.4). During the acute phase, potent steroids should be used to bring the situation under control. At times, systemic steroids are used to bring an acute flare-up under

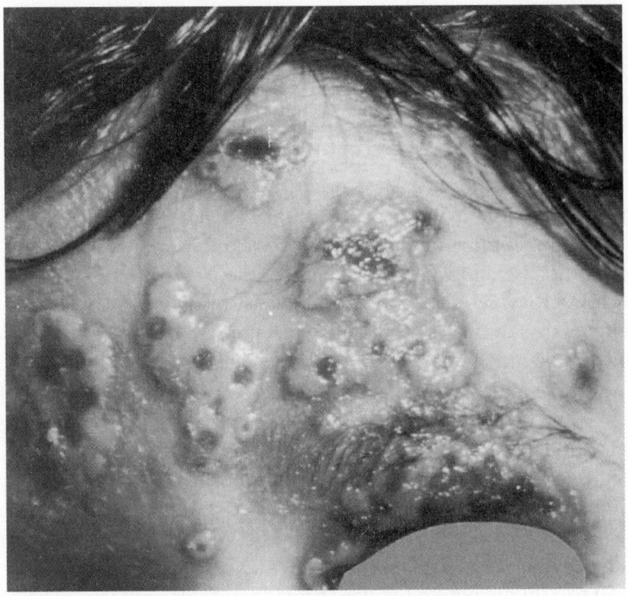

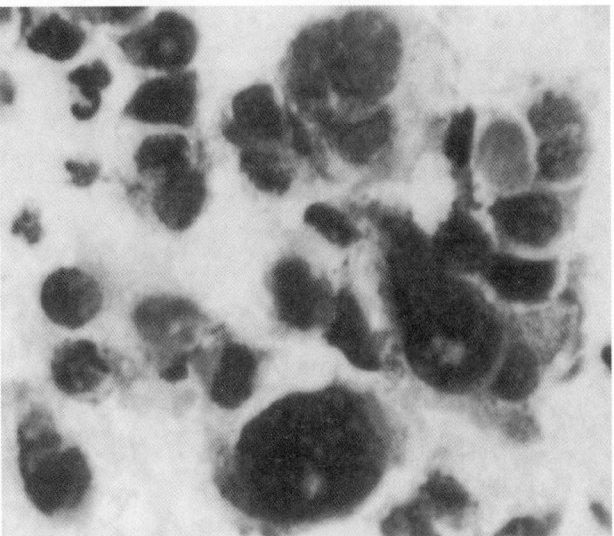

FIGURE 85.6 Eczema herpeticum.

FIGURE 85.7 Positive Tzanck test demonstrating multinuclear giant cells.

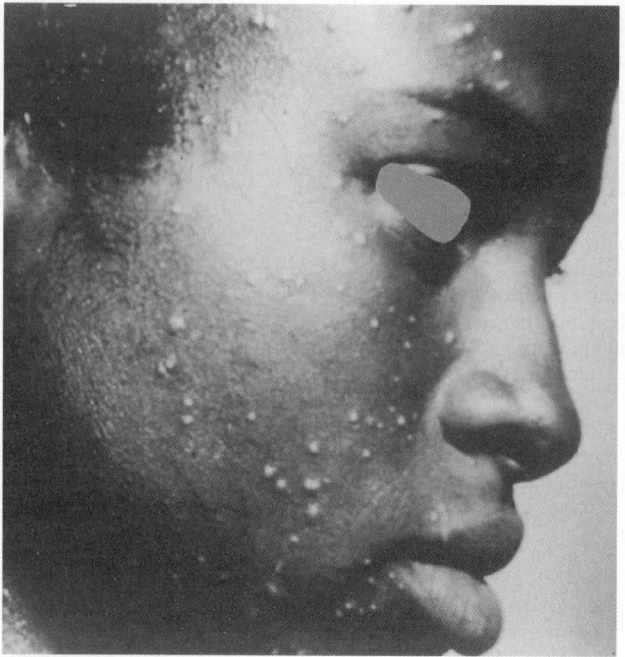

FIGURE 85.8 An atopic eczema patient whose face is covered with molluscum contagiosum.

TABLE 85.4

POTENCY OF TOPICAL STEROIDS[a]

Mild
Hydrocortisone 1%, 2.5%
Alclometasone ointment and cream 0.05%
Desonide ointment and cream 0.05%

Moderate
Aristocort® ointment 0.1% (triamcinolone acetonide)
Synalar® ointment and cream 0.025% (fluocinolone acetonide)
Dermatop® ointment and cream 0.1% (prednicarbate)
Cutivate® cream 0.05% (fluticasone)
Valisone® cream 0.1% (betamethasone valerate)

Potent
Diprosone ointment 0.05% (betamethasone dipropionate)
Lidex cream or ointment 0.05% (fluocinonide)
Topicort ointment and cream 0.25% (desoximetasone)

[a]Many of the synthetic preparations are fluorinated; hydrocortisone and prednicarbate are not.

control. Fortunately, this measure is rarely necessary. Once control is achieved, steroids of mild potency or steroid-sparing agents such as topical calcineurin inhibitors [pimecrolimus cream (Elidel®) for mild to moderate eczema or tacrolimus ointment (Protopic®) for moderate to severe eczema] or newer therapeutic emollients [MAS063DP cream (Atopiclair®), palmitoylethanolamine cream (Mimyx®), or a ceramide-based emollient (Epicream)] should be used and can often be applied less often. (Note: Steroids should not be used on the face for prolonged periods. Instead, the use of topical calcineurin inhibitors or therapeutic emollients is recommended because these appear to be safe and well tolerated on the face and periocular areas.)

Topical calcineurin inhibitors were first introduced in 2000 as a U.S. Food and Drug Administration (FDA)-approved

TABLE 85.3

ACUTE TREATMENT OF ATOPIC DERMATITIS

Reduction of Pruritus
Mild soaps   ⎫
Infrequent washing   ⎬ skin care
Skin lubrication   ⎭
Topical steroids (high potency)
Topical calcineurin inhibitor
Systemic steroids (rarely necessary)
Antihistamines (children >4 yr old)

Reduction of Inflammation
Skin care
Topical steroids (high potency)
Topical calcineurin inhibitor
Systemic steroids (rarely necessary)

Control of Infection
Penicillinase-resistant antibiotics

nonsteroidal drug for the management of atopic dermatitis. Topical tacrolimus (FK506) ointment and topical pimecrolimus cream bind to cytosolic macrolide receptors and act as intracellular calcineurin phosphatase inhibitors; by blocking the dephosphorylation of calcineurin, the production of proinflammatory cytokines contributing to atopic dermatitis is likewise inhibited. Unlike topical steroids, these agents lack the steroid-associated effects of hypothalamic-pituitary-adrenal (HPA) axis suppression, ocular cataracts or glaucoma, and cutaneous atrophy. Both agents appear to be safe and effective. The U.S. FDA has placed boxed warnings on these agents because animal data indicate that high doses applied topically or taken internally have been associated with immunosuppression and immunosuppression-related complications of lymphoma and skin cancers in animal studies. Ongoing patient registries (APPLES and PEER studies) designed to monitor this risk in humans have not to date identified an increased risk for these conditions in humans.

Maintenance with the least potent steroid, calcineurin inhibitor, or therapeutic emollient applied as infrequently as possible, is advisable. However, continued therapy is usually necessary. After control has been maintained for a fairly prolonged period, an attempt to discontinue topical pharmacologic therapy can be made. Protection of the skin against unknown irritants is best done by covering it. Long-sleeve polo shirts and leotards are helpful in preventing dust and pollens from coming in contact with the skin. Removal of known irritants is achieved by (i) environmental control (i.e., no stuffed toys, wool clothing or blankets, or pets), (ii) avoidance of harsh soaps, and (iii) keeping fingernails short. At times, hospitalization for control is advisable and certainly a more desirable alternative than systemic steroids.

Appropriate antibiotics are important in the treatment of secondary bacterial infections. A child who is not showing signs of systemic infection can often be treated orally in the home setting. When methicillin-sensitive staphylococcal organisms are involved, antibiotics such as erythromycin (40 mg per kg per day), dicloxacillin (50 mg per kg per day), or cephalexin (50 to 100 mg per kg per day) provide suitable coverage. These antibiotics also treat group A β-hemolytic streptococci that may be present. In places where MRSA is prevalent or when patients have had multiple hospitalizations for atopic dermatitis–related infection, clindamycin or trimethoprim-sulfamethoxazole may be indicated. When a child is toxic, inpatient intravenous (IV) therapy is advisable; although clindamycin, trimethoprim-sulfamethoxazole, or vancomycin is often employed as empiric therapy, antibiotic selection should be made on the basis of local antibiotic-resistance patterns.

Eczema herpeticum that is localized and has not produced toxicity in a child can be treated on an outpatient basis with oral antiviral therapy (acyclovir) and will usually clear in 2 to 3 weeks. With severe infection, especially in young infants, more aggressive therapy may be necessary. IV acyclovir dosed at 750 mg per m^2 per day divided q8h is advised for hospitalized patients. More localized primary or secondary infections can be treated orally at a dosage of 1,200 mg per m^2 per 24 hours in three divided doses for 7 to 10 days.

Patients with severe atopic dermatitis may be maintained on more intense therapies and may experience exacerbations that prompt evaluation in the emergency department. Ultraviolet light phototherapy can be extremely helpful in alleviating the pruritus and cutaneous manifestations of atopic dermatitis, but patients receiving this therapy should undergo gradual dose escalation or they may experience ultraviolet light burns. Systemic immunosuppressive and immunomodulating agents that have been used in more severe pediatric atopic dermatitis patients include cyclosporine, azathioprine, mycophenolate mofetil, and γ-interferon.

SEBORRHEIC DERMATITIS

Background

Seborrheic dermatitis is the term given to the salmon-colored patches with yellow, greasy scales occurring primarily in the so-called seborrheic areas (face, postauricular area, scalp, axilla, groin, presternal area). Seborrheic dermatitis is seen in infants or adolescents. Its onset occurs during the first 3 months of life and generally disappears shortly thereafter, only then reappearing in adolescence.

Pathophysiology

Although sebaceous gland dysfunction is often cited as a cause, the definite cause of this disorder has not been established. In fact, surface fat levels are normal in seborrheic dermatitis, but their ratio is altered. The presence of seborrheic dermatitis correlates strongly to concomitant emotional stress or neurologic disorders.

Clinical Manifestations

The two common locations of skin involvement during infancy are the scalp (cradle cap), as shown in the infant with seborrheic dermatitis in Fig. 85.9, and the diaper area. Most commonly, yellow, greasy scales are found over the anterior fontanel. Scaling is concentrated in this location because of the fear some mothers have about rubbing or scrubbing over the fontanel.

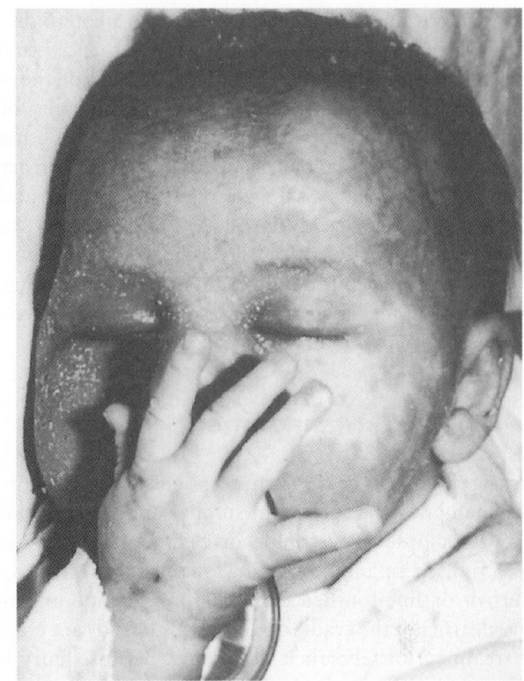

FIGURE 85.9 Seborrheic dermatitis.

Many times the scaling is limited to this area; however, occasionally, the scaling is spread to the forehead, eyebrows, nose, ears, and neck. The intertriginous and flexural areas may also become involved. This reaction is especially seen in the diaper area (Fig. 85.10). The child is not irritable, and pruritus does not seem to be present. The prognosis for clearing is excellent, and resolution usually occurs within several weeks to months.

Between the periods of infancy and adolescence, scaling of the scalp usually indicates causes other than seborrheic dermatitis (atopic dermatitis or tinea capitis). In fact, true seborrheic dandruff does not appear until puberty, when excessive production of sebum occurs. Most commonly, scalp scaling before puberty and after infancy indicates the presence of atopic dermatitis or tinea capitis (especially *Trichophyton tonsurans*). Differentiation is aided by clinical appearance, cultures, and response to therapy. Atopic dermatitis is often worsened with

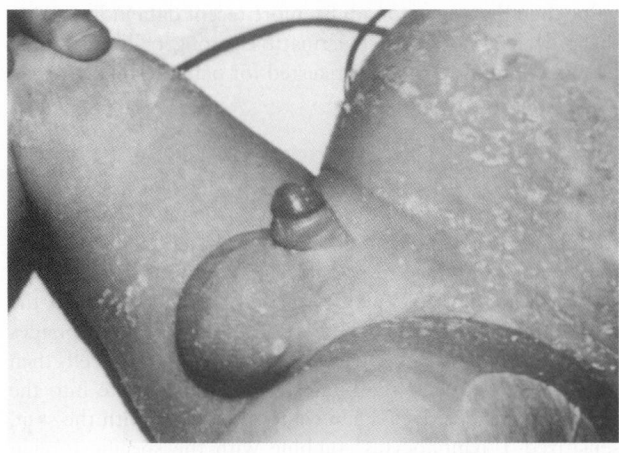

FIGURE 85.10 Infant with seborrheic diaper dermatitis.

harsh shampoos and responds slowly to topical steroids. The diagnosis of tinea capitis is best made with cultures. If steroids are used in the presence of tinea capitis, scaling of the scalp often increases secondary to suppressed local immunity of the skin and increased growth of the fungus. Seborrheic dermatitis of the scalp during the adolescent period is similar in nature to the condition in adults. Scaling in the scalp appears, and the seborrheic areas are variably involved. Erythema and scaling occur between the eyebrows, on the eyelid margins, and in the nasolabial creases, sideburns, beards, mustache, posterior auricular areas, and aural canals. Rarely, the patient may develop a secondary infection with monilia or bacteria.

Management

Seborrheic dermatitis of the scalp responds readily to antiseborrheic shampoos (i.e., selenium sulfide) and topical steroids such as fluocinolone acetonide or betamethasone valerate (Table 85.4). In infants, loosening of the scales with a soft toothbrush or fine-toothed comb before shampooing often hastens clearing of the cradle cap. Topical steroids are effective in the treatment of seborrheic dermatitis. Because hairy locations are commonly involved, steroid preparations in the form of solutions, lotions, or gels are advisable. The strength of the steroid and the frequency of application are determined by the response to therapy. Steroids should not be used for prolonged periods on the face because of potential damage to the skin in that area. Secondary infection with bacteria can be treated with appropriate antibiotics. If *Candida albicans* secondarily invades the lesions, agents such as topical nystatin or econazole cream, applied twice daily, are useful.

ALLERGIC CONTACT DERMATITIS

Background

Allergic contact dermatitis is a cell-mediated reaction to antigenic material in contact with the surface of the skin. Children younger than 1 year rarely respond to contactants and, until nearly 3 years of age, have a reduced incidence of contact dermatitis. While previous estimates had suggested that the incidence in children had been about 1.5%, a considerably lower value than that given for adults, more recent data indicate that the prevalence of contact dermatitis among children ranges from 25% to 60% of those referred for patch testing.

Pathogenesis

An allergen penetrates the stratum corneum (facilitated by trauma at times) and combines with a carrier protein to form the foreign substance responsible for initiating the sensitization process. This complex is carried via lymphatics to the regional lymph nodes where processing by macrophages occurs. Recognition by T lymphocytes follows; these cells then leave the node, enter the bloodstream, and migrate into the skin. When the antigen again comes in contact with the skin, sensitized T lymphocytes combine with the specific foreign material and release inflammatory lymphokines. The characteristic dermatitis occurs 6 to 18 hours later.

TABLE 85.5

REGIONAL PREDILECTION OF VARIOUS SUBSTANCES THAT CAUSE CONTACT DERMATITIS

Head and Neck
Scalp—hair dye, hair spray, shampoo
Ear canal—neomycin
Forehead—hat band
Eyelids—nail polish, volatile gases, false eyelash cement, mascara, eye shadow/cosmetics
Perioral—dentrifices, bubble gum, chewing gum
Ears—earrings, perfume

Trunk
Axilla—deodorant, clothing dye
Breasts—metal, elastic in bra

Arms
Wrist—cosmetic jewelry (nickel), leather (*p*-phenylenediamine, chrome)

Abdomen
Waistline—rubber dermatitis from elastic in pants, jockstrap (lower)
Lower abdomen—nickel dermatitis from metal snaps

Lower Extremities
Feet—shoe dermatitis

Clinical Manifestations

The acute onset of linear or geometric areas of erythema, edema, eczematization, and papulovesiculation usually indicates the presence of "an outside job" and frequently indicates an allergic contact dermatitis. Because skin involvement is limited to areas of contact, the distribution, pattern, and shape of the dermatitis provide important clues for the clinician (Table 85.5). Therefore, a round lesion on the back of the wrist would incriminate a wristwatch; a linear pattern encircling the waist points to the rubber in the waistband of a garment; linear lesions on exposed portions of the body indicate brushing against the leaves of a poison ivy plant (Fig. 85.11); and extensive involvement of exposed areas of skin suggests an airborne allergen, as with ragweed or vaporized oil transmitted in the

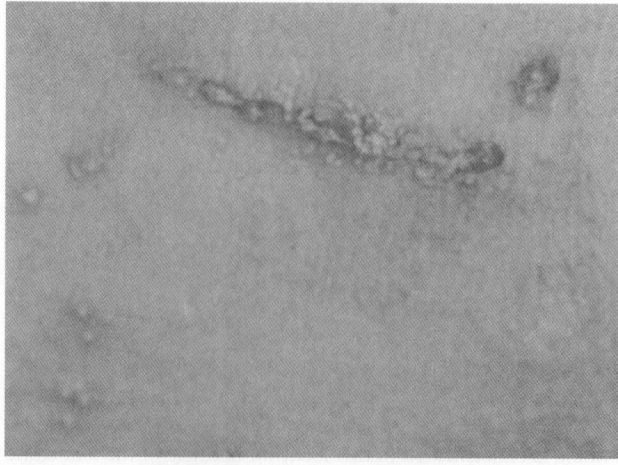

FIGURE 85.11 Typical linear pattern after exposure to the poison ivy plant.

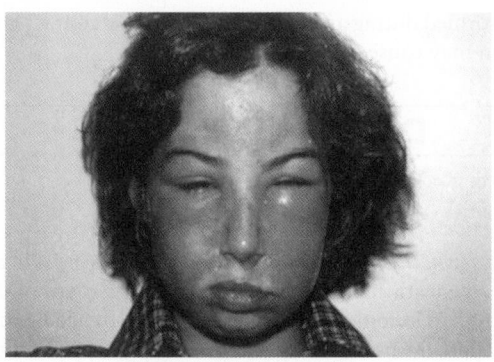

FIGURE 85.12 Facial edema and inflammation in response to exposure to airborne contact allergen (e.g., vaporized oil in smoke of burned poison ivy plants).

smoke of burning poison ivy (Fig. 85.12, see also color plate). Generally, the scalp, palms, and soles are less permeable to allergens and therefore are less often involved. Involvement of oral mucous membranes is uncommon. As previously mentioned, trauma or nonspecific factors such as pressure, heat, and perspiration may predispose the skin to allergic contact dermatitis.

The most common cause of contact dermatitis remains rhus (poison ivy, oak, sumac). However, a variety of other agents have been implicated as common causes of contact dermatitis in children: nickel, cobalt, thimerosal, fragrances, neomycin, rubber compounds, chromates, paraphenylenediamine, and colophony (rosin). Paraphenylenediamine, an agent commonly used in hair dye, has been encountered as an occasional cause of pediatric allergic contact dermatitis due to the frequent incorporation of paraphenylenediamine into commercial henna dyes used for temporary tattoos.

Rhus (Poison Ivy, Oak, Sumac)

Rhus dermatitis is the most common allergen involved in the production of contact dermatitis. The poison ivy plant (Fig. 85.13A) occurs in all parts of the United States as a shrub or vine, often on trees or fences. Poison oak (Fig. 85.13B), an upright shrub, appears only on the West Coast. Poison sumac (Fig. 85.13C) grows as a shrub or tree east of the Mississippi. Seventy percent of the population will become sensitized if exposed to the oleoresin, known as *urushiol*, contained on the leaf, stem, or root of the plant. The active ingredient in this oil is pentadecylcatechol. The oil can be carried on clothing and pets or by the wind.

Each plant produces an identical redundant eruption. From the time of exposure, the average time to appearance of the rash is 48 hours. At that time, onset of pruritus, inflammation, and grouped or linear papulovesicles or bullae occurs. With severe exposure, the face and eyelids become uniformly edematous. The eruption can last from 1 to 3 weeks. Occasionally, black, pseudonecrotic areas may be present on affected areas and indicate the presence of oxidized oleoresin shed from the poison plant, a phenomenon referred to as *black spot poison ivy*, and may clinically be mistaken for ecthyma gangrenosum. However, the intense itch of black spot poison ivy distinguishes it from ecthyma.

Avoidance of exposure is the best prophylaxis in treatment. Topical barrier agents such as the product that is used by forest rangers have been developed to prevent rhus dermatitis in high-risk individuals. However, at times, protection is impossible.

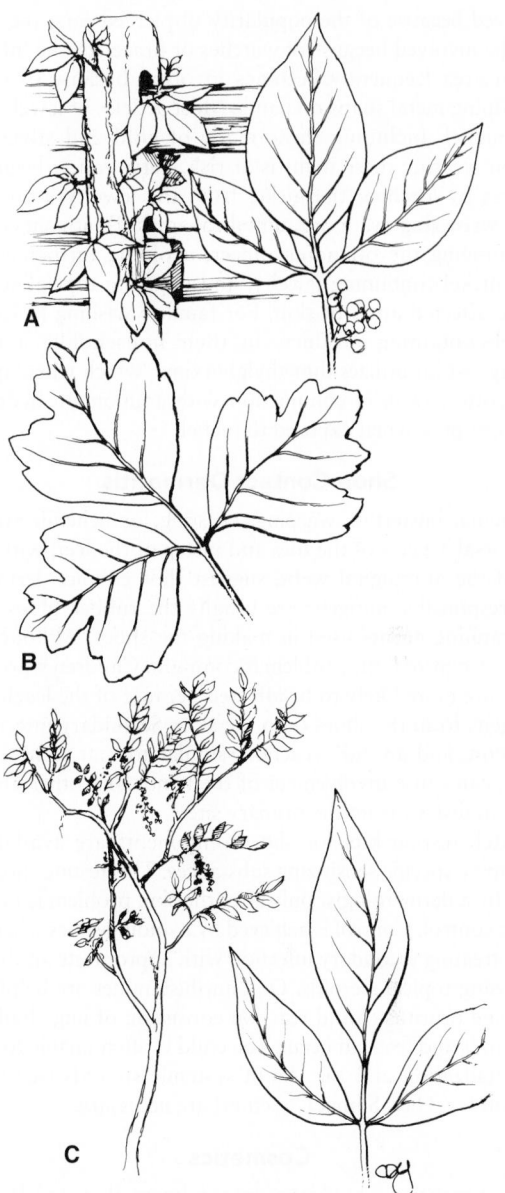

FIGURE 85.13 **A:** Poison ivy (*Rhus radicans*). **B:** Poison oak (*Rhus toxicodendron*). **C:** Poison sumac (*Rhus vernix*).

Once an individual is exposed, contaminated clothing should be removed and laundered and the body should be bathed with any soap as soon as possible, preferably within 5 to 10 minutes. Once the oil has been removed, spread does not occur, even from vesicular fluid. Although sequential outbreaks on various parts of the body suggest spread, lesions appearing later in time indicate initial exposure to a lesser dose of the offending oil.

Antipruritic lotions such as calamine are useful. Topical steroids are somewhat effective, but topical antihistamines and anesthetics should be avoided because they can themselves be sensitizers. Oral antihistamines can be helpful. With generalized reactions, oral prednisone 1 to 2 mg per kg once daily for 1 to 2 weeks, then tapered over the following week, is advisable.

Nickel Contact Dermatitis

Nickel dermatitis is seen commonly in children in response to nickel-containing jewelry or clothing. Earlobes are commonly involved because of the popularity of pierced ears; the wrists may be involved because of watches or bracelets; the infraumbilical area frequently becomes involved because of nickel-containing metal snaps on pants. Most articles of jewelry contain nickel, including those made of gold and silver. Any person wearing these items is at risk. Perspiration begins the process by leaching the nickel from the jewelry around the neck, wrist, fingers, or infraumbilical areas. Treatment consists of removing the offending object, avoiding further contact with nickel-containing jewelry, and applying topical steroids to the affected areas of skin. For families wishing to identify nickel-containing products in their households, a nickel allergy test kit utilizes dimethylglyoxime, which when applied to a cotton swab in conjunction with ammonium hydroxide will turn pink when exposed to nickel.

Shoe Contact Dermatitis

Erythema, blistering, weeping, crusting, or lichenification of the dorsal aspects of the toes and instep of the feet, with sparing of the interdigital webs, suggest shoe contact dermatitis. The responsible antigens are usually the rubber, glues, dyes, and tanning agents used in making the shoes. Although not often recognized, the problem is common. Children who sweat freely are more likely to be affected because of the leaching of allergens from the shoes onto the skin. Secondary infection is common, and an "id" reaction, similar to that seen in tinea pedis, can cause involvement of the hands and other areas of the skin distant from the primary site.

Patch testing kits for shoe components are available to determine specific sensitizing substances. This testing should be done by a dermatologist only after the skin problem is brought under control. Control is achieved by avoiding shoes when possible, treating secondary infection with appropriate antibiotics, and using topical steroids. Oral antihistamines are helpful for reducing pruritus. An id reaction consisting of huge bullae on the hands and feet can occur. The child is often unable to walk. Hospitalization and the use of systemic steroids [see "Rhus (Poison Ivy, Oak, Sumac)" section] are necessary.

Cosmetics

Many practicing physicians do not know that nail lacquers (containing sulfonamides and formaldehyde resins) or nail hardeners (containing formaldehyde) are a common cause of allergic reactions on the skin of the eyelids. The skin in this area is thin and permeable. Simply rubbing the eyes with fingernails that have polish on them can induce the problem. Paraphenylenediamine, which is contained in hair dyes, will also cause eczematous eruptions of the scalp and face.

Management

Elimination and avoidance of the causal antigen is the most effective preventive and therapeutic measure. Topical steroids and antihistamines help with inflammation and pruritus.

With localized involvement, moderate- to high-potency topical steroids can be helpful in reducing symptoms while the dermatitis clears. With generalized skin involvement, oral steroids (prednisone or prednisolone) are effective at a dosage of 1 to 2 mg per kg per day over 7 to 10 days then tapered over the next 7 days (rebound less likely). Patch testing should not be performed during an acute episode because contact with the allergen may cause worsening of the rash.

DIAPER DERMATITIS

Background

Diaper dermatitis is a general term used to describe skin abnormalities beneath the diaper secondary to a variety of causes. The problem is common in children 2 years of age or younger who require the use of a diaper. It generally disappears after toilet training.

Pathophysiology

The pathogenesis of the problem is multifactorial (Fig. 85.14) and not clearly defined. The possibilities include the concentration of bacteria or fungi, the action of organisms on the urine, and moisture itself.

No firm proof exists that bacteria play a major role. However, bacterial overgrowth does occur on moist skin with increasing time. Bacteria have been implicated in liberating ammonia from urine and raising urine pH. The rise in pH increases the activity of fecal proteases and lipases, which can damage skin. Bile salts can potentiate this damage.

C. albicans is found on the skin in 40% of infants with active diaper dermatitis within 72 hours of the appearance of the rash. Because studies show that this organism is present in less than 10% of infants without diaper dermatitis, *C. albicans* may be playing a significant role. Sources of *C. albicans* include the gastrointestinal (GI) tract and secondary implantation from a mother with candidal vaginitis.

Chronic exposure of the skin to moisture, especially under occlusion by the diaper, leads to maceration and alteration of the epidermal barrier with overgrowth of bacteria (including group A β-hemolytic streptococci) and *C. albicans*. If one major instigating factor exists, the effect of chronic exposure to moisture is critical to the development of diaper dermatitis.

Another consideration is the predisposition of certain individuals to react more easily and negatively to varying irritants. Generally, infants with an atopic or seborrheic background are at greater risk for the development and persistence of diaper dermatitis.

Clinical Manifestations

Differentiation of the various types of diaper dermatitis is difficult. Clues from the history and physical examination are necessary when characterizing the cause of this problem. The different types of diaper rashes include occlusion dermatitis, atopic dermatitis, seborrheic dermatitis, moniliasis, and mixed or not diagnosable rash.

Occlusion Dermatitis

Occlusion dermatitis (Fig. 85.15, see also color plate) results from two components. The first, friction, occurs mainly on those portions of the diaper area where contact with the diaper is greatest (inner thighs, lower abdomen, and prominent

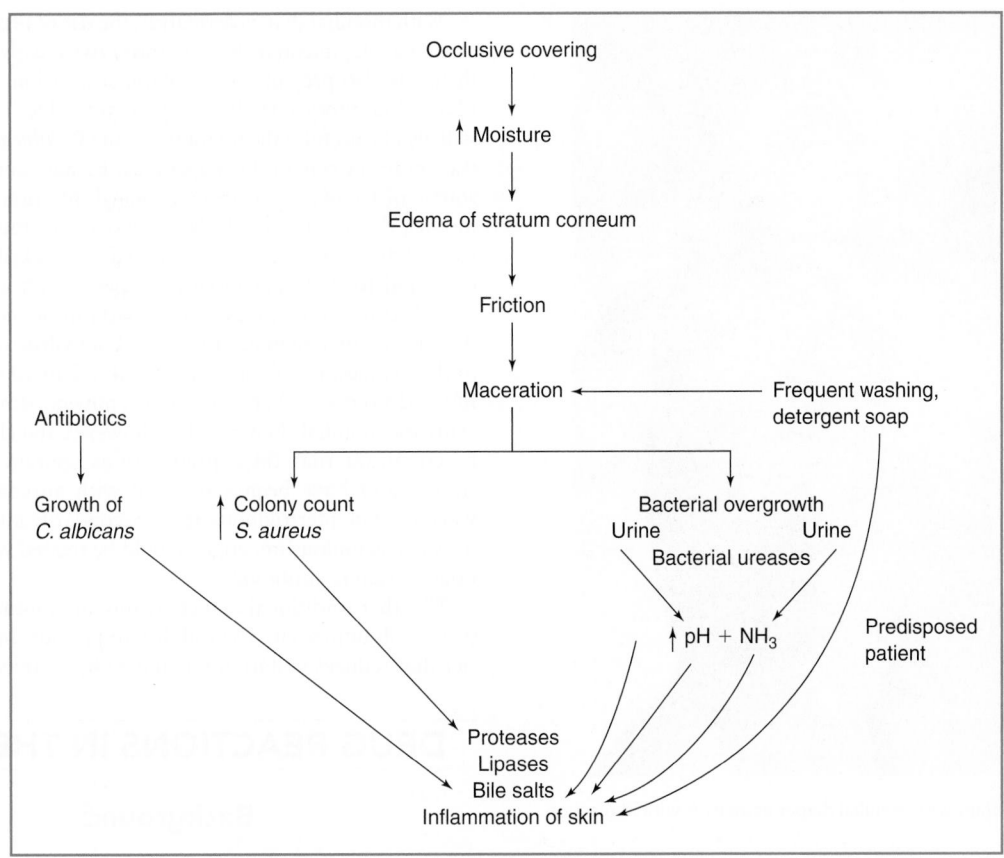

FIGURE 85.14 Proposed sequence of events producing skin inflammation in the diaper area.

surfaces of the genitalia and buttocks). The rash waxes and wanes and often has a shiny, glazed surface appearance. Occasionally, papules are associated with the rash. The second component, trapped moisture, causes the erythema and maceration that occurs in the intertriginous parts of the diaper area (inguinal, genital, intergluteal, and folds of the thighs). This problem is often associated with and precipitated by tightly applied diapers, commercial plastic diapers (especially those made with elastic edges to prevent leakage around the thighs), and rubber pants placed over cloth diapers. Such coverings increase friction and prevent the evaporation of moisture.

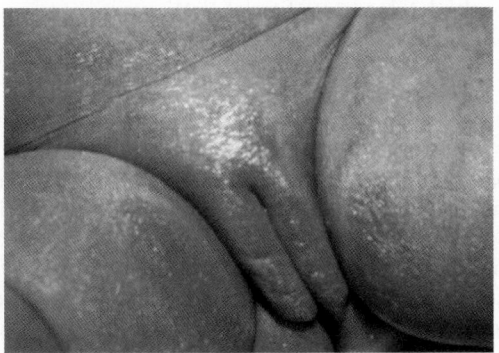

FIGURE 85.15 Infant with occlusion diaper dermatitis.

Atopic Dermatitis

The appearance of the rash in the diaper area is not different from occlusion dermatitis. It is, however, more chronic and difficult to treat. Examination may disclose lesions on other body surfaces (cheeks, antecubital and popliteal spaces) typical of atopic involvement, and a family history of atopy often exists.

Seborrheic Dermatitis

Generally, seborrheic dermatitis (Fig. 85.10) has an erythematous, salmon-colored base that is covered with yellow, greasy scaling. Similar involvement of other seborrheic locations such as the scalp, postauricular area, or other flexures helps establish the diagnosis. At times, a family history of seborrheic dermatitis exists.

Moniliasis

Moniliasis is the most characteristic of the diaper rashes. The skin in the diaper area has clusters of erythematous papules and pustules that coalesce into an intensely red confluent rash with sharp borders. Beyond these borders are satellite papules and pustules. At times, the infant has concomitant oral thrush. When the problem is chronic and recurrent, seeding from the GI tract or from a mother with monilial vaginitis should be considered.

On rare occasions an id reaction occurs (Fig. 85.16). Besides the primary monilial diaper rash lies an antigenic dissemination with involvement of the intertriginous areas and

MEDICAL EMERGENCIES

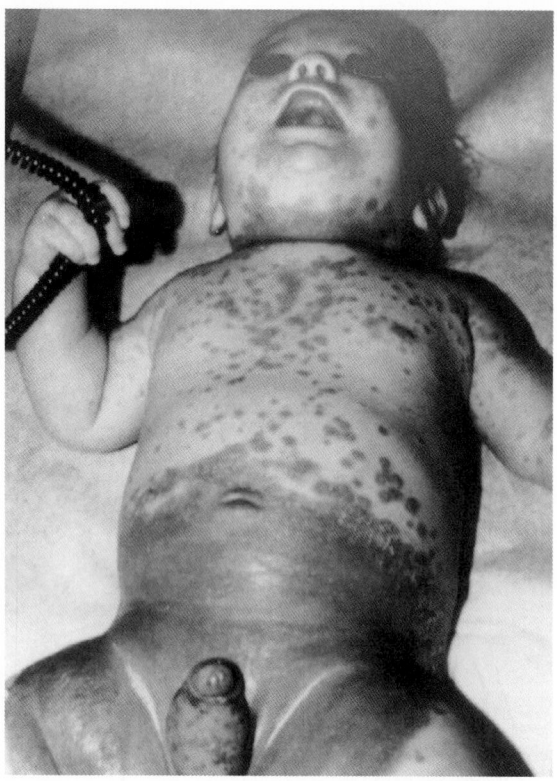

FIGURE 85.16 Infant with monilial diaper dermatitis with id reaction.

scattered small patches or plaques of scaling erythema on other parts of the skin surface. Generally, *C. albicans* cannot be cultured from these plaques.

Mixed or Not Diagnosable Rash

Mixtures of the previous categories of diaper dermatitis are often found on infants. A diagnosis is often difficult to make. Secondary invasion with *C. albicans* is common as mentioned. The potential for secondary bacterial infection exists. If blistering occurs, *S. aureus* infection should be considered. Foul-smelling areas of maceration within skin folds may also indicate group A β-hemolytic streptococcal intertrigo.

Management

Treatment is determined by the cause of the dermatitis. In general, proper skin care, which includes decreased frequency of washing, use of mild soaps, and keeping the diaper off as much as possible, will help resolve diaper dermatitis resulting from any cause. With occlusive dermatitis, avoidance of tightly fitting diapers, plastic-covered paper diapers, and rubber pants is important. When atopic dermatitis is present, the use of topical steroids is necessary. It is important to avoid fluorinated or other potent steroids in the diaper area because occlusion by the diaper enhances the steroid effect and is more likely to produce skin atrophy and striae. The newer antifungal–steroid combinations should also be avoided for these same reasons. Therefore, 1% hydrocortisone cream no more than twice daily over a short period is recommended. Hydrocortisone (1%) is also effective for seborrheic diaper dermatitis and can be used intermittently.

With monilial diaper dermatitis, the use of preparations such as econazole, miconazole or nystatin twice daily is effective. If thrush is also present, oral nystatin suspension, 200,000 units (2 mL) four times a day for 7 days, is advisable. This medication will also be useful if the infant is seeding *C. albicans* from the GI tract onto the skin of the diaper area. Because another potential source of *C. albicans* is from a vaginal infection in the infant's mother, the mother should be questioned for this problem; if a vaginal discharge is present, it should be checked by a gynecologist and treated appropriately. Patients with id reactions, as described previously, require oral nystatin or econazole on the diaper and intertriginous areas and 1% hydrocortisone applied to the plaques. Resolution usually takes 7 to 10 days. Mycolog II® and Lotrisone® creams are recommended by many physicians for monilial diaper rashes; however, the clinician should be cognizant that these preparations contain a fluorinated steroid and have been associated with adrenal suppression when used in intertriginous areas. Secondarily infected dermatitis, such as bullous impetigo, should be treated with the appropriate systemic antibiotics.

Whether traditional diaper creams and ointments are effective is still unproven. Their ability to provide an effective barrier that reduces irritation remains to be established.

DRUG REACTIONS IN THE SKIN

Background

When a drug is being taken by a child, any reaction of the skin that is not expected should be considered a drug reaction until proven otherwise. Hospitalized patients are more likely (30%) to have a reaction to a drug because of multiple exposures. Approximately 2% to 3% of these inpatients have cutaneous reactions. The rate of adverse effects depends on the particular drug. Arndt et al. showed that reactions occur at the rate of 59 per 1,000 drug courses for trimethoprim-sulfamethoxazole, whereas with the use of chloral hydrate, only 0.2 skin reactions per 1,000 courses occurred. When considering all drugs, they found skin reactions at a rate of 3 per 1,000 courses of therapy. In general, antibiotics, anticonvulsants, and blood products were responsible for most reactions.

When considering penicillin and its derivatives alone, allergies to these substances affect 1% to 10% of the population. Fatal anaphylaxis occurs in approximately 2 of 100,000 patients taking penicillin. Penicillin reactions appear less often in children, as is the case with any drug reaction. An increased risk for the development of anaphylactic reactions to penicillin is present in atopic individuals.

Pathophysiology

The pathogenesis of such reactions can be on an immune or nonimmune basis. When occurring on an immune basis, any of the four types of immunologic mechanisms (IgE-mediated, immune complex, cytotoxic, cell-mediated) can be involved. However, reactions also occur on the basis of overdose, specific toxicity, common side effects of a particular drug, and unusual drug interactions. Pathogenic mechanisms in specific situations often cannot be identified.

DRUGS COMMONLY ASSOCIATED WITH ALLERGIC
SKIN REACTIONS

Trimethoprim-sulfamethoxazole
Ampicillin
Semisynthetic penicillins (carbenicillin, cloxacillin,
    dicloxacillin, methicillin, nafcillin, oxacillin)
Sulfisoxazole
Penicillin G
Gentamicin
Cephalosporins
Dipyrone
Nitrazepam
Anticonvulsants (phenytoin, barbiturates, carbamazepine)
Nitrofurantoin
Glutethimide
Indomethacin

Clinical Manifestations

The appearance of drug reactions is nonspecific and may
mimic almost any known dermatosis. Therefore, the clinician
cannot make a diagnosis of a drug reaction based on the
appearance of the rash alone because the skin can react only in
a limited number of ways to many different stimuli. However,
certain patterns should raise suspicion of the presence of an
adverse reaction.

Laboratory analysis is usually not helpful in the diagnosis
of drug eruptions. Peripheral eosinophilia, believed to occur
commonly with adverse drug reactions, is actually uncommon.
Skin biopsy can be helpful.

Specific Reaction Patterns

Urticaria. Urticaria constitutes the most common expression
of drug sensitivity. Most commonly, reactions occur within 1
week of drug exposure. When an individual is on multiple
agents and has a reaction, the clinician should suspect those
agents that were most recently introduced or those medications
that are known to be commonly associated with drug reactions
(Table 85.6). When questioning for the use of medications, it is
important to ask not only about prescription items but also
about over-the-counter preparations. Occasionally, patients
who use aspirin, acetaminophen, laxatives, vitamins, or ear,
nose, or eye drops do not consider these substances to be medications or drugs.

Maculopapular Eruptions Similar to Those of a Viral Exanthem.
Maculopapular eruptions are the second most common of all
drug-induced rashes and may be caused by many different
agents. These eruptions are symmetric and consist of erythematous macules and papules with areas of confluence. Variable
involvement of the palms, soles, and mucous membranes, as well
as purpura, may occur. The presence and severity of pruritus are
variable. Ampicillin is a medication often associated with this
type of skin reaction, particularly in patients with infectious
mononucleosis.

Erythema Multiforme. Erythema multiforme is an acute and
often recurrent inflammatory syndrome often secondary to
drugs, particularly antibiotics and anticonvulsants (e.g., penicillins, sulfonamides, hydantoins, barbiturates, lamotrigine),
or infections. More recent observations suggest that a significant portion of idiopathic recurrent erythema multiforme
cases is likely caused by HSV. The skin findings include macules, papules, vesicles, and pathognomonic target or iris
lesions (Fig. 85.17) that tend to be more or less symmetrically
distributed. Bullous lesions may also be present. In the more
severe cases, constitutional symptoms occur; when mucous
membranes are involved, the terms *erythema multiforme
major* or *Stevens-Johnson syndrome* are used (Figs. 85.18 and
85.19, see also color plate). Erythema multiforme consists of
two lesion types: macular–urticarial and vesicular–bullous.
There is a predilection for the backs of the hands, palms, soles,
and extensor surfaces of the limbs. The lesions may begin at
these sites and then spread diffusely, or they may begin generalized. In 25% of the patients, the mucous membranes are
involved and, in fact, can be the sole site of involvement. The
usual sites of mucous membrane involvement are the lips, buccal mucosa, palate, conjunctivae, urethra, and vagina. With
severe involvement, the pharyngeal, tracheobronchial, and
esophageal mucous membranes are also affected. Less common sites are the anal and nasal mucosa. When the eyes are
involved, there may be simple conjunctivitis, severe keratitis,
or panophthalmitis. These changes may lead to blindness in
3% to 10% of these patients. Therefore, close attention to
involvement of the eyes is necessary. Lesions may continue to
erupt in crops for as long as 2 to 3 weeks. Again, drugs and certain infections, such as *Mycoplasma pneumoniae*, have been

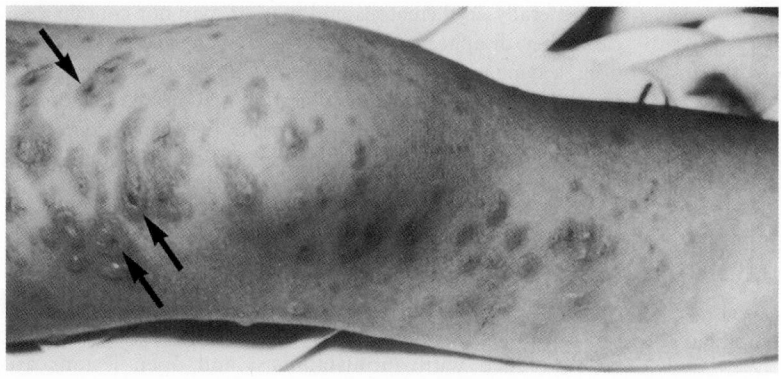

FIGURE 85.17 Iris or target lesions pathognomonic of
erythema multiforme.

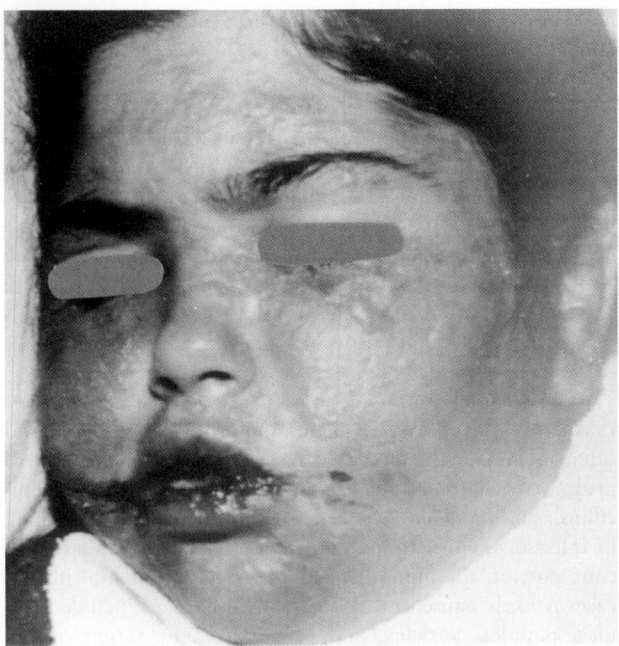

FIGURE 85.18 Adolescent with Stevens-Johnson syndrome secondary to sulfonamides. Note the involvement of mucous membranes of the mouth.

associated with Stevens-Johnson syndrome. Death occurs in 3% to 15% of patients with erythema multiforme major. Patients with Stevens-Johnson syndrome may also progress to toxic epidermal necrolysis (TEN). Avoidance of etiologic drugs, treatment of underlying infections, and supportive care have been the mainstay of therapy. Systemic corticosteroids have a limited role if treatment can be started early in the course of the reaction but should not be prolonged beyond 1 week, particularly if no benefit is seen. However, case reports and case series have suggested that IV immune globulin may significantly decrease morbidity and shorten the course of this syndrome and may be considered if organ function (such as vision) is at risk.

Toxic Epidermal Necrolysis. Drug-induced TEN is a life-threatening eruption characterized by a rapidly progressive, tender, red skin areas and skin sloughing and must be differ-

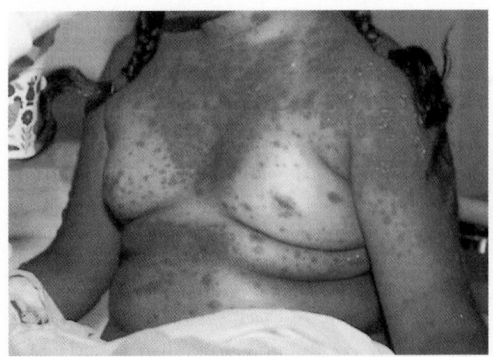

FIGURE 85.19 Same child as seen in Figure 85.18 with Stevens-Johnson syndrome secondary to sulfonamides. Note photo distribution of lesions.

entiated from the illness known as *staphylococcal scalded skin syndrome* (SSSS), caused by a circulating staphylococcal exotoxin. If a child who has TEN has been taking drugs long term or shortly before onset of the rash, is older than 6 years, or has a mixed rash (i.e., areas with the appearance of erythema multiforme and TEN), a biopsy must be performed to distinguish between the two disorders. With drug-induced TEN, dermal–epidermal separation is visible on histologic examination. If epidermolytic toxin has been released by staphylococci, epidermal cleavage occurs in the granular layer (Fig. 85.20). With extensive exfoliation of skin, fluid and electrolyte disturbances may occur and the potential for bacterial sepsis is present. Again, case reports and case series have suggested that IV immune globulin may significantly decrease morbidity and shorten the course of this syndrome.

Vasculitis. The classic lesions of vasculitis are palpable purpura. Although these lesions are characteristic, vasculitis may be manifest by erythematous macules, papules, urticaria, and hemorrhagic vesicles and bullae (Fig. 85.21, see also color plate). The diagnosis is made by a skin biopsy, which shows leukocytoclasis, endothelial cell necrosis, and destruction of dermal vessels.

Erythema Nodosum. The lesions of erythema nodosum appear as deep, tender, erythematous nodules or plaques of the extensor surfaces of the extremities (Fig. 85.22, see also color plate). They are believed to be hypersensitivity phenomena secondary to infections (e.g., streptococcal pharyngitis, tuberculosis, coccidioidomycosis, histoplasmosis), inflammatory bowel disease, sarcoidosis, malignancies, and occasionally, drugs. The exact immunologic mechanism has not been clarified.

Photosensitive Cutaneous Eruption. When a drug causes an exaggeration of the sunburn response, a phototoxic eruption should be considered. However, photoallergic eruptions usually do not occur on first exposure to a medication because immunologic induction must first occur. Because a hypersensitivity reaction is also involved, the eruption, although concentrated most heavily on sun-exposed areas, can also occur on non–sun-exposed areas. Tetracycline and sulfonamides can be involved in this reaction. Non-steroidal antiinflammatory agents and antifungals, such as voriconazole, may be associated with photosensitive eruptions (known as pseudoporphyria) in which blistering and skin fragility occur in photo-exposed areas.

Fixed Drug Eruption. Fixed drug eruption refers to a localized round or oval dermatitis that tends to recur at the same location each time there is exposure to the offending drug. The lesions are generally erythematous and may or may not contain vesicles. They disappear over 7 to 10 days after cessation of the drug, leaving various shades of postinflammatory hyperpigmentation in their place. The discoloration may persist for months or years. Initially, lesions are solitary but then can become multiple; they often involve the palms, soles, glans penis, and lips.

Management

Vital to the management of any suspected drug reaction is the identification and removal of the offending drug. Pruritus can be controlled with antihistamines, and open lesions are

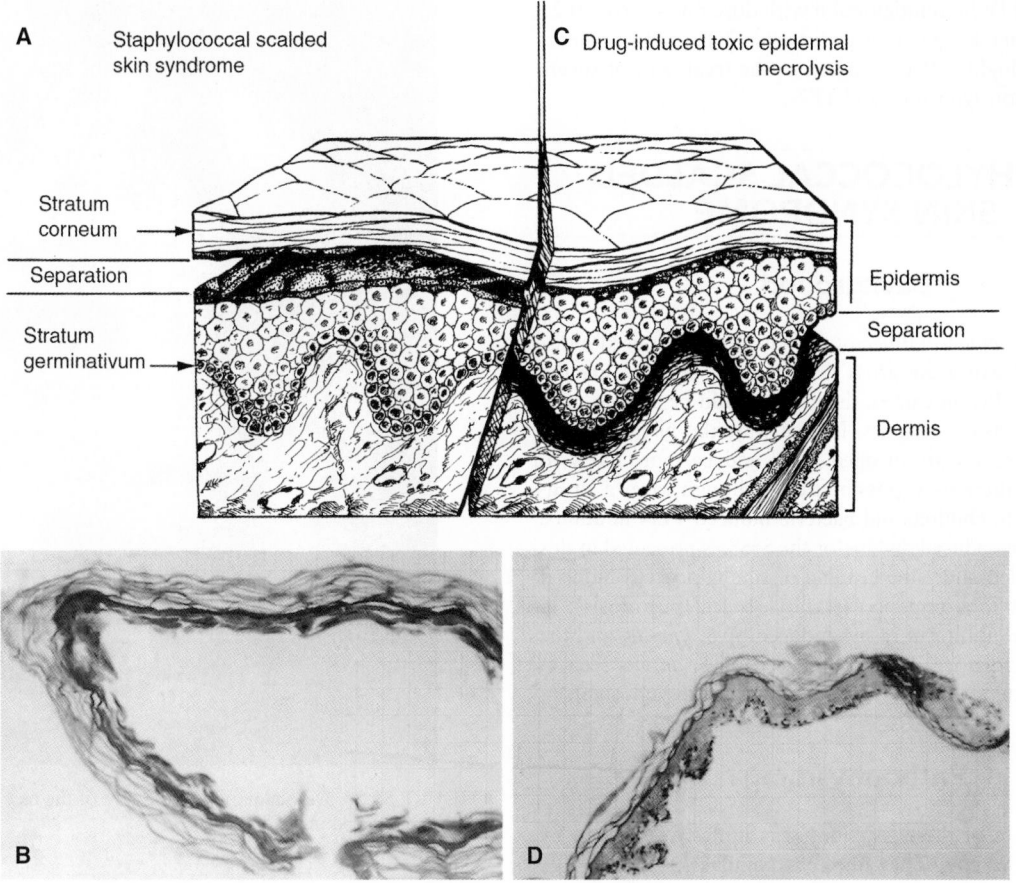

FIGURE 85.20 **A** and **B**: Pathology in staphylococcal scalded skin syndrome. **C** and **D**: Pathology in drug-induced toxic epidermal necrolysis.

responsive to compressing with Burow's solution and topical silver sulfadiazine. When extensive exfoliation occurs, attention to fluid and electrolyte balance and secondary infection is essential. Any patient with mucous membrane involvement should have an ophthalmologic examination to rule out the presence of corneal involvement. Hospitalization should be considered in any patient who has severe involvement of the skin, is toxic, or has extensive exfoliation.

The literature suggests that steroid therapy of Stevens-Johnson syndrome and drug-induced TEN is of no value, will prolong hospital stays, and may in fact be harmful. If used, steroids (i.e., an equivalent of prednisone 1 to 2 mg per kg per day) must be started within the first 2 days of the eruption to be effective. Progression of the reaction after 5 days of steroid therapy indicates that the medication is ineffective and should be discontinued. If skin denudation is greater than 20% of the child's body surface area, steroid therapy should be avoided. If denudation progresses to greater than 25% of body surface area, transfer to a burn unit should be considered. While the data are somewhat conflicting, recent investigations suggest

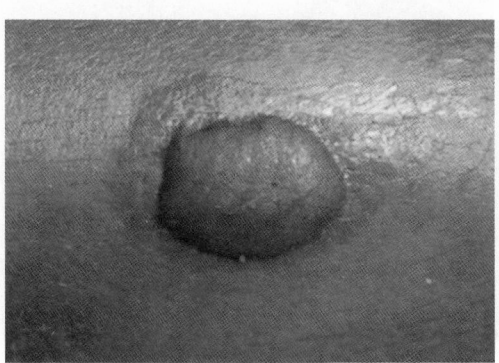

FIGURE 85.21 Hemorrhagic bulla in patient with vasculitis.

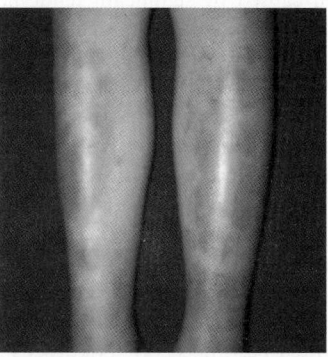

FIGURE 85.22 Extensor surface involved with lesions of erythema nodosum.

MEDICAL EMERGENCIES

that the use of IV immunoglobulin with dose ranges from 0.25 to 0.75 gm per kg per day given over 3 to 5 days shows promise as a highly effective agent in the treatment of severe Stevens-Johnson syndrome and TEN.

STAPHYLOCOCCAL SCALDED SKIN SYNDROME

Background

The term *toxic epidermal necrolysis* has often been used indiscriminately. Because the gross dermatologic changes are the same despite different causes, this term should be used to indicate only the visible changes. In this way, the physician will approach patients with an open mind and be more likely to consider the alternative possibilities: although rare, a drug-induced TEN in children and bacteria-induced TEN in adults. Staphylococcus-induced disease, or the SSSS, is presented in this section. Included under the heading of staphylococcus-induced disease are bullous impetigo (staphylococcal pustulosis); in newborns, scarlatiniform rashes induced by *S. aureus*; and the generalized exfoliative syndrome caused by *S. aureus* seen in newborns (Ritter's disease) or in children (Lyell's syndrome).

Pathophysiology

The mechanism of these reactions was initially described by Mellish and Glasgow. They injected coagulase-positive phage group II staphylococci into newborn mice, producing erythema and a positive Nikolsky's sign (denudation of skin with gentle rubbing) in 12 to 16 hours, followed by bullae and extensive exfoliation in 16 to 20 hours. Since then, phage group I and III staphylococci have also been implicated. The cellular basis was later elucidated by Amagai et al. Staphylococcal toxins (exfoliative toxins A and B) specifically cleave the superficial epidermal cellular adhesion molecule desmoglein 1. The disease is believed to occur primarily in children because they lack antibodies against the organism and are unable to metabolize and excrete the toxin as do adults.

Clinical Manifestations

The illness begins with malaise, fever, and irritability. The irritability is often caused by significant tenderness of the skin when touched. Mothers will relate that their infant does not want to be held and cries when handled. This is followed by a "sunburn" erythema, which begins and is most intense around the neck, intertriginous areas, and periorifically (especially around the eyes and mouth). The erythema spreads to varying portions of the skin surface, and the child may be very toxic. With mild involvement of the skin, superficial desquamation (flaking) then follows similar to the reaction that occurs after ordinary sunburn (Fig. 85.23). With severe involvement, large sheets of skin shear away, leaving a denuded, oozing surface similar to the reaction that occurs after a burn (Fig. 85.24). The skin can often be rubbed off (Nikolsky's sign). Vesicles, pustules, and bullae can also occur during the exfoliative phase. Often, a purulent discharge emits from the eyes, but no

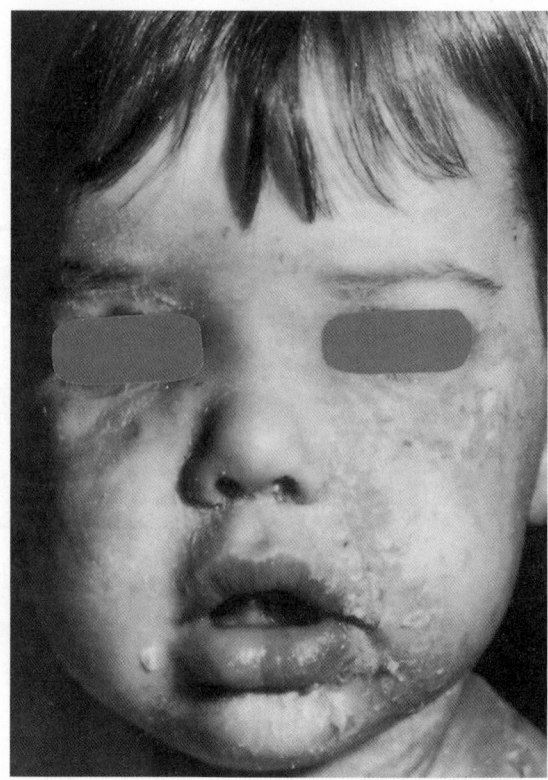

FIGURE 85.23 Desquamation of the skin of the face in the staphylococcal scalded skin syndrome.

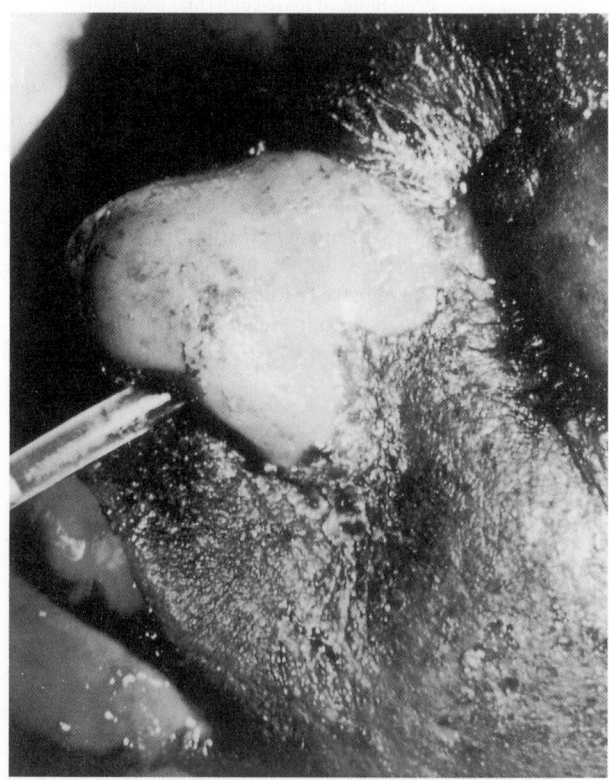

FIGURE 85.24 Denudation of skin of nose in child with staphylococcal scalded skin syndrome.

TABLE 85.7

TOXIC SHOCK SYNDROME

Fever
Toxic epidermal necrolysis-like rash
Desquamation (after 10 days)
Hypotension
Vomiting/diarrhea
Hyperemia of the mucous membranes
Sterile pyuria
Elevated bilirubin and enzyme levels
Low platelet count
Disorientation or alteration in consciousness

conjunctival injection is present. Mucous membranes are not involved. Most children do well, and clearing of the skin occurs in 12 to 14 days, leaving no residua.

Complete blood cell count and urinalysis are not helpful in the evaluation of such children. Although blood cultures should be performed, they are usually negative, as are cultures of intact vesicles or bullae. At times, *S. aureus* can be grown from exfoliating skin, the umbilicus, circumcision wounds, throat, eyes, ears, nose, or rectum. Histologic examination of the skin distinguishes between changes caused by staphylo-cocci or a drug. In SSSS, skin clippings or a shave or punch biopsy will show separation of the superficial layer of the epi-dermis subcorneally (Fig. 85.20A and 85.20B). Patients who have drug-induced TEN will have dermal–epidermal separa-tion (Fig. 85.20C and 85.20D). Children who are taking med-ications long term or shortly before the eruption of the rash, children older than 6 years, or children with a mixed rash (i.e., areas of TEN and erythema multiforme) should have a skin biopsy taken for differentiation.

Toxic shock syndrome (secondary to staphylococci and streptococci) has also been characterized (Table 85.7).

Causes other than *S. aureus* or drugs may produce a similar clinical picture of toxic erythema. These conditions include certain fumigants, lymphomas, aspergillosis, irradiation, and graft-versus-host reaction.

Management

Most of the time, SSSS is a self-limited disorder. Antibiotics probably ameliorate the course of the disease, but steroids have no beneficial effects. In fact, steroids may exacerbate the dermatitis by increasing the ability of the organisms to prolif-erate and produce greater amounts of epidermolytic toxin.

Neonates and children younger than 1 year should be admitted to the hospital and started on IV antistaphylococcal antibiotics (cefazolin, oxacillin) after blood cultures are obtained. The addition of IV clindamycin because of its effects on bacterial ribosome metabolism should also be considered to help decrease production of bacterial toxin in ill patients. In addition, any older child who is toxic or who has severe skin involvement with significant denudation should be admitted. Close attention should be paid to the child's state of hydration and electrolyte imbalances when a significant amount of skin is lost. Secondary infection, similar to a patient with a major burn, is an important consideration.

Older children with mild involvement limited to dry de-squamation, who are not toxic, can be managed on an outpa-tient basis. Depending on local bacterial antibiotic sensitivity profiles, these children can be started on oral dicloxacillin or erythromycin, cephalexin, clindamycin, or trimethoprim-sulfamethoxazole and followed closely. Skin care is nonspecific unless extensive denudation occurs, then the use of Silvadene® cream is warranted.

BITES AND INFESTATIONS (SEE ALSO CHAPTER 83)

Children are often bitten by insects (especially mosquitoes and fleas) and at times are infested by parasites. The papules, urticaria, blisters, and hemorrhagic lesions produced are com-monly misdiagnosed. The season of the year, area of the coun-try, grouping and appearance (central punctum) of the lesions, and distribution on exposed surfaces provide the clues neces-sary for diagnosis.

Mosquitoes and Fleas

Mosquitoes are probably the most common cause of insect bites in children, followed closely by fleas (Fig. 85.25). Bed-bugs have also become more common in various parts of the country. Mosquito bites are generally limited to the warm months of the year. In contrast, fleabites, which predominate from spring to fall, can also occur during the winter months as a result of cats and dogs living indoors. At times, fleabites occur without an animal living in the household. Generally, the clinician should ask for a history of visits to a household that has pets or whether the patient's family has recently moved into a home in which the prior owners had pets. In the latter situation, fleas can live in carpeting for a long time.

The distribution of lesions is a valuable clue in making the diagnosis of mosquito or fleabites. Insect bites generally involve the exposed surfaces of the head, face, and extremities. The lesions are usually urticarial wheals that occur in groups or along a line on which the insect was crawling. Some lesions may manifest a central punctum. On occasion, both mosquito bites and fleabites can cause blistering lesions. These lesions are not caused by secondary infection but rather by a violent

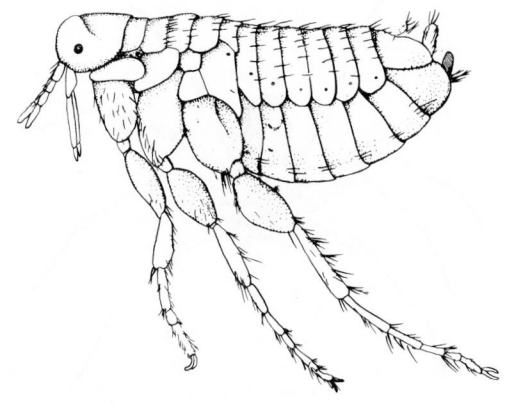

FIGURE 85.25 Flea (*Pulex irritans*).

immune response to the bite. Certainly, excoriation with resulting secondary infection with *S. aureus* or group A streptococci can complicate a simple bite.

A recurrent papular eruption called papular urticaria can occur in young children who become sensitized to insect bites. Although the lesions tend to occur on exposed parts of the body, with sensitization, they may appear at sites distant from the primary bite.

Unfortunately, no specific treatment exists for insect bites. Antihistamines, calamine lotion, or topical steroids have a limited or temporary effect. Prevention through the prophylactic use of insect repellents offers the best solution. Obviously, elimination of the biting insects by treatment of the homes with insecticides or treatment of the infested animals is important.

Tick Bites

Tick bites usually cause only local reactions. Rarely, they are associated with significant systemic illness, including Rocky Mountain spotted fever, tick paralysis, and Lyme arthritis.

When ticks are removed, it is important not to leave fragments of the mouthparts in the skin or to introduce body fluids containing infectious organisms. Various methods have been recommended for removal of ticks from the skin. The only safe method is to use a blunt curved forceps, tweezers, or fingers protected by rubber gloves. The tick is grasped close to the skin surface and pulled upward with a steady even force. The tick must not be squeezed, crushed, or punctured. If mouthparts are left in the skin, they should be removed.

Spider Bites

Loxosceles reclusus, or the brown recluse spider (Fig. 85.26), found most commonly in the south central United States (from southeastern Nebraska through Texas, east through southern Ohio and Georgia), is responsible for most skin reactions caused by the bite of a spider. This spider is small, the body being only 8 to 10 mm long, and bears a violin-shaped band over the dorsal cephalothorax. The venom contains necrotizing, hemolytic, and spreading factors.

The initial symptoms include mild stinging and/or pruritus. A hemorrhagic blister then appears, which can develop into a gangrenous eschar. Severe bites can cause a generalized erythematous macular eruption, nausea, vomiting, chills, malaise, muscle aches, and hemolysis. Treatment includes oral steroids within 6 to 12 hours after the bite, antibiotics to prevent secondary infection, the use of dapsone in selected cases, and surgical removal of the necrotic area to prevent spread of the toxin. An antivenom has been developed at the Vanderbilt School of Medicine.

Scabies Infestation

The cardinal symptom of any infestation with scabies is pruritus. Infants and children excoriate themselves to the point of bleeding. Two clues should be considered when attempting to make this diagnosis: (i) distribution (concentration on the hands, feet, and folds of the body, especially the finger webs, and genital areas) and (ii) involvement of other family members. It is important not only to ask other family members if they have pruritus but also to examine their skin. In contrast to adults, infants may develop blisters and exhibit lesions on the head and face.

The diagnosis is made by scraping involved skin and looking for mites under the 10× microscope objective (Fig. 85.27). The materials necessary to examine the skin for scabies are a glass slide, immersion or mineral oil, and no. 15 scalpel blade. A drop of mineral or immersion oil should be placed on the glass slide, and the no. 15 blade edge should be dipped into this oil. The best areas to scrape are the interdigital webs of the hands or tiny linear lesions that represent burrows caused by the mite. One procedure that may accentuate burrows involves the use of fountain pen ink applied to the suspected area of skin. After the surface ink is cleaned away, the mite burrows can be identified by means of the ink that has trickled into them. Also, local magnification with a dermatoscope or other magnifier may reveal the presence of air bubbles within burrows, which indicates the presence of live mites.

Once an infestation occurs, it usually takes 1 month for sensitization and pruritus to develop. The introduction of 5% permethrin cream (Elimite®) has obviated the need for lindane

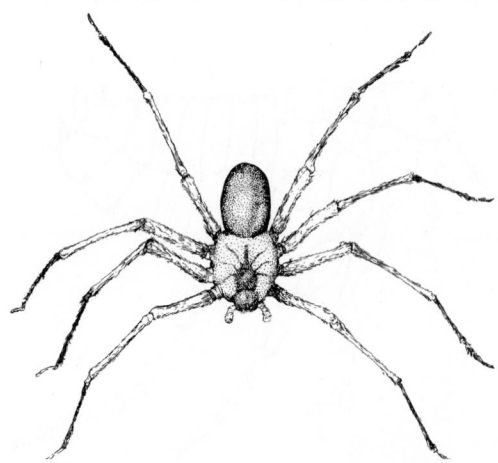

FIGURE 85.26 Brown recluse spider (*Loxosceles reclusus*).

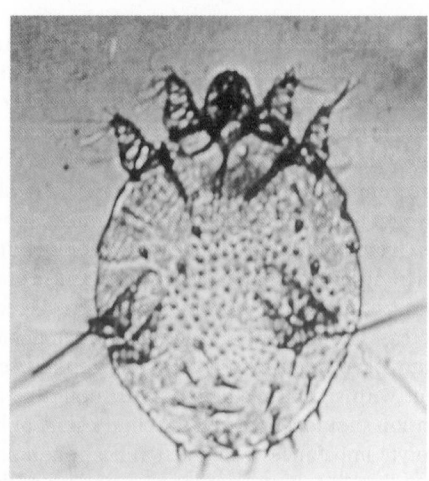

FIGURE 85.27 Mite that causes scabies (*Sarcoptes scabiei*).

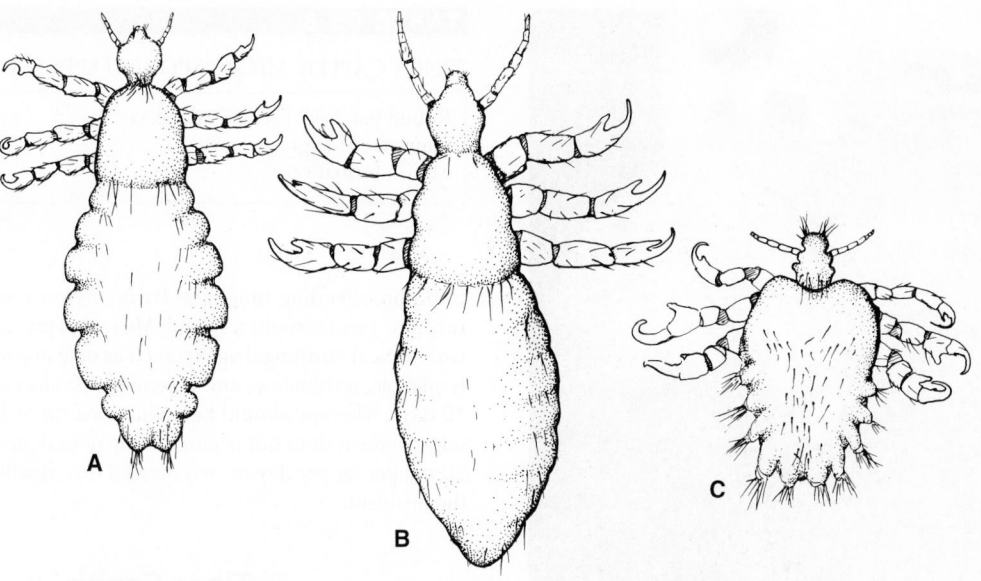

FIGURE 85.28 **A:** Head louse (*Pediculus humanus* var. *capitis*). **B:** Body louse (*Pediculus humanus* var. *corporis*). **C:** Pubic louse (*Phthirus pubis*).

and its potential toxicity. This cream should be applied from head to toe and left on for 8 to 14 hours. The preparation is then washed off with soap and water. All family members and close contacts (e.g., babysitters, grandparents) should be treated simultaneously. The safety of permethrin for use in pregnant women and very young infants has not been proven; these patients alternatively can be treated for four consecutive nights with precipitated sulfur (4%) compounded in petrolatum. The treatment should be repeated once 7 to 10 days later to eliminate any hatched eggs.

Louse Infestation

Three forms of lice infest humans: (i) the head louse, (ii) the body louse, and (iii) the pubic or crab louse (Fig. 85.28). The major louse infestation in children involves the scalp and causes pruritus. The female attaches her eggs to the hair shaft. The egg then hatches, leaving behind numerous nits (Fig. 85.29) that resemble dandruff. Secondary infection can occur from vigorous scratching. Body lice generally reside in the seams of clothing and lay their eggs there. They go to the body to feed, particularly the interscapular, shoulder, and waist areas. Red pruritic puncta that become papular and wheal-like then occur. Pubic lice occur in the genital area, lower abdomen, axillae, and eyelashes. Transmission is usually venereal. Blue macules (maculae caeruleae) that are 3 to 15 mm in diameter can be seen on the thighs, abdomen, or thorax of infested persons. These macules are secondary to bites.

Because the body louse resides in clothing, therapy consists mainly of disinfecting the clothing with steam under pressure. Pediculosis capitis is effectively treated with 1% permethrin or pyrethrin creme rinse (Nix®, Rid®, A-200®). The patient's hair should be shampooed, rinsed, and toweled dry. Enough medication to saturate the hair and scalp is applied. The medication is washed out after 10 minutes. Malathion has also

been recently made available again for the treatment of head lice. This agent is quite effective but carries the risks of flammability and potential toxicity of an organophosphate compound. Patients with resistant disease may also respond to topical petrolatum applied to hair and scalp nightly for 1 week as a lice suffocant or trimethoprim-sulfamethoxazole given for 5 to 7 days, which kills the symbiotic parasite present in the GI tract of head lice. Pediculosis pubis is best treated with the same permethrin or pyrethrin preparations used for head lice. Any nits are removed with a fine-toothed comb. The safest treatment for lice in the eyelashes is the application of Vaseline® twice daily for 8 days. The lice stick to the Vaseline®, cannot feed, and die. Another treatment alternative is physostigmine ophthalmic ointment, although it may carry more significant toxicity.

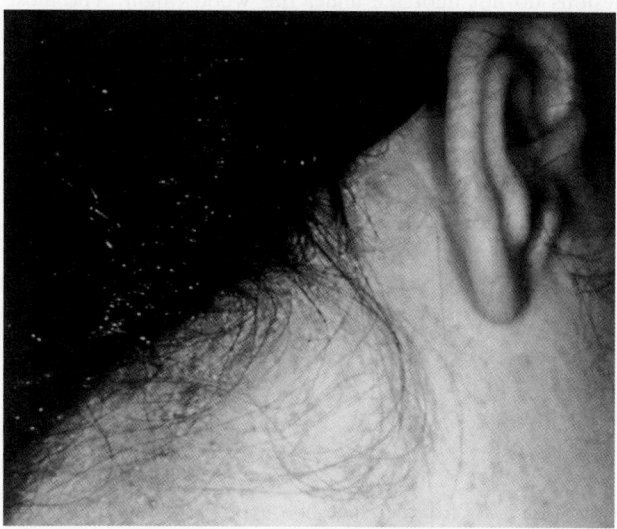

FIGURE 85.29 Nits in the hair of a child with head lice.

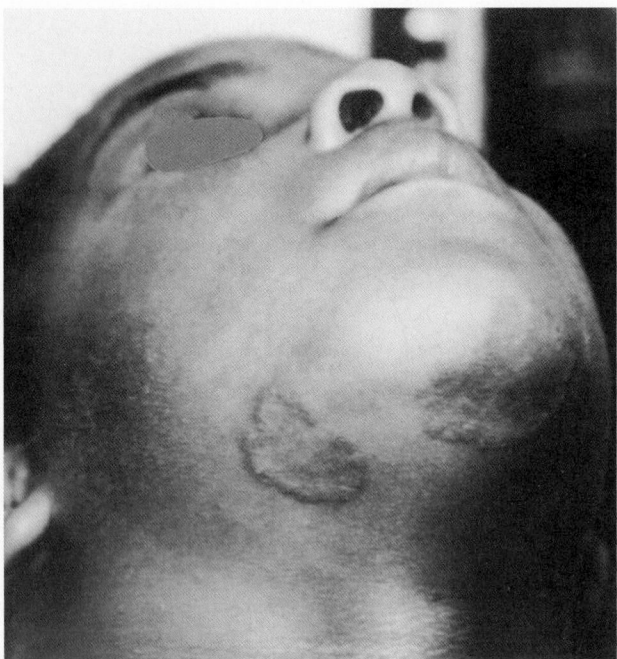

FIGURE 85.30 Child with tinea corporis.

SUPERFICIAL FUNGAL INFECTIONS OF THE SKIN

Tinea Corporis

Tinea corporis (Fig. 85.30) is characterized by one or more sharply circumscribed scaly patches. The center of the circular patch generally clears as the leading edge spreads out. The leading edge may be composed of papules, vesicles, or pustules. The lesions are most commonly confused with nummular eczema. The diagnosis can be made by scraping the active outer rim of papules and examining the scales with a potassium hydroxide (KOH) preparation under the microscope (Fig. 85.31). These lesions do not fluoresce under the Wood's light. The most

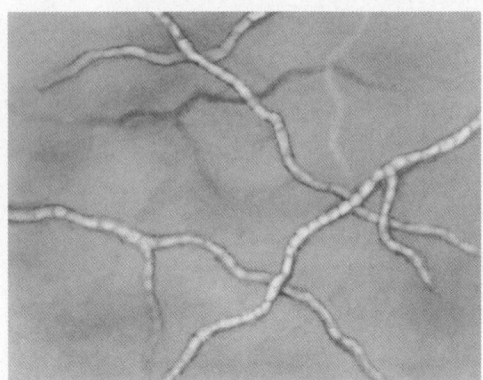

FIGURE 85.31 Characterization of a positive potassium hydroxide preparation demonstrating branching hyphae running across the microscope field.

TABLE 85.8

TINEA CAPITIS *MICROSPORUM* SPECIES

Round patches of scaling alopecia
Fluoresce blue-green
Kerion formation

common offending fungi are *Trichophyton* species (tonsurans, rubrum, mentagrophytes) and *Microsporum canis*. Treatment with topical antifungal agents such as clotrimazole, miconazole, econazole, terbinafine, and butenafine produces clearing in 7 to 10 days. Therapy should be maintained for at least 2 weeks. If improvement does not occur, treatment with griseofulvin (15 to 20 mg per kg per day in two divided doses) will usually resolve the problem.

Tinea Capitis

Although tinea capitis was commonly caused by the *Microsporum* species in the past, it usually results now from infection by *Trichophyton tonsurans*. The two forms have different clinical appearances. The *Microsporum* species (Table 85.8) generally causes round patches of scaling alopecia (Fig. 85.32). Illumination of a lesion with a Wood's lamp gives a blue-green fluorescence. Kerion formation can occur as a swollen, boggy abscess. The *Trichophyton* species (Table 85.9) usually causes scattered alopecia with seborrheic-like scaling, not always oval or rounded; the alopecia is irregular in outline with indistinct margins. Normal hairs grow within the patches

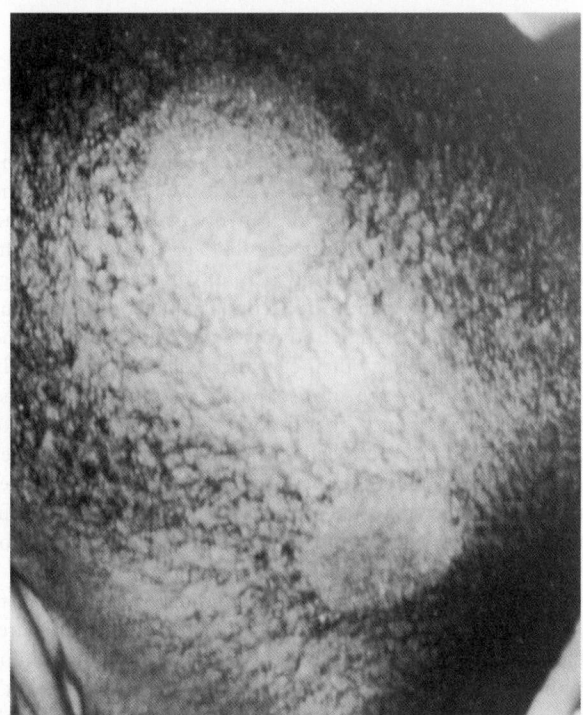

FIGURE 85.32 Tinea capitis secondary to infection with *Microsporum audouinii*.

TABLE 85.9

TINEA CAPITIS *TRICHOPHYTON* SPECIES

> Partial scattered alopecia—not always oval or rounded
> Alopecia irregular in outline with indistinct margins
> Normal hairs growing within patch of alopecia
> Black dots, diffuse scaling (dandruff)
> Nonfluorescent
> Folliculitis, suppuration, kerion formation

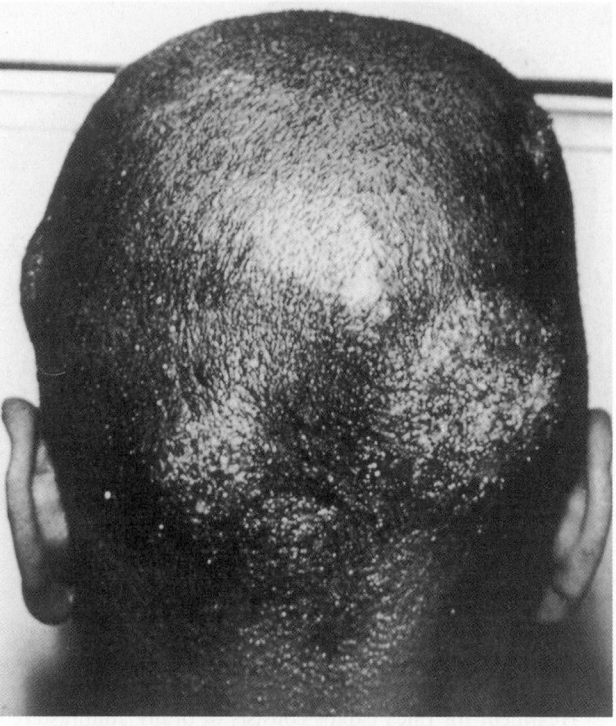

FIGURE 85.34 Patient with tinea capitis and multiple kerions.

of alopecia. At times, the hairs break off at the surface of the scalp, leaving a "black dot" appearance (Fig. 85.33). Diffuse scaling may simulate dandruff, and although minimal hair loss is present, it is not perceived. Wood's light examination of lesions caused by *Trichophyton* species does not produce fluorescence. The organism can cause a folliculitis, suppuration, and kerion formation (Fig. 85.34). Diagnosis is made by culturing the affected scalp area (Fig. 85.35). The clinician should consider the presence of tinea capitis when a nonresponsive seborrheic or atopic dermatitis of the scalp is present, black dots are seen, or increased scaling follows the use of topical steroids. With the use of dermatophyte test media, a color change occurs in the media (yellow to red) in the presence of a growing dermatophyte. If a kerion is present, the swelling (allergic reaction to the fungus) can be controlled by a combination of griseofulvin and prednisone.

In the differential diagnosis of patchy hair loss, as is seen in tinea capitis, the clinician should consider alopecia areata (Fig. 85.36). However, with alopecia areata, no inflammation or scaling of the scalp occurs. *Trichotillomania* (also *trichotillosis*), the term given to the habit children develop of rubbing, twirling, or playing with their hair to the point that the hair breaks and is lost in irregular sometimes geometric patches, should also be

considered. Hairs are characteristically of different length within the affected area, indicating breakage at different times. In addition, there is no scaling or inflammation typically seen. Traction alopecia occurs with certain hairstyles. Hair is lost at the margins of the hairline with the ponytail style or frequent use of hair rollers. Tight braiding or cornrowing can cause hair loss on any area of the scalp. At times, papules or pustules occur where the skin has been disrupted by the traction. Infants who

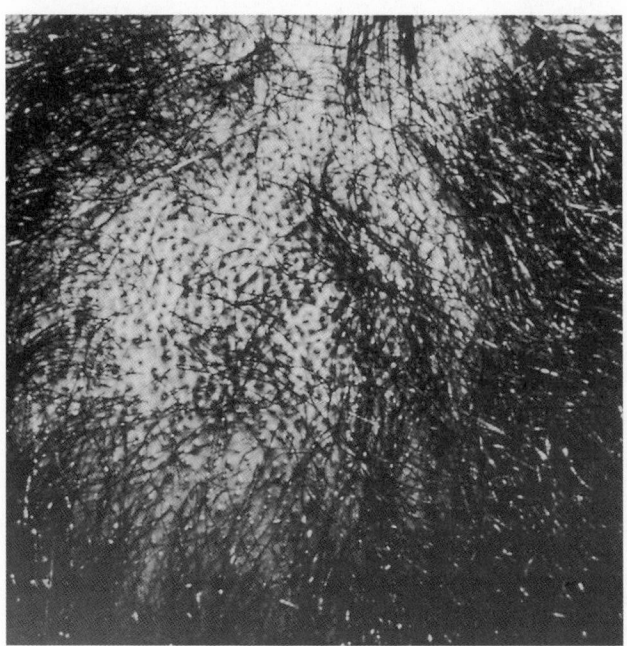

FIGURE 85.33 "Black dot" appearance of scalp infection with *Trichophyton tonsurans*.

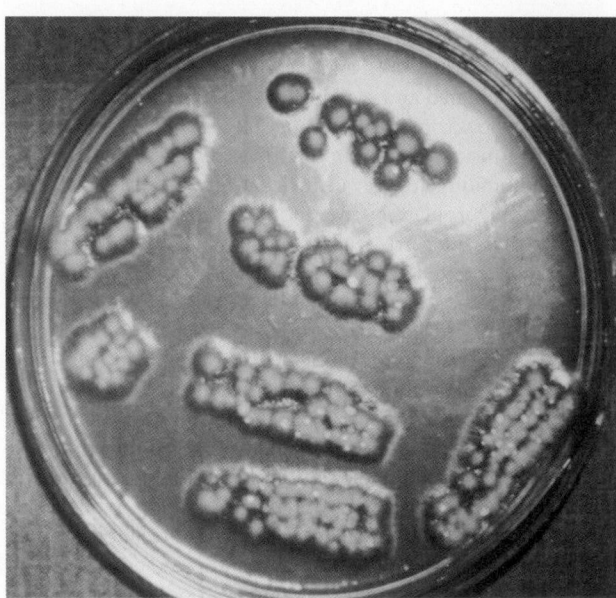

FIGURE 85.35 Toothbrush implants of scalp brushing that are growing fungus.

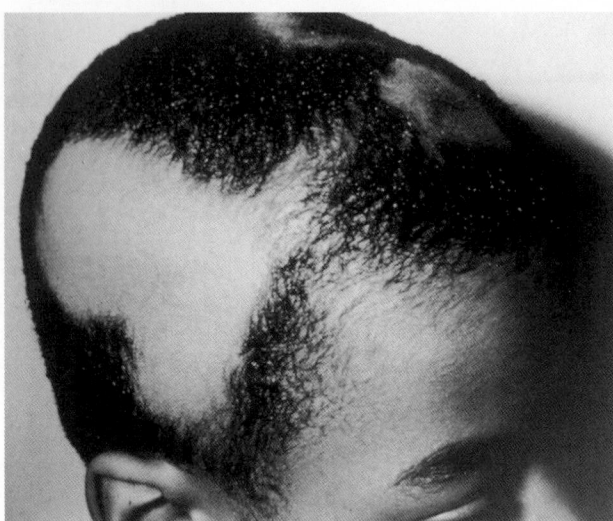

FIGURE 85.36 Child with alopecia areata.

are left on their backs for long periods may lose hair at the occiput from the constant friction in that area.

Treatment for tinea capitis consists of orally administered griseofulvin 15 to 20 mg per kg per day in two divided doses with a glass of whole milk or fatty food for 6 to 8 weeks. Adjunctive therapy includes the use of 2.5% selenium sulfide shampoo twice weekly. With the use of this shampoo, shedding of spores is decreased within 1 to 2 weeks. Terbinafine granules (5 to 8 mg per kg per day) have been approved by the U.S. FDA for use in tinea capitis, and this medication shows good efficacy, particularly for tinea capitis and can be used from 2 to 4 weeks. Fluconazole has been used for tinea capitis as well but has shown suboptimal efficacy rates.

Tinea Cruris

Tinea cruris begins as a small, red, scaling rash in the groin that spreads peripherally and clears centrally. The edges are sharply marginated and scalloped, extending down the thighs. Generally, the scrotum is not noticeably involved. This fungal infection is most common in semitropical regions where heat and high humidity are prevalent. Tight-fitting clothes also contribute to the problem by preventing evaporation. Other conditions to consider are seborrheic dermatitis (which usually can be differentiated by involvement of other areas of the body such as the ears, scalp, and eyelids), intertrigo (generally secondary to friction and maceration), contact dermatitis, candidiasis (which usually involves the inner thigh and causes the scrotum to appear bright red), and erythrasma (which will fluoresce under Woods' lamp). The clinician should always check the feet to ensure there is not fungal involvement in that area as well. In general, this condition affects only postpubertal children. Diagnosis is made by KOH preparation. Nonspecific measures for treatment include loose-fitting clothing, reducing the amount of perspiration by using dusting powders, and decreasing intake of caffeine-containing foods. Clotrimazole, miconazole, tolnaftate, and econazole are useful as topical antifungal agents. Oral griseofulvin may be needed in severe

cases. Again, commercially available compounded agents such as Mycolog II® and Lotrisone®, which include potent topical steroids, should be avoided in the intertriginous areas because of the risk of atrophy and HPA axis suppression.

Tinea Pedis

Tinea pedis is generally caused by *Trichophyton rubrum* or *Trichophyton mentagrophytes*. It occurs most commonly in postpubertal children. The cracking and peeling of the skin suggestive of tinea pedis in prepubertal children more often indicates the presence of atopic eczema or hyperhidrosis. Tinea pedis is a penalty of civilization in that it occurs primarily in those individuals who wear shoes. KOH preparation will demonstrate hyphae, especially when samples are taken from between the fourth and fifth interspaces of the toes. Clinically, the skin has a dry, white, hazy appearance and is often pruritic. When secondary bacterial infection is present, an odor occurs. At times, an inflammatory lesion (caused by *T. mentagrophytes*) causes blistering. The presence of an id reaction indicates dissemination of antigen to other parts of the body, especially the hands.

The differential diagnosis of tinea pedis includes simple maceration, contact dermatitis, and atopic eczema. Treatment consists of drying the feet thoroughly after washing; wearing dry, clean socks; avoiding caffeine-containing foods to decrease sweating; keeping shoes off as much as possible; and walking barefoot or in sandals. Topical antifungal agents (see "Tinea Cruris" section) and/or oral griseofulvin are used to treat this condition. Newer medications (see "Tinea Capitis" section) are being used for this problem with increasing frequency.

Tinea Versicolor

Tinea versicolor refers to a superficial infection of the skin caused by *Malassezia furfur*, which produces color changes of the skin, hypopigmentation, hyperpigmentation, and sometimes a salmon-colored redness (Fig. 85.37). Wood's light examination usually shows yellowish brown fluorescence. Because moisture promotes growth of the organism, exacerbations occur in warm weather or in athletes who sweat excessively. The infection is difficult to eradicate and recurs frequently. A KOH preparation

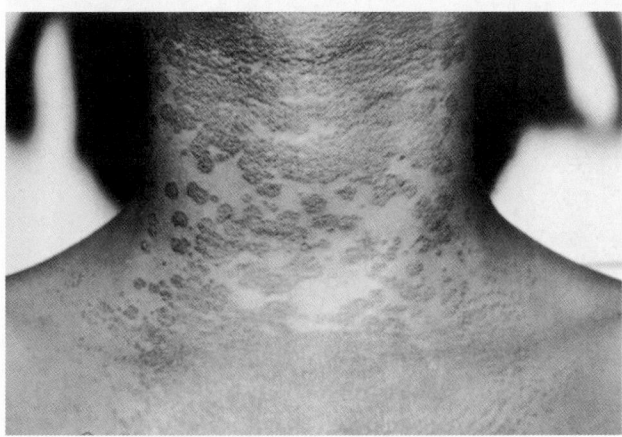

FIGURE 85.37 Adolescent with tinea versicolor.

shows short, stubby hyphae and large clusters of spores, often referred to as "spaghetti and meatballs."

Treatment consists of lathering the entire body with selenium sulfide shampoo (2.5% concentration) or ketoconazole shampoo after wetting the skin surface in a shower. The lather is left on for 20 minutes and is then showered off. This procedure is carried out daily during the first week, with decreasing frequency over the ensuing weeks. Maintenance therapy once weekly throughout the summer or warmer seasons is advisable because of the high incidence of recurrence. Localized areas of involvement can be treated with topical antifungal agents (e.g., econazole, ketoconazole topically). Adolescents can be treated with 400 mg of ketoconazole given as a single oral dose and then 200 mg at monthly intervals during the warm summer months or during a sports season when the patient sweats frequently. Because tinea versicolor tends to be a recurrent problem, retreatment in subsequent years may be necessary.

VASCULAR LESIONS

Pyogenic Granulomas

Pyogenic granulomas (Fig. 85.38A) are vascular nodules that develop rapidly at the site of an injury, such as a cut, scratch, insect bite, or burn. The histologic picture is that of proliferating

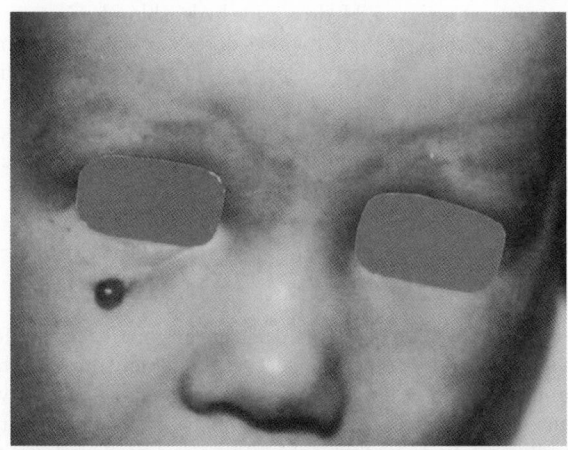

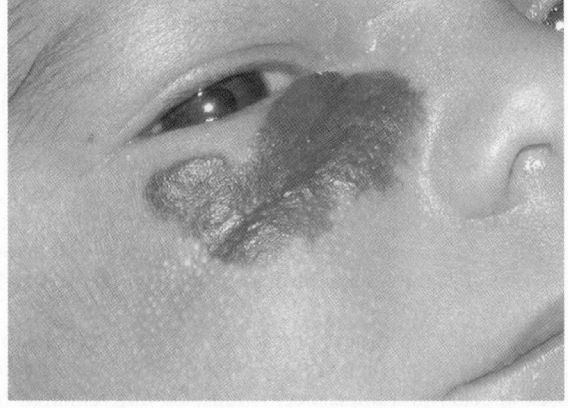

FIGURE 85.38 **A:** Pyogenic granuloma on the cheek of a child. **B:** Periocular hemangioma with risk of amblyopia.

capillaries in a loose stroma. Although this lesion was previously believed to be caused by infection of a small wound, the definite cause has not been established. Pyogenic granulomas occur commonly in children and young adults, usually on the fingers, face, hands, and forearms.

Clinically, the lesions are bright red to reddish brown or blue-black. The vascular nodules are pedunculated, ranging from 0.5 to 2 cm in size. Their surfaces are glistening, or raspberry-like, often becoming eroded and crusted. They bleed easily. Generally, they are asymptomatic. Because spontaneous disappearance is rare, the lesions must be removed by curettage, excision, electrosurgery, cryosurgery, laser surgery, or some combination of these various modalities.

Hemangiomas

Hemangiomas of infancy (infantile hemangiomas) represent benign vascular tumors that are present in approximately 3% of newborns and up to 10% of all infants. These are seen most frequently in premature and low-birth-weight infants and occur more commonly in girls (80%) than in boys. Superficial lesions possess a red color resembling a strawberry or raspberry. Deep lesions appear soft, compressible, and often are faintly bluish. Mixed lesions may show features of both superficial and deep hemangiomas. These lesions typically undergo a proliferative phase during the first 6 months, plateau in growth during the second 6 months, and then begin a slow process of involution. Although most lesions generally involute with little to no complications given time, certain hemangiomas pose potential risks based on their anatomic location.

Rapidly enlarging hemangiomas near the eyes (Fig. 85.38B) may result in amblyopia through obstruction of the visual axis (deprivation amblyopia) or because of the compression of the eyeball itself (strabismus or anisometropia) and require prompt intervention with systemic steroids or sometimes surgery. β-Blockers have recently been introduced in a small number of patients to treat severe hemangiomas of infancy with favorable responses. At present, limited data are available; so, caution should be taken particularly in light of potential complications such as bradycardia, hypotension, hypoglycemia, bronchospasm, and hypothermia. Hemangiomas in a "beard distribution"—around the mouth, preauricular areas, chin, or anterior neck—may indicate the presence of airway hemangiomas and warrant further evaluation by direct laryngobronchoscopy or radiologic imaging studies. Hemangiomas overlying the midline lower back may represent markers for spinal dysraphism or tethered cord syndrome and warrant imaging. Hemangiomas occurring in any area, but especially the oral or genital areas, may ulcerate and become secondarily infected, which may result in permanent scarring. Treatment with topical or oral antibiotics with nonadherent dressings can be helpful in managing these cases. Some may require treatment with a pulsed dye laser. Pain may also be an issue for these children. Finally, large, segmental facial hemangiomas have been associated with PHACE(S) syndrome, in which children suffer from posterior fossa malformations, arterial anomalies including coarctation of the aorta, structural cardiac malformations, endocrinologic and structural eye abnormalities, and midline sternal defects or supraumbilical raphe (Table 85.10). Intracranial vascular anomalies may predispose this subset of these children to an increased risk for stroke.

MEDICAL EMERGENCIES

TABLE 85.10

COMPLICATIONS RELATED TO HEMANGIOMAS

Anatomic location	Associated complication
Periocular	Amblyopia
Beard area	Airway involvement
Midline prevertebral	Tethered cord syndrome; spinal dysraphism
Genital area	Ulceration
Large, facial lesion	PHACES (posterior fossa malformation; large facial hemangioma; arterial anomalies; coarctation of the aorta or other cardiac malformation; eye abnormalities; midline sternal defects)

Some vascular tumors, including kaposiform hemangioendotheliomas and tufted angiomas, may resemble hemangiomas. These unusual vascular tumors may undergo sudden swelling with resulting hemolytic anemia, thrombocytopenia, and congestive heart failure, resulting in a life-threatening syndrome known as *Kasabach-Merritt phenomenon*. Patients with this syndrome may require high doses of systemic corticosteroid or other chemotherapeutic interventions to control these complications.

URTICARIA

Background

Urticaria as a symptom complex is often encountered in the pediatric population, occurring in 2% to 3% of all children. In most cases, no cause is identified. A small number of cases are caused by allergic reactions from the ingestion of drugs or foods (e.g., nuts, eggs, shellfish, strawberries). Urticaria also follows viral (e.g., Epstein-Barr virus, hepatitis), bacterial (streptococcal), or parasitic infections. Physical factors, including dermographism, cholinergic stimulation (induced by heat, exercise, and emotional tension), cold (acquired and familial), and solar exposure, can induce urticaria. Finally, urticaria may be caused by factors producing a vasculitis or other autoimmune phenomena (particularly thyroid diseases) and substances causing degranulation of mast cells (radiocontrast material). Episodes of urticaria that last less than 6 weeks are termed *transient* or *acute*. The most common causes of urticaria are infection, insect bites, drugs, and foods. Chronic urticaria is defined as that which lasts for more than 6 weeks. No cause is found in 90% of children. These cases include the physical urticarias or urticarial vasculitis.

Pathophysiology

The lesion itself follows vasodilation and leakage of fluid and red blood cells from involved vessels. The vascular damage can be caused by mediators such as histamine complement and immune complexes. IgE can attach to and cause degranulation

of mast cells in sensitized individuals, with resulting histamine release. Urticarias are usually acute and transient but at times become chronic and recurrent.

Clinical Manifestations

The typical urticarial lesions are familiar to all physicians. They can be localized or generalized (involving the entire body). At times, the lesions are giant with serpiginous borders. Individual wheals rarely last more than 12 to 24 hours. Most commonly, the lesions appear in one area for 20 minutes to 3 hours, disappear, and then reappear in another location. The total duration of an episode is usually 24 to 48 hours; however, the course can last 3 to 6 weeks. In young children, urticaria may have an annular or polycyclic (coalescent annular) or arcuate (partially annular) appearance and may be associated with edema of the hands or feet. Because this is frequently confused with erythema multiforme (which manifest with more fixed, targetoid lesions), this annular urticarial hypersensitivity has sometimes been referred to as *urticaria multiforme*.

Management

Acute relief can be accomplished with intramuscular epinephrine (1:1,000) 0.01 mL per kg (max 0.3 mL) in severe cases and intramuscular or IV diphenhydramine 1 mg per kg (max 50 mg). Oral antihistamines are useful for maintenance therapy for transient urticaria. Hydroxyzine hydrochloride (2 mg per kg per day in three to four divided doses) or diphenhydramine hydrochloride (5 mg per kg per day in three to four divided doses) should be prescribed for at least 10 days. Other longer-acting antihistamines include loratadine, desloratadine, cetirizine, levocetirizine, and fexofenadine, which are typically given once daily.

PITYRIASIS ROSEA

Pityriasis rosea can occur in all age groups but is seen predominantly in children older than 10 years and only rarely in those younger than 5 years. The cause is unknown; however, a viral cause is suspected. Less than 5% of cases occur in multiple family members. In 80% of children, a large, oval, solitary lesion known as the *herald patch* appears on the trunk (Fig. 85.39) before the eruption of subsequent lesions. Individual lesions are oval and slightly raised, pink to brown, with peripheral scaling. Because the lesions follow the cleavage lines (Fig. 85.40) of the skin, the backs of patients have a "Christmas or fir tree" appearance. Generally, the face, the scalp, and distal extremities are spared. On occasion, an inverse distribution occurs (lesions on the face and extremities with truncal sparing). The rash is pruritic early in the course but then becomes asymptomatic. It generally lasts 4 to 8 weeks.

The herald patch can be mistaken for tinea corporis, but a KOH preparation eliminates that possibility. When pityriasis rosea appears in adolescence, it must be differentiated from secondary syphilis. Clinical clues are helpful (Table 85.11), but serologic testing is necessary.

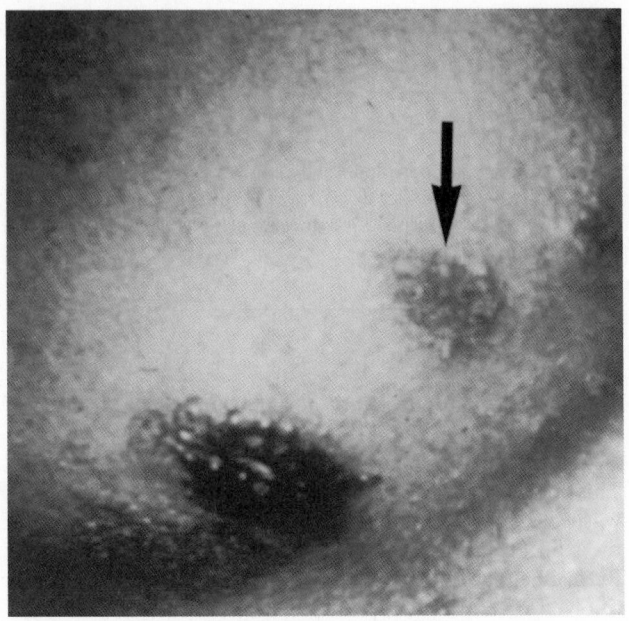

FIGURE 85.39 Herald patch (*arrow*) in adolescent with pityriasis rosea.

Treatment is symptomatic. Antihistamines and topical emollients can help alleviate the pruritus. Symptomatic patients may respond to a 14-day course of erythromycin or acyclovir to abbreviate the course of pityriasis rosea.

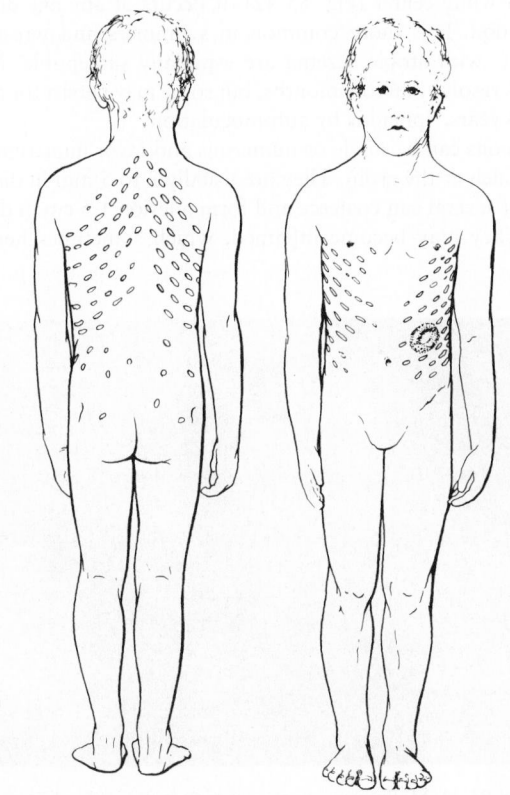

FIGURE 85.40 Typical distribution of pityriasis rosea.

TABLE 85.11

DIFFERENTIAL DIAGNOSIS

	Pityriasis rosea	Syphilis
Herald patch	+	−
Ovals follow dermatomes	+	−
Lymphadenopathy	−	+
Mucous membrane lesion	−	+

PANNICULITIS

Erythema Nodosum

Erythema nodosum seems to be a hypersensitivity reaction leading to inflammation of the subcutaneous fat and may be related to infection (streptococci, tuberculosis, coccidioidomycosis, histoplasmosis), inflammatory bowel disease, sarcoidosis, and drugs (such as oral contraceptive agents). The exact immunologic mechanism has not been clarified. The entity occurs predominantly in adolescents during the spring and fall. Women are affected more often than men.

The lesions of erythema nodosum appear as deep, tender, erythematous nodules or plaques on the extensor surfaces of the extremities (Fig. 85.22). The sedimentation rate is generally elevated and usually returns to normal with disappearance of the eruption, unless an underlying disease is present. The reaction usually lasts 3 to 6 weeks. Treatment should be directed toward the cause when and if established; otherwise, it is symptomatic (nonsteroidal antiinflammatory drugs and antihistamines). Hospitalization is unnecessary. Corticosteroids should not be used, except in severe cases after an underlying infection has been ruled out.

Cold Panniculitis

Cold panniculitis is secondary to cold injury to fat. During the cold of winter, infants and some older children develop red, indurated nodules and plaques on exposed skin, especially the face. The subcutaneous fat in infants and some children solidifies more readily at a higher temperature than that of an adult because of the relatively greater concentration of saturated fats. Infants who hold ice chips or popsicles in their mouths are also susceptible to this phenomenon (Fig. 85.41, see also color plate). The lesions gradually soften and return to normal over 1 or more weeks. Treatment is unnecessary.

WARTS AND MOLLUSCUM CONTAGIOSUM

Warts

Warts affect 7% to 10% of the population and are one of the most common dermatologic problems encountered in pediatrics. The peak incidence is during adolescence. Sixty-five percent of common warts disappear spontaneously within 2 years,

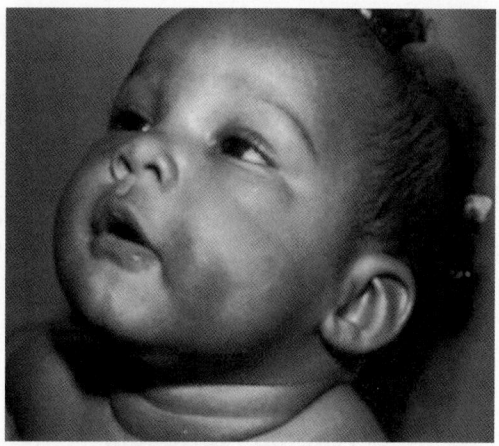

FIGURE 85.41 Infant with popsicle panniculitis of the cheek.

and 40% of plantar warts disappear within 6 months in prepubertal children. However, immunosuppressed patients may experience extensive spread of the lesions.

The common wart resembles a tiny cauliflower. Lesions disrupt the natural skin lines and may also manifest with small black dots, representing thrombosed capillaries. The shape of the wart varies with its location on the skin. They may be long and slender (filiform) on the face and neck or flat (verruca plana) on the face, arms, and knees. When located on the soles, they are called *plantar warts*, and when in the anogenital area, they are referred to as *condyloma acuminata*.

The tendency for recurrence of warts makes the treatment of this condition frustrating. Because most warts disappear spontaneously with time, procedures that are least traumatic for the child should be attempted first (Table 85.12). The simple, nontraumatic method of airtight occlusion with plain adhesive tape or duct tape for 1 month has been shown to be successful on many occasions. Topical application of 17% salicylic acid in flexible collodion (Duofilm®; Table 85.13) is good for home use, as are some of the over-the-counter preparations (e.g., Compound W®, Occlusal®). When simple methods are unsuccessful, touching the warts with liquid nitrogen or volatile cryogens such as dimethyl ether, propane, or isobutane (Verruca-Freeze®) for 10 to 30 seconds or surgical removal can be attempted on a 2- to 4-week schedule until the lesions clear completely. Both procedures are painful.

Plantar warts can be treated with 40% salicylic acid plaster. Circular pieces, slightly larger than the plantar wart, are cut from a sheet of this material. They are placed on the wart and kept in place continuously with adhesive tape for 1 to 2 weeks. At that point, the dead tissue is carefully pared away.

TABLE 85.12

MANAGEMENT OF WARTS

Decrease irritation—cover with waterproof or duct tape
  (1 to 2 mo)
Over-the-counter preparations, such as Compound W® (1 mo)
Salicylic in collodion (Duofilm®) (1 mo)
Refer to dermatologist

TABLE 85.13

USE OF DUOFILM®

1. Soak wart for 5 min.
2. Dry.
3. Surround with petroleum jelly.
4. Apply Duofilm® (let dry for few minutes).
5. Cover with waterproof or duct tape.
6. Repeat twice a day.
7. Pare dead skin.

Treatment is continued until normal skin is seen in place of the wart.

Anogenital warts can be treated with 20% podophyllin. This medication is carefully applied only to the wart and washed off in 4 to 6 hours (see Chapter 90). Severe burning of the skin occurs if the material is not completely removed. Retreatment every 1 to 2 weeks should be done until the warts resolve. Alternatively, topical preparations such as podophyllotoxin gel (Condylox®) or imiquimod cream (Aldara®) may be used at home. Podophyllotoxin gel is applied on the condylomata three consecutive nights each week while imiquimod is used every other night three times weekly. Both agents may be used for up to 3 months or so or until the warts clear. Child abuse should be considered in any child with genital warts.

Molluscum Contagiosum

The lesion, produced by the common poxvirus, is a papule with a white center (Fig. 85.42). It occurs at any age during childhood. It is more common in swimmers and wrestlers. Patients with atopic eczema are especially susceptible. Most lesions resolve in 6 to 9 months, but some may persist for more than 3 years. Spread is by autoinoculation.

Lesions can be single or numerous and favor intertriginous areas such as the groin. They are usually 2 to 5 mm in diameter, but several can coalesce and form a lesion 1.5 cm in diameter. They may become inflamed, which sometimes heralds

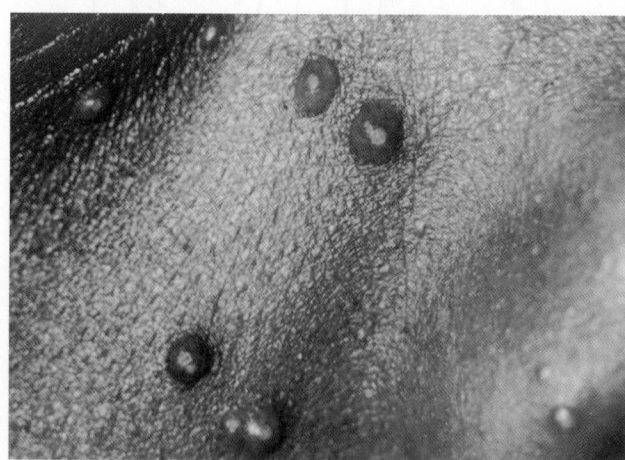

FIGURE 85.42 Molluscum contagiosum. Papules with white centers that contain the virus.

spontaneous disappearance. At times, an eczematous reaction occurs around some lesions, and they can sometimes become secondarily infected.

Since spontaneous resolution is common, treatment if elected should be gentle. Removal of the white core will cure the lesion. This treatment can be performed by applying a local anesthetic cream (e.g. EMLA® or LMX-4®) under occlusion to the lesion 1 to 2 hours before treatment. This procedure will anesthetize the area and allow the physician to prick the skin open over the core with a 26-gauge needle, and squeeze the core out with a comedone extractor. Multiple light touches with liquid nitrogen can also be effective. With widespread lesions, nonpainful procedures are preferable as multiple painful treatments will cause great fear in the patient and make future visits to a physician difficult for the family. Application of 0.1% tretinoin cream one to two times daily may induce enough inflammation to hasten the host's immune response or cause extrusion of the central core but caution should be observed since tretinoin may exacerbate secondary eczematization around molluscum lesions. A dilute formulation of cantharidin, a natural toxin derived from the blister beetle, can be used successfully to treat molluscum. Cantharidin can be applied to individual molluscum lesions for 1 to 4 hours and then washed off. The medication is generally painless when applied but may result in subsequent blistering of treated areas and should be avoided on the face or genital areas.

CONGENITAL HSV

Congenital HSV infection encompasses a broad clinical spectrum ranging from localized cutaneous and mucosal lesions to life-threatening central nervous system and internal organ involvements. Studies have shown that the prevalence of HSV-2 infection has increased by 30% from 1976 to 1994. The greatest increases occurred in white teenagers and white women in their twenties. The risk of acquiring HSV during pregnancy was 2% in susceptible women. The risk of acquiring the infection is similar in each trimester. Less than 10% of those who were seropositive gave a history indicating genital herpes infection. Other patients noted nonspecific genital urinary symptoms such as dysuria, leukorrhea, hematuria, and pelvic pain. If seroconversion occurs in the mother before delivery, the risk to the infant is small. However, if a primary infection occurs shortly before labor, neonatal HSV infection can occur in up to 50% of newborns. Whereas most infections are transmitted by direct contact with the infected birth canal during the second stage of labor, some evidence supports transplacental infection of the fetus.

The incubation period of congenital HSV infections ranges from 2 to 30 days after exposure. Lesions present at birth or shortly thereafter have been explained by transplacental passage of the virus. The clinical manifestations of congenital HSV infection are diverse, but more than 50% of infected neonates present with external involvement. In vertex deliveries, the scalp is a common site for the vesicles. Conversely, infants delivered by breech often develop lesions of the buttocks and perianal area initially. The lesions are not unlike those seen in older children or adults in that they are grouped tense vesicles arising on an erythematous base that may evolve into frank erosions. However, the infection may present on the

skin as individual vesicles, pustules, bullae, or denuded skin. Unfortunately, when infants have disease limited to the integument, HSV infection is often not considered as a possibility. Instead, these children are treated for "impetigo." The correct diagnosis may not be considered until constitutional symptoms such as fever, hypothermia, poor feeding, irritability, lethargy, and vomiting have appeared. By then, dissemination of the disease has occurred.

Diagnosis of congenital HSV infection should be suspected in any infant younger than 1 month who has a vesicular eruption on an erythematous base. A Tzanck preparation of the base of an unbroken vesicle is an easy and rapid diagnostic tool to aid in the recognition of this potentially lethal disease (Fig. 85.7). Giemsa, Papanicolaou, or hematoxylin-eosin stains of the smeared preparation of vesicles infected with HSV will reveal multinucleated giant cells, intranuclear inclusions, ballooning degeneration, or margination of nuclear chromatin. Rapid slide tests, using monoclonal antibodies, are also available for rapid diagnosis. Viral culture still remains the gold standard for proving that HSV is present, although many institutions are moving toward polymerase chain reaction–based systems.

The differential diagnosis of vesiculopustular lesions in the newborn includes bullous impetigo, congenital cutaneous candidiasis, congenital syphilis, neonatal pustular melanosis, and cytomegalovirus infection. Differentiation of these entities requires the use of Gram stains, KOH scrapings, serologic studies for syphilis, and appropriate cultures. Although many serologic tests are currently available to detect the presence of HSV antibodies, none of these studies is valuable in arriving at an early diagnosis of congenital infection. Direct culture of the herpes virus from a lesional vesicle takes 24 to 48 hours for identification.

All infants with suspected congenital HSV should be preferably treated with IV acyclovir. If not available, IV ganciclovir may also be used. Acyclovir should be given at a dosage of 60 mg per kg per day, divided every 8 hours (20 mg per kg per dose), in a 1- to 2-hour IV infusion.

DISORDERS OF PIGMENTATION

Hypopigmentation

A dominant form of partial albinism occurs in which localized areas of skin and hair are devoid of pigment. Ocular albinism is also seen. Two syndromes with albinism are Waardenberg's syndrome (white forelock, heterochromia of the iris, sensorineural hearing loss) and Chediak-Higashi syndrome (immunodeficiency, leukocytes with giant granules).

Loss of pigmentation can be a result of the absence of melanocytes as in vitiligo and halo nevi. Vitiligo is a symmetric, patchy loss of pigmentation. Hair located in areas of vitiligo is often white. Vitiligo can be associated with alopecia areata, pernicious anemia, Addison's disease, hypothyroidism, diabetes mellitus, hypoparathyroidism, and other endocrine disorders. Vitiligo and some of the diseases associated with it may be autoimmune disorders. Antibodies directed against melanocytes have been detected.

Suppression of melanocytic pigment production can cause loss of pigmentation as in postinflammatory hypopigmentation.

MEDICAL EMERGENCIES

An example of this condition is the white patch of hypopigmentation and scaling often seen on the face, trunk, or extremities of children with atopic eczema. The ash-leaf macule is a flat, hypopigmented (whitish) spot that is present in more than 90% of patients with tuberous sclerosis. In white patients, they are more easily seen by shining a Wood's lamp on the skin.

Hyperpigmentation

Diffuse hyperpigmentation is associated with Addison's disease, acromegaly, and hemochromatosis.

Pigment deep in the dermis appears gray or blue at the surface of the skin. Mongolian blue spots are an example. The nevus of Ota is dermal pigment in the distribution of the ophthalmic branch of the fifth nerve; this pigmentation can also involve the sclera and palate.

Certain syndromes, including neurofibromatosis, are associated with pigmented skin lesions. Patients with this disease have café-au-lait spots, which are flat, nonpalpable, coffee-colored lesions of varying size and shape. When six or more lesions are present, greater than 0.5 cm in size, neurofibromatosis should be considered. The Peutz-Jeghers syndrome is a dominantly inherited condition that includes freckle-like lesions of the lips, nose, buccal mucosa, fingertips, and subungual areas associated with polyps in the small intestine, stomach, or colon. Melena and intussusception are the chief complications that may develop, usually in the second decade of life. Albright's syndrome should be suspected when unilateral café-au-lait spots with irregular borders occur in the lumbosacral area. Included in this syndrome are bony abnormalities and precocious puberty. Children who have large, swirling areas of pigmentation following lines of Blaschko (lines representing planes of cutaneous embryogenesis) may have forms of cutaneous mosaicism as can be seen in linear and whorled nevoid hypermelanosis.

Single or multiple red-brown papules or nodules occurring on the extremities or face of children may have a confusing tissue structure. Although the lesions are benign, they have commonly been misdiagnosed as malignant melanoma. Therefore, the name *benign juvenile melanoma* has been assigned to this condition. Other names include *Spitz tumors* or *spindle-cell epithelioid nevi*. True malignant melanomas are rare in children. They usually arise from congenital pigmented nevi.

Suggested Readings

General

Eichenfield LF, Esterly NB, Frieden IJ. *Textbook of neonatal dermatology.* Philadelphia: Elsevier Health Sciences, 2008.
Harper J, Oranje A, Prose N. *Textbook of pediatric dermatology.* Oxford, England: Blackwell Science, 2000.
Hurwitz S. *Clinical pediatric dermatology,* 3rd ed. Philadelphia, PA: WB Saunders, 2005.
Odom RB, James WD, Berger TG. *Andrews' diseases of the skin,* 10th ed. Philadelphia, PA: WB Saunders, 2006.
Schachner LA, Hansen RC. *Pediatric dermatology,* 3rd ed. New York, NY: Churchill Livingstone, 2003.
Solomon LM, Esterly NB. Neonatal dermatology. In: *Major problems in clinical pediatrics.* Philadelphia: WB Saunders, 1973.
Weston WL, Lane AT, Morelli JG. *Color textbook of pediatric dermatology,* 4th ed. St Louis, MO: Mosby, 2007.
Wolff K, Goldsmith LA, Katz SI, et al. *Fitzpatrick's dermatology in general medicine,* 7th ed. New York, NY: McGraw-Hill, 2007.

Atopic Dermatitis

Akhavan A, Rudikoff D. Atopic dermatitis: systemic immunosuppressive therapy. *Semin Cutan Med Surg* 2008;27:151–155.
Hanifin JM. Atopic dermatitis in infants and children. *Pediatr Clin North Am* 1991;38:763–789.
Krakowski AC, Eichenfield LF, Dohil MA. Manangement of atopic dermatitis in the pediatric population. *Pediatrics* 2008;122:812–824.
Levy RM, Gelfand JM, Yan AC. The epidemiology of atopic dermatitis. *Clin Dermatol* 2003;21:109–115.
Leyden JJ, Baker DA. Localized herpes simplex infections in atopic dermatitis. *Arch Dermatol* 1979;115:311–312.
Nghiem P, Pearson G, Langley RG. Tacrolimus and pimecrolimus: from clever prokaryotes to inhibiting calcineurin and treating atopic dermatitis. *J Am Acad Dermatol* 2002;46:228–241.
Ong PY, Ohtake T, Brandt C, et al. Endogenous antimicrobial peptides and skin infections in atopic dermatitis. *N Engl J Med* 2002;347:1151–1160.
Rothe MJ, Grant-Kels JM. Atopic dermatitis: an update. *J Am Acad Dermatol* 1996;35:1–13.
Sampson HA, Scanlon SM. Natural history of food hypersensitivity in children with atopic dermatitis. *J Pediatr* 1989;115:23–27.
Suh L, Coffin S, Leckerman KH, et al. Methicillin-resistant *Staphylococcus aureus* colonization in children with atopic dermatitis. *Pediatr Dermatol* 2008;25:528–534.
Thygarajan A, Burks AW. American Academy of Pediatrics recommendations on the effects of early nutritional interventions on the development of atopic disease. *Curr Opin Pediatr* 2008;30:698–702.

Allergic Contact Dermatitis

Epstein WL. Topical prevention of poison ivy/oak dermatitis. *Arch Dermatol* 1989;125:499–501.
Gaul LE. Development of allergic nickel dermatitis from earrings. *JAMA* 1967;200:176–178.
Weston WL, Weston JA. Allergic contact dermatitis in children. *Am J Dis Child* 1984;138:932–936.

Diaper Dermatitis

Berg RW, Buckingham KW, Stewart RL. Etiologic factors in diaper dermatitis: the role of urine. *Pediatr Dermatol* 1986;3:102–106.
Buckingham KW, Berg RW. Etiologic factors in diaper dermatitis: the role of feces. *Pediatr Dermatol* 1986;3:107–112.
Honig PJ, Gribetz B, Leyden JL, et al. Amoxicillin and diaper dermatitis. *J Am Acad Dermatol* 1988;19:275–279.
Leyden JJ, Katz S, Stewart R, et al. Urinary ammonia and ammonia-producing microorganisms in infants with and without diaper dermatitis. *Arch Dermatol* 1977;113:1678.
Shaffer MP, Feldman SR, Fleisher AB Jr. Use of clotrimazole/betamethasone dipropionate by family physicians. *Fam Med* 2000;32:561–565.
Weston WL, Lane AT, Weston JA. Diaper dermatitis: current concepts. *Pediatrics* 1980;66:532–536.
Yan AC, Wahrman JE, Honig PJ. Clinical features and differential diagnosis of napkin dermatitis. In: Harper J, Oranje A, Prose N, eds. *Textbook of pediatric dermatology,* 2nd ed. Oxford, England: Blackwell Science, 2006:161–172.

Drug Reactions

Esterly NB. Corticosteroids for erythema multiforme? *Pediatr Dermatol* 1989;6:229–250.
Kramer MS, Hutchinson TA, Flegel KM, et al. Adverse drug reactions in general pediatric outpatients. *J Pediatr* 1985;106:305–310.
Metry DW, Jung P, Levy ML. Use of intravenous immunoglobulin in children with Stevens-Johnson syndrome and toxic epidermal necrolysis: seven cases and review of the literature. *Pediatrics* 2003;112:1430–1436.
Orton PW, Huff JC, Tonnesen JG, et al. Detection of herpes simplex viral antigen in skin lesions of erythema multiforme. *Ann Intern Med* 1984;101:48–50.
Prins C, Kerdel FA, Padilla RS, et al. Treatment of toxic epidermal necrolysis with high-dose intravenous immunoglobulins: multicenter retrospective analysis of 48 consecutive cases. *Arch Dermatol* 2003;139:26–32.
Shah KN, Honig PJ, Yan AC. "Urticaria multiforme": a case series and review of acute annular urticarial hypersensitivity syndrome in children. *Pediatrics* 2007;119:e1177–e1183.

Staphylococcal Scalded Skin Syndrome

Amagai M, Matsuyoshi N, Wang ZH, et al. Toxin in bullous impetigo and staphylococcal scalded-skin syndrome targets desmoglein 1. *Nat Med* 2000;6:1275–1277.
Amon RB, Diamond RL. Toxic epidermal necrolysis: rapid differentiation between staphylococcal and drug-induced disease. *Arch Dermatol* 1975;111:1433–1437.

Melish ME, Glasgow LA. The staphylococcal scalded-skin syndrome: development of an experimental model. *N Engl J Med* 1970;282:1114–1119.

Murono K, Fujita K, Yoshioka H. Microbiologic characteristics of exfoliative toxin-producing *Staphylococcus aureus*. *Pediatr Infect Dis J* 1988;7:313–315.

Stanley JR, Amagai M. Pemphigus, bullous impetigo and the staphylococcal scaled skin syndrome. *N Engl J Med* 2006;355:1800–1810.

Bites and Infestations

Davies HD, Sakuls P, Keystone JS. Creeping eruption. *Arch Dermatol* 1993;129:588.

Howard R, Frieden IJ. Papular urticaria in children. *Pediatr Dermatol* 1996;13:246–249.

Leone P. Scabies and pediculosis pubis: an update of treatment regimens and general review. *Clin Infect Dis* 2007;44:s153–s159.

Meinking TL, Serrano L, Hard B, et al. Comparative in vitro pediculicidal efficacy of treatments in a resistant head lice population in the United States. *Arch Dermatol* 2002;138:220–224.

Meinking TL, Taplin D, Hermida JL, et al. The treatment of scabies with ivermectin. *N Engl J Med* 1995;333:26.

Needham GR. Evaluation of five popular methods for tick removal. *Pediatrics* 1985;75:997.

Paller AS. Scabies in infants and small children. *Semin Dermatol* 1993;12:3–8.

Rees R, Campbell D, Rieger E, et al. The diagnosis and treatment of brown recluse spider bites. *Ann Emerg Med* 1987;16:945–949.

Rees RS, Altenbern DP, Lynch JB, et al. Brown recluse spider bites: a comparison of early surgical excision versus dapsone and delayed surgical excision. *Ann Surg* 1985;202:659–663.

Taplin D, Meinking BA, Porcelain SL, et al. Permethrin 5% dermal cream: a new treatment for scabies. *J Am Acad Dermatol* 1986;15:995–1001.

Vetter RS. Brown recluse spider bite diagnoses and lawsuits [letter]. *Pediatr Emerg Care* 2003;19(4):291–292.

Fungal Infections

Alston SJ, Cohen BA, Braun M. Persistent and recurrent tinea corporis in children treated with combination antifungal/corticosteroid agents. *Pediatrics* 2003;111:201–203.

Elewski BE, Caceres HW, DeLeon L, et al. Terbinafine hydrochloride granules versus oral griseofulvin suspension in children with tinea capitis: result of two randomized investigator blinded, multicenter, international controlled trials. *J Am Acad Dermatol* 2008;59:41–54.

Ghannoum MA, Wraith LA, Cai B, et al. Susceptibility of dermatophyte isolates obtained from worldwide terbinafine tinea capitis clinical trial. *Br J Dermatol* 2008;159:711–713.

Gupta AK, Sauder DN, Shear NH. Antifungal agents: an overview: part I. *J Am Acad Dermatol* 1994;30:677–698.

Gupta AK, Sauder DN, Shear NH. Antifungal agents: an overview: part II. *J Am Acad Dermatol* 1994;30(6):911–933.

Guzzo C, Honig PJ, Rabinowitz LG. Fungal infections from head to toe. *Patient Care* 1987;21:62.

Honig PJ, Caputo GL, Leyden JJ, et al. Microbiology of kerions. *J Pediatr* 1993;123:422.

Honig PJ, Caputo GL, Leyden JJ, et al. Treatment of kerions. *Pediatr Dermatol* 1994;11:69.

Hemangiomas

Enjolras O, Wassef M, Mazoyer E, et al. Infants with Kasabach-Merritt syndrome do not have "true" hemangiomas. *J Pediatr* 1997;130:631–640.

Leaute-Labreze C, Dumas de la Roque E, Hubiche T, et al. Propranolol for severe hemangiomas of infancy. *N Engl J Med* 2008;358:2649–2651.

Metry DW, Dowd CF, Barkovich AJ, et al. The many faces of PHACE syndrome. *J Pediatr* 2001;139:117–123.

Metry DW, Hebert AA. Benign cutaneous vascular tumors of infancy: when to worry, what to do. *Arch Dermatol* 2000;136:905–914.

Mussa A, Baldassare G, Rosaia De Santis L, et al. Four new cases of PHACES syndrome: variable phenotypic expression and endocrine features [published online ahead of print September 15, 2008]. *Acta Paediatr* 2008;97(12):1729–1733. doi:10.1111/j.1651-2227.2008.01032.x.

Rao RP, Drolet BA, Holland KE, et al. PHACES association: a vasculocutaneous syndrome. *Pediatr Cardiol* 2008;29:793–795.

Urticaria

Current management of urticaria and angioedema: proceedings of a round table: San Francisco, CA, December 7, 1989. *J Am Acad Dermatol* 1991;25(suppl, pt 2):145–204.

Ghosh S, Kanwar AJ, Kaur A. Urticaria in children. *Pediatr Dermatol* 1993;10:107.

Komarow HD, Metcalfe DD. Office-based management of urticaria. *Am J Med* 2008;121:379–384.

Schuller DE, Elvey SM. Acute urticaria associated with streptococcal infection. *Pediatrics* 1980;65:592.

Warts and Molluscum

Brown J, Janniger CK, Schwartz RA, et al. Childhood molluscum contagiosum. *Int J Dermatol* 2006;45:93–99.

Fit KE, Williams PC. Use of histamine2-antagonists for the treatment of verruca vulgaris. *Ann Pharmacother* 2007;41:1222–1226.

Focht DR, Spicer C, Fairchok FP. The efficacy of duct tape vs cryotherapy in the treatment of verruca vulgaris (the common wart). *Arch Pediatr Adolesc Med* 2002;156:971–974.

Gibbs S, Harvey I. Topical treatments for cutaneous warts. *Cochrane Database Syst Rev* 2006;3:CD001781.

Silverberg NB, Sidbury R, Mancini AJ. Childhood molluscum contagiosum: experience with cantharidin therapy in 300 patients. *J Am Acad Dermatol* 2000;43:503–507.

Smolinski KN, Yan AC. How and when to treat molluscum contagiosum and warts in children. *Pediatr Ann* 2005;34:211–221.

Congenital Herpes Simplex

Brown ZA, Selke S, Zeh J, et al. The acquisition of herpes simplex virus during pregnancy. *N Engl J Med* 1997;337:509–515.

Brown ZA, Vontver LA, Benedetti J, et al. Effects on infants of a first episode of genital herpes during pregnancy. *N Engl J Med* 1987;317:1246–1251.

Fleming DT, McQuillan GM, Johnson RE, et al. Herpes simplex virus type 2 in the United States, 1976 to 1994. *N Engl J Med* 1997;337:1105–1111.

Goodyear HM. Rapid diagnosis of cutaneous herpes simplex infections using specific monoclonal antibodies. *Clin Exp Dermatol* 1994;19:294–297.

Kimberlin DW. Herpes simplex virus infections in neonates and early childhood. *Semin Pediatr Infect Dis* 2005;16:271–281.

Kimberlin DW, Lin CY, Jacobs RF, et al. Natural history of neonatal herpes simplex virus infections in the acyclovir era. *Pediatrics* 2001;108:223–229.

Kimberlin DW, Lin CY, Jacobs RF, et al. Safety and efficacy of high-dose intravenous acyclovir in the management of neonatal herpes simplex virus infections. *Pediatrics* 2001;108:230–238.

Pityriasis Rosea

Chuh AA, Dofitasa BL, Comisel GG, et al. Interventions for pityriasis rosea. *Cochrane Database Syst Rev* 2007;2:CD005068.

Gonzalez LM, Allen R, Janniger CK. Pityriasis rosea: an important papulosquamous disorder. *Int J Dermatol* 2005;44:757–764.

Hartley AH. Pityriasis rosea. *Pediatr Rev* 1999;20:266–269.

Sharma PK, Yadav TP, Gautam RK, et al. Erythromycin in pityriasis rosea: a double-blind, placebo-controlled clinical trial. *J Am Acad Dermatol* 2000;42:241–244.

MEDICAL EMERGENCIES

CHAPTER 86 ■ ENDOCRINE EMERGENCIES

MICHAEL S.D. AGUS, MD

Because the symptoms and signs of endocrinologic disease are associated with a wide range of non-endocrinologic diseases, many endocrine conditions are not recognized in the emergency department (ED). However, to achieve a favorable outcome, endocrinologic causes should be included in the differential diagnosis of ill children and appropriate testing should be performed. In many cases, the results of specific diagnostic tests will not be available on an emergency basis, and management will have to be initiated based on a probable diagnosis. In this chapter, emphasis is placed on the clinical and laboratory findings that are helpful in recognizing endocrinologic emergencies and in effectively treating those emergencies. Table 86.1 summarizes the major clinical features, recommended investigations, and treatments of pediatric endocrine emergencies.

DIABETIC KETOACIDOSIS

Background

Severe ketoacidosis is a life-threatening complication of diabetes that is present in 20% to 40% of newly diagnosed type 1 (juvenile-onset) diabetic patients; it accounts for 65% of all admissions of diabetic patients younger than 19 years of age. The mortality rate for diabetic ketoacidosis (DKA) in children is 0.15%. Clinically significant cerebral edema is the most serious immediate risk to the child, occurring in 1% of cases, and it remains so during the first 24 hours of therapy, despite the more apparent issues of hypovolemia and acidosis. Reported mortality rates from cerebral edema are approximately 25%; however, 25% of survivors have significant morbidity. Characteristic biochemical findings of DKA include hyperglycemia and metabolic acidosis. DKA may be precipitated by acute infection, inadequate quantities of endogenous or exogenous insulin, or emotional factors. Recurrent or frequent episodes should lead to careful evaluation for this latter possibility. Nonketotic hyperosmolar coma, although rare in children, can be managed adequately using the principles outlined in the following sections.

Pathophysiology

Insulin deficiency initially leads to hyperglycemia that, once above the renal threshold of 180 mg per dL, leads to polyuria due to an osmotic diuresis. Without vigorous oral repletion at home, the child quickly becomes hypovolemic, prompting a stress response and elevations of the counterregulatory hormones glucagon, catecholamines, cortisol, and growth hormone. These hormonal changes produce significant insulin resistance that worsens the hyperglycemia, hypovolemia, and stress response, ultimately leading to further functional insulin deficiency to such a severe degree that adipose tissue is broken down in large quantities into free fatty acids, subsequently converted into ketoacids in the liver. Ketoacids readily dissociate in the blood to produce free hydrogen ions, and metabolic acidosis ensues. This reaction is partially compensated for by a respiratory alkalosis (hyperventilation), with a resultant lowering of PCO_2 and plasma bicarbonate (HCO_3-).

Intracellular potassium is depleted because of transcellular shifts of this ion brought about by the exchange of potassium with excess free hydrogen ions and extracellular dehydration. Protein catabolism secondary to insulin deficiency causes a negative nitrogen balance and results in additional efflux of potassium from cells. The potassium is then lost in the urine during the osmotic diuresis. Volume depletion causes secondary hyperaldosteronism, which further promotes urinary potassium excretion. Thus, total body depletion of potassium occurs, although the plasma potassium concentration may not reflect the loss at the time of presentation.

Clinical Manifestations

In cases of new-onset diabetes, the child usually has a history of polyuria and polydipsia for a few days or weeks before the acute decompensation. In fact, autoimmune destruction of the pancreatic beta cells has been underway at that point for many months. A prolonged history of polyuria, or hyperglycemia without acidosis, should raise the possibility of type 2 diabetes, particularly in obese children from ethnic and racial minorities. Significant weight loss often occurs despite a vigorous appetite. In children known to have diabetes, the prodrome may be less than 24 hours and precipitated by an intercurrent illness, inappropriate sick day management, or omission of insulin doses. Patients may complain of nausea, vomiting, and abdominal pain, and the parents may have noticed increasing listlessness. Less than 2% of children are in coma at the time of hospital admission, although a higher percentage has an altered state of consciousness. The history and physical examination usually suggest the diagnosis; however, particularly in the patient with new-onset diabetes, presenting clinical features can be misdiagnosed, especially in the infant or young child. For example, abdominal pain may be misinterpreted as appendicitis; hyperpnea may be mistaken as a sign of pneumonia or asthma; and polyuria may be incorrectly diagnosed as a urinary infection. Enuresis, polydipsia, and irritability are sometimes wrongly categorized as behavioral problems.

On physical examination, particular attention should be paid to the degree of dehydration, including skin turgor and

TABLE 86.1

SUMMARY OF CLINICAL FEATURES, INVESTIGATIONS, AND INITIAL TREATMENT OF PEDIATRIC ENDOCRINE EMERGENCIES

Condition	Major clinical features	Urgent investigations	Initial treatment
Diabetic ketoacidosis	Polyuria, polydipsia, dehydration, ketotic breath, hyperpnea, nausea, vomiting, abdominal pain, coma	Blood glucose, pH	0.9% saline 10–20 mL/kg in first 1–2 h IV; insulin infusion 0.1 Unit/kg/h; later, may need KAcetate 10–60 mEq/L and KPhos; 10–20 mEq/L
Hypoglycemia	*Older child:* hunger, sweatiness, dizziness, convulsions, coma *Neonate:* apnea, hypotonia, hypothermia, irritability, tremor, convulsions	Blood glucose Serum for growth hormone, cortisol, insulin; first voided urine for organic acids and toxin screen	25% dextrose 1–2 mL/kg IV bolus or 10% dextrose 5–10 mg/kg/min IV infusion, glucagon 0.5–1 mg IM stat (if hyperinsulinism)
Congenital adrenal hyperplasia	Ambiguous genitalia in females; poor feeding, weight loss, irritability, vomiting, dehydration	Plasma sodium, potassium, glucose, 17-hydroxyprogesterone; karyotype and pelvic ultrasound	0.9% saline 20 mL/kg in first hour IV; hydrocortisone 25 mg IV stat (neonatal dose)
Adrenal insufficiency	Nausea, vomiting, abdominal pain, weakness, malaise, hypotension, dehydration, hyperpigmentation	Plasma sodium, potassium, glucose, cortisol, and ACTH (for retrospective confirmation of diagnosis)	Hydrocortisone 100 mg IV stat; 10% dextrose in 0.9% saline 20 mL/kg in first hour
Hypercalcemia (hyperparathyroidism)	Headache, irritability, anorexia, constipation, polyuria, polydipsia, dehydration, hypertension	Plasma calcium, phosphate	0.9% saline at two to three times maintenance rate; furosemide 1 mg/kg
Hypocalcemia (hypoparathyroidism)	Cramps, carpopedal spasms, paresthesias, lethargy, apathy, convulsions, hypotension	Plasma calcium, phosphate, alkaline phosphatase	10% calcium gluconate 1 mL/kg IV over 15 min
Diabetes insipidus	Polyuria, polydipsia, dehydration, irritability, fever, drowsiness, coma	Paired plasma and urine osmolality and sodium	*Central:* IV fluids at two-thirds maintenance rate plus replete deficit over 48 h; pitressin 1–10 mUnit/kg per h IV *Nephrogenic:* IV fluids at urine output plus replete deficit over 48 h
Syndrome of inappropriate antidiuretic hormone secretion	Anorexia, headache, nausea, vomiting, irritability, seizures, coma	Paired plasma and urine osmolality and sodium	*Seizures:* 3% saline at 1–3 mL/kg IV; furosemide 1 mg/kg IV stat; benzodiazepines *Otherwise:* fluid restriction
Thyroid storm	Goiter, exophthalmos, high fever, tachycardia, congestive cardiac failure, delirium, stupor	Free T_4, TSH	Propranolol 10 μg/kg IV over 15 min; Lugol's iodine 9–15 drops/day orally; methimazole 20–30 mg q6–12 h (initially); tepid sponging
Neonatal thyrotoxicosis	Goiter, failure to gain weight, irritability, tachycardia, congestive cardiac failure	Free T_4, TSH	Propranolol 1 mg/kg TID orally; potassium iodide two drops bid orally; methimazole 0.5–0.7 mg/kg/day divided tid orally
Congenital hypothyroidism	Asymptomatic: hypothermia, hypoactivity, poor feeding, constipation, prolonged jaundice, large posterior fontanel	Free T_4, TSH	L-thyroxine 10–15 μg/kg/day orally
Hypopituitarism	See features listed for adrenal insufficiency and hypoglycemia		

IV, intravenous; IM, intramuscular; ACTH, adrenocorticotropic hormone; TSH, thyroid-stimulating hormone; tid, three times daily; bid, twice per day.

MEDICAL EMERGENCIES

dryness of mucous membranes. In severe cases, the child may exhibit signs of compensated shock, including a thready pulse and cold extremities, and rarely, as uncompensated shock with hypotension. The smell of ketones on the breath and the presence of deep, sighing (Kussmaul) respirations reflect the ketoacidosis. The patient's consciousness level, which may range from full alertness to deep coma, should be noted. The child may have exquisite abdominal tenderness with guarding and rigidity, which can mimic an acute abdomen. The ears, throat, chest, and urine should be examined because infection is often a precipitating factor. Careful attention should be paid to the skin exam because there have been several case reports of fasciitis copresenting with DKA. The presence of hyperpigmentation (acanthosis nigricans) on the posterior neck is a sign of long-standing insulin resistance and should alert the clinician to the possibility of noninsulin-dependent diabetes.

Diagnostic laboratory findings include plasma glucose greater than 200 mg per dL (commonly 400 to 800 mg per dL), the presence of glucose and ketones in the urine, acidosis (venous pH less than 7.3 and serum bicarbonate less than 15 mmol per L), high or normal plasma potassium, and slightly elevated blood urea nitrogen. Occasionally, DKA can occur with normoglycemia when persistent vomiting and decreased intake of carbohydrates are accompanied by continued administration of insulin or when patients have kept themselves particularly well hydrated with nonglucose-containing fluids. The measured serum sodium is usually low or in the low to normal range. Leukocytosis with a left shift may be noted but does not necessarily signify an underlying infection. Hyperglycemia in the absence of acidosis should cause the clinician to consider additional possibilities (see "Hyperglycemia" section).

Management

Careful clinical assessment and judgment are required. Children who have a recognized risk factor for cerebral edema (Table 86.3) require particularly meticulous attention to the details of their care. This section primarily focuses on the child who is significantly dehydrated, acidotic, and unable to take oral fluids because of vomiting or altered level of consciousness. Many cases of mild DKA can be managed with rehydration, either orally or intravenously, and with supplemental insulin either at home or in the ED. This possibility is addressed at the end of this section. For the severely dehydrated child, initial treatment is directed toward expansion of intravascular volume and administration of insulin. Subsequent treatment is directed at the normalization of the remaining abnormal biochemical parameters. Medical intervention carries significant risks of hypokalemia and cerebral edema (Tables 86.2 and 86.3).

Fluid and Electrolyte Replacement

Fluid replacement should be instituted promptly. In the first 1 to 2 hours, if hypovolemia is apparent, 10 to 20 mL per kg isotonic (0.9%) saline should be infused intravenously to establish an adequate intravascular volume and to improve tissue perfusion. This bolus may need to be repeated if the pulse rate and capillary refill rate do not improve, but rarely is more than 20 mL per kg required. The goal of this initial rehydration therapy is not euvolemia but adequate perfusion of end

---

TABLE 86.2

PRINCIPLES OF MANAGEMENT OF DIABETIC KETOACIDOSIS

Life-threatening Complications
Cerebral edema
Cardiovascular collapse
Profound metabolic acidosis
Hyperkalemia
Hypokalemia
Hypophosphatemia

Areas of Management Decisions

■ *Fluids.* Treat hypovolemia with crystalloid extracellular fluid expander. Use normal saline (0.9%) and infuse 10–20 mL/kg in the first 1–2 h. (Avoid hypotonic solutions initially because they are inefficient volume expanders and may contribute to cerebral edema.) Continue infusion at this rate until perfusion is improved and urine output is reestablished. After first 1–2 h, start half-normal saline—use greater tonicity, up to normal saline, if the initial serum sodium is less than 135 mmol/L or if the serum sodium falls with therapy. Total fluid administration in first 48 h should rarely exceed one and one-half to two times maintenance.

■ *Alkali.* Avoid bicarbonate therapy in DKA. Only consider if arterial pH <6.9 and impaired cardiac contractility and vascular tone, or if patient has life-threatening hyperkalemia.

■ *Potassium.* Start potassium therapy with administration of insulin. Starting concentration in fluid should be 40 mEq/L as a combination of potassium acetate and potassium phosphate. If the patient is hypokalemic (<4 mmol/L), a higher concentration of potassium, 60–80 mEq/L, may be necessary. Administer high concentrations of potassium only with electrocardiographic monitoring. If hyperkalemic (>6 mmol/L), decrease the concentration to 0–20 mEq/L.

■ *Insulin.* Should be given as a continuous IV infusion (0.1 Unit/kg/h).

■ *Glucose.* Add 5% glucose to solutions when plasma glucose is approximately 300 mg/dL. Continue adding glucose up to 12.5% in a peripheral IV in order to keep plasma glucose in target range of 200–300 mg/dL.

■ *Phosphate.* Add one-half of potassium in IVF as potassium phosphate up to 20 mEq/L, unless severe hypophosphatemia (PO_4 < 2 mmol/L).

Monitoring

■ *Clinical monitoring.* Blood pressure, pulse, respirations, neurologic status, and fluid intake and output. Continuous noninvasive $ETCO_2$ monitoring, if available.

■ *Laboratory monitoring.* Obtain initial glucose, electrolytes, blood gases, and blood urea nitrogen. Measure blood glucose every hour initially as guide to insulin dosage. Repeat electrolytes and pH measurements two to four times hourly as necessary, every hour if severe abnormalities.

■ *Use flow sheet.*

DKA, diabetic ketoacidosis; IV, intravenous; IVF, intravenous fluids; $ETCO_2$, end-tidal CO_2.

TABLE 86.3

RISK FACTORS FOR CEREBRAL EDEMA IN DIABETIC KETOACIDOSIS

Elevated blood urea nitrogen
Low P_{CO_2}
Treatment with bicarbonate
Failure of measured serum [Na^+] to rise steadily with correction of hyperglycemia
Age <3 yr
New-onset diabetes

organs. This may be best judged by monitoring mentation, capillary refill, and urine output.

Once adequate intravascular volume is established, the fluid deficit should be replaced over the next 48 hours. During the first 4 to 6 hours of this period isotonic fluids should be used with appropriate additional electrolyte supplementation as detailed below. The total body water deficit may be estimated based on a clinical estimate of dehydration, or intravenous (IV) fluid may be administered at a rate between one and one-half and two times maintenance fluid requirements (see Chapters 17 and 100). Ongoing urinary losses in excess of 5 mL per kg per hour (osmotic diuresis) should also be replaced.

The Na^+ deficit typically approximates 10 mEq per kg body weight and Na^+ maintenance is 3 mEq per 100 mL of maintenance fluid. From a practical point of view, half-normal (0.45%) saline can be started after the initial 4- to 6-hour period of isotonic fluids. The measured serum sodium should rise with initiation of therapy. If the initial serum sodium is less than 136 mmol per L, or if the serum sodium falls with therapy, the IV fluid should be changed to a more concentrated sodium stock, and the patient should be watched particularly closely. Serum sodium failing to rise with therapy has been identified as a risk factor for cerebral edema. Correcting the serum sodium for the degree of hyperglycemia may be useful in following the patient's total body sodium status:

$$\text{Corrected } [Na^+] = \text{measured } [Na^+] + [1.6 \times (\text{measured plasma glucose} - 100)/100]$$

If the corrected [Na^+] is less than 136 mmol per L or drops to less than 136 mmol per L during therapy, sodium concentration of the IV fluid should be increased to three-fourths normal (0.68%) or normal saline (0.9%). In addition, the serum sodium and the neurologic status of the patient should be followed more closely because this is a reported risk factor for cerebral edema (Table 86.3).

All children with DKA have total body potassium depleted (5 mEq per kg body weight); therefore, potassium replacement is an important part of therapy. If the initial serum [K^+] is 3 to 4.5 mmol per L, 40 mEq per L of potassium is added to the infusion after vascular competency has been established and the child has urinated. If the serum [K^+] is 4.6 to 5.0, only 20 mEq per L of potassium should be added, and if the [K^+] is above 5.0, potassium should be withheld in the initial fluids. Generally, K^+ is provided as potassium acetate (or chloride) and potassium phosphate in equal amounts. If the initial serum [K^+] is less than 4 mmol per L, potassium replacement

should be initiated promptly; if less than 3 mmol per L, IVF concentrations of K^+ of 60 mEq per L or greater may be necessary. With the higher concentrations of potassium, the phosphate component must be adjusted not to exceed the maximum rate. If the K^+ initial concentration is low, monitoring via an electrocardiogram (EKG) is indicated.

Phosphate depletion is almost universal in patients with DKA; however, the clinical significance of this reaction remains uncertain. As noted earlier, half of the K^+ replacement is with potassium phosphate, up to a maximum of 20 mEq potassium phosphate per liter except in the rare situation of severe hypophosphatemia (serum phosphate less than 2 mmol per L). Infusion of excess phosphate results in hypocalcemia, which may be complicated by tetanic seizures.

Alkali Therapy

In retrospective reviews of patients with DKA who developed significant cerebral edema, bicarbonate administration was identified as a significant risk factor (Table 86.3). This may be because the sickest patients are the ones most likely to have received bicarbonate therapy; however, without further clarification of the pathophysiology, bicarbonate therapy is reserved for patients with both severe acidosis (pH < 6.9) and secondary hemodynamic compromise that is unresponsive to inotropic agents.

A theoretical mechanism for the complications observed with alkali therapy is the development of a paradoxical acidosis of the central nervous system (CNS) and resultant cerebral depression. Paradoxical acidosis occurs because administered HCO_3^- combines with excess H^+ ions in the bloodstream to form H_2O and CO_2. Because the blood–brain barrier is relatively more permeable to CO_2 than to HCO_3^-, CO_2 accumulates in the CNS, resulting in further exacerbation of acidosis in this compartment, while acidosis is being corrected systemically.

Insulin and Glucose

Regular insulin is used for the treatment of ketoacidosis, but it should not be administered until the initial isotonic fluids have been administered for 1 hour. Insulin is initially necessary to stop ongoing ketone body production, the primary cause of the acidosis. Insulin should be started after 1 hour of initial fluid expansion to steadily correct the acidosis and may be either infused intravenously or, if necessary, injected intramuscularly at hourly intervals. Subcutaneous injections of insulin should be avoided because of the uncertainties of absorption in a dehydrated patient. The starting dose of insulin for continuous infusion is 0.1 Unit per kg per hour, infused by a regulated pump. Failure of the glucose to decrease in response to insulin suggests improper insulin preparation, inadequate hydration, or serious underlying disease (e.g., appendicitis or fasciitis with resultant significant increases in counterregulatory hormones). It is unnecessary and possibly detrimental to give an initial bolus of insulin. The dose for the hourly intramuscular (IM) injection, used if IV access cannot be obtained, is also 0.1 Unit per kg per hour.

Once the blood glucose approaches 300 mg per dL, glucose should be added to the IV fluids. As long as the child remains acidotic, insulin infusion should never be stopped; instead, the amount of glucose in the IV infusion should be increased in stepwise fashion up to a concentration of 12.5 g per dL to maintain the blood glucose between 150 and 250 mg per dL. If the blood glucose continues to drop, the rate of IV fluid administration should be increased to twice maintenance. If the blood glucose still cannot be maintained, the insulin infusion should be decreased by increments of 0.025 Unit per kg per hour.

When the child is able to eat and the anion gap has closed (normal = 10 to 12), IV infusion of insulin can be discontinued. Because IV insulin is metabolized rapidly, subcutaneous insulin must be given 30 minutes prior to the discontinuation of the infusion. The initial dose of subcutaneous insulin should be calculated based on a daily dose of 0.75 Unit per kg per day in the prepubertal child up to 1.0 Unit per kg per day in the pubertal child and beyond. If hourly IM injections are used, they should be continued until the blood glucose is less than 300 mg per dL and acidosis is correcting. By this time, perfusion is reestablished and subcutaneous insulin can be administered four times a day.

Cerebral Edema

Despite several investigations of the causes and risk factors for clinically significant cerebral edema in patients with DKA, and subsequent modifications in therapy, the incidence of the complication has not changed significantly during the past 20 years and remains at approximately 1%. Table 86.3 lists the leading risk factors published in more recent years. Clinical signs and symptoms of significant cerebral edema include abnormal motor or verbal response to pain, decorticate or decerebrate posturing, new cranial nerve palsy, and abnormal respiratory pattern. Other concerning signs are decrease or fluctuation in level of consciousness (e.g., Glasgow Coma Scale), age-inappropriate incontinence, vomiting, headache, and heart rate deceleration. If these signs are noted by the physician at the bedside, a clinical diagnosis of cerebral edema must be made and treatment initiated. The patient should receive mannitol 1 g per kg IV over 10 minutes. There is some evidence that hypertonic saline (3%) may be an appropriate substitute for mannitol; however, only case series data are currently available. Endotracheal intubation should be considered, primarily if the patient's mental status does not assure a safe airway, and secondarily if the patient is not able to maintain a respiratory alkalosis to partially compensate for the metabolic acidosis. If intubated, the patient should be initially hyperventilated to the P_{CO_2} he/she was maintaining prior to the neurologic decompensation (generally 10 to 20 mm Hg in the presence of significant ketoacidosis); this can be gradually reduced over several hours as the acidosis resolves and the cerebral edema is treated. Only after the patient is fully stabilized should a confirmatory computed tomography of the head be considered.

Monitoring

Close monitoring is mandatory, and a well-organized flow sheet ensures all parameters are being observed. Admission to an intensive care unit or specialized intermediate care unit should be considered if the patient is younger than 1 year of age, has a Glasgow Coma Scale score of less than 12, has an initial measured $[Na^+]$ of more than 145 mmol per L, or has an initial $[K^+]$ of less than 3 mmol per L. The patient should be maintained on continuous cardiorespiratory monitoring with hourly assessments of blood pressure and level of consciousness until the patient's trajectory of illness has been clearly established. Careful neurologic examination, with particular attention to arousability and pupillary reactivity, should be

performed frequently. The fluid input and output must be reviewed hourly to ensure appropriate rehydration is occurring. The IV fluids should be checked frequently so that pump failure or fluid leakage into the subcutaneous tissues can be corrected quickly. In the severely ill child, an EKG should be performed in the setting of hyperkalemia or hypokalemia.

The plasma glucose should be measured hourly until the blood glucose is stable and less than 300 mg per dL, and as long as the child is on an insulin infusion. Glucose measurement may be less frequent once the patient has been changed to subcutaneous insulin. Serum $[K^+]$ needs to be measured every 2 to 4 hours until the acidosis and hyperglycemia are normalized, or more frequently if hypokalemia is encountered or bicarbonate therapy is used. Calcium, phosphate, magnesium should be assessed initially and followed every 2 to 4 hours, more frequently if any are being actively replaced. With the advent of point-of-care ketone measurements, it may be advisable to follow serum ketone concentration every 2 to 4 hours, although continuous noninvasive capnography with nasal cannula end-tidal CO_2 ($etCO_2$) or transcutaneous CO_2 monitoring are also useful in tracking the degree of acidosis over time. Venous pH may be obtained to follow resolution of the acidosis if the above monitoring options are not available. Arterial sampling is not necessary for metabolic monitoring.

When the child is better hydrated and the acidosis resolves, mental alertness will improve and symptoms of nausea, vomiting, and abdominal pain should remit. If they do not resolve, an abdominal disorder should be considered. Some patients complain of blurred vision, which is caused by lens distortion resulting from fluid shifts of rehydration and correction of hyperglycemia—this should resolve within 24 hours of conclusion of therapy. When the anion gap has closed, most patients are able to tolerate oral fluids, at which point rehydration can be continued orally.

Mild Ketoacidosis

Some children with new-onset diabetes may also have hyperglycemia without ketoacidosis or with only mild acidosis. Generally, these patients are hospitalized for 24 to 48 hours to allow time to educate the family and stabilize the insulin dosage. These children require rehydration (as described in the next section) similar to patients with known diabetes and mild ketoacidosis. Insulin therapy can be initiated subcutaneously, at a total daily dose of 0.25 to 0.5 Unit per kg per day for the prepubertal child and 0.5 to 0.75 Unit per kg per day for the adolescent. There are two general regimens for dividing this total daily dose. In the conventional regimen, two-thirds of the total daily dose is administered in the morning, and one-third before dinner; two-thirds of the morning dose and evening dose should be as an intermediate-duration insulin (NPH, Lente), the remainder as rapid-acting insulin (lispro, aspart). Using the basal-bolus approach, one-half of the total daily dose is administered as insulin glargine or detemir, two 24-hour–acting analogs, and rapid-acting insulin (lispro, aspart) is dosed as a combination of coverage for ingested carbohydrates and as a correction for the degree of hyperglycemia above a chosen target—these initial dosages should be calculated along with the help of a consulting diabetes specialist.

Children with known diabetes often develop hyperglycemia and ketosis without significant acidosis (venous pH greater than 7.3 or bicarbonate greater than 15 mmol per L) during the course of intercurrent illness, especially gastroenteritis, or secondary to omission of insulin doses. Even the mildly dehydrated (5%) child with slight acidosis who presents to the ED benefits from an IV fluid bolus (10 to 20 mL per kg of normal saline); furthermore, this bolus will be given while awaiting laboratory test results. Once the laboratory results are available, the physician must decide whether to hospitalize the child, continue treatment in the ED, or send the child home. For purposes of definition, a patient does not have DKA if venous pH is greater than 7.3 and serum bicarbonate is greater than 15 mmol per L. Children who are significantly acidotic should be hospitalized and managed as outlined in the earlier section of this chapter. Several factors must be considered before sending a child home:

1. Is the child fully conscious and alert?
2. Can the child drink and retain oral fluids?
3. Can home glucose monitoring be done and are all related supplies available in the home?
4. Can ketones be measured at home, either in the urine with chemical test strips or in the serum with a point-of-care blood measurement device?
5. Will the child have competent supervision at home?
6. Does the family have access to both a telephone and transportation?
7. Is there a clinician available with whom the family can communicate by telephone?
8. Is the family comfortable with managing the mild acidosis at home?

If these questions can be answered in the affirmative, the child may be sent home.

Recommendations should be made to the family regarding fluid intake, insulin administration, and monitoring. Specific recommendations may vary with the age of the child and the experience of the family, but the following scheme may be helpful. Oral intake should be about the same as would be given intravenously to resolve the deficit and provide maintenance [e.g., the 10-year-old child (30 kg) would normally receive a 300-mL bolus followed by 100 to 140 mL per hour, for a total of up to 1 L during the first 6 hours intravenously if he/she was hospitalized; therefore, the physician should suggest that the family try to get in 150 to 180 mL of liquid every hour for the next 6 hours]. It is best if this liquid is taken in as sips.

Additional short-acting insulin will be required in addition to the patient's usual long-acting doses. In the ED, two decisions will need to be made regarding insulin: First, how much short-acting insulin (lispro or regular) should be given to the child before discharge? One way to dose additional insulin is using the 5–10% to 10–15% rule:

- If blood glucose is 250 to 400 mg per dL without urinary ketones, 5% of the child's usual total daily dose will suffice.
- If blood glucose is more than 400 mg per dL without ketones, or is 250 to 400 mg per dL with moderate or large ketones, 10% of the daily dose will be needed.
- If blood glucose is more than 400 mg per dL and ketones are moderate or large, the child will need 15% of the daily dose and admission to the hospital should be reconsidered.

Second, how much should be given at home and with what frequency? Once home, the preceding 5–10% to 10–15% rule is generally applicable and should be given every 4 hours, based on blood glucose and blood or urinary ketones. The family can begin using this algorithm once the child is able to return to a normal intake. For any child to be safely discharged home, however, he or she must be able to maintain adequate oral intake and have frequent contact with a clinician who is comfortable managing pediatric diabetes. Last, hourly monitoring of blood glucose, urine output, and ketones is recommended with the expectation that the blood glucose should decline, the urine output should fall, and the ketones should begin to clear.

HYPERGLYCEMIA

Background

According to American Diabetes Association guidelines, fasting laboratory plasma glucose of greater than 126 mg per dL or a random glucose greater than 200 mg per dL on two separate occasions is diagnostic of diabetes in an otherwise healthy person. These guidelines were developed primarily by specialists in adult diabetes and may not be completely applicable to the pediatric population.

Therefore, it is essential that any elevated glucose level be evaluated within the context of the ill child and that other factors, such as simultaneous medication administration, be considered.

Pathophysiology

As noted in the previous section on diabetes and the following section on hypoglycemia, glucose homeostasis reflects the balance between glucose input (from gut absorption, hepatic glycogen breakdown, or gluconeogenesis) and disposal (via storage or oxidation). With the exception of gut absorption, this process is largely regulated by insulin, although counterregulatory hormones also have a significant effect. Furthermore, tissue factors and medication also impact the insulin effect.

Clinical Manifestations

Plasma glucose concentrations in the 200 to 300 mg per dL range rarely result in symptoms. This level of hyperglycemia may be accompanied by intermittently increased frequency of urination; however, parents are rarely aware of their child's frequency of urination once the child is toilet-trained unless the frequency becomes disruptive (e.g., the child begins having "accidents" at school). Children and adolescents have no sense of what is the normal frequency of urination, so they rarely complain unless the frequent urination is accompanied by dysuria. Higher levels of glucose (greater than 300 mg per dL) may be associated with subtle clinical findings, such as blurring of vision or dryness of oral membranes.

Significant hyperglycemia may occur without significant symptoms and can be tolerated for a prolonged period without clinical signs. In the ED, hyperglycemia is likely to be seen in several different situations. First, the child may be known to have diabetes and present with an intercurrent illness or traumatic injury. Both illness and injury result in increased counterregulatory hormones, which may lead to relative insulin resistance and hyperglycemia. The second presentation is the child for whom diabetes is suspected because of classical symptoms of polyuria, polydipsia, and polyphagia accompanied by weight loss. Almost half of children with new-onset diabetes mellitus present to their pediatrician or to the ED in this way. Third, some medical conditions are associated with persistent hyperglycemia, such as recurrent urinary tract infections and vaginal yeast infections. Furthermore, type 2 diabetes is increasingly being reported in minority adolescents; in many, hyperpigmentation of the posterior neck and axilla (acanthosis nigricans) may be noted. Fourth, a laboratory panel obtained for some other reason (e.g., abdominal pain) may reveal hyperglycemia.

Management

In the child with diabetes, unless the child is clinically dehydrated or is unable to take oral fluids, hyperglycemia is not a crisis. Oral fluids should be encouraged, and supplemental short-acting insulin (lispro or aspart insulin) may be required; it can be dosed according to the 5–10% to 10–15% rule:

- If blood glucose is 250 to 400 mg per dL without urinary ketones, 5% of the child's usual total daily dose will suffice.
- If blood glucose is more than 400 mg per dL without ketones, or is 250 to 400 mg per dL with moderate or large ketones, 10% of the daily dose will be needed.
- If blood glucose is more than 400 mg per dL and ketones are moderate or large, the child will need 15% of the daily dose and admission to the hospital should be reconsidered.

Failure to respond to these simple measures, whether in the ED or at home, should lead to a consultation with the child's endocrinologist. If oral fluids must be restricted and the child is hyperglycemic (e.g., a child with traumatic injury requiring surgery), IV fluids without glucose should be used and glucose should be monitored frequently. As blood glucose concentration reaches 200 mg per dL, dextrose should be added to the IV fluid to maintain target blood glucose of 150 to 250 mg per dL. Additional supplemental insulin may be required, depending on when the child last received insulin and the response to simple hydration. Supplemental short-acting insulin should be dosed subcutaneously according to the 5–10% to 10–15% rule every 4 hours, and the child's usual long-acting insulin should be continued.

The child with classic symptoms merits further evaluation to determine whether he or she is dehydrated, hyperosmolar, or acidotic. If the child is simply hyperglycemic, hospitalization is often required for initiation of treatment and diabetes-related education; however, IV fluid resuscitation and intensive care are not indicated.

In children with classic signs or symptoms of hyperglycemia (i.e., polydipsia, polyuria), a plasma glucose should be obtained. If this test reveals hyperglycemia, as defined by the American Diabetes Association, the child should be referred for further evaluation and treatment of diabetes.

Last, if hyperglycemia is a coincidental finding, the diagnosis requires thoughtful consideration. How traumatic was the blood draw? How upset was the child? What medications or IV fluids were given to the child just before the phlebotomy? What was the child drinking while waiting to see the physician? Are the symptoms in any way related to the hyperglycemia? How sick is the child? The sicker the child is, the less

likely it is that hyperglycemia is reflective of diabetes. Three simple evaluations are helpful in determining whether the hyperglycemia is circumstantial or suggestive of diabetes. Brief hyperglycemia resulting from a stress response to phlebotomy or secondary to oral intake rarely results in significant glucosuria; therefore, a urine dip for glucose is often helpful. Second, in the absence of ongoing stress or input, glucose tends to fall over time. A fingerstick glucose is rarely stressful. Therefore, repeating a glucose measurement by fingerstick 1 to 2 hours after the original sample was sent is useful in separating disease from nondisease. Third, hyperglycemia secondary to these factors is usually mild (150 to 250 mg per dL). More significant hyperglycemia should raise the suspicion of diabetes, glucose intolerance, or an underlying medical illness that is producing a significant counterregulatory response.

HYPOGLYCEMIA

Background

Hypoglycemia is defined as plasma glucose of less than 50 mg per dL, regardless of whether symptoms are present. Hypoglycemia is a chemical finding that should lead to a diligent search for a cause. A differential diagnosis of hypoglycemia, as it may present in the ED, is provided in Table 86.4.

Hypoglycemia may be secondary to insulin therapy for diabetes. Excluding this category, almost all hypoglycemia in children occurs during periods of decreased or absent oral intake,

TABLE 86.4

CAUSES OF CHILDHOOD HYPOGLYCEMIA

Decreased Availability of Glucose
Decreased intake—fasting, malnutrition, illness
Decreased absorption—acute diarrhea
Inadequate glycogen reserves—defects in enzymes of glycogen synthetic pathways
Ineffective glycogenolysis—defects in enzymes of glycogenolytic pathways
Inability to mobilize glycogen—glucagon deficiency
Ineffective gluconeogenesis—defects in enzymes of gluconeogenic pathway

Increased Use of Glucose
Hyperinsulinism—islet cell adenoma or hyperplasia, ingestion of oral hypoglycemic agents, insulin therapy
Large tumors—Wilms' tumor, neuroblastoma

Diminished Availability of Alternative Fuels
Decreased or absent fat stores
Inability to oxidize fats—enzymatic defects in fatty acid oxidation

Unknown or Complex Mechanisms
Sepsis/shock
Reye's syndrome
Salicylate ingestion
Ethanol ingestion
Adrenal insufficiency
Hypothyroidism
Hypopituitarism

often coupled with increased energy demand (e.g., viral gastroenteritis with fever). Postprandial hypoglycemia is unusual in children, except in those who have had prior gastrointestinal surgery.

Pathophysiology

Because glucose is necessary for cellular energy production in most human tissues, the maintenance of an adequate blood glucose concentration is important for normal function. The plasma glucose reflects a dynamic balance among glucose input from dietary sources, glycogenolysis and gluconeogenesis, and glucose use by muscle, heart, adipose tissue, brain, and blood elements.

The liver plays a unique role in glucose homeostasis because it stores glucose as glycogen. With fasting, this glycogen is degraded to glucose, which is released into the bloodstream. In addition, the liver synthesizes new glucose from glycerol, lactate, and certain amino acids. During fasting, lipolysis occurs and the resultant fatty acids are used for the production of both energy and ketones (acetoacetate and β-hydroxybutyrate) by the liver. The energy generated from the metabolism of fatty acids is essential to sustain maximal rates of gluconeogenesis and ureagenesis in the liver. The ketones are an important auxiliary fuel for most tissues, including the brain.

Muscle contains significant quantities of glycogen and protein. Under fasting conditions, the glycogen is degraded and used endogenously but is not released as free glucose into the bloodstream. Certain amino acids, particularly alanine and glycine, are released from the muscle and subsequently used by the liver for gluconeogenesis. Muscle derives an increasing proportion of its energy requirement from fatty acids as fasting proceeds.

Brain tissue is highly dependent on glucose for its energy requirements. Under certain circumstances, it can extract a limited proportion of its energy requirement from other substrates (e.g., glycerol, ketones, lactate), although this process requires a period of adaptation and does not negate the need for a constant supply of glucose.

Insulin is the primary hormone that regulates the blood glucose level. Insulin stimulates the uptake of glucose and amino acids into skeletal, cardiac, and adipose tissue and promotes glycogen and protein synthesis. It inhibits lipolysis and glycogenolysis. The net effect of insulin action is to accelerate the removal of glucose and gluconeogenic substrates from the bloodstream. Opposing or modulating the effects of insulin are cortisol, glucagon, epinephrine, and growth hormone. The effects of these hormones include inhibition of glucose uptake by muscle, mobilization of amino acids for gluconeogenesis, activation of lipolysis, inhibition of insulin secretion, and induction of gluconeogenic enzymes. The net effect is to increase the availability of gluconeogenic substrates to the liver, and to increase the accessibility and use of nonglucose fuels by other tissues.

Clinical Manifestations

Prompt recognition of hypoglycemia is important because brain damage may result if the hypoglycemia is prolonged or recurs frequently. The acutely ill child warrants a glucose determination if the level of consciousness is altered because hypoglycemia may accompany an illness that interferes with oral intake. Historical evidence may aid in establishing the cause of hypoglycemia. Because hypoglycemia in children occurs after a period of fasting, a careful chronology of dietary intake during the preceding 24 hours should be obtained. The possibility of ingestion should be considered because ethanol, β-blockers, and oral hypoglycemic agents are in common use.

The symptoms and signs of hypoglycemia are nonspecific and are often overlooked, especially in the infant and young child. The clinical findings of hypoglycemia reflect both the decreased availability of glucose to the CNS and the adrenergic stimulation caused by decreasing or low blood glucose. Adrenergic symptoms and signs include palpitations, anxiety, tremulousness, hunger, and sweating. Irritability, headache, fatigue, confusion, seizure, and unconsciousness are neuroglycopenic symptoms. Any combination of these symptoms should lead to a consideration of hypoglycemia. Any child presenting with a seizure, other than a breakthrough seizure with known epilepsy, or unconsciousness should have a plasma glucose determination.

Management

If hypoglycemia is suspected, blood should be drawn, if at all possible, before treatment. An extra tube (3 mL, red top) should be obtained and refrigerated until the laboratory glucose is known. Rapid screening should be performed using a bedside glucose meter while awaiting definitive laboratory results. Therapy should be instituted if this screen is suggestive of hypoglycemia. This method may lead to some overtreatment because of error of bedside devices; however, treatment holds minimal risk. It is preferable to overtreat than to allow a child to remain hypoglycemic until definitive laboratory results are available. If the laboratory glucose confirms that the blood glucose was less than 50 mg per dL, the reserved serum can be used for chemical (β-hydroxybutyrate, acetoacetate, amino acid profile, acylcarnitine profile), toxicologic, and hormonal (insulin, growth hormone, cortisol) studies, and may provide the correct diagnosis without extensive additional testing. If adequate blood is obtained before correction, other metabolites to be considered are glucagon, c-peptide, lactate, and pyruvate. If blood is obtained with 15 minutes of glucose administration, it may still be helpful, although possibly not diagnostic.

The first voided urine after the hypoglycemic episode should be saved for toxicologic, organic acid evaluation, and acylglycine profile. In the ED, the urine should also be tested immediately for ketones. With hypoglycemia, ketones should be large. Failure to find large ketones in the presence of hypoglycemia strongly suggests either that fats are not being mobilized from adipose tissue, as might occur in hyperinsulinism, or that fat cannot be used for ketone body formation, as might occur in enzymatic defects in fatty acid oxidation. Both the urine and the serum results will be useful in determining the underlying cause of hypoglycemia. The preferred treatment for hypoglycemia is rapid IV administration of 0.25 g of dextrose per kg body weight (2.5 mL per kg of 10% dextrose, 1.0 mL per kg of 25% dextrose). The plasma glucose should then be maintained by an infusion of dextrose at a rate of 6 to 8 mg per kg per minute. Generally, this goal can be accomplished by providing 10% dextrose at one and one-half times maintenance rates. Glucagon (0.03 mg per kg up to a maximum of 1 mg intramuscularly) may be used to treat hypoglycemia that is known to be caused by hyperinsulinism but is not indicated as part of the routine therapy of hypoglycemia. Glucocorticoids should not be used because they have minimal acute benefit and may delay identification of the cause of hypoglycemia.

The adequacy of therapy should be evaluated both chemically and clinically. The plasma glucose should be monitored frequently and consistently until a stable level higher than 70 mg per dL is attained on more than one measurement. Adrenergic symptoms should resolve quickly. The resolution of CNS symptoms may be prolonged, particularly if the child was initially seizing or unconscious. Seizures that do not respond to correction of hypoglycemia should be managed with appropriate anticonvulsants (see Chapters 69 and 96). The mild acidosis (pH 7.25 to 7.35) usually seen in hypoglycemia will correct without specific intervention. Marked acidosis (pH less than 7.10) suggests shock or serious underlying disease and should be managed appropriately (see Chapter 3). Any child with documented hypoglycemia not secondary to insulin therapy should be hospitalized for careful monitoring and diagnostic testing.

HYPOPITUITARISM

Background

The term *hypopituitarism* generally applies to any condition in which more than a single pituitary hormone is deficient. This condition may include deficiencies resulting from a lack of hypothalamic-releasing factors, as well as deficiencies of anterior and posterior pituitary hormones. Diabetes insipidus (DI), the lack of antidiuretic hormone (ADH), may occur alone or in association with other hormonal defects and is discussed in a subsequent section.

Pathophysiology

Adrenocorticotropic hormone (ACTH) primarily affects adrenal glucocorticoid production; generally, it does not affect mineralocorticoid synthesis, which is primarily regulated by the renin–angiotensin system. A deficiency of ACTH production manifests as cortisol deficiency. Because cortisol plays a role as an insulin counterregulatory hormone, a lack of either ACTH or cortisol may result in hypoglycemia. Because the only identified role for thyroid-stimulating hormone (TSH) is the stimulation of thyroid hormone production, a deficiency of TSH is most likely to manifest as hypothyroidism. Luteinizing hormone (LH) and follicle-stimulating hormone (FSH) are involved in gonadal maturation, as well as the regulation of gonadal functions. LH and FSH play an important role in testicular descent and penile growth in the fetus, as well as affecting the onset of puberty in the adolescent. The circulating levels of these two pituitary hormones are low in children and have no demonstrable function. Prolactin is primarily involved in the maintenance of lactation and is of minimal significance in childhood. Growth hormone is a principal regulator of linear growth and an important insulin counterregulatory hormone. The absence of growth hormone may be associated with hypoglycemia, particularly in infants and young children.

Clinical Manifestations

The symptoms and signs of hypopituitarism depend on missing hormones. Isolated growth hormone deficiency is most likely to present with poor linear growth, although occasionally an infant or young child will present with hypoglycemia. The acute presentation of hypopituitarism is most likely to occur when the child is stressed by injury, illness, or fasting. The presentation may involve either an unusually rapid decompensation, reflecting the role of cortisol in adaptation to stress, or as hypoglycemia, mirroring the role of both cortisol and growth hormone in opposing the effects of insulin. In the older child, no specific symptoms or signs indicate a lack of LH and FSH. An association between a lack of these hormones and anosmia has been noted (Kallmann's syndrome). In the adolescent, a deficiency of LH and FSH may be evidenced as pubertal delay. No specific signs or symptoms have been associated with a deficiency of prolactin in childhood.

In the neonatal male, hypopituitarism may be accompanied not only by hypoglycemia, but also by micropenis (less than 2 cm, stretched length). This condition illustrates the role of LH and FSH in stimulating testicular function in utero. Significant liver dysfunction in the neonatal period may be associated with congenital hypopituitarism. Hypopituitarism is seen with various midline structural anomalies, including optic nerve hypoplasia, cleft palate, absence of the septum pellucidum, and spina bifida.

In the older child, intracranial mass lesions, particularly with craniopharyngioma and other pituitary abnormalities, may cause hypopituitarism. The presence of visual field abnormalities may aid in localizing the site of the lesion. A history of severe head trauma, surgery for CNS tumors, or CNS irradiation should increase the suspicion of hypopituitarism.

Management

The child with hypopituitarism may require any or all the following therapies. Adequate cortisol replacement is an absolute necessity in children with known or suspected secondary adrenal insufficiency (ACTH deficiency). Cortisol replacement under stress conditions (e.g., trauma, fever) should be the equivalent of 50 mg of hydrocortisone per m² per day (hydrocortisone IV infusion 12.5 mg per m² every 6 hours; hydrocortisone continuous IV infusion at 50 mg per m² per day; cortisone 50 mg per m² intramuscularly every 24 hours). A child with hypopituitarism presenting in extremis or with severe electrolyte abnormalities should immediately receive an initial rescue dose of 50 mg per m². In general, all cases of adrenal insufficiency should be treated with hydrocortisone because it is the only pharmacologic glucocorticoid that stimulates both the glucocorticoid receptor and the mineralocorticoid receptor. If a patient is known to have hypopituitarism, other steroids may be used in equipotent doses and the mineralocorticoid production can be assumed to be normal because it does not involve the pituitary.

Because both cortisol and growth hormone are insulin counterregulatory hormones, children with hypopituitarism are prone to hypoglycemia. If enteral intake is interrupted for prolonged periods, glucose should be supplied intravenously. Blood glucose should be monitored to ascertain the adequacy of therapy. Both adrenal insufficiency and diabetes insipidus can lead to fluid and electrolyte abnormalities; therefore, electrolytes should be determined at presentation and followed closely. Changes in IV therapy should be based on serum electrolytes. Judicious use of 1-desamino-8-D-arginine vasopressin (DDAVP) may be helpful in managing diabetes insipidus, as outlined subsequently; however, this treatment is usually unnecessary at the time of acute presentation.

Although both thyroid hormone and sex hormone(s) may need to be replaced, this treatment is not required in the ED. Growth hormone replacement therapy should only be initiated or continued in an inpatient if the child has a history of hypoglycemia and is not critically ill. Administration of growth hormone to critically ill adults has been shown to increase mortality, apparently as a result of hyperglycemia and increased incidence of sepsis, so it should generally be withheld in the critically ill patient.

Because hypopituitarism often results from intracranial lesions, the demonstration of a pituitary or a hypothalamic mass, or a history of a significant cranial insult, should lead to a diligent search for hormonal deficits. Similarly, documented pituitary deficits should lead to a thorough radiologic investigation of the cranial cavity.

ACUTE ADRENAL INSUFFICIENCY

Background

Acute adrenal insufficiency occurs when the adrenal cortex fails to produce enough glucocorticoid and mineralocorticoid in response to stress. Patients at risk of this life-threatening event include individuals with primary adrenal disease and those who have adrenal insufficiency secondary to hypothalamic-pituitary suppression (Table 86.5). This emergency has become more common with the widespread use of suppressive doses of corticosteroids in the treatment of chronic disease (e.g., nephrotic syndrome, acute lymphoblastic leukemia, asthma). Infection, trauma, or surgery in the susceptible patient generally precipitates the acute crisis. The diagnosis must be based primarily on clinical suspicion because prompt commencement of therapy is mandatory for survival and definitive diagnostic test results may not be available for days. Congenital adrenal hyperplasia is a

---

TABLE 86.5

COMMON CAUSES OF ACUTE ADRENAL INSUFFICIENCY IN CHILDREN

Primary Adrenal Insufficiency
Adrenoleukodystrophy (X-linked)
Congenital adrenal hyperplasia
Autoimmunity
Tuberculosis
Meningococcal septicemia
Adrenal hemorrhage

Secondary Adrenal Insufficiency
Suppression of adrenocorticotropic hormone by pharmacologic doses of glucocorticoid administration
Pituitary or hypothalamic tumors
Central nervous system surgery or irradiation
Structural abnormalities (septooptic dysplasia)
Congenital hypopituitarism

---

unique form of adrenal insufficiency that is discussed in a subsequent section of this chapter.

Pathophysiology

Because the production of corticosteroids by the adrenal cortex is under pituitary and hypothalamic control, adrenal insufficiency can result from either an adrenal (primary) or hypothalamic–pituitary (secondary) disorder. Specific adrenal problems resulting in adrenal insufficiency include inborn errors of hormonal biosynthesis (discussed in the "Congenital Adrenal Hyperplasia" section), autoimmune destructive processes, X-linked adrenoleukodystrophy, and adrenal hemorrhage. Hypothalamic–pituitary causes include CNS tumors, trauma, and radiation therapy for a variety of neoplastic disorders. Exogenous administration of glucocorticoids also suppresses the adrenal–pituitary axis, an effect that often lasts well beyond the cessation of corticosteroid therapy.

Glucocorticoids are essential for withstanding stress; therefore, adrenal insufficiency is most likely to be manifested during an intercurrent infection or after trauma. Mineralocorticoids, especially aldosterone, play an important role in salt and water homeostasis by promoting salt resorption in the distal renal tubules and collecting ducts. Mineralocorticoid production is primarily regulated by the renin–angiotensin system; thus, adrenal insufficiency resulting from hypothalamic–pituitary causes is rarely associated with a lack of aldosterone. However, aldosterone deficiency is a common feature in primary adrenal insufficiency. Because of the nature of the pituitary–adrenal axis, primary adrenal insufficiency is accompanied by significantly elevated ACTH levels.

Clinical Manifestations

The historical information suggestive of adrenal insufficiency depends on the cause. Children with a primary adrenal defect are more likely to have had a gradual onset of symptoms, such as general malaise, anorexia, fatigue, and weight loss. Salt craving and postural hypotension may also have been noted. Waterhouse-Friderichsen syndrome, acute adrenal infarction, should be considered in a patient with fulminant sepsis and hypotension unresponsive to vasopressors or inotropes, especially if due to meningococcemia. A child with secondary adrenal insufficiency is more likely to have a history of neurosurgical procedures, head trauma, CNS pathology, or chronic disease necessitating the prolonged use of glucocorticoids.

Findings on physical examination are more likely to be characteristic of the precipitating illness or trauma rather than specifically suggestive of adrenal insufficiency. Although a lack of glucocorticoid and aldosterone can be associated with hypotension and dehydration, a better clue to the possibility of adrenal insufficiency is inappropriately rapid decompensation in the face of metabolic stress. Hyperpigmentation may be present in primary adrenal insufficiency, especially of long duration. Red hair and peripheral eosinophilia may be noted in Addison's disease or autoimmune destruction of the adrenals.

Biochemical evidence suggestive of adrenal insufficiency includes hyponatremia, hyperkalemia, hypoglycemia, and hemoconcentration. Mild metabolic acidosis and hypercalcemia may be present. The definitive diagnosis depends on the demonstration of an inappropriately low level of cortisol in the serum. Blood should be obtained for the measurement of both cortisol and ACTH at baseline if the diagnosis is suspected, and then cortisol measurement is repeated 60 minutes after IV or IM administration of 0.25 mg of a synthetic ACTH preparation (i.e., cosyntropin). Results are unlikely to be available on an emergency basis.

Management

Treatment of adrenal crisis is based on rapid volume expansion and the administration of glucocorticoids. Immediate management consists of 50 to 100 mg of hydrocortisone intravenously. Subsequent management is hydrocortisone 50 mg per m^2 per 24 hours given intravenously continuously or divided every 6 hours. Volume expansion is accomplished with normal saline (20 mL per kg) in the first hour, followed by fluids appropriate for maintenance and replacement. Additional Na^+ may be needed in primary adrenal insufficiency because of ongoing urinary Na^+ losses. These fluids should contain 10% dextrose and should not contain potassium until the serum potassium is within the normal range.

Mineralocorticoid therapy is rarely important in the acute phase, provided fluid therapy is adequate; however, patients with primary adrenal insufficiency may need replacement with a mineralocorticoid for long-term management. Hydrocortisone acts at the mineralocorticoid receptor when dosed at stress levels of 50 mg per m^2 per day. Subsequent long-term therapy can be accomplished with fludrocortisone. Specific therapy directed toward correction of the hyperkalemia is rarely required unless cardiac EKG changes (peaked T wave, prolonged QRS duration) or arrhythmias are present. Hypoglycemia is remedied by the use of dextrose and by the hyperglycemic effects of glucocorticoids. The precipitating factor, such as infection, also requires appropriate therapy.

Improvement in peripheral circulation and blood pressure should occur quickly with therapy. Dramatic improvement often occurs in all parameters within hours after the first dose of glucocorticoid. Because adrenal crisis is commonly brought on by another stress such as infection, the symptoms of malaise, anorexia, and lethargy may take longer to resolve. Once instituted, high-dose glucocorticoid therapy should be continued for 48 hours, and adequate hydration should be maintained either orally or intravenously. The patient known to be at risk for adrenal insufficiency should wear an identifying bracelet to alert ED personnel to this possibility.

CONGENITAL ADRENAL HYPERPLASIA

Background

Inborn errors of adrenal steroid biosynthesis are grouped under the term *congenital adrenal hyperplasia* (CAH). Two major modes of presentation occur in early infancy and require prompt diagnosis and treatment: acute salt-losing crisis and ambiguous genitalia (Table 86.6). CAH may also present in children as precocious virilization. This form of CAH warrants investigation, but it does not require emergency management. The most common form of CAH presenting in infancy is 21-hydroxylase deficiency, which is recessively inherited and accounts for 90% of all cases. Clinically apparent salt wasting develops in approximately two-thirds of affected patients. In the United States, the incidence of 21-hydroxylase deficiency is approximately 1 in 15,000 live births.

Pathophysiology

The enzymes 21-hydroxylase, 11β-hydroxylase, 3β-hydroxysteroid dehydrogenase, and 20,22-desmolase are involved in the production of both cortisol and aldosterone (Fig. 86.1 and Table 86.6). Because the hypothalamic–pituitary axis is under feedback control by cortisol, the lack of production of this hormone caused by the enzyme deficiency results in a significant increase in ACTH. In turn, ACTH stimulates the adrenal to increase steroid hormone production. Because cortisol synthesis is impaired, the precursors of cortisol accumulate significantly. The symptoms and signs characteristic of each enzymatic deficiency reflect either the absence of cortisol or aldosterone or the accumulation of their precursors.

TABLE 86.6

CLINICAL AND LABORATORY FEATURES OF VARIOUS FORMS OF CONGENITAL ADRENAL HYPERPLASIA

	Clinical Features				
	Newborn with sexual ambiguity				
Enzyme deficiency	Female	Male	Salt wasting	Hypertension	Postnatal virilization
21-Hydroxylase					
Nonsalt wasting	Y	N	N	N	Y
Salt wasting	Y	N	Y	N	Y
11β-Hydroxylase	Y	N	N	Y	Y
3β-Hydroxysteroid dehydrogenase	Y	Y	Y	N	N
17α-Hydroxylase	N	Y	N	Y	N
Cholesterol desmolase	N	Y	Y	N	N
18-Hydroxylase	N	N	Y	N	N
17β-Hydroxysteroid dehydrogenase	N	Y	—	—	Y

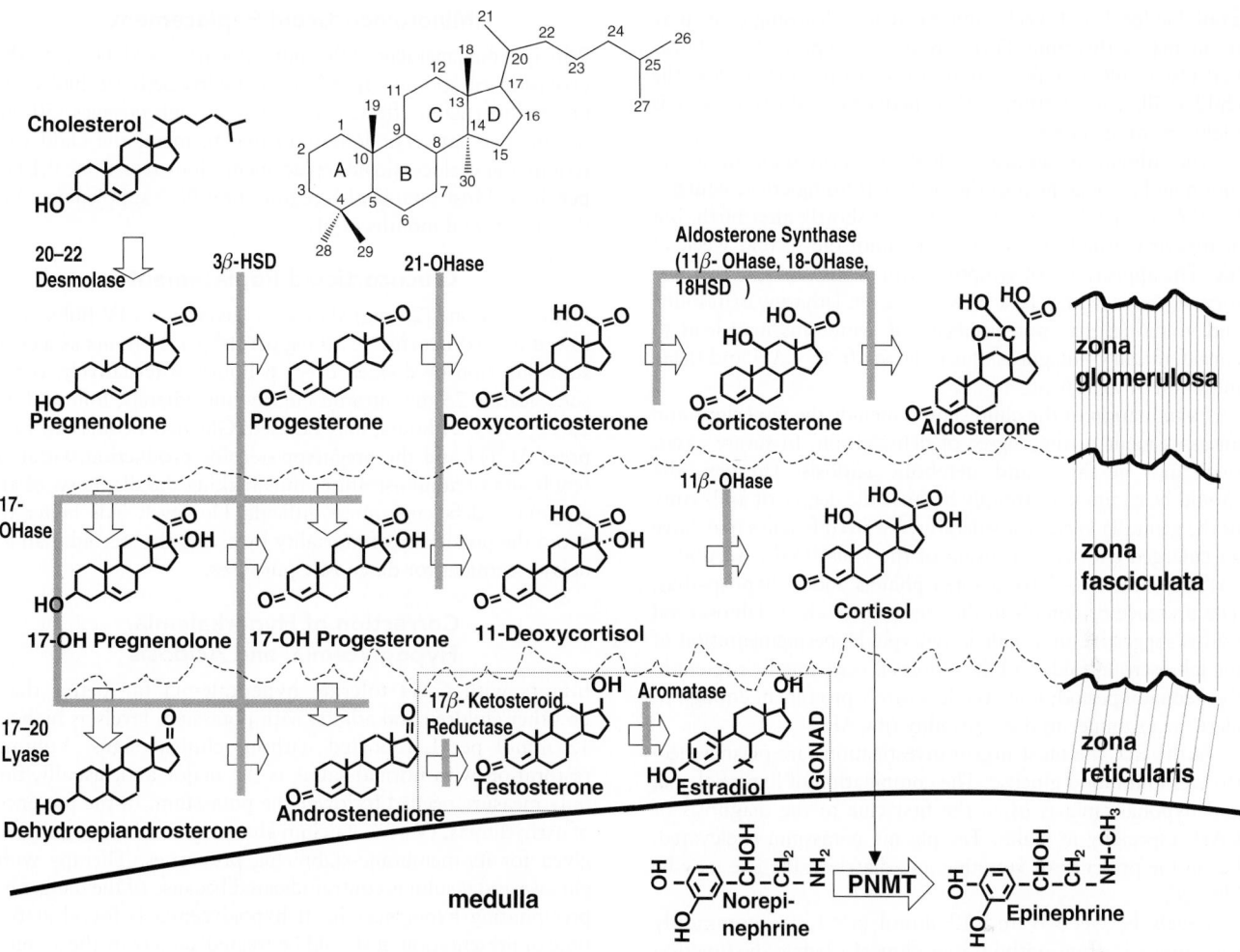

FIGURE 86.1 Adrenal steroid hormone biosynthesis. The pathways for the synthesis of adrenal steroid hormones (adrenal cortex) and catecholamines (adrenal medulla) are arranged from left to right. Synthesis of all compounds originates from cholesterol in the mitochondria of the adrenal cortex. Subsequent conversions are shown with enzyme names located next to *open arrows,* and *gray lines* indicating enzymatic blocks in the various forms of congenital adrenal hyperplasia (CAH). Mineralocorticoids (aldosterone) are produced in the zona glomerulosa, glucocorticoids (cortisol) in the zona fasciculata, and androgens (testosterone) and estrogens (estradiol) in the zona reticularis. Cortically produced cortisol is required for full induction of the medullary conversion of norepinephrine to epinephrine. (Courtesy of Joseph Majzoub, MD, Children's Hospital Boston.)

Impairment of mineralocorticoid synthesis by 21-hydroxylase, 3β-hydroxysteroid dehydrogenase, and 20,22-desmolase deficiency can result in salt wasting. Although 11β-hydroxylase deficiency also blocks aldosterone production, the immediate precursor to the block, desoxycorticosterone, has potent mineralocorticoid activity. Thus, instead of developing salt loss, patients with this enzyme defect often develop hypertension during childhood.

Androgenic compounds accumulate in 21-hydroxylase and 11β-hydroxylase deficiencies. Females with these defects are virilized in utero and are born with ambiguous genitalia; therefore, females are often identified in the newborn period. Some female infants are so virilized that they are mistaken as males with bilateral cryptorchidism. Males have normal genital development; therefore, the diagnosis is generally missed until they present with salt-wasting crisis during infancy or with evidence of precocious puberty during childhood. Deficiency of

3β-hydroxysteroid dehydrogenase leads to underproduction of testosterone. Boys with this deficiency are undervirilized because only weak androgens are produced, whereas girls are mildly virilized because of these weak androgens. Lack of cortisol renders the patient more susceptible to hypoglycemia and reduces the tolerance to severe stress, such as dehydration.

Clinical Manifestations

CAH may manifest at birth with the discovery of ambiguous genitalia, between 2 and 5 weeks of age when the baby presents with acute salt-losing crisis, or during childhood with the onset of precocious puberty. The affected child may come to the ED for any of these reasons. Caution is in order in considering newborn screening for CAH. Although many US states now screen newborns for CAH, the results may not be available for 3 to 4 weeks and the acute salt-losing crisis may occur before this time. Furthermore, the report of an abnormal test result may precipitate a visit to the ED: Unless the child is ill, consultation with a pediatric endocrinologist is highly recommended.

The subsequent discussion deals primarily with the recognition and management of the acute salt-losing crisis, which is life-threatening. Salt wasting is present shortly after birth, but acute crisis usually does not occur until the second week of life. The appearance of symptoms can be insidious, with a history of poor feeding, lack of weight gain, lethargy, irritability, and vomiting. The nonspecificity of symptoms may lead to consideration of diagnoses far removed from CAH and delay initiation of treatment.

Examination of the child should include the vital signs and an assessment of the degree of dehydration. In severe cases, there may be shock and metabolic acidosis. The genitalia should be examined carefully because the degree of ambiguity of the genitalia varies considerably. Virilized females may have an enlarged clitoris and fusion of the labial folds. An under-virilized male may have a small phallus and/or hypospadias. The presence of gonads in the inguinal canals or labioscrotal fold is suggestive of a male karyotype. Hyperpigmentation of the labioscrotal folds and the nipples is occasionally present in the neonatal period; however, it is rarely prominent enough to alert the examiner to the possibility of CAH.

In the ED, the most urgent investigations are plasma electrolytes and blood glucose. The combination of hyperkalemia and hyponatremia is often the first clue to the diagnosis of CAH, especially in males. The plasma potassium is elevated, but in the presence of vomiting and diarrhea, the rise may be blunted.

Levels between 6 and 12 mmol per L are commonly encountered, often without any clinical cardiac dysfunction or EKG changes. The plasma bicarbonate level is usually low, reflecting the metabolic acidosis that results from the retention of hydrogen ions in exchange for sodium loss. The blood glucose is usually normal; however, hypoglycemia may occur secondary to the lack of cortisol and the reduced caloric intake during the acute illness. Serum should be drawn for determination of an adrenal steroid profile to include cortisol, 17-hydroxyprogesterone, dehydroepiandrosterone, androstenedione, and testosterone. Ideally, blood should be obtained for these tests before the administration of hydrocortisone. In the child in crisis, the diagnosis must be based on physical findings and electrolyte abnormalities, and treatment must be instituted before the definitive adrenal steroid profile is available.

Management

Fluid and Electrolyte Replacement

If the child is dehydrated, fluid replacement is urgent. Volume expansion should be affected by the rapid infusion of 20 mL per kg normal saline in the first hour or more rapidly, if needed. Because the dehydration in salt-losing CAH represents urinary losses of isosmotic fluid, replacement should consist of normal saline (0.9%). The volume to be replaced should constitute the child's daily requirements and the estimated fluid loss. Fluid input and output should be monitored carefully.

Mineralocorticoid Replacement

Principal management of the mineralocorticoid deficit is by the provision of sodium. In addition, hydrocortisone has some mineralocorticoid effect, particularly at high dosages (50 mg per m^2 per day). For long-term management, the child will require mineralocorticoid replacement (fludrocortisone 0.1 mg per day). Most infants also require oral Na$^+$ supplements for the first several months of life.

Glucocorticoid Replacement

Hydrocortisone (25 mg) should be given in an IV bolus, followed by hydrocortisone 50 mg per m^2 per 24 hours as a constant infusion or divided every 6 hours. Alternatively, cortisone acetate 25 mg intramuscularly immediately, followed by 25 mg every 24 hours, may be used. Glucocorticoids can suppress ACTH and the precursor steroids production within a few hours of administration, thus making the diagnosis of an enzymatic deficiency more difficult. However, it is better to avoid the possibility of mortality by giving the steroid than to delay treatment for diagnostic purposes.

Correction of Hyperkalemia, Hypoglycemia, and Acidosis

Infants with CAH tolerate hyperkalemia far better than do other children and adults, with potassium levels as high as 12 mmol per L reported without clinical signs. Volume restoration with normal saline is the major and, usually, the only measure needed to lower the potassium. In the presence of arrhythmias, IV 10% calcium gluconate 1 mL per kg can be given for its membrane-stabilizing properties. Therapy with glucose and insulin is contraindicated because of the danger of precipitating hypoglycemia. If hypoglycemia is found at the time of presentation, it should be treated acutely by the administration of dextrose (0.25 g per kg) intravenously and by the subsequent inclusion of 10% dextrose in the infusate. Acidosis generally does not require specific treatment; however, the low serum bicarbonate may take days to fully correct. Bicarbonate therapy is reserved for patients with both severe acidosis (pH < 6.9) and secondary hemodynamic compromise that is unresponsive to inotropic agents.

Presentation of Known CAH to the ED

In patients with known CAH, or other forms of adrenal insufficiency, the inability to produce an adequate cortisol response to acute illness may only manifest once the acute illness has become severe. In these cases, the contribution of the CAH to the patient's pathology may become unclear to the physician at the bedside and treatment of adrenal insufficiency may be delayed. Emergency glucocorticoid therapy, delivered at the stress dose of hydrocortisone 50 mg per m^2 per day should be administered to any patient with known CAH or other form of adrenal insufficiency in the setting of temperature above 38.5°C, emesis and/or diarrhea, bony fracture of any type, or in the setting of altered mental status or shock. If the patient appears ill, and initial dose of hydrocortisone 50 mg per m^2 may be given either intramuscularly or intravenously, followed by that dose divided in four and given every 6 hours. If the patient is not ill-appearing and is tolerating oral fluids and medications, his/her usual daily dose may be tripled and given in three equal parts daily, or hydrocortisone 50 mg per m^2 per day may be given orally in three equal parts daily if the home dose cannot be readily established.

PHEOCHROMOCYTOMA

Background

Pheochromocytomas are functional tumors that arise in chromaffin tissues. In most children, these tumors are in the adrenal medulla, but they may be found in aberrant tissue along the sympathetic chain. Less than 5% of all pheochromocytomas occur in children. They are twice as common in males as in females, with the incidence of malignancy estimated to be 2% to 4%. Most information on pheochromocytoma is derived from adult studies, especially regarding signs and symptoms. Few detailed studies are available on children.

Pathophysiology

Catecholamines are low-molecular-weight substances produced in the CNS, the sympathetic nerves, the adrenal medulla, and the extraadrenal chromaffin cells. Catecholamines affect metabolic processes in most tissues of the body and have many effects, including accelerated heart rate, increased myocardial contraction, and changes in peripheral vascular resistance. Excessive production of catecholamines by a pheochromocytoma results in intensification of the normal physiologic effects.

Clinical Manifestations

The detection of a pheochromocytoma requires expert clinical awareness. Most patients are symptomatic, but the symptoms are nonspecific and, in the child, are likely to be attributed to other disease entities. The symptoms and signs are related to the excess production of catecholamines and can be explained on the basis of the pharmacologic effects of these substances. The most common symptoms are headache, palpitations, and excessive or inappropriate sweating. The headache, characteristically, is pounding and may be severe. The palpitations may be accompanied by tachycardia. Almost all patients will have one of the three symptoms listed, and most will have at least two. Other symptoms may include nervousness, tremor, fatigue, chest or abdominal pains, and flushing.

The most useful screening tool for pheochromocytoma is the blood pressure cuff because most pheochromocytomas are associated with hypertension.

Because this hypertension may be continuous or paroxysmal, frequent and repeated blood pressure determinations may be necessary. Hypertension is most likely to be found when the patient is symptomatic. A hypertensive patient who is asymptomatic is unlikely to have a pheochromocytoma. Paroxysmal symptoms and hypertension should lead to consideration of this diagnosis.

The diagnosis of a pheochromocytoma should also be considered in patients with malignant hypertension, in those who fail to respond or respond inappropriately to antihypertensive medications, and in those who develop hypertension during the induction of anesthesia or during surgery. Incidence of pheochromocytomas is increased among patients with neurofi-bromatosis and with the multiple endocrine neoplasia syndrome types II and III. Documentation of excess catecholamine in either the urine or serum confirms the diagnosis of pheochromocytoma. The most readily available and widely used test for this purpose remains the measurement of urinary catecholamines or their metabolites (3-methoxy-4-hydroxymandelic acid and total metanephrines) in a 24-hour urine collection accompanied by a patient symptom log. The finding of significant elevations of these substances is adequate confirmatory data. Some false-negative results may occur using urinary catecholamines. When the degree of suspicion is high, repeated specimens may be needed. Plasma metanephrine concentration has now been shown to be a superior screening and confirmatory test, however, and ought to be employed where available.

Once the diagnosis is confirmed, anatomic localization is necessary using either computed tomography or nuclear magnetic resonance imaging. Occasionally, arteriography with selective sampling for epinephrine production is necessary for localization.

Management

Pheochromocytoma is cured by the surgical removal of the tumor. The focus of ED management should be on controlling hypertension and hypertensive crisis that may occur before the surgical procedure. α-Adrenergic blocking agents are useful in controlling hypertension and in minimizing blood pressure fluctuations during the surgical procedure.

Preferred drugs for controlling hypertension are phenoxybenzamine (Dibenzyline®) and prazosin (Minipress®). Dosage schedules and quantity must be tailored to the individual for adequate control of hypertension. Hypertensive crisis may be appropriately managed with IV phentolamine (Regitine® 1 mg IV for children; 5 mg IV for adolescents) or sodium nitroprusside (0.5 to 8.0 μg per kg per minute). Beta blockade must be avoided because it may lead to unopposed alpha action on the part of secreted catecholamines and resultant severe hypertension.

DIABETES INSIPIDUS

Background

DI is caused by an inability of the kidneys to concentrate urine and is characterized clinically by polyuria and polydipsia. Either a deficiency of ADH secretion from the hypothalamus and posterior pituitary gland or renal unresponsiveness to ADH can cause this disease (Table 86.7). Most central causes of DI in children are acquired and can present at any age. In contrast, the most common cause of nephrogenic DI in children is X-linked recessive and manifests in males during early infancy. Renal lesions associated with nephrogenic DI can present in later childhood.

Pathophysiology

ADH is synthesized in the supraoptic and paraventricular nuclei of the hypothalamus. It is transported along nerve axons to the posterior pituitary gland, where it is stored. ADH

TABLE 86.7

CAUSES OF DIABETES INSIPIDUS IN CHILDREN

Antidiuretic Hormone Deficiency
Head injury
Meningitis
Idiopathic
Suprasellar tumors and their treatment by surgery and/or
    radiotherapy
    Craniopharyngioma
    Optic nerve glioma
    Dysgerminoma
Septooptic dysplasia
Association with midline cleft palate
Familial (dominant or sex-linked recessive)
Wolfram syndrome (diabetes insipidus, diabetes mellitus,
    optic atrophy, deafness)
Histiocytosis X (Hand-Schuller-Christian disease)

Nephrogenic Diabetes Insipidus
Sex-linked recessive
Renal disease
Polycystic kidneys
Hydronephrosis
Chronic pyelonephritis
Hypercalcemia
Hypokalemia
Toxins:
    Demeclocycline
    Lithium
Sickle cell disease
Idiopathic

is released in response to increased plasma osmolality, hypernatremia, and decreased right atrial pressure secondary to hypovolemia. The distal convoluted tubules and the collecting ducts of the kidneys respond to ADH by inserting a water channel (aquaporin) into the luminal membrane of the collecting duct and allowing water reabsorption along the medullary concentration gradient. Lack of ADH (central DI) can result from a wide variety of hypothalamic and pituitary lesions (Table 86.7). Conversely, in nephrogenic DI, ADH levels are normal or elevated because the defect resides in the renal collecting tubules, which are resistant to the action of ADH. In either case, failure of water reabsorption results in polyuria. A normal thirst mechanism contributes toward fluid balance by promoting adequate fluid intake; however, if this balance is not achieved, hypertonic dehydration ensues. If a hyperosmolar state develops abruptly, it may lead to dehydration of neural tissues, which can cause serious neurologic sequelae or result in death. The pons is particularly sensitive to this effect resulting in central pontine myelinolysis.

Clinical Manifestations

Urine excretion is increased in both volume and frequency in the child with DI. This condition may manifest as enuresis in the younger child. Provided the thirst mechanism is intact and fluids are accessible, the child can compensate for the water loss by drinking more. A history may be elicited of the child's awakening in the middle of the night to drink. If fluids are not

available or if fluid intake is interrupted because of an illness, dehydration rapidly ensues. In the young infant who is not provided with adequate fluids and consequently is chronically dehydrated, the child may fail to thrive or may have a history of intermittent low-grade fevers due to intermittent hypernatremia. However, if the cries of the infant are interpreted as hunger rather than thirst, the infant with DI may be obese.

Physical examination may be normal, or signs of dehydration, such as dryness of mucous membranes, decreased skin turgor, sunken eyes, and in an infant, a depressed anterior fontanel, may be present. Because of the hyperosmolarity, the degree of dehydration may be underestimated on physical examination. Hypothalamic or pituitary lesions can lead to other endocrine abnormalities such as secondary hypothyroidism and growth failure. A craniopharyngioma or optic nerve glioma may affect the visual fields or cause raised intracranial pressure, which is indicated by papilledema.

DI is diagnosed by demonstrating that the kidneys fail to concentrate urine when fluid intake is restricted. This condition can be difficult to prove in children. Criteria for the diagnosis of DI may be met by finding an elevated serum osmolality (greater than 300 mOsm per L) and an elevated serum [Na$^+$] (greater than 145 mmol per L) in the presence of dilute urine (osmolality less than 600 mOsm per L). Blood glucose and serum creatinine levels are normal.

In many cases, the diagnosis can be ruled out by the demonstration of appropriately concentrated urine and normal serum osmolality on specimens obtained upon awakening. The definitive diagnosis is made by a formal water deprivation test. This test is performed electively in cases in which the diagnosis is uncertain and should never be performed if the child is already dehydrated. The measurement of ADH by radioimmunoassay is available but generally is not useful in the diagnosis of DI.

Management

In most cases, a diagnosis of DI is not known at the time of presentation; therefore, the acute management is directed toward correction of the dehydration and the hyperosmolar state. The treatment of DI is similar to that described for hypernatremic dehydration (see Chapter 17), with the notable addition that the fluid required for the replacement of urinary fluid losses will be far greater. In fact, the high urinary output, despite significant dehydration, often provides the first and most convincing evidence for DI. If the child is hypotensive or if the serum [Na$^+$] is greater than 160 mmol per L, initial volume expansion is necessary, using 20 mL per kg normal saline during the first hour or more rapidly, if needed. Once an adequate intravascular volume has been achieved, further fluid replacement is accomplished slowly because overly rapid volume correction can cause cerebral edema, seizures, and death.

If the child is not hypotensive, or once the hypotension has been corrected, free water replacement is done over 48 hours. Calculations of appropriate fluids must include maintenance requirements, replacement needs, and ongoing urinary losses (see Chapter 17).

If DI is strongly suspected on the basis of discrepant serum and urine osmolality, DDAVP (10 μg intranasally or 0.2 to 0.4 μg per kg subcutaneously) may be a useful adjunct to IV fluid therapy. If DDAVP is not available or cannot be used for some reason, other antidiuretic agents are available. Aqueous pitressin may be administered as a continuous IV infusion starting at 1 mUnit per kg per hour and slowly (every 5 to 10 minutes) increasing the rate (maximum 10 mUnit per kg per hour) to decrease urine output to less than 2 mL per kg per hour.

DDAVP and pitressin act rapidly to promote tubular resorption of free H_2O; clinically, this response is apparent as decreased urinary output with increased osmolality within 15 minutes of administration. Once the patient has responded, however, extreme care must be used in subsequent fluid management because the patient can no longer excrete excess water. Therefore, baseline IV fluid administration must be maintained at 1 L per m^2 of body surface area per day (or roughly two-thirds maintenance fluids) using a low sodium infusate, such as 5% dextrose with one-fourth normal saline (0.23%), in addition to the fluid designed to replete the initial estimated free water deficit over 48 hours.

Failure to respond to either form of ADH suggests the possibility of tubular unresponsiveness to ADH (nephrogenic DI); however, more commonly, failure to respond results from improper administration of the medication or use of DDAVP that has lost its potency. Because of these factors, if cessation of diuresis is not noted within 2 hours of administration of the first dose, a second dose from a different bottle of DDAVP should be tried. The use of an ADH agonist generally simplifies management by reducing the quantity of fluid that must be infused; however, careful monitoring of input and output remains essential. Children who fail to respond to DDAVP are likely to have nephrogenic DI and must be acutely managed with fluid therapy alone. Hypercalcemia and renal failure are the most common causes of nephrogenic DI. Paradoxically, the thiazide diuretics have proven to be useful in the chronic control of nephrogenic DI.

The child should be closely observed for changes in level of consciousness, pulse rate, and blood pressure. Fluid input and output should be meticulously monitored. Serum osmolality and [Na^+] should be determined every 1 to 2 hours until the rate of their decline can be determined. Urine osmolality should be measured every 1 to 2 hours to determine the responsiveness of the renal tubule to DDAVP. Because large volumes of dextrose-containing fluids are used, the blood glucose should also be followed closely. If the blood glucose exceeds 160 mg per dL, the concentration of dextrose in the infusate should be decreased.

SYNDROME OF INAPPROPRIATE ANTIDIURETIC HORMONE SECRETION

Background

Excessive secretion of ADH accompanying normal or low plasma osmolality or [Na^+] is inappropriate because it further depresses the plasma osmolality and [Na^+]. Symptoms of excessive ADH secretion are not usually apparent until the plasma [Na^+] falls to less than about 125 mmol per L. The overall incidence of the syndrome of inappropriate ADH secretion (SIADH) in childhood is unknown, but it is common

in certain disease states. More than 50% of children with bacterial meningitis, about 20% of patients on positive-pressure ventilation, and about 70% of children with Rocky Mountain spotted fever develop some degree of SIADH.

Pathophysiology

ADH secretion is stimulated by hypertonicity of the fluid surrounding the hypothalamic osmoreceptors, volume receptors in the left atrium, and ill-defined nervous impulses from higher cortical centers. Disorders of the CNS (Table 86.8) may cause excessive ADH secretion by producing either a local disturbance of the hypothalamic osmoreceptors or some undetermined nervous stimuli. Many intrathoracic conditions are associated with SIADH, probably due to the vestigial ability of the lung to produce ADH. Physical and emotional stress, severe pain, and nausea are also potent stimuli of ADH secretion. Excessive secretion of ADH leads to water retention by the collecting tubules of the kidneys, a mechanism mediated by insertion of water channels into the luminal membrane of the collecting duct and allowing water reabsorption along the medullary concentration gradient. The retained water expands the intravascular compartment, dilutes all plasma constituents, and lowers the plasma osmolality.

TABLE 86.8

SOME CAUSES OF SYNDROME OF INAPPROPRIATE ANTIDIURETIC HORMONE SECRETION IN CHILDREN

Disorders of Central Nervous System
Infection (meningitis, encephalitis)
Trauma, postneurosurgery
Hypoxic insults, especially in the perinatal period
Brain tumor
Intraventricular hemorrhage
Guillain-Barré syndrome
Psychosis

Intrathoracic Disorders
Infection (tuberculosis, pneumonia, empyema)
Positive-pressure ventilation
Asthma
Cystic fibrosis
Pneumothorax
Patent ductus arteriosus ligation

Miscellaneous
Pain (e.g., after abdominal surgery)
Nausea
Severe hypothyroidism
Tumors (e.g., neuroblastoma)

Drug Induced
Increased antidiuretic hormone secretion
  Vincristine
  Cyclophosphamide
  Carbamazepine
  Adenine arabinoside
  Phenothiazines
  Morphine
Potentiation of antidiuretic hormone effect
  Acetaminophen
  Indomethacin

TABLE 86.9

CRITERIA FOR DIAGNOSIS OF SYNDROME
OF INAPPROPRIATE ANTIDIURETIC
HORMONE SECRETION

Hyponatremia, reduced serum osmolality
Urine osmolality inappropriately elevated (a urine osmolality
<100 mOsm/kg usually excludes the diagnosis)
Urinary Na$^+$ concentration that is excessive in comparison to
the degree of hyponatremia (usually >18 mmol/L)
Normal renal, adrenal, and thyroid function
Absence of volume depletion (euvolemic to hypervolemic
state)

Clinical Manifestations

Most patients with SIADH are asymptomatic until the plasma [Na$^+$] falls to less than 125 mmol per L. Symptoms associated with hyponatremia range from anorexia, headache, nausea, vomiting, irritability, disorientation, and weakness to seizures and coma, leading ultimately to death. Absence of edema and dehydration are significant clinical findings.

Laboratory investigations for diagnostic purposes must include concomitant serum and urine samples (Table 86.9). Hyponatremia, hypoosmolality (serum), and low blood urea nitrogen will be present. In contrast, the urinary osmolality and [Na$^+$] are inappropriately elevated for the hypotonicity of the serum. Due to the euvolemic or hypervolemic state, aldosterone is suppressed and urine potassium will be low. Radioimmunoassay for ADH is now available and has been helpful in defining this syndrome; however, the results of this test are unlikely to be available on an emergency basis. The underlying cause of the syndrome should be investigated according to the physician's clinical judgment. Hyperlipidemia may falsely lower laboratory measurement of [Na$^+$], leading to a factitious hyponatremia. Hyperglycemia and hypoproteinemia, however, lead to true hyponatremia. Renal salt wasting, secondary to adrenal insufficiency, should be accompanied by hyperkalemia and dehydration. Cerebral salt wasting may have laboratory parameters similar to SIADH but is characterized by hypovolemia and a high urine output as long as renal perfusion remains intact. The urine osmolality in water intoxication states is usually low compared with that found in SIADH.

Management

Severely Symptomatic Children

Patients with a persistent seizure attributable to severe hyponatremia and those who are severely lethargic or comatose need urgent treatment. Hypertonic (3%) saline is the preferred treatment. Infusing small amounts of 3% saline in the range of 3 mL per kg every 10 to 20 minutes until symptoms remit is likely the safest course of treatment. One milliliter per kilogram of 3% saline should raise the serum [Na$^+$] by approximately 1 mmol per L. A single dose of furosemide (1 mg per kg) also can be administered intravenously. Close monitoring of fluid balance, plasma and urinary sodium, potassium, and osmolality is essential. Seizures should be treated concomitantly with a standard emergency anticonvulsant protocol (see Chapters 69 and 96). Of note, phenytoin (Dilantin®) or fosphenytoin (Cerebryx®) intravenously (5 to 10 mg per kg) inhibits ADH release and may be helpful in the patient with seizures secondary to CNS causes of SIADH. The underlying cause of SIADH, such as meningitis or pneumonia, should be treated when possible; successful treatment is usually accompanied by remission of inappropriate antidiuresis.

Asymptomatic or Mildly Symptomatic Children

Asymptomatic or mildly symptomatic patients are treated by rigorous fluid restriction. If the patient is not vascularly compromised, fluid input should be sharply limited, often below insensible loss, until the [Na$^+$] and osmolality begin to rise. If the initial [Na$^+$] is less than 125 mmol per L, all fluids must be withheld. Frequent measurements of plasma electrolytes and osmolality, as well as close monitoring of fluid input and output, are essential. As the serum [Na$^+$] rises and urine osmolality falls, the rate of fluid administration can be gradually increased. The child with chronic or recurrent episodes of SIADH may require treatment with demeclocycline 10 mg per kg. The underlying cause should be identified, treated, and eliminated, if possible.

HYPERPARATHYROIDISM

Background

Hyperparathyroidism is most commonly recognized during the third, fourth, and fifth decades of life. It is uncommon in children.

Pathophysiology

The parathyroid glands are derived from the third and fourth pharyngeal pouch and are usually embedded in the posterior aspect of the thyroid gland. Occasionally, a gland may be found in the anterior mediastinum. Parathyroid hormone (PTH) is the primary hormone produced by the parathyroid glands. PTH is synthesized and released constitutively; its secretion is stimulated by low and suppressed by high serum ionized calcium concentration. Prolonged hypocalcemia, most commonly in the setting of renal failure, may lead to hypertrophy of the parathyroid glands and secondary hyperparathyroidism. PTH acts on the kidney to decrease the excretion of calcium, magnesium, and hydrogen, while increasing the excretion of phosphate, sodium, and bicarbonate. Many of the effects are mediated by cyclic adenosine monophosphate (cAMP), and an increased quantity of cAMP is present in the urine of patients with hyperparathyroidism. PTH also increases the formation of 1,25-dihydroxyvitamin D in the kidneys. PTH may increase intestinal absorption of calcium, although this effect is primarily mediated by 1,25-(OH)$_2$D. Both PTH and 1,25-(OH)$_2$D affect bone. PTH acts on bone to increase the release of calcium by increasing the number and activity of the osteoclasts, whereas vitamin D decreases calcium use in bone formation by decreasing the number of osteoblasts. The net effect of the actions of PTH and vitamin D is to increase serum calcium by decreasing renal calcium excretion, decreasing new bone formation, increasing bone resorption, and increasing intestinal absorption of calcium.

Clinical Manifestations

Hyperparathyroidism has two common presentations in children. The first presentation is the critically ill infant who is found to have severe hypercalcemia during the course of diagnostic investigations. The serum calcium level may be extremely high. The second presentation is a child in the early to midteens with nonspecific symptoms including nausea, constipation, unexplained weight loss, personality changes, and headaches. Diffuse bone pain or renal colic may be reported, although these symptoms are less common in children than in adults.

The physical findings of hypercalcemia are hypotonia, weakness, listlessness, anorexia, constipation, and vomiting, and in the neonate, respiratory distress and apnea. There may be hypertension, shortened QTc interval on EKG, polyuria (due to renal unresponsiveness to ADH), and rarely, encephalopathy with seizures. A palpable mass may occasionally be located in the parathyroid region. Certain characteristic features have been associated with idiopathic hypercalcemia in infancy, including hypertelorism, broad forehead, epicanthal folds, prominent upper lip, an underdeveloped nasal bridge, and a small mandible. Not surprisingly, these same features have been noted in infants with hyperparathyroidism.

A family history may be helpful because hyperparathyroidism has been associated with both multiple endocrine neoplasia types I and II, which are inherited as autosomal-dominant conditions. Hyperparathyroidism may also occur in infants of hypoparathyroid mothers. Radiologic findings consistent with hyperparathyroidism include evidence of demineralization and bone resorption (Figs. 86.2 and 86.3). Osteitis fibrosa cystica,

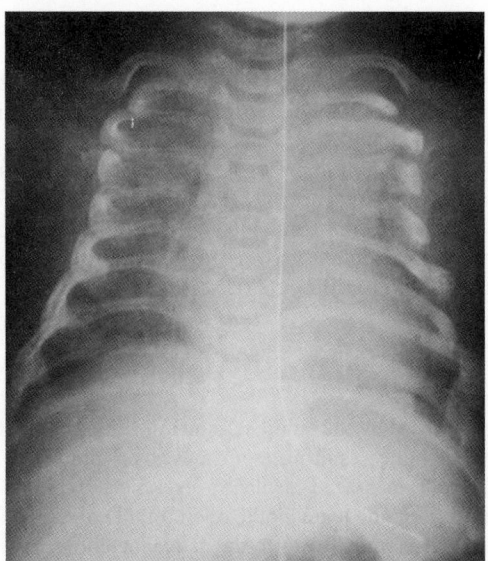

FIGURE 86.2 Primary hyperparathyroidism in a 3-day-old girl. Roentgenogram of the chest shows profound demineralization of the skeleton with loss of a well-defined cortical margin. Cystic changes in rib and subperiosteal bone resorption in humerus are seen. (Courtesy of Soroosh Mahboubi, MD, The Children's Hospital of Philadelphia.)

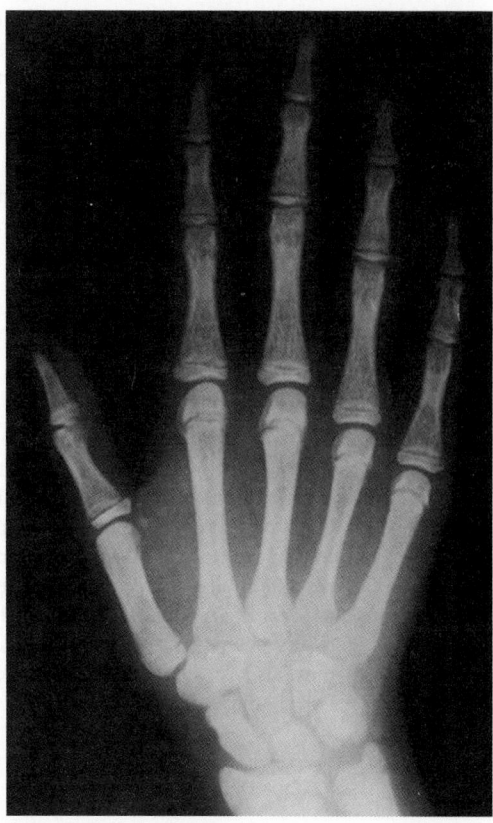

FIGURE 86.3 Secondary hyperparathyroidism in a 12-year-old girl with chronic pyelonephritis. There is moderate subperiosteal erosion on the radial side of the middle phalanges; note a lacy appearance of the periosteum and small-tuft erosion. Subperiosteal bone resorption is the most significant radiologic finding in hyperparathyroidism; subperiosteal bone resorption and tuft erosion are seen in both primary and secondary hyperparathyroidism. (Courtesy of Soroosh Mahboubi, MD, The Children's Hospital of Philadelphia.)

although highly suggestive of the diagnosis, is unusual in children.

The clinical laboratory is helpful in the recognition of hyperparathyroidism. Hypercalcemia is usually present but may be subtle or intermittent in mild cases. The serum inorganic phosphate level is usually low but may be normal, especially in patients with decreased renal function. Mild hyperchloremic acidosis may be present. Alkaline phosphatase level and urinary hydroxyproline excretion may be elevated secondary to increased osteoclast activity. Because PTH causes a significant increase in cAMP in the kidney tubule, the presence of excess cAMP in the urine is strongly suggestive of excess PTH production. The determination of PTH levels is critical for diagnostic purposes, and elevated levels of PTH, when the patient is hypercalcemic, are a definitive laboratory finding.

Management

Acute management of hyperparathyroidism is essentially the same as management of hypercalcemia (see Chapter 100). The specific management of hyperparathyroidism depends on the level of calcium and on the presence of signs and symptoms. In the asymptomatic patient with serum calcium of less than 12 mg per dL, careful follow-up with close attention to both bone mass and renal function is recommended. If the child is persistently hypercalcemic, parathyroid surgery is the preferred treatment. In the case of hyperplasia, the common reason for hyperparathyroidism in the infant, subtotal parathyroidectomy is indicated. If an adenoma is present, as is usually the case in the older child, simple removal of the involved parathyroid gland is adequate.

HYPOPARATHYROIDISM

Background

Hypoparathyroidism is rare in children. It may occur sporadically or be part of a familial syndrome consisting of combinations of several autoimmune diseases (e.g., Addison's disease, diabetes mellitus, lymphocytic thyroiditis, pernicious anemia, ovarian failure). Hypoparathyroidism is also associated with thymic aplasia and severe immunologic deficiencies (DiGeorge's syndrome). A transient form of hypoparathyroidism, lasting for as long as 1 year, has been reported in some infants. Hypoparathyroidism may also result from damage incurred during thyroid surgery or irradiation.

Pathophysiology

The basic actions of PTH are described in the preceding section on hyperparathyroidism. The lack of PTH, regardless of cause, has several deleterious effects on calcium homeostasis. Because PTH has significant effects on $1,25\text{-}(OH)_2D_3$ formation, the absence of PTH is magnified by a consequent reduction in $1,25\text{-}(OH)_2D_3$. The net effect of the lack of PTH (and decreased quantity of vitamin D) is a declining serum level of calcium, primarily caused by decreased intestinal absorption of calcium and decreased renal resorption of calcium.

Clinical Manifestations

The predominant historical features and clinical manifestations of hypoparathyroidism are the same as those of hypocalcemia (see Chapter 100). Unique historical information that may suggest the diagnosis of hypoparathyroidism includes other family members with autoimmune endocrine disease, recurrent episodes of serious infection in the affected child, and previous thyroid manipulations.

Most symptoms and signs of hypoparathyroidism are the same as those related to hypocalcemia. The particular symptoms and signs found depend on the age at disease onset, the chronicity of the disease, and the presence of other autoimmune or syndromic phenomena. Papilledema without hemorrhage may be seen during the initial examination and tends to resolve within several days after the initiation of therapy. Lenticular cataracts are common in hypoparathyroidism and are associated with long-standing hypocalcemia of any cause. Psychiatric and neurologic disorders occur in association with hypoparathyroidism. Subnormal intelligence occurs in about 20% of children with the idiopathic form of hypoparathyroidism, and the severity correlates closely with the period of

untreated hypocalcemia. Dry, scaly skin is a common finding, as is patchy alopecia. Psoriasis or mucocutaneous candidiasis may be found on occasion. Unusually brittle fingernails and hair are often found. Hypoplasia of tooth enamel may be seen if hypoparathyroidism was present at the time of dental development. Intestinal malabsorption and steatorrhea have been reported in association with hypoparathyroidism.

In most cases, the diagnosis of hypoparathyroidism is first considered when low serum calcium is found. If an elevated phosphate accompanies low calcium, low or normal serum alkaline phosphate, and normal blood urea nitrogen, hypoparathyroidism is a likely possibility. Finding a low or nonmeasurable level of PTH in the presence of hypocalcemia and hyperphosphatemia makes the definitive diagnosis. Because PTH increases cAMP levels in the urine, the excreted amount of cAMP in the urine is low in patients with hypoparathyroidism and rises briskly with the administration of exogenous PTH. The presence of antibodies in other endocrine tissues or organs may help in delineating the cause of the hypoparathyroidism.

Management

The acute management of hypoparathyroidism is essentially the management of the hypocalcemia (see Chapter 100). Long-term management consists of treatment with vitamin D, usually with one of its more active analogs—$1,25\text{-}(OH)_2D_3$ at 0.01 to 0.05 μg per kg per day. Supplemental oral calcium is almost always necessary. The goals of long-term therapy are to maintain the serum calcium in the lower range of normal and to avoid both vitamin D toxicity and hypercalcemia. Preparations of PTH are not available for the long-term management of hypoparathyroidism.

RICKETS

Background

Rickets describes a characteristic set of clinical features delineated centuries ago, which is now known to be predominantly caused by inadequate dietary vitamin D. With this awareness and the advent of vitamin D supplementation of foods, especially milk, the incidence of rickets has fallen significantly; however, rickets is still seen among certain ethnic groups, premature infants, children with severe malabsorption problems, and patients with serious renal disease.

Pathophysiology

Rickets is caused by the failure of mineralization of bone matrix in growing bone resulting from a lack of vitamin D. Consequently, unmineralized cartilage is excessive, and bone is soft. In addition to inadequate intake of vitamin D, the other causes of rickets are inability to form the active metabolite of vitamin D, excess phosphate excretion, and excess accumulation of acid.

Vitamin D may be obtained from dietary sources (especially animal fat) or synthesized from cholesterol via a complex pathway requiring the interaction of the precursor molecule with sunlight. Further hydroxylation of vitamin D in the liver

(25-hydroxylation) and kidney (1-alpha-hydroxylation) leads to the formation of the active metabolite 1,25-dihydroxyvitamin D. Therefore, failure to form 1,25-$(OH)_2D_3$ may result from inadequate intake of vitamin D or insufficient exposure to sunlight. This is a particular problem among ethnic groups that eat small quantities of animal meat and that are extensively clothed when outdoors. Because vitamin D is fat soluble, any problem leading to prolonged fat malabsorption can result in rickets. Diseases affecting kidney or liver function may also lead to inadequate production of 1,25-$(OH)_2D_3$. An inherited deficiency of the 1-alpha-hydroxylase in the kidney (vitamin D–dependency rickets) is known. Certain drugs, such as phenobarbital and phenytoin, affect liver metabolism of vitamin D and can lead to rickets. Premature infants are particularly prone to vitamin D deficiency because of their minimal stores of vitamin D and their limited capacity for vitamin D synthesis.

Phosphate is a critical component of bone formation. Excess excretion of phosphate may lead to clinical rickets. Conditions that lead to excess phosphate excretion include primary hyperphosphaturia, Lowe's syndrome, and Fanconi's syndrome. Vitamin D–resistant rickets is a misnomer because the primary defect is in the renal tubular resorption of phosphate and not a resistance to vitamin D. Both an X-linked recessive and an autosomal-dominant form of phosphate wasting are known.

Rickets may also occur in conditions leading to chronic acidosis because bone is resorbed to buffer the acid load. This condition is seen in patients with distal renal tubular acidosis and may be partially responsible for the rachitic changes associated with Fanconi's syndrome.

Clinical Manifestations

Children with rickets may come to medical attention because of specific physical abnormalities (bowed legs), limb pain and swelling, seizures, failure to thrive (renal tubular acidosis), biochemical abnormalities (hypocalcemia), or radiographic findings (broadened, frayed metaphysis). A thorough social and dietary history is helpful in delineating the probable cause and in sparing the patient an extensive and expensive evaluation. A family history may be useful in identifying the 1-hydroxylase deficiency or renal phosphate wasting. If the child has previously been treated with vitamin D, the reported response to that treatment may be helpful in identifying the likely site of defect.

The clinical findings in rickets may vary considerably, depending on the underlying disorder, the duration of the problem, and the child's age. Most features are related to skeletal deformity, skeletal pain, slippage of epiphyses, bony fractures, and growth disturbances. Muscular weakness, hypotonia, and lethargy are often noted. Failure of calcification affects those parts of the skeleton that are growing most rapidly or that are under stress. For example, the skull grows rapidly in the perinatal period; therefore, craniotabes is a manifestation of congenital rickets. However, the upper limbs and rib cage grow rapidly during the first year of life, and abnormalities at these sites are more common at this age (i.e., rachitic rosary, flaring of the wrist). Bowing of the legs is unlikely to be noted until the child is ambulatory. Dental eruption may be delayed, and enamel defects are common.

Radiography is the optimal way to confirm the clinical diagnosis because the radiologic features reflect the histopathology. Characteristic findings include widening and irregularity of the epiphyseal plates, cupped metaphyses, fractures, and bowing of the weight-bearing limbs (Figs. 86.4 and 86.5). The clinical laboratory is often helpful in correctly identifying the cause of rickets. Frank hypocalcemia (less than 7 mg per dL) is unusual in rickets. Calcium levels in the 7 to 9 mg per dL range are common and warrant careful attention because the initiation of vitamin D treatment increases bony deposition of calcium and may lead to a fall in serum calcium. Phosphate levels are often low. An amino aciduria is often present and may lead to some confusion of simple vitamin D deficiency with Fanconi's syndrome. Alkaline phosphatase levels are significantly increased, reflecting extremely active bony metabolism. Although PTH levels are elevated, the results of this test are unlikely to be available at the time initial clinical decisions are made. Chronic acidosis, liver disease, and renal disease should be ruled out.

Treatment

Treatment depends on the nature of the underlying disease. The response to treatment may be helpful in differentiating simple dietary vitamin D deficiency from more complex causes of rickets. In the absence of chronic disease, dietary rickets may be adequately treated with daily doses of 1,200 to 1,600 IU of vitamin D (ergocalciferol) until healing occurs. Alternatively, a single high IM dose to replenish stores may be administered as ergocalciferol 50,000 to 100,000 IU. Serum phosphate usually returns to normal within 1 to 2 weeks, and radiographic improvement is generally apparent by 2 weeks. Once healing is complete, the child should continue to be treated with 400 IU per day to prevent recurrence. If the initial serum calcium is borderline low or low, supplemental calcium should be initiated 48 hours before the institution of vitamin D, especially in the young child. Otherwise, the institution of vitamin D may cause a further decrease in serum calcium and elicit frank hypocalcemia. This presentation may occur naturally if the vitamin D–deficient patient has relatively low serum calcium concentration and then has prolonged exposure to the sun. This may lead to abrupt increases in vitamin D, ultimately leading to a rapid increase in bone recalcification (hungry bone syndrome) and severe hypocalcemia with possible seizures. This syndrome is seasonally termed "spring fits." Children with symptomatic hypocalcemia or with initial serum calcium of less than 7 mg per dL on presentation warrant hospitalization and frequent calcium determinations. Failure to respond to vitamin D treatment suggests that the child has a more complex cause of rickets, and consultation with a pediatric nephrologist or endocrinologist is recommended.

THYROID STORM

Background

Thyroid storm, or thyrotoxic crisis, is a fulminating intensification of the hyperthyroid state. Because hyperthyroidism uncommonly occurs in children and because thyroid storm occurs in only 1% of patients with hyperthyroidism, thyroid

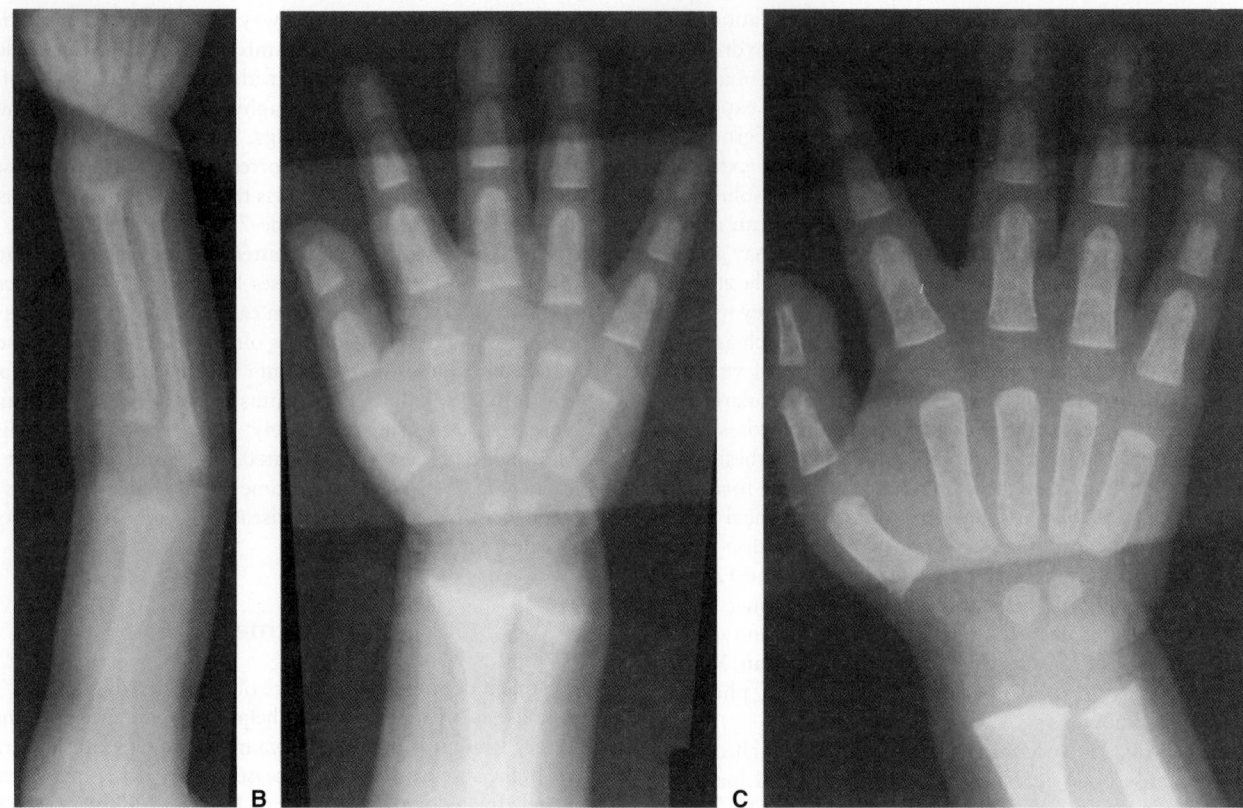

FIGURE 86.4 **A:** Rickets in an 11-month-old boy, breast-fed since birth. Roentgenogram of the upper extremity shows profound demineralization of the skeleton, with frayed, irregular cupping of the end of the metaphysis and poorly defined cortex. Note retardation of skeletal maturation. **B:** Same patient with some healing 4 weeks after supplemental vitamin D. Severe rachitic changes are noticeable. Periosteal cloaking, both of the metacarpals and of the radius and ulna, is evidence of healing. **C:** Complete healing of the rickets 8 months after treatment. Note the reappearance of the provisional zone of calcification. (Courtesy of Soroosh Mahboubi, MD, The Children's Hospital of Philadelphia.)

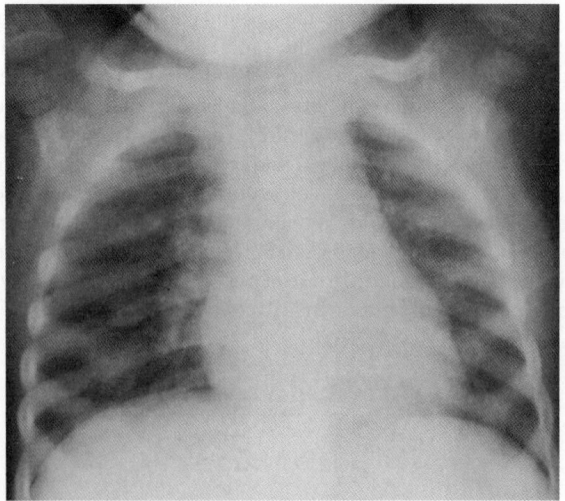

FIGURE 86.5 Rickets in an 11-month-old boy, breast-fed since birth. Roentgenogram of the chest shows demineralization of the skeleton with cupping of the distal end of ribs and humerus. (Courtesy of Soroosh Mahboubi, MD, The Children's Hospital of Philadelphia.)

storm is rare in children. Therefore, most information available on thyrotoxic crisis is derived from reports of this condition in adults. Precipitating factors include intercurrent infection, trauma, and subtotal thyroidectomy in an inadequately prepared patient. The mortality rate in adults may be as high as 20%; similar data are not available for children.

Pathophysiology

In thyroid storm, thyroid hormone is suddenly released into the circulation, which results in the uncoupling of oxidative phosphorylation and/or increased lipolysis, both of which contribute to excessive thermogenesis. Insensible fluid loss increases as a result of increased metabolism and sweating. Tachycardia is caused by both the hyperthermia and the direct action of thyroid hormones on the cardiac conduction system.

Clinical Manifestations

Almost all cases of thyroid storm occur in patients with known hyperthyroidism, although occasionally, a patient will present initially with thyroid storm. Most patients will have clinical findings characteristic of hyperthyroidism, including goiter (more than 95%), exophthalmos, tachycardia, bounding pulses, and systolic hypertension. Diastolic hypotension, tremulousness, restlessness, mania, delirium, or frankly psychotic behavior may be present. A primary feature that distinguishes thyroid storm from uncomplicated hyperthyroidism is the presence of high fever, often as high as 41°C (105.8°F). The marked increase in cardiac workload may result in high-output cardiac failure, in which case hypotension and pulmonary edema may be seen, rather than more classic hypertension.

Thyroid studies including serum-free thyroxine (T_4), free triiodothyronine (T_3), T_3 resin uptake, and TSH should be obtained. Many clinical laboratories can now perform free T_4 assays on an emergency basis, alternatively total T_4 or total T_3 are adequate indices; however, in many cases, therapy must be initiated on the basis of clinical evidence. Furthermore, the T_4 and T_3 values seen in thyroid storm overlap with those found in frank hyperthyroidism without storm. Serum electrolytes should be obtained but are unlikely to reveal any characteristic abnormalities, except for evidence of modest dehydration. A chest radiograph and EKG are helpful in evaluating and following cardiac status as treatment is initiated.

Management

Initial treatment is directed toward lowering the metabolic rate and reducing the cardiac workload. Subsequent treatment is directed toward controlling thyroid hormone production. Because many of the hypermetabolic effects of hyperthyroidism are mediated by the adrenergic system, a β-adrenergic antagonist (propranolol starting at 10 μg per kg intravenously over 10 to 15 minutes; or an esmolol infusion may be initiated with a loading doses of 500 μg per kg per minute over 1 minute with maximal infusion doses of 50 to 250 μg per kg per minute) is useful in the acute management of thyroid storm. Maintenance dosing of propranolol is 2 mg per kg per day divided every 6 hours in neonates and 10 to 40 mg every 6 hours in older children. EKG monitoring for heart rate and arrhythmias is recommended. Because the metabolic rate is increased about 10% for every degree of body temperature higher than 36.5°C (86.7°F), lowering body temperature is an effective means of reducing the metabolic rate in the patient with thyrotoxicosis. Tepid sponging, use of a cooling blanket, and administration of acetaminophen can accomplish this task. Aspirin should not be used because it is a potential uncoupler of oxidative phosphorylation that may exacerbate the hypermetabolic state.

Treatment of the hyperthyroidism in thyroid storm is accomplished by the use of iodide and an inhibitor of iodine oxidation in the thyroid gland such as methimazole 0.5 to 0.7 mg per kg per day divided into three oral doses, which blocks iodine's ability to combine with tyrosine to form thyroxine and triiodothyronine (T_3); of note neither medication inactivates circulating T_4 and T_3. Propylthiouracil was a first line agent, but due to its association with pediatric liver failure has now become contraindicated in children. Iodide rapidly terminates thyroid hormone release; however, this effect is overcome after 3 to 5 days of iodide therapy. Iodide also decreases

the vascularity of the thyroidal arterial supply and can be particularly useful as preoperative agent. Lugol's iodide (or SSKI) 3 to 5 drops once every 8 hours orally or sodium iodide 125 to 250 mg per day intravenously over 24 hours is the usual mode of iodide therapy. While iodide can reduce thyroid hormone secretion within 24 hours, methimazole's effects are minimally useful in acute management because the reduction in thyroid levels may take several days.

Adequate hydration is essential for effective treatment, and the estimate of fluid replacement should include a consideration of the significant increase in fluid requirements caused by fever and an accelerated metabolic rate. Glucocorticoids are useful in the acute presentation because they appear to inhibit thyroid hormone release from the thyroid and decrease the peripheral conversion of T_4 to T_3. Dexamethasone (0.2 mg per kg) or hydrocortisone (5 mg per kg) can be given parenterally during the acute phase. Because intercurrent infection may be the precipitating factor, it should be searched for and treated appropriately. Broad-spectrum antibiotics should be considered while awaiting the results of cultures, as there is a known association between thyrotoxicosis and pneumococcal bacteremia.

Improvement should be seen within a few hours after the initiation of treatment with propranolol, especially in terms of cardiovascular status. Full recovery and adequate control of the underlying thyroid disease take several days to achieve. For the patient presenting with thyroid storm, serious consideration should be given to permanent treatment of the hyperthyroidism, either by surgery or radioiodide ablation.

NEONATAL THYROTOXICOSIS

Background

Neonatal thyrotoxicosis is a life-threatening condition that may not be correctly diagnosed in the newborn nursery and that may be discovered only when the child presents in extremis in the ED. Neonatal thyrotoxicosis is found in 1% to 5% of infants born to mothers with a history of hyperthyroidism; however, the maternal disease does not have to be active during the pregnancy.

Pathophysiology

Neonatal thyrotoxicosis is caused by excessive thyroid hormone produced by the neonatal thyroid that has been stimulated by maternal thyroid-stimulating antibodies present in the immunoglobulin G (IgG) fraction that have crossed the placenta. TSH, T_4, and T_3 do not cross the placenta in significant quantities. In most cases, the disease is self-limiting, and hyperthyroidism remits within about 6 weeks. Occasionally, the disease may run a protracted course and arise in the absence of maternal thyroid-stimulating antibodies.

Clinical Manifestations

Goiter and exophthalmos are almost always present; however, a goiter may be difficult to appreciate in a small infant with a short neck. The child usually fails to gain weight despite a ravenous appetite. The child may also be irritable and have tachycardia, as well as signs of congestive heart failure. Laboratory investigations should include estimations of serum T_4, T_3, and TSH, and thyroid-binding capacity. Increased concentration of T_4 in the presence of suppressed TSH levels is consistent with the diagnosis. If the mother is taking antithyroid medication, thyroid function tests on the infant may be unreliable in the first days of life because of suppression of the fetal thyroid by transplacental passage of maternal antithyroid medication. The bone age may be advanced. In most cases, treatment must be initiated on the basis of historical and clinical findings.

For an infant who has an elevated level of T_4 but who has few, if any, symptoms or signs, consultation with a pediatric endocrinologist is strongly recommended. T_4 levels in all infants tend to be higher than those in older children because of increased TBG induced by maternal estrogen that crosses the placenta. Also, an elevated thyroxine may be seen with defects that alter the binding of T_4 to thyroid-binding globulin (TBG) or the end-organ sensitivity to T_4.

Management

Treatment is identical to that outlined for thyroid storm in older children. The duration of treatment is uncertain and should be based on serial thyroid function tests, especially TSH. It is anticipated that treatment need be continued only for 6 to 8 weeks in most cases because the causative agent is a subclass of IgG molecules with a serum half-life of about 2 weeks.

CONGENITAL HYPOTHYROIDISM

Background

Most westernized countries routinely screen infants in the first days of life for congenital hypothyroidism. The incidence of this problem is 1 in 3,500 live births. On occasion, notification of the parents by the screening program results in significant parental anxiety and leads to a visit to the ED. Emergency physicians should be knowledgeable about congenital hypothyroidism so they can appropriately educate parents and initiate therapy. Acquired hypothyroidism rarely results in urgent clinical problems that lead to ED visits.

Pathophysiology

The causes of congenital hypothyroidism are numerous; most cases (90%) are permanent. About 20% of patients have ectopic glands, and another 50% have hypoplastic or aplastic thyroid glands. Other causes are less common and include dyshormonogenesis, maternal ingestion of antithyroid medication, hypothalamic–pituitary disorders, and defects in thyroglobulin metabolism. The dyshormonogenic disorders are inherited as autosomal-recessive conditions. Congenital thyroid deficiency may result in impaired neurologic development if not treated before 1 month of age.

Clinical Manifestations

Clinical symptoms and signs of congenital hypothyroidism may be subtle and nonspecific, especially during the first month of life. Severely affected infants may be relatively large at birth, have a large posterior fontanel, manifest hypothermia and hypoactivity, feed poorly, tend to become constipated, and have prolonged jaundice. An enlarged tongue, coarse facies, and a hoarse cry may also be noted but are unusual in the first weeks of life. An umbilical hernia may be present. If treatment is not started, the physical characteristics become more prominent as the child grows older. Thyroid function tests beyond the first 2 days of life are most useful diagnostically. The TSH level is elevated in primary hypothyroidism, and the T_4 level is low or normal for age. A thyroid ultrasound or scan (^{123}I) may be helpful in identifying the particular type of primary hypothyroidism, but treatment should not be delayed to obtain this study. A low T_4 level in the absence of elevated TSH level may result from a deficiency of TBG, a pituitary deficiency of TSH, or prematurity.

Management

In term infants, treatment with L-thyroxine, 10 to 15 μg per kg per day should be instituted as soon as the relevant diagnostic tests are performed. In premature infants, 8 μg per kg per day can be administered. This dosage can be adjusted to maintain a TSH value that is normal for age; on appropriate replacement, the TSH will normalize within 4 weeks. Total T_4 and free T_4 concentrations should be maintained in the upper half of the normal range for age. Both undertreatment and overtreatment must be avoided. Careful follow-up on a monthly basis during the first several months, preferably by a physician who is accustomed to dealing with congenital hypothyroidism, is strongly recommended.

Suggested Readings

Diabetic Ketoacidosis

American Diabetes Association. Diagnosis and classification of diabetes mellitus. *Diabetes Care* 2004;27:S5–S10.

Burghen GA, Etteldorf JN, Fisher JN, et al. Comparison of high-dose and low-dose insulin by continuous intravenous infusion in the treatment of diabetic ketoacidosis in children. *Diabetes Care* 1980;3:15–20.

Butkiewicz EK, Liebson CL, Obrien PC, et al. Insulin therapy for diabetic ketoacidosis: bolus injection versus continuous insulin infusion. *Diabetes Care* 1995;18:1187–1190.

Dunger DB, Sperling MA, Acerini CL, et al. European Society for Paediatric Endocrinology/Lawson Wilkins Pediatric Endocrine Society consensus statement on diabetic ketoacidosis in children and adolescents. *Pediatrics* 2004;113:e133–e140.

Edge JA, Hawkins MM, Winter DL, et al. The risk and outcome of cerebral oedema developing during diabetic ketoacidosis. *Arch Dis Child* 2001;85:16–22.

Glaser N, Barnett P, McCaslin I, et al. Risk factors for cerebral edema in children with diabetic ketoacidosis. The Pediatric Emergency Medicine Collaborative Research Committee of the American Academy of Pediatrics. *N Engl J Med* 2001;344:264–269.

Jacobson AD, Hauser ST, Willett J, et al. Consequences of irregular versus continuous follow-up in children and adolescents with insulin dependent diabetes mellitus. *J Pediatr* 1997;131:727–733.

Klekamp J, Churchwell KB. Diabetic ketoacidosis in children: initial clinical assessment and treatment. *Pediatr Ann* 1996;25:387–393.

Krane EJ, Rockoff MA, Wallman JK, et al. Subclinical brain swelling in children during treatment of diabetic ketoacidosis. *N Engl J Med* 1985;312:1147–1150.

Lindsey R, Bolte RG. The use of insulin bolus in low-dose insulin infusion for pediatric diabetic ketoacidosis. *Pediatr Emerg Care* 1989;5:77–79.

Morris AD, Boyle DIR, McMahon AG, et al. Adherence to insulin treatment, glycaemic control and ketoacidosis in insulin dependent diabetes mellitus. *Lancet* 1997;350:1505–1510.

Thompson CJ, Cummings F, Chalmers J, et al. Abnormal insulin treatment behavior: a major cause of ketoacidosis in the young adult. *Diabet Med* 1995; 12:429–432.

Wolfsdorf J, Craig ME, Daneman D, et al. International Society for Pediatric and Adolescent Diabetes Clinical Practice Consensus Guidelines 2006–2007: diabetic ketoacidosis. *Pediatr Diabetes* 2007;8:28–42.

Hypoglycemia

Aynsley-Green A. Hypoglycaemia in infants and children. *Clin Endocrinol Metab* 1982;11:159–194.

Haymond MW. Hypoglycemia in infants and children. *Endocrinol Metab Clin North Am* 1989;18:211–252.

LaFranchi S. Hypoglycemia of infancy and childhood. *Pediatr Clin North Am* 1987;34:961–982.

Pagliara AS, Karl IE, Haymond M, et al. Hypoglycemia in infancy and childhood. Parts I and II. *J Pediatr* 1973;82:365–379, 558–577.

Stanley CA. Advances in diagnosis and treatment of hyperinsulinism in infants and children. *J Clin Endocrinol Metab* 2002;87:4857–4859.

Wolfsdorf JI, Weinstein DA. Glycogen storage diseases. *Rev Endocr Metab Disord* 2003;4:95–102.

Hypopituitarism

DeVile CJ, Stanhope R. Hydrocortisone replacement therapy in children and adolescents with hypopituitarism. *Clin Endocrinol* 1997;47:37–41.

Geffner ME. Hypopituitarism in childhood. *Cancer Control* 2002;9:212–222.

Lovinger RD, Kaplan SL, Grumbach MM. Congenital hypopituitarism associated with neonatal hypoglycemia and microphallus: four cases secondary to hypothalamic hormone deficiencies. *J Pediatr* 1975;87:1171–1181.

Rogol AD. Hypopituitarism. *Curr Ther Endocrinol Metab* 1994;5:26–29.

Stahnke N, Koehn H. Replacement therapy in hypothalamus-pituitary insufficiency: management in the adolescent. *Horm Res* 1990;4(suppl 33):38–44.

Willnow S, Kiess W, Butenandt O, et al. Endocrine disorders in septo-optic dysplasia: evaluation and follow-up of 18 patients. *Eur J Pediatr* 1996;155:179–184.

Acute Adrenal Insufficiency

August GP. Treatment of adrenocortical insufficiency. *Pediatr Rev* 1997;18:59–62.

Dorin RI, Qualls CR, Crapo LM. Diagnosis of adrenal insufficiency. *Ann Intern Med* 2003;139:194–204.

Lipiner-Friedman D, Sprung CL, Laterre PF, et al. Adrenal function in sepsis: the retrospective Corticus cohort study. *Crit Care Med* 2007;35:1012–1018.

New MI. Replacement doses of glucocorticoids. *J Pediatr* 1991;119:161.

Urban MD, Kogut MD. Adrenocortical insufficiency in the child. *Curr Ther Endocrinol Metab* 1994;5:131–135.

Congenital Adrenal Hyperplasia

Cutler GG Jr, Laue L. Congenital adrenal hyperplasia due to 21-hydroxylase deficiency. *N Engl J Med* 1990;323:1906–1913.

Levine LS. Congenital adrenal hyperplasia. *Pediatr Rev* 2000;21:159–170.

Miller WL. Congenital adrenal hyperplasia. *Endocrinol Metab Clin North Am* 1991;20:721–749.

Newfield RS, New MI. 21-Hydroxylase deficiency. *Ann N Y Acad Sci* 1997; 816:219–229.

Pang S. Congenital adrenal hyperplasia. *Endocrinol Metab Clin North Am* 1997; 26:853–891.

Pheochromocytoma

Bravo EL, Tagle R. Pheochromocytoma: state-of-the-art and future prospects. *Endocrinol Rev* 2003;24:539–553.

Caty MG, Coran AG, Geagen M, et al. Current diagnosis and treatment of pheochromocytoma in children. *Arch Surg* 1990;125:978–981.

Ein SH, Pullerits J, Crighton R, et al. Pediatric pheochromocytoma: a 36-year review. *Pediatr Surg Int* 1997;12:595–598.

Fonkalsrud EW. Pheochromocytoma in childhood. *Prog Pediatr Surg* 1991;26: 103–111.

Lenders JWM, Keiser HR, Goldstein DS, et al. Plasma metanephrines in the diagnosis of pheochromocytoma. *Ann Intern Med* 1995;123:101–109.

Werbel SS, Ober KP. Pheochromocytoma: update on diagnosis, localization and management. *Med Clin North Am* 1995;79:131–153.

Diabetes Insipidus

Buonocore CM, Robinson AG. The diagnosis and management of diabetes insipidus during medical emergencies. *Endocrinol Metab Clin North Am* 1993;22:411–413.

Harris AS. Clinical experience with desmopressin: efficacy and safety in central diabetes insipidus and other conditions. *J Pediatr* 1989;144:711–718.

Knoers N, Monnens LA. Nephrogenic diabetes insipidus: clinical symptoms, pathogenesis, genetics and treatment. *Pediatr Nephrol* 1992;6:476–482.

Lee YJ, Huang FY, Shen EY, et al. Neurogenic diabetes insipidus in children with hypoxic encephalopathy: six new cases and a review of the literature. *Eur J Pediatr* 1996;155:245–248.

Ober KP. Endocrine crisis: diabetes insipidus. *Crit Care Clin* 1991;7:109–125.

Schrier RW, Cadnapaphornchai MA. Renal aquaporin water channels: from molecules to human disease. *Prog Biophys Mol Biol* 2003;81:117–131.

Seckl JR, Dunger DB. Diabetes insipidus: current treatment recommendations. *Drugs* 1992;44:216–224.

Syndrome of Inappropriate Antidiuretic Hormone Secretion

Ganong CA, Kappy MS. Cerebral salt wasting in children: the need for recognition and treatment. *Am J Dis Child* 1993;147:167–169.

Kaplan SL, Feigin RD. Syndromes of inappropriate secretion of antidiuretic hormone in children. *Adv Pediatr* 1980;27:247–274.

Kappy MS, Ganong CA. Cerebral salt wasting in children: the role of atrial natriuretic factor. *Adv Pediatr* 1996;43:271–308.

Palmer BF. Hyponatremia in patients with central nervous system disease: SIADH versus CSW. *Trends Endocrinol Metab* 2003;14:182–187.

Hyperparathyroidism

Lawson ML, Miller SF, Ellis G, et al. Primary hyperparathyroidism in a paediatric hospital. *Q J Med* 1996;89:921–932.

Matsuo M, Okita K, Takemine H, et al. Neonatal primary hyperparathyroidism in familial hypocalciuric hypercalcemia. *Am J Dis Child* 1982;136:728–731.

Moe SM, Drueke TB. Management of secondary hyperparathyroidism: the importance and the challenge of controlling parathyroid hormone levels without elevating calcium, phosphorus, and calcium-phosphorus product. *Am J Nephrol* 2003;23:369–379.

Ross AJ, Cooper A, Attie MF, et al. Primary hyperparathyroidism in infancy. *J Pediatr Surg* 1986;21:493–499.

Hypoparathyroidism

Rosen JF, Fleischman AR, Finberg L, et al. 1,25-Dihydroxycholecalciferol: its use in the long-term management of idiopathic hypoparathyroidism in children. *J Clin Endocrinol Metab* 1977;45:457–468.

Taylor SC, Morris G, Wilson D, et al. Hypoparathyroidism and 22q11 deletion syndrome. *Arch Dis Child* 2003;88:520–522.

Winter WE, Silverstein JH, Maclaren NK, et al. Autosomal-dominant hypoparathyroidism with variable, age-dependent severity. *J Pediatr* 1983; 103:387–390.

Rickets

Chesney RW, Mazess RB, Rose P, et al. Long-term influence of calcitriol and supplemental phosphate in X-linked hypophosphatemic rickets. *Pediatrics* 1983;71:559–567.

Dwyer JT, Dietz WH, Hass G, et al. Risk of nutritional rickets among vegetarian children. *Am J Dis Child* 1979;133:134–140.

Lovinger RD. Rickets. *Pediatrics* 1980;66:359–365.

Mughal Z. Rickets in childhood. *Semin Musculoskelet Radiol* 2002;6:183–190.

Rajakumar K. Vitamin D, cod-liver oil, sunlight, and rickets: a historical perspective. *Pediatrics* 2003;112:e132–e135.

Wharton B, Bishop N. Rickets. *Lancet* 2003;362:1389–1400.

Thyroid Storm

Foley TP Jr. Thyrotoxicosis in childhood. *Pediatr Ann* 1992;21:43–49.

Foley TP Jr, Charron M. Radioiodine treatment of juvenile Graves' disease. *Exp Clin Endocrinol Diabetes* 1997;105(suppl 4):61–65.

Hung W. Graves' disease in children. *Curr Ther Endocrinol Metab* 1997;6: 77–81.

Rivkees SA, Mattison DR. Ending propylthiouracil-induced liver failure in children. *N Engl J Med* 2009;360:1574–1575.

Segni M, Gorman CA. The aftermath of childhood hyperthyroidism. *J Pediatr Endocrinol Metab* 2001;14(suppl 5):1277–1282.

Neonatal Thyrotoxicosis

Dirmikis SM, Munro DS. Placental transmission of thyroid-stimulating immunoglobulins. *Br Med J* 1975;2:665–666.

Foley TP Jr. Maternally transferred thyroid disease in the infant: recognition and treatment. *Adv Exp Med Biol* 1991;299:209–226.

Singer J. Neonatal thyrotoxicosis. *J Pediatr* 1977;91:749–750.

Congenital Hypothyroidism

Barsano CP, DeGroot LJ. Dyshormonogenetic goitre. *Clin Endocrinol Metab* 1979;8:145–165.

Burrow GN, Dussault JH. *Neonatal thyroid screening*. New York: Raven, 1980.

Fisher DA, Klein AH. Thyroid development and disorders of thyroid function in the newborn. *N Engl J Med* 1981;304:702–712.

New England Congenital Hypothyroidism Collaborative. Characteristics of infantile hypothyroidism discovered on neonatal screening. *J Pediatr* 1984;104:539–544.

Osborn DA. Thyroid hormones for preventing neurodevelopmental impairment in preterm infants. *Cochrane Database Syst Rev* 2001:CD001070.

CHAPTER 87 ■ ENVIRONMENTAL EMERGENCIES

MICHELE BURNS EWALD, MD, AND CARL R. BAUM, MD

DROWNING

Background

Drowning is defined as water submersion with resultant asphyxiation and death within 24 hours; *drowning* implies that resuscitation has extended survival beyond 24 hours. Each term is further classified according to whether aspiration has occurred.

In 2000, drowning was responsible for the deaths of more than 1,400 U.S. children younger than 20 years. Drowning affects all age groups and males two to three times more often than females. Individuals with epilepsy have a 15- to 19-fold higher risk of drowning when compared to the general population. Drowning is the major cause of death following water-related natural disasters such as Hurricane Katrina.

In more recent years, drowning was the second leading cause of injury death in children ranging from 1 to 14 years of age. Older infants and toddlers are disproportionately represented in these accidents, and their survival rates are lower. They are vulnerable to immersion in household buckets, baths and hot tubs, swimming pools, and other bodies of water near their homes. Young teenagers are also at greater risk because adult supervision decreases and impulsive behavior increases. However, coexisting trauma, drug or alcohol use, and suicidal intent must be considered in each case. The importance of continuous adult supervision and public safety measures, such as isolation (four-sided) fences around pools and swimming lessons, cannot be overemphasized.

Pathophysiology

When a child is submerged, either breath-holding or laryngospasm occurs. If hypoxemia follows, loss of consciousness and cardiovascular collapse may occur without aspiration of fluid. Alternatively, submersion and frantic struggling may result in gasping, with subsequent aspiration. If antecedent head trauma, drug ingestion, seizure activity, or cardiac arrhythmia impair consciousness and protective airway reflexes, aspiration is more likely to occur. Although most organs may become involved, the major morbidity occurs in the pulmonary and central nervous system (CNS).

Fresh water aspirated into the lungs is rapidly taken up into the circulation, resulting in a transient rise in circulating blood volume that is quickly redistributed through the body. In a canine study of fresh-water drowning, aspiration of fresh water caused body weight to increase an average of 16.5%

with concomitant hemodilution. Aspiration of salt water caused body weight to increase only 6% with hemoconcentration and diminished intravascular volume. In humans, changes in the hematocrit are not predictable, and those that occur are more closely related to coexisting trauma than to effects of hypertonic or hypotonic fluids. Occasionally, however, massive hemolysis may occur. Electrolyte abnormalities that occur after massive aspiration in laboratory animals rarely achieve clinical significance in either adult or child victims.

Even small (1 to 3 mL per kg) quantities of fresh water cause disruption of surfactant, a rise in surface tension in the lungs, and alveolar instability. Capillary and alveolar membrane damage allows fluid to leak into the alveoli with subsequent pulmonary edema.

Aspiration of salt water (osmolality greater than normal saline) does not denature surfactant but creates an osmotic gradient for fluid to accumulate in the lungs. This accumulated fluid greatly exceeds the volume that was aspirated and effectively removes surfactant from the alveolar–gas interface.

Both fresh- and salt-water aspiration decrease pulmonary compliance, increase airway resistance and pulmonary artery pressure, and diminish pulmonary flow. As nonventilated alveoli are perfused, an intrapulmonary shunt develops, leading to a drastic fall in partial pressure of arterial oxygen (PaO_2).

In other animal studies, aspiration of as little as 2.2 mL per kg of fresh water led to a fall in PaO_2 to about 60 mm Hg in 3 minutes, whereas a similar amount of sea water precipitated an even greater drop (to about 40 mm Hg). In humans, even lower levels of PaO_2 are seen; tissue hypoxia then leads to severe metabolic acidosis. The victim is usually able to correct a rise in partial pressure of arterial carbon dioxide ($PaCO_2$). Aspiration of bacteria, gastric contents, and foreign materials may cause additional trauma to the lungs.

Hypoxemia, whether secondary to upper airway obstruction (e.g., laryngospasm) or to impaired gas exchange after aspiration, results in loss of consciousness. If anoxia ensues, irreversible CNS damage begins after 4 to 6 minutes. Fear or cold may trigger the diving reflex (commonly encountered in infancy), which shunts blood to the brain and heart primarily and affords several minutes of additional perfusion. Experience with drowning victims and in cardiovascular surgery indicates that cold water is relatively protective of the CNS, but probably only if immersion hypothermia develops very rapidly or before compromise of oxygenation. Onset of hypothermia is more rapid in the victim who is younger (greater surface:volume ratio) or is struggling in or swallowing icy water. If, however, laryngospasm or aspiration occurs before a fall in core body temperature and cerebral metabolic rate, protection is probably minimal.

Cardiovascular effects are primarily those expected with myocardial ischemia, severe systemic acidosis, hypothermia, and intravascular volume changes. After aspiration of fresh water, the transient rise in intravascular volume later contributes to problems of cerebral edema and pulmonary function.

Clinical Manifestations

In the first moments after rescue, the appearance of the child who has nearly drowned may range from apparently normal to apparently dead. Body temperature is often low, even in temperate, warm-water environments. Respiratory efforts may be absent, irregular, or labored, with pallor or cyanosis, retractions, grunting, and cough productive of pink, frothy material. The lungs may be clear, or there may be rales, rhonchi, and wheezing. Infection may develop as a consequence of aspirated mouth flora or organisms in stagnant water, but this is not usually important in the first 24 hours.

Respiratory function may improve spontaneously or deteriorate rapidly as pulmonary edema and small airway dysfunction worsen. Alternatively, deterioration may ensue slowly over 12 to 24 hours. Intense peripheral vasoconstriction and myocardial depression may produce apparent or actual pulselessness.

Neurologic assessment may show an alert, normal child or any level of CNS compromise. A child may display agitation and combative behavior, blunted responsiveness to the environment, or profound coma with stereotypic posturing or flaccid extremities. Superficial evidence of head trauma may be noted in a few children whose submersion episode was a secondary event. Head CT most typically shows diffuse loss of gray–white differentiation and/or bilateral basal ganglia edema/infarction.

Pulmonary and neurologic damage need not occur together. Although extensive pulmonary destruction and resultant hypoxemia may cause neurologic damage, all combinations of mild and severe lung and brain damage are possible.

Management

The ultimate outcome of serious immersion accidents depends on the duration of submersion, the degree of pulmonary damage by aspiration, and in some cases, effectiveness of initial resuscitative measures. When all children who experience immersion accidents are considered as a group, most are salvageable, and all should receive the benefit of excellent cardiopulmonary resuscitation without delay at the scene, according to the principles elaborated in Chapter 1. In particular, children should be given the maximum concentration of supplemental oxygen possible (100%) in transport to an emergency facility. Even those rescued with spontaneous ventilation and minimal or no neurologic dysfunction should receive the benefit of supplemental oxygen to minimize the risk of progressive hypoxemia and acidosis with secondary myocardial and cerebral damage. Physical examination is notoriously insensitive to hypoxemia; a seriously hypoxemic child may be alert and talking. Once the child has arrived at an emergency facility (and cardiovascular stability is achieved), pulmonary and neurologic assessment should guide further treatment.

Several more recent pediatric studies have attempted to predict outcome in submersion accidents. One prospective inves-

tigation devised a prediction rule for children submerged in non-icy water who presented to the emergency department (ED) in a comatose state: lack of pupillary light reflex, male gender, and hyperglycemia were variables used to predict unfavorable outcome (vegetative state or death). A retrospective study of children presenting to the ED after warm-water submersion suggested that hemodynamic, rather than neurologic, status was more highly predictive of poor neurologic outcome.

Effective therapy of drowning depends on the reversal of hypoxemia and metabolic acidosis. The pulmonary status is assessed initially with a chest radiograph (Fig. 87.1) and with measurement of arterial oxygen saturation (SaO_2) and arterial blood gas (ABG), as in Figure 87.2. If oxygenation is normal on breathing room air, the child can be assumed to have suffered drowning without aspiration. Observation for 6 to 24 hours with repeat (SaO_2) or ABG determination should be sufficient to assess the possibility of late deterioration in gas exchange.

Other initial laboratory evaluation should include complete blood cell count (CBC), electrolytes, and urinalysis. Patients

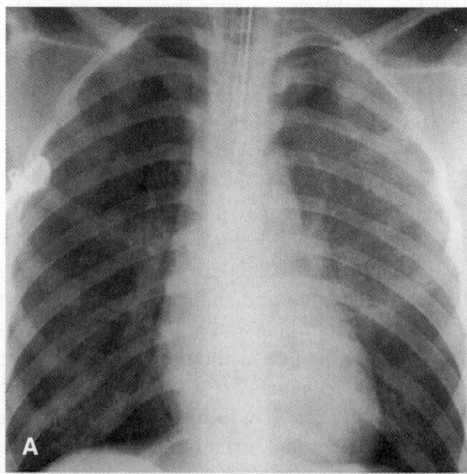
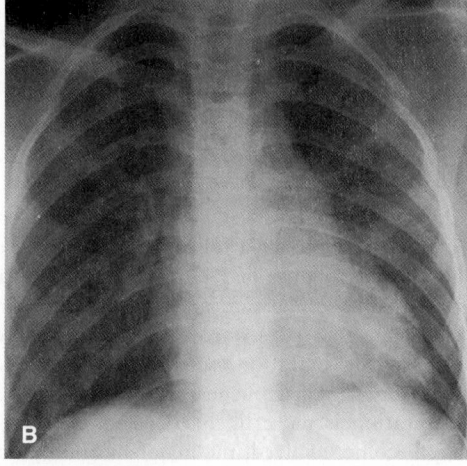

FIGURE 87.1 Drowning in a 4-month-old girl. **A:** There is bilateral disseminated alveolar pattern, more on the left than on the right, consistent with the pulmonary edema of drowning. This change may be the result of neurologic pulmonary edema rather than aspirated water. **B:** Two days later, the patient has been extubated and there is marked improvement in appearance of pulmonary edema secondary to drowning. (Courtesy of Soroosh Mahboubi, MD.)

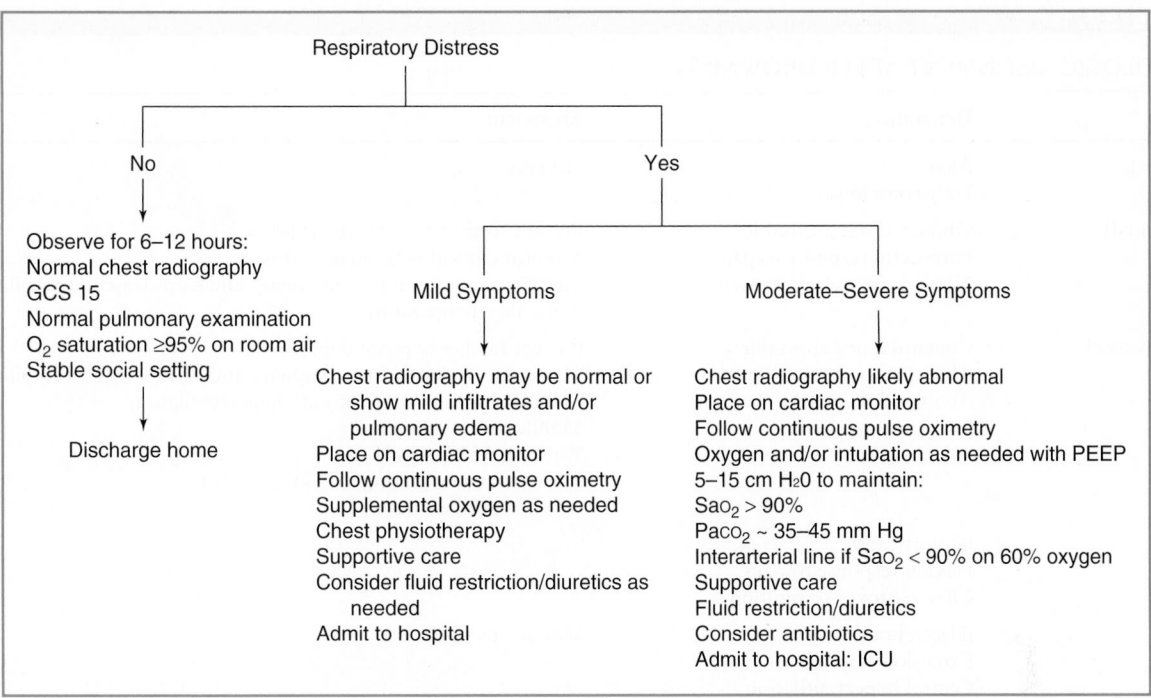

FIGURE 87.2 Algorithm for pulmonary assessment for drowning.

with abnormalities of gas exchange and acid–base status (but with normal chest radiographs) can usually be managed with supplemental oxygen, pulmonary physiotherapy, and bicarbonate therapy. Additional blood gas analysis should be done to document adequate oxygenation and reversal of metabolic acidosis. Any change in mental status or increase in respiratory distress may reflect arterial hypoxemia and should also prompt a repeat ABG determination. Continuous SaO_2 or serial PaO_2 measurements will guide the physician to continue conservative treatment or to intensify ventilatory support.

Patients with obvious respiratory distress, hypoxemia (SaO_2 less than 90% or PaO_2 less than 60 on 60% inspired oxygen), and extensive pulmonary edema or infiltration generally requires more vigorous treatment. All should be monitored for heart rate, cardiac rhythm, respiratory rate, and blood pressure (BP). Most will require frequent blood gas analysis and may be more easily monitored through arterial cannulation. Intubation, supplemental oxygen, and mechanical ventilation with positive end-expiratory pressure (PEEP; 5 to 15 cm H_2O) should be provided, as indicated.

Once BP is stabilized, fluid restriction (to approximately one-half the maintenance rate) and diuretic therapy (e.g., furosemide 0.5 to 1 mg per kg intravenously, usual maximum 20 mg/dose) may improve gas exchange. In the setting of extensive pulmonary damage, pulmonary and cardiovascular components of the disease are intimately entwined. Optimum management requires monitoring of blood gases and systemic arterial pressure.

The risk of pulmonary infection is always present, but retrospective studies have not demonstrated benefit from prophylactic antibiotics, which should be reserved for strongly suspected or proven bacterial infection. Exceptions may be made when grossly contaminated water is aspirated and, in the worst cases,

when maximal ventilatory support is required to provide any margin for survival. Most studies of bronchoalveolar lavage show no improvement. Steroids have no demonstrated benefit.

Renal function must be maintained. If significant hemoglobinuria exists, diuresis is required. Maintenance of an adequate hemoglobin level (more than 10 g per 100 mL) and normal electrolytes is obviously necessary. Specific problems vary from patient to patient in an unpredictable way, and an understanding of the principles outlined in Chapters 91 and 100 is essential.

The patient's clinical condition in the ED dictates further management and may provide prognostic clues. Patients may be assigned to one of three groups (Table 87.1). Those who are awake, alert, and fully responsive have survived the episode, presumably without CNS damage. One study suggests that if the child's GCS is greater than or equal to 13 with a normal physical exam/respiratory effort and room air oxygen saturations are more than 95%, the child could be discharged with a responsible guardian after 6 hours of observation. The second group includes those who are obtunded but able to be aroused and those who exhibit a normal respiratory pattern and purposeful responses to pain. These patients have suffered certain but reversible CNS hypoxia; the goal is to prevent further hypoxic damage through intensive management of cardiopulmonary disease. Repeated neurologic evaluation is essential, and fluid restriction and diuretic therapy within the limits of cardiovascular stability may decrease the risk of cerebral edema. There is no demonstrated value in the use of steroids in this setting (see Chapter 126). In both groups, temperature normalization should be prompt. If reversal of coexisting pulmonary damage is effective, neurologic recovery should be complete.

There is controversy over patients in a third group—those who have experienced severe CNS asphyxia. These children are

TABLE 87.1

NEUROLOGIC ASSESSMENT AFTER DROWNING

Group	Description	Treatment
A (alert)	Alert Fully conscious	Observe
B (blunted)	Obtunded but arousable Purposeful response to pain Normal respiratory pattern	Prevent further hypoxic damage Monitor clinical neurologic status Therapy as required for pulmonary and cardiovascular stability Normalize temperature
C (comatose)	Comatose, not arousable Abnormal response to pain Abnormal respiratory pattern	Prevent further hypoxic damage Therapy as required for pulmonary and cardiovascular stability Maintain normocapnia or mild hyperventilation Monitor core temperature Warm to 32°C (89.6°F) Allow passive warming to 37°C (98.6°F) Avoid hyperthermia
C.1	(Decorticate) Flexion response to pain Cheyne-Stokes respiration	
C.2	(Decerebrate) Extension response to pain Central hyperventilation	Monitor temperature
C.3	(Flaccid) No response to pain Apnea or cluster breathing	Consider withdrawal of support if no protection from hypothermia

not able to be aroused and can be further divided into three subcategories according to neurologic findings: (i) those with decorticate response to pain and Cheyne-Stokes breathing, (ii) those with decerebrate response to pain and central hyperventilation, and (iii) those who are flaccid with fixed, dilated pupils and apneustic breathing or apnea. Again, reversal of hypoxemia and acidosis is critical. Fluid resuscitation should be designed to prevent hyperglycemia. Avoiding hypercapnia and resultant cerebral hyperemia is generally accepted, but hyperventilation, barbiturate coma, and other measures initially believed to provide cerebral protection and prevent or treat elevated intracranial pressure have not been helpful in these patients.

Hypothermia does appear to have some protective value. Extreme hypothermia should be corrected to at least 32°C (89.6°F) to achieve hemodynamic stability and to minimize the risk of infection. The child should then be allowed to rewarm passively. Although data in humans are limited, animal studies suggest that maintenance of mild brain hypothermia may minimize reperfusion injury. Hyperthermia, a common result of active rewarming, should be avoided.

The prognosis for this group is certainly grimmer, with a much greater risk of death or severe anoxic/ischemic encephalopathy. Risk increases with depth of coma on presentation. Patients in the third subdivision (flaccid with fixed, dilated pupils) rarely survive intact regardless of treatment, although coexistent hypothermia has provided some remarkable exceptions.

More recent studies indicate that patients with asystole on arrival in the ED have uniformly poor neurologic outcomes. In each case, consideration should be given to the possibility that continued resuscitation will salvage only the cardiovascular system; in these cases, the physician may reasonably discontinue resuscitative efforts.

SMOKE INHALATION

Background

Among unintentional injuries, fires rank fifth in the United States. Although fire has been the cause of much death and misery throughout human history, the importance of smoke inhalation has been recognized only in the last 50 years. An analysis of fire deaths among Philadelphia children younger than 15 years revealed the following epidemiologic risk factors: low-income or single-parent households, housing built before 1939, and increased numbers of children younger than 15 years. A recent study suggests that personalized parent voice smoke alarms may be more effective than conventional residential tone smoke alarms for awakening children.

Respiratory complications of smoke inhalation rank with carbon monoxide poisoning (see "Pathophysiology" section) as a major cause of early death from fire. Although serious cutaneous injury may occur in the absence of pulmonary involvement, inhalation injury dramatically increases the morbidity and mortality associated with any given percent body surface area burn.

The severity of carbon monoxide inhalation and respiratory problems is related to the duration of exposure, the occurrence in a closed space (more likely in very young or elderly victims), the nature of materials involved, and the presence of products of incomplete combustion. Severe hypovolemic shock, massive tissue destruction, extensive fluid resuscitation, and infection further complicate direct inhalational trauma.

Pathophysiology

The relatively low heat capacity of dry air and the excellent heat exchange properties of the nasopharynx usually limit direct thermal injury to the upper airway. Dry air above 160°C (320°F) has little effect on the lower airway. The greater heat capacity of steam increases the risk of lower airway damage. In addition, continuing combustion of soot particles carried deeply into the lung may exacerbate thermal injury.

Chemical injury may occur at any level of the respiratory tract. Oxides of sulfur and nitrogen combine with lung water to form corrosive acids. Incomplete combustion of any carbon-containing material, such as wood, may produce carbon monoxide. Combustion of cotton or plastic generates aldehydes that cause protein denaturation and cellular damage. One example is acrolein, known to cause upper airway irritation at concentrations of 5.5 parts per million (ppm) and pulmonary edema within seconds at 10 ppm. Polyvinylchloride releases chlorine and hydrochloric acid, whereas polyethylene produces hydrocarbons, ketones, and other acids. Burning polyurethane may produce cyanide gas. Fire retardants that contain phosphorus may actually produce phosgene gas. The upper airway filters most soot particles, but those carried into the lung may adsorb various substances and cause reflex bronchospasm to further extend chemical damage.

Upper airway lesions include actual burns of varying severity as well as severe edema of the nose, mouth, pharynx, and laryngeal structures. A murine model of wood smoke inhalation suggests that combustion produces hydroxyl radicals in the gas phase of smoke that cause a reflex apneic response. In this investigation, a hydroxyl radical scavenger, applied to the larynx, attenuated the response. Upper airway edema increases inspiratory and expiratory resistance and causes a dramatic increase in the work of breathing. If airway narrowing is severe or complete, acute respiratory failure with hypercarbia and hypoxemia occurs and sets the stage for subsequent cardiovascular collapse.

Lower airway lesions depend on the toxin involved. A variety of features may aggravate pulmonary pathology, including circulatory, metabolic, and infectious complications, as well as therapeutic interventions such as endotracheal intubation, oxygen administration, mechanical ventilation, and fluid therapy.

Immediate effects of smoke inhalation on the lower airway include loss of ciliary action, mucosal edema, bronchiolitis, alveolar epithelial damage, and impaired gas exchange, particularly oxygenation. In addition, areas of atelectasis or air trapping worsen ventilation–perfusion mismatch and hypoxemia. Loss of surfactant activity exaggerates this phenomenon. Hours later, sloughing of tracheobronchial mucosa and mucopurulent membrane formation increase the degree of obstruction and poor gas exchange, as well as the likelihood of infection. Beyond the first 24 hours, pulmonary pathology that results from smoke inhalation is largely indistinguishable from adult respiratory distress syndrome, which arises from other insults.

Children who die from smoke inhalation may sustain serious respiratory damage in the absence of cutaneous injury. Necrosis of bronchial, bronchiolar, and alveolar epithelium; vascular engorgement and edema; and formation of membranes or casts of the airway produce small and large airway obstruction. Severe cutaneous injury increases alveolar capillary permeability, leading to pulmonary hemorrhage, edema, and hyaline membrane formation.

Clinical Manifestations

A history of exposure in a closed space should heighten concern for smoke inhalation. Need for cardiopulmonary resuscitation at the site implies significant carbon monoxide poisoning and/or hypoxia secondary to decreased ambient oxygen concentration or severe respiratory disease. The physician should also consider the types of material involved to determine the risk of poisoning from carbon monoxide or other toxins.

Physical examination that reveals facial burns, singed nasal hairs, pharyngeal soot, or carbonaceous sputum justifies a presumption of smoke inhalation. Any sign of neurologic dysfunction, including irritability or depression, should be presumed related to tissue hypoxia until proven otherwise. Signs of respiratory distress may be delayed for 12 to 24 hours, but tachypnea, cough, hoarseness, stridor, decreased breath sounds, wheezing, rhonchi, or rales may be detected on presentation.

Auscultatory findings often precede chest radiograph abnormalities by 12 to 24 hours. Radiographic changes may include diffuse interstitial infiltration or local areas of atelectasis and edema (Fig. 87.3). Acute respiratory failure may occur at any point. The cause may be asphyxia or carbon monoxide exposure and subsequent CNS depression initially, or airway obstruction or parenchymal dysfunction later. ABG analysis provides the ultimate assessment of effective respiratory function. Bronchoscopy can document the extent of inhalation injury and help remove debris but may worsen airway edema. In general, it is respiratory function, not the appearance of lesions, that guides supportive care; therefore, most patients can be treated effectively without bronchoscopy.

Management

Initial assessment and resuscitation at the scene of the fire should proceed according to the principles outlined in Chapter 1. Because of the likelihood of carbon monoxide exposure and the difficulty of assessing hypoxemia clinically, all victims should receive the maximum concentration of inspired oxygen possible in transport and in the ED until further evaluation is complete (Table 87.2).

Upon the patient's arrival in the ED, assessment of the airway and respiratory functions must proceed simultaneously with cardiovascular stabilization. Thermal injury to the nose, mouth, or face, or compromise of the upper airway (stridor, hoarseness, barking cough, retractions, delayed inspiration, or difficulty handling secretions) indicates the need for direct laryngoscopy. The presence of significant pharyngeal, supraglottic, or glottic edema mandates elective endotracheal intubation. Worsening edema over 24 hours may lead to respiratory arrest and a difficult emergency intubation through a

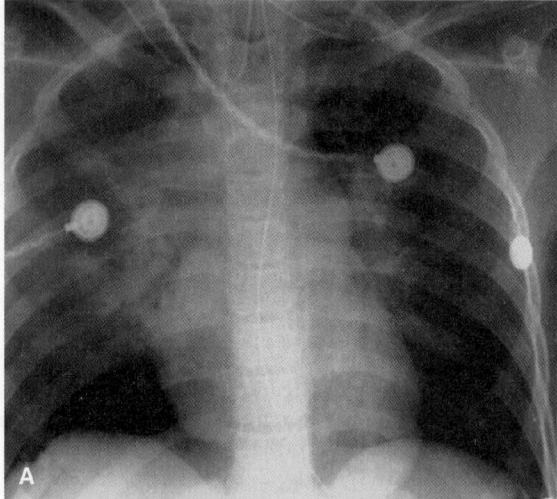

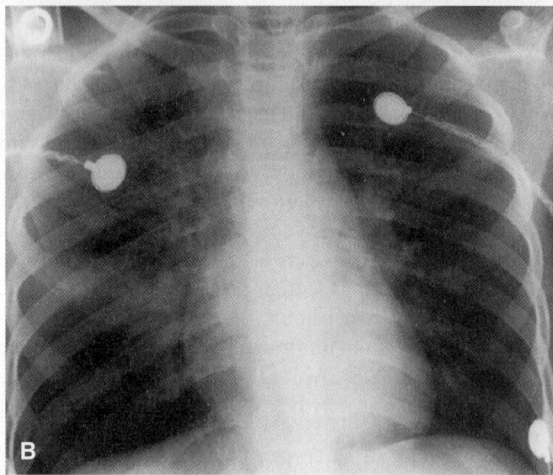

FIGURE 87.3 Smoke inhalation in a 9-year-old girl. **A:** There is bilateral central alveolar process consistent with acute smoke inhalation. **B:** A day later, the patient has been extubated and there is marked improvement in the appearance of pulmonary edema. (Courtesy of Soroosh Mahboubi, MD.)

distorted airway, and thus early endotracheal intubation cannot be overemphasized. Elective tracheostomy may be considered if placing or securing the endotracheal tube will further traumatize an edematous airway or severe facial burns. However, in the presence of extensive cutaneous burns, tracheostomy dramatically increases the risk of systemic and pulmonary infection.

Cardiovascular stabilization depends on fluid replacement, which is complex when major surface burns have occurred. The details of therapy are elaborated in Chapter 108, but in general, the goals are stabilization of cardiovascular function without fluid overload and compromise of gas exchange. Pulse rate and BP should guide administration of fluid volume. Maintenance of urine output of at least 0.5 mL per kg per hour should provide adequate tissue perfusion. Decreased urine output may respond to diuretics or inotropic agents. Although adequate fluid administration is essential, careful monitoring of renal and cardiovascular systems may prevent or minimize acute pulmonary edema and delayed pulmonary dysfunction secondary to late fluid mobilization and infection.

TABLE 87.2
MANAGEMENT OF SMOKE INHALATION

Initial Management
Remove from contaminated environment
Cardiopulmonary resuscitation as needed
Provide 100% supplemental oxygen
Insure patent airway

Laboratory Determinations
Arterial blood gas analysis
Carboxyhemoglobin level, troponin
Chest radiograph

Monitor
Heart rate, electrocardiogram, respiratory rate, blood
    pressure, SaO_2
Consider central venous pressure
Consider pulmonary artery catheterization

Fluids
5% dextrose in normal saline at maintenance rates or less to
    maintain urine output 0.5–1.0/mL/kg/h
Volume expansion in presence of cutaneous burns; normal
    saline, lactated Ringer's solution, or 5% albumin

Respiratory Management
Intubation for:
1. Upper airway obstruction
2. $PaO_2 < 60$ mm Hg on 60% oxygen
3. Central nervous system depression with loss of cough and
    gag reflexes. Continuous positive airway pressure 5–15 cm
    H_2O for $PaO_2 < 60$ mm Hg on 60% oxygen

Intermittent mandatory ventilation for:
1. Hypoxia unresponsive to continuous positive airway
    pressure or
2. $PaCO_2 > 50$ mm Hg
Humidification of inspired gases
Meticulous pulmonary toilette
Consider inhaled bronchodilators

Oxygen saturation and serial blood gas determinations should be obtained to guide oxygen supplementation and to assess adequacy of ventilation. Intubation is indicated if adequate oxygenation (SaO_2 greater than 90% or PaO_2 greater than 60 mm Hg) cannot be maintained with an inspired oxygen concentration of 40% to 60%, if $PaCO_2$ rises above 50 mm Hg, or if the work of breathing appears unsustainable. In the presence of small airway edema and disrupted surfactant activity, continuous distending airway pressure may improve oxygenation. Spontaneous ventilation with continuous positive airway pressure causes less cardiovascular interference, but in the patient with severe CNS depression or severe pulmonary parenchymal damage, mechanical ventilation with PEEP will likely be necessary. Maximally humidified oxygen should be delivered by mask or artificial airway to prevent inspissation of debris and occlusion of the airway. The patient with a natural airway should also receive humidified gas mixtures and be encouraged to take deep breaths and cough frequently. If an endotracheal tube is necessary, meticulous pulmonary toilette is essential, with frequent suctioning to remove edema fluid, mucus, and sloughed epithelium that may otherwise occlude the endotracheal tube.

A more recent study of lung mechanics in children with inhalation injury compared two modes of long-term ventilation in the intensive care unit. High-frequency percussive ventilation (hi-fi) was superior to conventional mechanical ventilation in reducing work of breathing. There is also evidence that extracorporeal membrane oxygenation (ECMO) may be useful in severely burned children.

After the first few hours, diuretic therapy (furosemide 0.5 to 1 mg per kg intravenously) within the limits of cardiovascular stability may also improve oxygenation and pulmonary compliance, leading to more effective ventilation. Chemical and particulate irritation of upper airway receptors may cause reflex bronchoconstriction and contribute to lower airway obstruction. Bronchodilators such as nebulized albuterol [2.5 mg in 2.5 mL, 0.9% sodium chloride (NaCl)] or intravenous (IV) terbutaline (load 10 $m$cg per kg per dose intravenously or subcutaneously; followed by a continuaus infusion of 0.4 to 6 $m$cg per kg per minute) may help reverse bronchospasm, but relief depends mostly on removal of secretions and debris from the respiratory tree.

Studies have not demonstrated a role for steroids in reducing airway edema or in decreasing the inflammatory response to smoke inhalation. When steroids are used, there is evidence that sodium and fluid retention increase, healing is delayed, and bacterial clearance from the lung is decreased. Little argument remains for their routine use.

Similarly, there is no value in the use of prophylactic antibiotics. Institution of antimicrobial therapy should await specific indications, which rarely occur in the first 24 hours.

CARBON MONOXIDE POISONING

Background

Each year, unintentional carbon monoxide poisoning claims about 500 lives and is largely responsible for early deaths related to fire. However, exposure may occur in a variety of other settings unrelated to accidental fires, including incomplete combustion of any carbon-containing fuel (i.e., propane-powered forklifts). Poisoning may occur with exposure to improperly vented wood- or coal-burning stoves, and to automobile exhaust in garages. In most reported cases, garage doors and windows were actually open. Passengers may be poisoned in vehicles or boats with open backs, or with faulty or blocked exhaust systems. During a 2005 snowstorm in Boston that resulted in numerous power outages, snow blocked the furnace pipes of a 7-year-old girl's home, leading to her death from carbon monoxide poisoning. Later that same year, Massachusetts passed "Nicole's Law" requiring carbon monoxide detectors in every home in the Commonwealth; other states are passing similar laws.

Pathophysiology

In the normal person, carboxyhemoglobin levels are less than 1%. In smokers, levels of 5% to 10% are common. Inhaled carbon monoxide has two important effects that conspire to cause tissue hypoxia: (i) it binds to hemoglobin with an affinity 200 to 300 times greater than that of oxygen, and (ii) it shifts the oxyhemoglobin dissociation curve to the left and changes the shape from sigmoidal to hyperbolic (Fig. 87.4). The first effect decreases oxygen content of the blood, whereas

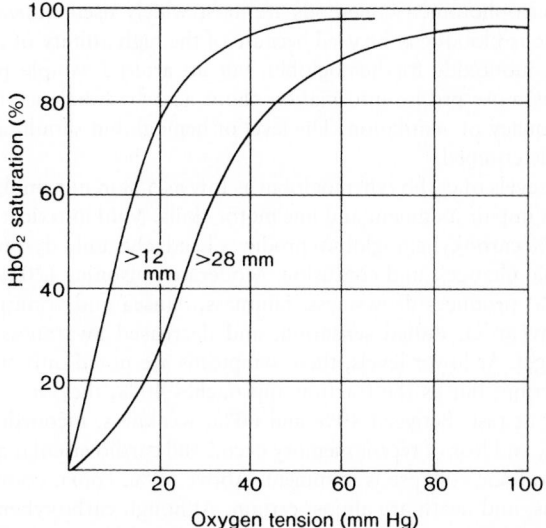

FIGURE 87.4 Carbon monoxide shifts the oxyhemoglobin dissociation curve to the left and changes its shape, making the unloading of oxygen in the tissues more difficult and provides an inadequate diffusion gradient. (*Left curve*, $P_{50} > 12$ mm; *right curve*, $P_{50} > 28$ mm.)

the second causes oxygen release at lower-than-normal tissue oxygen levels. Other endogenous (anemia) and exogenous (high altitude, or displacement of ambient oxygen during fires) factors contribute further to hypoxia. Although oxygen content of the blood is low, the PaO_2 remains normal. Because carotid body receptors respond to PaO_2, respiration may not be stimulated until late, when metabolic acidosis activates other centers. Tissue hypoxia increases cerebral blood flow, cerebrospinal fluid pressure, and cerebral capillary permeability, which predispose the patient to cerebral edema.

Carbon monoxide interacts with several other cellular proteins, including cytochrome oxidase. It appears to interfere with oxidative energy production and may generate free radicals, which exacerbate CNS dysfunction. Neuronal necrosis, as well as apoptosis, is seen in animal models in the frontal cortex, globus pallidus, and cerebellum, likely contributing to delayed cognitive effects such as deficits in learning, memory, and dementia. Carbon monoxide also binds to myoglobin; individuals, particularly with preexisting coronary disease, may develop cardiac ischemia and/or dysrhythmias.

Clinical Manifestations

History provides the most valuable clue to diagnosis. Carbon monoxide poisoning should be suspected in all fire victims and considered in children exposed to other hazards noted earlier. Presence or absence of the classically described "cherry red" skin color is of no diagnostic value. In fact, patients with thermal injury may appear red, whereas those with vasoconstriction may be quite pale. Both color and respiratory rate may be deceptive and may lead the physician away from recognition of severe tissue hypoxia. PaO_2 and arterial saturation as determined by pulse oximetry (SaO_2) are likely to be normal in carbon monoxide intoxication; low values reflect coexistent pulmonary dysfunction.

Determination of blood levels of carboxyhemoglobin may help document the diagnosis and may aid prognosis.

Spectrophotometric methods are most widely used clinically. Venous blood may be used because of the high affinity of carbon monoxide for hemoglobin, but an arterial sample provides more precise information about acid–base balance and adequacy of ventilation. The level of hemoglobin should also be determined.

Levels of carboxyhemoglobin as low as 5% in nonsmokers may impair judgment and fine motor skills. Mild intoxication (20% carboxyhemoglobin) produces headache, mild dyspnea, visual changes, and confusion. Moderate poisoning (20% to 40%) produces drowsiness, faintness, nausea and vomiting, tachycardia, dulled sensation, and decreased awareness of danger. At lower levels, these symptoms are noted only with exertion, but as the fraction approaches 40%, they are present at rest. Between 40% and 60%, weakness, incoordination, and loss of recent memory occur, and cardiovascular and neurologic collapse is imminent. Above 60%, coma, convulsions, and death are almost certain. Although carboxyhemoglobin levels and symptoms tend to follow the pattern just described, individual patients may be more or less symptomatic than predicted. An important caveat is that blood carboxyhemoglobin levels will fall rapidly with time and may not reflect cellular dysfunction, especially in high-demand tissues of the heart and CNS.

Patients with severe poisoning are peculiarly vulnerable to pressure trauma to skin, subcutaneous tissue, and muscle, especially at sites that support body weight or that are pinned under fallen objects. The history may suggest which sites are most vulnerable, and pain is an early symptom. Muscle breakdown and myoglobin deposition in renal tubular cells may precipitate acute renal failure.

A syndrome of delayed neuropsychologic sequelae (DNS) has been described in patients after exposure to carboxyhemoglobin. These patients develop neurologic symptoms acutely, appear to recover with treatment, and then exhibit a broad spectrum of neurologic and psychiatric abnormalities days to weeks after the exposure. Neuropsychiatric testing of children has obvious difficulties. Studies of DNS, many of which are methodologically flawed, have elucidated neither an exact mechanism nor a consensus on prevention and treatment.

Management

Most important and obvious is the immediate need to remove the victim from the contaminated environment (Table 87.3). Resuscitation should proceed according to general principles. As soon as possible, the patient suspected of suffering carbon monoxide poisoning should be provided 100% oxygen. If the patient is breathing spontaneously, this can be accomplished with a well-fitting mask supplied with nonrebreathing valves and a reservoir bag. Entrainment of room air precludes simple masks from providing more than 40% oxygen. The half-life of carboxyhemoglobin is approximately 4 hours in a patient breathing room air at sea level and approximately 1 hour if pure oxygen is inspired. The half-life is further reduced to less than 30 minutes if the patient has access to hyperbaric oxygen (HBO) at 2 to 3 atmospheres of pressure. There is no widespread agreement on indications for HBO, and transfer to a hyperbaric chamber should not jeopardize meticulous conventional cardiopulmonary stabilization. However, HBO administration

TABLE 87.3

MANAGEMENT OF CARBON MONOXIDE POISONING

Initial Management
Remove from contaminated environment
Cardiopulmonary resuscitation as needed
Provide 100% supplemental oxygen

Laboratory Determinations
Arterial blood gas analysis
Carboxyhemoglobin level, troponin
Complete blood cell count, electrolytes
Urinalysis for myoglobin

Monitoring
Heart rate, electrocardiogram, respiratory rate, blood pressure

Treatment
Correct anemia Hgb <10 g/dL
Continue supplemental oxygen until carboxyhemoglobin ≤5%
Decrease oxygen consumption with bed rest, avoid producing anxiety
Maintain urine output >1 mL/kg/h
Consider hyperbaric oxygen

may have effects beyond the mere reduction in carboxyhemoglobin half-life. Some studies in adults suggest a role for HBO in reducing the incidence of mortality and DNS. Well-controlled studies in children would have to be undertaken to answer these questions definitively, but would have obvious ethical and methodologic difficulties. In any case, early consultation with a poison control center or an HBO facility should be considered while the patient is receiving 100% oxygen (Table 87.4).

Severe metabolic acidosis, if present, should be treated with sodium bicarbonate, although adequacy of ventilation must be assessed to prevent paradoxical intracellular acidosis. The possibility of coexistent cyanide poisoning should be considered in patients involved in closed-space fires (especially where nitrogen-containing synthetic materials have burned) who have a persistent metabolic acidosis in the context of normal carboxyhemoglobin and methemoglobin. Cyanide has high mortality but a short half-life (approximately 1 hour), so empiric cyanide levels on patients who have survived the scene are not recommended generally unless confirmation is needed.

If cyanide poisoning is strongly suspected in an early-presenting patient, the cyanide antidote kit (formerly known as

TABLE 87.4

CONSIDERATIONS FOR HYPERBARIC OXYGEN THERAPY[a]

Neurologic symptoms or signs (syncope, seizure, coma) either on presentation or that persist despite normobaric oxygen
Signs of cardiac ischemia or metabolic acidosis
Pregnancy

[a]Consider early consultation with a poison control center or HBO facility.
HBO, hyperbaric oxygen.

the Lilly kit) may be considered. This two-step kit must be used with caution because the nitrite-containing first step induces methemoglobinemia. In case of doubt, the thiosulfate-containing second step, which is able to scavenge cyanide without significant additional toxicity, may be given alone. Anemia (hemoglobin less than 10 g per 100 mL) must be corrected to maximize oxygen-carrying capacity. Hydroxycobalamin (a synthetic form of vitamin B_{12}) was approved by the FDA in 2006 for use in cyanide poisoning. Its mechanism of action is that the hydroxyl group of the vitamin binds to free cyanide, forming the nontoxic cyanocobalamin. The dose is 70 mg/kg (max 5 grams) given over is minutes, with a repeat dose if necessary. The minimal side effects of hydroxocobalamin make this an attractive alternative to the traditional nitrite therapy.

If myoglobinemia or myoglobinuria is present, vigorous hydration and diuresis with furosemide (1 mg per kg intravenously) and/or mannitol (0.25 to 1 g per kg intravenously) with close attention to urine output may preserve renal function. If hydration and diuresis are ineffective, renal failure should be considered and fluids restricted accordingly (see Chapter 100).

The patient should be observed for at least 24 hours to identify other sequelae of smoke inhalation.

ENVIRONMENTAL AND EXERTIONAL HEAT ILLNESS

Background

Environmental and exertional heat illness occurs with excessive heat generation and storage. These conditions arise when high ambient temperature prevents heat dissipation by radiation or convection, and humidity limits cooling by sweat evaporation. The spectrum of illness is broad, including heat cramps, heat exhaustion, and heat stroke; the latter is an acute medical emergency with significant associated morbidity and mortality.

Heat illness is a serious tropical health hazard, but even in the United States, summer heat is responsible for significant morbidity and mortality. Heat waves, defined as more than 3 consecutive days of ambient temperatures greater than 32.2°C (90°F), may bring epidemic illness and death. During the period 1979 to 1999, more than 8,000 heat-related deaths were reported nationally, and nearly half were known to be weather related. During the California heat wave of 2006, it was estimated that for every rise in temperature by 10 degrees Fahrenheit, that there was a 9% increase in daily mortality for all counties as a whole. The elderly are most vulnerable (more than 80% of cases occur in people older than 50), but heat illness is also significant among healthy young people. Of the weather-related deaths noted previously for which the age of the decedent was recorded, 164 (4%) occurred in children younger than 15 years.

Military recruits, laborers, and athletes who work in a hot, humid atmosphere are notoriously vulnerable. Obesity, physical disability, heart disease, and alcohol and drug use increase risk. Pediatricians need to understand the special risk to children with cystic fibrosis or congenital absence of sweat glands, children receiving medications that cause oligohidrosis, infants left in automobiles on hot days, and young athletes. Heat stroke remains the third most common cause (after head injury

and cardiac disorders) of exercise-related mortality among U.S. high-school athletes, despite the fact that survival following acute heat stroke has improved over the last century from an estimated 20% to more than 90%.

Pathophysiology

Under normal conditions, body core temperature is maintained constant within 0.6°C (1°F) when the environment varies from 9.4°C to 60°C (49°F to 140°F) in dry air. This represents a remarkable balance between heat production and heat loss by the body. Heat is produced as (i) a byproduct of basal metabolism, (ii) a consequence of muscle activity (including shivering), and (iii) the effects of thyroxine and sympathetic stimulation on cellular processes. Heat is lost by (i) conduction to objects and air, (ii) convection through air or liquid that surrounds tissues, (iii) evaporation, and (iv) radiation of infrared energy.

Conduction to objects represents a small fraction (about 3%) of heat lost. Conduction to air and convection represent another 12% in still air. As air movement increases, the proportion of heat lost by these mechanisms may increase to nearly 60%. Evaporative losses normally account for 25% of heat lost, and radiant heat losses account for about 60%. However, the body gains heat by conduction and radiation when ambient temperature exceeds skin temperature and loses heat only by evaporation. High ambient humidity and absence of convection currents decrease the rate of evaporation.

Heat-sensitive centers of the posterior hypothalamus control sympathetic tone. This tone regulates vasoconstriction of arterioles and subcutaneous arteriovenous anastomoses, which, in turn, controls heat conduction from the body core to the skin. Flow through these areas may represent 0% to 30% of total cardiac output. High flow provides efficient heat transfer from the body core to the skin, which is an effective radiator. Low flow to the skin prevents radiation and allows only inefficient diffusion through the insulating skin and subcutaneous tissues.

When body temperature rises, blood in the preoptic area of the anterior hypothalamus is warmer than optimal. Impulses from this area increase and are conducted through autonomic pathways to the spinal cord and then, through cholinergic fibers to the sweat glands, where sweat is released. Exercise and certain emotional states release circulating epinephrine and norepinephrine to increase sweat production.

The sweat gland is composed of two portions. The deep, coiled portion actively elaborates a precursor secretion in response to cholinergic stimulation. At low rates of sweating, much of the NaCl contained in the precursor secretion is reabsorbed before the sweat is conducted through the straight portion to the skin. At higher rates, flow exceeds the capacity of the duct to reabsorb solute, and substantial total body NaCl depletion may occur.

In the unacclimatized adult, sweating may vary from negligible amounts at rest in a cool, dry environment to 1.5 L per hour during vigorous activity in hot weather. Long-term exposure to tropical weather results in a steady increase in sweating rate over approximately 6 weeks, to a maximum of about 4.0 L per hour. Initially, enormous salt losses may occur (15 to 20 g per day). However, aldosterone secretion rises and stimulates active reabsorption of NaCl in the ducts of sweat glands (as in the kidney), and salt losses decrease to a normal 3 to 5 g per day.

In humans, behavioral control over temperature regulation is probably as important as all other mechanisms. When body temperature changes, sensations of excessive warmth or cold prompt efforts to correct the situation. One moves out of the cold or into the shade, selects warmer or cooler clothing, initiates maneuvers that warm or cool the environment, or alters levels of activity. Light-colored clothing permeable to moisture but impervious to radiant heat from the environment prevents the formation of an insulating layer of air and allows for heat loss by evaporation.

Clinical Findings

Three types of heat illness are recognized and represent different physiologic disturbances (Table 87.5). Heat cramps refer to the sudden onset of brief, intermittent, and excruciating cramps in muscles after they have been subjected to severe work stress. Cramps tend to occur after the work is done, on relaxing, or on taking a cool shower. Occasionally, abdominal muscle cramps may simulate an acute abdomen. The usual victim is highly conditioned and acclimatized. Typically, these individuals can produce sweat in large quantities and provide themselves with adequate fluid replacement but inadequate salt replacement. Electrolyte depletion is probably the cause of cramps.

Most spasms last less than a minute, but some persist for several minutes, during which a rock-hard mass may be palpated in the affected muscle. Cramps often occur in clusters. Rapid voluntary contraction of a muscle, contact with cold air or water, or passive extension of a flexed limb may reproduce a cramp. Laboratory investigation reveals hyponatremia and hypochloremia and virtually absent urine sodium. The blood urea nitrogen (BUN) level is usually normal but may be mildly elevated.

Heat exhaustion is less clearly demarcated from heat stroke than are heat cramps. In most cases, water depletion predominates because individuals who live and work in a hot environment do not always voluntarily replace their total water deficit. Progressive lethargy, intense thirst, and inability to work or play progress to headache, vomiting, CNS dysfunc-

TABLE 87.5

CHARACTERISTICS OF HEAT ILLNESS

Illness	Who	When	Characteristic	Laboratory
Heat cramp	Highly conditioned Highly acclimatized Adequate water replacement Inadequate salt replacement	After severe work stress Usually when relaxing Triggered by cold	Excruciating cramps in affected muscle occurring in clusters (may simulate acute abdomen)	↓ Serum Na$^+$Cl$^-$↓↓ Urine Na$^+$ BUN nl or slightly ↑
Heat exhaustion A. Predominant water depletion	Generally unacclimatized Working in hot environment Inadequate water replacement	During periods of hot weather After physical exertion	T ≤ 39°C (102.2°F) Progressive lethargy Thirst Inability to work or play Headache Vomiting CNS dysfunction ↓ BP ↑ HR	Na, Cl ↑ Hct ↑ Urine-specific gravity ↑
B. Predominant salt depletion	Unacclimatized Inadequate salt replacement Cystic fibrosis	During periods of hot weather After physical exertion	T ≥ 39°C (102.2°F) Weakness, fatigue Headache GI symptoms exertion Prominent Muscle cramp ↑ HR Orthostatic hypotension	Na ↓ Hct ↑ Urine Na ↓↓
Heat stroke	Extremes of age Overdressed infants Infants in closed cars Extreme exertion (young athletes) Drug use (e.g., phenothiazines)	During heat waves After excessive exertion	T ≥ 41°C (105.8°F) Hot skin Circulatory collapse Severe CNS dysfunction Rhabdomyolysis Renal failure	Na, Cl nl or ↑ CPK ↑ Ca ↓

BUN, blood urea nitrogen; nl, normal; T, temperature; Hct, hematocrit; CNS, central nervous system; BP, blood pressure; HR, heart rate; GI, gastrointestinal; CPK, creatinine phosphokinase.

tion (including hyperventilation, paresthesias, agitation, incoordination, or actual psychosis), hypotension, and tachycardia. Hemoconcentration, hypernatremia, hyperchloremia, and urinary concentration are typical. Body temperature may rise but rarely to higher than 39°C (102.2°F). If unattended, heat exhaustion may progress to frank heat stroke.

Heat exhaustion may also occur secondary to predominant salt depletion. As in heat cramps, water losses are replaced but without adequate electrolyte supplementation. Symptoms include profound weakness and fatigue, frontal headache, anorexia, nausea, vomiting, diarrhea, and severe muscle cramps. Tachycardia and orthostatic hypotension may be noted.

Unlike heat cramp victims, these patients with heat exhaustion and salt depletion are typically unacclimatized. Hyponatremia, hemoconcentration, and significantly diminished urine sodium are consistent findings. Children with cystic fibrosis, particularly those who are young and unable to meet increased salt requirements, are at risk for electrolyte depletion because salt losses in their sweat apparently do not respond to acclimatization and aldosterone stimulation of the sweat gland.

Heat stroke (Table 87.5) is a life-threatening emergency. Classic signs are hyperpyrexia [41°C (105.8°F) or higher]; hot, dry skin that is pink or ashen, depending on the circulatory state; and severe CNS dysfunction. Often, but not invariably, sweating ceases before the onset of heat stroke.

The onset of the CNS disturbance may be abrupt, with sudden loss of consciousness. Often, however, premonitory signs and symptoms exist. These include a sense of impending doom, headache, dizziness, weakness, confusion, euphoria, gait disturbance, and combativeness. Posturing, incontinence, seizures, hemiparesis, and pupillary changes may occur. Any level of coma may be noted. Cerebrospinal fluid findings are usually normal. The extent of damage to the CNS is related to the time and extent of hyperpyrexia and to the adequacy of circulation. Once the body temperature is lowered, consciousness is usually restored quickly, but coma may persist for 24 hours or more.

Patients able to maintain cardiac output adequate to meet the enormously elevated circulatory demand are most likely to survive. Initially, the pulse is rapid and full, with an increased pulse pressure. Total peripheral vascular resistance falls as a result of vasodilation in the skin and muscle beds, and splanchnic flow diminishes. If hyperpyrexia is not corrected, ashen cyanosis and a thin, rapid pulse herald a falling cardiac output. The cause may be either direct thermal damage to the myocardium or significant pulmonary hypertension with secondary right ventricular failure. Even after body temperature is returned to normal, cardiac output remains elevated and peripheral vascular resistance remains low for several hours, resembling the compensatory hyperemia after ischemia noted in posttrauma, postshock, and postseptic states. Persistently circulating vasoactive substances probably account for this phenomenon.

Severe dehydration is not a necessary component of heat stroke but may play a role if prolonged sweating has occurred. Electrolyte abnormalities may occur, especially in the unacclimatized victim, if NaCl has not been replaced. In acclimatized persons, NaCl is conserved but often at the expense of a severe potassium deficit. Polyuria is sometimes noted, often vasopressin resistant and possibly related to hypokalemia. Acute

tubular necrosis may be seen in as many as 35% of cases and probably reflects combined thermal, ischemic, and circulating pigment damage. Hypoglycemia may also be noted.

Nontraumatic rhabdomyolysis and acute renal failure have been described as consequences of various insults, including hyperthermia and strenuous exercise in unconditioned persons. Clinically, there may or may not be musculoskeletal pain, tenderness, swelling, or weakness. Laboratory evidence includes elevated serum creatinine phosphokinase (CPK) (300 to 120,000 units) and urinalysis that is orthotolidine (Hematest)-positive without red blood cells and shows red-gold granular casts. Typically, serum potassium and creatinine levels rise rapidly relative to BUN. An initial hypocalcemia, possibly a consequence of deposition into damaged muscle, progresses to hypercalcemia during the diuretic phase a few days to 2 weeks later.

Management

Most cases of heat cramps are mild and do not require specific therapy. Rest and increased salt intake from liberally salted foods are sufficient. In severe cases with prolonged or frequent cramps, IV infusion of normal saline is effective. Approximately 5 to 10 mL per kg over 15 to 20 minutes should be adequate to relieve cramping. Oral intake of fluids and salted foods can then complete restoration of salt and water balance.

Heat exhaustion as a result of predominant water depletion is treated with rehydration and rest in a cooled or well-ventilated place. If the child is able to eat, he or she should be encouraged to drink cool liquids and be allowed unrestricted dietary sodium. If weakness or impaired consciousness precludes oral correction, IV fluids are given as in any hypernatremic dehydration.

Exhaustion caused by predominant salt depletion also requires rest in a cool environment. Alert, reasonably strong children can be given relatively salty drinks, such as tomato juice, and should be encouraged to salt solid foods. Hypotonic fluids (e.g., water, Kool-Aid®) should be avoided until salt repletion has begun. Patients with CNS symptoms or gastrointestinal (GI) dysfunction may be rehydrated with IV isotonic saline or Ringer's lactate. Initial rapid administration of 20 mL per kg over 20 minutes should improve intravascular volume with return of BP and pulse toward normal. Further correction of salt and water stores should be achieved over 12 to 24 hours. In especially severe cases with intractable seizures or muscle cramps, hypertonic saline solutions may be used. The initial dose of 3% saline solution is 5 mL per kg by IV over is minutes for seizures, more slowly over 30–60 minutes for cramping. An additional 5 mL per kg should be infused over the next 4 to 6 hours.

Treatment of heat stroke centers on two priorities: (i) immediate elimination of hyperpyrexia and (ii) support of the cardiovascular system (Table 87.6). Clothing should be removed and patients should be cooled actively. They should be transported to an emergency facility in open or air-conditioned vehicles. Ice packs may be placed at the neck, groin, and axilla. Although immersion in ice water may be a more efficient means of lowering body temperature, it may complicate other support and monitoring. Among the most efficient but invasive and rarely used methods is iced peritoneal lavage. Iced peritoneal lavage is contraindicated in the pregnant patient and those with a history of abdominal surgery. In addition, a canine model of heat stroke suggested that an evaporative

TABLE 87.6

MANAGEMENT OF HEAT STROKE

Initial Management
Remove clothing
Begin active cooling
Transport to cool environment
Cardiovascular support

Laboratory Determinations
Complete blood cell count, PT/PTT
Electrolytes, BUN, creatinine, CPK, Ca, P
Urinalysis including myoglobin
Arterial blood gas

Monitoring
Temperature
Heart rate, electrocardiogram, blood pressure
Peripheral pulses and perfusion
Urine output
Central nervous system function

Treatment
Active cooling
Fluids
   Maintenance: 5% dextrose in normal saline at maintenance
     rates
   Resuscitation: ≤20 mg/kg lactated Ringer's or 0.9%
     sodium chloride
   Additional fluids as determined by electrolytes, output, and
     hemodynamic status
Inotropic support
   Dobutamine 5–20 μg/kg/min or
Diuresis for myoglobinuria
   Maintain urine output >1 mL/kg/h
   Consider furosemide 1 mg/kg
   Consider mannitol 0.25–1 g/kg

PT, prothrombin time; PTT, partial thromboplastin time; BUN, blood
urea nitrogen; CPK, creatine phosphokinase.

technique in which fans blew room air over subjects sprayed
with 15°C (59°F) tap water was equally efficient. Temperature
should be monitored continuously with a rectal probe, and
active cooling should be discontinued when rectal temperature
falls to approximately 38.5°C (101.3°F). Sedation and paralysis of the patient can greatly augment the cooling process.

The severity of the patient's presentation determines the
degree of cardiovascular support. If the skin is flushed and BP
adequate, lowering body temperature with close attention to
heart rate and BP may be sufficient. Although severe dehydration and electrolyte disturbances are uncommon, these should
be assessed and corrected if necessary. Fluids cooled to 4°C
(39.2°F) hasten temperature correction but may precipitate
arrhythmias on contact with an already stressed myocardium.
Adult patients rarely have required more than 20 mL per kg
over the first 4 hours, but determinations of electrolytes,
hematocrit, and urine output, and clinical assessment of central vascular volume should guide precise titration of fluids
and electrolytes.

Patients with ashen skin, tachycardia, and hypotension demonstrate cardiac output insufficient to meet circulatory
demand and are in imminent danger of death. Monitoring of

the electrocardiogram (EKG) and arterial BP (with an
indwelling arterial line) should determine support.

Inotropic support may be required after a fluid challenge
(see Chapter 3). Dobutamine is probably most appropriate: its
β-agonist properties increase myocardial contractility and
maintain peripheral vasodilation. Isoproterenol has been used
successfully in the past but may cause myocardial oxygen consumption to exceed oxygen delivery. Additional fluid resuscitation may be necessary with the initiation of either dobutamine or isoproterenol to fill the effectively increased vascular
space. Normal saline or albumin should be given to maintain
the arterial BP in the normal range. Dopamine may also be
effective, infused at rates compatible with inotropic support
without vasoconstriction (i.e. 5–15 $m$cg/kg/min). In cases of
extreme hemodynamic instability, extracorporeal circulation
may provide both circulatory support and a means of rapid
temperature correction.

Agents with α-agonist characteristics (epinephrine and norepinephrine) are not recommended for initial management;
they cause peripheral vasoconstriction, interfere with heat dissipation, and may compromise hepatic and renal flow further.
Atropine and other anticholinergic drugs that inhibit sweating
should be avoided.

Renal function should be monitored carefully, especially in
patients who have been hypotensive or in whom vigorous exercise precipitated heat stroke. In general, BUN, creatinine, electrolytes, calcium, and urinalysis for protein and myoglobin
should be obtained. Once the patient's vascular volume has
been restored and arterial pressure normalized, hourly urine
output should be monitored. If urine output is inadequate (less
than 0.5 mL per kg per hour) in the face of normovolemia and
adequate cardiac output, furosemide (1 mg per kg by IV)
and/or mannitol (0.25 to 1 g per kg by IV) should be given. If
the response is poor, acute renal failure should be suspected,
and fluids should be restricted accordingly. Rapidly rising BUN
or potassium should prompt consideration of early dialysis.

ACCIDENTAL HYPOTHERMIA

Background

Elevated body temperature is a routine concern for most
physicians, especially pediatricians. However, hypothermia,
defined as core temperature at or less than 35°C (95°F), is
often overlooked. Reduced body temperature may be a consequence or cause of many disorders but is diagnosed only if
health-care providers maintain a high index of suspicion.

Hypothermia was responsible for nearly 14,000 deaths in
the United States from 1979 to 1998. Populations at high risk
for hypothermia are similar to those vulnerable to heat illness.
Neonates and the elderly are most often affected. Of the many
risk factors for hypothermia, vehicular breakdown is most relevant to young children. Physical disability, especially immobilizing conditions, and drug or alcohol ingestion increase risk
at any age. Healthy young people who work or play to
exhaustion in a cold environment are also at risk. The rising
popularity of cold weather sports is producing more cases of
accidental hypothermia. However, environmental conditions
need not be extreme, and the diagnosis should be considered
even in temperate climates.

Primary CNS dysfunction, endocrinopathies, sepsis, protein–calorie malnutrition, and various metabolic derangements may also depress core temperature.

Mortality rates, reported from 30% to 80%, depend more on the underlying disorder than on the degree of temperature depression.

Pathophysiology

Human core temperature is normally maintained within 0.6 °C (1°F). As described in the "Environmental and Exertional Heat Illness" section, this represents a fine balance between heat production and heat loss. When core temperature begins to fall to less than 37°C (98.6°F), physiologic mechanisms that produce and conserve heat are activated. Cooled blood stimulates the hypothalamus to increase muscle tone and metabolism (oxidative phosphorylation and high-energy phosphate production) and to augment heat production by 50% during nonshivering thermogenesis. When muscle tone reaches a critical level, shivering begins, and heat production increases two to four times basal levels.

Although the surface temperature of the body, especially of the extremities, may drop to nearly the environmental temperature, several mechanisms work to conserve heat and to protect blood and core structures from ambient air temperature, humidity, and wind. Sweating is abolished, decreasing heat loss by evaporation (unless there is external moisture), whereas vasoconstriction of cutaneous and subcutaneous vessels reduce losses further. Piloerection, which in many animal species traps an insulating layer of air next to the skin, occurs but is ineffective in humans.

When any component of the balance between heat production and loss is altered, the risk of hypothermia increases. Neonates, with large surface:volume ratios and small amounts of subcutaneous fat, conserve heat poorly and are unable to produce heat by shivering. The capacity for nonshivering thermogenesis—primarily metabolism of brown fat—is intact, but oxygen consumption is significantly increased. Hypoxemia may result, as well as metabolic acidosis, hypoglycemia, and hypocalcemia. Therefore, minor deviations in the thermal environment may produce hypothermia in neonates. More pronounced environmental stresses are required to overcome the greater compensatory capacity of older children.

Immersion in cold water causes the most rapid fall in body temperature. Struggling or swimming movements increase blood flow to the extremities and hasten hypothermia. Death occurs in 15 minutes in water at 0°C (32°F), but significant hypothermia may occur even in water at 21°C (69.8°F). Exposure to extreme cold is an obvious risk, taxing the body's ability to conserve and produce heat maximally. Voluntary motor activity produces heat, and physically fit, acclimatized persons may be able to increase activity to balance heat loss even in exceptionally cold environments. However, the metabolic cost of physical activity increases in the cold, and less fit persons quickly exhaust muscle glycogen supplies, are unable to maintain adequate heat production, and are likely to become hypothermic quickly. Wet, windy conditions hasten loss of body heat and may precipitate hypothermia even in temperate environments. Adolescents are psychologically less likely to conserve energy and to take preventive or corrective measures, thus increasing their risk of hypothermia.

Once homeostatic mechanisms fail and core temperature falls, predictable physiologic changes take place. If shivering does not occur, basal metabolic rate decreases steadily, reaching 50% of normal at 28°C (82.4°F). As a result, oxygen consumption and carbon dioxide production decline. The oxygen–hemoglobin dissociation curve shifts to the left.

Although respiratory depression occurs late, impaired mental status and cold-induced bronchorrhea predispose the patient to airway obstruction and aspiration. Acid–base balance follows no predictable pattern. Respiratory acidosis occurs, but tissue hypoxia, increased lactic acid production, and decreased lactate clearance by the liver produce metabolic acidosis.

Decreased heart rate contributes primarily to a drop in cardiac output. Peripheral vasoconstriction and an early increase in central vascular volume cause a transient rise in BP, which later falls to become clinically significant at less than 25°C (77°F). A variety of cardiac conduction abnormalities arise, including decreased sinus rate, T-wave inversion, prolongation of EKG intervals, and the appearance of pathognomonic J waves (Fig. 87.5), which may provide the first clue to the diagnosis. Atrial fibrillation may occur at temperatures less than 33°C (91.4°F) but is usually not hemodynamically significant. At less than 28°C (82.4°F), myocardial irritability increases dramatically, and ventricular fibrillation becomes likely.

Cold-induced vasoconstriction and elevated central blood volume and pressure contribute to a diuresis, which subsequently diminishes intravascular volume. At lower temperatures, tubular dysfunction allows salt and water loss. Acidosis causes potassium to shift from cells to the urine, where it is eliminated. Increased capillary permeability results in loss of fluid into the extracellular space.

Hematologic abnormalities may also occur. Plasma loss causes an increased hematocrit level, whereas splenic sequestration may be responsible for a fall in white blood cell and platelet counts. Disseminated intravascular coagulation is sometimes seen.

CNS abnormalities are progressive. Each fall of 1°C produces a 6% to 7% decline in cerebral blood flow. Plasma loss

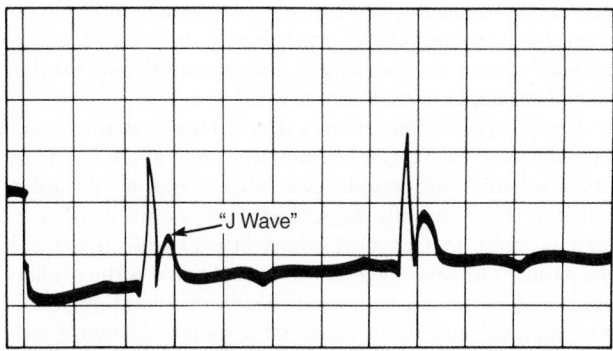

FIGURE 87.5 J wave (Osborn wave), pathognomonic of hypothermia. Rounded contour distinguishes it from an RSR′ pattern. It may also be confused with a T wave with a short Q-T interval. (Reprinted from Welton D, Mattox K, Miller R, et al. Treatment of profound hypothermia. *JAMA* 1978;240:2291–2292, with permission.)

increases blood viscosity, which further contributes to impaired cerebral microcirculation and mentation. Peripheral nerve conduction slows, and deep tendon reflexes decrease. Pupils dilate and react sluggishly, if at all, at less than 30°C (86°F). The electroencephalogram deteriorates progressively with falling temperature, from high-voltage slow waves, to burst suppression patterns, to electrical silence at 20°C (68°F).

GI motility decreases at less than 34°C (93.2°F). The liver's capacity for detoxification or conjugation of drugs and products of metabolism is poor. Insulin release abates, and serum glucose rises. Frank pancreatic necrosis may also occur, producing clinical evidence of pancreatitis.

Clinical Manifestations

The astute clinician must consider the possibility of hypothermia if the diagnosis is to be made in a timely manner. A history of sudden immersion in icy water or prolonged exposure to low environmental temperatures provides the obvious clue, but significantly low core temperatures may occur under much less suggestive circumstances. Examples include trauma victims found unconscious or immobile on a wet, windy, summer day; infants who are from inadequately heated homes or who are left exposed during prolonged medical evaluation; adolescents with anorexia nervosa; and patients with sepsis or burns. Severe hypothermia, coma, and cardiac arrest may present as the sudden infant death syndrome. Hypothermia may go undetected if the patient's temperature falls below the lower limit of the thermometer in use or if the thermometer is not shaken down adequately. Low-recording thermometers should be available in EDs and intensive care units. This diagnosis should be kept in mind for any patient with a suggestive history or coma of uncertain cause.

Physical examination reveals a pale or cyanotic patient. At mild levels of hypothermia, mental status may be normal, but CNS function is progressively impaired with falling temperature until frank coma occurs at approximately 27°C (80.6°F). BP also falls steadily at less than 33°C (91.4°F) and may be undetectable. Heart rate slows gradually unless atrial or ventricular fibrillation occurs. Intense peripheral vasoconstriction and bradycardia may render the pulse inapparent or absent. At less than 32°C (89.6°F), shivering ceases, but muscle rigidity may mimic rigor mortis. Pupils may be dilated and may not react. Deep tendon reflexes are depressed or absent. Evidence of head trauma or other injury, drug ingestion, and frostbite should be sought (Figs. 87.6 and 87.7).

Severe hypothermia mimics death. However, the significant decrease in oxygen consumption may allow life to be sustained for long periods, even after cessation of cardiac function. Signs usually associated with certain death (i.e., dilated pupils or rigor mortis) have little prognostic value. If the patient's history suggests that hypothermia is the primary event and not a consequence of death, resuscitation should be attempted and death redefined as failure to revive with rewarming.

Initial laboratory tests should include CBC, platelet count, clotting studies, electrolytes, BUN and creatinine, glucose, serum amylase, and ABGs corrected for temperature (Table 87.7). Urine should be sent for drug screening.

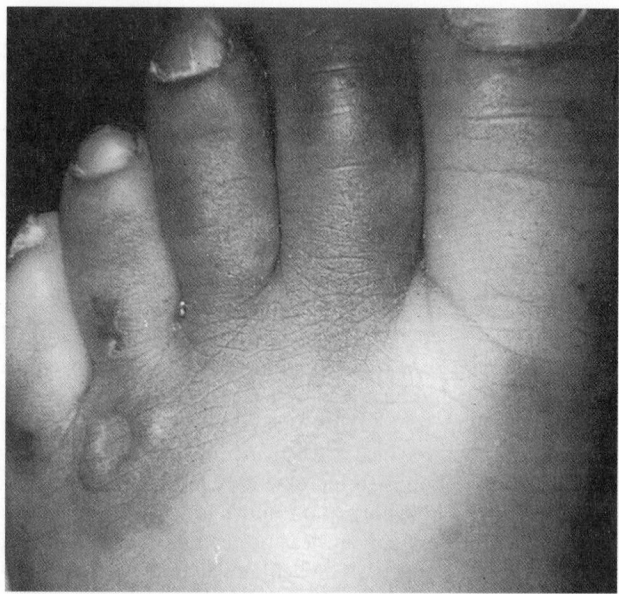

FIGURE 87.6 Frostbite of toes. Note the line of demarcation and ulcerative lesion.

Management

Therapy for hypothermia can be divided into two parts: general supportive measures and specific rewarming techniques (Table 87.8). Once hypothermia is diagnosed, temperature must be monitored continuously as treatment progresses.

All patients should be given supplemental oxygen. Patients with profuse secretions, respiratory depression, or impaired mental status should be intubated and mechanically ventilated. Intubation should be performed as gently as possible to minimize the risk of arrhythmias.

A decreased metabolic rate produces less carbon dioxide, and usual minute ventilation would produce respiratory alka-

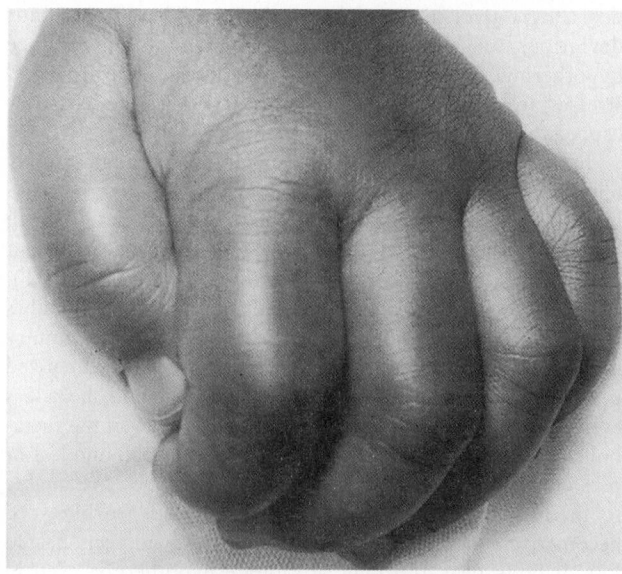

FIGURE 87.7 Swollen fingers of a child with cold exposure.

TABLE 87.7

EFFECT OF BODY TEMPERATURE ON ARTERIAL
BLOOD GASES MEASURED AT 37°C (98.6°F)

	For each elevation of 1°C	For each depression of 1°C
pH	−0.015	+0.015
$Paco_2$ (mm Hg)	+4.4%	−4.4%
Pao_2 (mm Hg)	+7.2%	−7.2%

losis, increasing the risk of dangerous arrhythmias. Therefore, ventilation should begin at approximately one-half the normal minute ventilation.

Assessment of acid–base status and ventilation in the hypothermic patient is the subject of considerable confusion. Blood gas machines heat the patient's blood sample to 37°C (98.6°F) before measuring pH and gas partial pressures [thus providing theoretical values if the patient were 37°C (98.6°F)]. If the patient's actual temperature is provided with the sample, the machine can correct the values according to the nomogram of Kelman and Nunn. (Table 87.7 shows one set of guidelines for appropriate correction.) However, it is most important to understand two concepts. The first is the ectothermic principle, which relies on the following aspect of physiology: disso-

TABLE 87.8

MANAGEMENT OF HYPOTHERMIA

Initial Management
Provide supplemental oxygen
Cardiopulmonary resuscitation for asystole, ventricular fibrillation

Laboratory Determinations
Arterial blood gas analysis corrected for temperature
Complete blood cell count, platelet count
Prothrombin time, partial thromboplastin time
Electrolytes, blood urea nitrogen, creatinine
Glucose, amylase
Urine drug screen

Monitoring
Heart rate, electrocardiogram, respiratory rate, blood pressure
Temperature
Consider central venous pressure

Treatment
Correct hypoxemia, hypercarbia
Correct hypokalemia
Correct hypoglycemia, 25% dextrose 1 g/kg IV
Tolerate hyperglycemia
Temperature
  ≥32°C (89.6°F): passive rewarming or simple external rewarming
  <32°C (89.6°F) (acute): external or core rewarming
  <32°C (89.6°F) (chronic): core rewarming
Fluid replacement
  (acute) 5% dextrose in normal saline at maintenance rates
  (chronic) normal saline, 5% albumin, and/or fresh-frozen plasma to maintain blood pressure

ciation of ions and partial pressures of gases are decreased in cooled blood. In hypothermia, therefore, neutral pH is higher, whereas "normal" Pco_2 is lower than is encountered at 37°C (98.6°F). For example, hypoventilation of the hypothermic patient with a pH of 7.5 would actually induce an undesirable respiratory acidosis. A second, more practical concept is that if the patient's blood volume is restored and oxygenation maintained, acidosis will be corrected spontaneously as the patient is warmed.

Heart rate and rhythm should be monitored continuously and the patient handled gently to avoid precipitation of life-threatening arrhythmias in an exquisitely irritable myocardium. Sinus bradycardia, atrial flutter, and atrial fibrillation are common but rarely of hemodynamic significance. Spontaneous reversion to sinus rhythm is the rule when temperature is corrected. Ventricular fibrillation may occur spontaneously or with trivial stimulation, especially at temperatures less than 28°C to 29°C (82.4°F to 84.2°F). Electrical defibrillation is warranted but frequently is ineffective until core temperature rises. Closed chest massage should be initiated and maintained until the temperature is higher than 30°C (86°F), when defibrillation is more likely to be effective. Drug therapy is rarely effective and fraught with hazards associated with decreased hepatic and renal metabolism.

Fluid replacement is essential. Relatively little plasma loss occurs in acute hypothermia (as it does after cold-water immersion), but losses may be great in hypothermia of longer duration. Normal saline or lactated Ringer's solution, warmed to about 43°C (109.4°F) in a blood-warming coil, is appropriate initially. Electrolyte determinations should guide further replacement. If clotting abnormalities occur, fresh-frozen plasma (10 mL per kg) is a useful choice for volume expansion (see Chapter 91). As temperature rises and peripheral vasoconstriction diminishes, hypovolemia is expected. Fluid volume should be sufficient to provide an adequate arterial BP.

Hypoglycemia, if present, is treated with glucose (0.5 to 1 g per kg by IV). Hyperglycemia, which may result from impaired insulin release in the hypothermic pancreas, should be tolerated to avoid severe hypoglycemia with rewarming.

A number of rewarming strategies exist (Fig. 87.8). Passive rewarming implies removal of the patient from a cold environment and use of blankets to maximize the effect of basal heat production. For patients with mild hypothermia [temperature higher than 32°C (89.6°F)], this may be adequate. As shown in the algorithm, the adequacy of perfusion and the degree of hypothermia are the major factors in the selection of rewarming strategies. For patients with an adequate pulse, passive rewarming is used as the initial strategy if the temperature is greater than 32°C and active core rewarming if the temperature is less than 32°C. Those with poor perfusion require active rewarming with a temperature greater than 32°C and ECMO, if available, with temperature less than 32°C.

Active rewarming is divided into external and core rewarming techniques. Electric blankets, hot-water bottles, overhead warmers, and thermal mattresses are simple, easily available sources of external heat. Immersion in warm-water baths is also possible but complicates monitoring or response to arrhythmias. These methods, however, cause early warming of the skin and extremities with peripheral vasodilation and shunting of cold, acidemic blood to the core. The well-known "afterdrop" of core temperature results. Severe

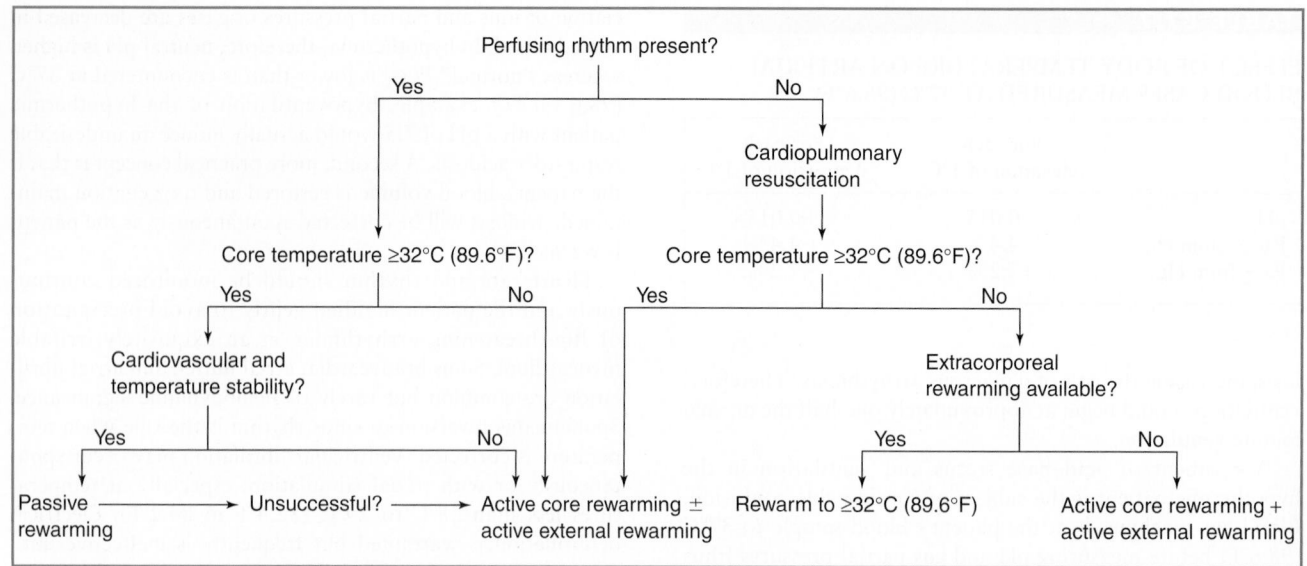

FIGURE 87.8 Algorithm for rewarming. (Adapted from Danzl DF, Pozos RS. Accidental hypothermia. *N Engl J Med* 1994;331(26):1756–1760.)

hypotension may also occur in chronic cases as vasodilation increases the effective vascular space. External rewarming techniques limited to the head and trunk may minimize vasodilation and afterdrop. In acute hypothermia, active external rewarming is appropriate, but there is some evidence that in chronic cases (more than 24 hours), mortality is higher if active external rewarming is used instead of simple passive techniques.

Core rewarming techniques are almost certainly more rapid and less likely to be associated with afterdrop, dangerous arrhythmias, or significant hypotension. These methods are especially valuable in the setting of severe chronic hypothermia [temperature less than 32°C (89.6°F)], where fluid shifts are most likely to occur. A nonshivering human model of severe hypothermia indicated that inhalation rewarming offered no rewarming advantage, whereas forced air warming (approximately 200 W) allowed a six- to tenfold increase in rewarming rate over controls. A canine study of experimental hypothermia found that heated aerosol inhalation alone contributed less heat than endogenous metabolism, but peritoneal lavage and pleural lavage had similar effect on rewarming (6°C per hour per m²). In humans, peritoneal dialysis with dialysate warmed to 43°C (109.4°F) is effective and requires only equipment routinely available in most hospitals. Limited clinical experience suggests that pleural lavage is a relatively simple and useful measure. Gastric or colonic irrigation has also been advocated, but placement of the intragastric balloon may precipitate dysrhythmias. Hemodialysis, extracorporeal blood rewarming, and mediastinal irrigation are effective but require mobilization of sophisticated equipment and personnel. Thus, new endovascular warming catheters, introduced after cannulization of the femoral vein and advancement to the inferior vena cava, use closed-loop circuitry to maintain the patient's temperature. In one case report, a woman's temperature increased by 2.8°C per hour, with a temperature of 37°C (98.6°F) achieved after 5 hours.

Each increment in core temperature produces a "new" patient who requires reassessment and appropriate management, but most children with hypothermia have a good prognosis. In patients with mild temperature depression [greater than 32°C (89.6°F)], external rewarming techniques, and supportive care based on vital signs, ABGs, and metabolic parameters such as glucose and calcium levels, should result in prompt recovery. Patients with temperatures less than 32°C (89.6°F), and especially those in whom hypothermia developed over 24 hours or more, require meticulous attention to continuously changing vital signs and metabolic needs. More elaborate core rewarming techniques are appropriate.

Frostbite, defined as injury or destruction of the skin and its underlying tissue, may result from extended exposure to freezing temperatures; the most typical body parts affected include the fingers, toes, ears and nose. The clinical presentation can range from superficial areas of pallor and edema to more severe hemorrhagic blisters and necrosis. Treatment can be broken into three phases. The initial prethaw period, usually performed by prehospital personnel, involves getting the patient out of the cold environment and then removing wet clothing. Soft padding should be applied to protect the affected area; care must be taken not to rub any of these tissues as this may cause further damage. The second phase, the actual rewarming process, will take place over the next 15 to 30 minutes with the affected area being immersed in water that is preheated to 40°C to 42°C. Because rewarming is quite painful, IV analgesics will likely be required. The third phase, the post-thaw period, involves careful wound management and application of loose, sterile dressings. Digits are typically separated with cotton, and extremities are splinted. Tetanus prophylaxis is warranted. Prophylactic antibiotic use is controversial; however, coverage for staphylococci, streptococci, and pseudomonas should be considered if there is any indication of an early infection. If amputation becomes a reality, long-term rehabilitation and possibly psychological support may be indicated.

HIGH-ALTITUDE ILLNESS

Background

Children may be exposed to higher altitudes through participation in sporting events, family vacations, and school activities. One source defines high altitude as 1,500 to 3,500 m (4,921 to 11,483 ft), very high altitude as 3,500 to 5,500 m (11,483 to 18,045 ft), and extreme altitude as greater than 5,500 m (18,045 ft). The diagnosis of altitude illness in children can be challenging, especially in the preverbal age group.

Factors that affect whether an individual gets sick include the altitude itself, rate of ascent, the altitude where sleeping occurs routinely, and the individual's physiology. Information regarding any potential genetic basis of high-altitude illness is limited, with no specific genetic polymorphisms identified to date. However, from an anatomical perspective, those who are able to tolerate brain swelling (i.e., the elderly whose brain size diminishes with age, or infants with their immature sutures and open fontanelles) are less susceptible to altitudes illnesses. A recent study from Switzerland finds the prevalence of acute mountain sickness (AMS) in both healthy children and adolescents to be 37.5%; fortunately, the symptoms were relatively mild and responded to supportive care without the need for descent.

Pathophysiology

Physiologic changes accompanying altitude may be attributed to hypobaric hypoxia. As altitude increases, barometric pressure decreases, with a subsequent reduction in the partial pressure of oxygen. Temperature also has an inverse relationship to altitude, with hypothermia compounding these hypoxic effects. The individual's response to hypoxia is to increase ventilation, which raises alveolar oxygen while reducing alveolar carbon dioxide simultaneously. Hypocapnia produces an alkalosis that, in turn, will serve as a "check and balance" for the body by limiting further increases in the respiratory rate. The pH returns to neutral as the kidneys excrete bicarbonate in response to this alkalosis. Acetazolamide (Diamox®) is used to inhibit carbonic anhydrase so carbon dioxide is not broken down; a metabolic acidosis is then created that allows the ventilatory rate to remain high and to maintain better oxygenation.

Clinical Manifestations

The four major illnesses seen with altitude include high-altitude headache (HAH), AMS, high-altitude cerebral edema (HACE), and high-altitude pulmonary edema (HAPE). Headache is typically the initial symptom upon climbing to higher altitudes; it may occur alone as in HAH or progress to AMS. AMS is defined as having a headache in the setting of at least one of four other symptoms: nausea/vomiting, fatigue, difficulty sleeping, and dizziness. Vasogenic edema is believed to explain the pathophysiology underlying AMS, with clinical progression to encephalopathy occurring as cerebral edema, or HACE, worsens. HAPE is the most common cause of death when exposed to high altitudes; younger individuals appear to be the most susceptible, especially children with upper respiratory symptoms. Pulmonary vascular leak leads to elevated pulmonary artery pressures.

Treatment

Treatment for HAH and mild AMS includes stopping the ascent and acclimatizing at the current altitude; acetazolamide given early will hasten this process. Analgesics, hydration, and antiemetics are also given for supportive care. Once AMS worsens, low-flow oxygen should be given in conjunction with acetazolamide and/or dexamethasone, and either HBO therapy with a portable compartment or immediate descent must occur. Therapy should be even more aggressive if HACE ensues, with dexamethasone administered in addition to oxygen, HBO, and immediate descent or even evacuation. The addition of the calcium-channel blocker nifedipine will reduce pulmonary vascular pressures in patients with HAPE. Exertion should be limited, oxygen provided, and either HBO or immediate descent arranged.

Prevention efforts may minimize an individual's chance of developing altitude illness. For example, different formulas exist regarding ideal ascent rates [i.e., above 3,000 meters (9,842 ft), sleeping elevations should not exceed the previous day by more than 300 to 500 meters and rest should occur every 3 days], following the mantra of "climb high, sleep low". If physically fit individuals follow such climbing guidelines, prophylaxis with acetazolamide is not typically required. However, because of the ease of getting to high elevations via car or airplane, individuals who ascend quickly, and/or have significant underlying diseases (hepatic, renal, or cardiopulmonary dysfunction in particular) may warrant acetazolamide prophylaxis. Most sources recommend using 250 mg twice daily, with pediatric dosing extrapolated from acetazolamide dosing for edema at 5 to 10 mg per kg per dose every 6 hours, not to exceed 1 g per day. Care should be taken in the individual with a sulfa allergy given acetazolamide contains a sulfa moiety; while the incidence of cross-reactivity is low at 7% to 10% in patients with a self-reported sulfa allergy, anaphylaxis has been reported and thus use of dexamethasone may be more prudent in these cases. More in-depth discussions of altitude illness and its prevention/treatment can be found in the references provided at the end of this chapter.

ELECTRICAL INJURIES

Background

Since the beginning of time, people have viewed lightning with fear and fascination. Cloud-to-ground lightning strikes occur 30 million times each year in the United States, primarily in afternoons and early evenings of the spring and summer, and in areas around the Gulf of Mexico. Lightning that strikes individuals carries a 30% risk of mortality and claims approximately 100 lives annually in the United States. The death rate is highest among children ranging from 15 to 19 years of age.

The last two centuries have witnessed the incorporation of controlled electricity into daily life and a better understanding of its properties and physiologic effects. Availability of electricity has also meant increased exposure to electrical hazards and accompanying injuries. Electrical injury is responsible for approximately 700 deaths per year, of which 10% are children. No federal safety standards exist for household electrical cords, the major cause of electrocution in children 12 years of age and younger. High-tension electrical injuries dominate in older children who climb on trees, buildings, or utility structures. Tasers and stun guns, which are high-voltage, low-current stimulators, cause pain due to involuntary muscle contractions. Young children may encounter them unintentionally if their caretakers are in law enforcement, or adolescents may feel their effects if they are being pursued by the police.

Pathophysiology

The spectrum of electrical injury is enormous, ranging from low-voltage household accidents to million-volt lightning strikes (Table 87.9). Appropriate management requires an understanding of the basic physical aspects of electricity, the physiologic responses to injury, and the potential for immediate and delayed damage.

The severity of electrical injury depends on six factors: (i) the resistance of skin, mucosa, and internal structures; (ii) the type of current (alternating or direct); (iii) the frequency of the current; (iv) the intensity; (v) the duration of contact; and (vi) the pathway taken by the current. Precise separation of the effect of these factors, which are interrelated, is impossible. Together, they produce either heat or current, and a variety of injuries result.

Resistance is a major factor determining the amount of current flow through tissue. Tissue injury is inversely related to resistance. Dry skin provides resistance of approximately 40,000 ohms, whereas thick, callused palms may provide up to 1×10^6 ohms. Thin, moist, or soiled skin lowers resistance to the 300- to 1,000-ohm range. The highly vascular, moist oral mucosa has even lower resistance.

Once surface resistance is overcome, current flows between points of contact, not necessarily along anatomic structures such as nerves or blood vessels. Although the resistance of various tissues is known, the voltage difference may determine the actual path taken. Low-voltage current usually follows the path of least resistance, whereas high-voltage current follows a more direct course to ground with less regard for tissue type. Assessment of the most likely current pathway does not reli-

ably predict injury. However, current that passes through the head or thorax may cause respiratory center or cardiac injury and increases the risk of cardiopulmonary arrest. Hand-to-hand flow carries risks of 60% mortality related to myocardial injury, spinal cord transection at C4 to C8, and tetanic contraction of thoracic muscles with suffocation. Hand-to-foot current passage is associated with cardiac arrhythmias but lower mortality (20%). Foot-to-foot injuries are rarely fatal.

The type of current is another important determinant of injury. Alternating current (AC) at low voltage is able to induce tetanic muscle contraction and is, therefore, more dangerous than direct current (DC). These contractions prevent the victim from releasing his grip ("locking-on"), thus extending the duration of contact. Normal household 60-Hz current changes direction 120 times per second, a frequency that induces an indefinite refractory state at neuromuscular junctions. Higher-frequency commercial currents are less likely to induce such a state and may be less harmful.

DC is used in medical settings for cardiac defibrillation, countershock, and pacing. Currents as low as 1 mA may trigger ventricular fibrillation, and high currents may damage the heart and conducting tissues directly. Lightning is another example of DC, discharged in a single, massive bolt that lasts 1/10,000 to 1/1,000 second. The brevity of exposure makes deep thermal injury unlikely.

In general, high-voltage injury is more dangerous than low-voltage injury. A higher voltage is more likely to cause "locking-on" and associated deep-tissue injury, although its tendency to throw victims from the source of current may mitigate this effect. The possibility of head and cervical spine injuries must be considered in these cases. The value of the current, or amperage, is of even greater importance than the voltage. Flow as low as 1 to 10 mA may be perceived as a tingling sensation. Progressively higher flows may paralyze muscles and ventilation, precipitate ventricular fibrillation, and cause deep-tissue burns.

Clinical Manifestations

Electrical injury may produce a variety of clinical pictures, ranging from local damage to widespread multisystem disturbances. Typically, deceptively small entry and exit wounds mask extensive damage to subcutaneous tissue, muscle, nerves, and blood vessels. Direct effects on the heart and

TABLE 87.9

LIGHTNING VERSUS HIGH-VOLTAGE ELECTRICAL INJURY

Factor	Lightning	High voltage
Duration	Brief	Prolonged
Energy level	100,000,000 V 200,000 amps	Much lower
Type of current	Direct	Usually alternating
Shock wave	Present	Absent
Cardiac	Asystole	Ventricular fibrillation
Burns	Superficial, minor	Deep, frequently obscured
Renal failures	Rare	Common secondary to myoglobinuria
Fasciotomy and amputation	Rare	Common, early, extensive

nervous system are particularly common, and injury to all other symptoms can occur. Much of the injury is revealed immediately, but late complications are often encountered.

Victims of the most severe accidents are commonly pulseless, apneic, and unresponsive. Current that passes directly through the heart may induce ventricular fibrillation. Brainstem (medullary) paralysis or tetanic contractions of thoracic muscles may result in cardiopulmonary collapse. Lightning injury is capable of inducing asystole, from which the heart may recover spontaneously, but the accompanying respiratory failure is commonly prolonged. Unless ventilation is initiated promptly, hypoxia leads to secondary ventricular fibrillation and death.

Other cardiac disorders, including arrhythmias and conduction defects, are common among survivors. Supraventricular tachycardia, atrial and ventricular extrasystoles, right bundle branch block, and complete heart block are most common. Complaints of crushing or stabbing precordial pain may accompany nonspecific ST-T wave changes. Some patients sustain myocardial damage or even ventricular wall perforation. Despite evidence of important cardiac injuries, patients without secondary hypoxic-ischemic injury usually regain good myocardial function.

Nervous system injury is also extremely common and may involve the brain, spinal cord, peripheral motor and sensory nerves, as well as sympathetic fibers. Loss of consciousness, seizures, amnesia, disorientation, deafness, visual disturbances, sensory deficits, hemiplegia, and quadriparesis occur acutely but may be transient. Vascular damage may produce subdural, epidural, or intraventricular hemorrhage.

Additional problems develop within hours to days after injury. The syndrome of inappropriate antidiuretic hormone secretion may precipitate herniation in rare cases. Electroencephalograms reveal diffuse slowing, epileptiform discharges, or burst suppression patterns, but they may not have prognostic significance. Spinal cord dysfunction yields more motor than sensory deficit. Peripheral neuropathies with patchy distribution may reflect direct thermal injury, vascular compromise, or current flow itself. A variety of autonomic disturbances may resolve spontaneously or persist as reflex sympathetic dystrophy.

Ocular damage is common, particularly after lightning strikes. Direct thermal or electrical injury, intensive light, and confusion contribute to the presentation. Findings include corneal lesions, hyphema, uveitis, iridocyclitis, and vitreous hemorrhage. Choroidal rupture, retinal detachment, and chorioretinitis occur less often. Autonomic disturbances in a lightning victim may cause fixed dilated pupils, which should not serve as a criterion for brain death without extensive investigation of other neurologic and ocular functions. Cataracts and optic atrophy are possible late developments.

Electrical injury may induce direct or indirect complications in other organ systems. Tetanic contractions may cause joint dislocations and fractures, especially of the upper-extremity long bones and vertebrae. Fractures of the skull and other long bones may occur when high-tension shock throws the victim from the site of contact. Early cardiopulmonary insufficiency, as well as direct renal effects, may cripple renal function. Damaged muscle releases myoglobin and CPK. As in crush injuries, myoglobin may induce renal tubular damage and kidney failure. Pleural damage may cause large effusions, whereas primary lung injury or aspiration of gastric contents may lead to pneumonitis. Gastric dilation, ileus, diffuse GI hemorrhage, and visceral perforation may occur immediately or later.

In addition to burns at the site of primary contact, burns are common where current has jumped across flexed joints. Such burns are most common on the volar surface of the forearm and across the elbow and axilla. Arcing current may also ignite clothing and produce typical thermal burns. Entry and exit wounds and arc burns are notoriously poor predictors of internal damage. Tissue that appears viable initially may become edematous and then ischemic or frankly gangrenous over several days. Diminished peripheral pulses may provide immediate evidence of vascular damage, but strong pulses do not guarantee vascular integrity. Blood flow falls to a minimum at about 36 hours, but current or thermal damage may lead to vasospasm, delayed thrombosis, ischemic necrosis, or aneurysm formation and hemorrhage weeks after the injury. Viable major arteries near occluded nutrient arteries may account for apparently adequate circulation and uneven destruction of surrounding tissues.

Young children are vulnerable to orofacial burns, especially of the lips (Fig. 87.9). These full-thickness burns of the upper and lower lips and oral commissure usually involve mucosa, submucosa, muscle, nerves, and blood vessels. The lesion usually has a pale, painless, well-demarcated, depressed center with surrounding pale gray tissue and erythematous border. After a few hours, the wound margin extends and marked edema occurs. Drooling is common. The eschar separates in 2 to 3 weeks and bleeding may occur at this time; granulation tissue gradually fills the wound. Scarring may produce lip eversion, microstomia, and loss of function. Damage to facial or even carotid arteries may result in delayed hemorrhage. Devitalization of deciduous and secondary teeth may occur.

Inadequately debrided burned or gangrenous tissue provides a medium for serious infection. Staphylococcal, pseudomonal, and clostridrial species are common pathogens in the extremities. Streptococci and oral anaerobic organisms may infect mouth wounds.

Management

The first step in emergency management (Table 87.10) is to separate the victim from the current source. The rescuer must be well insulated to avoid becoming an additional casualty. If the current cannot be shut off, wires can be cut with a wood-handled ax or appropriately insulated wire cutters. Contrary to popular myth, a lightning stroke victim does not remain "electrified" and presents no risk to another person.

Any victim in cardiopulmonary arrest should be resuscitated promptly following the guidelines discussed in Chapter 1. Prolonged efforts to restore adequate cardiopulmonary and cerebral function, especially in the lightning victim, may be appropriate in the context of bizarre neurologic phenomena that inhibit ventilatory efforts, consciousness, or pupillary function. The patient who fails to respond to resuscitative efforts over hours to days and meets standard brain death criteria can be pronounced dead with reasonable certainty.

Any patient who sustains electrical injury deserves a comprehensive physical examination. Bleeding or edema from orofacial burns may compromise the upper airway. The head, particularly eyes, and neck should be examined carefully for

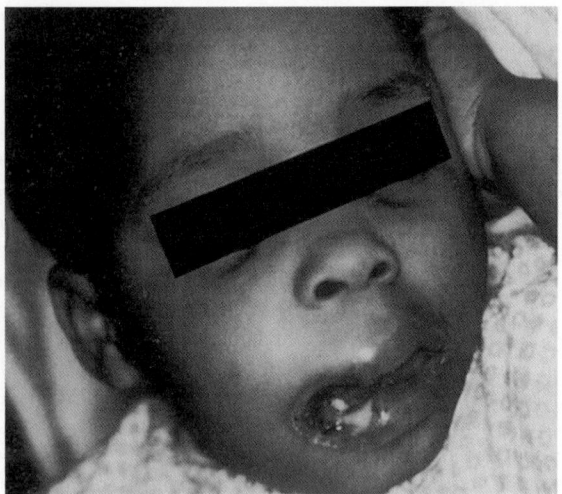
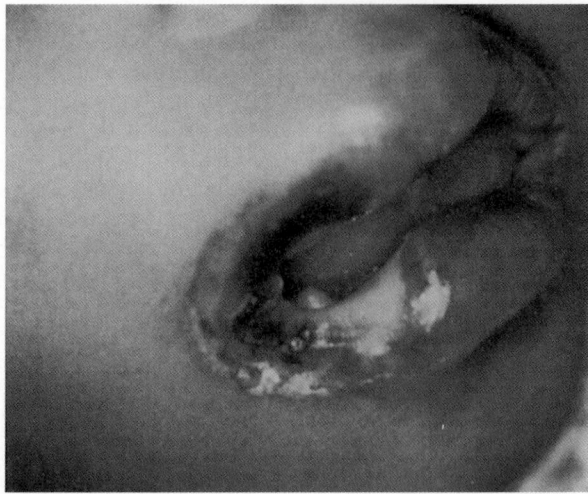

FIGURE 87.9 Patient with electrical burns to the corner of the mouth after biting on an electrical cord. (Courtesy of Evaline Alessandrini, MD.)

TABLE 87.10

MANAGEMENT OF ELECTRICAL INJURIES

Initial Management
Remove from source of current
Cardiopulmonary resuscitation as needed
Provide mechanical ventilation until spontaneous ventilation is adequate
Immobilize neck and spine

Clinical Assessment
Neurologic examination
Peripheral pulses and perfusion
Oral burns/edema
Chest wall injury
Abdominal distension
Eye or ear trauma
Cutaneous burns or bruises

Laboratory Determinations
Complete blood cell count
Blood urea nitrogen, creatinine, urinalysis including myoglobin
Electrolytes
Troponin
Electrocardiogram (EKG)
Consider skull, spine, chest, long bone radiographs
Consider computed tomography scan of brain
Consider electroencephalogram

Monitoring
Heart rate, EKG, respiratory rate, blood pressure

Management
Maintenance fluids: 5% dextrose in normal saline
Volume expansion in presence of thermal burns or extensive deep-tissue injury: 0.9% sodium chloride, lactated Ringer's solution, or 5% albumin
Fluid restriction for central nervous system injury
Maintain urine output >1 mL/kg/h
Treat arrhythmias
Treat seizures
Tetanus toxoid; consider penicillin/other antibiotics
Consider general, oral, or plastic surgical consultation

evidence of trauma. The skin should be examined carefully for burns and bruises. Limbs should be evaluated for pulses, perfusion, and motor and sensory function, as well as for soft-tissue swelling or evidence of fractures. Burns and deep-tissue injury may progress over hours to days, so repeated examination and monitoring are important.

Neurologic evaluation is especially important in all but the most minor, localized peripheral injuries. Level of consciousness and mental status should be assessed according to the child's developmental level. Cranial nerve, cerebellar, motor, and sensory evaluation are essential.

Children who have sustained minor household electrical injuries and are asymptomatic usually do not require laboratory evaluation, cardiac evaluation, or hospitalization. In one series, investigators were unable to assess the clinical significance of loss of consciousness, tetany, wet skin, or current flow across the heart, and recommended cardiac monitoring if any of these factors were present. If the history is one of a high-tension injury or lightning strike, laboratory evaluation should include EKG, CBC, CPK (with fractionation), BUN, creatinine, and urinalysis, including urine myoglobin. Physical examination that reveals evidence of bruises, bony tenderness, or distorted long bones should prompt appropriate radiographic studies.

Most children who sustain burns of the oral commissure (usually after biting an electrical cord) do not require extensive evaluation or admission. In cases of severe orofacial burns, use of an artificial airway should be considered before progressive edema leads to catastrophe. Mechanical ventilation may be necessary to overcome CNS depression or primary lung involvement.

Patients with persistent coma and loss of protective airway reflexes should be intubated to avoid aspiration. Good oxygenation and ventilation adequate to maintain a normal pH and $PaCO_2$ of 35 to 40 mm Hg must be ensured. Seizure activity should be treated as indicated (see Chapters 69 and 96).

Care of the CNS is of utmost importance. The neck and back should be immobilized if the patient was thrown from the site of injury. If the mechanism of injury was severe, a cervical collar should be maintained in place despite normal cervical spine radiographs. If a child fails to regain consciousness within a short time or shows signs of neurologic deterioration, a computed tomography scan will help exclude intracranial hemorrhage.

Any patient who has sustained cardiopulmonary arrest, loss of consciousness, or deep-tissue injury should be admitted to the hospital for evaluation and treatment. Heart rate, respiratory rate, and BP should be monitored regularly. Doppler evaluation may be helpful in cases of vasospasm, which may complicate assessment of BP and subsequent fluid management. True hypotension may require pressor support.

Cardiopulmonary support is nonspecific. Most patients resume circulatory stability unless severe hypoxia and ischemia have weakened the myocardium. Arrhythmias and acidosis should be treated along usual lines (see Chapters 84 and 100).

Patients struck by lightning require only maintenance fluids. Patients with ordinary thermal burns should be treated according to standard recommendations (see Chapter 108), although body surface area calculations may seriously underestimate fluid requirements. Extensive vascular and deep-tissue destruction may lead to extensive fluid sequestration. Isotonic fluid should be given in amounts to maintain normal pulse and BP. In all cases, fluids should be given with attention to possible CNS complications.

Cerebral edema may develop over hours to days after injury, especially after a lightning strike. If the child's neurologic status fails to improve or deteriorates, intracranial pressure monitoring and treatment, including hyperventilation, osmotic or loop diuretics, and sedation and neuromuscular blockade, may be necessary. Serum and urine electrolytes and osmolality should be followed closely to recognize promptly the syndrome of inappropriate antidiuretic hormone secretion.

Myoglobin in the urine is consistent with muscle breakdown and sets the stage for renal failure. Hydration and brisk diuresis with furosemide and/or mannitol may prevent renal damage but must be undertaken with caution if there is coexistent CNS injury. Extensive muscle damage after lightning injury is uncommon, however, and major CNS injury is common. Treatment should proceed with these relative risks in mind until definitive information is available.

Most burns associated with lightning injury are superficial. Although they may become more apparent after several hours, most remain first- or second-degree burns. Minor burns on the extremities can be treated with antibiotic ointment and should be allowed to slough and heal. Oral and plastic surgeons should evaluate children who sustain oral burns. In most cases, similar conservative management is recommended, but a removable stent may be necessary to minimize scarring.

High-voltage injuries commonly require more aggressive treatment. Fasciotomy may be necessary to restore adequate circulation to an injured extremity. The approach to debridement of wounds is controversial, but repeated examinations are considered most useful for detecting nonviable tissue. Approximately 30% of survivors of high-tension injuries ultimately require amputation of some part of an extremity.

The risk of infection in patients with deep-tissue injury is high. Any patient not clearly immunized against tetanus should be given tetanus toxoid. Prophylactic antibiotics have been recommended for oral injuries, but in general, antimicrobial therapy should be reserved for proven or strongly suspected infection.

Suggested Readings

Drowning

Baum CR. Environmental emergencies: weighing the ounce of prevention. *Clin Pediatr Emerg Med* 2003;4:121–126.

Bell GS, Gaitatzis A, Bell CL, et al. Drowning in people with epilepsy: how great is the risk? *Neurology* 2008;71:578–582.

Brenner RA, Committee on Injury, Violence, and Poison Prevention, American Academy of Pediatrics. Technical report: prevention of drowning in infants, children, and adolescents. *Pediatrics* 2003;12:440–445.

Brenner RA, Taneja GS, Haynie DL, et al. Association between swimming lessons and drowning in childhood: a case-control study. *Arch Pediatr Adolesc Med.* 2009;163:203–210.

Brunkard J, Namulanda G, Ratard R. Hurricane Katrina deaths, Louisiana, 2005. *Disaster Med Public Health Prep* 2008;2:215–223.

Causey AL, Tilelli JA, Swanson ME. Predicting discharge in uncomplicated near-drowning. *Am J Emerg Med* 2000;18:9–11.

Centers for Disease Control and Prevention. Nonfatal and fatal drownings in recreational water settings—United States, 2001–2002. *MMWR Morb Mortal Wkly Rep* 2004;53:447–452.

Cohen RH, Matter KC, Sinclair SA, et al. Unintentional pediatric submersion-injury-related hospitalizations in the United States, 2003. *Inj Prev* 2008; 14:131–135.

Modell JH. Drowning. *N Engl J Med* 1993;328:253–256.

Quan L, Cummings P. Characteristics of drowning by different age groups. *Inj Prev* 2003;9:161–163.

Rafaat KT, Spear RM, Kuelbs C, et al. Cranial computed tomographic findings in a large group of children with drowning: diagnostic, prognostic, and forensic implications. *Pediatr Crit Care Med* 2008;9:567–572.

Zuckerman GB, Conway EE. Drowning and near drowning: a pediatric epidemic. *Pediatr Ann* 2000;29:360–366.

Smoke Inhalation

Committee on Injury and Poison Prevention, American Academy of Pediatrics. Reducing the number of deaths and injuries from residential fires. *Pediatrics* 2000;5:1355–1357.

Dowd MD, Keenan HT, Bratton SL. Epidemiology and prevention of childhood injuries. *Crit Care Med* 2002;30:S385–S392.

Palmieri TL, Warner P, Mlcak RP, et al. Inhalation injury in children: a 10 year experience at Shriners Hospitals for Children. *J Burn Care Res* 2009;30:206–208.

Pierre EJ, Zwischengerger JB, Angel C, et al. Extracorporeal membrane oxygenation in the treatment of respiratory failure in pediatric patients with burns. *J Burn Care Rehabil* 1998;19:131–134.

Shai D, Lupinacci P. Fire fatalities among children: an analysis across Philadelphia's census tracts. *Public Health Rep* 2003;18:115–126.

Smith GA, Splaingard M, Hayes JR, et al. Comparison of a personalized parent voice smoke alarm with a conventional residential tone smoke alarm for awakening children. *Pediatrics* 2006;118:1623–1632.

Carbon Monoxide Poisoning

Chambers CA, Hopkins RO, Weaver LK, et al. Cognitive and affective outcomes of more severe as compared to less severe carbon monoxide poisoning. *Brain Inj* 2008;22:387–395.

Cho CH, Chiu NC, Ho CS, et al. Carbon monoxide poisoning in children. *Pediatr Neonatol* 2008;49:121–125.

Chou KJ, Fisher JL, Silver EJ. Characteristics and outcome of children with carbon monoxide poisoning with and without smoke exposure referred for hyperbaric oxygen therapy. *Pediatr Emerg Care* 2000;6:151–155.

Geller R, Barthold C, Saiers JA, et al. Pediatric cyanide poisoning: causes, manifestations, management, and unmet needs. *Pediatrics* 2006;118:2146–2158.

Martin JD, Osterhoudt KC, Thom SR. Recognition and management of carbon monoxide poisoning in children. *Clin Pediatr Emerg Med* 2000;1:244–250.

Weaver LK. Clinical Practice. Carbon Monoxide Poisoning. *N Engl J Med* 2009;360:1217–1225.

Weaver LK, Hopkins RO, Chan KJ. Hyperbaric oxygen for acute carbon monoxide poisoning. *N Engl J Med* 2002;347:1057–1067.

Environmental and Exertional Heat Illness

Centers for Disease Control and Prevention. Heat-related deaths—Chicago, Illinois, 1996–2001, and United States, 1979–1999. *MMWR Morbid Mortal Wkly Rep* 2003;52:610–613.

Hadad E, Rav-Acha M, Heled Y, et al. Heat stroke: a review of cooling methods. *Sports Med* 2004;34:501–511.

Klinenberg E. *Heat wave: a social autopsy of disaster in Chicago.* Chicago: University of Chicago Press, 2002.

Martin TJ, Martin JS. Special issues and concerns for the high school- and college-aged athletes. *Pediatr Clin North Am* 2002;49:533–552.

MEDICAL EMERGENCIES

Ostro BD, Roth LA, Green RS, et al. Estimating the mortality effect of the July 2006 California heat wave. *Environ Res* 2009;109:614–619.

Semenza JC, Rubin CH, Falter KH, et al. Heat-related deaths during the July 1995 heat wave in Chicago. *N Engl J Med* 1996;335:84–90.

Accidental Hypothermia

Centers for Disease Control and Prevention. Hypothermia-related deaths—Utah, 2000, and United States, 1979–1998. *MMWR Morbid Mortal Wkly Rep* 2002;51:76–78.

Danzl DF, Pozos RS. Accidental hypothermia. *N Engl J Med* 1994;331:1756–1760.

de Caen A. Management of profound hypothermia in children without the use of extracorporeal life support therapy. *Lancet* 2002;360:1394–1395.

Hughes A, Riou P, Day C. Full neurological recovery from profound (18.0 degrees C) acute accidental hypothermia: successful resuscitation using active invasive rewarming techniques. *Emerg Med J* 2007;24:511–512.

Kelman GR, Nunn JF. Nomograms for correction of blood pO_2, pCO_2, pH, and base excess for time and temperature. *J Appl Physiol* 1966;21:1484–1490.

Laniewics M, Lyn-Kew K, Silbergleit R. Rapid endovascular warming for profound hypothermia. *Ann Emerg Med* 2008;51:160–163.

Ulrich SA, Rathlev NK. Hypothermia and localized cold injuries. *Emerg Med Clin North Am* 2004;22:281–298.

High-altitude Illness

Basnyat B, Murdoch DR. High-altitude illness. *Lancet* 2003;361:1967–1974.

Bloch JC, Duplain H, Rimoldi SF, et al. Prevalence and time course of acute mountain sickness in older children and adolescents after rapid ascent to 3450 meters. *Pediatrics* 2009;123:1–5.

Hackett PC, Roach RC. High-altitude medicine. *N Engl J Med* 2001;345:107–114.

Kriemler S, Kohler M, Zehnder M, et al. Successful treatment of severe mountain sickness and excessive pulmonary hypertension treated with dexamethasone in a prepubertal girl. *High Alt Med Biol* 2006;7:256–261.

Luks AM, Swenson ER. Medication and dosage considerations in the prophylaxis and treatment of high-altitude illness. *Chest* 2008;133:744–755.

Moraga FA, Pedreros CP, Rodriguez CE. Acute mountain sickness in older children and their parents after rapid ascent to 3500 m (Putre, Chile). *Wilderness Environ Med* 2008;19:287–292.

Yaron M, Niermeyer S, Lindgren KN, et al. Physiologic response to moderate altitude exposure among infants and children. *High Alt Med Biol* 2003;4:53–59.

Electrical Injuries

Centers for Disease Control and Prevention. Lightning-associated deaths—United States, 1980–1995. *MMWR Morbid Mortal Wkly Rep* 1998;47:391–394.

Fish RM, Geddes LA. Effects of stun guns and tasers. *Lancet* 2001;358:687–688.

Garcia CT, Smith GA, Cohen DM, et al. Electrical injuries in a pediatric emergency department. *Ann Emerg Med* 1995;26:604–608.

Jumbelic MI. Forensic perspectives of electrical and lightning injuries. *Semin Neurol* 1995;5:342–350.

Kleinschmidt-DeMasters BK. Neuropathology of lightning-strike injuries. *Semin Neurol* 1995;5:323–328.

Matthews MS, Fahey AL. Plastic surgical considerations in lightning injury. *Am Plast Surg* 1997;39:561–565.

Nguyen BH, MacKay M, Bailey B, et al. Epidemiology of electrical and lightning related deaths and injuries among Canadian children and youth. *Inj Prev* 2004;10:122–124.

Rabban JT, Blair JA, Rosen CL, et al. Mechanisms of pediatric electrical injuries. *Arch Pediatr Adolesc Med* 1997;51:696–700.

CHAPTER 88 ■ INJURIES INVOLVING RADIATION

HENRY D. ROYAL, MD, JOANNA R. FAIR, MD, PHD, AND DAVID E. DRUM, MD, PHD

The radiation accident registry maintained at Oak Ridge, Tennessee, lists 432 accidents that have occurred worldwide from 1944 until June 2008. More than 3,000 people were exposed to significant amounts of radiation, and 127 persons died as a direct result. Most of the survivors had no permanent injury as a result of the accidents. The major issues for the survivors are a small increase in the risk of cancer and the psychological stress caused by their concerns and those of their community about the long-term effects of radiation exposure. Two hundred fifty of the accidents occurred in the United States, resulting in 26 fatalities. Worldwide, less than 10 fatalities have been reported in children. Thus, radiation accidents that result in medically significant injuries to children are quite uncommon.

Despite the rarity of medically significant radiation accidents, the emergency physician needs to be aware of the basic principles and management of radiation incidents for five major reasons. First, The Joint Commission requires plans for managing environmental events including those involving hazardous materials and terrorist events. Second, incidents in which radiation is perceived to have an important role are not rare. For instance, the discovery of a cardboard box with a radioactive label attached to it in a school play yard or public roadway is liable to cause great anxiety. Generally, the public believes radiation to be very hazardous and does not distinguish between amounts of radiation that we are exposed to every day from natural sources and amounts of radiation that have a measurable biological effect. If the emergency physician is knowledgeable about the effects of radiation, he or she can correctly counsel the patient and immediately help decrease the psychological trauma. Third, fear of radiation and lack of knowledge about its effects have led to the professional mismanagement of several individuals who were believed to be involved in a radiation accident. Fourth, the emergency physician needs to be informed about the effects of radiation because the rare radiation event is often not initially recognized. A review of radiation events that have occurred in the past should help physicians recognize situations in which radiation might be considered as etiologic. Frequent training and drills are essential to ensure that the emergency department (ED) staff have the knowledge, procedural skills, and supplies to deal with possible victims exposed to radiation accident. Finally, knowledge of radiation events will lead to better understanding of the effects of routine diagnostic radiation exposures.

PATHOPHYSIOLOGY

Types of Radiation

Radiation is a very general term used to describe energy that is emitted from a source (Fig. 88.1). Some forms of radiation may deposit a large amount of energy in a small volume of tissue. These energetic forms of radiation are called *ionizing radiation* because they deposit enough energy to strip electrons from atoms. X-rays are a type of ionizing radiation. Other types of radiation are less energetic (of longer wavelength) and are called *nonionizing radiation*. Examples of nonionizing radiation include visible light and infrared radiation. The distinction between ionizing and nonionizing radiation is important because their biological effects are very different; the latter primarily deposits heat in tissue.

Ionizing radiation can be further subdivided into types of radiation that have no associated mass (*nonparticulate*) and those that have mass (*particulate*). X-rays and gamma rays are nonparticulate types of radiation. This type of radiation can penetrate deeply into the body and affect radiation-sensitive tissues [e.g., bone marrow and the lining of the gastrointestinal (GI) tract]. X-rays are emitted by excited electrons, whereas gamma rays are emitted by excited or unstable nuclei (radioisotopes or radionuclides). Once x-rays or gamma rays have been emitted, they are indistinguishable.

Particulate radiation can be further divided into charged and uncharged particles. Neutrons, a type of particulate radiation that has no electrical charge, can penetrate the body to depths similar to x-rays and gamma rays. Because neutrons deposit their energy in a more concentrated area, they cause more biological damage than x-rays or gamma rays.

Alpha particles have a 2+ electrical charge and a large mass (two protons and two neutrons). Beta particles have a single negative charge and a small mass (one electron). Charged particles do not penetrate the body very well. Because of their larger mass and charge, alpha rays cannot penetrate even the dead layers of skin. For example, ^{239}Pu, an alpha emitter, is a biological hazard only when it is inhaled, ingested, or otherwise introduced into the body. Beta particles ("beta rays") are more penetrating and in high doses can severely damage the skin. Beta rays cannot damage the deep radiation-sensitive organs in the body unless the radioactive source is incorporated into the body. At the Chernobyl nuclear plant accident in Russia, some of the firefighters had severe skin damage due to intense beta particle exposure. This injury contributed to their deaths.

The words "radiation" and "radioactive" are often confused. An atom that is unstable spontaneously gives off energy as radiation and is radioactive. In contrast, an x-ray machine cannot spontaneously give off radiation: an external power source is needed. Therefore, an x-ray machine is not radioactive. A patient who has been exposed to radiation does not become radioactive. Patients emit radiation only if they have radioactive atoms on them (external contamination) or within them (internal contamination).

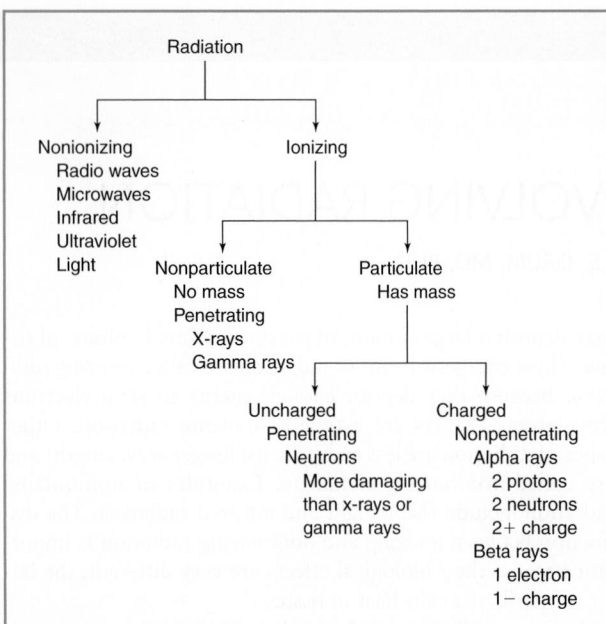

FIGURE 88.1 Types of radiation.

Amounts of Radiation

Although radiation cannot be perceived by the human senses, Geiger counters can easily measure amounts of radiation far below the levels that can be shown to have a measurable biological effect. Geiger counters are inexpensive and are readily available in the nuclear medicine department at most hospitals. Because a Geiger counter can detect and quantify immediately the radiation exposure rate, managing a radiation hazard can be easier than managing biological hazards such as bacterial meningitis or methicillin-resistant *Staphylococcus aureus* infection or managing hazardous chemical exposures.

Radiation exposure is commonly measured in three different units in the United States: roentgen, rad, and rem. However, new international units are being used by regulatory and professional organizations (Table 88.1). The roentgen (R) is a measure of radiation exposure in air. Absorbed dose in an organ is measured in grays (Gy); 1 Gy is equal to 100 rads. Effective dose, in sieverts (Sv), is a measure of overall risk to an individual when the irradiation is weighted for the sensitivity of each organ to late effects of radiation. One sievert is equal to 100 rems. Quantity of radiation is measured by becquerels (Bq), defined as 1 atomic disintegration per second. The former unit, the curie (Ci), is equal to 3.7×10^{10} Bq, and 1 mCi is equal to 37 MBq.

To put into perspective the magnitude of these units, it is helpful to recall that we are exposed to about 3 mSv of radiation each year from natural sources. During a 70-year lifetime, a person's total radiation exposure from natural sources will be more than 200 mSv, with no measurable biological effect of radiation. Typical radiation exposures that we encounter as part of our daily lives and in medicine are listed in Table 88.2.

In addition to the quantity of the radionuclide, the hazard posed by a radionuclide depends on its decay scheme, the energies of its emissions, its half-life, and on how long it stays in var-

INTERNATIONAL RADIATION UNITS

Metric	Definition
Exposure	Roentgen, R $R = 2.58 \times 10^{-4}$ C/kg air
Absorbed dose	Gray, Gy 1 Gy = 1 joule/kg 1 Gy = 100 rads
Effective dose	Sievert, Sv 1 Sv = 1 joule/kg, weighted for tissue sensitivity 1 Sv = 100 rems
Quantity	Becquerel, Bq 1 Bq = 1 disintegration/s 1 Ci = 3.7×10^{10} Bq 1 mCi = 37 MBq

ious organs in the body. For example, a radionuclide that decays by emitting only alpha particles is not a hazard if kept outside the body, since alpha particles cannot penetrate even the dead layers of the skin. However, some radionuclides (e.g., ^{131}I) that are readily absorbed by the body and/or are concentrated by an organ can be a hazard even when present in small amounts.

RADIATION SAFETY

The worst radiation accident involving a commercial nuclear power plant in the United States (Three Mile Island) resulted in a radiation dose to off-site medical personnel was of 0.14 mSv. Following the Chernobyl accident, the highest radiation dose to off-site medical personnel was tens of millisieverts, similar to the dose from one computed tomographic scan examination. These doses should reassure emergency personnel that it is extremely unlikely that a radiation event involving contamination would ever threaten their safety. Patients who have been exposed only to high doses of radiation, such as a patient after radiation therapy, are not radioactive and require no special precautions from radiation exposure.

Although the radiation doses to personnel involved in the care of a victim contaminated by radioactive material are likely to be very small, simple protective measures should be employed to minimize the doses. There are three methods of protection from radiation exposure: minimizing *time* of expo-

COMMON RADIATION DOSES

Sources	Effective dose
Roundtrip intercontinental air flight	20–30 μSv
Chest radiograph	50–100 μSv
Living in brick house	0.20 μSv/yr
Natural radiation	3 mSv/yr
Angiography	10 mSv
Abdominal computed tomographic scan	10–30 mSv

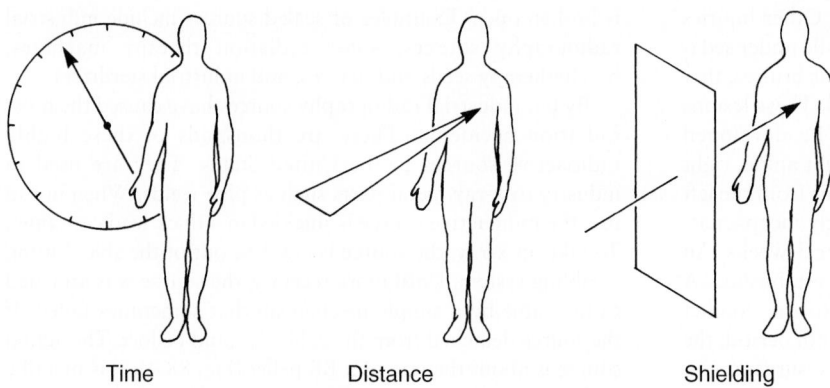

Time   Distance   Shielding

FIGURE 88.2 Three methods of reducing radiation exposure.

sure, maximizing *distance* from the material to the extent practical, and using *shielding* as appropriate (Fig. 88.2). The amount of exposure received is directly proportional to the time spent near the source of radiation. Distance is the most practical and effective method of reducing radiation exposure because the dose decreases by the square of the distance. In other words, doubling the distance from a source of radiation will reduce the dose by a factor of 4, and tripling the distance will reduce the dose by a factor of 9 (Fig. 88.3). This is known as the inverse square law. For shielding, the familiar lead aprons used in radiology departments, where the radiation comes from low-energy scattered radiation, are not generally useful in radiation event management. Lead aprons do not provide very effective protection against the higher-energy radionuclide emissions likely to be encountered with radioactive contamination.

CLINICAL MANIFESTATIONS AND EVALUATION

Recognizing Radiation Exposure

Radiation exposures can be recognized by understanding three questions: (i) Who is likely to be affected by a radiation expo-

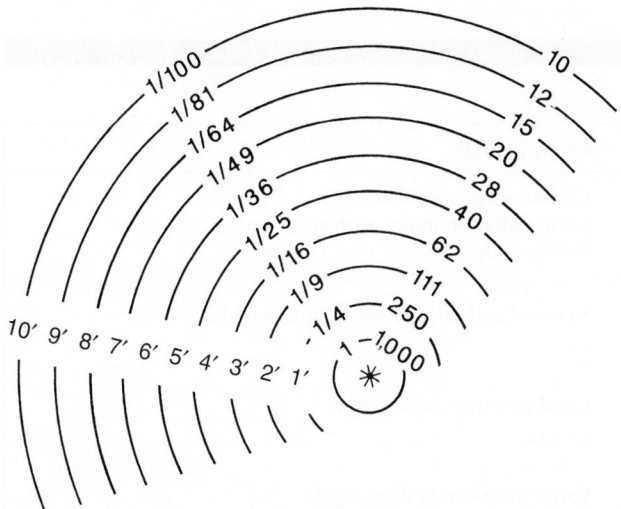

FIGURE 88.3 The effect of distance on radiation exposure from a point source of radiation.

sure or accident? (ii) What are the likely sources of radiation? and (iii) What are the likely injuries?

Types of Radiation Exposures

The people most likely to be involved in a radiation exposure event are individuals whose work involves radiation. Although these exposures are usually recognized, many work-related accidents were not initially appreciated. One valuable way to determine if a radiation accident has occurred is to contact the worker's supervisor and/or the radiation safety officer for the employer. In most instances, they will immediately recognize the possibility of a serious radiation exposure.

A second group of individuals who may be involved in a radiation exposure event are members of the general public who inadvertently come into contact with a radiation hazard. An example of this kind of exposure occurred in Goiana, Brazil, in September 1987. In that incident, a ^{137}Cs radiation therapy source was stolen from an abandoned medical clinic. The poachers brought the source to their home, exposing their family and friends to large doses of radiation. The exposure worsened when the victims broke open the ^{137}Cs source, subsequently contaminating their food, their living quarters, and the area surrounding their homes. As a result of this accident, four persons, including a 6-year-old girl, died. Hundreds of other people were exposed to nonlethal amounts of radiation. The accident was not recognized until 2 weeks after the source had been opened. When the individuals first became ill, their symptoms were diagnosed as gastroenteritis.

A more recent example of this second category is the striking increase in the prevalence of thyroid cancer (more than 2,000 cases) among children in the Ukraine and Belarus after the Chernobyl accident. Radionuclides, especially ^{131}I, were deposited by fallout and incorporated into foods and milk products. Those who were youngest at exposure had the greatest increase in prevalence, whereas there was a smaller increase in adolescents and no increase in those older than 20 years at the time of exposure.

A third group of individuals who may be involved in a radiation event are persons who are unknowingly intentionally exposed to radiation by another person. A 13-year-old boy was intentionally exposed to radiation by his father on multiple occasions during weekend visitations. The son later recalled occasionally finding "shiny silver pellets" in the ear pieces of headphones he was told to wear, in a pillow he was

MEDICAL EMERGENCIES

told to use, and in a sock he found on his bed. Other injuries suggested that he was exposed at other times while under sedation. The boy developed skin lesions, described as bruises, that gradually developed into reddish brown blisters. These lesions were attributed to infection. Subsequently, he developed lesions on the medial aspects of both thighs, right ankle, right hand, and left forehead. He also began losing hair from the left side of his head. The lesions became increasingly incapacitating, and the boy was admitted to a hospital for 3 weeks. An infectious etiology for the lesions could not be established. A psychiatrist suggested a neurodermatitis due to the conflict between the boy and his father. During a 20-month period, the boy was seen by 16 physicians. Finally, a plastic surgeon recognized the lesions as radiation necrosis.

The father, a petroleum engineer, had access to 74-GBq ^{137}Cs sources. The dose rate at contact for such a source is approximately 5 Gy per minute. However, at 1 cm, the dose rate drops to (0.3 Gy) per minute and is about 40 mGy per minute at 3 cm from the surface.

A fourth group of individuals who may be involved in a radiation exposure are patients who have undergone medical procedures (fluoroscopy or radiation therapy). Typical cases include one or more lengthy exposures to prolonged fluoroscopy, such as during an interventional cardiac catheterization. For example, a 17-year-old Spanish adolescent girl who underwent two lengthy cardiac radiofrequency ablations within 13 months developed chronic radiation dermatitis and associated limited range of motion of her right arm.

Types of Radiation Sources

To cause a significant radiation injury, an intense radiation source is needed. The four major types of possible intense radiation sources are listed in Table 88.3. Because of their various physical properties, different types of sources are likely to cause different types of radiation injuries.

Sealed sources contain a radioactive source in a leakproof container or capsule; hence, these accidents usually cause only radiation exposure. Contamination occurs only if the container

is broken open. Examples of sealed sources include industrial radiography sources, some radiation therapy machines, brachytherapy seeds and devices, and industrial sterilizers.

By far, industrial radiography sources have caused the most radiation accidents. There are thousands of these highly radioactive sources in the United States. They are used in industry to x-ray metal parts such as pipe welds. When not in use, the radioactive source is shielded in a thick lead container. To take an x-ray, the source is cranked out of the shield using a cabling system. Until more recently, the source was attached to the cable by a simple mechanism that sometimes failed. If the source detached from the cable, it could be lost. The actual source is about the size of a BB pellet (Fig. 88.4); it is metallic and appears innocuous. In the past, the source was not labeled; a passerby could find the source and not recognize it to be dangerous. Because this type of source is small, it usually causes a local radiation injury involving the hands (from picking up the source) or the buttocks (from putting the source in a pocket). Strict regulatory enforcement actions have markedly decreased the occurrence of this type of accident.

Sealed sources used in radiation therapy can be small (brachytherapy "seeds") or large (cobalt therapy machine). Industrial sterilizers use large, intense radiation sources to sterilize products (e.g., packaged food, medical supplies) that would be damaged by other methods of sterilization. Large, sealed sources are more likely to result in whole-body radiation exposure.

Unsealed sources, a second type of radiation source, consist of radioactive material in a form that is dispersed easily (e.g., liquid or powder). The likely injury caused by unsealed sources involves both external and internal contamination. Unsealed sources commonly found in hospitals include the radiopharmaceuticals used in nuclear medicine (e.g., ^{99m}Tc, ^{131}I, ^{18}F). Other industries or activities may use unsealed sources of ^{32}P, ^{241}Am, or ^{239}Pu. If these radioactive materials are kept outside the body (external contamination), they would not likely cause harm. Radioactive dirt can be washed from the skin with soap and water. If properly managed, external contamination is generally a nuisance rather than a serious health threat to the patient or medical staff. If the radioactive

TABLE 88.3

INTENSE RADIATION SOURCES

Type of source	Examples	Likely injuries
Sealed	Industrial radiography Brachytherapy Some radiation therapy machines Industrial sterilizers	Contamination unlikely Local radiation injury with small source Whole-body exposure with large source
Unsealed	Medical radionuclides (e.g., ^{131}I, ^{32}P) Accidental release by a reactor Radium dial painters	External and internal contamination likely
Radiation devices	Cyclotron Linear accelerator Fluoroscopy unit	Local radiation injury likely
Uncontrolled fission	Nuclear reactor Uranium enrichment Weapons production	Large whole-body doses likely On- and off-site contamination possible for nuclear reactors

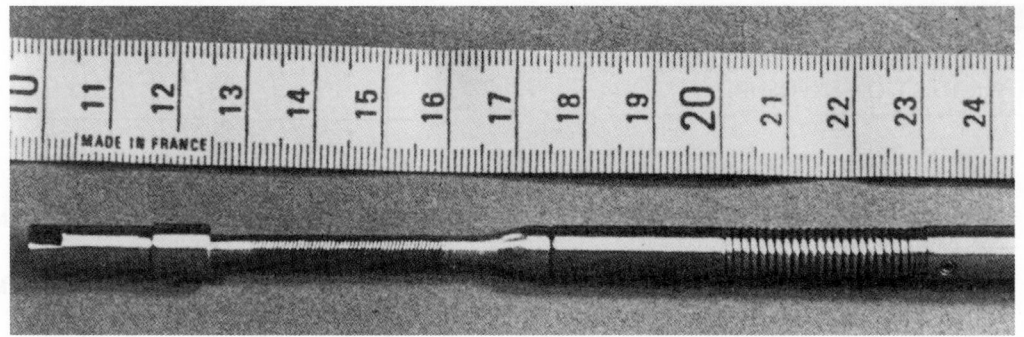

FIGURE 88.4 Source of radiation that affected two Algerian children in 1978.

dirt gets into the patient's body (internal contamination) by ingestion, inhalation, or absorption through the skin or a wound, minimizing the radiation dose is more difficult. Other examples of unsealed sources include radium ingested by radium dial painters and radionuclides such as those released during the accident at the Chernobyl nuclear power plant.

Radiation devices, the third potential radiation source listed in Table 88.3, are likely to cause a local radiation injury. Because these devices emit radiation when switched on but are not radioactive, it is highly unlikely that patients exposed to radiation from radiation devices will be radioactive should they present for treatment.

A fourth possible radiation source is an uncontrolled nuclear fission reaction (criticality accident). Usually, there is an intense radiation exposure and release of steam for a brief period of time. Criticality accidents have produced the largest whole-body radiation exposures resulting from radiation accidents. The largest portion of the dose is due to neutrons. These accidents can occur only at uranium enrichment facilities and nuclear reactors, where there is a critical mass of nuclear material. Fortunately, criticality accidents are very uncommon. Only two criticality accidents have occurred since the late 1960s; one of these was the 1986 accident at Chernobyl. The Chernobyl accident caused the deaths of 31 people who were at the nuclear power plant at the time of the accident. In addition, millions of people were exposed to low levels of radiation when hundreds of square miles of land was contaminated by radioactive fallout.

Types of Radiation Injuries

Perceived

There are three major types of radiation injury (Table 88.4). The first and by far the most common injury is the perceived radiation injury. Because of misconceptions about the possible health effects of radiation, members of the general public, fearful of having been exposed, may attribute almost any illness to radiation exposure. Unfortunately, these perceptions are often reinforced by physicians who are not knowledgeable about radiation effects. The psychological stress caused by misdiagnosis can be significant. Employers have a heavy burden to educate radiation workers to preempt such feelings. A threatened terrorist event or detonation of a "dirty bomb" could produce perceptions of radiation injury among the general

public. Health care workers educated about radiation risks should be able to anticipate these concerns.

Exposure

The second major type of radiation injury is exposure to radiation. Because these patients do not have radioactive dirt on them or in them, they are not radioactive and can be treated without any additional precautions on the part of health care workers. Two types of injury from radiation exposure are possible. A high dose of penetrating radiation over a short period of time to a large portion of the body (i.e., whole-body radiation) causes the acute radiation syndrome. Exposure to alpha or beta particles of any source would never cause this syndrome because these types of radiation are nonuniformly distributed and poorly penetrating. Large doses of radiation over a short period of time to a small portion of the body cause a local radiation injury. When only a small portion of the body is exposed, much larger doses of radiation can be tolerated. Analogous medical situations would be whole-body radiation as conditioning for bone marrow transplantation and localized radiation therapy for breast cancer.

Whole-body Exposure. The signs and symptoms of the acute radiation syndrome (Table 88.5) begin to appear after whole-body radiation doses of approximately 1 Gy. Organs with rapidly dividing cells (the bone marrow and the lining of the GI tract) are the most susceptible to radiation damage. The amount of damage that occurs is dependent both on the dose and on the dose rate. For example, a dose of 1 Gy received in

TABLE 88.4

TYPES OF RADIATION INJURIES

Perceived
Exposure
    Whole body
    Local
Contamination
    External
    Internal
Metal fragment
Hot particle
Terrorist event

TABLE 88.5

DOSE-EFFECT RELATIONSHIP AFTER ACUTE
WHOLE-BODY RADIATION EXPOSURE

Whole-body absorbed dose (Sv)	Comments
0.1	Asymptomatic (minimal detectable dose using cytogenetics)
0.5	Asymptomatic (minor depression of white blood cell and platelets)
1	Nausea and vomiting in approximately 15% of patients within 2 days of exposure
2	Nausea and vomiting in most patients
4	Nausea, vomiting, and diarrhea within 48 h; severe hematologic depression; 50% mortality without medical treatment
6	100% mortality within 30 days without medical treatment; 50% mortality with medical treatment
7	Gastrointestinal syndrome; survival unlikely; death in 2–3 wk
50	Neurovascular syndrome; death in 24–72 h

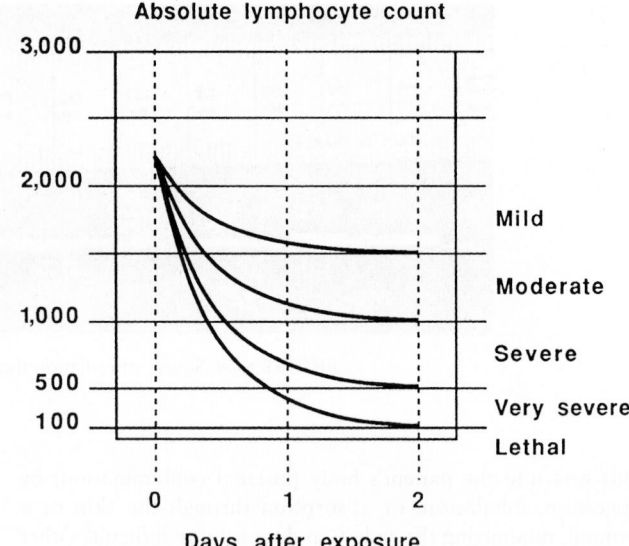

FIGURE 88.5 Effect of whole-body radiation on lymphocytes in the first 2 days after exposure.

1 minute would probably cause symptoms; however, 1 Gy received at a dose rate of 10 mGy per day for 100 days would likely be asymptomatic. Doses of about 4 to 6 Gy may be lethal in approximately 50% of people if they do not receive medical treatment. With maximum medical treatment, the dose of radiation that will kill 50% of people may be as high as 6.5 to 7 Gy.

The acute radiation syndrome consists of three distinct phases (Table 88.6). The *prodromal* phase begins minutes to hours after the radiation exposure and lasts for 2 to 3 days. During the prodromal phase, the patient may have nausea, vomiting, diarrhea, fatigue, and/or headache. The prodromal phase is followed by the *latent* phase, in which the patient is relatively asymptomatic. The latent phase generally lasts days or weeks after the exposure. The third and final phase is the *manifest illness* phase. During this phase, the patient is at greatest risk for infection and bleeding due to the bone marrow suppression and GI epithelial damage. As the radiation dose increases, the duration of the prodromal phase increases and the length of the latent phase decreases.

With doses of 2 to 4 Gy, the primary effect of the whole-body radiation is to depress the bone marrow. Although the absolute lymphocyte count (Fig. 88.5) decreases rapidly within the first 24 hours, there is no need for specific medical treatment. The patient will be at greatest risk 3 to 4 weeks after the radiation exposure when the white blood cell and platelet counts reach a nadir (Fig. 88.6). At this time, the patient is vulnerable to death from infection and bleeding. If the patient can be supported during this period of vulnerability and if the bone marrow is not irreversibly damaged, a recovery phase ensues (Fig. 88.7).

The GI syndrome occurs from absorbed doses of more than approximately 7 Gy. During the prodromal phase of this syndrome, there is prompt onset of severe nausea, vomiting, and diarrhea. There is a latent period of approximately 1 week and then recurrence of GI symptoms, sepsis, electrolyte imbalance, and likely death. The patient is susceptible to infection due to lack of granulocytes and because pathogens can readily enter the body across the damaged GI tract lining.

At dose levels of more than 50 Gy, the cardiovascular/central nervous system (CNS) syndrome predominates. There is almost immediate nausea, vomiting, prostration, hypotension, ataxia, and convulsions. The permeability of blood vessels increases. The patient suffers from CNS symptoms due to

TABLE 88.6

ACUTE RADIATION SYNDROME—SIGNS AND SYMPTOMS

Prodromal (0–2[a])	Latent (2–20[a])	Manifest illness (21–60[a])
Fatigue	Asymptomatic	Bone marrow depression
Nausea and vomiting		Sepsis
Diarrhea		Bleeding
Headache		Diarrhea
Dizziness		
Decreased lymphocyte count		

[a]Days after exposure.

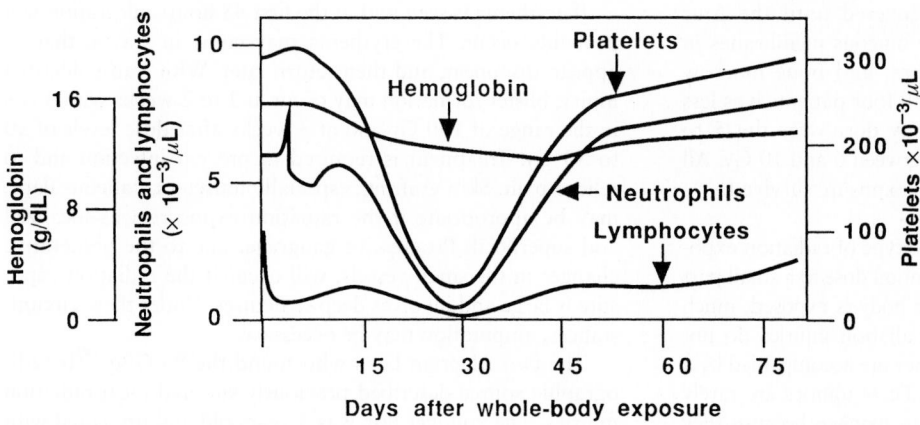

FIGURE 88.6 Effect of whole-body radiation on blood cell counts in the days after exposure.

brain edema and from hypotension caused by the difficulty of maintaining a normal intravascular space. Death usually occurs within 1 to 4 days.

Estimating the whole-body radiation dose may be difficult, especially when complicated by injuries that are not due to radiation. The signs and symptoms during the prodromal period are quite nonspecific except for a rapidly decreasing lymphocyte count. Nausea and vomiting are sensitive but nonspecific symptoms. Patients who do not have nausea and vomiting are unlikely to have been exposed to a radiation dose that is large enough to cause acute radiation syndrome. However, individuals may have nausea and vomiting for reasons other than exposure to radiation. The whole-body radiation dose from radia-

tion accidents is rarely uniform. The nonuniform nature of the radiation dose makes it more difficult to predict the biological effects of the exposure. Chromosome analysis (cytogenetic dosimetry) may be helpful in estimating the radiation dose, but the results may not be available for about 1 week.

A radiation accident involving whole-body exposure to four young (14 to 20 years old) women occurred in Algeria in 1978. A 93-GBq ^{192}Ir industrial radiography source (Fig 88.4) fell from a truck and was found by two young boys. They played with the source for several hours before taking it home. The source was taken away by their grandmother, who hid it in the kitchen. The source remained in the room for 5 to 6 weeks, irradiating several persons, including the four young

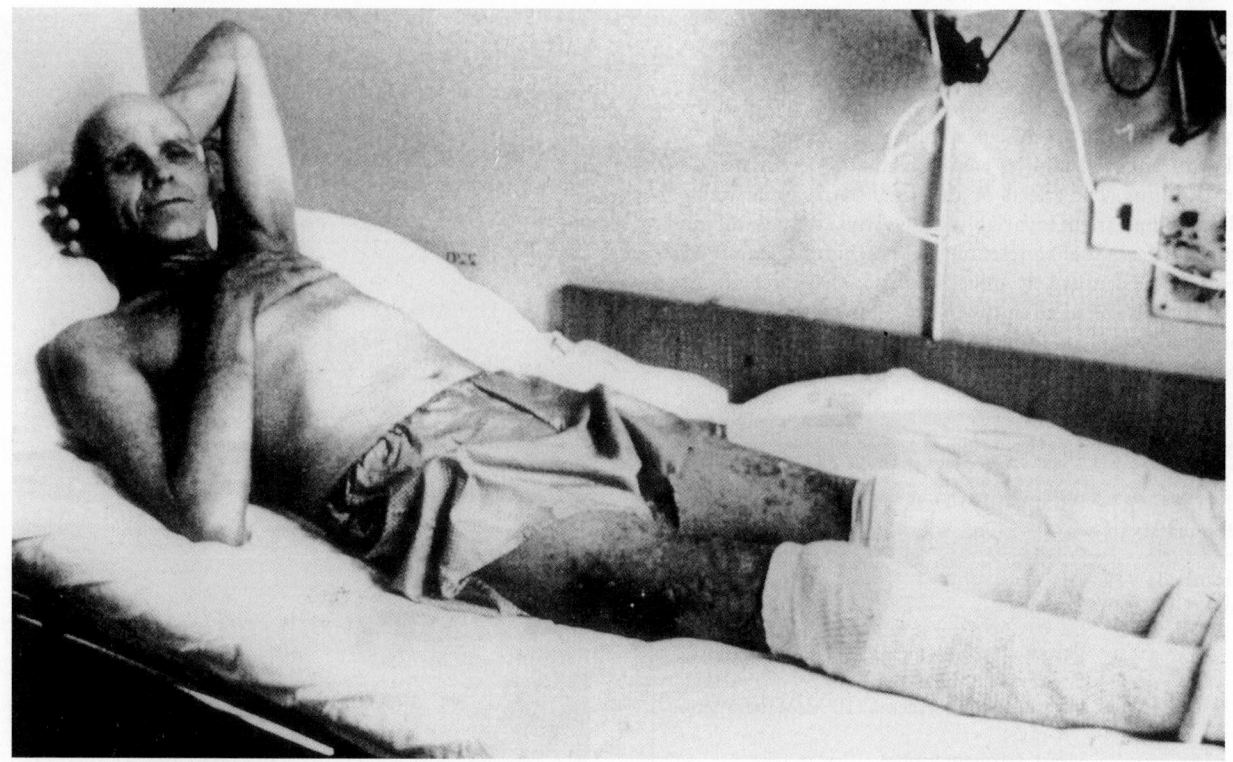

FIGURE 88.7 Chernobyl victim suffering from acute radiation syndrome a few weeks after the accident. Note the hair loss, indicating a radiation dose of 10 to 30 Gy. Also note injury to the skin of the lower extremities as a result of high, tens of grays, doses of beta (nonpenetrating) radiation. (Courtesy of A.M. Davis)

women. This accident was not discovered until the four women had severe bleeding from the mucous membranes in the mouth, anorexia, nausea, purpura, and bone marrow depression. The lymphocyte count in all four patients was less than 10% of normal. The whole-body dose over the 5 to 6 weeks was estimated to have been between 6 and 10 Gy. All four patients injured by this accidental exposure survived.

Local Radiation Exposure. The second type of radiation exposure that can occur involves a large radiation dose to a small part of the body. If only a small part of the body is exposed, much larger doses can be tolerated. Local radiation injuries do not cause bone marrow depression unless they are accompanied by a significant whole-body radiation dose. These injuries are rarely life threatening, but they are difficult to manage because they often cause a slowly progressive injury that takes months to years to fully evolve. The injury develops slowly because the radiation causes progressive fibrosis of the blood vessels, which, in turn, causes tissue necrosis. The ultimate extent of the injury may not be appreciated initially. Healing following amputation or reconstructive surgery is poor because of deficient blood supply.

The hand is the most common site for localized irradiation injuries. The next most common sites are the thighs and buttocks because individuals are likely to put things that they find into their pockets. A patient who has undergone a fluoroscopic procedure would have local radiation injury to the skin overlying the region imaged. For example, the radiation source is typically positioned posterior to a patient undergoing a cardiac catheterization and therefore a radiation burn would be on the back. Most industrial radiography sources deliver an extremely high dose on direct contact with the skin. For example, the 93-GBq ^{192}Ir source described previously has a surface dose rate of about 200 Gy per minute and will cause an absorbed dose of about 125 Gy per minute at 1-cm depth in tissue. In contrast, analytical x-ray crystallography machines, which emit x-rays of much lower energy than the photons of ^{192}Ir, are not likely to cause deep blood vessel injury.

Local radiation injuries can be readily differentiated from thermal burns. The effects of a thermal burn appear immediately, and the patient invariably knows when the painful injury occurred. If a patient presenting with a burnlike injury does not know the cause of the injury (realizing that carelessness on his or her part resulted in the injury), a local radiation injury should be suspected. Table 88.7 lists the dose-related findings expected after a local radiation exposure.

If erythema is seen within the first 48 hours, ulceration will probably occur. The erythema may come in waves, that is, appear, disappear, and then return later. With transepidermal injury, blister formation may occur at 1 to 2 weeks with doses in the range of 100 Gy and at 3 weeks after dose levels of 30 to 50 Gy. Treatment is required to prevent infection and to relieve pain. Skin grafting, especially musculocutaneous flaps, may be appropriate if the radiation exposure was localized and superficial. Progressive gangrene, due to the obliterative changes in the small vessels, will occur if the radiation exposure is large and involves deep structures. Under these circumstances, amputation may be necessary.

The two Algerian boys who found the 93-GBq ^{192}Ir radiographic source described previously suffered local radiation injuries. The younger boy was 3 years old and presented with lesions of the mouth and hands (Fig. 88.8). The boy apparently had sucked on the source, receiving an approximate dose of 25 Gy to the lip surface. The older boy (7 years old) had a necrotic deep ulceration in the hypothenar region of the right hand, apparently from using the source as a drumstick (Fig. 88.9). The estimated dose to the center of the lesion was estimated at 100 Gy, and at the periphery of the necrosis 15 Gy. Ultimately, the oral lesions in the young boy healed, whereas reconstructive surgery was required on the older boy.

Contamination

Contamination represents the third major type of radiation injury. Contamination occurs when radioactive dirt or liquid remains on the patient (external contamination) or, when inhaled or ingested, inside the patient (internal contamination).

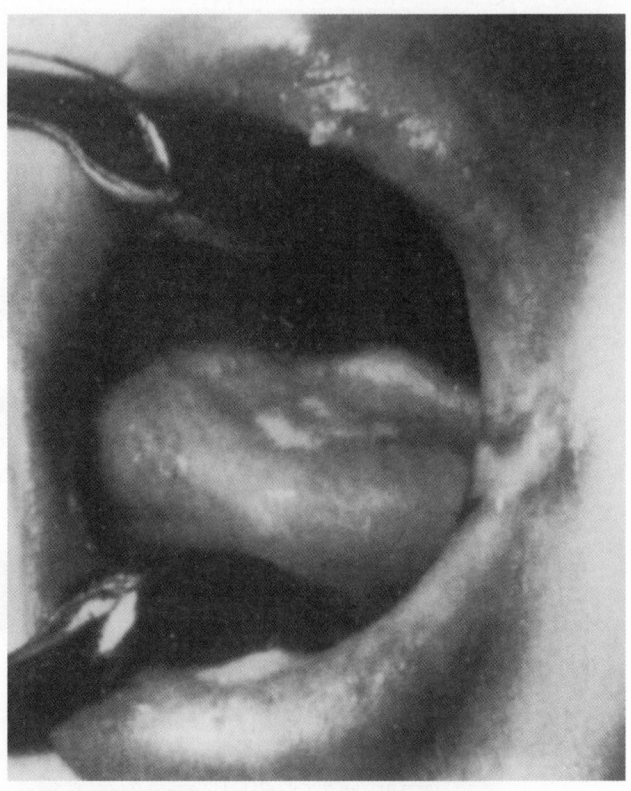

FIGURE 88.8 Mouth lesions caused by radiation of approximately 25 Gy. The lesions healed eventually.

TABLE 88.7

APPROXIMATE ABSORBED DOSE TO PRODUCE SKIN CHANGES

Absorbed dose (Gy)	Findings
3	Threshold for erythema (100 keV diagnostic x-rays)
6	Threshold for erythema (10 MeV therapeutic x-rays)
15	Moist desquamation
20	Skin ulceration with slow healing
>30	Gangrenous changes

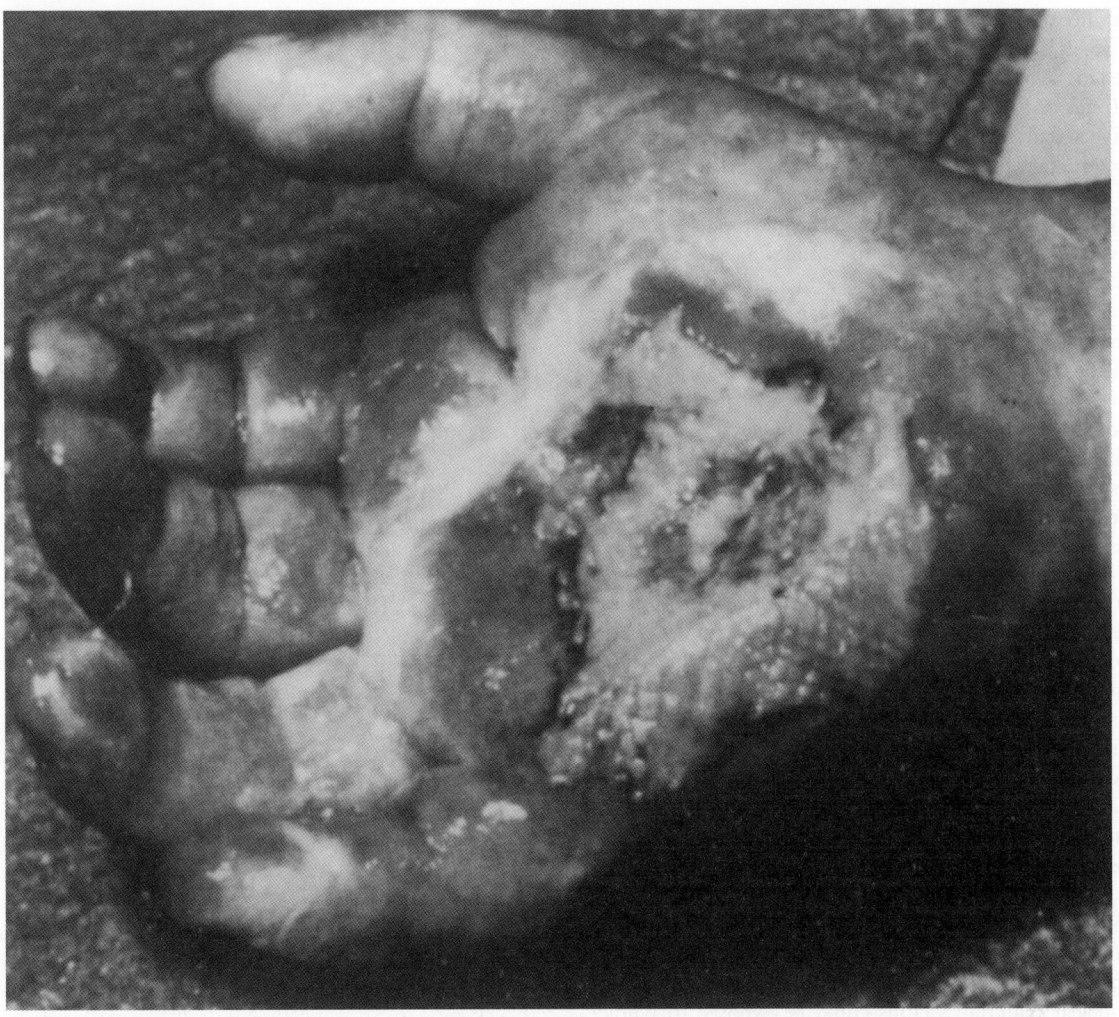

FIGURE 88.9 Radiation burns on the hand of the older Algerian child from a dose of 15 to 100 Gy. Reconstructive surgery was required.

Contamination is the only type of radiation injury that requires the medical staff to take any radiation-related precautions. It should be reemphasized that there is little danger to the medical staff when caring for a contaminated person once he or she has been transported to the hospital. However, medical personnel who respond to the accident site may be exposed to large, potentially life-threatening doses of radiation. For these rescue workers, 0.5 Gy is the voluntary limit suggested by the National Council on Radiation Protection and Measurements (NCRP) for lifesaving activities.

External Contamination. External contamination rarely is a significant medical problem. To prevent additional radiation exposure to the patient and unnecessary radiation exposure to the medical staff and the public, external contamination should be removed and dispersal of radioactive materials should be prevented. On the basis of the assumption that any radiation exposure is potentially harmful, the goal of the treatment of any contaminated patient is to keep radiation exposures "as low as reasonably achievable." This is called the ALARA principle and requires advance planning, specific supplies, and appropriate protective clothing. Preventing the dis-

persal of radioactive materials is accomplished by treating the patient in a single location, controlling access to that location, and by using standard contact precautions.

Internal Contamination. Internal contamination potentially is a more serious problem because it is more difficult to eliminate some long-lived radioactive materials from within the body than it is to remove radioactive dirt on the outside of the body. Death due to radiation from internal contamination is rare. A few deaths have been caused by medical misadministrations. Also, in the Goiana accident, a 6-year-old girl died from severe internal contamination with ^{137}Cs. Internal contamination, especially with ^{131}I, was a concern following the Chernobyl reactor accident. A familiar example of intentional, nonlethal internal contamination is the bone scan performed in a nuclear medicine department. Treatment of hyperthyroidism with ^{131}I also is, in a sense, planned internal contamination.

Metal Fragment. Another source of contamination that should be separately addressed is the radioactive metallic fragment. These could, in principle, be found if a "dirty bomb" were constructed with a radioactive metal source such as an ^{192}Ir radiographic source. Metallic fragments can be intensely radioactive. If a radioactive metal fragment is present (e.g., embedded in the patient's skin), it should never be touched with fingers. Tongs or forceps will increase the distance between the radioactive metal fragment and the fingers and thus greatly reduce any radiation dose to the health care worker.

Hot Particles. "Hot" particles are microscopic particles that can be highly radioactive. Typically, they contain ^{60}Co or fission products. These might be found on a nuclear reactor worker after a reactor accident. These particles can be difficult to localize and remove. They may give a large radiation dose to a small volume of tissues. If the particle is trapped under a nail or is in the fold of the skin, routine washings may not dislodge it. The particle can sometimes be localized by using a thick piece of lead. If the lead is placed between the particle and the radiation detector, the exposure rate should decrease substantially. Once the particle is localized, it can usually be removed by using simple mechanical means. Rarely, a punch biopsy of the skin may be necessary.

Terrorist Events. There are several scenarios in which nuclear materials may be used in a terrorist event. An intact sealed source could be placed in a populated area, generating whole-body exposures but no contamination. A radiological dispersal device, such as a conventional explosive combined with radioactive materials, the so-called "dirty bomb," could be employed to disseminate radioactive materials over a local or wide area. For example, a conventional explosive could be used in conjunction with a large sealed source or spent nuclear fuel to spread multiple radioactive metallic fragments or radioactive dirt. Victims of such an attack would likely have contamination in addition to local radiation exposures, as well as injuries from the explosion itself. An attack on a research or commercial power reactor could produce a large-scale dispersion of nuclear material; victims could be exposed to whole-body and localized radiation, as well as internal and external contamination. Transported nuclear materials such as radiopharmaceuticals or radioactive waste could be the subject of a terrorist attack. The effects would vary depending on whether the containers were breached—intact containers would produce only external exposures, whereas destruction of the containers and dispersal of their contents could also lead to contamination. A "dud" nuclear weapon that does not undergo a nuclear reaction would still disperse radioactive materials by the associated conventional explosion, leading to contamination in addition to effects from the conventional explosion itself. A nuclear weapon effectively detonated by a terrorist group might be relatively small scale but still capable of widespread damage, including thermal and blast effects from the denotation along with contamination and exposure of affected persons and equipment.

MANAGEMENT OF RADIATION INJURIES

General Measures

The principles governing the treatment of radiation injuries are similar to the principles governing the treatment of any medical condition, especially those arising from hazardous materials. Treatment objectives must be prioritized (Fig. 88.10).

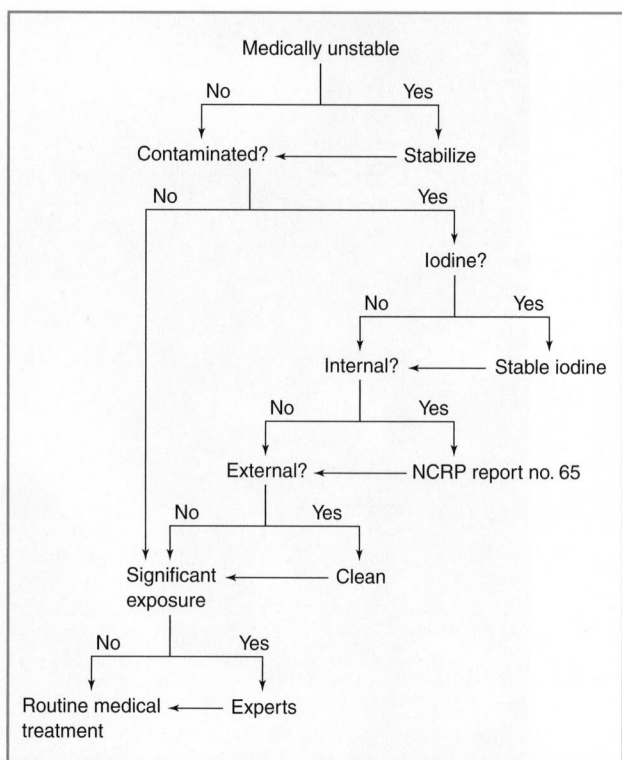

FIGURE 88.10 Treatment of radiation injuries. NCRP, National Council on Radiation Protection and Measurements.

Because no survivable radiation injury requires immediate life-saving treatment, the medical staff should focus their attention on the treatment of non–radiation-related life-threatening conditions. In the past, some medical personnel were so distracted by the radiation aspects of an accident that routine medical care was delayed.

Once the patient is stabilized, the radiation-related injuries can be addressed. Because there is no immediate treatment of radiation exposure, the problem of radioactive contamination should be addressed first. In most circumstances, a Geiger counter can be used to determine the presence of contamination. In addition, the probability of contamination can be assessed by obtaining an accurate description of the accident and the likely radiation source. If the patient is a radiation worker, finding his or her radiation badge and performing a "reenactment" of the accident may be critical for dose estimation.

Internal Contamination

Treatment of internal contamination is most effective if initiated promptly. The requirement for prompt treatment is a dilemma for the physician. First, it is difficult to determine if internal contamination is present until the external contamination has been removed. Moistened cotton Q-tips can be used to perform nasal swabs. If these show radioactivity, inhalation of radioactive materials is possible. The nature of the accident may provide clues to the possibility of internal contamination (e.g., a fire with smoke leading to the inhalation of radioactive particles). Second, the most effective treat-

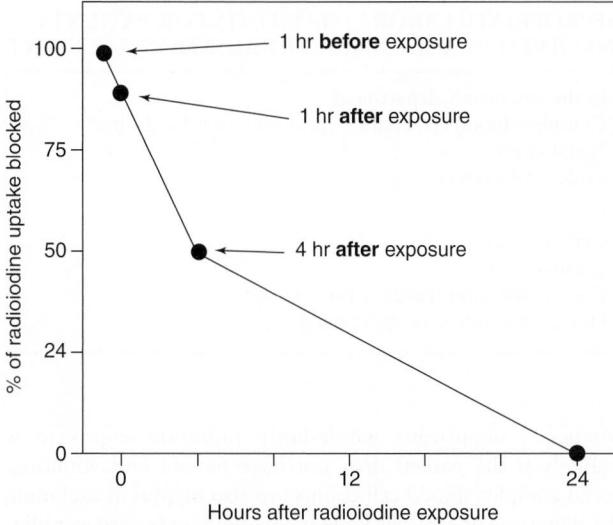

Effectiveness of stable iodine

FIGURE 88.11 Stable iodine is most effective if administered as soon as possible after the ingestion of radioactive iodine. Repeated daily doses would be appropriate only if there was potentially continuing ingestion or inhalation.

ment requires knowledge of the radionuclide involved and its chemical form. This information is usually not immediately available. Fortunately, there are simple general treatment measures that can be effectively instituted before the magnitude of the internal contamination is fully known.

If given soon after exposure, stable iodine is effective for preventing the uptake of radioactive iodine by the thyroid gland. Prompt administration of stable iodine should be considered if there is a possibility of external contamination with (or ingestion or inhalation of) radioactive iodine (Fig. 88.11 and Table 88.8). Because radioactive iodine is volatile, it is likely to be inhaled. If a contaminated child were brought to the ED after an accident with a radiopharmaceutical truck carrying radioactive iodine, administration of stable iodine would be appropriate. If further investigation revealed no radioactive iodine, little harm would have been done by having administered the stable iodine. A single dose of oral iodine is highly unlikely to cause any adverse reactions, even in persons who have serious reactions to iodinated contrast agents or seafood.

After a nuclear reactor accident that results in the release of a large amount of radioactive iodine, three steps can be taken to minimize the adverse effects on the public. First, the public should be sheltered or evacuated to prevent further exposure via fallout or gaseous materials. Second, potassium iodide (KI)

may be administered if available. However, it is important to note that many of nuclear reactors in the United States do not house radioactive iodine, making KI useless. Third, the food supply can be monitored carefully to prevent further ingestion of radioactive iodine or other radionuclides. If a reactor accident occurs that involves contamination of the public, understandable concern by members of the public will ensue. If this happens, emergency medical facilities should try to preserve their valuable resources for patients who need lifesaving medical treatment. Plans must be made to refer uninjured persons and persons with minor injuries to other facilities. Hospitals should not become decontamination centers.

Several simple steps can be taken to treat internal contamination nonspecifically. The goals of treatment are to prevent the absorption of the radionuclide and to enhance its excretion. Safe techniques that prevent the absorption of radionuclides include the administration of activated charcoal and alginate-containing antacids. Enhanced excretion can be achieved by hydration and administration of a purgative. Specific treatment of internal contamination depends on the radionuclide, its chemical and physical forms, and the route of internal contamination. Recommendations for many specific treatments can be found in the NCRP Report 65, titled *Management of Persons Accidentally Contaminated with Radionuclides*. This report ought to be available in every hospital ED and can be downloaded for a fee from the NCRP Web site (http://www.ncrponline.org). An updated version of this report is expected in 2009. Initiation of treatments that entail some risk to the patient (e.g., pulmonary lavage, intravenous chelating agents) should be undertaken only after consultation with experts; the benefits of the treatment should be significantly greater than the risks. The most effective treatment of internal contamination is preventing the internal contamination in the first place.

External Contamination

External contamination is treated in the same way as contamination by other hazardous chemical or biological agents. To make certain that the hazard is treated appropriately, it is easiest to imagine that the patient has been covered with an easily detectable noxious agent (e.g., sewage). Under this circumstance, the caregivers would wear gloves, a gown, shoe covers, and a mask. The purpose of wearing these garments is primarily to keep caregivers clean and to make cleanup easier. The garments do not decrease the exposure to penetrating radiation. The mask is recommended to prevent individuals from inadvertently touching their contaminated fingers to their nose or mouth. If available, film badges or other devices to measure radiation exposure should be worn by hospital staff who are in close contact with the patient.

If the external contamination is widespread, it may be helpful to cover the floor. If only a small area of contamination is present, spread can be prevented by simply wrapping the contaminated area until it can be cleaned. Because it is much easier to detect radioactive contamination than chemical or biological hazards, cleanup following a radiation accident will be much more effective and documentable. Precautions taken to prevent the inadvertent spread of contamination will make cleanup much easier.

MEDICAL EMERGENCIES

TABLE 88.8

DOSE OF STABLE IODINE (SSKI) BY AGE

Age	Dose (po)
<1 mo	16 mg
1 mo–3 yr	32 mg
3–18 yr	65 mg
>18 yr	130 mg

TABLE 88.9

DECONTAMINATION

Remove clothes	Cover clean wounds to prevent contamination
Wash with a damp cloth and tepid water	Prevent external contamination from becoming internal
Pay special attention to skin folds and fingernails	Do not abrade the skin

TABLE 88.10

APPROPRIATE LABORATORY TESTS FOR PATIENTS INVOLVED IN A SIGNIFICANT RADIATION ACCIDENT

In the emergency department
Complete blood cell count; repeat every 6 h for 24 h
Nasal swabs
Collect all excreta

Later
Cytogenetics
Sperm count
Eye examination (baseline for cataracts)
Human leukocyte antigen typing

External contamination is rarely a significant medical problem; however, logistic problems that must be addressed require preplanning. To minimize the chances of contaminating an unnecessarily large area of the ED, the patient should be admitted through a separate entrance. If this is not possible, the patient can be placed on a clean stretcher outside the ED and wrapped in a cloth (not plastic) sheet and then transported to the desired area of the hospital. Access to the treatment area should be controlled.

Removal of the patient's clothing will usually eliminate up to 90% of the external contamination (Table 88.9). Contaminated articles should be placed in labeled plastic bags. Residual contamination is likely to be on the hands, face, hair, and wounds. These should be washed with lukewarm water and soap. Cleaning the skin with damp washcloths is much better than cleaning with running water. The radioactive dirt on the damp washcloth can be contained by placing the cloth in a plastic bag. Radioactive dirt in wash water is much more difficult to control but, when necessary in the course of patient care, may be discharged to the sewer system by flushing. Shaving should not be performed because this may make small cuts and increase absorption through the skin. Excessive rubbing of the skin may also increase transdermal uptake.

Open uncontaminated wounds should be covered to prevent them from becoming contaminated. Contaminated wounds should be cleaned like any other dirty wound. All samples from the patient should be saved and labeled if there is any question about the identity of the radionuclides.

A Geiger counter should be used to monitor and document the progress of the decontamination efforts. If contamination persists, the source may be fixed to the skin or may be internal. Radiation experts should be consulted before more aggressive decontamination attempts are made. Some residual contamination may be acceptable.

Exposure

Other than symptomatic measures, there is no immediate treatment to reverse whole-body or local radiation exposure.

Medically significant whole-body radiation exposure is unlikely if the patient does not have nausea and vomiting. Serial complete blood cell counts are also helpful in excluding the diagnosis of a recent large whole-body exposure to radiation (Table 88.10). In the absence of other major trauma, the absolute lymphocyte count will rapidly fall in patients who have been exposed to a large radiation dose. If a patient has been exposed to a large dose of radiation, there is little in the way of specific medical treatment that needs to be done in the ED. The threat to the patient's life will occur within days to weeks after the exposure.

The diagnosis of a local radiation injury requires vigilance. The physician should consider the possibility of a local radiation injury whenever there is an unexplained painless "burn." A complete blood cell count to exclude an accompanying whole-body exposure is indicated. The prognosis of a local radiation injury depends on the dose. The dose can be estimated only by having a qualified physicist reconstruct the accident that led to the exposure.

Suggested Readings

American College of Radiology. *Disaster preparedness for radiology professionals: response to radiological terrorism.* Reston, VA: American College of Radiology, 2006.
Armed Forces Radiobiology Research Institute (AFRRI). *Medical management of radiological casualties,* 2nd ed. Bethesda, MD: AFRRI, 2003.
Gusev IA, Guskova AK, Mettler FA, eds. *Medical management of radiation accidents,* 2nd ed. Boca Raton, FL: CRC Press, 2001.
Mettler FA Jr, Voelz GL. Major radiation exposure—what to expect and how to respond. *N Engl J Med* 2002;345:1554–1561.
National Council on Radiation Protection and Measurements (NCRP). *Management of persons accidentally contaminated with radionuclides* (NCRP Report No. 65). Bethesda, MD: NCRP, 1980.
National Council on Radiation Protection and Measurements (NCRP). *Management of terrorist events involving radioactive material* (NCRP Report No. 138). Bethesda, MD: NCRP, 2001.
Ricks RC, Berger ME, O'Hara FM Jr, eds. *The medical basis for radiation—accident preparedness: the clinical care of victims.* Boca Raton, FL: Parthenon-CRC Press, 2002.

CHAPTER 89 ■ GASTROINTESTINAL EMERGENCIES

DENNIS R. DURBIN, MD, MSCE, CHRIS A. LIACOURAS, MD, AND JEFFREY A. SEIDEN, MD

GASTROINTESTINAL BLEEDING

Gastrointestinal (GI) bleeding is a common and occasionally life-threatening condition in infants and children. An orderly approach to this problem is essential and is outlined in Chapter 29. One of the most important initial steps in establishing the cause of GI bleeding in children is determining whether the source of bleeding is the upper or lower intestinal tract. The following discussion of general principles of management, as well as specific diagnoses, is therefore organized accordingly. Only those conditions most appropriately classified as medical diagnoses are described in this chapter. Additional causes of GI bleeding that are more appropriately classified as surgical diagnoses, including intestinal malrotation with volvulus, intestinal duplications, intussusception, and Meckel's diverticulum, are discussed in detail in Chapter 121.

General Principles of Management

In contrast to the adult experience, most children presenting to the emergency department (ED) with either upper or lower GI bleeding have not experienced significant blood loss. Many patients can be managed successfully with judicious laboratory investigation, conservative supportive care, and follow-up with a primary care provider or an appropriate subspecialist. A detailed discussion of pertinent laboratory evaluation and initial management of each of the most common causes of GI bleeding in children is provided in the following sections.

Severe GI bleeding should be considered a potentially life-threatening emergency that may require the cooperation of a team, including the emergency physician, surgeon, and gastroenterologist. Similar to the management of all potentially life-threatening conditions in children, the initial approach to the child with significant GI hemorrhage begins with an assessment of the child's airway, breathing, and circulation. A child with overt hemodynamic instability or suspected significant volume loss should have cerebral perfusion and oxygenation optimized by patient positioning, fluid resuscitation, and supplemental oxygen. For patients with hematemesis, airway protection is paramount to prevent pulmonary aspiration of blood. Positioning may be all that is needed, but in massive upper intestinal bleeding, endotracheal intubation may be lifesaving. The next priority is the insertion of two large-bore intravenous (IV) catheters (14 to 20 gauge in the child and at least 22 gauge in small infants). An intraosseous or central venous catheter should be placed if there is difficulty obtaining adequate peripheral venous access.

Immediate laboratory studies in any patient with severe GI bleeding should include (i) type and cross-match, (ii) complete blood cell (CBC) count, (iii) platelet count, (iv) prothrombin time (PT), and (v) partial thromboplastin time (PTT). Additional laboratory studies may be indicated on the basis of the differential diagnosis of the most likely cause of the patient's bleeding and are discussed later in this section. Arterial blood gases are also important parameters to follow in severe blood loss associated with shock. The hematocrit is an unreliable initial index of acute blood loss because it may be normal or only slightly decreased. Its subsequent fall will depend on (i) the rate and type of fluid replacement and (ii) the body's own hemostatic mechanisms, resulting in renal conservation of fluid and electrolytes and gradual shifts of fluid from extravascular to intravascular compartments.

IV therapy has two major objectives: (i) restoration of intravascular volume (reflected in blood pressure or pulse) and (ii) restoration of oxygen-carrying capacity (reflected in hemoglobin and hematocrit values). The former objective can be accomplished by both crystalloid and colloid solutions, whereas the latter can be accomplished solely by the infusion of blood. The practical limitations of time required to properly type and cross-match blood make crystalloid solutions the mainstay of early resuscitation. In the rare circumstance of massive, ongoing hemorrhage in which low oxygen-carrying capacity is believed to be an important factor at the onset of resuscitation, O-negative blood may be used. In most cases, proper type and cross-match can be performed whereas intravascular volume is restored by nonsanguineous solutions. The exact type of solution to be used is controversial. Studies in both animals and humans have shown a reduction in intravascular and extravascular volume in acute blood loss; therefore, the preferred method is manual infusion of crystalloid solutions, such as normal saline or Ringer's lactate, in 20 mL per kg boluses until intravascular volume is minimally restored as indicated by a decrease in the pulse rate, a rise in blood pressure level, and/or disappearance of clinical signs of peripheral vasoconstriction. Colloid solutions, such as albumin, plasma, or hetastarch, should be used only when blood loss is massive and continuous because in this situation, respiratory insufficiency or shock lung may develop with a fall in plasma oncotic pressure. Dextran is to be avoided because it may affect platelet function. Patients who are in shock at the time of admission should have the urinary bladder catheterized in the ED to accurately measure urine output and to allow for early detection of acute tubular necrosis.

Overexpansion of intravascular volume is potentially dangerous, particularly not only in bleeding varices but also in bleeding gastric or duodenal ulcers. Therefore, after correction of shock and restoration of urine flow, further IV volume replacement should be titrated to match continuing blood loss. The decision to begin transfusion depends on the hematocrit taken at the time of restoration of blood volume and on evidence of ongoing bleeding. For a patient who has stopped bleeding, blood transfusion may be given to allow some reserve in case of rebleeding. Under most circumstances, slow transfusion to return the hematocrit to approximately 30% is recommended to achieve this objective. In this case, packed red blood cells (10 mL per kg) are used to reduce the volume load for the patient. In addition, packed red blood cells contain considerably less ammonia than whole blood, an important factor for patients who have severe liver disease. For a patient who has continuous bleeding, ongoing blood transfusion is the only means of maintaining adequate oxygen-carrying capacity. In this case, the rate of bleeding determines the rate of transfusion. A sustained rate of transfusion is recommended and is best achieved with an electrical infusion pump, not by gravity. Potential complications of massive transfusions include hypercitrinemia, hyperlacticacidemia, hypocalcemia, decreased levels of clotting factors, and thrombocytopenia. The risks inherent in massive transfusions are definitively lowered by using packed red blood cells, fresh frozen plasma, proper filters, and blood warmers. Any patient with or without a history of liver disease who presents with GI bleeding associated with an abnormal PT should receive 5 to 10 mg of vitamin K (subcutaneously for non–life-threatening bleeding, intravenously for life-threatening bleeding) as soon as possible.

UPPER GASTROINTESTINAL BLEEDING

Background

Upper GI bleeding is generally regarded as originating proximal to the ligament of Treitz. Hematemesis or bloody gastric aspirates from a nasogastric (NG) tube may originate from the mouth, nasopharynx, esophagus, stomach, biliary tree, or duodenum. The most common causes of upper GI bleeding in children are mucosal lesions including esophagitis, gastritis, Mallory-Weiss tear, peptic ulcer disease, and duodenitis. Less common but important causes include bleeding esophageal varices and vascular lesions. Endoscopy, when performed by a well-trained physician, is the most sensitive and specific diagnostic procedure for determining the cause and site of upper GI bleeding. Specific diagnosis should be pursued in patients who have (i) active bleeding documented by NG lavage; (ii) evidence of severe hemorrhage (hemodynamic instability or equilibrated hemoglobin level less than 10 g per dL); (iii) conditions that affect healing or clotting, such as catabolic state or serious chronic disease; (iv) a history of unexplained gross or occult bleeding or unexplained iron deficiency anemia; or (v) a history of chronic dyspepsia (vomiting, abdominal pain, nausea, oral regurgitation, heartburn, dysphagia).

The pathophysiology, clinical manifestations, and specific management issues related to each of the most common causes of upper GI bleeding in children are discussed. As noted in Chapter 29, an upper tract source of GI bleeding is often indicated either by a history of hematemesis or by obtaining fresh (red) or old (coffee ground) blood via gastric lavage after the placement of an NG tube.

General Principles of Nasogastric Lavage

Not every child with a history of possible upper GI bleeding requires NG lavage. Patients who have acute, self-limited hematemesis of streaks of blood or a small amount of coffee-ground material in the context of forceful emesis, recurrent gastroesophageal reflux (GER), symptoms of infectious gastroenteritis, or epistaxis can often be managed presumptively without gastric lavage. However, lavage should be performed in all patients suspected of having significant GI bleeding that is indicated by either history or physical examination (e.g., pallor, unexplained tachycardia, poor perfusion). The purpose of gastric lavage is to confirm the level of bleeding and to estimate the rate of bleeding. There is no evidence that gastric lavage has any therapeutic role in controlling hemorrhage. It is important to realize that a clear NG aspirate does not exclude major bleeding from the upper GI tract.

Most patients can be effectively lavaged with an NG sump tube (12F in small children, 14F to 16F in older children). Verification of the location of the tube in the stomach by injection of air and auscultation over the stomach is essential. The recommended volume for each saline infusion depends on age: 50 mL for infants and 100 to 200 mL for older children. With the patient's head elevated to 30 degrees, the solution, at room temperature, is rapidly infused into the stomach, allowed to stand for 2 to 3 minutes, and then aspirated by gentle suction. Return volumes should approximate input volumes, and discrepancies should be recorded. If aspiration meets with significant resistance, the physician should reposition the tube, reposition the patient, or increase the amount of solution introduced. Saline lavage of the stomach should be performed ideally by two people. One person fills and empties the stomach, while the other person empties and fills the syringes.

Blood-flecked gastric aspirate or coffee-ground material indicates a low rate of bleeding. In contrast, bright red blood, especially if it does not clear with repeated lavage for 5 to 10 minutes, suggests a significant or ongoing hemorrhage. No benefit is derived from continuous lavage longer than 10 minutes if return is not clearing. The tube can be left to gravity or low suction and irrigated every 15 to 30 minutes to assess the activity of the bleeding. The presumed lesion causing the bleeding determines the subsequent management of the patient.

Nonspecific Mucosal Lesions

Background

GI bleeding may be a complication of all acute and chronic nonspecific upper GI mucosal lesions [esophagitis, gastritis, prolapse gastropathy (PG), Mallory-Weiss tears, and duodenitis].

Regardless of the cause, upper GI bleeding usually stops spontaneously, often by the time the patient arrives in the ED. Esophagitis as a result of GER is being diagnosed more often with improved pediatric fiber-optic endoscopes. The use of endoscopic biopsy has allowed physicians to document esophagitis as the cause of bleeding in many patients with clinically significant GER. Exposure to aspirin and nonsteroidal antiinflammatory drugs (NSAIDs; e.g., ibuprofen, naproxen) has also been associated with gastritis and mucosal ulceration. A more recent study suggests that clinically apparent upper GI bleeding from esophageal, gastric, and duodenal erosions and/or ulcerations may occur in as many as 1% of healthy, full-term newborns. Mallory-Weiss tears are mucosal lacerations of the gastric cardia or gastroesophageal junction induced by retching or vomiting. These lesions, however, are quite rare in children. While accounting for approximately 5% of cases of upper GI bleeding in adults, there are very few case reports of upper GI bleeding in children. On the other hand, PG is the more common postemetic condition that causes hematemesis in children. In one series, PG was found in approximately 25% of children undergoing upper endoscopy for hematemesis.

Pathophysiology

The upper GI mucosa bleeds when an ulcerating process erodes into a blood vessel, usually an artery in the base of the ulcer. In most cases, normal mechanisms of thrombosis and healing stop the bleeding and prevent recurrent bleeding. Erosion of larger arteries, however, in which blood flow exceeds the capacity of normal hemostasis, results in continuous hemorrhage. A more common scenario is that thrombosis temporarily stops the bleeding, but aneurysmal dilation of the artery in the recanal-ization process or continuing arteritis from the chemical irrita-tion of acid digestion facilitates recurrent hemorrhage. Acid and pepsin also produce profound adverse effects on platelet aggregation and plasma coagulation. The pathogenesis of Mallory-Weiss tears involves the production of transient large gradients between the intragastric and intrathoracic pressures at the gastroesophageal junction as a result of forceful retching. The gradient results in dilation of the gastroesophageal junc-tion and, thus, tears. PG is caused by repeated forceful emesis, in which the stomach prolapses through the lower esophageal sphincter causing mucosal injury.

Clinical Manifestations

Diagnosis of mucosal lesions is usually suspected by an antecedent history of vomiting and/or abdominal pain and the absence of physical findings suggestive of chronic liver disease or portal hypertension. Reflux esophagitis is suspected in infants, usually younger than 1 year, who have a history of recurrent nonprojectile emesis, "wet burps" after feeding, or a documented diagnosis of GER. Infants presenting with emesis that is blood streaked or contains a small amount of coffee-ground material. They may be fussy but consolable and may have been previously diagnosed with colic. Reflux esophagitis should also be suspected in infants with guaiac-positive stools or iron deficiency anemia. A history of repeated aspirin or NSAID use for control of fever and/or pain should also prompt suspicion for gastric mucosal lesions as the cause of upper GI bleeding. Clinical features of Mallory-Weiss tears and PG are similar, though bleeding in PG tends to be less severe. These entities should be suspected in children with a history of pro-tracted forceful vomiting and streaks of hematemesis appearing after several episodes of nonbloody emesis.

Management

For patients who have significant bleeding and for whom NG lavage was initiated, if gastric contents clear following initial saline lavage and immediate endoscopy is not planned, gastric irrigation should be performed every 15 minutes for 1 hour and then every hour for 2 to 3 hours. If the patient is hemody-namically stable and gastric return remains clear for the afore-mentioned period, the tube is electively removed. Persistent nausea or vomiting or the presence of ileus points to the need for continued drainage.

Patients with nonspecific mucosal lesions theoretically should benefit from neutralization of intragastric acidity by antacids, as well as reduction in gastric acid and pepsin secre-tion by H_2-receptor antagonists. For patients with significant symptoms or blood loss, H_2-antagonists may be given ini-tially by the IV route, switching to the oral route when the NG tube is removed. Ranitidine (1.0 mg per kg per dose intravenously three times a day or 2 to 4 mg per kg per dose orally two times a day initially) is an appropriate choice. IV proton pump inhibitors, such as pantoprazole (0.5 to 1 mg per kg per day once daily), have been prescribed for adults with good success. Studies are limited, but proton pump inhibitors appear to be safe and effective in children as well. In addition, sucralfate (40 to 80 mg per kg per day) in two or three divided doses may be prescribed for patients with mucosal lesions. Finally, children with acute discomfort may be given antacids via the NG tube. For patients who have acute, self-limited bleeding and who are not considered can-didates for endoscopy, oral H_2-antagonists are continued for 2 to 4 weeks, at which time they are empirically discontinued if the patient is asymptomatic.

In general, all patients with a history suggestive of signifi-cant upper GI bleeding should be admitted to the hospital for observation. A clear NG aspirate should never be used as an indication to discharge a patient from the ED if the history suggests significant bleeding. The main reason for admission is the unknown incidence of rebleeding from these lesions in children.

Esophageal Varices

Background

Portal hypertension may result from either extrahepatic presi-nusoidal obstruction (50% to 65% of cases in children) or hepatic parenchymal disorders. Extrahepatic obstruction (e.g., portal or splenic vein obstruction) is associated with omphali-tis, dehydration, sepsis, and umbilical vein catheterization. Hepatic parenchymal disease may result from biliary cirrhosis associated with biliary atresia, cystic fibrosis, hepatitis, α_1-antitrypsin deficiency, or congenital hepatic fibrosis. Persons with either type of portal hypertension are susceptible to GI hemorrhage both from bleeding esophageal varices and from congestive or hemorrhagic gastritis. After development of por-tal hypertension, the onset of esophageal varices can vary from a few months to many years.

Pathophysiology

Portal hypertension results from relative obstruction of portal venous blood flow, leading to the development of either portal systemic collateral veins or varices. Portal systemic collaterals develop in any area where veins draining the portal venous system are in close approximation to veins draining into the caval system (i.e., submucosa of the esophagus, submucosa of the rectum, and anterior abdominal wall). Esophageal and gastric fundal varices, connecting branches of the coronary veins with branches of the azygous vein, are the most likely site of spontaneous hemorrhage (Fig. 89.1).

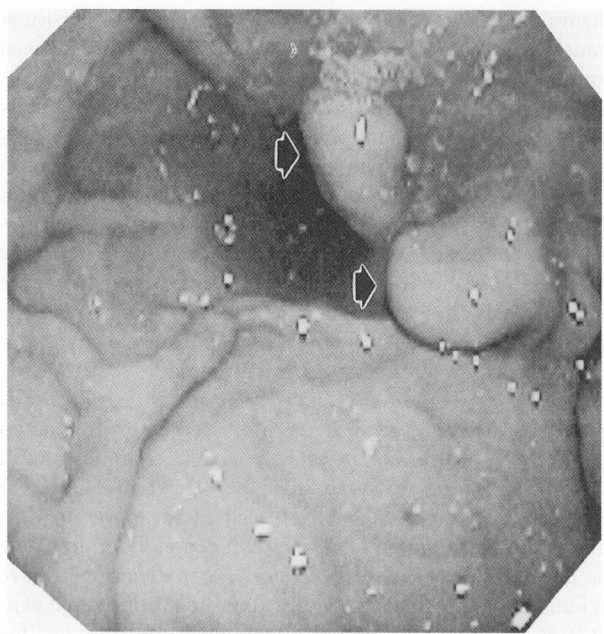

FIGURE 89.1 Gastric varices. The *arrows* represent two large blood-filled varices in the gastric cardia.

Clinical Manifestations

Patients with portal hypertension may have occult bleeding, but more commonly, the bleeding is brisk and patients will have melena and/or hematemesis. The possibility of bleeding esophageal varices should be considered in any patient with a history of jaundice (beyond the newborn period), hepatitis, blood transfusion, chronic right-sided heart failure, pulmonary hypertension, omphalitis, umbilical vein catheterization, or one of the hepatic parenchymal diseases previously noted. Accordingly, the physical examination may reveal stigmata of the underlying disease leading to portal hypertension, including jaundice, ascites, rectal hemorrhoids, and hepatosplenomegaly.

Management

The initial management of suspected variceal hemorrhage is identical to that of massive upper GI bleeding from any source. Fluid resuscitation to maintain adequate perfusion is warranted, but overexpansion of the intravascular volume should be avoided because it contributes to rebleeding. Coagulation abnormalities should be managed aggressively with IV vitamin K, fresh frozen plasma, and platelets. Bleeding varices may be the initial sign of sepsis in patients who have cirrhosis; therefore, any patient who has fever should be started on broad-spectrum antibiotics such as ampicillin (200 mg per kg per day) and gentamicin (5 to 7.5 mg per kg per day), pending results of blood cultures.

Suspicion of variceal bleeding is not a contraindication to pass an NG tube. An NG tube should be placed in a patient suspected of having upper GI bleeding. If bleeding ceases during the initial gastric lavage, the tube should be managed as previously described. Antacids and H_2-antagonists are given in the doses used for mucosal lesions. Pharmacologic therapy of acute variceal hemorrhage includes the splanchnic arterial constrictor vasopressin or somatostatin. Emergency flexible endoscopy should be arranged if the patient remains hemody-

namically unstable and should be performed as soon as possible once deemed safe. Alternatively, endoscopic treatment may be delayed until hemorrhage has been controlled by pharmacologic agents, especially if the endoscopist has difficulty obtaining a clear field of vision.

Vasopressin administration has been well documented to decrease blood flow and pressure through the portal circulation. The physician should begin infusing 0.002 units per kg per minute and titrate to effect up to 0.01 units per kg per minute. Adverse effects can be significant; thus, the child must be monitored carefully. Major complications include myocardial ischemia, life-threatening arrhythmias, and limb vasoconstriction or ischemia. Minor complications include water retention with sodium depletion, benign arrhythmias, and acrocyanosis. The vasopressin is usually given in 5% dextrose in water; the exact dilution is based on overall volumes of fluids being infused. Infusing vasopressin through a large-bore, preferably central venous, catheter is the safest method. The reported success rate of vasopressin infusion in adults is 50% to 70%. Because of the high rate of rebleeding, the drug should be continued at the dosage that controls bleeding for a minimum of 12 to 24 hours after all bleeding has stopped. This management plan stems from studies showing sustained vasoconstrictive effects of vasopressin on splanchnic vessels in dogs for more than 24 hours. However, this point is controversial because tachyphylaxis reportedly also develops with prolonged use of vasopressin.

Endoscopic techniques available for acute management of variceal bleeding include endoscopic variceal sclerotherapy, whereby a sclerosing agent such as sodium morrhuate is injected into the varix. In addition, endoscopic variceal ligation using an elastic band ligature device has also been widely used to control bleeding from varices and to prevent recurrences.

Gastroesophageal balloon tamponade is a high-risk procedure. It should be considered only for previously proven gastric or esophageal varices unresponsive to pharmacotherapy and when the patient cannot undergo endoscopic management in a timely fashion. Either a Sengstaken-Blakemore (S-B) tube or a Linton tube may be used. The S-B tube has both gastric and esophageal balloon tubes, whereas the Linton tube has a single lavage gastric balloon. A pediatric tube is used for children younger than 11 to 13 years; the adult tube can be used in adolescents. Gastroesophageal tamponade is reported to arrest bleeding initially in 50% to 80% of cases. However, the reported incidence of major complications from the use of the S-B tube ranges from 9% to 35%; such complications include rupture or erosion of the esophageal or gastric fundal mucosa, occlusion of the airway by the balloon, and aspiration of secretions resulting from inadequate drainage of the occluded esophagus. Death directly attributed to the use of the tube has been reported in 5% to 20% of patients in whom the tube was used.

Miscellaneous Causes of Upper Gastrointestinal Bleeding

In the first few days of life, or in breast-fed infants, *swallowed maternal blood* may be the cause of hematemesis or melena in an infant who otherwise appears healthy. Performing a guaiac test on expressed breast milk may suggest the diagnosis. An Apt-Downey test may be performed on a sample of emesis or

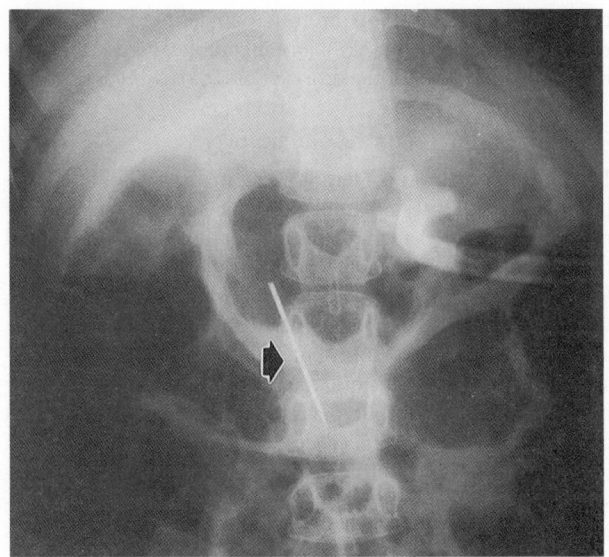

FIGURE 89.2 Gastric foreign body. This 6-year-old developmentally delayed patient ingested a large straight pin that caused bleeding of the gastric antrum. The *arrow* represents the foreign body. An opaque gastrostomy tube is also radiographically present.

NG aspirate to definitively diagnose the condition. Blood from the aspirate is placed on a filter paper and mixed with 1% NaOH. Adult hemoglobin will be reduced to give a rusty brown or yellow color. Fetal hemoglobin is resistant to denaturation and will retain a bright pink or red color.

A *Dieulafoy lesion* is an unusual cause of GI bleeding, in which massive hemorrhage occurs from a pinpoint nonulcerated arterial lesion, usually high in the fundus of the stomach. The bleeding results from an unusually large submucosal artery that travels a tortuous course through the submucosa and may erode through a mucosal defect. Its characteristic presentation is one of recurrent, massive hematemesis, usually without any prodromal symptoms. This diagnosis is primarily performed in adults, but patients as young as 20 months have been diagnosed with a Dieulafoy lesion, and most series contain a number of teenagers. Management is similar to that for any patient with a significant GI hemorrhage. Diagnosis can be made by endoscopy, during which the Dieulafoy lesion can usually be located.

Finally, swallowed foreign bodies can cause significant trauma and GI bleeding. Most swallowed foreign bodies, even those with sharp edges, will pass spontaneously and require no specific therapy. However, on occasion, a sharp foreign body may be the cause of GI bleeding (Fig. 89.2). Removal by endoscopy is indicated if significant bleeding occurs.

LOWER GASTROINTESTINAL BLEEDING

Background

Rectal bleeding is a relatively uncommon but worrisome complaint in the ambulatory or ED setting. A case series of children presenting with rectal bleeding to an urban, tertiary care ED indicated that rectal bleeding was the chief complaint of 0.3% of all ED visits during a 1-year period. The average age of patients was approximately 5 years, with nearly half of the patients younger than 1 year. No patient in the series was judged hemodynamically unstable in the ED, nor did any patient require a blood transfusion. The most common presentation was for hematochezia (98% of patients), with 10% of patients presenting with melena (some patients presented with both complaints). Diarrhea (37% of patients), abdominal pain (43%), and constipation (22%) were the most common associated symptoms, with only 2% of patients presenting with fever. Presumptive diagnoses were made in two-thirds of patients, most of which (81%) did not change with follow-up. Potentially life-threatening disorders (intussusception and Meckel's diverticulum) were found in 4% of cases.

The cause of lower GI bleeding varies with age. Among infants younger than 6 months, the most common diagnoses are milk-protein sensitivity (allergic colitis), anorectal fissures, and infectious gastroenteritis. Children 1 to 5 years of age are most likely to have infectious gastroenteritis, intussusception, Meckel's diverticulum, colonic polyps, and anorectal fissures. Older children typically have infectious gastroenteritis, inflammatory bowel disease (IBD), and hemorrhoids/rectal varices. The pathophysiology, clinical manifestations, and specific management indicated for the most common conditions causing lower GI bleeding in children are discussed in the following sections.

Anorectal Fissures and Hemorrhoids

Anal fissures are the most common cause of rectal bleeding in the first 2 years of life. Most occur in infants younger than 1 year. Anal fissures (pleural) may result from diarrhea, which causes perineal irritation, but it is more commonly associated with constipation. The fissure usually starts when passage of a hard stool tears the sensitive squamous lining of the anal canal. Subsequent bowel movements are associated with pain and/or bleeding. Bright red blood is seen coating the stool. The infant begins to withhold stool, leading to increasing constipation and a vicious cycle of hard stools, bleeding, and pain. Anal fissures (pleural) can be seen by spreading the perineal skin to evert the anal canal. Simply spreading the buttocks to view the anal opening is not sufficient. Treatment consists of local skin care combined with stool softeners. Malt extract (Maltsupex 1 to 3 tablespoons per day) or lactulose (1 to 4 tablespoons per day) can be given to soften the stool. Local care involves sitz baths four times a day, a perianal cleansing lotion (Balneol) after bowel movements, and an emollient protective ointment (Balmex) after each bowel movement.

Small varicosities of the external hemorrhoidal plexus (i.e., hemorrhoids) may occur in the healing process associated with anal fissure. They rarely cause pain or bleeding. Therapy is directed at the treatment of the anal fissure. The presence of external hemorrhoids does not imply associated internal hemorrhoids. The latter may develop in response to portal hypertension and may be a cause of painless rectal bleeding.

All patients with perianal excoriation, multiple anal fissures, recurrent anal fissure, or fissure resistant to conservative management should have perianal cultures for β-hemolytic streptococci. If this organism is recovered, the patient should receive a 7-day course of oral penicillin.

Polyps

There are two major types of polyps that may be diagnosed in infancy or childhood: hamartomatous and adenomatous. Hamartomatous polyps are generally benign and are the usual type of polyp found in juvenile polyps, juvenile polyposis coli, and Peutz-Jeghers syndrome. Adenomatous polyps are potentially premalignant and are found in a number of syndromes including familial adenomatous polyposis and Gardner's syndrome.

Juvenile polyps are the most common of the polyp syndromes in children, found in 15% of patients in one series who had colonoscopy for rectal bleeding (Fig. 89.3). More than one polyp may be found in more than 50% of cases of juvenile polyps. Most (75%) of the polyps are rectosigmoid or in the descending colon, 15% are found in the transverse colon, and 10% in the ascending colon. Autoamputation of juvenile polyps, especially in the rectum, occurs spontaneously in most cases. In juvenile polyposis coli, multiple juvenile polyps are found throughout the colon. Peutz-Jeghers syndrome is the association of mucocutaneous pigmented lesions and hamartomatous polyps. It has autosomal-dominant inheritance with a high degree of penetrance. The macular, melanin-containing pigmented lesions characteristically occur on the buccal mucosa, lips, face, arms, palms and soles, and perianal region. The polyps are typically located in the small intestine but can also be found throughout the GI tract.

Familial adenomatous polyposis is an autosomal-dominant inherited syndrome consisting of multiple adenomatous polyps that are generally confined to the colon but can also be found throughout the GI tract. A 6% incidence of malignant transformation of these lesions is present by 15 years of age, prompting recommendations for total proctocolectomy by 18 years of age. Gardner's syndrome is an autosomal-dominant inherited syndrome consisting of hereditary adenomatous polyps of the small and large intestine and soft tissue, as well as bony tumors. The tumors are often epidermoid cysts, fibromas, or osteomas of the skull and mandible and are often the initial manifestation of the disease.

Pathophysiology

Juvenile polyps are proliferations of mature colonic epithelium, with aggregates of lymphoid tissue and cystic dilation of normal glandular elements. This histopathology has prompted the use of other terms such as *retention, inflammatory,* or *hyperplastic polyps.* The surface epithelium is often ulcerated, with a loss of mucosal surface. Adenomatous polyps may appear grossly similar to juvenile polyps, although on microscopic examination, adenomatous polyps are distinguished by the amount of cellular atypia seen within colonic epithelial cells. More recently, detailed descriptions of the histology of juvenile polyps have indicated the presence of areas of dysplasia, typically associated with polyps larger than 1 cm in diameter. In addition, the presence of more than two colonic polyps raises concern about the possibility of juvenile polyps being capable of malignant transformation.

Clinical Manifestations

The most common presentation of juvenile polyps is painless rectal bleeding, often with blood streaking the outside of the stools. Most juvenile polyps occur in the first decade of life, with the peak incidence of presentation in preschool children, although they can also occur in older children and adolescents. The most common presenting manifestation is rectal bleeding, although prolapse of the polyp through the rectum may occur as a presenting symptom. The polyp may also form the "lead point" of an intussusception. All patients with rectal bleeding should have a careful rectal examination because 30% to 40% of polyps are palpable by rectal examination.

As noted, polyps may be a part of various inherited syndromes; therefore, a complete physical examination should be performed in any patient with rectal bleeding. A careful search for pigmented lesions or soft tissue and bony tumors may aid in the diagnosis of inherited polyposis syndromes as previously described.

Management

The initial ED management of patients who have suspected polyps is aimed at assessing the amount of blood loss and arranging the appropriate diagnostic study. Blood loss is rarely life threatening, but significant losses may be noted from chronic intermittent bleeding. All patients should have a CBC count performed, and if the history of blood loss is significant, a blood type and cross-match may also be indicated. Patients with suspected polyps should undergo elective colonoscopy. Only rarely will these patients require inpatient admission. Endoscopic removal of a polyp is safe and effective therapy even in a young child. For patients with brisk, painless hematochezia associated with a drop in hemoglobin level or vital sign instability and for whom rectal examination is negative for a palpable polyp, other causes for bleeding (e.g., Meckel's diverticulum) need to be considered. This possibility should prompt a decision to perform either red cell–labeled bleeding scan or a ^{99m}Tc radionucleotide (Meckel's) scan in an effort to identify the possible location of bleeding.

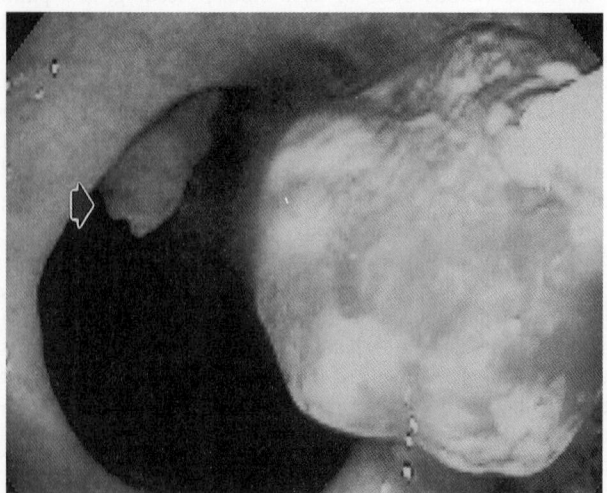

FIGURE 89.3 Juvenile polyp. The *arrow* demonstrates the cauterized polyp stalk.

Dietary Protein Sensitivity Syndromes ("Allergic Colitis")

Dietary proteins are capable of inducing significant bowel injury and may be the cause of several different types of enterocolitis presenting throughout childhood. Each condition, by definition, is induced by a dietary protein and resolves completely after the protein is eliminated from the diet. Immunologic responses may vary from classic allergic mast-cell activation to immune complex formation. The development of proctocolitis in response to cow's milk-protein exposure was among the first to be described. Subsequently, a similar condition has been described in response to soybean-based formula and among exclusively breast-fed infants, presumably in response to maternal dietary protein intake.

Pathophysiology

The appearance of the rectum and colon on colonoscopic examination characteristically consists of diffuse inflammation, friability, edema, and frequent focal ulcerations. Rectal biopsies demonstrate both acute and chronic inflammatory changes and eosinophilic infiltration is often present.

Clinical Manifestations

The typical presentation of milk-protein sensitivity colitis is that of acute onset of blood-streaked, mucoid diarrheal stools in an otherwise well-appearing infant younger than 6 months. Mean age of onset among 35 infants in one series was 4.3 ± 4.1 weeks. It is unusual to present within the first week of life. Blood loss is typically limited, so infants do not appear acutely ill or dehydrated. They are afebrile, and weight gain has typically been within normal limits since birth. The differential diagnosis includes anal fissures and infectious enterocolitis. External anal fissures can be ruled out by careful physical examination. Appropriate viral and bacterial cultures of stool may be indicated to rule out infectious causes.

Management

These patients are rarely hemodynamically unstable or seriously ill; therefore, initial ED management is focused on making a presumptive diagnosis based on history and physical examination, initiating appropriate dietary therapy, and arranging adequate follow-up with the patient's primary care physician or a pediatric gastroenterologist. One might consider basic laboratory testing to support the diagnosis, including a CBC count with white blood cell (WBC) differential to assess the hemoglobin level and check for leukocytosis and eosinophilia. Patients with histologically proven milk-protein sensitivity colitis have higher mean peripheral eosinophil counts than age-appropriate normal values. However, in the individual patient, a higher than normal eosinophil count is actually an insensitive marker (sensitivity = 10%) for histologically proven colitis. In addition, a serum albumin level should be considered because hypoalbuminemia has a sensitivity of approximately 80% for histologic colitis. Examination of stool for blood, fecal leukocytes, and routine bacterial culture should be performed on all infants. Infants who have milk-protein sensitivity colitis will characteristically have leukocytes seen on fecal smear, although eosinophils may not be present in the stool.

Treatment consists of elimination of the offending protein from the infant's diet. The diagnosis is typically confirmed by the resolution of symptoms within 72 hours of the dietary change, although histologic improvement may take 4 to 6 weeks. Infants receiving cow's milk-based or soy protein formulas should be changed to a formula containing casein hydrolysate as the protein source. Nutramigen®, Pregestimil®, and Alimentum® are currently available in the United States. Occasionally, in patients with severe allergic colitis, an amino acid–based elemental formula, such as Neocate® or Elecare®, is required. Gross symptoms of allergic colitis respond within a few days to elimination diet therapy, although guaiac-positive stools may persist for several weeks. In exclusively breast-fed infants, elimination of the offending protein from the mother's diet also leads to clinical improvement and breast-feeding can usually be continued. Persistent evidence of gross bleeding for 5 to 7 days following formula change is an indication for flexible proctosigmoidoscopy. Most infants who present for endoscopy have nodular lymphoid hyperplasia. Infants who respond to dietary elimination should not be rechallenged with a milk- or soy-based formula until 1 year of age. Parents should be counseled that symptoms of allergy might change with increasing age such that a positive challenge may evoke vomiting, diarrhea, or GI signs of allergy rather than recurrent rectal bleeding.

Infectious Enterocolitis

Infectious causes of GI bleeding are predominantly a result of bacterial pathogens including *Campylobacter*, pathogenic *Escherichia coli*, *Yersinia*, *Salmonella*, and *Shigella*. Less commonly, infection with *Giardia* or rotavirus is associated with heme-positive stools. A detailed discussion of the pathophysiology, clinical manifestations, and management of bacterial gastroenteritis can be found in Chapter 92.

Pseudomembranous colitis is a form of inflammatory colitis characterized by the pathologic presence of pseudomembranes consisting of mucin, fibrin, necrotic cells, and polymorphonuclear leukocytes. The entity develops as a result of colonic colonization and toxin production by the gram-positive obligate anaerobe *Clostridium difficile*, in most cases after normal bowel microflora have been altered by antibiotic therapy. All classes of antibiotics have been associated with pseudomembranous colitis. Patients usually present with profuse diarrhea, tenesmus, and crampy abdominal pain, usually beginning during the first week of antibiotic therapy. Frank hematochezia is rare. The diagnosis and management of pseudomembranous colitis are further discussed in Chapter 92.

Miscellaneous Causes of Lower Gastrointestinal Bleeding

Henoch-Schönlein purpura (HSP; see Chapter 100) is a systemic vasculitis that may cause edema and hemorrhage in the intestinal wall. Peak age of onset is between 3 and 7 years and the male:female ratio is 2:1. The presentation consists of the onset of a purpuric rash, typically confined to the buttocks and lower extremities, followed by arthralgias, angioedema, and diffuse abdominal pain. GI symptoms may precede the usual cutaneous symptoms and include abdominal pain (60% to 70%), occult bleeding (50%), gross bleeding (30%), massive hemorrhage (5% to 10%), and intussusception (3%). In a more recent series, thickening of the duodenal wall was noted by ultrasonography in 82% of children who had HSP, with multiple hemorrhagic duodenal erosions noted by endoscopy in two patients. All children with suspected HSP and GI symptoms should have a stool guaiac test performed, as well as a urinalysis to monitor for the onset of renal involvement (nephritis). Children with HSP limited to the involvement of the skin and joints can often be managed as outpatients. However, severe abdominal pain or GI hemorrhage is an indication for admission.

Hemolytic-uremic syndrome (HUS; see Chapter 100) is a disorder characterized by the triad of acute microangiopathic hemolytic anemia, thrombocytopenia, and oliguric renal failure. The disease is heralded by a prodrome of intestinal symptoms ranging from diarrhea (100%) to hemorrhagic colitis (80%). Fever (20% to 30%), vomiting (75% to 80%), and abdominal pain (60%) are also commonly seen. Acute infectious gastroenteritis or colitis secondary to infection with *E. coli* O157:H7 is now considered the most important initial causative event in both sporadic and epidemic cases of HUS.

All children with HUS require admission to the hospital. Laboratory studies should be obtained, including a CBC count, platelet count, PT, PTT, electrolytes, blood urea nitrogen (BUN), and creatinine. IV access needs to be secured immediately for the correction of dehydration and the administration of blood products. As with HSP, the GI manifestations of HUS resolve, usually without sequelae or the need for antibiotic treatment of the initial intestinal infection.

GI *vascular malformations*, including hemangiomas, angiodysplasia, and arteriovenous malformations (AVMs), are rare causes of GI bleeding in children and are often seen as a part of congenital syndromes. GI hemangiomas may be part of the Klippel-Trenaunay-Weber syndrome, which consists of a capillary or large vessel hemangioma on an extremity with hypertrophy of that limb. Diffuse visceral hemangiomatosis is rare, often fatal, and is always associated with cutaneous vascular lesions. GI hemangiomatosis should be suspected in any child with unexplained anemia and a syndrome of cutaneous hemangiomata.

Intestinal AVMs are rare in the pediatric age group, may occur both as solitary and as multiple AVMs, and are typically part of a congenital syndrome (e.g., Osler-Weber-Rendu disease). Many GI vascular malformations, particularly cavernous hemangiomas and AVMs, can be detected using computed tomographic (CT) scans with IV contrast. Intestinal angiography or tagged red blood cell scans are often used to identify the source of bleeding during an acute hemorrhage. ED management of patients with GI bleeding from vascular malformations is the same as for any patient with potentially significant blood loss. After initial stabilization, referral to an appropriate subspecialist for diagnosis and definitive treatment is warranted.

INFLAMMATORY BOWEL DISEASE

Background

IBD is used to designate two chronic intestinal disorders of unknown origin: (i) ulcerative colitis, characterized by inflammation and ulceration confined to the colonic mucosa; and

(ii) Crohn's disease, manifested by transmural inflammation and frequent granulomas that may affect any segment of the GI tract. The incidence of IBD has increased over the past few decades. In a recent study of IBD in California, the overall incidence of IBD among children younger than 18 years was 5.9 cases per 100,000 population. The incidence of Crohn's disease (3.0 per 100,000) was similar to that of ulcerative colitis (2.9 per 100,000). Other studies have reported higher rates for Crohn's disease than for ulcerative colitis. In a population-based survey of IBD in Wisconsin children, the median age at diagnosis was 15 years for both conditions and only 20% of diagnoses were made in children younger than 10 years. In this study, the incidence of IBD did not vary by population density or by race/ethnicity. Most (89%) newly diagnosed cases were nonfamilial.

Many clinical features are common to both disorders, including diarrhea, GI blood and protein loss, abdominal pain, fever, anemia, weight loss, and growth failure. Extraintestinal manifestations involving the joints (arthritis), skin (erythema nodosum), eyes (uveitis), and liver (chronic hepatitis and sclerosing cholangitis) are seen with both disorders, although they are generally more common with Crohn's disease.

Ulcerative colitis typically involves the rectum and extends proximally without skip areas (Fig. 89.4). In contrast, Crohn's disease has discontinuous, patchy involvement of the GI tract. In the study of IBD in Wisconsin, 25% of children had isolated ileal involvement, 32% had colonic disease, 29% had ileocolonic disease, and 14% had significant upper GI disease (Fig. 89.5). The onset of both ulcerative colitis and Crohn's disease is usually insidious, consisting of growth failure, weight loss, diarrhea, and occult rectal bleeding but may be more dramatic and extensive. The average time from onset of symptoms to diagnosis is typically 3 to 4 months.

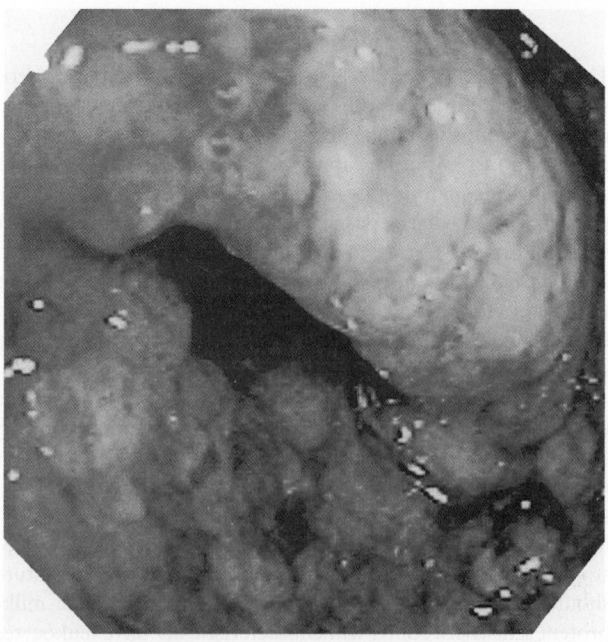

FIGURE 89.4 Severe ulcerative colitis. The mucosa appears granular, nodular, and edematous and is actively bleeding.

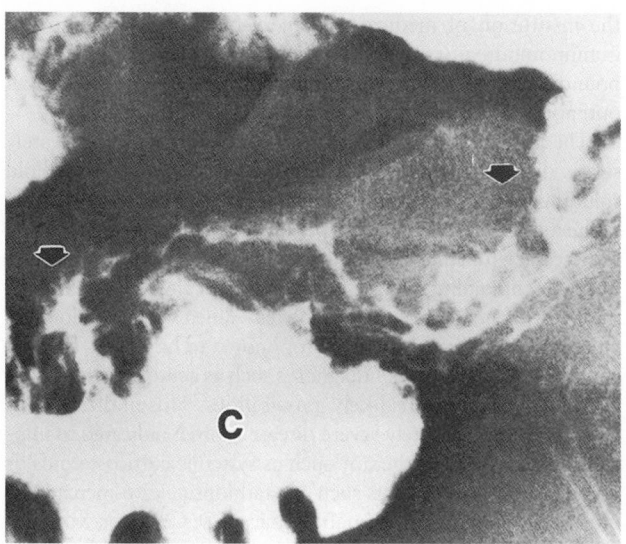

FIGURE 89.5 Crohn's disease of the terminal ileum demonstrated by severe narrowing of the terminal ileum (as shown between the two *arrows*). The cecum is represented by the "C."

Pathophysiology

IBD likely results from the inappropriate and ongoing activation of the GI mucosal immune system driven by the presence of normal bacterial flora. It is a disease that, for many patients, likely results from the interplay of an environmental precipitant affecting a genetically susceptible person. The cause of growth failure in patients with IBD is multifactorial, but inadequate nutrient intake is most likely the final common pathway. Growth failure is twice as likely in children who have Crohn's disease as it is in those who have ulcerative colitis. Malabsorption, especially with small bowel involvement of the disease, may lead to reduced assimilation of fats, vitamins, and minerals. Hematochezia, protein-losing enteropathy, and increased fecal losses of cellular constituents result from chronic inflammation and damage to the intestinal mucosa. The cause of diarrhea is also multifactorial, resulting from extensive mucosal dysfunction, bile acid malabsorption in terminal ileal disease, bacterial overgrowth secondary to strictures and disordered motility, and protein exudation from inflamed surfaces. Extraintestinal manifestations of the disease are often partially the result of a breakdown in the normal barrier and immunoregulatory functions of the GI tract as a result of chronic inflammation. This reaction enables bacterial products and inflammatory mediators (e.g., cytokines) to enter the circulation and subsequently to be deposited in various sites such as the eyes, skin, and joints, leading to localized inflammatory responses.

Clinical Manifestations

Clinical manifestations of IBD can be varied and related to either GI inflammation or the development of either GI tract or extraintestinal complications. Severe abdominal pain is among the most common complaints prompting an ED visit by the patient with IBD. Abdominal pain and diarrhea with or without occult blood are the most common symptoms at presentation. The pain is often colicky and, in Crohn's disease, may localize to the right lower quadrant or periumbilical area, prompting a consideration of acute appendicitis in the differential diagnosis. The abdominal examination may elicit guarding and rebound tenderness. Frank rectal bleeding occurs in fewer than 25% of all cases but is more common in ulcerative colitis. Interestingly, patients younger than 6 years are more likely to have rectal bleeding as the initial symptom of Crohn's disease. On the other hand, abdominal pain, weight loss, and/or fever are more common in older children and adolescents who are ultimately diagnosed with Crohn's disease. Perianal disease, including fissures, skin tags, fistulae, and abscesses, occurs in 15% of children with Crohn's disease. Perianal disease may precede the appearance of the intestinal manifestations of Crohn's disease by several years.

A low-grade fever and mild leukocytosis commonly occur. Approximately 10% of children with ulcerative colitis and a lesser percentage of those with Crohn's disease present with a fulminant onset of fever, abdominal cramps, and severe diarrhea with blood, mucus, and pus in the stools. A fulminant episode may also occur in the patient who has a known disease. There may be associated anemia and dehydration. IBD occasionally causes massive lower GI bleeding. Rarely, Crohn's disease causes complete intestinal obstruction. The patient always gives a history of antecedent abdominal pain, diarrhea, and weight loss. The presence of abdominal distension, accompanied by diminished or absent bowel sounds, should raise the suspicion of actual or impending perforation, even in the absence of severe pain. Perforation may occur even after minor abdominal trauma and must be ruled out when patients with known IBD complain of abdominal pain after trauma.

The development of massive colonic distension is a rare complication of both ulcerative colitis and Crohn's disease. Toxic megacolon represents a life-threatening emergency that has a reported mortality rate of as high as 25%. Although rare in children, nearly half of the cases occur with the first attack of IBD; another 40% are seen in patients receiving high-dose steroid therapy for fulminant colitis. Toxic megacolon almost always involves the transverse colon. The pathophysiology is believed to be an extension of the inflammatory process through all layers of the bowel wall, with resulting microperforation, localized ileus, and loss of colonic tone. The result is imminent major perforation, peritonitis, and overwhelming sepsis. Antecedent barium enema, opiates, or anticholinergics may all precipitate toxic megacolon. Clinical features include (i) a rapidly worsening clinical course usually associated with fever, malaise, and even lethargy; (ii) abdominal distension and tenderness usually developing over a few hours or days; (iii) a temperature of 38.5°C (101.3°F) or higher and a neutrophilic leukocytosis; and (iv) an abdominal radiograph showing distension of the transverse colon of more than 5 to 7 cm. In a recent case-control study of children with toxic megacolon, fever, tachycardia, dehydration, and electrolyte abnormalities were significantly more common than in age-matched controls with ulcerative colitis alone. The differential diagnosis of acute fulminant colitis includes acute bacterial enteritis, amebic dysentery, ischemic bowel disease, and radiation colitis.

Other potential clinical manifestations of IBD related to extraintestinal complications include thrombosis of cerebral, retinal, or peripheral vessels that may lead to coma, seizures, or focal visual or motor deficits; renal calculi leading to hematuria; and pancreatitis.

Management

The initial ED management of IBD is determined primarily by whether the patient is known to have been previously diagnosed with ulcerative colitis or Crohn's disease and by an assessment of the severity of GI symptoms and systemic toxicity. Several clinical classification systems are used, but in general, mild disease is associated with less than six stools passed per day and an absence of systemic signs such as fever and severe anemia. Moderate disease is characterized by more than six stools passed per day, fever [higher than 38°C (100.4°F)], hypoalbuminemia (serum protein concentration less than 3.2 g per dL), and anemia (hemoglobin concentration less than 10 g per dL). Severe disease is indicated by more than six stools passed per day, marked abdominal cramping and tenderness, fever, significant anemia (hemoglobin concentration less than 10 g per dL), leukocytosis (WBC count more than 15,000), hypoalbuminemia (3.0 mg per dL), and toxic megacolon.

Initial blood studies most commonly needed to evaluate patients who have known or suspected IBD include a CBC count, serum electrolytes, BUN, serum albumin and total protein, transaminases [alanine aminotransferase (ALT) and aspartate aminotransferase (AST)], and depending on the amount of suspected blood loss, a blood type and cross-match. The erythrocyte sedimentation rate can be a useful marker of inflammation; it is elevated in up to 80% of patients with newly diagnosed Crohn's disease and in 60% of those with newly diagnosed ulcerative colitis. A recent study of the utility of screening laboratory tests for IBD in children demonstrated that normal values do not rule out the diagnosis. Among children with newly diagnosed IBD, 21% of those with mild Crohn's disease and 54% of those with mild ulcerative colitis had a normal hemoglobin level, platelet count, serum albumin level, and erythrocyte sedimentation rate. These values were more likely to be abnormal in those with moderate or severe disease. The diagnostic yield of plain supine and upright or decubitus abdominal radiographs is relatively low (10% or less) in terms of positive findings of clinical relevance. Nevertheless, plain films can be useful in establishing the diagnosis of toxic megacolon, bowel obstruction, or perforation and should be strongly considered in the initial management of any patient with known or suspected IBD and who presents to the ED with abdominal pain or tenderness.

Stool examination for occult blood and fecal leukocytes may indicate the presence of active inflammation. For patients who have not been previously diagnosed with IBD, as well as during flare-ups in patients with a known diagnosis, stool should be obtained for culture to rule out infectious colitis, which may often either mimic IBD or complicate a known case. Noninfectious causes of rectal bleeding, including polyps, Meckel's diverticulum, HSP, and HUS, as discussed further in this and other chapters (see Chapters 100 and 121), may also be considered in some instances, with appropriate diagnostic evaluation tailored accordingly.

Patients with known or previously undiagnosed IBD, those who have mild manifestations of disease, and those whose initial laboratory and radiographic studies do not reveal significant abnormality can be discharged from the ED after arranging follow-up with an appropriate specialist (pediatric or general gastroenterologist). Further diagnostic studies such as sigmoidoscopy, colonoscopy, or air-contrast barium enema, as well as

the institution of medical management with corticosteroids, immunomodulators such as 6-mercaptopurine, or ASA compounds (mesalamine or sulfasalazine), can be arranged on an outpatient basis.

The goal of initial management of patients with moderately severe disease is supportive, and IV hydration with crystalloid solutions is often necessary to correct acute dehydration. Normal saline may be given as a 20 mL per kg bolus infusion and repeated as necessary to achieve hemodynamic stability. An infusion of a dextrose-containing electrolyte solution may then be initiated on the basis of initial serum electrolytes. When severe abdominal pain occurs in a patient who is not known to have IBD, surgical consultation is indicated if diagnoses such as acute appendicitis or bowel obstruction are likely possibilities. Hospitalization of patients with moderately severe disease is often indicated to initiate or modify specific therapy such as systemic corticosteroids or immunosuppressive agents such as azathioprine or 6-mercaptopurine. More recently, infliximab (Remicade®; Centocor, Malvern, Pennsylvania), a genetically engineered monoclonal antibody against tumor necrosis factor-α, has demonstrated effectiveness in reducing the need for steroids among children with Crohn's disease. Finally, improved nutritional intake, preferably via enteral means, is often necessary.

All patients with acute fulminant colitis should be admitted to the hospital. Oral intake should be discontinued and an IV infusion begun with normal saline until electrolyte and BUN levels are known. Opiate or anticholinergic drugs should be avoided because they may precipitate toxic megacolon. A fever, significant leukocytosis, or an ill-appearing child may suggest an abdominal abscess. In these cases, an abdominal/pelvic CT scan is warranted. If toxic megacolon is suspected, arrangements should be made for admission to an intensive care unit (ICU). The patient should discontinue all antidiarrheal and anticholinergic medicines. The first priority in the management of children with toxic megacolon is the treatment of intravascular dehydration and shock. Intensive IV therapy with normal saline, albumin, or blood must be sufficient to correct hypotension and ensure adequate urine flow. An NG tube, or preferably a Miller-Abbott tube for small bowel decompression, should be placed. Patients should be started on broad-spectrum antibiotics such as ampicillin (200 mg per kg per day), gentamicin (5 to 7.5 mg per kg per day), and clindamycin (40 mg per kg per day) in combination. Suitable alternative therapies include ampicillin/sulbactam, piperacillin/tazobactam, or cefoxitin in combination with gentamicin.

Management of significant GI bleeding should be performed as described earlier in this chapter. Emergency management of suspected intestinal obstruction includes gastric decompression with NG drainage and IV rehydration, initially with normal saline. Patients with fulminant colitis, suspected toxic megacolon, significant GI bleeding, or suspected intestinal obstruction should all receive prompt surgical consultation as part of their initial ED evaluation.

ULCER DISEASE

Background

The term *ulcer disease* describes a group of disorders, consisting of primary and secondary gastric and duodenal ulcers, as well as nodular gastritis. With increasing use of endoscopy in children, peptic ulcer disease is a more commonly recognized disorder, although it is still far less common than in adults. Reliable incidence data in children are generally lacking, although several studies have suggested that large pediatric referral centers diagnose approximately five new cases per year or 1 case per 2,500 hospital admissions.

In children younger than 10 years, ulcer disease is more common because of the use of noxious agents such as corticosteroids or NSAIDs or after major stresses such as burns, sepsis, or other systemic illness. Stress ulcers account for 80% of peptic disease in infancy and early childhood. These ulcers often present as medical emergencies as a result of perforation or hemorrhage and can be either gastric or duodenal in origin. In older children and adolescents, the clinical presentation and natural history of ulcer disease are more similar to those seen in adults, with duodenal ulcers far more common than gastric ulcers (Fig. 89.6). A family history of ulcer disease is typically present in 50% or more of children with duodenal ulcers.

The role of the bacterium *Helicobacter pylori* in the etiology of ulcer disease in children has been vigorously investigated. *H. pylori* infection is usually acquired in childhood, with earlier acquisition noted in developing countries. For example, infection rates among Bolivian children approach 70% by 10 years of age, with virtually everyone infected by 20 years of age. In contrast, seroprevalence rates in the southeastern United States are estimated at 12% to 15% by 9 years of age. Similarly, the prevalence of *H. pylori* infection diagnosed by urea breath test was 13.7% among healthy European preschool-aged children. There are higher prevalence rates among family members and institutionalized populations, suggesting person-to-person transmission via either an oral route or a fecal-to-oral route. Most children with *H. pylori* infections are asymptomatic. Available evidence to date shows a strong association between *H. pylori* infection and antral gastritis and duodenal ulcer disease in children. However, little to no evidence has been presented for an association with gastric

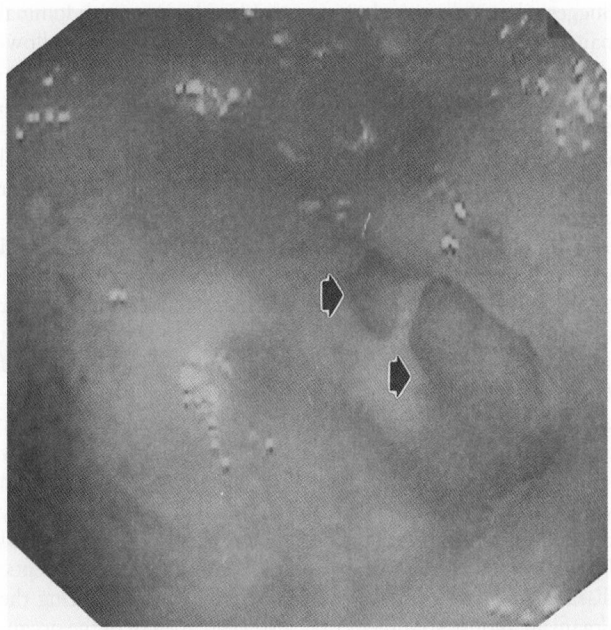

FIGURE 89.6 Duodenal bulb ulcers. The *arrows* show two individual duodenal nonbleeding ulcers.

ulcer or recurrent abdominal pain in children. The specific role of *H. pylori* in the pathogenesis and treatment of ulcer disease is discussed in the next section.

Pathophysiology

The pathogenesis of ulcer disease results from an imbalance between cytotoxic factors, such as acid, pepsin, medications such as NSAIDs, and infection with *H. pylori*, and cytoprotective factors, including the secretion of mucus and bicarbonate by superficial epithelial and mucus cells in the upper GI tract. Gastric acid is produced by parietal cells in the stomach and is controlled primarily by histamine, acetylcholine, and gastrin. The final common pathway for all acid secretion is the proton pump (H^+/K^+ ATPase). All agents that stimulate gastric acid secretion also stimulate pepsin secretion. Pepsins are enzymes that hydrolyze proteins, as well as gastric mucus glycoproteins, in an acid pH environment. They are secreted by gastric chief cells as pepsinogens and are converted to active pepsin by gastric acidity. The underlying mechanism of gastric ulcer formation is less well understood. Local blood flow, delayed gastric emptying, duodenal reflux, and other factors have all been suggested as important predictors of gastric ulceration. The exact interplay of gastric acid, *H. pylori*, local blood flow, and other factors in the pathogenesis of ulcer disease is the subject of intensive investigation but currently remains unclear.

H. pylori possesses a number of virulence factors that render it particularly pathogenic in the acidic gastric environment. *H. pylori* normally adheres only to gastric mucosa in vivo. It is a flagellated organism with the capacity for active motility, giving it the ability to penetrate the mucous layer overlying the gastric mucosa. It also possesses potent urease activity, converting urea, which is abundant in gastric epithelium, to ammonia and bicarbonate. This capacity has been proposed as both a survival mechanism for the organism (the bicarbonate may moderate the pH of the local environment of the organism) and a pathogenic mechanism (the ammonia functions as a gastric irritant). *H. pylori* invariably produces a localized inflammatory reaction that may contribute to epithelial damage either by direct toxic effect or via immunopathologic means (Fig. 89.7).

Clinical Manifestations

Symptoms of ulcer disease vary with the patient's age. Nonspecific signs and symptoms predominate among infants and preschool-aged children, with boys and girls affected equally. The older the child, the more specific (and similar to adult patterns of presentation) the signs and symptoms become. Among teenagers with ulcer disease, a male predominance is seen, with boys outnumbering girls nearly 4:1. Infants with ulcer disease (usually secondary to some other condition) may present either with nonspecific feeding difficulties and vomiting or more fulminantly with upper GI bleeding or perforation. Preschool-aged children often complain of poorly localized abdominal pain, vomiting, or GI hemorrhage and manifest as either hematemesis or melena. Older children and adolescents present almost invariably with abdominal pain, which is described as waxing and waning, sharp or gnawing, and localized to the epigastrium. It may awaken the child at

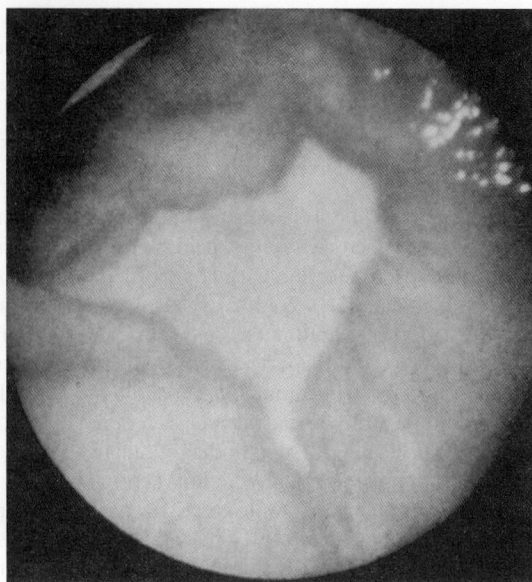

FIGURE 89.7 A large duodenal bulb ulcer secondary to *Helicobacter pylori* infection.

night or in the early hours of the morning. The presence of nocturnal pain may assist in distinguishing recurrent abdominal pain as a result of ulcer disease from functional abdominal pain, which rarely occurs at night. A careful history of the pain and a family history of ulcer disease will often suggest the diagnosis of peptic ulcer disease in the older child. History should also be obtained regarding the presence of predisposing factors such as smoking or regular use of NSAIDs.

Physical examination may reveal abdominal tenderness, poorly localized in young children and more commonly localized to the epigastrium or to the right of the midline in older children and adolescents. A rectal examination should be performed to evaluate the patient for the possible perianal disease that might suggest Crohn's disease in the differential diagnosis. Stool should be tested for occult blood, and the remainder of the physical examination should include an oral examination looking for dental enamel erosion, which would suggest chronic GER or recurrent emesis, and an examination of the lungs for wheezing, which also might suggest bronchospasm due to or exacerbated by reflux. Weight loss may be noted. If occurring in adolescent girls, it should also prompt suspicion for an eating disorder.

Differential Diagnosis

A number of conditions may mimic the presentation of ulcer disease. Abdominal pain is a common symptom during childhood, occurring in 10% to 15% of school-aged children. Most children with recurrent abdominal pain have a "functional" cause. These patients typically do not have any weight loss or vomiting and report that their pain is localized to the umbilical area. Further discussion regarding the differential diagnosis of abdominal pain can be found in Chapter 49. It should be noted that the prevalence of *H. pylori* infection in children who have recurrent abdominal pain varies widely in the literature, with most patients in published studies selected from

among those presenting to tertiary hospital gastroenterology clinics. Children with *H. pylori* infection are characteristically asymptomatic, and there does not appear to be an association between *H. pylori* infection and an increased prevalence of recurrent abdominal pain. Therefore, routine evaluation for *H. pylori* in patients without symptoms of acid-peptic disease is not indicated.

Gastritis, distal esophagitis, *giardiasis*, and pancreatitis may all cause epigastric pain and tenderness. Biliary tract disease and ureteropelvic junction obstruction may cause right upper quadrant tenderness. Children who have IBD, HSP, or diabetes mellitus may also present with abdominal pain, tenderness, or GI bleeding.

Diagnosis

Radiologic examination, with either single- or double-contrast (with air) barium upper GI series, is not an effective diagnostic tool to either confirm or rule out the presence of ulcer disease in children. These studies often do not detect superficial ulcers, and, conversely, barium trapped in a gastric or duodenal fold may falsely give the impression of an ulcer. However, radiologic examination may be used to rule out other conditions, such as malrotation with volvulus, or other structural anomalies of the GI tract.

Flexible fiber-optic esophagogastroduodenoscopy with mucosal biopsy is the most accurate method of diagnosing peptic ulcer disease in children. In most tertiary care referral centers, this procedure can be performed safely even on infants. It is typically not performed in the presence of active hemorrhage, although some centers are gathering experience with the use of therapeutic endoscopy to control significant bleeding. When performed, biopsy specimens should routinely be obtained from any area of endoscopic abnormality and from the distal esophagus, antrum, and second part of the duodenum. No clear guidelines exist to indicate which pediatric patients should undergo endoscopy for the evaluation of ulcer disease. Suggested guidelines include any child with chronic abdominal pain (longer than 3 months) associated with any of the following signs and symptoms: (i) hematemesis, (ii) a history of peptic ulcer disease in a first-degree relative, (iii) nocturnal pain, (iv) pain occurring within 1 hour of eating or relieved by eating, (v) recurrent vomiting, (vi) weight loss, or (vii) abdominal tenderness localized to the epigastrium (particularly in older children). In addition, endoscopy should be strongly considered in any patient presenting with significant acute upper GI bleeding or with any concern that *H. pylori* may be present.

All patients for whom an obvious cause of secondary gastric or duodenal ulceration (e.g., stress, sepsis, burns) does not exist should undergo diagnostic evaluation for the presence of *H. pylori* infection. *H. pylori* infection can be confirmed in a variety of ways in patients with primary ulcer disease. Histologic examination of biopsy specimens obtained during endoscopy should routinely be performed because *H. pylori* is readily seen with a variety of staining techniques. This is the diagnostic method currently recommended by the American Academy of Pediatrics for children with symptoms consistent with acid-peptic disease. In centers with appropriate facilities for culturing the organism, biopsy specimens may also yield growth of the organism, which can assist in the choice of appropriate antibiotic therapy, particularly in recalcitrant infections. A variety of commercially available assays take advantage of the urease activity of the organism for diagnostic purposes. A biopsy specimen is mixed with the assay, which typically contains urea and an indicator dye that changes color when the urea is converted to ammonia by the organism. The urease activity can also be detected through the use of breath tests, in which radiolabeled (^{13}C or ^{14}C) urea is ingested by the patient. Degradation of the urea by *H. pylori* results in the release of the radiolabeled carbon, which can be detected in the expired air. Finally, enzyme-linked immunosorbent assays are available for the detection of immunoglobulin G (IgG) antibodies to *H. pylori* in serum. Noninvasive tests, such as serology and breath tests, are useful but should not be promoted as the sole method of diagnosing *H. pylori*–associated ulcer disease in children because they cannot distinguish between incidental infection and the presence of ulceration. At this time, therefore, the presence of suspected ulcer disease should be confirmed by endoscopic examination according to the guidelines previously suggested.

Management

The focus of ED management of patients with suspected ulcer disease should be on the detection and stabilization of life-threatening complications such as perforation and major GI hemorrhage and on ruling out other potential serious or life-threatening conditions that may require urgent intervention. Depending on the suspected amount of blood loss, all patients with GI bleeding should have a CBC count and blood type and screen obtained. If vomiting has been prominent, electrolytes, BUN, creatinine, serum amylase, and lipase should also be determined. If physical examination findings suggest significant abdominal tenderness with guarding or rebound tenderness, plain radiographs of the abdomen should be obtained to rule out a perforation or bowel obstruction. IV access should be obtained in all patients who have significant emesis, dehydration, weight loss, or concerning abdominal examination findings. An initial bolus of normal saline (20 mL per kg) should be given and vital signs monitored frequently, with additional boluses given as needed to achieve hemodynamic stability.

A number of approaches are available for the treatment of ulcer disease in children. Therapies can be categorized as those that neutralize acid (i.e., antacids), block acid secretion, are cytoprotective, or are antiinfective. Antacids are a low-cost, safe, and effective means of treating peptic ulcer disease in children and can be prescribed for patients of any age. Adverse effects of antacids are related to the cation present in the preparation: magnesium-containing products cause diarrhea, whereas aluminum-containing products cause constipation. Some products are available combining the two to minimize these effects. The usual dosage for children is 0.5 mL per kg, given 1 hour after eating and before going to the bed. Patients with food-related or nocturnal abdominal pain without associated signs of serious illness can be started on empirical therapy with antacids, assuming good follow-up with a primary care physician. Referral to a pediatric gastroenterologist can then be made if the patient fails to respond to 2 weeks of therapy.

H$_2$-receptor antagonists are the most common agents used to block acid secretion and treat ulcer disease. Patients with significant GI bleeding, vomiting, or abdominal tenderness should be admitted to the hospital and begun on IV therapy with an H$_2$-receptor antagonist. Currently, most physicians with pediatric experience use ranitidine (2 to 4 mg per kg per day IV q6 to 8 h) or famotidine (1 mg per kg per day IV bid) for initial treatment. Both agents are competitive H$_2$-receptor antagonists that reduce gastric acid output, thereby raising gastric pH. Patients for whom initial outpatient therapy is appropriate can be prescribed an H$_2$-receptor antagonist following an ED visit, but this therapy is best done in consultation with either the patient's primary care physician or a pediatric gastroenterologist, who will establish appropriate follow-up for the patient. The proton pump inhibitors, omeprazole (0.6 mg per kg per day po qd) and lansoprazole (1 mg per kg per day po qd), are irreversible inhibitors of H$^+$/K$^+$ ATPase. Their potential adverse effects include headache, diarrhea, nausea, and vomiting. When initiating therapy, the emergency physician should arrange appropriate follow-up.

Sucralfate (40 to 80 mg per kg per day po q6h) is an aluminum salt that "coats" damaged gastric mucosa, effectively insulating it from further damage by acid, pepsin, or bile. It is typically given as a slurry and can be used with H$_2$-receptor antagonists, provided the drugs are given at least 1 hour apart.

Recurrences of *H. pylori*–associated ulcer disease are markedly reduced—from 65% to 5% at 1 year of follow-up—by treatment that includes eradication of the infection and acid suppression therapy. Most children with *H. pylori* infection are asymptomatic, and no convincing evidence that *H. pylori* causes symptoms in the absence of ulceration has been presented. Therefore, antimicrobial therapy is currently not recommended for children without ulcers or gastritis who harbor the organism. Current recommended protocols for first-line therapy include a proton pump inhibitor (for 1 month) plus two antibiotics (choosing two of the following: amoxicillin, clarithromycin, or metronidazole for 7 to 14 days). Compliance is an important consideration because it is a major determinant of the success of treatment.

REYE'S SYNDROME

Background

Reye's syndrome is a distinct, reversible, clinicopathologic syndrome occurring after an antecedent viral infection, characterized by severe noninflammatory encephalopathy and fatty degeneration of the liver. The incidence of Reye's syndrome peaked at 400 to 600 cases per year in the 1970s and early 1980s, when a series of case-control studies established a link between antecedent aspirin exposure and the onset of Reye's syndrome. The incidence has since declined to about two cases per year. Isolated case reports continue to be described, indicating the need to continue to consider Reye's syndrome when evaluating patients with the typical clinical presentation described in the next section.

Pathophysiology

The precise pathogenesis of Reye's syndrome remains unclear, but there is a primary mitochondrial injury in all tissues of the body, which results in disturbances of fatty acid and carnitine metabolism. Most of the clinical features of Reye's syndrome, including lactic acidosis, elevated fatty acids, nitrogen wasting, hyperammonemia, cellular fat accumulation, and cytotoxic cerebral edema, may be explained in the context of primary mitochondrial damage.

Clinical Manifestations

Reye's syndrome affects children of all ages. No gender difference is apparent. A biphasic clinical history is remarkably constant. First, the child has a history of a recent, usually febrile, illness that is waning or has resolved. Approximately 90% of the children have an antecedent upper respiratory tract infection. Varicella virus or influenza B infections have been characteristically associated with Reye's syndrome. The abrupt onset of protracted vomiting usually starts within 1 week following the prodromal illness. The vomiting is unresponsive either to restriction of oral intake or to antiemetic therapy.

Coincident with the onset of vomiting (or shortly thereafter), signs of encephalopathy appear. At first, encephalopathy may be manifested by unusual quietness or disinterest. However, a rapid sequential progression to irritability, combativeness, confusion, disorientation, delirium, stupor, and coma may occur. Seizures are a late sign in older children but may occur during early stages of encephalopathy in infancy (usually secondary to hypoglycemia).

In the ED, patients are usually afebrile. Tachycardia and hyperventilation commonly occur. At the initial presentation, only 50% of patients have hepatomegaly. The liver usually increases in size during the first 24 to 48 hours after the diagnosis is made. The absence of jaundice and scleral icterus is characteristic and is the major mitigating clinical sign against hepatic encephalopathy secondary to acute fulminant hepatitis. Despite evidence of encephalopathy, no focal neurological signs or signs of meningeal irritation are apparent.

The diagnosis of Reye's syndrome is suggested by the clinical presentation, supported by characteristic biochemical findings and confirmed by characteristic histologic findings on liver biopsy. The hallmark of the acute encephalopathy of Reye's syndrome is the associated evidence of liver abnormality. The levels of transaminases (ALT and AST) and blood ammonia are almost always elevated at the time of the onset of protracted vomiting. The range of transaminase elevation is highly variable and has not been shown to correlate well with severity of the disease. Ammonia levels more than 300 g per L have been shown to be an indicator of a poor prognosis. The PT is more than 50% of control in at least one-half of the patients, although clinical bleeding is rare and evidence of disseminated intravascular coagulation is absent. The level of serum bilirubin rarely exceeds 2 mg per dL. Hypoglycemia is rare, except in children who present in coma and in infants younger than 1 year, in whom the incidence is reported to be as high as 70% to 80%. Azotemia and ketonuria are common, secondary to starvation and dehydration from vomiting and poor oral intake. Patients most often have a mixed respiratory alkalosis and mild metabolic acidosis. The metabolic acidosis correlates with the level of ammonia elevation and reflects the degree of mitochondrial dysfunction.

Management

Once the diagnosis is made, immediate plans to admit the child to an ICU should be made, because the progression of the encephalopathy may be rapid, resulting in increased morbidity and mortality.

Despite the generalized nature of the mitochondrial insult in Reye's syndrome, the brain is the principal organ affected by the syndrome. Increased intracranial pressure (ICP) secondary to cerebral edema is the major factor contributing to morbidity and mortality in Reye's syndrome. With the ability to monitor ICP, numerous different invasive therapies have been introduced in an attempt to rapidly reduce and control cerebral edema. However, none of these therapies, including hyperventilation and muscle paralysis using neuromuscular-blocking drugs, hyperosmolar agents, high-dose barbiturates, exchange transfusions, or hypothermia, have been clearly proven to protect the brain from progressive ischemic insult. Ultimately, the management of Reye's syndrome is supportive because no specific curative therapy is currently available.

ACUTE BILIARY TRACT DISEASE

Background

Acute biliary disease occurs occasionally in children (more often in adolescents) and is associated with a wide spectrum of clinical manifestations. Acute cholecystitis is typically a complication of cholelithiasis, which is primarily associated in younger patients with hemolytic anemias (pigment stones) such as sickle cell disease and hereditary spherocytosis. Adolescent girls develop cholecystitis more often than do boys (cholesterol stones). Gallstones may be asymptomatic, and their prevalence increases with age. Acalculous cholecystitis, or acute inflammation of the gallbladder in the absence of gallstones, in children is actually more common than cholelithiasis and has been associated with bacterial enteric infections such as typhoid, shigellosis, and *E. coli* infection, parasitic infections, and other conditions such as leptospirosis, scarlet fever, pneumonia, Kawasaki disease, hepatitis, and polyarteritis nodosa. Acute cholangitis resulting from an ascending biliary infection or obstruction is seen primarily in the pediatric patient who has had surgical correction of congenital biliary tract obstruction (biliary atresia, choledochal cyst). Finally, hydrops of the gallbladder, causing jaundice and a right upper quadrant mass effect with pain, is a complication of Kawasaki disease.

Pathophysiology

Biliary colic results from acute transient obstruction of the cystic duct or common bile duct by gallstone(s). Cholecystitis is an aseptic inflammatory process that develops as a reaction to chemical injury triggered by obstruction to the cystic duct by a gallstone. This inflammation is mediated by (i) lysolecithin, which is formed from biliary lecithin by refluxed pancreatic enzyme phospholipase A; (ii) refluxed proteolytic pancreatic enzymes; and (iii) unconjugated bile salts. The cause of acalculous cholecystitis is unknown. The condition is commonly associated with gallbladder distension, called acute hydrops of the gallbladder. In infectious syndromes, inflammation of the cystic duct and/or enlargement of mesenteric lymph nodes may result in obstruction to bile flow. In vasculitis syndromes, such as mucocutaneous lymph node syndrome (Kawasaki disease) or polyarteritis nodosa, there may be a reactive serositis or vasculitis with increased mucus secretion by the gallbladder, which, when coupled with factors that contribute to bile stasis such as fever, prolonged fasting, ileus, or dehydration, may result in gallbladder distension that in turn may kink the cystic duct. Cholangitis results from secondary bacterial infection by enteric organisms in the face of biliary tract obstruction or after surgical manipulation of the biliary tract. Acute cholangitis may be mild and superficial, producing only short-lived symptoms, or it may be severe, causing suppurative cholangitis with septic shock and formation of hepatic abscesses.

Clinical Manifestations

The pain of biliary colic is acute in onset, often follows a meal, and is usually localized to the epigastrium or right upper quadrant. Some children may localize the pain to the periumbilical area. Characteristically, the pain increases to a plateau of intensity over 5 to 20 minutes, typically after meals, and persists for a variable duration, usually less than 4 hours (although less than 1 hour in 50% of patients). In contrast to the colicky pain of intestinal or ureteral origin, biliary colic does not worsen in relatively short cyclic paroxysms or bursts but instead is characterized by its sustained, intense quality. Unlike pancreatitis, the patient tends to move about restlessly and the pain is not improved by changes in position. In addition, referred pain is common, particularly to the dorsal lumbar back near the tip of the right scapula. Nausea and vomiting are commonly associated with biliary colic but are not severe and protracted as seen with pancreatitis. Mild jaundice occurs in 25% of patients, but the serum bilirubin rarely exceeds 4 mg per dL. An attack of acute cholecystitis begins with biliary colic, which increases progressively in severity or duration. Pain lasting longer than 4 hours suggests cholecystitis. As the inflammation worsens, the pain changes character, becoming more generalized in the upper abdomen and increased by deep respiration and jarring motions. The temperature is usually mildly elevated, ranging from 37.5°C to 38.5°C (99.5°F to 101.3°F).

In contrast, acute cholangitis should be suspected in the patient who has right upper quadrant abdominal pain, shaking chills with spiking fever [temperature higher than 39°C (102.2°F)], and jaundice (Charcot's triad). These patients usually have a history of abdominal surgery. A dangerous aspect of this disorder is that overwhelming sepsis can develop rapidly. Listlessness and shock are characteristic of advanced or severe cholangitis and usually reflect gram-negative septicemia. Cholangitis can evolve rapidly before the development of significant jaundice. Clinically apparent jaundice may be absent even in postsurgical biliary atresia patients. Hydrops of the gallbladder is associated with a palpable right upper quadrant mass and pain. Fever and jaundice generally do not occur.

In addition to scleral icterus, nonspecific physical findings that suggest gallbladder disease include right upper quadrant guarding, Murphy's sign (production of pain by deep inspiration or cough when the physician's fingers are depressing the abdomen below the right costal margin in the midclavicular line and abrupt cessation of inspiration because of pain), and production of pain or tenderness by a light blow applied with the ulnar surface of the hand to the subcostal area. In about one-third of patients with cholecystitis, the gallbladder is palpable as a sausage-shaped mass lateral to the midclavicular line. A rigid abdomen or rebound tenderness suggests local perforation or gangrene of the gallbladder.

Laboratory tests are typically nonspecific in cholecystitis. A CBC count and blood smear may show evidence of hemolysis. The leukocyte count averages 12,000 to 15,000 per mm^3 with a neutrophilic leukocytosis. Higher leukocyte counts suggest cholangitis. The level of serum bilirubin may be elevated but rarely exceeds 4 mg per dL. Higher values are more compatible with either complete common bile duct obstruction or cholangitis. The levels of serum transaminases (ALT and AST) and alkaline phosphatase may be mildly elevated but are often normal. Marked elevation in the levels of transaminases may occur with acute, complete common duct obstruction. Serum amylase levels may be mildly elevated without other evidence of pancreatitis. Abdominal flat and upright radiographs may show right upper quadrant calcification of gallstones, particularly in patients with hemolytic anemia (pigment stones), or a right upper quadrant mass. Abdominal radiographs are particularly important to rule out perforation. The erythrocyte sedimentation rate is often elevated in children with cholangitis, and organisms may be recovered from blood cultures.

Abdominal ultrasound is the most commonly used test to confirm gallbladder disease. This test is noninvasive, easily performed, and provides information on the surrounding organs such as the liver, pancreas, and kidneys. Ultrasound can determine the presence of most gallstones, dilated bile ducts, a thickened gallbladder wall or hydropic gallbladder, sludge, and hepatic abscesses. Other radiographic tests, such as cholecystograph or radionuclide testing, are not typically used in the emergency setting.

Other conditions to be considered in the differential diagnosis of biliary tract disease include perforated peptic ulcer, pneumonia, intercostal neuritis, pancreatitis, hepatitis, and hepatic and abdominal sickle cell crises. Therefore, evaluation should also include stool guaiac test, chest radiograph, amylase: creatinine ratio, and a peripheral blood smear.

Management

All patients with suspected acute biliary tract disease and acute symptoms should be admitted to the hospital. The exception is a patient with biliary colic that has resolved spontaneously, in which case an urgent outpatient evaluation by ultrasound can be pursued. Conditions associated with acalculous cholecystitis should be evaluated and treated if identified. General ED management includes discontinuation of oral intake, support with IV fluids, and surgical consultation. Cholecystitis and cholangitis associated with gallstones are general indications for surgery. The patient should be made NPO (nothing by mouth) and given IV fluids, pain medication, and antibiotics, if cholangitis is considered. Antibiotic coverage should include gram-negative organisms and enterococci. Ampicillin (200 mg per kg per day) and gentamicin (5 to 7.5 mg per kg per day) provide good coverage; ampicillin/sulbactam (dosed on ampicillin at 200 mg per

MEDICAL EMERGENCIES

kg per day) can also be used. Narcotics are useful to alleviate the pain and to reduce gallbladder mucosal secretion.

In all patients with suspected cholangitis, blood cultures should be drawn before antibiotics are administered. When possible, antibiotics should be withheld pending a liver biopsy for definitive culture. However, the exception is the clinically septic children in whom antibiotic coverage should be immediately instituted. In these cases, a liver biopsy performed after the institution of antibiotics may still show histologic evidence of cholangitis.

ACUTE PANCREATITIS

Background

Although uncommon, the diagnosis of pancreatitis is often overlooked because no specific pathognomonic symptoms are associated with the condition. Pancreatitis should be considered in any child with acute or chronic epigastric abdominal pain and vomiting, ascites of obscure origin, or following upper abdominal trauma. Table 89.1 lists the causes of pancreatitis. In 30% of cases, the precipitating factor is unknown. Approximately 50% of cases are associated with an infectious agent or blunt trauma. Mumps pancreatitis is seldom severe and rarely occurs in children younger than 5 years; clinical mumps is present in only 50% to 60% of cases. Most blunt injuries to the pancreas are the result of automobile crashes or falls from bicycles; however, because the pancreas is a fixed retroperitoneal structure, mild trauma from small pointed objects, such as sticks, handlebars, or fence posts, may transmit injury directly to the organ.

Pathophysiology

Regardless of the initiating event, the pathophysiology of acute pancreatitis is probably similar. Activation of the numerous pancreatic enzymes, including proteolytic enzymes, lipase, amylase, elastase, and phospholipase A, produces autodigestion of the gland. The process may be focal or diffuse. In mild cases, there is interstitial edema and inflammatory infiltrate without significant cell necrosis. This type of pancreatitis, called *acute edematous pancreatitis*, is by far the most common form seen in children; it is usually self-limiting and associated with complete recovery. When the autodigestive process intensifies with increased inflammation, fat necrosis, and hemorrhagic changes, it is called *necrotic* or *hemorrhagic pancreatitis*. This type of pancreatitis is associated with a 20% to 40% mortality rate and significant morbidity. It is unclear why the autodigestive process is arrested in some cases and not in others, but one factor may be the magnitude of the initial triggering mechanism.

The morbidity and mortality associated with pancreatitis is related to complications from the autodigestive process. Fat necrosis of neighboring tissue and saponification of calcium often result from the release of pancreatic lipase. Released proteolytic enzymes may extend the inflammatory process into the retroperitoneum and the peritoneal cavity. Proteolytic enzymes may activate kallikrein, a potent vasoactive polypeptide that may mediate systemic vasodilation and increase vascular permeability, producing severe hypotension, shock, and renal and/or pulmonary insufficiency that may prove fatal. Secondary infection may lead to abscess formation, and walling off the autodigestive process may result in pseudocyst formation.

Clinical Manifestations

Epigastric abdominal pain is the most consistent symptom of pancreatitis and may vary from tolerable distress to severe incapacitating pain. Symptoms may be chronic and insidious, but they typically progress rapidly, building to a crescendo over several hours. The pain is usually localized to the epigastrium and may radiate to the back (left or right scapula) or to the right or left upper quadrants. The pain is usually described as knifelike and boring in quality and is aggravated when the patient lies supine. Classically, the pain of pancreatitis is constant, as opposed to colicky pain, which waxes and wanes. Anorexia, nausea, and vomiting are the most common associated symptoms. Vomiting may be severe and protracted. Low-grade fever [temperature lower than 38.5°C (101.3°F)] is present in 50% to 60% of cases. In cases of severe necrotic pancreatitis, patients may complain of dizziness. Mental aberrations are common in necrotic pancreatitis; patients may act overtly psychotic or present in coma.

Early in the course of the disease, there may be a discrepancy between the severity of the patient's subjective pain and the objective physical findings. During the examination, patients are usually quiet and prefer sitting or lying on their side with knees flexed. The abdomen may be distended but is usually not rigid. There may be mild to moderate voluntary guarding in the epigastrium. A palpable epigastric mass suggests pseudocyst. Ascites is rare. Bowel sounds may be decreased or absent. Associated physical findings may include signs of parotitis, mild hepatosplenomegaly, epigastric mass, pleural effusions, and mild icterus. Although rare, rebound tenderness or a rigid abdomen is a poor prognostic sign if present. Similarly, a bluish discoloration around the umbilicus (Cullen's sign) or flanks (Grey Turner's sign) is rare in children but portends a poor prognosis and a diagnosis of hemorrhagic pancreatitis. Signs of overt hemodynamic instability are rarely

---

TABLE 89.1

CAUSES OF ACUTE PANCREATITIS IN CHILDREN

I	Trauma: blunt, penetrating, surgical
II	Infectious: mumps, coxsackievirus B infection, hemolytic *Streptococcus* infection, *Salmonella* infection, hepatitis A and B
III	Obstructive: cholelithiasis, ascaris infection, congenital duodenal stenosis, duplications, tumor, choledochal cyst
IV	Drugs: steroids, chlorothiazides, salicylazosulfapyridine, azothiaprine, alcohol, valproic acid, tetracyclines, borates, oral contraceptives
V	Systemic: systemic lupus erythematosus, periarteritis nodosa, malnutrition, peptic ulcer, uremia
VI	Endocrine: hyperparathyroidism
VII	Metabolic: hypercholesterolemia, cystic fibrosis, vitamin A and D deficiency
VIII	Hereditary
IX	Idiopathic

evident at initial presentation. It is particularly important to evaluate patients for clinical signs of hypocalcemia (Trousseau and Chvostek signs).

The clinical diagnosis is often tentative because the same constellation of symptoms (abdominal pain, vomiting, and low-grade fever) and signs (abdominal tenderness and guarding) may be mimicked by several other conditions including ulcer disease, gastritis, esophagitis, biliary colic, acute cholecystitis, intestinal obstruction, and appendicitis.

Currently, two easily attainable laboratory tests are used to make a diagnosis of pancreatitis: serum amylase and serum lipase. The combination of the aforementioned clinical symptoms and an elevation of the level of one or both of these enzymes strongly point to pancreatitis. In acute pancreatitis, the serum amylase increases hours after the onset of the autodigestive process. Generally, because amylase is rapidly cleared by the kidneys, serum amylase levels may return to normal after 3 to 5 days, even though pain persists. Elevated serum triglyceride levels may interfere with the assay and result in false-normal values. The degree of serum amylase elevation rarely corresponds to the severity of pancreatic inflammation. Although controversial in the past, lipase assays are now accurate and commonly used to diagnose pancreatitis. Serum lipase levels may remain elevated for up to 14 days after the onset of acute pancreatitis.

Elevated serum amylase and lipase levels are not pathognomonic for pancreatitis. Many situations, including penetrating or perforated ulcer, intestinal obstruction or infarction, Crohn's disease, pneumonia, hepatitis, liver trauma, acute biliary tract disease, salpingitis, salivary adenitis, renal failure, diabetic ketoacidosis, and benign macroamylasemia, can cause an amylase elevation. Other causes for an elevated serum lipase level include perforated peptic ulcer and bone fracture with pulmonary fat embolism.

Radiographically, the abdominal ultrasound provides a noninvasive, direct view of the pancreas and is probably the most useful test in diagnosing pancreatitis in the emergency setting. Ultrasound can assess pancreatic size, contour, and the presence of calcifications and pseudocyst formation. Ultrasound should be considered in all cases of suspected pancreatitis. Abdominal CT scan and endoscopic retrograde cholangiopancreatography (ERCP) are being used more often to assess the severity of pancreatitis and pseudocyst formation and to determine possible causes of pancreatitis. ERCP has the additional advantage of providing the option for therapeutic maneuvers such as stone removal or sphincterotomy. However, ERCP should not be performed in the acute phase or in patients with acute pseudocyst formation or pancreatic abscess formation but should be reserved for patients with chronic, recurrent pancreatitis. Rarely, ERCP may be indicated in acute pancreatitis if an obstructing gallstone is present in the common bile duct. More recently, magnetic resonance cholangiopancreatography has been considered equivalent to ERCP for the diagnosis of many pancreatic and biliary conditions. It is less invasive than ERCP, with reported sensitivity to detect common bile duct stones of 70% to 100%.

Management

All patients with evidence of pancreatitis or suspected pancreatitis should be admitted to the hospital. Treatment, however, should begin in the ED. The goals of medical treatment include suppression of pancreatic secretion and relief of pain. Morbidity and mortality in pancreatitis are directly related to complications that may already be present at the time of initial presentation. Therefore, aggressive early maintenance of intravascular volume and treatment of hypocalcemia, respiratory distress, and suspected infection are mandatory.

IV fluids should be immediately started, and the patient's oral intake should be discontinued. The patient should be assessed for hypotension. When the patient is judged stable, IV fluids should be administered at 1.5 times the maintenance rate. Vital signs and urine output should be monitored frequently. Continuous NG suction should be started; aspiration of gastric contents is based on the premise that the prevention of delivery of gastric acid into the duodenum will diminish hormonal stimulation of the pancreas. NG suction also relieves pain and prevents development of ileus. The use of anticholinergics or H_2-receptor antagonists to reduce gastric secretion is controversial and is not recommended in the initial management of patients. A crucial part of management is the treatment of abdominal pain. Traditionally, meperidine has been the analgesic of choice since morphine may increase spasm at the sphincter of Oddi. However, there is no evidence to support the assumption that morphine administration worsens pancreatitis, and repeated doses of meperidine may lead to neuromuscular irritation and seizures in rare instances.

Laboratory studies that should be performed in the ED include amylase, lipase, CBC count, electrolytes, BUN, calcium, glucose, AST, ALT, bilirubin, alkaline phosphatase, triglyceride, PT, and PTT. Arterial blood gases should be determined in patients with tachypnea. A chest radiograph should be obtained and evaluated for pleural effusion, interstitial pneumonic infiltrates, and basilar atelectasis. A flat and upright abdominal radiograph is needed to rule out perforation, ascites, and pancreatic calcifications. In severe cases or in cases of questionable diagnosis, an abdominal ultrasound should be performed.

In most cases, discontinuing enteral intake while maintaining intravascular volume and providing adequate analgesia will result in a rapid resolution of symptoms. Prognostic indicators of necrotizing or hemorrhagic pancreatitis include hypocalcemia (less than 8.0 mg per dL), hyperglycemia (more than 200 mg per dL), clinical shock, elevated hematocrit or BUN, ascites, and oxygen partial pressure of less than 60 mm Hg. Such patients should be admitted to an ICU, given sufficient colloid (e.g., albumin) to maintain normal intravascular volume, and have more extensive monitoring with an arterial catheter and a urinary catheter. A PaO_2 lower than 60 mm Hg is an indication for elective intubation. Early peritoneal dialysis should be started if rapid clinical deterioration occurs.

Antibiotics are not indicated in the initial management of pancreatitis. Pancreatic abscess should be considered if the patient's temperature is higher than 38.5°C (101.3°F). In those cases, broad-spectrum antibiotic coverage with ampicillin, gentamicin, and either clindamycin or metronidazole is indicated pending the results of blood cultures and diagnostic ultrasound. Emergency surgery is rarely necessary in acute pancreatitis; however, indications for surgery include active intraperitoneal bleeding, suspected abscess, biliary duct obstruction, and suspected traumatic transection.

MEDICAL EMERGENCIES

FULMINANT LIVER FAILURE

Background

Fulminant liver failure occurs when the vital functions of the liver fail, including the development of a coagulopathy, hypoglycemia, hyperbilirubinemia, hypoproteinemia, and encephalopathy. Liver failure can develop acutely, or it may be chronically progressive. The causes of liver failure are diverse and include infectious processes (e.g., viral hepatitis), metabolic diseases (e.g., Wilson's disease), pharmacologic agents, ischemia, and malignancy. Acute liver failure can be a life-threatening problem that causes a severe coagulopathy, hypoglycemia, and encephalopathy. Aggressive supportive medical management is required in most cases.

Pathophysiology

The pathogenesis of fulminant liver failure requires the progression of several key steps that lead to irreversible hepatocyte injury. The initiating step is the exposure of the susceptible person to the inciting agent, which leads to widespread hepatocyte injury. Hepatocyte necrosis may occur secondary to an infectious agent (viral hepatitis), a toxin (various pharmacologic substances), or a metabolic by-product.

Following hepatocyte death, the potentiation of the responsible agent is necessary to continue the hepatic destructive process. Normally, the liver is capable of regeneration; however, the regenerative process is inhibited in patients who develop liver failure. These steps may lead to terminal hepatic failure in which the liver becomes incapable of supporting those events required for life.

Although infectious agents (e.g., hepatitis A to E viruses) are responsible for most proven cases of liver failure (approximately 80% in most series), in many cases, no cause is determined. Common drugs and toxins that cause liver failure include acetaminophen, salicylates, solvents, valproic acid, amiodarone, isoniazid, NSAIDs, tetracycline, and chlorinated hydrocarbons. Rarely, metabolic diseases can lead to liver failure. These diseases include galactosemia, tyrosinemia, Wilson's disease, neonatal hemochromatosis, disorders of fatty acid oxidation, bile acid synthetic disorders, and hereditary fructose intolerance.

Clinical Manifestations

Many patients do not exhibit serious clinical features of acute liver failure. Typically, pediatric patients who develop acute liver failure were previously healthy and had no prior medical problems. Patients may initially complain of fatigue, nausea, vomiting, and diffuse abdominal pain. Occasionally, right upper quadrant pain may be severe. Commonly, a history of a prodromal viral illness can be elicited. The presence of jaundice usually initiates the first visit to the physician. As liver failure progresses, patients become more jaundiced and lethargic and develop tremors. In a short time, they become confused or somnolent and may have problems with easy bruising or bleeding.

The onset of encephalopathy occurs in conjunction with the severity and progression of liver failure. Encephalopathy is graded on a scale from I to IV. Grade I is manifested by a coherent individual who shows mild or episodic drowsiness, poor concentration, and impaired intellect. In grade II, the patient not only continues to be coherent and conversant but also becomes disoriented and fatigued. Agitation and aggressive behavior in conjunction with extreme drowsiness are manifested in grade III encephalopathy. Unresponsive patients who respond only to painful stimuli and who have evidence of cerebral edema are labeled as having grade IV encephalopathy. The clinical features of increased ICP include systemic hypertension, "decerebrate posturing," hyperventilation, abnormal pupillary responses, and impairment of brainstem reflexes. Cerebral edema is associated with increased mortality and requires aggressive supportive management. Finally, bleeding esophageal and gastric varices and ascites may rapidly develop secondary to increased portal hypertension.

Laboratory Findings

Because it may be difficult to diagnose patients clinically, biochemical evidence that provides evidence of liver failure may be collected. The liver plays an important role in hemostasis because the liver synthesizes a number of coagulation factors. An uncorrectable coagulopathy is usually the first laboratory manifestation of liver failure. Other factors may have a shorter half-life, but the PT is the most commonly used marker of the severity of liver disease. A prolonged PT despite IV supplementation of vitamin K should alert the physician to impending liver failure. Other laboratory markers suggestive of liver failure include evidence of increasing cholestasis manifested by a rising serum bilirubin level, hypoalbuminemia, and hypoglycemia.

It is also important to monitor serum transaminase levels. Falling transaminase levels usually indicate resolving liver disease, though in the setting of increasing jaundice and coagulopathy, this trend indicates hepatocyte death rather than hepatocyte repair. Serum fibrinogen is usually decreased in patients with liver failure. In cases in which the patient has splenomegaly, thrombocytopenia and leukocytopenia may be present.

Hypoglycemia almost always accompanies acute liver failure because the liver is the primary organ for gluconeogenesis, and this may complicate the signs of encephalopathy. Hepatorenal syndrome occurs in approximately 75% of patients who reach grade IV encephalopathy. The cause of hepatorenal syndrome is unclear; however, the result is oliguria in the presence of near normal intravascular pressures. Metabolic acidosis occurs in approximately 30% of patients who have liver failure, and the risk of sepsis is increased secondary to the patient's compromised immune function.

Management

All patients suspected of having liver failure should undergo a complete physical examination, including a thorough neurologic evaluation. Laboratory testing should include serum glucose, transaminases, total and direct bilirubin, albumin, PT, γ-glutamyl transpeptidase, CBC count with differential, electrolytes, blood culture, and fibrinogen. Patients with hypoglycemia should be administered IV fluids with 10% dextrose and should undergo frequent blood glucose monitoring (every 1 hour) until their blood glucose level stabilizes. Metabolic acidosis should be corrected; however, correction of hyponatremia should be gradual in patients with ascites. Patients who have a life-threatening coagulopathy should be given IV vitamin K (2.5 mg in infants; 5 mg in older children and adolescents). If the case of non–life-threatening coagulopathy, vitamin K should be given subcutaneously because of the risk of infusion reactions. A repeat PT should be performed 6 to 8 hours after administration. An uncorrectable PT is suggestive of severe hepatocyte damage. The management of bleeding esophageal varices has been previously discussed in this chapter. Therapeutic management of ascites should occur only in the face of respiratory distress or renal failure. In these cases, either direct paracentesis or IV 25% albumin (1g per kg) followed by IV furosemide can be used. Otherwise, the introduction of a diuretic (e.g., spironolactone) to achieve a slow, gradual change in ascites is all that is initially required.

Patients with encephalopathy should be frequently monitored for changes in neurologic function. In cases in which the patient has developed cerebral edema, management consists of an intensive care setting, insertion of a subdural transducer, mechanical ventilation (hyperventilation), and administration of mannitol to maintain near normal levels of ICP.

ACUTE VIRAL HEPATITIS

Background

The existing alphabet of viral hepatitis is now up to E, with new variants awaiting discovery. Hepatitis A (HAV), the cause of "infectious" or epidemic hepatitis, is transmitted by the fecal-oral route. On a worldwide scale, fewer than 5% of cases are clinically recognized. HAV is a rare cause of fulminant hepatitis. No chronic carrier state exists. The virus is maintained in the human population through person-to-person transmission. Hepatitis B (HBV) is endemic in the human population. Although predominantly transmitted by the parenteral route or sexual contact, the high incidence of infection in family contacts suggests that the virus may also spread by saliva or breast milk. The ability of HBV to produce a chronic carrier state in 5% to 10% of infected subjects allows maintenance of an infectious pool without serial transmission. Hepatitis C (HCV) accounts for about 95% of hepatitis infections in recipients of blood transfusion and 50% of cases of sporadic non-A, non-B hepatitis. Most of these patients will progress to chronic hepatitis, and about 20% will develop cirrhosis. Hepatitis D (HDV) requires hepatitis B helper functions for the propagation in hepatocytes and may occur either simultaneously with hepatitis B infection (coinfection) or as superinfection in chronic hepatitis B carriers. Hepatitis E is an enterically transmitted virus responsible for large epidemics of acute hepatitis in Asia, the Middle East, and parts of Africa.

Clinical Manifestations

Most childhood cases of acute hepatitis produce minimal symptoms, are anicteric, and, unless suspected by palpation of tender hepatomegaly, are usually confused with a GI flu-like illness. Clinical hepatitis classically consists of a 5- to 7-day prodrome of variable constitutional symptoms (low-grade fever, anorexia, nausea, vomiting, malaise, fatigue, and epigastric or right upper quadrant abdominal pain), followed by acute onset of scleral icterus, jaundice, and passage of dark urine. Pruritus and diarrhea are rare. Physical examination after the onset of jaundice may reveal tender hepatomegaly. Mild splenomegaly is present in 25% to 50% of patients. HBV patients may also present with extrahepatic signs and symptoms such as arthralgia, arthritis, or papular acrodermatitis (on face, buttocks, and extensor surfaces of arms and legs). When the rash is associated with lymphadenopathy and fever, it is called the Gianotti-Crosti syndrome. Onset of the icteric phase of acute hepatitis most commonly is temporarily associated with improvement in the constitutional symptoms. In up to 15% of cases, severe fatigue, anorexia, nausea, and vomiting persist. The icteric period usually lasts 1 to 4 weeks. Occasionally, the jaundice is prolonged for 4 to 6 weeks, with increasing pruritus at 2 to 3 weeks.

Differential Diagnosis

A number of infectious agents may mimic a viral hepatitis-like illness. The most common are Epstein-Barr virus (EBV; infectious mononucleosis) and cytomegalovirus (CMV). Both agents rarely produce clinical jaundice, and high fever and diffuse adenopathy are more characteristic. Less common agents include herpes, adenovirus, coxsackievirus, rheovirus, echovirus, rubella, arbovirus, leptospirosis, toxoplasmosis, and tuberculosis.

Diagnostic Evaluation

The following laboratory tests are usually performed in all cases of suspected viral hepatitis: serum transaminases (AST and ALT), alkaline phosphatase, total and direct bilirubin, CBC count, PT, electrolytes, BUN, glucose, total protein, albumin, globulin, and, in patients who are older than 5 years, ceruloplasmin. AST and ALT are the best indicators of ongoing hepatocellular injury. Alkaline phosphatase levels are usually less than two times the upper limit of normal for age. Levels greater than three times normal should raise suspicions of EBV or CMV hepatitis or biliary tract disease. Hepatitis classically produces direct fractions of serum bilirubin in excess of 30% of total, indicating definite liver disease. Hyperbilirubinemia may be present in the absence of scleral icterus or jaundice because these signs usually cannot be appreciated until levels of total bilirubin exceed 3 to 4 mg per dL. Serum bilirubin levels peak 5 to 7 days after the onset of jaundice. The initial biochemical screen may reveal several indicators of severe hepatocellular injury, including (i) total bilirubin level more than 20 mg per dL, (ii) serum transaminase levels that exceed 3,000 units per L, (iii) WBC count more than 25,000 per mm³, (iv) elevated PT, and (v) hypoglycemia.

Serum albumin and globulin are usually within normal levels. Decreased albumin or increased globulin levels should suggest an acute flare of chronic liver disease. Serum ceruloplasmin levels should be drawn in all patients older than 5 years who have suspected hepatitis to rule out Wilson's disease. A chest

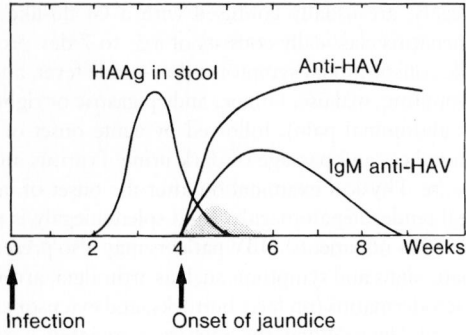

FIGURE 89.8 Serologic changes in hepatitis A. HAAg, hepatitis-associated antigen; HAV, hepatitis A virus.

radiograph may reveal cardiomegaly if any suspicion of low cardiac output states exists. Figures 89.8 and 89.9 contrast the sequence of clinical, biochemical, and serologic events in typical HAV and HBV infection. The serodiagnosis of acute hepatitis is best approached by first testing for anti-HAV IgM, HB surface antigen, HB e antigen, HB serum DNA (quantitative), anti-HB core Ab, anti-HCV, hepatitis C serum polymerase chain reaction (PCR) (quantitative), anti-CMV, and EBV serology. The finding of serum IgM anti-HAV is diagnostic of acute HAV infection because the antibody is present at the time of clinical symptoms. A positive HB surface antigen suggests the diagnosis of HBV in a symptomatic patient. A positive HB e antigen or anti-HB core Ab is helpful in the rare patient who rapidly clears HB surface antigen from the serum. It is also important to note that in long-term HB surface antigen carriers who have HDV superinfection, the suppression of HBV replication may lead to a transient absence of HBV markers in the serum; unless HDV markers in the serum are sought, the diagnosis may be missed. Anti-HCV does not appear in the patient's circulation until 1 to 3 months after the onset of acute illness, and in rare cases, detectable levels may not be demonstrated for up to 1 year. Thus, unless the acute presentation is actually a flare of chronic HCV, serodiagnosis of an HCV infection (Hep C PCR) will await long-term follow-up.

Management

No specific treatment of acute viral hepatitis is available. Most patients can be managed at home. No restrictions in diet or ambulation are necessary. The traditional recommendations of a low-fat, high-carbohydrate diet and bed rest are now recognized to have no effect on the symptoms or duration of the disease. Parents should be told that anorexia and fatigue are common symptoms. Small, frequent feedings may be helpful. Drugs should be strictly avoided. The key for both the patient and other household contacts is personal hygiene. Infants and children should avoid contact with the patient even after they have received immunoprophylaxis. In HAV, shedding of the virus may occur for up to 2 weeks after the onset of jaundice. Patients should be kept at home during this time. After this, they may return to school. Indications for hospitalization of a patient who has acute hepatitis include (i) dehydration secondary to anorexia and vomiting, (ii) bilirubin levels more than 20 mg per dL, (iii) abnormal PT, (iv) WBC count more than 25,000 per mm^3, or (v) levels of transaminases more than 3,000 units per L.

Patients who have acute hepatitis and who are hospitalized should be isolated. Follow-up studies of all patients with acute hepatitis should be performed to document biochemical resolution. Follow-up serology may also establish a specific cause in cases of apparent non-A, non-B hepatitis (fourfold increase in CMV serology, development of anti-HCV). Reevaluation of patients with HBV is especially important either to ensure clearance of HB surface antigen or to recognize the development of the HB surface antigen carrier state.

Postexposure Prophylaxis

Hepatitis A

The mean incubation period for HAV infection is about 4 weeks (range = 15 to 45 days). Conventional immune serum globulin (ISG; 0.02 mL per kg IM) confers passive protection against clinical HAV infection if given within 2 weeks of exposure. Seventy-five percent of this group will develop detectable levels of anti-HAV IgM, suggesting passive-active immunity. Postexposure immunoprophylaxis is suggested for (i) household and close personal contacts, (ii) institutionalized contacts, and (iii) contacts within a day care facility. Grade school classroom contacts of an isolated case and routine play contacts do not require ISG. However, a second case within a class is an indication for immunoprophylaxis of the rest of the class. An alternative method for determining who should receive ISG is to test high-risk contacts for anti-HAV IgG. Importantly, current guidelines recommend preexposure prophylaxis via routine HAV immunization for all children. Recently, studies have shown that immunizing patients postexposure with the hepatitis A vaccine is as effective as providing immune globulin.

Hepatitis B

Prophylactic treatment to prevent infection after exposure to HBV should be considered in the following situations seen in the ED: (i) sexual exposure to the HBV surface antigen–positive patient, (ii) inadvertent percutaneous or permucosal exposure to HBV surface antigen–positive blood, and (iii) household exposure of an infant younger than 12 months to a primary caregiver who has acute HBV. Before treatment in the first two situations, testing for susceptibility is recommended if it does not delay treatment beyond 14 days postexposure. Testing for anti-HBV core Ab is the most efficient prescreening procedure. All susceptible persons should receive a single dose

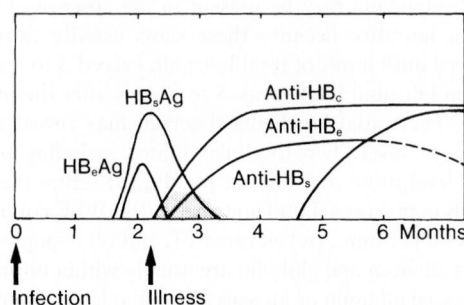

FIGURE 89.9 Serologic changes in hepatitis B. HB$_s$Ag, hepatitis B$_s$ antigen; HB$_e$Ag, hepatitis B$_e$ antigen; HB$_c$, hepatitis B$_c$; HB$_e$, hepatitis B$_e$; HB$_s$, hepatitis B$_s$.

of hepatitis B immunoglobulin (0.06 mL per kg) intramuscularly and hepatitis B vaccine in recommended doses.

CELIAC DISEASE

Background

Celiac disease (also known as celiac sprue and gluten-sensitive enteropathy) is an immune-mediated enteropathy triggered by the ingestion of gluten-containing grains such as wheat, rye, and barley in genetically susceptible persons. Nearly all patients with celiac disease carry either the human leukocyte antigen (HLA)-DQ2 or HLA-DQ8 haplotype. More recent prevalence data generated on large, population-based samples of subjects from the United States and Europe indicate that the disease is far more common than originally thought. Data from 32 U.S. states suggest that the prevalence among asymptomatic, not-at-risk persons is 1 in 133. Among at-risk groups such as first- or second-degree relatives or symptomatic patients, the prevalence varied from 1 in 56 to 1 in 22. The protean clinical manifestations with which celiac disease may present, as well as increasing recognition of its prevalence, require emergency physicians to maintain a high degree of suspicion for the disorder when evaluating patients with a variety of complaints.

Pathophysiology

Celiac disease is a classic disorder in which the interplay of genes and environment (gluten) leads to disease. There is undisputed evidence regarding the role of gluten as the triggering agent. It abnormally passes into the lamina propria in susceptible persons and is then deamidated by tissue transglutaminase and subsequently recognized by antigen-presenting cells bearing the HLA-DQ2 or HLA-DQ8, thereby triggering the autoimmune reaction of celiac disease. The hallmark findings resulting from autoimmune damage are crypt hyperplasia, epithelial lymphocytosis, increased plasma cells, and villous atrophy. In the continued presence of gluten, celiac disease is self-perpetuating.

Clinical Manifestations

In its classic form, the disease is characterized by malabsorption and failure to thrive. Other common GI symptoms include diarrhea, constipation, and recurrent abdominal pain. However, more recently, several non-GI symptoms have been increasingly appreciated as presentations for celiac disease. Anemia, joint pain, arthritis, chronic fatigue, irritability, and other behavioral changes can all be the presenting symptoms of celiac disease. These nonspecific signs and symptoms in part explain the observation that the average time from onset of symptoms to diagnosis in U.S. children is typically several years.

Laboratory Findings

The gold standard for making the diagnosis of celiac disease is the typical pattern of villous atrophy and crypt hyperplasia demonstrated on a small bowel biopsy specimen. Villous height and crypt depth are measured and a ratio of villous height to crypt depth is calculated. A ratio of less than two is considered indicative of celiac disease.

The advent of new serologic tests has dramatically changed the way celiac disease is initially diagnosed. Serum antigliadin antibodies, antiendomysial antibodies (EMAs), and tissue transglutaminase antibodies can now be measured. They have been used to evaluate symptomatic patients and in large-scale screening of asymptomatic persons. Currently, EMA is the most sensitive test. A CBC count should also be considered in the evaluation of patients with suspected celiac disease to check for anemia. In the ED setting, it is more likely that a physician may suspect celiac disease and initiate this workup but not have results of serologic tests available in a timely fashion. Proper referral to the patient's primary care physician and/or gastroenterologist is paramount for any patient suspected to have celiac disease.

Management

The only effective treatment of celiac disease is the complete avoidance of gluten-containing grains. Early diagnosis of the disease and dietary elimination of gluten are currently the only ways to avoid complications of the disease that may manifest in adulthood, including intestinal lymphoma and diabetes mellitus. Beside the obvious sources of gluten—wheat, barley, rye, and oats—many processed foods contain gluten as a stabilizer or thickener. Gluten content of foods is not typically provided on product labels, complicating the already challenging task of providing a gluten-free diet.

Suggested Readings

Gastrointestinal Bleeding

Bishop PR, Nowicki MJ, Parker PH. Vomiting-induced hematemesis in children: Mallory-Weiss tear or prolapse gastropathy? *J Pediatr Gastroenterol Nutr* 2000;30(4):436–441.

Celinska-Cedro D, Teisseyre M, Woynarowski M, et al. Endoscopic ligation of esophageal varices for prophylaxis of first bleeding in children and adolescents with portal hypertension: preliminary results of a prospective study. *J Pediatr Surg* 2003;38(7):1008–1011.

Gilger MA. Gastroenterologic endoscopy in children: past, present, and future. *Curr Opin Pediatr* 2001;13:429–434.

Latt TT, Nicholl R, Domizio P, et al. Rectal bleeding and polyps. *Arch Dis Child* 1993;69:144–147.

Lazzaroni M, Petrillo M, Tornaghi R, et al. Upper GI bleeding in healthy full-term infants: a case-control study. *Am J Gastroenterol* 2002;97(1):89–94.

Leung AK, Wong AL. Lower gastrointestinal bleeding in children. *Pediatr Emerg Care* 2002;18(4):319–323.

Teach SJ, Fleisher GR. Rectal bleeding in the pediatric emergency department. *Ann Emerg Med* 1994;23(6):1252–1258.

Vinton NE. Gastrointestinal bleeding in infancy and childhood. *Gastroenterol Clin North Am* 1994;23(1):93–122.

Wu JC, Sung JJ. Update on treatment of variceal hemorrhage. *Dig Dis* 2002; 20(2):134–144.

Colitis

Hirsch BZ. Breast milk-induced allergic colitis. *J Pediatr Gastroenterol Nutr* 1995;20(4):480.

Kelso JM, Sampson HA. Food protein-induced enterocolitis to casein hydrolysate formulas. *J Allergy Clin Immunol* 1993;92:909–910.

Machida HM, Catto Smith AG, Hall DG, et al. Allergic colitis in infancy: clinical and pathologic aspects. *J Pediatr Gastroenterol Nutr* 1994;19(1):22–26.

Moon A, Kleinman RE. Allergic gastroenteropathy in children. *Ann Allergy Asthma Immunol* 1995;74(1):5–12.

Odze RD, Wershil BK, Leichtner AM, et al. Allergic colitis in infants. *J Pediatr* 1995;126(2):163–170.

MEDICAL EMERGENCIES

Inflammatory Bowel Disease

Benchimol EI, Turner D, Mann EH, et al. Toxic megacolon in children with inflammatory bowel disease: clinical and radiographic characteristics. *Am J Gastroenterol* 2008;103:1524–1531.

Grand RJ, Ramakrishna J, Calenda KA. Inflammatory bowel disease in the pediatric patient. *Gastroenterol Clin North Am* 1995;24(3):613–632.

Gupta N, Bostrom AG, Kirschner BS, et al. Presentation and disease course in early-compared to later-onset pediatric Crohn's disease. *Am J Gastroenterol* 2008;103:2092–2098.

Herrinton LJ, Liu L, Lewis JD, et al. Incidence and prevalence of inflammatory bowel disease in a northern California managed care organization, 1996-2002. *Am J Gastroenterol* 2008;103:1998–2006.

Kugathasan S, Judd RH, Hoffmann RG, et al. Epidemiologic and clinical characteristics of children with newly diagnosed inflammatory bowel disease in Wisconsin: a statewide population-based study. *J Pediatr* 2003;143(4):525–531.

Levine JB, Lukawski-Trubish D. Extraintestinal considerations in inflammatory bowel disease. *Gastroenterol Clin North Am* 1995;24(3):633–646.

Mack DR, Langton C, Markowitz J, et al. Laboratory values for children with newly diagnosed inflammatory bowel disease. *Pediatrics* 2007;119:1113–1119.

Podolsky DK. Inflammatory bowel disease. *N Engl J Med* 2002;347(6):417–429.

Ulcer Disease

Bode G, Rothenbacher D, Brenner H, et al. *Helicobacter pylori* and abdominal symptoms: a population-based study among preschool children in southern Germany. *Pediatrics* 1998;101(4):634–637.

Chelimsky G, Czinn S. Peptic ulcer disease in children. *Pediatr Rev* 2001;22(10):349–355.

Chelimsky G, Czinn SJ. *Helicobacter pylori* infection in children: update. *Curr Opin Pediatr* 2000;12(5):460–462.

Gold BD. *Helicobacter pylori* infection in children. *Curr Probl Pediatr Adolesc Health Care* 2001;31(8):247–266.

Kelly DA. Do H$_2$ receptor antagonists have a therapeutic role in childhood? *J Pediatr Gastroenterol Nutr* 1994;19(3):270–276.

Macarthur C, Saunders N, Feldman W. *Helicobacter pylori*, gastroduodenal disease, and recurrent abdominal pain in children. *JAMA* 1995;273(9):729–734.

Mezoff AG, Balistreri WF. Peptic ulcer disease in children. *Pediatr Rev* 1995;16(7):257–265.

Sherman P, Czinn S, Drumm B, et al. *Helicobacter pylori* infection in children and adolescents: Working Group Report of the First World Congress of Pediatric Gastroenterology, Hepatology, and Nutrition. *J Pediatr Gastroenterol Nutr* 2002;35(suppl 2):S128–S133.

Sherman PM. Peptic ulcer disease in children: diagnosis, treatment and the implication of *Helicobacter pylori*. *Gastroenterol Clin North Am* 1994;23(4):707–725.

Reye's Syndrome

Bhutta AT, Van Savell H, Schexnayder SM. Reye's syndrome: down but not out. *South Med J* 2003;96(1):43–45.

da Silveira EB, Young K, Rodriguez M, et al. Reye's syndrome in a 17-year-old male: is this disease really disappearing? *Dig Dis Sci* 2002;47(9):1959–1961.

Glasgow JF, Middleton B. Reye syndrome—insights on causation and prognosis. *Arch Dis Child* 2001;85(5):351–353.

McGovern MC, Glasgow JF, Stewart MC. Lesson of the week: Reye's syndrome and aspirin: lest we forget. *BMJ* 2001;322(7302):1591–1592.

Schrör K. Aspirin and Reye syndrome. *Pediatr Drugs* 2007;9(3):195–204.

Acute Biliary Tract Disease

Holcomb GW Jr, O'Neill JA, Holcomb GW III. Cholecystitis, cholelithiasis, and common duct stenosis in children and adolescents. *Ann Surg* 1980;191:626.

McEvoy CF, Suchy FJ. Biliary tract disease in children. *Pediatr Clin North Am* 1996;43(1):75–98.

Narkewicz MR. Biliary atresia: an update on our understanding of the disorder. *Curr Opin Pediatr* 2001;13(5):435–440.

Acute Pancreatitis

DeBanto JR, Goday PS, Pedroso MR, et al. Acute pancreatitis in children. *Am J Gastroenterol* 2002;97:1726–1731.

Jackson WD. Pancreatitis: etiology, diagnosis, and management. *Curr Opin Pediatr* 2001;13(5):447–451.

Lopez MJ. The changing incidence of acute pancreatitis in children: a single institution perspective. *J Pediatr* 2002;140:622–624.

Nydegger A, Couper RTL, Oliver MR. Childhood pancreatitis. *J Gastroenterol* 2006;21:499–509.

Yachha SK, Chetri K, Saraswat VA, et al. Management of childhood pancreatic disorders: a multidisciplinary approach. *J Pediatr Gastroenterol Nutr* 2003;36(2):206–212.

Liver Failure

Kirsh BM, Lam N, Layden TJ, et al. Diagnosis and management of fulminant hepatic failure. *Compr Ther* 1995;21:166–171.

Lidofsky SD. Fulminant hepatic failure. *Crit Care Clin* 1995;11:415–430.

Poddar U, Thapa BR, Prasad A, et al. Natural history and risk factors in fulminant hepatic failure. *Arch Dis Child* 2002;87(1):54–56.

Tissieres P, Prontera W, Chevret L, et al. The pediatric risk of mortality score in infants and children with fulminant liver failure. *Pediatr Transplant* 2003;7(1):64–68.

Whitington PF. Fulminant hepatic failure in children. In: Suchy FJ, ed. *Liver disease in children.* St Louis, MO: Mosby, 1994:180–213.

Whitington PF, Alonso EM. Fulminant hepatitis in children: evidence for an unidentified hepatitis virus. *J Pediatr Gastroenterol Nutr* 2001;33(5):529–536.

Viral Hepatitis

Alter MJ. Prevention of spread of hepatitis C. *Hepatology* 2002;36(5)(suppl 1):S93–S98.

Balistreri WF. Viral hepatitis. *Pediatr Clin North Am* 1988;35:375.

Broderick AL, Jonas MM. Hepatitis B in children. *Semin Liver Dis* 2003;23(1):59–68.

NIH consensus statement on management of hepatitis C. *NIH Consens State Sci Statements* 2002;19(3):1–46.

Solal EM, Bortolotti F. Update on prevention and treatment of viral hepatitis in children. *Curr Opin Pediatr* 1999;11(5):384–389.

Celiac Disease

Fasano A. Celiac disease—how to handle a clinical chameleon. *N Engl J Med* 2003;348(25):2568–2570.

Fasano A, Berti I, Gerarduzzi T, et al. Prevalence of celiac disease in at-risk and not-at-risk groups in the United States: a large multicenter study. *Arch Intern Med* 2003;163(3):286–292.

Maki M, Mustalahti K, Kokkonen J, et al. Prevalence of celiac disease among children in Finland. *N Engl J Med* 2003;348(25):2517–2524.

McManus R, Kelleher D. Celiac disease—the villain unmasked? *N Engl J Med* 2003;348(25):2573–2574.

CHAPTER 90 ■ PEDIATRIC AND ADOLESCENT GYNECOLOGY

JOELI HETTLER, MD

INTRODUCTION

Evaluation of Premenarcheal Girls

Among premenarcheal girls with gynecologic complaints, the most commonly encountered specific entities are vaginal infections, urethral prolapse, trauma, and suspected sexual abuse. Many other patients have nonspecific genital irritation. In assessing any child with a gynecologic complaint, the physician must be alert to the possibility that sexual abuse is the underlying problem.

The premenarcheal girl should not receive a standard pelvic examination, including the use of a speculum and vaginoabdominal palpation, because such an examination is uncomfortable and unnecessary for diagnosis. An exception to this rule is the girl with vaginal bleeding caused by an injury. If an external source for the bleeding cannot be identified, speculum examination of the vaginal vault under procedural sedation or anesthesia is warranted to allow visualization of the injury. Some major vaginal lacerations produce only mild pain or minimal bleeding. For most premenarcheal girls, the history, a general physical examination including inspection of the vulva (Fig. 90.1) and visualization the vagina, and culture of a vaginal discharge, if one is present, will lead to a diagnosis.

Most young children will cooperate readily for initial inspection of the external genitalia either on the examining table or while held on a parent's lap. The child should be placed in the supine position with flexed hips and knees and with heels touching (Fig. 90.2). In most cases, the examiner can obtain a good view of the child's vaginal vestibule by grasping the labia majora firmly and exerting gentle laterocaudal traction. For inspection of the vaginal vault, the knee-chest position is helpful. Most children older than 4 years can cooperate for this maneuver. The child is first asked to "get up on your hands and knees like you are going to crawl." She is then instructed to rest her head on her folded arms, facing her parent. The examiner or an assistant gently presses the child's buttocks and labia upward and outward. If the child relaxes her abdominal muscles and back at this point, her vagina will usually fall open, permitting inspection of the vault, using an otoscope for magnification and illumination (Fig. 90.2). If the child has a vaginal discharge or bleeding, she should then be returned to the supine position so that specimens for culture can be obtained, using either a soft plastic medicine dropper or a cotton-tipped swab moistened with nonbacteriostatic saline solution. A rectal examination should be performed if there is abdominal pain or a lower abdominal mass. Rectoabdominal palpation may be helpful if a hard vaginal foreign body is suspected, but nearly all vaginal foreign bodies are composed of toilet tissue and are therefore not palpable. On rectal examination, a child's cervix is normally felt as a firm, midline button of tissue, but the uterus and ovaries should not be palpable.

Evaluation of Adolescent Girls

The differential diagnosis of gynecologic symptoms and signs in an adolescent girl who has had sexual intercourse includes a number of major entities [e.g., pregnancy, pelvic inflammatory disease (PID), tuboovarian abscess] that do not pertain to the teenager who is not sexually experienced. Therefore, the emergency physician evaluating an adolescent girl must routinely inquire about sexual activity and, if the response is positive, about contraceptive use, prior sexually transmitted infections (STIs), pregnancies, and abortions. A detailed menstrual history—age at menarche, characteristics of the menstrual cycle, date of last menstrual period, presence or absence of dysmenorrhea—should be obtained from every adolescent patient.

Obtaining a candid history of sexual activity from adolescent girls is not always a simple matter, but the emergency physician can maximize honest reporting by using some basic interviewing principles. First, the teenage girl who asks for a female physician is stating directly what will make her more comfortable. Her request should therefore be honored if possible. Second, questions to the teenager about sexual activity (as well as other potentially sensitive subjects such as contraception, sexual orientation, and substance abuse) should not be asked when a parent or sexual partner is present. Third, before any questions are asked, it is helpful to assure the teenager that if she wants, her answers will be kept confidential.[1] Finally, the physician who adopts an empathetic, nonauthoritarian interviewing style is most likely to win the teenager's trust.

---

[1] All 50 states and the District of Columbia allow most minors to consent to testing and treatment of sexually transmitted infections (STIs), and many explicitly include testing and treatment of HIV. Many states, however, allow physicians to inform parents that the minor is seeking or receiving STI services when they deem it in the best interests of the minor. Twenty-one states and the District of Columbia explicitly allow all minors to consent to contraceptive services, and 35 states require some type of parental involvement in a minor's decision to have an abortion. Emergency physicians should familiarize themselves with the relevant current laws of their own states. From www.guttmacher.org/statecenter/spibs/index.html. Accessed October 9, 2008.

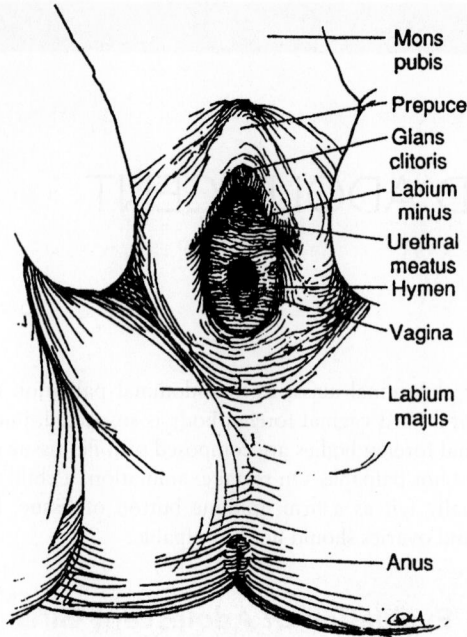

FIGURE 90.1 Anatomy of the normal female external genitalia.

Most virginal adolescents with menstrual cramps, mittelschmerz, or vaginal discharge do not require full pelvic examinations because the likelihood that occult pelvic pathology will be found is small. Rectoabdominal palpation can be used to evaluate the virginal patient with undiagnosed lower abdominal pain or a mass. However, trauma and vaginal bleeding are indications for pelvic examination, even among patients who have never been sexually active.

Every sexually experienced adolescent girl who comes to the emergency department (ED) for abdominal pain or a gynecologic complaint must receive a pelvic examination because such patients have high rates of pregnancy and STIs. Before the examination, the patient should be given a chance to empty her bladder. If urine nucleic acid amplification testing for *Neisseria gonorrhoeae* or *Chlamydia trachomatis* is planned, she should be instructed to void without cleaning the periurethral area and save the first 30 mL of urine in a specimen cup. A female chaperone is necessary when the examining physician is male and recommended when she is female. The examiner should take care to explain the examination and answer any questions because many sexually active adolescents have never had a pelvic examination. After the patient is situated in the lithotomy position and draped, her vulva is inspected and a narrow speculum is inserted for visualization of her vagina and cervix. A sterile cotton-tipped swab is used to collect endocervical secretions for culture of *N. gonorrhoeae*. A second endocervical specimen is obtained to test for *C. trachomatis* antigen. If nucleic acid amplification testing is performed, endocervical secretions or urine may be used. After a sample of vaginal discharge for microscopic examination has been taken with a third swab, the speculum is removed. If the physician suspects gonococcal infection, urethral and rectal swabs may also be taken. The endocervical specimens should be obtained before bimanual palpation is done because lubricating jelly can inhibit growth of *N. gonorrhoeae*. During the bimanual examination, the cervix is assessed for softness, patency of the os, and pain elicited by lateral cervical movement. The size and consistency of the uterus are determined, and the adnexal areas are palpated for masses and tenderness. Finally, rectovaginal palpation is performed, checking again for masses and local tenderness.

In addition to providing treatment of the patient's current problem, the emergency physician should determine the source of the patient's routine outpatient gynecologic care. The ED should maintain a list of local programs that provide health care to adolescents so that referral can be made easily. Many communities have specialized services for teenagers sponsored by hospitals, health departments, or private agencies. Similarly, because previously unrecognized pregnancy is a common ED diagnosis, procedures should be established to facilitate prompt referral of teenagers who need counseling, prenatal care, and therapeutic abortion to the appropriate services.

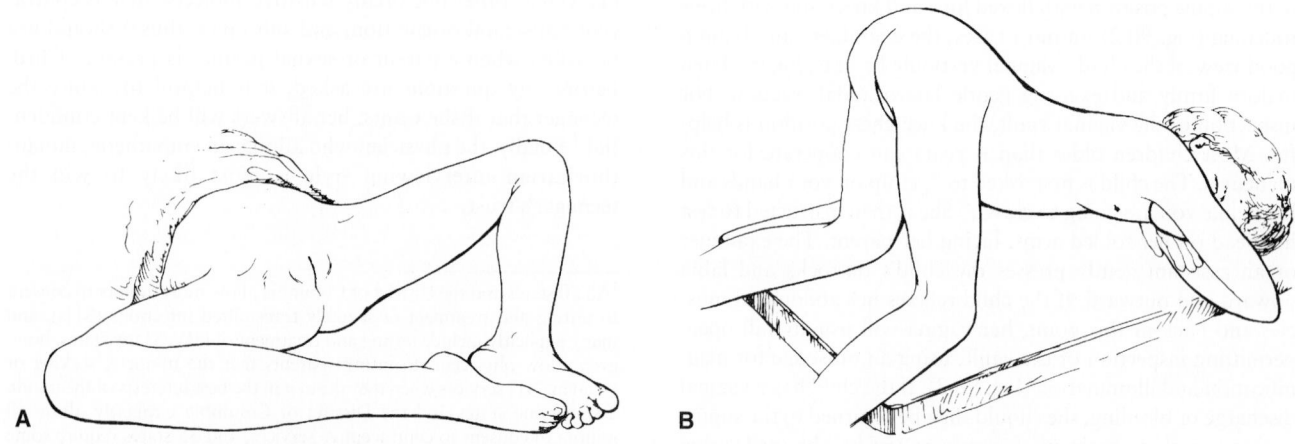

FIGURE 90.2 A: Girl in the frog-leg position for the examination of the external genitalia. **B:** Girl in the knee-chest position with exaggerated lordosis and relaxed abdominal muscles. The examiner can inspect the interior of her vagina by gently separating her buttocks and labia, using an otoscope without an attached speculum for illumination.

GYNECOLOGIC DISORDERS OF CHILDHOOD

Congenital Vaginal Obstruction

Background

Definition. In normal females, the vagina provides an outlet for genital secretions and menstrual blood. If the vagina is obstructed, accumulating fluid will eventually distend it, causing symptoms to develop either during infancy or after menarche. During infancy, vaginal distension with mucus secreted as a result of stimulation by maternal hormones is called hydrocolpos or mucocolpos. If the volume of secretions is so large that the uterus is also distended, this condition is called hydrometrocolpos. If an obstructing congenital malformation is not recognized before menarche, menstrual blood will gradually fill the vagina, producing hematocolpos or, less commonly, hematometrocolpos.

Etiology

For hydrocolpos or one of its variations to arise, a female must have vaginal obstruction, a uterus, and a patent cervix. The two most common anomalies with these features are transverse vaginal septum (sometimes called vaginal atresia) and imperforate hymen. These malformations are probably produced between the 16th and 20th weeks of gestation if the developing vaginal plate fails to perforate at its junction with either the fused paramesonephric (Müllerian) ducts proximally or the urogenital sinus caudally. Most patients with complete agenesis of the vagina (Rokitansky-Küster-Hauser syndrome) have rudimentary uteri or none at all, so hydrocolpos does not occur. Transverse vaginal septum occurs sporadically, with an estimated incidence of 1 in 4,000 to 5,000 girls. Imperforate hymen occurred in 0.1% of term female neonates.

Clinical Manifestations

Infancy. Although vaginal obstruction should be properly identified during the initial examination of the newborn female, infants with hydrocolpos often go unrecognized until days or weeks later when they develop the three hallmarks of this condition: (i) a lower abdominal mass, (ii) difficulty with urination, and (iii) a visible bulging membrane at the introitus. In more severe cases, infants may also have constipation, hydronephrosis, edema of the lower extremities, and hypoventilation. Inspection of the perineum should immediately indicate the proper diagnosis.

Adolescence. The girl with congenital vaginal obstruction that escapes notice during infancy will not come to attention until late in puberty when she presents with either primary amenorrhea or lower abdominal pain. She will have had satisfactory pubertal development until her menarche apparently fails to occur. Accumulating menstrual blood will then eventually produce vague lower abdominal pain that is not necessarily cyclic. As the hematocolpos grows, it will finally interfere with comfortable micturition, producing symptoms of urgency, frequency, or dysuria. The history of amenorrhea and the finding of a lower abdominal mass may lead the physician to suspect a tumor or even pregnancy, but the char-

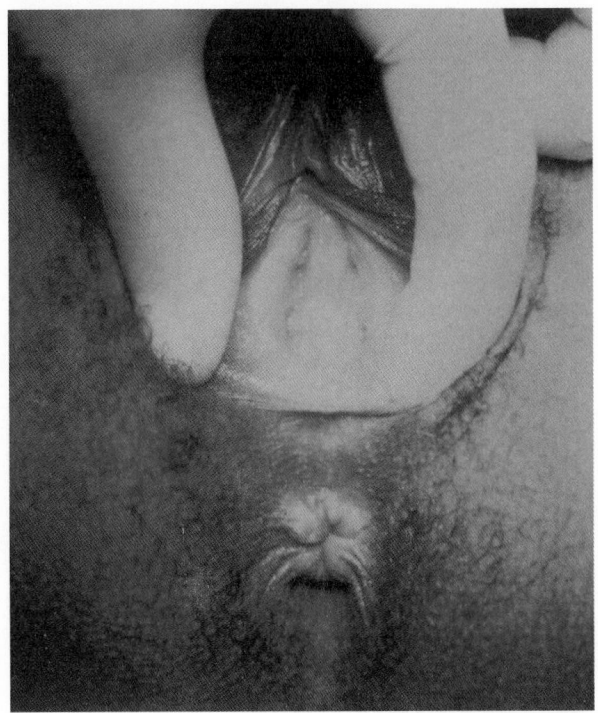

FIGURE 90.3 Hematocolpos in a 15-year-old patient with an imperforate hymen. The membrane bulges at the introitus underneath the labia minora (see also Fig. 90.4).

acteristic appearance of the introitus covered by a bluish bulging membrane is diagnostic of hematocolpos with imperforate hymen (Fig. 90.3). Patients with a high transverse vaginal septum will not be so easily diagnosed because the introitus will appear normal. However, palpation of the vagina will promptly show that it is obstructed and that the cervix cannot be felt.

Complications

The complication of congenital vaginal obstruction most likely to require urgent attention among both infants and adolescents is acute urinary retention. Patients without complete urethral obstruction can instead have variable degrees of hydroureter or hydronephrosis as a result of the chronic extrinsic pressure. Rarely, an infant may have respiratory insufficiency or inferior vena caval obstruction because of the large mass. Imperforate hymen is usually an isolated anomaly, but other types of obstruction, chiefly transverse vaginal septum, are regularly associated with renal malformations, including hypoplastic or single kidneys, and duplicated or ectopic collecting systems. Endometriosis can be a late complication of severe hematocolpos.

Differential Diagnosis

The differential diagnosis of hydrocolpos and its variations includes patients with either a lower abdominal mass or a pelvic mass but no vaginal obstruction and patients with apparent vaginal obstruction. In the former category, the physician simply needs to demonstrate that the patient has a patent genital tract. The latter group includes girls with microperforate hymen, labial adhesions, Gartner's (mesonephric) duct cysts,

MEDICAL EMERGENCIES

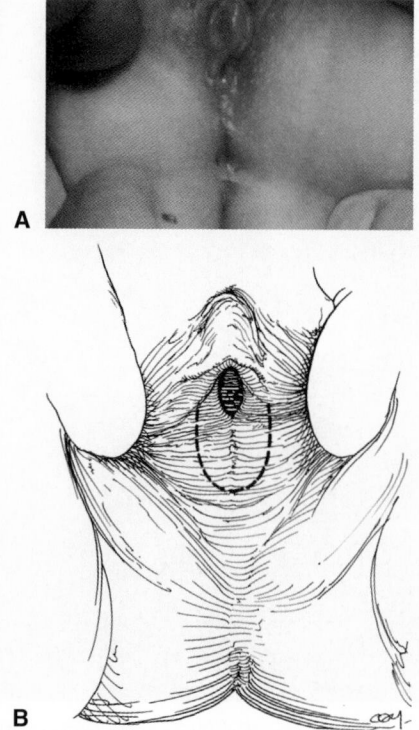

FIGURE 90.4 **A:** Labial adhesion in an asymptomatic 3-year-old girl. **B:** A flat surface, a dense central line of fusion, and an opening below the clitoris are characteristic features of labial adhesions, which cover the introitus (see also Fig. 90.3).

and, rarely, complete agenesis of the vagina and testicular feminization. The microperforate hymen has a tiny orifice just below the urethra and requires only careful inspection for its diagnosis. Adhesions of the labia minora are superficial to the plane of the hymen and are characterized by a central vertical line of fusion (Fig. 90.4). A large vaginal Gartner's duct cyst can resemble an imperforate hymen, but it can be seen to protrude through the hymenal ring, which is itself patent. Patients with complete agenesis of the vagina have only a rugated dimple or shallow indentation at the introitus. A short blind vagina also occurs in testicular feminization, a disorder characterized by end-organ insensitivity to androgen. These patients are phenotypic females with an XY karyotype who undergo breast development at puberty but lack pubic hair and female reproductive organs.

Management

Patients with congenital vaginal obstruction need surgical treatment. The management of simple imperforate hymen can be modified according to the patient's age. Surgery should be scheduled promptly for adolescents but can be performed electively for asymptomatic infants and children.

Labial Adhesions

Background

Labial adhesions are an acquired attachment of the medial surfaces of the labia minora to each other. The terms *labial fusion*,

synechiae, and *agglutination* are also often used to describe this condition. Labial adhesions are a common gynecologic condition, occurring in approximately 0.6% to 7% of girls between the ages of 3 months and 6 years.

Pathophysiology

The etiology of labial adhesions are unclear, but conditions that lead to irritation of the vulva in the prepubertal girl with normally low levels of estrogen are thought to contribute to the fusion of the edges of the labia minora. The line of fusion usually advances anteriorly from the posterior frenulum of the labia minora.

Clinical Manifestations

Most labial adhesions are asymptomatic, being noted by a parent at home or a physician during the child's routine physical examination. The diagnosis of labial adhesions can be made by simple inspection of the child's genitalia. When the labia majora are gently retracted laterally, a flat plane of tissue marked by a central vertical line of adhesion obstructs the view of the introitus within (Fig. 90.4B). This thin vertical raphe is pathognomonic of labial adhesions. It is occasionally difficult to detect if the child's adhesions are old and dense. The length of the adhesions is variable, and they can be perforated. They are usually thickest posteriorly and stop below the clitoris. Even when adhesions appear to have closed the vulva completely, a pinpoint opening generally permits the egress of urine.

While most girls with labial adhesions have no symptoms, a few may have associated dysuria, frequency, or refusal to void that may be a result of either the obvious mechanical obstruction or concurrent urinary tract infection. Whether associated urinary tract infections are a cause or an effect of adhesions is uncertain, but these are recognized complications of the condition. For girls with urinary tract infections, urine cultures should be performed and appropriate medical follow-up provided. Because vaginal infection is not associated with adhesions, vaginal cultures are not indicated except in patients who have concurrent vaginal discharge. Asymptomatic girls need no laboratory evaluation.

Management

Treatment is not indicated for asymptomatic girls with labial adhesions because the condition spontaneously remits early in puberty as a result of increasing endogenous estrogen. Some parents, however, prefer that their daughters be treated. Of girls with labial adhesions, 90% can be treated successfully with a small amount of estrogen cream (Premarin® or Dienestrol) dabbed onto the adhesions at once or twice a day for 2 to 4 weeks. Parents should be warned specifically that prolonged use of the hormone could stimulate breast growth in children. Vulvar hyperpigmentation is a common, transient adverse effect of treatment. Labial adhesions should never be manually separated. The procedure is painful and usually results in relapse when the raw, newly separated labia adhere again. As recurrence rates vary from 15% to 40%, care after separation is important. Proper hygiene is recommended, as well as daily application of a bland emollient (petroleum jelly).

Urethral Prolapse

Background

Urethral prolapse is the protrusion of the distal urethral mucosa outward through its meatus, with a cleavage plane between the longitudinal and circular–oblique smooth-muscle layers of the urethra. Most happen spontaneously, but a sudden or recurrent increase in intraabdominal pressure (severe coughing, seizure, constipation, lifting heavy objects) has been noted to precede some cases. The prolapsed segment is constricted at the meatus and venous blood flow is impaired, so the involved tissue becomes swollen, edematous, and dark red or purplish. If the process is not corrected, the tissue can become thrombosed and necrotic.

About half of affected females are prepubertal children, and the majority of the remainder is postmenopausal women. Most prolapses during childhood occur in girls between the ages of 2 and 10 years. Of girls with urethral prolapse, the vast majority are African American.

Clinical Manifestations

Vaginal bleeding or spotting is the chief complaint of 90% of children with significant urethral prolapses. The bleeding is painless, occasionally misinterpreted as hematuria or menstruation, and accompanied by urinary frequency or dysuria in about one-fourth of cases. Only a minority of girls or their parents are aware of the presence of a vulvar mass. However, it is not rare for the physician simply to note a small prolapse during the routine examination of an asymptomatic child.

On examination of the child's vulva, a red or purplish, soft, doughnut-shaped mass is seen (Fig. 90.5). Most prolapses are not tender and measure 1 to 2 cm in diameter. By retracting the labia majora posterolaterally, the examiner can often demonstrate that the mass is separate from and anterior to the vaginal introitus, but this process may be difficult if the prolapse is large. A small central dimple in the mass indicates the urethral lumen. This dimple can be missed if lighting is inadequate, bleeding is active, or mucosal edema is significant. In most cases, the appearance of the prolapse is diagnostic. However, if the diagnosis is in doubt, sterile straight catheterization of the bladder through the mass can be performed to demonstrate the anatomic relationships safely and rapidly. No other test is needed. If urinalysis is performed on a spontaneously voided specimen, red blood cells are likely to be found, but urine cultures are routinely sterile. Urethral polyps, prolapsed uterocele, sarcoma botryoides, and urethral carcinoma may be included in the differential diagnosis, but these entities are rare in children and lack the characteristically annular appearance of a urethral prolapse.

Management

For the symptomatic patient with a small segment of prolapsed mucosa that is not necrotic, warm moist compresses or sitz baths, combined with a 2-week course of topical estrogen cream, may be prescribed. Most patients treated in this way have improved within 10 to 14 days and remained normal thereafter, thus avoiding surgery. Patients with dark-red or necrotic mucosa should be treated surgically within several days by reduction of the prolapse and/or excision of necrotic tissue. After the diagnosis is confirmed by cystoscopy, the prolapse is excised and the cut edges are sutured together.

GYNECOLOGIC DISORDERS OF ADOLESCENCE

Dysmenorrhea

Background

Definition. Primary dysmenorrhea is painful menstruation that cannot be attributed to a specific pelvic abnormality such as endometriosis, PID, or a uterine malformation. Menstrual pain resulting from an underlying disorder is termed secondary dysmenorrhea.

Epidemiology

Among adolescents, primary dysmenorrhea is far more common than secondary dysmenorrhea. The incidence of primary dysmenorrhea is estimated to be 60% to 70%, with 15% of adolescents reporting symptoms severe enough to interrupt with daily activities. The prevalence of dysmenorrhea increases with increasing chronologic and gynecologic (postmenarcheal) age, reflecting the strong association of dysmenorrhea with ovulatory menstrual cycles. At gynecologic age 1, approximately 30% of girls have dysmenorrhea. By gynecologic age 5, the proportion increases to nearly 70%. Risk factors for dysmenorrhea include early menarche, cigarette smoking, and possibly low fish consumption.

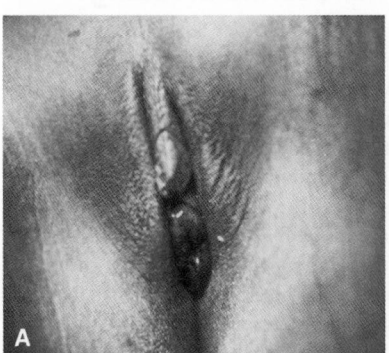

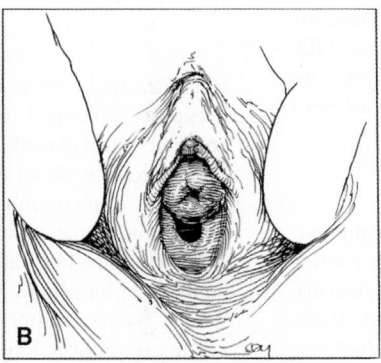

FIGURE 90.5 **A:** Urethral prolapse in a 6-year-old girl with "vaginal" bleeding. The vaginal orifice cannot be seen. **B:** The smooth doughnut shape and central lumen are characteristic features of a urethral prolapse, which, if large or swollen, often conceals the vagina below it.

MEDICAL EMERGENCIES

Pathophysiology

The end of ovulatory menstrual cycles, prostaglandins $F_{2\alpha}$ and E_2 are synthesized by and released from endometrial tissue. The prostaglandins cause increases in both the uterine resting tone and the amplitude and frequency of myometrial contractions. Uterine contractions that exceed systolic blood pressure produce tissue ischemia and perceptible pain. Intravenous (IV) administration of prostaglandins can reproduce the systemic discomforts—vomiting, diarrhea, and headache—that often accompany dysmenorrhea. A dose–response relationship has been demonstrated in studies comparing the prostaglandin content of menstrual fluid from women with and without dysmenorrhea and from individual women during painful and pain-free cycles.

The role of ovarian hormones in endometrial prostaglandin production is not completely understood. Progesterone or its withdrawal appears to enhance prostaglandin synthesis during ovulatory cycles. Conversely, progesterone-impregnated intrauterine devices (IUDs) and the inhibition of ovulation by birth control pills are associated both with decreased prostaglandin production and with relief from dysmenorrhea.

The most common explanation for menstrual cramping is the overproduction of prostaglandins. Before menstruation, as progesterone withdrawal occurs, arachidonic acid (an omega-6 fatty acid) is released, prompting a cascade of prostaglandins and leukotrienes. This mediates the inflammatory response that causes both cramping and systemic symptoms. In particular, prostaglandin $F_{2\alpha}$ (a cyclooxygenase metabolite of arachidonic acid) causes potent vasoconstriction and myometrial contractions. The specific role of leukotrienes in dysmenorrhea is still under investigation.

Clinical Manifestations

Typical primary dysmenorrhea consists of cramping, dull, midline, or generalized lower abdominal pain at the onset of a menstrual period. The pain may coincide with the start of bleeding or may precede the bleeding by several hours. Many women have associated symptoms including backache, thigh pain, bloating, diarrhea, nausea or vomiting, and headache. The discomfort usually abates within 48 hours. Because dysmenorrhea is a hallmark of ovulation, adolescents characteristically do not experience dysmenorrhea until after several months of painless, anovulatory cycles. Menstrual pain that begins either at menarche or more than 4 years after regular cycles have been established is less common.

When pain is chronic (lasting throughout the cycle), begins at menarche, or is associated with dysparunia or metrorrhagia, causes of secondary dysmenorrhea should be considered. The most common cause of secondary dysmenorhea in adolescents is endometriosis. Other causes include adhesions, PID, abscess, ectopic pregnancy, miscarriage, ovarian cyst, and reproductive tract anomalies such as rudimentary uterine horn and obstructed genital duplications.

Diagnosis

Patients with straightforward dysmenorrhea have normal physical examinations and no associated abnormalities on routine laboratory evaluation. The virginal adolescent with a typical history of dysmenorrhea should undergo a routine physical examination, but a pelvic examination is unnecessary. However, virginal patients with atypical or severe pain should undergo rectoabdominal or one-finger vaginoabdominal palpation. Sexually experienced adolescents with pelvic pain cannot be adequately evaluated without a complete pelvic examination to screen for pelvic infection and unsuspected pregnancy. In most cases, no specific laboratory or radiologic evaluation is needed for otherwise healthy virginal adolescents. Qualitative serum or urine β-human chorionic gonadotropin (β-hCG) should be considered in these allegedly virginal adolescent females with severe pain, vaginal bleeding, or signs of shock because a history of never being sexually active, provided by a teenage girl, does not completely rule out the possibility of pregnancy. Pelvic ultrasound or laparoscopy may be helpful in the assessment of patients either with uncertain diagnoses or with pain unresponsive to adequate treatment.

Management

Nonsteroidal antiinflammatory drugs (NSAIDs) are the treatment of choice for patients with moderate or severe dysmenorrhea, providing pain relief for 60% to 80% of symptomatic women. Treatment is most effective when initiated 1 to 2 days before the onset of menses and is recommended until the dysmenorrhea resolves, typically by day 2 or 3 of the menstrual period. Examples of commonly used NSAID treatment regimens are as follows:

- Mefenamic acid: 500 mg once orally, followed by 250 mg four times a day
- Ibuprofen: 400 to 600 mg orally four times a day
- Naproxen sodium: 550 mg once orally, followed by 275 mg three times a day
- Celecoxib: 500 mg once orally, followed by 200 mg twice a day

Patients should be instructed to take NSAIDs with food and to drink adequate fluids. Celecoxib is prescribed for those with risk factors for gastrointestinal (GI) bleeding. It is approved for dysmenorrhea in women older than 18 years.

Patients who do not respond to NSAIDs administered for at least 3 menstrual periods should be offered a combination estrogen and progestin pill. All patients who smoke should be offered smoking cessation support. Some practitioners recommend increasing dietary intake of omega-3 polyunsaturated fatty acid. Other agents commonly recommended in the past for the treatment of dysmenorrhea—acetaminophen, caffeine, and propoxyphene—lack specific antiprostaglandin action and have only limited effectiveness.

Dysfunctional Uterine Bleeding

Background

Dysfunctional uterine bleeding (DUB) is best characterized as irregular, prolonged, or excessive menstrual bleeding associated with anovulation and unrelated to pregnancy. Ovulatory cycles occur in about 20% of adults with DUB, but this phenomenon is uncommon during the teenage years. Terms often used to categorize patterns of DUB are *metrorrhagia* (irregular or acyclic bleeding) and *menorrhagia* (excessive duration or quantity of bleeding). Menstrual bleeding that persists beyond 9 days, recurs at intervals of fewer than 21 days, or produces anemia is abnormal and warrants attention.

DUB is prevalent at the beginning and end of the reproductive years, paralleling the times when anovulatory cycles are most common. In girls during the first year after menarche, about half of menstrual cycles are anovulatory. This proportion decreases gradually, so only 5% of cycles are anovulatory 10 years or more after menarche. Of course, most adolescents with anovultory cycles experience self-limited, reasonably cyclic bleeding episodes.

Pathophysiology

From the standpoint of ovarian function, the normal ovulatory menstrual cycle is divided into an initial follicular and a subsequent luteal phase. The parallel phases of endometrial development are termed, respectively, *proliferative* and *secretory*. At the start of an ovulatory cycle, pituitary follicle-stimulating hormone (FSH) promotes the growth of ovarian follicles. In turn, the rising concentration of estradiol from these follicles stimulates the proliferation of endometrial stroma and glands and induces a midcycle surge of luteinizing hormone (LH) that triggers ovulation. The duration of the preovulatory phase of the menstrual cycle is variable but generally lasts about 14 days. After ovulation has occurred, the ruptured ovarian follicle forms a corpus luteum that secretes progesterone and estradiol and levels of both FSH and LH gradually decline. Although progesterone limits the ultimate thickness of the endometrium, it also promotes further growth of the endometrial secretory glands and spiral blood vessels, so they become coiled and tortuous. At the end of the corpus luteum life span (a highly consistent 14 days unless conception occurs), it degenerates, and circulating levels of both estrogen and progesterone fall, eventually stimulating a resurgence of LH and FSH. As hormonal support wanes, blood flow to the secretory endometrium diminishes, and the spiral arterioles constrict and relax rhythmically under the influence of local prostaglandins. The resulting progressive ischemia leads to endometrial necrosis and menstrual sloughing.

In contrast, during intervals of anovulation, luteal progesterone is not present either to limit the endometrium thickness or to promote its structural integrity. Parts of the endometrial surface undergo growth and sloughing sporadically, without cyclic coordination. The amount of estrogen secreted by ovarian follicles fluctuates unpredictably, and bleeding can occur either because of a fall in estrogen level (withdrawal bleeding) or despite a sustained level of production (breakthrough bleeding). Relatively constant low levels of estrogen tend to produce intermittent spotty bleeding (metrorrhagia). Larger amounts of estrogen cause greater endometrial proliferation and a cyclic pattern of amenorrhea followed by profuse bleeding (menorrhagia) whenever either the endometrial vessels and glands outstrip their stromal support or hormone levels spontaneously fall. Compared with the 35 to 80 mL of blood lost during a normal menstrual period, dysfunctional bleeding often results in the loss of 100 to 200 mL each month, which may produce iron deficiency and anemia.

Clinical Manifestations

DUB has a substantial capacity to disrupt the everyday lives of adolescents who may have unpredictable, urgent need for bathroom facilities due to risk of visible blood stains. Large amounts of bleeding often provoke considerable fear in both patients and their parents. These concerns can overshadow the history of the bleeding itself, but the details of the problem's chronology and an estimate of blood loss (in pads per day) will help the physician assess the severity of the bleeding, follow the patient's clinical course, and gauge her prognosis. The symptoms that characteristically accompany only ovulatory menstrual cycles—mittelschmerz, premenstrual breast tenderness, bloating, mood changes, and dysmenorrhea—should be absent. DUB is classically painless, but occasionally, a patient with active bleeding may experience crampy pain if a large quantity of blood is passed rapidly. Weakness or fainting should alert the examiner to the possibility of significant blood loss. Pertinent questions should include whether the patient is pregnant, whether she uses contraception if she has been sexually active, and whether she has an underlying platelet disorder (e.g., thrombocytopenia, von Willebrand's disease).

The physical examination starts with the measurement of the patient's vital signs, including a check for orthostatic changes in the pulse and blood pressure. Pertinent signs, including pallor, petechiae or bruises that might indicate a bleeding disorder, and hirsutism or obesity consistent with the polycystic ovary syndrome, should be noted. The pelvic examination is likely to be normal except for the presence of bleeding but should be performed to evaluate the patient for pelvic infections, previously unrecognized pregnancy, and functional ovarian cysts. If necessary, rectoabdominal palpation can be substituted for the standard bimanual examination. Ovarian enlargement is an uncommon finding even among adolescent patients with clear-cut polycystic ovary syndrome. The differential diagnosis of DUB is discussed at greater length in Chapter 76.

Management

A determination of the hemoglobin or hematocrit is essential for the emergency evaluation of patients with DUB because historical estimates of blood loss are imprecise. A platelet count should also be obtained because thrombocytopenia is the most common hematologic disorder that produces menorrhagia. The history and physical examination should be used to guide the choice of additional laboratory tests. Sexually active adolescents should receive a pregnancy test and an antigen-detection test for chlamydial infection and gonorrhea because STI-associated endometritis is a common cause of otherwise unexplained uterine bleeding. Patients with menorrhagia beginning at menarche, severe hemorrhage, or a history of bleeding problems should undergo further evaluation for possible disorders of platelet number or function.

For patients with brisk hemorrhage or hypotension, prompt volume resuscitation and hospitalization are necessary (see Chapter 3). Control of the bleeding itself is accomplished with hormonal treatment (Table 90.1). Regimens vary according to the severity of bleeding and individual preference, but each is designed first to stop the bleeding, second to convert the unstable proliferative uterine endometrium to the secretory state, and finally to allow a self-limited endometrial slough under controlled conditions. Pregnancy must be excluded in every case before hormonal treatment is begun. Estrogen is used to support the endometrium for short term and to stop the bleeding. A progestational agent must be administered simultaneously to produce a secretory endometrium; otherwise, the problem will recur predictably whenever the estrogen is stopped. Any of the oral contraceptive pills with 35 or 50 g

TABLE 90.1

MANAGEMENT OF DYSFUNCTIONAL UTERINE BLEEDING

Clinical situation	Treatment
Acute hemorrhage with shock	Volume resuscitation Rarely, red blood cell transfusion Conjugated estrogens 25 mg IV every 4 h until bleeding stops (up to six doses) Rarely, curettage if IV estrogen fails When able to take oral medications: Iron 60 mg/day Progestin 10–20 mg/day Antiemetics as needed
Severe bleeding Hb < 10 mg/dL	Estradiol 50 μg/norgestrel (0.5 mg) orally[a]: Every 4 h until bleeding stops (usually within 24 h) qid for 4 days tid for 3 days bid for 2 weeks Iron 60 mg/day Antiemetics as needed
Moderate bleeding Hb 10–12 mg/dL	Estradiol 50 μg/norgestrel (0.5 mg) orally[a]: tid until bleeding stops (usually within 48 h) bid for 5 days Daily to complete 21 days Iron 60 mg/day Antiemetics as needed
Not currently bleeding Hb > 12 mg/dL	Consider combined estrogen/ progesterone hormonal contraception Iron 60 mg/day

qid, four times a day; tid, three times a day.
[a]Many different regimens of combination oral hormonal therapy appear to be equally effective.

of either ethinyl estradiol or mestranol and a progestin provides a convenient means of administering the two hormones together. Nausea is a common side effect of estrogen in each of these regimens and can be treated symptomatically. Vomiting rarely precludes oral therapy. Progestins alone in higher dosages can be used if estrogen is contraindicated or not tolerated, but the resulting hemostasis is less prompt and less predictable.

After the cessation of treatment, a self-limited, heavy menstrual period will follow within 2 to 3 days. The family must be forewarned so they anticipate this episode and do not misinterpret it as a recurrence of DUB. This withdrawal bleeding will stop spontaneously within several days. Subsequent therapy must be tailored to the individual patient. For sexually active adolescents and for those with chronic or recurrent DUB, long-term use of combined oral contraceptive pills is an excellent therapeutic choice.

Adolescents with severe, chronic, or recurrent DUB should receive diagnostic investigation to address the question of an underlying endocrinologic disorder (see Chapter 47). Iron supplementation is prudent for all patients with DUB; those without frank anemia are likely to have depleted marrow stores of iron. Patients should be encouraged to maintain a menstruation calendar to aid her clinician in future visits. Finally, outpatient follow-up is an essential component of management because treatment may be needed for months or years and because chronic anovulation is a risk factor for both infertility and the late development of endometrial carcinoma.

Sexual Abuse and Assault

The five major gynecologic aspects of treating a girl who has been sexually abused or assaulted are (i) collection of evidence, (ii) the management of injury, (iii) screening and treatment of STIs, (iv) prevention of pregnancy, and (v) referral for medical and psychological follow-up. The overall management of sexually abused children is discussed in Chapter 132.

Physical Examination and Evidence Collection

Police and prosecutors ask physicians to document observations and collect evidence that may corroborate a patient's history of sexual assault or abuse. This evidence may consist of a child's exact statement concerning the abuse; the finding of prostatic acid phosphatase in vaginal secretions, indicating the presence of seminal fluid; a small bruise on the labia majora; or the discovery of leaf or grass fragments in the underwear of a child who states that she was assaulted outdoors. In prepubertal children, physical evidence collection is usually recommended up to 72 hours after any sexual contact; however, most evidence is found when it is collected within 24 hours of the contact. In adolescents, some recommend evidence collection up to 120 hours after sexual contact. While some evidence collection kits are designed for use with children, most general collection kits involve the collection of specimens that are unlikely to yield usable evidence (e.g., pubic hair sample, fingernail scrapings) because they are rarely relevant to the circumstances of victimized children. Which types of samples to collect should be determined on a case-by-case basis. In cases involving prepubertal children, extra care should be taken to submit underwear and any involved bed linens because these materials may be more likely to yield evidence of abuse than samples taken from the genital area. If material is collected that may be used in court, its movement from the physician's possession to locked storage or a police officer's custody should be documented with signatures, times, and dates to preserve the chain of evidence that will allow the material's origin to be verified in court. When, as is often the case, a sexually abused child is not examined until several weeks after the most recent episode of sexual contact, the likelihood of the physician's finding physical evidence is very low.

The likelihood of identifying genital injury in an adolescent sexual assault victim depends on the nature of the assault, the time elapsed since the event, and whether magnification is used during examination. Most young women are sexually assaulted by acquaintances and do not sustain any injury, genital or otherwise. Genital injuries that do occur are usually located on the posterior fourchette or the labia minora. Any injuries noted should be clearly described, drawn, and, if possible, photographed.

Few girls sustain serious physical injuries as a result of sexual abuse or assault. Any sexually abused girl who has vaginal bleeding that cannot be attributed to a clearly visible injury or infection must be examined carefully to determine the source of the bleeding. This will usually require the use of sedation or general anesthesia in premenarcheal girls. The management of girls with vaginal bleeding is discussed at greater length in Chapter 76.

Laboratory Evaluation

STIs are seen in about 5% of abused children, generally mirroring their relative prevalence in the adult population. The most prevalent clinically evident STIs found in sexually abused children are gonorrhea, chlamydial infection, and genital warts. Rarely, syphilis and HIV can be transmitted by sexual abuse. Although common in adults, trichomoniasis is rarely seen in prepubertal abused girls because trichomonads do not proliferate in the absence of an estrogenic milieu.

For prepubertal children, STI testing should be limited to high-risk cases, including those (i) with a history of an STI or a sibling with an STI, (ii) victimized by multiple assailants or by an assailant known to have an STI, or (iii) exhibiting signs of infection (vaginal, urethral, or rectal discharge) or genital injury indicating history of vaginal or rectal penetration.

While there is agreement that adolescents are at higher risk of acquiring STIs and developing PID, some advocate for all adolescents to be tested while others prefer to treat presumptively for gonorrhea, chlamydial infection, and trichomoniasis without testing.

Because of the legal and psychosocial consequences of a false-positive diagnosis, only tests with high specificities should be used. Culture is the only acceptable method of testing for gonorrhea and chlamydial infection in sexually abused children; any positive indirect test (Gram stain, antigen testing) needs to be confirmed by culture.

Testing for other STIs, including syphilis, hepatitis C, and HIV, is based on signs and symptoms of disease, patient/family preference, and the overall risk-assessment of the case. Hepatitis B screening should be offered for those who have not completed a hepatitis B vaccination series. HIV pretest counseling, including implications of an unexpected positive result and importance of follow-up testing, should be performed before any child is screened for HIV.

Treatment

Antibiotic prophylaxis after sexual abuse is best limited to children victimized in high-risk situations (including any child with signs or symptoms of infection) and adolescents. The antibiotic regimen should include coverage for both chlamydial infection and gonorrhea. Adolescents should also be covered for trichomonasis and bacterial vaginosis. Those not immunized against hepatitis B should be given the first vaccine dose (followed in 1 and 6 months by the subsequent doses) and hepatitis B immune globulin (HBIG).

HIV Postexposure Prophylaxis

In adults, the risk for HIV transmission per episode of receptive penile-anal sexual exposure is estimated at 0.1% to 3%; the risk per episode of receptive vaginal exposure is estimated at 0.1% to 0.2%. Factors to consider and discuss with the family are (i) local rates of HIV/AIDS, (ii) the likelihood the perpetrator is infected, (iii) circumstances of the assault that may predispose to HIV transmission, (iv) the toxicity of recommended medications, and (v) unknown efficacy of the regimen. Postexposure prophylaxis (PEP) is believed to be most effective if given within 24 hours of the assault (Fig. 90.6). PEP is not typically recommended for cases in which the exposure occurred more than 72 hours before seeking care. However, in unusual circumstances in which the potential benefits outweigh the risks, PEP may be considered for exposure that occurred more than 72 hours before seeking care.

While both failures and successes have been reported, there are no data regarding the efficacy of PEP after sexual assault. Adverse effects, some of them serious, often limit the ability to complete the recommended 28-day course. The theoretic advantage of improved efficacy with a three-drug regimen needs to be considered against the lower toxicity and increased compliance with a two-drug regimen (a combination of two reverse transcriptase inhibitors). Prophylaxis offers a benefit only when the risk of transmission is high, therapy can be

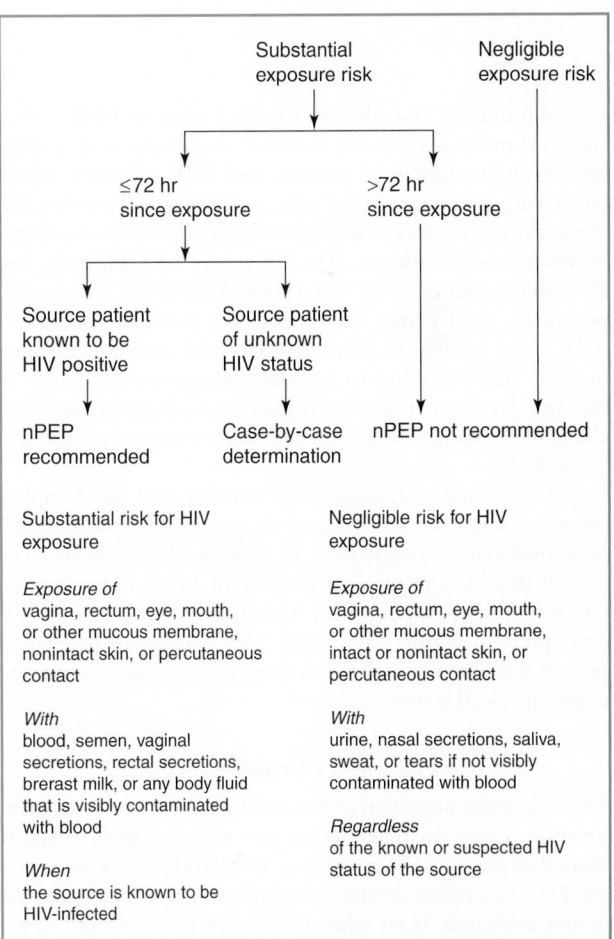

FIGURE 90.6 Algorithm for the evaluation and treatment of possible nonoccupational HIV exposure. nPEP, nonoccupational postexposure prophylaxis (Adapted from Centers for Disease Control and Prevention. Antiretroviral postexposure prophylaxis after sexual, injection-drug use, or other nonoccupational exposure to HIV in the United States. *MMWR Morb Mortal Wkly Rep* 2005;54(RR-2):1–20).

MEDICAL EMERGENCIES

TABLE 90.2

SUGGESTED GUIDELINES FOR POSTEXPOSURE PROPHYLAXIS FOLLOWING SEXUAL ASSAULT

Prepubertal

Zidovudine[a] 10 mg/mL 100 mg capsule 300 mg tablet	240 mg/m^2/dose Max 300 mg/dose	Orally, twice daily for 28 days
Lamivudine[a] 10 mg/mL 150 mg tablet	4 mg/kg/dose Max 150 mg/dose	Orally, twice daily for 28 days
Kaletra (lopinavir/ritonavir) Liquid: 80/20 mg/mL Regular tablet 200/50 mg/tablet Pediatric tablet 100/25 mg/tablet	Dosing based on lopinavir: If 7–15 kg: 12 mg/kg/dose If 15–40 kg: 10 mg/kg/dose Max 400 mg/dose	Orally twice daily for 28 days

Pubertal

Truvada (300 mg tenofovir/200 mg emtricitabine)	1 tablet	Orally, once daily for 28 days
Kaletra (lopinavir/ritonavir) Regular tablet: 200/50 mg/tablet Pediatric tablet: 100/25 mg/tablet	25–35 kg: 3 pediatric tablets >35 kg: 2 adult tablets	Orally, twice daily for 28 days Orally, twice daily for 28 days

[a]Zidovudine/lamivudine (Combivir) available in 300/150 mg tablet.

started promptly, and adherence to the regimen is likely. When standard protocols are not available, a clinician with experience in the treatment of persons with HIV infection should participate in starting PEP. Current recommendations regarding medication regimens and associated toxicities can be found at www.aidsinfo.nih.gov. The University of California–San Francisco operates a hot line (1-888-HIV-4911) that is supported by the Centers for Disease Control and Prevention (CDC) and staffed 24 hours a day to aid clinicians through decision pathways and to provide information on choice of therapy. Recommendations regarding medication regimens change frequently. One set of PEP recommendations is listed in Table 90.2.

If PEP is initiated, baseline measurement of the complete blood cell count, creatinine, and alanine transaminases should be considered in anticipation of possible drug toxicity. The patient should be given a starter pack of 3 days of medication and a follow-up appointment with a pediatric infectious disease specialist within 2 to 3 days. This allows for the evaluation of medication side effects, drug toxicity, and assessment of psychosocial status.

Pregnancy Prophylaxis

The emergency physician must consider the possibility of pregnancy in every postmenarcheal girl who has been sexually abused or assaulted. A pregnancy test should be conducted in the ED to ascertain whether the patient is pregnant when she is first evaluated. If an adolescent is not pregnant and is not using hormonal contraception, her risk of becoming pregnant as a result of rape must be assessed. The risk of pregnancy from one occurrence of unprotected coitus at midcycle is estimated to be 15%. The risk from coitus occurring more than 6 days before or after ovulation is negligible. Plan B (two 0.75 mg pills of levonorgestrel given after intercourse) is the most

commonly prescribed regimen. Plan B is 90% effective if used within 24 hours, 75% effective if used within 72 hours, and 60% effective if used within 120 hours. It is not recommended more than 5 days after intercourse. The patient can expect to have her next menstrual period within 21 days after treatment.

Patient Follow-up

Many victims of sexual assault experience guilt, shame, and grief. They may blame themselves for the assault. Discussion of common reactions to sexual assault and referral to psychological counseling to specifically address these feelings will give the patient the best chance for a full psychological recovery.

Many victims of sexual assault remember little of what was said during the short-term evaluation. Important information such as medications given, medications to be taken at home, and follow-up instructions should be given in verbal and written form to the patient. A visit to a primary care physician within 2 to 3 days of the assault is warranted in most cases and is necessary when PEP for HIV is initiated. Serologic tests for syphilis should be repeated 4 to 6 weeks after the assault. HIV testing should be repeated at 4 to 6 weeks, 3 months, and 6 months.

GENITAL TRACT INFECTIONS

Vaginitis

Background

Definition. Vaginitis, or inflammation of the vagina, can be produced by chemical and mechanical irritants, foreign bodies, and a variety of infectious agents including viruses, chlamydial species, bacteria, fungi, protozoa, and helminths. During childhood, vaginitis is characterized by the presence of vaginal discharge, bleeding, or both. After puberty has begun,

TABLE 90.3

TREATMENT OF VAGINITIS

Infection	Drug	Dose, route
Bacterial vaginosis	Metronidazole	500 mg orally bid for 7 days
	Metronidazole gel 0.75%	One full applicator vaginally daily for 5 days
	Clindamycin 300 mg	One orally twice daily for 7 days
Vulvovaginal candidiasis	Intravaginal agents	
	Butoconazole 2% cream[a]	5 g intravaginally for 3 days
	Butoconazole 2% cream (butaconazole 1-sustained release)	Singe intravaginal application
	Clotrimazole 1% cream[a]	5 g intravaginally for 7–14 days
	Clotrimazole 100 mg vaginal tablet	One vaginally daily for 7 days
	Clotrimazole 100 mg vaginal tablet	2 tablets vaginally for 3 days
	Miconazole 2% cream[a]	5 g intravaginally for 7 days
	Miconazole 100 mg vaginal suppository[a]	One vaginally daily for 7 days
	Miconazole 200 mg vaginal suppository[a]	One vaginally daily for 3 days
	Miconazole 1,200 mg vaginally suppository[a]	Once vaginally
	Nystatin 100,000-unit vaginal tablet	One vaginally daily for 14 days
	Ticonazole 6.5% ointment[a]	5 g intravaginally daily for 7 days
	Terconazole 0.4% cream	5 g intravaginally daily for 7 days
	Terconazole 0.8% cream	5 g intravaginally daily for 3 days
	Terconazole 80 mg vaginal suppository	One vaginally daily for 3 days
	Oral agent: fluconazole 150 mg	Once orally
Trichomoniasis	Metronidazole	2 g orally as single dose
	Tinidazole	2 g orally as single dose

[a]Over-the-counter preparations.
Adapted from Centers for Disease Control and Prevention. Sexually transmitted diseases treatment guidelines, 2006. *MMWR Morb Mortal Wkly Rep* 2006;55(RR-11):76–78. Alternative regimens are available at: http://www.cdc.gov/std/treatment/2006/vaginal-discharge.htm.

girls normally have an asymptomatic vaginal discharge; vaginitis is then indicated by the discomfort it produces or by a change in the character of the discharge. The etiology, clinical manifestations, diagnosis, and treatment of common vaginal infections are presented in this chapter. For a review of the differential diagnosis of vaginal bleeding and discharge, see Chapters 76 and 77. Table 90.3 summarizes the treatment of common vaginal infections. Infections with *N. gonorrhoeae* and *C. trachomatis* are discussed in Chapter 92.

Epidemiology

At least half of all symptomatic premenarcheal girls with vaginal discharge visible on physical examination will prove to have specific vaginal infections that warrant antimicrobial treatment. Among prepubertal girls in the United States, *N. gonorrhoeae* causes the greatest number of these specific infections. Less common offenders include *Shigella* species, *Streptococcus pyogenes*, and in infants and after puberty has begun, *Trichomonas vaginalis*. Although staphylococci and *Haemophilus influenzae* usually colonize the lower genital tract without producing symptoms, they are associated with vaginal discharge in only a small proportion of patients. *Candida albicans* is the most common vaginal pathogen among both pubertal (but premenarcheal) and postmenarcheal girls.

The relative prevalence of vaginal infections in a population of postmenarcheal adolescents depends primarily on how many of them are sexually active. Bacterial vaginosis is found commonly and nearly exclusively among sexually active adolescents. Diabetes mellitus, pregnancy, immunodeficiency, and the use of broad-spectrum antibiotics and corticosteroids predispose patients to developing *Candida* vulvovaginitis, but the infection is most often seen in patients who lack any of these risk factors. Trichomoniasis is transmitted vertically or by sexual contact. Up to one-third of patients with trichomoniasis have concurrent gonorrhea, but there is no increased rate of infection with *C. trachomatis*.

Trichomonal Vaginitis

Clinical Manifestations

A small proportion of vaginally delivered female neonates acquire trichomonal vaginitis from their infected mothers. Infants harboring only a few trichomonads may never develop clinical disease, but the remainder will have a thin whitish or yellowish vaginal discharge that appears within 10 days after birth and may persist for several months if untreated. Infected babies may be irritable but are otherwise well.

The classic vaginal discharge of trichomonal vaginitis after puberty is pruritic, frothy, and yellowish. However, many infected women do not complain of excessive discharge and the discharge may be scant or nondescript. The so-called strawberry cervix with multiple punctate areas of hemorrhage is pathognomonic for trichomoniasis but is visible without colposcopy in only about 2% of infected patients.

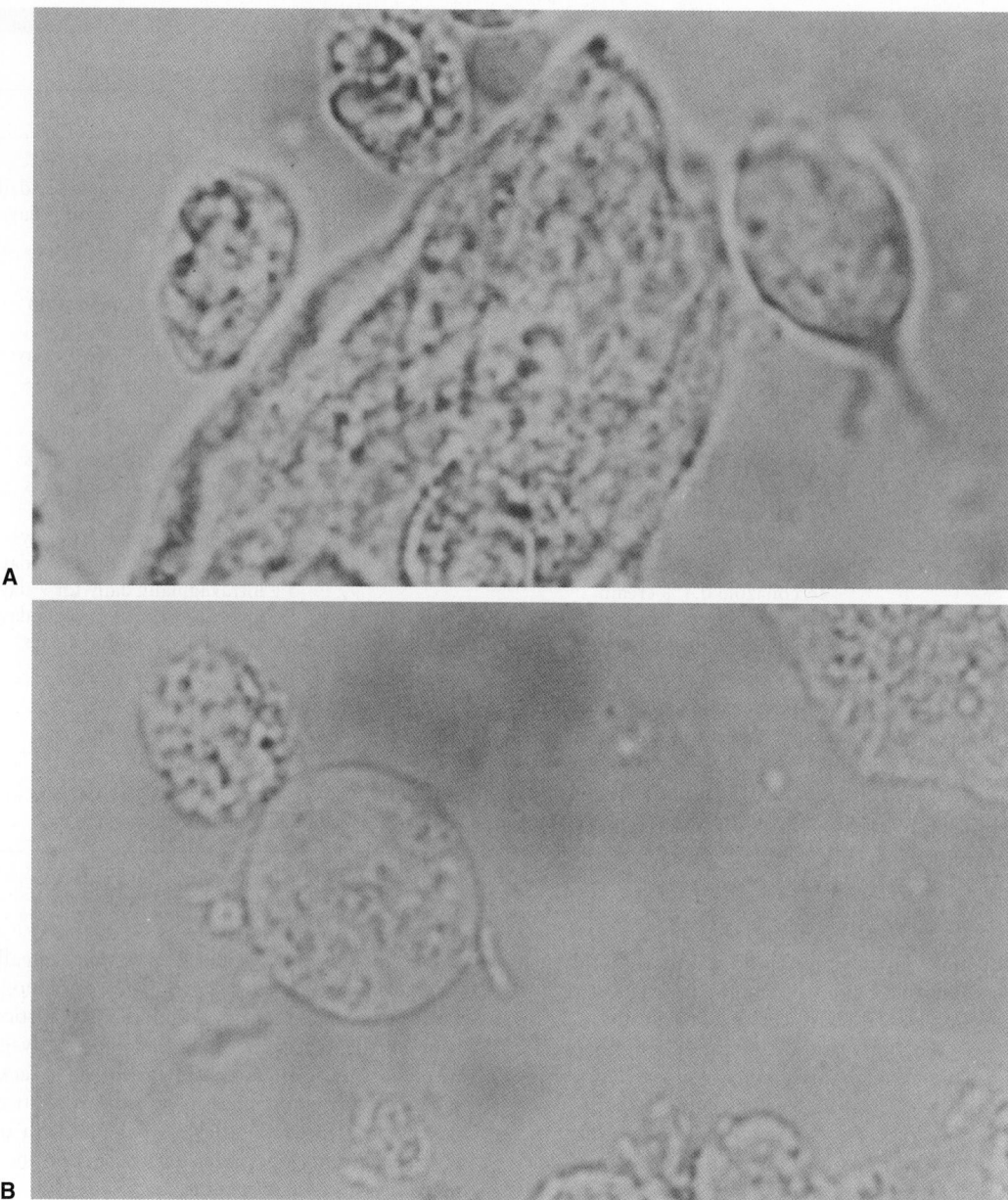

FIGURE 90.7 **A:** Trichomonad in the vaginal discharge of a 17-year-old patient with gonococcal pelvic inflammatory disease. The flagellated protozoan is elliptical and somewhat larger than the adjacent polymorphonuclear leukocytes (×225 magnification). **B:** After suspension in saline solution for microscopy, trichomonads gradually become swollen and immobile. This balloon-shaped trichomonad is barely recognizable (×225 magnification).

For patients of all ages, the diagnosis is made easily and rapidly if characteristically motile, flagellated trichomonads are seen in a saline suspension of discharge examined microscopically within about 15 minutes after the specimen has been obtained (Fig. 90.7). If a longer delay occurs, the organisms will gradually lose their mobility and normal shape, making them much more difficult to identify. The sensitivity rate for wet mount examinations is 50% to 70%. Cultures from a specialized parasite medium have a sensitivity of 85% to 95%, but results are delayed. Newer diagnostic methods such as DNA probes, monoclonal antibody kits, and poly- merase chain reaction techniques provide rapid and more accurate results.

Management

Metronidazole is effective for the treatment of vaginal trichomoniasis. The dosage for infants is 15 mg per kg per day orally in two to three divided doses for 7 days. Recommended treatment of adolescents include metronidazole 2 g orally in a single dose or tinadazole 2 g orally in a single dose. Because trichomoniasis is a sexually transmitted disease, the adolescent patient's partner(s) must also be referred for treatment.

Nausea and an unpleasant taste are common side effects of nitroimidazoles. Alcohol should be avoided during treatment to prevent the occurrence of more severe abdominal pain, vomiting, flushing, and headache (disulfiram reaction). Recent data indicate that metronidazole is not a teratogen, but many clinicians prefer to postpone treatment of pregnant patients until the second trimester. Intravaginal clotrimazole (two intravaginal tablets at bedtime for 7 days) can provide symptomatic relief for pregnant patients but will cure only 10% to 20%.

Shigella Vaginitis

Clinical Manifestations

Shigella flexneri, *Shigella sonnei*, *Shigella boydii*, and *Shigella dysenteriae* can produce vaginal infections in infants and children but do not appear to cause genital disease after puberty. The vaginitis is characterized by a white to yellow discharge that is bloody in three-fourths of cases. Associated pruritus and dysuria are uncommon. One-third of patients have diarrhea that precedes, accompanies, or follows the vaginal discharge. On inspection, the vulvar mucosa is often inflamed or ulcerated. The diagnosis is established by culture of a specimen of vaginal discharge. Rectal cultures are positive for *Shigella* species in some cases.

Management

Patients with *Shigella* vaginitis should be treated with oral antibiotics chosen on the basis of sensitivity testing. If the antibiotic sensitivity is unknown, trimethoprim-sulfamethoxazole (8 mg per kg per day orally of trimethoprim in two divided doses for 5 days) should be used.

Streptococcal Vaginitis

Clinical Manifestations

S. pyogenes can be identified in cultures of vaginal specimens taken from about 14% of prepubertal girls with scarlet fever. Most of these vaginal infections produce either no symptoms or minor discomfort, but a few patients develop outright vaginitis with a purulent discharge. Streptococcal vaginitis can accompany or follow symptomatic pharyngitis and occurs uncommonly in girls with neither symptomatic pharyngitis nor scarlet fever. Most of these latter patients are pharyngeal carriers of the organism. Streptococcal vaginitis causes genital pain or pruritus and can mimic candidal or gonococcal vaginitis. A swab of the patient's discharge should be cultured to verify the clinical diagnosis, as well as to exclude gonococcal infection.

Management

As for any other infection with group A β-hemolytic streptococci, penicillin is the preferred antibiotic. Intramuscular benzathine penicillin G is an alternative if poor compliance with oral treatment is anticipated. Oral erythromycin ethylsuccinate or azithromycin can be prescribed for children who are allergic to penicillin.

Candidal Vulvovaginitis

Clinical Manifestations

C. albicans frequently colonizes the vagina after the onset of puberty when estrogen stimulates local increases in glycogen stores and acidity that both appear to enhance its growth. If the ecologic balance of the vagina is changed by inhibition of the normal bacterial flora, impaired host immunity, or an increase in the availability of nutrients (broad-spectrum antibiotics, immunodeficiency states, corticosteroids, diabetes mellitus, pregnancy), the resulting proliferation of *Candida* will produce symptoms in a fraction of affected patients. However, most patients with candidiasis have no identifiable predisposing risk factor for infection. Because of the importance of estrogen in promoting fungal growth, candidal vulvovaginitis is rare among prepubertal girls.

The most common clinical manifestation of vulvovaginal candidiasis is vulvar pruritus. In severe infections, vulvar edema and erythema can occur. "External" dysuria is produced when urine comes in contact with the inflamed vulva. Vaginal discharge is variable in quantity and appearance. In severe cases, the vaginal vault is red, dry, and has a whitish, watery, or curd-like discharge that may be relatively scanty. Patients with mild disease may have only intermittent itching and an unimpressive discharge.

Microscopic examination of a sample of vaginal discharge suspended in 10% potassium hydroxide solution to clear the field of cellular debris can provide a rapid diagnosis of candidiasis if hyphae are seen (Fig. 90.8). However, in as many as 50% of cases, wet mounts are falsely negative. Gram-stained smears of discharge are somewhat more sensitive because hyphae and yeast cells are gram positive and more easily visible. Culture can only corroborate or fail to corroborate the clinical impression of candidiasis because the vaginal flora includes *C. albicans* in up to 25% of young women who have no symptoms or signs of infection. Similarly, cultures from patients with classic signs of candidal infection may yield only a light growth of the organism, making heavy growth an inadequate criterion for diagnosis. From these considerations, it is apparent that, although the presence of *C. albicans* can be confirmed by laboratory tests, the diagnosis and subsequent treatment of this infection should be guided by the presence or absence of clinical disease.

Management

Topical imidazoles will promptly cure 80% to 90% of patients with candidal infections. Most are available without prescription. The creams are packaged with intravaginal applicators, but many premenarcheal and virginal girls can be treated adequately and more comfortably by applying cream to the vulva alone. Effective, nonprescription, short-course treatments of patients with mild to moderate candidal vulvovaginitis include butoconazole 2% cream (one full applicator at bedtime for three nights), clotrimazole 500-mg tablets (one tablet intravaginally as a single dose), miconazole 200-mg suppositories (one suppository at bedtime for three nights), and tioconazole 6.5% ointment (one full applicator as a single dose). For patients with severe discomfort, one of the 5- or 7-day formulations of a topical agent is likely to be more effective. Creams and suppositories in this regimen are oil-based and might

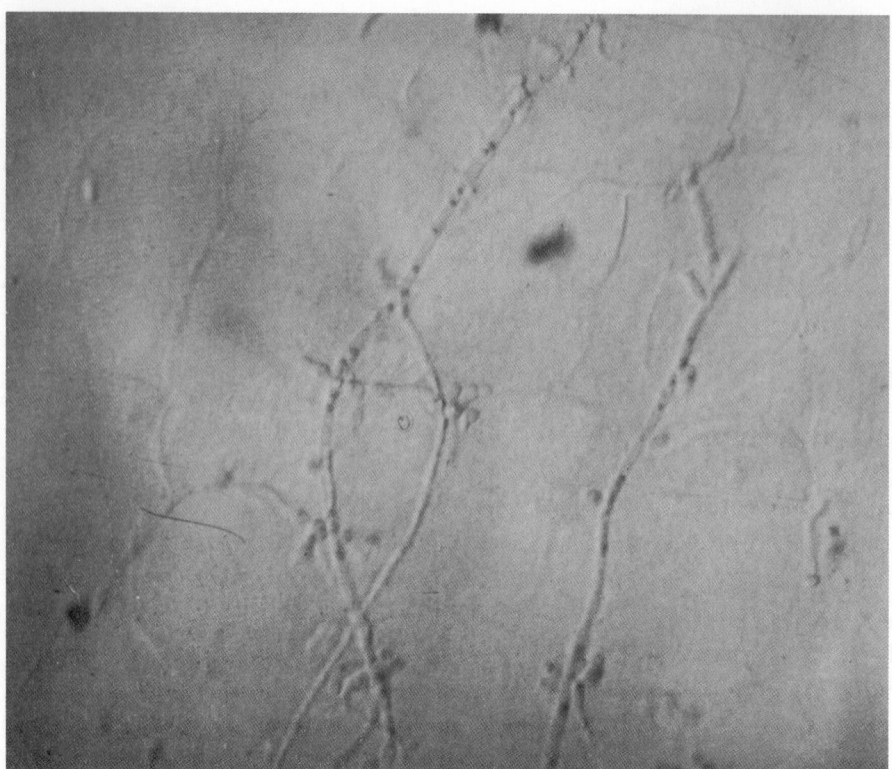

FIGURE 90.8 Branching hyphae of *Candida albicans* in vaginal discharge suspended in 10% potassium hydroxide solution. Ghosts of vaginal epithelial cells are also visible (×100 magnification).

weaken latex condoms and diaphragms. Patients should be referred to condom product labeling for more information. Fluconazole, 150 mg oral tablet in a single dose, cures candidal vulvovaginitis as effectively as the topical preparations, and many patients prefer oral to topical treatment. However, the potential for promoting fungal resistance and the risks, albeit low, of systemic toxicity and allergy are important disadvantages of oral antifungal agents.

Nonspecific Vaginitis in Children

Clinical Manifestations

The term *nonspecific vaginitis*, referring to a disorder of prepubertal girls, encompasses a variety of genitourinary symptoms and signs that are sometimes caused by poor perineal hygiene but that in other cases have no readily identifiable cause. Genital discomfort, discharge, itchiness, and dysuria are relatively common childhood complaints. When a girl with such symptoms has either a normal vulva and vagina or only mild vulvar inflammation on physical examination, a specific vaginal infection is unlikely, and other possible explanations for the complaint—smegma, pinworms, urinary tract infection, a local chemical irritant, or sexual abuse, for example—should be sought with appropriate questions and laboratory tests. (It should be noted that commercially available bubble bath is not often the culprit.) If, however, a vaginal discharge is present on physical examination, the specific vaginal infections discussed in this chapter are diagnostic possibilities and cultures should therefore be obtained. In a reported series of premenarcheal girls with vaginitis who have been systematically evaluated, between 25% and 75% are ultimately categorized as having nonspecific vaginitis. The diagnosis should not

be made until other entities have been excluded. (A more comprehensive discussion of the differential diagnosis of genital complaints is presented in Chapters 76 and 77.)

Management

General measures to promote cleanliness and comfort should be initiated for the girl with nonspecific vaginitis. Daily soaking in a bath of warm water, either plain or with some baking soda added, gentle perineal cleaning with a soft washcloth, and the use of cotton underwear can be recommended. The girl should be taught to wipe toilet paper anteroposteriorly. Using these suggestions, most girls with perineal irritation will show improvement within 2 weeks. The remaining patients should be reevaluated to exclude any specific but previously unrecognized disorder. If none is found, these girls may benefit from a brief course of topical estrogen cream (a small amount dabbed onto the vulva nightly for 2 to 4 weeks) to stimulate thickening of the vaginal mucosa so that it is more resistant to local irritation. Parents should be cautioned that estrogen cream is capable of producing breast growth if it is used for a prolonged period of time.

Bacterial Vaginosis

Background

Bacterial vaginosis is a syndrome characterized clinically by the presence of three of the following four signs: (i) a homogeneous, white adherent vaginal discharge; (ii) vaginal pH above 4.5; (iii) a fishy, amine-like odor released when 10% potassium hydroxide solution is added to a sample of the discharge; and (iv) the presence of clue cells (Amsel criteria). The syndrome occurs when lactobacilli that normally predominate in the genital tract are displaced by an overgrowth of mixed flora, including *Gardnerella vaginalis*, *Mobiluncus* species, other anaerobes, and *Mycoplasma hominis*. What accounts for this change in the vaginal microflora is not understood. The high prevalence of the syndrome in sexually active women and in women attending STI clinics suggests that a wide range of epidemiologic and microbiologic factors may contribute to its pathogenesis.

Clinical Manifestations

The symptoms of bacterial vaginosis—malodor and discharge—are not distinctive and can resemble those of trichomonal infection. A complaint of dysuria or pruritus goes against the diagnosis. As many as half of women who have signs of vaginosis are asymptomatic. The vaginal discharge is moderate or copious, grayish-white, and homogeneous. On examination, the vulva, vagina, and cervix are not inflamed, but concomitant infection with trichomonas or gonococci can complicate this picture.

Compared with the composite Amsel criteria, the use of single tests (e.g., pH, clue cells, or whiff test alone) produces lower positive and negative predictive values for the diagnosis of bacterial vaginosis. When a wet mount of vaginal discharge is examined, epithelial cells are seen to be studded with large numbers of small bacteria and have a granular appearance with shaggy borders (Fig. 90.9). The ratio of epithelial cells to polymorphonuclear leukocytes in the discharge is 1 or higher. Lactobacilli (long rods) are sparse. Gram stain can be used to confirm the presence of clue cells and the scarcity of long gram-positive rods (lactobacilli). Because 35% to 55% of women without bacterial vaginosis have positive cultures for *G. vaginalis*, culture is not a useful diagnostic test. Trichomonal infection is the major diagnostic alternative for patients suspected of having bacterial vaginosis.

Management

The standard treatment of bacterial vaginosis is oral metronidazole, 500 mg twice daily for 7 days. Treatment of patients' sexual partners does not reduce the recurrence rate and is not recommended. Common side effects of metronidazole include GI upset, headache, and a metallic taste. Metronidazole in standard doses is not a human teratogen; however, some

clinicians prefer to postpone treatment of pregnant women until the second trimester. Intravaginal clindamycin cream (2%, 5 g) and metronidazole gel (0.75%, 5 g) are alternative treatment options for nonpregnant women. Oral clindamycin (300 mg twice a day for 7 days) is an alternative treatment regimen for pregnant patients with bacterial vaginosis.

Gonococcal and Chlamydial Infections

Refer to Chapter 92 for information on gonococcal and chlamydial infections.

Bartholin Gland Abscess and Cyst

Background

Abscesses and symptomatic cysts of the Bartholin glands are relatively uncommon disorders during adolescence. The Bartholin glands lie at about the 4 and 8 o'clock positions in the vestibule and drain through ducts that open into folds between the hymen and the labia minora. Many Bartholin gland cysts are asymptomatic and need no treatment. The clinical distinction between a symptomatic cyst and an abscess can be arbitrary in some cases.

Clinical Manifestations

The patient with a Bartholin gland abscess presents with a painful, tender, fluctuant mass bulging on the involved side of the vestibule inferior to the labium minus. Pus can sometimes be milked upward from the gland to the duct orifice. Cultures of pus from abscessed glands yield *N. gonorrhoeae* in 10% to 50% of cases. Most of the remaining cases contain mixed growths of facultative, aerobic, and anaerobic organisms, often including *Bacteroides* species. Cultures from a small number of abscesses yield *C. trachomatis*, and in 15% to 30% of cases, the pus is sterile. The patient with a cyst complains of vulvar discomfort; the unilateral mass is typically 1 to 3 cm in diameter and mildly tender. Cyst fluid is usually sterile.

Management

Abscesses and symptomatic cysts are treated similarly, with placement of a Word catheter (Fig. 90.10), marsupialization, or a "window operation." Each procedure opens the cyst cavity widely and facilitates prolonged drainage. Many experts recommend against simple incision and drainage because of the high recurrence rate associated with this procedure. All patients with abscesses or purulent exudate should be treated for presumed gonorrhea (as outlined in Chapter 92), and their sexual partners should be referred for concurrent treatment. Complications of Bartholin gland abscess after treatment include slow healing, persistent discomfort, dyspareunia, and recurrence.

Pelvic Inflammatory Disease

Background

Definition. PID is a polymicrobial inflammatory condition of the upper genital tract, variably involving the endometrium, fallopian tubes, ovaries, adjacent structures, and pelvic peritoneum. The following discussion concerns acute PID caused

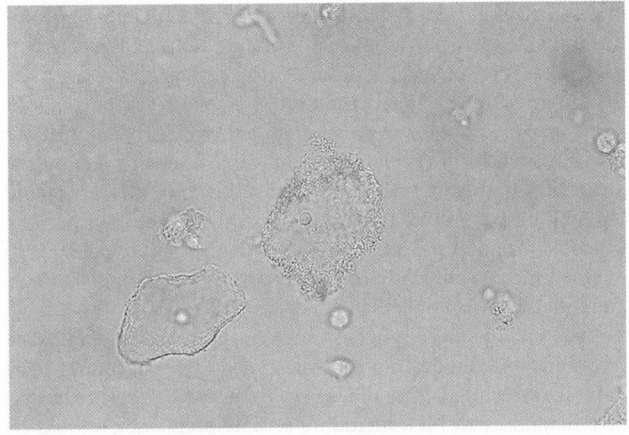

FIGURE 90.9 A clue cell. The vaginal epithelial cell on the right has shaggy borders obscured by coccobacilli (×100 magnification).

MEDICAL EMERGENCIES

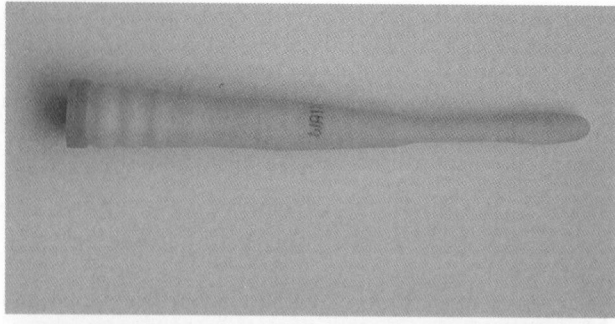

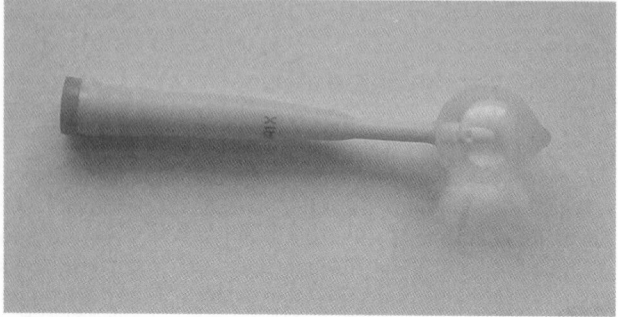

FIGURE 90.10 Word catheter before and after instillation of 3 mL of sterile water.

by sexually transmitted microorganisms ascending from the cervix and excludes infections associated with childbirth, spontaneous abortion, or pelvic surgery.

Epidemiology

PID disproportionately affects adolescents and young adults. An estimated one in eight sexually active adolescent girls develop PID before reaching 20 years of age. Young age, a large number of sexual partners, and nonbarrier contraceptive methods are risk factors for infection with *N. gonorrhoeae* and *C. trachomatis*, the microorganisms responsible for initiating most cases of acute PID. Recent douching is also a likely risk factor for the development of PID, but the mechanism by which it increases risk is unknown. Other risk factors include cigarette smoking, bacterial vaginosis, previous gynecologic surgery, and HIV infection. Compared with no contraceptive method, barrier methods—male and female condoms, diaphragms, and spermicides—decrease the overall risk of acquiring gonococcal and chlamydial cervicitis. Oral contraceptive pills decrease the likelihood that users with cervical gonorrhea will develop ascending infection. The effect of oral contraceptives on chlamydial disease is less uniform. The increased cervical ectropion produced by oral contraceptives increases the likelihood of chlamydial cervicitis, but the thickened cervical mucus and reduced menstrual flow appear to inhibit ascending infection. Patients with an IUD have an increased risk of developing PID within the first 3 weeks of device placement.

The sequelae of PID—chronic and recurrent pelvic pain, dyspareunia, tuboovarian abscesses, ectopic pregnancy, and involuntary infertility—affect large numbers of women. It has been estimated that 20% of women with PID will have chronic pelvic pain. It is estimated that half of all ectopic pregnancies result from tubal damage produced by PID. Women with a

history of PID have a 10-fold risk of infertility. Repeated bouts of PID substantially increase the likelihood of infertility.

Etiology

Most episodes of PID in adolescents are the result of gonococcal or chlamydial infection, or both, ascending from the cervix. If lower genital tract infection is not treated, approximately 10% to 40% of women with gonococcal cervicitis and 20% to 40% of women with chlamydial cervicitis will eventually develop PID. Microorganisms that comprise the vaginal flora (e.g., anaerobes, *G. vaginalis*, *H. influenzae*, enteric gram-negative rods, and *Streptococcus agalactiae*) have been associated with PID. In addition, cytomegalovirus (CMV), *M. hominis*, *Ureaplasma urealyticum*, and *Mycoplasma genitalium* might be associated with some cases of PID.

Clinical Manifestations

Although the constellation of symptoms and signs associated with PID—abdominal pain, irregular uterine bleeding, abnormal vaginal discharge, and lower abdominal and pelvic tenderness—is well known, no single symptom or sign or a combination of symptoms and signs is both sensitive and specific. Clinical findings that improve the specificity of the diagnosis of PID (i.e., increase the likelihood that the diagnosis is correct) do so only at the expense of sensitivity (i.e., exclude patients who do in fact have PID). Criteria for the diagnosis of PID suggested by the CDC are shown in Table 90.4. Because the diagnosis of PID is imprecise, and the potential for damage to the reproductive health of the patient, even by mild disease, is great, providers should maintain a low threshold for the diagnosis of PID.

Complications

Perihepatitis (Fitz-Hugh-Curtis syndrome), consisting of right upper quadrant pain and tenderness produced by inflammation of the liver capsule in association with PID, occurs in 4% to 30% of cases of PID and is more likely to occur with gonococcal infection and more severe diseases. On transvaginal ultrasonography, about one-third of patients with PID will have visible fallopian tubes and about one-fifth will have a demonstrable tuboovarian abscess (Fig. 90.11).

A complication of PID that warrants prompt diagnosis is ruptured tuboovarian abscess. About 15% of tuboovarian abscesses rupture spontaneously. The symptoms and signs of a ruptured abscess may be mild if only a small amount of pus has leaked out, but the usual clinical picture includes peritonitis and shock. A pelvic mass is palpable in less than one-half the cases. Prompt surgical intervention can be lifesaving.

Laparoscopy confirms the diagnosis of PID in only about 60% of patients who are suspected, either by gynecologists or by primary care physicians, on clinical grounds of having the disease. Conditions most often mistaken for PID are acute appendicitis, endometriosis, hemorrhagic and nonhemorrhagic ovarian cysts, and ectopic pregnancy. In up to 25% of women judged clinically to have PID, no abnormality can be identified laparoscopically.

The emergency physician must consider the possibility of pregnancy in adolescents with presumed PID. Ascending genital tract infection is rare during pregnancy. As a result, alternative diagnoses to PID, including ectopic pregnancy, should be considered. Hospitalization is recommended for all pregnant patients with PID.

MEDICAL EMERGENCIES

TABLE 90.4

DIAGNOSTIC CRITERIA FOR PELVIC
INFLAMMATORY DISEASE

Minimum criteria	Sexually active patient with pelvic or lower abdominal pain, no cause other than PID identified, *and* one of the following: Cervical motion tenderness *or* Uterine tenderness *or* Adnexal tenderness
Additional criteria	These findings enhance the specificity of the minimum criteria and support a diagnosis of PID: Oral temperature > 101°F (>38.3°C) Abnormal cervical or vaginal mucopurulent discharge Abundant numbers of white blood cell on saline microscopy of vaginal secretions Erythrocyte sedimentation rate >15 mm/h Elevated C-reactive protein Documented gonococcal or chlamydial cervical infection
Specific criteria	These findings offer a definitive diagnosis of PID Endometrial biopsy with histopathologic evidence of endometritis Laparoscopic abnormalities consistent with PID Transvaginal sonography or magnetic resonance imaging techniques showing thickened, fluid-filled tubes or tuboovarian complex, or Doppler studies showing tubal hyperemia

PID, pelvic inflammatory disease.
Adapted from Centers for Disease Control and Prevention. Sexually transmitted diseases treatment guidelines. MMWR *Morb Mortal Wkly Rep* 2006;55(RR-11):76–78.

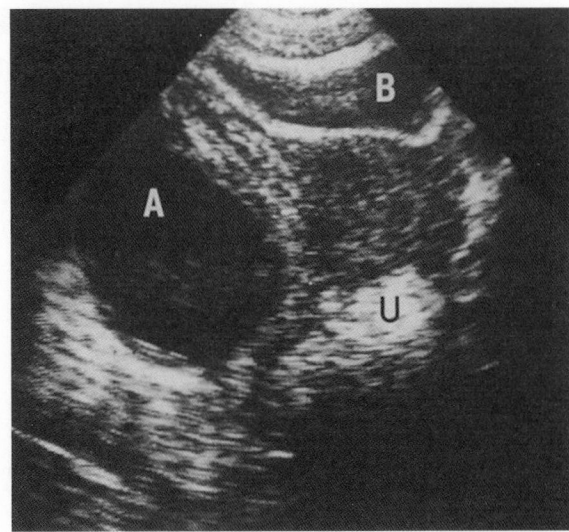

FIGURE 90.11 Transverse real-time sonogram of the pelvis of a 15-year-old patient with gonococcal salpingitis, demonstrating a 6 × 8-cm right tuboovarian abscess *(A)* containing a fluid-debris level. U, uterus; B, bladder.

providing rather than withholding antibiotic treatment, and diagnostic specificity for women with relatively severe illness, focusing on the consideration of major competing diagnoses.

Management

The 2006 CDC guidelines for the treatment of PID are summarized in Table 90.5. The antibiotics listed were selected for their effectiveness in combination against *N. gonorrhoeae*, *C. trachomatis*, and the aerobes and anaerobes responsible for polymicrobial PID. Hospitalization is recommended for any patient with PID whose diagnosis is uncertain, particularly if

An important pathophysiologic irony is the observation that tubal occlusion is associated more often with a relatively unimpressive clinical presentation of PID (i.e., long duration of symptoms, no signs of peritonitis, normal peripheral leukocyte count) than with a "hot" clinical disease (i.e., short duration of symptoms, fever, peritoneal signs, leukocytosis). Similarly, chlamydial PID is associated with both a longer duration of pain at patient presentation and a higher risk of infertility than is gonococcal PID. Thus, if the diagnosis of PID is allowed to depend substantially on patients' appearance—as either "well" or "sick"—clinicians may be tempted to reject the diagnosis of PID and to withhold antibiotic treatment of those patients at highest risk of subsequent ectopic pregnancy and infertility.

The Kahn approach to the clinical diagnosis of PID is recommended for the emergency physician (Fig. 90.12). This strategy emphasizes diagnostic sensitivity for women with relatively mild illness, encouraging clinicians to err on the side of

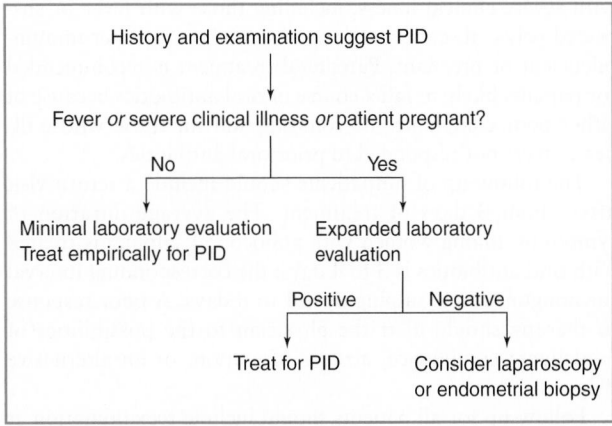

FIGURE 90.12 Strategy for diagnosis of pelvic inflammatory disease (PID). Minimal laboratory evaluation should include tests for gonococcal and chlamydial cervicitis. Expanded laboratory investigation may include, in addition to the minimal evaluation, complete blood cell count, C-reactive protein or erythrocyte sedimentation rate, and pelvic or transvaginal ultrasonography. (Adapted from Kahn JG, Walker CK, Washington E, et al. Diagnosing pelvic inflammatory disease. *JAMA* 1991;266:2594–2604.)

TABLE 90.5

TREATMENT REGIMENS FOR PELVIC INFLAMMATORY DISEASE

	Initial therapy	Subsequent therapy	Comments
Regimen A Extended parenteral treatment	Cefotetan 2 g IV every 12 h *or* Cefoxitin 2 g IV every 6 h *with* Doxycycline 100 mg po or IV every 12 h	Doxycycline 100 mg po bid to complete 14 days of therapy	Oral doxycycline is preferred to avoid infusion pain Parenteral treatment may be stopped 24 h after clinical improvement
Regimen B[a] Extended parenteral treatment	Clindamycin 900 mg IV every 8 h *with* Gentamicin 2 mg/kg and then 1.5 mg/kg IV or IM every 8 h (single daily dosing may be substituted)	Doxycycline 100 mg po bid *or* Clindamycin 450 mg po qid to complete 14 days of therapy	Clindamycin is preferred for oral treatment of tuboovarian abscess Parenteral treatment may be stopped 24 h after clinical improvement
Regimen C Combined parenteral/oral treatment	Ceftriaxone 250 mg IM *or* Cefoxitin 2 mg IM with probenecid 1 g po	Doxycycline 100 mg po bid for 14 days	Ceftriaxone has better coverage than cefoxitin against *Neisseria gonorrhoeae* Adding metronidazole (500 mg orally twice a day for 14 days) will treat the bacterial vaginosis associated with many cases of PID and will enhance anaerobic coverage

IV, intravenous; IM, intramuscular; po, orally; bid, twice a day; qid, four times daily.
[a]Fluoroquinolones are no longer recommended for the treatment of gonococcal infections.
Adapted from Centers for Disease Control and Prevention. Sexually transmitted diseases treatment guidelines, 2006. MMWR MMWR *Morb Mortal Wkly Rep* 2006;55(RR-11):76–78. Alternative regimens are available at: www.cdc.gov/STD/treatment/2006/updated-regimens.htm. Accessed November 2008.

ectopic pregnancy or appendicitis seems likely; for patients with severe clinical illness, including those with fever or suspected pelvic abscess; and for patients who are either immunodeficient or pregnant. Parenteral treatment is recommended for patients likely to fail a course of oral antibiotics because of either poor compliance or vomiting and for those whose illnesses have not responded to prior oral antibiotics.

The follow-up of outpatients should include a return visit after about 3 days of treatment. The average duration of symptoms among women with gonococcal salpingitis treated with oral antibiotics is 3 to 4 days; the corresponding interval for nongonococcal salpingitis is 4 to 6 days. A poor response to therapy should alert the physician to the possibilities of inadequate compliance, abscess formation, or an alternative diagnosis.

Follow-up for all patients should include reexamination at the end of antibiotic therapy to check for residual pelvic tenderness and adnexal masses. To identify patients with persistent or repeated infection resulting from noncompliance with antibiotics or an untreated sexual partner, follow-up tests for gonococcal and/or chlamydial cervicitis should be scheduled 4 to 6 weeks after the end of treatment. All patients with gonococcal and chlamydial infections should be counseled about

the HIV infection and offered serologic screening for both syphilis and HIV infection.

The importance of identifying and treating sexual partners of women with PID cannot be overemphasized. About 25% of such men have asymptomatic urethritis and are unlikely to seek treatment on their own. If these men are not treated, they become part of the reservoir of undetected carriers of STIs. The success of various patient referral strategies conducted by public health care personnel to achieve treatment of partners ranges from 29% to 59%. The success rate of patient-initiated partner treatment is unknown.

Expedited Patient Therapy

When medical evaluation, counseling, and treatment of partners cannot be reliably done, the CDC recommends the consideration of expedited patient therapy (EPT), in which partners of infected patients are treated without previous medical evaluation or prevention counseling. Medications and/or prescriptions should be accompanied by treatment instructions, appropriate warnings about taking medications, and advice that partners should seek personal medical evaluations.

EPT is believed to be a useful option for male partners of women with chlamydial infection or gonorrhea but has a limited role in partner management for trichomoniasis. Currently, EPT is not feasible in many settings because of legal and operational barriers. As of 2008, EPT is legal in 15 states, potentially allowable in 24, and prohibited in 11. An up-to-date discussion of legal issues with state-by-state restrictions can be viewed at www.cdc.gov/std/ept/legal/default.htm.

Genital Warts

Background

Genital warts, or condylomata acuminata, are multicentric, exophytic tumors on anogenital skin (Fig. 90.13) caused by the DNA-containing human papillomavirus (HPV), most commonly by HPV types 6 and 11. Although HPV infections are not reportable, many venereologists believe they are the most common STIs in the United States. There are 5.5 million new cases of HPV infection every year, and approximately 20 million Americans are infected. Most HPV infections are subclinical. The HPV types that produce most anogenital warts are considered to have low potential for malignant change. HPV infection of the cervix, which is associated with cervical dysplasia and cancer, occurs at an annual incidence of 9% to 20% in college-aged women. An HPV vaccine that targets subtypes 6, 11, 16, and 18 has been recently introduced into the general population.

Although HPV type 2 (associated with cutaneous, common warts) has been identified in anogenital warts in children, suggesting autoinoculation or heteroinoculation, nearly all genital warts in adolescents and adults, and some in children, are transmitted from person to person by sexual contact. The time from contact with an infected partner to the appearance of genital warts is estimated to be 1 to 3 months. However, the concept of an incubation period does not apply readily to the large number of infections that remain subclinical for long periods.

Pathophysiology

Grossly, genital warts are hyperplastic lesions that occur on squamous epithelium. On microscopic examination, the stratum granulosum contains foci of vacuolated cells. Acanthosis, parakeratosis, and hyperkeratosis are characteristic findings. The presence on Papanicolaou smear of koilocytes—intermediate, often multinucleated squamous cells with perinuclear halos, pyknotic nuclei, and dense peripheral cytoplasm—indicates cervical HPV infection.

Clinical Manifestations

Most patients with genital warts either have no complaint or report noticing "bumps" in the genital area. Uncommonly, large perianal warts can be painful and interfere with defecation. Prepubertal girls with vulvovaginal warts may have a bloody vaginal discharge. Because HPV infection in males is so consistently asymptomatic, most female patients are not aware of their exposure to an infected partner.

Warts can occur anywhere on the perineum, but their growth seems to be encouraged by moisture. The most common locations in females are the posterior fourchette, adjacent areas of the labia minora and majora, and the lower vagina (Fig. 90.13). Single warts, 1 cm or more in diameter, and clusters of seedlings, each a few millimeters across, are both common. Warts can be velvety and flat or papillomatous. Large warts often contain distinct cauliflower-like lobulations. On the cervix, acetowhite infected areas are usually seen only with a colposcope. Immunodeficient patients are particularly susceptible to extensive or severe disease with an increased risk of malignant change. Genital warts must be differentiated from condylomata lata, a contagious manifestation of secondary syphilis (Fig. 90.14) and molluscum contagiosum.

The diagnosis of genital warts is easy to make in patients with obvious lesions but can be more difficult in patients with flat warts or "microwarts" of the vulva. A magnifying lens or colposcope can be used to inspect suspicious areas that have been soaked in 5% acetic acid for 5 minutes. Infected skin, areas of nonspecific inflammation, and skin treated with

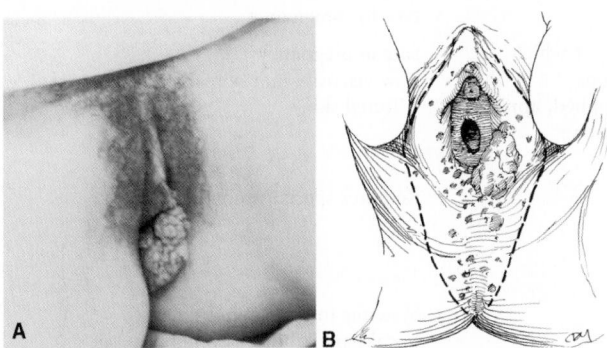

FIGURE 90.13 **A:** Large vulvar and perianal genital warts in a 15-year-old patient. **B:** In females, genital warts are most commonly located along the posterior margin of the introitus, inside the vagina, and on the labia minora.

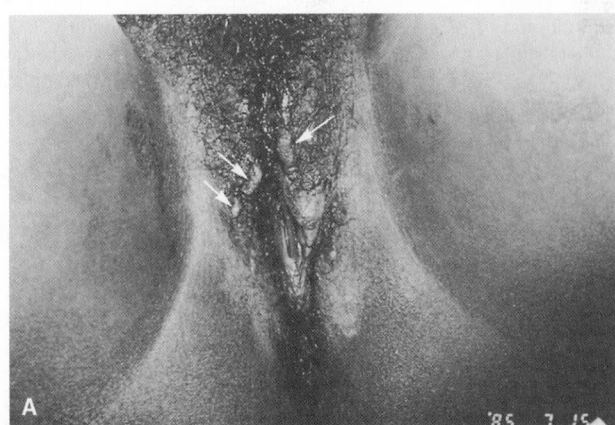

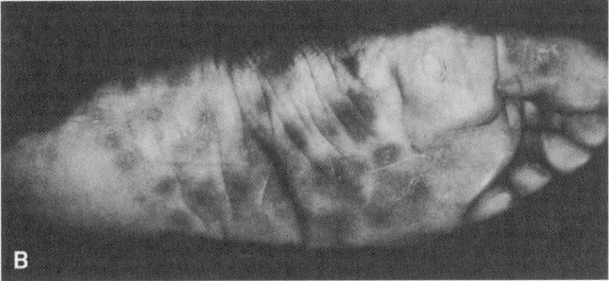

FIGURE 90.14 **A:** Vulvar condylomata lata of secondary syphilis in a 15-year-old patient. **B:** Macular rash on the sole of foot of same patient.

podophyllin will turn white after soaking. No data support the use of HPV nucleic acid tests in the routine diagnosis or management of visible genital warts. To exclude syphilis, patients should also receive serologic screening.

Management

Treatment of genital warts should be guided by the preference of the patient, the available resources, and the experience of the health care provider. Eradicating visible lesions does not end the viral infection. Whether it reduces contagiousness is uncertain. Spontaneous improvement or resolution of genital warts occurs in a minority of patients, so an acceptable alternative for some persons is to forego treatment and wait for spontaneous resolution.

Common recommended treatment options for genital wart removal are listed in Table 90.6. Recurrence rates for most therapies are relatively high, and treatment requirements or side effects limit some otherwise effective regimens. Each of the several available treatment methods has advantages and disadvantages; none is more than about 50% to 60% effective, and recurrences are common.

For extensive or recurrent disease or when repeated applications of podophyllin, trichloroacetic acid, or imiquimod are not successful, alternative treatment options include surgical removal, cryotherapy, and intralesional interferon. All women with genital warts should be referred to a primary care clinician for gynecologic care, including Papanicolaou screening.

Although anogenital warts in young children can result from vertical transmission or nonsexual contact with common warts, sexual abuse is another possible source of infection. The management of a child with genital warts should include either consultation with an expert in child abuse and neglect or a report to the state child protective service agency (see Chapter 132). Parents of children with genital warts should be examined for both common and genital warts. Excisional biopsy is preferred to ablative treatment of warts in children because histologic examination of the biopsy tissue can confirm the clinical diagnosis. Viral typing of anogenital warts in children may suggest abuse if a condylomatous HPV type is identified, but cannot exclude sexual contact if a cutaneous type is found because fondling is a common manifestation of child sexual abuse.

TABLE 90.6

TREATMENT REGIMENS FOR EXTERNAL GENITAL WARTS

	Dosing Info	Comments
Patient applied		
Podofilox[a] 0.5% solution or gel	Apply with a cotton swab twice daily for 3 days Follow by 4 days of no therapy Repeat cycle as needed up to 3 more times	Not for >10-cm² area Use < 0.5 mL/day Not for pregnancy
Imiquimod 5% cream	Apply cream nightly 3×/wk for 16 wk Area should be washed with soap and water 6–10 h after the application.	Not for pregnancy Local itching, erythema, and burning
Provider administered		
Cryotherapy Liquid nitrogen Cryoprobe	Apply to warts Repeat every 1–2 wk as necessary	
Podophyllin[a] resin 10%–20% in compound tincture of benzoin	Apply to each wart and allow to air dry May repeat weekly Wash area 1–4 hr after application	Each session, application should be limited to: <0.5 mL of podophyllin on <10-cm² area Not for use with open lesions near treatment area Not for pregnancy
Trichloroacetic acid 80%–90% Bichloroacetic acid 80%–90%	Apply to warts and allow to dry, at which time a white "frosting" develops If an excess amount of acid is applied, apply sodium bicarbonate or liquid soap May be repeated weekly	Safe in pregnancy Low viscosity may spread easily to unaffected skin
Surgical removal	Tangential scissor excision Tangential shave excision Curettage Electrosurgery	Requires special training
Interferon	Injected intralesionally	Systemic interferon not effective Local pain/irritation common Not recommended as primary modality

[a]Systemic absorption of podophyllin can produce bone marrow suppression, peripheral neuropathy, coma, and death.
Adapted from Centers for Disease Control and Prevention: Sexually transmitted diseases treatment guidelines. *MMWR Morb Mortal Wkly Rep* 2006;55(RR-11):76–78.

TABLE 90.7

RISK FACTORS FOR ECTOPIC PREGNANCY

High risk factors	Moderate risk factors	Weak association
Previous ectopic pregnancy Exposure to diethylstilbesterol Prior tubal surgery Current IUD in place History of > 2 episodes of chlamydial infection	History of PID History of chlamydial or gonorrhea infection Endometriosis Infertility	More than 1 sexual partner History of IUD History of threatened abortion Cigarette smoking Vaginal douching Previous pelvic surgery

IUD, intrauterine device.

Ectopic Pregnancy

Background

Ectopic pregnancy occurs in nearly 1% of pregnancies in North American women aged 15 to 24 years and is a leading cause of maternal mortality in the first trimester. Although the overall incidence of ectopic pregnancy in teenagers is low, this group has the highest mortality rate, largely caused by delays in seeking care. Despite improved methods of detection, ectopic pregnancy is misdiagnosed in up to 40% of patients on the initial ED visit and is an important cause of emergency medicine malpractice risk.

Risk factors of ectopic pregnancy are associated with conditions that inhibit normal transport of the blastocyst through the fallopian tube. In nearly half of ectopic pregnancies, a history of acute salpingitis is present. Other risk factors for ectopic pregnancy are listed in Table 90.7. The absence of risk factors is not reassuring, however, because 40% to 50% of those with ectopic pregnancy have no identifiable risk factors.

Pathophysiology

Ectopic pregnancy is any pregnancy in which the fertilized ovum implants in a location other than the intrauterine cavity. More than 95% of ectopic pregnancies occur in the fallopian tubes. Less common places for ectopic pregnancy include cornua of the uterus, cervix, ovary, and abdominal cavity. A heterotopic pregnancy is an ectopic pregnancy that coexists with an intrauterine pregnancy. Heterotopic pregnancies occur in 1 in 4,000 to 8,000 patients not treated with fertility agents.

After implantation in any of these extrauterine sites, β-hCG values rise, the uterus begins to enlarge, the patient is amenorrheic, and symptoms are similar to those of normal early pregnancy. Inevitably, the gestation begins to fail because of inadequate blood supply in the implantation site. β-hCG produced by trophoblastic tissue plateaus or declines. The endometrium of pregnancy, known as decidua, loses its hormonal support and begins to bleed and slough in a process analogous to menstruation. Occasionally, the decidua sloughs as one piece and passes as tissue, known as a decidual cast. Eventually, the placenta may erode through blood vessels or rupture the wall of the tube. Intraperitoneal hemorrhage, which may be gradual or catastrophic, may result.

Clinical Manifestations

The most common symptoms of ectopic pregnancy are amenorrhea, abdominal pain, and vaginal bleeding. However, this classic triad is nonspecific for ectopic pregnancy and is actually more commonly a presentation of threatened miscarriage. Incidence of common signs and symptoms of ectopic pregnancy is listed in Table 90.8.

The physical examination in any patient with suspected ectopic pregnancy should focus on the vital signs and the abdominal and pelvic examination. It should be noted that, although 50% of women with ectopic pregnancies have an adnexal mass, it is on the opposite side of the ectopic pregnancy in 20% to 30% of cases.

Laboratory evaluation should begin with testing for β-hCG. The standard urine pregnancy test is 99% sensitive and 99% specific for pregnancy. False-negative results can occur with urine testing, especially if the urine is very dilute. Therefore, when there is a high index of suspicion of pregnancy and a negative urine pregnancy test, a more sensitive, serum β-hCG measurement should be done.

In the patient with tachycardia, hypotension, or an acute abdomen, two large-bore IV catheters should be placed and blood should be sent for hematocrit, Rh and ABO typing and cross-matching, and quantitative serum β-hCG measurements. Serial serum β-hCG measurements will help the obstetrician to monitor the resolution of the ectopic pregnancy after surgery.

TABLE 90.8

SIGNS AND SYMPTOMS OF ECTOPIC PREGNANCY

Symptoms	% of patients with symptom
Abdominal pain	90–100
Amenorrhea	74–95
Vaginal bleeding	50–80
Dizziness/fainting	20–35
Urge to defecate	5–15
Pregnancy symptoms	10–25
Passage of tissue	5–10

Signs	% of patients with sign
Adnexal tenderness	75–98
Abdominal tenderness	80–95
Adnexal mass	10–50
Uterine enlargement	20–30
Orthostatic changes	10–15
Fever	5–10

MEDICAL EMERGENCIES

When the β-hCG gives a positive result and the patient has any signs or symptoms of ectopic pregnancy, the emergency physician must differentiate between an intrauterine pregnancy (IUP) and an ectopic pregnancy. See Chapter 76 for discussion of the distinction between spontaneous abortion and ectopic pregnancy. Abdominal ultrasonography should be able to identify a gestational sac when the serum β-hCG is higher than 6,500 mIU per mL. Similarly, transvaginal ultrasonography should allow visualization of an IUP at β-hCG levels between 1,000 and 1,500 mIU per mL (correlating to 4.5 to 5 weeks' gestation). When ultrasonography cannot identify an IUP and β-hCG levels are greater than those listed previously, an ectopic pregnancy is very likely. The only true ultrasound finding diagnostic of an ectopic pregnancy is the visualization of a gestational sac outside the endometrial cavity.

Management

Findings consistent with ectopic pregnancy mandate obstetric consultation in the ED. Any Rh-negative pregnant female with vaginal bleeding or ectopic pregnancy should receive RhoD immune globulin (RhoGAM).

Care directed by the obstetrician may include either emergent laparotomy for unstable patients or laparoscopy to perform a linear salpingostomy. Expectant management (allowing resolution without intervention) or medical management with chemical agents (most commonly methotrexate) has been successfully used in certain cases in which the level of β-hCG is low and the ectopic mass is small; however, outpatient management is not appropriate for most adolescents with ectopic pregnancy.

Suggested Readings

General

Centers for Disease Control and Prevention. Sexually transmitted diseases treatment guidelines. *MMWR Morb Mortal Wkly Rep* 2006;55(RR-11):76–78.
Emans SJH, Laufer MR, Goldstein DP. *Pediatric and adolescent gynecology*, 4th ed. Philadelphia, PA: Lippincott Williams & Wilkins, 1998.
Hatcher RA, Trussell J, Stewart F, et al. *Contraceptive technology*, 18th ed. New York, NY: Irvington, 2005.
Neinstein LS. *Adolescent health care: a practical guide*, 4th ed. Baltimore, MD: Williams & Wilkins, 2002.

Congenital Vaginal Obstruction

Heller DS. Lower genital tract disease in children and adolescents—a review. *J Pediatr Adolesc Gynecol* 2005;18:2.
Heller DS. Diseases manifesting in the upper genital tract in children and adolescents: a review. *J Pediatr Adolesc Gynecol* 2006;19(1):3–9.

Imperforate Hymen

El-Messidi A. Congenital imperforate hymen and its life-threatening consequences in the neonatal period. *J Pediatr Adolesc Gynecol* 2006;19(2):99–103.
Pillai M. Genital findings in prepubertal girls: what can be concluded from an examination? *J Pediatr Adolesc Gynecol* 2008;21(4):177–185.

Labial Adhesions

Bacon JL. Prepubertal labial adhesions: evaluation of a referral population. *Am J Obstet Gynecol* 2002;187:2.
Kumetz LM, Quint EH, Fisseha S, et al. Estrogen treatment success in recurrent and persistent labial agglutination. *J Pediatr Adolesc Gynecol* 2006;19:6.

Urethral Prolapse

Leslie JA. Pediatric urologic emergencies and urgencies. Pediatr Clin North Am 2006;53(3):513–527.

Lowe FC, Hill GS, Jeffs RD, et al. Urethral prolapse in children: insights into etiology and management. *J Urol* 1986;135:100–103.
Shurtleff BT. Urethral prolapse: four quadrant excisional technique. *J Pediatr Adolesc Gynecol* 2002;15(4):209–211.
Valerie E, Gilchrist BF, Frischer J, et al. Diagnosis and treatment of urethral prolapse in children. *Urology* 1999;54(6):1082–1104.

Dysmenorrhea

Doty E, Attaran M. Managing primary dysmenorrhea. *J Pediatr Adolesc Gynecol* 2006;19(5):341–344.
Klein JR, Litt IF. Epidemiology of adolescent dysmenorrhea. *Pediatrics* 1981;68:661–664.
Zeev H. Dysmenorrhea in adolescents and young adults: etiology and management. *J Pediatr Adolesc Gynecol* 2006;19(6):363–371.

Dysfunctional Uterine Bleeding

Bayer SR, DeCherney AH. Clinical manifestations and treatment of dysfunctional uterine bleeding. *JAMA* 1993;269:1823–1828.
Casablanca Y. Management of dysfunctional uterine bleeding. *Obstet Gynecol Clin North Am* 2008;35(2):219–234.
Matysyna LA. Dysfunctional uterine bleeding in adolescents: concepts of pathophysiology and management. *Prim Care* 2006;33(2):503–515.
Slap GB. Menstrual disorders in adolescents. *Best Pract Res Clin Obstet Gynaecol* 2003;17(1):75.
Strickland JL, Wall JW. Abnormal uterine bleeding in adolescents. *Obstet Gynecol Clin North Am* 2003;30(2):321–335.

Sexual Abuse and Assault

American Academy of Pediatrics. *Red Book 2006: Report of the Committee on Infections Diseases.* Elk Grove Village, IL: American Academy of Pediatrics; 2006.
American Academy of Pediatrics Committee on Adolescence. Care of the adolescent sexual assault victim. *Pediatrics* 2001;107:1476–1479.
American College of Emergency Physicians. *Evaluation and management of the sexually assaulted or sexually abused patient.* Dallas, TX: American College of Emergency Physicians, 1999. http://www.acep.org/library/index.cfm/id/2101. Accessed October 12, 2008.
Atabaki S, Paradise JE. The medical evaluation of the sexually abused child: lessons from a decade of research. *Pediatrics* 1999;104:178–186.
Centers for Disease Control and Prevention. Antiretroviral postexposure prophylaxis after sexual, injection-drug use, or other nonoccupational exposure to HIV in the United States. *MMWR Morb Mortal Wkly Rep* 2005;54(RR-2):1–20.
Christian CW, Lavelle JM, De Jong AR, et al. Forensic evidence findings in prepubertal victims of sexual assault. *Pediatrics* 2000;106(1, pt 1):100–104. http://childabusemd.com/index.shtml. Accessed November 2008.
Havens PL, Committee on Pediatric AIDS. Postexposure prophylaxis in children and adolescents for nonoccupational exposure to human immunodeficiency virus. *Pediatrics* 2003;111(6):1475–1489.
Kellogg N, American Academy of Pediatrics Committee on Child Abuse and Neglect. The evaluation of sexual abuse in children. *Pediatrics* 2005;116: 506–512.
Olshen E, Hsu K, Woods ER, et al. Use of human immunodeficiency virus postexposure prophylaxis in adolescent sexual assault victims. *Arch Pediatr Adolesc Med* 2006;160(7):674–680.
Paradise JE, Finkel MA, Beiser AS, et al. Assessments of girls' genital findings and the likelihood of sexual abuse. *Arch Pediatr Adolesc Med* 1997;151:883–891.

Vaginitis

Centers for Disease Control and Prevention. Sexually transmitted diseases treatment guidelines. *MMWR Morb Mortal Wkly Rep* 2006;55(RR-11):76–78.
Hellberg D, Nilsson S, MDrdh PA. The diagnosis of bacterial vaginosis and vaginal flora changes. *Arch Gynecol Obstet* 2001;265:11–15.
Kingston MA, Bansal D, Carlin EM. "Shelf life" of *Trichomonas vaginalis*. *Internet J STD AIDS* 2003;14:28–29.
Nyirjesy P, Sobel JD. Vulvovaginal candidiasis. *Obstet Gynecol Clin North Am* 2003;30:671–684.
Paradise JE, Campos JM, Friedman HM, et al. Vulvovaginitis in premenarcheal girls: clinical features and diagnostic evaluation. *Pediatrics* 1982;70:193–198.
Shapiro RA, Schubert CJ, Siegel RM. *Neisseria gonorrhea* infections in girls younger than 12 years of age evaluated for vaginitis. *Pediatrics* 1999;104:e72.
Tasker GL, Wojnarowska F. Lichen sclerosus. *Clin Exp Dermatol* 2003;28: 128–133.

Bartholin Gland Abscess and Cyst

Anderson PG, Christenson S, Detlefsen GU, et al. Treatment of Bartholin's abscess: marsupialization versus incision, curettage and suture under antibiotic cover—

a randomized study with 6 months' follow-up. *Acta Obstet Gynecol Scand* 1992;71:59–62.

Bleker OP, Smalbraak DJ, Schutte MF. Bartholin's abscess: the role of *Chlamydia trachomatis*. *Genitourin Med* 1990;66:24–25.

Downs MC, Randall HW. The ambulatory surgical management of Bartholin duct cysts. *J Emerg Med* 1989;7:623–626.

Hill DA, Lense JJ. Office management of Bartholin gland cysts and abscesses. *Am Fam Phys* 1998;57:1611–1616.

Pelvic Inflammatory Disease

Banikarim C, Chacko MR. Pelvic inflammatory disease in adolescents. *Adolesc Med Clin* 2004;15(2):273–285.

Beckmann KR, Melzer-Lange MD, Gorelick MH. Emergency department management of sexually transmitted infections in US adolescents: results from the National Hospital Ambulatory Medical Care Survey. *Ann Emerg Med* 2004;43(3):333–338.

Centers for Disease Control and Prevention. *Sexually Transmitted Diseases Surveillance, 2001*. Atlanta, GA: US Department of Health and Human Services, 2002:51–57.

Centers for Disease Control and Prevention. Sexually transmitted diseases treatment guidelines. *MMWR Morb Mortal Wkly Rep* 2006;55(RR-11):76–78. http://www.cdc.gov/std/EPT/legal/EPTLegalMatrix10-07-2008.pdf. Accessed October 14, 2008

Centers for Disease Control and Prevention. *Expedited partner therapy in the management of sexually transmitted diseases*. Atlanta, GA: US Department of Health and Human Services, 2006.

Jacobson L, Westrom L. Objectivized diagnosis of acute pelvic inflammatory disease. *Am J Obstet Gynecol* 1969;105:1088–1098.

Kahn JG, Walker CK, Washington E, et al. Diagnosing pelvic inflammatory disease. *JAMA* 1991;266:2594–2604.

Laufer MR, Goitein L, Bush M, et al. Prevalence of endometriosis in adolescent girls with chronic pelvic pain not responding to conventional therapy. *J Pediatr Adolesc Gynecol* 1997;10:199–202.

Risser WL. Impact of new diagnostic criteria on the prevalence and incidence of pelvic inflammatory disease. *J Pediatr Adolesc Gynecol* 2004;17(1):39–44.

US National Library of Medicine, National Institutes of Health. Pelvic inflammatory disease Updated September 19, 2006. http://www.nlm.nih.gov/medlineplus/ency/article/000888.htm. Accessed October 12, 2008.

Genital Warts

Diaz ML. Human papilloma virus: prevention and treatment. *Obstet Gynecol Clin North Am* 2008;35(2):199–217.

Ho GYF, Bierman R, Beardsley L, et al. Natural history of cervicovaginal papillomavirus infection in young women. *N Engl J Med* 1998;338:423–428.

Hollier LM. Treatment of sexually transmitted infections in women. *Infect Dis Clin North Am* 2008;22(4):665–691.

Trigg BG. Sexually transmitted infections and pelvic inflammatory disease in women. *Med Clin North Am* 2008;92(5):1083–1113.

Ectopic Pregnancy

Barnhart KT, Sammel MD, Gracia CR, et al. Risk factors for ectopic pregnancy in women with symptomatic first-trimester pregnancies. *Fertil Steril* 2006;86(1):36–43.

Della-Giustina D. Ectopic pregnancy. *Emerg Med Clin North Am* 2003;21(3):565–584.

Mukul LV. Current management of ectopic pregnancy. *Obstet Gynecol Clin North Am* 2007;34(3):403–419.

Silva C, Sammel MD, Zhou L, et al. Human chorionic gonadotropin profile for women with ectopic pregnancy. *Obstet Gynecol* 2006;107(3):605–610.

MEDICAL EMERGENCIES

CHAPTER 91 ■ HEMATOLOGIC EMERGENCIES

COLIN A. SIEFF, MD, AND JENNIFER C. KESSELHEIM, MD, M.ED

Hematologic emergencies arise in children who have been previously well, who have known blood disorders, or who have systemic diseases. Although the particular setting in which a serious blood abnormality occurs affects some facets of emergency care, the initial measures of support, diagnosis, and treatment are based on general principles that often cross the boundaries between the usual categories of blood disorders. This chapter emphasizes these principles as they apply to disorders of red blood cells, white blood cells, platelets, and coagulation. The initial evaluation and treatment of life-threatening disorders are described in detail. When controversy exists regarding specific management problems, alternative approaches are presented.

DISORDERS OF RED BLOOD CELLS

Severe anemia is a pediatric emergency that requires rapid evaluation and treatment to prevent hypoxia, congestive heart failure, and death. The classification of causes of anemia according to (i) blood loss, (ii) increased red blood cell destruction, and (iii) decreased red blood cell production is familiar to most physicians and provides an excellent starting point for the evaluation of the anemic child. In the next section, the same classification is applied to the emergency management of specific hematologic disorders.

Blood Loss

Trauma (see Chapters 104 and 105) is the leading cause of major hemorrhage in children. Every emergency physician must be prepared to act quickly and systematically when confronted with an actively bleeding child. The initial approach often requires the joint effort of a team of doctors and nurses to accomplish numerous tasks simultaneously. Within the first few minutes, the nature of the accident, an estimate of blood loss, and the presence of major current or chronic illnesses, including bleeding disorders, should be determined. The adequacy of the airway must be ensured. Vital signs should be measured frequently to detect early signs of hypovolemic shock. All clothing should be removed, and the child should be examined for sites of bleeding other than those found on initial inspection. In cases of significant hemorrhage, standard protocols recommend the insertion of two large-bore catheters, preferably in peripheral veins, with at least one being placed above the diaphragm. Blood samples should be drawn for cross-matching of donor blood, a complete blood cell (CBC) count (including platelet count), and screening coagulation studies [prothrombin time (PT)

and partial thromboplastin time (PTT)]. A spun hematocrit should be measured immediately in the emergency department (ED) if a CBC count cannot be obtained quickly. If bleeding is brisk and sustained or if there is any suggestion of hypovolemic shock, volume expanders should be infused. Both colloid preparations, such as 5% blood (O negative when necessary), and crystalloids, such as saline or Ringer's lactate, are effective for the maintenance of intravascular volume, but the latter solutions may be more readily available and should be used initially.

After immediate stabilization has been achieved and external hemorrhage has been slowed or stopped, the child, who had sustained blunt trauma, should be evaluated for internal hemorrhage. This evaluation is especially important when the nature of the trauma is unclear or when multiple areas of the body may have been involved, as in automobile or bicycle accidents. The importance of suspecting and identifying internal hemorrhage is underscored by the occurrence of hypovolemic shock and death in the child whose skin lacerations were sutured but whose ruptured spleen went undetected. Suspicion of internal bleeding should be raised in the presence of a continuously falling hematocrit or continuing signs of hypovolemic shock, despite control of external bleeding and the replacement of seemingly adequate volume. Respiratory compromise, a protuberant abdomen, or changing sensorium may be further clues to the presence of internal hemorrhage. Further studies, including radiographs of the chest and abdomen, computed tomography (CT) of the head and/or abdomen, and rarely peritoneal lavage, should be instituted when appropriate.

Gastrointestinal (GI) bleeding and other forms of nontraumatic hemorrhage can also be life threatening. In some cases, the severity of bleeding is accentuated by the combination of an anatomic lesion and a related bleeding disorder, such as esophageal varices with a coagulopathy caused by liver failure. Unexplained severe anemia requires a careful search for bleeding in the GI tract, retroperitoneal space, or elsewhere.

The approach to blood transfusion (Table 91.1) can be divided into three levels of intervention, depending on the clinical findings and the laboratory data:

1. If bleeding has been controlled, vital signs are stable, the hemoglobin/hematocrit level remains above 7 g per dL, and further bleeding is considered unlikely, the initially cross-matched blood should be held for at least 24 hours and then released for other use if no longer required for this patient.
2. If bleeding has led to hypovolemic shock but tissue oxygenation is not critically affected, intravascular volume should be supported with crystalloid or colloid solutions until a cross-match has been performed and compatible

TABLE 91.1

GUIDELINES FOR TRANSFUSION THERAPY

Blood component	Indication	Dose
Whole blood	Immediate restoration of blood volume and red blood cell mass after trauma or surgery; exchange transfusion	Calculation of red blood cell transfusion requirements[a]
Packed RBCs	For all nonemergency transfusions or emergency restoration of red blood cell mass (may be combined with saline or fresh-frozen plasma for volume expansion or exchange transfusion)	Calculation of red blood cell transfusion requirements[a]
Leukoreduced RBCs	Same indications as packed RBCs but contains few leukocytes; helpful in preventing febrile transfusion reactions and platelet alloimmunization	Calculation of red blood cell transfusion requirements[a]
White blood cells	Recommended only for some severely neutropenic patients with documented or strongly suspected sepsis	One unit daily (each unit should contain at least 10^{10} granulocytes)
Platelets	For hemorrhagic complications caused by thrombocytopenia or abnormal platelet function	5–10 mL/kg
Fresh-frozen plasma	To provide multiple coagulation factors	10–20 mL/kg/dose

RBC, red blood cell.
[a]Calculation of RBC transfusion requirements:
Required volume of packed RBCs = blood volume × [(desired hematocrit − present hematocrit)/hematocrit of packed RBCs].
Blood volume (mL) = weight (kg) × 70 mL/kg.
Packed RBCs usually have a hematocrit of 60%–75%; whole blood has a hematocrit of 44%–48%.

donor blood is available. If necessary, group and Rh-type-specific but noncross-matched blood can be used. A similar approach should be used if the hemoglobin/hematocrit level slowly falls to a level less than 6 g per dL or if the hematocrit remains stable at a low level, but further bleeding is considered likely (e.g., esophageal varices).

3. Only when bleeding is life-threatening should noncross-matched group O, Rh-negative blood be administered. Transfusion of blood with minor blood group incompatibilities may result in immediate hemolysis and renal failure or, more commonly, may result in sensitization of the recipient to red blood cell antigens, making future blood compatibility testing difficult. The determination of the patient's ABO or Rh blood group can be performed within a few minutes, so selection of ABO- and Rh-compatible donor units is almost always feasible.

A common pitfall in the assessment and treatment of the bleeding patient is the underestimation of the amount of blood loss. Neither the history of bleeding nor the initial hemoglobin level may accurately reflect the severity of hemorrhage. For example, a child with upper GI tract bleeding may have a modest amount of hematemesis or melena and hemoglobin of 8 g per dL when initially evaluated in the ED. However, within an hour, the child may pass a large amount of tarry stool and the hemoglobin level may fall to 3 g per dL. Tachycardia or hypotension in a patient with only a moderate degree of anemia should serve as a warning that intravascular blood loss is out of proportion to the hemoglobin level and that early replenishment of intravascular volume is essential.

Increased Red Blood Cell Destruction

Membrane Disorders

The underlying anemia in disorders of the red blood cell membrane (hereditary spherocytosis, hereditary elliptocytosis, stomatocytosis, liver disease) is rarely severe enough to constitute a hematologic emergency. However, the hemoglobin level may fall even further when red blood cell destruction increases (hemolytic crisis) or red blood cell production slows (aplastic crisis). Hemolytic crises are usually associated with acute infections and are self-limiting. Most aplastic crises accompany parvovirus infection; anemia may be the only manifestation of the infectious process.

The hemoglobin level and reticulocyte count should be routinely checked when children with known disorders of the red blood cell membrane develop increasing jaundice or pallor associated with an infectious illness. The hemolytic crisis is characterized by worsening jaundice, falling hemoglobin level, and increasing reticulocyte count. In contrast, the aplastic crisis is associated with slowly increasing pallor, worsening anemia, and low or absent reticulocytes. In children whose underlying red blood cell membrane disorder is associated with brisk hemolysis (hemoglobin level less than 8 to 9 g per dL and reticulocytes greater than 5% to 7%), these crises may produce acute symptoms of anemia. If the hemoglobin level falls below 3 to 4 g per dL or if cardiovascular stability is threatened, red blood cell transfusions may be necessary. One unit or less of red blood cells is usually sufficient to support the patient until the hemolytic or aplastic crisis is over.

For some children, an aplastic crisis may be the first clinical manifestation of an undiagnosed membrane disorder or other chronic hemolytic anemia. The low hemoglobin level and reticulocyte count may suggest a pure problem of red blood-cell production, such as transient erythroblastopenia of childhood or Diamond-Blackfan anemia (DBA). However, a careful history for features such as neonatal jaundice or splenectomy in other family members, a thorough physical examination to assess spleen size, and a review of the peripheral smear to look for spherocytes or other abnormalities may identify the underlying hemolytic anemia.

The need for transfusions in an aplastic crisis should be considered carefully because the relatively slow development of the anemia usually allows adequate time for compensatory physiologic responses to the anemia. An increase in cardiac output keeps the patient hemodynamically stable even at very low hemoglobin levels. Moreover, many patients with aplastic crises are already beginning to resume red blood cell production when the crises are recognized, and the reemergence of reticulocytes in the peripheral blood or the presence of mature erythrocyte precursors in the bone marrow often precludes the need for red blood cell transfusions.

Older children and adolescents with red blood cell membrane disorders may develop gallstones because of increased red blood cell destruction and bilirubin release. Cholelithiasis or cholecystitis in affected patients should be managed the same way as in patients without underlying hematologic disease (see Chapter 89).

Metabolic Abnormalities

Like the red blood cell membrane disorders, erythrocyte metabolic abnormalities usually do not cause severe anemia. However, episodes of acute and sometimes life-threatening hemolysis can occur in many variants of glucose-6-phosphate dehydrogenase (G6PD) deficiency, including the A⁻ variant found in 10% of African-American boys, after exposure to drugs or chemicals (Table 91.2) or during an infectious illness. Ingestion of naphthalene-containing mothballs is the most common cause of severe hemolysis in American children with G6PD deficiency, and parents should be asked about the presence of mothballs as part of the evaluation of any child with an acute hemolytic anemia. The acute intravascular hemolysis of G6PD deficiency usually occurs within 1 to 3 days of oxidant exposure and is characterized by pallor, malaise, fever, scleral icterus,

TABLE 91.2

DRUGS AND SUBSTANCES ASSOCIATED WITH ACUTE HEMOLYSIS IN CHILDREN WITH GLUCOSE-6-PHOSPHATE DEHYDROGENASE (G6PD) DEFICIENCY

Antimalarials (primaquine)
Sulfonamides (including sulfasalazine and trimethoprim-sulfamethoxazole)
Nalidixic acid and nitrofurantoin
Naphthalene (mothballs)
Fava beans
Aspirin (does not cause acute hemolysis with G6PD deficiency in African Americans when used in therapeutic doses)

abdominal and back pain, and dark urine. The anemia is accompanied by an increased reticulocyte count, and diagnostic "bite" or "blister" cells are present on the peripheral smear as well as the transient presence of Heinz bodies after supravital staining with methyl violet. Hematologic changes may be minimal or absent in the first 24 hours after ingestion. Careful monitoring of the patient should continue for at least another day. Treatment should include removal of the offending agent and fluid administration to prevent renal tubular damage. When hemolysis is severe, red blood cell transfusions may be required. However, if the diagnosis is uncertain, a pretransfusion blood sample should be saved for the measurement of specific enzyme levels. Because enzyme levels are higher in younger red blood cells, the diagnosis of G6PD or other enzyme deficiencies may be obscured at the time of acute hemolysis and a high reticulocyte count.

Aplastic crises may occur in more severe variants of G6PD deficiency and other red blood cell metabolic disorders such as pyruvate kinase deficiency that are associated with chronic hemolysis. Diagnosis and treatment of this complication are the same as described in the previous section regarding membrane disorders.

Autoimmune Hemolytic Anemia

Background. One of the most serious causes of severe anemia in children is autoimmune hemolytic anemia (AIHA). This antibody-mediated disorder occurs most commonly in young children. Affected erythrocytes are lysed intravascularly or removed prematurely from the circulation by macrophages of the reticuloendothelial system. AIHA may be associated with infections, drugs, inflammatory diseases, or malignancies, but a specific cause is rarely identified in pediatric patients.

Clinical Manifestations. Although this disorder may occasionally be indolent and may go undetected for days or weeks, AIHA is usually associated with the sudden onset of pallor, jaundice, and dark urine. The hemoglobin level may be as low as 1 to 2 g per dL at the time of diagnosis. When the anemia is this severe, the child may appear moribund and desperately ill. Signs of congestive heart failure may be prominent.

The anemia is usually accompanied by reticulocytosis, although the reticulocyte count may be below 5% during the first few days of the illness. Occasionally, patients remain reticulocytopenic for prolonged periods. Spherocytes are often found on the peripheral smear, and red blood cell agglutination may be present. If there is intravascular hemolysis, free hemoglobin in the urine produces a positive dipstick reaction for blood in the absence of red blood cells on microscopic urinalysis; when hemolysis is severe enough to exceed the renal clearance of hemoglobin, the plasma will be pink, and careful inspection of the plasma layer of a spun hematocrit may provide an early diagnostic clue. Unfortunately, it is often not easy to get this simple procedure done, but if available, it can be very useful. The direct antiglobulin (Coombs) test using broad-spectrum Coombs serum (IgG, IgM, and complement) is usually positive in childhood AIHA. Acute hemolysis is most commonly associated with a warm (37°C)-reactive IgG antibody with or without complement that is usually panreactive or reactive with the proteins of the Rhesus complex. This type of hemolysis is usually extravascular (spleen). IgM-mediated cold agglutinin disease is less common in children than in adults, but can occur following *Mycoplasma* (anti-I) or infectious mononucleosis (anti-i). These antibodies bind to red blood cells in the cold and characteristically cause intravascular hemolysis, as complement is bound and activated at warmer temperatures. Cold-reactive IgG antibodies (Donath-Landsteiner test) cause paroxysmal cold hemoglobinuria (PCH), which in children frequently follows a virus infection. The direct antiglobulin test can be negative or positive for complement only, and the antibody can be demonstrated by the Donath-Landsteiner test on a blood specimen maintained at 37°C during transport to the laboratory [a cup of warm (not hot!) water is the best method].

Management

The management of the child with AIHA should be aggressive because the hemoglobin level may fall precipitously (Table 91.3). Hospitalization for careful observation and treatment is usually necessary. In patients with warm-reactive AIHA or PCH, the immediate institution of corticosteroid therapy (methylprednisolone 1 to 2 mg per kg administered intravenously every 6 to 8 hours) may prevent or reduce the need for red blood cell transfusions. Alternatively, the patient may be treated with intravenous γ-globulin (IVIG) 1 g per kg. For life-threatening AIHA, the use of steroids and IVIG should be considered. Patients with cold-reactive IgM antibodies do not respond as favorably to steroids and IVIG as those with warm-reactive antibodies (most IgG antibodies), but a trial of either therapy is still warranted in the severely anemic patient. These parents must be kept warm. The response to steroids or IVIG in AIHA usually occurs within a few hours or days.

Red blood cell transfusions are hazardous in patients with AIHA and should be reserved for children with severe anemia and signs of hypoxia or cardiac failure. The presence of a nonspecific antibody in the patient's serum makes it difficult to find a unit of donor blood compatible in the major cross-match (donor cells and patient serum) and sufficient serum and cells must be obtained well in advance of the anticipated transfusion if possible. The finding of an apparently compatible unit may

TABLE 91.3

TREATMENT OF SEVERE AUTOIMMUNE HEMOLYTIC ANEMIA

Maintain normal or increased urine output with intravenous fluids.
Immediately begin corticosteroid therapy with prednisone 2–4 mg/kg/day or a parenteral preparation in an equivalent dose. Alternatively, administer γ-globulin 1 g/kg administered intravenously, alone or in combination with corticosteroid.
Administer red blood cell transfusions when severe anemia is accompanied by signs of hypoxia or cardiac failure:
Give first 5 mL in 10–15 min and observe for symptoms of acute hemolysis.
Check plasma layer of a spun hematocrit for pink color indicative of hemolysis of the transfused red blood cells.
If the antibody is cold-reactive, the blood should be warmed.
If symptoms or signs of worsening hemolysis are present, try a different unit of red blood cells.
If hemoglobin level does not increase after these measures, including transfusion:
Begin plasmapheresis or exchange transfusion; *or*
Perform splenectomy.

pose even greater danger because the physician is lured into a false sense of confidence when, in fact, an undetected antibody may still cause a severe hemolytic transfusion reaction. The use of the "least incompatible" unit is a common practice, although data to support this approach are lacking. Fortunately, acute transfusion reactions are infrequent, but the best policy is to avoid transfusion when possible. If red blood cells are required and a compatible donor unit can be found, this unit should be used. Otherwise, ABO- and Rh-compatible units should be administered despite the incompatibility in vitro. The recognition of the risks of transfusion in children with AIHA should not lead to the withholding of "incompatible" blood when transfusion therapy is required to prevent severe morbidity or death.

Whether the unit of red blood cells appears compatible or incompatible on the basis of serologic studies, special precautions should be taken during the actual transfusion. The first 5 mL should be administered in 10 to 15 minutes, and the patient should be observed closely for malaise, back pain, fever, and other signs of acute hemolysis. If any of these findings is present, the transfusion should be stopped and normal saline should be administered until a new unit can be prepared. If the patient is asymptomatic and the plasma is clear, the remainder of the unit should be given with continuing close observation. Blood administered to patients with cold antibodies should be infused through a warmer.

In rare instances, the hemoglobin level continues to fall despite steroids, IVIG, and red blood cell transfusion, necessitating alternative therapeutic attempts to sustain life. Plasmapheresis may remove sufficient antibody to reduce the destruction of the patient's erythrocytes and to allow improved survival of transfused red blood cells. If this measure fails, emergency splenectomy may be required. Immunosuppressive agents are useful in the long-term management of refractory AIHA but do not have a role in the emergency management of this disorder.

Nonimmune Acquired Hemolytic Anemia

Acute hemolytic anemia in children may be caused by infections, chemicals, or drugs that damage the red blood cell directly. These disorders resemble AIHA in their clinical presentation and should be considered in the child with acquired hemolytic anemia and a negative antiglobulin test result. Infectious agents that may induce hemolytic anemia include malaria (which is of particular importance in immigrants from, and travelers to, Southeast Asia and Africa), other protozoa, and a wide variety of gram-positive and gram-negative organisms. Treatment is directed at the elimination of the offending agent. Red blood cell transfusions are usually unnecessary unless anemia is severe (hematocrit less than 15%) or accompanied by signs of cardiovascular compromise.

Erythrocyte Fragmentation Syndromes

Red blood cells undergo fragmentation and lysis when subjected to excessive physical trauma within the cardiovascular system. Hemolytic anemias as a result of red blood cell fragmentation have been associated with abnormalities of the heart (valve homografts, synthetic prostheses, or uncorrected valvular disease), great vessels (coarctation of the aorta), small vessels [hemolytic-uremic syndrome, thrombotic thrombocytopenic purpura (TTP), collagen vascular disease, giant hemangiomas in infancy (Kasabach-Merritt syndrome)], and bone marrow transplantation.

Physical findings are related to the underlying disorder. The presence of red blood cell fragments on the peripheral smear strongly suggests mechanical damage to the erythrocyte. When small vessels are involved, thrombocytopenia may also be present. Hemolytic anemia associated with valvular or great vessel disease rarely causes severe anemia. However, iron deficiency as a result of intravascular lysis and urinary excretion of hemosiderin in renal tubular epithelial cells may aggravate the hemolytic anemia. Oral iron supplementation may obviate the need for transfusions. When hemolysis is a result of small vessel disease, treatment of the underlying disorder (e.g., collagen vascular disease) or primarily affected organs (e.g., renal failure in hemolytic-uremic syndrome) is the first priority. The diagnosis of TTP is important and should be considered in the presence of fever, neurological abnormalities, renal abnormalities, thrombocytopenia, and microangiopathy. Serum lactate dehydrogenase is frequently markedly increased. TTP is due to either mutation in the gene for or antibodies to the ADAMTS13 protease that cleaves large multimers of von Willebrand factor (VWF). The prompt institution of plasma exchange can be lifesaving. Red blood cell transfusions should be reserved for the treatment of symptomatic anemia. Because the hemolysis is caused by extracorpuscular factors, survival of transfused cells may be markedly shortened. The management of intravascular coagulation associated with several of these disorders is discussed later in this chapter.

Decreased Red Blood Cell Production

Disorders of red blood cell production, unless accompanied by shortened red blood cell survival, are characterized by a slowly progressive anemia. Consequently, the physician does not often encounter many of the difficulties associated with acute, life-threatening hemolysis or severe bleeding. However, the insidious onset of anemia when erythropoiesis is impaired may delay recognition of the disorder, and severe anemia and cardiac failure may be present at the time of diagnosis. Tissue oxygenation may be inadequate because of the low hemoglobin level, and conditions that increase the cardiac rate or output (fever, exercise) may precipitate congestive heart failure in the previously compensated patient. In addition, anemia secondary to diminished red blood cell production may be associated with an underlying, severe illness such as leukemia, neuroblastoma, or aplastic anemia in which other life-threatening hematologic abnormalities (severe neutropenia or thrombocytopenia) may be present. Thus, the patient with impaired production of erythrocytes may be as ill as the patient with acute hemolysis.

The important role of the history, physical examination, and laboratory studies in the initial evaluation of the child with decreased red blood cell production is described in Chapter 58. Initial management should include basic support of cardiorespiratory function and identification and treatment of conditions such as fever that may be compounding the problems of severe anemia. The patient with hypoxia or cardiac failure requires red blood cell transfusions. As described earlier, the urgency of the clinical situation rarely dictates the need to abbreviate the standard cross-matching procedures. A pretransfusion anticoagulated blood sample and a serum sample should always be saved for further diagnostic studies, as well as for the determination of the patient's red blood cell antigen profile should long-term

transfusion therapy be necessary. The initial transfusion should be given as a small aliquot of packed red blood cells. In many instances, the symptoms of severe anemia will be relieved after the hemoglobin level has risen to only 1 or 2 g per dL. The administration of additional blood is rarely necessary in the early stages of therapy. Furthermore, the added volume may precipitate cardiac failure in the face of a preexisting high-output state. A helpful rule is to administer a number of milliliters per kilogram of packed red blood cells equivalent to the hemoglobin level. For example, in a child with aplastic anemia, a hemoglobin level of 3 g per dL and early signs of cardiovascular compromise would indicate that 3 mL per kg of packed red blood cells should be given. Some physicians routinely administer diuretics (e.g., furosemide 1 mg per kg per dose) during the transfusion in a severely anemic patient. An alternative approach is to reserve diuretic therapy for those patients who develop signs of increasing cardiac compromise during the transfusion.

Aplastic and Hypoplastic Anemias

The differential diagnosis of aplastic and hypoplastic anemias is discussed in Chapter 58. Most of these disorders have a protracted course and, after initial stabilization of the patient, require intensive diagnostic evaluation and careful assessment of long-term therapy rather than emergency management. Transfusion should be used with particular caution in the initial management of patients with hypoplastic and aplastic anemias because exposure to human leukocyte antigen (HLA) and other antigens may adversely affect engraftment of transplanted bone marrow in patients who might otherwise have benefited from this procedure. If transfusions are required for severe anemia and signs of cardiac failure or poor oxygenation, the goal of treatment should be relief of symptoms, not restoration of a normal hemoglobin level. When possible, leukoreduced red blood cells should be used to reduce the likelihood of alloimmunization. Cytomegalovirus (CMV)-negative products should be used unless the patient is known to be CMV positive, or stem-cell transplantation is not a treatment option. First-degree relatives should not be chosen as blood donors to avoid allosensitization to family minor HLA antigens.

Patients with pure red blood cell aplasia most likely have DBA or transient erythroblastopenia of childhood (TEC). In DBA, the level of red blood cell adenosine deaminase is frequently elevated, and blood for this test should be obtained before transfusion. For patients with a hypoplastic anemia suggestive of TEC, a bone marrow aspirate may be helpful in predicting the course of the disease during the next few days and, in particular, the likelihood that red blood cell transfusions will be required later. For example, a patient with TEC has a hemoglobin level of 4 g per dL and the absence of reticulocytes at the time of diagnosis. If examination of the bone marrow reveals only an occasional pronormoblast, a further decrease in the hemoglobin concentration should be anticipated and red blood cell transfusions will almost certainly be required. However, if the bone marrow aspirate shows numerous erythrocyte precursors progressing through all levels of red blood cell maturation, a peripheral reticulocytosis can be expected within 24 hours and red blood cell transfusions may be unnecessary.

Nutritional Anemias

Nutritional anemias in children constitute more of a public health problem than a hematologic emergency. However, on occasion, the hemoglobin level may be very low at the time of diagnosis. Severe iron deficiency occurs mainly in 1- to 2-year-old children who drink 1 quart (32 fl oz or 1 L) or more of cow's milk daily and have little room for other foods richer in iron. Adolescent girls make up another group at high risk for iron deficiency because a diet normally marginal in iron content becomes totally inadequate in the face of menstrual blood losses. The presenting complaint in severe iron-deficiency anemia is usually pallor, lethargy, irritability, or poor exercise tolerance. In megaloblastic anemias such as vitamin B_{12} deficiency in an infant exclusively breast-fed by a vegetarian mother or in folic acid deficiency caused by impaired folate absorption, non-hematologic symptoms such as diarrhea, slowed development, or coma may be more prominent than the symptoms of anemia.

Stabilization and improvement can usually be achieved with replacement of the deficient nutrient. Nucleated red blood cells or reticulocytes usually appear within 48 hours of replacement therapy in folic acid or vitamin B_{12} deficiency and within 72 hours of therapy in severe iron-deficiency anemia. Because of this rapid response, red blood cell transfusions are rarely required unless symptoms associated with the anemia pose a serious threat. A response to replacement therapy should not preclude further investigation of the origin of the anemia, especially when the dietary history is inconclusive. For example, iron-deficiency anemia may result from repeated small pulmonary hemorrhages or chronic bleeding from an intestinal lesion rather than from inadequate iron intake. Similarly, megaloblastic anemias may be caused by deficient intrinsic factor or abnormalities of folic acid transport rather than from a seriously altered diet.

Iron replacement therapy consists of 3 to 6 mg per kg per day of elemental iron given orally as ferrous sulfate at night on an empty stomach as a single daily dose. Intramuscularly administered iron is painful and should be avoided. Intravenously administered iron has been associated with anaphylaxis, but such reactions are infrequent, and preparations such as iron-dextran can be given after a small test dose. Other IV iron preparations (iron-sucrose or iron-gluconate) are also safe and can be used if noncompliance with or poor tolerance of oral iron therapy is an issue. The hematologic response to parenterally administered iron is no faster than the response to orally administered iron. When considering replacement of folic acid or vitamin B_{12}, traditional replacement doses of 1 mg of folic acid and 100 μg of vitamin B_{12} daily are undoubtedly excessive, but their common use reflects the safety and concentrations of the available compounds.

The administration of supplemental iron, vitamin B_{12}, or folic acid should not be considered a substitute for adequate dietary intake when nutritional deficiency is recognized. Unlike most hematologic emergencies, the rapid improvement after treatment of these disorders may reduce the likelihood of further visits despite attempts to ensure adequate follow-up care. Therefore, a strong effort to restructure the diet should begin at the time of the initial contact.

DISORDERS OF HEMOGLOBIN STRUCTURE AND PRODUCTION

The disorders of hemoglobin structure and production that are most often encountered in a pediatric ED are the sickle hemoglobin syndromes [e.g., sickle cell anemia, hemoglobin S–hemoglobin C (SC) disease, hemoglobin S-β-thalassemia]. Thalassemia major and methemoglobinemia occur much less commonly than the sickling disorders. Lack of familiarity and vigilance with these diseases may delay recognition of serious illness, resulting in severe morbidity and even death. In the section that follows, particular attention is paid to the recognition of unusual but serious diseases and the management of the many and diverse complications associated with the hemoglobinopathies.

Sickle Hemoglobin Disorders

The sickling disorders are responsible for a large percentage of hematologic emergencies and a major proportion of total visits for any reason in many urban pediatric EDs. Although the basic molecular lesion in these disorders is well defined, treatment of the numerous complications is often unsatisfactory. Early recognition and aggressive management of specific problems may alleviate unnecessary suffering and prevent much of the morbidity and mortality associated with the sickling disorders. Optimal long-term care should be provided at a center with specialists who are familiar with sickle cell disease and its complications. The long-term management of many of the complications of sickle cell disease is beyond the scope of this chapter. In most instances, a thorough knowledge of the patient's clinical course and previous laboratory data are necessary for correct management of the hematologic complications presenting in the ED. Therefore, the treatment of hematologic emergencies in children with sickle cell disease is accomplished best in the center that also provides comprehensive care to affected patients.

Many complications of sickle cell disease include red blood cell transfusion, either simple or exchange, as part of their management. The indications for red blood cell transfusions are discussed in the following text with the complications of sickle cell disease. But, in general, in considering transfusions in this patient population, it is important to remember that patients with sickle cell disease may receive many transfusions throughout life. They are therefore at risk for developing new alloantibodies that may cause them to hemolyze if incompatible blood is given. As a result, extended red blood cell antigen testing is to be performed early in the course of the disease before the first transfusion and after each subsequent transfusion by hematologists as a routine part of sickle cell disease management. This is intended to screen for the development of new antibodies to donor blood, which would affect the type of blood the patient can receive in the future. The ED need not obtain this testing but should inform the blood bank when ordering blood for a frequently transfused patient so that the blood bank can consult this patient's transfusion history and immune profile. Attention should be paid to whether patients with sickle cell disease need premedications before red blood cell transfusions. Because these patients have likely required blood transfusions before, the history in the ED should include asking whether the patient has had a transfusion reaction and whether premedication with acetaminophen, diphenhydramine, and/or hydrocortisone may be needed. When administering a simple blood transfusion, clinicians should consider the following:

1. Whether the patient's long-standing anemia could have impacted his or her cardiac function, which might make patient sensitive to standard volumes of blood (10 to 15 mL

per kg up to 40 to 50 kg of body weight at which point the dose becomes 2 units). When needed, smaller aliquots can sometimes be used to restore tissue oxygenation without causing symptoms of cardiac failure or fluid overload.

2. Whether it is possible to administer an adequate volume of red blood cells while exposing the patient to as few donors as possible, in an effort to limit allosensitization.

3. Exchange transfusion is a special type of red blood cell transfusion that can be useful in multiple clinical settings. Sometimes exchange transfusions are needed to manage patients with sickle cell disease. This usually occurs when the patient experiences significant complications from sickling disorders, such as acute chest syndrome or stroke, in the setting of a hematocrit that is near the patient's baseline. A simple transfusion that would elevate the hematocrit much higher than the patient's baseline level should be avoided, as this would increase blood viscosity and lead to further complications. In this setting, exchange transfusion should be considered, in collaboration with the blood bank specialists, to decrease the percentage of sickled cells in the patient's circulation without increasing the hematocrit overall. Exchange transfusions require the same precautions as simple transfusions with regard to blood typing, screening for antibodies, and premedications. In addition, the following considerations apply:

   a. Should sophisticated blood banking services be unavailable, serious consideration should be given to transferring the patient to such a center if it is considered safe to do so.

   b. This procedure requires adequate IV access to both remove and transfuse blood and often requires a pheresis machine. Infants may be exchange transfused with simple syringes, but this too should occur in consultation with a hematologist.

DIAGNOSING SICKLING DISORDERS IN THE EMERGENCY DEPARTMENT

Clinical Manifestations/Management

Newborn screening for sickling disorders is now performed throughout the United States. However, newborns may occasionally elude testing or may rarely be misidentified as having sickle trait. Regardless, the information regarding the newborn screening is frequently unavailable at the time of the ED visit.

It is important to identify the ill child with an undiagnosed or unrevealed sickling disorder so that appropriate therapy is instituted. The diagnosis of sickle cell disease should be considered in African–American children with unexplained pain or swelling (especially of the hands or feet), pneumonia, meningitis, sepsis, neurologic abnormalities, splenomegaly, or anemia. The hemoglobin level and reticulocyte count are inadequate screening tests for the sickle hemoglobinopathies because values in affected patients (especially those with hemoglobin SC disease and S-β-thalassemia) may overlap with normal values. Similarly, the peripheral smear may be devoid of sickled cells. Definitive testing for sickling disorders is not usually performed in the ED. Hemoglobin electrophoresis should be performed on all patients with hematologic or nonhematologic emergencies

that may be related to sickle cell disease. Because the results of the electrophoresis will take several days, it is imperative that adequate follow-up is ensured, either with the patient's primary care provider or with a hematology specialist.

The major complications of sickle cell disease include infections, sickle cell crises, which may be vasoocclusive, sequestration or aplastic, and chronic organ damage, which will not be fully considered further here, except for complications that may present to the ED.

Sepsis. Impaired immunologic functions, including early loss of normal splenic activity, contributes to the significantly increased frequency of sepsis in patients with sickle cell disease. The risk of bacterial sepsis in the patient with sickle cell disease is increased several hundredfold in comparison with the normal population. *Streptococcus pneumoniae* and *Haemophilus influenzae* are the most common pathogens in young children, although *Escherichia coli* and *Salmonella* are more frequent causes of bacteremia in older children. Mortality from bacteremic episodes may be as high as 20% to 30%. While patients with hemoglobin SC disease have a lower incidence of bacteremia and a lower mortality rate from these episodes, their risk of sepsis is still much elevated over the general population. The period of greatest risk is between the ages of 6 months and 5 years, when development of protective antibodies is limited and splenic function is diminished or absent. Children with hemoglobin SC or SS disease are prescribed prophylactic penicillin (or erythromycin should a penicillin allergy be present) through age 5 years to prevent *S. pneumoniae* sepsis. Immunization with pneumococcal and *H. influenzae* vaccines and administration of prophylactic penicillin through age 5 years help prevent serious infections but certainly do not eliminate this complication of sickling disorders.

The common occurrence of fever with no obvious source in young children with sickle cell disease makes the distinction between serious bacterial infections and benign, self-limiting viral disorders a particularly frustrating problem. Unfortunately, no single physical finding or laboratory test (other than blood culture) can accurately identify the septic patient. ED management of the febrile patient with a sickling disease must include a through history and physical examination, consideration of laboratory and radiographic tests, a decision about the use of antibiotics, and careful deliberation about patient disposition. The history should focus on whether the patient has experienced symptoms, beyond the fever, that could indicate a serious bacterial infection. A complete physical examination should investigate sources of the fever and should include auscultation of the lungs, abdominal examination looking for splenomegaly or tenderness, and a skin examination to assess pallor or jaundice. All patients with fever and sickle cell disease should receive a basic laboratory evaluation including a CBC count, blood culture, urine analysis, and, in some cases, cultures of the urine and throat. A lumbar puncture to look for meningitis need not be routinely performed (see the following text). The emergency physician should have a low threshold for obtaining a chest radiograph to screen for new infiltrates.

In deciding about antibiotic use and patient disposition, the physician must choose among several options, including routine admission, prolonged observation, or outpatient management. In many centers, children with sickle cell disease and fever who do not appear to be seriously ill, but who nonetheless are at increased risk for sepsis, continue to be admitted to the hospital for at least 48 hours. During these hospital stays, ampicillin or a third-generation cephalosporin is usually administered intravenously until the culture results are confirmed to be negative. As an alternative to conventional inpatient management, other centers treat selected children with sickle cell disease and fever in short-stay units or as outpatients. This approach is usually restricted to children who do not appear acutely ill and who, on physical examination, do not have findings such as pallor, rales, or increased spleen size that indicate additional problems.

Some centers employ additional criteria such as age, previous history, temperature, and white blood cell count. Young children (younger than 2 years) are at higher risk of bacterial sepsis and may be more difficult to assess for early signs of sepsis than older children. A history of bacterial infection may be a risk factor for a subsequent episode. Temperatures greater than 39°C to 40°C may suggest an increased likelihood of sepsis, although lesser degrees of elevation do not guarantee negative blood culture results.

Those children who do not appear to be seriously ill and who, on the basis of physical findings and results of laboratory tests, are judged to be at low risk for bacteremia are treated in the ED with a long-acting cephalosporin such as ceftriaxone (50 to 75 mg per kg) and then most commonly discharged or admitted for 4 to 24 hours. Further therapy after discharge from the short-stay unit or ED varies among centers but may include 1 to 3 days of an oral antibiotic such as amoxicillin. A key component of the outpatient management of children with sickle cell disease and fever is a return visit or telephone report within 24 hours after discharge from the ED or short-stay unit. Inpatient care should be strongly considered for children whose families are unlikely to comply with this follow-up.

No matter which option for patient disposition is selected, the goal is to be certain that all children with sickle cell disease and sepsis receive appropriate antimicrobial therapy. Thus, the cornerstone of management in the ED is rapid initiation of antibiotics after obtaining appropriate cultures. Differences in subsequent management should not detract from the importance of this early step.

The treatment of the very ill-appearing child with sickle cell disease, fever, and probable sepsis should include the rapid institution of antibiotic therapy and aggressive management of septic shock. As in other patients with reduced or absent splenic function, clinical deterioration may be extremely rapid. The patient who is alert on arrival to the ED may be moribund and hypotensive 30 minutes later. Because of the emergence of penicillin-resistant strains of *S. pneumoniae*, children in whom sepsis is strongly suspected should receive a third-generation cephalosporin (cefotaxime or ceftriaxone), and vancomycin. Septic shock should be treated in the same way as in patients without hematologic disorders (see Chapter 70). Simple red blood cell transfusions or exchange transfusions may be needed to correct severe anemia or to reduce the likelihood of secondary organ damage caused by massive sickling in the presence of hypoxia, stasis, and acidosis.

Because unexplained fever is somewhat uncommon in children older than 10 years in general, the diagnosis of bacterial sepsis should be strongly considered in the older child with sickle cell anemia and fever. A careful assessment of the child's clinical condition should take into account the factors noted earlier. If the child appears toxic with pallor or cyanosis, inconsolable irritability, poor capillary refill, tachypnea, or tachycardia, admission for antibiotic treatment is advisable even in the absence of high fever or leukocytosis. Once again, good follow-up care must be ensured if the patient is managed as an outpatient.

Other Infections. Children with sickle cell disease are affected more often with infections other than sepsis in comparison with their hematologically normal counterparts. Meningitis, pneumonia, septic arthritis, and osteomyelitis may be responsible for substantial morbidity and mortality unless promptly recognized and appropriately treated. The level of suspicion for meningitis should be particularly high in the young, irritable child with sickle cell disease and unexplained fever. A lumbar puncture should be performed on toxic children and anyone with signs or symptoms for meningitis. Antibiotic therapy for meningitis is similar to that recommended for hematologically normal children with this disorder (see Chapter 92) and should include ceftriaxone and vancomycin. Exchange transfusion to lower the percentage of sickle hemoglobin may reduce the risk of intracerebral sickling and infarction in areas of local swelling and possible red blood cell sludging. When hemoglobin S is less than 30% of the total hemoglobin, sickling is unlikely, allowing fluid management to be dictated by the central nervous system (CNS) findings as opposed to the need to ameliorate sickling. Septic arthritis and osteomyelitis present particularly difficult diagnostic problems in children with sickle cell disease because the clinical findings so closely resemble those found in infarctions of the bone. A careful physical examination and judicious use of laboratory tests help the physician weigh the relative likelihood of infection and infarction. Diagnostic imaging with a ^{99m}Tc-diphosphonate bone scan, gallium scans, radiolabeled white blood cell scans, or magnetic resonance imaging (MRI) usually cannot distinguish between osteomyelitis and bone infarction secondary to vasoocclusion. Frequently, these studies yield results that do not point unequivocally to any one diagnosis. When possible, closed or open bone aspiration should precede the institution of antibiotic therapy in the patient with suspected osteomyelitis. Similarly, aspiration of an affected joint should be performed if septic arthritis is strongly suspected. In most instances, swollen, warm, and tender joints are caused by local infarction. The presence of other sites of concurrent infarction and the patient's description of the pain as typical "crisis pain" may be helpful in identifying the cause as vasoocclusion. The total white blood cell count and differential count of the joint fluid may be similar in both septic arthritis and sterile effusion secondary to infarction. Therefore, the Gram stain and culture are especially important. Septic arthritis of the hip deserves special mention because delayed intervention may result in necrosis of the femoral head. Children with this complication usually appear quite ill and hold the limb in a "frog-leg" position. Confirmation of septic arthritis of the hip by joint aspirate should be followed as soon as possible by surgical decompression.

Acute chest syndrome. Acute chest syndrome, which includes pneumonia as well as pulmonary infarction, is one of the most common reasons for hospital admission of children with sickle cell anemia. The affected patient is usually tachypneic, even after antipyretic therapy. Rales, rhonchi, and physical findings of lobar consolidation may be present. However, in some children, particularly those who are somewhat dehydrated, physical findings may be far less striking. Rales may be heard only after several hours of rehydration. Because acute chest syndrome may escape detection on physical examination, a chest radiograph should be obtained in children with sickle cell disease and unexplained fever or chest pain. A decrease in oxygen saturation, readily measured in the ED and compared with baseline values, may identify patients with early acute chest syndrome.

The problem of identifying a responsible pathogen in patients with sickling disorders and acute chest syndrome is similar to that encountered in hematologically normal children with pneumonia (see Chapter 93). Although pneumonia caused by *Mycoplasma pneumoniae, S. pneumoniae, Chlamydia trachomatis,* and gram-negative organisms is more common in sickle cell disease, a causative organism is rarely identified in cultures of the blood and sputum. The initial white blood cell count and differential count are usually not helpful in distinguishing patients with bacterial pneumonia from those with viral pneumonia or pulmonary infarction. The hemoglobin level is more likely to fall and the fever is more likely to persist during the course of bacterial pneumonia, but this information is not yet known, of course, when the patient is first seen in the ED.

Because a responsible organism for acute chest syndrome is rarely known at the outset, treatment is begun with intravenously administered ampicillin or a third-generation cephalosporin and modified according to the clinical response. Azithromycin or another macrolide antibiotic is usually added to cover atypical bacterial pneumonia, as it is more common in this patient population. In the very ill child, the identification of the causative organism should be pursued more vigorously with tracheal aspirate or aspiration of pleural fluid when present. Oxygen should be administered to children with acute chest syndrome who have evidence of respiratory distress or hypoxia. Red blood cell transfusions or exchange transfusion should be performed very early in the course when the patient is severely anemic (e.g., hemoglobin less than 5 g per dL), is hypoxic, or has radiologic or other evidence of severe or rapidly progressive disease. Therapy with corticosteroids is not usually indicated unless the patient has a history of asthma or a reactive lower airway that is further complicating their respiratory picture.

Vaso-Occlusive crises/Pain crises. Infarction of bone, soft tissue, and viscera may occur as a result of intravascular sickling and vessel occlusion. Physiologic or environmental factors that initiate the process of vasoocclusion and pain are rarely identified, although swimming in cold water may be one important cause of painful crisis. Children may have only pain or may have symptoms related to the affected organ (e.g., right upper quadrant pain and jaundice in hepatic infarct). Initial management usually centers on control of pain, general supportive measures, and differentiation of vasoocclusion and disorders unrelated to the hematologic abnormality.

The treatment of the child with a painful crisis requires an objective assessment of the severity of the discomfort and an appropriate use of analgesic therapy (Table 91.4). Once non-sickling disorders have been ruled out, hydration should be undertaken with D51/4 normal saline solution (D5W 1/4 NS) or D51/2 NS at a rate of 1.5 maintenance fluid requirements (see Chapter 17). The choice of analgesic is aided by familiarity with the patient's previous crises. Hesitancy to use parenteral narcotics may result in inadequate pain relief, mounting anxiety, and a loss of trust between physician and patient.

This is a particularly common occurrence when the patient has had repeated visits to the ED and physicians are suspicious of the stated degree of discomfort. For moderate or severe vasoocclusive pain, morphine sulfate (0.1 to 0.15 mg per kg) should be administered intravenously, and further therapy should be based on the degree of pain and the duration of pain control. Use of IV ketorolac or another NSAID should also be instituted in the ED as the antiinflammatory properties of these medications are of definite value in treating vasoocclusive pain. Admission to the hospital is necessary if continuing parenteral analgesic therapy is required, fluid intake is inadequate, or the child has had several visits for the same problem. Repeated prolonged stays in the ED often leave the child and family exhausted and rarely prevent hospital admission. Timely and efficient use of pain control early in the crisis has been shown to decrease the length of hospital stays. One strategy may include initiation of PCA (patient controlled analgesia) in appropriate patients while still in the ED.

Several specific areas of vasoocclusion deserve special attention. Between 6 and 24 months of age, dactylitis is a common manifestation of sickle cell disease. Infarction of the metacarpals and metatarsals results in swelling of the hands and feet. These episodes recur frequently. Pain usually resolves after several days, but swelling may persist for 1 or 2 weeks. Treatment is similar to that described for a painful crisis.

Infarction of abdominal and retroperitoneal organs may produce clinical findings that closely resemble the findings in a variety of nonhematologic diseases. The distinction between occlusion of the mesenteric vessels and appendicitis or other causes of an acute abdomen is, at times, particularly difficult. Physical findings and laboratory studies are remarkably similar. The onset and quality of the pain may be familiar to the patient and readily recognized as typical "crisis pain." The patient may describe the symptoms as distinctly different from episodes of infarction, however, giving support to the diagnosis of an acute abdomen. Because painful crises occur far more often than appendicitis and other causes of acute abdomen, a period of careful observation is warranted unless the patient is severely ill (e.g., peritonitis or other convincing signs of perforated appendix). Repeated assessment of the abdominal examination and the clinical response to fluid therapy help identify the child with an acute abdomen and reduces unnecessary and risky emergency surgical procedures in children with sickle cell disease. Hepatic infarction may also create a diagnostic dilemma because the acute onset of jaundice and abdominal pain that characterize this disorder are similar to the symptoms of hepatitis, cholecystitis, and biliary obstruction. In addition, vasoocclusion elsewhere in the abdomen that causes right upper quadrant pain may mimic biliary tract disease. The distinction between infarction and cholecystitis or biliary obstruction is particularly important because recurrent gallbladder disease is an indication of cholecystectomy. In both hepatic infarction and biliary obstruction, the alanine aminotransferase and direct bilirubin levels may be increased. Ultrasonography of the abdomen often shows a dilated common bile duct or the presence of stones in the duct in children with biliary tract disease when the study is performed shortly after the onset of symptoms. In many instances, however, biliary tract disease and vasoocclusion cannot be definitively distinguished, and the clinician must depend on a pattern of recurrence for additional information. The initial management

TABLE 91.4

SIGNIFICANT COMPLICATIONS OF SICKLE CELL ANEMIA

Complication	Symptoms	Management	Comments

Vasoocclusive crisis	1. Pain derived from sickling and vasoocclusion in bone, soft tissue, or viscera
	2. Patients aged 6–24 mo may manifest dactylitis
	3. Vasoocclusion in the abdomen or retroperitoneum may mimic an acute abdomen
		1. Mild or moderate pain
		■ Oral or IV hydration at 1½ times maintenance volume
		■ Analgesia
		  ■ Oral medications such as acetaminophen with codeine or oxycodone may be sufficient for some patients
		  ■ IV (intermittent) doses of morphine or hydromorphone
		  ■ NSAIDs
		■ Consider admission if pain worsens, oral fluid intake is inadequate, or repeat visits to the emergency department have occurred.
		2. Severe pain
		■ IV hydration at 1½ times maintenance volume
		■ Analgesia
		  ■ IV (intermittent) doses of morphine or hydromorphone
		  ■ Patient controlled analgesia with morphine or hydromorphone
		  ■ NSAIDs
		■ Admit unless pain markedly reduced and patient tolerates oral fluids
			IV fluid can be D5 ½ normal saline solution
			NSAID may be ibuprofen or ketorolac and should continue after discharge until pain resolves
			Patient controlled analgesia may include a continuous infusion of opioid

Priapism	1. Prolonged erection lasting more than 4 h 2. Pain 3. May experience difficulty urinating	1. Oral or IV hydration at 1½ times maintenance volume for 24–48 h 2. Analgesia as needed to control pain 3. Consider simple red blood cell transfusion to raise hemoglobin to 9–10 g/dL. 4. If simple transfusion not helpful or feasible, consider exchange transfusion to reduce HbS to <30% total hemoglobin 5. Consult with urology 6. Admit to the hospital for hydration and analgesia	Urology may consider aspiration of the corpora
Splenic sequestration	1. Left upper quadrant pain 2. Pallor 3. Lethargy 4. Splenomegaly 5. May have altered vital signs (tachycardia, hypotension) 6. Worsened anemia with elevated reticulocytes and mild to moderate thrombocytopenia	1. Immediate volume replacement ■ IV fluids ■ Simple red blood cell transfusion 2. Admission to hospital	Onset of symptoms is often sudden Usually occurs before age 5 years but may develop later in patients with hemoglobin SC disease
Acute chest syndrome	1. Oxygen saturation below patient's baseline 2. Symptoms of respiratory distress 3. New finding on chest radiograph 4. Fever is often present	1. Antibiotic therapy ■ Third-generation cephalosporin ■ Macrolide 2. Consideration of red blood cell transfusion ■ Simple transfusion if hematocrit has fallen ■ Exchange transfusion to decrease % HbS without raising hematocrit	Therapy with steroids not usually needed unless patient has a history of asthma and signs of an asthma exacerbation

IV, intravenous; NSAID, nonsteroidal antiinflammatory drug.

MEDICAL EMERGENCIES

of these disorders is similar to that described for vasoocclusive crises (i.e., fluids, analgesics).

Priapism. Priapism is an unusually painful and frightening complication of sickle cell disease. The penis becomes swollen, edematous, and very tender. Urination may be difficult. The initial treatment consists of fluid therapy and analgesics (Table 91.4). Once again, red blood cell transfusions or exchange transfusion may promote resolution, but these forms of therapy should be reserved for patients without a rapid response to other measures. Early aspiration of the corpora has been recommended to abort the course of priapism and preserve later potency. The relationship between the duration of priapism and later potency in boys with sickle cell disease is still unclear, adding to the uncertainty of when to use particular therapies. However, the trend is toward more aggressive treatment to promote earlier resolution. Priapism should be managed in the ED with an involvement of a hematologist and an urologist.

Stroke. Infarction of the CNS is a catastrophic complication that affects about 7% of children with sickle cell disease. Early detection of cerebral vascular disease using transcranial Doppler screening may reduce the frequency of stroke by allowing the preemptive use of long-term transfusion therapy. The initial presentation varies from the mild and fleeting symptoms of a transient ischemic attack to seizures, hemiparesis, coma, and death. Physical findings usually define, and CT usually confirms, the area of cortical infarction. Supportive therapy should be instituted immediately. A 1.5- or 2-volume exchange transfusion should begin as soon as the blood is ready. This procedure reduces the likelihood of further intravascular sickling and may prevent extension of cortical damage. Long-term transfusion therapy designed to maintain HbS to less than 30% is the standard of care, since the risk of recurrence is reduced from 70% within 3 years to 10% to 15% with therapy. Transfusion therapy carries the risks of allosensitization, infection, and iron overload, but recurrence rate for stroke is high after stopping transfusion. Other approaches to be considered include stem-cell transplantation and maintenance therapy with hydoxyurea, which increases the level of HbF, has prevented secondary stroke in one study, and is under evaluation in a randomized prospective trial.

Cerebral aneurysms occur with increased frequency in patients with sickle cell disease. The origin of this complication, which is usually detected in teenagers or adults, remains obscure but may be related to local vessel damage. Unfortunately, the aneurysm often escapes detection until after major, and often fatal, subarachnoid or intracerebral bleeding. The severe morbidity and high mortality associated with ruptured cerebral aneurysms require careful evaluation of patients with sickle cell disease and headaches or other neurologic findings (vertigo, syncope, nystagmus, ptosis, meningismus, or photophobia). If the aneurysm is accessible and bleeding persists, surgical intervention should follow radiologic confirmation.

Splenic Sequestration. The sudden enlargement of the spleen with resulting sequestration of a substantial portion of the blood volume is a life-threatening complication of sickle cell disease. Because this crisis requires the presence of vascularized splenic tissue, it usually occurs before 5 years of age in patients

with hemoglobin SS disease but may occur much later in children with milder sickling disorders, such as hemoglobin SC or S-β^0-thalassemia, in which splenic vasculature may remain viable for a greater number of years. The patient undergoing a severe sequestration crisis may first complain of left upper quadrant pain (Tables 91.4). Within hours, the patient becomes very pale, lethargic, and disoriented and appears ill. The physical examination shows evidence of cardiovascular collapse; hypotension and tachycardia are often present. The level of consciousness decreases. The hallmark of a severe sequestration crisis is a spleen that is significantly enlarged in comparison with previous examinations and is unusually hard. The hematocrit or hemoglobin level is much lower than during routine visits, and the reticulocyte count is usually increased. Mild neutropenia or thrombocytopenia may be present.

Recognition of this complication should be immediate so that lifesaving therapy is begun without delay. The rapid infusion of large amounts of normal saline or albumin is necessary to restore intravascular volume. Although a sufficient number of red blood cells to relieve tissue hypoxia may be released by the spleen after initial fluid resuscitation, transfusion with packed red blood cells (5 to 10 mL per kg, beginning carefully with 2 to 3 mL per kg) is often required in more severe cases and relieves the dual problems of intravascular volume depletion and impaired tissue oxygenation. Reversal of shock and a rising hematocrit signal improvement of a sequestration crisis. The spleen gradually becomes less firm and smaller.

Aplastic Crisis. Under normal circumstances, increased bone marrow erythroid activity (as reflected by the elevated reticulocyte count and presence of nucleated red blood cells in the peripheral blood) partially compensates for the shortened red blood cell survival in sickle cell anemia and other hemolytic disorders. If erythropoiesis slows or ceases, this precarious balance is disturbed and the hemoglobin level may gradually fall. The event that most commonly causes erythroid aplasia is a parvovirus infection. Progressive pallor is unaccompanied by jaundice or other signs of hemolysis. Severe anemia may result in dyspnea and changes in the level of consciousness. The hemoglobin level is unusually low, and reticulocytes are decreased or absent. If a red blood cell transfusion is required because of symptomatic anemia in the absence of reticulocyte response, a small aliquot is usually sufficient to raise the hemoglobin concentration to a level that ensures adequate oxygenation until red blood cell production recovers.

Papillary Necrosis. Papillary necrosis in the kidneys causes hematuria that is usually sudden and painless and that is often persistent. A history of recent trauma, streptococcal infection, or recurrent urinary tract infection should alert the physician to other causes of hematuria. Similarly, hypertension suggests the presence of nephritis rather than simple vasoocclusion. In papillary necrosis, microscopic examination of the urine shows numerous red blood cells but red blood cell casts are rarely seen. Pyuria and proteinuria in excess of what might be attributed to the blood in the urine are not found in papillary necrosis but may indicate nephritis. The hematocrit or hemoglobin level should be measured because the hematuria, if persistent or severe, may markedly worsen the chronic anemia. In many instances, however, admission to the hospital is required for IV hydration. When hematuria is severe, red blood cell transfusions are sometimes required for the treatment of anemia. Transfusions or exchange transfusions may also be useful in shortening the course of persistent hematuria.

Hepatobiliary. Cholelithiasis is the most common hepatic and biliary tract complication in children with sickle cell disease, with an incidence of around 12% in 2- to 5-year-olds and approximately 40% by the age of 15 to 18 years. Patients can present with acute right upper quadrant pain and tenderness, hyperbilirubinemia, and elevated liver enzyme levels. The optimal treatment is elective laparoscopic cholecystectomy after adequate preparation for surgery (transfusions) once the acute inflammation has subsided. Acute cholecystectomy is associated with a significant risk of complications.

More rarely, acute intrahepatic sickling or viral hepatitis can result in a similar clinical presentation with massive hyperbilirubinemia and elevated enzyme levels. Fulminant hepatic failure with hepatic encephalopathy and shock can also occur as a rare, often fatal, syndrome that may be amenable to exchange transfusion.

Femoral Avascular Necrosis. The most common cause of avascular necrosis of the femoral head in children is sickle cell disease, and this complication is even more common in patients with SS and coexisting α-thalassemia. It is also more common if the hematocrit is high and the clinical course severe, with frequent painful crises. Treatment options are limited, with bed rest and core decompression the initial approaches. Total hip replacement may eventually be necessary.

Thalassemias

Background

The thalassemias are disorders characterized by mutations in globin genes that diminish or abolish production of either the α- or β-globin chains of hemoglobin. The β-thalassemia gene mutations occur most commonly in countries that border the Mediterranean, parts of the Middle East, Southeast Asia, India, and Indonesia. In β-thalassemia major, the most common of the homozygous thalassemia syndromes, the affected child produces little (β^+) or no (β^0) hemoglobin A and usually presents only after 2 to 3 months of age with the switch from γ- to β-globin chain production. Although most of the problems associated with thalassemia major are the result of long-term transfusion therapy, severe anemia at the time of diagnosis may constitute a hematologic emergency. Other thalassemic disorders that may be associated with severe anemia include hemoglobin E-β^0-thalassemia and hemoglobin C-β^0 thalassemia. Although some patients with these disorders (especially E-β^0-thalassemia) are transfusion dependent, many with β^+ alleles require transfusions only for acute exacerbations of their anemia and are characterized as having thalassemia intermedia. The α-thalassemia mutations are also found in the Mediterranean basin, but gene frequencies are even higher in parts of West Africa and are very high in Southeast Asia. Loss of one or two of the four α-globin genes is clinically trivial and manifests as a silent carrier or α-thalassemia trait, respectively. Loss of three α-globin genes causes hemoglobin H disease, which is usually associated with a moderate anemia with chronic hemolysis and the thalassemia intermedia phenotype.

Loss of all four α-globin genes results in hydrops fetalis (stillborn or death soon after birth).

Clinical Manifestations

Children with β-thalassemia major usually develop a sallow complexion and increasing fatigue between the ages of 6 and 24 months. Weight gain and linear growth may be retarded. Physical examination shows pallor and enlargement of the liver and spleen. The hemoglobin level may be as low as 3 or 4 g per dL, and the mean corpuscular volume is often low. The red blood cells are hypochromic and microcytic, with striking variation in size and shape; nucleated red blood cells are present in the peripheral smear. Thalassemia major is readily distinguishable from severe nutritional iron deficiency. In the latter disorder, the dietary history is grossly abnormal, organomegaly is uncommon, changes in red blood cell morphology are less impressive, and nucleated red blood cells are rarely seen in the peripheral smear. The diagnosis of thalassemia major should be considered in a child with severe microcytic anemia and an appropriate ethnic background.

Children and adolescents with thalassemia intermedia have a moderate hemolytic anemia, with hemoglobin levels usually between 7 and 10 g per dL. Other findings often include scleral icterus and splenomegaly. Because of their constant dependence on a compensatory increase in red blood cell production, patients with thalassemia intermedia are subject to exacerbations of their anemia during febrile or other illnesses, perioperatively, or during pregnancy. In addition, in hemoglobin H disease, the increased sensitivity of red blood cells to oxidative damage makes acute exacerbations of the anemia during febrile illnesses or as a result of oxidant drugs, both common and serious. For some patients, the acute exacerbation may bring the thalassemia disorder to initial medical attention.

Management

The moderate anemia usually apparent at the presentation of thalassemia major allows sufficient time for a careful diagnostic evaluation and outpatient transfusion therapy. However, when anemia is severe and congestive heart failure is present or imminent, the need for red blood cell transfusion may be urgent. In such instances, pretransfusion blood should be saved for appropriate diagnostic studies (hemoglobin electrophoresis) and initial red blood cell antigen typing. If transfusion is necessary, small aliquots of red blood cells (3 to 5 mL per kg) should be given slowly. The administration of a rapid-acting diuretic (furosemide 1 mg per kg per dose, maximum 20 mg per dose) may diminish the risk of fluid overload. Because patients with thalassemia major have a lifelong dependence on red blood cell transfusions, the use of noncross-matched blood should be scrupulously avoided at the time of presentation to prevent sensitization to foreign red blood cell antigens. The use of leukoreduced red blood cells is important for the prevention of febrile reactions and to reduce the likelihood of CMV infection in patients who may later be candidates for stem-cell transplantation.

Patients with thalassemia intermedia most commonly present to the ED when their hemoglobin level falls during an acute illness. The decision regarding transfusion with red blood cells in this situation depends on the severity of the anemia and the status of the underlying illness. If the hemoglobin level is mildly decreased from baseline levels and the patient has no evidence of cardiovascular compromise, transfusion may be unnecessary. However, transfusion of red blood cells is appropriate when there is a more significant fall in the hemoglobin level during a serious illness. The balance tips toward transfusion even more readily in hemoglobin H disease because the tissue oxygen deficit from the worsening anemia is aggravated further by the inability of HbH to deliver oxygen normally.

Methemoglobinemia

Background

Methemoglobinemia is an uncommon cause of cyanosis in infants and children but is capable of causing severe problems and even death. Cyanosis results from a disproportionate amount of heme iron being present in the ferric rather than ferrous state. Under these conditions, oxygen binding of hemoglobin is severely impaired. The diagnosis of methemoglobinemia should be considered when cyanosis occurs in the absence of demonstrable cardiac or pulmonary disease.

The disturbance in the usual balance between ferrous and ferric iron may be a result of inherited alterations of hemoglobin structure (hemoglobin M) or abnormalities of red blood cell enzymes (cytochrome b5 reductase), or acquired conditions such as acute infectious illnesses [in particular, gastroenteritis in infancy (nitrite generation)] or exposure to oxidant drugs (nitrates, primaquin) or chemicals. Infants are particularly susceptible to acute methemoglobinemia because of the relative immaturity of the NADH-dependent enzyme system required to maintain hemoglobin iron in a reduced state (cytochrome b5 reductase and cytochrome b5 itself).

Clinical Manifestations

Symptoms depend on the concentration of methemoglobin. Only when methemoglobin constitutes approximately 10% to 30% of total hemoglobin does cyanosis occur. As the level rises to 30% to 50%, dyspnea, tachycardia, dizziness, fatigue, and headache may be noted. Severe lethargy and stupor are often present when the methemoglobin concentration exceeds 50%, and death may occur at concentrations greater than 70%. If anemia is present, oxygen delivery is further compromised and toxicity may be more severe at lower concentrations of methemoglobin.

Accurate diagnosis and rapid therapy prevent serious damage. The diagnosis should be strongly suspected when a cyanotic patient has a normal arterial Po_2 from an arterial blood gas and when the oxygen saturation as reported on pulse oximetry (usually more than 85%) is significantly less than that calculated from the arterial blood gas analysis. For patients with methemoglobinemia, oxygen administration fails to affect the cyanosis and the blood typically appears brown when dried on a filter paper.

Management

The treatment of methemoglobinemia depends on the clinical severity. In all cases, an attempt should be made to identify an oxidant stress and, once identified, to remove the causative substance. If symptoms are mild after oxidant exposure, therapy is unnecessary. Red blood cells with normal metabolism will reduce the methemoglobin in several hours. If the symptoms are severe, 1 to 2 mg per kg of methylene blue as a 1%

solution in saline should be infused intravenously over 5 minutes, as it can reduce Hb Fe^{3+} to Fe^{2+} in an NADPH-dependent manner (hexose monophosphate shunt). A second dose can be given if symptoms are still present 1 hour later. Because methylene blue can act as an oxidant at high dosages, the total dosage should not exceed 7 mg per kg. Failure of methylene blue to improve the course of methemoglobinemia may be a result of concomitant G6PD deficiency because the therapeutic effect requires an intact hexose monophosphate shunt. For patients with G6PD deficiency, ascorbic acid (500 mg orally) may be of some value, but if symptoms are severe, exchange transfusion or hyperbaric oxygen may be required. Even if treatment with methylene blue or ascorbic acid in the ED is successful, any child with symptomatic methemoglobinemia should be admitted to the hospital for close observation and further evaluation of the underlying abnormality or causative agent.

DISORDERS OF WHITE BLOOD CELLS

Infection is the most significant complication associated with quantitative or qualitative white blood cell disorders. In some children, death may follow a single episode of acute, overwhelming sepsis. In others, repeated local infections may cause severe organ damage or may culminate in a fatal, disseminated fungal infection. The appropriate emergency management of the child with white blood cell abnormalities and fever or other signs of infection may have a profound impact on the length and quality of the patient's life.

Neutropenia

The most common forms of neutropenia and abnormal neutrophil function are listed in Table 91.5. Neutropenia is usually defined as an absolute neutrophil count below 1,000 to 1,500 per μL. When the neutrophil count falls below 500 per μL, the patient exhibits an increased susceptibility to infections caused by normal skin, respiratory, or GI tract flora. Between 500 and 1,000 per μL, susceptibility to infection is less significant but the host's ability to combat more typical infections is impaired. However, management of the patient cannot be based on the absolute neutrophil count alone because other factors contribute to the severity of the clinical course. For example, serious, recurrent bacterial infections are common in severe congenital neutropenia, and in the absence of treatment with growth factors, death often occurs in early childhood. Similarly, severe morbidity and substantial mortality may be the result of infection in children with leukemia undergoing chemotherapy. In contrast, serious infection is unusual in immune-mediated neutropenia, although the absolute neutrophil count may be less than 500 per μL.

The management of localized infection or unexplained fever in the child with neutropenia depends in large part on the underlying disorder and on the patient's history of infection. In neutropenic states associated with repeated, severe infections, an aggressive attempt to identify a causative organism should be undertaken. Blood and urine cultures, along with appropriate cultures from identified areas of infection (e.g., skin abscess, cellulitis), should be obtained. The cerebrospinal fluid

TABLE 91.5

CAUSES OF NEUTROPENIA AND DISORDERS OF
NEUTROPHIL FUNCTION IN CHILDREN

Inherited neutropenia
Severe congenital neutropenia, includes autosomal dominant
  [neutrophil elastase (ELA2) mutation], autosomal recessive
  Kostmann disease (HAX1 mutation)
Cyclic neutropenia (ELA2)
Dyskeratosis congenita (DKC1 X-linked), TERC, TERT, or
  TINF2 mutations)
Shwachmann-Diamond syndrome (SBDS mutation in 90%)
Congenital neutropenia associated with pigmentation and or
  immune disorders—Chediak-Higashi syndrome, Griscelli
  syndrome, Hermansky Pudlak syndrome type 2 and p14
  mutation
Reticular dysgenesis, myelokathexis/WHIM syndrome
Other neutropenias—Metaphyseal chondrodysplasia or
  cartilage-hair hypoplasia, Barth syndrome, glycogen
  storage type 1b

Acquired neutropenias
Drugs and chemical toxins
Infection (bacterial, viral, rickettsial, protozoal)
Bone marrow infiltration or failure (leukemia, aplastic
  anemia)
Nutritional deficiencies (starvation; anorexia nervosa; vitamin
  B_{12}, folate, and copper deficiencies)
Immune neutropenias (collagen vascular diseases, Felty's
  syndrome, neonatal isoimmune neutropenia, autoimmune
  neutropenia including chronic benign neutropenia of
  childhood)

Disorders of neutrophil function
Abnormal adhesion (leukocyte adhesion deficiency)
Abnormal chemotaxis (hyperimmunoglobulin E syndrome)
Abnormal opsonization and ingestion (complement
  deficiency, leukocyte adhesion deficiency)
Abnormal degranulation (Chediak-Higashi syndrome)
Abnormal oxidative metabolism (chronic granulomatous
  disease, myeloperoxidase deficiency)
Acquired disorders of phagocytic dysfunction (malnutrition,
  malignancies, severe burns)

should be examined and cultured when CNS infection is suspected. If the child appears ill or toxic, broad-spectrum IV antibiotic therapy should be instituted with modification of therapy when culture results are available. Initial treatment should include antibiotics effective against *Staphylococcus aureus* and other gram-positive organisms as well as gram-negative bacteria, including *Pseudomonas aeruginosa* (e.g., vancomycin and ceftazidime). If no source of fever is identified and the child appears well, observation in the hospital or close follow-up without antibiotic therapy may be considered.

Decisions regarding admission to the hospital and treatment are often more difficult in children with significant fever (more than 101.4°F) and a more benign neutropenic state. Although infections are usually mild and localized in these patients, severe infections may rarely occur. A white blood cell count with differential and a blood culture is valuable. As a practical approach, if the absolute neutrophil is less than 500 per μL and the child is well, ceftriaxone can be given intramuscularly or intravenously with follow-up the next day; if the child appears

ill, admission for IV antibiotics is necessary. If the ANC is more than 500 per μL, the child can be managed as one would a non-neutropenic patient. In some children, the white count will rise to normal or near normal levels during acute infection.

A particularly perplexing problem arises when a child is first found to be neutropenic during an evaluation of fever. In most instances, both the fever and neutropenia are results of a viral illness. Under these circumstances, serious secondary bacterial infections are unlikely to occur, and admission to the hospital and antibiotic therapy are probably unnecessary. However, because the neutropenia usually cannot be attributed with certainty to a viral illness, other causes of neutropenia should be carefully sought. The patient or parents should be questioned about the use of drugs associated with neutropenia (e.g., penicillins, cephalosporins, phenothiazines, phenytoin). The family history should be explored for recurrent infections or deaths in early childhood that might suggest a congenital neutropenia. Underlying disorders such as malignancies or nutritional disturbances should be considered. If the child appears even moderately ill, admission to the hospital for further evaluation is appropriate.

Disorders of Neutrophil Function

Numerous disorders of neutrophil function have been described. These disorders are associated with serious infections to a variable extent. Therefore, the evaluation and treatment of the patient with abnormal neutrophil function should be based on the specific cause and the history of serious infection. Guidelines for the management of febrile illnesses are generally similar to those for the management of patients with neutropenia. However, particular attention should be paid to disorders such as chronic granulomatous disease, which have characteristic differences at the site of infection (liver, bones, GI tract) and causative organisms (*Aspergillus* species, *Pseudomonas cepacia*, *Serratia marcescens*).

DISORDERS OF PLATELETS

The clinical course and management of patients with platelet abnormalities are determined primarily by the cause of the underlying disorder. For example, at the same level of thrombocytopenia, bleeding is more common in disorders of platelet production than in immune-mediated disorders of platelet survival. Consequently, the treatment of bleeding should be more aggressive in the former disorder. In this section, emphasis will be placed on the management of bleeding in accordance with the underlying causes.

Idiopathic Thrombocytopenic Purpura

Background

Idiopathic thrombocytopenic purpura (ITP) is the most commonly encountered platelet disorder in children. Serious bleeding is rare, occurring in only 2% to 4% of cases. This low incidence is particularly remarkable because the disease is most common between the ages of 1 and 4 years, when children are particularly prone to trauma as they learn to walk, run, and climb. The risk of serious bleeding decreases sharply after the first week of illness, reflecting the presence of newly formed platelets with greater hemostatic capability.

Clinical Manifestations

The diagnosis of ITP is made readily in the well-appearing child with newly acquired petechiae and ecchymoses, thrombocytopenia, normal or increased megakaryocytes in the bone marrow, and the absence of any underlying disease. The children with this diagnosis are usually without major systemic illness and have a physical examination that is entirely normal except for the bleeding. Epistaxis, gum bleeding, and hematuria occur less commonly than simple bruising and petechiae, but when persistent, these hemorrhagic manifestations can lead to moderate or even severe anemia. In teenage girls with ITP, heavy and prolonged menstrual bleeding can also cause a severe fall in the hemoglobin level. Fortunately, the development of anemia in children with ITP is gradual; acute, massive blood loss is extremely rare.

The major life-threatening complication of ITP is intracranial hemorrhage. This rare but catastrophic problem may occur within a few days of diagnosis of the platelet disorder or months later. Although a history of head trauma in a child with ITP should alert the physician to the possibility of intracranial bleeding, the absence of any recognized injury is surprisingly common in patients with this complication. The symptoms of intracranial hemorrhage may be subtle, such as persistent mild headache, or they may be dramatic, such as severe headache, vomiting, and generalized or localized weakness. Intracranial bleeding in ITP is unusual once the platelet count has risen above 20,000 per μL unless a significant injury has occurred or platelet function is also impaired (e.g., as in the patient who has received aspirin).

Management

Controversy continues to surround the management of the patient with newly diagnosed ITP who has no serious bleeding. Not every physician considers it necessary to treat all patients newly diagnosed with ITP. The usually benign course of this disease must be weighed against the potential side effects and cost of the various therapeutic options. In patients older than 1 year, with no active bleeding, for whom close follow-up is ensured, treatment may entail observation alone. Aspirin and nonsteroidal drugs that interfere with platelet function should be avoided and activities limited while the platelet count is very low. Specific therapy may be reserved for patients with sufficient bleeding to cause moderate or severe anemia, for patients who remain severely thrombocytopenic (platelet count less than 10,000 per μL) several weeks after diagnosis, for patients younger than 1 year, or for patients whose physical activities cannot be effectively restricted. Decisions about whether and how to treat a patient with ITP should be made in collaboration with a hematologist.

One of the traditional approaches to the treatment of the stable patient with ITP is a 4-day course of prednisone, at 4 mg per kg per day, divided into two daily doses. Steroids, especially at these high doses, can cause side effects such as gastritis, emotional lability, hyperphagia, hypertension, and hyperglycemia. Whether a bone marrow aspiration and biopsy should be performed to confirm the diagnosis of ITP before beginning therapy with steroids remains the subject of debate. If a patient with

acute leukemia is mistakenly diagnosed as having ITP and treated with steroids, the correct diagnosis of leukemia may be delayed and long-term outcome may be affected adversely. For patients with a classic presentation of ITP, in the common age range and without associated anemia, neutropenia, abnormalities on the peripheral blood smear, or abnormalities on physical examination, a bone marrow aspirate to confirm the diagnosis of ITP may be unnecessary. However, careful examination of the peripheral blood smear by a hematologist is certainly indicated before initiation of steroid therapy to identify the large platelets characteristic of ITP and to be certain no signs of leukemia are evident on the smear. Table 91.6 provides complete guidelines for when a bone marrow aspirate and biopsy should be included in the management of ITP.

A second option for the treatment of acute ITP is the administration of antibody directed against the D-antigen of red blood cells. The antibody-coated erythrocytes are sacrificed to the reticuloendothelial system so that antibody-coated platelets can continue to circulate. The effect of anti-D (WinRho), usually given at a dosage of 50 to 75 μg per kg administered intravenously, is slightly delayed compared with γ-globulin, and the peak platelet count may be somewhat lower. However, anti-D has the advantage of being administered over minutes rather than hours, and it causes severe headache less commonly than γ-globulin. Mild to moderate hemolysis may follow the administration of anti-D, with a fall in hemoglobin level of 0.5 to 2.0 g per dL; occasionally, the hemolysis is more severe. This therapy is effective only in Rh-positive patients and should be used with caution if patients are anemic (hemoglobin $<$ 10 g per dL) at presentation.

Some patients with ITP are treated with IVIG at a dosage of 0.8 to 1 g per kg, with a second dose 24 hours later if the platelet count remains below 40,000 to 50,000 per mm^3. This therapy is effective in raising the platelet count in the majority

---

TABLE 91.6

INDICATIONS FOR PERFORMING A BONE MARROW ASPIRATE/BIOPSY IN THE SETTING OF IDIOPATHIC THROMBOCYTOPENIC PURPURA

History findings
■ Age $<$ 1 yr
■ Adolescent patients
■ Complaints of systemic illness (e.g., fever, weight loss, anorexia, fatigue)

Physical examination findings
■ Splenomegaly
■ Hepatomegaly
■ Lymphadenopathy
■ Clinical signs suggesting possibility of mass in chest, abdomen, pelvis, extremity

Peripheral blood findings
■ Anemia
■ Elevated mean corpuscular volume
■ Leukopenia
■ Neutropenia
■ White blood cell differential with blasts or immature forms (e.g., metamyelocytes)
■ Nucleated red blood cells
■ Red blood cells with tear drop morphology

of patients with acute ITP. However, the low incidence of serious hemorrhagic complications of ITP, such as intracranial bleeding, has made it impossible to ascertain the overall benefits of this or other therapies. Unfortunately, one of the more common side effects of IVIG is headache, and when this symptom persists despite slowing the rate of infusion, imaging studies of the brain may be necessary to investigate possible intracranial bleeding. Also, IVIG requires patients to be exposed to donor blood product that can carry with it risks such as allergic reaction, transfusion reactions, and a theoretical risk of viral transmission. Symptoms such as fever, chills, flushing, and rash can develop in the setting of IVIG.

For the patient with ITP and active bleeding, local therapeutic measures may be of additional help until corticosteroids, infusions of γ-globulin, or anti-D raise the platelet count to a hemostatic level or when these drugs are ineffective. Nasal packing and topical phenylephrine are useful for persistent epistaxis. Excessive menstrual bleeding may require hormonal therapy. If bleeding does not stop despite these measures, plasmapheresis should be undertaken and, if necessary, followed by a transfusion of 5 to 10 mL per kg (0.2 units per kg) of platelets. The removal of antiplatelet antibody by plasmapheresis may increase the survival of transfused platelets sufficiently to stop or retard active bleeding, as outlined in Table 91.7.

Intracranial hemorrhage in the setting of ITP is extremely rare (incidence less than 0.5%), but it is also the major cause of death in ITP and therefore requires immediate recognition and therapy. Table 91.7 provides guidelines for managing head trauma in the setting of ITP. In general, management of head trauma in a patient with ITP hinges on whether the trauma was mild or severe and whether the patient demonstrates neurologic findings.

Alloimmune Neonatal Thrombocytopenia

Serious bleeding may occur in the newborn or young infant with isoimmune thrombocytopenia or in the infant born to a mother with ITP. A discussion of the pathophysiology and diagnosis of these disorders is beyond the scope of this section. However, because mortality may be high in these disorders, particularly in isoimmune thrombocytopenia, the management of actual or potential bleeding deserves special emphasis. The brain is the major site of serious bleeding, perhaps because of trauma sustained during vaginal delivery. IV administration of γ-globulin raises the platelet count in infants with isoimmune thrombocytopenia or alloimmune thrombocytopenia caused by maternal ITP. Steroid therapy may also be effective. In isoimmune thrombocytopenia, transfusion of random donor platelets is usually ineffective; the platelets are destroyed rapidly because of the presence of the same offending antigen as that found on the infant's platelets. However, the blood bank may be able to provide platelets free of the offending antigen. Maternal platelets will survive normally and may be used for the affected infant after the removal of the maternal plasma, which contains the offending antibody. Transfusion of the thrombocytopenic infant born to a mother with ITP is more difficult because survival of all donor platelets is significantly shortened. However, serious bleeding is unusual in this disorder. If signs of generalized bleeding are present or if vital

TABLE 91.7

MANAGEMENT OF HEAD TRAUMA IN IDIOPATHIC THROMBOCYTOPENIC PURPURA

Mild head trauma without neurologic findings	
Management	Comments
1. Carefully observe and consider hospitalization 2. CT of the head 3. Check platelet count 4. Assess for signs of spontaneous bleeding 5. Initiate ITP-directed therapy if bleeding is evident 6. Evaluate certainty of follow-up	Even if the head CT is negative, inpatient management encouraged for patients with platelet count <20,000, for spontaneous bleeding (especially of the head or neck), and when follow-up is uncertain

Severe head trauma or neurologic abnormalities	
Management	Comments
1. Hydrocortisone 8–10 mg/kg administered intravenously 2. ITP directed therapy as appropriate 3. CT of the head 4. Platelet transfusion 10 mL/kg	ITP-directed therapy such as intravenous γ-globulin or WinRho may be selected on the basis of risk–benefit profile for the particular patient

Clinical status deteriorating due to ongoing bleeding	
Management	Comments
1. Consider splenectomy 2. Exchange transfusion of plasmapheresis followed by platelet transfusion 10 mL/kg (0.2 units/kg)	Full recovery unlikely in this situation

CT, computed tomography; ITP, idiopathic thrombocytopenic purpura.

organs are impaired by local hemorrhage, and if IVIG fails to raise the platelet count, a 2-volume exchange transfusion should be performed to remove a portion of the circulating antiplatelet antibody. A platelet transfusion should be administered immediately after completion of the exchange transfusion.

The recognition of immune-mediated neonatal thrombocytopenia is important for the counseling of the parents and for the preparation for future deliveries, as well as for the treatment of the affected child. In some instances, maternal ITP has been recognized only after the delivery of a thrombocytopenic newborn. In isoimmune thrombocytopenia, accurate diagnosis allows appropriate counseling regarding the risk to infants born of subsequent pregnancies and the management of the mother and the affected fetus. If necessary, maternal platelets can be prepared just before future deliveries so that they are available for immediate transfusion if required. These factors make it imperative for the physician to obtain appropriate diagnostic studies in the thrombocytopenic infant.

Heparin-Induced Thrombocytopenia

Children treated with heparin are at risk for developing heparin-induced thrombocytopenia (HIT), although this is more common in adults. This diagnosis becomes relevant to the clinician in the ED because HIT is high on the list of differential diagnosis for isolated thrombocytopenia and because missing this diagnosis can cause significant harm to the patient.

Interactions between heparin and platelet factor 4 (PF-4) creates a new antigen that provokes the development of an IgG antibody in patients with HIT. The IgG mediates destruction of platelets and thrombocytopenia results. Platelet levels may not become very low, but may fall to less than 100,000 per μL or below 50% of baseline counts. Importantly, these patients do not often bleed but instead clot, and thromboses of the arterial or venous circulation can become life or limb threatening in these patients.

HIT more frequently develops in the setting of unfractionated heparin use but can evolve in patients receiving low-molecular-weight heparin (Lovenox®) as well. The immune response emerges 5 to 10 days after heparin is initiated, unless the patient has received heparin before, in which case antibodies can form in 2 days time. The antibody can be detected using an HIT assay, which may include either enzyme-linked immunosorbent assay or serotonin release. In patients exposed to heparin whose platelets counts have fallen below 100,000 per mm^3 or below 50% of the previous baseline levels, testing for HIT should be sent. While this testing is pending, the patients should be given no more lovenox or unfractionated heparin. Anticoagulation should change to alternative agents such as lepirudin, argatroban, and danaparoid in consultation with a hematologist.

Nonimmune Thrombocytopenia

Although thrombocytopenia in the pediatric setting is often immune-mediated, nonimmune thrombocytopenias do exist. These are usually due to deficient platelet production, platelet sequestration, or bone marrow replacement. Platelet production deficits result from insults to the bone marrow that can be due to infections (typically viral), but serious bacterial infections and sepsis can also suppress thrombopoiesis, toxins, or side effects from a medication. Rarely, bone marrow failure processes can present with isolated thrombocytopenia. Examples include idiopathic acquired aplastic anemia, the thrombocytopenia with absent radii syndrome or congenital amegakaryocytic thrombocytopenia. Wiskott-Aldrich syndrome is an X-linked inherited immunodeficiency that also causes thrombocytopenia, and peripheral blood smear reveals characteristically small platelets. Bone marrow replacement, most commonly due to a malignancy such as leukemia or another cancer that has metastasized to the marrow compartment, does not usually present with isolated thrombocytopenias but instead is usually accompanied by other abnormalities in the physical examination or the CBC count. Platelet sequestration is most commonly due to splenomegaly.

Serious bleeding as a result of decreased platelet production usually responds rapidly to the transfusion of platelets (0.4 units per kg or 20 mL per kg, maximum 8 units of random donor platelets prepared from whole blood or 1 unit of single-donor platelets prepared by apheresis).

However, unless they are part of a program of prophylactic therapy, transfusions should be reserved for severe or persistent bleeding or for significant trauma. Many affected patients have chronic disorders and require repeated transfusion. The excessive use of platelet transfusions, whether prepared from multiple, single, or HLA-matched donors, may contribute to the early formation of antiplatelet antibodies, making future transfusions more difficult and, in many instances, less effective. Single-donor transfusions should be carried out whenever possible. The use of leukocyte-depleted blood products reduces the risk of alloimmunization and is strongly recommended in this setting.

DISORDERS OF COAGULATION

Coagulation abnormalities are responsible for a large proportion of hematologic emergencies. Indeed, parents of children with hemophilia may use the ED as their primary source of acute care facility because bleeding episodes often require immediate evaluation and treatment at times when other health care facilities are closed. This section places particular emphasis on the prevention and management of bleeding that poses a direct threat to life or to normal, long-term organ function in children with common inherited and acquired coagulopathies. The more rare inherited disorders of coagulation are not discussed in detail. Bleeding episodes are usually similar to those found in the more common disorders. Appropriate replacement products are listed in Table 91.8.

TABLE 91.8

SPECIFIC FACTOR DEFICIENCIES AND REPLACEMENT THERAPY

Factor deficiency	Replacement therapy
Fibrinogen (I) (also dysfibrinogenemias)	Cryoprecipitate, fresh-frozen plasma
Prothrombin (II)	Fresh-frozen plasma Prothrombin complex concentrate
Factor V	Fresh-frozen plasma
Factor VII	Factor VIIa (recombinant) concentrate
Factor VIII	Factor VIII concentrates (recombinant and plasma derived), DDAVP if mild
Factor IX	Factor IX concentrates (recombinant and plasma derived) Prothrombin complex concentrates
Factor X	Fresh-frozen plasma Prothrombin complex concentrates
Factor XI	Fresh-frozen plasma
Factor XIII	Cryoprecipitate
von Willebrand disease	DDAVP Factor VIII concentrates high in von Willebrand factor

Approach to the Patient with Abnormal Coagulation Studies

Coagulation studies such as PT and PTT are sometimes obtained for children by their primary care pediatricians. Sometimes this occurs because of a parent of family member expressing concern for bleeding or bruising in the child and other times these laboratory tests are performed because of a family history of a bleeding problem. Whatever the reason, screening coagulation studies will at times be performed and children may be referred to the ED when the results of these studies are abnormal. The ED physician should therefore develop an initial approach to these patients (Table 91.8).

A thorough history should reveal whether the patient has experienced any significant bleeding and whether the family history truly reveals concern for a bleeding disorder. A physical examination should also be performed to determine whether there is evidence of bleeding. The usual initial screening tests include quantitation of platelets, examination of the peripheral blood smear, PT, and activated partial thromboplastin time (aPTT), thrombin time (TT), and fibrinogen. These studies should be performed to confirm or dispute the findings of the laboratory test results leading to the patient's referral to the ED. If a bleeding disorder is still suspected on the basis of these results, and the patient is not actively bleeding, further workup can occur in the setting of a hematology consultation. If active bleeding is present, or an imminent threat, further evaluation and possible treatment may be needed in the ED.

Of note, proper collection of the blood sample is essential for interpreting the results of clotting tests. Blood for coagulation tests should not be drawn from an existing heparinized indwelling catheter. A cleanly drawn venipuncture sample without air bubbles or tissue fluid contamination is the most appropriate sample for coagulation tests, and the citrate tube must be filled exactly to the appropriate mark.

Inherited Bleeding Disorders

Background

The most common inherited bleeding disorders are factor VIII deficiency (hemophilia A), factor IX deficiency (hemophilia B), and von Willebrand disease (VWD). The severity of bleeding in the hemophilias can usually be predicted from the level of factor coagulant activity. If less than 1% of the functional factor is present (severe hemophilia), bleeding episodes occur frequently and are often unrelated to trauma. If the factor level is between 1% and 5% (moderate hemophilia), spontaneous hemorrhage is less common, but bleeding often occurs in response to minor trauma. If the factor level is greater than 5% (mild hemophilia), significant trauma is usually required to induce bleeding. VWD is a dominantly inherited bleeding disorder characterized by loss of both VWF, important for platelet adhesion to subendothelium, and stability of the protein that it carries in plasma, factor VIII (FVIII:C). VWF is measured both by its antigen level (VWF:Ag) and by its function, most commonly as a cofactor for ristocetin-induced platelet aggregation (VWF:RCo). Most patients (70% to 80%) have type 1 VWD, which is characterized by a quantitative moderate decrease in

VWF:Ag, VWF:RCo, and FVIII:C; levels of 20% to 30% are usual. Because of variable penetrance and overlap with normal individuals, especially those of blood type O, assays in the 30% to 50% range are referred to as low normal, not VWD; only a subset of patients is likely to experience clinically relevant bleeding problems, which are often mucocutaneous in character. Type 2 patients have various functional defects in VWF, and type 3 patients, who are rare and often referred to as autosomal recessive, have compound heterozygous inheritance of a VWF null allele and no detectable VWF.

The classification of inherited bleeding disorders according to severity is important in assessing patients who have sustained trauma or who have signs of active bleeding. For example, after mild head trauma, the patient with severe hemophilia is at greater risk of developing intracranial bleeding than the patient with mild hemophilia and therefore must be managed more aggressively. When extensive hemorrhage is seen in a child with mild hemophilia, however, significant trauma has probably occurred and injury to deeper organs should be suspected.

Many children and young adults with severe hemophilia now receive regular infusions of factor VIII or IX in programs of prophylaxis designed to reduce the frequency of bleeding. In general, these programs maintain the minimum factor VIII or IX level above 1% to 2% so that bleeding should be no worse than would be expected in moderate hemophilia. At times, the level of factor may be normal. Unfortunately, at the time of trauma, it may be difficult to predict the degree of hemostatic protection conferred by prophylaxis. Thus, patients on prophylaxis who have head trauma or other types of injuries that may lead to serious complications should be treated as patients with severe disease at high risk of hemorrhage.

Clinical Manifestations and Management

Joint Bleeding. Hemarthrosis is the most common complication in hemophilia and may occur in the absence of known trauma in severe disease. The knees, ankles, and elbows are the most commonly affected joints. Initial replacement therapy should be designed to raise the factor level to 50% to 70%, and the cornerstone of management is to treat as early as possible. Patients with severe hemophilia are often aware of a bleed long before clinical signs are evident, and so the patient must be believed! Many centers treat all joint bleeds with one or two additional doses of factor replacement, whereas others reserve further treatment of patients with persistent pain or increasing swelling. When the involved joint has been the site of recurrent hemorrhages, several doses of replacement therapy are usually required. Initial immobilization of the joint is often helpful and can be easily accomplished with a splint that extends to the next joint distally. The pain associated with joint bleeding usually resolves within a few hours of treatment; therefore, only short-term, orally administered analgesics are necessary. Rarely, pain is severe and analgesic therapy should be given parenterally. Aspirin must not be used because its inhibitory effect on platelet function may further aggravate the clotting disorder. Acetaminophen, either alone or in combination with codeine, is usually sufficient.

The role of arthrocentesis in the management of a hemarthrosis varies from center to center. Although removal of the blood from a joint has been helpful in allowing early mobilization and maintaining normal range of motion, arthrocentesis is generally unnecessary and should only be considered after consultation with a hematologist and an orthopedist.

Muscle Bleeding. Most muscle bleeding is superficial and, if treatment is deemed necessary, can be easily controlled with a single dose of replacement therapy to achieve 30% to 50% correction. However, emergencies may arise when substantial blood loss occurs or when nerve function is impaired. Extensive hemorrhage is most commonly found in retroperitoneal bleeds (e.g., ileopsoas) or thigh bleeds. Retroperitoneal bleeds are often accompanied by lower abdominal pain. A mass is sometimes palpable deep in the pelvis, and sensation in the distribution of the femoral nerve may be diminished. Loss of the psoas shadow may be seen on an abdominal radiograph, and a hematoma may be demonstrated by ultrasonography. The hemoglobin level should be measured initially and, if bleeding persists, at regular intervals thereafter. Treatment consists of hospitalization, bed rest, initial correction to 70% to 100%, and maintenance of a 30% to 50% factor level until pain has resolved and ambulation has been successfully achieved.

Subcutaneous Bleeding. Hemorrhage under the skin may cause extensive discoloration but is rarely dangerous and usually requires no therapy unless compression of critical organs occurs. However, pressure on the airway from a subcutaneous bleed of the neck may be life threatening, requiring steps to ensure airway patency, such as placement of an endotracheal tube, in addition to correction of the factor level to 100%.

Infants with undiagnosed hemophilia may present to the ED with prolonged bleeding from the site of circumcision. A careful family history may lead to a specific diagnosis in patients with an affected relative (see Chapter 65). A PTT should be measured and interpreted carefully because of the wide normal range in healthy newborns. Additional blood should be saved for assays of specific factors. If bleeding is not severe, correction can await determination of the type of hemophilia so that a treatment product specific for the identified deficiency can be used. If immediate replacement therapy is necessary, fresh-frozen plasma should be used because it will correct both factor VIII and factor IX deficiency, as well as less common inherited clotting factor deficiencies.

Oral Bleeding. Mouth bleeds are particularly common in young children with hemophilia. The presence of fibrinolysins in saliva may lead to persistent oozing in the absence of aggressive management. The site of bleeding should be identified. If a weak or redundant clot is present, it should be removed and dry topical thrombin placed on the site. Initial correction should be 70% to 100%. Often, one or more additional treatment options are necessary to achieve adequate clot formation and to prevent rebleeding when the clot falls off. The antifibrinolytic agent, ϵ-aminocaproic acid (Amicar), is a useful adjunct in the treatment of oral bleeding. Amicar should be administered orally for 5 days at a dosage of 100 mg per kg every 6 hours, with a maximum of 24 g per day. Because children with oral bleeding may swallow a substantial amount of blood, the actual amount and duration of blood loss may be underestimated by the patient or family and measurement of the hemoglobin level is helpful. As in bleeds of the neck muscles, careful evaluation of airway patency is essential. Complete airway obstruction may result from extensive bleeding in the tongue.

Gastrointestinal Bleeding. Hemorrhage from the GI tract is rarely severe in hemophilia unless an anatomic lesion such as a duodenal ulcer or diverticulum is present. Maintenance of the factor level above 30% to 50% for 2 or 3 days after initial correction to 70% to 100% is usually sufficient. If bleeding persists, appropriate diagnostic studies are necessary.

Urinary Tract Bleeding. Atraumatic, painless hematuria is the most common manifestation of renal bleeding in children with hemophilia. If bleeding is persistent, moderate to severe anemia may develop and the hemoglobin level should be carefully monitored. In the absence of trauma of a demonstrable lesion, one or more doses of factor replacement (70% to 100%) are used in combination with bed rest for at least 24 hours after gross hematuria has ceased. A brief course of orally administered prednisone may also be effective.

Although approaches to the treatment of painless hematuria differ, most clinicians agree about the potential hazard of Amicar in affected patients. The strong, antifibrinolytic activity of this drug may cause the formation of ureteral clots and outflow obstruction and should therefore be avoided.

When the child with hemophilia develops hematuria or flank tenderness after trauma, a more aggressive approach to diagnosis and treatment is required. Ultrasonography, MRI, or IV pyelography should be performed as soon as possible to look for subcapsular or intrarenal bleeding or an obstructive clot at the pelvic–ureteral junction. To prevent parenchymal damage and deterioration of renal function, replacement therapy to achieve a level of 70% to 100% should be administered immediately. If a lesion is demonstrated using the techniques already noted, replacement therapy should be continued for 5 to 10 days. If no lesion has been identified, a shorter course of therapy is usually sufficient, using resolution of pain and hematuria as an end point. The hemoglobin level and renal function tests should be followed carefully.

Intracranial Hemorrhage. Bleeding within the cranial vault is the most common cause of death in hemophilia, justifying the concern, anxiety, and urgency attached to it. In practical terms, however, head trauma in children with hemophilia is common, whereas intracranial hemorrhage is comparatively rare. Thus, the physician must be able to recognize and treat the child at risk without exposing other patients to unnecessary hospitalization, diagnostic studies, or therapy.

The management of the hemophiliac child with head trauma, but no neurologic signs, requires careful attention to the severity of the bleeding disorder, type of trauma, history of intracranial bleeding, and likelihood of close follow-up. Children with seemingly insignificant trauma may develop the first obvious signs of intracranial bleeding several days later when concern has diminished. If the trauma is mild (e.g., a light bump on the forehead), patients may be observed at home for the usual signs of intracranial hemorrhage or increased intracranial pressure. When the trauma is somewhat more substantial (e.g., falling down two or three carpeted stairs), the child with severe hemophilia must be evaluated by a physician, given replacement therapy to achieve a level of 70% to 100%, observed for several hours in the office or ED, and, if well, discharged. The child with mild hemophilia usually does not need replacement therapy under these circumstances, whereas the child with moderate hemophilia needs particularly careful attention to the type of trauma and bleeding history for the physician to decide whether to use replacement therapy.

A CT scan is extremely important in identifying intracranial bleeding that requires more intensive and prolonged treatment. A normal neurologic examination in a child with hemophilia who has sustained significant head trauma does not preclude the presence of an intracranial bleed or, therefore, the need for a CT scan. Equally important, the imaging study should not be used to decide on the administration of an initial dose of replacement factor. Patients undergoing CT scans for the assessment of possible intracranial bleeding should always receive factor replacement therapy before the study in order to avoid unnecessary delays in the treatment of potentially devastating bleeding.

If more severe trauma (e.g., hitting the head on the dashboard, falling off a changing table onto a hard floor) has occurred in any hemophiliac child, hospital admission and repeated doses of replacement therapy are essential. The initial dose of replacement should be administered as soon as it is available. A CT scan should be performed after initial correction to search for intracranial bleeding and help determine the duration of treatment.

The management of the patient with hemophilia who has neurologic findings in the presence or absence of head trauma begins with replacement therapy and those measures required for life support and treatment of increased intracranial pressure. Levels of the appropriate factor should be raised to 100%. The indications for surgery are similar to those for children without coagulation disorders, provided an appropriate correction of clotting abnormalities has been achieved.

Preparation of the Hemophiliac for Emergency Surgery. The child with hemophilia is subject to the surgical emergencies that affect children with normal hemostasis (e.g., appendicitis, compound fractures), as well as those hemorrhagic complications that require immediate operative intervention. When the need for surgery has been definitely established, correction up to 100% should be given and the PTT should be measured to ensure its normalization. Because the PTT may be normal when the factor VIII or IX level is as low as 20% to 30%, the measurement of factor coagulant level is needed to assess the adequacy of response to treatment when levels above 30% are desired. This test cannot always be performed before surgery but is essential in the postoperative management of the patient with hemophilia. Therefore, surgery in a child with hemophilia should rarely, if ever, be undertaken in a hospital without appropriate laboratory facilities.

Von Willebrand Disease. The sites of bleeding in mild VWD resemble those found in patients with platelet disorders. Bruising, epistaxis, oral bleeding, and menorrhagia are common, whereas joint bleeding is very unusual. Seventy to eighty percent of patients have type 1 VWD. Children affected with more severe form of VWD (type 3), in which the factor VIII level is very low, may have bleeding problems that resemble those found in both hemophilia and VWD. Massive or persistent GI bleeding with angiodysplasia of the bowel is an unusual complication of VWD that requires prolonged factor replacement therapy and, in some cases, surgical resection of the involved area.

1-Deamino-8-D-Arginine Vasopressin. After the administration of DDAVP (desmopressin), levels of factor VIII coagulant activity, von Willebrand antigen, and ristocetin cofactor activity increase by about twofold in most people with type 1 VWD. This activity makes DDAVP an excellent alternative to blood products for the treatment of minor bleeding episodes in patients with mild hemophilia and for the treatment of most bleeding episodes in patients with the common form (type 1) of VWD and some forms of type 2; it should not be prescribed to patients of type 2B, whose VWF binds spontaneously to platelets, as DDAVP can exacerbate the mild thrombocytopenia that these patients often have. Because some patients with these disorders do not respond to DDAVP, it is strongly recommended that children with mild hemophilia or type 1 VWD receive a trial dose of DDAVP to assess individual responses to this therapy before needing treatment of a bleeding episode. The dose of DDAVP is 0.3 μg per kg, administered intravenously over 30 minutes. Side effects include facial flushing, headache, and, rarely, hypertension, hypotension, and water retention. Hyponatremic seizures have occurred, and the patient should avoid excessive water intake. Patients younger than 2 years should not be given DDAVP. Subsequent doses may be less effective because the drug acts by releasing factors VIII and VWF from stores rather than by increasing their synthesis. In patients with severe factor VIII deficiency, DDAVP is ineffective. This is also true for many patients with type 2 and 3 VWD.

DDAVP is also available as a concentrated nasal spray that should be distinguished from the more diluted form used for enuresis or diabetes insipidus. For patients who have been previously shown to respond adequately to this form of therapy, the nasal spray is an alternative to an IV administration. However, the nasal spray is designed primarily for use at home. DDAVP-responsive patients who come to the ED may have already tried the intranasal spray unsuccessfully or may have bleeding that requires other therapy.

Replacement Products

The products commonly used for the treatment of children with hemophilia and VWD are recombinant factor concentrates or plasma-derived factor concentrates (Table 91.9). Fresh-frozen plasma and cryoprecipitate are rarely used in the management of hemophilia and VWD because alternative products are safer and more potent.

Most patients are accustomed to receiving a particular product in their regular hemophilia care, and parents often bring their prescribed factor concentrate with them when they come to the ED. The treating physician should pay careful attention to the patient's treatment plan as developed by the hemophilia treatment center. The ED is rarely the place to alter the long-term treatment program for a patient with hemophilia. A particularly important situation is the treatment of a child with a previously undiagnosed bleeding disorder. Whenever possible, the diagnosis should be established before treatment is begun. For example, the diagnosis of factor VIII or IX deficiency might save a child a one-time exposure to a plasma product. However, establishment of a diagnosis of a specific factor deficiency should not take precedence over the timely management of a serious bleeding episode.

Factor Concentrates. In more recent years, the development of new factor concentrates has dramatically improved the care of children with hemophilia. Recombinant factor VIII and IX products are presently prescribed for almost all children and adolescents with hemophilia in the United States.

TABLE 91.9

EVALUATION OF A PROLONGED PROTHROMBIN TIME (PT) OR ACTIVATED PARTIAL THROMBOPLASTIN TIME (APTT)

PT	aPTT	Causes of laboratory findings	Next steps in evaluation in addition to hematology referral
Prolonged	Normal	■ Inherited 　■ Factor VII deficiency ■ Acquired 　■ Acquired factor VII deficiency 　■ Inhibitor to factor VII 　■ Vitamin K deficiency 　■ Liver disease 　■ Warfarin (Coumadin)	Mixing study Factor VII level Liver function testing
Normal	Prolonged	■ Inherited 　■ Deficiency in factors VIII, IX, or XI 　■ von Willebrand disease 　■ Deficiency in factor XII, prekallikrein, or high-molecular-weight kininogen ■ Acquired 　■ Heparin administration 　■ Inhibitor to factors VIII, IX, or XI 　■ Acquired von Willebrand disease 　■ Lupus anticoagulant	Factor VIII, IX, and XI levels von Willebrand panel Mixing study Lupus anticoagulant
Prolonged	Prolonged	■ Inherited 　■ Deficiency in factor V or X, prothrombin, fibrinogen ■ Acquired 　■ Liver disease 　■ Disseminated intravascular coagulation 　■ Supratherapeutic doses of warfarin or heparin 　■ Combined administration of warfarin and heparin 　■ Inhibitor to factor V or X, prothrombin, fibrinogen	Factor V, X, prothrombin levels Mixing study D-dimer Liver function testing

For children with VWD who do not achieve hemostasis after treatment with DDAVP or are not appropriate candidates for DDAVP, treatment of bleeding episodes with plasma-derived, intermediate purity factor VIII concentrates with VWF is indicated. Dosing is based on the ristocetin cofactor activity, and vials of the concentrate are labeled with the content of VWF:RCo activity. One IU of VWF:RCo per kg body weight raises the plasma level by 1.5% to 2.0%. For minor bleeding episodes, raising the VWF:RCo level above 50% should provide adequate hemostasis. For more serious bleeding or for the prevention of surgical bleeding, an initial dose calculated to raise the VWF:RCo to 100%, followed by repeat dosing every 12 hours, is recommended. Prothrombin complex concentrates are used primarily both for the treatment of patients with hemophilia and inhibitors and for the treatment of the relatively rare disorders of factor II and X deficiency. The use of this product for factor VII and IX deficiency has diminished since plasma-derived and recombinant factor IX concentrates and recombinant factor VII concentrates became available.

Calculation of Dosage for Factor VIII and IX Replacement. A formula commonly used for determining the number of units of factor VIII or IX necessary to achieve a specific level:

Factor VIII:
One unit of recombinant or plasma-derived factor VIII per kg raises the measured factor level by 2% [number of units = desired level × weight of patient (kg) × 0.5].

Factor IX:
One unit of recombinant factor IX per kg raises the measured factor IX level by 0.83% for recombinant product [number of units = desired level × weight of patient (kg) × 1.2) or by 1% for plasma-derived factor IX number of units = desired level × weight of patient (kg)].

In the treatment of major hemorrhages, the achieved level of factor activity should be measured directly because the recovery in vivo varies widely among patients and because inadequate hemostasis may lead to severe morbidity or death. In addition, the dose of plasma-derived factor VIII required in children to achieve a particular factor VIII level may be 50% to 100% greater than in adults. If a minor bleed fails to respond to conventional dosing, a pre- and posttreatment factor level should be measured to be certain that the desired level is being achieved.

Fresh-frozen Plasma. Fresh-frozen plasma contains all plasma clotting factors and is therefore particularly useful when a child with a previously undiagnosed bleeding disorder presents to the ED with a hemorrhage that requires therapy before the specific factor deficiency can be ascertained. Its use is generally restricted to the treatment of an unknown inherited factor deficiency or a deficiency of a factor, such as factor XI, for which there is no available factor concentrate. Although the average concentration of factor in fresh-frozen plasma is 1 unit per mL, the actual concentration in a particular unit may vary widely (0.5 to 1.5 unit per mL) and is rarely measured. A typical dose for fresh frozen plasma is 15 mL per kg.

Cryoprecipitate. When plasma is frozen and then slowly thawed, the precipitate that forms contains enriched factor VIII coagulant activity, VWF, fibrinogen, and factor XIII. However, like fresh-frozen plasma, the actual amount of these clotting factors in a single unit depends on the level in the donor and may vary. The usual content in a 10-mL bag or "unit" is only 100 units of factor VIII and 200 mg of fibrinogen. A typical dose for cryoprecipitate is 1 to 2 units for every 10 kg of body weight. However, this product is not the first choice in the treatment of hemophilia since purified factor VIII concentrates have become available but may be used in areas of the world where concentrates are unavailable.

Management of Patients with Inhibitors

Neutralizing inhibitors against factors VIII and IX occur in 20% to 30% of children with factor VIII deficiency and 3% to 5% of patients with factor IX deficiency. The treatment of bleeding episodes in the child with hemophilia and antibodies against the missing or diminished factor is difficult and requires consultation with the hematology service. Extensive resources, experience, and ingenuity are necessary to achieve hemostasis. For serious bleeding in patients with factor VIII deficiency and relatively low inhibitor titers (less than 10 Bethesda units), large doses of factor VIII may overwhelm the antibody and raise the factor VIII level to hemostatic levels. Doses as high as 100 to 200 units per kg may be necessary. However, those patients who are "high responders" to the factor VIII antigen will develop rising titers of antibody within 3 to 5 days, reducing or eliminating the usefulness of further therapy with factor VIII. Despite the subsequent rise in inhibitor titer, this brief period of initial factor VIII therapy may be sufficient to stop bleeding in critical organs such as the brain. In contrast, factor VIII replacement should not be used as initial therapy for a minor bleed in a patient with a high-responding inhibitor because the anamnestic antibody response may impair the management of a later, more serious bleed.

If the initial inhibitor titer in a patient with critical bleeding is too high to warrant a trial of factor VIII therapy or if no response to factor VIII is obtained, alternative approaches should be initiated. Recombinant factor VIIa concentrate has assumed a prominent role in the treatment of bleeding in children with high-titer inhibitors. This product has proven effective in achieving hemostasis in most patients with inhibitors. However, factor VIIa is expensive and must be administered every 2 hours because of its very short half-life. The success of treatment must be judged clinically rather than by changes in laboratory values. Another approach to the treatment of serious bleeding in the patient with factor VIII deficiency and inhibitors is the administration of activated prothrombin complex concentrate (aPCC). These products presumably are effective because of their ability to bypass factor VIII through the presence of factors II, VII, and X. The relative efficacy of aPCC and factor VIIa is uncertain. Treatment with aPCC, such as treatment with factor VIIa, cannot be monitored by the PTT or factor levels but by clinical response. Factor VIIa and aPCC should not be administered simultaneously because of the potential for developing thrombosis.

Occasionally, the condition of the patient with inhibitors will worsen despite factor therapy. For example, the child with an intracranial hemorrhage may have continued bleeding and neurologic deterioration despite high-dose factor VIII or VIIa. In such instances, plasmapheresis may remove sufficient antibody to allow a response to factor VIII administration. However, because 50% of the IgG inhibitor is tissue bound and will rapidly return to the plasma, further infusions of factor VIII will be unsuccessful unless preceded by additional plasmaphereses.

The treatment of patients with factor IX deficiency and inhibitors employs high-dose factor IX therapy, factor VIIa, and aPCCs in approaches that are similar to those used for patients with factor VIII inhibitors. However, the treatment of patients with factor IX inhibitors is particularly challenging because of the risk of anaphylaxis and proteinuria on further exposure to products containing factor IX, even if similar problems did not occur prior to the development of the inhibitor. Patients with factor IX inhibitors who are receiving their first dose of either aPCCs or factor IX concentrate after the development of an inhibitor should be monitored carefully for adverse reactions. Exchange transfusion followed by infusion of factor IX concentrate may also be useful if the hemorrhage is severe or life threatening.

The recognition of a newly developed inhibitor may be equally important as the treatment of choice for a patient with a known inhibitor. With the development of an inhibitor, patients with severe hemophilia often experience no change in their pattern of bleeding. However, the response to previously effective therapy is usually noted to be less satisfactory. Patients with moderate hemophilia who develop inhibitors have more bleeding and an inadequate response to treatment. If an inhibitor is suspected at the time of emergency therapy, a PTT should be measured after therapy because, in the presence of a strong inhibitor, a level of factor activity adequate to normalize the PTT (20% to 30% factor VIII) is rarely achieved. An inhibitor screen can also be performed by mixing the patient's plasma with normal plasma and by demonstrating a prolonged PTT compared with normal plasma mixed with saline. The level of inhibitor should be measured using more sophisticated techniques. Although the PTT need not be measured after routine treatment of minor hemorrhages, it should always be used to demonstrate an appropriate response in vitro to the treatment of major hemorrhage because a failure to respond to initial therapy may compromise organ function or life itself.

Inherited Hypercoagulable Conditions

Background

Hemostasis is a balance between the activities of proteins that promote and inhibit clotting. Deficiencies of the factor that promote clotting, such as factors VIII and IX, lead to abnormal bleeding, and the recognition and emergency treatment of the hemophilias and related disorders are familiar to many physicians. Deficiencies of the factors that inhibit coagulation lead to local and sometimes disseminated thrombosis. In contrast to bleeding disorders, the identification and emergency management of these unusual hypercoagulable disorders are likely to be unfamiliar to many clinicians. In fact, the role of these inhibitory proteins is only now being fully characterized.

Clinical Manifestations

The three major proteins that serve as brakes on the coagulation pathway are antithrombin (formerly called antithrombin III), protein C, and protein S. Antithrombin inactivates the serine proteases that normally promote hemostasis. Patients heterozygous for antithrombin deficiency have an increased risk of developing deep vein thrombosis and pulmonary embolus. Protein C, with its cofactor protein S, is activated (APC) by thrombin binding to vascular thrombomodulin, and inactivates activated factors V and VIII. Persons heterozygous for protein C or protein S deficiency have an increased risk of venous thrombosis. Clinical findings in heterozygotes usually appear during adolescence or adulthood. In contrast, homozygous protein C deficiency causes widespread thrombosis in the neonatal period; homozygous protein S deficiency is uncommon but may have similarly severe and early clinical manifestations. This syndrome of purpura fulminans, sometimes accompanied by cerebral thrombosis, is a dire emergency that requires immediate intervention to preserve any chance of a good outcome.

The most common inherited cause of thrombosis, factor V Leiden (FVL), is a single gene mutation that alters the amino acid composition of factor V and makes this coagulation protein resistant to the antithrombotic activity of activated protein C. Heterozygosity for FVL is found in 3% to 6% of the Caucasian population in the United States, but it is rare in those of African-American or Asian descent. Heterozygosity carries a 2- to 7-fold increased relative risk of venous thromboembolism compared with normal individuals, whereas the risk for homozygotes is 80-fold. FVL may be a risk factor for both venous and arterial thrombosis in ill neonates. Other inherited conditions that may increase the risk of developing thrombosis include the prothrombin 20210 gene mutation (threefold), dysfibrinogenemias, severe hyperhomocystinemia, and elevated levels of lipoprotein (a). An important acquired condition associated with an increased risk of venous or arterial thrombosis is the antiphospholipid antibody syndrome, which is more common in teenagers than in young children.

Management

Patients who develop a deep venous thrombosis, in the presence or absence of a discernible underlying risk factor, should be treated initially either with unfractionated heparin (UFH) by IV bolus or low-molecular-weight heparin (LMWH) given subcutaneously. Treatment with UFH is usually initiated with a bolus injection of 75 units per kg body weight followed by a constant infusion of 20 units per kg per hour for children older than 1 year and 28 units per kg for neonates and infants. The UFH dose should be adjusted to maintain an anti-factor Xa level of 0.3 to 0.7 units per mL according to readily available nomograms. Anticoagulation with LMWH is equal in safety and efficacy to UFH. The initial dose of LMWH for the treatment of DVT is 1 mg per kg every 12 hours by subcutaneous injection. Young children may require higher doses, generally 1.5 mg

per kg every 12 hours. The anti-factor Xa assay is used to monitor treatment with LMWH, generally arranged 4 hours after the second or third dose. The therapeutic goal is an anti-factor Xa level of 0.5 to 1 units per mL. Once this level is achieved, further monitoring is usually unnecessary. The PTT is suboptimal as a monitoring assay, particularly in children younger than 1 year.

Once adequate anticoagulation with heparin or LMWH has been achieved, long-term therapy with subcutaneously administered LMWH or orally administered warfarin should begin. Warfarin inhibits synthesis of the vitamin K–dependent clotting factors. However, in the first few days of therapy, warfarin may disproportionately inhibit the synthesis of protein C, which is also vitamin K dependent and short lived, leading to the paradoxical effect of increased hypercoagulability. Thus, the use of warfarin as initial therapy (i.e., without heparin) should be avoided because it may cause increased clotting, which manifests as skin necrosis.

Newborns with homozygous protein C deficiency and purpura fulminans should receive fresh-frozen plasma 8 to 12 mL per kg of body weight every 12 hours. Both recombinant and plasma-derived protein C concentrates are now available. Long-term therapy includes regular infusions of fresh-frozen plasma or oral anticoagulation. Cryoprecipitate plays an analogous role in the short- and long-term therapy for homozygous protein S deficiency.

In many instances, a venous thrombosis is diagnosed in a patient without previous knowledge of an inherited hypercoagulable condition. The family history should be carefully reviewed for the occurrence of venous thrombosis or pulmonary embolus, in otherwise healthy adults, for strokes, and also for frequent miscarriages. Pretreatment plasma should be obtained for the measurement of antithrombin, protein C, and protein S. Because levels of these proteins may be transiently decreased after a large thrombosis, the diagnosis of a specific deficiency may be difficult.

It is important to understand that most pro- and anticoagulant factors are reduced at birth and only approach normal adult levels by 6 months of age. Measurement of antithrombin, protein C, and protein S levels in both parents may help clarify the diagnosis of both a possible thrombosis and a possible inherited hypercoagulable condition in the child. Molecular analysis for the FVL mutation and prothrombin mutation can be performed before or after treatment.

When venous or arterial thrombosis results in extensive thrombosis or occlusion of blood flow that poses a threat to a patient's life or to the integrity of a limb or vital organ, infusion of a thrombolytic agent can result in the dissolution of the thrombus and reestablishment of blood flow. Thrombolytic agents such as tissue plasminogen activator (tPA), streptokinase, and urokinase have been used extensively in adult practice for three decades, but tPA is the agent of choice in pediatric patients. For maximum effectiveness in the appropriate clinical setting, tPA is given as soon as possible after the symptoms begin and the extent of vascular occlusion is documented. However, thrombolysis may still be successful days to weeks after thrombus formation. Therapy can be administered systemically or directed to the distal end of the thrombosis by catheter placement. Most clinicians use tPA, 0.1 to 0.5 mg per kg per hour. Unanswered questions regarding thrombolysis in children include whether concomitant heparin infusion is safe, how long therapy can be safely administered, and how to best

shock. This condition demands vigorous fluid resuscitation with normal saline. The response to an initial bolus of 20 mL per kg saline determines the need for further therapy, such as the use of vasopressor agents (see Chapter 3). The urgency to provide adequate perfusion to the vital organs by expanding the intravascular volume takes precedence over concerns about edema in the CNS.

Hyponatremia often accompanies meningitis, resulting from water retention because of inappropriate secretion of antidiuretic hormone (SIADH). Occasionally, the oral administration of hypotonic solutions by the parents during the preceding prodromal illness may produce fluid overload and a low serum sodium (Na). If the child is believed to have seizures on the basis of acute hyponatremia, the physician may give 3% NaCl (see Chapter 100) 5 mL/kg over 15 minutes until seizure abates remainder to be infused over 1 hour. A repeat dose may be required.

After the correction of dehydration or shock, the rate of fluid administration to the child with meningitis should generally not exceed maintenance requirements (see Chapter 100). Generally, D51/2NS (dextrose and half normal saline) is used for this purpose. Failure of the serum Na to rise in the hyponatremic child mandates further restriction on hydration. The ongoing measurement of patient weight and serum electrolytes and urine specific gravity and electrolytes can be used to evaluate the need for fluid restriction.

Hypoglycemia occurs as a reaction to septicemia and stress. It is a more common concomitant of meningitis in the first 3 months of life. If the blood glucose is less than 50 mg per dL, glucose, usually as a 10–25% solution, should be given at a dosage of 0.25 to 1 g per kg. This bolus is followed by an infusion of 5% glucose and monitoring of the response. Occasionally, 10% glucose will be necessary to maintain an acceptable serum level.

Seizures occur in 20% of children with bacterial meningitis and, occasionally, in those with viral infections of the CNS, such as meningoencephalitis due to herpes simplex virus (HSV). One should always be suspicious of derangement of the glucose or sodium as a cause of convulsive activity. However, most seizures are caused by irritation of the brain from the infectious process. They are controlled in the usual fashion with diazepam or lorazepam, fosphenytoin, and phenobarbital (see Chapters 69 and 96).

Subdural effusion and, less often, empyema occur in 20% to 40% of young children with meningitis but usually appear later in the course and remain asymptomatic. In the rare case of an infant with herniation caused by a subdural collection, percutaneous drainage relieves the pressure on the brain and produces significant improvement.

Occasional children with meningitis manifest signs of increased intracranial pressure (ICP), which requires appropriate supportive therapy. Although a few preliminary studies have suggested that measures directed specifically at lowering elevated ICP may be beneficial, this approach is not part of standard therapy.

Some studies have found that dexamethasone at a dosage of 0.15 mg per kg per dose given every 6 hours to children older than 2 months mitigates the sequelae of bacterial meningitis, particularly sensorineural hearing loss. The mechanism of action has been postulated to involve inhibition of cytokine production in the CSF. Although many clinicians choose to administer dexamethasone to patients beyond the first 2 months of life in whom the diagnosis of bacterial meningitis appears highly likely, contradictory evidence exists in the literature and expert panels have withheld a definitive endorsement. If the decision is made in favor of administration, the drug should be given before or shortly after antibiotic administration, when possible, because it appears to lose its theoretical benefit after an interval or more than 4 hours.

Aseptic Meningitis

Background

The aseptic meningitis syndrome is defined here as an inflammation of the meninges that occurs in the absence of bacterial growth on routine culture media. A child whose initial CSF findings suggest an aseptic meningitis may turn out to have a purulent infection because bacteria do not always elicit a marked polymorphonuclear leukocytosis early in the course of the disease. In addition, bacteria with unusual growth requirements, inhibited by subtherapeutic concentrations of antibiotics, or sequestered in pockets adjacent to but not directly communicating with the CSF, may produce an aseptic meningitis syndrome. Last, rare patients diagnosed initially with aseptic meningitis progress over time to develop clinical signs of encephalitis.

Both infectious and noninfectious diseases cause the aseptic meningitis syndrome (Table 92.11). By far, the most common

TABLE 92.11

ASEPTIC MENINGITIS SYNDROME

Infectious
Viruses
  Early or partially treated
    Bacterial meningitis
  Parameningeal infection
  Unusual bacteria
    Leptospirosis
    Syphilis
    Tuberculosis
    Ehrlichia canis
    Borrelia burgdorferi (Lyme)
    Bartonella henselae (Cat scratch)
Mycoplasma
Rickettsia
Fungi
  Cryptococcus
  Candida
Parasites
  Trichinosis
  Toxoplasmosis
  Cysticercosis
  Malaria
  Naegleria

Noninfectious
Neoplasm
Hemorrhage
Hypersensitivity reactions
Heavy metal poisoning
Collagen vascular disease
Sarcoidosis
Kawasaki disease (? infectious)

cause is viral meningitis; however, the clinician should be alert to Lyme disease in endemic regions and to unusual pathogens in patients who are immunocompromised or who show atypical clinical features. Despite underreporting, the Centers for Disease Control and Prevention (CDC) notes about 5,000 cases annually in the United States.

Aseptic meningitis occurs throughout the year. Because the incidence of enteroviral infections, which are responsible for a large number of the cases, peaks in the summer in temperate regions, outbreaks of aseptic meningitis are more often seen in the warm months.

Pathophysiology

The multiple causes of aseptic meningitis syndrome produce inflammation of the meninges by different mechanisms. Even among the viral infections, the pathogenesis varies considerably. Some viruses lead to an immune reaction in the CNS, whereas others invade the neural tissue directly. Access to the meninges is usually hematogenous but may be achieved by ascension along peripheral nerves.

Clinical Manifestations

The signs and symptoms of aseptic meningitis resemble those of bacterial infections of the CNS but are not usually as severe. The infant shows only lethargy and irritability, whereas the older child complains of a headache, photophobia, and stiff neck. Vomiting may occur and may be persistent. There is often a history of a concomitant upper respiratory or GI viral illness. Fever usually occurs. The infant may appear toxic, but the older child may remain remarkably well. Nuchal rigidity in a patient who is alert and conversant suggests aseptic, rather than bacterial, meningitis. Shining a flashlight in the eyes often elicits photophobia. The fontanel of the infant generally maintains a normal configuration but may bulge rarely. Aside from occasional positive Kernig and Brudzinski signs, the neurologic examination often shows no abnormalities. An altered level of consciousness or focal neurologic deficit points to meningoencephalitis rather than aseptic meningitis (see Chapter 96).

Management

In addition to the routine CSF studies, children with aseptic meningitis usually require a CBC count, electrolytes, and a BUN. In regions where Lyme disease is endemic, consideration should be give to serologic testing for Borrelia. Most patients need no further tests, but in atypical situations, consideration should always be given to nonviral causes that may mandate additional diagnostic steps or specific therapy. If tuberculosis is suspected based on family contacts, a low CSF glucose with lymphocytic predominance, or pulmonary findings, then a Mantoux test and chest radiograph are useful for confirmation. In endemic areas, serologic studies for Lyme disease and antibiotic therapy may be indicated based on exposure history and time of year. A computed tomography (CT) scan provides essential information about patients with symptoms or signs of a parameningeal infection, HSV encephalitis, or CNS tumors and hemorrhages. Immunosuppressed patients develop infections with a wide variety of unusual bacteria, fungi, and parasites that can be identified in many cases with appropriate examination and culture of the CSF (India ink and acid-fast stains, cryptococcal antigen testing, fungal and mycobacterial cultures). In particular when dealing with infants in the first month of life, the physician must remain alert to the possibility of a HSV infection and consider both obtaining a PCR for HSV and initiating acyclovir therapy (60 mg per kg per day IV in three divided doses).

Therapy for the common viral infections does not currently extend beyond supportive care. Dehydration from prolonged emesis may necessitate IV fluid administration. After any deficit has been corrected, the rate should be set to provide 75% to 100% of the daily maintenance requirement to avoid overhydration and the possible aggravation of cerebral edema in the child who develops an encephalitic component.

Because the CSF findings in aseptic meningitis overlap those in bacterial infections, hospital admission is usually warranted until the CSF culture results are available. However, the experienced clinician may choose to follow the older child as an outpatient if the family is reliable and nonviral causes (e.g., Lyme Disease, tuberculosis, cryptococcosis) are clinically unlikely. Generally, to qualify for discharge with aseptic meningitis, a patient must have all CSF parameters pointing away from bacterial infection, for example, less than 500 cells per mm^3, less than 50% polymorphonuclear leukocytes, protein less than 100 mg per dL, and glucose greater than 30 mg per dL.

UPPER RESPIRATORY TRACT INFECTIONS

Infections in children involve the upper respiratory tract more often than any other region of the body. Included in this category are nasopharyngitis (common cold), stomatitis, pharyngitis, sinusitis, otitis, peritonsillar abscess, retropharyngeal and parapharyngeal abscesses, laryngotracheobronchitis (croup), and epiglottitis. The most common causative organism varies between sites as does the diagnostic and therapeutic approach. As a result it is useful to divide these infections into specific anatomic diagnoses to guide the clinician in further management.

Nasopharyngitis

Nasopharyngitis (URI), or the common cold, is a viral illness of the upper respiratory tract in children. The most commonly isolated organisms are the rhinoviruses and coronaviruses. Prospective family studies have shown that five or six episodes occur yearly during childhood. The illness is characterized by a fever lower than 39°C (102.2°F) and coryza. There may be a mild conjunctivitis and infection of the pharynx. Although the tympanic membranes may show a dull appearance and decreased mobility, the characteristic features of acute purulent OM (erythema, loss of the landmarks, and bulging) are absent. Therapy is limited to a recommendation for rest, adequate hydration, and antipyretic agents. Neither antibiotic nor decongestant therapy prevent secondary bacterial infections such as acute purulent OM. The use of antiviral agents or immunomodulatory therapy is not recommended.

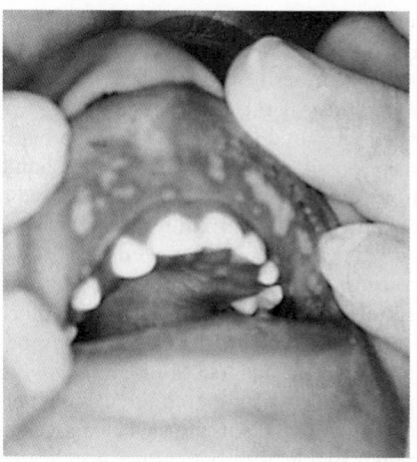

FIGURE 92.4 Lesions of herpetic stomatitis.

Stomatitis

Stomatitis, an infection of the mouth, is caused by herpes simplex and the coxsackieviruses at any age and by *Candida albicans* ("thrush") in the infant (see Chapters 122 and 123) or in the immunosuppressed child. Viral infections cause vesicular lesions initially (Fig. 92.4) and ulcerations and plaques subsequently. Some coxsackieviruses may involve the hands and feet (Fig. 92.5A) as well as the mouth (coxsackievirus hand-foot-mouth syndrome), and herpetic stomatitis may be complicated by spread of infection to the digits, which is called herpetic whitlow (Fig. 92.5B). For otherwise healthy patients, treatment is limited to systemic antipyretic and analgesic drugs and the local application of topical analgesics, such as 2% viscous Xylocaine® (do not exceed 3 mg/kg/dose) or the combination of Maalox® and diphenhydramine. IV or oral acyclovir, oral valacyclovir or oral famciclovir minimally shorten the course of disease in immunocompetent patients with stomatitis due to

HSV if started within the first 24 hours of onset but should not be used routinely. Unless adequate hydration is ensured (typically the admitted patient receiving parenteral fluids) there is an increased risk of renal toxicity with these drugs. Therapy with one of these agents is recommended for HSV stomatitis in immunosuppressed patients but again hydration must be ensured.

C. albicans produces white plaques on the mucosa that bleed if scraped. Nystatin swish and swallow suspension (200,000 units four times daily) leads to a prompt resolution of this condition. Oral fluconazole is also an effective treatment but is not routinely indicated for the immunocompetent host.

Pharyngitis

Pharyngitis (see Chapter 71) is an infection of the throat (including the tonsils). In the immunocompetent child, several viruses, perhaps *Mycoplasma pneumoniae*, *Chlamydophyla pneumoniae*, and *Arcanobacterium haemolyticum*, and only a few bacteria cause pharyngitis. Common viral isolates include the adenoviruses, influenza viruses, enteroviruses (including coxsackievirus), parainfluenza viruses, and the Epstein-Barr virus (EBV). Although many bacteria may cause pharyngitis, only three organisms (group A streptococci, *Corynebacterium diphtheriae,* and *Neisseria gonorrhoeae*) have well-defined roles. Of these, only group A streptococcal infections have relevance to most clinical situations in children.

Pharyngitis is a common infection in children. Moffet et al. reported that 128 of 230 visits to an infirmary by youngsters of school age at a children's home were for pharyngeal infections. Group A streptococcus causes almost 50% of such infections between 5 and 15 years of age but is uncommon in the first 3 years of life. In one study of 50 children younger than 3 years old with exudative pharyngitis, only 7 had illness from group A streptococci.

For practical purposes, isolated pharyngitis can be considered as streptococcal (bacterial) or nonstreptococcal (viral).

MEDICAL EMERGENCIES

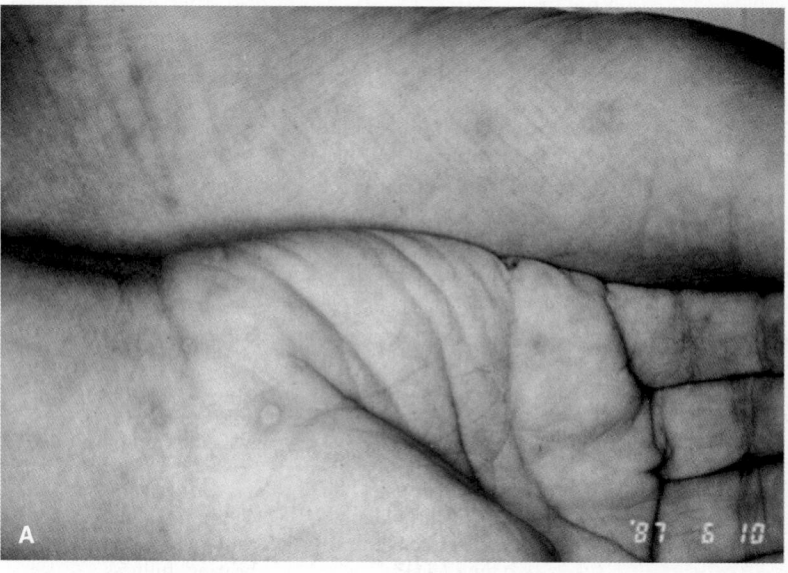
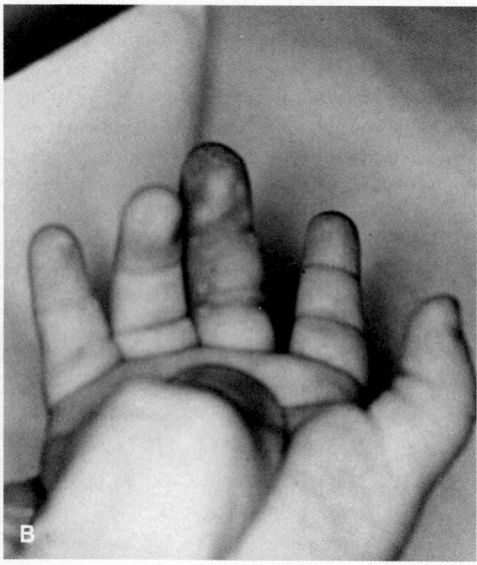

FIGURE 92.5 **A:** Vesicles in coxsackievirus hand-foot-mouth syndrome. **B:** Herpetic whitlow.

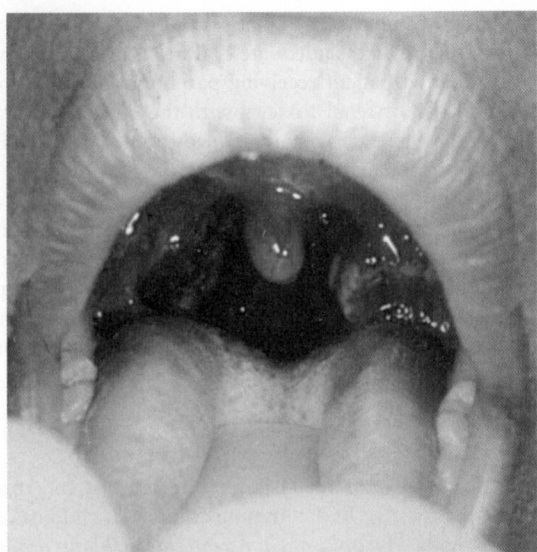

FIGURE 92.6 Examination of the pharynx in a child with streptococcal infection shows enlarged, erythematous tonsils with exudate.

Because the symptoms of the two types overlap, the physician can reliably distinguish the more important streptococcal infections only with the aid of the laboratory. However, certain clinical features favor a bacterial cause. Group A streptococcal pharyngitis is more likely to have an abrupt onset with fever and sore throat; whereas cough and coryza are uncommon. Examination of the pharynx reveals an erythematous pharyngeal mucosa, enlarged tonsils and exudate (Fig. 92.6) occasionally with petechiae on the posterior palate. In addition, the anterior cervical lymph nodes often become enlarged and tender.

Although unusual, complications may occur with bacterial pharyngitis; both suppurative and nonsuppurative sequelae can result from streptococcal infections. The latter category includes acute rheumatic fever and glomerulonephritis. Viral pharyngitis resolves spontaneously in 2 to 5 days with the exception of EBV, as discussed under the "Infectious Mononucleosis" section.

In the ambulatory setting, a tonsillar swab for antigen detection by latex agglutination or optical immunoassay should be obtained from children with pharyngeal inflammation and those who complain of sore throat, unless the diagnosis of a generalized viral syndrome can be confidently established on clinical grounds. If the test for antigen is positive the child is treated with penicillin. Although a single intramuscular injection of benzathine penicillin (600,000 units if less than 28 kg and 1.2 million units if 28 kg or more) obviates all prob-

lems with compliance, oral penicillin VK (250 mg per dose for children and 500 mg per dose for adolescents, given two to three times per day) prescribed for 10 days serves as standard therapy. Amoxicillin (40 mg per kg per day, given in two divided doses) may be used in place of penicillin but offers no advantage except possibly improved taste in the liquid preparation. Erythromycin (40 mg per kg per day) is used for penicillin-allergic children; azithromycin for 5 days (12 mg per kg once daily for 5 days, maximum single dose 500 mg) represents a more expensive alternative. Unlike the penicillins, resistance to macrolides may occur with group A streptococci and the rates of resistance, while generally low, may be high in some areas. Antipyretic agents, fluids, and adequate rest should be recommended. Among children with pharyngitis suggestive of streptococcal disease for which antigen detection is negative or unavailable, a throat culture is indicated. While awaiting the results of culture, one may choose to treat presumptively children with severe pharyngitis characteristic of streptococcal disease and those unable to reliably return for follow-up. Because antibiotics shorten the course of acute course of streptococcal pharyngitis only minimally, there is no reason to give these drugs hastily before confirming a bacterial cause. The prevention of nonsuppurative complications is generally accomplished even if treatment awaits confirmation by culture. Institution of a liquid diet and acetaminophen provide some symptomatic relief. In selected circumstances special culture methods should be employed, e.g. when *N. gonorrhoeae*, group C or group G streptococci are considered. *N. gonorrhoeae* should be considered in the sexually active adolescent and group C and group G streptococci may be considered in local outbreaks of pharyngitis where group A streptococci is known not to be the cause.

Otitis Media

Background

Otitis media refers to suppuration and inflammation within the middle ear. The disease can be further classified according to the associated clinical symptoms, specific otoscopic findings, duration, and occurrence of complications. Currently, the disease is divided into two broad categories (Table 92.12): acute otitis media (AOM) and otitis media with effusion (OME). AOM (formerly called acute purulent otitis media) is caused by an acute bacterial (or occasionally viral) infection, has a sudden onset, and usually causes symptoms. However, OME (formerly called serous otitis media) is not primarily bacterial in origin, has a more gradual onset, and often remains asymptomatic. A great deal of overlap exists between these two entities, such that clinical differentiation at a single

TABLE 92.12

CLASSIFICATION OF OTITIS MEDIA

Type	Duration	Bacteriology	Tympanum	Signs and symptoms
Acute otitis media	Days to weeks	Isolates in 70%	Erythematous or purulent, bulging	Fever (30%), earache (older child), irritability
Otitis media with effusion	Weeks to months	Occasional isolates	Dull, retracted, fluid level	Asymptomatic, decreased hearing, fullness

point in time may not be possible. The bacterial flora of middle ear infections varies somewhat with age. Although gram-negative enteric bacilli and *S. aureus* cause 15% to 20% of AOM during the first month of life, *S. pneumoniae*, *H. influenzae*, and *Branhamella catarrhalis* predominate at all ages, even in the neonate. *S. pneumoniae* can be recovered from about 40% and *H. influenzae* and *B. catarrhalis* each from 20% of children with AOM between 1 month and 10 years of age. Among older children and adolescents, *H. influenzae* decreases in frequency but remains a significant pathogen. More than 90% of the *H. influenzae* that cause AOM are nontypeable,. Most *H. influenzae* and *Moraxella catarrhalis* are resistant to ampicillin and thus penicillin and amoxicillin. Among pneumococci, the incidence of penicillin resistance varies geographically and continues to evolve; at present, on average, 10% to 30% of these organisms exhibit decreased susceptibility to beta lactam antibiotics.

AOM concerns the emergency physician to a far greater extent than OME. It is the most common bacterial infection in children, affecting an estimated 9 million children annually. Howie et al. found at least one episode of OM in two-thirds of 2-year-old children in their practice, and one in seven children had more than six episodes. Teele et al. reported an average of 0.4 to 1.2 episodes of OM annually among children from birth to age 7 years. AOM is more common in the winter in temperate climates. This is presumably related to the higher incidence of URIs during the colder months.

Pathophysiology

Any discussion of the pathophysiology of OM provokes great controversy among pediatricians and otolaryngologists alike. However, it appears that abnormal function of the eustachian tube contributes to the development of OM in most cases. Possible mechanisms for obstruction of the eustachian tube include hypertrophied nasopharyngeal lymphoid tissue or intrinsic abnormalities of the various components of this structure. Whatever the cause, blockage impairs ventilation of the middle ear, leading to an accumulation of fluid behind the tympanic membrane. This effusion then provides a fertile environment for the proliferation of bacteria from the heavily colonized nasopharynx.

Clinical Manifestations

Studies by Howie, Paradise, Klein, and others showed the variable spectrum of OM. An infection in the middle ear may produce no symptoms, being detected only on examination, or it may cause obvious localizing pain. In the young child, the initial manifestation is often not otologic but rather fever, irritability, or diarrhea. Children older than the age of 3 years generally, but not invariably, complain of pain in the ear. Less common symptoms include vertigo and hearing impairment.

Fever occurs in 25% to 35% of children with AOM. The diagnosis of AOM rests in the usual clinical settings on the accurate interpretation of the otoscopic findings, a skill gained only by experience with the pneumatic otoscope (Fig. 92.7). If cerumen obscures the tympanic membrane, a sufficient quantity must be cleared to allow adequate visualization. Either a blunt curette or an apparatus for irrigation adequately removes such material in most cases.

The tympanic membrane in AOM typically bulges out at the examiner as a result of the positive pressure generated by the production of purulent material in the middle ear cavity. Although the drum is sometimes red, it may appear white or yellow because of the exudate behind it. A convex contour of the drum secondary to an effusion in the child suspected of having AOM is sufficient to make this diagnosis, regardless of the color of the membrane. The diffuse injection of the normal tympanum, which is often exaggerated by crying, should not be confused with the intense erythema of infection.

Difficulty arises in differentiating AOM from OME and in diagnosing "early" AOM, particularly in the child with a pre-existing middle ear effusion. The tympanic membrane has decreased mobility in both AOM and OME; however, it is usually retracted in the latter condition. During the course of a single examination, the physician may be unable to differentiate with any certainty; in such cases, it is safest to assume a bacterial cause.

The WBC count, not indicated in a routine case, usually falls within the normal range or shows a mild leukocytosis, when obtained. Tympanocentesis, when performed, yields an organism in 60% to 70% of cases. Blood cultures are not more or less likely to reveal a pathogen among children with AOM compared to children with comparable fever without AOM. Acute complications occur only occasionally with AOM, subsequent to the advent of effective antibiotics. Local suppuration may involve the mastoids and rarely leads to meningitis, epidural or subdural abscess or brain abscess. Perforations of the tympanic membrane generally heal spontaneously (see Chapter 110). A child with OM in the first year or two of life may develop dehydration from vomiting and diarrhea associated with the infection.

Management

Uncomplicated AOM in the child older than 1 month should be treated with oral antibiotic therapy on an outpatient basis. Amoxicillin (90 mg per kg per day in two or three divided doses for 10 days) is the drug of choice in the United States. The most reasonable alternatives include (i) high concentration amoxicillin with clavulanic acid in a 14:1 formulation (90 mg per kg per day of amoxicillin in two divided doses for 10 days); (ii) cefdinir [14 mg per kg per day (maximum single dose 600 mg) given once daily for 10 days]; (iii) azithromycin [30 mg per kg (maximum 1,500 mg) as a single dose]; and (iv) ceftriaxone (50 mg per kg intramuscularly as a single dose). Cefuroxime axetil (30 mg per kg per day in two divided doses for 10 days) is an additional choice. Cephalosporins and azithromycin can be used in children with a history of penicillin allergy, but the latter agent has not been extensively studied. Intramuscular ceftriaxone has an advantage in children with persistent vomiting and perhaps in those at high risk of occult bacteremia, and also obviates the issue of compliance in high-risk social situations. Whether the course of therapy must be 10 days (except for single-dose ceftriaxone and azithromycin) or can be shortened is controversial. Most authorities believe antibiotics administered for 5 days are sufficient in children older than 2 years with uncomplicated AOM but prefer the longer course in infants. Antihistamines and decongestants have not hastened the resolution of AOM in published studies and are thus not indicated. It should not be forgotten that there is often pain associated with AOM and, therefore, the use of analgesics should be considered as well.

If AOM persists during therapy with amoxicillin or recurs within 2 days of its discontinuance, ampicillin-resistant

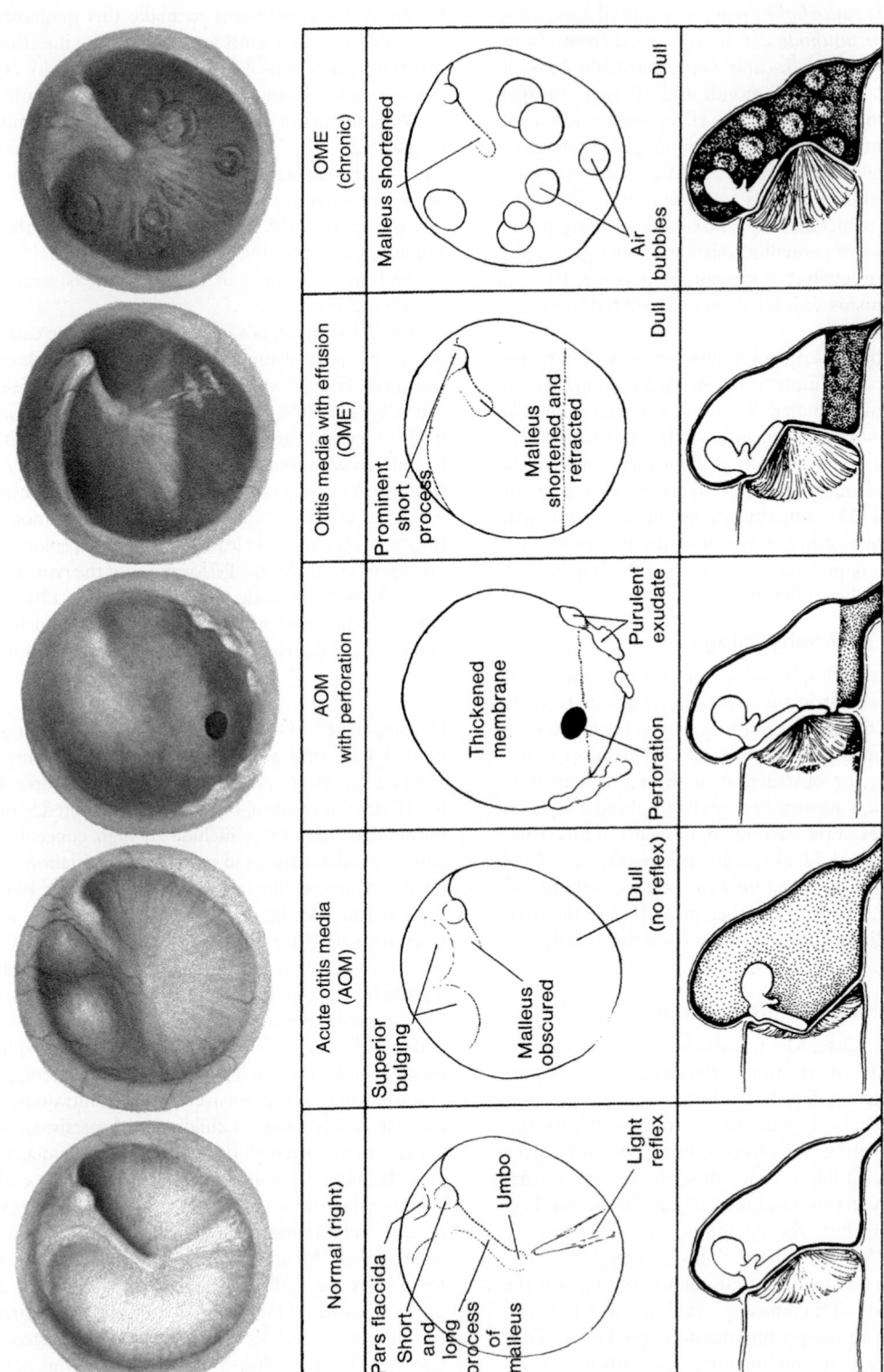

FIGURE 92.7 Appearance of the tympanic membrane in different types of otitis media.

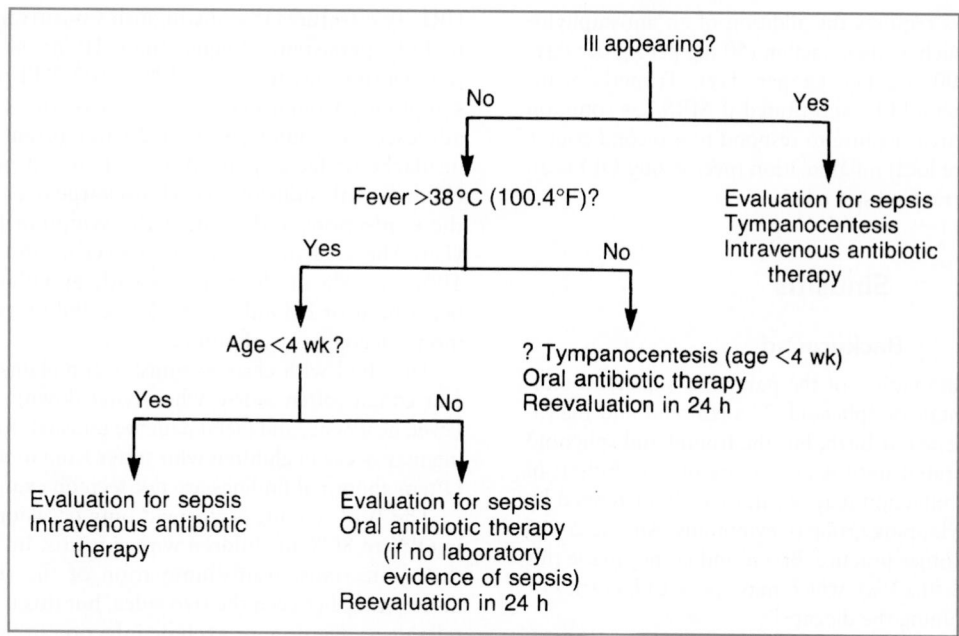

FIGURE 92.8 Diagnostic approach for the management of acute otitis media in the very young infant.

organisms are likely the cause of the infection if compliance with medication is assured. The alternatives to amoxicillin represent reasonable agents for a second course, and no compelling data favor any particular regimen. Failure of such a second course of antibiotics to eradicate the infection necessitates a third course of antibiotic therapy and merits consideration of a tympanocentesis for culture.

The management of AOM in the first month of life has provoked controversy because of (i) the occurrence of gram-negative enteric bacilli and *S. aureus* in middle ear infections in these children, and (ii) the decreased ability of the neonate to resist infection (Fig. 92.8). If a child younger than 1 month presents with fever or irritability and is found to have OM, in the opinion of many, admission for IV antibiotic therapy provides the safest course pending the outcome of cultures of the blood, urine, and CSF. Afebrile infants in the first month of life may be treated as outpatients with the usual oral antibiotics used for older patients and with careful follow-up.

Infants between 4 and 12 weeks of age with OM can be managed as outpatients because *S. pneumoniae, H. influenzae,* and *B. catarrhalis* are the predominant organisms. However, other sources of infection, including meningitis, must be excluded in the febrile child before attributing the source of a temperature elevation to OM alone.

Otitis Externa

Otitis externa (OE), or swimmer's ear, is an infection of the auditory canal and external surface of the tympanic membrane that spares the middle ear. Multiple organisms, particularly *Pseudomonas aeruginosa,* play a role in this disease. There is usually a history of recent swimming, but occasional cases are seen in children whose only submersion occurs during normal bathing. The first symptom is itching of the ear canal. The child complains subsequently of an earache that may be uni-

lateral or bilateral, and purulent material often drains from the ear. Fever is never present unless cellulitis or another illness is associated. Unlike AOM, pulling on the ear lobe to straighten the canal in preparation for otoscopic examination elicits marked tenderness. A cheesy white or gray-green exudate fills the canal in more than 50% of patients, often obscuring the tympanum.

OE is at times confused with AOM. Although both may cause earache (see Chapter 54), the signs and symptoms usually make an exact diagnosis possible. Occasionally, the physician cannot distinguish OE from AOM with perforation and must treat for both disorders.

Treatment consists of removing the inflammatory debris from the ear canal, eliminating pathogenic bacteria, providing symptomatic relief, and controlling predisposing factors. Usually, dry mopping of the exudate with a cotton-tipped wire applicator cleanses the canal adequately; occasionally, gentle suction is also necessary. The patient should be given commercially available otic drops and a mild analgesic, such as aspirin or acetaminophen. Acetic acid solutions (Otic-Domeboro® or Vosol®) and the combination antibiotic–corticosteroid preparations (Cortisporin®, Lidosporin®), four drops instilled four times daily, or fluoroquinolines (ofloxacin and ciprofloxacin) are effective. The fluoroquinolines are more expensive but offer the advantages of fewer local allergic reactions and once daily administration. In cases with known or suspected perforations, suspensions (but not solutions) are preferred. For the occasional case of a patient with an edematous canal and thick exudate, a wick of cotton or gauze should be inserted 10 to 12 mm into the canal after cleansing to facilitate entry of the medications. All patients should be instructed to avoid swimming or to wear appropriately fitted earplugs until cured.

Children who return without improvement after initial therapy should be examined to be certain they have OE. If this diagnosis is confirmed, the canal should be cleansed again and an alternate medication prescribed. The occurrence of a local cellulitis or adenitis requires the addition of an antistaphylo-coccal antibiotic, such as dicloxacillin (50 mg per kg per day) or cephalexin (100 mg per kg per day). Trimethoprim-sulfamethoxazole should be substituted if MRSA is common in the geographic area. Failure to respond to a second course of therapy or severe local inflammation (necrotizing OE) is an indication for referral to a specialist.

Sinusitis

Background

Sinusitis is an inflammation of the paranasal sinuses: maxillary, ethmoid, frontal, or sphenoid. The ethmoid and maxillary sinuses are present at birth, but the frontal and sphenoid do not become aerated until 4 or 7 years of age. Either an acute or a chronic infection may occur, each characterized by a different but overlapping group of symptoms. Among 2,613 patients seen in an office practice, Breese and Disney made this diagnosis in only 6 (0.23%), which may speak to its rarity or difficulty in ascertaining the diagnosis.

Wald et al. studied the bacteriology of sinusitis in children using cultures of material obtained by antral puncture. They recovered 47 organisms from 30 children: 17, *S. pneumoniae*; 11, nontypeable *H. influenzae*; 9, *M. catarrhalis*; 2, *Streptococcus viridans*; 7, group A streptococcus; and 1, *Moraxella* species. Hamory et al. found a similar spectrum of pathogens in adults with maxillary sinusitis. Although anaerobic organisms and *S. aureus* have been reported occasionally, they do not play a role in most of these infections seen in children. *H. influenzae* type b formerly caused ethmoiditis and periorbital cellulitis with great frequency but now occurs rarely.

Pathophysiology

Infection of the sinuses arises in a fashion similar to that described for AOM. Organisms ascend from the nasopharynx and cause disease if the mucosal barrier of the sinus or the normal pattern of drainage has been altered.

Clinical Manifestations

The presentation of acute sinusitis varies in some respects with the child's age. Usually, the infection follows a viral URI. Two features that distinguish sinusitis from a viral URI include persistent (longer than 10 days) and/or severe [temperature greater than 39°C (102.2°F) beyond 3 days] symptoms. Cough occurs in 75% of the patients. Unlike adolescents, young children do not often complain of a headache or facial pain. A fever is noted in about half of children with sinusitis. Nasal discharge occurs in almost all these infections and is often the symptom that prompts a visit. The area of the face that overlies the sinus swells in 10% to 20% of the patients with maxillary disease, and periorbital or orbital edema and cellulitis even more commonly accompany ethmoiditis.

The child with chronic sinusitis complains only of persistent cough (often worse when lying down) and rhinorrhea. Fever, headache, and facial pain are unusual. Recurrent wheezing may occur in children who suffer from underlying asthma. Often, abnormal findings are not seen on examination.

The WBC count, performed only occasionally, is normal in 60% to 80% of children with sinusitis. In 10% to 30% of these infections, transillumination of the sinuses shows a discrepancy between the two sides, but this is not sufficiently reliable to diagnose or exclude infection in the sinuses. Plain radiographs are abnormal in almost every child with sinusitis (Fig. 92.9); there may be an air–fluid level, complete opacification, or mucosal thickening (greater than 4 mm). Of 60 sinuses in 30 children evaluated radiographically by Wald et al., 4 were normal, 38 showed complete opacification, 15 showed mucosal thickening, and 3 showed an air–fluid level. Hamory et al. obtained radiographs on 43 patients with 58 episodes of sinusitis. Eighteen had an air–fluid level, 18 had opacification, 12 had mucosal thickening, and 10 had no abnormalities. A CT scan is more sensitive for diagnosis than plain radiograph but is not needed in routine cases. Unfortunately sinuses may be opacified with simple viral upper respiratory tract infections and, therefore, an abnormal radiographic study may be seen without bacterial sinusitis.

Although sinusitis usually responds to oral antibiotic therapy, serious complications occasionally result from the local spread of the suppuration. These include orbital infection, brain abscess, epidural or subdural empyema, and cavernous sinus thrombosis. Proptosis and paralysis of the extraocular muscles point to the accumulation of purulent material within

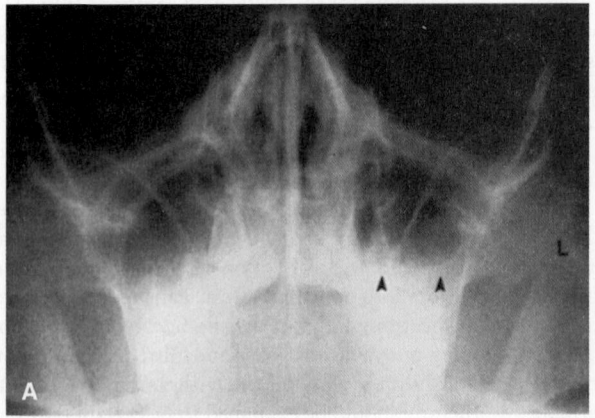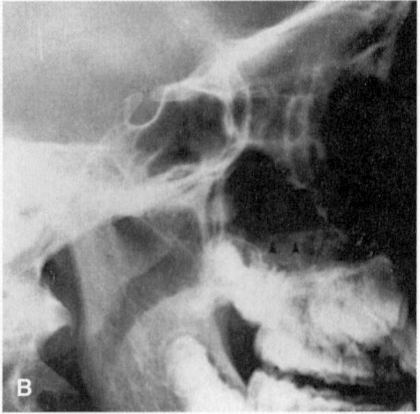

FIGURE 92.9 Anteroposterior (**A**) and lateral (**B**) radiographs show an air–fluid level in the left maxillary sinus *(arrowheads)* and mucoperiosteal thickening on the right side.

the orbit. After intracranial extension, the child appears toxic and usually has a detectable neurologic deficit.

Management

Children suspected of having acute sinusitis with severe symptoms or an uncertain clinical picture should have a radiograph evaluation of their sinuses. Among this group of patients clinically believed to be at risk for an infection, any abnormality (air–fluid level, opacification, or mucosal thickening) suffices to confirm the diagnosis. Afebrile children with chronic sinusitis diagnosed on the basis of persistent nasal discharge need no laboratory or radiographic evaluation. Possible indications for antral puncture and aspiration of the sinus include (i) associated life-threatening infection, (ii) immunocompromise, (iii) persistent illness despite therapy, and (iv) unusually severe disease. Amoxicillin (90 mg per kg per day divided into two or three daily doses) effectively treats the common pathogens, *S. pneumoniae* and nontypeable *H. influenzae*, in most cases. Current recommendations call for antibiotic therapy for 10 days although patients with chronic symptoms or underlying risk factors may require 14 to 21 days of therapy. Alternative drugs for penicillin-allergic children and those with recurrent disease are the same as for OM. Children with acute sinusitis require admission if they appear ill, have facial swelling and tenderness, or develop any complications.

Peritonsillar Abscess

A peritonsillar abscess, or "quinsy," results from the accumulation of purulent material within the tonsillar fossa. Adolescents develop this condition more often than younger children. Group A streptococci, various anaerobic organisms, and occasionally *S. aureus* are isolated from these lesions, which are unusual when compared to the frequency of uncomplicated tonsillopharyngitis.

The complaints of trismus and difficulty in speaking separate a peritonsillar abscess from the far more common pharyngitis. The voice sounds muffled, and the child drools profusely. Both tonsils may swell, but the enlargement of one is typically much more pronounced. Usually, the abscessed tonsil becomes sufficiently large to push the uvula to the opposite side of the pharynx, and the examiner may be able to palpate a fluctuant mass intraorally. The WBC count is often elevated but not needed for diagnosis.

All children with a peritonsillar abscess should have the lesion drained in the ED or, if admitted, after admission to the hospital followed by treatment with antibiotics. Amoxicillin (40 mg per kg per day divided into three daily doses) or amoxicillin-clavunate (40 mg per kg per day of amoxicillin component divided into three daily doses) are common oral selections. Ampicillin-sulbactam (200 mg per kg per day IV divided into four daily doses) or clindamycin (30 mg per kg per day IV divided into four daily doses) represent typical initial therapy. In the unusual case of a child with respiratory compromise, aspiration or drainage of the abscess can be life saving. This is accomplished by using an 18-gauge needle mounted on a 10-mL syringe or with a scalpel (see Chapter 123).

Cervical Lymphadenitis

Background

Cervical lymphadenitis is a bacterial infection of the lymph nodes in the neck. This condition must be distinguished from lymphadenopathy, an enlargement of one or more lymph nodes that occurs with viral infections, or as a reaction to bacterial disease in structures that drain to the nodes.

S. aureus and group A streptococci are the cause of acute suppurative lymphadenitis in most children with an identifiable pathogen. Of 74 children with this condition, Barton and Feigin isolated *S. aureus* from 27 (36%) and group A streptococci from 19 (26%). Other organisms that play a role in more chronic cases include mycobacteria and *Bartonella henselae* [cat-scratch disease (CSD)]. Rare causes include *Yersinia pestis* (plague), gram-negative bacilli, *H. influenzae* type b, *Francisella tularensis*, *Actinomyces*, and *Nocardia*.

Pathophysiology

The causative organisms in cervical adenitis initially colonize the nares or pharynx, or less commonly are inoculated transcutaneously. Dental abscesses may also be a source of pathogens. Regardless of whether they produce a local infection at the portal of entry, the bacteria can spread to the lymph nodes in the neck. If not contained by the immune system, they proliferate within the node and evoke an inflammatory response.

Clinical Manifestations

The child with cervical lymphadenitis is usually noted to have swelling in the neck. If sufficiently old, he or she will complain of pain. Fever occurs only occasionally, more often in children younger than 1 year. The infected node may vary in size from 2 cm to more than 10 cm. Initially, it has a firm consistency, but fluctuance (Fig. 92.10) develops in about 25% of the infected nodes. The skin overlying the node becomes erythematous, and there may be associated edema.

The WBC count is usually normal but may be elevated in the younger, febrile child. Aspiration of the node often identifies the organism by both Gram stain and culture, even if fluctuance is

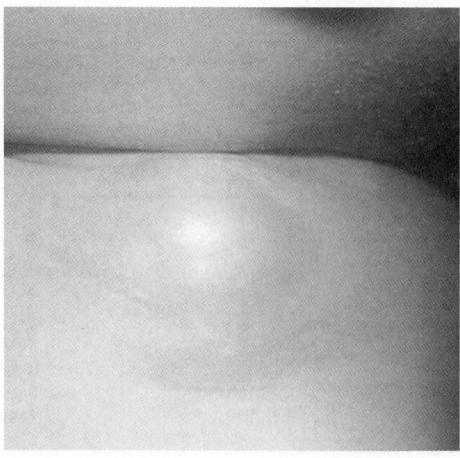

FIGURE 92.10 Lymphadenitis in the inferior cervical chain. The node appears fluctuant.

not appreciated. Children with infections from *Mycobacterium tuberculosis* usually react to the standard purified protein derivative (PPD-S) skin test and may have changes compatible with tuberculosis seen on chest radiograph.

Complications of bacterial adenitis are unusual. Organisms such as *S. aureus* and group A streptococci can spread locally if unchecked. A draining sinus tract may develop in untreated children with atypical mycobacterial adenitis. Recurrence of infection suggests a local anatomic abnormality (e.g., branchial cleft cyst) or immunocompromising conditions such as chronic granulomatous disease.

Management

Figure 92.11 outlines the management of the child with cervical lymphadenitis. Children with cervical adenitis who are otherwise healthy should receive an antibiotic effective against *S. aureus* and the group A streptococci. Agents such as dicloxacillin (50 mg per kg per day) and cephalexin (50 mg per kg per day) have activity against both organisms. In more severe infections, oxacillin (100 to 200 mg per kg per day in four divided doses) can be administered intravenously. If the node is fluctuant, aspiration provides useful etiologic information and speeds the rate of resolution. All children with lymphadenitis should have a PPD skin test and be followed until the infection subsides. Clindamycin (15 to 25 mg per kg per day in three divided doses PO or 30 mg per kg per day IV) or vancomycin (40 mg per kg per day in four divided doses IV) offers alternatives in the face of penicillin and/or cephalosporin allergy or in geographic areas where coverage for methicillin-resistant *S. aureus* (MRSA) must be considered.

Children younger than 3 months and those who appear toxic or who have developed a draining sinus are best managed in the hospital. A failure to improve with oral antibiotic therapy or a positive skin test for tuberculosis necessitates subsequent hospitalization.

Retropharyngeal and Lateral Pharyngeal Abscess

A retropharyngeal abscess fills the potential space between the anterior border of the cervical vertebrae and the posterior wall of the esophagus. The usual pathogens are group A streptococci, anaerobic organisms, and occasionally *S. aureus*. These infections occur most often in children younger than 4 years. A lateral pharyngeal (or parapharyngeal) abscess occurs in the deep soft-tissue space of the neck, but not in the midline, and is less common than a retropharyngeal infection.

The child with a retropharyngeal abscess may develop a clinical picture similar to that seen with epiglottitis, with a change in voice, high fever and a toxic appearance, but the onset is less abrupt; as purulent material collects, the fluctuant mass obstructs the larynx and esophagus, leading to stridor and drooling. Findings in less acute presentations include sore throat, neck pain, especially with movement of the neck from side to side, cervical lymphadenopathy, and, less commonly, torticollis. Inflammation surrounding the abscess may lead to meningismus; thus, this diagnosis should be considered in the child with nuchal rigidity but no pleocytosis in the CSF.

Although a retropharyngeal infection can rarely be seen as a midline swelling on examination of the pharynx, it is usually difficult to observe this finding in the uncooperative child. If the diagnosis is suspected and the airway is not threatened, a lateral neck radiograph or CT scan should be obtained. The radiograph shows an increase in the width of the soft tissues anterior to the vertebrae and, on occasion, an air–fluid level. In the child without retropharyngeal infection, the width of the retropharyngeal space is less than the width of the adjacent vertebral body in the young child at the upper cervical vertebrae (C2, C3) if the examination is performed with the neck properly extended. For children approaching school age and beyond the width of this space is typically less than half of the adjacent vertebral body at the mid cervical spine if the neck is properly extended.

A lateral pharyngeal abscess causes virtually identical symptoms to an infection in the retropharyngeal area. One important difference is that a lateral pharyngeal abscess, which is not well visualized by radiograph, requires a CT scan for confirmation. If sedation is to be given to facilitate CT imaging then consideration should be given to the possible need to secure the airway.

A retropharyngeal or lateral pharyngeal abscess poses a risk to the patency of the airway. All children with this infection should have careful monitoring in the ED and then be hospitalized in consultation with an otolaryngologist. Unless the airway is in immediate jeopardy, IV access should be secured and treatment given with either clindamycin (30 mg per kg per day in four divided doses) or ampicillin/sulbactam (ampicillin 200 mg per kg day in four divided doses). In the event of respiratory compromise, intubation or, less commonly, tracheotomy becomes necessary. Patients with smaller abscesses or phlegmon may be treated with antibiotic therapy alone; those with larger collections or persistent fever despite

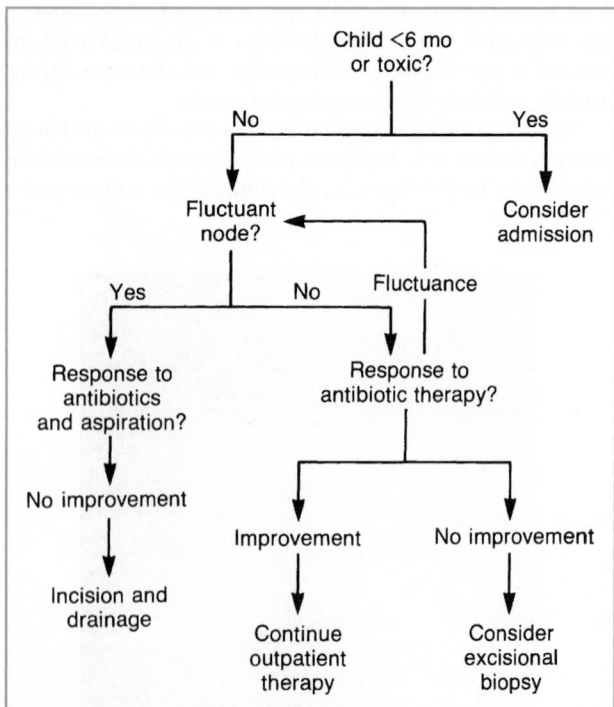

FIGURE 92.11 Diagnostic approach for the management of the child with presumed bacterial lymphadenitis.

therapy will require drainage, either transcutaneously with ultrasound guidance or at surgery.

Laryngotracheobronchitis (Croup)

Background

Croup, or laryngotracheobronchitis, is a viral infection that involves the larynx and may extend into the trachea and bronchi. It is a common infection, with thousands of cases of croup to every one of epiglottitis. Although most children with croup are treated as outpatients, some develop more pronounced respiratory distress and require hospitalization. Hoekelman reported that 3 (1.2%) of 246 healthy term infants in a pediatric practice developed croup during their first year of life. This infection is the most common cause for stridor in the febrile child (see Chapter 72).

Parainfluenza virus can be recovered from about 60% of children with croup. Additional causes of the disease are influenza, adenoviruses, measles, and respiratory syncytial virus (RSV). Bacteria play no role.

Croup occurs more commonly in the winter months. Children between the ages of 6 months and 3 years are most often affected. The diagnosis of croup in a child older than 3 years should arouse the suspicion of an underlying anatomic abnormality or foreign body.

Pathophysiology

The viral pathogens that eventually produce croup invade the epithelium of the pharynx initially. Spread occurs downward to the larynx and occasionally further along the respiratory tract. The infection causes endothelial damage, production of mucus, loss of ciliary function, and edema. Erythema and swelling of the vocal cords and the subglottic larynx are present. A fibrinous exudate partially occludes the lumen of the trachea.

Clinical Manifestations

Croup begins insidiously with the onset of fever and coryza. During the next 1 to 2 days, the infection spreads farther along the airway, producing signs of upper respiratory obstruction. Inspiratory stridor develops at this stage of the illness, and a barking cough is heard. The child may be unable to maintain adequate oral intake.

Although the severity of croup varies, most children appear mildly to moderately ill in contrast to the toxic patients with epiglottitis or retropharyngeal abscess. The fever usually ranges from 38°C to 39°C (100.4°F to 102.2°F). Tachycardia and tachypnea are evident, but the respirations rarely exceed 40 breaths per minute. Suprasternal and subcostal retractions often accompany croup. On auscultation of the chest, the examiner may hear either stridor alone in mild disease or rhonchi and wheezes with more extensive involvement of the respiratory epithelium. Cyanosis occurs only in the minority of children with severe croup.

Ancillary studies are indicated only occasionally. The WBC count is generally normal or mildly low; lymphocytosis may occur as with other viral infections. The lateral and anteroposterior neck radiographs may show subglottic narrowing ("steeple" sign) from soft-tissue edema in severe disease. However, most of the radiographic studies of the airway are normal or disclose only ballooning of the hypopharynx. Rather than confirm the diagnosis of croup, radiographic examination more often excludes other illness such as epiglottitis or retropharyngeal abscess. Although rarely indicated, analysis of ABG levels, which are normal in mild cases, may show hypoxia and/or hypercarbia, as respiratory fatigue ensues.

Both dehydration and upper airway obstruction may complicate croup. Because of the respiratory distress and the toxicity associated with a febrile illness, the ability to maintain normal hydration will decrease in some children. Dehydration then occurs in the face of increased fluid losses through the pulmonary and cutaneous routes.

Occasionally, a child with croup develops significant upper airway obstruction. Signs suggestive of impending respiratory failure include (i) hypotonicity, (ii) marked retractions, (iii) decreased or absent inspiratory breath sounds, (iv) depressed level of consciousness, (v) tachycardia out of proportion to the fever, and (vi) cyanosis. Although an ABG is not needed in the evaluation of children with mild croup, this study may play a role in deciding on the therapy in more severe cases. Respiratory failure is defined as a partial pressure of arterial carbon dioxide ($PaCO_2$) of 60 mm Hg or higher or a partial pressure of arterial oxygen (PaO_2) of less than 50 mm Hg in 100% oxygen. However, significant respiratory compromise is present in croup when the $PaCO_2$ rises over 45 mm Hg and the PaO_2 falls to less than 70 mm Hg in room air.

Management

Croup is usually apparent from the history and physical examination. Soft-tissue radiographs of the neck are needed only if the diagnosis is uncertain. Although visualization of the posterior pharynx/epiglottis is not advised routinely when epiglottitis is suspected, this examination may be performed to confirm the absence of tonsillar infection or an obviously enlarged epiglottis in cases in which one is confident that the diagnosis is croup.

Many children with croup are never taken to seek medical attention. Of those who come to the ED, most can be managed as outpatients. Clear indications for admission are dehydration and/or significant respiratory compromise. If any of the signs of respiratory failure are noted, hospitalization becomes necessary. Use of a scoring system may be helpful in deciding on disposition (Table 92.13). Neck radiographs and an ABG may be obtained in cases in which the clinical picture is inconclusive. In addition, the physician should consider the social milieu of the family. Hospitalization provides the safest course for the child when there is a concern about the ability of the family to return reasonably promptly with worsening symptoms.

Mist therapy serves as one of the traditional remedies for croup, but more recent studies have been unable to demonstrate the effectiveness of this modality. Because the viral origin of this disease has been well established, antibiotics play no role.

Racemic epinephrine, or L-epinephrine, is indicated for children with moderate to severe croup who will be hospitalized or for whom admission is being considered. The dose is 0.25 mL of racemic epinephrine, mixed with 3 to 5 mL of saline, delivered by nebulization. If a response is noted and discharge to home is contemplated, the child should be observed for at least 2 hours to be certain that the respiratory symptoms do not recur.

TABLE 92.13

SCORING SYSTEM FOR ASSESSING SEVERITY OF CROUP

	Croup Score			
	0	1	2	3
Stridor	None	Only with agitation	Mild at rest	Severe at rest
Retraction	None	Mild	Moderate	Severe
Air entry	Normal	Mild decrease	Moderate decrease	Marked decrease
Color	Normal	Not applicable	Not applicable	Cyanotic
Level of consciousness	Normal	Restless when disturbed	Restless when undisturbed	Lethargic

Croup Severity[a]		
Score	Degree	Management
All severity scores	Mild to severe	Most patients in the ED with croup should receive a single oral or intramuscular dose of 0.6 mg/kg dexamethasone (max 10 mg)
4	Mild	Outpatient—mist therapy
5–6	Mild to moderate	Outpatient if child improves in emergency department after mist, is older than 6 mo, and has a reliable family
7–8	Moderate	Admitted—racemic epinephrine
≥9	Severe	Admitted—racemic epinephrine, oxygen, intensive care unit

[a]Any one category with score of 3 leads to classification as severe disease.
Modified from Taussig LM, Castro O, Beaudry PH, et al. Treatment of laryngotracheobronchitis (croup): use of intermittent positive pressure breathing and racemic epinephrine. *Am J Dis Child* 1975;129:790–793.

Corticosteroids have long been mentioned as potential aids to the treatment of croup, but the early controlled studies on these agents failed to substantiate the early anecdotal successes. Subsequently, Leipzig et al. found dexamethasone effective in a controlled study in 1979, and a meta-analysis of the literature in 1989 supported the use of corticosteroids for hospitalized patients.

Therapy should be tailored to the severity of illness. In rare cases with inadequate gas exchange, management of the airway, at times with endotracheal intubation, takes precedence; tracheal edema may make passage of a tube with the usual diameter impossible, and the physician should be prepared with one a size smaller than typically expected. Patients in the ED who have concerning upper airway obstruction should receive prompt therapy with epinephrine by nebulization and parenteral dexamethasone at 0.6 mg per kg (maximum 10 mg). Patients with impending respiratory failure should receive epinephrine IM 0.01 mL/kg of the 1:1000 concentration (maximum 0.3 mL). For children with moderately severe croup, while hospitalization is being arranged, should also receive epinephrine by nebulization and parenteral (intramuscular or IV) or oral dexamethasone therapy. Patients with mild to moderate croup may be managed with an initial trial of mist, which has never been shown to have any efficacy, and either oral or intramuscular dexamethasone. Last, the majority of patients, who are only very mildly ill, require only instructions for antipyresis, oral hydration, and observation at home.

Epiglottitis

Background

Epiglottitis, or supraglottitis, is a life-threatening bacterial infection of the epiglottis and the surrounding structures.

Rarely, trauma such as thermal injury to the epiglottis may cause swelling and clinical findings similar to those seen with infection.

Before the advent of a vaccine against Hib, epiglottitis occurred with regularity in children, accounting for 1 of every 1,000 pediatric admissions in the United States. It is now a rare disease in the pediatric population. Occasional cases are caused by the group A streptococcus. Although more common in the winter months, epiglottitis may occur throughout the year. The peak incidence during an era of greater prevalence fell between the ages of 3 and 7 years; however, infants and adults with epiglottitis have been well described.

Pathophysiology

The pharynx of normal children is often colonized with potentially pathogenic microorganisms such as *H. influenzae* and *S. pneumoniae*. Occasionally, these bacteria penetrate the mucosal barrier and invade the bloodstream. During the course of bacteremia, focal infection may occur at several sites, including the epiglottis and surrounding structures. Infection causes inflammatory edema, beginning on the lingual surface of the epiglottis, where the submucosa is loosely attached. The swelling progresses rapidly to involve the aryepiglottic folds, the arytenoids, and finally, the entire supraglottic larynx. Tightly bound epithelium on the vocal cords halts the spread at this level. The tremendous reduction in the caliber of the airway results in turbulent air flow on inspiration, appearing clinically as stridor.

Two possible mechanisms may explain the sudden respiratory arrest that can sometimes complicate this disease. The swollen epiglottis may be drawn into the glottis, acting like a plug to obstruct the flow of air, but this seems unlikely because the edematous, inflamed tissues of the supraglottic region become relatively tense. More likely, aspiration of oropharyngeal secretions occludes an already narrowed laryngeal inlet.

TABLE 92.14

EPIGLOTTITIS AND CROUP: A COMPARISON

	Epiglottitis	Croup
Anatomy	Supraglottic	Subglottic
Etiology	Bacterial (formerly *H. influenzae*)	Viral: parainfluenza
Age range	3–7 yr, adults	0.5–3 yr
Onset	6–24 h	24–72 h
Toxicity	Marked	Mild to moderate
Drooling	Frequent	Absent
Cough	Unusual	Frequent
Hoarseness	Unusual	Frequent
White blood cell count	Leukocytosis	Normal

Clinical Manifestations

Epiglottitis has an abrupt onset. The duration of illness before presentation is often as short as 6 hours and rarely exceeds 24 hours. Generally, parents first note the onset of fever. Shortly thereafter, the child develops stridor and labored respirations. As the disease progresses, the supraglottic edema interferes with the ability to swallow secretions; thus, drooling is a complaint in 60% to 70% of cases. Among children with epiglottitis, 50% complain of a sore throat. Aphonia, hoarseness, and cough are uncommon. Although both croup and epiglottitis manifest with stridor in a febrile child, the examiner can usually differentiate these two illnesses on the basis of the clinical features (Table 92.14).

The anxious appearance of most children with epiglottitis strikes the examiner immediately (Fig. 92.12). To maximize air entry, these children assume a sitting position with their jaws thrust forward. Cyanosis may occur in the later stages of the illness. The temperature, almost always elevated, often reaches a level of 40°C (104°F). Tachycardia is a constant feature. Although the patients are universally tachypneic, the respiratory rate rarely exceeds 40 breaths per minute. Stridor can be heard without a stethoscope, but auscultation of the lungs reveals no other adventitious sounds. Marked retractions are seen, predominantly involving the suprasternal and subcostal musculature.

As discussed under the "Management" section, rigorous attempts to visualize the epiglottis are hazardous and should

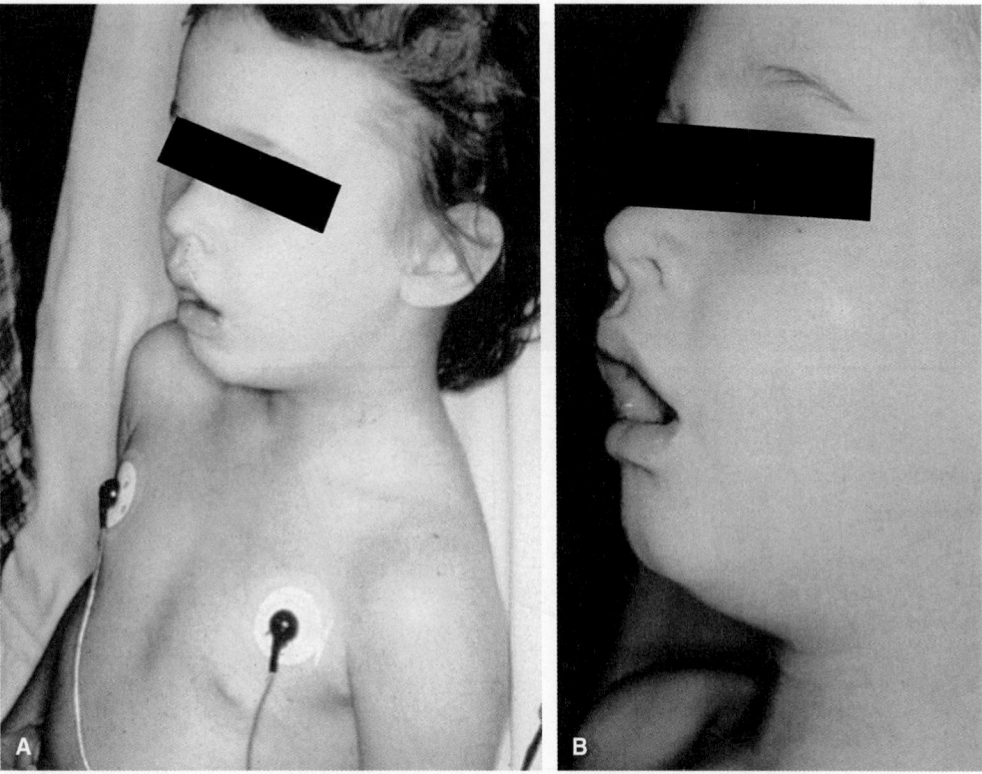

FIGURE 92.12 A 3-year-old girl with epiglottitis has an anxious appearance, assumes the "sniffing" position (**B**), and prefers to remain sitting (**A**).

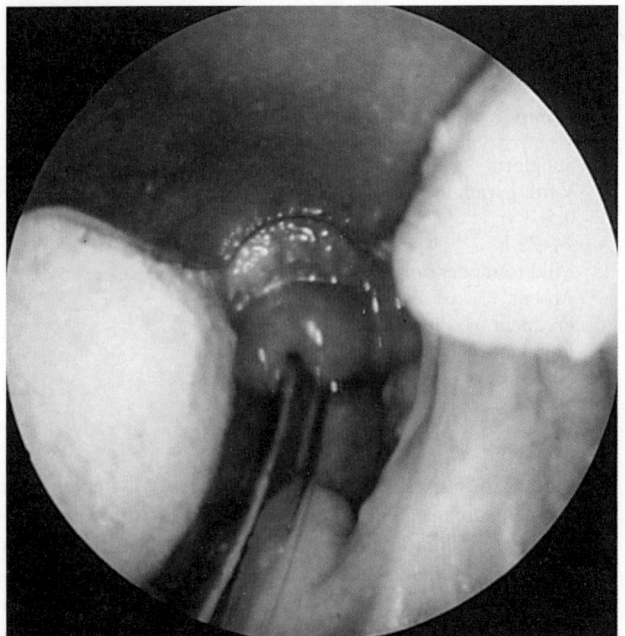

FIGURE 92.13 A swollen, erythematous epiglottis after endotracheal intubation of a child with epiglottitis.

be avoided in the child with suspected epiglottitis. However, the examiner may view the pharynx without the use of a tongue depressor. The mucosa is seen to be erythematous, and pooled secretions are present in about half the children. Occasionally, a swollen, cherry red epiglottis (Fig. 92.13) pro-

trudes above the base of the tongue and is visible without instrumentation.

Collection of laboratory specimens is usually delayed until the airway has been secured. The WBC count is elevated in most children with epiglottitis. Reports in the literature, addressing children with infections due to *H. influenzae* type b, describe a leukocytosis in the range of 15,000 to 25,000 per mm^3 and positive blood cultures in 80% to 90% of cases.

A lateral neck radiograph is pathognomonic of epiglottitis. There are three characteristic features: (i) a swollen epiglottis, (ii) thickened aryepiglottic folds, and (iii) obliteration of the vallecula (Fig. 92.14). The normal epiglottis has a thin, curved silhouette that has been likened to a bent finger, convex on one side and concave on the other. As a result of inflammatory edema from infection, it swells and assumes a configuration that is convex on both sides. This has been called the "thumb sign." The airway below the level of the vocal cords appears normal on the lateral neck radiograph of a child with epiglottitis.

The most serious complication of epiglottitis is sudden respiratory obstruction. This may occur unpredictably at any point in the illness, before seeking medical attention, in the ED, or after hospitalization. Although a child with minimal respiratory distress may occasionally have a total obstruction, marked retractions and labored breathing should serve as warning of an impending airway catastrophe. An additional complication of this illness is extraepiglottic spread of the infection. During the course of the bacteremia, seeding may involve the meninges, lungs, pericardium, synovial membranes, and soft tissues. Thus, the initial examination should attempt to elicit signs of infection at these additional sites.

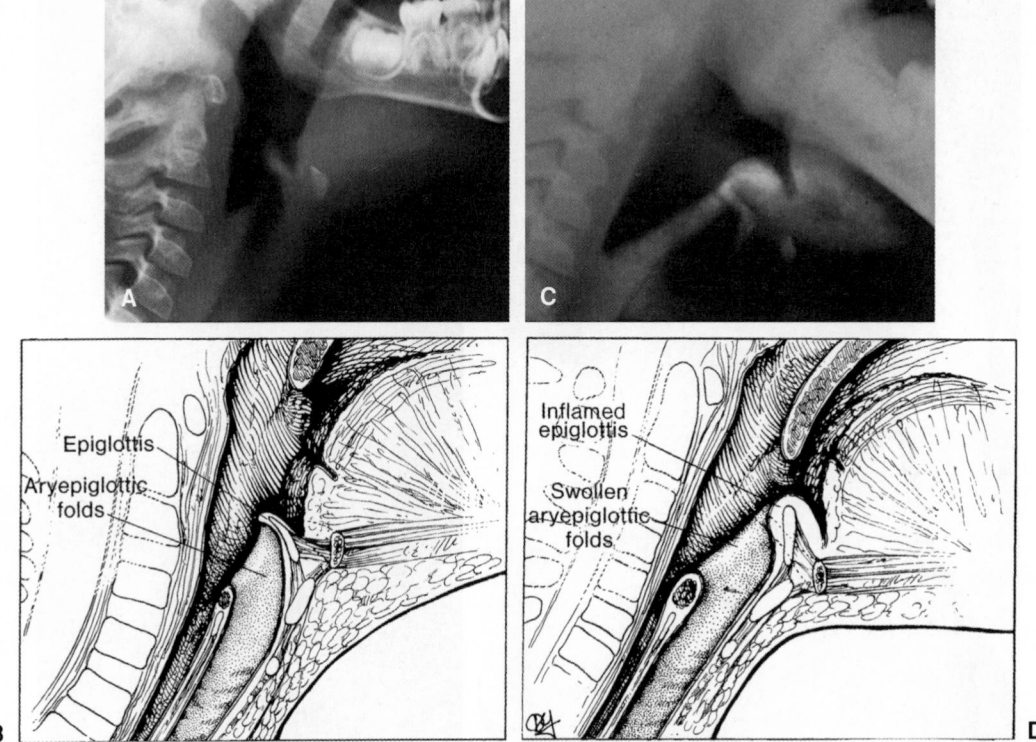

FIGURE 92.14 Appearance of the lateral neck region in a normal child (**A** and **B**) and a child with epiglottitis (**C** and **D**).

Management

When a child is suspected of having epiglottitis, the thrust of the management plan is to make a definitive diagnosis and institute therapy before the onset of airway obstruction. The major pitfall in this process is the vigorous examination of the posterior pharynx without having considered the possibility of supraglottic infection. Such manipulation may rarely initiate laryngeal obstruction in a small number of children with epiglottitis.

The initial steps in management are based on the degree of respiratory distress and the likelihood of epiglottitis, as judged from the clinical features (Fig. 92.15). Some children with epiglottitis have total or nearly total airway obstruction as the initial presentation of their disease. In this situation, treatment precedes any diagnostic evaluation and steps to maintain an adequate exchange of air are taken (see Chapters 1 and 5).

The majority of children, however, manifest lesser degrees of stridor and respiratory compromise with fever. The clinician must decide whether the constellation of historical and physical features points to croup or epiglottitis. In most children with stridor, the history will favor croup, which is the more common of the two diseases. The child will not appear toxic or show signs of air hunger. In such situations, a lateral neck radiograph is not indicated. Rather, the pharynx may be visualized directly with a tongue depressor to confirm the absence of a swollen, inflamed epiglottis.

When the findings weigh in favor of epiglottitis, however, further examination should be postponed and immediate preparation should be made for the insertion of an artificial airway; this includes collecting the necessary equipment and summoning additional personnel as needed. Anesthesiologists and otorhinolaryngologists alike, if available, should be involved in the care of children with epiglottitis, in addition to

TABLE 92.15

IMMEDIATE MANAGEMENT OF EPIGLOTTITIS

Insure adequate ventilation
Gain peripheral venous access, if tolerated by the child
Endotracheal intubation (or tracheostomy), providing
    bag-mask ventilation as needed
Defer laboratory studies until airway is secured

the staff in the ED. Following the appropriate preparations, a physician should accompany the child to the radiology department for a lateral neck radiograph, or a portable radiograph may be obtained. An IV infusion using a plastic cannula may be started in the cooperative patient. However, if the child becomes agitated or the procedure lengthy, the radiograph must be obtained quickly, assuming the airway has not been compromised, rather than persisting with attempts to gain IV access. The lateral neck radiograph either confirms or disproves the clinical diagnosis. If epiglottitis is verified radiographically, a skilled physician next performs endotracheal intubation, most often in the operating suite. If intubation is not possible, a surgical approach to the airway is necessary (Table 92.15).

A review of the mortality statistics in epiglottitis emphasizes the importance of an artificial airway in the management of this illness. Rapkin described a fatal outcome in 20% of the children treated with antibiotics and observation alone. In 1978, Cantrell et al. summarized 749 cases of epiglottitis. The mortality varied with the method of airway management as follows: tracheostomy, 3 deaths in 348 children (0.86%); endotracheal intubation, 2 in 216 (0.92%); no artificial airway, 13 in 214 (6.1%).

Ceftriaxone (100 mg per kg per day in one or two divided doses) and cefotaxime (200 mg per kg per day in four divided doses) provide appropriate antibacterial coverage. Vancomycin (45 mg per kg per day in three divided doses) and aztreonam (120 mg per kg per day in three divided doses) offers an alternative for patients allergic to penicillins or cephalosporins. Steroids have not been shown to play a role in epiglottitis.

Bacterial Tracheitis

Infections of the trachea, presumed to be bacterial, were originally described in the period from 1920 to 1940. Although an uncommon and, in the past, occasionally disputed entity, increasing reports of bacterial tracheitis confirm that this disease represents an occasional concern. The etiologic agents are *S. aureus* and *H. influenzae* type b, the latter occurring rarely at this point in time. Patients may range from infants to young children.

Clinical Manifestations

Published reports indicate that the signs and symptoms of bacterial tracheitis mimic those of acute epiglottitis but with a somewhat slower onset. The fever is usually greater than 39°C (102.2°F), and the patients are stridorous. Toxicity and respiratory distress occur as a rule. On radiograph, there is tracheal narrowing, and a pseudomembrane may be visible within the tracheal lumen; the supraglottic area is normal.

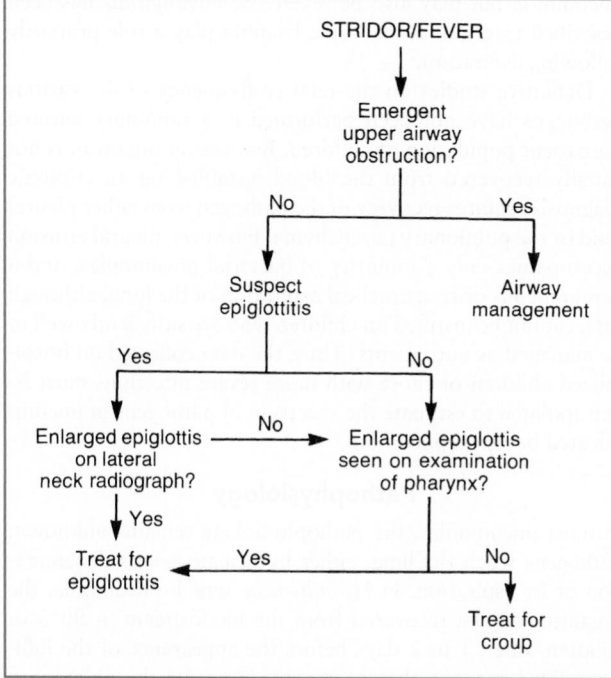

FIGURE 92.15 Diagnostic approach to the child with suspected epiglottitis.

Management

Children with bacterial tracheitis are often diagnosed initially as having severe viral croup or epiglottitis. Their management is as outlined for these conditions. The first priority is to secure an adequate airway. If bacterial tracheitis is suspected on the basis of a lateral neck radiograph or the findings at laryngoscopy, intravenous antibiotic therapy should be initiated with vancomycin (45 mg per kg per day in three divided doses) and ceftriaxone (100 mg per kg per day in one or two divided doses) or ampicillin–sulbactam (200 mg per kg per day of ampicillin in four divided doses). Aztreonam (120 mg per kg per day in three divided doses) offers an alternative for penicillin-allergic patients. Admission to an ICU is essential.

LOWER RESPIRATORY TRACT INFECTIONS

The most common lower respiratory tract infections in children include bronchiolitis and pneumonia, which may be caused by various bacteria or viruses, *Chlamydia trachomatis*, *M. pneumoniae*, or *C. pneumoniae*. Approximately 1 of 50 children in the United States has pneumonia annually. In a 12-year study of approximately 125,000 patients enrolled in the Group Health Cooperative of Puget Sound, the incidence of childhood pneumonia from all causes averaged 19 per 1,000 per year. Occasional episodes of pertussis and pulmonary tuberculosis are also seen. More recently described agents are rare but can be remarkably severe and include *Hantavirus*, which occurs in patients with exposure to rodents; the coronavirus causing severe acute respiratory syndrome (SARS), and influenza.

Pneumonia is an inflammation of the lung tissue that may follow a noninfectious or an infectious insult. In the ED, the febrile child with an acute onset of pneumonia almost always has an infection. The causative organisms in pneumonia vary according to the age of the child (Table 92.16). Although viral agents account for 60% to 90% of pneumonia, bacteria, particularly *S. pneumoniae*, play a major role. *M. pneumoniae* increases in frequency after 4 years of age. Unusual causes of pneumonia in the immunocompetent child include *Legionella pneumophilia* (Legionnaires' disease), *M. tuberculosis*, *Hantavirus*, coronavirus (SARS), rickettsia (Q fever), fungi, and protozoa. Children with neoplasms, HIV, and other forms of immunocompromise show susceptibility to a variety of unusual pathogens, including *Pneumocystis carinii*, *Candida*, *and Aspergillus species* (see Chapters 93 and 97).

Bacterial Pneumonia

Background

Bacterial pneumonia is an inflammation of the pulmonary parenchyma caused by a bacterial pathogen. In the first weeks of life, the group B streptococcus and gram-negative bacilli cause most such infections (Table 92.16). Between 2 weeks and 2 months of age, viruses and *C. trachomatis* are most common but group B streptococcus and *S. pneumoniae* are the cause of many cases requiring hospitalization. Among the bacteria, *S. pneumoniae* predominates at every age beyond the

TABLE 92.16

LOWER RESPIRATORY TRACT INFECTIONS

Age	Infecting organism
<3 wk	Bacteria 　Group B streptococcus 　Gram-negative bacilli (*E. coli*, Klebsiella) 　*S. aureus* Viruses (CMV, rubella, herpes, RSV)
3 wk–3 mo	*Chlamydia trachomatis* Viruses (RSV, parainfluenza, adenovirus, influenza) Bacteria 　*S. pneumoniae* 　*S. aureus* 　*H. influenzae*
3 mo–5 yr	Viruses (RSV, parainfluenza, adenovirus, influenza) Bacteria 　*S. pneumoniae* 　*S. aureus* 　*H. influenzae*
5 yr–19 yr	Viruses (adenovirus, influenza) Bacteria 　*S. pneumoniae* 　*M. pneumoniae*

newborn period. *H. influenzae* type b formerly ranked second to pneumococcus in children 2 months to 3 years of age but now occurs rarely in countries utilizing the conjugate Hib vaccine. *S. aureus* causes a severe, rapidly progressive but uncommon pneumonia in young children; 60% of these infections occur in the first year of life. Group A streptococcus is also uncommon but may also be severe, *N. meningitidis* has been described rarely, and anaerobic bacteria play a role primarily following aspiration.

Definitive studies on the relative frequency of the various pathogens have not been performed in a randomly selected outpatient population of children. Because an organism is not usually recovered from the blood, establishing an etiologic diagnosis requires recovery of the pathogen from either pleural fluid or the pulmonary parenchyma. However, pleural effusion accompanies only a minority of bacterial pneumonias, and a percutaneous or transtracheal aspiration of the lung, although safe, cannot be justified on children who are sufficiently well to be managed as outpatients. Thus, the data collected on hospitalized children or those with more severe infections must be extrapolated to estimate the spectrum of pathogens in uncomplicated bacterial pneumonia.

Pathophysiology

In most pneumonias, the pathophysiology remains unknown. Pathogens reach the lung, either by hematogenous dissemination or by aspiration. In *H. influenzae* type b pneumonia, the organism can be recovered from the bloodstream in 90% of children, often 1 to 2 days before the appearance of the infiltrate. This suggests that bacteremia precedes the pulmonary infection. However, bacteremia is found in only 5% of pediatric pulmonary infections with *S. pneumoniae* at the time of diagnosis. Thus, aspiration must play a greater role in the pathogenesis of infections with this organism or else the preceding bacteremia resolves before the development of pneumonia.

Following invasion of the pulmonary tissue by bacteria, an acute inflammatory reaction ensues. There is an exudation of fluid and polymorphonuclear leukocytes, followed by the deposition of fibrin. Several days later, macrophages appear in the alveoli. The accumulation of fluid in a lobe of the lung leads to the characteristic lobar consolidation seen on the chest radiograph.

Clinical Manifestations

Bacterial pneumonia generally has an abrupt onset with fever, often accompanied by chills. A cough is a common but non-specific complaint. The young child reacts to bacterial infection in the chest with lethargy and/or a decreased appetite. Occasionally, pleuritic involvement produces pain with respiratory effort.

The observation of the child at rest before the examination often provides the key to the diagnosis of pneumonia. Tachypnea out of proportion to the fever is sometimes the only sign, particularly in the first year of life. The infant who breathes at a normal rate, to the contrary, is much less likely to have a bacterial infection of the lung. A hasty effort at auscultation that disturbs the quiet infant obscures this finding.

Fever is almost universally present, ranging from 38.5°C to 41°C (101.2°F to 105.8°F). Grunting respirations in a young child should arouse a strong suspicion of pneumonia. Localized findings, more often seen in the child older than 1 year, include inspiratory rales, decreased breath sounds (sometimes the only abnormality), and less often, dullness to percussion. Gastric dilation may accompany pneumonia. Patients with lower-lobe pneumonia may present with abdominal pain; occasionally, the abdominal findings in pulmonary infections mimic appendicitis. With upper lobe pneumonia, the pain may radiate to the neck, causing meningismus; the diagnosis of pneumonia must, therefore, be considered in the child with nuchal rigidity and normal CSF.

In the ED, a chest radiograph often assists in the management of a child suspected of having bacterial pneumonia. Although a patient who is dehydrated with pneumonia occasionally may not have an infiltrate, the radiographic evaluation confirms or denies the diagnosis of bacterial pneumonia in most cases. This is important in a clinical setting not conducive to continuity of care. In addition, the radiograph may provide information on the disease process. A lobar consolidation is assumed to be of bacterial origin, needing treatment with antibiotics (Fig. 92.16), whereas a minimal, diffuse interstitial infiltrate in a previously healthy toddler suggests a viral infection that can be managed with symptomatic therapy or, in an adolescent, *M. pneumoniae*, calling for treatment with erythromycin or azithromycin. Bilateral involvement, pleural effusion, and pneumatoceles point to more severe disease.

Further laboratory studies are obtained only on specific indications. A WBC count may be helpful in differentiating viral from bacterial disease or in assessing the likelihood of bacteremia in the young child; the count often exceeds 15,000 per mm³ and occasionally rises above 30,000 per mm³ with bacterial invasion of the pulmonary parenchyma or the bloodstream. An elevated CRP correlates with the bacteremia and lobar infiltrates more closely than the WBC count but is rarely needed. A blood culture can be helpful when positive.

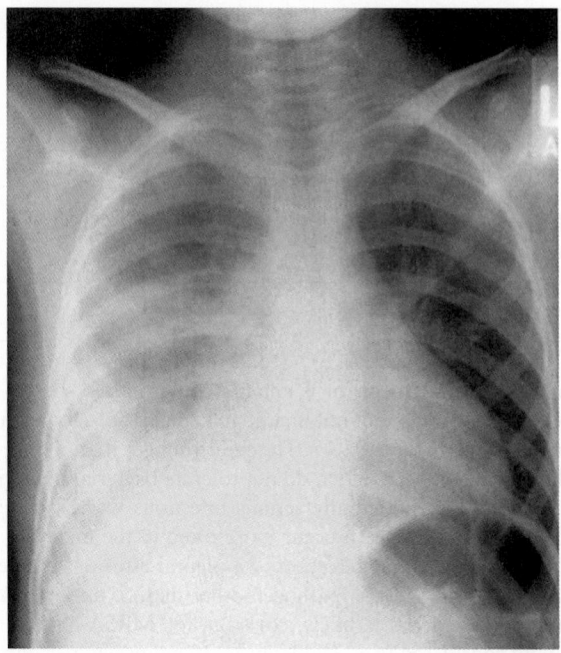

FIGURE 92.16 Radiograph showing lobar consolidation and pleural effusion in a child with bacterial pneumonia.

The most common complication of pneumonia is dehydration, particularly in young children. Electrolytes and a BUN are useful in assessing the degree of fluid loss in a child who appears ill or exhibits dry skin and/or mucosa. Rarely, extensive pulmonary involvement compromises ventilation, leading to respiratory failure. ABGs should be considered for any child with significant respiratory distress or transcutaneous oxygen saturation below 90%. A pleural effusion accumulates in many infections with *S. aureus* and *H. influenzae*, less often with *S. pneumoniae*. Bacteremia may result in additional foci of infection, including meningitis, pericarditis, epiglottitis, and septic arthritis.

Management

The large majority of healthy children with pneumonia respond to outpatient antibiotic therapy.

Because most of the bacterial pneumonias are caused by *S. pneumoniae*, amoxicillin (90 mg per kg per day given orally in three divided doses) has been the mainstay of therapy. Ceftriaxone (50 mg per kg) may be administered intramuscularly at the time of diagnosis, especially if there is any concern about oral intake during the first 24 hours. Alternatively, macrolides, including erythromycin (40 mg per kg per day in four divided doses) or azithromycin (10 mg per kg as a single dose on the first day and 5 mg per kg as a single dose on days 2 to 5), may be used in penicillin-allergic children or when mycoplasmal infection is suspected on the basis of age or radiographic findings.

Supportive therapy includes antipyretics and adequate hydration. Antitussives have no place in the treatment of pneumonia. Ill children should return within 24 to 48 hours for a second evaluation; patients who do not clinically improve and become afebrile should be evaluated carefully for admission to the hospital.

TABLE 92.17

INDICATIONS FOR ADMISSION IN CHILDREN
WITH PNEUMONIA

Age <1 yr (lobar infiltrate)	Failure to respond to antibiotic therapy within 24–48 h
Respiratory compromise	Dehydration
Pleural effusion	
Pneumatocele	

Any child who appears to be toxic (on the basis of the physician's clinical judgment) or is immunocompromised should be hospitalized. Firmer, but not unarguable, indications for admission are listed in Table 92.17. The child younger than 1 year, as well as those who are older, do not tolerate bacterial pneumonia. In addition, potentially serious infections with *S. aureus* and *H. influenzae* type b occur more often in the first year of life. The radiographic detection of a pleural effusion or pneumatocele also suggests a pathogen other than *S. pneumoniae*. Whenever *S. aureus* is likely, coverage for MRSA should be strongly considered (e.g., clindamycin 30 mg per kg per day in three divided doses or, in severely ill patients, vancomycin 45 mg per kg per day in three divided doses per day). Effusions should be cultured by thoracentesis (see Procedures in Section VII), when possible, which requires subsequent observation of the child in the hospital. Although a persistent elevation of the temperature is well described in children with pneumococcal pneumonias that subsequently respond to penicillin, failure of the fever to defervesce within 24 to 48 hours after the administration of antibiotics suggests a greater likelihood of more virulent pathogens or a viral etiology.

Viral Pneumonia

Background

A number of viruses are able to infect the lungs of children and adolescents. Respiratory syncytial and parainfluenza viruses are the most common isolates, particularly in the first year of life. Other viruses, including influenza, adenoviruses, enteroviruses, rhinoviruses, measles, varicella, rubella, herpes simplex, cytomegalovirus, EBV (rare), metapneumovirus, coronavirus (SARS), and *Hantavirus*, can cause pneumonia. Pulmonary disease complicates infections with influenza and varicella more often in the adolescent. The annual incidence of viral pneumonia peaks in the first 5 years of life at 40 per 1,000, and then declines with advancing age.

Pathophysiology

Most viruses that cause pneumonia initially invade the epithelium of the upper respiratory tract and spread locally to the lungs. The infection evokes an inflammatory response that consists primarily of mononuclear cells. After infection, the epithelial cells slough into the airway and obstruct the bronchi, producing the hyperinflation characteristically seen on chest radiograph.

A few viruses may reach the lungs by hematogenous dissemination. These include measles, varicella, rubella, cytomegalovirus, herpes simplex, and EBV.

Clinical Manifestations

Viral pneumonia generally has its onset over a 2- to 4-day period, being more gradual than with bacterial infection. Cough, coryza, and low-grade fever commonly occur. Particularly with RSV infections in the first 3 months of life, an apneic spell may be the first sign to draw attention to the illness.

Fever in viral pneumonia is usually lower than 39°C (102.2°F). As with bacterial infections, tachypnea in the undisturbed child may be the only physical finding. Rales are often audible diffusely throughout the chest, and wheezing may also be present. With more severe disease, the child shows signs of respiratory failure: grunting, cyanosis, and changes in mental status.

The WBC count varies widely in viral pneumonia. Although leukocytosis over 15,000 per mm^3 may occur in some cases, such elevated counts should arouse suspicion of bacterial disease.

The radiographic examination provides useful clues to the type of pathogen that causes a pneumonia but can never confirm a viral infection or rule out a bacterial cause. Most typically, the radiograph in a child with viral pneumonia shows bilateral air trapping and peribronchial thickening. A diffuse increase in the interstitial markings is also commonly seen. However, the findings can vary from barely detectable increases in volume to segmental infiltrates. Decubitus films occasionally detect small effusions. Because of the limitations in obtaining reliable cultures for bacteria, it is safest to presume a bacterial cause in the child with clinical evidence of pneumonia and a lobar infiltrate, a pleural effusion, a temperature greater than 39°C (102.2°F), or signs of clinical toxicity. Particularly in a dehydrated child, the chest radiograph may fail to show a lobar consolidation early in the course of a bacterial pneumonia.

Most viral pneumonias resolve without specific therapy. Potential complications include dehydration, apnea, and local progression of the infection. Apnea may occur in the first 3 months of life.

Occasional patients initially appear to have an uncomplicated viral pneumonia and then go on to develop systemic manifestations. This picture of marked deterioration suggests pathogens such as *Hantavirus* or coronavirus (SARS).

Management

The physician must attempt to make an etiologic diagnosis in pneumonia on the basis of the clinical and radiographic findings without the benefit of definitive laboratory tests. A WBC count should be obtained if there is uncertainty about the likely cause. In such cases, a leukocytosis over 15,000 per mm^3 would weigh against a viral infection. In individuals with signs of systemic involvement for whom less common pathogens are being considered, a more extensive laboratory evaluation is merited.

If an uncomplicated viral pneumonia is strongly suspected, no specific therapy need be given. An example of such a situation would be a well-hydrated 5-year-old child with a gradual onset of cough, a temperature of 38°C (100.4°F), scattered bilateral rales, WBC count of 8,000 per mm^3 with predominantly lymphocytes, and the finding of hyperaeration on chest radiograph. Treatment in this case could be limited to antipyresis and hydration with a follow-up visit in 24 hours.

Because the infant younger than 3 months may become apneic during the course of viral pneumonia, these young children may benefit from observation in the hospital.

Mycoplasma Pneumonia

Background

M. pneumoniae is one of the most common causes of pneumonia among children older than 5 years. In younger children, infections with this organism are often limited to the upper respiratory tract or, occasionally, to the bronchial tree, although one study has implicated this organism as a common cause of pneumonia in children as young as 18 months. By the end of adolescence, 90% of the population has antibodies to *M. pneumoniae.*

Pathophysiology

The initial infection with *M. pneumoniae* occurs on the surface of the respiratory epithelium. Destruction of these cells causes them to slough into the lumen of the bronchi. The infection evokes an inflammatory response, primarily by mononuclear leukocytes.

Clinical Manifestations

Pneumonia caused by *M. pneumoniae* begins insidiously with fever, myalgias, headache, and malaise. After 3 to 5 days, the child develops a nonproductive cough, hoarseness, sore throat, and in one-quarter of cases, chest pain. Fever is almost invariably present and may reach a level of 40°C (104°F). Children seldom develop much respiratory distress, with the exception of those who are younger than 5 years old or also have sickle cell anemia or an immunodeficiency. Rales are heard in 75% of these infections, often bilaterally. The pharynx may appear inflamed, and some investigators have noted ear infections, particularly bullous myringitis, in association with pneumonia caused by *M. pneumoniae*. In 10% of patients, a maculopapular or, less often, a vesicular rash occurs; rarely, erythema multiforme, urticaria, or petechiae are seen.

The total WBC count is often normal in infections with this pathogen. A cold agglutinin titer of 1:32 or higher is found in most patients with lobar infiltrates from an *M. pneumoniae* infection but may also occur, although less often, with viral and bacterial illnesses. While not routinely indicated, the organism may be recovered from oropharyngeal specimens by culture or PCR. Alternatively antibody titers in acute and convalescent sera may be used to confirm the diagnosis. The radiographic findings show considerable variation. Between 10% and 25% of children will have lobar consolidation. Scattered segmental infiltrates, interstitial disease, and combinations of all these patterns may be seen. Pleural effusions occur in 5% of cases.

Numerous complications are described in association with *M. pneumoniae* infections, but they occur rarely. These include hemolytic anemia, arthritis, encephalitis, meningitis, and neuropathy.

Management

The diagnosis of mycoplasmal pneumonia is presumptively based on the clinical and radiographic findings and, in unusual cases, on the cold agglutinin titer or specific serologic testing. An older child or adolescent with the gradual onset of a mild bilateral pneumonia should be treated for this infection. However, a lobar infiltrate in a 5-year-old child is usually assumed to be of bacterial origin regardless of the level of the cold agglutinins. The results of cultures and specific serologic assays entail too great a delay to be useful to the clinician in the ED. Erythromycin (40 mg per kg per day in three to four divided doses) or azithromycin (10 mg per kg as a single dose on day 1, followed by 5 mg per kg daily as a single dose for four additional days) provide effective therapy for *M. pneumoniae* infections. The response is more pronounced in the older child with lobar disease than in the younger child with a diffuse infiltrate.

Chlamydia trachomatis Pneumonia

Background

C. trachomatis is the most commonly recovered pathogen from children with afebrile pneumonias between 4 and 12 weeks of age.

Pathophysiology

Among infants born to pregnant women with vaginal colonization by *C. trachomatis,* one-third to one-half acquire the organism. These infants are at risk for the subsequent development of pneumonitis. Pathologic examination in chlamydial pneumonitis shows a mononuclear consolidation with occasional eosinophils and neutrophils and marked necrotic changes in the bronchioles.

Clinical Manifestations

Infancy. Infants with chlamydial pneumonia usually have a dry staccato cough that may resemble the paroxysms seen in pertussis but is usually less prolonged. In 50% of cases, conjunctivitis precedes the onset of respiratory symptoms. Pneumonia with this organism only rarely produces a fever. Mild retractions, hyperresonance, and diffuse rales are noted on examination of the chest. Hyperaeration of the lungs depresses the liver, allowing the edge to be palpated 1 to 2 mm below the right costal margin. Because of the increased work of breathing these infants may not gain weight as expected.

Although the WBC count is usually in the normal range, the eosinophil count rises slightly (400 per mm^3, or 5% to 10%) in 75% of these patients. Elevated immunoglobulin levels, although nonspecific, often occur with chlamydial infections, but seldom with viral illnesses. Mild hypoxemia is common. The chest radiograph shows hyperaeration of the lungs and a diffuse increase in the interstitial markings. Lobar consolidations and pleural diffusions are not seen.

Although usually a mild illness, chlamydial pneumonia may be complicated by the occurrence of mucous plugging of the bronchi, apnea, and severe impairment of oxygenation. It is impossible to predict which infants with an initially mild course will have a stormy one.

Management

Because of the difficulty in making a definitive etiologic diagnosis and the potential for complications, young infants with presumed chlamydial pneumonia should be considered for admission to the hospital. Azithromycin (10 mg per kg on day 1 and 5 mg per kg per day as a single daily dose for four additional doses) may shorten the course and should be given.

Chlamydophyla Pneumonia

Two species of *Chlamydophyla* cause pneumonia: *Chlamydia psittaci* and *Chlamydia pneumoniae* (TWAR). Psittacosis, a severe pneumonia caused by *C. psittaci*, is rare but should be suspected in patients with unusual avian exposures. *C. pneumoniae* causes pneumonia primarily in children older than 5 years. In a study from Seattle, the attack rate for this agent was approximately 0.5 to 1 case per 1,000 children (5 to 14 years old) per year, compared with 4 to 5 cases per 1,000 for *M. pneumoniae*.

Pathophysiology

C. pneumoniae spreads within families, day care centers, and schools.

Clinical Manifestations

The spectrum of infection ranges from asymptomatic to severe. Most children have seroconversion as evidence of infection that did not require any medical intervention. Adolescents are more likely to have signs of pneumonia than younger children, who may have clinical findings confined to the upper respiratory tract. Pneumonia is often preceded by sore throat and hoarseness, usually with a brief fever. By the time pneumonia has developed, the fever often resolves. Patients usually have a cough and scattered rales on auscultation. As for the clinical syndrome, the chest radiograph picture resembles that seen with *M. pneumoniae*, consisting of subsegmental lesions rather than lobar consolidation. Leukocytosis is not seen. No specific diagnostic testing is routinely available.

Management

C. pneumoniae infections in older children respond to therapy with macrolide antibiotics, including erythromycin (40 mg per kg per day in three to four divided doses) or azithromycin (10 mg per kg as a single dose on day 1, followed by 5 mg per kg daily as a single dose for 4 additional days).

Bronchiolitis

Background

Bronchiolitis is a pulmonary infection of young children characterized by wheezing. RSV causes most of these illnesses, but other viruses, particularly parainfluenza, influenza, and metapneumovirus may also cause bronchiolitis. In addition, *M. pneumoniae* has been reported as a rare cause of bronchiolitis.

The epidemiology of bronchiolitis primarily follows the pattern of its principal pathogen, RSV. Most of these infections occur in the winter and affect children between 2 and 8 months of age. Although some authorities do not accept the diagnosis of bronchiolitis after the age of 1 year, others believe that the disease occurs until the second birthday.

Pathophysiology

RSV, the most common cause of bronchiolitis, invades the epithelial cells of the nasopharynx and spreads to the mucosa of the lower respiratory tract by cell-to-cell transfer. The infection causes death of the cells that line the bronchi, which then slough into the lumen. The production of mucus increases, and mononuclear cells infiltrate the area. Clumps of necrotic epithelium and mucus initially decrease the diameter of the bronchi, causing turbulent air flow, particularly on expiration when the luminal diameter normally decreases. Eventually, plugging of the bronchi produces hyperinflation and atelectasis.

Clinical Manifestations

Bronchiolitis begins as a URI with cough and coryza. Over 2 to 5 days, signs of respiratory distress appear. The parents can often hear the child wheezing. Fever occurs in two-thirds of children with bronchiolitis. They often appear ill on overall assessment. The respiratory rate climbs to at least 40 breaths per minute and may reach 80 to 100 breaths per minute. Nasal flaring and retractions of the intercostal and supraclavicular muscles are noted and increase as the disease progresses. In bronchiolitis and other lower respiratory tract infections, the intercostal retractions are more pronounced than the supraclavicular, the opposite of the findings in croup and epiglottitis. Wheezes and a prolonged expiratory phase are heard in all children with bronchiolitis, at times without a stethoscope, and rales are usually minimal. As the ventilatory muscles fatigue, the child will have grunting respirations; only in the most severe cases does cyanosis occur.

The total WBC count in bronchiolitis is most often normal. Usually, the chest radiograph shows only hyperaerated lungs and peribronchial cuffing, but there may occasionally be areas of atelectasis. If respiratory failure supervenes, the PaO_2 decreases and carbon dioxide is retained.

The complications of bronchiolitis include apnea, dehydration, respiratory failure, and rarely, bacterial superinfection. Pneumothorax and pneumomediastinum are rarely seen. The increased respiratory effort in bronchiolitis may prevent an infant from maintaining an adequate oral intake. Careful attention should be paid to the details of fluid balance when taking a history. Of infants with bronchiolitis, 10% to 20% develop significant respiratory compromise. Cyanosis (or an oxygen saturation less than 91%), decreased inspiratory breath sounds, and lethargy on examination point to ventilatory failure. Bacterial superinfection is uncommon in the early stages of the illness, occurring occasionally in hospitalized infants. However, lobar consolidation seen on the chest radiograph suggests a potential bacterial pneumonia, although areas of atelectasis may be confused with infiltrates.

Apnea has been a particular concern to pediatricians and emergency physicians because it has been considered to be unpredictable. In a more recent study by Willwerth and colleagues, 19 of 691 (2.7%) infants hospitalized with bronchiolitis developed apnea, but all had one of three high-risk criteria: full-term birth and age younger than 1 month; preterm birth (less than 37 weeks) and less than 48 weeks postconception; or report of a suspected apneic episode at home.

Management

In the management of children with suspected bronchiolitis in the ED, a chest radiograph should be considered to help exclude other entities such as lobar pneumonia or a foreign body. Pulse oximetry provides an estimate of the degree of hypoxia. A WBC count, ABG, and/or electrolytes are obtained only if the diagnosis is uncertain or the clinical picture suggests that complications have occurred.

Children with bronchiolitis may benefit from nebulized bronchodilators, although most recent studies suggest minimal, if any, efficacy from albuterol, salbutamol, or epinephrine. For the child with moderate to severe distress, a trial of nebulized broncholidators is reasonable, starting at 0.1 to 0.3 of a 0.5% solution of albuterol or using 3 to 4 mL of 1:1,000 epinephrine and reassessing after three treatments spaced 20 minutes apart. Patients who show a favorable response to nebulized therapy are candidates to receive further nebulized treatments. Oral albuterol solution has no proven efficacy.

Corticosteroids are not indicated for the treatment of patients with bronchiolitis. In general, it is difficult to differentiate asthma from bronchiolitis during the first 2 years of life; thus, corticosteroids may be given occasionally to some children who may have bronchiolitis or asthma, in accordance with the guidelines for the latter disease.

For the patient who does not respond to nebulized bronchodilator agents, therapy is limited to antipyretics, the encouragement of adequate oral intake, and reevaluation after 24 to 48 hours. Dehydration, secondary bacterial infection, and significant respiratory distress necessitate admission to the hospital. Although not validated in infants with bronchiolitis, a score of 4 or more on the asthma scale (see Chapter 82) suggests significant respiratory compromise. A transcutaneous oxygen saturation less than 91% to 93% or an arterial PaO_2 less than 70 mm Hg in room air at sea level also suggests a need for hospitalization. In addition, children with underlying cardiac or pulmonary disease and those with high-risk factors for apnea should be considered for admission.

Pertussis

Background

Pertussis, or whooping cough, is an infection of the respiratory tract caused by *Bordetella pertussis*. Occasionally, a similar clinical syndrome is caused by *Bordetella parapertussis*, the adenoviruses, or *C. trachomatis*. Usually, young children most often contract pertussis, but the incidence in adolescents has increased more recently. Although vaccination has contributed to the significant decrease in the frequency of this disease, several thousand cases occur yearly in the United States among unvaccinated children and, to a lesser degree, among those who have received vaccine.

Pathophysiology

Following inhalation, *B. pertussis* organisms attach to the epithelial cells of the respiratory tract. Multiplication of the bacteria leads to infiltration of the mucosa with polymorphonuclear leukocytes and lymphocytes. Inflammatory debris in the lumen of the bronchi and peribronchial lymphoid hyperplasia obstruct the smaller airways, causing atelectasis.

Clinical Manifestations

Although pertussis can be divided into three stages for discussion, a clinically distinct syndrome does not evolve until the disease has progressed to the second stage. Initially, the symptoms mimic a viral URI. This first stage (catarrhal), characterized by a mild cough, conjunctivitis, and coryza, lasts for 1 to 2 weeks. An increasingly severe cough heralds the onset of the second stage (paroxysmal), which continues for 2 to 4 weeks. After a prolonged spasm of coughing often involving 10 or more coughs in succession, the sudden inflow of air produces the characteristic whoop (young infants lack the ability to generate sufficient negative inspiratory pressure and may, therefore, not whoop). Vomiting often occurs after such an episode. When not coughing, the child has a remarkably normal physical examination, except for an occasional subconjunctival hemorrhage. During the third stage (convalescent), the intensity of the cough wanes. At times, pertussis may present as a chronic cough without other signs of infection (see Chapter 15).

The WBC count in children usually reaches a level of 20,000 to 50,000 per mm³ with a marked lymphocytosis, but such changes are not often seen in infants younger than 3 to 6 months. Although a chest radiograph occasionally shows the characteristic "shaggy" right heart border, more often the lung fields appear clear. *B. pertussis* can be identified by PCR of nasopharyngeal secretions, or less commonly, recovered by culture of this material if the specimen is obtained in the first or early second phase of the illness.

The fatality rate for pertussis is approximately 1% for patients in the first month of life and 0.3% for those between age 2 and 12 months. Complications often occur during a bout of pertussis. The most immediately life-threatening complication is complete obstruction of the airway by a mucous plug, leading to respiratory arrest. Although secondary bacterial pneumonia has a more insidious onset, it occurs in 25% of children with pertussis and accounts for 90% of the fatalities. Seizures are seen in 3% of patients, and encephalitis in 1%. Sudden increases in intrathoracic pressure can cause intracranial hemorrhages, rupture of the diaphragm, and rectal prolapse.

Management

The initial diagnosis of pertussis rests on clinical grounds. Children with an unmistakable paroxysmal cough followed by a whoop should be assumed to have the disease. When the clinical picture is unclear, a WBC count and chest radiograph may be useful. The radiograph helps eliminate other causes of a severe cough (e.g., foreign body, bacterial pneumonia, cystic fibrosis, tuberculosis), and the WBC count provides confirmatory evidence if a leukocytosis with marked lymphocytosis is found. Because of the grave risk of complications, all children younger than 3 to 6 months diagnosed firmly as having pertussis should be considered for observation in the hospital. While paroxysms typically resolve spontaneously, the younger child may have cyanosis and bradycardia at the end of paroxysms and seem to benefit from gentle stimulation often given as pats on the back. Older children who show signs of respiratory compromise, such as cyanosis during paroxysms of coughing, or who develop complications also require admission. Treatment includes erythromycin (40 mg per kg per day for 14 days) or azithromycin (10 mg per kg as a single dose on day 1, followed by 5 mg per kg per day as a single dose on days 2 to 5),

MEDICAL EMERGENCIES

maintenance of adequate hydration, and a level of respiratory support appropriate to the severity of the disease. Household and other close contacts require chemoprophylaxis with erythromycin (40 mg per kg per day for 14 days) or azithromycin (10 mg per kg per day for 5 days). Children younger than 7 years who are unimmunized or have received fewer than four doses of pertussis vaccine should have their pertussis immunization initiated or continued as soon as possible after exposure. Children who are fully immunized for age but have received only three doses require a fourth dose. Those who have had four doses need a booster unless the last dose has been within 3 years or they are older than 6 years. DT$_a$P is preferred. For adolescents and adults requiring a tetanus booster, one should be given as Tdap to ensure adequate protection against pertussis.

Tuberculosis

Background

In the United States, tuberculosis is caused almost exclusively by *M. tuberculosis* and occurs in childhood in several clinical forms. Although currently an unusual infection in developed countries the disease should be kept in mind as an occasional, treatable cause of morbidity and mortality. At particular risk are children in urban, low-income areas and recent immigrants from underdeveloped countries. In addition, the emergency physician must be concerned about tuberculosis when either the patient or close contacts are infected with HIV (see Chapter 93).

Pathophysiology

Tubercle bacilli enter the body through the respiratory tract, producing an initial focus in the lungs. This lesion usually remains subclinical but may progress locally, resulting in a primary tuberculous pneumonia. During the primary infection, the organisms can disseminate hematogenously. Such spread may remain quiescent or, in a young child, may lead to miliary tuberculosis. Seeding of various organs occurs and may produce focal infections, a particularly serious concern with meningeal involvement.

Usually, the immune system limits the initial infection. However, reactivation of these foci may cause disease years later at any site involved during dissemination. Pulmonary lesions reactivate to produce tuberculous pneumonia in adults and adolescents much more often than in children.

Clinical Findings

Most infections by *M. tuberculosis* in children never cause any significant symptoms. Among the many possible clinical presentations, three stand out as particular concerns to the emergency physician: primary pneumonia, miliary tuberculosis, and meningitis. Pneumonia is by far the most common. Of note, these infections may develop despite prior vaccination against tuberculosis with Bacillus Calmette-Guerin vaccine.

The onset of primary tuberculosis pneumonia resembles that of bacterial infections of the lungs. It begins with fever and tachypnea; rales and an area of dullness are found on examination of the chest. The WBC count may be elevated with a shift to the left, and the chest radiograph shows a lobar consolidation, often accompanied by hilar adenopathy and less often by pleural effusion or cavitation. Although the primary pneumonia often resolves spontaneously, the child occasionally follows a downhill course caused by local progression. In addition to the epidemio-

logic risks described, clinical findings that should arouse a suspicion of tuberculous pneumonia in the child otherwise believed to have a bacterial infection of the lung include pleural effusion, cavitation, toxicity, and a failure to respond to antibiotic therapy.

Miliary tuberculosis begins with an abrupt rise in temperature but a paucity of other physical findings; it may mimic sepsis. Subsequently, respiratory symptoms and enlargement of the liver, spleen, and superficial lymph nodes occur. The WBC count is usually in the range of 15,000 per mm^3. Although the chest radiograph initially shows no lesions, a diffuse mottling of the lung fields appears 1 to 3 weeks after the fever. Miliary tuberculosis is a consideration in a child with a persistent fever and hepatosplenomegaly.

Tuberculous meningitis comes on insidiously with a low-grade fever, apathy, and in 50% of patients, vomiting. After 1 to 2 weeks of nonspecific illness, neurologic signs appear, including cranial nerve deficits, drowsiness and nuchal rigidity; if untreated, the child lapses into coma. The CSF shows a mononuclear pleocytosis, an elevated protein concentration, and eventually, a low glucose level. A CSF glucose level greater than 30 mg per dL would be distinctly unusual in a child with tuberculosis meningitis. Cranial CT imaging with contrast will typically reveal evidence of a basilar meningitis.

Management

A child suspected of having pneumonic, meningeal, or miliary tuberculosis should be admitted to the hospital for evaluation and possible chemotherapy. Among inner-city populations, where the risk of tuberculosis is greatest, the routine placement of a tuberculous skin test (Mantoux test) in children with lobar pneumonia should be considered. The Mantoux test must be interpreted in accordance with the child's age and the presence of risk factors (Table 92.18). Current treatment for tuberculosis

---

TABLE 92.18

DEFINITION OF POSITIVE CRITERIA FOR THE STANDARD MANTOUX SKIN TEST (5 TUBERCULIN UNITS OF PPD) IN CHILDREN[a]

Induration >5 mm
Children in close contact with known or suspected cases of active tuberculosis, if adequate and timely treatment cannot be verified
Children suspected to have tuberculosis based on a consistent chest radiograph or clinical findings
Children immunosuppressed on the basis of therapy or disease

Induration >10 mm
Children <4 years
Children with chronic illness, including lymphoma, diabetes mellitus, renal failure, and malnutrition
Children born in or traveling to regions of the world with a high prevalence of tuberculosis or exposed to adults likely to be infected

Induration >15 mm
Children ≥4 years without any risk factors

[a]Applies regardless of previous BCG vaccination.
Modified from Committee on Infectious Diseases. *2006 RedBook*. Elk Grove Village, IL: American Academy of Pediatrics, 2006.

consists of two to four or more drugs (isoniazid, rifampin, pyrazinamide, ethambutol, streptomycin, capreomycin, ciprofloxacin, cycloserine, ethionamide, kanamycin, ofloxacin, paraaminosalicylic acid) for a minimum of 6 months.

Hantavirus

The *hantavirus* pulmonary syndrome was described in 1994 among 17 adults, of whom 13 died with severe pneumonia and hypotension. In a subsequent series, 8 of 100 patients were 16 years old or younger. Rodents serve as the reservoir for the hantaviruses, of which several varieties infect humans. The syndrome begins with fever, cough, and myalgias, followed shortly thereafter by tachypnea, tachycardia, dyspnea, and finally, hypotension. A marked leukocytosis is common along with thrombocytopenia and elevated clotting studies. The initial chest radiograph shows an interstitial more often than an alveolar infiltrate, with changes starting or becoming bilateral in the majority of cases.

Pleural effusions occur in about one-fourth of the patients. The diagnosis should be considered when a severe pneumonia occurs in combination with systemic deterioration and can be confirmed subsequently by specific viral serology. Treatment is supportive.

Severe Acute Respiratory Syndrome

SARS affects predominantly adults, although a few cases have occurred in patients younger than 15 years. It is caused by a coronavirus and has an incubation period that typically ranges from 2 to 7 days. The illness begins generally with a prodrome of fever, which may be accompanied by headache, malaise, and myalgias. Some patients have mild respiratory syndromes and occasionally diarrhea is noted. After 3 to 7 days, a lower respiratory phase ensues with cough and then dyspnea, which may progress to hypoxemia and respiratory failure. Chest radiographs may either be normal or show focal interstitial infiltrates. Although the CBC count is usually normal initially, approximately 50% of patients develop leucopenia and thrombocytopenia at the peak of the respiratory illness. Elevated creatinine kinase (CK) levels and hepatic transaminases occur commonly. Treatment is primarily supportive. Although efficacy is unproven, ribavirin may be considered in patients with significant respiratory symptomatology.

GASTROINTESTINAL INFECTIONS

Gastroenteritis is an inflammation of the alimentary tract that, in its acute form, is overwhelmingly infectious in origin. Viruses are the organisms most commonly found in children with diarrhea in the United States and can be isolated from 30% to 40% of patients. In 10% to 15% of patients, bacteria are recovered, including *Salmonella, Shigella, Campylobacter, Yersinia,* and pathogenic *E. coli; Aeromonas hydrophila* and vibrio species, such as *Plesiomonas shigelloides,* are occasional pathogens. *Clostridium difficile,* which elaborates a toxin, may cause colitis, particularly after the use of antibiotics. Parasitic infestations rarely lead to diarrhea in developed countries. *Giardia lamblia* and *Cryptosporidium* should be considered, particularly in outbreaks in day care centers, and

Entamoeba histolytica, among immigrants or travelers from tropical areas; cryptosporidiosis also commonly affects patients with HIV. Current diagnostic techniques are unable to identify an etiologic agent in most of the remaining episodes.

In the United States, GI infections rank second in frequency to respiratory tract infections during childhood. An estimated 30,000,000 children with gastroenteritis receive treatment at home each year, 3,000,000 visit a physician, and 200,000 require hospitalization. Approximately 12% of all hospitalizations of children 1 month through 4 years of age include diarrhea among one of the top three positions on the list of discharge diagnoses. Almost 400 children die annually in the United States from infections of the GI tract.

Viral hepatitis is covered in Chapter 89. Bacterial infections of the liver and bacterial cholangitis, almost exclusively abscesses, are rare in otherwise healthy children; more commonly, they complicate either an anatomic malformation or an immunosuppressive condition, or they affect the neonate.

Because calculi in the bile ducts rarely occur before adolescence, cholecystitis occurs much less often in children than in adults. Occasionally, episodes are seen in teenagers or children predisposed to stone formation, as in the chronic hemolytic anemias. Less commonly, salmonellosis, leptospirosis, Kawasaki disease, or drug therapy produces acalculous cholecystitis.

In childhood, peritonitis almost invariably reflects an intraabdominal catastrophe that requires surgical intervention. However, the accumulation of ascitic fluid in children with diseases such as nephrosis and cirrhosis allows the development of a primary infection of the peritoneum.

Viral Gastroenteritis

Background

Viral gastroenteritis occurs primarily in two forms caused by different pathogens. The human calciviruses (norovirus and sapovirus) produce an illness characterized by an explosive onset and vomiting, more severe than the diarrhea that accompanies it. The symptoms are self-limiting, resolving in 2 to 3 days. Infections occur in epidemics, most often in the winter, and affect predominantly school-age children. Rotavirus, however, produces a prolonged diarrheal illness of varying severity. It occurs more often in young children, although older family members may be affected. Other viruses, including enteroviruses, coronaviruses, and adenoviruses, may play a role in gastroenteritis.

Viral gastroenteritis is common. Among U.S. families, it trails only the common cold in frequency. Rotaviruses are the most commonly isolated pathogens, particularly among children who develop dehydration. Viral infections of the GI tract cause considerable loss of time from school and occasionally require treatment in the hospital.

Pathophysiology

Rotaviruses invade the intestinal epithelial cells, where they can be visualized by electron microscopy. The histology of the mucosal layer is disturbed during the active infection and for 3 to 8 weeks afterward. Functional abnormalities accompany the morphologic changes, including depressions of disaccharidase levels. Although calcivirus may invade the mucosal lining of the intestine, they have not been detected intracellularly. Histologic changes occur and persist for 2 weeks, and disaccharidase levels decline during the infection.

Clinical Findings

Children with viral gastroenteritis develop diarrhea and/or vomiting. The numbers of stools may vary from 2 or 3 to 15 or 20 daily. Most commonly, there are 6 to 8 bowel movements in a 24-hour period; the stools range from semisolid in consistency to watery. Although hematochezia may occasionally occur in viral infections, the presence of blood in the stool should suggest a bacterial gastroenteritis. Vomiting may accompany diarrhea or be the sole manifestation of a viral gastroenteritis. The daily frequency of emesis varies in the same range as for diarrhea. After forceful emesis, streaks of blood may be present in the vomitus. Many children with viral gastroenteritis older than the age of 2 or 3 years complain of crampy abdominal pain. Parents may relate a history of decreased oral intake and, in more severe cases, oliguria.

Children with viral gastroenteritis are usually febrile, occasionally highly so. However, in the child older than 3 years, a temperature higher than 39°C (102.2°F) may suggest a bacterial enteritis. Tachycardia, hypotension, and lethargy may reflect dehydration in moderate to severe episodes. Whereas the respiratory rate is usually normal, tachypnea occurs when acidosis and/or dehydration are present. The abdomen is soft and nondistended in most cases. Although the child may perceive palpation as uncomfortable, this maneuver does not elicit localized or rebound tenderness. Auscultation reveals hyperactive bowel sounds. The skin turgor is decreased and the mucous membranes are dry, when gastroenteritis leads to clinically detectable dehydration (see Chapters 17, 18, and 100).

No laboratory studies are indicated in the uncomplicated case of gastroenteritis. The CBC count, electrolytes, and BUN usually fall within the normal range. If oral intake fails to keep pace with the efflux of fluids from the alimentary tract, dehydration occurs. The sodium, usually normal, may drop as low as 110 mEq per L or rise to 170 mEq per L, and the bicarbonate is often low. With mild dehydration, the serum bicarbonate hovers just below the normal level at 18 to 20 mEq per L; however, values of 10 to 12 mEq per L may be found in the face of prolonged diarrhea. The BUN reflects the state of hydration and the adequacy of the recent intake of protein. It may climb rarely as high as 50 to 60 mg per dL in children who lose 10% to 15% of their body weight, although mild elevations (20 to 30 mg per dL) occur more commonly. In a child who has been maintained on clear liquids, however, the BUN will not accurately indicate the degree of dehydration because urea arises as a breakdown product during protein metabolism. Although the hemoglobin and WBC count are usually normal in the child with viral gastroenteritis, hemoconcentration may occur with dehydration.

Management

Uncomplicated viral gastroenteritis usually remits in 2 to 5 days and does not require treatment in the hospital. All children should be weighed, preferably with minimal clothing, to provide a baseline for follow-up. The vomiting will generally respond to a brief cessation of oral intake. After 2 to 4 hours of abstinence, the diet should be resumed gradually. The diarrhea may persist for several days, but hydration can usually be maintained orally after the vomiting has subsided.

Current recommendations for oral therapy emphasize the use of appropriately balanced glucose and electrolyte solutions, as well as the early reintroduction of feedings. Generally, rehydration is initiated, particularly in infants younger than 1 year, with a solution that contains 75 to 90 mEq per L sodium in a ratio with glucose of 1:1 (e.g., Rehydralyte®). Older children often tolerate juices and sodas. Some studies have advocated the use of glucose polymers (e.g., Ricelyte®) instead of glucose as a means to reduce diarrhea, but significant advantages have yet to be demonstrated for these products. Preparation at home of fluids that contain salt notoriously leads to errors, and this procedure is to be condemned. Similarly, the physician should avoid the use of boiled skim milk, a hypertonic solution that may produce hypernatremia.

The antiemetic ondansetron may be helpful in selected children coming to the ED for care. By providing some improved ability of the child to tolerate oral intake, there may be more opportunity to manage these children as outpatients. Ondansetron can be administered orally, as an orally disintegrating tablet or intravenously (0.15 mg per kg, maximum 8 mg, as a single dose or an age based regimen [see drug formulary section]) to improve the ability of the child to maintain hydration. Trimethobenzamide (Tigan®) appears to be ineffective as an antiemetic in children. The phenothiazine compounds reduce emesis somewhat, but they occasionally produce adverse side effects, such as extrapyramidal reactions or oculogyric crises that limit their usefulness. Antidiarrheal medications to reduce stool output are not commonly used in children, as some of these drugs may carry significant risks to infants, especially those with bacterial enteritis. Loperamide (0.5 mg per kg per day) has been shown to reduce the severity of diarrhea in conjunction with oral rehydration therapy, but is indicated only for unusually severe or prolonged cases of gastroenteritis after excluding a cause that would respond to specific therapy. Although administration of the combination of diphenoxylate and atropine (Lomotil®) may be successful in adults, toxic reactions in children limit its usefulness. A few studies have suggested a small benefit from bismuth subsalicylate (Pepto-Bismol®), but this agent is not recommended for routine cases.

Dehydration is the only significant complication of viral gastroenteritis. If the physician suspects that a child has developed more than 5% to 10% dehydration, electrolytes and a BUN should be obtained. These tests establish the degree of acidosis and the presence of hyponatremia or hypernatremia.

Most children with gastroenteritis tolerate oral rehydration. In underdeveloped countries, even patients with severe dehydration are often managed successfully by using the oral route. However, in the ED, treatment for children with moderate to severe dehydration is usually initiated intravenously. As a rule, all patients with dehydration estimated to be greater than 10%, and many cases falling in the range of 5% to 10%, receive IV fluids.

When IV therapy is chosen, a bolus of fluid, such as 10 to 20 mL per kg normal saline or normal saline with 5% dextrose, may be administered over 1 hour, or more rapidly if needed (see Chapter 3). As some children with moderate to severe dehydration develop mild hypoglycemia, it is reasonable to perform a rapid test of serum glucose and administer a bolus of dextrose (0.5 to 1 g per kg) or use glucose-containing solutions, when indicated. If rehydration is achieved and the child is capable of subsequent oral intake, treatment may be continued at home (as in the milder cases).

Children who are more than 5% dehydrated or have alterations in the serum sodium (less than 130 mEq per L or more than 145 mEq per L) may require hospitalization. IV therapy should be started in the ED, particularly if there is evidence of vascular instability (see Chapters 3, 17, 18, and 100).

Bacterial Gastroenteritis

Background

Five bacterial pathogens commonly produce gastroenteritis: *Salmonella, Shigella, Yersinia, Campylobacter,* and pathogenic *E. coli.* Together, these organisms cause 10% to 15% of the diarrheal illnesses seen in children coming to the ED (Fig. 92.17). In underdeveloped countries and occasionally in the United States, *Vibrio* species must also be considered. In addition, *A. hydrophila* has been associated occasionally with diarrheal illnesses in children. *C. difficile* causes toxin-associated colitis, particularly in patients who receive antibiotics.

Salmonella, Shigella, Yersinia, and *Campylobacter* do not normally inhabit the alimentary tract. Thus, recovery of one of these organisms suffices for the diagnosis of gastroenteritis. *E. coli,* however, is part of the normal bowel flora, only occasionally assuming a pathogenic role. Serotyping is useful for detecting *E. coli* O157, which along with related strains is capable of inducing hemolytic uremic syndrome, but identification of other disease-producing strains is not readily available to the clinician.

Pathophysiology

Salmonella species gain access to the small intestine following ingestion. Gastric acid is usually lethal to the organism, but large numbers of bacteria may overcome this defense mechanism. Patients with gastrectomies (or taking agents that inhibit the production of gastric acid) are more susceptible to *Salmonella* infection than those with an intact, normally functioning stomach. *Salmonella* can penetrate the epithelial layer to the level of the lamina propria and evoke a leukocyte response. Generally, the infection extends no further, but bacteremia may occur, especially in young children. Several species, notably *Salmonella choleraesuis* and *Salmonella typhi,* readily enter the circulation through the lymphatics. *Salmonella* produce diarrhea by multiple mechanisms. Several toxins have been identified; in addition, prostaglandins that stimulate the active secretion of fluids and electrolytes may be released.

Certain *Shigella* attach to binding sites on the surface of the intestinal mucosal cells. The organisms penetrate the cells and proliferate within them. Intraepithelial multiplication destroys the cell and produces mucosal ulcerations. Invasion of the epithelium evokes an intense inflammatory response. At the base of the ulcerated lesions, erosion of blood vessels may lead to bleeding. Other species of *Shigella* elaborate exotoxins that can produce diarrhea. These toxins result in increased secretion of fluid and electrolytes by the intestinal mucosa.

Although the pathophysiology of infection from *Yersinia enterocolitica* has not been completely elucidated, clues are available from animal models and occasional pathologic specimens. The organisms are believed to produce terminal ileitis; inflammatory changes and ulcerations have been visualized with endoscopy. The infection elicits a neutrophilic response, particularly around the Peyer's patches. It then extends to the mesenteric lymph nodes, which are destroyed by microabscess formation and may enlarge considerably. Occasionally, further dissemination occurs with involvement of the liver and spleen.

Campylobacter utilize mobility and chemotaxis to navigate the gastrointestinal epithelial surface, appear to produce adhesins and cytotoxins and possess the ability to survive within macrophages, monocytes, and epithelial cells but predominantly within vacuoles. At present the mechanism by which diarrhea results is not known. Mesenteric lymphadenitis and ileocolitis are common. Extraintestinal complications or bloodstream invasion is rare among patients with intact humoral immunity and phagocytosis.

E. coli may produce diarrhea on the basis of several characteristics. Disease-producing strains have been classified as enteropathogenic, enterotoxic, enteroinvasive, enteroaggregative, enteroadherent, and enterohemorrhagic. The risk of developing hemolytic uremic syndrome after infection with *E. coli* O157 is estimated to be 10% to 15% in children.

Clinical Manifestations

Signs and Symptoms. A careful epidemiologic history often provides a clue to the diagnosis of Salmonella infections. Foodborne outbreaks usually occur in the summer. After an

MEDICAL EMERGENCIES

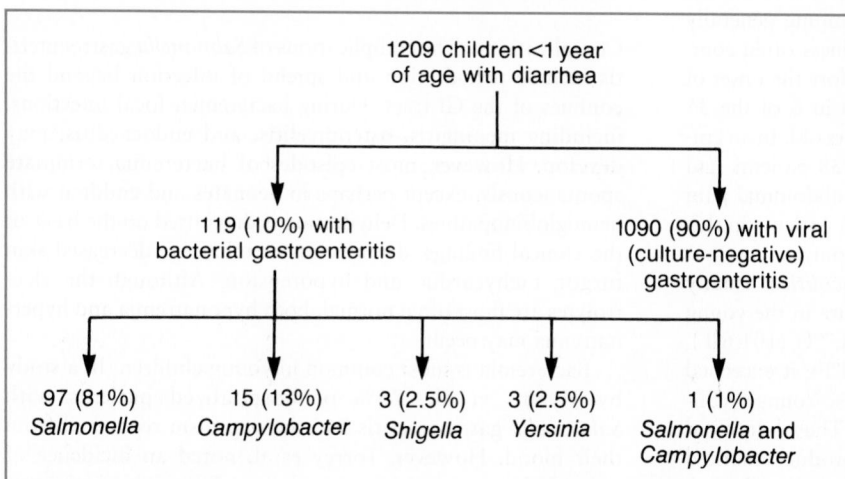

FIGURE 92.17 Etiology of gastroenteritis among consecutively cultured infants younger than 1 year in an urban emergency department. (Reprinted from Torrey S, Fleisher G, Jaffe D. Incidence of *Salmonella* bacteremia in infants with *Salmonella* gastroenteritis. *J Pediatr* 1986; 108:718, with permission.)

incubation period of 8 to 48 hours, the child experiences crampy abdominal pain and nausea. The stools are watery and may contain blood, but this is not the rule. Fever is noted in most children. Unless protracted diarrhea has led to clinically apparent dehydration, the physical examination is unremarkable. Abdominal tenderness and distension are occasional findings. The leukocyte count is usually 10,000 to 15,000 per mm³. Methylene blue staining of the stool may show the presence of polymorphonuclear leukocytes but not in sheets as seen with *Shigella*. A single rectal swab leads to isolation of *Salmonella* from more than 90% of children with this infection.

Shigella may cause an asymptomatic infection, mild gastroenteritis, or bacillary dysentery. Mild illnesses are more common. Children affected in this way complain of frequent watery stools but few constitutional symptoms. The temperature remains normal in many cases, and the physical examination is unremarkable.

Bacillary dysentery from *Shigella* begins suddenly with fever and abdominal pain. Diarrhea begins shortly thereafter. The stools, which may average 10 to 12 daily, contain mucus and blood, and tenesmus is common. Children with this form of shigellosis have a fever, often in the range of 39°C to 40°C (102.2°F to 104°F). Palpation of the abdomen often elicits diffuse tenderness but no evidence of peritoneal irritation.

Occasionally, a *Shigella* infection may produce CNS irritation because of the release of toxin before the onset of diarrhea. Thus, shigellosis must be considered in the differential diagnosis of meningismus in the absence of a pleocytosis in the CSF. A seizure may actually be the first manifestation of the illness.

Certain laboratory abnormalities strongly suggest *Shigella* as the cause of gastroenteritis. The leukocyte count often shows many band forms that exceed the mature neutrophils in number. One study described this phenomenon in 85% of 123 children between the ages of 2 months and 8 years with shigellosis. The total WBC count may show a leukopenia or a leukocytosis but most commonly hovers in the normal range. Because *Shigella* invades the intestinal mucosa, this infection elicits a profound inflammatory response. The exudation of white cells leads to the finding of sheets of neutrophils in the stool after methylene blue staining. A single rectal swab suffices for the isolation of *Shigella* from most children with this illness. Children with gastroenteritis caused by *Y. enterocolitica* usually have an abrupt onset of diarrhea. The stools are often watery and may contain blood, but vomiting generally remains inconsequential. Patients with this illness often complain of severe abdominal pain, sometimes before the onset of diarrhea. Delorme et al. noted this symptom in 6 of the 35 children studied, half of whom were 1 to 5 years old. In an epidemic in a school in New York State, 37 of 38 patients had abdominal pain; the potential severity of the abdominal pain in this disease is illustrated by the fact that 16 patients in this outbreak mistakenly underwent an appendectomy.

Gastrointestinal infection with *Y. enterocolitica* usually elicits a febrile response. The mean temperature in the young adolescents reported by Black et al. was 38.7°C (101.6°F), with a range of 37.2°C to 40°C (99°F to 104°F); it exceeded 37.8°C (100°F) in more than 95% of patients. Younger children appear to develop a fever less often. The abdominal examination is usually benign, but palpation produces marked tenderness in the subset of patients with mesenteric adenitis.

Arthritis and skin rashes occur in 5% to 10% of patients with this disease.

The mean WBC count in children with yersiniosis is usually normal, although leukocytosis with a shift to the left occurs occasionally. The electrolytes and BUN are normal except in the face of dehydration. Examination of stool stained with methylene blue reveals polymorphonuclear neutrophils. The organism can be recovered from stool culture but requires enrichment techniques. Although a single specimen is diagnostic in 70% to 80% of illnesses, a second sample should be obtained in the face of a previous negative culture when the clinical suspicion of disease remains strong.

Campylobacter enteritis is characterized by the abrupt onset of fever and abdominal pain, followed shortly by diarrhea. The temperature often remains normal in children younger than 3 months old, but ranges up to 40°C (104°F) in the older child. Vomiting occurs uncommonly and resolves rapidly. Two-thirds of children complain of abdominal pain, which may be severe. The number of stools varies from 2 to 20 daily; they are watery and contain blood in at least 50% of cases. The physical examination is generally unremarkable. Although the abdominal pain occasionally simulates appendicitis, palpation of the abdomen elicits minimal tenderness. Signs of dehydration are found only rarely.

The WBC count in *Campylobacter* enteritis usually remains below 12,000 per mm³, the highest being 22,500 per mm³ in one study; on occasion, there may be a shift to the left. The electrolytes and BUN are usually normal. Maki et al. found fecal leukocytes in four of five patients with enteritis caused by *Campylobacter*. The organism is not often isolated from the blood but can be recovered easily from the stool by using appropriate media. When available, phase contrast microscopy can demonstrate the organism in fresh stool specimens.

The clinical picture of diarrhea caused by *E. coli* varies. This organism is suspected most often in the setting of a specific outbreak.

In general, features suggestive of a bacterial rather than a viral gastroenteritis include (i) more than ten stools per day or diarrhea lasting for more than 4 days, (ii) blood in the stool, (iii) fever of 39.5°C (103°F) or higher, (iv) clinical toxicity, and (v) polymorphonuclear leukocytes in the stool. The presence of these findings enhances the likelihood that a bacterial pathogen is involved, although a viral gastroenteritis is not necessarily ruled out.

Complications. The complications of *Salmonella* gastroenteritis include dehydration and spread of infection beyond the confines of the GI tract. During bacteremia, focal infections, including meningitis, osteomyelitis, and endocarditis, may develop. However, most episodes of bacteremia terminate spontaneously, except perhaps in neonates and children with hemoglobinopathies. Dehydration is diagnosed on the basis of the clinical findings: dry mucous membranes, decreased skin turgor, tachycardia, and hypotension. Although the electrolytes are most often normal, both hyponatremia and hypernatremia may occur.

Bacteremia is most common in young children. In a study by Hyams et al., 25% of hospitalized patients with *Salmonella* gastroenteritis had the organism recovered from their blood. However, Torrey et al. noted an incidence of only 6% in an ambulatory population. Although a high fever usually accompanies spread to the circulation, the physical examination is often devoid of any signs of serious illness. In addition, infants in the first 3 months of life often remain afebrile in the face of bacteremia. The WBC count is greater than 15,000 per mm^3 in 80% to 90% with bacteremia, and culture of the blood leads to recovery of the organism.

Enteric fever also occurs from the dissemination of certain serotypes of *Salmonella*; if *S. typhi* is isolated, the illness is called typhoid fever. The disease is characterized by chills and fever, often rising in a steplike pattern to 40°C (104°F). Diarrhea does not necessarily precede or coexist with the systemic illness. A relative bradycardia in relation to the height of the temperature is a hallmark of enteric fever. Splenomegaly and a macular rash, or rose spots, are detectable in 20% to 30% of patients. Leukopenia characterizes the hematologic picture. Both blood and stool cultures may be negative.

Invasion of the bloodstream may lead to various focal diseases. Meningitis most commonly affects the youngest children. The features are identical to those observed in CNS infections with other purulent organisms. Children with sickle cell hemoglobinopathies have a peculiar predilection for bone and joint involvement. Endocarditis is less commonly seen.

The complications of shigellosis include dehydration, bacteremia, seizures, and colonic perforation. Dehydration often accompanies dysenteric infections and is diagnosed on the basis of the usual clinical findings. Bacteremia and perforation are both rare, occurring in far fewer than 1% of GI infections.

Most episodes of gastroenteritis with *Yersinia* are self-limiting, resolving before dehydration develops. Appendicitis occasionally results from obstruction of the appendiceal lumen by swollen lymphoid tissue. The incidence is unknown, but 5 of 38 patients in the aforementioned New York State epidemic underwent removal of appendices that were suppurative. Bacteremia and focal infection follow gastroenteritis almost exclusively in the compromised host, particularly in association with thalassemia.

Campylobacter infections occasionally lead to dehydration, but less often than is seen with the other bacterial pathogens in the GI tract. Rarely, bacteremic or focal infections occur.

Management

Salmonella gastroenteritis is usually a self-limiting illness. In most cases, the disease is not sufficiently distinct or severe enough to suggest to the clinician the need for a diagnostic evaluation. However, serious complications occur on occasion in very young infants and in children with sickle cell hemoglobinopathies.

The treatment of *Salmonella* gastroenteritis should be directed toward the maintenance of adequate hydration. As with viral infections, limitation of the diet to electrolyte solutions ("clear liquids") suffices in most children. Antibiotic therapy neither ameliorates the course of the gastroenteritis nor eradicates the organism from the intestinal tract in the immunocompetent host. In fact, several studies have suggested prolonged carriage after the administration of antibiotics.

Potential indications for admission of a child with diarrhea suspected or proved to be caused by *Salmonella* species are (i) dehydration not responsive to treatment, (ii) focal infection or bacteremia/sepsis, (iii) age younger than 3 months or temperature higher than 39°C (102.2°F) in a child younger than 12 months (unless blood culture is known to be sterile),

(iv) sickle cell anemia, or (v) immunosuppressive conditions such as HIV. If bacteremia is suspected, IV therapy with ceftriaxone (50 mg per kg per day in one daily dose) or cefotaxime (100 mg per kg per day in two divided doses) should be initiated. Fluoroquinolones (ciprofloxacin, ofloxacin) or azithromycin provides an alternative for cephalosporin-allergic patients. When oral therapy is indicated trimethoprim-sulfamethoxazole (8 mg per kg per day of trimethoprim in two divided doses) is the drug of choice for susceptible strains.

Shigellosis stands alone as the only form of bacterial gastroenteritis for which antibiotics have proved efficacious. Antimicrobial therapy shortens the course of the illness and the duration of excretion of the organisms in the stool. Treatment alleviates the symptoms and signs of the gastroenteritis and limits transmission of the disease. Trimethoprim-sulfamethoxazole (8 mg of trimethoprim and 40 mg of sulfamethoxazole per kilogram per day) is the initial drug of choice while the results of sensitivity tests are pending. Fluoroquinolones and ceftriaxone are alternatives.

Supportive therapy is an important aspect of the management of shigellosis. The initial oral intake should be limited to solutions with physiologic concentrations of glucose and electrolytes. As the diarrhea begins to abate, solid foods can be added. Dietary manipulation leads to resolution of the disease in some children before the isolation of the organism. Antibiotic therapy may be omitted in such cases, unless there is a particular concern about spread in a closed population.

As with other varieties of infectious gastroenteritis, most medications designed to provide symptomatic relief from diarrhea have no demonstrated efficacy. In particular, paregoric or combinations of diphenoxylate and atropine (Lomotil®) are contraindicated. Dupont and Hornick showed that diarrhea persisted longer in infected volunteers treated with antibiotics and diphenoxylate/atropine than with those who received only antibiotics.

Most episodes of shigellosis can be handled on an outpatient basis. Potential indications for admission include (i) age 6 months or younger, (ii) dehydration, and (iii) bacteremia (rare). Before the definitive diagnosis of shigellosis, particularly with significant bleeding, hospitalization may be required because of a concern about noninfectious entities such as a Meckel's diverticulum.

Most children with yersiniosis can be treated as outpatients. Initially, the diet may be limited to electrolyte solutions (clear liquids). Although *Y. enterocolitica* is usually sensitive in vitro to tetracycline, chloramphenicol, colistin, gentamicin, and kanamycin, current studies have demonstrated no benefit from antibiotic therapy of uncomplicated gastroenteritis. However, persistent diarrhea may respond to antimicrobial treatment. Suspected or proven sepsis merits IV administration of antibiotics such as gentamicin (5 to 7.5 mg per kg per day in one to three divided doses, beyond the neonatal period). Potential indications for admission include dehydration, severe abdominal pain suggesting appendicitis, and underlying diseases such as thalassemia.

Campylobacter enteritis is a self-limited but prolonged illness; diarrhea persists for more than 1 week in one-third of children. These organisms exhibit almost universal sensitivity to erythromycin, which can be given orally at a dosage of 40 mg per kg per day; ciprofloxacin is an alternative for adolescents. However, antimicrobial therapy has not proved to decrease the duration of diarrhea.

MEDICAL EMERGENCIES

Antibiotic-associated Colitis

Background

Children who take antibiotics often develop diarrhea, which varies from mild to severe. For most of the mild cases, no specific diagnosis is established. A small subset of patients, usually with more severe illnesses, manifest pseudomembranous colitis, caused by *C. difficile*. Although antibiotics are the most important precipitating factor for pseudomembranous colitis, the disease was recognized in the preantibiotic era and still occurs occasionally in the absence of prior antibiotic therapy. Almost every antibiotic has been reported to be associated with pseudomembranous colitis. Clindamycin, lincomycin, and the broad-spectrum β-lactam agents in particular predispose to overgrowth of *C. difficile,* but because these drugs are rarely used for children on an outpatient basis, widely prescribed medications, such as amoxicillin, are more often implicated in the pediatric age group.

Pathophysiology

C. difficile, the etiologic agent in pseudomembranous colitis, is a gram-positive anaerobic bacillus that may be part of the normal intestinal flora, particularly during the first year of life. Even a short course of antibiotic therapy may lead to overgrowth of this organism. Colitis results from toxin production by *C. difficile* within the intestinal lumen; the two major toxins are known as A and B. These toxins attack the membranes or microfilaments of cells and produce hemorrhage, necrosis, and inflammation.

Clinical Manifestations

Colitis with *C. difficile* varies widely in severity. Typically, profuse watery or mucoid diarrhea begins after several days of antibiotic therapy. Many older children complain of crampy abdominal pain. On examination, the usual findings include fever and diffuse abdominal tenderness. Often, the WBC count rises above 15,000 per mm^3. The stool may be guaiac-positive or frankly bloody; leukocytes are found on smears from approximately 50% of patients. An etiologic diagnosis requires the identification of *C. difficile* toxin in the stool; recovery of the organism on culture is suggestive but not sufficient.

If *C. difficile* colitis goes unrecognized and untreated, complications, including toxic megacolon, perforation, and peritonitis, may develop. Case fatality rates as high as 10% to 20% were described before the introduction of specific treatments.

Management

The treatment for children with colitis caused by *C. difficile* depends on the severity of the disease. Mild cases respond to cessation of antibiotic treatment and supportive therapy with fluids and electrolytes. In particular, children seen with a small amount of diarrhea on oral antibiotics for a minor infection, and in whom the suspicion of pseudomembranous colitis is low, do not need an extensive diagnostic investigation or institution of specific antimicrobial therapy.

Patients with more severe or persistent antibiotic-associated diarrhea should be evaluated for *C. difficile* with a test for toxin in the stool. Oral metronidazole (30 mg per kg per day in four divided doses) or oral vancomycin (40 mg per kg per day, with a usual maximum of 125 mg per dose, in four divided doses) is prescribed most commonly. Although used with some success in the past, cholestyramine does not have the same efficacy as oral antibiotics, but it may be tried in patients who fail treatment with vancomycin and metronidazole. Antidiarrheal agents should be avoided. When possible, the precipitating antibiotic should be discontinued, but cessation is not essential once specific therapy has been initiated. Children with more pronounced clinical illnesses, particularly those receiving antibiotic therapy, may merit hospitalization.

Gastritis

Background

Gastritis is an inflammation of the lining of the stomach. Most cases are noninfectious; however, *Helicobacter pylori*, a gram-negative rod that is capable of surviving in the acid milieu of the stomach, is the cause in some patients. Infection rates with this organism are low in young children but increase in adolescence. Chronic infection with *H. pylori* is associated with peptic ulcer and gastric carcinoma.

Clinical Manifestations

Gastritis caused by *H. pylori* manifests in older children and adolescents with persistent epigastric pain, nausea, and vomiting. Often, the stool will test positive for blood. More severe cases are characterized by hematemesis. In younger children and infants unable to verbalize or localize pain reliably, irritability may be the primary manifestation.

H. pylori can be diagnosed by culture of gastric tissue obtained at biopsy, breath testing, serology, and stool antigen assays. Only serology and stool assay have applicability in the setting of the ED. Sensitivity for these two tests has been reported to range from 80% to 95%, with greater accuracy being observed in older children; specificity hovers around 90%.

Management

In most cases, the clinician cannot diagnose *H. pylori* infection in the ED with sufficient certainty to warrant the initiation of treatment with antibiotics. Effective therapies require two or three drugs, an inhibitor of acid secretion along with one or two antibiotics, administered for 10 to 14 days. For adolescents, a frequently used regimen includes omeprazole (20 mg twice daily), clarithromycin (500 mg twice daily), and amoxicillin (1 g twice daily) for 10 days.

SKIN, SOFT-TISSUE, AND BONE INFECTIONS

The major infections of the skin, soft tissues, and bones include impetigo, cutaneous abscesses, lymphadenitis, cellulitis, fasciitis, pyomyositis, septic arthritis, and osteomyelitis. Additionally mastitis and omphalitis occur in the neonate. Chapter 117 deals with cutaneous abscesses. Among the disorders in this group, impetigo and cellulitis are both common complaints in the ED. Although children with bone and joint infections are seen only occasionally, the differential diagnosis of several common complaints (e.g., fever, limp) often includes these conditions. Thus, the emergency physician who deals

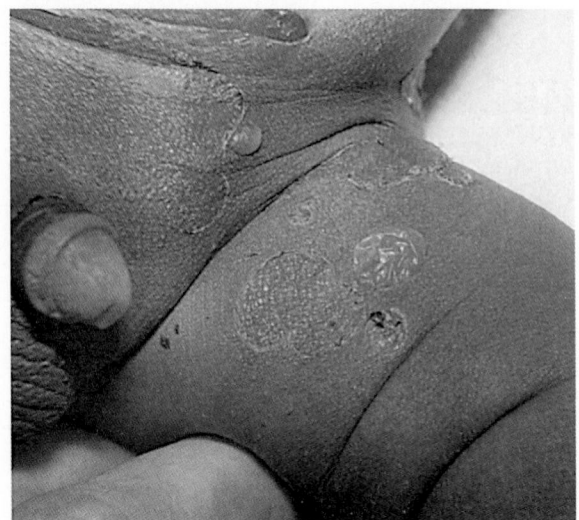

FIGURE 92.18 Bullous impetigo.

with children should be familiar with such infections, particularly because a prolonged delay in the institution of therapy can result in appreciable morbidity.

Impetigo

Background

Impetigo is a bacterial infection of the skin confined to the epidermis. A deeper variety of impetigo, ecthyma, also involves the dermis. Pustules larger than 1 cm in diameter (Fig. 92.18) characterize bullous impetigo. Impetigo is a common infection in children, particularly during the summer months. It occurs in epidemics during the warm weather in confined populations of children.

Any strain of group A streptococcus, including nephritogenic varieties, can infect the skin and cause impetigo. *S. aureus,* the primary agent in bullous impetigo is a common cause of nonbullous impetigo as well.

Pathophysiology

The intact epidermis forms a relatively impervious barrier to bacteria. However, a breach in the integument, even if too small to be noticed by the patient or parents, may allow the entry of pathogens and the development of impetigo. In streptococcal infections, toxins, such as streptolysins, elaborated by the organism, promote local spread of the process. Different toxins produced by *S. aureus* lead to the accumulation of purulent material and the evolution of bullae.

Clinical Manifestations

Impetigo is more common in young children, particularly those younger than 6 years. Typically, a parent will bring a child to the ED complaining of sores on the body. No systemic ailments, such as fever or malaise, are associated. Physical examination shows a healthy child with a normal temperature. The lesions usually ooze serous fluid but may be bullous or crusted as well (Fig. 92.18). Surrounding erythema is minimal, and the regional lymph nodes often do not enlarge noticeably.

Laboratory studies are not routinely obtained in children with impetigo. Cultures of the lesions, performed only if there is any doubt about the diagnosis, will yield group A streptococci or *S. aureus* in most cases. The WBC count is normal.

The complications of impetigo include spread of the infection locally and remote nonsuppurative disease. Occasionally, impetigo may progress to cellulitis. If the lesions are caused by nephritogenic streptococci, glomerulonephritis may develop 7 to 14 days later. The attack rate for glomerulonephritis has been as high as 1% in certain epidemics, but the incidence is far less in the usual clinical setting.

Management

A single course of antibiotic therapy cures impetigo in 95% of children. Erythromycin (40 mg per kg per day in four divided doses) provides effective oral treatment for the usual pathogens. Other acceptable oral drugs include dicloxacillin (50 mg per kg per day) or cephalexin (50 mg per kg per day). For cases of impetigo due to MRSA, trimethoprim-sulfamethoxazole (8 mg per kg per day of TMP) or clindamycin (30 mg per kg per day) may be prescribed. Mupirocin (Bactroban®) applied locally is able to eradicate most cases of impetigo, particularly if the disease is limited in distribution. Combination topical and systemic therapy is unnecessary. Vigorous scrubbing does not hasten the resolution, and routine cleanliness is sufficient. Even when systemic antibiotic therapy eliminates the infection, the incidence of glomerulonephritis has not been demonstrated to decrease.

Lymphadenitis

Lymph nodes in any region of the body may become infected. Regardless of the site of involvement, the same considerations apply as discussed under cervical lymphadenitis. *S. aureus* and group A streptococci are the most common pathogens. The finding of inguinal or axillary adenitis should prompt a meticulous search for a portal of entry for bacteria on the extremities. Locating an impetiginous lesion or other breech in the integument provides reassurance that the lymph node enlargement is caused by infection rather than by neoplasm. History should be requested regarding a cat scratch or bite as a possible etiologic focus. Particularly in the adolescent, inguinal adenitis suggests a need to look for sexually transmitted pathogens. The child with lymphadenitis should be treated with antibiotic therapy and drainage with culture, if fluctuation occurs. Dicloxacillin (50 mg per kg per day) and cephalexin (50 mg per kg per day) are effective against the usual pathogens except for community acquired MRSA where clindamycin or the addition of trimethoprim sulfamethoxasole should be used.

Cellulitis

Background

Cellulitis is an infection of the skin and subcutaneous tissues. Any anatomic area may be involved, but the body can be divided, for etiologic considerations, into two regions: (i) the face and (ii) the scalp, neck, trunk, and extremities.

Facial cellulitis includes buccal, periorbital, and less often, orbital lesions. Before the introduction of a vaccine against Hib, *H. influenzae* type b caused 50% of these infections. At present, the organisms involved most commonly are *S. aureus*, group A streptococci, and *S. pneumoniae*. Bacteremia is present in 90% of the cases of disease caused by *S. pneumoniae* and *H. influenzae* type b. Alternatively, a dental abscess may serve as the source for an apparent cellulitis, in which case treatment relies almost exclusively on drainage of the abscess.

S. aureus causes most nonfacial cellulitis and has been reported to be recovered from 70% of extremity lesions with an identifiable origin, either as the sole pathogen or in combination with group A streptococci. Nonfacial cellulitis very rarely results from infection with *H. influenzae*, although when this organism is involved, as with facial lesions, it usually invades the bloodstream.

Cellulitis occasionally occurs among immunosuppressed patients. In these cases, unusual organisms, including *P. aeruginosa*, gram-negative enteric rods, and anaerobic bacteria, must be considered. Even when initial examination suggests minimal inflammation, an extensive infection may exist, because neutropenia often masks the depth of the lesion.

Cellulitis is a common infection that is more often seen in temperate climates when the weather is warm. Precise statistics on the incidence of cellulitis are not available; however, in one study during the summer months, this infection accounted for approximately 1 of every 500 visits to the ED of a children's hospital.

Pathogenesis

Cellulitis follows either hematogenous dissemination of a pathogenic organism or local invasion.

Surgical or traumatic wounds may serve as a portal of entry for bacteria. This is the route by which *S. aureus* and group A streptococci usually gain access to the subcutaneous tissue; subsequently, toxins produced by these organisms allow for local spread. Alternatively, invasion of the bloodstream may precede the appearance of cellulitis. The periorbital and facial lesions seen occasionally with *H. influenzae* and *S. pneumoniae* follow a bacteremia, and these organisms often are recovered from the blood. *S. aureus* and group A streptococcus are less often spread by this mechanism.

Clinical Manifestations

The child with cellulitis develops a local inflammatory response (Fig. 92.19) at the site of infection with erythema, edema, warmth, pain, and, when an extremity is involved, limitation of motion. There may be a history of a prior wound or insect bite. Facial infections are more common during the first 5 years of life. Fever is unusual, except in bacteremic infections or when the lesions are extensive. Only 10% to 20% of children with cellulitis manifest a fever. The lesion itself is erythematous and tender, and may be indurated but is not fluctuant; red streaks may radiate proximally along the course of the lymphatic drainage. The regional lymph nodes usually enlarge in response to the infection.

With cellulitis caused by *S. aureus* or group A streptococci, the WBC count is normal in most children. More extensive lesions or bacteremia, seen only occasionally with these organisms, evoke a leukocytosis. A culture obtained from the central

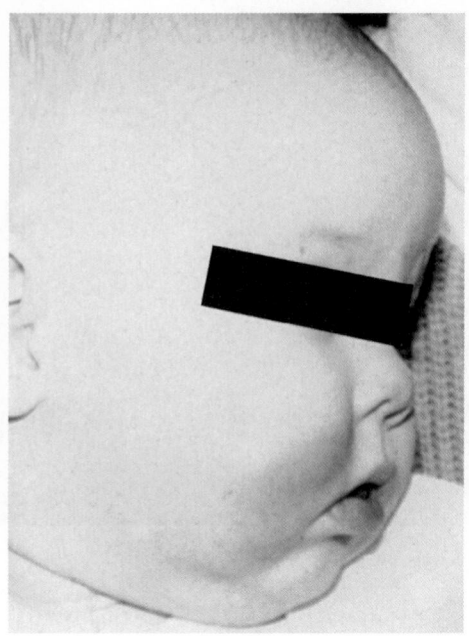

FIGURE 92.19 Infant with buccal cellulitis caused by *Haemophilus influenzae*.

area of the cellulitis by needle aspiration or biopsy will yield a pathogen in 50% of cases, even though cultures of the blood usually remain sterile.

Bacteremia accompanies cellulitis caused by *H. influenzae* or *S. pneumoniae;* these organisms are isolated from the blood in 90% of infected patients. The WBC count is greater than 15,000 per m^3 as a rule, usually with a shift to the left.

The complications of cellulitis, although uncommon, include local and metastatic spread of infection. The organisms may invade deeper tissues, producing septic arthritis or osteomyelitis. During the course of bacteremia with *H. influenzae*, *S. pneumoniae*, or rarely other organisms, there may be involvement of the meninges, pericardium, epiglottis, or synovial membranes. Multifocal areas of cellulitis should arouse a suspicion of hematogenous dissemination. Occasionally, cellulitis provides a clue to an infection that originates in deeper anatomic structures. As an example, a lesion on the abdominal wall may be a sign of peritonitis.

Management

Most children with nonfacial cellulitis can receive antibiotic therapy as outpatients, as long as bacteremic disease is unlikely (Fig. 92.20). Because *S. aureus* and group A streptococci are most commonly isolated, treatment should be directed at these organisms. Acceptable alternatives include a semisynthetic penicillin, such as dicloxacillin (50 mg per kg per day), cephalexin (50 mg per kg per day), or amoxicillin–clavulanic acid (50 mg per kg per day of amoxicillin); even methicillin-susceptible *S. aureus* will generally be resistant to penicillin and ampicillin. In areas where community-acquired MRSA are common the use of clindamycin or a combination of a semisynthetic penicillin, such as dicloxacillin, or cephalexin and trimethoprim-sulfamethoxazole may be needed. A CBC count, blood culture, and aspirate culture are not necessary in afebrile patients.

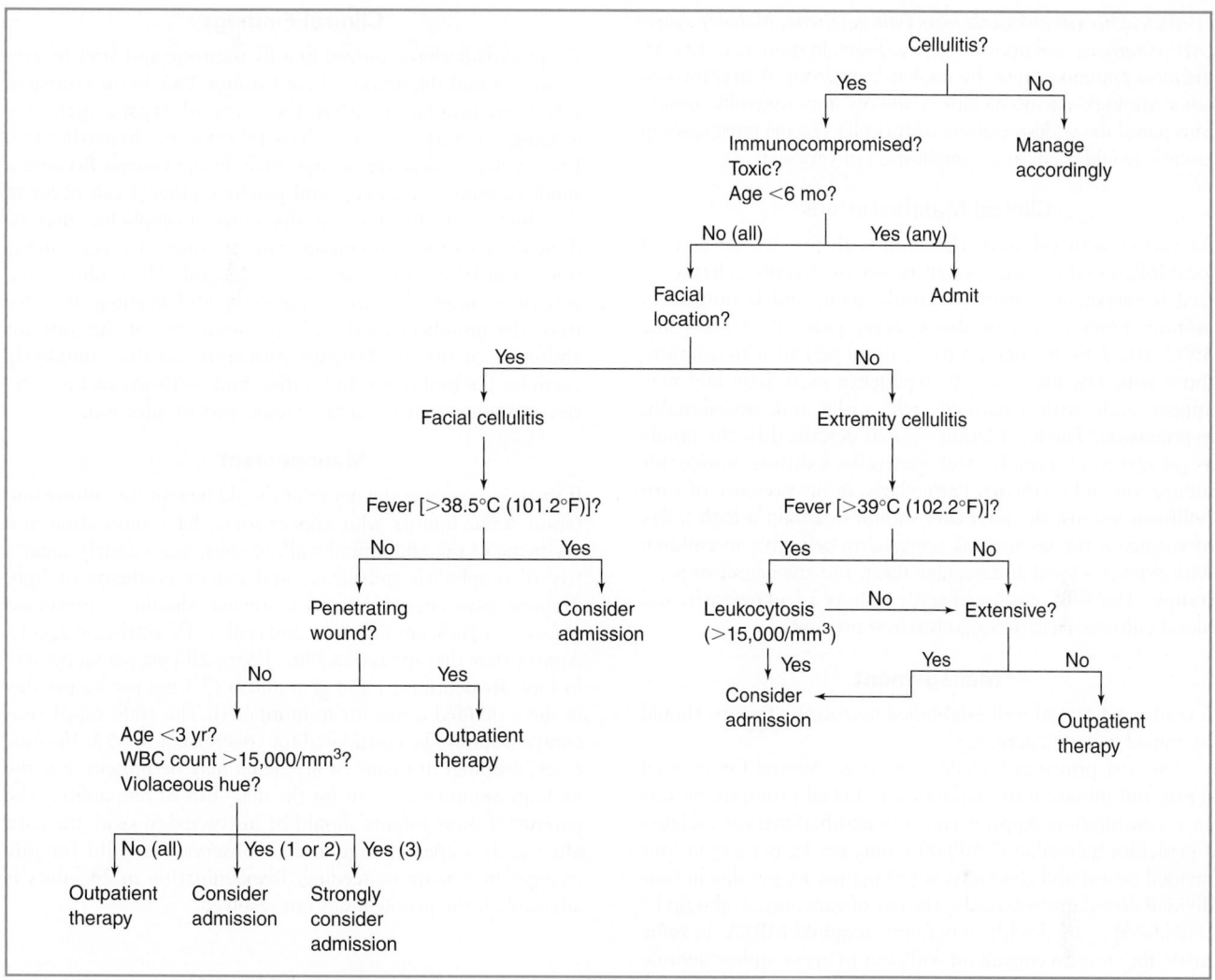

FIGURE 92.20 Diagnostic approach for the management of the child with soft-tissue swelling and possible cellulitis. WBC, white blood cell.

If a child with a nonfacial cellulitis has a high fever [39°C (102.2°F) or higher], the likelihood of a bacteremic infection or lymphangitic spread remains low but increases. A WBC count and culture of the blood should be obtained, along with consideration of a culture from the lesion. In cases in which the patient is well-appearing, little evidence of lymphangitic spread is seen and the WBC count is below 15,000 per mm³, antibiotic therapy is given as described for afebrile children, with a plan to have the patient reevaluated the following day. An ill-appearing patient, rapid spread, or a leukocytosis in association with a fever of 39°C (102.2°F) or higher should result in strong consideration for IV treatment, usually on an inpatient basis, with oxacillin (100 to 200 mg per kg per day in four divided doses) or cefazolin (100 mg per kg per day in three divided doses). Where rates of MRSA are high, intravenous clindamycin (40 mg per kg per day in four divided doses) or vancomycin (45 mg per kg per day in three divided doses) may be needed. For children not immunized against Hib, consider therapy with cefotaxime (200 mg per kg per day in four divided doses), ceftriaxone (100 mg per kg per day in a single dose), or ampicillin sulbactam acid (200 mg per kg per

day of ampicillin in four divided doses). Children allergic to penicillins and cephalosporins can be given clindamycin (40 mg per kg per day in four divided doses). When *H. influenzae* type b is a concern a quinolone or aztreonam should be added.

Children with facial cellulitis and fever are particularly likely to be bacteremic, in most cases with *S. pneumoniae* or, less commonly, *H. influenzae* type b, and are at risk for local complications. Thus, most should receive IV therapy as listed previously. Those who are afebrile may be managed as outpatients if they do not have risk factors for bacteremic disease—age younger than 3 years, spontaneous cellulitis without a preceding wound, and violaceous discoloration (Fig. 92.20).

Fasciitis

Background

Fasciitis is a deep soft-tissue infection. Unlike cellulitis, it involves the fascial and muscle layers, as well as the skin and subcutaneous tissues, but it does not extend per se to the bones or joints. Terms used to refer to this condition include *necrotizing*

MEDICAL EMERGENCIES

fasciitis, acute streptococcal hemolytic gangrene, Meleney synergistic gangrene, and *necrotizing erysipelas.* In more recent years, the most common cause, by far, has been group A streptococci; other etiologic agents include *S. aureus* and anaerobic organisms. Until the widespread use of varicella vaccine most cases of fasciitis would occur as a complication of varicella.

Clinical Manifestations

As occurs with cellulitis, the child with fasciitis develops a local inflammatory response at the site of infection, characterized by erythema, edema, warmth, pain, and limitation of motion. Fever occurs in almost every case, often exceeding 39°C (102.2°F). In contrast to the usual patient with cellulitis, those with fasciitis generally experience more pain and may appear toxic with a marked tachycardia and, occasionally, hypotension. The local lesion is often described by the family as progressing rapidly and generally exhibits noticeable induration and erythema. Particularly, in the presence of varicelliform lesions, the physician should maintain a high index of suspicion for fasciitis, as opposed to cellulitis, in children with extensive local disease, high fever, and any degree of prostration. The WBC count generally reflects a leukocytosis, and blood cultures yield an organism in most cases.

Management

A confirmed case of well-established necrotizing fasciitis should be considered an emergency.

The first priorities include supportive therapy for signs of sepsis and initiation of antibiotics, followed promptly by surgical consultation. Appropriate antimicrobial therapy includes a penicillin (penicillin G 500,000 units per kg per day in four divided doses) and clindamycin (40 mg per kg per day in four divided doses) intravenously. The use of vancomycin should be considered in areas with community acquired MRSA. In some cases, the surgical consultant will elect to incise and/or debride the lesions.

Omphalitis

Background

Omphalitis is an infection of the umbilical cord and surrounding tissues. Although formerly an important cause of neonatal mortality, the disease is now rare in developed countries because of advances in antisepsis and local care of the umbilical cord stump. Home delivery and low birth weight represent risk factors. When infection occurs, the usual pathogen is *S. aureus*; group B streptococci, *Streptococcccus pyogenes* (group A streptococci), and gram-negative enteric rods may also be isolated. Children are at risk during the first 2 weeks of life.

Pathophysiology

After ligation at delivery, the umbilical stump undergoes necrosis as a result of interruption of its blood supply. Bacterial colonization follows soon after birth. In rare cases, because of colonization by virulent bacteria or ill-defined host factors, colonizing organisms may invade the umbilical cord stump and surrounding tissues. The initial infection is cellulitis, but peritonitis, liver abscess, and/or sepsis may ensue in short order.

Clinical Findings

Omphalitis is characterized first by drainage and later by erythema around the umbilical cord stump. Late in the course of infection, infants manifest the signs of sepsis, including lethargy, irritability, and hypothermia or hyperthermia. Laboratory studies are normal early in the course. Because a small amount of drainage and patchy erythema can occur in the absence of infection, the diagnosis of omphalitis may be difficult. There are no definite clinical criteria for early infections, and laboratory tests are not helpful. The findings suggestive of omphalitis are (i) purulent, foul-smelling drainage from the umbilical cord with any erythema of the anterior abdomen; or (ii) any drainage with erythema that completely encircles the umbilicus. Induration and erythema of the anterior abdomen wall are definite indicators of infection.

Management

If there is drainage, the material should be sent for culture and Gram stain. Infants who appear toxic, have induration and erythema of the abdominal wall, or show signs clearly suggestive of omphalitis (purulence and patchy erythema or light drainage plus circumferential erythema) should be presumed to have a significant infection and require IV antibiotic agents. Appropriate therapy is oxacillin (100 to 200 mg per kg per day in four divided doses) and gentamicin (7.5 mg per kg per day in three divided doses for term infants). The addition of vancomycin should be considered for coverage of MRSA. In some cases, minimal drainage or erythema may be present, but the findings are not sufficient for the diagnosis of omphalitis. The parents of these infants should be instructed to swab the cord after each diaper change and to observe the child for any changes in activity or feeding. Reexamination in 24 hours is advisable if the problem has not resolved.

Neonatal Mastitis

Background

Mastitis is an infection of the breast tissue that affects prepubertal children only during the first 2 to 5 weeks of life. In most cases, *S. aureus* is the usual offending organism, although 5% to 10% of the infections are caused by gram-negative enteric bacteria. Girls are affected twice as commonly as boys.

Pathophysiology

Maternal hormones cross the placenta during gestation and stimulate hypertrophy of neonatal breast buds in both males and females. Usually, the enlargement subsides within 2 weeks. In occasional cases, bacteria are able to invade the hypertrophied glandular tissue, leading to abscess formation. Manipulation of the breast to excrete "witch's milk" may be a predisposing factor.

Clinical Manifestations

The primary finding in neonatal mastitis is a warm, erythematous, enlarged breast bud (Fig. 92.21). With disease progression, purulent drainage from the nipple may occur and there is tenderness to palpation. Only 25% of infants are febrile or appear ill. Mastitis in the infant must be distinguished from physiologic hypertrophy, which resolves spontaneously. The

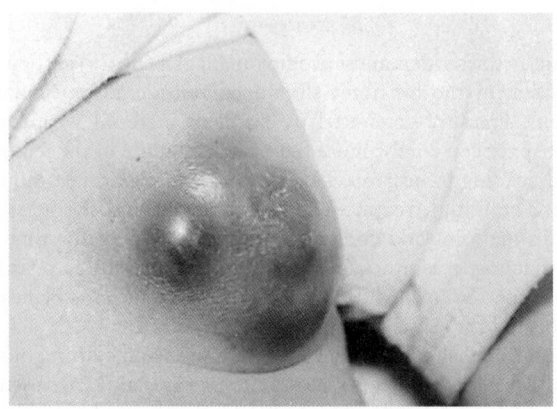

FIGURE 92.21 A 2-week-old infant with mastitis, characterized by erythema and induration.

normal breast bud that enlarges in response to stimulation by maternal hormones is neither red nor tender; if any drainage is present, the material is milky white, rather than yellow, and does not contain polymorphonuclear leukocytes or bacteria on Gram stain. Culture of the purulent drainage yields the pathogen in most cases, but the blood is usually sterile. Because these infections are well localized, the WBC count is usually in the normal range.

Management

Occasionally, an infant will appear septic and require appropriate supportive therapy, as described earlier in this chapter. The remainder will nonetheless require IV antibiotics, pending the results of cultures. Oxacillin (100 to 200 mg per kg per day in four divided doses) and gentamicin (7.5 mg per kg per day in three divided doses) provide appropriate coverage for the expected pathogens. The addition of vancomycin should be considered for coverage of MRSA. Incision and drainage is advisable in the case of local fluctulance, with careful attention to avoiding injury to the developing breast bud, which is already at risk of damage from the infectious process and may lead to cosmetic issues of the breast first noted at adolescence.

Septic Arthritis

Background

Septic arthritis is defined as a bacterial infection within a joint space. The incidence of this infection is low at an estimated 5 per 100,000 children per year for pyogenic bacteria. As opposed to adults, children who develop septic arthritis are generally otherwise healthy. Boys are affected twice as often as girls.

The bacterial cause of septic arthritis varies with age. During the first 2 months of life, group B streptococcus and *S. aureus* predominate. Gram-negative enteric bacilli, *Candida* species, and *N. gonorrhoeae* are seen sporadically.

Between 3 months and adolescence, *S. aureus* emerges as the single most common pathogen, being isolated from 80% to 90% of children with septic arthritis. The incidence of disease caused by *H. influenzae* type b has declined significantly since the introduction of the conjugated vaccine, but this organism remains a concern in children in this age range who have not been immunized against this pathogen. Group A streptococci and *S. pneumoniae* cause occasional cases.

The incidence of gonococcal arthritis in teenagers has varied in different reports, depending on the prevalence of sexual activity in the population studied. In most studies, *N. gonorrhoeae* has been the most common cause of septic arthritis among adolescents, trailed closely by *S. aureus*.

Many other organisms occasionally invade the joint space, some only in special circumstances. *P. aeruginosa* shows a peculiar predilection for septic arthritis after trauma as is seen in the foot after puncture wounds. In the child with sickle cell anemia, *Salmonella* species may cause septic arthritis. With the exception of Kingella, the gram-negative bacilli are almost never recovered from previously healthy children but are seen in immunosuppressed patients. *M. tuberculosis* is a rare causative agent but may be isolated at any age. In endemic areas, Lyme arthritis merits consideration.

Pathophysiology

Septic arthritis generally results from the hematogenous dissemination of an organism, into either the joint or the bony metaphysis. Except in circumstances of osteomyelitis, trauma, or recent surgery, it is rare for pediatric patients to have the pathogen gain access to the joint by direct inoculation or spread from a contiguous site of infection as is seen in adults. Although many children have a history of recent trauma, the role played by injury remains unknown. In gonococcal arthritis, the initial site of infection may be the genitals, pharynx, or rectum. Dissemination from the cervix follows menstruation when shedding of the organism is highest.

Bacteria in the joint space evoke an inflammatory response with an infiltration of neutrophils. The accumulation of purulent material distends the joint capsule, producing the physical and radiographic findings. *S. aureus* septic arthritis is associated with long-term joint morbidity in approximately 25% of patients.

Clinical Features

Infection within a joint produces pain and limitation of motion. Thus, the site of the arthritis determines the specific complaint. Ninety percent of children have a monoarticular arthritis that involves the lower extremity (hip, knee, and ankle). Thus, limp (see Chapter 42) is the most common initial manifestation. If a joint in the arm is involved, mobility of the upper extremity will be decreased (see Chapter 35).

With infections in deeper joints, the pain may radiate to contiguous anatomic structures. Children with a septic hip often complain of an ache at the knee, and sacroiliac arthritis may mimic appendicitis, pelvic neoplasm, or UTIs. Although the duration of symptoms in septic arthritis is less than 3 days in more than 50% of children with these conditions, the delay in diagnosis may reach 3 to 4 weeks with sacroiliac arthritis.

The findings are often vague in the first 6 months of life. Pyoarthritis may cause paradoxical irritability and an increase in crying on being fondled, as seen with meningitis. The infant with a septic hip usually lies quietly, holding the leg abducted and externally rotated.

Of children with septic arthritis, 60% to 70% have a temperature of 38.5°C (101.2°F) or higher. The absence of fever occurs most commonly in the adolescent with a gonococcal infection or in the neonate. Infants with infections caused by

H. influenzae, rare since the advent of the conjugated vaccine, almost invariably have high fever. An erythematous swelling may surround a superficial joint that is infected. Although a temperature difference exists between the affected and unaffected sites, it can be difficult to discern in the febrile child. Inflammation within the joint distends the capsule and produces pain with movement. If a child allows the physician to manipulate an extremity through a full range of motion, septic arthritis is unlikely.

The ESR and CRP are the most consistently abnormal laboratory study. Molteni observed an elevated ESR in 32 of 37 (86%) children with septic arthritis; the median value was 50 mm. The peripheral WBC count usually varies from less than 5,000 to more than 20,000 per mm^3. Although a leukocytosis with a shift to the left commonly occurs, as many as 20% of children will have a WBC count less than 10,000 per mm^3. If septic arthritis is diagnosed early, a radiograph of the joint will not show any pathologic changes. The first radiographic alteration to be noted is edema of the adjacent soft tissues, which is not pathognomonic of inflammation in the joint. Later, distension of the capsule becomes visible, and bony destruction may be seen late in the course of the infection.

The thickness of the tissues that surround the hip joint makes the detection of an effusion difficult by physical examination. A radiograph of the hip should generally be obtained if infection in this joint is possible. Early in the course, the tendon of the obturator internus is displaced as the muscle passes over the distended hip capsule. Continued accumulation of an inflammatory exudate forces the femoral head laterally and upward, disrupting the arc formed by the femoral head and the pelvis (Shenton's line). The hip may actually dislocate with intraarticular infection in the young infant, but this is an unusual radiographic finding in older children. Ultrasound examination is useful for the detection of an effusion not apparent on radiograph and to direct diagnostic aspiration.

No constellation of laboratory and radiographic results can rule out the diagnosis of septic arthritis; an analysis of the joint fluid is mandatory if the index of suspicion is high (see Procedures in Section VII). Infection causes an infiltration of polymorphonuclear leukocytes into the joint space. Although intraarticular WBC counts greater than 100,000 per mm^3 are traditionally associated with infection, a lesser cellular response is often noted. Nelson found a WBC count in the joint fluid of less than 25,000 per mm^3 in 9 (34%) of 31 children with proven bacterial arthritis. The joint fluid glucose is reduced to less than 40 mg per dL in only 25% to 50% of patients, but the Gram stain of the synovial fluid shows organisms in 75%. In part because inflammatory exudates have bacteriostatic properties, cultures of joint fluid yield an organism in only 60% of cases. A pathogen is recovered from the bloodstream in 40% of children with septic arthritis, more commonly if *H. influenzae* type b or *S. pneumoniae* is the cause of the disease.

The complications of septic arthritis include both local and distant spread of the infection. Osteomyelitis often accompanies joint infections in the first year of life because of the location of the metaphysis within the joint capsule. During the process of hematogenous dissemination, bacteria may invade sites other than the joint. Simultaneous infections may occur in the meninges, pericardium, or the soft tissues; these are particularly common with *H. influenzae.* Lyme arthritis is an important consideration in areas where it is endemic.

Management

Septic arthritis demands prompt management; in particular, infection in the hip joint should be considered particularly urgent. Pressure generated by purulent material within the joint space can compromise the vascular supply of the femoral head, leading to necrosis and eventual loss of normal ambulation. The initial treatment is aimed at relieving the pressure within the joint and controlling the infection. At the time of the diagnostic aspiration, as much purulent fluid as possible should be removed. Prompt surgical intervention is typically advocated for septic arthritis of the hip.

Joint fluid should be sent for Gram stain and culture, blood should be sent for routine aerobic culture, and in endemic areas blood testing for Lyme should also be performed routinely. With the widespread emergence of community-acquired MRSA, some now advocate routine nasal culture for MRSA, which, if positive, supports the need to provide coverage for MRSA if *S. aureus* is suspected.

All children with septic arthritis require admission to the hospital for IV antibiotic therapy. Because *S. aureus* is common at all ages, the addition of clindamycin, trimethoprim-sulfamethoxazole, or vancomycin (in children who appear ill) to the suggested regimens below should be considered for coverage of MRSA where these organisms are prevalent. Otherwise, the initial choice of antimicrobials depends on the child's age and the Gram stain. If no organisms are apparent on examination of the joint fluid, presumptive antibiotic therapy is determined by the age of the patient. For infants 2 months of age or younger, the usual therapy is oxacillin 100 to 200 mg per kg per day in four divided doses and gentamicin 7.5 mg per kg per day in three divided doses. In children older than 2 months to younger than 3 years, choices include oxacillin 100 to 200 mg per kg per day in four divided doses or, for children not fully immunized against Hib, either cefotaxime 200 mg per kg per day in four divided doses or ampicillin/sulbactam 200 mg per kg per day of ampicillin in four divided doses. In cases of penicillin allergy, clindamycin 40 mg per kg per day in four divided doses with the possible addition of aztreonam 120 mg per kg per day in three divided doses if Kingella or Hib are suspected. For children between 3 and 12 years of age, oxacillin 100 to 200 mg per kg per day up to a maximum of 6 g per day suffices as a single agent, with clindamycin available with penicillin allergy. Adolescents at risk for gonococcal infections require ceftriaxone, 50 to 100 mg per kg per day once daily.

Osteomyelitis

Background

Osteomyelitis is an infection of the bone; a variant, discitis, affects the intervertebral disc space. An estimated 1 in 10,000 children per year develop osteomyelitis. Approximately 10 children with bone infections were admitted yearly to the pediatric service at Parkland Memorial Hospital in Dallas between 1959 and 1973.

S. aureus causes osteomyelitis in most cases, regardless of age. During the neonatal period, group B streptococcus is the second most common isolate; *N. gonorrhoeae* and gram-negative enteric bacilli are also found. Group A streptococcus causes 5% to 10% of osteomyelitis in children. Other pathogens are recovered rarely, including *S. pneumoniae, H. influenzae, Y. enterocolitica, Brucella* species, anaerobic organisms, *M. tuberculosis,* and *Actinomyces* species.

P. aeruginosa may infect the bones of the foot after a puncture wound. In children with sickle cell hemoglobinopathies, *Salmonella* species account for almost half the cases of osteomyelitis. Unusual pathogens may be recovered from immunocompromised children.

Pathophysiology

In most children with osteomyelitis, bacteria reach the bone through the bloodstream. Occasional infections follow the direct inoculation of pathogens or spread from a contiguous focus. During hematogenous dissemination, organisms lodge in the sinusoidal vessels of the metaphysis at the site of sludging or thrombosis. Bacterial proliferation evokes an inflammatory exudate. Within the confined space of the bone, the pressure generated by the accumulation of purulent material can necrose the cortex and elevate or rupture the periosteum. If the metaphysis is contained within the joint capsule, as at the hip, septic arthritis may ensue.

Clinical Features

Osteomyelitis causes bone pain as the infection progresses. The site of the osteomyelitis determines the presentation of the disease. In 90% of cases, a single bone is involved. The femur and tibia are the most common bones infected, making limp (see Chapter 42) a common presentation. In a study of 100 consecutive children with a limp seen at the ED of The Children's Hospital of Philadelphia, osteomyelitis was diagnosed in 2%. Osteomyelitis affects the bones of the upper extremity in 25% of cases. These children complain of pain on motion of their upper extremities (see Chapter 35).

The multiplicity of bones that may be involved leads to a wide spectrum of chief complaints. Vertebral osteomyelitis manifests as backache, torticollis, or stiff neck, and involvement of the mandible causes painful mastication. Infection of the pelvis is particularly elusive and may masquerade as appendicitis, septic hip, neoplasm, or UTI. Infants with osteomyelitis localize the symptoms less well than older children. Initially, irritability may be the only complaint.

Fever exceeds 38.5°C (101.2°F) in 70% to 80% of children with osteomyelitis. The infant with a long bone infection often manifests pseudoparalysis, an unwillingness to move the extremity. Movement may also be decreased in the older child, but to a lesser degree. Point tenderness is seen commonly in osteomyelitis; however, it is found in other conditions, such as trauma, may be difficult to discern in the struggling infant, and does not always occur early in the course of the infection. Percussion of a bone at a point remote from the site of an osteomyelitis may elicit pain in the area of infection.

When purulent material ruptures through the cortex, diffuse local erythema and edema appear. This finding occurs often in infants, but late in the course, and is confined primarily to children in the first 3 years of life (before the cortex thickens sufficiently to contain the inflammatory exudate). Weissburg et al. noted swelling of the extremity in 14 of 17 patients with osteomyelitis who were younger than 1 month.

The ESR or CRP provides a useful screening test for osteomyelitis because bony infection almost always leads to an elevation. Nelson found an ESR less than 15 mm per hour in only 4 of 88 children with osteomyelitis, and the mean value was 70 mm per hour. Although the WBC count may reach a level of 20,000 per mm^3, it falls within the normal range in two-thirds of cases. Cultures from the blood yield an organism in 50% and from the bone in 60% of children with osteomyelitis.

If osteomyelitis is suspected, radiographs of the affected area should always be obtained, even though they are often normal early in the course. The first change, noted after 3 to 4 days, is deep soft-tissue swelling seen as a subtle shift of the lucent deep-muscle plane away from the bone. Within 3 to 10 days, the muscles swell and obliterate the lucent planes that usually separate them radiographically. Visualization of osseous destruction requires the loss of 40% of the bony matrix in an area at least 1 cm in diameter. This amount of demineralization occurs only after 10 to 14 days of infection. At this stage, lytic lesions and periosteal elevation are apparent on the radiograph (Fig. 92.22).

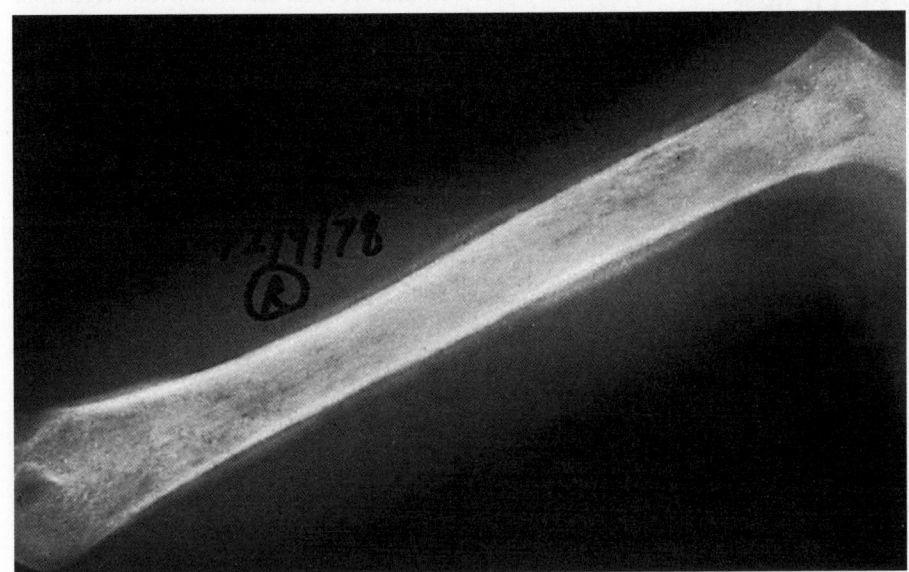

FIGURE 92.22 Radiograph showing lytic lesions and periosteal elevation with osteomyelitis.

MEDICAL EMERGENCIES

Radionuclide scanning provides a useful diagnostic tool for the clinician. Uptake of compounds such as technetium is seen at sites of increased osteoblast activity, which occurs in an infection before sufficient bony destruction has occurred to be seen on conventional radiographs. If scintigraphy is available, the patient who is strongly suspected of having osteomyelitis despite a normal radiograph should have this study. However, the absence of increased uptake does not preclude bony infection. Some patients will have decreased uptake because the accumulation of purulent material lessens the flow of blood to the site; occasionally, in children, the scan may be entirely normal early in the course. When scintigraphy is not diagnostic and clinical suspicion persists, magnetic resonance imaging (MRI) is useful, although some authorities prefer MRI as an initial alternative to a technetium scan. MRI should be used routinely in suspected spinal or pelvic osteomyelitis as associated abscesses are common or pose specific risk.

The complications of osteomyelitis include the spread of infection, either locally or to remote sites, chronic infection, and irreparable bony destruction.

Management

Children strongly suspected or known to have osteomyelitis require admission to the hospital for initial IV antibiotic therapy. Those with a low likelihood of bony infection should have a blood culture obtained and can be reevaluated in 24 hours at which time a technetium scan or MRI can be performed if the clinical findings are not definitive. The emergency physician should withhold antibiotics until the orthopedic surgeon has been contacted about culturing the bone at the site of infection. Infants should subsequently receive oxacillin (100 to 200 mg per kg per day in four divided doses) and gentamicin (7.5 mg per kg per day in three divided doses); older children can be treated with either oxacillin or, in the case of penicillin allergy, clindamycin (40 mg per kg per day in three to four divided doses) alone. The addition of clindamycin, trimethoprim-sulfamethoxazole, or vancomycin (in children who appear ill) should be considered for coverage of MRSA in areas where MRSA are prevalent.

GENITOURINARY INFECTIONS

UTIs in the child are discussed in this section and in Chapter 53. Chapter 93 addresses the range of sexually transmitted diseases, including HIV, and Chapter 90 focuses on issues in the female.

Urinary Tract Infection

Background

Infections occur along the urinary tract from the tip of the urethra to the renal parenchyma. Clinical syndromes that may accompany infections include urethritis, cystitis, and pyelonephritis. *Bacteriuria* refers to the presence of bacteria in the urine, arising from any site in the urinary tract, with or without symptoms. Significant bacteriuria describes the presence of bacteria in sufficient quantity such that infection is more likely than contamination or colonization. Significant bacteriuria may be asymptomatic, and the clinical syndromes mentioned previously may occur in the absence of infection. Because cystitis and pyelonephritis may coexist or be difficult to distinguish clinically and share a similar etiology, they are discussed together, using the generic term *urinary tract infection*.

The predominant pathogen isolated in UTIs is *E. coli*, which is recovered in 90% of cases. Next in frequency are other members of the *Enterobacteriaceae* family, including *Enterobacter* and *Klebsiella*. Among the gram-positive organisms, enterococci are seen at all ages, staphylococcal species (*Staphylococcus saprophyticus*) occur most often in adolescents, and group B streptococci are recovered primarily in infants and during pregnancy. *P. aeruginosa*, *C. albicans*, and a number of other bacteria and fungi infect patients with immunocompromise, anatomic obstruction, or indwelling catheters. Cystitis may be caused, in addition, by adenoviruses. *S. aureus* is not a common pathogen unless there is bacteremia, urinary tract abnormality, or indwelling hardware.

The frequency of infections of the urinary tract varies by age, gender, and race. Overall, infections occur commonly in neonates, decrease in frequency during childhood, and then rise in incidence after puberty in sexually active females. Males are more commonly infected than females in the first 6 months of life, in part because of a higher incidence of congenital urinary tract anomalies, but they rarely acquire infections beyond this period unless uncircumcised and then these infections are uncommon beyond a year of age. Females have a rather high incidence of symptomatic infection between 6 months and 2 years of age and of asymptomatic bacteriuria throughout childhood. Bachur and Harper (Table 92.19) recently described an incidence of UTI that decreased from 6.9% in febrile infants younger than 1 month to 0.8% in children between 18 and 24 months of age.

Pathophysiology

Bacteria may invade the urinary tract by ascension or hematogenously. In most cases, the organisms colonize the urethral area and ascend to the bladder. The higher incidence of UTI in girls is often attributed to the shorter female urethra. Hematogenous spread to the kidney may occur at times in neonates but rarely thereafter.

Those organisms that cause UTIs have certain distinct properties. In comparison to other gram-negative rods, the few strains of *E. coli* that are most commonly recovered from the urine share recognized virulence factors, including increased adherence to uroepithelial cells and higher quantities of K antigen.

Children with UTIs have a higher incidence of genitourinary anomalies than the general population, although in most infections, no anatomic or functional abnormalities are identified. Lesions that obstruct the flow of urine and/or predispose to incomplete emptying of the bladder contribute to an increased risk of infection. Additional host factors that play a role include an alkaline urinary pH and glucosuria.

Clinical Manifestations

The manifestations of UTIs vary with age, being particularly nonspecific in infancy. During a neonatal onset, a septic appearance (see Chapter 70) or fever is often the only finding. UTIs in infants may also cause vomiting, diarrhea, irritability, and, reportedly, meningismus.

Beyond 2 to 3 years of age, symptoms more often point to the urinary tract. For all practical purposes, strict differentiation

TABLE 92.19

PREVALENCE OF URINARY TRACT INFECTIONS IN FEBRILE CHILDREN
YOUNGER THAN 24 MONTHS

Age (mo)	Prevalence (%)	Females: Prevalence (%)	Males: Prevalence %
0–1	6.9	5.1	8.5
>1–3	5.5	5.9	5.3
>3–6	3.6	5.1	2.5
>6–9	2.1	3.7	0.8
>9–12	1.4	2.3	0.7
>12–18	0.8	1.4	0.4
>18–24	0.8	1.4	0.3

Modified from Bachur R, Harper M. Reliability of the urinalysis for predicting urinary tract infections in young febrile children. *Arch Pediatr Adolesc Med* 2001;155:60–65.

between upper and lower tract disease in children is not feasible for the clinician in most cases, and children who are febrile [greater than or equal to 38.5°C (101.2°F)] should be assumed to have pyelonephritis. However, some patients will have typical syndromes that localize disease to the upper or lower tract. Typically, children with cystitis appear relatively well and complain of dysuria and suprapubic pain. On examination, they have a lower-grade fever and tenderness on the suprapubic area. In contrast, patients with pyelonephritis may be toxic and usually have additional symptoms, including vomiting and flank pain. The physician is often able to elicit tenderness to percussion in the costovertebral area, either unilaterally or bilaterally.

The mainstays of diagnosis are the urinalysis and culture of the urine, both of which require the clinician to make an interpretation that is influenced by the method of collection and processing, as well as the clinical syndrome exhibited by the patient.

Urine is analyzed directly using both a chemical reagent strip (dipstick) and microscopy, looking most specifically, in regard to infection, for the presence of leukocyte esterase,

nitrites, WBCs, and bacteria. Either spun or unspun urine may be studied through the microscope, with or without the aid of a Gram stain. Spinning should be done in accordance with a standardized protocol. When a clean urine specimen is centrifuged at 2,000 rpm for 5 minutes and examined under high power, each leukocyte [per high power field (hpf)] represents 5 to 10 cells per mm^3, with 10 to 50 WBC per mm^3 (5 to 10 per hpf) being the upper limit of normal. One organism per high-power field seen on Gram stain of a spun specimen correlates with a colony count of 10^5 organisms or more.

In interpreting a urine culture in children, the physician must keep in mind that the guidelines for positivity were developed based on data in adults and that the significance of colony counts applies most explicitly to voided specimens. Given these caveats, it is generally accepted that a colony count of greater than 10^5 on a single sample indicates a probability of infection of greater than or equal to 80% to 90% for a specimen obtained by suprapubic aspiration, transurethral catheterization, or clean void technique. Table 92.20 presents more specific guidelines.

TABLE 92.20

CRITERIA FOR DIAGNOSIS OF AN INITIAL URINARY TRACT INFECTION BY CULTURE

Method of collection	Colony count (pure culture)	Probability of infection
Suprapubic aspiration	Gram-negative rods: any Gram-postive cocci: $\geq 10^3$	99%
Transurethral catheterization	$\geq 10^5$ 10^4–10^5 10^3–10^4 $\leq 10^3$	95% Infection likely Suspicious: repeat Infection unlikely
Clean void: boy	$\geq 10^4$	Infection likely
Clean void: girl	3 specimens $\geq 10^5$ 2 specimens $\geq 10^5$ 1 specimen $\geq 10^5$ 5×10^4–10^5 10^4–5×10^4 $< 10^4$	95% 90% 80% Suspicious; repeat Symptomatic: suspicious; repeat Asymptomatic: infection unlikely Infection unlikely

Modified from American Academy of Pediatrics. Practice parameter: the diagnosis, treatment, and evaluation of the initial urinary tract infection in febrile infants and young children. *Pediatrics* 1999;103:843–852.

In general, a single negative finding on one parameter of the urinalysis does not exclude a UTI. Taken together, however, negative testing for both leukocyte esterase and nitrites by dipstick alone, or even more so in combination with a microscopic examination that shows the absence of pyuria, makes the diagnosis of a UTI (as opposed to asymptomatic bacteriuria) in a male infant older than 6 months or a female older than 2 years highly unlikely. A schema for the use of urinalysis and urine culture is presented in Fig. 92.23. As illustrated for selected children who are somewhat older but not yet toilet

trained, in the absence of a high likelihood of UTI a priori, the urinalysis may be collected using a bag. However, if the urinalysis is positive, a specimen for culture should preferably be obtained by catheterization or suprapubic aspiration.

Bacteremia accompanies UTIs primarily during the first 6 to 12 months of life. In the very young infant, bacteremia may be present in the absence of fever and should be suspected in any child during the first year of life with a temperature greater than or equal to 39°C (102.2°F) or higher. Indications for a CBC count and blood culture with a suspected UTI include (i)

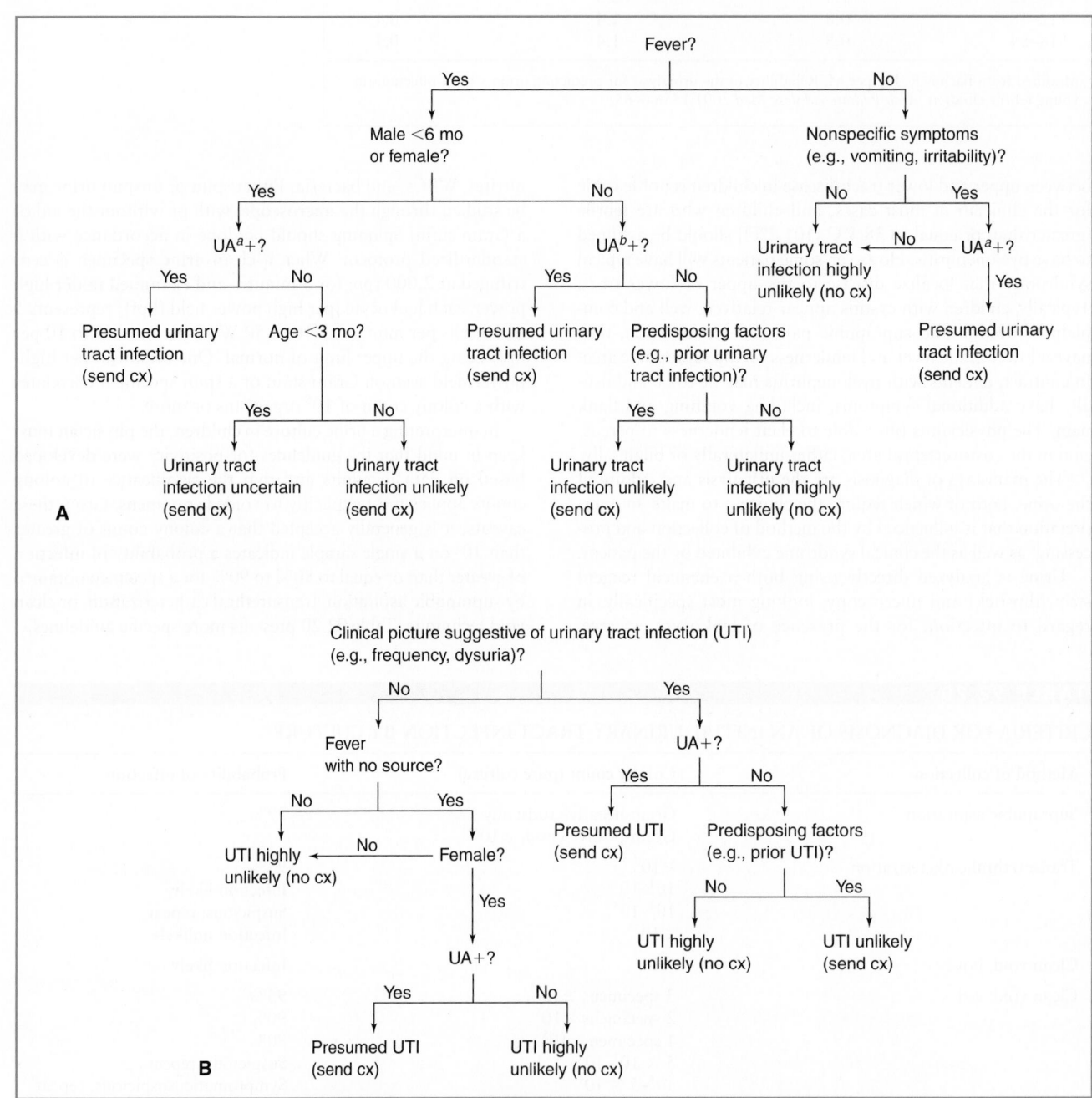

FIGURE 92.23 Diagnostic approach to infants and children with fever, symptoms specifically suggestive of urinary tract infection (UTI), and/or nonspecific symptoms and signs compatible with UTI. Use of urinalysis (UA) and culture (cx) in the diagnosis of UTI (**A**) in children age 2 years or younger and (**B**) in those older than 2 years. [a]UA obtained by catheterization or suprapubic aspiration. [b]UA (only) may be obtained using a urine collection bag.

signs of clinical toxicity (extreme tachycardia, low blood pressure, shaking chills); (ii) age younger than 3 months; and (iii) age 3 months to 1 year and temperature greater than or equal to 39°C (102.2°F). Children with dehydration or likely pyelonephritis (as opposed to cystitis) require measurement of electrolytes, BUN, and creatinine.

Management

When the diagnosis of UTI has been established as a result of earlier urine culture or is presumed based on the clinical syndrome and findings on urinalysis, antibiotic therapy is indicated. The clinician may choose to await the results of culture before prescribing antibiotic therapy, when the combination of clinical symptomatology and urinalysis is suggestive but not strongly presumptive. If available, the results of susceptibility testing should guide the selection of antimicrobial agent. In all other cases, an antibiotic is chosen to cover the most likely pathogens.

Most patients respond to oral antibiotic therapy. Indications for IV administration of antibiotics include (i) clinical toxicity; (ii) age younger than 2 months; (ii) vomiting, refusal to drink, or other factors making the delivery of oral medications unreliable; (iv) adverse anatomic factors, such as an obstruction to urinary flow; and (v) a known positive culture for a pathogen not susceptible to oral agents.

For ill-appearing patients, IV ampicillin (200 mg per kg per day in four divided doses) plus gentamicin (5 to 7.5 mg per kg per day in a single dose, adjusted for gestation age and weight; Table 92.4) are given. Cefotaxime (150 mg per kg per day divided into three 50 mg per kg daily IV doses) provides an alternative. Options for oral therapy in children, given for a 7- to 10-day course, include cefdinir (14 mg per kg per day as a single dose), cefixime (8 mg per kg per day as a single dose), or trimethoprim-sulfamethoxazole (8 mg per kg per day of trimethoprim in two divided doses), if the regional prevalence of resistance to this antibiotic is low. Fluoroquinolones, such as ciprofloxacin (500 mg twice daily), offer an alternative for adolescents. As 20% to 30% of the strains of *E. coli* demonstrate resistance to ampicillin, the physician should not choose this drug or amoxicillin for oral therapy, unless local patterns of susceptibility dictate otherwise.

SPECIFIC INFECTIONS

Viral Syndrome

The term *nonspecific viral syndrome* is used to refer to a generalized illness, presumed clinically to be caused by a virus and characterized by malaise and, usually, fever. Numerous agents, including influenza, enteroviruses, and herpesvirus (roseola), have been implicated. Nonspecific viral syndromes and viral URIs account for most of the febrile visits made by children to the ED.

Usually, a viral syndrome begins with malaise and fever. The temperature varies from 37°C (98.6°F) to more than 40°C (104°F), greater elevations occurring particularly in children younger than 2 years. Children who are older and able to verbalize their discomfort complain of diffuse aching, especially with influenza. There may be a cough or occasional bout of emesis. Signs of mild inflammation may be seen in the upper respiratory tract.

The physician arrives at a diagnosis of a nonspecific viral syndrome by excluding other diseases on the basis of the history and physical examination. Particularly in children younger than 6 months and/or not fully immunized against bacterial pathogens, a WBC count may help the physician determine whether the young child with a high fever is at risk for occult bacteremia (see "Bacteremia" section). Treatment is limited to antipyresis with acetaminophen (15 mg per kg per dose, maximum 4000 mg per day) or ibuprofen (10 mg per kg per dose, maximum 800 per dose), for patients who do not respond to acetaminophen, and the maintenance of an adequate oral intake. Antibiotics will not prevent secondary bacterial infections and are not to be prescribed routinely. Generally, parents should seek further care for their children if fever persists for more than 48 hours, although additional testing or therapy will only occasionally be needed. When fever persists for more than 5 days in infants and young children, at least passing consideration should be given to occult bacterial infections, such as UTI, and to Kawasaki disease.

Influenza

Influenza viruses A and B produce annual outbreaks of disease during the winter months that involve 10% to 40% of healthy children during each cycle. Infection may produce a generalized viral syndrome, predominant respiratory symptomatology, or less commonly, other syndromes, including a sepsislike picture in young infants, croup, bronchiolitis, pneumonia, diffuse myositis, and rarely Reye's syndrome (usually following the administration of aspirin). Older children with influenza classically manifest sudden onset of fever, chills, malaise, headache, a nonproductive cough, and diffuse myalgia. Some may develop nasal congestion, sore throat, and occasionally conjunctivitis. Myositis may be sufficiently severe as to cause an inability/refusal to walk and tenderness of palpation of the muscles, particularly in the calf.

Influenza may be diagnosed on the basis of rapid testing of nasopharyngeal material for antigen, viral culture of the nasopharynx, or the collection of acute and convalescent sera for serology. With myositis, serum CPK levels may be elevated. In the ambulatory setting, the rapid tests have the greatest utility, although sensitivity is only in the 50% to 70% range. Specific therapy is available for some strains of influenza but is generally reserved for (i) patients with underlying conditions, such as chronic lung disease or immunosuppression, that place them at risk for prolonged or severe infection; (ii) healthy children with unusually severe illness; and (iii) individuals with special social or family situations for which ongoing illness would be detrimental; (iv) circumstances where there are newly circulating strains with increased rates of morbidity or mortality (e.g., H1N1 flu, avian flu). The specific antivirals recommended (e.g., oseltamivir, zanamivir, rimantidine) will depend on the susceptibility of circulating strains. The CDC posts regular updates regarding influenza activity and treatment recommendations at http://www.cdc.gov/flu. Vaccination and chemoprophylaxis are occasionally advised in the acute care setting, and standard references are available with specific indications and dosage schedules.

Erythema Infectiosum (Fifth Disease)

Erythema infectiosum, or fifth disease, is an exanthematous illness of childhood caused by parvovirus B19. It occurs most commonly between 2 and 12 years of age. The appearance of a rash marks the onset of the disease; fever or other prodromal symptoms are uncommon. The rash involves the face initially, conferring on the child a "slapped-cheek" appearance. Maculopapular lesions erupt 24 hours later, initially on the upper portion of the extremities, and they then spread both proximally and distally. Fading of the central portion of the lesions gives a lacelike appearance to the rash. Adolescents in particular may develop arthralgia or arthritis, and patients with chronic hemolytic anemias, such as sickle cell disease, are at risk for aplastic crisis. During pregnancy, infection with parvovirus B19 causes fetal hydrops in approximately 10% of cases. There is no specific therapy in the normal host, but immunocompromised patients may benefit from IV gamma globulin.

Infectious Mononucleosis

Background

Infectious mononucleosis (IM) is a disease characterized by malaise, fever, pharyngitis, lymphadenopathy, and splenomegaly. In 1968, Henle and Henle identified EBV as the cause of this illness. EBV infections are common, but usually relatively asymptomatic, during the first years of life. In children, sporadic infections occur, and IM is occasionally diagnosed. By late adolescence, 50% to 90% of all people are seropositive. In lower socioeconomic groups infections are most common in the preschool age where infections are typically mild. Children in higher socioeconomic groups are commonly infected in adolescence and young adulthood; half of these will experience the clinical manifestations of IM.

Pathophysiology

EBV is shed in oropharyngeal secretions, which represent the major source of infectious virus. The virus infects B lymphocytes that may spread to the various lymphoid tissues in the body. The atypical lymphocytes seen in the circulation represent activated, EBV-specific cytotoxic (CD8)-suppressor T lymphocytes, which destroy the infected B cells and limit the production of virus. Natural killer lymphocytes also play a role and together these changes result in a transient general depression of cellular immunity.

Clinical Manifestations

IM begins insidiously with fever and malaise. Three-fourths of children with this illness complain of a sore throat. Although a child may recover from IM in 7 to 10 days, the symptoms usually last for 2 to 4 weeks. This persistence of symptoms separates the patient with IM from those with pharyngitis caused by group A streptococci or other viruses. Occasionally, the onset resembles that of infectious hepatitis.

The symptomatic child with IM is febrile in 90% of cases at presentation. The fever often persists for several days and low-grade fevers may persist for 2 weeks or more. Enlarged lymph nodes are uniformly palpable. Although the lymphadenopathy may be limited to the cervical region, involvement of the axillary and inguinal areas is common. Pharyngitis caused by any pathogen produces an increase in the size of the anterior cervical nodes, but EBV characteristically affects the posterior cervical and submental glands as well (Fig. 92.24). In 75% of

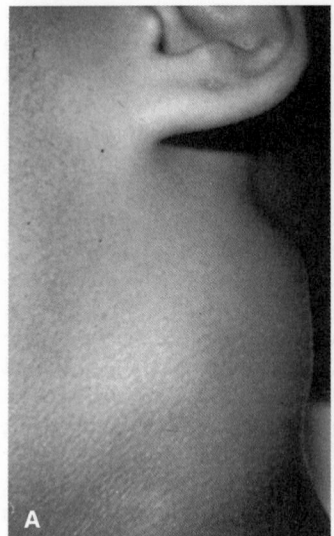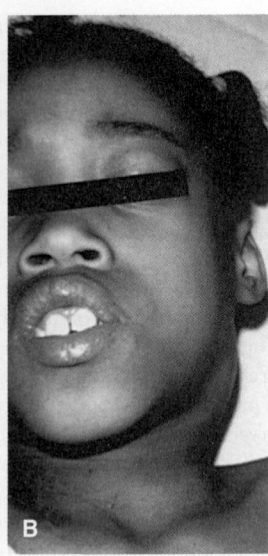

FIGURE 92.24 Posterior cervical adenopathy in a child with infectious mononucleosis. **A:** Close-up of posterior adenopathy. **B:** Anterior and posterior cervical node enlargement.

cases, the pharynx is inflamed, often with an exudate. The spleen enlarges in 60% of children typically in the second week of illness and the hepatomegaly occurs in 25%. Some elevation of liver transaminases (AST and ALT) occur in 80%. Periorbital edema and a diffuse maculopapular rash are seen occasionally.

The hemoglobin and hematocrit are normal in the uncomplicated disease. Although the total WBC count does not often increase much beyond 15,000 per mm^3, levels up to 30,000 per mm^3 are seen in 10% to 15% of children. A higher leukocyte count casts some doubt on the diagnosis of IM. There is an absolute lymphocytosis with many atypical mononuclear cells; however, 16% of children presenting with IM in one series had fewer than 10% atypical lymphocytes, and 50% had fewer than 20% of such cells. The mainstay for the diagnosis of IM in the adult is the heterophil antibody test, but these antibodies reach levels detectable by routine assays in only 50% of young children. Confirmation of a heterophil-negative case of IM is typically by EBV-specific serologic assays. Serum PCR tests for EBV are available and may be useful in selected circumstances.

The most worrisome complications of IM in the immunocompetent host for the emergency physician are splenic rupture and airway obstruction. Even minor trauma can cause a rent in the capsule of the enlarged spleen seen in IM; these children manifest the usual signs of intraperitoneal hemorrhage. Occasionally, massive lymphoid hyperplasia of the tonsils occludes the airway, leading to stridor and retractions. The site of narrowing is easily visualized on examination. Less common complications include encephalitis, pneumonia, myocarditis, hemolytic anemia, and thrombocytopenia.

Patients with immunosuppression related to transplantation (visceral, liver, kidney, lung, cardiac, stem cell) receiving agents such as antithymocyte globulin, cyclosporine, and tacrolimus are at risk for EBV-related posttransplant lymphoproliferative disorders (PTLD). Patients with AIDS may experience EBV related lymphocytic interstitial pneumonitis (LIP), lymphoma. EBV is also associated with the development of X-linked lymphoproliferative syndrome and infection-associated hemophagocytic syndrome (HLH). These latter entities occur among patients with specific defects in regulating EBV proliferation and/or the immunologic response to infection.

Management

A WBC count and heterophil antibody titer usually suffice for the confirmation of the clinical diagnosis. EBV-specific antibodies are indicated only for heterophil-negative cases. Specific therapy is not available. Adequate rest and nutrition should be maintained, and antipyretic agents will increase the child's comfort. Children with airway compromise can be treated with oral corticosteroids, which will almost always dramatically shrink the enlarged tonsils. Prednisone is given at 2 mg per kg for the first few days and tapered, once improvement has occurred, over 5 to 7 days. Antivirals such as acyclovir or ganciclovir do not have demonstrated efficacy in immunocompetent hosts. Consultation with an infectious diseases specialist should be considered for management of EBV infection or its complications in the immunocompromised host.

Measles (Rubeola)

Background

Measles is a disease caused by a specific myxovirus and is characterized by fever, cough, coryza, conjunctivitis, and rash. Since the widespread introduction of effective vaccines, the incidence of this disease has decreased significantly. In 2001, just over 100 cases were reported to the CDC.

Pathophysiology

Measles virus enters the body through the upper respiratory tract, where local replication is believed to occur. A transient viremia ensues, and virus spreads to the reticuloendothelial system. A secondary viremia then follows, producing the clinical disease.

Clinical Findings

Fever and malaise herald the onset of measles. During the course of the illness, the temperature often rises to 40°C (104°F). Within 24 hours, coryza, conjunctivitis, and cough develop. Koplik's spots appear on the buccal mucosa by the third day of fever. These are seen as fine white spots on an erythematous background and have been likened to grains of sand. The rash erupts on the fourth or fifth day. The exanthem is maculopapular in appearance and begins on the face and neck. The lesions are heaviest on the upper portion of the body, often coalescing. As the rash advances down the trunk, the prodromal findings (cough, coryza, conjunctivitis) and the Koplik's spots resolve. The rash involves the extremities on its third day but has already begun to fade on the face. A leukopenia and lymphopenia accompanies uncomplicated measles. Specific antibodies, initially absent from the serum, reach detectable levels 2 weeks after the onset of illness.

Complications, which are unusual, fall into two categories: (i) extension of the viral infection and (ii) secondary bacterial infection. The virus itself may produce inflammation of the lower respiratory mucosa, leading to laryngotracheitis, bron-

chitis, and/or pneumonia. Encephalitis occurs in 1 of every 1,000 cases of measles; this is a debilitating illness with a mortality rate of 15%. Thrombocytopenia and corneal ulcerations are rarely seen. Lymphoid hyperplasia in the bowel can occlude the lumen of the appendix, leading to inflammation of this organ; histologic examination of surgically removed tissue confirms the diagnosis of measles on the basis of the characteristic giant cells. Acute purulent OM is the most common bacterial complication of measles, and cervical adenitis occasionally occurs. Pneumonia, although usually viral, may have a bacterial etiology.

Management

Clinical clues, gathered from the history and physical examination, suffice for the diagnosis of measles by the experienced clinician. However, most U.S. physicians are no longer familiar with this disease. As a result, and for epidemiologic purposes, serologic studies are used to confirm the cause, particularly among the first few children seen in sporadic outbreaks. Ordinarily, acute and convalescent titers drawn 1 to 2 weeks apart are used for a determination, but a single specimen positive for measles-specific IgM antibodies is sufficient.

Measles runs a self-limited course. Bed rest and antipyretic therapy help keep the child comfortable. Antitussives, antihistamines, and topical ophthalmic preparations have no role. Prophylaxis against secondary bacterial infections with antibiotics is not warranted. Children with uncomplicated measles or superficial secondary infections such as otitis and cervical adenitis can be treated as outpatients. Hospitalization is required when significantly severe laryngotracheobronchitis is evident, as discussed earlier in this chapter. Lower respiratory tract or CNS involvement necessitates admission to the hospital.

Measles is a preventable disease. Otherwise healthy, susceptible contacts should receive intramuscular immune serum globulin, 0.25 mL per kg; the dose is increased to 0.5 mL per kg for immunocompromised patients. Unless the patient is younger than 6 months or immunocompromised, vaccine is also indicated within 72 hours of exposure (see Appendix D).

Roseola

Roseola infantum, or exanthem subitum, is a common, self-limiting, viral infection of infants caused in most cases by human herpesvirus 6; and only occasionally by human herpesvirus 7. The child, usually younger than 3 years, presents with a high fever, ranging up to 40.5°C (104.9°F), and a paucity of physical findings. Mild irritability may occur, half have some URI, mild pharyngeal erythema and may have red tympanic membranes. There is typically no bulbar conjunctivitis but some mild palpebral redness may be seen. A bulging fontanelle is seen in 25% of young infants and neurologic complications can be seen (most commonly seizure). After 2 to 4 days of illness, the fever drops precipitously and a rash appears. The lesions are discrete, pink maculopapules, 2 to 3 mm in diameter. They fade with pressure and do not coalesce. The exanthem appears on the trunk initially and spreads outward. Roseola resolves without complications other than an occasional febrile convulsion. The diagnosis of roseola is made on the basis of the clinical course, often in retrospect. If a WBC count is obtained, it is typically low for age. CSF when obtained is typically normal. Specific testing is not typically warranted. Treatment is symptomatic and generally limited to antipyretic agents except in cases of reactivation in severely immunocompromised patients.

Rubella

Background

Rubella is a childhood infection caused by a specific togavirus. Before the advent of vaccination, epidemics occurred every 6 to 9 years; 488,796 cases were reported to the CDC in the United States in 1964, the year of the last outbreak in this country. In contrast, the CDC reported only 18 cases in 2002. Rubella traditionally affects children 5 to 9 years of age. The initial site of inoculation is the upper respiratory tract, where local replication occurs. A viremia ensues, disseminating the virus to the skin.

Clinical Manifestations

Only 10% of children experience prodromal symptoms such as fever, malaise, cough, and mild conjunctivitis. However, these complaints are often voiced by the adolescent. The rash begins on the face and spreads downward, reaching the extremities by the end of the second day. The lesions are pink maculopapules that may coalesce. The lymph nodes in the postauricular, suboccipital, and posterior cervical chains enlarge and become somewhat tender. During the first 2 days of illness, the temperature usually rises, but remains less than 39°C (102.2°F). The WBC count often decreases in rubella, and a few atypical lymphocytes may appear. A fourfold rise in specific antibodies occurs after 10 to 14 days.

Complications of rubella are rare in children but include encephalitis, thrombocytopenia, and arthritis or arthralgia. Painful and/or swollen joints often occur in adolescents. Encephalitis has an incidence of 1 in 6,000 cases of rubella and usually resolves spontaneously.

Management

Rubella is difficult to diagnose clinically because of its rare occurrence and the plethora of exanthems that have a similar appearance. Situations that require a definite etiologic diagnosis, such as pregnancy in an adolescent, demand serologic confirmation. Children with rubella can be managed as outpatients with antipyretic therapy. Only the rare child with encephalitis or thrombocytopenia requires admission to the hospital.

Varicella/Zoster

Background

Herpesvirus varicellae causes two clinical illnesses, varicella (chickenpox) and zoster (shingles). Varicella occurs during a primary infection, and zoster occurs after a reactivation of latent virus.

With introduction of a vaccine in 1995, varicella has become a relatively uncommon infection in children but cases continue to be seen with the CDC reporting approximately 10,000 cases in 2008. Varicella is highly contagious: Almost 90% of susceptible household contacts of an index case develop the disease. By adolescence, serologic surveys have shown a seropositive rate of 70% to 80%. Zoster, however, affects adults predominantly. More than 60% of cases occur in persons older than 45 years.

Pathophysiology

The virus typically enters the body on inhalation of virus exhales by patients with chickenpox or contact with skin lesions of patients with varicella or shingles. The virus is then thought to spread to regional lymph nodes and cause a primary viremia infecting cells of the reticuloendothelials cells of the liver and it is the secondary viremia that causes the skin lesions seen in primary infection. During an episode of varicella, the virus invades sensory nerve endings and ascends to the dorsal root ganglion where it becomes latent. Zoster follows reactivation of the latent virus.

Clinical Findings

Varicella. A mild prodrome that lasts 1 to 3 days often precedes the exanthem of varicella; however, the first sign of illness may be the rash. Most children develop fever, usually less than 39.5°C (103.1°F) and may complain of malaise. The fever usually has subsided within 24 hours of the appearance of the skin lesions. Recurrence of significant fever should serve as a warning sign for suspicion of complications. Lesions erupt initially on the upper trunk, neck, or face and spread centripetally. Pruritus is universal.

The abnormal findings on physical examination are limited to the elevated temperature and the skin and mucous membrane lesions. Initially, the exanthem consists of erythematous papules that evolve into vesicles and then pustules over 6 to 8 hours (Fig. 92.25). The early vesicles have a diameter of 2 to 4 mm and a "dewdrop-like" appearance. Because new lesions erupt in crops for 2 to 4 days, papules, vesicles, and pustules are usually seen together. An exanthem involves the mucosa of the oropharynx and, occasionally, the vagina. The severity of the cutaneous manifestations varies widely, and there may be from 1 to more than 1,000 lesions.

Previously vaccinated children may experience breakthrough varicella infection following exposure to wild-type virus. The illness is usually mild without much fever and typically few skin lesions that may remain maculopapular rather than becoming vesicular. Because of its atypical presentation diagnosis frequently depends on an exposure history. Not all cases of breakthrough varicella are mild and a minority of patients will have clinical features similar to those occurring in unvaccinated patients. These children, especially if immunocompromised, should be considered for treatment as they would if unvaccinated.

There are few laboratory derangements in varicella. The WBC count occasionally shows a leukocytosis, and the AST and ALT may be mildly elevated. In adolescents, the chest radiograph reveals an interstitial infiltrate in 5% to 10% of patients, even though there may be no respiratory symptoms.

Varicella runs a self-limited course in most cases but is occasionally a more serious illness. Fleisher et al. reviewed 96 children hospitalized with complications of this disease during a 5-year period at The Children's Hospital of Philadelphia. Of the group, 81 were immunocompetent children older than 1 month; they experienced complications, including encephalitis (20),

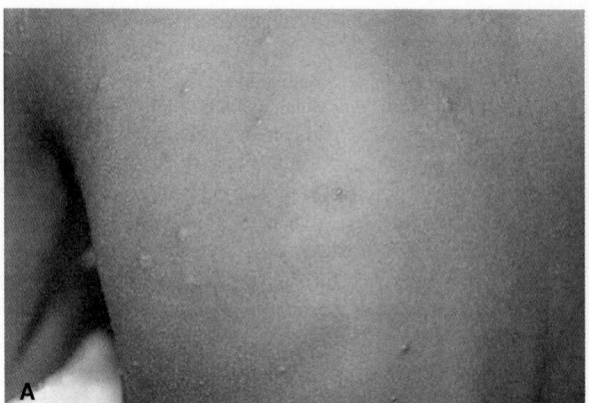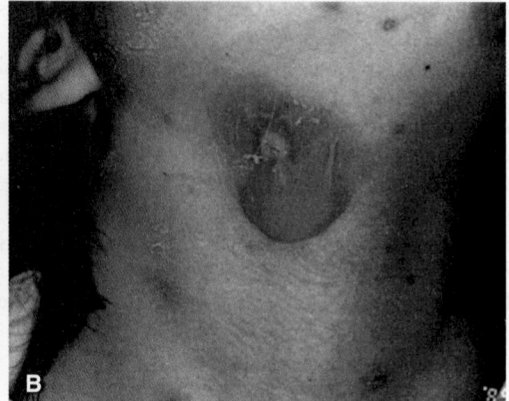

FIGURE 92.25 **A:** Typical lesions of varicella. **B:** Bullous varicella.

pneumonia (5), hepatitis (8), bacterial superinfection (22), Reye's syndrome (17), unusual cutaneous manifestations (5), medication overdoses (5), exacerbation of an underlying disease (2), and dehydration (1). Simultaneous streptococcal pharyngitis can also occur.

Encephalitis takes two forms: (i) a diffuse cerebritis with coma and seizures, and (ii) a cerebellitis with ataxia. Both varieties may occur before, during, or after the cutaneous eruption. Because bacterial meningitis can also complicate varicella, an analysis of the CSF should be considered even if viral encephalitis is suspected. There will often be a mild pleocytosis (10 to 300 cells) and a slight elevation of the protein (40 to 80 mg per dL). If the encephalopathy is believed to be related to Reye's syndrome, a serum ammonia should be obtained.

Starting in approximately 1990, a number of authors reported an increasing incidence of group A streptococcal complications with varicella, including primarily sepsis and necrotizing fasciitis. The diagnosis of streptococcal sepsis should be considered in patients who appear toxic, remain febrile for 5 days or more, or develop a fever after being afebrile for more than 48 hours.

Zoster. Zoster appears suddenly in most children without any warning symptoms (pain or pruritus). The lesions are grouped vesicles on an erythematous base in a dermatomal distribution. In 15% to 20% of cases, extradermatomal cutaneous dissemination is seen. However, spread to the viscera does not occur in the immunocompetent child. If the eruption follows the ophthalmic branch of the trigeminal nerve, the cornea may be involved. The appearance of vesicles on the tip of the nose should evoke a suspicion of ocular involvement that can be best seen after fluorescein staining of the eye. Zoster in childhood occurs most commonly among children who had varicella in the first 1 to 2 years of life; it may affect vaccinated patients.

Management

Visual inspection suffices for the diagnosis of varicella; no laboratory studies are indicated. Acetaminophen is given to control the fever, and antihistaminic drugs provide some relief from the pruritus. Aspirin is contraindicated because of an association with Reye's syndrome. Although some investiga-

tors have speculated about a relationship between the use of ibuprofen and the development of fasciitis, this remains unproven. Diphenhydramine (5 mg per kg per day), hydroxyzine (2 mg per kg per day), or other antihistamines may be used to decrease pruritus. The child is excluded from attending school for 1 week after the eruption of the first lesion.

Immunosuppressed children with varicella should be treated with acyclovir (30 mg per kg per day IV in three divided doses per day), or oral famciclovir, or oral valacyclovir (note the doses are higher than required for HSV infections, with the exception of HSV encephalitis). Complications that mandate admission to the hospital for immunocompetent patients include fasciitis, Reye's syndrome, pneumonia, and encephalitis, except in the mildest cases. Superficial bacterial infections such as impetigo, cellulitis (if fasciitis is believed to be unlikely), and adenitis can be treated with oral antibiotic therapy such as dicloxacillin, cephalexin, clindamycin, and/or trimethoprim sulfamethoxazole as discussed previously in this chapter. Children with deeper bacterial infections (i.e., septic arthritis) should receive IV antimicrobials.

For immunocompetent children, oral acyclovir (80 mg per kg per day in four divided doses) given within 24 hours of the onset of the rash reduces the duration of fever and the number and duration of skin lesions. Indications for use have not been formalized, but consideration is warranted for patients who are at some risk for a particularly severe course: infants younger than 6 months old, adolescents (older than 12 years), children receiving long-term aspirin therapy or being treated with oral/inhaled steroid, patients with chronic cutaneous (e.g., atopic dermatitis) or pulmonary (e.g., cystic fibrosis) disorders, and those with fever above 40°C (104°F) and a large number of lesions noted as early as the first day of the eruption (particularly if case follows a household contact). Oral acyclovir should be considered for the pregnant adolescent, but its use remains controversial in this situation.

Zoster (or shingles) is typically treated with oral famciclovir or valacyclovir in adults with the primary goal of reducing postherpetic neuralgia. Postzoster pain syndromes are, fortunately, uncommon in children and efficacy has not been demonstrated in this group. Antipruritic and antipyretic agents provide symptomatic relief. Immunocompromised children should be treated with acyclovir, famciclovir or valacyclovir with the goal to prevent dissemination and shorten the duration of new lesion formation. Ocular involvement merits consultation with an ophthalmologist.

Anyone likely to experience a severe episode of varicella should receive prophylaxis after a significant exposure to a patient contagious for varicella-zoster virus (household or close contact for more than 1 hour in a closed environment). Varicella-zoster immunoglobulin, one vial (125 units) per 10 kg, is indicated for susceptible normal adults, pregnant women, and immunocompromised children. Newborns whose mothers have had onset of varicella within 5 days before or 2 days after delivery should receive 125 units, as soon as possible (see Appendix D).

MISCELLANEOUS INFECTIONS

Babesiosis

Babesia species, particularly *Babesia microti*, are protozoa, transmitted by the bite of an *Ixodes* tick, which also serves as a vector in Lyme disease. Cases of this infection have been reported with increasing frequency along both coasts and in the upper Midwest. The majority of infected children are asymptomatic or experience only mild symptoms. However, the clinical picture of babesiosis can resemble that of malaria and is characterized by anorexia; malaise; fatigue; and intermittent chills, sweats, and fevers (Fig. 92.26) as high as 40°C (104°F). Other than an elevated temperature, physical findings are absent or limited to mild hepatosplenomegaly. Patients with asplenia are susceptible to severe, or even life-threatening, disease, especially with *Babesia divergens* (more often seen in Europe). Laboratory findings include hemolytic anemia with reticulocytosis, a normal or slightly decreased leukocyte count, mild thrombocytopenia, and elevated liver enzymes. Microscopic examination of a peripheral smear confirms the presence of intracellular and extracellular ring forms, similar

to those of *Plasmodium falciparum*. The degree of parasitemia is generally less than 20% in patients with functional spleens but can exceed 85% in asplenic patients. Specific serologic assays are also available, but the results are often delayed for several weeks and do not distinguish between acute infection and asymptomatic seropositivity. Therapy is reserved for patients with symptomatic infections or a predisposition to severe disease. The treatment of choice is clindamycin (30 mg per kg per day in three divided doses) plus quinine (25 to 30 mg per kg per day in three divided doses) orally or atovaquone (40 mg per kg per day in two divided doses) plus azithromycin (12 mg per kg once daily) orally for 7 days. The latter combination (atovaquone and azithromycin) is associated with fewer adverse reactions.

Botulism

Background

Botulism is a paralytic illness produced by neurotoxins elaborated by *Clostridium botulinum*. The disease may result from the ingestion of preformed toxin or from the elaboration of toxin by organisms in a wound or in the GI tract. Of particular concern to the physician who cares for children is infantile botulism caused by toxin formed in the intestines. In the United States, the CDC reports approximately 100 cases of infantile and 20 cases of foodborne botulism annually.

During growth, *C. botulinum* releases neurotoxins that are the most potent poisons known on a weight basis. They interfere with neurotransmission at peripheral cholinergic synapses by blocking the release of acetylcholine.

Clinical Manifestations

Botulism from the ingestion of toxin, which affects children and adolescents, as opposed to infants, causes vomiting in 50% of cases. The patients complain of weakness and a dry

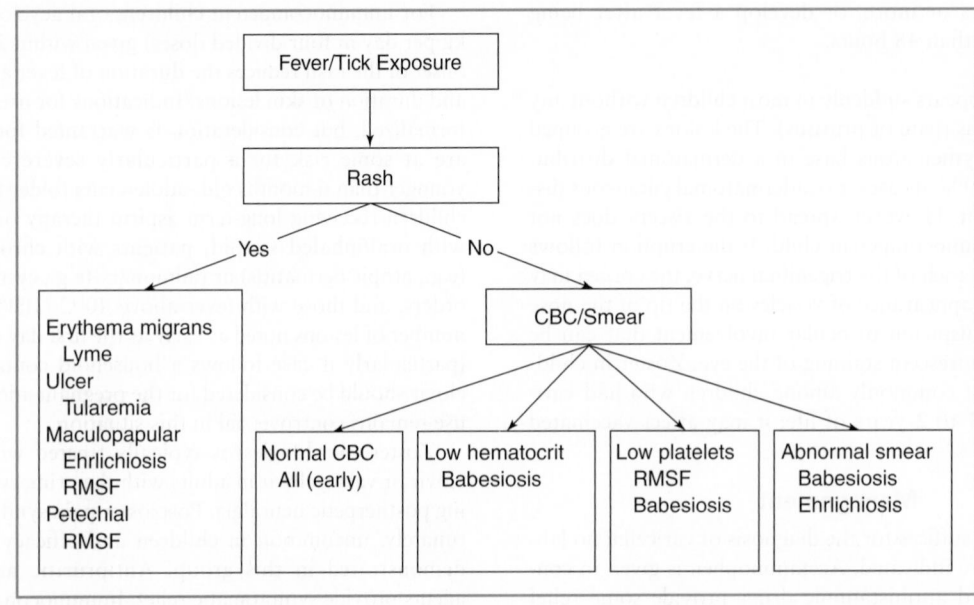

FIGURE 92.26 Approach to the febrile child with an exposure to ticks. CBC count, complete blood cell count; RMSF, Rocky Mountain spotted fever.

mouth; constipation and urinary retention may occur. Paralysis is noted within 3 days, usually affecting the cranial nerves first and then the extremities. The patients are alert and afebrile. Abnormalities of the neurologic examination include ptosis, extraocular palsies, fixed dilated pupils, symmetric weakness, and hyporeflexia. Both the ileus and urinary retention seen in this disease may lead to abdominal distension.

Infantile botulism occurs in children in the first 6 months of life who are otherwise healthy. The duration of symptoms before hospitalization ranges from 1 to 20 days. Breastfed, Caucasian infants from middle-class families are primarily affected. Constipation is the first symptom of the disease but may not be sufficiently severe to draw attention to any underlying illness. After several days, mild lethargy, weakness, and a decreased appetite are noted. Occasionally, the onset of lethargy and weakness may be so precipitous as to resemble bacterial sepsis or meningitis.

On examination, the infant is quiet, with little discernible movement, and has a weak cry. Fever is not a part of this syndrome. The child sucks on a nipple with difficulty and may be unable to swallow. The absence of a gag reflex, profound hypotonia, and hyporeflexia in infantile botulism helps distinguish this illness from bacterial sepsis.

The WBC count is normal in botulism. Organisms may be recovered by anaerobic culture techniques from the GI tract in infantile or wound botulism, but identification of the toxins requires the specialized facilities of the public health department. Children with botulism have an electromyogram that shows a characteristic pattern of brief duration, small amplitude, overly abundant motor unit action potentials (BSAP).

Respiratory failure is a potential life-threatening complication in botulism of any variety, and ventilatory support is often required. The profound bulbar weakness in infantile botulism often prevents an adequate fluid intake; dehydration occurs frequently.

Management

Because no test is immediately available to diagnose infantile botulism, the initial evaluation of these infants aims at excluding other causes of lethargy and weakness such as sepsis, poliomyelitis, myasthenia gravis, neuropathy, and drug ingestion. A lumbar puncture is often performed in the ED to rule out meningitis. Electrolytes and a BUN are useful to assess hydration.

The children all require admission to the hospital (Table 92.21). Monitoring of pulse and respiratory rate should start in the ED. An IV line should be started for the administration of fluids to correct dehydration and in anticipation of a possible respiratory arrest. Neither antibiotics nor antitoxin ameliorate

TABLE 92.21

INFANTILE BOTULISM: IMMEDIATE MANAGEMENT

Ensure adequate ventilation.	Achieve venous access and maintain hydration.
Administer oxygen, as indicated.	Obtain laboratory studies.
Initiate cardiorespiratory monitoring.	Administer botulism immune globulin (BIG) as soon as available

the course of infantile botulism. Because they may potentiate the neuromuscular blockade, aminoglycoside antibiotics should be avoided when treating for possible sepsis when there is a concomitant concern for botulism.

Children with foodborne and wound botulism also require admission to the hospital. All children suspected clinically of having botulism should be treated with a single dose of human botulism immune globulin IV (BIG-IV or BabyBIG) while awaiting confirmation by testing. Such treatment has been documented to substantially reduce length of stay, need for mechanical ventilation, and the need for parenteral nutrition or nasogastric feeds. However, because of the notable expense and difficulty obtaining of this therapy, consultation with a *toxicologist or infectious diseases specialist* is typically warranted. Information on obtaining the drug is available at http://www.infantbotulism.org/

Cat-scratch Disease

CSD is an infection caused by *B. henselae*. Approximately 80% of cases occur in patients younger than 20 years. Traditionally, this disorder has been thought of primarily as an infection of regional lymph nodes (typical CSD), but the spectrum of the disease has been expanded to include infections of other organ systems by *B. henselae* (atypical CSD). In addition, this same agent causes severe infections (bacillary angiomatosis and peliosis hepatis) in patients with HIV (see Chapter 93).

More than 90% of children with typical CSD have a history of exposure to cats. The most complete form of the illness begins with the appearance of a pustule at the site contact, 7 to 10 days after exposure. Lymphadenopathy follows within 1 to 6 weeks. The regional nodes enlarge and become mildly to moderately tender on palpation. In one-third of cases, the glands become fluctuant. The epitrochlear, axillary, inguinal, and cervical nodes are commonly affected.

Manifestations of atypical CSD include encephalitis, aseptic meningitis, neuroretinitis (blindness and stellate macular lesions of the retina), Parinaud's syndrome (conjunctivitis and preauricular adenitis), hepatitis, osteolytic lesions, and fever of unknown origin.

In typical cases with a history of exposure, particularly to a kitten, and characteristic lymph node enlargement, no specific diagnostic studies are needed. In atypical disease or with lymphadenopathy that is not characteristic, serologies should be sent.

Various antibiotics have been reported to have some efficacy for CSD, including rifampicin, TMP-SMZ, ciprofloxacin, and azithromycin. The only controlled study of patients with typical CSD found that azithromycin (10 mg per kg in a single dose on day 1, followed by 5 mg per kg once daily on days 2 through 5) shortened the duration of adenopathy. Although not definitive, some current authorities recommend this antibiotic at 12 mg per kg daily for 5 days. Nodes that persist and become fluctuant usually resolve after needle aspiration.

Ehrlichiosis and Anaplasmosis

Ehrlichia chaffeensis causes human monocytic ehrlichiosis and *Ehrlichia ewingii* can also cause disease. *Anaplasma phagocytophilum* causes a disease known as human granulocytic anaplasmosis. These three infections are transmitted by a number of tick vectors. The disease they produce may resemble Rocky Mountain spotted fever (RMSF) with symptoms of fever, chills, malaise, myalgias, nausea and headache. Additional symptoms may include vomiting, diarrhea, cough, arthralgias and confusion. Unlike RMSF, rash may develop late in the illness and occurs in only 60% of patients with human monocytic ehrlichiosis and rarely with human granulocytic anaplasmosis. The infection may spread to involve the meninges or cause the typical complications of septic shock. Laboratory findings may include anemia, thrombocytopenia, leukopenia, lymphopenia, hyponatremia, and mildly elevated liver enzymes. Examination of the peripheral smear may show inclusions (morulae) in monocytes or granulocytes (depending on the species) but these not uniformly seen. A definitive diagnosis relies on serology, detection of Ehrlichia or anaplasma DNA by PCR, antigen detection by immunohistochemical methods, or isolation in cell culture any of which is available only from reference laboratories. The treatment of choice is doxycycline (3 mg per kg per day in two divided doses), even for children younger than 8 years; chloramphenicol (75 to 100 mg per kg per day in four divided doses) offers an alternative.

Malaria

Malaria is a protozoal infection that occurs in humans and is caused by four species: *P. falciparum, Plasmodium vivax, Plasmodium ovale,* and *Plasmodium malariae.* Although one of the most common infections in the world, malaria is rare in the United States; about 1,000 cases occur annually. This illness should be considered particularly in recent immigrants from tropical areas and in travelers, but there have been a handful of indigenously acquired cases since 1990, including transmission in the northeastern part of the country. At times, malaria may be fatal, particularly with infections from *P. falciparum.*

Pathophysiology

Plasmodia gain access to the bloodstream when a person is bitten by a female anopheline mosquito or, rarely, by transfusion or transplacentally. The sporozoites invade liver parenchymal cells that subsequently release merozoites. The merozoites enter the erythrocytes and eventually cause their destruction. Subsequent cycles of infection account for the recurrent nature of the illness.

Clinical Manifestations

Fever characterizes malarial infections. Although specific patterns may occur, chaotic elevations of the temperature are more common because of multiple broods of parasites. The typical attack starts with a chill and tachycardia. Within 1 hour, the fever rises to 40°C (104°F) or higher. A profuse diaphoresis follows and lasts for several hours. Hepatosplenomegaly is a common finding. The febrile episodes may be accompanied by hypotension and jaundice. Laboratory findings include anemia, leukocytosis, thrombocytopenia, and hyperbilirubinemia.

Complications of malaria resulting from *P. falciparum* include massive hemolysis (blackwater fever), renal failure, pulmonary edema, and cerebral dysfunction. Neurologic signs of cerebral malaria include decreased level of consciousness, behavioral changes, hallucinations, seizures, and rarely, focal signs. The CSF is usually normal.

Management

Malaria must be suspected in any febrile child recently in an endemic area and in febrile neonates born to women who are recent immigrants from such regions. Thick and thin blood smears should be performed and, if positive, will confirm the diagnosis. However, these smears may be negative in some infections and are often not easily interpreted except by experienced personnel. In such circumstances, a CBC count is helpful. Thrombocytopenia often occurs in children during febrile episodes; the platelet count usually falls in the range of 50,000 to 100,000 per mm^3.

Children with suspected or proven malaria from areas without resistant *P. falciparum* (representing only about 10% of the disease diagnosed in the United States and occurring at present only in the Middle East, Eastern Europe, Central America north of the Panama Canal, and Haiti/Dominican Republic) should be given chloroquine phosphate [initial dose is 10 mg per kg of base (maximum 600 mg), followed by 5 mg per kg at 6, 24, and 48 hours] plus either doxycycline [3 mg per kg per day (maximum 200 mg) once daily for 3 days] or a single dose of sulfadoxine-pyrimethamine (Fansidar®; younger than 1 year old, one-fourth tablet; 1 to 3 years, one-half tablet; 4 to 8 years, one tablet; 9 to 14 years, two tablets; older than 14 years, three tablets). Fansidar should not be used in patients with known sensitivity to sulfa drugs. (Updated information on the geographic prevalence of resistance is available from the CDC at www.CDC.gov.) Patients who are seriously ill or unable to take oral medication require IV quinidine, beginning with a loading dose of 10 mg per kg over 1 hour, followed by a continuous infusion of 0.02 mg per kg per minute, with cardiac monitoring. Uncomplicated infections with chloroquine-resistant *P. falciparum* can be treated with oral quinine sulfate (25 to 30 mg per kg per day in three divided doses) plus oral pyrimethamine-sulfadoxine, as previously discussed. An alternative regimen for chloroquine-resistant *P. falciparum* is atovaquone-proguanil (Malarone®), dosed once daily for 3 days according to weight (11 to 20 kg: one adult tablet; 21 to 30 kg: two adults tablets; 31 to 40 kg: three adult tablets; greater than 40 kg: four adult tablets).

Children with nonfalciparum malaria from any area can be treated with chloroquine, as previously discussed. For *P. vivax* and *P. ovale,* primaquine [0.6 mg base per kg per day (maximum 30 mg)] for 14 days is indicated after chloroquine for the prevention of relapse, in patients who are not G6PD deficient.

Parasitic Infestations of the Gastrointestinal Tract

A variety of parasites can infest the GI tract or invade the body via this route. These infestations may be asymptomatic, being detected on screening examination of the stool. In the ED, the diagnosis is usually entertained when a parent reports observing a worm (pinworm, *Enterobius vermicularis*) or in acute diarrheal diseases, particularly among patients who are immunosuppressed or recently in underdeveloped countries. Two pathogens deserve particular consideration in the United States among immunocompetent children. *Cryptosporidium parvum,* first reported as a cause of human disease in 1976 and well known as a pathogen in children with HIV, has been reported to be the responsible pathogen in 2% to 5% of cases

TABLE 92.22

PARASITIC DISEASES

Parasite	Disease	Clinical manifestations	Treatment (uncomplicated disease)
Ancylostoma braziliense	Cutaneous larval migrans	Serpiginous rash	Thiabendazole topically or 50 mg/kg/day in two divided doses
Ascaris lumbricoides	Ascariasis	Abdominal pain, passage of large (20 cm) worm	Mebendazole 100 mg twice daily for 3 days
Balantidium coli	Balantidiasis	Abdominal pain, vomiting, bloody diarrhea	Metronidazole 35–50 mg/kg/day in three divided doses
Cryptosporidium parvum	Cryptosporidiosis	Diarrhea	Nitrozoxanide 12–47 mo: 100 mg (5 mL) q12h for 3 days 4–11 yr: 200 mg q12h for 3 days
Entamoeba histolytica	Amebiasis	Abdominal pain, bloody diarrhea, extraintestinal abscesses	Metronidazole 35–50 mg/kg/day in three divided doses
Enterobius vermicularis	Enterobiasis (pinworms)	Perianal pruritus Observation of small (1 cm) worm	Mebendazole 100 mg once; repeat in 2 weeks
Giardia lamblia	Giardiasis	Diarrhea, malabsorption, abdominal pain	Furazolidone 8 mg/kg/day in four divided doses or metronidazole 15 mg/kg/day in three divided doses or nitrozoxanide 12–47 mo: 100 mg (5 mL) q12h for 3 days 4–11 yr: 200 mg q12h for 3 days
Necator americanus	Hookworm	Initial pedal rash, then diarrhea and eosinophilia, later anemia	Mebendazole 100 mg twice daily for 3 days
Taenia saginatum/solium	Taeniasis (adult)/ cysticercosis (larvae)	Diarrhea, tapeworm segment in stool, seizures (cysticercosis)	Taeniasis: praziquantel 10 mg/kg as a single dose Cysticercosis: praziquantel 100 mg/kg/day in three divided doses for 1 day then 50 mg/kg/day in 3 divided doses for 29 days. Seizure control and steroids should be considered.
Toxocara canis	Visceral larva migrans	Hepatosplenomegaly	Thiabendazole 50 mg/kg/day in two divided doses
Trichinella spiralis	Trichinosis	Abdominal pain, vomiting, myalgias, periorbital edema, eosinophilia	Mebendazole 300 mg three times daily

of nonspecific, watery diarrhea and has been implicated in several large, waterborne outbreaks, one affecting an estimated 400,000 persons in Milwaukee, Wisconsin, in 1993. *G. lamblia* is also a waterborne parasite that can survive even in running waters and has been described as a cause of diarrhea among campers and hikers who have ingested water from streams. Both cryptosporidiosis and giardiasis merit consideration in day care settings. Table 92.22 summarizes the clinical symptoms and treatment of GI parasites in children.

Rabies

Rabies is a viral infection of the brain that is almost invariably fatal. Although the actual disease is rare in the United States, potential exposure in the form of animal bites commonly occurs. Dogs bite 1 million to 2 million people per year, and 75% of the victims are children.

The decision whether to give prophylaxis for rabies is influenced by the species of animal, the condition of the animal, the ability to study the animal, the type of exposure, and the prevalence of rabies in the region (Fig. 92.27). The incidence of rabies in the area should be available from the local health department. If a sleeping or preverbal child has had close exposure to a bat in an area where rabies is endemic in this species, prophylaxis is indicated even in the absence of a visible bite wound because of the occurrence of several pediatric cases in this circumstance. When the physician determines that prophylaxis is necessary, human rabies immune globulin (HRIG) 20 units per kg and human diploid cell vaccine (HDCV) are used. After cleaning the wound, as much of the HRIG as possible is given locally and the remainder at a distant site. Vaccine must be given in the deltoid muscle (not the thigh or buttock) in a different extremity than that used for the HRIG (see "Practical Information" in Appendix D).

MEDICAL EMERGENCIES

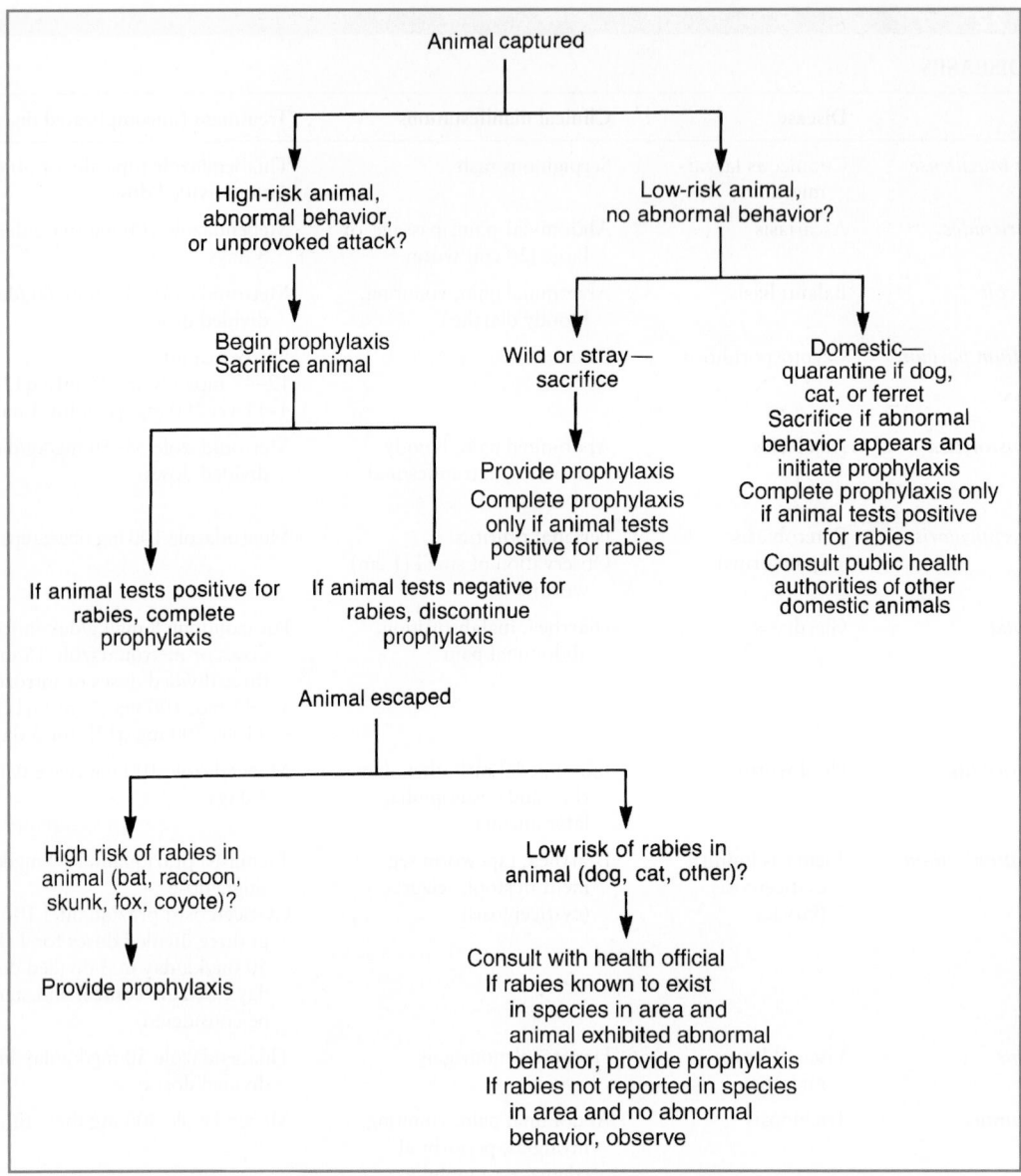

FIGURE 92.27 Diagnostic approach for the management of the child with a mammalian bite wound.

Rocky Mountain Spotted Fever

Background

RMSF is an infection caused by *Rickettsia rickettsii*. It is the most commonly occurring rickettsial disease in the United States. Ticks harbor the organism and transmit it to humans during blood sucking. Although the disease is named for the area of the country in which the causative agent was discovered, most cases of RMSF occur in the states along the eastern coast of the United States. The incidence of the disease peaks during the warmer months. It affects persons of all ages, but two-thirds of the victims are children and adolescents. Each year, approximately 1,000 cases are reported to the CDC.

Pathophysiology

Rickettsiae are inoculated during blood sucking by a tick and replicate locally. In animal models, the organisms disseminate hematogenously and invade the endothelial lining of the small blood vessels. The infection induces an inflammatory reaction in these cells that leads to swelling, necrosis, thrombosis, and finally, occlusion of the vascular lumina. The diffuse vasculitis underlies the widespread clinical manifestations that may involve almost every organ.

Clinical Manifestations

The incubation period of RMSF ranges from 2 to 10 days but usually lasts 1 week. The initial symptoms of headache and malaise are followed by fever (Fig. 92.28). The rash erupts on the third or fourth day of illness. In more than half the cases reviewed by Vianna and Hinman, the exanthem appeared first on the wrists and ankles and then spread inward toward the trunk. The initial lesions are maculopapular but become hemorrhagic in the ensuing 24 to 48 hours if the disease remains unchecked (Fig. 92.28).

Septic Arthritis

Chusid MJ, Jacobs WM, Stay JR. Pseudomonas arthritis following puncture wounds of the foot. *J Pediatr* 1979;94:429–431.

Dagan R. Management of acute hematogenous osteomyelitis and septic arthritis in the pediatric patient. *Pediatr Infect Dis J* 1993;12:88–93.

Del Beccaro MA, Champoux AN, Bockers T, et al. Septic arthritis versus transient synovitis of the hip: the value of screening laboratory tests. *Ann Emerg Med* 1992;21:1418–1422.

Kocher MS, Mandiga R, Zurakowski D, et al. Validation of a clinical prediction rule for the differentiation between septic *arthritis* and transient synovitis of the hip in children. *J Bone Joint Surg Am* 2004;86-A(8):1629–1635.

Kunnamo I, Kallio P, Pelkonen P, et al. Clinical signs and laboratory tests in the differential diagnosis of arthritis in children. *Am J Dis Child* 1987;141:34–40.

Memon IA, Jacobs NM, Yeh TF, et al. Group B streptococcal osteomyelitis and septic arthritis. Its occurrence in infants less than 2 months old. *Am J Dis Child* 1979;133:921–923.

Molteni RA. The differential diagnosis of benign and septic joint disease in children. Clinical, radiologic, laboratory, and joint fluid analysis, based on 37 children with septic arthritis and 97 with benign aseptic arthritis. *Clin Pediatr* 1978;17(1):19–23.

Nelson JD. The bacterial etiology and antibiotic management of septic arthritis in infants and children. *Pediatrics* 1972;50(3):437–40.

Pittard WB, Thullen JD, Fanaroff AA. Neonatal septic arthritis. *J Pediatr* 1976; 88:621–624.

Schaad UB, McCracken GH, Nelson JD. Pyogenic arthritis of the sacroiliac joint in pediatric patients. *Pediatrics* 1980;66:375–379.

Volberg FM, Sumner TE, Abramson JS, et al. Unreliability of radiographic diagnosis of septic hip in children. *Pediatrics* 1984;74:118–120.

Willis AA, Widmann RF, Flynn JM, et al. Lyme arthritis presenting as acute septic arthritis in children. *J Pediatr Orthop* 2003;23:114–118.

Osteomyelitis

Capitanio MA, Kirkpatrick JA. Early roentgen observations in acute osteomyelitis. *Am J Roentgenol Radium Ther Nucl Med* 1970;108:488–496.

Correa AG, Edwards MS, Baker CJ. Vertebral osteomyelitis in children. *Pediatr Infect Dis J* 1993;12:228–233.

Dich PQ, Nelson JD, Haltallin KC. Osteomyelitis in infants and children: a review of 163 cases. *Am J Dis Child* 1975;129:1273–1278.

Edward MS, Baker CJ, Wagner ML, et al. An etiologic shift in infantile osteomyelitis: the emergence of the group B *Streptococcus. J Pediatr* 1978;93:578–583.

Fleisher GR, Paradise JE, Plotkin SA, et al. Falsely normal radionuclide scans for osteomyelitis. *Am J Dis Child* 1980;134:499–502.

Granoff DM, Sargent E, Jolivette D. *Haemophilus influenzae* type B osteomyelitis. *Am J Dis Child* 1978;132:488–490.

Jacobs FR, Adelonan L, Sack CM, et al. Management of *Pseudomonas* osteochondritis complicating puncture wounds of the foot. *Pediatrics* 1982;69:432–435.

Jacobs RF, McCarthy RE, Elser JM. *Pseudomonas* osteochondritis complicating puncture wounds of the foot in children: a 10-year evaluation. *J Infect Dis* 1989;160:657–661.

Meulen DC, Majd M. Bone scintigraphy in the evaluation of children with obscure skeletal pain. *Pediatrics* 1987;79:587–592.

Minnefor AB, Olson MI, Carver DH. *Pseudomonas* osteomyelitis following puncture wounds of the foot. *Pediatrics* 1971;47:598–601.

Trevis S, Khettry J, Broker FH, et al. Osteomyelitis: early scintigraphic detection in children. *Pediatrics* 1976;57:173–186.

Unkila-Kallio L, Kallio MJ, Eskola J, Peltola H. Serum C-reactive protein, erythrocyte sedimentation rate, and white blood cell count in acute hematogenous osteomyelitis of children. *Pediatrics* 1994;93:59–62.

Waldvogel FA, Papageorgiou PS. Osteomyelitis: the past decade. *N Engl J Med* 1980;303:360–370.

Weissburg ED, Smith AL, Smith DH. Clinical features of neonatal osteomyelitis. *Pediatrics* 1974;53:505–510.

Zaoutis T, Localio AR, Leckerman K, et al. Prolonged intravenous therapy versus early transition to oral antimicrobial therapy for acute osteomyelitis in children. *Pediatrics* 2009:123:636–642.

Urinary Tract Infections

American Academy of Pediatrics. Practice parameter: the diagnosis, treatment, and evaluation of the initial urinary tract infection in febrile infants and young children. *Pediatrics* 1999;103:843–852.

Bachur R, Caputo GL. Bacteremia and meningitis among infants with urinary tract infections. *Pediatr Emerg Care* 1995;11:280–284.

Bachur R, Harper M. Reliability of the urinalysis for predicting urinary tract infections in young febrile children. *Arch Pediatr Adolesc Med* 2001;155:60–65.

Crain EF, Gershel JC. Urinary tract infections in febrile infants younger than 8 weeks of age. *Pediatrics* 1990;86:363–367.

Downes SM. Technical report: urinary tract infection in febrile infants and young children. *Pediatrics* 1999;103:e54.

Hewitt IK, Zucchetta P, Rigon L, et al. Early treatment of acute pyelonephritis in children fails to reduce renal scarring: data from the Italian Renal Infection Study Trials. *Pediatrics* 2008;122:486–490.

Hoberman A, Chao HP, Keller DM, et al. Prevalence of urinary tract infection in febrile infants. *J Pediatr* 1993;123:17–23.

Hoberman A, Charron M, Hickey RW, et al. Imaging studies after a first febrile urinary tract infection in young children. *N Engl J Med* 2003;348:195–202.

Hoberman A, Wald ER, Hickey RW, et al. Oral versus initial intravenous therapy for urinary tract infections in febrile young children. *Pediatrics* 104;1999:79–86.

Hoberman A, Wald ER, Reynolds EA, et al. Pyuria and bacteriuria in urine specimens obtained by catheter from young children with fever. *J Pediatr* 1994;124:513–519.

Hoberman A, Wald ER, Reynolds EA, et al. Is urine culture necessary to rule out urinary tract infection in febrile young children. *Pediatr Infect Dis J* 1996;15:304–309.

Kuppermann N, Bank DE, Walton EA, et al. Risks for bacteremia and urinary tract infections in young febrile infants with bronchiolitis. *Arch Pediatr Adolesc Med* 1997;151:1207–1214.

Lohr JA, Portilla MG, Geuder TG, et al. Making a presumptive diagnosis of urinary tract infection by using a urinalysis performed in an on-site laboratory. *J Pediatr* 1993;122:22–25.

Neuhaus TJ, Berger C, Buechner K, et al. Randomised trial of oral versus sequential intravenous/oral cephalosporins in children with pyelonephritis. *Eur J Pediatr* 2008;167:1037–1047.

Shaw KN, Gorelick M, McGowan KL, et al. Prevalence of urinary tract infection in febrile young children in the emergency department. *Pediatrics* 1998;102:e16.

Viral Syndrome and Influenza

Chiu SS, Lau YL, Chan KH, et al. Influenza related hospitalizations among children in Hong Kong. *N Engl J Med* 2002;347:2097–2103.

Finelli L, Fiore A, Dhara R, Brammer L, et al. Influenza-associated pediatric mortality in the United States: increase of *Staphylococcus aureus* coinfection. *Pediatrics.* 2008;122:805–11.

Krugman S, Ward R, Katz S. *Infectious disease of children.* St. Louis, MO: Mosby, 1981.

Monto AS, Pichichero ME, Blanckenberg SJ, et al. Zanamivir prophylaxis: an effective strategy for the prevention of influenza types A and B within households. *J Infect Dis* 2002;186:1582–1588.

Newland, JG, Laurich, VM, Rosenquist, AW, et al. Neurologic complications in children hospitalized with influenza: characteristics, incidence, and risk factors. *J Pediatr* 2007;150:306–310.

Peltola, V, Reunanen, T, Ziegler, T, et al. Accuracy of clinical diagnosis of influenza in outpatient children. *Clin Infect Dis* 2005;41:1198–1200.

Ploin, D, Gillet, Y, Morfin, F, et al. Influenza Burden in Febrile Infants and Young Children in a Pediatric Emergency Department. *Pediatr Infect Dis J* 2007;26:142–147.

Poehling, KA, Edwards, KM, Weinberg, GA, et al. The underrecognized burden of influenza in young children. *N Engl J Med* 2006;355:31–40.

Uyeki TM. Influenza diagnosis and treatment in children: a review of studies on clinically useful tests and antiviral treatment for influenza. *Pediatr Infect Dis J* 2003;22:164–177.

Updated information for health professionals regarding flu activity and recommended antiviral therapy available at http://www.cdc.gov/flu/

Erythema Infectiosum

Bell LM, Naides SJ, Stoffman P, et al. Human parvovirus B19 infection among hospital staff members after contact with infected patients. *N Engl J Med* 1989;321:485–491.

Nunuoe T, Okochi K, Mortimer PP, et al. Human parvovirus (B19) and erythema infectiosum. *J Pediatr* 1985;107:38–40.

Infectious Mononucleosis

Alpert G, Fleisher GR. Complications of EBV infection during childhood. *Pediatr Infect Dis J* 1984;3:304.

Fleisher GR, Henle W, Henle G, et al. Primary Epstein-Barr virus infections in American infants: clinical and serological observations. *J Infect Dis* 1979; 139:553.

Fleisher GR, Lennete ET, Henle G, et al. Incidence of heterophil antibody responses in children with infectious mononucleosis. *J Pediatr* 1979;94:723.

Fleisher GR, Paradise J. Atypical lymphocytosis in children. *Ann Emerg Med* 1981;10:424.

Fleisher GR, Paradise JE, Lennette ET. The leukocyte response in childhood infectious mononucleosis. *Am J Dis Child* 1981;135:699.

Peter J, Ray CG. Infectious mononucleosis. *Pediatr Rev* 1998;19:276–279.

van der Horst C, Joncas J, Ahronheim G, et al. Lack of effect of peroral acyclovir for the treatment of acute infectious mononucleosis. *J Infect Dis* 1991;164:788.

Measles

Barkin RM. Measles mortality: analysis of the primary cause of death. *Am J Dis Child* 1975;129:307.

Farizo KM, Stehr-Green PA, Simpson DM, et al. Pediatric emergency room visits: a risk factor for acquiring measles. *Pediatrics* 1991;87:74–79.

MEDICAL EMERGENCIES

Mason WH, Ross LA, Lanson J, et al. Epidemic measles in the postvaccine era: evaluation of epidemiology, clinical presentation and complications during an urban outbreak. *Pediatr Infect Dis J* 1993;12:42–48.

Roseola (Exanthem Subitum)

Lyall EG. Human herpesvirus 6: primary infection and the central nervous system. *Pediatr Infect Dis J* 1996;15:693–696.
Suga S, Yoshikawa T, Nagia T, et al. Clinical features and virological findings in children with primary human herpesvirus 7 infection. *Pediatrics* 1997; 99:E4.
Yoshikawa T, Suga S, Asano Y, et al. Distribution of antibodies to a causative agent of exanthem subitum (human herpesvirus-6) in healthy individuals. *Pediatrics* 1989;84:675–677.

Varicella

Centers for Disease Control. Decline in annual incidence of varicella-selected states, 1990–2001. *MMWR Morb Mortal Wkly Rep* 2003;52:884–885.
Cameron JC, Allan G, Johnston F, et al. Severe complications of chickenpox in hospitalised children in the UK and Ireland. *Arch Dis Child* 2007;92: 1062–1066.
Doctor A, Harper MB, Fleisher GR. Group A beta-hemolytic streptococcal bacteremia: historical overview, changing incidence, and recent association with varicella. *Pediatrics* 1995;96:428–433.
Dunkle LM, Arvin AM, Whitley RJ, et al. A controlled trial of acyclovir for chickenpox in normal children. *N Engl J Med* 1991;325:1539–1544.
Fleisher GR, Henry W, McSorley M, et al. Life-threatening complications of varicella. *Am J Dis Child* 1981;135:896–899.
Galil K, Lee B, Strine T, et al. Outbreak of varicella at a day-care center despite vaccination. *N Engl J Med* 2002;347:1909–1915.
Weinstein L. Failure of chemotherapy to prevent the bacterial complications of measles. *N Engl J Med* 1955;253:679–683.

Babesiosis

Krauss PJ, Feder HM. Lyme disease and babesiosis. *Adv Pediatr Infect Dis* 1994;9:183–209.
Krauss PJ, Telford SR, Pollack RJ, et al. Babesiosis: an underdiagnosed disease of children. *Pediatrics* 1992;89:1045–1048.

Botulism

Centers for Disease Control. Infant botulism—New York City, 2001–2002. *MMWR Morb Mortal Wkly Rep* 2003;52:21–24.
Grover W, Peckham G, Berman P. Recovery following cranial nerve dysfunction and muscle weakness in infancy. *Dev Med Child Neurol* 1974;16: 163–171.
Johnson RO, Clay SA, Arnon SS. Diagnosis and management of infant botulism. *Am J Dis Child* 1979;133:586–593.
Long SS, Gajewski JV, Brown LW, et al. Clinical, laboratory, and environmental features of infant botulism in southeastern Pennsylvania. *Pediatrics* 1985; 75:935–941.
Pickett J, Berg B, Chaplin E, et al. Syndrome of botulism in infancy: clinical and electrophysiologic study. *N Engl J Med* 1976;295:770–772.
Sobel J. Botulism. *Clin Infect Dis* 2005;41:1167–1173.
Underwood K, Rubin S, Deakers T, et al. Infant botulism: a 30-year experience spanning the introduction of botulism immune globulin intravenous in the intensive care unit at Childrens Hospital Los Angeles. *Pediatrics* 2007; 120:e1380–e1385.

Cat-Scratch Disease

Bass JW, Freitas BC, Freitas AD, et al. Prospective randomized double blind placebo-controlled evaluation of azithromycin for treatment of cat-scratch disease. *Pediatr Infect Dis J* 1998;17:447–452.
Demers DM, Bass JW, Vincent JM, et al. Cat scratch disease in Hawaii: etiology and seroepidemiology. *J Pediatr* 1995;127:23–26.
Margileth AM. Cat scratch disease: nonbacterial regional lymphadenitis. *Pediatrics* 1969;42:803–818.

Ehrlichiosis

Bakken JS, Dumler S. Human granulocytic anaplasmosis. *Infect Dis Clin North Am* 2008; 22:433–448.
Barton LL, Rathore MH, Dawson JE. Infection with *Ehrlichia* in childhood. *J Pediatr* 1992;120:998–1001.

Goodman JL, Nelson C, Vitale B, et al. Direct cultivation of the causative agent of human granulocytic ehrlichiosis. *N Engl J Med* 1996;334:209–215.
Schutze G, Jacobs RF. Human monocytic ehrlichiosis in children. *Pediatrics* 1997;100:E10.
Stone JH, Dierberg K, Aram G, Dumler JS. Human monocytic ehrlichiosis. *JAMA* 2004;292:2263–2270.

Malaria

Greenwood BM, Bojang K, Whitty CJ, et al. Malaria. *Lancet* 2005;365: 1487–1498.
Griffith KS, Lewis LS, Mali S, et al. Treatment of malaria in the United States: a systematic review. *JAMA* 2007;297:2264–2277.
McCaslin RI, Pikis A, Rodriquez WJ. Pediatric *Plasmodium falciparum* malaria: a ten year experience from Washington, DC. *Pediatr Infect Dis J* 1994; 13:709–715.
Stauffer W, Fischer PR. Diagnosis and treatment of malaria in children. *Clin Infect Dis* 2003;37:1340–1348.
Updated information for health professionals regarding malaria diagnosis and treatment available at: http://www.cdc.gov/malaria

Parasites, Intestinal

Committee on Infectious Diseases. *2009 Redbook*. Elk Grove Village, IL: American Academy of Pediatrics, 2009.

Rabies

Mann JM. Systematic decision-making in rabies prophylaxis. *Pediatr Infect Dis J* 1983;2:162–167.
Plotkin SA, Wiktor TJ, Koprowski H, et al. Immunization schedules for the new human diploid cell vaccine. *Am J Epidemiol* 1976;103:75–80.
Wilde H, Briggs DJ, Meslin FX, et al. Rabies update for travel medicine advisors. *Clin Infect Dis* 2003;37:96–100.

Rocky Mountain Spotted Fever

Abramson JS, Givner LB. Should tetracycline be contraindicated for therapy of presumed Rocky Mountain spotted fever in children less than 9 years of age? *Pediatrics* 1990;86:123–124.
Bradford WD, Hawkins HK. Rocky Mountain spotted fever in childhood. *Am J Dis Child* 1977;131:1228–1232.
Cunha BA. Clinical features of Rocky Mountain spotted fever. *Lancet Infect Dis* 2008;8:143–144.
Fleisher G, Lennette ET, Honig P. Diagnosis of Rocky Mountain spotted fever by immunofluorescent identification of *Rickettsia rickettsii* in skin biopsy tissue. *J Pediatr* 1979;95:63–65.
Hattwick MA, Retailliau H, O'Brien RJ, et al. Fatal Rocky Mountain spotted fever. *JAMA* 1978;240:1499–1503.
Vianna NJ, Hinman AR. Rocky Mountain spotted fever in Long Island. Epidemiologic and clinical aspects. *Am J Med* 1971;51:725–730.
Wilfert CM, MacCormack JN, Kleeman K, et al. The prevalence of antibodies to *Rickettsia rickettsii* in an area endemic for Rocky Mountain spotted fever. *J Infect Dis* 1985;151:823–831.
Woodward TE, Pederson CE, Oster CN, et al. Prompt confirmation of Rocky Mountain spotted fever: identification of rickettsiae in skin tissues. *J Infect Dis* 1976;134:297–301.

Tetanus

Brand DA, Acampora D, Gottlieb LD, et al. Adequacy of anti-tetanus prophylaxis in six hospital emergency rooms. *N Engl J Med* 1983;309:636–640.
Freelander FC. Tetanus neonatorum. *J Pediatr* 1951;39:448.
Turner TB, Velasco-Joven EA, Prudovsky S. Studies on the prophylaxis and treatment of tetanus. II. Studies pertaining to treatment. *Bull Johns Hopkins Hosp* 1958;102:71–84.
Weinstein L. Tetanus. *N Engl J Med* 1973;289:1293–1296.

Toxic Shock Syndrome

Davis JP, Chesney PJ, Wand PJ, et al. Toxic shock syndrome: epidemiologic features, recurrence, risk factors, and prevention. *N Engl J Med* 1980;303: 1429–1435.
Todd J, Fishant M, Kapral F, et al. Toxic-shock syndrome associated with phagegroup-1 staphylococci. *Lancet* 1978;2:1116–1118.
Wiesenthal AM, Todd JK. Toxic shock syndrome in children aged 10 years or less. *Pediatrics* 1984;74:112–117.

CHAPTER 93 ■ INFECTIOUS DISEASE EMERGENCIES—SEXUALLY TRANSMITTED DISEASES

MARVIN B. HARPER, MD

Sexually transmitted diseases (STDs) are the most commonly reported infections in the United States and represent an important pediatric problem, particularly during infancy or adolescence. This chapter focuses on infections due to gonorrhea, chlamydia, syphilis, and human immunodeficiency virus (HIV). A myriad of social issues necessarily interpose themselves with regard to the management of these patients. Sexual abuse as a general topic is handled in Chapter 132, but the emergent antimicrobial postexposure prophylaxis of sexual assault is also discussed here. Issues of adolescent sexuality and pelvic inflammatory disease are discussed in Chapter 90. The pathogens causing STDs are described separately in this chapter, but the risk episodes leading to infection with these organisms, as well as the nature of the infections and their lesions, will commonly result in coinfections. Therefore, any patient identified as having one of these pathogens should be considered to possibly have infection with any or all the others.

GONORRHEA

Congenital

Background

The epidemiology of congenital infection depends entirely on the prevalence of gonorrhea among pregnant women and the prenatal care, testing, and treatment they receive. Infection occurs from infected mothers via ascending infection, possibly including chorioamnionitis, with ruptured membranes prior to delivery or during passage through the birth canal.

Clinical Manifestations

Among infants, the most common site for infection is the eye. This is not a commonly seen complication in the United States because of the success of neonatal ocular prophylaxis; however, no strategy is uniformly applied or completely effective and cases do occur. In the neonatal period, generally day of life 2 to 5, an initial simple conjunctivitis rapidly comes to develop a thick mucopurulent discharge (see color plate 127.7). Gram-stained smears of the exudates often reveal gram-negative intracellular diplococci, distinguishing gonococcal conjunctivitis from other causes.

Management

This infection must be treated promptly and aggressively because corneal ulceration and perforation may occur and iridocyclitis may also develop. The usual treatment is ceftriaxone 125 mg intramuscular (IM) and hospitalization commonly in consultation with an ophthalmologist. In addition to conjunctivitis, focal gonococcal infections or sepsis may occur as a result of direct inoculation (e.g., at scalp electrode site) or hematogenous seeding. Infants born to a mother with untreated gonorrhea should receive postexposure prophylaxis (PEP) with a single dose of parenteral ceftriaxone (50 mg per kg to a maximum of 125 mg) in an effort to prevent dissemination. Specific focal infections such as meningitis require therapy with intravenous (IV) penicillin. Testing and treatment of the infant and/or mother for chlamydia must also be considered.

Acquired

Background

Gonorrhea decreased in incidence by 75% from 1975 to 1996, but this rate has been steady at approximately 120 per 100,000 population in the United States since. It remains the second most commonly reported communicable disease. Rates are highest in the southeastern states, among minorities, and among adolescents of all racial and ethnic groups. The peak age incidence overall is in the 15- to 19-year age group.

Pathophysiology

Humans are the only host for this organism, which causes infections of mucous membranes, most often in the genitourinary tract. Infections of the conjunctivae, pharynx, and rectum occur less frequently than infections of the sites lined with a columnar epithelium, such as the urethra, prostate, or epididymis in males; and the urethra, Skene's and Bartholin's glands, cervix, and fallopian tubes in females. Because *Neisseria gonorrhoeae* cannot invade stratified squamous epithelium, the postpubertal vagina and the external genitalia are not infected, whereas these sites may be involved in prepubertal females. The incubation period is very short at 2 to 7 days.

Clinical Findings

The most common gonococcal infection of young children is vulvovaginitis, which usually occurs as a result of sexual abuse (see Chapter 132). In adolescence, the typical presentation is with urethritis or cervicitis, although some may have clinically asymptomatic disease. Prostatitis, epididymitis, and pelvic inflammatory disease are also relatively common. Approximately 1% of patients with gonococcal infections will develop disseminated disease. This disseminated gonococcal infection

TABLE 93.1

SUMMARY OF TREATMENT REGIMENS FOR LOWER GENITAL TRACT GONORRHEA
AND CHLAMYDIAL INFECTION

Patient circumstance	Drug	Dose, route	Comments
Treatment for Gonorrhea			
In children <45 kg	Ceftriaxone	125 mg, IM	
In children >45 kg and adolescents	Ceftriaxone *or* cefixime *or* ciprofloxacin *or* ofloxacin	125 mg, IM 400 mg PO 500 mg PO 400 mg PO	Regimens other than ceftriaxone may not treat incubating syphilis
Penicillin allergy			
In children	Spectinomycin	40 mg/kg, IM	Maximum dose 2 g
In adolescents	Spectinomycin	2 g, IM	May not treat incubating syphilis
Treatment for Chlamydial Infection			
All ages	Azithromycin	20 mg/kg in a single dose to maximum 1 g	Single-dose regimen obviates compliance problems
Alternative for those ≥8 years of age	Doxycycline	100 mg PO bid for 7 d	
During pregnancy	Erythromycin base *or* erythromycin ethylsuccinate	500 mg PO qid for 7 d 800 mg PO qid for 7 d	Efficacy of this therapy to eradicate organism estimated 80%

usually presents with an inflammatory polyarthropathy and dermatitis (discrete papules and pustules, sometimes hemorrhagic), often with bacteremia. This phase may resolve spontaneously but is often followed by the development of a purulent arthritis (commonly the knee). When this disease is suspected, all mucosal sites (cervix, rectum, pharynx) should be cultured to improve the yield of the organism recovery from approximately 50% from blood or synovial fluid to at least 80% when mucosal sites are also cultured. Other manifestations of infection include gonococcal perihepatitis (Fitz-Hugh-Curtis syndrome), conjunctivitis, pharyngitis, proctitis, and pelvic inflammatory disease (see Chapter 90).

The diagnosis of gonorrhea relies primarily on culture from an infected site or antigen detection, either from the site or from a urine specimen. Newly introduced nucleic acid amplification tests have proven highly sensitive and specific; however, false-positive tests can occur, so these methods should not be used in low-risk populations or in legal cases where culture methods that can confirm *N. gonorrhoeae* are preferred. In addition, the nucleic acid amplification tests are not approved for testing from vaginal, rectal, or pharyngeal swabs although in preliminary reports they appear to have improved sensitivity as compared with that of culture. These tests can, however, conveniently be used on voided urine specimens from symptomatic sexually active adolescents seeking care for urethritis, epididymitis, cervicitis, or pelvic inflammatory disease.

Culture for *N. gonorrhoeae* requires the use of selective media and prompt placement into a CO_2-enriched environment, avoiding notable temperature changes and drying. It is also important to alert the microbiology laboratory of the specimen source because this will be important for distinguishing nonpathogenic *Neisseria* organisms, which can represent normal flora from *N. gonorrhoeae*.

Penicillin, tetracycline, and quinolone resistance are all reported problems with gonococcal infections in various parts of the world. However, in the United States, treatment with a

single 50 mg per kg IM dose (maximum of 125 mg, regardless of age or weight) of ceftriaxone (Table 93.1) is effective for most mucosal forms of gonorrhea (higher or more prolonged doses are recommended for conjunctivitis, disseminated disease, arthritis, meningitis, and endocarditis). In the penicillin-allergic postpubertal patient, the use of fluoroquinolones is no longer recommended unless susceptibility has been confirmed in culture. Azithromycin as a single 2-g oral dose is an option but concerns about emerging resistance prevent its routine use. Only parenteral cephalosporins have been studied and can therefore be recommended for use in prepubertal children. Patients with documented gonococcal infections should be evaluated for other STDs (hepatitis B virus, syphilis, *Chlamydia trachomatis*, and HIV) and empirically treated for *C. trachomatis*. Sexual partners should also be evaluated.

SYPHILIS

The *Treponema pallidum* causes syphilis. This thin, slowly growing helical organism cannot be grown on artificial media. Natural host immunity can suppress but does not eradicate infection that, untreated, may persist for life.

Congenital Syphilis

Background

A sustained reduction in the incidence of congenital syphilis in the United States has occurred during the last decade, with 10.5 cases reported per 100,000 live births in 2007. Congenital infection occurs via transplacental transfer of spirochetes from the mother's bloodstream or during birth. Pregnant mothers with diagnosed syphilis should be treated as early as possible during gestation and evaluated for reinfection regularly to help prevent congenital transmission.

Clinical Manifestations

Clinical findings early in congenital syphilis can range from very profound (stillbirth) to initially asymptomatic. The rate and the severity of infection correlate with the staging in the mother. Women with untreated early syphilis are estimated to have a 40% rate of spontaneous abortion. The rate of transmission to the fetus is very high in maternal secondary syphilis but decreases for mothers with latent or tertiary syphilis. The most common neonatal symptoms include hepatosplenomegaly, jaundice (conjugated hyperbilirubinemia), bony changes seen on radiographs (osteochondritis or periostitis), rhinitis (snuffles), and rash (small red maculopapules that persist for 1 to 3 months). Less commonly, fever, lymphadenopathy, and nephritis or nephrosis may occur. A reactive cerebrospinal fluid (CSF) venereal disease research laboratory (VDRL), elevated CSF white blood cell (WBC) count, or elevated CSF protein are unfortunately not highly sensitive or specific for diagnosing congenital syphilis or the presence of treponemal organisms in the CSF. Late findings of congenital syphilis include changes in the teeth, bones, eyes (interstitial keratitis), hearing loss, and rarely neurosyphilis, which can be seen years or even decades after birth.

Diagnosis and Management

The diagnosis of the infant with congenital syphilis is made difficult by the frequent lack of symptoms initially and the presence of maternal IgG antibodies used in serologic testing (Table 93.2). Therefore, cautious management is recommended. Any infant whose mother has inadequately treated syphilis, or the infant with any symptoms consistent with congenital syphilis and positive serologic tests for syphilis, should be managed as a presumptive case. Definitive diagnosis can be made when spirochetes are identified by microscopic dark field or direct fluorescent antibody testing of the placenta or umbilical cord. Treatment of the newborn with syphilis is with penicillin G, either as 50,000 units per kg penicillin G procaine given intramuscularly once per day for 10 days or as aqueous penicillin G 50,000 units per kg per dose given intravenously every 12 hours during the first 7 days of life and dosed every 8 hours thereafter until 10 days of treatment is completed. If one or more days of therapy are missed, the treatment course is restarted.

Acquired Syphilis

Background and Pathophysiology

The population rate of syphilis is low but rising, especially among males, in the last decade. In 2007, primary or secondary syphilis was diagnosed in 3 per 100,000 in the teen population with a peak incidence in the young adult male population of 15 per 100,000. Sporadic outbreaks among adolescents have been reported.

Acquisition is by direct contact with an ulcerative lesion of an infected individual. The incubation period to primary syphilis is 10 to 90 days.

Clinical Manifestations

Acquired syphilis infections are divided into three stages. Primary syphilis is characterized by the presence of a well-

---

TABLE 93.2

CRITERIA FOR DIAGNOSIS OF NEONATAL AND EARLY CONGENITAL SYPHILIS

I. Diagnostic Criteria
  A. Absolute
    1. *Treponema pallidum* seen by dark-field microscopy
  B. Major
    1. Condylomata
    2. Osteochondritis, perichondritis
    3. Snuffles
  C. Minor
    1. Fissures of lips
    2. Cutaneous lesions
    3. Mucous patches
    4. Hepatomegaly, splenomegaly
    5. Lymphadenopathy
    6. CNS signs
    7. Hemolytic anemia
    8. Elevated cell count or protein level in spinal fluid
  D. Serologic
    1. Reactive serologic test for syphilis
    2. Reactive immunoglobulin M (FTA-ABS) fluorescent treponemal antibody absorption test
    3. Nonreactive serologic test for syphilis
    4. Reactive serologic test for syphilis STS that does not revert to nonreactive within 4 mo
    5. Rising titer over 3 mo
II. Certainty of Diagnosis
  A. Definite: absolute clinical criterion
  B. Probable: any of the following: (i) serologic criterion 4 or 5; (ii) one major or two or more minor clinical criteria and serologic criterion 1 or 2; (iii) one major and one minor clinical criterion
  C. Possible: serologic criterion 1 or 2 with only one minor or no clinical criterion
  D. Unlikely: (i) serologic criterion 3; (ii) maternal history of adequate treatment for syphilis during pregnancy

CNS, central nervous system; STS, serologic test for syphilis.
Modified from Mascola L, Pelosi R, Blount JH, et al. Congenital syphilis revisited. *Am J Dis Child* 1985;139:575–580.

---

defined, rounded, firm, painless localized ulcer (chancre) at the site of acquisition, which is most commonly the genitalia (Fig. 93.1). This ulcer forms within weeks of infection (most commonly about 3 weeks) and persists for several weeks.

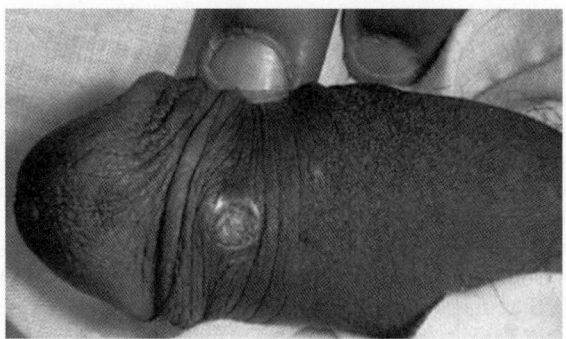

FIGURE 93.1 Chancre in an adolescent with serologically confirmed syphilis.

MEDICAL EMERGENCIES

TABLE 93.3

TREATMENT RECOMMENDATIONS FOR SYPHILIS

Syphilis stage	Recommended treatment
Primary, secondary, or early latent (infection acquired within the previous year) syphilis	A single dose of 50,000 units/kg benzathine penicillin IM (maximum is the adult dose of 2.4 million units)
Late latent (>1 year since acquisition), latent syphilis of unknown duration, or tertiary syphilis	Three separate single doses given at 1-wk intervals of 50,000 units/kg benzathine penicillin IM (maximum single dose is the adult dose of 2.4 million units)
Neurosyphilis or congenital syphilis	Aqueous penicillin G 200,000–300,000 units/kg/day (to maximum adult dose of 24 million units total per day) as 50,000 units/kg/dose every 4 to 6 h for 10–14 day An alternative for adults: procaine penicillin G 24 million units given IM daily with probenicid 500 mg four times per day for 10–14 day

The penicillin-allergic nongravid adult may be treated with twice daily 100-mg oral doses of doxycycline daily for 14 days with primary, secondary, or early latent syphilis, and for 4 weeks with late latent or latent syphilis of unknown duration.

Secondary syphilis occurs several weeks to months after the primary phase and is characterized by a diffuse rose pink rash that involves to include the palms and soles, generalized adenopathy, malaise, fever, headache, and pharyngitis. Condylomata lata (warts), splenomegaly, and mucocutaneous lesions may be seen. The rash in this stage may resemble pityriasis rosea. This phase generally resolves within 1 to 3 months.

Late syphilis is extremely uncommon in children because it is the manifestation of many years of infection that typically presents as neurosyphilis, cardiovascular disease (e.g., aortic aneurysm), or gummas.

It should be noted that the manifestations of syphilitic stages may not occur in the usual manner in immunocompromised patients. In particular, neurosyphilis can occur at any stage of infection among patients with HIV.

Diagnosis and Management

In primary syphilis, dark-field examination or a direct fluorescent antibody test for *T. pallidum* in exudates or tissue from the lesion can confirm the diagnosis. Specimens for testing should be obtained after washing the ulcer with saline and then by scraping and squeezing the lesion to express serum, which is sent for testing. Aspirated material from regional lymph nodes may also be sent. Serologic tests should also be sent, although the diagnosis may be missed if only a serum nontreponemal test (RPR, VDRL, or antiretroviral therapy) is ordered because it may be too early for reliable response. In this circumstance, the laboratory should perform a treponemal test (FTA-ABS or TP-PA), regardless of the nontreponemal result. Serologic tests of either type are reliably positive in later stages of syphilis. Confirmation of infection from serologic testing is best when both nontreponemal and treponemal tests are positive because false-positive test results can occur with each. Treponemal tests generally remain positive for life and are therefore not helpful in diagnosing reinfection. When neurosyphilis is suspected, CSF should be evaluated and sent for VDRL testing and for routine testing for CSF protein and cell count. Patients with documented syphilitic infections should also be evaluated for other STDs (hepatitis B virus, *N. gonorrhoeae*, *C. trachomatis*, and HIV).

The preferred treatment is always with penicillin G, unless the patient is allergic. The dose, dosage form, and the duration of therapy depend on the stage and form of the illness (Table 93.3). Oral forms of penicillin and combination forms of benzathine plus procaine penicillin are not considered acceptable alternatives to aqueous crystalline penicillin, aqueous procaine penicillin, or benzathine penicillin. Sexual partners will require clinical and serologic evaluation.

CHLAMYDIA

Congenital Chlamydia

Background

Pregnant women with an active chlamydia infection at the time of vaginal delivery have a 50% chance of transmitting the organism to the newborn. Transmission to infants born by cesarean section delivery with intact membranes is rare. Of infants colonized with *C. trachomatis*, it is estimated that 25% to 50% will develop conjunctivitis and 5% to 20%, pneumonia.

Clinical Manifestation

Infants exposed to chlamydia in the birth canal are likely to acquire infection at one of several sites. The best sources to culture are the conjunctivae, nasopharynx, rectum, and vagina. Symptoms depend on the site infected, and the timing of onset varies by site. Conjunctivitis will generally occur within the first 2 weeks of life (and is the most common identifiable cause of conjunctivitis at this age) and will last for 1 to 2 weeks but can, in some cases, when left untreated, persist for weeks or months. Approximately half of infants with conjunctivitis will have colonization of the nasopharynx. Nasopharyngeal colonization with chlamydia can persist for 2 to 3 years and will lead to pneumonia in one-third of cases. The pneumonia presents as nasal congestion, dry cough, and tachypnea without fever. Symptoms will appear within the first 4 months and most commonly in the second or third month of life. Rales and wheezing may be heard on auscultation of the chest but are uncommon. Chest radiographs are nonspecific but often reveal hyperinflation and/or increased interstitial markings and infiltrates. Diagnostic testing should be performed, using culture methods from the nasopharynx and/or conjunctivae, to confirm the need for treatment of the infant as well as mother and her partner(s). Treatment of congenital chlamydia infections is with erythromycin base or ethylsuccinate 50 mg per kg per day orally divided into four doses daily for 14 days. Infants treated with erythromycin should be followed for signs and symptoms of pyloric stenosis because of a possible association of this condition with the use of erythromycin. Azithromycin 20 mg per kg per day for 3 days is an alternative to erythromycin in cases where the development of pyloric stenosis is of particular concern. It must be noted that even with appropriate dosing of erythromycin, there is a relapse rate of approximately 20%; therefore, follow-up should be arranged and a second course of therapy may be required. The addition of topical therapy for chlamydia conjunctivitis is not necessary or recommended.

Acquired Chlamydia

Background

There has been a large increase in the reported cases of chlamydia infections in the United States, with the Centers for Disease Control and Prevention (CDC) reporting a rate among women of 370 cases per 100,000 population in 2007. This is more than triple the reported incidence of gonorrhea. The highest reported rates are among adolescents with a prevalence of 4.8% among a nationally representative sample of 18 to 26 year olds. Recurrence within months of treatment is common.

Acquisition is by direct contact of mucous membranes with an infected source. This can include the pharynx, cervix, vagina, and rectum. The incubation period is generally at least 1 week.

Clinical Manifestations

Infected males can present with clinically evident urethritis, but most will be asymptomatic and do not seek care. Chlamydia infections account for a large proportion of nongonococcal urethritis in men. There is much variability in the clinical symptoms of males, but generally, cases of chlamydial urethritis are less purulent than gonococcal infections. However, testing will reveal more than 15 WBCs per high-powered field in the spun urine sediment of a first void urine sample. Overall, *C. trachomatis* causes 50% of epididymitis among men 15 to 34 years of age. Homosexual or bisexual males practicing anal receptive intercourse can present with a chlamydia proctitis.

Infected females can present with mucopurulent cervicitis, but most remain asymptomatic. Infections when left untreated can last for months or even years. Women can also develop acute or chronic pelvic inflammatory disease with the subsequent risks for infertility or ectopic pregnancy (see Chapter 90).

Diagnosis

When testing urethral (male), vaginal, or endocervical swab specimens or first void urine specimens, nucleic acid amplification tests are more sensitive than other diagnostic methods and are generally preferred over culture. False-positive tests can occur; therefore, in certain circumstances (e.g., evaluation for sexual abuse), it is advisable to obtain cultures or a second type of nonculture test. Although not Food and Drug Administration (FDA)-cleared for use, nucleic amplification testing is offered by some laboratories for testing of rectal swab specimens. Nucleic amplifications tests are not recommended for detection of *C. trachomatis* from the pharynx at this time. Patients with documented chlamydia infections should also be evaluated for other STDs (hepatitis B virus, syphilis, *N. gonorrhoeae*, and HIV).

Treatment of acquired *C. trachomatis* infections is with 20 mg per kg (maximum 1 g) of oral azithromycin given as a single dose (Table 93.1). Alternatives include doxycycline (100 mg orally twice per day for 7 days), ofloxacin (300 mg orally twice per day for 7 days), or levofloxacin (500 mg orally once per day for 7 days), but the age of the child and possibility of pregnancy must be considered. Sexual partners should also be evaluated.

The treatment of acute salpingitis and pelvic inflammatory disease is discussed elsewhere (see Chapter 90).

HERPES SIMPLEX VIRUS

Herpes simplex virus (HSV) can infect the genitals and other anatomic sites. Although the most common cause of genital ulceration seen among adolescents and adults at venereal disease clinics, this entity is unusual in prepubertal children.

Genital pain is a frequent complaint with infections caused by herpes simplex and may precede the appearance of the lesions. Characteristically, the virus produces grouped vesicles on an erythematous base (Fig. 93.2); however, erosion of the overlying skin often leaves only painful ulcers at the time of the first visit. Particularly with a primary infection, the inguinal lymph nodes enlarge. HSV-2 is nearly always the result of anogenital infection. HSV-1 most commonly causes oropharyngeal infections but is an increasing cause of anogenital infections as well. National data on seroprevalence suggest

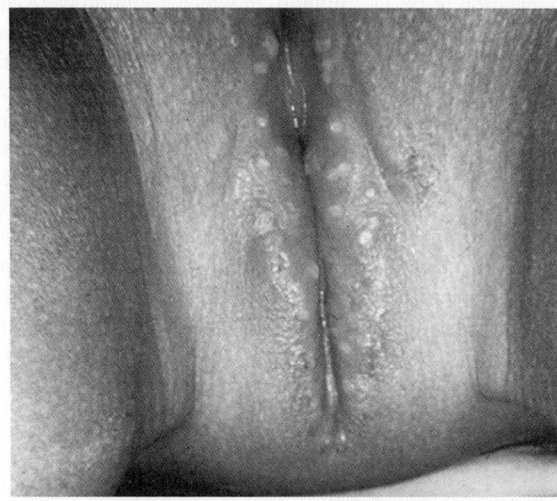

FIGURE 93.2 Genital herpetic lesions in a young girl who was sexually abused. (Courtesy of Stephen Ludwig, MD)

a decrease in rates of HSV-2 to 17% in the years 1999 to 2004 from 21% a decade earlier. Fewer than one-fourth of patients seropositive for HSV-2 report having been diagnosed with genital herpes.

Visual inspection often suffices for the initial diagnosis in the adolescent presenting to the emergency department (ED). However, specific testing, typically by culture, to confirm the diagnosis as due to HSV-1 or HSV-2 is warranted as this impacts subsequent prognosis for recurrences and therefore impacts counseling. Cellular change as seen with a Tzanck smear (Chapter 85) positive for giant cells lends further weight to the clinical impression but has poor sensitivity for detection of disease; either immunofluorescent staining of a scraping from the base of a vesicle or a viral culture can also verify the diagnosis. In the setting of negative HSV cultures but clinical suspicion of HSV disease or known positive partner with HSV, it may be prudent to obtain type specific serologic testing that distinguishes between HSV-1 and HSV-2 antibody. In children, a culture should always be obtained because the disease is seen rarely and needs medicolegal confirmation. Serologic tests for syphilis and HIV and cultures for gonorrhea and chlamydia are appropriate to rule out coexisting sexually transmitted infections. Although it is occasionally spread by nonsexual contact, the physician must explore the possibility of sexual abuse when herpes genitalis occurs before puberty. Oral acyclovir therapy is indicated for primary infections; the dose is 80 mg per kg per day in four divided doses (or for postpubertal patients, 400 mg orally three times per day for 7 to 10 days). Alternatives include famciclovir 250 mg orally three times per day for 7 to 10 days or oral valacyclovir 1 g orally twice per day for 7 to 10 days.

HIV INFECTION

Epidemiology

HIV, the etiologic agent for acquired immunodeficiency syndrome (AIDS), has been present in humans for decades. As a worldwide problem, in 2007, the number of people living with HIV infection was estimated by the World Health Organization to be 33.2 million, of which 2 million were children younger than 15 years. It is estimated that more than 1,000 children are infected each day (370,000/year). In the United States, improved prenatal testing and perinatal treatment and blood product testing has made acquisition of infection rare with fewer than 200 newly acquired HIV infections per year among children younger than 13 years. Unfortunately, adolescents continue to be infected, with 19,200 new cases among 13- to 29-year-old adolescents and young adults in 2006. Eighty percent of new HIV infections among female population are acquired via heterosexual contact (20% by injection drug use). Males are more likely to acquire infection by male-to-male sexual contact (three quarters) with only 13% from heterosexual exposure.

Pathophysiology

HIV is a ribonucleic acid (RNA) retrovirus. After gaining entrance to the body, it binds to helper T lymphocytes, mono-

cytes, macrophages, dendritic and glial cells, and intestinal endothelial cells and enters the cell. There, viral RNA is transcribed to deoxyribonucleic acid (DNA) by reverse transcriptase and is incorporated into the host cell DNA. The viral DNA may remain dormant for long periods but can be stimulated at any time to transcribe itself into messenger RNA, which, in turn, leads to protein synthesis, assembly, and release of virus and virus particles. Abnormalities develop in both the cellular and humoral immune systems as HIV replication continues. Most circulating cells showing HIV infection are CD4 helper lymphocytes, and the number of circulating CD4 lymphocytes has been shown to be a useful marker of risk for opportunistic infection; early in childhood, this is not reliably the case. Children often have an abnormal polyclonal activation of B cells that can result in notable hypergammaglobulinemia; however, these children do not respond with appropriate antibodies to new antigens and often produce autoantibodies.

The likelihood of acquiring infection depends on the amount of infectious virus in the body fluid and the extent of contact with that body fluid. The risk of perinatal acquisition increases with increasing maternal viral load and decreased maternal immunity. Viral load will depend on many factors but most importantly the use of antiretroviral therapy. Untreated, infected infants often have high levels of viremia; this is also common very early and late during the course of infection among affected individuals.

Blood and genital secretions (seminal, vaginal) are the most likely media to transmit HIV. Other fluids such as saliva, urine, sweat, amniotic fluid, synovial fluid, feces, and tears contain no virus or only low levels of virus and are not important sources of virus transmission. The likelihood of HIV infection after a single exposure to an HIV-positive source has been estimated to be less than 1% for most exposures (Table 93.4). Breast-feeding is also associated with an increased risk of transmission of HIV to the infant. Therefore, in areas such as the United States where alternatives to breast-feeding are safe, HIV-infected women should be counseled not to breast-feed.

TABLE 93.4

APPROXIMATE RISK OF HUMAN IMMUNODEFICIENCY VIRUS ACQUISITION AFTER A SINGLE EXPOSURE LISTED BY SOURCE

Exposure	Risk of infection (per 10,000)
Transfusion with positive blood unit	950
Intravenous drug use	67
Percutaneous exposure (needlestick)	30
Receptive anal intercourse	50
Receptive penile-vaginal intercourse	10
Insertive anal intercourse	10
Insertive penile-vagnial intercourse	5
Receptive oral sex	1
Insertive oral sex	0.5

Detection of virus can now be accomplished in commercial laboratories by culture, quantitative HIV RNA and HIV DNA polymerase chain reaction (PCR) techniques, and antigen testing. Commercially available quantitative HIV RNA PCR techniques allow detection of viral RNA to levels as low as 50 copies per milliliter.

Clinical Manifestations

Initial Presentation of Children with HIV

Most perinatally infected infants develop symptoms progressively over time, and although lymphadenopathy, hepatosplenomegaly, and failure to thrive are common clinical features, any organ system can be affected (Table 93.5). Many children show signs of abnormal humoral immune function such as recurrent or persistent bacterial infection. Children lack preexisting antibodies to bacterial pathogens at the time they are infected with the HIV virus, which makes them vulnerable to infection by these organisms. Some children show early defects in cellular immunity, exhibited by persistent candidiasis, chronic diarrhea, or opportunistic infections. Still others, especially with antiretroviral therapy, remain relatively asymptomatic for long periods (6% completely asymptomatic at 5 years).

Untreated, approximately 50% of infants infected perinatally will develop clinical signs or symptoms within the first 12 months of life. Among adolescents with acquired infection, the initial presentation may represent acute HIV infection. Within days to weeks of initial exposure to HIV, an acute syndrome occurs that almost always includes fever. Approximately 70% will have lymphadenopathy, pharyngitis, or a rash that can be a maculopapular (can involve palms and soles) or have mucocutaneous ulcerations. Almost 30% to 50% will experience myalgias, arthralgias, headache, nausea, vomiting, and/or diarrhea. Finally, 10% to 15% will have hepatosplenomegaly, weight loss, thrush, or neurologic signs or symptoms (e.g., meningoencephalitis or aseptic meningitis, peripheral neuropathy or radiculopathy, facial palsy, Guillain-Barré syndrome, brachial neuritis, cognitive impairment, or psychosis). During this acute phase, many patients also develop leukopenia and thrombocytopenia.

Although some patients with acute HIV infection will seek care, few are diagnosed with acute HIV unless a specific history of HIV exposure is given because of the common occurrence of these symptoms with other viruses. The diagnosis of acute HIV infection cannot be made with standard serologic tests [enzyme-linked immunosorbent assays (ELISAs) or Western blot] because these tests first become positive 3 to 4 weeks after acute infection. Early detection, when indicated, is possible through the use of plasma HIV RNA testing but should be confirmed within 2 to 4 months after the initial testing by ELISA and Western blot serology. Follow-up testing and counseling should be arranged.

Fever

Background. The evaluation of the HIV-infected child with fever requires a careful history, thorough physical examination, and often, laboratory testing. Fever in HIV-infected children can represent simple childhood viral infections, but because of the humoral immunodeficiency of these children, they also commonly suffer from acute bacterial infections. Otitis media, sinusitis, pneumonia, adenitis, bacteremia, and skin and soft-tissue infections are common. In addition, opportunistic infections must be considered. It is important to inquire about any previous opportunistic infection or the use of prophylactic medications for the prevention of *Pneumocystis jiroveci* pneumonia (PCP), Mycobacterium avium intracellulare (MAI), or cytomegalovirus (CMV), because these may be markers for poor immune function. Some adolescents or parents may be able to provide a recent CD4 count, but laboratory data that reflect the status of the immune system are frequently unavailable to the emergency physician.

The clinical appearance of the patient is the starting point for determining ED management (Fig. 93.3). Identification of a focal source, particularly in the well-appearing children, plays a key role in determining management.

Evaluation of the Well-appearing, Febrile, HIV-positive Child. The HIV-infected child who appears well and does not have an obvious source of infection presents a more difficult problem than the child with an obvious localized infection. The first step is to decide on an appropriate evaluation. Several studies have demonstrated that HIV-positive children have an increased incidence of bacteremia. They are also more susceptible to serious viral infections such as disseminated CMV. However, it appears that serious bacterial, viral, or opportunistic infections are relatively uncommon among well-appearing HIV-positive children who present to the ED with fever.

Whenever a child with HIV infection presents with high-grade fever (temperature higher than 39°C or 102.2°F), a complete blood cell count (CBC) with differential and blood culture is recommended. If the child is still in diapers, a urine sample should be obtained for analysis and culture. Older children who are toilet-trained usually complain of dysuria or frequency if they have a urinary tract infection. If the child has any respiratory signs or symptoms, including isolated tachypnea, or if the CBC has an elevated leukocyte count with a shift to left, regardless of the presence of respiratory signs, pulse oximetry and a chest radiograph should be ordered. The WBC count is best evaluated in relation to baseline counts because many HIV-infected children have some degree of leukopenia. If it is known that the child is not leukopenic or the baseline is not available, a WBC count of 15,000 per mm^3 or more should be considered suggestive of bacterial infection. These patients may

---

TABLE 93.5

SIGNS AND SYMPTOMS OF HUMAN
IMMUNODEFICIENCY VIRUS INFECTION
IN CHILDREN

Lymphadenopathy	Recurrent fevers
Hepatomegaly	Splenomegaly
Failure to thrive	Chronic or recurrent diarrhea
Bacteremia	Wasting syndrome
Oral thrush	Developmental delay
Chronic or recurrent parotitis	Acquired microcephaly
Opportunistic infections	Spastic paresis

MEDICAL EMERGENCIES

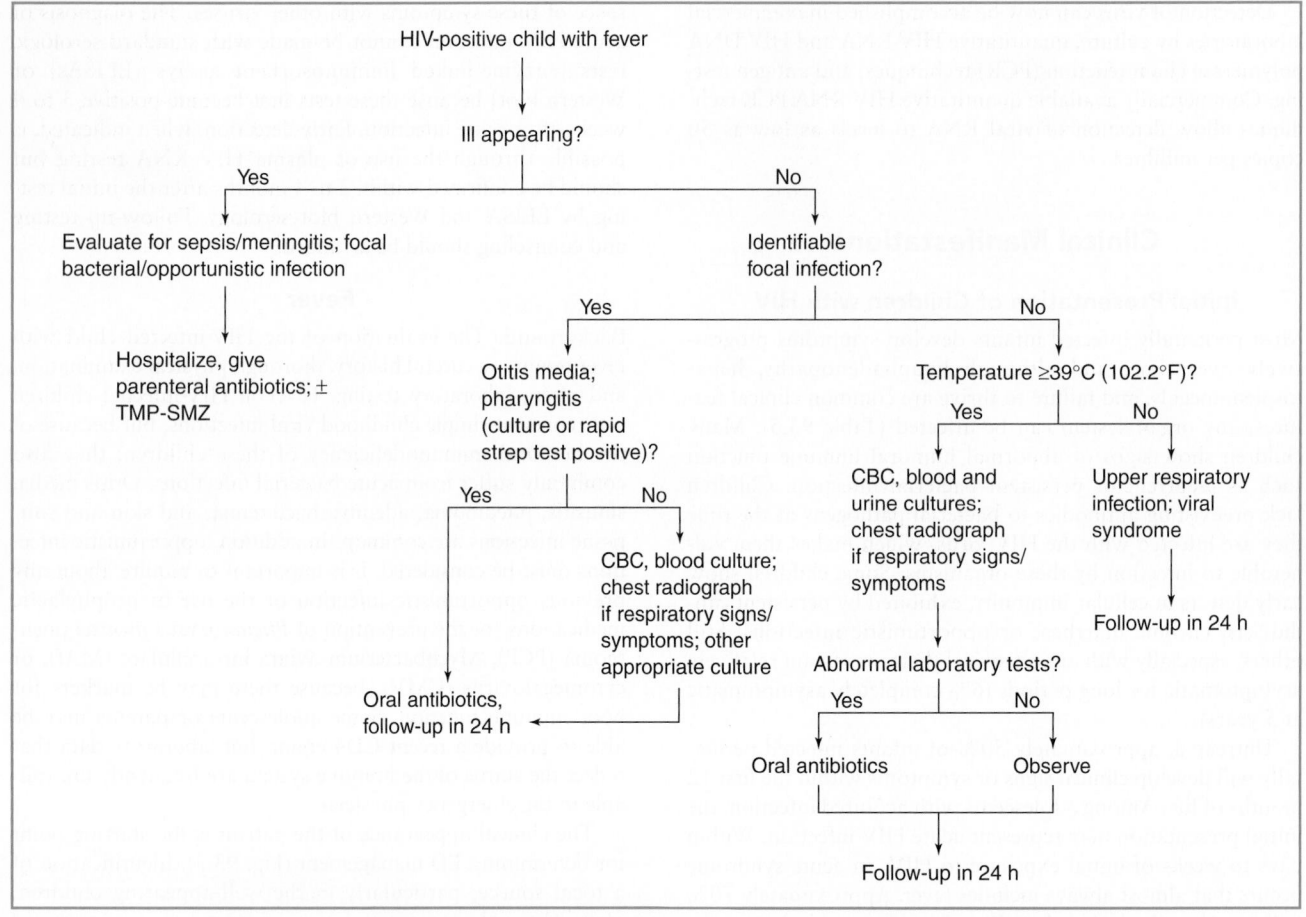

FIGURE 93.3 Evaluation of the HIV-positive child with fever. TMP-SMZ, trimethoprim–sulfamethoxazole; CBC, complete blood cell count. (Adapted from Dorfman D, Crain E, Bernstein L. Care of febrile children with HIV infection in the emergency department. *Pediatr Emerg Care* 1990;6:308.)

be started on empiric antibiotic treatment such as high-dose amoxicillin, amoxicillin-clavulanic acid (Augmentin®), or IM ceftriaxone (Rocephin®), pending the results of culture(s).

If the child appears well and the evaluation has not revealed a source for the fever that requires hospitalization, the child may be sent home (if the child's caregiver can be easily contacted and has the means to return if necessary) with instructions to return if symptoms worsen or if the patient develops lethargy or will not take adequate amounts of fluids. A follow-up evaluation by telephone or a revisit to the child's regular provider or the ED should be scheduled for the next day.

Evaluation of the Ill-appearing, Febrile, HIV-positive Child. HIV-positive patients with fever who appears ill should be treated like other ill-appearing, febrile children because they are likely to be infected with the same types of organisms that infect immunocompetent children. A lumbar puncture is indicated for those with meningismus, change in mental status, or an underlying abnormal mental status makes assessment difficult. If a child is believed to be so unstable that lumbar puncture is not safe, it can be delayed. In either case, the child should be started on parenteral broad-spectrum antimicrobials. Ceftriaxone (100 mg per kg per day divided every 12 hours) is an appropriate choice because it covers the organisms that most commonly cause sepsis in children. In young chil-

dren, because of the possibility of PCP presenting with fever and ill appearance, trimethoprim-sulfamethoxazole (TMP-SMZ) (5 mg per kg per dose of trimethoprim every 6 hours) should be considered if there are respiratory symptoms, with or without a positive chest radiograph. Treatment for suspected PCP should not be delayed because of fear of interfering with the diagnostic workup. Fungal infections, with the exception of oral thrush, are uncommon in HIV-infected children. However, candidal sepsis should be considered in hospitalized patients who do not improve with antibiotics.

Evaluation of the HIV-positive Child with Persistent Fever. Chronic fever is common in HIV-infected children. It can have many causes, and the evaluation of children with fever of unknown origin is often difficult and not always revealing. The major focus of such an evaluation in the ED is to rule out acute bacterial infection. A careful history and physical examination should be followed by a CBC, urinalysis, chest and sinus films, and blood, urine, and stool cultures. Recurrent otitis media is commonly seen, and some children may have recurrent parotitis or sinusitis. If no source is recognized on examination and the initial testing is negative, more unusual infections need to be considered. Tuberculosis, although common among HIV-infected adults, is uncommon in children but may be more likely among adolescents. MAI may cause chronic fevers in HIV-infected children. This pathogen is often associated with anemia secondary to bone marrow infiltration and can be cultured from blood, stool, and bone marrow. Numerous viruses can cause chronic infections associated with fever in these children. Epstein-Barr virus (EBV) and CMV are among the more common, with CMV often presenting with chronic hepatitis and bloody diarrhea. It may also cause pneumonia and retinitis. A blood buffy coat specimen can be sent for quantitative CMV-antigen detection. Most HIV-positive children with fever of unknown origin are hospitalized to facilitate the diagnostic process. The possibility of drug fever must also be considered.

Soft-tissue Infections

Clinical Manifestations. Cervical adenitis and cellulitis are common and may be accompanied by fever. Both cervical adenitis and cellulitis may be secondary to alterations in the child's immune status or may occur on a mechanical basis as a secondary infection of already-enlarged lymph nodes (in the case of cervical adenitis) or disruption of the normal skin by other lesions such as condylomata, molluscum, or vesicular and follicular eruptions. Acute bacterial adenitis in these patients is usually caused by *Staphylococcus aureus* or group A streptococci. *Bartonella*, the agent of cat-scratch disease, which can also cause bacillary angiomatosis and trench fever in these patients, should be considered.

Parotitis is a common soft-tissue infection that occurs in HIV-positive children who can have chronic enlargement of the parotid glands secondary to lymphocytic infiltration (Fig. 93.4). In these children, the parotid glands are enlarged and firm but nontender, and the overlying skin is not erythematous. With acute suppurative parotitis, these children develop fever, tenderness over the parotid, and purulent drainage from Stenson's duct. *S. aureus* is the most likely offending organism.

Management. If the child appears well and the infection is well circumscribed and does not impinge on a critical structure

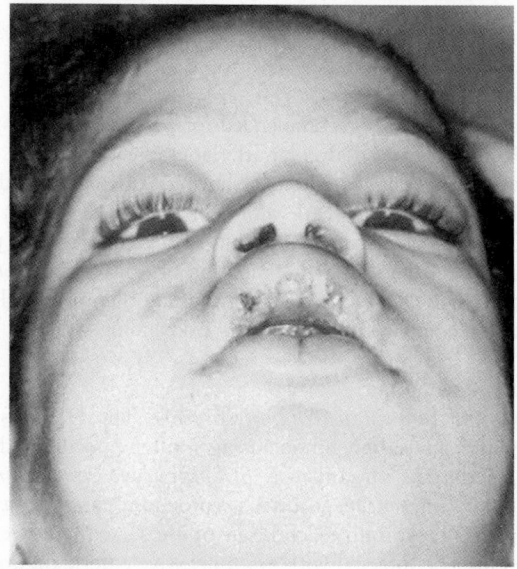

FIGURE 93.4 Chronic parotitis in an HIV-positive child. (Courtesy of Dr. A. Rubenstein.)

such as the airway, outpatient antibiotic therapy active against *S. aureus* and *Streptococcus pyogenes* (e.g., cephalexin 60 to 80 mg per kg per day, divided four times daily) is appropriate as long as it appears that the caregiver can adhere to the regimen and the child can be reevaluated within 24 to 48 hours. Coverage for community acquired methicillin resistant *S. aureus* may be warranted if the prevalence in the community is higher than 10% to 20%. In most cases, a blood culture should be obtained, particularly if the child has fever, has a history of an opportunistic infection, or does not appear well. In addition, the need for drainage of an infected lymph node (needle aspiration or surgical) must be considered. Children who are sent home must have close outpatient follow-up.

Pulmonary Manifestations

Just as respiratory complaints are common among immunocompetent children, so are respiratory conditions in patients and children with HIV infection. They deserve special attention, however, because they are the most common cause of mortality in these patients. Documentation of oxygenation by pulse oximetry or arterial blood gas, blood culture for bacterial pathogens, nasopharyngeal specimens for rapid viral diagnosis, and viral culture should all be considered in any HIV-positive patient with respiratory symptoms (Fig. 93.5). Chest radiographs should be obtained and can be helpful in determining the cause (Fig. 93.6). Decisions regarding sputum induction or bronchoscopy do not usually need to be made in the ED.

Pneumocystis jiroveci Pneumonia (formerly *Pneumocystis carinii* pneumonia)
Background. PCP is the most common serious opportunistic infection in HIV-infected children. Although PCP can occur at any age, in children, it develops most often between the ages of 2 and 8 months and may be the first presentation of HIV infection. Moreover, the first episode is often acute in onset and may be fatal.

For the most part, the results of immunologic studies are not available to the emergency physician. However, particularly relevant differences between adults and children should be noted in case the CD4 lymphocyte counts are known. Among adults, absolute CD4 lymphocyte counts are associated with the risk of acquiring PCP. In young children, CD4 counts cannot be used to exclude the risk of PCP. For indications for PCP prophylaxis (and prophylaxis of other infections complicating HIV), see Table 93.6.

Clinical manifestations. PCP presents as an acute or subacute illness. The infant or child typically is febrile, with marked tachypnea, wheezing, rhonchi, and diminished breath sounds. Rales are not usually part of the PCP picture, and cough may be absent. When coughing is present, it is typically dry and nonproductive. Over hours to days, the patient develops hypoxia and increased respiratory distress.

Management. When PCP is suspected, the physician should intervene to maintain the airway as necessary, obtain an arterial blood gas or room air pulse oximetry, and provide supplemental oxygen. A chest radiograph and a serum lactate dehydrogenase (LDH) evaluations should be ordered. The patient typically has a high (greater than 30 mm Hg) alveolar-arterial oxygen gradient and low oxygen saturation, and generally

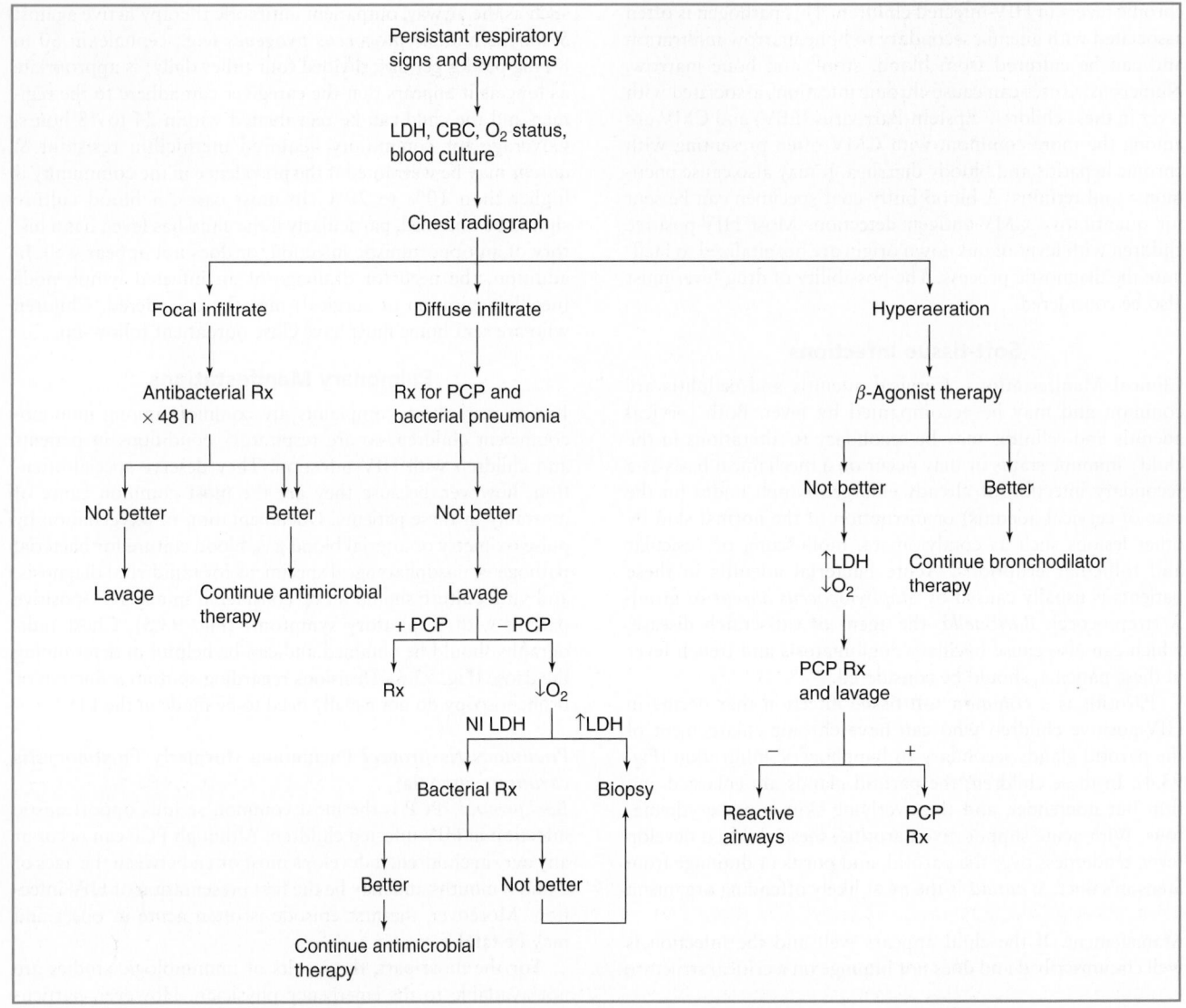

FIGURE 93.5 Evaluation of persistent respiratory signs and symptoms. LDH, lactate dehydrogenase; CBC, complete blood cell count; Rx, treatment; PCP, *Pneumocystis jiroveci* pneumonia. (Modified from Cunningham SJ, Crain EF, Bernstein LJ. Evaluations of the HIV-infected child with pulmonary signs and symptoms. *Pediatr Emerg Care* 1991;7:32–37.)

shows a marked (greater than 500 IU) elevation of the serum LDH. Radiographic findings typically consist of a diffuse interstitial ("ground glass") pattern, but infants may develop patchy infiltrates or complete opacification of the lung fields. Occasionally, however, the lung fields may be clear with hyperinflation suggestive of bronchiolitis, and in 5% to 10% of patients with PCP, the chest radiograph appears normal.

It is often difficult to make the diagnosis of PCP in the ED. If PCP is suspected on the basis of the history, physical examination, or the results of the laboratory investigation, it is appropriate to start IV TMP-SMZ at a dosage of 20 mg per kg per day of TMP divided every six hours. The child should be hospitalized for close observation and further evaluation as needed. In general, patients with PCP do not respond rapidly to antibiotic therapy. Patients intolerant of TMP-SMZ can be treated with pentamidine (4 mg per kg per day as a single daily dose) or atovaquone, but these should be considered second-line agents. Corticosteroid therapy in children with severe PCP improves sur-

vival and is generally recommended for patients with PaO$_2$ less than 70 mm Hg or an alveolar-arterial gradient of greater than 35 mm Hg. Patients suspected of having PCP should undergo bronchoalveolar lavage (BAL) although an induced sputum may be sufficient in older patients. Results of BAL may remain positive for 3 to 4 days after the initiation of TMP-SMZ therapy. Therefore, if PCP is suspected, appropriate therapy should be started immediately and not be withheld pending lavage.

Bacterial Pneumonia
Background and clinical manifestations. The HIV-positive child with bacterial pneumonia is most often infected with the usual pediatric organisms: *Streptococcus pneumoniae, Hemophilus influenzae,* group A streptococcus, and *Moraxella catarrhalis.* Hospitalized children or those with indwelling devices may be infected with gram-negative enteric organisms or *S. aureus.* In addition, these children often present with coinfection by respiratory viruses.

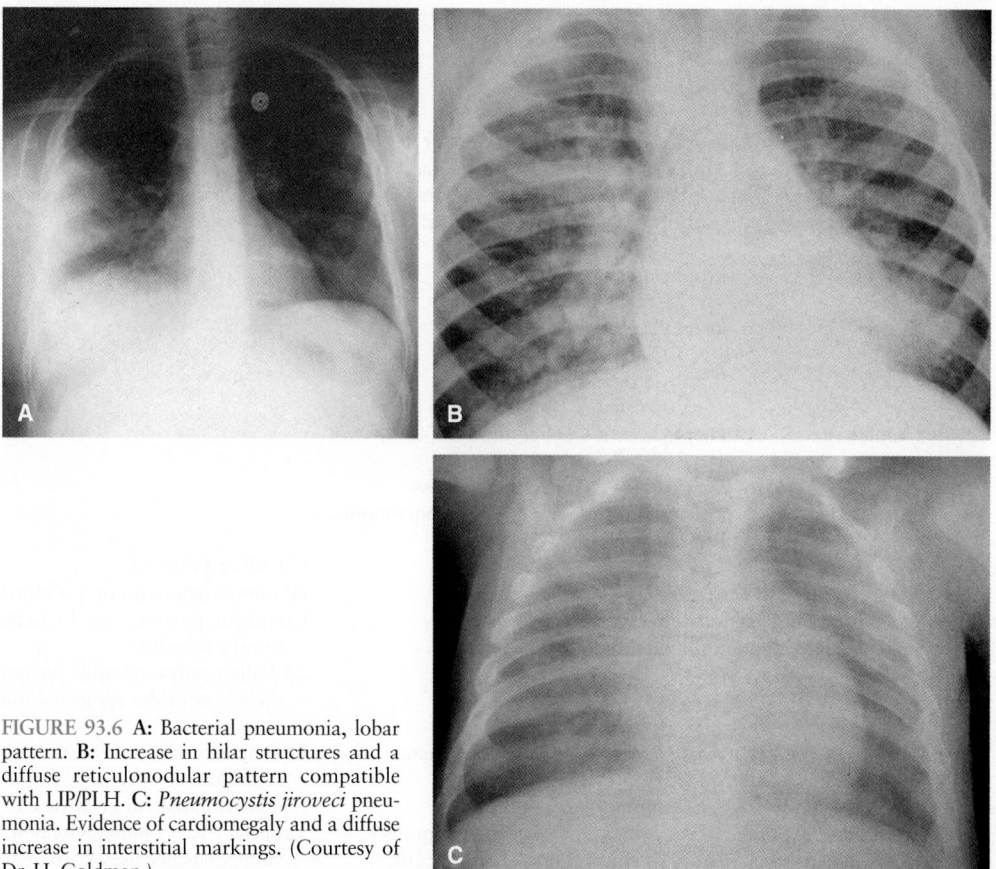

FIGURE 93.6 **A:** Bacterial pneumonia, lobar pattern. **B:** Increase in hilar structures and a diffuse reticulonodular pattern compatible with LIP/PLH. **C:** *Pneumocystis jiroveci* pneumonia. Evidence of cardiomegaly and a diffuse increase in interstitial markings. (Courtesy of Dr. H. Goldman.)

Management. A chest radiograph should be part of the evaluation of the HIV-positive child with fever of unknown origin or with respiratory signs or symptoms. The radiograph can help distinguish bacterial pneumonia (Fig. 93.6) from PCP or pulmonary lymphoid hyperplasia, and in fact, a chest radiograph compatible with bacterial pneumonia in an otherwise well-appearing child suggests that outpatient therapy may be possible if other criteria are met (Table 93.7).

The chest radiograph in bacterial pneumonia typically reveals a lobar or segmental infiltrate, and the peripheral WBC count is often more than 20,000 per mm³. However, because many of these children are leukopenic when not infected, it may be difficult in the ED to determine what constitutes leukocytosis. For example, a child whose normal WBC count is 2,000 per mm³ may mount a WBC of 8,000 to 10,000 per mm³ in response to a bacterial infection, but this would go unnoticed without knowledge of the child's baseline. Because it is rare to be confident that pneumonia is not bacterial in origin, children with pulmonary signs and symptoms, especially associated with fever, are commonly given antimicrobial therapy against the common respiratory pathogens.

Other Pulmonary Infections. Other infections associated with respiratory signs and symptoms in HIV-positive children include viral illnesses, particularly, CMV pneumonia, *Mycobacterium tuberculosis*, and MAI. Except for *M. tuberculosis*, which is surprisingly rare in HIV-infected children as compared with adults, there has been little documentation of

the frequency of the other infections. Adults and some children with environmental exposures have also had problems with coccidioidomycosis, blastomycosis, and histoplasmosis.

Wheezing.

Background and clinical manifestations. Reactive airway disease is the most likely diagnosis in an HIV-positive child with wheezing, with or without fever. If the wheezing is associated with rales, however, the physician needs to consider the possibility of PCP, lymphoid interstitial pneumonitis (LIP), acute pneumonia, or congestive heart failure. Congestive heart failure is rarely a presenting sign of HIV infection; instead, HIV-positive children with cardiomyopathy can develop congestive heart failure when under additional stress caused by an infection or fever. Physical examination may reveal the constellation of tachycardia, tachypnea, rales, and a palpable liver. However, these findings commonly occur in HIV-positive children without congestive heart failure.

Management. After a rapid but thorough physical examination to evaluate the degree of wheezing and air movement, the presence and location of retractions, and any other focus for fever, note whether the child responds to bronchodilator therapy. If so, reactive airway disease is the likely diagnosis, and the child can be treated accordingly. Pulse oximetry should be performed before the patient is discharged. Steroid therapy should be used as it would for an immunocompetent child with the same clinical findings.

MEDICAL EMERGENCIES

TABLE 93.6

PROPHYLAXIS OF INFECTIONS IN HUMAN IMMUNODEFICIENCY VIRUS (HIV)-INFECTED PATIENTS[a]

Pathogen	Indication	Treatment
Pneumocystis jiroveci	Birth–4 wk — No prophylaxis	
	4–6 wk to 12 mo — Prophylaxis is recommended for all HIV-infected infants, as well as all HIV-exposed infants in the first year of life, until HIV infection can be reasonably excluded	Trimethoprim-sulfamethoxazole (TMP-SMZ) with secondary choices of dapsone, atovaquone, or pentamidine (aerosolized or IV)
	1–2 yr — Prophylaxis if CD4 count <750 cells/μL or <15%	
	2–5 yr — Prophylaxis if CD4 count <500 cells/μL or <15%	
	≥6 yr — Prophylaxis if CD4 count <200 cells/μL or <15%	
	Adult — Prophylaxis if CD4 count <200 cells/μL or <14%, or history of AIDS defining illness	
	Any age — Previous episode of *P. jiroveci* pneumonia Rapidly declining CD4 count	
Bacterial infections	Neutropenia	G-CSF or GM-CSF
	Recurrent invasive bacterial infections	IV immunoglobulin or antibiotic prophylaxis
Streptococcus pneumoniae	All patients unless already received vaccine as per schedule with good immune function at the time	Conjugate pneumococcal vaccine as per routine schedule
	>2 yr	23-Valent polysaccharide pneumococcal vaccine consider revaccination at 5-yr intervals
Influenza	>6 mo of age, on a yearly basis before influenza season (generally recommended)	Influenza vaccine, alternative rimantidine or amantadine
Varicella zoster virus (VZV)	Age >12 mo with good immunity	Live-attenuated varicella vaccine
	Significant exposure to varicella and no primary immunity (no documented history of chicken pox or shingles or, if available, negative VZV antibody)	Varicella zoster immunoglobulin; if within 96 hr, consider use of attenuated vaccine, consider preemptive acyclovir
Mycobacterium avium complex (MAC)	<1 yr: CD4 count <750 cells/μL 1–2 yr: CD4 count <500 cells/μL 2–6 yr: CD4 count <75 cells/μL ≥6 yr: CD4 count <50 cells/μL Any age: previous MAC disease	Clarithromycin, azithromycin, or rifabutin
Mycobacterium tuberculosis	Positive diagnostic test for latent tuberculosis (TB) infection without treatment or contact with case of active TB or history of inadequately treated TB	Recommendation varies according to likely antibiotic susceptibility
Herpes simplex	Very frequent or severe recurrences	Acyclovir, famciclovir, or valganciclovir
Candida	Frequent or severe recurrences; generally can discontinue when CD4+ count >200 cells/μL	Topical—nystatin, clotrimazole Oral—fluconazole, ketoconazole, itraconazole
Toxoplasma gondii	Positive IgG antibody to *Toxoplasma* and CD4 count <100 cells/μL	Primary prophylaxis—TMP-SMZ, dapsone with pyrimethamine, or atovaquone ± pyrimethamine
	Prior toxoplasmic encephalitis	Pyrimethamine plus sulfadiazine plus leucovorin, or pyrimethamine plus leukovorin
Cryptococcus neoformans	Documented cryptococcal disease; May discontinue if CD4+ >200 cells/μL for > 6 mo in response to antitretroviral therapy	Fluconazole or itraconazole
Coccidiodis immitis	Documented coccidiodal disease; or CD4+ count <250 cells/μL and Positive IgM or IgG serologic test	Fluconazole or itraconazole
Histoplasma capsulatum	Documented disease or live in highly endemic area and CD4 count <150 cells/μL	Itraconazole
Human papillomavirus (HPV)	Women aged 15–26 yr	HPV quadravalent vaccine
Hepatitis A	>2 yr old and high risk for exposure or chronic liver disease (e.g., hepatitis b or c)	Hepatitis A vaccine ×2
Hepatitis B	All susceptible patients	Hepatitis B vaccine ×3

Criteria for discontinuing prophylaxis among patients with immune reconstitution on antiretroviral therapy are not presented.

IV, intravenous; G-CSF, granulocyte colony-stimulating factor; GM-CSF, granulocyte-macrophage colony-stimulating factor.

[a]It is assumed that patients will receive routine hepatitis B, diphtheria, pertussis, tetanus, haemophilus influenzae type b, polio, measles, mumps, and rubella vaccinations but have not yet received varicella vaccination.

Modified from CDC guidelines. *MMWR Morbid Mortal Wkly Rep* 51 (RR-8):1–60.

TABLE 93.7

GENERAL GUIDELINES FOR ELECTING OUTPATIENT THERAPY OF HUMAN IMMUNODEFICIENCY VIRUS-POSITIVE CHILDREN WITH PNEUMONIA

Age >6 mo
Able to tolerate oral fluids and medication
Absence of signs of respiratory distress (e.g., flaring or retractions)
Respiratory rate
   <45 Respirations/min if age <2 yr
   <30 Respirations/min if age >2 yr
Oxygen saturation ≥93%
Has not already worsened while receiving oral antibiotic
Close clinical follow-up available and patient able to return
Pneumocystis jiroveci pneumonia should be considered unlikely

If the child has a high fever [temperature higher than 39°C (102.2°F)], a chest radiograph should be obtained to look for an infiltrate or evidence of PCP or congestive heart failure. The febrile child with wheezing and rales or evidence of pneumonia on chest radiograph who otherwise appears well enough for outpatient therapy may be given oral amoxicillin (80 to 100 mg per kg per day) or IM ceftriaxone (50 mg per kg) in addition to bronchodilator therapy.

Children with clinical or radiographic evidence of PCP or congestive heart failure should be hospitalized. A first dose of IV TMP-SMZ should be given to infants suspected of having PCP, and congestive heart failure should be treated with afterload reducers and diuretics in addition to bronchodilators (see Chapter 84).

Lymphocytic Interstitial Pneumonitis

Background. LIP or pulmonary lymphoid hyperplasia is common among pediatric HIV-infected patients with pulmonary disease. It is believed to be an infiltrative lymphoproliferative disorder associated with HIV, EBP, and HTLV type 1 infections.

Clinical manifestations. LIP is an insidious condition that causes a slowly progressive hypoxia typically in children who are older than 1 year. Most children present to the ED with chronic cough, mild tachypnea, marked lymphadenopathy, and may have intermittent rales, occasional wheezing, and marked hypoxia and clubbing of the digits. Definitive diagnosis requires bronchoscopy with transbronchial biopsy or open lung biopsy.

Management. Rarely is intervention required to maintain the airway in children with LIP. Most HIV-positive children with a cough should undergo chest radiography. Chest radiography commonly reveals an interstitial nodular pattern that can be diagnostic. Occasionally, bronchiectasis develops, and these children may become superinfected with bacterial or viral pathogens and have fever. Fever is an important differentiating point in the management of HIV-positive children believed to have LIP. Therapy may be with highly active antiretroviral therapy (HAART), but in acute respiratory compromise, empiric corticosteroid therapy may be warranted. If the PaO$_2$ is less than 65 mm Hg, LIP is treated with 1 to 2 mg per kg per day of prednisone to a maximum of 60 mg for 2 to 4 weeks and subsequently tapered as necessary to maintain the PaO$_2$ above 70 mm Hg. If the patient is febrile, tuberculosis or MAI must be ruled out before beginning steroid therapy.

Gastrointestinal Manifestations

Chronic or recurrent oral thrush or esophageal candidiasis are common and can be treated with nystatin, clotrimazole, or fluconazole.

Diarrhea

Background. The gastrointestinal tract generally shows only subtle changes in histology in HIV infection unless there are secondary infections. In addition to the common causes of diarrhea that affect immunocompetent children, HIV-positive children are prone to parasitic (*Giardia*, *Microsporidium*, *Cryptosporidium*), chronic viral (CMV), mycobacterial, and serious bacterial infections of the gastrointestinal tract (Table 93.8). Malnutrition is a common problem in HIV infection and, in children, requires careful monitoring of growth parameters.

Clinical Manifestations and Management. The general evaluation of the child with diarrhea is described in Chapter 18. Because diarrhea has many potential etiologies in HIV-infected children, the physician should seek to identify the cause. A stool test for blood, a stool smear for polymorphonuclear leukocytes, and a stool culture (for *Salmonella*, *Shigella*, *Yersinia*, *Campylobacter*, *Escherichia coli*) should be obtained, with consideration given to sending stool for parasites and *Clostridium difficile* toxin. The child who is afebrile, appears to be well hydrated, and has no blood or leukocytes in the stool can be treated symptomatically with dietary management and close follow-up. If the child attends a day care program and is still in diapers, the parents/guardians should be instructed to keep the child home until the illness has resolved and the culture is tested negative.

In febrile children with gastroenteritis, although viral causes are still most common, *Salmonella* is the primary bacterial pathogen of concern and is a major cause of bacteremia in HIV-positive children. If there is blood or more than five leukocytes per high-power field on examination of the stool smear but the child has normal vital signs and looks well, he or she should be treated with TMP-SMZ and reevaluated the next day. Oral ampicillin is an alternative drug, but in many

TABLE 93.8

ORGANISMS ASSOCIATED WITH ACUTE DIARRHEA IN HUMAN IMMUNODEFICIENCY VIRUS-POSITIVE CHILDREN

Viral agents	*Shigella*
Rotavirus	*Escherichia coli*
Adenovirus	*Clostridium difficile*
Norwalk agent	*Giardia lamblia*
Cytomegalovirus	*Cryptosporidium*
Salmonella species	*Isospora*
Yersinia enterocolitica	*Microsporidia*
Campylobacter	

areas, 20% to 30% of *Salmonella* species are resistant to ampicillin. The child who appears dehydrated or ill should be admitted for IV hydration and parenteral antibiotic therapy.

If the patient remains symptomatic in the face of a negative stool culture and dietary management, a total of at least three stool specimens should be sent for ova and parasite evaluation and two samples tested for *C. difficile* toxin. If no cause is identified, endoscopy or colonoscopy should be considered, depending on the severity of symptoms.

Hematologic Manifestations

Hematologic abnormalities are common and can be the result of HIV infection itself (occurring early or late in the illness) or secondary to concomitant infections (mycobacteria, CMV, parvovirus B19, fungal infections), lymphoma, or medication toxicities. Anemia redominates, especially with zidovudine therapy; erythropoietin levels may be low, identifying patients likely to benefit from erythropoietin therapy. Nutritional deficiencies are frequent and may also contribute to the anemia. Neutropenia is common and may be accentuated by medications (e.g., zidovudine, ganciclovir, TMP-SMZ) but is generally mild. If necessary, granulocyte colony-stimulating factor or granulocyte—macrophage colony-stimulating factor can be given with improvement of the neutropenia. Thrombocytopenia is a typical part of the acute HIV infection and can persist or worsen over time. Improvement is often seen with antiviral therapy. If the thrombocytopenia is severe, it can generally be managed along the same lines as for non–HIV-infected patient with idiopathic thrombocytopenia (steroids, Rhogam®, or gamma globulin) (see Chapter 91).

Rash

Background and Clinical Manifestations. Of all the categories of dermatologic manifestations of HIV infection in children, seborrheic dermatitis and infections are by far the most common. Neoplasms with skin manifestations such as Kaposi's sarcoma are not often seen in children. Measles can be particularly severe in HIV-positive children. This illness may be associated with the characteristic clinical signs and symptoms of generalized rash, coryza, conjunctivitis, cough, and Koplik's spots, or it may occur without the typical rash. The HIV-infected child with measles must be evaluated carefully for signs of dehydration and respiratory distress. If the child is taking liquids well and breathing comfortably, he or she may be sent home with careful instructions to return for reevaluation if status worsens. All HIV-positive children who have been exposed to measles should receive gamma globulin (0.5 mL per kg with maximum of 15 mL given intramuscularly), regardless of whether they have been vaccinated against measles.

Varicella can also cause severe illness in the immunocompromised host. Varicella zoster immunoglobulin should be given to HIV-infected children after exposure to chicken pox (1 vial containing 125 units for each 10 kg of body weight with any opened vial used completely, maximal dose is five vials). Once clinical illness has started, these children should initially be treated with IV acyclovir (10 mg per kg every 8 hours). Children with local single dermatome zoster infection may be treated with oral acyclovir (20 mg per kg per dose given every 6 hours). These children must be followed closely to ensure the infection does not disseminate.

More than 10% of children infected with HIV will have thrombocytopenia associated with high levels of circulating immune complexes and antiplatelet antibodies that may manifest as petechiae or easy bruising. Patients with platelet count more than 50,000 per mm^3 should be considered for admission and treatment. Febrile or toxic-appearing HIV-positive children with petechiae must be considered to have septicemia (see Chapter 92). After a rapid assessment of the airway, breathing, and circulation, these patients should undergo a full evaluation for sepsis, including lumbar puncture, and they should receive parenteral antibiotics pending culture results.

Syphilis screening should be performed for any HIV-infected child whose syphilis serology at birth is unknown because women with HIV have a high rate of coinfection with syphilis.

Molluscum contagiosum is a viral infection of the skin that presents as single or grouped small, firm, skin-colored papules. The appearance of these papules over scattered areas of the body is common among immunocompromised patients. Finally, medication-related adverse reactions including rashes are common among HIV patients as well (Table 93.9).

Neurologic Manifestations

Background. Once transmitted to the central nervous system (CNS), a neurotropic HIV strain emerges. In the early 1980s, a progressive dementia was reported in adults with AIDS. A syndrome analogous to the adult AIDS dementia complex was described in HIV-infected children in 1985 and was called *AIDS encephalopathy*. As it turns out, AIDS encephalopathy is common and does not require other manifestations of full-blown AIDS. Untreated, a large proportion of children with HIV infection will have neurologic involvement, and the possibility of HIV infection should be considered in the differential diagnosis of developmental delay or loss of milestones. With treatment, the proportion with neurologic involvement decreases substantially to about 20%.

HIV-infected children are at increased risk of meningitis (including cryptococcal, although less commonly than in adults, and tuberculous meningitis), encephalitis (including that caused by *Toxoplasma*), stroke and cerebral infarcts, progressive multifocal leukoencephalopathy (caused by human polyomavirus JC), and a variety of vasculopathies.

Clinical Manifestations. Children with AIDS encephalopathy exhibit developmental delay or developmental regression, acquired microcephaly, and pyramidal tract signs. Although growth and development are often affected by any serious illness in a child, AIDS encephalopathy may occur in patients with no signs of opportunistic infections and few signs of immunodeficiency. It may manifest itself as a static, progressive, or indolent encephalopathy with periods of plateaus in cognitive and motor development. Static encephalopathy is defined by the presence of nonprogressive cognitive or motor deficits. Progressive encephalopathy usually begins within 2 months to 5 years after initial exposure to HIV. It is characterized initially by deterioration of play and progressive apathy. Developmental delay ensues, with loss of developmental milestones, including deficits in socially adaptive language and in fine and gross motor skills. As the condition progresses, there may be spastic diplegia and quadriparesis. Patients develop extrapyramidal and cerebellar signs, including rigidity,

TABLE 93.9

ADVERSE EFFECTS OF DRUGS USED IN TREATING HUMAN IMMUNODEFICIENCY VIRUS, PREVENTING OPPORTUNISTIC INFECTIONS, OR IN TREATING COMMONLY ACQUIRED INFECTIONS[a]

Adverse effect—drug(s)

Bone marrow suppression—amphotericin B, cidofovir, dapsone, enfuvirtide, foscarnet, flucytosine, ganciclovir, hydroxyurea, interferon alpha, linezolid, peginterferon alpha pyrimethamine, rifabutin, ribavirin, sulfadiazine, trimethoprim-sulfamethoxazole, trimetrexate, valganciclovir, zidovudine

Diarrhea—atovaquone, didanosine, clindamycin, nelfinavir, ritonavir, lopinavir/ritonavir, tenofovir

Hepatotoxicity—atovaquone, azitrhomycin, clarithromycin, fluconazole, isoniazid, itraconazole, ketoconazole, pyrazinamide, rifabutin, rifampin, trimethoprim-sulfamethoxazole, voriconazole, most antiretrovirals; hepatic failure can be seen with nevirapine.

Nephrotoxicity—acyclovir, adefovir, amphotericin B, cidofovir, foscarnet, indinavir, pentamidine, tenofovir

Ocular effects—didanosine, cidofovir, ethambutol, rifabutin, voriconazole

Pancreatitis—didanosine, lamivudine, pentamidine, ritonavir, stavudine, trimethoprim-sulfamethoxazole, zalcitabine

Peripheral neuropathy—didanosine, isoniazid, linezolid, stavudine, zalcitabine

Neurotoxicity—high-dose acyclovir, quinolones

Skin rash—abacavir, amprenavir, atovaquone, dapsone, delavirdine, efavirenz, nevirapine, primaquine, pyrimethamine, ribavirin, sulfadiazine, trimethoprim-sulfamethoxazole, voriconazole

[a]Adapted from *2001 USPHS/IDSA guidelines for the prevention of opportunistic infections in persons infected with human immunodeficiency virus and the guidelines for the use of antiretroviral agents in HIV-1-infected adults and adolescents.* For more related information see *Guidelines for the Use of Antiretroviral Agents in HIV-1-Infected Adults and Adolescents.* http://aidsinfo.nih.gov/guidelines.

dystonic posturing, and ataxia. Seizures, although uncommon, may occur.

Another group of children present with indolent encephalopathy. These patients experience variable plateaus in their development during which there is little or no further cognitive growth. Either new milestones are not obtained or the rate of acquisition of new skills deviates from the norm and the child's initial rate of developmental progress. Many of these children may go on to develop the progressive form of AIDS encephalopathy.

Physical examination of the patient with AIDS encephalopathy often reveals microcephaly. Younger children will be hypotonic with persistence of the Moro or tonic neck reflexes after 4 months of age. Older children may have symmetric ankle clonus and extensor plantar responses. As the condition progresses, pyramidal signs of varying severity, including a pure spastic quadriparesis with signs of pseudobulbar palsy, dysphagia, and dysarthria, are seen. Ataxia may be seen in children old enough to walk.

Management. The diagnosis of AIDS encephalopathy involves obtaining a history suggestive of developmental delay or regression in an HIV-infected child. Management is more complicated when these children come to the ED with fever because it may be difficult to evaluate their mental status. Commonly, a lumbar puncture is necessary to rule out bacterial meningitis, unless the physician can be confident on a clinical basis that the child is behaving at baseline and that the fever is not secondary to CNS infection.

Cancers

Cancers have been seen less frequently in children than in adults. The most common malignancies of children with AIDS are non-Hodgkin's lymphomas. The next most common are leiomyomas and leiomyosarcomas in the gastrointestinal tract. These are associated with EBV infection. Some other malignancies have also been linked to specific viral infections. Kaposi's sarcoma is associated with human herpes virus-8

infection, some peripheral lymphomas and most primary to the brain contain EBV, and anal cancers and cervical carcinomas are linked with human papilloma virus infections.

Management of HIV

Overview of Anti-HIV Medications

Many effective anti-HIV medications are now available. At present, these can be divided into several general classes.

Entry inhibitors such as enfuvirtide (Fuzeon®) or maraviroc (Selzentry®) work by blocking the entry of the HIV virus into human cells.

Nucleoside (and nucleotide) reverse transcriptase inhibitors are nucleoside (nucleotide) analogs that compete with the viral reverse transcriptase and include abacavir (Ziagen®), apricitabine (in trials), didanosine (Videx®, ddI), emtricitabine (Emtriva®, FTC®), lamivudine (Epivir®, 3TC®), stavudine (Zerit®, d4T), tenofovir DF (Viread®), zidovudine (Retrovir®, AZT, ZDV), and combinations of the above medications: Combivir® (lamivudine and zidovudine), Trizivir® (abacavir, lamivudine, and zidovudine), and Epzicom® (abacavir and lamivudine).

Nonnucleoside reverse transcriptase inhibitors also block the viral reverse transcriptase enzyme and include delavirdine (Rescriptor®), efavirenz (Sustiva®), and nevirapine (Viramune®).

Protease inhibitors block protease enzymes responsible for cleaving viral proteins into functional units. Medications in this class include atazanavir (Reyataz®), darunavir (Prezista®), fosamprenavir (Lexiva®), indinavir (Crixivan®), lopinavir/ritonavir (Kaletra®), nelfinavir (Viracept®), ritonavir (Norvir®), saquinavir (Fortavase®, Invirase®), and tipranavir (Aptivus®). Because of poor tolerability at full dose, ritonavir is predominantly used in low dose to reduce the metabolic clearance and thus increase the levels of another concurrently given protease inhibitor.

MEDICAL EMERGENCIES

Integrase inhibitors interfere with the ability of the integrase enzyme to insert the DNA, produced by reverse transcription of the virus RNA, into the human cell DNA. The first FDA-approved drug of this class is raltegravir (Intelence®) and trials are underway with a second in the class, elvitegravir.

Because HIV has the capacity to rapidly develop resistance to individual antiviral drugs, combination therapy using three to four agents has now become the treatment standard. As a result combinations of different classes of medications have been introduced to reduce the number of separate pills that must be taken simultaneously. Such medications include Atripla® (efavirenz, emtricitabine, and tenofovir) and Truvada® (emtricitabine and tenofovir).

Unfortunately, drug therapy does not eradicate infection. The efficacy of these antivirals in various tissues that may (i) harbor virus, (ii) be important in the spread of virus, or (iii) be important to symptomatology (e.g., lymph nodes, brain, testes, mucosal surfaces) is not always known. These drugs also commonly cause significant side effects and drug interactions that may bring patients to the ED for attention. These most often include rash, headache, nausea, diarrhea, pancreatitis, fatigue, anemia, granulocytopenia, peripheral neuropathy, renal stones, decreased absorption of other medications, and increased or decreased metabolism of other medications (Table 93.9). Significant advances have been made in drug therapy with the ability to monitor drug and quantitative viral levels in the clinical setting. In addition, these patients frequently require antimicrobials for treatment or prophylaxis against bacterial, fungal, mycobacterial, and viral infections, management of malignancies, neuropathic pain, and/or metabolic, hematologic, and endocrine derangements. All of these medications may result in important interactions or toxicities. The emergency physician must therefore also consider the patient's medications as a possible culprit for acute presentations in these patients.

Prevention of HIV Acquisition

Development of an effective and safe vaccine for the prevention of HIV is a high priority, but progress has been disappointing. Until such a vaccine is available, current strategies for postexposure prevention of HIV infection take advantage of the finding that it may take several hours after exposure (or possibly, in some cases, days) for HIV infection to become established. During this time, antiviral medications can be given to prevent the transmitted virus from causing an established infection. Prevention of perinatal acquisition through the use of anti-HIV medications during the last trimester of pregnancy and the first days or weeks of infancy has been successful in significantly reducing the risk of infection. The introduction of antiviral therapy has resulted in an impressive reduction in perinatally acquired HIV cases currently seen in the United States. Unfortunately, the cost of this treatment is prohibitive in the countries where 90% of HIV infections occur. The risks of acquisition from exposures to HIV are listed in Table 93.4.

Postexposure HIV Prophylaxis

Community Exposures: Consensual Sex and Needlesticks. Sexual contact is the most common means of transmitting HIV infection, and reducing exposure is the mainstay of public health efforts. Prophylaxis after sexual intercourse or sharing needles could potentially decrease transmission, although efficacy has not yet been demonstrated and is not likely to be practical where repeated exposure is likely. A patient with a significant exposure to HIV, such as receptive or penetrative anal or vaginal sex, receptive oral intercourse with ejaculation, or needle sharing involving a partner who is HIV positive or who is in a known risk group should be considered for PEP. The patient who has had an isolated high-risk episode of consensual sex with an individual known to have HIV in which safe sex practices were not followed (or failed, e.g., broken condom) should also be offered HIV prophylaxis and risk-reduction counseling.

Accidental community-acquired needlestick exposures also require attention. HIV has been detected and infectious virus has been recovered from syringes obtained from high-risk community sources. Most discarded syringes will not have any recoverable HIV, and if complete drying of the syringe has occurred, there will be no infectious HIV. Thus far, no report exists of transmission of HIV from a discarded syringe left in a public place. Therefore, the risk of transmission of HIV from an accidental needlestick from a needle/syringe found in a public place is likely very low. Prophylaxis should not be routinely recommended, but because the risk is not zero, careful discussion with the family should include the need for subsequent monitoring and testing of the patient. Voluntary sharing of needles among IV drug abusers would pose a substantially higher risk because immediate use of the needle would result in a greater likelihood of infectious virus being transmitted. A prophylaxis strategy in this situation would demand the patient discontinue ongoing exposures that carry a continued risk for acquiring HIV.

Health-care Worker Exposures. An increased risk for HIV infection after percutaneous or mucous membrane exposures to HIV-infected blood is associated with the quantity of blood, as indicated by visible contamination of the device with the patient's blood, its use directly in a vein or artery, or a deep injury to the health-care worker. It is likely to increase with a higher viral load in the patient's blood. Finally, the risk of acquiring HIV is decreased by an estimated 80% by the prompt postexposure use of effective antiretrovirals. Each health-care institution should have a system to evaluate their employees' occupational exposures and offer treatment. As of December 2002, the CDC was aware of 57 health-care workers who had documented seroconversion after occupational exposures and another 139 HIV-positive health-care workers who are likely to have acquired infection after an occupational exposure.

Sexual Assault

Evaluation of the victim of sexual assault is a multidisciplinary process and will involve medical, psychological, and legal issues (Table 93.10). Medical issues to consider include acute trauma care, postexposure pregnancy prophylaxis, and postexposure infection prophylaxis. The discussion that follows is limited to issues of infection prophylaxis. The most commonly acquired infections after sexual assault are chlamydia, gonorrhea, trichomoniasis, and bacterial vaginosis. Other less commonly acquired but important infections include HIV; hepatitis viruses A, B, and C; human papillomavirus condylomata

TABLE 93.10

ISSUES TO CONSIDER IN CASES OF SEXUAL ASSAULT

Medical
Obtain medical history
Evaluate and treat physical injuries: genital/nongenital (consider EUA)
Obtain cultures/serology/clinically indicated tests
   –Culture: gonorrhea, chlamydia (sites based on contact), others as indicated
   –Serology: RPR, HIV ELISA, hepatitis B surface antibody, hepatitis C antibody
   –Clinically indicated tests: pregnancy, hematocrit, toxicology screen
Treat preexisting infection
Offer postcoital contraception (Plan B or Ovral®) if postpubertal
Evaluate risk for transmission of STDs
Consider and offer postexposure prophylaxis to postpubertal patients for bacterial infections
   –Gonorrhea: ceftriaxone
   –Chlamydia: azithromycin
   –Bacterial vaginosis or *Trichomonas*: metronidazole (Flagyl®)
Consider antiviral prophylaxis
   –Hepatitis B: vaccine
Less commonly indicated (see text)
   –HIV: specific recommendations vary based patient age, local HIV resistance patterns and
    exposure risk for acquisition of infection but two or three drug regimens are typical.
Depending on injuries consider tetanus: vaccine ± tetanus immunoglobulin
Arrange medical follow-up within 1 wk if feasible
Provide and/or arrange counseling with very specific follow-up instructions
Recommend sexual abstinence until STD prophylaxis completed

Legal
Record events accurately
Document injuries; photo as indicated, clothes, semen, etc.
Collect forensic specimens
Preserve chain of evidence
Determine need to contact civil authorities (police, child protective services)

EUA, examination under anesthesia; STD, sexually transmitted disease; HIV, human immunodeficiency virus. See also: http://www.cdc.gov/std/treatment/ and http://www.aidsinfo.nih.gov/Guidelines/ under Guidelines > Nonoccupational Exposure Considerations, for the most up-to-date recommendations.

acuminata; syphilis; and herpes simplex. Finally, pubic lice, scabies, and sexually transmitted infections that are rare in developed countries will be seen occasionally or identified in follow-up. Depending on the form of the sexual assault and risk of acquiring infection, empiric PEP is generally discussed and offered. For patients without a contraindication, treatment with 1 g azithromycin for *C. trachomatis* prophylaxis, 125 mg IM ceftriaxone for gonorrhea prophylaxis, and 2 g metronidazole for bacterial vaginosis prophylaxis are offered. Hepatitis B vaccination with follow-up doses at 1 to 2 months and 4 to 6 months should be given if the victim has not previously been vaccinated and known to have an adequate response.

Generally, postexposure prophylaxis for HIV is not required but should be discussed in circumstances where the risk of transmission is high. The possibility of HIV transmission with such contacts should be discussed with the victim, the risk of transmission assessed, and PEP offered or recommended if appropriate. Risk increases with ejaculation without effective condom use, multiple assailants, injuries that involve blood, evidence to suggest illicit drug use on the part of the assailant(s), and/or threats or suggestions that the assailant(s) is HIV positive.

Treatment with antiretrovirals should be considered when the patient presents within 72 hours after a single event where there is exposure of vagina, rectum, mouth, or other mucous membrane with blood, semen, vaginal secretions, rectal secretions, breast milk, or any blood-contaminated fluid or percutaneous contact where bleeding is present. Exposures to urine, nasal secretions, saliva, sweat, or tears when not visibly blood-contaminated are not considered sufficient to warrant postexposure prophylaxis. The drug of choice will depend on local HIV susceptibility patterns and perhaps knowledge regarding the assailant, but as of this printing, the preferred regimens typically contain at least two and more often three drugs. Preferred regimens as per the CDC include: (i) Efavirenz® or Kaletra® (lopinavir/ritonavir); plus (ii) lamivudine or emtricitabine; plus (iii) zidovudine or tenofovir. An infectious diseases consultant can assist in drug selection. The decision regarding the use of postexposure prophylaxis for HIV should be made as early as possible, and discussion with the patient must include the limited data for efficacy and the potential toxicities and requirement for close outpatient follow-up.

When considered appropriate (Fig. 93.7), PEP should be instituted as quickly as possible after exposure. Most would limit PEP to exposures within 72 hours of exposure (preferably less than 24 hours). Patients receiving PEP should receive first doses of medication in the ED, if available, and need

MEDICAL EMERGENCIES

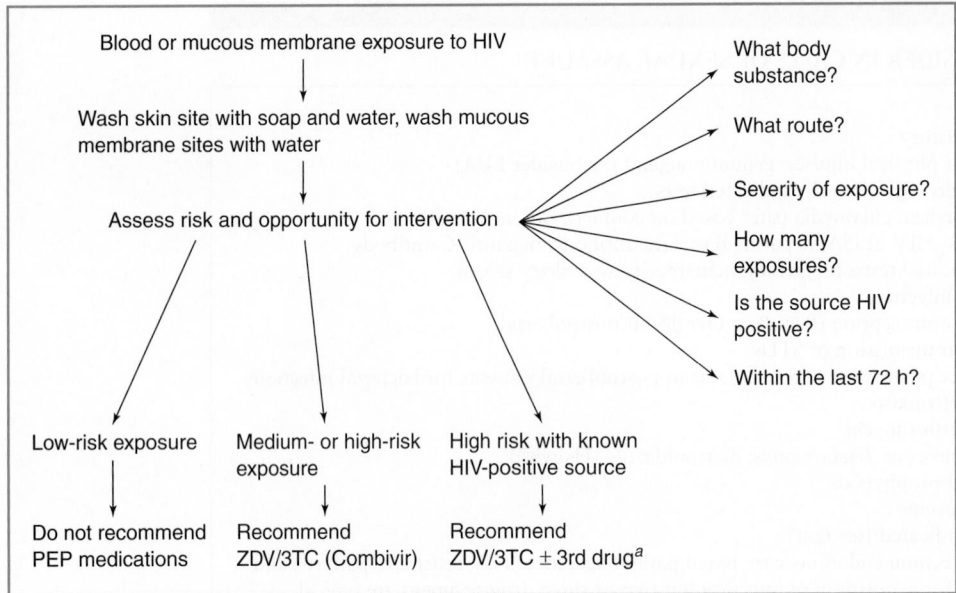

FIGURE 93.7 Postexposure prophylaxis (PEP) for possible community-acquired exposures to human immunodeficiency virus (HIV). When available, additional information regarding the source individual may alter recommendations. [a]3rd drug; commonly recommended: indinavir, nelfinavir, efavirenz or abacavir; other drugs only with expert consultation.

follow-up with clinicians knowledgeable about antiviral therapies and able to provide intensive emotional and behavioral counseling to help cope with the immediate event and to help them avoid situations likely to result in future exposure. Studies have demonstrated that compliance with these medications is poor. The antiviral medications, generally recommended to be taken for 4 weeks, can have significant side effects.

Suggested Readings

Sexually Transmitted Diseases

Ackerman AB, Goldfaden G, Cosmides JC. Acquired syphilis in early childhood. *Arch Dermatol* 1972;106:92–93.

Bell TA. Major sexually transmitted diseases of children and adolescents. *Pediatr Infect Dis* 1983;2:153–161.

Branch G, Paxton R. A study of gonococcal infection among infants and children. *Public Health Rep* 1965;80:347–352.

Centers for Disease Control and Prevention. Sexual assault and STDs. http://www.cdc.gov/std/treatment/2006/sexual-assault.htm.

Centers for Disease Control and Prevention. Sexually transmitted diseases: treatment guidelines. http://www.cdc.gov/std/treatment/.

Finelli L, Crayne EM, Spitalny KC. Treatment of infants with reactive syphilis serology, New Jersey: 1992 to 1996. *Pediatrics* 1998;102:E27.

Fleisher G, Hodge D, Cromie W. Penile edema in childhood gonorrhea. *Ann Emerg Med* 1980;9:314–315.

Hare M, Mowla A. Genital herpesvirus infection in a prepubertal girl. *Br J Obstet Gynaecol* 1977;84:141–142.

Henretig FM. Acute urinary retention secondary to severe gonococcal balanoblennorrhea. *Pediatrics* 1981;67:734–736.

Ingram DL, Everett VD, Flick LAR, et al. Vaginal gonococcal cultures in sexual abuse evaluations: evaluation of selective criteria for preteenaged girls. *Pediatrics* 1997;99:E8.

Kaplan KM, Fleisher GR, Paradise E, et al. Social relevance of genital Herpes simplex in children. *Am J Dis Child* 1984;138:872–874.

Mascola L, Pelosi R, Blount JH, et al. Congenital syphilis revisited. *Am J Dis Child* 1985;139:575–580.

Moyuer VA, Schneider V, Yetman R, et al. Contribution of long-bone radiographs to the management of congenital syphilis in the newborn infant. *Arch Pediatr Adolesc Med* 1998;152:353–357.

Siegel RM, Schubert CJ, Myers PA, et al. The prevalence of sexually transmitted diseases in children and adolescent evaluated for sexual abuse in Cincinnati:

rationale for limited STD testing in prepubertal girls. *Pediatrics* 1995;96:1090–1094.

Tomeh MO, Wilfert CM. Venereal disease of infants and children at Duke University Medical Center. *N C Med J* 1973;34:109–113.

HIV (General)

AIDSinfo. Offering information on HIV/AIDS treatment, prevention, and research. http://aidsinfo.nih.gov/.

American Academy of Pediatrics. *Red book: 2009 report of the Committee on Infectious Diseases*, 28th ed. Elk Groove Village, IL: American Academy of Pediatrics, 2009.

Centers for Disease Control and Prevention, Division of Healthcare Quality Promotion. HIV in healthcare settings. http://www.cdc.gov/ncidod/dhqp/bp_hiv.html.

Centers for Disease Control and Prevention, Divisions of HIV/AIDS Prevention, National Center for HIV, STD, and TB Prevention. HIV/AIDS. http://www.cdc.gov/hiv/dhap.htm.

HIV InSite. Comprehensive, up-to-date information on HIV/AIDS treatment, prevention, and policy from the University of California San Francisco. http://hivinsite.ucsf.edu/.

Joint United Nations Programme on AIDS. Uniting the world against AIDS. http://www.unaids.org/en/.

Kaiser Family Foundation. HIV/AIDS. http://www.kff.org/hivaids/.

Evaluation of the Febrile HIV-infected Child

Andiman WA, Mezger J, Shapiro E. Invasive bacterial infections in children born to women infected with human immunodeficiency virus type 1. *J Pediatr* 1994;124:846–852.

Dayan PS, Chamberlain JM, Arpadi SM, et al. Streptococcus pneumoniae bacteremia in children infected with HIV: presentation, course, and outcome. *Pediatr Emerg Care* 1998;14:194–197.

Dorfman DH, Crain EF, Bernstein LJ. Care of febrile children with HIV infection in the emergency department. *Pediatr Emerg Care* 1990;6:305–310.

Farley JJ, King JC Jr, Nair P, et al. Invasive pneumococcal disease among infected and uninfected children of mothers with human immunodeficiency virus infection. *J Pediatr* 1994;124:853–858.

Krasinski K, Borkowsky W, Bonk S, et al. Bacterial infections in human immunodeficiency virus-infected children. *Pediatr Infect Dis J* 1988;7:323–328.

Mao C, Harper M, McIntosh K, et al. Invasive pneumococcal infections in human immunodeficiency virus-infected children. *J Infect Dis* 1996;173:870–876.

Principi N, Marchisio P, Tornaghi R, et al. Occurrence of infections in children infected with human immunodeficiency virus. *Pediatr Infect Dis J* 1991;10:190–193.

Neurologic Manifestations of the HIV-infected Child

Zuckerman G, Metrou M, Bernstein LJ, et al. Neurologic disorders and dermatologic manifestations in HIV-infected children. *Pediatr Emerg Care* 1991;7:99–105.

Prevention of HIV Acquisition

Panlilio AL, Cardo DM, Grohskopf LA, et al. Updated U.S. Public Health Service guidelines for the management of occupational exposures to HIV and recommendations for postexposure prophylaxis. *MMWR Recomm Rep* 2005;54(RR-9):1–17.

Perinatal HIV Guidelines Working Group. Public Health Service Task Force recommendations for use of antiretroviral drugs in pregnant HIV-infected women for maternal health and interventions to reduce perinatal HIV transmission in the United States. http://aidsinfo.nih.gov/ContentFiles/PerinatalGL.pdf. Published April 29, 2009.

Smith DK, Grohskopf LA, Black RJ, et al. Antiretroviral postexposure prophylaxis after sexual, injection-drug use, or other nonoccupational exposure to HIV in the United States: recommendations from the U.S. Department of Health and Human Services. *MMWR Recomm Rep* 2005;54(RR-2):1–20.

Antiviral Medications

Department of Health and Human Services Panel on Antiretroviral Guidelines for Adults and Adolescents. Guidelines for the use of antiretroviral agents in HIV-1-infected adults and adolescents. http://www.aidsinfo.nih.gov/ContentFiles/AdultandAdolescentGL.pdf. Published November 3, 2008.

Working Group on Antiretroviral Therapy and Medical Management of HIV-Infected Children. Guidelines for the use of antiretroviral agents in pediatric HIV infection. http://aidsinfo.nih.gov/ContentFiles/PediatricGuidelines.pdf. Published February 23, 2009.

CHAPTER 94 ■ METABOLIC EMERGENCIES

DEBRA L. WEINER, MD, PHD

INTRODUCTION

Recognition and understanding of inborn errors of metabolism (IEMs) in the acutely ill child in the emergency department (ED) is critical for appropriate, and possibly lifesaving, management. Individually, metabolic diseases are rare, but collectively they are common. In the United States, the incidence is approximately 1 in every 4,000 newborns. IEMs usually manifest in the neonatal period or infancy but can present at any age, even during adulthood. Many IEMs are now diagnosed by newborn screen (NBS) performed using tandem mass spectrometry (MS/MS). Nearly all states screen for a core set of IEMs, additional IEMs screened for varies by state, results may not be available in the first days to weeks of life, and false negatives and false positives occur. Clinical diagnosis and management do not require an extensive knowledge of individual metabolic diseases or biochemical pathways. An understanding of the clinical manifestations of IEMs provides the basis for knowing when they should be considered. Most important in making the diagnosis of metabolic disease is a high index of suspicion. Successful emergency treatment of suspected and known IEMs depends on prompt institution of therapy to correct and prevent further metabolic derangement. The goals of this chapter are to provide insights into when the diagnosis of an IEM should be considered, the tests necessary to make the diagnosis, and the appropriate initial management of patients with suspected or known IEM, as well as evaluation and management of the asymptomatic neonate with a positive NBS.

PATHOPHYSIOLOGY

IEMs are usually caused by single gene defects that result in abnormalities in protein, carbohydrate, fat, or complex molecule metabolism. Most are due to a defect in, or deficiency of, an enzyme, enzyme cofactor, or transport protein that results in a block in a metabolic pathway. Clinical effects are the consequence of toxic accumulations of substrates before the block or intermediates from alternative metabolic pathways and/or defects in energy production and utilization due to a deficiency of products beyond the block. Toxic accumulation of substances results from disorders of protein metabolism (i.e., amino acidopathies, organic acidemias also referred to as *organic acidurias*, urea cycle defects), carbohydrate intolerance (e.g., galactose, fructose intolerance), and lysosomal storage (i.e., mucopolysaccharidoses, glycoproteinoses, sphingolipidoses, mucolipidoses). Defects in energy production or utilization result from disorders of glycogenolysis and gluconeogenesis (e.g., glycogen storage disorders), fatty acid oxidation

defects, mitochondrial disorders (i.e., Kreb's cycle disorders, pyruvate dehydrogenase deficiency, electron transport chain disorders). Peroxisomal disorders (e.g., Zellweger syndrome, Refsum disease, adrenoleukodystrophy) are a diverse group of IEMs caused by defects of single or multiple peroxisomal enzymes, or of peroxisomal biogenesis that result in toxic accumulations, energy deficiency, and/or defects in biosynthesis of complex molecules. Other categories include disorders of metal metabolism (e.g., Wilson's disease, Menkes syndrome, acrodermatitis enteropathica, hemochromatosis); purine and pyrimidine biosynthesis (e.g., Lesch-Nyan syndrome); cholesterol biosynthesis (e.g., Smith-Lemli-Opitz syndrome); bone metabolism (e.g., hypophosphatasia); heme, bile acid, and bilirubin metabolism (e.g., porphyrias, Dubin-Johnson syndrome, Crigler-Najjar syndrome, Gilbert's disease); lipoprotein metabolism (hyperlipidemia, hypertriglyceridemia, hypercholesterolemia); and glycosylation (i.e., congenital disorders of glycosylation). Congenital adrenal hyperplasia is classified as an endocrine disorder and described in Chapter 86.

UNKNOWN SUSPECTED IEM

Background

An understanding of the clinical manifestations of IEMs provides the basis for knowing when IEM should be considered. Most important in making the diagnosis of metabolic disease is a high index of suspicion. Diseases involving the same metabolic pathways usually share similar features. In the ED, evaluation and management of patients with undiagnosed suspected IEM is usually guided by the potential metabolic category of disease and does not require a specific diagnosis. Prompt emergency treatment of physiologic and metabolic derangements, as well of precipitant causes of decompensation, is critical for optimizing outcome.

Clinical Manifestations

History

For a patient with an undiagnosed IEM, the history often provides clues that should prompt consideration of an IEM. Poor feeding, frequent vomiting, failure to thrive, lethargy in the morning before feeding or with delayed feeding, and onset of symptoms with change in diet and/or unusual dietary preferences, particularly protein or carbohydrate aversion, are concerning for possible IEM. Symptoms may be episodic in an otherwise apparently normal child. Physiologic stressors such as fasting, illness, or surgery may precipitate symptoms, especially if the stressor induces a catabolic state. Intercurrent infection may result in decompensation out of proportion to the illness. A history of multiple hospitalizations for lethargy and dehydration with improvement following intravenous (IV) fluids and glucose is common. Psychomotor developmental delay, especially with loss of milestones, is also concerning for an IEM. Some patients, particularly those with developmental delay, may already have been labeled as having other conditions, commonly cerebral palsy. It is now recognized that many patients with a history of Reye syndrome have a previously undiagnosed IEM. Patients with what is thought to be idiopathic cardiomyopathy may also have an undiagnosed IEM. Certain findings suggest particular categories of IEMs. Vomiting occurs with many IEMs but is a prominent feature of organic acidemias and urea cycle defects. Diarrhea is also a common feature of many IEMs, particularly disorders of carbohydrate intolerance and mitochondrial disorders. Lethargy progressing to coma is common with organic acidemias, urea cycle defects, fatty acid oxidation defects, and certain disorders of carbohydrate intolerance. IEM should also be considered in any child with unexpected, unexplained sudden death, even without other history suggestive of IEM. Most IEMs are autosomal recessive in their inheritance, but they may be X-linked, mitochondrial, or uncommonly autosomal dominant. A history of suggestive findings; death due to neurologic, cardiac, and/or hepatic dysfunction; sepsis; or unexplained neonatal or sudden infant deaths in siblings or maternal male relatives is also concerning. Maternal illness during pregnancy, particularly acute fatty liver of pregnancy or HELLP (hemolysis, elevated liver enzymes, low platelets) syndrome, may be due to maternal heterozygosity for a fatty acid oxidation defect, specifically 3-hydroxyacyl-CoA dehydrogenase deficiency. Parental consanguinity increases the likelihood of autosomal recessive IEM because relatives are more likely to carry the same defective gene. Certain IEMs are more prevalent in particular ethnic or religious groups. A negative family history does not rule out an IEM because most carriers have no clinical manifestations of disease. A negative NBS does not exclude the possibility of an IEM. A report prepared by the American College of Medical Genetics for the Maternal and Child Health Bureau in 2005, recommend that states screen for a core panel of 29 conditions, 22 of which are IEMs, and an additional 25 conditions that are considered secondary targets on the basis of more mild symptoms and/or absence of treatment options, of which 24 are IEMs. Most, but not all states, now screen for core conditions, and at least some of the secondary targets (http://genes-r-us.uthscsa.edu/nbsdisorders.pdf).

False-negative results occur, most commonly due to screening too soon after birth, especially within the first 24 hours, prematurity, particularly in neonates less than 1,500 g, neonatal illness, medications, transfusions, inadequate sample and inappropriate sample handling. Results are often not available in the first several days of life. In addition, in some states, parents have the option of not having their child tested.

Physical Examination

Clinical manifestations of IEMs vary from those of acute life-threatening decompensation to subacute progressive degenerative disease (Table 94.1). Nearly all IEMs have several variants that differ in age of clinical onset and severity. Clinical manifestations may even vary among family members. Life-threatening diseases tend to present clinically during the neonatal period or infancy, whereas those with intermittent decompensation or insidious onset and slow progression tend to become apparent during infancy, childhood, adolescence, or even adulthood.

Disease onset and severity may be influenced by environmental factors such as changes in dietary intake; poor intake or sudden onset, intercurrent illness; surgery; or trauma. IEMs can affect any organ system, and often affect multiple organ systems, and therefore should be considered in patients who present with altered level of consciousness, cardiac failure, hepatic failure, skeletal muscle myopathy, and/or neuropsychiatric disturbance. Physical examination results may be normal, have subtle and/or nonspecific findings (as is often the case with disorders of amino acid metabolism; fatty acid oxidation defects; and disorders of carbohydrate intolerance, gluconeogenesis, or glycogenolysis), or have findings that provide more specific diagnostic information (most commonly with lysosomal, mitochondrial, or peroxisomal disorders) (Table 94.2). Findings tend to be related to abnormal anatomic proportion (i.e., size and shape), rather than to major structural defects and usually become more pronounced over time. Patients tend to have characteristic facies, short stature, organomegaly, and/or musculoskeletal abnormalities. Unrelated, affected individuals with IEMs who have characteristic physical findings usually look more alike than do patients and their unaffected siblings. It is also now recognized that some genetic diseases classically categorized as dysmorphic syndromes, and presumed due to disruption of morphogenesis, are actually IEMs, such as Smith-Lemli-Opitz syndrome. IEMs within each major category are listed in Table 94.3. Features of specific IEMs can be found in texts referenced at the end of this chapter and on various Web sites, including the National Center for Biotechnology Information's Online Mendelian Inheritance in Man Web site (http://www.ncbi.nlm.nih.gov/entrez/query.fcgi?db=OMIM).

Neonate. IEMs should be considered in any neonate who is critically ill. Most of the IEMs that are acutely life-threatening present during the neonatal period, usually as acute encephalopathy and/or hepatic disease. Among the most common life-threatening IEMs to present in the neonate are amino acidopathies, organic acidemias, urea cycle defects, galactosemia, and hereditary fructose intolerance. In neonates, clinical features of IEMs are usually nonspecific, especially at the onset of symptoms. Manifestations may include poor feeding, vomiting, diarrhea, dehydration, temperature instability, tachypnea or apnea, cyanosis, respiratory failure, bradycardia, poor perfusion, hiccups, jaundice, hepatomegaly, pseudoobstruction, irritability, lethargy, coma, seizures, involuntary movements (e.g., tremors, myoclonic jerks, boxing, pedaling), posturing (e.g., opisthotonus), and abnormal tone (e.g., hypertonia or central hypotonia). These same symptoms are also manifestations of sepsis, congenital viral infections, respiratory illness, cardiac disease, gastrointestinal obstruction, hepatic dysfunction, renal disease, central nervous system (CNS) problems, and drug withdrawal. The presence of these conditions does not rule out the possibility of an IEM. In term infants who develop symptoms of

TABLE 94.1

COMMON PRESENTATIONS OF INBORN ERRORS OF METABOLISM[a]

Acute Neonatal Catastrophe
Septic appearing
Temperature instability
Apnea, tachypnea, cyanosis, respiratory failure
Bradycardia, poor perfusion
Irritability, lethargy, coma
Seizures
Poor feeding, vomiting
Hypertonia, hypotonia
Sudden infant death

Neurologic Disturbance
Developmental delay, usually progressive, with or without loss of milestones
Autism
Learning disabilities, behavioral and/or emotional disturbances
Hallucinations, delirium
Ataxia, dizziness, headache
Lethargy, coma
Encephalopathy
Seizures
Movement disorder, posturing
Peripheral neuropathy
Stroke, stroke-like episode
Vision, hearing, speech impairment
Dementia

Cardiac Failure/Myopathy
Failure w/cardiomegaly ± skeletal muscle weakness
Cardiac arrhythmia, syncope, sudden death
Pericardial tamponade, effusion

Gastrointestinal/Hepatic Dysfunction, Failure
Poor feeding, food intolerances/aversion, failure to thrive
Chronic intermittent vomiting, decompensation out of proportion to illness
Chronic diarrhea
Abdominal pain
Pseudoobstruction
Acute pancreatitis
Hepatomegaly
Liver failure/hepatocellular dysfunction—jaundice (direct and/or indirect), coagulopathy, elevated liver function tests

Myopathy
Muscle weakness, pain, cramping
Exercise intolerance

Psychiatric Disturbance
Anxiety
Psychosis
Personality changes
Behavioral disturbances
Depression
Obsessive compulsive disorder
Delirium, hallucinations, schizophrenia

Biochemical Disturbance
Acidosis—chronic or acute recurrent
Hyperammonemia with or without alkalosis
Hypoglycemia with or without ketonuria, hypoketosis

[a]Findings may be in isolation or combination and may be either intermittent or progressive over time.

sepsis without known risk for sepsis, metabolic disease may be nearly as common as sepsis. Sepsis may in fact be the earliest recognized clinical manifestation of an IEM, occurring within the first days to weeks of life, even prior to availability of NBS results. *Escherichia coli* sepsis in galactosemia is the classic example. Other IEMs with increased risk of sepsis are, most notably, the organic acidemias and glycogen storage disorders.

One of the most important clues to an IEM in the neonate is a history of deterioration after an initial period of apparent good health ranging from hours to weeks, usually following an uncomplicated pregnancy and delivery in a term infant. For neonates with IEMs of protein metabolism and carbohydrate intolerance disorders, onset of symptoms occurs after there has been significant accumulation of toxic metabolites following the initiation of feeding. Onset of symptoms is usually between 2 and 5 days of life but may occur within hours. Absence of a symptom-free period does not exclude the possibility of an IEM, especially if there were unrelated perinatal complications. Initial symptoms often are poor feeding, vomiting, irritability, and lethargy. In the neonatal period, jaundice occurs most commonly with tyrosinemia, galactosemia, and hereditary fructose intolerance. Progression to coma, multisystem organ failure, and death is usually extremely rapid, although often somewhat fluctuating, usually occurring within 24 hours of symptom onset. Neonates with

tyrosinemia may present with intracranial or pulmonary hemorrhage due to coagulopathy. Patients with organic acidemias may have recurrent or chronic subdural hemorrhages, sometimes mistakenly attributed to child abuse. Fatty acid oxidation disorders, particularly very long chain acyl-CoA dehydrogenase deficiency, may present during the neonatal period. Many of the peroxisomal disorders and some of the mitochondrial and lysosomal disorders also present in the neonatal period. Neonates with these disorders are less likely to have coma as an early manifestation and are more likely to have dysmorphic features, brain abnormalities, skeletal malformations, cardiopulmonary compromise, organomegaly, hepatic dysfunction, myopathy, and/or severe generalized hypotonia, usually evident at birth. Intractable seizures due to pyridoxine or folinic acid responsive disorders usually begin within the first few days of life, and biotin responsive multiple carboxylase deficiency may present within the first few days.

Infant and Young Child (1 Month to 5 Years). Infants or children with potentially acute life-threatening IEMs, most commonly partial deficiency of the urea cycle enzyme ornithine transcarbamylase, fatty acid oxidation defects, disorders of carbohydrate intolerance, and disorders of gluconeogenesis and glycogenolysis, typically present during infancy with recurrent episodes of vomiting and lethargy,

TABLE 94.2

CLINICAL AND LABORATORY FINDINGS OF INBORN ERRORS OF METABOLISM

	AA	OA	UCD	FAOD	CID	CPUD	LSD	MD	PD
Clinical Findings[a]									
Episodic decompensation	±	+	++	+	+	±	−	±	−
Poor feeding, vomiting, failure to thrive	±	+	++	±	+	±	+	+	+
Dysmorphic features and/or skeletal or organ abnormalities	±	±	−	±	−	±	+	+	+
Abnormal hair and/or dermatitis	−	±	±		−	−	±	−	±
Ophthalmologic (cataracts, corneal clouding, retinopathy, glaucoma, subluxed lens, optic atrophy, abnormal extraocular motion)	−	−	−		±	±	±	±	±
Cardiomegaly and/or arrhythmia, structural defect	−	±	−	±		±	+	±	±
Hepatomegaly and/or splenomegaly	±	+	+	+	+	+	+	±	±
Developmental delay ± neuroregression	+	+	+	±	±	±	++	+	+
Lethargy or coma	±	++	++	++	+	±	−	±	−
Seizures	±	±	+	±	±	±	+	±	+
Hypo- or hypertonia, weakness	+	+	+	+	+	±	±	±	+
Ataxia	−	±	+	±	±	±	±	±	±
Abnormal odor[b] (urine, sweat, cerumen, breath, and/or saliva)	±	±	±	−	−	−	−	−	−
Laboratory Findings[a]									
Primary metabolic acidosis	±	++	−	±	+	±	−	±	−
Primary respiratory alkalosis	−	−	+	−	−	−	−	−	−
Hyperammonemia	±	+(+)	++	±	−	−	−	−	−
Hypoglycemia	±	±	−	+	+	+	−	±	−
Liver dysfunction	±	±	±	+	+	±	±	±	±
Reducing substances	±	−	−	−	+	−	−	−	−
Ketones	A/H	H	A/H	L	A/H	A/H	A	A/H	A

AA, amino acidopathies; OA, organic acidemias; UCD, urea cycle defects; FAOD, fatty acid oxidation defects; CID, carbohydrate intolerance disorders; CPUD, carbohydrate production/utilization disorders (glycogenolysis, gluconeogenesis); LSD, lysosomal storage disorders; MD, mitochondrial disorders; PD, peroxisomal disorders; ±, sometimes present; +, usually present; ++, always present; −, usually absent; A, appropriate; H, inappropriately high; L, inappropriately low/absent. Urine[b] or body odors: boiled cabbage or rancid butter—tyrosinemia; musty—phenylketonuria; sulfur—cystinuria; maple syrup—maple syrup urine disease; fruity—propionic acidemia, methylmalonic academia; sweaty feet—isovaleric acidemia, glutaric aciduria type II; tomcat urine—3-methylcronylCoA carboxylase deficiency, multiple carboxylase deficiency; ammonia—urea cycle defects.

[a]Within disease categories, not all diseases have all findings. For disorders with episodic decompensation, clinical and laboratory findings may be present only during acute crisis. For progressive disorders, findings may not be present early in the course of disease.

[b]Urine odor best detected by drying urine on filter paper or by opening container of urine kept at room temperature for a few minutes.

Adapted from Weiner DL. Inborn errors of metabolism. In: Aghababian RV, ed. *Emergency medicine: the core curriculum*. Philadelphia, PA: Lippincott-Raven, 1999:702.

MEDICAL EMERGENCIES

which may progress to ataxia, seizures, coma, and even death. Some of the amino and organic acidopathies also present during infancy, usually with progressive neurologic deterioration. Most of the lysosomal storage disorders, as well as some of the mitochondrial disorders and peroxisomal disorders, also become apparent in infancy and early childhood, usually presenting with increasingly apparent dysmorphism or coarse features, organomegaly, myopathy, and/or neurodegeneration. More subtle and/or progressive findings in infants and children with IEMs include failure to thrive, chronic dermatoses, dilated or hypertrophic cardiomyopathy, liver dysfunction, hepatomegaly, pancreatitis, musculoskeletal weakness, hypotonia and/or cramping, impairments of hearing and vision, and developmental delay, sometimes with loss of milestones. With routine illnesses, children with IEMs may be more symptomatic, develop symptoms more quickly, or take longer than unaffected children to recover. Children with disorders of protein metabolism, even disorders that usually present in neonates, may present when changed from breast milk to cow milk formula, particularly if the breast-feeding mother is a vegetarian and the child has not yet started solid food or the solid food diet is low in protein. Fructose intolerance often manifests between ages 4 and 8 months when fruits are introduced into the diet. Disorders with decreased tolerance for fasting, particularly fatty acid oxidation defects and defects of gluconeogenesis and glycogenolysis, often manifest when children have poor intake due to illness or surgery and when infants begin to have longer overnight fasts, commonly between 7 and 12 months of age. The length of fast that produces symptoms is usually in the 6- to 8-hour range but may be less than 3 hours for disorders of glyconeogenesis and glycogenolysis,

TABLE 94.3

SPECIFIC INBORN ERRORS OF METABOLISM BY CATEGORY[a]

Amino Acidopathies
Alkaptonuria
Cystinuria types I–III
Hartnup disease
Hawkinsinuria
Histidinemia
Homocystinuria types Ia, Ib, II
Nonketotic hyperglycinemia
Phenylketonuria
Tyrosinemia types I–III

Organic Acidemias[b]
3-Hydroxy-3-methylglutaric aciduria
3-Methylcronylglycinuria
3-Methylglutaconic aciduria types I–IV
Biotinidase deficiency
Glutaric acidemia type I
Holocarboxylase synthetase deficiency
Hydroxyglutaric aciduria
Isovaleric acidemia
Maple syrup urine disease
Methylmalonic acidemia
Propionic acidemia types I, II
β-Ketothiolase deficiency

Urea Cycle Defects and Disorders of Ammonia Detoxification
Urea Cycle Defects
Argininemia
Arginosuccinic aciduria
Carbamyl phosphate synthetase deficiency
Citrullinemia
N-acetyl glutamate synthetase deficiency
Ornithine transcarbamylase deficiency
Hepatic Amino Acid Transport
Homocitrullinuria, hyperonithinemia, and hyperammonemia
(HHH) syndrome
Lysinuric protein intolerance

Fatty Acid Oxidation Defects
Carnitine palmitoyltransferase deficiency types I, II
Carnitine transporter deficiency
Carnitine-acylcarnitine translocase deficiency
Hydroxymethylglutonyl-CoA (HMG-CoA) lyase deficiency,
HMG-CoA synthetase deficiency
Long chain 3-hydroxyacyl-CoA dehydrogenase deficiency
(LCHAD)
Medium chain 3-ketoacyl thiolase deficiency (MCKAD)
Medium chain acyl-CoA dehydrogenase deficiency (MCAD)
Short chain 3-hydroxyacyl-CoA dehydrogenase deficiency
(SCHAD)
Short chain acyl-CoA dehydrogenase deficiency (SCAD)
Very long chain acyl-CoA dehydrogenase deficiency (VLCAD)

Disorders of Carbohydrate Metabolism
Carbohydrate Intolerance Disorders
Galactosemia
Galactokinase deficiency
Hereditary fructose intolerance
Fructosuria
Fructose-1,6-diphosphatase deficiency

Carbohydrate Production/Utilization Disorders
Glycogen storage disorder types 0, Ia (von Gierke), Ib/c, Ic,
II (Pompe), IIb, III (Cori or Forbes), IV (Anderson), V
(McArdle), VI (Hers), VII (Tarui), VIII, IX, X, XI

Lysosomal Storage Disorders
Mucopolysaccharidoses (MPS)
MPS IH (Hurler), IH/S (Hurler-Scheie), IS (Scheie), MSII
(Hunter), IIIA-D (Sanfilippo), IVA, B (Morquio), VI
(Maroteaux-Lamy), VII (Sly)
Sphingolipidoses
Canavan's disease
Fabry's disease
Farber's disease
Gaucher's disease types I–III
GM1 gangliosidosis types 1–3
GM2 gangliosidosis types 1 (Tay-Sachs), 2 (Sandhoff)
GM3 gangliosidosis
Krabbe's disease
Metachromatic leukodystrophy—infantile, juvenile, adult
Multiple sulfatase deficiency
Neimann-Pick disease—types IS, IC, IIA, IIS, IIC
Oligosaccharidoses (Glycoproteinoses)
Asparylglucosaminuria
Fucosidosis types I, II
Galactosialidosis
Mannosidosis α types I, II, β
Pycnodysostosis (Maroteau-Lamy III)
Schindler's disease
Sialidosis types I, II (previously mucolipidosis I)
Sialolipidosis
Mucolipidosis
Mucolipidosis types II (I-cell), III (pseudo-Hurler), IV

Mitochondrial Disorders
2-Ketoglutarate dehydrogenase complex deficiency
Freidrich ataxia
Fumarase deficiency
Glutaric acidemia type II
Kaerns-Sayre syndrome
Leigh's disease
Mitochondrial encephalopathy lactic acidosis stroke-like episodes
Myoclonic epilepsy, ragged red-fiber disease
Pearson syndrome
Phosphoenopyruvate carboxylase deficiency
Pyruvate carboxylase deficiency
Pyruvate dehydrogenase complex deficiency
Succinate dehydrogenase deficiency

Peroxisomal Disorders
Adenomyeloneuropathy
Adrenoleukodystrophy neonatal, adult
Catalase deficiency
Glutaric acidemia type III
Leber's hereditary optic neuropathy
Refsum disease infantile, adult
Rhizomelic chondroplasia punctata
Wolfram syndrome
Zellweger syndrome

[a]Disease list is not comprehensive. Some diseases can be categorized in more than one category.
[b]Disease category and most diseases terms aciduria and acidemia are used interchangeably.

most commonly glycogen synthetase deficiencies, and 12 to 24 hours for fatty acid oxidation defects. When patients with these disorders present with vomiting, they are often initially indistinguishable from patients without IEM who are vomiting, but the severity of illness, particularly the lethargy, is usually out of proportion to the duration of illness and the amount of vomiting. Ketotic hypoglycemia, believed to be due to a noninherited condition commonly seen in children ages 1 to 5 years, has been shown, in some cases, to be due to fatty acid oxidation defects and less commonly due to amino acidopathies or organic acidemias. It is now recognized that Reye syndrome-like symptoms are more commonly attributable to an IEM, most often a fatty acid oxidation defect, particularly medium chain acyl-CoA dehydrogenase deficiency, or less commonly a urea cycle defect, particularly ornithine transcarbamylase deficiency, than actual Reye's syndrome, especially now that aspirin is rarely used in children. Mortality for those with a previously undiagnosed fatty acid oxidation defect may be more than 40% with the first clinical decompensation, depending on the specific disease. IEMs also explain sudden infant death syndrome (SIDS) in approximately 5% to 10% of cases, most commonly fatty acid oxidation defects that cause cardiac arrest due to arrhythmia and/or cardiomyopathy. The most common of these is medium chain fatty acyl-coA dehydrogenase deficiency, with SIDS occurring in 25% of the approximately 1 in 10,000 patients with this disorder. Other fatty acid oxidation defects, organic acidemias, and congenital adrenal hyperplasia account for most of the remainder of SIDS cases attributable to genetic defects.

Older Child, Adolescent, or Adult (Older than 5 Years).

In the older child, adolescent, or even adult, undiagnosed metabolic disease should be considered in individuals with subtle neurologic or psychiatric abnormalities. Many will have had long-term manifestations believed to be due to other causes. Most typically, these children are diagnosed as having birth injury, behavioral problems, attention deficit hyperactivity disorder, psychiatric disorders, or atypical forms of medical diseases such as multiple sclerosis, migraines, epilepsy, or stroke. The more common findings include mild to profound developmental delay, autism, learning disabilities, irritability, aggressiveness, agitation, anxiety, emotional liability, social withdrawal, panic attacks, delirium, hallucinations, paranoia, insomnia, seizures, dizziness, ataxia, peripheral neuropathy, muscle weakness, and exercise intolerance. Hormonal changes associated with puberty may initiate or exacerbate symptoms. Manifestations may be intermittent, precipitated by the stress of illness or by dietary changes or fast, especially as teens take more control over their own diet, or may be progressive, with worsening over time. Most IEMs diagnosed in this age group are not immediately life-threatening. However, even a patient with a late-onset, presumably milder, form of an IEM that classically presents earlier in childhood may die with a first or subsequent metabolic crisis. An example is partial ornithine transcarbamylase deficiency, which can manifest at this time as a life-threatening encephalopathy. This is seen particularly in adolescent females with a history of protein aversion, migraine-like headaches, vomiting, abdominal pain, lethargy, and behavioral problems, particularly following protein ingestion. Fatty acid oxidation defects may also present at this time

with sudden death or life-threatening cardiac arrhythmia, hypoketotic hypoglycemia, and/or rhabdomyolysis. Glycogen storage disorders that manifest as exercise intolerance, muscle weakness, cramping, and/or rhabdomyolysis often present in adolescents because of their greater participation in sports during these years. Some mitochondrial disorders present during adolescence or adulthood with loss of vision and/or hearing, cardiac dysfunction, myopathy, neurologic degeneration, and endocrine disturbances. Stroke or stroke-like episodes with or without encephalopathy may occur with amino acidopathies, in particular homocystinuria, urea cycle defects, organic acidemias, disorders of carbohydrate metabolism, and mitochondrial disorders, most notably MELAS (mitochondrial encephalomyelopathy, lactic acidosis, stroke-like episodes). Disorders in which psychiatric disturbances may be the initial presenting manifestation include homocystinuria; urea cycle defects, especially partial ornithine transcarbamylase deficiency; lysosomal storage disorders; peroxisomal disorders; and Wilson's disease, a disorder of copper metabolism. Patients with phenylketonuria who are no longer on a low-protein diet may also manifest psychiatric symptoms.

Studies

Laboratory Findings. Initially, evaluation for possible IEM, particularly those that are potentially acutely life-threatening, can usually be accomplished in the acute setting with a few screening tests. Along with laboratory studies, these may include imaging studies and electrophysiologic. In the patient with potentially life-threatening symptoms, evaluation for possible IEM should be initiated as soon as it is considered, not after other etiologies have been ruled out.

Laboratory studies to evaluate for possible IEM should be performed in all patients with suggestive history, physical examination, and/or consistent abnormalities of routine laboratory tests.

Initial laboratory findings in the acutely ill patient that may suggest an IEM include a complete blood cell count (CBC) that reveals neutropenia, anemia, and/or thrombocytopenia; serum electrolytes and blood gas analysis that detect electrolyte imbalances, an increased anion gap, and/or acid-base status abnormalities; blood urea nitrogen (BUN) and creatinine levels that reveal impaired renal function; total and direct bilirubin, aspartase (AST) and alanine (ALT) transaminases, prothrombin time (PT), partial thrombin time (PTT), and/or ammonia that indicate hepatic dysfunction or failure; hypoglycemia, particularly with low or absent urine ketones, that suggests inability to appropriately metabolize fatty acids or carbohydrates; or urine-reducing substances that suggest carbohydrate intolerance (Table 94.4). Complete metabolic screen may also reveal abnormalities in uric acid, calcium, phosphate, and/or magnesium. In addition to these studies, patients with history or physical examination suggestive of myopathy should have lactate dehydrogenase, aldolase, creatinine kinase, and urine myoglobin measured as part of their initial screen.

If a metabolic disease is suspected, consultation with an IEM specialist and/or the laboratory may be helpful in guiding further laboratory evaluation and assisting with appropriate collection and processing of specimens. Blood should be collected and, based on results of initial studies, sent for plasma amino acids and acylcarnitine profile, which reflect fatty acid oxidation and organic acid, and, indirectly, amino acid metabolisms

INITIAL LABORATORY STUDIES[a]

Test	Laboratory abnormality metabolic diseases[a]	Indications, comments
Blood		

CBC (plasma)	Neutropenia (± vacuoles), anemia, and/or thrombocytopenia
	    Organic acidemias
	    Urea cycle defects
	    Carbohydrate intolerance disorders
	    Carbohydrate production/utilization disorders
	    Lysosomal storage disorders
	    Mitochondrial disorders
		Neutropenia may be masked by infection. Patients with certain IEMs are at increased risk of infection; infection can also precipitate metabolic crisis
		Anemia hemolytic, megaloblastic, or normocytic, depending on specific IEM

Glucose (serum)	Hypoglycemia
	    Amino acidopathies
	    Organic acidemias
	    Fatty acid oxidation defects
	    Carbohydrate intolerance disorders
	    Carbohydrate production/utilization disorders
	    Mitochondrial disorders
		Hypoglycemia may be due to primary defect of gluconeogenesis or glucose consumption that exceeds production

Test of acid-base status (serum)
  Electrolytes
  Anion gap
  pH (arterial or venous)
	Primary metabolic acidosis
	    Amino acidopathies
	    Organic acidemias
	    Fatty acid oxidation defects
	    Carbohydrate intolerance disorders
	    Carbohydrate production/utilization disorders
	    Mitochondrial disorders
	Primary respiratory alkalosis
	    Urea cycle defects
		Na^+, K^+, Cl^- usually normal unless abnormal secondary to vomiting, which may produce hyperchloremic metabolic acidosis, or with rhabdomyolysis, which may result in hyperkalemia
		Normal bicarbonate does not rule out amino or organic acidemias

Ammonia (plasma)	Hyperammonemia
	    Amino acidopathies
	    Organic acidemias
	    Urea cycle defects
	    Fatty acid oxidation defects
		Obtain if altered consciousness, persistent or recurrent unexplained vomiting, recurrent dizziness or ataxia, primary metabolic acidosis with increased anion gap, primary respiratory alkalosis in the absence of toxic ingestion.
		Must be free-flow venous (no tourniquet) or arterial. Arterial preferred because skeletal muscle releases ammonia, ice sample immediately, assay promptly
		Newborns 90–150 μg/dL, children 40–120 μg/dL, adults 18–54 μg/dL, (www.pediatriccareonline.org/pco/ub/view/Pediatric-drug-Lookup/153930/0/Normal-Laboratory-Values-for-Children)
		Normal <100 μg/dL neonate, <80 μg/dL >1 month
		False positives—valproic acid

Liver function tests (serum)
  Bilirubin
  Transaminases
  Clotting factors
	Hyperbilirubinemia
	    Amino acidopathies (tyrosinemia)
	    Carbohydrate intolerance disorders
	Elevated transaminases
	    Amino acidopathies
	    Organic acidemias
	    Urea cycle defects
	    Fatty acid oxidation defects
	    Carbohydrate intolerance disorders
	    Carbohydrate production/utilization disorders
	    Lysosomal storage disorders
	    Mitochondrial disorders
	    Peroxisomal disorders
		Obtain if vomiting, jaundice, and/or hepatomegaly
		Hyperbilirubinemia predominantly conjugated, except galactosemia first few days may be unconjugated

(continued)

TABLE 94.4

CONTINUED

Test	Laboratory abnormality metabolic diseases[a]	Indications, comments
Muscle function tests (serum) Lactate dehydrogenase Aldolase Creatine kinase	Abnormal muscle enzymes Carbohydrate production/utilization disorders Fatty acid oxidation defects Mitochondrial disorders	Obtain if muscle weakness, tenderness, cramping, atrophy, exercise intolerance Carnitine deficiency due to carnitine transport disorders or secondary to organic acidemias, fatty acid oxidation defects
Urine		
Reducing substances (Clinitest®)	Amino acidopathies (tyrosinemia, alkaptonuria) Carbohydrate intolerance disorders	Clinitest® positive for reducing substances and dipstick negative for glucose (glucose oxidase reaction) False positives—penicillins, salicylates, ascorbic acid, drugs excreted as glucuronides Absence of reducing substances does not eliminate possibility of IEM
Ketones (Ketostix®, Acetest®)	Elevated ketones Amino acidopathies Organic acidemias Carbohydrate intolerance disorders Carbohydrate production/utilization disorders Mitochondrial disorders Absent ketones, hypoketosis Fatty acid oxidation defects	Ketones detected by Ketostix®, Chemstix®, Acetest® Inappropriate ketones: Ketonuria in neonates Ketonuria, normal glucose beyond neonate Low/absent ketones, hypoglycemia beyond neonate
Myoglobin	Myoglobin present Organic acidemias Carbohydrate production/utilization disorders Mitochondrial disorders	Not always present, even with rhabdomyolysis, especially if creatinine kinase <10,000 IU

IEM, inborn error of metabolism.
[a]Within disease categories, not all diseases have the laboratory abnormality. In disorders of protein metabolism, carbohydrate metabolism and fatty acid oxidation defects and abnormality may be present only during acute crisis.
Adapted from Weiner DL. Inborn errors of metabolism. In: Aghababian RV, ed. *Emergency medicine: the core curriculum*. Philadelphia, PA: Lippincott-Raven, 1999:705.

(Table 94.5). In neonates younger than or at 7 to 14 days of age, blood on NBS filter paper can be used for tandem mass spectrometry and should be considered not only if tandem mass spectrometry was not initially performed but also if the initial screen was negative. Urine should be collected for potential analysis of organic acids, acylglycine, and/or orotic acid. Additional blood and urine for possible further testing should be obtained, aliquoted, and stored. Cerebral spinal fluid (CSF), if obtained, should be collected at the same time as plasma and immediately frozen and stored for possible further testing for neurometabolic disorders, most commonly nonketotic hyperglycinemia, disorders of serine biosynthesis, and/or neurotransmitter disorders. Measurement of lactate and pyruvate in the acute setting may be of limited value, particularly in the patient with hypoxia, poor perfusion, and/or sepsis. Plasma-free fatty acids, ketones, endocrine studies, and disease-specific tests may also be appropriate. Laboratory abnormalities are often transient, particularly if fluids and/or glucose are administered; therefore, normal values do not rule out an IEM. It is critical to obtain pretreatment specimens, if possible. If pretreatment specimens were not obtained, as is often the case because many IEMs are first suspected based on results of

routine laboratory studies, discarded pretreatment samples are likely to be more informative than those collected after therapy. Studies may need to be repeated during future episodes of illness. Collection of samples during acute illness is usually preferred to provocative testing by metabolic challenge performed when the child is otherwise well because this method may not yield diagnostic specimens and may be dangerous.

The confirmatory specific diagnosis of most IEMs requires additional specialized tests for detection of abnormal metabolites or abnormal concentrations of metabolites in plasma, urine, and/or cerebral spinal fluid; histochemical light and/or electron microscopic evaluation of affected tissues; and chromosome, DNA, and/or enzyme analysis in red blood cells, leukocytes, skin fibroblasts, and/or tissues from affected organs.

In the child who has died, it is still extremely important to attempt to diagnose an IEM because of the possibility that asymptomatic siblings, and with a few diseases, parents, are presently affected or that future children are at risk of being affected. Routine autopsy is usually not informative for the definitive diagnosis of IEM but may rule out other causes of death and offer clues. IEMs can be diagnosed in the child who

TABLE 94.5

SECONDARY TESTS

Test	Laboratory abnormality metabolic diseases[a]	Indications, comments
Blood		
Amino acids—quantitative (plasma or serum)	Amino acidopathies Organic acidemias Urea cycle defects Mitochondrial disorders	Tandem mass spectrometry, requires minimum 1 mL blood, 3 mL ideal,[b] heparin, or EDTA tube Obtain if metabolic catastrophe, neurologic, cardiac, GI/hepatic, musculoskeletal, psychiatric symptoms suggestive of possible IEM, metabolic acidosis, elevated anion gap, hypoglycemia, inappropriate ketonuria, hyperammonemia
Acylcarnitine profile (plasma or serum)	Organic acidemias Fatty acid oxidation defects Mitochondrial disorders Primary carnitine deficiency	Carnitine deficiency may be due to primary defect in carnitine or carnitine transporter, or secondary due to organic acidemia or fatty acid oxidation defect; can also occur in normal children during dehydration Free and total carnitine may also be helpful if carnitine deficiency is suspected
Lactate, pyruvate (deproteinized blood)	Disorders carbohydrate utilization Mitochondrial disorders	Samples must be free flow, deproteinized at bedside—1 mL into tubes with 2 mL perchloric or trichloroacetic acid, transport on ice Evaluate lactate, pyruvate, and ratio Lactate also increased in patient with hypoxia, poor perfusion, sepsis
Urine		
Organic acids	Amino acidopathies Organic acidemias Fatty acid oxidation defects Mitochondrial disorders Peroxisomal disorders	Urine best source for organic acids, minimum 2–5 mL, 10–20 mL ideal without preservative[c] Obtain if metabolic catastrophe, neurologic, cardiac, GI/hepatic, musculoskeletal, psychiatric, symptoms suggestive of possible IEM, metabolic acidosis, elevated anion gap, hypoglycemia, inappropriate ketonuria, hyperammonemia
Acylglycines	Organic acidemias Fatty acid oxidation defects	Should be performed only in conjunction with serum or plasma carnitines, minimum 2–5 mL without preservative[c]
Orotic acid	Urea cycle defects (ornithine transcarbamylase deficiency)	Send if hyperammonemia, minimum 1 mL without preservative
Cerebral Spinal Fluid		
Glucose, protein, lactate, pyruvate, glycine, serine, alanine, organic acids, neurotransmitters, folate, pterins, other disease-specific metabolites	Amino acidopathies Organic acidemias Mitochondrial disorders Nonketotic hyperglycinemia Neurotransmitter disorders	1–4 mL, freeze –20°C or –70°C

EDTA, ethylenediaminetetraacetic acid; GI, gastrointestinal; IEM, inborn error of metabolism.

[a]Within disease categories, not all diseases have the laboratory abnormality. In disorders of protein metabolism, carbohydrate metabolism and fatty acid oxidation defects and abnormality may be present only during acute crisis.

[b]Samples, quantities required, collection method, preparation, and storage are institution dependent. Tandem mass spectrometry measures amino acids and acylcarnitines, derived from carnitine, which combines with acyl-CoA derived from fatty acids and organic acids (which may have been derived from amino acids). Tandem mass spectrometry may be used as a screen for amino acidopathies, organic acidemias, and fatty acid oxidation defects. Confirmation of diagnosis usually requires further testing, including plasma amino acids, urinary organic acids, histologic examination, DNA analysis, and enzyme and/or biochemical assays.

[c]Total minimum is 4 mL for organic acids and acylglycines.

has just died, by collecting the appropriate specimens (Table 94.6). Specimens should be collected as soon after death as possible, ideally within the first 1 to 2 hours, before organ autolysis precludes the opportunity to obtain informative specimens. If not already collected during the resuscitation attempt, blood and urine should be obtained in the ED. Specimens to be collected at autopsy include additional blood, urine, and cerebral spinal fluid, and if not already obtained, skin biopsy, organ biopsies (brain, heart, liver, kidney, spleen, skeletal muscle), and bile. Aqueous humor from the anterior chamber of the eye, particularly if blood is not available, may be helpful. Photographs of children with dysmorphic features and imaging studies may be performed as part of the autopsy and are indicated if skeletal or organ abnormalities are suspected. If permission for an autopsy is not granted by the family, seek permission for aqueous humor aspiration, skin biopsy, and needle tissue biopsy,

TABLE 94.6

POSTMORTEM SPECIMENS COLLECTED AT AUTOPSY[a]

Postmortem specimens	Analyses	Comments on collection, storage
Blood[a] 10-mL EDTA tube 4–6 filter paper spots 5-mL heparinized tube	Chromosome analysis DNA analysis (requires PCR amplification) Tandem mass spectrometry for organic acidemias, urea cycle defects, fatty acid oxidation defects, Acylcarnitines Amino acids Bile acids	Obtain blood by vascular access or intracardiac puncture For filter paper spots, apply free-flow blood to filter paper, saturate through to back, do not layer drops. Air-dry 3–4 h, do not heat, place in envelope, refrigerate Freeze plasma at –20°C or –70°C, store erythrocytes at 4°C
Urine[a] Urine 10 mL in 1–2-mL aliquots	Amino acids Organic acids Acylcarnitines Bile acids	Collect by bladder catheterization, suprapubic aspiration. If unsuccessful, irrigate bladder with 20 mL normal saline and collect or perform intrabladder swabs at autopsy Freeze at –20°C or –70°C
Cerebral Spinal Fluid (CSF) CSF 3–5 mL in 1-mL aliquots	Glucose Lactate, pyruvate Glycine, serine Neurotransmitters Organic acids	If not collected for clinical care, may be appropriate to collect postmortem Freeze at –20°C or –70°C
Aqueous Humor Aqueous humor	Organic acids	May be appropriate if blood not available Collect by intraocular puncture at autopsy Freeze at –20°C or –70°C
Skin Biopsy[a] Skin—2 samples, 3-mm diameter each	Chromosome analysis DNA analysis Enzyme activity	Best collected premortem or immediately postmortem, usually viable 2–3 days, maybe 1 wk may be helpful to discuss with specialist Skin, punch, or incisional biopsy, sterile technique, 2 sites—flexor surface forearm, anterior thigh, transport in sterile tube completely filled with tissue culture media, viral culture media, (do not use culture media if planing for microscopic studies), normal saline without preservative, or normal saline-soaked sterile gauze in sterile tube, freeze at –70°C Fibroblast culture provides unlimited specimen
Organ Biopsy Brain[b] Heart muscle[b] Liver[a] 1 cm³, 10–20 mg, ≤0.5 cm thick Kidney[b] Spleen[b] Skeletal muscle 20–50 mg, ≤0.5 cm thick	Histochemical light and/or electron microscopy Enzyme activity Biochemical metabolites Mitochondrial studies	Biopsy potentially affected organs, collect within 1–2 h after death Needle or open incisional biopsy, sterile technique, wrap in aluminum foil, dry ice, freeze at –70°C, screw-top airtight vial. Some assays may need to be performed on fresh specimens
Bile Bile 2 mL	Bile acids Acylcarnitines	

EDTA, ethylenediaminetetraacetic acid; PCR, polymerase chain reaction; ED, emergency department.

[a]If autopsy refused by family or if unable to obtain autopsy within hours of death, collect blood, urine, and CSF; perform punch or open incisional biopsy of skin and needle biopsy of liver and skeletal muscle; take photographs if dysmorphic features; and obtain radiologic studies to evaluate for neurologic, cardiac, or skeletal abnormalities. Obtain parental permission. Tests that are not accurate using postmortem specimens are those for serum amino acids, lactate, pyruvate, and total and free carnitine assessment. Consider developing postmortem specimen collection kit for ED that contains necessary equipment, specimen containers, and institution-specific instructions.

[b]Obtain at autopsy if autopsy permission granted.

particularly of the liver as appropriate. Most IEMs can be categorized based on findings of initial laboratory evaluations. Nearly all patients with IEMs that present as acute life-threatening disease will have hypoglycemia, metabolic acidosis, and/or hyperammonemia. These initial findings will guide immediate treatment and further evaluation. Important exceptions are nonketotic hyperglycinemia, which usually presents within 48 hours of birth with lethargy, coma, seizures, hypotonia, spasticity, hiccups, and apnea, and pyridoxine deficiency and folinic acid responsive disorders, which present with intractable seizures with or without encephalopathy as early as the first day of life. Hypoglycemia, metabolic acidosis, and hyperammonemia are also usually not seen in lysosomal storage and peroxisomal disorders.

Hypoglycemia. Serum glucose level of less than 40 mg per dL in the neonate and less than 45 to 50 mg per dL at all ages beyond the neonatal period should be considered abnormally low. Even with poor oral intake and/or metabolic stressors, hypoglycemia with glucose less than 45 mg per dL is unusual in the normal child. Hypoglycemia may cause a decreased level of consciousness, ranging from lethargy to confusion to coma as well as irritability, and seizures. Newborns may also have a high-pitched cry, hypothermia, cyanosis, and poor feeding. In the older child or adult, symptoms may include headache, blurred vision, repeated yawning, diaphoresis, pallor, and nervousness. Hypoglycemia most commonly occurs with fatty acid oxidation defects, disorders of carbohydrate metabolism, and hyperinsulinemic states. Low serum glucose can also be seen with amino acidopathies and organic acidemias due to inhibition of hepatic gluconeogenesis in these disorders. In patients with hypoglycemia, inappropriate ketonuria is highly suggestive of a fatty acid oxidation defect, especially along with elevated anion gap, blood urea nitrogen, uric acid, creatine kinase, and liver transaminases. Ketonuria when present in the hypoglycemic neonate is always abnormal. Beyond the neonatal period, hypoglycemia with inappropriately low or absent ketones is also always abnormal. The presence of urinary ketones in a patient with hypoglycemia beyond the neonatal period does not rule out an IEM, particularly short chain fatty acid oxidation defects, organic acidemias, disorders of carbohydrate production or utilization, or ketotic hypoglycemia of childhood. Hypoketosis, if not evident from the urine, can be determined by measuring ketones (3-hydroxybutyrate and acetoacetate) and free fatty acids in blood. Normal glucose and appropriate ketonuria also does not rule out IEM. In patients with hypoglycemia, in addition to plasma amino acids and acylcarnitine and urine organic acids and acylglycines, serum cortisol and insulin should be sent, as well as liver function tests (LFTs) and ammonia, if not previously sent. Serum lactate, pyruvate and ketones, free and total carnitine and specialized blood, urine, fibroblast, and/or tissue tests may be helpful. Growth hormone is not an informative test in the acute setting. Causes of hypoglycemia other than IEM most commonly include liver diseases, hyperinsulinemia, and toxic ingestions of salicylates, β-blockers, ethanol or polyethylene glycol, maternal diabetes/gestational diabetes, prematurity or small for gestational age, asphyxia, and/or sepsis.

Metabolic Acidosis. IEMs must be considered in patients with metabolic acidosis with or without acidemia. Clinical manifes-

tations of acidosis include vomiting and tachypnea. Primary metabolic acidosis is diagnosed by a low pH, low PCO_2, and low bicarbonate. Urine pH higher than or equal to 5.5 suggests bicarbonate loss due to renal tubular acidosis but does not rule out IEM, particularly disorders of energy metabolism. Metabolic acidosis may also be due to bicarbonate loss in stool, but this also does not eliminate the possibility of an IEM because diarrhea is a prominent feature of many IEMs. In neonates believed to have pyloric stenosis, the diagnosis of IEM, particularly an organic acidemia, should be considered if the patient has metabolic acidosis rather than metabolic alkalosis. The anion gap ($[Na] - [Cl + HCO_3]$) should be determined in any patient with low serum bicarbonate, particularly if the value is out of proportion to the clinical presentation because an elevated anion gap acidosis (greater than 16 mmol per L) is characteristic of acute metabolic crisis with many IEMs. An elevated anion gap with a normal chloride usually reflects excess acid production, most often of lactate, ketone bodies, and/or other organic acids. Metabolic acidosis, usually severe, with marked ketonuria, with or without hyperammonemia or hypoglycemia, is a hallmark of organic acidemias. Fatty acid oxidation disorders may also present with metabolic acidosis, but usually with hypoglycemia and absent ketones or hypoketosis. The IEMs in which a primary lactic acidosis is the cause of the metabolic acidosis include disorders of gluconeogenesis and mitochondrial disorders of oxidation. Anion gap in renal tubular acidosis and acidosis from stool bicarbonate loss is usually normal. The absence of acidosis does not preclude an IEM. In patients with metabolic acidosis, concentration of serum ammonia and glucose, and presence or absence of urine ketones and reducing substances will also help direct further metabolic workup. Plasma amino acids, acylcarnitines and urine organic acids, and acylglycines should be measured. Measurement of serum lactate, pyruvate, ketones, and organic acids, specific metabolites or enzymes, and DNA analysis may also be helpful. Other causes of metabolic acidosis are hypoxia, poor perfusion, sepsis, seizures, Reye syndrome, diabetic ketoacidosis, uremia, and toxins, most notably, salicylates, ethanol, methanol, ethylene glycol, isoniazid, iron, and arsenic.

Hyperammonemia. Early manifestations of hyperammonemia are anorexia and irritability. Children and adolescents may report headache, abdominal pain, and fatigue. Progression to vomiting, lethargy, seizures, coma, and death may occur within hours. In addition to brain stem dysfunction, hyperammonemia can cause cerebral edema and intracranial hemorrhage. Some patients with chronic hyperammonemia adapt to their elevated ammonia level and may appear to have no overt symptoms despite ammonia concentrations above normal. Ammonia is an intermediary in the catabolism of nitrogen-containing compounds, particularly amino acids. Normally, ammonia is converted in the liver to either urea by the urea cycle or to glutamine by glutamine synthetase. Hyperammonemia is the hallmark of urea cycle defects. Plasma amino acids and urine orotic acid should be sent to establish the diagnosis of a urea cycle defect. Hyperammonemia also occurs with organic acidemias and fatty acid oxidation defects as a consequence of inhibition of the urea cycle. Normal ammonia levels are less than 100 μg per dL in neonates and less than 80 μg per dL beyond the neonatal period. Proper collection and handling of blood for ammonia determination is critical to prevent falsely elevated values. Abnormal levels should be confirmed by immediate stat repeat by using proper technique for drawing and sending because inappropriate technique can result in values elevated several fold of normal. Ammonia levels are typically highest in urea cycle defects and may exceed 1,000 μg per dL. Ammonia levels in organic acidemias are usually less than 500 μg per dL during decompensation but may exceed 1,000 μg per dL. Hyperammonemia in fatty acid oxidation defects, if present, is usually less than 250 μg per dL. Transient hyperammonemia of the newborn should be considered in the differential diagnosis, particularly if hyperammonemia is present on the first day of life. Hyperammonemia directly stimulates the respiratory center, resulting in tachypnea. Ammonia level higher than 250 μg per dL with respiratory alkalosis in the absence of metabolic acidosis is highly suggestive of a urea cycle defect. Patients with urea cycle defects may have compensatory metabolic acidosis. Patient with organic acidemias and fatty acid oxidation defects and hyperammonemia have primary metabolic alkalosis usually without respiratory alkalosis. Patients with hyperammonemia due to organic acidemias usually have marked ketosis and normal glucose level, whereas those with fatty acid oxidation defects usually have hypoketotic hypoglycemia. Even during minor illnesses, protein catabolism may result in hyperammonemia. Normal ammonia level does not eliminate the possibility of an IEM, particularly in a patient who is dehydrated with decreased renal urea excretion and/or has an IEM with a partial enzyme defect. In patients with hyperammonemia, liver function should be evaluated. Mild elevation of transaminases may be seen in metabolic disorders in each category. Plasma should be sent for amino acids and acylcarnitines evaluation, and urine for organic acids, acylglycines, and orotic acid evaluation. For many disorders, leukocytes, fibroblasts, or organ tissue, most often liver, is required for confirmatory enzyme or molecular assay. Liver dysfunction due to causes other than IEM, including primary liver disease, hepatic infection, toxic insult, sepsis, and asphyxia, may also cause hyperammonemia.

Imaging Studies. In the ED, imaging studies may be useful to guide management of potential acutely life-threatening organ system failure, particularly cerebral edema, hemorrhagic or thrombotic stroke, or cardiac failure. Imaging studies to aid in diagnosis and long-term management are rarely appropriate in the ED setting.

Chest and abdominal radiographs may reveal cardiomegaly, an abnormal cardiac silhouette, pulmonary effusion or hemorrhage, and/or hepatomegaly. Head computed tomography (CT) scan, magnetic resonance imaging (MRI), or ultrasound (US) in the neonate may show structural and functional abnormalities of the brain (most commonly of the corpus callosum, basal ganglia, cerebellum, and/or gray–white matter), cerebral edema, intracranial hemorrhage and/or stroke, and stroke-like episodes. CT and US can be used to evaluate for organomegaly, pleural effusion, and/or ascites. Echocardiography (ECHO) can be performed to evaluate abnormalities in cardiac structure, pericardial fluid, and impaired cardiac function.

Electrophysiologic Studies. Electrocardiogram (EKG) should be performed as clinically indicated to evaluate for possible cardiomegaly, cardiomyopathy, structural heart disease, arrhythmia, and/or effusion. Electroencephalogram (EEG) may be informative to determine whether patients are having seizures and may suggest specific IEMs based on brain wave patterns and anatomic focus. EEG rarely needs to be performed emergently. Other electrophysiologic studies that may be informative but not indicated as part of the ED evaluation include electromyelogram (EMG) to differentiate between muscular and neural pathology in patients with myopathy and/or nerve conduction studies to distinguish between peripheral and axonal nerve degeneration in patients with concern of neuromuscular disorders, as well as evoked potential studies to evaluate visual and auditory function.

Management

Initial treatment of IEMs is aimed at correcting acute metabolic abnormalities. Even the apparently stable patient with mild symptoms may deteriorate rapidly with progression to death within hours. Failure to administer immediate, appropriate treatment for IEMs can result in long-term neurologic sequelae or death. For patients with IEMs of amino acid metabolism or carbohydrate intolerance, treatment is aimed at elimination of toxic metabolites. For disorders of fatty acid oxidation or gluconeogenesis and glycogenolysis, therapy is aimed at correcting the energy deficiency. With appropriate therapy, patients with these acutely life-threatening disorders may recover completely. In patients with lysosomal, mitochondrial, and peroxisomal disorders, emergent treatment is aimed at ameliorating the effects of organ dysfunction and usually involves temporizing measures that do not have long-term impact on the inevitable progressive, degenerative course of these disorders. As always, airway, breathing, and circulation must be addressed first. Treatment for a potential IEM should be started empirically as soon as the diagnosis is considered (Table 94.7).

Fluids

All oral intake should be stopped to prevent the introduction of potentially harmful protein or sugars. Fluid bolus(es), as clinically indicated, should be normal saline, 10 mL per kg for neonates or patients with concern of heart failure and 20 mL per kg for infants and children. Ringer's lactate should be avoided because it can worsen acidosis. Normal saline bolus fluid should contain 10% dextrose unless the patient is hypoglycemic.

Hypoglycemia

Hypoglycemia, if present, should be corrected by dextrose bolus instead of adding D_{10} to bolus fluid; 0.25 to 1 g per kg, D_{10} for neonates, D_{10} or D_{25} for those beyond the neonatal period. Hydration after fluid/dextrose bolus should be with D_{10} to D_{15} in ½ normal saline at 1 to 1.5× maintenance to provide 8 to 12 mg per kg per minute of glucose and maintain serum glucose level at 120 to 170 mg per dL, with the goal of preventing catabolism. Large, rapid fluctuations in glucose level should be avoided. Although controversial and rarely

MEDICAL EMERGENCIES

TABLE 94.7

EMERGENT TREATMENT

Access and establish airway, breathing, circulation
  Fluid boluses normal saline, avoid lactated Ringer's. Avoid hypotonic fluid load due to risk of cerebral edema, particularly if hyperammonemia.
Discontinue intake of offending agents, provide adequate glucose to prevent catabolism
  NPO (especially no protein, galactose, or fructose).
  Glucose for hypoglycemia, 0.25–1 g/kg (i.e., D_{10} neonates; D_{10} or D_{25} infant, child).
  D_{10} to D_{15} with electrolytes: 8–12 mg/kg/min IV at 1–1.5× maintenance to maintain serum glucose level at 120–170 mg/dL).
  If necessary, treat hyperglycemia with **insulin** (0.2–0.3 U/kg/h) to further prevent hyperglycemia.
Correct metabolic acidosis (pH < 7.0–7.22) slowly, cautiously
  Sodium bicarbonate and/or potassium acetate: 0.25–0.5 mEq/kg/h (up to 1–2 mEq/kg/h) IV; if intractable acidosis, consider hemodialysis (peritoneal dialysis, hemofiltration, exchange transfusion much less effective).
Eliminate toxic metabolites
  Hyperammonemia therapy:
  For organic acidopathies, fatty acid oxidation defects, hyperammonemia is usually corrected by **treatment of dehydration, acidosis, and hypoglycemia. Hemodialysis** should be considered for persistent hyperammonemia for this conditions or suspected IEM.
  For urea cycle defects, recommendations of the New England Consortium dialysis for ammonia >300 μg/dL if concentration is rising, transfer to a facility/unit with dialysis capability for ammonia >200–250 μg/dL. If dialysis not immediately available or levels >100–125 μg/dL, use **sodium phenylacetate, sodium benzoate** as Ammonul® (Ucyclyd Pharma, 1-888-829-2593). If <20 kg load 250 mg/kg (2.5 mL/kg) in 10% glucose via central line over 90 to 120 min, then 250 mg/kg/day (2.5 mL/kg/day) in 10% glucose via central line continuous infusion, if ≥20 kg 5.5 g/m² (55 mL/m²) over 90 to 120 min, then 5.5 g/m²/day (55 mL/m²/day) via central line; **arginine HCl** 600 mg/kg (6 mL/kg) IV in 10% glucose over 90 to 120 min, then 600 mg/kg/day IV continuous infusion. Ammonul® must be given by central line. Arginine HCl can be mixed with Ammonul®. Can decrease arginine HCl doses to 200 mg/kg if carbamyl phosphate deficiency, ornithine transcarboxylase deficiency. L-carnitine conjugates with and inactivates sodium benzoate; therefore, it must not be given with Ammonul®. Has also been used for **neonatal hyperammonemic coma of unknown etiology.**
Administer cofactors if indicated:
  Pyridoxine (B_6) 100 mg IV for possible pyridoxine-responsive disorder (seizures unresponsive to conventional anticonvulsants).
  Folinic acid as leucovorin; 2.5 mg IV for possible folate-responsive disorder (seizures unresponsive to conventional anticonvulsants)
  Biotin 10–40 mg NG tube for possible biotin-responsive disorder (seizures unresponsive to conventional anticonvulsants)
  L-**carnitine** 25–50 mg/kg over 2–3 min or as an infusion added to the maintenance fluid, followed by 25–50 mg/kg over 24 h, max 100 mg/kg not to exceed 3 g/day for presumed carnitine deficiency if life-threatening manifestations. Use is controversial, consultation with an IEM specialist is recommended.

Adapted from Weiner DL. Inborn errors of metabolism. In: Aghababian RV, ed. *Emergency medicine: the core curriculum.* Philadelphia, PA: Lippincott-Raven, 1999:707.

---

necessary in the ED, insulin (0.2 to 0.3 units per kg per hour) can be administered to prevent hyperglycemia rather than decreasing the concentration of glucose administered below 10%. Correction of hypoglycemia with glucose will improve most conditions with the exception of primary lactic acidosis due to disorders of gluconeogenesis involving pyruvate metabolism.

Metabolic Acidosis

For the immediate treatment of metabolic acidosis, sodium bicarbonate may be administered but must be given cautiously. Sodium bicarbonate should not be given unless it has been determined that the patient has metabolic acidosis and is maintaining adequate ventilation. Rapid and/or overcorrection of acidosis may have adverse CNS effects. In the patient with hyperammonemia, alkalinization of the blood favors the conversion of NH_4^+ to NH_3, which crosses the blood–brain barrier more readily and may cause cerebral edema and/or hemorrhage. Furthermore, alkalinization of the urine decreases excretion of ammonia. The pH for which sodium bicarbonate should be administered and the dose are controversial because data are lacking. Conservative guidelines rec-

ommend that sodium bicarbonate therapy be given for a pH of less than or equal to 7.0 at a dose of 0.25 to 0.5 mEq per kg per hour, but following these guidelines does not guarantee that complications from sodium bicarbonate therapy will be avoided. More aggressive guidelines recommend treatment of a pH of less than or equal to 7.2 with 1 to 2 mEq per kg per hour of bicarbonate. Continued administration of sodium bicarbonate is titrated based on acid-base status. Sodium bicarbonate may cause hypernatremia, which can in part be prevented by giving potassium as potassium acetate, which may decrease the need for bicarbonate. When using potassium acetate, however, the infusion rate must be no more than 0.1 to 0.25 mEq per kg per hour of potassium and requires frequent analyses of serum level. Definitive treatment of acidosis requires removal of the abnormal metabolites either by restricting intake of substances, primarily protein, or in severe cases, by dialysis, preferably hemodialysis.

Hyperammonemia

Significant hyperammonemia is life-threatening and must be treated immediately on diagnosis. Treatment protocols for hyperammonemia in neonates and infants and children are detailed on the New England Consortium Web site and as per their site are meant to be used in consultation with an IEM specialist: http://www.childrenshospital.org/newenglandconsortium/NBS/neonate2.html and http://www.childrenshospital.org/newenglandconsortium/NBS/infant_child.html, for neonates and infants, respectively. The goals of emergent treatment of hyperammonemia are to eliminate protein intake, prevent catabolism, and enhance the elimination of ammonia. Intake of protein should be stopped. Fluid containing D_{10} or D_{15} at a rate of 1 to 1.5× maintenance to deliver 8 to 12 mg per kg per minute of dextrose and maintain serum glucose level at 120 to 170 mg per dL should be administered to prevent catabolism and enhance elimination of ammonia. If a urea cycle defect is the likely etiology of hyperammonemia, D_{10} at a rate to deliver 6 to 8 mg per kg per minute of dextrose should be adequate, since these urea cycle defects do not usually cause hypoglycemia. Use of insulin can be administered to prevent hyperglycemia. Colloids can be considered but should be used cautiously because they increase nitrogen load. Hypotonic fluid overload should be avoided, particularly in patients with hyperammonemia, because this could result in cerebral edema. Increased intracranial pressure in patients with hyperammonemia should not be treated with steroids or mannitol. Steroids increase catabolism and can therefore worsen hyperammonemia. Mannitol has not been shown to be effective.

Hemodialysis is the most rapid and effective method for removing ammonia. Extracorporeal membrane oxygenation (ECMO) is the most effective form of dialysis but has higher risks than other forms of dialysis, particularly in neonates. ECMO, which can reduce ammonia levels by more than 600 μg per dL in 1 to 2 hours, is up to 20 times more effective than hemofiltration and up to nearly 70 times more effective than peritoneal dialysis. Exchange transfusion is not effective. Consensus on ammonia concentration for which hemodialysis is indicated is lacking. Dialysis is most effective for ammonia concentrations higher than 300 to 350 μg per dL. Recommendations of the New England Consortium are to consider dialysis for ammonia level higher than 300 μg per dL if concentration is rising and transfer to a facility/unit with dialysis capability for ammonia level higher than 200 to 250 μg per dL. If dialysis is not immediately available or levels are higher than 100 to 125 μg per dL but lower than 200 μg per dL, pharmacologic agents for ammonia removal should be administered to patients with known or suspected urea cycle defect. Sodium phenylacetate and sodium benzoate, available in combination as the preparation Ammonul®, 100 mg each per mL (Ucyclyd Pharma, Inc, Scottsdale, AZ; 1-888-829-2593) eliminates nitrogen by an alternative pathway that does not rely on an intact urea cycle. Ammonul® does not remove ammonia rapidly enough to serve as primary therapy in patients with severe hyperammonemia. As per the package insert (http://www.medicis.com/products/pi/pi_ammonul.pdf), Ammonul® is "indicated as an adjunctive therapy for the treatment of acute hyperammonemia and associated encephalopathy in patients with deficiencies in enzymes of the urea cycle." It has also been used to treat neonatal hyperammonemic coma of unknown etiology. The dose is 2.5 mL per kg (250 mg per kg) for patients weighing less than 20 kg and 55 mL per m² (5.5 g per m²) for those weighing more than 20 kg. This dose must be diluted in at least 25 mL per kg of 10% dextrose and administered as a bolus via central line over 90 to 120 minutes. The same dose in at least 25 mL per kg of 10% dextrose is then also given as a 24-hour infusion via central line. Arginine, which enhances urea cycle activity in patients with most urea cycle defects, should be administered using arginine HCl 10% at a dose of 600 mg per kg IV over 90 to 120 minutes, followed by the same dose over 24 hours. Arginine HCl can be mixed with Ammonul®. If Ammonul®/arginine HCl are being administered, the hourly infusion rate of maintenance fluids should be reduced by the volume of Ammonul®/arginine HCl being given. Given the high concentration of sodium in Ammonul® and chloride in arginine HCl, extreme caution must be taken if administering other sodium chloride–containing fluids. Sodium phenylacetate may deplete potassium. Potassium should be replaced as potassium acetate. Ondansetron (0.15 mg per kg up to every 8 hours) should be administered for vomiting and/or prophylactically if treating with Ammonul®. To assess patient response to treatment, ammonia should be monitored every 4 hours, plasma amino acids daily, and electrolytes, anion gap and acid base status every 4 hours to daily depending on last values. Usually, 2 to 3 days of therapy are necessary.

Other Treatment

L-carnitine may be administered in acutely life-threatening situations for disorders associated with carnitine deficiency, but its use is controversial and consultation with an IEM specialist is recommended. L-carnitine is given at a dose of 25 to 50 mg per kg over 2 to 3 minutes or as an infusion added to the maintenance fluid, followed by 25 to 50 mg per kg over 24 hours, up to 100 mg per kg per day, maximum 3 g per day. For seizures unresponsive to conventional anticonvulsants, empiric therapy with pyridoxine (B_6; 100 mg IV), folinic acid (leucovorin; 2.5 mg IV), and/or biotin (10 to 40 mg delivered by nasogastric tube) should be considered particularly in neonates, and also in infants, to treat a possible cofactor-responsive IEM. While there are other disease-specific pharmacologic agents, their administration is rarely indicated in the ED. Given that some IEMs are associated with increased risk of infection and that serious bacterial infection can precipitate metabolic crisis, antibiotics should be considered for any patient of concern for possible serious bacterial infection. Fresh-frozen plasma may be indicated for patients with coagulopathy.

KNOWN IEM

Background

Early recognition of acute metabolic decompensation and the potential for precipitous life-threatening deterioration is critical for the effective management of patients with a known IEM. A history of physiologic stress, such as intercurrent illness or recent surgery, and/or noncompliance with diet and/or therapeutic agents may precipitate symptoms. Manifestations and need for hospitalization with previous decompensations can provide insights into severity of disease and guide appropriate ED treatment and disposition.

Principles of evaluation and management are similar to those for patients with undiagnosed IEM as detailed in the

TABLE 94.8

LABORATORY ABNORMALITIES, EMERGENT TREATMENT OF KNOWN IEMS

IEM category	Laboratory abnormalities	Abnormalities to treat emergently (see Table 94.7 for specifics)[a]
Amino acidopathies	Hypoglycemia Metabolic acidosis ± Increased anion gap ± Elevated lactate Elevated transaminases	Hypoglycemia Acidosis
Organic acidemias	Ketonuria Neutropenia, anemia thrombocytopenia ± Hypoglycemia Metabolic acidosis Increased anion gap ± Elevated lactate ± Hyperammonemia Elevated transaminases Ketosis, ketonuria	Hypoglycemia Acidosis Hyperammonemia
Urea cycle defects, disorders of ammonia detoxification	Myoglobinuria	
Fatty acid oxidation defects	Hyperammonemia with respiratory alkalosis ± Elevated transaminases Hypoketotic hypoglycemia ± Hyperammonemia	Hyperammonemia Hypoglycemia Acidosis
Disorders of carbohydrate intolerance	± Elevated transaminases Hypoglycemia Hyperchloremic metabolic acidosis Direct hyperbilirubinemia	Hypoglycemia Acidosis
Disorders of carbohydrate production/utilization	Urinary reducing substances Hypoglycemia Metabolic acidosis ± Increased anion gap ± Increased lactate, pyruvate ± Hyperammonemia ± Elevated transaminases Hyperuricemia Ketonuria	Hypoglycemia Acidosis

IEM: inborn error of metabolism.
[a]Treatment must also include management of airway, breathing, circulation, life-threatening organ failure, and intercurrent illness including sepsis, which is associated with galactosemia, congenital adrenal hyperplasia, and certain organic acidemias and glycogen storage disorders.

section of this chapter on Management of Suspected IEM. Specifics of evaluation and treatment should be tailored to the IEM and the patient. Additional studies and treatment are indicated based on current clinical manifestations. Results should be interpreted relative to previous studies as available. Management for specific categories of disease is discussed below and presented in Table 94.8. The family may have an emergency treatment plan with them developed by an IEM specialist, specifically for their child. Families may also have a plan detailing desired resuscitation measures if resuscitation is necessary. Families without such plans should be encouraged to work with their IEM physician to develop and modify plans as appropriate on an ongoing basis. Some EDs that routinely care for specific patients maintain copies of these plans or have access to them through electronic medical records. Use of clin-

ical pathways for treatment of patients with an IEM in the ED has been shown to improve timeliness and effectiveness of care.

Patients most likely to present to an ED with acute decompensation due to their IEM are those with the amino acidopathy tyrosinemia, organic acidemias, urea cycle defects, fatty acid oxidation defects, and galactosemia (Table 94.3).

Amino Acidopathies

Most amino acidopathies do not cause acute decompensation. Important exceptions include tyrosinemia type I and maple syrup urine disease. Maple syrup urine disease, while categorized as an amino acidopathy on NBS, has manifestations more similar to organic acidemias and is therefore discussed below, under "Organic Acidemias." Tyrosinemia type I, a disorder of phenylalanine and tyrosine metabolism that results initially in liver failure and later in hepatocellular carcinoma, usually presents in early infancy but can present in the neonatal period. Clinical features include lethargy, vomiting, diarrhea, failure to thrive, hypoglycemia, jaundice, ascites, edema, bleeding, and renal tubular acidosis. Patients, particularly neonates, may have sepsis. Infants and children, in addition to manifestations seen in the neonate, may also have hepatosplenomegaly, rickets, hypotonia, and neurologic deficit. Some patients are asymptomatic until they develop hepatocellular carcinoma. Emergent treatment requires dietary elimination of tyrosine and phenylalanine. To treat dehydration, normal saline bolus(es), 10 mL per kg for neonates and 20 mL per kg for infants and children should be administered. Bolus fluid should also contain D_{10}, unless the patient is hypoglycemic, in which case dextrose should instead be administered as a bolus of 0.25 to 1 g per kg as D_{10} for neonates and D_{10} or D_{25} for infants and children. After administration of bolus fluid, D_{10} to D_{15} in ½ normal saline should be continued at 1 to 1.5× maintenance to provide glucose at 8 to 12 mg per kg per minute. Insulin 0.2 to 0.3 units per kg per hour can be administered as necessary to maintain serum glucose levels at 120 to 170 mg per dL. CBC, electrolytes, glucose, phosphate, calcium, albumin, PT, PTT, and blood gas levels should be evaluated and derangements corrected. As clinically indicated, cultures to evaluate for sepsis should be sent and antibiotics administered. Liver and renal transplant may be necessary. Ongoing treatment with nitisinone [NTBC; 2-(2-nitro-4-trifluor-methylbenzoyl)-1,3-cyclohexaanedione], which blocks metabolism of phenylalanine and tyrosine, can prevent manifestations in some patients if started at time of diagnosis.

Organic Acidemias

Organic acids are intermediary products of protein, fat, and carbohydrate metabolism. Their accumulation results in metabolic acidosis, which is often very severe and usually associated with elevated anion gap. Hypoglycemia is common because metabolic stress increases metabolic demand, which induces degradation of glucose, and because toxic accumulations of organic acids inhibit gluconeogenesis. Increased metabolism of fatty acids results in ketosis in certain organic acidemias, while others are characterized by hypoketotic hyperglycemia. Hyperammonemia results from inhibition of the urea cycle by organic acids. Organic acids also cause bone marrow toxicity that inhibits leukocyte and platelet maturation, resulting in neutropenia and thrombocytopenia. Organic acidemias most likely to be associated with acute decompensation are carnitine palmitoyltransferase deficiency types I and II, and carnitine uptake deficiency, glutaric academia type I, holocarboxylase synthase deficiency, HMG-CoA lyase deficiency maple syrup urine disease, methylmalonic acidemia, and propionic acidemia. Biotinidase deficiency, categorized on NBS as other disease rather than organic acidemia, results from a defect of biotin metabolism, the cofactor required by holocarboxylase synthase for metabolism of branch chain amino acids and therefore has manifestations similar to organic acidemias. Neonatal onset forms of organic acidemias usually present within the first week with life-threatening metabolic decompensation. Clinical features include lethargy and/or encephalopathy progressing to obtundation, feeding problems, vomiting, hepatomegaly, metabolic acidosis, hyper-

ammonemia, and neutropenia. Several of the organic acidemias result in a characteristic urine or body odor (Table 94.2 footnote). Infantile, late-onset forms tend to have a more insidious presentation with failure to thrive, seizures, spasticity, hypotonia, and developmental delay. Affected individuals may have episodic metabolic decompensation with rapid progression to coma, particularly with physiologic stressors. Many of the clinical features can be prevented by initiation of disease-specific formula free of offending metabolites, and/or disease-specific vitamin therapy for vitamin-responsive disorders, as soon as the diagnosis is made.

Evaluation of patients with organic acidemias should include assessment of vital signs, temperature, and levels of cardiovascular stability electrolytes, glucose, calcium, ammonia, aspartate aminotransferase (AST), alanine aminotransferase (ALT), alkaline phosphatase, prothrombin time (PT), partial thromboplastin time (PTT), plasma amino acids, serum carnitine, blood gas, CBC, differential, platelets, urine specific gravity and ketones, urine organic acids, and as clinically indicated, analysis of blood, urine, cerebrospinal fluid (CSF), throat, and secretions for infection. Note that CBC may not be a reliable indicator of infection because of bone marrow suppression. If considering a lumbar puncture, recognize that patients may be hemodynamically unstable and/or may have cerebral edema due to toxic concentrations of organic acids and/or ammonia.

Goals of treatment are to stabilize cardiorespiratory status, restore and maintain hydration, correct metabolic derangements, decrease organic acid production, enhance elimination of organic acids, and treat precipitating causes, such as infection. All protein intake should be stopped for 48 to 72 hours in the acutely ill child. To treat dehydration, normal saline bolus(es), 10 mL per kg for neonates and 20 mL per kg for infants and children should be administered. Bolus fluid should contain D_{10}, unless the patient is hypoglycemic in which case dextrose should instead be administered as a bolus of 0.25 to 1 g per kg; D_{10} is given for neonates, and D_{10} or D_{25} for infants and children. Ringer's lactate should not be used. After administration of bolus fluid, D_{10} to D_{15} in ½ normal saline should be continued at 1 to 1.5× maintenance to provide glucose at 8 to 12 mg per kg per minute. Insulin, 0.2 to 0.3 units per kg per hour can be administered as necessary to maintain serum glucose level at 120 to 170 mg per dL. Because of the potential for severe metabolic acidosis in these patients due to accumulation of organic acids, treatment of acidosis needs to be more aggressive than with many other types of IEMs. Sodium bicarbonate, as much as 1 to 2 mEq per kg should be administered to correct acidosis, pH less than 7.2 or bicarbonate less than 14 to 16 mmol per L, and should be titrated based on acid-base status. Patients with organic acidemias may require as much as 10 to 15 mEq per kg per day of sodium bicarbonate. Potassium given as potassium acetate may decrease the amount of sodium bicarbonate required thus decreasing the risk of hypernatremia. Treatment of acidosis and hypoglycemia usually corrects hyperammonemia. Hemodialysis is indicated to hasten clearance of metabolic toxins in the obtunded or comatose patient and to correct persistent metabolic acidosis, hyperammonemia, and/or severe electrolyte abnormalities. L-carnitine (25 to 50 mg per kg over 2 to 3 minutes or as an infusion added to the maintenance fluid, followed by 25 to 50 mg per kg over 24 hours, up to

MEDICAL EMERGENCIES

100 mg per kg per day, maximum 3 g per day) may benefit some patients with an organic academia, but its use is controversial and consultation with an IEM specialist is recommended. Glycine (150 to 300 mg per kg per day IV or PO), which enhances secretion of organic acids, should be considered for patients with isovaleric acidemia. Patients with holocarboxylase synthase or biotinidase deficiency may improve with biotin (10 to 40 mg per day given PO or NG), those with maple syrup urine disease may benefit from hydroxycobalamin (vitamin B12; 1 mg IM). It is usually not imperative that these cofactor therapies be administered in the ED. Antibiotics should be administered as clinically indicated for infection. Administration of an oral, broad-spectrum antibiotic (e.g., neomycin) to reduce gut flora, a significant source of organic acids, may be beneficial but usually is not initiated in the ED. Efficacy of emergent treatment is monitored by ongoing assessment of mental status, fluid and cardiovascular status, signs of bleeding, and measurement of electrolytes, glucose, ammonia, and blood gas levels every 4 to 6 hours until the patient is stabilized. Resolution of metabolic crisis usually takes days to weeks.

Urea Cycle Defects

Disorders of the urea cycle result in toxic accumulation of ammonia generated by the catabolism of protein. Urea cycle disorders include carbamyl phosphate synthetase deficiency, ornithine transcarboxylase deficiency, citrullinemia, arginosuccinate lyase deficiency, and arginosuccinic aciduria. All except ornithine transcarboxylase deficiency, which is X-linked in its inheritance pattern, are autosomal recessive. Ammonia, in excess, is a neurotoxin that results in cerebral edema as well brain stem dysfunction. Those with severe enzyme deficiency present within the first few days of life, following consumption of protein in breast milk or formula. Others with partial deficiency present within the first few months of life, or even as adults, after intake of a quantity of protein that exceeds their metabolic capacity. Arginase deficiency typically presents later in life, ranging from infancy to adulthood, as a neurologic syndrome with developmental delay and progressive neurologic abnormalities and usually less severe hyperammonemia. Ornithine transcarboxylase deficiency, is the most common urea cycle defect, and in males, it is the most severe. Female carriers for ornithine transcarboxylase deficiency may manifest clinical disease due to disproportionate inactivation of their normal X chromosome (lyonization), but usually present later, including during adolescence. The other urea cycle defects, of which carbamoyl phosphate synthetase deficiency is the most common, affect males and females similarly. Presentation even later in life can be acute, severe, and even life-threatening. Acute manifestations are lethargy, irritability, vomiting, hepatomegaly, ataxia, seizures, progressing to coma, and death without appropriate emergent treatment. Duration of coma is a better predictor of outcome than is serum ammonia concentration. With late-onset forms, symptoms, although similar, are usually episodic and/or less severe and may include subtle findings such as failure to thrive in infants and learning and attention deficits, personality and behavioral disturbances, and migraine-like headaches in school-age children and adolescents. Level of alertness and cardiorespiratory status must be assessed and stabilized. Potential precipitating factors, such as infection, should be investigated and treated. Hyperammonemia is a brain stem respiratory stimulant that results in tachypnea. Increased intracranial pressure due to hyperammonemia may produce bradycardia and elevated blood pressure. Electrolytes, blood gas, glucose, AST, ALT, alkaline phosphatase, bilirubin, ammonia, and plasma amino acids levels, as well as CBC, urinalysis, and cultures to evaluate for infection, as clinically indicated, should be evaluated. Respiratory alkalosis is common, sometimes with secondary metabolic acidosis. Hepatotoxicity due to hyperammonemia may result in elevated LFTs. Even patients who are not lethargic may have significant hyperammonemia, masked by acclimatization to chronic elevations of ammonia.

Goals of acute therapy are to eliminate protein intake, avoid protein catabolism, and remove ammonia. Patients should be treated aggressively with fluids to correct dehydration and maintain hydration, glucose to prevent catabolism, and dialysis and/or sodium benzoate, sodium phenylacetate (Ammonul®), and arginine to correct hyperammonemia as described for suspected IEM (p. 989). Patients with urea cycle defects are usually not hypoglycemic, which is not usually the case for patients with a urea cycle defect. Arginine HCl should be given to all patients with urea cycle defect, except those with arginase deficiency because arginine is in excess in these patients. For patients with ornithine transcarbamylase deficiency or carbamyl phosphate synthetase deficiency, the arginine HCl dose is 200 mg per kg per day administered as a 10% solution. For patients with citrullinemia and arginosuccinic acidemia, the arginine HCl dose is 600 mg per kg per day as a 10% solution. In patients with OTC and CPS, enteral citrulline may be beneficial for enhancing elimination of ammonia, but it is not imperative that it be administered in the ED and should not be administered with patients who are vomiting and/or have decreased level of consciousness. Citrulline should not be administered to patients with citrullinemia or arginosuccinic aciduria because they already have excess citrulline. Although patients with urea cycle defects have low levels of carnitine and may be taking L-carnitine as a routine medication, patients should not receive L-carnitine while being treated with Ammonul® because it conjugates and inactivates sodium benzoate. For treatment of seizures, valproic acid should be avoided because it decreases urea cycle activity and may therefore worsen hyperammonemia.

Fatty Acid Oxidation Defects

Disorders include enzyme deficiencies involving metabolism of short, medium, long and very long chain fatty acids and carnitine transport defects. Medium chain acyl-CoA dehydrogenase deficiency is not only the most common fatty acid oxidation defect but also one of the most common IEMs with an incidence of approximately 1 per 10,000. Patients with a fatty acid oxidation defect usually present in infancy between ages 3 months and 2 years due to longer overnight fasts as the infant begins sleeping through the night or due to increased metabolic demand caused by intercurrent illness, often gastroenteritis, recent surgery or, particularly in children and adolescents, vigorous exercise. Hypoglycemia results in catabolism of fatty acids. Accumulation of fatty acid metabolites inhibits gluconeogenesis and has hepatotoxic effects. Initial clinical manifestations of fatty acid oxidation defects may also occur in the neonatal period, childhood, or adulthood. Sibs and even parents of patients with certain fatty acid oxidation defects, particularly medium and short chain acyl-CoA dehydrogenase deficiency and carnitine uptake defect, should be tested even if they have been asymptomatic because severe decompensation, and even death, can occur with the initial crisis. Early manifestations of decompensation may include lethargy, dehydration, vomiting and/or diarrhea, hepatomegaly, and, usually but not always, hypoglycemia with absent or inappropriately low ketones, except in patients with short chain acyl-CoA deficiency who most often produce ketones with hypoglycemia. Decompensation may progress within hours to encephalopathy, coma, cardiac dysfunction, liver dysfunction, hypotonia, seizures, metabolic acidosis, and hyperammonemia. Patients with very long chain acyl-CoA dehydrogenase deficiency or long chain L-3-hydroxyacyl-CoA dehydrogenase deficiency may have exercise-induced rhabdomyolysis. Patients may be normal between episodes of decompensation or may have chronic manifestations of disease that can include failure to thrive, developmental delay, chronic peripheral neuropathy and/or motor deficits (with long chain L-3-hydroxyacyl-CoA dehydrogenase deficiency), retinitis pigmentosa (with glutaric academia type II, also known as multiple acyl-CoA deficiency, carnitine palmatoyl transferase deficiency, and carnitine/acylcarnitine translocase deficiency), and/or dysmorphic facial features. Patients with a fatty acid oxidation defect are at risk for SIDS and cardiac arrest due to hypertrophic cardiomyopathy and/or cardiac arrhythmia. Women who are pregnant with a fetus affected with long chain L-3-hydroxyacyl-CoA dehydrogenase deficiency are at risk for HELLP syndrome.

Laboratory assessment should include electrolytes, BUN, creatinine, blood gas, blood glucose, AST, ALT, alkaline phosphatase, PT, PTT, bilirubin, ammonia, carnitine, creatinine kinase in patients with muscle weakness, and as clinically indicated blood, urine and CSF, to evaluate for infection. Chest x-ray, EKG, and possibly ECHO to evaluate for cardiac failure, cardiomegaly, and/or pericardial effusion are indicated in all patients with long chain L-3-hydroxyacyl-CoA dehydrogenase deficiency and very long chain acyl Co-A dehydrogenase deficiency, as well as any patient with a fatty acid oxidation defect who manifests cardiac dysfunction. Fluids, glucose and acidosis are managed as described for suspected IEM (p. 983–985).

In patients with fatty acid oxidation defects, correction of acidosis and hypoglycemia usually corrects hyperammonemia. Administration of L-carnitine to patients with a fatty acid oxidation defect is controversial because in excess, long chain acylcarnitine may produce cardiac arrhythmias. Use of L-carnitine should be decided on a case-by-case basis based on the recommendation of the metabolic specialist. Underlying physiologic stressors should be treated. Drugs that induce hypoglycemia and epinephrine, which stimulates lipolysis, should be avoided, and if they must given, glucose concentration should be maintained with dextrose. Clinical and laboratory parameters should be monitored until the patient is stabilized and tolerating fluid well. Long term, patients may be on a high-carbohydrate, low-fat diet that includes a complex carbohydrate such as cornstarch to avoid hypoglycemia. Siblings and even parents of patients with a fatty acid oxidation defect, particularly medium or short chain acyl-CoA dehydrogenase deficiency, should be tested, even if they have never had symptoms, but especially if they have a history of "idiopathic cardiomyopathy."

Carbohydrate Disorders

Disorders of Carbohydrate Intolerance

Galactosemia. Classic galactosemia, characterized by less than 1% galactose-1-phosphate uridyltransferase activity, results in clinical symptoms usually within the first week of life, often within the first 2 to 3 days and may be rapidly fatal. Manifestations include poor feeding, vomiting, diarrhea, failure to thrive, bulging fontanelle lethargy that may progress to coma, jaundice and coagulopathy due to liver disease, and/or sepsis, classically with *E. coli*, which may be the initial manifestation. Most newborns will have cataracts although they may only be appreciated by slit lamp examination.

Urine dip will be positive for nonglucose reducing substances, that is, positive Clinitest®, and have negative or trace glucose with glucose oxidase strip, that is, Clinistix® or Glucostix®. CBC will reveal hemolysis. Electrolytes may be remarkable for hyperchloremic metabolic acidosis due to renal tubular dysfunction. LFTs are expected to reveal markedly elevated bilirubin level, initially indirect and after 1 to 2 weeks direct, alkaline phosphate and mild to moderately elevated AST and ALT, and markedly elevated PT and PTT. Given that most patients present as neonates, those with known diagnosis will likely have received the diagnosis based on NBS. Definitive diagnosis requires measurement of erythrocyte enzyme activity, and particularly in patients with less severe presentation, it may reveal more benign forms.

In addition to correction of dehydration, metabolic derangements, and infection, treatment requires complete lifelong exclusion of galactose from the diet. In neonates, breast and cow milk must be replaced with lactose-free soy formula, for example, Nutramigen®, Progestimil®. Even when galactose-free diet is initiated early, those who survive the neonatal period often have developmental delay or learning disabilities.

Disorders of Carbohydrate Production or Utilization

Glycogen storage disorders. Glycogen storage disease type 0 is most likely to present with acute decompensation. Presentation, evaluation, and management are similar to that for fatty acid oxidation defects.

NEONATE WITH POSITIVE NBS

Background

All neonates with a positive NBS require evaluation and confirmatory testing. Those with NBS positive for a condition that may result in decompensation in the neonatal period require emergent evaluation even if they appear to be asymptomatic. Most neonates with a positive NBS will have a false-positive result. To minimize the number of false-negative NBS results, cutoff values have been deliberately set low with a national goal of an overall 0.3% false-positive rate and a 20% positive predictive value. This has resulted in 12 to 60 false positives for every true positive, depending on the IEM. False positives also occur because of maternal IEM, which, in some cases is undiagnosed. Even in the asymptomatic neonate, a false positive cannot be assumed. Evaluation should include history, physical examination, and routine laboratory tests to reveal clinical manifestations of disease or confirm absence of manifestations. In addition, confirmatory testing is required for all neonates with a positive screen. The IEMs most likely to cause acute decompensation in neonates include certain forms of tyrosinemia, organic acidemias, urea cycle defects, galactosemia, and, less commonly, biotinidase deficiency. Manifestations and treatment of these conditions is detailed in the section of this chapter on known IEMs. Patients with NBS positive for congenital adrenal hyperplasia (Chapter 86), considered an endocrine disorder, should also be evaluated emergently. Evaluation and management of neonates with positive NBS should be in consultation with a metabolic specialist, or an endocrinologist in the case of congenital adrenal hyperplasia, guided by NBS condition specific ACTion sheets developed by the American College of Medical Genetics (http://www.acmg.net/resources/policies/ACT/condition-analyte-links.htm), which provide an overview about the condition and information about potential clinical manifestations, and appropriate routine and confirmatory laboratory tests. The sheets also provide links to Web-based disease-specific information and resources. The New England Consortium Web site includes descriptions of some of the diseases (http://www.childrenshospital.org/newenglandconsortium/NBS/Disease_Descriptions.html) and analyte concentrations associated with probable versus possible disease (http://www.childrenshospital.org/newenglandconsortium/NBS/NBS_Protocols.html).

Clinical Manifestations

History

History should focus on details of pregnancy and delivery, including gestational age, complications, medications, exposures, route of delivery, Apgar scores, and complications; medications; family history of affected relatives, stillbirths, SIDS; and postnatal history, including fever, lethargy, feeding, vomiting, diarrhea, jaundice, abnormal movements, and abnormal odors. History may be unremarkable.

Physical Examination

Examination should take note of level of activity, vital signs, temperature, weight, height, head circumference, dysmorphic features, skin color, fontanelle, red reflex, cataracts, heart sounds, perfusion, respiratory distress, abdominal distension, bowel sounds, hepatomegaly, splenomegaly, ambiguous genitalia, cryptorchidism, suck, grasp, Moro, deep tendon reflexes, tone, symmetry, and seizures. Physical examination may be normal.

Studies

Laboratory evaluation should be disease specific. Routine tests may include electrolytes, BUN, creatinine, glucose, ammonia, AST, ALT, bilirubin, PT, PTT, CBC, differential, platelets, blood gas, and as indicated, blood, urine, and CSF to evaluate for infection. Appropriate tests for confirmation of the NBS condition for which the patient is positive should

be sent, even if all routine laboratory tests are normal. In some cases, further testing is limited, at least initially, to repeat NBS, which may include measurement of standard analytes, as well as additional analytes, while in other cases, specialized tests including enzyme assays and/or molecular tests are indicated.

Management

Specifics of management depend not only on the condition for which the patient screened positive but also on the likely variant(s) of that condition, the concentration of the metabolite on NBS interpreted in the context of age at time of screening, and others factors that could modify test results. Cardiopulmonary abnormalities and metabolic derangements must be corrected. Dietary modification, vitamin cofactors, and/or medication may be appropriate and, in many cases, can prevent clinical manifestations. Patients with any abnormality should, in most cases, be admitted to the hospital. For patients who are discharged, a plan for very close follow-up and genetic counseling, even though confirmatory testing may rule out true disease, should be established.

SUMMARY

Collectively IEMs are not rare, and clinical manifestations are often nonspecific. Therefore, a high index of suspicion is essential for diagnosis. A few routine tests will serve as an informative screen for most IEMs. Evaluation and treatment of patients with known IEM should be disease specific. All neonates with positive NBS, even if asymptomatic, require evaluation and confirmatory testing, and if at risk for acute decompensation emergent initiation of treatment. Rapid initiation of appropriate treatment for patients with suspected or known IEM or positive NBS may not only be lifesaving but is also critical for optimizing long-term outcome.

Suggested Readings

ACMG Newborn Screening Work Group; Metabolic Disorders. Newborn screening ACT sheets and confirmatory algorithms. http://www.acmg.net/resources/policies/ACT/condition-analyte-links.htm. Accessed January 30, 2009.[a]

Acute Illness Protocols. New England Consortium of Metabolic Programs at Children's Hospital Boston. http://www.childrenshospital.org/newengland-consortium/NBS/Emergency_Protocols.html. Accessed January 30, 2009.[a]

Arn PH, Valle DL, Brusilow SW. Inborn errors of metabolism: not rare, not hopeless. *Contemp Pediatr* 1988;5:47–63.

Blau N, Duran M, Gibson KM, et al., eds. *Physicians guide to the laboratory diagnosis of metabolic diseases*, 2nd ed. Heidelberg, Germany: Springer, 2002.

Burton BK. Inborn errors of metabolism in infancy: a guide to diagnosis. *Pediatrics* 1998;102(6):E69.

Calvo M, Artuch R, Macia E, et al. Diagnostic approach to inborn errors of metabolism in an emergency unit. *Pediatr Emerg Care* 2000;16(6):405–408.

Chace DH, Kalas TA, Naylor EW. Use of tandem mass spectrometry for multianalyte screening of dried blood specimens from newborns. *Clin Chem* 2003;49(11):1797–1817.

Chow SL, Gandhi V, Krywawych S, et al. The significance of a high plasma ammonia value. *Arch Dis Child* 2004;89(6):585–586.

Clarke JTR. *A clinical guide to inherited metabolic diseases,* 2nd ed. Cambridge, United Kingdom: Cambridge University Press, 2002.

Enns GM, Packman S. Diagnosing inborn errors of metabolism in the newborn: clinical features. *Neoreviews* 2001;2:e183–e190.

Fernandes J, Saudubray JM, Van den Berghe G, et al. *Inborn metabolic diseases: diagnosis and treatment*, 4th ed. Heidelberg, Germany: Springer Medizin Verlag, 2006.

Garganta CL, Smith WE. Metabolic evaluation of the sick neonate. *Semin Perinatol* 2005;29(3):164–172.

Goodman SI. Inherited metabolic disease in the newborn: approach to diagnosis and treatment. *Adv Pediatr* 1986;33:197–223.

Hoffman GF, Nyhan WL, Zschocke J. *Inherited metabolic diseases*. Philadelphia, PA: Lippincott Williams & Wilkins, 2002.

James PM, Levy HL. The clinical aspects of newborn screening: importance of newborn screening follow-up. *Ment Retard Dev Disabil Res Rev* 2006;12:246–254.

Kwon KT, Tsai VW. Metabolic emergencies. *Emerg Med Clin North Am* 2007;25(4):1041–1060, vi.

Marsden D, Larson C, Levy HL. Newborn screening for metabolic disorders. *J Pediatr* 2006;148(5):577–584.

McKusik VA. OMIM Online Mendelian Inheritance in Man [database online]. http://www.ncbi.nlm.nih.gov/omim. Accessed January 30, 2009.[a]

National Newborn Screening and Genetics Resource Center. United States table of newborn screening tests performed by state. http://genes-rus.uthscsa.edu/nbsdisorders.pdf. Canadian table of newborn screening tests performed by province and territory. http://genes-r-us.uthscsa.edu/nbsdisorders.pdf. Accessed January 30, 2009.[a]

Pagon RA. Gene Tests. http://www.ncbi.nlm.nih.gov/sites/GeneTests/?db=GeneTests Accessed November 10, 2009.

Rinaldo P, Zafari S, Tortorelli S, et al. Making the case for objective performance metrics in newborn screening by tandem mass spectrometry. *Ment Retard Dev Disabil Res Rev* 2006;12(4):255–261.

Scriver CR, Sly WS, Barton C, et al., eds. *The metabolic and molecular basis of inherited disease*, 8th ed. New York, NY: McGraw-Hill, 2001.

Seashore MR, Wappner RS. *Genetics in primary care and clinical medicine*. Stamford, CT: Appleton & Lange, 1996.

Soldin JS, Rifai N, Hicks J. *Biochemical basis of pediatric disease*, 2nd ed. Washington, DC: AACC Press, 1995.

Summar M. Current strategies for the management of neonatal urea cycle disorders. *J Pediatr* 2001;138:S30–S39.

The Urea Cycle Disorders Conference Group. Consensus statement from a conference for the management of patients with urea cycle disorders. *J Pediatr* 2001;138:S1–S5.

Waisbren SE. Expanded newborn screening: information and resources for the family physician. *Am Fam Physician*. 2008;77:987–994.

Ward JC. Inborn errors of metabolism of acute onset in infancy. *Pediatr Rev* 1990;11(7):205–216.

Weinstein DA, Butte AJ, Raymond K. High incidence of unrecognized metabolic and endocrinologic disorders in acutely ill children with previously unrecognized hypoglycemia. *Pediatr Res* 2001;49:103A#578.

[a]Consider adding these URLs as bookmarks on computers where this information is needed.

MEDICAL EMERGENCIES

CHAPTER 95 ■ PROBLEMS IN THE EARLY NEONATAL PERIOD

AMEER P. MODY, MD, MPH, AND BENJAMIN K. SILVERMAN, MD

INTRODUCTION

The evaluation and treatment of newborn infants in the emergency department (ED) setting can be an anxiety-provoking experience for all parties involved. Emergency physicians must be able to not only manage serious neonatal concerns, such as possible sepsis, complications of congenital heart disease, and bowel obstruction but also identify and manage variations in newborn physiology and behavior, such as jaundice and feeding problems (Table 95.1). This chapter serves as a guide to evaluating and managing the parents' concerns in the ED during the first week to 10 days with their new baby.

Many of the problems will be insignificant and can be dealt with by judicious reassurance, but it must be kept in mind that seriously ill newborns may present with only subtle, nondescript symptoms. The parents' expressed complaint may be only a clue to a serious problem far removed from their area of concern; so, a relevant perinatal history should be queried and, in most instances, a thorough physical examination performed.

The chapter is structured to allow the physician quick access to the complaint that precipitated the emergency visit. For conciseness and for easier access to information, the description of the presenting complaints is divided into subsections, based on physical, behavioral, and etiologic concerns. In most subsections, there is a delineation of those findings that are normal variants, those that might need further evaluation, and those that call for immediate attention. References are made to other chapters in this book where the more complicated problems are discussed in greater detail.

HISTORY

The emergency physician must be able to elicit relevant information needed to make decisions regarding diagnosis and management within a relatively short period. Time constraints, level of acuity within the ED, and the absence of long-term relationships can make communication in this setting particularly challenging. In the newborn period, not only is it essential to evaluate the health and physiologic stability of the baby, but often it is equally important to assess the psychosocial, emotional, and physical well-being of the caretaker; the ability and confidence in caring for the baby; the adequacy of support systems for the mother and family; and the access to follow-up care.

Because current concerns may have their origins in issues related to pregnancy or parturition, knowledge of the immediate history, a review of the events of labor and delivery, history of prior and current pregnancies, and a review of the family history are all essential components of the newborn history. Neonatal mortality is defined as the death of an infant between birth and 1 month of age. The leading causes of neonatal mortality—congenital anomalies, disorders related to short gestation and low birth weight, respiratory distress syndrome, and maternal complications of pregnancy—all have an association with pregnancy or parturition. Disclosure or identification of certain maternal, pregnancy, or infant-related factors (Table 95.2) may place the newborn at increased risk and should alert the practitioner to the potential for morbidity and mortality.

Certain points should be included in the history of all newborn infants, regardless of the presenting complaint. Always query regarding the infant's birth weight and gestational age because size of an infant at birth does not necessarily reflect gestational age. An infant who is born "small for gestational age" (SGA) or with "intrauterine growth retardation" (IUGR) is at higher risk for morbidity and mortality than an infant of the same gestational age who is "appropriate for gestational age" (AGA). An infant whose birth weight is below the 10th percentile for gestational age is SGA. SGA infants have a more than fourfold increase in perinatal mortality than AGA infants of the same gestational age. Conversely, an infant whose birth weight is above the 90th percentile for gestational age is "large for gestational age" (LGA). The most common causes for LGA infants are familial, infants of diabetic mothers, and overgrowth syndromes such as the Beckwith–Wiedemann syndrome. Hypoglycemia, hyperbilirubinemia, hypocalcemia, and polycythemia are all associated acute complications that may be seen in the macrosomic infant.

The clinician should inquire regarding the infant's general level of alertness, diet, and elimination patterns. Inadequate alimentation or infrequent urination may be clues to more serious problems. Parental concern about excessive crying or inability to soothe their infant requires attention because this excessive fussiness may have an underlying organic origin (see Chapter 16). Nonspecific complaints such as increased crying, sleepiness, and decreased appetite are sometimes the only symptoms of serious illness in the newborn.

More recently, there has arisen concern regarding the increasing number of infants delivered "near term" (late preterm). This refers primarily to infants who are scheduled to deliver by induction or by caesarian section 1 to 4 weeks before term (36- to 39-week gestation). Although not quantified, these infants are at increased risk for all potential problems in the

TABLE 95.1

FREQUENT PRESENTING COMPLAINTS AND FREQUENT DIAGNOSES OF NEWBORNS YOUNGER THAN 8 DAYS PRESENTING TO THE EMERGENCY DEPARTMENT

Most Frequent Presenting Complaints
Jaundice
Difficulty breathing
Feeding problem
Irritability
Abnormal bowel movement frequency
Lethargy

Most Frequent Diagnoses
Normal newborn
Jaundice
Feeding problem
Query sepsis
Dehydration

Adapted from Millar KR, Gloor JE, Wellington N, et al. Early neonatal presentations to the pediatric emergency department. *Pediatr Emerg Care* 2000;16:145–150.

TABLE 95.2

HIGH-RISK FACTORS FOR NEONATAL MORBIDITY AND MORTALITY

Demographic/Socioeconomic
Teenage pregnancy or advanced maternal age (age <16 or >40 yr)
Alcohol, tobacco, or illicit drug use
Poverty

Previous Pregnancies
History of prematurity, intrauterine fetal demise, or neonatal death
Previous infants with congenital malformations
Rh or other blood group sensitization

Current Pregnancy
Lack of prenatal care
Preexisting medical conditions: diabetes, hypertension, thyroid diseases, systemic lupus erythematosus
Gestational complications: preeclampsia, gestational diabetes, vaginal bleeding, multiple gestation
Infectious diseases: sexually transmitted diseases, HIV infection, group B streptococcal colonization of the cervix, TORCHES infections
History of alcohol, tobacco, or illicit drug use

Delivery/Intrapartum
Predates or postdates delivery (<37 wk or >42 wk)
Prolonged rupture of membranes
Meconium-stained amniotic fluid
Nuchal cord
Delivery: cesarean section, forceps delivery, breech presentation
Low Apgar scores

Newborn
Low birth weight (weight <2,500 g)
LGA (large for gestational age)
IUGR (intrauterine growth retardation)/SGA (small for gestational age)
Birth asphyxia
Congenital malformations
Prolonged neonatal jaundice
Prolonged hospitalization
Apnea
History of poor weight gain

HIV, human immunodeficiency virus; TORCHES, toxoplasmosis, rubella, cytomegalovirus, herpes virus, syphilis.

early neonatal period, including significant jaundice, respiratory problems, and feeding difficulties. Many of these infants are presenting to the ED with a variety of respiratory and neurological and feeding difficulties related to their immaturity.

Additional history should be guided by and focused specifically on the presenting complaint. Relevant historical suggestions are included in each of the "presenting complaint" subsections.

VITAL SIGNS

Growth

Weight gain serves as an important indicator of general well-being during the newborn period. Failure of a newborn to gain weight appropriately may be a sign of underfeeding or significant underlying illnesses such as heart disease, metabolic problems, or malabsorption. Weight gain, according to age-specific norms, can be one of the best indicators that the infant is well, despite nondescript symptoms, such as fussiness. Weight at presentation should be quantified as accurately as possible, preferably unclothed.

The average newborn infant weighs **3,400 g (7 lb, 8 oz)**, is **about 50 cm (20 in.)**, and has a head circumference of **35 cm (14 in.)**. The newborn will lose about 5% to 10% of his or her birth weight during the first several days of life and then regain this weight by 10 to 14 days of age. Typically, formula-fed infants will return to their birth weight before breast-fed infants. Thereafter, the newborn should gain about 25 to 35 g per day (roughly 1% of the birth weight per day). **The average newborn takes 60 to 90 mL (2 to 3 oz) of formula (the equivalent of about 10 minutes on each breast) every 2 to 3 hours. Elimination increases with each day of life to an average of 10 to 12 wet diapers and one to three bowel movements per day (as often as once after each feeding for breast-fed infants).** Because breast milk is easier to digest and passes out of the stomach quicker than formula (on average 1.5 hours vs. up to 4 hours for formula), the breast-fed infant will want to feed more frequently, with an increased number of nighttime feedings as well.

Temperature

The young infant's immature autonomic thermoregulatory responses, larger body surface area to mass ratio, immature sweating response, and limited ability to move away from or modify adverse environments all limit his or her thermoregulatory ability. Temperature instability, either *hypothermia* or *hyperthermia,* may be the only sign of significant infectious illness. It is unusual to see high temperatures in the newborn.

Even a septic newborn may develop only a slight elevation in temperature or will present with hypothermia. Therefore, any temperature higher than 38°C (100.4°F) should be regarded as a fever in the newborn and receive appropriate evaluation (see Chapters 27 and 92). A rectal temperature is the preferred method of temperature determination. The use of warm blankets or warming lights during evaluation and treatment of vulnerable infants can be helpful in avoiding iatrogenic hypothermia.

Heart Rate (See Chapter 84)

Normal resting heart rate is between 120 to 160 beats per min. It varies with respiration (increasing with inspiration) and activity (increasing significantly with crying and appreciably slowing during sleep). Cardiac output in the infant is primarily increased by increasing the heart rate rather than stroke volume. Sinus *tachycardia* (heart rate more than 180 beats per min) is a common response to many types of stress, such as pain, hypovolemia, fever, or cardiac disease (see Chapter 74). *Sinus tachycardia* may be differentiated from *paroxysmal supraventricular tachycardia (SVT)* (see Chapter 84) when the electrocardiogram (EKG) demonstrates a narrow QRS complex tachycardia with a P wave preceding each QRS complex. SVT is usually associated with a more rapid heart rate (usually more than 220 beats per min) than is sinus tachycardia and the P wave may be obscured or absent. SVT is commonly a fixed tachycardia, whereas the heart rate in sinus tachycardia will vary with crying or manipulation (beat to beat variability). Infants may tolerate SVT for a variable period, but eventually they develop irritability, tachypnea, poor feeding, and poor perfusion. The development of *bradycardia* (heart rate less than 80 beats per min) usually signals the presence of significant cardiorespiratory compromise and is an ominous sign that requires immediate attention (see Chapters 2 and 3).

Respiratory Rate

Normal resting respiratory rate is usually between 40 to 60 breaths per min. During sleep, most newborn infants will exhibit some degree of *periodic breathing*, in which normal respiration is interrupted with short pauses. This breathing pattern is especially common in premature infants. Periodic breathing must be differentiated from *pathologic apnea* (see Chapter 9).

In the simplest of terms, *apnea* is an absence of respiration that can have a central, obstructive, or mixed cause. Short periods of central apnea (less than 15 seconds) can be normal at all ages. However, pathologic apnea is a prolonged respiratory pause (more than 20 seconds) or a shorter pause associated with cyanosis, pallor, bradycardia, or hypotonia. Underlying disorders that must be considered in the evaluation of the apneic infant, include septicemia, severe anemia, intracranial hemorrhage, seizures, central hypoventilation, gastroesophageal reflux, metabolic disturbances such as hypoglycemia, and infant or maternal ingestion of narcotics or other central nervous system (CNS) depressants. The occurrence of apnea due to any of the above causes may result in an apparent life-threatening event.

Varying degrees of *expiratory grunting, chest retractions, nasal flaring, crackles,* or *rales* are all signs of respiratory distress in the newborn. In addition to a primary pulmonary cause, respiratory distress in the newborn can also be a presenting sign of *congestive heart failure.* Among term infants, especially those born by cesarean section, a common cause of respiratory distress presenting within the first 24 hours, usually beginning between 2 and 6 hours after birth, is *transient tachypnea of the newborn* (TTN). TTN is believed to be caused by a delay in the resorption of the normal fetal lung fluid. The differential diagnosis of TTN includes meconium aspiration pneumonitis, respiratory distress syndrome (less likely in the term newborn), pneumonia, and bronchiolitis. Symptoms of TTN typically resolve within 72 hours.

Blood Pressure

Normal systolic blood pressure in the term newborn after the first few days of life ranges between 60 and 90 mm Hg. Blood pressure may be lower during the first few days of life and in premature infants is related to weight and gestational age. Congenital renal abnormalities, renal tumors, and complications of umbilical artery catheters are some of the more common causes of *hypertension* (see Chapter 34) in the neonatal period. *Coarctation of the aorta* may be diagnosed by the combination of increased upper-extremity blood pressure, with lowered blood pressure or diminished pulses in the lower extremities.

Pulse Oximetry

Pulse oximetry measures the degree of oxygen-saturated hemoglobin in the arterial circulation and is an indirect measure of the partial pressure of arterial oxygen. It should be measured in any neonate in whom there is suggestion of respiratory distress, is febrile, appears cyanotic, is mottled, or has unusual cardiac or CNS findings. Normal pulse oximetry reading should be between 94% and 100%. Decreased oxygen saturation can indicate a wide variety of pathologies including sepsis, respiratory conditions, or cardiac disease in neonates.

COLOR CHANGES

Normal Variants

Racial and ethnic factors may result in variation of the baby's skin color. Comparison of the baby's color with the parents' pigmentation may offer assurances that the baby's color is appropriately normal. The skin of a normal Caucasian early neonate is a pink, flushed color. This in itself may be a cause for alarm to some parents but can be dismissed with reassurance if the remainder of the history and physical examination is not remarkable. A hemoglobin or hematocrit determination offers assurance that the baby is not abnormally polycythemic.

Alterations of the appearance to blue, deep yellow, orange, or pale may precipitate an ED visit. Evaluation and management of these changes are discussed here.

Cyanosis/Acrocyanosis (See Chapter 15)

The presenting complaint may be that "the baby is blue." Relevant questions to be asked include the following: When was the blueness first noted? Is it persistent or does it come and go? Does it involve all of the body or only the distal extremities and lips? Does it increase or lessen with crying or feeding? Is there emesis or diarrhea?

Physical examination should be complete. The distribution of the blueness should be carefully noted; particularly, check the color of the tongue. Does the intensity of the blueness decrease or increase with crying or with effort? Are the vital signs normal for a neonate? Is the baby responsive to stimulation? Is mottling present? Is there a cardiac murmur? Are respirations labored? Are the lungs clear? Is the liver enlarged? Are the femoral pulsations palpable?

The degree of cyanosis should be documented by pulse oximetry. The more likely causes are discussed in the following sections.

Acrocyanosis

An otherwise healthy baby with acrocyanosis appears cyanotic only in the hands, feet, and lips. The tongue is pink; pulse oximetry is normal. The transient color change may be associated with cool ambient temperature. Parent(s) should be reassured that the acrocyanosis is self-limited.

Cyanotic Congenital Heart Disease (See Chapters 15, 32, and 84)

Cyanosis is diffusely distributed and increases with crying. Pulse oximetry shows diminished saturation at rest, worsening with crying; cyanosis responds only minimally to oxygen therapy. A cardiac murmur is usually, but not necessarily, present. EKG, chest radiography, and echocardiography, if accessible, should be performed. Neonates with cyanotic heart disease only rarely go into cardiac failure, but lesions associated with obstructed pulmonary or systemic flow may cause extreme hypoxemia and shock. Consideration should be given to maintaining ductal patency with prostaglandin E1 (0.1 μg per kg per min), if cardiac consultation is not immediately available, with the knowledge that prostaglandin E1 infusions can result in apnea requiring intubation and airway management. Very early neonates with a strong suspicion of cyanotic cardiac defect should be admitted or transferred to an appropriate facility if cardiac consultation is not readily available and definitive diagnosis is uncertain.

Congestive Cardiac Failure (See Chapters 32 and 84)

Cyanosis is diffusely distributed, and pulse oximetry shows desaturation but improves somewhat with oxygenation. The infant is tachypneic, with or without increased respiratory effort. Rales may be apparent in lung fields. Cardiac murmur may be present or femoral pulsations may be absent. The liver is enlarged. Chest radiography and echocardiography should be performed, if available. If there is suggestion of obstructed systemic flow, consideration should be given to maintaining ductal patency with prostaglandin E1. Emergency treatment and admission are indicated.

Respiratory Distress (See Chapters 15, 68, and 98)

Respiratory disease is associated with tachypnea, noisy respirations, and possibly retractions. Pulse oximetry shows desaturation but usually improves significantly with rest, crying, and oxygenation. The clinician should think of respiratory infection or congenital intrathoracic defect. A chest radiograph should be obtained. After appropriate emergency treatment, the patient should be admitted. Laryngomalacia or tracheomalacia may simulate respiratory distress with noisy respirations originating in the upper airway, but oxygen saturation and chest radiographs are normal. If laryngomalacia is present, prone position across the examiner's arm will resolve the distress and/or stridor and can assist in making the diagnosis.

Primary Pulmonary Hypertension of the Newborn (PPHN)

This entity is becoming increasingly recognized in the cyanotic neonate with respiratory distress. It is more common in the larger baby, particularly the large postmature baby. The constriction of the pulmonary arterial vasculature results in hypertension of the right heart. This in turn causes right-to-left shunting of unoxygenated blood through the patent ductus or foramen ovale, resulting in hypoxia and severe cyanosis, not responding to oxygenation. When pulse oximetry readings are taken separately in each of the four extremities, oxygenation will be about 10% higher in the right arm, the preductal extremity. Aggressive treatment of PPHN, including extracorporeal membrane oxygenation, may be life-saving.

Hypovolemia, Acidosis, and Shock (See Chapters 3 and 70)

Hypovolemia, acidosis, and shock are characterized by cyanosis accompanied by mottling in an extremely lethargic, hypotonic baby with marked tachycardia and possibly hypotension. Pulse oximetry is desaturated. After appropriate emergency workup, including early treatment with hydrating parenteral fluids, the patient should be admitted.

Methemoglobinemia (See Chapter 102)

Methemoglobinemia is characterized by a cyanotic-appearing infant without underlying cardiac or pulmonary disease. The infant will look diffusely cyanotic to gray in color, with a factitiously almost normal-appearing pulse oximetry reading 85% or more. Supplemental oxygen also will not alter the color (an indication that the cyanosis is not from a primary pulmonary process). Acquired methemoglobinemia in infants is most commonly associated with diarrheal illnesses and dehydration. Methemoglobinemia may be confirmed by venous or capillary blood gas sampling or by the persistent chocolate-brown color of a drop of blood on filter paper. Volume resuscitation should first be initiated in infants with normal saline and dextrose.

If the methemoglobinemia persists, a dose of 1 mg per kg of methylene blue, should be considered. An infant with methemoglobinemia should be admitted.

Blue Sclerae

Blue color confined to the sclerae may be associated with osteogenesis imperfecta. The neonate's sclerae commonly may be normally blue although the intensity is less. If in doubt, the clinician should take a careful family history and examine for fractures of the extremities, ribs, and pelvis.

Jaundice (See Chapters 40, 41)

The parent may be concerned because the newborn appears yellow or orange. Because this may be a normal variant in Pacific rim or Native American racial or ethnic groups, the parents' coloring should be compared with the baby's.

Bilirubin is formed by the catabolism of hemoglobin and may accumulate when there is excessive hemolysis, failure of conjugation with glucuronic acid in the liver, or inadequate excretion through the liver canaliculi or the bile ducts. Bilirubin that has not been conjugated in the liver, tests as indirect and is related to excessive hemolysis of red cells; conjugated bilirubin is reported as direct and is elevated when excretion is obstructed.

If jaundice is identified, relevant questions to be asked should include the following: When was the jaundice first noticed? What is the color of stools and urine? What type of feeding is being used (breast or formula)? Are feedings adequate? What are the mother's and baby's blood types, if known? Has the infant vomited? Is there a family history of jaundice? Is the mother diabetic?

The most precise clinical method for determining whether the color change is truly jaundice is by examining the sclerae—yellow color of the sclerae is jaundice. A complete physical examination should be performed, with emphasis on vital signs, intensity and distribution of icterus, presence of cephalohematoma, or hepatosplenomegaly.

The intensity of jaundice is determined by the level of bilirubin in the blood and by its distribution. As a rule, jaundice is not discernible in infants at levels less than 5 mg per dL. Jaundice is usually first discerned in the face and becomes more obvious caudally as the total serum bilirubin (TSB) level increases. In each patient, a TSB level and a complete blood cell count (CBC) with blood smear should be performed. If subsequent TSB levels are indicated in the baby, the direct bilirubin level should be determined at least once.

Physiologic Jaundice (See Chapter 40)

Physiologic jaundice is icterus that is not pathologic. Discernible jaundice in the first 24 hours of life of a healthy term newborn is probably pathologic, so a cause must be sought and therapy inaugurated. Beyond the first day, however, if the CBC and smear are not abnormal and the physical examination is not remarkable, a degree of jaundice not exceeding the published standard can be assumed to be physiologic. Infants of diabetic mothers and babies with congenital hypothyroidism or those with resorption from large cephalohematomata may have higher levels of icterus than one would expect physiologically.

Management and disposition can be governed by the recommendations in Table 104.3 and will vary with the baby's age and the bilirubin level. Babies with TSB nearing the levels at which therapy is suggested should be followed with at least one repeat determination within 24 hours to get a sense of the rate of rise.

Breast Milk Jaundice (See Chapter 40)

In breastfed babies, jaundice may arise early because of inadequate caloric intake and the dehydration that may occur before there is sufficient milk. Later onset of jaundice associated with breast-feeding occurs for unknown reasons, probably related to undiscovered hormonal changes or excessive reuptake from the gastrointestinal tract. If TSB is not approaching levels at which phototherapy needs to be considered, breast-feeding should be continued and even encouraged more frequently. Higher TSB levels should be followed with at least one additional determination.

Blood Type Incompatibility (See Chapters 40 and 91)

If the TSB level is at or near levels requiring therapy (Table 95.3) and particularly if the jaundiced baby has a lower hemoglobin than expected, direct Coombs' test should be conducted. Mother and baby should be blood-typed for ABO and Rh factors. If there is an incompatibility and if the bilirubin is rising rapidly despite phototherapy, blood should be prepared for possible exchange transfusion. Rh incompatibility is uncommon in those mothers who have had ongoing obstetric care. ABO incompatibility is usually more insidious in onset

TABLE 95.3

MANAGEMENT OF HYPERBILIRUBINEMIA IN THE HEALTHY TERM INFANT ACCORDING TO TSB AND BABY'S AGE[a]

Age (h)	Initiate phototherapy[b] (mg/dL)	Exchange transfusion if intensive phototherapy fails[c] (mg/dL)
<25	8–10	17–20
25–48	12–15	19–22
49–72	17–19	22–25
>72	20–21	25

TSB, total serum bilirubin.

[a]These guidelines apply to well neonates of gestational age equal to or more than 35 weeks. The lower ends of the above TSB ranges apply to the youngest in each age range.

[b]Lower bilirubin levels than the above would warrant initiation of phototherapy in infants who have any of the following risk factors: shorter gestation, isoimmune hemolytic disease, glucose-6-phosphate dehydrogenase deficiency, asphyxia, significant ● lethargy, respiratory distress, temperature instability, sepsis, acidosis, or albumin level higher than 3.0 g per dL. Consult neonatology and/or hematology regarding possible need for exchange transfusion or alternative therapy if levels significantly exceed these numbers or if the bilirubin is predominately conjugated (direct).

[c]Intensive phototherapy should produce a decline of TSB of 1 to 2 mg per dL within 4 to 6 hours, and the TSB level should continue to fall and remain below the threshold level for exchange transfusion. If this does not occur, it is considered a failure of phototherapy.

Adapted from American Academy of Pediatrics, Subcommittee on Neonatal Hyperbilirubinemia. Management of hyperbilirubinemia in the newborn infant 35 or more weeks of gestation. *Pediatrics* 2004;114:297–316.

and less severe than Rh. Other minor red cell incompatibilities may also result in hyperbilirubinemia.

Sepsis (See Chapters 70 and 92)

Sepsis need not be a consideration in the alert, well-appearing, jaundiced newborn. If the jaundiced baby is lethargic or extremely irritable, hypotonic, febrile, or excessively tachycardiac and has been feeding poorly, sepsis and/or urinary tract infection should be considered. The bilirubin may be indirect or direct.

Congenital Red Cell Defects (See Chapters 40 and 92)

Careful examination of the blood smear may provide a clue to red cell membrane defects. These babies may have indirect bilirubinemia and anemia and may have a positive family history for spherocytosis or elliptocytosis. More severe forms of glucose-6-phosphate dehydrogenase deficiency also may present with early jaundice and anemia, especially if the mother has received possibly precipitating drugs during late pregnancy. Elevated reticulocytes with a negative Coombs' test would heighten suspicion.

Other Congenital Problems (See Chapters 40 and 41)

The group of congenital infections that falls under the acronym of TORCHES (toxoplasmosis, rubella, cytomegalovirus, herpes virus, syphilis) may present with jaundice. These should be thought of in the baby with elevated direct bilirubin who presents with microcephaly, jitteriness, seizures, organomegaly, or petechiae. Elevated direct bilirubin also may be an early manifestation of galactosemia and cystic fibrosis.

Babies with the severe form of congenital glucuronyl transferase deficiency defined as Crigler–Najjar syndrome may present with extremely high levels of unconjugated bilirubin, which may rise despite phototherapy. This defect is mostly confined to geographical areas where conjugal-related marriage is more common.

The presence of gray-colored (acholic) stool and/or direct hyperbilirubinemia should raise the concern for obstructive jaundice. The differential diagnosis includes extrahepatic biliary atresia, intrahepatic biliary atresia (Alagille's syndrome), hepatitis secondary to TORCHES infections, or metabolic disorders. The presence of extrahepatic biliary atresia necessitates immediate admission or transfer to a specialty pediatric center for definitive management.

Pallor

The neonate may be brought to the physician because the neonate appears pale to the parents. A careful history and physical examination should be conducted to consider the possibilities of septic or cardiogenic shock, severe chemical or electrolyte imbalance, or significant anemia.

Questions should be asked regarding the mother's perinatal history, the baby's suck and feeding, the occurrence of vomiting or diarrhea, fever, and the baby's responsiveness. Physical examination should include a thorough evaluation of the vital signs. Is the baby extremely lethargic? The clinician should look at the inner palpebral conjunctivae and check the skin for petechiae or rashes. Is there a large cephalohematoma? Is there hepatosplenomegaly?

A CBC should be conducted and consideration given to a stat glucose and electrolyte panel and TSB level. Normal levels at this age for hemoglobin are in the range of 13 to 20 g per dL with a mean of 16 g per dL; for hematocrit, 42% to 65%, with a mean of 50%. Diagnostic considerations include the topics discussed in the following sections.

Fair Complexion

If the vital signs and the physical examination are normal and the CBC does not indicate anemia, the presenting concern probably relates to the baby's normal fair-skinned coloring. Offer appropriate explanation and discharge home.

Anemia (See Chapters 58 and 91)

Anemia in the neonate is not usually recognized as pallor until the hemoglobin level falls below 10 g per dL. It is most commonly, but not always, related to excessive hemolysis of the red cells and often is accompanied by jaundice. Possible etiologies might include the following:

- *Hemolytic disease of the newborn:* Complete maternal and neonate blood typing should be performed, as well as a Coombs' test. Depending on the degree of anemia and the baby's functional status, crossmatching for possible packed cell or exchange transfusion should be initiated.
- *Congenital erythrocyte membrane defects:* These defects can usually be suggested by careful evaluation of the blood smear.
- *Malignancy:* Congenital leukemia is a rare entity that should be discernible on the blood smear.
- *Congenital and aplastic anemias:* Diamond–Blackfan syndrome, transient erythroblastopenia of childhood, sickle cell disease, and Fanconi's syndrome do not usually manifest in the very early neonatal period.
- *Blood loss:* Blood loss can occur through the gastrointestinal tract (Meckel's diverticula; bleeding disorder) and should be suspected if a stool is positive for gross blood. Imaging evaluation is indicated. Significant blood loss can also occur into a large cephalohematoma or an intracranial hemorrhage in an infant.
- *Disseminated intravascular coagulopathy (DIC):* DIC may occur in association with bacterial sepsis, viremia (especially herpes simplex), and shock, accompanied by petechiae and purpura. Platelet count is significantly diminished in these ill children. Evaluation is directed at finding a cause and therapy at replacing deficient elements (see Chapters 3, 65, and 91).

Ill Children (See Chapter 3)

Pallor may be the most striking presenting complaint in the neonate who is ill. Children in septic or cardiogenic shock may appear pale because of poor perfusion, without necessarily being anemic. Hypoglycemic infants and those with severe electrolyte disturbances may also present with pallor. Rapid diagnosis and emergency administration of glucose and volume restoration are essential.

Mottling

Mottling in the neonate is the patchy appearance of the body surface, resulting from prominent dilation of the superficial

MEDICAL EMERGENCIES

veins showing through the thin skin and causing a mosaic-like, patchy appearance. Mottling may be a normal variant when it appears in an otherwise normal baby, undressed in a cool ambient temperature. It is more likely to appear in a preterm baby with thin skin.

However, mottling can be an ominous diagnostic sign in a neonate. It may be indicative of hypovolemia and poor perfusion in a baby in shock or a septic baby. A careful history and complete physical examination with cautious evaluation of the vital signs need to be done. If there is doubt about the baby's status, a CBC, an electrolyte panel, and stat glucose should be drawn. Treatment of the underlying cause and restoration of hemodynamic stability should be inaugurated in the ED.

SKIN FINDINGS

The quality of the newborn's skin varies with the gestational age. The premature infant's thin, almost-translucent skin is in sharp contrast to the dry, cracked, peeling skin of the postterm infant. The term infant's skin is usually pale pink in color, with some diffuse superficial peeling noted at several days of age. Normal peeling of the superficial layers of the skin should be differentiated from the full-thickness skin loss that is associated with *staphylococcal scalded skin syndrome*. *Excoriations* when noted in an irritable or jittery infant, especially when they are located primarily on the nose or knees, may be a sign of withdrawal in an infant exposed to narcotics prenatally.

Seborrheic dermatitis (see Chapter 85) is a localized scaling or crusting eruption that most commonly involves the scalp (cradle cap), forehead, and area behind the ears. Occasionally, the diaper area may be involved. The eruption may have a greasy appearance and the lesions are generally nonpruritic.

Hair

Soft, downy, fine body hair, lanugo, located primarily on the back and shoulders, is a normal finding. However, a tuft of coarse, dark hair located in the midline lumbosacral region may be associated with spina bifida occulta.

Papular Rashes (See Chapters 63, 64, 65)

A variety of papular rashes may be observed in the healthy newborn. Characteristic body distribution patterns and age at appearance of these typical rashes may help differentiate them from more worrisome conditions.

Milia are small 1 to 2 mm ivory or yellow papules located primarily on the forehead, nose, and cheeks of the newborn. Milia are keratin retention cysts that require no treatment because they will spontaneously rupture and disappear during the first 3 to 4 weeks of life.

Erythema toxicum is a more generalized eruption of small papules or pustules on an erythematous base that may occur anywhere on the body. Usually presenting during the first 3 to 4 days of life, these lesions may be noted as late as 2 weeks of age. *Herpes simplex* infections, although usually vesicular (see below), and *impetigo*, usually pustular or crusted, may be entertained in the differential diagnosis of this eruption. If the diagnosis of erythema toxicum is in question, a smear of the papular contents will show a predominance of eosinophils, with a relative absence of neutrophils and no organisms.

Erythematous papules or pustules (rarely comedones) confined primarily to the cheeks, chin, and forehead are characteristic of *neonatal acne*. Lesions are secondary to the influence of circulating maternal hormones and usually appear at 3 to 4 weeks of age and disappear within a few weeks.

Vesicular Rashes (See Chapter 67)

The most important condition to consider when evaluating a vesicular eruption is a herpes simplex virus (HSV) infection because it has the most significant associated morbidity and mortality. Most neonatal *HSV infections* are caused by HSV type 2, although either type 1 or type 2 may be implicated. Although transplacental transmission of HSV can occur, the vast majority of neonatal disease is acquired from infection of the maternal genitourinary tract. Primary maternal infection at the time of delivery is associated with a 40% to 50% risk of disease transmission to the newborn, whereas recurrent maternal disease has a much lower risk of transmission (less than 5%). Therefore, most infected newborns are from mothers that are unaware of their own HSV infection. Clinical disease in the newborn includes (1) localized infection of skin, eyes, and mouth; (2) infection of the CNS with fever, seizures, and alteration of consciousness; or (3) disseminated viremia with multisystem involvement and shock. The infant generally appears well at birth but then becomes ill at any time from day 2 of life to day 28 (usually between days 4 and 7), at which time a vesicular eruption may be noted. Unfortunately, not all HSV-infected infants have the typical vesicular eruption, making early diagnosis difficult. Small (1- to 2-mm) vesicles on an erythematous base, which may become pustular in 24 to 48 hours, are the most common lesions. At times, only 1 or 2 vesicles may be present; lesions are noted most often on the scalp and face, the presenting part of the infant in a normal delivery. Early diagnosis and prompt initiation of antiviral therapy can improve morbidity and mortality.

Neonatal varicella may develop when maternal varicella infection occurs during the last 2 to 3 weeks of pregnancy or the first few days postpartum. The severity of neonatal disease depends on the timing of the maternal infection. If maternal disease onset is 5 or more days before delivery, the infection in the newborn is usually mild because of the transplacental passage of maternal varicella IgG antibody. In contrast, if maternal disease onset is within 5 days before delivery or within 48 hours after delivery, the neonate is at risk of developing severe infection with up to a 30% mortality, usually caused by pulmonary or visceral involvement. Diagnosis can usually be made by the history and the characteristic rash or vesicles on an erythematous base (dew drops on a rose petal). The primary differential diagnosis includes HSV-1 or HSV-2 infection. Acyclovir may be considered for moderate or severe cases of neonatal varicella. Varicella-zoster immunoglobulin is recommended for uninfected infants born to mothers whose onset of chickenpox was within 5 days before to 2 days after delivery.

Incontinentia pigmenti is an X-linked dominant disorder with both skin and systemic lesions (affecting the eyes, CNS, and bone). It presents at birth or shortly thereafter with an inflammatory vesicular or bullous rash that develops in crops over the trunk and extremities. The cutaneous lesions have four phases (inflammatory vesicles or bullae, verrucous lesions, whorled hyperpigmentation, and hypopigmented patches) that may overlap and occur in an irregular sequence. Suspected cases should be referred to a dermatologist for evaluation because of the potential for systemic involvement.

Miliaria, or neonatal prickly heat, is caused by sweat retention and is characterized by easily ruptured, tiny (1- to 2-mm) vesicles located primarily on the face, chest, and back.

Impetigo appears as superficial vesicular, pustular, or bullous lesions on an erythematous base. In the newborn, lesions tend to occur primarily in the diaper area, folds of the neck, or axillae.

Vascular Lesions

The *salmon patch (nevus simplex)* is the most common vascular lesion of infancy. It is a pale pink macular lesion that is found most commonly on the nape of the neck (often called a *stork bite*), forehead, nasolabial region, or upper eyelids. With the exception of the lesions on the nape of the neck, most will fade within the first year of life.

Nevus flammeus (port-wine stain) consists of mature dilated dermal capillaries and presents at birth as pink to purple macular lesions that can vary tremendously in size, sometimes involving a significant portion of the body (Klippel–Trenaunay–Weber syndrome should be considered when the port-wine stain involves a lower limb). Unilateral facial port-wine stains in a trigeminal nerve distribution may be associated with the Sturge–Weber syndrome (seizures, intracranial calcifications, and hemiparesis). These lesions generally will not fade with time. Some are amenable to laser therapy.

Although *capillary hemangiomas (strawberry hemangiomas)* may be present at birth, most develop during the first few weeks of life. Lesions may occur anywhere on the body and typically begin as small, well-demarcated telangiectatic macules that subsequently develop into raised bright red or purple tumors with distinct borders. Most lesions will go through a period of rapid growth over the first 6 months of life, followed by a static period and then spontaneous involution, usually by 5 years of age.

Cavernous hemangiomas are deep-seated capillary hemangiomas that usually present at birth as a diffuse swelling with little change in the color of the overlying skin or a bluish hue. Most involute spontaneously with time.

Hemangiomas that may require intervention during the neonatal period are those that by location or size may compromise vital structures such as the eyes, nares, or auditory canals; lesions that by their size or location (e.g., perianal or labial lesions) are susceptible to trauma, ulceration and secondary infection; and large, rapidly enlarging hemangiomas associated with thrombocytopenia and a consumption coagulopathy (Kasabach–Merritt syndrome).

Pigmentary Changes

Mongolian spots are poorly circumscribed blue-black, gray, or brown large macular lesions generally located over the lumbosacral region, buttocks, and lower limbs in more than 80% to 90% of African American, Native American, Hispanic, or East Asian infants. The incidence is less than 10% in Caucasian infants. Lesions will usually fade during the first few years.

Café-au-lait macules are round or oval, brown macular lesions varying in size from less than 1 cm to more than 20 cm. Although normal individuals may have these lesions, they may be a sign of neurocutaneous disease, most commonly neurofibromatosis, particularly if multiple (more than 4) or large (larger than 1 to 2 cm).

Ash-leaf macules are irregular hypopigmented macules, often with an oval or "ash-leaf" appearance found in 70% to 90% of individuals with tuberous sclerosis. This is an autosomal dominant condition characterized by CNS lesions, seizures (infantile spasms), retinal lesions, cardiac rhabdomyomas, and renal lesions (hamartomas or cystic kidneys).

HEAD AND NECK PROBLEMS

Head Size and Shape

Shape, size, and symmetry are factors that must all be considered in the evaluation of the neonate's head. *Microcephaly* refers to a head circumference that is larger than 2 standard deviations below the mean, or smaller than the third percentile for age and sex. Microcephaly is usually a sign of a severe underlying abnormality of brain growth or development and is often associated with mental retardation. It may be secondary to a variety of causes, including Down syndrome, congenital TORCHES infections, and fetal alcohol syndrome. *Macrocephaly* is a head circumference that is larger than 2 standard deviations above the mean, or larger than the 97th percentile for age and sex. An excessively large head may be familial or suggestive of hydrocephalus, storage disease, or intracranial hemorrhage.

Molding of the skull bones during the vaginal delivery process is a common cause of temporary asymmetry and scalp edema, *caput succedaneum*. Caput succedaneum is an ill-defined, generalized swelling of the soft tissues of the scalp that extends across suture lines. Generally, both caput succedaneum and skull molding spontaneously resolve by 7 to 10 days of age. Trauma during the birth process may produce a *cephalohematoma*, a subperiosteal hemorrhage, distinguished from a caput by the fact that the swelling never crosses suture lines. However, the diagnosis can be difficult in the immediate newborn period if overlying scalp edema is present. Most commonly, a cephalohematoma is unilateral, but it can be bilateral. Cephalohematomas resolve slowly over 4 to 6 weeks, possibly with calcification and the formation of a hard bump on the scalp that may be a source of great concern to parents. Fetal scalp monitoring probes used during delivery may also leave a residual eschar or small bump on the scalp. Occasional complications resulting from the breakdown and resorption of large hematomas are jaundice or anemia.

Overriding cranial sutures, caused by the pressures exerted on the skull during its descent through the pelvis, may be noted for the first several days of life. Overriding sutures that are palpable beyond this time may be a sign of underlying brain pathology and deserve further evaluation. Ridging or

MEDICAL EMERGENCIES

prominence of cranial sutures may be a sign of *craniosynostosis*, a premature fusion of cranial sutures. Overriding sutures are ballottable, but if the sutures are rigid and have a heaped-up solid closure, radiographs or even a computed tomography scan should be conducted to rule out craniosynostosis. Soft areas, *craniotabes*, are occasionally found on palpation of the parietal bones during the first several days of life, especially in premature infants. Soft areas noted in the occipital region may be suggestive of osteogenesis imperfecta or other syndromes and should be investigated.

At birth, the newborn has two *fontanels*. The anterior fontanel, situated at the junction of the coronal and sagittal sutures, usually measures about 2 cm × 2 cm (can be up to 5 to 6 cm in its largest diameter) and normally closes between 9 and 18 months. The posterior fontanel, situated at the junction of the lambdoidal and sagittal sutures, generally measures between 0.5 and 1 cm (may be closed at birth in some cases) and usually closes to palpation by 3 to 4 months of age. Enlarged fontanels may be associated with a variety of conditions, including prematurity, hypothyroidism, or hydrocephalus. Increased intracranial pressure produces a full or bulging fontanel, whereas dehydration produces a depressed fontanel. A fontanel that appears full while the infant is supine or crying should be reassessed while the infant is held upright and sleeping or feeding before it is determined to be full or bulging.

Face

Facial asymmetry is usually secondary to in utero position. Commonly, when the face and neck are pressed against the shoulder in utero, a characteristic flattening of the face and angle of the jaw is noted on that side because of displacement of the mandible. This facial asymmetry will resolve spontaneously in a few weeks.

Neck (See Chapters 44 and 45)

Congenital muscular torticollis is a positional abnormality of the neck, resulting in abnormal tilting and rotation of the head. It is believed to be secondary to intrauterine positioning or trauma to the soft tissues of the neck during delivery, with resulting ischemia of the sternocleidomastoid muscle secondary to venous occlusion. This leads to edema and degeneration of the muscle fibers with eventual fibrosis of the muscle body. Although congenital muscular torticollis may be noted at birth, it usually manifests at 2 to 4 weeks of age. The incidence is increased in breech presentations and difficult deliveries. Unilateral contracture and fibrosis of the sternocleidomastoid muscle results in a characteristic head tilt toward the affected side and the chin pointing toward the opposite side. On examination, a firm, nontender mass may be felt within the body of the sternocleidomastoid muscle. Treatment consists of passive stretching exercises of the neck and repositioning toys and mobiles in the crib to stimulate the infant to look toward the side opposite the preferred gaze. Occipitocervical spine anomalies, such as the Klippel–Feil syndrome (congenital fusion of two or more cervical vertebrae; clinical triad of short neck, limited neck motion, and low occipital hairline), are rare causes of torticollis that present in the newborn period.

Congenital neck lesions may present during infancy or sometimes much later in childhood. The most common lesions include, *thyroglossal duct cysts* (midline in the neck and inferior to the hyoid bone), *branchial cleft cysts* (along the lateral neck), and *cystic hygromas* (usually located behind the sternocleidomastoid muscle in the supraclavicular fossa; two-thirds of cystic hygromas are present at birth).

Redundant skin on the back of the neck or webbing in a female infant are suggestive of Turner's syndrome and may be associated with lymphedema of the dorsum of the hands and feet in the newborn.

EYE PROBLEMS

The newborn is very nearsighted at birth, with a visual acuity of about 20/400. The eyelids are closed most of the time, and any attempt to force them open usually meets with marked resistance and causes blepharospasm. Darkening the examination room, holding the infant upright and gently swaying him or her from side to side or up and down often induces the eyes to open spontaneously. Neonatal ophthalmologic concerns include leukokoria, neonatal conjunctivitis, excessive tearing, scleral and subconjunctival hemorrhages, and uncoordinated eye movements.

Leukokoria

The pupillary light reflex is a simple test that takes only moments and should be performed on all newborns. In the normal newborn, a "red reflex" is seen when the ophthalmoscope is held 10 to 12 in. in front of the eyes. A white pupillary light reflex, or leukokoria, is never normal in the newborn. Leukokoria may be a sign of several conditions of variable severity and prognosis such as colobomas, cataracts, retinal detachment, retinopathy of prematurity, or retinoblastoma [the most common signs are leukokoria (60%) and strabismus (20%)]. Therefore, all infants with an abnormal pupillary light reflex should be referred to an ophthalmologist for a prompt evaluation.

Conjunctivitis (See Chapters 23 and 127)

The major causes of *neonatal conjunctivitis*, or *ophthalmia neonatorum*, are chemicals, chlamydia, bacteria, and virus. The time of onset of symptoms after birth can help identify the causative agent. Mild inflammation of the conjunctivae that begins 12 to 24 hours after birth is typically caused by the prophylactic eyedrops instilled at birth. This *chemical conjunctivitis* usually resolves by 48 hours of age. *Neisseria gonorrhoeae* conjunctivitis generally appears 2 to 5 days after birth, whereas conjunctivitis caused by *Chlamydia trachomatis* presents between 5 and 14 days after birth because of its longer incubation period. Gonococcal infection may be delayed beyond 5 days of age because of partial suppression by the prophylactic drops instilled at birth. Gonococcal infection usually manifests as marked inflammation of the eyelids, chemosis, and copious purulent discharge. Presentation of chlamydial infection, which is primarily localized to the palpebral conjunctiva, can vary from mild inflammation to severe swelling of the eyelids with copious discharge. Of neonates with chlamydial conjunctivitis, 10% to 20% have chlamydial pneumonia, which can either occur simultaneously with the eye infection or up to 4 to 6 weeks later. Gonococcal conjunctivitis is considered a medical emergency because the infection can spread to the cornea, producing corneal ulceration and perforation. HSV is a less common cause of neonatal conjunctivitis. The presence of characteristic skin lesions can help in the diagnosis. Gram stain and cultures are essential in the evaluation of neonatal conjunctivitis. Treatment is discussed in detail in Chapters 24 and 120.

Excessive Tearing
(See Chapters 23 and 127)

Congenital obstruction of the nasolacrimal duct, *dacryostenosis*, is the most common cause of excessive tearing in the newborn. Dacryostenosis should be differentiated from *congenital* or *infantile glaucoma*, a serious but fortunately rare cause of excessive tearing. Most cases of infantile glaucoma presenting during the first 3 months of life are bilateral, whereas dacryostenosis is usually unilateral.

Increased wetness of the affected eye relative to the normal eye, excessive tearing, mucoid eye discharge, and crusting along the eyelid margins are the usual presenting symptoms of dacryostenosis. Gentle pressure along the medial canthal region over the lacrimal sac may produce a reflux of tears or purulent material onto the surface of the eye, confirming the diagnosis. Infants with glaucoma, in addition to excessive tearing, also present with rhinorrhea, photophobia, and corneal haziness. The cornea may be inspected after instillation of fluorescein dye to rule out a *corneal abrasion* as the reason for the excessive tearing. Uncomplicated cases of nasolacrimal duct obstruction should be managed with gentle cleansing of the eyes, followed by local massage of the nasolacrimal duct, several times per day. Topical ophthalmologic antibiotic ointments should be prescribed if there is associated conjunctivitis or purulent discharge. Suspected cases of infantile glaucoma require immediate ophthalmologic evaluation.

Scleral and Subconjunctival Hemorrhage

Scleral and subconjunctival hemorrhage are often noted in the newborn, secondary to birth trauma. These lesions are common and spontaneous resolution within 1 to 2 weeks is the rule. When the funduscopic examination is performed, similar hemorrhages may be noted on the retina in about 25% of newborns. The presence of retinal hemorrhages should also raise the possibility of intentional trauma. Specifically, the *shaken baby syndrome* has been associated with flame-shaped retinal hemorrhages and subdural hematomas (see Chapter 132).

Transient Neonatal Strabismus
(See Chapter 24)

Intermittent esotropia or exotropia may be noted in normal infants during the first 2 to 3 months of life. These deviations are believed to be secondary to neuromuscular immaturity and generally resolve spontaneously by 4 months of age. If such eye devi-

ations are constant instead of intermittent, the infant should be referred for an ophthalmologic examination. In many infants, a broad, flat nasal bridge and prominent epicanthal folds may obscure a medial portion of the sclera near the nose and create the appearance of esotropia. This *pseudostrabismus*, or apparent deviation of the eyes, is an illusion that can be dispelled by the finding of symmetric bilateral pupillary light reflexes.

MOUTH PROBLEMS (SEE CHAPTER 48)

Normal Findings

Common normal findings in the oropharynx include natal teeth and benign gingival cysts. The incidence of *natal teeth* (teeth present at birth) is about 1 in every 3,000 live births. The mandibular central incisors are the most commonly affected teeth. Because most natal teeth are primary teeth that have erupted early, they should be extracted only if they are loose and pose a danger of aspiration, cause discomfort to the mother or child during nursing, or are confirmed to be supernumerary by focused radiographic examination.

Benign gingival cysts (see Chapter 122) are found in 75% of newborns. *Epstein's pearls* are usually single, small, white, keratin-filled cysts found along the midline of the palate. *Bohn's nodules* are mucous gland cysts that appear as multiple, firm, grayish white lesions along the gums and occasionally on the palate. *Dental lamina cysts* are formed by remnants of dental lamina epithelium and appear as small, cystic lesions along the crests of the mandibular and maxillary mucosa. They are usually larger and more lucent than both Epstein's pearls and Bohn's nodules. These cysts generally disappear by 4 weeks of age.

Thrush

Thrush is caused by *Candida albicans*. Diagnosis may be based on clinical examination. Creamy white plaques located on the buccal mucosa or tongue that are difficult to remove and may cause bleeding when scraped are characteristic of candidiasis. Treatment consists of local application of nystatin oral suspension four times a day. Topical application of nystatin ointment to the mother's nipples may be indicated in recurrent or refractory cases if the infant is breast-feeding.

Lip and Palate Defects

Defects in the formation of the lip (harelip) are obvious on even casual visualization. Possibility of defects of the palate should be considered in any neonate with feeding difficulties. The defect may vary in size. These infants should be referred for eventual surgical repair and for monitoring of feeding techniques.

CHEST AND BACK FINDINGS

This section discusses those external lesions on the thorax and back of the neonate for which a parent may bring the baby to emergency care. Intrathoracic lesions and diseases that present

MEDICAL EMERGENCIES

with secondary symptomatology are discussed in detail in other contexts elsewhere in this book (see Chapters 68, 98, and 118).

Normally, the term newborn's thorax is symmetric and barrel-shaped. It is graced with two nipples anteriorly, each about 10 mm in diameter and slightly elevated and stippled. Respiratory excursion should be symmetric and accompanied by simultaneous movement of the abdomen. In the midline of the back, the tips of the vertebrae can be palpated but not visualized. The rib cage is not flared or depressed. There are a number of variations of the apparent normal anatomy, some normal and some not, which may be striking enough for a parent to bring the child to the ED.

Respiratory Excursion (See Chapters 68, 92, and 98)

Intrathoracic disease or anomaly may be suggested by variations in the normal symmetric excursion of the thorax. If thoracic excursion is asymmetric or if there is significant tachypnea or retraction accompanied by grunting and either excessive or paradoxical excursion of the abdomen, pulse oximetry should be checked and a chest radiograph is warranted.

Fractured or Absent Clavicle(s)

In the course of vaginal delivery, the clavicle may be fractured, resulting in asymmetry at the shoulder girdle area. Palpation of the clavicle may reveal a "drop-off" in the continuity of the bone and possible crepitation when gentle pressure is applied. A confirmatory radiograph should be taken and appropriate reassurance offered for the healing process. Much more rarely, clavicles may be absent bilaterally with resultant low positioning of the shoulders. This positioning may be indicative of the dominant genetic defect known as *cleidocranial dysostosis* and requires orthopedic and genetic evaluation.

Pectus Excavatum

Relative depression of the lower sternum and rib cage is usually a normal variant unless accompanied by signs of respiratory distress.

Xiphoid Process

Parents may feel a firm, small mass in the midline at the distal end of the sternum. This is the xiphoid process angled outwardly and is a normal variant.

Breast (See Chapters 11 and 84)

Supernumerary Nipples

A round, possibly slightly elevated or slightly depressed lesion, about 10 mm in diameter, lighter in shade than the nipple, and located about 2 to 3 cm below, is a supernumerary nipple. This is a normal variant and will remain permanently. Uncommonly,

these may be associated with renal lesions, but that possibility need not be investigated in a child who is otherwise well.

Breast Buds

Prominent, nontender breast tissue in the neonate of either sex is a normal variant, probably related to maternal estrogen. This subsides with time, and no therapy is indicated. Often, colostrum-like material can be extruded, but efforts to do this should be gentle and conducted under hygienic conditions.

Breast Cellulitis/Abscess

Breast tissue that is hypertrophied, reddened, and tender is probably infected. The child may or may not be febrile. Warm compresses and intravenous antibiotic treatment, including coverage for probable staphylococcal origin, should be inaugurated after appropriate cultures are taken. The baby should be admitted for continuing therapy.

Absent

An absent nipple may be associated with an ipsilateral absent pectoralis muscle. Chest radiograph should be taken and the baby referred for genetic and orthopedic evaluation.

Spinal Column Defects

Spina Bifida

A grossly apparent spina bifida lesion, complete with lower-extremity flaccidity and meningeal extrusion in the midline of the back, obviously should not have been missed in the hospital nursery. The baby delivered at home, however, may be referred into the ED for initial management. Sterile, moist dressing should be applied and the baby admitted for neurosurgical, orthopedic, and urologic management. If the home delivery occurred under less than sterile conditions, cultures should be taken and inauguration of appropriate antibiotic therapy considered.

Sacral Dimple

A midline dimple of the lower back, with or without a tuft of hair, or a lipomatous intracutaneous or subcutaneous lesion in that area may be clues to the presence of spina bifida occulta, a less obvious form of spina bifida. This may or may not be associated with lower-extremity deformity. The dimple may also be the external manifestation of a sinus tract connecting to the intradural space without vertebral anomaly, which would leave the infants susceptible to meningeal infection. On the other hand, the dimple may be a normal skin indentation. An infant with an open lesion requires admission for further workup of the dimple. A closed lesion can be referred for further imaging studies, such as ultrasound or magnetic resonance imaging.

ABDOMINAL AND PERINEAL FINDINGS

The neonatal abdomen is full but is neither distended nor scaphoid. The liver is normally palpable 2 to 3 cm below the right costal margin; the spleen is not usually palpable; the lower edges of the kidneys may be felt with deep palpation.

There should be no palpable extraneous masses. Constipation, meconium passage, and vomiting are discussed in Chapters 13, 78, 99, and 121. This section discusses those external findings in the abdomen and perineum that might cause a parent to bring the new baby to the ED.

Umbilicus

The umbilical cord is tied or clamped at the time of delivery and usually sloughs off by the 10th day. Umbilical care consists of gentle hygienic measures and cleansing with isopropyl alcohol several times a day. Still, the umbilical area may be a source of concern for parents, who may appear in the ED with their neonate.

Discharge

Discharge from the umbilical area may occur and is benign if it is clear or yellow-tinged and thin. Reassurance and instruction in hygienic measures are all that is necessary. A thick, purulent discharge accompanied by intense redness and apparent tenderness is omphalitis, a serious bacterial infection with the potential to spread into the abdominal wall and systemically. The infant should be admitted, cultures from the blood as well as the discharge should be obtained, and the intravenous antibiotics should be administered.

Granuloma

Granulation tissue, lumped into a small ball about 1 cm across and attached in the umbilical area, can be cauterized with a silver nitrate stick. Extreme caution should be used when applying silver nitrate, as severe burns have resulted, requiring skin graft. The parents should be forewarned that the area will turn transiently black. Often, this treatment has to be repeated in a week or so.

Umbilical Hernia

Umbilical hernia is a result of incomplete merging of the recti muscles at the ring through which the cord had been protruding. It is often accompanied by a larger rectus diastasis extending superiorly, sometimes to as high as the xiphoid process. The size can vary from as little as a few millimeters to as much as 4 or 5 cm. It is covered by skin. With crying or straining, portions of the intestine and omentum can be palpated, but not visualized, within the hernia. No treatment is necessary in the neonatal period because these almost always close as the baby becomes ambulant and strengthens the rectus muscles. Abdominal bandages are unnecessary. Rarely, at a later age, an umbilical hernia may strangulate and require surgery.

Omphalocele

An omphalocele is essentially a large hernia into the base of the umbilical cord, but it is covered only by peritoneum, not skin. It contains a significant amount of intestine and, rarely, a lobe of the liver. The child should be admitted for early surgery.

Genital Area

The penis should be at least 1 cm in length, with a urethral opening at the tip. The testes are usually palpable within the scrotal sac. The labia majora overlie and cover the labia minora.

Vaginal Discharge and Bleeding (See Chapters 76 and 77)

White mucoid discharge, which may be thick, in the vaginal opening is a normal finding. Vaginal bleeding after the first day or two and during the first week is also a normal occurrence. It is the result of postpartum estrogen withdrawal.

Inguinal Mass

A mass palpable in the scrotum may be an inguinal hernia or a hydrocele or a combination of the two. Hernias are usually easily reducible in the neonate. Hydroceles are fluid-filled and transilluminate readily. A mass within the labia majora is most likely ovary or intestine that has passed through an inguinal hernia. These are somewhat more likely to incarcerate than hernias in males.

Hypospadias

When the urethral opening is not at the tip of the penis but on the glans, the baby has first-degree hypospadias. When the opening is on the shaft, it is second-degree and on the perineum, third-degree. Infants with second- and third-degree hypospadias should be referred for urologic evaluation and imaging of the genitourinary tract.

Ambiguous Genitalia

The possibility of ambiguous genitalia should be considered in a male neonate if the apparent penis is small and there is third-degree hypospadias with a cleft in the scrotum; in the female neonate, genitalia are ambiguous if there appears to be an unusually long clitoris with partial or complete fusion of the labia majora and if there is a firm mass in the labia. In the female neonate, but not in the male neonate, such pseudohermaphroditism may be associated with *congenital adrenal hyperplasia*, with or without "salt-losing" symptomatology (see Chapter 86). To establish gender identity and to evaluate for the possibility of congenital adrenal hyperplasia, electrolyte, imaging, and chromosomal studies need to be conducted early in the child's neonatal period under the supervision of a urologist and geneticist and possibly an endocrinologist.

Imperforate Anus

An imperforate anus may not be obvious on external examination. The finding of an anus located considerably more anteriorly than expected might suggest a fistula from the lower rectum to the skin, detouring around an imperforate anus. Meconium may actually pass through this fistula, simulating normal rectal passage. The area should be examined carefully, looking for the normal perianal-anal puckering, which will not be present if the anteriorly placed opening is a fistula. The rectal examination should be performed gently. Imaging studies and surgical referral should be considered.

ORTHOPEDIC CONCERNS

Most neonatal orthopedic problems are deformities secondary to intrauterine positioning. Some problems (e.g., metatarsus adductus) require only parental reassurance and expectant management, whereas others (e.g., congenital clubfoot and hip dysplasia) require early orthopedic attention.

Developmental Hip Dysplasia

Developmental dysplasia of the hip (DDH) applies to a range of hip pathology, from instability to frank dislocation, that may either be present at birth or develop during infancy. With the baby in the supine position and with hips and knees slightly flexed, abduct both thighs simultaneously. If both knees can be brought to touch the examining table without undue pressure, there is no dysplasia of the hips.

The time-tested Ortolani and Barlow maneuvers also may be used in the neonatal period to evaluate for hip instability. Both tests are performed with the infant in a supine position and the hips and knees flexed to 90 degrees. Each leg is examined separately, not simultaneously. In the Ortolani maneuver, gentle abduction and lifting of the femoral head anteriorly produces a palpable "thunk" or "clunk" as the examiner relocates a dislocated hip. Nonpathologic processes such as ligamentous snapping can produce hip clicks that differ from the pathologic "clunk" associated with DDH. In the Barlow maneuver, the examiner attempts to dislocate the hip by gentle adduction and posterior axial pressure on the thigh. If in doubt, confirmatory ultrasound should be performed and orthopedic consultation obtained in a timely manner.

Intoeing

The differential diagnosis of intoeing is guided by the age at presentation. In the newborn period, the most common causes of intoeing are metatarsus adductus and clubfoot. *Metatarsus adductus* is a functional deformity, resulting from intrauterine positioning, in which the forefoot is in adduction with respect to the hindfoot. Most cases resolve spontaneously by 3 to 6 months of age. If the forefoot cannot be brought into the neutral position either by stroking the lateral border of the foot or by gently straightening it, referral to an orthopedic surgeon for cast correction is indicated.

Congenital clubfoot is a pathologic deformity consisting of three components: forefoot varus, heel varus, and ankle equinus. Clubfoot may either be an isolated deformity or seen in association with other neuromuscular anomalies such as arthrogryposis, cerebral palsy, myelomeningocele, or amniotic band syndrome. Orthopedic treatment should begin in the first week of life.

Brachial Plexus Injuries (See Chapter 35)

Lateral traction on the head and neck during delivery can result in injury to the brachial plexus. Clinical signs relate to the site of the traumatic injury. *Erb's palsy*, the most common birth injury of the brachial plexus, results from injury to the upper plexus affecting the C5 and C6 roots, the upper trunk, or its divisions. The affected arm is held with the shoulder adducted and internally rotated, the elbow in extension and pronation, and the wrist in flexion (waiter's tip posture). On examination, the Moro reflex (allowing the infant's head to

drop back suddenly) is asymmetric. On the affected side, there is abduction and upward movement of the arms, followed by adduction and flexion. There is weakness of shoulder abduction, flexion, and supination; the biceps reflex is decreased; and there is slight weakness of wrist and finger extensors. In addition, when the C4 root is also involved, ipsilateral hemidiaphragmatic paralysis may be appreciated by ultrasound examination.

Klumpke's paralysis results from injury to the lower plexus, affecting the C8 and T1 roots, the lower trunk, or its divisions. The injury primarily affects the muscles of the hand. The infant presents with clawing of the affected hand [hyperextension at the metacarpophalangeal (MCP) joints and flexion of the interphalangeal joints], the elbow is held in flexion and the wrist is usually held in extension, unless there is injury to the middle trunk. On examination, the palmar grasp and the triceps reflex are decreased.

Treatment consists of immobilization and appropriate positioning to prevent contractures. Orthopedic referral is indicated.

NEUROLOGIC CONCERNS

Neonatal Seizures (See Chapters 69 and 96)

Neonatal seizures may be difficult to recognize clinically, because it is rare for newborns to have symmetric, generalized tonic-clonic convulsions. It is much more common to see seizure episodes that present as focal abnormalities or subtle findings. Subtle seizures can be difficult to distinguish from the normal spectrum of newborn behaviors, jitteriness, or benign myoclonic movements. Benign myoclonic movements are isolated jerky movements of an extremity that occur primarily during sleep. Jitteriness may be differentiated from seizures by its disappearance when the affected extremity is touched or held (Table 95.4).

Four clinical seizure types are recognized in the newborn (Table 95.5): subtle, tonic, clonic, and myoclonic. Generalized tonic-clonic seizures tend not to occur in the first month of life because the newborn's immature nervous system is unable to produce and sustain this type of activity. Not all neonatal seizure types are associated with electroencephalogram (EEG) seizure activity (Table 104.5). It has been hypothesized that these seizures may be originating from areas of the CNS that cannot be detected by surface electrodes (e.g., brainstem or spinal cord).

TABLE 95.4

CLINICAL DIFFERENTIATION OF NEONATAL SEIZURES FROM JITTERINESS

Clinical characteristic	Seizure	Jitteriness
Stimulus sensitive	No	Yes
Movement ceases with restraint	No	Yes
Accompanied by autonomic changes	Yes	No
Speed of movements	Slower	Faster
Abnormal eye movements	Common	No

TABLE 95.5

CLASSIFICATION OF NEONATAL SEIZURES

Seizure type	Electroencephalogram seizure correlation
Subtle	
Sucking or chewing motion	Uncommon[a]
Lip smacking	
Bicycling of legs	
Apnea	
Eyelid fluttering	
Eye deviations	
Laughter	
Tonic posturing	
Tonic	
Focal	Common
Generalized	Uncommon
Clonic	
Focal	Common
Multifocal	Common
Myoclonic	
Focal	Uncommon
Multifocal	Uncommon
Generalized	Common

[a]Except for tonic eye deviation, which often has an electroencephalographic correlation.

Subtle seizures, perhaps the most common type of neonatal seizures, are stereotypical repetitive movements such as eye blinking, eye deviations, chewing motions, lip smacking, and bicycling or pedaling movements. Most subtle seizures, especially in term infants, are not consistently associated with EEG seizure activity.

Focal *tonic seizures* present as sustained posturing of a limb, whereas generalized tonic seizures are characterized by either tonic extension of all extremities (simulating decerebrate posturing) or, less commonly, flexion of the upper extremities with extension of the lower extremities (simulating decorticate posturing). These seizures may be seen in association with severe hypoxic brain injury or with intraventricular hemorrhage, not uncommon in premature infants but may also be seen in term infants.

A *clonic seizure* involves rhythmic jerking of one or more parts of the body. Clonic seizures can be focal (affecting only one extremity or both the upper and lower extremities on one side of the body) or multifocal (clonic activity in one extremity that randomly migrates to another part of the body—e.g., left arm jerking followed by right leg jerking). Although focal clonic seizures can result from focal brain lesions, they can also be caused by a generalized metabolic disturbance such as hypoglycemia.

Benign myoclonic jerks are often noted in sleeping infants, especially premature infants, during the first 6 months of life. Unlike this benign sleep-related phenomenon, *myoclonic seizures* occur during waking and are single or repetitive rapid jerks of either the entire body or a particular extremity. They are distinguished from clonic seizures by their more rapid speed and a predilection for flexor muscle groups. These seizures usually indicate severe underlying brain pathology or

injury such as hypoxic brain injury. Infants with these seizures may later develop infantile spasms. Focal myoclonic seizures typically involve the upper extremity. Multifocal myoclonic seizures are characterized by asynchronous twitching of several areas of the body, whereas generalized myoclonic seizures present as bilateral flexion jerks of the upper extremities and sometimes also the lower extremities.

Although there are a variety of causes for neonatal seizures (Table 95.6), only a few causes (perinatal asphyxia, intracranial hemorrhage, metabolic disturbances, and infection or malformations of the brain) account for most cases. Benign or idiopathic neonatal seizures occur, but this diagnosis should be made only after other causes are thoroughly investigated.

Perinatal asphyxia is the most common cause of neonatal seizures. During the first several days to weeks of life, signs of acute *hypoxic-ischemic encephalopathy (HIE)* are lethargy, hypotonia, and decreased spontaneous movements. Mild asphyxia is often marked by a transient state of hyperalertness and irritability. Seizures, if they occur, generally begin within the first 24 hours of life and may be difficult to control. The diagnosis of HIE should be strongly considered in a hypotonic infant with increased deep tendon reflexes.

Intracranial hemorrhage is the second most common cause of neonatal seizures. Intraventricular hemorrhages are seen primarily in premature infants, whereas subarachnoid or subdural hemorrhages are more likely in large, term infants and may be associated with birth trauma.

A variety of metabolic disturbances are associated with neonatal seizures. SGA infants and infants of diabetic mothers are at risk for hypoglycemia during the first 24 hours of life. These infants may have a variety of findings, ranging from jitteriness to seizures. Infants of diabetic mothers are also at risk for hypocalcemic seizures during the first 24 hours. Premature infants and infants with perinatal asphyxia are also at risk for early-onset (within the first 2 days of life) hypocalcemia. Late-onset hypocalcemic seizures (after day 2 to 3 of life) may be caused by an imbalance in dietary intake, hypomagnesemia, or hypoparathyroidism. Inborn errors of metabolism, pyridoxine dependence, and mitochondrial disorders are less common

TABLE 95.6

COMMON CAUSES OF NEONATAL SEIZURES BY GESTATIONAL AGE

First 24 h
Hypoxic-ischemic encephalopathy
Infection (meningitis, TORCHES infection, sepsis)
Direct drug effects (inadvertent anesthetic injection)
Metabolic (hypoglycemia, hypocalcemia)
Intracranial hemorrhage (preterm—intraventricular hemorrhage; term—subdural/subarachnoid hemorrhage)
Pyridoxine dependency

>24 h
Infection (meningitis, sepsis, herpes simplex virus)
Intracranial hemorrhage
Metabolic [inborn errors of metabolism, hypocalcemia (dietary)]
Intracranial malformations
Drug withdrawal

metabolic causes of seizures in the newborn. Inborn errors of metabolism should be suspected when seizures are associated with vomiting, failure to thrive, hepatomegaly, and altered tone or consciousness.

Several bacterial and viral CNS infections can cause seizures in the newborn. Common bacterial causes are group B *Streptococcus* and *Escherichia coli* infections. HSV encephalitis is an important viral source that must be considered. A newborn with a history of a seizure associated with fever requires a comprehensive evaluation for the cause and should not be diagnosed with simple febrile seizures.

The evaluation of newborn seizures should include a detailed history of prenatal, perinatal, and postnatal events. The examination should be directed toward identifying treatable causes, such as infectious or metabolic disturbances. Minimal laboratory evaluation for all newborns with seizures includes a CBC; both rapid bedside and laboratory measurement of serum glucose level; serum electrolytes level, including calcium, phosphorus, and magnesium; blood culture; and cerebrospinal fluid analysis and culture. Cranial ultrasound is especially useful in identifying suspected intraventricular hemorrhages. Measurements of serum ammonia, serum amino acids, and urine organic acids levels should be obtained if a metabolic defect is suspected. Urine testing with the Clinitest reagent (detects excess excretion of both galactose and glucose) can screen for galactosemia.

Appropriate *medical management* includes early correction of metabolic abnormalities and consideration of empiric antibiotic therapy. If the results of serum glucose and calcium measurements will not be available in a timely manner, empiric chemical therapy may be instituted if the infant is actively seizing. Hypoglycemia (serum glucose level less than 40 mg per dL) is treated with a 5 to 10 mL per kg bolus over 20 minutes of a 10% dextrose solution. More concentrated forms of dextrose (25% or 50%) should be avoided to prevent sclerosis to infant peripheral veins. Treat symptomatic hypocalcemia (serum calcium level less than 8 mg per dL) with 100 to 200 mg per kg (1 to 2 mL per kg) of elemental calcium as a 10% calcium gluconate solution further diluted by slow intravenous drip.

For seizures, empiric anticonvulsant therapy may be instituted while awaiting consultation with a neurologist. Subtle seizures or patients who present with a history of seizure but a normal neurologic examination should not be treated with anticonvulsants before consultation. The anticonvulsant of choice for neonates is lorazepam, given intravenously at a dose of 0.1 mg per kg. Intramuscular administration can be considered, although absorption and clearance are more erratic. Diazepam may alternatively be used at a dose of 0.05 to 0.25 mg per kg. Careful monitoring of cardiorespiratory status and avoidance of hypoxia are essential at presentation and during therapy. Phenobarbital 10 to 20 mg per kg is the secondary drug of choice if the seizure persists beyond the second dose of benzodiazepine. Alternatively, phenytoin or fosphenytoin may be added although the kinetics are notoriously unpredictable. If the infant continues to actively seize, a trial of pyridoxine (50 to 100 mg intravenously) may be considered. If a second agent is required, particularly phenobarbital, significant respiratory depression must be considered and preparation to provide airway support with endotracheal intubation should be made.

Hypotonic Infant (See Chapter 96)

A healthy term newborn normally moves his or her extremities spontaneously and has a dominance of flexor tone. Compared with the term *newborn's tone*, the premature infant's tone is relatively hypotonic, so corrected gestational age must be taken into consideration during evaluation.

Decreased spontaneous movements, poor head and trunk control, and a preponderance of extensor tone are all characteristics of the hypotonic infant. The healthy, term newborn when supported by the trunk in an outstretched prone position, also known as *ventral suspension*, will flex all extremities against gravity, keep the back straight, and support the head in a neutral position with relation to the rest of the body. In the hypotonic and preterm infant, the forces of gravity may allow the back and head to droop downward and the extremities to hang in extension. When held by the axillae in vertical suspension, the hypotonic infant will "slip through" the hands of the examiner instead of reflexively flexing the upper extremities to maintain position. Because weakness is often associated with hypotonia, the newborn may present with resultant weak cry, poor suck, or respiratory effort. Weakness should also be suspected if the infant does not briskly withdraw a limb that is subjected to a forceful stimuli.

The causes of hypotonia depend on the level of the nervous system that is affected (Table 95.7). Motor dysfunction at any level from the CNS to the muscle itself may result in hypotonia. Central hypotonia involves pathology of the cerebral cortex down to the level of the lower motor neuron or can be caused by systemic disease affecting motor function. Neuromuscular disease can be caused by dysfunction at any of four anatomic sites: anterior horn cell (lower motor neuron), peripheral nerve, neuromuscular junction, and muscle.

Central Hypotonia

If muscle weakness is not a significant accompanying feature, a central source for the hypotonia should be considered. Features characteristically associated with central hypotonia include a decreased level of alertness, seizures, and a weak cry; muscle bulk is normal, and deep tendon reflexes are either normal or increased. Perinatal asphyxia and intracranial hemorrhage are the two most common CNS causes of hypotonia that presents in the neonatal period. Depressive symptoms are usually present during the first 1 to 2 days of life in these conditions. An infant who is normal at birth and then develops lethargy, hypotonia, vomiting, or seizures at several days of age after ingestion of milk protein and carbohydrate may have an inborn error of metabolism (Chapter 94). Metabolic diseases should always be taken into consideration in the evaluation of the hypotonic infant, especially when the clinical presentation does not readily fit into any distinct diagnosis. Occasionally, unusual odors (Chapter 46) of the infant or urine are noted (e.g., mustiness—phenylketonuria, sweaty feet—isovaleric acidemia, maple syrup—maple syrup urine disease).

Disorders of the Lower Motor Neuron

Disorders of the lower motor neuron are characterized by hypotonia, muscle weakness, and hypoactive to absent deep tendon reflexes in an otherwise alert infant. Spinal muscular

TABLE 95.7

DIFFERENTIAL DIAGNOSIS OF NEONATAL HYPOTONIA

Central Nervous System Disease
Perinatal asphyxia (hypoxic-ischemic encephalopathy)
Intracranial hemorrhage
Infection
Hyperbilirubinemia
Neonatal drug withdrawal
Metabolic diseases
  Organic and aminoacidemias
  Hypercalcemia
Chromosomal abnormality
  Down syndrome
  Prader–Willi syndrome
Neuromuscular Disease
Anterior horn cell diseases (lower motor neuron)
  Type I spinal muscular atrophy (Werdnig–Hoffman disease)

Neonatal poliomyelitis
Type II glycogen storage disease (Pompe's disease)
Peripheral nerve diseases
  Leukodystrophies
  Guillain–Barre syndrome
Neuromuscular junction diseases
  Infantile botulism
  Neonatal myasthenia gravis (congenital or acquired
    transient myasthenia)
Muscle diseases
  Congenital myopathies
  Mitochondrial myopathies
  Glycogen storage disease
  Hypothyroidism

atrophy (Werdnig–Hoffman disease) is the most common of the lower motor neuron diseases. In the classic, early-onset form of the disease, infants may present at birth or during the first several weeks of life with generalized weakness, absent deep tendon reflexes, muscle atrophy, fasciculations, and cranial nerve abnormalities, including disordered sucking and swallowing. Infants have a characteristic posture with flaccid tone, abducted limbs, and little spontaneous movement. Respiratory distress may be present. The disease is unfortunately rapidly progressive, and death usually occurs in most patients by 3 years of age.

Disorders of the Neuromuscular Junction

Disorders of the neuromuscular junction are important to recognize because supportive and therapeutic interventions are available. Infants with neuromuscular disorders have hypotonia and weakness like infants with lower motor neuron disease, but infants with neuromuscular disease have normal muscle bulk and normal deep tendon reflexes. Infantile botulism (see Chapter 92) is a toxic abnormality of the neuromuscular junction that is seen in infants younger than 12 months. It is caused by the ingestion of *Clostridium botulinum* spores (from soil, honey, or corn syrup), which germinate in the gastrointestinal tract and produce botulinum toxin. Early symptoms include constipation and poor feeding as a result of poor sucking and swallowing. A descending paralysis develops over the next several days, with development of ptosis, loss of head control, weak cry, flat facial expression, and eventually, generalized hypotonia. Treatment with botulinum antitoxin should be considered. Supportive nutritional and electrolyte care are essential; ventilatory support may be required for respiratory failure.

Disorders of Muscle

A variety of primary muscle disorders may present during the neonatal period, with the nonspecific features of hypotonia, weakness, decreased muscle bulk, and normal to decreased deep tendon reflexes. Metabolic myopathies are caused by abnormal energy metabolism in the muscle and include disorders of the mitochondria and carnitine metabolism. A mitochondrial myopathy should be considered in a hypotonic infant with lactic acidosis.

Laboratory evaluation of hypotonia is guided by the level of the nervous system believed to be affected. If CNS disease is suspected, brain imaging, an EEG, and endocrine and metabolic determinations may be appropriate. When neuromuscular disease is suspected, muscle enzyme determinations, nerve conduction velocities, electromyography, and nerve or muscle biopsies can be conducted on a scheduled basis.

Most importantly, it is essential to consider the possibility that hypotonia is really lethargy related to shock or sepsis.

Neonatal Screening

Screening for congenital metabolic disorders through tandem mass spectrometry has significantly increased the number of patients diagnosed with these disorders. This technology is now available in 47 states. Tandem mass spectrometry detects amino acid and urea cycle disorders, fatty acid oxidation disorders, and organic acid disorders. Blood samples are generally taken prior to discharge from the nursery and become available in the first 2 weeks of life. States require physician notification of positive screening results. Families may be directed to the ED (or they may come of their own volition) upon notification of a positive newborn screen. Confirmatory testing and disposition should be performed in conjunction with the designated metabolic specialist and/or referring physician.

CONGENITAL INFECTIONS

There are a group of transplacentally transmitted congenital infections, often referred to jointly by the acronym TORCHES, which vary in their postpartum presentation according to the time during the pregnancy when they were acquired and with the intensity of the inoculum. These include toxoplasmosis, rubella, cytomegalovirus, herpes virus infections (herpes simplex and varicella), and syphilis.

Fetal infection with these agents acquired in midpregnancy may result in a neonate born with a complex of findings that may include low birth weight or SGA; jaundice, purpura, and thrombocytopenia; hypotonia; microcephaly;

cataracts; microphthalmia; chorioretinitis; hepatosplenomegaly; intracerebral calcifications; congenital heart disease; hypoplastic limbs; hearing loss; cicatricial scarring of the skin; and seizures. Obviously, not all, not even most, of these findings will be present in any one affected infant, but their presence should at least arouse suspicion for the TORCHES syndrome.

Clinically, it is often difficult to distinguish one of these infections from the other. Rubella is more likely to be associated with cataracts and cardiac lesions; toxoplasmosis with chorioretinitis and cerebral calcifications; herpes simplex and varicella with vesicular or cicatricial skin lesions; cytomegalovirus with hearing loss; and syphilis with bone lesions, snuffles, and palm and hand bullae. However, symptoms overlap. The essentials in management include a careful maternal history and appropriate serologic testing and culturing of both mother and infant.

The clinician should keep in mind the possibility, however, that aspects of this symptom complex, particularly purpura and jaundice in a hypotonic baby, may be associated with an active acute septic infection.

Infants may acquire human immunodeficiency virus (HIV) vertically from mothers transplacentally, through delivery, or through breast-feeding. At birth, infants may test negative for infection by traditional assays and may not appear ill. Infected infants commonly have no symptoms. Symptomatic infants may have failure to thrive, recurrent thrush, hepatosplenomegaly, lymphadenopathy, diarrheal illness, or recurrent lower respiratory tract infections. Chapter 93 describes the care of HIV-infected children in detail.

NEONATAL DRUG WITHDRAWAL

Maternal substance abuse during pregnancy places the newborn at risk for a variety of medical, developmental, behavioral, and psychosocial problems. The particular effects on the newborn infant depend on the type of drug or drugs, the timing of the exposure during gestation, and the frequency of the exposure. In addition to illicit drugs, many infants are exposed to cigarettes and alcohol.

■ *Narcotics:* Prenatal exposure to heroin and methadone results in physiologic addiction in the newborn. The symptoms of withdrawal are nonspecific and may not be detected in the newborn nursery, especially when the maternal history of drug abuse is unknown or when the infant is discharged home within 24 hours of delivery. Narcotic antagonists such as naloxone may precipitate withdrawal and should be avoided at the time of delivery. Heroin has a short serum half-life, so clinical signs of withdrawal are generally apparent on the first day of life, whereas clinical signs of methadone withdrawal seldom occur before 24 to 48 hours of age because of its longer half-life. Symptoms of narcotic withdrawal include irritability, jitteriness, tremors, seizures, disorganized suck and poor feeding, vomiting, diarrhea, sweating, and sneezing. Additional signs of withdrawal that may be noted in the older infant include failure to gain weight and abraded marks along the nose, shins, or occiput caused by the infant's tremulousness and irritability.

■ *Cocaine:* In utero cocaine exposure has been associated with an increased incidence of abruptio placentae, low birth weight, and preterm delivery. Classically, the cocaine-exposed infant is not so much jittery as he or she is disorganized in sleeping and feeding. These infants are lethargic and poorly responsive but are easily overstimulated and become irritable when awake, making feeding a challenge for many of them. Gavage feeding may be necessary in some instances. Any history of feeding intolerance, vomiting, or abdominal distension needs to be investigated because necrotizing enterocolitis has been noted in term, cocaine-exposed infants. Stool occult blood may be positive, secondary to bowel necrosis caused by the vasoconstrictive actions of cocaine. Small CNS bleeds have been described in the basal ganglia and frontal lobes.

■ *Amphetamines:* Methamphetamine-exposed infants are often described as being too quiet and may need to be awakened regularly for feedings. Prolonged sleep, depression, and voracious appetite when awakened are characteristic of amphetamine withdrawal. Infants born to methamphetamine-abusing mothers are frequently born small for gestational age and are at increased risk for future neurodevelopmental problems.

■ *Selective serotonin reuptake inhibitors* (SSRIs), commonly used for maternal depression, readily cross the placenta and can cause a neonatal withdrawal or discontinuation syndrome in infants exposed during the third trimester in utero. Although SSRIs do not appear to increase teratogenic risk, there have been several reports of neonatal complications, possibly caused by their common discontinuation syndrome. Symptoms, including irritability, constant crying, shivering, increased tone, eating and sleeping difficulties, and seizures, have been noted within a few days after birth and lasting up to 1 month after birth.

Evaluation

In general, toxicologic screening can be performed on infants on medical grounds without parental consent. Metabolites of cocaine can be detected for 1 to 2 days after use in the adult and 5 to 7 days in the newborn; amphetamine is present for 1 to 2 days in the adult; and marijuana can be detected in the urine for up to 7 days after use. Most urine toxicology screens use immunoassays and are inexpensive and sensitive but not specific (e.g., antihistamines can cross-react with amphetamines). Using infant hair or meconium samples to check for the presence of illicit drugs, especially cocaine, provide a broader window on drug use during pregnancy and are able to document the presence of drugs in the time before delivery.

The *Neonatal Abstinence Score* (NAS) developed by Finnegan is an objective way of assessing the severity of narcotic withdrawal symptoms (Table 95.8). Infants should be scored at 4-hour intervals for the first several days of life. Three consecutive scores higher than 8 or two scores higher than 12 are an indication for pharmacologic therapy. The NAS can also be used to guide effectiveness of pharmacologic therapy.

Management

Swaddling and minimizing sensory stimulation are two of the simplest and most effective techniques in managing neonatal

TABLE 95.8

NEONATAL ABSTINENCE SCORE

Signs and symptoms	Score
Central Nervous System	
High-pitched cry (excessive or continuous)	2 or 3
Sleeps <1, 2, or 3 h after feeding	3 or 2 or 1
Moro reflex (hyperactive or significantly hyperactive)	2 or 3
Tremors when disturbed (mild or moderate to severe)	1 or 2
Tremors undisturbed (mild or moderate to severe)	3 or 4
Increased muscle tone	2
Excoriations	1
Myoclonic jerks	3
Generalized convulsions	5
Vasomotor/Respiratory	
Sweating	1
Fever (99–101°F or >101°F; 37.2–38.3°C)	1 or 2
Frequent yawning (>3–4 times/interval)	1
Mottling	1
Nasal stuffiness	1
Sneezing (>3–4 times/interval)	1
Nasal flaring	2
Respiratory rate (>60/min or >60/min with retractions)	1 or 2
Gastrointestinal	
Excessive sucking	1
Poor feeding	2
Regurgitation or projectile vomiting	2 or 3
Stools (loose or watery)	2 or 3

Modified from Finnegan LP. Neonatal abstinence. In: Nelson NM, ed. *Current therapy in neonatal-perinatal medicine.* Philadelphia, PA: BC Decker, 1990:314–320.

drug withdrawal. A blanket or sheet can be draped over the infant's bed to minimize light exposure. Often, these infants do well when placed in a "snugly or front pack" over the mother's chest and abdomen. The mother's regular, monotonous cardiorespiratory sounds can be soothing. Demand feeding with hypercaloric formula (24 to 27 cal per oz) may be necessary to maintain weight.

Indications for pharmacologic therapy for neonatal abstinence syndrome are seizures, poor feeding, diarrhea and vomiting resulting in excessive weight loss and dehydration, irritability interfering with sleeping or feeding, and hypothermia or hyperthermia. Other causes of these symptoms, such as infection, hypoglycemia, hypocalcemia, hypomagnesemia, hyperthyroidism, CNS hemorrhage, and anoxia must be excluded before initiating treatment. Benzodiazepines for alcohol withdrawal and methadone for opioid withdrawal are the only agents approved by the U.S. Food and Drug Administration for the treatment of drug withdrawal. However, several agents, such as tincture of opium, paregoric, morphine, clonidine, phenobarbital, chlorpromazine, and diazepam, have shown favorable effectiveness in neonatal narcotic withdrawal. Infants presenting with neonatal abstinence syndrome to the ED should be admitted for stabilization and initiation of pharmacologic therapy.

Prognosis

Drug-exposed infants are at increased risk for abuse and neglect because of a combination of environmental (chaotic family environments, limited financial resources, and limited parenting skills because of the impact of the substance abuse) and infant risk factors (poor attachment, high-pitched cry, irritability, difficult to console, and poor feeding).

ACKNOWLEDGMENT

The authors thank Dr. Geeta Grover, MD, Behavior/Developmental Department, Children's Hospital of Orange County, California, for essential contributions to this chapter.

Suggested Readings

American Academy of Pediatrics. Herpes simplex. In: Pickering LK, et al. *Red book 2006 report of the Committee on Infectious Diseases,* 27th ed. Elk Grove Village, IL: American Academy of Pediatrics, 2006:361–371.

American Academy of Pediatrics. Human immunodeficiency virus. In: Pickering LK, et al. *Red book 2006 report of the Committee on Infectious Diseases.* 27th ed. Elk Grove Village, IL: American Academy of Pediatrics, 2006:378–400.

American Academy of Pediatrics, Committee on Drugs. Neonatal drug withdrawal. *Pediatrics* 2006;101:1079–1088.

American Academy of Pediatrics, Subcommittee on Neonatal Hyperbilirubinemia. Management of hyperbilirubinemia in the newborn infant 35 or more weeks of gestation. *Pediatrics* 2004;114:297–316.

Babbitt CJ, Garrett JS. Diarrhea and methemoglobinemia in an infant. *Pediatr Emerg Care* 2000;16:416–417.

Bale JF. Congenital infections. *Neurol Clin* 2002;20:1039–1060.

Booth D, Evans DJ. Anticonvulsants for neonates with seizures. *Cochrane Database Syst Rev* 2004:CD004218. doi:10.1002/14651858.CD004218.pub2.

Clemmens MR, Bell L. Infant botulism presenting with poor feeding and lethargy: a review of 4 cases. *Pediatr Emerg Care* 2007;23:492–494.

Costei AM, Kozer E, Ho T, et al. Perinatal outcome following third trimester exposure to paroxetine. *Arch Pediatr Adolesc Med* 2002;156:1129–1132.

Dennery PA. Pharmacological interventions for the treatment of neonatal jaundice. *Semin Neonatol* 2002;7:111–119.

Dick EA, de Bruyn R. Ultrasound of the spinal cord in children: its role. *Eur Radiol* 2003;13:552–562.

Donnelly V, Foran A, Murphy J, et al. Neonatal brachial plexus palsy: an unpredictable injury. *Am J Obstet Gynecol* 2002;187:1209–1212.

Fraser N, Davies BW. Neonatal omphalitis: a review of its serious complications. *Acta Paediatr* 2006;95:519–522.

Freishtat RJ, Chamberlain JM, Johns CM, et al. A cross-sectional ED survey of infantile subclinical methemoglobinemia [letter to the editor]. *Am J Emerg Med* 2005;23:574–576.

Fuerst RS. Use of pulse oximetry. In: Henretig FM, King C, eds. *Textbook of pediatric emergency procedures.* Baltimore, MD: Lippincott Williams & Wilkins, 1996:823–828.

Gartner LM. Jaundice and breastfeeding. *Pediatr Clin North Am* 2001;48:389–395.

Gersony WM. Major advances in pediatric cardiology in the twentieth century. *J Pediatr* 2001;139:328–333.

Greenough A, Khetriwal B. Pulmonary hypertension in the newborn. *Paediatr Respir Rev* 2005;6:111–116.

Johnson K, Gerada C, Greenough A. Treatment of neonatal abstinence syndrome. *Arch Dis Child Fetal Neonatal Ed* 2003;88:F2–F5.

Kandall SR. Treatment strategies for drug-exposed neonates. *Clin Perinatol* 1999;26:231–243.

Kappas A. A method for interdicting development of severe jaundice in newborns by inhibiting production of bilirubin. *Pediatrics* 2004;1:119–123.

Kimberlin DW. Herpes simplex virus infections of the newborn. *Semin Perinatol* 2007;31:19–25.

King C. Evaluation and management of febrile infants in the emergency department. *Emerg Med Clin North Am* 2003;21:89–99.

Lehmann HP, Hinton R, Morello P, et al. Developmental dysplasia of the hip—practice guideline: technical report. Committee on Quality Improvement and Subcommittee on Developmental Dysplasia of the Hip. *Pediatrics* 2000;105:E57.

Levene M. The clinical conundrum of neonatal seizures. *Arch Dis Child Fetal Neonatal Ed* 2002;86:F75–F77.

MEDICAL EMERGENCIES

Millar KR, Gloor JE, Wellington N, et al. Early neonatal presentations to the pediatric emergency department. *Pediatr Emerg Care* 2000;16: 145–150.

O'Malley PJ, Brown K, Krug SE; Committee on Pediatric Emergency Medicine. Patient- and family-centered care of children in the emergency department. *Pediatrics* 2008;122:e511–e521.

Rosen TS, Bateman DA. Infants of addicted mothers. In: Fanaroff AA, Martin RJ, eds. *Neonatal-perinatal medicine*, 7th ed. St Louis, MO: Mosby, 2002:661–673.

Shaw KN, Gorelick MH, McGowan KL, et al. Prevalence of urinary tract infection and occult bacteremia in febrile young children in the emergency department. *Arch Pediatr Adolesc Med* 1996;150:37.

Silverstein FS, Jensen FE. Neonatal seizures. *Ann Neurol* 2007;62:112–120.

Smith L, Yonekura ML, Wallace T, et al. Effects of prenatal methamphetamine exposure on fetal growth and drug withdrawal symptoms in infants born at term. *J Dev Behav Pediatr* 2003;24:17–23.

Smith LM, LaGasse LL, Derauf C, et al. The infant development, environment, and lifestyle study: effects of prenatal methamphetamine exposure, polydrug exposure, and poverty on intrauterine growth. *Pediatrics* 2006;118:1149–1156.

Stenmark KR. Primary pulmonary hypertension in the neonate. In: Rudolph CD, Rudolph AM, eds. *Rudolph's pediatrics*, 21st ed. New York, NY: McGraw Hill, 2003:181–184

Stevenson DK. Prediction of hyperbilirubinemia in near-term and term infants. *Pediatrics* 2001;108:31–39.

Teoh DL, Reynolds S. Diagnosis and management of pediatric conjunctivitis. *Pediatr Emerg Care* 2003;19:48–55.

Wasibren SE. Expanded newborn screening: information and resources for the family physician. *Am Fam Physician* 2008;77:987–994.

Yager JY, Vannucci RC. Seizures in neonates. In: Fanaroff AA, Martin RJ, eds. *Neonatal-perinatal medicine*, 7th ed. St Louis, MO: Mosby, 2002:887–899.

Zorc JJ, Kanic Z. A cyanotic infant: true blue or otherwise? *Pediatr Ann* 2001;30:597–601.

CHAPTER 96 ■ NEUROLOGIC EMERGENCIES

MARC H. GORELICK, MD, MSCE, AND CHARLES D. BLACKWELL, MD

Signs and symptoms of neurologic dysfunction in children either are produced by primary nervous system disorders or are secondary to systemic disease. The differential diagnosis of many such neurologic findings can be found in the second section of this book (Chapters 10, 12, 20, 26, 55, 69, and 73). This chapter focuses on the management of conditions primarily involving the various parts of the nervous system, including the brain, spinal cord, and peripheral nerves. The illnesses are classified by their most prominent clinical manifestations: seizures, altered mental status, headache, weakness, disorders of balance, abnormal movements, and cranial nerve dysfunction.

SEIZURES (SEE ALSO CHAPTER 69)

Seizures are among the more common neurologic symptoms that lead to an emergency department (ED) visit. Epidemiologic studies indicate that from 3% to 6% of children will have at least one seizure in the first 16 years of life; most of these are simple febrile seizures, discussed in the following section. Fortunately, recurrent seizures or other signs of neurologic dysfunction occur in only a small number of these children. However, the first seizure is always frightening and produces anxiety.

A *seizure* is defined as a transient, involuntary alteration of consciousness, behavior, motor activity, sensation, and/or autonomic function caused by an excessive rate and hypersynchrony of discharges from a group of cerebral neurons. The term *convulsion* is often used to describe a seizure with prominent motor manifestations. *Epilepsy*, or seizure disorder, is a condition of susceptibility to recurrent seizures.

Most seizures are brief, lasting for less than 10 to 15 minutes. *Status epilepticus (SE)* refers to seizures that are continuous for 30 minutes or longer or to repetitive seizures between which the patient does not regain consciousness. Many authorities now consider that seizures lasting for longer than 5 minutes or multiple seizures with no return to baseline in between constitute early SE.

Pathophysiology

The basic pathophysiologic abnormality common to all seizures and convulsions is the hypersynchrony of neuronal discharges. Many precipitating factors, including metabolic, anatomic, and infectious abnormalities (see Chapter 69), may produce seizures. Seizures that result from an identified precipitant are called *symptomatic*, or provoked, *seizures*, whereas those with no precipitating factor are called *idio-*

pathic or *cryptogenic*. Febrile seizures (seizures occurring in association with a febrile illness, without evidence of intracranial infection or other identified cause) are a particular type of provoked seizure seen in children between the ages of 6 months and 6 years. The exact cause of febrile seizures remains elusive. Elevated body temperature lowers the seizure threshold, and the immature brain appears to have a particular susceptibility to seizures in response to fever. It is unclear whether height of fever or rate of temperature rise is more important in inducing febrile seizures, but individual predisposition plays an important role.

During a seizure, cerebral blood flow, oxygen and glucose consumption, and carbon dioxide and lactic acid production increase. If the patient remains well ventilated, the increase in cerebral blood flow is sufficient to meet the increased metabolic requirements of the brain. Brief seizures rarely produce lasting deleterious effects on the brain; however, prolonged and serial seizures, especially SE, may be associated with permanent neuronal destruction.

Clinical Manifestations

When the physician is examining a child with an acute paroxysmal event, the first step is to distinguish seizures from other nonepileptic phenomena. If the event is indeed a seizure, it may be classified according to type. Finally, a specific causative factor should be sought. The extent of the emergency evaluation is determined by the clinical scenario; some of the diagnostic assessment may be deferred. Of course, when a child is actively seizing, the first priority is to provide necessary resuscitation measures and control the seizures (see Chapter 69 and the following sections).

Nonepileptic Paroxysmal Events

Paroxysmal events other than seizures that involve changes in consciousness or motor activity are common during childhood and may mimic epilepsy (Tables 69.2 and 96.1). Breath-holding spells occur in children 6 months to 4 years of age. Breath-holding spells take two forms: cyanotic and pallid. In the cyanotic form, the infant begins crying vigorously, often in response to an inciting event, then holds his or her breath and becomes cyanotic. After approximately 30 to 60 seconds, the child becomes rigid. As the spell ends, the child becomes limp and may have a transient loss of consciousness and twitching or jerking of the extremities, but the child quickly returns to full alertness. A pallid breath-holding spell may follow a seemingly insignificant trauma. The child may start to cry, but then turns pale and collapses. There is a brief period of apnea and limpness, followed by rapid recovery. In both types of

TABLE 96.1

NONEPILEPTIC EVENTS THAT MAY MIMIC SEIZURES

Breath-holding spells
Syncope
Migraine
Jitteriness
Benign myoclonus
Shuddering attacks
Tics
Acute dystonia
Gastroesophageal reflux
Night terrors
Sleep paralysis
Narcolepsy
Pseudoseizures

breath-holding spells, the typical history and lack of postictal drowsiness help determine the diagnosis. Breath-holding spells may be recurrent but disappear spontaneously before school age.

Syncope is a brief, sudden loss of consciousness and muscle tone. There are numerous causes of syncope, many of which can be detected on the basis of historical information, physical examination, and simple laboratory tests (see Chapter 73). A syncopal episode can usually be distinguished from a seizure on the basis of the description. The child is typically upright before the event and often senses a feeling of light-headedness or nausea. The child then becomes pale and slumps to the ground. The loss of consciousness is brief, and recovery is rapid. On awakening, the child is noted to have signs of increased vagal tone, such as pallor, clammy skin, dilated pupils, and relative bradycardia. Patients with narcolepsy also experience sudden alterations in alertness, with sleep occurring suddenly and uncontrollably during the daytime. In about half of the patients, narcolepsy is associated with cataplexy, an abrupt loss of muscle tone brought on by a sudden emotional outburst. Narcolepsy is far less common than syncope; both occur more often in adolescents than in younger children.

Single episodes of staring, involuntary movements, or eye deviation have been found to occur commonly in the first months of life, although they rarely lead to the parent seeking medical attention. In some children, however, these episodes occur frequently. Children with benign shuddering attacks have episodes of staring and rapid tremors involving primarily the arms and head, sometimes associated with tonic posturing. The episode lasts only a few seconds, and afterward, the child resumes normal activity. Acute dystonia, usually seen as a side effect of certain medications, can mimic a tonic seizure. The child having a dystonic reaction, however, does not lose consciousness and has no postictal drowsiness.

Several paroxysmal events are associated with sleep. Night terrors (see Chapter 131) usually begin in the preschool years. The sleeping child wakes suddenly, is confused and disoriented, and appears frightened, often screaming and showing signs of increased autonomic activity (tachycardia, tachypnea, sweating, dilated pupils). Such episodes typically last only a few minutes, and the child does not usually recall the event. Benign myoclonus is characterized by self-limited episodes of

sudden jerking of the extremities, usually upon falling asleep. There is no alteration of consciousness. In sleep paralysis, there is a transient inability to move during the transition between sleeping and waking, also with no change in the level of consciousness.

Pseudoseizures are occasionally seen, often in patients with an underlying seizure disorder or with a relative with epilepsy. Some features suggestive of pseudoseizures are suggestibility; lack of coordination of movements; moaning or talking during the seizure; lack of incontinence, autonomic changes, or postictal drowsiness; and poor response to treatment with anticonvulsant agents.

The most important diagnostic test in distinguishing nonepileptic events from seizures is a careful history, including a detailed description of the event from the person who witnessed it. In atypical or unclear cases, referral for electroencephalogram (EEG) or video EEG monitoring may help in establishing the diagnosis.

Types of Seizures

Clinically, seizures may be divided into partial and generalized seizures (Table 96.2). Generalized tonic-clonic seizures (previously called *grand mal seizures*) are the type most often seen in acute pediatric care. The onset of generalized tonic-clonic seizures is usually abrupt, although 20% to 30% of children may experience a sensory or motor aura. If sitting or standing, the child falls to the ground. The face becomes pale, the pupils dilate, the eyes deviate upward or to one side, and the muscles contract. As the increased tone of the thoracic and abdominal muscles forces air through the glottis, a grunt or cry may be heard. Incontinence of urine or stool is common. After this brief tonic phase (10 to 30 seconds), clonic movements occur. The child is unresponsive during the seizure and remains so postictally for a variable period. After the seizure, there may be weakness or paralysis of one or more areas of the body (Todd's paralysis). In atonic, or akinetic, seizures (drop attacks), there is abrupt loss of muscle tone and consciousness. *Myoclonic seizures* are characterized by a sudden dropping of the head and flexion of the arms (jackknifing); however, extensor posturing may also occur. The episodes occur quickly and frequently, as often as several hundred times daily.

Absence (petit mal) seizures are generalized seizures, marked by sudden and brief loss of awareness, usually lasting 5 to 30 seconds. With typical absence seizures, there is no loss

TABLE 96.2

SEIZURE TYPES

Generalized	Partial (focal)
Absence (petit mal)	Simple (no impaired consciousness)
Typical	Motor
Atypical	Sensory
Tonic-clonic (grand mal)	Autonomic
Clonic	Psychic
Tonic	Complex (impaired consciousness)
Myoclonic	Partial seizures becoming partially
Akinetic/atonic	generalized
(drop attacks)	

of posture or tone and no postictal confusion. There may be a minor motor component such as eyelid blinking.

The child with simple partial (focal) seizures has unimpaired consciousness. Motor signs are most common in children, although sensory, autonomic, and psychic manifestations are possible. The motor activity usually involves the hands or face and spreads in a fixed pattern determined by the anatomic origin of the nerve fibers that innervate the various muscle groups. Focal seizures may become secondarily generalized, in which case there will be alteration of consciousness. Complex partial seizures, also called *psychomotor* or *temporal lobe seizures*, exhibit a diverse set of clinical features, including alterations of perception, thought, and sensation. In children, they are usually marked by repetitive and complex movements with impaired consciousness and postictal drowsiness.

Establishing an Underlying Cause

The first steps in the evaluation of seizures are a thorough history and a physical examination, the results of which are helpful in determining the direction of the search for a specific cause (see Table 69.1 and Fig. 69.1). Important historical items to elicit include fever, trauma, underlying illnesses, current medications, and possible toxic ingestions. A complete neurologic assessment to evaluate for signs of increased intracranial pressure (ICP), focal deficits, or signs of meningeal irritation is also essential.

An important distinction is whether the seizure is associated with fever. Simple febrile seizures are those that are single, brief (lasting less than 15 minutes), and generalized. Approximately 20% of febrile seizures are complex, meaning they are focal, are prolonged (last for more than 15 minutes), or occur multiple times during the same illness. In children older than 12 months with a typical simple febrile seizure and no evidence of meningeal signs, no further evaluation of the seizure is generally required. However, lumbar puncture (LP) is mandatory if meningitis is suspected on the basis of physical findings. An LP should be considered in children younger than 12 months, in whom signs of meningitis may be subtle, such as irritability and poor feeding, when the febrile seizure is complex, or if there has been pretreatment with antibiotics. In addition, LP should be considered for children with prolonged fever before the seizure, particularly those who have sought medical care in the previous 48 hours, as a prior visit is associated with a higher risk. Other laboratory tests discussed in the next paragraph have been found to have little yield in the child with a typical febrile seizure and are unnecessary. Appropriate diagnostic tests to determine the source of the fever are determined by other features such as the intensity of fever and child's age, because the frequency of specific infections such as occult bacteremia is not increased in children who have experienced a febrile seizure.

For the child who presents with a first-time, nonfebrile seizure, laboratory or radiologic evaluation to search for a specific treatable cause of the seizure may be indicated. There is little utility in extensive, routine workups; rather, ancillary test selection should be guided by the results of the history and physical examination. In young infants, children with prolonged seizures, and those with a suggestive history or physical examination, determination of serum glucose, sodium, and calcium levels is indicated. Other ancillary tests that may be

indicated, depending on the clinical picture, include serum magnesium, hepatic transaminases, ammonia, serum or urine toxicology tests, electrocardiogram (EKG), and computed tomography (CT) scan of the brain. LP is rarely emergently necessary in the afebrile child without meningeal signs, although it should be considered in neonates even without fever.

In children with a known seizure disorder, subtherapeutic anticonvulsant levels are the most common reason for recurrent seizures. The name and dosage of anticonvulsant medications used should be elicited, as well as the time of the last dose given, any missed doses, the last change in dosage, and recent levels if known. Intercurrent illness may also play a role because the metabolism of some medications is affected by systemic illness. Such children should have blood drawn for measurement of anticonvulsant levels. Although many drugs have a standard therapeutic range (Table 96.3), individual patients may require levels outside that range for adequate seizure control; conversely, dose-dependent toxic effects may be observed in some children even at typically therapeutic levels.

CT and magnetic resonance imaging (MRI) allow detailed visualization of the gross anatomy of intracranial structures by a noninvasive technique. Presently, CT is more available on an emergent basis in most institutions. It is also a shorter procedure, and patient monitoring is usually easier. CT (or MRI, if available) is indicated in the emergency evaluation of prolonged or focal seizures, when focal deficits are present, when there is a history of trauma, when the child has a ventriculoperitoneal shunt, or when there are associated signs of increased ICP. For other children, an imaging study may be useful in identifying structural anomalies and determining prognosis, but such studies may be deferred to a follow-up visit. Cranial imaging is not indicated in the evaluation of simple febrile seizures.

EEG is also helpful in the evaluation of children with nonfebrile seizures. It is rarely beneficial in acute management, but children with nonfebrile seizures should be referred for outpatient testing.

Management

Resuscitation and Supportive Care

The administration of nasal oxygen and maintenance of an adequate airway are vital parts of the initial management of the unconscious, actively convulsing child (see Chapter 69). Trismus often occurs in generalized seizures but is transient. If the teeth are tightly clenched, even the placement of the airway should be deferred until it can be inserted without undue trauma during a phase of relaxation. Seizure-associated hypoventilation and apnea are common with prolonged seizures, often as a side effect of anticonvulsant medications, and providers caring for such children should be prepared to offer assisted ventilation. Intravenous (IV) access should be established promptly; however, because of the potential for increased ICP, fluid therapy should be used judiciously until a more thorough evaluation is performed. The child with active convulsions should be protected from trauma. There is no benefit of placing objects in the child's mouth to prevent tongue biting.

TABLE 96.3

COMMONLY USED ANTICONVULSANT AGENTS

Drug	Seizure type	Daily dose (mg/kg)	Oral dosage forms	Serum half-life (h)	Therapeutic blood levels (μg/mL)
Carbamazepine (Tegretol)	Generalized motor, partial, complex partial	10–30	Tablets: 100, 200 mg Suspension: 100 mg/5 mL	8–24	4–12
Phenytoin (Dilantin)	Generalized motor, partial, complex partial	3–10	Capsule: 100 mg Chewable tab: 50 mg Suspension: 125 mg/5 mL	10–36	10–20
Phenobarbital	Generalized motor, partial, complex partial	3–6	Tablets: 15, 30, 60, 100 mg Elixir: 20 mg/5 mL	24–96	15–40
Valproate (Depakote)	Absence, myoclonic, partial complex, generalized motor	20–40	Tablets: 125, 250 mg Sprinkles: 125 mg Syrup: 250 mg/5 mL	6–18	50–100
Ethosuximide (Zarontin)	Absence	20–40	Capsule: 250 mg Syrup: 250 mg/5 mL	20–60	40–100
Lamotrigine (Lamictal)	Partial, atonic, myoclonic, mixed types	10–15	Tablets: 25, 100, 150 mg	24	1–5
Clonazepam (Klonopin)	Atonic, myoclonic, generalized motor	0.05–0.2	Tablets: 0.5, 1, 2 mg	18–50	0.02–0.08 (20–80 ng/mL)
Topiramate (Topamax)	Partial, Lenox–Gastaut syndrome	6–15	Tablets: 25, 100, 200 mg	19–23	Not known
Oxcarbazepine (Trileptal)	Partial	10–40	Suspension: 300 mg/5 mL Tablets: 150, 300, 600 mg	9	Not known
Tiagabine (Gabritril)	Partial	Not established for <12 yr	Tablets: 2, 4, 12, 16 mg	2–10	Not known
Gabapentin (Neurontin)	Partial, generalized	25–35	Solution: 250 mg/5 mL Tablets: 600, 800 mg Capsules: 100, 300, 400 mg	5	Not known

Stopping the Seizure

It is unusual for the child with a brief seizure to arrive in the ED actively convulsing because, by definition, such seizures last for less than 15 minutes. Therefore, the actively convulsing child is usually already in a prolonged or serial seizure state, and pharmacologic intervention to terminate the seizure is required (Fig. 96.1).

IV access is established, and blood is drawn for diagnostic studies. If hypoglycemia is documented by rapid glucose assay or if rapid determination is unavailable, IV glucose is given most commonly in a dose of 2 to 4 mL per kg of 25% dextrose in water, although 10% and 50% glucose in equivalent doses may also be used (D10W should be used in infants). In neonates or in children with suspected isoniazid toxicity, IV pyridoxine 100 mg may be administered.

In most situations, benzodiazepines are the first drug of choice for acute seizures because of their rapidity of action. Lorazepam (Ativan) is the historically preferred agent. Given in a dose of 0.05 to 0.1 mg per kg IV (usual maximum 4 mg per dose), it has an onset of action of 2 to 5 minutes, and the duration of anticonvulsant effect is 12 to 24 hours. The dose may be repeated after 5 to 10 minutes. An alternative is diazepam (Valium), 0.2 to 0.4 mg per kg IV (usual maximum 10 mg per dose), which has a similarly rapid onset of action but a much shorter duration of anticonvulsant activity, usually less than 30 minutes. Thus, if diazepam is used, another agent for longer-term control, such as fosphenytoin (Cerebyx), may be needed to prevent seizure recurrence. If IV or intraosseous

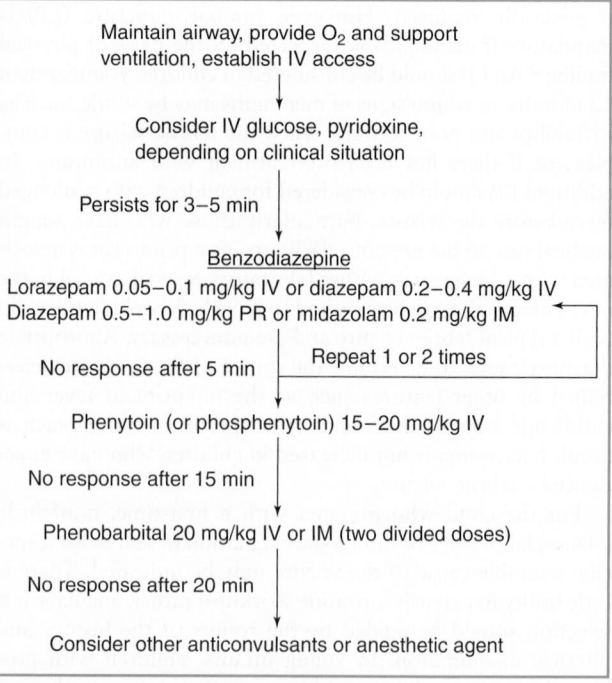

FIGURE 96.1 Treatment of status epilepticus. O₂, oxygen; IV, intravenous; PR, per rectum; IM, intramuscular.

access cannot be established, diazepam may be administered rectally in a dose of 0.5 mg per kg (maximum 20 mg per dose), instilling the IV formulation with a slip-tip syringe (remove needle) or by using a specific rectal gel preparation. Intramuscular (IM) midazolam (Versed) has also been shown to be effective in a dose of 0.2 mg per kg (maximum 7 mg per dose). IV midazolam may also be given ; the intranasal and buccal routes have also been described and appear to have promising initial results.

All the benzodiazepines can cause sedation and respiratory depression. Equipment for establishing an airway and supporting respiration must be available, especially if repeated doses are used. Sedation and respiratory depression may persist for hours, particularly with diazepam. Hypotension is uncommon but may be a problem with multiple doses or when barbiturates are administered concomitantly.

If the seizures have not been controlled within 10 minutes with benzodiazepines, phenytoin or fosphenytoin should be given. Fosphenytoin is a prodrug of phenytoin, which is rapidly metabolized to the active form. It offers several advantages over phenytoin, including more rapid administration and fewer local and systemic side effects. Fosphenytoin may also be given IM, unlike phenytoin. The dose of the two drugs is identical; fosphenytoin doses are expressed as phenytoin equivalents. The loading dose of fosphenytoin is 15 to 20 mg phenytoin equivalents (PE) per kg IV, at a rate of 2 mg PE per kg per min to a maximum of 150 mg per min. In the absence of any clinical effect, an additional 10 mg per kg IV may be administered. Cardiac monitoring is required because rapid IV infusion may lead to hypotension, QT prolongation, and cardiac dysrhythmias. (If phenytoin is used instead, the maximum rate of administration is 50 mg per min.) In patients known to be taking phenytoin chronically, a smaller dose of 5 to 10 mg per kg should be used initially unless the serum level is known to be very low. Each 1 mg per kg of phenytoin administered raises the serum level by approximately 1 μg per mL, although phenytoin kinetics are notoriously unpredictable. Phenytoin is highly lipid soluble and reaches therapeutic levels in the brain within 10 to 20 minutes, with duration of action of 12 to 24 hours. Unlike other anticonvulsant medications, phenytoin does not cause sedation or respiratory depression.

Phenobarbital is the next agent often added if phenytoin is not effective or contraindicated (e.g., allergy, known therapeutic level). The loading dose of phenobarbital is 20 mg per kg, sometimes given in two divided doses. The drug is given over 5 to 10 minutes IV (maximum 30 mg per min), or IM in the absence of IV access. Onset of action is usually within 15 to 20 minutes and lasts more than 24 hours. Phenobarbital, like other barbiturates, may cause significant sedation and hypotension.

IV valproate (VPA) and IV levetiracetam (Keppra) may also serve as an alternative to phenobarbital or phenytoin in the treatment of SE. A recent study demonstrated that valproic acid may be particularly useful for patients with a known seizure disorder, who are currently using VPA, when low serum concentrations are suspected. Effective loading doses in one study were 10 mg per kg IV when subtherapeutic levels were suspected and 25 mg per kg IV when the patient was not being treated with VPA. In this study, no adverse effects related to hypotension or heart rate were observed.

Similarly, IV levetiracetam may also serve as an alterative therapy in the treatment of SE that is refractory to benzodi-azepines. In a recent report, levetiracetam was used for 18 episodes of benzodiazepine refractory focal SE in 16 patients. SE was controlled in all patients by the given combination of drugs, with no adverse events such as hemodynamic instability. However, further study is still needed to investigate the efficacy of IV levetiracetam for the use in treatment of SE.

Patients with SE that lasts for more than 30 to 60 minutes present a special problem. Further management should be done, when possible, in conjunction with a neurologist and with EEG monitoring. Continuous infusion of benzodiazepines may be used. Previously, paraldehyde and lidocaine hydrochloride have been used to treat SE. However, these medications have not demonstrated any advantage over the conventional therapies already discussed and have more serious side effect profiles. In addition, paraldehyde is no longer available in the United States. Other agents potentially useful in the management of refractory SE include continuous infusion pentobarbital or midazolam and general anesthetics such as isoflurane, etomidate, and propofol.

With prolonged seizures, the duration of postictal drowsiness and confusion may also be protracted. However, the child who fails to arouse within 15 to 30 minutes after cessation of seizures should be evaluated carefully to rule out nonconvulsive SE. Children with SE, even if successfully treated in the ED, should be admitted to the hospital for monitoring and observation.

Rarely, a child may enter the ED in absence status. In this case, the child may be sitting in a confused or dreamy state. Such attacks may last for hours or even days. The drug of choice in the treatment of absence status is lorazepam or diazepam at the dosages already outlined.

At times, a child may present with continual focal seizure activity (with or without clouding of consciousness), a condition known as *epilepsia partialis continua*. The treatment for partial seizures is less urgent than that for generalized seizures, and such seizures are often intractable to anticonvulsant medication. In such cases, fosphenytoin in a dose of 15 to 20 mg per PE per kg can be infused slowly. All such patients should be admitted to the hospital for further observation and evaluation. Other pharmacologic attempts to control these focal seizures should be performed in the hospital.

Initiating Anticonvulsant Medication

Nonfebrile Seizures. The decision to initiate long-term prophylactic therapy with anticonvulsant medications is based on a consideration of a number of factors, including the patient's age, type of seizure, risk of recurrence, coexisting medical conditions, and family factors. The consequences of further seizures must be balanced against the potential side effects of the anticonvulsant agents. Treatment is seldom started after a single, uncomplicated nonfebrile seizure because most such patients will not experience a seizure recurrence. However, a patient who has had two or more such seizures should generally receive anticonvulsant therapy. When possible, it is preferable for long-term treatment decisions to be made in conjunction with the provider who will be responsible for ongoing follow-up of the patient, either a neurologist or the child's primary care physician. Sometimes, it may be necessary to begin prophylactic treatment in the ED, pending a more complete outpatient evaluation.

A number of drugs are effective in preventing seizures (Table 96.3). Some are better for certain types of seizures, and all have different profiles of adverse effects. The following principles should guide selection of an anticonvulsant medication:

1. Choose a drug that is effective for the particular type of seizure. When more than one agent is available, choose the least toxic one. Initial therapy should be with a single agent.
2. Start at the low end of the dosage range.
3. Arrange for a serum level of the drug to be measured, when appropriate. This is done after a steady state is anticipated, usually five times the half-life of the drug.
4. If a child is already taking an anticonvulsant medication and has an adequate level, consider adding another agent.

Carbamazepine (Tegretol). Carbamazepine is effective against generalized tonic-clonic seizures as well as simple and complex partial seizures. The effective serum concentrations of carbamazepine range between 4 and 12 μg per mL, but with this drug there is a variable correlation among clinical efficacy, toxicity, and the serum concentration. Initial dose is 5 to 10 mg per kg per day; recommended maintenance dosages range between 10 and 35 mg per kg per day, divided into three daily doses. The administration of a total maintenance dose to a previously untreated patient often results in drowsiness, blurred vision, and at times, severe lethargy; so, this drug should be initiated by gradual increases in dosage (10 mg per kg per day to start, increased by 5 mg per kg per day every 3 to 4 days) until a full maintenance level is reached. Note that carbamazepine induces its own metabolism around day 14, and levels may suddenly become subtherapeutic and should be monitored closely. Unlike several other agents, it is not available in an IV form. Concomitantly administered medications that may lead to toxic carbamazepine levels include macrolide antibiotics (e.g., erythromycin), isoniazid, cimetidine, verapamil, and diltiazem.

Carbamazepine may cause hepatic and hematologic toxicity but causes little, if any, cognitive dysfunction in most patients. Therefore, it is often the drug of choice for children with generalized seizures.

Phenobarbital. Phenobarbital is another broad-spectrum anticonvulsant useful for generalized tonic-clonic and partial (simple and complex) seizures. It remains a commonly used initial drug, primarily because of its low cost and low toxicity. The effective serum concentration ranges between 15 and 40 μg per mL. This serum level can usually be maintained with a dosage of 3 to 6 mg per kg per day in children and 1 to 2 mg per kg per day in adolescents, administered in divided doses twice daily. A loading dosage of approximately twice the maintenance dosage (6 to 10 mg per kg per day in children and 2 to 4 mg per kg per day in adolescents) for 2 to 3 days brings the serum concentration to the therapeutic range within 48 to 72 hours. Such loading dosages are usually associated with considerable transient drowsiness. There is a wide margin between the anticonvulsant and soporific effects of phenobarbital, and drowsiness rarely persists at the recommended dosages. Decreased attention, hyperactivity, and alterations of mood occur in 30% to 50% of children maintained on phenobarbital. These behavioral changes are the most commonly encountered side effects and are often sufficiently undesirable to force the change to another drug. Possible associated long-term cognitive effects also makes phenobarbital problematic, and many clinicians do not consider it a first-line drug. Primidone (Mysoline) and mephobarbital (Mebaral) are related drugs.

Phenytoin (Dilantin). Phenytoin is another agent effective in the treatment of several seizure types, including generalized motor seizures and both simple and partial complex seizures. The effective serum concentration of phenytoin is between 10 and 20 μg per mL. The usual maintenance dosage is 7 to 10 mg per kg per day in children weighing less than 20 kg, 5 to 7 mg per kg per day in children weighing between 20 and 40 kg, and 5 mg per kg per day in children weighing more than 40 kg, given in once or twice daily doses. However, there is considerable variation in metabolism among patients. Saturation of biotransforming enzyme systems often occurs between serum levels of 10 and 20 μg per mL, so small changes in a dose in this range may lead to relatively large changes in serum levels.

Loading dosages of four times the daily dosage (maximum 20 mg per kg per day) on the first day and two times the daily dosage for the next 2 days will bring serum levels into the therapeutic range within 24 hours; side effects rarely occur with this loading dosage. Gingival hyperplasia is a common side effect and may be seen with phenytoin concentrations in the therapeutic range; this cosmetic side effect and the drug's tendency to cause hirsutism and coarsening of facial features often limit long-term use, especially in girls. Drowsiness, ataxia, nystagmus, and seizures are dose-dependent toxic effects rarely seen with levels in the therapeutic range. Other adverse effects include drug rashes (Stevens–Johnson syndrome) and hematologic and hepatic side effects. Several medications may cause increased phenytoin levels: cimetidine, estrogens, chlorpromazine, chloramphenicol, and isoniazid.

Valproate (Depakote). VPA is highly effective in the treatment of generalized epilepsy, including especially absence and myoclonic seizures, as well as simple and complex partial seizures. Doses of 20 to 40 mg per kg usually result in therapeutic levels of 50 to 100 μg per mL, although doses of up to 100 mg per kg per day may be necessary when combined with other enzyme-inducing antiepileptics. However, serum drug levels may not be highly predictive of efficacy or toxicity. The primary side effects include gastrointestinal upset and drowsiness; hepatic, renal, pancreatic, and hematologic dysfunction are also seen. Carnitine is often prescribed for patients receiving doses higher than 50 mg per kg per day, in attempt to avoid hepatotoxicity. Children younger than 2 years are at particular risk of idiosyncratic fatal hepatotoxicity. Therefore, VPA is rarely the initial drug of choice for young children with generalized seizures.

Clonazepam (Klonopin). Clonazepam is used to control myoclonic and atonic seizures. The usual dosage is 0.05 to 0.2 mg per kg per day, given in two to four divided doses. The therapeutic range is 0.02 to 0.08 μg per mL (20 to 80 ng per mL). Patients taking clonazepam may experience drowsiness, ataxia, and drooling.

Ethosuximide (Zarontin). Ethosuximide is indicated for the management of absence seizures. It is given at a dosage of 20 to 40 mg per kg per day, divided into twice-daily doses, with a usual therapeutic level of 40 to 100 μg per mL. Side effects include headache, nausea, and vomiting; erythema multiforme and a lupus-like syndrome have also been reported.

Lamotrigine (Lamictal). Lamotrigine is indicated for treatment of partial seizures, atonic and myoclonic seizures, and intractable mixed seizures (Lennox–Gastaut syndrome). The usual dosage is 10 to 15 mg per kg per day, which is reduced to 5 mg per kg per day when given in conjunction with VPA. Initial doses are substantially lower, starting at 0.6 mg per kg per day and 0.2 mg per kg per day, respectively. Drowsiness, vomiting, nystagmus, ataxia, and life-threatening drug rashes (including Stevens–Johnson syndrome) are reported side effects. If the patient develops a rash while on lamotrigine, particularly in the first 3 months of therapy, the drug should be stopped immediately and not rechallenged without consultation with a pediatric neurologist.

Topiramate (Topamax). Topiramate is available for adjunctive therapy in the treatment of refractory partial epilepsy and Lennox–Gastaut syndrome. The usual dosage is initiated at 0.5 to 1.0 mg per kg per day, in two divided doses for 1 week. This may then be increased by 0.5 to 1.0 mg per kg per day per week until an effective dose is achieved. The usual minimum effective dose is 6 mg per kg per day, in two divided doses. Side effects can include drowsiness and impairment of physical and speech coordination. It should be used with caution in patients having renal dysfunction or previous allergic reactions to sulfa-based medications.

Oxcarbazepine (Trileptal). Oxcarbazepine is used for treatment of partial epilepsy. Like many other anticonvulsants, it is metabolized in the liver by the cytochrome p450 pathway; concomitant administration with inducers or inhibitors of this pathway may alter serum levels. The usual dose range is 10 to 40 mg per kg per day. Adverse effects include somnolence, anxiety, rash, hyponatremia, and hypersensitivity. There is a 25% to 30% incidence of cross-hypersensitivity with carbamazepine.

Diazepam (Diastat-R). Diazepam rectal gel has been used intermittently to successfully stop seizure activity in the outpatient setting. The most effective use is in a selected group of patients with refractory epilepsy who are on stable regimens of antiepileptic drugs. In this setting, the most common side effect is sedation.

Levetiracetam (Keppra). Levetiracetam is a newer anticonvulsant that is indicated for adjunctive therapy of partial-onset seizures in children older than 4 years, as well as treatment for generalized tonic-clonic seizure in those older than 6 years and juvenile myoclonic seizures in those older than 12 years. The usual dose begins at 20 mg per kg per day, divided in 2 doses. Adverse effects can include dizziness, somnolence, and headache.

Other Agents. Several other antiepileptic medications are available but are generally reserved as add-on therapy prescribed in consultation with a pediatric neurologist. These include gabapentin (Neurontin), tiagabine (Gabitril), and zonisamide (Zonegran). Several new agents are more recently available in the United States or are currently under investigation, notably lacosamide (Vimpat), pregabalin (Lyrica), and rufinamide (Banzel). Another new agent, fluorofelbamate, is under development as a derivative of an older medication, felbamate (Felbatol). Felbamate is restricted to use in children with intractable seizures refractory to other treatment due to the risk of severe hepatotoxicity. The new compound was created to avoid the production of the metabolite thought to cause this side effect. Vagus nerve stimulation is a novel nonpharmacologic approach to the management of children with intractable seizures. Intermittent electrical stimulation is delivered to the cervical vagus nerve trunk by an implanted device. The lead is typically located on the left side of the neck, and the generator is implanted in the chest wall. In addition to the programmed impulses, patients with an aura of an impending seizure may trigger additional impulses with a handheld magnet. Adverse effects are generally mild and include hoarseness, cough, and paresthesias. If the device needs to be inactivated temporarily, this is accomplished noninvasively with a telemetry wand.

Febrile Seizures. For children with febrile seizures, the issue of chronic prophylactic medication is more controversial. Presumptive antipyretic therapy for a nonspecific illness does not appear to reduce the risk of seizure recurrence, although it may give the parent a sense of "doing something." Phenobarbital was widely used in the past for children with recurrent febrile seizures, but this practice is much less common now because of concerns about adverse cognitive and behavioral effects of the medication. To be effective, phenobarbital must be given continuously. Other commonly used anticonvulsant agents such as phenytoin and carbamazepine appear to be ineffective. More recently, some clinicians have used diazepam, administered intermittently during febrile illnesses (0.33 mg per kg every 8 hours), to prevent febrile seizures. One controlled trial showed this treatment to be effective, albeit with a high incidence of side effects; while other studies have failed to confirm the effectiveness of this approach, largely as a result of poor compliance or inadequate recognition of fever. With little evidence that febrile seizures (even febrile SE) cause permanent neurologic damage or that their control results in a lower incidence of subsequent epilepsy, there is little need to treat most patients. In carefully considered individual cases, long-term continuous therapy with phenobarbital or intermittent therapy with diazepam may be considered. This should usually be done in conjunction with the child's primary care provider.

Disposition. Hospital admission is generally required for children who have had a prolonged seizure requiring acute treatment with anticonvulsant medication. With the exception of very young infants, other children, even those with a first-time seizure, can generally be followed as outpatients if they appear well after the seizure, follow-up can be ensured, and the parents are comfortable with home management. Seizure first aid should be explained to the family before discharge. Some practitioners may choose to prescribe rectal diazepam until a decision is made about instituting chronic anticonvulsant therapy.

MEDICAL EMERGENCIES

After a simple febrile seizure, hospitalization is seldom necessary, and children may be followed by their primary physician. Some useful information can be given to parents after a first febrile seizure. First, they should be informed of the benign nature of the convulsions and the lack of evidence that they cause any type of neurologic injury. Approximately one-third of children with a first febrile seizure will have another one. Of recurrences, 75% occur within 1 year, and they are uncommon beyond 2 years; fewer than 10% of children with febrile seizures have more than three. The recurrence rate is lower if the seizures begin after the first year of life, and the risk is also reduced in children with higher temperature and longer duration of fever before the initial febrile seizure. For example, the recurrence risk is about 35% when the first seizure occurs at a temperature of 38.5°C (101.3°F), compared with a risk of 13% with a temperature of 40°C (104°F). Having a complex first febrile seizure (even febrile SE) does not increase the risk of recurrence, nor does it increase the chance that a recurrent seizure, if it occurs, will be complex.

Many parents are concerned that febrile seizures will lead to future epilepsy. A child who has had a febrile seizure but no other risk factors for epilepsy may have a slightly increased risk of future nonfebrile seizures, but the magnitude of this increase is still extremely small: 1% to 2% lifetime risk versus a 0.5% to 1% lifetime risk in the general population. Several risk factors that increase the likelihood of a child experiencing future nonfebrile seizures have been identified. These risk factors include a family history of epilepsy, a complex febrile seizure, and the presence of an underlying neurologic or developmental abnormality. Importantly, even with two or more of these risk factors, the risk of epilepsy is only 10%. Thus, for most children with no risk factors, the parents may be reassured that future epilepsy, although possible, is extremely unlikely. Furthermore, there is no association between febrile seizures and any type of developmental or learning disabilities.

DISORDERS THAT PRESENT WITH ENCEPHALOPATHY (SEE ALSO CHAPTER 12)

Encephalopathy is an imprecise term that implies diffuse brain dysfunction with or without alterations in the level of consciousness. The emergency physician often must decide whether the child's degree of irritability, uncooperativeness, and lethargy is proportionate to the degree of systemic illness; whether it is caused by fear; or whether it represents cortical dysfunction. Encephalopathy may be a sign of numerous systemic disorders, or it may result from primary disorders of the central nervous system (CNS), the most common of which is encephalitis.

Encephalitis

Background

Encephalitis is an inflammation of the brain parenchyma. When there is an associated leptomeningeal involvement (as often occurs), the term *meningoencephalitis* may be applied, whereas *encephalomyelitis* implies involvement of the spinal

---

TABLE 96.4

AGENTS OF VIRAL ENCEPHALITIS

Arboviruses
Eastern equine encephalitis
Western equine encephalitis
St. Louis encephalitis
Japanese encephalitis
California (LaCrosse) encephalitis
West Nile
Herpesviruses
Herpes simplex
Varicella-zoster
Epstein-Barr
Cytomegalovirus
Mumps
Measles
Enteroviruses
Rabies

---

cord as well. CNS dysfunction is caused by direct invasion of brain by a pathogen, most often a virus, or is secondary to immunologic mechanisms, as in postinfectious encephalomyelitis.

Viral encephalitides are caused by a wide variety of viruses that lead to clinically similar illnesses (Table 96.4). Currently, an etiology is not identified in most cases, even with an extensive laboratory evaluation. Mumps was the most common cause of meningoencephalitis before the introduction of vaccination, with up to 50% of patients with mumps parotitis having cerebrospinal fluid (CSF) pleocytosis. Classically, the illness occurs several days to 2 weeks after the onset of parotitis but may precede the onset of systemic illness or occur without parotitis and tends to be mild. Measles encephalitis is less common since the advent of widespread live immunization. The onset usually occurs during the prodromal period or after the rash has appeared. Ataxia is the most common neurologic abnormality, and sequelae occur in up to 30% of cases. Varicella encephalitis occurs 2 to 9 days after the onset of the rash; severe infections are uncommon, except in the immuno-suppressed host.

The arthropodborne encephalitides—including St. Louis, Western equine, Eastern equine, and California encephalitis—occur in sporadic and epidemic forms, often in late summer or early fall, and tend to cluster in localized geographic areas. Sequelae may be severe and mortality high, especially in Eastern equine encephalitis. West Nile virus is another agent in this family that first appeared in the United States in 1999. Since then, it appears to have become endemic in large parts of North America, although infections in children are uncommon.

Herpes simplex virus (HSV) is a relatively common cause of sporadic encephalitis. Disease in neonates is usually caused by HSV type 2, acquired from perinatal transmission. In previously healthy older children and adults, encephalitis more often results from infection with HSV type 1 and may be a complication of acute primary infection or reactivated latent infection. Recognition of herpes encephalitis is often difficult early in the course but is important because specific antiviral therapy reduces the substantial morbidity and mortality of this disease.

Infection with rabies virus, although rare in the United States, is an important cause of encephalitis worldwide. Nonviral pathogens, including *Mycoplasma pneumoniae*, Lyme disease, and rickettsiae, may also cause encephalitis.

Postinfectious encephalitis may follow infection with numerous viruses, including measles, varicella, influenza, and Epstein-Barr virus. The CNS involvement may be confined to a specific area, as in acute cerebellar ataxia after varicella infection, or may be widespread. The latter condition is often designated *acute disseminated encephalomyelitis*. A particularly virulent form with high mortality is known as *acute hemorrhagic leukoencephalitis*. A clinical syndrome of encephalopathy after immunization, particularly with whole-cell pertussis vaccine, is also described, although more recent epidemiologic evidence has called into question the association with pertussis immunization.

Pathophysiology

Viral encephalitis usually follows a viremia, although direct spread can occur less commonly via peripheral nerves or the nasal mucosa. Upon reaching the CNS, viral replication in neural cells interferes with cellular function and may lead to cell death. Cerebral edema may result from capillary leakage, with subsequent increased ICP. The degree and extent of neuronal dysfunction depends in part on the pathogen involved and also on host factors, especially immunocompetence. In general, the incidence of overt neurologic findings and sequelae is higher in children younger than 1 year.

Postinfectious encephalitis is presumed to be an immune-mediated phenomenon, involving the white matter of the CNS. Demyelination, the pathologic hallmark of the disease, may be focal or widespread.

Clinical Manifestations

The clinical picture of viral encephalitis ranges from a mild febrile illness associated with headache and minimal changes in mentation to a severe, fulminant presentation with coma, seizures, and death. The onset of encephalitis may be abrupt or insidious. Typical features consist of fever, headache, vomiting, and signs of meningeal irritation. Altered consciousness, ataxia, and seizures are also seen. Focal neurologic deficits may occur in certain types of encephalitis, particularly HSV. Flaccid paralysis may be seen in cases of encephalomyelitis, and rarely, respiratory or cardiac dysfunction results from brain stem involvement. Rash or mucous membrane lesions are often seen with the exanthematous viruses such as measles and varicella; however, cutaneous findings are uncommon with HSV encephalitis.

Laboratory assessment is often nonspecific. The peripheral blood count usually shows a mild polymorphonuclear or mononuclear leukocytosis. With viral encephalitides, CSF pleocytosis is variable and, if present, is usually fewer than 500 cells per cubic millimeter. These cells may be predominantly polymorphonuclear early in the course of the illness; however, a mononuclear predominance is common later. Red blood cells are present in the CSF in approximately 50% of children with herpes encephalitis. Spinal fluid protein and glucose levels are usually normal with viral encephalitis, but the protein level may be greatly elevated in postinfectious encephalomyelitis.

Virus isolation from the CSF may be difficult but should be attempted, as should viral isolation from other body sites, including the nasopharynx, skin lesions, urine, and feces. Serologic evidence for viral infection based on acute and convalescent IgG titers, although useful later, gives little help in making an immediate diagnosis. Infection with arboviruses may be established more rapidly by detecting virus-specific IgM in CSF or serum.

Herpes simplex poses a special problem because early diagnosis is important in instituting effective therapy. Although not usually available with rapid turnaround time, polymerase chain reaction testing of CSF yields rapid evidence of viral nucleic acid and is relatively sensitive and specific. Imaging studies, although less sensitive, may also be useful. Either CT or MRI may demonstrate focal parenchymal involvement or edema of the temporal lobes (Fig. 96.2). MRI is more sensitive than CT, although both may show normal results in the early stages of disease. Similarly, EEG may demonstrate focal slowing or epileptiform discharges localized to the temporal lobes, but absence of such findings does not rule out herpes encephalitis.

Management

Presently, the treatment of nonherpes viral encephalitis is primarily supportive. Children with aseptic meningitis and mild manifestations may be followed at home, but those with encephalitis should be hospitalized for observation and monitoring of neurologic status, treatment of increased ICP if present, and fluid restriction and monitoring of urine output and serum sodium because of the risk for inappropriate antidiuretic hormone secretion.

Herpes simplex encephalitis causes death or neurologic sequelae in more than 70% of patients. Treatment with acyclovir (60 mg per kg per day divided q8h daily for 14 to 21 days) has resulted in a decrease in mortality and some improvement in morbidity. Obviously, treatment should be initiated as early as possible after deciding that HSV is a reasonably likely diagnosis (although institution of therapy in the first 24 to 48 hours has never been shown to convey a statistically significant advantage over late treatment). Thus, acyclovir should be considered in all patients suspected of having herpes encephalitis on the basis of clinical or epidemiologic grounds (e.g., oral vesicles, focal neurologic or radiographic findings); because clinical features and laboratory tests are not perfectly sensitive, initial presumptive treatment may be indicated even in the absence of corroborating evidence.

DISORDERS THAT PRESENT WITH HEADACHE

Headaches of varying character, severity, and origin affect patients of all ages. Much of the CNS, including the brain parenchyma, is devoid of pain sensors. However, headache may result from compression, inflammation, or distortion of a number of pain-sensitive cranial structures, including the proximal portions of the large cerebral arteries, the arteries of the dura and scalp, the intracranial venous sinuses, the dura, the facial sinuses, orbits, teeth, scalp, muscles, and cervical roots of the spinal cord. A full discussion of the differential diagnosis of headache is given in Chapter 55.

MEDICAL EMERGENCIES

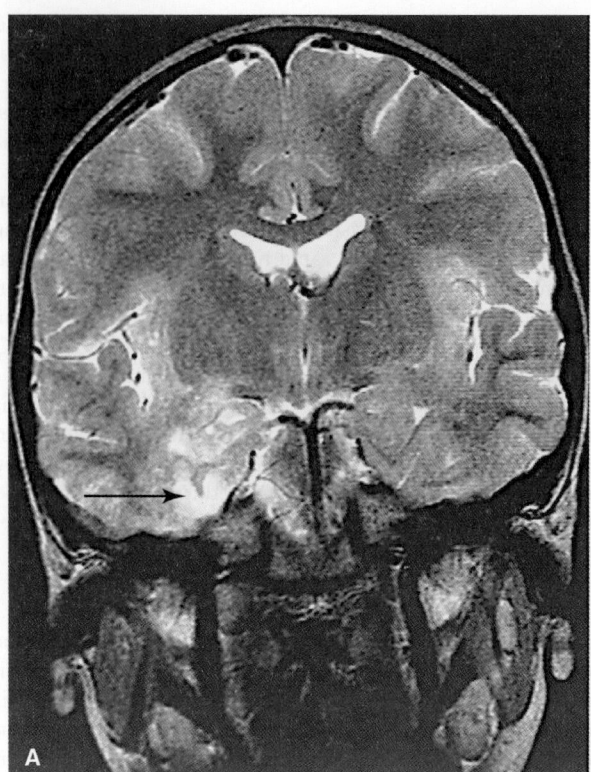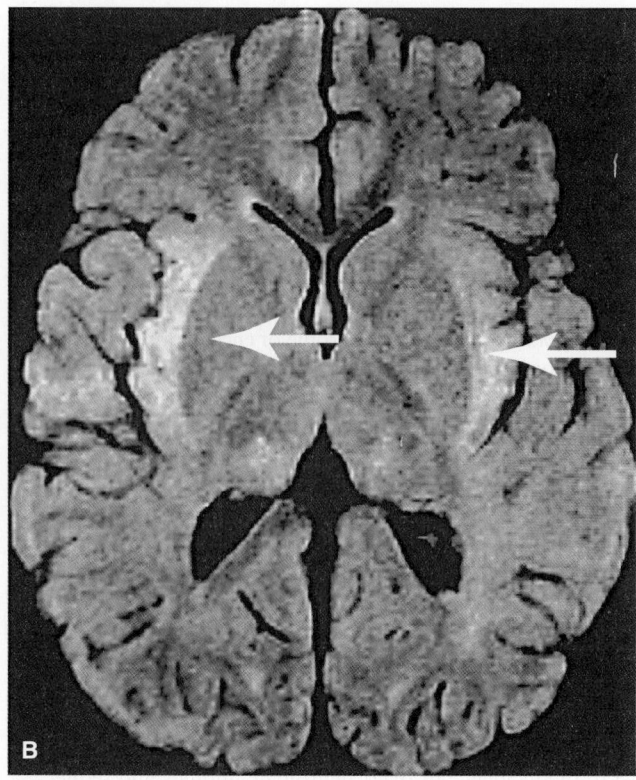

FIGURE 96.2 Coronal (**A**) and axial (**B**) T$_2$-weighted magnetic resonance images showing multifocal areas of abnormal signal in the medial aspects of both temporal lobes *(large arrow)* and left posterior parietal lobe *(small arrow)* in a patient with herpes simplex encephalitis.

Migraine

Background

Migraine—recurrent headaches separated by long, symptom-free intervals—is probably the most common specific cause of episodic headaches in afebrile children. In epidemiologic studies, prevalence estimates for migraine in children range from 3% to 10%. A number of forms of migraine are recognized. Migraine is considered "classic" when the headache is well localized and preceded by an aura and considered "common" when it is not. The common form of migraine predominates in children. Basilar migraine is a migraine variant that involves the posterior cerebral circulation in which brain stem symptoms, possibly including transient loss of consciousness, predominate. Cluster headaches, which are unilateral, occur in runs and are associated with autonomic changes. They represent a rare migraine variant in childhood. Cyclic vomiting, a syndrome of recurrent, discrete attacks of abdominal pain, nausea, vomiting, and pallor, is also believed to be a migraine variant, sometimes called *abdominal migraine*.

Pathophysiology

Migraine is a result of an underlying hyperexcitable cerebral cortex. In a genetically predisposed individual, a variety of stimuli can trigger episodes of "cortical spreading depression," a slowly propagating wave of neuronal hyperpolarization followed by depolarization. This in turn triggers a neuronally-mediated vascular instability that results in intracranial hypoperfusion (which may produce the migraine aura of premonitory motor, visual, or sensory symptoms), followed by vasodilation and a sterile, neurogenic inflammation, which are responsible for the headache.

Clinical Manifestations

Prolonged (up to 24 to 48 hours), moderate to severe headache is characteristic of migraine. The headaches may be pulsating and unilateral but assume this pattern less often in children than in adults. Migraine is commonly associated with nausea, vomiting, abdominal pain, and photophobia or phonophobia. Auras occur in less than half of children who experience migraines. During the headaches, standard, oral analgesics may be relatively ineffective, and children seek a quiet, dimly lit area to rest or sleep. Occasionally, the attacks awaken the children from sleep. The physical examination usually shows no focal neurologic deficits, although hemiplegia and ophthalmoplegia may occur in complicated migraine. Unless these episodes have occurred previously, their presence warrants further neurologic evaluation, usually in the form of CT or MRI scanning.

A family history of migraine is helpful in diagnosis, and a disproportionate number of children who experience migraines have episodes of motion sickness, dizziness, vertigo, or frank paroxysmal events. Common trigger factors for migraine in children include emotional stress, lighting changes, and minor head trauma. Particularly in adolescents, it is useful to screen for depression or other psychosocial stressors that may warrant separate treatment. Foods, such as lunch meats, which contain nitrates, and cheeses, which contain tyramine, are less common but important triggers.

The diagnosis of migraine is based almost exclusively on the history and is supported by the absence of abnormalities on examination. There are no diagnostic laboratory tests or imaging studies. Given an accurate history, differentiation from tension headaches, sinusitis, and headaches secondary to intracranial lesions is usually possible; studies such as EEG, CT, and MRI are rarely indicated. Of children who experience migraines, 20% to 90% have been reported to have nonspecific EEG abnormalities, but the EEG is usually not helpful in diagnosis.

Management

A number of agents are available for the treatment of acute migraine (Table 96.5). For many children, mild oral analgesics such as acetaminophen or ibuprofen combined with bed rest may provide sufficient relief and should be considered the first-line agents of choice. Ketorolac (Toradol), a nonsteroidal anti-inflammatory agent for parenteral use, may be used when nausea or vomiting limits oral intake. A short course of a narcotic analgesic such as oxycodone may occasionally be needed if nonnarcotic agents have failed, especially if the headache prevents sleep.

When nausea and vomiting are severe, antiemetic medications such as metoclopramide (Reglan), prochlorperazine (Compazine), and promethazine (Phenergan) are useful. In addition to their antiemetic effect, these agents often provide some relief of the headache as well and may permit the use of other oral medications. All these agents have the potential to produce dystonic reactions. Due to fewer side effects, ondansetron (Zofran) and granisetron (Kytril) have also become first-line agents in the treatment of nausea and vomiting for migraine headaches.

Sumatriptan succinate (Imitrex) is a serotonergic agent available for oral, intranasal, or subcutaneous administration. Its effectiveness in relieving symptoms of acute migraine has been demonstrated in clinical trials in children and adults, but it has not been approved by the U.S. Food and Drug Administration for use in younger children. The dose for children 12 years and older is 6 mg subcutaneously or 100 mg orally. Sumatriptan is generally well tolerated; side effects include irritation at the injection site, flushing, tachycardia, disorientation, and chest tightness that lasts for several minutes after parenteral administration. In one trial, adverse effects were more common in younger children. A reasonable approach is to use sumatriptan after a trial of analgesics in an older child, although older children or adolescents with recurrent migraine and a history of successful treatment with sumatriptan in the past may benefit from earlier use of this agent. Other agents in this family include rizatriptan (Maxalt), zolmitriptan (Zomig), and naratriptan (Amerge).

Ergot preparations act primarily as cerebral vasoconstrictors and are specifically indicated for aborting acute migraine attacks. Ergotamine tartrate is administered orally or sublingually, but it must be used early in the headache to be effective, preferably at the outset of the prodrome. Because most young children cannot identify an aura, their use is limited before adolescence. Common side effects of ergot preparations include nausea, vomiting, cramps, and distal paresthesias, all of which may intensify the symptoms of migraine. Dihydroergotamine (DHE) is an injectable ergot derivative with fewer side effects. Ergot preparations should not be used concomitantly with triptans. For acute migraine, DHE can be given to older children and adolescents in an initial dose of 0.5 mg IM or IV (no milligram-per-kilogram dose has been established). The initial dose of DHE may be repeated in 1 hour if necessary. One study in adults reported that 3 mg administered intranasally is also effective. Antiemetics may be useful to control the nausea and vomiting that often occur after DHE administration.

If migraines are frequent and severe, prophylactic treatment is possible. Many drugs have been used, but because some require close, serial examination and have no effect on the acute attack, generally they should not be started in the ED. Among the medications used for chronic suppressive therapy are propranolol, tricyclic antidepressants, cyproheptadine (Periactin), valproic acid, and calcium channel blockers. More

TABLE 96.5

AGENTS FOR ACUTE TREATMENT OF MIGRAINE

Drug	Usual dose
Analgesics	
Acetaminophen	10–15 mg/kg/dose PO or PR q4h
Ibuprofen	5–10 mg/kg/dose PO q6h
Ketorolac (Toradol)	30 mg initial dose, then 15–30 mg/dose (0.5 mg/kg) IV or IM, or 10 mg/dose PO, q4–6h
Codeine	0.5–1 mg/kg/dose PO q4–6h
Antiemetics	
Metoclopramide (Reglan)	0.5–2 mg/kg/dose PO or IV q4–6h
Prochlorperazine (Compazine)	0.1 mg/kg/dose PO, IM, or IV q6h
Promethazine (Phenergan)	0.25–1.0 mg/kg/dose PO, PR, IV, or IM q4–6h
Specific Antimigraine Agents	
Dihydroergotamine	0.5–1.0 mg/dose IV or IM; may repeat after 1 h
Sumatriptan (Imitrex)	6 mg SC or 100 mg PO

PO, orally; PR, per rectum; IV, intravenously; IM, intramuscularly; SC, subcutaneously.

recent studies of antiepileptic medications have shown some efficacy in preventing migraine headaches in adult patients, including gabapentin, topiramate, lamotrigine, and tiagabine. However, pediatric studies regarding prevention of migraine with antiepileptic drugs have not been conducted.

Idiopathic Intracranial Hypertension (Pseudotumor Cerebri)

Background and Pathophysiology

Idiopathic intracranial hypertension (IIH), also called *pseudotumor cerebri*, is a poorly understood condition of increased ICP. It may occur at any age during childhood but is more common in adolescents, especially in obese individuals. The female population is more commonly affected. A number of other conditions have been reported in association with IIH; these include infections (otitis media, mastoiditis, Lyme disease), endocrinologic conditions (hyperthyroidism, Addison's disease), medications (steroid withdrawal, tetracycline, hypervitaminosis A), and mild head trauma. However, a causal relationship remains unproved, and in most cases of IIH, no cause is identified. The mechanism of increased ICP in IIH remains unknown, although several hypotheses have been postulated, including vasogenic brain edema and impaired reabsorption of CSF by the arachnoid villi.

Clinical Manifestations

Headache of variable severity and duration is the most common presenting symptom. It is typically worse in the morning. Nausea, vomiting, dizziness, and double or blurred vision also occur. If the process is long-standing, decreased visual acuity or visual field deficits can result. Infants often have nonspecific symptoms of lethargy or irritability. Papilledema is seen in virtually all cases. Other neurologic symptoms and signs are often absent; however, cranial nerve palsies, particularly affecting the cranial nerve VI, may be seen.

Diagnosis should be considered when a child with a prolonged history of headache is found to have evidence of papilledema without other neurologic findings. Pseudotumor cerebri is a diagnosis of exclusion, and mass lesions and infectious processes must be ruled out. Because posterior fossa tumors and obstructive or nonobstructive hydrocephalus may mimic pseudotumor early in the course of disease, CT or MRI scan should be obtained in all children with this constellation of findings. In cases of IIH, the ventricles will appear normal or small. If no mass lesion is present, an LP should be performed with a manometer to measure opening pressure. The patient must be recumbent with legs extended to ensure an accurate reading of the opening pressure. Children with primary pseudotumor (e.g., not secondary to Lyme infection or other causes) have elevated opening pressure (greater than 200 mm H_2O) but normal CSF cell count, protein, and glucose. In children with intermittent symptoms, the opening pressure may be normal when the headache is waning, even though papilledema may persist for several weeks.

Management

Removal of sufficient CSF to normalize ICP usually leads to relief of symptoms. Treatment may then be started with acetazolamide (Diamox) to decrease CSF production (60 mg per kg per day divided four times daily). Although recommended by some authorities, corticosteroids have not been proven to be effective in the management of this condition. However, in cases of IIH following withdrawal of steroid therapy, a course of prednisone or dexamethasone may be beneficial. Patients with mild symptoms and good response to LP may be discharged to home with close follow-up arranged. Children with severe or persistent symptoms or those with visual changes may require hospital admission. Intracranial hypertension may be recurrent or chronic, and long-term monitoring, particularly of visual function, is important.

DISORDERS OF MOTOR FUNCTION (SEE ALSO CHAPTER 79)

Every level of the neural axis is involved in the performance of motor tasks. Anatomic localization is usually possible after evaluation of the distribution and character of the deficit (Table 96.6). Paresis refers to partial or complete weakness of a part of the body.

Various clinical designations are used to describe some patterns of weakness: paraplegia (or paraparesis), affecting the

TABLE 96.6

LOCALIZING LEVEL OF NEUROMOTOR DYSFUNCTION

	Tone	Distribution	Reflexes	Babinski	Other
Upper motor neuron	Increased (may be decreased acutely)	Pattern (e.g., hemiparesis, paraparesis) Distal > proximal	Increased (may be decreased acutely)	Extensor	Cognitive dysfunction possible
Anterior horn cell	Decreased	Variable, asymmetric	Decreased to absent	Flexor	Fasciculations; no sensory involvement
Peripheral nerve	Decreased	Nerve distribution	Decreased to absent	Flexor	Sensory involvement
Neuromuscular junction	Normal	Fluctuating	Usually normal	Flexor	
Muscle	Decreased	Proximal > distal	Decreased	Flexor	Tenderness, signs of inflammation possible

lower half of the body; quadriplegia, affecting all limbs; and hemiplegia, referring to weakness of one side of the body. Paraplegia most often results from spinal cord involvement, whereas hemiparesis is most often a sign of cortical disease. Some of the common conditions affecting various levels of the neuromotor system that may present with acute motor dysfunction are discussed next.

Stroke/Cerebrovascular Accident

Background

Stroke is defined as a syndrome of acute onset of focal neurologic deficit that persists for more than 24 hours, although some pediatric neurologists include more transient deficits. Stroke is relatively rare in healthy children but may complicate a number of other pediatric medical conditions. For example, among children with sickle cell disease, the incidence of stroke has been reported to be 6% to 9%. Others at risk are those with various forms of cardiac disease, which is one of the most common causes of stroke in children. Table 96.7 lists some of the common causes of stroke, as well as some more uncommon conditions in which stroke is a prominent clinical feature.

TABLE 96.7

CAUSES OF STROKE IN CHILDREN

Vascular	**Drugs**
Arteriovenous malformation	Cocaine
Aneurysm	Amphetamine
Moyamoya disease	Oral contraceptives
Fibromuscular dysplasia	Ergot poisoning
Cardiac	**Metabolic**
Valvular heart disease (including endocarditis)	Homocystinuria
	Fabry's disease
Right-to-left shunts	Mitochondrial encephalopathies
Atrial tumors	(MELAS syndrome)
Arrhythmia	Organic acidemias
Cardiomyopathy	Hyperlipidemias
Infectious	**Hematologic/Autoimmune**
Meningitis (especially tuberculous)	Sickle cell disease
	Coagulopathies (e.g., hemophilia)
Mycotic aneurysm	Anticoagulant deficiency (protein C, protein S, antithrombin III)
Mastoiditis, otitis media, or sinusitis leading to venous sinus thrombosis	
	Polycythemia
	Acute myelogenous leukemia
Trauma	Systemic lupus erythematosus
Intracranial hemorrhage	
Cervical trauma with vertebral artery injury	**Neurocutaneous Syndromes**
Intraoral trauma with carotid injury	Neurofibromatosis
	Tuberous sclerosis
Brain tumor	Sturge–Weber syndrome

Pathophysiology

Generally, stroke is classified as either primarily ischemic (including embolic phenomena) or hemorrhagic. In ischemic stroke, there is focal reduction in cerebral blood flow, with hypoxic damage to brain parenchyma, leading to neuronal injury and death. Further damage ensues from reperfusion of ischemic areas. More recently, attention has focused on secondary factors that play an important part in determining the extent of damage after acute ischemia; these include excess accumulation of excitatory amino acids and generation of free radicals. Hemorrhagic strokes are relatively more common in children than adults, accounting for 30% to 60% of pediatric stroke.

Clinical Manifestations

The presentation of stroke in children is highly variable, influenced by the portion of the cerebral vasculature affected and the child's age. Hemiparesis is most often observed, with facial weakness either ipsilateral or contralateral to weakness in the rest of the body. Involvement of the anterior cerebral artery leads primarily to lower-extremity weakness, whereas compromise of the middle cerebral artery circulation produces hemiplegia with upper limb predominance, hemianopsia, and possibly dysphasia. Less commonly, the posterior circulation is affected, which results in vertigo, ataxia, and nystagmus, as well as hemiparesis and hemianopsia. Older children often have concomitant headache, whereas children younger than 4 years are more likely to have associated seizures. The child with a stroke may also have a diminished level of consciousness.

Investigations in a child with acute hemiparesis should be directed at confirming the diagnosis of stroke and attempting to identify an underlying cause if none is known. Imaging studies are useful. Cranial CT without contrast is the study of choice for identifying acute hemorrhage. However, CT scan may be normal in the first 12 to 24 hours after an ischemic stroke; MRI, in contrast, may show changes as early as 6 hours after infarction. A usual approach is to obtain a noncontrast CT, followed by MRI with magnetic resonance angiography if no hemorrhage is seen.

In a child without a known predisposing condition, ancillary tests may be revealing of the cause of the stroke. Studies worth considering in such patients, depending on the clinical picture, are listed in Table 96.8. In one large series of 129 children with ischemic stroke, no cause was found in 35%.

Management

Initial treatment after an acute stroke is focused on stabilization and supportive care, including control of any seizures. Several aspects require special attention. Although evident hypotension should be treated with volume expansion, administration of free water should be restricted because of the potential for edema formation. Hypertension, if present, must be treated cautiously, and the blood pressure lowered gradually. Both hypoglycemia and hyperglycemia can exacerbate ischemic stroke, so careful monitoring of serum glucose level and judicious use of insulin are important. Fever, which can occur in children with stroke, may also contribute to ischemic damage and should be controlled with antipyretics.

Further therapy is determined by the type of stoke. With hemorrhagic stroke, neurosurgical intervention may be required

STUDIES TO CONSIDER IN THE EVALUATION
OF THE CHILD WITH ACUTE STROKE

Brain Imaging
Computed tomography (noncontrast)
Magnetic resonance imaging
Angiography (standard or magnetic resonance)

Cardiac
Electrocardiogram
Echocardiogram

Hematologic
Complete blood cell count
Prothrombin and partial thromboplastin times
Fibrinogen
Erythrocyte sedimentation rate
Hemoglobin electrophoresis
Protein C and S quantification
Antithrombin III level

Chemistry
Blood urea nitrogen
Cholesterol and triglycerides
Hepatic transaminases
Serum amino acids
Urine organic acids
Toxicology screen
Lactate

Lumbar Puncture

to evacuate a hematoma or control a bleeding arteriovenous malformation (AVM). Catheter-directed embolization may also be possible in cases of AVM. Children with sickle cell disease and stroke should have acute transfusion to decrease the level of hemoglobin S to less than 30%. Thrombolytic and anticoagulant therapies have been shown to be effective in adults with ischemic stroke but remain untested in children. Similarly, novel therapies such as calcium channel blockers and free radical scavengers have not been studied in pediatric patients; their use remains experimental.

Overall, prognosis for children with stroke is better than that in adults. However, regardless of treatment, long-term morbidity of stroke in children is high, with more than 75% of affected children experiencing sequelae such as hemiparesis, seizures, and learning difficulties.

Spinal Cord Dysfunction

Background

Dysfunction of the spinal cord may result from any of a variety of disorders, either intrinsic or extrinsic to the spinal cord, with a great deal of overlap in their clinical presentation. *Transverse myelitis* is an intramedullary disorder, involving both halves of the cord over a variable length, with involvement of motor and sensory tracts. It occurs in children and adults, although it is rare in the first year of life. Transverse myelitis is believed to be a localized form of acute disseminated encephalomyelitis, discussed previously. Like the latter disorder, transverse myelitis may occur after a number of infections; among those commonly

reported are Epstein-Barr virus, cytomegalovirus, measles, mumps, *Campylobacter jejuni*, and *M. pneumoniae*. Transverse myelitis may also result from systemic autoimmune disorders such as lupus erythematosus or scleroderma. In some older children and adolescents, transverse myelitis is a first manifestation of multiple sclerosis.

Acute spinal cord compression in children is usually caused by trauma, infection, or cancer. Spinal trauma may lead to contusion or concussion of the cord with hemorrhage, edema, and local mass effect or to development of a spinal epidural hematoma.

Parenchymal injury usually presents acutely, but an epidural hematoma may develop over several days after the antecedent trauma. Epidural abscess is the most common infectious cause of spinal cord compression. It is usually caused by hematogenous spread of bacteria, with *Staphylococcus aureus* being the most common pathogen. Neoplastic causes include both primary intraspinal tumors (ependymoma and astrocytoma) and extrinsic lesions such as neuroblastoma or lymphoma.

Pathophysiology

Transverse myelitis is believed to be caused by an autoimmune process, with demyelinating lesions found in the spinothalamic and pyramidal tracts and posterior columns of the spinal cord. During the course of the illness, the initial area or areas of spinal cord inflammation may extend rostrally and caudally to involve an extensive portion of the spinal cord.

Mass lesions may cause damage by direct compression of spinal cord tissues or, secondarily, by interference with the tenuous arterial (or, less commonly, venous) blood flow to the spine with resultant spinal infarction.

Clinical Manifestations

Spinal cord dysfunction from any cause is characterized by paraplegia and hyporeflexia below the level of involvement; sensory symptoms, such as band-like pain at the level of compression; and sensory loss or paresthesias below the area of damage. If the lower spinal cord is involved (the conus), there is usually early loss of bowel and bladder control. Compression of the cauda equina usually results in asymmetric symptoms, radicular pain, and focal lower-extremity motor and sensory abnormalities.

Transverse myelitis may affect any level of the spinal cord, but thoracic involvement is the most common. Initial symptoms include lower-extremity paresthesia, local back pain, unilateral or bilateral lower-extremity weakness, and urinary retention. A preceding respiratory or gastrointestinal illness is usually reported, and at the time of diagnosis, fever and meningismus are sometimes seen in children. Characteristically, the insidious onset of paresthesia or weakness of the lower extremities progresses over days or, rarely, weeks and then is replaced by the abrupt occurrence of static paraplegia or quadriplegia and, in the cooperative child, a detectable sensory level. In other children, the course of progression may be less than 12 hours. The sensory loss generally involves all modalities, although a spinothalamic deficit (pain) may occur without posterior column dysfunction (vibration). The weakness is usually symmetric but may be asymmetric. After a variable interval, initial flaccidity may be replaced by spasticity. Sphincter disturbance of the bowel and bladder occurs in most patients, bladder distension being the most common initial sign of damage.

Traumatic and infectious spinal lesions are usually accompanied by relatively acute onset of local back pain, which is exacerbated by direct percussion of the area. Pain from an infectious cause occasionally may precede other symptoms for days. With tumors, however, there may be weakness in the absence of pain. Patients with epidural abscess often have systemic signs of infections such as fever, headache, vomiting, and, perhaps, neck stiffness. Bony tenderness in such a patient may indicate vertebral osteomyelitis or discitis, which can also present with weakness, although usually less severe than is seen with actual spinal cord involvement.

Prompt diagnosis of spinal cord lesions requires a high level of suspicion. Detailed neurologic examination is essential, with particular attention to the quality of deep tendon reflexes, any asymmetry of reflexes or strength, evaluation for a sensory level, and assessment of anal tone and cremasteric reflexes (in male patients). Note also any point percussion tenderness.

Diagnosis is confirmed by emergency neuroimaging, with precautions to immobilize the patient with the possibility of an unstable lesion. Plain spine films are useful initially in trauma. MRI of the spine is the procedure of choice to detect compressive mass lesions, but if not immediately available, plain or CT myelography is an alternative. In transverse myelitis, the cord may be widened at the level of involvement. This is easier to detect with MRI, which in some cases may also reveal evidence of focal intramedullary demyelination.

LP alone should not be performed if a diagnosis of spinal cord compression is entertained. If no mass lesion is noted and transverse myelitis is a diagnostic possibility, LP may be useful, showing a normal or slightly elevated opening pressure and a mild CSF pleocytosis in the CSF in nearly 50% of patients at the time of presentation. The CSF protein level is often elevated and may demonstrate oligoclonal bands or increased myelin basic protein, but the glucose level is usually normal.

Management

Treatment of children with spinal injury from trauma begins with splinting and immobilization of the spine. If trauma is likely, some experts recommend high-dose methylprednisolone, which was shown in one study, when given within 8 hours of injury at an IV dose of 30 mg per kg followed by infusion at 5.4 mg per kg per hr for 23 hours, to improve the quality of neurologic outcome. Neurosurgical consultation should be obtained as soon as possible; however, early surgical attempts to decompress the swollen spine (laminectomy or midline myelotomy) have proven ineffective and, possibly, detrimental.

In cases of possible epidural abscess or tumor-related mass, IV dexamethasone at a loading dose of 2 mg per kg (up to a maximum of 100 mg) should be given, followed by 1 to 2 mg per kg per day IV in four divided doses over the next 24 hours. In patients with a presumed infectious cause and those with cancer of unknown origin, surgical decompression is indicated on an emergent basis to alleviate pressure and pinpoint diagnosis. Further treatment depends on the organism or exact tumor type found.

Treatment of transverse myelitis is supportive, and some degree of recovery occurs in approximately 80% of cases. All children with this syndrome should be hospitalized. Although

there are no controlled trials of their efficacy, there is a consensus supporting the use of systemic corticosteroids. Some experts have also recommended IV immunoglobulin, again without supportive evidence from clinical trials.

Acute Polyneuritis (Guillain–Barré Syndrome)

Background and Pathophysiology

Acute polyneuritis, also called *Guillain–Barré syndrome*, is characterized by symmetric ascending paralysis. Pathologically, the hallmark of this disease is primary demyelination of motor and sensory nerves, believed to be secondary to autoimmune mechanisms. It occurs in children in all age groups but is uncommon before 3 years of age. An antecedent respiratory or gastrointestinal infection or immunization precedes the onset of illness by 1 to 2 weeks in more than 75% of childhood cases.

Clinical Manifestations

Weakness, commonly with an insidious onset, is the usual presenting complaint. Paresthesias or other sensory abnormalities such as pain or numbness are prominent in up to 50% of cases, particularly in older children. The paresthesias and paralysis are usually symmetric and ascending, although variations may occur. Early in the course of illness, distal weakness is more prominent than proximal weakness. Deep tendon reflexes are depressed or absent at the time of diagnosis. Affected children often have an ataxic gait. Similar clinical findings may be seen in West Nile virus infection.

Cranial nerve abnormalities occur during the illness in 30% to 40% of cases and may be the predominant finding, especially in the Miller-Fisher variant of this syndrome, which is characterized by oculomotor palsies, ataxia, and areflexia without motor weakness of the extremities. The most common cranial nerve deficit is VII (facial) nerve palsy, followed in decreasing frequency by impairment of cranial nerves IX, X, and XI and oculomotor abnormalities. Autonomic dysfunction occurs commonly and results in blood pressure lability, postural hypotension, and cardiac abnormalities; it is a disproportionate cause of morbidity and mortality. Urinary retention, if it occurs, is usually seen late in the illness. As the paralysis ascends, muscles of breathing may become involved, leading to respiratory embarrassment.

The primary aid in diagnosis is LP, which demonstrates an elevated protein level, normal glucose level, and fewer than 10 white blood cells per cubic millimeter—the so-called albuminocytologic disassociation. The protein elevation occurs in almost all cases but may be delayed for weeks, usually peaking in the second or third week of illness. Electrophysiologic evidence for Guillain–Barré syndrome is the presence of nerve conduction velocity delay, which is usually not demonstrable until the second or third week of illness. Emergency electromyography (EMG) and nerve conduction velocity testing are not indicated.

Management

Because of the potential for progression to life-threatening respiratory compromise, the child with Guillain–Barré syndrome should be hospitalized and observed closely. Impending respiratory distress must be anticipated, and routine respiratory monitoring should be aided by specific measures of respiratory function, particularly measurement of negative inspiratory force. Because autonomic dysfunction is common, blood pressure must be monitored closely and abnormalities treated vigorously.

Acute polyneuritis is generally self-limiting, with more than 90% of children in most series having complete or near-complete recovery. In mild cases, in which children retain the ability to ambulate, only supportive care is required. However, immunomodulatory therapy may be of benefit in more severely affected children. Plasmapheresis and IV immunoglobulin both have been used. Although well-controlled, blinded studies of these treatments in children are lacking, the available data suggest that both are effective in reducing the duration and severity of illness in those most severely affected, especially when begun early in the course of the disease. Corticosteroids have not been shown to be beneficial in acute Guillain–Barré syndrome; a recent metaanalysis demonstrated that oral corticosteroids actually delayed recovery.

Myasthenia Gravis

Background and Pathophysiology

In myasthenia gravis, antibodies directed against the acetylcholine receptor protein of the postsynaptic neuromuscular junction cause intermittent failure of neuromuscular transmission and fluctuating weakness. Myasthenia manifests as fluctuating weakness of cranial and skeletal musculature, exacerbated by exertion. More commonly a disease seen in adults, myasthenia gravis occurs in children in three major forms: transient neonatal, infantile (congenital), and juvenile (most common).

Clinical Manifestations

The juvenile form of myasthenia clinically mimics the adult disease. The mean age of onset is 8 years, with a female predominance of approximately 4:1. The onset of symptoms may be insidious or acute. Most cases affect the cranial nerves, and any cranial nerve can be involved in combination or isolation. Bilateral ptosis is the most common cranial nerve deficit, followed in incidence by oculomotor impairment. Generalized truncal and limb weakness is present at onset in up to half of cases and eventually develops in most children with myasthenia. The diagnosis should be suspected if there is a history of worsening weakness during continual activity or if fatigability of muscle strength is demonstrable. Illnesses confused with myasthenia include the muscular dystrophies, congenital myopathies, inflammatory myopathies, acute and chronic polyneuropathies, and in the infant, botulism.

The Tensilon test is useful in ED diagnosis. In this procedure, the anticholinesterase drug edrophonium (Tensilon), which has a 30-second onset and approximately a 5-minute duration of action, is given slowly IV at a dosage of 0.2 mg per kg, up to a maximum dose of 10 mg. Atropine should be immediately available to treat potential severe cholinergic reactions (e.g., bradycardia). Initially, one-tenth of the total dose is given, and if no hypersensitivity or severe reactions are noted, the remainder of the dose is administered. Because

edrophonium is short-lived, interpretation of the response requires close monitoring of a muscle or muscle group in which improvement can be seen clearly, such as the eyelid elevators. In small children, this is often impossible and longer-acting anticholinesterases, such as neostigmine (0.125 mg in an infant and 0.04 mg per kg in an older child), can be used. EMG provides electrophysiologic evidence for myasthenia gravis, with a decremental response to repetitive nerve stimulation, but may be negative when the disease is confined to the cranial nerves.

Management

Although myasthenia gravis is potentially life-threatening, specific management can usually be delayed until after diagnosis is made. If there is evidence of respiratory compromise, ventilatory support is mandatory. Treatment is begun with the use of cholinesterase inhibitors to prolong the availability of acetylcholine at the neuromuscular junction. At present, the anticholinesterase of choice is pyridostigmine (Mestinon) at a starting dosage of 1 mg per kg by mouth every 4 hours, adjusted according to the clinical response. If there is any concern about respiratory compromise or if severe weakness is present, the child should be hospitalized immediately.

Myasthenia has a fluctuating, unpredictable course that can be exacerbated by intercurrent illness and by certain drugs, particularly the aminoglycoside antibiotics. In a known myasthenic, rapid worsening and respiratory compromise (myasthenic crises) may be difficult to differentiate from deterioration secondary to overdose of anticholinesterases (cholinergic crises) because the muscarinic side effects of the anticholinesterases, such as nausea, vomiting, cramps, and muscle fasciculations, may be absent. At times, differentiation can be made by giving 1 to 2 mg of IV edrophonium after ensuring respiratory sufficiency. This should result in rapid improvement in the patient with a myasthenic crisis. This procedure may be falsely positive, however, and if the diagnosis is unclear, the patient should be withdrawn from all anticholinesterases and, if necessary, maintained on mechanical respiration for 48 to 72 hours. Cholinergic crises require the immediate withdrawal of all anticholinesterases. Myasthenic crises respond variably to additional anticholinesterases, and plasmapheresis or steroid therapy may be particularly useful in this situation. Both myasthenic and cholinergic crises mandate admission to the hospital.

Botulism (See Also Chapter 92)

Background and Pathophysiology

Infantile botulism is a cause of acute weakness in previously well infants younger than 6 months. The illness is secondary to intestinal colonization by *Clostridium botulinum*, which produces a neurotoxin that impairs acetylcholine release from the nerve terminal. Spores of *C. botulinum* are of ubiquitous origin, found in soil and agricultural products. Honey has been found to be a particularly significant reservoir. Although infant botulism occurs throughout the United States, the incidence is highest in certain areas; approximately half the cases reported have been from California, Utah, and Pennsylvania. The various host factors that predispose certain infants to intestinal colonization are poorly understood.

Clinical Manifestations

The initial symptom of infantile botulism is usually constipation, followed insidiously by lethargy and feeding difficulties. Physical findings at the time of presentation are hypoactive deep tendon reflexes, decreased suck and gag, poorly reactive pupils, bilateral ptosis, oculomotor palsies, and facial weakness. Differential diagnosis includes all the potential causes of lethargy and poor feeding in infancy, and infants are often misdiagnosed initially. Laboratory test results, including the leukocyte count and LP, are normal. The diagnosis is confirmed by identification of *C. botulinum* toxin (usually type A or B) in the feces or isolation of the organism in stool culture, which is less sensitive. EMG may supply immediate information. Characteristic EMG findings are brief, small-amplitude action potentials; posttetanic facilitation; and normal nerve conduction velocity.

Management

Affected infants require hospitalization to observe for respiratory compromise. In one large series of 57 patients, 77% required endotracheal intubation because of loss of protective airway reflexes, and 68% received mechanical ventilation for some period. Nasogastric or nasojejunal feedings are usually needed as well.

Human botulism immunoglobulin, with activity against type A and B toxins, is approved for use in infant botulism (often referred to as BabyBIG). Trials have shown a decrease in duration of illness in treated infants. Equine botulinum antitoxin has a high rate of anaphylactic reaction in infants and is not recommended. The use of cathartics or other laxatives to reduce the amount of *C. botulinum* present in the intestine has not proved beneficial. Antibiotics such as penicillin, although widely used, have not been shown to eradicate the organism from the bowel or result in clinical improvement. Aminoglycosides, which can cause neuromuscular blockade, should be avoided.

Periodic Paralysis

Background and Pathophysiology

Familial periodic paralysis is a rare illness, inherited in an autosomal-dominant fashion that results in episodes of severe weakness associated with an abnormality of circulating potassium during attacks. Two major forms of illness—hyperkalemic and hypokalemic—are recognized. (A third type, normokalemic, has been described but most likely represents a rare variant of the hyperkalemic variety.) Other disorders that can produce weakness and electrolyte abnormalities, such as use of corticosteroids or diuretics, thyrotoxicosis, hyperaldosteronism, and renal insufficiency, may mimic the periodic paralyses. The serum potassium abnormalities in familial periodic paralysis are believed to be epiphenomena of yet undelineated muscle membrane abnormalities.

Clinical Manifestations

Many of the clinical features are common to the various forms of periodic paralysis. Characteristically, a previously well patient develops a flaccid weakness in his or her trunk and upper thighs, and the weakness gradually involves the remainder of the skeletal muscles. Deep tendon reflexes are diminished. The attacks last from hours to days, and between the attacks, muscular strength is usually normal, although a minority of patients have residual muscular weakness.

Hypokalemic periodic paralysis, the most common type, occurs primarily in adolescents and young adults. Trigger factors include vigorous exercise, heavy carbohydrate meals, alcohol, and the cold. During an attack, potassium levels are usually 2 to 2.5 mEq per L, and electrophysiologic examination demonstrates unstimulatable muscles. The hyperkalemic form usually begins in the first decade of life, and attacks occur predominantly during the period of rest after vigorous exercise or after fasting. The episodes are more common than in hypokalemic paralysis but often last less than a few hours. Myotonia is usually associated with the illness. During the attack, plasma potassium level is moderately elevated, although it is often in the upper normal range. In both forms of periodic paralysis, EKG changes consistent with the serum potassium abnormality may be noted and cardiac arrhythmias may rarely arise.

Management

Emergency treatment of hypokalemic periodic paralysis includes oral, or rarely IV, potassium. Prophylactically, patients should avoid precipitants such as vigorous exercise or large carbohydrate loads. Recurrences may be prevented with spironolactone or acetazolamide.

Attacks of hyperkalemic periodic paralysis are often brief enough that acute treatment is unnecessary. In severe attacks, inhaled albuterol and IV calcium gluconate may be helpful. Acetazolamide, thiazide diuretics, and albuterol have been used for prevention of recurrences.

DISORDERS OF BALANCE (SEE CHAPTER 10)

Acute Cerebellar Ataxia

Background and Pathophysiology

Acute cerebellar ataxia, characterized by the acute onset of unsteadiness in a previously well child, is the most common cause of ataxia in young children. It is seen primarily between the ages of 1 and 4 years but can occur at any time during childhood. The exact cause of the illness is unclear; however, it is believed to be a parainfectious or postinfectious demyelinating phenomenon and likely represents a localized form of postinfectious encephalitis. Acute cerebellar ataxia occurs most commonly after primary varicella. Other infections implicated include infectious mononucleosis, enteroviruses, HSV, influenza, *Mycoplasma,* and Q fever. Ataxia is usually seen 5 to 10 days after the onset of illness, although symptoms may be delayed for up to 3 weeks, and there are some reports of cerebellar ataxia preceding the rash of chickenpox.

Clinical Manifestations

The child develops acute truncal unsteadiness with a variable degree of distal motor difficulty, such as tremor and dysmetria. Dysarthria and nystagmus are variably present. Some children have nausea and vomiting, presumably caused by vertigo. Headache is rare.

When acute ataxia follows varicella in a child with no other neurologic findings, the diagnosis may be made on clinical grounds. In atypical cases, CT or MRI may be necessary to rule out a cerebellar mass. LP is not usually necessary in typical cases; if performed, it reveals a mild CSF pleocytosis in approximately half of the cases.

Management

Treatment is supportive. Resolution of symptoms is complete in most children within 2 weeks of onset, but mild residual neurologic deficits have been reported in 10% to 30% of cases. Varicella-associated cases appear to have the most benign prognosis.

Benign Paroxysmal Vertigo

Benign paroxysmal vertigo is an illness that affects children primarily between 1 and 4 years of age, although it can occur any time during the first decade. It manifests with acute episodes of dizziness and imbalance, lasting seconds to minutes. Between episodes, the child is asymptomatic. During the spell, the child characteristically becomes frightened and pale but does not lose consciousness. He or she may have associated nausea, vomiting, or visual disturbance. The physical examination is usually normal except for nystagmus, which may be present. Although the cause of this illness is unknown, it is believed to be a migraine variant. Many children go on to develop more typical migraine headaches later, and there is often a family history of migraine disease. As the name suggests, the course of benign paroxysmal vertigo is self-limiting and benign, and treatment is supportive.

MOVEMENT DISORDERS

Involuntary movements are components of many CNS disorders and tend to be complex. A classification into specific subtypes, based on the character, predominant anatomic localization, rhythmicity, and frequency, is arbitrary but useful in deducing the cause of the disorder (Table 96.9). Movements such as chorea, athetosis, dystonia, ballismus, and certain types of tremors suggest dysfunction of the extrapyramidal nervous system. Involuntary movements are also caused by damage to the cerebellum or its outflow tract, especially static (on maintaining fixed position) and intention tremors. Myoclonus may occur secondary to cerebral cortex, brain stem, or spinal cord disease. Tics, another form of involuntary movement, may be extremely difficult to distinguish from chorea and are best differentiated by their stereotypic character. They probably represent the most common involuntary movement disorder but are not true neurologic emergencies. Many illnesses may present with involuntary movements and are diagnosed by associated neurologic findings.

Acute Dystonia

Dystonia is marked by involuntary, sustained muscle contractions, typically of the neck and trunk, that cause twisting movements and abnormal postures. In generalized dystonia, the head is usually deviated to the side and there is grimacing of the face. Acute dystonia in children is nearly always the result of exposure to an antidopaminergic agent such as a neuroleptic, antiemetic, or metoclopramide. Chronic dystonias are rare but may be seen as an isolated disorder or as a manifestation of cerebral palsy. Dystonia must be differentiated from torticollis, an abnormal tilt of the head and neck usually resulting from irritation or spasm of the sternocleidomastoid muscle. Another clinically similar condition is Sandifer's syndrome, which describes intermittent arching of the back and neck, observed in infants with gastroesophageal reflux.

Acute dystonia resulting from exposure to antidopaminergic drugs is treated with diphenhydramine [1 mg per kg per dose IV, orally (PO), or IM] or benztropine (Cogentin; 1 to 2 mg per dose IM). Because the half-life of many of the precipitating agents is fairly long, treatment should be continued for 24 to 48 hours.

Sydenham's Chorea

Background

Sydenham's chorea, the most common form of acquired chorea seen in children, occurs primarily between the ages of 3 and 13 years. Marked by involuntary movements, coordination difficulties, and emotional lability, its onset may be abrupt

---

TABLE 96.9

CATEGORIZATION OF MOVEMENT DISORDERS

Movement	Character	Location	Speed	Rhythmicity	Stereotype
Chorea	Jerky	Anywhere, may be universal	Rapid	Irregular	No
Athetosis	Writhing	Primarily distal	Slow	Irregular	At times
Dystonia	Writhing	Primarily proximal	Slow	Irregular	At times
Ballismus	Flailing	Proximal	Rapid	Irregular	No
Tremor	May be resting, static, or intention	Primarily distal	Variable	Regular	Yes
Myoclonus	Jerky	Anywhere	Rapid	Irregular	Variable
Tic	Jerky	Anywhere (especially face, neck, hands)	Rapid	Variable	Yes

or insidious. Sydenham's chorea is believed to be a poststreptococcal disease and may occur months after the primary bacterial infection. It is one of the major diagnostic criteria for rheumatic fever (see Chapter 92).

Clinical Manifestations

The involuntary movements may be subtle at first and exacerbated by stress. Initially, the movements classically affect the face and distal portion of the upper extremities and consist of rapid, involuntary random jerks. This results in the "milkmaid hand," in which the child's hand cannot maintain a uniform strength while grasping the examiner's hand. The involuntary movements disappear during sleep. There is usually associated muscular hypotonia and marked coordination difficulties and speech is often jerky. Hemichorea, in which the abnormal movements are predominantly unilateral, occurs in some cases. The deep tendon reflexes are normal, although occasionally, the patellar reflex is said to be "hung up." There is no evidence for upper motor neuron disease.

Serologic evidence for preceding streptococcal infection is absent in up to 25% of cases, and only one-third of patients have associated manifestations of rheumatic fever at the time of diagnosis. In the absence of such confirmatory evidence of a poststreptococcal cause, other disorders that may present with chorea must be considered in the differential diagnosis. These include atypical seizures, drug intoxication, choreoathetoid cerebral palsy, familial choreas, chorea gravidarum, collagen vascular disease, Wilson's disease, and Lyme disease.

Management

Initially, all patients should have a hematologic profile, sedimentation rate, and serologic tests performed for streptococcal infection. An EKG should also be performed to look for evidence of rheumatic carditis (e.g., prolonged P-R interval). If there is a question concerning diagnosis, further tests, such as CT, MRI, LP, and serologic evaluation for collagen vascular disease, might be helpful, but they are not usually necessary on an urgent basis.

The success of any treatment is hard to evaluate because the course is so unpredictable. Haloperidol (0.5 to 1 mg PO twice daily) has been reported to result in improvement within 2 to 3 days. Valproic acid and carbamazepine have also been used. In patients with severe symptoms refractory to these agents, methylprednisolone, IV immunoglobulin, and plasmapheresis have all been described, in case series. Because patients with Sydenham's chorea have an increased incidence of rheumatic carditis, prophylactic penicillin should be used unless another specific cause is determined for the chorea.

DISORDERS OF CRANIAL NERVE FUNCTION

Optic Neuritis

Background

Optic neuritis is an acute inflammation or demyelination of the optic nerve, characterized by an impairment of vision, progressing over hours or days and associated with tenderness of the eyeball exacerbated by eye movement. The disease is primarily unilateral but an increased incidence of bilateral involvement is found in children. Optic neuritis in children is most commonly presumed to be on an autoimmune basis following a viral disease, including the childhood exanthems. At times, a contiguous sinusitis may cause the illness. Of patients with unilateral optic neuritis, 20% will develop multiple sclerosis at a later date, but there is little reason to make this diagnosis before the development of other symptoms of neurologic dysfunction.

Clinical Findings

On examination, decreased visual acuity and decreased color vision are associated with a relative afferent pupillary deficit to light and a central scotoma in the affected eye. The relative afferent pupil defect is demonstrated by the swinging flashlight maneuver, during which the pupil of the affected eye constricts briskly when light is shone into the contralateral eye (the consensual light reflex) and dilates when light is immediately shone into the affected eye. With bilateral disease, the change in pupillary reflexes may not be apparent. Funduscopic examination discloses a hyperemic, swollen optic disc; in the rare cases of retrobulbar optic neuritis, funduscopic examination is normal.

Optic neuritis must be distinguished from papilledema, secondary to increased ICP. Papilledema is almost always bilateral and associated with normal vision and normal pupil reactivity until late in the disease. In cases of bilateral optic neuritis, differentiation may be impossible because funduscopic findings are identical in the two illnesses. If any doubt of increased ICP persists, the patient should undergo evaluation by CT or MRI of the brain and, if normal, CSF analysis. In optic neuritis, the opening pressure is normal, but there may be a mild lymphocytic pleocytosis or elevated CSF protein level.

Management

The course of the illness is variable, with most patients recovering to normal or near normal vision over 4 to 5 weeks. Treatment with high-dose systemic corticosteroids has not been shown to improve the ultimate prognosis but may result in a slightly faster resolution of symptoms.

Facial Nerve Palsy

Background

Weakness in the distribution of the cranial nerve VII (facial) may be produced by either central (upper motor neuron) or peripheral (lower motor neuron) dysfunction. Peripheral disease is most common in children, particularly when the facial weakness is an isolated finding. Bell's palsy refers to peripheral facial nerve weakness with no identifiable underlying cause. It is believed to be secondary to edema of the facial nerve as it passes through the facial canal within the temporal bone. There is often a history or preceding upper respiratory tract infection, and in at least a subset of patients, there is evidence of reactivation of infection with Epstein-Barr virus or HSV. Seventh nerve palsy may occur in association with otitis media, in which case it may indicate the presence of mastoid involvement. Facial palsy may also be a manifestation of early-disseminated Lyme disease. It usually occurs in isolation, although there may be other signs of CNS disease. Although in general most cases of facial nerve palsy in children are of the idiopathic (or viral reactivation) type, in endemic areas, Lyme disease may be the most common cause.

Clinical Manifestations

Facial weakness may be partial or complete. On the affected side, there is flattening of the nasolabial fold at rest, and the child has difficulty closing the eye or raising the corner of the mouth to smile. In many cases, pain localized to the ear precedes the paralysis. With upper motor neuron involvement, there will be some residual capacity to furrow the brow because of crossed innervation, whereas the entire face is involved with peripheral disease. There may be bilateral involvement in Lyme disease, in contrast to Bell's palsy, which is always unilateral.

In children with facial nerve palsy caused by Lyme disease, other manifestations, such as erythema migrans, are rarely seen (27% in one series). Thus, even in the absence of other findings, serologic evidence for systemic Lyme infection should be sought in all children with isolated cranial nerve VII paresis in endemic areas, although only about 50% of affected children will have elevated titers at the time of diagnosis. An LP should be performed if there is other evidence of meningoencephalitis such as headache; however, the need for LP in a child at risk for Lyme disease with isolated facial nerve palsy is controversial. Other associated neurologic abnormality, specifically in the other cranial nerves, or concomitant otitis media, necessitates further evaluation, including CT or MRI.

Management

Symptomatic treatment for facial nerve palsy consists of protection of the cornea by the instillation of bland ointments (e.g., Lacri-Lube). For patients with facial nerve palsy due to Lyme disease, oral antibiotic treatment is indicated as for other manifestations of early-disseminated Lyme disease (see chapter 101). Parenteral antibiotics are reserved for those with findings of meningitis.

Specific treatment for facial nerve palsy not associated with Lyme disease is somewhat controversial, but steroids may be beneficial when started early in the course of the disease. Although earlier studies are mixed, a recent large controlled trial demonstrated greater long-term improvement in adults with Bell's palsy treated with prednisolone. Only one trial has included children, and all patients in that study recovered regardless of treatment. However, based on adult studies, many authors have recommended a course of prednisone (1 to 2 mg per kg per day) over 7 to 10 days if the patient is seen within the first 72 hours of disease. Studies in adults suggest that antiviral agents combined with prednisone may provide additional benefit, with valacyclovir showing greater efficacy than acyclovir. However, studies have been mixed, and the lack of evidence for antiviral therapy in children mandates against routine administration.

Regardless of treatment, complete recovery is seen in 60% to 80% of children, beginning during the second to third week of illness. Those with partial paralysis generally have a better prognosis. During the recovery period, special care should be taken to protect the cornea by the instillation of bland ointments (e.g., Lacri-Lube). The child should be referred for reexamination to ensure a recovery during the expected time period.

Children with clinical or serologic evidence of Lyme-associated facial nerve palsy should be treated with oral antibiotics (amoxicillin, tetracycline, or erythromycin) for 21 to 28 days. The effectiveness of steroids in such patients has not been evaluated. Parenteral antibiotic treatment is recommended for children who also have evidence of meningitis. Peripheral facial nerve palsy in association with otitis media may require myringotomy.

Suggested Readings

Seizures

Abend NS, Huh JW, Helfaer MA, et al. Anticonvulsant medications in the pediatric emergency room and intensive care unit. *Pediatr Emerg Care* 2008;24:705–718.

Armon K, Stephenson T, MacFaul R, et al. An evidence and consensus based guideline for the management of a child after a seizure. *Emerg Med J* 2003;20(1):13–20.

Bhatia MS, Sapra S. Pseudoseizures in children: a profile of 50 cases. *Clin Pediatr* 2005;44(7):617–621.

Bye A, Kok D, Ferenschild F. Paroxysmal non-epileptic events in children: a retrospective study over a period of 10 years. *J Paediatr Child Health* 2000; 36(3):244–248.

Chapman MG, Smith M, Hirsch NP. Status epilepticus. *Anaesthesia* 2001;56(7): 648–659.

French JA, Kanner AM, Bautista J, et al. Efficacy and tolerability of the new antiepileptic drugs, II: treatment of refractory epilepsy: report of the Therapeutics and Technology Assessment Subcommittee and Quality Standards Subcommittee of the American Academy of Neurology and the American Epilepsy Society. *Neurology* 2004;62:1261–1273.

Harden CL, Huff JS, Schwartz TH, et al. Reassessment: neuroimaging in the emergency patient presenting with seizure (and evidence-based review): report of the Therapeutics and Technology Assessment Subcommittee of the American Academy of Neurology. *Neurology* 2007;69:1772–1780.

Hesdorffer DC, Logroscino G, Cascino GD, et al. Recurrence of afebrile status epilepticus in a population-based study in Rochester, Minnesota. *Neurology* 2007;69(1):73–78.

Kanazawa O. Shuddering attacks—report of four children. *Pediatr Neurol* 2000;23(5):421–424.

Knake S, Gruener J, Hattemer K, et al. Intravenous levetiracetam in the treatment of benzodiazepine refractory status epilepticus. *J Neurol Neurosurg Psychiatry* 2008;79(5):588–589.

Loddenkemper T, Wyllie E. When is routine video-EEG monitoring in children warranted? *Nat Clin Pract Neurol* 2005;1(2):78–79.

Manno EM. New management strategies in the treatment of status epilepticus. *Mayo Clin Proc* 2003;78:508–518.

Pellock JM. Safety of Diastat®, a rectal gel formulation of diazepam for acute seizure treatment. *Drug Saf* 2004;27(6):383–392.

Rainbow J, Browne GJ, Lam LT. Controlling seizures in the prehospital setting: diazepam or midazolam? *J Paediatr Child Health* 2002;38:582–586.

Rivello JJ, Ashwal S, Hirtz D, et al. Practice parameter: diagnostic assessment of the child with status epilepticus (an evidence-based review): report of the Quality Standards Subcommittee of the American Academy of Neurology and the Practice Committee of the Child Neurology Society. *Neurology* 2006;637:1542–1550.

Valencia I, Sklar E, Blanco F, et al. The role of routine serum laboratory tests in children presenting to the emergency department with unprovoked seizures. *Clin Pediatr* 2003;42(6):511–517.

Vilke GM, Sharieff GQ, Marino A, et al. Midazolam for the treatment of out-of-hospital pediatric seizures. *Prehosp Emerg Care* 2002;6:215–217.

Yu K, Mills S, Thompson N, et al. Safety and efficacy of intravenous valproate in pediatric status epilepticus and acute repetitive seizures. *Epilepsia* 2003; 44(5):724–726.

Febrile Seizures

Berg AT, Shinnar S, Hauser WA, et al. A prospective study of recurrent febrile seizures. *N Engl J Med* 1992;327:1122–1127.

Chungath M, Shorvon S. The mortality and morbidity of febrile seizures. *Nat Clin Pract Neurol* 2008;4(11):610–621.

Committee on Quality Improvement, Subcommittee on Febrile Seizures. Practice parameter: long-term treatment of the child with simple febrile seizures. *Pediatrics* 1999;103(6):1307–1309.

Offringa M, Moyer VA. Evidence based paediatrics: evidence based management of seizures associated with fever. *BMJ* 2001;323:1111–1114.

Rantala H, Tarkka R, Uhari M. Preventive treatment for recurrent febrile seizures. *Ann Med* 2000;32(3):177–180.

Shah S, Alpern E, Zwerling L, et al. Low risk of bacteremia in children with febrile seizures. *Arch Pediatr Adolesc Med* 2002;156(5):469–472.

Warden CR, Zibulewsky J, Mace S, et al. Evaluation and management of febrile seizures in the out-of-hospital and emergency department settings. *Pediatrics* 2003;41:215–222.

Waruiru C, Appleton R. Febrile seizures: an update. *Arch Dis Child* 2004; 89(8):751–756.

Encephalitis

Alper G, Schor NF. Toward the definition of acute disseminated encephalitis of childhood. *Curr Opin Pediatr* 2004;16:637–640.

Campbell GL, Marfin AA, Lanciotti RS, et al. West Nile virus. *Lancet Infect Dis* 2002;2:519–529.

Carstairs SD, Carstairs KL. Emergency department presentation of acute disseminated encephalomyelitis. *Pediatr Emerg Care* 2007;23:109–111.

Leake JA, Albani S, Kao AS, et al. Acute disseminated encephalomyelitis in childhood: epidemiologic, clinical and laboratory features. *Pediatr Infect Dis J* 2004;23:756–764.

Lewis P, Glaser CA. Encephalitis. *Pediatr Rev* 2005;26:353–363.

Murthy SN, Faden HS, Cohen ME, et al. Acute disseminated encephalomyelitis in children. *Pediatrics* 2002;110:e21.

Richer LP, Sinclair DB, Bhargava R. Neuroimaging features of acute disseminated encephalomyelitis in childhood. *Pediatr Neurol* 2005;32:30–36.

Silvia MT, Licht DJ. Pediatric central nervous system infections and inflammatory white matter disease. *Pediatr Clin North Am* 2005;52: 1107–1126.

Whitley RJ, Kimberlin DW. Viral encephalitis. *Pediatr Rev* 1999;20:192–198.

Migraine

Annequin D, Tournaire B, Massiou H. Migraine and headache in childhood and adolescence. *Pediatr Clin North Am* 2000;47:617–631.

Bailey B, McManus BC. Treatment of children with migraine in the emergency department: a qualitative systematic review. *Pediatr Emerg Care* 2008;24: 321–330.

Brousseau DC, Duffy SJ, Anderson AC, et al. Migraine headaches: a randomized, double-blinded trial of prochlorperazine versus ketorolac. *Ann Emerg Med* 2004;43:256–262.

Callenbach PM, Pels LP, Mulder PG, et al. Sumatriptan nasal spray in the acute treatment of migraine in adolescents and children. *Eur J Paediatr Neurol* 2007;11:325–330.

Damen L, Bruijn JK, Verhagen AP, et al. Symptomatic treatment of migraine in children: a systematic review of medication trials. *Pediatrics* 2005;116: e295–e302.

Detsky ME, McDonald DR, Baerlocher MO, et al. Does this patient with headache have a migraine or need neuroimaging? *JAMA* 2005;296:1274–1283.

Eiland LS, Jenkins LS, Durham SH. Pediatric migraine: pharmacologic agents for prophylaxis. *Ann Pharmacother* 2007;41:1181–1190.

Frazee LA, Foraker KC. Use of intravenous valproic acid for acute migraine. *Ann Pharmacother* 2008;42:403–407.

Lewis DW. Pediatric migraine. *Pediatr Rev* 2007;28:43–53.

Li BU. Cyclic vomiting syndrome: age-old syndrome and new. *Semin Pediatr Neurol* 2001;8:13–21.

Lindley KJ, Andrews PL. Pathogenesis and treatment of cyclical vomiting. *J Pediatr Gastroenterol Nutr* 2005;41(suppl 1):S38–S40.

Logan P, Lewis D. Towards evidence based emergency medicine: best BETs from the Manchester Royal Infirmary: chlorpromazine in migraine. *Emerg Med J* 2007;24:297–300.

McCrory DC, Gray RN. Oral sumatriptan for acute migraine. *Cochrane Database Syst Rev* 2003;(3):CD002915.

Silver S, Gano D, Gerretsen P. Acute treatment of paediatric migraine: a meta-analysis of efficacy. *J Paediatr Child Health* 2008;44:3–9.

Stickler GB. Relationship between cyclic vomiting syndrome and migraine. *Clin Pediatr* 2005;44:505–508.

Tanen DA, Miller S, French T, et al. Intravenous sodium valproate versus prochlorperazine for the emergency department treatment of acute migraine headaches: a prospective, randomized, double-blind trial. *Ann Emerg Med* 2003;41:847–853.

Idiopathic Intracranial Hypertension

Friedman DI. Pseudotumor cerebri. *Neurosurg Clin North Am* 1999;10: 609–621.

Hartel C, Schilling S, Neppert B, et al. Intracranial hypertension in neuroborreliosis. *Dev Med Child Neurol* 2002;44:641–642.

Zemel L. Lyme disease and pseudotumor. *Mayo Clin Proc* 2000;75:315.

Stroke

Atkinson DS Jr. Computed tomography of pediatric stroke. *Semin Ultrasound CT MR* 2006;27:207–218.

Calder K, Kokorowski P, Tran T, et al. Emergency department presentation of pediatric stroke. *Pediatr Emerg Care* 2003;19:320–328.

Carlin TM, Chanmugam A. Stroke in children. *Emerg Med Clin North Am* 2002;20:671–685.

deVeber G, Roach ES, Riela AR, et al. Stroke in children: recognition, treatment, and future directions. *Semin Pediatr Neurol* 2000;7:309–317.

Jordan LC, Hillis AE. Hemorrhagic stroke in children. *Pediatr Neurol* 2007; 36:73–80.

Seidman C, Kirkham F, Pavlakis S. Pediatric stroke: current developments. *Curr Opin Pediatr* 2007;19:657–662.

Wang WC. Central nervous system complications of sickle cell disease in children: an overview. *Child Neuropsychol* 2007;13:103–119.

Winrow N, Melhem ER. Sickle cell disease and stroke in a pediatric population: evidence-based diagnostic evaluation. *Neuroimaging Clin N Am* 2003;13: 185–196.

Spinal Cord Dysfunction

Andronikou S, Albuquerque-Jonathan G, Wilmshurst J, et al. MRI findings in acute idiopathic transverse myelopathy in children. *Pediatr Radiol* 2003;33: 624–629.

Baylor P, Garoufi A, Karpathios T, et al. Transverse myelitis in 2 patients with Bartonella henselae infection (cat scratch disease). *Clin Infect Dis* 2007; 45:e42–e45.

Defresne P, Hollenberg H, Husson B, et al. Acute transverse myelitis in children: clinical course and prognostic factors. *J Child Neurol* 2003;18:401–406.

Defresne P, Meyer L, Tardieu M, et al. Efficacy of high dose steroid therapy in children with severe acute transverse myelitis. *J Neurol Neurosurg Psychiatr* 2001;71:272–274.

Pohl D. Epidemiology, immunopathogenesis and management of pediatric central nervous system inflammatory demyelinating conditions. *Curr Opin Neurol* 2008;21:366–372.

Acute Polyneuritis

Agrawal S, Peake D, Whitehouse WP. Management of children with Guillain-Barré syndrome. *Arch Dis Child Educ Pract Ed* 2007;92:ep161–ep168.

Hughes RA, Raphael JC, Swan AV, et al. Intravenous immunoglobulin for Guillain-Barré syndrome. *Cochrane Database Syst Rev* 2006;(1): CD002063. doi: 10.1002/14651858.CD002063.pub3.

Hughes RAC, Swan AV, van Koningsveld R, et al. Corticosteroids for Guillain-Barré syndrome. *Cochrane Database Syst Rev* 2006;(2):CD001446. doi: 10.1002/14651858.CD001446.pub2.

Hughes RAC, Wijdicks EFM, Barohn R, et al. Practice parameter: immunotherapy for Guillain-Barré syndrome: report of the Quality Standards Subcommittee of the American Academy of Neurology. *Neurology* 2003;61:736–740.

Raphael JC, Chevret S, Hughes RAC, et al. Plasma exchange for Guillain-Barré syndrome. *Cochrane Database Syst Rev* 2002;(2):CD001798.

Myasthenia Gravis

Andrews PI. Autoimmune myasthenia gravis in childhood. *Semin Neurol* 2004;24:101–110.

Hetherington KA, Losek JD. Myasthenia gravis: myasthenia vs. cholinergic crisis. *Pediatr Emerg Care* 2005;21:546–548.

Botulism

Fox CK, Keet CA, JB Strober. Recent advances in infant botulism. *Pediatr Neurol* 2005;32:149–154.

Francisco AMO, Arnon SS. Clinical mimics of infant botulism. *Pediatrics* 2007;119:826–828.

Long SS. Infant botulism. *Pediatr Infect Dis J* 2001;20:707–709.

Periodic Paralysis

Finsterer J. Primary periodic paralyses. *Acta Neurol Scand* 2008;117:145–158.

Jurkat-Rott K, Lehmann-Horn F. Paroxysmal muscle weakness—the familial periodic paralyses. *J Neurol* 2006;253:1391–1398.

Venance SL, Cannon SC, Fialho D, et al. The primary periodic paralyses: diagnosis, pathogenesis and treatment. *Brain* 2006;129:8–17.

Acute Cerebellar Ataxia

Davis DP, Marino A. Acute cerebellar ataxia in a toddler: case report and literature review. *J Emerg Med* 2003;24:281–284.

Nussinovitch M, Prais D, Volovitz B, et al. Post-infectious acute cerebellar ataxia in children. *Clin Pediatr* 2003;42:581–584.

Ryan MM, Engle EC. Acute ataxia in childhood. *J Child Neurol* 2003;18(5): 309–316.

MEDICAL EMERGENCIES

Benign Paroxysmal Vertigo

Tusa RJ, Saada AA, Niparko JK. Dizziness in childhood. *J Child Neurol* 1994;9: 261–274.

Movement Disorder

Dooley JM. Tic disorders in childhood. *Semin Pediatr Neurol* 2006;13: 231–242.

Rodnitzky RL. Drug-induced movement disorders in children and adolescents. *Expert Opin Drug Saf* 2005;4:91–102.

Sanger TD. Pediatric movement disorders. *Curr Opin Neurol* 2003;16:529–535.

Uddin MK, Rodnitzky RL. Tremor in children. *Semin Pediatr Neurol* 2003;10: 26–34.

Weiner SG, Normandin PA. Sydenham chorea: a case report and review of the literature. *Pediatr Emerg Care* 2007;23:20–24.

Wolf DS, Singer HS. Pediatric movement disorders: an update. *Curr Opin Neurol* 2008;21:491–496.

Optic Neuritis

Beck RW, Trobe JD, Moke PS, et al. High- and low-risk profiles for the development of multiple sclerosis within 10 years after optic neuritis: experience of the optic neuritis treatment trial. *Arch Ophthalmol* 2003;121:944–949.

Boomer JA, Siatkowski RM. Optic neuritis in adults and children. *Semin Ophthalmol* 2003;18:174–180.

Zeid NA, Bhatti MT. Acute inflammatory demyelinating optic neuritis: evidence-based visual and neurological considerations. *Neurologist* 2008;14: 207–223.

Facial Nerve Palsy

Ashtekar CS, Joishy M, Joshi R. Best evidence topic report: do we need to give steroids in children with Bell's palsy? *Emerg Med J* 2005;22:505–507.

Hato N, Matsumoto S, Kisaki H, et al. Efficacy of early treatment of Bell's palsy with oral acyclovir and prednisolone. *Otol Neurotol* 2003;24:948–951.

Hato N, Yamada H, Kohno H, et al. Valacyclovir and prednisolone treatment for Bell's palsy: a multicenter, randomized, placebo-controlled study. *Otol Neurotol* 2007;28:408–413.

Kitsko DJ, Dohar JE. Inner ear and facial nerve complications of acute otitis media, including vertigo. *Curr Allergy Asthma Rep* 2007;7:444–450.

Nigrovic LE, Thompson AM, Kimia A. Clinical predictors of Lyme disease among children with a peripheral facial palsy at an emergency department in a Lyme-disease endemic area. *Pediatrics* 2008;122:e1080–e1085.

Riordan M. Investigation and treatment of facial paralysis. *Arch Dis Child* 2001;84:286–287.

Salman MS, MacGregor DL. Should children with Bell's palsy be treated with corticosteroids? A systematic review. *J Child Neurol* 2001;16:565–568.

Singhi P, Jain V. Bell's palsy in children. *Semin Pediatr Neurol* 2003;10:289–297.

Sullivan FM, Swan IRC, Donnan PT, et al. Early treatment with prednisolone or acyclovir in Bell's palsy. *New Engl J Med* 2007;357:1598–1607.

White N, McCams KM. Facial paralysis secondary to acute otitis media. *Pediatr Emerg Care* 2000;16:343–345.

CHAPTER 97 ■ ONCOLOGIC EMERGENCIES

AMY L. BILLETT, MD, AND JENNIFER C. KESSELHEIM, MD, M.ED

INTRODUCTION

Every year in the United States, approximately 12,000 children and adolescents are diagnosed with cancer and 2,300 children die of their disease or side effects of treatment. Both cancer and treatment can cause significant morbidity for children. This chapter is organized in three major sections. The first section addresses the diagnosis and initial care of a child who presents to the emergency department (ED) at the time of new cancer diagnosis or at recurrence of disease. While this first section is organized by both the kind of cancer and by location of initial signs or symptoms, it does not address how to complete a diagnostic workup for cancer or initiate a definitive treatment plan. The second section addresses complications of treatment that may lead to an ED visit. The section is organized by the organ system affected. The final section addresses pain management and end-of-life care.

In general, when considering the pediatric oncology patient in the ED, the approach outlined in Table 97.1 will help the practitioner obtain historical information that is often unique to this patient population. A detailed medication history is critical because patients may be on multiple medications whose side effects may be contributing to the cause of the current ED visit. The antibiotic history should explore if the medication is being given to prevent an infection, to treat a known infection, or to suppress colonization. When taking a history from a pediatric oncology patient, we emphasize the paramount importance of the patient/parent point of view. While we as clinicians do have significant knowledge, the patient and family experiencing the cancer diagnosis are truly the experts. Exploring the perspective of the patient and parents about what the potential cause of the problem and how the patient is doing is a crucial step in the evaluative process. One last introductory principle is to consider always the extreme psychosocial stress that a pediatric cancer diagnosis places on a family. The care of these patients therefore requires the highest level of compassion and professionalism from clinicians.

INITIAL CARE OF THE CHILD WITH NEW OR RECURRENT CANCER

Childhood cancer can present with nonspecific signs and symptoms that can overlap with those of many childhood illnesses (Table 97.2). This is common with hematologic malignancies or with widely metastatic solid tumors. Even when the chief complaint is a localized symptom, disseminated disease may be present. Thus, the diagnosis of possible cancer in the ED may require not only a thorough history and physical

examination but also an initial laboratory and radiologic workup.

In general, once the diagnosis of cancer is suspected, a child should be referred to a center skilled in the management of childhood cancer and whose staff includes a pediatric oncologist as well as other subspecialists such as pediatric surgeons and radiation oncologists. Supportive care for life-threatening complications may need to be initiated in the ED prior to referral. In general, the specific workup, including obtaining tissue for diagnosis, should be carried out under the direction of a pediatric oncologist so that optimal information can be obtained. Histologic slides and paraffin blocks from a standard biopsy are often insufficient because viable tissue is essential for critical immunologic, cytogenetic, and molecular testing necessary to categorize the disease and choose the appropriate treatment. A number of studies have shown improved outcome for older adolescents and young adults when treated by pediatric oncologists using pediatric treatment programs. This information should be considered when referring a patient with a new or presumed diagnosis of cancer for further care. No patient should be discharged from the ED without a specific plan for definitive diagnosis and management.

The emergency physician should describe the findings and concern about possible cancer to the patient and family. It is appropriate to reassure them that most childhood cancer is curable. Specific details about diagnosis, treatment, and prognosis are best deferred to the pediatric oncologist to address once definitive information is available. The possibility of a cancer diagnosis usually causes fear and distress and requires empathic care and support from the health-care team in the ED.

Leukemia

Leukemia is a cancer of white blood cells (WBCs), and their precursors, that proliferate in excess within the bone marrow and other hematopoietic tissues. The presentations of childhood leukemia that a clinician in the ED may encounter are varied and, in some cases, the diagnosis of leukemia is not at all obvious (Table 97.2). Symptoms are usually secondary to bone marrow replacement or from infiltration of leukemic blast cells into tissues outside of the bone marrow. Leukemia is the most common childhood malignancy accounting for 29% of all cancer diagnoses in children from 0 to 14 years of age. Approximately 3,500 children are diagnosed with leukemia each year in the United States. Leukemias are classified as either acute or chronic. More than 95% of pediatric leukemias are acute, and acute lymphoblastic leukemia (ALL) accounts for the vast majority. ALL includes B-precursor ALL and T-lineage ALL. The other leukemias seen in children in order of decreasing

HISTORICAL DATA NEEDED FOR EVALUATION OF
PEDIATRIC ONCOLOGY PATIENTS IN THE
EMERGENCY DEPARTMENT

Category	Specific history to explore

Primary diagnosis	Tumor type
	Primary or metastatic
	   Where are sites of metastatic
	     disease?
	Date of diagnosis
	Status of disease
	   In remission, on treatment
	   In remission, off treatment
	   Relapsed

Surgical history	Date of surgical procedures Surgical complications Extent of tumor resections

Recent treatments	Chemotherapy
	   Drugs included in current
	     treatment plan
	   Dates of last chemotherapy
	     doses
	Radiation therapy
	   Doses of radiation used
	   Location of radiation field(s)
	   Dates of radiation therapy
	Stem cell transplant
	   Autologous or allogeneic
	   Use of immunosuppressants
	   History of graft-versus-host
	     disease

Central venous access	Type History of infections in line

Current medications	Chemotherapy:
	Prophylaxis for *Pneumocystis*
	   jiroveci or other infections
	Growth factors
	Pain treatment
	Supportive care medications
	   such as
	   Antiemetics
	   GI acid blockade
	   Bowel regimen
	   Antihypertensives

Patient/family perspective	How is the patient acting?
	Has this problem happened
	   before?
	Are symptoms getting worse
	   or better?
	What does parent or patient
	   believe to be cause of the
	   problem?

frequency include acute myeloid leukemia (AML), chronic myelogenous leukemia (CML), and chronic myelomonocytic leukemia (CMMoL). Specific classification is based on morphology, immunologic surface markers, and cytogenetic abnormalities from the bone marrow aspirate. Children with trisomy 21 are at increased risk of transient myeloproliferative disorder of the newborn, AML (younger than 4 years), and ALL (older than 1 year).

Leukemia presents in a variety of ways. As the leukemia proliferates in the bone marrow, normal hematopoietic elements are decreased leading to anemia, thrombocytopenia, and neutropenia. This is most common in the setting of leukemia but can occur with solid tumors, such as neuroblastoma and rhabdomyosarcoma with marrow metastasis. Anemia can be mild or severe but is often asymptomatic because of its slow development. Anemia with associated clinical signs or symptoms should be treated with a red cell transfusion. Thrombocytopenia can present with mucocutaneous bleeding such as epistaxis, gingival bleeding, petechiae, and ecchymosis. Concurrent nonsteroidal antiinflammatory drugs (NSAIDs) can increase the bleeding manifestations. The risk of bleeding may also be compounded by coagulopathy from the leukemia itself or from disseminated intravascular coagulation (DIC) related to sepsis.

Tumor lysis syndrome (TLS) is a metabolic complication resulting from the rapid death and destruction of tumor cells. As dying leukemic cells release their intracellular contents into the blood, potassium, phosphate, and uric acid rise. The elevated phosphate complexes with calcium and leads to hypocalcemia. The resulting calcium phosphate crystals can then deposit in the renal tubules causing renal insufficiency or in other tissue sites. Urate crystals can precipitate in the acidic renal tubular environment, causing an obstructive uropathy and renal insufficiency. TLS is common with acute leukemias and lymphomas but can also occur with neuroblastoma or other solid tumors with a very high tumor burden. The risk of TLS is highest in advanced Burkitt's lymphoma and ALL with hyperleukocytosis. Screening and preemptive therapy with hydration and allopurinol is appropriate for all patients at risk of TLS. The use of allopurinol or rasburicase (Elitek®) to decrease uric acid levels is often driven by institutional protocol.

Management of TLS relies on protecting the function of the kidneys while preventing severe metabolic derangements (Table 97.3). Alkaline hydration should be initiated to achieve brisk, dilute urine output with a pH 7 to 7.5 as long as the patient is not expected to receive rasburicase. If using rasburicase, hydration without alkalinization should be given. Alkalinization of the urine helps dissolve uric acid crystals but the pH should be kept below 8 to avoid increasing the probability of calcium phosphate crystal deposition in the kidney. In addition to IV hydration, all patients should either receive therapy with allopurinol (10 mg per kg per day with maximum dose 300 mg) or rasburicase. Allopurinol is a xanthine oxidase inhibitor that impairs the production of uric acid. Rasburicase, a recombinant urate-oxidase enzyme, causes direct lysis of uric acid and leads to a rapid drop in uric acid levels. The usual starting dose is 0.2 mg per kg IV. Rasburicase is indicated in patients who are at higher risk of TLS complications such as patients who present with compromised renal function or an extremely elevated uric acid level (e.g., greater than 12); who have advanced Burkitt's lymphoma; who cannot tolerate hydration [e.g., central nervous system (CNS) hemorrhage], or whose uric acid is rising despite allopurinol. There is no need to alkalinize the urine when rasburicase is used. Rasburicase is contraindicated in glucose-6-phosphate dehydrogenase (G6PD) deficiency as it can result in oxidative stress and hemolysis.

Of note, not all electrolyte abnormalities in the setting of TLS should be corrected (Table 97.3). Hyperphosphatemia can be treated using aluminum hydroxide as frequently as every 2 to 4 hours. Hypophosphatemia should not be corrected unless it is

TABLE 97.2

COMMON PRESENTING SYMPTOMS AND SIGNS OF PEDIATRIC CANCER

Symptoms and signs	Acute leukemia[a]	Lymphoma	Histiocytic diseases	Wilm's tumor	Neuroblastoma	Hepatic tumors	Ovarian tumors	Testicular tumors	Soft tissue sarcomas	Bone tumors	Central nervous system tumors
Abdominal mass		+		+	+	+	+		+		
Anorexia	+	+	+		+	+			+		±
Back pain	+	+	+		+				+	+	+
Cord compression	±	±	±				±			+	+
Cranial nerve palsies	+	+	+		+				±		+
Diarrhea			+								
Diplopia					+						+
Epistaxis	±	±	±								
Fever	+	±	+		+	+				±	±
Failure to thrive	+	+	+		+						+
Gait abnormality	+	+			+					+	+
Gastrointestinal bleeding											
Headache	±	+	+								+
Head/neck mass	±	±	±						+		
Hepatomegaly	+	+	+		+	+					
Hypertension				+	+						+
Irritability	+		+	+	+					±	+
Limp	+	+	+		+					+	±
Lymphadenopathy	+	+	+		+				+		+
Malaise	+	+	+		±				+		
Nasal obstruction									+		
Pallor	+	+	+	+	+						+
Petechiae	+	±	+		+						
Proptosis	±	±	±		+				+		+
Respiratory distress					+				+		
Scrotal/testicular abnormality					±			+	+		
Seizures			+								+
Splenomegaly	+	+									
Vomiting	+	+	+		+	+					+
Weight loss		+	+		+	+			+	+	±

[a]Patients with solid tumors invading the marrow may have symptoms and signs similar to those seen in leukemia.

MEDICAL EMERGENCIES

TABLE 97.3

EMERGENCY DEPARTMENT CARE OF PATIENT WITH PROBABLE OR CERTAIN ACUTE LEUKEMIA

Diagnostic Evaluation for All Patients
Detailed medical history and complete physical examination
CBC count with manual differential and peripheral blood smear
Electrolytes, including potassium, calcium, phosphorus
Uric acid
Assessment of renal function with BUN and creatinine
Coagulation studies, PT, PTT
Blood group type, antibody screen
Liver function tests
Chest x-ray to assess for mediastinal mass

Supportive Care for All Patients
Results of CBC count should be examined to determine if patient has anemia or thrombocytopenia requiring transfusion
 (please see below)
IV fluids should run at approximately 1½ times maintenance and should be alkalinized with $NaHCO_3$ to ensure a urine pH of 7–8
Allopurinol

Specific Problems that Require Immediate Intervention

Problem	Required data/findings	Therapy/management

Tumor lysis syndrome	Frequent lab monitoring (q 4–6 h)
	  Uric acid
	  Electrolytes
	  BUN and Creatinine
	  Ca and PO_4
	  Follow urine output
		Preemptive Management of patients at risk for tumor lysis syndrome[a]
		  IV fluids 1.5–2× maintenance with $NaHCO_3$ 40 mEq/L
		    Target urine pH 7–8
		    Target urine output >1 mL/kg/h
		  No potassium in IV fluids
		  Allopurinol
		Treatment of patients with TLS[b]
		  IV fluids as above
		  Allopurinol or rasburicase
		    Rasburicase, if renal function is impaired at presentation, if uric acid levels are rapidly rising or extremely high, or if there is a contraindication to hyperhydration
		    No alkalinization needed if rasburicase given
		  Replacement of phosphorus for serum level <1
		  Hyperkalemia: furosemide, insulin/glucose, kayexalate
		  Hypokalemia: No replacement of potassium unless critical level with high risk of cardiac arrhythmia
		  Hypocalcemia: no calcium replacement unless symptomatic hypocalcemia
		  Consider whether renal function or metabolic derangements may necessitate dialysis

Hyperleukocytosis	WBC count >100,000/mL	Ensure IV fluids are being given at maximum tolerated volume Avoid transfusion of packed red blood cells, which can increase viscosity Monitor for leukostasis
Leukostasis (occurs in some patients with hyperleukocytosis)	Clinical symptoms of respiratory distress or change in neurologic status Chest x-ray findings may be present	Urgent leukopheresis to decrease viscosity Continue IV fluids Proceed with caution if PT or PTT elevated
Mediastinal mass	Chest x-ray and/or chest CT scan Assessment of respiratory status while upright and supine Peak flow	Mass will likely shrink quickly in response to chemotherapy Support respiratory mechanics No sedation/anesthesia
Fever	Blood culture Additional culture from any site with localizing symptoms Avoid lumbar puncture	All patients should be assumed neutropenic, even if ANC >500 Empiric broad-spectrum antibiotics (see Figure 97.4) Tylenol, no NSAIDs

(continued)

TABLE 97.3

CONTINUED

Problem	Required data/findings	Therapy/management
Anemia	Hemoglobin <7 g/100mL Symptoms related to low red blood cell mass	Please see Table 97.7 for special guidelines for transfusions in the oncology population Avoid red cell transfusions in the setting of hyperleukocytosis If severe anemia, transfuse slowly to avoid precipitating congestive heart failure
Thrombocytopenia	Platelet count <150,000/mL	Please see Table 97.7 for special guidelines for transfusions in the oncology population
Coagulopathy	PT, PTT, fibrinogen, D-dimer	Fresh frozen plasma 10 mL/kg If hypofibrinogenemia exists in isolation, treat with cryoprecipitate, 1–2 U/10 kg Platelet transfusion if count <50,000/mL Leukopheresis and lumbar puncture may be contraindicated until coagulopathy corrected
CNS symptoms	Neurologic examination WBC count to screen for hyperleukocytosis PT, PTT, fibrinogen, D-dimer to assess risk for CNS hemorrhage Serum electrolytes Lumbar puncture with cell count and cytology Head and/or spinal cord imaging with CT or MRI	Leukopheresis to decrease viscosity and leukostasis, if WBC >100,000/mL and symptomatic Correct coagulopathy 　Fresh frozen plasma 10 mL/kg 　Cryoprecipitate 1–2 U/10 kg 　Platelet transfusion if count <50,000/mL Manage TLS as above to minimize electrolyte abnormalities Initiation of chemotherapy is best management for CNS leukemia or chloroma Consultation with radiation oncology in the setting of spinal cord compression

q, every; IV, intravenous; BUN, blood urea nitrogen; TLS, tumor lysis syndrome; WBC, white blood cells; PT, prothrombin time; PTT, partial thromboplastin time; CT, computed tomography; ANC, absolute neutrophil count; NSAIDs, nonsteroidal antiinflammatory drugs; CNS, central nervous system; MRI, magnetic resonance imaging.
[a]Patients with possible acute leukemia, advanced lymphoma. Consider for patients with likely neuroblastoma or rhabdomyosarcoma and high tumor burden.
[b]Patients with hyperuricemia, hyperkalemia, hyerphosphatermia, hypocalcemia, or elevated Cr.

in a critically low range (less than 1 mEq per L). Serum potassium levels must be aggressively monitored. Hyperkalemia in the setting of TLS should be managed as it would in other disease states (see Chapter 100) with Kayexelate®, insulin, and glucose, and dialysis, if needed. Hypokalemia should not be corrected unless the patient's serum potassium falls in a critically low range (less than 2 mEq per L) or EKG changes develop. Hypocalcemia should remain uncorrected as well, unless clinical signs or symptoms of hypocalemia develop. Supplemental calcium may increase the risk of formation of calcium phosphate precipitates in the kidney.

Hyperleukocytosis is defined as WBC count above 100,000 per mm³. When hyperleukocytosis is present, the clinical findings of leukostasis may develop from sludging of WBCs in the capillary beds. The most vulnerable beds are those in the lungs and CNS where increased viscosity can cause either thrombosis or hemorrhage. Leukostasis is much more common with myeloid leukemia than with ALL. In the setting of hyperleukocytosis, hydration should be initiated immediately to reduce viscosity. Transfusion of red blood cells and diuretics should be avoided to prevent further increases in blood viscosity. Platelet transfusions should be given to reduce the risk of CNS hemorrhage. Leukocytopheresis, a technique to reduce blood viscosity acutely, should be initiated immediately whenever even mild

respiratory or neurologic symptoms are present. The use of prophylactic leukocytopheresis when the WBC count exceeds 100,000 per mm³ in AML or greater than 300,000 per mm³ in lymphoid leukemias is controversial and should be considered only in consultation with a pediatric oncologist. Since new onset leukemia may have an associated coagulopathy, we recommend obtaining coagulation studies to determine the risk of bleeding during leukocytopheresis.

As leukemia develops, malignant cells can infiltrate tissue outside of hematopoietic locations. It is possible for these extramedullary sites of disease to cause the leukemia to come to clinical attention. Anterior mediastinal masses occur primarily with T-lineage ALL and can lead to life-threatening airway compromise and/or superior vena cava (SVC) syndrome. The approach to the presentation and management of anterior mediastinal masses is discussed in more detail in the section on thoracic tumors. Chloroma, a mass of leukemic blasts in the soft tissue, can occur in body part. Chloromas are much more common with AML than ALL. When this mass develops and rapidly expands near the spinal cord, compression of the cord can result (see "Tumors In and Around the Spinal Cord" section). Adenopathy, hepatomegaly, and splenomegaly are very common manifestations of leukemia. Leukemic involvement in the spinal fluid can cause meningeal symptoms, cranial

MEDICAL EMERGENCIES

nerve palsy, headache, seizure, increased intracranial pressure (ICP), or visual disturbances (from retinal infiltrates). Boys can present with testicular enlargement. There may also be skin lesions due to leukemia cutis (more common in monocytic leukemias and infant leukemia) and (in the case of AML) gingival hypertrophy due to leukemic infiltration.

Fever is common at the time of presentation with acute leukemia. Management is summarized in Table 97.3. Rarely, patients present with sepsis at the time of diagnosis or relapse. The increased risk of sepsis may be because of neutropenia and or immune dysfunction caused by the leukemia itself. Management of sepsis in the setting of leukemia is not unique and the principles are similar to those described more thoroughly in Chapter 91. For some patients, limp or a refusal to walk or bear weight on the legs is the first sign of the leukemia. In fact, it is not uncommon for a patient to receive diagnoses such as osteomyelitis or septic hip, and even receive IV antibiotics, before the diagnosis of leukemia is uncovered. It is essential for the emergency physician to ensure that a refusal to walk is not because of cord compression from chloroma as discussed above. Pain in the legs, or other bones, is usually because of replacement of the bone marrow with leukemic cells that are rapidly proliferating, thereby causing strain on the marrow spaces. Pathologic fractures may develop in children with leukemia as the expanding marrow compartments but strain on and weaken the bony cortex.

Tables 97.3 includes management guidelines for leukemia in the ED. The evaluation should begin with a thorough history and physical examination. The history should focus on the time frame in which symptoms developed and should screen for the complications described above. The physical examination should include assessment of airway, breathing, and circulation as well as an evaluation for lymphadenopathy and hepatosplenomegaly. Evidence for soft tissue infiltration by leukemia cells should be explored, such as a skin infiltration (leukemia cutis) or testicular enlargement in male patients. A thorough neurologic examination is also essential to screen for cord compression and CNS effects of the leukemia. Any abnormalities on the neurologic examination warrant CNS imaging to determine whether a neurologic complication of the leukemia has occurred.

Laboratory evaluation should begin with a complete blood cell (CBC) count, WBC differential, and peripheral blood smear to be reviewed by a hematologist-oncologist or pathologist. Automated differentials might count leukemic blasts as either atypical lymphocytes or monocytes so abnormal numbers of these cell types should raise concern for leukemia. It is possible for leukemia to present without peripherally circulating blasts, as is often the case in T-cell ALL. The ED can also send a sample of peripheral blood for flow cytometry analysis. This testing can provide important clues as to what kind of leukemia a patient has by analyzing the proteins of the blast cell surface. Specific diagnosis requires a bone marrow aspirate, which is not routinely performed in the ED and should be done only in consultation with an oncologist.

In constructing a differential diagnosis, it is helpful to consider whether leukemic blasts are present in the peripheral circulation. If blasts are present in substantive quantities (greater than 20%), then leukemia is the most likely diagnosis. However, a smaller percentage of blasts could indicate a myelodysplastic syndrome, a myeloproliferative disorder,

recovery from an aplastic process, or a leukemoid reaction. If blasts are not evident on the CBC count, and the patient has pancytopenia, one must consider leukemia but also bone marrow failure, which can be because of aplastic anemia, infections (usually viral), and marrow replacement by a solid tumor involving bone marrow. If the patient is not pancytopenic and if only one to two cell lines seem to be affected, the clinician must consider the differential diagnoses for each cytopenia individually (see Chapter 91).

Assess airway patency, which may be compromised in the setting of a mediastinal mass. A chest x-ray should also be obtained to screen for the presence of a mediastinal mass. Assessment of the patient's breathing should include attention to the respiratory rate and oxygenation with O_2 saturation, both of which can become compromised in the setting of anemia, leukostasis, congestive heart failure, and pulmonary infection. To attend to the patient's circulation, the clinician must establish intravascular access and assess for signs or symptoms of SVC syndrome. The patient should not be allowed to eat or drink in case sedation or anesthesia will be needed for the diagnostic evaluation or treatment. In addition to the laboratory investigations needed to diagnose the leukemia, the evaluation should screen for TLS by checking serum chemistries, including potassium, calcium, magnesium, phosphorus, and uric acid. Renal function should be assessed with a blood urea nitrogen (BUN) and creatinine. The results of the CBC should be reviewed to assess needs for transfusions of blood products and a prothrombin time (PT) and partial thromboplastin time (PTT) should be checked to look for coagulopathy (Table 97.3). The patient should receive alkalinized intravenous hydration and allopurinol or non-alikalinized hydration and rasburicase as described in Table 97.3.

It is not uncommon for patients with leukemia to be febrile at presentation. Although the fever may be an inflammatory reaction driven by the leukemia itself, serious infection must be explored. It is essential to determine if the patient is neutropenic in the setting of the fever. If absolute neutrophil count (ANC) is less than 500, broad spectrum antibiotics intended to empirically cover gram-positive and -negative bacteria as well as pseudomonas should be administered in the ED. If localizing signs of a bacterial infection are evident, or if high fevers are present (greater than 39°C), empiric therapy should be initiated even if the patient is not neutropenic.

Histiocytic Diseases

Histiocytic diseases are a complex and sometimes confusing group of disorders for two reasons. First, several different disease entities make up this group, although efforts have been made to simplify the terminology for these various diagnoses. Second, significant clinical heterogeneity exists between the major disease entities in this category. Histiocyte is a term referring to several different cells that are thought to derive from a common CD34+ progenitor in the bone marrow. Depending on the cytokines to which the progenitors become exposed, the differentiation can yield tissue macrophages, dermal/interstitial dendritic cells, or Langerhans cells (see Fig. 97.4). In general, disorders involving histiocytes are rare; of the group, the most common is Langerhans cell histiocytosis (LCH), which has an incidence of three to five cases per million children. The most significant histiocyte disorders include LCH and hemophagocytic lymphohistiocytosis (HLH).

LCH has clinical heterogeneity and the locations involved in the disease have implications for therapy and prognosis. Low-risk LCH may present at any age and systemic symptoms (e.g., weight loss or fever) are rare. The organs usually involved in these cases are skin, bone, lymph nodes, or a combination of these. Skin involvement can present as a red papular rash, resembling a candidal diaper rash, that may appear on the groin, abdomen, back, or chest. There may also be seborrheic flaking of the scalp, often misdiagnosed as "cradle cap" in infants, draining otitis externa, or ulcerative lesions behind the ears, on the scalp, or in the genital region. Boney involvement may be asymptomatic or the patient may complain of pain in a localized area of bone. A lytic lesion of the skull that presents as a tender mass is the most common but any bone may be involved. Loose teeth from involvement of the jaw occur. Certain sites of disease have become known as "risk" organs because their involvement implies more aggressive disease. These patients are often very young with disease that involves the lung, liver, spleen, and/or bone marrow. Lung involvement is rare but worrisome and usually manifests first as hypoxia, in which case imaging with chest x-ray or chest CT scan is needed. Liver and spleen involvement is usually accompanied by enlargement of those organs, although hepatic dysfunction may also be present. Bone marrow involvement usually presents with cytopenias, which should prompt a bone marrow aspirate and biopsy.

Diabetes insipidus (DI) is the most frequent endocrine abnormality in LCH; some patients may present with an apparent "idiopathic" presentation of DI before other lesions are identified. DI is caused by involvement of the posterior pituitary. A few patients may present with diarrhea or malabsorption as colitis related to LCH has been described. In these cases, endoscopic examination with biopsies are needed.

HLH is a very rare, severe, and life-threatening systemic disease with rapid progression from presentation to death without appropriate intervention. Thus, consideration of this diagnosis in the ED can be critical to outcome. For these reasons, it is essential for the emergency physician to have some familiarity with this disorder. Congenital HLH presents in infants and very young children. Other forms of HLH develop secondary to Epstein-Barr virus (EBV) infection, malignancy, or severe rheumatologic disorders or without a specific trigger. Regardless of etiology, HLH presents with fever, hepatosplenomegaly, adenopathy, and rash. Laboratory analysis reveals a markedly high serum ferritin as well as transaminitis, hypertriglyceridemia, hypofibrinogenemia, and cytopenias. Bone marrow evaluation may show characteristic hemophagocytosis.

All patients with suspected histiocytic disorders need thorough history and physical examination as well as overall assessment of whether they are systemically ill or not. Patients with HLH may have significant systemic illness with organ dysfunction and even vital sign instability and will require inpatient management, often in an ICU. On the other extreme, patients with a single site suspected to be LCH may require little to no intervention in the ED but need only close follow-up with oncology.

Laboratory evaluation should include CBC count, liver function testing, electrolytes to screen for DI, and inflammatory markers such as erythrocyte sedimentation rate (ESR) and C-reactive protein (CRP). If HLH is suspected, ferritin and triglycerides should be obtained. Pulse oximetry should be checked to screen for hypoxia if LCH is suspected, and consideration given to a chest x-ray if hypoxia is detected. Consultation with oncology can be useful to guide the evaluation and management of systemically ill patients, as in the case of HLH, or allow for careful follow-up of more stable patients with LCH.

Tumors of the Central Nervous System

Tumors of the CNS, most commonly affecting the brain, represent the most common solid tumor in the pediatric population and the second most common pediatric cancer overall. There are approximately 2,000 new malignant brain tumors diagnosed annually in children. These tumors can affect children and adolescents of any age group but the peak incidence is in school-aged children, 5- to 10-year old. The risk of developing a pediatric brain tumor is increased in certain syndromes, such as neurofibromatosis type I, which is associated with gliomas. Brain tumors in children are usually primary, not metastatic. Since tumor location usually drives presenting signs and symptoms, this is the most useful categorization for the ED (Table 97.4). Supratentorial tumors are more common in children younger than 1 year and older than 10 years. Infratentorial lesions are more common between ages 1 and 10 years.

Some of the symptoms of brain tumors in children are nonspecific and nonlocalizing complaints can be present for a variety of tumor types. Examples include headache, altered behavior, vision changes, altered growth or weight, somnolence, and altered school performance. The diagnosis of brain tumor may be delayed in these patients whose presentation is not specific. Once patients develop signs and symptoms more easily referred to the CNS, their presentations tend to hinge on the tumor's location (Table 97.4).

Infratentorial tumors may present with cranial nerve deficits, such as facial nerve palsies, dysphagia, or paresis of cranial nerve VI, causing diplopia or strabismus. Alternatively, ependymomas of the fourth ventricle may present with hydrocephalus and increased ICP. Cerebellar lesions can elicit truncal ataxia and a reeling gait when located on the midline. When only one cerebellar hemisphere is involved, patients may display an ipsilateral hypotonia, resulting in falling to the affected side. An example is medulloblastoma involving the cerebellar vermis. Herniation of the cerebellar tonsil can cause head tilt toward the tumor and neck pain or stiffness. Astrocytomas may present in infratentorial locations.

In contrast, supratentorial masses may present with signs and symptoms derived from the involved anatomic locations. Supratentorial tumors unassociated with the ventricles are often glial tumors, of which a wide variety exists. Tumors near the optic chiasm may present with vision deficits. Craniopharyngiomas, located in the pituitary gland, can cause visual disturbances, headache, and alterations in the endocrine function. Growth hormone deficiency or hypothyroidism may cause delayed growth and DI or syndrome of inappropriate antidiuretic hormone (SIADH) may cause derangements in the serum sodium levels. Pineal tumors may cause hydrocephalus by obstructing the aquaduct of Sylvius or can cause Perinaud's syndrome (deficits in upward gaze, convergence nystagmus,

TABLE 97.4

TUMORS AFFECTING THE CENTRAL NERVOUS SYSTEM

Location	Specific tumor types	Presenting signs and symptoms	Comments

Supratentorial hemispheric	Low grade gliomas
	  Pilocytic
	  Fibrillary
	High grade glioma
	Mixed neuronal-glial
	  Neoplasms
	  Ganglioglioma
	Ependymoma
	Choroid plexus Tumors
	Primitive neuroectodermal
	  tumor (PNET)
		Varies with site
		  Hemiparesis
		  Hemisensory deficits
		  Seizure
		  Hemianopsia
			Outcome for these tumors usually
			  improved by extensive resection

Supratentorial midline	Chiasmatic/hypothalamic
	  glioma
	Craniopharyngioma
	Germinoma/malignant germ
	  cell Tumors
	Pineoblastoma
	PNET
		Vision deficits
		Diencephalic syndrome
		Neuroendocrine symptoms
		Hydrocephalus
		Parinaud's syndrome
			Germinoma and germ cell tumors
			  require bx as treatment,
			  usually just chemotherapy, not
			  surgery

Infratentorial	Medulloblastoma
	Cerebellar astrocytoma
	Ependymoma
	Diffuse malignant brainstem
	  glioma
	Benign focal brainstem glioma
		Cranial nerve palsies
		Cerebellar signs
		  Ataxia
		  Dysmetria
		Brainstem signs
		  Weakness
		  Unsteady gait
		Increased intracranial pressure	

bx, biopsy

and impaired papillary response). Hypothalamic tumors may cause diencephalic syndrome, which includes failure to thrive, wasting, and unusual euphoria. If a tumor is located near the third ventricle, hydrocephalus and symptoms of increased ICP can result. Masses within the cerebral hemispheres themselves usually present with focal motor dysfunction or seizure.

The spinal cord may be the site of a primary tumor or, in some cases, can be affected by a "dropped metastasis" from a primary lesion within the brain. These can present with focal neurologic deficits attributable to areas of the spinal cord inferior to the lesion (see "Tumors In and Around the Spinal Cord" section).

Brain tumors can cause increased ICP by blocking CSF drainage. The symptoms of increased ICP can vary based on patient age. Infants with an open fontanelle can sometimes present with bulging of the fontanelle as well as seizure, vomiting, irritability, or loss of acquired skills. Older children often have headache and early morning vomiting. Sixth nerve palsies are common. Sometimes increased ICP is detected only on imaging of the brain that reveals enlargement of the ventricles or effacement of the gyri. Whether the diagnosis of increased ICP is made radiographically or by history, its management is the same. First, if ICP is known or suspected to be elevated, a lumbar puncture should be avoided, as this theoretically may precipitate a rapid change in ICP followed by herniation of the brain. The pressure may be relieved using steroids such as dexamethasone at a dose of 2 to 4 mg every 6 hours. Mannitol mannitol may be useful in bringing down the ICP. In some situations, intubation may be needed to allow for hyperventilation as the low P_{CO_2} works to ameliorate swelling in

the brain. Neurosurgical consultation can address the appropriateness of a ventriculostomy or debulking procedure.

Seizures developing in the setting of a child with cancer, whether due to a CNS tumor or another malignancy, should be managed as described in Chapter 69. Brain tumors should be considered in the differential diagnosis of new onset seizures.

Patients with brain tumors are at risk for several metabolic complications, which may lead to the initial presentation in the ED. The presence of an intracranial tumor may be a cause for cerebral salt wasting or SIADH. Also, DI can result from tumor involvement of the pituitary gland. Patients should be screened for these abnormalities with serum chemistries. However, these complications are not managed uniquely because of the brain tumors. Chapter 135 provides guidelines on evaluation and management.

After ensuring the patient has stable airway, breathing, and circulation, the evaluation in the ED should focus on a thorough history and physical examination. The history should assess for any neurologic symptoms and should screen for complications of brain tumors described above. A complete physical examination should follow including a thorough ophthalmologic and neurologic assessment. Physical examination should also include evaluation of the patient's external genitalia for precocious puberty or virilization, since some pediatric brain tumors may be hormone secreting. A rectal examination to evaluate the anal "wink" is also useful as a screen for spinal cord compression. If the history or physical examination raises concern for increased ICP or spinal cord compression, then therapy should be initiated as described above. Imaging is an important component of the evaluation with a CT scan being useful to rule out hemorrhage and assess for increased ICP. A CT scan can sometimes be used to visualize a brain tumor; however, the study may miss infratentorial masses. In most cases, an MRI (magnetic resonance imaging) with gadolinium will ultimately be needed. Laboratory evaluation should include serum electrolytes to ensure that the patient exhibits neither SIADH, salt wasting, nor DI. A CBC count is also useful to ensure the patient's hematocrit and platelet count are adequate for any upcoming procedures.

The decision about whether to admit a patient with a newly diagnosed brain tumor hinges mostly on the neurologic status. Patients may have altered airway, breathing, or circulation due to the tumor compressing the brainstem. Cranial nerve dysfunction may compromise a patient's ability to eat normally. The tumor may cause symptoms such as headache, nausea, or vomiting, which require inpatient management. Or the neurologic examination may be compromised leading to functional deficits making discharge problematic. In any of these cases, patients should be admitted to the hospital either to a neurosurgical service or, in some cases, to the operating room directly. Prompt consultation with pediatric oncology, pediatric neurology, and pediatric neurosurgery is essential to ensure that patients are referred to experienced centers for definitive management.

Tumors of the Head and Neck

Children can present with intraorbital tumors, which may involve any of the tissues contained by the orbit including bone, muscle and soft tissue (further distinguished by whether the tumor has an intraconal or extraconal location), and the globe itself. Masses in these regions have a wide differential diagnosis, which includes benign etiologies such as infections (periorbital and orbital cellulitis), orbital myositis, benign germ cell tumors, or cystic lesions such as a dermoid cyst. The most common malignancies affecting the boney orbit are LCH and neuroblastoma. Presenting symptoms usually include proptosis or strabismus. Soft tissue tumors with intraconal locations usually include rhabdomyosarcomas and germ cell tumors, whereas extraconal tumors are likely to be rhabdomyosaromas as germ cell tumors occur more rarely in this location. Here again, presenting symptoms usually include proptosis and strabismus. Vascular tumors including capillary hemangiomas of the orbit may present with red or purple nodular lid lesion or proptosis.

Retinoblastoma is the most common intraocular malignancy in children. It occurs in 1 in 23,000 births and is usually diagnosed by age 2 years. Retinoblastoma occurs in both a hereditary and sporadic form. Two-thirds of patients present with a white pupil (leukocoria) noted by parents. This is the tumor as seen through the vitreous. Children with leukocoria should have an ophthalmologic examination under anesthesia to help differentiate retinoblastoma from other possible etiologies such as congenital cataract, coloboma, idiopathic retinal detachment, and others. Other ophthalmologic complaints such as hyphema, red painful eye, strabismus, fixed pupillary dilation, and proptosis are all possible. Direct extension via the optic nerve into the meninges and spinal fluid is a possible but unlikely complication of the tumor. Presentations are usually local and therefore cured by enucleation, but chemotherapy, cryotherapy, laser therapy, and insertion of radioactive plaques are all being explored to preserve vision. Leukemia and lymphoma can infiltrate the retina. Ocular melanoma is very rare in children. Management of retinoblastoma hinges on the probability of useful vision in the affected eye. Ophthalmology should be consulted early to determine if the patient's visual acuity has already been affected by the mass and to plan the urgency of examination under anesthesia. Management of intraorbital tumors may be possible on an outpatient basis, in conjunction with an experienced pediatric ophthalmologist, if the mass is unlikely to affect vision quickly or if vision is already profoundly impaired in the affected eye.

Tumors of the aerodigestive tract include sarcomas, lymphoid tumors, and carcinomas. While the latter are commonly seen in the adult population, carcinoma is rare in pediatrics. Masses in this region may also be benign, infectious, or reactive in etiology. Regardless of the tissue of origin, these masses usually present with symptoms related to their anatomic position. Oropharyngeal tumors can cause snoring and obstructive sleep apnea as well as chronic otitis media and unilateral tonsillar hypertrophy, in the case of lymphomas such as Burkitt's. Gingival hypertrophy may be a sign of a monocytic leukemia. LCH or Burkitt's lymphoma of the mandible can present with loose teeth. Rhabdomyosarcoma of the salivary or parotid gland often presents with pain or a visible/palpable facial mass. Malignant tumors of the nose, nasopharynx, and sinuses can present with purulent or bloody rhinorrhea, epistaxis, or sinusitis. Nasopharyngeal carcinoma tends to have a long duration of symptoms before diagnosis because symptoms are rarely specific. Malignant tumors of the sinuses and base of the skull can present with cranial neuropathies such as deviation of the eyes due to compression of the cranial nerves by the tumor. Rhabdomyosarcoma of the middle ear can present with persistent otitis, pain, or cranial neuropathy. The external ear canal can be affected by LCH leading to otorrhea and otitis externa.

The clinician in the ED should carefully assess airway, breathing, and circulation as tumors in some of these locations can threaten vital structures within the head or neck. Following this, a complete history and physical examination are necessary. Often radiographic imaging and laboratory evaluation is not needed. However, in the case of suspected leukemia or lymphoma, laboratory studies should be obtained to assess for hyperleukocytosis, cytopenias and TLS (see preceding discussion on leukemia). Radiographic imaging should be pursued if more information is needed about the tumor's position in relationship to the patient's airway and other vital structures of the head and neck. Management of these tumors can sometimes occur on an outpatient basis, in conjunction with a pediatric oncologist and a specialist, such as a dentist or otorhinolaryngologist with expertise in the anatomic region of the tumor. However, specific symptoms such as uncontrolled pain, difficulty with oral hydration, TLS, or any evolving threat to the airway would make inpatient management essential.

Neck masses due to benign, congenital anomalies of the neck such as branchial cleft cysts or cystic hygromas can cause masses, which may grow suddenly, as a result of infection or bleeding, prompting an ED visit. Neck masses are commonly because of enlarged lymph nodes. Lymphadenopathy in children is common and usually benign and either reactive or infectious in etiology. Bilateral nodes may be associated with

MEDICAL EMERGENCIES

viral infections such as EBV or cytomegalovirus (CMV). Unilateral lymphadenopathy, especially in infants and young children, may be associated with *Staphylococcus aureus* or group A streptococcus infections. Even lymph node enlargement with a chronic time course is still most likely infectious (e.g., mycobacteria, cat scratch disease, toxoplasma). Lymph nodes can appear large even without infection or malignancy, as observed in Castleman's, Kikuchi's, and Rosai-Dorfman syndromes. Enlarged lymph nodes in the neck due to malignancy can be from lymphoma or leukemia or can be because of metastasis from an adjacent solid tumor such as rhabdomyosarcoma, neuroblastoma, or nasopharyngeal carcinoma. It can be difficult to distinguish the primary tumor mass from a lymph node in these circumstances.

Children with neck tumors, regardless of etiology, must be evaluated for impact on the airway, breathing, and circulation. If any of these are at risk, inpatient management will be needed. Clinicians should explicitly consider the following:

- Does the mass impinge on or compress the airway?
- Does the patient experience respiratory distress or any compromise to his or her breathing due to the mass?
- Does the mass interfere with circulation of the head and neck leading to SVC syndrome (discussed in section on "Thoracic Tumors")?
- Does the tumor threaten to compress the cervical spine (see "Tumors In and Around the Spinal Cord" section)?

Following this assessment, a careful history should address the duration the mass has been present and its rate of growth, any recent infectious illnesses, the patient's immunization status, cat exposure, medications, and the presence or absence of systemic systems. Physical examination should screen for other masses or lymphadenopathy in the body. In evaluating nodes of the neck, infected or reactive nodes are often small, mobile and soft, or, if enlarged, the enlargement is often accompanied by redness and tenderness. Characteristics that make malignancy more likely are nontender masses, very firm/hard texture, diameter more than 3 cm, adherence to other structures, irregular margins, and absence of signs or symptoms of infection.

Diagnostic evaluation in the ED should focus on defining the relationship between the mass and the airway and major vessels of the neck. A CT scan is often helpful in establishing the neck anatomy in this way. In addition, a chest x-ray should be obtained to explore whether the disease could include a mass in the anterior mediastinum. Laboratory evaluation should include a CBC count with differential, ESR and lactate dehydrogenase (LDH) (which may be elevated in certain lymphomas), testing for any relevant infectious etiologies, and consideration of thyroid function testing.

Tumors of the Thorax

Thoracic tumors can be caused by a number of childhood cancers. While hematologic malignancies are common, embryonal neoplasms such as neuroblastoma, sarcomas such as PNET, and carcinomas can also present in the chest. In general, there are no specific predisposing conditions or factors. The most critical decision making and care in the ED is the differentiation of emergent from nonemergent. This difference is frequently driven by tumor location.

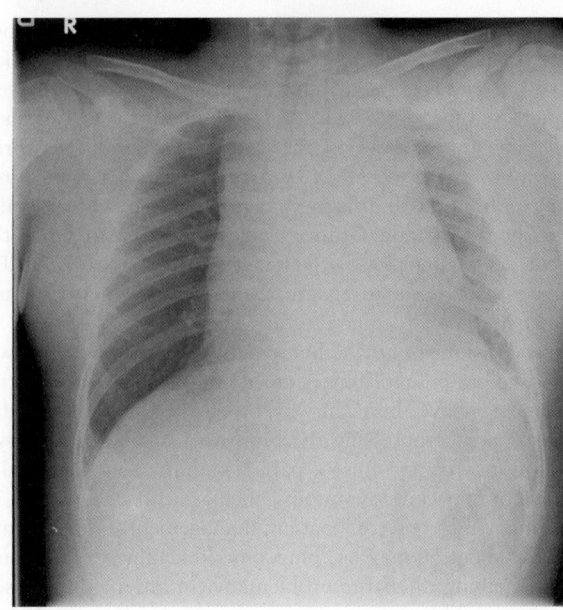

FIGURE 97.1 Chest radiograph demonstrating a large, homogenous anterior mediastinal mass. Patient presented with persistent cough and progressive orthopnea.

Tumors that arise in the anterior and middle mediastinum often present with respiratory symptoms ranging from mild cough to severe respiratory distress (Fig. 97.1). These tumors can compress the great vessels and cause SVC syndrome. They also may be "asymptomatic" and identified during evaluation for nonspecific systemic symptoms or, less commonly, an asymptomatic presentation on a chest radiograph performed for another reason. In contrast, posterior mediastinal masses are frequently identified on a chest radiograph performed for another reason. They may, however, cause local pain from nerve root involvement and/or cord compression (see "Tumors In and Around the Spinal Cord" section).

The differential diagnosis is also usually based on location. The "4 Ts" of the anterior medastinal tumors include "terrible lymphoma," "teratoma," "thymoma," and "thyroid carcinoma." The latter three are rare. Nonmalignant conditions with anterior mediastinal masses include adenopathy associated with infection, sarcoid, and normal thymus (especially if the chest radiograph is interpreted by a radiologist unfamiliar with children). Common lymphomas (Table 97.5) in the anterior mediastinum include T-cell lymphoblastic lymphoma (or T-cell ALL with an associated anterior mediastinal mass), Hodgkin's lymphoma, and diffuse B-cell large cell lymphoma. Lymphoma can also occur in the middle mediastinum, which can also be the site of masses associated with pulmonary sequestration and other developmental anomalies. "Teratoma" of the mediastinum includes benign and malignant germ cell tumors. Posterior mediastinal masses include neuroblastoma and other neurogenic tumors such as malignant peripheral nerve sheath tumors (especially in patients with neurofibromatosis, type 1), or benign lesions such as schwannoma.

The initial focus should include a thorough assessment of airway, breathing, and circulation, all of which may be compromised by an anterior mediastinal mass. Since an anterior mediastinal mass may compress the airway below the level of the carina, intubation can be ineffective to manage respiratory fail-

TABLE 97.5

LYMPHOMA PRESENTATIONS AND CONSIDERATIONS IN THE ED

Lymphoma	Typical presentation	Potential complications at diagnosis and considerations for ED management

Hodgkin's disease—Classical	Painless, hard adenopathy: neck and supraclavicular common
	AMM common, with or without symptoms
	Pleural effusions uncommon
	May have "B" symptoms
	    Fevers
	    Night sweats
	    Weight loss
		Superior vena cava (SVC) syndrome
		Tracheal obstruction

Hodgkin's disease—nodular lymphocyte predominant	Painless, hard adenopathy: often neck or supraclavicular. Can be inguinal. Often at a single site B symptoms rare AMM rare	SVC syndrome Tracheal obstruction (very rare)
Lymphoblastic lymphoma	Painless, hard adenopathy at any site Respiratory symptoms from rapidly, growing mediastinal mass, often with pleural effusions (T-lineage, advanced stage) GI tract involvement rare	Tumor lysis syndrome SVC syndrome Tracheal obstruction Pleural effusions

Burkitt's lymphoma	Single site of enlarged lymphoid tissue(low stage)
	    Incidental finding on appendectomy
	    Asymmetric enlarged tonsil
	    Lead point for intussusception in >3 yr
	    A single, painless enlarged node
	Painless, hard adenopathy with rapid growth (usually advanced stage)
	Rapidly progressing abdominal distension with diffuse involvement of the GI tract/liver with ascites and pleural effusions (advanced stage)
		Rapid assessment for tumor lysis syndrome (TLS): High risk of severe tumor lysis, even prior to treatment (advanced stage)
		First dose rasburicase in ED if uric acid >8 and low-risk for G6PD deficiency
		Urgent consultation with oncology
		Admission to center with available pediatric dialysis

Diffuse large B-cell lymphoma	Painless, hard adenopathy at any site, neck/supraclavicular common AMM common, symptoms variable (advanced) Symptom progression can be rapid (advanced stage) Systemic symptoms of malaise, weight loss common with advanced disease GI symptoms/abdominal mass from GI tract and mesenteric nodes involvement	TLS SVC syndrome Tracheal obstruction
Anaplastic large cell lymphoma	Painless, hard adenopathy at any site Skin/subcutaneous nodules GI symptoms/abdominal mass from GI tract and mesenteric node involvement Systemic symptoms (fevers, night sweats, weigh loss, malaise) common with advanced disease	TLS

AMM, anterior mediastanial mass; G6PD, glucose-6-phosphate dehydrogenase.

MEDICAL EMERGENCIES

ure. Management must focus on prevention of respiratory failure through such strategies as oxygen therapy and maximizing respiratory mechanics via keeping the patient calm and upright. Do not put the patient in a supine position if evidence of respiratory distress. Do not sedate or anesthetize the patient. Do not start empiric steroids without a discussion with an oncologist to ensure that steroids will not interfere with ability to establish the diagnosis subsequently. If there is evidence of SVC syndrome with plethora, facial edema, and jugular venous distension, ensure adequate intravascular volume to support systemic return, the patient should not receive anesthesia as it can lead to severe cardiovascular collapse. Diuresis should not be attempted either since tumors of the thorax can grow toward the spinal column, a careful neurologic history and examination is needed to assess for possible cord compression (see "Tumors In and Around the Spinal Cord" section).

There may be useful clues to the diagnosis from the history and physical examination. A recent history of new onset asthma in an older child that responded to a course of steroids but has now returned is consistent with partial treatment of lymphoblastic leukemia or lymphoma. Many lymphomas can also present with nonspecific systemic symptoms such as weight loss, fatigue, unexplained fevers, night sweats, and malaise. Itching can be a paraneoplastic phenomenon associated with Hodgkin's lymphoma. The pace of symptom development and severity of current symptoms should be used to determine the rate at which subsequent workup must occur. Examination should include assessment of all nodal groups (including axilla and supraclavicular) to both aid in the differential diagnosis and establish a site for possible biopsy. Of note, almost all pediatric lymphomas are high grade and have an acute to subacute course.

Diagnostic workup in the ED should always include a chest radiograph, including a lateral view, to help establish the location of the mass. Chest CT scan should only be performed in a patient who can lie flat comfortably. A CT contrast should not be given without verifying adequate renal function since TLS can occur with lymphoma (see "Leukemia" section). Laboratory evaluations should include CBC to assess for evidence of marrow replacement and to identify circulating blasts, and metabolic screening for possible TLS. Patients with symptoms from an anterior mediastinal mass must be admitted to a center with pediatric oncology expertise and may frequently require ICU admission. Those with minimal or no symptoms from the mass and no metabolic disturbances may be discharged to the care of a pediatric oncologist for further workup as an outpatient.

Primary lung tumors are vanishingly rare in childhood but presentation of lung metastasis at diagnosis or relapse is not uncommon. The initial complaints may include respiratory insufficiency, postobstructive infection, foreign body–type symptoms, or hemoptysis. Presentation may also involve the discovery of pulmonary nodules on a chest radiograph performed for a different reason. Primary lung tumors in children include pleuropulmonary blastoma that may be associated with congenital cystic adenomatoid malformation or very small bronchogenic carcinomas. Most of these latter are asymptomatic. Many pediatric sarcomas, some lymphomas, germ cell tumors, Wilm's tumor, and rarely neuroblastoma can present or recur with lung metastasis. These typically involve multiple small or large lung nodules in the pulmonary parenchyma or are pleural-based. In children, infection is a more common cause of lung nodules than cancer. In general, there are no emergency management issues unique to lung tumors versus other lung problems. Patients who are systemically ill require admission for further evaluation and management. Askin's tumor (PNET or primitive neuroectodermal tumor) is a unique chest wall tumor that occurs in children and young adults. If the tumor is relatively exophytic, it may present as a chest wall mass with or without pain. More commonly, it presents with respiratory symptoms from an effusion as described below.

Pulmonary effusions can be the presenting sign of childhood cancer. Effusions can be caused by malignant cells in the pleural space or from obstruction of lymphatic drainage. Effusions are common with anterior mediastinal masses due to leukemia or lymphoma and can also occur with posterior mediastinal neuroblastoma, lung metastasis, and chest wall tumors. They may be symptomatic or asymptomatic. The effusion may obscure a mass on both chest x-ray and chest CT scan. Malignant pericardial effusions are most often associated with leukemias and lymphomas. For general diagnosis and management of pulmonary and pericardial effusions (see Chapters 84 and 98). If fluid is drained from either space in the ED for relief of symptoms, a fluid sample should be sent to pathology for cytology if malignancy is suspected. In general, patients who are not compromised by a malignant effusion should not have fluid drained for diagnostic purposes while in the ED.

Tumors of the Hepatobiliary Tree

Tumors of the hepatobiliary tree in children are more likely to include tumors that metastasize to liver than primary tumors of the liver (Table 97.6). Of the primary tumors, hepatoblastoma (HB) and hepatocellular carcinoma (HCC) are the most common (Fig. 97.2). HB usually occurs in patients younger than 6 years and is associated with such risk factors as overgrowth syndromes (e.g., Beckwith-Wiedmann), prematurity, and familial adenomatosis poli. In contrast, HCC starts to become more common in patients older than 6 years, particularly in children older than 10 years. Risk factors include chronic liver injury from inborn errors of metabolism such as tyrosinemia, glycogen storage disease type I, chronic hepatitis, chronic iatrogenic androgen exposure, or cirrhosis for any reason. In general, these latter risk factors rarely lead to cancer in childhood.

Typical presenting symptoms include abdominal mass, abdominal pain, and very rarely acute abdomen from massive hepatomegaly or tumor rupture. Other primary liver masses include embryonal sarcoma (extremely rare), vascular lesions that are nonmalignant such as infantile hemangioendothelioma, and malformations such as hamartoma. Focal nodular hyperplasia can cause a mass on liver imaging but rarely has associated symptoms or hepatic enlargement. Metastatic disease usually is characterized by diffuse nontender enlargement of the liver or multiple small nodules rather than a single dominant mass. Neuroblastoma and advanced hematologic malignancies such as ALL, AML, lymphoblastic lymphoma, and Burkitt's commonly metastasize to the liver. Although tumors may block biliary drainage, hepatic synthetic function is rarely affected by malignancy in the liver.

Emergent management is rarely required except in the extremely rare setting of liver failure (see Chapter 89), tumor rupture that may require rapid repletion of intravascular volume and blood loss while consulting surgery, or severe coagulopathy (see Chapter 91). History may elicit a risk factor or systemic symptoms such as malaise and anorexia that are more common with HCC than HB. Pain does not help with the differential diagnosis but requires management. Jaundice is most common with HCC but can occur with all liver tumors.

Initial workup in the ED should include AST, ALT, bilirubin total and direct, CBC count with platelets, PT, PTT, and fibrinogen. Alpha fetoprotein (AFP) can be elevated in both HB and HCC. It is also important to note that normal AFP values are high in the first months of life, especially in premature infants. Initial diagnostic imaging in the ED should include an ultrasound, which can help identify if the palpable mass is likely to be hepatic in origin and if the liver contains one or multiple masses. If a CT scan is done in the ED, it is important to give intravenous contrast to look for intravascular extension of tumor from the hepatic veins, into the inferior vena cava, and possibly into the right atrium. Renal function should be checked before giving intravenous contrast. Since HB can metastasize to the lungs, consider if a chest CT scan should be performed at the same time in patients younger than 10 years who have a primary liver tumor.

Tumors of the Kidney

There are several different causes of renal tumors in children, some malignant and some benign. Wilm's tumor, the most common pediatric renal tumor, arises from embryonic renal blastemal cells. Overgrowth syndromes such as Beckwith-Wiedemann, Soto syndrome, hemihypertrophy, and Denys-Drash syndrome also predispose to embryonal tumors such as Wilm's. There are 500 cases of Wilm's diagnosed annually in United States with peak incidence between the ages of 2 and 3 years. Eighty percent of cases are diagnosed by age 5 years.

Wilm's tumors most commonly present with a painless mass found incidentally by either the parents or pediatrician in a child who is otherwise well-appearing (Fig. 97.2). Masses are deep in the flank, smooth, and either firm or soft. Wilm's tumor may have more serious or life-threatening presentations including

- hypertension, due to increased rennin secretion from renal artery compression, in <15% of cases;
- gross hematuria in less than 25% of cases (although microscopic hematuria is very common);
- hematologic complications such as anemia, tumor thrombus in the renal veins with or without extension into the inferior vena cava; and
- abdominal compartment syndrome from a massive renal tumor in a very small child.

The differential diagnosis of a pediatric renal mass also includes benign lesions such as hydronephrosis, multicystic or polycystic kidneys, and mesoblastic nephroma. The age of the patient can help clarify the likely etiology of a renal mass. For example, a neonatal mass is less likely to be malignant and more likely a congenital malformation of the genitourinary (GU) tract. Both neuroblastoma and Wilm's tumor most commonly develop in the 1 to 5 year age range. Other malignant tumors, less common than Wilm's, include rhabdoid tumor of the kidney, clear cell sarcoma, and mesoblastic nephroma. Carcinomas, including medullary carcinoma and renal cell carcinoma, are extremely rare. Hematologic malignances often metastasize to the kidney but rarely present with a solitary lesion.

A thorough history and physical examination is needed, including assessment of measured blood pressure against normal values for age. Because Wilm's tumor can be associated with other syndromes, such as Beckwith-Wiedemann syndrome and WAGR (Wilm's tumor, aniridia, GU anomalies, mental retardation) syndrome, the physical examination should screen for physical anomalies that may signal that the renal mass is part of a larger picture. The clinician should screen for signs and symptoms of pain and treat pain as needed. Laboratory evaluation should include a CBC to look for evidence of bleeding, a urinalysis, and liver and renal function testing (BUN and creatinine). Serum calcium should also be measured as this value may be elevated in rhabdoid tumor of the kidney or congenital mesoblastic nephroma.

Radiographic evaluation can be helpful in further defining the tumor. Ultrasound can define the anatomic position of the mass, explore whether it has cystic or solid components, and assess for any hydronephrosis or ureteral obstruction. The radiologist should assess for tumor thrombus in renal veins or inferior vena cava. Centers skilled in pediatric imaging may elect to perform a CT scan with intravenous con-

trast. If it is certain that the mass is renal in origin, it is appropriate to include the chest to evaluate for presence of lung metastasis.

As in adrenal tumors discussed above, the initial management of renal masses should focus on a determination of how ill the patient is and consultation with a pediatric oncologist or pediatric surgeon. Well-appearing patients without evidence of bleeding, may be discharged to home if appropriate follow-up with a pediatric oncologist or surgeon is arranged.

Tumors of the Lower Genitourinary Tract

While tumors of the lower GU tract in adults are most commonly carcinomas, in the pediatric population these tumors are more likely to be sarcomas. Their presentation is determined by their location. Vaginal tumors are most commonly rhabdomyosarcomas of the botryoid histology. These tumors classically present protruding from the vagina, accompanied by a mucous/bloody discharge. Uterine tumors more commonly present in adolescent girls and may cause a palpable mass or vaginal discharge. Tumors of the bladder may present with hematuria, urinary obstruction, or extrusion of tumor tissue from the urethra. Bladder tumors, most common in children younger than 4 years, are usually within the lumen of the bladder. Prostate tumors are usually rhabdomyosarcomas that can cause constipation, urinary obstruction, or a large pelvic mass. Paratesticular tumors present as painless unilateral scrotal enlargement or swelling (see section on "Gonadal Tumors" for details on testicular tumors).

The management of patients presenting with these tumors should begin with a thorough history and physical examination. Children are not usually acutely ill at the time of presentation. Most of the evaluation can be done on an outpatient basis, in consultation with a pediatric oncologist. The clinician in the ED should ensure adequate bowel, bladder, and renal function as well as good analgesia. An ultrasound may be useful to determine where the tumor is located. The most common reason for admission is management of urinary obstruction.

Gonadal Tumors

In children, most gonadal tumors are derived from malignant transformation of the primordial germ cells, although other tissues within the gonads may be the source of malignant cells. Presentation of these tumors varies based on the gender of the patient and the stage of development (i.e., the maturity) of the germ cell when the malignancy begins. During embryonic development, germ cells migrate to the gonads, but aberrant migration in the setting of malignancy can lead to extragonadal germ cell tumors. This section will focus on tumors located within the gonads themselves.

The gonads contain three different cell types, all of which can experience malignant transformation.

- Germ cells: Many histologic subtypes exist for ovarian and testicular germ cell tumors. Tumors range from benign teratomas (mature and immature) to a number of malignant histologies including germinoma (also called dysgerminoma), embryonal carcinoma, endodermal sinus tumor (also called yolk sac tumor), choriocarcinoma, and mixed germ cell tumors, which include two or more germ cell histologies. Dysgenesis of the gonad increases the risk of developing a germ cell tumor.

■ Sex cords: Cells can develop into ovarian granulosa cell tumors or testicular Sertoli or Leydig cell tumors.

■ Epithelia: These neoplasms are seen mostly in adults and are extremely uncommon in children.

Tumors of the ovary are rare and account for only 1% of pediatric cancers overall. While they may occur at any age, the incidence begins to increase at 8 to 9 years and peaks at 19 years of age. Two-thirds of pediatric ovarian tumors are germ cell tumors. Abdominal pain is the most common presenting symptoms, occurring in 80% of patients. Pain may be chronic or acute, mimicking an acute abdomen, as the tumor can cause ovarian torsion. Other presenting signs and symptoms include a palpable abdominal mass, dysfunction of the bowel or bladder, or menstrual changes. Some ovarian tumors may cause precocious puberty or virilization.

If a patient has a known or possible ovarian mass, the history and physical examination should include a thorough menstrual history as well as assessment of any virilization or precocious puberty. Laboratory evaluation should include a CBC count, chemistries, quantitative β-HCG (beta human chorionic gonadotropin) (obtained from the serum), AFP, LDH, and CA-125. Ultrasound can clarify whether the tumor is cystic or solid as well as location. Further imaging should generally be carried out only in conjunction with the managing oncologist or surgeon and rarely needs to be performed in the ED.

Differential diagnosis should include benign etiologies, such as an ovarian cyst or torsion, as well as malignant causes of the mass. Malignant masses are most commonly germ cell derived. Of these, the more common are dysgerminoma, which may be bilateral in 20% of cases, and endodermal sinus tumor (yolk sac tumor), which presents with an elevated AFP. Malignant tumors may also be derived from nongerm cell ovarian tissue or from nonovarian tissues, as is the case for ovarian involvement in leukemia or lymphoma.

Tumors of the testicle are rare and account for only 2% of solid neoplasms in boys. While they may occur at any age, testicular tumors seen in adolescents are similar to those found in adult males but prepubertal boys have tumors with unique clinical manifestations and different prognostic implications. The major risk factor for the development of a testicular tumor is the presence of an undescended testicle, even after repair. Approximately 75% of pediatric testicular tumors are germ cell tumors (as compared with more than 90% in the adult population).

Testicular tumors commonly present as irregular, nontender scrotal masses that do not transilluminate. They may have minimal to no associated symptoms, which may cause a delay in diagnosis. At the time of diagnosis, 20% of patients will also have an inguinal hernia and another 20% will have a hydrocele. About 75% of these tumors are localized at diagnosis, but sites of potential metastases include retroperitoneal lymph nodes and the chest.

Testicular tumors usually present with an enlarged testicle. The clinician in the ED should perform a thorough history and physical examination looking for evidence of virilization or precocious puberty as occurs with functional tumors. Laboratory evaluation should include a CBC count, chemistries, quantitative β-HCG (obtained from the serum) and AFP. Imaging of the mass should begin with an ultrasound that can clarify whether the tumor is cystic or solid and whether it is derived from the testicle itself or paratesticular tissues.

When evaluating scrotal enlargement, it is critical to distinguish testicular tumors from paratesticular tumors from other etiologies such as varicocele or scrotal edema. Almost all paratesticular tumors are rhabdomyosarcomas. Malignant tumors in the testis itself include germ cell tumors of all histologies, sex cord tumors, leukemia, lymphoma, and neuroblastoma. Teratomas, representing 10% of testicular tumors, develop mostly in children younger than 4 years. Embryonal carcinoma, the testicular tumor most commonly seen in adults, is rare in the pediatric population until late adolescence.

Tumors In and Around the Spinal Cord

Tumors can come into contact with the spinal cord through various mechanisms. Those derived from tissues in close proximity to the spinal cord can grow into and impinge upon the cord. Primary tumors from either adjacent bone (see "Tumors of Bone" section) or adjacent parameningeal soft tissues, as in neuroblastoma or soft tissue sarcomas (STS), or from the spinal cord itself (gliomas, ependymomas) can cause cord compression. The same tumors when present at another site can also metastasize to tissue in or around the spinal cord. Tumors in the fourth ventricle can have drop metastases that grow and compress the spinal cord. Neuroblastoma, in particular, is known for its ability to spread through spinal foramina and then expand within the spinal canal. In addition, leukemic blasts can infiltrate the paraspinal soft tissues to form a chloroma, which can enlarge to compress the spinal cord as well (see "Leukemia" section).

Evaluation of spinal cord compression, regardless of the tumor type causing the compression, begins with a thorough history during which the clinician should explore whether the patient has had pain or focal neurologic symptoms including weakness or paresis, which could indicate cord compression. More subtle complaints such as urinary retention, fecal incontinence, or constipation could indicate compression of the spinal cord. A thorough neurologic examination should follow and any asymmetry or focality detected on that examination should provoke neuroimaging with, in most cases, a spine MRI. Findings could include loss of reflexes, focal or asymmetric weakness, sensory deficits, or an upgoing Babinski reflex. Percussion tenderness of the posterior vertebral elements should be assessed. Management of cord compression should include analgesia, as patients are frequently in extreme pain. Glucocorticoids usually improve the pain within several hours, but most patients require opiate analgesics to tolerate the physical examination and necessary diagnostic studies. Management of the compression begins with steroids, most commonly dexamethasone at a starting dose of 0.25 to 0.5 mg per kg IV (maximum dose is usually 10 mg as an initial dose followed by doses of 4 mg every 6 hours thereafter). Multispecialty consultation with neurosurgery, radiation oncology, and pediatric oncology is optimal when choosing among surgical decompression, radiation therapy, and chemotherapy. Decisions must consider both

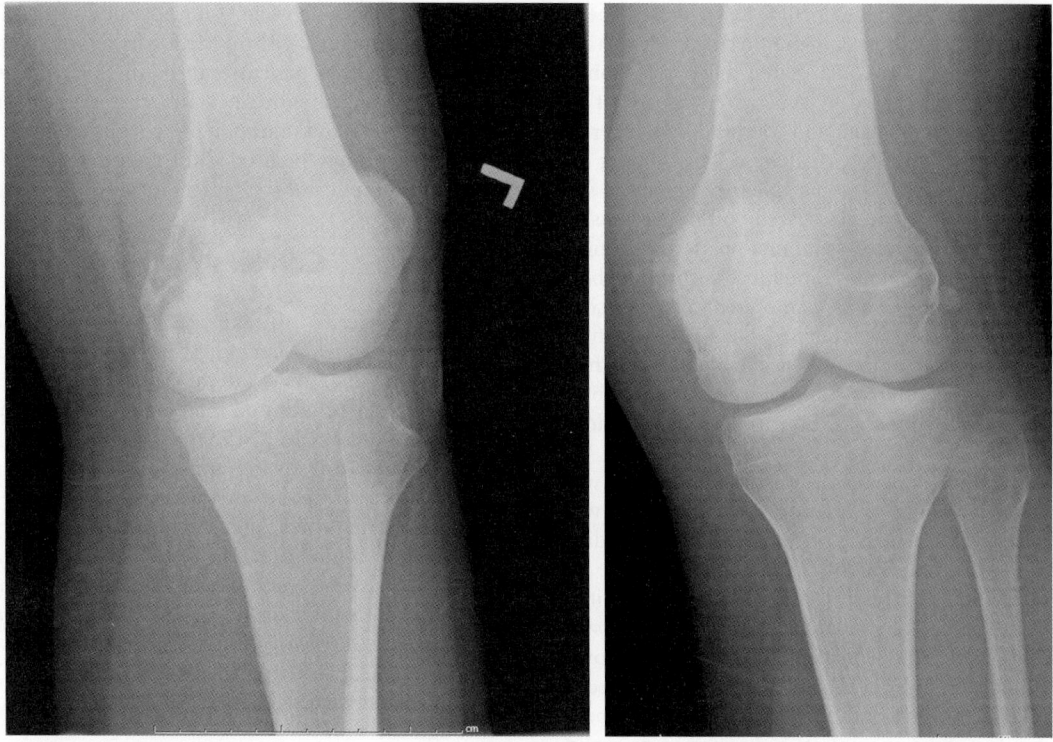

FIGURE 97.3 Two plain radiographs demonstrating osteosarcoma of the distal femur.

the short-term efficacy of the treatment to relieve the compression as well as the long-term consequences.

Tumors of Bone

Primary bone tumors are uncommon pediatric malignancies, representing the sixth most common neoplasm in children. However, bone tumors are the third most frequent malignancy of adolescent and young adults. In the United States, it is estimated that 2,400 primary bone tumors are diagnosed annually in children. Presentation commonly includes pain at the tumor site (present in 80% to 90% of cases), soft-tissue swelling, and/or a painful limp. The pain may wake the patient at night in some cases (less than 25%).

The differential diagnosis of a bony mass includes both benign and malignant entities. Subacute osteomyelitis can present with fever, elevated inflammatory markers, pain and swelling over the involved bone, as well as a bone scan with increased uptake of tracer. Benign tumors of bone account for half of the bone tumors in children and include entities such as giant cell tumor of bone, eosinophilic granuloma, and aneurysmal bone cysts. Benign lesions usually have smooth, well-defined borders on plain radiographs and rarely have associated soft tissue masses. Osteosarcoma and Ewing sarcoma are the most common primary malignant bone tumors. Osteosarcoma is characterized by its production of immature bone or osteoid. It is the most common malignant bone tumor in children and adolescents, presenting most often in the second and third decades of life. Although Ewing sarcoma is second to osteosarcoma in overall frequency, it affects children and

adolescents of all ages and is more common than osteosarcoma in children younger than 10 years. Leukemia, lymphoma, LCH, and metastases from neuroblastoma, sarcomas, and other childhood tumors can all cause bone pain and abnormalities on radiograph (Fig. 97.3).

Diagnostic evaluation in the ED should include a thorough history and physical examination. There is frequently a history of trauma. Pain in retrospect may be intermittent and nondescript for weeks or months. Constitutional symptoms or signs, such as fever, fatigue, and weight loss may occur with Ewing sarcoma/PNET. If tumor is present in an extremity, a hard mass may be felt. Osteosarcoma usually involves the metaphyseal end of long bones, most commonly around the knee or proximal humerus. Ewing can occur in any bone but tends to involve the diaphysis when in a long bone. Pelvic lesions often produce no specific physical findings. Lesions of the vertebral body may evoke neurologic symptoms such as neuropathic pain or cord compression. In this setting, a careful history of bowel and bladder function should be taken and a thorough neurologic examination performed. Any focal neurologic deficits should prompt immediate imaging of the spinal cord to determine if compression is present. Should the bony mass be in an extremity, that extremity should be completely examined in terms of pulses, perfusion, range of motion, and sensation for compartment syndrome due to swelling or bleeding within the mass.

Laboratory evaluation should include a CBC count, evaluation of renal and liver function, inflammatory markers such as ESR and CRP, and serum LDH. Diagnostic imaging should being with a plain radiograph of the affected region. Characteristic findings of primary bone tumors include a lytic lesion with cortical destruction. Early changes include loss of soft-tissue fat planes and periosteal elevation (Codman triangle), which has been associated with osteosarcoma. Later, there is an "onion skin" periosteal reaction caused by repetitive episodes of the lesion pushing out the periosteum and followed by the periosteum responding by laying down calcium. This finding has been associated with Ewing sarcoma. Neither finding is specific. With osteosarcoma, the associated soft tissue mass is sometimes ossified in a radial or "sunburst" pattern. "Benign" bone tumors such as eosinophilic granuloma, aneurysmal bone cysts, and giant cell tumor of bone can present as lytic lesions that tend to have smooth, well-defined borders. Plain films should always be assessed for the presence of a pathologic fracture. A large lesion with a thin cortex in a weight-bearing bone may require immediate immobilization to prevent pathologic fracture.

Often patients with bony masses can be discharged with follow-up securely arranged with an orthopedic surgeon with oncology expertise or a pediatric oncologist for further diagnostic workup and initiation of appropriate therapy. An improperly performed biopsy may prevent subsequent limb-sparing surgery. A plan for analgesia should be established prior to discharge. Patients with tumors affecting the lower extremities should refrain from bearing weight on the affected limb so as to avoid causing a pathologic fracture. Weight bearing activity should not resume unless so directed by an orthopedic surgeon. Inpatient management may also be needed for pain control or if cord compression or compartment syndrome complicates the presentation.

Tumors of the Soft Tissues

Tumors of the soft tissues present the clinician with a very broad differential diagnosis. Many of these lesions may be benign. Rhabdomyosarcoma is the most common soft-tissue sarcoma in children. There are many other types of STS that collectively account for less than 1% of all pediatric cancer. They can arise in any anatomic location because connective tissue is located throughout the body. Masses are frequently painless and asymptomatic. Any presenting symptoms are usually because of invasion of nerves locally leading to pain or weakness. Systemic symptoms are rare. The histologic variants of rhabdomyosarcoma tend to have characteristic presentations. Botryoid tumors tend to grow in potential spaces such as the bladder and vagina, present in young children and have a very good prognosis. Embryonal tumors often occur in GU tract, the orbit and head, the neck, and the parameningeal locations. Alveolar tumors often present in the extremities and have a worse prognosis. Rhabdomyosarcoma can metastasize to local lymph nodes, lungs, bone, and rarely bone marrow.

There are many benign causes of soft tissue masses in children but the emergency physician needs to consider cancer as a possible cause. Diagnostic evaluation in the ED should include a thorough history and physical examination. The history should focus on symptoms caused by the mass and other systemic or constitutional symptoms that may be present. When a reasonable suspicion for cancer exists, laboratory evaluation should include a CBC count, renal and liver function tests, and serum LDH. A plain radiograph of the affected area can be useful to look for bone destruction or fracture

from an underlying bone lesion. A true soft tissue mass, however, is best imaged with an MRI, which is often not performed in the ED. Often patients can be discharged with follow-up securely arranged with a pediatric oncologist for further diagnostic workup and initiation of appropriate therapy. Inpatient management may be needed for pain control or if cord compression complicates the presentation.

Cancers of the Skin

Primary cancers of the skin, such as squamous or basal cell carcinoma or melanoma, are seen in the adult practice setting but rarely occur in children. Melanoma accounts for less than 3% of all childhood malignancies but occurs occasionally in adolescents 15 to 19 years old. There may be increased risk in the setting of immunosuppression, immunodeficiencies, history of radiation therapy or stem cell transplant, giant congenital nevi, giant congenital melanocytic nevi, or xeroderma pigmentosum. Other pediatric cancers may involve the skin, such as leukemia, which may produce leukemia cutis (particularly in infant ALL or in AML). Rash may be part of the presentation of histiocytic disorders, such as HLH or LCH. Neuroblastoma does not affect the skin but may present with subcutaneous pigmented nodules visible through the skin.

Skin abnormalities can result from the presence of a cancer even if the cancer itself does not affect or involve the skin. Petechiae, purpura, or bruising can indicate malignant replacement of the bone marrow due to a primary cancer of the marrow (i.e., leukemia) or metastatic disease of the marrow. Pallor may indicate anemia either due to marrow replacement or bleeding into a mass. The skin may appear jaundiced if there is a mass obstructing biliary flow.

Management in the ED should begin with a thorough history and physical examination. The examination should be used to screen for other skin lesions, lymphadenopathy, hepatosplenomegaly, masses, other signs of malignancy that might be related to the skin findings. If the history and physical examination suggest a particular diagnosis, then further laboratory or radiographic evaluation may be helpful. If not, and if the patient appears to be stable without signs or symptoms of systemic illness, then the patient can be discharged to home with follow-up secured with either oncology or dermatology. When cancer is suspected, a biopsy will likely be needed to help make a diagnosis and involvement from a dermatopathologist with pediatric experience will be essential. Some melanocytic lesions in children may appear malignant to pathologists without sufficient experience with the pediatric population.

COMPLICATIONS OF CANCER TREATMENT

Introduction

This section focuses on the complications of cancer treatment that are likely to lead to an ED visit for care. Complications that tend to occur only in patients who are already hospitalized are not covered in this section. The review of management focuses on the initial care of the patient and does not address the more detailed evaluation and management needed subsequently. A detailed oncology history, as described in Table 97.1, is critical to all patients coming to the ED during or shortly after treatment.

Hematologic Complications of Cancer Treatment

Most but not all chemotherapy causes reversible myelosuppression. Neutrophils have a very short half-life and thus their numbers may drop rapidly but also may recover quickly. Platelets have a slightly longer half-life and thus tend to drop and recover slightly more slowly. Because red blood cell half-life is over 100 days, chemotherapy effects tend to be more chronic than acute. The nadir blood counts usually occur 7 to 10 days after start of treatment and recovery usually occurs 10 to 14 days after start of treatment. Many factors can influence the pattern of myelosuppression in terms of depth, duration, or specific cell line effect. The pattern of myelosuppression differs by chemotherapy regimen. For example, most solid tumor regimens allow for complete recovery within 10 to 14 days, while acute myelogenous leukemia regimens may delay recovery until 4 to 6 weeks after treatment. Even within a given regimen, there is variation both between patients and between cycles for one patient. In general, recovery is slower for patients who have already received many cycles of chemotherapy, whose course has been complicated by infection, or whose bone marrow has been extensively replaced by tumor. Radiation to the marrow cavity, especially including the spine or pelvis, can also cause myelosuppression during treatment and/or delayed recovery after treatment.

Significant neutropenia is usually defined as an ANC below 500 cells per μL. The ANC is calculated by multiplying the percentage of WBCs that are neutrophils or bands by the total WBC count. The absolute phagocyte count (APC) includes monocytes as well as neutrophils and bands. It is less widely used than the ANC as a measure of neutropenia. Patients with an ANC below 500 have an increased risk of bacterial infections related to insufficient numbers of phagocytic cells to fight bacteria. The risk increases dramatically when the ANC is below 100. Patients may develop infections with bacteria that are not pathogens in normal hosts. There is also a risk of fungal infections. The incidence of fungal infections increases with prolonged (more than 21 days) and severe (ANC below 500) neutropenia. The infectious risks of neutropenia are increased by a number of contributing factors. Indwelling foreign bodies such as central lines, ventriperitoneal shunts, and bone allografts provide a foreign surface that increases the likelihood of infection and the difficulty of treatment. The mucosal injury that typically accompanies myelosuppression increases the risk of bacteria entering the circulation. Immunosuppression decreases phagocytic function as well.

Neutrophil and/or monocytic specific growth factors can decrease the duration but not the depth of neutropenia. The short-acting growth factors are filgrastim (G-CSF, Neulasta®) and sargramostim (GM-CSF, Leukine®). These drugs are usually given daily by subcutaneous injection starting 1 day after the end of chemotherapy and continued until adequate ANC recovery after the expected nadir. There may be a temporary rise in the WBC and ANC prior to the expected nadir, then a fall, and subsequent recovery. PEG-filgrastim (Neulasta®), a long-acting form of filgrastim that is given 24 to 72 hours after chemotherapy is complete, has a usual duration of action of 10 to 14 days. Its usage is usually limited to near adult-sized patients on solid tumor regimens with expected ANC recovery by 14 days.

There is no specific management of neutropenia itself but careful attention must be paid to the associated infectious risks (see "Infectious Complications of Cancer Treatment" section). Neutropenic patients should be isolated from the potential infectious exposures that can occur in an ED by rapid triage and placement in a private room. In addition, the assessment should avoid increasing the risk of bacteremia by routine procedures such as a rectal examination or urinary catheterization. When neutropenia is present in the setting of sepsis, the literature does not support starting or increasing the dose of growth factor although this is the practice at some institutions. There is also an inconclusive literature about the use of WBC transfusions in neutropenic patients with bacteremia, if the neutrophil recovery is expected within the next 7 to 10 days.

Thrombocytopenia is defined as a platelet count of less than 150,000 per μL, but the risk of bleeding at a given platelet count may vary (Table 97.7). There are no commercially available growth factors to prevent chemotherapy-induced thrombocytopenia. The urgency of the need for platelet transfusion varies with the circumstance. In the ED, it may be more expedient to give platelets during a procedure rather than transfusing in advance and rechecking a platelet count prior to the procedure. Institutional guidelines should prevail regarding AB matching, use of anti-D products in males, and prophylactic transfusion criteria. In a patient with active life-threatening bleeding, transfusion should not be delayed to await apheresis platelets. If there is severe bleeding in a patient who is refractory to platelet transfusions, the blood bank should be consulted to arrange a continuous infusion of platelets.

Anemia is very common in oncology patients and tends to be a chronic problem due to underproduction. The need for transfusion in the ED varies with the severity of the anemia and clinical circumstances (Table 97.7). Additional information on transfusions in the actively bleeding patient and administration guidelines can be found in Chapter 91.

Most chemotherapy causes immunosuppression that affects WBC function, independent of WBC count. The immunosuppression persists throughout treatment, and for 6 to 12 months after completion of chemotherapy. The severity of immunosuppression varies by chemotherapy regimen. The impact of immunosuppression may be more profound in the patient younger than 1 year because of the immaturity of the immune system. Stem cell transplant recipients have very severe immunosuppression (see "Complications of Hematopoietic Stem Cell Transplant" section).

One of the infectious risks attributable to the immunosuppression of chemotherapy is *Pneumocystis jiroveci* (formerly known as *Pneumocystis carinii*) pneumonia. Patients younger than 1 year and those receiving treatment for leukemia or high-stage lymphoma are at increased risk. Most, if not all, pediatric oncology patients are thus treated with prophylactic trimethoprim-sulfamethoxazole to prevent infection. Those who do not tolerate trimethoprim-sulfamethoxazole are on second-line agents such as atovaquone, dapsone, aerosolized pentamidine, or intravenous pentamidine.

Prophylaxis for other infections is more variable in usage. Fungal prophylaxis is increasingly common with specific regimens that are associated with a high frequency of fungal disease. For example, many patients with acute myelogenous leukemia take prophylactic voriconazole throughout their treatment. Respiratory syncytial virus (RSV) prophylaxis with RSV immunoglobulin Palvizumab® may be used in children younger than 1 year on highly immunosuppressive regimens.

Bleeding complications are common in oncology patients. Aside from thrombocytopenia, bleeding may occur because of coagulopathy resulting from a number of different factors. Leukemia itself may cause coaguloapathy. Asparaginase, a chemotherapy drug, impairs protein synthesis and leads to abnormal coagulation parameters on testing that cause both a bleeding and a clotting diathesis. Many patients are also on anticoagulation therapy for previous clotting problems. Any bleeding risk from the anticoagulation may be exacerbated by intercurrent thrombocytopenia. Bleeding in and around solid tumors tends to be more common at diagnosis and with relapse. Bleeding can also occur after biopsy or tumor resection. Mucosal injury from treatment can contribute to bleeding throughout the GI tract.

The management of bleeding is outlined in Chapter 91. The oncology-specific history is critical to identify contributing factors. The platelet count should always be checked immediately and transfusion given as indicated (Table 97.7). Reversal of any anticoagulation (see Chapter 91) should be considered in a patient with significant bleeding.

Cancer patients have an increased risk of clotting due to a number of factors such as compression of vessels by tumor, disturbance of flow from central lines, asparaginase-induced deficiency of endogenous anticoagulants such as protein C and protein S, decreased physical activity, and immobilization due to surgery. Catheter-related clots may present with line dysfunction, obvious or subtle signs of edema in the head or one upper extremity, or collateral vessels visible on the upper chest.

Other thrombotic complications may include pulmonary emboli (PE), deep venous thromboses (DVT), or central venous sinus thrombosis, a rare complication in patients on asparaginase chemotherapy. The presentation of central venous sinus thrombosis usually consists of vague and/or nonspecific symptoms including seizure, headache, nausea, and vomiting. Physical examination may or may not have focal neurologic findings, altered mental status, or papilledema. If a clot is suspected, the CBC count, PT, PTT, and fibrogen should be checked. CT scans may not be sensitive enough to diagnose a central venous sinus thrombosis, but MRI is generally reliable. Once the diagnosis is established, management consists of supportive care and initiation of anticoagulation. Of note, for patients on asparaginase receiving anticoagulation for a thrombus, the antithrombin level must be monitored regularly. Since asparaginase usually depletes antithrombin, a protein required for the proper function of heparin (unfractionated or fractionated), a level above 50% must be maintained. Should levels fall below 50%, antithrombin III should be repleted. To calculate the replacement dose, the following formula can be used:

$$\text{Dose (IU)} = \{[\text{Desired Level} - \text{Patient's Level}] \times [\text{Weight (kg)}]\}/1.4$$

Infectious Complications of Cancer Treatment

Infection is an extremely common problem in oncology patients due to the neutropenia and immunosuppression associated with treatment. Identification of infection can be challenging because typical symptoms may be absent or decreased. Nonetheless, prompt initiation of appropriate management is critical to optimal outcome.

Fever in a neutropenic patient is a true emergency, even in a well appearing patient (Fig. 97.4). The depth and duration of neutropenia helps to predict the risk of serious infections. All patients with an ANC below 500 or with a rapidly falling ANC that will shortly be below 500 should be considered at risk. Although fever itself can be a manifestation of some cancers, this is a diagnosis of exclusion, particularly in a patient with neutropenia. While fever should certainly raise concern for infection, the absence of fever should not overly reassure the clinician. Fever may be absent or minimized in patients on high-dose steroids and/or patients with hypothalamic dysfunction from tumor. In addition, localizing signs of infection may be blunted because the lack of neutrophils prevents many of the usual manifestations such as pus, significant local erythema, or edema.

Certain elements of the history can be very helpful. Patients or family members may know if the patient is already neutropenic. Specific questions to elicit any focal pain can direct the physical examination and empiric treatment decisions since this may be the only evidence of a localizing infection. The presence of any indwelling devices such as a central line, ventriculoperitoneal shunt, or metal hardware used for bone tumors can also help with the differential diagnosis and/or empiric antibiotic coverage. Since antibiotic allergies may be common in this population, a thorough allergy history is critical to avoid prescribing inappropriately.

The physical examination of the patient must be detailed and meticulous with careful attention paid to all mucocutaneous surfaces to elicit any focal tenderness, erythema, or edema, which may be slight. Sites to examine include any central venous access devices including both the skin entrance site and/or subcutaneous reservoir, as well as along the subcutaneous line tract, nails beds on both fingers and toes, and a thorough external rectal examination with circumferential palpation. Do not perform an internal rectal examination as it may increase the risk of bacteremia.

Diagnostic testing should include a stat CBC count with differential and blood culture from all line lumens or via venipuncture in patients without a line. Institution-specific guidelines should be followed regarding the need for peripheral blood cultures in addition to line cultures and if additional orders or specimens are needed for anaerobic cultures. Additional diagnostic testing can be obtained as needed after empiric antibiotics are started. A chest radiograph should only be obtained in patients with respiratory symptoms. A urine analysis is not valuable for screening for infection since there are too few WBCs for the leukocyte esterase to be of value. A urine culture should be obtained as long as it does not delay start of antibiotics or require catheterization, which may also increase the risk of bacteremia. If the patient has a history of urinary tract infections, the risk of urinary catheterization may

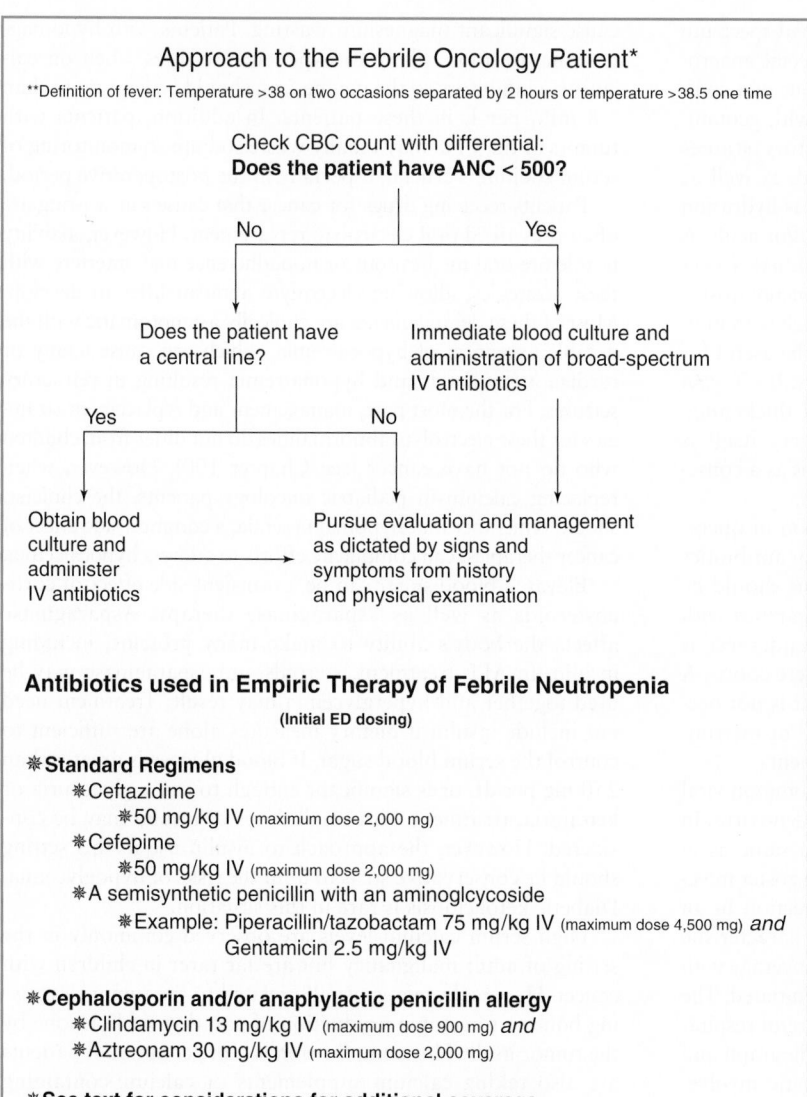

Approach to the Febrile Oncology Patient*

**Definition of fever: Temperature >38 on two occasions separated by 2 hours or temperature >38.5 one time

Check CBC count with differential:
Does the patient have ANC < 500?

No — Yes

Does the patient have a central line?

Immediate blood culture and administration of broad-spectrum IV antibiotics

Yes — No

Obtain blood culture and administer IV antibiotics

Pursue evaluation and management as dictated by signs and symptoms from history and physical examination

Antibiotics used in Empiric Therapy of Febrile Neutropenia

(Initial ED dosing)

❋**Standard Regimens**
  ❋Ceftazidime
    ❋50 mg/kg IV (maximum dose 2,000 mg)
  ❋Cefepime
    ❋50 mg/kg IV (maximum dose 2,000 mg)
  ❋A semisynthetic penicillin with an aminoglcyoside
    ❋Example: Piperacillin/tazobactam 75 mg/kg IV (maximum dose 4,500 mg) *and* Gentamicin 2.5 mg/kg IV

❋**Cephalosporin and/or anaphylactic penicillin allergy**
  ❋Clindamycin 13 mg/kg IV (maximum dose 900 mg) *and*
  ❋Aztreonam 30 mg/kg IV (maximum dose 2,000 mg)

❋**See text for considerations for additional coverage**

FIGURE 97.4 Management guidelines for the febrile oncology patient. Risk assessment and management hinges substantially on whether the absolute neutrophil count (ANC) is below 500, whether the patient has localizing signs or symptoms, and whether an indwelling catheter is present.

be justified. Throat cultures may be of value if there are focal findings involving only the pharynx and/or tonsils but are rarely informative in a patient with diffuse mucositis. Specific imaging may be of value based on physical findings.

Treatment should be initiated within 1 hour of patient arrival with the institutional standard regimen. Regimens need to cover both gram-positive and gram-negative organisms, including opportunistic pathogens (Fig. 97.4). Specific coverage, in addition to empiric therapy, is indicated for several clinical settings. Third-generation cephalosporins may have inadequate gram-positive coverage for patients with a soft-tissue site infections and consideration should be given to a semisynthetic penicillin and an aminoglycoside or the addition of vancomycin, given the rising incidence of MRSA. With signs or symptoms of sepsis, double coverage for gram-negative organisms should be added in addition to vancomcyin to cover for possible Streptococcus viridans, especially in patients with advanced hematologic malignancies. Fungal coverage is often added for patients in shock. All pediatric patients with fever and neutropenia less than 500 to 1,000 per mm³ should be admitted to

the hospital unless there is an institutional management guideline that includes a specific follow-up plan for outpatient management of low-risk fever and neutropenia. In the case of sepsis or septic shock, acute management as described in Chapter 92 should be followed for oncology patients, with the empiric antibiotic coverage described above for neutropenia. Stress-dose steroids should be considered in patients who have received prolonged steroids recently either as part of cancer treatment or management of nausea and vomiting.

Typhlitis, also known as neutropenic colitis, is a potentially life-threatening infection that occurs in patients with neutropenia and GI mucosal injury. This infection occurs in the watershed regions of the cecum, appendix, and terminal ileum. It is much more common in patients with advanced hematologic malignancies but can occur in patients with solid tumors. Initial symptoms can mimic appendicitis with periumbilical pain preceding right lower quadrant pain. As the infection progresses, abdominal pain can become severe and examination findings include distension and persistent right lower quadrant tenderness. Empiric antibiotics should be started as soon as the diagnosis is

MEDICAL EMERGENCIES

suspected. Antibiotic coverage should include broad-spectrum coverage of gram-negative enteric flora as well as specific anaerobic coverage. Typical regimens are a carbapenem alone or a combination regimen such as piperacillin/tazobactam with gentamicin or ceftazidime with metronidazole. Laboratory studies should include coagulation studies and lactic acid, as well as CBC with differential and basic chemistries to assess hydration and renal function. Uncontrolled coagulopathy and/or acidosis are consistent with necrotic bowel. Serial abdominal x-rays should be performed to look for intramural air (pneumatosis), which is a hallmark of this diagnosis, or free air, which is an indication for surgery. A CT scan of the abdomen can be useful for better delineation of the degree of bowel wall injury. If CT scan is unavailable, ultrasound can show bowel wall thickening. Early surgical consultation is appropriate. Surgery itself is reserved for uncontrollable coagulopathy or acidosis as a consequence of bowel necrosis or evidence of perforation.

Clostridium difficile colitis is relatively common in oncology patients due to treatment with broad-spectrum antibiotics that eradicates normal bowel flora. This diagnosis should be considered in patients with abdominal pain and diarrhea with or without abdominal distension. Abdominal tenderness is generally minimal except in patients with very severe colitis. A CT scan can confirm involvement of the colon but is not necessary for most patients. Either vancomycin (oral) or metronidazole (parenteral or oral) can be used for treatment.

Pediatric oncology patients are also at risk for common viral infections such as RSV, CMV, EBV, influenza, and adenovirus. In general, the presentation of these infections is the same as in immunocompetent hosts. Of note, primary varicella zoster infection can rapidly progress to a life-threatening infection in an immunocompromised patient. Thus as soon as characteristic vesicles on an erythematous base are seen, empiric coverage with acyclovir 10 mg per kg IV every 8 hours should be initiated. The patient should be assessed for pneumonitis with careful respiratory examination, oxygen saturation, and chest radiograph and liver enzymes should be checked for possible hepatic involvement (see "Skin Complications of Cancer Treatment" section).

Metabolic Complications of Cancer Treatment

Complications affecting metabolic balance and the endocrinologic system are common in children with cancer. These may be because of the neoplastic disease itself, as has been addressed in the sections on newly diagnosed cancer, or to complications due cancer therapy. TLS is probably the most noteworthy example of metabolic derangement in the setting of cancer (see "Leukemia" section). TLS can be present at the time of diagnosis or may be subsequently induced as chemotherapy is initiated and tumor cells begin to die in response.

Renal tubular dysfunction is common in oncology patients. Patients may waste electrolytes such as potassium, calcium, magnesium, and phosphorus through their kidneys as a result of specific treatment exposures or prior renal injury. Ifosfamide, cisplatin, and carboplatin all are likely to cause salt wasting. Antifungal agents such as amphotericin and ambisome cause potassium wasting, which may have clinical significance. Calcineurin inhibitors, such as tacrolimus or cyclosporine, which may be used after stem cell transplantation, can cause significant magnesium wasting. Patients with hypomagnesemia are more likely to experience seizures when on calcineurin inhibitors so the magnesium should be kept more than 1.8 mEq per L in these patients. In addition, patients with tumors of the CNS may renally waste sodium so monitoring of serum sodium is crucial, especially in the postoperative period.

Patients receiving drugs for cancer that cause salt wasting are often prescribed oral electrolyte replacement. However, inability to tolerate oral medications or nonadherence may interfere with these strategies, allowing electrolyte abnormalities to develop. Most of these derangements are clinically asymptomatic with the notable exception of hypocalcemia, which can cause tetany or cardiac arrhythmias and hyponatremia resulting in refractory seizures. For the most part, management and replacement strategies for these electrolyte abnormalities do not differ from children who do not have cancer (see Chapter 100). However, when replacing calcium in pediatric oncology patients, the clinician should remember that hypomagnesemia, a common side effect of cancer therapies, can complicate efforts to address hypocalcemia.

Elevated blood sugar can be a transient side effect of corticosteroids as well as asparaginase therapy. Asparaginase affects the body's ability to make many proteins, including insulin. In ALL treatment, steroids and asparaginase may be used together and hyperglycemia may result. Treatment need not include insulin if dietary measures alone are sufficient to control the serum blood sugar. If blood glucose is greater than 250 mg per dL or is significant enough to cause glycosuria or ketonuria, treatment with small doses of insulin may be considered. However, the approach to insulin use in this setting should be conservative so as to limit the risks of hypoglycemia. Diabetic ketoacidosis is rare in this situation.

High serum calcium levels are observed commonly in the setting of adult malignancy but are far rarer in children with cancer. Hypercalcemia is usually related to the tumor destroying bone or to ectopic production of parathyroid hormone by the tumor itself. This complication is more common if patients are also taking calcium supplements or calcium-containing medications such as antacids. If asymptomatic, hypercalcemia does not always require intervention. When present, symptoms may include nausea/vomiting, constipation, altered mental status, and renal failure. Management in these cases is similar to strategies to address hypercalcemia outside of the oncology setting (see Chapter 91). However, steroids should be avoided in patients with known or suspected leukemia or lymphoma. In addition, control of the underlying malignancy is the best way to address the hypercalcemia.

Although the SIADH can develop as a result of some cancers themselves, particularly those involving the lungs or CNS, treatment with vincristine and cyclophosphamide can be associated with SIADH. Management of this complication, which hinges on fluid restriction, does not differ from that of SIADH developing in other settings (see Chapter 91).

Pain

Unfortunately, pain is a common symptom in oncology patients with data showing that more than 30% of pediatric cancer patients have experienced pain in the last week. When pain leads to visits to the ED, it requires careful and immediate management. Severe pain is a true emergency, in and of itself, and also may be particularly upsetting for cancer patients who may have already confronted significant pain as part of their cancer diagnosis, who may anticipate or fear future pain, and who may worry (usually needlessly) that their pain is a sign of progressive cancer.

In some cases, pain may be related to the tumor itself and therefore often will respond to chemotherapy or other cancer-directed therapies. Tumors can cause neuropathic pain when they directly invade local nerves or when they cause local edema that affects the nerves in the vicinity. Tumor infiltrating an organ may cause ill-defined pain as the organ capsule becomes stretched. Bone pain may signify a pathologic fracture from a tumor weakening the bone, as can occur with Ewing sarcoma or osteosarcoma. The bones may also hurt due to tumor invading the bone marrow space. Pain in the head and neck may result from increased ICP or tumor involvement of the meninges/cerebrospinal fluid (most common in hematologic malignancies).

On the other hand, pain may be related to cancer treatment. In these cases, the patient or family may report that this particular pain has been historically linked to a specific therapy. Patients may complain of pain secondary to surgical procedures they have experienced. Such cases are very common and are not substantially different from postoperative pain in children without cancer. A particularly challenging example of this is the phantom pain that can occur after limb amputation. In addition, oncology patients may experience pain of the mouth, GI tract, or even urethra as part of mucositis. Pain could also represent a focal infection, complicating the patient's compromised immune system. Bony pain may reflect recent therapy with hematopoietic growth factors to stimulate neutrophil recovery after chemotherapy. Radiation therapy can induce local tissue injury, which may be very painful.

Abdominal pain is a common complaint in cancer patients and can arise from several sources. The differential diagnosis may be very wide including pancreatitis, hepatitis, cholecystitis, constipation, mucosal injury, intraabdominal infection, and bowel obstruction (see "Hepatic and Gastrointestinal Complications of Cancer Treatment" section).

An important first step in management is to explicitly address pain when taking the patient's history. Even patients who come to the ED for other reasons may have pain complicating their presentation. Pain should be assessed with an age-appropriate scale.

Upon determining that a patient is in pain, according to the patient's report as opposed to the clinician's assessment, the emergency physician must initiate immediate pain treatment. The remainder of the history and physical examination should be used to identify the cause of the pain and to explore specific treatment for that cause.

Acetaminophen is a useful analgesic with minimal side effects for most patients, remembering to avoid the rectal route if the patient is neutropenic. NSAIDs and aspirin may be effective as pain relievers but are generally avoided in this patient population due to their antiplatelet effect in the setting of frequent thrombocytopenia. Opioids represent the mainstay of pain treatment for the pediatric oncology patient. General principles of dosing include the following:

- A dose that is commonly used as a standard starting dose may be insufficient to provide adequate pain relief if the patient is not opioid-naïve.

- Far more important than the actual dose is the dose to *effect*. Patients may need repeated doses in order to get control of their pain and repeated doses should not be limited when analgesia has not yet been attained.
- A patient-controlled analgesia (PCA) pump is frequently needed for several types of pain, particularly mucositis where oral intake can be limited. Such pumps may be initiated in the ED using morphine, fentanyl or hydromorphone, institutional standard permitting. Small children and infants may benefit from nursing-controlled analgesia (NCA), should they not be old enough to handle a PCA. Parents should not control analgesic pumps except in the setting of end-of-life care, per institutional policy.
- Long-acting opioids, such as MS Contin®, Oxycontin®, and methadone, may be appropriate in the setting of chronic pain. These medications should not be used in the setting of acute pain and are rarely initiated in the ED unless in consultation with a pain expert.

Careful consideration must be given to decisions about whether patients in pain may be discharged to home. If oral medications seem to be relieving the pain, then it is generally acceptable to discharge the patient after ensuring that he/she has an adequate supply of the analgesics for use at home. If the pain is inadequately controlled on oral medications and parenteral administration is required, then the patient will need to be admitted.

Neurologic Complications of Cancer Treatment

Neurologic complications in children with cancer are extremely common and may relate to disease, cancer treatment, or supportive care medications. Drug-related side effects are extremely frequent. Many of the common problems are fully reversible but a few can lead to permanent neurologic injury. The cancer-specific history is critical to identify the likely causes of neurologic problems. The diagnosis and management of neurologic problems in children is covered in Chapter 96. This section focuses on the unique considerations in the pediatric cancer patient.

Both motor and sensory peripheral neuropathies are common in children with cancer. Vincristine and vinblastine, two chemotherapy agents used to treat many kinds of childhood cancer, both cause reversible neuropathy affecting motor, sensory, and autonomic nerves. Thalidomide can also cause peripheral neuropathy, which may or may not be fully reversible.

Initial management tends to focus on establishing the diagnosis by the cancer-directed history and physical examination. Pain responds best to agents with efficacy against neuropathic pain such as gabapentin. Such drugs rarely have immediate effect and thus narcotics may be needed in the short run.

There is a wide differential to consider when evaluating a pediatric cancer patient with new onset cranial nerve palsy. Symmetric involvement may reflect vincristine-induced neuropathy, particularly when it involves ptosis. Increased ICP from shunt malfunction or tumor progression should also be considered. Asymmetric involvement can occur with fatigue or vincristine-induced exacerbation of baseline weakness. Vincristine can also cause asymmetric ptosis in some patients, but this tends to be a diagnosis of exclusion. Increased ICP should be suspected in a child with a sixth nerve palsy. Carcinomatous meningitis should be considered in patients with a history of tumors likely to involve the cerebrospinal fluid or meninges, such as leukemia, lymphoma, parameningeal sarcomas, and meningeal seeding brain tumors, such as medulloblastoma. Patients treated with a scopolamine patch for nausea may develop pupillary asymmetry as scopolamine transferred by fingertip from the patch to the eye can elicit unilateral mydriasis.

Management in the ED requires an appropriate oncology-directed history and physical examination to establish the potential differential. Unless drug effect can be established as the most likely cause, a head CT scan to rule out increased ICP may be required. The CT scan findings may also direct the specific ED and post-ED management. Admission for observation may be required for some patients where the diagnosis or trajectory is uncertain.

The most common cause of proximal muscle weakness in pediatric cancer patients is prolonged steroid exposure as part of cancer treatment or management of side effects. Diagnosis can usually be established by the appropriate history and physical examination. Patients with very severe symptoms whose families cannot manage care at home may require admission for respite care or initiation of rehabilitation.

Altered mental status in pediatric cancer patients has an extremely broad differential (Table 97.8). Cerebrovascular accident (CVA) as a cause of altered mental status should be considered in patients with risk factors such as thrombocytopenia, DIC, asparaginase-induced coagulopathy. Cytarabine can cause cerebellar dysfunction that in severe forms can progress to coma. This usually only occurs with doses of at least 1 g per m^2 given over several hours or less. Onset usually occurs within hours of treatment and thus would be more likely to be identified in an inpatient rather than during an ED visit after discharge. Ifosfamide can cause an acute neurologic syndrome including confusion, inappropriate laughter, somnolence, or psychosis. Onset is usually within hours of treatment but can occur several days later. Thalidomide can also cause somnolence, especially at times of dose escalation. Somnolence can be a side effect of many supportive-care medications such as narcotics, gabapentin, antihistamines, some antiepileptics, and antidepressants. Cranial radiation causes somnolence syndrome 6 to 12 weeks after treatment that may last several weeks in duration. Typical manifestations are extreme amounts of sleep (up to 20 hours per day) with normal mental status and function when awake.

An oncology-directed history, with particular attention to a detailed medication history, is critical to narrowing the differential diagnosis. Physical examination should look for other findings such as papilledema or focal neurologic findings that may also narrow the differential diagnosis. Laboratory evaluation should be carried out as recommended in Chapter 96. If a drug-related cause is suspected, specific drug levels when available may be helpful. If a lumbar puncture is planned to look for malignant cells or an infectious etiology, the risk of herniation and the resultant need for imaging should be assessed. Imaging studies may also be appropriate if an intracranial lesion is suspected or when the diagnosis is unclear. A CT scan without contrast can be useful to identify midline shift, increased ventricular size, or a hemorrhaghic stroke. A CT scan with contrast can identify likely carcinomatous meningitis or a supratentorial mass lesion. MRI can identify mass lesions anywhere in the CNS, including below the tentorium; ischemic stroke; hypertensive encapalopathy; or encephalitis.

TABLE 97.8

ETIOLOGY OF ACUTE ALTERATION IN MENTAL STATUS IN CHILDREN WITH CANCER

Tumor
  Primary CNS tumor
  Metastatic tumor
  Leukemic or carcinomatous meningitis
  Hyperleukocytosis
Infection
  Meningitis—bacterial, fungal
  Viral encephalitis
  Brain abscess
  Septic shock
Cerebrovascular accident
Seizure/postictal state
Increased intracranial pressure
  Shunt malfunction
  All transretinoic acid (Tretinoin)
Treatment
  Cytotoxic chemotherapy
    Methotrexate
    Cytosine arabinoside
    Ifosfamide
    Thalidomide
  Supportive care
    Narcotics
    Benzodiazepines
    Gabapentin
    Anticonvulsants
    Tricyclic antidepressants
    Antihistamines
    Dronabinol
Leukoencephalopathy
Metabolic derangements
  Hyponatremia/SIADH
  Hypo/hyperglycemia
  Hypomagnesemia
  Uremia
Postradiation therapy somnolence syndrome
Hypo/hypertension
Hypoxia
Liver failure
Depression

SIADH, syndrome of inappropriate antidiuretic hormone.

Management of drug-related altered mental status usually involves withholding the offending agent and supporting the patient until resolution. If narcotic-related, avoid rapid reversal with standard doses of naloxone, which could cause excrutiating pain that will be unresponsive to further narcotics for 2 to 3 hours. Supportive care such as stimulation should be tried prior to reversal. If reversal is required, the appropriate dose of naloxone (0.1 mg per kg) should be diluted in 10 mL of normal saline and then administered in 1 mL aliquots while titrating to effect. Alternatively, dosing can be initiated at 1 mcg/kg for mild respiratory depression and 10 mcg/kg for reversal of moderate to severe respiratory depression as needed. Laboratory evaluation of hepatic and renal function may identify contributing factors to increased drug effect. If ifosfamide neurotoxicity is suspected, many recommend methylene blue treatment using dosages that have been extrapolated from other settings. The usual dose for adolescents and adults is 50 mg administered orally or by slow IV push. There is no clear dosage for younger children but there are case reports using 1 to 2 mg per kg as in the treatment for methemoglobinemia. For management of hypertensive encephalopathy, see Chapter 34.

Patients with improvement of symptoms in the ED for whom a likely cause of altered mental status has been established may be discharged to home. Most others will require admission for further evaluation and/or observation.

The presentation and management of increased ICP is not unique to pediatric cancer patients (see Chapter 96). The differential diagnosis includes tumor (see the "Tumors of the Central Nervous System" section) or shunt malfunction more often than treatment effect. Tretinoin (all transretinoic acid), an agent uniquely used in the treatment of APML causes increased ICP. Children are particularly sensitive to this side effect. For patients with severe symptoms attributable to tretinoin, a diagnostic and therapeutic lumbar puncture may be needed. Opening pressure should be measured and cerebrospinal fluid should be withdrawn to reduce the pressure (see Chapter 96).

Children with cancer are at increased risk of seizures from the causes summarized below. Severe metabolic disturbances can result from SIADH (a side effect of vincristine and high-dose cyclophosphamide) or from renal tubular wasting of electrolytes (see "Metabolic Complications of Cancer Treatment" section). Seizures can also be caused by primary brain tumors, particularly supratentorial, CNS metastasis of refractory solid tumors, or carcinomatous meningitis. Some chemotherapy agents such as intrathecal administration or high-dose systemic administration of methotrexate or cytarabine can cause seizures. New onset seizures can be a sign of a bacterial abscess (more likely with *Bacillus cereus* bacteremia), fungal abscess, or a viral encephalitis such as those caused by herpes simplex virus or CMV. The approach to seizure management is not unique in patients with cancer and is addressed in Chapter 96. Specific consideration should be given to assess and correct problems with metabolic abnormalities.

Children with cancer are at increased risk of CVAs. Specific causes in children with cancer include sagittal sinus thrombosis (a potential complication of asparaginase chemotherapy) and intracranial bleeding with contributing factors of hypertension, coagulopathy, thrombocytopenia, intracranial tumor, prior surgery, and radiation. Spontaneous intracranial hemorrhage is extremely rare except when the platelet count is less than 5,000 per μL (see "Hematologic Complications of Cancer Treatment" section). The approach to diagnosis and management is addressed is Chapter 96. Specific consideration should be given to assess and correct problems with coagulopathy and/or thrombocytopenia.

Side effects of some supportive-care medications can include extrapyramidal reactions. Symptoms of such reactions can range from oculogyric crisis with mild repetitive eye deviation and/or neck motion to severe torticollis and eye deviations. Reactions can also include tardive dyskinesia ("frozen") and akathisia (restless/agitation). The key to diagnosis involves not only a thorough physical examination but also a thorough medication history. Dopamine-receptor antagonists used as antiemetics are the most common trigger in cancer patients. Such drugs include high-dose metoclopramide; phenothiazines such as compazine, chlorpromazine (thorazine), and thiethylperazine (torecan); and butyrophenones such as droperidol and haldol. Since more effective antiemetics, such as serotonin-receptor antagonists, have become available, the use of these drugs has decreased along with the incidence of this side

effect. If an extrapyramidal reaction is suspected, management should include diphenhydramine 1 mg per kg IV (maximum dose 50 mg). If symptoms are refractory to diphenhydramine, benztropine (Cogentin®) should be given at a dosage of 0.02 mg per kg (maximum 1 mg) IV. If symptoms do not remit or diagnosis remains unclear, patients should be admitted.

Cardiovascular Complications

Cancer treatment can affect cardiac function in patients both on active treatment and long after completion of therapy.

Anthracycline-induced cardiomyopathy is the most common cause of cardiac damage in pediatric oncology patients although only a small percentage of them are affected. Anthracycline chemotherapy is widely used in the treatment of leukemia, lymphoma, sarcoma, and embryonal tumors such as neuroblastoma and Wilm's tumor. The most commonly used anthracyclines include doxorubicin (Adriamycin®) and daunorubicin (Daunomycin®). Other drugs included in this category are epirubicin, idarubicin, and mitoxantrone. These drugs injure and potentially kill individual cardiomyocytes and can cause acute cardiomyopathy during and up to one year after the end of treatment. Late cardiomyopathy may develop 8 or more years after completion of therapy. Typical findings on echocardiogram include decreased shortening fraction/ejection fraction and/or increased afterload. Specific risk factors include high total dose (greater than 300 mg per m^2), high dose rate, very young age at treatment, and trisomy 21. Most regimens today are designed to minimize the risk of cardiomyopathy by limiting total dose and dose rate and/or giving dexrazoxane, a cardioprotectant.

Patients exposed to substantial doses of anthracycline are screened with echocardiograms to look for early cardiac dysfunction. Early-onset cardiomyopathy usually presents as acute cardiac failure or cardiac dysfunction out of proportion to a stressor such as sepsis. Late onset cardiomyopathy is generally a slowly progressive process that may be detected on screening. Both forms may be associated with arrhythmias. The initial management of this problem follows the standard regiment for cardiac failure (see Chapter 84).

Radiation to the heart can cause long-term injury to the endothelial surfaces leading to early onset atherosclerotic vessel and/or valve disease. The heart is exposed in mantle radiation for Hodgkin's disease and total body irradiation as part of a transplant preparative regimen.

Hypertension may occur in pediatric oncology patients. Contributing factors include steroid exposure, salt overload, and renal injury from treatment. Most hypertension is not an emergency and is better addressed by the treating oncologist as part of long-term management. Hypertensive emergencies (see Chapter 34) are rare in pediatric oncology patients.

Hepatic and Gastrointestinal Complications of Cancer Treatment

Cancer treatment frequently affects the GI tract and liver. The majority of complications are minor and fully reversible. A few complications are potentially severe and/or have long-term consequences. Chemotherapy frequently impairs the ability of the mucosal lining of the GI tract to regenerate itself. Severity varies with different chemotherapy regimens. Time to occurrence is similar to the timing of myelosupression with onset 7 to 10 days after treatment and recovery by 14 days. Radiation also causes temporary injury to any areas of mucosa included in the radiation field. This injury becomes evident after several weeks of treatment and will persist/worsen until treatment is complete.

Initial assessment must include a thorough oncology history to elicit chemotherapy or radiation exposures as well as localizing symptoms and a complete physical examination. Chemotherapy-induced mucositis can affect part or all of the GI tract from oropharynx to the rectum and may be manifest as oral ulceration, throat pain, esophagitis, gastritis, enteritis, or rectal ulceration. Radiation-induced mucosal injury is often associated with skin manifestations in the treatment field. Oropharyngeal involvement usually includes pain and visible mucosal injury ranging from irregular mucosal surfaces to scattered ulcerations to severe diffuse ulceration with swelling of the lips and inability to open the mouth. Esophagitis may be evident only by refusal to swallow and/or retrosternal pain. Enteritis, common with radiation fields that include the intestines, may be evident with crampy watery diarrhea. Mucosal injury to the rectum leads to pain with defecation, tenesmus, or rectal pain. There may be obvious perirectal erythema or ulceration. Do not do an internal rectal examination, which may cause an increased likelihood of bacteremia.

Management of moderate to severe mucositis usually requires pain control with parenteral narcotics. Cancer patients may require higher than standard starting doses, especially if already on narcotics at home. Patients and their families should be asked whether they have preferences based on prior episodes of pain which narcotic works best. PCA with both continuous and bolus dosing should be initiated in the ED if available. Do not use NSAIDs for pain control since they usually have platelet inhibitory effects and thrombocytopenia frequently coincides in time with mucositis. Avoid regular use of acetaminophen, which may mask fever since neutropenia also often occurs at the same time. Assess hydration and provide intravenous support as needed. Patients with adequate oral pain control and oral hydration can be discharged to home. Others will need to be admitted for pain control and/or hydration until the mucositis resolves.

Nausea and vomiting are common symptoms in oncology patients. It is critical to consider the differential diagnosis and not just attribute all such symptoms to chemotherapy-induced nausea and vomiting (CINV). CINV can be divided into three categories: acute, delayed, and anticipatory. Acute symptoms occur within 24 hours of emetogenic treatment. Delayed symptoms occur 2 to 5 days after treatment and are particularly common with cisplatin. Anticipatory symptoms are conditioned symptoms that occur without emetogenic treatment with a variety of emotional or sensory triggers. These anticipatory symptoms can become chronic in some patients. Despite appropriate prophylactic therapy, almost all cancer patients experience some nausea and vomiting. Radiation to the GI tract or the CNS is also emetogenic. Other causes of nausea and vomiting include GI injury from a variety of causes such as gastritis from steroids, obstipation/constipation, medication side effects (e.g., narcotics), pancreatitis (from asparaginase), GI obstruction (e.g., adhesions from prior surgery), or superior mesenteric artery syndrome in patients with severe malnutrition.

Initial management should focus on developing an appropriate differential diagnosis based on the patient's oncology-specific history, medication history, and physical examination. Symptoms may also be multifactorial. Specific evaluations should be carried out based on the differential diagnosis. An abdominal x-ray can be quite helpful if obstruction or obstipation/constipation is suspected. Amylase and lipase should be measured in patients who are being treated with asparaginase.

A strategy for symptom management for CINV (or radiation-induced) is outlined in Table 97.9. As with pain management, all medications are less effective when treating established symptoms. Standard hydration and electrolyte management should be considered for all patients with severe nausea/vomiting.

Obstipation and constipation are very common in oncology patients. Contributing factors included decreased GI motility from vinca alkaloids, narcotics, poor oral intake, decreased activity, and/or withholding due to rectal pain from mucositis. Patients may present with complaints of nausea/vomiting, abdominal discomfort and/or abdominal distension. The evaluation should include a detailed history to elicit any of the contributing factors as well as a specific bowel history. Physical examination should *not* include an internal rectal examination due to potential increased risk of bacteremia. Abdominal x-ray may be helpful in establishing the amount of stool. Treatment of constipation in oncology patient should include only those agents that can be given by mouth. Rectal suppositories and enemas should be avoided except in extreme circumstances. Patients with severe symptoms may need to be admitted for clean out.

Transaminitis with elevations in AST and/or ALT are common in pediatric cancer patients. Many chemotherapy agents cause a mild reversible transaminitis. Elevations as high as $10\times$ normal can occur 1 to 3 days after the administration of high-dose methotrexate. Treatment-related transaminitis is usually a laboratory-only finding without any clinical correlate. Transfusion-associated viral transaminitis can also occur in the highly transfused oncology population. The incidence of viral transmission has been reduced by both direct and indirect screening of donor blood. Immunosuppression from treatment can also increase the risk of CMV and EBV. Isolated transaminitis may be noted during an evaluation in the ED but rarely is an indication for a laboratory evaluation.

Mild, reversible elevations in bilirubin are common during cancer treatment and should rarely require an ED evaluation. Such elevations are likely multifactorial and may relate to chemotherapy, transfusion, or subclinical liver injury. Isolated mild hyperbilirubinemia may be noted but rarely needs further testing.

Diarrhea in an oncology patient may be triggered by a variety of causes including radiation injury as noted above. Oncology patients may be at increased risk of Clostridia difficile colitis due to prolonged hospitalizations and/or use of broad-spectrum antibiotics. Irinotecan chemotherapy can cause two forms of diarrhea. The first is an acute effect that occurs during or immediately after infusion. It is mediated via a cholinergic effect and should be treated with loperamide. Prophylaxis with atropine should be given with subsequent cycles. Delayed diarrhea (more than 24 hours after infusion) also occurs and should also be treated with loperamide. Typical dosing regimens use loperamide 4 mg po at onset of diarrhea followed by 2 mg po every 2 hours until resolution of diarrhea. Prophylaxis with subsequent courses includes cefixime to eliminate aerobic gut flora that deglucuronidate the SN-38G metabolite of irinotecan.

Veno-occlusive disease of the liver (VOD) is a rare but important complication to recognize. Risk factors include exposure to actinomycin-D chemotherapy and liver radiation. Manifestations

TABLE 97.9

MANAGEMENT OF CHEMOTHERAPY-INDUCED NAUSEA AND VOMITING (CINV)

Agents with a high therapeutic index			
Drug class	**Specific drug**	**Pediatric dosage and frequency (usual adult maximum)**	**Route**

Drug class	Specific drug	Pediatric dosage and frequency (usual adult maximum)	Route	Comment
Serotonin-S3 receptor antagonists	Ondansetron	0.15 mg/kg (8 mg) q 8 h or 0.45 mg/kg (24 mg) q 24 h	IV/PO	There are limited data that there may be incomplete cross-resistance between agents.
	Granisetron	10–40 µg/kg (1 mg) q 24 h	IV/PO	
	Dolasetron	1.8 mg/kg (100 mg) q 24 h	IV/PO	
Steroid	Dexamethasone	10 mg/m² (10 mg) q 12–24 h	IV/PO	■ Should not be used in patients with steroid-sensitive malignancies without consultation with oncologist (e.g., ALL, lymphoma ■ Use should be avoided/minimized in patients at high risk of infection or if at increased risk of mucosal toxicity from chemotherapy (e.g., AML, advanced lymphomas, ALL during induction)
NK receptor antagonist	Aprepitant		PO	There are minimal pediatric data with this drug. There are no published data using this drug for established symptoms. Thus, we do not recommend using this drug in the ED setting.
Other	Scopolamine	1.5 mg fixed-dose transdermal patch for patients >40 kg	Transdermal	Avoid concurrent use of anticholinergic drugs such as diphenhydramine

Agents with a low therapeutic index			

Drug class	Specific drug	Pediatric dosage and frequency (usual adult maximum)	Route	Comment
Benzodiazepine	Lorazepam	0.05 mg/kg (1 mg) q 6 h	IV/PO	Overdosage may be common with weight-based dosing strategies. Thus, also consider 0.25 mg for <25 kg, 0.5 mg for ≥25–50 kg, and 1 mg for ≥50 kg. More potent as an anxiolytic than as an antiemetic.
Dopamine antagonist	Metoclopramide	0.5 mg/kg q 6 h	IV/PO	■ Children are at high risk of extrapyramidal reactions. □ Must be given with diphenhydramine prophylaxis. □ If more than 1 mg/kg of metoclopramide given in 24 h, recommend diphenhydramine coverage for 24 h after the last dose of metoclopramide.
	Prochlorperazine	Complex dosing guidelines, consult appropriate source.	IV	
	Prochlorperazine		PO	
	Prochlorperazine		PR	
	Thiethylperazine			
	Haloperidol			We do not recommend usage in the ED setting unless the prescriber is experienced with the use of this drug.
Other	Dronabinol	5 mg/m²	PO	No data in use younger than 5 yr

IV, intravenous; PO, per os; ALL, acute lymphoblastic leukemia; AML, acute myeloid leukemia; NK, neurokinin; ED, emergency department; PR.

MEDICAL EMERGENCIES

include hepatomegaly, transaminitis, thrombocytopenia, and ascites. The thrombocytopenia is frequently more than what would be expected from the chemotherapy alone or may occur at the wrong timing relative to chemotherapy. Once the diagnosis is suspected, a hepatic ultrasound with Doppler assessment of hepatic vein flow should be performed. Reversal of flow in the small hepatic veins establishes the diagnosis in the appropriate clinical setting. Management is supportive until the problem resolves on its own. Most patients will require admission for both observation and support.

For a discussion of typhlitis, see section on "Infectious Complications of Cancer Treatment."

RENAL COMPLICATIONS OF CANCER TREATMENT

Renal injury from cancer treatment is very common and some degree of renal dysfunction is frequently present even in patients with normal creatinine for age. Other patients will have documented renal dysfunction based on elevated creatinine, decreased glomerular filtration rate (GFR), or decreased 24-hour creatinine clearance. Renal complications may also lead to metabolic disturbances (see "Metabolic Complications of Cancer Treatment" section). Contributing factors are listed below.

- Urate-acid nephropathy can occur in patients with very high cell turnover (see "Leukemia" section).
- Drug-induced renal injury is common in oncology patients.
  - □ Administration of high-dose methotrexate (dosage greater than 500 mg per m^2) very rarely causes acute renal failure, typically manifested as brisk urine output and a rapidly rising creatinine. Onset is usually within 24 hours of treatment. The renal failure itself is usually fully reversible and is managed with supportive care only.
  - □ High-dose cisplatin given in dosages of greater than 50 mg per m^2 per course causes chronic renal insufficiency manifested as decreased glomerular filtration and tubular wasting. Tubular wasting of magnesium is prominent and many patients require magnesium supplementation both on treatment and for months after completion.
  - □ Ifosfamide exposure causes renal injury manifested as Fanconi's syndrome with proximal tubular dysfunction and wasting of phosphate, glucose, potassium, and bicarbonate.
- Radiation injury to the kidney may cause renal insufficiency as well as radiation nephritis, 3 to 6 months after treatment. Typical findings include the manifestations of vasculitis with hemolytic-uremic syndrome (HUS). Oncology patients are also at risk for medical renal disease associated with poor perfusion (secondary to sepsis), exposure to multiple nephrotoxic agents, and hypertension.

Since renal injury is common, it is appropriate to check BUN, creatinine, electrolytes, calcium, magnesium, and phosphate in all systemically ill oncology patients. If significant abnormalities are noted, the oncology-specific history should be reviewed to determine specific risk factors or exposures that may help explain the problem. In general, the management of significant abnormalities is not unique to patients with cancer and should follow the guidelines in Chapter 100. Consider the possibility of a decreased GFR (whether known or not) when starting antibiotics and other medications excreted via the kidney.

Genitourinary Complications of Cancer Treatment

The most common form of bladder injury in cancer patients is hemorrhagic cystitis, a potential complication of exposure to cyclophosphamide or ifosfamide. Both of these drugs have an acrolein metabolite that is directly toxic to the bladder mucosa. Prevention of drug-induced hematuria usually includes hydration, frequent voiding, and administration of mesna, a drug that binds the toxic metabolite. Manifestations include dysuria, suprapubic pain, and microscopic or gross hematuria with onset within 24 hours of drug administration. Other causes of toxicity to the GU tract include infection, bladder radiation, tumor resection, or ongoing presence of tumor in the GU tract.

If a patient is complaining of bladder-related symptoms or the urinalysis shows evidence of hematuria, the oncology-specific history should be reviewed to help develop an appropriate differential diagnosis in addition to the usual causes (such as infection) that would be considered in a patient without cancer. Initial management should include initiation of one and one-half times to twice maintenance hydration and frequent voiding. Laboratory evaluation should include a urine analysis, CBC count to look for anemia or thrombocytopenia, and coagulation studies. Any contribution from coagulopathy and/or thrombocytopenia should be corrected. If severe bleeding or bladder outlet obstruction from clots occurs, an urologist should be consulted. A bladder catheter large enough to be used for irrigation should be placed and bladder washing initiated in consultation with urology. Packed red blood cell transfusion may be needed. In very rare cases, bleeding can be life-threatening and bladder sclerosis is indicated. Mesna (2-mercaptoethane sulfonate sodium) has no utility once the offending drug has cleared from the system. Pain management with oxybutynin chloride and narcotics should be initiated as needed.

Skin Complications of Cancer Treatment

Various cancer treatments are known to have cutaneous toxicities.

- High does of cytarabine may cause erythroderma, often limited to the plantar surfaces, with subsequent desquamation. Treatment is supportive.
- Radiation induces dermatitis in the treatment field that can range from mild to severe, based on the total dose and any concurrent radiation sensitizers. The presentation may vary from a mild erythroderma, similar to a sunburn, to severe desquamation in the treatment field. Any topical treatment must be prescribed in conjunction with the treating radiation oncologist because certain topical agents may increase the radiation dose to the skin.
- Drug rashes are very common in oncology patients. Because any one patient tends to be on many drugs at one time, it may be difficult to identify the specific culprit. Management of a drug reaction is not unique to oncology patients. However, consultation with the oncologist may be needed to discuss if alternate treatment is needed.

Infections may be accompanied by cutaneous manifestations (see Chapter 92). Although not unique to oncology patients, certain infections affecting the skin may be more common in this patient group. Immunosuppressed patients are at increased risk for herpes simplex and herpes zoster. Any skin lesions in a dermatomal distribution, with or without associated pain and whether or not the lesions are "classic," should be considered herpes zoster until proven otherwise. Immunocompromised patients with herpes zoster have an increased risk of disseminated disease and should be placed in respiratory isolation. Evaluation should include chest radiograph and liver function tests. If there is vesicular lesion, it should be scraped and sent for both rapid testing and culture for herpes simplex and varicella zoster. Empiric therapy should be started with either acyclovir or one of its derivatives. Admission for intravenous therapy is indicated for evidence of dissemination, ophthalmologic involvement or failure to respond to oral therapy. Oral home therapy can be considered in consultation with oncology after considering extent of involvement, degree of underlying immunosuppression, likelihood of medication compliance at home, and ability to follow up.

COMPLICATIONS OF HEMATOPOIETIC STEM CELL TRANSPLANT

Bone marrow transplantation is an increasingly utilized therapy aimed at treating various hematologic, oncologic, metabolic, or immunologic diseases. In hematologic malignancies, allogeneic marrow transplantation may follow initial remission induction or disease relapse. The allogeneic donor may be related, usually a sibling, or unrelated to the recipient. In solid tumors and some lymphomas, patients may receive aggressive chemotherapy and radiation and then have their own stem cells infused as a "rescue" to help reconstitute their immune system following therapy. Knowledge of the type of transplant a patient received (Table 97.1) can help the clinician to anticipate what complications might ensue. In general, patients who have had a stem cell transplant represent a fragile patient population at risk for many complications.

In approaching these patients, substantial immunosuppression should be presumed for at least 6 months following the transplant. For patients still receiving immunosuppressing medications, the period of immune dysfunction may be much longer. Regardless of the WBC and neutrophil counts, immune function following a stem cell transplant can be profoundly impaired.

Graft-versus-host disease (GVHD) may develop in the setting of allogeneic stem cell transplants as newly engrafted immune cells of the donor react against tissue antigens of the recipient that are perceived to be foreign (Table 97.10). The risk of developing GVHD is higher if the degree of HLA (human leukocyte antigen) matching between the donor and recipient was less optimal and if donors and recipients are unrelated. Acute GVHD occurs in the first 100 days post transplant, often when patient is still in hospital, and typically involves the skin, GI tract, or liver. Chronic GVHD presents after 100 days and is accompanied by severe immunologic dysfunction.

The management in the ED of patients with known or suspected GVHD following an allogeneic stem cell transplant begins with a history to explore whether the patient could be dehydrated or anemic due to colitis or whether he/she is experiencing dyspnea due to lung involvement. Physical examination should explore the skin for rash, fibrosis, or jaundice,

liver size and tenderness, and oxygen saturation. Assessment should focus on screening for organ dysfunction serious enough to require intervention in the ED. Clinicians should have a low threshold for admitting such patients for inpatient management due to overall fragility of this patient population.

Therapy for GVHD is primarily immunosuppressive using corticosteroids, cyclosporine, and other agents directed against T cells. Specialists in hematopoietic stem cell transplant decide whether to pursue such agents and when. Often a biopsy (skin, bowel, liver, etc.) is required to diagnose GVHD on histopathology.

The management of infectious complications for patients following stem cell transplant is not different from infections in the oncology population overall, but the relevant organisms may vary and the clinician's level of suspicion may need to be higher (Table 97.10). Infections in these patients result from the extreme immunosuppression achieved by myeloablation, cutaneous and mucosal barrier damage intrinsic to the transplant process, and the immunologic immaturity of the transplanted marrow. Exacerbating the risk is the presence of central lines in these patients.

Importantly, the types of infections patients tend to develop after hematopoietic stem cell transplant can vary based on how many days have elapsed since the transplant.

- In the first month after the transplant, as patients are hospitalized and awaiting engraftment of their bone marrow, they are vulnerable to gram-positive and -negative bacteria, anaerobic bacteria, respiratory viruses and reactivation of herpes simplex virus, and fungal infection with candida and aspergillus.
- After engraftment, from day 30 to 100 after the transplant, patients remain at risk for bacterial infections, particularly those related to their central lines. Aspergillus and respiratory viruses continue to be a concern. However, CMV becomes more of a threat at this point as can infections with pneumocystis and toxoplasma.
- More than 100 days after the transplant, patients are at risk for encapsulated bacteria, especially if they are simultaneously affected by GVHD or on ongoing immunosuppression. Aspergillus, pneumocystis, and toxoplasma continue to be a concern. Viral infections with varicella zoster virus, CMV, EBV, and respiratory viruses are also a large threat for these patients.

When patients present to the ED with fever following a hematopoietic stem cell transplant, empiric coverage with antibiotics should be instituted at once while cultures of the blood and urine are pending. While gram-negative organisms have historically been of primary concern, gram-positive bacteria have more recently become more threatening, particularly with the emergence of MRSA in some regions. Antibiotic regimens need to broadly cover gram-positive and -negative bacteria (e.g., piperacillin/tazobactam and gentamicin) as well as MRSA when relevant.

Rarely seen as a complication of stem cell transplant, TTP (thrombotic thrombocytopenic purpura) can present in this patient population manifesting the classic pentad of fever, neurologic symptoms, hemolytic anemia, thrombocytopenia, and renal compromise (Table 97.10). The disorder seems to be associated with immunosuppression with cyclosporine or FK506 in the posttransplant period. In some patients, TTP

TABLE 97.10

COMPLICATIONS OF HEMATOPOIETIC STEM CELL TRANSPLANT

Complication	Clinical findings	Management

Graft versus host Disease (GVHD)	Acute
	  Skin
	    Erythematous rash
	    Classic involvement of palms and soles
	  GI tract
	    Colitis, sometimes bloody diarrhea
	    Abdominal pain
	  Liver
	    Elevated bilirubin, alkaline phosphatase, transaminases
	    Hepatomegaly
	    Right upper quadrant tenderness
	Chronic
	  Pulmonary
	    Hypoxia
	    Shortness of breath
	  Liver (as above)
	  Eye dryness
	  Mouth dryness
	  Skin
	    Sclerodermatous changes
	    Contractures
		Immunosuppressive medications chosen only in consultation with experts in stem cell transplant
		Aggressive management of infections and fevers given immunosuppression intrinsic to Graft-versus-host disease (GVHD)
		Hydration as needed for dehydration from colitis
		Assessment of anemia secondary to bloody diarrhea
		Caution using drugs metabolized in the liver if hepatic GVHD present

Infection	Bacterial
	  Bacteria
	    Gram positive
	    Gram negative
	Viral
	  Endogenous
	    Varicella zoster
	    Herpes simplex
	    Epstein-Barr virus
	    Cytomegalovirus
	    Adenovirus
	  Exogenous
	    Influenza
	    Parainfluenza
	    Respiratory syncytial virus
	    Adenovirus
	Fungal
	  Disseminated candidemia
	  Invasive aspergillosis
		Empiric broad spectrum antibiotics for fever
		All patients to be considered functionally neutropenic and immunocompromised until they have been off all immunosuppressive medications for at least 6 mo
		Aggressive imaging to follow-up and localizing signs or symptoms elicited through history and physical examination
		Bacterial and fungal cultures as well as viral studies of blood, urine, sputum
		Spinal tap not required

Thrombotic thrombocytopenic purpura	Acute form displays classic pentad
	  Fever
	  Hemolytic anemia
	  Thrombocytopenia
	  Renal failure
	  Neurologic symptoms
	Rarely can evolve into chronic hemolytic-uremic syndrome–like picture
		Manage as TTP would be managed outside of the stem cell transplant setting

may evolve into a more chronic picture with abnormal renal dysfunction and a clinical picture more consistent with HUS.

Care of Patients with Advanced Cancer

Pediatric palliative care has seen major changes in recent decades and these developments clearly impact care for children with cancer. Children with incurable cancer may still receive treatment that may be life prolonging and options for managing symptoms related to advanced disease have expanded. Also noteworthy is the increased role for the patient and family members in decisions in the setting of advanced disease. Finally, options for patients to receive care outside of the hospital, either in hospice or at home, have greatly evolved.

Central to the mission of the emergency physician approaching a child with advanced cancer should be establishing the current goals of care. This can occur in two major ways:

- The preferences of the patient and/or family members may already be documented in the medical record. Often, these preferences have been explored during previous hospitalizations or clinic appointments with the patient's primary oncology team. In many cases, the outcome of such discussions may now be written in the form of a Do-Not-Resuscitate (DNR) order, a Seven Wish Document, or an outpatient/home form or order meant to establish limits for resuscitation. The use of these latter orders/forms are increasing in prevalence. Insight into the patient's and family's goals of care may be gained by direct communication with the oncology provider who knows the patient best.
- During the visit to the ED, the clinician should ask the patient/family open-ended questions to allow for an open expression of preferences. During this conversation, if the patient has any documented preferences already expressed in the medical record, the clinician should inquire whether there have been any recent changes to these preferences. Changes sometimes occur and medical staff unacquainted with the patient often feel uncomfortable embarking upon these discussions, even though patients and family members usually welcome the opportunity to communicate in this way.

Approaching patients with advanced cancer requires the clinician to acknowledge that sometimes patient/family preferences do not seem well aligned with those of the health-care team. For example, the physician may encounter a patient who is clearly within hours or days of death but who still "wants everything done," including cancer-directed therapy and aggressive management such as intubation or resuscitation. On the other hand, the clinician may instead face a patient with seemingly good functional status and quality of life who declines further disease-directed treatments. Cases may also exist anywhere in between these two extremes. It is the clinician's responsibility to provide honest and complete information and elicit the patient's beliefs and wishes to facilitate decision making that most reflects the individual wishes of the patient and family. Once decisions are made, it is then the duty of the clinician to help carry out those wishes.

Initiation of a management plan intended to reduce symptoms is always an appropriate step. The kind of intervention best able to reduce symptoms must be chosen based on the goals of care. Patients with advanced cancer have often received large amounts of opioids in the past and may therefore require larger doses of pain medications than routinely administered to children in the ED (see the "Pain" section). It is imperative for the clinician to increase the opioid dose until an efficacious dose is reached. Opioids may also be used to treat shortness of breath or other respiratory symptoms.

Diagnostic workup and specific management beyond symptom control should be undertaken in a manner consistent with the goals of care. If the patient's focus is only on comfort, then a diagnostic workup should be considered only if it will help identify a reasonable strategy to optimize that comfort. Consider, for example, a patient who presents for pain management but who is also cachectic and dehydrated. The clinician may wonder whether checking serum electrolytes and initiating rehydration are indicated. If the stated goals of care are comfort, then these measures should be omitted since electrolyte disturbances rarely cause pain/discomfort and hydration often will prolong the suffering associated with severe pain at the end of life. Indeed, hydration could increase edema or secretions that would actually decrease quality of life. As an additional example, consider a patient presenting with a malignant pleural effusion causing severe respiratory distress. Under other circumstances, the management of a large effusion might be immediate placement of chest tube. In this case, the clinician might instead ask him or herself "how will a chest tube help *this* patient and does it match what he/she wants?" This change in thought process is often extremely hard for health-care providers whose experience and training do not include care of patients with advanced disease but it is an essential element of their care.

Patients with advanced cancer may have clear preferences regarding admission to the hospital. While some patients and families may have adequate services in place to remain in their homes, some will still desire inpatient management as a form of respite.

Suggested Readings

General

Golden CB, Feusner JH. Malignant abdominal masses in children: quick guide to evaluation and diagnosis. *Pediatr Clin North Am* 2002;49:1369–1392.
Nicolin G. Emergencies and their management. *Eur J Cancer* 2002;38:1365–1377. discussion 1378–1379.
Zojer N, Ludwig H. Hematological Emergencies. *Ann Oncol* 2007;18:i45–i48.

Leukemia

Blum W, Porcu P. Therapeutic apheresis in hyperleukocytosis and hyperviscosity syndrome. *Semin Thromb Hemost* 2007;33:350–354.
Kaspers GJ, Zwaan CM. Pediatric acute myeloid leukemia: towards high-quality cure of all patients. *Haematologica* 2007;92:1519–1532.
Pieters R, Carroll WL. Biology and treatment of acute lymphoblastic leukemia. *Pediatr Clin North Am* 2008;55:1–20.
Pui CH, Robison LL, Look AT. Acute lymphoblastic leukaemia. *Lancet* 2008;371:1030–1043.
Rubnitz JE, Gibson B, Smith FO. Acute myeloid leukemia. *Pediatr Clin North Am* 2008;55:21–51.
Tiu RV, Mountantonakis SE, Dunbar AJ, et al., Tumor lysis syndrome. *Semin Thromb Hemost* 2007;33:397–407.
Tosi P, Barosi G, Lazzaro C, et al. Consensus conference on the management of tumor lysis syndrome. *Haematoligica* 2008;93:1877–1885.

Histiocytic Diseases

Janka GE. Hemophagocytic syndromes. *Blood Rev* 2007;21:245–253.
Weitzman S, Egeler RM. Langerhans cell histiocytosis: update for the pediatrician. *Curr Opin Pediatr* 2008;20:23–29.

Tumors of the Central Nervous System

Packer RJ, MacDonald T, Vezina G. Central nervous system tumors. *Pediatr Clin North Am* 2008;55:121–145.
Ullrich NJ, Pomeroy SL. Pediatric brain tumors. *Neurol Clin* 2003;21:897–913.

Tumors of the Thorax

Gross TG, Termuhlen AM. Pediatric non-Hodgkin's lymphoma. *Curr Oncol Rep* 2007;9:459–465.
Olson MR, Donaldson SS. Treatment of pediatric Hodgkin lymphoma. *Curr Treat Options Oncol* 2008;9:81–94.
Perger L, Lee EY, Shamberger RC. Management of children and adolescents with a critical airway due to compression by an anterior mediastinal mass. *J Pediatr Surg* 2008;43:1990–1997.
Schwartz CL. The management of Hodgkin disease in the young child. *Curr Opin Pediatr.* 2003;15:10–16.
Yu JB, Wilson LD, Detterbeck FC. Superior vena cava syndrome–a proposed classification system and algorithm for management. *J Thorac Oncol* 2008;3:811–814.

MEDICAL EMERGENCIES

Tumors of the Hepatobiliary Tree

Emre S, McKenna GJ. Liver tumors in children. *Pediatr Transplant* 2004;8: 632–638.
Litten JB, Tomlinson GE. Liver tumors in children. *Oncologist* 2008;13:18–20.

Neuroblastoma

De Bernardi B, Pianca C, Pistamiglio P, et al., Neuroblastoma with symptomatic spinal cord compression at diagnosis: treatment and results with 76 cases. *J Clin Oncol* 2001;19:183–190.
Kim S, Chung DH. Pediatric solid malignancies: neuroblastoma and Wilm's tumor. *Surg Clin North Am* 2006;86:469–487.
Park JR, Eggert A, Caron H. Neuroblastoma: biology, prognosis, and treatment. *Pediatr Clin North Am* 2008;55:97–120.

Tumors of the Kidney

Kaste SC, Dome JS, Babyn PS, et al. Wilm's tumour: prognostic factors, staging, therapy, and late effects. *Pediatr Radiol* 2008;38:2–17.
Kim S, Chung DH. Pediatric solid malignancies: neuroblastoma and Wilm's tumor. *Surg Clin North Am* 2006;86:469–487.
Siegel MJ, Chung EM. Wilms' tumor and other pediatric renal masses. *Magn Reson Imaging Clin N Am* 2008;16:479–497.

Gonadal Tumors

Billmire DF. Germ cell tumors. *Surg Clin North Am* 2006;86:489–503.
Schneider DT, Calaminus G, Koch S, et al. Epidemiologic analysis of 1,442 children and adolescents registered in the German germ cell tumor protocols. *Pediatr Blood Cancer* 2004;42:169–175.

Tumors in and Around the Spinal cord

Kwok Y, DeYoung C, Garofalo M, et al. Radiation oncology emergencies. *Hematol Oncol Clin North Am* 2006;20:505–522.
Pollono D, Tomarchia S, Drut R, et al. Spinal cord compression: a review of 70 pediatric patients. *Pediatr Hematol Oncol* 2003;20:457–466.

Tumors of Bone and Soft Tissue Tumors

Albritton KH. Sarcomas in adolescents and young adults. *Hematol Oncol Clin North Am* 2005;19:527–546.
Loeb DM, Thornton K, Shokek O. Pediatric soft tissue sarcomas. *Surg Clin North Am* 2008;88:615–627.
Marec-Berard P, Philip T. Ewing sarcoma: the pediatrician's point of view. *Pediatr Blood Cancer* 2004;42:477–480.

Hematologic Complications

Athale UH, Chan AK. Hemorrhagic complications in pediatric hematologic malignancies. *Semin Thromb Hemost* 2007;33:408–415.

Wiernikowski JT, Athale UH. Thromboembolic complications in children with cancer. *Thromb Res* 2006;118:137–152.

Infectious Complications

Bremer CT, Monahan BP. Necrotizing enterocolitis in neutropenia and chemotherapy: a clinical update and old lessons relearned. *Curr Gastroenterol Rep* 2006;8:333–341.
Davila ML. Neutropenic enterocolitis. *Curr Opin Gastroenterol* 2006;22:44–47.
Elihu A, Gollin G. Complications of implanted central venous catheters in neutropenic children. *Am Surg* 2007;73:1079–1082.
Hughes WT, Armstrong D, Bodey GP, et al. 2002 guidelines for the use of antimicrobial agents in neutropenic patients with cancer. *Clin Infect Dis* 2002;34:730–751.
McCarville MB, Adelman CS, Li C, et al. Typhlitis in childhood cancer. *Cancer* 2005;104:380–387.
Rosen GP, Nielsen K, Glenn S, et al. Invasive fungal infections in pediatric oncology patients: 11-year experience. *J Pediatr Hematol Oncol* 2005;27:135–140.

Pain

Brislin RP, Rose JB. Pediatric acute pain management. *Anesthesiol Clin North America* 2005;23:789–814.
Galloway KS, Yaster M. Pain and symptom control in terminally ill children. *Pediatr Clin North Am* 2000;47:711–746.

Neurologic Complications

Sul JK, Deangelis LM. Neurologic complications of cancer chemotherapy. *Semin Oncol* 2006;33:324–332.

Cardiovascular Complications

Appel JM, Nielsen D, Zerahn B, et al. Anthracycline-induced chronic cardiotoxicity and heart failure. *Acta Oncol* 2007;46:576–580.

Hepatic and Gastrointestinal Complications

Hesketh PJ. Chemotherapy-induced nausea and vomiting. *N Engl J Med* 2008; 358:2482–2494.

Complications of Stem Cell Transplantation

Barfield RC, Kasow KA, Hale GA. Advances in pediatric hematopoietic stem cell transplantation. *Cancer Biol Ther* 2008;7:1533–1539.

Palliative Care

Collins JJ. Palliative care and the child with cancer. *Hematol Oncol Clin North Am* 2002;16:657–670.
Himelstein BP, Hilden JM, Boldt AM, et al. Pediatric palliative care. *N Engl J Med* 2004;350:1752–1762.
Mack JW, Wolfe J. Early integration of pediatric palliative care: for some children, palliative care starts at diagnosis. *Curr Opin Pediatr* 2006;18:10–14.

CHAPTER 98 ■ PULMONARY EMERGENCIES

JOSHUA NAGLER, MD

ACUTE RESPIRATORY FAILURE

Background

Respiratory disease accounts for almost 10% of pediatric emergency department (ED) visits. Most cases are benign and self-limited, requiring no intervention. However, respiratory illnesses also contribute to a significant proportion of morbidity and mortality in pediatrics, including approximately 20% of hospital admissions and 3% to 5% of deaths in children. Importantly, respiratory failure often precedes cardiopulmonary arrest in children, unlike in adults where primary cardiac disease is often responsible. Therefore, prompt recognition and treatment of pediatric patients with pending respiratory failure can be lifesaving.

Many different disease processes can lead to respiratory failure (Table 98.1), including primary pulmonary diseases as well as disorders outside the respiratory tract (see Chapter 68). This section discusses the pathophysiology and clinical manifestations of respiratory failure, as well as a general approach to initiating treatment in the emergency setting. The management of specific disorders can be found in subsequent sections of this chapter, as well as in Chapters 82, 92, and 128, and other areas of the text.

Pathophysiology

By definition, respiratory failure indicates an inability of the respiratory system to provide sufficient oxygen for metabolic needs or to excrete the CO_2 produced by the body. The former can be further categorized as *hypoxemic* respiratory failure and the latter as *ventilatory* failure. Alternatively, causes of acute respiratory failure can be categorized by etiology (Table 98.1), each of which is reviewed here.

The nervous system plays a major role in the control and maintenance of respiration. Therefore, either reversible or irreversible causes of central nervous system (CNS) disease can affect respiratory function. CNS disease may result in depressed respiratory drive or inability to maintain protective airway reflexes. In addition, neurologic disease may directly affect the peripheral nerves or muscles, leading to either airway obstruction or inadequate excursion of the chest wall and diaphragm. The result is inadequate gas exchange and ventilation-perfusion (V̇/Q̇) mismatch.

Untreated upper airway obstruction in children can also lead to respiratory failure. Pediatric airways are intrinsically small; therefore, further narrowing or collapse can have a profound effect on airflow. Edema from infectious, allergic, or caustic etiologies; foreign material in the airway; or obstruction by enlarged or compressing anatomic structures can contribute to airway obstruction. These may occur in isolation or in combination. For example, patients with severe static encephalopathy or anatomic head and neck problems may have only partial compromise of the airway when well, but they may develop increased obstruction during respiratory infection, a seizure, or other acute medical problems.

Lower airway disease is a common cause of acute respiratory failure. Asthma accounts for the largest percentage of this group, but infections such as bronchiolitis or viral pneumonia are also common and predominantly impact the small airways. Foreign-body aspiration in the lower airway can present acutely with obstruction or may be a delayed diagnosis, following the development of secondary postobstructive atelectasis or pneumonia (Fig. 98.1).

Chest wall deformities and mechanical impairments can play a role in respiratory failure. Inability to fully expand the chest leads to restrictive disease and lowers the vital capacity. The decreased expansion of the thoracic cavity leads to decreased minute ventilation and resultant hypercapnia, while the extra energy expended by the inefficient respiratory pattern can lead to hypoxemia. As with airway obstruction described above, many of these patients are able to maintain near normal respiratory function until additional physiologic compromise occurs, often from illness as minor as an upper respiratory tract infection.

Parenchymal lung disease can lead to acute respiratory failure, most commonly in children younger than 1 year. While the majority of cases do not result in failure, patients with underlying cardiopulmonary disorders [e.g., bronchopulmonary dysplasia (BPD) or congenital heart disease] are particularly susceptible. In such cases, the additional respiratory embarrassment from acute pulmonary infection can induce respiratory failure.

Finally, numerous nonrespiratory conditions may precipitate respiratory failure. Although with varied underlying pathophysiology, the diseases listed in Table 98.1 each alter the balance of O_2 consumption and CO_2 production such that gas exchange cannot be maintained by the respiratory system, leading to secondary respiratory failure.

Clinical Manifestations

Acute respiratory failure represents the severe end of the spectrum of respiratory disease. Although the onset can be hyperacute (e.g., complete airway obstruction from foreign-body aspiration or traumatic injury to the phrenic nerve with complete loss of respiratory effort), respiratory failure more

TABLE 98.1

CAUSES OF ACUTE RESPIRATORY FAILURE IN CHILDREN

Neurologic Disease			**Airway Obstruction**	
Central nervous system	Status epilepticus		Lower	Reactive airway disease (asthma)
	Severe static encephalopathy			Bronchiolitis
	Acute meningoencephalitis			Foreign-body aspiration
	Brain abscess, hematoma, tumor			Cystic fibrosis
	Brain stem insult			Bronchiectasis
	Arnold–Chiari crisis			Tracheobronchomalacia
	Drug intoxication			Bronchopulmonary dysplasia
	General anesthesia			α_1-Antitrypsin deficiency
Spinal/anterior horn cell	Transverse myelitis			Hydrocarbon aspiration,
	Poliomyelitis			aspiration syndromes
	Polyradiculitis (Guillain–Barré)			Congenital lobar emphysema
	Spinal muscle atrophy type 1		**Chest Wall Deformity**	Diaphragmatic hernia
	(Werdnig–Hoffmann syndrome)		**Disorders**	Kyphoscoliosis (severe)
Neuromuscular junction	Myasthenia gravis			Restrictive lung disease secondary
	Botulism (e.g., infantile,			to chest deformity
	food-borne, wound)		**Pulmonary Diseases**	Infectious pneumonias (bacterial,
	Tetanus			viral, fungal, and other)
	Myopathy			Tuberculosis
	Neuropathy			Pertussis, parapertussis syndrome
	Drugs (e.g., succinylcholine,			Cystic fibrosis
	curare, pancuronium,			Drug-induced pulmonary disease
	organophosphates)			Vasculitis, collagen vascular disease
				Pulmonary dysgenesis
Airway Obstruction				Pulmonary edema
Upper	Acute epiglottitis			Pneumothorax, hemothorax,
	Laryngotracheobronchitis (croup)			chylothorax
	Bacterial tracheitis			Near drowning
	Foreign-body aspiration		**Other Diseases**	Cardiac disease
	Adenotonsillar hypertrophy			Anemia (severe)
	Retropharyngeal abscess			Acidemia (e.g., renal failure, diabetic
	Subglottic stenosis, web, or			ketoacidosis, hepatic disease)
	hemangioma			Oxygen dissociation (e.g.,
	Laryngomalacia			methemoglobinemia, carbon
	Laryngeal edema			monoxide, or cyanide poisoning)
	Congenital anomalies			Hypothermia, hyperthermia
	Static encephalopathy			Sepsis
				Obstructive sleep apnea syndrome

commonly results from a progression of respiratory illness and distress. Therefore, recognizing the signs and symptoms of *impending* respiratory failure is as important as establishing criteria for failure. By identifying patients (i) at increased risk (e.g., neonates, those with underlying lung or cardiac disease), (ii) who show signs of significant distress (e.g., grunting, gasping, retracting), and (iii) with a worrisome trajectory based on observation and response to therapy over time (e.g., evidence of tiring), aggressive intervention can sometimes avert progression to failure. For those patients whose respiratory compromise is more advanced, clinical, laboratory, and physiologic criteria for respiratory failure are outlined in Table 98.2.

Management

Table 98.3 outlines an approach to management for acute respiratory failure. Resuscitation and basic life support measures

are discussed in Chapter 1. Immediate therapeutic interventions aim at increasing oxygen delivery, assisting ventilation, and identifying and treating specific underlying etiologies wherever possible.

All patients in acute respiratory failure should receive supplemental oxygen to improve arteriolar oxygen concentration. For spontaneously breathing patients who do not require assisted ventilation, utilizing high-flow oxygen through a non-rebreather mask will provide maximal oxygen delivery. The goal is to achieve a minimal acceptable PaO_2, generally greater than 60 mm Hg (SaO_2 greater than 90%). If hypoxemia persists despite passive supplemental oxygen administration, assisted ventilation should be initiated. A mask seal using a flow-inflating resuscitation bag delivers continuous positive airway pressure (CPAP), which can improve oxygen delivery. Importantly, CPAP cannot be delivered though a self-inflating (Ambu) bag. Positive-pressure breaths utilizing either a self-inflating or flow-inflating bag will further increase oxygen delivery. Endotracheal intubation provides the most effective

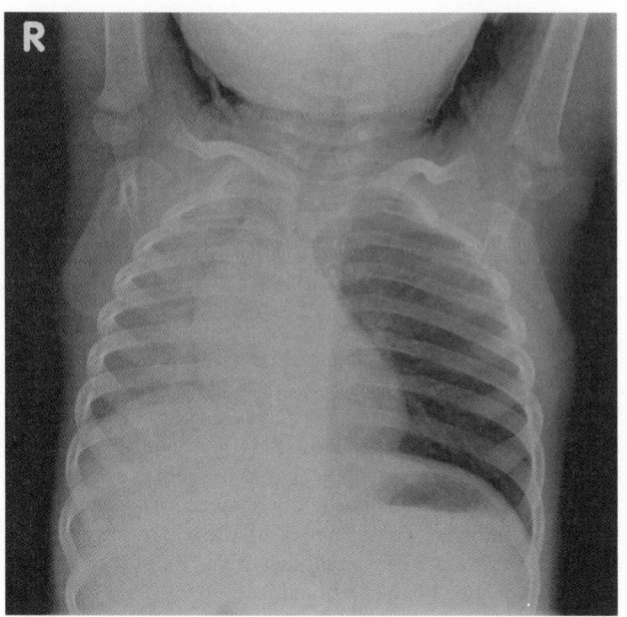

FIGURE 98.1 Foreign body aspiration. This 2-year-old girl presented in significant respiratory distress after choking on a peanut. The chest film shows hyperinflation of the left lung, tracheal deviation and mediastinal shift, and compression atelectasis of the right lung, consistent with air trapping secondary to foreign body aspiration (FBA).

TABLE 98.2

DIAGNOSIS OF ACUTE RESPIRATORY FAILURE FROM PULMONARY CAUSES IN CHILDREN

Clinical findings
Vital signs: tachycardia, tachypnea or bradypnea, hypoxemia
General appearance: cyanosis, diaphoresis, confusion, restlessness, fatigue, shortness of breath, apnea, grunting, stridor, retractions, decreased air entry, wheezing
Blood gas abnormalities
$Pa_{CO_2} > 50$ mm Hg with acidosis (pH < 7.25)
$Pa_{CO_2} > 40$ mm Hg with severe distress
$Pa_{O_2} < 60$ mm Hg (or $Sa_{O_2} < 90\%$) on 0.4 F_{IO_2}
Pulmonary function abnormalities
Vital capacity (<15 mL/kg)
Inspiratory pressure (<25–30 cm H_2O)

means of increasing Pa_{O_2} and is required for patients with persistent hypoxemia despite other interventions.

In addition to improving oxygen delivery, assisted ventilation may be required to correct alveolar hypoventilation.

Adequacy of ventilation should be assessed clinically by chest wall expansion and confirmed with either end-tidal carbon dioxide ($EtCO_2$) or serum Pa_{CO_2}. New recommendations suggest this can often be achieved with a tidal volume of 7 to 10 mL per kg, although this will vary based on lung compliance and underlying disease. Using a manometer within the airway circuit can provide valuable information regarding appropriate airway pressures and help prevent unnecessary barotrauma.

Specific ventilatory strategies will vary based on underlying disease. In children with acute respiratory failure but normal lung function (e.g., CNS depression), standard airway pressures and respiratory rates are adequate. CPAP or positive end-expiratory pressures (PEEP) may be useful where alveolar recruit-

TABLE 98.3

MANAGEMENT OF ACUTE RESPIRATORY FAILURE

Primary hypoxemia	1. High flow supplemental oxygen (e.g., nonrebreather mask), titrate for cyanosis, or by pulse oximetry or Pa_{O_2} 2. Use CPAP or PEEP to further improve oxygenation 3. Consider endotracheal intubation when persistent hypoxemia on $F_{IO_2} > 0.6$ or when decreased lung compliance and $F_{IO_2} > 0.4$ 4. Use assisted ventilation to improve gas exchange (increased inspiratory time, normal respiratory rates, tidal volume: 10–15 mL/kg; pressure cycle ventilation if wt. < 10 kg, volume cycle ventilation if wt. > 10 kg). If inspiratory pressure exceeds 40 cm H_2O, consider use of permissive hypercapnia to reduce barotrauma. 5. Treat underlying cause

Primary hypoventilation	1. Supplemental oxygen (as above)
	2. Support ventilation
	   a. Oral/nasal pharyngeal tube or endotracheal intubation
	   b. Bag-mask ventilation with high-flow oxygen
	   c. Use assisted ventilation (normal to increased respiratory rates, increased expired time, increased flow rates)
	   d. Use increased tidal volume (pressure) with obstructive airway disease or with atelectasis
	   e. Monitor carefully for side effects of ventilation

Adjunctive therapy	1. Intravenous fluid to achieve normal vascular volume (less fluid for child with interstitial lung disease) 2. Diuretics such as furosemide (1 mg/kg) for acute pulmonary edema or fluid overload 3. Sedatives/analgesics—morphine sulfate (0.1–0.2 mg/kg) every 1–2 h intravenously; midazolam (0.1–0.2 mg/kg every 2–4 h intravenously) 4. Muscle relaxants—vecuronium bromide, starting at 0.1 mg/kg every 1–2 h or alternative 0.1–0.2 mg/kg/h drip

CPAP, constant positive airway pressure; PEEP, positive end-expiratory pressure.

MEDICAL EMERGENCIES

ment is important to improve gas exchange (e.g., atelectasis). By increasing the end-expiratory lung volume or functional residual capacity, PEEP shifts lungs to a position on the pressure–volume curve that improves alveolar ventilation while minimizing the risk of barotrauma. In patients with decreased lung compliance due to either stiff lungs (e.g., fibrosis) or hyperinflation (e.g., bronchiolitis or asthma), higher pressures must be generated to sufficiently ventilate the child. The inspiratory:expiratory (I:E) ratio can also be tailored to the disease process. Increased I:E ratios of 1:5 to 1 should be utilized in alveolar or interstitial disorders to improve oxygenation. A normal or decreased I:E ratio is used in obstructive lower airway disease to extend exhalation time to better allow elimination of CO_2.

Although past practice aimed to achieve normocapnia, recent recommendations suggest that permissive hypercapnia may be advantageous. That is, accepting slightly elevated PCO_2 values is acceptable as long as pH is maintained. This may allow for pressure-limited ventilation, which will reduce the risk of barotrauma.

Fluid management is also a key component to tailored therapy in respiratory failure. Patients with increased work of breathing generate high negative intrathoracic pressures, which increase venous return. When these patients are intubated, the transition to positive pressure ventilation rapidly decreases venous return and may precipitate cardiovascular collapse. Therefore, unless clinical circumstances mandate more immediate action, rapid intravascular repletion prior to intubation is prudent. In contrast, for patients with interstitial disease or pulmonary capillary leak, a slightly reduced intravascular volume may improve the mechanics necessary for effective ventilation. As a result, the FIO_2 requirement may be decreased and airway pressures minimized. Beyond such circumstances, other clinical indicators should guide fluid management. In general, however, fluids should be titrated to maintain normal intravascular volume as determined by observation of heart rate, blood pressure, peripheral perfusion, and urine output. In severely ill or complex patients, the measurement of central venous pressure may provide a more precise guide for monitoring fluid status.

Sedation is also an important adjunct to efficient assisted ventilation. In neurologically depressed children, sedation may not be required. However in most circumstances, parenteral sedation is utilized to reduce anxiety and to increase tolerance to the presence of a tracheal tube and assisted ventilation. Morphine sulfate dosed 0.1 to 0.2 mg per kg every 1 to 2 hours or as a continuous infusion of 0.1 mg per kg per hour is often used. This is frequently combined with a benzodiazepine, for example, midazolam 0.1 to 0.2 mg per kg every 1 to 2 hours or as a continuous infusion. Muscle relaxants may be helpful to optimally ventilate children with severe respiratory failure. This may be necessary for children with stiff lungs (e.g., severe interstitial pneumonia) or a stiff chest wall (e.g., status epilepticus). Muscle relaxants improve chest wall compliance and reduce oxygen consumption. Vecuronium may be given initially in doses of 0.1 mg per kg every 1 to 2 hours or as a continuous infusion at 0.05 to 0.1 mg per kg per hour (see Chapter 5). Some children, particularly younger infants, will metabolize vecuronium quickly and require either more frequent dosing or a higher infusion rate, titrated to movement.

Beyond the ED, other innovative ventilatory options in respiratory failure that may reduce risk of ventilation-associated

barotrauma include use of helium–oxygen (heliox) gas mixtures, prone positioning, high-frequency oscillation, extracorporeal membrane oxygenation (ECMO), nitric oxide, and liquid ventilation. Detailed description of these critical care processes may be found in the references at the end of the chapter.

BRONCHOPULMONARY DYSPLASIA

Background

Bronchopulmonary dysplasia is a cause of chronic respiratory disease in infants and children. BPD is a clinical diagnosis, defined as the need for supplemental oxygen at a prescribed postconceptual or chronologic age, with associated radiographic findings. The specifics of these parameters have changed over time. The current definitions for graded severity of BPD as defined by the National Institute of Child Head and Human Development are presented in Table 98.4.

The etiology of BPD is thought to be multifactorial. While newer data suggest a genetic predisposition, previously defined risk factors include immaturity, supplemental oxygen therapy, positive-pressure ventilation, and inadequate nutrition. Pathophysiologically, the disease process is thought to stem from inflammation and injury to the lung, with resultant arrest of alveolar septation and impaired microvascular development. This occurs most commonly in infants with hyaline membrane disease or other acute perinatal lung disease. Infants with apnea, congenital heart disease, or other illnesses requiring prolonged ventilation in the first weeks of life are also at risk. Utilization of improved ventilation strategies, as well as antenatal glucocorticoids, surfactant, and improvement in nutrition, has improved outcomes. However, with these advances in neonatal care has also come the survival of large number of infants born at earlier gestational age and lower birthweights. As a result, the overall incidence of BPD has not changed significantly over time.

In emergency medicine, BPD becomes important because these patients may present with acute exacerbations of their

| TABLE 98.4 |

DEFINITION OF BPD FOR INFANTS BORN LESS THAN 32 WEEKS' GESTATIONAL AGE[a]

Mild	Room air at 36 weeks postmenstrual age (PMA) or discharge
Moderate	Need for <30% oxygen at 36 weeks PMA or discharge
Severe	Need for ≥30% oxygen and/or positive pressure (ventilation or CPAP) at 36 weeks PMA

BPD, bronchopulmonary dysplasia; CPAP, constant positive airway pressure.
[a]All patients with BPD require supplemental oxygen for the first 28 days of life and have characteristic findings on chest X-ray.
Adapted from Walsh MC, Szefler S, Davis J, et al. Summary proceedings from the bronchopulmonary dysplasia group. *Pediatrics* 2006;117:S52–S56.

chronic lung disease and because BPD is a risk factor for increased severity of other respiratory illnesses.

Clinical Manifestations

Signs and symptoms of patients with BPD will vary based on severity; therefore, recognizing interim worsening of disease requires an understanding of baseline examination findings and pulmonary function. This is most commonly elicited from parents although referral to findings from prior visits can also be helpful.

Children with BPD are typically tachypneic, with some degree of retractions that worsen with even mild respiratory or febrile illnesses. Findings on auscultation can include crackles, wheezes, or decreased breath sounds. Failure to thrive often results from concomitant nutritional issues, or from increased energy expenditure secondary to chronic increased work of breathing. Chest radiographs (Fig. 98.2) demonstrate varying amounts of hyperinflation; several patterns occur, including cystic areas with signs of fibrosis, which are often confused with congenital lobar emphysema, severe cystic fibrosis, or new infiltrates.

Management

Emergency physicians most often will evaluate children with BPD when their underlying disease is worsened by intercurrent acute respiratory infections. More than 50% of infants with BPD require admission within a year of their diagnosis for respiratory illness. Of particular importance is respiratory syncytial virus (RSV) infection, which typically causes bronchiolitis with fever, tachypnea, crackles, and wheezing. Patients with RSV can also present with apnea, without significant acute pulmonary change, particularly in younger infants and those with a history of prematurity. Patients with BPD who develop RSV bronchiolitis are prone to more severe courses, including higher rates of intensive care unit admission, need for mechanical ventilation, and mortality.

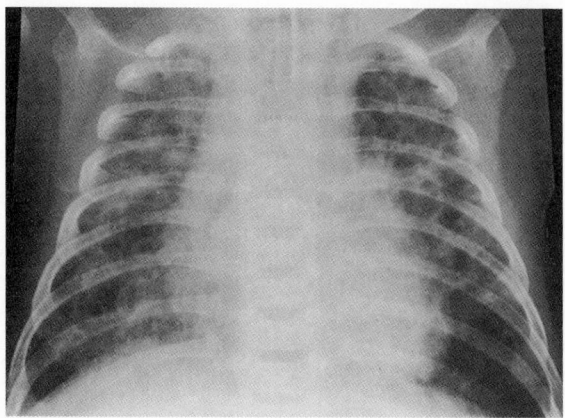

FIGURE 98.2 Bronchopulmonary dysplasia. This 2-month-old child was treated with mechanical ventilation during the first days of life for hyaline membrane disease. The chest film shows generalized overaeration and coarse nodularity with multiple cystlike areas throughout both lung fields.

Pulse oximetry can be beneficial in assessing for hypoxemia. Arterial, venous, or capillary blood gas is indicated when signs and symptoms suggest hypercapnia or when cyanosis, respiratory distress, or deterioration from baseline cannot be easily reversed. Arterial blood gas measurements may be misleading because decreases in PaO_2 may reflect hypoxia from crying or breath-holding during the painful procedure rather than worsening pulmonary function. A chest radiograph is helpful in most episodes; however, given baseline abnormalities, these often need to be compared with prior films.

Management of children with BPD and intercurrent respiratory illnesses is primarily limited to supportive care. Although some patients can be treated as outpatients, care must be taken to first assess the severity of the episode. If the acute exacerbation is mild, outpatient therapy may be indicated with frequent follow-up every 1 to 2 days. In infants with moderate to severe BPD, even mild deterioration may herald early respiratory failure. Ensuring hydration by oral or intravenous (IV) routes, addressing hypoxemia, and, when necessary, providing assisted ventilation for hypercarbia and respiratory acidosis are the mainstays of therapy.

Bronchodilators, inhaled corticosteroids, and diuretics may also be helpful. Most children with BPD have had trials of β-agonist therapy. Although the use of metered dose inhalers for β-agonists is effective in older infants with asthma, the evidence for their use in young infants with BPD is less clear. Although most acute episodes are from viral infection, antibiotic therapy should be considered when the risk of bacterial infection appears higher. Indications for admission include a respiratory rate above 70 to 80 breaths per minute or significant change from baseline, increasing hypoxia or hypercarbia, poor feeding, apnea, or new radiographic infiltrates. Parental fatigue and stress are also important factors to consider.

Prevention of BPD exacerbations is challenging. Although routine viral illnesses may not be avoidable, RSV and influenza are the leading preventable causes of rehospitalization in patients with BPD. Monoclonal antibody against RSV (palivizumab, Synagis®) has largely replaced RSV-IGIV prophylaxis in preventing or lessening disease secondary to RSV. Such immunoprophylaxis is recommended for children less than 2 years of age with BPD who have required medical therapy within 6 months of the start of RSV season. Patients with more severe BPD who continue to require medical therapy may also benefit from prophylaxis during a second RSV season, although supporting data here are limited. Influenza vaccination should also be considered each winter for children older than 6 months of age with BPD. Two doses separated by at least 1 month, ideally prior to December, are recommended for the first immunization season. After the first year, subsequent influenza vaccinations require only one dose.

INTERSTITIAL LUNG DISEASE

Background

Childhood interstitial lung disease (ILD) comprises a heterogeneous group of pulmonary disorders, characterized by diffuse infiltrates and impaired gas exchange. Although data are limited, the overall incidence is a fraction of that seen in the adult population. In addition, while the nomenclature is similar,

TABLE 98.5

CAUSES OF INTERSTITIAL LUNG DISEASE

Environmental irritants	Sarcoidosis
Inorganic dusts	Inherited disorders
Organic dusts (hypersensitivity)	Neurofibromatosis
Noxious gases	Miscellaneous causes
Drugs	Celiac disease
Radiation	Whipple's disease
Collagen vascular disease	Weber–Christian disease
Rheumatoid arthritis	Histiocytosis
Scleroderma	Hermansky–Pudiak
Systemic lupus erythematosus	syndrome

there are significant differences between pediatric and adult ILD with regard to etiology, management, and outcome.

There are numerous causes for the group of conditions that are included as ILD (Table 98.5). Either primary pulmonary diseases or systemic disorders with pulmonary involvement can be responsible. These may be inherited or may result from lung insult, for example, secondary to infection or environmental exposures. Importantly, many of the included entities are distinct to infants and young children. Therefore, adult-based classification schemes may not be fully applicable. As a result, a novel classification system based on etiology and pathology has been introduced for children. It will not be fully reviewed here but can be found in the reference at the end of the chapter.

Idiopathic interstitial pneumonias, defined by their histology, make up an important subgroup of ILD. Although similar nomenclature is used in adults and children, many of these disease processes are quite different. Usual interstitial pneumonia (UIP) is the pathologic correlate of idiopathic pulmonary fibrosis and is a relatively common cause of ILD in adults. Although defined in children, no pediatric case has described the fibroblastic foci, which are thought to be the defining histologic feature. In addition, children reported to have UIP are reported to have a nonprogressive course, different than their adult counterparts. Desquamative interstitial pneumonitis (DIP) also occurs rarely in children. Histology tends to show cellular rather than fibrotic infiltrates. In adults, smoking has been associated, whereas in children gene mutations are felt to be responsible. DIP tends to be responsive to steroids, particular in the adult population. Lymphoid interstitial pneumonia (LIP) has a lymphocytic infiltrate. In children, it is commonly associated with HIV infection, including up to 30% of perinatally transmitted disease (see Chapter 93).

Clinical Manifestations

Congenital ILD may present in infants or young children; however, the pneumonic processes are more likely to manifest in older children. Immunocompromised children are at risk at all ages. Infants may present with tachypnea or hypoxemia, while older children are more likely to complain of chronic cough or dyspnea on exertion. Patients with more severe or advanced cases will frequently have dyspnea even at rest. Systemic symptoms including weight loss, anorexia, and fatigue may also occur. Occasionally, hemoptysis or a "spontaneous" pneumothorax may be the primary clinical event. Physical findings may include tachypnea and tachycardia, often with shallow excursions and bibasilar rales. In severe cases, digital clubbing and cyanosis may be present.

Oxygen saturation or PaO_2 generally correlate with severity; initially they are reduced only during exercise but with disease progression, they eventually become compromised at rest. The $PaCO_2$ usually remains normal until late in the course. Polycythemia may be present secondary to hypoxemia in severe cases.

Management

Evaluation of patients with suspected ILD should focus on assessing for the primary etiology as well as the extent and severity of disease. A systematic approach that combines historical and examination findings with noninvasive and invasive studies is required. Because the diagnostic workup can be extensive, the child with characteristic history and physical findings will need admission to the hospital and consultation with a pediatric pulmonologist.

Laboratory evaluation is generally limited. A complete blood cell count can detect polycythemia and abnormal white blood cell differentials may suggest immunodeficiencies. Arterial blood gas may be performed to assess PaO_2 if oxygen saturation testing is felt to be inadequate. Focused testing may be performed based on specific concerns, for example, antinuclear antibody and serum immunoglobulins to detect vasculitis and genetic mutations testing, which can identify certain etiologies of ILD.

Noninvasive evaluation can include pulmonary function testing and radiologic imaging. In older children who are able to cooperate, pulmonary function testing with diffusion capacity and exercise testing generally shows a pattern of restrictive lung disease. Specifically, the forced expiratory volume in 1 second (FEV_1) and forced vital capacity (FVC) are both reduced, with a normal FEV_1:FVC ratio. Chest radiographs (Figs. 98.3 and 98.4) typically show a diffuse reticulonodular infiltrate, especially in the lower lobes. As disease progresses,

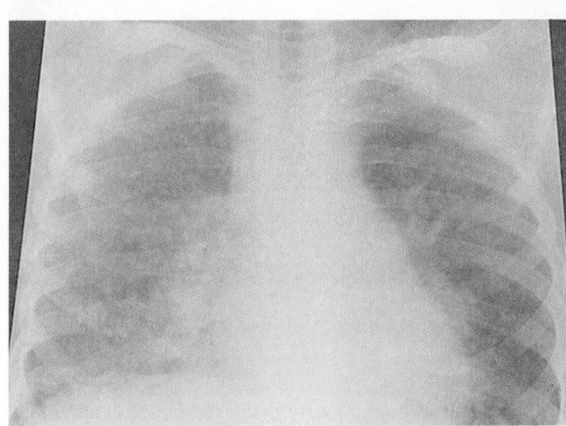

FIGURE 98.3 Sarcoid. A 9-year-old child with hepatosplenomegaly but no pulmonary complaints. The chest film shows interstitial lung disease with hilar adenopathy.

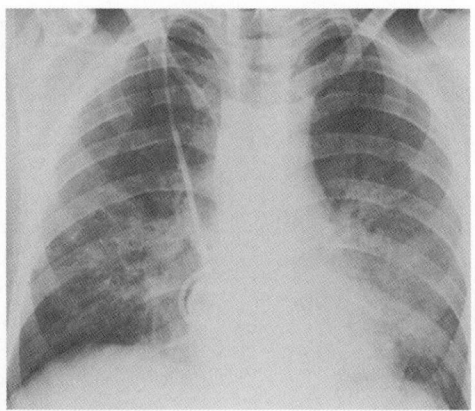

FIGURE 98.4 Idiopathic interstitial pneumonia. An 18-year-old boy with chronic granulomatous disease, after bone marrow transplant, with insidious onset of shortness of breath. The chest film shows bilateral interstitial disease in the lower lung field more on left side.

decreased lung volume and pulmonic changes may result in a cystic "honeycomb" appearance. High resolution computed tomography (HR-CT) has become the primary imaging modality for ILD. It can confirm the diagnosis, characterize findings to help identify underlying etiology, and localize areas amenable to biopsy. A method known as *controlled ventilation HR-CT* can be employed to reduce motion artifact and improve lung detail in tachypneic children.

Invasive testing employed during the evaluation of children with suspected ILD might include bronchoalveolar lavage (BAL) and lung biopsy. Bronchoscopy with BAL can identify cellular and biochemical components of alveolar-lining fluids, which may be helpful in understanding the etiology. For example, lipid-laden or hemosiderin-laden macrophages, alveolar proteinosis, and surfactant deficiency may be suggestive of select diagnoses. Similarly, staining and culture may identify infectious causes, including *Pneumocystis carinii*, in patients with possible LIP in an immunocompromised host or HIV-infected patient. Historically, there has been a reluctance to perform biopsies in children because of the associated morbidity and the low diagnostic yield. However, the acceptance of a thoracoscopic approach to biopsy coupled with better-defined ILD syndromes in children has led to increased willingness to obtain tissue from pediatric patients.

Treatment of the child with suspected or known ILD will vary based on the underlying etiology. Acutely, patients should be evaluated and treated for hypoxemia. Systemic illnesses, for example, systemic lupus erythematosus (SLE) or HIV, should be treated, and antimicrobial therapy initiated when infectious etiologies are of concern. Corticosteroids have also become a mainstay of therapy. Patients with biopsy-proven disease known to be steroid-responsive should be treated. For those who have not undergone biopsy or whose diagnosis remains unclear, an empiric trial of steroids can be considered; however, risks and benefits need to be weighed in such cases. Alternative steroid-sparing immunosuppressants have also been used with some success. Unfortunately, ILD may progress despite aggressive therapy. In such circumstances, lung transplantation may become the only viable treatment option for some patients. Outcomes for transplanted patients have been similar to those for patients with cystic fibrosis and pulmonary hypertension.

ASPIRATION PNEUMONIA

Background

Aspiration of foreign material into the lung can result in inflammation and impaired lung function. Chemical injury to lung tissue, often from sterile gastric contents, results in *aspiration pneumonitis*. Infection following inhalation of foreign material, commonly from the oropharynx, is termed *aspiration pneumonia*. Infectious pneumonia may result from aspiration of viral or bacterial pathogens, as described in Chapter 92; however, the term *aspiration pneumonia* denotes infection following inhalation of foreign material.

Two groups of patients at risk for aspiration pneumonia are those with neurological impairment and those with inadequate gastrointestinal motility. Children with altered consciousness and CNS disorders that impair normal swallowing or protective airway reflexes are at risk for aspiration. This is particularly true for chronically impaired, institutionalized children, although healthy children who are transiently depressed from procedural sedation or during seizures can also aspirate. Likewise, children with decreased esophageal or intestinal motility or delayed gastric emptying are at increased risk of regurgitation of stomach contents and therefore possible aspiration. Dysmotility may be secondary to underlying disease, trauma, or medications such as opiates or those with anticholinergic properties. Similarly, anatomic narrowing or obstruction along the gastrointestinal tract can also increase the risk of aspiration.

Pathophysiology

The pathophysiology of pulmonary disease secondary to aspiration can be classified based on the source of the foreign material. In humans, aspirate contents with a pH of less than 2.5 are considered acidic. Such material causes a severe chemical pneumonitis with direct injury to alveolar-capillary membranes. A hemorrhagic, granulocytic, necrotizing reaction generally follows. Effects from the initial injury can occur within minutes to hours, and may include reflex airway closure, destruction of surfactant resulting in atelectasis, exudation of fluid and protein across damaged membranes creating interstitial and alveolar edema, and alveolar hemorrhage and consolidation.

Aspirates with a pH greater than 2.5 are considered nonacidic. These may come from the oropharynx or from the stomach in patients on H_2 blockers or proton-pump inhibitors. The early pathophysiologic response is similar to that seen with acidic injury, with the exception of reduced alveolar neutrophilic infiltration and necrosis. The extent of lung damage from nonacid aspirates varies depending on the composition of the aspirate; clear liquid aspiration resolves quickly while sizable food particles are likely to lead to a prolonged pathologic response. Repeated aspirations occurring over an extended period may result in radiographic evidence of granuloma formation similar to that of miliary tuberculosis. Aspiration of hydrocarbons is covered separately in Chapter 102.

Most physicians agree that infection plays little role in the initial pulmonary complications that result from aspiration. However, pathogenic bacterial from the oropharynx may accompany foreign material, resulting in direct inoculation of lung tissue. Alternatively, following acid aspiration, the injured lung is vulnerable and secondary bacterial infection may occur in up to half of these cases.

For those who develop infection, two distinct patterns are possible. A localized necrotizing bacterial pneumonia, abscess, or empyema may result from a heavily infected inoculum. Although opinions vary, anaerobic organisms, either alone or as polymicrobial infection with aerobes, are likely culprits in such cases. The second pattern of infection is that which follows large aspirates, usually of the acidic type. Aerobic rather than anaerobic organisms predominate here; gram-negative organisms, such as *Pseudomonas aeruginosa*, and gram-positive organisms, such as staphylococci, may be isolated.

Clinical Manifestations

Aspiration pneumonia should be considered in any at-risk child who has signs of respiratory distress. Occasionally, an aspiration event will be witnessed or vomitus will be present in the vicinity, suggesting the possibility of this diagnosis. However, not uncommonly, particularly in cognitively compromised children, no triggering episode is witnessed.

The clinical manifestations of pneumonia are discussed in Chapter 92. With aspiration, a very brief latent period occurs before the onset of respiratory signs and symptoms, and more than 90% of patients are symptomatic within 1 hour. Fever, tachypnea, and cough are often seen. Hypoxia is common, whereas apnea and shock are less likely but possible. Sputum production is usually minimal.

The physical findings in patients with aspiration pneumonia are not dissimilar from those in patients with pulmonary infections resulting from community- or hospital-acquired bacterial or viral causes. Focal or diffuse crackles and wheezing are common. Cyanosis appears with progression or more severe disease. Chest radiographs (Figs. 98.5A and B) may show either localized or diffuse infiltrates, which may be unilateral or bilateral. The chest x-ray of a patient who has aspirated may evolve from normal to complete bilateral opacification within several hours.

Management

The suspicion of aspiration should be confirmed with a chest radiograph. Children with significant aspiration pneumonia, diagnosed either by clinical suspicion or radiograph, require admission to the hospital. Table 98.6 outlines therapeutic modalities that may be useful. Some children who aspirate may have relatively normal radiographs early in the course but significant symptomatology. Conversely, radiographs may be significantly abnormal in the face of minimal clinical symptoms in patients with aspiration of hydrocarbon or other volatile agents.

In the acute care setting, children who aspirate require primarily supportive care. Specifically, prevention of further aspiration by gastric decompression, oropharyngeal suctioning, and proper positioning should be utilized. Supplemental oxygen should be administered as needed, based on pulse oximetry or direct measurement of oxygenation with an arterial blood gas. Endotracheal intubation is indicated if airway

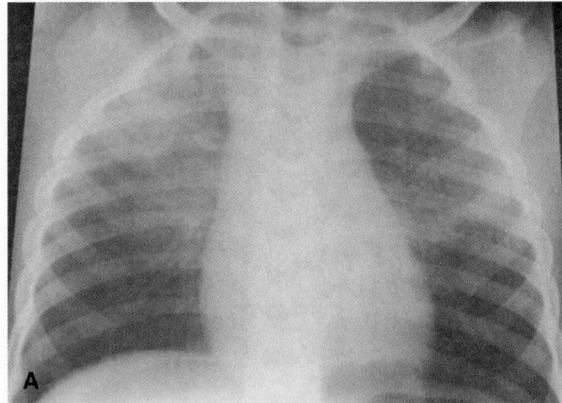

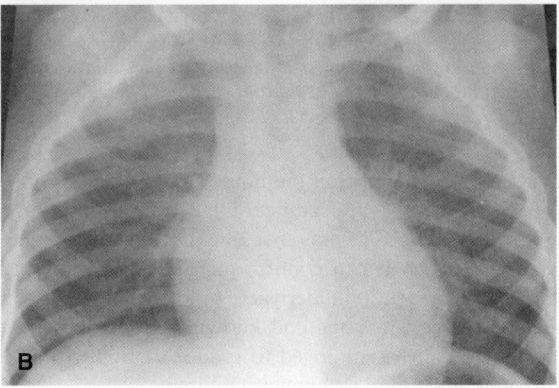

FIGURE 98.5 **A:** Blood aspiration. A 3-year-old boy with tachypnea 1 day after surgery for enlarged adenoids/tonsils. Chest film shows an infiltrate in the right upper lobe and left lower lobe. **B:** Blood aspiration (see **A**). The chest film 2 days later shows clearing of the infiltrate in the right upper lobe and left lower lobe.

reflexes are inadequate or for severe cases with impending respiratory failure.

The use of corticosteroids in the treatment of aspiration pneumonia is controversial. Because experimental evidence indicates minimal benefit at best and because the concomitant immunosupression may contribute the development of secondary bacterial pneumonia, their administration is not usually indicated in the ED.

The decision whether or not to initiate antibiotic therapy is challenging. There is no strong data to suggest that prophylactic antibiotic therapy will prevent subsequent infection in a patient with chemical pneumonitis. However, fever, purulent sputum, leukocytosis, and pulmonary infiltrates may result from chemical inflammation alone; therefore, the distinction from infectious aspiration pneumonia can be difficult. A reasonable initial approach is to defer antibiotic treatment in

TABLE 98.6

INITIAL TREATMENT OF ASPIRATION PNEUMONIA

Proven measures	Optional modalities
Suction	Corticosteroids
Airway protection	Antibiotics
Oxygen	

favor of careful observation in a well-appearing child and empirically treat only those with a tenuous respiratory status or compelling clinical evidence of infection.

For those who receive antimicrobial therapy, the choice of antibiotics can be guided by both the clinical setting and the results of properly obtained specimens for culture. Aspiration pneumonias developing outside the hospital generally involve anaerobes and are adequately treated with ampicillin or clindamycin, whereas nosocomial infections require broader aerobic and anaerobic coverage. Clindamycin with gentamicin, or ampicillin/sulbactam, are often used. In neurologically impaired children, with either aspiration or tracheostomy-associated pneumonia, antibiotics effective against penicillin-resistant anaerobic bacteria and *P. aeruginosa* have been shown to produce superior clinical and microbiologic responses.

PULMONARY EMBOLISM

Background

Pulmonary embolism (PE) is the partial or complete obstruction of the pulmonary artery or branches from detachment of all or part of a thrombosis from within the systemic venous system. In adults, it contributes to significant morbidity and mortality, with reported incidence of 2% to 5% of the population and up to 300,000 deaths per year. The epidemiology in children is less well defined because of limited available pediatric data, although one series reports an incidence of 0.7 per 10,000 children. This is likely an underestimate, however, as newer diagnostic modalities are increasingly recognizing subclinical disease. In addition, improved survival of children with illnesses and injuries that predispose to PE may also be leading to increased risk of thomboembolic events.

Children with PE very commonly have underlying medical conditions that predispose them to thromboembolic events. Central venous catheters have been identified as the most common precipitant for PE in pediatric patients. Other underlying conditions include malignancy, congenital heart disease, collagen vascular disease, significant trauma/surgery, and severe infection/sepsis. Available data suggest that more than 90% of children diagnosed with PE will have at least one of these risk factors. In addition, a minority of children with PE will be diagnosed with a congenital prothrombotic condition, although data estimating the risk of thrombophilia are varied. Traditional "adult" risk factors, including oral contraceptives, elective abortion, prolonged immobilization, IV drug use, rheumatic heart disease, smoking, and obesity, may also play a role in some older pediatric patients.

Pathophysiology

Virchow identified stasis, venous injury, and hypercoagulabilty as the three factors that contribute to thrombogenesis. A combination of environmental and genetic factors may contribute to each of these. One potential complication of such thromboses is the embolization of all or part of the clot into the pulmonary vasculature. The degree of anatomic obstruction of the arterial vessel will dictate the degree of hemodynamic compromise. Increases in right-sided afterload can lead to pulmonary hypertension or, with comcomitant reductions in left-sided cardiac output, can result in cardiovascular collapse, particularly in patients with preexisting heart or lung disease. In addition to direct vascular obstruction from PE, release of vasoactive and bronchoconstrictive cytokines may also lead to further V̇/Q̇ mismatching and intrapulmonary shunting, which may contribute to the hyoxemia seen in more than 80% of cases.

Clinical Manifestations

The challenge in recognizing PE in children stems from the relative infrequency of the condition coupled with the nonspecific signs and symptoms in most patients (Table 98.7). While the presentation of massive PE with severe circulatory compromise in a patient at high risk may be easily recognized, making the diagnosis in a patient with common respiratory complaints may not. Dyspnea, pleuritic chest pain, cough, and hemoptysis are the most common symptoms of PE in both adults and children; however, children with these symptoms are much more likely to have alternative diagnoses. Less frequent symptoms such as apprehension, fever, sweats, and palpitations are similarly nonspecific. Current literature suggests that 25% of adults with PE will be asymptomatic, which further complicates recognition. The extent of asymptomatic disease in children has not been similarly reported; however, this may reflect different methodologies in available pediatric registries and studies, which have not screened for subclinical disease in pediatric populations.

Physical examination findings are often absent with PE. Tachycardia, rales, and tachypnea are the most common signs in those with findings, although again each is nondiscriminating. Significant vascular obstruction that results in pulmonary hypertension may lead to distended neck veins, a prominent S$_2$, or a ventricular gallop. Similarly, in cases where embolism results in large pulmonary infarction, there may be decreased resonance over the lung fields and a pleural friction rub. Breath sounds may be distant or absent, and crackles may be heard. The presence of hypoxemia not clearly explained by an underlying disease process or clinical state may also suggest the possibility of PE.

To help quantify the risk of PE, clinical prediction scores that combine historical risk factors with physical findings have been created. Both the Wells criteria and the Geneva score have been shown to be useful in categorizing pretest probability for PE in adults and have been integrated into management schemes, as described below.

To supplement an initial assessment based on the history, physical examination, and possible risk factors, additional studies may help qualify the likelihood of PE.

An electrocardiogram (EKG) should be obtained; although similar to history and examination findings, abnormalities are rare and, when present, are nonspecific (Table 98.7). Sinus tachycardia is the most common but least specific finding. Conversely, right axis deviation, right bundle branch block, and the classic "S1, Q3, T3" are all consistent with cor pulmonale, which is usually seen only with massive PE but may also occur in nonembolic disease including pneumothorax.

Arterial blood gases will commonly indicate hypoxemia with a reduced partial pressure of oxygen, which may be

MEDICAL EMERGENCIES

TABLE 98.7

CLINICAL MANIFESTATION OF PULMONARY EMBOLISM

	Nonspecific	Suggestive	Diagnostic
Symptoms	Syncope	Dyspnea out of proportion to degree of abnormal findings	
	Sweating	Hemoptysis	
	Pleuritic pain		
	Dyspnea		
	Cough		
	Apprehension		
Signs	Tachypnea	Pleural friction rub	
	Tachycardia	Unexplained cyanosis	
	Distant or absent breath sounds	Accentuated S_2	
	Crackles		
	Fever		
Laboratory/radiography findings	Decreased PaO_2	Wedged infiltrate with ipsilateral elevated hemidiaphragm	CT angiography
		Abnormal ventilation-perfusion scan	Abnormal pulmonary angiography
EKG abnormalities	Right axis deviation	S_1-Q_3-T_3 pattern	
	ST-T wave changes		
	Right bundle branch block		

EKG, electrocardiogram.

supportive but nondiagnostic of PE. In addition, because 15% of patients will have a PaO_2 greater than 80 mm Hg and 5% of patients greater than 90 mm Hg, the negative predictive value of a normal gas may not justify the use of this painful and occasionally difficult procedure in the diagnostic evaluation in children.

The laboratory study, which has traditionally played the most significant role in the evaluation of adult patients with suspected PE, is the D-dimer. Measurement of degradation products produced when plasmin splits cross-linked fibrin is a sensitive marker for intravascular clot. Such biomarkers will be positive as early as 1 hour after thrombus formation, with a circulating half-life of 4 to 6 hours. However, with continued PE fibrinolysis, plasma D-dimer levels are commonly elevated for at least 1 week. Many different enzyme-linked immunosorbent assays (ELISAs) are available to detect D-dimers in the circulation. Newer-generation assays have reported sensitivities of 96% to 98% and reasonable turnaround times. Nonetheless, because of the presence of wide variability in performance of each assay, it is important for practitioners to be aware of the characteristics within their laboratory when incorporating results into their medical decision making. The applicability of D-dimer testing to evaluation and management of pediatric patients with suspected PE is discussed below. Radiographic studies are an important part of the evaluation of patients with possible PE. Chest radiographs are recommended because they are relatively noninvasive although they are rarely diagnostic. The presence of a segmental pulmonary infiltrate with an ipsilateral elevated hemidiaphragm is suggestive of a PE; however, even these radiographic findings are not pathognomonic. Occasionally, however, chest films will uncover an alternative diagnosis for a patient's symptoms, obviating the need for further evaluation in low-risk patients.

For years, $\dot{V}/\dot{Q}$ scans were the mainstay of imaging in patients with concern for PE. For patients without preexisting cardiopulmonary disease, some $\dot{V}/\dot{Q}$ studies can effectively rule in or out the diagnosis. A characteristic pattern of normal ventilation in a poorly perfused area of lung is considered high probability and effectively establishes the diagnosis of PE. Similarly, a normal $\dot{V}/\dot{Q}$ scan essentially excludes the diagnosis. However, many patients have underlying structural lung disease or the scans are reported as low or intermediate probability, making results nondiagnostic. In fact, the majority of patients ultimately diagnosed with embolic disease are classified as low or intermediate rather than high probability, based on $\dot{V}/\dot{Q}$ scanning alone.

In recent years, computed tomography angiography (CTA) has become the most common imaging modality for diagnosis of PE. Compared with $\dot{V}/\dot{Q}$ scanning, it is more rapid, more readily available, and has the advantage of characterizing nonvascular structures as well. Utilizing pulmonary angiography as the diagnostic standard, initial adult studies investigating the utility of spiral CT scanning reported sensitivities of 64% to 93% and specificities of 89% to 100%. The test performance in more recently available multidetector scanners is likely even higher. Still, CTA is likely less sensitive for emboli beyond main, lobar, or segmental pulmonary arteries. Therefore, at present, a negative scan cannot absolutely rule out PE, especially in any patient considered to be at high risk.

Management

Utilizing available data from history and physical examination, as well as adjunctive testing modalities described above, forms the basis for decision making regarding management of patients with suspected PE. The challenge is to accurately and rapidly identify the minority of presenting patients with the disease from the multitude without PE who present with overlapping nonspecific complaints and findings. Toward these ends, algorithms for adult patients have suggested a dichotomous approach.

Patients deemed to have low pretest probability by Wells criteria or Geneva scores and a negative D-dimer are felt to have a low likelihood of PE and, therefore, may not need further evaluation. This may exempt one-third of presenting adult patients from requiring additional workup and has been shown to have a negative predictive value of 99% in select populations. Patients with high pretest probability or an abnormal D-dimer should have additional imaging performed. On the basis of this protocol, a negative CTA in these patients was found to have an observed risk of missed diagnosis nearly identical to that identified by pulmonary arteriography (less than 2%).

There are a number of differences in PE in children and adults; and therefore, utilizing a similar evaluative approach in children may not be straightforward. While the Wells criteria and Geneva scores may accurately stratify adult patients into risk categories, this may not be true for children. Risk factors in these assessments include age more than 65 years and heart rate more than 100 beats per minute, which are clearly less applicable in pediatrics. In addition, the majority of emboli in children originate in the upper venous system as a result of central venous catheters, which differs dramatically from adults where more than 75% of clots originate in the legs and pelvis, suggesting the need for different weighting for risk factors in children than in adults. In fact, all children in whom PE is being entertained as a diagnosis might need to be considered high risk. Therefore, the prospect of linking pretest probability screening with D-dimer results as an initial screen may not be applicable, as a negative D-dimer in a patient who cannot be considered low risk may still not reliably exclude the possibility of PE. More data are needed before this or any other evaluative algorithm can be used safely in children. Nonetheless, the concept of utilizing available information from multiple sources to determine probability of disease in children is important. When clinical suspicion is low, and all the aforementioned tests are normal and the patient's clinical condition permits, the patient may be discharged with close follow-up. If abnormalities are uncovered, further diagnostic workup (e.g., additional imaging studies such as magnetic resonance angiography/venography (MRA/MRV) or pulmonary arteriography) and admission to the hospital should be considered. Regardless of the results, if the clinical suspicion is high, the patient should be admitted for initiation of definitive treatment.

Initial therapy for patients with presumed or proven PE includes supplemental oxygen, achievement of vascular access, and ventilatory support as indicated. Anticoagulation remains the mainstay of definitive therapy for PE because its onset of action is immediate and it is rapidly metabolized. Although unfractionated heparin has been the traditional approach, low-molecular-weight heparin (LMWH) may be advantageous. It has more predictable dosing and requires minimal monitoring, which is particularly important in children in whom phlebotomy may be challenging and painful. In addition, LMWH has a reduced risk of heparin-induced thrombocytopenia.

Heparin therapy is recommended for a minimum of 5 days. Longer-term anticoagulation can be accomplished either with continuation of LMWH or with oral anticoagulation with warfarin. Oral anticoagulation may be initiated either at the time of initial treatment with heparin or 1 to 2 days thereafter (Table 98.8). The required daily dose varies, depending on concomitant medical illness and other drug ingestion. The dose is adjusted to maintain the INR at 2.0 to 3.0. Anticoagulant therapy is usually continued for 3 to 6 months beyond the time of diagnosis.

For the rare massive PE with hemodynamic compromise, fluid and inotropic support as well as immediate anticoagulation are the mainstays of therapy. Thombolytic therapy may prove helpful in cases of cardiogenic shock; however, the risk of intracranial or other life-threatening hemorrhage is not insignificant and the clinical utility in children is unknown (Fig. 98.6).

MEDICAL EMERGENCIES

TABLE 98.8

TREATMENT FOR FIRST-TIME DVT/PE IN CHILDREN

	First line	Therapeutic goal	Duration	Notes
Immediate Therapy	IV heparin	aPTT corresponding to anti-Factor Xa level 0.3–0.7 U/mL	5–10 days	Longer duration recommended for massive PE or extensive DVT
	Alternatively: LMWH	Anti-Factor Xa level 0.5–1.0 U/mL	5–10 days	
Ongoing Therapy	Warfarin	INR 2.5 (2.0–3.0)	3–6 mo	Minimum 6 mo if thromboembolic event is idiopathic.
	Alternatively: LMWH	Anti-Factor Xa level 0.5–1.0 U/mL	3–6 mo	For CVL-related DVT, following initial 3 mo therapy, continuation of low-dose anticoagulation (INR 1.5–1.8 or anti-Factor Xa levels 0.1–0.3) until catheter is removed

DVT, deep vein thrombosis; PE, pulmonary embolism; IV, intravenous; aPTT, activated partial thromboplastin time; LMWH, low-molecular-weight heparin; INR, international normalized ratio; CVL, central venous line.
Adapted from Monagle P, Michelson AD, Bovill E, et al. Antithrombotic therapy in children. *Chest* 2001;119:344–370.

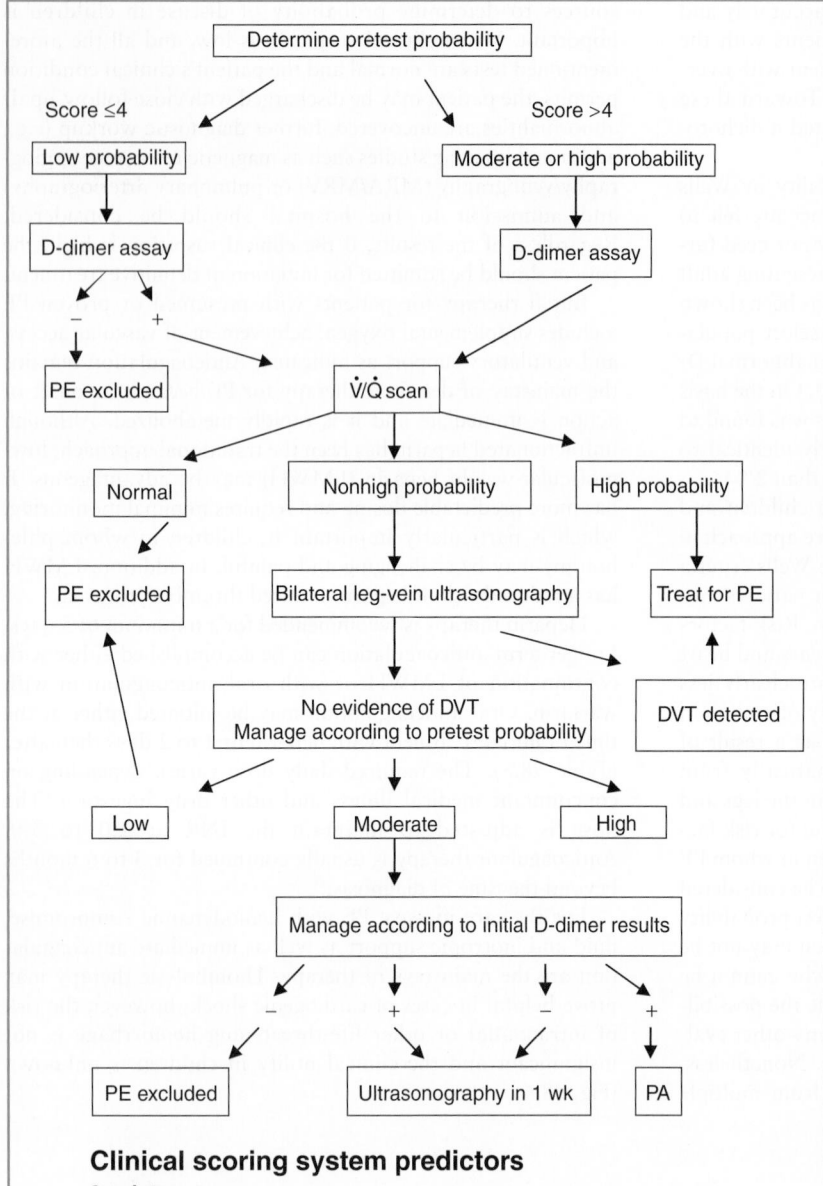

Clinical scoring system predictors

3 points

- Clinical signs of leg DVT
- Pulmonary embolism most likely diagnosis, based on clinical impression + evaluation of EKG and chest X-ray

1.5 points
- Heart rate > 100 bpm
- Immobilization for >3 day
- Surgery within previous 4 wk
- Previous objectively diagnosed PE/DVT

1 point
- Malignancy: patient with cancer who is receiving treatment, or treatment stopped within 6 months, or receiving palliative care
- Hemoptysis

FIGURE 98.6 Management scheme for suspected PE. PE, pulmonary embolism; V̇/Q̇, ventilation-perfusion; DVT, deep vein thrombosis; PA, pulmonary angiography; EKG, electrocardiogram; bpm, beats per minute. *Note:* This is an updated version of Wells' predictor, presented by the author on May 19, 2002, at a panel discussion in St. Louis during the annual meeting of the Society for Academic Emergency Medicine. The algorithm remains the same as when published in 1998. (From Wells PS, Ginsberg JS, Anderson DR, et al. Use of a chemical model for safe management of patients with suspected pulmonary embolism. *Ann Intern Med* 1998;129:997–1005.)

PULMONARY EDEMA

Background

Pulmonary edema refers to the abnormal accumulation of fluid within the alveolar spaces and bronchioles. In the healthy lung, intravascular and interstitial hydrostatic and plasma oncotic pressures are relatively balanced, resulting in minimal fluid flux into the interstitium and alveoli. However, alterations in these pressures or changes in permeability of fluid-exchanging membranes in the lungs can lead to pulmonary edema.

The differentiation between cardiogenic pulmonary edema, which results from increases in pulmonary capillary hydrostatic pressure and noncardiogenic edema, originates from the adult population where coronary artery disease and resultant pump failure are highly prevalent. In pediatrics, because the etiologies are more varied, it is more effective to categorize the disease by the underlying pathophysiology.

Pathophysiology

Pulmonary edema can result from increased pulmonary vascular hydrostatic pressures. In adults, this most commonly results from left-sided heart failure. In children, this can be secondary to congenital cardiac abnormalities such as hypoplastic left heart syndrome, cor triatriatum, mitral stenosis, severe aortic stenosis, coarctation of the aorta, or acquired myocardial disease. Overcirculation within the pulmonary vasculature secondary to left-to-right vascular shunting is seen in patent ductus arteriosus, ventricular septal defects, and iatrogenic cardiac shunts. These processes increase pulmonary vascular blood flow and can also lead to pulmonary edema. Beyond cardiac disease, increased hydrostatic pressures from overaggressive administration of IV fluids can be causative.

Intracranial pathology or insult can result in neurogenic pulmonary edema. This can be seen with seizure activity or increased intracranial pressure. Although the mechanism is not entirely understood, it likely results also from increased capillary hydrostatic pressures. Experimental evidence supports an acute sympathetic discharge in these patients. The increase in sympathetic tone leads to profound generalized vasoconstriction with increased venous return and simultaneous pulmonary vasoconstriction. The resultant surge in the pulmonary-capillary pressure can lead to pulmonary edema. The possibility of concomitant capillary leak in neurogenic pulmonary edema has also been proposed.

Decreased plasma oncotic pressure is also associated with pulmonary edema. This condition is seen with lowered levels of circulating plasma proteins, such as occurs with nephrosis, protein-losing enteropathies, massive burns, and severe malnutrition.

Any breakdown in the alveolar-capillary barrier can result in accumulation of protein-rich fluid in the interstitium. This is the major and initial manifestation of ARDS. Lung insult leads to targeting of pulmonary vasculature by inflammatory cells, with resultant tissue destruction from chemical mediators such as prostaglandins, histamine, and bradykinin. The damaged endothelial and epithelial cells create increased permeability of the alveolar-capillary membrane.

In addition to ARDS, a variety of other clinical conditions can similarly lead to capillary leak syndromes. Circulating toxins, such as snake venom and endotoxins from gram-negative sepsis, are examples. In addition, altered permeability is the most common pathophysiology behind pulmonary edema from asthma, hypersensitivity pneumonitis, Goodpasture's syndrome, and systemic lupus erythematosus. Inhaled environmental exposures can have a similar effect. Noxious gases from fires, hydrocarbons, oxides from sulfur and nitrogen, and inhalation of some herbicides (e.g., paraquat) can denature proteins and cause cellular damage with development of pulmonary edema.

Postobstructive pulmonary edema, also known as *negative-pressure pulmonary edema*, is associated with upper airway obstruction (Figs. 98.7A, B, and C). It is thought to result from exaggeration of the transmural pulmonary vascular hydrostatic pressure gradient. The highly negative pleural pressures that accompany upper airway obstruction lead to increased venous return, which increases pulmonary vascular volume and may impair cardiac output. In addition, the negative pressures cause highly negative pulmonary interstitial pressures. All of these mechanisms can contribute to transudation of fluid across pulmonary capillaries.

Finally, pulmonary edema can result from travel to high altitudes. This characteristically affects young people who are exposed to altitudes above 2,700 m. It generally occurs soon after arrival and can occur in those who are new to such elevations or those who have returned from time spent nearer to sea level. Although the precise mechanism is unclear, cardiac catheterizations have suggested that the cause is not related to increased hydrostatic pressures.

Clinical Manifestations

The onset of pulmonary edema is variable depending on etiology but can occur rapidly (i.e., flash pulmonary edema). Cough is the most common symptom and may produce frothy, pink-tinged sputum. Patients may also endorse dyspnea, shortness of breath, orthopnea, and chest pain. On physical examination, the child may appear pale or cyanotic and frequently has a rapid pulse. Tachypnea is almost universally present. Grunting often occurs in an effort to stent open small airways and airspaces and prevent lung collapse. Auscultatory findings include decreased breath sounds and moist crackles, particularly at the bases; however, these are often absent with small amounts of edema. Indeed, physical examination and radiographic findings may not manifest until the interstitial and extravascular fluid has doubled or tripled in volume.

Chest radiographs are often diagnostic, although findings may lag behind the acute clinical process. Lymphatic and interstitial fluid accumulations may be visible as Kerley A and B lines (septal lines; Fig. 98.8). These lines represent interstitial edema, tangential to the radiograph beam. The B lines, which lie in the periphery, are often the first findings. Unlike blood vessels, these radiopacities will reach the lung edge. As edema progresses, Kerley A lines near the hilum may occur, and ultimately, a butterfly pattern with a central predominance of shadows can be seen. Although these findings are not specific, transient changes in an appropriate clinical context usually signify edema.

MEDICAL EMERGENCIES

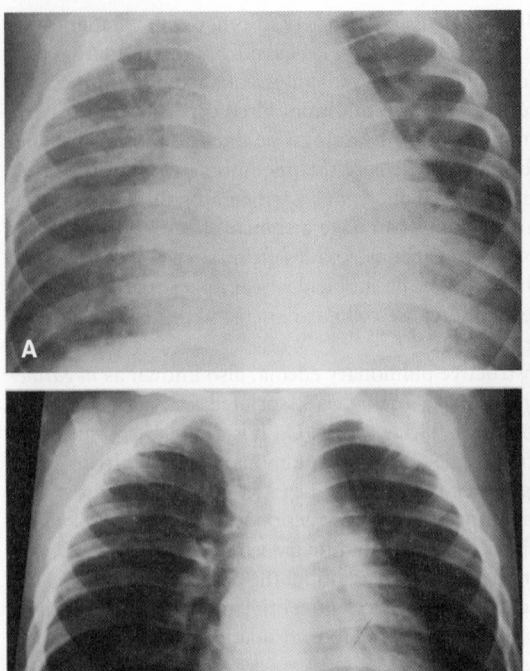

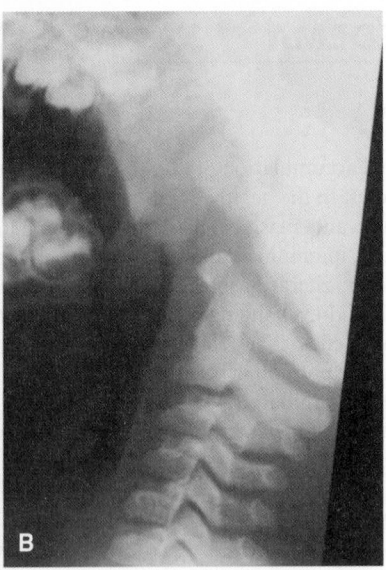

FIGURE 98.7 Cor pulmonale secondary to upper airway obstruction. **A:** This is a 2-year-old boy with tachypnea and dyspnea. The chest film shows a large heart and mild interstitial edema. **B:** The lateral view of the neck shows obstructing enlarged adenoids and tonsils. **C:** The chest film 2 days after adenoidectomy shows a decreased heart size and improvement in interstitial edema.

The distribution, symmetry, and extent of radiographic findings may also provide helpful information regarding possible etiology and severity of edema. Patterns of radiographic findings in particular can be helpful in identifying underlying cause. Cardiac size and increased prominence of pulmonary vasculature may suggest increased hydrostatic pressure or cardiogenic edema. Conversely, presence of air bronchograms,

peribronchial cuffing, and increased lung volume may suggest primary lung injury with resultant capillary leak.

It should be kept in mind that if pulmonary edema is superimposed on another pulmonary process, the clinical and radiographic findings may be obscured by those of the primary illness. Similarly, once pulmonary edema is severe enough, it may be difficult to separate edema, atelectasis, and inflammation on the chest film.

Management

The management of patients with pulmonary edema includes supportive therapies and correction of the underlying disorder. Initial efforts (Table 98.9) should be directed toward correction of hypoxemia through the administration of supplemental oxygen. In addition to satisfying the patient's oxygen demands,

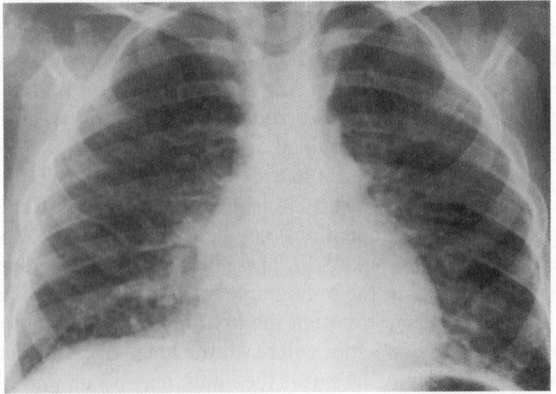

FIGURE 98.8 Interstitial fluid from volume overload. This is a 2-year-old child with paraspinal sarcoma removed 6 months earlier. Before chest radiation, he received a large fluid load. The chest film shows interstitial edema with Kerley's lines and small pleural effusions.

TABLE 98.9

TREATMENT OF PULMONARY EDEMA

Oxygen	Afterload reduction
Diuresis	Morphine 0.1 mg/kg IV
Furosemide 1 mg/kg IV	Digitalis (see Table 82.7, for dosage)

IV, intravenous.

reversal of hypoxemia is often useful in relieving chest pain and is important to the metabolism of vasoactive mediators that affect microvascular permeability.

In severe cases, CPAP or mechanical ventilation may be warranted. Assisted ventilation has several beneficial effects for patients with pulmonary edema. It reduces oxygen consumption by decreasing work of breathing. Oxygenation is also improved through prevention of alveolar collapse. In addition, positive intrathoracic pressures decreases pulmonary vascular volume and reduced fluid filtration in the lung.

In healthy lungs, there is a small fluid flux from pulmonary capillaries into the interstitium. This fluid is actively drained by a sodium transporter in the alveolar epithelium and reenters the vascular system as lymph. This process can be actively enhanced and alveolar fluid clearance augmented with β-adrenergic agonists, which may be utilized in some clinical circumstances.

Other therapeutic measures should be tailored to fit the patient's underlying disease process. When ventricular failure is the cause of pulmonary edema, diuretics can be used to decrease plasma volume, and inotropes can improve contractility. Morphine helps physiologically by dilating the venous system and may also relieve anxiety and dyspnea. Afterload reducers such as milrinone may also be helpful.

When decreased plasma oncotic pressure is primary, administration of colloid such as albumin is indicated. Slow infusion and concomitant diuretic use will help minimize resultant increases in pulmonary vascular pressure.

The management of ARDS is beyond the scope of this chapter. Management is focused on addressing underlying illness and supportive ventilatory strategies. Clinical studies have shown that the use of systemic steroids does not improve outcome and may in fact increase the incidence of secondary infections and subsequent mortality.

PULMONARY HEMORRHAGE

Background

Pulmonary hemorrhage, or bleeding into the lung, manifests clinically with hemoptysis. Although relatively uncommon, this can be dramatic and life-threatening. Therefore, early evaluation and treatment is paramount.

The incidence of pulmonary hemorrhage is difficult to ascertain. Underreporting is probably uncommon, given that children with hemoptysis are unlikely to forego medical evaluation. However, the relative frequency of causative etiologies will vary significantly by the population being evaluated, making estimation of incidence of disease difficult.

Table 98.10 provides a differential diagnosis for pulmonary hemorrhage by category. The initial supportive management for the hemoptysizing patient will be similar regardless of etiology; however, subsequent management is tailored to the underlying disease process. Therefore, evaluative efforts are aimed at identifying a specific diagnosis whenever possible.

Clinical Manifestations

Hemoptysis is the most common presentation of pulmonary hemorrhage. It may be necessary to distinguish this from hematemesis or blood from the nose, tonsils, or upper airway. Findings may be mild with blood-streaked sputum, or patients may present with massive blood loss. Hypoxia and shortness of breath sometimes occur. Apprehension is not uncommon in these children as dyspnea is compounded by the visualization of loss of blood. Children with recurrent intrapulmonary

TABLE 98.10

CAUSES OF PULMONARY HEMORRHAGE IN CHILDREN

Primary	Associated with other organ dysfunction	Secondary	Airways	Parenchymal	Nonlung sources
Cow's milk allergy Hiener's syndrome	Goodpasture's	Congestive heart failure	Bronchitis	Trauma (including nonaccidental)	Hematemesis/GI bleeding
Idiopathic pulmonary hemosiderosis	Wegener's granulomatosis	Pulmonary hypertension	Bronchiectasis/cystic fibrosis	Infection— tuberculosis, other	Nasal or tonsillar bleeding
Acute idiopathic pulmonary hemorrhage (AIPH) among infants	Henoch–Schönlein purpura	Clotting disorders	Airway anomalies	Infarction	Factitious hemoptysis
	Systemic lupus erythematosus (SLE) and collagen vascular disease	Malignancy	Vascular anomalies, (hemangioma and arteriovascular malformation (AVM's))	Neoplasm	
		Alveolar injury (e.g., drugs, radiation, smoke, acid aspiration)	Foreign body	Cavitary lesion	

Modified from Boat TF. Pulmonary hemorrhage and hemoptysis. In: Chernick V, Boat TF, eds. *Kendig's disorders of the respiratory tract in children*, 6th ed. Philadelphia, PA: WB Saunders, 1998:624.

bleeding are more likely to be anemic. As a result, they may also present with fatigue and poor weight gain.

Examination findings are often nonspecific and include: tachypnea, tachycardia, and hypoxia. Crackles may be appreciated over the affected area, although isolating the location of the bleeding by auscultation is rare. For older patients, identifying the affected area may be best accomplished by asking the patient where they feel changes. Other signs on examination may be helpful in elucidating an underlying diagnosis, such as abnormal cardiac sounds with heart failure, rash or joint involvement with collagen vascular disease, or external signs of thoracic injury in trauma patients. Cardiorespiratory decompensation can occur in children with severe anemia or shock from severe hemorrhage.

Characteristic laboratory findings include a microcytic, hypochromic anemia in patients with recurrent hemorrhage. Elevated reticulocytes may be present except in hyperacute cases and if not suppressed by underlying disease or reduced iron stores. Chronically affected patients may develop secondary restrictive lung with subsequent retention of CO_2. Additional laboratory findings will vary based on underlying disease, such as eosinophilia with immune-mediated disease or elevated inflammatory markers with vasculidities. Coagulation and hematologic studies will be abnormal in patients with bleeding diatheses.

Radiographs (Fig. 98.9) will vary depending on etiology. Alveolar infiltrates may be transient localized processes or diffuse and chronic. In idiopathic pulmonary hemosiderosis, diffuse alveolar changes are usually symmetric and spare the apices and costophrenic angles.

Because most children swallow their sputum, a presumptive diagnosis can be made by finding hemosiderin-laden macrophages in nasogastric washings; these macrophages will stain blue with the Prussian blue reaction. More definitive diagnosis, however, requires bronchoscopy and BAL. Finding similar macrophages from BAL is diagnostic, and direct visualization of the airways provides an opportunity to potentially localize the site and assess the activity of bleeding. Lung biopsy is required only for patients with recurrent bleeding in whom no diagnosis can be made on a clinical basis and alternative systemic diseases cannot be excluded.

Pulmonary function testing may reveal an obstructive pattern secondary to bronchial irritation from blood. Chronically, however, patients with systemic disease frequently develop scarring and fibrosis and may develop a restrictive or mixed pattern.

Management

Immediate management of any patient with presumed pulmonary hemorrhage is supportive. Supplemental oxygen to correct hypoxia and intravascular volume repletion should be initiated. For those with chronic disease or large acute blood losses with resultant anemia, anticipating the need for blood transfusions is important. Occasionally, pulmonary hemorrhage is so severe that it causes respiratory insufficiency or hypotension. Aggressive fluid resuscitation followed by positive-pressure ventilation with PEEP is the preferred treatment in this situation. In these severe cases, platelets and fresh-frozen plasma can also provide volume replacement and help with hemostasis.

Bronchoscopy can be diagnostically useful, usually to determine infectious causes rather than to localize a source of bleeding and control it, which is unusual. Occasionally, for brisk bleeding in a patient with a known or likely source, such as in bronchiectasis from cystic fibrosis or a known vascular malformation, embolization of vessels may be employed to rapidly stop the hemorrhage.

Additional treatment is tailored to the underlying etiology of disease. In allergic, vasculitic, and idiopathic hemorrhage, the administration of methylprednisolone (2 mg per kg per day IV divided in three to four divided doses) is indicated. When hemorrhage is caused by infection, especially tuberculosis, antimicrobial therapy should be instituted and steroids avoided. Admission is necessary until the cause of the bleeding has been determined and the hemorrhage has been controlled.

PLEURITIS

Background

Pleuritis or *pleurisy* refers to inflammation of the pleural membranes, resulting from primary pleural, adjacent pneumonic, or systemic disease. This inflammation may be associated with minimal or considerable accumulation of fluid in the pleural space. Specific references to the incidence of pleural effusions in various respiratory infections are made in Chapter 92, and the surgical approach to pleural effusions is reviewed in Chapter 128.

There exist a wide spectrum of illnesses and injuries that lead to pleural inflammation (Table 98.11). Infectious etiologies are most common and may include viruses (e.g., Coxsackie virus, Epstein-Barr virus, herpes zoster), mycoplasma, bacteria (e.g., *Staphylococcus aureus*, *Streptococcus pneumoniae*, *Haemophilus influenzae*, group A streptococcus, *Mycobacterium tuberculosis*), and fungi (e.g., histoplasmosis, coccidioidomycosis). Infections from pulmonary, subdiaphragmatic, or more distant sites may all eventually involve the pleura.

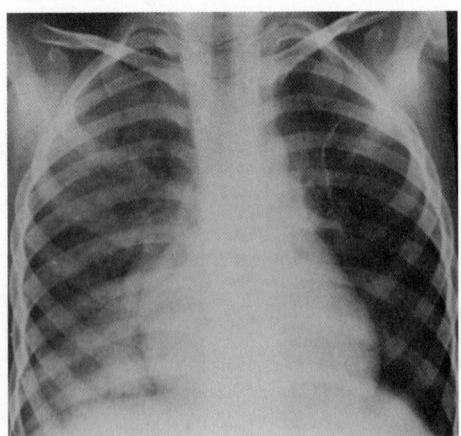

FIGURE 98.9 Idiopathic pulmonary hemosiderosis. A 5-year-old child with repeated bouts of pulmonary hemorrhage. The chest film shows diffuse radiopacities throughout both lungs (more on right side), with a well-defined alveolar opacity in the right lower lobe. Note the surgical sutures in left upper lobe.

TABLE 98.11

DIFFERENTIAL DIAGNOSIS OF PLEURAL EFFUSION

Transudative Pleural Effusions
Congestive heart failure
Cirrhosis
Nephrotic syndrome
Acute glomerulonephritis
Myxedema
Peritoneal dialysis
Hypoproteinemia
Meigs' syndrome
Sarcoidosis
Vascular obstruction
Ex vacuo effusion

Exudative Pleural Effusions
Infectious diseases
   Tuberculosis
   Bacterial infections
   Viral infections
   Fungal infections
   Parasitic infections
Neoplastic diseases
   Mesotheliomas
   Metastatic disease
Collagen vascular diseases
   Systemic lupus erythematosus
   Rheumatoid pleuritis
Pulmonary infarction/embolization
Gastrointestinal diseases
   Pancreatitis
   Esophageal rupture
   Subphrenic abscess
   Hepatic abscess
   Whipple's disease
   Diaphragmatic hernia
   Peritonitis
Trauma
   Hemothorax
   Chylothorax
Drug hypersensitivity
   Nitrofurantoin
   Methysergide
Miscellaneous diseases
   Asbestos exposure
   Pulmonary and lymph node myomatosis
   Uremia
   Postmyocardial infarction syndrome
   Trapped lung
   Congenital abnormalities of the lymphatics
   Postradiation therapy
   Drug reactions

From Light RW. Pleural effusions. *Med Clin North Am* 1977;61:
1339–1352. (See text for transudate/exudate criteria.)

Neoplastic involvement may also be primary or metastatic. When oncologic lesions obstruct the lymphatic drainage, accumulation of pleural fluid can occur. PE may cause pleural inflammation with or without effusion as a result of focal parenchymal necrosis. Trauma, both accidental and following diagnostic and therapeutic procedures in the chest, can irritate the pleura and lead to secondary infection. Pleuritis with or without effusion is seen in more than half of patients who have a systemic vasculitis such as systemic lupus erythematosus or sarcoidosis.

Pathophysiology

The pleura is a double-layered, thin membrane that separates the lung from the chest wall, diaphragm, and mediastinum. The outer parietal pleura is adherent to the chest wall, and the inner visceral pleura completely covers the lungs except at the hili. In the healthy child, the two layers of pleura are apposed, separated by only a thin physiologic layer of serous fluid. This pleural fluid is constantly being turned over, entering from the parietal pleura and exiting via the lymphatics and vasculature of the visceral pleura.

Abnormal pleural fluid accumulation can result from changes in hydrostatic or oncotic pressures or diseases of the pleural surface that alter capillary permeability or affect lymphatic reabsorption. The underlying pathophysiology will determine if an effusion will be transudative or exudative. Transudates occur as a consequence of increased capillary hydrostatic pressure such as congestive heart failure or decreased oncotic pressure such as hypoproteinemic states. Exudates result from diseases of the pleural surface that produce increased capillary permeability or lymphatic obstruction, such as pleural infection or tumor.

The determination of the nature of pleural fluid may be helpful from a diagnostic perspective (Table 98.11). Light's criteria for classifying pleural fluid is the most reliable for distinguishing exudative from transudative effusions. These criteria include a pleural fluid:serum protein ratio greater than 0.5, a pleural fluid:serum lactate dehydrogenase (LDH) ratio greater than 0.6, and a pleural LDH concentration more than two-thirds the normal upper limit for serum. If any one of these values is exceeded, the effusion is classified as exudative. Recent efforts at utilizing additional markers such as pleural C-reactive protein and adenosine deaminase levels have also shown promise, although their clinical use is not yet widespread.

In adult populations, where the high frequency of congestive heart failure, cirrhosis, and renal disease make transudative effusions common, differentiating effusion type is helpful. In pediatrics, however, because the majority of effusions are exudative, classification focuses instead on whether pleural fluid collections are infectious or noninfectious.

Clinical Manifestations

The hallmarks of pleural disease are pain, shortness of breath, fever, and an abnormal chest radiograph. Pain with respirations, or pleuritic chest pain, is the most characteristic symptom with pleural inflammation. Most patients also describe some degree of dyspnea. Additional symptoms vary depending on the primary cause. In "dry" pleurisy, which is usually caused by a minor pulmonary infection, the patient is often febrile with an irritating, nonproductive cough. With oncologic etiologies, weight loss, night sweats, and fatigue may be present.

On examination, pressure over the involved area may elicit tenderness, and a coarse vibration may sometime be appreciated on palpation. A pleural friction rub is most apt to be heard when pleural inflammation is associated with little or no effusion. The sound has been described as low pitched, sometimes with a grating or squeaking quality. It is usually loudest on inspiration, but often it may also be audible during expiration. Sometimes, the rub is confused with low-pitched rhonchi, produced by secretions partially blocking the airway. A vigorous cough will eliminate these secretions and sounds but will not affect the pleural friction rub. Grunting may occur, although related to pain rather than respiratory distress in most patients with dry pleurisy.

For patients with pleural effusions, characteristic physical findings include restriction of movement of the chest wall on the affected side, dullness to percussion, diminished to absent tactile and vocal fremitus, and decreased or absent breath sounds. These signs are similar to patients with large areas of atelectasis or collapse, although pleural effusions decrease the available space within the hemithorax, causing the trachea to deviate away from the diseased side. Conversely, atelectasis causes the trachea to deviate toward the diseased side.

Radiographs may be used to evaluate for pleural thickening or pleural effusion, as well as to help determine underlying etiology. Pleural inflammation alone can be difficult to appreciate on chest films. Instead, effusion is the most common radiographic manifestation of pleural disease. The first radiographic sign of a pleural effusion is usually blunting of the costophrenic angles, producing wedgelike menisci that extend upward along the lateral chest wall. Similar collections can be seen in the posterior costophrenic angles on lateral views. Larger effusions may be seen to extend up the entire lateral chest wall or retrosternally.

Pleural effusions may alternatively present with apparent prominence or thickening of the interlobar fissures or by wedge-shaped accumulations of fluid at either end of these fissures. The latter may be mistaken for focal infiltrates or segmental atelectasis on some views.

Although small effusions are easily overlooked on radiograph, with proper technique, collections as small as 25 mL have been identified. In adults, pleural effusions are visible on lateral chest radiographs at a volume of approximately 50 mL. At a volume of 200 mL, the meniscus can be identified on the posteroanterior radiograph, whereas at a volume of 500 mL, the meniscus obscures the hemidiaphragm.

Management

The management of pleural disease is aimed at determining the cause, treating the primary disorder, and relieving associated functional disturbances. When no effusion is present, relief of chest pain is the most pressing issue. Antiinflammatory therapy and rest are indicated. Pleurisy can be significant in some children, and constant aggravation with respiration can be frustrating. Irritability and restlessness can result, and mild sedatives may be helpful.

For patients with increased accumulation of pleural fluid, pain is usually less significant; however, respiratory compromise is more likely. Thoracentesis is indicated when fluid accumulation is extensive enough to cause dyspnea and/or for diagnostic purposes (Fig. 98.10). Sonographic guidance is not mandatory but can simplify and enhance the success of this procedure, particularly with small or loculated effusions. Complications of thoracentesis include pneumothorax, hemo-

thorax, reexpansion pulmonary edema, and, rarely, air embolism. The recommended technique for thoracentesis is provided in Section VII, and details of management of fluid in the pleural space are reviewed in Chapter 128.

Additional means of draining pleural fluid are also available. Thoracostomy using small "pigtail" tubes placed by Seldinger technique is minimally more invasive than needle thoracentesis and allows for ongoing drainage as needed. Again, ultrasound guidance can be utilized at the bedside, or the location of maximal fluid can be marked prior to drainage. Image-guided catheter drainage is most effective in patients with short duration of symptoms, free-flowing or unilocular effusions, absence of thick pleural peel, and fluid collections that can be easily reached. Other approaches for more advanced disease include surgical tube thoracotomy; video-assisted thoracosopic surgery, which allows directed chest tube placement and debridement; and minithoracotomy with open pleural decortication.

Diagnostic tests of pleural fluid should include gross and microscopic examination; Gram stain; protein, glucose, LDH, and pH determinations; and cytology if malignancy is known or suspected. Gross examination can be suggestive of fluid content. For example, frank pus can be diagnostic of empyema, chylous effusions are milky white, and exudative fluid with high content of protein and cells is usually turbid. However, oftentimes, classification of pleural fluid by visual appearance alone will not be feasible or accurate. Therefore, concomitant blood and pleural fluid protein and LDH determinations are required.

For patients with exudative effusions, pleural fluid pH measurement is helpful in guiding decisions regarding drainage. In adult patients, pH values of greater than 7.2 to 7.3 are generally found in sterile pleural fluid that does not require further drainage. One exception is *Proteus mirabilis* infection, which causes an elevated pleural fluid pH. In contrast, a pH of less than 7.0 is seen only in empyema, collagen vascular disease, or esophageal rupture. Therapeutically, a pleural fluid pH of less than 7.2 suggests that the effusion will likely require chest tube drainage.

A pleural fluid:serum glucose ratio less than 0.5 has a similar differential diagnosis as low pleural fluid pH. In animal studies, both leukocytes and bacteria have been shown to use glucose anaerobically, resulting in reduced glucose concentration. Diseases associated with low pleural fluid glucose (less than 60 mg per dL) include infectious causes, collagen vascular diseases, malignancies, and esophageal rupture.

Although pleural fluid white blood cell count is routinely obtained, rarely will findings influence management. While blood cell counts are generally higher in children with purulent effusions than in those with transudative effusions, values overlap considerably. In large series of both adult and pediatric patients, pleural fluid white blood cell counts have not been helpful in narrowing the differential diagnosis or in determining the need for or duration of chest tube drainage.

OBSTRUCTIVE SLEEP APNEA

Background

Sleep-disordered breathing refers to the group of respiratory disorders that occur or are exacerbated by sleep. These include

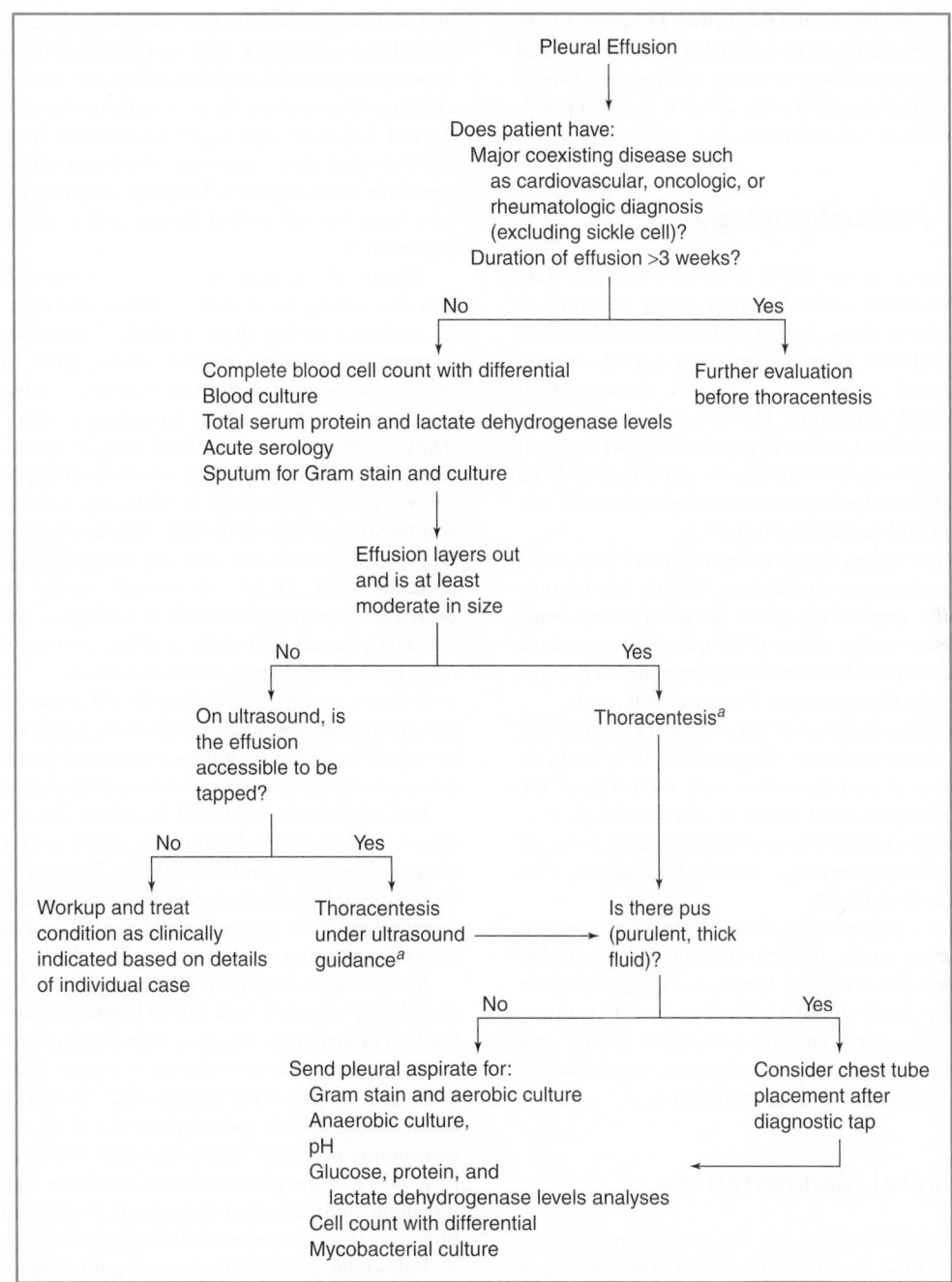

FIGURE 98.10 Approach to pleural effusion. [a]Consider simultaneous placement of small gauge (8F to 10F) chest tube by Seldinger technique for large, free-flowing effusions.

those disease processes that result in central or obstructive apnea or hypoventilation. Of those with obstructive etiologies, primary habitual snoring is the most common, but also the least worrisome. On the other end of the spectrum is obstructive sleep apnea syndrome (OSAS), which can have long-term consequences, including neurocognitive deficits and cardiovascular morbidities.

Obstructive sleep apnea was first described nearly a century ago when William Osler coined the term *Pickwickian*, referring to obese hypersomnolent patients. Subsequent accounts of sleep apnea associated with obesity emerged. For years, however, confusion in nomenclature and incomplete under-

standing of the overlapping pathophysiology of these reported disorders prevented the recognition of a unified syndrome. In 1996, the American Thoracic Society defined OSAS in children as a disorder of breathing during sleep, characterized by prolonged upper airway obstruction or intermittent complete obstruction that disrupts normal ventilation during sleep and normal sleep patterns.

Although the reported incidence varies depending on the data collection methodology and inclusion criteria, most studies suggest that OSAS occurs in 1% to 5% of children. It is more common in boys than in girls. The peak incidence is in children between 2 and 8 years of age, paralleling the prominence of

MEDICAL EMERGENCIES

growth of lymphoid tissues around the airway. However, OSAS can occur in any age. Craniofacial anomalies and neurological disorders affecting upper airway structure and tone predispose infants to OSAS, while obesity is often a factor in the development of the syndrome in older children.

Pathophysiology

The exact pathophysiology of OSAS is unclear. Available data suggest that upper airway resistance, from either anatomic or dynamic airway obstructions, leads to variable and abnormal breathing patterns during sleep. Complete or partial obstruction leads to limited airflow that prompts electrocortical arousal and autonomic activation. This response stimulates an increased respiratory effort and tachypnea in an effort to maintain normal gas exchange. Collectively, the result is disordered sleep patterns that have downstream consequences on the cardiovascular system and on daytime behaviors.

In the majority of cases, adenotonsillar hypertrophy is the major precipitant of airway obstruction. Obesity has become another precipitant, particularly given the growing epidemic of childhood obesity in this country. Of note, obese patients with OSAS tend to require less tonsillar hypertophy to become symptomatic than do their younger, thinner counterparts.

Children with craniofacial anomalies are also at higher risk for obstruction, oftentimes beginning shortly after birth. In children whose craniofacial anomalies reduce the size of the nasal cavity, nasopharynx, or oropharynx, the normal pharyngeal tissues or minimal hyperplasia of the lymphoid tissue of Waldeyer's ring can cause varying degrees of obstruction. This obstruction can result in OSAS.

Children with neuromuscular diseases are also prone to obstruction and sleep apnea. In these children, impaired pharyngeal tone allows posterior soft tissues to collapse into the airway during sleep. Such children with neuromuscular disorders are likely to also have chronic pulmonary disease and impaired ability to clear pharyngeal secretions, which further complicates their evaluation and management.

Clinical Manifestations

Snoring and difficulty breathing are the most common complaints in children (and parents) with OSAS. The snoring is described as loud, often with interspersed pauses, snorts, or gasps. Retractions are frequently noted while the child is sleeping. Episodes of obstruction may be witnessed, many of which are terminated by gasping, movement, or awakening. Children will frequently appear restless throughout the night, naturally repositioning themselves to promote airway patency. Increased autonomic tone frequently results in nighttime diaphoresis and may contribute to enuresis. Chronic nighttime cough may also be observed as a result of intermittent aspiration of small amounts of pharyngeal secretions.

Although symptoms including nasal voice and mouth breathing may be noticeable during the daytime, many children exhibit no evidence of airway compromise when awake. However, because of disrupted sleep, children with OSAS may demonstrate excessive somnolence, although this is much less common in younger children than in teens and adults. Behavioral and neurocognitive changes are relatively common, however, resembling symptoms seen in patients with attention deficit hyperactivity disorder. Other commonly associated behavioral abnormalities include fighting with peers, crying easily, withdrawal behavior, and rapid fluctuations in alertness. Older children may also experience decreased school performance, especially with regard to language acquisition. These changes may result from disrupted sleep as well as chronic, intermittent hypoxemia.

Abnormal physical findings on examination are unusual. Tonsillar enlargement may be noted; however, it is often mild to moderate rather than marked. A normal oropharyngeal examination does not exclude OSAS, given the potential for other soft tissue structures or dynamic changes to cause the airway obstruction. Other nonspecific signs might include delayed growth or impaired weight gain, from chronic increased work of breathing, intermittent hypoxia, and limited caloric intake secondary to difficulty eating and breathing comfortably at the same time. Alternatively, obesity is a risk factor for disease and may be noted particularly in older patients with OSAS. Abnormal facies or systemically decreased tone may be found as etiologies, and a loud S_2 can occur in patients with long-standing disease who have developed pulmonary hypertension as a result.

Initial screening for snoring should occur at routine health care maintenance visits. If a history of nightly snoring is elicited, or a child has other symptoms concerning for OSAS, a comprehensive history and physical examination should be performed. A detailed account of labored breathing during sleep, observed apnea, restless sleep, diaphoresis, enuresis, cyanosis, excessive daytime sleepiness, and behavior or learning disorders should be obtained. Formal questionnaires are available, although differentiating OSAS from primary habitual snoring based on self- or family-reported results may be difficult.

Soft-tissue radiographs of the lateral neck taken with the child lying on his/her back can be helpful but are not a definitive method of diagnosis. Much as with physical examination of the pharynx, static images cannot replicate potential dynamic changes that may occur during sleep. Standardized recordings of breathing sounds, videotaping of a child while sleeping, or continuous overnight pulse oximetry can occur either in the hospital or in the patient's home. Evidence suggests that these screening tools can have reasonable positive predictive value; however, absence of abnormal findings cannot exclude OSAS.

Polysomnography is the current gold standard and the diagnostic test of choice for evaluating apnea and should be performed on children with historical and physical findings associated with OSAS. It can distinguish primary snoring from OSAS and can determine the severity of OSAS. Although polysomnography can be performed satisfactorily in children of any age, it requires appropriate equipment and appropriately trained staff. Therefore, availability is often limited. Abbreviated or nap polysomnography in the hospital or unattended home polysomnography have been utilized in place, but as with other screening tools, these have limited negative predictive value.

Management

Children with concern for significant apnea may warrant hospitalization until a diagnosis and severity can be determined.

Historical clues will be most important in making this determination, as children with OSAS do not usually appear in extremis during wakeful periods. However, some well-appearing children may be at risk for repeated apnea and subsequent hypoxemia while sleeping. During hospitalization, airway obstruction should be managed according to basic life support protocols, with airway maneuvers such as repositioning, jaw thrust, and head-tilt chin lift to open the upper airway as necessary. Nasal trumpets may also be helpful.

Supplemental oxygen therapy is sometimes recommended to alleviate nocturnal hypoxemia. However, it does not prevent sleep-related upper airway obstruction, sleep fragmentation, or increased work of breathing. In addition, patients with long-standing disease may chronically retain CO_2; therefore, aggressive correction of hypoxia may depress respiratory drive and potentially worsen hypoventilation. Assessing a serum HCO_3 or blood gas level may be helpful in identifying such patients.

In addition to a thorough general medical evaluation, children with OSAS will usually require otolaryngologic consultation for airway evaluation and, if needed, planning for relief of obstruction.

Numerous methods of management of OSAS have been suggested and studied. Patients with hyperplasia of the tonsils and adenoids as the primary cause for obstruction may be trialed on high-dose nasal steroids, although those who improve may not have sustained benefit. Most of these patients will have dramatic relief of symptoms following surgical resection. Postoperative polysomnography shows resolution of OSAS in 75% to 100% of patients. Patients with craniofacial anomalies and with neuromuscular disorders also usually have significant improvement after adenotonsillectomy or other targeted surgical procedures.

Patients with obesity-hypoventilation syndrome (Pickwickian syndrome) may benefit from maintained weight reduction. Unfortunately, weight loss in these patients is often either difficult to achieve or only temporarily successful. Because many obese children will be adequately treated with adenotonsillectomy, it is generally the first-line therapy for these patients.

Oral appliances have been shown to improve snoring and reduce apnea and hypopnea in adults by modifying the upper airway by changing the posture of the mandible and tongue. Although some tolerate such devices well, oral discomfort probably decreases compliance rates, which may be as low as 50% in adults and would likely be even lower in children. For some OSAS patients, nasally administered CPAP successfully alleviates hypoventilation, although again this may be less well tolerated in pediatric population. Rarely, patients require artificial airway placement and/or supplemental ventilation.

SARCOIDOSIS

Background

Sarcoidosis is a rare, chronic, granulomatous disease of unknown cause. Lungs are the most affected organs although joints, skin, eyes, lymph nodes, liver, spleen, muscle, and brain can all be involved. Involved organs have accumulations of T lymphocytes and mononuclear phagocytes, noncaseating epithelioid granulomas, and derangements of normal tissue architecture. Although the exact cause of sarcoidosis is unknown, evidence suggests a multifactorial etiology; both environmental and genetic factors result in an exaggerated cellular immune response to an unclear antigen.

The incidence of sarcoidosis varies with age, race, and geography. The majority of those affected are adults between the ages of 20 and 40 years. Although cases of patients less than 1 year of age have been reported, most pediatric cases present in the second decade. The disease is often acute or subacute and self-limiting. However, in many, it is chronic, with waxing and waning symptoms over many years.

Clinical Manifestations

The most common initial symptoms in children and young adults are nonspecific and may include malaise, fatigue, fever, and weight loss. Organ-specific symptoms vary by age. Children younger than 5 years most commonly have skin, eye, and joint involvement, whereas older children are more likely to report symptoms related to lung involvement or enlarged lymph nodes. The presence of cough and dyspnea usually indicates pulmonary involvement. However, extensive pulmonary disease can be present without clinical findings. Hoarseness, dyspnea, and dysphagia can result from laryngeal involvement. Arrhythmia or congestive heart failure can also present as initial findings of cardiac disease. Other symptoms vary depending on affected systems and may include bone and joint pain, visual acuity impairment, ocular swelling or pain, parotid gland enlargement, headache, and unexplained fever.

On physical examination, lymph node enlargement is the most frequently detected abnormality. Intrathoracic nodes including hilar, paratracheal, or mediastinal chains are enlarged in 75% to 90% of patients. When present, hilar adenopathy is usually bilateral and symmetric. Peripheral adenopathy is also common, particularly in cervical, axillary, and inguinal regions. Affected lymph nodes are firm, nontender, mobile, and nonulcerative. Some patients have a skin rash that is similar in appearance to erythema nodosum. Plaques, subcutaneous nodules, and maculopapular eruptions can also be seen. Uveitis is present in up to 25% of patients. Small yellow nodules are frequently found on the conjunctiva in these patients. Hepatosplenomegaly and joint effusions can also be present.

Laboratory test abnormalities in patients with sarcoid tend to be nonspecific. Hyperproteinemia, elevated erythrocyte sedimentation rate, hypercalciuria, eosinophilia, and rarely hypercalcemia can be seen. Although not pathognomonic, an elevated serum angiotensin-converting enzyme level in patients in whom sarcoid is suspected is strongly supportive. On chest radiograph, between 40% and 60% of symptomatic children will have hilar adenopathy alone or in combination with parenchymal infiltrates. Pulmonary function testing usually reveals restrictive lung disease.

Diagnosis of sarcoid in children is challenging because it is extremely rare and oftentimes findings are subtle. For pediatric patients with multisystem complaints, however, sarcoid should be considered. In particular, pulmonary disease associated with rash, uveitis, or arthritis is suggestive. However, because lung disease can remain clinically silent, respiratory complaints need not be present at the time of initial presentation.

MEDICAL EMERGENCIES

Alternatively, unexplained intrathoracic adenopathy may prompt further investigation, leading to the diagnosis.

The diagnosis is ultimately made histologically. Biopsy of a lymph node or other easily accessible organ will demonstrate noncaseating epithelioid cell granulomas. These findings may need to be further differentiated from other rheumatologic or infectious diseases that can have similar histopathology.

Management

Glucocorticoid treatment is the most commonly used therapy for sarcoidosis. However, because the disease resolves spontaneously in a substantial proportion of patients, there is often debate about who requires steroids. Patients with significant lung or eye lesions are most commonly treated. In addition, those with cardiac, CNS, or multiorgan system involvement usually warrant therapy. Corticosteroids seem to be effective as acute therapeutic agents but have little effect on permanent organ derangements, including chronic lung disease.

For many, the prognosis in sarcoidosis is favorable, although clinical and genetic factors are important factors. Most patients with an acute presentation improve gradually over months and are left with no sequelae. However, some develop progressive cystic emphysema, bronchiectasis, or severe restrictive pulmonary disease with exercise-induced hypoxemia. Younger children and those with multiorgan system involvement tend to have less favorable outcomes. In addition, all patients require close monitoring during and after treatment because relapses are not uncommon.

SEVERE ACUTE RESPIRATORY SYNDROME

Background

An epidemic of a newly defined respiratory illness, severe acute respiratory syndrome (SARS), occurred in 2002/2003. Index cases in Hong Kong appeared to transport the illness to Singapore, Vietnam, Canada, Ireland, and the United States, resulting in widespread infection, totaling more than 3,000 cases with 10% mortality reported throughout 27 countries. Laboratory and epidemiologic studies revealed SARS-associated coronavirus as the etiologic agent. The small droplets, which serve as vectors for transmissibility, allowed for easy spread, even in relatively protected environments.

Clinical Presentation

In adults, clinical features include fever, cough, shortness of breath, and varying degrees of respiratory distress. Associated laboratory findings may include leukopenia, thrombocytopenia, liver function abnormalities, and coagulation abnormalities. Patients with more significant disease have bilateral pulmonary infiltrates on radiographs and may progress to ARDS and multiorgan system failure.

Pediatric patients diagnosed with SARS tend to have less severe illness, although most adolescents require more aggressive therapy than do younger children. Similar to adults, pediatric

patients with confirmed SARS-associated coronavirus infection present most commonly with fever, cough, malaise, coryza, and other nonspecific symptoms. Some children show no evidence of lower respiratory tract infection, yet others have clinical signs such as inspiratory crackles, chest radiographs suggestive of alveolar infiltrates, or occasionally CT findings confirming parenchymal lung involvement. The most common laboratory abnormalities tend to be mild and may include leukopenia; thrombocytopenia; elevated alanine aminotransferase, aspartate aminotransferase, and lactate dehydrogenase levels; and prolonged aPTT (activated partial thromboplastin time).

Because the signs and symptoms of SARS are nonspecific and immediately available laboratory testing could be supportive but not diagnostic, incorporation of careful investigation into potential exposures was crucial during the epidemic. Evaluation of symptomatic patients required investigation for SARS as well as more common etiologies for community-acquired pneumonia. Nasopharyngeal swab for PCR for coronavirus, serum antibody to SARS-CoV (SARS coronavirus), and clinical specimen for isolation in cell culture are all acceptable testing methodologies.

Little is known about the potential transmission from child to child. However, of greater importance was the reduction of potential spread from children to higher risk adults by isolation during the viremic phase.

Management

In addition to supportive therapy with supplemental oxygen, nutrition, and symptomatic therapy, ribavirin was used in a number of cases. The benefits are unclear, although there exists a theoretical benefit in treatment of RNA viruses such as coronavirus. Many patients received pulse steroids for 3 to 5 days, particularly those with radiographic findings and hypoxemia.

There have been no recurrent epidemics of SARS since 2003. Depending on future epidemiology, more may be elucidated regarding this particular pulmonary infection in pediatrics. For now, however, the SARS outbreak serves as an example of the important interaction between epidemiologic and clinical investigation during the development of new, severe illnesses in children and the general population.

Suggested Readings

Acute Respiratory Failure

Hansell DR. Extracorporeal membrane oxygenation for perinatal and pediatric patients. *Respir Care* 2003;48(4):352–352.
Heulitt MJ, Wolf GK, Arnold JH. Mechanical ventilation. In: Nichols DG, ed. *Textbook of pediatric intensive care,* 4th ed. Baltimore, MD: Lippincott Williams & Wilkins, 2008:508–531.
Marraro GA. Innovative practices of ventilatory support with pediatric patients. *Pediatr Crit Care Med* 2003;4(1):8–20.
Mellins RB, Stripp B, Taussig LM. Pediatric pulmonology in North America—coming of age. *Am Rev Respir Dis* 1986;134:849–853.
Murray JF. *The normal lung,* 3rd ed. Philadelphia, PA: WB Saunders, 1986.
Shann F, Barker J, Poore P. Clinical signs that predict death in children with severe pneumonia. *Pediatr Infect Dis J* 1989;8:852–855.

Bronchopulmonary Dysplasia

Abman SH, Davis JM. Bronchopulmonary dysplasia. In: Chernick V, Boat TF, Wilmott RW, et al., eds. *Kendig's disorders of the respiratory tract in children,* 7th ed. Philadelphia, PA: WB Saunders, 2006:342–358.

Carpenter TC, Stenmark KR. Predisposition of infants with chronic lung disease to respiratory syncytial virus-induced respiratory failure: a vascular hypothesis. *Pediatr Infect Dis J* 2004;23:S33–S40.

Groothuis JR, Gutierrez KM, Lauer BA. Respiratory syncytial virus infection in children with bronchopulmonary dysplasia. *Pediatrics* 1988;82:199–203.

Jobe AH. The new BPD. *Neoreviews* 2006;7:e531–e545.

Jobe AH, Bancalari E. Bronchopulmonary dysplasia. *Am J Respir Crit Care Med* 2001;163:1723–1729.

Meissner HC, Long SS, and the Committee on Infectious Diseases and Committee on Fetus and Newborn. Revised indications for the use of palivizumab and respiratory syncytial virus immune globulin intravenous for the prevention of respiratory syncytial virus infections. *Pediatrics* 2003;112:1447–1452.

Myers MG, McGuinness GA, Lachenbruch PA, et al. Respiratory illness in survivors of infant respiratory distress syndrome. *Am Rev Respir Dis* 1986; 133:1011–1018.

Northway WJ Jr, Rosan RC, Porter DY. Pulmonary disease following respiratory therapy of hyaline membrane disease. *N Engl J Med* 1967;276: 357–368.

Walsh MC, Szefler S, Davis J, et al. Summary proceedings from the bronchopulmonary dysplasia group. *Pediatrics* 2006;117:S52–S56.

Interstitial Lung Disease

Bokulic RE, Hilman BC. Interstitial lung diseases in children. *Pediatr Clin North Am* 1994;41:543–567.

Carrington CB, Gaensler EA, Contu RE, et al. Natural history and treated course of usual and desquamative interstitial pneumonia. *N Engl J Med* 1978;298:801–809.

Deutsch GH, Young LR, Deterding RR. Diffuse lung disease in young children: application of a novel classification scheme. *Am J Respir Crit Care Med* 2007;176:1120–1128.

Fan LL, Detering RR, Langston C. Pediatric interstitial lung disease revisited. *Pediatr Pulmonol* 2004;38:369–378.

Fan LL, Lung MC, Wagener JS. The diagnostic value of bronchoalveolar lavage in immunocompetent children with chronic diffuse pulmonary infiltrates. *Pediatr Pulmonol* 1997;23:8–13.

Hauger SB, Powell KR. Infectious complications in children with HIV infection. *Pediatr Ann* 1990;19:421–433.

Nicholson AG, Bush A. Classification of diffuse lung disease in infants: the reality of groups. *Am J Respir Crit Care Med* 2007;176:1060–1061.

Rothenberg SS, Wagener JS, Chang JH, et al. The safety and efficacy of thoracoscopic lung biopsy for diagnosis and treatment in infants and children. *J Pediatr* 1996;31:100–103.

Wolff LJ, Bartlett MS, Baehner RL, et al. The causes of interstitial pneumonitis in immunocompromised children: an aggressive systematic approach to diagnosis. *Pediatrics* 1977;60:41–45.

Aspiration Pneumonia

Boesch RP, Daines C, Willging JP, et al. Advances in the diagnosis and management of chronic pulmonary aspiration in children. *Eur Respir J* 2006;28: 847–861.

Brook I. Aspiration pneumonia in institutionalized children: a retrospective comparison of treatment with penicillin G, clindamycin and carbenicillin. *Clin Pediatr* 1986;20:117–122.

Brook I. Treatment of aspiration of tracheostomy-associated pneumonia in neurologically impaired children: effect of antimicrobials effective against anaerobic bacteria. *Int J Pediatr Otorhinolaryngol* 1996;35:171–177.

Brook I, Finegold SM. Bacteriology of aspiration pneumonia in children. *Pediatrics* 1980;65:1115–1120.

Bynum LJ, Pierce AK. Pulmonary aspiration of gastric contents. *Am Rev Respir Dis* 1976;114:1129–1136.

Downs JB, Chapman RL, Modell JH, et al. An evaluation of steroid therapy in aspiration pneumonitis. *Anesthesiology* 1974;40:129–135.

Marik PE. Aspiration pneumonitis and aspiration pneumonia. *N Engl J Med* 2001;344:665–671.

Marik PE, Careau P. The role of anaerobes in patients with ventilator associated pneumonia and aspiration pneumonia: a prospective study. *Chest* 1999;115: 178–83.

Mier L, Dreyfuss D, Darchy B, et al. Is penicillin G an adequate initial treatment for aspiration pneumonia? A prospective evaluation using a protected specimen brush and quantitative cultures. *Intensive Care Med* 1993;19: 279–284.

Murray HW. Antimicrobial therapy in pneumonia aspiration. *Am J Med* 1979;66:188–190.

Platxker ACG. Gastroesophageal reflux and aspiration syndromes. In: Chernick V, Boat TF, Wilmott RW, et al., eds. *Kendig's disorders of the respiratory tract in children,* 7th ed. Philadelphia, PA: WB Saunders, 2006:592–609.

Weir K, McMahon S, Barry L, et al. Oropharyngeal aspiration and pneumonia in children. *Pediatr Pulmonol* 2007;42:1024–1031.

Wynne JW, Modell JH. Respiratory aspiration of stomach contents. *Ann Intern Med* 1977;87:466–474.

Pulmonary Embolism

Bernstein D, Coupey S, Schonberg SK. Pulmonary embolism in adolescents. *Am J Dis Child* 1986;140:667–671.

Buck JR, Connors RH, Coon WW, et al. Pulmonary embolism in children. *J Pediatr Surg* 1981;16:385–391.

Chan AK, Deveber G, Monagle P, et al. Venous thrombosis in children. *J Thromb Haemost* 2003;1:1443–1455.

Goddard R, Scofield RH. Right pneumothorax with $S_1Q_3T_3$ electrocardiogram pattern usually associated with pulmonary embolus. *Am J Emerg Med* 1997;15:310–312.

Johnson AS, Bolte RG. Pulmonary embolism in the pediatric patient. *Pediatr Emerg Care* 2004;20:555–560.

Kutinsky I, Blakely S, Roche V, et al. Normal D-dimer levels in patients with pulmonary embolism. *Arch Intern Med* 1999;159:1569–1572.

McBride WJ, Gadowski GR, Keller MS, et al. Pulmonary embolism in pediatric trauma patients. *J Trauma* 1994;37:913–915.

Monagle P, Michelson AD, Bovill E, et al. Antithrombotic therapy in children. *Chest* 2001;119:344–370.

Mullins MD, Becker DM, Hagspiel KD, et al. The role of spiral volumetric computed tomography in the diagnosis of pulmonary embolism. *Arch Intern Med* 2000;160:293–298.

Nguyen LT, Laberge J. Spontaneous deep vein thrombosis in childhood and adolescence. *J Pediatr Surg* 1986;21:640–643.

Nuss R, Hays T, Chudgar U, et al. Antiphospholipid antibodies and coagulation regulatory pattern in children with pulmonary embolism. *J Pediatr Hematol Oncol* 1997;19:202–207.

Sadosty AT, Goyal DG, Boie ET, et al. Emergency department D-dimer testing. *J Emerg Med* 2001;21:423–429.

Tapson VF. Acute pulmonary embolism. *N Engl J Med* 2008;358:1037–1052.

Task Force on Pulmonary Embolism, European Society for Cardiology. Guidelines on diagnosis and management of acute pulmonary embolism. *Eur Heart J* 2000;21:1301–1336.

Value of the ventilation/perfusion scan in acute pulmonary embolism: results of the prospective investigation of pulmonary embolism (PIOPED): the PIOPED investigators. *JAMA* 1990;263:2753–2759.

van Belle A, Büller HR, Huisman MV, et al. Effectiveness of managing suspected pulmonary embolism using an algorithm combining clinical probability, D-dimer testing, and computed tomography. *JAMA* 2006;295: 172–179.

van Ommen CH, Heijboer H, Buller HR, et al. Venous thromboembolism in childhood: a prospective two-year registry in the Netherlands. *J Pediatr* 2001;139:676–681.

van Strijen MJ, de Monyé W, Schiereck J, et al. Single-detector helical computed tomography as the primary diagnostic test in suspected pulmonary embolism: a multicenter clinical management study of 510 patients. *Ann Intern Med* 2003;138:307–14.

Victoria T, Mong A, Altes T, et al. Evaluation of pulmonary embolism in a pediatric population with high clinical suspicion. *Pediatr Radiol* 2009;39:35–41.

Wells PS, Ginsberg JS, Anderson DR, et al. Use of a chemical model for safe management of patients with suspected pulmonary embolism. *Ann Intern Med* 1998;129:997–1005.

Pulmonary Edema

Carter EP, Matthay M. Resolution of pulmonary edema: recent advances. In: George RB, Campbell GD, Jenkinson SG, et al., eds. *Current pulmonary and critical care medicine,* vol. 17. St. Louis, MO: Mosby, 1996:351–376.

Hopkins RL, Levine SD. Severe pulmonary edema in meningococcemia. *Clin Pediatr (Phila)* 1983;22:452–454.

Kanter RK, Watchko JF. Pulmonary edema associated with upper airway obstruction. *Am J Dis Child* 1984;138:356–358.

Mulroy JJ, Mickell JJ, Tong TK, et al. Postictal pulmonary edema in children. *Neurology* 1985;35:403–405.

O'Brodovich H. Pulmonary edema. In: Chernick V, Boat TF, Wilmott RW, et al., eds. *Kendig's disorders of the respiratory tract in children,* 7th ed. Philadelphia, PA: WB Saunders, 2006:622–638.

Robin ED, Coss CE, Zelis R. Pulmonary edema. *N Engl J Med* 1973;288:292.

Scoggin CH, Myers TM, Reeves JT, et al. High-altitude pulmonary edema in the children and young adults of Leadville, Colorado. *N Engl J Med* 1977;297: 1269–1272.

Sofer S, Jacob B, Scharf SM. Pulmonary edema following relief of upper airway obstruction. *Chest* 1983;83:401–403.

Theodore J, Robin ED. Speculations on neurogenic pulmonary edema (NPE). *Am Rev Respir Dis* 1976;113:405–411.

Pulmonary Hemorrhage

Boat TF. Pulmonary hemorrhage and hemoptysis. In: Chernick V, Boat TF, Wilmott RW, et al., eds. *Kendig's disorders of the respiratory tract in children,* 7th ed. Philadelphia, PA: WB Saunders, 2006:676–685.

MEDICAL EMERGENCIES

Brown CM, Redd SC, Damon SA. Acute idiopathic pulmonary hemorrhage among infants: recommendations from the Working Group for Investigation and Surveillance. *MMWR Recomm Rep* 2004;53:1–12.

Dearborn DG. Pulmonary hemorrhage in infants and children. *Curr Opin Pediatr* 1997;9:219–224.

Godfrey S. Pulmonary hemorrhage/hemoptysis in children. *Pediatr Pulmonol* 2004;37:476–484.

Levy J, Wilmott RW. Pulmonary hemosiderosis. *Pediatr Pulmonol* 1986;2: 384–390.

Susarla SC, Fan LL. Diffuse alveolar hemorrhage syndromes in children. *Curr Opin Pediatr* 2007;19:314–320.

Pleuritis

Bechamps GJ, Lynn HB, Wenzl JE. Empyema in children: review of Mayo Clinic experience. *Mayo Clin Proc* 1970;45:43–50.

Blackmore CC, Black WC, Dallas RV, et al. Pleural fluid volume estimation: a chest radiograph prediction rule. *Acad Radiol* 1996;3:103–109.

Freij BJ, Kusmiesz H, Nelson JD, et al. Parapneumonic effusions and empyema in hospitalized children: a retrospective review of 227 cases. *Pediatr Infect Dis* 1984;3:578–591.

Heffner JE, Brown LK, Barbieri CA. Diagnostic value of tests that discriminate between exudative and transudative pleural effusions. *Chest* 1997;111: 970–980.

Klein JS, Schultz S, Heffner JE. Interventional radiology of the chest: image-guided percutaneous drainage of pleural effusions, lung abscess, and pneumothorax. *Am J Roentgenol* 1995;164:581–588.

Light RW. Pleural effusions. *Med Clin North Am* 1977;61:1339–1352.

Light RW, MacGregor MC, Luchsinger PC, et al. Pleural effusions: the diagnostic separation of transudates and exudates. *Ann Intern Med* 1972;77: 507–513.

McLaughlin FJ, Goldmann DA, Rosenbaum DM, et al. Empyema in children: clinical course and long-term follow-up. *Pediatrics* 1984;73:587–593.

Mitri RK, Brown SD, Zurakowski D, et al. Outcomes of primary image-guided drainage of parapneumonic effusions in children. *Pediatrics* 2002;110; e37–e43.

Montgomery M, Sigalet D. Air and liquid in the pleural space. In: Chernick V, Boat TF, Wilmott RW, et al., eds. *Kendig's disorders of the respiratory tract in children*, 7th ed. Philadelphia, PA: WB Saunders, 2006:368–387.

Sahn SA. The pathophysiology of pleural effusions. *Ann Rev Med* 1990;41: 7–13.

Vives M, Porcel JM, de Vera MV, et al. A study of Light's criteria and possible modifications for distinguishing exudative from transudative pleural effusions. *Chest* 1996;109:1503–1507.

Obstructive Sleep Apnea

American Academy of Pediatrics, Section on Pediatric Pulmonology, Subcommittee on Obstructive Sleep Apnea Syndrome. Clinical practice guideline: diagnosis and management of childhood sleep apnea syndrome. *Pediatrics* 2002;109:704–712.

American Thoracic Society. Standards and indications for cardiopulmonary sleep studies in children. *Am J Respir Crit Care Med* 1996;153:866–878.

Boxer GH, Bauer AM, Miller BD. Obesity-hypoventilation in childhood. *J Am Acad Child Adolesc Psychiatry* 1988;27:552–558.

Guilleminault C, Korobkin R, Winkle R. A review of 50 children with obstructive sleep apnea syndrome. *Lung* 1981;159:275–287.

Lumeng JC, Chervin RD. Epidemiology of pediatric obstructive sleep apnea. *Proc Am Thorac Soc* 2008;5:242–252.

Muzumdar H, Arens R. Diagnostic issues in pediatric obstructive sleep apnea. *Proc Am Thorac Soc* 2008;5:263–273.

Schmidt-Nowara W, Lowe A, Wiegand L, et al. Oral appliances for the treatment of snoring and obstructive sleep apnea: a review. *Sleep* 1995;18: 501–510.

Sarcoidosis

Consensus conference: activity of sarcoidosis. Third WASOG meeting, Los Angeles, USA, September 8–11, 1993. *Eur Respir J* 1994;7:624–627.

Crystal RG, Bitterman PB, Rennard SI, et al. Interstitial lung disease of unknown cause: disorders characterized by chronic inflammation of the lower respiratory tract (first of two parts). *N Engl J Med* 1984;310:154–156.

Fauroux B, Clement A. Paediatric sarcoidosis. *Paediatr Respir Rev* 2005;6: 128–133.

Iannuzzi MC, Rybicki BA, Teirstein AS. Sarcoidosis. *N Engl J Med* 2007;357: 2153–2165.

Nagai S, Izumi T. Pulmonary sarcoidosis: population differences and pathophysiology. *South Med J* 1995;88:1001–1010.

Pattishall EN, Strope GL, Spinola SM, et al. Childhood sarcoidosis. *J Pediatr* 1986;108:169–177.

Sharma OP. Pulmonary sarcoidosis and corticosteroids. *Am Rev Resp Dis* 1993;147:1598–1600.

Severe Acute Respiratory Syndrome

Bitnun A, Allen U, Heurter H, et al. Children hospitalized with severe acute respiratory syndrome-related illness in Toronto. *Pediatrics* 2003;112(4):e261.

Chiu W-K, Cheung PCH, Ng KL, et al. *Pediatr Crit Care Med* 2003;4(3): 279–283.

Lee TWK, Kwek T-K, Tsi D, et al. Acute respiratory distress syndrome in critically ill patients with severe acute respiratory syndrome. *JAMA* 2003; 290(3):374–380.

Leung C, Kwan Y, Ko P, et al. Severe acute respiratory syndrome among children. *Pediatrics* 2004;113;e535–e543.

Update: severe acute respiratory syndrome—United States. *MMWR Morbid Mortal Wkly Rep* 2003;52(16):359–360.

Wong GWK, Li AM, Ng PC, et al. Severe acute respiratory syndrome in children. *Pediatr Pulmonol* 2003;36:261–266.

CHAPTER 99 ■ EMERGENCIES IN CYSTIC FIBROSIS

EVA LEDER, MD, AND HENRY L. DORKIN, MD

INTRODUCTION

Cystic fibrosis (CF), previously known in Europe and first described in the American literature by Anderson, is a relatively common recessive genetic disease, predominantly seen in the Caucasian population. The basic defect, an abnormal cystic fibrosis transmembrane conductance regulator (CFTR) protein, was not elucidated until 1989. In the late 1970s, 50% expected survival was in the 16- to 18-year-old range. However, with the advent of new therapies directed at the pulmonary and gastrointestinal (GI) manifestations of the disease, survival has dramatically improved. Currently, of the approximately 24,000 CF patients listed in the Registry of the Cystic Fibrosis Foundation (CFF), 45% are older than 21 years, with the 50% expected survival now at 39 years of age in the United States. The improved survival, coupled with opportunities for leisure travel and college enrollment far away from their usual health-care providers, means that the presentation in the emergency department (ED) of acute illness in CF patients is likely to increase. While some of these encounters are manifestations of common complaints applicable to the general pediatric population, the setting in the CF patient changes the paradigm. An understanding of the disease and its emergent presentations is important to address these issues and avoid complications arising from unappreciated aspects of CF. Where treatment varies little from that of the same complaint in the non-CF patient, the reader may refer to the appropriate chapters elsewhere in this textbook.

The common emergency presentations can be grouped as systemic, pulmonary, or GI processes. Some of these are single events, while other complaints are recurrent (with similar findings on representation). Knowledge of successful treatment for a previous episode can be quite instructive in understanding how to manage a repeat event.

BACKGROUND

CF, an autosomal, recessively inherited disease, results from genetic mutation on the long arm of chromosome 7. This code for a 1,479 amino acid protein, is the CFTR. The first defect identified was a deletion of phenylalanine at the 508th position (df508). Since that discovery more than 1,500 different defects, variably represented in various ethnic groups, have been elucidated. In addition, modifier genes have been proposed that accentuate or mitigate the expression of the major CF genes, thus possibly explaining phenotypic variability beyond that conveyed by the CF genotype. These defects have maximal impact on cells lining the respiratory tract, the pancreatic exocrine system, the sweat glands, and the intrahepatic biliary epithelium. The defect leads to impaired chloride transport, with resultant altered water movement across the epithelial boundaries. In the respiratory and GI tracts, this leads to dehydrated secretions that are difficult to mobilize. In the sweat duct, it produces highly concentrated sweat. The former leads to inflammation and (in the respiratory tract) chronic infection. The latter results in the loss of electrolyte-concentrating abilities causing excessive electrolyte loss and dehydration.

SYSTEMIC PRESENTATIONS

Hyponatremic, hypochloremic dehydration, while more common in the era before widespread environmental temperature control, still occurs. The mechanism is the loss of electrolyte with sweat, where concentrations of sodium and chloride can be as high as 130 to 140 mEq per L (as compared with 10 to 30 mEq per L in non-CF patients). In the heat of the summer, infants and athletes are most at risk, although such dehydration can occur at any age. It has, in fact, also presented in swaddled babies in the wintertime. Exclusively breastfed infants, whose sodium chloride (NaCl) intake may be lower than that of formula-fed infants, may be even more susceptible. In an earlier era before newborn screening, dehydration was commonly the first presentation of CF and should still raise suspicion of the diagnosis whenever encountered in patients not known to have CF. Signs of dehydration (loss of skin turgor, dry mucus membranes, tenting, irritability, etc.) are usually seen and respond appropriately to standard fluid resuscitation. For those patients without a previous CF diagnosis, it is imperative that electrolyte normalization be achieved before considering diagnostic testing with pilocarpine iontophoresis. Sweat chlorides may not be in the diagnostic range in the setting of electrolyte depletion and may render false results below the diagnostic range. Modest NaCl supplementation can prevent recurrence and is usually given as ~1/7th level teaspoon of salt daily, distributed in an infant's feeds over the course of the day. Older children can be given salt containing foods and educated that the salt intake restrictions that the non-CF population use as part of good health diets must not be applied to them.

RESPIRATORY/CHEST PRESENTATIONS

Chest Pain

Chest pain is a common complaint in patients with CF and can stem from a variety of underlying processes (Table 99.1). When evaluating such a patient in the ED, it is important to formulate

TABLE 99.1

CHEST PAIN IN CYSTIC FIBROSIS PATIENTS

Common	Uncommon	Rare
Costochondritis	Rib fracture	Cardiac disease
Pleurisy/pleuritis	Pulmonary embolism	
Pneumothorax		
Esophagitis		
Minor trauma		

a differential diagnosis based on age, disease severity, and associated symptoms. As always, the underlying cause should be treated rather than simply masking the pain with analgesics. Where such analgesia is needed, care must be taken to avoid untoward side effects. CF patients, through years of aminoglycoside exposure and other nephrotoxic therapies, may not have normal renal function. Renally excreted analgesics therefore should not be used long term without assessment of renal function. Furthermore, narcotic analgesics can cause decreased GI motility. This may, in turn, lead to constipation and bowel obstruction, which can have other implications (vide infra).

Pneumothorax

Spontaneous pneumothorax is a well-known complication in CF patients and is far more common than in the general population. Occasionally a first presentation of CF, it occurs in approximately 1:167 patients yearly; nearly 3.5% of all CF patients will experience a pneumothorax at some point in their lives. Risk of recurrence, on both the ipsilateral and contralateral sides of the hemithorax, is also significantly increased at 20%.

The principal risk factor is the severity of disease, with a mean age of first pneumothorax in the late teens to early 20s. Mucous plugging and air trapping impose increased intrapulmonary air pressure differentials on fibroelastic lung structures weakened from chronic inflammation. Classic symptoms include sudden or subacute onset of sharp chest pain, often referred to the shoulder. Depending on the size of the pneumothorax as well as the patient's respiratory reserve, there can be varying degrees of dyspnea, tachypnea, hypoxemia, and cyanosis. Large pneumothoraces can be appreciated by visual assessment of the chest wall, with differential hyperexpansion of the affected hemithorax. Auscultation for all but small pneumothoraces will demonstrate decreased breath sounds. In the absence of loculation, the altered auscultation will be most evident high in the axilla and in the supraclavicular region. Listening alternately from one hemithorax to the other is the best way to appreciate this physical finding.

Confirmation should be sought with a chest radiograph (CXR), which should include frontal and lateral views (Fig. 99.1). If age is appropriate, inspiratory and expiratory views can also be helpful to define the extent of the extraaveolar air collection. Supine films should be avoided as they are more likely to miss less than a moderate or severe pneumothorax.

While consensus guidelines are currently being developed by the CFF, at present, every CF patient with a newly diagnosed, first pneumothorax should be hospitalized and

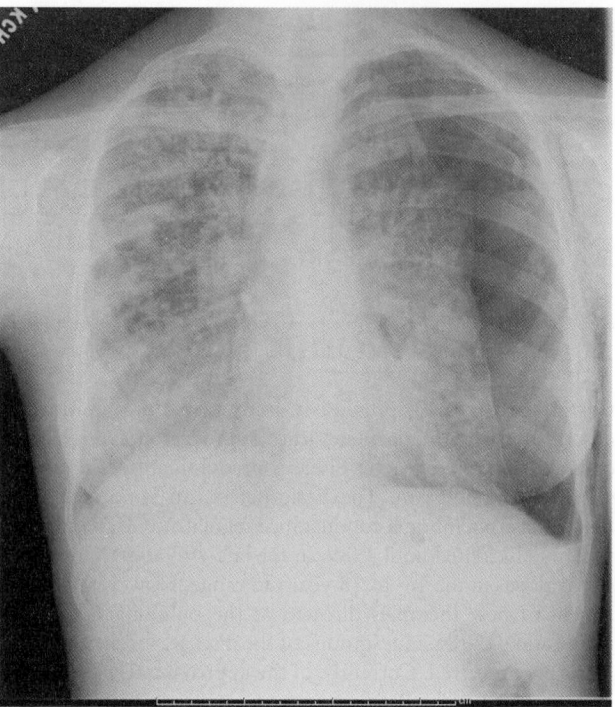

FIGURE 99.1 Chest radiograph showing pneumothorax.

observed for a minimum of 24 hours. A minimally asymptomatic patient with a small pneumothorax (less than 1 cm from apex to parietal pleural surface) and no increase in the size of the pneumothorax, auscultatory asymmetry, or pain/dyspnea over the next 24 hours can then be followed as an outpatient until spontaneous resolution. If the patient is symptomatic or the pneumothorax appears to be more than 1 cm from apex to parietal pleural surface, a chest tube should be inserted. The tube may be a pigtail catheter, placed over a guide wire. Negative pressure of up to −20 cm of water should be applied. Very large pneumothoraces are best managed by applying modest suction initially and letting the lung reexpand slowly to avoid reinflation pulmonary edema of the affected tissue (admittedly a rare occurrence).

After chest tube insertion, a new CXR should be obtained to confirm placement and at least partial resolution of the extraalveolar air. There are no current data to support the use of 100% oxygen via face mask to increase the rate of pneumothorax reabsorption in CF patients. Supplemental oxygen should therefore only be used as needed to optimize oxygenation and patient comfort, avoiding excess oxygen exposure in those patients with advanced disease and hypoxic ventilatory drive.

Needle aspiration is indicated only when patients are severely compromised upon presentation and require immediate intervention (e.g., tension pneumothorax). This should be followed by chest tube insertion. In recurrent or persistent cases, the patient should be evaluated for pleurodesis, by personnel from the CF center. While this may prevent recurrence, such intervention may have implications for lung transplant eligibility and should be discussed with physicians having experience in either CF or lung transplantation.

Daily CF therapies, such as chest percussion and postural drainage, oscillatory percussive vest therapy, other airway clearance techniques (e.g., positive expiratory pressure (PEP) mask, flutter valve), inhalation of dornase alfa, and pulmonary function testing, should be suspended transiently to avoid exacerbating the pneumothorax. Where needed, inhalational therapy with bronchodilators and/or inhaled corticosteroids may be continued with nebulization. The usual inhalational maneuvers with metered dose inhalers probably should be avoided until the pneumothorax is no longer an issue. Timing for reimplementation of the other therapies is determined by observation of pneumothorax resolution/extension and discussion with the patient's CF physician.

Gastroesophageal Reflux Disease

While many patients with CF are on acid suppression [e.g., H2 blocker or protein pump inhibitor (PPI)] for enhancement of exogenous pancreatic enzyme function, the incidence of gastroesophageal reflux disease (GERD) in children with CF is actually as high as 55% in some studies. Acute exacerbations of reflux can cause symptoms of gastritis and esophagitis including significant chest pain in the epigastrium and retrosternal regions. Medications, such as nonsteroidal antiinflammatory drugs (NSAIDs), recent dietary changes and stress and ethanol may exacerbate preexisting GERD. Clinical entities such as hiatal hernia or pulmonary hyperinflation may also predispose the patient to reflux. An empiric trial of acid control may be warranted, but all patients with recurrent symptoms of GERD, including regurgitation and chest pain, should be followed closely after ED discharge. In refractory cases, this leads to referral of the patient to a gastroenterologist for a formal evaluation including upper GI series, pH/impedance probe study, and/or endoscopy with biopsy.

Costochondritis

Costochondritis can be a common cause of chest pain in CF patients with increased intensity and frequency of cough or with certain viral infections with focal, inflammatory effects. The pain is described as sharp, exacerbated by coughing, and readily elicited either by palpation of the costochondral joints directly or by compression of the chest wall/sternum in an anteroposterior or lateral dimension. There is no curative therapy for this self-limited entity. A short course of analgesia can be considered, but care should be taken to inquire about baseline bowel and renal function, as concomitant CF medications may (synergistically with the analgesic) affect these organ systems.

Pleuritis

Pleuritic chest pain can present in CF patients during acute/subacute bacterial exacerbations of CF lung disease or with concomitant viral infection and, where possible, should be differentiated from costochondritis. Such pain is phasic with respiration. It is caused by pleural irritation secondary to inflammation of underlying lung tissue, with visceral pleura rubbing against the parietal pleural surface. The pain usually improves with antibiotic treatment of the underlying infectious process (if bacterial) and oral analgesia, the latter only necessary until the underlying infectious/inflammatory cause is resolving.

Cardiac Pain

Chest pain of cardiac origin is rare in the pediatric CF population, although they are as susceptible as any pediatric patient to entities such as viral pericarditis. While cardiac pain is more common outside the pediatric patient age group, the rare pediatric CF patient with severe pulmonary disease, nonpulmonary pain, and borderline secondary right heart dysfunction should be evaluated with a careful cardiac examination, electrocardiogram, CXR, and echocardiogram. Such patients with chest pain should be admitted for appropriate evaluation and management in consultation with a cardiologist.

Pulmonary Embolism

There is no current literature to suggest an increased incidence of pulmonary embolism (PE) in CF patients. As in any other patient with chest pain, shortness of breath, tachypnea, and possibly pleural effusion, one should entertain this etiology in the differential diagnosis. Depending on the extent of the underlying CF lung disease, even the use of PE protocol computed tomography (CT) scanning may not allow one to unequivocally confirm or refute this entity. Coupled with the propensity of CF patients to have hemoptysis, the risks in using anticoagulation or thrombolytic therapy with more than mild pulmonary disease are not trivial, and these therapies should always be performed in the inpatient setting. Once confirmed, standard management of pulmonary embolism is appropriate (while considering the confounders noted above).

Trauma/Rib Fracture

Schoolyard play and sports can lead to mild thoracic trauma or musculoskeletal injury as in children without CF. However, in patients with malnutrition, rib fracture can occur secondary to predisposing osteopenia. This can also happen in CF patients with overly aggressive chest percussion and postural drainage. Superficial ecchymoses, point tenderness along the rib margin, and evidence for scant subcutaneous fat tissue are suggestive of this entity. Diagnosis can be confirmed radiologically. Treatment is complicated by the need to at least temporarily limit airway clearance, which can lead to increasing airway obstruction. History of fracture or suspicious behavior should also raise the question of child abuse.

Shortness of Breath and Cough in the Absence of Chest Pain

As CF is characterized by impaired mucociliary clearance with concomitant chronic bacterial colonization and infection, recurrent bronchitis/pneumonia is common. Current standard of CF care is to use early maintenance airway clearance coupled with frequent culturing of the airway secretions and appropriate antibiotic therapy. However, most patients have difficulty fully clearing pathogens from the airways and experience chronic, recurrent pulmonary infections and chronic inflammation despite their daily maintenance therapies. An increase in a symptom such as cough or shortness of breath may simply be the sign of an acute viral respiratory tract infection but can also be caused by several other etiologies [e.g., acute exacerbation of progressive CF bacterial lung disease, allergic bronchopulmonary aspergillosis (ABPA), asthma].

Viral Respiratory Tract Infection

Simple viral respiratory infections, as common in the CF patient as in the general population, are often the inciting event for a pulmonary exacerbation. CF patients will be more likely to suffer increased/prolonged symptoms due to impaired mucociliary clearance and decreased respiratory reserve. It is important to check baseline oxygen saturation and (depending on findings from physical examination) obtain a CXR. Ideally the CXR should be compared with prior studies to differentiate new infiltrates from chronic changes. Even in patients with stable vital signs, oxygenation, and CXR, one may consider a short outpatient course of oral antibiotics if there is suspicion of exacerbation of the underlying CF lung disease (vide infra). It should be explained that such therapy is not directed at the viral infection but only at the superimposed chronic bacterial colonization, so that the parents do not automatically expect an antibiotic with any viral presentation.

Pulmonary Exacerbations of CF Bacterial Lung Disease

The pathophysiological triad of CF lung disease with inflammation, impaired mucociliary clearance, and subsequent chronic airway infection is the starting point for all pulmonary exacerbations. These events are usually associated with decline of lung function and acute worsening of respiratory symptoms. Clinical features of an exacerbation may include any or all of the following: increased cough, change of sputum quality or quantity, shortness of breath, increased work of breathing, loss of appetite, fatigue, and low-grade fever. On examination, the presence of new crackles/wheezes, increased tactile fremitus, and increased hyperinflation may be present. Lung function test changes usually associated with an exacerbation are decrease in forced vital capacity (FVC) and/or forced expiratory volume in 1 second (FEV_1) as compared with the patient's best values in the previous 12 months. In the ED setting, basic vital signs, including pulse oximetry, CXR, and sputum cultures, as well as baseline chemistries and blood counts should be obtained. Oxyhemoglobin saturation is often decreased from baseline values. Frequently, there is leukocytosis. CXR should ideally be compared with prior studies to assess for new infiltrates.

Treatment varies from oral/inhaled antibiotics to parenteral antibiotic treatment, either route being coupled with an increase in aggressive airway clearance. Other medications used chronically for maintenance of lung health may be continued or even increased during treatment of an acute exacerbation of pulmonary disease. Depending on the severity of symptoms, treatment options range from home therapy to hospital admission. Candid assessment of the family's ability to provide the increased care at home must be made. It is important to consider the recent overall course, home situation/adherence, and nutritional history in addition to the acute presentation.

In the case of a mild exacerbation, the patient can be managed at home with a 10- to 14-day course of antibiotics covering the usual organisms affecting CF patients. Here, the knowledge of organisms recovered from the patient in the CF center maintenance program may allow a choice of antibiotics directed against known pathogens specific to the individual patient. Common CF pathogens such as *Haemophilus influenzae* and *Staphylococcus aureus* (including methicillin-resistant *S. aureus*), *Pseudomonas aeruginosa*, *Stenotrophomonas maltophilia*, *Achromobacter xylosoxidans*, and *Burkholderia cepacia* complex require oral, inhaled, or combination therapy. It is important to ensure that the patient has a good airway clearance regimen in place at home, as antibiotics alone will not necessarily achieve the desired improvement.

In the case of a severe exacerbation, intravenous (IV) antibiotics should be initiated and the patient admitted either for a stabilizing period before home therapy completion or for the duration of intense treatment. Antibiotic coverage should be based on prior respiratory culture results and should include double coverage for *Pseudomonas* to limit the chance for the development of drug resistance to a single agent. An increased airway clearance regimen should be initiated. Special attention should be given to the patient's nutritional status and caloric requirements, both of which may deteriorate during acute illness. In patients with endocrine pancreatic insufficiency and CF-related diabetes, blood glucose levels can be more difficult to control during acute exacerbations. While dehydration is to be avoided, judicious fluid use is necessary to avoid mild pulmonary edema, which can easily occur in the setting of hyperinflation, poor oncotic pressure, and multiple IV administrations. Where possible, antibiotics should be concentrated to the smallest volume necessary for administration.

Whether in the ED or in the hospital, care must be given to infection control. Cross infection with various organisms has been demonstrated in many studies, and policies of the CFF have been promulgated to decrease the chance for such transmission. Early acquisition of organisms such as *Pseudomonas* have led to more rapid decline in lung function, and chance acquisition from another patient in the ED would be most unfortunate. Gown and gloves are the minimum standard precautions for CF patient care, with mask added as required for droplet precautions in suspected viral settings.

Wheezing

Wheeze on expiration is a common presentation in the pediatric ED, with acute viral processes, asthma, foreign bodies, and extrinsic airway compression from enlarged nodes/masses high in the differential diagnosis. With the CF patient, the list must include ABPA. ABPA occurs in 1% to 15% of patients with CF. ABPA is an exaggerated type I hypersensitivity reaction to the ubiquitous organism *Aspergillus fumigates*. CD4+ Th2 cells are activated and excess IgE and IgG1 are produced, all of which drive an inflammatory response in the airways. Clinically, patients present with (i) chronic wheeze that is difficult to control, (ii) decline in lung function, (iii) chronic cough, and (iv) transient infiltrates on CXR. Symptoms typically respond well to oral steroids. Any CF patient with recurrent wheezing and cough as well as changes on CXR and decline in lung function not responsive to antibiotic therapy and airway clearance should be evaluated for ABPA. Diagnostic criteria for CF patients include elevated total serum IgE level, positive skin reactivity to *Aspergillus*, and positive specific serum antibodies to *Aspergillus*. Treatment consists of a prolonged course of oral steroids (prednisone or prednisolone), usually starting at a dose of 2 mg per kg per day, with subsequent taper and close follow-up. IgE levels should be followed at regular intervals both as indication of response to therapy and as a warning of reexacerbation. There are no current studies to suggest a clear benefit of antifungal therapy along with steroids, although some physicians use concomitant oral itraconazole therapy in the hope that the course of oral steroids may be shortened.

Hemoptysis

Mild Hemoptysis

Blood streaking of the sputum is common in CF patients and requires no specific treatment other than observation to resolution. Persistent streaking may indicate the onset of a pulmonary exacerbation requiring antibiotic treatment. Other factors such as chronic use of medications with antiplatelet function activity (e.g., aspirin) or coagulopathy secondary to decreased vitamin K levels should be ruled out and treated accordingly. Other sources of bleeding, such as posterior epistaxis or hematemesis, should be ruled out as they require different approaches.

Moderate/Severe Hemoptysis

The CFF's Guidelines for Management of Hemoptysis define hemoptysis as mild (less than 60 cm³ daily), moderate (more than 60 and less than 240 cm³ daily), and severe (more than 240 cm³ daily or more than 100 mL per day for more than 2 days). Severe episodes can be life-threatening due to asphyxiation from airway obstruction, hypotension to the point of overt shock, chronic anemia, and/or chemical pneumonitis. Approximately 1% of CF patients experience an episode of major bleeding per year, the majority of patients being 16 years or older. The bleeding usually originates from enlarged and tortuous bronchial arteries, two-thirds of which arise from the ventral surface of the aorta. The remaining third come from the internal mammary and intercostals arteries. Onset is often unheralded. After initial stabilization of the patient, it is essential to differentiate true hemoptysis from extrathoracic upper airway tract or GI tract bleeding. A history may help to localize a pulmonary bleed as many CF patients notice localized gurgling or other unusual sensation in specific sites. Physical examination may reveal new, localized pulmonary findings or bleeding from an upper airway site such as the nasopharynx. Placing a nasogastric tube or performing endoscopy may become necessary in differentiating GI from pulmonary sources. A CXR can help determine localized changes from previous chest studies, as well as other unusual findings which could explain the bleeding (e.g., a new thick-walled cystic lesion suggesting infection with atypical mycobacterium). Unfortunately, often the CXR is not helpful in localizing the affected site.

The following laboratory tests should be obtained: complete blood cell count/differential, prothrombin time, partial thromboplastin time, liver function tests, arterial blood gas levels, emergency type and cross match, and sputum culture. Bronchoscopy may be necessary to localize the site of bleeding. However, not only can the procedure destabilize the patient further but also it is not always successful. Often, either the patient has stopped bleeding or massive hemorrhage prevents adequate visualization of the main stem/segmental bronchi. The majority of severe pulmonary bleeds in CF are self-limited and can be dealt with by using intensive care unit (ICU) monitoring, vitamin K, blood products, and antibiotics. Nonemergent bronchoscopy is indicated when bleeding appears to be progressive or persistent, and either surgery or local vascular therapy with arterial embolization will be necessary. In that situation, both rigid and flexible bronchoscopy should be available during the procedure in the operating room or ICU.

Ongoing management after hemodynamic stabilization is aided by reassuring and calming the patient. Drugs that could interfere with coagulation including aspirin, NSAIDs, inhaled drugs such as N-acetylcysteine, dornase alfa, and aerosolized antibiotics should be discontinued. Coagulation defects should be corrected with Vitamin K, fresh frozen plasma, or specific factors as indicated. Acute blood loss should be corrected with transfusions as clinically indicated, keeping in mind that patients with severe lung disease may be awaiting lung transplantation at some future date. Care should be taken when possible to obtain blood products prepared in a manner to minimize the risk of posttransplant complications.

As a majority of major bleeds are associated with pulmonary exacerbations, treatment with IV antibiotics may need to be initiated. Placing the lung that appears to be bleeding in the dependent position may help to prevent aspiration into the as yet uninvolved lung. IV therapies to halt bleeding, such as pitressin or octreotide, should be discussed with the pulmonologist or intensivist who will be accepting the admission. Local airway treatment may be indicated in acutely life-threatening situation, such as therapies including endobronchial tamponade, selective double lumen intubation, and iced saline lavage. Timely embolization or access to surgery needs to be organized. When a patient with major hemoptysis is admitted, a surgeon and interventional radiologist should be notified and should be readily available. If that is not possible, referral to another center should be considered.

Respiratory Failure

Thickened airway secretions with bacterial infection, mucus hypersecretion, bronchoconstriction, mucosal edema, inflammation, and fibrosis contribute to respiratory muscle fatigue and can lead to the development of respiratory failure in CF. Patients will present with hypoxia and/or hypercapnia associated with obstructive airway disease. The goal of treatment is to correct gas exchange and acid–base status, which are most likely occurring in the setting of concomitant pulmonary hypertension and cor pulmonale. The initial therapeutic approach should include intensification of antibacterial and airway clearance therapy. The patient should also be evaluated for comorbidities (e.g., atypical infections, ABPA, pneumothorax), which can be precipitating events for acute or subacute decompensation.

Long-term supplemental oxygen therapy should be initiated for patients with chronic hypoxemia. Usually noted first by desaturation while asleep, patients with daytime hypoxia (PaO_2 less than 55 torr or ~88%) need continuous supplemental oxygen therapy to limit development of pulmonary hypertension and right heart failure. Patients with daytime oxygen saturation of more than 88% but less than 92% or early signs of pulmonary hypertension with/without right heart failure should be evaluated for nocturnal desaturation. In any event, supplemental oxygen therapy needs to be introduced with caution in patients with chronic CO_2 retention, to avoid suppressing hypoxic ventilator drive. Initiation of Continuous Positive Airway Pressure or Bi-level Positive Airway Pressure via mask can be helpful in situations of acute decompensation or chronic fatigue and can be very effective when overnight relief is needed. Intubation with assisted ventilation is appropriate when there are reversible causes of respiratory failure, such as infection, or when lung transplantation is imminent. CF patients with progressive respiratory failure who are not lung transplant candidates and have been aggressively treated with standard therapy in a CF center have very poor chances of survival after intubation and mechanical ventilation is initiated and should be counseled accordingly.

ABDOMINAL PRESENTATIONS

GI problems account for a significant number of primary and secondary problems in patients with CF. Even in this era of CF prenatal diagnosis and neonatal screening, newborn meconium ileus may be the first symptom that leads to the diagnosis of CF. Similarly, in the young child, rectal prolapse or failure to thrive may first bring a patient to medical attention, and these may be first noted in the ED. In older children, recurrent bowel obstructive symptoms may lead to repeated ED visits and hospitalization. Despite the high incidence of CF-specific GI symptoms in this patient population, it is important to maintain a high suspicion for other etiologies such as appendicitis or intussusceptions (vide infra).

Abdominal Pain

Appendicitis

Appendicitis is often difficult to diagnose in patients with CF. Symptoms may be mild or severe, and the presentation may be altered concurrent with respiratory infection antibiotic use. Other etiologies are often considered first and lead to delay in diagnosis. This in turn may lead to an increased incidence of complications such as perforation and periappendiceal abscess formation (Table 99.2). Appropriate attention to the rectal examination and the widespread availability of abdominal CT scan (Fig. 99.2) in the ED makes earlier determination of appendicitis possible in this patient population.

Constipation/Meconium Ileus/Distal Intestinal Obstructive Syndrome

Constipation can be an intermittent or chronic problem in CF patients with pancreatic insufficiency. The earliest manifestation is meconium ileus, which may present to the ED in infants discharged too early (e.g., before passing a stool) from the birthing hospital. Abdominal distension, irritability, and failure to feed in a neonate raise the possibility. More likely, however,

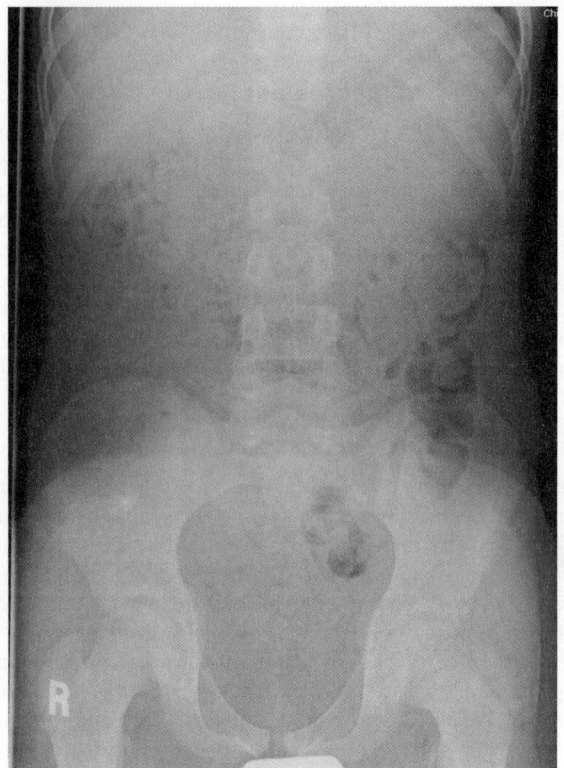

FIGURE 99.2 Radiograph showing constipation.

this will present in an older infant with a history of stooling, possibly with frequent diarrhea and other manifestations of CF that had not yet been diagnosed.

The consistency of the stool in CF constipation is not that of "rock hard" inspissated stool. Rather, it is a sticky, tenacious material that is very adherent to the bowel wall. Some stool may actually pass by the initial intermittent obstruction, so history of recent stooling should not deter one from considering this diagnosis. In addition, the softer consistency of the stool is such that more frequently than not, no stool is palpable on examination. Thus, a soft abdomen does not rule out constipation and stool retention.

Diagnosis is best made with supine and upright abdominal films (Fig. 99.3), although it should also be evident on CT scan. Localization of the stool retention will help guide therapy (vide infra). In the more advanced case, air–fluid levels, marked distension, and severe abdominal pain may denote the presence of DIOS, or distal intestinal obstruction syndrome. This latter represents a more extensive constipation event and invariably leads to admission despite any initial improvement in the ED.

First treatment should include adequate (although not excessive) hydration. If the stool is predominantly in the descending or transverse colon, a simple enema in the ED may begin removal of the obstruction. After distal stool removal, or in the face of a predominantly ascending colon obstruction, a poorly absorbable hypertonic solution such as GoLYTELY® should be administered. While some older children will drink this, the most reliable method is to pass an nasogastric tube for administration as clearance is much more gradual if the rate of administration is too slow. N-acetylcysteine enemas may be

TABLE 99.2

ABDOMINAL PAIN IN CYSTIC FIBROSIS PATIENTS

Common	Uncommon	Rare
Malabsorption	Appendicitis	Intussusceptions
Constipation	Cholecystitis	Inflammatory
GERD		bowel disease
DIOS		
Pancreatitis		

GERD, gastroesophageal reflux disease; DIOS, distal intestinal obstruction syndrome.

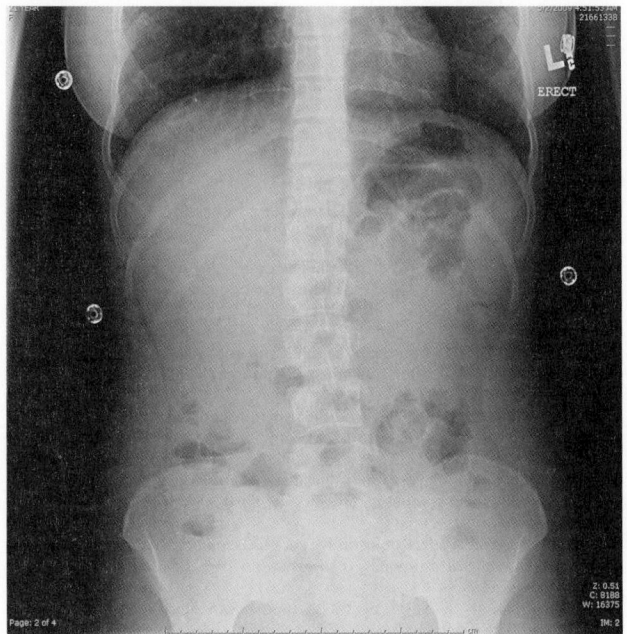

FIGURE 99.3 Radiograph showing distal intestinal obstructive syndrome.

beneficial in some patients. For patients with DIOS, a retrograde, hyperosmolar contrast enema under fluoroscopic guidance from the radiologist may be needed. In this setting, it may be prudent to notify the abdominal surgeon of the case so that in the (unlikely) event of perforation, surgical resources may be mobilized rapidly.

Depending on the degree of obstruction and the rapidity of response, the patient may need to be admitted. Refeeding before complete clearance of stool from the KUB (plain frontal supine radiograph of the abdomen) radiograph may lead to reaccumulation of feces and the need to start the process all over again. It is important to try and determine what led to the obstruction. Did the patient fail to take their oral enzymes? Are the enzyme supplements outdated or damaged (exposed to excessive heat)? Has there been an alteration in diet to more constipating foods? Have sports or summer heat led to relative dehydration or limited access to toilet facilities? Does the patient need the intermittent use of stool-hydrating agents or cathartics? Failure to appreciate such etiologies may lead to representation to the ED a few days or weeks later.

Pancreatitis

Historically, it was thought that acute pancreatitis only occurred in CF patients who were clinically pancreatic insufficient (PI). We now appreciate, however, that even the presence of one CF allele predisposes to a statistically higher incidence of pancreatitis in the general population, and that pancreatitis can occur in PI patients with enough functioning pancreatic tissue to become obstructed and inflamed. Precipitating events are not very different from those of non-CF patients, and this is complicated by the fact that CF patients are often on high-fat diets to promote weight gain. Elevations of amylase and lipase levels are usually noted, although because of preexisting pancreatic insufficiency, the levels reached may be lower than expected in non-CF pancreatitis. As patients age and have recurrent episodes of pancreatitis, both the intensity of symp-

toms and the levels of lipase/amylase elevation decline. Eventually, the exocrine pancreas is completely destroyed to the point where the patient no longer has enough functioning tissue to be symptomatic from pancreatitis.

Gastroesophageal Reflux with Esophagitis

Reflux, often clinically asymptomatic, has been recognized in CF patients since the early 1980s. It is not surprising, given the hyperinflation, increased coughing with resultant elevated intraabdominal pressures, and use of agents that may decrease lower esophageal tone. When pain presents, it will be either as chest pain or as subxiphoid pain. It is usually not influenced by phase of respiration but can be excruciating. If considered, one can treat with an antacid preparation to see if there is transient relief. Assuming no GI bleeding is active at the time of presentation, appropriate management with H2 blockers or PPIs can be started. At the present time, many CF patients are already on such agents because of the improvement in exogenous pancreatic enzyme supplement function. Routinely, if CF patients require higher doses of supplemental enzymes to resolve their steatorrhea and gain weight, such agents are added to alkalinize the duodenal environment. Presence of such an agent in the patient's medication list should not of itself remove the diagnosis from consideration. Some patients are not as consistent in taking these medications as they should be, and not all specific PPIs work well in individual CF patients. Sometimes several different PPIs have to be tried before the desired response is noted.

Cholecystitis

Thirty percent of all CF patients have a small, hypotrophic gall bladder filled with sludge. This is due in part to the intrahepatic biliary epithelium defect for CFTR transport, the same defect seen in airway and pancreatic cells. The stones are often difficult to visualize and may require discussion with the radiologist as to how best to visualize them. In older patients (both with and without CF), medical treatment is only symptomatic and frequent manifestation of cholecystitis often leads to cholecystectomy.

Other Causes of Abdominal Pain

Patients with CF are no more, and no less, likely to develop adhesions postoperatively than are others. Occasionally, patients with a history of meconium ileus surgery earlier in life may develop signs of intestinal obstruction either without stool retention or unresponsive to therapy directed at such a cause. Abdominal CT scan may be useful in ascertaining whether this or other less common causes of CF abdominal pain (intussusception, inflammatory bowel disease, etc.) may be etiologic. Treatment, either medical or surgical as indicated, does not differ from that of the non-CF population.

GI Bleeding

Although not common in CF patients, GI bleeding can occur in a subset of the patient population. Because of malabsorption of vitamin K, some patients do not have normal clotting function. While this usually manifests as either frequent ecchymoses or airway hemorrhage, a few patients may have minor bleeding from GI sources (e.g., esophagitis). However, a small fraction of CF patients have cirrhosis and develop bleeding varices or hemorrhoids. The etiology is the CFTR defect in the intrahepatic biliary epithelium, which leads to bile stasis and fibrosis. Onset of CF liver disease can be subtle and missed despite CFF mandated quarterly abdominal examinations and yearly phlebotomy. Sometimes the first presentation is an enlarging spleen, or even a GI bleed.

Such hemorrhage can be quite significant, and any evaluation of GI bleeding for common causes has to include evaluation for cirrhosis with varices. Any CF patient with GI bleeding needs to have the cause elucidated, and in the ED, this may require complete blood cell count/differential, prothrombin time, partial thromboplastin time, fat-soluble vitamin levels (to evaluate absorption in general), and either CT scan or abdominal ultrasound. Standard approaches for blood replacement and hemodynamic stabilization with admission to the ICU are appropriate. Immediate and long-term follow-up with the gastroenterologist/hepatologist, if not already part of the patient's care profile, should be in place. Endoscopy, either investigative or for treatment of esophageal varices, is often necessary.

FOLLOW-UP CARE

The majority of CF patients in the United States are followed in CFF approved and supported CF centers. All centers' contact information is available at the CFF Web site (http://www.cff.org). Close contact between emergency physicians and the CF center team caring for this patient population facilitates continuity of care and hopefully diminishes representation to the ED for recrudescence of the presenting problem. Transmission of radiographs, laboratory results, and evaluation summaries will be much appreciated by the CF care team. At the same time, CF center physicians are on call and always available to provide information about their patients to the physicians in the ED providing acute care.

Suggested Readings

Anderson DH. Cystic fibrosis of the pancreas and its relation to celiac disease: clinical and pathological study. *Am J Dis Child* 1938;56:344–399.

Bartlett JR, Friedman KJ, Ling SC, et al. Genetic modifiers of liver disease in cystic fibrosis. *JAMA* 2009;302(10):1076–1083.

Bishop MD, Freedman SD, Zielenski J. The cystic fibrosis transmembrane conductance regulator gene and ion channel function in patients with idiopathic pancreatitis. *Hum Genet* 2005;118:372–381.

Button BM, Roberts S, Kotsimbos TC, et al. Gastroesophageal reflux (symptomatic and silent): a potentially significant problem in patients with cystic fibrosis before and after lung transplantation. *J Heart Lung Transplant* 2005;24(10):1522–1529.

Columbo C, Battezzati PM. Hepato-biliary manifestations of cystic fibrosis. *Eur J Gastroenterol Hepatol* 1996;8:748–754.

Donaldson SH, Bennett WD, Zeman KL, et al. Mucus clearance and lung function in cystic fibrosis with hypertonic saline. *New Engl J Med* 2006;354(3):241–250.

Flume PA. Pulmonary complications of cystic fibrosis. *Respir Care* 2009;54(5):618–627.

Flume PA, Mogayzel PJ Jr, Robinson KA, et al. Cystic fibrosis pulmonary guidelines: treatment of pulmonary exacerbations. *Am J Respir Crit Care Med* 2009;180:802–808.

Flume PA, Strange C, Ye X, et al. Pneumothorax in cystic fibrosis. *Chest* 2005;128:720–728.

Houwen RH, van der Doef HP, Sermet I, et al. Defining DIOS and constipation in cystic fibrosis with a multicentre study on the incidence, characteristics, and treatment of DIOS. *J Pediatr Gastroenterol Nutr* 2009 Jun 9. (Epub ahead of print).

Ramsey BW, Boat TF. Outcome measures for clinical trials in cystic fibrosis: summary of a Cystic Fibrosis Foundation Consensus Conference. *J Pediatr* 1994;124:177–192.

Rommens JM, Ianuzzi MC, Bat-Sheva K, et al. Identification of the CF gene: chromosome walking and jumping. *Science* 1989;8:1059–1065.

Saiman L, Siegel J. Cystic Fibrosis Foundation. Infection control recommendations for patients with cystic fibrosis: microbiology, important pathogens, and infection control practices to prevent patient-to-patient transmission. *Infect Control Hosp Epidemiol* 2003;24:S6–S52.

Schidlow DV, Taussig LM, Knowles MR. Cystic Fibrosis Foundation Consensus Conference report on pulmonary complications of cystic fibrosis. *Pediatr Pulmonol* 1993;15:187–198.

Stevens DA, Moss RB, Kurup VP, et al. Allergic bronchopulmonary aspergillosis in cystic fibrosis—state of the art: Cystic Fibrosis Foundation Consensus Conference. *Clin Infect Dis* 2003;37(suppl 3):S225–S264.

CHAPTER 100 ■ RENAL AND ELECTROLYTE EMERGENCIES

NANCY M. RODIG, MD

DEHYDRATION/HYPOVOLEMIA

Background

Clinically significant hypovolemia occurs more commonly in children than in adults, and this is predicted given characteristics specific to the pediatric patient. Predisposing factors include a higher frequency of acute gastroenteritis (AGE) in children when compared to adults, a higher surface area-to-volume ratio in children with proportionally higher insensible losses, and the inability to access adequate fluids to replenish losses given developmental limitations. Volume depletion will develop as fluid lost from the extracellular space is inadequately replaced. Losses may ensue from the gastrointestinal tract, skin, or kidneys. Far less frequently, volume depletion may result when fluid intake is inadequate to provide maintenance requirements necessitated by caloric intake without excessive losses, which may occur in those who are supported with enteral tube feedings.

Gastrointestinal loss is the most common cause of pediatric hypovolemia, and viral AGE accounts for the majority of cases. Database analysis studying disease burden in the United States and Europe reveals that diarrhea was associated with approximately 4% of emergency department visits. Rotavirus-positive AGE is generally more severe than rotavirus-negative AGE, resulting in more significant dehydration and increased need for emergency room assessment and hospitalization. Rotavirus-associated diarrhea has been estimated to be associated with 4% to 5% of all childhood hospitalizations.

Clinical Manifestations

The initial assessment of a child with hypovolemia will include history and thorough physical examination. A careful history should establish the cause of hypovolemia, duration of illness, and approximate volume and composition of fluid taken in and retained. Inquiries regarding urine production, one indication of intravascular volume, should be made. Potential causes of increased insensible losses, such as fever and tachypnea, should be accounted for.

The physical assessment should include an accurate weight, and the weight should be remeasured if ongoing losses are significant and difficult to quantify. A change in weight from a recent healthy baseline, if available, would provide an objective account of the degree of depletion. Assessment of intravascular volume should include the pulse quality and rate, blood pressure,

hydration of mucous membranes, skin turgor, mental status, and activity. Mild hypovolemia (3% to 5% volume loss) may be associated with minimal or absent clinical signs. Moderate hypovolemia (6% to 9% volume loss) will have clinical signs apparent, which may include tachycardia, fall in blood pressure with orthostatic accentuation, dry mucous membranes, and delayed capillary refill time. A systematic review of published data reported by Steiner et al. revealed that the most useful individual signs for predicting 5% hypovolemia in children were delayed capillary refill time, abnormal skin turgor, and deep respiratory pattern. A combination of examination signs provided the best predictive data. In the setting of severe dehydration (greater than or equal to 10% volume loss), evidence of shock may be apparent. Severe hypovolemia requires immediate attention with aggressive isotonic fluid resuscitation and the reader is referred to Chapter 3 to review the management of shock. Clinical dehydration scales have been published and recently validated for children with AGE.

Though laboratory assessment has been shown to be less useful than physical findings when predicting the degree of volume depletion, laboratory testing can identify associated electrolyte and acid–base abnormalities. Classification of the type of hypovolemia based upon the serum sodium (Na) may impact subsequent fluid therapy and monitoring. The serum Na concentration is determined by the ratio between total body solutes and total body water (TBW). Solute is primarily composed of sodium salts in the extracellular fluid (ECF) and potassium salts in the intracellular fluid (ICF). The presenting serum Na in the child with hypovolemia results from the loss of solute relative to water during the illness. Determinants of the serum Na include the type of fluid lost, the composition of fluid provided prior to presentation, and the ability to excrete water during the illness.

Hyponatremic hypovolemia (serum Na less than 135 mEq per L) reflects the net loss of solute in excess of water. Solute is never lost in excess of water in any physiologic fluid, as losses can never be hypertonic to plasma. Hyponatremia results when water taken in is retained due to the effect of antidiuretic hormone (ADH), which is secreted due to the stimulation of volume receptors for ADH release. Additional stimuli of ADH secretion identified in children with gastroenteritis include vomiting, hypoglycemia, and stress. Isonatremic hypovolemia (serum Na 135 to 145 mEq per L) results when solute is lost in proportion to water, and hypernatremic hypovolemia (serum Na greater than 145 mEq per L) reflects net loss of water in excess of solute. The sodium plus potassium concentration of diarrheal fluid in viral gastroenteritis is typically less than 100 mEq per L, representing relatively hypotonic losses. Despite the relatively dilute losses, the majority of cases of hypovolemia caused by viral gastroenteritis are isonatremic.

Other biochemical abnormalities that may develop during hypovolemia include disorders of potassium homeostasis, acid–base abnormalities, and increased blood urea nitrogen and creatinine, reflecting a decline in glomerular filtration rate (GFR). Though hyperkalemia may result, hypokalemia is more commonly seen in children with gastroenteritis given the loss of potassium in diarrheal fluid and urine. Urine losses of potassium may be generous and driven by aldosterone. The effect of aldosterone is to conserve urinary sodium to maintain effective intravascular volume and promote potassium excretion. Alternatively, marked acidosis may favor the development of hyperkalemia due to transcellular shift of potassium ions. During acidosis hydrogen ions enter the intracellular space to be buffered, and potassium moves to the extracellular space to maintain electroneutrality. If a child presents with hypovolemia and acidosis, one may expect that the serum potassium will fall with correction of the acidosis. Therefore, if hypokalemia and acidosis are concurrent abnormalities at presentation, hypokalemia may worsen with resolution of acidosis, or hypokalemia may develop despite initial normal serum potassium concentration. Physicians should be prepared to provide supplemental potassium if appropriate. If the patient is oligoanuric or renal function is significantly compromised, excessive potassium supplementation may cause hyperkalemia.

Management

The treatment of children with dehydration should be guided by the following inquiries: (i) Is there need for emergent fluid therapy? (ii) Is there an abnormality of the serum Na? (iii) Should fluid be provided by the oral or intravenous route? The aims of treatment are to restore perfusion and maintain adequate volume in the face of ongoing losses. Approaching fluid management with a plan for initial repletion therapy followed by ongoing maintenance therapy may be useful. The repletion phase may require emergent fluid resuscitation, and therefore may be considered in two phases if necessary—emergent repletion and ongoing repletion.

Oral therapy, when tolerated, is recommended by the American Academy of Pediatrics as the preferred treatment of fluid and electrolyte losses in children with mild to moderate diarrhea. The following will focus on intravenous fluid therapy, and the reader is referred to Chapter 17 for more extensive discussion regarding recommendations for oral rehydration therapy (ORT). In general, limitations to ORT include severe dehydration, altered mental status, abdominal ileus or disorders that limit intestinal absorption, severe and persistent vomiting, excessive stool losses and severe electrolyte abnormalities.

Emergent Fluid Repletion

Patients who have moderate or severe hypovolemia will have compromised effective circulating volume, and rapid volume resuscitation is required to restore perfusion and avoid tissue damage. Emergent intravenous fluid therapy should be provided with a rapid infusion of 20 mL per kg of isotonic crystalloid, such as 0.9% sodium chloride (NS) or NS with 5% dextrose (D5% NS). Assessment of the patient's perfusion during and at completion of the intravenous bolus is imperative in

order to determine if additional bolus therapy is indicated. Isotonic crystalloid fluid is the only solution recommended for emergent fluid repletion, and the use of hypotonic or hypertonic crystalloid solutions in emergent resuscitation is not recommended. Currently, there is inadequate data to support the use of colloid-containing solutions during resuscitation in the general population. However, patients with decreased oncotic pressure due to illnesses such as nephrotic syndrome or cirrhosis may benefit from a colloid solution if they present with hypovolemia. In these patients, initial bolus therapy with 5% albumin may be beneficial. In addition to monitoring the physical exam for evidence of adequate perfusion, establishment of urine flow would be reassuring. The urine flow in response to therapeutic interventions should be clearly documented.

Ongoing Repletion and Maintenance Therapy

Once effective circulating volume has been adequately restored, the second phase of fluid therapy corrects persistent deficits, replaces ongoing losses, and provides maintenance fluids. In cases of hypotonic or isotonic hypovolemia, there are various approaches to this phase of therapy, including the traditional "deficit" therapy for which the composition of the fluid is based upon estimates of depletion and therapy based upon isotonic intravenous fluid. Deficit therapy is a method of replacing previous fluid losses while providing the expected maintenance requirements for water and electrolytes. The water deficit may be estimated by the fall in body weight, and this estimate is most accurate if a recent baseline weight is known. The Na deficit can be estimated by the following equation using the serum Na concentration and estimates of TBW:

$$\text{Na deficit} = [\text{TBW(n)} \times 140 \text{ mEq/L}] - [\text{TBW(c)} \times \text{serum Na}]$$

In this calculation, TBW(n) is the estimated normal TBW, TBW(c) is the estimated current TBW, and serum Na is the serum Na concentration. The normal TBW in term neonates, toddlers, and older or pubertal children is approximately 75% to 80%, 65% to 70%, and 60% of body weight, respectively. The current body water is estimated by considering the degree of dehydration. For example, if a healthy child's TBW content is approximately 60% of weight, then in the setting of severe dehydration, the current body water may be 50% of weight. The maintenance requirement for water in children is based upon the estimated caloric expenditure of hospitalized children at bed rest as described in Holliday and Segar's landmark paper published in 1957. The calculations based upon this are outlined in Table 100.1 and can serve as a starting point to provide maintenance needs.

TABLE 100.1

WEIGHT-BASED DAILY MAINTENANCE FLUID FOR CHILDREN

Body weight (kg)	Daily fluid requirements
3.5–10 kg	100 mL/kg/day
11–20 kg	1,000 mL + 50 mL/kg (for each kg >10), maximum 1,500 mL/day
>20 kg	1,500 mL + 20 mL/kg (for each kg >20), typical maximum 2,400 mL/day

Though common practice has been to provide hypotonic maintenance fluids based upon deficit calculations and maintenance requirements, recent reports have highlighted the potential risks of acquired hyponatremia. Of note, some reports pointing to this risk have included postoperative patients. A group of children who presented to a tertiary pediatric hospital with hypovolemia due to presumed gastroenteritis were randomly assigned to receive hypotonic (0.45% NS with 2.5% dextrose) or isotonic fluid (0.9% NS with 2.5% dextrose). Hyponatremia was a common finding, noted in 36% of patients at presentation. Of the children presenting with hyponatremia, the serum Na was unchanged with hypotonic solution and increased from approximately 132 to 134 mEq per L with isotonic solution after 4 hours of rehydration. Of the children who presented with isotonic hypovolemia, the serum Na fell approximately 2 mmol per L after hydration with hypotonic fluid and was unchanged after hydration with isotonic solution. Nonosmotic stimuli for ADH release would predispose to positive water balance and hyponatremia. Some have proposed that isotonic fluid be continued in the ongoing repletion and maintenance phase of therapy with periodic assessment of serum Na to determine if further adjustment in fluid composition is warranted. The risks of sodium excess, inadequate free water provision during ongoing hypotonic losses, and hypernatremia must be considered. Rapid rehydration schemes have been put forth for cases of moderate or severe hypovolemia and recommend expanding the ECF with 40 mL per kg over 1 to 2 hours utilizing lactated Ringer's solution or normal saline. Additional isotonic therapy of 20 to 40 mL per kg over 1 to 2 hours is provided if warranted by physical assessment of perfusion. The potential benefits of rapid rehydration include restoration of the ECF with improved gastrointestinal and renal perfusion. Improved gastrointestinal perfusion may allow earlier oral hydration. Currently there are inadequate data to support the use of isotonic solution as the new "standard of care" for ongoing fluid repletion and maintenance therapy in hypovolemia. Further studies are needed to compare the efficacy and safety of differing fluid regimens.

Of importance is the recognition of potential potassium deficit when planning fluid therapy. Potassium is the principal cation of the ICF and contributes to the maintenance of intracellular tonicity. The ICF contains approximately 98% of the body potassium, and the serum potassium concentration does not adequately reflect total body stores. There is no practical means of calculating the potassium deficit. When calculating the Na deficit as outlined above, this actually reflects *total cation* (Na^+ and K^+) deficit lost from the extracellular and intracellular compartments. The majority of patients with hypovolemia will present after a brief illness, which typically has persisted for less than 1 week. If the illness has been ongoing for less than 3 days, historical estimates suggest that 75% to 100% fluid losses arise from ECF (primarily sodium loss). As the duration of the illness lengthens to beyond 3 days, a greater proportion of fluid is lost from the ICF (primarily potassium loss) with approximately 60% to 75% lost from the ECF.

The following tables (Tables 100.2 through 100.4) provide examples of isonatremic, hyponatremic, and hypernatremic hypovolemia and outline an approach to fluid therapy. The examples assume that the duration of illness has been brief,

---

TABLE 100.2

ESTIMATED DEFICITS AND INTRAVENOUS THERAPY: 10 kg CHILD WITH 10% HYPOVOLEMIA AND SERUM SODIUM 140 mEq/L

Water and sodium (Na) deficits
Water deficit: 10 kg × 10% = 1 L
Na deficit: 1 L × 140 mEq/L = 140 mEq

Emergent fluid repletion with NS or D5% NS
20 mL/kg × 10 kg = 200 mL (200 mL water and ≈30 mEq sodium)

Ongoing repletion and maintenance requirements
Remaining water deficit: 1,000 mL − 200 mL = 800 mL
Daily maintenance water requirement: 100 mL/kg/day × 10 kg = 1,000 mL/day
800 mL + 1,000 mL = 1,800 mL/24 h = 75 mL/h
Remaining Na deficit: 140 mEq − 30 mEq = 110 mEq
Maintenance sodium requirement: 3 mEq/100 mL water × 1,000 mL/day = 30 mEq/day
110 mEq + 30 mEq = 140 mEq/24 h
140 mEq/1,800 mL ≈ 0.45% sodium chloride (½ NS)
Maintenance potassium requirement: 3 mEq/100 mL water × 1,000 mL/day = 30 mEq/day
30 mEq/1,800 mL ≈ 15–20 mEq/L
Intravenous fluid based upon deficit calculations:
D5% 1/2 NS with 20 mEq/L KCl at 75 mL/h

Ongoing losses
Extrarenal losses should be replaced mL-for-mL if volumes are significant.
The sodium content of the fluid lost should be estimated or measured in order to select the appropriate replacement fluid.

---

and therefore, potassium losses from the ICF are relatively small compared to sodium losses from the ECF. For illnesses of longer duration, 20% to 40% of the total cation deficit may be potassium and would require less sodium and more potassium repletion. For the examples of isotonic and hypotonic hypovolemia, the deficit is corrected over the first 24 hours. Traditional schemes of replacing one half of the remaining deficit over the first 8 hours and the remainder over the next 16 hours for isotonic hypovolemia and replacing about two thirds of the deficit in the first 24 hours for isonatremic hypovolemia may be applied.

Isonatremic Hypovolemia

Table 100.2 outlines the estimated deficits and therapeutic approach of a 10-kg child with isotonic hypovolemia. In this example, the isotonic deficit is corrected by an initial bolus of isotonic saline followed by ongoing repletion. The traditional approach of deficit calculation and therapy is outlined. Replacement of ongoing extrarenal losses should be provided if the volume of losses is significant and increased free water provision may be necessary should ongoing gastrointestinal losses be significant in order to avoid hypernatremia. The importance of strict monitoring of fluid balance is emphasized and repeated assessment of the serum Na may be indicated on the basis of losses and duration of intravenous therapy.

TABLE 100.3

ESTIMATED DEFICITS AND INTRAVENOUS THERAPY:
10 kg CHILD WITH 10% HYPOVOLEMIA AND
SERUM SODIUM 125 mEq/L

Water and sodium deficits
Water deficit: 10 kg × 10% = 1 L
Sodium deficit: [TBW(n) × 140 mEq/L] − [TBW(c) × 125 mEq/L]
TBW(n) = 10 kg × 65% = 6.5 L
TBW(c) = TBW(n) − water deficit = 6.5 L − 1 L = 5.5 L
Sodium deficit: (6.5 L × 140 mEq/L) − (5.5 L × 125 mEq/L) ≈ 220 mEq

Emergent fluid repletion with NS or D5%NS
20 mL/kg × 10 kg = 200 mL (200 mL water and ≈30 mEq sodium)

Ongoing repletion and maintenance requirements
Remaining water deficit: 1,000 mL − 200 mL = 800 mL
Daily maintenance water requirement: 100 mL/kg/day × 10 kg = 1,000 mL/day
800 mL + 1,000 mL = 1,800 mL/24 h = 75 mL/h
Remaining sodium deficit: 220 mEq − 30 mEq = 190 mEq
Maintenance sodium requirement: 3 mEq/100 mL water × 1,000 mL/day = 30 mEq/day
190 mEq + 30 mEq = 220 mEq
220 mEq/1,800 mL ≈120 mEq/L
Maintenance potassium requirement: 3 mEq/100 mL water × 1,000 mL/day = 30 mEq/day
30 mEq/1,800 mL ≈15–20 mEq/L KCl
Intravenous fluid based upon deficit calculations:
D5% with 120 mEq/L NaCl and 20 mEq/L KCl at 75 mL/h
Given the availability of standard solutions in emergency departments, D5%NS *with added potassium* could be provided for the initial half of the total volume and completed with D5%1/2 NS *with added potassium.*

Ongoing losses
Extrarenal losses should be replaced mL-for-mL if volumes are significant.
The sodium content of the fluid lost should be estimated or measured in order to select the appropriate replacement fluid.

TABLE 100.4

ESTIMATED DEFICITS AND INTRAVENOUS THERAPY:
10 kg CHILD WITH 10% HYPOVOLEMIA AND
SERUM SODIUM 155 mEq/L

Water and sodium deficits
Total water deficit: 10 kg × 10% = 1 L
TBW(c) = TBW(n) − 1 L = (10 kg × 65%) − 1 L = 5.5 L
Free water deficit: TBW(c)[(155/140) − 1] = 5.5[(155/140) − 1] = 0.59 L
Isotonic deficit = total water deficit − free water deficit = 0.41 L
Sodium deficit: 0.41 L × 140 mEq/L ≈ 60 mEq

Emergent fluid repletion with NS or D5%NS
20 mL/kg × 10 kg = 200 mL (200 mL water and ~30 mEq sodium)

Ongoing repletion and maintenance requirements
Remaining total water deficit: 1,000 mL − 200 mL = 800 mL, plan to replace over 36–48 h or 400 mL/day × 2 days
Daily maintenance water requirement: 100 mL/kg/day × 10 kg = 1,000 mL/day
1,000 mL + 400 mL = 1,400/24 h or ≈60 mL/h
Remaining sodium deficit: 60 mEq − 30 mEq = 30 mEq
Maintenance sodium requirement: 3 mEq/100 mL water × 1,000 mL/day = 30 mEq/day
Total sodium requirement: 30 mEq + 30 mEq = 60 mEq
60 mEq/1,400 mL or ≈0.225% sodium chloride
Maintenance potassium requirement: 3 mEq/100 mL water × 1,000 mL/day = 30 mEq/day
30 mEq/1,400 mL ≈20 mEq/L KCl
D5% 1/4 NS with 20 mEq/L KCl at 60 mL/h for ~36–48 h

Ongoing losses
Extrarenal losses should be replaced mL-for-mL if volumes are significant.
The sodium content of the fluid lost should be estimated or measured in order to select the appropriate replacement fluid.

Hyponatremic Hypovolemia

Children with mild to moderate hyponatremia should be provided isotonic or near-isotonic fluids to both complete the repletion phase and continue the maintenance phase of intravenous fluid therapy. Providing hypotonic fluid in the setting of persistent decreased intravascular volume and acute illness with osmotic and nonosmotic stimuli for ADH secretion may perpetuate or worsen hyponatremia. Isotonic saline will correct the volume depletion and raise the serum Na concurrently. When intravascular volume is restored, the volume stimulus for ADH secretion will be removed and will allow the renal excretion of free water. The therapy of asymptomatic hyponatremia requires gradual correction of the serum Na with a target increase of less than 10 to 12 mEq per L per day.

Table 100.3 estimates the sodium and water deficits and outlines a plan for fluid management of a child with hyponatremic hypovolemia and serum Na of 125 mEq per L. As in the previous example, the deficits are replaced by an initial bolus and then completed over the next 24 hours. Of note, the composition of the intravenous fluid based upon deficit calculations with added potassium chloride (120 mEq per L Na$^+$ + 20 mEq per L K$^+$) is an isotonic fluid. Potassium is osmotically active, and infused potassium will move to the intracellular space in exchange for sodium to the extracellular space, promoting an increase in the serum Na concentration. Therefore, if the rate of rise of the serum Na is greater than targeted (10 to 12 mEq per L per day), the concentration of sodium in the intravenous fluids should be reduced. The need for serial assessment of serum Na concentration in order to make appropriate adjustments to fluid composition is again emphasized.

For children with severe hyponatremia (i.e., serum Na less than 125 mEq per L) and hypovolemia, volume resuscitation should proceed with isotonic solution to restore effective circulating volume. However, given mechanisms of cellular adaptation to maintain normal cell volume in brain cells, rapid correction of the serum Na should be avoided. The therapy of severe hyponatremia or symptomatic hyponatremia is discussed further in the section "Hyponatremia."

Hypernatremic Hypovolemia

In children who present with hypernatremic hypovolemia, the total fluid deficit is composed of both a free water deficit and an isotonic deficit. A pure water deficit is consistent with dehydration. Hyperosmolality initially promotes water movement out of the cells, including brain cells. Over several days, idiogenic osmols are generated within the brain cells, prompting water movement into the intracellular space and restoring normal brain volume. Once cerebral adaptation has occurred, rapid correction of the serum Na can result in cerebral edema and severe neurologic consequence. The goal of therapy in children with a serum Na concentration above 150 mEq per L is to correct the hypernatremia at a rate of less than 10 to 12 mEq per L in 24 hours. The total fluid deficit can be inferred by the estimated weight loss. Calculation of the free water deficit is based upon the serum Na and estimated current body water,

$$\text{Free water deficit} = \text{TBW(c)} \times [(\text{serum Na}/140) - 1]$$

The difference between the total fluid deficit and the free water deficit is the estimated isotonic deficit. After the patient has received the initial isotonic fluid bolus to emergently restore intravascular volume, subsequent therapy should correct the remaining isotonic deficit, free water deficit, ongoing losses, and maintenance requirements. Depending on the acuity and severity of the process, the free water deficit should be replaced gradually to allow judicious correction of the serum Na at the desired rate. Table 100.4 estimates the sodium and water deficits and outlines a plan for fluid management of a child with hypernatremic hypovolemia and serum Na of 155 mEq per L. The Na deficit is calculated on the basis of the isotonic deficit. Alternatively, the Na deficit can be calculated using the serum Na and estimates of TBW as previously reviewed.

ELECTROLYTE DISORDERS

Disorders of Sodium Homeostasis

Sodium salts are the predominant solutes in the extracellular space. The serum Na concentration is directly related to the total body solute content and inversely related to the TBW. Given this relationship, the plasma sodium concentration will vary depending on changes of the either total body sodium or TBW. All body compartments are freely permeable to water, and water will move along an osmotic gradient. Sodium is cell membrane permeable, though remains predominantly in the extracellular space due to the action of Na^+–K^+-ATPase.

Hyponatremia

Background. Hyponatremia is commonly defined as a measured serum Na concentration less than 135 mEq per L. When approaching a patient with hyponatremia, it is necessary to estimate the patient's total body sodium and water based on history and physical exam. Gastroenteritis is a common cause of hyponatremia presenting for pediatric urgent or emergent care, which would be a state of total body sodium deficiency relatively greater than TBW deficiency. However, as outlined in Table 100.5, there are numerous causes of hyponatremia associated with normal or increased total body sodium, including states of impaired water excretion such as renal failure and the syndrome of inappropriate antidiuretic hormone (SIADH) secretion. It is critical to assess for underlying causes associated with increased total body sodium and water, as in the edema-forming states. In these clinical circumstances, providing supplemental sodium would aggravate the state of volume excess.

Appropriate evaluation to determine the cause of hyponatremia begins with a thorough physical examination in order to estimate the child's volume status. History may reveal obvious sources of sodium loss or raise the concern for water intoxication. Laboratory tests should include serum electrolytes, osmolality, and assessment of renal function. Concomitant urine studies should include osmolality, urine sodium, and urinalysis. In children with hyponatremia and concentrated urine, the urine sodium may distinguish between states of decreased effective circulating volume and euvolemic hyponatremia, such as the SIADH. In the setting of decreased effective circulating volume, the urine sodium concentration is generally less than 25 mEq per L, which is an appropriate renal response to maintain perfusion. Patients with SIADH have impaired free water excretion, though urine sodium handling is intact and dependent on sodium intake. In patients with SIADH, the urine sodium concentration is generally greater than 40 mEq per L. Further studies to investigate the underlying cause of hyponatremia are guided by clinical assessment and consideration of the differential diagnosis.

MEDICAL EMERGENCIES

TABLE 100.5

CAUSES OF HYPONATREMIA BASED UPON TOTAL BODY SODIUM CONTENT

Low total body sodium	Normal total body sodium	High total body sodium
Diarrhea	SIADH	Congestive heart failure
Vomiting	Adrenal insufficiency	Nephrotic syndrome
Ostomy losses	Hypothyroidism	Liver failure (cirrhosis)
Bleeding	Acute renal failure	Multiorgan dysfunction
Diuretic use	Water intoxication	
Mineralocorticoid deficiency	Psuedohyponatremia	
Salt wasting renal disease		
Cystic fibrosis		
Marathon running		

Clinical Manifestations. The symptoms attributable to hyponatremia are primarily neurologic and due to water movement into brain cells. The symptoms mirror the severity of cerebral edema, which in turn is related to the degree of hyponatremia and the acuity of the process. The mechanisms of cellular adaptation include movement of intracellular electrolytes to the extracellular space, which can occur within minutes. Over hours to days, organic solutes move to the extracellular space. Given the ability for cerebral adaptation, the degree of cerebral edema and neurologic symptoms are less severe in chronic hyponatremia. Early neurologic symptoms include nausea and malaise, and may be seen when the serum Na concentration falls below 125 mEq per L. With progressive derangement of cerebral cell volume, symptoms of headache, altered mental status, lethargy, ataxia, and psychosis may ensue. Signs of severe cerebral edema include seizures, coma, and respiratory depression.

Management. For children with hyponatremia associated with hypovolemia, isotonic solutions should be provided to restore intravascular volume. In cases of severe hyponatremia (i.e., serum Na less than 125 mEq per L), symptoms of neurologic dysfunction due to cerebral edema may evolve. Children with symptomatic hyponatremia require urgent treatment to avoid progressive neurologic complications. Symptoms are more likely to develop if hyponatremia evolves rapidly, as water will move along an osmotic gradient from the extracellular space to the intracellular space. Given the effect of cell volume regulatory mechanisms, an important goal is to control the rate of rise in serum Na to prevent rapid fluid shifts into the extracellular space and avoid the development of osmotic demyelination. The general recommendation for a child with severe hyponatremia is to increase the serum Na no more rapidly than 12 mEq per L in the first 24 hours or an average of 0.5 mEq per L per hour. An exception to this guideline would be symptomatic hyponatremia and evolving cerebral edema. Symptomatic hyponatremia would call for a more aggressive initial correction of the serum Na of approximately 2 mEq per L per hour for 2 to 3 hours, which should result in clinical improvement. This can be achieved with hypertonic or 3% saline (513 mEq per L of sodium). As an example, the calculation for the dose of sodium required to increase the serum Na by 4 mEq per L in a symptomatic patient is

$$Na \ (mEq) = TBW(c) \times 4 \ mEq/L$$

Once the dose of sodium is estimated, the volume of 3% saline can be calculated as each mL contains approximately 0.5 mEq of sodium. After the initial correction is achieve, the goal for the daily correction remains approximately 12 mEq per L in the first 24 hours (including the initial emergent correction). Frequent assessment of serum Na is necessary to avoid rapid correction, which may lead to the osmotic demyelination syndrome.

Patients who have asymptomatic hyponatremia and euvolemia do not require urgent intervention. The care of these patients should be carefully planned and based upon the underlying diagnosis with the aim of gradual correction. If hyponatremia is associated with an edema-forming state, providing supplemental sodium will worsen the state volume excess, and the goal of therapy would be to achieve negative water balance in excess of negative sodium balance. To achieve this effectively, the underlying pathophysiology must be considered, though initial water restriction is generally indicated. Sodium restriction and diuretic therapy may also be warranted. The treatment of SIADH begins with water restriction, though this may be insufficient. Some cases of SIADH require the administration of salt supplements and loop diuretics to achieve the desired negative water balance. Loop diuretics interfere with the countercurrent concentrating mechanism in the loop of Henle and impair the renal responsiveness to ADH.

Hypernatremia

Background. Hypernatremia is defined as a serum Na greater than 145 mEq per L. An increase in the serum Na can result from an increase in the total body solutes, a decrease in body water, or a reduction of body water relatively greater than a concurrent reduction in total body solutes. Protective mechanisms to prevent the development of hypernatremia include the stimulation of thirst and the ability to excrete concentrated urine, thereby minimizing free water loss. For these mechanisms to be effective, there must be adequate access to and the ability to retain free water. Given the potential for limited access to water, infants and the elderly are predisposed to hypernatremic dehydration. The causes of hypernatremia based on total body sodium are outlined in Table 100.6. Hypernatremia due to isolated water deficit is termed dehydration. If both salt and water deficits are present, this condition is termed hypovolemia.

Diarrhea is a common cause of hypernatremia in the urgent or emergent care setting. Though the degree of Na deficit may vary, generally children who present for care have

---

TABLE 100.6

CAUSES OF HYPERNATREMIA BASED UPON TOTAL BODY SODIUM CONTENT

Low total body sodium	Normal total body sodium	High total body sodium
Diarrhea	Increased insensible losses	Salt poisoning
Vomiting	Fever	Inappropriately mixed formula
Ostomy losses	Prematurity	Salt water drowning
Osmotic diuresis	Phototherapy	NaHCO₃ given with CPR
Immature renal	Radiant warmers	
conservation	Tachypnea	
(prematurity)	Nephrogenic DI	
	Central DI	

NaHCO₃, sodium bicarbonate; CPR, cardiopulmonary resuscitation; DI, diabetes insipidus.

true hypovolemia. Though hypernatremia due to salt excess is rare, this can occur with the improper mixing of infant formulas or iatrogenic administration of a salt load. The latter can result after sodium bicarbonate infusion during cardiopulmonary resuscitation or during therapy of refractory metabolic acidosis. Hypernatremia secondary to nearly pure water loss may develop if replacement of insensible water loss from the skin and respiratory tract is inadequate. Central diabetes insipidus is due to insufficient release of ADH from the hypothalamic nuclei, and nephrogenic diabetes insipidus is due to a renal resistance to the effect of ADH. Most children affected with these disorders have normal thirst and free access to water and are able to maintain acceptable water balance. However, infants who do not have free access to water and children with intercurrent illness precluding adequate intake of free water are at risk for the development of hypernatremic dehydration.

The cause of hypernatremia is usually evident from the presenting history. In formula fed infants, an accurate account of formula preparation should be pursued to evaluate for inappropriate mixing, which would result in increased renal osmotic load. Inquiries of urine volume should also be made, as the production of significant urine in a child who presents with apparent hypernatremic dehydration would be suggestive of diabetes insipidus. The physical examination should assess weight, perfusion, and mental status. During hypernatremic hypovolemia, water moves from the intracellular to the extracellular space. Given the relative preservation of the extracellular volume, this may delay the objective signs of volume depletion typically noted by clinicians. Laboratory studies should include serum electrolytes, serum osmolality, BUN, and renal serum creatinine. If the underlying diagnosis remains in question, urine studies may be informative. Urine osmolality should be compared to serum osmolality and would be elevated if renal concentrating mechanisms are intact. If the urine osmolality is inappropriately low when compared to the serum osmolality, then central or nephrogenic diabetes insipidus should be considered. The urine sodium concentration may also assist diagnosis. During hypernatremic hypovolemia, the urine sodium is generally less than 25 mEq per L due to the effect of aldosterone to maintain perfusion. If hypernatremia is due to salt excess, the appropriate renal response is to excrete sodium, and the urine sodium concentration would be elevated.

Clinical Manifestations. Similar to hyponatremia, the clinical manifestations of hypernatremia are primarily neurologic. The rise in the plasma osmolality causes water movement out of the brain. The decrease in brain volume may lead rupture of the blood vessels contained in the membranes that tether the brain to the overlying skull and elsewhere. Early clinical manifestations can include lethargy, weakness, fever, and irritability. More severe manifestations include seizures and coma. Symptoms are more likely if the disturbance is acute and rapid. If hypernatremia evolves more slowly, there is cerebral adaptation to protect brain cell volume. Adaptive mechanisms include movement of cerebrospinal fluid into the brain, uptake of sodium and potassium into the cells, followed by intracellular accumulation of osmolytes.

Management. During sustained hypernatremia, cerebral adaptation occurs over several days to restore brain cell volume. Rapid correction of the serum Na after cerebral adaptation occurs results in osmotic movement of water into the brain and cerebral edema. Data suggest that the plasma sodium concentration should be lowered by less that 0.5 mEq per L per hour and no more than 12 mEq per L per day. In children with hypernatremia due to salt loading, treatment should facilitate renal excretion of sodium. This is typically achieved with salt restriction and free water and may be facilitated with diuretics. If intravenous fluids are required, the sodium plus potassium concentration of the fluid provided should be less than the sum of these electrolytes in the urine, and the fluid should be given at a rate sufficient to achieve positive water balance. Adequate intravascular volume should be assured to allow renal excretion of sodium. The therapy of children with hypernatremic hypovolemia (sodium and water deficit) was previously reviewed. In summary, children with clinical signs of decreased effective circulating volume should be provided isotonic saline to restore perfusion. Once intravascular volume is restored, hypotonic fluids should continue to allow judicious restoration of the estimated free water deficit. If hypernatremia is due to nearly pure water deficit (hypernatremic dehydration), replacement of free water should be provided at a rate to allow correction of the serum Na at an acceptable rate.

Disorders of Potassium Homeostasis

Potassium is the most abundant intracellular cation in the body with only approximately 2% of total body stores present in the extracellular space. Among a variety of vital cellular functions, high cytosolic potassium concentration is required for growth, metabolism, cell division, and protein synthesis. Maintenance of the cytosolic potassium concentration and transcellular gradient is dependent on the function of the basolateral cell membrane enzyme, Na^+–K^+-ATPase. This enzyme is physiologically regulated by insulin, thyroid hormone, catecholamines, aldosterone, and plasma potassium concentration. Hormonal and metabolic dysregulation may result from conditions present in ill children and result in abnormalities of potassium homeostasis.

Hypokalemia

Background. Hypokalemia is defined as a measured serum potassium concentration below 3.5 mEq per L. Hypokalemia may result from total body deficit, transcellular shift of potassium to the intracellular space, or a combination of both processes. There are numerous causes of hypokalemia including renal loss, extrarenal loss, and increased cellular uptake, which are outlined in Table 100.7. The common causes of hypokalemia seen in pediatric emergency departments are due to gastrointestinal loss, diuretic use, and diabetic ketoacidosis (DKA).

Loss of gastric or intestinal secretions from any cause will predispose a child to the development of hypokalemia by both direct and indirect mechanisms. The potassium concentration of lower intestinal fluids is relatively high, ranging from 20 to 50 mEq per L, and diarrhea may result in significant potassium loss. The potassium content of gastric fluid is lower at approximately 5 to 10 mEq per L, and hypokalemia associated with vomiting is not primarily due to enteral loss but increased renal excretion of potassium. Gastrointestinal losses resulting in volume contraction will stimulate the secretion of aldosterone,

TABLE 100.7

CAUSES OF HYPOKALEMIA

Decreased potassium intake
Increased renal excretion
   Diuretics
   Metabolic alkalosis (chloride deficient)
   Diabetic ketoacidosis
   Increased mineralocorticoid effect
   Nonreabsorbable anions
   Renal tubular acidosis (type 1 and type 2)
   Bartter's syndrome
   Gitelman's syndrome
   Magnesium depletion

Increased gastrointestinal losses
   Diarrhea
   Laxatives
   Ostomy losses

Increased cellular uptake (redistributive)
   Acute alkalosis
   Insulin therapy
   Elevated β-adrenergic activity
   Increase in bone marrow cell production
   Hypokalemic periodic paralysis

which promotes sodium conservation and increased potassium excretion in the distal nephron. Gastric losses associated with metabolic alkalosis will increase the delivery of sodium and water to the aldosterone-sensitive site and facilitate this exchange. Metabolic alkalosis will also promote transcellular shift of potassium to the intracellular space to maintain electroneutrality. For every approximately 0.1 U rise in blood pH, the anticipated reduction of extracellular potassium concentration of approximately 0.4 to 0.6 mEq per L.

Potassium homeostasis is complex and dynamic in the setting of DKA. Urinary losses of potassium are high due to osmotic diuresis, hypovolemia-induced hyperaldosteronism, and the presence of β-hydroxybutyrate in the glomerular filtrate. β-Hyroxybutyrate is a nonreabsorbable anion and obligates cation loss, which includes both sodium and potassium. Patients with DKA generally have total body potassium depletion at presentation. However, the combination of insulin deficiency, which reduces the activity of the Na^+–K^+-ATPase, and hyperosmolality, which draws water and potassium out of the cells, may result in normal or elevated serum potassium at presentation. Hypokalemia in child who presents with DKA would suggest significant potassium depletion and need for supplementation with close monitoring.

The cause of hypokalemia may be inferred after a careful history is obtained. This should include a thorough account of medications taken, such as diuretics, laxatives, and beta agonists. The laboratory assessment of hypokalemia should include serum electrolytes, magnesium, calcium, serum bicarbonate, renal function, and glucose. In addition to urinalysis and urine pH, urine electrolytes and osmolality should be submitted to assess the renal response to hypokalemia. If the urine potassium concentration is less that 15 mEq per L, this would suggest extrarenal losses, though would be misleading if the child was polyuric. Calculation of the transtubular potassium

gradient (TTKG) estimates the tubular potassium concentration at the end of the cortical collecting duct, permitting estimation of the aldosterone effect. This calculation is relatively accurate as long as the urine sodium concentration is greater than 25 mEq per L and the urine osmolality is greater than the plasma osmolality:

$$TTKG = [(\text{urine K/serum K}) \div (\text{urine osmolality/serum osmolality})]$$

If the TTKG is less than 3, this would be consistent with low urine excretion and extrarenal cause of hypokalemia.

Clinical Manifestations. The clinical manifestations of hypokalemia are generally proportionate to the severity and duration of the disorder and result from hyperpolarization of the cell membrane. Unless the serum potassium falls rapidly or is associated with digitalis use, symptoms are typically not apparent until the serum level is below 2.5 mEq per L. Symptoms may also vary dependent on the concentration of other ions, including calcium, magnesium, and hydrogen. Clinically relevant signs and symptoms of hypokalemia relate to abnormal neuromuscular function and cardiovascular effects, and monitoring of muscle strength and electrocardiogram (EKG) are indicated to assess the functional consequences of hypokalemia. Neuromuscular dysfunction typically manifests as skeletal muscle weakness in an ascending pattern with worsening hypokalemia. Lower extremity muscles are initially affected with progression to the trunk and upper extremities. Respiratory weakness may develop and lead to respiratory failure. Smooth muscle dysfunction can lead to nausea, vomiting, constipation, and voiding dysfunction with urinary retention. Significant hypokalemia produces characteristic changes on the EKG. As the plasma K drops, T-wave amplitude declines, U waves develop, and ST segment depression may result. With more profound hypokalemia the QRS complex may widen and the PR interval may prolong. Supraventricular and ventricular dysrhythmias may develop, the likelihood being greater for patients taking digitalis and in patients with congestive heart failure and coronary ischemia. Renal effects of hypokalemia include a defect in the ability to concentrate urine, an acquired form of nephrogenic diabetes insipidus.

Management. The therapeutic approach to hypokalemia must take into consideration numerous factors including severity, acuity, associated clinical signs, comorbid conditions, and the expectation for ongoing loss. In general, potassium replacement is indicated when there has been potassium loss. If hypokalemia is redistributive in nature but associated with either severely depressed levels or clinical signs, supplementation may be required. However, supplementation during a redistributive process should proceed with close monitoring given the risk of rebound hyperkalemia. In cases when potassium has been lost, there is no strict correlation between serum level and total body stores, and potassium deficit can only be approximated. In clinical scenarios when potassium loss is accompanied by acid–base disturbance, a redistribution effect should be factored when losses are estimated. Magnesium supplementation is indicated in hypokalemia associated with hypomagnesemia. In all cases of significant hypokalemia, monitoring for EKG changes and muscle strength is imperative, and if abnormalities are present, immediate replacement is warranted.

The choice of oral or intravenous replacement will depend on the severity of the disorder and the ability to tolerate enteral salts. If the child is clinically well, oral therapy is preferable and can be provided two to four times per day as potassium chloride. Dosing may start at 2 to 5 mEq per kg per day and be adjusted on the basis of serial laboratory assessment. If there is concurrent metabolic acidosis, potassium citrate or bicarbonate can be provided. If the child is unable to take oral medications or is symptomatic, intravenous potassium should be provided. If the child is not symptomatic, potassium can be added to the maintenance fluids. If intermittent infusion is indicated, this can begin with an intravenous dose of 0.5 to 1 mEq per kg (typical maximum 30 to 40 mEq per dose). In order to avoid insulin secretion, which promotes transcellular shift of potassium into the intracellular space, potassium should be provided in a dextrose-free solution. Potassium chloride or potassium phosphate may be used, though the use of phosphate salt is typically limited to the treatment of DKA or documented severe hypophosphatemia. The reader is referred to Chapter 86 for further discussion regarding potassium replacement in the setting of DKA. Potassium acetate or its equivalent should be used if there is metabolic acidosis. The infusion rate for clinically stable patients should provide 0.25 mEq per kg per hour, though emergent conditions may warrant the maximal rate of 0.5 to 1 mEq per kg per hour (maximum 15 to 40 mEq per hour depending on local policy) with continuous EKG monitoring.

Hyperkalemia

Background. Hyperkalemia is typically defined as serum potassium concentration exceeding 6 mEq per L in neonates or 5.5 mEq per L in children or adults. Serum potassium concentration is determined by the interplay of potassium intake, distribution between the intracellular and extracellular space, and renal excretion. In normal subjects, ingestion of a large potassium load is initially handled by cellular uptake driven by increased activity of the Na^+–K^+-ATPase. The activity of this enzyme is increased by insulin and β_2-adrenergic stimulation. Potassium is subsequently excreted by incremental increase in serum potassium concentration and increased aldosterone effect, which promotes potassium excretion in the distal nephron. This effect of aldosterone is dependent on the delivery of sodium and water to the distal secretory site, which may be compromised in states of decreased intravascular volume. Hyperkalemia can therefore result from excessive load, transcellular shift, decreased renal excretion, or a combination of these factors.

If hyperkalemia develops, both endogenous and exogenous sources of potassium should be considered. Potential sources of exogenous potassium include large volume packed red blood cell transfusion, medicines with significant potassium content, such as Penicillin G potassium (1.7 mEq K per 1 million units), and potassium salt infusions. Given improvements in blood bank procedure, hyperkalemia is less common with transfusion of red cells. Endogenous sources of potassium may result from tissue damage, including burns, trauma, rhabdomyolysis, hemolysis, tumor lysis, and gastrointestinal bleeding with enteral reabsorption. Clinical scenarios associated with extracellular shift include metabolic acidosis, hyperosmolarity, insulin deficiency, and the use of β-adrenergic receptor antagonists. Reduced renal excretion of potassium may occur

TABLE 100.8

MEDICATIONS ASSOCIATED WITH HYPERKALEMIA

NSAIDs
ACE inhibitors
Angiotensin II receptor blockers
Amiloride
Spironolactone
Eplerenone
Tacrolimus
Cyclosporine
Propranolol
Digitalis

in acute or chronic renal insufficiency, hypovolemia, mineralocorticoid deficiency, inherited or acquired renal tubulopathy, and due to the use of certain medications (Table 100.8).

Evaluation begins with a thorough history with specific inquiries regarding injuries, muscle pain, history of renal disease, and medications taken. Laboratory studies should include serum electrolytes, calcium, phosphorus, bicarbonate, and renal function. Serum creatinine kinase should be submitted if there is suspicion for rhabdomyolysis. Urine electrolytes and osmolality should be obtained to calculate the TTKG to estimate the aldosterone effect. The TTKG would be greater than 10 to 11 in a normal subject provided a potassium load, reflecting appropriate aldosterone effect. A value below 5 to 7 would be suggestive of hypoaldosteronism. An EKG should be obtained to monitor for cardiac effect.

Clinical Manifestations. The clinical features associated with hyperkalemia are a consequence of altered cellular transmembrane potassium gradient, which reduces the resting membrane potential. Initially this increases membrane excitability, which is followed by a sustained reduction in excitability. Unless the rise is rapid, symptoms or signs generally do not become apparent until the serum potassium concentration exceeds 7.0 mEq per L. Clinical features predominantly involve cardiac conduction and neuromuscular disturbance. Cardiac dysrhythmias are the most serious consequence, and toxicity is exacerbated by a rapid rise in potassium concentration, acidosis, hyponatremia, and hypocalcemia. Early EKG changes include narrow peak T waves with shortened QT interval, which is followed by progressive lengthening of the PR interval and widening of the QRS complex. There may be loss of P-wave amplitude and eventual "sine wave" pattern when the QRS merges with the T wave. This is typically followed by ventricular fibrillation or standstill. Neuromuscular effects are rarely evident at potassium concentrations less than 8 mEq per L and include paresthesias, skeletal muscle weakness, and ascending flaccid paralysis. Respiratory muscles are typically spared.

Management. Strategies to prevent complications from hyperkalemia include (i) removing potassium from the body, (ii) shifting potassium to the intracellular space, and (iii) antagonizing the cell membrane effects of hyperkalemia (Table 100.9). The urgency of care should be based upon the degree of hyperkalemia and evidence of cardiac or neuromuscular effect. Should there be EKG changes consistent with hyperkalemia,

THERAPIES FOR HYPERKALEMIA

Intravenous calcium to stabilize cardiac membrane
Calcium gluconate 10% solution, 50–100 mg/kg (0.5–1 mL/kg); typical adult dose 1,000 mg, max 2,000–3,000 mg
Infuse over 2–5 min, central access is preferred, may repeat in 10 min if needed
Patient must be on cardiac monitor
Effect is immediate in onset though transient (~30 min)

Measures to redistribute potassium into the intracellular space
Insulin and dextrose:
Give dextrose 1 g/kg and provide insulin 0.2 U/g of dextrose
Monitor blood glucose
Time to onset is ~15–30 min, duration is 2–6 h

β_2 Agonists:
2.5–5 mg nebulized albuterol
Time to onset is 20–30 min, duration 2–4 h

Sodium bicarbonate:
1–2 mEq/kg IV over 5–15 min
Minimal effect if the child is not acidemic
Time to onset ~15–30 min, duration ~2 h

Measures to remove potassium from the body
Cation exchange resins:
Sodium polystyrene sulfonate 1 g/kg orally or per rectum, may repeat dose after 4 h
Do not give retention enema with sorbitol
Do not give if within 1 wk of surgery (postoperative ileus)
Time to onset is 1–2 h

Loop diuretics:
1–2 mg/kg furosemide IV, higher doses may be required in renal insufficiency
To avoid hypovolemia, provide appropriate non-potassium–containing fluids
Time to onset 15–60 min

Dialysis:
To be employed if conservative measures fail after discussion with nephrology consultant

the patient should be placed on cardiac monitor and intravenous calcium should be provided to stabilize cardiac membranes. It has been recommended that calcium is indicated only in instances of significant EKG changes, such as widening of the QRS or loss of the P wave but is not indicated in isolated peaked T waves. The effect of calcium is nearly immediate but also transient and should be coupled with other measures to shift potassium to the intracellular space and remove potassium from the body. Calcium gluconate (10% solution) 50 to 100 mg per kg IV or calcium chloride (10% solution) 20 mg per kg IV infused over 2 to 5 minutes with continuous cardiac monitoring. The usual adult dose of calcium gluconate is 1,000 mg and calcium chloride is 500 to 1,000 mg. Calcium is irritating to veins and can result in tissue necrosis; therefore, central vein access is preferable for both the gluconate and chloride salts and strongly recommended if calcium chloride is infused. In patients taking digitalis, an immediate cardiac consultation should be obtained prior to administration if possible as calcium therapy may precipitate other dysrhythmias.

Several therapies are aimed at shifting potassium into the intracellular space and are outlined in Table 100.6. Increasing the effect of insulin enhances the activity of the Na^+–K^+-ATPase in skeletal muscle, driving the K^+ into the cell. Enzyme activity can be increased by intravenous dextrose infusion, though a greater effect is anticipated with the combination of insulin and dextrose. The time of onset is 15 to 30 minutes, peak effect at approximately 60 minutes, and duration of several hours. Providing sodium bicarbonate raises the systemic pH and promotes hydrogen movement out of the cells accompanied by potassium movement into the cells. This is most effective in patients with metabolic acidosis. The time of onset is approximately 15 to 30 minutes and persists for several hours. β_2-adrenergic agonists increase Na^+–K^+-ATPase activity and promote transcellular shift, and therefore, nebulized albuterol may provide further benefit.

Though slower in onset than measures applied to shift potassium into the intracellular space, efforts to remove potassium are necessary. This is essential in cases of total body potassium excess. Sodium polystyrene sulfonate (Kayexalate®) is a commonly used ion exchange resin. Within the intestinal lumen, the resin takes up potassium in exchange for sodium. To a lesser extent, the resin will also exchange for calcium and magnesium, and therefore, electrolytes should be monitored with frequent or prolonged dosing. Oral doses may be provided in sorbitol, which tends to precipitate osmotic diarrhea and augments enteral potassium loss. The pediatric oral dose is 1 g per kg provided every 4 to 6 hours as necessary. Adults are typically provided 15 to 30 g orally. Rectal doses of 1 g per kg every 2 to 6 hours may be given without sorbitol, though the dose must be retained for 15 to 30 minutes to be effective. Kayexalate should not be provided to patients within 1 week of surgery due to risk of intestinal necrosis. In patients who have acceptable renal function, providing isotonic saline and loop diuretics may increase potassium excretion. Isotonic expansion may be particularly effective in patients who are hypovolemic with decreased effective renal perfusion. In cases of hypovolemia, diuretics should only be provided once volume status is restored to avoid prerenal insult. Thereafter, close monitoring of volume balance will allow appropriate adjustment of fluid rate and diuretic dosing. In those patients with significantly impaired renal function, dialysis may be indicated. Hemodialysis provides more rapid clearance of potassium, though peritoneal dialysis may be more practical depending on the size of the child, center preference, and comorbidities such as cardiovascular instability or congenital heart disease.

Disorders of Calcium Homeostasis

Calcium is the most abundant cation in the body with approximately 99% of calcium present in the skeleton in the form of hydroxyapatite. The small fraction remaining in the soft tissue and ECF compartment plays a pivotal role in cellular processes. The intracellular calcium concentration (approximately 10^{-7} mmol per L) is very low when compared to ECF concentration (approximately 1.25 mmol per L), and this concentration gradient is maintained by activity of calcium ATPase. A well-regulated ECF calcium concentration is critical for cell function and survival. The ECF calcium is approximately 40% bound to plasma proteins, approximately 12% complexed with other ions, such as phosphate and citrate, and approximately 48% free or ionized. It is the ionized fraction of calcium that exerts physiologic effect and is under physiologic regulation. Of note, the fraction of calcium bound to plasma proteins is affected by the extracellular pH. During acidemia, hydrogen ions will displace calcium from proteins and increase ionized calcium levels, and alkalemia will promote the opposite effect.

Calcium homeostasis is dependent on endocrine control of three primary organ systems: intestines, kidneys, and the skeletal system. The parathyroid gland allows for the rapid regulation of ionized calcium concentration via the calcium-sensing receptor (CaSR). The CaSR is highly expressed in the parathyroid gland and is activated by low concentrations of ionized calcium, thereby stimulating parathyroid hormone (PTH) secretion. PTH will increase serum calcium levels through several mechanisms: (i) mobilize calcium from the bone, (ii) increase calcium reabsorption in the distal renal tubule, (iii) stimulate the conversion of 25-hydroxyvitamin D to 1,25-dihydroxyvitamin D, the active metabolite of vitamin D. 1,25-Dihydroxyvitamin D promotes calcium and phosphorus absorption from the gastrointestinal tract and reabsorption from the renal tubules. Calcitonin is a hormone produced by the parafollicular cells of the thyroid when calcium levels are high. Calcitonin inhibits osteoclastic activity and promotes movement of calcium from the blood into the skeletal system.

Hypocalcemia

Background. Hypocalcemia has many causes, which include PTH deficiency or resistance, vitamin D deficiency or resistance, extravascular deposition, and abnormal magnesium metabolism (Table 100.10). Abnormal serum calcium should be confirmed by repeat measurement and if confirmed, ionized serum calcium should be measured. As approximately 90% of protein-bound calcium is bound to albumin, the serum albumin concentration should also be determined. For each 1 g per dL reduction in serum albumin, the total calcium concentration will be lowered by approximately 0.8 mg per dL. Hypoalbuminemia does not effect the ionized calcium concentration, which is under hormonal regulation. If available, previous calcium levels should be reviewed to determine if this is an acute or chronic process. Though results will not be available during an urgent or emergent assessment period, a serum PTH level must be performed in all patients with confirmed hypocalcemia. Measurement of serum phosphate, magnesium, and creatinine should also be performed. Hyperphosphatemia increases the risk for calcium phosphate precipitation in tissues and may lead to hypocalcemia. Magnesium is required for PTH release, and hypomagnesemia results in hyporesponsiveness to the effect of PTH in target organs. Hypocalcemia is common in renal failure and is due to phosphate retention and insufficient production of 1,25-dihydroxyvitamin D. As timely serum PTH levels may not be available for review, urine calcium, phosphate, and creatinine should be submitted to assess renal tubular handling, which may suggest the PTH effect. Vitamin D metabolites should be performed in selected patients if clinically indicated.

Clinical Manifestations. The clinical manifestations of hypocalcemia are dependent on the severity of the abnormality, the rate of decline in serum calcium, and the chronicity of the underlying process. Other factors affecting the development of symptoms include acid–base balance and hypomagnesemia. Classic acute manifestations of hypocalcemia include neuromuscular instability or tetany, which effects both sensory and muscular function. Early or mild symptoms include paresthesias of the perioral region, hands and feet, and muscle cramps. More severe symptoms include seizure, laryngospasm and bronchospasm. Classic physical findings in patients with neuromuscular instability include Trousseau's sign and Chvostek's sign. A positive Trousseau's sign is the precipitation of carpopedal spasm by inflation of a sphygmomanometer above systolic blood pressure for 3 minutes. A positive Chvostek's sign is contraction of the ipsilateral facial muscle induced by tapping of the facial nerve in front of the ear. Of note, Chvostek's sign may be present in up to 10% of normal subjects. In addition to neuromuscular findings, acute hypocalcemia may result in significant cardiovascular disturbance, including hypotension, congestive heart failure, prolonged QT interval, and dysrhythmias. Papilledema may also be present and resolves with correction of hypocalcemia.

Management. Numerous forms of calcium salts are available, and therefore, attention to the salt form is critical when dosing to determine the elemental calcium dose. Calcium may be provided by either oral supplementation or intravenous solution. The appropriate choice is guided by pertinent clinical findings. In general, intravenous calcium is indicated if the patient has prolonged QT, significant symptoms (tetany, seizures, carpopedal spasm), or acute decrease in serum corrected calcium to less than or equal to 7.5 mg per dL regardless of symptoms. Oral supplementation is more appropriate when symptoms are absent or mild and corrected calcium is greater than or equal to 7.5 mg per dL. In patients with asymptomatic chronic hypocalcemia associated with chronic kidney disease (CKD), oral calcium supplementation is preferred with concomitant

---

TABLE 100.10

CAUSES OF HYPOCALCEMIA

Precipitation or altered binding
  Hyperphosphatemia
  Metabolic alkalosis
  Citrated products
  Pancreatitis

Vitamin D deficiency
  Nutritional
  Malabsorption
  Impaired synthesis
    Hepatic dysfunction
    Renal dysfunction
  Impaired metabolism
    Vitamin D–dependent rickets

Hypoparathyroidism
  Impaired synthesis
    DiGeorge Syndrome
    Activating mutations of the calcium-sensing receptor
  Psuedohypoparathyroidism

Other
  Hypomagnesemia
  Hungry bone syndrome
  Fluoride poisoning

replacement of 1,25-dihydroxyvitamin D. If hypocalcemia is associated with metabolic acidosis, correction of the acidosis will reduce the ionized calcium level. Therefore, if metabolic acidosis is not causing clinical compromise, priority should be given to increasing the serum calcium. If hypocalcemia is associated with severe hyperphosphatemia, the provision of calcium may result in the precipitation of calcium and phosphate in the tissues, a disorder known as calciphylaxis. In patients with associated hypomagnesemia, magnesium supplements should be provided, as persistent hypomagnesemia will hinder the correction of hypocalcemia.

Prompt treatment of symptomatic or severe acute hypocalcemia should be initiated intravenously with either calcium chloride or calcium gluconate. Central access is necessary for calcium chloride infusions, though emergent situations may indicate peripheral infusion. Central access is preferred for calcium gluconate, though this salt can be infused peripherally via a large vein. The use of calcium gluconate is usually favored as it is less likely to result in tissue damage if extravasation occurs. As concentrated forms are irritating to veins, calcium salts should be diluted in dextrose and water or saline. The final concentration of calcium gluconate should be 50 mg per mL, and calcium chloride should be diluted to 20 mg per mL. Calcium should not be prepared or infused with fluids containing phosphate or bicarbonate given the risk of precipitation of insoluble salts. The dose for intravenous bolus of calcium gluconate in the setting of cardiac disturbance is 50 to 100 mg per kg per dose infused over 3 to 5 minutes and for tetany is 100 to 200 mg per kg per dose infused over 5 to 10 minutes. Intravenous calcium should not be infused more rapidly given the risk for cardiac arrhythmia, bradycardia, and arrest. Cardiac monitoring and serial monitoring of the serum calcium level should be performed. Repeat boluses should be provided until the symptoms resolve, and then a slower infusion should be continued.

For patients with either chronic hypocalcemia or milder degrees of acute hypocalcemia without severe symptoms, oral calcium is preferred. Numerous forms of oral calcium salts are available. Calcium carbonate is readily available and well tolerated. If either hypoparathyroidism or vitamin D deficiency is suspected, vitamin D replacement should be provided to optimize enteral absorption. The overall management goal of chronic hypocalcemia is to achieve acceptable serum calcium while avoiding hypercalcemia and excessive hypercalciuria.

Hypercalcemia

Background. Hypercalcemia results when the influx of calcium into the extracellular space exceeds the rate of deposition into bone or renal capacity for excretion. This may occur due to excessive absorption from the gastrointestinal tract, accelerated bone resorption, or decreased renal excretion. Excessive exposure to vitamin D will increase intestinal calcium and phosphate absorption and would be associated with a depressed PTH level. In addition to exogenous sources of vitamin D, granulomatous disorders may be associated with unregulated activity of monocytic 1-α-hyroxylase with conversion of 25-hydroxyvitamin D to the more active 1,25-dihydroxyvitamin D and promote absorptive hypercalcemia. Accelerated bone resorption would be anticipated in primary, secondary, and tertiary hyperparathyroidism. Jansen's syndrome, a genetic disorder of the PTH receptor, renders the receptor constitutively active. Children with Jansen's syndrome present with hypercal-

cemia, undetectable levels of PTH, and skeletal changes consistent with hyperparathyroidism. Immobilization, particularly in rapidly growing adolescents, may result in significant bone resorption and hypercalcemia. Malignancy is a rare cause of hypercalcemia in children. Decreased renal excretion occurs in familial hypocalciuric hypercalcemia (FHH), an autosomal dominant disorder affecting the CaSR. FHH is characterized by mild, asymptomatic hypercalcemia, increased tubular reabsorption of calcium, and inappropriately normal PTH. Medications associated with hypercalcemia include thiazide diuretics and lithium.

The evaluation of hypercalcemia begins with a thorough assessment of symptoms, diet, medication, medical history, and family history. Laboratory evaluation should include ionized calcium, electrolyte, phosphorus, magnesium, renal function, serum albumin, and acid–base assessment. Review of previous laboratory studies, if available, should be performed. Though results will not be available to the emergency department physicians, PTH level is critical to ultimately differentiate the underlying cause. If the PTH is not elevated, vitamin D metabolites should be submitted. Assessment of urine calcium excretion via random urine calcium to creatinine ratio may also be informative. Calcium excretion is high in hyperparathyroidism but low in FHH and with thiazide therapy.

Clinical Manifestations. Hypercalcemia is associated with a number of signs and symptoms depending on the acuity and severity of the disorder. Patients with mildly elevated calcium (less than 11.5 to 12 mg per dL) are often asymptomatic, especially if the elevation is chronic in onset. Patients with moderate hypercalcemia (12 to 14 mg per dL) may experience anorexia, irritability, abdominal pain, constipation, and weakness. An important renal manifestation of hypercalcemia is polyuria due to an inability to concentrate urine, an acquired form of nephrogenic diabetes insipidus. Should polyuria be associated with gastrointestinal symptoms and decreased fluid intake, dehydration will ensue and aggravate the existing hypercalcemia by reducing renal excretion of calcium. If hypercalcemia is severe, progressive weakness, confusion, seizures, and coma may develop.

Management. When hypercalcemia is mild, no specific therapy is warranted and efforts should focus on identifying the underlying condition. Chronic moderate hypercalcemia (12 to 14 mg per dL) may be well tolerated and not require immediate intervention, though thorough evaluation should be pursued. If hypercalcemia is severe (greater than 14 mg per dL) or associated with clinically significant symptoms, prompt intervention is warranted. Given the gastrointestinal and renal manifestations associated with hypercalcemia, patients may present with hypovolemia. Initial efforts should focus on restoring adequate intravascular volume with isotonic intravenous fluids, which will increase GFR and increase renal excretion of calcium. Once intravascular volume is restored, attempts to promote continued calcium excretion with intravenous saline and loop diuretics (furosemide 1 to 2 mg per kg) should be employed. Loop diuretics inhibit tubular reabsorption of calcium and enhance excretion, an effect that is optimized when adequate tubular sodium is present. The rate of intravenous fluid will depend upon the urine flow rate and volume status, and meticulous attention to fluid balance and serial assessment of weight is warranted. If renal function and urine flow are preserved, hydration at a rate of 2,000 to 3,000 mL per m^2 per day will likely be well tolerated. If the patient is in renal failure or efforts with saline diuresis are not sufficient, contacting a pediatric nephrology or endocrinology consultant is advised. Therapeutic options for cases not responsive to conventional therapies include calcitonin, bisphosphonates, and renal replacement therapy (RRT), if clinically indicated.

Disorders of Acid–Base Homeostasis

When compared to the extracellular sodium ion concentration, normally ranging between 135 and 145 mEq per L, the extracellular hydrogen ion (H$^+$) concentration is precisely maintained within narrow limits to achieve a concentration of 40 nanoEq per L or 0.00004 mEq per L. This underscores the impact of H$^+$ concentration on cellular function. Once a derangement of H$^+$ concentration occurs, several homeostatic responses are activated in a stepwise fashion to restore normal acid–base balance. Within minutes chemical buffers begin to neutralize the derangement, followed by an appropriate adjustment in pulmonary ventilation, and finally renal mechanisms are activated to adjust acid–base excretion. The effect of pulmonary ventilation and renal control of acid–base excretion on systemic pH can be predicted by applying the Henderson-Hasselbalch equation,

$$pH = 6.10 + \log ([HCO_3^-] \div [0.03 \times pCO_2]).$$

Metabolic Acidosis

Background. Metabolic acidosis is a process that tends to lower extracellular pH and results from either a net gain of H$^+$ ions or a net loss of bicarbonate (HCO$_3^-$) ions. Acidemia is a state of low extracellular pH. The two classes of physiologic acids are volatile acids and nonvolatile acids. The excretion of volatile acid is achieved by pulmonary ventilation, and the elimination nonvolatile acid is achieved by renal excretion. Children typically produce 2 to 3 mEq per kg per day of nonvolatile acids, primarily sulfuric acid derived from the metabolism of sulfur-containing amino acids. Nonvolatile acids are initially buffered by bicarbonate in the extracellular space and by proteins and phosphates in the intracellular space. The net effect is a fall in serum HCO$_3^-$, which is restored by renal excretion of the daily acid load. There are two basic steps involved in this process: (i) reabsorption of the filtered HCO$_3^-$ and (ii) tubular secretion of H$^+$ ion, which combines with either titratable acid (primarily phosphate) or ammonia to generate ammonium. The net effect of secreting a H$^+$ is the generation of a HCO$_3^-$ ion. The secreted H$^+$ ion is derived from the breakdown of water and generates a hydroxyl ion (OH$^-$). OH$^-$ combines with carbon dioxide (CO$_2$) within the cell and generates a new HCO$_3^-$ ion, which is returned to the systemic circulation and replaces the HCO$_3^-$ ion loss in the initial buffering reaction. When there is a significant increase in the daily acid load, the kidney compensates largely by increasing ammonium excretion.

Clinical Manifestation. The clinical manifestations of metabolic acidosis are variable and will depend on the underlying etiology and severity. Children may be asymptomatic or present with a variety of acute or chronic manifestations such as tachypnea, abdominal pain, vomiting, lethargy, neurologic abnormalities, and failure to thrive. Inquiries regarding the presence and duration of symptoms such as diarrhea, polyuria, and poor growth should be included in the historical assessment. The physical examination should include an assessment of perfusion and measurement of growth parameters to determine if growth has been impaired.

Evaluation of metabolic acidosis ideally begins with an assessment of the arterial or venous blood gas, which defines systemic pH, pulmonary compensation, and may identify the presence of complex acid–base disorders (mixed acid–base disorders). The serum bicarbonate is typically measured indirectly by blood gas or directly by adding a strong acid to venous blood and observing the amount of CO$_2$ generated. Once metabolic acidosis is diagnosed, assessment of respiratory compensation can be performed. The arterial partial pressure of CO$_2$ (pCO$_2$) normally falls an average of 1.2 mmHg for every 1 mEq per L reduction in the serum HCO$_3^-$ to a minimum pCO$_2$ of 10 to 15 mmHg. The Winter's formula can also approximate the expected arterial pCO$_2$,

$$\text{Arterial pCO}_2 = (1.5 \times \text{measured HCO}_3^-) + 8 \pm 2$$

If the fall in pCO$_2$ is significantly different than the expected value, a mixed acid–base disorder is likely present.

Patients with metabolic acidosis can be classified in two groups based on the serum anion gap (AG), and this determination may facilitate the diagnosis of the underlying cause. Serum electrolytes should be obtained to calculate the AG using the following formula:

$$\text{AG (mEq/L)} = Na^+ - (Cl^- + HCO_3^-)$$

The normal AG typically ranges between 7 and 13 mEq per L, and an AG greater than 14 to 16 mEq per L is elevated. In normal subjects, the AG is primarily due to negative charges from plasma proteins, particularly albumin. An elevated AG is most often due to an unmeasured anion, though can also result from a low concentration of serum cations (K$^+$, Ca^{2+}, Mg^{2+}). A low AG can result from an increase in serum cations or low serum albumin. For every 1 g per dL reduction in serum albumin level, the AG would be expected to be reduced by approximately 2.5 mEq per L. The causes of metabolic acidosis based on elevated or normal AG are outlined in Table 100.11. In addition to serum electrolytes and serum albumin, initial laboratory studies should include serum glucose, BUN, creatinine, and urinalysis with urine pH. A higher than expected urine pH in the setting of acidosis may suggest renal tubular acidosis (RTA). Further studies are based upon clinical suspicion.

Management. The management of metabolic acidosis should focus on the identification and treatment of the underlying cause and to ensure adequate perfusion. The immediate therapy of metabolic acidosis in the emergency department generally depends on the severity of the disorder. In children with severe acidemia (serum pH less than 7.10), bicarbonate therapy is generally indicated. The basis for correcting severe acidosis is the negative impact severe acidemia has on cardiac function, including impaired cardiac contractility and increased risk for cardiac arrhythmias. An exception would include metabolic acidosis in patients with DKA, as lower thresholds for pH are allowed before bicarbonate is provided given the expected

TABLE 100.11

CAUSES OF METABOLIC ACIDOSIS WITH RESPECT TO THE ANION GAP

> **Elevated anion gap**
> Lactic acidosis
>   Hypoperfusion
>   Inborn errors of carbohydrate metabolism
>   Mitochondrial disorders
> Diabetic ketoacidosis
> Inborn errors of metabolism
>   Organic acidemias
>   Fatty acid oxidation defects
> Ingestions
>   Methanol, ethanol, ethylene glycol, salicylates
> Renal failure
>
> **Normal anion gap**
> Renal tubular acidosis
> Diarrhea
> Enteric fistulae
> Ureterosigmoidostomy
> Early renal failure

TABLE 100.12

CAUSES OF METABOLIC ALKALOSIS

> **Renal hydrogen loss**
> Loop or thiazide diuretics
> Posthypercapnic alkalosis
> Mineralocorticoid excess
> Bartter's and Gitelman's syndromes
>
> **Gastrointestinal hydrogen loss**
> Vomiting
> Nasogastric suction
>
> **Alkali therapy**
> **Contraction alkalosis**
> Loop or thiazide diuretics
> Cystic Fibrosis
> Congenital chloridorrhea
>
> **Intracellular movement of hydrogen**
> Hypokalemia

metabolism of ketoacid into bicarbonate with insulin and fluid repletion. The reader is referred to Chapter 86 for further discussion regarding emergent treatment of DKA. The role of alkali therapy remains controversial in hypoperfusion lactic acidosis and is yet to be resolved. The aim of treatment in hypoperfusion lactic acidosis is to restore intravascular volume and perfusion in a timely fashion, which will allow metabolism of lactate anions to bicarbonate. The potential complications of alkali therapy in metabolic acidosis include hypercarbia, hypernatremia, transcellular shift of potassium ion into the intracellular space resulting in hypokalemia, and alkalosis. Furthermore, alkalosis or an increase in blood pH may precipitate tetany by promoting binding of calcium to albumin, which reduces the ionized calcium concentration.

When bicarbonate therapy is to be given, estimating the necessary dose may prove to be challenging. The apparent bicarbonate space reflects total body buffering capacity, which includes extracellular bicarbonate, intracellular proteins, and bone carbonate. The bicarbonate distribution space rises from 50% of body weight to 100% of body weight with progressive acidemia. Given the difficulty in accurately estimating the bicarbonate deficit, bicarbonate can be given at an initial dose of 0.5 to 1 mEq per kg if clinically indicated with the aim of increasing the systemic pH to more than 7.20. Further alkali therapy will depend upon the response and subsequent disease course. If the patient is asymptomatic, the underlying process can be controlled (e.g., diarrheal dehydration), and tissue perfusion can be assured, alkali therapy may not be required. In the setting of asymptomatic chronic metabolic acidosis, such as RTA and CKD, consultation with an appropriate specialist would be reasonable to guide oral therapy and avoid complications such as electrolyte derangements and volume excess.

Metabolic Alkalosis

Background. Metabolic alkalosis is characterized by a rise in the plasma bicarbonate concentration, and causes include hydrogen loss from the gastrointestinal tract or kidneys, volume contraction around a relatively constant amount of extracellular bicarbonate (contraction alkalosis), and the administration of bicarbonate. Given the renal capacity to excrete excess bicarbonate, clinical circumstances must be present that impair bicarbonate excretion and sustain the disorder. Therefore, when approaching the patient with metabolic alkalosis, identification of both the inciting cause and the clinical factors allowing persistence of the disorder must be pursued.

Though there are many causes (Table 100.12), metabolic alkalosis in children most commonly results from diuretic therapy and H^+ loss from gastrointestinal secretions. Diuretics are prescribed to children for a variety of chronic and acute disorders. Renal acid excretion requires adequate delivery of both sodium and water to the distal tubule and is promoted by the effect of aldosterone. By increasing Na^+ reabsorption in the distal nephron, aldosterone creates a lumen-negative potential difference and favors H^+ movement into the lumen. Furthermore, aldosterone directly stimulates the H^+-ATPase, enhancing H^+ secretion into the tubular lumen. Loop and thiazide diuretics increase distal delivery of both sodium and water and predispose to volume contraction, thereby stimulating aldosterone secretion. Gastrointestinal causes of metabolic alkalosis include vomiting or nasogastric suction. Gastric secretions have high concentrations of hydrogen chloride and a lesser amount of potassium chloride (5 to 10 mEq per L), and gastric losses will predispose to the development of metabolic alkalosis. In addition, if gastrointestinal losses are significant and inadequately replaced, intravascular depletion may ensue with resultant increase in aldosterone secretion.

In normal subjects, the renal capacity to excrete bicarbonate prevents the development of metabolic alkalosis. The persistence of metabolic alkalosis implies a limitation of renal bicarbonate excretion, and the most common perpetuating cause is effective circulating volume depletion. A central mechanism to preserve intravascular volume is renal tubular reabsorption of Na^+, stimulated by aldosterone as described above. To maintain electroneutrality, bicarbonate will be reabsorbed with Na^+. During sustained volume depletion, the adaptive tubular reabsorptive capacity for bicarbonate will increase steadily and may exceed 35 mEq per L.

In addition to volume depletion, chloride depletion will also limit renal bicarbonate excretion and is associated with gastric fluid loss and diuretic therapy. Low renal tubular concentration of chloride favors both bicarbonate reabsorption and decreases bicarbonate excretion. Distal bicarbonate secretion is dependent upon the Cl^-–HCO_3^- exchanger located in the luminal membrane, which transports chloride into the intercalated cells of the cortical collecting tubule and excretes bicarbonate into the tubule lumen. A fall in the tubular lumen chloride will diminish the favorable gradient for ion exchange and bicarbonate excretion. Hypokalemia also directly increases bicarbonate reabsorption, which is in part due to intracellular acidosis induced by the entry of H^+ into the cell in exchange for K^+ movement out of the cell. Intracellular acidosis induces renal acid excretion and promotes net bicarbonate reabsorption.

Management. The cause of metabolic alkalosis is generally evident from the history. The evaluation of metabolic alkalosis should include a thorough history to identify gastrointestinal losses and an account of medications taken, specifically diuretics and antacids. Serum studies should include assessment of renal function and electrolyte balance to evaluate for concurrent abnormalities such as hypokalemia, hypercalcemia, and abnormalities in serum magnesium, which may support a renal tubulopathy such as Gitelman's syndrome. Urine electrolytes may also be informative. In patients with metabolic alkalosis and volume contraction, the urine sodium and chloride concentrations may be dissociated. If the serum bicarbonate exceeds the renal capacity to conserve, some of the excess bicarbonate will be excreted with sodium and potassium. This loss of cations will worsen the Na deficit and may lead to potassium depletion. Despite metabolic alkalosis, the conservation of chloride is intact, and a urine chloride concentration less than 25 mEq per L would be consistent with volume depletion. A urine chloride concentration greater than 40 mEq per L in the setting of metabolic alkalosis would be consistent with disorders such as primary mineralocorticoid excess, Bartter's syndrome, Gitelman's syndrome, or continued diuretic therapy.

The treatment of metabolic alkalosis is supportive, and reversible underlying cause should be addressed. The focus of therapy should aim at restoring adequate circulating volume and correcting chloride and potassium deficits. Providing isotonic sodium chloride will restore intravascular volume, remove the stimulus for sodium retention, and increase distal chloride delivery. Once these results have been achieved, there will be decreased bicarbonate reabsorption, increased bicarbonate excretion, and correction of the metabolic alkalosis. Potassium chloride should be provided if depletion is suspected with close monitoring to avoid excessive replacement. Though the extracellular concentration of K^+ may be low during metabolic alkalosis due to transcellular shift to the intracellular space, true potassium depletion may be present. Potassium can be lost due to impaired renal absorption from diuretic therapy, aldosterone effect associated with volume depletion, and obligatory wasting of cations (Na^+ and K^+) associated with bicarbonate excretion. In patients with metabolic alkalosis and edematous states, providing sodium chloride may be hazardous. Therapy should take into account the underlying condition and planned in concert with appropriate subspecialty care if possible.

ACUTE KIDNEY INJURY

Background and Pathophysiology

Previously termed acute renal failure, acute kidney injury (AKI) defines an abrupt decrease in GFR with impairment of nitrogenous waste product excretion. Depending on the severity of the injury, there may be altered water and electrolyte excretion and disturbance of metabolic and acid–base regulation. In mild cases, nonoliguric AKI may be asymptomatic and only detected when serum laboratory studies are performed. When severe, oliguric AKI may result in profound derangements of electrolyte and volume balance and necessitate the initiation of RRT.

Due to various definitions, the incidence and prevalence of AKI in the pediatric population is difficult to ascertain. However, the incidence appears to be rising and causation changing with the advancement of medical and surgical practice. This trend is most apparent in tertiary care centers and was illustrated in a retrospective study from a large pediatric tertiary center, which reviewed the course of AKI in approximately 250 children. Approximately two thirds of these children had underlying comorbid conditions, and only 7% of cases of AKI were due to primary renal disease. The most common causes of AKI were renal ischemia (21%), nephrotoxic agents (16%), and sepsis (11%). Infants with congenital heart disease requiring cardiopulmonary bypass and recipients of stem cell transplants appear to be particularly vulnerable populations. In contrast to the underlying causes of AKI in tertiary centers, primary renal disease is more likely to cause AKI in community hospital and less developed countries. In 2004, the Acute Dialysis Quality Initiative proposed a consensus definition for AKI: the RIFLE criteria. This was modified and validated in pediatric patients and renamed the pediatric RIFLE criteria. These criteria define five levels of AKI based upon degree of creatinine elevation, urine output, and requirement for dialysis. As a research tool, this standardized definition will advance our understanding of AKI with respect to incidence and outcome and potentially allow the identification of modifiable risk factors.

AKI may be classified as prerenal, intrinsic renal, and postrenal. Prerenal AKI may result from intravascular volume depletion or reduced effective circulating volume. Uncontrolled bleeding, gastrointestinal losses, diuretic therapy, osmotic diuresis, and cutaneous losses are potential causes of intravascular depletion. Intravascular volume depletion also develops when fluid shifts out of the vascular space into the interstitial space and occurs with hypoalbuminemia and during systemic inflammatory response syndrome (SIRS). Decreased effective circulating volume may be present in heart failure and during systemic vasodilation. Intrinsic renal disease may result from insults to the renal vasculature, glomeruli, interstitium, and tubular mass. Of note, a sustained prerenal state may result in acute tubular necrosis (ATN), an intrinsic renal disease not immediately reversible with restoration of effective intravascular volume. Causes of postrenal AKI include bilateral ureteral obstruction (stones, masses), unilateral obstruction in a solitary kidney, and functional or anatomic bladder outlet obstruction. Posterior urethral valves are the most common cause of postrenal failure and commonly detected during gestation given the routine practice of fetal ultrasounds during prenatal care.

Management

A thorough physical exam and history is a necessary starting point to reveal the underlying etiology of AKI. Prerenal physiology is not an uncommon finding in emergency departments and often due to gastrointestinal losses. A detailed history of fluid balance should be obtained, and the physical exam should assess hydration status and perfusion. An account of medications taken prior to presentation should also be performed to identify the potential for drug-induced nephrotoxicity. Important classes of medications increasing the risk for AKI include nonsteroidal antiinflammatory drugs (NSAIDs), angiotensin-converting enzyme (ACE) inhibitors, angiotensin II receptor blockers (ARBs), and calcineurin inhibitors. Physical exam may also reveal signs of systemic vasculitis associated with nephritis, such as rashes or arthritis. Any patient who presents with anuria should have a thorough abdominal exam to assess for palpable bladder or masses, which may be compressing the urinary tract.

Laboratory assessment of AKI should serve two purposes. First, it should determine the severity of renal dysfunction and identify associated metabolic or hematologic abnormalities, which may require urgent intervention. Second, a focused investigation should begin to elucidate the underlying cause of AKI. For any child who presents with AKI, initial serum laboratory studies should include serum creatinine, electrolytes, and complete blood cell counts. Serial assessment of renal function and electrolytes will be required to determine the disease course and to monitor for the development of electrolyte derangements. Other laboratory tests should be considered based on the clinical presentation of the patient and should be pursued at a tempo reasonable for the clinical course. In cases of suspected glomerulonephritis, serum complements, antistreptococcal antibodies, and antinuclear antibodies should be considered. If there is rapid deterioration of renal function consistent with rapidly progressive glomerulonephritis (RPGN), antineurophil cytoplasmic antibodies (ANCA) and anti–glomerular basement (GBM) antibodies should be submitted. RPGN would necessitate prompt evaluation by a pediatric nephrologist.

Initial urine studies submitted during the evaluation of AKI must include urinalysis with microscopic assessment. An elevated urine-specific gravity may be consistent with prerenal physiology. Results of the urine dipstick may reveal nitrite or leukocyte esterase, a sign of urinary tract infection. Detection of large heme by dipstick is found in glomerulonephritis and pigment nephropathy, and differentiation between these two disorders relies upon the presence or absence of red blood cells in the urine sediment, respectively. Heavy proteinuria by dipstick, which detects albumin excretion, would be suggestive of glomerular disease and should be followed by a quantitative urine protein to creatinine ratio (normal less than 0.2, nephrotic range greater than 2 to 3). Microscopic examination of the urine sediment may be normal or nearly normal, consistent with prerenal AKI and some cases of ATN. ATN may also be associated with granular, muddy brown, and/or tubuloepithelial cell casts. The finding of red blood cell casts is pathognomonic of glomerulonephritis, and concomitant white blood cells or white blood cell casts would be consistent with an exudative nephritis such as postinfectious glomerulonephritis or renal vasculitis. The urine sediment associated with acute interstitial nephritis (AIN) varies and include microscopic hematuria, sterile pyuria, and white blood cell casts. The degree of proteinuria associated with AIN is also variable, though is typically not severe. A notable exception is NSAID-induced AIN, which may be associated with nephrotic range proteinuria. If interstitial nephritis is suspected, urine eosinophils should be submitted, though sensitivity and specificity of urine eosinophilia is limited.

An assessment of urine chemistries may also be useful in distinguishing prerenal AKI from ATN, and initial studies to consider include urine electrolytes and urine creatinine. The fractional excretion of sodium (FENa) is calculated as follows:

$$FENa\ (\%) = (urine\ sodium \times serum\ creatinine/$$
$$serum\ Na \times urine\ creatinine) \times 100$$

A value below 1% suggests prerenal disease and reflects reabsorption of almost all of the filtered sodium to maintain intravascular volume, an appropriate response to decreased renal perfusion. A value greater than 2% is consistent with ATN or other tubular disorders. Of note, the FENa may be less than 1% in normal subjects and reflects normal tubular handling of sodium in the setting of relatively low sodium intake. The fractional excretion of urea is similarly calculated as the FENa with substitution of urine urea nitrogen and blood urea nitrogen and is generally less than 35% in prerenal states. Diuretics increase urine sodium excretion, though have less effect on urea excretion. Therefore, the FENa may be less reliable and the fractional excretion of urea more informative if diuretics have been provided prior to the collection of urine.

Radiographic assessment should be considered in all patients with AKI of unclear etiology. This is most certainly true in those who present with acute anuria, as urinary tract obstruction is a possible etiology and would require intervention. Given its safety and general availability, ultrasonography of the kidneys and urinary tract should be considered in all children with AKI. Ultrasound provides timely and valuable data, including assessment of renal parenchymal mass and may identify conditions of acquired or congenital obstruction of the urinary tract. Doppler investigation of the renal vessels should be performed if there is concern for vascular compromise or thrombosis, though further imaging may be necessary, given the limitations of this modality.

The initial management of AKI in the emergency department is largely supportive and aimed at addressing fluid or electrolyte abnormalities and avoiding further renal insult. If prerenal physiology is suspected, appropriate volume resuscitation with isotonic fluids should be provided with frequent assessment of perfusion and urine flow. Normal saline bolus therapy provided at 5 to 10 mL per kg is warranted with reassessment to determine if further resuscitation is indicated. Though prerenal physiology should be corrected, prevention of fluid overload should be emphasized. This balance is most challenging in those patients who present critically ill with sepsis associated with capillary leak and in those with heart failure and ineffective circulating volume. Potassium supplementation should be withheld until urine flow is established and results of serum electrolytes are available. Electrolyte and acid–base disturbances should be addressed as previously reviewed.

TABLE 100.13

ESTIMATION OF GFR BY THE SCHWARTZ FORMULA

$C_{cr} = k \times L/S_{cr}$

C_{cr} = creatinine clearance in mL/min/1.73 m^2

k = proportionality constant

L = length (cm)

S_{cr} = serum creatinine (mg/dL)

k values
  Low birth weight infants during the first year of life = 0.33
  Full term babies during first year of life = 0.45
  Children and adolescent girls = 0.55
  Adolescent boys = 0.7

Adapted from Schwartz GJ, Feld LG, Langford DJ. A simple estimate of glomerular filtration rate in full-term infants during the first year of life. *J Pediatr* 1984;104:849–854; Schwartz GJ, Gauthier B. A simple estimate of glomerular filtration rate in adolescent boys. *J Pediatr* 1985;106:522–526; Schwartz GJ, Haycock GB, Edelmann CM Jr, et al. A simple estimate of glomerular filtration rate in children derived from body length and plasma creatinine. *Pediatrics* 1976;58:259–263.

If AKI is associated with oligoanuria, the child may present in a state of volume excess. If severe, hypertension and pulmonary edema may be present and would warrant a trial of diuretic therapy. Intravenous furosemide given at a dose of 1 to 2 mg per kg should be provided if volume excess is causing cardiopulmonary compromise. Hypertension can be treated with either oral or intravenous agents. Oral calcium channel blockers and hydralazine are well tolerated and would not worsen renal function, unlike ACE inhibitors and ARB therapy. If intravenous agents are required, intermittent doses of hydralazine or labetalol are often effective. If the child remains oligoanuric despite diuretic challenge and has clinical evidence of volume excess, a pediatric nephrologist should be consulted given the potential need for RRT and ultrafiltration. If medications are indicated, such as antibiotics, the need for dose adjustment based on decreased renal function must be considered. The Schwartz formula allows estimation of the GFR based on serum creatinine and patient length and has gained widespread clinical use in North America (Table 100.13). This formula tends to overestimate GFR, and this overestimation increases with decreasing GFR.

Rhabdomyolysis

Background

Rhabdomyolysis accounts for approximately 3% of all cases of AKI in children and causes include both traumatic and nontraumatic. Traumatic etiologies include crush injuries, vascular occlusions, and acute lower extremity compartment syndrome. Nontraumatic causes include extreme exertion, prolonged seizure, malignant hyperthermia, DKA, hypokalemia, hypophosphatemia, and metabolic myopathies. Rhabdomyolysis has also been associated with a variety of infections, including influenza A and B, parainfluenza, Coxsackie virus, Epstein-Barr virus, herpes simplex virus, varicella zoster, human immunodeficiency virus, and sepsis. Both prescribed and illicit drugs can

cause rhabdomyolysis and include lipid lowering drugs (primarily statins), colchicines, alcohol, cocaine, ecstasy, and amphetamines. In a retrospective study of approximately 190 children presenting to the emergency department of a tertiary pediatric hospital, the most common causes of pediatric rhabdomyolysis were viral myositis (38%) and trauma (26%). Of this group, none of the children with urinary heme dipstick of less than 2+ developed acute renal failure. In general, if the serum creatinine kinase level is less than 15,000 to 20,000 U per L at presentation, the risk for AKI is relatively low but not negligible. Clinical factors increasing the risk for AKI at lower concentrations of serum creatinine kinase include dehydration, metabolic acidosis, and sepsis.

Clinical Manifestations

The classic symptoms of rhabdomyolysis include myalgias, weakness, and red or brown discolored urine, though these findings are not consistently reported by those affected. The serum studies reflect the release of myocyte contents and include elevated serum creatinine kinase. Unlike hemoglobin, myoglobin is a monomer and is freely filtered into the urine. The severity of rhabdomyolysis ranges from asymptomatic elevations in serum muscle enzymes to oliguric renal failure associated with life-threatening electrolyte abnormalities. Electrolyte abnormalities include hyperkalemia and hyperphosphatemia, which result from the endogenous load released from damaged muscle cells and limited excretion if renal function is impaired. Hypocalcemia may also develop due to calcium phosphate precipitation into injured muscle tissue. AKI during rhabdomyolysis is often multifactorial, and insults include prerenal physiology, tubular cell damage, and tubular obstruction. Decreased intravascular volume and prerenal physiology develop secondary to fluid sequestration within damaged muscle and intrarenal vasoconstriction. Tubular cell injury results from tubular obstruction with heme pigment casts and lipid peroxidation from hydroxyl radicals generated by heme and free iron. The urine sediment may reveal pigmented granular casts and a red to brown discoloration of the urine supernatant.

Management

The mainstay of therapy for rhabdomyolysis includes early vigorous hydration to ensure adequate intravascular volume and promote urine flow. The benefit of high urine flow is the removal of obstructing, pigmented casts, which initiate the cytotoxic insults. Children should be provided isotonic saline to ensure adequate renal perfusion, and intravenous fluids should continue to optimize urine flow. The intravenous fluid rate will depend on urine flow rate and should be reevaluated regularly to avoid volume excess. Guidelines for adults suggest targeting urine flow rate at approximately 3 mL per kg per hour. Should the urine flow be low despite adequate volume status, a trial of furosemide 0.5 to 1 mg per kg IV would be reasonable and should be continued (i.e., every 6 to 8 hours) if effective. If diuretics are used, meticulous attention should be given to volume balance and perfusion to avoid prerenal insult. Some have advocated the use of a forced alkaline or mannitol diuresis, though the clinical benefits are not proven. Should metabolic acidosis develop, this should be treated with addition of bicarbonate to intravenous fluids. The risk of providing bicarbonate is excessive alkalinization and reduction of ionized calcium in patients with evolving hypocalcemia. For those with severe AKI associated with oligoanuria and electrolyte disturbance, dialysis may be required until renal recovery is achieved.

GLOMERULAR DISEASES

Glomerular diseases encompass a variety of disorders, including both acute and chronic processes. Moreover, they may be due to a primary renal disorder or reflect renal involvement in a systemic disease or infection. The differential diagnosis of glomerular disease is broad, and Table 100.14 lists some of the more common forms of glomerular disease seen in the pediatric population. Depending on the underlying disorder, the clinical course may be mild and self-limited with full recovery or severe with progression to renal insufficiency. Glomerulonephritis is the leading cause of acquired chronic renal failure during childhood. The following will review the clinical presentations and management of postinfectious glomerulonephritis, Henoch-Schönlein purpura (HSP), and hemolytic uremic syndrome (HUS).

Postinfectious Glomerulonephritis

Background

Postinfectious glomerulonephritis is the leading cause of glomerulonephritis in children and has been associated with a host of bacteria, viruses, and parasites. In children, however, nephritogenic strains of group A β-hemolytic streptococci are the most frequently implicated organisms. Currently nephritis-associated streptococcal plasmin receptor and streptococcal pyrogenic exotoxin B are considered the major putative nephritogens. The classic preceding illnesses are streptococcal pharyngitis and cellulitis. The latent period from pharyngitis and cellulitis to acute poststreptococcal glomerulonephritis (APSGN) averages 10 days and 21 days, respectively. APSGN may be sporadic or occur during an

TABLE 100.14

GLOMERULAR DISEASES IN CHILDHOOD

Primary
  IgA nephropathy
  Focal segmental glomerulosclerosis
  Membranoproliferative glomerulonephritis
  Membranous glomerulonephritis

Associated with systemic disease
  Henoch-Schönlein purpura
  Hemolytic uremic syndrome
  Systemic lupus erythematosus
  Wegner granulomatosis
  Goodpasture syndrome
  Microscopic polyarteritis

Infectious
  Poststreptococcal glomerulonephritis
  Hepatitis B and C associated nephritis
  Shunt nephritis
  Subacute bacterial endocarditis

Inherited
  Benign familial hematuria
  Alport syndrome

endemic and more commonly affects school age children. During an epidemic of pharyngitis, the incidence of clinically detectable APSGN is approximately 5% to 10%. In recent decades, the prevalence of APSGN has declined in most industrialized nations, though persists at high rates in some developing countries.

Clinical Manifestations

The clinical presentation of APSGN may vary from asymptomatic microscopic hematuria to an abrupt onset of the nephritic syndrome, which can be associated with gross hematuria, proteinuria, oliguria, edema, and hypertension. Hypertension can be severe and evolve into hypertensive emergency, which typically affects the central nervous system (CNS) in children and manifests as seizure activity. Given the potential morbidity, hypertension at presentation would be an indication for admission. In a small minority of children (less than 1%) the course will be consistent with RPGN and warrant renal biopsy. Generally, the clinical symptoms of ASPGN begin to improve after 1 to 2 weeks. If reduced renal function and edema are evident at presentation, renal function begins to normalize and diuresis ensues within this several week period. Gross hematuria will fade rapidly, though microscopic hematuria may persist for 6 months or longer. Proteinuria typically improves quickly and resolves within 6 months.

Laboratory studies during a typical episode of ASPGN reflect a nephritic process with activation of the alternative complement pathway. Subendothelial immune deposits with activation of complement will result in an influx of inflammatory cells, leading to a proliferative glomerulonephritis. The urine sediment will demonstrate glomerular erythrocytes and leukocytes, and may contain red cell casts. Proteinuria is not uncommon, though not typically in the nephrotic range. Serum studies may demonstrate reduced renal function. Associated electrolyte abnormalities include hyponatremia, reflecting inability to excrete water, and hyperkalemia. The majority of patients will have a low total hemolytic complement, low C3 complement, and a normal C4 complement. The C3 level typically recovers in 6 to 8 weeks. Serologic testing to document recent streptococcal infection is helpful but does not prove causation, as a significant number of children are asymptomatic carriers. In addition, it is important to recognize that antibiotic therapy may blunt the increase in antibody titers. Serologic tests available include antistreptolysin O, antideoxyribonuclease B, and hyaluronidase. If the C3 remains depressed after 3 months or the C4 is low, diagnostic considerations include chronic forms of glomerulonephritis, including membranoproliferative glomerulonephritis (MPGN) and lupus nephritis. If the complement levels are normal at presentation, this would make ASPGN less likely, and IgA nephropathy would be a consideration.

Management

Therapy for APSGN is largely supportive. Given the underlying glomerular inflammation and generally intact tubular function, there is a propensity for salt and water retention leading to edema and increased blood pressure. Therefore, weight should be measured daily and blood pressure checked regularly during the early acute illness. Children with hypertension or decreased renal function should be considered for admission. If edema or hypertension is present, salt and fluid restriction should be initiated and diuretic therapy considered. Furosemide can be provided at doses of 0.5 to 1 mg per kg once to four times daily to optimize fluid balance. If the child is hypertensive, short or long acting calcium channel blockers can be initiated while awaiting recovery. If the blood pressure is significantly elevated, intravenous hydralazine 0.1 mg per kg can be given every 4 to 6 hours with appropriate dose adjustment until other supportive measures are effective. If a child demonstrates persistent hypertension and proteinuria and if his renal function has been stable, ACE inhibitors or ARBs can be considered with close monitoring of serum creatinine and potassium. In a child whose course is consistent with RPGN, an immediate renal biopsy is warranted to provide histologic diagnosis and guide therapy.

In the absence of RPGN, the prognosis for complete recovery from the initial episode is good, which is true even for those who presented with renal insufficiency or hypertension. However, studies evaluating the long-term prognosis reveal residual signs of chronic kidney damage in some patients decades after the initial course. Late complications include proteinuria, hypertension, and decreased renal function. This underscores the importance of routine monitoring of blood pressure and urinalyses as part of health maintenance in those who have a history of ASPGN.

Henoch-Schönlein Purpura

Background

HSP is a multisystem IgA-mediated vasculitis predominantly affecting the skin, joints, gastrointestinal tract, and kidneys. Despite concerted research efforts, the exact pathogenesis of HSP remains unclear. Though HSP can occur at any age, most cases affect children between 3 and 15 years with a peak incidence at 4 to 7 years of age. In pediatric cases, there has been a male predominance noted with reported male-to-female ratio as high as 1.8:1. Presentation during adolescence or adulthood may predict a worse prognosis. The disease is more prevalent during autumn, winter, and early spring. The onset is usually sudden and frequently preceded by an acute illness, often involving the mucosal upper respiratory tract.

Clinical Manifestations

The clinical manifestations of HSP reflect the small-vessel vasculitis of affected organs. The hallmark signs and symptoms include nonthrombocytopenic purpuric rash, arthralgias, nonerosive arthritis, abdominal pain, and nephritis. The rash, often the most distinctive feature of the disease, characteristically involves the buttocks and extensor surfaces of the lower extremities. Purpura and joint pain are the most common presenting symptoms, though studies have revealed that abdominal symptoms may precede the rash in as many as 15% to 35% of cases. Overall, gastrointestinal symptoms occur in approximately half of children with HSP, and the most common abdominal symptoms are periumbilical pain, vomiting, diarrhea, and hematochezia. Surgical emergencies develop in 1% to 5% of patients and include intussusception and bowel perforation. The intussusception is confined to the small bowel in the majority of cases. The acute morbidity of HSP typically stems from severe gastrointestinal manifestations.

Though the acute illness may be overshadowed by gastrointestinal symptoms, the long-term prognosis for children with HSP depends upon the extent of the renal involvement.

The exact prevalence of HSP nephritis is unknown, though rates as high as 54% have been reported. If nephritis develops, 90% of cases present within 6 weeks after the onset of systemic symptoms, and it is rare for nephritis to develop later than 6 months after presentation. Generally, if the urinalyses remain normal during the initial 6-month period, there is no need to screen for renal disease thereafter. Most children who develop nephritis will have relatively mild renal involvement. Signs of mild renal involvement include asymptomatic hematuria, mild proteinuria, and preserved or mildly and transiently impaired renal function. These patients are expected to have a favorable long-term prognosis. A subset of children will develop more severe renal involvement and develop nephritic syndrome or combined nephritic-nephrotic syndrome. Severe disease can be associated with decreased renal function, hypertension, hypoalbuminemia, and edema, and severe acute involvement would increase the risk for long-term renal sequelae. Histologically, children with severe clinical disease are more likely to have extensive involvement, such as crescentic changes in the majority of the glomeruli sampled.

Management

Most patients with HSP and associated nephritis receive supportive care, which includes ensuring hydration and comfort. If hypertension is present, short or long acting calcium channel blockers can be used. If the patient has significant nephritis, ACE inhibitors or ARB therapy should be used with caution as these agents may result in decreased renal function, which would be difficult to distinguish from a progressive case of HSP nephritis. Patients with HSP nephritis should undergo regular evaluation to screen for signs of progressive renal disease, such as worsening proteinuria, decreasing renal function, and hypertension.

Once HSP has developed, there are conflicting reports regarding the efficacy of early prednisone therapy to prevent significant nephritis. More recently, two randomized controlled studies have been performed to evaluate the effect of glucocorticosteroids on changing the risk of developing renal involvement with HSP. The first study included 40 children followed for 1 year. The treatment group received prednisone 2 mg per kg daily for 1 week followed by weaning doses over the second week. At 1 year there was no difference in the rate of renal involvement. The second study included 171 children who were followed over a 6-month period. The treatment group received 1 mg per kg daily of prednisone for 2 weeks followed by weaning over the subsequent 2 weeks. Prednisone did not prevent renal involvement, though appeared to improve the course of the nephritis with resolution of renal symptoms more rapidly when compared to the placebo group. This effect was most apparent in children older than 6 years who developed renal symptoms early in the course. However, spontaneous resolution also occurred in the placebo group and most children did well long-term with or without any steroid therapy. Further studies are required to determine if there is a role for steroids in HSP nephritis, either provided early in the acute course to reduce the incidence of renal involvement or prescribed after nephritis manifests to impact the course of renal involvement. The relatively infrequent occurrence of HSP nephritis and the overall favorable renal outcome has hindered research efforts, especially those involving medications such as steroids with significant clinical sequelae.

MEDICAL EMERGENCIES

The optimal treatment of children with extensive renal disease remains controversial. Prior to initiating therapy, a renal biopsy should be obtained to determine the extent of crescent formation, as this appears to be the best indicator of prognosis. Cases with greater than 50% crescentic change have a guarded prognosis. Though data are limited given the rarity of severe HSP nephritis, aggressive therapy may be beneficial in patients with severe disease. Numerous uncontrolled trials have shown benefit when patients are treated with steroids with or without other agents such as azathioprine, cyclophosphamide, and anticoagulants. However, controlled trial of oral cyclophosphamide for 6 weeks without steroids did not demonstrate a difference in outcome after a mean follow up of nearly 7 years.

The short-term outcome of childhood HSP nephritis is favorable with 94% of children demonstrating complete recovery at a mean follow up of nearly 20 months. Recurrence of HSP is common and occurs in up to one third of patients and may not predict worse long-term outcome. The long-term outcome depends on the extent of renal involvement. A longitudinal study of 270 children with HSP followed over a mean of more than 8 years reported an optimistic outcome. Fifty-five children were found to have initial evidence of HSP nephritis at presentation and two thirds had mild renal disease (isolated hematuria or hematuria with mild proteinuria). Of those affected by mild disease, all recovered completely and had no evidence of persistent kidney disease at follow up. Of those with more severe nephritis, all had normal renal function and less than 20% had persistent urinary abnormalities at follow up. Other studies have demonstrated a guarded prognosis for those with severe HSP nephritis as evidenced by nephritic syndrome, combined nephritic-nephrotic syndrome, or more than 50% crescent formation on biopsy. Long-term follow-up of these patients reveal chronic renal sequelae such as hypertension or CKD in as many as 44% of patients.

Hemolytic Uremic Syndrome

Background and Pathophysiology

HUS is characterized by the clinical triad of microangiopathic hemolytic anemia, thrombocytopenia, and AKI. HUS can be broadly divided into typical forms associated with prodromal diarrhea or atypical cases distinguished by the absence of diarrhea. Typical HUS accounts for approximately 90% of pediatric cases and is frequently due to infection with enterohemorrhagic *Escherichia coli* (EHEC), which produce Shiga toxin. Atypical HUS is a heterogenous disorder and may be precipitated by numerous triggers, including drugs, bone marrow transplantation, and nonenteric infections such as those due to *Streptococcus pneumoniae* and human immunodeficiency virus. Evidence for a pathologic role of the alternative complement pathway has been revealed, and an increasing number of genetic mutations associated with atypical HUS have been described. Given that the majority of cases of HUS in children follow diarrhea, the subsequent discussion will focus on typical or diarrhea-associated HUS.

Typical Hemolytic Uremic Syndrome

Although outbreaks of diarrhea-associated HUS are dramatic and draw considerable public attention, only approximately 10% of cases in children arise from epidemics. A variety of organisms have been implicated in the pathogenesis, including *Shigella dysenteriae* type 1, *Salmonella*, and *Yersinia*. However, EHEC that produce a Shiga toxin accounts for the majority of cases, and *E. coli* serotype O157:H7 has been isolated in more than 80% of cases in the United States. EHEC may be carried in the intestines of asymptomatic cattle, and higher carriage rates have been noted in the summer months and early fall, mimicking the seasonal variation of human disease that peaks from June through September. Ground beef, vegetables, unpasteurized milk or juice, and water all serve as possible vectors of disease via contamination with bovine feces. Rarely, human-to-human transmission occurs via oral-fecal contamination. Although children of all ages can develop typical HUS, this principally affects children younger than 5 years. Approximately 10% to 15% of children who develop culture confirmed *E. coli* O157:H7 gastroenteritis progress to HUS. Measures to prevent progression to postdiarrheal HUS have been unsuccessful, and the use of antibiotics and antimotility agents appear to increase the risk of subsequent HUS.

Pathophysiology. Central to the pathogenesis of typical HUS is microvascular endothelial cell injury induced by Shiga toxin. Once the integrity of the intestinal mucosal barrier is disrupted by the inciting pathogen, cytotoxin gains access to the circulation and extragastrointestinal sites. After binding to the cell surface receptor glycosphingolipid globotriosyl ceramide, which is highly expressed on renal endothelium, a subunit of the toxin inactivates the 60S ribosome and suppresses protein synthesis leading to cellular dysfunction. The hematologic abnormalities reflect the underlying microangiopathic process and microthrombi formation.

Clinical Manifestations. The clinical manifestations of HUS are generally apparent 5 to 10 days after the onset of colitis. The colitis begins with watery diarrhea and evolves to hemorrhagic colitis in the majority of patients. The intestinal involvement may be associated with vomiting and severe abdominal pain and mimic other diseases such as ulcerative colitis, regional enteritis, intussusception, and appendicitis. Gastrointestinal complications include bowel wall necrosis, toxic megacolon, intussusception, and rectal prolapse. HUS generally becomes apparent as the diarrhea is resolving, and the evolution of the clinical signs may be abrupt. The child may present pale and listless with laboratory studies showing microangiopathic anemia and thrombocytopenia. Jaundice is present in approximately one third of patients. Given symptoms of severe diarrhea and vomiting, the child may present with hypovolemia. Alternatively, if oral intake has been maintained in the face of oliguric renal failure, signs of volume excess may be apparent, including edema and hypertension.

Laboratory studies show decreasing hemoglobin, increased reticulocytes, increased lactate dehydrogenase, and thrombocytopenia. Assessment of the blood smear demonstrates fragmented erythrocytes and schistocytes. Coagulation studies are generally normal, distinguishing HUS from sepsis and disseminated intravascular coagulation. The indirect and direct Coomb's test should be negative.

The severity of the renal involvement in typical HUS varies widely. AKI may be mild and self-limited, associated with microscopic hematuria, mild proteinuria, and preserved renal function. When renal microangiopathy is severe, fulminant oligoanuric renal failure may ensue and necessitate RRT. In a retrospective review of typical HUS in Utah over a 20-year period, 60% of children experienced anuria or oliguria lasting a median of 6 days, and dialysis was performed in 43% of cases. Age less than 2 years, anuria before admission, and leukocytosis on admission predicted more severe disease. Hypertension was present in two thirds of children but was mild and typically resolved at the time of discharge.

Microangiopathic injury of organs other than the kidneys and intestine may occur. Pancreatic involvement can be associated with transient or rarely permanent diabetes mellitus. Liver injury manifests as hepatomegaly and elevated transaminases. Clinical evidence of microangiopathy of the myocardium or lung is not usually apparent, though cases of circulatory collapse due to decreased ventricular function have been reported. Involvement of the CNS can result in significant morbidity and is the most common cause of death in children. The majority of children demonstrate some degree of encephalopathy as irritability and somnolence. More significant manifestations are apparent in up to 20% of children with typical HUS and include seizures, coma, stroke, hemiparesis, and cortical blindness. Seizures and cerebral infarct occur in 10% and 4% of children, respectively and predict a poorer prognosis.

Management. The mainstay of therapy for typical HUS is meticulous supportive care. As children often present after several days of gastrointestinal losses and poor oral intake, intravascular volume may be depleted, increasing the risk for prerenal AKI to compound the microvascular disease. Fluid resuscitation with isotonic saline should be provided with repeated assessment of volume status. Once the intravascular volume status has been restored, further fluid management should be guided by renal function and urine flow. If oligoanuria is present, a trial of furosemide (1 to 2 mg per kg per day) may be provided to establish urine flow. If oligoanuria persists, fluids should be provided at a rate to ensure adequate intravascular volume but avoid volume excess. Both intravenous and oral intake should match the total of measurable output (urine and gastrointestinal losses) and insensible water losses, estimated at 300 mL per m^2 per day. Frequent monitoring of fluid balance, weight, and vital signs is essential. If hypertension develops and is sustained, therapy should be provided. Vasodilators such as hydralazine or calcium-channel blockers are effective and preferred over ACE inhibitors and ARBs given ongoing kidney injury.

The anemia associated with typical HUS can be fulminant. Packed red blood cell transfusions should be provided for symptomatic anemia or vigorous hemolysis with anticipated or actual hematocrit less than 18% to 20%. If the patient is oligoanuric, this should be performed while on dialysis to avoid volume excess and hyperkalemia. During microangiopathy, transfused platelets will be consumed quickly and not result in sustained increase in the platelet count. Platelet transfusion is only indicated in patients with active bleeding or when a surgical procedure is intended.

Approximately 40% to 60% of children with typical HUS will require RRT. Indications for dialysis include progressive azotemia, clinically significant volume overload, and hyperkalemia or acidosis that is refractory to conservative medical therapy. Dialysis is also indicated to safely provide blood products and nutritional support in the setting of persistent oligoanuria. The modality of dialysis depends on the expertise of the center. However, if there is a severe abdominal complication requiring surgical intervention, hemodialysis will be necessary as peritoneal dialysis will be contraindicated. Plasma exchange can be considered in children with severe CNS involvement such as stroke and seizures based upon reported benefits in adults with thrombotic thrombocytopenic purpura and severe neurologic dysfunction.

Nephrotic Syndrome

Background and Pathophysiology

Nephrotic syndrome results when there is increased permeability across the glomerular filtration barrier and is characterized by massive proteinuria exceeding 50 mg per kg per day leading to hypoproteinemia, edema, and hyperlipidemia. Nephrotic syndrome is the clinical expression of a variety of glomerular diseases and can be classified as primary or secondary. Primary nephrotic syndrome includes idiopathic nephrotic syndrome and nephrotic syndrome associated with primary glomerulonephritis. Idiopathic nephrotic syndrome is typically associated with bland urine sediment and no significant glomerular inflammation on renal pathology, and underlying causes include minimal change disease (MCD) and primary focal segmental glomerulosclerosis (FSGS). Nephrotic syndrome associated with primary glomerulonephritis, such as IgA nephropathy and MPGN, is generally associated with an active urine sediment and inflammation on renal pathology. Secondary nephrotic syndrome is associated with systemic disorders such as infection with the human immunodeficiency virus, systemic lupus erythematosus, and HSP. Intrauterine infections with syphilis, toxoplasmosis, and other organisms have been associated with congenital nephrotic syndrome.

In children younger than 16 years, the annual incidence of nephrotic syndrome is approximately 2 per 100,000. Presentation within the first year of life is uncommon, and nephrotic syndrome within the first 3 months of life should raise the suspicion for congenital nephrotic syndrome. Idiopathic nephrotic syndrome is the most common form of childhood nephrosis. Children typically present between the ages of 2 and 6 years, and the reported ratio of boys to girls who are diagnosed at a younger age is as high has 2:1. The gender ratio is closer to 1:1 in those who present later in childhood or as adolescents. When children with primary nephrotic syndrome underwent renal biopsy at presentation during the 1960s and 1970s as part of the International Study of Kidney Disease in Children, it was revealed that MCD was the most common histopathology accounting for 77% of cases. MPGN and FSGS accounted for 8% and 7%, respectively. Other pathologies included proliferative nephritis, mesangial proliferation, and membranous glomerulonephropathy. Contemporary data have documented an increased incidence of FSGS, a disorder less responsive to glucocorticoid therapy and more likely to progress to renal failure.

Most patients with MCD (greater than 90%) will respond to glucocorticoid therapy. Clinical findings at presentation suggestive of MCD include age younger than 6 years; normal renal function, blood pressure, and complement levels; and benign urine sediment. Given the high frequency of MCD as the cause of idiopathic nephrotic syndrome and the favorable response of MCD to glucocorticoid therapy, an empiric trial of glucocorticoid therapy without confirmatory pathology is often provided to prepubertal children with suggestive clinical characteristics. Adolescents are also considered for empiric therapy, though obtaining a renal biopsy prior to therapy or after a defined period of glucocorticoid therapy without response would be reasonable given the increased occurrence of FSGS, MPGN, and membranous nephropathy in this age group. Patients with idiopathic nephrotic syndrome are further classified on the basis of their response to glucocorticoid therapy: glucocorticoid-responsive, glucocorticoid-dependent, and glucocorticoid-resistant nephrotic syndrome. Patients with responsive disease have a favorable long-term prognosis, and those with resistant pattern have a more guarded prognosis.

Nephrotic syndrome diagnosed within the first 3 months and first year of life is termed congenital nephrotic syndrome and infantile nephrotic syndrome, respectively. Most of these children have a genetic basis for the renal disease with mutations affecting nephrin (NPHS1), podocin (NPHS2), WT1, and laminin beta-2 (LAMB2). Nephrin is a key component of the slit diaphragm, and podocin is a protein that interacts with nephrin at the slit diaphragm. WT1 encodes a protein involved in kidney development, and LAMB2 encodes a component of the glomerular basement membrane. In a European study analyzing these genes in 89 children and 80 families with nephrotic syndrome in the first year of life, it was found that approximately 85% of the families with congenital onset and 44% of those with infantile onset were explained by known mutations. Mutations in nephrin and podocin were by far the most common. As predicted by their structural or developmental roles, infants with causative mutations in any of these four genes did not respond to glucocorticoid therapy. Congenital nephrotic syndrome may also be due to intrauterine infection, such as congenital syphilis, toxoplasmosis, cytomegalovirus, human immunodeficiency virus, and other organisms. Evaluation should be pursued for these treatable infectious diseases.

Clinical Manifestations and Complications

Edema is one of the major clinical manifestations of nephrotic syndrome and represents excessive salt and water retention. Periorbital edema is often the initial finding and may be misdiagnosed as signs of allergy. Prominent upper eyelid edema should prompt evaluation for nephrotic syndrome. The edema is gravity dependent and therefore will vary in location based on patient position and activity. Upon awakening, edema may be more marked in the face and then shift to the lower extremities with ambulation. Anasarca, or generalized and massive edema, may develop and is characterized by marked peripheral edema, vulvar or scrotal edema, ascites, abdominal distention, and pleural effusions with respiratory compromise.

Two major processes have been proposed to be the cause of edema formation: arterial underfilling because of low oncotic pressure (hypoalbuminemia) and primary renal sodium retention. Evidence has supported both mechanisms, and it is likely that both processes contribute to varying degrees in individual patients. To be able to determine which is most relevant may impact clinical care. Diuretic therapy would be effective in reducing edema and indicated if the primary process is renal sodium retention. However, if hypoalbuminemia leads to decreased plasma volume via movement of fluid from the vascular space to the interstitium, diuretic therapy may aggravate arterial underfilling. As it may be difficult to determine intravas-

cular volume in patients with nephrotic syndrome, clinical characterics that may predict intravascular volume status include GFR and serum albumin level. Patients with reduced GFR and higher plasma albumin concentrations (greater than 2 g per dL) may be more likely to have elevated intravascular volume and tolerate diuretics with less risk of precipitating clinically significant arterial underfilling. Patients who are more likely to have underfilling are those with severe hypoalbuminemia (less than 1 g per dL) or those with rapid onset of nephrosis.

In addition to volume excess, complications resulting from nephrotic syndrome include infection, thromboembolism, and hypovolemia. Children with nephrotic syndrome are at increased risk of developing serious bacterial infection, particularly infections with encapsulated bacteria, given urinary losses of immunoglobulins and alternative complement pathway factor B and factor D. Children who are treated with immunosuppressive agents will have additional risks. Furthermore, ascites and pleural effusions will increase the risk for peritonitis, pneumonia, and empyema. The reported rates of peritonitis are approximately 2% to 6%. Other infections include sepsis, meningitis, cellulitis, urinary tract infection, upper respiratory tract infection, and severe AGE. A retrospective review of 24 episodes of peritonitis in children with idiopathic nephrotic syndrome prior to the current practice of vaccination with pneumococcal vaccine revealed *Streptococcus pneumoniae* was the most common isolated pathogen (50%). *Escherichia coli* was also commonly isolated, accounting for 25% of cases. Children with nephrotic syndrome who are receiving immunosuppression may also develop life-threatening viral infections, and varicella may result in significant morbidity and mortality.

Thromboembolic complications are reported in approximately 2% to 3% of children with nephrotic syndrome and may occur in either the arterial or venous circulation. The risk may be higher in children with steroid-resistant disease and persistent of nephrotic syndrome. Nephrotic syndrome results in a hypercoagulable state due to urinary losses of antithrombin, protein S, and plasminogen. Additional risk factors include hemoconcentration, thrombocytosis, infection, and immobility. Though many embolic events are silent, as has been documented by ventilation-perfusion scan abnormalities detected in asymptomatic subjects, pulmonary embolism and renal vein thrombosis may result in significant morbidity. Though a much less frequent occurrence in children than in adults with nephrotic syndrome, renal vein thrombosis should be suspected in cases of sudden onset macroscopic hematuria and flank pain.

Though children with nephrotic syndrome and edema have total body sodium and water excess, some will present with evidence of intravascular depletion. This is more likely to occur in those with severely depressed serum albumin and will be exacerbated by diuretic use, gastrointestinal losses, and restricted intake. Signs of decreased effective circulating volume include tachycardia, peripheral vasoconstriction, and oliguria. Laboratory studies may demonstrate renal insufficiency, which may be acute and transient due to intravascular depletion, secondary to the underlying renal pathology, or due to a combination of these factors.

Management

The initial assessment of a child with nephrotic syndrome should focus on the adequacy of intravascular volume and perfusion, respiratory status, and assess for evidence of infection.

As some patients with nephritis will have concomitant nephrotic syndrome (secondary nephrotic syndrome), accurate measurement of blood pressure should be documented to screen for associated hypertension. There should be a thorough assessment of recent fluid balance, with specific inquiries to diuretic use, urine output, and gastrointestinal losses.

The intent of laboratory investigation should include confirmation of nephrotic syndrome, identification of associated electrolyte abnormalities, and a determination if the disorder is associated with glomerulonephritis or systemic disease. The serum albumin should be less than 2.5 g per dL to fulfill the criteria for nephrotic syndrome and may be profoundly depressed (less than 1 g per dL). A freshly obtained urine sample should confirm heavy proteinuria by dipstick and be inspected for the presence of macroscopic hematuria, which may suggest glomerulonephritis. Nephrotic range proteinuria in children is defined as protein excretion greater than 50 mg per kg per day, though this would depend upon a timed 24-hour urine collection, which is prone to inaccuracies and may not be feasible in a young child. Alternatively, a urine protein to creatinine ratio can be submitted on a spot urine sample to quantify the degree of proteinuria. A normal ratio is less than 0.5 in children younger than 2 years and less than 0.2 in older children and adults. Generally, a ratio more than 2 to 3 is consistent with nephrotic range proteinuria. Serum electrolytes may reveal hyponatremia, which is not uncommon and secondary to decreased intravascular volume and stimulation of ADH release. Hyponatremia in the edematous child does not reflect total body sodium depletion but water excess greater than sodium excess. Renal function studies may be abnormal and reflect decreased intravascular volume or the underlying renal disease. Complete blood cell counts may demonstrate elevated hemoglobin and hematocrit due to hemoconcentration. Studies to distinguish the cause of nephrotic syndrome should be considered based on the patient's presentation. Serum complements may identify disorders associated with complement consumption such as postinfectious glomerulonephritis, MPGN, and lupus nephritis. Additional studies to be considered include serum antinuclear antibodies, antibodies to double-stranded DNA, and hepatitis B and C serologies.

Children with nephrotic syndrome who present to the emergency department with the primary complaint of edema are generally provided supportive care. Therapy of edema and volume excess should begin with sodium restriction. Optimally, children are restricted to approximately 2 to 3 mEq per kg per day of sodium or up to a maximum of 2,000 mg per day in older children and adolescents. Edematous children who have adequate intravascular volume and mild to moderate hyponatremia should not be provided supplemental sodium, as they are in a state of sodium excess. Water restriction should be initiated, given the release and action of ADH resulting in dilutional hyponatremia. Though diuretics are commonly provided to adults with nephrotic syndrome, the risks of aggravating intravascular volume depletion in children should be considered and discussed with a pediatric nephrologist if possible. Children who present with severe edema should be admitted and may be treated with furosemide and salt-poor albumin (e.g., 25% albumin) to achieve diuresis. Albumin (0.5 to 1 g per kg) infused over 4 hours with one to two doses of furosemide (0.5 to 1 mg per kg per dose) should result in fluid mobilization. Providing albumin will bolster the intravascular oncotic pressure and safeguard against volume depletion during fluid mobilization. The effect of albumin and furosemide will be transient given ongoing urinary losses of albumin and should be coupled with sodium restriction and education. Should renal function be diminished, albumin infusions may result in hypertension and pulmonary congestion due to limited ability to excrete salt and water despite improved intravascular volume, and these risks must be considered.

Children with nephrotic syndrome who present with evidence of inadequate intravascular volume should be provided isotonic intravenous fluid. Due to the increased risk of infection, any evidence of sepsis physiology should be addressed promptly. Normal saline can be infused as bolus therapy to restore perfusion. If readily available, 5% albumin would provide the additional benefit of oncotic support should the serum albumin be severely depressed. Once the intravascular volume is adequately restored, sodium and water restriction should be tailored to the individual need in order to avoid progressive volume excess and respiratory compromise. Admission for close volume management should be strongly considered if evidence of hypovolemia is apparent at presentation or uncontrolled fluid loss is anticipated (i.e., gastroenteritis) given the risk for thromboembolic complications and prerenal kidney injury.

Children with nephrotic syndrome are at increased risk for infectious complications, and overwhelming infection carries a mortality rate of 1.5%. As these children are predisposed to infections with *Streptococcus pneumoniae* and gram-negative bacterial infections, appropriate antibiotic coverage should be provided. Pneumococcal vaccination with the 23-valent and heptavalent conjugated pneumococcal vaccine is recommended, though data do not support the routine use of prophylactic antibiotics. Children with nephrotic syndrome who require immunosuppressive therapy are also at increased risk for developing severe varicella infection. Prophylactic treatment with varicella zoster immune globulin (VZIG) is recommended in cases of exposure to nonimmune children with nephrotic syndrome who are taking immunosuppressive treatments and should be administered within 96 hours of the exposure. In addition, acyclovir can be considered an adjunctive measure to VZIG in exposed patients on immunosuppressive therapy. Acyclovir should be initiated promptly in any patient exhibiting any signs of varicella infection. Varicella vaccine should be administered to children with nephrotic syndrome, if not immune. Ideally, it should be administered when the child is on alternate day or off corticosteroid therapy and should not be given within 5 months of VZIG.

Though children with nephrotic syndrome are at risk for thromboembolic complications as discussed above, most clinicians do not give prophylactic therapy initially given the lack of randomized controlled clinical trials supporting this practice. Some, however, will treat high-risk patients based on their coagulation profile with warfarin, low-dose aspirin, or dipyridamole. Supportive measures to reduce the risk of thromboembolism include mobilization and avoiding intravascular volume depletion (hemoconcentration). If thrombosis does occur, heparin is provided with the expectation that infusions of antithrombin III may be required to be effective. In children with a history of thrombotic complications and ongoing nephrosis, warfarin should be initiated to prevent future events.

MEDICAL EMERGENCIES

In addition to the management of acute complications of nephrotic syndrome in emergency care settings, management of chronic complications requires regular outpatient visits and monitoring. Therapy for hyperlipidemia, persistent proteinuria, chronic hypertension, and dietary guidance is provided, though full discussion is beyond the scope of this chapter.

Urolithiasis

Background

Urolithiasis accounts for 1 in every 1,000 to 7,600 admissions to pediatric hospitals annually throughout the United States, which is approximately one fiftieth to one seventy-fifth of that reported in adults. Furthermore, the incidence over the last decade may be increasing. In the United States, urolithiasis occurs more commonly in the southeastern region, and Caucasian children are most often affected. Boys may demonstrate an increased risk for renal stone formation when compared to girls, with reported male-to-female ratios of 1.4:1 to 2:1. In 75% to 85% of children affected, an identifiable risk factor is revealed. The most common underlying factors are metabolic predisposition and structural urinary tract abnormalities, accounting for approximately 50% and 32% of cases, respectively. The most common metabolic risk factors are hypercalciuria, hypocitraturia, and hyperoxaluria. Renal and urinary tract anomalies associated with urinary stasis include neurogenic bladder, ureteropelvic junction obstruction, medullary sponge kidneys, and autosomal dominant polycystic kidney disease. As in adults, the majority of stones in children are calcium based with approximately 45% calcium oxalate and approximately 25% calcium phosphate reported at analysis.

Clinical Manifestations

Flank pain and hematuria due to renal colic are commonly experienced in adults who present with nephrolithiasis. Though many children present with classic symptoms, approximately 15% to 20% are asymptomatic at presentation, and these tend to be younger children. In one series, 94% of adolescents presented with pain or hematuria. In children from birth to 5 years, 56% presented with these symptoms. The age-related difference in the symptoms may be due to stone location. Young children are more likely to have renal rather than ureteral stones. Ureteral stones causing obstruction would produce renal colic, whereas renal stones may be asymptomatic and found incidentally. Gross hematuria has been reported in up to 55% of children and can occur with pain or in isolation. Dysuria and urgency has also been reported and may be due to mechanical irritation of the lower urinary tract or concomitant urinary tract infection. Urease-producing bacteria are strongly associated with urolithiasis. Hydrolysis of urea will produce ammonium and bicarbonate ions and increases the risk for magnesium ammonium phosphate (struvite) stones. Urease-producing bacteria include *Proteus, Klebsiella, Providencia, Pseudomonas, Enterobacter,* and *Ureaplasma urealyticum.*

The evaluation of a child with urolithiasis includes a thorough personal and family history. Inquiries regarding previous urolithiasis, recurrent urinary tract infections, and underlying urologic abnormalities should be pursued. Given the high proportion of children with and underlying metabolic predisposi-

tion, specifically hypercalciuria, the history should account for periods of immobilization, vitamin D supplementation, and treatment with loop diuretics. Children with fat malabsorption are at risk for increased enteric absorption of oxalate and hyperoxaluria, and therefore, gastrointestinal history should include symptoms consistent with inflammatory bowel disease, pancreatic insufficiency, and history of bowel resection. Patients with cystic fibrosis have numerous potential risk factors for calcium oxalate stones, including pancreatic disease, vitamin D supplementation, altered bowel flora, and low urine volume. Physical examination should include documentation of temperature, careful abdominal exam, and growth measurements. Poor growth may be a sign of chronic renal disease, such as distal RTA, which may be associated with urolithiasis.

Management

The initial laboratory evaluation should include urinalysis with urine pH and assessment of the urine sediment, which may reveal crystals. Urine culture should be submitted to evaluate for urinary tract infection, especially in children with known abnormality of the urinary tract given the risk for chronic urinary tract infection. Serum studies should include measurement of electrolytes, including calcium and phosphorus, bicarbonate, magnesium, uric acid, and creatinine. Depending on the results of the initial laboratory screen, other studies to be considered include PTH and vitamin D metabolites. Given the frequency of metabolic predisposition, urine studies to be performed in the nonurgent setting include a timed 24-hour assessment of urinary solutes (e.g., calcium, oxalate, uric acid, citrate, magnesium, cystine), urine creatinine, and urine volume. This should also be pursued in children with known urologic tract abnormalities, as approximately 35% of children with urologic malformation and urolithiasis were found to have metabolic risk factors. If the child's age or development is not permitting for a daily collection, assessment of solute excretion based upon random urine samples should be submitted. If the stone is available, this should be submitted for analysis, which may guide future preventative therapy.

Diagnostic imaging techniques available to evaluate for urolithiasis include abdominal plain radiography, ultrasonography, and noncontrast helical computed tomography (CT). Abdominal radiograph may detect radiopaque stones (e.g., calcium, cysteine, and struvite stones) though will not reveal radiolucent stones (e.g., uric acid stones). Plain radiograph may miss small stones and stones overlying bony structures, and one center reported a sensitivity of 57%. Furthermore, radiograph will not assess the urinary tract for obstruction. Ultrasonography is widely available, avoids radiation, and will assess for urinary obstruction. Ultrasonography can detect radiolucent stones, though may not identify small papillary, calyceal, or ureteral stones. Noncontrast helical CT scan is the most sensitive modality to detect urolithiasis, especially ureteral or small calculi and provides the most anatomic detail of the urinary tract. Performance of CT scan will result in radiation exposure, and this must be considered. However, adjustments of scanning technique appropriate for the size and weight of the child can be made to reduce radiation exposure.

The management of urolithiasis will be based on the severity of symptoms and likelihood of spontaneous passage of the stone. Children with significant acute renal colic, urinary tract obstruction, and potentially infected stones should be evaluated in concert with a urologist. Children with smaller stones (less than 5 mm) and mild symptoms may be appropriately managed as an outpatient with hydration and NSAIDs. Hydration will increase urine flow and may facilitate passage. Increased hydration may also minimize stone growth and decrease the risk for recurrent stone disease. In adults, medications prescribed to facilitate the passage of ureteral stones include antispasmodic agents, calcium channel blockers, and alpha blockers. Studies evaluating these therapies in children are not currently available. Instructions to strain the urine should be provided, and any retrieved fragments should be submitted for analysis. Reliable follow up should be assured. Children with significant pain, vomiting, or concern for urinary tract infection should be admitted for appropriate care.

Urologic intervention may be required and indications include unremitting severe pain, persistent obstruction despite conservative management, urolithiasis in a solitary kidney with obstruction or risk of obstruction, larger stones that are unlikely to pass spontaneously (e.g., greater than 5 mm), renal insufficiency, and urosepsis. Though open surgical repair remains an option, other procedures have been adapted for use in children and have reduced the need for surgical intervention. These procedures include extracorporeal shock wave lithotripsy (ESWL), percutaneous nephrostolithotomy, and ureterostomy. The procedure utilized is determined by the experience of the clinician, the stone size and location, and anatomic abnormalities. Stone composition, if known, is also considered. Stones of harder composition, such as cystine and calcium oxalate monohydrate, are less likely fragmented with ESWL.

Recurrence of urolithiasis in children and adolescents is common with reported rates of 30% to 65%, underscoring the need for referral to a pediatric urologist or nephrologist for metabolic evaluation and appropriate preventive care. Children with an identified metabolic abnormality are at the highest risk for recurrence. Preventive measures should be pursued in all children with urolithiasis to reduce the risk of recurrence. The importance of increased fluid intake to increase the urine flow rate and lower urine solute concentration must be emphasized. Recommended fluid intake is based upon age and desired 24-hour urine volume (Table 100.15). For children with hypercalciuria, additional measures should include low-sodium diet and avoidance of supplemental vitamin D. Low sodium intake enhances renal tubular absorption of both sodium and calcium, thereby reducing calcium excretion. Dietary calcium should meet the RDA but not be excessive. Limiting calcium intake was found to increase oxalate excre-

tion in adults. If the response to supportive measures is insufficient based upon repeat assessment of urinary solutes or recurrent disease, thiazide diuretics to reduce calcium excretion should be considered. For patients with hypocitraturia, supplemental potassium citrate can be provided. Citrate inhibits stone formation by forming a soluble complex with calcium. Specific preventive measures for other disorders, including hyperoxaluria, hyperuricosuria, and cystinuria should be pursued, though discussion is beyond the scope of this chapter. Monitoring should include imaging to follow the size of existing stones and to identify the development of new stones. Ultrasonography is generally the favored modality given the lower radiation exposure and availability.

CHRONIC KIDNEY DISEASE

Background

The definition of CKD is based upon persistent structural or functional abnormalities, which may be associated with reduced or normal GFR. When reviewing registry data of children with CKD, the most common primary diseases were congenital and included obstructive uropathy (20.7%); renal aplasia, hypoplasia, and dysplasia (17.3%); and reflux nephropathy (8.4%). FSGS, which is an acquired glomerulopathy, accounted for 8.7% of diagnoses. The natural history of CKD is variable and depends upon the severity of the underlying kidney damage. When kidney damage is significant, there is progressive loss of functioning nephron mass leading to end-stage renal disease (ESRD). In 2002, the National Kidney Foundation Kidney Disease Outcomes Quality Initiative put forth definition criteria and a classification scheme to define the stages of CKD in patients older than 2 years (Table 100.16). Emphasis is placed on early detection and intervention, as measures to retard the progression of renal dysfunction include treating hypertension and reducing proteinuria when it is significant. For children who progress to ESRD, therapies include chronic hemodialysis, peritoneal dialysis, and renal transplantation. Renal transplantation is recognized as the preferred treatment for children with ESRD, as restoration of normal renal physiologic function can greatly improve the child's quality of life.

Clinical Manifestations

The clinical presentation of CKD will depend upon the severity of the renal dysfunction and the underlying cause. Children with mild CKD (stage 1 and 2) and no other comorbidities may be asymptomatic. Children with more severe CKD are at increased likelihood for associated symptoms and signs such as fatigue, anorexia, and poor growth. Furthermore, these children may present for emergent care with a variety of complaints directly related to renal dysfunction including hypertension, volume excess, anemia, and severe electrolyte or acid–base abnormalities. They may also present with illness attributable to the underlying disorder, such as urinary tract infection in those with complex urologic disease and symptoms of systemic inflammation in those with systemic vasculitis. Children with CKD have limited renal reserve and are susceptible to AKI

TABLE 100.15

UROLITHIASIS: TARGET DAILY URINE VOLUME BASED ON AGE

Infants	>750 mL/day
Children <5 yr	>1,000 mL/day
Children 5–10 yr	>1,500 mL/day
Children >10 yr, adolescents, adults	>2,000 mL/day

From Milliner D. Urolithiasis. In: Avner ED, Harmon WE, Niaudet P, ed. *Pediatric Nephrology*. 5th ed. Philadelphia: Lippincott Williams & Wilkins, 2004:1104.

TABLE 100.16

STAGES OF CHRONIC KIDNEY DISEASE

Stage	Description	GFR (mL/min/1.73 m^2)
1	Kidney damage with normal or increased GFR	$\geq$90
2	Kidney damage with mildly decreased GFR	60–89
3	Moderately decreased GFR	30–59
4	Severely decreased GFR	15–29
5	Kidney failure	<15 (or dialysis)

Chronic kidney disease is defined as either kidney damage of GFR <60 mL/min/1.73 m^2 or $\geq$3 mo. Kidney damage is defined as pathologic abnormalities or makers of damage, including abnormalities in blood or urine tests or imaging studies.
Adapted from Hogg RJ, Furth S, LemLey KV, et al. National Kidney Foundation's Kidney Disease Outcomes Quality Initiative clinical practice guidelines for chronic kidney disease in children and adolescents: evaluation, classification, and stratification. *Pediatrics* 2003;111:1416–1421.

superimposed on chronic insufficiency, which will increase the risk for metabolic derangements and volume excess.

Though many children with CKD who present for emergent care have a known history of renal disease, some will present with newly diagnosed CKD. For those with a new diagnosis, the physician should inquire about previous episodes of urinary tract infection and signs of concentrating defect or urologic disease, such as polyuria, polydipsia, and enuresis. To evaluate for signs consistent with chronic glomerulonephritis, history of gross hematuria, edema, unusual rashes, or evidence of systemic inflammation should be sought. A review of the family history should include inquiries of urologic disease, vesicoureteral reflux, progressive kidney disease, cystic kidney disease, and early onset hypertension.

Management

The initial evaluation of a child with CKD must include accurate assessment of blood pressure, cardiopulmonary exam, volume status, and growth parameters. Initial laboratory studies should be guided by the presenting complaint and history, though assessment of blood counts, electrolytes (including calcium and phosphorus), acid–base status, and renal function should be performed. The GFR may be estimated by using the Schwartz formula (Table 100.13), which takes into account the serum creatinine and the patient's height and gender. This formula is convenient for use at the bedside, though tends to overestimate GFR due to the tubular secretion of creatinine. This overestimation increases with decreasing GFR, and newer equations are being developed but need validation. Urinalysis should also be submitted as it may provide useful clinical data. Most patients with congenital dysplasia or reflux nephropathy will have bland urine sediments and modest amounts of proteinuria. Significant hematuria, heavy proteinuria, and active urine sediment with glomerular hematuria and cellular casts would be consistent with glomerular disease. Further laboratory studies should be guided by the presentation of illness and clinical suspicion.

For all children with newly diagnosed CKD of unknown etiology and for many children with known urologic disease, a renal ultrasound is indicated. This is a safe and readily available radiographic study and can provide valuable assessment of the renal parenchyma and the urologic tract. Ultrasound

can detect such disorders as renal dysplasia, renal cortical thinning consistent with reflux nephropathy, cystic kidney disease, urinary tract obstruction, and screen for renal vascular disease. If the kidneys appear relatively normal but enlarged, this is more suggestive of an acute or reversible process. Small kidneys would be consistent with a chronic process and parenchymal scarring. Of note, the use of gadolinium has been associated with nephrogenic systemic fibrosis (NSF), a recently identified severe fibrosing disorder found only in patients with renal failure. Gadolinium should be avoided in patients with acute or chronic renal failure, and this includes those patients on hemodialysis and peritoneal dialysis. If gadolinium is thought to be necessary, then the risks and benefits should be discussed, the lowest possible dose of gadolinium should be provided, and consideration should be given to the preparation of gadolinium as some may result in increased risk for the development of NSF. Furthermore, hemodialysis immediately after gadolinium exposure may reduce the risk of NSF, though this is not proven effective.

The treatment of children with CKD can range from routine care to intensive management. If a child with CKD presents to the emergency department with a significant illness, treatment should be coordinated with a pediatric nephrologist when possible. The initial approach should identify reversible causes of decreased renal function, such as intravascular volume depletion and use of nephrotoxic medications (i.e., NSAIDs). Children who have decreased effective circulating volume should be provided intravenous isotonic fluid if oral hydration is expected to be insufficient or not well tolerated. Bolus intravenous fluid can be provided at 5 to 10 mL per kg and should be followed by repeated assessment to determine if further intravenous fluid is warranted. Subsequent fluid rates should be provided on the basis of ongoing losses and urine flow to ensure adequate perfusion and avoid volume excess.

With severe decline in GFR, sodium and water retention may develop and lead to clinical signs if volume overload. Children with CKD may present with edema, hypertension, and pulmonary congestion. Diuretic therapy should be trialed for treatment of clinical volume overload, though may not be adequately effective. Furosemide at a dose of 1 to 2 mg per kg intravenously may be given, recognizing that higher doses may be required to achieve the desired effect for those with more severe renal dysfunction. For children with sustained hypertension, therapy will depend on the degree and the chronicity of elevation. Severe hypertension with end-organ dysfunction or concern for impending end-organ dysfunction should be treated with short acting intravenous antihypertensive medications, and commonly used agents include hydralazine and labetalol. The aim of therapy is to lower the blood pressure by 20% to 30% or to a range that is not acutely dangerous within the first 2 to 3 hours. Blood pressure can then be controlled gradually over the next several days or longer. ACE inhibitor and ARB therapy are generally well tolerated in early stages of CKD and may slow the progression of CKD over time, especially in those with proteinuria. However, in more severe CKD, these agents may result in unacceptable elevations in serum potassium and decreased GFR. For those children with CKD and on ACE inhibitor or ARB therapy chronically, these agents may need to be temporarily held during periods of acute deterioration of renal function.

Electrolyte and acid–base abnormalities are common in CKD and include hyperkalemia, hypocalcemia, hyperphosphatemia, and metabolic acidosis. The therapy of these electrolyte and acid–base disturbances were previously discussed. Of note, the metabolic disturbances associated with CKD generally develop gradually, and therefore, immediate correction may not be warranted and may, in fact, be deleterious. Given the potential for cardiac dysrhythmias, hyperkalemia should be addressed urgently. In clinically stable patients with concurrent hypocalcemia and acidosis, the potential risk for tetany with alkali therapy should be considered. If clinically reasonable, hypocalcemia should be treated initially, and this can be achieved with oral calcium if the patient is asymptomatic.

For some children with severe CKD or AKI superimposed on CKD, supportive medical management will be insufficient and RRT will be required. Accepted indications for RRT include severe fluid overload, refractory hyperkalemia, and severe uremia. Modalities of dialysis include continuous renal replacement, intermittent hemodialysis, and peritoneal dialysis. The modality utilized will depend on the clinical circumstances, local resources, and clinician preference.

Suggested Readings

Hypovolemia and Disorders of Sodium Homeostasis

Goldman RD, Friedman JN, Parkin PC. Validation of the clinical dehydration scale for children with acute gastroenteritis. *Pediatrics* 2008;122:545–549.

Holliday MA, Friedman AL, Segar WE, et al. Acute hospital-induced hyponatremia in children: a physiologic approach. *J Pediatr* 2004;145:584–587.

Holliday MA, Segar WE. The maintenance need for water in parenteral fluid therapy. *Pediatrics* 1957;19:823–832.

Hoorn EJ, Geary D, Robb M, et al. Acute hyponatremia related to intravenous fluid administration in hospitalized children: an observational study. *Pediatrics* 2004;113:1279–1284.

King CK, Glass R, Bresee JS, et al. Managing acute gastroenteritis among children: oral rehydration, maintenance, and nutritional therapy. *MMWR Recomm Rep* 2003;52:1–16.

Malek MA, Curns AT, Holman RC, et al. Diarrhea- and rotavirus-associated hospitalizations among children less than 5 years of age: United States, 1997 and 2000. *Pediatrics* 2006;117:1887–1892.

Moritz ML, Ayus JC. Prevention of hospital-acquired hyponatremia: a case for using isotonic saline. *Pediatrics* 2003;111:227–230.

Moritz ML, Ayus JC. Preventing neurological complications from dysnatremias in children. *Pediatr Nephrol* 2005;20:1687–1700.

Neville KA, Verge CF, O'Meara MW, et al. High antidiuretic hormone levels and hyponatremia in children with gastroenteritis. *Pediatrics* 2005;116:1401–1407.

Neville KA, Verge CF, Rosenberg AR, et al. Isotonic is better than hypotonic saline for intravenous rehydration of children with gastroenteritis: a prospective randomised study. *Arch Dis Child* 2006;91:226–232.

Practice parameter: the management of acute gastroenteritis in young children. American Academy of Pediatrics, Provisional Committee on Quality Improvement, Subcommittee on Acute Gastroenteritis. *Pediatrics* 1996;97: 424–435.

Steiner MJ, DeWalt DA, Byerley JS. Is this child dehydrated? *JAMA* 2004;291: 2746–2754.

Disorders of Potassium and Calcium Homeostasis

Benjamin RW, Moats-Staats BM, Calikoglu's A, et al. Hypercalcemia in children. *Pediatr Endocrinol Rev* 2008;5:778–784.

Karet FE. Mechanisms in hyperkalemic renal tubular acidosis. *J Am Soc Nephrol* 2009;20:251–254.

Schaefer TJ, Wolford RW. Disorders of potassium. *Emerg Med Clin North Am* 2005;23:723–747, viii-ix.

Schwartz GJ. Potassium. In: Avner ED, Harmon WE, Niaudet P, eds. *Pediatric nephrology*. 5th ed. Philadelphia: Lippincott Williams & Wilkins, 2004: 147–176.

Singh J, Moghal N, Pearce SH, et al. The investigation of hypocalcaemia and rickets. *Arch Dis Child* 2003;88:403–407.

Weisberg LS. Management of severe hyperkalemia. *Crit Care Med* 2008;36: 3246–3251.

Disorders of Acid–Base Homeostasis

Chan JC, Mak RH. Acid-Base Homeostasis. In: Avner ED, Harmon WE, Niaudet P, eds. *Pediatric nephrology*. Philadelphia: Lippincott Williams & Wilkins, 2004:189–202.

Galla JH. Metabolic alkalosis. *J Am Soc Nephrol* 2000;11:369–375.

Kraut JA, Kurtz I. Use of base in the treatment of severe acidemic states. *Am J Kidney Dis* 2001;38:703–727.

Rose BD, Post TP, eds. *Clinical physiology of acid-base and electrolyte disorders*. 5th ed. New York: McGraw-Hill, 2001:551–571.

Acute Kidney Injury

Akcan-Arikan A, Zappitelli M, Loftis LL, et al. Modified RIFLE criteria in critically ill children with acute kidney injury. *Kidney Int* 2007;71:1028–1035.

Andreoli SP. Acute renal failure. *Curr Opin Pediatr* 2002;14:183–188.

Andreoli SP. Acute kidney injury in children. *Pediatr Nephrol* 2009;24:253–263.

Flynn JT. Choice of dialysis modality for management of pediatric acute renal failure. *Pediatr Nephrol* 2002;17:61–69.

Huerta-Alardin AL, Varon J, Marik PE. Bench-to-bedside review: Rhabdomyolysis—an overview for clinicians. *Crit Care* 2005;9:158–169.

Hui-Stickle S, Brewer ED, Goldstein SL. Pediatric ARF epidemiology at a tertiary care center from 1999 to 2001. *Am J Kidney Dis* 2005;45:96–101.

Luck RP, Verbin S. Rhabdomyolysis: a review of clinical presentation, etiology, diagnosis, and management. *Pediatr Emerg Care* 2008;24:262–268.

Mannix R, Tan ML, Wright R, et al. Acute pediatric rhabdomyolysis: causes and rates of renal failure. *Pediatrics* 2006;118:2119–2125.

Watanabe T. Rhabdomyolysis and acute renal failure in children. *Pediatr Nephrol* 2001;16:1072–1075.

Zepeda-Orozco D, Ault BH, Jones DP. Factors associated with acute renal failure in children with rhabdomyolysis. *Pediatr Nephrol* 2008;23:2281–2284.

Glomerular Diseases

Ahn SY, Ingulli E. Acute poststreptococcal glomerulonephritis: an update. *Curr Opin Pediatr* 2008;20:157–162.

Andreoli SP, Trachtman H, Acheson DW, et al. Hemolytic uremic syndrome: epidemiology, pathophysiology, and therapy. *Pediatr Nephrol* 2002;17:293–298.

Chartapisak W, Opastiraku S, Willis NS, et al. Prevention and treatment of renal disease in Henoch-Schonlein purpura: a systematic review. *Arch Dis Child* 2009;94:132–137.

Dillon MJ Henoch-Schonlein purpura: recent advances. *Clin Exp Rheumatol* 2007;25:S66–S68.

Foster BJ, Bernard C, Drummond KN, et al. Effective therapy for severe Henoch-Schonlein purpura nephritis with prednisone and azathioprine: a clinical and histopathologic study. *J Pediatr* 2000;136:370–375.

Gerber A, Karch H, Allerberger F, et al. Clinical course and the role of shiga toxin-producing Escherichia coli infection in the hemolytic-uremic syndrome in pediatric patients, 1997–2000, in Germany and Austria: a prospective study. *J Infect Dis* 2002;186:493–500.

Huber AM, King J, McLaine P, et al. A randomized, placebo-controlled trial of prednisone in early Henoch Schonlein purpura [ISRCTN85109383]. *BMC Med* 2004;2:7.

Narchi H. Risk of long term renal impairment and duration of follow up recommended for Henoch-Schonlein purpura with normal or minimal urinary findings: a systematic review. *Arch Dis Child* 2005;90:916–920.

Noris M, Remuzzi G. Hemolytic uremic syndrome. *J Am Soc Nephrol* 2005;16: 1035–1050.

Rodriguez-Iturbe B, Musser JM. The current state of poststreptococcal glomerulonephritis. *J Am Soc Nephrol* 2008;19:1855–1864.

Ronkainen J, Koskimies O, Ala-Houhala M, et al. Early prednisone therapy in Henoch-Schonlein purpura: a randomized, double-blind, placebo-controlled trial. *J Pediatr* 2006;149:241–247.

Weiss PF, Feinstein JA, Luan X, et al. Effects of corticosteroid on Henoch-Schonlein purpura: a systematic review. *Pediatrics* 2007;120:1079–1087.

Yang YH, Hung CF, Hsu CR, et al. A nationwide survey on epidemiological characteristics of childhood Henoch-Schonlein purpura in Taiwan. *Rheumatology (Oxford)* 2005;44:618–622.

Nephrotic Syndrome

Eddy AA, Symons JM. Nephrotic syndrome in childhood. *Lancet* 2003;362: 629–639.

Furth SL, Arbus GS, Hogg R, et al. Varicella vaccination in children with nephrotic syndrome: a report of the Southwest Pediatric Nephrology Study Group. *J Pediatr* 2003;142:145–148.

Gipson DS, Massengill SF, Yao L, et al. Management of childhood onset nephrotic syndrome. *Pediatrics* 2009;124:747–757.

Hinkes BG, Mucha B, Vlangos CN, et al. Nephrotic syndrome in the first year of life: two thirds of cases are caused by mutations in 4 genes (NPHS1, NPHS2, WT1, and LAMB2). *Pediatrics* 2007;119:e907–e919.

Hogg RJ, Portman RJ, Milliner D, et al. Evaluation and management of proteinuria and nephrotic syndrome in children: recommendations from a pediatric nephrology panel established at the National Kidney Foundation conference on proteinuria, albuminuria, risk, assessment, detection, and elimination (PARADE). *Pediatrics* 2000;105:1242–1249.

Niaudet P. Genetic forms of nephrotic syndrome. *Pediatr Nephrol* 2004;19: 1313–1318.

Ulinski T, Leroy S, Dubrel M, et al. High serological response to pneumococcal vaccine in nephrotic children at disease onset on high-dose prednisone. *Pediatr Nephrol* 2008;23:1107–1113.

Urolithiasis

Borghi L, Schianchi T, Meschi T, et al. Comparison of two diets for the prevention of recurrent stones in idiopathic hypercalciuria. *N Engl J Med* 2002;346:77–84.

Coward RJ, Peters CJ, Duffy PG, et al. Epidemiology of paediatric renal stone disease in the UK. *Arch Dis Child* 2003;88:962–965.

Milliner D. Urolithiasis. In: Avner ED, Harmon WE, Niaudet P, ed. *Pediatric nephrology*. 5th ed. Philadelphia: Lippincott Williams & Wilkins, 2004:1091–1105.

Nicoletta JA, Lande MB. Medical evaluation and treatment of urolithiasis. *Pediatr Clin North Am* 2006;53:479–491, vii.

VanDervoort K, Wiesen J, Frank R, et al. Urolithiasis in pediatric patients: a single center study of incidence, clinical presentation and outcome. *J Urol* 2007;177:2300–2305.

Chronic Kidney Disease

Hogg RJ, Furth S, LemLey KV, et al. National Kidney Foundation's Kidney Disease Outcomes Quality Initiative clinical practice guidelines for chronic kidney disease in children and adolescents: evaluation, classification, and stratification. *Pediatrics* 2003;111:1416–1421.

Perazella MA. Current status of gadolinium toxicity in patients with kidney disease. *Clin J Am Soc Nephrol* 2009;4:461–469.

Schwartz GJ, Munoz A, Schneider MF, et al. New equations to estimate GFR in children with CKD. *J Am Soc Nephrol* 2009;20:629–637.

Wong H, Mylrea K, Feber J, et al. Prevalence of complications in children with chronic kidney disease according to KDOQI. *Kidney Int* 2006;70:585–590.

Wuhl E, Schaefer F. Therapeutic strategies to slow chronic kidney disease progression. *Pediatr Nephrol* 2008;23:705–716.

CHAPTER 101 ■ RHEUMATOLOGIC EMERGENCIES

AMY L. WOODWARD, MD, MPH, AND ROBERT P. SUNDEL, MD

Pediatric rheumatologic conditions are relatively rare, affecting less than 0.5% of children in the United States. Further, pediatric autoimmune diseases are most commonly chronic conditions with an indolent onset rather than acute conditions likely to bring a child to the emergency department (ED). Nonetheless, arthritis, lupus, and vasculitis [especially Kawasaki disease (KD)] may have acute and life-threatening manifestations requiring rapid initiation of appropriate therapy. These plus the conditions that must be distinguished from them are quite prevalent; for example, up to 20% of urgent visits to pediatricians involve musculoskeletal complaints. Thus, arthritis, vasculitis, and other inflammatory and autoimmune conditions of childhood must be considered if clinicians are to recognize and treat the far more common infectious and traumatic complaints likely to bring children to their attention. Finally, treatment of rheumatologic disorders is becoming more sophisticated and more specialized, involving combinations of antiinflammatory, immunosuppressive, and biologic agents with a wide spectrum of intended and undesired effects. For all of these reasons, familiarity with rheumatologic conditions and their treatments is essential if children are to receive high-quality emergency care.

JUVENILE RHEUMATOID ARTHRITIS

Background

Juvenile rheumatoid arthritis (JRA) is now the most common pediatric rheumatologic disease in the developed world, having replaced acute rheumatic fever. JRA occurs in all races and ethnic groups, with a reported prevalence that varies from 30 to 400 per 100,000 children depending upon the population studied and the diagnostic techniques used. In the United States alone, JRA affects at least 100,000 children.

Arthritis is a clinical finding of persistent joint swelling or restriction of joint movement by pain. A variety of different classification systems exist, but in the absence of a clear-cut understanding of the pathogenesis of arthritis, these systems do not differ practically. Accordingly, we will continue to use the American College of Rheumatology criteria used in previous editions of this textbook. Persistent unexplained arthritis of one or more joints lasting more than 6 weeks in children younger than 16 years of age will be referred to as JRA (Table 101.1). The differences from other nomenclature systems are largely irrelevant to ED evaluations (Table 101.2). In all cases, because there are no laboratory abnormalities specific for JRA, the diagnosis is made clinically after exclusion of other infectious, inflammatory, and traumatic conditions.

Pathophysiology

The etiology of JRA is not known. It may be triggered by infections including borrelia, parvovirus, or Epstein-Barr virus (EBV), or by trauma, but most cases develop without identifiable precipitants. The presence of rheumatoid factor (RF) in the serum of some children with JRA, a lowered level of complement in the synovial fluid, and activated lymphocytes in the synovial tissue suggest that immunologically mediated injury plays a role in the pathogenesis of this disease. There may also be genetic factors, as suggested by the association of JRA with particular histocompatibility antigens and cytokine alleles.

It is useful conceptually to divide the pathogenesis of JRA into an initiating phase and a perpetuating phase. Various events, particularly viral infections, may trigger articular inflammation. For a variety of reasons related to both the host and the inciting event, a process that is self-limited in most children leads to ongoing inflammation in others. This inflammation is characterized by abnormal tissue and circulating levels of proinflammatory cytokines [including interleukin (IL)-1, IL-6, tumor necrosis factor (TNF), and interferon-γ] leading to activation of lymphocytes and infiltration of synovium. In fact, conditions labeled as JRA most likely represent a final common pathway for many different types of synovitis in view of the widely disparate characteristics of the different subtypes of JRA.

Pathologically, synovial vasculitis is prominent in early lesions. In established cases of arthritis, light microscopy of the synovium shows fibrin deposits, hyperplasia and hypertrophy of synovial lining cells, and an inflammatory cell infiltrate. Increased secretion of synovial fluid results in joint effusions. In uncontrolled and persistent arthritis, synovial villi project into the joint, so-called pannus formation. Fronds of synovium may spread from the edges of the joint and overgrow the cartilage, causing damage to the articulation and eventually to the underlying bone.

Clinical Manifestations

JRA is characterized by wide demographic and clinical variety, so the condition has been divided into subtypes based on these factors and on the pattern of the disease during the first 6 months following onset (Table 101.1). These varieties, in turn, are treated in different ways, and are associated with different complications. While the term JRA will likely be familiar to practitioners in the United States, a classification scheme with the umbrella term juvenile idiopathic arthritis (JIA) has become widely used in the rheumatologic literature. Until better means of classifying and distinguishing these subtypes of JRA become available, what is likely to be several discrete

TABLE 101.1

SUBGROUPS OF JUVENILE RHEUMATOID ARTHRITIS

Subgroup	At onset % of JRA	Gender ratio	Age at onset	Joints affected	Serologic and genetic test[a]	Extraarticular manifestations	Prognosis
Rheumatoid-positive polyarticular	15	90% female	Late childhood	Any joints, especially hands, wrists	ANA 75% RF 100%	Low-grade fever, anemia, malaise, rheumatoid nodules	>50% Severe arthritis
Rheumatoid-negative polyarticular	20	70% female	Younger onset	Any joints	ANA 50%	Low-grade fever, mild anemia, malaise, growth retardation	20%–40% Severe arthritis
Type 1 pauciarticular	45	80% female	Early childhood	Few large joints (hips and sacroiliac joints spared)	ANA 50%	Few constitutional complaints, chronic iridocyclitis in 50%	Severe arthritis uncommon; 10%–20% ocular damage from iridocyclitis if untreated
Type 2 pauciarticular	5	90% male	Late childhood	Few large joints (hip and sacroiliac involvement common)	ANA negative, HLA-B27 75%	Few constitutional complaints, acute iridocyclitis in 5%–10% during childhood	Clinically similar to spondyloarthritis
Systemic onset	15	50% female	Any age	Any joints	ANA negative, RF negative	High fever, rash, organomegaly, polyserositis, leukocytosis, growth retardation	30% Severe arthritis

ANA, antinuclear antibody; RF, rheumatoid factor; HLA-B27, histocompatibility antigen-B27.

TABLE 101.2

CLASSIFICATION SYSTEMS FOR JUVENILE ARTHRITIS

Comparison of current classification systems for chronic arthritis in children, showing differing names for similar types of arthritis in parallel columns.

ACR	ILAR	EULAR
Juvenile rheumatoid arthritis	Juvenile idiopathic arthritis	Juvenile chronic arthritis
Systemic onset	Systemic arthritis	Systemic onset
Polyarticular onset	RF-negative polyarthritis	Polyarticular onset
	RF-positive polyarthritis	Juvenile rheumatoid arthritis
Pauciarticular onset	Oligoarthritis	Pauciarticular onset
Type 1	Persistent	
	Extended	
	Psoriatic arthritis	Juvenile psoriatic arthritis
Type 2	Enthesitis-related arthritis	Juvenile ankylosing spondylitis
	Undifferentiated arthritis	

ACR, American College of Rheumatology; ILAR, International League of Associations for Rheumatology; EULAR, European League Against Rheumatism.

conditions will continue to be grouped on the basis of purely clinical features. The remainder of this chapter will utilize the traditional JRA classification scheme.

Pauciarticular arthritis, synovitis involving four or fewer joints, is the most common subtype of JRA and accounts for approximately half of all cases. Type 1 pauciarthritis occurs more often in young girls, typically causing swelling, pain, and limitation of movement in one or more large joints. Antinuclear antibodies (ANAs) are detectable in the sera of more than 50% of these children, and their presence correlates with a higher risk for developing iridocyclitis. Type 2 pauciarticular JRA occurs more often in preadolescent boys. Although they are often classified as having JRA, the predilection for axial involvement is more typical of spondyloarthritis. In fact, some of these children may develop ankylosing spondylitis on long-term follow-up. Typical of spondyloarthritis, the risk for developing chronic iridocyclitis is negligible, but 5% to 10% of these children may develop acute anterior uveitis.

Polyarticular arthritis (both RF positive and RF negative) occurs more commonly in girls. It is characterized by the insidious onset of symmetric synovitis in both large and small joints, accompanied by low-grade fever, morning stiffness, and malaise (Fig. 101.1). The presence of antibodies to native immunoglobulins in the serum (RF) corresponds to an increased risk of severe, erosive arthritis, as well as to the development of vasculitic complications and subcutaneous nodules. Cervical spine involvement occurs in approximately 30% to 50% of patients with this variety of arthritis, resulting in neck pain, stiffness, and torticollis. Unlike pauciarticular JRA, in which ocular involvement is the cause of the most significant morbidity, polyarticular disease may result in severe musculoskeletal disability. Thus, involvement of the temporomandibular joint may result in restricted ability to open the mouth, involvement of the hips may permanently affect ambulation, and small joint arthritis of the hands may compromise manual dexterity.

MEDICAL EMERGENCIES

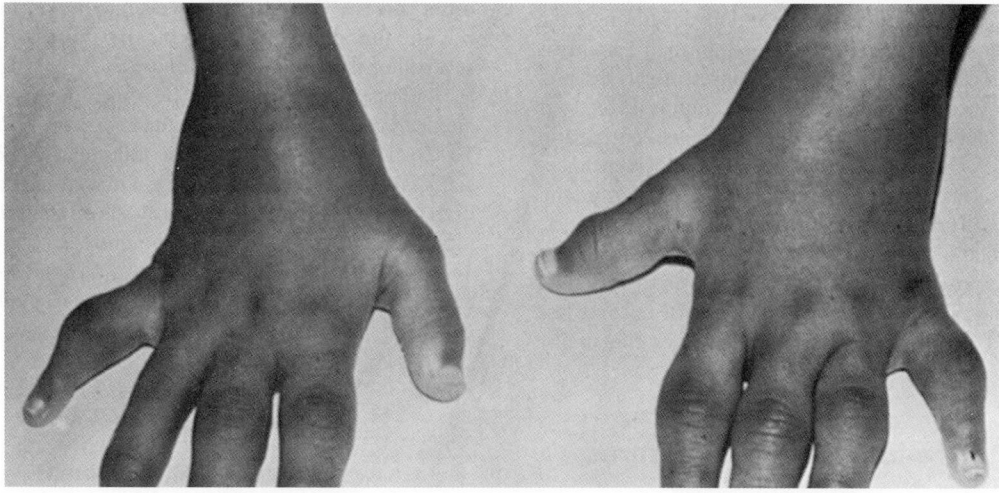

FIGURE 101.1 Symmetric involvement of large and small joints of the hands in a child with polyarticular arthritis.

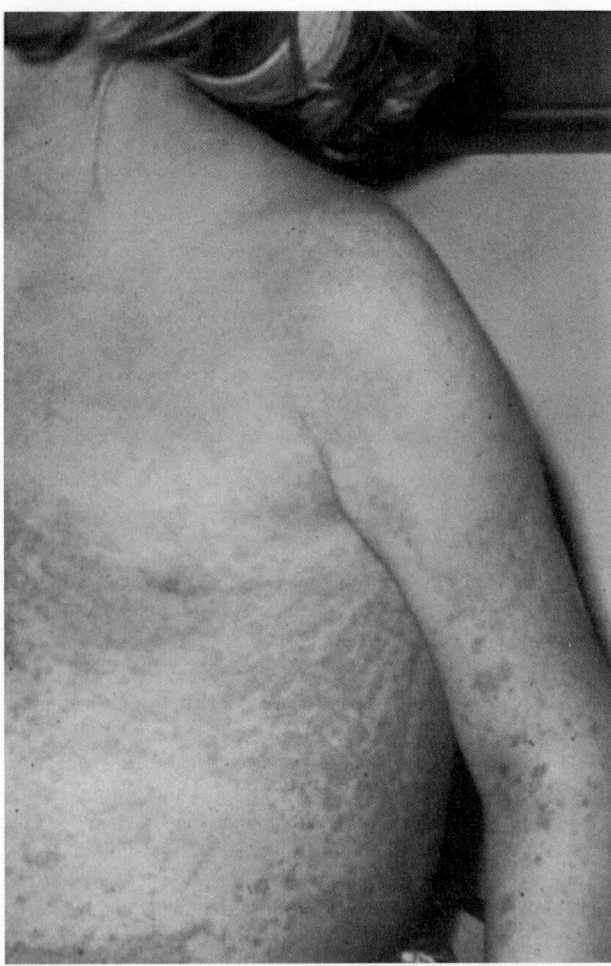

FIGURE 101.2 Macular rash in a child with systemic type of juvenile rheumatoid arthritis.

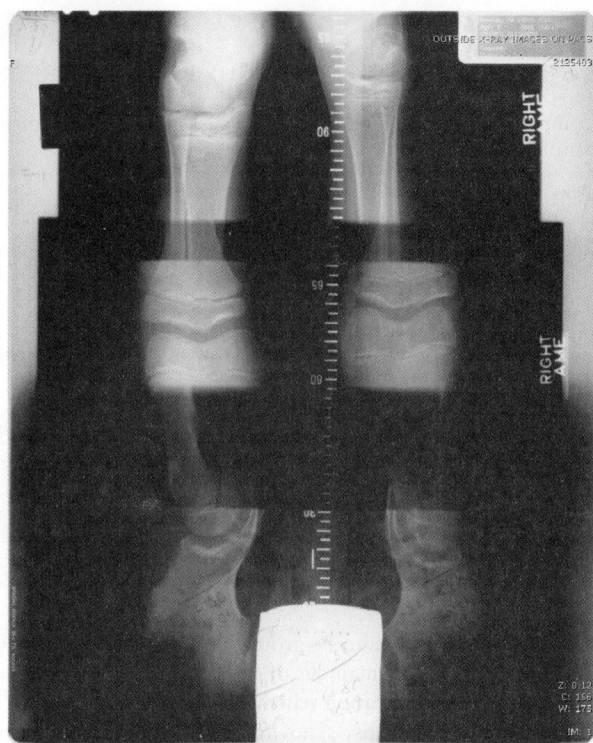

FIGURE 101.3 Radiograph showing features of juvenile rheumatoid arthritis, including soft-tissue swelling, bony overgrowth, and periarticular osteopenia adjacent to affected joints.

The least common subtype of JRA is systemic-onset or Still disease. This subtype occurs most often in boys younger than 5 years of age, although it has been reported even in adults. Clinically, these children often present with a fever of unknown origin; they may have high spiking temperatures (39°C to 41°C) for several weeks or months. Although the child often feels stiff and does not move normally, arthritis may not be a prominent feature at the onset of the disease. Diagnosis therefore generally involves excluding infectious and malignant conditions, especially sepsis, leukemia, and neuroblastoma. A characteristic salmon-pink evanescent maculopapular rash (Fig. 101.2), diffuse lymphadenopathy, and hepatosplenomegaly may also be present in the early stages, offering clues to the diagnosis. Arthralgias and myalgias are common, and pericarditis occurs most typically in this subtype of JRA. With time, systemic features of the disease become less prominent, and polyarticular arthritis becomes the major focus of management.

Laboratory and Radiologic Features

No laboratory test is diagnostic of JRA. Rather, it is a clinical condition diagnosed on the basis of characteristic findings on history and physical examination, although some laboratory studies may be suggestive of the diagnosis. In polyarticular JRA, one subgroup shows RF in the serum; no other pediatric rheumatologic disease typically has this marker. Mild to moderate anemia is common in all subtypes, particularly the systemic type. The white blood count is often elevated, again most typically in the systemic type, in which leukemoid reactions may be seen. Platelet counts are often elevated, and urinalysis is usually normal. There is elevation of levels of acute-phase reactants in the serum, often in proportion to the number of joints involved, and most prominently in systemic-onset disease. Complement levels may be normal or elevated, but immunoglobulins are typically increased, leading to a reversal of the albumin:globulin ratio.

Radiographic features of JRA include soft-tissue swelling and periarticular osteopenia adjacent to affected joints (Fig. 101.3). Later, narrowing of the joint spaces, bony cysts, erosions, subluxations, and ankylosis may be seen. In rare children in whom physical examination is difficult or inconclusive, ultrasonography may confirm the presence of a joint effusion, and magnetic resonance imaging (MRI) with gadolinium enhancement may show both synovial proliferation and increased fluid in the joint space.

Management

General Management

The major goal of therapy in children with JRA is to help both the child and the family maintain as normal a life as possible.

Emotional support, including the information that most children with this disease are able to lead a normal life with few long-term problems, provides reassurance. Simple measures, such as warm tub baths and the use of electric blankets at night, help control morning stiffness. For children with minimal joint involvement, regular daily activities, including participation in physical education classes, are to be encouraged, although direct impact on inflamed joints should be avoided. In the presence of muscle wasting, weakness, or restricted range of motion in any joint, an active physical therapy program is indicated. Splinting may be used to rest actively inflamed, painful joints and to prevent worsening of deformities, though complete disuse should be avoided in order to minimize atrophy and loss of motion.

Medications. The pharmacologic management of JRA has changed dramatically over the past two decades due both to therapeutic advances and improved understanding of the natural history of synovitis. Contrary to old teachings, children do not tend to "outgrow" JRA. Rather, in the absence of therapy, most children continue to have active synovial inflammation for decades, often leading to disruption of normal growth and compromised functioning of involved joints. Accordingly, modern therapy aims not only for relief of symptoms of pain and stiffness, but also for joint protection through suppression of synovial inflammation. Although the regimen necessary for disease control varies from child to child, the trend is for more children to receive a broader spectrum of medications. Consequently, physicians caring for these children must be familiar with the intended and unintended effects of a wide variety of drugs.

Nonsteroidal antiinflammatory drugs (NSAIDs) are the initial agents used in most children with JRA. Aspirin, formerly the preferred agent, has fallen into disfavor because of concerns about Reye syndrome and the need for doses every 4 to 6 hours. Other NSAIDs that are approved for use in children include naproxen, ibuprofen, tolmetin sodium, and meloxicam (Table 101.3). COX-2 inhibitors such as celecoxib are antiinflammatory drugs that are specific for the inducible isotype of the cyclooxygenase enzyme. This specificity results in fewer gastrointestinal (GI) side effects than traditional mixed COX-1 and COX-2 inhibitors. One long-acting COX-2 inhibitor, rofecoxib, was withdrawn from the market in 2004 after it was associated with an increased relative risk of cardiovascular events in middle-aged men. No such effect has been seen in children, however, and in fact celecoxib was approved by the FDA in 2006 for use in JRA patients age 2 years and older. This medication should be avoided in children sensitive to sulfonamides, in whom it may precipitate Stevens-Johnson syndrome.

For children who respond inadequately to NSAIDs, so-called disease-modifying antirheumatic drugs (DMARDs) must be added to control symptoms and prevent long-term complications of the arthritis. Several agents are available, including sulfasalazine, hydroxychloroquine, leflunomide, and methotrexate (Table 101.4). Practitioners choose among these agents based on a child's age, the severity of the synovitis, and the subtype of arthritis. Sulfasalazine is most often used in children with inflammatory bowel disease and spondyloarthropathies, but it also has a role in milder cases of JRA. It is typically administered 40 to 70 mg per kg per day divided in two or three doses. Neither sulfasalazine nor hydroxychloroquine, an antimalarial agent with mild immunomodulatory effects, can prevent joint damage in aggressive disease. Doses of hydroxychloroquine should never exceed 7 mg per kg per day, in order to minimize the risk of potentially irreversible ocular toxicity.

Methotrexate is the most commonly used second-line agent in JRA, and the first shown to prevent erosive changes. Doses of 0.5 to 1.0 mg per kg given once per week are usually employed in arthritis. This is several orders of magnitude lower than chemotherapeutic doses, so most of the toxicity generally associated with this agent in patients with cancer is not seen in children with JRA. Leflunomide inhibits de novo pyramidine synthesis, especially in activated lymphocytes. It is taken as a 10- or 20-mg tablet once daily. The side effects of

TABLE 101.3

NSAIDs USED IN THE TREATMENT OF ARTHRITIS IN CHILDREN

Drug	Doses/day	Dose (mg/kg/day)	Side effects
Ibuprofen (Motrin, Advil, Pediaprofen)	3–4	30–40 (maximum 2,400 mg/day)	Gastric irritation, chemical hepatitis
Naproxen (Naprosyn, Aleve)	2	10–20 (maximum 1,000 mg/day)	Gastric irritation, behavioral changes, headache, photosensitivity
Meloxicam (Mobic)	1	0.25 (maximum 15 mg/day)	Gastric irritation, headache, fever
Indomethacin (Indocin)	3	1.5–3 (maximum 200 mg/day)	Gastric irritation, headache, chemical hepatitis
Celecoxib (Celebrex)	2	10–25 kg: 50 mg/dose (maximum 100 mg/day) >25 kg: 100 mg/dose (maximum 200 mg/day) >40 kg: 200 mg/dose (maximum 400 mg/day)	Gastric irritation, cough, rash (including Stevens-Johnson syndrome)

NSAIDs, nonsteroidal antiinflammatory drugs.

TABLE 101.4

DMARDs USED IN THE TREATMENT OF JRA

Drug	Dosing schedule	Dose	Side effects
Methotrexate	Weekly	10–15 mg/m^2 (maximum 25 mg/wk)	Nausea, hair loss, chemical hepatitis, hypersensitivity, pneumonitis
Leflunomide	Once a day	<20 kg: 5 mg >20 kg: 10 mg (maximum 20 mg/day)	Nausea, diarrhea, chemical hepatitis
Sulfasalazine	Twice a day	30–50 mg/kg/day (maximum 3 g/day)	Gastric irritation, photosensitivity, behavioral changes, hypersensitivity reaction, neutropenia
Hydroxychloroquine	Once a day	<7 mg/kg/day (maximum 400 mg/day)	Abdominal pain, diarrhea, retinitis

DMARDs, disease-modifying antirheumatic drugs; JRA, juvenile rheumatoid arthritis.

leflunomide are similar to those of methotrexate. It is teratogenic, and in view of the prolonged half-life of its active metabolite, women of childbearing age should allow sufficient washout time (potentially up to 2 years) before conceiving.

The newest agents in the arthritis armamentarium are the biologic response modifiers, medications that specifically target inflammatory cytokines, cellular receptors, and adhesion molecules, but which are generally more immunosuppressive than conventional DMARDs. The most widely used biologic agents are TNF inhibitors. Etanercept, a TNF-receptor fusion protein, was the first biologic approved for the treatment of JRA, particularly polyarticular disease inadequately controlled with methotrexate. The route of administration is via subcutaneous injection once per week or in two divided doses, depending on the size of the child. The most common side effects reported with etanercept are generally mild, including injection site reactions, upper respiratory tract infections, and abdominal complaints. Adalimumab, an anti-TNF monoclonal antibody, has also been approved for use in JRA. This, too, is given by subcutaneous injection, generally every 1 to 2 weeks. Infliximab is a third TNF inhibitor, a chimeric mouse–human monoclonal antibody. While it is not FDA approved in JRA, it is used widely in children. Infliximab is administered via intravenous (IV) infusion rather than fixed-dose injection so the potential dosing range is broader, but it carries the risk of infusion reactions. Additional anti-TNF monoclonals currently undergoing review include certolizumab, a pegylated antibody, and golimumab. Both were recently approved by the FDA for treatment of adult RA.

Newer biologic response modifiers target other components of the immune response. Abatacept is a fusion protein consisting of the extracellular domain of cytotoxic T lymphocyte–associated antigen 4 linked to the Fc portion of human IgG1 (CTLA4-Ig). It is a costimulatory inhibitor that interferes with T-cell activation. Abatacept has been FDA approved for use in polyarticular JRA patients age 6 years and older. Rituximab, a B cell–depleting agent, is approved for use in adult RA, though data concerning a potential role in JRA are minimal. With all of these agents, major concerns involve an increased risk of developing infection, as well as a possibility of increased risk of malignancy. Abatacept may also pose particular risk for patients with chronic obstructive pulmonary disease (COPD), while adults receiving rituximab rarely have developed pro-gressive multifocal leukoencephalopathy, an invariably fatal slow viral infection of the central nervous system (CNS).

Corticosteroids must be employed judiciously in JRA due to the significant toxicity associated with their use. Systemic steroids are typically reserved for children with severe systemic symptoms, pericarditis, or pleuritis, during brief flare-ups of severe arthritis, or while waiting for slower-acting agents to take effect. Topical steroids are also effective for localized manifestations of JRA. Intraarticular steroids may be used in patients with pauciarthritis, or in children with polyarticular disease in whom selected joints require particularly aggressive management. Ocular steroids are the lynchpin of therapy for iridocyclitis.

Drug Toxicity. Almost all drugs used for the treatment of JRA have the potential for serious toxicity. If a child with JRA on treatment develops a new symptom, drug toxicity must always be considered as a possible cause. Tables 101.3 and 101.4 list the common adverse reactions reported with NSAIDs and DMARDs typically used in the treatment of JRA. Though new medications are more targeted in their effects on the immune system, most advanced therapies for arthritis cause at least a mild degree of immunosuppression. Accordingly, physicians caring for children with JRA should be particularly vigilant for evidence of infections.

For the nonsteroidal antiinflammatory agents, GI toxicity is the most common side effect. Nonetheless, significant NSAID gastropathy is unusual in children, and gastric or intestinal perforations, a significant problem in older adults, are rare. Antacids and H$_2$-blockers do not reduce the risk of GI complications. They may actually delay diagnosis of gastritis or ulceration by ameliorating symptoms. Prostanoids, on the other hand, do provide a degree of gastroprotection for children on NSAIDs, and the COX-2–specific agent celecoxib also appears to carry less risk of GI toxicity.

NSAIDs may also cause various other side effects. Reversible CNS complaints, particularly headaches, dizziness, and fatigue, occur in about 5% of children. Hepatotoxicity, manifested primarily as elevation of transaminases, and nephrotoxicity, including proteinuria and renal papillary necrosis, are rare but potentially dangerous if overlooked. Friability of the skin and a porphyria-like blistering of sun-exposed areas may be seen with these agents, especially naproxen when used in fair-skinned children.

Unlike salicylates, NSAIDs rarely cause tinnitus or hyperventilation. Reye syndrome, although far less common than with salicylates, has been reported in children receiving NSAIDs; therefore, it is prudent to consider suspension of these agents in children with influenza or varicella. Salicylates must be carefully avoided in children who are even exposed to these viruses. In any child using salicylates or other NSAIDs, development of pernicious vomiting and/or alteration in mental status warrants consideration of Reye syndrome.

Each of the second-line agents used in the treatment of JRA also has the potential to cause specific forms of toxicity. As methotrexate is now the most commonly used advanced medication for JRA, questions of potential side effects are most likely to involve this drug. Doses used for JRA are much lower than those employed for treating malignancies, typically 0.3 to 1 mg per kg per week, and the degree of immunosuppression appears to be minimal. Live viral vaccines are nonetheless generally avoided in children receiving methotrexate, but reported cases of opportunistic or unusually severe infections are rare.

Despite its favorable therapeutic profile, methotrexate is an antimetabolite with the potential to cause oral ulcers, nausea, and abdominal pain. These adverse effects may be minimized by supplementation with folic acid. Children must be monitored regularly for evidence of hepatic toxicity; persistent elevation of hepatic transaminases identifies those at risk for hepatic fibrosis or cirrhosis. Methotrexate may also cause lymphopenia, especially with prolonged use, or even pancytopenia due to bone marrow suppression. Ten percent of children receiving methotrexate for arthritis may develop mild hypogammaglobulinemia, but there is no evidence that this is clinically significant. Concurrent use of other dihydrofolate reductase inhibitors, such as trimethoprim–sulfamethoxazole (Bactrim®), potentiates these risks and should be avoided.

Rarely, use of methotrexate is associated with the development of pulmonary hypersensitivity. This most commonly occurs during the first 6 to 12 months of use and may be marked by dyspnea, cough, fever, and fluffy infiltrates on chest x-ray. Although such symptoms may be conclusively distinguished from viral pneumonitis only by lung biopsy, suspicion of this complication necessitates discontinuation of methotrexate and institution of treatment with systemic corticosteroids. Failure to stop the drug, or rechallenge with methotrexate, may cause fatal respiratory failure.

The newest pharmaceuticals used to treat arthritis are the biologic response modifiers. Agents of this class are generally well tolerated, but as with all medications that target the immune response as a way of controlling inflammation, biologics are immunosuppressive. Although these effects are more limited than those of traditional cytotoxic agents, defenses against various infections are definitely impaired. The infectious risk appears to increase significantly with use of more than one biologic agent at a time, so use of combinations of biologics should be avoided. Although most people note only an increased frequency of mild upper respiratory tract illnesses, treatment with TNF inhibitors also increases susceptibility to potentially serious mycobacterial, bacterial, fungal, and herpes viral infections. Patients should therefore be screened with a purified protein derivative (PPD) before initiating anti-TNF therapies. Screening for histoplasmosis in endemic areas is also recommended. Doses of TNF inhibitors should be withheld during febrile illnesses. In addition, as with methotrexate, live viral vaccines are generally avoided while children are receiving biologic agents.

MedWatch screening suggests that use of TNF-inhibitors increases the risk of developing malignancies, and they now carry a black box warning to this effect. Current FDA mandated postmarketing surveillance programs should provide more precise information concerning infectious and malignant risks of these agents within the next few years.

The long-term effects of altering the immune response with anti-TNF medications are not known. In adults, new autoantibodies may develop [including ANA and anti–double-stranded DNA (anti-ds DNA)], and rarely patients may develop multiple sclerosis–like CNS abnormalities. These associations should be kept in mind if a patient on anti-TNF therapy develops new neurologic or rheumatologic complaints.

Sulfasalazine is a sulfa drug, and its most severe side effects are typical of this class of medications. Headache and GI upset—especially with preparations that are not enterically coated—occur most commonly. Although rare, more concerning are bone marrow suppression, agranulocytosis, photosensitive eruptions, and hypersensitivity reactions, including Stevens-Johnson syndrome. Sulfasalazine is contraindicated in children with known intolerance of sulfa drugs, as well as in children younger than 2 years of age, in whom neurotoxicity may occur.

Antimalarial agents such as hydroxychloroquine must be administered judiciously because of their ability to cause irreversible ocular toxicity at high doses. Even at lower doses, children may develop rashes, gastric upset, or reversible visual disturbances secondary to altered accommodation. Finally, children with glucose-6-phosphate deficiency who receive hydroxychloroquine may develop hemolytic anemia, especially during intercurrent infections.

The long list of potential side effects of systemic corticosteroids is enumerated elsewhere. In the acute setting, immunosuppressive effects of systemic steroids are most salient. It is important to remember that these agents dramatically increase susceptibility to herpes viruses (especially disseminated varicella) and intracellular pathogens, such as mycobacteria and listeria. Although they have little effect on susceptibility to other bacterial pathogens, their antiinflammatory effects tend to mask clinical signs of infection, accentuating the need for attentiveness on the part of clinicians.

Various other agents are rarely used in the United States, although occasional patients receiving intramuscular or oral gold, or D-penicillamine, may present for evaluation. The major side effects from gold compounds are skin rash, bone marrow suppression with cytopenias, and proteinuria. D-penicillamine may cause skin rash, bone marrow suppression, nephrotoxicity, myasthenia gravis, and Goodpasture syndrome. In view of their low benefit-to-risk ratios and prolonged duration of action, these agents should be discontinued whenever toxicity is suspected. If subsequent investigations identify another explanation for an apparent drug reaction, the drug may be restarted.

Management of Complications and Emergencies (Table 101.4)

Fever. Marked elevation of body temperature is characteristic of systemic JRA, whereas a lower-grade fever often accompanies polyarticular disease. The diagnosis of systemic JRA is one of exclusion and fever is a common symptom, so diligent efforts should be made to rule out infectious diseases and malignancies. This may require hospitalization for a diagnostic evaluation, particularly in infants and young children. Appropriate cultures should be obtained, including cultures of cerebrospinal fluid (CSF) if indicated. A bone marrow examination to rule out malignancy is necessary in many patients with systemic JRA because acute lymphoblastic leukemia may cause joint pain and swelling, fever, lymphadenopathy, and hepatosplenomegaly that are indistinguishable from findings in JRA.

In a patient being treated for known systemic JRA, the appearance of fever is always of concern. Fever may represent recurrence of JRA, or it may be because of an intercurrent infection. Fevers in Still disease typically follow the classic double quotidian pattern, with two peaks above 39°C daily, as well as periods at or below normal without use of antipyretic medications. If there are no localizing signs of infection, if the complete blood cell (CBC) count shows the leukocytosis, thrombocytosis, and anemia typical of JRA, and if the urinalysis is normal, the child may be treated for a presumed JRA flare-up. On the other hand, a child with evidence of a specific infection (e.g., otitis media or urinary tract infection), should receive appropriate antibiotics. Children being treated with immunosuppressive medications may require empiric antibiotics or observation in the hospital until negative culture results allow infections to be excluded. If the patient has received more than 20 mg of prednisone daily for more than 6 weeks within the previous 12 months, appropriate coverage with stress dosages of steroids (three times the physiologic dose) is indicated while the infection is being treated.

Fever in systemic JRA, especially within 6 months of disease onset, occasionally may be caused by macrophage activation syndrome (MAS). This life-threatening complication is characterized by disseminated intravascular coagulopathy with diffuse microthromboses, hemophagocytosis causing cytopenias, hepatic inflammation, and CNS changes progressing to seizures or coma. The cause of MAS is unknown, but it does occur more commonly during intercurrent viral illnesses, as well as in children receiving NSAIDs or DMARDs (particularly sulfasalazine) as treatment. Differentiation from sepsis or a flare-up of JRA may be difficult, although a sudden rise in hepatic enzymes, ferritin, and triglycerides or a sudden drop in platelets, red blood cells, or erythrocyte sedimentation rate (ESR) (due to consumption of cellular elements and fibrinogen) are suggestive. Early diagnosis and a high level of suspicion are essential. Treatment with pulse-dose methylprednisolone (30 mg per kg, maximum 1.5 g) and/or cyclosporine, as well as general support measures for disseminated intravascular coagulation (DIC), often lead to full recovery. Delayed diagnosis, in contrast, is accompanied by a reported mortality rate of 20% to 50%.

Pericarditis, Myocarditis, and Cardiac Tamponade. Cardiac involvement is an important feature of systemic-onset JRA but is uncommon in other subtypes of juvenile arthritis. Pericarditis, like other systemic manifestations of Still disease, most often occurs during the first 2 years of the illness. Common symptoms are fever, chest pain, dyspnea, and inability to lie flat in bed, although at times pericardial effusions may be asymptomatic. On physical examination, a parasternal

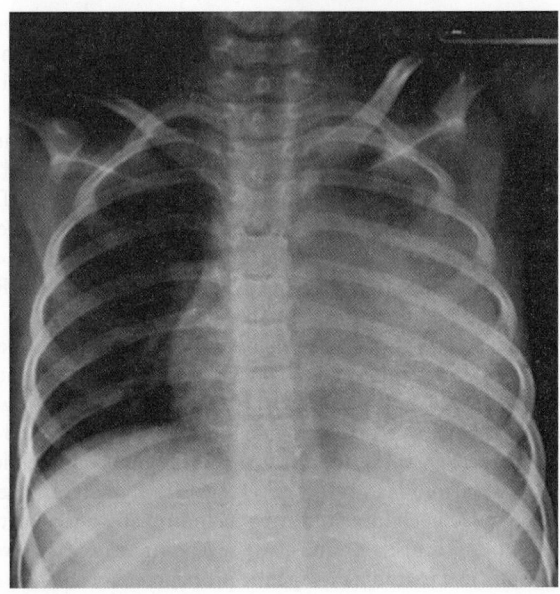

FIGURE 101.4 Pericardial and pleural effusions in a child with systemic type of juvenile rheumatoid arthritis.

pericardial friction rub may be heard over the left second and third intercostal spaces, especially with the patient supine. If the child has a moderate to large effusion (Fig. 101.4), one may not hear the friction rub but should look for the following signs of pericardial fluid: edema, tachycardia, weak pulse, distended neck veins, distant heart sounds, palpation of the apical impulse within the border of cardiac dullness, and hepatomegaly. Occasionally, the effusion may be massive, as suggested by a pulsus paradoxus of more than 20 mm Hg. Fortunately, pericardial effusions in JRA rarely lead to cardiac tamponade.

Other types of cardiac involvement are unusual. Valvulitis is not typical of JRA and should suggest the possibility of acute rheumatic fever or bacterial endocarditis. Myocarditis is rare but may be seen. Tachycardia out of proportion to the elevation of temperature, arrhythmias, and congestive heart failure (CHF) are the usual clinical indicators of myocarditis.

If pericarditis or myocarditis is suspected, the child should be admitted and observed closely. Diagnostic studies should include electrocardiogram (EKG), chest x-ray, and echocardiogram. Typical EKG changes that may be noted in children with pericarditis or myocarditis include tachycardia, elevated ST segment, and arrhythmias. Radiographs of the chest may show straightening of the left border of the heart and cardiac enlargement. Echocardiogram should be performed to confirm the presence of a pericardial effusion, as well as to quantify ventricular function, particularly if cardiac tamponade or myocarditis is suspected.

Bed rest and therapy with an NSAID should be adequate for the treatment of mild to moderate pericarditis due to JRA. Corticosteroids (prednisone 1 to 2 mg per kg per day, maximum 60 to 80 mg) are indicated for the treatment of noninfectious myocarditis, for massive pericarditis causing compromise of cardiac output, or if significant symptoms persist despite therapy with NSAIDs. In the presence of tamponade or progressive deterioration, pericardiocentesis provides temporary relief, whereas antiinflammatory medications are used to prevent reaccumulation of fluid. If the child is acutely ill, requiring IV fluid support, care should be taken to avoid fluid overload, and diuretics should be added to the regimen.

Pulmonary Emergencies. Pleural effusions are a recognized manifestation of systemic JRA (Fig. 101.4). Other pleuropulmonary complications include pneumonitis, diffuse interstitial disease, lymphoid bronchiolitis, and pulmonary arteritis. Occasionally, pleural fluid collections may be massive, resulting in respiratory distress. The usual clinical features of pleural effusion are chest pain, cough, and dyspnea. On physical examination, there is dullness to percussion and diminished breath sounds on auscultation over the area of fluid. Chest x-rays, including lateral decubitus views (involved side down), may be used to document the extent of the effusion. Thoracentesis is indicated for diagnostic purposes, especially to rule out infectious processes, and in severe cases, removing pleural fluid may help relieve respiratory compromise. Otherwise, treatment is aimed at the underlying disease process, primarily involving control of inflammation with NSAIDs or corticosteroids. Children with pleural effusions often require admission in order to address the overall severity of systemic features of the disease, if not to ameliorate the cardiopulmonary effects of the pleural effusion.

Iridocyclitis. Iridocyclitis (inflammation of the iris and ciliary body) occurs in approximately 10% to 20% of all children with JRA. This can be of acute or chronic onset. The chronic type of iridocyclitis occurs primarily in young children with pauciarticular JRA, and it is virtually universal in girls with pauciarthritis and a positive ANA. In contrast, acute iridocyclitis occurs most often in older boys with pauciarticular disease.

The onset of chronic iridocyclitis is insidious and asymptomatic. Late signs are decreased visual acuity, unequal pupils, and band keratopathy. These reflect irreversible damage to the eye and so represent a missed opportunity for prevention. Therefore, all children with JRA, particularly those at high risk for iridocyclitis, should have a routine eye examination as soon as the diagnosis is made and at frequent (3- to 6-month) intervals thereafter. The physician in the ED may be able to recognize evidence of established iridocyclitis, such as posterior synechiae or cataracts using a +8 or +10 diopter lens in the ophthalmoscope. Early anterior chamber inflammation due to chronic uveitis, however, cannot be identified without a slit-lamp examination.

Acute iridocyclitis, in contrast, is characterized by sudden onset of redness, tearing, pain, and photophobia, and urgent management may be required to preserve vision. Consultation with an ophthalmologist is essential. The usual treatment includes topical corticosteroids and mydriatics.

Flare-up of a Single Joint in a Patient with JRA. In a patient known to have JRA and receiving antiinflammatory medication, acute swelling with pain and limitation of range of movement of a single joint raises a common management problem. Potential causes of such an acute monoarthritis include a flareup of JRA versus infectious arthritis, and careful attention to physical examination and historical features are essential to avoid misdiagnosis.

Physical findings characteristic of infection of a joint are extreme pain, tenderness, erythema, and warmth over the joint. The affected joints of JRA, while often swollen, warm, and stiff, are rarely red. There is usually pronounced splinting of an infected joint due to pain; the slightest movement may cause muscle spasm. In contrast, some range of motion is usually possible even with severely inflamed joints of JRA. If the patient is taking an immunosuppressive medication, physical findings of inflammation and/or infection may be masked.

If infection cannot be excluded with confidence, joint fluid must be aspirated, and the fluid sent for cell count, Gram stain, and culture. Synovial fluid is bacteriostatic and some fastidious organisms, such as *Kingella*, may be particularly difficult to culture, so joint fluid samples should be inoculated into blood culture bottles to optimize sensitivity. If there is any doubt about the diagnosis, it is best to also obtain a blood culture (which increases diagnostic yield, as the organisms causing septic arthritis are generally spread hematogenously) and then to initiate treatment for septic arthritis.

For the acute swelling and pain in a single joint caused by a JRA flare, resting the involved extremity for 2 to 3 days may be adequate. After infection has been excluded, local injection of the joint with a topical steroid preparation such as triamcinolone hexacetamide (1 mg per kg, maximum 40 to 60 mg) may provide rapid and sustained relief.

Ruptured Popliteal Cyst. There are six bursae around the knee joint. Of these, the gastrocnemius-semimembranosus bursa is the one that most often communicates with the synovial space. Consequently, in the presence of effusion in the knee joint, fluid may enter the bursa and produce a popliteal cyst (Baker cyst). Patients with popliteal cysts have a palpable and visible enlargement in the popliteal area, best seen while the patient is standing with knees extended.

Rupture of a popliteal cyst with drainage of fluid into the calf muscles may present as an emergency. Affected patients complain of sudden pain in the calf associated with swelling in the leg. On physical examination they have induration, erythema, warmth, and tenderness of the calf, as well as ankle edema. An effusion in the knee joint and evidence of synovial thickening are often present. Homan sign may be positive, but other signs of venous thrombosis, including palpable venous cords, dilation of collateral veins, or arterial spasm, are usually absent.

Differentiation of a ruptured popliteal cyst from thrombophlebitis may be difficult, though the latter are very rare in otherwise healthy children, and the former relatively common in children with arthritis. Elevated D-dimers and other evidence of a consumptive coagulopathy characterize venous thrombosis, while most children with systemic JRA do not have such abnormalities. Ultimately, ultrasonographic or MRI imaging may be needed to establish the diagnosis. Intraarticular administration of steroids (triamcinolone hexacetamide, 1 mg per kg) is the recommended initial treatment for a ruptured Baker cyst. If there is an inadequate response or if the syndrome is chronic, surgical excision of the cyst may be necessary.

Cervical Spine Involvement. This complication usually is seen in children with established severe polyarticular JRA. Although cervical spine involvement is known to occur in 30% to 50% of patients with JRA, subluxation of the

MEDICAL EMERGENCIES

atlantoaxial (AA) joint or the lower cervical spine are less common in children than adults. Clinical evidence of pressure on the spinal cord is seen in 23% to 65% of adults with radiologic evidence of AA subluxation. Similar figures are not available for children.

Neck stiffness that is worst in the morning is the most common symptom of cervical spine involvement in JRA. Occasionally, torticollis may be the presenting manifestation of cervical arthritis. Severe pain in the neck and referred pain over the occipital and retro-orbital areas also may occur. The pain has a dull, aching quality and is often aggravated by neck movement. On physical examination, torticollis and/or loss of lordosis of the cervical spine, as well as limitation of range or movement of the neck, are the typical findings.

Paresthesia of the fingers is the most common symptom of spinal cord compression. Weakness of the arms and legs and inability to control the bladder are other complaints that should suggest spinal cord compression. During the initial stages, exaggerated deep tendon reflexes and an extensor plantar reflex are noted. Chronic myelopathy results in muscle atrophy and loss of deep tendon reflexes. Lateral radiographs of the neck in flexion and in extension are required for complete evaluation of the cervical spine. The patient should be asked to actively and slowly flex and extend the neck to tolerance without discomfort; care should be taken not to force these movements. Tomograms and an open-mouth view of the odontoid process may be helpful. On some occasions, computed tomography (CT) or MRI may be indicated.

The distance between the anterior surface of the odontoid and the posterior surface of the anterior arch of atlas when measured in a lateral flexion film is usually 4 mm or less. In the presence of AA subluxation, this may be as wide as 10 to 12 mm (Fig. 101.5). Other radiologic abnormalities characteristic of cervical spine involvement in JRA include loss of curvature, osteoporosis, erosions and sclerosis of joints, disc space narrowing, and altered height-to-width ratio of the vertebral bodies.

Although most children with AA subluxation do not have evidence of spinal cord compression, the physician must be wary of its occurrence with excessive movement, as occurs during endotracheal intubation. Regular use of a light plastic cervical collar is often all that is required to relieve pain and prevent excessive anterior flexion, particularly during automobile rides. In the presence of spinal cord compression with muscle weakness and atrophy, surgical stabilization may be required.

Cricoarytenoid Arthritis. The cricoarytenoid joint is a diarthroidal joint with a synovial membrane. In patients with known polyarticular JRA, cricoarytenoid arthritis rarely may lead to acute airway obstruction. Clinical features of cricoarytenoid arthritis include stridor and hoarseness. The inspiratory stridor may wax and wane, and may be present only when the patient is asleep. Some of these patients also may complain of pain in the throat while swallowing, and pain in the ears. Many of these symptoms and signs are similar to those of severe acute laryngotracheobronchitis, which at times may be excluded only by direct laryngoscopy. Redness and swelling of the arytenoid eminences may be observed in cricoarytenoid arthritis, rather than the airway inflammation of croup.

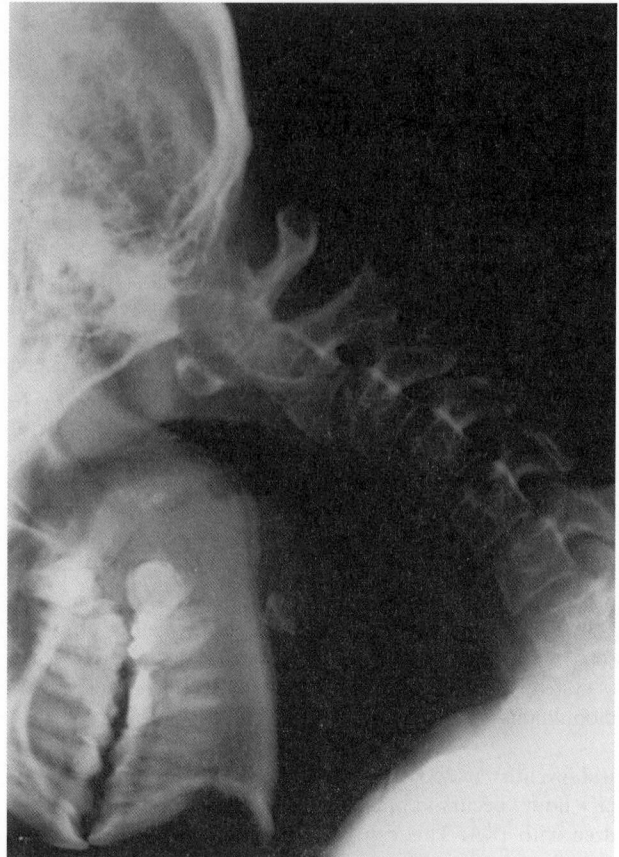

FIGURE 101.5 Atlantoaxial sublocation in a child with juvenile rheumatoid arthritis. (The distance between the anterior arch of the atlas and the odontoid process in the original radiograph was 5 mm.)

Increasing airway obstruction with severe inspiratory retractions demands urgent treatment with respiratory support. Large doses of corticosteroids (methylprednisolone, 2 mg per kg per day IV) may control acute inflammation of the joints, avoiding emergency tracheostomy. If significant obstruction occurs, intubation should be attempted to establish an airway until swelling decreases; occasionally, emergency tracheostomy may be necessary. Even if tracheostomy is done, corticosteroid therapy is indicated so the tracheostomy may be closed as quickly as possible.

SYSTEMIC LUPUS ERYTHEMATOSUS

Background

Systemic lupus erythematosus (SLE) is a multisystem disease that is both pleomorphic in its presentation and variable in its clinical course. In many ways, it is the archetypal autoimmune disease, with antibodies to cellular constituents causing immune-mediated attack on various organs. The diagnosis of SLE is based on classification criteria established by the American College of Rheumatology (ACR). The 1971 preliminary criteria were revised in 1982 to include the presence of ANA and antibodies to native DNA; in 1997, a subcommittee

TABLE 101.7

COMPLICATIONS OF SYSTEMIC LUPUS ERYTHEMATOSUS

	Symptoms and signs	Laboratory	Treatment[a]
Fever	Malaise	CBC, urinalysis, ESR, anti-DNA antibodies CH_{50}, C3 Cultures (blood, urine, CSF, stool and appropriate secretions) Chest radiograph Gallium scan	Prednisone 1–2 mg/kg/day
Infection	Fever, headache, seizure, cough, sputum, skin lesions, arthritis, disease flare, weight loss	Same as above	Intravenous antibiotics (broad spectrum) Reevaluate prednisone dose
Renal disease	Dehydration, fever, weight gain, hypertension, decreased urine output	Urinalysis, urine culture, 24-h urine protein Serum creatinine Creatinine clearance Anti-DNA CH_{50}, C3, C4 CBC, ESR, platelets Electrolytes, BUN	Prednisone "pulse therapy" (as needed) Cytotoxic agents (azathioprine PO or cyclophosphamide IV) Plasmapheresis
Hemolytic anemia	Fatigue, malaise, pallor, dyspnea, edema	CBC, Coombs', reticulocyte count, haptoglobin Peripheral smear Total bilirubin	Prednisone 2 mg/kg/day Transfusion, if acute emergency
Central nervous system	Seizures, coma, cranial nerve palsies, papilledema, hypertension psychosis	EEG, MRI, CT scan CSF—opening pressure, cell count, Gram and special stains, cultures	ICU admission Prednisone 2 mg/kg/day or pulse therapy Plasmapheresis Cytotoxic agents
Pleural effusion	Fever, chest pain, dyspnea, decreased breath sounds, splinting	Chest radiograph Thoracentesis—cell count, Gram stain, protein, glucose, culture, cytology	Thoracentesis, if indicated Oxygen, prednisone, cytotoxic agents
Peritonitis	Abdominal pain, fever, vomiting, diarrhea, tenderness, rigidity, hypoactive bowel sounds, melena	Radiograph (abdominal flat plate, cross-table, upright and/or lateral decubitus) Peritoneal aspiration—cell count, special stains, cultures CBC, electrolytes, ESR, ANA Test for occult blood in gastric contents and stool, nuclear scan	Surgical consult, NPO, IV hydration, NG tube, antacids, transfusion Prednisone Interventional radiology (if available)
Pancreatitis	Same	Serum amylase Amylase clearance ratio	IV hydration, NPO, adjust steroid dose, hyperalimentation
Pericarditis	Fever, chest pain, distended neck veins, decreased heart sounds, hepatomegaly	Chest radiograph, EKG Echocardiogram-2D CBC, ESR, blood culture, ANA	NSAIDs Perdnisone 2 mg/kg/day Pericardiocentesis as needed
Raynaud's phenomenon	Triple color change of fingers and/or toes; pain, swelling in digits	CBC, ESR, ANA, cryoglobulins Doppler flow studies	Protection from cold, biofeedback, analgesia, prednisone Calcium channel blockers Sympathetic ganglion block
Ocular	Blurring or loss of vision, headache	Funduscopic examination CT scan	Lumbar puncture (caution), prednisone
Traverse myelitis	Paraplegia, paraparesis, pain, sensory level	CT, MRI, LP (once epidural abscess excluded), antiphospholipid antibody, lupus anticoagulant	Pulse dose methylprednisolone, cytotoxic agents, anticoagulation

[a]Treatment regimens (except for infectious category) assume that an infectious etiology has been excluded. CBC, complete blood count; ESR, erythrocyte sedimentation rate; CSF, cerebrospinal fluid; BUN, blood urea nitrogen; PO, orally; IV, intravenously; EEG, encephalogram; MRI, magnetic resonance imaging; CT, computed tomography; ICU, intensive care unit; ANA, antinuclear antibody; NPO, nothing by mouth; NG, nasogastric; EKG, electrocardiogram; NSAIDs, nonsteroidal antiinflamatory drugs; LP, lumbar puncture.

given antibiotics pending culture results; abnormal splenic function places them at increased risk of rapid development of bacteremia and overwhelming sepsis.

Renal Complications. Renal disease is a major cause of morbidity in SLE, so it is important to establish its presence and severity at the time of diagnosis, and to regularly monitor renal function thereafter. Clinical manifestations of lupus nephritis are often minimal. Gross hematuria or headache resulting from hypertension may be warning signs. In the presence of nephrotic syndrome, the child may be edematous. Laboratory evidence of renal disease includes proteinuria, hematuria, hyposthenuria, casts, and elevated levels of BUN and creatinine. The presence of these findings in a patient with known SLE requires a more thorough investigation that should include estimation of the protein in a 24-hour urine collection; creatinine clearance; measurement of C3, ANA, and anti-ds DNA antibodies; as well as renal biopsy. In a patient with SLE and documented renal disease, hospitalization is necessary in the presence of rapidly worsening renal status, hypertensive crisis, or severe complications of therapy.

Treatment of renal disease is aimed at preserving renal function while minimizing medication toxicity. Selection of therapeutic agents depends on biopsy results and classification of renal involvement according to the World Health Organization classification. Active disease often may be managed with pharmacologic doses of corticosteroids (prednisone 1 to 2 mg per kg per day). In the presence of progressive renal failure, the patient should be hospitalized for more aggressive therapy. This generally includes divided doses of IV corticosteroids with or without an immunosuppressive agent such as cyclophosphamide. "Pulse" therapy with methylprednisolone (30 mg per kg in 50 mL of 5% dextrose in water, 1,500 mg maximum) may be indicated in the presence of rapidly progressive renal disease. Plasmapheresis has been used in the treatment of severe lupus nephritis, especially in patients who fail to respond to conventional therapy with corticosteroids and cytotoxic agents. Although this modality appears to have little effect on long-term outcome, acute disease flare-ups may be rapidly controlled by removing pathogenic autoantibodies, immune complexes, and cytokines. Such therapy may be associated with significant toxicity, so its use should be limited to centers experienced in the care of acutely ill children with SLE.

Hematologic Complications. Anemia is common in SLE and may have many causes. Most typically, patients have a nonspecific normocytic, normochromic anemia of chronic disease. Microcytic anemia, in contrast, may be caused by GI blood loss secondary to vasculitis or gastritis. These patients often have symptoms of GI distress and occult blood in the stool. They require further investigation, with the urgency dependent on the severity of the bleeding and the patient's overall well-being. Hemolytic anemia in SLE may be related to the disease itself (antierythrocyte antibodies) or to medications. Patients with hemolytic anemia often present with pallor, fatigue, jaundice, splenomegaly, and dark-colored urine. Occasionally, these patients develop symptoms of cardiorespiratory distress and CHF after severe hemolysis and a rapid fall in hemoglobin.

Laboratory investigation of anemia in SLE should include CBC count, reticulocyte count, and examination of the blood smear for red cell size and shape, nucleated red cells, and frag-

mented red cells. Serum levels of iron, iron-binding capacity, haptoglobin, and bilirubin may be helpful when the anemia is more severe or otherwise more concerning. The antibody responsible for autoimmune hemolytic anemia is of the "warm" variety, most commonly of the IgG type; IgM-type antibody is present in only a small percentage of cases. These red cell–bound antibodies may not be demonstrated by the standard Coombs' test, so more sensitive assays may have to be employed.

Mild to moderate anemia of any etiology may be managed using oral iron preparations and by treatment of the primary disease. Children with a hematocrit of less than 20% or compromised cardiac function often require admission to the hospital. Corticosteroids are the most effective agents for the control of autoimmune hemolytic anemia in SLE. Prednisone at 2 mg per kg per day is the initial treatment of choice.

Transfusion may be needed for children with a rapidly dropping hemoglobin concentration or CHF due to hemorrhage. In the case of hemolytic anemia, additional therapy is also mandatory to ensure that red blood cells are not lysed as rapidly as they are infused.

Leukopenia occurs in about 50% of patients with SLE. It may be caused by a reduction in granulocytes, lymphocytes, or both. Granulocytopenia may be secondary to drugs used in the treatment of SLE or less commonly to disease-related destruction of granulocytes. As with all cases of neutropenia, febrile children with absolute granulocyte counts of less than 1,000 per mm^3 are at higher risk of severe infections and should be admitted for empiric antibiotic coverage pending results of further studies.

Thrombocytopenia occurs in approximately 25% of patients with SLE; conversely, more than 5% of children presenting with ITP eventually develop SLE. The usual causes of thrombocytopenia are circulating antibodies to platelets or drug-induced bone marrow suppression. Infection should always be considered as a possible cause, so the presence of purpura and ecchymoses requires immediate investigation. Significant hemorrhage, a sudden drop in hemoglobin, and platelet counts of less than 20,000 per mm^3 are the usual indications for admission to the hospital. Studies should include CBC count, examination of the peripheral blood smear, and appropriate cultures. At times, bone marrow examination and testing of serum for antiplatelet antibodies may be helpful in determining the cause of reduced platelet counts. Patients with SLE are at risk of bleeding from any mucosal surface due to vasculitic ulceration, impaired hemostasis, thrombocytopenia, or a combination of these factors. Patients with life-threatening *epistaxis* may require local packing and platelet replacement in addition to high-dose corticosteroids. Severe *pulmonary hemorrhage* may necessitate general supportive measures such as transfusions, ventilatory assistance, and bronchial lavage. Once infections have been excluded, treatment of the underlying condition with high-dose corticosteroids, immunosuppressive agents, and/or plasmapheresis is essential. Treatment of GI hemorrhage is described in the "Gastrointestinal Complications" section.

Although less common than in systemic JRA, DIC associated with MAS may occur in SLE, with or without an associated infection. Therefore, patients with thrombocytopenia and severe bleeding should be investigated with prothrombin time, partial thromboplastin time (PTT), fibrin split products, and examination of the peripheral smear. Lupus also appears to predispose to a particularly malignant form of thrombotic thrombocytopenic purpura. Reported mortality rates are extremely high, despite general support in ICUs and aggressive treatment with pheresis and immunosuppression. Outcomes are optimal when the diagnosis is suspected early and treatment is initiated rapidly.

The presence of a circulating *lupus anticoagulant* does not lead to a bleeding diathesis unless associated with significant thrombocytopenia; on the contrary, these patients are at increased risk of deep venous or arterial thrombosis. Prolongation of PTT and chronic false-positive serologic tests for syphilis are the usual clues to the presence of these autoantibodies. Specialized studies such as mixing assays and the Russell viper venom test may confirm the diagnosis. Significant thrombosis or pulmonary embolus in a child with SLE is an indication for immediate anticoagulation with heparin, followed by oral warfarin or subcutaneous low-molecular-weight heparin, pending assays for these circulating anticoagulants.

Neurologic Complications. *Seizures* (see Chapter 69) and altered states of consciousness (see Chapters 12 and 96) are the most common manifestations of CNS involvement in SLE. Other possible causes of seizures in patients with SLE include hypertension (from the disease itself or as a complication of corticosteroid therapy), infection (meningitis, encephalitis, or abscess), and uremia. Coma is not a primary manifestation of SLE but may result from meningitis or CNS hemorrhage secondary to thrombocytopenia. Therefore, patients with SLE who develop seizures or altered states of consciousness require admission for evaluation. They should have repeated examinations with special attention to blood pressure and neurologic findings, as well as the following investigations: CBC count with differential and platelet counts, PT/PTT, electrolytes, BUN, creatinine, and urinalysis. Once space-occupying lesions have been excluded, lumbar puncture (including measurement of opening pressure) should be performed, with CSF sent for routine studies as well as special stains to look for opportunistic organisms such as fungi and acid-fast bacilli.

No study is perfectly sensitive for detecting lupus cerebritis. Measurement of the IgG index [(CSF IgG/serum IgG)/(CSF albumin/serum albumin)] may allow estimation of IgG synthesis within the blood–brain barrier. Although this is increased in various chronic infections, it also typically rises in active CNS lupus. In addition, an electroencephalogram (EEG), MRI study, and CT scan with contrast may facilitate elucidation of the cause of CNS signs in children with lupus. Patients with CNS lupus also demonstrate abnormalities on single photon emission CT scanning, but a potential role for this modality in diagnosis and management is not proven.

IV lorazepam (0.1 mg per kg) is the drug of choice for the initial management of seizures, followed by phenytoin or fosphenytoin (20 mg per kg) for maintenance of seizure control. Phenytoin is preferred over phenobarbital because the latter may alter mental status acutely. If CNS manifestations are considered secondary to active vasculitis, IV corticosteroid therapy should be initiated. In the presence of deteriorating mental function, "pulse" methylprednisolone (30 mg per kg in 50 mL of 5% dextrose in water, 1.5 g maximum), IV cyclophosphamide, or plasmapheresis may be beneficial.

Other manifestations of CNS involvement, such as psychosis, also may need inpatient evaluation. *Listeria monocytogenes* may cause indolent meningitis that is clinically indistinguishable from organic brain syndromes. Similarly, it may be difficult to determine whether psychosis is secondary to corticosteroid therapy; steroids are most likely to induce an altered sensorium in patients with underlying psychiatric disease. Clinicians should not hesitate to aggressively pursue a diagnostic evaluation, including lumbar puncture and imaging procedures, so appropriate therapy may be instituted as expeditiously as possible. When psychosis due to SLE is suspected, psychotropic drugs (e.g., haloperidol 0.025 to 0.05 mg per kg per day in divided doses) may be used along with large doses of corticosteroids for 1 to 2 weeks. If there is no improvement, the steroid dose may be reduced gradually in an attempt to rule out steroid-induced psychosis.

Transverse myelitis is a rare complication of SLE believed to result from vascular compromise of the spinal cord. Patients note acute onset of pain and weakness, and they may develop incontinence. Physical examination is remarkable for weakness or flaccid paralysis below the level of the functional transection. In a high percentage of cases, the process is associated with a circulating lupus anticoagulant or antiphospholipid antibodies. Prognosis is related to the duration of symptoms prior to initiation of therapy, and favorable outcomes are only possible with urgent intervention. Thus, once infection, epidural abscess, and hematoma are excluded with appropriate imaging procedures and lumbar puncture, pulse doses of IV methylprednisolone (30 mg per kg over 1 to 2 hours), plus anticoagulation with IV heparin, are begun. Immunosuppressive agents such as cyclophosphamide, 500 to 750 mg per m^2 IV, must be added in short order.

Pulmonary Complications. *Pleural effusion* is the most common pulmonary manifestation of SLE. However, pulmonary infections and hemorrhage present more acute management issues. Pleural effusion is often bilateral and small, although occasionally it may be massive. The child is often ill with acute manifestations of systemic disease, such as fever, fatigue, and poor appetite. Symptoms may be minimal (cough, chest pain, and mild tachypnea) or absent. Chest pain aggravated by deep breathing or coughing is suggestive of pleurisy, although pain may be absent. In the presence of a moderate or large effusion, the patient may have dyspnea and tachypnea. The presence of fluid is easily demonstrated clinically (diminished breath sounds and dullness to percussion), and radiographs of the chest establish the extent of the effusion.

If the child has a previous history of pleurisy and there are no concerns about infection, hospitalization may not be necessary. Increasing the corticosteroid dose or adding an NSAID such as indomethacin (0.5 to 2 mg per kg per day) may be adequate therapy, but arrangements must be made for close follow-up. Thoracentesis is often necessary (i) to relieve symptoms, (ii) for diagnosis, or (iii) to reveal any underlying lesions obscured by the effusion. Pleural effusions caused by SLE usually are exudative, with elevated protein levels and cell counts and decreased levels of lactic dehydrogenase. Patients with large effusions should be admitted to the hospital for further observation and management.

Pulmonary hemorrhage is a potentially catastrophic complication of SLE, particularly in the pediatric age group. Early recognition and treatment are critical. A hemorrhage may be related to the disease itself (e.g., pulmonary vasculitis), to the treatment (e.g., drug-induced thrombocytopenia), or to an infection (e.g., aspergillosis). Clinical features of patients with pulmonary hemorrhage include hemoptysis, tachypnea, tachycardia, and dyspnea; respiratory function may deteriorate rapidly if the process is not controlled.

Evaluation of patients with unexplained respiratory symptoms should include a chest x-ray. In cases of pulmonary hemorrhage, this shows fluffy infiltrates resembling pulmonary edema. CBC counts often reveal a dramatic drop in hemoglobin and a low platelet count. Diagnosis of a pulmonary hemorrhage may be confirmed by PFT, including DLCO. Intraalveolar blood increases CO absorption, making it one of the few conditions that results in an abnormally high DLCO. Bronchoalveolar lavage or lung biopsy still may be needed in some patients in whom *Pneumocystis* or *Aspergillus* infection remains a concern.

Management should include support with blood products as needed, plus high doses of IV corticosteroids. If bleeding is related to thrombocytopenia, platelet transfusion is indicated. Tracheal lavage with epinephrine, oxygen therapy, and intubation with positive end-expiratory pressure ventilation may be necessary, depending on the severity and progression of the process.

Occasionally, children with lupus may develop interstitial pneumonitis. Such patients are often ill with high fever, chest pain, cough, and dyspnea. On examination, rales may be heard throughout the chest. Radiographs show a diffuse alveolar infiltrate, unilateral or bilateral, with or without effusion. Cultures of the blood and respiratory secretions, bronchial washings, transtracheal aspirate, or lung biopsy may be necessary to exclude opportunistic infections. Supportive therapy should include increased concentrations of oxygen, adequate pulmonary toilet, and antipyretic drugs. Measures employed to control other manifestations of SLE, including corticosteroids or immunsuppressive agents, may lead to dramatic improvement once infections have been excluded.

Gastrointestinal Complications. Peritonitis and GI hemorrhage are emergencies associated with SLE. Drug-induced gastric ulcer and pancreatitis also occur. Often it is difficult to determine the nature of an intraabdominal catastrophe. Plain radiographs of the abdomen, ultrasonogram, MRI, CT scanning, peritoneal aspiration, and rarely even exploration, may be required to distinguish between possible etiologies.

Peritonitis may be a feature of the disease itself (serosal inflammation) or may be caused by secondary infection or visceral perforation. Patients with SLE and peritonitis should be admitted to the hospital at once. Symptoms and signs associated with peritonitis are pain in the abdomen, fever, vomiting, diarrhea, abdominal distension, diffuse tenderness, rigidity of the anterior abdominal wall, and hypoactive or absent bowel sounds on auscultation. It is important to remember, however, that these findings of peritoneal irritation may be masked by corticosteroid therapy.

A radiograph of the abdomen may show dilatation of intestinal loops with edema of the wall of the intestines, free air in the peritoneal cavity, or evidence of ileus or obstruction. Aspiration of the peritoneal fluid under strict aseptic conditions is essential if the cause of the peritoneal effusion is in doubt. The fluid should be sent for Gram stain and culture. Cell counts higher than 300 per mm^3 should be considered indicative of infection. Peritonitis secondary to GI perforation should be treated aggressively with surgery and IV antibiotics. Peritonitis due to serositis, a feature of SLE, may be treated with one of the NSAIDs; corticosteroids may be added if there is an inadequate response to the antiinflammatory medication or if there is additional evidence of active systemic disease. Prolonged use of both NSAIDs and corticosteroids should be avoided, however, as it increases the risk of GI irritation and/or ulceration.

An *acute abdomen* in SLE may be the result of bowel ischemia, infarction, or perforation, in addition to the occasional unrelated occurrence of intussusception or appendicitis. Symptoms of an acute abdomen include sudden onset of abdominal pain, vomiting, and diarrhea that may be bloody, although corticosteroids may obscure all signs and symptoms. The patient may go into shock rapidly. There is often localized abdominal tenderness, guarding, and rigidity with absent bowel sounds. Rectal examination should be performed to localize tenderness, palpate any masses, and obtain stool for occult blood testing. The patient should be well hydrated and shock promptly treated in an intensive care setting. A CBC count, serum electrolytes, and serum amylase determination should be obtained at once. A plain radiograph of the abdomen may show air–fluid levels or free air under the diaphragm. Abdominal ultrasound or CT may allow greater diagnostic precision. Paracentesis may help rule out infection or hemorrhage. Gram stain and culture of peritoneal fluid, in addition to blood culture, should be obtained immediately. Infection should be treated aggressively, and the ischemic or perforated area of intestine surgically repaired.

Pancreatitis must be considered in children with SLE and abdominal symptoms. SLE is the most common medical cause of *pancreatitis* in children, and corticosteroids are the medication most often associated with this complication. Whether pancreatitis is truly caused by steroids or merely tends to occur in sick patients receiving steroids for the underlying disease is not entirely clear; recent evidence supports the latter possibility. Accordingly, if the serum amylase is normal and pancreatitis is suspected, one should obtain an amylase clearance. An amylase/creatinine clearance ratio of greater than 5 suggests pancreatitis. In most cases it is prudent to assume that pancreatitis is secondary to active SLE and to increase immunosuppression in order to treat it. Recovery may be protracted, during which time the patient may have to be maintained on parenteral hyperalimentation.

GI hemorrhage may be secondary to NSAIDs (stomach), vasculitis of the GI tract (small intestines), or thrombocytopenia. Symptoms include abdominal pain, hematemesis, and melena if the bleeding is in the upper GI tract, and abdominal pain with hematochezia or occult blood in the stool if bleeding is from the lower GI tract. The patient may develop massive bleeding leading to shock. Immediate studies to be obtained in the ED include hematocrit, CBC count, serum electrolytes, and blood type and cross-match. Stool obtained by rectal examination should be tested for occult blood, even if the stool appears frankly bloody. If bleeding from a gastric ulcer is suspected, endoscopy can confirm the diagnosis. Therapy for a bleeding gastric ulcer includes volume replacement, hourly antacid administration, and H$_2$-blockers (e.g., cimetidine 20 to 40 mg per kg per day, maximum 1,200 mg per day).

If active bleeding due to vasculitis is suspected, celiac axis angiography or endoscopy with deep intestinal biopsies is required for confirmation. GI vasculitis is rare in pediatric lupus, but when it develops, it most commonly occurs in the setting of chronically active disease. Children typically have an associated peripheral neuropathy, as well as chronic weight loss, anorexia, and inanition.

Cardiac Complications. Pericarditis and myocarditis are two of the important cardiac complications of SLE that may require emergency care. The features of lupus *pericarditis* are similar to those described in JRA and include chest pain, dyspnea, inability to lie flat, and pericardial friction rub. In the presence of cardiac tamponade, additional signs supervene (weak pulse, distended neck veins, distant heart sounds, and pulsus paradoxus of more than 20 mm Hg). Pericarditis without significant hemodynamic effects may be managed with NSAIDs or corticosteroids. Massive effusion leading to tamponade requires pericardiocentesis, in addition to treatment with corticosteroids, which may be injected directly into the pericardium at the time of pericardiocentesis.

Myocarditis is characterized by resting tachycardia out of proportion to fever, cardiomegaly without an effusion, CHF, ST-T wave changes on EKG, and arrhythmias. Infarction of papillary muscles or damage to aortic or mitral leaflets may lead to rapid development of valvular insufficiency. These patients should be on strict bed rest with monitoring. In addition to treatment of the basic disease, digoxin and diuretic therapy are often indicated.

Raynaud Phenomenon. Raynaud phenomenon (RP) is characterized by triphasic color changes of the extremities upon exposure to cold. These color changes proceed from cyanosis to blanching due to microcirculatory compromise, and resolve with erythema caused by reactive hyperemia. Severe episodes of RP may cause excruciating pain in the extremities, or even digital ulceration and autoamputation. Poor circulation impairs wound healing and clearing of infections, so patients with paronychia or digital cellulitis in the setting of acral ischemia may require admission for IV antibiotics.

Prophylactic techniques to improve digital circulation (avoidance of cold exposure, biofeedback) are the cornerstones of treatment of RP. Calcium-channel blockers (e.g., slow-release nifedipine, 30 to 180 mg daily) may decrease the frequency and severity of attacks, whereas oral (e.g., prazosin, sildenafil) and topical (e.g., nitroglycerine) vasodilators or medical or surgical sympathetic blockade may be necessary during severe episodes. Cases of impending gangrene may also be treated with prostacylin analogs such as Iloprost. These medications may cause dramatic vasodilation and result in pulmonary edema or cardiac arrythmias; therefore, they should only be used by experienced clinicians.

Hypertension. Hypertension may be a result of effects of SLE on systemic vasculature, a concomitant of renal involvement, or secondary to steroid therapy. Mild to moderate hypertension is usually controlled by combinations of diuretics, vasodilators, and α- or β-blockers, whereas angiotensin-converting enzyme (ACE) inhibitors are effective for renovascular hypertension. Hypertensive encephalopathy requires emergency therapy with nitroprusside, diazoxide, calcium-channel blockers, or other potent, rapidly acting agents.

Headaches. Up to 80% of patients with SLE develop headaches, many migrainous, and they may experience acute, incapacitating exacerbations. Meningitis (both septic and aseptic), hypertension, and pseudotumor cerebri must be ruled out in children with severe headaches. They should have appropriate investigations including an exhaustive neurologic evaluation and examination of the CSF once a space-occupying lesion has been excluded. If the headache is accompanied by blurring or loss of vision, an ophthalmologic consultation should be obtained to exclude other complications such as retinal vasculitis or retinal vascular occlusion. Gradual periodic release of CSF pressure is the immediate treatment of choice for pseudotumor cerebri. High-dose corticosteroid therapy should be added if the intracranial hypertension is believed to be because of SLE, whereas it should be tapered if the pseudotumor is secondary to steroid toxicity. If other causes are excluded, a child with a severe headache may be treated for a suspected acute migraine with analgesics, antiemetics, and ergot preparations or sumatriptan (Chapter 96).

JUVENILE DERMATOMYOSITIS

Background

Juvenile dermatomyositis (JDMS) is a rare rheumatic disorder characterized by inflammation of the skin and striated muscle. The annual incidence rate is roughly 3 cases per 1 million children in the United States. Girls are more often affected than boys (~2:1), as is typical of most autoimmune conditions. The mean age of onset is estimated at 6.9 years in the United States, with almost 20% of patients diagnosed at 4 years of age or younger. Prior to the availability of steroid therapy, as many as one-third of patients died of the disease, whereas another one-third developed permanent disabilities. More recently, the introduction of more effective therapies, particularly use of potent immunomodulators earlier in the disease course, has led to improved outcomes. The mortality rate may now be as low as 1.5% in the United States, and drug- and disease-related morbidity are also improving. Despite these advances, however, JDMS remains a serious disease that requires the care of physicians experienced with its management.

As with other idiopathic rheumatic diseases of childhood, diagnosis of JDMS depends on fulfillment of clinical criteria. Bohan and Peter's criteria for dermatomyositis (DM)/polymyositis (PM) in adults are typically used for diagnosing this condition, and they are given in Table 101.8. In fact, the condition in children differs significantly from that in adults: it includes a more prominent degree of vascular inflammation, less commonly involves detectable autoantibodies, and rarely accompanies malignancies. Further, in children, the appearance on MRI is essentially diagnostic because other causes of inflamed muscle and soft tissue are not seen in this age group (Fig. 101.8). New pediatric criteria are being developed, but until they are validated, Bohan and Peter's criteria remain the gold standard for classification of children with inflammatory myopathies.

TABLE 101.8

CRITERIA FOR DIAGNOSIS OF DERMATOMYOSITIS
(DM)/POLYMYOSITIS (PM)*

1. Symmetric weakness of the proximal limb muscles and
   anterior neck flexors
2. Evidence of necrosis of type I and II fibers on muscle
   biopsy
3. Elevation of serum levels of skeletal muscle enzymes—
   creatine phosphokinase and aldolase
4. Short, small, polyphasic motor unit potentials with fibrillation; insertional irritability; and high-frequency repetitive
   discharges on electromyography
5. Skin rash—characteristic heliotrope rash, scaly erythematous rash over extensor aspects of the joints, and periungual erythema

Definite: 4 criteria (PM)
Probable: 3 criteria (PM)
Possible: 2 criteria (PM)

*N Eng J Med 1975;292:344–347

Pathophysiology

Microscopically, the skin in JDMS shows dermal atrophy,
obliteration of appendages, and lymphocytic infiltration. The
muscle typically demonstrates a mixture of degenerating and
regenerating muscle fibers, variations in muscle fiber size,
perivascular lymphocytic infiltration, and perifascicular atrophy of muscle fibers. Small arteries, venules, and capillaries of
the skin, muscle, fat, and GI tract characteristically reveal
angiopathy. Viral infections, particularly Coxsackie B, vasculitis caused by immune complex deposition, and cell-mediated
cytotoxicity against muscle fibers, have been implicated in the
pathogenesis of JDMS. Certain HLA haplotypes, especially
HLA-B8/DR3, may predispose to the disease. Synthesizing
these findings, JDMS is thought to represent an as-yet unexplained perpetuation of muscle inflammation in susceptible
hosts following what is typically a self-limited illness in most
children.

Clinical Manifestations

JDMS has a wide clinical spectrum, from a mild form involving
mainly the skin to a severe vasculitic type with a rapidly fulminating course. JDMS may be conceptualized as passing through
four overlapping phases that typically last for 2 to 5 years but
may persist indefinitely: (i) a prodromal phase of nonspecific
aches and pains, (ii) a phase of progressive muscle and skin
inflammation characterized by weakness and rash, (iii) a phase
of persistent active disease and cumulative tissue damage, and
(iv) an indolent phase with development of contractures and
calcinosis but minimal ongoing inflammation. The goal of
therapy is to compress this natural history into a shorter time
period that ends before irreversible sequelae occur.

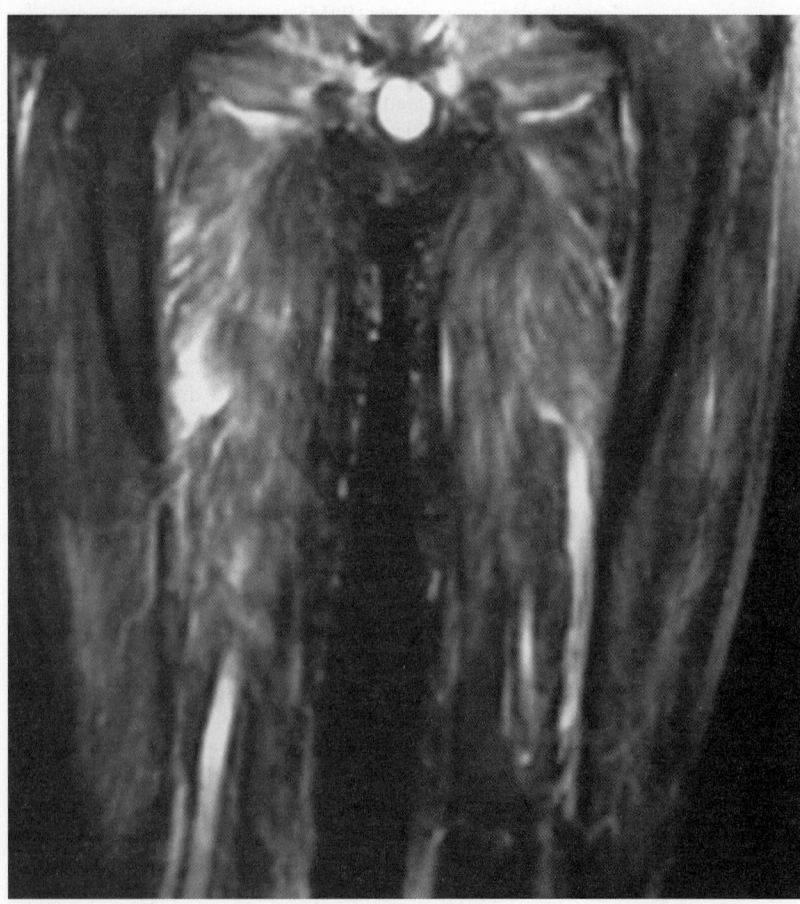

FIGURE 101.8 Coronal fast multiplanar inversion
recovery image of the thighs shows areas of
increased signal intensity, especially in the adductor
muscle groups, in a patient with dermatomyositis.

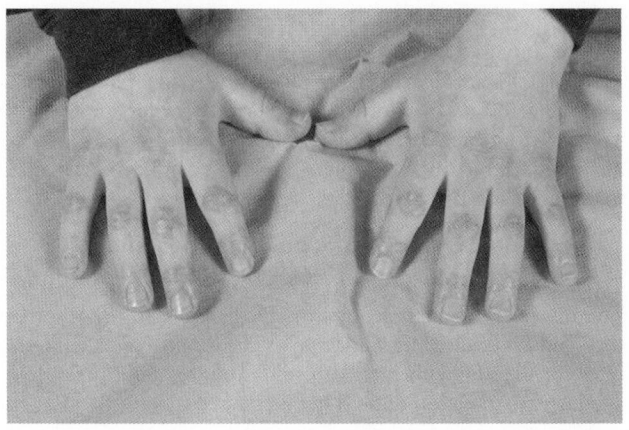

FIGURE 101.9 Gottron papules in juvenile dermatomyositis (JDMS). (Courtesy of Lisa Rider, MD.)

The onset of JDMS is often insidious, with aches and pains in the limbs, malaise, low-grade fever, and edema of the hands, feet, and eyelids. There may be a diffuse and nonspecific rash. This prodromal stage evolves into the acute phase, when the characteristic features of JDMS become evident. Classical skin manifestations include a violaceous heliotrope rash in the periorbital region and occasionally on the forehead; dusky red or atrophic lesions over the extensor aspects of the knees, elbows, and knuckles (Gottron papules); and periungual erythema (Fig. 101.9, see also color plate). Skin findings may precede or follow the onset of muscle weakness. Ulcerative skin lesions and anasarca are rare presenting manifestations of JDMS associated with a particularly severe disease course.

Muscular involvement in JDMS is characterized by pain, tenderness, and weakness of proximal muscles in a symmetric fashion. Strength of the anterior neck flexors and abdominal muscles is particularly affected, while facial muscles are spared. The disease may progress to involve the muscles of the palate and pharynx, resulting in regurgitation, nasal voice, and aspiration. Weakness of the respiratory muscles can lead to a poor cough, pneumonia, and respiratory failure. Risk of GI hemorrhage and perforation are increased at this stage and are associated with abdominal pain, hematemesis, and melena.

The clinical course of JDMS is variable. Traditionally, patterns such as "limited" or "monocyclic," with a single period of disease activity, were differentiated from a "chronic" or "polycyclic" pattern of exacerbations and remissions. It now appears that these distinctions are an artifact of inadequate therapy, however. With newer approaches to treatment, disease manifestations may be controlled within a few months in the vast majority of patients.

Children who continue to have florid or smoldering muscle inflammation for more than 6 to 12 months are at risk of developing late complications of JDMS. These include pronounced muscle wasting, contractures, lipodystrophy, and pigmentary changes of the skin. The rash over the extremities often becomes dry, scaly, and atrophic. Subcutaneous calcifications historically have occurred in up to 30% of children during this phase, although aggressive treatment of inflammation from the onset of JDMS dramatically lowers this figure. Calcifications are most typically discrete nodules around large joints, but at times they may take the form of a diffuse encasement of the soft

tissues, known as calcinosis universalis. Occasionally, children pass through the early stages insidiously and come to the attention of physicians only when they develop contractures and calcinosis.

Although skin and striated muscle are the primary targets of the inflammatory process in JDMS, typically other organ systems are also involved. Up to one-third of children develop arthritis, which may be present at diagnosis or may develop months into the disease process. The arthritis of JDMS is generally nonerosive and often improves as the primary disease is treated, although some children require specific therapy for their arthropathy. Neurologic manifestations of JDMS are extremely rare, but peripheral polyneuropathy, seizures, psychosis, and one case of suspected brainstem vasculopathy have been reported.

Laboratory Studies

Weakness is a consistent manifestation of JDMS, but it is a late, variable, and subjective clinical sign. Objective evidence of muscle inflammation should also be sought by measuring serum levels of muscle enzymes that are released into the circulation when myocytes are injured. A wide variety of enzymes may be elevated in JDMS, including creatine kinase (CK), aldolase, lactate dehydrogenase (LDH), and transaminases (ALT and AST). These markers must be interpreted with caution, however, because none is specific for muscle. Elevated levels may be derived from damage to a variety of other tissues, including hepatocytes, brain cells, and the GI tract. Further, for unknown reasons many children do not reliably demonstrate elevated muscle enzymes despite significant myositis. This is particularly true during later stages of the disease, when subtle increases in LDH and aldolase may herald a disease flare-up, but CK levels often remain normal.

Because JDMS is a microangiopathic process, active disease is also characterized by elevated levels of von Willebrand factor antigen (vWF:Ag), which is released by damaged endothelial cells. In contrast, evidence of systemic inflammation may be absent, and acute-phase markers (including ESR and CRP) and CBC counts are typically normal. In particularly difficult cases, MRI of the thighs may be the most sensitive method of documenting muscle inflammation (Fig. 101.8). Evidence of cardiac involvement should also be sought, particularly with an EKG and an echocardiogram. Serologic markers of myocardial involvement are unreliable because both the CK-MB fraction and the troponin level are elevated in JDMS due to myoblast proliferation in skeletal muscles.

Management

General Management

The sine qua non of treating JDMS is aggressively controlling muscle inflammation. The more rapidly markers of myocyte damage such as CK and aldolase can be normalized, the less the chance that acute and chronic complications will occur. During the initial evaluation of JDMS, it is essential to monitor the function of the palatopharyngeal and respiratory muscles; palatal weakness increases the risk of aspiration. Eating only in the upright position, frequent suctioning, or placement of a nasogastric tube may be necessary to avoid aspiration. Support of weak muscles, such as wearing a soft neck collar while riding in automobiles, helps minimize the risk of complications until children regain their strength.

Recognition of the importance of expeditious disease control is leading to modifications in the medical management of JDMS. Thus, virtually all children with clinical or biochemical evidence of muscle inflammation begin treatment with pulsed doses of IV methylprednisolone (30 mg per kg, maximum 1.5 g) infused over 1 to 2 hours. Oral prednisone is then started at a dose of 1 to 2 mg per kg per day. If muscle enzymes, weakness, or GI symptoms do not rapidly improve, steroid-sparing agents such as methotrexate (0.75 to 1.25 mg per kg per week), IV immune globulin (2 g per kg per month) or cyclosporine A (2 to 4 mg per kg per day) are introduced within 4 to 8 weeks. In more recalcitrant cases, it may be necessary to add imunosuppressive drugs such as cyclophosphamide (10 to 20 mg per m^2 every 2 to 4 weeks) or azathioprine (1 to 3 mg per kg per day). A potential role for biologic agents, including infliximab and rituximab, is currently the subject of multicenter studies. Parenteral administration of medications is generally preferable in order to bypass the GI tract, where absorption of orally administered medications may be impaired because of vasculitis. Plasmapheresis may be beneficial in particularly severe cases. Under all circumstances, the goal is to rapidly control disease activity while minimizing toxicity from medications. Fortunately, active disease generally does not recur if a complete remission can be induced and maintained for 1 to 2 years.

Management of Complications and Emergencies (Table 101.9)

The most serious emergencies in JDMS relate to the respiratory and GI tracts. In addition, complications may occur as a result of therapy with corticosteroids and immunosuppressive agents (e.g., infection and GI hemorrhage).

Respiratory Complications. Respiratory emergencies seen in childhood DM have diverse etiologies. Entities to be considered include (i) aspiration pneumonia secondary to weakness of velopalatine muscles; (ii) atelectasis and pneumonia secondary to difficulty in clearing secretions as respiratory muscles become involved; (iii) respiratory failure secondary to profound involvement of respiratory musculature, including the

TABLE 101.9

COMPLICATIONS OF JUVENILE DERMATOMYOSITIS

Clinical entity	Symptoms and signs	Investigations	Treatment
Respiratory failure	Air hunger, tachypnea, cyanosis, shallow respiration, alteration in mental status	Chest radiograph Arterial blood gas	Oxygen Mechanical ventilatory support Corticosteroids and immunosuppressives, plasmapheresis Antibiotics if evidence of aspiration pneumonia
Pneumothorax	Chest pain Breathlessness, tachypnea, cyanosis, diminished breath sounds, increased resonance to percussion	Chest radiograph	Chest tube
Velopalatine weakness	Pooling of secretions, drooling Nasal voice Aspiration pneumonia—recurrent	Careful barium cineradiographic study Chest radiograph	Corticosteroids Nasogastric feedings Tracheostomy
Gastrointestinal hemorrhage	Abdominal pain, nausea, vomiting Guarding, diminished bowel sounds (may be masked by corticosteroids) Hematemesis, melena, hematochezia	CBC; type and cross Abdominal radiograph: flat plate and upright Endoscopy Angiography Nuclear scan	NPO, NG tube Support of circulatory volume Antacids Corticosteroids Surgical consult Interventional radiology
Gastrointestinal perforation	May be silent (corticosteroids) or associated with abdominal pain, distension, vomiting	Abdominal radiographs: flat plate and upright	NPO, NG tube Surgical consult
Calcinosis	Swelling resembling cellulitis around large joints Fever	CBC Radiograph Aspiration	Antibiotics if superinfection suspected Pain control
Carditis	Dyspnea, tachycardia, arrhythmias	Chest radiograph EKG Echocardiogram	Digoxin, diuretics Antiarrhythmics Corticosteroids

CBC, complete blood count; NPO, nothing by mouth; NG, nasogastric; EKG, electrocardiogram.

diaphragm; (iv) progressive interstitial lung disease; and (v) opportunistic infection (tuberculosis, fungi, viruses, or *Pneumocystis*) in the immunosuppressed host.

The history should provide clues for differentiating between these possibilities. On physical examination, the child with a respiratory complication is often acutely ill with an elevated temperature. Because fever also may occur with active DM, it is necessary to differentiate pyrexia caused by infection from that caused by underlying disease. The patient with respiratory complications is often dyspneic and tachypneic, and has a weak cough with impaired production of sputum. Pooling of secretions in the mouth and a nasal voice should suggest the presence of palatal weakness. Each breath is shallow, with poor air entry on auscultation. The child cannot complete a sentence in one breath and often pauses between words. On auscultation, crackles may be heard. Cyanosis and alteration of consciousness imply impending respiratory failure.

Children with JDMS who develop respiratory problems are usually hospitalized for observation and diagnosis. Those at risk of developing respiratory failure should be cared for in an ICU. Preliminary investigations should include a CBC count, urinalysis, serum electrolytes, measurement of muscle enzymes (including CK, aldolase, AST, ALT, and LDH), and chest x-ray. Depending on the seriousness of the symptoms and the cooperativeness of the child, blood gas analysis, pulmonary function studies, and high-resolution chest CT may be obtained. These latter studies should be compared with baseline PFTs obtained previously on the same child because more than two-thirds of children with DM show restrictive disease and a diffusion abnormality.

If the etiology of the respiratory deterioration remains in doubt, more sensitive tests of disease activity, including vWF:Ag and MRI of the thigh muscles, may be necessary to determine whether more aggressive control of the underlying myositis is necessary. Corticosteroids are an essential component of the armamentarium for treating weakness of respiratory muscles and interstitial lung disease. If the weakness seems to be worsening, maximum efficacy may be obtained with pulsed-dose methylprednisolone. During this pulse therapy, blood pressure and cardiac rhythm should be monitored and the infusion stopped if there is sudden hyper- or hypotension or a rhythm disturbance. Plasmapheresis is reserved for children who deteriorate even after pulse steroid therapy. At best this provides temporary respite, so pheresis must be accompanied by institution of a long-term immunosuppressive regimen. Frequent suctioning, nasogastric feeding, and, occasionally, tracheostomy, may be necessary to avoid aspiration pneumonia. Conventional or high-frequency ventilation may be needed as supportive measures, and the use of extracorporeal membrane oxygenation (ECMO) has been reported in a particularly severe case of JDMS.

Aspiration pneumonia can be recognized on the basis of clinical and radiographic data. A chest x-ray with a severe interstitial or reticulonodular pattern may indicate progression of underlying lung disease or opportunistic infection. Lung biopsy may be helpful in such situations. If pulmonary problems are suspected to result from infection, treatment with IV antibiotics should be initiated after appropriate cultures are obtained. In addition, sufficient corticosteroids (three times physiologic need) are given to compensate for potential iatrogenic adrenal insufficiency if the child has recently received high doses of steroids.

Pneumothorax is another complication known to occur during the course of childhood DM. The usual symptoms are sudden onset of chest pain and tachypnea. Physical examination shows deviation of the trachea to the opposite side of the chest and increased resonance and diminished breath sounds on the affected side. A radiograph of the chest shows air in the pleural cavity. A chest tube should be placed and connected to underwater seal.

GI Complications. Vasculitic changes, characterized by intimal hyperplasia and arteriolar occlusion by fibrin thrombi, are characteristic of severe or poorly controlled JDMS. Arteries and veins of the skin, muscles, and GI tract may be involved. Resultant ulcerations and perforations may occur anywhere from the esophagus to the large intestine, and they may disrupt the integrity of the integument. Symptoms and signs of these complications depend on the site of the lesion. For example, bleeding from the esophagus is not common, but perforation may cause mediastinitis. In contrast, bleeding from ulceration of the stomach or duodenum typically leads to abdominal pain with vomiting and melena. If the bleeding is severe, hematemesis with a sudden drop in the hemoglobin will be the presenting manifestation. Laboratory studies to be obtained include a CBC count, electrolytes, and BUN. Endoscopy may prove useful in locating the site of bleeding. Treatment of upper intestinal hemorrhage includes support of circulatory volume and hematocrit, antacids, and H_2-blockers (e.g., cimetidine 20 to 40 mg per kg per day, maximum 1,200 mg).

Evidence of bleeding from the lower portion of the GI tract includes abdominal distension and pain, vomiting, and melena or bright red blood in the stool. The hematocrit may fall precipitously, and radiographs of the abdomen may show free air in the peritoneum. If there is active bleeding, a technetium scan to locate the area of hemorrhage is the initial step. This may be followed by an angiogram to localize the actual vessel that is bleeding. The details of the management of hemorrhage from the GI tract are discussed under SLE and in Chapters 29 and 89.

In a patient with JDMS, intestinal perforation may go unnoticed and present with pneumatosis intestinalis. This finding also may precede clinical perforation and pneumoperitoneum. Thus, any patient with JDMS and persistent abdominal pain should be examined radiographically for the presence of gas in the bowel wall. In the presence of acute perforation, usual physical findings are tenderness and guarding of the abdomen, and distant or absent bowel sounds. It should be stressed that corticosteroids may mask these physical findings. Supine and erect abdominal radiographs are indicated to demonstrate intramural gas or subdiaphragmatic air. Patients with this diagnosis require admission to the hospital and emergent surgical evaluation, although resolution with only supportive care may occur.

Calcinosis. During the period of formation of subcutaneous calcification, children with JDMS may develop high fever, chills, and one or more areas of swelling under the skin. The inflammation caused by the subcutaneous calcium deposit may be indistinguishable from that of cellulitis or abscess formation, with warmth, erythema, and tenderness. Eventually, the lesion may spontaneously extrude calcium, at which time the fever often subsides. Although this is the natural history of subcutaneous calcifications, it is often hard to exclude an infectious etiology for the swelling. If doubt exists, needle aspiration of the site may be performed and the fluid examined for calcium crystals and organisms. In the face of uncertainty, it is best to treat for infection with antibiotics until culture reports are available. Incision and drainage or surgical debridement should be avoided, as the inflamed skin rarely heals satisfactorily. Complete control of the underlying disease offers the best hope for resolution of calcinosis, although this may be incomplete or require many years.

Cardiac Emergencies. Although EKG abnormalities may be seen in up to 50% of children with JDMS, development of myocarditis is uncommon. Tachycardia out of proportion to fever may be the earliest evidence of this complication. Involvement of the conduction system by edema and fibrosis leads to electrical abnormalities and arrhythmias. All patients with myocarditis should be admitted for an evaluation that includes an EKG, chest x-ray, and echocardiogram. Supportive management includes judicious and careful use of diuretics and cardiotonic drugs while aggressively treating the primary disease.

SCLERODERMA

Background

Scleroderma, or hardening of the skin, is most commonly a process restricted to the skin and subcutaneous tissues in children. The far more serious systemic form, systemic sclerosis (SS), is also far rarer, occurring in less than 1,000 children nationwide. Various conditions are included within the category of scleroderma, as listed in Table 101.10.

Pathophysiology

The most characteristic microscopic feature of affected areas of the skin is increased thickness and density of collagen in the dermis. In addition, flattening of rete pegs, mononuclear cell infiltrate around small blood vessels, obliteration of skin appendages, and hyalinization and fibrosis of arterioles are seen.

The etiology of this disease is unknown. Increased collagen production by fibroblasts, perhaps in response to disordered immune regulation and cytokine release, appears to be a final common pathway for a clinical entity with numerous genetic and environmental triggers. Similarities between this disorder and graft-versus-host disease after bone marrow transplantation, and to chronic LD (acrodermatitis chronica atrophicans), have stimulated many areas of research. Clear understanding of the underlying abnormalities in scleroderma, however, remains elusive.

Clinical Manifestations

Localized scleroderma is more common in children than in adults. The lesions may be one of three types. *Morphea* is a focal ivory-white patch with a violaceous or erythematous rim; it is often a single lesion on the trunk, although generalized morphea also occurs in children. *Linear scleroderma* causes scarring, fibrosis, and atrophy that crosses dermatomes.

TABLE 101.10
CLASSIFICATION OF SCLERODERMA AND RELATED CONDITIONS

Systemic Sclerosis
  Scleroderma
  CREST syndrome
  Overlap connective tissue diseases
    SLE
    Mixed connective tissue disease (MCTD)
Localized scleroderma
  Morphea
  Linear (include *"en coup de sabre"*)
  Eospinophic fasciitis
Toxin-mediated conditions
  Eosinophilia-myalgia
  Polyvinyl chloride
  Toxic oil syndrome
  Pentazocine
  Bleomycin
  Graft-versus-host disease
Pseduoscleroderma
  Edematous
    Myxedema
    Scleredema
  Indurative
    Porphyria cutanea tarda
    Pheylketonuria
    Acromegaly
Atrophic
  Progeria
  Acrodermatitis chronica atrophicans

Involved skin develops a "hidebound" appearance due to tethering of the subcutaneous tissues to deeper structures. It may extend to involve an entire extremity (Fig. 101.10) and to affect underlying muscle and bone, leading to flexion contractures, leg-length discrepancies, and atrophy of an extremity. A variant affecting the forehead is called *scleroderma en coup de sabre;* this form may involve underlying skull and nervous tissue, as well as the skin. Although localized forms of scleroderma are generally not associated with internal organ involvement, one large pediatric cohort found nearly a quarter of patients to have at least one extracutaneous manifestation. In addition, though rare, progression to SS is reported. Therefore, complications related to SS should be considered if a child with localized scleroderma presents with acute clinical decompensation.

SS often presents with cutaneous changes such as RP (90% of patients), edema, induration, increased pigmentation, and tightening of the skin. Some of these children may also develop arthritis resembling JRA, muscle weakness resembling JDMS, and nodules along tendon sheaths. If these features are seen, one should consider the possibility of undifferentiated or overlap connective tissue disease, in which features of SLE, SS, JDMS, and JRA intermingle.

Serious illness and death can occur in SS. Severe, uncontrolled hypertension and rapidly progressive renal failure (scleroderma renal crisis) have been a major source of mortality, although introduction of ACE inhibitors has dramatically

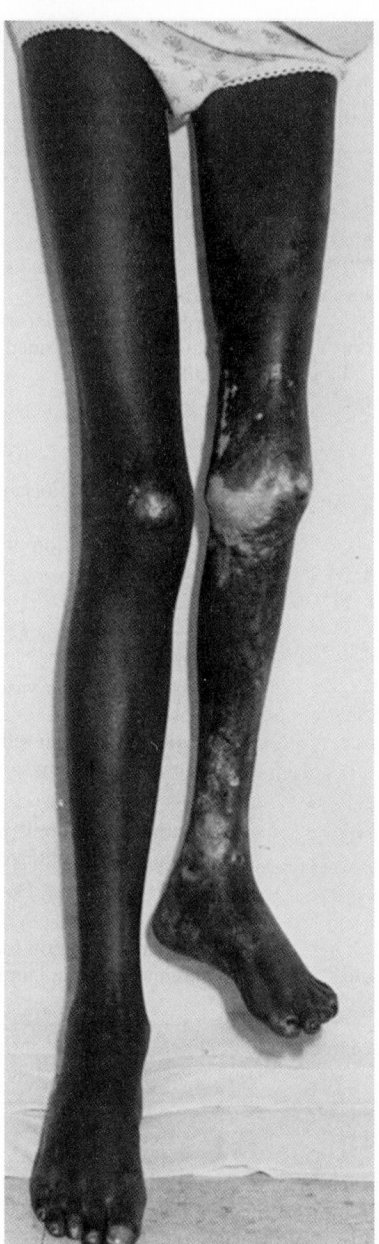

FIGURE 101.10 Linear scleroderma involving left lower extremity in a 12-year-old girl.

improved short-term survival. Primary myocardial disease with conduction disturbances, pericarditis, and intractable CHF, as well as pulmonary hypertension secondary to fibrosis, remain significant sources of morbidity and mortality. Additional complications of SS include (i) digital gangrene and nonhealing ulcers most frequently involving the fingers, elbows, and malleoli secondary to vascular occlusion; (ii) disordered motility of the distal esophagus with dysphagia and reflux esophagitis (60% of affected children); (iii) malabsorption syndrome; (iv) thrombocytopenia with subsequent cerebral hemorrhage; (v) interstitial lung disease; and (vi) cranial nerve involvement with trigeminal sensory neuropathy, facial weakness, and tinnitus.

Management

General Management

Specific therapy for SS is nonexistent at present. Virtually every medication, from antihistamines to potent immunosuppressives, has been used in patients with this disease, though none shows clear benefit. During the inflammatory, prefibrotic stages of interstitial lung disease and pulmonary vascular involvement, corticosteroids (prednisone 2 mg per kg per day or the equivalent) are indicated. Cyclophosphamide appears to forestall pulmonary fibrosis if added early to the treatment regime. If the esophageal sphincter is involved, patients should be advised to sleep with the head comfortably elevated, and an antacid may be prescribed.

Minor episodes of Raynaud syndrome are managed with prophylactic measures such as the avoidance of cold exposure and the use of warm clothing. Biofeedback training and calcium-channel blockers such as nifedipine may be helpful in decreasing the frequency of attacks. Aggressive physical therapy is indicated to prevent contractures and to maintain normal function. Despite these measures, linear scleroderma with involvement of deep structures may lead to contractures of the extremities requiring surgery. Juvenile onset SS carries an approximate 5-year mortality rate of 10%.

Management of Complications and Emergencies (Table 101.11)

Cardiac Complications. Signs and symptoms of myocardial fibrosis are essentially those of a cardiomyopathy with dyspnea, orthopnea, and fatigue. Angina pectoris and myocardial infarction also occur. Fibrosis of the conduction system may result in arrhythmias, presenting as palpitations, syncope, or sudden death. Pericarditis is usually silent and valvular involvement in scleroderma is rare. Even in the absence of symptoms or physical findings, cardiac involvement eventually develops in the majority of patients with SS, and sensitive imaging or functional studies reveal some cardiac involvement early in the course of disease in the majority of cases. Management of cardiac dysfunction is symptomatic, including inotropic support and afterload reduction. Extensive diuresis should be avoided because of potential adverse effects on renal cortical perfusion. No specific drugs are available to arrest the progress of cardiac involvement.

Pulmonary Complications. Pulmonary involvement in SS may have three manifestations: pleurisy, interstitial lung disease, or pulmonary artery fibrosis. Diffuse interstitial lung disease is often asymptomatic. A dry cough may be the first symptom. Early in the course of the disease, even before symptoms appear, pulmonary function tests in these patients show a restrictive pattern and diffusion abnormalities. Later, radiographs of the chest show increased reticulation, a so-called "honeycombed" appearance, mainly basilar and bilateral. Other diagnostic modalities, including high-resolution CT scanning, bronchoalveolar lavage, and lung biopsy, may identify earlier, prefibrotic states of disease more responsive to anti-inflammatory therapy. With progression of the disease, cough and dyspnea become prominent. On examination, crackles over both sides of the chest, particularly over the infrascapular area, may be the only finding. Development of right-sided heart

TABLE 101.11

COMPLICATIONS OF SYSTEMIC SCLEROSIS

Clinical entity	Symptoms and signs	Investigations	Treatments
Myocardial fibrosis	Exertional dyspnea, orthopnea, angina pectoris Distant heart sounds, gallop rhythm, arrhythmias	Chest radiograph EKG Echocardiogram Gated nuclear-ventricular scans	Digoxin Diuretics Antiarrhythmics
Pulmonary interstitial fibrosis	Cough, dyspnea Dry crackles Cor pulmonale	Chest radiograph, EKG Pulmonary function tests, including CO diffusion High-resolution CT, bronchoalveolar lavage Lung biopsy	Corticosteroids Oxygen, bronchodilators Treatment of right-sided heart failure
Pulmonary hypertension	Acute dyspnea Increased P_2 and widely split S_2	Chest radiograph EKG Echocardiogram Right-sided heart catheterization Lung biopsy	Corticosteroids Calcium channel blockers ACE inhibitors Direct PA installation of vasodilators
Scleroderma renal crisis	Severe headache, blurred vision, congestive heart failure, seizures Malignant hypertension, retinopathy	Electrolytes, BUN Creatinine Plasma renin activity	Captropril and other ACE inhibitors Minoxidil and other vasodilators, β-blockers Diuretics, dialysis; in refractory cases, nephrectomy
Impending gangrene	Pain, loss of sensation in distal digits Trophic changes	Cryoglobulins Doppler flow studies	Topical vasodilators Sympathetic ganglionic blockade (digital, regional), prostaglandin E_1 infusion
Esophagitis	Restrosternal pain, pyrosis, melena	CBC Barium swallow Esophageal pH probe and manometry	Antacids/cimetidine Surgical manipulation for chronic unremitting complaints

EKG, electrocardiogram; CO, carbon monoxide; CT, computed tomography; ACE, angiotensin-converting enzyme; PA, posteroanterior; BUN, blood urea nitrogen; CBC, complete blood count.

failure is heralded by increasing dyspnea, although edema of the lower extremities may not be appreciated because of hidebound skin. Patients with right-sided heart failure generally require admission and symptomatic management.

Patients with irreversible pulmonary fibrosis and chronic respiratory failure may also need admission. They have diminished respiratory reserve, so such patients must be treated promptly when they contract intercurrent respiratory infections. Supplemental oxygen, bronchodilators, and corticosteroids may be helpful. If residual inflammation is demonstrable after further investigations such as those noted previously, these patients should receive corticosteroids (prednisone 2 mg per kg per day) for 6 to 8 weeks, although the value of this therapy is doubtful in established fibrosis. In addition, treatment of right-sided overload is indicated.

Pulmonary hypertension is the most common cause of dyspnea in patients with SS. On auscultation, there is a wide or fixed splitting of the second heart sound and the pulmonic component is accentuated. The EKG shows right ventricular hypertrophy. Echocardiography and right heart catheterization may be necessary to differentiate cardiac from pulmonary

etiologies of respiratory deterioration. Corticosteroids and cyclophosphamide (50 mg per day orally or 500 to 750 mg per m² by monthly IV infusion) are the treatment of choice in patients without established interstitial fibrosis, in addition to supportive measures. Endothelin-1 receptor antagonists such as bosentan, calcium-channel blockers, ACE inhibitors, and prostaglandin analogs (e.g., epoprostenol) may provide temporary improvement in individual cases.

Renal Complications. Sclerodermatous involvement of the vessels of the kidney is the most common cause of renal failure in adults with SS. Proteinuria, hypertension, rapid progression of skin thickening early in the illness, anemia, pericardial effusion, and CHF are all markers of the patient at risk for renal scleroderma. The development of a microangiopathic hemolytic anemia suggests imminent renal failure. These complications appear to be less common in children than in adults.

Renal failure may develop gradually or acutely in a patient with known renal disease, and use of corticosteroids may precipitate its appearance. The combination of rapidly progressing azotemia with malignant hypertension (scleroderma renal crisis) requires hospitalization and urgent management. Characteristically, a patient displays a sudden rise in blood pressure to levels as high as 150 to 200 mm Hg diastolic, often with minimal or no symptoms (such as a headache). Evaluation reveals hypertensive retinopathy (flame hemorrhages, cotton wool exudates, and papilledema), elevated plasma renin activity, and rapid deterioration of renal function. Immediate investigation should include urinalysis, measurement of urine output and urinary electrolytes, serum electrolytes, BUN, creatinine, and plasma renin level.

A major advance in the pharmacologic management of scleroderma renal crisis has been the use of ACE inhibitors such as captopril. Patients who fail to respond to this drug may still respond to potent vasodilators such as minoxidil, along with β-blockers and diuretics; regimens involving multiple drugs may also be necessary (see Chapter 34). Renal dialysis and rarely bilateral nephrectomy may be indicated in hypertension unresponsive to pharmacologic therapy. Because most patients with severe scleroderma renal disease have a component of myocarditis and ventricular stiffness, maintenance of blood volume is essential to ensure adequate preload to support the circulation.

Peripheral Vascular Complications. RP can often be incapacitating, particularly in cold weather. Symptoms include severe pain in the extremities and loss of sensation in the tips of the digits. Treatment with calcium-channel antagonists such as slow-release nifedipine (30 to 180 mg daily) may decrease the frequency or severity of attacks. In urgent cases with impending gangrene, systemic or topical vasodilators (e.g., nitroglycerine paste or intraarterial reserpine) or sympathetic ganglion block may be tried, although these forms of therapy have not been validated in well-constructed studies. Excessive peripheral vasodilation may also precipitate cardiovascular collapse due to a "steal syndrome," so caution must be exercised to ensure cardiac filling pressures are maintained. Consequently, these procedures should be performed only with intensive monitoring. If gangrene has set in, it is best left alone if there is no infection. Spontaneous separation of the tips of the digits will occur and carries less risk and morbidity than surgical amputation.

GI Complications. Abnormal esophageal motility with reflux may result in esophagitis. The major symptom of this condition is retrosternal pain that is made worse by certain foods and recumbent positioning. The pain may be severe and incapacitating, and the risk of aspiration is increased. Although children with the complaint of retrosternal pain do not require admission to the hospital, they need an evaluation of their lower esophageal sphincter with esophageal manometry. Those with mild pain and objective manifestations of reflux (lower esophageal sphincter pressure of less than 10 mm Hg, evidence of esophagitis on endoscopy) are usually treated with simple measures, such as antacids 1 hour after meals and 1 hour before bedtime and elevation of the head during sleep. If symptoms are severe, H_2-blockers such as cimetidine (20 to 40 mg per kg per day, maximum daily dosage 1,200 mg) or protein pump inhibitors such as lansoprazole (15 to 30 mg once or twice daily) may be prescribed. Any patient with scleroderma who develops acute respiratory symptoms in association with reflux must be evaluated for possible aspiration pneumonia.

VASCULITIS

Although the pathologic process in vasculitis is limited to the blood vessels, the presence of vasculature in every organ of the body means that virtually any symptom could be a presentation of vasculitis. Vascular inflammation and damage can lead to anything from numbness to pain, thrombosis to bleeding, aneurysm formation to vascular obstruction. Pediatric vasculitides are very rare, however, so this section will be limited to a general overview of situations in which the diagnosis should be considered, followed by discussions of the two most prevalent chronic vasculitides found in children, polyarteritis nodosa (PAN), and KD.

Diagnosis

Early in the course of a vasculitis, findings are generally nonspecific, primarily reflecting systemic inflammation (fever, malaise, fatigue, failure to thrive, elevated acute-phase reactants). As vascular damage progresses, evidence of vascular compromise characteristic of the particular vessels involved becomes evident on physical examination. Although these findings are often consistent with vasculitis, they are seldom part of a routine screening evaluation, so a physician must consider the diagnosis of vasculitis before its manifestations are pathognomonic. Should the diagnosis be delayed beyond this stage, irreversible tissue damage may occur; it is important that therapy be initiated while the findings remain subtle.

Despite the extreme variability of the manifestations of vasculitis, certain specific symptoms are particularly suggestive of vascular inflammation. Involvement of large- or medium-sized muscular arteries, as may be seen in Takayasu arteritis (TA) or PAN, initially causes symptoms related to the severity of the inflammatory response. As vascular compromise progresses, symptoms of arterial insufficiency begin to dominate. Involvement of large vessels to the extremities, such as the subclavian or femoral arteries, typically leads to claudication, whereas involvement of visceral vessels causes hypertension (renal arteries), abdominal pain (mesenteric and celiac axes), chest pain (aortic or coronary artery involvement), or neurologic symptoms (focal neurologic deficits or neuropathic pain).

Inflammation of smaller arteries and arterioles leads to symptoms in richly vascularized organs. Skin involvement—livedo reticularis, purpuric (generally palpable) or nonblanching lesions, and palmar or plantar rashes—is most suggestive of vascular inflammation. Pulmonary, renal, and GI arterial beds are often involved as well. Consequently, hemoptysis, hematuria, hypertension, abdominal pain, or melena may signify vascular involvement. Capillary and venous inflammation typically involves the same organs, although the lower volume of blood flow through these vessels tends to make capillaritis and venulitis less of an acute emergency than arteritis.

Whenever vasculitis is considered as a diagnosis, a thorough history and careful general physical examination should be augmented by focus on clinical features of vascular disease. History should include recent illnesses, in particular infections, other exposures (including prescription and over-the-counter drugs), travel, and family history. All pulses must be palpated carefully, and bilateral Allen tests should be performed to confirm patency of the radial and ulnar arteries and volar arch. The neck, abdomen, and proximal extremities should be auscultated for bruits, and blood pressures in all four extremities should be compared for asymmetry. The skin should be examined carefully for lesions that are nodular or do not blanch, and the two other windows on small vessel abnormalities—ocular fundi and nailbed capillaries—should be assessed as well.

Laboratory studies specific for the diagnosis of vasculitis are not yet available. When vasculitis is being considered, laboratory investigation should include a CBC count and acute-phase reactants (especially ESR and CRP) for evidence of systemic inflammation. Ongoing immune activation leads to hypergammaglobulinemia in many cases of systemic vasculitis. Certain small-vessel diseases (especially Wegener granulomatosis and Churg-Strauss syndrome) are characterized by antinuclear cytoplasm antibodies (ANCA). von Willebrand factor antigen is released by damaged vascular endothelium, so it is elevated in small-vessel vasculitides but also in other conditions that cause vessel damage, including stroke, trauma, and severe infections.

Imaging procedures should be used to confirm a clinical suspicion of vasculitis, not to hunt blindly for a diagnosis. When pulmonary involvement is suspected, pulmonary function tests and imaging of the lungs with radiographs or CT are often useful. Vascular imaging must be selected on a case-by-case basis, based on clinical and laboratory data. Doppler ultrasound studies and CT or MRI angiograms are adequate for resolving abnormalities in large- or medium-sized vessels, but conditions involving smaller vessels often can be visualized only by use of conventional angiography. Even in the hands of interventional radiologists experienced in pediatric procedures, these procedures are potentially morbid, so careful attention to history and physical examination should be relied upon to minimize the number of unnecessary studies.

The reference standard for diagnosing vasculitis remains histopathologic demonstration of vascular inflammation, although tissue specimens may not be available in many cases because of the inaccessibility of lesions or patchiness of the vascular involvement. When skin lesions are present, deciding to obtain a biopsy is relatively easy; when inaccessible structures such as the brain are involved, calculating the risks and benefits of a biopsy is significantly more complicated.

POLYARTERITIS NODOSA

Background

The annual incidence of PAN in adults is approximately 0.3 per 100,000; no comparable data are available for children. Prior to the introduction of corticosteroids for the treatment of PAN, mortality rates as high as 100% were reported; today, less than one in five cases is believed to have a fatal outcome.

Pathophysiology

PAN is characterized by focal, panmural, necrotizing inflammation of small- and medium-sized muscular arteries. As the name implies, vessels affected by PAN typically develop nod-

ules in the walls of muscular arteries. Sites of bifurcation are particularly prone to involvement, presumably because of hemodynamic turbulence at these points. Biopsies reveal a cellular infiltrate initially predominated by polymorphonuclear leukocytes and fibrinoid necrosis. As lesions mature, mononuclear cells, thrombosis, and recanalization mark the healing process.

The etiology of PAN is unknown, although it is considered to be an archetype of immune complex–mediated vascular damage. Most children with PAN have serologic evidence of an antecedent streptococcal infection; up to one-third of adults have chronic hepatitis B or C, with viral proteins demonstrable in the circulating and fixed immune complexes. The incidence of hepatitis-associated PAN in children is significantly lower, particularly in Western countries.

Clinical Manifestations

Childhood PAN occurs in both cutaneous and generalized forms, and distinguishing between them may be difficult. Both types display systemic manifestations, including fever, malaise, and myalgias. However, generalized PAN is significantly more likely to also involve the renal, GI, and central nervous systems. Common to both are rashes, although these are more likely to be nodular or lacy (so-called livedo reticularis) in the cutaneous form, and urticarial, petechial, or ischemic in the systemic form. Renal involvement (including proteinuria, abnormal urinary sediment, and hypertension), abdominal pain (often a manifestation of gut vasculitis), arthritis, mononeuritis multiplex, and CNS involvement (seizures, hemiparesis) typify generalized PAN. Less commonly, children may have cardiac disease (pericarditis, cardiomegaly, EKG changes, myocardial infarction) or pulmonary involvement (diffuse infiltrates, pulmonary hemorrhage, or hemothorax). A rare subtype of PAN, Cogan syndrome, is characterized by interstitial keratitis and sensorineural hearing loss.

Laboratory Studies

Laboratory findings in polyarteritis are nonspecific. Most children have white blood cell counts higher than 15,000 per mm^3, hemoglobin less than 10 g per dL, broadly elevated acute-phase reactants, and hypergammaglobulinemia. Complement levels are usually normal or increased, and ANA and RF levels are elevated only slightly, if at all. Some children have evidence of ANCAs, although other autoantibodies are usually absent.

Diagnosis of PAN generally requires tissue confirmation. Acute necrotizing inflammation of small- and medium-sized arteries is demonstrable in renal, cutaneous, muscular, or GI tissues. At times, biopsy may not be practical, and angiographic visualization of aneurysms may provide an acceptable alternative. Other findings include visceral perfusion defects, especially in the kidneys, development of collateral arteries, and a "beaded" appearance of involved vessels as a result of alternating areas of constriction and dilatation. Performance and interpretation of these studies requires the expertise of a radiologist experienced in pediatric angiography.

Management

Prognosis in PAN is better in patients with less disease-related organ damage, so therapy should be initiated as early as possible. Absence of tissue confirmation need not delay therapy, but in most cases, empiric therapy for a presumed diagnosis of PAN should be avoided; most therapies for severe systemic vasculitis have unacceptably severe toxicities to use in unconfirmed cases. Thus, clinicians must balance a high level of suspicion and willingness to employ invasive diagnostic procedures when indicated, against a recognition that vasculitis in children is very rare.

The initial management of PAN should include corticosteroids (generally divided doses of prednisone, 2 mg per kg per day, to a maximum of 60 mg daily). Rash and constitutional symptoms improve first, followed by control of end-organ involvement. Pulse doses of methylprednisolone (30 mg per kg in 50 mL of 5% dextrose in water by IV infusion over 1 to 2 hours, maximum dose 1,500 mg) may offer an alternative for the treatment of acute exacerbations, provided that blood pressure and cardiac rhythm are closely monitored.

Cutaneous PAN may require lower doses of steroids to suppress disease activity, or alternative agents such as methotrexate, dapsone, or colchicine may adequately control the rash. Use of intravenous immunoglobin (IVIG) has also been reported in cutaneous PAN. In contrast, children with systemic PAN may not tolerate a reduction in their steroid dosage or may not respond adequately to steroids. In such cases, addition of immunosuppressive agents (e.g., oral or IV cyclophosphamide) or biologic response modifiers (e.g., infliximab 5–10 mg per kg monthly) may improve the outcome or allow tapering of steroids without a disease flare. Other pharmacologic agents, including NSAIDs for fever and arthritis, anticonvulsants, antihypertensives, and physical therapy, should be employed when appropriate.

Management of Complications and Emergencies (Table 101.12)

The most serious emergencies in childhood polyarteritis are (i) renal insufficiency; (ii) severe hypertension; (iii) cardiac complications such as CHF, myocardial infarction, and dysrhythmias; (iv) GI vasculitis resulting in bowel infarction, intestinal perforation, or cholecystitis; and (v) CNS manifestations, such as seizures and cranial nerve palsies.

Renal Emergencies. Although medical management of PAN has resulted in a significantly improved prognosis, azotemia and hypertension at the time of diagnosis continue to identify children with extremely aggressive disease. Arteritis of medium-sized vessels of the kidney may lead to renal infarction and ischemia or to glomerulonephritis manifested by hematuria, hypertension, and uremia. Sudden flank pain associated with gross hematuria, falling blood pressure, and an expanding abdominal mass suggest the possibility of aneurysmal dilatation and rupture, with renal artery hemorrhage.

Serial urinalyses, measurements of BUN and creatinine levels, and determination of creatinine clearance are essential components of the investigation of all patients with PAN. Management of renal failure includes correction of fluid and electrolyte abnormalities, as well as high doses of corticosteroids to control the underlying disease process (e.g., prednisone 2 mg per kg per day). Rupture of a renal artery aneurysm is initially managed with treatment of shock and replacement of volume, followed by surgical repair of the aneurysm once the patient is stabilized.

Hypertension. A mild to moderate elevation of blood pressure is noted in more than 90% of children with generalized PAN. Management follows the general rules for treating renovascular hypertension (Chapter 34). Severe hypertension associated with encephalopathy or CHF requires inpatient management.

Cardiac Emergencies. *Pericarditis* may be asymptomatic. Alternatively, chest pain (particularly in the recumbent position), shortness of breath, pericardial friction rub, and pulsus paradoxus may be present. EKG may reveal depression of the ST segment and T-wave inversion, and chest x-ray may demonstrate globular enlargement of the cardiac silhouette. Echocardiographic demonstration of pericardial fluid, however, is the most sensitive means of confirming the presence of pericarditis.

Chest pain with tachycardia, arrhythmia, and dyspnea may herald the occurrence of *myocardial infarction* in a patient with PAN involving the coronary arteries. Pericardial tamponade caused by a ruptured coronary aneurysm may present similarly. Occasionally, a patient with coronary artery disease may present with CHF. Characteristic EKG changes (deep Q waves) and areas of ischemia on myocardial nuclear scanning may be seen. Echocardiography is indicated to study the function of the myocardium and the status of the valves. Coronary arteriography is essential to establish the size, location, and extent of aneurysms and occlusions.

Patients with CHF, myocardial ischemia, and arrhythmias will require continuous monitoring and urgent management in an intensive care setting. Patients with pericarditis without effusion may be treated with bed rest, careful monitoring, and corticosteroids. Pericardiocentesis is indicated in the presence of tamponade or if infection is suspected. Patients with myocardial infarction need careful monitoring, pain relief (morphine), treatment of shock, antiarrhythmic agents, and treatment of CHF (Chapter 84). A radiograph of the chest, EKG, and echocardiogram should be obtained as soon as possible; thallium scan and coronary angiography may be indicated in certain patients.

Supportive medical management includes careful monitoring of cardiorespiratory status, judicious use of IV fluids, diuretics, and cardiotonics when needed. Treatment of the primary disease with steroids and immunosuppressive agents should be continued as described. If hypertension does not respond to diuretic therapy, other antihypertensive agents may have to be added. Serum electrolytes should be monitored because most patients will be taking high doses of steroids, diuretics, and antihypertensive agents, and electrolyte imbalances increase the risk of toxicity.

GI Complications. Abdominal pain is the most common manifestation of GI involvement in PAN. It may be diffuse and nonspecific or localized and severe. Hematemesis and melena suggest ulceration and hemorrhage. Patients with persistent

TABLE 101.12

COMPLICATIONS OF POLYARTERITIS NODOSA

Clinical entity	Symptoms and signs	Investigations	Treatment
Renal failure	Usually insidious; no symptoms until uremia sets in	Urinalysis (serial); BUN; creatinine; creatinine clearance; serum electrolytes	Fluid, electrolyte management Treatment of hypertension Peritoneal dialysis Hemodialysis
Renal infarction	Flank pain High blood pressure	Urinalysis; BUN; creatinine Renal arteriogram	Management of renal failure as given above, hemodialysis
Renal artery aneurysm with hemorrhage	Severe, sudden flank pain; gross hematuria; shock; palpable abdominal mass	Serial hematocrit Renal arteriogram	Management of shock Surgical consult
Hypertension	Asymptomatic or headache; retinal changes; encephalopathy	Serial measurement of BP; BUN; creatinine, creatinine clearance; IVP (or) renal arteriogram	Diuretics Antihypertensive agents
Pericarditis	Chest pain; pericardial rub; pulsus paradoxus (if tamponade)	EKG; radiograph chest; echocardiogram; removal of fluid for analysis	Rest, steroids, removal of fluid (if tamponade) *Caution:* if tamponade is sudden, it may be caused by ruptured aneurysm with blood in pericardium
Myocardial infarction	Sudden chest pain; shock; arrhythmia; dyspnea; congestive failure	EKG (continuous monitor); echocardiogram; thallium scan; coronary arteriography	Pain relief; oxygen Circulatory support Heparin, thrombolytic agents
Gastrointestinal hemorrhage	Abdominal pain; vomiting; melena, hematemesis, or hematochezia; shock; tenderness and guarding of abdomen; bowel sounds absent	Plain radiograph abdomen Peritoneal aspiration Endoscopy Celiac arteriogram	Treat shock; block bleeding vessel during angiography; surgical ligation
Gastrointestinal perforation	Sudden abdominal pain; shock; guarding, tenderness, and rigidity of abdomen; absent bowel sounds	Plain radiograph abdomen (upright)	Treat shock Surgical repair
Aneurysm with rupture (intraabdominal)	Abdominal pain (chronic) with acute exacerbation Palpable mass Sudden onset of shock	Ultrasound Celiac arteriogram	Treat shock Surgical repair
Central nervous system lesions	Convulsions; gradual onset of loss of consciousness; hemiparesis	Exclude hypertensive encephalopathy CT scan, MRI Carotid arteriography	Supportive care Control BP Anticonvulsants High-dose corticosteroids and/or immunosuppressives

BUN, blood urea nitrogen; BP, blood pressure; IVP, intravenous pyelogram; EKG, electrocardiogram; CT, computed tomography; MRI, magnetic resonance imaging.

abdominal pain, hematemesis, and melena require immediate admission.

Visceral perforation should be suspected in cases of active systemic disease and unrelenting abdominal pain. Tenderness on palpation of the abdomen, guarding of the abdominal wall, and absent bowel sounds are the usual physical findings, although they may be masked by steroid therapy. Arteritis involving specific organs may lead to cholecystitis, pancreatitis, appendicitis, or hepatitis. These complications are generally manifested by vomiting and localized abdominal pain and tenderness.

Mesenteric thrombosis with infarction of the bowel may present with sudden abdominal pain, vomiting, hematemesis or hematochezia, and shock. Exquisite tenderness of the abdomen and absent bowel sounds are the major findings. Hemorrhage from a ruptured aneurysm (mesenteric, hepatic, or renal) with hemoperitoneum is heralded by sudden onset of severe pain, vomiting, tachycardia, and shock. The abdomen is tender and tense, and bowel sounds are diminished or absent.

Initial management of each of these GI catastrophes includes volume replacement, gastric decompression, and stress doses of corticosteroids. All such patients will require measurement of intake and output, as well as serial determination of hematocrit, BUN, and electrolytes. Abdominal x-rays (supine and upright), abdominal ultrasound, technetium scan, angiography of the celiac axis vessels, and peritoneal aspiration may be indicated in some cases. In selected instances, direct examination of the GI tract by endoscopy may yield valuable information concerning the nature, location, and extent of lesions. Surgical consultation should be obtained immediately, and in the presence of bleeding aneurysms or infarcted bowel, exploratory laparoscopy or laparotomy should be performed as soon as the patient can be stabilized.

CNS Complications. Clinical signs of CNS disease are less frequent than those of peripheral nervous system involvement. Seizures and hemiparesis are the most common manifestations of CNS involvement in PAN and require immediate hospitalization. A complete neurologic evaluation should be performed, including measurement of blood pressure, and fundoscopic examination for evidence of hypertension or intracranial bleeding. CT and/or carotid angiography may help localize the lesion.

Management of hypertensive encephalopathy and increased intracranial pressure are described elsewhere (see Chapters 34 and 96). Surgical correction of a ruptured aneurysm should be undertaken if the bleeding vessel can be localized and is accessible.

Miscellaneous Complications. As with all vasculitides, PAN may involve testicular vessels, leading to acute scrotal pain and purpura and accompanying dysuria. Once other causes of scrotal pain are excluded, including epididymitis and testicular torsion, treatment may proceed with steroids and immunosuppressive medications.

BEHÇET DISEASE

Behçet disease (BD) is a vasculitis that is rare in children, especially in nonendemic areas such as the United States. First described by the Turkish dermatologist Hulusi Behçet in 1937, the classical description of BD is a clinical triad consisting of recurrent buccal aphthous ulcers, recurrent genital ulcers, and uveitis with hypopion. In addition to these cardinal features of BD, there are a host of associated clinical manifestations, including arthritis, neurologic involvement, GI manifestations, vascular/thrombotic disease, and various dermatologic lesions including erythema nodosum and necrotic folliculitis. Thus, BD may resemble a large number of other conditions, and should be included in the differential diagnosis of various complaints evaluated in EDs.

Since Dr. Behçet's original description, there have been various revisions of the clinical criteria. The diagnostic criteria formulated by the International Study Group for Behçet Disease in 1990 have become fairly standard. This diagnostic schema requires recurrent oral ulceration observed by a physician at least three times in 12 months, plus two of the following four clinical manifestations: recurrent genital ulceration, ocular disease, skin lesions, and positive pathergy test. A pathergy test is considered positive if the patient develops an erythematous nodule or pustule greater than 2 mm in diameter 24 to 48 hours after the skin of the forearm is pricked with a sterile needle.

Because of the rarity of BD in children, most published clinical series are small. Overall, the clinical manifestations in children are similar to those in adult BD. Recurrent oral ulcerations are the most common presenting sign and ongoing manifestation of pediatric BD. Ulcerative mucocutaneous lesions are far from specific for BD; however, unlike those associated with inflammatory bowel disease, SLE, chronic oral aphthosis, and Sweet syndrome, oral lesions in BD tend to scar. In the United States, many children have so-called "incomplete Behçet disease," meeting only partial diagnostic criteria, but remaining at risk for complications of the disease.

Although oral and genital ulcers can certainly be painful for the patient and problematic from a management standpoint, there are other less common but more serious complications of BD that may lead to severe morbidity and even mortality. Ocular disease can be devastating, ultimately resulting in blindness. GI disease can result in perforation. Neurologic complications are varied, including headache, meningoencephalitis, pseudotumor cerebri, and quadriparesis. Psychiatric symptoms including depression, personality changes, and memory loss are also reported. Vascular/thrombotic complications are a particularly ominous development in BD patients; these can include dural sinus thrombosis and arterial lesions. In one multinational pediatric BD series, large vessel thrombosis was the leading cause of death, carrying a 30% mortality rate.

The general treatment of BD is similar to other forms of vasculitis discussed in this chapter, consisting of antiinflammatory/immunosuppressive agents. Topical corticosteroid preparations may be helpful for oral and genital lesions; steroid drops may be necessary for ocular disease. Colchicine can be an effective systemic agent for relatively mild mucocutaneous symptoms and can be helpful in preventing episodes of uveitis. Dapsone is also used for mucocutaneous disease. Thalidomide is particularly effective for oral and genital ulcers, although it must be used with extreme caution, given the potential for teratogenicity and neurologic disturbances. Cyclosporin A is often used for BD uveitis. Emerging data suggest that anti-TNF agents are often very effective for treating severe manifestations of BD.

Life-threatening cases of BD may require high-dose systemic corticosteroids and cyclophosphamide. Thrombotic disease requires formal anticoagulation, in addition to aggressive immunosuppressive therapies.

KAWASAKI DISEASE

Background

Mucocutaneous lymph node syndrome was first described by a Japanese pediatrician in 1967, and it is now known as KD in his honor. In fact, the condition certainly predates this description: A preserved heart from the 19th century shows pathologic changes characteristic of KD, and the entity of "infantile polyarteritis" probably represents the same syndrome. KD is an idiopathic vasculitis of small- and medium-sized vessels, which has surpassed acute rheumatic fever to become the leading cause of acquired heart disease in children in the developed world. Incidence estimates in the continental United States range from 9 to 19 per 100,000 children; the incidence in Asia may be up to ten times as high. KD is 50% more common in boys than in girls, and it usually affects children younger than 5 years. However, pediatricians must remain vigilant in all age groups because the disease may be more difficult to diagnose, but more likely to cause chronic sequelae in infants and adolescents.

Characteristically, children with KD have fever, conjunctivitis, rash, mucosal inflammation, lymphadenopathy, and extremity changes. The major morbidity of KD, however, occurs in the heart. Coronary artery aneurysms or ectasia develop in approximately 15% to 25% of untreated children and may lead to myocardial infarction, sudden death, or chronic coronary artery insufficiency. IVIG decreases the incidence of coronary artery aneurysms by three- to fivefold if given within 10 days of disease onset. Management of children with suspected KD, therefore, requires accurate and expeditious diagnosis and close monitoring of the cardiovascular system.

Pathophysiology

In KD as in other vasculitides, blood vessel damage appears to result from an aberrant immune response leading to endothelial cell injury and vessel wall damage. A direct cell-mediated attack on endothelial cells, either because they are infected with an as-yet unidentified infectious agent, or simply as innocent bystanders, may underlie the vascular injury. Humoral factors, such as antiendothelial cell antibodies or circulating immune complexes, may also play a role. The reason that KD preferentially involves coronary arteries is unknown.

The pathologic changes of coronary arteries in KD have been classified by Fujiwara and Hamashima into four stages, depending on the duration of illness at the time of examination (Table 101.13). Initially, endothelial swelling is accompa-

nied by a neutrophilic infiltrate. Lymphocytes and plasma cells replace polymorphonuclear cells by the subacute stage (beginning 2 weeks after onset), accompanied by destruction of the internal elastic lamina; coronary artery aneurysms characteristic of KD first become apparent at this time. Finally, during the convalescent state of KD, healing of the vascular lesions occurs with fibromuscular proliferation and scar formation, along with expansion of aneurysms due to hemodynamic forces.

Many lines of evidence point toward a role of infections in the causation of KD. The fact that the disease often occurs in epidemics, that boys are more susceptible than girls, and that household contacts of children with KD are at increased risk for developing the disease in Japan, all point to a transmissible agent. Nonetheless, although many putative etiologies have been proposed during the past four decades, suggestions that certain viruses (EBV, human coronavirus, parvovirus, HIV-2) or bacterial toxins (streptococcal erythrogenic toxin, staphylococcal toxic shock toxin) account for the majority of cases have not been substantiated. Many researchers now believe that KD represents a final common pathway of immune-mediated vascular inflammation in genetically susceptible children triggered by any one of a variety of common infections.

Clinical Manifestations

KD is a clinical syndrome diagnosed on the basis of fever and four of five signs of mucocutaneous inflammation (Table 101.14). These criteria were established by Tomisaku Kawasaki in 1967, and they remain the sine qua non for diagnosing KD. Nonetheless, as with all clinical guidelines, these should be regarded as imperfect, with less than 100% sensitivity and specificity. Children who do not meet criteria may indeed have KD, whereas some children with other conditions may nonetheless manifest five or six criteria of KD. Acknowledgement of this fact was made explicit in 2004 when an expert panel published revised criteria for diagnosing and treating children suspected to have KD.

TABLE 101.13

PATHOLOGY OF KAWASAKI DISEASE[a]

Stage I—Disease duration <10 days
Acute perivasculitis of coronary arteries
Microvascular angiitis of coronary arteries and aorta
Pancarditis with pericardial, myocardial, endocardial
  inflammation
Inflammation of the atrioventricular conduction system

Stage II—Disease duration 12–28 days
Acute panvasculitis of coronary arteries
Coronary artery aneurysms present
Coronary obstruction and thrombosis
Myocardial and endocardial inflammation less intense

Stage III—Disease duration 28–45 days
Subacute inflammation in coronary arteries
Coronary artery aneurysms present
Myocardial, endocardial inflammation much decreased

Stage IV—Disease duration >50 days
Scar formation, calcification in coronary arteries
Stenosis and recanalization of coronary vessel lumen
Myocardial fibrosis without acute inflammation

IVIG, intravenous immunoglobin.
[a]Duration of each stage may be decreased by prompt treatment with IVIG.

TABLE 101.14

DIAGNOSTIC CRITERIA FOR KAWASAKI DISEASE

Fever ≥5 days unresponsive to antibiotics
If the fever disappears because of intravenous gamma-globulin
  therapy before the fifth day of illness, a fever of <5 days'
  duration fulfills fever criterion for case definition.
At least four of the five following physical findings with no
  other more reasonable explanation for the observed clinical
  findings:
1. Bilateral conjunctival injection
2. Changes in the oropharyngeal mucous membranes (erythematous and/or fissured lips, strawberry tongue, injected pharynx)
3. Changes of peripheral extremities, including erythema and/or edema of the hands or feet (acute phase) or periungual desquamation (convalescent phase) (Fig. 101.12)
4. Polymorphous rash, primarily truncal; nonvesicular
5. Cervical lymphadenopathy ≥1.5-cm diameter

Fever is probably the most consistent manifestation of KD. It reflects the elevated levels of proinflammatory cytokines (e.g., TNF, IL-1), which are also believed to mediate the underlying vascular inflammation. A diagnosis of KD should be considered in all children with prolonged, unexplained fever, irritability, and laboratory signs of inflammation, especially in the presence of mucocutaneous inflammation. Conversely, the diagnosis must be suspect in the absence of fever.

The remaining cardinal manifestations of KD vary considerably in frequency. Up to one-half of children with KD do not have cervical lymphadenopathy, especially children younger than 2 years of age. When present, lymphadenopathy tends to involve the anterior cervical nodes overlying the sternocleidomastoid muscle. Diffuse lymphadenopathy, as well as other signs of reticuloendothelial involvement such as splenomegaly, should prompt a search for an alternative diagnosis.

Bilateral, nonexudative conjunctivitis is present in more than 90% of patients. A predominantly bulbar injection typically begins within days of the onset of fever, and eyes eventually develop a brilliant erythema, which spares the limbus. Children are also frequently photophobic, and five out of six patients have evidence of anterior uveitis during the first week of illness. Consequently, in ambiguous cases, slit-lamp examination may be helpful in confirming a diagnosis of KD.

Cracked, red lips and a strawberry tongue are characteristic of the mucositis typically seen during the first week of KD (Fig. 101.11). Discrete oral lesions, such as vesicles or ulcers, and tonsillar exudate, are suggestive of a viral or bacterial infection rather than KD. The cutaneous manifestations of KD are polymorphous. The rash typically begins as perineal erythema and desquamation, followed by macular, morbilliform, or targetoid lesions of the trunk and extremities. Vesicular or bullous lesions are rare. Changes in the extremities are generally the last clinical manifestation of KD to develop. Children demonstrate an indurated edema of the dorsum of their hands and feet, and a

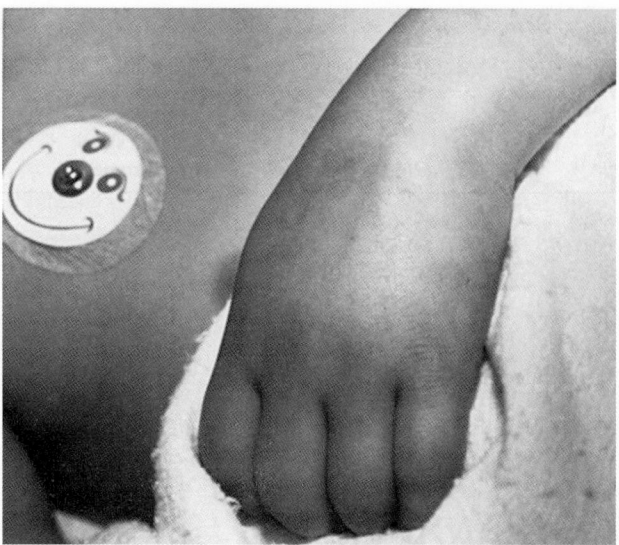
FIGURE 101.12 Brawny edema of dorsum of hand and small joint polyarthritis in Kawasaki disease.

diffuse erythema of their palms and soles (Fig. 101.12). During the convalescent phase of KD, sheetlike desquamation that begins in the periungual region of the hands and feet is characteristic (Fig. 101.13, see also color plate). Linear nail creases known as Beau lines are also common late manifestations of KD.

As a systemic vasculitis, KD may cause a variety of other clinical manifestations. Pulmonary involvement may lead to symptoms such as cough and infiltrates, peribronchial cuffing, and pleural effusions on chest radiographs. GI signs may range from emesis and diarrhea to findings suggestive of an acute surgical abdomen. Neurologic involvement including seizures, facial nerve palsies, ataxia, hemiplegia, and severe encephalopathy is also reported. In general, as with other vasculitides, manifestations of KD may be protean, so clinicans should not exclude the possibility solely on the basis of atypical features.

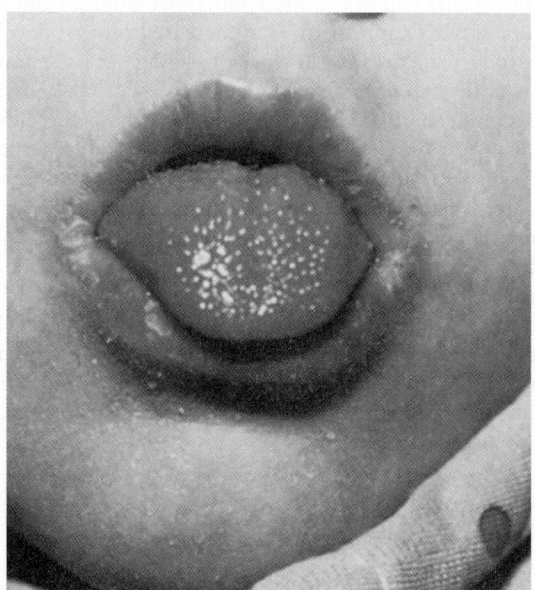
FIGURE 101.11 Cracked, erythematous lips and "strawberry" tongue in Kawasaki disease.

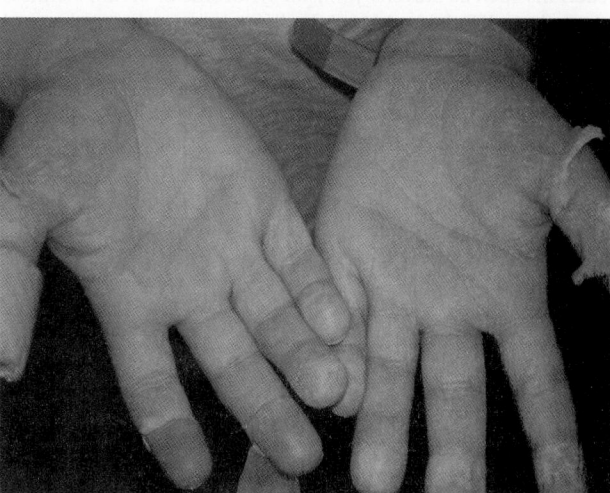
FIGURE 101.13 Periungual desquamation during the convalescent phase of Kawasaki disease.

MEDICAL EMERGENCIES

TABLE 101.15

DIFFERENTIAL DIAGNOSIS OF KAWASAKI DISEASE

	Kawasaki disease	Toxic shock syndrome	Streptococcal scarlet fever	Stevens-Johnson syndrome	Systemic juvenile rheumatoid arthritis
Age	<5 yr	>10 yr	2–8 yr	All ages	2–5 yr
Fever	≤12 days	<10 days	Variable	Prolonged	Prolonged
Eyes	Nonexudative conjunctivitis, limbal sparing, anterior uveitis	Conjunctivitis	Normal	Exudative conjunctivitis, keratitis	Normal
Oral mucosa	Erythema, "strawberry tongue"	Erythema	Pharyngitis, "strawberry tongue," circumoral pallor	Erythema, ulcerations, pseudomembrane formation	Normal
Extremities	Erythema of palms and soles, indurative edema, periungual desquamation	Peripheral edema	Fine flaking desquamation	Normal	Arthritis
Rash	Polymorphous; targetoid or purpuric in 20%	Erythroderma	Erythroderma, Pastia's lines	Target lesions	Transient, salmon pink
Lymph nodes	Single anterior lymph node	Normal	Painful, diffuse cervical nodes	Normal	Diffuse
Other	Arthritis	Shock, coagulopathy, mental status changes	Positive throat culture	Arthralgia, associated herpes virus infection (30%–50%)	Pericarditis

KD is most commonly confused with exanthematous infections of childhood (Table 101.15). Measles, echovirus, and adenovirus may share many of the signs of mucocutaneous inflammation, but they typically have less evidence of systemic inflammation, and generally lack the extremity changes seen in KD. Toxin-mediated illnesses, especially β-hemolytic streptococcal infection and toxic shock syndrome, generally lack the ocular and articular involvement typical of KD. Finally, drug reactions such as Stevens-Johnson syndrome or serum sickness may mimic KD but with subtle differences in the ocular and mucosal manifestations.

The conventional diagnostic criteria are particularly useful in preventing overdiagnosis, but they may result in failure to recognize incomplete forms of the illness. It should be emphasized that children who do not fulfill formal diagnostic criteria are still at risk of cardiac complications. Depending on the series, between 10% and 60% of children who develop coronary aneurysms never meet clinical criteria for KD. The guidelines of the American Heart Association Council on Cardiovascular Disease in the Young provide a useful framework for managing children with suspected KD who do not meet criteria for the diagnosis (see Fig. 101.14 and also section on Incomplete KD below).

Clinical manifestations of KD tend to be most incomplete and atypical in the youngest patients, the subgroup at highest risk for development of coronary artery abnormalities. Infants younger than 6 months are at particularly high risk. Thus, KD should be considered in any infant with prolonged, unex-plained fever. In contrast, alternative explanations for the child's symptoms must be carefully excluded before treating empirically with IVIG. Consideration should be given to referring children to a regional KD center for further evaluation when the diagnosis is unclear.

At the other end of the spectrum, older children and adolescents with KD appear to be at increased risk for developing coronary aneurysms; however, older age at presentation is also associated with delayed diagnosis, which is known to incur significant risk. Unlike infants, in whom the clinical findings of KD are often incomplete, older children appear to present with fairly typical manifestations. Diagnosis may be delayed because clinicians are less likely to consider the diagnosis in older patients because most cases involve young children. Further, children older than 8 years of age frequently exhibit GI and meningeal symptoms, potentially clouding the diagnostic picture. In any event, whether KD is indeed more aggressive in older children, or simply because diagnosis is more likely to be delayed, pediatricians must consider KD as a possible cause of prolonged fever in children of any age.

Laboratory Studies

No laboratory studies are included among the diagnostic criteria for KD, but certain findings may support the diagnosis. Most characteristic is systemic inflammation, with widespread

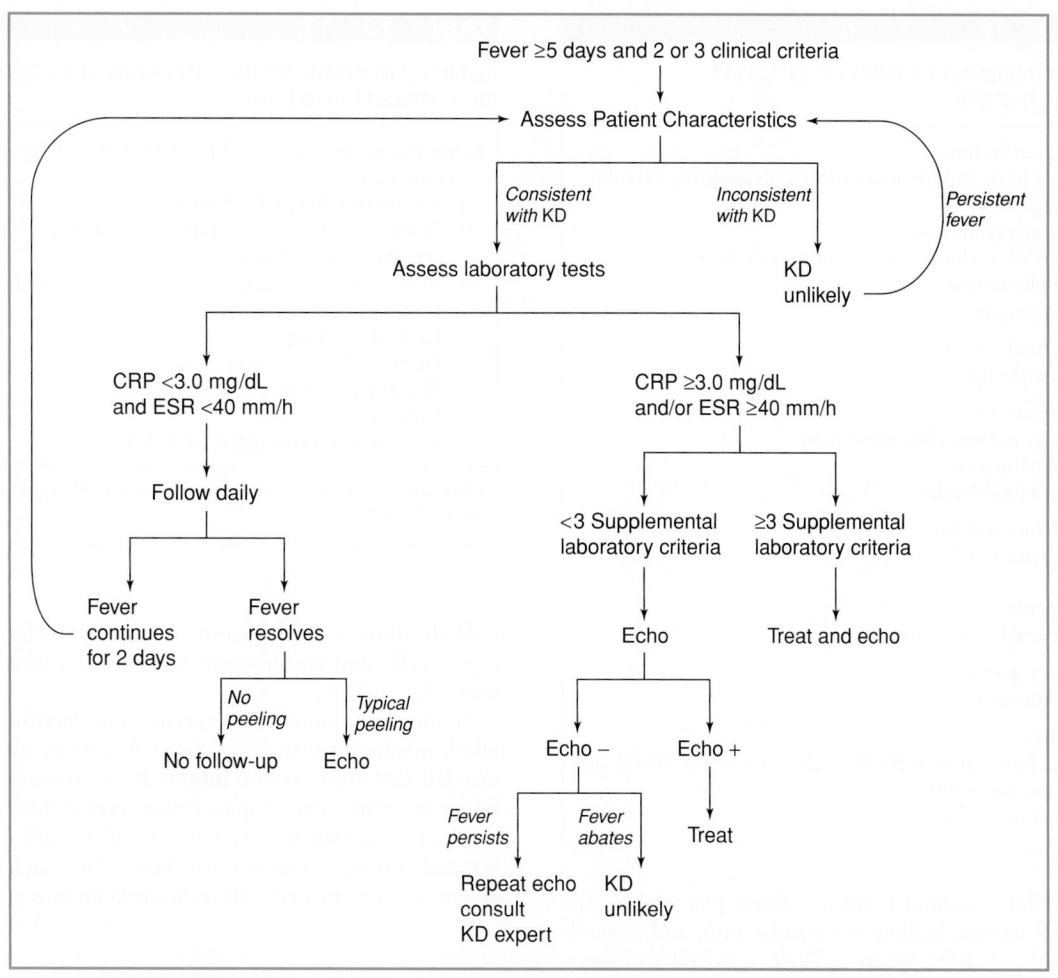

FIGURE 101.14 Evaluation of suspected incomplete Kawasaki Disease (KD). (From Newburger JW, Takahashi M, Gerber M, et al. diagnosis, treatment, and long-term management of Kawasaki disease: a statement for health professionals from the Committee on Rheumatic Fever, Endocarditis, and Kawasaki Disease, Council on Cardiovascular Disease in the Young, American Heart Association. *Pediatrics* 2004;114:1708–1733.)

elevation of acute-phase reactants (including CRP and ESR), leukocytosis, and a left shift in the white blood cell count. By the second week of illness, platelet counts also rise, reaching 1,000,000 per mm³ in the most severe cases.

Children with KD often present with a normocytic, normochromic anemia; hemoglobin concentrations more than two standard deviations below the mean for age are noted in approximately one-half of patients within the first 2 weeks of illness. Urinalysis commonly reveals white blood cells on microscopic examination; the cells are mononuclear, and so are not detected by dipstick tests for leukocyte esterase. They also originate in the urethra, so they will be missed on urinalyses obtained by bladder tap or catheterization. Measurement of liver enzymes often reveals elevated transaminase levels or mild hyperbilirubinemia due to intrahepatic congestion. In addition, a minority of children may develop obstructive jaundice from hydrops of the gallbladder. If sampled, other body fluids demonstrate inflammation as well: CSF typically displays a mononuclear pleocytosis (less than 100 cells per mm³) with normal glucose and protein concentrations, whereas

arthrocentesis of involved joints demonstrates 50,000 to 300,000 white blood cells per mm³, primarily neutrophils.

Assessment of Incomplete KD

The limitations of the classical criteria for KD have long posed challenges for clinicians, particularly in those cases of "incomplete" or "atypical" KD. In 2004, the American Heart Association (AHA) put forth an algorithm suggesting an approach for evaluation of possible incomplete KD (Fig. 101.14). Unlike the classical criteria, this algorithm takes into account laboratory studies and findings on echocardiogram.

Prolonged fever is still the cardinal manifestation of KD under the AHA algorithm. Children with 5 or more days of fever and 2 or 3 clinical criteria in whom KD is being considered should be evaluated further for incomplete KD. This starts with a full assessment for possible characteristics suggesting KD, including those outlined in Table 101.16. Characteristics suggestive of an alternative diagnosis are considered as well,

TABLE 101.16

CLINICAL FINDINGS CONSISTENT WITH
KAWASAKI DISEASE

Cardiovascular findings
  Congestive heart failure, myocarditis, pericarditis, valvular
    regurgitation
  Coronary artery abnormalities
  Aneurysms of medium-size noncoronary arteries
  Raynaud phenomenon
  Peripheral gangrene

Musculoskeletal system
  Arthritis, arthralgia

Gastrointestinal tract
  Diarrhea, vomiting, abdominal pain
  Hepatic dysfunction
  Hydrops of gallbladder

Central nervous system
  Extreme irritability
  Lethargy
  Aseptic meningitis
  Sensorineural hearing loss

Genitourinary system
  Urethritis/meatitis

Other findings
  Erythema, induration at Bacille Calmette-Guerin (BCG) site
  Anterior uveitis (mild)
  Desquamating rash in groin

TABLE 101.17

ECHOCARDIOGRAPHIC CRITERIA SUGGESTIVE
OF KAWASAKI DISEASE

Echocardiogram considered positive if any of the three crite-
  ria are met
  I. z score of LAD or RCA of ≥2.5
  II. Coronary arteries meet Japanese Ministry of Health
      criteria for aneurysms
  III. If three or more suggestive features are present
      Perivascular brightness
      Lack of tapering
      Decreased LV function
      Mitral regurgitation
      Pericardial effusion
      z scores in LAD or RCA of 2–2.5

LAD, left anterior descending coronary artery; RCA, right coronary
artery; LV, left ventricle.

including exudative conjunctivitis, exudative pharyngitis, discrete intraoral lesions, bullous or vesicular rash, and generalized adenopathy. If KD appears unlikely, watchful waiting is employed, but ongoing reassessment is recommended if fevers persist. If the clinical picture is consistent with KD, laboratory tests are evaluated. If inflammatory markers are relatively unimpressive (CRP less than 3 mg per dL, ESR less than 40 mm per hour), this is less suggestive of KD, though the child should be followed daily, and formally reassessed if fevers persist. Even in children with unimpressive inflammatory markers whose fever resolves, an echocardiogram should be considered if typical peeling of the skin develops.

In those children with a clinical picture consistent with KD and significantly elevated inflammatory markers (CRP greater than or equal to 3.0 mg per DL, ESR greater than or equal to 40 mm per hour), supplemental laboratory criteria are taken into consideration. Supplemental lab criteria include albumin less than or equal to 3.0 g per dL, anemia for age, elevated alanine aminotransferase, platelets greater than or equal to 450,000 per mm^3 after 7 days of illness, white blood cell count greater than or equal to 15,000 per mm^3, and urine greater than or equal to 10 white blood cells per high-power field. If the child has more than three supplemental lab criteria, treatment for KD is recommended, and can be started before an echocardiogram is performed. In children with less than three supplemental lab criteria, an echocardiogram is recommended, with treatment to follow if the echocardiogram is positive (Table 101.17); treatment is recommended even if the child is past day 10 of fever, if there are clinical and laboratory signs of continued inflammation. If the echocardiogram is negative and the fever subsides, KD is considered to have been

unlikely. If the echocardiogram is negative and fever persists, a repeat echo and consultation with a KD expert are recommended.

It should be noted that special consideration is given to febrile infants less than or equal to 6 months of age. It is recommended that these young infants have laboratory studies if febrile for more than or up to 7 days, even if there are no other clinical manifestations of KD present. If systemic inflammation is found, it is recommended that those infants undergo echocardiogram and be treated if the echocardiogram is positive.

Management

Intravenous Immune Globulin

IVIG has revolutionized the care of children with KD; treatment within 10 days of onset significantly shortens disease duration and minimizes the incidence of complications. Overall, prompt diagnosis and appropriate therapy prevent aneurysm formation in approximately 95% of children and result in rapid symptomatic improvement in about 90%. Studies in Japan were the first to suggest relative protection from coronary artery aneurysms when IVIG is administered early in the course of KD. Since then, further trials in the United States and Japan have confirmed this finding and documented the safety of high-dose infusions of immunoglobulin. At present, a single large infusion of IVIG (2 g per kg) administered over 8 to 12 hours is the standard of care for KD. This is somewhat more effective and equally as safe as multiple smaller infusions, and it also significantly shortens the duration of hospitalization.

Therapy with IVIG also has other benefits. Treatment results in a reduced prevalence of giant aneurysms, the most serious form of coronary abnormality caused by the disease. It also accelerates normalization of abnormalities of left ventricular systolic function and contractility. Finally, high-dose IVIG reduces fever and laboratory indices of inflammation, suggesting a rapid, generalized antiinflammatory effect in addition to specific cardioprotective effects. Different preparations of IVIG purified in different manners are available, but data are insufficient to determine whether all are equally effective.

Despite its advantages, IVIG is an expensive and potentially toxic intervention. The greatest long-term concern is the possible transmission of blood-borne pathogens. Elaborate sterilization procedures, including lyophilization, pasteurization, and addition of solvent detergents, are generally effective in rendering the product free of infectious agents. Nonetheless, technical errors apparently led to more than 100 cases of hepatitis C in recipients of a single brand of IVIG in 1994, although none were children with KD. Overall, however, significant toxicity is rare, and benefits clearly outweigh risks in children with confirmed KD.

Aspirin

Aspirin was the first medication to be used for treatment of KD, both for its antiinflammatory and its antithrombotic effects. High-dose (greater than 80 mg per kg per day) and lower-dose regimens (30 mg per kg per day) are still used in conjunction with IVIG during the acute phase of the illness despite the fact that meta-analyses demonstrate no additive protection from coronary artery aneurysms from aspirin. Once fever resolves, patients are generally switched to antiplatelet doses of aspirin (3 to 5 mg per kg per day). Unless coronary artery abnormalities are detected by echocardiogram, aspirin is discontinued once laboratory studies return to normal, usually within 2 months of the onset of KD.

The risks of aspirin appear to be similar to those reported in other settings: transaminitis, chemical hepatitis, transient hearing loss and, rarely, Reye syndrome. These risks may even be increased in KD: Aspirin-binding studies have suggested that the hypoalbuminemia of children with KD predisposes them to toxic-free salicylate levels despite measured (bound) values within the therapeutic range. At least one case of Reye syndrome has been reported after 6 days of aspirin therapy for KD. Alternative antipyretic and antiinflammatory agents, such as ibuprofen, may be used for treatment of arthralgias, and aspirin should be rapidly discontinued whenever varicella or influenza are concerns.

Management of Complications and Emergencies

Cardiovascular. Cardiac abnormalities dominate the pathology of KD. Clinical examination is often remarkable for tachycardia and gallop rhythms that are more prominent than expected from the degree of fever and anemia. The EKG in acute KD may show mild abnormalities consistent with myocarditis, most commonly a prolonged PR interval and nonspecific ST- and T-wave changes. Echocardiographic evaluation of myocardial function early in the course of the disease frequently reveals reduced left ventricular function and contractility. Rarely, myocardial inflammation may progress to frank CHF. The severity of myocarditis does not correlate with the risk of coronary artery aneurysms or with other complications such as pericardial effusion, which may develop during the second week of illness. The effusion rarely progresses to tamponade and resolves spontaneously in most instances. Valvulitis presenting as either aortic or mitral regurgitation is seen in a percentage of children during the early phases of KD. Late-onset mitral regurgitation, from papillary muscle dysfunction or myocardial infarction, may also complicate the clinical course.

Most characteristic of KD is inflammation of the coronary arteries. This progresses to ectasia or aneurysm formation in 15% to 25% of untreated children. Male gender, age less than 1 year, prolonged fever, dramatic elevation of CRP and absolute band count, and pronounced depression of albumin level, identify children at greatest risk for developing coronary artery aneurysms. Dilatation of coronary arteries may be detected by echocardiography as early as 6 days after the onset of fever and usually peaks 3 or 4 weeks into the course of the illness. Cardiac catheterization need not be performed in patients with normal echocardiograms and EKGs throughout the disease course because the likelihood of finding unsuspected lesions is negligible.

Coronary aneurysms in early KD usually occur in the proximal segments of the major coronary vessels; abnormalities that occur distally are almost always associated with proximal coronary dilatation. Aneurysms may also occur in arteries outside the coronary system, most commonly the subclavian, brachial, axillary, iliac, or femoral vessels, and occasionally in the abdominal aorta and renal arteries. For this reason, abdominal aortography and subclavian arteriography are often performed in patients undergoing coronary angiograms for KD. For unknown reasons, visceral vessels are almost never involved.

Myocardial Disease. Myocardial infarction caused by thrombotic occlusion of an aneurysmal and/or stenotic coronary artery is the principal cause of death in KD. Rarely, dilated and weakened coronary arteries may rupture. Mortality due to KD has decreased from almost 2% to less than 0.1% as a result of improved treatment. Nonetheless, most deaths continue to occur during the first 6 months after disease onset, when myocardial and coronary artery inflammation are greatest. A Japanese registry of 195 children with myocardial infarction revealed that almost 40% infarcted within 3 months of disease onset, and 74% had their infarctions during the first year after KD. About two-thirds of myocardial infarctions were associated with symptoms (shock, crying, chest or abdominal pain, vomiting, dyspnea, or arrhythmia), but only three patients had a history of antecedent angina.

Treatment with thrombolytic agents in adults with myocardial infarction results in decreased mortality and improved function. In children with KD and coronary artery thrombosis, thrombolytic agents—mainly urokinase and streptokinase, either IV or intracoronary—have been used with variable success. Thrombolytic therapy for coronary artery thrombosis is most effective if begun within 3 to 4 hours of symptom onset. Immediately following clot lysis, systemic heparin is begun in combination with aspirin. Maintenance of reperfusion then requires chronic oral antithrombotic therapy (e.g., warfarin with dipyridamole), although the ideal regimen has not been established.

CHF may rarely complicate the acute phase of KD. When this is because of myocarditis, routine treatment with IVIG generally results in rapid clinical improvement. Although IVIG therapy involves infusing large volumes of isotonic solution—2 g per kg of 5% IVIG delivers 40 cm^3 per kg over 8 to 12 hours—improvements in myocardial contractility compensate for the volume load, and treatment rarely leads to circulatory deterioration. By the second week of illness, and especially in children with coronary artery dilatation, ischemia or infarction must be excluded as causes of new myocardial dysfunction. Characteristic electrocardiographic and echocardiographic changes allow this distinction to be made rapidly in most patients.

Vascular Obstruction. Children with severe KD, especially infants or those in whom treatment is delayed, may develop other complications related to arterial occlusion. Peripheral obstruction leading to ischemia and gangrene most typically occurs in children with other manifestations of critical disease such as giant coronary artery aneurysms or aneurysms in peripheral arteries. Various therapies may restore circulation, although control of vascular inflammation with sufficient IVIG and/or other medications (e.g., corticosteroids and anti-TNF agents) is an essential prerequisite to arterial reperfusion. Thereafter, treatments may include thrombolytic therapy if arterial thrombosis is present, or vasodilators if tissue viability is primarily threatened by vasospasm. Peripheral arterial obstruction may be corrected by thrombolysis with urokinase, streptokinase, or tissue-type plasminogen activator, after which perfusion is maintained with heparin followed by a chronic oral anticoagulant regimen.

Other Complications. *Arthritis* occurs in approximately one-third of children with KD. Because it is rare in many of the conditions that may mimic KD, the presence of synovitis adds supportive evidence for the diagnosis in ambiguous cases. The arthritis tends to involve the small joints of the extremities during the acute phase of illness and the large joints during the second and third weeks. The arthritis of KD is always non-deforming and self-limited, generally resolving within 30 days. Antiinflammatory medications such as ibuprofen are usually effective in relieving symptoms until spontaneous resolution occurs.

KD may *recur* in 1% to 2% of children within 12 months of diagnosis, and an additional 5% to 10% may respond poorly to IVIG treatment during the initial bout of illness. In fact, patients who fail to respond completely to IVIG pose the greatest therapeutic dilemma. Prolonged fever itself correlates with increased risk of developing coronary artery abnormalities, and fever lasting for more than 14 days identifies a group of children at risk for developing giant coronary artery aneurysms (internal diameter greater than 8 mm), the group that is most susceptible to infarction and sudden death.

In cases of persistent, recurrent, or recrudescent KD, most clinicians retreat with IVIG, 2 g per kg over 8 to 12 hours. The risk of additional IVIG seems to be minimal, and several studies show a dose response to IVIG in KD. It is, however, extremely important to confirm the diagnosis; it must be remembered that failure to respond to IVIG might indicate that the child has a different source of fever, such as a bacterial or viral infection, or a chronic inflammatory disease.

Approximately two-thirds of children with KD who fail to respond to an initial dose of IVIG improve with a second course. A small number seem to be resistant to IVIG, and approaches to these children vary. One regimen that appears to be safe and effective is the use of pulse doses of methylprednisolone, as employed in PAN and other vasculitides. A multicenter randomized double-blind placebo-controlled trial of pulse dose methylprednisolone in conjunction with IVIG and ASA as initial therapy did not find a significant difference in coronary outcome between the steroid and placebo groups. In those children who required retreatment with IVIG, however, there was improved coronary outcome in the steroid compared to the placebo group. This suggests perhaps that those children who are at risk for IVIG-resistant disease at baseline might benefit from initial use of corticosteroids.

LYME DISEASE

Background

Current knowledge of LD is the result of discoveries that have spanned most of the twentieth century. Afzelius (1921) in Sweden first described the chronic migrating erythematous skin rash of LD in 1909, in association with an ixodid tick bite. Twenty-one years later, Bannworth (1944) reported a tick-borne syndrome of lymphocytic meningitis, neuritis, radicular pain, and an expanding erythematous rash (erythema migrans). In 1975, an outbreak of arthritis in Lyme, Connecticut, allowed identification of the tick vector associated with late disease. Finally, in 1981, the spirochete that is transmitted by ticks and causes the illness, *Borrelia burgdorferi*, was characterized.

LD is now the most common tick-borne illness in the United States. The Centers for Disease Control and Prevention report a steady increase in the incidence of LD. There were 248,074 cases from the 50 states, the District of Columbia, and U.S. territories reported to the CDC between 1992 and 2006, representing a 101% increase over the course of those 15 years (9,908 cases in 1992 compared to 19,931 cases in 2006). The northeastern and north-central states remain the most endemic for LD, with 92.6% of all cases reported from 10 states (Connecticut, Delaware, Massachusetts, Maryland, Minnesota, New Jersey, New York, Pennsylvania, Rhode Island, and Wisconsin). The highest rate of LD was found in children aged 5 to 9 years (8.6 cases per 100,000), with a second peak at 55 to 59 years (7.8 cases per 100,000). While cases occurred year-round, the summer months of June, July, and August saw the highest reported incidence of LD.

Clinical Manifestations

Symptoms of *B. burgdorferi* infection may be classified into three stages, similar to the progression of syphilis. Stage 1 or early disease consists of a localized erythema migrans rash (Fig. 101.15). This begins as a small, red, indurated papule at the site of the tick bite, and then expands centrifugally for a period of days or weeks. Lesions ultimately may reach an average diameter of 15 cm and may be accompanied by mild flu-like symptoms, including fever, regional lymphadenopathy, and malaise.

Stage 2 of LD results from hematogenous dissemination of the spirochete. Integumental, musculoskeletal, and central nervous systems are most commonly affected. Approximately one-half of patients develop secondary annular skin lesions similar to erythema migrans but smaller and without central punctae. Debilitating fatigue may accompany myalgias and migratory arthralgias, followed in somewhat more than 50% of patients by a large-joint oligoarthritis. Severe headache and meningismus, cranial neuritis (especially seventh nerve palsy), and peripheral radiculoneuropathy may supervene. Finally, approximately 5% of patients demonstrate cardiac involvement, including conduction abnormalities or, more rarely, pancarditis. These symptoms generally resolve within weeks or months, but they may recur or persist.

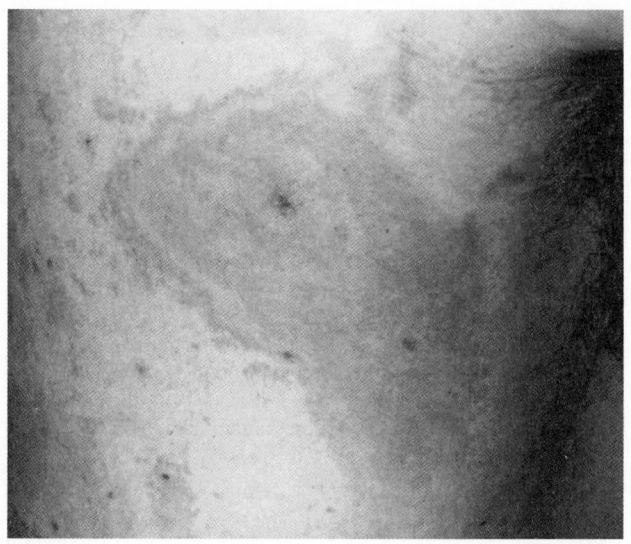

FIGURE 101.15 Primary erythema migrans lesion in Lyme disease. (Courtesy of James Leyden, MD.)

Stage 3 disease is characterized by persistent infection and symptoms of prolonged latency. A scleroderma-like skin rash, acrodermatitis chronica atrophicans, is seen most commonly in Europe. A potentially erosive chronic oligoarthritis may be seen months to years following the tick bite. Subtle neurologic findings, including peripheral neuropathies and organic brain syndromes, may become apparent long after other manifestations of spriochete infestation have resolved.

Particularly in the later states of the infection when the classic erythema migrans rash is not present, the diagnosis of LD requires the clinician to be familiar with its protean manifestations. This is particularly important for the pediatric ED physician because children and adolescents presenting to the ED are less likely to exhibit an erythema migrans rash than those evaluated in a primary care setting. Studies done in an LD-endemic area in Connecticut found that either single or multiple erythema migrans lesions were seen in 89% of LD patients presenting to pediatric practices, whereas only 24% of LD patients presenting to the Yale-New Haven Pediatric Emergency Department exhibited such a rash.

Laboratory Studies

B. burgdorferi is extremely difficult to grow in culture, and spirochetes generally cannot be identified in infected tissues. Diagnosis of LD is therefore made on the basis of characteristic clinical features accompanied by confirmatory serologic markers. Two caveats accompany serologic testing for LD. First, these tests are relatively difficult to perform, and standardization has been difficult to achieve. Many laboratories are plagued by both false-positive and false-negative results, so only experienced reference labs, preferably state or regional centers, should be employed. Second, serologic tests for LD are dependent on the patient's antibody response. Titers may not be measurable until the second month after a tick bite in up to 85% of cases, and they may be abrogated by early antibiotic therapy. Early LD is thus a clinical condition characterized by

a typical EM rash, and serology should not be relied on to confirm the diagnosis.

Current recommendations for testing employ a two-step approach to optimize efficiency and accuracy. Patients are screened using an enzyme immunoassay or immunofluorescent assay. If these are negative, generally no further testing is indicated. Positive results by these methods, however, require confirmation because various viral illnesses and autoimmune conditions may cause false-positive results.

The second level of serologic evaluation involves Western or immune blotting. Any positive or equivocal antibody screening study should be confirmed by demonstrating the presence of at least 5 IgG bands directed against discrete *B. burgdorferi* proteins. This test is not foolproof, and false-positive studies may be seen in the setting of EBV and HIV infections, and in SLE. In addition, up to 10% of residents of endemic regions have positive Lyme titers without evidence of true infection. Consequently, only those with compatible clinical findings and positive serologies should be treated.

Other laboratory data are not specific for LD. Hemoglobin, white blood cell counts, and platelet counts are generally normal. ESR is elevated in approximately 50% of cases. ANA and RF are negative. Serum IgM is elevated in one-third of cases and correlates with the severity and chronicity of illness; IgM cryoglobulins are similarly associated. Immune complexes may be demonstrated in serum and synovial fluid.

In Lyme arthritis, synovial fluid analysis typically reveals elevated leukocyte counts ranging from 2,000 to 100,000 cells per mm^3. Polymorphonuclear leukocytes usually predominate, but LD is one of the few conditions in which a significant number of eosinophils may be identified in the synovial fluid. Total protein is elevated. Synovial biopsy reveals nonspecific synovial hypertrophy and mononuclear cell infiltration. In cases of neuroborreliosis, CSF analysis may reveal a mononuclear pleocytosis ranging from 25 to 500 cells per mm^3. At times, however, CSF may be entirely normal despite the presence of neurologic symptoms; even PCR testing might fail to reveal evidence of borrelial DNA. In such cases, MRI of the brain may be useful, although other causes of the symptoms must also be considered. Suspected involvement of the heart may be confirmed by electrocardiography, which reveals varying degrees of atrioventricular (AV) block and nonspecific ST-T-wave changes in children with Lyme carditis.

Management

General Management

The cornerstone of treatment of LD is antibiotics. Oral antibiotic therapy is beneficial in early stages of the infection, whereas IV medications have a lower failure rate in chronic LD. Late manifestations of LD may represent a host autoimmune response rather than direct effects of the spirochete, but antibiotics may nonetheless be beneficial.

Current treatment guidelines are shown in Table 101.18. Patients with erythema migrans should be treated with 14 to 21 days of doxycycline (100 mg bid). Pregnant women and children younger than the age of 8 years should receive amoxicillin (25 to 50 mg per kg per day, divided bid, maximum 2 g per day). For penicillin-allergic patients, cefuroxime axetil and azithromycin are alternative therapies, although the macrolides

TABLE 101.18

TREATMENT OF LYME DISEASE

Disease stage	Organ system	Treatment
Acute (stage 1)	General malaise, flulike symptoms Skin: erythema migrans	Oral regimens: doxycycline 100 mg bid for 14–21 days Children <8 yr old: amoxicillin 25–50 mg/kg/day divided tid (maximum 2 g/day) for 14–21 days
Chronic (stage 2)	Skin: multiple erythema migrans Neurologic: facial palsy Musculoskeletal: migratory arthralgias and arthritis	Oral regimen as for early disease, but for 21–28 days
Persistent (stage 3)	Skin: acrodermatitis chronica atrophicans Neurologic: meningitis, encephalitis Cardiac: heart block, myocarditis Musculoskeletal: chronic arthritis	Parenteral regimen: ceftriaxone 75–100 mg/kg IV or IM qd (maximum 2 g/day) for 14–28 days, or penicillin 300,000 U/kg/day IV divided q 4 h (maximum 20 million U/day) for 14–28 days

appear to be somewhat less effective. Therapy of early constitutional symptoms is supportive and includes bed rest, analgesics, and antipyretics. As with other spirochetal infections, a Jarisch-Herxheimer reaction may be seen after initial antibiotic therapy.

Management of Complications and Emergencies

Neurologic Complications. The presentation of neuroborreliosis is varied and may be categorized according to duration of infection. Early neurologic involvement, occurring during the first month after exposure, is seen in approximately 15% of untreated patients. Symptoms of aseptic meningitis and encephalitis are most notable, including severe headache, stiff neck, nausea and vomiting, photophobia, lethargy, and poor memory. Kernig and Brudzinski signs are generally negative. Cerebellar ataxia is also reported as a presenting manifestation of pediatric LD.

Facial nerve palsy is the most common cranial neuropathy of early neuroborreliosis. This is most often unilateral, but may be bilateral in up to one-third of cases. Facial nerve involvement due to *B. burgdorferi* must be distinguished from that of viral, autoimmune, and idiopathic Bell palsy, although in endemic regions up to 50% of cases of seventh nerve palsy are because of LD. A retrospective single-center study of patients with peripheral facial palsy presenting to the ED of a tertiary care pediatric center in Massachusetts identified (i) presentation during peak LD season (defined as June through October), (ii) no previous herpetic lesions, (iii) fever, and (iv) headache as independent predictors of LD in this endemic area. Lyme-induced facial nerve symptoms tend to resolve spontaneously, but oral antibiotics are recommended to prevent dissemination and late sequelae. If a lumbar puncture is performed, it will be abnormal in the majority of cases of LD, typically showing a lymphocytic pleocytosis with or without elevated protein. A CSF index, obtained by comparing the ratio of albumin to Lyme antibody levels centrally and peripherally, is currently the most sensitive marker of neuroborreliosis. Evidence of intrathecal production of antiborrelial antibodies may be found in 80% to 90% of patients with Lyme meningoencephalitis and is treated with parenteral ceftriaxone or penicillin for 14 to 21 days. In general, lumbar puncture is not recommended in cases of isolated facial palsy because it

will not facilitate diagnosis, and long-term neuropsychologic outcomes of children with Lyme-induced facial nerve palsies are generally excellent with oral antibiotic therapy.

Some patients may develop late or chronic peripheral neuropathies months or years after infection. These manifest as symmetric or asymmetric paresthesias; radicular pain and muscle weakness are generally less intense than in early neuroborreliosis. Treatment with IV antibiotics, generally for 2 to 4 weeks, usually results in gradual improvement.

Most vexing of the late neurologic sequelae of LD is chronic Lyme encephalopathy. Symptoms are largely nonspecific, including debilitating fatigue, cognitive slowing, memory impairment, sleep disturbances, and depression. Distinction from idiopathic chronic fatigue syndrome or psychiatric conditions is extremely difficult. In cases attributable to LD on the basis of positive serologic markers of borrelial infection in addition to antibody, PCR, or MRI evidence of CNS involvement, symptoms often improve gradually with IV antibiotic therapy. In general, such cases are best cared for by physicians familiar with late LD, not in the ED.

Cardiac Complications. Lyme carditis may present weeks to months after the initial infection in 5% to 10% of untreated children. AV block is the most common manifestation; pericarditis, intraventricular conduction disturbances, and heart failure also may be seen. Patients may be asymptomatic with low-grade AV block, but 50% or more develop higher-grade conduction disturbances accompanied by dyspnea, chest pain, palpitations, dizziness, or syncope. In such cases, physical signs include those of CHF with gallop rhythm, bibasilar crackles, and hepatojugular reflux, or those of pericarditis with friction rub and pulsus paradoxus (greater than 10 mm Hg). The heart rate may be elevated in the face of myocarditis or congestive failure; bradycardia as low as 30 beats per minute can be seen in patients with conduction abnormalities. EKG reveals varying degrees of AV block and ST-T-wave changes. Chest radiographs may reveal cardiomegaly. Echocardiography is useful in documenting small pericardial effusions and ventricular dysfunction.

Treatment decisions are made on the basis of the severity of the carditis. Symptomatic patients or those with high-grade conduction disturbances should be admitted to the hospital for close monitoring with telemetry. This course should also be considered for those with significant prolongation of the PR interval. Placement of a temporary pacemaker may be necessary in patients with complete heart block. There is no evidence that antibiotic therapy speeds recovery from Lyme carditis, but these agents are nonetheless employed to eradicate infection and prevent additional complications. Oral antibiotics are used in early or mild cases, while IV regimens are indicated for more severe or chronic disease. Antiinflammatory therapy with either aspirin (80 to 100 mg per kg per day) or occasionally prednisone (1 to 2 mg per kg per day) is recommended in cases of cardiomegaly, high-grade heart block, or markedly prolonged PR interval (more than 300 milliseconds) due to LD. The prognosis of all forms of cardiac involvement is excellent, with very few patients left with chronic sequelae.

Arthritis. Lyme arthritis occurs in more than 50% of untreated children, making it the most common late manifestation of borrelial infection. The classic presentation is a pattern of intermittent episodes of joint swelling beginning weeks to months after exposure. Approximately one-third of children develop an acute arthritis indistinguishable from bacterial infection, with joint pain, swelling, and erythema accompanied by fever. This presentation can be particularly vexing for the ED physician who must make a fairly immediate decision regarding the possibility of a septic joint. A small study focusing on the knee from a pediatric center in a Lyme endemic area suggests that MRI may be helpful in distinguishing between septic arthritis and LD; the presence of myositis and lymphadenopathy, and lack of subcutaneous edema, were statistically more common in LD than in septic arthritis.

Alternatively, synovitis might be migratory, simulating serum sickness or a postinfectious process, or chronic and persistent as in JRA. There is a propensity for large joint involvement, and often there is relatively little discomfort for the degree of swelling. The knee is affected in approximately 90% of cases, whereas more than two joints, or joints other than the knee, hip, ankle, or wrist, are involved in fewer than 2% of cases.

Lyme arthritis is clinically indistinguishable from JRA, septic arthritis, and postinfectious reactive synovitis, and it should be diagnosed only in the presence of convincing serologic evidence of borrelial infection. Current guidelines recommend initial treatment with oral antibiotics. Joint symptoms may only gradually improve over several weeks, but if joint pain and swelling persist for more than 2 months despite treatment, patients should be changed to IV therapy. Adjunct treatment with NSAIDs and physical therapy are important means of minimizing disability and accelerating recovery from Lyme arthritis. However, a small minority of patients develop a chronic inflammatory arthritis that must be treated in the same way as JRA.

Suggested Readings

Juvenile Rheumatoid Arthritis

Adams A, Lehman TJA. Update on the pathogenesis and treatment of systemic onset juvenile rheumatoid arthritis. *Curr Opin Rheumatol* 2005;17: 612–616.

Athreya BH, Doughty RA, Bookspan M, et al. Pulmonary manifestations of juvenile rheumatoid arthritis. A report of 8 cases and review. *Clin Chest Med* 1980;1:361–374.

Bland JH. Rheumatoid arthritis of the cervical spine. *J Rheumatol* 1974;1: 319–341.

Bray VJ, Singleton JD. Disseminated intravascular coagulation in Still's disease. *Semin Arthritis Rheum* 1994;24:222–229.

Cassidy JT, Petty RE. Juvenile rheumatoid arthritis. In: *Textbook of pediatric rheumatology*. 3rd ed. Philadelphia: WB Saunders, 1995.

Cron RQ, Sherry DD, Wallace CA. Methotrexate-induced hypersensitivity pneumonitis in a child with juvenile rheumatoid arthritis. *J Pediatr* 1998; 132:901–902.

Cunnane G, Doran M, Bresnihan B. Infections and biological therapy in rheumatoid arthritis. *Best Pract Res Clin Rheumatol* 2003;17:345–363.

De Silva B, Banney L, Uttley W, et al. Psuedoporphyria and nonsteroidal antiinflammatory agents in children with juvenile idiopathic arthritis. *Pediatr Dermatol* 2000;17:480–483.

Duffy CM, Colbert RA, Laxer RM, et al. Nomenclature and classification in chronic childhood arthritis. Time for a change? *Arthritis Rheum* 2005;52: 382–385.

FDA Consumer. Celebrex approved for juvenile arthritis. 2007;41:3.

Hashkes PJ, Laxer RM. Update on the medical treatment of juvenile idiopathic arthritis. *Curr Rheumatol Rep* 2006;8:450–458.

Ilowite NT. Current treatment of juvenile rheumatoid arthritis. *Pediatrics* 2002;109:109–115.

Ilowite NT. Update on biologics in juvenile idiopathic arthritis. *Curr Opin Rheumatol* 2008;20:613–618.

Jacobs JC, Hui RM. Cricoarytenoid arthritis and airway obstruction in juvenile rheumatoid arthritis. *Pediatrics* 1977;59:292–294.

Keenan GF, Giannini EH, Athreya BH. Clinically significant gastropathy associated with nonsteroidal antiinflammatory drug use in children with juvenile rheumatoid arthritis. *J Rheumatol* 1995;22:1149–1151.

Kelly A, Ramanan AV. Recognition and management of macrophage activation syndrome in juvenile arthritis. *Curr Opin Rheumatol* 2007;19:477–481.

Lee J, Slifman NR, Gershon SK, et al. Life-threatening histoplasmosis complicating immunotherapy with tumor necrosis factor alpha antagonists infliximab and etanercept. *Arthritis Rheum* 2002;46:2565–2570.

Lindsley CB. Uses of nonsteroidal anti-inflammatory drugs in pediatrics. *Am J Dis Child* 1993;147:229–236.

Lovell DJ, Reiff A, Ilowite NT, et al. Safety and efficacy of up to eight years of continuous etanercept therapy in patients with juvenile rheumatoid arthritis. *Arthritis Rheum* 2008;58:1496–1504.

Lovell DJ, Ruperto N, Goodman S, et al. Adalimumab with or without methotrexate in juvenile rheumatoid arthritis. *N Engl J Med* 2008;359:810–820.

Martinez-Cordero E, Orozco Barocio G, Martinez Miranda E. Evaluation of disease activity by laboratory tests in juvenile rheumatoid arthritis. *J Investig Allergol Clin Immunol* 1995;5:216–220.

Mouy R, Stephan JL, Pillet P, et al. Efficacy of cyclosporine A in the treatment of macrophage activation syndrome in juvenile arthritis: report of five cases. *J Pediatr* 1996;129:750–754.

Murray K, Thompson SD, Glass DN. Pathogenesis of juvenile chronic arthritis: genetic and environmental factors. *Arch Dis Child* 1997;77:530–534.

Padeh S, Passwell JH. Intraarticular corticosteroid injection in the management of children with chronic arthritis. *Arthritis Rheum* 1998;41:1210–1214.

Ramanan AV, Whitworth P, Baildam EM. Use of methotrexate in juvenile idiopathic arthritis. *Arch Dis Child* 2003;88:197–200.

Ruperto N, Lovell DJ, Cuttica R, et al. A randomized, placebo-controlled trial of infliximab plus methotrexate for the treatment of polyarticular-course juvenile rheumatoid arthritis. *Arthritis Rheum* 2007;56:3096–3106.

Ruperto N, Lovell DJ, Quartier P, et al. Abatacept in children with juvenile idiopathic arthritis: a randomized, double-blind, placebo-controlled withdrawal trial. *Lancet* 2008;372:383–391.

Schneider R, Passo MH. Juvenile rheumatoid arthritis. *Rheum Dis Clin North Am* 2002;28:503–530.

Van Rossum MA, Fiselier TJ, Franssen MJ, et al. Sulfasalazine in the treatment of juvenile chronic arthritis: a randomized, double-blind, placebo-controlled, multicenter study. *Arthritis Rheum* 1998;41:808–816.

Yancey CL, Doughty RA, Cohlan BA, et al. Pericarditis and cardiac tamponade in juvenile rheumatoid arthritis. *Pediatrics* 1981;68:369–373.

Systemic Lupus Erythematosus

Ardoin SP, Sandborg C, Schanberg LE. Management of dyslipidemia in children and adolescents with systemic lupus erythematosus. *Lupus* 2007;16:618–626.

Avcin T, Silverman ED. Antiphospholipid antibodies in pediatric systemic lupus erythematosus and the antiphospholipid syndrome. *Lupus* 2007;16:627–633.

Benseler SM, Silverman ED. Neuropsychiatric involvement in pediatric systemic lupus erythematosus. *Lupus* 2007;16:564–571.

Brunner HI, Silverman ED, To T, et al. Risk factors for damage in childhood-onset systemic lupus erythematosus. *Arthritis Rheum* 2002;46:436–444.

Buratti S, Szer IS, Spencer CH, et al. Mycophenolate mofetil treatment of severe renal disease in pediatric onset systemic lupus erythematosus. *J Rheumatol* 2001;28:2103–2108.

Caramaschi P, Riccetti MM, Pasini AF, et al. Systemic lupus erythematosus and thrombotic thrombocytopenic purpura. Report of three cases and review of the literature. *Lupus* 1998;7:37–41.

MEDICAL EMERGENCIES

Carreno L, Lopez-Longo FJ, Gonzalez CM, et al. Treatment options for juvenile-onset systemic lupus erythematosus. *Pediatr Drugs* 2002;4:241–256.

Carreno L, Lopez-Longo FJ, Monteagudo I, et al. Immunological and clinical differences between juvenile and adult onset of systemic lupus erythematosus. *Lupus* 1999;8:287–292.

Connolly B, Manson D, Eberhard A, et al. CT appearance of pulmonary vasculitis in children. *AJR Am J Roentgenol* 1996;167:901–904.

Esdaile JM, Abrahamowicz M, Joseph L, et al. Laboratory tests as predictors of disease exacerbations in systemic lupus erythematosus. Why some tests fail. *Arthritis Rheum* 1996;39:370–378.

Friedman DM, Lazarus HM, Fierman AH. Acute myocardial infarction in pediatric systemic lupus erythematosus. *J Pediatr* 1990;117:263–266.

Green L, Vinker S, Amital H, et al. Pseudotumor cerebri in systemic lupus erythematosus. *Semin Arthritis Rheum* 1995;25:103–108.

Hiraki LT, Benseler SM, Tyrrell PN, et al. Clinical and laboratory characteristics and long-term outcome of pediatric systemic lupus erythematosus: a longitudinal study. *J Pediatr* 2008;152:550–556.

Hoch S, Schur PH. Methylprednisolone pulse therapy for lupus nephritis: a follow-up study. *Clin Exp Rheumatol* 1984;2:313–320.

Iqbal S, Sher MR, Good RA, et al. Diversity in presenting manifestations of systemic lupus erythematosus in children. *J Pediatr* 1999;135:500–505.

Klein-Gitelman M, Reiff A, Silverman ED. Systemic lupus erythematosus in childhood. *Rheum Dis Clin North Am* 2002;28:561–577.

Lacks S, White P. Morbidity associated with childhood systemic lupus erythematosus. *J Rheumatol* 1990;17:941–945.

Lee T, von Scheven E, Sandborg C. Systemic lupus erythematosus and antiphospholipid syndrome in children and adolescents. *Curr Opin Rheumatol* 2001;13:415–421.

Lehman TJ, Sherry DD, Wagner-Weiner L, et al. Intermittent intravenous cyclophosphamide therapy for lupus nephritis. *J Pediatr* 1989;114:1055–1060.

MacDermott EJ, Adams A, Lehman TJA. Systemic lupus erythematosus in children: current and emerging therapies. *Lupus* 2007;16:677–683.

McCune WJ, Golbus J, Zeldes W, et al. Clinical and immunologic effects of monthly administration of intravenous cyclophosphamide in severe systemic lupus erythematosus. *N Engl J Med* 1988;318:1423–1431.

Mok CC, Lau CS, Chan EY, et al. Acute transverse myelopathy in systemic lupus erythematosus: clinical presentation, treatment, and outcome. *J Rheumatol* 1998;25:467–473.

Parikh S, Swaiman KF, Kim Y. Neurologic characteristics of childhood lupus erythematosus. *Pediatr Neurol* 1995;13:198–201.

Platt JL, Burke BA, Fish AJ, et al. Systemic lupus erythematosus in the first two decades of life. *Am J Kidney Dis* 1982;2:212–222.

Ranchin B, Fargue S. New treatment strategies for proliferative lupus nephritis: keep children in mind! *Lupus* 2007;16:684–691.

Ravelli A, Martini A. Antiphospholipid antibody syndrome in pediatric patients. *Rheum Dis Clin North Am* 1997;23:657–676.

Roldan CA, Shively BK, Crawford MH. An echocardiographic study of valvular heart disease associated with systemic lupus erythematosus. *N Engl J Med* 1996;335:1424–1430.

Saab S, Corr MP, Weisman MH. Corticosteroids and systemic lupus erythematosus pancreatitis: a case series. *J Rheumatol* 1998;25:801–806.

Sibbitt WL, Brandt JR, Johnson CR, et al. The incidence and prevalence of neuropsychiatric syndromes in pediatric onset systemic lupus erythematosus. *J Rheumatol* 2002;29:1536–1542.

Silverman ED, Lang B. An overview of the treatment of childhood SLE *Scand J Rheumatol* 1997;26:241–246.

Stahl NI, Klippel JH, Decker JL. Fever in systemic lupus erythematosus. *Am J Med* 1979;67:935–940.

Tucker LB, Uribe AG, Fernandez M, et al. Adolescent onset of lupus restuls in more aggressive disease and worse outcomes: results of a nested matched case control study within LUMINA, a multiethnic US cohort (LUMINA LVII). *Lupus* 2008;17:314–322.

Uziel Y, Laxer RM, Silverman ED. Persistent pulmonary hemorrhage as the sole initial clinical manifestation of pediatric systemic lupus erythematosus. *Clin Exp Rheumatol* 1997;15:697–700.

Ward MM, Pyun E, Studenski S. Causes of death in systemic lupus erythematosus. Long-term follow up of an inception cohort. *Arthritis Rheum* 1995;38:1492–1499.

Yell JA, Mbuagbaw J, Burge SM. Cutaneous manifestations of systemic lupus erythematosus. *Br J Dermatol* 1996;135:355–362.

Dermatomyositis

Banker BQ, Victor M. Dermatomyositis (systemic angiopathy) of childhood. *Medicine (Baltimore)* 1966;45:261–289.

Bohan A, Peter JB. Polymyositis and dermatomyositis. *N Engl J Med* 1975;292:344–347, 403–407.

Bowyer SL, Blane CE, Sullivan DB, et al. Childhood dermatomyositis: factors predicting functional outcome and development of dystrophic calcification. *J Pediatr* 1983;103:882–888.

Cooper MA, Willingham DL, Brown DE, et al. Rituximab for the treatment of juvenile dermatomyositis. A report of four pediatric patients. *Arthritis Rheum* 2007;56:3107–3111.

Crowe WE, Bove KE, Levinson JE, et al. Clinical and pathogenetic implications of histopathology in childhood polydermatomyositis. *Arthritis Rheum* 1982;25:126–139.

Fisler RE, Liang MG, Fuhlbrigge RC, et al. Aggressive management of juvenile dermatomyositis results in improved outcome and decreased incidence of calcinosis. *J Am Acad Dermatol* 2002;47:505–511.

Gonzalez-Lopez L, Gamez-Nava JI, Sanchez L, et al. Cardiac manifestations in dermato-polymyositis. *Clin Exp Rheumatol* 1996;14:373–379.

Huber A, Feldman BM. Long-term outcomes in juvenile dermatomyositis: How did we get here and where are we going? *Curr Rheumatol Rep* 2005;7:441–446.

Huemer C, Kitson H, Malleson PN, et al. Lipodystrophy in patients with juvenile dermatomyositis—evaluation of clinical and metabolic abnormalities. *J Rheumatol* 2001;28:610–615.

Kim S, El-Hallak M, Dedeoglu F, et al. Complete and sustained remission of juvenile dermatomyositis resulting from aggressive treatment. *Arthritis Rheum* 2009;60:1825–1830.

Laxer RM, Stein LD, Petty RE. Intravenous pulse methylprednisolone treatment of juvenile dermatomyositis. *Arthritis Rheum* 1987;30:328–334.

Magill HL, Hixson SD, Whitington G, et al. Duodenal perforation in childhood dermatomyositis. *Pediatr Radiol* 1984;14:28–30.

Mamyrova G, Kleiner DE, James-Newton L, et al. Late-onset gastrointestinal pain in juvenile dermatomyositis as a manifestation of ischemic ulceration from chronic endarteropathy. *Arthritis Rheum* 2007;57:881–884.

Mendez EP, Lipton R, Ramsey-Goldman R, et al. US incidence of juvenile dermatomyositis, 1995–1998: results from the National Institute of Arthritis and Musculoskeletal and Skin Diseases Registry. *Arthritis Rheum* 2003;49:300–305.

Mitchell JP, Dennis GJ, Rider LG. Juvenile dermatomyositis presenting with anasarca: a possible indicator of severe disease activity. *J Pediatr* 2001;138:942–945.

Pachman LM. Juvenile dermatomyositis: immunogenetics, pathophysiology, and disease expression. *Rheum Dis Clin North Am* 2002;28:579–602.

Pachman LM, Hayford JR, Hochberg MC, et al. New-onset juvenile dermatomyositis: comparisons with a healthy cohort and children with juvenile rheumatoid arthritis. *Arthritis Rheum* 1997;40:1526–1533.

Ramanan AV, Campbell-Webster N, Ota S, et al. The effectiveness of treating juvenile dermatomyositis with methotrexate and aggressively tapered corticosteroids. *Arthritis Rheum* 2005;52:3570–3578.

Ramanan AV, Feldman BM. Clinical features and outcomes of juvenile dermatomyositis and other childhood onset myositis syndromes. *Rheum Dis Clin North Am* 2002;28:833–857.

Rider LG, Miller FW. Classification and treatment of the juvenile idiopathic inflammatory myopathies. *Rheum Dis Clin North Am* 1997;23:619–655.

Riley P, Maillard SM, Wedderburn LR, et al. Intravenous cyclophosphamide pulse therapy in juvenile dermatomyositis. A review of efficacy and safety. *Rheumatology(Oxford)* 2004;43:491–496.

Riley P, McCann LJ, Maillard SM, et al. Effectiveness of infliximab in the treatment of refractory juvenile dermatomyositis with calcinosis. *Rheumatology(Oxford)* 2008;47:877–880.

Rouster-Stevens KA, Gursahaney A, Ngai K, et al. Pharmacokinetic study of oral prednisolone compared with intravenous methylprednisolone in patients with juvenile dermatomyositis. *Arthritis Rheum* 2008;59:222–226.

Singsen BH, Tedford JC, Platzker ACG, et al. Spontaneous pneumothorax: a complication of juvenile dermatomyositis. *J Pediatr* 1978;92:771–774.

Tse S, Lubelsky S, Gordon M, et al. The arthritis of inflammatory childhood myositis syndromes. *J Rheumatol* 2001;28:192–197.

Zeller V, Cohen P, Prieur AM, et al. Cyclosporin A therapy in refractory juvenile dermatomyositis. Experience and long-term follow-up of 6 cases. *J Rheumatol* 1996;23:1424–1427.

Zulian F, Toldeo MMM, Amigoni A, et al. Successful use of extracorporeal membrane oxygenation for severe interstitial lung disease in a child with dermatomyositis. *Intensive Care Med* 2007;33:1663–1666.

Vasculitis/Polyarteritis Nodosa

Besbas N, Ozen S, Saatci U, et al. Renal involvement in polyarteritis nodosa: evaluation of 26 Turkish children. *Pediatr Nephrol* 2000;14:325–327.

Blau EB, Morris RF, Yunis EJ. Polyarteritis nodosa in older children. *Pediatrics* 1977;60:227–234.

Brogan PA, Davies R, Gordon I, et al. Renal angiography in children with polyarteritis nodosa. *Pediatr Nephrol* 2002;17:277–283.

Camilleri M, Pusey CD, Chadwick VS, et al. Gastrointestinal manifestations of systemic vasculitis. *Q J Med* 1983;52:141–149.

Chalopin JM, Rifle G, Turc JM, et al. Immunological findings during successful treatment of HBs-Ag-associated polyarteritis nodosa by plasmapheresis. *Br Med J* 1980;280:368.

Cheung YF, Brogan PA, Pilla CB, et al. Arterial distensibility in children and teenagers: normal evolution and the effect of childhood vasculitis. *Arch Dis Child* 2002;87:348–351.

Dahlberg PJ, Lockhart JM, Overholt EL. Diagnostic studies for systemic necrotizing vasculitis. Sensitivity, specificity, and predictive value in patients with multisystem disease. *Arch Intern Med* 1989;149:161–165.

Chapter 101: Rheumatologic Emergencies **1169**

Dedeoglu F, Sundel RP. Vasculitis in Children. *Pediatr Clin North Am* 2005; 52:547–575.

Dillon MJ. Rare vasculitic syndromes. *Ann Med* 1997;29:175–179.

Fauci AS, Doppman JL, Wolff SM. Cyclophosphamide-induced remissions in advanced polyarteritis nodosa. *Am J Med* 1978;64:890–894.

Fink CW. Vasculitis. *Pediatr Clin North Am* 1986;33:1203–1219.

Gillespie DN, Burke EC, Holley KE. Polyarteritis nodosa in infancy: a diagnostic enigma. *Mayo Clin Proc* 1973;48:773–775.

Gunal N, Kara N, Cakar N, et al. Cardiac involvement in childhood polyarteritis nodosa. *Int J Cardiol* 1997;60:257–262.

Magilavy DB, Petty RE, Cassidy JT, et al. A syndrome of childhood polyarteritis. *J Pediatr* 1977;91:25–30.

Moore PM, Cupps TR. Neurological complications of vasculitis. *Ann Neurol* 1983;14:155–167.

Ozen S, Anton J, Arisoy N, et al. Juvenile polyarteritis: results of a multicenter survey of 110 children. *J Pediatr* 2004:145:517–522.

Reimold EW, Weinberg AG, Fink CW, et al. Polyarteritis in children. *Am J Dis Child* 1976;130:534–541.

Sack M, Cassidy JT, Bole GG. Prognostic factors in polyarteritis. *J Rheumatol* 1975;2:411–420.

Smoller BR, McNutt NS, Contreras F. The natural history of vasculitis. What the histology tells us about pathogenesis. *Arch Dermatol* 1990;126:84–89.

Sundel R, Szer I. Vasculitis in childhood. *Rheum Dis Clin North Am* 2002; 28:625–654.

Ting TV, Hashkes PJ. Update on childhood vasculitides. *Curr Opin Rheumatol* 2004;16:560–565.

Uziel Y, Silverman ED. Intravenous immunoglobulin therapy in a child with cutaneous polyarteritis nodosa. *Clin Exp Rheumatol* 1998;16:187–189.

Kawasaki Disease

Barron KS. Kawasaki disease: etiology, pathogenesis, and treatment. *Cleve Clin J Med* 2002;69:SII69–SII78.

Beiser AS, Takahashi M, Baker AL, et al. A predictive instrument for coronary artery aneurysms in Kawasaki disease. US Multicenter Kawasaki Disease Study Group. *Am J Cardiol* 1998;81:1116–1120.

Burns JC, Mason WH, Glode MP, et al. Clinical and epidemiologic characteristics of patients referred for evaluation of possible Kawasaki disease. US Multicenter Kawasaki Disease Study Group *J Pediatr* 1991;118:680–686.

Centers for Disease Control and Prevention (CDC). Outbreak of hepatitis C associated with intravenous immunoglobulin administration—United States, October 1993–June 1994. *MMWR Morb Mortal Wkly Rep* 1994; 43:505–509.

Dengler LD, Capparelli EV, Bastian JF, et al. Cerebrospinal fluid profile in patients with acute Kawasaki disease. *Pediatr Infect Dis J* 1998;17: 478–481.

Durongpisitkul K, Gururaj VJ, Park JM, et al. The prevention of coronary artery aneurysm in Kawasaki disease: a meta-analysis on the efficacy of aspirin and immunoglobulin treatment. *Pediatrics* 1995;96:1057–1061.

Fujiwara H, Hamashima Y. Pathology of the heart in Kawasaki disease. *Pediatrics* 1978;61:100–107.

Fukushige J, Takahashi N, Ueda Y, et al. Incidence and clinical features of incomplete Kawasaki disease. *Acta Paediatr* 1994;83:1057–1060.

Fukushige J, Takahashi N, Ueda K, et al. Long-term outcome of coronary abnormalities in patients after Kawasaki disease. *Pediatr Cardiol* 1996;17:71–76.

Holman RC, Curns AT, Belay ED, et al. Kawasaki syndrome hospitalizations in the United States, 1997 and 2000. *Pediatrics* 2003;112:495–501.

Horrigome H, Sekijima T, Miyamoto T. Successful thrombolysis with intracoronary administration of tissue plasminogen activator in an infant with Kawasaki disease. *Heart* 1997;78:517–518.

Kato H, Sugimua T, Akagi T, et al. Long-term consequences of Kawasaki disease. A 10- to 21-year follow up study of 594 patients. *Circulation* 1996;94:1379–1385.

Kawasaki T, Kosaki F, Okawa S, et al. A new infantile acute febrile mucocutaneous lymph node syndrome (MLNS) prevailing in Japan. *Pediatrics* 1974;54:271–276.

Levy M, Koren G. Atypical Kawasaki disease: analysis of clinical presentation and diagnostic clues. *Pediatr Infect Dis J* 1990;9:122–126.

Nakamura Y, Yanagawa H, Harada K, et al. Mortality among persons with a history of Kawasaki disease in Japan: the fifth look. *Arch Pediatr Adolesc Med* 2002;156:162–165.

Naoe S, Takahashi K, Masuda H, et al. Kawasaki disease with particular emphasis on arterial lesions. *Acta Pathol Jpn* 1991;41:785–797.

Newburger JW, Sanders SP, Burns JC, et al. Left ventricular contractility and function in Kawasaki syndrome. *Circulation* 1989;79:1237–1246.

Newburger JW, Sleeper LA, McCrindle BW, et al. Randomized trial of pulsed corticosteroid therapy for primary treatment of Kawasaki disease. *N Engl J Med* 2007;356:663–675.

Newburger JW, Takahashi M, Beiser AS, et al. A single intravenous infusion of gamma globulin as compared with four infusions in the treatment of acute Kawasaki syndrome. *N Engl J Med* 1991;324:1633–1639.

Newburger JW, Takahashi M, Burns JC, et al. The treatment of Kawasaki syndrome with intravenous gamma globulin. *N Engl J Med* 1986;315:341–347.

Newburger JW, Takahashi M, Gerber MA, et al. Diagnosis, treatment, and long-term management of Kawasaki disease: a statement for health professionals from the Committee on Rheumatic fever, Endocarditis, and Kawasaki disease, Council on Cardiovascular Disease in Young, American Heart Association. *Pediatrics* 2004;114:1708–1733.

Rosenfeld EA, Corydon KE, Shulman ST. Kawasaki disease in infants less than one year of age. *J Pediatr* 1995;126:524–529.

Smith LB, Newburger JW, Burns JC. Kawasaki syndrome and the eye. *Pediatr Infect Dis J* 1989;8:116–118.

Stockheim JA, Innocentini N, Shulman ST. Kawasaki disease in older children and adolescents. *J Pediatr* 2000;137:250–252.

Sundel RP. Update on the treatment of Kawasaki disease in childhood. *Curr Rheumatol Rep* 2002;4:474–482.

Sundel RP, Baker AL, Fulton DR, et al. Corticosteroids in the initial treatment of Kawasaki disease: report of a randomized trial. *J Pediatr* 2003;142: 611–616.

Von Planta M, Fasnacht M, Holm C, et al. Atypical Kawasaki disease with peripheral gangrene and myocardial infarction: therapeutic implications. *Eur J Pediatr* 1995;154:830–834.

Zulian F, Falcini F, Zancan L, et al. Acute surgical abdomen as presenting manifestation of Kawasaki disease. *J Pediatr* 2003;142:731–735.

Behçet Disease

Eldem B, Onur C, Ozen S. Clinical features of pediatric Behçet's disease. *J Pediatr Ophthalmol Strabismus* 1998;35:159–161.

Kone-Paut I, Yurdakul S, Bababri SA, et al. Clinical features of Behçet's disease in children: an international collaborative study of 86 cases. *J Pediatr* 1998;132:721–725.

Krause I and Weinberger A. Behçet's disease. *Curr Opin Rheumatol* 2008;20: 82–87.

Sakane T, Takeno M, Suzuki N, et al. Behçet's disease. *N Engl J Med* 1999; 341:1284–1291.

Sfikakis PP, Markomichelakis N, Alpsoy E, et al. Anti-TNF therapy in the management of Behcet's disease—review and basis for recommendations. *Rheumatology(Oxford)* 2007;46:736–741.

Uziel Y, Brik R, Padeh S, et al. Juvenile Behçet's disease in Israel. *Clin Exp Rheumatol* 1998;16:502–505.

Yazici H, Yurdakul S, Hamuryudan V. Behçet's Syndrome. *Curr Opin Rheumatol* 2001;13:18–22.

Scleroderma

Alstaedt HO, Berzewski B, Breddin HK, et al. Treatment of patients with peripheral arterial occlusive disease Fontaine stage IV with intravenous iloprost and PGE1: a randomized open controlled study. *Prostaglandins Leukot Essent Fatty Acids* 1993;49:573–578.

Armstrong GP, Whalley GA, Doughty RN, et al. Left ventricular function in scleroderma. *Br J Rheumatol* 1996;35:983–988.

Athreya BH. Juvenile scleroderma. *Curr Opin Rheumatol* 2002;14:553–561.

Condliffe R, Kiely DG, Peacock AJ, et al. Connective tissue disease-associated pulmonary arterial hypertension in the modern treatment era. *Am J Respir Crit Care Med* 2009;179:151–157.

Denton CP, Humbert M, Rubin L, et al. Bosentan treatment for pulmonary arterial hypertension related to connective tissue disease: a subgroup analysis of the pivotal clinical trials and their open-label extensions. *Ann Rheum Dis* 2006;65:1336–1340.

Fine LG. Systemic sclerosis: current pathogenetic concepts and future prospects for targeted therapy. *Lancet* 1996;347:1453–1458.

Foeldvari I. Update on pediatric systemic sclerosis: similarities and differences from adult disease. *Curr Opin Rheumatol* 2008;20:608–612.

Fujita Y, Yamamori H, Hiyoshi K, et al. Systemic sclerosis in children: a national retrospective surgery in Japan. *Acta Paediatr Jpn* 1997;39:263–267.

Garty BZ, Athreya BH, Wilmott R, et al. Pulmonary functions in children with progressive systemic sclerosis. *Pediatrics* 1991;88:1161–1167.

Haber PL. Clinical manifestations of scleroderma. *Pediatr Rev* 1995;16:49.

Harrison NK, Glanville AR, Strickland B, et al. Pulmonary involvement in systemic sclerosis: the detection of early changes by thin section CT scan, bronchoalveolar lavage and 99mTc-DTPA clearance. *Respir Med* 1989;83: 403–414.

Harrison NK, Myers AR, Corrin B, et al. Structural features of interstitial lung disease in systemic sclerosis. *Am Rev Respir Dis* 1991;144:706–713.

Laxer RM, Zulian F. Localized scleroderma. *Curr Opin Rheumatol* 2006;18: 606–613.

Martini G, Foeldvari I, Russo R, et al. Systemic sclerosis in childhood. Clinical and immunologic features of 153 patients in an international database. *Arthritis Rheum* 2006;54:3971–3978.

Mayorunjk FJ, McCurley TL, Levernier JE, et al. Progression of childhood linear scleroderma to fatal systemic sclerosis. *J Rheumatol* 1994;21:1955–1957.

Medsger TA Jr, Steen V. Systemic sclerosis and related syndromes. In: Schumacher HR, ed. *Primer on the rheumatic diseases.* 10th ed. Atlanta: Arthritis Foundation, 1993.

Murray KJ, Laxer RM. Scleroderma in children and adolescents. *Rheum Dis Clin North Am* 2002;28:603–624.

Roberts NK, Cabeen WR, Moss J, et al. The prevalence of conduction defects and cardiac arrhythmias in progressive systemic sclerosis. *Ann Intern Med* 1981;94:38–40.

Rodeheffer RJ, Rommer JA, Wigley F, et al. Controlled double-blind trial of nifedipine in the treatment of Raynaud's phenomenon. *N Engl J Med* 1983;308:880–883.

Seely JM, Jones LT, Wallace C, et al. Systemic sclerosis: using high resolution CT to detect lung disease in children. *AJR Am J Roentgenol* 1998;170: 691–697.

Sjogren RW. Gastrointestinal motility disorders in scleroderma. *Arthritis Rheum* 1994;37:1265–1282.

Steen VD, Costantino JP, Shapiro AP, et al. Outcome of renal crisis in systemic sclerosis: relation to the availability of angiotensin converting enzyme (ACE) inhibitors. *Ann Intern Med* 1990;113:352–357.

Teasdall RD, Frayha RA, Shulman LE. Cranial nerve involvement in systemic sclerosis (scleroderma): a report of 10 cases. *Medicine(Baltimore)* 1980;59: 149–159.

Uziel Y, Feldman BM, Krafchik BR, et al. Methotrexate and corticosteroid therapy for pediatric localized scleroderma. *J Pediatr* 2000;136:91–95.

Vancheeswaran R, Black CM, David J, et al. Childhood-onset scleroderma: is it different from adult-onset disease? *Arthritis Rheum* 1996;39:1041–1049.

Zulian F, Vallongo C, Woo P, et al. Localized scleroderma in childhood is not just a skin disease. *Arthritis Rheum* 2005;52:2873–2881.

Lyme Disease

Afzelius A. Erythema chronicum migrans. *Acta Derm Venerol* 1921;2:120–125.

Albisetti M, Schaer G, Good M, et al. Diagnostic value of cerebrospinal fluid examination in children with peripheral facial palsy and suspected Lyme borreliosis. *Neurology* 1997;49:817–824.

American Academy of Pediatrics. Lyme disease. In: Pickering LK, ed. *Red book: 2006 report of the Committee on Infectious Diseases*. 27th ed. Elk Grove Village, IL: American Academy of Pediatrics, 2006:428–433.

Athreya BH, Rose CD. Lyme disease. *Curr Probl Pediatr* 1996;26:189–207.

Bannworth A. Zur Klinik und pathogenese der "chronischen lymphozytaren Meningitis." *Arch Psychiatr Nervenkr* 1944;117:161–185.

Centers for Disease Control and Prevention. Surveillance for Lyme Disease— United States, 1992–2006. *MMWR Surveill Summ* 2008;57:1–9.

Coyle PK, Schutzer SE. Neurologic aspects of Lyme disease. *Med Clin North Am* 2002;86:261–284.

Dattwyler RJ, Halperin JJ, Volkman DJ, et al. Treatment of late Lyme borreliosis—randomised comparison of ceftriaxone and penicillin. *Lancet* 1988;1:1191–1194.

Dedeoglu F, Sundel RP. Emergency department management of Lyme disease. *Clin Pediatr Emerg Med* 2004;5:54–62.

Ecklund K, Vargas S, Zurakowski D, et al. MRI Features of Lyme Arthritis in Children. *AJR Am J Roentgenol* 2005;184:1904–1909.

Gerber MA, Shapiro ED. Diagnosis of Lyme disease in children. *J Pediatr* 1992;121:157–162.

Gerber MA, Zemel LS, Shapiro ED. Lyme arthritis in children: clinical epidemiology and long-term outcomes. *Pediatrics* 1998;102:905–908.

Kaplan RF, Jones-Woodward L. Lyme encephalopathy: a neuropsychological perspective. *Semin Neurol* 1997;17:31–37.

Klempner MS, Nu L, Evans J, et al. Two controlled trials of antibiotic treatment in patients with persistent Lyme disease. *N Engl J Med* 2001;345:85–92.

Nigrovic LE, Thompson AD, Fine AM, et al. Clinical predictors of Lyme disease among children with a peripheral facial palsy at an emergency department in a Lyme disease endemic area. *Pediatrics* 2008;122:e1080–e1085.

Pinto DS. Cardiac manifestations of Lyme disease. *Med Clin North Am* 2002;86:285–296.

Seltzer EG, Gerber MA, Cartter ML, et al. Long-term outcome of persons with Lyme disease. *JAMA* 2000;283:609–616.

Sigal LH. Lyme arthritis: lessons learned and to be learned. *Arthritis Rheum* 1999;42:1809–1812.

Steere AC. Lyme disease. *N Engl J Med* 2001;345:115–125.

Steere AC, Malawista SE, Snydman DR, et al. Lyme arthritis: an epidemic of oligoarticular arthritis in children and adults in three connecticut communities. *Arthritis Rheum* 1977;20:7–17.

Vazquez M, Sparrow SS, Shapiro ED. Long-term neuropsychologic and health outcomes of children with facial nerve palsy attributable to Lyme disease. *Pediatrics* 2003;112:e93–e97.

Williams CL, Strobino B, Lee A, et al. Lyme disease in childhood: clinical and epidemiologic features of ninety cases. *Pediatr Infect Dis J* 1990;9:10–14.

Willis AA, Widmann RF, Flynn JM, et al. Lyme arthritis presenting as acute septic arthritis in children. *J Pediatr Orthop* 2003;23:114–118.

CHAPTER 102 ■ TOXICOLOGIC EMERGENCIES

KEVIN C. OSTERHOUDT, MD, MS, MICHELE BURNS EWALD, MD, MICHAEL SHANNON, MD, MPH, AND FRED M. HENRETIG, MD

POISONED CHILD

Poisoning represents one of the most common medical emergencies encountered by young children and accounts for a significant fraction of emergency department (ED) visits in the adolescent population.

Estimates of poisoning episodes annually in the United States range in the millions. Poisonings may be unintentional or intentional. Unintentional or exploratory exposures to poisons make up 80% to 85% or more of all reports, whereas intentional poisonings comprise the other 10% to 15%. Persons in this latter group have much higher rates of treatment in the ED, hospitalization, and intensive care. Among children 5 years and younger, most poisoning exposures are related to exploratory behavior or result from willful child abuse. Although less common, the physician must also consider the possibility of environmental exposures, suicide attempts in children, and neonates exposed to toxicants in utero.

The exploratory ingestion of a drug or chemical by a toddler represents a complex interplay of host, agent, and environmental factors and may be considered a subset of the modern traumatic injury model. In this model, each factor contributes, more or less, in a given context to the probability of the injury occurring. Some children are more at risk because of peak age of 1 to 4 years, male gender, temperament that leans toward hyperactivity, and increased finger–mouth activity and/or pica. Some agents are more culpable because of ease of access, attractiveness/palatability, and toxic potential. Two classic examples are iron tablets, which may look like candy, are widely available, and are toxic in significant overdose; and mouthwash, which has a bright color, as well as a pleasant taste and smell, is often packaged in large volumes without child-safety caps, and may have surprisingly high ethanol content (15% to 25%). Typical environmental factors include an acute stressor, such as a recent move or new baby in the household, and chronic issues, such as parental illness/disability. The young child's exploratory encounter with a poison should not be viewed as an "accident," as the concordance of child, agent, and environmental factors may lead predictably to the statistical likelihood of toddler ingestion. Pediatricians have led the way in poisoning prevention strategies by modifying these risk factors with traditional anticipatory guidance and by spearheading the lobby for child-safety caps on particularly dangerous medications and household products. Although these efforts have resulted in a dramatic decrease in childhood poisoning morbidity and mortality since the 1970s, such poisonings continue to occur and demand the emergency physician's attention.

The scope of toxic substances involved in poisonings is broad, requiring a wide range of knowledge. Table 102.1 presents the categories of substances most commonly reported in human exposures in the United States for the year 2007. Table 102.2 presents the 10 most common toxic exposures involved in human deaths for the year 2007. The former listing much more closely approximates the profile of pediatric poisonings, whereas the latter is more typical of intentional adult exposures. The most important difference between the pediatric and the adult profile by type of agent is in the higher percentage of cases in which psychopharmacologic drugs (sedatives, tranquilizers, and antidepressants) cause poisoning in adults and the much higher frequency of exposures to household and personal care products and plants in children.

There are six basic modes of exposure to poisons: ingestion, ocular exposure, topical exposure, envenomation, inhalation, and transplacental exposure. Poisonings may be the result of acute or chronic exposures. Most poisonings treated in EDs are acute, and the patients are typified by the child who surreptitiously invades the medicine cabinet or the storage area for household cleaners or the adolescent or adult who takes a massive number of pills in a fit of despair. *Chronic poisoning* refers to toxicity produced over time in which a substance accumulates in the body, producing toxic results; it is best exemplified by environmental exposure to lead or other heavy metals. In the drug category, chronic toxicity can also exist. Acetaminophen hepatotoxicity that occurs in infants and small children or aspirin poisoning in older adults as a result of salicylate accumulation after administration of too much drug for too long is typical of chronic toxicity. Chronic toxicity is a special problem for the clinician because the source is not always apparent, the toxicity is not always clear, and the toxic process is not often obvious until serious clinical derangements occur.

GENERAL APPROACH TO THE POISONED CHILD

Following the analogy between unintentional poisoning and traumatic injury, a similar model may be used in formulating a management approach. The poisoned patient often represents an acute-onset emergency with a broad spectrum of multiorgan system pathophysiology that shares many features with the multiple trauma patient. In essence, poisoning might be viewed as a multiple chemical trauma. The concept of a brief window of opportunity to make critical diagnostic and management decisions is likewise analogous. One may conceptualize a management

TABLE 102.1

SUBSTANCES MOST OFTEN REPORTED IN
HUMAN EXPOSURES

Substance	Percentage of total exposures
Analgesics	12.5
Cosmetics/personal care products	9.1
Cleaning substances	8.7
Sedatives/hypnotics/ antipsychotics	6.2
Foreign bodies/toys	5.1
Topical preparations	4.5
Cough and cold preparations	4.5
Antidepressants	4.0
Pesticides	3.9
Cardiovascular drugs	3.5

Adapted from Bronstein AC, Spyker DA, Cantilena LR, et al. 2007
Annual report of the American Association of Poison Control Centers'
National Poison Data System. *Clin Toxicol* 2008;46:927–1057.

approach that attempts to prioritize critical assessment and, at
times, simultaneous management interventions (Table 102.3).
The initial phase (or primary survey) addresses the traditional
airway, breathing, and circulation (ABCs) of airway securement
and cardiorespiratory support, with a slight additional emphasis
on emergent toxicologic considerations. The more specific evaluation and detoxification phase (or secondary survey) is aimed at
simultaneously initiating generic treatment while assessing the
actual extent of intoxication (in cases of known or presumed
exposures) and/or identifying the actual toxicants involved (in
unknown but highly suspected intoxications).

Initial Life Support Phase

The general approach to recognition and support of vital airway and cardiorespiratory functions (or ABCDs) is well
known to most readers and is covered in detail in Chapter 1.
In the context of the poisoned child, a few points deserve special emphasis. In addition to the usual signs of airway obstruction, the physician must pay special attention to evidence of

TABLE 102.2

TOXIC EXPOSURES ASSOCIATED WITH THE
MOST DEATHS

Nonprescription analgesics	Sedatives-hypnotics, antipsychotics
Antidepressants	
Stimulants and street drugs	Cardiovascular drugs
Anticonvulsants	Alcohols
Muscle relaxants	Gases and fumes
	Antihistamines

Adapted from Bronstein AC, Spyker DA, Cantilena LR, et al. 2007
Annual report of the American Association of Poison Control Centers'
National Poison Data System. *Clin Toxicol* 2008;46:927–1057.

disturbed airway protective reflexes. Many poisoned patients
will vomit, and some may be administered charcoal, which
poses an aspiration risk. Elective endotracheal intubation (see
Chapter 5) may thus be indicated at a slightly lower threshold
in this context than in another child with comparable central
nervous system (CNS) depression.

It is also particularly important to anticipate imminent respiratory failure in the deeply comatose poisoned child.
Cyanosis and overt apnea are late findings with progressive
drug-induced medullary depression. Thus, clinical or laboratory assessment of early ventilatory insufficiency is critical in
such patients to avoid the chaos of a precipitous respiratory
arrest. Likewise, it is far easier to establish intravenous (IV)
access in a child with normal circulatory status than in a child
in shock; early efforts to obtain a secure IV line in symptomatic
overdose patients are thus well worth the time and effort.

After securing the airway, ensuring effective breathing, and
supporting circulation, it is important to evaluate poisoned
patients for neurological "disability," and the need for empiric
"*drug*" treatment, and emergent "*decontamination.*" Level of
consciousness may be assessed rapidly with a semiquantitative
scale such as the Glasgow Coma Scale or the AVPU (spontaneously *a*lert, response to *v*erbal stimulation or *p*ain, or *u*nresponsive) scale. Pupillary size and reactivity may be quickly
noted. Rapid changes in mental status are common in serious
intoxications and may herald precipitous cardiorespiratory
failure.

Empiric "drug" treatment is warranted for most symptomatic poisoned children with altered mental status. All such
patients may initially be given humidified *oxygen* and their
blood oxyhemoglobin saturation monitored, if possible, by
pulse oximetry. If available, rapid bedside blood glucose testing
may be used; if low, or not readily available, a trial dosage of
0.25 to 1 g per kg glucose as 10% to 25% solution should be
infused. It should be noted that drug- or toxicant-induced
hypoglycemia does not present uniformly with coma or
seizures. Almost any neuropsychiatric picture may predominate, including aphasia; slurred, dysarthric speech; and focal
neurologic signs. Adrenergic signs, such as diaphoresis and
tachycardia, are not uniformly present. Hypoglycemia is a
complication seen in ingestions of ethanol, oral hypoglycemics,
β-blockers, salicylates, and, of course, insulin injection. As
basic as this intervention seems, in our experience, it is still one
of the most often missed (or more accurately, *delayed*) critical
treatments in the management of the poisoned patient.

Thiamine (100 mg IV), although routinely administered to
adult overdose patients who receive hypertonic glucose to obviate precipitating Wernicke's encephalopathy, is not generally
necessary in the pediatric population. Perhaps it should be considered in adolescent patients who may be thiamine deficient
secondary to eating disorders, chronic disease (e.g., inflammatory bowel disease), or alcoholism. Last, empiric naloxone
therapy is just as important in potentially poisoned toddlers
with altered mental status as it is in adults. Although substance
abuse is admittedly uncommon in the average 2-year-old child,
it is amazing how many narcotics find their way into the
curious child's mouth. Many households contain a variety of
oral opioid analgesic agents, as well as cough medicines
(codeine, dextromethorphan), antidiarrheal agents (paregoric,
diphenoxylate), and partially naloxone-responsive antihypertensive agents such as clonidine. In addition, the possibility of

TABLE 102.3

GENERAL APPROACH TO THE KNOWN OR SUSPECTED INTOXICATION

Initial Life Support Phase
Airway: Maintain patency, assess protective reflexes
Breathing: Adequate tidal volume?
   ABG or ETCO$_2$?
Circulation: Secure IV access, assess perfusion
Disability: Level of consciousness (AVPU or GCS)
   Pupillary size, reactivity
Drugs: Dextrose (rapid bedside test)
   Oxygen
   Naloxone
   (Other ALS medications)
Decontamination: Ocular—copious saline lavage
   Skin—copious water, then soap and water
   GI—consider options

Evaluation and Detoxification Phase
History—Brief, focused
   Known toxicant: Estimate amount
               Elapsed time
               Early symptoms
               Home treatment
               Significant underlying conditions
   Suspected but unknown toxicant—consider poisoning if:
   Patient: Acute onset of illness
        Pica-prone age
        History of pica, ingestions
        Current household "stress"
        Multiorgan system dysfunction
        Significantly altered mental status
        Puzzling clinical picture
   Family: Medications at home
        Recent illness (under treatment)
   Social: Grandparents visiting
        Holiday parties, other events

Physical Examination
   Vital signs
   Level of consciousness, neuromuscular status
   Eyes—pupils, extraocular movements, fundi
   Mouth—corrosive lesions, odors
   Cardiovascular—rate, rhythm, perfusion
   Respiratory—rate, chest excursion, air entry
   GI—motility, corrosive effects
   Skin—color, bullae or burns, diaphoresis, piloerection
   Odors
Laboratory (individualize)
   CBC, cooximetry
   ABG, serum osmolarity
   EKG/cardiac monitor
   Chest radiograph, abdominal radiograph
   Electrolytes, BUN/creatinine, glucose, calcium, liver
      function panel
   Urinalysis
   Rapid overdose toxicologic screen
   Quantitative toxicology tests (especially acetaminophen)
Assessment of Severity/Diagnosis
   Clinical findings
   Laboratory abnormalities (with consideration of anion,
      osmolar gaps)
   Toxidromes (see Table 102.5)
Specific Detoxification
   Reassess ABCDs
   Institute appropriate GI decontamination (if not
      already under way)
   Urgent antidotal therapy
   Consider excretion enhancement
   Continue supportive care

ABG, arterial blood gas; ETCO$_2$, end-tidal carbon dioxide; AVPU, *a*lert, *v*erbal, *p*ain, *u*nresponsive; GCS, Glasgow Coma Scale; ALS, advanced life support; GI, gastrointestinal; CBC, complete blood cell count; EKG, electrocardiogram; BUN, blood urea nitrogen.

exploratory ingestion of a "stash" of illicit opioids does exist. Thus, naloxone should be used as a therapeutic/diagnostic trial when there is a reasonable possibility that altered mental status is drug induced. Previous recommendations have based dosing on weight (e.g., 0.01 to 0.1 mg per kg); however, many authorities now prefer a unified pediatric dose of 0.4 to 2 mg for acute overdose patients of all ages (outside the neonatal period). Such an approach conceptualizes naloxone dosing as based on total narcotic load and number of opioid receptors that require competition for binding sites. In general, this latter approach is easier to remember and has not been associated with complication in the ED. Adolescent patients with a strong clinical picture for opioid intoxication (without habituation) may receive 2-mg bolus doses every 2 minutes, up to a total dose of 8 to 10 mg, before abandoning hope of benefit because several congeners of morphine (e.g., propoxyphene, illicit fentanyl derivatives, pentazocine) may require such large doses. If chronic abuse is suspected, lower initial doses (0.2 to 0.4 mg) are warranted. Administration of flumazenil to adolescents exhibiting depressed consciousness after an unknown drug overdose is not recommended by the authors (see "Central Nervous System Sedative-Hypnotics" section).

The rationale for decontamination of the poisoned child is discussed in the next section. This treatment phase may begin urgently, after or in concert with attention to the ABCDs. At times, a decision to perform gastric decontamination through the preferred technique can be made almost immediately upon presentation and, if so, should be instituted as soon as possible in light of the patient's clinical status and the number of hands available to assist in management. For example, a toddler with coma, shock, and massive hematochezia who is rushed into the ED by the rescue squad—and for whom there is witnessed or strong circumstantial evidence of massive iron overdose—requires a concerted team effort directed toward resuscitation, stabilization, and urgent gastric decontamination. However, an apparently asymptomatic adolescent who admits to ingesting 10 g of acetaminophen 1 hour before arrival at the ED may be more fully evaluated in a timely but orderly manner (as outlined in the next section) and within short order can be considered for less emergent gastric decontamination—in this case, possibly an oral dose of activated charcoal. Significant dermal or ocular exposures require immediate copious lavage, and precautions should be taken to protect the health-care providers tending to the patient from exposure.

At the completion of this initial life support phase, the poisoned patient should have been assessed for compromise of vital airway and cardiorespiratory function and for global neurologic status and should have had resuscitative measures instituted. Patients with significant altered mental status have been critically evaluated for respiratory status, have had IV access secured, and have had their therapeutic trials of oxygen, glucose, and naloxone. Other advanced life support interventions such as anticonvulsants or antiarrhythmics have been instituted as necessary. Consideration of decontamination options has begun.

Evaluation and Detoxification Phase

History

A brief and focused *historical evaluation* should be addressed as soon as the life support phase has been completed. The primary goal is to determine the potential severity of the exposure. This assessment requires poison and patient-related data alike.

For a known or highly suspected toxic exposure, an attempt is made to estimate the total amount ingested (number of pills missing, ounces left in the bottle, dosage of pills, concentration of alcohol, and so forth). The best estimate of time elapsed since ingestion is also sought. Parents should be questioned regarding early symptoms noted at home or en route to the ED and any treatments administered before arrival. Certain underlying medical conditions may be relevant [e.g., glucose-6-phosphate dehydrogenase (G6PD) deficiency for mothball ingestions]; thus, any significant medical history should be noted.

Often, children who are poisoned do not come to the ED with a clear history of exposure followed by onset of symptoms. Rather, they develop signs and symptoms that mimic other diseases and give no history of toxic exposure. Thus, the ED staff must always consider the possibility of ingestion when treating young children.

General historical features that suggest the possibility of poisoning include (i) acute onset; (ii) age range of 1 to 5 years or adolescence; (iii) history of pica or known exposure to a potential toxicant; (iv) substantial environmental stress, either acute (e.g., arrival of a new baby, serious illness in a parent) or chronic (e.g., marital conflict, parental disability); (v) multiple organ system involvement; (vi) significant alteration in level of consciousness; and (vii) a clinical picture that seems especially puzzling.

Certain family and social history variables are also important. Medications used by other household members, particularly new medications introduced into the home environment by virtue of recent illnesses or visits from grandparents and other relatives, are a common source of ingested drugs. Changes in routine and large family gatherings (e.g., holiday parties, moving to a new home) are particularly risky occasions for decreased parental supervision and new (or less carefully guarded) potentially toxic medications or household products.

Physical Examination

The focused physical examination should begin with a reassessment of vital functions and complete recording of vital signs, including core temperature. With secure airway and cardiorespiratory function confirmed, the examination should then focus on the central and autonomic nervous systems, eye findings, changes in the skin and/or oral and gastrointestinal (GI) mucous membranes, and odors (see Chapter 46) on the breath or clothing of the patient. These features represent those areas most likely affected in toxic syndromes and, when taken together, often form a constellation of signs and symptoms referred to as toxidromes (Tables 102.4 and 102.5). Such toxidromes may be so characteristic as to provide guidance for early therapeutic management before precise historical or laboratory confirmation of a specific exposure is available.

Laboratory Evaluation

Laboratory studies may be helpful in confirming diagnostic impressions or in demonstrating toxicant-induced metabolic aberrations. However, there is no "tox panel" that is uniformly helpful or necessary. Most poisonings can be managed appropriately without extensive laboratory studies, and in particular, the reflex ordering of rapid overdose toxicology "screens" has rarely been found to be helpful in acute patient management. They have important, nonemergent roles (e.g., in resolving medicolegal issues or considering drug-induced causes of behavioral changes in a psychiatric patient). In toddlers with a known or strongly suspected specific ingestion, rapid drug screens are rarely indicated. In the adolescent intentional overdose patient who is not critically ill or who does not have a particularly puzzling clinical picture, the drug screen again is rarely helpful, although the finding of an unexpected toxic level of acetaminophen (which may have been omitted in the history) may impact management, and some authors recommend that quantitative acetaminophen levels (in lieu of "tox screens") be sought in such patients.

The labor-intensive comprehensive urine drug screen may be useful for patients who are seriously ill with an occult ingestion or for the occasional intentional overdose adolescent patient whose clinical picture does not fit with the stated history. Often of greater help is the critical interpretation of routine measurements of serum chemistries and osmolality in patients with altered mental status. The presence of hypoglycemia or aberrations of serum electrolytes may provide crucial information about the poisoned patient. In certain circumstances, tests of liver or renal function, urinalysis, creatine phosphokinase levels, and other select tests may be useful. Metabolic acidosis with a high anion gap is found in many clinical syndromes and toxidromes, reflected by the often-cited mnemonic *MUDPILES*, for *m*ethanol and *m*etformin; *u*remia; *d*iabetic and other ketoacidoses; *p*araldehyde; *i*soniazid, *i*ron, and *i*nborn errors of metabolism; *l*actic acidosis (seen with hypoxia, shock, carbon monoxide, cyanide, and many drugs that cause compromised cardiorespiratory status or prolonged seizures); *e*thylene glycol; and *s*alicylates. Differences between calculated and measured serum osmolarity [calculated = 2 (serum Na mEq per L) + blood urea nitrogen (BUN) mg per dL ÷ 2.8 + glucose mg per dL ÷ 18; with normal osmolarity ~290 mOsm per kg] may suggest intoxication with ethanol, isopropanol, or more rarely in pediatric patients, methanol or ethylene glycol. Blood collection tubes containing ethylene diamine tetraacetic acid (EDTA) should not be used to send samples to the laboratory because the osmolal gap will be falsely elevated.

TABLE 102.4

CLINICAL MANIFESTATIONS OF POISONING

Vital Signs

Pulse

Bradycardia

Digoxin, opioids, organophosphates, plants (lily-of-the-valley, foxglove, oleander), clonidine, β-blockers, calcium channel blockers

Tachycardia

Alcohol, amphetamines and sympathomimetics, anticholinergic agents, tricyclic antidepressants, theophylline, salicylates, phencyclidine, cocaine

Respirations

Slow, depressed

Alcohol, barbiturates (late), narcotics, clonidine, sedative-hypnotics

Tachypnea

Amphetamines, barbiturates (early), methanol, salicylates, carbon monoxide

Blood Pressure

Hypotension

Cellular asphyxiants (methemoglobinemia, cyanide, carbon monoxide), antipsychotics, tricyclic antidepressants, barbiturates, iron, theophylline, clonidine, narcotics, β-blockers, calcium channel blockers

Hypertension

Amphetamines/sympathomimetics, phencyclidine, monoamine oxidase inhibitors (MAOIs), antihistamines, anticholinergic agents, clonidine

Temperature

Hypothermia

Ethanol, barbiturates, sedative-hypnotics, opioids, phenothiazines, antidepressants, clonidine, cabamazepine

Hyperpyrexia

Sympathomimetics, anticholinergics, salicylates, neuroleptics, inhalational anesthetics, succinylcholine, serotonin reuptake inhibitors, withdrawal from sedatives

Neuromuscular

Coma

Narcotic depressants, sedative-hypnotics, anticholinergics (antihistamines, antidepressants, phenothiazines, atropinics, OTC sleep preparations), alcohols, anticonvulsants, carbon monoxide, salicylates, organophosphate insecticides, clonidine, γ-hydroxybutyrate

Delirium/Psychosis

Alcohol, phenothiazines, drugs of abuse (phencyclidine, LSD, peyote, mescaline, marijuana, cocaine, heroin, methaqualone), sympathomimetics and anticholinergics (including prescription and OTC cold remedies), steroids, heavy metals, dextromethorphan

Convulsions

Alcohol, amphetamines, cocaine, phenothiazines, antidepressants, antihistamines, camphor, boric acid, lead, organophosphates, isoniazid, salicylates, plants (water hemlock), lindane, lidocaine, phencyclidine, carbamazepine

Ataxia

Alcohol, barbiturates, carbon monoxide, anticonvulsants, heavy metals, organic solvents, sedative-hypnotics, hydrocarbons

Paralysis

Botulism, heavy metals, plants (poison hemlock), ticks, paralytic shellfish poisoning

Eyes

Pupils

Miosis

Opioids, organophosphates, ethanol, barbiturates, phenothiazines, phencyclidine, clonidine

Mydriasis

Amphetamines, anticholinergic agents, barbiturates (if comatose), botulism, cocaine, methanol, glutethimide, LSD, marijuana, phencyclidine, antihistamines, antidepressants

Nystagmus

Phenytoin, sedative-hypnotics, carbamazepine, glutethimide, phencyclidine (both vertical and horizontal), barbiturates, ethanol, MAOIs, ketamine, phencyclidine, dextromethorphan

Skin

Jaundice

Carbon tetrachloride, acetaminophen, naphthalene, phenothiazines, plants (mushrooms, Fava beans), heavy metals (iron, phosphorus, arsenic)

Cyanosis (unresponsive to oxygen, as a result of methemoglobinemia)

Aniline dyes, nitrites, benzocaine, phenacetin, nitrobenzene, phenazopyridine, dapsone

Pinkness to Redness

Atropinics and antihistamines, alcohol, carbon monoxide, cyanide, boric acid

Odors

Acetone: acetone, isopropyl alcohol, phenol, salicylates

Alcohol: ethanol (alcoholic beverages)

Bitter almond: cyanide

Garlic: heavy metal (arsenic, phosphorus, thallium), organophosphates

Oil of wintergreen: methylsalicylates

Hydrocarbons: hydrocarbons (gasoline, turpentine)

OTC, over the counter; LSD, lysergamide.

Adapted from Mofenson HC, Greensher J. The unknown poison. *Pediatrics* 1974;54:336.

MEDICAL EMERGENCIES

An immediate determination of quantitative levels is helpful in making management decisions for some drugs, and these are outlined in Table 102.6. Furthermore, many important causes of coma and altered vital signs are not detected on even the most sophisticated "comprehensive" toxicology panels (which are usually biased toward psychoactive medications and illicit drugs). An overview of such agents is presented in Table 102.7. An electrocardiogram (EKG) should be per-

formed in all seriously ill patients in whom poisoning is being considered. Detectable conduction delays may provide diagnostic direction and impact management by predicting imminent life-threatening cardiac rhythm disturbances.

Assessment of Severity and Diagnosis

At this juncture, most intoxicated patients may be readily stratified by specific toxicant or category of drug(s) ingested

TABLE 102.5

TOXIDROMES

	Sympathomimetics (amphetamines, cocaine)	Anticholinergics (antihistamines, many others)	Organophosphates (insecticides, nerve gases)	Opioids/ clonidine	Barbiturates/ sedative-hypnotics	Salicylates	Theophyline
Mental status/CNS	Agitation, delirium, psychosis, convulsions	Delirium, psychosis, coma, convulsions	Confusion, fasciculations, coma	Euphoria, somnolence, coma	Somnolence, coma	Lethargy, convulsions	Agitation, tremor, convulsions
Heart rate	Increased	Increased	Decreased (or increased)	Decreased	—	—	Increased
Blood pressure	Increased	Increased	—	Decreased	Decreased	—	Decreased
Temperature	Increased	Increased	—	Decreased	Decreased	Increased	—
Respirations	—	—	Increased	Decreased	Decreased	Increased	Increased
Pupils	Large, reactive	Large, sluggish	Small	Pinpoint	—	—	—
Bowel sounds	Present	Diminished	Hyperactive	—	—	—	—
Skin	Diaphoresis	Flushed, dry	Diaphoresis[a]	—	—	—	—
Miscellaneous	—	—	SLUDGE[a]	—	—	Vomiting	Vomiting

CNS, central nervous system; —, minimal direct effect.
[a]SLUDGE is a mnemonic representing salivation, lacrimation, urination, defecation, gastric cramping, and emesis.

TABLE 102.6

FREQUENTLY USEFUL QUANTITATIVE TOXICOLOGY TESTS IN PEDIATRIC PATIENTS

Drug/toxin	Optimal time after ingestion (h)
Acetaminophen	4
Carbamazepine	2–4
Carboxyhemoglobin	Immediate
Digoxin	4–6
Ethanol	½–1
Ethylene glycol	½–1
Iron	4
Lithium	2–4[a]
Methanol	½–1
Methemoglobin	Immediate
Phenobarbital	1–2
Phenytoin	1–2
Salicylate	2–4[a]
Theophylline	1–2[a]
Valproate	2–4

[a]Repeat levels over 6 to 12 hours may be necessary with sustained-release preparations.
Adapted from Weisman RS, Howland MA, Flomenbaum NE. The toxicology laboratory. In: Goldfrank LR, Flomenbaum NE, Lewin NA, et al., eds. *Toxicologic emergencies*. Norwalk, CT: Appleton & Lange, 1990.

and some judgment made as to the potential or current severity of the exposure. For some children, clinical features of a complex illness of acute onset may suggest intoxication without a specific history of such ingestion. In a few cases, some laboratory confirmation of clinical suspicion will be available on an immediate basis. Using all the clinical clues available and with some familiarity of the "toxidrome" approach to differential diagnosis as detailed previously (Tables 102.4 and 102.5) and, at times, with help from the laboratory, the emergency physician must now establish a working diagnosis and proceed with consideration of options for specific detoxification.

TABLE 102.7

IMPORTANT DRUGS AND TOXICANTS NOT DETECTED BY MOST DRUG SCREENS

Coma causing	Hypotension causing
Bromide	β-Blockers[a]
Carbon monoxide	Calcium channel blockers[a]
Chloral hydrate	Clonidine[a]
Clonidine	Colchicine
Cyanide	Cyanide
γ-Hydroxybutyrate	Digitalis[a]
Organophosphates	Iron
Tetrahydrozoline (in over-the-counter eyedrops)	

[a]Hypotension is often seen with bradycardia.
Adapted from Wiley JF II. Difficult diagnoses in toxicology: poisons not detected by the comprehensive drug screen. *Pediatr Clin North Am* 1991;38:725–737.

Specific Detoxification

Again, the proviso that the patient be continually reassessed and managed for impaired vital function is addressed. All decisions about further decontamination and/or specific antidotal therapy involve a complex interplay between the toxicant(s) ingested and the patient's condition.

GI Decontamination. The effort to "get the poison out" has long been a mainstay of the traditional discussion of toxicologic management. However, gastric emptying measures have fallen out of favor over the past 15 years, and the routine use of activated charcoal as a poison adsorbent has been subjected to increased academic scrutiny. Unfortunately, young children have been underrepresented in clinical studies of GI decontamination. It is likely that as further research is conducted, particularly as directed toward the pediatric population, current dogma regarding optimal GI decontamination will evolve. For the sections that follow, several appropriate techniques for gastric decontamination are reviewed, all of which may be useful under certain circumstances. An approach to the overall decision process in a given patient is then offered.

Simple dilution. Dilution may be indicated only when the toxicant produces local irritation or corrosion. Water or milk is an acceptable diluent. Dilution for caustic agents is controversial; dilution may be used in the first few minutes after an exposure but only if there is no evidence of airway compromise or significant abdominal pain/vomiting. For drug ingestion, however, dilution alone should not be used because it may increase absorption by increasing dissolution rates of the tablets or capsules or it may promote more rapid transit into the lower GI tract.

Gastric emptying. The goal of gastric emptying is to rid the stomach of remaining poison to prevent further local effect or systemic absorption. The utility of gastric emptying diminishes with time and is most effective if done early after ingestion when unabsorbed drug is still present within the stomach (operationally, within the first 30 minutes to 1 hour). In certain circumstances, such as the delayed gastric emptying accompanying intoxication with anticholinergic drugs, benefit may be noted longer after ingestion. *Emesis* was once a favored means of gastric emptying, but the American Academy of Pediatrics has issued a policy statement recommending that syrup of ipecac no longer be used routinely for the poisoned patient in the home or health-care facility.

Studies addressing the efficacy of ipecac-induced emesis in reducing bioavailability of ingested drug have widely varying results with ranges from 0% to 70% decrease in absorption. Individuals with eating disorders and those with Munchausen syndrome by proxy can abuse syrup of ipecac. Furthermore, a more recent study of U.S. Poison Centers suggested no improvement in patient outcome or reduction in resource utilization when ipecac was used in the home. Finally, despite a long history of use, it has been difficult to prove improved clinical outcome in poisoned patients given ipecac compared with patients treated with activated charcoal alone, and ipecac has been found to delay the time to administration of activated charcoal and some specific antidotes.

An alternative to ipecac-induced emesis for emptying the stomach is *gastric lavage*. This procedure is usually reserved for patients who have ingested a potentially life-threatening amount of poison, in cases where the procedure can be performed safely very early after ingestion and charcoal alone is not believed to be adequate. To carry out a satisfactory lavage, the patient should be on his or her left side, head slightly lower than feet, and the largest orogastric lavage tube that can reasonably be passed should be used (e.g., 24F orogastric tube for a toddler, 36F orogastric tube for an adolescent). A smaller caliber nasogastric (NG) tube is sufficient only for some liquid toxins. Gastric contents should be aspirated initially before any lavage fluid is introduced. Normal saline aliquots of 50 to 100 mL in young children and 150 to 200 mL in adolescents can be lavaged repeatedly until the return is clear. Like induced emesis, gastric lavage's efficacy in reducing drug absorption has been reviewed critically in more recent studies. Again, the efficacy has been highly variable and lavage has not been demonstrated to improve outcome in poisoned patients. Several important risks are associated with gastric lavage, including oxygen desaturation, aspiration, and mechanical trauma to the oropharynx and esophagus. Gastric lavage is rarely recommended anymore but might be considered for patients presenting very early after very dangerous ingestions (of toxicants such as colchicine or arsenic). Contraindications to the procedure include caustic or corrosive ingestions, impending loss of airway protection, and the presence of cardiac arrhythmia.

Activated charcoal. Activated charcoal minimizes absorption of drugs by adsorbing them onto its surface. Charcoal administration has become the decontamination strategy of choice to prevent pediatric poisoning after toxicant ingestion and is most effective when used in the first hour after ingestion. Therefore, if activated charcoal is considered as a treatment option, quick triage of an exposed patient may be necessary to allow charcoal administration in a timely fashion. A number of notable compounds, such as iron and lithium, do not adsorb well to activated charcoal (Table 102.8). The usual dose of activated charcoal is 1 g per kg; adolescents and adults should receive 50 to 100 g. Most activated charcoal is now available premixed with water to make a slurry that can be taken orally or administered by NG tube. Simply adding soda or another nonparticulate flavoring agent to the charcoal can improve palatability.

Activated charcoal was "rediscovered" by the toxicology community during the 1980s, with several studies finding its use to be superior to gastric emptying alone and, at least, equivalent to the combination of gastric emptying plus charcoal administration. The use of charcoal alone is less invasive and less likely to be associated with complications in the clinical setting than is gastric emptying. Aspiration of charcoal can be a serious concern among patients with poor airway protec-

TABLE 102.8

SUBSTANCES POORLY (OR NOT) ADSORBED BY ACTIVATED CHARCOAL

Common electrolytes
Iron
Mineral acids or bases
Alcohols
Cyanide
Most solvents
Most water-insoluble compounds (e.g., hydrocarbons)

tive reflexes, and vomiting remains the most common difficulty associated with its use. The use of an NG tube, which renders the esophagogastric sphincter patent, may also increase aspiration risk. Charcoal is contraindicated in patients with an unprotected airway or a disrupted GI tract (e.g., after severe caustic ingestion) or in patients in whom charcoal therapy may increase the risk and severity of aspiration (e.g., hydrocarbons). The use of multiple doses of activated charcoal to achieve enhanced drug elimination is addressed later in this chapter.

Catharsis. Two types of osmotic cathartics have most commonly been used to treat poisoned patients: the saccharide cathartics (e.g., sorbitol) and the saline cathartics (e.g., magnesium citrate, magnesium sulfate). *Whole bowel irrigation (WBI)* with a high-molecular-weight polyethylene glycol solution is discussed in the next section. Little evidence exists to suggest that standard cathartics accomplish their goal of reducing drug absorption by decreasing GI transit time. It is still unclear whether cathartics administered with activated charcoal reduce subsequent constipation, and some believe cathartics increase the incidence of vomiting. Repetitive doses of osmotic cathartics are associated with considerable diarrhea and cramping, and hypernatremic dehydration has been reported in young infants. A single dose of premixed charcoal/sorbitol is safe for most pediatric ingestions, but this preparation should be used with caution in young infants. Mineral oil or stimulant cathartics such as castor oil are discouraged because they may be aspirated, increase absorption of some poisons, or unnecessarily extend the cathartic effect.

Whole bowel irrigation. An additional technique of cathartic GI decontamination is that of intestinal irrigation with large volumes and flow rates of a polyethylene glycol-balanced electrolyte solution such as GoLYTELY® or Colyte®. Typically, these solutions are not significantly absorbed nor do they exert an osmotic effect, so the patient's net fluid/electrolyte status is unchanged. They have a long safety track record in patient populations such as infants and in those surgical patients requiring application of preoperative bowel preparation. WBI has been found to be particularly useful in pediatric iron overdoses, in which gastric lavage may be limited by tube size, the fact that metals do not bind to charcoal, and the possibility that the ingestion is not a recent one. It has been used for other metal ingestions (e.g., lead), overdoses of sustained-release medications (e.g., lithium, theophylline), ingested pharmaceutical patches, and ingestions of vials or packages of illicit drugs. It might also be useful in particularly massive and/or late-presenting overdoses for which the efficacy of gastric emptying and/or charcoal is expected to be suboptimal. The technique may be used by mouth in cooperative patients or by NG tube; the usual recommended dosing is 500 mL per hour in toddlers and 2 L per hour in adolescents and adults.

GI Decontamination Strategies

It should be apparent that no unique approach to GI decontamination of all poisoned patients is optimal in every case. Factors to be considered include the expected degree of toxicity from the drug, the physical nature of the drug, the current location of the drug within the body, and the presence of contraindications or alternatives. A risk–benefit decision must be made before the institution of any decontamination strategy.

Syrup of ipecac was used primarily as first aid treatment of potentially toxic ingestions in the home. However, the American Academy of Pediatrics no longer recommends routine use in the home, and induced emesis is not favored in the ED. The use of gastric lavage as a decontamination strategy has become more limited in recent years. If it still has a role, it is only in patients with recent ingestions of extremely toxic substances that put them at risk for a lethal course, especially when those substances do not bind well to charcoal. Likewise, patients with truly massive overdoses may benefit from gastric lavage because standard charcoal preparations may have diminished effectiveness when the charcoal-to-drug ratio is less than 10:1. The correct technique for gastric lavage requires that careful attention be given to prevent aspiration and anatomic trauma.

Overall, the mortality from acute poisoning is less than 1%. Suicidal overdoses in adolescents typically have more inherent lethality than unintentional overdoses in toddlers. If a GI decontamination strategy is to be used, the administration of activated charcoal or WBI are now the favored procedures. Some of the patients in question will have undergone endotracheal intubation during the initial life support phase of management, as detailed previously, or they may be strong candidates for such airway protection because of borderline mental status and in anticipation of their ensuing critical course. Others may be awake, alert, and cooperative, with normal airway protective reflexes, and thus given activated charcoal without prior endotracheal intubation. The combative, agitated patient poses a dilemma and must be carefully managed on an individualized basis.

An attempt to summarize these considerations is diagrammed in Fig. 102.1; however, it should be reiterated that all decisions regarding gastric decontamination involve multiple patient and toxic agent-related factors and should not be made with a "cookbook" approach.

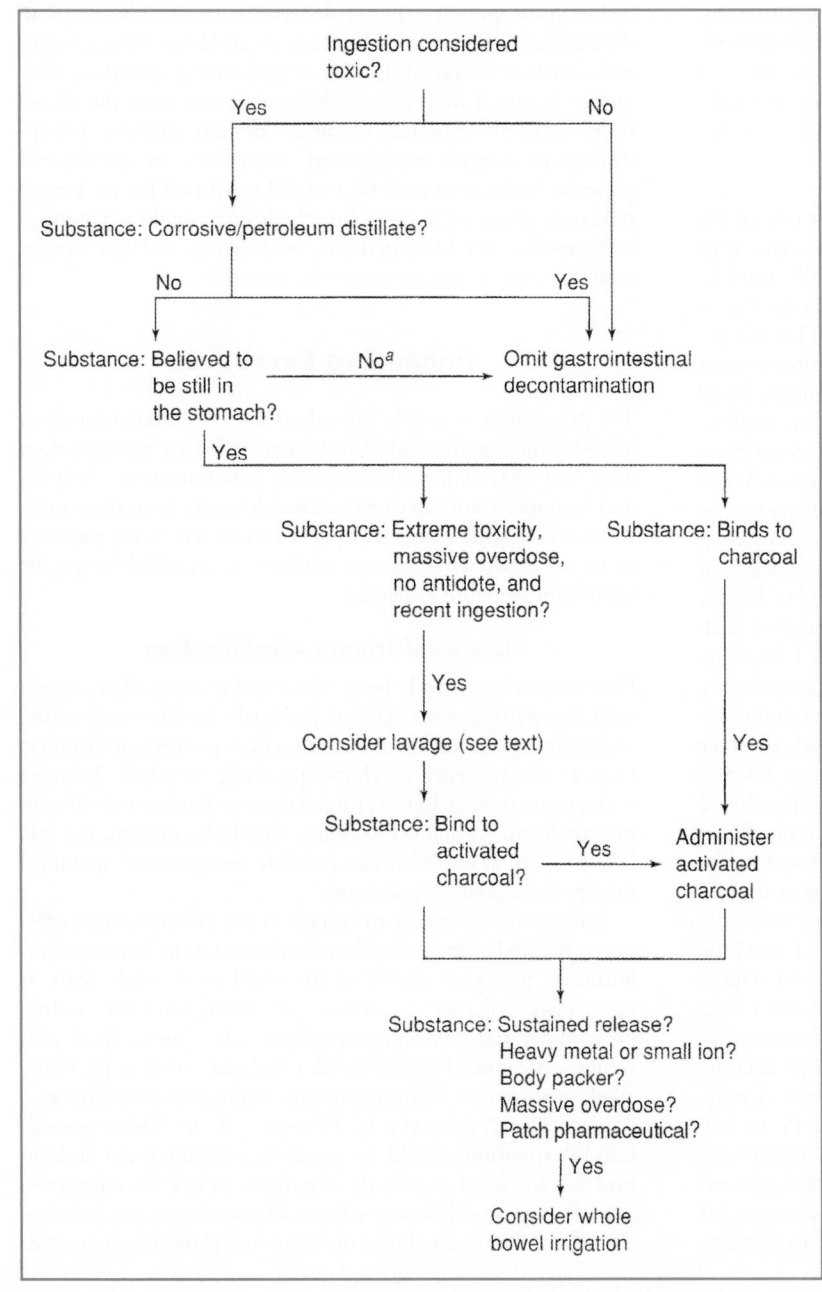

FIGURE 102.1 Approach to gastrointestinal decontamination. [a]For patients in whom the toxicant is no longer believed to be in the stomach, whole bowel irrigation might still be a valid consideration.

MEDICAL EMERGENCIES

Antidotal Therapy. Beyond the setting of acetaminophen overdose, the overall number of toxic ingestions for which a specific antidote is necessary or available is small. When a specific antidote can be used, it is vital that it be administered as early as possible and in an appropriately monitored dose. Those antidotes that should be available for immediate administration include sodium bicarbonate (tricyclic antidepressants), sodium nitrite/sodium thiosulfate or hydroxocobalamin (cyanide), atropine and pralidoxime (cholinesterase inhibitors), ethanol or fomepizole (ethylene glycol and methanol), deferoxamine (iron), dextrose (ethanol, salicylates, oral hypoglycemics), methylene blue (methemoglobinemic agents), oxygen (carbon monoxide), flumazenil (benzodiazepines), pyridoxine (isoniazid and *Gyromitra* mushrooms), digoxin immune Fab (digoxin), and naloxone (opioids). Other antidotes usually do not require such urgent administration and may be given subsequent to initiation of other management modalities. Even when available, antidotes do not diminish the need for meticulous supportive care or other therapy. Indiscriminant use of antidotes without other forms of management should be discouraged. Table 102.9 summarizes a list of commonly used antidotes, suggested doses, and their indications for use. Because of its frequent use, naloxone is discussed further here.

Naloxone. Naloxone, a pure opioid antagonist, is one of the broadest-acting, safest, and most effective of any true antidotes now available. It is effective against all opioids. Naloxone is a synthetic congener of oxymorphone but is devoid of morphine agonist or depressant effects. It has no significant side effects in the treatment of acute overdose except narcotic withdrawal symptoms in the addicted patient. These symptoms include GI upset, tachycardia, hyperpnea, mydriasis, rhinorrhea, diaphoresis, sialorrhea, increased blood pressure, anxiety, restlessness, discomfort, and hyperalgesia. These symptoms are not usually life-threatening to teenagers and adults but can be fatal to an infant born to an addicted mother. Withdrawal symptoms secondary to naloxone, if observed during acute overdose treatment, would be expected to last no more than 30 minutes and should generally be treated with supportive care. The serum half-life of naloxone is 1 hour; its duration of action 1 to 4 hours. Initial reversal of narcosis may then revert to coma, requiring ongoing reassessment and readministration of naloxone. There are a few case reports of other adverse effects, including hypertension, pulmonary edema, ventricular irritability, and seizures after naloxone-induced reversal of narcosis in the perioperative setting, typically in patients with underlying cardiopulmonary disease and in the presence of additional medications or anesthetic agent use.

The mechanism of action of naloxone is by competitive displacement of narcotic analgesics at central opioid receptor sites. It can be used as a diagnostic test when faced with a questionable history. Current dosage recommendations reflect the proven safety of naloxone in large doses and the necessity of such doses to reverse effects of synthetic opioids such as propoxyphene and pentazocine. If severe respiratory depression is present, the initial dose should be 2 mg IV in any patient. Repeat doses may be given every 2 minutes until 10 mg has been administered for adolescent patients with suspected opioid overdose who fail to respond to the lower dosages. Of course, concomitant airway management is vital. In patients without respiratory depression, an initial dose of 0.4 to 1 mg can be used. In adolescents suspected of chronic opiate abuse, smaller initial doses (e.g., 0.2 to 0.4 mg) are warranted. Again, if there is no response but a strong clinical suspicion, 2-mg doses can be repeated up to a total of 10 mg before concluding that further dosing will be of no benefit. Naloxone can also be given intramuscularly (IM), sublingually, or by endotracheal tube if no IV access is available.

If a lightening response occurs, naloxone will have to be repeated at the effective total dose every 20 to 60 minutes. An alternative approach is to provide a continuous IV infusion; generally about two-thirds of the total reversal dose will need to be infused per hour initially, with subsequent adjustments as necessary.

Nalmefene and naltrexone are longer-acting opioid antagonists that may have use in some clinical situations in which a longer duration of action (4 to 6 hours for nalmefene, 24 hours for naltrexone) is deemed beneficial, such as in reversal of procedural/postoperative opioid depression or as aids in opioid detoxification programs. However, as antidotes for acute opioid overdose in the adolescent or pediatric population, their longer duration may be problematic in assessing the actual time course for resolution of clinical toxicity and/or in precipitating prolonged withdrawal symptoms in habituated patients. Nalmefene may be a useful substitute for prolonged naloxone infusions in cases for which such opioid antagonism is necessary, but little pediatric experience and few dosing guidelines for its use are currently available.

Enhancing Excretion

The procedures available for enhancing the elimination of an absorbed poison that have the greatest value are multiple-dose activated charcoal, diuresis/urinary alkalinization, dialysis, and hemoperfusion. Because some risk is involved, these measures are indicated only in those cases in which the patient's recovery would be otherwise unlikely or in which a specific significant benefit is expected.

Diuresis/Urinary Alkalinization

Diuresis has historically been advocated in cases of poisoning with agents that are excreted primarily by the renal route. Although it is important to maintain high glomerular filtration rates in the presence of rhabdomyolysis or when chelating with agents such as EDTA, forced diuresis has limited value in the treatment of acute poisoning. Similarly, diuretic use has fallen out of favor with the possible exception of mannitol therapy for ciguatera poisoning.

Ionized diuresis takes advantage of the principle that excretion is favored when a drug is in its ionized state. Urinary alkalinization promotes excretion of salicylate (a weak acid). It may also enhance clearance of phenobarbital, chlorpropamide, and chlorophenoxy herbicides, but in these poisonings, it cannot be considered a mainstay of therapy. Urine alkalinization can be initiated with sodium bicarbonate at a dose of 1 to 2 mEq per kg IV over a 1- to 2-hour period. Careful attention should be given to total fluid and sodium load administered, especially in patients at risk for congestive heart failure or pulmonary edema. Hypokalemia can interfere with the ability to alkalinize the urine and should be corrected.

TABLE 102.9

SUMMARY OF ANTIDOTES

Poison	Antidote
Acetaminophen	N-acetylcysteine; intravenous (IV)—150 mg/kg over 1 h, then 12.5 mg/kg/hr for 4 h, then 6.25 mg/kg/hr; enteral—140 mg/kg, then 70 mg/kg every 4 h.
Anticholinergics	Physostigmine (adult, 0.5 to 2 mg; child, 0.02 mg/kg) slow IV; may repeat in 15 min until desired effect is achieved; subsequent doses every 2–3 h PRN (*Caution: May cause seizures, asystole, cholinergic crisis; see text*)
Anticholinesterases	Atropine, 2–5 mg (adults); 0.05–0.1 mg/kg (children) intramuscular (IM) or IV, repeated every 10–15 min until atropinization is evident
Organophosphates	Pralidoxime chloride 1–2 g (adults); 25–50 mg/kg (children) IV; repeat dose in 1 h PRN, then every 6–8 h for 24–48 h (consider also constant infusion; see text)
Carbamates	Atropine, as above; pralidoxime for severe cases (see text)
Benzodiazepines	Flumazenil, 0.01 mg/kg IV (estimated pediatric dose; see text)
β-Adrenergic blockers	Glucagon, 0.1 mg/kg IV, followed by 0.05 mg/kg/h
Calcium channel blockers	Calcium chloride 10%, 10 mL (adult); 0.2 mL/kg (pediatric) IV Insulin (see text) Or Calcium gluconate 10%, 30 mL (adult); 0.6 mL/kg (pediatric) IV
Carbon monoxide	Oxygen 100% inhalation, consider hyperbaric for severe cases
Cyanide—cyanide antidote kit	*Adult:* Amyl nitrite inhalation (inhale for 15–30 s every 60 s) pending administration of 300 mg sodium nitrite (10 mL of a 3% solution) IV slowly (over 2–4 min); follow immediately with 12.5 g sodium thiosulfate (2.5–5 mL/min of 25% solution) IV *Children* (Na nitrite should not exceed recommended dose because dangerous methemoglobinemia may result):

Hemoglobin	Initial dose 3% Na nitrite	Initial dose 25% Na thiosulfate IV
8 g	0.22 mL (6.6 mg)/kg	1.10 mL/kg
10 g	0.27 mL (8.7 mg)/kg	1.35 mL/kg
12 g (normal)	0.33 mL (10 mg)/kg	1.65 mL/kg
14 g	0.39 mL (11.6 mg)/kg	1.95 mL/kg

Poison	Antidote
Cyanide— hydroxocobalamin	*Adult:* 5g IV; *Child:* 70 mg/kg IV.
Digitalis	Fab antibodies (Digibind): dose based on amount ingested and/or digoxin level (see text, package insert)
Fluoride	Calcium gluconate 10%, 0.6 mL/kg IV slowly until symptoms abate, serum calcium normalizes; repeat PRN
Heavy metals (usual chelators)	BAL (British Anti-Lewisite; dimercaprol): 3–5 mg/kg/dose deep IM every 4 h for 2 days, every 4–6 h for an additional 2 days, then every 4–12 h for up to 7 additional days
Arsenic (BAL)	EDTA (ethylene diamine tetraacetic acid): 50–75 mg/kg/24 h deep IM or slow IV infusion given in 3–6 divided doses for up to 5 days; may be repeated for a second course after a minimum of 2 days; each course should not exceed a total of 500 mg/kg body weight (see text)
Lead (BAL, EDTA, penicillamine, DMSA)	(see text and Table 102.14)
Mercury (BAL, DMSA)	*Penicillamine:* 100 mg/kg/d (max 1 g) by mouth (PO) in divided doses for up to 5 days; for long-term therapy, do not exceed 40 mg/kg/d *DMSA (succimer):* 350 mg/m^2 (10 mg/kg) PO every 8 h for 5 days, followed by 350 mg/m^2 (10 mg/kg) PO every 12 h for 14 days
Iron	Deferoxamine: 5–15 mg/kg/h IV; use higher dosage for severe symptoms (see text) and decrease as patient recovers
Isoniazid (INH)	Pyridoxine 5%–10%, 1 g per gram of INH ingested (70 mg/kg up to 5 g if dose unknown) IV slowly over 30–60 min

MEDICAL EMERGENCIES

(continued)

TABLE 102.9

SUMMARY OF ANTIDOTES (CONTINUED)

Poison	Antidote
Methanol/ ethylene glycol	Fomepizole: load 15 mg/kg; maintenance 10 mg/kg q12h 4 doses, then 15 mg/kg q12h (dose should be adjusted during dialysis; ethanol may be used if fomepizole unavailable) Ethanol loading dose: 0.75 g/kg infused over 1 h (fomepizole is preferred) Ethanol maintenance: 0.1–0.2 g/kg/h infusion; adjust as needed with target level 100 mg/dL Folate 1 mg/kg IV every 6 h (methanol) Thiamine 0.5 mg/kg and pyridoxine 2 mg/kg (ethylene glycol)
Methemoglobinemic agents	Methylene blue 1%, 1–2 mg/kg (0.1–0.2 mL/kg) IV slowly over 5–10 min if cyanosis is severe or methemoglobin level >40%
Opioids	Naloxone 0.4–2 mg IV, IM, sublingual or by ETT; may repeat up to total 8–10 mg in adolescent/adult (see text)
Phenothiazines (dystonic reaction)	Diphenhydramine, 1–2 mg/kg IM or IV; or Benztropine, 1–2 mg IM or IV (adolescents)
Sulfonylureas	Octreotide 1–2 μg/kg/dose subcutaneous (SC) or IV every 6–12 h
Tricyclic antidepressants	Sodium bicarbonate, 1–2 mEq/kg IV
Warfarin (and "superwarfarin" rat poisons)	Vitamin K_t 10 mg (adult); 1–5 mg (pediatric) IV, IM, SC, PO
Animals	Antivenin[a] For envenomation (see Chapter 91)
Snake, Crotalidae (all North American rattlers and moccasins)	Crotalidae polyvalent immune Fab (Savage)
Snake, coral	Antivenin (*Micrurus fulvius*), monovalent (Wyeth)
Spider, black widow	Antivenin *Latrodectus mactans* (Merck, Sharp & Dohme)

[a]See package insert for dosage and administration.

The rate of bicarbonate infusion can be adjusted to maintain a urinary pH of 7.5 to 8.5. Urinary acidification is never indicated because it may lead to serious side effects such as systemic acidosis and exacerbation of renal impairment in the context of myoglobinuria.

Dialysis

Dialysis is indicated for selected cases of severe poisoning or when renal failure is present. Indications for dialysis depend on patient- and drug-related criteria. Patient-related criteria include (i) anticipated prolonged coma with the high likelihood of attendant complications, (ii) development of renal failure or impairment of normal excretory pathways, and (iii) progressive clinical deterioration despite careful medical supervision. Drug-related criteria are (i) satisfactory membrane permeability, (ii) a correlation between plasma drug concentration and drug toxicity of the agent, (iii) plasma levels in the potentially fatal range or the presence of a significant quantity of an agent that is normally metabolized to a toxic substance, and (iv) significant enhancement of clearance. Those xenobiotics with low volumes of distribution (less than 1 L per kg), low molecular weight (less than 500 Da), and low protein binding are the most amenable to enhanced clearance with dialysis. Hemodialysis is the most effective means of dialysis. Because it requires highly technical skills, as well as a physician and a technician, it is not always available; however,

it is an essential consultative service for units that manage severe poisoning cases. The emergency physician should be aware that most typical dialysis patients are hypervolemic but most toxicology dialysis patients (poisoning with salicylate, ethylene glycol, methanol, etc.) are hypovolemic; it is incumbent upon the ED care provider to try to achieve euvolemia prior to hemodialysis.

Hemoperfusion

Hemoperfusion, the process of passing blood through an extracorporeal circuit and a cartridge containing an adsorbent after which the detoxified blood is returned to the patient, is also effective in drug removal. However, with newer "high flux" dialysis membranes, this technology is less commonly needed and less widely available. Indications for use are similar to those for hemodialysis. Table 102.10 summarizes the generally accepted common drugs and drug concentrations for which hemodialysis and hemoperfusion should be considered, in light of the previous discussion regarding clinical criteria.

Multiple-Dose Activated Charcoal (GI Dialysis)

Several studies have shown significant increase in clearance for a number of drugs when repeated doses of 0.5 to 1 g per kg of activated charcoal are given every 4 to 6 hours. By using a nearly continuous stream of fresh charcoal that descends through the intestinal tract, a constant concentration gradient

TABLE 102.10

A PARTIAL LISTING OF DRUGS AND THEIR PLASMA CONCENTRATIONS FOR WHICH HEMODIALYSIS OR HEMOPERFUSION SHOULD BE CONSIDERED

Hemodialysis	Hemoperfusion
Lithium (acute), 4.0 mEq/L	Phenobarbital, 100 mg/L
Lithium (chronic), 2.5 mEq/L	Theophylline, 60–100 mg/L
Ethylene glycol, 50 mg/dL	Paraquat, 0.1 mg/dL
Methanol, 50 mg/dL	
Salicylates, 60 (chronic) to 80 (acute) mg/dL	

Adapted from Winchester JF. Active methods for detoxification. In: Hadded LM, Shannon MW, Winchester JF, eds. *Clinical management of poisoning and drug overdose*, 3rd ed. Philadelphia: WB Saunders, 1998:175–187.

is maintained that favors the back diffusion of free drug from periluminal capillary blood into the intestinal lumen, where it may be bound immediately to the newer charcoal, so the free drug concentration in the intestinal lumen remains low. In addition, enterohepatic recirculation of some drugs may be interrupted as reabsorption from bile is prevented. To be safe and effective, this technique requires active peristalsis and an intact gag reflex or a protected airway. Common pediatric poisonings for which repetitive charcoal dosing may be considered include phenobarbital, carbamazepine, phenytoin, digoxin, salicylates, and theophylline. Cathartics, such as sorbitol, should be administered no more frequently than every third dose.

Supportive Care

The final step in optimizing treatment for the poisoned child is the direction of scrupulous attention to supportive care, including continued close monitoring of ABCDs, fluid and electrolyte status, urine output, and level of consciousness. The value of these efforts usually far outweighs that which may be ascribed to any specific toxicologic interventions in most cases. Severely symptomatic patients are most properly cared for in specialized facilities that have skilled pediatric critical care staff and access to toxicology consultation.

NONTOXIC INGESTION

Often, the emergency provider will be asked about a childhood ingestion of some common household products, many of which are nontoxic unless taken in huge amounts. The availability of a list of such nontoxic products often leads to immediate relief of parental anxiety and avoids the institution of unnecessary noxious interventions. Before using such a list, however, several precautions need to be kept in mind. The fact that an ingestion is nontoxic does not necessarily mean that it has no medical significance. Ingestions often occur in the context of a suboptimal environment. There may be poor supervision or unusual family stresses surrounding the incident, or the ingestion may not have been purely exploratory in nature. Several criteria have been suggested to qualify an ingestion as "nontoxic." These include the assurance that only one identifiable product is ingested in a well-approximated amount, that the product label includes no cautionary signal word, that the child is symptom free and younger

than 5 years, and that an appropriate mechanism is available for telephone follow-up. When used with these criteria, Table 102.11 provides an updated list of nontoxic ingestions. In certain cases, consultation with a regional poison control center (in the United States, the phone number 1-800-222-1222 may be used nationwide) is often helpful.

PEDIATRIC OVERDOSES

The following section highlights selected agents that are ingested by children. They have been chosen for inclusion because of their common occurrence, because they represent the potential for serious or life-threatening toxicity, and because timely recognition and appropriate treatment may be lifesaving.

Acetaminophen

Background

Acetaminophen, *N*-acetyl-*p*-aminophenol (APAP), is the most popular pediatric analgesic-antipyretic and has now become one of the most common pharmaceutical preparations ingested by young children. It is also one of the 10 most common drugs used by adolescents and adults in intentional self-poisoning. Acetaminophen also occasionally turns up as an unreported coingestant in intentional overdoses. Fortunately, exploratory ingestion in young children has been associated with low morbidity, although occasional cases of hepatotoxicity occur, particularly in the context of inadvertent repetitive overdosing.

Pathophysiology

The major toxicity of APAP is severe hepatic damage. Acetaminophen is metabolized in three ways by the liver: (i) glucuronidation, (ii) sulfation, and (iii) metabolism through the cytochrome P-450 pathway to form a potentially toxic intermediate, which conjugates with glutathione. In a massive overdose, glutathione becomes depleted, thus allowing the undetoxified intermediate to bind to hepatocytes, leading to cellular necrosis. This damage is reflected by rising levels of liver enzymes, by hepatic dysfunction, and in severe poisonings, by hepatic failure and death. The use of *N*-acetylcysteine as an antidote relates in part to this molecule's ability to act as a glutathione precursor.

Clinical Findings

Initially, the signs and symptoms of APAP ingestion are vague and nonspecific but include nausea and vomiting, anorexia, pallor, and diaphoresis. These manifestations usually resolve within 12 to 24 hours, and the patient appears well for 1 to 4 days. During this latent period, levels of liver enzymes may rise, and jaundice with liver tenderness may ensue. Most patients have a gradual resolution of their hepatic dysfunction, although without antidotal treatment about 2% to 4% of intoxications that develop toxic plasma levels will go on to hepatic failure and death. Such patients with severe toxicity develop further clinical evidence of hepatic disease at 3 to 5 days after ingestion, and some develop renal damage. Anorexia, malaise, and abdominal pain may progress to signs of liver failure with hepatic coma.

TABLE 102.11

PRODUCTS THAT ARE NONTOXIC WHEN INGESTED IN SMALL AMOUNTS

Abrasives	Hand lotions and creams
Adhesives	Hydrogen peroxide (medicinal 3%)
Antacids	Incense
Antibiotics	Indelible markers
Baby product cosmetics	Ink (black, blue)
Ballpoint pen inks	Laxatives
Bath oil	Lipstick
Bathtub floating toys	Lubricating oils
Bleach (less than 5% sodium hypochlorite)	Magic Markers
Body conditioners	Matches
Bubble bath soaps	Mineral oil
Calamine lotion	Newspaper (black and white pages)
Candles (beeswax or paraffin)	Paint (indoor, latex)
Caps	Pencil (graphite)
Chalk	Perfumes
Cigarettes (less than 3 butts)	Petroleum jelly
Clay (modeling)	Phenolphthalein laxatives (Ex-Lax)
Colognes	Porous-tip marking pens
Contraceptive pills	Putty (less than 2 oz)
Corticosteroids	Rubber cement
Cosmetics	Shampoos (liquid)
Crayons (marked AP, CP)	Shaving creams and lotions
Dehumidifying packets (silica or charcoal)	Soap and soap products
Detergents (phosphate)	Suntan preparations
Deodorants	Sweetening agents (saccharin,
Deodorizers (spray and refrigerator)	cyclamates)
Elmer's Glue	Teething rings (water sterility)
Etch-A-Sketch	Thermometers (mercury)
Eye makeup	Thyroid tablets
Fabric softener	Toothpaste
Fertilizer (if no insecticides or herbicides	Vitamins (without iron)
added)	Warfarin (rat poison; excludes
Glues and pastes	"superwarfarins")
Grease	Watercolors
Hair products (dyes, sprays, tonics; excludes	Zinc oxide (Desitin)
"relaxers")	Zirconium oxide

Adapted from Mofenson HC, Greensher J. The unknown poison. *Pediatrics* 1974;54:336.

The potential severity of an acute intoxication may be predicted by the amount ingested, if accurately known, and the plasma level of APAP. APAP in single doses of less than 200 mg per kg in young children is likely to be harmless. Severe toxicity in adolescents or adults usually occurs with overdoses of at least 7.5 g. Initial GI symptoms, although vague, are generally more pronounced when the overdose is large. However, the only reliable indication of the potential severity of the hepatic damage is the plasma APAP level, taken at least 4 hours after ingestion. After a single acute overdose at a known time of ingestion, a nomogram (Fig. 102.2) is available for using the serum APAP level in the prediction of likely toxicity. We recommend use of the lower line of the nomogram, plotted 25% below the possible toxicity line, to err on the safe side in making therapeutic decisions. Importantly, the nomogram is not validated for chronic APAP toxicity.

Management

The basic toxicologic principles of preventing absorption apply to APAP overdoses, and it is important to note that both immediate- and extended-release preparations exist. Activated charcoal therapy may be used for adsorption of gastric APAP. Many APAP-poisoned patients will benefit from the use of the oral antidote N-acetylcysteine (NAC), and some have speculated that activated charcoal might decrease the bioavailability of the NAC. However, studies have demonstrated clinically insignificant decreases in NAC absorption, even when using large doses of charcoal. For most cases of acetaminophen overdose per se, and particularly for those typically seen early after ingestion, charcoal alone is probably effective and should not significantly alter the ability to use NAC several hours later. In cases that present after 4 hours have elapsed, gastric decontamination is usually not warranted.

NAC, given orally or IV, is most effective at ameliorating hepatotoxicity when instituted within 8 hours of ingestion. It also lessens the severity of hepatic damage if used in the setting of clinical presentation beyond 8 hours. The major adverse reaction associated with IV NAC is the occurrence of anaphylactoid reaction, which typically occurs during the relatively higher dose loading infusion. Clinicians administering IV NAC should be skilled at recognizing and treating anaphylactoid reactions

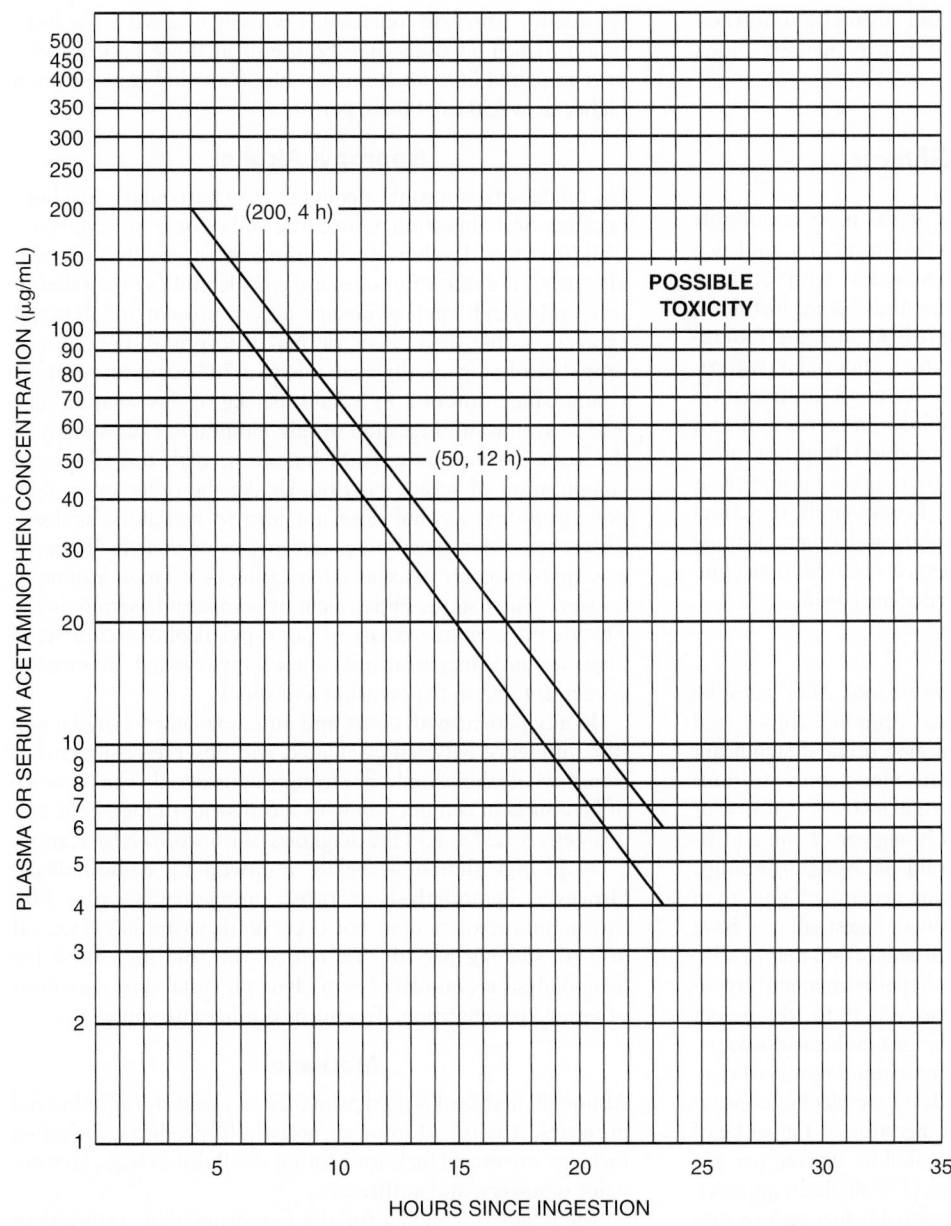

FIGURE 102.2 Nomogram for estimating severity of acute acetaminophen poisoning. (Modified from Rumack BH, Matthew H. *Pediatrics* 1975;55:871–876. Copyright 1975, American Academy of Pediatrics. Reprinted by permission.)

MEDICAL EMERGENCIES

and should be particularly cautious when using this route in patients with a history of asthma. The inhalational form of NAC can be administered enterally and can be mixed with fruit juice or soda to disguise its foul smell, or it can be administered by NG tube. Only mild GI side effects result from its use, but persistent vomiting is an occasional obstacle to completing the course of therapy. This may be obviated by giving the dose slowly or by NG or duodenal tube infusion. Antiemetic therapy with metoclopramide or ondansetron may also be helpful.

The protocol for NAC therapy may be summarized as follows:

1. Consider GI decontamination options as already noted.
2. If patient presents less than 4 hours after a single acute ingestion, wait to draw 4-hour level and base therapeutic decision on nomogram (assumes rapid turnaround time so level will be available by 6 hours after ingestion); if necessary, initiate treatment as described next. For extended-release preparations, McNeil Consumer Products Co. (Fort Washington, Pennsylvania), a manufacturer of acetaminophen, suggests a second APAP level drawn 4 hours after the first; antidotal therapy is to be instituted if either level suggests possible toxicity.
3. If patient presents more than 6 to 8 hours after ingestion, initiate NAC therapy, obtain level and base subsequent course of therapy on nomogram.
4. If level plots out above the lower line on the nomogram, admit the patient to hospital and continue NAC until APAP is not detectable in the blood and liver function is either normal or clearly recovering. Monitor complete blood cell count (CBC) and renal and liver function tests.
5. Treatment for patients who present more than 24 hours after ingestion is controversial, as is treatment for patients with subacute, repetitive overdosing over several days. We consider children who receive more than 150 mg per kg per day for 1 to 2 days to be at risk; again, a combination

of a nondetectable APAP level and normal aminotransferases identifies a patient at low risk of hepatic injury from APAP.

Alcohols and Glycols

The alcohols and glycols are some of the most commonly found organic compounds in the environment. Ethanol is a commonly encountered solvent and is used as a topical antiseptic, chemical intermediate, beverage, and in some instances, a rubbing alcohol. It is also an ingredient in some mouthwashes and many perfumes, colognes, and toilet waters. Methanol, or methyl alcohol, functions as an antifreeze (in windshield washers/deicers and gasoline antifreeze) and as a solvent in many industrial and home products. Isopropyl alcohol serves as a rubefacient. Ethylene glycol is used primarily as a deicer or antifreeze. A related class of compounds, the glycol ethers, is widely used in rug shampoos and other cleaning compounds. The toxicity of these agents is believed to be comparable to (if not more severe than) ethylene glycol.

Ethanol

The most commonly ingested alcohol is ethanol. After ingesting ethanol, children may develop nausea, vomiting, stupor, and ataxia. Coma and death from apnea may occur if significant quantities are consumed. In adolescents, blood concentrations of less than 50 mg per dL rarely result in overt sensory or motor impairment. Values of 80 to 150 mg per dL are consistent with intoxication and cause mild neurologic findings. Lethal blood alcohol concentrations are generally higher than 500 mg per dL. Infants and toddlers who ingest ethanol have a clinical course that is significantly different from that in adolescents and adults; a triad of coma, hypothermia, and hypoglycemia appears once ethanol levels exceed 50 to 100 mg per dL. This triad may be accompanied by metabolic acidosis.

The amount of an ethanol-containing liquid that is of concern when ingested by a child depends on the alcohol concentration. However, a rough rule is that ingestion of 1 g per kg of ethanol is sufficient to raise blood alcohol to 100 mg per dL. Therefore, for a beverage such as beer (5% alcohol), approximately 10 to 15 mL per kg must be ingested before serious toxicity results. Similar estimates are 4 to 6 mL per kg for wine (14% alcohol) and 1 to 2 mL per kg for 80-proof liquor (40% alcohol).

The management of ethanol ingestion in children begins with prompt recognition and evaluation of blood glucose level. Airway or ventilatory compromise should be treated with endotracheal intubation. If seizures result from hypoglycemia, they should be promptly treated with 10% to 50% (0.25 to 1 g per kg) IV dextrose. Warming techniques should be instituted to increase core temperature. Because ethanol is rapidly absorbed from the gut and is not adsorbed by activated charcoal, there is rarely a role for GI decontamination.

Alcohol is metabolized by the hepatic enzyme alcohol dehydrogenase; its elimination rate is dose dependent. This means that the higher the blood alcohol concentrations, the longer the elimination process because the capacity of the body to produce alcohol dehydrogenase is limited. The rate of reduction in blood alcohol concentration varies from 10 to 25 mg per dL per hour. Although hemodialysis effectively enhances

elimination (three- to fourfold), it is rarely necessary. The institution of hemodialysis may be useful in those patients who have impaired liver function or a blood alcohol concentration higher than 450 to 500 mg per dL.

Isopropyl Alcohol

Poisoning with isopropyl alcohol may be particularly insidious because oral ingestion is not the only route of exposure. Children may develop severe intoxication, including coma, after topical application of isopropyl alcohol for the relief of fever (although such exposure may represent inhalational exposure rather than direct, dermal absorption). Because isopropyl alcohol is usually available in a 70% concentration by volume, ingestion of 2 to 2.5 mL per kg of this solution may lead to symptoms. Ingestion of this compound causes many of the same features as ethanol ingestion, with the additional complication of severe gastritis. Unlike the other toxic alcohols, isopropyl alcohol does not lead to metabolic acidosis. This is because its metabolite, acetone, is not an acid. However, it is approximately twice as intoxicating as ethanol, leading to greater mental status impairment at comparable serum levels. The life-threatening toxicity of isopropyl alcohol is cardiac; at high serum concentrations, direct myocardial depression occurs, leading to hypotension and shock.

In any patient with coma and an unexplained osmolal gap (the difference between calculated and observed osmolarity), isopropyl alcohol should be strongly considered. The presence of ketonuria in conjunction with the absence of metabolic acidosis effectively makes the diagnosis of isopropyl intoxication.

Isopropyl alcohol is easily removed by hemodialysis. However, hemodialysis is rarely necessary because life-threatening toxicity does not occur until serum levels exceed 400 to 500 mg per dL. Therefore, the sole indication for hemodialysis is considered hemodynamic instability, regardless of serum concentration. Treatment is otherwise supportive.

Methanol

Although methanol is used primarily as a solvent for industrial purposes, it is found in other household products, including fuels for stoves, gel fuels for heating small dishes (e.g., Sterno), paint removers, and antifreezes.

Methanol is a model for the few drugs that, rather than being detoxified, become more toxic as they are metabolized. Thus, although methanol has little or no inherent toxicity, its metabolism by alcohol and aldehyde dehydrogenase to form formaldehyde and formic acid creates highly toxic compounds. Formic acid is a potent organic acid that results in severe metabolic acidosis and ocular toxicity. Fortunately, because methanol is metabolized slowly, toxicity appears after some delay, permitting time for intervention. Ingestions approaching 100 mg per kg should be considered dangerous.

The clinical effects of methanol ingestion usually occur after a latent period of 8 to 24 hours. This delay occurs as the result of the metabolic conversion of methanol to its toxic by-products. In large ingestions, acute methanol poisoning may cause severe CNS depression, metabolic acidosis, and a number of reversible or irreversible optic changes. In the early stages of intoxication, funduscopic examination may be remarkable for hyperemia. However, if left untreated, methanol intoxication results in blindness, with the appearance of a pale, avascular retina. In subacute ingestions, the nonspecific neurologic symptoms of methanol intoxication resemble those of ethanol with a "hangover," malaise, headache, and dizziness. During recovery from a mild ingestion, occasional paresthesias of the extremities may develop.

The most immediately significant clinical concern from methanol ingestion is severe metabolic acidosis. This acidosis is primarily the result of formic acid production. The metabolic acidosis may be intractable and results in multiorgan dysfunction, which includes cardiac arrhythmias, seizures, and pancreatitis. The ophthalmologic abnormalities that develop during methanol intoxication may be temporary or permanent. These include blurred or double vision, changes in color perception, and sharply reduced visual acuity. Permanent abnormalities may include diminished pupillary light reaction or frank blindness. The occurrence of permanent visual defects correlates directly with the degree of metabolic acidosis, the duration of the acidosis, and the quantity of methanol ingested.

Management. The treatment of methanol ingestion consists of supportive care, administration of specific therapies, and enhancement of elimination. Activated charcoal does not adsorb methanol effectively and is unnecessary.

Laboratory assessment includes serial blood gases, electrolytes, BUN, creatinine, glucose, serum osmolality, and methanol level analyses. Serum methanol concentration in milligrams per deciliter can be estimated by the formula (osmolar gap × 3).

There are three specific treatments for methanol intoxication: sodium bicarbonate, folic acid, and fomepizole (or ethanol). Sodium bicarbonate should be administered aggressively to correct metabolic acidosis. Folate is provided because of its role in formic acid disposition within the tetrahydrofolate cycle. Customary doses are 1 mg per kg IV every 6 hours.

Because serum methanol levels of 20 mg per dL or higher are associated with toxicity if untreated, higher levels require treatment to prevent its metabolism and/or interventions to enhance its elimination. Ethanol, which has a higher affinity for alcohol dehydrogenase than methanol, may be provided to "block" further production of toxic metabolites. Fomepizole, another alcohol dehydrogenase antagonist, is more expensive than ethanol, but the simplicity of fomepizole therapy has led to its rapid and widespread therapeutic acceptance.

An alcohol dehydrogenase inhibitor should be instituted if the calculated or measured methanol concentration is 20 mg per dL or higher. The loading dose of fomepizole is 15 mg per kg, which may be given IV or orally. The maintenance dose is 10 mg per kg every 12 hours for four doses, then 15 mg per kg every 12 hours thereafter. More frequent dosing is required during hemodialysis.

If fomepizole in unavailable, ethanol is administered with the goal of maintaining serum ethanol concentrations of at least 100 mg per dL. Ethanol may be given by continuous IV infusion (600 mg per kg bolus followed by 110 mg per kg per hour) or by oral administration. During dialysis, ethanol dosing may need to be doubled to maintain sufficient blood ethanol content to effectively block the metabolism of methanol. IV ethanol is preferred but has the problems of being often unavailable and hyperosmolar (precluding its administration in small veins) and of requiring large fluid volumes. When the oral route is used, it must be remembered that proof designation of a beverage is twice the alcohol concentration expressed as a percentage (e.g., 80 proof equals 40% alcohol). Children must be closely monitored for the complications of ethanol administration, including mental status depression, hypoglycemia, and hypothermia.

Hemodialysis should be strongly considered for children with a blood methanol concentration of 50 mg per dL or higher, after alcohol dehydrogenase inhibition has been achieved. When alcohol dehydrogenase is blocked, methanol has a very long time to elimination, primarily via exhalation.

Ethylene Glycol

The ingestion of ethylene glycol, although uncommon, causes significant morbidity and occasional mortality in adolescents and young adults. The toxicity of ethylene glycol, like that of methanol, is the result of drug toxification; ethylene glycol has virtually no toxicity in its parent state. However, metabolism by alcohol dehydrogenase produces several toxic intermediates, including glycolaldehyde, glycolic acid, and oxalate. These metabolites result in severe metabolic acidosis and deposition of calcium oxalate crystals in all vital organs. Therefore, ethylene glycol intoxication is associated with more systemic toxicity than that of methanol poisoning. Also, because ethylene glycol is metabolized more rapidly than methanol (elimination half-life approximately 3 hours), toxicity appears rapidly after ingestion.

The clinical syndrome of ethylene glycol intoxication appears in three different stages. The first stage consists predominantly of CNS manifestations and is accompanied by a profound metabolic acidosis. In this early stage, mild hypertension, tachycardia, and leukocytosis are often present. Nausea and vomiting commonly occur, and with larger doses, coma and convulsions may appear within a few hours. Another common finding is the presence of hypocalcemia. This is believed to result from the widespread formation of calcium oxalate. Hypocalcemia may be severe enough to cause tetany and cardiac conduction disturbances. Urinalysis usually reveals a low specific gravity, proteinuria, microscopic hematuria, and crystalluria. The second distinct state is ushered in by coma and cardiopulmonary failure; it is usually the result of acidosis and hypocalcemia. The third stage usually occurs after 24 to 72 hours. Here, renal failure emerges as the dominant problem. Usually, a picture of acute tubular necrosis develops with either polyuria or anuria. Urine sediment contains blood, protein, and casts. Patients often require dialysis for extended periods and may be left with permanent renal insufficiency.

Consideration of ethylene glycol poisoning should be based either on the history or, in the absence of diabetic ketoacidosis, the presence of any of the following criteria: (i) alcohol-like intoxication without the odor of alcohol, (ii) large anion-gap metabolic acidosis, (iii) an elevated osmolar gap in the absence of ethanol or methanol ingestion, or (iv) a urinalysis that demonstrates oxalate crystals. Another diagnostic tool is to perform a Wood's lamp examination of urine. If the ingested substance is radiator antifreeze, the fluorescein dye that it contains will be excreted in urine and may fluoresce under Wood's lamp. Serum chemistries or blood gas levels should be obtained frequently because of the rapid evolution of metabolic acidosis. The availability of ethylene glycol levels varies by institution.

Activated charcoal negligibly adsorbs ethylene glycol and is unnecessary. As with methanol intoxication, treatment of ethylene glycol poisoning falls into three areas: supportive care, administration of pharmacologic agents, and enhancement of elimination. Supportive care includes close monitoring of vital signs and anticipation of life-threatening events, particularly cardiac arrhythmias secondary to hypocalcemia. An EKG should be obtained, and the patient should be placed on a cardiac monitor. Intubation and mechanical ventilation should be provided as needed for control of acid–base balance.

Pharmacologic therapy is subdivided into four areas: administration of sodium bicarbonate, calcium, pyridoxine with thiamine, and fomepizole or ethanol. Correction of acidosis should begin immediately with the administration of sodium bicarbonate and appropriate ventilation. Hypocalcemia may present as skeletal muscle disturbances (tetany) or cardiac dysfunction (prolonged Q-T interval). These may be alleviated by the prompt institution of calcium (e.g., 10% calcium gluconate, 0.3 to 0.6 mL per kg). Thiamine and pyridoxine are vitamins that act as cofactors in the nontoxic metabolic pathways of ethylene glycol and, theoretically, divert its metabolism toward formation of nontoxic metabolites. Therefore, thiamine (0.25 to 0.5 mg per kg) and pyridoxine (1 to 2 mg per kg) are recommended for the first 24 hours of treatment.

Fomepizole (or ethanol) administration is an option to inhibit ethylene glycol metabolism by alcohol dehydrogenase (previously discussed under "Methanol"). Inhibition should be initiated as soon as possible to interrupt further formation of organic acids. As with methanol, alcohol dehydrogenase inhibition is indicated for ethylene glycol concentrations of 20 mg per dL or higher. If a serum ethylene glycol cannot be obtained in a timely fashion, it can be estimated by the formula (osmolar gap × 6), assuming no other alcohols are contributing to the osmolar gap. Hemodialysis is indicated if there is renal failure or severe electrolyte disturbances, regardless of the serum ethylene glycol concentration. Hemodialyis may be considered for patients who are stable hemodynamically but who have very elevated blood ethylene glycol levels. The cost–benefit analysis of hemodialysis versus continued, prolonged fomepizole therapy is currently being investigated; however, recent case reports indicate that fomepizole alone can be effective for ethylene glycol ingestions when the acid–base status and renal function are normal at the time of presentation.

Antihistamines

Antihistamines are used to treat children with allergic diseases, as sedatives and antinauseants, and to prevent motion sickness. They are present in many cough syrups, available both over the counter (OTC) and by prescription. Antihistamines may also be found in combination with analgesics, sympathomimetic amines, and caffeine for the symptomatic relief of the common cold. They are combined with analgesics, such as salicylamide, and an anticholinergic drug, such as scopolamine, for use as a nonprescription sleep medication. Finally, they are included in some liquid cough and cold preparations that may also contain ethanol as the solvent.

Antihistamines may depress or stimulate the CNS. Used therapeutically, CNS depression is most commonly seen as drowsiness or dizziness. With increasing doses, stimulation results in insomnia, nervousness, and restlessness. In antihistamine overdose, the CNS stimulatory effects of the drug predominate. In children, CNS stimulation causes excitement, tremors, hyperactivity, hallucinations, and with higher dosages, tonic-clonic convulsions. Children are also more likely to have signs and symptoms of anticholinergic poisoning: flushed skin, fever, tachycardia, and fixed dilated pupils. The nonsedating antihistamines terfenadine and astemizole (both no longer available in the United States) have caused cardiac arrhythmia after overdose and as a result of drug–drug interactions. Cetirizine, loratadine, and fexofenadine have not produced this complication. Death from antihistamine ingestion in children is usually the result of uncontrolled seizures that progress to coma and cardiorespiratory arrest.

The treatment of antihistamine poisoning requires an accurate history of the time of ingestion and the type and quantity of drug consumed. Of particular importance is the type of drug ingested because numerous sustained-release antihistamine products are available on the market. Options for GI decontamination include the use of activated charcoal, and overdoses with the sustained-release preparations may benefit from WBI.

Patients with seizures (see Chapters 69 and 96) require anticonvulsant therapy immediately. Preferably, short-term control may be gained by using diazepam, in a dose of 0.1 to 0.2 mg per kg IV. Severely agitated patients with a clear anticholinergic toxidrome may have improved sensorium after administration of physostigmine. This is usually administered in an initial dose of 0.02 mg per kg (not to exceed 0.5 mg per dose) IV slowly over 3 minutes. The dose may be repeated every 10 to 15 minutes (adult maximum 2 mg) to establish the effective total dose. This minimal effective dose may be repeated in several hours, if necessary. It should be noted that when administered too rapidly or in too large of a dose, physostigmine might precipitate seizures or asystole. Physostigmine would be particularly dangerous to use in the context of any coingestants that might affect intracardiac conduction, such as tricyclic antidepressants. A 12-lead EKG should be examined for conduction delays before physostigmine is given. Cardiac rhythm should be monitored closely during antidote infusion, and atropine should be available to reverse severe cholinergic effects that may also occur with physostigmine use. The potential risks encountered with physostigmine may favor use of a benzodiazepine for treatment of anticholinergic delirium.

Meticulous attention to supportive care is critical. Some patients may develop extreme hyperthermia and thus require aggressive measures to reduce core body temperature, including ice water baths or misting and fans. There is little evidence for therapeutic efficacy of dialysis or hemoperfusion because of the high plasma protein binding and large volumes of distribution for most of these agents.

Aspirin

Background

Aspirin continues to be a common cause of poisoning in children and adolescents. Salicylism is the result of acute ingestion in about 60% of cases and chronic ingestion in the remaining 40%. Clinical features of acute versus chronic salicylate intoxication often require a different management approach, depending on the manner of intoxication.

Several factors work in concert to make chronic salicylate intoxication so common. The primary factor is aspirin's elimination pattern. As serum salicylate concentrations increase, the ability of the liver to metabolize the drug diminishes until predictable, first-order elimination kinetics are replaced by unpredictable, dose-dependent, zero-order elimination. Thereafter, increments in dose are associated with disproportionate increases in serum salicylate concentration. Also, much of aspirin elimination is through urinary excretion of unchanged drug. Therefore, in the face of dehydration and decreased glomerular filtration, drug clearance is impaired even more. Finally, because aspirin is often prescribed for illnesses that may be associated with hepatic dysfunction, reduced biotransformation initiates the spiraling increase in serum concentration. Unfortunately, because chronic salicylism is associated with nonspecific symptoms (e.g., fever, vomiting, tachypnea), diagnosis may be delayed until more striking signs of intoxication appear.

Pathophysiology

The direct effects of aspirin on metabolism are multiple. Aspirin stimulates the medullary respiratory center, which leads to tachypnea and respiratory alkalosis—its hallmark. Metabolic disturbances are widespread and include CNS hypoglycemia, as well as abnormalities in lipid and amino acid metabolism. Inhibition of Krebs cycle enzymes and uncoupling of oxidative phosphorylation in conjunction with lipid disturbances create the combined lactic and ketoacidosis responsible for metabolic acidosis (which leads to the mixed respiratory alkalosis and metabolic acidosis found on the arterial blood gas). In addition to inhibiting platelet function, aspirin intoxication is associated with disturbances in vitamin K-dependent and vitamin K-independent clotting factors, resulting in a significant coagulopathy. Mild elevations in liver enzymes are also common. Other features of aspirin intoxication include leukocytosis and electrolyte disturbances, particularly hypokalemia. Physical manifestations include fever, tachypnea, nausea, vomiting, lethargy, slurred speech, and seizures. Children with chronic salicylism are more likely to present with severe metabolic acidosis and seizures than those with acute intoxication.

The combination of respiratory alkalosis with metabolic acidosis produces an arterial blood gas that is almost pathognomonic for salicylism. Serum pH typically ranges from 7.41 to 7.55, except in severe cases in which metabolic acidosis combined with respiratory acidosis from severe CNS depression leads to pH less than 7.35, and Pco_2 is generally less than 30 mm Hg. Serum bicarbonate is mildly depressed, often ranging from 15 to 20 mEq per L. However, although adults may continue to hyperventilate for extended periods when poisoned with salicylates, children with mild to moderate poisoning quickly lose this respiratory drive and are more likely to present with metabolic and respiratory acidosis.

As mentioned, glucose homeostasis is seriously altered in acute aspirin poisoning. Early in the course, hyperglycemia usually occurs because of glycogenolysis and decreased peripheral use. Later, hypoglycemia may supervene as glucose stores are depleted. High rates of oxidative metabolism in the CNS may lead to low CNS glucose concentration even in the presence of peripheral hyperglycemia.

Fluid and electrolyte disturbances are multifactorial, resulting in dehydration, hyponatremia or hypernatremia, and hypokalemia. Among contributing factors are increased insensible water losses through both skin and lungs, emesis, and increased renal water and potassium loss. The patient with severe salicylate poisoning may lose 4 to 6 L of water per square meter.

Clinical Findings

The initial clinical signs and symptoms, the estimate of dose ingested, and the measurement of salicylate levels all serve to gauge the severity of a given acute aspirin poisoning. However, in cases of chronic therapeutic salicylism, the clinical picture is the most useful guideline. Because of the nonspecific nature of symptoms with salicylism, the initial differential diagnosis is broad and may include diabetic ketoacidosis, iron intoxication, and ethylene glycol ingestion.

Signs and symptoms of salicylism depend on the method and severity of intoxication. Acute ingestion of amounts of 150 to 300 mg per kg are associated with mild symptoms, 300 to 500 mg per kg are associated with moderate toxicity, and more than 500 mg per kg are associated with death. With mild toxicity (serum concentrations 30 to 50 mg per dL), manifestations may be confined to GI upset, tinnitus, and mild tachypnea. With moderate salicylate poisoning (serum level 50 to 100 mg per dL), more visible signs of toxicity—fever, diaphoresis, and agitation—appear. After severe salicylate poisoning (serum concentrations higher than 100 mg per dL), signs and symptoms are primarily neurologic and consist of dysarthria, coma, and seizures. Pulmonary manifestations, particularly pulmonary edema, may appear in severe cases. In patients of chronic salicylism, these same conditions appear at significantly lower serum salicylate concentrations. Death from salicylism results from severe CNS toxicity with complete loss of function in cardiorespiratory centers, leading to respiratory and/or cardiac arrest. The severity of salicylate intoxication is best assessed by physical examination, electrolytes, and blood gas level analyses rather than through use of a nomogram.

Management

Assessment of the patient of salicylate intoxication begins with an accurate history that identifies the patient as having acute or chronic poisoning. Laboratory assessment is extensive and includes serum salicylate concentration, electrolytes and arterial blood gas levels, liver function tests, CBCs, prothrombin and partial thromboplastin times, urinalysis, and an EKG. In the case of intentional ingestions by adolescents, attention to a serum acetaminophen measurement is important (because many OTC analgesics contain aspirin and acetaminophen in combination).

Supportive care includes assessment of ventilatory function, cardiac monitoring, and vascular access. Because aspirin overdose is associated with delayed gastric emptying and drug coalescence to form bezoars, GI decontamination should receive careful consideration in those patients who present within 4 to 6 hours of ingestion. In patients who present more than 6 hours after ingestion or in those with chronic salicylism, activated charcoal might still be administered because it may enhance postabsorptive elimination of salicylates (through GI dialysis).

Health-care providers are cautioned to be wary of sedating or mechanically ventilating aspirin poisoned patients, as depressing the spontaneous ventilation rate may worsen aspirin-induced neurotoxicity. Specific therapeutic goals in salicylate intoxication include correction of fluid and electrolyte disturbances and the enhancement of salicylate excretion.

MEDICAL EMERGENCIES

Fluid therapy should be aimed at restoring hydration and electrolyte balance, preventing distribution of salicylate to the brain, and promoting renal salicylate excretion. Aggressive restoration of intravascular volume is advisable; however, fluids should be given prudently to prevent precipitation of pulmonary edema, particularly in patients with severe intoxication. The blood pH should be kept alkaline, pH 7.45 to 7.5. For patients with symptomatic salicylate intoxication, urine alkalinization should be combined with fluid resuscitation. The administration of sodium bicarbonate, by increasing urinary pH, ionizes filtered aspirin, increasing tubular secretion and inhibiting its tubular reabsorption (ion trapping). The initial fluid is, therefore, designed to replace both sodium and bicarbonate losses as well as promote urine alkalinization. It should contain 5% dextrose with 100 to 150 mEq per L of sodium bicarbonate. Because hypokalemia impairs the ability of the kidney to create alkaline urine and is exacerbated by administration of sodium bicarbonate, potassium must be added to IV fluids. Forced diuresis does not appear to enhance salicylate excretion more than the clearance accomplished by alkalinization alone. Therefore, fluids are given as needed to restore normal hydration and to produce 1 to 2 mL per kg per hour of urine. Calcium homeostasis should also be monitored during therapy with exogenous bicarbonate. Both urine alkalinization and repetitive oral charcoal (up to every 4 hours) should be continued until salicylate concentration falls below 30 to 40 mg per dL and symptoms resolve.

Salicylate elimination can also be enhanced by hemodialysis or hemoperfusion. Although hemoperfusion results in superior clearance technique, hemodialysis is usually preferred because it permits correction of fluid and electrolyte imbalances. Hemodialysis should be reserved for seriously ill patients. Hemodialysis might be considered for patients with serum salicylate levels higher than 100 mg per dL after acute ingestion or 60 mg per dL or higher after chronic salicylism. Specific indications for hemodialysis include (i) severe acidosis or other electrolyte disturbance, (ii) renal failure, (iii) persistent neurologic dysfunction, (iv) pulmonary edema, and/or (v) progressive clinical deterioration despite standard treatment.

Cardiac Drugs

β-Adrenergic Blockers and Calcium Channel Blockers

The approaches to overdoses of these two categories of cardiovascular agents are discussed together because of similarities of clinical presentation and management approach. They both are commonly prescribed to adult patients with a variety of cardiovascular disorders, including angina and past myocardial infarction, hypertension, and arrhythmias. As such, experience with pediatric overdoses has been increasing in more recent years.

β-Blockers (BBs) vary considerably in terms of receptor specificity and pharmacokinetics, but most overdose experience is with propranolol. Similarly, the calcium channel blockers (CCBs) most commonly used in the United States (verapamil, diltiazem, nifedipine, amlodipine, etc) are chemically dissimilar and have varied degrees of effect on vasodilation, myocardial contractility, and sinoatrial (SA)-atrioventricular (AV) node function.

Both BBs and CCBs may present with fulminant cardiovascular and neurologic findings after a large overdose. Typical presentations of both agents include marked bradycardia and hypotension; particularly with the CCBs, common additional findings are those of abnormal AV node conduction, with AV block or accelerated junctional rhythm. The CNS may also be affected, with coma and/or convulsions that occur in either category of overdoses. Metabolic disturbances include hypoglycemia with BBs and hyperglycemia and metabolic acidosis with CCBs. Bronchospasm may further complicate BB toxicity in patients with underlying reactive airway disease.

Management begins with aggressive gastric decontamination for both types of agents. Activated charcoal/cathartic should be administered to patients presenting soon after ingestion. Sustained-release preparations may cause prolonged effects, and WBI may be considered in this context. Bradycardia and hypotension may improve with standard treatment such as atropine, fluid boluses, and pressors; however, many cases prove resistant to these measures.

Additional therapy includes calcium infusion for the CCBs, with the recommended adult initial dose being 10 mL of 10% calcium chloride or 30 mL of 10% calcium gluconate, which may be repeated two or three times as necessary (e.g., an initial pediatric dose of approximately 0.2 mL per kg calcium chloride or 0.6 mL per kg of calcium gluconate). Serum calcium should be monitored. Glucagon increases intracellular cyclic adenosine monophosphate (cAMP) by a mechanism independent of β receptors and has been used with success to improve heart rate and blood pressure in overdoses of BB agents. The usual adult dosing regimen is 3 to 5 mg by IV bolus, which may be repeated to a total dose of 10 mg, followed by infusion at 2 to 5 mg per hour. Such dosing translates to 50 to 150 μg per kg boluses and similar amounts per hour for pediatric patients.

For hemodynamically significant overdose of a CCB, hyperinsulinemia–euglycemia therapy is currently in favor; this therapy should be guided by a clinician or poison control center consultant familiar with its use. Severe cases may also benefit from pacemaker insertion and consideration of aortic balloon pump and/or cardiopulmonary bypass. (Lipid emulsion infusion has shown promise in animal studies of verapamil toxicity but is unproven in humans as of this writing.) It is unlikely that hemodialysis or hemoperfusion would benefit most of these cases.

Clonidine

Clonidine is an antihypertensive that appears to have growing popularity, part of which comes from its efficacy in illnesses other than hypertension, including nicotine withdrawal and attention deficit disorder. Also, the advent of clonidine in transdermal patches has become a convenient and somewhat unique vehicle for drug administration.

Clonidine exerts its antihypertensive effect through stimulation of CNS α_2-adrenergic receptors. These receptors are located on presynaptic neurons in cardiorespiratory centers of the midbrain. Their stimulation results in decreased secretion of catecholamines into the synaptic cleft, resulting in decreased pulse and blood pressure. In addition, clonidine appears to interact with or modulate CNS opiate receptors; this interaction has been used to explain clonidine's efficacy in opiate withdrawal and the picture of coma and miosis that accompanies clonidine intoxication. An imidazoline compound, clonidine is related to other medications, including tetrahydrozoline and oxymetazoline—common vasoconstrictors found in nasal decongestants and ophthalmic agents.

Clonidine is an extremely potent drug with typical doses of 100 to 200 μg in adults. Therefore, ingestions of small amounts can potentially lead to significant toxicity in children. Initial toxic manifestations include altered mental status that may range from lethargy to coma. Patients may also develop significant hypothermia. In severe intoxications, coma, miosis, and respiratory depression may appear. The cardiovascular changes that accompany clonidine intoxications may range from profound hypotension and bradycardia to hypertension. Clonidine-induced hypertension occurs uncommonly and is believed to result from α-adrenergic effects at peripheral vascular receptors that override the central, antihypertensive effect. The clinical picture of clonidine intoxication typically lasts 8 to 24 hours.

Management. The treatment of clonidine intoxication requires immediate assessment of the ABCs. Because patients with severe intoxication often have coma and respiratory depression, emergency endotracheal intubation may be necessary. Also, because of blood pressure instability, vascular access should be achieved immediately for better hemodynamic control. Hypotension should be treated with fluids and vasopressors as needed. Hypertension is generally uncommon, is very transient, and would rarely require specific treatment.

Activated charcoal binds clonidine. In addition to supportive care measures, other pharmacologic interventions may be effective. Naloxone has been suggested as a specific antidotal agent after clonidine intoxication, based on case reports of improved mental status and cardiorespiratory function after its administration. However, in reported case series, there have not been consistent improvements after naloxone administration.

Because naloxone is a benign agent and may potentially improve mental status to the extent that intubation becomes unnecessary, a trial dose of 1 to 2 mg should be administered. Large amounts of naloxone (up to 8 mg) must be provided before it can be concluded that the intoxication is not responsive to this therapy. If effective, repeat doses or a continuous infusion of naloxone may be useful. Other pharmacologic agents that have been used include yohimbine, tolazoline, and phentolamine; but specific efficacy from these agents has not been demonstrated, and they are not considered important in the treatment of clonidine intoxication.

Digoxin

Digoxin is still widely used in young infants with congenital heart disease and elderly patients with congestive heart failure. This continued popularity, its narrow therapeutic index, and the appealing color of digoxin elixir make it a source of many childhood poisoning episodes annually. Also, related agents, particularly the foxglove and oleander plants, are occasionally ingested by children, leading to a clinical picture identical to that of digoxin.

Digoxin's primary pharmacologic action is to inhibit activity of sodium-potassium adenosine triphosphatase (ATPase), which is responsible for maintaining the electrical potential of excitable tissues through transmembrane concentration of electrolytes. Therefore, the effects of digoxin are largely related to disturbances in this action.

In all patients of digoxin poisoning, two distinct pictures of toxicity exist: acute and chronic. These pictures have several differences: The patient of acute digoxin ingestion is typically a toddler who ingests a relative's medication. The toddler is generally healthy with no underlying cardiac disease. The child with chronic digoxin poisoning, however, by definition has preexisting heart disease and is likely to be taking other medications known to modulate the effects of digoxin poisoning (e.g., diuretics). Therefore, it is the latter patient who is more likely to have severe toxic manifestations after digoxin intoxication.

Digoxin pharmacokinetics are complex. After ingestion, absorption is complete within 2 to 4 hours. However, after peak serum levels are achieved, the drug is rapidly redistributed, resulting in dramatic falls in serum concentration. This has particular importance with the patient of acute digoxin intoxication who may have an initial serum digoxin concentration (SDC) in the highly toxic range that falls to the therapeutic range within a matter of hours. After redistribution, digoxin elimination occurs primarily through renal excretion of unchanged drug. Therefore, any condition associated with decreased renal function may be associated with the insidious development of intoxication.

The therapeutic SDC is less than 2 ng per mL. A concentration in the slightly higher range often does not correlate with clinical manifestations and may be of limited value. However, when SDC exceeds 4 ng per mL, some evidence of intoxication usually appears. This toxicity is influenced by many host factors, including patient age; underlying illness; and disturbances in serum potassium, magnesium, and calcium.

With significant intoxication, the symptoms of digoxin poisoning include nausea, vomiting, and visual disturbances. With more severe intoxication, additional symptoms, including lethargy, disorientation, electrolyte disturbances, and cardiac disturbances, appear. The hallmark of severe acute digoxin toxicity is hyperkalemia, the result of profound inhibition of sodium-potassium ATPase activity. The typical pattern of cardiac toxicity with digoxin overdose initially is prolonged atrioventricular dissociation that appears as heart block that ranges from first to third degree. These conduction disturbances can lead to the development of ventricular or supraventricular escape rhythms. In patients with chronic digoxin intoxication, these symptoms may be more striking than in those with acute, single digoxin overdoses. In fact, children with acute digoxin intoxication rarely develop life-threatening illness if their peak SDC remains below 10 ng per mL.

Management. The management of the patient with digoxin intoxication begins with evaluation of the vital signs, particularly hemodynamic status. Patients should have an EKG performed, followed by continuous cardiac monitoring. If significant cardiac arrhythmias are already present, they are treated initially according to advanced cardiac life support protocols.

GI decontamination should include administration of activated charcoal. Clinical assessment typically includes an EKG, electrolytes (including magnesium and calcium) level, urinalysis, and SDC. Electrolyte disturbances should be treated aggressively because they will aggravate any digoxin-induced arrhythmias.

Digoxin-specific antibody fragments have become specific antidotal therapy for reversing the toxic manifestations. These fragments are the result of sheep-derived immunoglobulin that is cleaved to extract only the Fab fragment. This low-molecular-weight antibody fragment is capable of avidly binding free digoxin so a gradient results that favors digoxin removal from receptor sites into interstitial water. The effect of this gradient is that sodium-potassium ATPase function is immediately restored. The digoxin–antibody complex is then rapidly excreted in the urine. Of note, after digoxin antibody fragments are administered, SDC increases astronomically, reflecting bound, inactive digoxin that has diffused into the vascular compartment.

These antibody fragments are indicated in the following circumstances after digoxin poisoning: (i) progressive signs and symptoms of intoxication, (ii) life-threatening cardiac arrhythmias, or (iii) severe hyperkalemia (defined as a serum potassium level of 5.5 mEq per L or higher). The dose of antibody fragments is calculated on the basis of ingested digoxin dose (in the case of acute intoxication) or on the basis of SDC (in the case of chronic intoxication). Each 40-mg vial of digoxin-Fab will bind 0.6 mg of digoxin. The total dose of Fab needed (in vials) may be estimated by dividing a known ingested dose by 0.6, or calculated for the steady-state context as body load of digoxin:

$$\text{No. of vials} = \frac{\text{SDC (ng/mL)} \times \text{wt (in kg)}}{100}$$

Complications from the administration of antibody fragments are low and consist of an allergic reaction (in approximately 0.6% of patients), precipitation of congestive heart failure (secondary to the abrupt loss of digoxin's inotropic action), and rebound hypokalemia. These complications should be anticipated and treated accordingly. Infusions should be given over 30 minutes, and some prefer to use a 0.22 μm in-line filter. If the patient is in cardiac arrest, the antibody fragments may be infused over 5 minutes.

Disc Batteries

The development and widespread use of disc batteries in home toys and appliances has led to a burgeoning increase in the rate of disc battery ingestions in young children. A somewhat unusual feature of these ingestions is the frequency among children 4 to 8 years of age who often ingest them inadvertently or out of curiosity. Children with hearing aids form another group at particular risk.

Disc batteries contain a number of potentially toxic substances, including mercury, lithium, and potassium hydroxide. However, their toxic potential is primarily confined to their corrosive action when they are in contact with a mucosal surface for an extended time. Thus, disc batteries that are placed in nasal or aural cavities should be removed immediately.

With the history of disc battery ingestion, all patients should receive an immediate chest radiograph. This is because disc batteries that are retained in the esophagus act as local corrosives, leading to esophageal injury or perforation. If the disc battery is found in the esophagus, it must be removed immediately. If the battery is beyond the esophagus, the patient may be discharged and followed as an outpatient.

The natural history of disc battery ingestion is that the object is usually expelled within 72 hours of ingestion without inducing symptoms. Therefore, the treatment of these inges-

tions involves no intervention. Rather, parents are asked to monitor stools for 3 days to document passage of the battery. In the event the battery is not passed within that time, an abdominal radiograph might be obtained to confirm that the battery has not been incarcerated in a bowel loop. If the battery is still in the gut, there is continued observation. Surgical removal of these objects is almost never necessary.

Foods/Fish

In addition to drugs and medications and household products and plants, toxic ingestions may occur through normal diet when the ingested product contains a toxin that is preformed by microorganisms. The largest class of such toxins is the enterotoxins produced by organisms that include *Shigella*, *Salmonella*, *Yersinia*, *Escherichia coli*, *Staphylococcus*, *Bacillus cereus*, *Clostridium*, *Vibrio*, and *Clostridium botulinum*. After this large group of toxins, the next most common cause of foodborne intoxications results from the ingestion of contaminated marine life.

The general approaches to the patient with diarrhea and infectious causes of the gastroenteritis syndrome are discussed in Chapters 18 and 89, respectively. The association of hemolytic-uremic syndrome with GI infection by *E. coli* O157:H7 is discussed in Chapters 89 and 100. Plant toxicity is discussed later in this chapter, under its own heading. Here, the common causes of acute bacterial toxin-induced food poisoning are outlined, followed by a discussion of marine-related illness.

When similar GI symptoms occur in a group of persons who share the same meal or the same food on separate occasions, the emergency physician may consider the possibility of foodborne disease. Detailed epidemiologic investigations are usually beyond the capacity of the ED setting, but the hospital infection control officer and/or local health department can often be helpful.

Staphylococcal food poisoning is probably the most common cause of such cases in the United States. The heat-stable toxins typically produce acute abdominal pain, nausea, vomiting, and diarrhea within 1 to 6 hours of eating the contaminated meal. The illness is usually self-limiting, although occasionally, patients develop severe symptoms and dehydration.

Other bacterial toxin-induced diarrheal food poisonings include those secondary to *Bacillus cereus*, *Clostridium perfringens*, and *Vibrio* species. The onset of clinical illness and usual food sources of these and staphylococcal disease are outlined in Table 102.12. All these illnesses are generally self-limiting, and treatment is supportive, with careful attention given to fluid and electrolyte status in unusually severe cases (e.g., the rare occurrence of cholera in the United States).

Infant botulism shares many pathophysiologic and clinical features with foodborne botulism (it is discussed in detail in Chapter 96). The etiology of the foodborne disease differs, of course, in that preformed toxin is ingested at the time of consuming contaminated food, typically improperly home-canned, low-acidity vegetables (e.g., potatoes, onions, beans) or poorly refrigerated pot pies or meats. The incubation period is usually 12 to 36 hours, with initial GI symptoms soon followed by weakness, malaise, and then cranial nerve symptoms, particularly diplopia, dysphagia, and dysarthria. The neurologic examination is notable for normal mental status

TABLE 102.12

COMMON CAUSES OF DIARRHEAL FOOD POISONING IN THE UNITED STATES

Organism	Onset (h)	Effect of heat	Typical sources
Staphylococcal	1–6	Stable	Meats, potato/egg salads, cream-filled desserts
Bacillus cereus			
Emetic type	1–6	Stable	Fried rice
Diarrheal type	12–16	Labile	Cooked meats
Clostridia	12–24	Spores, stable Toxin labile	Meats/poultry[a]
Cholera/other *Vibrio* spp.	12–24	Toxin labile	Raw shellfish

[a]In context of inadequate refrigeration.

and symmetric ocular findings, such as ptosis, lateral rectus weakness, and pupillary abnormalities.

Diagnosis should be suspected clinically and may be buttressed with positive serum or stool analyses for botulinum toxin and suggestive electromyelograph findings. The management of foodborne botulism shares with infant botulism the requirement for meticulous, intensive supportive care, with special attention to airway and ventilatory status. In addition, unlike the case in infant botulism, administration of bivalent antitoxin is recommended for all symptomatic patients. This antitoxin and details regarding its optimal use are available from the Centers for Disease Control and Prevention, which should be contacted through a state health department.

Scombroid Poisoning

Scombroid poisoning is an intoxication that occurs shortly after ingestion of spoiled fish from the Scombroidea family (e.g., tuna, bonita, skipjack), as well as ingestion of non-Scombroidea fish (e.g., bluefish, mahi mahi). The ingested toxin(s) has not been completely characterized, but large quantities of histamine-like compounds are invariably found in these fish when tissue histidine decomposes.

The clinical picture of scombroid poisoning consists of sudden-onset headache, facial flushing, a peppery taste in the mouth, dizziness, nausea, and vomiting. An urticarial eruption with pruritus may develop. In its extreme, patients may develop tachycardia, bronchospasm, respiratory distress, and hypotension.

In patients with severe symptoms, treatment is directed toward ensuring adequate ventilation and hemodynamic stability. Fluids and vasopressor support may be needed to treat hypotension. Pharmacologic treatment of scombroid poisoning includes administration of antihistamines, corticosteroids, and if necessary, adrenergic agents. Both diphenhydramine and cimetidine have been used successfully to treat the symptoms of scombroid poisoning. In the event of severe bronchospasm, other bronchodilators, including inhaled β_2 agonists may be necessary adjuncts.

Ciguatera

Ciguatera is an illness endemic to the South Pacific but is considerably less common in the continental United States, where it is largely confined to the lower Atlantic states. However, because it does occasionally appear in the United States or may occur in recent visitors from endemic areas, its clinical manifestations should be recognized.

Ciguatera results from ingestion of a toxin elaborated by the dinoflagellate, *Gambierdiscus toxicus*. This parasite is ingested by small fish, which begin to concentrate the toxin. As predators ingest those small fish, the toxin ascends the food chain until ingested by humans. The fish that most commonly harbor ciguatoxin include barracuda, grouper, red snapper, and parrot fish. The physiologic actions of ciguatoxin are primarily neurologic. The toxin decreases CNS concentrations of γ-aminobutyric acid (GABA) and dopamine. This action occurs in conjunction with sodium channels being "locked open," permitting unrestricted sodium ingress.

The clinical picture of ciguatera poisoning begins 4 to 36 hours after ingestion of contaminated fish. After a brief period of nausea and vomiting, patients develop paresthesias, particularly perioral, or weakness. A hallmark of ciguatera toxin is the reversal of hot–cold sensation. In severe cases, CNS dysfunction, including coma, may appear. Toxic manifestations may persist for days to months after significant exposure.

The diagnosis of ciguatera intoxication is clinical, based on the history of ingestion of a fish known to carry this toxin. Because symptoms appear many hours after ingestion of contaminated fish, there is no clear role for GI decontamination.

Management of ciguatera is supportive. Primary attention should be paid to CNS status and its effects on airway and ventilation. IV mannitol has shown great promise in reversing many of the neurologic manifestations, particularly coma. It is administered in a dose of 0.5 to 1 g per kg via an in-line filter.

Paralytic Shellfish Poisoning

The dinoflagellate *Gonyaulax* is responsible for elaborating the toxin (saxitoxin) that causes paralytic shellfish poisoning (PSP). The name "red tide" is based on the characteristic red pigment of the *Gonyaulax*. PSP appears in large bloom between the months of May and October and is found primarily along the eastern seaboard (although blooms have increased across the world in more recent years and may be found on either U.S. coast). The animals that ingest and concentrate this toxin are primarily bivalve shellfish, including mussels, clams, oysters, and uncommonly, scallops. The toxin, saxitoxin, is capable of reversibly binding neuronal sodium channels, resulting in depolarization disturbances. The toxin is heat stable.

After ingestion of contaminated shellfish, patients quickly develop GI distress with nausea and vomiting. This is followed by generalized paresthesias, cranial nerve disturbances, and weakness. In severe intoxications, cardiorespiratory failure may ensue.

Treatment of PSP is supportive. Patients may require ventilatory support until the intoxication resolves over hours to days.

Household Cleaning Products and Caustics

Household Cleaning Products

Background. Until the early 1950s, cleaning products used for home laundering, household maintenance, and personal hygiene were usually some form of soap. However, soap has the disadvantage of forming an insoluble precipitate that clings to surfaces such as skin, bathtubs, clothes, and dishes. Most products today use synthetic detergents that do not form such precipitates. Soap is one type of surface-active agent (surfactant). A "detergent" is any cleansing product. However, in common use, the word *detergent* has come to mean a household cleaning product that is based on nonsoap surfactants, used mainly for laundering and dishwashing. Other cleaning products include disinfectant cleaners; cleaners for drains, ovens, and toilet bowls; bleaches; and ammonia. These agents are of concern because their accessibility to children makes them commonly involved in human ingestions. Furthermore, animal studies and clinical observations have shown some of these products to be injurious after topical applications.

Each year, about 8% of reported pediatric exploratory ingestions involve household cleaning substances. Most of these cases involve children younger than 5 years, of whom only 1% to 2% of those ingesting noncorrosive products are hospitalized. Most such exposures occur inside the home while the product is in use. In almost half of these cases, the product had been transferred out of its original container, often unfortunately, to an empty glass or soda bottle.

Caustics

Background and Pathophysiology. Many agents possess corrosive potential when they are placed in direct contact with biological tissues.

These agents, collectively referred to as *corrosives*, may be acidic, alkaline, or rarely, have neutral pH (e.g., silver nitrate, concentrated hydrogen peroxide). Essentially all corrosives found in the home are acids or alkalis. Strong alkalis and acids cause direct destruction of tissue but with differing histopathologic patterns. Acids produce coagulation necrosis that usually causes superficial damage, rather than deep, penetrating burns. Alkalis, in contrast, cause a deep and penetrating liquefaction necrosis, which often has severe consequences, such as esophageal perforation. Such deep burns are often associated with severe scarring and, ultimately, with stricture formation (Fig. 102.3). Acid corrosives include the mineral acids, such as hydrochloric, sulfuric, nitric, and hydrofluoric acids. Common

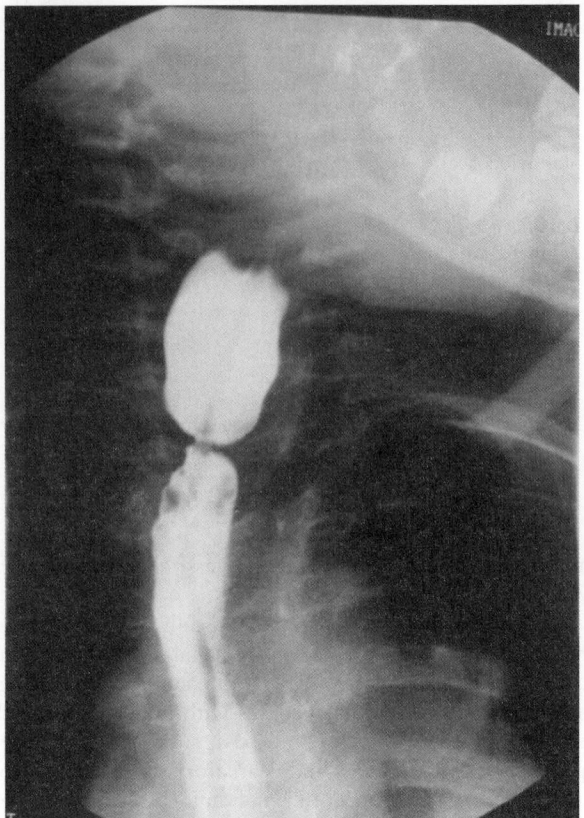

FIGURE 102.3 Barium swallow radiograph demonstrating esophageal stricture in a boy subsequent to ingestion of drain cleaner.

household products that contain acid corrosives include toilet bowl and drain cleaners. However, many home incidents involve acids brought home (often in unmarked food containers) by parents from the workplace.

Alkali caustics are found in several household products. Sodium hydroxide (lye), which is available in crystalline and liquid forms, is used primarily as an oven cleaner or drain pipe cleaner. Other products may contain alkaline corrosives, including powdered laundry and dishwasher detergents.

Clinical Findings. Ingestions of acid and alkali corrosives cause immediate severe burning of exposed surfaces, usually with intense dysphagia. Associated glottic edema may cause airway obstruction and asphyxia. Severe acid ingestions most often cause gastric necrosis and may be complicated by gastric perforation and peritonitis. With alkalis, severe damage is more commonly found in the esophagus; deep-tissue injury may quickly lead to esophageal perforation, mediastinitis, and death. As already noted, alkalis also produce severe esophageal strictures in survivors.

Management. The initial step in the management of a caustic ingestion is to determine whether the agent is, in fact, corrosive and, if so, whether it is an alkaline or acid corrosive. Many products that are believed to have corrosive potential (e.g., household bleach) are simple irritants and do not require intervention. Identification of ingredients and their corrosive potential can be found through consultation with a regional poison control center.

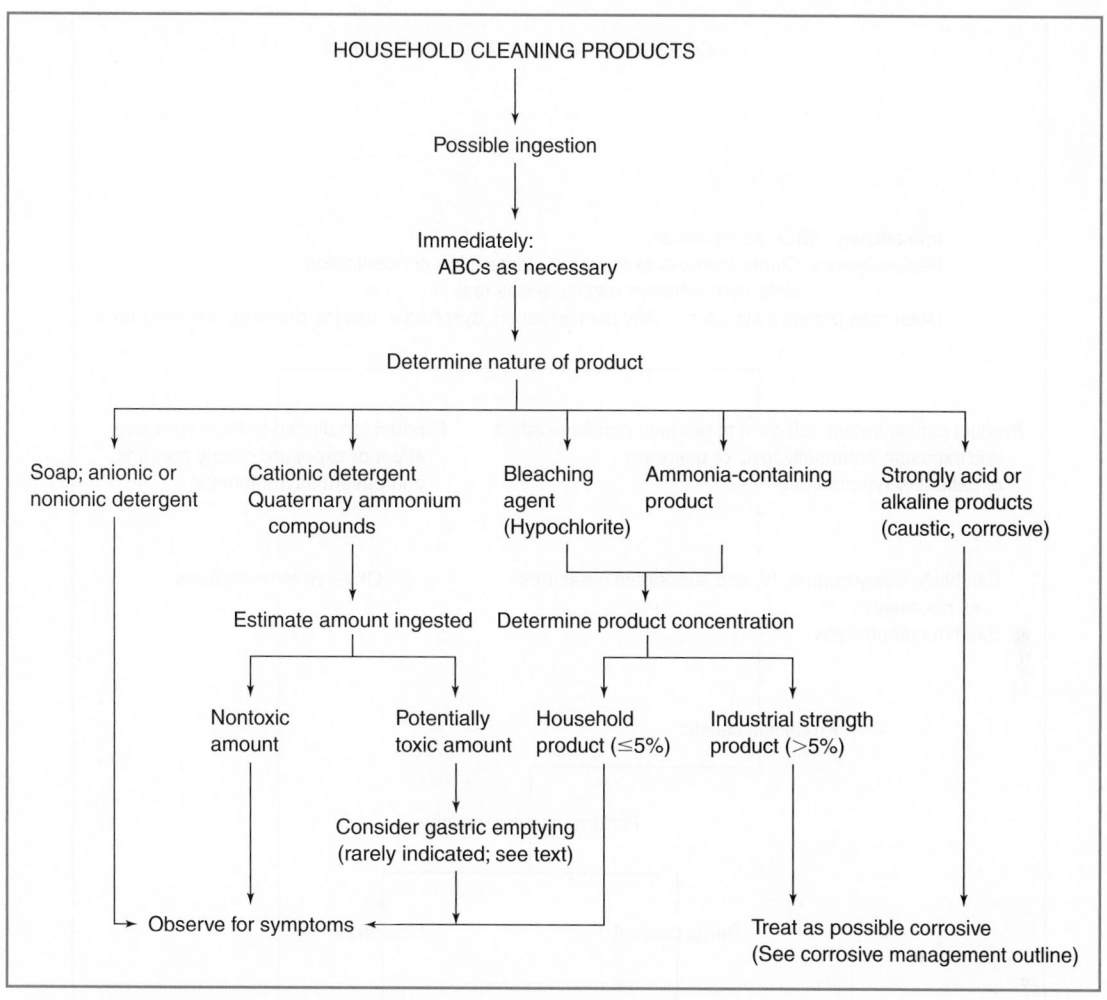

HOUSEHOLD CLEANING PRODUCTS

↓

Possible ingestion

↓

Immediately:
ABCs as necessary

↓

Determine nature of product

- Soap; anionic or nonionic detergent
- Cationic detergent Quaternary ammonium compounds
- Bleaching agent (Hypochlorite)
- Ammonia-containing product
- Strongly acid or alkaline products (caustic, corrosive)

Estimate amount ingested   Determine product concentration

- Nontoxic amount
- Potentially toxic amount
- Household product (≤5%)
- Industrial strength product (>5%)

Consider gastric emptying
(rarely indicated; see text)

Observe for symptoms ←

Treat as possible corrosive
(See corrosive management outline)

FIGURE 102.4 Algorithm for management of household cleaning product ingestion. ABC, airway, breathing, circulation. (Modified with permission from Temple AR, Lovejoy FH Jr. *Cleaning products and their accidental ingestion.* New York, NY: Soap and Detergent Association, 1980.)

MEDICAL EMERGENCIES

The approach to management of cleaning products and caustic ingestions, as outlined in Figs. 102.4 and 102.5, begins with rapid clinical assessment of cardiorespiratory function, neurologic status, and evidence of GI hemorrhage. Life support measures may be needed emergently to secure the airway and to treat shock or metabolic acidosis. As noted previously, most patients with significant exposures develop symptoms early and may appear critically ill. However, even patients with minimal symptoms and the absence of oral lesions may have significant esophageal injury; thus, all patients with a convincing history of significant exposure to a caustic substance merit esophagoscopy to be evaluated fully for the presence of esophageal burns.

Simple dilution has been suggested as being safe and potentially diagnostic. However, there are several reasons why this should only be recommended as first aid in mildly symptomatic children. First, in the event esophageal injury or perforation has occurred, fluids may extravasate, inducing severe mediastinitis. Also, because esophagoscopy is the diagnostic procedure of choice in establishing the extent of injuries, an empty stomach is necessary for minimizing the risks of anesthesia. Finally, if administered fluids are alkaline or acidic, an exothermic reaction

may occur that also can worsen esophageal injury. No GI decontamination is conducted after the ingestion of corrosive agents.

If the eyes are involved (something that should always be considered if a caustic has splashed on the face), copious irrigation should be provided and carried out for at least 15 minutes, with longer periods for crystalline caustics. The physician should perform pH testing of fluids in the ocular cul-de-sac after irrigation to confirm that corrosives have been neutralized; the normal pH of tears is 7. Alkali eye injuries require urgent ophthalmologic consultation. Skin contamination also deserves prolonged rinsing with water and removal of contaminated clothing. Irrigation should continue until the skin is free of alkali, as determined by disappearance of the soapy sensation.

The next phase of management calls for further evaluation. All exposed surfaces, especially the oropharynx, should be examined scrupulously. A CBC and chest radiograph should be obtained; the latter particularly if any respiratory signs or symptoms are noted. Immediate referral should also occur.

Analgesic therapy may be necessary for severe pain. An IV line should be established if not previously done for basic life support. Conflicting data regarding the role of corticosteroids in the treatment of corrosive esophageal injury exist.

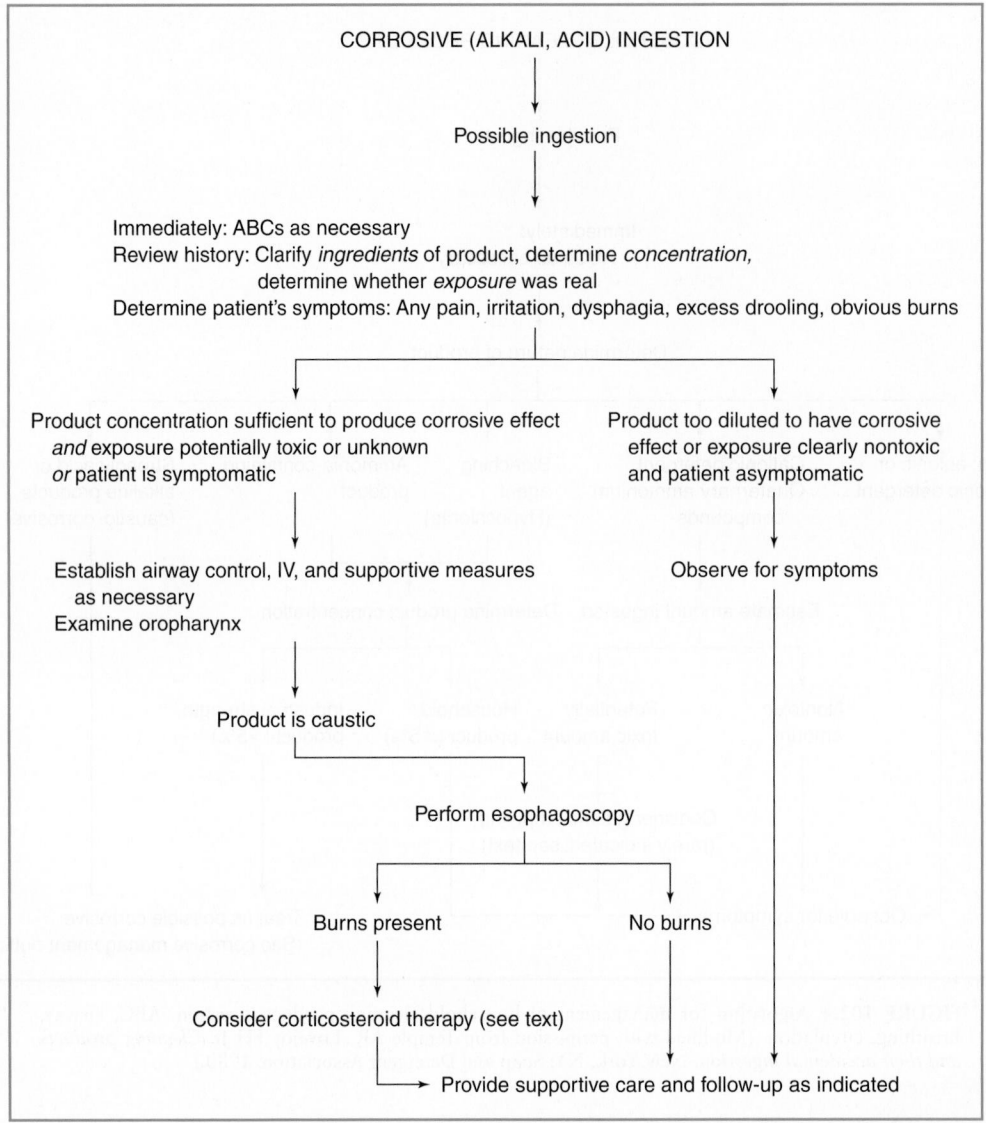

FIGURE 102.5 Algorithm for management of corrosive ingestion. ABC, airway, breathing, circulation; IV, intravenous. (Modified with permission from Temple AR, Lovejoy FH Jr. *Cleaning products and their accidental ingestion.* New York, NY: Soap and Detergent Association, 1980.)

First-degree burns typically heal without long-term sequelae. Circumferential second-degree burns may be less likely to stricture after steroid administration; therefore, corticosteroids with empiric antibiotics may be considered in this scenario. Third-degree burns are likely to scar despite treatment, and administration of steroids in this situation may provide more risk than benefit. The consulting otolaryngologist or surgeon may elect to administer steroids in select patients on the basis of endoscopic findings. All patients are admitted for supportive care and monitoring for acute complications such as mediastinitis, pneumonitis, and peritonitis.

The long-term management of survivors with severe caustic esophageal burns and stricture formation is complex, involving many surgical, medical, and psychologic stresses to the patient. Years of repeated bougienage may be necessary, and some patients will require esophagectomy with colonic interposition in an effort to replace the destroyed esophagus.

The patient may be incapable of tolerating solid foods for prolonged periods.

Hydrocarbons

Hydrocarbons are carbon compounds that become liquid at room temperature. The term *hydrocarbons* is somewhat confusing and is often used interchangeably with the term *petroleum distillates.* However, whereas all petroleum distillates are hydrocarbons, not all hydrocarbons are petroleum distillates (e.g., pine oil). Hydrocarbons can be found in solvents, fuels, household cleaners, and polishes.

Hydrocarbons are typically divided into three categories: the aliphatic hydrocarbons, the aromatics, and the "toxic" hydrocarbons. The aliphatic hydrocarbons are petroleum distillates and are found in such household products as furniture polish, lamp oils, and lighter fluids. The aromatic hydrocarbons are cyclic structures and include toluene, xylene, and benzene. These agents are found in solvents, glues, nail polish, paints, and paint removers. The "toxic" hydrocarbons consist of a broad class of substances that possesses no specific profile of toxicity. These agents include halogenated hydrocarbons and hydrocarbons that serve as vehicles for toxic substances such as pesticides.

The major toxicity of hydrocarbons varies from class to class. However, the feature that these agents have in common is a low viscosity and surface tension that permits them to spread freely over large surface areas, such as the lungs, when ingested. This property (plus their solvent actions) leads to a necrotizing, potentially fatal chemical pneumonitis (Fig. 102.6) when these compounds are aspirated. The high volatility of these substances is responsible for alterations in mental status, including narcosis, inebriation, and frank coma. In addition to these toxicities, the solvents possess additional toxicities (see "Inhalants" section), including the risk of bone marrow injury (in the case of benzene). Finally, with the toxic hydrocarbons, additional toxicities may occur as a result of actions such as cardiotoxicity or as a result of the pharmacologic properties of the other agents contained within these compounds. The major toxicity of hydrocarbons is classified in Table 102.13.

The amount of a hydrocarbon that has been ingested by a pediatric patient is often difficult to quantify. However, any degree of aspiration results in signs, including coughing, gagging, or tachypnea. Less than 1 mL of some compounds, when aspirated directly into the trachea, may produce severe pneumonitis and eventual death. When ingested, these compounds are poorly absorbed from the GI tract.

The major aspiration hazard associated with hydrocarbons can be quantified by their viscosity. Products with a viscosity of 150 to 250 Saybolt seconds units (SSU), such as oils, pose a small risk of chemical pneumonitis; those with a viscosity less

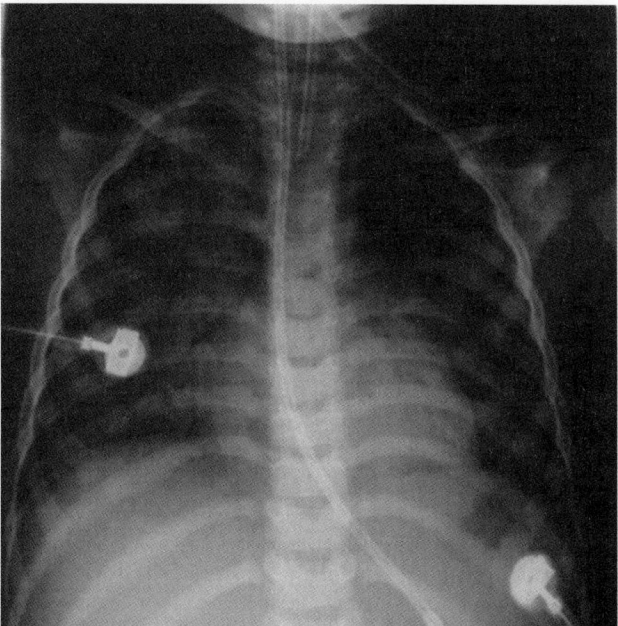

FIGURE 102.6 Chest radiographic findings in a young girl subsequent to lamp oil ingestion.

TABLE 102.13

CLASSIFICATION OF HYDROCARBONS

Nontoxic (Unless Complicated by Gross Aspiration)
Asphalt, tars
Mineral oil
Liquid petrolatum
Motor oil, axle grease
Baby oils, suntan oils

Systemic Toxicity
Halogenated (carbon tetrachloride, trichloroethane)
Aromatic (benzene, toluene, xylene)
Additives (camphor, organophosphates, heavy metals)

Aspiration Hazard (Without Significant Systemic Toxicity
  Unless Ingested in Massive Quantity)
Lamp oil/torch oil
Turpentine
Gasoline
Kerosene
Mineral seal oil (furniture polish)
Charcoal lighter fluid
Cigarette lighter fluid
Mineral spirits

than 60 SSU, such as furniture oils or polishes, have a high aspiration hazard.

Clinical manifestations of hydrocarbon ingestion depend largely on the specific profile of toxicity of the ingested substances. These agents cause significant GI irritation that may be associated with nausea and bloody emesis. CNS effects may range from inebriation to coma. Hemolysis with hemoglobinuria has been reported after significant ingestions. Finally, hydrocarbon ingestion may be associated with the development of fever and leukocytosis in up to 15% of patients in the absence of clinically evident pneumonitis.

Because most hydrocarbons cause clinical toxicity only when aspirated, the mainstay of treatment is to leave ingested compounds in the gut (when possible) and to prevent emesis or reflux. Gastric emptying is generally reserved only for those compounds with the potential for systemic toxic effects (Table 102.13). These compounds include the halogenated hydrocarbons (e.g., trichloroethane, carbon tetrachloride) and aromatic hydrocarbons (e.g., toluene, xylene, benzene). In addition, some petroleum distillates contain dangerous additives, such as heavy metals or insecticides.

Patients who have aspirated may exhibit immediate choking, coughing, and gagging as the product is swallowed and then vomited after ingestion. Aspiration of the product may also occur at the time of the initial swallowing. ED management of these patients is outlined in Fig. 102.7. If the patient has any cough or respiratory symptoms upon arrival to the ED, a chest radiograph should be obtained immediately. Because there is a gradual evolution of abnormal radiographs, an initially negative chest radiograph should be repeated at 4 to 6 hours after ingestion. All patients with abnormal chest radiographs or persistent respiratory symptoms after 4 to 6 hours of ED observation warrant further medical observation. Patients who are asymptomatic after this period of observation may be discharged. Because pneumonitis occasionally appears

MEDICAL EMERGENCIES

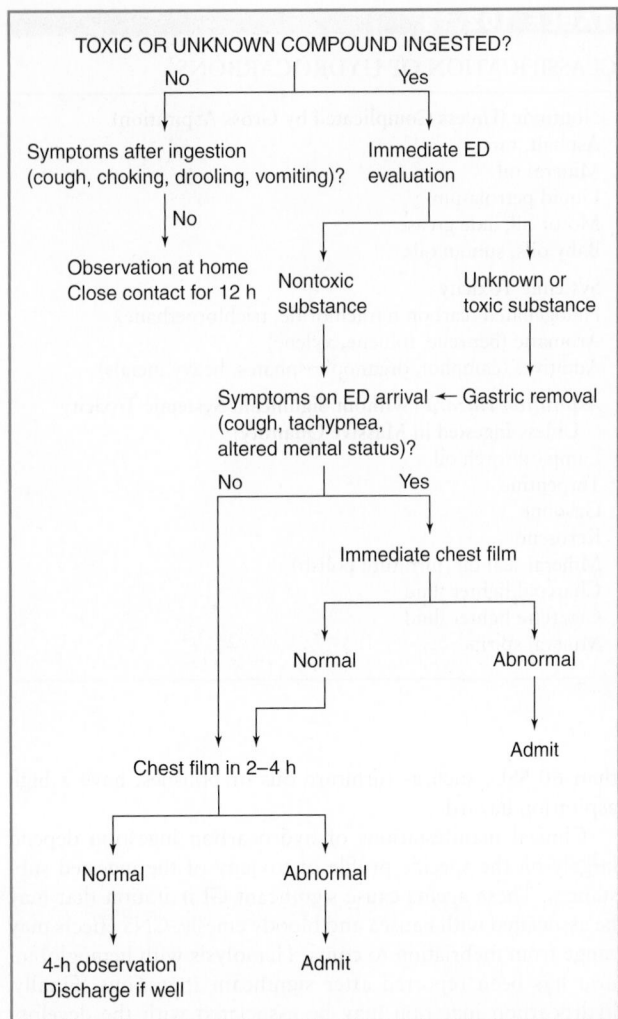

TOXIC OR UNKNOWN COMPOUND INGESTED?

No — Symptoms after ingestion (cough, choking, drooling, vomiting)?

Yes — Immediate ED evaluation

No — Observation at home Close contact for 12 h

Nontoxic substance

Unknown or toxic substance

Symptoms on ED arrival ← Gastric removal (cough, tachypnea, altered mental status)?

No — Immediate chest film — Yes

Normal / Abnormal

Abnormal → Admit

Chest film in 2–4 h

Normal → 4-h observation Discharge if well

Abnormal → Admit

FIGURE 102.7 Management of petroleum distillate ingestion. ED, emergency department.

12 to 24 hours after exposure, detailed instructions should be provided for warning signs of respiratory dysfunction.

Treatment of hydrocarbon pneumonitis consists of airway control if there is mental status depression and mechanical ventilation if ventilation is impaired. Adult respiratory distress syndrome may ensue, and heroic measures such as extracorporeal membrane oxygenation have been successfully employed. Antibiotics should not be used prophylactically but should be reserved for specific infections if they develop. The use of corticosteroids in the treatment of aspiration from hydrocarbons has been associated with increased morbidity and is not recommended. In the event of hypotension or bronchospasm, epinephrine is contraindicated because hydrocarbons are known to cause ventricular irritability and predispose to fibrillation, an effect that is exacerbated by catecholamines.

Iron

Background

In the 1990s, iron poisoning was one of the most common, potentially fatal intoxications in children. Most serious childhood poisonings result from ingestion of prenatal vitamins or ferrous sulfate tablets (which unfortunately often look much like candy) that were intended for adults. A common scenario is that the patient is a toddler whose mother has just had a new baby; the increased demands on the mother's attention and almost universal prescription of iron to postpartum women combine to set the stage for this ingestion. In addition, numerous exposures result from ingestion of iron-fortified children's vitamins, but these tend to be far less toxic.

Sufficient data to define a safe lower limit for toxic iron ingestions are not available. As little as 20 mg per kg of elemental iron has caused toxicity, whereas ingestions of more than 50 mg per kg often produce toxic effects. Of course, it is often impossible to know the exact number of tablets ingested. As few as ten 300-mg $FeSO_4$ tablets have been fatal to a young child. Furthermore, the elemental iron content of whole bottles of chewable vitamins is usually about 1,200 mg. Industry standards typically lead to the use of child resistant caps for vitamin bottles that contain more than 250 mg of elemental iron. Unit dose (blister) packaging has been advised for pills with high iron content. These measures have led to a dramatic reduction in deaths due to exploratory iron poisoning.

Pathophysiology

Iron toxicity results from direct caustic effect on the GI mucosa and the presence of free iron in the circulation. Pathologic changes include hemorrhagic necrosis of stomach and intestinal mucosa and lesions in the liver that range from cloudy swelling to areas of complete necrosis. Occasionally, pulmonary congestion and hemorrhage are noted. Excess free iron is believed to act as a mitochondrial poison, particularly in the liver, with resulting changes in cellular energy metabolism and the production of metabolic acidosis.

Clinical Manifestations

The clinical effects of iron poisoning are classically divided into four phases. Phase I represents the effects of direct mucosal injury and usually lasts 6 hours. Vomiting, diarrhea, and GI blood loss are the prominent early signs; when severe, the patient may lapse into early coma and shock caused by volume loss and metabolic acidosis.

Phase II, which lasts from 6 to 24 hours after ingestion, is marked by diminution of the GI symptoms. With appropriate therapy to replace fluid and/or blood losses, the child may seem relatively well and often goes on to full recovery without any subsequent symptoms. However, this remission may be transient and may be followed by phase III, characterized by metabolic acidosis, coma, seizures, and intractable shock. This phase is believed to represent hepatocellular injury with consequent disturbed energy metabolism; elevated levels of lactic and citric acids are noted in experimental iron poisoning before cardiac or respiratory failure occurs. Jaundice and elevated transaminases are noted in this phase. A phase IV has been described in survivors of severe iron poisoning, marked by pyloric stenosis that results from scarring and consequent obstruction.

Laboratory abnormalities often associated with severe iron intoxication include metabolic acidosis, leukocytosis, hyperglycemia, hyperbilirubinemia and increased liver enzymes, and a prolonged prothrombin time. If fluid loss is significant, there will be hemoconcentration and elevated BUN. Abdominal films may show radiopaque material in the stomach, but the absence of this finding does not indicate a trivial ingestion.

Management

All children alleged to have ingested iron are potentially at significant risk for life-threatening illness. However, severe iron poisoning is uncommon compared with the number of children who develop only mild symptoms or remain entirely asymptomatic. Thus, the emergency physician needs an approach that encompasses the response to the severely poisoned child and to most who will remain well.

As noted earlier, the amount of iron ingested is often hard to quantify, and minimal "safe" amounts are not well established. Serum iron levels have been shown to correlate with the likelihood of developing symptoms (usually a reflection of the serum iron that exceeds the iron-binding capacity and results in free-circulating iron). Usually, when drawn 3 to 5 hours after ingestion, iron levels lower than 350 μg per dL predict an asymptomatic course. Patients with levels in the 350 to 500 μg per dL range often show mild phase I symptoms but rarely develop serious complications. Levels higher than 500 μg per dL suggest significant risk for phase III manifestations. However, the serum iron determination is not always available on a stat basis.

Although serum iron levels are useful, toxicity from iron overdose remains a clinical diagnosis. Ill patients require vigorous hydration and support. Children who are completely asymptomatic 6 hours after ingestion are unlikely to develop systemic illness. Among laboratory studies, the presence of metabolic acidosis or acidemia probably best correlates with toxicity. Radiopaque material on abdominal radiograph also suggests potential for significant absorption of iron (Fig. 102.8). Measurement of the total iron-binding capacity is no longer believed to be useful in acute management. With these observations in mind, it is possible to construct a protocol for the triage and initial management of the patient who has ingested a possibly toxic amount of iron (Fig. 102.9).

Categorization

Patients who arrive with severe early symptoms, including vomiting, diarrhea, GI bleeding, depressed sensorium, or circulatory compromise merit urgent, intensive treatment in the ED. The first priority is to obtain venous access. Simultaneously, blood is drawn for CBC, blood glucose, electrolytes, BUN, liver function tests, serum iron, and type and cross-match analyses. GI decontamination is begun as detailed in the following section. Blood pressure should be supported with normal saline. Specific chelation therapy with IV deferoxamine is begun immediately in all severely poisoned patients. An abdominal radiograph should be obtained as soon as possible after GI decontamination to determine its efficacy and to investigate for the presence of iron pill concretions.

Patients with only mild vomiting and diarrhea in the early postingestion period still need urgent treatment but usually do well. Again, GI decontamination strategies should be promptly addressed. Blood studies, as previously noted, are drawn, and parenteral deferoxamine therapy is begun.

If serum iron levels are available, blood should be sent for this study, an abdominal radiograph should be obtained, and the patient should be observed for 6 hours. An iron level of less than 350 μg per dL taken 3 to 5 hours after ingestion in an asymptomatic patient with a normal radiograph suggests that the patient is at minimal risk and may be discharged. Iron levels higher than 500 μg per dL, the development of any symptoms, or a positive radiograph should lead to admission and management as previously described for the mild to moderately ill patient.

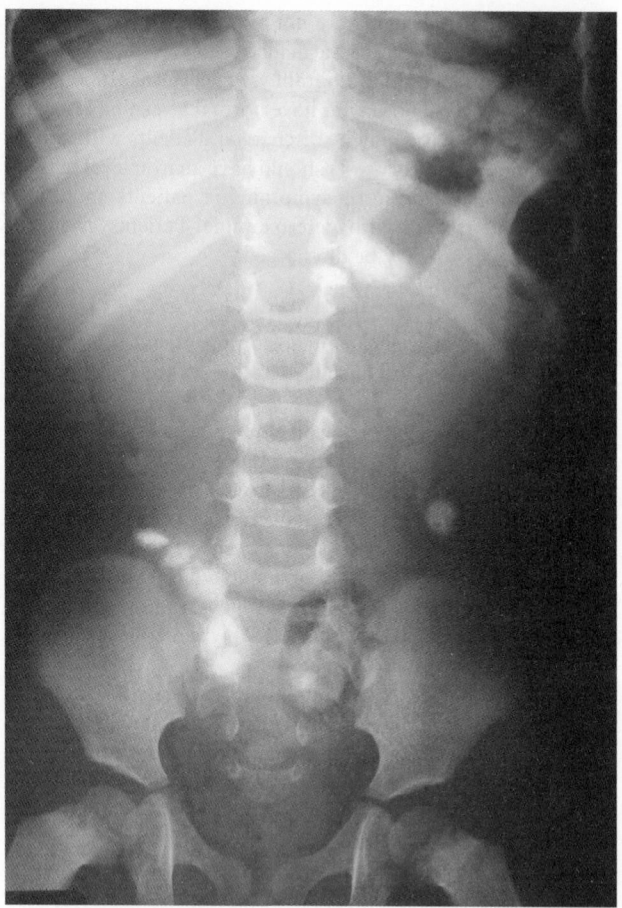

FIGURE 102.8 Intestinal iron pills evident upon abdominal radiography.

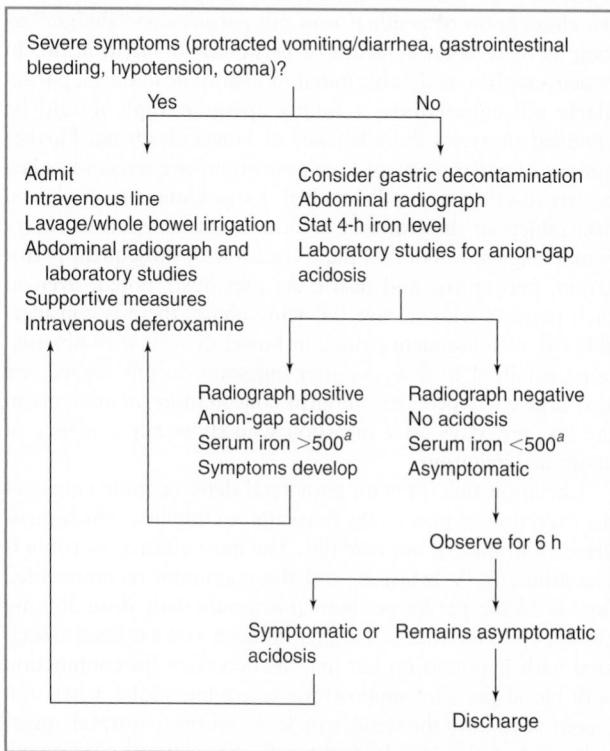

FIGURE 102.9 The initial approach to the patient ingesting a possibly toxic dose of iron. [a]Iron levels expressed in μg per dL.

When serum iron levels are not available on an emergency basis, clinical decisions must be made based on symptoms, electrolytes, and abdominal radiography. Patients are observed for 6 hours in the ED. Those who have normal screening tests and remain asymptomatic may be discharged. Patients with abnormal screening laboratory tests should have an iron level sent for later reference. Acidotic or symptomatic patients should be admitted and treated with deferoxamine. Patients asymptomatic after 6 hours may be discharged.

Treatment

The treatment for acute iron poisoning includes efforts to decrease absorption and hasten excretion, as well as appropriate supportive care.

Most children with toxic iron exposures will exhibit spontaneous vomiting. Administration of ipecac may interfere with the clinical interpretation of early signs of iron toxicity, as detailed previously. Activated charcoal is not effective in binding iron salts. For serious poisonings, gastric lavage with normal saline can be considered in patients who present early, in the hope of minimizing any direct mucosal injury caused by residual particulate matter and possibly contributing to the dissolution of pill concretions.

The mainstay of GI decontamination currently for iron-poisoned patients is the early and aggressive use of WBI. This approach is believed to be effective in decreasing iron absorption and in breaking up pill concretions that might be a risk for direct mucosal injury. As noted previously, an abdominal radiograph should be obtained early in the evaluation of symptomatic patients. If this study demonstrates significant radiopaque material and the patient's condition allows it, WBI should be instituted for at least 4 to 6 hours. A few hours of WBI (until rectal effluent is clear) may be indicated in symptomatic cases even without definite radiographic findings to hasten elimination of residual iron pill particles or "sludge," as long as there is no evidence of peritonitis or perforation. In patients with considerable initial radiographic findings, particularly pill concretions, a follow-up radiograph should be obtained to assess the adequacy of bowel cleansing. Further options of gastroscopy or even gastrotomy are reserved as last resorts to effect iron pill removal. Large clumps of coalesced iron tablets in the stomach or duodenum have led to severe hemorrhagic infarction of these viscera with subsequent perforation, peritonitis, and death. As previously noted, even in such patients who survive the acute phase, there is considerable risk of subsequent pyloric or bowel stenosis with obstruction, usually 4 to 6 weeks after ingestion. In this regard, we also urge early pediatric surgical consultation for patients in the first few days after ingestion who show any evidence of peritoneal irritation.

Chelation therapy with parenteral deferoxamine enhances the excretion of iron as the feroxamine complex, which turns urine an orange or *vin rose* tint. The most efficacious route is a continuous IV infusion, and the maximum recommended dose is 15 mg per kg per hour (maximum daily dose 360 mg per kg, up to 6 g total). A higher infusion rate has been associated with hypotension but may be necessary (in conjunction with blood pressure support) for severe ingestions. Chelation is continued until the serum iron level returns to normal, metabolic acidosis has resolved, the patient is clinically improved, and the urine color returns to normal. The dose of deferoxam-ine may be titrated down in concert with the patient's clinical response and fall in iron levels.

Once the patient has been stabilized initially, further problems may include hypotension, profound metabolic acidosis, hypoglycemia or hyperglycemia, anemia and colloid loss caused by GI hemorrhage (after equilibration), renal shutdown resulting from shock, and hepatic failure with an associated bleeding diathesis. The maintenance of an adequate urine output is critical to prevent renal failure and to foster excretion of the feroxamine complex. If renal failure supervenes, chelation may be continued with concurrent dialysis because the complex is dialyzable.

Isoniazid

Isoniazid (INH) is an important treatment for tuberculosis. Even when taken appropriately, INH has many actions that can lead to clinical toxicity. These include hepatic dysfunction and interactions with foods such as those containing tyramine. However, its greatest toxicity appears after acute single ingestions of more than 20 mg per kg in children or more than 1.5 g in an adult.

INH's mechanism of toxicity involves its potent effect at reversing the biological activity of vitamin B_6 (pyridoxine). This action, as well as other effects on the synthesis of catecholamines and the neurotransmitter GABA, provides an explanation for the epileptogenic toxicity of the drug. INH also prevents hepatic conversion of lactate to pyruvate.

In overdose, the hallmark of INH poisoning is the triad of seizures, metabolic acidosis, and coma. Seizures induced by INH are typically generalized and appear to have a rhythmic recurrence. They are generally difficult to treat; patients usually remain comatose between seizures. The metabolic acidosis of INH can be severe; pH values of as low as 6.4 have been reported. This places INH on the list of substances associated with the development of high anion gap metabolic acidosis (see MUDPILES mnemonic). Of all these drugs, only INH possesses seizures as a prominent characteristic. Interestingly, in animal models of INH poisoning, metabolic acidosis does not occur if seizures are prevented through paralysis. Finally, the coma of INH intoxication can be severe and prolonged.

Because of the striking clinical picture of INH poisoning, diagnosis is often easily made on the basis of demographic characteristics and clinical manifestations. INH is not usually detected on routine toxicology laboratory screens, and serum concentrations are of little value in acute management. Laboratory tests that are important in initial assessment include arterial blood gas levels, electrolytes level, liver function tests, creatine kinase level, and urinalysis.

Management

Management of INH intoxication begins with advanced life support. Because of seizures and coma, airway protection and ventilation are typically necessary. Cardiac monitoring should be initiated to monitor for the development of cardiac arrhythmias (resulting from severe metabolic acidosis).

Although of unproven benefit, orogastric lavage might be considered within 30 minutes of ingestion. Activated charcoal may also be considered if it can be given safely. Theoretically, giving multiple doses of activated charcoal to enhance postabsorptive elimination of INH may be advantageous.

Pharmacologic treatment for INH intoxication includes sodium bicarbonate, anticonvulsants, and pyridoxine. Sodium bicarbonate is provided as needed to restore serum pH to normal. In treating seizures, effective anticonvulsants include the benzodiazepines or phenobarbital (both of which are GABA agonists). Either diazepam (0.1 to 0.3 mg per kg) or lorazepam (0.1 mg per kg) should be administered IV to terminate seizures.

Administration of pyridoxine has been shown to provide specific antidotal therapy for INH poisoning. After administration of vitamin B_6, seizures and metabolic acidosis promptly resolve. Pyridoxine is given as an IV dose that equals the estimated dose of INH in milligrams. In cases in which the ingested amount is unknown, a single dose of 5 g (70 mg per kg in children) of pyridoxine is administered. Rarely, repeat administration is necessary.

Although INH clearance can be enhanced by hemodialysis or hemoperfusion, these techniques are rarely necessary if pyridoxine, activated charcoal, and aggressive supportive care are provided.

Lead

Background

Although lead poisoning is usually the result of chronic ingestion by pica-prone children or of occupational exposure in adults, patients with lead poisoning may come to the ED with varied complaints of recent onset that often mimic diverse acute illnesses. Fortunately, severe lead encephalopathy is now rare, attributable in large part to widespread screening programs and early treatment of asymptomatic or mildly ill children. However, the risk of lead intoxication still exists, and emergency physicians and pediatricians in every community must maintain an index of suspicion.

Sources of Lead

The major source of excess lead absorption in children is lead-based paint, widely used in home interiors through the 1950s. In addition to the ingestion of macroscopic-size chips of paint, inner-city children are often exposed to house dust with a high lead content that results from finely crumbled paint particles, which gets on their hands and toys. Repetitive mouthing can lead to increased lead exposure even in the absence of observable pica. Although classically a disease of poor inner-city residents, the more recent phenomenon of young, middle socioeconomic level families moving into older sections of large cities and renovating town houses has led to an expanded population at risk. This is because the sanding, stripping, and burning of lead-based paint from woodwork in such houses has also been associated with lead intoxication in the occupants. Other unusual sources of lead exposure include the burning of battery casings for heat, soft well water carried by outdated lead pipes, improperly home-glazed ceramics, drinking glass-glazed decals, and dust or dirt alongside heavily traveled roads (resulting from auto emissions in communities still using leaded gasoline). Infants have also developed elevated lead levels when parents prepare formula with first-draw tap water or when they boil the water before mixing.

Pathophysiology

Absorption of lead occurs through GI and pulmonary routes, although the former is predominant in pediatric intoxications. Lead is then compartmentalized into three main areas: bone, soft tissues, and blood. Excretion occurs slowly through urine, feces, and sweat. Children are probably at double jeopardy as compared with adults in that there is experimental evidence that younger animals have increased absorption and also a heavier distribution into soft tissues (including the brain). Concomitant nutritional deficiency, especially low dietary iron and calcium, may enhance intestinal lead absorption. Unfortunately, the same children at greatest risk for lead poisoning by virtue of age and residence are also likely to be at risk for dietary deficiency, especially iron.

Lead exerts its toxic effect principally by two mechanisms: by interference with calcium function at the cellular level and by enzyme inhibition, particularly on enzymes rich in sulfhydryl groups. In humans, the most obvious effects are on neurologic function and on the heme synthesis pathway, which is interrupted at several points, resulting in abnormally high levels of porphyrins and their precursors.

Clinical Findings

Early signs and symptoms of plumbism are notably vague and nonspecific. Abdominal complaints, including colicky pain, constipation, anorexia, and intermittent vomiting, are common; of course, these same symptoms are often ascribed to relatively normal 2-year-old children by their parents. The child with early plumbism may also show listlessness and irritability. When encephalopathy begins, the child develops persistent vomiting and becomes drowsy, clumsy, or frankly ataxic. As encephalopathy worsens, the level of consciousness deteriorates further, and seizures commonly occur. Pathologic examination of brains of children who have died of lead encephalopathy shows severe cerebral edema with vascular damage; intracranial pressure is often, although not invariably, increased during the encephalopathy. When spinal fluid is examined, it often reveals a picture similar to that of aseptic meningitis with a mononuclear pleocytosis and elevated protein; however, lumbar puncture should be avoided if possible because of the risk of subsequent herniation. Peripheral neuropathy often occurs in adults with lead poisoning but is rare in children, although it is seen occasionally in those with an underlying hemoglobinopathy. Other organs may be damaged by lead. The kidneys may develop disturbances that range from slight aminoaciduria to a full Fanconi's syndrome with glycosuria and phosphaturia (in addition to aminoaciduria). High blood lead level (BLL) is also associated with a microcytic anemia that results from a defect in hemoglobin synthesis. However, much of the anemia seen in children with excess BLL may be caused by concurrent iron deficiency. A moderately sensitive laboratory measure of lead effect on heme synthesis is the evaluation of erythrocyte protoporphyrin (EP), a heme precursor. Moderately elevated EP levels are seen in iron deficiency, but levels above 250 to 300 μg per dL are almost always the result of chronic lead poisoning.

Management

The asymptomatic child discovered to have a BLL in the 20 to 44 μg per dL range, particularly if the EP level is higher than 250 μg per dL, deserves immediate referral to a pediatrician or toxicologist. Such children warrant environmental investigation, clinical evaluation, and case management to reduce lead exposure as expeditiously as possible. Chelation therapy may be considered in some such children. All symptomatic children and those with BLL higher than 44 µg per dL need urgent treatment as outlined next, as well as pediatric consultation to ensure adequate postchelation follow-up.

The remainder of this discussion is addressed primarily to the early recognition and treatment of plumbism, including acute lead encephalopathy. This single aspect of chronic childhood lead poisoning is focused on because it represents a true medical emergency.

Recognition

As stated previously, to recognize mildly symptomatic patients with lead poisoning (or asymptomatic children with high lead levels, who are at great risk to soon become symptomatic) requires a high index of suspicion. All children between 1 and 5 years of age are suspect if they have (i) persistent vomiting, listlessness or irritability, clumsiness, or loss of recently acquired developmental skills; (ii) afebrile convulsions; (iii) a strong tendency to pica, including a history of acute exploratory ingestions or aural or nasal foreign body; (iv) a deteriorating pre-World War II house or a parent with industrial exposures; (v) a family history of lead poisoning; (vi) iron-deficiency anemia; or (vii) evidence of child abuse or neglect.

The child between ages of 1 to 5 years who comes to the ED with an acute encephalopathy and the above-cited risk factors presents the physician with a dilemma: lead intoxication requires urgent diagnosis, but confirmation with a BLL is usually not available on an immediate basis. A constellation of historical features of lead poisoning increases the likelihood of the diagnosis. These features include (i) a prodromal illness of several days' to weeks' duration (suggestive of mild symptomatic plumbism); (ii) a history of pica; and (iii) a source of exposure to lead. Several nonspecific laboratory findings make lead poisoning likely enough to warrant presumptive chelation therapy until confirmation by lead levels is available. These findings include (i) microcytic anemia; (ii) elevated EP level, especially if higher than 250 µg per dL (conversely, a normal or minimally elevated EP level, less than 50 µg per dL, would make lead encephalopathy caused by chronic lead paint exposure unlikely); (iii) basophilic stippling of peripheral erythrocytes or, if feasible, of red blood cell precursors on bone marrow examination; (iv) glycosuria; (v) aminoaciduria; (vi) radiopaque flecks on abdominal radiographs; and (vii) dense metaphyseal bands on radiographs of knees and wrists (lead lines—Fig. 102.10).

Abnormalities on examination of cerebrospinal fluid (CSF) are also indicative of lead encephalopathy, including a lymphocytic pleocytosis, elevated protein level, and increased pressure. However, a lumbar puncture should not be performed if lead encephalopathy is strongly suspected because the risk of herniation is considerable. If CSF must be examined to rule out bacterial meningitis, the minimal amount (less than 1 mL) necessary should be obtained. Alternatively, one might institute treatment for presumed meningitis, perform a determination of BLL, and consider a delayed lumbar puncture after several days if the BLL is normal.

Treatment

The treatment of lead poisoning involves relocation of the child to a lead-free environment, chelation therapy, and

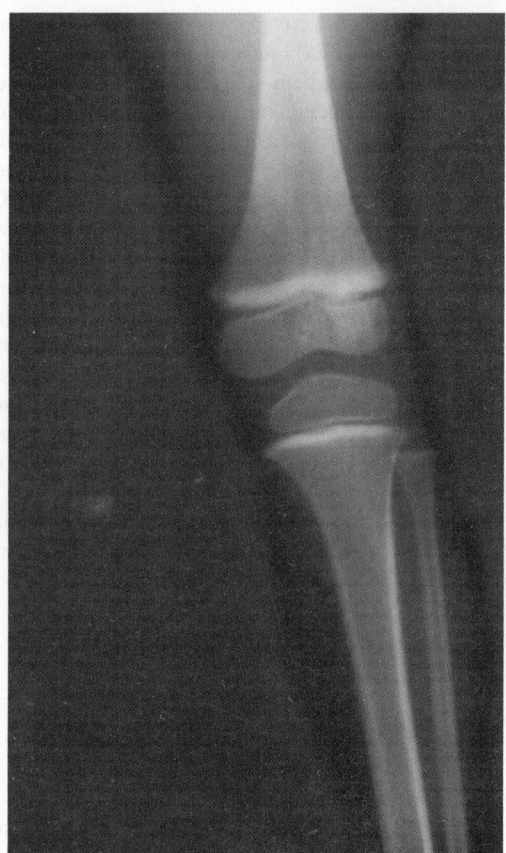

FIGURE 102.10 Knee radiograph demonstrating increased calcium deposition at metaphysis—the so-called "lead lines." Reproduced with permission from Henretig FM. A toddler in status epilepticus. In: Osterhoudt KC, Perrone J, DeRoos F, et al., eds. *Toxicology pearls.* Philadelphia, PA: Hanley & Belfus, 2004:S2–S5.

appropriate supportive care. Symptomatic patients are at risk of developing encephalopathy with subsequent death or neurologic sequelae. In addition, asymptomatic patients with high BLL (especially higher than 100 µg per dL) are also at significant risk for developing CNS involvement and might require urgent treatment.

The specific chelating drugs commonly used for symptomatic lead intoxication are edetate calcium disodium (CaEDTA) and 2,4-dimercaptopropanol [British Anti-Lewisite (BAL); Table 102.14]. Side effects of CaEDTA include local reactions at injection sites, fever, hypercalcemia, and renal dysfunction manifested by rising BUN and abnormal urine sediment with proteinuria, hematuria, and/or epithelial cells. The major side effects of BAL include nausea and vomiting, so for the first day or two of BAL therapy, it is prudent to maintain the patient on IV fluids and clear liquids or nothing by mouth. BAL is formulated in peanut oil, is given only by IM injection, and also induces hemolysis in patients with G6PD deficiency. Its use is hazardous if the patient has severe hepatic dysfunction, and it forms a toxic complex if given concurrently with iron. Succimer [dimercaptosuccinic acid (DMSA)] has been approved for pediatric use in cases in which BLL exceeds 45 µg per dL (Table 102.14). This water-soluble analog of BAL may be taken orally, and several studies have found such use to be as effective as CaEDTA given parenterally. Some centers use D-penicillamine as an enteral form of chelation for elevated BLLs.

TABLE 102.14

GUIDELINES FOR CHELATION THERAPY OF LEAD POISONING

Condition, BLL	Regimen[a]	Comment
Encephalopathy	BAL 450 mg/m²/d + CaNa₂EDTA 1,500 mg/m²/d	75 mg/m² IM every 4 h for 5 days Continuous infusion, or 2–4 divided IV doses, for 5 days (start 4 h after BAL)
Symptomatic, and/or BLL > 70	BAL 300–450 mg/m²/d + CaNa₂EDTA 1,000–1,500 mg/m²/d	50–75 mg/m² every 4 h for 3–5 days (see text) Continuous infusion, or 2–4 divided IV doses, for 5 days (start 4 h after BAL)
Asymptomatic, BLL 45–69	Succimer 700–1,050 mg/m²/d or CaNa₂EDTA, 1,000 mg/m²/d	350 mg/m² TID for 5 days, then BID for 14 days Continuous infusion, or 2–4 divided IV doses, for 5 days

BLL, blood lead level (µg/dL); BAL, British Anti-Lewisite; IM, intramuscular; IV, intravenous.
[a]Doses expressed in mg/kg: BAL 450 mg/m² (24 mg/kg), 300 mg/m² (18 mg/kg); CaNa₂EDTA 1,000 mg/m² (25–50 mg/kg), 1,500 mg/m² (50–75 mg/kg); Succimer 350 mg/m² (10 mg/kg).
Adapted from American Academy of Pediatrics, Committee on Drugs. Treatment guidelines for lead exposure in children. *Pediatrics* 1995;1996: 155–160; and Henretig FM. Lead. In: Goldfrank LR, Flomenbaum NE, Lewin NA, et al., eds. *Goldfrank's toxicologic emergencies,* 9th ed. New York, NY: McGraw-Hill, 2009.

Asymptomatic children found to have BLL of 45 to 69 µg per dL should have urgent referral and treatment with oral DMSA (typically a 19-day course) or parenteral CaEDTA for 5 days (Table 102.14). If the BLL is higher than 69 µg per dL, combination therapy is initiated with both BAL and EDTA; the BAL may be discontinued in many cases after 2 to 3 days, but CaEDTA is continued for 5 days. Supportive care includes adequate hydration to promote good urine output. Symptomatic children without frank encephalopathy should receive chelation therapy with a combination of BAL for 3 to 5 days and CaEDTA for 5 days. Supportive care includes close monitoring for signs of encephalopathy and, again, maintenance of urine flow.

Patients with encephalopathy require combination chelation therapy with higher dose CaEDTA and BAL for 5 days, as well as intensive supportive care. Fluid therapy is critical and must be individualized. Adequate urine flow is needed to excrete the lead–chelate complexes; however, fluid overload must be avoided so that cerebral edema is not exacerbated. A reasonable goal is to supply basal water requirements, maintaining urine production at 0.35 to 0.5 mL per kcal per 24 hours. Basal water needs in children average 1 mL per kcal and may be calculated as 100 kcal per kg for 0 to 10 kg, plus 50 kcal per kg for 10 to 20 kg, plus 20 kcal per kg for each kilogram above 20 kg.

Seizures commonly occur in acute encephalopathy and should be controlled with anticonvulsant drugs (see Chapter 96). Hypothetical precautions have been made about the use of phenobarbital in lead encephalopathy (i.e., synergistic disturbances in porphyrin metabolism), but its clinical use has not been associated with any noticeable deleterious effect.

Recent advances in the management of cerebral edema and increased intracranial pressure (see Chapter 126 have not been evaluated in a controlled fashion in the context of lead encephalopathy. However, it seems reasonable that noninvasive measures such as prevention of hypoxia and hypercarbia with tracheal intubation and controlled ventilation, seizure treatment and prophylaxis, maintenance of adequate cerebral perfusion pressure, mild hyperventilation with PCO₂ of 30 to 35 mm Hg, and neutral head positioning with head of bed elevation to 30 degrees might have a beneficial effect. Mannitol administration

may be helpful in deteriorating patients. Whether more aggressive measures, such as acute hyperventilation for impending herniation, intracranial pressure monitoring, ventricular CSF drainage, induced hypothermia, or barbiturate coma, would enhance survival or decrease morbidity further is unknown.

Oral Hypoglycemics

Although almost all juvenile diabetics require insulin therapy for control, the frequent prescription of oral hypoglycemic agents for patients with non–insulin-dependent, adult-onset diabetes has made the availability and, consequently, the ingestion of these medications commonplace among toddlers. The scenario typically involves visits to a grandparent's home (or conversely, a visit by the grandparent to the child's home). The sulfonylureas (chlorpropamide, glipizide, glyburide) are capable of inducing significant hypoglycemia in a toddler after the ingestion of a single tablet. In addition, the onset of hypoglycemia may be delayed up to 16 to 24 hours after ingestion. Thus, prudent management of such exposures generally implies prolonged close observation and a challenge period of fasting. Excretion of chlorpropamide may be enhanced by urinary alkalinization. The biguanides (e.g., metformin) are unlikely to create hypoglycemia but may promote metabolic acidosis.

Maintenance of euglycemia is usually accomplished in symptomatic patients with the infusion of hypertonic glucose (e.g., 10% to 20%) solutions, supplemented as necessary by bolus doses. Occasionally, patients may still exhibit hypoglycemia, requiring additional treatment. Octreotide, a somatostatin analog that antagonizes insulin release, has been used effectively in cases of refractory hypoglycemia at a suggested dose of 1 to 2 µg per kg per dose every 6 to 12 hours via either an IV or subcutaneous route. Occasionally, patients require glucose infusion for several days; as their condition improves, the glucose load may be tapered gradually with frequent monitoring. Historically, diazoxide has been a useful adjunct in correcting refractory drug-induced hypoglycemia, but its use has largely been replaced by octreotide.

Organophosphates

Background

Organophosphates are lipid-soluble insecticides that are commonly applied in sprayed dust or emulsion formulations. These compounds are found in agricultural and home use, and they form the basis of "nerve gases" in chemical warfare agents (see Chapter 7). Organophosphates are readily degraded in the environment and metabolized in mammals by hydrolic cleavage. Some of these chemicals are "systemic" insecticides, meaning that they are taken up by the roots of the plants and translocated into foliage, flowers, and/or fruits.

Pathophysiology

Compounds of this class can be absorbed by inhalation, ingestion, and skin penetration. They irreversibly phosphorylate the enzyme acetylcholinesterase in tissues, allowing acetylcholine accumulation at cholinergic junctions in autonomic effector sites (causing muscarinic effects), in skeletal muscle or autonomic ganglia (causing nicotinic effects), and in the CNS.

Clinical Findings

The symptoms of acute poisoning usually develop during the first 12 hours of contact. These include findings related to the CNS (dizziness, headache, ataxia, convulsions, and coma); nicotinic signs, including sweating, muscle twitching, tremors, weakness, and paralysis; and muscarinic signs characterized by the SLUDGE mnemonic (including *s*alivation, *l*acrimation, *u*rination, *d*efecation, *g*astrointestinal cramping, and *e*mesis). In addition there may be miosis, bradycardia, bronchorrhea, and wheezing; in severe cases, pulmonary edema develops. Severe intoxications may also cause a toxic psychosis that resembles alcoholism.

A history of exposure to organophosphates and the clinical manifestations already discussed are the best clues to an organophosphate poisoning. A depression of plasma or red blood cell cholinesterase activity provides the best laboratory marker of excessive absorption of organophosphates, although it is rarely available on a stat basis. A decrease in the cholinesterase activity of the red blood cells is more specific for organophosphate inhibition than is the plasma assay. Although plasma cholinesterase is depressed by liver injury from various causes and a small percentage of the population has a genetically determined deficiency of plasma cholinesterase activity, a depression of 25% or more is a strong evidence of excessive organophosphate absorption. However, it is important that treatment not be delayed until confirmation of plasma cholinesterase is obtained. Note that children may also encounter acetylcholinesterase inhibitors if they ingest an adult's medication for Alzheimer's or Parkinson's disease (i.e., rivastigmine, donepezil, tacrine, and galantamine).

Management

The management of a patient who has ingested organophosphates must always include safeguards against exposure for the persons who treat the patient because the organophosphates are readily absorbed through the skin and mucous membranes. Patients who have been poisoned by the topical application of organophosphates should receive a thorough scrubbing with a soap solution on admission to prevent further absorption of organophosphates. In addition, all contaminated clothing must be removed and stored in a plastic bag to protect the institutional personnel.

After decontamination, antidotal therapy begins with the administration of atropine sulfate given in a dose of 0.05 to 0.1 mg per kg to children and 2 to 5 mg for adolescents and adults. This dose should be repeated every 10 to 30 minutes or as needed to obtain and maintain full atropinization, as indicated by an end point of clearing bronchial secretions and pulmonary rales. Therapy is continued until all absorbed organophosphate has been metabolized and may require 2 mg to more than 2,000 mg of atropine over the course of a few hours to several days. After atropinization has been instituted, severe poisonings should be treated with the addition of pralidoxime. This drug is particularly useful in poisonings characterized by profound weakness and muscle twitching. A dose of 25 to 50 mg per kg should be administered in 100 mL of saline by infusion over approximately 30 minutes; adults may receive 1 to 2 g by IV. In life-threatening situations, 50% of the initial pralidoxime dose may be infused over 2 minutes, followed by the remainder of the dose over 30 minutes. After loading, a 1% concentration may be infused continuously at the rate of 500 mg per hour in adolescents and adults, or approximately 10 mg per kg per hour in children, and can be titrated to clinical effect. Occasionally, patients may require more than 48 hours of therapy; the end point should be persistent relief of neurologic and cholinergic signs.

Organophosphates are usually dissolved in hydrocarbon bases; thus, the clinician should be prepared to treat hydrocarbon pneumonitis if it develops. Also, bronchopneumonia that complicates the pulmonary edema has been observed in acute poisonings.

Because the organophosphates cause elevated levels of acetylcholine in the plasma, compounds that affect the uptake of acetylcholine and/or its release should be avoided in the management of these patients. Specifically, aminophylline and phenothiazines are contraindicated. In situations in which identification of the ingested insecticides is difficult, consultation may be obtained from the National Insecticide/Pesticide Hotline (800-858-7378). This hotline provides an around-the-clock consultation service for advice on pesticides.

Carbamate insecticides have a similar mechanism of action to organophosphate insecticides but the phosphorylation of acetylcholinesterase is reversible and temporary. Pralidoxime therapy is generally regarded as unnecessary after poisoning from carbamates.

Phenothiazines/Antipsychotics

Background and Pathophysiology

The phenothiazines are commonly prescribed major tranquilizers. Phenothiazines are also often used to treat nausea and vomiting in young children. The toxic effects of this drug class primarily involve the three components of the nervous system: central, autonomic, and extrapyramidal.

The three subgroups of phenothiazines—aliphatic, piperazine, and piperidine—vary in their effects on the different components of the CNS. In general, the aliphatic group (e.g., chlorpromazine) may cause sedation and hypotension in overdose. The piperazine group (e.g., prochlorperazine) is more likely to create extrapyramidal side effects. Several new classes of nonphenothiazine antipsychotic agents are now widely prescribed.

Clinical Findings

The manifestations of phenothiazine toxicity may be dose dependent or dose independent (idiosyncratic). These have significantly different features.

With dose-dependent effects, the manifestations of intoxication after acute ingestion vary from mild to severe. In mild intoxication, CNS signs such as sedation, ataxia, and slurred speech occur. The anticholinergic effects of these drugs may cause constipation, urinary retention, and blurred vision. Because phenothiazines have potent actions on the temperature-regulating center of the hypothalamus, temperature disturbances occur in up to 30% of patients and may consist of hypothermia or hyperthermia. Orthostatic hypotension, the probable result of peripheral vasodilation, may also be noted with mild intoxication.

In moderate intoxications, the patients may have significant depression in the level of consciousness. Extrapyramidal effects become notable at this level of intoxication with muscle stiffness or "cogwheel" rigidity seen on passive movement of the neck, biceps, or quadriceps. Anticholinergic manifestations are severe and include acute urinary retention and paralytic ileus; hypotension may be profound. Cardiac conduction disturbances may make their appearance and are often heralded by a prolonged Q-T interval.

In severe overdoses patients are unarousable. Deep tendon reflexes may be hyperactive. Dystonic reactions may occur, involving the head and neck and the cranial nerves (torticollis and opisthotonos). Arrhythmias and shock may result in death.

The dose-independent effect of the phenothiazines is the dystonic reaction. This striking clinical occurrence consists of episodic spasm of voluntary muscles, particularly those of the head and neck. Patients may develop torticollis, bruxism, tongue protrusion, or oculogyric crisis. Dystonic reactions are unrelated to the amount of ingested phenothiazine. They may or may not occur after the first dose. Their onset is 8 to 40 hours after ingestion of a single dose of phenothiazine. This marked delay between ingestion and clinical manifestations often interferes with obtaining an accurate history of ingestion. Fortunately, although painful and distressing, dystonic reactions are rarely life-threatening and usually resolve quickly after administration of anticholinergics.

The clinical chemistry of the newer antipsychotic agents is varied and complex. CNS depression, seizures, prolongation of the Q-T interval, and α-adrenergic blockade–mediated hypotension are common.

Management

Treatment of acute phenothiazine intoxication hinges on the severity of ingestion. The autonomic signs and symptoms are most often transient and require no treatment. In patients with moderate or severe overdoses, the potential for life-threatening manifestations requires prompt evaluation of vital signs, GI decontamination (if ingestion was within an hour of ED arrival), vascular access, and cardiac monitoring. Pressors such as norepinephrine (see Chapter 3) may be used to correct the hypotension. In those rare instances of hypertension, the use of nitroprusside (see Chapter 34) may be indicated. Severe arrhythmias should be treated aggressively, as detailed later under "Tricyclic Antidepressants" and in Chapter 84. Attention should be directed to the treatment of temperature instability and other autonomic disturbances.

Dystonic reactions are effectively controlled by the IM or IV administration of diphenhydramine in a dose of 1 to 2 mg per kg (max 50 mg per dose). This dose may be repeated within 15 to 20 minutes if no effect is noted. An alternative agent is benztropine mesylate (1 to 2 mg for an older child/adolescent). This agent reportedly causes less sedation than diphenhydramine. Another potential alternative, especially in younger children, is diazepam (0.1 to 0.2 mg per kg). After resolution of the dystonic reaction, oral treatment should be continued for an additional 24 to 72 hours to prevent recurrences.

Plants/Mushrooms

Plant Toxicity

Plants are among the more commonly reported exploratory ingestions in children. Most such ingestions involve common house and garden plants. Fortunately, of the many varieties of such plants, only a small fraction poses a serious toxic hazard (Tables 102.15 and 102.16).

TABLE 102.15

COMMON NONTOXIC PLANTS

Abelia	Eugenia
African daisy	Gardenia
African palm	Grape ivy
African violet	Hedge apples
Airplane plant	Hens and chicks
Aluminum plant	Honeysuckle
Aralia	Hoya
Asparagus fern (may cause dermatitis)	Impatiens
Aspidistra (cast iron plant)	Jade plant
Aster	Kalanchoe
Baby's tears	Lily (day, Easter, or tiger)
Bachelor buttons	Lipstick plant
Begonia	Magnolia
Bird's nest fern	Marigold
Blood leaf plant	Monkey plant
Boston ferns	Mother-in-law tongue
Bougainvillea	Norfolk Island pine
Cactus—certain varieties	Peperomia
California holly	Petunia
California poppy	Prayer plant
Camelia	Purple passion
Christmas cactus	Pyracantha
Coleus	Rose
Corn plant	Sansevieria
Crab apples	Schefflera
Creeping Charlie	Sensitive plant
Creeping Jennie, moneywort, lysima	Spider plant
Croton (house variety)	Swedish ivy
Dahlia	Umbrella
Daisies	Violets
Dandelion	Wandering jew
Dogwood	Weeping fig
Donkey tail	Weeping willow
Dracaena	Wild onion
Easter lily	Zebra plant
Echeveria	

TABLE 102.16

COMMON PLANT TOXIDROMES

Gastrointestinal Irritants
  Philodendron
  Diffenbachia
  Pokeweed
  Wisteria
  Spurge laurel
  Buttercup
  Daffodil
  Rosary pea
  Castor bean

Digitalis Effects
  Lily-of-the-valley
  Foxglove
  Oleander
  Yew

Nicotinic Effects
  Wild tobacco
  Golden chain tree
  Poison hemlock

Atropinic Effects
  Jimsonweed (thorn apple)
  Deadly nightshade

Epileptogenic Effects
  Water hemlock

Cyanogenic Effects
  Prunus species (chokecherry, wild black cherry, plum,
    peach, apricot, bitter almond)
  Pear (seeds)
  Apple (seeds)
  Crab apple (seeds)
  Hydrangea
  Elderberry

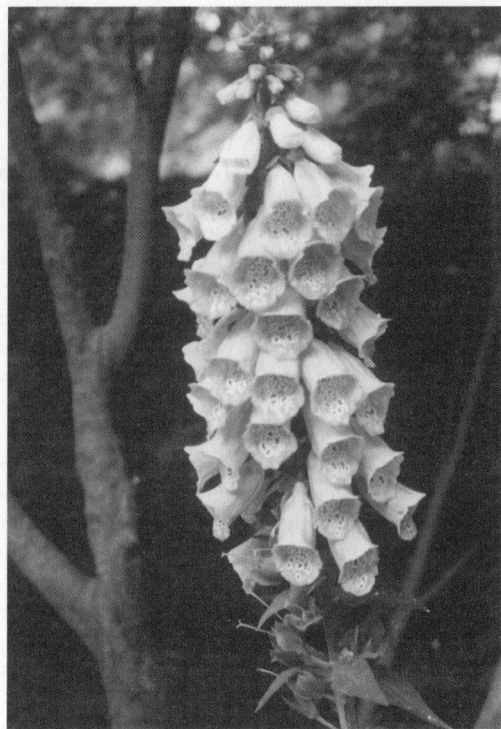

FIGURE 102.11 The foxglove plant *(Digitalis purpurea)*.

When a child visits the ED after plant ingestion, a general evaluation should be performed. Activated charcoal may be useful in adsorbing plant toxins. The child who remains asymptomatic after a period of observation may then be discharged and observed at home. Children who develop symptoms or for whom there is strong suspicion or confirmation that the ingested plant poses a potentially serious intoxication should be admitted for further observation and specific or supportive treatment.

Specific Categories of Plant Toxidromes

Plants with GI Irritation. Plants that cause GI irritation account for most plant poisonings in the United States. The range of symptoms extends from mild oral burning to a severe gastroenteritis syndrome. Representative species include *Philodendron* and *Dieffenbachia* species (leaves), which cause minor mouth and throat burning; pokeweed (roots, stem), Wisteria (seeds), spurge laurel (berries), buttercup (leaves), and daffodil (bulbs, accidentally substituted for onions), which cause severe vomiting, colicky abdominal pain, and diarrhea; and the toxalbumin-containing plants such as rosary pea and castor bean (seeds), which can cause a violent hemorrhagic gastroenteritis that leads to profound dehydration and circulatory collapse when the seeds are chewed up. The management of this group of ingestions consists essentially of fluid and electrolyte therapy.

Plants with Digitalis Effects. Several common garden or wildflowers contain digitalis, and they have been responsible for fatal ingestions. Instances of chewing on leaves or flowers or swallowing the berries of lily-of-the-valley, foxglove (Fig. 102.11), red squill, and oleander all have led to such poisonings. Intoxication has even occurred when water from a vase that contained these flowers was ingested. Early after ingestion, the child may complain of intestinal symptoms such as mouth irritation, vomiting, and diarrhea. As the digitalis is absorbed, typical digitalis effects may ensue, with conduction defects and, at times, serious arrhythmias. Treatment may include administration of digoxin-specific antibody fragments as was previously discussed.

Plants with Nicotinic Effects. Several species of plants contain nicotine or closely related alkaloids. Ingestion of wild tobacco (leaves), golden chain tree (seeds), and poison hemlock (leaves, seeds) usually leads to spontaneous vomiting within 1 hour. Salivation, headache, fever, mental confusion, and muscular weakness may follow, and the child may deteriorate to convulsions, coma, and death from respiratory failure. Charcoal may be useful in adsorbing these nicotinic alkaloids. Further treatment consists of intensive supportive care, with anticonvulsants and ventilatory assistance.

Plants with Atropinic Effects. The most common atropine-containing plant in the United States is jimsonweed, which is widely distributed. Cases most commonly occur in rural areas but have been seen even in inner-city children who managed to find this weed growing in their neighborhoods, where flora in general is scarce.

Symptoms and signs are those of atropinization (Table 102.7) and include visual blurring, dilated pupils, dryness of the mouth, hot and dry skin, fever, delirium, and psychosis. Convulsions and coma may follow. Treatment consists of supportive care and, in severe cases, physiologic antagonism with physostigmine (Table 102.4).

Plants That Cause Convulsions. Convulsions represent the principal toxic effect of some plants. Water hemlock, with its potent cicutoxin, is the main species to cause convulsions in the United States. Within 1 hour after ingestion, nausea, vomiting, and profuse salivation occur. These initial symptoms are followed by tremors, muscle rigidity, and multiple major motor seizures. Treatment is with anticonvulsants, as for status epilepticus (see Chapters 69 and 96).

Plants That Contain Cyanogenic Glycosides. Many plants and particularly fruit seeds (pits) contain the cyanogenic glycoside amygdalin (Table 102.16). However, these glycosides are relatively protected within the seeds and would be unlikely to cause illness after an exploratory ingestion by a young child.

Symptoms and signs after ingestion are those of cyanide poisoning, with resultant cellular hypoxia. Initially, there is CNS stimulation and headache, with tachypnea, hypertension, and reflex bradycardia. Anxiety and excitation may progress to opisthotonus and seizures. Respiratory depression, with cyanosis, tachycardia, and hypotension, follows. An odor of bitter almonds may be detected. Treatment is initiated with 100% oxygen and cardiopulmonary resuscitation as necessary. Antidotal therapy for cyanide poisoning, with hydroxocobalamin, or with nitrates and sodium thiosulfate, is detailed in Table 102.9 and in Chapter 7.

Mushrooms

Mushrooms cause an estimated 50% of all deaths from plant and fungi poisoning in the United States. The difficulty in accurate identification of mushrooms makes reliance on such identification for appropriate management of ingestions extremely hazardous in the ED.

Two main groups of mushrooms can be characterized on the basis of the time interval between ingestion and symptom onset: those with the immediate onset of symptoms and those with delayed onset. Regardless of the mushroom, the initial management for all suspected poisonings includes consideration of activated charcoal and other GI decontamination strategies.

Onset of symptoms within 6 hours of ingestion usually confers a benign prognosis, although careful attention to fluid and electrolyte management is critical. Most mushrooms have GI effects. There are several general classes of mushrooms in this group, each possessing a unique toxicologic feature. Some "early-onset" mushrooms cause muscarinic effects, usually within 15 minutes, such as sweating, salivation, colic, and pulmonary edema. This syndrome responds to atropine therapy. Other early-onset mushrooms cause anticholinergic effects, including drowsiness, followed by mania and hallucinations. Another subgroup of early-onset mushrooms produces a severe gastroenteritis syndrome. Hallucinogenic mushrooms such as those containing psilocybin make up another class of mushrooms with early-onset symptoms. Finally, some mushrooms precipitate a disulfiram-like reaction if they are coingested with alcohol. Management for all these agents consists of supportive care and careful monitoring of fluid status.

The second, more important, category of mushrooms that are responsible for 90% of mushroom-related deaths are those associated with onset of symptoms that occur more than 6 hours after ingestion. The most important members of this group are those mushrooms that belong to the *Amanita phalloides* species. With these mushrooms, after a latent period of many hours, GI upset appears. Approximately 24 hours after ingestion, hepatic dysfunction appears, which may progress to fulminant hepatic failure. Without liver transplantation, such patients generally die.

Two compounds are known to produce the toxic effects of *A. phalloides*. Phallotoxin acts first, causing GI symptoms, including nausea, vomiting, abdominal pain, and diarrhea. Fever, tachycardia, and hyperglycemia may also occur during this stage. The other toxin, amatoxin, causes renal tubular and hepatic necrosis.

Treatment of the gastroenteric phase includes fluid and electrolyte replacement. If renal failure develops, dialysis may be necessary. Hepatic damage after *A. phalloides* ingestion may be attenuated by early use of repetitive activated charcoal, which appears to interrupt enterohepatic recirculation of amatoxin.

Additional therapies have shown mixed results in the treatment of *A. phalloides* poisoning. High-dose penicillin, cimetidine, *n*-acetylcysteine, thioctic acid, silibinin, prophylactic charcoal hemoperfusion, and other modalities await further investigation. A regional poison control center may offer guidance with experimental therapies, but multiple-dose activated charcoal and vigorous attention to supportive care remain the standard. For patients with poor prognosis, early referral for liver transplantation may be lifesaving.

In management of mushroom ingestions in which the specific mushroom cannot be identified, GI decontamination, including activated charcoal, should always be provided. Identification of the agent may be possible through consultation with a local mycologist, although mushroom cohabitation makes classification uncertain even if a fragment of mushroom is brought for direct inspection.

Tricyclic Antidepressants

Background

The ingestion of tricyclic antidepressant compounds is a significant problem in pediatric patients. The availability of these compounds in the household may be the result of therapy for depression for a parent or a grandparent or of treatment for enuresis in the patient or a sibling.

Clinical Findings

The ingestion of 10 to 20 mg per kg of most tricyclic antidepressants represents a moderate to serious exposure, with coma and cardiovascular symptoms expected. The ingestion of 35 to 50 mg per kg may result in death. Children have been reported to be more sensitive than adults to tricyclic antidepressants and often have symptoms at lower dosages.

Cyclic antidepressants have many pharmacologic effects. Anticholinergic activity causes altered sensorium and sinus tachycardia. α-Adrenergic blockade may lead to hypotension. However, the more severe cardiovascular effects are primarily caused by the membrane-depressant or "quinidine-like" effects that depress myocardial conduction and may lead to multiple focal premature ventricular contractions and ventricular tachycardia. It has been shown that a QRS interval over 0.1 second is associated with a significant morbidity and mortality in these patients; this delay in conduction may progress to complete heart block and cardiac standstill and/or the previously mentioned ventricular arrhythmias. Another typical electrocardiographic finding suggestive of cyclic antidepressant poisoning is the finding of an R wave of greater than 3-mm amplitude in the QRS complex in lead aVR.

Neurologic findings include lethargy, disorientation, ataxia, hallucinations, and with severe overdoses, coma, and seizures. Fever is commonly present initially, but hypothermia may occur later. Additional anticholinergic symptomatology includes decreased GI motility, which delays gastric emptying time, and urinary retention. Muscle twitching has been observed and may be associated with increased deep tendon reflexes. Although the pupils may be dilated, they usually respond to light.

Management

Severe tricyclic antidepressant overdoses warrant gastric decontamination. Because tricyclic antidepressants decrease GI motility, unabsorbed drug may be left in the stomach for prolonged periods. Seizures should be treated aggressively with benzodiazepines and/or barbiturates, or even with neuromuscular paralysis if needed to prevent acidosis. Significant conduction delays or arrhythmias resulting from tricyclic antidepressants may benefit from alkalinization of the blood. A sodium bicarbonate bolus of 1 to 2 mEq per kg can be given during continuous EKG monitoring. Bicarbonate infusion can then be used to keep the serum pH at 7.45 to 7.55. These therapeutic maneuvers likely serve to decrease drug binding to the myocardium. Additional bolus doses of sodium bicarbonate may be required if the QRS interval is noted to widen. An additional benefit of the sodium cation may be to partially overcome the sodium channel blockade that is believed to represent the biomolecular substrate of the membrane depressant effect of these agents. If arrhythmias persist, appropriate antiarrhythmic therapy should be instituted, perhaps using lidocaine (see Chapters 1 and 84). Quinidine or procainamide should be avoided because each may increase heart block in this situation. Physostigmine, although previously recommended for its antidotal effects on the anticholinergic aspects of these poisonings, has the potential to worsen ventricular conduction defects and to lower the seizure threshold. Its use is considered to be contraindicated in cyclic antidepressant overdoses, particularly in the setting of an abnormal EKG. In the presence of hypotension, many clinicians have advocated the use of norepinephrine infusions (0.1 to 0.3 μg per kg per minute). This is based on the observation that the hypotension is the result of norepinephrine depletion secondary to the block of catecholamine uptake, caused by tricyclic antidepressants. Other clinicians have reported that dopamine is as effective; however, the occurrence of ventricular arrhythmias has been reported with dopamine. A novel potential therapy, the infusion of lipid emulsion, has shown promise in animal studies of cyclic antidepressant toxicity, as well as for calcium antagonists as noted previously. Several clinical cases of its efficacy in refractory local anesthetic cardiotoxicity and one in bupropion overdose are reported, although most experts would not recommend its use as yet, except as a last resort in patients facing refractory cardiotoxicity despite adequate efforts at cardiopulmonary resuscitation. During the recovery period, serum electrolyte levels should also be monitored because the infusion of bicarbonate may cause hypokalemia, which may aggravate tricyclic antidepressant-induced cardiac arrhythmias. It must be remembered in the treatment of such antidepressants that these compounds have long half-lives and slow elimination rates; therefore, the therapy for these ingestions is often protracted and intensive.

Other Antidepressants

Besides the tricyclic antidepressants, numerous agents designed to elevate mood are prescribed. The chemical structure of these agents and their profile of toxicity are diverse. Major groupings of nontricyclic antidepressants include (i) the selective serotonin reuptake inhibitors (SSRIs; e.g., fluoxetine, sertraline), (ii) the monoamine oxidase inhibitors (MAOIs; e.g., phenelzine, tranylcypromine), and (iii) other atypical antidepressants (e.g., amoxapine, venlafaxine, bupropion).

SSRIs most commonly produce CNS depression in overdose. Seizures may occur after large ingestions. Life-threatening events from acute overdose of these compounds rarely occur. The serotonin syndrome, manifested by the triad of autonomic instability, neuromuscular changes (myoclonus, rigidity especially in the lower extremities), and altered mental status, is potentially lethal. Amoxapine has anticholinergic activity but is best known for its convulsant properties and the tendency for patients to present with status epilepticus. Bupropion, prescribed perhaps most commonly in smoking-cessation programs, prevents reuptake of biogenic amines, is highly seizurogenic, and in large overdose, may cause QRS widening and life-threatening cardiotoxicity. The α-adrenergic antagonism of trazodone may lead to hypotension.

The MAOIs, although pharmacologically effective and therapeutically important, are some of the most toxic medications known. Acute single overdoses of as little as 6 mg per kg have been associated with a fatal outcome. In addition, because of their irreversible inhibition of the enzyme monoamine oxidase, which is responsible for the degradation of most biogenic amines, MAOIs possess several important interactions with foods and other medications that can lead to severe toxicity, even in the patient who takes them in appropriate doses. There are three important clinical pictures of MAOI toxicity. First, because GI tract activity of monoamine oxidase is also inhibited by these drugs, patients who take them appropriately and then ingest foods that contain biogenic amines (e.g., tyramine in wines, cheeses, or soy sauce) may develop severe hypertension with subsequent headache, seizures, or stroke. The second picture of MAOI toxicity appears when those who take the drug therapeutically are given certain sympathomimetic or serotonergic agents causing the serotonin syndrome. Important examples of such drugs include common agents in OTC cough and cold preparations such as dextromethorphan, analgesics such as meperidine, and psychotropic medications such as clomipramine and fluoxetine or other SSRIs. In these patients, this drug combination may quickly lead to hyperpyrexia, skeletal muscle rigidity, cardiac arrhythmias, and death. This is one of the few fatal drug interactions known. Finally, those with acute MAOI overdoses develop a clinical syndrome that includes blood pressure instability, hyperpyrexia, skeletal muscle rigidity, opsoclonus, seizures, and death.

Because of the toxicity of these agents and the frequent delay in their onset of activity (up to 24 hours), all patients with a history of MAOI ingestion, regardless of symptoms, should be admitted to the hospital for 24 hours. Management of the patient with MAOI toxicity is largely dictated by the specific toxic manifestations. In those with hypertensive reactions, treatment consists of the immediate administration of an antihypertensive. The ideal agent may be nitroprusside because its brief duration of action permits titration of effect. In the treatment of hyperpyrexia, cooling measures are promptly instituted. Because hyperpyrexia is often accompanied by skeletal muscle rigidity and rhabdomyolysis, serum creatine kinase level should be measured and close attention should be paid to the urine for any signs of myoglobinuria. Benzodiazepines are often helpful in this situation and neuromuscular blockade may be beneficial in patients who have severe muscle rigidity with hyperthermia. In the patient with acute overdose, treatment is directed to hemodynamic stability. Because blood pressure changes occur quickly and consist of hypotension and hypertension, hypertension should be treated with short-acting agents (see Chapter 34) and hypoten-

sion with fluid and vasopressor support (see Chapter 3). Intensive care unit admission is mandatory for these patients because of their clinical instability.

Drugs Dangerous in Small Doses

Toddlers often are brought to EDs for evaluation after possibly having ingested one or two doses of a medication. This can be a particularly vexing problem. Most often these children will be fine with little treatment beyond reassurance. There are circumstances, however, when this situation can be life-threatening and proper intervention can be lifesaving. A large list of chemicals and poisons can be extremely toxic in small amounts; but, this is beyond the scope of this discussion. However, it is wise to be familiar with a modest list of pharmaceuticals that may cause dangerous toxicity to young children with just one or two doses (Table 102.17). Many of these agents have been discussed earlier in this chapter. The actual incidence of life-threatening

---

TABLE 102.17

MEDICATIONS DANGEROUS TO TODDLERS IN ONE TO TWO DOSES[a]

Agent	Minimal potential fatal dose[b]	Maximal dose size	Potential fatal dose	Major toxicity
Benzocaine	<20 mg/kg	10% gel 20% spray	~2 mL Baby Oragel	Methemoglobinemia, seizures
β-Blockers (propranolol)	Unclear	160 mg	1–2 tablets	Bradycardia, hypotension, seizures, hypoglycemia
Calcium antagonists (verapamil)	<40 mg/kg	240 mg	1–2 tablets	Bradycardia, hypotension
Camphor	<100 mg/kg	1 g/5 mL	1 tsp camphorated oil 2 tsp Campho-Phenique 5 tsp Vicks Vaporub	Seizures, CNS depression
Chloroquine	<30 mg/kg	500 mg	1 tablet	Seizures, arrhythmia
Clonidine	Unclear	0.3-mg tablet 7.5-mg patch	1 tablet 1 patch	Bradycardia, CNS depression
Diphenoxylate (Lomotil)	<1.2 mg/kg	2.5 mg/tablet or tsp	2 tablets/tsp	CNS and respiratory depression
Hypoglycemics, oral (glyburide)	~1 mg/kg	5 mg	2 tablets	Hypoglycemia
Lindane	~6 mg/kg	1% lotion	2 tsp	Seizures, CNS depression
Methyl salicylate	~200 mg/kg	1.4 g/mL	½ tsp oil of wintergreen 2 tsp Icy Hot Balm	Seizures, cardiovascular collapse
Opioids	Variable by potency	Variable	1–2 tablets	CNS and respiratory depression
Phenothiazines (chlorpromazine)	~20 mg/kg	200 mg	1 tablet	Seizures, arrhythmia
Quinidine	~50 mg/kg	300 mg	2 tablets	Seizures, arrhythmia
Quinine	~80 mg/kg	650 mg	2 tablets	Seizures, arrhythmia
Theophylline	~50 mg/kg	500 mg	1 tablet	Seizures, arrhythmia
TCAs (imipramine)	~20 mg/kg	150 mg	1–2 tablets	Seizures, arrhythmia, hypotension

CNS, central nervous system; TCAs, tricyclic antidepressants.
[a]A long list of commonly-encountered, highly toxic, *non*pharmacologic agents can be severely poisonous in 1 to 2 doses. These are not included here.
[b]For the purposes of this table, a "dose" refers to a single pill or roughly a 5-cc swallow. Calculations are based on a previously healthy toddler of 10-kg body weight.

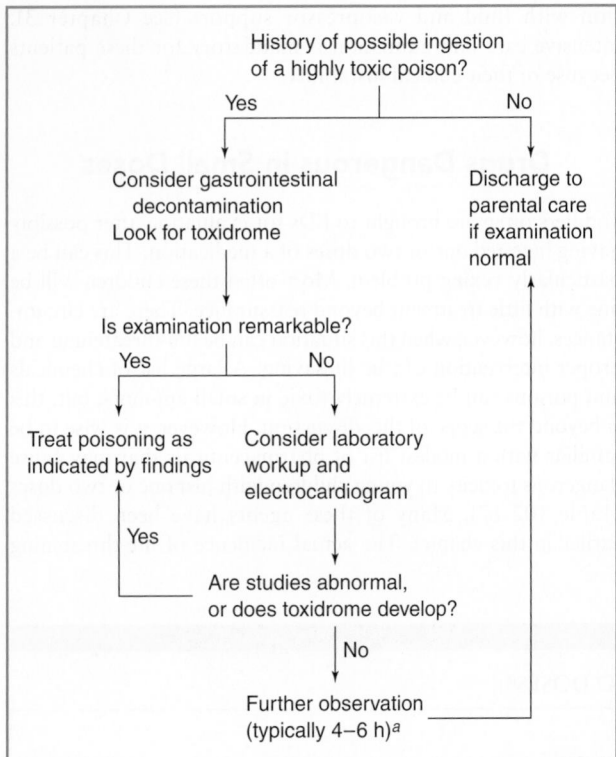

FIGURE 102.12 Algorithmic approach to a toddler having ingested one to two doses (1 to 2 pills or 5- to 10-cc swallow) of a drug. [a]Medications notorious for their ability to have delayed onset in toxicity, beyond 4 to 6 hours, include oral hypoglycemic agents, sustained-release preparations, monoamine oxidase inhibitors, drugs taken concomitantly with anticholinergic agents, and acetaminophen.

toxicity of each of these drugs, when just one or two doses have been ingested, is as yet undefined.

A systematic approach to these patients includes a careful history, an examination with attention to the presence of toxidromes (Table 102.5), and a guided laboratory assessment. This approach may allow narrowing of the differential diagnosis and may allow a determination of the possible severity of the ingestion. If the differential diagnosis includes any of the drugs listed in Table 102.17, it may be prudent to consider decontamination and prolonged observation. An algorithmic approach to this situation is provided in Fig. 102.12.

SUBSTANCE ABUSE

As a special category of pediatric toxicology, exposures to psychoactive drugs are outlined in this section. In a discussion of substance abuse, three distinct age populations in the pediatric group may be placed at risk from such exposures: (i) the adolescent or preadolescent who abuses drugs for their mind-altering effects (and, in the case of women, may do so when pregnant); (ii) the neonate who is exposed to substances of abuse during gestation and manifests signs of intoxication or abstinence after birth; and (iii) the infant or toddler who becomes exposed to drugs of abuse through either active administration by a caregiver (chemical child abuse), the ingestion of a drug left in an accessible place (e.g., the coffee table), or passive exposure

created by being in an environment where drugs of abuse are used (e.g., marijuana, cocaine, phencyclidine (PCP), methamphetamine). In any of these circumstances, the exposure can be sufficient to produce severe intoxication. Thus, knowledge of the epidemiology and manifestations of substance abuse become important in the management of children of all ages.

Further discussion regarding the general phenomenon of chronic adolescent drug abuse and addiction, including alcoholism, is found in Chapter 130.

Clinical Manifestations

The drug-abusing child or adolescent may present to the ED after an unintentional overdose, a suicidal gesture, suicide attempt, sudden bizarre behavior, or multiple trauma (e.g., assault, motor vehicle collision). Often, the history of drug exposure is undeclared and may not be diagnosed unless there is a high index of suspicion and appropriate diagnostic tests are performed. In such cases, the patient's mental status can range from fully awake and responsive to comatose; physical examination can be without any signs of drug exposure or with overt signs of toxicity (e.g., seizures). Table 102.18 provides a summary of the common drugs of abuse, their typical routes of administration, associated symptoms, toxic levels, and duration of action.

Initial history from the patient, family, or friends must specify drugs taken and estimate quantities when an ingestion is suspected. In the absence of a history of exposure, it is important to inquire whether the patient has used any psychoactive drugs in the past. In many cases, the patient may admit to using a drug but may identify it by a street name. Although drug terminology tables are often available in pharmacology or toxicology texts as well as the Internet, temporal and regional changes in street drug terminology generally make such tables of limited value.

Management

Primary attention is paid toward assessment of vital signs and life support as needed to provide a patent, secure airway; to ensure adequate respiratory function; and to treat seizures, shock, or cardiorespiratory arrest. A key, but often overlooked, feature in the assessment of such patients is an accurate temperature because many drug intoxications are associated with hyperpyrexia. If there is any suspicion of hyperthermia, a rectal temperature must be obtained. In the agitated patient, physical and/or chemical restraint may be necessary to obtain vital signs. Chemical restraint should be used liberally to prevent patients from harming themselves or others. The preferred agents in such cases are diazepam (0.1 to 0.3 mg per kg IV) or midazolam (0.05 to 0.1 mg per kg IV). Haloperidol (0.05 mg per kg) given IM is also effective but reduces heat-dissipating capability and lowers the seizure threshold. Droperidol received an U.S. Food and Drug Administration (FDA) "black box" warning in 2001 due to concerns about QTc prolongation; subsequently, this medication is used less commonly in the agitated toxicology patient.

Management must also include consideration of the need for GI decontamination. It is common with psychoactive drug use where several distinct routes of exposure are possible (e.g.,

TABLE 102.18

DRUG ABUSE: SUMMARY OF TOXICITY

Drug of abuse	Symptoms and signs of drug abuse	Diagnosis	Toxic dose	Toxic serum level	Half-life
Cannabis Group (marijuana; hashish; Δ9-THC; hash oil)	Pupils unchanged; conjunctiva injected; blood pressure (BP) decreased on standing; heart rate increased; increased appetite, euphoria, anxiety; sensorium often clear; dreamy; fantasy state; time–space distortions; hallucinations rare. Significant airway obstruction with heavy smoking, decreased forced expiratory volume, and decreased vital capacity. Major psychiatric toxic effects: Panic reaction most common Psychotic reactions (especially in patients with underlying psychopathology) Toxic delirium (disorientation, confusion, memory impairment) in heavy users	Blood, urine levels	20 mg Δ9-THC or 1 g cigarette of 2% Δ9-THC produces effects on mood, memory, motor coordination, cognitive ability sensorium, time sense		*1st phase,* minutes, distribution in lipid-rich tissues; *2nd phase,* 1½–2 days, until mobilized from lipid-rich tissue
Hallucinogens	Pupils dilated (normal or small with PCP); BP elevated, heart rate increased, hyperactive tendon reflexes, increased temperature, flushed face, euphoria, anxiety or panic, paranoid thought disorder, inappropriate affect, time and visual distortions, visual hallucinations, depersonalization.				
LSD	Psychosis with hyperalertness; changes in body image; sense of profound significance, delusions; hallucinations (also with amphetamines), visual perceptual distortions caused by peripheral effects of LSD on visual system.	Blood, urine levels	20–25 μg produce CNS effects; 0.5–2 μg/kg produce somatic symptoms; between 1 and 16 μg/kg intensity of pathophysiologic effects proportional to dose	Variable	3 h
PCP	Cyclic coma, extreme hyperactivity, violent outbursts, bizarre behavior, amnesia, analgesia, nystagmus, gait ataxia, muscle rigidity. Dystonic reactions, grand mal seizures, tardive dyskinesia, athetosis, bronchospasm, urinary retention, diaphoresis, hypoglycemia. Increased uric acid, increased creatine phosphokinase, increased creatinine, increased hepatic transaminases heralds onset of rhabdomyolysis (risk of renal failure).	Blood, gastric contents, urine (but level does not correlate with toxicity)	1 cigarette (PCP) = 1–100 mg. Psychosis may last several weeks after a dose. Fatal dose = 1 mg/kg; <5 mg = hyperactivity; 5–10 mg = stupor, coma; >10 mg = respiratory depression, convulsions	Individual variability (~0.1 μg/mL)	1–3 d

(continued)

TABLE 102.18

DRUG ABUSE: SUMMARY OF TOXICITY (CONTINUED)

Drug of abuse	Symptoms and signs of drug abuse	Diagnosis	Toxic dose	Toxic serum level	Half-life
CNS Stimulants					
Amphetamines	Pupils dilated and reactive. Increased BP, pulse, temperature, cardiac arrhythmias; dry mouth; sweating; tremors; sensorium hyperacute or confused; paranoid ideation; impulsivity; hyperactivity; stereotypy; convulsions; exhaustion.	Blood level, urine test	1. Variable 2. Rare under 15 mg 3. Severe reactions have occurred at 30 mg 4. 400–500 mg not uniformly fatal 5. Tolerance is striking; chronic user may take 1,700 mg/day without ill effects	Variable	3 h
Cocaine	1. Excitement, restlessness, euphoria, garrulousness. 2. Increased motor activity, physical endurance because of decreased sense of fatigue. 3. Increased tremors, convulsive movements. 4. Increased respiration, pulse, BP, temperature, chills.	Urine, serum	Fatal dose may be as low as 30 mg; ingested cocaine less toxic than by other routes		1 h (after PO or nasal route)
CNS Sedatives (barbiturates, chlordiazepoxide, diazepam, flurazepam, glutethimide, meprobamate, methaqualone)	Pupils normal or small (dilated with glutethimide); BP decreased, respirations depressed; drowsy, coma, lateral nystagmus, confusion, ataxia, slurred speech, delirium; convulsions or hyperirritability with methaqualone overdosage; serious poisoning rare with benzodiazepines alone.	Serum level			
Barbiturates (Secobarbital) (Seconal)	As above.	Serum level	100 mg per dose	30 μg/mL	19–34 h
Chlordiazepoxide (Librium)	As above.	Serum level	25 mg	8 μg/mL	8–25 h
Diazepam (Valium)	As above.	Serum, urine	15 mg or greater		20–90 h
Flurazepam (Dalmane)	As above.	Serum, urine		0.12 μg/mL (fatal)	47–100 h
Glutethimide (Doriden)	As above.	Serum level	>500 mg (acute intoxication, 3 g)	2 mg/100 mL (but even below, full ICU support may be required)	5–22 h
Meprobamate	As above.	Serum level	>800 mg	150 μg/mL	6–17 h

Drug	Symptoms	Specimen	Dose	Serum level	Duration
Methaqualone (Parest, Somnafae)	As above.	Serum level	200–400 mg	10 μg/mL	20–60 h
Narcotics	Pupils constricted (may be dilated with meperidine or extreme hypoxia); respiration depressed to absent with cyanosis; BP decreased, sometimes shock; temperature reduced; reflexes diminished to absent, stupor or coma; pulmonary edema; constipation; convulsions with propoxyphene or meperidine; arrhythmia with propoxyphene.	Serum, urine			
Heroin	As above.	Serum, urine	—	—	1½ h[c]
Morphine	As above.	Serum	60 mg = toxic[b] 200 mg = fatal dose[b]	—	3 h[c]
Codeine	As above.	Serum	800 mg = fatal dose[b]	1.1 μg/mL	2 h[c]
Methadone	As above.	Serum	100 mg = fatal dose[b]	1.6 μg/mL (fatal)	18–97 h[c]
Propoxyphene	As above.	Serum	500 mg = fatal dose[b]	2 μg/mL (fatal)	3–12 h
Anticholinergics (atropine, belladonna, henbane, scopolamine, trihexphenidyl, tricyclic antidepressants, benzotropine mesylate)	Pupils dilated and fixed, heart rate increased, temperature increased, BP increased; drowsy, coma, flushed, dry skin and mucous membranes, erythematous skin, amnesia, disoriented, visual hallucinations, body image alterations.	Urine test			
Atropine	As above.		5 mg		24 h
Belladonna	As above.		5 mg		24 h
Scopolamine	As above.		5 mg		24 h
Imipramine (Tofranil)	As above.		500 mg		8–16 h
Amitriptyline (Elavil)	As above.		>500 mg	5 μg/mL	32–40 h
Desipramine	As above.		1 g	10 μg/mL	12–54 h

LSD, lysergamides; ICU, intensive care unit.
[a]Dose is amount given subcutaneously that produces same analgesic effect as morphine 10 mg subcutaneously.
[b]Higher doses given for addicts.
[c]Duration is for subcutaneous dose. Intravenous dose peak is more pronounced and overall effects have shorter duration.
Adapted from Dreisbach RH. *Handbook of poisoning.* Los Altos, CA: Lange Medical Publications, 1980.

MEDICAL EMERGENCIES

1213

ingestion, inhalation, injection, and/or nasal insufflation). Therefore, GI decontamination is not always necessary or appropriate.

However, because those who abuse drugs almost invariably use more than one drug, decontamination should be considered if there is any possibility of an ingestion, utilizing the same guiding principles regarding toxin and patient characteristics detailed earlier in this chapter. In the event that decontamination seems appropriate, assessment of the patient's mental status and gag reflex must be performed; in the presence of obtundation or a diminished gag reflex, airway protection by endotracheal intubation should be accomplished before decontamination measures.

Disposition

In the case of the adolescent who presents with intentional drug abuse, after initial assessment and medical stabilization, an evaluation must be made of the severity of the drug use problem. Although issues of patient confidentiality may require the physician to provide limited information to parents, obtaining a thorough psychosocial evaluation is necessary for complete management of the acute event. Such discussions may require or may be facilitated by an interview with a social services or psychiatry consultant. Once the severity of the drug problem has been established, referral to a treatment program should be discussed. Primary care physicians may be comfortable managing those patients who have no long-standing histories of drug abuse. Compulsive users or anyone who presents with a drug abstinence syndrome must be referred for intensive rehabilitation. Family therapy is often a vital component of this rehabilitation.

SPECIFIC DRUGS

The major categories of drugs of abuse that require the physician's familiarity with the whole spectrum of their physiologic effects are (i) hallucinogens [phencyclidine, ketamine, lysergic acid diethylamide, marijuana], (ii) stimulants (amphetamines, cocaine), (iii) central anticholinergics, (iv) sedatives (benzodiazepines, barbiturates), (v) opioids (morphine, codeine, heroin, methadone, buprenorphine, oxycodone, and hydrocodone), (vi) inhalants, and (vii) alcohol. (Acute alcohol overdose is discussed in the previous section; chronic alcoholism in teenagers is discussed in Chapter 130.)

Hallucinogens (Psychedelics)

No single characteristic distinguishes psychedelics from other classes of centrally active drugs such as anticholinergics, cocaine, and amphetamines. These drugs can produce a number of mental status changes, including illusions, hallucinations, delusions, and paranoid ideation. However, the psychedelic state is characteristically described as consisting of vivid and unusual visual experiences with diminished control over what is experienced. Images and sensations take on profound meaning, and the ability to differentiate oneself from the environment is decreased. Most drugs in this category are related to the indolealkylamines [psilocybin, dimethyltryptamine (DMT), diethyltryptamine], lysergamides (LSD), or phenylethylamines [mescaline, methylenedioxymethamphetamine (MDMA, Ecstasy)].

Phencyclidine, Ketamine, and Dextromethorphan

Identification. PCP was developed in the 1950s as a general anesthetic. It rapidly fell into disuse because of disturbing emergence syndromes that developed in postoperative patients. Sporadic abuse occurred in the 1960s, but its popularity peaked in the 1970s. The drug remains common in several metropolitan areas as does ketamine, a PCP analog with approximately one-tenth the potency and a shorter duration of action. Ketamine is discussed in detail in Chapter 4. Another drug with related structure, but milder effects, is dextromethorphan, which is popular with adolescents because of its ready availability as a legal, OTC cough suppressant. PCP is easily synthesized and is often sold on the streets misrepresented as LSD, mescaline, or marijuana. It is well absorbed across all mucous membranes and is most popularly used by inhalation (often mixed into cigarettes or marijuana "joints"), but it can be ingested, injected, or insufflated.

Chemically, PCP is an arylcyclohexylamine. This group of drugs has a range of CNS actions that range from hallucinations with smaller doses, to stimulation with moderate doses (occasionally associated with seizures), to profound CNS depression with respiratory arrest with large doses.

Pharmacodynamics. There is great variability in the metabolism of PCP. In general, 0.1 μg per mL is considered a toxic serum level. One cigarette may contain 1 to 100 mg. A dose of 5 to 10 mg may produce stupor and coma; with doses exceeding 10 mg, respiratory depression and convulsions occur. A fatal dose is in the range of 1 mg per kg. Because PCP has a long elimination half-life (18 hours), clinical symptoms may last for more than 12 hours; also, patients may have cyclic symptoms because the drug undergoes enterohepatic recirculation.

Pharmacologically, PCP acts as a dissociative anesthetic, meaning that it interferes potently with association pathways that link the cerebral cortex with deeper structures in the brain, thus diminishing the ability to integrate sensory input into meaningful behavior. Its anesthetic actions also lead to a marked diminution of pain sensation. In conjunction with bizarre behavior, this often leads patients to have feelings of invulnerability and to attempt life-threatening actions (e.g., stepping into automobile traffic).

Clinical Symptoms. Small doses of PCP produce signs and symptoms of inebriation with staggering gait, slurred speech, and nystagmus (vertical or rotatory). Users may also be diaphoretic and have catatonic muscular rigidity with a blank stare. Having sympathomimetic actions, it is often associated with hypertension and tachycardia. Dextromethorphan toxicity resembles the syndrome of low-dose PCP exposure; nystagmus and myoclonus may help distinguish this toxidrome from alcohol or sedative toxicity, and the urine drug screen may be falsely positive for PCP. Moderate doses of PCP cause other signs of intoxication, including hypersalivation, pyrexia, repetitive movements, and muscle rigidity. Larger doses can cause seizures, coma, or respiratory arrest. The typical "high" from a single dose lasts 4 to 6 hours and is followed by an extended "coming down"; PCP-induced psychotic states may be long lasting and may recur (flashbacks). Tolerance develops to the behavioral and toxic effects of the drug. Chronic users report persistent difficulties with recent memory, speech, and thinking that last from 6 months to 1 year after the last dose; they also may be left with personality changes such as withdrawal, isolation, anxiety, nervousness, and depression.

Management. PCP is easily detected through a qualitative analysis of urine. Serum levels are rarely available and do not correlate with clinical manifestations. Therefore, management must often be based solely on a history of exposure or index of suspicion. Initial treatment is directed at stabilizing vital signs and treating life-threatening events such as seizures. If exposure is the result of ingestion, GI decontamination should be performed by administration of activated charcoal. A quiet room may be helpful, although the ability to monitor the patient cannot be compromised. Physical restraints should be avoided if possible because they may lead to significant rhabdomyolysis with resulting myoglobinuria and renal injury. For chemical restraint diazepam (0.1 to 0.3 mg per kg IV) or lorazepam (0.1 mg per kg IV) may be effective, although a major tranquilizer (e.g., haloperidol) is often necessary.

Although urine acidification (pH less than 5.0) enhances the urinary excretion of PCP, it should never be performed in these patients because it exacerbates metabolic acidosis and may promote deposition of myoglobin in renal tubules. In a review of 27 confirmed cases of PCP poisoning, 3 patients developed rhabdomyolysis and 2 progressed to acute renal failure. Both patients had received acidification measures before diagnosis. If tests for muscle enzymes and/or renal function are abnormal and the urine has a positive test for hemoglobin without red blood cells, the patient should be assumed to have rhabdomyolysis and should be treated accordingly (see Chapter 86).

LSD (Blotter, Acid)

Pathophysiology. LSD and related psychedelic drugs such as psilocybin, mescaline, and DMT have actions at multiple sites in the CNS (from the cortex to the spinal cord). In addition, dozens of congeners of these agents exist in mushrooms or have been synthesized, and they also cause signs and symptoms similar to those of LSD. The pharmacologic action that these drugs seem to have in common is as agonists of presynaptic serotonin-2 receptors (which modulate serotonin release into the synaptic cleft). Most of these agents have structural similarities to serotonin (5-hydroxytryptamine).

Pharmacodynamics. In humans, the somatic symptoms of dizziness, weakness, drowsiness, nausea, and paresthesias may be observed after one oral dose of 0.5 to 2 μg per kg. Between the dose range of 1 to 16 μg per kg, the intensity of LSD's psychoactive effects is proportional to the dose. A typical LSD "hit" is 200 to 400 μg. A high degree of tolerance to the behavioral effects develops after three to four daily doses, with sensitivity returning after a drug-free interval. Deaths directly attributable to LSD are virtually unknown, although fatal accidents and suicides have occurred during states of intoxication.

Clinical Symptoms. In general, the somatic effects of hallucinogens are sympathomimetic and include pupillary dilation, hypertension, tachycardia, hyperreflexia, and hyperpyrexia. Doses as low as 20 to 25 μg can produce CNS effects such as euphoria, visual perceptual distortions, alteration of subjective

time so time passes slowly, lability of mood, or even an acute panic episode. Hallucinations and psychosis with hyperalertness are commonly seen. The clinical duration of action of LSD is somewhat dose dependent but averages 6 to 12 hours. The psychedelic state includes a heightened awareness of sensory input, often accompanied by an enhanced sense of clarity but a diminished control over what is experienced. There is often a feeling that one part of the self is a passive observer while another part receives vivid sensory input. The ability to separate one object from another or to separate self from the environment is diminished. There is an enhanced sense of oneness with humanity.

Management. LSD intoxication is rarely associated with life-threatening events. However, vital signs should be assessed to ensure that the patient is stable in the event there has been drug coingestion. Because LSD is ingested in minuscule doses and onset of symptoms occurs hours after ingestion, GI decontamination is unnecessary, unless coingestion is suspected.

Clinical management involves placing the patient in a quiet room. Someone who knows the patient may be able to quietly "talk down" and reassure the patient. The patient's loss of boundaries and fear of fragmentation or self-disintegration create a need for a structuring or a supportive environment. Both benzodiazepines (e.g., diazepam 0.1 to 0.3 mg per kg IV or midazolam 0.05 to 0.1 mg per kg IV) and haloperidol (0.05 mg per kg IM) are effective tranquilizers in the event that anxiety or agitation persists.

Marijuana (Pot, Reefer, Smoke, Grass, Hemp)

Pathophysiology. With the exception of ethanol, marijuana remains the most popular psychoactive drug of abuse. It is typically sold in "nickel" bags that produce two to three joints. Marijuana is occasionally laced with other psychoactive substances, including PCP and cocaine. Hashish is the concentrated resin of marijuana.

The flowering tops of the female marijuana plant contain the highest concentration of the active constituent, tetrahydrocannabinol (THC). In the 1970s, most marijuana contained approximately 1% to 2% THC by weight. More recently, cultivated seedless varieties of marijuana (sensimilla) have become popular, and they contain 5% to 8% THC by weight. Therefore, a joint is now likely to lead to a greater degree of altered mental status than previously.

Within minutes of smoking this material, perceptual, behavioral, and emotional states become altered for several hours. Patients often have the appearance of inebriation with dysarthria and ataxia. However, violence, hallucinations, and agitation are uncommon after marijuana use.

Pharmacodynamics. It is estimated that no more than 50% of the THC inhaled in a marijuana cigarette is actually absorbed. Pharmacologic effects begin immediately. In contrast, the onset of effects after oral ingestion occurs in 30 minutes to 1 hour, and peak effects may not occur until the second and third hours after ingestion; THC is three times more potent when smoked than when taken by mouth.

Clinical Symptoms. The most prominent effects in humans are on the CNS and cardiovascular system. In doses of up to 20 mg, THC produces effects on mood, memory, motor coordination, cognitive ability, sensorium, time sense, and self-perception.

MEDICAL EMERGENCIES

There is an increased sense of well-being or euphoria accompanied by feelings of relaxation or sleepiness when subjects are alone. With greater intake of THC, short-term memory is impaired, and the capacity to carry out tasks that require multiple mental steps to reach a specific goal deteriorates. This effect on memory-dependent, goal-directed behavior has been called *temporal disintegration* and is correlated with a tendency to confuse past, present, and future. Depersonalization, a sense of strangeness, and unreality about one's self also occur. Marijuana smokers often report a voracious appetite (the munchies), dry mouth and throat, more vivid visual imagery, and a keener sense of hearing. Altered time perception is a consistent effect of cannabinoids, so minutes seem like hours. Larger doses of THC can produce frank hallucinations, delusions, and paranoid feelings. Thinking becomes confused and disorganized. Anxiety that reaches panic proportions may replace euphoria, often as a feeling that the drug-induced state will never end. Because of the rapid onset of effects when marijuana is smoked, most users can regulate their intake to avoid the excessive doses that produce these unpleasant effects. Marijuana may cause an acute exacerbation of symptoms in stabilized schizophrenics. Cardiovascular effects include tachycardia, hypertension, and marked conjunctival injection. Chronic smoking of marijuana and hashish is associated with bronchitis and asthma, even though THC is a mild bronchodilator.

Infants and toddlers passively exposed to marijuana may develop profound lethargy or coma, occasionally with tachycardia.

Management. In general, the only treatment required is discontinuation of the drug. In the adolescent patient with a psychotic reaction or acute toxic delirium, a sedative such as diazepam, 5 to 10 mg by mouth or 0.1 mg per kg IV, may be necessary. These acute symptoms should improve with drug abstinence over 4 to 6 hours.

Stimulants

Amphetamines (Crank, Speed)

Pathophysiology. Amphetamines have powerful CNS stimulant actions, in addition to peripheral adrenergic actions. Unlike epinephrine, amphetamines are effective after oral administration. However, they are often taken by injection and nasal insufflation. Amphetamines have been used medically to treat narcolepsy, obesity, fatigue, and nasal congestion. Several decongestant nasal inhalers continue to add amphetamine agents that may be extracted and ingested by drug-seeking adolescents. The pharmacologic effects of amphetamines include increased blood pressure, occasionally with a reflex slowing of heart rate, contraction of bladder sphincter, and dramatic CNS stimulation. Like other indirect sympathomimetics, amphetamines act by releasing endogenous biogenic amines from the presynaptic neurons.

Methamphetamine is the most commonly abused of these drugs, reportedly because its greater lipid solubility is associated with more potent CNS effects.

Abuse patterns of amphetamines have changed in more recent years because these drugs have begun to approach cocaine as widely abused stimulants. In fact, the National Institute on Drug Abuse reports a 58% increase in ED visits due to one type of amphetamine, Ecstasy, between 1999 and 2001. This increase has paralleled government interdiction efforts that have reduced the illegal entry of cocaine. Many drug users prefer amphetamines over cocaine because the clinical duration of action is considerably longer than that of cocaine. Also, the smokable form of methamphetamine (ice) is associated with more striking and prolonged alterations in CNS function. Children may be exposed to a myriad of dangerous chemicals when living with adults who operate clandestine meth laboratories. Finally, amphetamines have become a popular substance of abuse in pregnant women, leading to increases in neonatal intoxication or abstinence syndromes.

Pharmacodynamics. The therapeutic dose of dextroamphetamine in adolescents is typically 5 mg three times daily. The toxic dose is variable but is rarely less than 15 mg. Severe reactions have been reported at 30 mg, yet doses up to 400 to 500 mg may cause only mild symptoms. Tolerance is striking, with chronic users taking 10 to 15 g daily without ill effects. The elimination half-life of the amphetamines is about 3 hours, with much of the drug being excreted in the urine unchanged.

Clinical Symptoms. The psychic effect of amphetamines depends on the dose, mental state, and personality of the drug user. In general, 10 to 30 mg cause wakefulness, alertness, a decreased sense of fatigue, and an elevation of mood. Other behavioral changes may include increased initiative, self-confidence, ability to concentrate, elation, euphoria, and increased motor and speech activity. Physical performance in athletes may be improved. Prolonged use of large doses is followed by depression and fatigue. Amphetamines have an appetite-suppressant effect through an action on the lateral hypothalamic feeding center. However, tolerance to this effect also develops; thereafter, the effect is insufficient to reduce weight for a sustained period.

The acute toxic effects of amphetamine are usually extensions of its therapeutic actions. The central effects induce euphoria, restlessness, dizziness, tremor, hyperactive reflexes, talkativeness, irritability, weakness, insomnia, and fever. In addition, confusion, assaultiveness, anxiety, delirium, paranoid hallucinations, panic states, and suicidal or homicidal tendencies can occur, especially in patients who have underlying mental illnesses. However, these psychotic effects may occur in anyone who chronically abuses amphetamines. Cardiotoxic effects include palpitations, anginal pain, and rarely, hypertensive crisis or circulatory collapse. GI effects include anorexia, nausea, vomiting, diarrhea, and abdominal cramps. Severe overdoses may cause convulsions, coma, and cerebrovascular accidents. Both psychological and physical dependence occurs with chronic use. Chronic amphetamine abuse causes symptoms similar to many of those seen after acute overdose. The most common serious effect is a psychotic reaction with vivid hallucinations and paranoid delusions, often mistaken for schizophrenia. Recovery may or may not occur after withdrawal of the drug. In patients with persistent psychotic symptoms, it has been theorized that the amphetamine has hastened the onset of incipient schizophrenia. Chronic amphetamine abuse is also associated with the development of cerebral vasculitis.

An amphetamine derivative, MDMA, or Ecstasy, is popular among drug-abusing college students and may find its way into the high school scene. It is a drug with mildly hallucinogenic effects. In larger doses, it causes perceptual distortions, hallucinations, and agitation.

Management. Treatment of intoxication after ingestion of these agents should include GI decontamination. For severe agitation, specific treatment consists of administration of a benzodiazepine (e.g., diazepam 0.1 to 0.2 mg per kg IV) or haloperidol (0.01 to 0.05 mg per kg IM). Severe hypertension unresponsive to benzodiazepines may be treated with such agents as phentolamine, hydralazine, or IV sodium nitroprusside. Because up to 45% of amphetamines are excreted in the urine unchanged, ample fluids are beneficial.

Cocaine

Pathophysiology. Cocaine occurs in the leaves of *Erythroxylon coca* and other species of *Erythroxylon* trees indigenous to Peru and Bolivia, where the leaves have been used for centuries by the natives to increase endurance and to promote a sense of well-being. Chemically, cocaine is benzoylmethylecgonine. Ecgonine is an amino alcohol base closely related to tropine, the amino alcohol in atropine. Cocaine may be used by injection, inhalation (in the form of cocaine alkaloid or "crack"), nasal insufflation, and rarely, ingestion. Although oral ingestion is uncommon, there are two circumstances under which cocaine may be ingested in toxic quantities: the "body packer" and the "body stuffer." In the body packer, large quantities of cocaine are enclosed in plastic and ingested in an attempt to smuggle the drug, usually across international boundaries. In the case of the body stuffer, the person in fear of being found with the substance suddenly ingests cocaine. Body stuffers are typically at greater risk of cocaine intoxication because they do not take sufficient care to guarantee that the cocaine does not leach from the bag.

Cocaine is reportedly used in up to 15% of women during pregnancy. This gestational use has led to epidemic increases in the number of "cocaine babies" who are often preterm, small for age, irritable, and show neurodevelopmental delay. Beyond the postnatal age, passive cocaine exposure in infants and toddlers has been associated with severe intoxication, including the development of convulsions.

Pharmacodynamics. The relief from fatigue that occurs with cocaine use results from central stimulation that masks the sensation of fatigue. Cocaine potentiates the excitatory and inhibitory responses of sympathetically innervated organs to norepinephrine and epinephrine by blocking the reuptake of catecholamines at adrenergic nerve endings. This explains why cocaine, unlike other local anesthetics, produces vasoconstriction and mydriasis. The most important pharmacologic action is its ability to block the initiation or conduction of the nerve impulse after local application. Cocaine is still occasionally used as a local anesthetic for ophthalmologic or otorhinolaryngologic procedures. It also can be used as a topical anesthetic for laceration repair in the form of TAC (tetracaine, adrenaline, cocaine), although this formulation has largely been replaced by the less toxic combination of lidocaine, epinephrine, and tetracaine.

Although fatalities have been associated with cocaine doses as low as 30 mg, 1 to 2 g is generally the lethal dose in adults. Ingested cocaine is less toxic than that taken by other routes because of its prolonged absorption by this route. The

elimination half-life of cocaine is approximately 1 hour. Cocaine metabolism is complex and consists of nonenzymatic degradation to form benzoylecgonine and metabolism by plasma cholinesterases to form ecgonine methyl ester. A small fraction of cocaine is also metabolized through the cytochrome P-450 enzymes to form norcocaine. Individuals with congenital deficiencies in plasma cholinesterase are believed to have exaggerated responses to cocaine; cocaine abusers have been known to ingest inhibitors of cholinesterases or P-450 3A4 enzymes (e.g., organophosphate insecticides, cimetidine) to enhance the effect of the cocaine. Cocaine metabolites are readily detected in urine for approximately 3 days after exposure.

Cocaine is absorbed from all sites of application, including GI mucosa. Body packing may lead to severe toxicity (seizures and cardiorespiratory collapse) if the container ruptures. If smuggling is suspected, a flat plate may show opaque densities within the bowel highlighted by a gas halo.

In addition to nasal application, cocaine can be used by injection or inhalation. The latter is called *freebase* (crack) and is a dangerous practice. In making crack, street cocaine (which is in the form of cocaine hydrochloride) is converted to cocaine alkaloid by removal of the salt moiety. This reaction is accomplished by mixing the cocaine with water and sodium bicarbonate. The crack is then separated from the water by filtration and drying. The paste hardens and is cut into chips that resemble soap. It is then smoked in a pipe or sprinkled onto a cigarette or joint. A small piece, called a *quarter rock*, produces a 20- to 30-minute high when smoked in a water pipe. Probably because of its enhanced lipid solubility, crack crosses the blood–brain barrier rapidly, causing an intense rush of pleasure. This habit is highly addictive. Presently, crack is primarily used by older teenagers and persons in their early 20s, in part because it is relatively inexpensive (approximately $5 to $10 per rock).

Clinical Symptoms. Cocaine's most dramatic clinical effect is CNS stimulation. In humans, this manifests in a feeling of well-being and euphoria, often accompanied by gregariousness, restlessness, excitement, and a sense of clarity. However, as the dose is increased, tremors, forced speech, agitation, and even tonic-clonic convulsions may result from excessive stimulation.

Initially, small doses (1 to 1.5 mg per kg) may slow the heart rate through central vagal stimulation. After moderate doses, pulse increases, the result of both central and peripheral adrenergic effects. Hypertension may appear abruptly and lead to cerebrovascular accidents. Fortunately, hypertension is generally short lived. Larger doses of cocaine may cause hypertension that may be followed quickly by cardiovascular collapse, often the result of myocardial ischemia and infarction. Myocardial injury that ranges from angina pectoris to massive infarction can be seen in young adults after acute cocaine exposure. With chronic cocaine use, a cardiomyopathy may develop that results in depressed cardiac function and death.

Rhythm disturbances are also characteristic of acute cocaine intoxication. These may consist of ventricular or supraventricular tachyarrhythmias and may be intractable. Arrhythmias are the most common cause of death after severe cocaine exposure.

Use of crack has been associated with a number of pulmonary disturbances, including bronchospasm, hemoptysis, pneumothorax, and pneumomediastinum. These lesions are believed to result from the barotrauma associated with inhalation of hot, particulate matter, followed by a Valsalva maneuver.

Cocaine has been associated with other syndromes of organ dysfunction, including hyperpyrexia and renal failure. *Coke fever* (or *pyrexia*) is a common occurrence after acute cocaine use. It is often associated with muscle rigidity (resembling neuroleptic malignant syndrome) or rhabdomyolysis (the result of agitation and/or physical restraint). Rhabdomyolysis may result in subsequent myoglobinuric renal failure if not promptly recognized and treated. Recent reports of cocaine adulterated with levamisole, a veterinary antihelminth that potentiates cocaine's euphoric effects, describe patients presenting with fever and reversible agranulocytosis.

Infants exposed to cocaine may also exhibit CNS excitation that includes hyperactivity, dystonic posturing, altered mental status, or frank seizures.

Management. Among substances of abuse, cocaine is the most likely to create the unstable patient with life-threatening manifestations. Therefore, this intoxication requires rapid, thorough assessment and management. Immediate attention should be paid to the vital signs, including temperature (which should be obtained rectally). The patient who develops seizures requires immediate airway control as well as anticonvulsant therapy. Benzodiazepines (e.g., diazepam 0.1 to 0.3 mg per kg) are considered the anticonvulsants of choice because of their rapid onset of action and because animal data have associated their use with decreased mortality from cocaine intoxication. Benzodiazepines should also be administered liberally to the patient with mild to moderate toxicity (agitation, hypertension, tachycardia) because of their efficacy in reversing many of these clinical manifestations.

Because circulatory function can range from hypertensive crisis to cardiovascular collapse, early vascular access is important. Blood pressure instability should be anticipated and treated accordingly. For treatment of hypertensive crises, liberal benzodiazepine use may be combined with a short-acting antihypertensive (e.g., nitroprusside). Immediate treatment of hypertension is recommended because it may lead to cerebrovascular or myocardial injury, although the use of IV β-blockers alone is contraindicated. Cardiac arrhythmias are treated according to advanced cardiac life support protocols (see Chapters 1 and 82).

Hyperthermia must be recognized and treated promptly to prevent its complications. Management is discussed in Chapter 89. IV fluids should be used aggressively if urinalysis is suggestive of myoglobinuria.

Patients with CNS depression or a lateralizing neurologic examination should receive cranial tomography to rule out an intracranial vascular event.

Because cocaine is rarely ingested, the need for GI decontamination is confined to body packers/stuffers or when drug coingestion is suspected. With body stuffers, because bag leakage can lead to abrupt onset of severe intoxication and possibly death, activated charcoal should be administered immediately. Gastric emptying maneuvers and endoscopic removal of cocaine bags are relatively contraindicated because of the risk of bag rupture. Instead, decontamination is confined to administration of activated charcoal and WBI. Multiple-dose activated charcoal may be recommended to maximize the opportunity for cocaine to be adsorbed by the charcoal. Because

cocaine bags and crack vials are radiopaque in up to 50% of cases, an abdominal radiograph is recommended to determine the location and extent of retained packets after decontamination has been initiated. A contrast study or computed tomography scan may be considered to improve detection.

In the event of severe intoxication or ingestion of more than 1 to 2 g of cocaine, transfer to the intensive care unit is essential for appropriate monitoring.

Central Anticholinergics

Pathophysiology

Increasingly, drugs, plants, and mushrooms with anticholinergic properties are ingested for their psychoactive effects. Because antidepressants, antihistamines, antispasmodics, and belladonna alkaloids are in widespread use, these compounds are more readily available than illicit psychoactive substances. Also, many OTC drugs having anticholinergic activity are available without prescription and are ingested to get "high." These agents are competitive antagonists with acetylcholine at the neuroreceptor site (Table 102.19). The major effects of these drugs are on the myocardium, CNS, smooth muscle, and exocrine glands. These effects include tachycardia, mydriasis, facial flushing, hyperpyrexia, cardiac arrhythmias, urinary retention, dry mucous membranes, decreased sweating, and decreased or absent bowel sounds. CNS effects include delirium, anxiety, hyperactivity, visual hallucinations, illusions, and disorientation. These signs and symptoms lead to the common mnemonic, "Mad as a hatter, red as a beet, dry as a bone, blind as a bat, and hot as a hare." In excess, anticholinergics may lead to severe toxicity that includes cardiac arrhythmias, seizures, and death.

Pharmacodynamics

The effects of anticholinergics vary according to the specific drug ingested, particularly because the many classes of drugs

---

TABLE 102.19

DRUGS AND CHEMICALS THAT MAY PRODUCE THE CENTRAL ANTICHOLINERGIC SYNDROME

Antidepressants: amitriptyline (Elavil), imipramine (Tofranil), doxepin (Sinequan, Adopin)
Antihistamines: chlorpheniramine (Ornade, Teldrin), diphenhydramine (Benadryl), orphenadrine (Norflex)
Ophthalmologic Preparations: cyclopentolate (Cyclogel), tropicamide (Mydriacyl)
Antispasmodic Agents: propantheline (Probanthine), clidinium bromide (Librax)
Antiparkinson Agents: trihexyphenidyl (Artane), benztropine (Cogentin), procyclidine (Kemadrin)
Proprietary Drugs: Sleep-Eze (scopolamine, methapyrilene), Sominex (scopolamine, methapyrilene), Asthma-Dor (belladonna alkaloids), Excedrin-PM (methapyrilene)
Belladonna Alkaloids: atropine, homatropine, hyoscine, hyoscyamus, scopolamine
Toxic Plants: mushroom (*Amanita muscaria*), bitter-sweet (*Solanum dulcamara*), Jimsonweed (*Datura stramonium*), potato leaves and sprouts (*Solanum tuberosum*), deadly nightshade (*Atropa belladonna*)

lead to secondary actions that are independent of anticholinergic actions. An important universal anticholinergic effect, however, is decreased GI motility. This is associated with delayed absorption of drug and, if GI decontamination is not performed, the appearance of severe toxicity may be delayed 12 to 24 hours after ingestion.

Management

The management of a patient with a known central anticholinergic syndrome is a challenge, particularly because one must also be prepared for the other distinct toxicities of the ingested drug or plant. Also, most plants and many drugs are not detected on toxicology screens, so the diagnosis must rely on history and clinical suspicion. Along similar lines, serum drug levels do not predict the degree of anticholinergic symptoms.

GI decontamination may be valuable beyond an hour after anticholinergic poison ingestion because of the likelihood of drug persistence in the gut lumen for an extended time. Once again, activated charcoal remains the drug of choice.

On the basis of presenting signs and symptoms, the patient may require sedation and monitoring in an intensive care unit setting to provide ventilatory support for coma, anticonvulsants for seizures, and antiarrhythmic drugs for cardiac arrhythmias. Adequate sedation may be achieved with titrated doses of benzodiazepines. Physostigmine, a potent anticholinesterase, is a recognized antidote for anticholinergic-induced mental status alterations; however, its use is controversial. Physostigmine can produce bronchospasm, bradycardia, hypotension, and seizures. It is therefore reserved for those who have normal EKGs and mental status dysfunction confined to hallucinations or severe agitation. The adult dose is 1 to 2 mg via slow IV infusion over 5 minutes. The trial dose can be repeated in 10 to 15 minutes up to a maximum of 4 mg. The pediatric dose is 0.5 mg IV administered slowly, with repeat every 10 minutes up to a maximum of 2 mg. The smallest effective dose may be repeated every 30 to 60 minutes if symptoms recur over 6 to 8 hours. The muscarinic toxicity of physostigmine may be treated with IV atropine at one-half the physostigmine dose given; physostigmine-related seizures may be treated with benzodiazepines.

Central Nervous System Sedative-Hypnotics

Pathophysiology

The sedative-hypnotics reversibly depress the activity of all excitable tissues. For most of these agents, CNS effects occur with little action on skeletal, cardiac, or smooth muscle. Uncommonly, serious depression in cardiovascular and other functions may occur. The prevalence of abuse of these agents was formerly exceeded by opioid abuse. However, with the increasing popularity of cocaine, these agents have become the preferred choice in treating cocaine-induced tension and anxiety. Many of these agents, including glutethimide, meprobamate, methaqualone, and barbiturates, are uncommonly available and have been replaced by the benzodiazepines. Because they have retained some popularity and still make periodic appearances on the streets, however, they should be included in discussions of such drugs.

Pharmacodynamics

The sedative-hypnotics have tranquilizing, euphoriant effects that may be similar to morphine. With all these agents—prescribed for this tranquilizing action—it is difficult to draw the line between appropriate use, abuse, habituation, and addiction. However, for all, tolerance is common and physical dependence quickly develops. Therefore, their abuse potential is considered high.

The pharmacologic characteristics of each drug are largely determined by their specific chemical nature. For example, all barbiturates are bound by plasma proteins. These characteristics have important implications in affecting their renal elimination and the effectiveness of extracorporeal drug removal techniques (hemodialysis, hemoperfusion).

For all sedative-hypnotics, patterns of abuse vary, ranging from infrequent sprees of intoxication to compulsive daily use. Introduction to these drugs may be through street use or drug trade (which is most common in adolescents), but, commonly, exposure is initiated through a physician's prescription to a parent for insomnia or anxiety. Because tolerance develops to most of the actions of these drugs, no signs of chronic use may be apparent.

Clinical Symptoms

After sedative-hypnotic use, the adolescent may exhibit sluggishness, difficulty in thinking, dysarthria, poor memory, faulty judgment, emotional lability, and short attention span. Irritability and lability are common. With chronic use, these drugs also lead to dependence, so a picture of abstinence may appear after their disuse, with clinical manifestations of apathy, weakness, tremulousness, agitation, or frank convulsions. In its mildest form, the abstinence syndrome may consist only of rebound increases of rapid eye movement sleep, insomnia, or anxiety.

Management

With patients of acute sedative-hypnotic ingestion, attention should be directed to ensuring a patent airway and an intact gag reflex. Cardiovascular disturbances are rare after sedative use, but because of the possibility of drug coingestion, thorough hemodynamic assessment is necessary. Most sedative-hypnotics are detectable on comprehensive toxin screens, so specimens of serum and urine may be sent for analysis; however, these "send out" screens rarely come back in real time, thus minimizing their importance at the bedside. GI decontamination should be considered and can typically be confined to administration of activated charcoal. Repeated doses of charcoal have been shown to enhance clearance of certain barbiturates and benzodiazepines. Urinary alkalinization aids in the excretion of phenobarbital. In extreme cases, charcoal hemoperfusion should be considered.

Optional treatment of sedative overdose includes continuous monitoring in an intensive care unit with intubation and ventilator support as indicated. Flumazenil, a benzodiazepine antagonist, can be administered in cases of suspected benzodiazepine ingestion. Its pediatric dose is 0.01 to 0.02 mg per kg IV (max 0.2 mg per dose) and may be repeated to a max of 0.05 mg per kg or 1 mg, whichever is less. Indications for flumazenil administration may be (i) to reverse a witnessed, unintentional benzodiazepine overdose in a young child or (ii) to prevent airway intubation after an iatrogenic overdose. Flumazenil must not be given empirically in unknown or intentional overdoses for which induction of seizures may be life-threatening.

Opioids (Morphine, Codeine, Heroin, Methadone, Propoxyphene, Oxycodone, and Hydrocodone)

Epidemiology. In the United States, three distinct groups who abuse opioids have been described: (i) those who are prescribed an opioid as medical treatment and then go on to become dependent and develop drug-seeking behaviors (this group constitutes a minority of opioid abusers), (ii) those who begin with recreational drug use and quickly progress to regular use, and (iii) women who abuse opioids when pregnant. Such women and their offspring are at risk for a number of adverse pregnancy outcomes. For the patient who abuses opiates through injection, other consequences include the risk of hepatitis, endocarditis, acquired immunodeficiency syndrome (AIDS), and vasculitis.

In the past decade, recreational abuse of insufflated heroin and ingested prescription opioid analgesics (particularly oxycodone and hydrocodone) has risen to epidemic proportions in the United States and may be partly responsible for the first increase in overall drug-related mortality in a generation. In addition, some opioid-related deaths are likely inadvertent and represent inappropriate misuse of combinations of alcohol, sedative-hypnotic agents, and prescription analgesics. The significant rate of opioid abuse has also given rise to the common treatment of opioid addiction by the outpatient prescription of opioid antagonists such as buprenorphine, which has resulted in the relatively common occurrence of an opioid syndrome in toddlers due to exploratory ingestion of this agent.

Toxicology. The opioids produce their major effects by combining with receptors in the brain and other tissues. Effects include analgesia, drowsiness, change in mood, respiratory depression, decreased GI motility, nausea, and vomiting. The opiate receptors appear to be the normal sites of action of several endogenous opioid-like substances (e.g., the endorphins).

Generally, the toxic opioid dose for a person who is not addicted depends on the particular drug. For example, with morphine, clinical toxicity (excessive sedation) may appear with doses that exceed 5 mg in the adolescent. Tolerance rapidly develops to many CNS effects. However, death may occur as a result of marked respiratory depression and consequent anoxia. In particular, those individuals who are ultrarapid metabolizers of codeine through CYP2D6 may have increased morbidity and mortality. Other toxicities of opiates include (neurogenic) pulmonary edema, mast cell degranulation (which leads to histamine release and an "anaphylactoid" reaction), cardiac disturbances (with propoxyphene intoxication), and neurotoxicity with seizures (with meperidine intoxication).

Clinical Symptoms. Opioids invariably cause miosis, even after development of tolerance. Respiration may be depressed because of decreased responsiveness of brain stem respiratory centers to increases in carbon dioxide tension. Therapeutic doses of morphine have no effect on blood pressure or cardiac rate or rhythm. When blood pressure changes occur, they result from histamine release. Because histamine dilates capacitance blood vessels and decreases the ability of the cardiovascular system to respond to gravitational shifts, sitting or standing may produce orthostatic hypotension.

Many opioids have extensive effects on the GI tract. They decrease the secretion of hydrochloric acid, GI motility, and pancreatic secretions while increasing colonic tone to the point of spasm. In addition, the tone of the anal sphincter is augmented. Therapeutic doses of morphine and codeine can also increase biliary tract pressure, producing epigastric distress and biliary colic.

Management. The presence of coma, pinpoint pupils, and depressed respiration should suggest opioid poisoning in the absence of history. The finding of needle marks on the body further suggests this diagnosis. To confirm the diagnosis, toxicologic analysis of urine and/or serum should be conducted (of note, however, several important synthetic or semisynthetic opioids such as methadone, fentanyl, and oxycodone may not be detected on routine urine drug screens).

The first management step with opioid intoxication is to ensure adequate ventilation of the patient. Endotracheal intubation may be necessary if there is severe respiratory depression or pulmonary edema. If appropriate, GI decontamination should be performed. The narcotic antagonist naloxone (1 to 2 mg) should be given by IV. If there is no response despite the suspicion of opiate intoxication, the naloxone dose should be repeated (up to 8 to 10 mg), depending on effect and level of suspicion. Naloxone can precipitate an abstinence syndrome in those who have developed physical dependence; in such patients, smaller initial doses of 0.2 to 0.4 mg, with upward titration as needed, are preferable.

When patients who are addicted to opiates are hospitalized, small doses of an opiate may be necessary to prevent severe withdrawal. Methadone substitution is the preferred agent, because in small doses, it is less euphorigenic and its long elimination half-life permits once- or twice-daily dosing. With the patient under observation, 10 to 20 mg of methadone are given, ideally before the appearance of withdrawal symptoms (insomnia, irritability, agitation, piloerection). Other agents, such as buprenorphine and clonidine, are also being explored.

γ-Hydroxybutyrate, γ-Hydroxybutyrolactone, and 1,4-Butanediol

The related agents, γ-hydroxybutyrate (GHB), γ-hydroxybutyrolactone (GBL), and 1,4-butanediol (1,4 BD), have become popular substances of abuse among teenagers and young adults. GHB is an endogenous compound with neurotransmitter and/or neuromodulator function and interacts with dopamine, serotonin, GABA, and endogenous opioid-based neural systems. GHB and its congeners, when used for human consumption, can be considered a schedule I drug by the FDA. In the 1990s, it had been widely available through the purchase of kits (e.g., by mail order, via the Internet) that allow its home synthesis; access to these may be more limited currently. GBL is actually a precursor to GHB and is the primary ingredient of such kits and has also been sold in health food stores. However, GBL is rapidly metabolized in vivo to GHB, and the clinical effects of ingesting either agent are nearly indistinguishable. 1,4 BD is also metabolized to GHB via alcohol dehydrogenase. These agents are used for a variety of reasons, but primarily as euphoriants and aphrodisiacs at parties or all-night dance clubs (raves). GHB has gained a particular notoriety as a date-rape agent. This class also has a reputation in the body-builder community as growth hormone stimulants and thus enhancers of muscle development and fat loss.

GHB, GBL, and 1,4 BD are CNS depressants that cause rapid onset of deep sleep that can progress to coma and respiratory depression. Patients who have overdosed may have transient seizure activity and are often hypothermic and bradycardic. The coma is usually relatively short in duration, on the order of 1 to 2 hours. During emergence, transient delirium and vomiting are often observed. Depressed respiratory effort and airway-protective reflexes are common in the more severe cases, although aspiration pneumonia as a complication has been rare. Many patients are surprisingly responsive to stimulus, and attempts at laryngoscopy to effect endotracheal intubation in a seemingly deeply comatose patient may result in an angry, combative patient who sits up and swears at the endoscopist.

Most patients with acute overdose can be managed with the provision of ambient oxygen, suctioning, and attention to the airway. A nasal trumpet is helpful in some cases, and endotracheal intubation may be required occasionally, although it may necessitate rapid sequence induction for the reasons previously noted. Atropine has been used for severe bradycardia with success. Blood pressure support is rarely necessary.

Inhalants

The High School Senior Survey, conducted by the National Institute on Drug Abuse, has suggested that the abuse of inhalants is relatively common in adolescents, with a lifetime prevalence rate of up to 20%. Additional data suggest that these psychoactive agents are even more common in school-aged children and preadolescents. The prevalence of inhalant abuse among young children has been related to the ready availability of these products. Patterns of abuse are also strikingly region-specific, with the highest rates of abuse in the southwestern and southeastern United States.

The psychoactive inhalants can be placed into three broad categories: (i) hydrocarbons, (ii) nitrous oxide, and (iii) nitrites. The hydrocarbons can be subdivided further into the aliphatic hydrocarbons, the halogenated hydrocarbons, and solvents. Regardless of the class, all inhalants possess the pharmacologic property of narcosis, leading to euphoria and light-headedness after inhalation. Typically, the agents are abused by "huffing" or "bagging." In huffing, the agent is placed into a rag or handkerchief, held under the nose, and then deeply inhaled. With bagging, a common method of abuse at parties, the compound is placed into a large bag (e.g., garbage bag) with the drug user placing his or her head into the bag.

Several distinct profiles of toxicity have been described after inhalant abuse. The inebriation that these agents produce may be associated with mental status changes that include coma with respiratory arrest or aspiration. The halogenated hydrocarbons all possess potent cardiotoxicity, leading to myocardial irritability and cardiac arrhythmias. This action has been associated with many reports of spontaneous ventricular fibrillation in adolescents during a binge. Finally, the act of bagging is associated with the risk of simple asphyxia. A syndrome known as *sudden sniffing death* has been described in adolescents who abuse inhalants. This syndrome may be the result of any of these previously described toxicities. Finally, acute exposure to those inhalants that contain nitrites may lead to methemoglobinemia, often severe.

Other toxicities are associated with chronic inhalant abuse. The solvents, particularly toluene, may lead to a syndrome that includes abdominal pain, muscle wasting, electrolyte disturbances (hypokalemia), and renal tubular acidosis. Patients of chronic solvent abuse may also develop a leukoencephalomalacia with cerebral atrophy.

Management

Because inhalant abuse may lead to the development of life-threatening symptoms, close attention should be directed to the vital signs and their stability. Patients with depressed levels of consciousness may require airway support and ventilation. Because of the risk of cardiac arrhythmias when halogenated hydrocarbons are abused, vascular access should be established early. Arrhythmias should be treated according to the standard protocol (see Chapters 1 and 82); however, the use of epinephrine is relatively contraindicated because it has been associated with worsening of rhythm disturbances. As a part of the evaluation, a complete metabolic panel that includes electrolyte levels, with calcium, phosphate, and magnesium; amylase level; liver function tests; creatine phosphokinase level; and urinalysis should be obtained.

Treatment of methemoglobinemia is discussed in Chapter 91.

Suggested Readings

Reference Toxicology Textbooks

Erickson T, Ahrens W, Aks S, et al., eds. *Pediatric toxicology: diagnosis and management of the poisoned child.* New York, NY: McGraw-Hill, 2005.

Flomenbaum NE, Goldfrank LR, Hoffman RS, et al., eds. *Goldfrank's toxicological emergencies,* 8th ed. New York, NY: McGraw-Hill, 2006.

Osterhoudt KC, Perrone J, DeRoos F, et al. *Toxicology pearls.* Philadelphia, PA: Hanley & Belfus, 2004.

Shannon MW, Borron SW, Burns MJ, eds. *Haddad and Winchester's clinical management of poisoning and drug overdose,* 4th ed. Philadelphia, PA: Saunders Elsevier, 2007.

General Approach and Management

Abbruzzi G, Stork CM. Pediatric toxicologic concerns. *Emerg Med Clin North Am* 2002;20(1):223–247.

Albertson TE, Dawson A, de Latorre F, et al. TOX-ACLS: toxicologic-oriented advanced cardiac life support. *Ann Emerg Med* 2001;37(4)(suppl):S78–S90.

American Academy of Pediatrics, Committee on Injury, Violence, and Poison Prevention. Policy statement: poison treatment in the home. *Pediatrics* 2003;112:1182–1185.

Bond GR. The role of activated charcoal and gastric emptying in gastrointestinal decontamination: a state-of-the-art review. *Ann Emerg Med* 2002;39(3):273–286.

Bronstein AC, Spyker DA, Cantilena LR, et al. 2007 Annual report of the American Association of Poison Control Centers' National Poison Data System (NPDS): 25th Annual Report. *Clin Toxicol (Phila)* 2008;46:927–1057.

Bryant S, Singer J. Management of toxic exposure in children. *Emerg Med Clin North Am* 2003;21(1):101–119.

Burns MM. Activated charcoal as the sole intervention for treatment after childhood poisoning. *Curr Opin Pediatr* 2000;12(2):166–171.

Dart RC, Borron SW, Caravati EM, et al. Expert consensus guidelines for stocking of antidotes in hospitals that provide emergency care. *Ann Emerg Med* 2009;54:386–394.

Eldridge DL. Van Eyk J, Kornegay C. Pediatric toxicology. *Emerg Med Clin North Am* 2007;25:283–308.

Erickson TB, Thompson TM, Lu JJ. The approach to the patient with an unknown overdose. *Emerg Toxicol Clin North Am* 2007;25:249–281.

Franklin RL, Rodgers GB. Unintentional child poisonings treated in United States hospital emergency departments: national estimates of incident cases, population-based poisoning rates, and product involvement. *Pediatrics* 2008;122:1244–1251.

Hoffman RJ, Nelson L. Rational use of toxicology testing in children. *Curr Opin Pediatr* 2001;13(2):183–188.

Litovitz TL, Manoguerra A. Comparison of pediatric poisoning hazards: an analysis of 3.8 million exposure incidents (a report from the American Association of Poison Control Centers). *Pediatrics* 1992;89:999–1006.

Osterhoudt KC, Durbin D, Alpern ER, et al. Risk factors for emesis after therapeutic use of activated charcoal in acutely poisoned children. *Pediatrics* 2004;113:806–810.

Shannon MW. Ingestion of toxic substances by children. *N Engl J Med* 2000; 342(3):186–191.

Acetaminophen

Betten DP, Cantrell FL, Thomas SC, et al. A prospective evaluation of shortened course oral N-acetylcysteine for the treatment of acute acetaminophen poisoning. *Ann Emerg Med* 2007;50:272–279.

Harrison PM, Keays R, Alexander GJ, et al. Improved outcome of paracetamol-induced fulminant hepatic failure by late administration of acetylcysteine. *Lancet* 1990;335:1572–1573.

Heard KJ. Acetylcysteine for acetaminophen poisoning. *N Engl J Med* 2008; 3593:285–292.

Henretig FM, Selbst SM, Forrest C, et al. Repeated acetaminophen overdosing causing hepatotoxicity in children. *Clin Pediatr (Phila)* 1989;28:525–528.

Rumack BH, Peterson RG. Acetaminophen overdose, incidence, diagnosis and management in 416 patients. *Pediatrics* 1978;62(suppl):898–903.

Alcohols and Glycols

Barceloux DG, Bond GR, Krenzelok EP, et al. American Academy of Clinical Toxicology practice guidelines on the treatment of methanol poisoning. *J Toxicol Clin Toxicol* 2002;40(4):415–446.

Bestic M, Blackford M, Reed M. Fomepizole: a critical assessment of current dosing recommendations. *J Clin Pharmacol* 2009;49:130–137.

Brent J. Fomepizole for ethylene glycol and methanol poisoning. *N Engl J Med* 2009;360:2216–2223.

Brown MJ, Shannon MW, Woolf A, et al. Childhood methanol ingestion treated with fomepizole and hemodialysis. *Pediatrics* 2001;108(4):E77.

George M, Al-Duaij N, Becker ML, et al. Re: ethylene glycol ingestion treated only with fomepizole. *J Med Toxicol* 2008;4:67.

George M, Al-Duaij N, Nikkanen H, et al. Mouthwash—time for policy change. *Pediatr Emerg Care* 2009;25:58–59.

Lepik KJ, Levy AR, Sobolev BG, et al. Adverse drug events associated with the antidotes for methanol and ethylene glycol poisoning: a comparison of ethanol and fomepizole. *Ann Emerg Med* 2009;53:439–450.

Lynd LD, Richardson KJ, Purssell RA, et al. An evaluation of the osmole gap as a screening test for toxic alcohol poisoning. *BMC Emerg Med* 2008;8:5.

Roy M, Bailey B, Chalut D, et al. What are the adverse effects of ethanol used as an antidote in the treatment of suspected methanol poisoning in children? *J Toxicol Clin Toxicol* 2003;41(2):155–161.

Youssef GM, Hirsch DJ. Validation of a method to predict required dialysis time for cases of methanol and ethylene glycol poisoning. *Am J Kidney Dis* 2005;46:509–511.

Antihistamines

Baker AM, Johnson DG, Levisky JA, et al. Fatal diphenhydramine intoxication in infants. *J Forensic Sci* 2003;48(2):425–428.

Frascogna N. Physostigmine: is there a role for this antidote in pediatric poisonings? *Curr Opin Pediatr* 2007;19:201–205.

Nine JS, Rund CR. Fatality from diphenhydramine monointoxication: a case report and review of the infant, pediatric, and adult literature. *Am J Forensic Med Pathol* 2006;27:36–41.

Ten Eick AP, Blumer JL, Reed MD. Safety of antihistamines in children. *Drug Saf* 2001;24(2):119–147.

Aspirin Poisoning

Greenberg MI, Hendrickson RG, Hofman M. Deleterious effects of endotracheal intubation in salicylate poisoning. *Ann Emerg Med* 2003;41:583–584.

O'Malley GF. Emergency department management of the salicylate poisoned patient. *Emerg Med Clin North Am* 2007;25:333–346.

Stolbach AI, Hoffman RS, Nelson LS. Mechanical ventilation was associated with acidemia in a case series of salicylate-poisoned patients. *Acad Emerg Med* 2008;15:866–869.

β-Adrenergic Blockers

Belson MG, Sullivan K, Geller RJ. Beta-adrenergic antagonist exposures in children. *Vet Hum Toxicol* 2001;43(6):361–365.

Kerns W. Management of beta-adrenergic blocker and calcium channel antagonist toxicity. *Emerg Med Clin North Am* 2007;25:309–331.

Calcium Channel Blockers

Belson MG, Gorman SE, Sullivan K, et al. Calcium channel blocker ingestions in children. *Am J Emerg Med* 2000;18(5):581–586.

Durward A, Guerguerian AM, Lefebvre M, et al. Massive diltiazem overdose treated with extracorporeal membrane oxygenation. *Pediatr Crit Care Med* 2003;4(3):372–376.

Kerns W. Management of beta-adrenergic blocker and calcium channel antagonist toxicity. *Emerg Med Clin North Am* 2007;25:309–331.

Megarbane B, Karyo S, Baud FJ. Hyperinsulinaemia/euglycaemia therapy in acute calcium channel antagonist and beta-blocker poisoning. *Toxicol Rev* 2004;23:215–222.

Ranniger C, Roche C. Are one or two dangerous? Calcium channel blocker exposure in toddlers. *J Emerg Med* 2007;33:145–154.

Salhanick SD, Shannon MW. Management of calcium channel antagonist overdose. *Drug Saf* 2003;26(2):65–79.

Clonidine

Eddy O, Howell JM. Are one or two dangerous? Clonidine and topical imidazolines exposure in toddlers. *J Emerg Med* 2003;25:297–302.

Osterhoudt KC. Clonidine poisoning. In: Rose BD, ed. *UpToDate*. Waltham, MA: UpToDate, 2008.

Seger DL. Clonidine toxicity revisited. *J Toxicol Clin Toxicol* 2002;40(2):145–155.

Digoxin

Thacker D, Sharma J. Digoxin toxicity. *Clin Pediatr* 2007;46:276–279.

Woolf AD, Wenger T, Smith TW, et al. The use of digoxin-specific Fab fragments for severe digitalis intoxication in children. *N Engl J Med* 1992;326:1739–1744.

Disc Batteries

Bartlett D. Button battery ingestions in children. *J Emerg Nurs* 2006;32:189–190.

Litovitz T, Schmitz BF. Ingestion of cylindrical and button batteries: an analysis of 2382 cases. *Pediatrics* 1992;89:747–757.

Foodborne Intoxications

Friedman MA, Fleming LE, Fernandez M, et al. Ciguatera fish poisoning: treatment, prevention, and management. *Mar Drugs* 2008;6:456–479.

Guly HR, Grant IC. Case of the month: lesson of the week: don't forget scombroid. *Emerg Med J* 2006;23:955–956.

Horowitz BZ. Botulinum toxin. *Crit Care Clin* 2005;21:825–839.

Lawrence DT, Dobmeier SG, Bechtel LK, et al. Food poisoning. *Emerg Med Clin North Am* 2007;25:357–373.

Household Cleaning Products and Caustics

Salzman M, O'Malley RN. Updates on the evaluation and management of caustic exposures. *Emerg Med Clin North Am* 2007;25:459–476.

Hydrocarbons

Chyka PA. Benefits of extracorporeal membrane oxygenation for hydrocarbon pneumonitis. *J Toxicol Clin Toxicol* 1996;34:357–363.

Iron

Anderson BD, Turchen SG, Manoguerra AS, et al. Retrospective analysis of ingestions of iron containing products in the United States: are there differences between chewable vitamins and adult preparations? *J Emerg Med* 2000;19(3):255–258.

Fine JS. Iron poisoning. *Curr Probl Pediatr* 2000;30(3):71–90.

Henretig FM, Drott HR, Osterhoudt KC. Acute iron poisoning. In: Shaw LM, ed. *The clinical toxicology laboratory: contemporary practice of poisoning evaluation.* Washington, DC: AACC Press, 2001:401–409.

Tenenbein M. Unit-dose packaging of iron supplements and reduction of iron poisoning in young children. *Arch Pediatr Adolesc Med* 2005;159: 593–595.

Isoniazid

Geib AJ, Shannon MW. Isoniazid. In: Shannon MW, Borron SW, Burns MJ, eds. *Haddad and Winchester's Clinical management of poisoning and drug overdose,* 4th ed. Philadelphia, PA: Saunders Elsevier, 2007:919–926.

Morrow LE, Wear RE, Schuller D, et al. Acute isoniazid toxicity and the need for adequate pyridoxine supplies. *Pharmacotherapy* 2006;26:1529–1532.

Orlowski FP, Paganini EP, Pippenger CE. Treatment of a potentially lethal dose isoniazid ingestion. *Ann Emerg Med* 1988;17:73–76.

Lead

American Academy of Pediatrics. Lead exposure in children: prevention, detection, and management. *Pediatrics* 2005;116:1036–1046.

Canfield RL, Henderson CR, Cory-Slechta DA, et al. Intellectual impairment in children with blood lead concentrations below 10 mcg per deciliter. *N Engl J Med* 2003;348(16):1517–1526.

Henretig FM. Lead. In: Goldfrank LR, Flomenbaum NE, Lewin NA, et al., eds. *Goldfrank's toxicologic emergencies*, 9th ed. New York, NY: McGraw-Hill, 2009.

Rogan WJ, Dietrich KN, Ware JH, et al. The effect of chelation therapy with succimer on neuropsychological development in children exposed to lead. *N Engl J Med* 2001;344(19):1421–1426.

Shannon MW. Lead. In: Shannon MW, Borron SW, Burns MJ, eds. *Haddad and Winchester's Clinical management of poisoning and drug overdose*, 4th ed. Philadelphia, PA: Saunders Elsevier, 2007:1129–1146.

Wolf AD, Goldman R, Bellinger DC. Update on the clinical management of childhood lead poisoning. *Pediatr Clin North Am* 2007;54:271–294.

Oral Hypoglycemics

Calello DP, Kelly A, Osterhoudt KC. Case files of the medical toxicology fellowship training program at The Children's Hospital of Philadelphia: a pediatric exploratory sulfonylurea ingestion. *J Med Toxicol* 2006;2:19–24.

Rowden AK, Fasano CJ. Emergency management of oral hypoglycemic drug toxicity. *Emerg Med Clin North Am* 2007;25:347–356.

Phenothiazines and Other Neuroleptics

Heng Tan H, Hoppe J, Heard K. A systematic review of cardiovascular effects after atypical antipsychotic medication overdose. *Am J Emerg Med* 2009;27:607–616.

James LP, Abel K, Wilkinson J, et al. Phenothiazine, butyrophenone, and other psychotropic medication poisonings in children and adolescents. *J Toxicol Clin Toxicol* 2000;38(6):615–623.

Reilly TH, Kirk MA. Atypical antipsychotics and newer antidepressants. *Emerg Med Clin North Am* 2007;25:477–497.

Organophosphates

Bond RG, Pieche S, Sonicki Z, et al. A clinical decision aid for triage of children younger than 5 years and with organophosphate or carbamate insecticide exposure in developing countries. *Ann Emerg Med* 2008;52:617–622.

Lai MW, Moen MM, Ewald MB. Pesticide-like poisoning from a prescription drug. *N Engl J Med* 2005;353:317–318.

Reigart JR, Roberts JR. Pesticides in children. *Pediatr Clin North Am* 2001;48(5):1185–1198, ix.

Rotenberg JS, Newmark J. Nerve agent attacks on children: diagnosis and management. *Pediatrics* 2003;112(3, pt 1):648–658.

Vates C, Osterhoudt KC. Give me three steps. *Pediatr Emerg Care* 2008;24:389–391.

Plants/Mushrooms

Beno S, Osterhoudt KC, Meaney P. An exceedingly agitated patient. *Pediatr Emerg Care* 2004;20:845–848.

Enjalbert F, Rapior S, Nouguier-Soule J, et al. Treatment of amatoxin poisoning: 20-year retrospective analysis. *J Toxicol Clin Toxicol* 2002;40(6):715–757.

Froberg B, Ibrahim D, Furbee RB. Plant poisoning. *Emerg Med Clin North Am* 2007;25:375–433.

Richardson WH, Slone CM, Michels JE. Herbal drugs of abuse: an emerging problem. *Emerg Med Clin North Am* 2007;25:435–457.

Savluc P, Danel V. New syndromes in mushroom poisoning. *Toxicol Rev* 2006;25:199–209.

Tricyclic Antidepressants/Other Antidepressants

Belson MG, Kelley TR. Bupropion exposures: clinical manifestations and medical outcome. *J Emerg Med* 2002;23(3):223–230.

Liebelt EL. An update on antidepressant toxicity: an evolution of unique toxicities to master. *Clin Pediatr Emerg Med* 2008;9:24–34.

Osterhoudt KC, Mistry R. A boy with tremor, diaphoresis, and altered behavior. *Pediatr Emerg Care* 2007;23:419–421.

Sirianni AJ, Osterhoudt KC, Calello DP, et al. Use of lipid emulsion in the resuscitation of a patient with prolonged cardiovascular collapse after overdose of bupropion and lamotrigine. *Ann Emerg Med* 2008;51:412–415.

Zorc JJ, Ludwig S. A 12-year-old girl with altered mental status and a seizure. *Pediatr Emerg Care* 2004;20:613–616.

Drugs Dangerous in Small Doses

Osterhoudt KC. The toxic toddler: drugs that can kill in small doses. *Contemp Pediatr* 2000;17:73–89.

Substance Abuse

Aaron CK. Sympathomimetics. *Emerg Med Clin North Am* 1990;8:513–526.

Baldridge EB, Bessen HA. Phencyclidine. *Emerg Clin North Am* 1990;8:541–550.

Bateman KA, Heagarty MC. Passive freebase cocaine ("crack") inhalation by infants and toddlers. *Am J Dis Child* 1989;143:25–27.

Blum RW. Adolescent substance use and abuse. *Arch Pediatr Adolesc Med* 1997;151:805–808.

Ford M, Hoffman RS, Goldfrank LR. Opioids and designer drugs. *Emerg Med Clin North Am* 1990;8:495–512.

Gasche Y, Daali Y, Fathi M, et al. Codeine intoxication associated with ultrarapid CYP2D6 metabolism. *N Engl J Med* 2004;351:2827–2831.

Geib AJ, Babu K, Ewald MB, et al. Adverse effects in children after unintentional buprenorphine exposure. *Pediatrics* 2006;118:1746–1751.

Hall AJ, Logan JE, Toblin RL, et al. Patterns of abuse among unintentional pharmaceutical overdose fatalities. *JAMA* 2008;300:2613–2620.

Henretig F. Inhalant abuse in children and adolescents. *Pediatr Ann* 1996;25:47–52.

Henretig FM, Slap GB. A guide to acute medical management of intoxication in adolescents. *Am Acad Pediatr Adolesc Health Update* 1994;6:1–7.

Illegal meth labs: cleanup raises health and environmental concerns. *J Environ Health* 2003;65:50.

Kulig K. LSD. *Emerg Med Clin North Am* 1990;8:551–558.

Li J, Stokes SA, Woeckener A. A tale of novel intoxication: a review of the effects of gamma-hydroxybutyric acid with recommendations for management. *Ann Emerg Med* 1998;31(6):729–736.

Ling W, AmassL, Shoptaw S, et al. A multi-center randomized trial of buprenorphine-naloxone versus clonidine for opioid detoxification: findings from the National Institute on Drug Abuse Clinical Trials Network. *Addiction* 2005;100:1090–1100.

LoVecchio F, Curry SC, Bagnasco T. Butyrolactone-induced central nervous system depression after ingestion of RenewTrient, a "dietary supplement" [letter]. *N Engl J Med* 1998;339:847–848.

Mueller PD, Benowitz NL, Olson KR. Cocaine. *Emerg Med Clin North Am* 1990;8:481–494.

Osterhoudt KC. A Cadillac ride to the emergency department. *Pediatr Emerg Care* 2005;21:877–879.

Osterhoudt KC. Children and drug smuggling [letter]. *Arch Pediatr Adolesc Med* 2003;157:703.

Osterhoudt KC. Experiencing ecstasy: is it all the rave? *Pediatr Case Rev* 2002;2:126–129.

Osterhoudt KC, Henretig FM. Comatose teenagers at a party: what a tangled "web" we weave. *Pediatr Case Rev* 2003;3:171–173.

Perry HE, Shannon MW. Diagnosis and management of opioid- and benzodiazepine-induced comatose overdose in children. *Curr Opin Pediatr* 1996;8:243–247.

Prosser JM, Naim M, Hlefaer MA. A 14-year-old girl with agitation and hyperthermia. *Pediatr Emerg Care* 2006;22:676–679.

Shannon MW. Methylenedioxymethamphetamine (MDMA, "Ecstasy"). *Pediatr Emerg Care* 2000;16:377–380.

Shieh-Czaja A, Calello DP, Osterhoudt KC. Sick sisters. *Pediatr Emerg Care* 2005;21:400–402.

Tancredi DN, Shannon MW. Case records of the Massachusetts General Hospital: weekly clinicopathological exercises: case 30-2003: a 21-year old man with sudden alteration of mental status. *N Engl J Med* 2003;349:1267–1275.

Traub SJ, Hoffman RS, Nelson LS. Body-packing: the internal concealment of drugs. *N Engl J Med* 2003;349:2519–2526.

Zhu NY, LeGatt DF, Turner AR. Agranulocytosis after consumption of cocaine adulterated with levamisole. *Ann Intern Med* 2009;150:287–289.

Zvosec DL, Smith SW, McCutcheon R, et al. Adverse events, including death, associated with the use of 1,4-butanediol. *N Engl J Med* 2001;344:87–94.

MEDICAL EMERGENCIES

CHAPTER 103 ■ EVALUATION OF THE ILL RETURNING TRAVELER

MARK L. WALTZMAN, MD, AND RICHARD MALLEY, MD

The world is a book, and those who do not travel read only one page.

Augustine of Hippo (354–430)

Trips do not end when you return home—usually this is the time when in a sense they really begin.

Agnes E. Benedict and Adele Franklin (*The Happy Home*)

In the United States, outbound travel by residents has increased from less than 52 million people in 1995 to more than 63.5 million in 2005. Approximately 20% to 70% report some illness associated with their travel. While most illnesses are mild, between 1% and 5% of travelers seek medical attention either during or immediately after travel and 1 in 100,000 travelers die secondary to travel-related illness. An estimated 1.9 million children from the United States travel internationally each year. While some travel health concerns are similar for children and adults, international pediatric travelers may experience unique problems related to their developing immune systems and different age-based behaviors. As with non–travel-related illness and injury, a newly ambulating toddler will have different health risks than a "high-risk" taking adolescent. Although data about the incidence of pediatric illnesses associated with international travel are limited, there are studies that report serious morbidity and mortality in pediatric travels. The most common reported health problems are diarrheal illnesses, malaria, motor vehicle accidents, and water-related injuries. There are differences in preventative medicine options for children, as several travel-related vaccinations and medications indicated for adults are not licensed or recommended for pediatric use.

Pediatric travelers may be classified into at least two groups: tourists and travelers visiting friends and relatives (VFR). In general, VFR travelers are predominantly immigrants and their children returning to their home countries for vacations, to maintain family ties, or to visit sick relatives. This latter group of travelers may have an increased risk of illness, as family and relatives who are living in developing countries may be more likely to have endemic infectious diseases that are contagious, such as intestinal parasites and tuberculosis. In addition, travelers visiting friends and relatives are less likely to seek pretravel preventive care.

There are several schemata that have been proposed for the evaluation of the returning traveler who is ill. A systematic approach beginning with the chief complaint allows for a rational and stepwise method of developing a differential diagnosis. Ill patients returning from international travel tend to have complaints that fall into one of three categories:

1. Fever
2. Diarrheal/ gastrointestinal complaints
3. Dermatologic issues

FEVER

Fever in the returning traveler is not uncommon. Nearly 3% of travelers returning even from brief international trips (less than 1 month) report fever. The initial assessment should include a detailed history of travel itinerary (including visits to all rural areas, irrespective of the length of time spent in those regions). This will allow for the determination of the likely incubation period as well as possible exposures to infectious agents. It will also allow for the determination of the length (duration) and characteristics of the fever [fever profile including height of the fever, characteristics of the fever (i.e., waxing and waning)], immunization status, and whether appropriate antimalarial prophylaxis was utilized and, if so, whether the medication was taken at appropriate dose, intervals, and proper length of time after leaving the endemic area. The degree of illness, exposure history, time course of illness, and associated signs and symptoms all contribute to the degree of intensity of the evaluation. Some causes of fever in the returning travel are benign, while others are potentially fatal, and still others may pose a public health concern.

The timing of onset of symptoms will vary by causative agents. Knowledge of the incubation period of the infectious causes of fever will allow the clinician to perform a more focused evaluation (Table 103.1). For example, if a fever begins less than 2 weeks after a traveler's return from a short international trip, then tuberculosis, leishmaniasis, and schistosomiasis are unlikely almost regardless of the exposure history.

Although there will be some overlap, further classification of the type of fever may help focus the differential diagnosis. A categorization of fever into the following groups can be useful: undifferentiated (isolated) fever, fever associated with hemorrhage, respiratory complaints, eosinophilia, or central nervous system (CNS) involvement.

Undifferentiated Fever

Malaria

Worldwide there are more than 2.5 million deaths per year caused by malaria, with approximately 1 million deaths in children younger than 5 years. Official estimates of mortality

TABLE 103.1

INFECTIOUS CAUSES OF UNDIFFERENTIATED FEVER IN THE RETURNING TRAVELER

Disease	Distribution	Incubation period
Incubation < 14 days		
Malaria	Most tropical and subtropical areas; some temperate areas	6 days to years
Dengue	Tropics and subtropics, including urban areas	4–8 days (3–14 days)
Spotted fever (rickettsiae)	Worldwide	Few days to 2–3 wk
Scrub typhus (*Orientia tsutsugamushi*)	Widespread in Asia; also in Australia	10 days (6–21 days)
Leptospirosis (*Leptospira interrogans*)	Widespread; most common in tropics	7–12 days (2–26 days)
Campylobacteriosis, salmonellosis, shigellosis	Widespread, most common in developing countries	2–6 days (1–20 days)
Typhoid fever (*Salmonella enterica* serotype *typhi*)	Developing countries, especially Indian subcontinent	7–18 days (3–60 days)
Acute HIV infection	Worldwide	Acute illness, 10–28 days (10 days–6 wk) (may also lead to asymptomatic infection)
East African trypanosomiasis (*Trypanosoma brucei rhodesiense*)	Sub-Saharan East Africa, with focal distribution	Acute illness, 5–16 days (3–21 days); chronic illness, months to years
Incubation 14 days to 6 wk		
Malaria	See malaria above	
Typhoid fever	See typhoid fever above	
Hepatitis A	Widespread	28–30 days (15–50 days)
Hepatitis E	Widespread; outbreaks in Asia, Africa, and Latin America	26–42 days (2–9 wk)
Acute schistosomiasis (Katayama fever)	Parts of Africa, Asia, and Latin America	Katayama fever, 4–8 wk
Amebic liver abscess (*Entamoeba histolytica*)	Widespread; most common in developing countries	Weeks to months
Leptospirosis	See leptospirosis above	
Acute HIV infection	See HIV infection above	
East African trypanosomiasis	See East African trypanosomiasis above	
Incubation > 6 wk		
Malaria	See Malaria above	
Tuberculosis	Worldwide; common in parts of Africa, Asia, Latin America, Eastern Europe, and Russia	Primary, weeks; reactivation, years
Hepatitis B	Worldwide; chronic infection common in parts of Asia, Africa, and Latin America	60–90 days (45–180 days; rarely 9 mo)
Visceral leishmaniasis (*Leishmania donovani, L. chagasi*, others)	Many parts of Africa, Asia, South America, and the Mediterranean basin, especially rural	2–6 mo (10 days to years)
Lymphatic filariasis (*Wuchereria bancrofti* and other filariae)	Widespread in tropical areas	3–6 mo or longer
Schistosomiasis	See acute schistosomiasis above	
Amebic liver abscess	See amebic liver abscess above	
Chronic mycosis	Worldwide	1 wk to years
African trypanosomiasis (*T. brucei rhodesiense, T. brucei gambiense*)	Sub-Saharan Africa, with focal distribution	Chronic illness, months to years

among children younger than 5 years in sub-Saharan Africa in 2002 show that 22% of all deaths were related to malaria, 16% to acute respiratory infections, 14% to diarrheal illness, 13% to "neonatal deaths," 8% to measles and HIV infection, and 19% to "all other causes." Malaria has varied presenta-

tions and outcomes that are largely based on the infecting plasmodium species. VFR travelers are at particular risk since many fail to take the necessary precautions either to avoid insect exposure or to take prophylaxis. Approximately 40% of the reported cases of malaria in the United States are from

VFR travelers. Infections with *Plasmodium falciparum* can progress rapidly, some fatally, and must be considered in the differential diagnosis in all febrile children who have recently visited an endemic region. Approximately 90% of *P. falciparum* infections are acquired in sub-Saharan Africa, and up to 90% of travelers who are infected begin to have symptoms within 1 month after their return. In contrast to *P. falciparum* infections, travelers infected with *Plasmodium vivax* and *P. ovale* may show symptoms several months to years after exposure. Seventy percent of *P. vivax* infections are acquired in Asia or Latin America.

Chloroquine-sensitive malaria exists in Central America as well as the Caribbean and limited parts of South America. There are regions that have developed chloroquine and mefloquine resistance (specifically in Southeast Asia). It is vital for the clinician to ask about not only malaria prophylaxis but also the type and how it has been taken. Both chloroquine and mefloquine kill the parasite only in the hematogonous phase; it is thus vital to take these medications for 4 weeks upon leaving the endemic region. Early termination of these medications could result in malaria even in someone who was "taking prophylaxis."

Malaria infections in children typically present with fever; however, 10% to 40% may be afebrile at the time of the initial evaluation. The fever pattern of malaria, when present, is usually continuously elevated in *P. falciparum* infection.

The life cycle of the malarial parasites begin when the *sporozoites* are inoculated into humans by the bite of an *Anopheles* mosquito and invade hepatic parenchymal cells. The parasites undergo asexual multiplication or *schizogony* (where the parasites are known as *trophozoites*); in this tissue phase, it is also referred to as the exoerythrocytic schizogony. After a period of development (7 to 10 days for *P. falciparum*, *P. ovale*, and *P. vivax* and 10 to 14 days for *P. malariae*), *merozoites* emerge to invade the erythrocytes and begin the symptomatic phase of illness. The last few hours of the erythrocytic stage of the parasite's life cycle, where the parasite is called a *schizont*, comprise the actual replicative phase in which the parasite undergoes mitosis, subdivides, and differentiates into merozoites. It is the subsequent rupture and release of merozoites that lead to fever and other malarial symptoms. If infections are synchronized, there periodicity of symptoms is 48 hours in *P. ovale* and *P. vivax* malarial infection, whereas it is 72 hours in *P. malariae* infections. While periodicity may be every 48 hours in *P. falciparum* infections, it often is irregular. Parasite populations do not become synchronized until at least the second week of clinical illness in the benign malarias, so that it is unusual to see the classical 48- or 72-hour cyclic pattern of fever produced by simultaneous lysis of erythrocytes and release of merozoites. The parasite's reproductive cycles often are not synchronized with any of the species and the absence of periodicity does not rule against malaria being the cause of fevers. Other symptoms at presentation include sweats, rigors, nausea, vomiting, abdominal pain, headache, and malaise. The malaria species and degree of parasitemia will affect the types and degree of symptoms that are displayed. Given the constellation of symptoms, malaria should be considered in all febrile travelers almost regardless of their clinical presentation.

The blood smear is considered the "gold standard" in the diagnosis of malaria. Both thick and thin smears should be obtained. Thick smears allow for a much larger volume of blood to be examined and thus for the detection of smaller numbers of parasites (leading to increased sensitivity), while the thin smear will allow for the identification of the species and the percentage of affected red blood cells. If the initial blood films are negative for malaria and the disease is still clinically suspected, examination of the thick and thin smears should be repeated at least once within 12 to 24 hours after the initial evaluation. Thrombocytopenia without leukocyctosis is a characteristic feature of malaria as is splenomegaly.

In 2007, the U.S. Food and Drug Administration approved a rapid test for the detection of malaria. The Binax NOW® is an immunochromatographic test that detects *P. falciparum*–specific HRP2 antigen to a panmalaria aldolase common to all malaria species. The assay has 94% sensitivity for the detection of *P. falciparum* (up to 96% for pure *P. falciparum* infection) and 87% sensitivity for pure *P. vivax* infection.

Malaria is a reportable disease to the U.S. Center for Disease Control and Prevention (CDC). Empiric treatment should be decided upon in consultation with an infectious disease specialist and the CDC. Drugs of choice usually include quinidine or chloroquine (dependent upon the resistance patterns in the visited areas and the use of prophylactic medications) with the addition of primaquine for *P. vivax* or *P. ovale* infections. Both chloroquine and quinidine are available in intravenous preparations from the CDC.

Dengue Fever

Dengue is caused by one of four strains of the mosquito-borne flavovirus. It has become one of the major infectious disease threats in the tropical and subtropical areas of the world, accounting for approximately 50 million cases and at least 12,000 deaths annually. Seasonal epidemics of dengue occur frequently in many tropical and subtropical regions, with recent outbreaks in Rio de Janeiro, Singapore, Puerto Rico, Haiti, and the Dominican Republic. It has become a common cause of fever in recently returned travelers and, in contrast to malaria, is often acquired during urban travel. Dengue is most often transmitted during daylight hours because of the feeding preferences of its vector, the *Aedes aegypti* mosquito.

The incubation period of dengue is typically 4 to 7 days, with symptoms manifesting most often as a mild influenza-like illness with fever, headache, and myalgia, but sometimes as high fever, severe retroorbital headache, and severe muscle pain (breakbone fever). The fever usually lasts 5 to 7 days. A rash, typically macular or maculopapular and often confluent with the sparing of small islands of normal skin, has been reported in approximately 50% of patients. This rash typically appears near the time of defervescence, often lasts for 2 to 4 days, and may be accompanied by scaling and pruritus. Other signs and symptoms may include flushed facies (typically in the first 24 to 48 hours), lymphadenopathy, injected conjunctivae, inflamed pharynx, and mild respiratory and gastrointestinal symptoms.

Dengue shock syndrome and dengue hemorrhagic fever are uncommon in travelers, as is death from dengue; however, two deaths were reported in a series of more than 200 cases of dengue imported to the United States between 1993 and 2000. The risk of dengue hemorrhagic fever is more than 4 times higher in immigrants and in VFR travelers to areas where the disease is endemic than in general travelers to the same area.

This is likely because dengue shock syndrome and dengue hemorrhagic fever develop as a result of antibody-dependent enhancement (overstimulation of the immune response to an infection with a prior serotype) in individuals who have had pervious infections. Thus, in contrast to malaria, dengue infection may result in more severe disease in previously exposed individuals.

Dengue fever is typically diagnosed on the basis of clinical suspicion and confirmed by comparing serum antibody titers during acute and convalescent phases. The most commonly used test is the IgM capture ELISA; however, this test is often gives negative results early in the course of the disease and therefore should optimally be performed at least 4 to 5 days after the onset of symptoms. Primary infections are characterized by an increase in the dengue-specific IgM antibodies 4 to 5 days after the onset of fever and increase in the IgG antibodies only after 7 to 10 days. A test for capillary fragility, the tourniquet test, gives positive results if 20 or more petechiae appear in a 1-in^2 (6.25-cm^2) patch on the forearm after inflation and deflation of a blood pressure cuff. This test has been incorporated in the WHO clinical case definition of dengue hemorrhagic fever, but the definition differentiates poorly between dengue and dengue hemorrhagic fever and is not very specific.

Treatment of dengue is symptomatic. Appropriate administration of intravenous fluids is associated with marked reductions in the rates of death due to dengue shock and dengue hemorrhagic fever Avoidance of nonsteroidal antiinflammatory medications and aspirin is recommended because of the thrombocytopenia and increased risk of bleeding.

Typhoid Fever

Typhoid fever is not an uncommon cause of fever in children or adults returning from travel. It is caused by fecal-oral transmission of *Salmonella typhi* or *S. paratyphi*, which are gram-negative bacteria. More than 70% of cases of typhoid fever in the United States are associated with international travel, with most occurring in travelers who have visited family or friends on the Indian subcontinent, in the Philippines, or in Latin America. Common manifestations include fever, headache, abdominal pain, and initial diarrhea followed by constipation. Frequently patients will manifest a "relative bradycardia" (a heart rate that is not as high as one would expect with the height of the fever), although this finding is not specific for typhoid fever and can be associated with other infections by other intracellular organisms such as *Plasmodium*, *Legionella*, and *Babesia*. Other physical examination findings of typhoid fever include a toxic appearance, hepatosplenomegaly, "rose spot" rash, as well as CNS manifestations such as altered mental status and syndrome of inappropriate release of antidiuretic hormone. Bowel perforation can occur in the second week of illness, accompanied by leukocytosis.

The diagnosis of typhoid fever relies on a combination of physical examination findings and serological and microbiological tests. The "Widal" test evaluates the presence of somatic (O) and flagellar (H) agglutinins to *S. typhi* in the patient's serum using suspensions of O and H antigens. The historical recommended method of performing the Widal test is the tube agglutination technique, in which serial twofold dilutions of the subject's serum from 1:20 to 1:1,280 are tested. Subsequent improvements of the test resulted in a rapid slide test. Although this test is widely used in developing countries, it is not commonly used in the United States, as it has been found to be neither sensitive nor specific. Isolation of *Salmonella* from blood or stool is the current standard in the developed world. Initial blood cultures are up to 70% sensitive, whereas the stool culture is rarely positive during the first week of illness. As the disease advances, the stool culture becomes increasingly sensitive, whereas the blood culture loses sensitivity, dropping to less than 30% sensitivity during the second week of illness. The most sensitive test to confirm typhoid is the bone marrow aspirate, with a sensitivity of up to 93%. If typhoid fever is suspected, empiric therapy with a fluoroquinolone or a third-generation cephalosporin antibiotic for 10 to 14 days may be considered. Shorter courses of third-generation cephalosporins have resulted in relapse. Because of the difficulty in diagnosing typhoid fever and its potential seriousness, prevention of the disease is critical. Prophylactic measures, including carefully observing food and water precautions, consuming only commercially bottled or boiled water, and eating only cooked foods or raw foods that can be pealed, aid in prevention. Furthermore, vaccination is indicated for at-risk travelers. The current options for vaccines include the injectable Vi-polysaccharide vaccine (with reported rates of efficacy up to 70%). However, because it is a pure polysaccharide vaccine, it is only indicated in patients older than 2 years. This vaccine has an estimated duration of protection of 2 to 3 years. The live oral Ty21a vaccine is licensed for patients older than 6 years. This oral vaccine has efficacy rates that are similar to that of the Vi polysaccharide but has a duration of protection estimated around 3 to 5 years. Protein–Vi conjugate vaccines have been developed, shown to be effective in the prevention of typhoid fever in children and would theoretically induce long-lasting immunity even if given in infancy but are not commercially available at this time.

Rickettsial Diseases

Fever, headache, and myalgia in persons who have recently traveled should prompt the consideration of rickettsial infections. These infections include African tick typhus (*Rickettsia africae*), Mediterranean tick typhus (*R. conorii*), and scrub typhus (*Orientia tsutsugamushi*). Rickettsiae are transmitted by arthropods, and the detection of a painless eschar at the inoculation site ("site of the bite of the mite") can be an important diagnostic clue. High-risk travelers include those that have been hiking, camping, or traveling on safari in grassy or scrubby regions. Regional lymphadenopathy, rash, leukopenia, and thrombocytopenia are often present, although rash is frequently absent in African tick typhus. The diagnosis of rickettsial infection is generally made on the basis of clinical suspicion, which should prompt treatment (generally with tetracycline antibiotics) pending serologic confirmation.

Leptospirosis

Leptospira interrogans are motile, finely coiled, catalase-producing spirochetes that infect humans through intact mucous membranes or disrupted skin, invade the bloodstream, and can disseminate rapidly to multiple organs. The usual incubation period is approximately 10 days (range = 7 to 14 days), although symptoms can be seen in as short as 2 days and as long as 25 days. The clinical manifestations are divided into the initial "septicemic" phase and the subsequent "immune" phase.

Anicteric leptospirosis may begin abruptly with a viral-like illness marked by fever, myalgia, and headache. Abdominal pain, vomiting, diarrhea, anorexia, and conjunctival suffusion may be present. Symptoms usually last 4 to 7 days and resolve spontaneously. Some patients experience a second, immune phase of the illness that begins 1 to 3 days later that may or may not be accompanied by a low-grade fever. During this phase, patients usually have headache, myalgia, rash, and conjunctival suffusion, as well as hepatomegaly. Typically, the headache is severe and may be associated with nuchal rigidity. Interstitial nephritis is common; renal involvement can range from incidental pyuria, hematuria, and proteinuria to renal failure. The rash of leptospirosis is immune-mediated and nonspecific. It can be macular, maculopapular, urticarial, petechial, or purpuric. The more severe, icteric form of leptospirosis, also called Weil syndrome, is indistinguishable in the early phase from the benign, anicteric form. The hallmarks of Weil syndrome are jaundice, azotemia, and hemorrhage, becoming evident 4 to 6 days after the onset of symptoms and may progress through the second week of illness. Weil syndrome has a mortality of 5% to 10%.

A history of exposure to fresh water (rafting or kayaking or wading through flooded streets) in a person with relevant symptoms should suggest the diagnosis of leptospirosis. Antibiotics such as penicillin and tetracycline are effective, and the diagnosis is usually confirmed serologically by a fourfold or greater increase in antibody titers between serum samples obtained during the acute and convalescent phases.

Fever Associated with Hemorrhage

There are several treatable infections that may affect travelers that manifest as fever with hemorrhage. These include meningococcemia, malaria, leptospirosis, and rickettsial infections. There are a handful of viral infections (in addition to dengue and yellow fever) that are also associated with fever and hemorrhage; these, however, are rarely acquired by travelers. Viral hemorrhagic fevers (such as Lassa fever and Ebola fever) need to be considered in travelers who present with fever and hemorrhage; these diseases also have important infection control and public health concerns. Epidemiologic clues include history of visits to rural areas or recent contact with ill persons in areas where the viral hemorrhagic fevers are endemic. Most patients with viral hemorrhagic fevers note the onset of fever within 3 weeks after exposure to infected persons, contaminated water, or infected insects/vectors.

There is currently no specific treatment available for the viral hemorrhagic fevers. Supportive care with special attention to careful fluid and electrolyte management is indicated. Endothelial dysfunction makes hydration challenging; pulmonary edema occurs rapidly with intravenous hydration. To prevent agitation, analgesia and sedation may be useful.

Of special consideration is the yellow fever virus. This flavivirus is transmitted to humans primarily by infected *Aedes* and *Haemogogus* mosquitoes in tropical areas of Africa and South America. There have been sporadic human infections occurring following exposure to the enzootic mosquito vectors (*Haemogogus* species in South America and *Aedes africanus*, *A. furcifer*, *A. vittatus*, *A. luteocephalus*, and *A. simpsoni* in Africa). These mosquitoes acquire the yellow fever virus from infected monkeys and transmit the virus to humans.

There is a 3- to 6-day incubation period, followed by the development of symptoms, including headache, fever, chills, and myalgia, often accompanied by photophobia, back pain, anorexia, vomiting, and restlessness. During this phase, patients are viremic. Viremia usually clears about 4 days following the onset, as fever and other symptoms subside ("period of remission"). Although patients may remain anicteric and then fully recover, approximately 15% to 20% of patients enter a "period of intoxication," characterized by return or persistence of fever, development of jaundice, nausea, vomiting, epigastric tenderness, oliguria, and hemorrhage. Viral invasion of the CNS is rare, but neurologic manifestations can include delirium, convulsions, and coma. The case fatality rate of severe disease ranges from 20% to 50%. Laboratory abnormalities include elevated aspartate and alanine aminotransferases, proteinuria, thrombocytopenia, leucopenia, and abnormal blood coagulation studies.

Patients with confirmed or suspected yellow fever require intensive supportive care with careful attention to optimizing fluid and metabolic balance. Secondary bacterial infections should be treated with appropriate antibiotics.

The live-attenuated yellow fever vaccine has been available since 1937 and is recommended for persons who travel to yellow fever endemic areas. It is currently contraindicated in persons younger than 6 to 9 months, those with allergy to egg or egg products, patients who are pregnant, or those who have underlying immunocompromised disease. The effective duration is approximately 10 years.

Fever Associated with Respiratory Findings

Respiratory symptoms in a febrile returning traveler should suggest the presence of common agents such as influenza and other respiratory viruses, *Mycoplasma*, *Streptococcus pneumoniae*, and *Legionella pneumophila*, the etiologic agent of legionnaires disease. *L. pneumophila* has been documented as a source of infection by travelers on cruise ships or those spending times in spas or hotels. Another important consideration is tuberculosis, an infection that is becoming more prevalent in travelers, although its presentation can occur months or years later. In travelers to regions of Mexico, consideration should be given as well to histoplasmosis and coccidioidomycosis.

The constellation of fever, pneumonia, and hepatitis should prompt consideration of *Coxiella burnetti* (Q fever), particularly if there has been exposure to farm animals. Cough, nonspecific pulmonary infiltrates, and peripheral eosinophilia should lead one to the consideration of Löffler's syndrome, which results from a transient migration of larval helminths (ascaris, hookworm, or *Strongyloides*) through the alveolar spaces.

Fever with Associated Eosinophilia

Elevated eosinophil counts are associated with a myriad of illnesses, including allergic reactions, drug reactions, and hematologic and neoplastic conditions. Infections with HTLV-1 and HIV, as well as *Bartonella*, *Mycobacterium tuberculosis* or *M. leprae*, streptococci (during recovery), and diseases such as syphilis, coccidiomycosis, and acute bronchopulmonary aspergillosis can all induce eosinophilia. A useful mnemonic for diseases associated with eosinophilia is "worms, wheezes, and weird diseases." It is important to note that, in consideration of eosinophilia, the absolute eosinophil count is probably more important than the percentage of eosinophils present. A total peripheral white blood cell count of 5,000 with 5% eosinophils is quite different than a patient with a total peripheral white blood cell count of 25,000 with 5% eosinophils. Although these cutoffs are somewhat arbitrary, it is useful to consider an absolute eosinophil count of less than 400 as normal, 400 to 1,000 as moderate, and greater than 1,000 as more consistent with parasitic infections. Although fever in association with peripheral eosinophilia of greater than 400 may be due to hematologic conditions or acute allergic reactions, the presence of both fever and eosinophilia in a pediatric traveler should prompt consideration of an infectious cause. Peripheral eosinophilia is characteristically associated with helminthic infections in which the worms dwell in or migrate through tissues. In the febrile traveler with eosinophilia, diagnoses to be considered include acute hookworm, ascaris, or *Strongyloides* infections; acute schistosomiasis (Katayama fever); visceral larva migrans (toxocariasis); lymphatic filariasis; and acute trichinosis. The initial evaluation of travelers with eosinophilia should include examination of several stool specimens for ova and parasites, serologic tests for strongyloidiasis, schistosomiasis, or other helminthic infections, and examination of blood smears or skin biopsy to detect microfilariae, all dictated by the geographic regions traveled and the clinical findings.

Fever Associated with Central Nervous System Involvement

There are numerous processes that may cause fever associated with neurologic changes; however, special consideration should be given to specific etiologies in the returning traveler. Malaria, tuberculosis, typhoid fever, rickettsial infections, leptospirosis, poliomyelitis, rabies, and the viral encephalitides (including Japanese encephalitis, West Nile encephalitis, and tick-borne encephalitis) are possible infections that affect the CNS. Travelers to the "meningitis belt" regions in Africa (during the months of December to June) and those who travel to the Arab world around the time of the annual pilgrimage to Mecca for the *Hajj* are at increased risk for developing meningococcal meningitis. CNS involvement with eosinophilia should also raise the possibility of coccidioidomycosis and angiostrongyliasis (the latter caused by invasion of the meningeal space by the rat lungworm *Angiostrongylus cantanensis*). Rare causes of CNS involvement in travelers also deserve mention. East African trypanosomiasis (the so-called "African sleeping sickness") is transmitted through the bite of the tsetse fly. It manifests as an erythematous swelling or chancre at the site of the fly bite, intermittent high fevers, headache, myalgia, and myocarditis, which can be fatal. These symptoms precede the meningoencephalitis. During the acute phase, trypanosomes are often detectable on smears of peripheral blood. Early treatment is essential because the prognosis is poor once CNS involvement has occurred. In the absence of CNS disease, suramin and eflornithine are the drugs of choice. Suramin sodium is useful only in the treatment of early *Trypanosoma brucei gambiense* and *T. brucei rhodesiense* infections because

it does not cross the blood–brain barrier. Melarsoprol (a combination of melarsen oxide and dimercaprol) and eflornithine are the most effective compounds for the treatment of the second stage of the disease since they can cross the blood–brain barrier. Neither agents are commercially available in the United States, and treatment would need to be coordinated with the CDC.

DIARRHEAL AND GASTROINTESTINAL COMPLAINTS

Many children who travel to developing countries develop diarrhea. Most episodes of traveler's diarrhea resolve during or shortly after the travel. Five to 10% of travelers report diarrhea that lasts for 2 weeks or longer and 1% to 3% have diarrhea that lasts 4 weeks or longer. In the majority of cases, the etiologic agent of traveler's diarrhea cannot be isolated. However, among cases in which a pathogen is isolated, 50% to 75% are identified within 2 weeks of developing symptoms. As the duration of the diarrhea increases (typically greater than 2 weeks), the likelihood of identifying a specific bacterial cause decreases; in contrast, the likelihood of identification of a parasitic cause increases. The most commonly identified parasitic infections include *Giardia lamblia*, *Cryptosporidium parvum*, *Entamoeba histolytica*, and *Cyclospora cayetanesis*, although even these are detected in less than one-third of travelers with chronic diarrhea and in only 1% to 5% of travelers with acute diarrhea. Infected children are predominantly asymptomatic, but bloody or nonbloody diarrhea, hepatobiliary symptoms, and failure to thrive may occur.

Viral hepatitis should be considered when evaluating a child with nonspecific gastrointestinal symptoms, particularly when jaundice is present. Hepatitis A is prevalent in both developed and developing nations and is acquired through contaminated food and water. Hepatitis A is usually asymptomatic or manifests as mild symptoms in young children. Hepatitis E must be considered because it is a common etiology of acute hepatitis in developing countries. Although rarely presenting acutely, hepatitis B and C are common in the developing world and should be considered in any adolescent or young adult who is sexually active or has had a tattoo or body piercing while traveling.

Invasive or inflammatory enteropathy (e.g., dysentery) should be suspected in persons with bloody diarrhea, fever, or leukocytes detected in the mucous portion of the stool. Invasive enteropathy has a fairly abrupt onset (over a period of hours generally) and may be complicated by metastatic infections, reactive arthropathy, or, in the case of infection with *Campylobacter jejuni*, the Guillain-Barré syndrome. Amoebic dysentery, caused by *E. histolytica* among other amoebae, often presents slowly over the course of days and may be complicated by hepatic abscess formation.

Prolonged diarrhea with malabsorption should prompt consideration of a protozoal infection of the small bowel (such as *G. lamblia*) as well as tropical sprue. Tropical sprue is a syndrome characterized by acute or chronic diarrhea, weight loss, and malabsorption of nutrients. It occurs in residents of or visitors to the tropics and subtropics. The exact causative factor is unknown, but an intestinal microbial infection is believed to be the initiating insult. The infection results in enterocyte injury, intestinal stasis, and possible bacteria overgrowth. Villous destruction and demonstrable nutrient malabsorption occur in varying degrees. Folate, vitamin B_{12}, and iron are the most common nutrient deficiencies. Tropical sprue is pathologically indistinguishable from nontropical sprue (i.e., gluten-sensitive enteropathy or celiac disease), but it is not associated with antigliadin and antiendomysial antibodies and does not respond to removal of gluten from the diet. Useful therapeutic interventions involve treatment with antibiotics and replacement of nutrients (e.g., folic acid, vitamin B_{12}, iron), deficient fluid, and sometimes blood. The use of antibiotics to treat tropical sprue is controversial. Despite success in some regions, studies in southern India have not suggested any benefit on outcomes. The general recommendation is to consider a combination of antibiotics (tetracycline is recommended for children older than 8 years) and folic acid for patients for 3 to 6 months.

There are several common noninfectious causes of chronic diarrhea in travelers including postinfectious disaccharidase deficiency and irritable bowel syndrome. Importantly, a diarrheal illness that develops more than 1 month after travel is not likely due to travel exposure.

Returning travelers with diarrhea should have stool samples cultured for enteric pathogens and examined microscopically for ova and parasites if there is evidence of an invasive enteropathy, if the diarrhea is persistent, if the diarrhea is unresponsive to empirical therapy, or if the infected person is immunocompromised. Assays for the detection of *Clostridium difficile* toxins may also be indicated. The routine microbiologic techniques often times cannot detect many of the bacteria associated with persistent diarrhea. The sensitivity of a single stool specimen for the detection of ova and parasites varies, depending on the parasite, but it rarely exceeds 80%. The likelihood of identifying a parasite may be increased by examining additional stool samples (three samples obtained on separate occasions increase the sensitivity to more than 90%).

In many cases of persistent diarrhea, no causative agent can be identified. In these cases, some experts recommend empiric antimicrobial therapy such as a fluoroquinolone or a macrolide for suspected bacterial diarrhea. Metronidazole (or a related agent) is recommended for presumed giardiasis, since *G. lamblia* is the most commonly identified intestinal parasite in travelers. Multiple courses of antimicrobial agents should be avoided. For travelers whose diarrhea persists, endoscopic examination and biopsy should be considered to exclude entities such as tropical sprue and inflammatory bowel disease.

DERMATOLOGIC CONDITIONS

Dermatologic conditions are common among persons who have recently traveled. The location of the lesions, the lesion type (macular, papular, urticarial, etc.), and the presence or absence of associated symptoms (i.e., pain, pruritus, fever) are helpful in establishing the diagnosis. The skin can be affected through a primary process or secondary to a systemic disease.

Papular Lesions and Urticaria

There are numerous causes of urticaria, including allergic, viral, bacterial, medication-induced, or parasitic exposure. The para-

sites commonly associated with urticaria include *Strongyloides stercoralis* and *Schistosoma* species. Bites from insects (such as bedbugs and fleas) are the most common cutaneous finding in the returning traveler. These lesions cause pruritic, papular lesions that generally occur in clusters or in a linear distribution. *Sarcoptes scabiei* is the parasite that causes scabies and is common in the developing world. Seabather's eruption is a pruritic, papular rash that is generally confined to the skin covered by a bathing suit or wet suit. It is caused by larval forms of sea anemones such as *Edwardsiella lineate* as well as jellyfish such as *Linuche unguiculata* that become trapped under the fabric after exposure to salt water. Fresh water exposure–related causes of rashes include cercarial dermatitis, which results from penetration of the skin by schistosomal cercariae from fresh water (swimmer's itch) or from coastal water (digger's itch). Acute schistosomiasis, known as Katayama fever, typically occurs several weeks after exposure to freshwater in an endemic area (typically sub-Saharan Africa) and presents with high fever, urticaria, and eosinophilia. Long-term travelers returning from Africa may develop a pruritic, papular rash due to onchocerciasis (caused by *Onchocerca volvulus*).

Papular/Nodular/Ulcerative Lesions

Cutaneous larva migrans is the most frequent serpiginous lesion among travelers. It results from the migration of animal hookworms (e.g., *Ancylostoma braziliense* and *A. canium*) in superficial tissues. It is typically acquired after direct contact of the skin with soil or sand that has been contaminated with dog or cat feces. The lesions, which may initially be papular or vesicular, are pruritic and commonly found on the foot or buttock. *S. stercoralis* larvae may be rapidly mobile (moving approximately 5 cm per hour) and produce a cutaneous track (larva currens) that is often perianal. These are often acquired in travelers to Mexico or the Caribbean islands.

Furuncular myiasis, also known as Tumbu fly or botfly (*Dermatobia hominis*), are commonly found in Central and South America (mainly in wooded and forest margins of the lowlands and river valleys). The larvae are parasitic and undergo their development in the skin of animals such as cattle, dogs, swine, and, inadvertently, humans. When the female botfly is ready to lay eggs, she captures other *Diptera* (and less commonly ticks) and "glues" the eggs to the bottom of their abdomen. The embryos hatch in 5 to 15 days and abandon them while in contact with a warm-blooded host. If the carrier is a blood-sucking fly or mosquito, the botfly embryo can utilize the puncture site to gain entry into the host tissue; otherwise, the embryo penetrates the host through a hair follicle or a break in the epidermis. Once in the skin, the larva develops a boil-like pocket that has an opening to the outside (punctum) that allows the larvae to breathe. Conditions that may mimic botfly infestation include cellulitis, sebaceous cyst, folliculitis, cutaneous leishmaniasis, staphylococcal boil, and less commonly atopic dermatitis. Treatment is centered on the removal of the larva. The most common and invasive method is surgical excision. The main difficulties include risk of dissecting the larvae during the excision, which can result in an incomplete removal. Another option involves injecting each individual larval cavity with lidocaine and then removing the parasite with forceps once they appear at the punctum.

Similar to the botfly, tungiasis is an infestation by the burrowing flea *Tunga penetrans* or related species. It is also known as chigoe flea, jigger, pigue, nigua, pico, and bicho de pie (bug of the foot). Tungiasis was first reported in crewmen who sailed with Christopher Columbus. The flea is indigenous to the West Indies/Caribbean region, but has spread to Africa, India, Pakistan, and Latin America. Travelers to endemic areas may import cases to other countries, including the United States. To reproduce, the flea requires a warm-blooded host. In addition to humans, reservoir hosts include cattle, sheep, horses, mules, rats, mice, dogs, pigs, and other wild animals. The main habitat is warm, dry soil and sand of beaches, stables, and stock farms. Upon contact, the fleas invade unprotected skin. The most common site of involvement is the feet (interdigital skin and subungual area). Both the male and the nonfertilized female flea feed intermittently on warm-blooded hosts. Once impregnated, however, the female flea anchors herself to the skin by using biting mouthparts and painlessly burrows into the epidermis. The flea expands, often reaching 1 cm in diameter. The head is down into the upper dermis feeding from blood vessels, whereas the caudal tip of the abdomen is at the skin surface, often forming a punctum or an ulcer. The flea breathes through this opening. In many cases, this is described as a white patch with a black dot.

Over 1 to 2 weeks, more than 100 eggs, which fall to the ground, are individually released from this exposed orifice. Afterward, the flea dies and is slowly sloughed by the host. The eggs hatch on the ground in 3 to 4 days, go through larval and pupal stages, and become adults in 2 to 3 weeks. The complete life cycle lasts approximately 1 month. Reported topical treatments include cryotherapy or electrodesiccation of the nodules. Topical ivermectin, metrifonate (not available in the United States), and thiabendazole have also been reported as effective. Occlusive petrolatum may suffocate the organism; however, these organisms breathe infrequently and the effectiveness of this modality has been questioned. Topical treatments do not remove the flea from the skin and therefore do not result in relief from painful lesions. The flea may be gently removed with a needle or forceps. A number of surgical treatment methods are available, including removal of the flea from its cavity with sterile instruments, but this is more difficult when the flea is engorged. The orifice needs to be enlarged, and the entire nodule should be curetted or excised. An antibiotic ointment may be applied, along with systemic antibiotic therapy when indicated for superinfection. Aggressive treatment of secondary infection and tetanus prophylaxis are important.

Ulcers and Eschars

Ecthyma (pyoderma) is the most frequent cutaneous ulcer among travelers. These lesions are shallow, painful, and purulent ulcers of ecthyma often as a result of skin trauma or bites that have become secondarily infected with pyogenic organisms such as *Staphylococcus aureus* or group A streptococci. Less commonly, ulcers may be due to cutaneous leishmaniasis; however, these are important to recognize. These ulcers are painless and typically enlarge slowly and have a granulomatous or crusted base with raised margins. New World leishmaniasis, caused by *Leishmania* (*Viannia*) *braziliensis*, may progress to form destructive localized recrudescences on mucosal surfaces. New World leishmaniasis refers to infections acquired in Latin America, whereas Old World leishmaniasis is associated with travel to Central Asia. Leishmaniasis is occasionally manifested as isolated lymphadenopathy or as lymphocutaneous changes that can also resemble sporotrichosis or *M. marinum* infections. Eschars may be seen in rickettsial disorders such as Mediterranean spotted fever, scrub typhus, and African tick typhus. An eschar at the site where a rickettsia-transmitting arthropod has fed is usually small (less than 1 cm in diameter), asymptomatic, and is often overlooked by the patient or family.

The ill returning pediatric travel poses a number of diagnostic issues for the clinician. These can be addressed by taking a stepwise approach toward the chief complaint. Important clues to consider regarding the ill returning pediatric traveler include where they traveled to, how long they were there, when the symptoms began relative to their travel, and whether the patient was seen for pretravel counseling by a travel medicine specialist. Travel medicine specialists make recommendation for vaccinations and prophylactic medications based on the proposed travel itinerary. Vaccinations commonly used for travel prophylaxis include hepatitis A, hepatitis B, typhoid (both oral and Vi polysaccharide), meningococcal, Japanese encephalitis, inactivated poliovirus, and yellow fever. In addition to pretravel vaccination, prophylactic medications for malaria (either weekly chloroquine or mefloquine or daily atovoquone/proquanil) should be considered in the evaluation of the febrile returning patient. If appropriate vaccinations were given and chemoprophylaxis was complied as prescribed, the diagnosis may possibly be narrowed.

Suggested Readings

Introduction

Fenner L, Weber R, Steffen R, et al. Imported infectious disease and purpose of travel, Switzerland. *Emerg Infect Dis* 2007;13(2):217–222.
Steffen R, deBernardis C, Banos A. Travel epidemiology—a global perspective. *Int J Antimicrob Agents* 2003;21(2):89–95.
Steffen R, Rickenbach M, Wilhelm U, et al. Health problems after travel to developing countries. *J Infect Dis* 1987;156(1):84–91.
U.S. Department of Commerce ITA, Office of Travel and Tourism Industries. *U.S. resident travel to Canada, Mexico and overseas countries historical visitation outbound: 1995–2005.* Published data on the Internet. Washington, DC: U.S. Department of Commerce, International Trade Administration, 2006.

Fever

Barat LM, Zucker JR, Barber AM, et al. Malaria surveillance—United States, 1993. *MMWR CDC Surveill Summ* 1997;46(2):27–47.
Bigaillon C, Fontan E, Cavallo JD, et al. Ineffectiveness of the Binax NOW malaria test for diagnosis of Plasmodium ovale malaria. *J Clin Microbiol* 2005;43(2):1011.
Centers for Disease Control and Prevention. Imported dengue—United States, 1993–1994. *MMWR Morb Mortal Wkly Rep.* 1995;44(18):353–356.
Centers for Disease Control and Prevention. Imported dengue—United States, 1995. *MMWR Morb Mortal Wkly Rep.* 1996;45(45):988–991.
Centers for Disease Control and Prevention. Imported dengue—United States, 1996. *MMWR Morb Mortal Wkly Rep.* 1998;47(26):544–547.
Centers for Disease Control and Prevention. Imported dengue—United States, 1997 and 1998. *MMWR Morb Mortal Wkly Rep.* 2000;49(12):248–253.
Centers for Disease Control and Prevention. Imported dengue—United States, 1999 and 2000. *MMWR Morb Mortal Wkly Rep.* 2002;51(13):281–283.
Dung NM, Day NP, Tam DT, et al. Fluid replacement in dengue shock syndrome: a randomized, double-blind comparison of four intravenous-fluid regimens. *Clin Infect Dis* 1999;29(4):787–794.
Farcas GA, Zhong KJ, Lovegrove FE, et al. Evaluation of the Binax NOW ICT test versus polymerase chain reaction and microscopy for the detection of malaria in returned travelers. *Am J Trop Med Hyg* 2003;69(6):589–592.
Freedman DO, Kozarsky PE, Weld LH, et al. GeoSentinel: the global emerging infections sentinel network of the International Society of Travel Medicine. *J Travel Med.* 1999;6(2):94–98.

MEDICAL EMERGENCIES

Freedman DO, Woodall J. Emerging infectious diseases and risk to the traveler. *Med Clin North Am* 1999;83(4):865-83, v.

Hill DR. Evaluation of the returned traveler. *Yale J Biol Med.* 1992;65(4):343–356.

Hill DR. Health problems in a large cohort of Americans traveling to developing countries. *J Travel Med.* 2000;7(5):259–266.

Hoffner RJ, Slaven E, Perez J, et al. Emergency department presentations of typhoid fever. *J Emerg Med* 2000;19(4):317–321.

Hoffman SL, Edman DC, Punjabi NH, et al. Bone marrow aspirate culture superior to streptokinase clot culture and 8 ml 1:10 blood-to-broth ratio blood culture for diagnosis of typhoid fever. *Am J Trop Med Hyg* 1986;35(4):836–839.

Jelinek T. Dengue fever in international travelers. *Clin Infect Dis* 2000;31(1):144–147.

Jensenius M, Fournier PE, Raoult D. Rickettsioses and the international traveler. *Clin Infect Dis* 2004;39(10):1493–1499.

Jensenius M, Fournier PE, Vene S, et al. African tick bite fever in travelers to rural sub-Equatorial Africa. *Clin Infect Dis* 2003;36(11):1411–1417.

Kachur SP, Reller ME, Barber AM, et al. Malaria surveillance—United States, 1994. *MMWR CDC Surveill Summ* 1997;46(5):1–18.

Kain KC, Keystone JS. Malaria in travelers. Epidemiology, disease, and prevention. *Infect Dis Clin North Am* 1998;12(2):267–284.

Lin FY, Ho VA, Khiem HB, et al. The efficacy of a *Salmonella typhi* Vi conjugate vaccine in two-to-five-year-old children. *N Engl J Med* 2001;344(17):1263–1269.

Long SS, Pickering LK, Prober CG. *Principles and practice of pediatric infectious diseases*, 3rd ed. Philadelphia, PA: Churchill Livingstone/Elsevier, 2008.

Malik AS. Complications of bacteriologically confirmed typhoid fever in children. *J Trop Pediatr* 2002;48(2):102–108.

Martone WJ, Kaufmann AF. Leptospirosis in humans in the United States, 1974–1978. *J Infect Dis* 1979;140(6):1020–1022.

McCaslin RI, Pikis A, Rodriguez WJ. Pediatric *Plasmodium falciparum* malaria: a ten-year experience from Washington, DC. *Pediatr Infect Dis J* 1994;13(8):709–715.

Mulholland EK, Adegbola RA. Bacterial infections—a major cause of death among children in Africa. *N Engl J Med* 2005;352(1):75–77.

Nazarian S, Stauffer W, Kamat D. Index of suspicion. Case 1. Typhoid fever. *Pediatr Rev* 1997;18(10):357–358.

O'Brien D, Tobin S, Brown GV, et al. Fever in returned travelers: review of hospital admissions for a 3-year period. *Clin Infect Dis* 2001;33(5):603–609.

Peter G. Leptospirosis: a zoonosis of protean manifestations. *Pediatr Infect Dis* 1982;1(4):282–288.

Phuong CX, Nhan NT, Kneen R, et al. Clinical diagnosis and assessment of severity of confirmed dengue infections in Vietnamese children: is the World Health Organization classification system helpful? *Am J Trop Med Hyg* 2004;70(2):172–179.

Reid D, Cossar JH. Epidemiology of travel. *Br Med Bull* 1993;49(2):257–268.

Ryan ET, Wilson ME, Kain KC. Illness after international travel. *N Engl J Med* 2002;347(7):505–516.

Schwartz E, Mendelson E, Sidi Y. Dengue fever among travelers. *Am J Med* 1996;101(5):516–520.

Schwartz E, Mileguir F, Grossman Z, et al. Evaluation of ELISA-based serodiagnosis of dengue fever in travelers. *J Clin Virol* 2000;19(3):169–173.

Shah S, Filler S, Causer LM, et al. Malaria surveillance—United States, 2002. *MMWR Surveill Summ* 2004;53(1):21–34.

Vaughn D, Green S. *Hunter's tropical medicine and emerging infectious diseases.* Philadelphia, PA: Saunders, 2000.

Vaughn DW, Green S, Kalayanarooj S, et al. Dengue in the early febrile phase: viremia and antibody responses. *J Infect Dis* 1997;176(2):322–330.

Warrell DA. Management of severe malaria. *Parasitologia* 1999;41(1–3):287–294.

Watt G, Jongsakul K, Chouriyagune C, et al. Differentiating dengue virus infection from scrub typhus in Thai adults with fever. *Am J Trop Med Hyg* 2003;68(5):536–538.

Wilder-Smith A, Schwartz E. Dengue in travelers. *N Engl J Med* 2005;353(9):924–932.

Diarrheal and Gastrointestinal Complaints

Castelli F, Pezzoli C, Tomasoni L. Epidemiology of travelers' diarrhea. *J Travel Med* 2001;8(suppl 2):S26–S30.

Cook GC. Aetiology and pathogenesis of postinfective tropical malabsorption (tropical sprue). *Lancet* 1984;1(8379):721–723.

DuPont HL, Capsuto EG. Persistent diarrhea in travelers. *Clin Infect Dis* 1996;22(1):124–128.

Klein JL, Millman GC. Prospective, hospital based study of fever in children in the United Kingdom who had recently spent time in the tropics. *BMJ* 1998;316(7142):1425–1426.

Nield LS, Stauffer W, Kamat D. Evaluation and management of illness in a child after international travel. *Pediatr Emerg Care* 2005;21(3):184–195; quiz 96–98.

Rees JH, Soudain SE, Gregson NA, et al. *Campylobacter jejuni* infection and Guillain-Barre syndrome. *N Engl J Med* 1995;333(21):1374–1379.

Thielman NM, Guerrant RL. Persistent diarrhea in the returned traveler. *Infect Dis Clin North Am* 1998;12(2):489–501.

Dermatologic Conditions

Caumes E, Carriere J, Guermonprez G, et al. Dermatoses associated with travel to tropical countries: a prospective study of the diagnosis and management of 269 patients presenting to a tropical disease unit. *Clin Infect Dis* 1995;20(3):542–548.

Czachor JS, Elder BL, Sutherin SR. Travelers beware the bot fly! *J Travel Med* 1995;2(4):264–266.

Freudenthal AR, Joseph PR. Seabather's eruption. *N Engl J Med* 1993;329(8):542–544.

MacPherson DW. Intestinal parasites in returned travelers. *Med Clin North Am* 1999;83(4):1053–1075.

McCarthy JS, Ottesen EA, Nutman TB. Onchocerciasis in endemic and nonendemic populations: differences in clinical presentation and immunologic findings. *J Infect Dis* 1994;170(3):736–741.

Raoult D, Fournier PE, Fenollar F, et al. *Rickettsia africae*, a tick-borne pathogen in travelers to sub-Saharan Africa. *N Engl J Med* 2001;344(20):1504–1510.

SECTION IV ■ TRAUMA

GARY R. FLEISHER

CHAPTER 104 ■ AN APPROACH TO THE INJURED CHILD

LOIS K. LEE, MD, MPH, AND GARY R. FLEISHER, MD

Injuries are commonly seen in the emergency department (ED), and clinicians taking care of children and adolescents in the emergency setting should be prepared to manage these patients who may present with a range of injuries. Although pediatric trauma victims have needs distinguishing them from adults, it is only since the mid-1990s that investigators have begun to systematically look at the care of the injured child. The goal of this chapter is to help prepare ED clinicians for the triage, assessment, and initial management of pediatric trauma patients from the spectrum of minor to life-threatening injuries.

The leading cause of death in children 1 to 19 years old in the United States is injury, which account for more than 50% of all childhood deaths. In 2005, more than 15,000 children and adolescents younger than 19 years died from unintentional and nonaccidental trauma in the United States. Injuries also lead to more than 10 million primary care office visits, more than 9 million ED visits, and more than 500,000 hospitalizations yearly in the United State. Injuries are the leading cause of ED visits and account for approximately one-third of all visits for children younger than 15 years. It has been estimated that the cost of unintentional pediatric injuries is $347 billion every year: $17 billion in medical costs, $72 billion in future work lost, and $257 billion in lost quality of life.

Motor vehicle crashes continue to be the most common cause of death due to injury resulting in more than 6,000 deaths in 2005. Homicide and suicide remain the second and fourth leading causes of death in children and adolescents 1 to 19 years old in the United States. In black teenagers, homicide from firearms is the leading cause of death. Although less fatal, falls, drowning, poisoning, and fire/burn injuries are significant causes of morbidity.

This chapter provides a framework for secondary prevention, after the "impact" has occurred causing the injury, with the goal of decreasing morbidity and mortality. Secondary prevention is performed in the field by emergency medical services providers or after arrival to the hospital. General principles of management are outlined for patients with multiple and local injuries ranging from mild to severe. Although most of the injuries are mild to moderate in severity, the ED clinician caring for these patients should be prepared to rapidly and systematically evaluate and manage those who present with serious and life-threatening injuries.

SPECTRUM OF TRAUMA AND INITIAL TRIAGE

Trauma causes injuries that range from minimal to fatal, from the splinter lodged in the sole of the foot to a victim of a motor vehicle crash with multiple injuries. To assist in the initial triage and diagnostic process, several categorizations of injury are useful: (1) extent—multiple or local; (2) nature—blunt or penetrating; and (3) severity—mild, moderate, or severe (Table 104.1).

Trauma can be multiple or local. From a surgical point of view, *multiple trauma* is defined as significant injury to two or more body areas (e.g., the head and abdomen, the chest and extremities, or other combinations). Although this definition serves a useful purpose in comparing outcomes retrospectively among various centers, it does not suit the needs of emergency physicians who must evaluate and treat children before all diagnostic information has become available. For the purpose of triage in the ED, *multiple trauma* is defined as apparent injury to two or more body areas. Thus, the child who fell from a bicycle, sustaining a forehead laceration and a forearm fracture, would be classified in the ED as having multiple trauma (head and extremity), even though the completed evaluation may not uncover any additional or serious injuries. Multiple trauma is common, given the child's small and immature body habitus. Localized trauma involves only one anatomic region of the body: head, neck, chest, abdomen/pelvis, back, or extremities. Again, during ED triage, the designation of local trauma is assigned initially on the basis of even superficial injuries in a given anatomic area, despite the fact that subsequent evaluation might not detect any deeper involvement.

The initial diagnostic task confronting the emergency physician is to decide whether trauma is local or multiple. In some cases, the distinction between local and multiple trauma is obvious. The 13-year-old boy who twisted his ankle coming down with a rebound has a local musculoskeletal injury. The 2-year-old boy who is cyanotic, pulseless, and apneic after a plunge from a ninth story window has sustained critical multiple trauma.

At times, however, the distinction between local and multiple trauma may not be straightforward. A 7-year-old girl who flies over the handlebars of her bicycle onto the sidewalk and is brought to the ED covered with blood, thrashing and screaming

TABLE 104.1

CATEGORIZATION OF TRAUMA

Extent: local or multiple
Nature: blunt or penetrating
Saverity: mild, moderate, or severe

at every touch, may be judged initially to have serious multiple trauma. After complete and rapid assessment, she may instead have only a superficial forehead laceration and an acute anxiety reaction. The next child with the same history and a constellation of symptoms may have a concussion and a ruptured spleen. A third child in a similar scenario may have a rib fracture leading to a pneumothorax; a fourth child may have a buckle fracture of the radius and a depressed skull fracture.

The distinction between local and multiple trauma may be difficult to ascertain initially because (1) some serious injuries are occult in their early phase; (2) some children are difficult to examine because they are nonverbal, uncooperative, frightened, or in pain; (3) some parents might have played a role in the trauma (i.e., child abuse) and will try to conceal the extent of the injury; and (4) some children, particularly adolescents, may be under the influence of drugs or alcohol. Differentiation between local and multiple trauma is thus a dynamic process, and the emergency physician's first impression may change as new evidence accumulates. Generally, it is best to consider trauma as multiple until proven otherwise; when the skin is contused over several body parts, the patient is categorized as having multiple trauma until it is known that all the injuries are superficial.

Once it has been decided that multiple trauma has or has not occurred, the emergency physician should then focus on the specific anatomic region(s) involved. For each region, it is important to ascertain whether the injury is the result of blunt or penetrating trauma and to determine the severity of the wound. Trauma may be caused by either blunt or penetrating forces. Although most civilian injuries, particularly during childhood, result from blunt trauma, some trauma centers have seen as much as 15% of serious trauma related to gunshots, stabbings, and other penetrating wounds. The distinction between these two mechanisms of injury is important because it will determine the evaluation based on the expected internal injuries. In this chapter, the management of blunt and penetrating trauma is reviewed for each specific anatomic region.

Finally, the seriousness of injury may vary from mild to severe. Table 104.2 provides a review of a classification of severity based on history and physical examination, as well as a general schema for disposition of the child with trauma, based on the general extent of the evaluation with laboratory tests and imaging required to diagnose or manage the trauma. Whereas only a few patients with penetrating injuries are considered to have mild wounds, most of the more common blunt injuries seen in the ED are minor. The first categorization by severity depends initially on the history of the incident and the physical examination. An important factor is that a history of a significant or critical force applied during impact increases the index of severity. The schema varies somewhat for each anatomic region; thus, Table 104.2 provides only a general overview. Assessment of severity is essential in the ED because it will determine whether the child requires immediate intervention, undergoes a diagnostic evaluation, is discharged after an examination, or receives further observation. The more laboratory and imaging studies required for the assessment and management of the trauma victim, the more likely a child will need admission.

GENERAL PRINCIPLES OF MANAGEMENT

The child who has sustained more than a trivial injury must be considered at risk for decompensation; therefore, an immediate decision must be made regarding the severity of the trauma (Table 104.2). The American College of Surgeons has standardized and disseminated an approach to the initial management of the trauma patient through the Advanced Trauma Life Support (ATLS) program. The goals of the initial trauma management for the trauma victim are to rapidly assess the injuries, determine the management priorities, and provide critical interventions. A systematic and logical approach to the trauma patient is required to assess and address any physiologic threats to life, followed by a complete evaluation. The clinical approach includes the following: (1) primary assessment; (2) resuscitation of vital functions (initial treatment); (3) more comprehensive secondary assessment; and (4) transition to definitive care. The assessment and management may occur simultaneously in patients with significant injuries. For example, while the primary assessment is being performed, an intravenous (IV) catheter can be placed and fluid resuscitation initiated. This approach provides a set of principles for

TABLE 104.2

CLASSIFICATION AND DISPOSITION OF TRAUMA BY SEVERITY

| Category | History | Physical examination | | Laboratory radiographic studies | Probable disposition |
		Vital signs	Local findings		
Mild	Minimal force	Normal	Superficial only	Few	Discharge
Moderate	Significant force	Normal	Suspicious for internal injury	Intermediate	Evaluate
Severe	Critical force	Abnormal	Indicative of internal injury	Many	Immediate therapy; admit

efficiently diagnosing and treating life-threatening conditions without neglecting less severe but important injuries.

The primary assessment includes evaluating the vital signs and quickly reviewing the essential functions of all organs. The emphasis is on discovering treatable injuries and preventing complications (e.g., paralysis from an unstable cervical spine fracture). Concomitantly, resuscitation (initial treatment) is attempted to normalize vital functions and prevent further deterioration from conditions such as hypoxia or blood loss. Primary assessment and resuscitation occupy the first 5 to 10 minutes of the encounter in most cases. As soon as possible, a thorough reassessment of the patient (secondary assessment) should take place to fine-tune the details of management. The secondary assessment is the head-to-toe, front-to-back physical assessment that includes the screening radiographs and stat laboratory tests. To be effective, physical examinations must be repeated serially and then compared. Although resuscitation of unstable patients is critical and requires a strong team approach, the close surveillance of the apparently stable patient at risk of single or multiorgan trauma is paramount and may be even more challenging in terms of the early detection of occult injuries. Definitive care includes stabilization of specific local injuries, preparation of the patient for the operating room, and surgery, as indicated. At the completion of care for trauma patients, a tertiary survey is performed. This is a last thorough check for occult injuries. It is done prior to discharge from the ED, when a patient either goes home after being assessed and treated or moves to the next stage of care in the hospital.

MULTIPLE TRAUMA

Classification

Multiple trauma (see Chapter 105), as defined for the emergency physician, may vary from mild to severe (Table 104.3). The child with a history of injury caused by minimal force and a physical examination that shows only superficial lesions in two or more areas of the body would be assigned to the mild category—for example, a 7-year-old child who fell while running and is found to have abrasions on the forehead and right elbow and tenderness of the right flank. On examination, signs suggestive of deeper injury would place the child in at least the moderate category. Detection of a serious injury or abnormal vital signs (unrelated to anxiety alone) elevates the classification to severe. Unfortunately, the classification of injury by mechanism alone is not a uniformly useful predictor in blunt trauma in children or adults.

Management

Mild Multiple Trauma

The major goal in the management of a child with apparent mild multiple trauma is to confirm the initial impression of lack of severity of the injuries. If there is any question of more severe injury, a large-bore peripheral IV catheter should be inserted and appropriate laboratory studies obtained. However, in cases that obviously seem to involve minimal trauma, the physician can proceed directly to the examination. Initially, the vital signs should be obtained. Subsequent examination includes a complete assessment with special attention to the level of consciousness; tenderness or limitation of motion of the cervical spine; auscultation of the heart and lungs; palpation of the abdomen, back, and pelvis; and tenderness of the extremities. The complete physical examination should include vital signs with capillary refill; Glasgow Coma Scale (GCS) score; inspection and palpation of the head for injuries, pupillary reactions, extraocular muscle function, nasal tenderness and/or septal hematoma, and dental/oral trauma; cervical spine motion (if the child is alert, not in a cervical collar, and without complaint of tenderness); neck vein distension; auscultation of the breath and heart sounds; inspection and palpation of the chest; evaluation of bowel sounds; inspection and palpation of the abdomen; palpation and inspection of the back, flank, and pelvis; rectal and genital examination; evaluation of extremities for deformity or tenderness; palpation of peripheral pulses; neurologic evaluation; and careful survey of the skin and soft tissues.

A child with a history of minimal multiple trauma and a normal examination may require no laboratory or radiographic studies. If there is any concern for intraabdominal injury, a complete blood cell (CBC) count and urinalysis should be obtained.

Moderate Multiple Trauma. The child with multiple trauma categorized as moderate requires immediate intervention and a thorough diagnostic evaluation. A child in this category has an obvious history of involvement of several areas of the body but initially may only have evidence of musculoskeletal or several superficial local injuries. A 3-year-old child who has been hit by an automobile and has a significantly deformed femur and a few ecchymoses on the upper extremities, or an older child who fell off a second-story roof but appears well, may fit this group. As a first step, a minimum of one large-bore peripheral IV catheter should be placed. If the child is in respiratory distress, supplemental oxygen should be administered. Any suggestion

TABLE 104.3

SEVERITY OF MULTIPLE TRAUMA

| Category | History | Physical examination | |
		Vital signs	Local findings
Mild	Minimal force	Normal	Abrasions/contusions
Moderate	Significant force	Normal	Refer to Tables 104.7–104.9 by anatomic region
Severe	Critical force	Abnormal	Refer to Tables 104.7–104.9 by anatomic region

of cervical spine injury mandates immobilization of the neck with a semirigid collar or foam head immobilizers. If the vital signs and primary survey are normal for age, the physician should then proceed with a thorough examination, as outlined in mild multiple trauma.

Most patients with moderate multiple trauma require ancillary studies as part of their evaluation. These might include a CBC count, urinalysis, amylase/lipase, and/or liver function tests and radiographs of the chest, cervical spine, and/or pelvis. A type and screen for red blood cells (RBCs) is indicated. Depending on the history and physical examination, computed tomographic (CT) scans of the head, abdomen, pelvis, and/or spine may be indicated. In fully awake patients, a completely normal examination may be relied upon to exclude the need for all screening studies. Many patients in this category require admission to the hospital. However, an older child with a history of a moderately severe impact, who has an unremarkable examination and normal studies, may be discharged from the ED after observation for several hours.

Severe Multiple Trauma. The management of the child with severe multiple trauma demands immediate action. The initial approach assumes either obvious life-threatening injury or a reasonable likelihood that such an injury exists. An alteration of vital signs (hypotension, tachycardia), diaphoresis, or depressed consciousness automatically categorizes the injury as severe. Although helpful as an initial guide, mechanism alone (e.g., a fall from a two-story building) is not a highly accurate predictor of the risk of sustaining significant injuries. To adequately manage the child with severe multiple trauma, the physician must understand the need to institute treatment before completing a full examination and to continually intersperse detailed reassessments into an intensive treatment protocol. Table 104.4 provides an outline for organizing the initial approach to severe multiple trauma in the ED. It uses a four-pronged strategy: assessment, treatment, monitoring, and diagnostic testing. The protocol is laid out over time in an idealized fashion; obviously, limitations in the number of personnel or unusually difficult technical procedures may slow the progression of the evaluation and management.

LOCALIZED HEAD TRAUMA

Classification

Head trauma (see Chapters 38 and 105) can be divided into penetrating and nonpenetrating. Cases that involve penetration of the cranial vault entail severe injuries and often require operative intervention. Nonpenetrating (blunt) head trauma can be classified as mild, moderate, or severe (Table 104.5).

Management

Penetrating Trauma

Wounds limited to the scalp and not entering the cranial vault are appropriate for primary repair in the ED. Minor wounds from sharp objects, when the likelihood of penetration is high, should have radiologic evaluation and local exploration before primary closure. All other penetrating injuries require

initial stabilization and neurosurgical consultation, as discussed in the "Blunt Trauma—Severe" section. Protruding objects should be left in place until definitive management.

Blunt Trauma—Mild

Most children seen in the ED have sustained mild head trauma, arrive awake, and primarily in need of a thorough physical examination. The head should be palpated for evidence of local injury, assessing for evidence of a depressed fracture. Bruises around the eyes or behind the ear or a hemotympanum suggest a basilar skull fracture. The pupils will be equal and reactive and the extraocular muscle function intact, unless the severity of injury has been misjudged. Although the finding of focal neurologic abnormalities is unlikely, a careful neurologic examination is mandatory. Skull radiographs and CT scans are generally unnecessary but may be indicated in selected situations such as palpation of a potentially depressed fracture or in infants in the first year of life (see Chapter 38). Although uncommon, misclassification of a patient as mild may occur in selected situations, such as when children sustain a significant direct impact to their temporoparietal skull, which is not readily appreciated, or when the history is either not available or deliberately misrepresented, as in cases of child abuse.

Patients with minor head trauma may be discharged from the ED with specific instructions to watch for changes indicative of increased intracranial pressure (ICP) or hemorrhage. Albeit unlikely, these symptoms include depression of mental status, progressive vomiting (more than 4 to 6 hours from the trauma), worsening headache, visual disturbances, ataxia, or seizures. Postconcussive seizures are unusual but may occur within a few days of mild head injury. In general, they are not prognostic for recurrent seizures.

Blunt Trauma—Moderate

Moderate head injury includes any clear-cut prolonged loss of consciousness (1 to 5 minutes) or a history suggesting a severe injury, even without specific physical findings to confirm it. This category would include those who have sustained a concussion with an alteration in their level of consciousness but not necessarily loss of consciousness. Once again, a thorough examination is required to search for signs of intracranial hemorrhage. The most important feature of the examination is a serial evaluation of the neurologic status, including the GCS score or AVPU testing (A, alert and spontaneous responsiveness; V, responds to voice; P, responds to painful stimuli; and U, unresponsive). The initial score serves as the baseline for the detection of subsequent deterioration. Radiographs are reserved for the same indications as for mild trauma. CT scanning is often, but not necessarily, performed in awake patients on arrival, however, it becomes mandatory upon deterioration in mental status, in the presence of focal abnormalities, or with more than a brief loss of consciousness (more than 1 to 5 minutes). Because of the small chance of subsequent intracranial hemorrhage or worsening cerebral edema, prolonged observation in the ED or admission is warranted in many cases with moderate injury.

Blunt Trauma—Severe

The child with severe head trauma is at risk for sudden intracranial catastrophe, acute respiratory insufficiency, or a secondary insult (e.g., brain swelling) to the central nervous system. After initial steps to assess the adequacy of the airway,

TABLE 104.4

MANAGEMENT OF SEVERE MULTIPLE TRAUMA

Time (min)	Phase	Action	Phase description
0	1	A	Airway, respiration, pulse, active hemorrhage, capillary refill, level of consciousness (AVPU or GCS score)
		T	Airway management with stabilization of cervical spine (bag-valve-mask, endotracheal intubation) (Surgical airway PRN)
			Ventilation with $F_{IO_2} = 1.00$, mild hyperventilation
			Cardiac compression (cardiopulmonary resuscitation) as needed
			Intravenous access/volume infusion
			Decompress pneumothorax/thoracostomy, tube placement as needed
			Relieve tamponade, control major hemorrhage
			Elevated head of bed to 30 degrees if no signs of shock
			Exposure—remove all clothing
			Wrap/bind pelvis
		M	Respiratory rate, pulse oximetry
			Heart rate (electrocardiogram)
			Blood pressure (mercury or Doppler)
		D	Complete blood cell count, type and cross-match, chemistries (glucose, amylase, alanine transaminase, aspartate transaminase)
5	2	A	Adequacy of airway, breathing, and circulation
			Level of consciousness (AVPU or GCS score)
			Temperature
			Penetrating wounds
		T	Nasogastric tube (orogastric if suspected midface fracture)
			Intravenous access, intraosseous, central catheter, or cut down as needed
			Thoracotomy or thoracostomy tube as needed
			Pericardiocentesis as needed
			Drug therapy (e.g., epinephrine)
			Blood transfusion/volume
			Prevent or treat increased ICP
		M	Heart rate, respiratory rate, pulse oximetry, blood pressure
			ET_{CO_2} if intubated
			Temperature (especially infants)
		D	ABGs PRN
10	3	A	Adequacy of airway, breathing, and circulation
		T	Additional venous access PRN/volume
			Urinary catheter (except in suspected urethral disruption)
			Arterial access as needed
			Thoracotomy as needed
			Drug therapy, including for pain management
			Avoid hypothermia
			Operating suite as needed
		M	Heart rate, respiratory rate, pulse oximetry, blood pressure
			ET_{CO_2} if intubated
			Temperature (especially infants)
		D	ABGs PRN
20	4	A	Adequacy of airway, breathing, and circulation
			GCS score, neurologic assessment
			Repeat full examination
		T	Cervical traction as needed
			Splint fractures
			Drug therapy (e.g., tetanus toxoid or tetanus immune globulin, antibiotics)
		M	Heart rate, respiratory rate, pulse oximetry, blood pressure
			Consider ICP bolt if severe head injury
		D	Repeat laboratory studies PRN

A, assessment; T, treatment; M, monitoring; D, diagnostics; AVPU, *a*lert, *v*erbal stimuli response, *p*ainful stimuli response, *u*nresponsive; GCS, Glasgow Coma Scale; ICP, intracranial pressure; ET_{CO_2}, end-tidal carbon dioxide; ABG, arterial blood gas; PRN, as needed.

TABLE 104.5

SEVERITY OF BLUNT HEAD TRAUMA

		Physical examination	
Category	History	Vital signs	Local findings
Mild	Minimal force No/momentary LOC	Normal	GCS score = 15 Abrasions/contusions
Moderate	Significant force LOC 1–5 min	Normal	GCS score ≥ 13 Drowsiness
Severe	Critical force LOC >5 min	Abnormal	GCS score ≤ 12 Focal neurologic abnormalities

GCS, Glasgow Coma Scale; LOC, loss of consciousness.

breathing, and circulation, these functions should be supported as necessary. The cervical spine should managed as if there is a presumed injury and should be stabilized with a semirigid collar or foam head immobilizers. Gentle opening of the airway with maintenance of the head in the neutral position allows the patient's passive ventilation to become adequate in many instances. If intubation is required immediately, extension of the neck should be avoided and an assistant should stabilize the cervical spine during the procedure. In less urgent situations, intubation may be deferred until a cross-table lateral radiograph of the cervical spine is obtained. In all cases, supplemental oxygen should be administered and two large-bore IV cannulas inserted. Most children with serious head injury will hyperventilate spontaneously if their airway is patent, and this will decrease their cerebral blood flow, helping to maintain normal ICP. Intubated, apneic children should be hyperventilated manually to achieve a $PaCO_2$ of 30 to 35 mm Hg. Ideally, continuous, noninvasive end-tidal CO_2 monitoring with an arterial blood gas analysis obtained to assess CO_2 correlation should be the goal in the ED. An arterial catheter can be placed as needed. Corticosteroids have not been shown to be beneficial and are not recommended by most authorities. Osmotic agents are not used prophylactically, but mannitol (0.5 to 1 g per kg of a 20% solution) is occasionally necessary to decrease ICP when acute herniation is suspected or proven.

Standard skull radiographs provide little useful information for the patient with serious head injury. More efficient management calls for an immediate CT scan to evaluate the intracranial space. Rarely, neurosurgical intervention must precede imaging of the cranial contents. See Chapter 105 for more specific management.

LOCALIZED NECK TRAUMA

Classification

The larynx and trachea, carotid arteries, jugular veins, spinal cord, and esophagus all pass within the confined anatomic space of the neck. Thus, both penetrating and nonpenetrating insults can cause devastating injuries. All penetrating trauma, with the exception of tangential wounds superficial to the platysma muscle, should be considered serious and be referred promptly for surgical evaluation and possible exploration. Weapons or objects protruding from the neck should be left in place. Children with neck trauma (see Chapter 115) should be carefully examined in the ED for thoracic injuries such as pneumothorax.

Isolated blunt trauma to the neck does not occur often in children. However, the potential for major disruptions of the airway or large vessels demands a thorough evaluation. The examiner should palpate for crepitus, unequal carotid pulses, an acute hematoma that carries a risk of expansion, and cervical spine tenderness. On the basis of the history and physical findings, an estimate of the severity of the injury can be made (Table 104.6). A thorough neurologic examination, with

TABLE 104.6

SEVERITY OF BLUNT NECK TRAUMA

		Physical examination	
Category	History	Vital signs	Local findings
Mild	Minimal force	Normal	Abrasions/contusions
Moderate	Significant force	Normal	Refusal to move head Cervical spine tenderness
Severe	Critical force	Abnormal	Crepitus Expanding hematoma Unequal carotid pulses Paralysis or sensory loss

particular emphasis on determining if there may be spinal cord injury, is essential.

Management

Penetrating Trauma

Wounds clearly superficial to the platysma muscle are appropriate for repair in the ED. Children with penetrating injuries deep to the platysma require stabilization and subsequent surgical evaluation. Initial measures are directed at establishing a patent airway, providing adequate ventilation, controlling hemorrhage, and restoring the circulation. Protruding objects should be left in place by the physician in the ED. Neck exploration is recommended for the following: continued bleeding from the wound, blood in the aerodigestive tract, subcutaneous emphysema, stridor, hoarseness/aphonia, or neurologic deficits.

Blunt Trauma—Mild

If the history is one of a minimal force and no physical findings are indicative of trauma to the deeper structures, the child may be symptomatically treated and discharged from the ED. Exceptions may include patients with underlying illnesses, such as hemophilia, who are at potential risk for delayed complications. Follow-up after discharge should be clearly defined to ensure intervention if symptoms indicate a worsening situation, before compromise to internal structures occurs.

Blunt Trauma—Moderate

The child with an apparent moderate injury to the neck by definition has no evidence of respiratory or vascular compromise. However, either the history of the amount of force involved or the local findings may raise the possibility of cervical spine or other injuries. Such patients require immobilization of the cervical spine with a semirigid collar or foam head immobilizers and a meticulous neurologic examination. As a first step, a cross-table lateral radiograph of the cervical spine should be obtained with the child immobilized, often in the ED. If this first radiograph shows all seven cervical vertebrae to be intact and properly aligned, a complete radiologic evaluation of the cervical spine can be performed, which may include antero-posterior, oblique, and open-mouth views. The discovery of a bony or ligamentous injury requires consultation with appropriate specialists. A focused CT scan over the suspected area of injury may be considered for further evaluation of vertebral injury. Spinal cord injury without radiographic abnormality (SCIWORA) may be present and should be pursued when symptoms or signs are suggestive. A magnetic resonance imaging may be required to evaluate injuries to the spinal cord or adjacent soft tissues. The neurologically intact child with a normal cervical spine evaluation and no other neck trauma who remains well on repeat physical examination may be discharged after observation. If there are particular concerns, the child should have follow-up scheduled within several days with a specialist to assess for ligamentous neck injury.

Moderate trauma to the anterior neck requires careful evaluation for possible disruption of the major vessels, trachea, and esophagus. Cervical spine radiographs may outline the airway adequately. However, it is important to pay attention to the alignment of the larynx and trachea and to check for air in the soft tissues resulting from a tear in the airway or esoph-agus. The carotid triangle must be palpated carefully. If there is a hematoma or abnormality of the pulse, referral for possible a CT angiogram should be made.

Blunt Trauma—Severe

Classification of blunt neck trauma as severe indicates concern for overt injury to the airway, the major vessels, or the spinal cord. The initial goals of management are establishment of a patent airway, stabilization of the cervical spine, and IV access. The first choice for the establishment of the airway is orotracheal intubation, with maintenance of the patient's head in the neutral position. The inability to intubate a critical airway requires an immediate surgical approach to the trachea. Blood should be sent for a type and cross-match; if vascular injury is suspected, multiple units of blood should be made available. A surgical consultant should decide whether to proceed with an exploration in the operating room or to rely on further diagnostic studies such as bronchoscopy, CT angiography, and/or esophagoscopy.

LOCALIZED THORACIC TRAUMA

Classification

Penetrating chest injuries (see Chapter 118) are extremely relevant to physicians in the ED because they may be rapidly life threatening if untreated, yet usually respond to fairly straightforward therapeutic maneuvers. Any object that enters the thoracic cavity will result in significant injury. Patients with large open wounds or with instability of vital signs should be considered to have sustained life-threatening trauma.

Blunt chest trauma is seen more often than penetrating injury in civilian practice in general and in children in particular. Although there are no studies on the percentage of chest injuries classified as mild in childhood, statistics are available for older patients. Newman et al. found that 53% of chest injuries sustained by adults in motor vehicle accidents were merely bruises or abrasions. As with trauma to other anatomic regions, blunt thoracic trauma can be divided into mild, moderate, and severe categories (Table 104.7).

Management

Penetrating Trauma

Patients with mild injury, in which the wound clearly entered only the superficial tissues and not the thoracic cavity, may need only ED management. However, for any knife or gunshot injuries, it is advisable to have an experienced physician explore the wound and to obtain radiographs to determine the extent of injury.

Patients with deeper wounds require chest radiography, a CBC count, and blood type and cross-match. A CT angiogram may be necessary in the stable patient with a suspected aortic injury. An open pneumothorax should be covered with an occlusive dressing sealed on three sides and then a chest tube thoracostomy should be placed away from the dressing. A tube thoracostomy should also be performed to drain a hemothorax. Hemorrhage can be managed starting with crystalloid, followed by blood replacement. For the child sustaining a

TABLE 104.7

SEVERITY OF BLUNT CHEST TRAUMA

		Physical examination	
Category	History	Vital signs	Local findings
Mild	Minimal force	Normal	Abrasions/contusions
Moderate	Significant force	Tachypnea	Splinting
		Normal pulse and blood pressure	Bony tenderness
			Decreased breath sounds
Severe	Critical force	Abnormal pulse or blood pressure	Flail chest
			Distant heart tones
			Absent breath sounds

cardiopulmonary arrest while in the ED after a penetrating thoracic injury, immediate resuscitative thoracotomy may be lifesaving.

Blunt Trauma—Mild

The child with a history of a minimal blow to the chest, normal vital signs, and no local signs of trauma other than abrasions or contusions has sustained a mild injury. The combination of absent or minimal bony tenderness, a normal respiratory rate, symmetric breath sounds, and normal heart rate obviates the need for radiologic evaluation of the thoracic cage or its contents.

Blunt Trauma—Moderate

If the history indicates significant force, significant bony tenderness is elicited, or there is a question of abnormal breath or cardiac sounds, a chest radiograph, an electrocardiogram (EKG), and a CBC count are indicated. Particularly in children, a pneumothorax may follow blunt injury with or without a rib fracture. Widening of the mediastinum on chest radiograph suggests disruption of the aorta. The detection of a solitary rib fracture is not important per se because no specific treatment is necessary. However, it raises the suspicion of visceral or vascular disruption, given the force required to cause a rib fracture, particularly in a younger child. Fracture of the first rib is correlated in adults with injuries to the great vessels. Although the data are scant in pediatrics, an injury to the first rib may require the patient to have a CT angiogram. The chest radiograph may provide a clue to the diagnosis of pericardial hemorrhage (by showing a slightly enlarged cardiac silhouette), but it is more often normal in this condition. Bleeding into the pericardial space leading to tamponade will invariably manifest on the physical examination at some point; findings include tachycardia, followed by pulsus paradoxus, hypotension, distended neck veins, and muffled heart tones. A pulmonary contusion or aspiration may produce a consolidation on chest radiograph. The EKG is obtained as an aid in the diagnosis of myocardial contusion; elevated ST segments are characteristic of this entity. A troponin level may be considered in the evaluation of cardiac injury. Although it may be elevated in patients with minor injury, a normal troponin level and EKG indicate that a significant myocardial injury is unlikely.

In the setting of moderate blunt chest injury, it is advisable to achieve venous access and order a blood type and crossmatch. Sophisticated diagnostic studies, such as CT angiogram, are reserved for children with abnormal findings on the prelim-

inary evaluation. Admission for observation is often warranted; however, the child who shows improvement on examination over the observation interval with normal vital signs and does not have an abnormal chest radiograph, EKG, or CBC may often be discharged.

Blunt Trauma—Severe

The child with abnormal vital signs or local findings indicative of internal injuries has sustained an immediate life-threatening injury. Initial therapy includes airway management, the institution of two large-bore IV catheters, and the administration of supplemental oxygen. Depending on the condition of the child, chest tube insertion may be necessary for the treatment of hemopneumothorax before radiographic studies are obtained. In selected circumstances, resuscitative thoracotomy in the ED may be beneficial, although in blunt trauma to the chest, the outcome is almost uniformly poor if there has been cardiopulmonary arrest. Admission to the hospital is mandatory, and a full diagnostic evaluation should be performed to ascertain the need for surgical intervention.

LOCALIZED ABDOMINAL TRAUMA

Classification

Penetrating abdominal injuries (see Chapters 107 and 112) often cause moderate to severe trauma. However, the physician may cautiously define a small category of mild injuries, depending on the weapon involved.

All gunshot wounds must be considered at least moderate because almost all penetrate the peritoneum. Of those that penetrate the peritoneum, most cause visceral injury. If the vital signs are abnormal after a gunshot, the trauma should be considered severe.

Stab wounds, in contrast, may be superficial to the peritoneum. The patient with stable vital signs and an apparent superficial stab wound may be judged to have a mild injury if local exploration confirms the clinical impression. Stab wounds that violate the peritoneum should be considered moderately serious, and the patient should be referred for immediate surgical consultation. By definition, stab wounds that lead to unstable vital signs have produced severe trauma.

Overall, blunt abdominal trauma is much more common than penetrating injury in children. Most children evaluated in the ED for blunt trauma to the abdomen will have relatively minor injuries.

Management

Penetrating Trauma

All gunshot wounds are of at least moderate severity. Thus, these children require two large-bore IV catheters (preferably inserted above the diaphragm); a nasogastric tube; radiographs of the abdomen and chest; and laboratory studies, which may include CBC count, urinalysis, amylase, aspartate transaminase (AST), and alanine transaminase (ALT) concentrations, and blood type and cross-match. In the child with unstable vital signs, appropriate resuscitation should be initiated and laparotomy urgently considered. A decubitus or upright abdominal radiograph may be obtained to evaluate for free air under the diaphragm. Otherwise in a stable patient, an initial CT scan may be preferable to delineate the extent and location of internal injury. All patients will require hospitalization.

Stab wounds produce variable degrees of internal injury, and the approach to management differs among institutions. Patients with abnormal vital signs require stabilization in the ED, including appropriate resuscitative measures, IV access, a nasogastric tube, radiographs, and laboratory studies. Transfer to the operating room may be necessary on an urgent basis. Patients whose vital signs are stable are evaluated further by local exploration or laparotomy.

Blunt Trauma—Mild

Mild blunt abdominal injuries often occur when there is contusion of the abdominal wall from local trauma (e.g., a punch from a fist, a short fall). After a careful history and physical examination, the patient may be discharged home if there is no abdominal tenderness and no emesis. If there is suspicion for kidney injury, usually only a urinalysis for RBCs is required.

Blunt Trauma—Moderate

Moderate blunt abdominal trauma is often seen in patients with multiple injuries or those in whom there has been an isolated but forceful blow to the abdomen. These patients should have laboratory studies that include a CBC count, amylase, AST and ALT, and blood type and cross-match. At least one IV catheter should be inserted, preferably in veins of the upper extremities that are above the level of the injury. A CT scan for the evaluation of intraabdominal injury may be indicated for patients with abdominal tenderness, low systolic blood pressure, elevated ALT and/or AST, hematocrit less than 30%, or urinalysis with more than 5 RBCs per high-power field. In addition, a CT scan of the abdomen may be considered for patients with a GCS score of 13 or less. In many cases, hospitalization or prolonged observation in the ED is indicated. Other imaging studies, such as IV pyelography, are obtained in selected situations (see Chapters 107 and 112).

Blunt Trauma—Severe

Severe blunt abdominal trauma often warrants prompt surgery after an initial stabilization of the vital signs. In general, patients who have stable vital signs after initial fluid resuscitation may be evaluated with CT scanning to define intraabdominal injuries and bleeding. The scans help define the need for surgery, especially if a hepatic or splenic injury producing limited hemorrhage is identified. A Focused Assessment Sonography for Trauma (FAST) examination may be useful, especially in the hypotensive trauma patient who may be too unstable for immediate CT evaluation of the abdomen. The FAST examination may also be used in the setting in which an unstable patient with a decreased level of consciousness requires a CT scan of the brain, and potential operative intervention, to determine the presence of possible intraabdominal bleeding that may require laparotomy.

In the presence of significant hematuria or strong suggestion of renal injury, a CT scan should be performed (see Chapter 112). In symptomatic patients with severe blunt trauma, the absence of RBCs in the urine is not by itself sufficient evidence of an intact genitourinary tract. Avulsion of the renal pedicle may occur without hematuria.

EXTREMITY TRAUMA

Classification

Most injuries to the extremities of children (see Chapter 115) seen in the ED are mild. A few injuries are of moderate extent, and occasionally, extremity trauma may be life or limb threatening. Both penetrating (Table 104.8) and nonpenetrating (Table 104.9) trauma can range in their severity. With penetrating

TABLE 104.8

SEVERITY OF PENETRATING EXTREMITY TRAUMA

| Category | History | Physical examination | |
		Vital signs	Local findings
Mild	Minimal force	Normal	Laceration
Moderate	Significant force (e.g., stab)	Normal	Laceration of tendon or nerve Significant venous hemorrhage
Severe	Critical force (e.g., gunshot)	Abnormal	Partial/complete amputation of arm or leg Arterial hemorrhage Open fracture

TRAUMA

TABLE 104.9

SEVERITY OF BLUNT EXTREMITY TRAUMA

		Physical examination	
Category	History	Vital signs	Local findings
Mild	Minimal force	Normal	Contusions/point tenderness
Moderate	Significant force	Normal	Obvious dislocation of major joint
	Crush injury		Displaced fracture
Severe	Critical force	Abnormal	Decreased or absent pulses

wounds, the major immediate concern is hemorrhage, although impairment of neurovascular or musculoskeletal integrity with concomitant loss of long-term function is also a consideration. In contrast, nonpenetrating trauma may cause vascular insufficiency without external bleeding.

Management

Penetrating Trauma

The child with mild penetrating trauma requires appropriate wound care and tetanus prophylaxis (see Appendix D) in the ED. A radiograph is indicated if a radiopaque foreign body (including glass) is suspected in the wound. Moderate injuries require careful physical examination and often local exploration to define the extent of the trauma and the degree of functional impairment. At times, prompt surgical consultation or follow-up with a specialist is indicated. Some injuries require repair in the operating room; however, others—even extensive lacerations or extensor tendon disruptions—may be handled, time permitting, in the ED by an experienced physician. Surgical referral is mandatory for children in the severe category, and it is important to proceed as rapidly as possible when vascular damage is suspected.

Blunt Trauma—Mild

Children with mild nonpenetrating injuries often require a radiograph to detect underlying fractures. Particularly, when there is tenderness at the end of long bones, careful consideration should be given to radiologic evaluation for growth plate (physeal) injuries, keeping in mind that a normal radiograph does not exclude a nondisplaced Salter-Harris type I fracture.

Blunt Trauma—Moderate

Obvious dislocations should be repositioned as expeditiously as possible, usually after radiographs confirm the diagnosis. Dislocations of large joints, such as the knee, hip, and elbow, can impeded the vascular supply if not promptly reduced. Depending on the joint involved, discharge is acceptable after reduction and radiologic reevaluation (e.g., shoulder, patella, metacarpal-phalangeal, or interphalangeal joints). Crush-type injuries may initially manifest with pain and swelling. Of particular concern is the possibility that crush injury may lead to a compartment syndrome over the ensuing 6 to 24 hours, necessitating observation. Fractures with an obvious deformity should be treated with the appropriate pain medications, and the extremity should be splinted in a position of comfort as long as there is no vascular compromise. If vascular compromise is apparent with decreased pulses in the injured extremity, the fracture should be reduced and then splinted.

Blunt Trauma—Severe

Extremity injury associated with hemodynamic disturbances or disruption of the vascular supply is categorized as a severe injury. These include degloving and crush (i.e., wringer-type) injuries, as well as some long-bone fractures with high-energy transfer (i.e., femur fractures in pedestrians struck by high-speed automobiles). Patients with severe extremity injuries should receive a rapid but thorough overall assessment, followed by prompt surgical consultation.

SUMMARY

Injuries, ranging from mild to severe, frequently present to the ED, and the challenge lies in executing a thorough evaluation so that injuries are not missed while obtaining the appropriate radiologic and/or laboratory studies. The approach to the injured child requires great care and clinical acumen to establish the extent of the trauma and institute appropriate treatment. Loss of life from occult internal hemorrhage or neurologic sequelae from a missed unstable cervical spine injury is devastating. Yet, physicians in the ED must also know when children need only a careful physical examination and when laboratory testing or admission is unwarranted. This chapter describes a brief schema for providing appropriate care to children with trauma in such a way that specific issues about management can be approached reasonably by the emergency physician. The subsequent chapters in this section further describe the specific management of traumatic injuries for each anatomic area of the body.

Suggested Readings

Abujamra L, Joseph MM. Penetrating neck injuries in children: a retrospective review. *Pediatr Emerg Care* 2003;19:308–313.

American College of Surgeons Committee on Trauma. *Advanced trauma life support for doctors.* Chicago, IL: American College of Surgeons, 2004.

Bowman S, Zimmerman F, Christakis DA, et al. Hospital characteristics associated with management of pediatric splenic injuries. *JAMA* 2005;294:2611–2617.

Cantor RM, Laeming JM. Evaluation and management of pediatric major trauma. *Emerg Med Clin North Am* 1998;16:229–256.

Capraro AJ, Mooney D, Waltzman ML. The use of routine laboratory studies as screening tools in pediatric abdominal trauma. *Ped Emerg Care* 2006;22:480–484.

Cervical spine immobilization before admission to the hospital. *Neurosurgery* 2002;50:S7–S17.

Cotton BA, Nance ML. Penetrating trauma in children. *Semin Pediatr Surg* 2004;13:87–97.

Dormans JP. Evaluation of children with suspected cervical spine injury. *J Bone Joint Surg* 2002;84-A:124–132.

Eppich WJ, Zonfrillo MR. Emergency department evaluation and management of blunt abdominal trauma in children. *Curr Opin Pediatr* 2007;19: 265–269.

Holmes JF, Gladman A, Chang CH. Performance of abdominal ultrasonography in pediatric blunt trauma patients: a meta-analysis. *J Pediatr Surg* 2007;42: 1588–1594.

Holmes JF, Sokolove P, Brant WE, et al. Identification of children with intra-abdominal injuries after blunt trauma. *Ann Emerg Med* 2002;39: 500–509.

Jaffe D, Wesson D. Emergency management of blunt trauma in children. *New Engl J Med* 1991;324:1477–1483.

Kuppermann N, Holmes JF, Dayan PS, et al., for the Pediatric Emergency Care Applied Research Network (PECARN). Identification of children at very low risk of clinically-important brain injuries after head trauma: a prospective cohort study. *Lancet* 2009;374:1160–1170.

Lloyd-Thomas AR. Paediatric trauma: primary survey and resuscitation, part I. *BMJ* 1990;301:334–336.

Mutabagani KH, Beaver BL, Cooney DR, et al. Penetrating neck trauma in children: a reappraisal. *J Pediatr Surg* 1995;30:341–344.

National Center for Injury Prevention and Control. *Injury Fact Book I, 2001–2002.* Atlanta, GA: Centers for Disease Control and Prevention, 2001.

National Center for Injury Prevention and Control. Web-based Injury Statistics Query and Reporting System (WISQARS). www.cdc.gov/ncipc/wisqars. Accessed October 15, 2008.

Newman RS, Jones IS. A prospective study of 413 consecutive car occupants with chest injuries. *J Trauma* 1984:24:129–135.

Palchak MJ, Holmes JF, Vance CW, et al. A decision rule for identifying children at low risk for brain injuries after blunt head trauma. *Ann Emerg Med* 2003;42:492–506.

Rees MJ, Aickin R, Kolbe A, et al. The screening pelvic radiograph in pediatric trauma. *Pediatr Radiol* 2001;31:497–500.

Schafermeyer R. Pediatric trauma. *Emerg Med Clin North Am* 1993;11:187–205.

Slack SE, Clancy MJ. Clearing the cervical spine of paediatric trauma patients. *Emerg Med J* 2004;21:189–193.

Stafford PW, Binman TA, Nance ML. Practical points in evaluation and resuscitation of the injured child. *Surg Clin North Am* 2002;82:273–301.

TRAUMA

CHAPTER 105 ■ MAJOR TRAUMA

MARK L. WALTZMAN, MD, AND DAVID P. MOONEY, MD

It's not the speed which kills, it's the sudden stop.

A. L. Moseley, Crash Investigator, Harvard University

Between the years 1950 and 1993, the overall annual death rate for children in the United States younger than 15 years declined substantially owing to the decreases in deaths associated with pneumonia, influenza, cancer, and congenital anomalies. In 2005, in the United States, unintentional injury, homicide, and suicide were the first, second, and fourth leading causes of death among persons aged 1 to 19 years, respectively. Injury continues to account for nearly one-half of all deaths in children from the ages of 1 to 14 years, with more than 7,000 fatalities per year in the United States. Nearly 22 million children are injured each year in the United States, surpassing all major diseases in children and young adults. Two of three childhood injuries occur in males. The peak age range is between 4 and 12 years, with the highest frequency at age 8 years. In the year 2000 alone, there were 37,115 injury-related emergency department (ED) visits by children being struck by a moving motor vehicle while in the street. Unintentional injury also accounts for approximately 30% of infant deaths. Data from the National Electronic Injury Surveillance System All Injury Program (NEISS-AIP), during July 2000 to June 2001, estimate 4.3 million sports- and recreation-related injuries treated in U.S. hospital emergency departments. This comprises 16% of all unintentional injury-related ED visits. Rates were highest among children 10 to 14 years of age. In 1996, the Consumer Products Safety Commission reported 116,800 nonfatal, toy-related, unintentional injuries requiring ED care; 56% involved children aged 0 to 4 years. The societal impact of years of life lost from childhood unintentional injury is staggering.

Along with unintentional injuries, data have demonstrated that between 1950 and 1993, the rates for childhood homicide tripled and the rates for childhood suicide quadrupled. In 2005, among children aged 1 to 4 years, homicide was the fourth leading cause of death, responsible for 375 deaths. In children 5 to 14 years of age, homicide was once again the fourth leading cause of death and suicide was the fifth. Data from 26 high-income countries with populations of 1 million or more contain 2,872 deaths among children younger than 15 years for a period of 1 year. Homicides accounted for 1,995 of those deaths (59% in males). The homicide rate was five times higher for children in the United States than in the other 25 countries combined (2.57 per 100,000 compared with 0.51).

Firearms were reported to be involved in 2,154 deaths among children in 2005. Sixty-five percent were reported as homicides, 27.8% as suicides, and 7.1% as unintentional.

The mortality rate for children hospitalized after an accident is less than 1% in many pediatric trauma centers, but that is in part because 80% of all childhood trauma deaths occur either at the scene or in the hospital ED. The most common preventable cause of death in injured children is failure to secure the airway. As many as 18% of hospital trauma deaths are avoidable if a correct diagnosis is made and a treatment regimen is instituted. The most common cause of death in injured children is brain injury, which alone or in association with other injuries is responsible for 80% of trauma mortality. More than 50% of major injuries have associated injuries of the head, chest, and musculoskeletal system. Such multisystem injuries require the use of multiple medical disciplines, with varied diagnostic and treatment modalities, to achieve optimal care. These problems clearly place a large burden on the emergency physician to effect an improvement in outcome from childhood trauma.

A critical factor that influences outcome for the pediatric trauma patient is the recognition that a child's physiologic needs are not the same as those of an adult. Although the child will usually mount an appropriate physiologic and endocrinologic response to stress, the difference in response, such as enhanced peripheral vasoconstriction, may mask significant underlying derangement, such as impending circulatory collapse. Also, the greater surface area relative to body size results in greater susceptibility to body heat loss and insensible fluid loss. Water, minerals, trace elements, fat, and vitamins are all needed in greater maintenance portions in the child. Critically, the growing child has a significantly higher energy requirement than that of an adult. Equally important to proper tissue repair are greater total protein and essential amino acid nitrogen requirements, which are age dependent. Whether reversal of the malnourished state will influence morbidity and mortality in childhood trauma is speculative and the nutritional requirements during the acute phase on injury remain much less well defined in children than in adults. However, if data examining this question for adults are applicable to the child, attention to the patient's nutritional status is certainly important.

CAUSES OF MAJOR TRAUMA

The predominant mechanism of major injury in children is blunt trauma, with only 10% to 20% of children suffering a penetrating injury. Motor vehicle crashes accounted for more than 60% of all trauma deaths from ages 1 to 18 in 2005. Motor vehicle occupant death rates begin to climb steeply at age 13 years and peak at 18 years. Falls from heights and falls against fixed objects are the most frequent reasons for hospital admission; however, in 2005, it accounted for only 1.3% of deaths while drownings accounted for 11% and burns 5%.

Societal violence as a cause of death in children is increasing at an alarming rate. An estimated 8,625 child maltreatment fatalities occurred in the 50 states and the District of

Columbia from 1999 to 2002. Homicide rates in children have two peaks: from age 0 to 3 years and from 14 to 18 years. Death by homicide afflicts African-American citizens most severely. Presently, 1 of every 28 African-American males born today will die as a result of homicide.

In infancy, the most common causes of unintentional death are aspiration, suffocation, and motor vehicle crashes. In a 10-year period, more than 50,000 unintentional deaths will be reported in children younger than 5 years. Annually, there will be more than 70,000 injuries as a result of automobile crashes in the same population. Crash mortality statistics show that the youngest occupant in an automobile is the most vulnerable to injury.

Children from 5 to 9 years of age are most likely to be pedestrian injury victims. Overall, pediatric pedestrian injury accounts for 46% of motor vehicle fatalities. Boys in densely populated urban areas represent the largest group at risk. Injury from bicycle crashes is particularly common in children 6 to 16 years. There were 203 bicycle crash deaths, principally from head injury, in this age group alone in 1998.

Because the United States is a nation in which vehicles are driven on the right side of the road, injuries to the left side of the pedestrian are the most common. The resulting frequency of injured organs includes, in order, the spleen, genitourinary tract, gastrointestinal tract, liver, pancreas, pelvis, and major vessels.

ORGANIZATION OF THE TRAUMA SERVICE

The regionalization of trauma care in the United States has progressed but is still in an evolutionary stage. In many areas hospitals have been stratified on the basis of both their capability and their desire to care for the multiply injured child, but in other areas, no such stratification has occurred. The goal of trauma center verification, under the guidance of the American College of Surgeons' Committee on Trauma, is the triage of injured children to appropriate, qualified facilities. Because of the relative scarcity of pediatric trauma centers, approximately 70% of injured children still receive their care in adult facilities. The availability of rapid pediatric transport services may accelerate the regionalization of pediatric trauma care.

The effective management of pediatric trauma requires the integration of a multidisciplinary team, including surgeons, emergency physicians, critical care physicians, emergency and intensive care nurses, respiratory therapists, radiologists, and various subspecialty services (neurosurgery, orthopedic surgery, etc.), as well as the ready availability of laboratory and operating room facilities. Each institution must develop its own organizational response plan for pediatric trauma with a well-established chain of command with an appropriately designated leader, a responsibility that may change hands as additional personnel arrive for resuscitation in the ED. The role of this leadership position in a hospital trauma service is to accept responsibility for patient care and organize the multiple specialists needed to care for the patient with multisystem injury. Such organization begins at the scene of an injury and includes transport, patient triage after initial

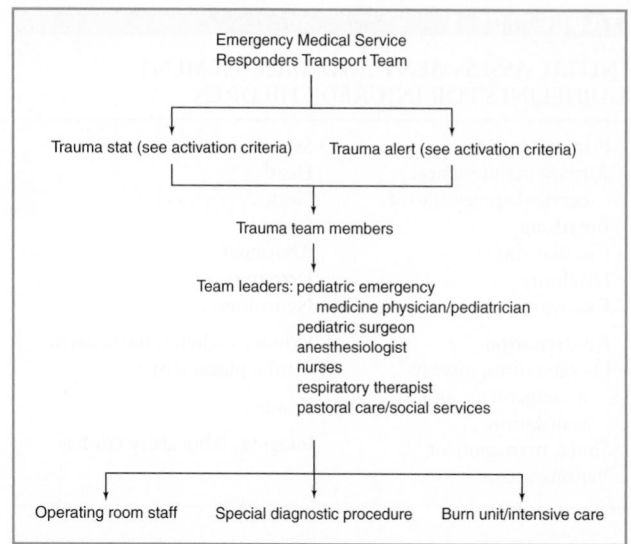

FIGURE 105.1 Sample flow diagram of a response from the emergency medical services team that is placed into action when or before a victim of serious trauma arrives in the emergency department.

evaluation, and care once the patient arrives in the hospital ED. Subsequently, the decision to transfer the child to a hospital with a higher level of capability, admit the child to the ward or to the intensive care unit, or take the child straight to the operating room will be made by the team leader after consultation with the specialists involved. If it becomes clear that the predominant injury is to a single-body system, it may be appropriate for the team leader to transfer patient care responsibility to the designated head of a given subspecialty. Figure 105.1 demonstrates a flow diagram of a response to the traumatized child, an example of organizational schema put into action when or before a victim of serious trauma arrives in the ED. The trauma team should conduct mock resuscitations to be prepared for the unusual critically injured child.

ASSESSMENT AND MANAGEMENT

Initial Evaluation

Guidelines for the evaluation and management of trauma victims have been well established by the American College of Surgeons. A list of priorities needs to be established in advance for the logical approach to the trauma victim—priorities that are similar to those for severely ill ED patients. It is also imperative that during injury assessment, a simultaneous patient management protocol be initiated in a logical sequence. After prehospital evaluation and care, the injured child is transported to the hospital. A rapid and reproducible schema of immediate, simultaneous, and subsequent evaluation and treatment principles should be applied to every child who may potentially have major or multiple trauma (Table 105.1). This initial assessment includes a primary survey,

TABLE 105.1

INITIAL ASSESSMENT AND MANAGEMENT
GUIDELINES FOR INJURED CHILDREN

Primary survey	Secondary survey
Airway maintenance, cervical spine control	Head
	Neck
Breathing	Chest
Circulation	Abdomen
Disability	Extremities
Exposure	Neurologic
Resuscitation	**Urinary catheter, nasogastric tube placement**
Oxygenation, airway management, and ventilation	
	Triage
Shock management	**Imaging, laboratory studies**
Venous access	

TABLE 105.2

CRITERIA FOR TRAUMA ACTIVATION

Trauma stat
Physiologic
Cardiopulmonary arrest
Hypotension per age
Respiratory distress
Neurologic failure (Glasgow Coma Scale score <8)
Trauma score <12
Anatomic
Penetrating (gunshot or stab) wound to head, chest, or abdomen
Facial/tracheal injury with potential airway compromise
Burn >30% BSA; inhalation airway burn
Major electrical injury

Trauma alert
Mechanism
Ejected from motor vehicle
Extrication time of >20 min
Fatality of another passenger in motor vehicle accident
Intrusion of vehicle ≥20 in by collision
Vehicle traveling at ≥20 mph in pedestrian accident or passenger unrestrained in motor vehicle accident (≥35 mph restrained)
Fall >20 ft
Run over by vehicle
Lightning
Anatomic
Significant injuries both above and below the diaphragm
Two or more proximal long bone fractures
Burn of 15%–30% BSA (second/third degree)
Traumatic amputation of limb proximal to wrist or ankle
Crush injury of torso
Spinal injury with paralysis

BSA, body surface area.

resuscitation, secondary survey, and subsequent triage. Two key principles must be followed in the initial assessment of the trauma patient. First, if any physiologic threat to the patient is identified, this threat must be treated immediately. The order of priority is airway, breathing, and then circulation (ABC). For example, a problem with breathing, such as relief of a tension pneumothorax, is addressed before proceeding with intravenous (IV) access. Second, if at any point in the patient's secondary survey or subsequent care there is unexpected physiologic deterioration, the primary survey is rapidly repeated in order of priority (ABC). An organized team of trained responders, when available, should be activated on notification of the impending arrival or simultaneously on the unexpected arrival of a child with multiple injuries. All participants of the trauma care team should fulfill their role in this initial evaluation and treatment of the patient (Fig. 105.1). The indication for team activation may vary depending on local personnel but should minimally include all children with anatomic or physiologic signs of significant injury, as listed in Table 105.2. Trauma team activation based solely on mechanism of injury criteria has been proven inaccurate and may lead to high rates of unnecessary activation. The principles of crisis resource management should be utilized to guide the flow of the evaluation and resuscitation.

Primary Survey

The first priority in assessment and management is to secure an adequate airway while concomitantly stabilizing the neck to protect the cervical spinal cord, using the chin-lift or jaw-thrust maneuver and clearing the oropharynx of accumulated foreign debris and secretions. A cervical spine injury should be assumed to be present in all patients with major trauma, especially those injured above the clavicle. Therefore, the neck should be neither hyperextended nor hyperflexed while securing the airway. All patients with major trauma should receive supplemental oxygen therapy. Before any effort at intubation, artificial ventilation should be established using a bag-valve-mask device (see Chapter 1). Cricoid pressure

should be performed while preparations are made for an artificial airway. This maneuver prevents possible aspiration of gastric content caused by passive regurgitation and/or increased intragastric pressure. It is imperative to anticipate the "difficult airway" before attempting intubation. Findings suggestive that endotracheal intubation may be difficult include patients with a small mouth, inability to open the mouth, temporomandibular joint abnormalities, narrow receding mandible, protuberant maxilla (overbite), large tongue, less than 6-cm distance between the mandible and thyroid prominence, inability to place in the "sniffing position" (such as with suspected cervical spine injury), or patients with a short, full, or bull neck, or those patients with the presence of a neck mass such as a large hematoma. If the airway is deemed "highly" difficult, airway management with bag-valve-mask ventilation may be preferred until a definitive airway can be established more safely. In patients with significant facial trauma, the laryngeal structures are often surprisingly preserved and at least one attempt at visualization of the airway should be attempted prior to a surgical airway. In children younger than 8 years, the choice of surgical airway is most often a needle cricothyroidotomy.

Breathing is evaluated once a patent airway has been secured and comprises adequate air exchange with normal oxygen saturation and carbon dioxide excretion. The early use of oxygen saturation monitoring is important. Compromise of ventilatory function in an injured child most often occurs secondary to a depressed sensorium. It may also be caused by airway occlusion, restriction of lung expansion, and direct pulmonary injury (see Chapter 18). Ventilatory function in both the intubated and nonintubated patients may be accurately assessed via end-tidal CO_2 detection and the evaluation of the capnogram. Compromise of diaphragmatic excursion is a special hazard in children because of the increased importance of their diaphragms in ventilation. Gastric distension, a common event in an injured child, may significantly limit diaphragmatic excursion. Therefore, the early use of a nasogastric or an orogastric tube to decompress the stomach may be considered. If the child is obtunded or comatose, ventilation may require the use of a bag-valve device that is connected to a mask or an endotracheal tube to produce an appropriate rise in the chest and adequate oxygen saturation. Prompt recognition of and attention to a hemothorax or pneumothorax, especially with mediastinal shift secondary to tension, is essential for the management of breathing (see "Secondary Survey" section). Thoracic subcutaneous emphysema in an injured child should be considered a sign of a pneumothorax until determined otherwise.

Circulation is initially assessed by examining the pulse, skin color, and capillary refilling time. From this information, the peripheral perfusion and oxygenation may be estimated. A palpable peripheral pulse will generally correlate with a pressure greater than 80 mm Hg; an absent peripheral pulse but a palpable central pulse indicates a pressure greater than 50 to 60 mm Hg. In a normovolemic patient, the capillary refilling time, as assessed by color return after blanching, will be within 2 seconds. External hemorrhage should be controlled by direct pressure or pneumatic splints, but the application of an extremity tourniquet to bleeding, while becoming

TABLE 105.3

AVPU METHOD FOR ASSESSING LEVEL OF CONSCIOUSNESS

A—*A*lert	P—*P*ainful stimuli, responds to
V—*V*oice, responds to	U—*U*nresponsive

more common in adult trauma patients, remains to be evaluated in children.

To assess patient disability, a rapid neurologic examination is completed to establish the level of consciousness, as well as pupillary size and reaction. Table 105.3 provides a list of the AVPU (*a*lert, *v*erbal stimuli response, *p*ainful stimuli response, *u*nresponsive) method of assessing the level of consciousness, in addition to pupillary assessment as previously mentioned. The Glasgow Coma Scale (GCS; Table 105.4) provides a quantitative measure of the level of consciousness and may be useful for following the progression of the injury.

To facilitate both assessment and treatment, the patient should be fully undressed and exposed; however, careful attention must be paid to the maintenance of body heat. Radiant warmers, air shields, and IV fluid warmers are useful tools in maintaining adequate temperature control in the pediatric patient.

Resuscitation

Vascular access is an early necessity in resuscitation. Percutaneous cannulation of bilateral upper extremity veins with two large-bore cannulas is ideal. However, the size of the available veins may guide the choice of cannulas. In a hypovolemic child, the visible veins may be small. Successful placement of a 22- or 20-gauge cannula is preferable to a failed attempt to place a larger cannula. In a small child, one can give

TABLE 105.4

PEDIATRIC COMA

	Glasgow coma scale	Infant coma scale	Score
Eye opening	Spontaneous	Spontaneous	4
	To voice	To voice	3
	To pain	To pain	2
	None	None	1
Verbal response	Oriented	Coos, babbles	5
	Confused	Irritable cry, consolable	4
	Inappropriate	Cries to pain	3
	Garbled	Moans to pain	2
	None	None	1
Motor response	Obeys commands	Normal movements	6
	Localizes pain	Withdraws to touch	5
	Withdraws to pain	Withdraws to pain	4
	Flexion	Flexion	3
	Extension	Extension	2
	Flaccid	Flaccid	1

TRAUMA

relatively large volumes (per kilogram body weight) of fluids and blood through a small cannula. Improvement in vascular volume may then permit the placement of a larger cannula at an alternative site. Early resuscitation may also be begun by intraosseous infusion into the tibial marrow space by a transtibial needle, which has been simplified by the development of intraosseous insertion devices. Cannulation of antecubital veins is preferred, but the greater saphenous vein at the ankle offers a reasonable alternative. In a hypotensive child in whom peripheral access is quickly found to be unsuccessful, the femoral vein provides a safe site for the insertion of a central catheter, often accomplished rapidly using the Seldinger guide wire technique. However, a long, narrow, standard central catheter may be less effective than a large peripheral IV catheter for fluid resuscitation. Rapid cutdown access is best done on a basilic vein at the elbow or the saphenous vein either at the ankle or in the groin just below the saphenofemoral junction. Central vein cannulation above the diaphragm, although necessary at times, is not a preferred emergency access route and, in children, should be done only by experienced personnel.

At cannulation, blood should be sent for a type and crossmatch and a hematocrit, and a tube of blood should be held for chemical parameters if they are needed on the basis of physical findings (Table 105.5). Shock after major trauma usually occurs secondary to the acute loss of a 40% or more of the blood volume, although it may less often be cardiogenic or secondary to spinal cord injury. Shock secondary to an isolated brain injury is more common than previously believed, but other etiologies must be excluded first. The presence of shock must be assessed by appreciating whether inadequate organ perfusion exists. Any injured patient who has cold skin and tachycardia is in shock until proven otherwise. Reliance on the hematocrit alone may prove unreliable because an initial near-normal hematocrit level does not exclude the possibility of significant blood loss.

To quantify the extent of the problem and decide on treatment priorities, hemorrhagic shock can be classified according to severity (Table 105.6). Class I hemorrhage occurs with an up to 15% acute blood volume loss (up to a 250-mL blood loss in a 20-kg child), and physiologic changes will be minimal. A single 20 mL per kg IV fluid bolus should stabilize the circulation. Class II hemorrhage, 15% to 30% blood loss (approximately 250- to 500-mL blood loss in a 20-kg child), is associated with tachycardia and tachypnea along with a fall in pulse pressure, as catecholamine release produces elevation in peripheral vascular resistance. Such patients may have impaired capillary refilling, and they may develop early signs of poor mentation. These patients would typically be stabilized by one or two 20 mL per kg boluses of IV crystalloid. Class III hemorrhage is physiologically more significant, with 30% to 40% blood loss corresponding to 500 to 650 mL of blood in a 20-kg child. These patients have obvious signs of shock with altered mental status, tachycardia, tachypnea, and measurable diminution in systolic pressure.

Crystalloid resuscitation should begun promptly, and some patients will also require blood products. Class IV hemorrhagic shock, involving more than 40% blood loss, is immediately life threatening. Patients are mentally depressed, cold, and pale; they have profound tachycardia and tachypnea, the

pulse pressure is narrow, and there is no urine output. After rapid transfusion, such patients often require prompt operative intervention to stop ongoing blood losses.

Cardiogenic shock after major childhood injury is rare, but it could be a result of cardiac tamponade or myocardial contusion. Dilated neck veins in a patient with a decelerating injury, sternal contusion, or penetrating thoracic trauma should arouse such suspicion (see Chapters 84 and 118). Neurogenic shock classically presents with hypotension without tachycardia or vasoconstriction. Also, isolated head injuries may produce shock, though other causes of hypovolemia should always be sought in such patients. Septic shock rarely occurs immediately after injury, even in the face of abdominal contamination.

Crystalloid isotonic solution, preferably Ringer's lactate or normal saline solution, is the initial resuscitative fluid of choice for the patient in hypovolemic shock. The American College of Surgeons has specific recommendations for the management of hemorrhagic shock resulting from trauma. The initial crystalloid infusion is given as rapidly as possible in a dose of 20 mL per kg with careful monitoring of patient physiologic response. Table 105.6 emphasizes the anticipated fluid needs, depending on the degree of shock, and the formulation is based on the premise that the patient will require 300 mL of crystalloid for each 100 mL of blood loss. A simplified rule of thumb would be if shock is present, give 20 mL per kg of crystalloid; if no response, give another 20 mL per kg of crystalloid; and if there is no response, give a third 20 mL per kg of crystalloid or 10 mL per kg of packed red blood cells (RBCs). In adults with hemorrhagic shock, this resuscitation strategy is inferior to a blood plus fresh-frozen plasma resuscitation, though this therapy has not yet been evaluated in children. No response to three-bolus infusion in children suggests the need for operative intervention. The restoration of perfusion may be clinically assessed, although in unusual situations, invasive monitoring with elective placement of a central venous catheter may be helpful. A most useful practical guide is the monitoring of urinary output; 1 mL per kg per hour is optimum, although for children younger than 1 year, preferred output should approach 2 mL per kg per hour.

There are currently a number of published studies on "low-volume" fluid resuscitation (LVFR). In patients with *uncontrolled hemorrhagic shock* (which refers to an injury that can only be managed operatively, such as intrathoracic or intraabdominal trauma), the use of LVFR appears indicated. Several animal studies have confirmed the intuitive arguments raised for LVFR. These arguments include the one that, because internal hemorrhage cannot be controlled by external means, the body effectively tamponades (especially venous injuries) hemorrhage. IV fluid boluses, under these circumstances, raise central venous pressure, disrupt clots, dilute clotting factors, and worsen hemorrhage. As a result, end-organ oxygen delivery suffers. A prospective clinical trial by Bickell et al. randomized 598 adults older than 15 years with prehospital systolic blood pressures of 90 mm Hg to immediate versus delayed fluid resuscitation. They concluded that delaying aggressive administration of IV fluids to hypotensive patients with penetrating injuries to the torso until the time of operative intervention may improve outcome. Teach et al. retrospectively studied

TABLE 105.5

RAPID APPROACH TO PEDIATRIC TRAUMA PATIENTS

Time interval patient priority	System assessment	Initial therapy	System monitor	Diagnostic study
First 5 min Primary survey	Respiration	Cervical spine stabilization (sand bags, collar) Airway (bag-valve-mask, intubation)	End-tidal CO_2 monitor	Arterial blood gas
		Ventilation with 100% oxygen	Pulse oximetry	Arterial blood gas
	Pulse	Cardiac compression	Heart rate (electrocardiogram) Blood pressure	
	Ventilation	Needle/tube thoracostomy—tension pneumothorax Dressing to sucking chest wound		
	External hemorrhage	Compression		
Second 5 min Resuscitation	Perfusion	Intravenous/intraosseus needle access; 20 mL/kg crystalloid Needle pericardiocentesis Thoracotomy, aortic cross clamping	Perfusion Pulse Blood pressure PO_2, PCO_2, pH	Type and cross-match Complete blood cell count
	Level of consciousness	Nasogastric tube Urinary catheter Drugs	Temperature	Blood gas Urinalysis
Third 5 min Secondary survey	Ventilation Perfusion Head Neck Chest	Venous access Type specific blood Crystalloid Tube thoracotomy—pneumothorax, hemothorax	Perfusion Pulse Blood pressure Arterial line Foley catheter	Lateral neck film Chest radiograph
	Abdomen	Nasogastric tube		Plan for abdominal pelvic CT scan
	Pelvis Neurologic Extremities	Bony pelvis reconstruction Pelvic binder		Urgent intravenous pyelogram
Fourth 5 min Triage	Ventilation Perfusion Neurologic status	Splint fractures Drugs for intracranial pressure Type specific blood Intensive care unit Radiograph Operating room	Perfusion Pulse Blood pressure Temperature	Blood gas Head CT scan Intracranial pressure bolt

CT, computed tomography.

prehospital fluid therapy in 50 pediatric trauma patients and assigned them to one of three groups: (i) IV therapy detrimental, (ii) IV therapy inconsequential, and (iii) IV therapy beneficial. The authors found that IV therapy was inconsequential in 47 of 50 cases, potentially beneficial in 2 cases (children with external stab wounds whose bleeding was controlled at the scene), and potentially detrimental in 1 case (a child with a head injury). Data from the Iraq conflict reveal that delay in high-volume resuscitation may be beneficial in patients with a normal sensorium and a palpable peripheral pulse.

Blood transfusion preferably is done with fully cross-matched, warmed blood passed through a 160-m macropore filter. In the face of a transient or absent response to a rapid crystalloid infusion, fully cross-matched, type-specific, or type O-negative blood should be given as a whole-blood transfusion. In summary, fluid and blood are given rapidly enough to maintain stable vital signs and adequate urine output. Vasopressors, steroids, and sodium bicarbonate do not play a role in the initial treatment of hypovolemic shock. In massive transfusion situations in adults, resuscitation with a ratio of fresh-frozen plasma to packed RBCs of 1:1 leads to the best survival.

TABLE 105.6

THERAPEUTIC CLASSIFICATION OF HEMORRHAGIC SHOCK IN PEDIATRIC PATIENT

	Class I	Class II	Class III	Class IV
Blood volume loss[a]	Up to 15%	15%–30%	30%–40%	≥40%
Pulse rate	Normal	Mild tachycardia	Moderate tachycardia	Severe tachycardia
Blood pressure	Normal/increased	Normal/decreased	Decreased	Decreased
Capillary blanch test	Normal	Positive	Positive	Positive
Respiratory rate	Normal	Mild tachypnea	Moderate tachypnea	Severe tachypnea
Urine output	1–2 mL/kg/h	0.5–1.0 mL/kg/h	0.25–0.5 mL/kg/h	Negligible
Mental status	Slightly anxious	Mildly anxious	Anxious/confused	Confused/lethargic
Fluid replacement (3:1 rule)	Crystalloid	Crystalloid	Crystalloid % blood	Crystalloid % blood

[a]Assume blood volume to be 8%–9% of body weight (80–90 mL/kg).

While resuscitation is underway, a urinary catheter should be placed in patients who need ongoing close monitoring of organ perfusion. Urethral injuries are rare in children. However, urinary catheterization should not be attempted before a retrograde urethrogram has proven urethral integrity if blood has been noted at the urethral meatus or in the scrotum, or if there is abnormal prostate placement on rectal examination. The urinary specimen should be immediately analyzed for the presence of gross or microscopic blood. Patients with significant abdominal injury and those with inadequate airway protection should have a nasogastric or orogastric tube placed. In the presence of a basilar skull fracture, care must be taken in inserting a nasogastric tube to avoid passage into the brain through a cribriform plate fracture. An orogastric tube is preferred in such patients.

Secondary Survey

A rapid, systematic assessment of organ systems must be performed after securing the ABC. A pertinent history should at least include allergies, medications, past illnesses, time of last meal, and events preceding the injury.

A head examination includes evaluation of pupillary size and reactivity, a conjunctival and fundoscopic examination for hemorrhage or penetrating injury, and a quick assessment of visual acuity. Visualization of blood in the external auditory canal or behind the tympanic membrane raises suspicion for a basilar skull fracture. Thorough palpation of skull and mandible may detect fractures and dislocations, but if the airway is secure, further evaluation of maxillofacial bony trauma is of lesser priority in the total treatment plan.

Injury to the cervical spine is uncommon in children (see Chapter 115), but risk of injury must always be considered. This is especially true for any child with trauma above the clavicles. It is also true for young children who fall one or more floors, are hit by a motor vehicle at 30 mph or more, and who are unrestrained or poorly restrained occupants of a motor vehicle involved in a significant crash. In older children, sports injuries are the second most common cause of cervical spine injury. In a child with low risk for cervical spine injury (e.g., a fall when running), the "neck can be cleared" with a normal clinical examination in the fully awake, cooperative patient, similar to the adult NEXUS criteria. In the patient who is neurologically intact and has no tenderness over the cervical vertebrae, the clinician should actively maneuver the neck in controlled flexion, extension, and rotatory motion. If there are no symptoms or signs of spasm, guarding, pain, or tenderness, a decision can be made with a high degree of certainty that there is no fracture, ligamentous instability, or cord injury. Otherwise, adequate cervical spine radiographs are required to evaluate for a bony injury. Ligamentous disruption and dislocations of the cervical spine without radiographic evidence of bony injury are not uncommon in children because of the weakness of the soft tissue of the neck and the incomplete development of the bony spine. In approximately 30% of children with a spinal cord injury, no radiologic abnormality is present (SCIWORA). In patients with a high-risk mechanism of trauma, it is best to obtain anteroposterior, odontoid (in older children), and lateral views before "clearing" the neck. If the patient has an altered sensorium, a semirigid cervical collar should be left in place even if the three survey radiographs show negative findings. When the patient recovers sufficiently to permit a full evaluation of the neck, the collar can be removed. For unconscious patients not expected to awaken, the following should be performed: normal plain radiographs and the addition of either a normal cervical spine magnetic resonance imaging within 48 hours or normal flexion and extension views with simultaneous brain stem evoked potentials may serve to clear the spine and allow removal of the cervical collar.

Two situations require further discussion. First, if a seriously injured child has had an endotracheal tube placed, one can get a computed tomographic (CT) scan of C1 and C2 when getting a head CT scan, in place of the standard odontoid view. Second, if a patient is brought to the hospital with a helmet on (e.g., football or motorcycle) and there is no respiratory distress or other problem requiring immediate intubation, an initial cervical spine radiographic series can be performed before helmet removal (these helmets are designed to allow for adequate penetration of the x-ray beam). If it is necessary to remove the helmet before the neck is cleared, a two-person technique ensuring neck immobilization should be used.

Visual inspection of the chest may identify a rare sucking chest wound, best treated by immediate application of a sterile occlusive dressing; even more rarely, a major flail component, treated by splinting or endotracheal intubation; or a penetrating wound (see Chapter 115). Auscultation may not reveal a pneumothorax or hemothorax secondary to the broad transmission of breath sounds in a child. A prompt chest radiograph may be helpful in disclosing these conditions in stable patients. They should be treated by tube thoracostomy. Cardiac tamponade may be detected by muffled heart sounds, distended neck veins, and a narrow pulse pressure and should be relieved by prompt pericardiocentesis (see Section VII: Procedures). If the patient is stable, echocardiography may be used in making the diagnosis and in performing the procedure. A diagnosis of tension pneumothorax is supported by observing a contralateral tracheal shift and distended neck veins, in addition to diminished breath sounds. Anterior needle thoracostomy should provide relief, but tube thoracostomy should follow, with the placement of the tube to suction. If an impaled object is protruding from the chest or any part of a patient, it is best debrided from surrounding clothing and left in place until definitive operation. If the history suggests a severe deceleration injury and the chest radiograph demonstrates a widened mediastinum with or without a fractured first rib, a thoracic aortic injury is suggested. In the stable patient, a thoracic CT angiogram is promptly indicated.

The secondary abdominal examination establishes whether visceral injury exists (see Chapters 104 and 107); it is not meant to provide an exact diagnosis. Visceral injury should be suspected in the presence of abdominal wall contusion, distension, abdominal or shoulder pain, signs of parietal peritoneal irritation, gross hematuria, and/or shock. Hemodynamically stable patients with the previous findings should undergo an abdominal CT scan as soon as possible. Gastric distension may lead to left upper quadrant tenderness, even in patients with injuries remote to their abdomen. The passage of a nasogastric or orogastric tube may relieve this condition and prevent the need for imaging. Diagnostic peritoneal lavage (DPL), previously a mainstay of emergency trauma evaluation, should be considered only with blunt trauma in the patient who remains unstable despite resuscitation and in whom the diagnosis of abdominal injury is unclear. However, DPL has been supplanted by focused abdominal sonography for trauma, the focused abdominal sonography for trauma (FAST) examination, which may sensitively demonstrate intraperitoneal free fluid. The large majority of children with documented intraabdominal or retroperitoneal injury who remain stable or rapidly become so do not require surgery, rendering the findings of peritoneal RBCs much less helpful. The performance of a DPL prior to abdominal CT scan may introduce air, decreasing the ability of CT to diagnose this life-threatening condition.

A rectal examination is still essential, assessing sphincter tone, rectal integrity, prostatic position, pelvic fracture, and the presence of gross blood in the stool. The finding of microscopic blood on rectal examination adds little to the evaluation, and guaiac testing need not be performed.

A thorough extremity examination should assess deformity, contusions, abrasions, penetration, and perfusion, including pulse palpation. Although the presence of a distal extremity pulse does not exclude a concomitant proximal arterial injury, the presence of equal Doppler blood pressures makes it much less likely. Soft-tissue injuries should be thoroughly inspected both for wound foreign bodies and for the presence of devitalized tissue. Long bones should be palpated with rotational or three-point pressure for tenderness, crepitance, or abnormal movement, and pressure should be applied to the pubis and anterior iliac spines to assess for the presence

of pelvic instability. Sensation should be assessed in all limbs. Severe extremity angulations should be straightened and immobilized, and traction splints should be applied after an examination of distal neurological function and perfusion. Compound fracture sites should be covered with sterile dressings. Generous irrigation and debridement of open wounds not associated with fractures or joint injuries are beneficial in early wound care to minimize contamination before considering primary or delayed wound closure (see Chapter 124).

Hypothermia is a special risk in injured children, since a child has relatively more surface area than an adult. Hypothermia can develop in the prehospital setting and then worsen in the ED, where proper assessment and treatment may require full exposure of the patient. The dangers of hypothermia are impaired circulatory dynamics, impaired coagulation, increased peripheral vascular resistance, and increased metabolic demand. The use of overhead radiant warmers, warm blankets, and warmed IV solutions are important measures in combating the deleterious effects of hypothermia. These measures should be used as soon after arrival in the ED as possible when hypothermia is a concern. There has been increasing literature on the use of "controlled" mild hypothermia (32°C to 35°C) in the first hours after an ischemic event, which may prevent or mitigate permanent injuries. This effect has been shown most clearly for postanoxic brain injury but could also apply to other organs such as the heart and kidneys. Hypothermia has also been used as a treatment of traumatic brain injury, stroke, hepatic encephalopathy, myocardial infarction, and other indications.

The child with burn injury needs to have an initial appraisal of burn severity, including the depth, location, and type of burn (Table 105.7); an appraisal of the extent of the burned area, using the percentage of surface area for children up to or older than 10 years as defined in Table 105.8; and a determination of whether the injury also includes pulmonary, soft-tissue, or bony damage. Burns may be classified in the following categories:

- *Critical:* an inhalation injury; second-degree burns exceeding 30% of body surface area (BSA); third-degree burns exceeding 10% to 20% of the BSA; a complicating fracture or soft-tissue injury; extensive electrical burns; or extensive deep acid burns.

TABLE 105.7

BURN WOUND ASSESSMENT: BODY SURFACE ESTIMATION (ADULT VS. CHILD)

Anatomic area	Percentage adult surface (age >10 yr)	Percentage infant surface
Head	9	16
Right upper extremity	9	9
Left upper extremity	9	9
Right lower extremity	18	13
Left lower extremity	18	13
Anterior trunk	18	18
Posterior trunk	18	18
Neck	1	4
Total	100	100

TABLE 105.8

BURN INJURY

Classification	Morphology	Appearance	Cause
First degree	Superficial epidermis devitalized; vasodilation and vasocongestion	Erythema: blanches on pressure	Ultraviolet exposure; short flash
Second degree	Epidermal destruction; coagulation necrosis with congestion and fluid collection; skin elements remain viable for regeneration	Painful, erythematous, weeping, blisters, bullae; skin elements white, soft, and dry	Short flash or spill scald
Third degree	All skin elements destroyed; coagulation necrosis of subdermal plexus; capillary thrombosis	Dry, hard, inelastic with visible vein thrombosis	Flame, scald immersion; contact electrical

■ *Moderate:* 10% to 30% BSA second-degree burns; from 1% to 10% BSA third-degree burns and no involvement of the hands, feet, or genitalia.

■ *Minor:* less than 10% BSA second-degree burns and less than 1% BSA third-degree burns.

The burn victim should be undressed, and sterile covers should be placed over the burn wounds. IV fluid resuscitation is necessary promptly if the burn exceeds 20% of BSA (see Chapters 1 and 108). Referral to a burn center should be considered in critical burns, burns of the hands, feet or perineum, or cases with the possibility of devastating cosmetic and functional deficits.

Neurologic assessment includes a reevaluation of the level of consciousness, a repeat pupillary examination, and a thorough sensorimotor examination. Not only is serial reassessment critical but also quantification of the findings using a GCS is of benefit to detect early changes (Table 105.4; see Chapter 116). Any evidence of paralysis or paresis suggests a major neurologic injury and should be carefully documented. Until spinal cord injury is determined or ruled out in any patient with signs of central nervous system injury, maintain the patient in a semirigid cervical collar and immobilize him or her on a firm surface.

Supplemental studies (including regular and contrast imaging studies; biochemical analyses of liver, pancreatic, and renal function; and electrocardiographic analysis of cardiac function) may be performed after the secondary survey, as indicated by a history and physical examination. The routine use of a broad laboratory "panel" is unlikely to add to patient evaluation. Tetanus prophylaxis should be considered (see Chapters 92 and 104), and antibiotics should be administered if specifically indicated.

Imaging the Pediatric Trauma Patient

In any child with major trauma caused by a blunt mechanism, a basic radiographic survey series should be considered. Traditionally, this survey included cervical spine, chest, and pelvic radiographs. More recent studies have demonstrated that patients with a GCS score of 15, no distracting injury, no pain in the pelvic region, and a normal physical examination of their pelvis have a low incidence of pelvic fractures. In these patients, the routine use of pelvic radiographs is not necessary

and is also rarely helpful in the short-term initial management of the traumatized child. In a stable, cooperative patient, the clinician examines the cervical spine and then proceeds with radiographs as necessary. Additional survey radiographs of the thoracolumbar spine and extremities depend on clinical findings and the mechanism of trauma.

The primary or secondary survey may suggest a need for more definitive imaging studies. For example, any patient who is normotensive but has an abnormal GCS score should undergo a CT scan of the head. Other indications for a head CT scan include a history of posttraumatic seizures, prolonged lethargy or loss of consciousness, or an underlying medical risk factor such as hemophilia. A CT scan of the abdomen is indicated in a hemodynamically stable victim of blunt trauma who has physical signs of intraabdominal injury, gross hematuria, or a worrisome mechanism of trauma in the presence of neurologic compromise. Most CT scans of the abdomen for trauma should be performed with IV contrast alone. Double contrast (enteral and IV) may delay the process and increase the risk for aspiration. If a Foley catheter is in place, it should be clamped during the abdominal CT scan to provide information about the bladder. Because of the potential for injury to the liver or spleen in children with blunt abdominal trauma, an abdominal CT scan is more comprehensive in evaluating a patient with significant hematuria than an IV pyelogram.

The likelihood of positive findings in abdominal CT scans is significantly increased if three or more of the following indicators are present: (i) gross hematuria, (ii) lap belt injury, (iii) assault or abuse as a mechanism of trauma, (iv) abdominal tenderness, and (v) trauma score 12 or less. However, certain indicators alone, such as positive abdominal findings, worrisome mechanism of trauma (e.g., ejected from a motor vehicle), and neurologic compromise (e.g., GCS score of less than 10), warrant obtaining an abdominopelvic CT scan to document possible intraabdominal or retroperitoneal injury. In general, the accuracy of CT scans in diagnosing intraperitoneal or retroperitoneal injuries is 95% or better. The use of ultrafast and multiplanar CT scans increases the diagnostic accuracy of CT scans because of less motion artifact and better contrast enhancement. Ultrasound has been used successfully in the evaluation of the adult trauma patient using the FAST examination. In the hands of an experienced examiner, it can be performed in the ED and will document approximately 70% of the injuries to the liver, spleen, and/or kidneys

TABLE 105.9

PEDIATRIC TRAUMA SCORE[a]

Component	Category		
	+2	+1	−1
Size	>20 kg (40 lb)	10–20 kg	<10 kg
Airway	Normal	Maintainable	Unmaintainable
Systolic blood pressure	>90 mm Hg	50–90 mm Hg	<50 mm Hg
Central nervous system	Awake	Obtunded/loss of consciousness	Coma/decerebrate
Skeletal	None	Closed fracture	Open/multiple fractures
Cutaneous	None	Minor	Major/penetrating sum (pediatric trauma score)

[a]Pediatric trauma score for prehospital and in-hospital use.
From Tepas JJ III, Ramenofsky ML, Mollitt DL, et al. The pediatric trauma score as a predictor of injury severity: an objective assessment. *J Trauma* 1988;28:425–429. Copyright Lippincott Williams & Wilkins. Reprinted with permission.

through the demonstration of free intraperitoneal fluid. This may be an alternative when emergency CT scans of the abdomen are not available; however, its utility in the pediatric trauma patient has not been fully evaluated.

The major limitations of CT scans of the abdomen in trauma patients are in the diagnosis of hollow viscus injuries such as perforation of the bowel and bladder. Free intraperitoneal air is seen in only 25% of patients with a bowel perforation. Other signs, free fluid in the abdomen without solid organ injury, bowel wall thickening, and a mesenteric hematoma are also seen on CT scan in a minority of patients with documented bowel injury. In alert patients, serial abdominal examinations and serial CT scans may be helpful. In unconscious patients, DPL may be useful, although false-negative studies have been reported if this maneuver is done early after injury.

Finally, selective urologic contrast studies are indicated in two situations. First, a patient with gross blood at the meatus, especially if clinical and radiographic studies suggest a pelvic fracture, should undergo a retrograde urethrogram. Gross blood at the meatus often correlates with clinical and/or radiologic evidence of a pelvic fracture. If the urethra is damaged, a surgical or urologic consultation is essential. If the urethra is not damaged, a cystogram may be performed after carefully advancing the catheter into the bladder. Second, if a patient with blunt or penetrating abdominal trauma is too unstable for a CT scan, a one-shot IV pyelogram may be performed in the operating room during laparotomy. After IV administration of a bolus of 2 to 4 mL per kg of 50% diatrizoate sodium (Hypaque; Winthrop Laboratories), the clinician should obtain a survey film of the abdomen 5 minutes after injection. This study will usually confirm the function or malfunction of both kidneys and occasionally the upper ureters.

Triage

Definitive care may occur in the prehospital setting (e.g., endotracheal intubation), in the ED (e.g., chest tube placement), or in the intensive care unit or operating room. Triage is a process of patient assessment, prioritization of treatment, and selection of appropriate treatment location. In the early stages of

patient assessment, the precise diagnosis of anatomic injury is often impossible. To identify patients with a potential for major morbidity or at risk of dying, various physiologic scoring systems have been developed. In pediatric trauma, the most useful are the GCS score, the trauma score (TS), which uses the GCS (Table 105.4), and the pediatric trauma score (PTS) (Table 105.9). For the purposes of prehospital triage, admission to a designated pediatric trauma center is indicated in any patient with a GCS score of 12 or less, a TS of 12 or less, or a PTS of 8 or less. Field studies of the TS showed that at night, it is difficult to assess capillary refill and respiratory effort. Therefore, the most common tool used in prehospital triage is the revised trauma score (RTS), which deletes these two variables. Admission to a pediatric trauma center is then indicated for any of the following criteria: (i) GCS score of 12 or less, (ii) low systolic blood pressure per age, or (iii) abnormal respiratory rate per age. In the ED setting, a complete TS or PTS is usually obtained, but for trauma outcome studies, the RTS is the most commonly used tool.

The PTS is designed to give added emphasis to the importance of patient size and airway control in injured children. Indeed, studies confirm the validity of the PTS as a predictor of outcome: 9% mortality for PTS above 8 and 100% mortality for PTS of 0 or less. From 8 to 0, there is a linear relationship between decreased PTS and an increasing potential for mortality. Nevertheless, studies comparing TS, RTS, and PTS do not show any statistical advantage of PTS over the other two for the purposes of triage. In addition, many children with significant solid organ injuries were found to have a normal PTS. Therefore, whichever physiologic scoring system is selected, it should be used consistently and sequentially. For example, a repeat TS 1 hour after baseline TS shows how the patient is responding to treatment. Alternatively, it may reveal any delayed deterioration of the patient's condition and may suggest the need for more urgent intervention.

SUMMARY

Tables 105.5 and 105.10 describe a rapid approach to the patient. Over a 20- to 40-minute interval, the patient may be

TRAUMA

TABLE 105.10

EMERGENCY DEPARTMENT ASSESSMENT AND MANAGEMENT PLAN FOR INJURED CHILD

Assessment	Diagnosis	Management	Evaluation study
Airway/breathing		Clear airway Ventilate Intubate	
Cardiac function		External cardiac massage	Cardiorespiratory monitor
Shock	External hemorrhage Internal hemorrhage	Direct pressure Trendelenburg position Establish intravenous/ intraosseous access	CBC count CBC count
Head/neck injury	Closed head injury Possible cervical spine fracture	Normal perfusion, ventilation Cervical spine immobilization	CT scan, head Lateral neck radiograph
Chest injury	Cardiac contusion Hemopneumothorax Flail chest Sucking wound	Pericardiocentesis Tube thoracostomy Intubation/ventilation Sterile dressing	Chest radiograph Electrocardiogram Oxygen saturation monitor Arterial blood gas
Abdominal injury	Penetrating injury Blunt injury	Wound exploration Operating room Serial examination Paracentesis with lavage	Triple-contrast CT scan Laparoscopy Abdominal CT scan FAST examination Amylase/liver function tests Serial CBC count
Renal/urinary injury	Renal contusion/laceration Bladder/urethral injury	Bladder catheterization Delayed catheterization	Urinalysis Abdominal CT scan Retrograde urethrogram Voiding cystourethrogram
Musculoskeletal injury	Dismembered part Compound fracture Bony injury	Salvage, irrigate, and cool Sterile dressing; splint Splint, traction	Extremity radiographs Operating room Distal neurologic assessment Distal perfusion assessment
Soft-tissue injury		Irrigate, debride Primary vs. delayed repair	Radiograph to exclude foreign body

CBC count, complete blood cell count; CT, computed tomography.

sequentially and simultaneously assessed, treated, monitored, and subjected to further diagnostic study while the format of primary survey, resuscitation, secondary survey, and triage is followed. Each physician dealing with the injured child should have such a format within his or her armamentarium. With these treatment formats well in hand, the clinician can optimize the subsequent care of the patient.

Suggested Readings

General

American College of Surgeons. Advance trauma life support program. Chicago, IL: American College of Surgeons, 1997.

American College of Surgeons, Committee on Trauma. Multiple trauma: early management in the emergency department. *Bull Am Coll Surg* 1980;65(2):19–21.

Baker SP, O'Neill B, Ginsburg M, et al. *The injury fact book*, 2nd ed. New York, NY: Oxford University Press, 1992.

Bickell WH, Wall MJ, Pepe PE, et al. Immediate versus delayed fluid resuscitation for hypotensive patients with penetrating torso injuries. *N Engl J Med* 1994;331:1105–1109.

Centers for Disease Control and Prevention. Toy-related injuries among children and teenagers–United States, 1996. *MMWR Morb Mortal Wkly Rep* 1997;46:1185–1189.

Eichelberger MR. Pediatric trauma. In: Trunkey DD, Lewis FR, eds. *Current therapy of trauma*, 3rd ed. St Louis, MO: BC Decker Mosby—Year Book, 1991:21–39.

Jaffe D, Wesson D. Emergency management of blunt trauma in children. *N Engl J Med* 1991;324:1477–1482.

Kaback KR, Sanders AB, Meislin HW. MAST suit update. *JAMA* 1984; 252:2598–2603.

Karwacki JJ, Baker SP. Children in motor vehicles: never too young to die. *JAMA* 1979;242:2848–2851.

Kaufman CR, Rivara FP, Maier RV. Pediatric trauma: need for surgical management. *J Trauma* 1989;29:1120–1126.

Kowalenko T, Stern S, Dronen S, et al. Improved outcome with hypotensive resuscitation of uncontrolled hemorrhagic shock in a swine model. *J Trauma* 1992;33:349–353.

Kronick JB, Kisson N, Frewen TC. Guidelines for stabilization of the critically ill child before transfer to a tertiary care facility. *Can Med Assoc J* 1988;139: 213–220.

Lloyd-Thomas AR. ABC of major trauma. Paediatric trauma: primary survey and resuscitation, parts I and II. *BMJ* 1990;301:334–336, 380–382.

Mayer T, Matlak ME, Johnson DG, et al. The modified injury severity scale in pediatric multiple trauma patients. *J Pediatr Surg* 1980;15:719–726.

Moulton SL, Lunch FP, Peterson B. Resuscitation of the pediatric victim. In: Mancini ME, Klein J, eds. *Decision making in trauma management: a multidisciplinary approach*. Philadelphia, PA: BC Decker, 1991:214–219.

National Center for Health Statistics. *Health, United States, 1994*. Hyattsville, MD: Public Health Service, 1995. www.cdc.gov/nchs/data/hus/hus94.pdf.

Nonfatal sports- and recreation-related injuries treated in emergency departments—United States, July 2000–June 2001. *MMWR Morb Mortal Wkly Rep* 2002;51(33):736–740.

Pokorny WJ, Haller JA. Pediatric trauma. In: Moore EE, Mattox KL, Feliciano DV, eds. *Trauma*, 2nd ed. Norwalk, CT: Appleton & Lange, 1991:689–702.

Robertson LS. Present status of knowledge in childhood injury prevention. In: *Preventing childhood injuries.* Report of the Twelfth Ross Roundtable on Critical Approaches to Common Pediatric Problems. Columbus, OH: Ross Laboratories, 1982.

Sadow KB, Teach SJ. Prehospital intravenous fluid therapy in the pediatric trauma patient. *Clin Pediatr Emerg Med* 2001;2:23–27.

Singh GK, Yu SM. US childhood mortality, 1950–1993: trends and socioeconomic differentials. *Am J Public Health* 1996;86:505–512.

Tanz RR, Christoffel KK. Pedestrian injury, the next motor vehicle injury challenge. *Am J Dis Child* 1985;139:1187–1190.

Teach SJ, Antosia RE, Lund DP, et al. Prehospital fluid therapy in pediatric trauma patients. *Pediatr Emerg Care* 1985;11:5–8.

Templeton JR Jr, O'Neill JA Jr. Pediatric trauma. *Emerg Med Clin North Am* 1984;2(4):899–912.

Thierbach AR, Lipp MDW. Airway management in trauma patients. *Anesthesiol Clin North Am* 1999;17(1):66–81.

U.S. Department of Health and Human Services, Children's Bureau. *Child maltreatment 1996: reports from the states to the National Child Abuse and Neglect Data System.* Washington, DC: U.S. Government Printing Office, 1998. http://www.acf.dhhs.gov/programs/cb/publications/ncands96/index.htm.

Wetzel RC, Burns RC. Multiple traumas in children: critical care overview. *Crit Care Med* 2002;30(11):468–477.

World Bank. *World development report.* New York, NY: Oxford University Press, 1994:251–252.

Diagnostic Peritoneal Lavage

Hawkins ML, Scofield WM, Carraway RP, et al. Diagnostic peritoneal lavage in blunt trauma. *South Med J* 1988;81:293–296.

Rothenberg S, Moore EE, Marx JA, et al. Selective management of blunt abdominal trauma in children—the triage role of peritoneal lavage. *J Trauma* 1987; 27:1101–1106.

Radiographic Imaging of the Trauma Patient

Beaver BL, Colombani PM, Fal A, et al. The efficacy of computed tomography in evaluating abdominal injuries in children with major head trauma. *J Pediatr Surg* 1987;22:1117–1122.

Bond SJ, Gotschall CS, Eichelberger MR. Predictors of abdominal injury in children with pelvic fracture. *J Trauma* 1991;31:1169–1173.

Brody AS, Seidel FG, Kuhn JP. CT evaluation of blunt abdominal trauma in children: comparison of ultrafast and conventional CT. *AJR Am J Roentgenol* 1989;153:803–806.

Haftel AJ, Lev R, Mahour GH, et al. Abdominal CT scanning in pediatric blunt trauma. *Ann Emerg Med* 1988;17:684–689.

Jones TK, Walsh JW, Maull KI. Diagnostic imaging in blunt trauma of the abdomen. *Surg Gynecol Obstet* 1983;157:389–398.

Kane NM, Cronan JJ, Dorfman GS, et al. Pediatric abdominal trauma: evaluation by computed tomography. *Pediatrics* 1988;82:11–15.

Loiselle JM. Focused abdominal sonography for trauma (FAST) in children with blunt abdominal trauma. *Ann Emerg Med* 2001;37(6):902–906.

Mahboubi S. Abdominal trauma in children: role of computed tomography. *Pediatr Emerg Care* 1985;1:37–39.

Rees MJ, Aickin R, Aolbe A, et al. The screening pelvic radiograph in pediatric trauma. *Ann Emerg Med* 2003;41(2):497–500.

Sivit CJ, Taylor GA, Bulas DI, et al. Blunt trauma in children: significance of peritoneal fluid. *Radiology* 1991;178:185–188.

Sivit CJ, Taylor GA, Newman KD, et al. Safety-belt injuries in children with lapbelt ecchymosis: CT findings in 61 patients. *AJR Am J Roentgenol* 1991; 157:111–114.

Taylor GA, Eichelberger MR. Abdominal CT in children with neurologic impairment following blunt trauma. *Ann Surg* 1989;210:229–233.

Taylor GA, Eichelberger MR, O'Donnell R, et al. Indications for computed tomography in children with blunt trauma. *Ann Surg* 1991;213:212–218.

Taylor GA, Fallat ME, Potter BM, et al. The role of computed tomography in blunt abdominal trauma in children. *J Trauma* 1988;28:1660–1664.

Trauma Scoring and Triage

American College of Surgeons, Committee on Trauma. Appendix E to hospital resources document. Field categorization of trauma patients and hospital trauma index. *Bull Am Coll Surg* 1980;65(2):28–33.

Aprahamian C, Cattey RP, Walker AP, et al. Pediatric trauma score. Predictor of hospital resource use? *Arch Surg* 1990;125:1128–1131.

Champion HR, Sacco WJ, Copes WS. Trauma scoring. In: Moore EE, Mattox KL, Feliciano DV, eds. *Trauma*, 2nd ed. Norwalk, CT: Appleton & Lange, 1991:47–65.

Eichelberger MR, Gotschall CS, Sacco WJ, et al. A comparison of the trauma score, the revised trauma score, and the pediatric trauma score. *Ann Emerg Med* 1989;18:1053–1058.

Kaufman CR, Maier RV, Kaufman EJ, et al. Validity of applying adult TRISS analysis to injured children. *J Trauma* 1991;31:691–698.

Kaufman CR, Maier RV, Rivara FP, et al. Evaluation of the pediatric trauma score. *JAMA* 1990;263:69–72.

Nayduch DA, Moylan J, Rutledge R, et al. Comparison of the ability of adult and pediatric trauma scores to predict pediatric outcome of following major trauma. *J Trauma* 1991;31:452–458.

Tepas JJ, Ramenofsky ML, Mollitt DL, et al. The pediatric trauma score as a predictor of injury severity: an objective assessment. *J Trauma* 1988;28:425–429.

CHAPTER 106 ■ MINOR TRAUMA—LACERATIONS

STEVEN M. SELBST, MD, AND MAGDY W. ATTIA, MD

LACERATIONS

Each year an estimated 12 million wounds are treated in emergency departments (EDs) in the United States. Lacerations account for 30% to 40% of all injuries for which care is sought in a pediatric ED. Broken glass, wooden furniture, asphalt or concrete, or other sharp objects cause most of these lacerations. Animal bites also account for many lacerations. More than 40% of the wounds involve a fall. Boys are injured twice as often as girls. The mechanism of injury varies with the patient's age. Household items, fences, and trees most likely injure preschoolers; older children sustain injuries in violent encounters.

Two-thirds of the injuries occur during warm weather months, although half of the injuries in an urban environment occur indoors. Deaths from minor lacerations are rare; however, complications occur in about 8%. Complications include infection, hypertrophic scarring or keloid formation, and poor cosmetic results.

Pathophysiology

Wound Healing

Normal skin is under constant tension, produced, in part, by underlying joints and muscles. The amount of tension varies by anatomic location and position of a body part. For example, skin overlying a joint will vary in tension, depending on whether the joint is flexed or extended. Lacerations that run parallel to joints and normal skinfolds usually heal more quickly and with better cosmetic results. Wounds under a large amount of tension, crossing joints, or perpendicular to wrinkle lines often heal with wide, unattractive scars. When skin is injured, sutures may be placed to provide temporary support until the skin can regenerate and overcome tension to allow wound closure.

A wound such as a laceration regains about 5% of its previous strength 2 weeks after injury and 30% after 1 to 2 months. It reaches full tensile strength 6 to 8 months after the original injury. Many factors, such as infection, tissue edema, and poor nutrition, may delay this progression.

All wounds deeper than the dermis have the potential for scar formation. Scar formation involves the laying down of collagen, which is a complex process essential in restoring tensile strength of the skin. Collagen synthesis begins within 48 hours of the injury and reaches a peak within the first week afterward. Anything that interferes with collagen synthesis, such as infection, may lead to wound dehiscence at this time. Wound contraction is expected with all healing wounds through the action of fibroblasts. Therefore, eversion of suture lines is desired at the time of repair so that the skin will contract to a flat wound during healing. Remodeling may occur for up to 12 months. Thus, the scar may fade and recede over the first 3 months, and the final appearance of the scar may not be apparent until 6 months after injury.

Wound Infection

Wound infection plays a major role in wound healing. Bacteria inhabit normal intact skin. This is the usual source of infection when skin tissue is disrupted. The amount of bacteria on the skin varies by anatomic location. High counts of bacteria are in moist areas such as the axilla and perineum. Low counts of bacteria are in dry areas such as the back, chest, and abdomen. High bacteria counts can also be expected in areas of exposed skin such as the hands, face, and feet. Areas colonized with high bacterial contamination are most prone to infection. Wounds in regions of high vascularity, such as the scalp and face, more easily resist bacterial infection despite the high bacteria count. Certainly, the oral cavity is highly contaminated with bacteria, and this is an important source of infection when a child sustains a bite wound.

Wounds inflicted by shearing forces with a sharp object such as a knife cause minimal devitalization of adjacent areas and thus are less likely to lead to infection. Wounds caused by a blunt object striking the skin at an angle of less than 90 degrees result in a tension injury such as an avulsion or flap. These injuries involve a larger force applied to the skin than that of a shearing injury, and there is more devitalized tissue. They are more likely to become infected than shearing injuries and are often more difficult to repair. Finally, compression injuries from blunt trauma to the skin at about a 90-degree angle cause the most tissue disruption and devitalization. They are characterized by ragged edges and lead to the highest infection rates and unacceptable scarring.

Clinical Manifestations

History

In the evaluation of a laceration, it is important to learn the *mechanism* of the injury because this may radically change management plans. For instance, if the wound is caused by an animal bite, the likelihood of devitalized tissue and infection is higher and repair may be omitted (see Chapter 83). Also, a wound caused by a blunt object may be associated with an underlying fracture or crush injury. Certain crush injuries, such as wringer injuries, are inherently more complicated and may require surgical consultation and hospital admission. A wound caused by a sharp object may have injured deeper tissues. Determine the *age* of the wound, as well as the possibility of a *foreign body*, in the wound.

Also, consider the *location* of the wound. If the wound is in the neck area, the physician should consider possible extension through the platysma muscle, with potential for a serious injury to underlying structures. If the wound involves the chest, the physician should look for crepitance in the subcutaneous tissue, suggesting injury to the underlying lung. An injury to the lower extremities is more likely to result in infection because of the relatively poor blood supply. Likewise, a wound overlying a joint space can be complicated if the joint cavity is violated. Injury to distal body parts such as the ear, nose, and fingers may threaten the viability of more distal tissues because of vascular compromise. Conversely, in areas where the vascular supply is good, such as the face, scalp, and tongue, the infection rate is low regardless of the mechanism of injury.

Assess the *environment* in which the injury occurred. If the injury occurred on the street, it is possible that small particulate matter may be embedded in the wound. If this debris is left in place, tattooing of the skin could result, leaving an unfavorable appearance to the healed wound. Injuries that occurred in a field, farm, or a wet, swampy area may have high bacterial loads.

The patient's *health status* should be addressed. If the patient has diabetes, immunosuppression, malnutrition, or other chronic conditions such as cyanotic heart disease, chronic respiratory problems, or renal insufficiency, higher infection rates may be anticipated. Bleeding disorders and current medications should be determined because some drugs, such as ibuprofen and corticosteroids, may affect the wound. Ascertain *allergies* to latex, antibiotics, and local anesthetics, as well as the child's *tetanus status*.

Physical Examination

A careful physical examination is essential before local anesthesia is given. First, determine whether there is an associated injury distant from the obvious wound. Wound management should not preempt care of more life-threatening injuries. It is important to assess the wound for *vascular damage* and to control bleeding if present. Brisk flow of blood may indicate injury to a major vessel. These vessels can usually be safely tamponaded and later ligated or sutured. The bleeding site must be identified, although it is often obscured by profuse bleeding. Pressure applied to the site or temporary use of a tourniquet or inflated blood pressure cuff (less than 2 hours) controls hemorrhage and allows identification of the bleeding vessel. Blind clamping of an artery should be avoided except in the scalp. Palpation of pulses and capillary refill distal to the site of injury must be checked.

Next, potential *nerve damage* must be assessed. In an older, cooperative child, the physician should always test the median and ulnar nerves of an injured upper extremity. If a young child does not permit this, pinprick sensation may be tested. Fortunately, when sensation is intact, motor function of the nerve is also usually intact.

Next, the wound must be evaluated for possible *tendon injury*. The superficial location of extensor tendons of the dorsum of the hand predisposes them to injury. Tendon injuries are sometimes visible if the wound is wide and deep. For example, a torn tendon on the flexor surface of the forearm may be seen when the patient with a laceration to the wrist is asked to flex the hand and wrist. Unless the tendon injury is obvious, wounds over joints and tendons should be put through a full range of motion. A young patient may be too

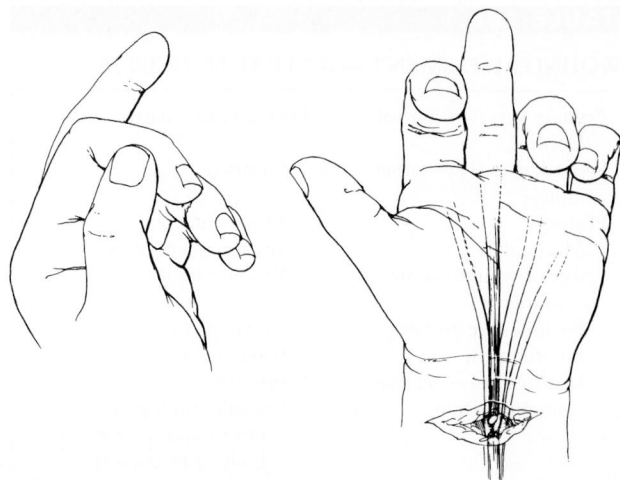

FIGURE 106.1 A seemingly superficial laceration at the wrist might be treated simply by closure of the subcutaneous tissue and skin, unless one appreciates the abnormal posture of the middle finger when the hand is at rest. The loss of normal flexor tone as a result of a divided superficial tendon results in the involved finger lying in a position of relative extension.

uncooperative to flex and extend the fingers on command. Therefore, it is important to inspect the resting position of the injured hand in a young child to note a flexor tendon injury to the finger. One digit may be found extended at rest, while the other uninjured digits are flexed (Fig. 106.1). Applying a noxious stimulus and noting inability to withdraw the finger that is tested may show injury to the extensor tendons.

Determine whether there is *foreign material* in the wound. If the history or physical examination suggests a radiopaque foreign body, consider obtaining a radiograph or an ultrasound of the area for confirmation. This is especially important in assessing a wound caused by glass. A deeply embedded piece of glass may be missed without radiographs or ultrasound. Some recommend obtaining plain radiographs in all cases in which glass is involved, except for the most superficial wounds. Ultrasound is sensitive in detecting and localizing foreign bodies and is most helpful for those which are nonradiopaque, such as plastic and wood. Further inspect for foreign material after the wound is anesthetized.

Finally, *bones* near the wound should be palpated for crepitance, tenderness, or deformity, which may suggest a fracture. Obtain radiographs to confirm suspicious findings. Wounds overlying a fracture may constitute an open fracture and deserve consultation with a specialist for possible repair in the operating room. Table 106.1 summarizes general principles of wound assessment.

Patients with vascular, nerve, or tendon injury or deep, extensive wounds to the face merit consideration for referral to a surgical specialist for possible repair in the operating room.

Decision to Close the Wound

Children are less likely to get wound infections than do adults. In children, the infection rate is about 2% for all sutured wounds. Thus, most wounds may be closed primarily, meaning that the wound edges are approximated as soon

TABLE 106.1

WOUND ASSESSMENT—GENERAL PRINCIPLES

Primary survey—control bleeding	Physical examination
Secondary survey—other injury?	Location
History	
Mechanism	Muscle function
Age of wound—time of injury	Tendon involvement
	Vascular injury
Possible foreign body	Nerve injury
Environment	Foreign material
Health status—tetanus immunization	Laboratory
	Consider radiographs or ultrasound if a foreign body or fracture is suspected

after the injury as possible to speed healing and improve the cosmetic result. If primary closure is long delayed, the risk of subsequent infection increases. However, the length of time before the risk of infection becomes significant is variable. Some authors suggest that the "golden period" for wound closure is 6 hours. However, wounds at low risk for infection (e.g., a clean kitchen knife injury) can be closed even 12 to 24 hours after the injury. In a study from a developing country where patients presented with wounds after variable delays in care, it was found that wounds of the face and scalp heal well in more than 90% of cases, regardless of the time from injury to repair.

Most wounds of the face are best closed, primarily, even up to 24 hours after injury to achieve an optimal cosmetic effect. If the wound is extensive or has a high potential for infection (e.g., a dog bite on the face), thorough irrigation is essential. On the contrary, wounds at high risk for infection such as those in anatomic locations with poor blood supply, contaminated or crush wounds, and those involving immunocompromised hosts should be closed promptly within 6 hours of injury. Some contaminated wounds (animal or human bites or those occurring in a barnyard) in an immunocompromised host should not be sutured, even if the patient presents immediately for care. Thus, the decision to close a wound must be individualized.

Some wounds should be allowed to heal by *secondary intention* (secondary closure), although scar formation may be more unsatisfactory. Infected wounds, ulcers, and many animal bites are best left to heal by granulation and reepithelialization. Human bites over the metacarpophalangeal joints (clenched-fist bites) are especially prone to infection and should not be closed. Puncture wounds to the foot, with only a small laceration and a low concern for cosmetic results, may also be left open. A small sterile wick of iodoform gauze may be placed inside the wound to separate the edges. This gauze can be removed after 2 to 3 days, and the subsequent granulation tissue will aid healing.

If a wound is not closed initially, *delayed primary closure* (tertiary closure) should be considered after the risk of infection decreases, about 3 to 5 days later. This is recommended for selected heavily contaminated wounds and those associated with extensive damage, such as high-velocity missile

injuries, crush injuries, explosion injuries of the hand, and selected bite wounds. The wound should be cleaned and debrided and covered at the time of initial presentation and then reassessed in a few days for infection. It is believed that a contaminated but healing wound gradually gains sufficient resistance to infection to permit uncomplicated closure at a later time. This may still reduce discomfort and lead to a better cosmetic result than that with no repair. Tertiary closure is used rarely in pediatrics because children have few severely contaminated wounds from farm or industrial injuries.

Management of Lacerations

Preparing the Child and Family

It is important to reassure the child and the family that everything will be done to care for the wound appropriately and to relieve the patient's pain and anxiety. In many cases, early removal of blood and foreign material from the surface of the wound is reassuring. Also, carefully chosen words will reduce fear and pain from the procedure. The physician must honestly warn the patient of an impending painful stimulus but may leave open the possibility that it may not hurt as much as the child thinks. Appearing unhurried and confident, giving the child some control of the situation, and explaining the upcoming procedure seem to help reduce anxiety and pain. The parent(s) and the child should be informed that steps would be taken to make the procedure as quick and painless as possible, such as with the use of topical anesthetics. The clinician should provide an age-appropriate empathic explanation, rather than give cold, impersonal instructions about a painful procedure to reduce anxiety. Prepare frightening instruments, such as needles and scalpels, away from the child. Allow the child to listen to music or view age-appropriate, entertaining videos during the procedure because this may serve as a distraction (see Chapter 4).

When parents are inclined to remain in the room during the procedure, they should be encouraged to do so. Inviting the parent to be in the room increases their level of confidence in the physician and can improve their overall satisfaction with the visit. Most parents want to be present during wound repair in the ED, and most can be a stabilizing force if properly oriented. The parent can reassure or distract the child with a story while maintaining physical contact under necessary drapes and restraints. It is usually best if the parent is sitting down and focusing on the child, rather than directly observing the procedure.

Appropriate use of *sedation* and *local anesthetics* is essential for successful repair of lacerations in children and will reduce the need for restraint devices (see Chapter 4). Not all children will receive sedation and some children younger than 4 years will need to be placed in a restraining device, such as a papoose board, for better immobilization. Restraint is needed to ensure the child's safety, protect him or her from self-injury, and allow for more rapid completion of the procedure. Because the child may get excessively warm while in the papoose board, it is important to ensure proper ventilation and assess the child's comfort during the restraint process. A caring, but firm, nurse or assistant is often needed to further immobilize the injured body part and complete the procedure successfully. It is better to use such hospital personnel instead of parents to immobilize a child. A school-aged child can usually cooperate without restraint.

Preparing the Wound

Hair near the wound usually creates minimal difficulty during repair and generally does not need to be removed. In any case, nearby hair should not be closely shaved because this may damage hair follicles and increase infection. Instead, the hair should be clipped with scissors when necessary. Alternatively, petroleum jelly can be used to keep unwanted scalp hair away from the wound while suturing. Hair over the eyebrows should not be removed because this may lead to abnormal or slow regrowth.

It is essential to *clean the wound periphery* at the time of wound evaluation. Povidone-iodine solution (a 10% standard solution) is often used because it is a safe and effective antimicrobial agent with little tissue toxicity. This solution may be diluted with saline 1:10 to create a 1% solution. Use of chlorhexidine or povidone-iodine surgical scrub preparations, hydrogen peroxide, or alcohol in the wound itself is not recommended. These may irritat tissues and may increase infection by damaging white blood cells.

Wound irrigation is extremely important to reduce bacterial contamination and prevent subsequent infection. It is often necessary to anesthetize the wound before thoroughly cleansing. Taking universal precautions, the wound should be irrigated with normal saline, about 100 to 200 mL for the average 2-cm laceration. More may be needed if the wound is unusually large or contaminated. Use a large syringe (20 to 50 mL) with a splash-guard (20-gauge bore) attached to the end to reduce splatter during the irrigation. With the splash-guard almost touching the skin surface and the tip of the syringe about 2 cm from the wound, the clinician should apply firm pressure to the plunger. This technique is usually capable of generating 5 to 8 lb psi of pressure, which is considered the ideal pressure for wound irrigation. Consider warming the saline before irrigation because this may be more comfortable. Tap water has been used instead of saline and is equally effective at irrigating wounds without increasing the risk of infection. Soaking the injured body part should be avoided because this may lead to maceration of the wound and edema.

Scrubbing the wound should be reserved for particularly "dirty" wounds in which contaminants are not effectively removed with irrigation alone. Use topical or infiltrative anesthetics for pain control before scrubbing. It may be necessary to extract some foreign material with fine forceps if it remains adherent after copious irrigation. This will avoid tattooing of the skin and reduce the risk of infection.

In rare cases, the wound must be extended with a scalpel to allow proper exploration and cleaning. The physician should trim irregular lacerations and excise necrotic skin but should not make dramatic changes in the wound on a routine basis. Devitalized tissue should be removed only if it looks ischemic or is otherwise clearly indicated. Only an experienced physician should attempt to remove more than a small amount of tissue. Subcutaneous fat can be safely and easily removed if it seems to interfere with wound closure. It is wise to remove such fat carefully, in small quantities, to avoid disruption of small vessels and cutaneous nerve branches. Debridement is advantageous because it creates well-defined wound edges that can be more easily apposed. However, excessive removal of tissue can create a defect that is difficult to close or may increase tension at the wound margin such that scarring is more likely. Avoid removal of facial fat because this may leave an unsightly depression.

Examine the wound further after cleansing and debridement. After exploration, it is wise to reevaluate the decision to close the wound primarily. When proceeding further, the clinician should wash hands carefully before donning sterile gloves. Although some studies report no increased risk of infection with nonsterile gloves, most still recommend using latex-free, nonpowder, sterile gloves for wound repair. Sterile masks are not helpful in reducing wound infections, but a facial splash-shield is useful to protect the clinician. The area surrounding the wound should be appropriately draped before surgical repair. However, if a young child is particularly upset by facial drapes, they can be omitted. Proper cleaning of the wound is more important to uncomplicated healing than meticulous attempts to avoid introduction of small numbers of bacteria by preserving a sterile field.

Wound Closure

Equipment

Suture material must have adequate strength while producing a little inflammatory reaction. Nonabsorbable sutures such as monofilament nylon (Ethilon) or polypropylene (Prolene) retain most of their tensile strength for more than 60 days and are relatively nonreactive. Thus, they are appropriate for closing the outermost layer of a laceration. With monofilament nylon, it is important to secure the knot adequately with at least four to five throws per knot. Polypropylene is useful for lacerations on the scalp or eyebrows because it is more visible and thus easier to remove, although it is somewhat more difficult to control while suturing. Silk is rarely used now because of increased tissue reactions and infection.

In many cases, it is appropriate to use fine, absorbable (synthetic) sutures such as Dexon®, Monocryl®, or Vicryl® in deeper, subcuticular layers. These materials may elicit an inflammatory response and may extrude from the skin before they are absorbed if they are placed too close to the skin. When subcuticular sutures are used, they should be placed on the deeper surface of the dermis and epithelial margins may be approximated with tape strips. Synthetic absorbable sutures are less reactive than chromic gut and retain their tensile strength for long periods, making them useful in areas with high dynamic and static tensions. Absorbable sutures are advantageous for intraoral lacerations. Some recommend using rapidly absorbable sutures (fast-absorbing gut) for skin closure of facial or scalp wounds in children because suture removal is avoided. Equally acceptable cosmetic results are found with absorbable sutures compared with nonabsorbable sutures in pediatric facial laceration repair.

A 3-0 suture is recommended for tissues with strong tension, such as fascia, and a 4-0 suture is recommended for deep tissues with light tension, such as subcutaneous tissue. Skin is best closed with 4-0 to 7-0 sutures and oral mucosa with 3-0 to 4-0 sutures. The physician should use the finest sutures (6-0) for wounds of the face; heavier sutures for scalp, trunk, and extremities (4-0 or 5-0); and 3-0 or 4-0 for thick skin, such as the sole of the foot, or over large joints, such as the knee.

Needles are available in various forms, including cuticular, plastic, and "reverse cutting." The reverse cutting needle is used most for laceration repair. Its outer edge is sharp so as to allow for atraumatic passage of the needle through the relatively tough dermis and epidermal layers; this minimizes cutting of the skin where suture tension is greatest. A higher-grade plastic needle (designated P or PS) should be used for repairs on the face. A small needle (e.g., P3) should be used for wounds that require fine cosmesis. Needles come in various sizes such as 3/8 and 1/2 circle. Clinicians may develop a preference for a specific needle. However, in general, a 3/8 reverse cutting needle satisfies most needs.

General Principles

Perhaps, the two most important goals of suturing are to match the layers of the injured tissues and to create eversion of the wound margins so that they will flatten as the wound heals. Layers on one side of a wound should be sutured to the corresponding, matching layers on the other side. First, all layers of skin that have been injured should be identified. Then, an attempt should be made to appose each layer (muscles, fascia, subcutaneous tissue, and skin) as nearly as possible back to its original location. This is achieved by carefully matching the depth of the bite taken on each side of the wound when suturing.

Proper *suture placement* should result in slight eversion of the wound so that there is no depressed scar when remodeling takes place. Eversion may be achieved by slight thumb pressure on the wound edge as the needle is entering the opposite side. Sutures should take equal bites from both wound edges so that one margin does not overlap the opposite margin when the knot is tied. Wound-edge eversion is best achieved by taking proper bites while suturing, not by pulling the knot tightly (Fig. 106.2).

Suture placement may be deep or superficial. Deep sutures reapproximate the dermal layers of skin and do not penetrate the epidermis. They help relieve skin tension and improve the cosmetic appearance by reducing the width of the scar. They should be avoided in wounds prone to infection because they will further increase the risk of infection. To secure a deep suture, the needle is placed at the depth of the wound and removed at a more superficial level. The needle is then inserted superficially into the opposite side of the wound and exit out deeply so that the knot is buried within the wound. The needle end and free end of the suture should be on the same side of the loop before the knot is tied (Fig. 106.3). The simple interrupted technique (described next) with absorbable suture material should be used.

Superficial or percutaneous sutures are passed through the dermis and the epidermis and leave the knot visible at the skin surface. Skin should be closed with a minimal amount of tension. Sutures should be pulled tightly enough to approximate the wound edges but not so tightly that they cause tissue necrosis. Sutures that seem well placed initially may begin to cut into the tissue in the next few days because of swelling and inflammation. There is no need to tightly close the skin if other layers have been well sutured. Scalp wounds are an exception. They are under considerable tension, and the knots in this location should be pulled firmly to keep the skin together. The wound will be hidden by hair, so the skin can be pulled more tightly than elsewhere. Firm, but not strangulating, apposition of the wound will also help with hemostasis.

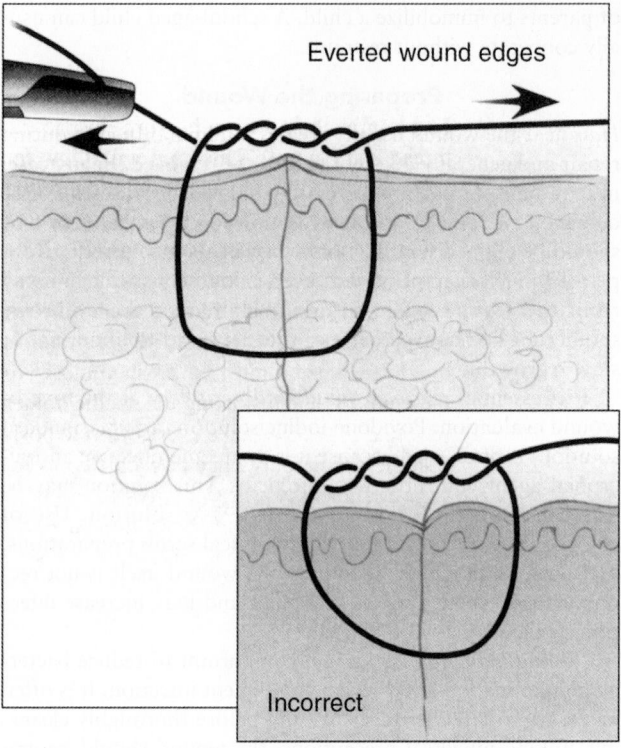

FIGURE 106.2 Suturing technique for wound-edge eversion.

To ensure proper alignment, the first suture may be placed at the midpoint of the wound, with subsequent sutures then placed in a bisecting fashion lateral to the midpoint. Use of forceps to hold tissue should be encouraged because this allows the operator to precisely pass the needle through the desired points alongside the wound edge. However, forceps use should be kept to a minimum during the repair to avoid tissue damage.

Suture Technique

Skin wounds can generally be repaired using interrupted suturing. To place a *simple interrupted suture*, the needle is held upside down and the wrist is pronated as the needle enters the skin at a 90-degree angle. The needle tip will then move farther away from the wound margin and penetrate deeply. Thus, more tissue is at the depth of the wound, and this causes the wound to evert. Sutures should be placed about 2-mm apart and 2 mm from the wound edge on delicate areas such as the face. More sutures placed closer together decrease wound tension and leave a less noticeable scar. Larger bites should be used for body parts where cosmesis is less important.

Use an instrument tie to secure the suture (Fig. 106.4). The knots should ideally be placed on one side of the wound. Knots placed directly over the wound increase inflammation and scar formation. On the first throw, the physician should wrap the needle holder twice to create a surgeon's knot and then wrap subsequent throws a single time. The first and second throws should be snug enough to approximate the wound edges but not so tight that tissue is strangulated. All subsequent knots are squared to maintain the closure. Four or five throws are usually required to keep the knot from unraveling.

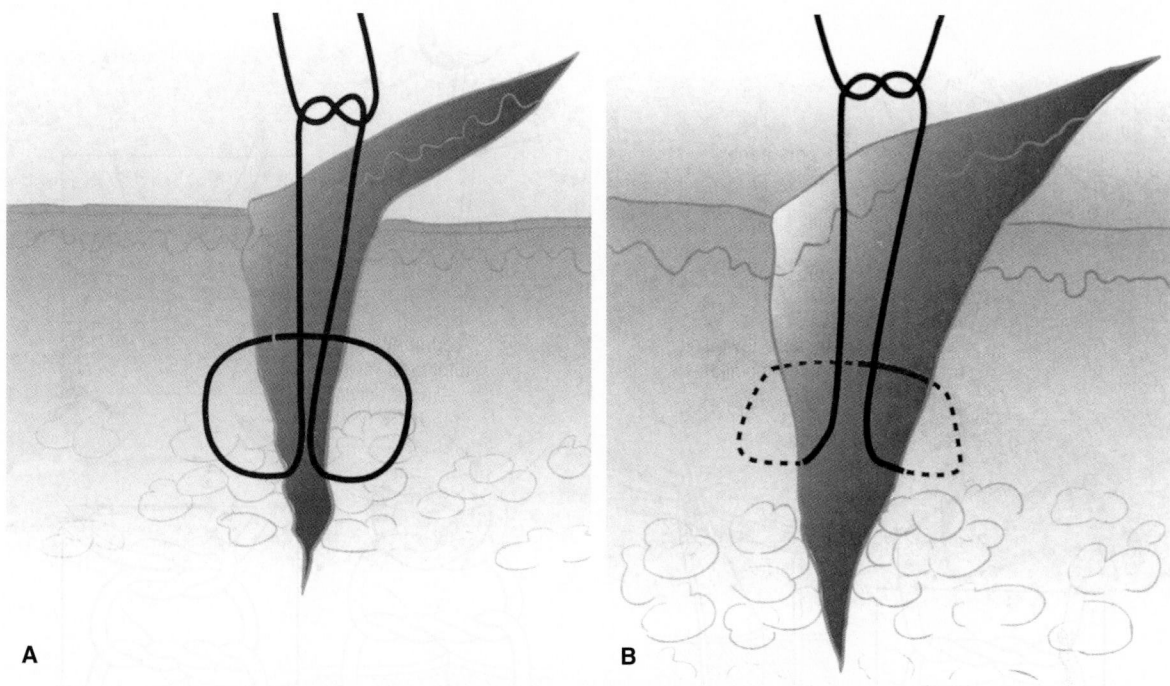

FIGURE 106.3 **A:** The buried subcutaneous suture. **B:** The horizontal dermal stitch.

A "loop knot" is effective in apposing the wound edge with minimal tension. This involves placing a surgeon's knot, using the instrument tie, followed by a loop. The surgeon's knot will "give" slightly should edema develop subsequently. The loop knot allows easier, painless removal of sutures because it creates a free space between the suture and the skin (Fig. 106.5).

Running or *continuous sutures* can be applied rapidly to close large, straight wounds or multiple wounds. In this technique, the suture is not cut and tied with each stitch. The first suture is placed at one end of the wound and a knot is tied, cutting only the end of thread not attached to the needle. The next loop is placed a few millimeters away and continuous loops of equal bites are made to close the wound. On the final loop, because the suture is not completely pulled through, a small loop remains on the opposite side of the wound. Now, the knot can be tied using the preceding loop of suture (Fig. 106.6). This type of stitch is more likely to leave suture marks if not removed in 5 days. Apposition of the edges and eversion are more difficult to achieve with this stitch, and the entire suture line can unravel if the suture breaks anywhere along the repair. However, the technique gives the advantage of having equal tension on the wound edges.

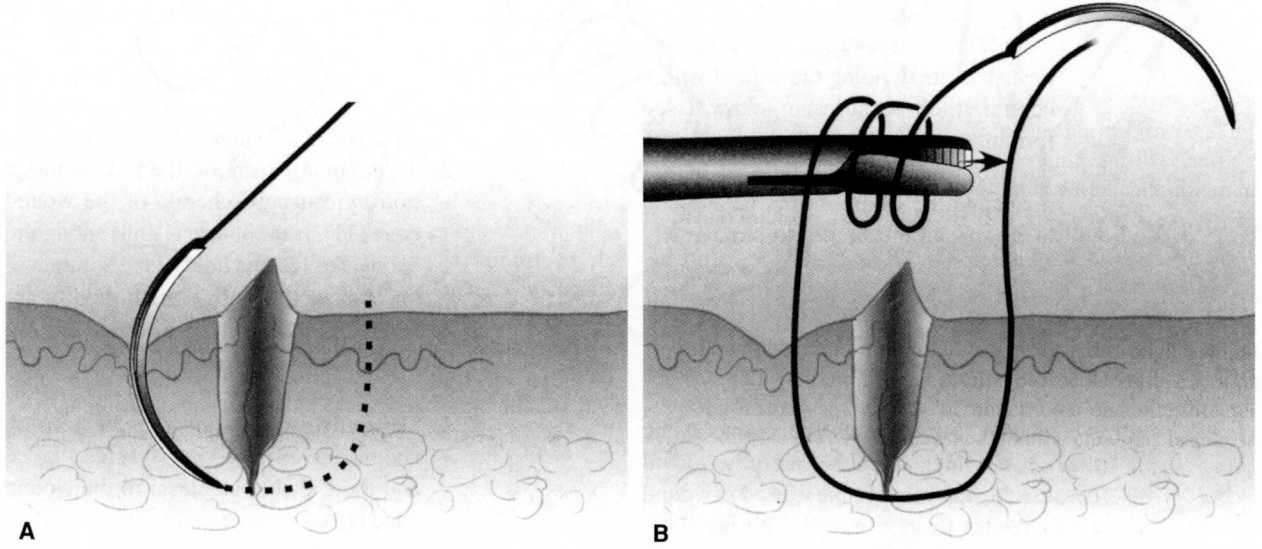

FIGURE 106.4 Simple interrupted skin suture secured with instrument tie.

TRAUMA

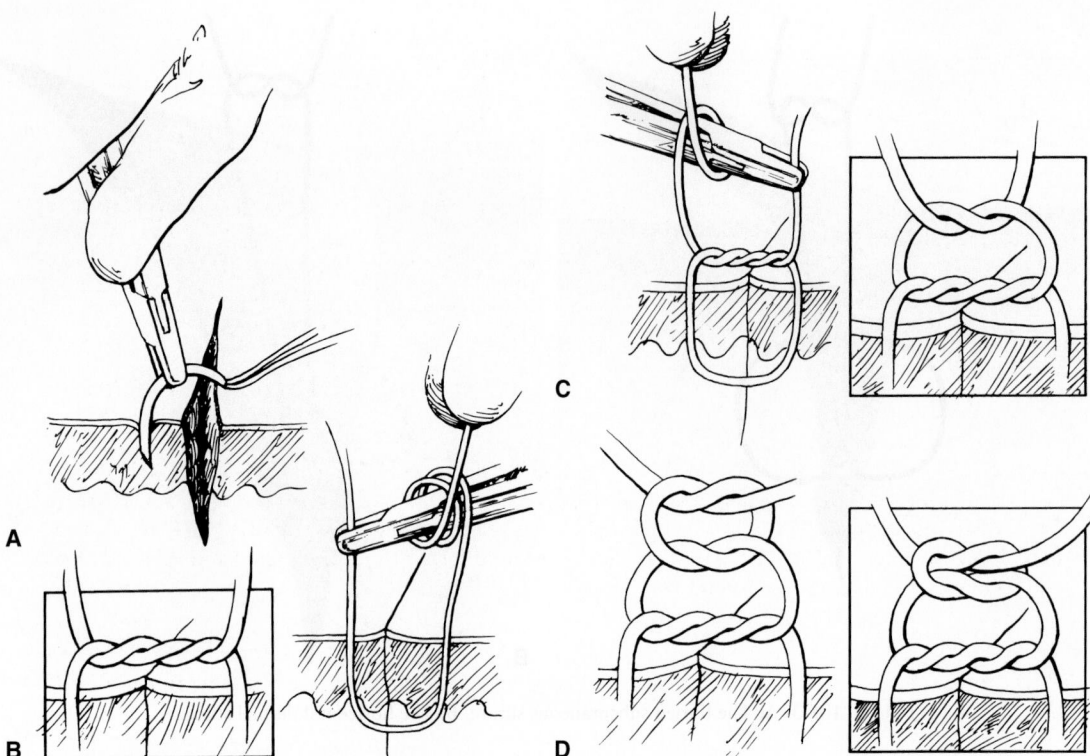

FIGURE 106.5 Placement of a "loop knot" in conjunction with simple sutures of the skin using an eversion technique. **A:** The needle enters the skin at a right angle in a way that allows somewhat less skin and more subcutaneous tissue to be caught in the passage of the needle. The needle should incorporate the same amount of skin and subcutaneous tissue on each side. The ideal suture material for placing a "loop knot" is 4-0 nylon. One can also use 5-0 nylon. **B:** The first knot should be a surgeon's knot drawn down gently to barely coapt the skin edges. **C:** The second tie should be placed to produce a square knot but should be drawn to produce an approximate 2- to 3-mm loop. **D:** The third tie should be placed to produce a square knot. This third tie can be secured tightly against the second tie, preserving the loop and allowing for some spontaneous loosening of the surgeon's knot as later edema develops.

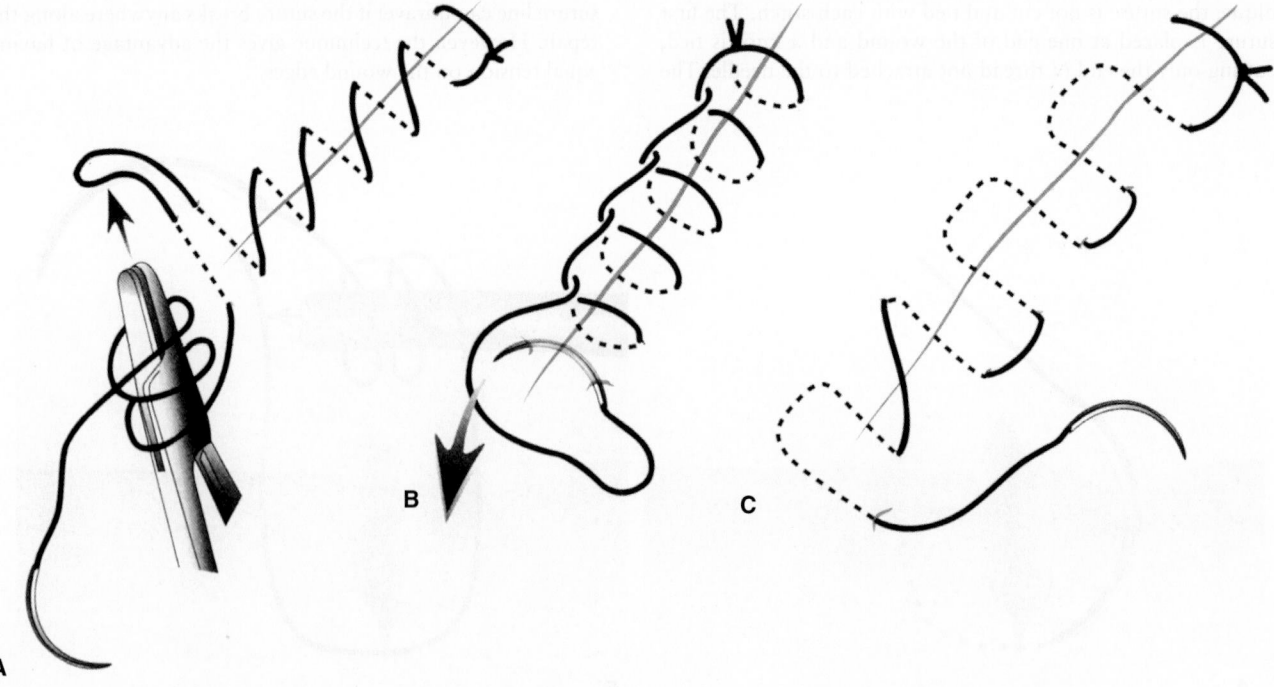

FIGURE 106.6 Continuous skin sutures. **A:** The simple continuous running stitch. **B:** The continuous interlocking skin stitch. **C:** The running lateral mattress stitch or continuous half-buried horizontal mattress stitch.

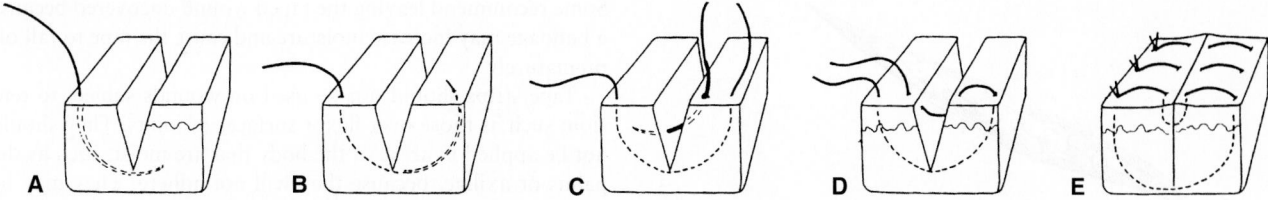

FIGURE 106.7 **A–E:** The vertical mattress suture. After initially placing a simple interrupted stitch with a somewhat larger bite, make a backhand pass across the wound, taking small, superficial bites. When the knot is tied, the edges of the laceration should evert slightly. (Adapted from Grisham J. Wound care. In: Dieckmann RA, Fiser DH, Selbst SM, eds. *Illustrated textbook of pediatric emergency & critical care procedures.* St. Louis, MO: Mosby, 1997:676. Reprinted with permission.)

The *vertical mattress stitch* is useful for deep wounds in which it may be difficult to tie a simple, deep, interrupted suture. It reduces tension on the wound and may close dead space within the wound. It essentially combines a deep and superficial stitch in one suture. The needle is placed deep within the wound (about 3 mm from the wound edge) and brought out to the opposite skin surface. It is then brought across the epidermis to approximate the epidermal edges (Fig. 106.7). This stitch takes more time to accomplish and produces more cross marks, but it provides excellent wound eversion and apposition of the wound edge. Too tight a knot will pucker the wound.

The *horizontal mattress stitch* reinforces the subcutaneous tissue and effectively relieves tension from the wound edges. It does not provide wound-edge approximation as well as the vertical mattress stitch. The needle is passed 0.5 to 1 cm away from the wound edge deeply into the wound. It is then passed through the opposite side and reenters the wound parallel to the initial suture. To avoid "buckling" and to provide some eversion of the wound edges, the skin must be entered perpendicularly and the wound must be entered and exited at the same depth (Fig. 106.8).

The *modified horizontal mattress stitch* (half-buried) is often used to close a flap. It is also called the corner stitch. It relieves intrinsic tension and vascular compromise when approximating the tip of the flap. Using 5-0 or 6-0 nylon, the needle should enter the intact skin across from the apex of the flap and exit the wound just below the subcuticular plane. The needle should be brought to the tip of the flap, entering and exiting at the subcuticular plane. Then, the needle is brought across the edge of the flap in the subcuticular plane and exit out of the skin. A knot should be tied in the usual manner and the tip of the flap brought to the apex of the wound (Fig. 106.9).

Placing the needle in the flap edge first can also repair wounds with flaps. The edge of the flap can then be moved back and forth until proper alignment with the opposite fixed side is obtained. After the tip of the flap is sutured, the sides of the flap are brought together. For wounds with several stellate flaps, subcuticular or subcutaneous sutures should be used to hold the tips of the flap together. Then, a single suture at the tip will provide good apposition without further damaging the tip of the flap. Other interrupted sutures can be placed on the lateral margins of the wound to provide further support. If the wound has many narrow-base stellate flaps or necrotic flap tips, the wound may be better managed with excision and simpler repair (Fig. 106.10).

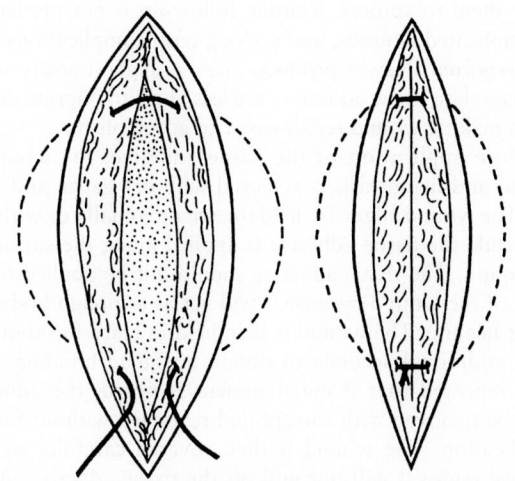

FIGURE 106.8 The horizontal mattress stitch is useful for closing the deep layer in shallow lacerations and in body areas with little subcutaneous tissue. Certain dyed suture materials may cause a tattooing of the skin if placed in such a shallow position. (Adapted from Grisham J. Wound care. In: Dieckmann RA, Fiser DH, Selbst SM, eds. *Illustrated textbook of pediatric emergency & critical care procedures.* St. Louis, MO: Mosby, 1997:678. Reprinted with permission.)

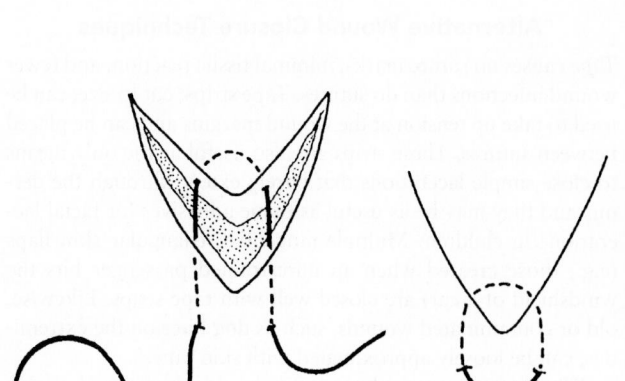

FIGURE 106.9 **A** and **B:** The corner stitch. Also called the half-buried horizontal mattress stitch, this technique allows repair of flap-type lacerations without further compromising blood flow. Place additional simple interrupted sutures along the sides of the flap if necessary. (Adapted from Grisham J. Wound care. In: Dieckmann RA, Fiser DH, Selbst SM, eds. *Illustrated textbook of pediatric emergency & critical care procedures.* St. Louis, MO: Mosby, 1997:676. Reprinted with permission.)

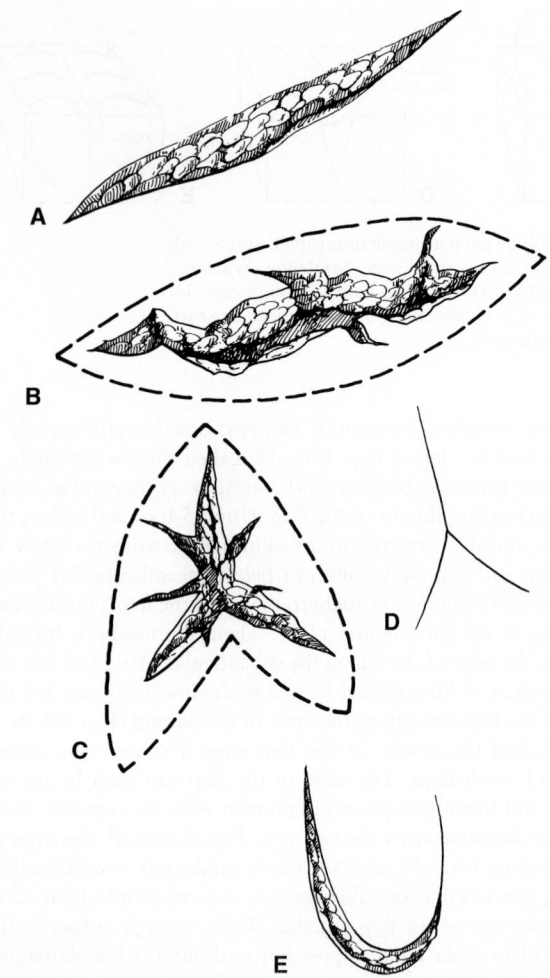

FIGURE 106.10 Variation in laceration injuries and suggestions for management: simple laceration (**A**), elliptical excision of damaged wound margins (**B**), excision and closure of stellate laceration (**C** and **D**), and flap-type laceration (**E**).

Alternative Wound Closure Techniques

Tape causes no suture marks, minimal tissue reaction, and fewer wound infections than do sutures. Tape strips, cut to size, can be used to take up tension at the wound margins and can be placed between sutures. These strips are also useful as the only means to close simple lacerations that barely extend through the dermis and they may be as useful as tissue adhesives for facial lacerations in children. Multiple tangential, triangular skin flaps (e.g., those created when an unrestrained passenger hits the windshield of a car) are closed well with tape strips. Likewise, old or contaminated wounds, such as dog bites on the extremities, can be loosely approximated with skin tape.

When tape is used, the wound should be cleansed as any other wound. Care must be taken to properly realign the dermis and the epithelium. If the tape is pulled too tightly, the margins of the wound may overlap, causing the wound to heal with a raised ridgelike area where the overlap occurred. The tape is applied perpendicularly across the wound with some space between to allow the wound to drain. In some cases, an adhesive such as benzoin is applied to the adjacent skin (not the wound) to keep the tape strips more securely in place.

Some recommend leaving the taped wound uncovered because a bandage may increase moisture and cause the tape to fall off prematurely.

Tape strips should not be used on wounds subject to tension, such as those over flexor surfaces of joints. They should not be applied in areas of the body that are moist, such as the palms or axillae, because they will not adhere. They may be impractical for small children, who may inadvertently remove them from the face.

Staples can be applied more rapidly than sutures and have a lower rate of infection, with less of a foreign-body reaction. They are best for wounds of the scalp, trunk, and extremities when saving time is important. Therefore, they are particularly helpful when treating mass casualties. Staples are left in place for the same length of time as sutures. They are somewhat more painful to remove and should be removed with a specially designed instrument to avoid tissue damage. Staples do not allow for meticulous cosmetic repair, as do sutures. Thus, they should not be used for lacerations of the face, neck, hands, or feet. They should not also be used if the patient requires magnetic resonance imaging or computed tomographic scanning.

Tissue adhesives, or skin glues, such as octylcyanoacrylate, have been used to close wounds for many years. They allow rapid and painless closure of wounds. Anesthesia is unnecessary, unless painful irrigation or exploration of the wound is anticipated. No removal is needed because the adhesives slough off after 7 to 10 days. They provide an excellent cosmetic result in comparison with sutures. One study using plastic surgeons blinded to the method of repair ranked the wounds repaired with tissue adhesives to be cosmetically equal to sutured wounds at 2-month and 1-year follow-up visits.

Tissue adhesives act to decrease wound infections because they have antimicrobial effects against gram-positive organisms. Dehiscence rates (1% to 3%) are similar to that of sutured wounds. They are less expensive than sutures because little equipment is needed and personnel time is reduced. Studies have noted that patients and families of small children prefer them to sutures. Routine follow-up is not needed for uncomplicated wounds, and no long-term complications have been reported. Newer products such as high-viscosity octyl-cyanoacrylate tissue adhesives are less likely to migrate during repair, making wound repair easier to accomplish.

Before application of the tissue adhesive, the wound is cleaned and hemostasis is achieved with dry gauze and pressure. The wound edges are held together manually or with forceps while the tissue adhesive is applied along the surface of the wound. The tissue adhesive should not be applied to the inside of the wound because it will act as a foreign body and inhibit healing. The wound is then held in place for about 20 to 30 additional seconds to obtain adequate bonding. One study reported that if malalignment is noted, the adhesive could be removed with forceps and reapplied without further complication. The wound is then covered carefully so that bandage removal will not pull off the tissue adhesive. Avoid routine application of antibiotic ointments by parents, as these will dissolve the adhesive and cause dehiscence. However, this interaction is beneficial when adhesive (available over the counter) is inadvertently applied to areas such as the eyelashes. Any antibiotic ophthalmic ointment can be used to dissolve the adhesive when needed.

TABLE 106.2

COMMON TECHNIQUES OF WOUND CLOSURE

Technique	Advantages	Disadvantages
Sutures	Greatest tensile strength Meticulous closure Low dehiscence rate	Painful Removal needed Slow application Increased tissue reaction Risk of needle stick (clinician)
Staples	Rapid application Low cost Low tissue reaction	Not for use on the face (less meticulous closure)
Tissue adhesive	Rapid application Painless No removal needed Low cost No risk of needle stick (clinician)	Lower tensile strength Not for use on joints
Tape strips	Rapid application Painless Low cost Low infection risk Least tissue reaction	High risk of dehiscence Not for use in moist areas, young children

Tissue adhesives should be used only to close skin of superficial wounds. For many lacerations, deep absorbable sutures will also be needed because the glue has less strength than most sutures. Skin glues should not be used for wounds subject to great tension, such as on the hands or joints.

Table 106.2 summarizes advantages and disadvantages of several techniques available for wound closure.

Dressings

Dressings protect the wound from further injury and contamination. They also help absorb secretions (not likely with small wounds) and immobilize the injured part. Some use a nonadherent sterile dressing (e.g., Telfa, Xeroform) to cover the wound. This prevents the wound edges from sticking to the dressing. Then, a second layer of absorbent gauze is applied and a third layer of gauze wrap or tape is used to stabilize the other two. This protects and immobilizes the area while absorbing exudate from the wound surface.

For most simple wounds, it is adequate to cover the wound with dry sterile gauze after applying topical antibacterial ointment. Some studies indicate that topical antibiotic ointments may reduce infection and prevent scab formation by lubricating the wound edges. This allows for more rapid epithelialization of the wound.

For the face and trunk, a large bulky dressing is not practical. Thus, for small wounds in these areas, a clear plastic adhesive such as Tegaderm should be used to secure the bandage. Rolls of cotton or stretchable tube gauze can be used for larger wounds to keep the sterile dressing in place. This keeps young children from touching the wound. Scalp wounds are usually not dressed. Patients can generally wash their hair gently after 24 hours.

For children who are active, it may be best to keep the wound covered until sutures are removed. The dressing should remain in place for 24 to 48 hours after which epithelialization is usually sufficient to keep the wound from gross contamination. Then, the bandage should be changed daily and the wound inspected. Any dressing should be changed if it becomes soiled, wet, or saturated with drainage because the wet dressing may be a source of infection.

It may be advisable to splint the wound if it overlies a joint. This is most important for active children who will likely resume full activity soon after the injury. Some even recommend splinting nearby joints for any large laceration of an extremity to reduce stress across the wound even if it does not involve a joint itself. This should be done for no more than 72 hours to facilitate function. The injured extremity should be elevated to provide comfort and reduce edema.

Systemic Antibiotics

Use of prophylactic systemic antibiotics for wound management is controversial. Studies demonstrating proven benefit to the use of antibiotics are lacking. They may lead to allergic reactions, growth of resistant organisms, and unnecessary expense. Thus, they are not recommended for routine use. Decontamination with proper irrigation is more efficacious than the use of antibiotics to prevent wound infection. Consider antibiotics for heavily contaminated wounds that are at greater risk for infection. They are often used for human and cat bites (see Chapter 83), crush injuries, stellate lacerations, and very large wounds (exceeding 5 cm). Other high-risk wounds include intraoral lacerations and wounds of the hands, feet, and perineum. Similarly, open fractures, exposed joints and tendons, and any tetanus-prone wound may benefit from antibiotics. Likewise, wounds that result in exposed cartilage of the nose or ears or extensive facial wounds that may involve contamination from adjacent nasal passages are often treated with antibiotics. It may also be reasonable to use

TABLE 106.3

TETANUS PROPHYLAXIS, CHILDREN ≥ 7 YEARS OLD

Prior tetanus toxoid immunization (doses)	Clean minor wound	All other wounds
Uncertain (or <3)	Td or Tdap	Tdap or Td and TIG
Three or more (most recent >10 yr ago)	Td or Tdap	Td or Tdap
Three or more (most recent within past 5 yr)	None	None
Three or more (most recent between 5 and 10 yr)	None	Td or Tdap

Tdap, tetanus toxoid, reduced diptheria toxoid, and acellular pertussis; Td, adult formulation of diphtheria, tetanus toxoid; TIG, tetanus immunoglobulin (dose: 250–500 units intramuscularly).

antibiotics for wounds (other than scalp lesions) when repair takes place more than 12 hours after injury. They may be justified for wounds that occurred in a contaminated environment, such as a farm or roadside. Injured immunocompromised patients may warrant antibiotics.

Usually, a first-generation cephalosporin or penicillinase-resistant penicillin is used to cover staphylococci and streptococci. Amoxicillin-clavulanic acid is recommended for wounds created by mammalian bites (see Chapter 83). Additional coverage for gram-negative organisms with an aminoglycoside may be worthwhile for heavily contaminated open fractures.

Tetanus

Immunization status of all injured patients should be documented in the medical record. If the wound is clean and minor and the patient has received three previous doses of tetanus toxoid, a booster of tetanus toxoid is given only if 10 or more years have passed since the last dose. If a patient has received three or more previous tetanus immunizations but the wound is not a clean, minor laceration, tetanus toxoid is indicated if the last dose was given more than 5 years earlier.

In many cases, the tetanus immunization record is unknown. If tetanus status is unknown and the wound is not clean or minor, tetanus toxoid and tetanus immunoglobulin (TIG) are indicated. Wounds involving massive tissue destruction and contamination may also require TIG. Patients with such wounds should be admitted to the hospital (Table 106.3).

Discharge Instructions and Suture Removal

Careful discharge instructions, regarding wound care, covering the wound, when to get the wound wet, and how to dry it, are extremely important. The family should be warned about signs of infection. Specifically, they should be told to return for medical care if the wound develops increasing pain, redness, edema, and/or wound discharge, or if the child develops a fever. Analgesics may be given for minor pain, but worsening pain should always prompt a wound check. The family should also be informed that the wound was inspected for a foreign body but that there is still a possibility of a retained foreign body or an undetected injury that may require further treatment. Parents should be told that no matter how skillful the operator is, every laceration leaves some scar. The appearance

of the scar will change during the next several months, and the scar's appearance will not be complete for about 6 to 12 months. Patients and parents should be advised to keep the injured part elevated when possible. A sling can be provided to accomplish elevation of the upper extremities. Some recommend that healing skin should not be exposed to sunlight for 6 months after injury because this could lead to permanent hyperpigmentation.

Follow-up care should be arranged for 24 to 48 hours in all but very simple wounds. The wound can then be reinspected for signs of infection, and healing can be assessed.

Wounds closed with tape strips do not require removal of the tape because these will fall off spontaneously. Skin glue also sloughs spontaneously. However, nonabsorbable sutures should be removed at the appropriate time, depending on the location of the injury. The importance of timely removal should be stressed to the patient and the family. Sutures should be removed when fibroblastic proliferation at the wound interface is strong enough to take the place of sutures. Removing sutures too early may lead to dehiscence and widening of the scar. Sutures left in too long may create an unnecessary tissue reaction and result in visible cross-hatching ("railroad ties").

Wounds on the scalp or face are nourished by a better blood supply and generally exhibit more rapid healing. Sutures in these areas are removed more quickly than those at other locations to avoid unsightly tracts.

When sutures are subject to considerable tension (over joints and on the hands), they should be left in place longer (Table 106.4). After the removal of sutures, it is often necessary to reinforce the healing wound with tape strips to prevent dehiscence.

In the first 24 to 48 hours, wound dressings should be changed only if wet or soiled. After that, bathing can be permitted as long as the wound is present and then patted dry and

TABLE 106.4

TIMELY SUTURE REMOVAL

Wound location	Time of removal (days)
Neck	3–4
Face, scalp	5
Upper extremities, trunk	7–10
Lower extremities	8–10
Joint surface	10–14

covered again. There is no proven harm to exposing the sutures to soap and water for short periods.

Table 106.5 summarizes an approach to reduce risk in managing wounds in the ED.

CARE FOR COMMON WOUNDS

The principles of wound care discussed earlier should be applied in repairing any of the wounds discussed in this section. These principles include evaluation of the wound by history, physical examination, and when indicated, radiographic examination. After the wound is evaluated, the feasibility of closure and the possible need for consultation with a surgeon should be addressed. The following section discusses some of the commonly encountered wounds in children.

Facial and Oral Wounds

Forehead Lacerations

Forehead lacerations are common in early childhood. Most of these injuries occur secondary to falls on objects or furniture such as coffee tables. Most of these lacerations are simple and not associated with any other significant injuries. However, complete evaluation of the head and neck should be carried out. Superficial transverse lacerations of the forehead are easy to manage, and the outcome is usually favorable. Closure with simple or continuous cuticular sutures using 6-0 nonabsorbable material is recommended. Deeper transverse lacerations involving the deep fascia, the frontalis muscle, or the periosteum should be repaired in layers. Absorbable 5-0 material such as coated Vicryl or catgut can be used. If the deeper tissue plains are not closed, the function of the frontalis muscle, eyebrow elevation, may be hampered. Other facial expressions can also be affected because the skin may tether to the scar tissue, bridging the unrepaired gaping tissues.

Vertical forehead lacerations tend to have a wider scar because they traverse the tension lines. Complex forehead wounds, such as stellate lacerations from windshield impact and those with tissue loss, particularly secondary to animal bites, may require consultation with a plastic surgeon. Forehead lacerations are rarely associated with skull fractures, but facial or intracranial injuries should be ruled out.

Lacerations of the Eyebrow

Eyebrow lacerations are common. Repairing an eyebrow laceration is complicated by the presence of hair. It is advisable not to shave the eyebrow for wound preparation because it serves as a landmark during repair. Also, eyebrow regrowth is unpredictable; it may be either slow or incomplete, potentially leading to poor cosmetic outcome. Debridement, if required, should be minimal and along the same axis of the hair shafts to avoid damage to hair follicles; otherwise, alopecia of the brow will result. Closure with simple interrupted stitches using nonabsorbable material is usually sufficient. Attention must be paid to avoid inverting the hair-bearing edges into the wound. It is also important to pay attention to proper alignment of both ends along an eyebrow wound.

Lacerations of the Eyelid

Most eyelid lacerations are simple transverse wounds of the upper eyelid just inferior to the eyebrow. Repairing these wounds does not require any special skills. Some lacerations in the transverse crease of the eyelid will heal just fine if left alone. However, recognizing complicated eyelid lacerations is crucial for proper repair and good outcome. Vertical lacerations involving the lid margin require precision in approximation to avoid deformity and malfunction of the eyelid. Injuries potentially involving the levator palpebrae muscle, medial canthal ligament, or lacrimal duct should be considered for ophthalmologic referral. A high index of suspicion for lacrimal duct injury is particularly important when evaluating a medially positioned lower eyelid laceration. If not repaired, inferior duct injury may lead to chronic tearing, as the lower lacrimal duct is the main drain of tears from the conjunctival sac. Evaluation for an associated injury of the globe is a must, particularly if periorbital fat is exposed or tarsal plate penetration is present.

Lacerations and Blunt Trauma of the External Ear

Although the ears are subject to trauma because of their exposed position, lacerations involving the ears are rather rare. To obtain the best results in caring for injuries involving the external ear (auricle or ear lobe), attention must be paid to certain anatomic and physiologic facts. The auricle contains a cartilaginous structure that provides the framework for the complex shape of the ear. The perichondrium covering the cartilage provides it with nutrients and oxygen. Separation of the cartilage from the perichondrium because of trauma may lead to necrosis of the cartilage, leaving the auricle deformed. The overlying skin, although thin and with no or little subcutaneous tissue, is well vascularized. Skin flaps with small pedicles often survive and should not be hastily debrided.

Simple auricular lacerations can be repaired without difficulty. To avoid chondritis, approximation of the skin is important so that no cartilage is exposed. Occasionally, debridement of the cartilage is needed to obtain complete coaptation of the wound; however, cartilage debridement should be kept to a minimum. It is imperative to avoid catching the auricular cartilage with the needle tip because the skin and the perichondrium are in close proximity to each other.

Complex auricular lacerations with significant skin damage and involvement of the auricular cartilage can be difficult to repair and may require consultation with a plastic surgeon. In general, when repairing auricular cartilage, a few 5-0 absorbable sutures should be used to approximate the edges. Landmarks of the auricle should be used for proper alignment. The perichondrium should be included in the sutures so that the suture material does not tear through the friable cartilage and also to

TRAUMA

ensure restoration of nutrient and oxygen supply. For the same reason, excessive tension should be avoided. Closure of the skin should follow as described previously. If the laceration involves the anterior and posterior aspects of the ear, closure of the posterior aspect first is recommended.

To avoid a deep scar line (notching) in repairing the ear lobe or the auricular rim, the skin edges should be everted at the time of closure because fibrotic tissue will eventually pull the scar line down, leading to notching.

For *partial avulsion* or *total amputation of the ear*, make every effort to reattach the amputated part because tissue survival and cosmetic outcome are usually favorable. Furthermore, blunt ear trauma can lead to a simple contusion or a significant *subperichondrial hematoma* that can compromise the auricular cartilage. Classically, a significant perichondrial hematoma is tense and appears as smooth ecchymotic swelling that disrupts the normal contour of the auricle. This injury is particularly common among wrestlers. Auricular hematoma should be promptly drained to avoid necrosis of the cartilage and deformed auricle or cauliflower ear.

After repair of ear lacerations or evacuation of an auricular hematoma, a pressure dressing should be applied. Follow-up in 24 hours to evaluate vascular integrity to the area is recommended.

Lacerations of the Nose

Unlike blunt injuries, lacerations to the nose are unusual. When a laceration results from blunt trauma, careful evaluation of underlying nasal bones and examination for a nasal septal hematoma are essential. Other associated injuries, such as facial bone fractures or injuries to the orbit, should also be ruled out.

The skin overlying the nose is taut and stiff. Approximating the edges of simple, nongaping nasal wounds, mostly along the upper half of the nose, is usually straightforward. Wounds with any gaping, commonly in the lower part of the nose, can be difficult to coapt because of the nature of the skin in this location. The suture material can tear through the skin easily. Absorbable subcutaneous stitches are recommended before skin closure to relieve tension and prevent tearing through the wound edges. Skin closure should be with simple interrupted 6-0 nonabsorbable material. Early removal of the sutures is advised for the same reason.

Full-thickness nasal lacerations involving the alae nasi or entering the vestibule require layered closure. The procedure should begin with the nasal mucosa, using absorbable material, and finished with the skin, preferably using continuous subcuticular intradermal suture technique.

The nasal cartilage, when involved, rarely requires sutures. When alignment is difficult, a few fine sutures (Vicryl or plain catgut) will help hold it in place. When the free rim of the nares is involved, precise alignment is imperative for good cosmetic outcome. For complex nasal lacerations, lacerations associated with fractures, or when there is tissue loss, consultation with an otolaryngologist or a plastic surgeon is recommended.

Lacerations of the Lip

Lip lacerations are a particular concern because of the importance of the lip as a facial landmark. The lip is a vascular structure with multiple layers. The vermilion border, the junction of the dry oral mucosa and the facial skin, serves as an important landmark for proper repair when involved. The relative pallor of the vermilion border to the lip and to the skin easily identifies it. Therefore, the use of epinephrine with local anesthesia should be avoided so the landmark is not obscured. When parted, the vermilion border should be precisely reapposed using a 6-0 suture. The buccal mucosal surface is then closed with 5-0 absorbable material, followed by the skin, using 6-0 nonabsorbable sutures. The parents should be warned that, while the lip is still anesthetized, there is a chance that the child will bite the sutures off and that they should distract the child from doing so. Typically after the local anesthesia has worn off, the site is sore enough so that the child will not attempt to manipulate the area.

In general, lip lacerations should be closed in layers, depending on the depth of the wound. In full-thickness lacerations, a three-layer repair is required. The physician should begin with the oral mucosa, using 5-0 absorbable material, followed by the orbicularis oris muscle layer to include the inner and outer fibrofatty layers, and finish with the skin, using 6-0 nonabsorbable interrupted sutures. Small wounds, less than 2 cm in length, on the inner aspect of the lip without communication to the skin surface need not be repaired. External lip wounds not communicating with the mucosal surface can be sutured by single- or double-layer closure, depending on the depth and degree of gaping of the wound. Absorbable sutures (5-0) for the subcutaneous layer and nonabsorbable (6-0) sutures for closure of the skin can be used.

Extensive lip injuries with tissue loss or those caused by electric burns, especially those that involve the angle of the mouth, should be referred to a plastic surgeon. Associated injuries such as dental trauma, mandibular fractures, and closed head injuries should be ruled out.

Lacerations of the Cheeks

When managing lacerations involving the cheeks, the physician must evaluate the integrity of the underlying structures. The parotid gland and duct, the facial nerve, and the labial artery are in close proximity of the surface of the skin and can be injured often as a result of an animal bite. If parotid gland or duct injury is identified, consultation with a surgeon is advised. Puncture wounds resulting from animal bites should be debrided and irrigated thoroughly. Some of these puncture wounds are better off left without closure to reduce infection rate, especially if the cosmetic outcome is not compromised. Otherwise, simple interrupted 6-0 nonabsorbable sutures can be used to close uncomplicated lacerations of the cheeks.

Lacerations of the Tongue

The tongue is a vascular and muscular organ. Tongue lacerations often hemorrhage excessively in the beginning, but the bleeding usually ceases quickly as the lingual muscle contracts. Lacerations of the tongue can pose a challenge to repair not only because of their inaccessibility but also because of the controversy surrounding the indications for closure.

Most tongue lacerations can be left alone with good results. However, large lacerations involving the free edge may heal with a notch causing dysfunction of the tongue. Generally, this type of laceration should be repaired. Large flaps and lacerations that continue to bleed should also be repaired. Assess patients with tongue lacerations requiring repair for potential airway problems, as well as the need for sedation or even general anesthesia. Often, local or regional anesthesia is sufficient. The mouth should be retained open by using a padded tongue depressor placed on the side between the upper and lower teeth or by using a Denhardt-Dingman side mouth gag. The tongue can be maintained in the protruded position by a gentle pull using a towel clip or by placing a suture through the tip. Interrupted 4-0 absorbable suture, with full-thickness bites to include the two mucosal surfaces and the lingual muscle between, will close the tongue wound and provide hemostasis. Multiple knots and inverted sutures are recommended to prevent the untying of the sutures. Some authors suggest that only deep muscle closure is required because the mucosal surface heals rapidly. As in lip lacerations, children may chew off the stitches. Parents must be warned of this possibility and should attempt to distract the child at least until the local anesthesia wears off.

Lacerations of the Buccal Mucosa

Small, isolated lacerations of the buccal mucosa, mostly from impaction of teeth following falls, require no suturing. Lacerations 2 to 3 cm in length or with flaps are best closed with simple interrupted absorbable material. Coated Vicryl (4-0) on a round needle is preferred because it is less irritating to the child and is easier to work with than with chromic gut. Closure of the mucosal surface in through-and-through lip lacerations should be carried out before closure of the muscle and skin layers. After repair, a soft diet and avoidance of irritating foods should be advised, as well as vigilant mouth hygiene. Evaluation for associated injuries of the teeth or the alveolar margin is imperative.

Fingertip Injuries

Fingertip Avulsions

Fingertip injuries are rather common in children. In young children, most of these injuries are blunt and secondary to entrapment of the finger in closing doors. Most of these injuries are contused lacerations or partial avulsions. Complete amputation of the fingertips is not as common. Sharp injuries are more common in older children and less likely to be associated with fractures. Fingertip injuries should be evaluated clinically for an associated nail bed injury and radiographically for possible fractures of the phalanges. In general, this type of injury is manageable by the emergency physician, especially in preadolescent children, because tissue regeneration is remarkable and management is mostly conservative.

The management of amputations of fingertips (distal to the distal interphalangeal joint) can be approached on the basis of the absence or presence of bone exposure. If no or minimal bone is exposed, conservative management is advised. The wound should be cleansed, dressed in nonadherent gauze, and splinted for protection. Frequent dressing changes and appropriate follow-up should be planned. Antibiotic coverage is recommended. When a significant amount of bone is exposed, consultation with a surgeon should be considered. The treatment of choice usually involves shortening of the distal phalanx and covering the tip with volar skin flap. However, some hand surgeons advocate for various skin-grafting procedures to avoid permanent shortening and deformity. Consider microscopic reimplantation by a surgeon for amputations proximal to the distal interphalangeal joint.

Nail Bed Injuries

Trauma to the distal fingers is often associated with nail and nail bed (matrix) injuries. Nail avulsion can be partial or complete and may or may not be associated with nail bed laceration. An underlying fracture of the distal phalanx may also be present. Injury to the fingertip is often associated with subungual hematoma. In evaluating these injuries, the emergency physician should determine the need to explore the nail bed for a laceration. Unrepaired nail bed lacerations may permanently disfigure the growth of the new nail from the cicatrix nail bed. If the nail is partially avulsed but is firmly attached to its bed, exploring the nail bed is difficult and is probably not warranted. Good outcome is expected because the nail holds the underlying lacerated nail bed tissues in place.

If a subungual hematoma exists, it should be drained (see the following text). When the nail is completely avulsed or is attached loosely, remove the nail and assess the nail bed for laceration. If the nail bed is lacerated, repair it using 6-0 absorbable material. After cleansing and trimming its soft proximal portion, replace the nail between the nail bed and the nail fold (eponychium) and then anchor it in place with a few stitches. This will splint the nail fold away from the nail bed, which will prevent the obliteration of the space between the nail bed and the nail fold. By preserving this space, the new nail is allowed to grow undisturbed. Some have used tissue adhesive (skin glue) instead of sutures to secure the nail. The preferred method of local anesthesia for nail bed repair is digital block, and the use of a finger tourniquet during the repair allows a bloodless field. Application of a finger splint or a bulky dressing after repair, especially if there is an associated fracture, is recommended.

Subungual Hematoma

Subungual hematoma is the collection of blood in the interface of the nail and the nail bed. It is commonly seen with blunt fingertip injuries. The usual presentation is throbbing pain and discoloration of the nail. Subungual hematoma may be associated with nail bed injury or fracture of the distal phalanx.

Usually, drainage of the hematoma provides relief from the symptoms. Generally, no local anesthesia is required for a simple trephination by cauterization of the nail. After drainage, care for simple subungual hematoma includes elevation of the hand and warm soaks for a few days. Inform the family about the possibility of nail deformity in the future. When the injury is more involved, digital block is advised. If the hematoma is large and extends to the tip of the nail, consider separating the nail from the nail bed using a sharp or blunt method to allow drainage. Outcomes with nail trephination and nail removal are similar. In the presence of a distal phalangeal fracture, the physician has to be concerned about transforming a closed fracture to an open one by communicating the subungual, and hence the fracture hematoma, to the exterior surface of the nail. If there is a possibility of an underlying fracture, consider antibiotic coverage and ensure close follow-up.

Suggested Readings

American Academy of Pediatrics Committee on Infectious Diseases. Tetanus. In: Pickering LK, ed. *Red book*, 28th ed. Elk Grove Village, IL: American Academy of Pediatrics, 2009:655–660.

TRAUMA

Bansal BC, Wiebe RA, Perkins SD, et al. Tap water for irrigation of lacerations. *Am J Emerg Med* 2002;20:469–472.

Boutros S, Weinfeld AB, Friedman JD. Continuous versus interrupted suturing of traumatic lacerations—a time, cost, and complication rate comparison. *J Trauma* 2000;48:495–497.

Brancato JC, Schamban N, Wiley JF. Minor wound preparation and irrigation. *UpToDate.* Last literature review version 16.2. May 2008.

Brown DJ, Jaffe JE, Henson JK. Advanced laceration management. *Emerg Med Clin North Am* 2007;25:83–99.

Callahan JM, Baker MD. General wound management. In: Henretig FM, King C, eds. *Textbook of pediatric emergency procedures*, 2nd ed. Philadelphia, PA: Wolters Kluwer/Lippincott Williams & Wilkins, 2008: 1005–1017.

DeBoard RH, Rondeau DF, Kang CS, et al. Principles of basic wound evaluation and management in the emergency department. *Emerg Med Clin North Am* 2007;25:23–29.

Dingeman RS, Mitchell EA, Meyer EC, et al. Parent presence during complex invasive procedures and cardiopulmonary resuscitation: a systematic review of the literature. *Pediatrics* 2007;120:842–854.

Ernst AA, Gershoff L, Miller P, et al. Warmed versus room temperature saline for laceration irrigation—a randomized clinical trial. *South Med J* 2003; 96:436–439.

Holger JS, Wnadersee SC, Hale DB, et al. Cosmetic outcomes of facial lacerations repaired with tissue adhesive, absorbable and non-absorbable sutures. *Am J Emerg Med* 2004;22:254–257.

Karounis H, Gouin S, Eisman H, et al. A randomized control trial comparing long-term cosmetic outcomes of traumatic pediatric lacerations repaired with absorbable plain gut versus non-absorbable nylon sutures. *Acad Emerg Med* 2004;11:730–735.

Khan ANGA, Dayan PS, Miller S, et al. Cosmetic outcome of scalp wound closure with staples in the pediatric emergency department: a prospective, randomized trial. *Pediatr Emerg Care* 2002;18:171–173.

Mark DG, Granquist EJ. Are prophylactic oral antibiotics indicated for the treatment of intraoral wounds? *Ann Emerg Med* 2008;52:368–372.

Mattick A, Clegg G, Beattie T, et al. A randomized controlled trial comparing a tissue adhesive (2-octylcyanoacrylate) with adhesive strips (Steristrips) for paediatric laceration repair. *Emerg Med J* 2002;19:405–407.

McNamara R, DeAngelis M. Laceration repair with sutures, staples and wound closure tapes. In: Henretig FM, King C, eds. *Textbook of pediatric emergency procedures*, 2nd ed. Philadelphia, PA: Wolters Kluwer/Lippincott Williams & Wilkins, 2008:1018–1044.

Orlinsky M, Bright AA. The utility of routine x-rays in all glass-caused wounds. *Am J Emerg Med* 2006;24:233–236.

Perelman VS, Francis GJ, Rutledge T, et al. Sterile versus nonsterile gloves for repair of uncomplicated laceration in the emergency department: a randomized controlled trial. *Ann Emerg Med* 2004;43:362–370.

Singer AJ, Dagum AB. Current management of acute cutaneous wounds. *N Engl J Med* 2008;359:1037–1046.

Singer AJ, Giordano P, Fitch JL, et al. Evaluation of a new high viscosity octylcyanoacrylate tissue adhesive for laceration repair: a randomized, clinical trial. *Acad Emerg Med* 2003;10:1134–1137.

Singer AJ, Mach C, Thode HC Jr, et al. Patient priorities with traumatic lacerations. *Am J Emerg Med* 2000;18:683–686.

Singer AJ, Quinn JV, Clark RE, et al. Closure of lacerations and incisions with octylcyanoacrylate: a multicenter randomized controlled trial. *J Fam Pract* 2002;51:517.

Singer AJ, Quinn JV, Thode HC Jr, et al. Determinants of poor outcome after laceration and surgical incision repair. *Plast Reconstr Surg* 2002;110:429–435.

Strauss EJ, Weil WM, Jordan C, et al. A prospective randomized controlled trial of 2-octylcyanoacrylate versus suture repair for nail bed injuries. *J Hand Surg* 2008;33:250–253.

Templeton JM. Minor trauma. In: Fleisher GR, Ludwig S, eds. *Textbook of pediatric emergency medicine*, 3rd ed. Baltimore, MD: Williams & Wilkins, 1993:1288–1297.

Valente JH, Forti RJ, Freundlich LF, et al. Wound irrigation in children: saline solution or tap water? *Ann Emerg Med* 2003;41:609–616.

Weinberger LN, Chen EH, Mills AM. Is screening radiography necessary to detect retained foreign bodies in adequately explored superficial glass-caused wounds? *Ann Emerg Med* 2007;51:666–667.

Zehtabchi S. The role of antibiotic prophylaxis for prevention of infection in patients with simple hand lacerations. *Ann Emerg Med* 2007;49:682–689.

Zempsky WT, Parotti D, Grem C, et al. Randomized controlled comparison of cosmetic outcomes of simple facial lacerations closed with Steri-Strip skin closures or Dermabond tissue adhesive. *Pediatr Emerg Care* 2004;20:519–524.

CHAPTER 107 ■ ABDOMINAL TRAUMA

RICHARD A. SALADINO, MD, AND DENNIS P. LUND, MD

Trauma is the most common cause of death in children between 1 and 18 years of age in the United States; more than 10,000 children die each year from injuries. Blunt trauma accounts for more than 90% of childhood injuries; the most common associated mechanisms are falls and motor vehicle–related trauma. Although injury to the abdomen accounts for only 10% of injuries in children with trauma, it is the most common unrecognized cause of fatal injuries. Therefore, a compulsive and systematic approach to identification and treatment is necessary.

Children are at greater risk than adults for intraabdominal injuries after blunt trauma because of their immature musculoskeletal system. The overlying muscles and associated skeleton is much weaker than for adults and, therefore, less protective. In addition, children have a higher abdominal organ-to-body mass ratio. A given force delivered to the abdomen is distributed over a smaller body surface area, increasing the likelihood of injury to the underlying structures.

APPROACH

The assessment of any trauma patient always begins with the ABCs (airway, breathing, and circulation). Priorities in evaluation and treatment include recognition and relief of airway obstruction, appropriate protection of the cervical spine, and management of life-threatening chest injuries and shock. Once resuscitation and cervical spine stabilization have begun, evaluation of the abdomen is included in both the primary and secondary surveys.

The evaluation for intraabdominal injuries in children starts with a determination of the mechanism of trauma, elicited from witnesses, caregivers, and emergency medical personnel. Blunt injuries account for most of the morbidity and mortality of childhood trauma, although the frequency with which penetrating injuries occur is increasing. Penetrating trauma is usually evident on careful inspection of both the anterior and posterior torsi. In contrast, blunt abdominal trauma must be suspected from both historical information and careful physical examination. Children with severe multiple trauma are obviously at risk for intraabdominal injuries, but sufficient energy to injure may also be present in apparently minor falls, direct blows to the abdomen from balls, bats, bicycle handlebars, and countless toys, and during contact sports.

Life-threatening abdominal injuries may be occult or manifest in several ways: abdominal ecchymoses or distension, shock, or external hemorrhage (e.g., from a penetrating injury). Historical information or physical examination findings are often subtle or lacking. Children have the capacity to maintain a normal blood pressure level in the face of signifi-

cant blood loss and hence may mask major intraabdominal bleeding. The examining physician must always keep in mind that the abdomen is a large potential reservoir for blood loss.

Physical Examination

A traumatized child is often difficult to examine; pain associated with extraabdominal injuries may obscure abdominal findings. In addition, the results of physical examination may be subtle or unreliable in an unconscious, intoxicated, agitated, or fearful child. Vital signs, including blood pressure and pulse, may be normal for age, especially in children with isolated injuries of the liver and spleen. Furthermore, external signs of injury, abdominal tenderness, and absent bowel sounds seldom differentiate pediatric patients who require laparotomy from those who do not.

Careful serial examinations are critically important in maintaining the index of suspicion necessary to proceed with more sophisticated testing when appropriate. Inspection should note abrasions, lacerations, ecchymoses, penetrating wounds (including missile entry and exit sites), and telltale markings (e.g., seat belt marks, tire tracks). Attention should be paid to the anterior and posterior abdomen and to both flanks, as well as to the lower thorax, when considering abdominal injuries. Abdominal distension may be caused by hemoperitoneum or peritonitis but most often results from gastric distension from air swallowed by the crying child. Early gastric decompression may assist the abdominal examination and prevent vomiting with aspiration of gastric contents. The presence or absence of bowel sounds is generally not of much significance in the initial evaluation, but prolonged ileus may be a sign of intraabdominal pathology. Tenderness upon palpation, percussion, or shaking may be caused by abdominal wall contusion or may indicate intraabdominal injuries. Pelvic stability is evaluated by gently compressing and distracting the ileac wings.

Digital rectal examination should be performed; the presence of blood may indicate perforation of the bowel. A boggy or high-riding prostate, blood at the urethral meatus, or a distended bladder may be present with urethral disruption and preclude bladder catheterization until a retrograde urethrogram has been performed (see Chapter 112). Diminished or absent rectal sphincter tone may indicate a spinal cord injury.

Laboratory Data

Blood should be obtained and sent for immediate baseline hemoglobin measurement and typing and cross-matching, not only in all instances of multiple trauma but also if isolated intraabdominal injury is suspected. The blood bank at a trauma center not only should be able to provide type-specific blood in a short time frame but must also have O-negative packed red blood cells (RBCs) ready for resuscitation if needed.

Routine multipanel laboratory testing (so-called "trauma panels") has historically been standard for patients with trauma, but more recent studies have called into question this undifferentiated approach. Nonetheless, common additional laboratory studies include measurement of liver transaminases, amylase, and lipase and urinalysis.

Many recent studies indicate that, in combination with the presence of physical examination findings, abnormal laboratory findings contribute to the identification of children with intraabdominal injuries. Elevated serum liver transaminase levels may be associated with intraabdominal trauma, especially hepatic injuries. Screening for intraabdominal injuries by evaluating transaminase levels is not universally accepted because sensitivity and specificity vary widely in the literature, but some data suggest that elevated transaminase levels [as low as aspartate aminotransferase more than 200 U per L and alanine aminotransferase more than 125 U per L] correlate well with hepatic injuries. Using thresholds such as these may allow for more judicious use of computerized tomographic (CT) scan of the abdomen for children with blunt abdominal trauma.

Examination of the urine may also play a role in an increased suspicion for intraabdominal injury after blunt force trauma to the abdomen. Grossly bloody urine indicates likely injury to the kidneys and has been shown to be associated with nonrenal intraabdominal injuries in pediatric patients with trauma. The predictive capacity of microscopic hematuria is controversial. In one study, microscopic examination of urine that revealed more than 50 RBCs per high-powered field (hpf) was 100% sensitive and 64% specific for the presence of an intraabdominal injury (see Chapter 112). A more recent study suggests consideration of CT scan of the abdomen in the context of a urinalysis demonstrating as few as 5 or more RBCs per hpf when the history indicates a significant force has been applied to the abdomen. In addition, clinicians must remember that major trauma may cause complete disruption of a renal pedicle without any hematuria.

Hyperamylasemia may be present with pancreatic injury, but its absence does not preclude injury. In one study, elevations of amylase level more than 200 U per L and lipase level more than 1,800 U per L were markers of possible major pancreatic ductal disruption. In a more recent retrospective study, elevations of amylase and lipase levels were infrequently detected in patients with blunt abdominal trauma (4% and 7%, respectively), and neither the sensitivity nor negative predictive values of elevated measurements were sufficient to be used as screening tools for pancreatic injury. Pancreatic injury is difficult to diagnose, particularly since a CT scan of the abdomen is only 60% to 70% accurate in identifying pancreatic injury.

INITIAL MANAGEMENT PRINCIPLES

Basic Principles of Management

Airway management and cervical spine stabilization are first priorities (Fig. 107.1). Supplemental oxygen should be admin-

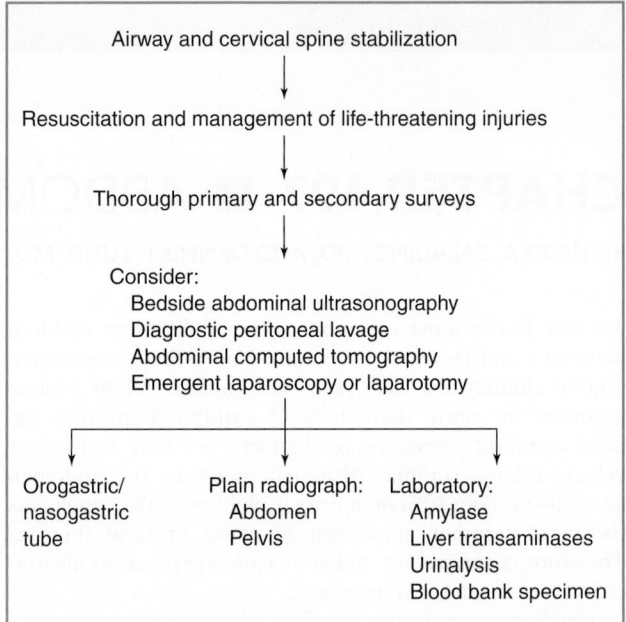

FIGURE 107.1 Initial evaluation and treatment of the child with abdominal trauma.

istered to any child with significant injuries, regardless of whether obvious signs of shock are present. Intravenous or intraosseous access should be obtained while the primary survey is completed. Immediate life-threatening injuries should be treated promptly. Hemorrhagic shock should be addressed with rapid infusion of isotonic crystalloid solution. A first intravenous administration of a bolus of 20 mL per kg may be given rapidly, followed by a second bolus of 20 mL per kg, if the pulse and blood pressure remain outside the physiologic range. If hemodynamic instability persists after 40 mL per kg of crystalloid, ongoing bleeding should be suspected and administration of blood strongly considered. Large-bore catheters are preferable, whether in the upper or lower extremities, to allow rapid infusion of large volumes of fluid during resuscitation. Accessing the femoral vein is acceptable and in fact is a preferred site in children for central access.

The American College of Surgeons currently recommends that aggressive fluid resuscitation be pursued. Although some animal data and a single clinical study suggest that less rigorous (hypotensive) fluid resuscitation may improve survival by limiting hemorrhage into the peritoneal space, application to the management of children is still controversial and not part of the approach to the injured child with hypotension.

As the initial evaluation proceeds, the priorities of management depend on the extent of multisystem injuries and the condition of the patient (Fig. 107.2). Patients who are unstable as a result of ongoing blood loss or an expanding intracranial hemorrhage require operative intervention early in the evaluation phase.

The Unstable Patient

Immediate life-threatening injuries, such as airway obstruction, tension pneumothorax, pericardial tamponade, and obvious sources of external blood loss, must be treated promptly upon detection. The role of emergency department (ED)

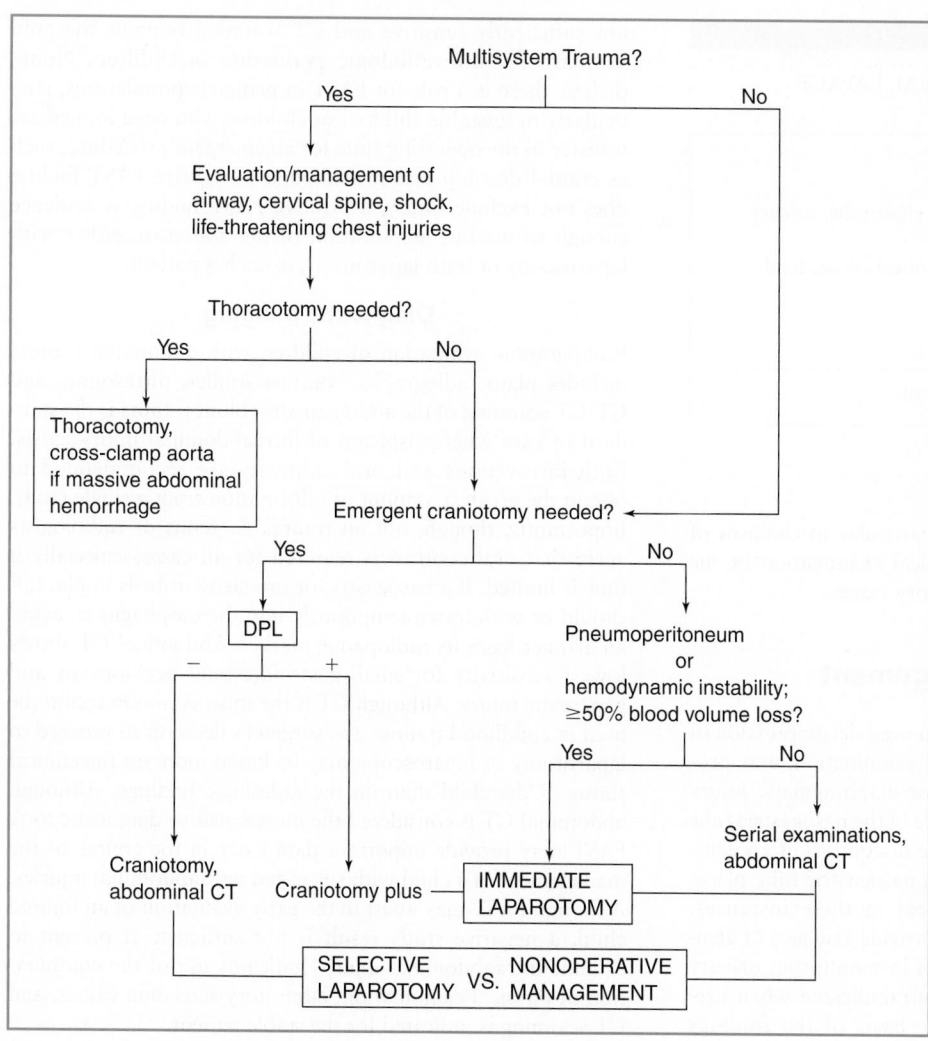

FIGURE 107.2 Management of blunt abdominal trauma. DPL, diagnostic peritoneal lavage; CT, computed tomography (see Table 107.2).

thoracotomy is controversial in children; its use should be confined to situations in which control of intrathoracic bleeding is needed (e.g., with lung or heart lacerations) or in patients in whom previously detected vital signs are lost. If emergent thoracotomy is performed in the latter instance for presumptive intraabdominal hemorrhage, the aorta is cross-clamped at a level just above the diaphragm.

If significant head trauma has occurred, a determination must be made regarding the need for immediate neurosurgical intervention. A rapidly performed CT scan of the head is usually sufficient to determine the presence of a hematoma, which can be evacuated surgically. If hemodynamic instability or the need for immediate craniotomy exists and does not allow for CT evaluation of the abdomen (Table 107.1), a diagnostic peritoneal lavage (DPL) should be performed either in the ED or in the operating suite. In the presence of a positive DPL finding (Table 107.2), laparotomy and craniotomy proceed simultaneously. Finally, if neither thoracotomy nor craniotomy is indicated, emergent laparotomy is performed when pneumoperitoneum is noted on a plain radiograph or when the patient remains hemodynamically unstable in the face of historical or physical evidence of abdominal trauma (Fig. 107.2).

The Stable Patient

Commonly, the injured child can be stabilized in the ED with proper airway and cervical spine management, and with intravenous fluid therapy and blood transfusion. A careful secondary survey should then be performed. On the basis of history and careful, serial abdominal examinations, CT is indicated when intraabdominal injuries are suspected (Table 107.1). Children who have had only moderate injuries should be examined serially in the ED. At times, an abdominal CT scan is merited based

TABLE 107.1

INDICATIONS FOR ABDOMINAL COMPUTED TOMOGRAPHIC SCAN IN PEDIATRIC TRAUMA PATIENTS

1. Mechanism of injury suggesting abdominal trauma
2. Slowly declining hematocrit
3. Unaccountable fluid or blood requirements
4. Neurologic injury precluding accurate abdominal examination
5. Hematuria
6. Acute "need to know" (e.g., before general anesthesia)

TRAUMA

TABLE 107.2

POSITIVE DIAGNOSTIC PERITONEAL LAVAGE
CRITERIA

1. >5 mL of gross blood
2. Obvious enteric contents (e.g., bile)
3. Peritoneal lavage fluid exiting from chest tube, urinary bladder catheter
4. Positive laboratory analysis of peritoneal lavage fluid
   a. >100,000 RBCs/mm^3
   b. >500 WBCs/mm^3
5. Elevated amylase in effluent

RBCs, red blood cells; WBCs, white blood cells.

solely on severe force inherent in a particular mechanism of injury, despite an unremarkable physical examination or the absence of abnormal screening laboratory values.

Additional Management

Children with abdominal trauma often need decompression of the stomach; this procedure facilitates examination, may provide information concerning gastric or diaphragmatic injury (bloody aspirate, radiographic evidence of the nasogastric tube in the thoracic cavity), and relieves the discomfort of an ileus. Major maxillofacial trauma precludes nasogastric tube placement, but an orogastric tube suffices in these instances. Urinary bladder catheterization may provide evidence of genitourinary system injury and is helpful in monitoring urinary output. Bladder catheterization is contraindicated when urethral disruption is suspected on the basis of the findings described previously.

Focused Abdominal Sonography for Trauma

Ultrasound screening (FAST: focused abdominal sonography for trauma) of the abdomen has been routinely utilized in adult trauma patients for many years with excellent sensitivity and specificity. FAST is typically performed in the ED during the secondary survey. The operator looks at four windows in the abdomen: the left upper quadrant, the right upper quadrant, the pericardium via a subxiphoid window, and the pelvis. The purpose of the scan is simple: the identification of free fluid. Free fluid in any of these areas indicates the need for further evaluation and treatment.

Review of several studies of adults with blunt abdominal trauma suggests that the immediate use of FAST may reduce the use of CT for unstable patients with a positive ultrasound finding. The predominance of the more recent literature suggests that FAST may support a decision to proceed to laparotomy without the need to undergo DPL or CT. In the unstable patient, free fluid points toward the need for operative intervention, whereas in the stable patient, further evaluation with CT scan is indicated.

The utility of FAST in the management of pediatric patients remains controversial. The literature for pediatric patients with intraabdominal injuries suggests that, to date, FAST is

not sufficiently sensitive and CT scanning remains the gold standard for the radiologic evaluation in children. Nonetheless, there is a role for FAST in pediatric populations, particularly in unstable children or children who need immediate transfer to the operating suite for an emergent procedure, such as cranial decompression. Although a negative FAST finding does not exclude injury, a positive FAST finding is evidence enough to warrant exploration of the abdomen, either with laparoscopy or with laparotomy, in such a patient.

Diagnostic Imaging

Radiographic evaluation of children with abdominal trauma includes plain radiographs, contrast studies, ultrasound, and CT. CT scanning of the abdomen after blunt trauma is the standard of care when suspicion of intraabdominal injury exists. Both intravenous and oral contrasts are recommended to obtain the greatest amount of information from a single study. Importantly, though, not all trauma surgeons or radiologists agree that oral contrast is required for all cases, especially if time is limited. If a nasogastric or orogastric tube is in place, it should be withdrawn temporarily into the esophagus to avoid an artifact from its radiopaque marker. Abdominal CT shows lowest sensitivity for small gastrointestinal perforations and pancreatic injury. Although CT is the most common technique used in childhood trauma, the surgeon's decision to proceed to laparotomy or laparoscopy may be based more on the clinical status of the child than on the radiologic findings. Although abdominal CT is considered the most sensitive diagnostic tool, FAST may provide important data early in the course of the management of a child with suspected intraabdominal injuries. Although FAST may assist in the early evaluation of an injured child, a negative study result is not sufficient at present to exclude intraabdominal injury. Judicious use of the combination of physical examination, laboratory screening values, and CT scanning is indicated for the stable patient.

Diagnostic Peritoneal Lavage

DPL is occasionally a helpful adjunct to the management of children with abdominal trauma. The disadvantages of DPL include the introduction of air and fluid into the abdomen (subsequent radiologic evaluations are less helpful) and peritoneal irritation caused by the procedure (subsequent physical examinations are less reliable).

It is rarely necessary to perform laparotomy on children with free intraperitoneal blood. DPL, which effectively detects small volumes of blood, is often too sensitive in children. The primary indication for DPL in children is an urgent "need to know" with regard to the status of the peritoneal cavity, such as in the child who is hemodynamically unstable or requires immediate craniotomy and cannot be delayed for abdominal CT. If the technology is available, however, this need can be met with FAST or laparoscopy.

The technique for DPL in children is similar to that in adults, although in young children, a small supraumbilical incision is preferred over the usual infraumbilical approach to avoid the bladder. If a nasogastric tube and a urinary bladder catheter have not been placed, they should be inserted before peritoneal lavage is performed. Warm Ringer's lactate solution (10 mL per kg, maximum 1,000 mL) is instilled into the peritoneal cavity over 10 minutes and then removed for analysis.

TABLE 107.3

INDICATIONS FOR IMMEDIATE LAPAROTOMY FOR CHILDREN WITH ABDOMINAL TRAUMA

Multisystem injuries with indications for craniotomy in the presence of a positive diagnostic peritoneal lavage, free peritoneal fluid on ultrasonography, or strong historical, physical, or radiographic evidence of abdominal injury

Persistent and significant hemodynamic instability with evidence of abdominal injury in the absence of extraabdominal injury

Penetrating wounds to the abdomen

Pneumoperitoneum

Significant abdominal distension associated with hypotension

Criteria for the presence of a positive lavage are shown in Table 107.2.

Emergent Versus Selective Laparotomy

The indications for immediate laparotomy are limited in blunt abdominal trauma (Table 107.3). In most cases of childhood trauma (Fig. 107.2), emergency laparotomy is not necessary and further diagnostic studies direct either elective (selective) laparotomy or observation and monitoring. Most children with blunt abdominal trauma require only in-hospital observation and monitoring after delineation of the site and extent of their injury by abdominal CT.

The indications for emergent laparotomy in children with penetrating trauma are illustrated in Fig. 107.3. Any gunshot wound to the abdomen mandates immediate exploration. Other types of penetrating wounds in the presence of unexplained hemodynamic compromise, evisceration, pneumoperitoneum, or any evidence of violation of the peritoneum require prompt laparotomy.

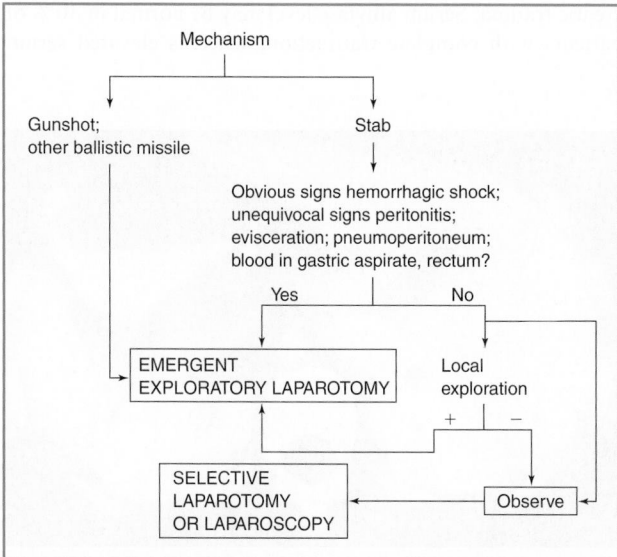

FIGURE 107.3 Management of penetrating abdominal trauma.

BLUND ABDOMINAL TRAUMA

Abdominal Wall Contusions

Many children have minor trauma to their abdomen in the course of play and as a result of minor accidental events. Balls, bats, swings, toys, and contact with other children may cause contusions of the abdominal wall.

Children subjected to minor forces without signs of intraabdominal pathology (e.g., distension, tenderness on deep palpation, peritoneal irritation) can be sent home. Those with a troubling history or any worrisome signs should receive a diagnostic laboratory evaluation and should be observed in consultation with a surgeon. Suspicion for more serious intraabdominal injuries is based on the mechanism of injury and careful abdominal examination. Bilious or bloody vomiting, persistent vomiting, abdominal distension, any signs of peritoneal irritation, and rectal blood or hematuria suggest possible visceral injury, as does an elevation in amylase or liver transaminase levels in cases in which a clinical decision is made to obtain these studies. A low threshold for the use of abdominal CT should be maintained. Children with even minor contusions of the liver, spleen, pancreas, or hollow viscera should be hospitalized.

Solid Organ Injuries

The spleen is the most commonly injured intraabdominal organ, followed by the liver. Most of these injuries are the result of automobile-pedestrian trauma, although falls and bicycle accidents are also common mechanisms. The potential morbidity and mortality result from the highly vascular anatomy of this organ and hemorrhage into the large potential space of the peritoneal cavity.

Patients who have splenic injuries may present with either diffuse abdominal pain or localized tenderness. Subphrenic blood may cause referred left shoulder pain (Kehr's sign). Percussion and palpation tenderness is usually of greatest magnitude in the left upper quadrant of the abdomen. Abdominal radiographs occasionally reveal a medially displaced gastric bubble. CT scan will identify the extent of injury (Figs. 107.4 and 107.5).

Management of splenic injuries has evolved during the last three decades since the recognition of the postsplenectomy sepsis syndrome, resulting from the influence of both clinical and diagnostic advances. Nonoperative management of splenic injuries has largely replaced the traditional treatment, which included splenectomy or splenorrhaphy. The safety measure in nonoperative management for most childhood spleen injuries has been well documented, and the incidence of postsplenectomy sepsis has declined. The availability of noninvasive diagnostic CT also has allowed for greater confidence in the nonoperative approach to splenic trauma.

Blunt liver trauma is the most common fatal abdominal injury (Fig. 107.6). Mechanisms of injury are those that are common to splenic trauma. Diffuse abdominal tenderness may be a result of hemoperitoneum, but maximal tenderness is elicited in the right upper quadrant of the abdomen. Right shoulder pain is an occasional complaint.

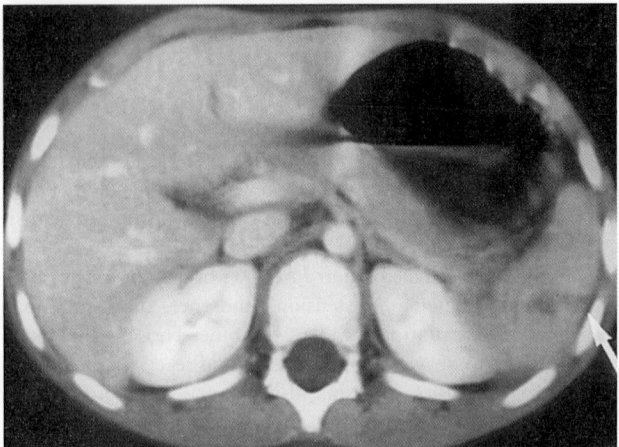

FIGURE 107.4 Abdominal computed tomography of a 13-year-old girl who fell from a horse onto her left side, showing a splenic laceration.

As with trauma to the spleen, nonoperative management of blunt hepatic injuries has become more common and is now the rule rather than the exception. Nonoperative management of isolated spleen and liver injuries without blood transfusion is the standard of care in pediatric trauma care facilities and is successful in 95% and 90% of cases, respectively. The American Pediatric Surgical Association Trauma Committee has published the guidelines for the nonoperative management of isolated solid visceral injuries in children, as listed in Table 107.4. These recommended practices are the result of a retrospective analysis of surgeon practices, national data on outcomes, and a prospective multicenter trial.

Pancreatic Injuries

Blunt abdominal injuries, particularly from bicycle handlebars, are the most common cause of pancreatic pseudocyst formation in children, although this injury is infrequent. Diagnosis is often delayed because of the nonspecific nature of subjective complaints and physical examination findings.

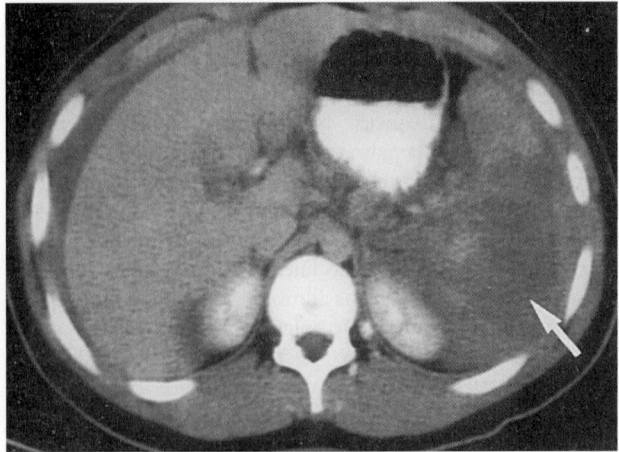

FIGURE 107.5 Abdominal computed tomography of a 10-year-old boy struck by a motor vehicle while crossing a street, showing massive splenic rupture and hemoperitoneum.

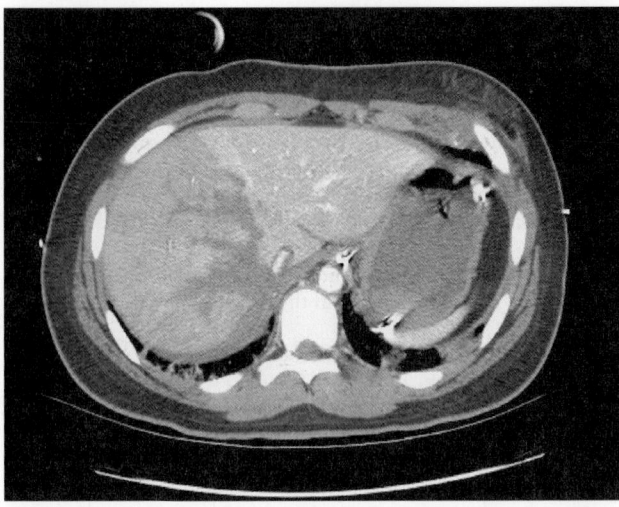

FIGURE 107.6 Abdominal computed tomography of an unrestrained 13-year-old girl in a rollover motor vehicle collision. A liver fracture is evident with differential perfusion of the lobes of the liver. Additional injuries included lung contusion.

The classic triad of epigastric pain, a palpable abdominal mass, and hyperamylasemia are detected only rarely in children and may develop slowly. The pancreas is relatively well protected and associated trauma such as hepatic and intestinal injuries is commonly present when injury to the pancreas has occurred. Abdominal ultrasound and contrast CT (often serial examinations) are used to make the diagnosis (Fig. 107.7); however, acute pancreatic injuries may not be apparent on the initial CT scan.

Severe injury of the pancreas is rare, but when it occurs, blood loss and leakage of enzyme-laden secretions may result in hypovolemia and peritonitis. Blunt abdominal trauma may also injure the ductal elements of the pancreas, and diagnosis depends on a high index of suspicion, consideration of the mechanism of injury, physical examination, serum amylase determination, and diagnostic imaging. Of note, however, is that the absence of hyperamylasemia does not preclude pancreatic trauma. Serum amylase level may be normal in 30% of patients with complete transaction, whereas elevated serum

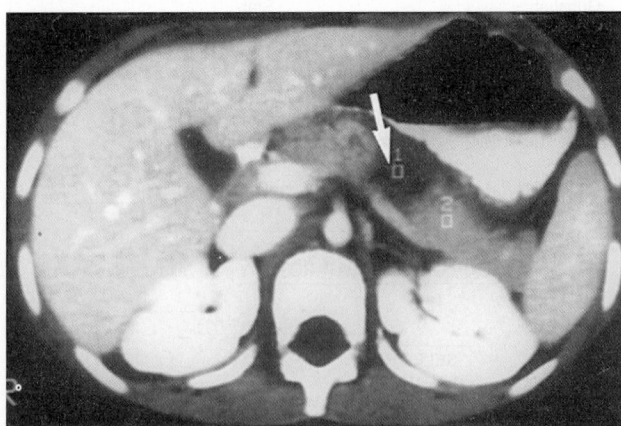

FIGURE 107.7 Abdominal computed tomography of a 6-year-old boy who fell onto the handlebar of his bicycle, showing a pancreatic hematoma and pseudocyst formation.

TABLE 107.4

GUIDELINES FOR MANAGEMENT IN CHILDREN WITH ISOLATED SPLEEN OR LIVER INJURIES

Computed tomography grade	I	II	III	IV
Intensive care unit days	None	None	None	1
Hospital days	2	3	4	5
Predischarge imaging	None	None	None	None
Postdischarge imaging	None	None	None	None
Time of restricted activity (wk)	3	4	5	6

amylase level is detected in 14% to 80% of cases of blunt injury. Elevated serum amylase level should suggest the possibility of pancreatic involvement, but the absolute value does not correlate with the degree of injury. Elevation of the amylase level in fluid returned from DPL suggests injury to bowel or pancreatic ductile elements.

Nasogastric decompression and bowel rest are indicated when pancreatic injury is suspected. Nonoperative therapy is normally used initially for children with isolated pancreatic pseudocyst caused by blunt trauma. Maturation of the pseudocyst may necessitate surgical drainage, although spontaneous resolution may occur in 25% of children. Experience with percutaneous drainage of pancreatic pseudocysts in children is increasing, but the traditional approach has been to use surgical internal drainage once a pseudocyst has persisted beyond 6 weeks. When severe pancreatic crush or transection is suspected, the surgeon may elect to perform immediate exploration and resection or drainage.

Hollow Abdominal Viscera Injuries

Intestinal perforation caused by blunt abdominal trauma is rare in the pediatric age group, but the most common causes of this injury are automobile-pedestrian trauma, automobile lap belt injuries, and child abuse. The mechanisms of injury usually involve rapid acceleration or deceleration of a structure near a point of anatomic fixation (e.g., ligament of Treitz), or trapping of a piece of bowel between two unyielding structures such as a lap belt and the spine. Hollow visceral injury may be difficult to diagnose because physical findings may be minimal and/or nonspecific for the first few hours, and abdominal CT is not particularly sensitive in this situation. However, succus entericus, bile, and activated pancreatic enzymes are extremely irritating to the peritoneum over time. The development of fever or worsening peritonitis on serial physical examinations should alert the examining physician to the possibility of bowel perforation.

Plain radiographs of the abdomen demonstrate free intraabdominal air in only 30% to 50% of cases. Similarly, pneumoperitoneum or leakage of gastrointestinal contrast is only rarely seen on the CT scan. DPL, which is rarely performed because of limited indications, may demonstrate bile or amylase in the effluent and is sensitive for bowel perforations (see Fig. 107.2 and Table 107.2). Most perforations or transections of bowel are found during laparotomy, which the surgeon has chosen to perform because of advancing peritoni-

tis or unexplained persistent fever. Management depends on the site and extent of structural injury.

A significant percentage (up to 25%) of hollow visceral injuries may not be apparent on the initial CT scan of a child with blunt injury. Therefore, evaluating the mechanism of injury should lead to a high index of suspicion for this type of injury. A significant lap belt sign is a harbinger of possible bowel injury. Similarly, free fluid in the abdomen on CT scan should be very carefully evaluated and consideration should be given for laparoscopy or laparotomy.

Late Presentations of Intraabdominal Trauma

Some children with abdominal trauma do not have evidence of intraabdominal pathology on initial evaluation but may return days or weeks later with abdominal distension and/or pain, persistent emesis, or hematochezia. In particular, three injuries are characterized by late presentations: (i) pancreatic pseudocyst (previously discussed), (ii) duodenal hematoma, and (iii) hematobilia.

Intramural duodenal hematoma is an uncommon injury that results from a direct blow to the epigastrium (blunt force delivered by a small-diameter instrument such as a broom handle or the toe of a boot) or from rapid deceleration (e.g., in the lap belt syndrome) and may cause partial or complete gastric outlet obstruction. Bleeding into the wall of the duodenum causes compression and therefore symptoms of intestinal obstruction, including pain, bilious vomiting, and gastric distension.

Diagnosis is made by ultrasonography or a contrast upper gastrointestinal study, revealing the "coiled spring sign." Injury of the pancreas must be suspected when duodenal hematoma is considered. Nonoperative management includes nasogastric decompression and parenteral nutrition for up to 3 weeks.

Rupture of the gallbladder is rare and is almost always associated with severe blunt trauma to the liver. Likewise, hematobilia is associated with hepatic trauma and is a result of pressure necrosis from an intrahepatic hematoma or direct injury to the biliary tree. Children with hematobilia present several days after a blunt abdominal trauma with abdominal pain and upper gastrointestinal tract bleeding. Cholangiography confirms the diagnosis. Embolization is used to achieve hemostasis, but partial hepatic resection is necessary when this treatment fails.

PENETRATING ABDOMINAL TRAUMA

Penetrating abdominal trauma is much less common than blunt trauma in the pediatric age group and accounts for less than 10% of pediatric trauma injuries. However, the evolution of a more heavily armed society has resulted in a worrisome increase in the frequency with which children sustain penetrating injuries.

The high morbidity and mortality associated with penetrating trauma to the abdomen is a result of the destructive force of ballistic missiles and fragments, rapid hemorrhage of vascular structures and solid organs after missile and stab injuries, difficulty in surgical repair of grossly injured intraabdominal organs, and postoperative complications. Intraabdominal organs are at risk for penetrating trauma, depending on their size and location. The colon and small bowel are large in volume and are the most commonly injured structures, followed by the liver, spleen, and major vessels. Hypovolemia and/or signs of peritonitis are then the result of brisk hemorrhage and spillage of enteric contents into the peritoneal space.

The approach to these patients includes management of all life-threatening injuries and treatment of hemorrhagic shock. The need for laparotomy must be determined quickly, and broad-spectrum antibiotics, such as cefoxitin 25 mg per kg, should be given.

Gunshot Wounds

The destructive energy of ballistic missiles and fragments is related to mass and velocity (kinetic energy $= \frac{1}{2}MV^2$, where M is the mass and V is the velocity), and more than 90% of gunshot wounds to the abdomen are associated with significant injuries. Hollow viscera and large vessels are often involved, and solid organs such as the liver and the spleen may demonstrate burst injuries. Therefore, laparotomy is mandated in virtually all gunshot wounds to the abdomen.

Stab Wounds

Stab wounds to the abdomen carry potential for devastating injury, depending on which intraabdominal structures are involved. The extent of the injury also depends on the type, size, and length of the weapon and on the trajectory. Major vascular injuries pose the greatest threat; commonly injured vessels include the intraabdominal aorta, the inferior vena cava, the portal vein, and the hepatic veins.

Anterior stab wounds are explored via laparotomy if hemodynamic instability or signs of peritonitis are present, if blood is noted in the gastric aspirate or on rectal examination, or if pneumoperitoneum or evisceration is noted (Fig. 107.3). Local exploration is needed to rule out penetration of the peritoneum, even in minor stab wounds. In cases in which the exploration cannot rule out peritoneal penetration, laparoscopy will delineate the injury and many minor injuries can be repaired without open surgery.

Stab wounds to the flank or back are less readily and less quickly diagnosed than do anterior wounds; the retroperi-toneal structures are more protected by paraspinal musculature, and bleeding is often tamponaded in this area. Dorsal stab wounds are sometimes managed nonoperatively unless hemodynamic instability or signs of peritonitis are present, although selective laparotomy is a common surgical strategy.

LAP AND SHOULDER BELT AND AIR BAG INJURIES

Children who are too small for adult seat belts are at increased risk for injuries. In particular, children restrained only by lap belts in motor vehicles involved in rapid deceleration crashes are at risk to sustain Chance fractures (compression or flexion-distraction fractures of the lumbar spine) in association with intraabdominal injuries (the lap belt complex). As many as one-half the children with Chance fractures have intraabdominal injuries, including duodenal perforation, mesenteric disruption, transection of small bowel, and bladder rupture (Fig. 107.8). Therefore, a high index of suspicion must be maintained to detect such injuries. The hallmark of the lap belt complex is abdominal or flank ecchymosis in the pattern of a strap or belt (Fig. 107.9). This is accompanied by abdominal and back pain. A normal abdominal CT scan does not rule out ruptured viscus, and laparoscopy or laparotomy should be considered for children in whom the lap belt complex is suspected strongly (Fig. 107.10). Carotid injuries caused by high-riding shoulder restraints in motor vehicle collisions are much less common.

Although it is well publicized that children younger than 12 years or less than 5 feet in height should not ride in the front seat of a vehicle that has functioning air bag restraints, significant injuries and deaths continue to occur. Life-threatening injuries caused by air bag deployment are typically related to cervical spine injuries and closed head trauma. Less severe air bag injuries include abrasions to the face, neck, and chest;

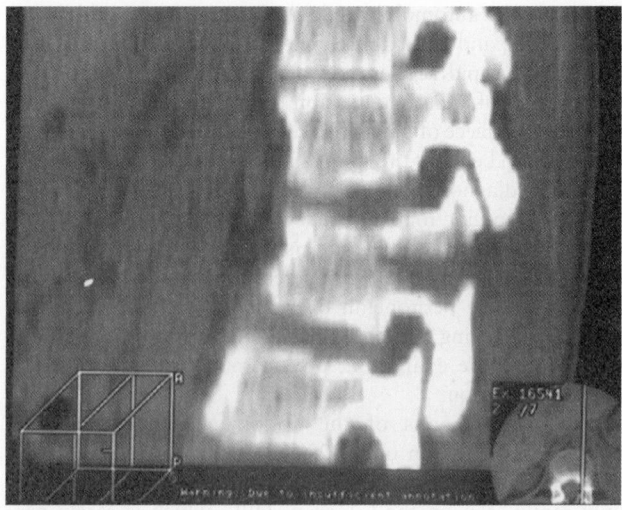

FIGURE 107.8 Magnetic resonance imaging scan of the lumbar spine of a 12-year-old girl involved in a high-speed motor vehicle collision. An anterior compression of L2 is seen, with disruption of the posterior elements. The lap belt complex in this patient also included loss of her small bowel secondary to thrombosis of the superior mesenteric artery.

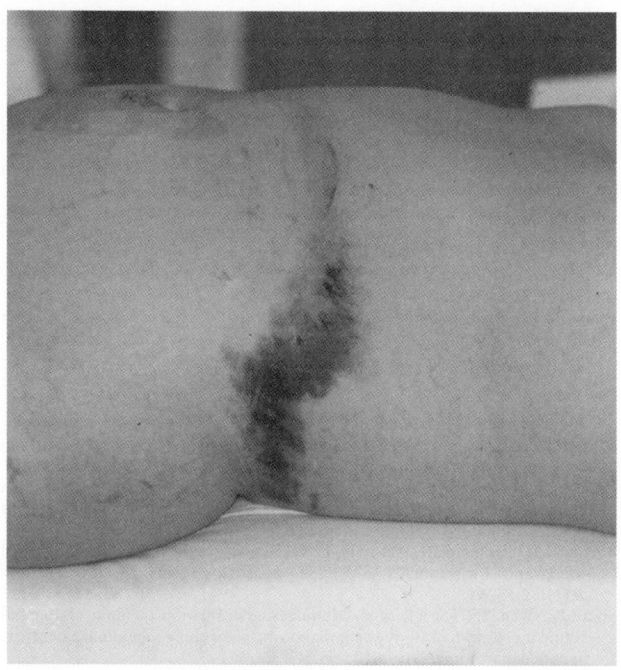

FIGURE 107.9 Eleven-year-old girl with classic abdominal and flank ecchymosis in the pattern of a lap belt. Her injuries included colon perforation and a Chance fracture.

minor burns to the upper extremities; blunt ocular trauma; and chemical keratitis.

CHILD ABUSE

At least 1.6 million children are abused or neglected every year in the United States. Major blunt abdominal trauma resulting from physical abuse is uncommon but highly fatal in children;

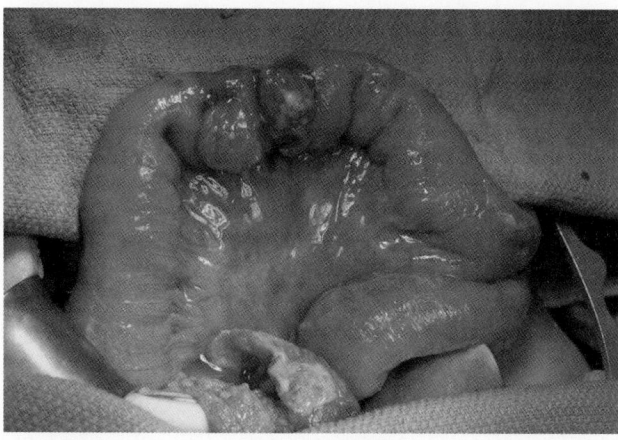

FIGURE 107.10 Intraoperative photograph of a segment of small bowel of a 15-year-old boy who was a lap and shoulder belt–restrained back seat passenger in a motor vehicle collision. Initial examination revealed ecchymosis below the umbilicus and significant tenderness upon palpation of the lower abdomen. Findings at laparotomy included near transaction of the terminal ileum with devitalized tissue at the edges of the injury.

mortality rates are as high as 50%. This high fatality rate is the result of the unfortunate but typical delay with which parents or caregivers who abuse children seek treatment.

Children who are seriously injured because of physical abuse commonly have more than one site of trauma; some of the injuries can be occult, and others may have been inflicted at different times. Abdominal injuries are usually inflicted by fists, feet, or small handheld objects and are rarely penetrating. The diagnosis of blunt abdominal injury caused by battering is difficult to make unless a high index of suspicion for child abuse is maintained. An important clue is often an implausible historical account for the seriousness of the injury. As with abdominal trauma caused by other mechanisms, physical examination findings may not be obvious. Laboratory analyses and abdominal CT may be necessary to confirm the diagnosis. Less obvious intraabdominal injuries may be suspected by the use of a Wood lamp. Enhanced visualization of bruising not otherwise seen in normal light may be apparent under ultraviolet (Wood lamp) illumination. Such bruising on the abdomen or flanks should increase the suspicion for occult intraabdominal injuries.

Severe injuries may present with obtundation and shock, abdominal distension, and tenderness. Intraabdominal injuries most commonly involve the liver and the spleen, as well as the pancreas-duodenum-jejunum region. In all such cases in which child battering is suspected, a child protection consultant should be involved early.

Suggested Readings

Adesanya AA, da Rocha-Afodu JT, Ekanem EE, et al. Factors affecting mortality and morbidity in patients with abdominal gunshot wounds. *Injury* 2000;31:397–404.
Akgur FM, Aktug T, Olguner M, et al. Prospective study investigating routine usage of ultrasonography as the initial diagnostic modality for the evaluation of children sustaining blunt abdominal trauma. *J Trauma* 1997;42:626–628.
Arkovitz MS, Johnson N, Garcia VF. Pancreatic trauma in children: mechanisms of injury. *J Trauma* 1997;42:49–53.
Bensard DD, Beaver BL, Besner GE, et al. Small bowel injury after blunt abdominal trauma: is diagnostic delay important? *J Trauma* 1996;41:476–483.
Benya EC, Lim-Dunham JE, Landrum O, et al. Abdominal sonography in examination of children with blunt abdominal trauma. *Am J Radiol* 2000;174:1613–1616.
Bickell WH, Wall MJ Jr, Pepe PE, et al. Immediate versus delayed fluid resuscitation for hypotensive patients with penetrating torso injuries. *N Engl J Med* 1994;331:1105–1109.
Bond SJ, Eichelberger MR, Gotschell CS, et al. Nonoperative management of blunt hepatic and splenic injury in children. *Ann Surg* 1996;223:286–289.
Boyle EM, Maier RV, Salazar JD, et al. Diagnosis of injuries after stab wounds to the back and flank. *J Trauma* 1997;42:260–265.
Branney SW, Moore EE, Cantrill SV, et al. Ultrasound based key clinical pathway reduces the use of hospital resources for the evaluation of blunt abdominal trauma. *J Trauma* 1997;42:1086–1090.
Capraro AJ, Mooney DP, Waltzman ML. The use of routine laboratory studies as screening tools in pediatric abdominal trauma. *Pediatr Emerg Care* 2006;22:480–484.
Carillo EH, Bergamini TM, Miller FB, et al. Abdominal vascular injuries. *J Trauma* 1997;43:164–171.
Coley BD, Mutabagani KH, Martin LC, et al. Focused abdominal sonography for trauma (FAST) in children with blunt abdominal trauma. *J Trauma* 2000;48:902–906.
Cooper A, Floyd T, Barlow B, et al. Major blunt abdominal trauma due to child abuse. *J Trauma* 1988;28:1483–1487.
Durbin DR, Arbogast KB, Moll EK. Seat belt syndrome in children: a case report and review of the literature. *Pediatr Emerg Care* 2001;17:474–477.
Emery KH, McAneney CM, Racadio JM, et al. Absent peritoneal fluid on screening trauma ultrasonography in children: a prospective comparison with computed tomography. *J Pediatr Surg* 2001;36:565–569.
Ford E, Hardin W, Mahour G, et al. Pseudocyst of the pancreas in children. *Am Surg* 1990;56:384–387.

Gaines BA, Ford HR. Abdominal and pelvic trauma in children. *Crit Care Med* 2002;30:S416–S423.

Georgi B, Massad M, Obeid M. Ballistic trauma to the abdomen: shell fragments versus bullets. *J Trauma* 1991;31:711–716.

Hackam DJ, Potoka D, Meza M, et al. Utility of radiographic hepatic injury grade in predicting outcome for children after blunt abdominal trauma. *J Pediatr Surg* 2002;37:386–389.

Hennes H, Smith D, Schneider K, et al. Elevated liver transaminase levels in children with blunt abdominal trauma: a predictor of liver injury. *Pediatrics* 1990;86:87–90.

Holmes JF, Brant WE, Bond WF, et al. Emergency department ultrasonography in the evaluation of hypotensive and normotensive children with blunt abdominal trauma. *J Pediatr Surg* 2001;36:968–973.

Holmes JF, Sokolove PE, Brant WE, et al. Identification of children with intra-abdominal injuries after blunt trauma. *Ann Emerg Med* 2002;39:500–509.

Isaacman DJ, Scarfone RJ, Kost SI, et al. Utility of routine laboratory testing for detecting intraabdominal injury in the pediatric trauma patient. *Pediatrics* 1993;92:691–694.

Karaduman D, Sarioglu-Buke A, Kilic I, et al. The role of elevated liver transaminase levels in children with blunt abdominal trauma. *Injury* 2003;34:249–252.

Keller MS, Stafford PW, Vane DW. Conservative management of pancreatic trauma in children. *J Trauma* 1997;42:1097–1100.

Ladd AP, West KW, Rouse TM, et al. Surgical management of duodenal injuries in children. *Surgery* 2002;132:748–753.

Lieu TA, Fleisher GR, Mahboubi S, et al. Hematuria and clinical findings as indications for intravenous pyelography in pediatric blunt renal trauma. *Pediatrics* 1988;82:216–222.

Lutz N, Arbogast KB, Cornejo RA, et al. Suboptimal restraint affects the pattern of abdominal injuries in children involved in motor vehicle crashes. *J Pediatr Surg* 2003;38:919–923.

McKinley AJ, Mahomed AA. Laparoscopy in a case of pediatric blunt abdominal trauma. *Surg Endosc* 2002;16:358.

Meyer D, Thal E, Weigelt J. The role of abdominal computed tomography in the evaluation of stab wounds to the back. *J Trauma* 1989;29:1226–1229.

Nadler EP, Gardner M, Schall LC, et al. Management of blunt pancreatic injury in children. *J Trauma* 1999;47:1098–1103.

Nagy KK, Krosner SM, Joseph KT. A method of determining peritoneal penetration in gunshot wounds to the abdomen. *J Trauma* 1997;43:242–246.

Nance ML, Peden GW, Shapiro MB. Solid viscus injury predicts major hollow viscus injury in blunt abdominal trauma. *J Trauma* 1997;43:618–623.

Newman KD, Bowman LM, Eichelberger MR, et al. The lap belt complex: intestinal and lumbar spine injury in children. *J Trauma* 1990;30:1133–1140.

Nichol PF, Helin M, Zdeblick TA, et al. Traumatic near-hemicorpectomy by a seat belt injury in an 11-year-old girl. *J Trauma* 2002;53(4):777–779.

Okamoto K, Norio H, Kaneko N, et al. Use of early-phase dynamic spiral computed tomography for primary screening of multiple trauma. *Am J Emerg Med* 2002;20:528–534.

Oldham K, Guice R, Kaufman R, et al. Blunt hepatic injury and elevated hepatic enzymes: a clinical correlation in children. *J Pediatr Surg* 1984;19:457–461.

Partrick DA, Bensard DD, Moore EE, et al. Nonoperative management of solid organ injuries in children results in decreased blood utilization. *J Pediatr Surg* 1999;34:1695–1699.

Patel JC, Tepas JJ. The efficacy of focused abdominal sonography for trauma (FAST) as a screening tool in the assessment of injury children. *J Pediatr Surg* 1999;34:44–47.

Patton JH, Syden SP, Croce MA, et al. Pancreatic trauma: a simplified management guideline. *J Trauma* 1997;43:234–241.

Peitzman AB, Ford HR, Harbrecht BG, et al. Injury to the spleen. *Curr Probl Surg* 2001;38:932–1008.

Potoka DA, Schall LC, Ford HR. Risk factors for splenectomy in children with blunt splenic trauma. *J Pediatr Surg* 2002;37:294–299.

Puranik SR, Hayes JS, Long J, et al. Liver enzymes as predictors of liver damage due to blunt abdominal trauma in children. *South Med J* 2002;95:203–206.

Richards JR, Derlet RW. Computed tomography and blunt abdominal injury: patient selection based on examination, haematocrit and haematuria. *Injury* 1997;28:181–185.

Richards JR, Schleper NH, Woo BD, et al. Sonographic assessment of blunt abdominal trauma: a 4-year prospective study. *J Clin Ultrasound* 2002;30:59–67.

Rose JS, Levitt MA, Porter J, et al. Does the presence of ultrasound really affect computed tomographic scan use? A prospective randomized trial of ultrasound in trauma. *J Trauma* 2001;51:545–550.

Sahdev P, Garramone R, Schwartz R, et al. Evaluation of liver function tests in screening for intra-abdominal injuries. *Ann Emerg Med* 1991;20:830–841.

Saladino R, Lund D, Fleisher G. The spectrum of liver and spleen injuries in childhood: failure of the pediatric trauma score and clinical signs to predict isolated injuries. *Ann Emerg Med* 1991;6:636–640.

Soudack M, Epelman M, Maor R, et al. Experience with focused abdominal sonography for trauma (FAST) in 313 pediatric patients. *J Clin Ultrasound* 2004;32:53–61.

Shih HC, Wen YS, Ko TJ, et al. Noninvasive evaluation of blunt abdominal trauma: prospective study using diagnostic algorithms to minimize nontherapeutic laparotomy. *World J Surg* 1999;23:265–270.

Stalker HP, Kaufman PR, Sledge K. The significance of hematuria in children after blunt trauma. *AJR Am J Roentgenol* 1990;154:569–571.

Stylianos S, APSA Liver/Spleen Trauma Study Group. Compliance with evidence-based guidelines in children with isolated spleen or liver injury: a prospective study. *J Pediatr Surg* 2002;37:453–456.

Stylianos S, Jacir NN, Hoffman MA, et al. Experimental volume replacement through lower extremity veins. *J Trauma* 1993;35:666–670.

Subcommittee on Advanced Trauma Life Support of the American College of Surgeons Trauma Committee. *Advanced trauma life support for doctors*, 8th ed. Chicago, IL: American College of Surgeons, 2008.

Taylor GA, Eichelberger MR, Potter BM. Hematuria: a marker of abdominal injury in children after blunt abdominal trauma. *Ann Surg* 1988;208:688–693.

van der Sluis CK, Kingma J, Eisma WH, et al. Pediatric polytrauma: short-term and long-term outcomes. *J Trauma* 1997;43:501–506.

Vogeley E, Pierce MC, Bertocci GE. Experience with Wood lamp illumination and digital photography in the documentation of bruises on human skin. *Arch Pediatr Adolesc Med* 2002;156:265–268.

West K, Grosfeld J. Post-splenectomy sepsis: historical background and current concepts. *World J Surg* 1985;9:477–483.

Zantut LF, Ivatury RR, Smith RS, et al. Diagnostic and therapeutic laparoscopy for penetrating abdominal trauma: a multicenter experience. *J Trauma* 1997;42:825–831.

CHAPTER 108 ■ BURNS

MARK D. JOFFE, MD

BACKGROUND

Children in modern society will inevitably be exposed to thermal energy that has the potential to cause injury. While preventive efforts are paramount in importance, all clinicians who care for injured children must be able to assess and begin treatment of both minor and severe burns. Burns and related injuries are the third leading cause of death in childhood, killing approximately 2,500 children per year. Children suffering morbidity from serious burns are three times as numerous as those who die. Medical care is sought for burn injuries more than 250,000 times per year in the United States, generating costs that exceed $1 billion per year. Competent management of minor burns can optimize cosmetic results and minimize functional morbidity for children, a benefit that is difficult to express in dollars.

The past 40 years has seen major advances in burn treatment and improved outcomes. A recent study reported a mortality rate of only 39% for children with burns of more than 80% of body surface area (BSA). Factors associated with hospital care were much more predictive of survival than injury characteristics or time to resuscitation, so every child, regardless of the extent and severity of burns, should be aggressively resuscitated by prehospital and emergency care providers.

Only 3% to 5% of all burns in children are life threatening. Most burns are minor scalds, accounting for about 80% of all thermal injuries. Flames produce 13% of burns and with associated smoke inhalation result in the majority of deaths. Electrical or chemical burns account for 2% to 3% of injuries and pose special challenges in management.

Males and children younger than 5 years are at highest risk of thermal injury. Bathing-related scalds are a particular risk during infancy. Hot liquid spills are common in toddlers. School-aged children are often injured as a result of playing with matches, with high morbidity and mortality to the child and his or her family. Burns related to high-voltage electrical lines are seen primarily in teenagers.

Several preventive strategies can reduce the risk of thermal injury to children. Lowering the temperature of water heaters from more than 130°F (54.4°C) to 120°F (48.9°C) increases the time for full-thickness scalding from less than 30 seconds to 10 minutes. Burn centers have noted a decrease in full-thickness flame burns since the introduction of flame-resistant children's sleepwear. Cigarette misuse is responsible for more than 30% of house fires. Childproof lighters and "fire-safe" cigarettes have the potential to reduce the frequency of these often-deadly events. Smoke detectors and sprinkler systems can greatly reduce deaths, but only if installed and maintained properly. Advances in burn prevention can have a far greater impact on public health than refinements in burn management.

PATHOPHYSIOLOGY

The skin is a complex organ performing many vital functions that are often unappreciated until it is severely injured. Skin preserves body fluids, efficiently regulates heat loss to the environment, and acts as a barrier to infectious pathogens. It is composed of an outer, mostly nonviable epidermis, and a dermis. The outer layer of the epidermis, the stratum corneum, prevents passive water loss and is lethal to most viruses and gram-negative bacteria. It has a fatty acid film that is fungistatic and bacteriostatic. The dermal–epidermal junction prevents loss of macromolecules through the skin. Eccrine sweat glands in the dermis secrete fluid to increase evaporative heat loss. Vasodilation and vasoconstriction of blood vessels in the dermis regulate radiant heat loss, affecting a 100-fold variation in skin perfusion. Therefore, children with extensive burns have difficulty retaining body fluids and regulating temperature (Fig. 108.1).

Major systemic physiologic effects are seen in children with burns of more than 20% of BSA. Burn injury causes increased capillary permeability and the release of osmotically active molecules to the interstitial space resulting in extravasation of fluid. Protein is lost from the vascular space to the interstitium during the first 24 hours. In patients with large burns, vasoactive mediators are released to the circulation and result in systemic capillary leakage. Edema develops in both burned and noninjured tissues. Circulating factors that depress myocardial function decrease cardiac output. Acute hemolysis of up to 15% of red blood cells may occur both from direct heat damage and from a microangiopathic hemolytic process. The profound circulatory effects of severe burns can result in life-threatening shock early after injury.

Hair follicles, sweat glands, and sebaceous glands in the dermis play a crucial role in the healing of partial-thickness burns. After an inflammatory phase characterized by leukocyte infiltration, cytokine release, and complement activation, epithelial cells in these structures undergo metaplasia to produce a stratified squamous epithelial cell layer that is required for healing of skin. Neovascularization and fibroblast migration occur 1 to 3 weeks after partial-thickness burns. Overproduction of collagen can result in hypertrophic scarring. In full-thickness and deep partial-thickness burns, the absence of sufficient dermal appendages precludes reepithelialization by this mechanism and necessitates skin grafting.

Thermal energy damages the skin structures in proportion to the intensity and duration of exposure. Hot grease and

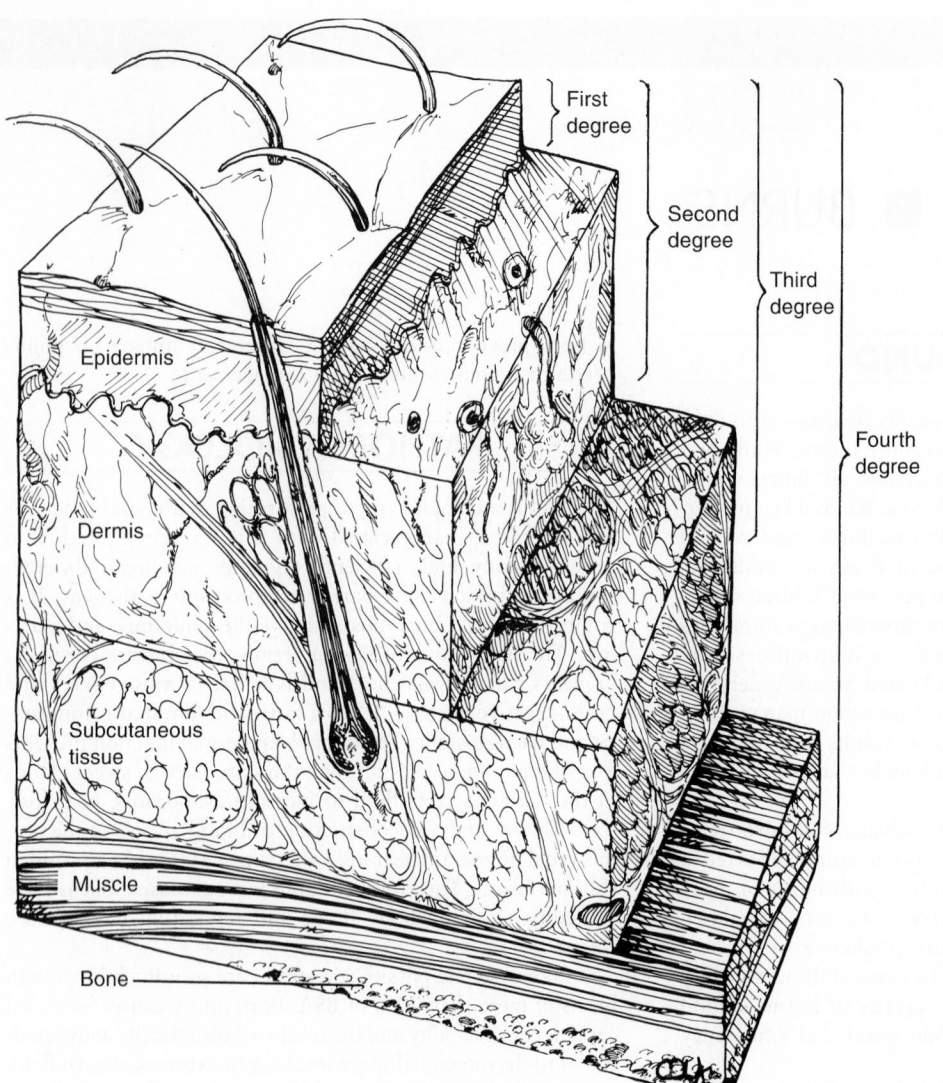

FIGURE 108.1 Degree of burn wound depth. First degree involves only the epidermis, second degree extends into the dermis, third degree into subcutaneous tissue, and fourth degree to muscle, tendons, or bone.

thick soups and cereals cause deeper injuries because they cling to the skin longer than scalding water, affording more time for transfer of the thermal energy. Ignition of synthetic fabrics often causes melting and adherence to the skin, resulting in more serious burns than ignition of cotton garments. Skin thickness is also a variable in the severity of injury with a given thermal exposure. Submersion of the hand may result in deep burns of the dorsum, with relative sparing of the thick skin of the palm. The thinner skin of young children accounts for deeper burns than those in adults with similar heat exposure.

A first-degree burn is characterized by redness and a mild inflammatory response confined to the epidermis, without significant edema or bulla formation. First-degree burns are not included in the calculation of burn surface area used for therapeutic decisions. These minor burns may be painful and resolve in 3 to 5 days without scarring.

Most burns treated in emergency departments (EDs) are partial-thickness or second-degree burns. Superficial second-degree burns involve destruction of the epidermis and less than half of the dermis. Blistering is often present. Increased capillary permeability, resulting from direct thermal injury and local mediator release, results in edema. These injuries are usually painful because intact sensory nerve receptors are exposed. The capillary network in the superficial dermis gives these burns a pink-red color and moist appearance. Healing occurs in about 2 weeks, and scarring is usually minimal.

Deep partial-thickness burns involve destruction of the epidermis and most of the dermis. Edema can lessen the exposure of sensory nerve receptors, making some partial-thickness burns less painful and tender. Deep partial-thickness burns have a paler, drier appearance than superficial injuries, at times making them difficult to distinguish from full-thickness injury. Thrombosed vessels often give deep partial-thickness burns a speckled appearance. Burns evaluated immediately may appear to be partial-thickness injuries and subsequently become full-thickness injuries, especially if secondary damage from infection, trauma, or hypoperfusion ensues. Deep partial-thickness burns can take many weeks to heal completely. Unacceptable scarring is common and skin grafting may be necessary to optimize cosmetic results.

Full-thickness or third-degree burns involve destruction of the epidermis and the entire dermis. They usually have a pale or charred color and a leathery appearance. Destruction of the cutaneous nerves in the dermis makes them nontender, although surrounding areas of partial-thickness burns may be painful. Full-thickness burns cause a loss of skin elasticity. The burned skin cannot expand as tissue edema develops during the first 24 to 48 hours of fluid therapy. Circumferential or near-circumferential burns can therefore cause respiratory distress, abdominal compartment syndrome, and vascular insufficiency of the distal extremities. Full-thickness burns cannot reepithelialize and can heal only from the periphery. Most require skin grafting. Fourth-degree burns are those full-thickness injuries that also involve underlying fascia, muscle, or bone.

Heat causes coagulation necrosis of tissue, producing a protein-rich medium that nourishes bacterial growth. Burns become colonized with potentially pathogenic organisms, primarily from the skin and intestinal flora of the patient with burn injury and not from exogenous sources. Cleansing and debridement reduce substrate for bacterial proliferation and topical antimicrobial therapy reduces the number of microorganisms, but burns are never completely sterilized so that the risk of secondary infection is always present.

FIRST AID AND PREHOSPITAL CARE

Emergency physicians may be consulted about the immediate care of minor burns. Early cooling is accomplished by running cold water over the injured area. If performed in the first 30 minutes after injury, it not only stops ongoing thermal damage but also prevents edema, reducing progression to full-thickness injury. Applying ice directly to the wound is painful, and the extreme cold can worsen the injury. Parents should be reminded not to put grease, butter, or any ointment on the burn because these substances do not dissipate heat well and may contribute to the contamination. Intact blisters should not be broken during the prehospital phase. The burn should be covered with a clean cloth or bandage.

Small burns from mechanisms unlikely to cause full-thickness injury can be managed at home with a topical antibiotic and a bandage. Burns of larger size and burns involving the face, hands, feet, or perineum should be evaluated promptly by a physician. Telephone advice, without the benefit of physical examination, should always err on the side of caution with recommendation for a medical evaluation.

The concerns for children with major burns are different. Prehospital care providers should initially forget about the burn and focus on airway, breathing, and circulation, as they would for any other trauma victim. Rapid transport to a hospital setting is crucial. Oxygen should be administered. The trachea should be intubated if there are signs of upper airway obstruction, apnea, or severe hypoventilation. If transport time is likely to be prolonged, intravenous fluids should be started. Inadequate prehospital fluid resuscitation has been associated with preventable deaths in children with burns.

MAJOR BURNS

Evaluation and Management

During the first few seconds after arrival, the physician must determine if a patient with burn injury requires aggressive therapy for major burns (more than 20% of BSA) (Fig. 108.2). In children with severe injuries, the evaluation and initial management take place simultaneously. Smoldering clothing or other sources of continued burning must be removed. Information about the circumstances of the burn and the potential for associated injuries should be sought from prehospital care providers, police, or family members, but this should not delay the initial treatment.

Airway

Improper airway management has been implicated in some deaths of children with severe burns. Most life-threatening burns are the result of house fires. The inhalation of hot gases can burn the upper airway, leading to progressive edema and airway obstruction. Any child with burns of the face, singed facial hairs, or hoarseness is at high risk, but airway burns can occur in the absence of these signs. Edema of the burned airway will worsen over the first 24 to 48 hours. Knowledge of the time course of airway swelling justifies intubation of the trachea for subtle signs of airway compromise that occur shortly after the injury. Early intubation may circumvent a difficult intubation later in the course of a child with severe pharyngeal and airway edema. Endotracheal tubes of smaller diameter than expected for age should be available in anticipation of a narrowed airway. Increasingly, cuffed endotracheal tubes are used to decrease air leaks, even in children younger than 8 years.

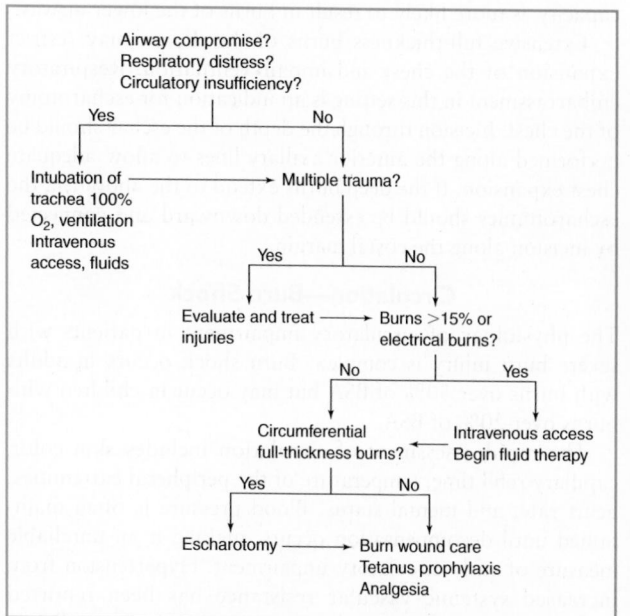

FIGURE 108.2 Diagnostic approach to the patient with burn injury.

TRAUMA

Children who have jumped or fallen in house fires, been burned in motor vehicle accidents, or been burned by explosions are at risk for associated cervical spine and other traumatic injuries. A history of trauma may not be available at the time of airway management. Physicians should manage the airway with the neck in a neutral position, avoiding any flexion or extension. Radiographs can be obtained later to help exclude cervical spine injury (see Chapter 115). Children with severe burns may have depressed levels of consciousness for many reasons. Airway obstruction from the loss of pharyngeal tone is not uncommon. A chin-lift maneuver is now recommended for all lay rescuers, but the jaw-thrust maneuver is preferred in patients with possible cervical spine injury.

Breathing

A rapid assessment of ventilation includes respiratory effort, chest expansion, breath sounds, and color. Pulse oximetry is useful, but patients with significant levels of carboxyhemoglobin will look pink and have "normal" oxygen saturation as measured by a pulse oximeter. Children with severe burn injury should receive 100% oxygen. Arterial blood gases with CO-oximetry should be obtained promptly. Careful assisted ventilation is recommended for patients whose ventilatory status is questionable. Avoidance of high inflating pressures and application of cricoid pressure can minimize gaseous distension of the stomach and reduce the risk of regurgitation with pulmonary aspiration.

Children burned in house fires or in any closed space are at high risk of inhalation injury. Facial burns, singed facial hairs, and carbonaceous sputum are not always present in children with significant inhalation injury. Chest radiographs may be normal initially, even if pulmonary injury has occurred. Smoke is responsible for most of the lower airway abnormalities in patients with burn injury, and management of smoke inhalation is covered in Chapter 87. The efficient heat-exchange function of the upper airway can dramatically reduce the temperature of inspired dry gases, protecting the lower airway from thermal injury. Inhalation of steam, with its higher heat capacity, is more likely to result in burns of the lower airway.

Extensive full-thickness burns of the thorax may restrict expansion of the chest and impair ventilation. Respiratory embarrassment in this setting is an indication for escharotomy of the chest. Incision through the depth of the eschar should be performed along the anterior axillary lines to allow adequate chest expansion. If the deep burns extend to the abdomen, the escharotomies should be extended downward and connected by incision along the costal margin.

Circulation—Burn Shock

The physiology of circulatory impairment in patients with severe burn injury is complex. Burn shock occurs in adults with burns over 30% of BSA but may occur in children with burns over 20% of BSA.

The rapid assessment of circulation includes skin color, capillary refill time, temperature of the peripheral extremities, heart rate, and mental status. Blood pressure is often maintained until decompensation occurs, making it an unreliable measure of early circulatory impairment. Hypertension from increased systemic vascular resistance has been reported immediately after severe burns, particularly in pediatric patients, and must not discourage proper fluid therapy.

Vascular access should be obtained soon after arrival of the child with severe burn injury. Peripheral, large-bore intravenous catheters are favored because they have the lowest resistance. Catheters placed in the upper extremity through intact skin are preferred because they are easier to secure, but access through burned areas may be necessary. Anticipating the need for hyperalimentation, sites for central catheter placement should be saved, if possible. Attention to aseptic technique when starting intravenous catheters in the ED can prevent infectious complications during subsequent care. Circumferential taping is dangerous because the swelling that occurs during the first 24 hours can cause circulatory insufficiency distal to the constriction. Urine output is the most important means of monitoring fluid status, but in patients with severe burns with associated inhalation injury, central venous pressure monitoring may be useful in the first few hours.

An initial bolus of 20 mL per kg of Ringer's lactate solution is recommended while assessment of the extent of the burns takes place. Fluid volume from initial boluses should be counted when calculating fluid volumes during the first 24 hours of treatment. A urinary catheter should be placed early in the management because there are often several hours of monitoring during transport or in the ED during which urine production can provide clinicians with information about fluid status. Major burns cause decreased splanchnic blood flow and ileus. After ensuring that the airway is protected by an endotracheal tube or an adequate gag reflex, the clinician should place a nasogastric tube. Hypothermia can occur rapidly in small children, especially in those whose skin injury impairs normal thermoregulation. Core temperature should be monitored and the child kept covered, except as necessary for examination and burn assessment. Children younger than 7 years who are not fully immunized, or if immunization status is unknown, should receive DTap patients 7 years and older who require tetanus prophylaxis should receive Td or Tdap (not immunized, unknown status 5 years or longer since last tetanus-containing vaccine dose); unimmunized and underimmunized patients also require tetanus immune globulin.

Peripheral circulation may require assessment with a Doppler device because the usual methods of assessment, including capillary refill and temperature, are difficult in a child with severe burn injury. First, all jewelry and watches should be removed because these may restrict distal flow of the blood. For extensive, deep upper extremity burns, the radial, ulnar, and palmar arch pulses should be checked by Doppler ultrasound. Posterior tibial and dorsalis pedis pulses are assessed when the lower extremity is involved. Absence of flow or progressive diminution of the pulse is an indication for escharotomy through the depth of the eschar on the medial and lateral aspects of the extremities, including the hands. Finger escharotomies are seldom necessary and should be undertaken only after consultation with a burn center surgeon. It is especially important to extend escharotomy incisions across the joints because at these locations, the skin is tightly adhered to the underlying fascia where vascular obstruction is likely to occur. The procedure does not require anesthesia because the wounds are full thickness and therefore insensate. Pulses assessed by Doppler ultrasound should immediately improve after escharotomy. If improvement is not immediate, hypovolemia should be suspected. Reperfusion of the extremities after escharotomy may abruptly reduce intravascular volume and require prompt adjustment of fluid therapy.

Assessment

After stabilization of vital functions in the primary survey, a systematic evaluation of the surface area and depth of burns follows. The rule of nines used to estimate burn surface area in adults cannot be applied to children because they have different body proportions. Young children have relatively larger heads and smaller extremities. Areas of partial- and full-thickness injuries should be recorded on an anatomic chart (Fig. 108.3) and then total percentage burn surface area computed using age-appropriate proportions. First-degree burns are not included. A child's palm including the fingers is approximately 1% of BSA and can be used to estimate the extent of scattered, smaller burns (Fig. 108.3).

BSA calculations are inexact, and some first-degree burns may progress to second-degree burns over time, so BSA estimates should be reassessed.

Fluid Therapy

Rapid treatment of the hypovolemia that occurs early in children with severe thermal injuries is of prime importance. The fluid status of children with burn injury is a dynamic process that requires careful reevaluation and therapeutic adjustments. Extravasation of water, sodium, and protein through abnormally permeable capillaries continues for about 24 hours after injury. Capillary integrity then improves and intravascular volume stabilizes. Most burn centers recommend crystalloid during

Area	Birth–1 yr	1–4 yr	5–9 yr	10–14 yr	15 yr	Adult
Head	19	17	13	11	9	7
Neck	2	2	2	2	2	2
Anterior trunk	13	13	13	13	13	13
Posterior trunk	13	13	13	13	13	13
Right buttock	2½	2½	2½	2½	2½	2½
Left buttock	2½	2½	2½	2½	2½	2½
Genitalia	1	1	1	1	1	1
Right upper arm	4	4	4	4	4	4
Left upper arm	4	4	4	4	4	4
Right lower arm	3	3	3	3	3	3
Left lower arm	3	3	3	3	3	3
Right hand	2½	2½	2½	2½	2½	2½
Left hand	2½	2½	2½	2½	2½	2½
Right thigh	5½	6½	8	8½	9	9½
Left thigh	5½	6½	8	8½	9	9½
Right leg	5	5	5½	6	6½	7
Left leg	5	5	5½	6	6½	7
Right foot	3½	3½	3½	3½	3½	3½
Left foot	3½	3½	3½	3½	3½	3½
						Total

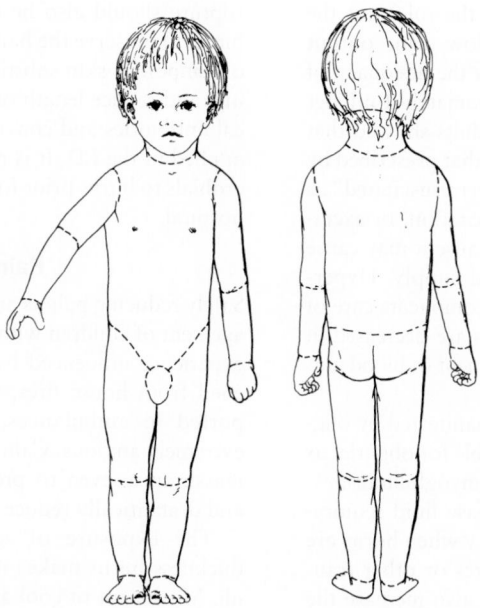

FIGURE 108.3 Estimation of surface area burned on the basis of age. This modification by O'Neill of the Brooke Army Burn Center diagram shows the change in surface of the head from 19% in an infant to 7% in an adult. Proper use of this chart *(above)* provides an accurate basis for subsequent management of the child with burn injury.

TABLE 108.1

FLUID RESUSCITATION FORMULAS

Parkland: 4 mL/kg/% of BSA second- and third-degree burns, half in the first 8 h following injury, half in the next 16 h. Add maintenance with 5% dextrose in children <5 years old
Galveston Shriners: 5,000 mL/m²/% of BSA second- and third-degree burns, half in the first 8 h, half in the next 16 h. Add 2,000 mL/m²/day maintenance with 5% dextrose

the first 24 hours because colloid may extravasate through the leaky capillaries and worsen interstitial edema. Once capillary integrity is restored, colloid is useful for volume expansion and for restoration and maintenance of serum oncotic pressure. The sodium ion is critical for maintaining adequate intravascular volume, so isotonic crystalloid solutions are recommended in the resuscitation phase. Hyperosmolar therapy with 3% saline appears to have little benefit and increased risk. Potassium is released from damaged cells and may elevate measured serum levels shortly after injury; therefore, potassium replacement is not recommended during the early phase of fluid therapy.

Several formulas for the calculation of initial fluid therapy exist (Table 108.1). The Parkland formula recommends 4 mL per kg/% of BSA of crystalloid over the first 24 hours, half during the first 8 hours from the time of injury and half during the next 16 hours. This formula underestimates the fluid needs of young children, who are also at greater risk for hypoglycemia. Maintenance requirements are added for patients with burns who are younger than 5 years using isotonic solutions with 5% dextrose. The Galveston Shriners formula uses BSA rather than weight to calculate fluid therapy. Galveston Shriners recommends 5,000 mL per m²/% of BSA, half during the first 8 hours from the time of injury and half during the next 16 hours, plus 2,000 mL per m² per day as maintenance. The calculated volume requirements are useful in choosing an initial rate of fluid infusion. Adjustments of infusion rates are the rule, not the exception. Most pediatric burn centers follow urine output rather than central venous pressure to assess the adequacy of fluid therapy. Children should produce approximately 1 mL per kg per hour of urine. A study of burns in adults showed that most patients receive more fluid volume than that prescribed by the Parkland formula, and almost half are "overresuscitated" as defined by excessive urine output. Overresuscitation, or excessive fluid administration, is to be avoided because it may cause tissue edema that compromises local blood supply. Hyperglycemia may cause an osmotic diuresis and complicate care of the patient with burn injury. Before infusions are decreased in response to excessive urine output, a measurement of blood glucose should be made.

Inadequate fluid resuscitation is usually manifested by oliguria. Rarely, intrinsic renal disease is responsible for oliguria, as may occur after electrical injuries because of myoglobinuria.

Trauma associated with burns may increase fluid requirements. Additional fluids may also be necessary when burns are associated with an inhalation injury. Fractures or other traumatic lesions causing blood loss and edema also increase the need for fluids. Neurogenic shock from unrecognized cervical spine or head injury may cause hypotension, usually with a relative bradycardia. Toxins, such as cyanide, ingested before the burn or inhaled during the fire can depress myocardial function or vascular tone. Any patient with shock that appears out of proportion to the extent of the burn injury, or who is poorly responsive to fluid therapy, should have an aggressive diagnostic workup for concurrent problems.

Antibiotics

Burn sepsis continues to be the major cause of mortality after the period of resuscitation despite improvements in topical and systemic antimicrobials. Meticulous antiseptic techniques can lessen colonization of burns with potential pathogens. Topical antibiotics further reduce bacterial number. Early streptococcal cellulitis is less common than in years before the development of topical antibiotics for burns, and most burn centers do not routinely treat patients with prophylactic penicillin. Pediatric patients, however, may have greater risk than adults, and some pediatric burn centers administer intravenous penicillin for the first 3 to 5 days after injury.

Broad-spectrum antibiotics should not be used prophylactically because of the increased likelihood of inducing resistant organisms. Frequent examination of healing burns for signs of infection and cultures to monitor colonization can direct specific antibiotic therapy for documented infections.

Care of the Burn Wound

Early surgical management of some partial-thickness and most full-thickness burns with excision and grafting has been an important advance in burn treatment. Initially, burns should be covered loosely with clean sheets during the resuscitation phase in severe injuries. Once cardiorespiratory status is stabilized, the wounds are uncovered and assessed for size and depth. The goals of burn wound care are to promote rapid healing and prevent infection. Cleansing with large volumes of lukewarm sterile saline or chlorhexidine gluconate reduces contamination. Loose tissue can often be wiped away with sterile gauze, simplifying and expediting burn debridement. Bullae larger than 2 cm and those at locations that are likely to rupture should also be debrided. Smaller bullae may be left intact to preserve the barrier to bacterial invasion. Application of temporary skin substitutes may reduce pain, expedite healing, and reduce length of hospitalization compared with topical antibiotics and conventional dressings but are usually not applied in the ED. It is not necessary to apply topical antimicrobials to burns prior to transfer to a burn center or children's hospital.

Pain Management

Safely reducing pain is an important consideration in the management of children with burns of all sizes. Pain is a subjective experience influenced by the preceding events. Children rescued from house fires, separated from their parents, transported in ambulances, and brought to EDs are usually extremely anxious. Calm, developmentally appropriate verbal reassurance, even to preverbal children, can reduce anxiety and dramatically reduce the perception of pain.

The exposure of sensory nerve receptors in partial-thickness burns makes them sensitive to environmental stimuli. Movement of cool air across burned tissue increases pain significantly. The simple measure of covering burns with a clean sheet, only exposing them when necessary for burn assessment, is an extremely effective and safe analgesia.

Many children will still have significant pain after nonpharmacologic measures are taken. Narcotic analgesics are useful when administered appropriately. Morphine may reduce the blood pressure, especially in patients who are hypovolemic. Fentanyl causes less cardiovascular effect than morphine but has a short half-life. Clinicians should be reluctant to use narcotics until adequate circulation is reliably established.

Analgesic medications administered intravenously are preferred in patients with severe burns because they are more effective and predictable. Intramuscular injections or oral doses should not be given to patients with significant burns because circulation to muscle and gut is reduced, and absorption of medication will be delayed and unpredictable. Morphine (0.1 to 0.15 mg per kg (2.5 mg–5 mg max)) is the drug of choice for most patients with severe burns. In children who do not respond well to the initial dose of morphine, a careful assessment for other causes of pain or agitation should be sought. Compartment syndrome, hypoxemia, early shock, and occult injuries should be excluded before repeating doses of analgesics. Analgesic administration just before debridement of the burn wound is recommended.

Disposition

Guidelines for admission must be individualized when treating children with burns. Hospitals, physicians, and parents have varying capabilities for managing pediatric patients with burns. In general, admission is recommended for children with burns of smaller percentages of BSA than adults, especially patients younger than 2 years.

Children with partial-thickness burns of more than 5% to 10% of BSA should be considered for admission to a hospital. Partial-thickness injury over 10% of BSA warrants admission to a children's hospital or burn center. Full-thickness burns over 2% of BSA require inpatient treatment. Burns in certain locations are at higher risk for disability or poor cosmetic outcome and should be considered for treatment in the hospital. These include more than 1% of BSA burns of the face, perineum, hands, and feet; circumferential burns; or burns overlying joints. Children with inhalation injury or associated trauma require admission with burns involving lesser percentages of BSA. Any time the physician suspects that the burns cannot be adequately cared for in the home, admission to the hospital is warranted.

OUTPATIENT MANAGEMENT OF BURNS

A small minority of all burns in children require therapy in the hospital. Once a careful assessment has led to a decision to manage a burn as an outpatient, preparations for treatment at home should begin. Parents become the physician's partner in this context and need to be instructed carefully.

A first-degree burn usually does not require therapy. Moisturizers and acetaminophen or ibuprofen can be given as needed. Partial-thickness burns are first cleansed with mild soap and water, povidone-iodine solution at one-fourth strength, chlorhexidine gluconate, or saline alone. Devitalized tissue can usually be removed by wiping with gauze. Bullae larger than 2 cm are likely to rupture and should be debrided. Clean partial-thickness burns less than 2% of BSA can be dressed with petrolatum gauze. Topical antibiotics are recommended for larger or more contaminated burns. Silver sulfadiazine cream (Silvadene) and bacitracin are the topical antibacterial agents of choice at most burn centers. A $\frac{1}{16}$- to $\frac{1}{8}$- in layer of silver sulfadiazine is applied to the burn with a sterile tongue blade or gloved hand. Silver sulfadiazine is soothing to the burn, has few side effects, and kills many gram-positive and gram-negative bacteria and *Candida* species. Mild bleaching of the skin may occur with silver sulfadiazine, so bacitracin is often chosen for burns of the face. About 5% of children are allergic to sulfa drugs and can be treated with bacitracin or povidone-iodine ointment. Leukopenia has also been reported in patients treated with silver sulfadiazine. Mafenide acetate (Sulfamylon) is a topical antimicrobial agent that is more penetrating than silver sulfadiazine. It causes pain when applied, cannot be used in sulfa drug–sensitive patients, and inhibits carbonic anhydrase, which can cause a metabolic acidosis. Some experts recommend mafenide acetate for burns overlying cartilaginous structures such as the ear and nose.

A loose gauze dressing should be placed over the burn and secured with tape. Burns of the face can be treated with an open technique. Dressings should be changed twice each day. The parent should rinse off residual antibacterial cream with warm water and inspect the wound. Signs of infection, such as redness and tenderness around the margin of the burn, warrant immediate evaluation by a physician. A gray-greenish material formed by serous drainage from the burn mixing with the silver sulfadiazine cream is often mistaken for purulence. If the burn is healing well, the parent should reapply the antibiotic cream and dress the wound as demonstrated by the physician or nurse in the ED. Burns should be examined by a physician every 2 or 3 days until healing is well under way. Large burns or burns of the hands, feet, perineum, or overlying joints that are managed as an outpatient should be referred for follow-up to a burn specialist and evaluated more frequently. Prophylactic antibiotics are not recommended.

A new method for managing burns as an outpatient involves dressings composed of carboxymethylcellulose fibers impregnated with silver. Fluid from the burn surface interacts with the dressing to form a firm bandage with an antimicrobial contact layer. These dressings continue to release antimicrobial agent to the burn surface for 1 to 2 weeks and do not require daily dressing changes. They are as effective as silver sulfadiazine at reducing microbial counts and greatly simplify the management of outpatient burns, but long-term data on outcomes are not yet available.

INFLICTED BURNS—CHILD ABUSE

Child abuse must be considered in patients with specific patterns of burn injury. Between 10% and 20% of burns in children are inflicted, accounting for 10% of child abuse cases. Most inflicted burns are scalds. Forced submersion of the hands or feet often causes burns that are deep, have a clear line of immersion, and are symmetric. Scald burns of the buttocks and thighs in toddlers are frequently the result of forcible submersion in a tub of hot water as punishment for toilet-training mishaps. Inflicted contact burns also have characteristic patterns. Small, round, deep burns result from cigarettes intentionally applied to the skin. Deep injuries with distinctive patterns may be noted in children held against portable heaters or burned with irons.

In many children with inflicted burns, the pattern of injury is nonspecific and a history of abuse is not offered. A deep wound with a geometric pattern and sharply demarcated borders suggests a contact burn. Scald burns usually have scattered splash lesions. In burns from spilled hot beverages, there is often a pattern of injury spreading downward from the falling liquid. Physicians should make a judgment whether the characteristics of a burn correspond with the reported mechanism in a plausible way. Identifying suspicious injuries and notifying the appropriate authorities can prevent subsequent injuries.

ELECTRICAL BURNS

Burns that result when electrical current passes through the body have unique characteristics. Each year there are more than 4,000 ED visits caused by electrical injuries mostly in children (see Chapter 87). Electrical burns account for 3% of burn center admissions and are increasing in number. Most injuries occur in young children from contact with low-voltage (less than 120 V) alternating household current, often from mouthing plugs or extension cords. Severe high-voltage (more than 500 V) injuries are also seen, often in adolescent boys as a consequence of risk-taking behaviors.

Thermal energy is released in proportion to the amount and duration of electrical current that passes through tissue. Current flows preferentially through tissues of low electrical resistance, such as blood vessels, nerves, and muscles. Moisture on the skin decreases resistance, accounting for the greater severity of injury in the antecubital, axillary, popliteal, and inguinal areas in patients of electrical burns. Current arcing through the skin can ignite clothing and cause severe thermal burns in addition to the electrical injury. In some direct current electrical burns, a depressed entrance wound and a blown out exit wound can be identified. If the current traverses the heart, which occurs more often when the flow is arm to arm, a myocardial injury may occur. Current through the heart at certain points of the cardiac cycle can induce ventricular fibrillation or asystole. Electrical injury, especially by alternating current, can cause tetany of the musculature that may prolong the contact with the high-voltage source. Tetany of the respiratory muscles can lead to suffocation.

The initial approach to patients of electrical burns is similar to that in other children with severe burns. Electrical burns are usually more severe than they appear. Significant deep and internal injuries may occur in patients with relatively small external burns. Fluid requirements are higher than those predicted by formulas based on percentage of BSA because a larger portion of the injury is internal. Destruction of muscle often causes myoglobinuria, so serum creatine kinase and urine for myoglobin should be tested. Renal failure can usually be prevented with forced diuresis and alkalinization. Electrical injury and edema within fascial compartments can cause a compartment syndrome requiring fasciotomy. Patients with a normal electrocardiogram (rate and rhythm) in the ED do not appear to be at significant risk for later development of arrhythmias. Severe electrical injuries require extensive evaluation for internal injuries, which should be done at a children's hospital or regional burn center.

A common electrical injury occurs to the lips and mouth of toddlers who suck on plugs or extension cords. Deep burns at the corner of the mouth require specialized attention to prevent severe scarring and contracture. Bleeding from the labial artery 1 to 2 weeks after injury, when the eschar separates, can result in a significant blood loss. In previous years, children with electrical injuries were hospitalized for 2 weeks, but some burn specialists now manage these children as outpatients after giving careful instructions to children's caregivers. See Chapters 87 and 109 for additional discussion of electrical burns, including lightning strikes.

CHEMICAL BURNS

More than 25,000 different caustic products are in use in the United States. Most are either acidic or alkaline. Acids cause coagulation of tissue proteins, which limit the depth of penetration. Alkali results in liquefaction and deeper injury. Some organic compounds, including petroleum products, damage tissue by dissolving the fats in cell membranes. Caustic chemicals on the skin cause a prolonged period of burning compared with most thermal burns, making immediate irrigation especially important in limiting the extent of injury. Edema of the underlying tissue can make full-thickness injuries appear deceptively superficial. Treatment of caustic burns, regardless of the substance involved, requires copious irrigation to dilute and remove the chemical to stop the burning process. Attempts at neutralization are usually ineffective and should be avoided. The pH of the effluent can be monitored to help determine whether irrigation has been adequate. A thorough examination is necessary to identify other areas of skin exposed from splashes or contact that also require irrigation. Consultation with a burn specialist and admission are recommended at smaller percentages of BSA with chemical burns than with thermal injuries. Chemical burns to the eye can threaten vision and, after starting irrigation, require prompt consultation with an ophthalmologist (Chapter 127).

Suggested Readings

Barret JP, Diewulski P, Ramzy PI. Biobrane versus 1% silver sulfadiazine in second degree burns. *Plast Reconstr Surg* 2000;105(1):62–65.

Carvajal HF. Fluid resuscitation of pediatric burn victims: a critical appraisal. *Pediatr Nephrol* 1994;8(3):357–366.

Jeschke MG, Chinkes DL, Finnerty CC, et al. Pathophysiologic response to severe burn injury. *Ann Surg* 2008;248(3):387–401.

Mozingo DW, ed. *Advanced burn life support provider manual*. Chicago, IL: American Burn Association, 2007.

O'Brien SP, Billmire DA. Prevention and management of outpatient pediatric burns. *J Craniofac Surg* 2008;19(4):1034–1039.

Pizano LR, Davies J, Corallo JP, et al. Critical care and monitoring of the pediatric burn patient. *J Craniofac Surg* 2008;19(4):929–932.

Sheridan RL, Remersnyder JP, Schnitzer JJ, et al. Expectation for survival in pediatric burns. *Arch Pediatr Adolesc Med* 2000;154(3):245–249.

Spies M, Herndon DN, Rosenblarr JI, et al. Prediction of mortality from catastrophic burns in children. *Lancet* 2003;361(9362):989–994.

Walker AR. Emergency department management of house fire burns and carbon monoxide poisoning in children. *Curr Opin Pediatr* 1996;8(3):239–242.

CHAPTER 109 ■ DENTAL TRAUMA

LINDA P. NELSON, DMD, MSCD, HOWARD L. NEEDLEMAN, DMD, AND BONNIE L. PADWA, DMD, MD

ASSESSMENT OF TRAUMATIC DENTAL EMERGENCIES

The care of pediatric patients with oral and maxillofacial and dental trauma should follow the basic tenets of emergency medicine. An initial general assessment includes evaluation of airway, breathing, and circulation (ABCs). Control of bleeding, assessment of the degree of shock, evaluation of neurologic status, and notation of other injuries must be done sequentially.

Life Support

The most common cause of airway obstruction in a child with facial injuries is the accumulation of blood in the oral cavity and pharynx. Unconscious children may be unable to clear their airway by coughing or swallowing. A tooth aspirated by a child can block the airway. A fractured mandible may cause the tongue to fall posteriorly and create obstruction. The mouth should be gently suctioned clean. If the tongue of an unconscious child is causing obstruction, the mandible can be pulled forward by pressure at the angles or an oropharyngeal or nasopharyngeal airway can be placed. Chapter 1 details the procedures for establishing a patent airway. If endotracheal intubation fails, a surgical airway must be obtained with either a cricothyrotomy or a tracheostomy.

The soft tissues and bones of the lower and midface are well vascularized and bleed profusely when injured. Hemorrhage is best controlled both by direct pressure and by ligating any vessels that are easily seen. However, vessels of the face often retract when severed, making them difficult to visualize. If there is extensive blood loss, the patient should be assessed for signs of shock (see Chapter 3).

History

A thorough history and physical examination are important to any treatment considerations. Traumatic orofacial injuries can be dramatic, making the history difficult to obtain, and informants other than the patient may have to be questioned. The practitioner should always be alert to the possibility of "nonaccidental" trauma (i.e., child abuse) if the history is not consistent with the observed injury. Many traumatic facial injuries occur with concomitant soft-tissue injuries, and the need for tetanus prophylaxis is based on the history of immunization. Antibiotics may be indicated before treatment is indicated in children with congenital heart defects to prevent bacterial endocarditis (see Chapter 84 and Table 84.25) and in children who have certain hematologic, oncologic, or endocrine disorders (e.g., sickle cell disease, leukemia, diabetes). The history should also give the physician an indication of the preinjury and postinjury neurologic status. A thorough neurologic assessment must be made as early as clinically possible because the concurrent risk of neurologic injury is high in patients with head and neck trauma.

Physical Examination

Children with facial injuries are usually frightened and apprehensive, requiring an authoritative and reassuring manner during the initial contact. The examination should be organized to include inspection and palpation of extraoral and intraoral structures.

Extraoral Examination

Inspection. The extraoral examination should start with noting the symmetry of the face in the anterior and profile views. A loss of symmetry is often associated with swelling as the result of trauma. The clinician should carefully note the location and nature of any swollen or depressed structures, the color and quality of the skin, and the presence of lacerations, hematomas, ecchymoses, foreign bodies, or ulcerations. The child should be asked to open and close his or her mouth while facing the clinician to see whether the mandible deviates during function. If the child is unable to open or close his or her mouth because of pain, the action should not be forced because it may increase the extent of injury. The clinician should inspect for lip competency (the ability of the lips to cover the teeth) because loss of competency may indicate displacement of the teeth from trauma.

Palpation. Gentle bilateral digital palpation of the temporomandibular joints (TMJs) should be the next point of the examination. The clinician should feel the TMJs as the child opens and closes his or her mouth. There should be equal movement on both sides without major deviations. The infraorbital rims should be palpated to ensure it is continuous and intact all the way to the inner canthus of the eye. Examination continues across the zygoma to the nose, palpating for crepitus or mobility. Attention should focus on the mandible, feeling along the posterior border of the ramus and moving anteriorly along the body to the symphysis, palpating for any discontinuity, mobility, swellings, or point tenderness. The child should be questioned and examined for any evidence of paresthesia or hypoesthesia (numbness) of the lips, nose, and cheeks, which may indicate a fracture through the bony foramen in which the nerve exits. Figure 109.1 shows the main nerve supply to facial structures.

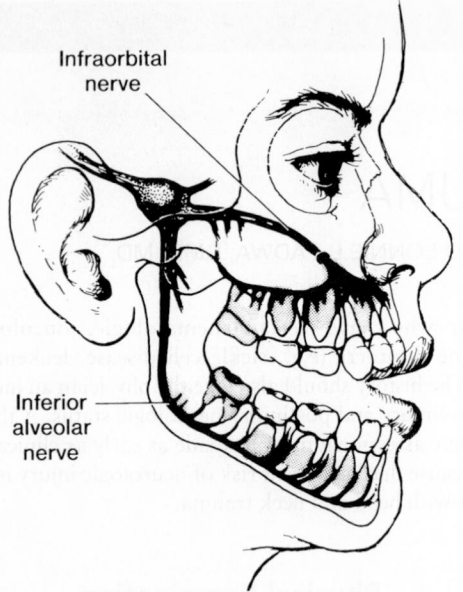

FIGURE 109.1 Infraorbital and inferior alveolar main nerve supplies the teeth.

Intraoral Examination

Inspection. A good light is essential for the intraoral examination to inspect the color and quality of the lips, gingiva (gums), buccal mucosa, floor of the mouth, tongue, and palate. The gingiva should be pink, firm, and stippled (like a grapefruit skin). The mucosa of the cheeks and floor of the mouth should be pink, moist, and glassy in appearance. Any soft-tissue swelling that is blue as a result of ecchymoses and/or hematoma should be noted. Hematomas or mucosal ecchymoses at the floor of the mouth or vestibular area are highly suggestive of mandibular fractures. Any inflamed, ulcerated, or hemorrhagic areas, as well as any foreign bodies or denuded areas of bone, should be documented.

Teeth are labeled according to their position. For older children with secondary dentition, the examiner begins on the upper right at the third molar with #1, precedes clockwise across the top to #16, and then continues on the lower left with the third molar from #17 across the bottom to #32. A similar process in young child with primary teeth starts with A in the upper right and proceeds clockwise across the top to J picks up on the bottom left from K to T.

Traumatically displaced teeth often result in malocclusion (complaint that the child's teeth do not fit together when he or she bites on the back teeth). This should not be confused with a similar complaint, which may be expressed by a child when a primary tooth is mobile and about to exfoliate. Figure 109.2 shows key eruption times for primary and secondary teeth. Exfoliation of primary teeth can be confused with traumatic dental injuries, and clarification can be made with an intraoral radiograph if necessary. The child should be examined for any damaged teeth and if a tooth is chipped or missing, the clinician should check for any fragments of teeth or foreign bodies in the adjacent soft tissues. If the child's teeth are missing yet no bloody socket is present, the eruption/exfoliation timetables (Tables 109.1 and 109.2) can be helpful in determining whether the loss

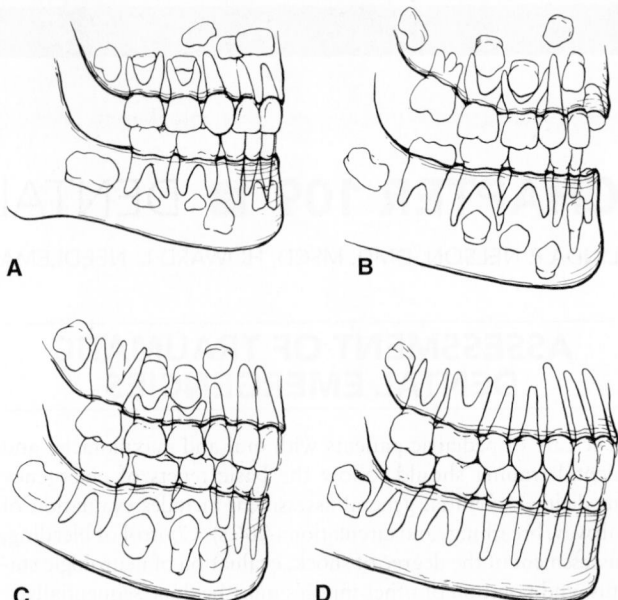

FIGURE 109.2 **A:** At age 3 years, 20 primary teeth should be erupted. The permanent teeth are in various stages of calcification underneath and behind the primary teeth. **B:** At age 6 years, 16 primary teeth should be present. The permanent 6-year molars should be erupting distal to the last primary molars. The permanent anterior central incisors should be erupting. **C:** At age 9 years, 8 to 12 primary teeth should still be present. The permanent 6-year molars should be totally erupted and in occlusion. The permanent anterior central and lateral incisors are totally erupted and are most prone to fracture at this time. **D:** At age 12 years, 28 permanent teeth should be present. Only teeth not present should be third molars (wisdom teeth).

TABLE 109.1

CHRONOLOGY OF ERUPTION OF PRIMARY AND PERMANENT DENTITION

	Maxillary	Mandible
Primary[a]	**Mean age (mo)**	**Mean age (mo)**
Central incisor	10 (8–12)	8 (6–10)
Lateral incisor	11 (9–13)	13 (10–16)
Canine	19 (16–22)	20 (17–23)
First molar	16 (13–19 boys) (14–19 girls)	16 (14–18)
Second molar	29 (25–33)	27 (23–31)
Permanent[b]	**Mean age (yr)**	**Mean age (yr)**
Central incisor	7–7.5	6–6.5
Lateral incisor	8–8.5	7.2–7.7
Canine	11–11.6	9.7–10.2
First premolar	10–10.3	10–10.7
Second premolar	10.7–11.2	10.7–11.5
First molar	6–6.3	6–6.2
Second molar	12.2–12.7	11.7–12.0
Third molar	20.5	20–20.5

[a]Mean age in months ±1 standard deviation. (From Lunt RC, Law DB. *J Am Dent Assoc* 1974;89:878. Reprinted with permission.)
[b]From Baudi AR. The development and eruption of the human dentitions. In: Forrester DJ, Wagoner ML, Fleming J, eds. *Pediatric dental medicine*. Philadelphia, PA: Lea & Febiger, 1981. Reprinted with permission.

TABLE 109.2

SEQUENCE OF PRIMARY TOOTH EXFOLIATION

Rank	Mandibular arch	Maxillary arch	Mean age[a] (yr, mo)	
			Boys	Girls
First	Central incisors		6.0	5.7
Second		Central incisors	6.10	6.7
Third	Lateral incisors		7.2	6.10
Fourth		Lateral incisors	7.10	7.5
Fifth	Canines		10.5	9.7
Sixth	First molars		10.8	10.2
Seventh		First molars	10.11	10.6
Eighth		Canines	11.3	10.7
Ninth	Second molars	Second molars	11.9	11.5

[a]Ages are for the right side of the mouth; however, exfoliation is generally bilaterally symmetric.
From Ripa LW, Lesks GS, Sposanto AL, et al. Chronology and sequence of exfoliation of primary teeth. *J Am Dent Assoc* 1982;105:641. Reprinted with permission.

is normal. In addition, intraoral and/or extraoral dental radiographs, such as a panoramic view, can be diagnostic.

Palpation. Using the thumb and index finger, the clinician should palpate the alveolar ridge in all four quadrants for any swelling, discontinuity, or mobility of the soft tissues, and underlying bone. The palate should be examined for any swelling or tenderness. The masseter muscle should be palpated with fingers placed intraorally and extraorally, and rolling the muscle between the two. Using a gauze pad, the clinician should hold the tongue and lift it gently to better view and examine its dorsal, ventral, and lateral surfaces and the floor of mouth. The lips should be palpated for any swelling or nodules, and the quality of the swelling should be noted (i.e., fluctuance vs. induration). The teeth should be assessed for mobility, tenderness, or fracture, and the gums should be palpated for erupting teeth, noting any purulent exudate.

Percussion. The teeth should be percussed individually with the end of a mouth mirror handle or tongue depressor. Mobile, abscessed, vertically fractured, or traumatized teeth may be sensitive and sound dull on percussion.

Radiographs are a valuable supplement to the clinical examination. However, obtaining a diagnostic radiographic survey in a child with acute orofacial/dental injuries may be difficult.

OROFACIAL/DENTAL TRAUMA

Dental trauma occurs in various forms that can be confusing to the primary care provider. The emergency physician needs to know which injuries can be managed without dental consultation, which need follow-up care with a dentist, and which need emergency dental care. In a survey at an urban pediatric emergency department, trauma represented 21.7% of the chief complaints and 29.2% of the diagnoses. Several factors, including age, occlusion, and agility in sports, predispose pediatric patients to orofacial trauma. Traumatic dental injuries occur as the toddler becomes ambulatory (ages 1 to 3), as the child

enters school (ages 7 to 10), and as the older adolescent (ages 16 to 18) engages in athletic activities. In addition, proclined or prominent maxillary anterior teeth are more susceptible to being displaced or fractured. Early orthodontic treatment to retract prominent incisors can reduce the risk of trauma to these teeth. Also, the use of a preformed ("boil and bite") or custom-made mouth guard in children with prominent maxillary incisors is helpful in reducing the chance of these accident-prone teeth sustaining traumatic injuries. This section details the management of dental injuries that are most commonly seen in the pediatric emergency patient.

Soft-tissue Lacerations

Management of soft-tissue injuries of the oral cavity follows the same emergency care principles used for injuries at other sites. Injuries to the lip result in significant swelling after minor trauma. Lacerations of the tongue and frenum bleed profusely because of the richness of their vascularity. However, ligating specific vessels is usually unnecessary because bleeding almost always stops with direct pressure and careful suturing. Frenum lacerations heal spontaneously and, therefore, do not require suturing. The injured area should be thoroughly examined for a foreign body, including obtaining a radiograph before suturing when a foreign body is suspected. If chipped teeth are present, radiograph examination is imperative to rule out the presence of the missing piece in the soft tissues. When a laceration in the oral cavity is more than a few hours old, primary closure depends on the relative risk of secondary infection (see Chapter 122).

Suturing the lip must be done carefully to achieve a precise approximation of the edges of the vermilion border to avoid a disfiguring scar. If necessary, the lip must be sparingly debrided and the skin closed with 5-0 or 6-0 nylon sutures. Deep lip lacerations require closure in multiple layers, beginning with approximation of the obicularis oris muscle using 4-0 chromic and then 5-0 or 6-0 nylon for the skin and vermilion. If the lip laceration is through and through, debridement may be necessary. In children younger than 5 years, 4-0 chromic on the deeper mucosal aspects of the lip and 6-0 chromic on the superficial aspects are preferred. In children older than 5 years, 4-0 chromic is used on the deeper mucosal aspects of the lip and 5-0 or 6-0 nylon on the superficial edges. Most superficial tongue lacerations heal without suturing; however, deep lacerations or those that create a flap need to be sutured. When necessary, tongue lacerations are usually sutured with 4-0 chromic in superficial wounds and with 3-0 chromic in deeper wounds. With tongue lacerations, it is important to consider the excessive muscular movements that pull at the sutures; therefore, tongue sutures should be made deep into the musculature.

Injuries to the Teeth

Traumatic dental injuries can be categorized into two groups: (i) injuries to the teeth—hard dental tissues and pulp; and (ii) injuries to the periodontal structures—periodontal ligament and alveolar bone. Figure 109.3A indicates the relative positions of these structures. Injuries to the teeth can be further categorized into complicated and uncomplicated fractures.

Injuries to Hard Dental Tissues and Pulp

Uncomplicated tooth fractures are confined to the hard outer dental tissue (enamel) and the underlying (dentin). The fracture line may appear deep, but no sign of bleeding from the central core (pulp) of the tooth is apparent. The child may complain of sensitivity, especially to cold air and fluids. Emergency treatment is aimed at decreasing sensitivity of the involved tooth and protecting the pulp, even if no frank pulp exposure is noted. The child should be seen by a dentist within 48 hours to place a dressing of calcium hydroxide or glass ionomer over the exposed dentin for thermal and chemical insulation to minimize the chance of (pulpal) necrosis. A temporary restoration is then placed to prevent the insulation material from dissolving. At some later date, an aesthetic resin acid-etched restoration can be placed (Figs. 109.3B and 109.3C). The prognosis for uncomplicated tooth fractures is good.

A complicated tooth fracture involves not only the enamel and dentin but also the pulp of the tooth. Often, bleeding is noted from the central core of the tooth. To best preserve the viability of that tooth, dental pulpal treatment must be initiated immediately. Prognosis depends on the size of the exposure (less than 1 mm carry the best prognosis), the time interval between the trauma and therapy (less than 48 hours carries the best prognosis), and the maturity (root development) of the involved tooth. Thus, calling the dental consultant as soon as possible to institute pulpal therapy is important. Root fractures are generally seen after the tooth has reached full root formation, which is approximately 2 to 3 years after eruption begins (Table 109.1). Root fractures most commonly involve maxillary anterior teeth. Diagnosis depends on intraoral dental radiographs; therefore, immediate dental consultation is necessary. Treatment involves reduction if the segments are not aligned, followed by splinting. Pulpal therapy of the involved teeth may be necessary if healing of the fragments does not occur.

In any injury resulting in fragmentation of teeth, the emergency physician should attempt to account for all the fragments. Soft-tissue lacerations, especially of the lower lip and tongue, should be evaluated clinically and, if necessary, radiographically to rule out embedded tooth fragments. Infection and poor wound healing are the sequelae of such an oversight.

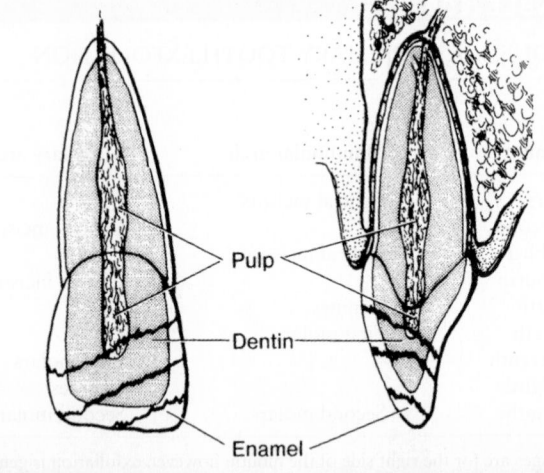

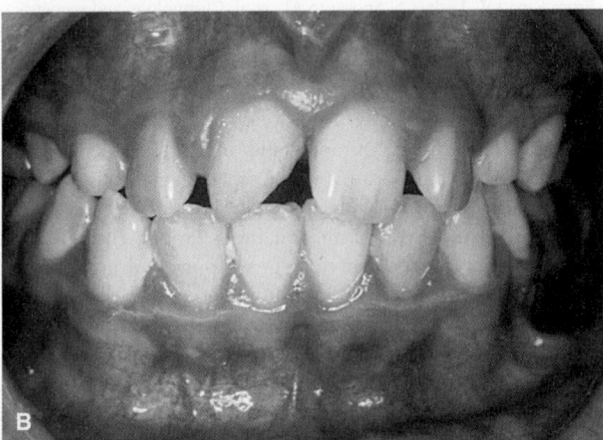

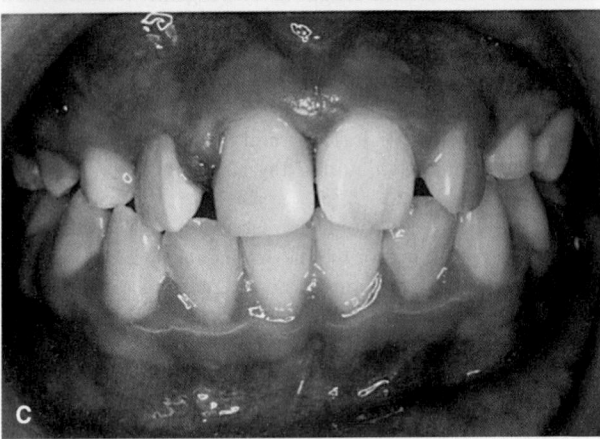

FIGURE 109.3 **A:** The anatomy of a tooth should be considered during a traumatic injury: enamel fracture, no emergency treatment; dentin fracture, emergency treatment as soon as convenient; and pulpal fracture, emergency treatment as soon as possible. **B:** Enamel and dentin fracture of a permanent incisor. **C:** The same child after bonded restoration.

Displaced Teeth

The tooth is held in the socket by slender elastic and collagen fibers collectively known as the periodontal ligament. These fibers are easily injured or severed with trauma to the teeth. Clinically, the physician may note either an increase or a decrease mobility, depending on the extent of the cortical plate fracture and/or displacement of the affected teeth. If asked, the child will be able to point to an injured tooth because of the tooth's heightened sensitivity. Periodontal injuries may be further subdivided into five clinical types: (i) concussion, (ii) subluxation, (iii) intrusion, (iv) extrusion/lateral luxation, and (v) avulsion, as noted in Fig. 109.4.

Concussion is usually caused by minor damage to the periodontal ligament, resulting in slight edema. Teeth sustaining concussive injuries exhibit no displacement or excessive mobility. They are, by definition, percussion sensitive when tapped with the blunt end of an instrument such as an intraoral mirror. No emergency treatment is indicated for such injuries, although baseline radiographs are needed at a subsequent dental consultation to rule out more serious involvement. The prognosis for concussion injuries is good, although pulpal necrosis is possible over time.

Subluxation is more damaging to the periodontal ligament because of increased edema. There is excessive mobility in the horizontal and/or vertical direction, but no displacement within the dental arch. The tooth is sensitive to percussion. The child may complain that his or her teeth feel like they do not meet when biting down. Because subluxated teeth, especially in the permanent dentition, may require stabilization with a bonded resin splint, this type of injury should be referred to the dental service as soon as possible.

Intrusion, although more commonly seen in the primary dentition, can be seen in the permanent dentition with high-velocity or high-force injuries. Intruded teeth are teeth displaced directly into the socket. Intruded teeth may not be visible and thus give the false appearance of being avulsed. To confirm complete intrusion and to rule out avulsion, an intra-oral dental radiograph must be obtained when this condition is suspected. An intruded primary tooth must be evaluated by a dental consultant for its proximity to the developing permanent tooth. The prognosis for pulpal tissues of an intruded tooth is poor because of pulpal compression and severance, which occurs on impact. Intruded primary teeth can be either extracted or allowed to spontaneously reerupt, depending on the severity of the intrusion and condition of the surrounding bone and soft tissues. Intrusive injuries in the permanent dentition usually require repositioning and splinting. Pulpal treatment (endodontics) is almost always needed because the pulp is rendered nonvital as a result of trauma, which can cause root resorption and periapical infection. Compression fractures of the alveolar socket and anterior nasal spine may be seen radiographically.

Extrusion/lateral luxation injuries are manifested clinically as displacement of the tooth or teeth from the alveolar socket in an extrusive or lateral direction. Most commonly, the anterior maxillary teeth are involved. These teeth are extruded and displaced lingually, causing a fracture of the labial cortical plate of the alveolar socket. Luxated permanent teeth must be realigned and immobilized with a splint as soon as possible. Endodontic treatment is often needed in the long term. Extrusive/lateral luxations of the primary dentition usually necessitate extraction to allow children to fully occlude their teeth and to avoid potential injury to the permanent tooth bud during realignment or as a result of eventual pulpal necrosis.

Avulsion is the term used to describe a tooth that has been completely displaced from its socket. Radiographs may show the tooth to be actually intruded, ingested, or aspirated. The

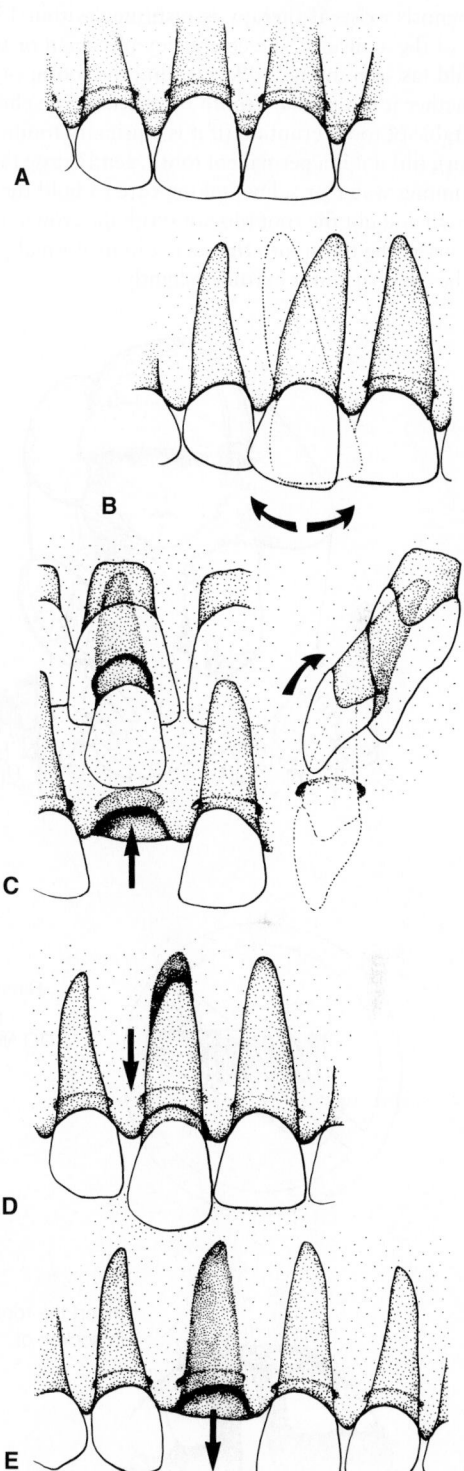

FIGURE 109.4 The various types of trauma to the periodontal structures. Concussion/subluxation (**A**); lateral luxation (**B**); intrusion (if primary tooth is intruded note location of developing permanent tooth bud) (**C**); extrusion (**D**); and avulsion (**E**). Refer emergencies (**B**) through (**E**) to the dental staff as soon as possible.

best prognosis exists if therapy is instituted within 15 to 30 minutes of the avulsion. The emergency physician or the parent should (as seen in Fig. 109.5) (i) find the tooth; (ii) determine whether it is a primary tooth by checking the child's age and the table of tooth eruption (if it is a primary tooth, do not reimplant); (iii) if it is a permanent tooth, gently rinse the tooth under running water or saline, taking care to hold the crown of the tooth and not the root (do not scrub the crown or root); and (iv) insert the tooth into the socket in its normal position (do not be concerned if it extrudes slightly).

If on-site reimplantation is impossible, the optimal storage to preserve the vitality of the periodontal ligament of the root surface is a cell culture medium such as ViaSpan or Hank's balanced salt solution. A commercial product such as the 3M Save-a-Tooth Emergency Tooth Preserving System (Smart Practice, Phoenix, AZ) containing Hank's solution is available to place the tooth into during transportation to the dental office. If none of these products are available, milk is an excellent alternative transport medium. Although saliva or saline are not ideal, they are alternative mediums that are preferred

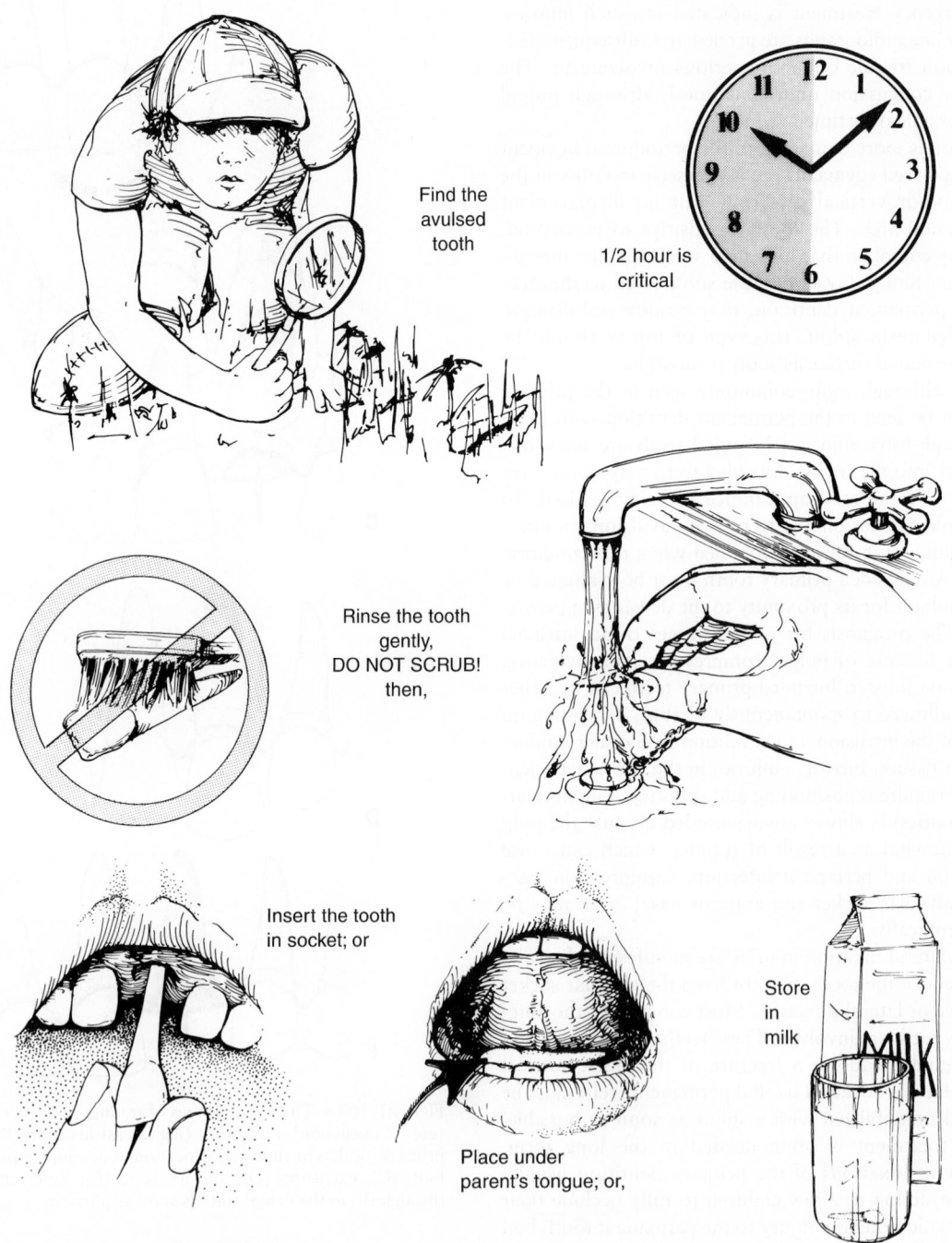

Find the avulsed tooth

1/2 hour is critical

Rinse the tooth gently, DO NOT SCRUB! then,

Insert the tooth in socket; or

Place under parent's tongue; or,

Store in milk

FIGURE 109.5 If a child loses or avulses a tooth, find the tooth and determine whether it is a primary or permanent tooth by checking Table 109.1. If it is a primary tooth, *do not reimplant.* Gently rinse under running water or with saline, but do not scrub the tooth. Insert the tooth back into the socket or place in milk or Hank's balanced salt solution and take immediately to the dentist. Remember, you have only 15 to 30 minutes to preserve the vitality of the tooth.

over allowing the root surface to air dry. The patient should go directly to the dentist for immobilization (splint). Dental follow-up is mandatory to prevent resorption of the root. Prophylactic pulpal therapy (endodontics) helps improve the prognosis by limiting pulpal necrosis and thus root resorption. Avulsed primary teeth are generally not reimplanted because of the close proximity of the permanent tooth and possible negative effects on development of this tooth.

Orthodontic Trauma

Young patients are frequently undergoing orthodontic treatment, and trauma results in loosening of wires or ligatures that are attached to orthodontic brackets or bands. These emergencies should be seen by the dental service as soon as possible to alleviate any discomfort and soft-tissue trauma. If dental treatment is unavailable, the physician can bend or cut the wire away from the soft tissues with a hemostat. Softened wax can be molded over the loose wire as a temporary method or to allow the traumatized soft tissues to heal. If no discomfort is noted and no loose foreign bodies are present, definitive treatment can be delayed until an orthodontic specialist can see the patient.

Mandibular Fractures/Dislocations

Although the incidence of facial fractures in children is low, the most common facial fractures are those of the nasal bones, followed by the mandible. The emergency physician should be knowledgeable in the diagnosis and management of mandibular fractures. History, physical, and radiographic examination should be used to establish the diagnosis of mandibular fracture.

The mandible can be compared with an archery bow, which is strongest at its center and weakest at its ends. Thus, most fractures occur at the neck of the condyles. Other areas of the jaw that are predisposed to fracture include the angle of the mandible where deep impacted teeth or unerupted 6-year molars make the mandible more vulnerable. The clinician should examine the teeth for any changes in occlusion and any raised or depressed fragments. Areas of bleeding, gingival/mucosal tears, or sublingual ecchymoses are also clues. Pain when opening the mouth, especially if the child is unable to open it fully, often indicates mandibular fracture. A unilateral condylar fracture should be suspected if the mandible deviates toward the affected side on opening.

A panoramic radiograph or preferably a computed tomographic scan should be obtained. In the pediatric patient, a mandibular fracture generally necessitates hospital admission. The appropriate consulting service should be called to stabilize the fracture, using either open or closed reduction.

Mandibular dislocation occurs when the capsule and TMJ ligaments are sufficiently stretched to allow the condyle to move to a point anterior to the articular eminence during opening. Dislocation can be unilateral or bilateral and often accompanies a history of extreme mouth opening (e.g., deep yawn) or occurs after a long dental appointment. The muscles of mastication enter a tonic contraction state, and the patient is unable to move the condyle back into the glenoid fossa and close his or her mouth. Gentle downward and backward pressure should be applied by the physician's thumb (wrapped in gauze) on the occlusal surfaces of the posterior teeth

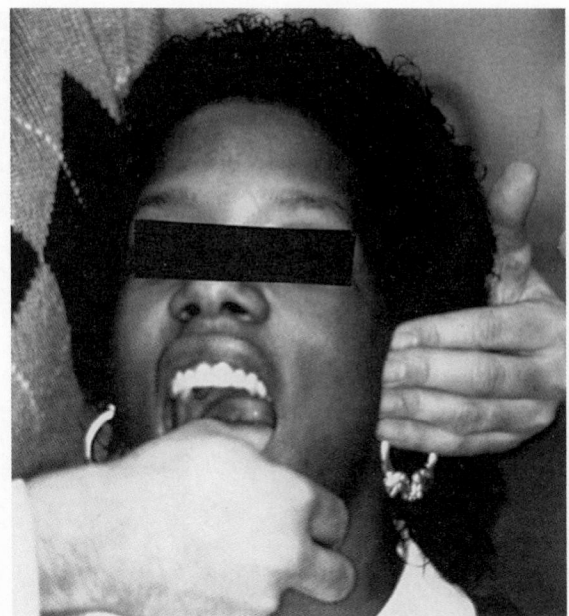

FIGURE 109.6 Position for the reduction of a dislocated mandible.

(Fig. 109.6). The downward pressure moves the dislocated condyle below the articular eminence; subsequent backward pressure on the molars shifts the condyle posteriorly into the mandibular fossa. If this approach fails, intravenous diazepam (0.2 mg per kg, maximum 10 mg) can be administered as an adjunct before relocating the condyles. Figure 109.7 shows the anatomic landmarks and repositioning of the TMJ.

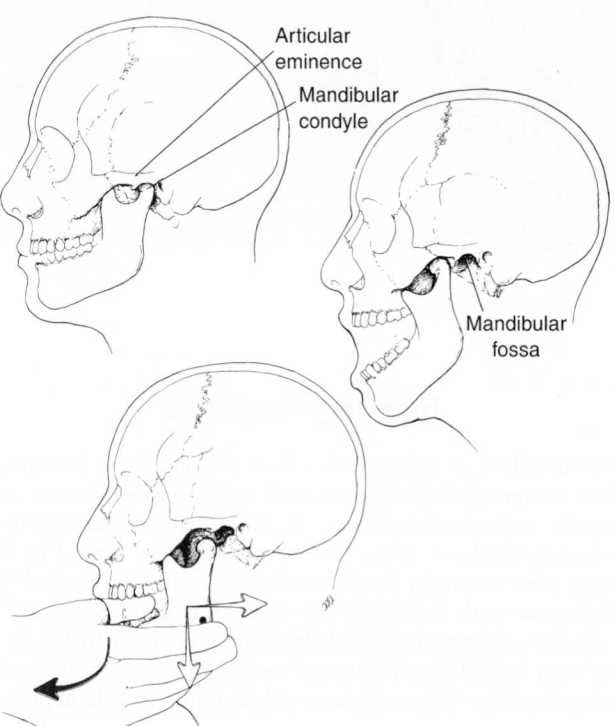

FIGURE 109.7 Dislocation of the temporomandibular joint occurs when the mandibular condyle moves to a point anterior to the articular eminence during opening. Reduction is accomplished by pushing downward and backward on the occlusal surfaces of the posterior teeth.

TRAUMA

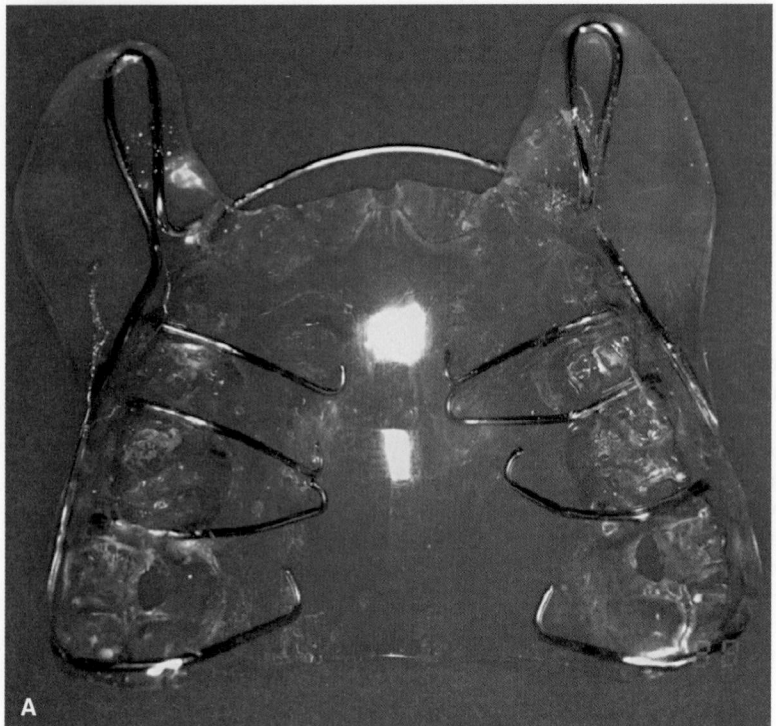

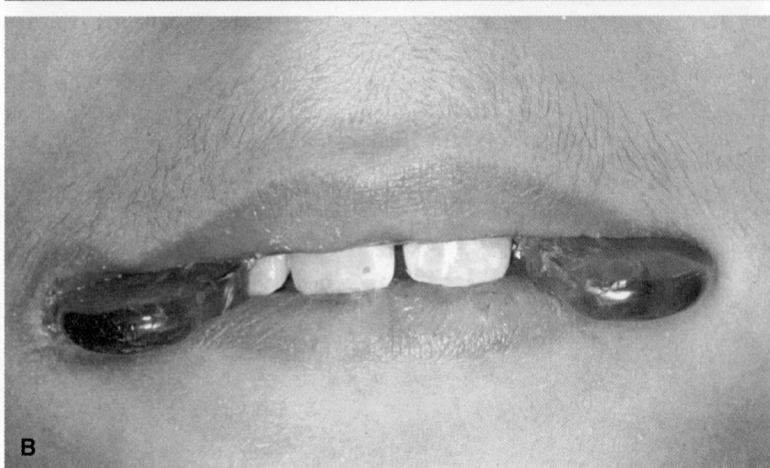

FIGURE 109.8 **A:** Removable maxillary intraoral acrylic appliance with extraoral commissure extensions. **B:** Appliance in place, separating the upper and lower lips with electrical burns at the commissure.

Maxillary Fractures

Premaxillary or anterior maxillary alveolar bone fractures are a common finding associated with the displacement or avulsion of maxillary anterior teeth. By gentle digital manipulation, the labial plate of bone can often be guided back into position under local anesthesia. Infiltration with 2% lidocaine with 1:100,000 epinephrine is commonly used. The bone fragment can be held in place temporarily by aluminum foil (three thicknesses) molded over the teeth and alveolar ridge. This emergency splint should be held in place by having the child bite down. A dental consultant should be contacted as soon as possible for fabrication of a more permanent dental splint. Splinting the loose teeth and suturing the gingival tissue holds the bone fragments in place.

Mandibular and other facial fractures are covered in greater detail in Chapter 111.

Electrical Burns

Electrical burns of the mouth occur when children bite on electrical cords. The saliva in the mouth acts as a conductor to complete the circuit. In the emergency department, the first consideration is the patient's respiratory status. Next, the patient should be assessed for the presence of shock or other injuries. Although the commissure of the mouth is most likely affected, the tongue, alveolar ridge, and floor of the mouth are occasionally involved. Most children with these injuries can be managed as an outpatient. A bland, soft, cold diet is initially recommended. If refusal of food and dehydration are problems, the child requires admission to the hospital for the administration of intravenous fluids. Meticulous oral hygiene using a toothbrush with or without toothpaste must be performed three to four times per day, as well as hydrogen peroxide and water (1:1) rinses. With severe burns of the lips and mouth, arterial bleeding may occur 5 to 8 days after the injury. The clinician should instruct the parent on the method for digitally compressing the labial artery or consider admission to the hospital for wound management. To prevent scarring down of the commissure, electrical burns of this area require the fabrication of an intraoral or extraoral device to separate the upper and lower segments during healing (Figs. 109.8A and 109.8B).

Suggested Readings

Andreason JO, Andreason FM. *Textbook and color atlas of traumatic injuries to the teeth,* 4th ed. Boston, MA: Wiley-Blackwell, 2007.

Croll T, Brooks EB, Schut L, et al. Rapid neurologic assessment and initial management for the patient with traumatic dental injuries. *J Am Dent Assoc* 1980;100:530–534.

Kaban L, Troulis M. *Pediatric oral and maxillofacial surgery.* Philadelphia, PA: Saunders, 2004.

Schultz RC. *Facial injuries,* 3rd ed. Chicago, IL: Year Book, 1988.

Trope M. Clinical management of the avulsed tooth: present strategies and future directions. *Dent Traumatol* 2002;18:1–11.

CHAPTER 110 ■ OTOLARYNGOLOGIC TRAUMA

KEN KAZAHAYA, MD, MBA

In children, the head and neck regions are common sites for trauma; therefore, emergency medicine specialists must be familiar with injuries to these regions as they will often be called upon to evaluate these areas. Although the presenting complaints may seem extremely distressing to the patient and cause considerable anxiety for the parents, the conditions prompting the visit are rarely life-threatening. While many injuries may be isolated to the head, ear, nose, mouth, or throat, associated trauma (e.g., eye, dental, central nervous system, thorax) is also common and must be considered and detected when evaluating and treating patient's suffering from otolaryngologic trauma.

Evaluation of the patient with otolaryngologic trauma requires a careful and thorough examination of the head and neck. The specific methods of examination of each anatomic area are detailed in a separate chapter in this textbook.

EAR

Foreign Bodies

Foreign bodies in the external auditory canal (EAC) are common in children Solid objects, such as stones, beads, foam, silicone wax, or paper, are the most commonly encountered foreign bodies, but live insects may also enter the EAC. Foreign bodies should be removed as soon and as safely as possible. Evaluation and manipulation of the foreign body should be done with good illumination, and often, magnification, such as a microscope, is required. Most objects can be gently rolled out of the external meatus with an ear curette or grasped and removed with an otologic forceps. If a disk battery is in the EAC, it should be removed expediently to avoid caustic injury to the EAC. Round or occluding objects may be removed by irrigation of the canal with body-temperature water. The stream is directed along the side of the foreign body, forcing it to the external meatus. Irrigation, however, should not be performed if a tympanic membrane (TM) perforation is suspected or if a ventilating tube is in place. Furthermore, organic foreign bodies should not be irrigated, to avoid absorption of the fluid and expansion of the material in the EAC. If a disc battery is present in the EAC, irrigation is not recommended. Insects should be killed by filling the ear canal with alcohol or mineral oil before they are removed from the ear canal by the techniques already described. Objects resting against the TM are best removed by irrigation to avoid injury and pain from manipulation.

Care must be taken to remove the foreign material without causing pain or trauma to the external canal. The medial portion (bony portion) of the EAC and TM are exquisitely sensitive and easily traumatized. Topical anesthetic emulsions are available and have been used to decrease the sensitivity of the ear canal skin. Unfortunately, it may be difficult to get the emulsion past the foreign body, and it requires time for optimal performance. Furthermore, in the event there is a TM perforation, the anesthetic may cause nausea and vomiting as a result of direct effect upon the vestibular system. If removal of the foreign body is not easily performed, it may be prudent to seek consultation from an otolaryngologist before the child becomes averse to allowing anyone near their ear. If the removal is unsuccessful, an otolaryngologist may elect to proceed to the operating room and remove the foreign body while the patient is under general anesthesia. If an excoriation or trauma of the EAC occurs, use of an ototopical antibiotic drop, such as a fluoroquinolone, for example, ofloxacin, may prevent development of otitis externa.

Trauma

External Ear Trauma

External ear trauma is common in children because the pinna is in an exposed position on the side of the head. Reflex turning of the face to the side to avoid a blow or a fall places the ear directly in the line of injury. External blunt trauma is often secondary to an athletic injury, a fall, or a direct blow to the ear. The injury may result in ecchymosis or it may disrupt perichondrial blood vessels with subsequent hematoma or seroma formation. These collections usually form a smooth, bluish-colored mass on the lateral surface of the auricle that obscures the normal contours of the helix and antihelix. Hematomas and seromas must be evacuated expeditiously to prevent cartilage necrosis and potentially a cauliflower ear. After drainage of the collection, sutures are used through the pinna to hold bolsters in place on both sides of the pinna to prevent recollection. Lacerations of the pinna should be closed by using the same surgical principles applied to repairing lacerations in other end-organ areas of the body. Earrings in pierced ears may be torn from the lobule. These lacerations should be closed like all skin lacerations, reestablishing the normal anatomy—care should be taken to avoid notching the lobule at the laceration site. The skin edge should be everted.

Thermal injury of the external ear commonly occurs because the ear protrudes from the head and is exposed to burns and cold. The external ears frequently become exposed to environmental conditions such as excessive sun or subfreezing air. Burns of the ear should be treated in the same manner as burns of other parts of the body. Care should be taken to observe for sign of development of a chondritis. Frostbite is suspected when the ear is pale and is usually painful on warming. The frostbitten ear should be rewarmed rapidly by applying warm soaked cotton pledgets at 38°C to 40°C (100.4° to 104°F); the ear should be completely thawed and never recooled.

Middle Ear Trauma

Perforations of the TM may result from acute otitis media. These perforations are typically small and heal readily. Traumatic perforations of the TM may also occur as a result of a slap to the side of the head (by a hand or a breaking wave) from the sudden compression of the air in the EAC; however, traumatic perforations of the drum are more often a consequence of poking an object into the ear canal. The structures of the middle ear may also be damaged by the penetrating object. The ossicles may be fractured or dislocated, resulting in a conductive hearing loss, or a perilymph fistula may be created if the footplate of the stapes is disrupted or dislodged from the oval window. A perilymph fistula typically presents with immediate vertigo, nystagmus, and sensorineural hearing loss. The facial nerve may be injured and may result in facial paralysis from injury in the horizontal portion of the facial nerve as it courses horizontally over the oval window. Traumatic perforations of the TM must be examined carefully, ideally under magnification, to be certain that the edges of the perforation do not fold into the middle ear. If this occurs, skin may grow into the middle ear and a cholesteatoma may develop. Clean perforations with margins that do not fold into the middle ear usually heal spontaneously in 2 to 3 weeks. The perforation should be kept clean and dry. If the ear is draining, topical antibiotic drops (e.g. ofloxacin or ciprofloxacin) should be used for 10 days. Systemic antibiotics are usually unnecessary. Any perforation that does not heal within 3 weeks should be referred to an otolaryngologist for evaluation and management. Traumatic perforations associated with vertigo, sensorineural hearing loss, or facial nerve paralysis requires urgent consultation and possible exploration of the middle ear by an otolaryngologist.

Barotrauma to the ear may occur any time there is a significant change in ambient pressure on one side of the TM that is not compensated by a change in pressure on the other side. This may occur during an airplane trip, while scuba diving or sometimes even diving in the deep end of a swimming pool. These injuries are more common if a child has eustachian tube dysfunction—as can occur with an acute upper respiratory tract infection. The eustachian tube provides communication between the middle ear and the nasopharynx, normally permitting prompt equalization of pressure on both sides of the TM. If the eustachian tube is obstructed or nonfunctioning, changes in ambient pressure may not be transmitted to the middle ear, and barotrauma can result. It is proposed that, as the one descends in an airplane (or during an underwater dive), the increased ambient pressure is transmitted to the cardiovascular system and thus to the vessels of the mucosal lining of the middle ear. The vessels become engorged and the mucosa becomes edematous. If the eustachian tube is obstructed and has not equalized the air pressure, a large differential pressure occurs between the middle ear mucosa and its air-filled cavity. This condition results in a rupture of the blood vessels within the mucosa and bleeding into the middle ear. Serous fluid may also accumulate in the middle ear secondary to eustachian tube obstruction. Rarely, perforation of the TM occurs. These injuries usually resolve spontaneously over several weeks. Antimicrobials may be prescribed to prevent infection of the middle ear fluid/blood. The rare case that does not respond to this regimen should be referred to an otolaryngologist for further evaluation and treatment. Persistent symptomatic fluid may require myringotomy and ventilation tube placement. Barotrauma with acute sensorineural hearing loss and/or vertigo may indicate the presence of a perilymph fistula (previously described). Persistence of these symptoms requires urgent middle ear exploration to close the fistula.

Inner Ear Trauma

Concussive injuries to the head may cause inner ear trauma by disrupting the delicate intracochlear membranes. Sensorineural hearing loss and/or vertigo may occur as a result of such an injury. Occasionally, the losses from these injuries can improve spontaneously but most are permanent. Temporal bone fractures (especially transverse) have a high incidence of otic capsule and cochlear disruption.

The presence of enlarged vestibular aqueducts (EVA's) may predispose an affected individual to sudden sensorineural hearing loss from minor head trauma, such as a blow or jarring the head or sudden dramatic pressure changes (such as scuba diving or skydiving). EVA is the most common congenital ear anomaly causing sensorineural hearing loss in children. EVA can be diagnosed with high-resolution, thin-cut computed tomography (CT) or magnetic resonance imaging scans of the temporal bones. Typical radiologic criteria consider more than 1.5 mm at the midpoint of the vestibular aqueduct or more than 2 mm at the internal opening of the vestibular aqueduct as an EVA.

Constant exposure to loud noise or amplified sound may cause a progressive high-frequency sensorineural hearing loss. Loud blasts from explosions or other sudden loud noises may cause sudden permanent sensorineural hearing loss.

Temporal Bone Fractures

Temporal bone fractures are usually the result of an impact to the head, such as from a motor vehicle collision, a fall, or an object striking the head. Typically, significant forces are required to fracture the temporal bone. Temporal bone fractures have been traditionally classified as longitudinal or transverse. Eighty percent of temporal bone fractures are usually classified as longitudinal and are most commonly the result of impact to the side of the head. Typically, longitudinal temporal bone fractures stay extralabyrinthine—the fracture line usually parallels the internal auditory canal and may disrupt the bony annulus of the TM. Hemotympanum and ossicular disruption may occur. Bleeding from an external ear canal laceration or TM disruption is not uncommon. Facial paralysis is uncommon.

Transverse fractures of the temporal bone occur less frequently and are usually the result of severe impact to the front or back of the head. There is typically disruption of the otic capsule, the internal auditory canal, the facial nerve, and the auditory-vestibular nerve (cranial nerve VIII). Fifty percent of transverse temporal bone fractures have facial nerve involvement. It is important to document the status of the facial nerve function in head trauma cases, especially in cases where a temporal bone fracture is suspected. Sensorineural hearing loss is common.

TRAUMA

Cerebrospinal fluid (CSF) leaks are more common with transverse fractures, which may present with CSF rhinorrhea.

Cerebrospinal Fluid Otorrhea

CSF otorrhea may be secondary to a temporal bone (usually longitudinal) fracture that results in a fracture through the inner ear and ruptures the TM. Transverse fractures have a higher incidence of CSF leak; however, since there is typically an intact TM, otorrhea is usually not present. Manipulation or instrumentation of the EAC in the presence of CSF otorrhea is discouraged because it could introduce bacteria and contribute to the development of meningitis. If CSF otorrhea is suspected, the child should be placed at bed rest with the head elevated and neurosurgical consultation should be obtained. The use of prophylactic antimicrobials in CSF otorrhea is controversial. CSF in the middle ear space should be suspected in cases of temporal bone fractures and a persistent effusion. CSF leaks from temporal bone fractures may sometimes present as clear rhinorrhea or a persistent salty postnasal drip. A CSF leak should be considered if a patient develops recurrent bouts of meningitis.

Facial Nerve Paralysis

Facial nerve paralysis may occur as a result of temporal bone trauma. The functional status of the facial nerve should be documented as early as possible after head trauma, especially in cases where temporal bone fracture may be possible. Transverse fractures of the temporal bone can cause disruption of the facial nerve in its intratemporal segment. Longitudinal fractures are less likely to cause facial nerve paralysis. Usually, if facial paralysis is incomplete or delayed in onset, there is less chance that the nerve has been transected. Sudden loss of facial motion may signify disruption. Patients with traumatic facial nerve paralysis should be referred to the otolaryngologist for evaluation, management, and possible exploration and nerve repair.

NOSE AND PARANASAL SINUSES

Nasal Trauma

General Principles/Nasal Fracture

Facial trauma often occurs in children as a result of play activities, contact sports, and automobile accidents. Most of these injuries are minor. Nevertheless, any child with facial trauma should be assessed for associated, possibly more serious, injuries to the cervical spine, eyes, central nervous system, and chest.

Because of its prominent position on the face, the nose is subject to frequent trauma and accounts for most facial injuries in children. It is important, however, to realize that nasal trauma may also be associated with ocular injury, such as hyphema or retinal detachment, or orbital bony fractures. If the initial survey suggests a serious ocular injury, an ophthalmologic consultation must be obtained.

In children, the nasal architecture is different from that of adults as it is has more of a prominent soft cartilaginous portion. The cartilage will bend easily, allowing the force of the blow to dissipate across the midface, and may result in signifi-

cant edema and ecchymosis. This soft-tissue swelling can make examination of the facial bones and nasal structure difficult.

A direct blow to the nose can fracture the nasal skeleton with resultant deviation and/or depression of the nasal bones and septum. The deformity may be readily apparent by clinical examination, but the postinjury edema may prevent its recognition for several days until the swelling has subsided (Fig. 110.1). A step-off or bony irregularity may often be detected in these patients. Radiographs of the nose are notoriously unreliable in the evaluation of nasal injuries and are not recommended in the routine management of simple nasal fractures. Even in cases where there may appear to be a fracture on plain radiographs, if there is no significant displacement of the nasal bones, no intervention would be warranted. Epistaxis commonly accompanies nasal trauma but usually has stopped by the time the child reaches the emergency department (ED). Persistent or severe bleeding may require local pressure, topical vasoconstrictors, or nasal packing.

In assessing the nasal injury, the emergency physician must determine the nature and extent of trauma to the overlying skin, the nasal skeleton, and the nasal septum. A septal hematoma (see below), if present, requires emergent incision and drainage. The amount of nasal deviation and/or depression should be noted. Because this condition can be masked by postinjury edema, it may be best to examine the child again in 3 to 4 days when the swelling has subsided, to allow an accurate determination of nasal deviation and/or depression. Orbital and nasoethmoid fractures should always be suspected when a child appears to have suffered from significant facial injuries.

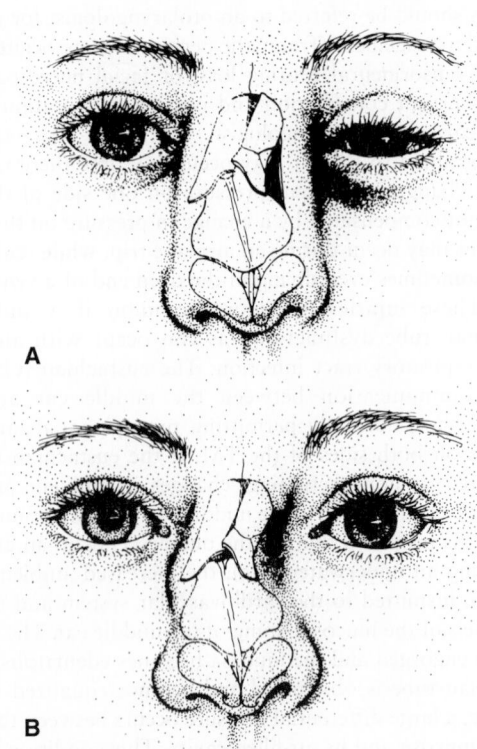

FIGURE 110.1 **A:** Postinjury edema may mask underlying nasal bone deformity. **B:** Nasal deformity manifests as edema subsides.

If no septal hematoma or associated ocular or intracranial injuries are present, then the deviated nose and septum can be reduced by the otolaryngologist when the swelling has subsided enough to permit an accurate evaluation of the nasal deformity. If more than 7 to 10 days elapse between the time of injury and the attempt at reduction, the fracture fragments begin to form a strong fibrous union in their deviated positions, making reduction difficult. Antimicrobials (such as amoxicillin 25 to 50 mg per kg per day for 7 days) are generally administered to these patients to prevent complications from occurring in what is almost always a compound fracture (i.e., open into the nasal cavity).

Septal Hematoma

The presence of a septal hematoma must be recognized as soon as possible after the injury. A septal hematoma appears as a bulging of the nasal septum into one or both sides of the nasal cavity. The septal hematoma results from the disruption of the septal perichondrium from the cartilage when it is deformed by trauma. Bleeding from the inner aspect of the perichondrium accumulates between the septal cartilage and its overlying mucoperichondrium, depriving the cartilage of its blood supply. Immediate nasal obstruction following injury should be suspect for a septal hematoma. Septal hematomas will not vasoconstrict with topical nasal decongestants. Otolaryngologic consultation should be obtained as quickly as possible if a septal hematoma is suspected. The hematoma should be drained as soon as possible and the mucoperichondrium packed back against the septal cartilage to restore its blood supply. If the hematoma is left for any duration, septal abscess may develop and cartilage destruction may occur. If there is loss of septal cartilage, a saddle nose deformity may result.

Cerebrospinal Fluid Rhinorrhea

A clear, watery rhinorrhea occurring after nasal trauma may be CSF rhinorrhea, which would indicate a skull fracture, usually through the cribriform plate. Less commonly, the CSF originates from a temporal bone fracture and enters the nasopharynx through the eustachian tube. If the patient leans forward, allowing the nasal drainage to drip onto a piece of paper, a characteristic target pattern will often appear, with a bloodstain in the center of the drop and a clear halo of CSF around it. CSF is high in glucose content, which may be detected with the use of a glucose oxidase test paper (used in urinalysis). Care must be taken in interpreting these tests because normal nasal mucus can look like CSF and the oxidizing substances present in nasal and lacrimal secretions may give a false-positive reaction. If traumatic CSF rhinorrhea is suspected by history or clinical examination, the child should be admitted and restricted to bed rest with his or her head elevated about 30 degrees in an attempt to decrease and seal the leak. Frequently, traumatic CSF leaks will heal spontaneously with rest and conservative management. If possible, some of the fluid should be collected and tested for β-2-transferrin (found specifically in CSF). Otorhinolaryngology and neurosurgery consultations should be obtained. The use of prophylactic antimicrobials in CSF rhinorrhea is controversial. Further diagnostic studies, such as CT scans and isotope scans, can be performed to confirm the diagnosis of CSF leak.

Sinus Trauma

Fractures of the paranasal sinuses may occur as isolated injuries or in association with trauma to the nose and orbital structures. Fractures of the ethmoid sinus or anterior wall of the maxillary sinus usually occur as a result of blunt trauma to the nose or cheek, respectively. The otolaryngologist should assist the emergency physician in evaluating these injuries. Subcutaneous crepitance may be felt in the cheek or around the eye. Radiographs may demonstrate air in the cheek or orbit or air-fluid levels in the sinus cavities. After determining the absence of potential associated ocular injury, the patient is usually placed on oral antimicrobials (usually amoxicillin 25 to 50 mg per kg per day for 7 days) and observed as an outpatient until the crepitance resolves. Displaced anterior maxillary sinus wall fractures rarely require intervention.

Facial Trauma

Blunt facial trauma can result in focal injuries and fractures or more generalized fractures involving much of the midface. Blunt trauma to the orbit may result in the force being transmitted through the globe to break the orbital floor (roof of maxillary sinus) or the medial orbital wall (lamina papyracea of the ethmoid sinus). These blowout fractures are discussed in detail in other chapter in this textbook.

Midface fractures include fractures of the malar bone, which affect both the orbital floor and the maxillary sinus. A complete malar (incorrectly called *trimalar* or *tripod*) fracture is present when the malar bone fractures at the infraorbital rim, zygomatic arch, and zygomaticofrontal suture line. Isolated malar fractures can also occur at the zygomatic arch or the lateral wall of the maxillary sinus. (For more detail regarding sequential steps and examination for facial fractures, see Chapter 111.) Severe midface injuries often require multidisciplinary cooperation among specialists in otolaryngology, ophthalmology, plastic surgery, oral surgery, and neurosurgery.

Sinus Barotrauma

A direct open communication between the paranasal sinuses and the nasal cavities normally permits prompt equalization of changes in ambient pressure. If a sinus ostia is obstructed, however, changes in ambient pressure may not be transmitted to the affected sinus cavity (most commonly the maxillary sinus, although the frontal sinus may be affected in older children and adolescents), and barotrauma can result. As the child descends in an airplane or during an underwater dive (even to the depth of the deep end of a swimming pool), the increased ambient pressure is transmitted to the cardiovascular system and, thus, to the vessels of the mucosal lining of the sinus. The vessels become engorged and the mucosa becomes edematous. If the sinus is obstructed and has not equalized the air pressure, a large differential pressure occurs between the sinus mucosa and its air-filled cavity. This condition results in a rupture of the blood vessels within the mucosa and bleeding into the sinus. The child usually complains of cheek pain and may have epistaxis. Treatment for this condition involves amoxicillin 25 to 50 mg per kg per day for 7 days (to prevent infection of the

TRAUMA

blood-filled sinus), antihistamine–decongestant therapy and topical nasal sprays to restore the normal physiologic communication between the sinus and the nasal cavities, and the avoidance of further barotrauma. The rare case that does not respond to this regimen should be referred to an otolaryngologist for further evaluation and treatment.

Foreign Bodies

Nasal foreign bodies are common in children. These children are usually brought to the ED with the history of putting an object into the nose, but the presence of a foreign body may often be unsuspected and may be discovered only during evaluation of a child with persistent, unilateral, foul-smelling, purulent rhinorrhea. This mode of presentation for these problems is so common that any child with a foul-smelling unilateral nasal discharge (even without a history of placing an object in the nose) should be considered to have a nasal foreign body until proven otherwise. The foreign body is usually visible on anterior rhinoscopy. However, suctioning of purulent secretions from the nasal cavity may be required before the object is seen. If the foreign object has been present for a while, there may be granulation tissue around the object and may bleed. Radiographs are of limited value because most of the foreign bodies are radiolucent (e.g., paper, cloth, sponge, food).

If the object is located in the nasal vestibule, the emergency physician may attempt to remove it. The child should be adequately restrained, and the necessary equipment, including a nasal speculum, directed light, suction, small hooks, and forceps, should be available. Otologic instruments are often very useful in the removal of nasal foreign bodies. Vasoconstriction with a topical nasal decongestant, such as oxymetazoline, plus a few drops of 4% lidocaine, for topical anesthesia, can be placed in the nostril before attempting the removal of the foreign body. An otolaryngologist should be consulted if the foreign body cannot be removed easily.

Hygroscopic foreign bodies, such as beans, may swell with nasal secretions and become difficult to remove. Disk batteries can be extremely caustic and need to be removed emergently, as they may cause a septal perforation and/or scarring; if they cannot be easily removed, an otolaryngologist should be immediately consulted. A foreign body should never be pushed or irrigated into the nasopharynx, where it could be aspirated by the struggling child. Antimicrobials (usually amoxicillin 25 to 50 mg per kg per day for 7 days) are administered to prevent (or treat) an infection (rhinitis, sinusitis) in this already traumatized area, especially after removal of a long-standing foreign body.

ORAL CAVITY, PHARYNX, AND ESOPHAGUS

Trauma

A common etiology of oral cavity trauma is biting the inside of the cheek or tongue; this is painful and can cause result in a laceration or hematoma formation. Treatment of self-inflicted bites is rarely needed, but a laceration may require suturing if it bleeds excessively, has a significant soft-tissue flap (trap-door flap), or is severe enough to alter intraoral anatomy or

physiology (i.e., breathing, deglutition, or speech). Oral hygiene with warm saline for irrigation or over-the-counter oral rinses, such as Peroxyl™, can be considered. These lesions rarely require oral antibiotic therapy. Topical analgesic preparations can be used for pain relief.

Children may suffer oropharyngeal lacerations or puncture wounds when they fall with an object, such as a stick, in their mouths. If the injury is restricted to the central portion of the palate, damage to vascular or neural structures of the head and neck is unlikely. These children are usually safe to send home after confirmation of absence of any retained foreign body (see the following section). However, trauma to the lateral aspects of the palate or the posterior pharyngeal wall may be associated with vascular injuries of the carotid artery or the jugular vein. Expanding hematoma of the neck or pharynx, continued intraoral bleeding, diminished pulses in the neck, or neurologic changes are all signs of serious vascular injury. These children need to be admitted and have an urgent angiogram/ venogram performed (such as conventional angiography, computed tomography angiogram [CTA], or magnetic resonance imaging arteriogram/venogram [MRA/MRV]), and possibly require surgical exploration. If a lateral pharyngeal or palatal puncture injury is present without signs of vascular injury, the child should be observed closely in the hospital or at home for signs of neurologic deterioration.

In treating puncture wounds of the pharynx, it is imperative to determine whether the foreign body has been recovered intact or if a portion of the foreign body may have been left in the palatal tissues. A portion of pencil lead left in the palatal tissue can cause a chronic foreign body reaction if it is not removed at the time of initial treatment and repair. Plain radiographs may not be useful in determining whether a foreign body has been left in the wound because most of the objects are radiolucent and/or too small to be seen. Inspecting the actual object that caused the wound, to make sure that it is intact, is more important. If a retained portion of the foreign body is suspected, CT scan may be required, followed by exploration of the wound, usually under general anesthesia. Clean puncture injuries or simple lacerations do not require surgical repair and usually heal by secondary intention. Large gaping injuries may require exploration, debridement, and a formal layered closure to restore normal function to the palate.

Caustic Injuries

Caustic substances (lye or acid) may be ingested, causing burns anywhere from the lips to the stomach. Burns of the oral mucosa appear as patches of erythema, blebs, or ulcerated areas. Although caustic burns are usually visible in the oral cavity and pharynx, large skip areas may exist. Therefore, the absence of oral or pharyngeal burns does not rule out esophageal injury. If a history of significant caustic ingestion exists, an esophagoscopy should be performed 6 to 12 hours later to establish the presence of esophageal burns, regardless of the condition of the oral cavity and pharynx. Because burns occur rapidly after ingestion, the child need not be given any oral antidote in the ED. In fact, emesis should not be induced because it only re-exposes the esophagus to the caustic substance; induced emesis also carries the risk of aspiration of the caustic material.

Caustic substances may burn the larynx when ingested and can cause rapidly progressive edema and respiratory distress. Endotracheal intubation for acute airway management should be performed in the ED if necessary. A tracheotomy should be considered as soon as possible after intubation to minimize the possibility of laryngotracheal stenosis.

Foreign Bodies

Foreign bodies in the oral cavity and pharynx are uncommon because of the child's protective reflexes. The tongue is sensitive and can detect sharp foreign objects that are then spat out. The gag reflex often expels foreign material from the pharynx, but sharp objects, such as fish bones, pins, and pieces of plastic, may get stuck in the oral mucosa, tonsils, or pharynx (Fig. 110.2). If a foreign body is visible and the patient is cooperative, the object may be removed in the ED with a clamp or forceps.

Objects of all types may lodge in the hypopharynx or esophagus. Esophageal foreign bodies generally lodge at the areas of natural narrowing of the esophagus. The most common sites are the cricopharyngeal area, thoracic inlet, arch of the aorta, and the gastroesophageal junction. If the child can

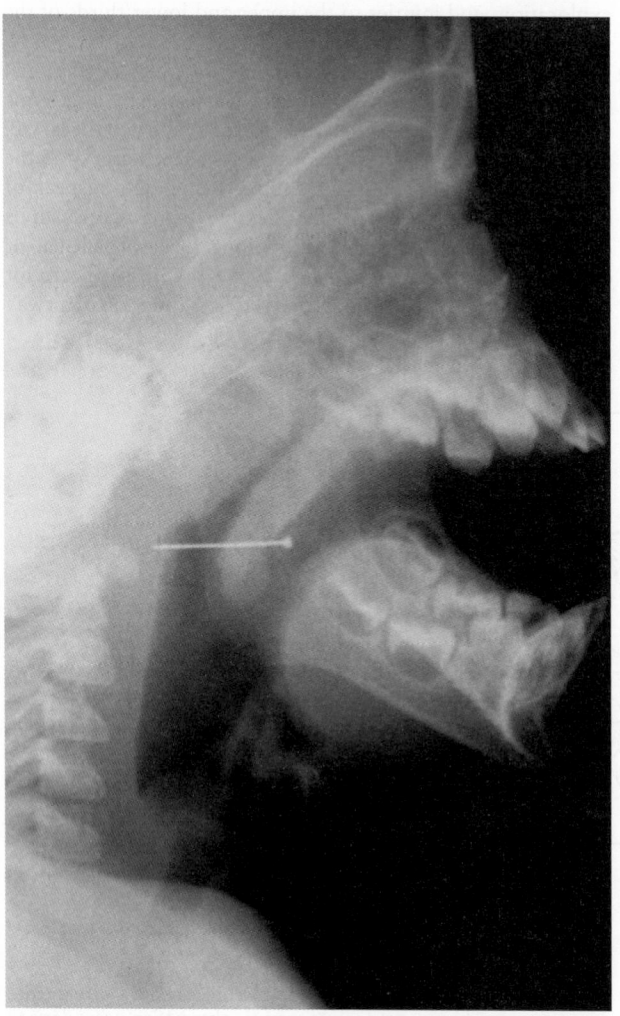

FIGURE 110.2 Lateral neck radiograph of a straight pin lodged in posterior pharyngeal wall.

breathe and talk, no attempt should be made to remove the object in the ED. The safest method of removal is under direct visualization while a child is under a general anesthetic. If the child is gagging and unable to breathe, the Heimlich maneuver may be used. If this method is not effective, emergency intubation or tracheotomy may be required to bypass the obstructing object.

Lateral neck and chest radiographs reveal radiopaque hypopharyngeal and esophageal foreign bodies. Plastic and other nonradiopaque objects cause the same foreign body sensation (something stuck in the throat) but are not visible on radiograph. Young children often have dysphagia and drooling because of painful swallowing.

Although ingestion of a foreign body usually causes gagging and choking that last for several seconds, these symptoms often subside. In addition, the initial episode may have taken place unobserved by an adult. Thus, unexplained dysphagia or drooling should initiate a search for a possible foreign body.

If a child presents to the ED with a history of swallowing an object, such as a toy or a fish bone, and complains of a foreign body sensation, a careful examination of the oral cavity and hypopharynx must be performed. If no foreign body is seen, plain radiographs of the neck should be obtained. Barium esophagrams are rarely helpful in pinpointing sharp foreign bodies in the esophagus but may be useful to confirm esophageal obstruction from an impacted foreign body such as a bolus of food. Foreign bodies easily seen in the oral cavity may be removed by the emergency physician. Consultation with an otolaryngologist (or similarly skilled specialist) should be obtained if a foreign body is detected in the pharynx or esophagus because removal usually requires endoscopic examination under anesthesia.

If the physical examination and radiographs fail to detect a foreign body, management is determined by the child's symptoms. If the child is having significant pain, the otolaryngologist should be consulted to perform esophagoscopy in the operating room. If the pain is mild, the child can swallow his or her own saliva, and no evidence of respiratory distress is present, the foreign body sensation may be secondary to a mucosal scratch from a foreign body that has passed into the stomach. In that instance, it may be appropriate to send the child home to return the next day if the sensation persists, which would indicate the potential presence of a persistent foreign body and require further evaluation.

Particular attention should be observed when there is disk-like foreign object on a plain film—it should be carefully examined to determine whether the object is coin or a disk battery. The anteroposterior (AP) and lateral views should be carefully scrutinized—looking for the presence of a double ring on the AP view and/or a step-off on the lateral view (Fig. 110.3). Disk battery ingestion must be emergently managed as disk batteries can cause significant caustic injury to the esophageal mucosa.

LARYNX AND TRACHEA

Trauma

Laryngeal trauma can occur in a variety of ways. Blunt or penetrating injuries of the larynx can result in mucosal lacerations, laryngeal hematomas, vocal cord paralysis, or fractures

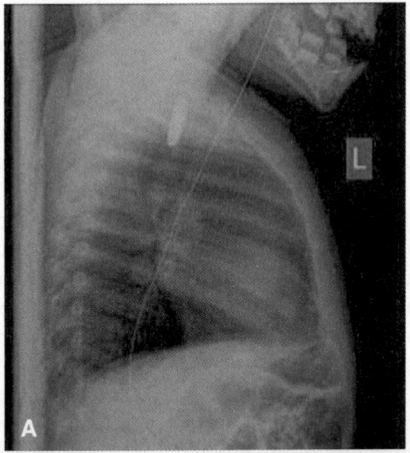

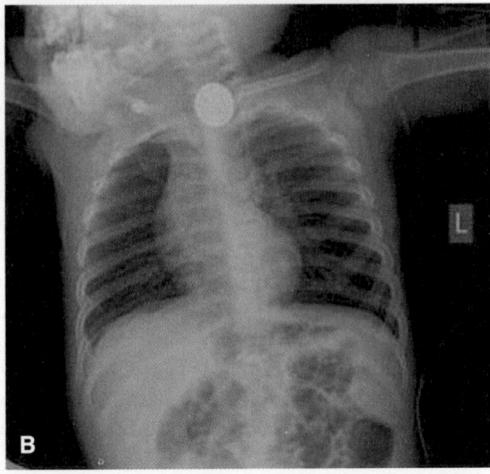

FIGURE 110.3 Chest radiographs of child with esophageal foreign body. **A:** AP film with round radiopaque foreign object—double ring makes this object suspect for a disc battery. **B:** Lateral film—note the step-off along the anterior edge of the foreign object, once again concerning for a disc battery. AP, anteroposterior.

of the thyroid and cricoid cartilages. Burn injuries can result from inhaling hot air or smoke from fires, or chemical burns may arise from caustic ingestion. Proper treatment requires prompt recognition of the presence and nature of a laryngeal injury and protection of the airway. Patients with laryngeal trauma present with varying degrees of neck pain, hoarseness, hemoptysis, and airway obstruction. Physical examination of a child with blunt trauma can reveal anterior neck tenderness, crepitance, and absence of the normal prominence of the thyroid cartilage or "Adam's apple" (Fig. 110.4). The otolaryngologist (or similarly skilled specialist) may be needed to perform an indirect examination of the larynx on the child with a suspected laryngeal injury. A direct laryngoscopy may be required when the child is in respiratory distress. The otolaryngologist should be prepared to intervene with intubation, rigid bronchoscopy, tracheotomy, and/or surgical exploration of these laryngeal injuries. If a child has a stable airway, radiologic imaging may help assess the airway for laryngeal, thyroid cartilage or tracheal injury. Penetrating neck injuries may require angiography or MRA/MRV to evaluate the vasculature of the neck for site of potential damage, including assessment for intimal damage, thrombus, or pseudoaneurysm formation. Even if the patient is stable, penetrating injuries of the central third of the neck should be considered for surgical exploration, and injuries to the upper and lower thirds of the neck should be imaged.

Home fires are the most common etiology of inhalational injury to the airway. Any child who was involved in a home fire should be assessed for possible thermal injury to the larynx and airway. Soot or carbonaceous debris at the nares or in the oral cavity and oropharynx should make one suspect of inhalation of hot gases. Typically, flexible laryngoscopy can be performed to assess the larynx, looking for soot, edema, or evidence of thermal injury to the larynx. If there is concern for thermal injury to the larynx, prophylactic intubation of airway

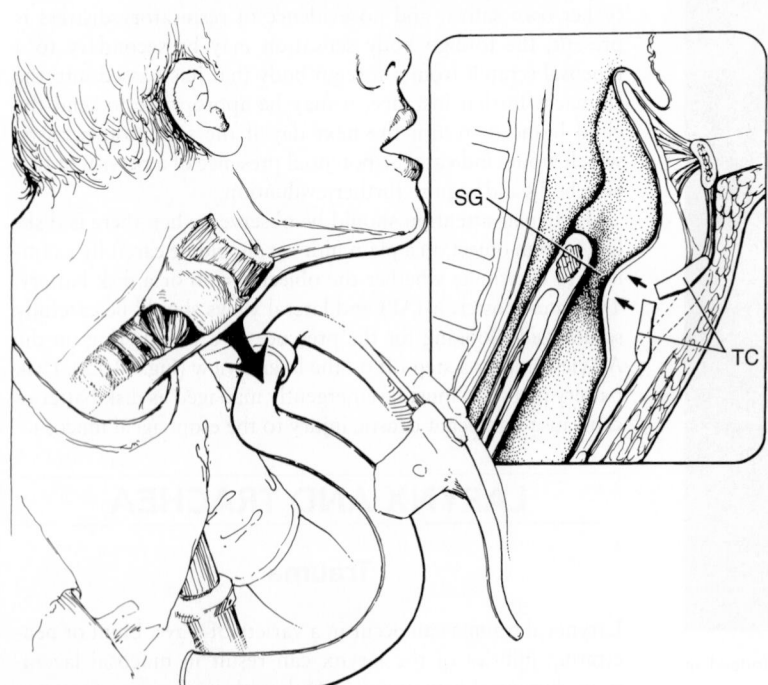

FIGURE 110.4 Loss of thyroid cartilage prominence and associated acute airway obstruction secondary to laryngeal fracture. *SG,* narrowed subglottic space; *TC,* fracture of thyroid cartilage.

may be considered to protect the airway prior to the onset of significant swelling.

Ingestion of caustic substances can cause severe burns of the larynx and pharynx; airway obstruction may occur secondary to the edema related to this injury. Laryngeal burns should be suspected in the child who has hoarseness or stridor after caustic ingestion. The child should be hospitalized, and otolaryngologic consultation should be obtained. If signs of respiratory distress (e.g., tachypnea, stridor) occur, the child should be taken to the operating room, where endoscopy can be performed and an artificial airway, usually a tracheotomy, can be established.

Foreign Bodies

Foreign bodies may become trapped in the laryngeal inlet, causing acute upper airway obstruction. The child usually presents with severe coughing, hoarseness, and significant respiratory distress. If the child is able to phonate, air is moving through his or her larynx, indicating only partial obstruction. "Back blows" or the Heimlich maneuver should not be performed in these children because this action may cause the foreign body to lodge more firmly in the larynx and convert a partial obstruction into a complete one. The child should be taken immediately to the operating room, where the otolaryngologist (or similarly skilled specialist) can perform the direct laryngoscopy necessary to remove the foreign body. In contrast, if the child is unable to speak, the foreign body may be causing total obstruction. In this case, back blows or the Heimlich maneuver may be lifesaving. Care must be taken in performing the Heimlich maneuver in young children because of the potential hazard of liver laceration. Emergency laryngoscopy, intubation, or tracheotomy is rarely required, and only if the previously described maneuvers are unsuccessful.

Foreign bodies that pass the larynx to lodge in the trachea or proximal bronchi can present problems in diagnosis and management. A history of coughing or choking on food (e.g., a peanut, raw carrot) or a toy is usually obtained. The child is often in no acute distress but may demonstrate a mild cough and/or wheezing. Inspiratory and expiratory stridors are characteristic of tracheal foreign bodies. Unilateral wheezes and decreased, or even absent, breath sounds are often seen with unilateral bronchial obstruction. Because most of the foreign bodies are radiolucent, they are not identifiable on radiographs. However, a radiographic difference in aeration of the lungs often helps detect the presence and identify the site of bronchial obstruction. Volume decrease, atelectasis, and infiltrate on the involved side may be seen on plain chest radiographs if the bronchus is completely occluded by the foreign body. Hyperaeration (air trapping) secondary to a ball-valve effect of a foreign body that is partially blocking the bronchus is best seen by comparing inspiration and expiration films (Fig. 110.5). If the child will not cooperate to obtain these views, right and left lateral decubitus films can often demonstrate the same phenomenon. Although differentiating hyperaeration and contralateral volume loss from atelectasis and compensatory contralateral lung expansion may help predict the location of a possible foreign body, this distinction is not as important as recognizing that any radiographic asymmetry signals a possible foreign body and requires endoscopy. A normal chest

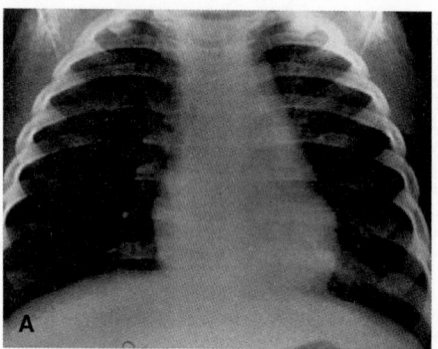
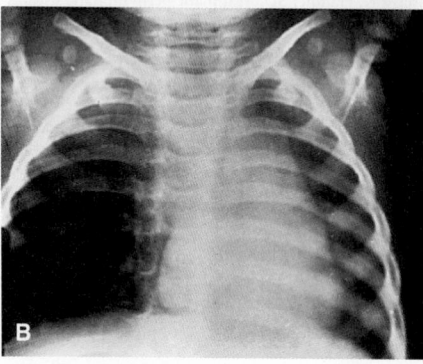

FIGURE 110.5 Chest radiograph of child with bronchial foreign body. **A:** Inspiratory film demonstrates only subtle hyperaeration of right lung. **B:** Expiratory film shows accentuated hyperaeration on the right side secondary to air trapping ("ball-valve" phenomenon) by the foreign body in the right mainstem bronchus. In addition, the mediastinum is displaced to the left.

radiograph, however, does not rule out the possibility of a foreign body. If a foreign body is suspected (by history or clinical examination), the child should be admitted and otolaryngologic consultation should be obtained to consider performing the endoscopy necessary for the prompt and safe removal of the foreign object.

Suggested Readings

Abujamra L, Joseph MM. Penetrating neck injuries in children: a retrospective review. *Pediatr Emerg Care* 2003;19(5):308–313.

Amadsun JE. An observational study of the management of traumatic tympanic membrane perforations. *J Laryngol Otol* 2002;116:181–184.

Bressler K, Shelton C. Ear foreign-body removal: a review of 98 consecutive cases. *Laryngoscope* 1993;103(4, pt 1):367–370.

Canty PA, Berkowitz RG. Hematoma and abscess of the nasal septum in children. *Arch Otolaryngol Head Neck Surg* 1996;122(12):1373–1376.

Colvin IB, Beale T, Harrop-Griffiths K. Long-term follow-up of hearing loss in children and young adults with enlarged vestibular aqueducts: relationship to radiologic findings and Pendred syndrome diagnosis. *Laryngoscope* 2006;116(11):2027–2036.

Darrouzet V, Duclos JY, Liguoro D, et al. Management of facial paralysis resulting from temporal bone fractures: our experience in 115 cases. *Otolaryngol Head Neck Surg* 2001;125(1):77–84.

Darrow DH, Holinger LD. Aerodigestive tract foreign bodies in the older child and adolescent. *Ann Otol Rhinol Laryngol* 1996;105(4):267–271.

De Jong AL, Macdonald R, Ein S, et al. Corrosive esophagitis in children: a 30-year review. *Int J Ped Otorhinolaryngol* 2001;57:203–211.

Duval EL, Geraerts SD, Brackel HJ. Management of blunt tracheal trauma in children: a case series and review of literature. *Eur J Pediatr* 2007;166:559–563.

Edmonds C, Lowry C, Pennefather J, et al. Diving and subaquatic medicine, 4th ed. New York, NY: Arnold, 2002.

Fernandes SV. Nasal fractures: the taming of the shrew. *Laryngoscope* 2004; 114:587–592.

TRAUMA

Ferreira PC, Amarante JM, Silva PN, et al. Retrospective study of 1251 maxillofacial fractures in children and adolescents. *Plast Reconstr Surg* 2005;115(6):1500–1508.

Hawkins DB. Removal of blunt foreign bodies from the esophagus. *Ann Otol Rhinol Laryngol* 1990;99:935–940.

Healy GB. Management of tracheobronchial foreign bodies in children: an update. *Ann Otol Rhinol Laryngol* 1990;99:889–891.

Hester TO, Campbell JP. Diagnosis and management of nasal trauma for primary care physicians. *J Ky Med Assoc* 1997;95(9):386–392.

Jackler RK, De La Cruz A. The large vestibular aqueduct syndrome. *Laryngoscope* 1989;99:1238–1243.

Kadish HA, Corneli HM. Removal of nasal foreign bodies in the pediatric population. *Am J Emerg Med* 1997;15(1):54–56.

Kadish HA, Schunk JE. Pediatric basilar skull fracture: do children with normal neurologic findings and no intracranial injury require hospitalization? *Ann Emerg Med* 1995;26(1):37–41.

Kim SH, Kazahaya K, Handler SD. Traumatic perilymphatic fistulas in children: etiology, diagnosis, and management. *Int J Ped Otorhinolaryngol* 2001; 60(2):147–153.

Lima JA. Laryngeal foreign bodies in children: a persistent, life-threatening problem. *Laryngoscope* 1989;99:415–420.

Lin CY, Lin SL, Kao CC, et al. The remediation of hearing deterioration in children with large vestibular aqueduct syndrome. *Auris Nasus Larynx* 2005;2:99–105.

Lin VYW, Daniel SJ, Papsin BC. Button batteries in the ear, nose and upper aerodigestive tract. *Int J Pediatr Otorhinolaryngol* 2004;68:473–479.

Liu-Shindo M, Hawkins DB. Basilar skull fractures in children. *Int J Pediatr Otorhinolaryngol* 1989;17:109–117.

Losee JE, Afifi A, Jiang S, et al. Pediatric orbital fractures: classification, management, and early follow-up. *Plast Reconstr Surg* 2008;122(3):886–897.

Lusk RP, Muntz HR. Introduction to pediatric rhinology. In: Wetmore RF, Muntz HR, McGill TJI, eds. *Pediatric otolaryngology: principles practice pathways.* New York, NY: Theime, 2000:439–452.

Madnani DD, Steele NP, deVries E. Factors that predict the need for intubation in patients with smoke inhalation injury. *Ear Nose Throat J* 2006;85(4): 278–280.

Mori T, Westerberg BD, Atashband S, et al. Natural history of hearing loss in children with enlarged vestibular aqueduct syndrome. *J Otolaryngol Head Neck Surg* 2008;37(1):112–118.

Potsic WP. Management of trauma of the external ear. In: English G, ed. *Otolaryngology.* New York, NY: Harper & Row, 1990.

Reilly JS, Cook SP, Stool D, et al. Prevention and management of aerodigestive foreign body injuries in childhood. *Pediatr Clin North Am* 1996;43(6):1403–1411.

Senders CR. Pediatric facial trauma. In: Wetmore RF, Muntz HR, McGill TJI, eds. *Pediatric otolaryngology: principles practice pathways.* New York, NY: Theime, 2000:497–512.

Singh B, Kantu M, Har-El G, et al. Complications associated with 327 foreign bodies of the pharynx, larynx, and esophagus. *Ann Otol Rhinol Laryngol* 1997;106(4):301–304.

Soose RJ, Simons JP, Mandell DL. Evaluation and management of pediatric oropharyngeal trauma. *Arch Otolaryngol Head Neck Surg* 2006;132:446–451.

Toback S. Nasal septal hematoma in an 11-month-old infant: a case report and review of the literature. *Pediatr Emerg Care* 2003;19:265–267.

Tong MC, Ying SY, van Hasselt CA. Nasal foreign bodies in children. *Int J Pediatr Otorhinolaryngol* 1996;35(3):207–211.

CHAPTER 111 ■ FACIAL TRAUMA

MARK I. NEUMAN, MD, MPH

BACKGROUND

Soft-tissue injuries and lacerations account for the majority of facial trauma in children. Common mechanisms of facial injury in children include falls, sports-related injuries, assaults, and motor vehicle accidents. Children account for approximately 15% of all facial fractures, with children younger than 5 years comprising only 5% of this total. The majority of facial fractures in children occur in teenagers, with a 2.5:1 male predominance.

This low prevalence of facial fractures in children is multifactorial. The face of a child is relatively small compared with the head and thus most fractures in young children tend to involve the upper face and skull. In addition, the face is much stronger because the sinus cavities are poorly developed and the proportion of cancellous to cortical bone is greater, providing more elasticity. Young children are also afforded some protection by large fat pads, particularly the buccal fat pad in the malar region. Children are also less likely than adults to be exposed to occupational trauma, assaults, and major trauma associated with motor vehicle accidents.

INITIAL MANAGEMENT

Injuries sustained as a result of facial trauma are rarely, in and of themselves, life threatening. However, patients who have sustained enough force to cause significant facial injury may have occult injuries elsewhere and a complete trauma evaluation is usually warranted. In rare instances, these life-threatening injuries have been overlooked, likely due to the profound appearance of some facial injuries. In particular, care should be taken when examining the face and head until an injury to the cervical spine is excluded. In some series, up to 10% of patients with maxillofacial trauma have an associated cervical spine injury. Patients with tenderness of the cervical spine, impaired sensorium, focal neurologic deficits, or major distracting injury elsewhere should be placed in a hard cervical collar until an injury to the cervical spine can be excluded.

Stabilization of the airway is the primary concern in the management of facial injuries in children. Patients can have airway obstruction resulting from various factors, including blood, loose teeth, the tongue, and pharyngeal edema; therefore, the airway should be cleared and examined for patency. Loss of support of subglottic musculature can result from severe mandibular fractures, and the tongue can fall posteriorly and occlude the airway in a comatose patient. Oral or nasal airway may serve as an adjuvant to positioning in order to achieve airway patency. Tracheal intubation may be required if the airway remains unstable. Cricothyrotomy or tracheostomy may be necessary if these measures fail to secure the airway. These should be attempted only as a last resort because of the technical difficulty and complications associated with such procedures.

Difficulties in decision making in the initial management of patients with facial trauma often revolve around whether subspecialist input is warranted, and if so, which particular subspecialist to involve. Plastic surgeons, ophthalmologists, otorhinolaryngologists, and oral and maxillofacial surgeons have expertise and interest in the management of patients with facial trauma. Once it is determined that subspecialist input is warranted, the decision of which subspecialist to involve will depend largely on availability and expertise of such individuals within the institution. Although most facial injuries can be managed without involving a subspecialist, many of the injuries detailed in this chapter do require such input.

HISTORY

Special attention must be paid to the mechanism of injury in order to determine the facial injuries one is likely to encounter. In addition, the timing and location of the injury are important factors to consider when determining the course and prognosis, particularly related to infection. Often in the child with serious facial trauma, the history may need to be obtained from a bystander, emergency medical services personnel, or family members. In the alert and verbal child, key questions should include (i) Where does it hurt? (ii) Do you have blurry or decreased vision? (iii) Do you have any numbness of a particular region of your face? and (iv) Does it hurt when you open or close your mouth? Responses to these questions will help focus the examination. In the case of facial lacerations, it is important to ascertain whether the mechanism of injury was likely to result in a retained foreign body or whether it poses a high risk of infection. Finally, one must ensure the child's tetanus immunizations are up to date.

PHYSICAL EXAMINATION

Examination for specific bony injuries begins with the observation for deformity and asymmetry, which should be carried out in all projections. Malar eminences and zygomatic arches are visualized well when standing behind the patient and looking down over the forehead. Asymmetry can take the form of swelling or loss of projection or flattening.

Next, systematic palpation of the facial bones should be performed (Fig. 111.1). Tenderness, crepitus, and "step off" are signs of underlying fracture. Particular attention should be

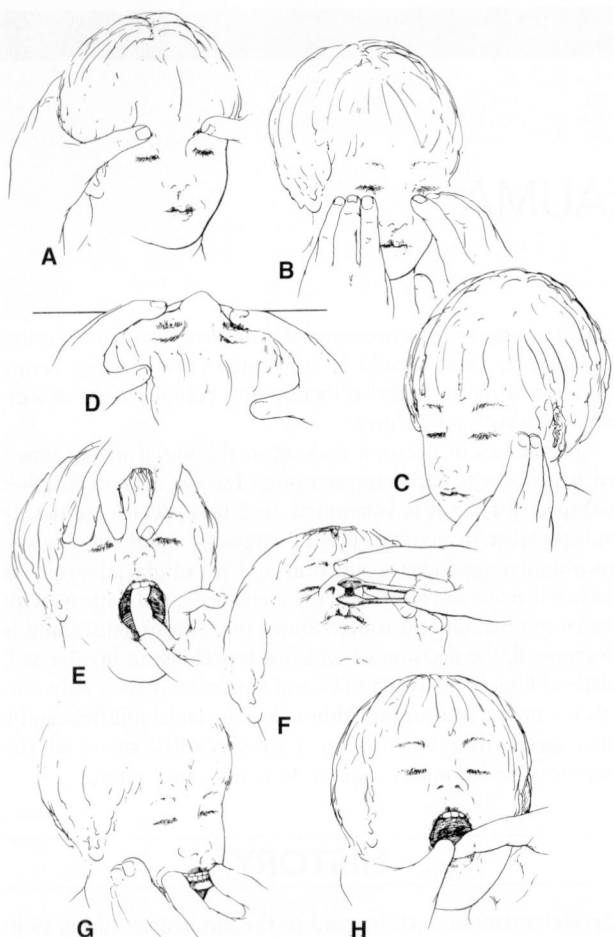

FIGURE 111.1 Sequential steps in examination for facial fractures.
A: The supraorbital ridges are palpated while keeping the patient's
head steady. B: The infraorbital ridges are palpated using the index,
middle, and ring fingers to assess for areas of point tenderness. C: The
zygomatic arch is palpated on each side to determine continuity and
the possible presence of displaced fractures. D: The infraorbital rims,
zygomatic bodies, and maxilla are palpated and examined from the
top of the head to determine depressions and fracture displacement.
E: The nasal bone and maxilla are examined for stability and possible
fracture displacement. F: The nose is examined intranasally to determine the placement of the nasal septum and the possible displacement
of nasal bones or disruption of nasal mucosa. G: The occlusion is
observed to determine any disturbances of normal teeth relations.
H: The mandible is palpated and then retracted to determine sites of
discomfort and possible mandibular fractures.

paid to the malar eminences, zygomatic arches, and superior
and inferior orbital rims. Assessment for a fracture of the maxilla can be performed by grasping and attempting to move the
upper central teeth. Any laxity of the maxilla or crepitus is
suggestive of fracture. External and intraoral palpation of the
mandibular symphysis, body, angle, and ramus can help diagnose fractures in these areas.

Inspection of the mouth and oral cavity should be performed to assess for injury to the maxilla and mandible.
Occlusal disharmony is an indication of mandibular and/or
maxillary displacement. Older children will be able to tell the
examiner if their bite "feels normal." Opposing teeth that do
not come together, but that exhibit wear facets (smoothing of

mamillations along the incisal surfaces of the teeth), suggest a
traumatic malocclusion. An inability to hold a tongue blade
between occluded teeth on each side of the mouth is suggestive
of a mandibular fracture.

Examination of the eyes should include the assessment of
pupillary reactivity and size and examination of extraocular
movements, visual acuity, and surrounding orbital injuries.
Direct trauma to the globe should be excluded. Orbital dystopia
and/or enophthalmos are suggestive of a fracture of the orbit.
An ophthalmologist should be consulted if any of these abnormalities are suspected (see Chapter 117). Examination of the
nose should include documentation of focal tenderness, swelling
and asymmetry, bleeding, or other nasal discharge, as well as the
presence or absence of a septal hematoma.

Neurologic examination of the face should include evaluation of both sensory and motor functions. All three branches
of the trigeminal nerve should be evaluated for sensation.
Anesthesia of the cheek suggests injury to the infraorbital
nerve, whereas anesthesia of the lower teeth and lower lip suggest inferior alveolar nerve involvement. The facial nerve
should be evaluated by asking the patient to wrinkle the forehead, close and open the eyes fully, smile, show his or her
teeth, and close the mouth tightly. Pure motor injuries to the
facial nerve are quite amenable to microsurgical repair if
detected and repaired in a timely fashion. Therefore, all suspected motor nerve injuries warrant appropriate surgical consultation to allow for the best functional recovery.

IMAGING STUDIES

The use of radiography in the evaluation and management of
children with facial trauma should be considered if there is a
concern of fracture based on history and physical examination. Because of the occult nature of pediatric facial fractures,
as well as the inability of many young children to communicate, one should have a low threshold for radiographic evaluation. The complexity of bony and soft-tissue facial structures
can make the interpretation of plain radiographs difficult. In
addition, plain radiographs are often inadequate to determine
whether a patient requires operative intervention. Computed
tomography (CT) has mainly replaced plain radiographs in the
definitive assessment of bony facial injuries because it has a
greater ability to detect fractures and associated displacement,
as well as a greater ability to visualize soft-tissue structures.

Despite their limitations, plain radiographs obtained in the
emergency department during the initial evaluation can provide useful information about suspected bony injuries, are less
expensive and easier to obtain than CT scans in most institutions, and do not require the use of sedation. The Waters view
(occipitomental) is used to visualize the midface region—the
orbital rims and floor of the orbit, nasal bones, zygoma, and
maxilla. This view may be particularly useful in patients suspected of having a blowout fracture of the orbit, as well as for
detecting fluid in the maxillary sinus. The Caldwell view supplements the Waters view for the evaluation of the upper two-
thirds of the face, including visualization of the superior
orbital rim, frontal sinuses, and nasoethmoid complex; however, the orbital floor is often obscured. The lateral view is useful for the detection of fractures to the anterior wall of the
frontal sinus, the anterior and posterior walls of the maxillary

sinus, and the nasal bones. The submentovertex view provides visualization of the zygomatic body and arch. Posterior–anterior, right and left lateral oblique, and Townes views are used to detect fractures of the mandible; however, fractures of the symphysis may be difficult to discern. Panorex views provide visualization of the entire mandible and lower teeth.

With the development of high-resolution scanners, CT has become the most frequently used imaging modality for the evaluation of suspected facial fractures. Axial views demonstrate fractures of the anterior and posterior walls of the frontal sinus, medial and lateral orbital walls, posterior wall of the maxillary sinus, zygomatic arches, and mandible. Coronal views demonstrate fractures of the ethmoid, sphenoid, and paranasal sinuses; orbital floors and infraorbital rims; the nasoethmoid region; and mandibular condyles and symphyses. Coronal imaging requires hyperextension of the neck and thus requires prior exclusion of a cervical spine injury. Three-dimensional CT imaging can help guide operative repair.

SPECIFIC INJURIES

Bony Injuries

In general, fractures of the upper face are managed with the goal of restoring anatomic alignment. Unless there is evidence of nerve or muscle entrapment, most surgical reductions of facial fractures do not need to be performed immediately. Generally, repairs occur a few days after the injury to allow for proper radiographic evaluation, as well as time for the swelling to subside. Because bony healing is relatively rapid in children, anatomic reduction becomes more difficult when healing in the displaced position has occurred, and early treatment (within 4 to 5 days) is preferred. There is an increasing trend toward early repair to facilitate a rapid recovery. Patients who are unable to drink, either because of pain or because of inability to open the mouth, require hospitalization.

Mandible Fractures

Fractures of the mandible can occur in one or more of the following regions: the symphysis, body, angle, ramus, and condyle (Fig. 111.2). The mechanism of injury often determines the site of potential fracture in patients with trauma to the mandible. Motor vehicle collisions and falls tend to cause fractures of the condyles and symphysis because the force is directed against the chin, whereas assaults tend to produce injuries to the body

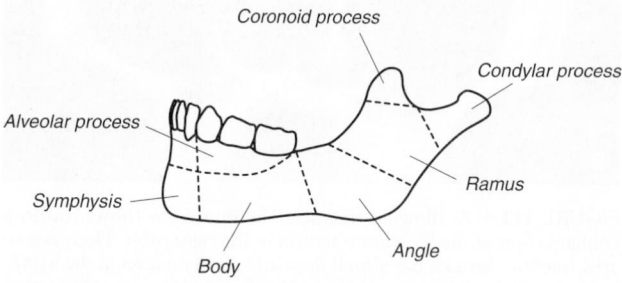

FIGURE 111.2 Anatomy of the mandible. Common sites of fracture include the condyle and subcondylar region, as well as the angle, body, and symphysis of the mandible.

or angle of the mandible at the point of impact. Patients with parasymphyseal fractures resulting from falls often have an associated fracture in the opposite subcondylar region. Pain and difficulty with mouth opening are usually present with mandibular fractures. Numbness of the lip and chin may also suggest a mandibular fracture because the inferior alveolar nerve courses through the center of the mandible, from the middle of the ramus, to its exit at the mental foramen. Mandibular fractures may result in airway obstruction due to hemorrhage either from the floor of the mouth or from a disruption in the bony support structure for the tongue.

Powerful muscles of mastication apply distracting forces to the fractured mandibular segments, often resulting in bony displacement and occlusal disharmony. The growth center for the mandible is located in the area of the condyle, and damage to this area from a fracture can cause significant growth disturbances, especially if sustained before the age of 3 years. Therefore, the clinical evaluation of any chin laceration should include palpation of the mandible, particularly the condyles. Malalignment of the lower central incisors (i.e., step off in dentition) suggests a mandibular fracture at the symphysis. Unilateral condyle fractures will most often result in the deviation of the jaw toward the side of the fracture upon mouth opening.

Because of concern regarding mandibular growth retardation and injury to permanent tooth buds, mandibular fractures in children are treated by more conservative measures than those in adults. A majority of fractures can be managed conservatively with closed reduction and maxillomandibular fixation. A soft or liquid diet is recommended. The remaining fractures are treated by open reduction, internal fixation, or the use of splints. Antibiotics are usually warranted because these fractures are often in communication with the oral cavity.

Temperomandibular joint dislocation may not only result from a direct blow to the chin but also occur while yawning or opening the mouth widely. With dislocation, the condyle of the mandible is displaced anteriorly and is prevented from sliding back into place by spasm of the jaw muscles. Preauricular swelling and inability to close the mouth fully are the key features on physical examination. Reduction of such dislocations often requires the use of procedural sedation and may be facilitated with a benzodiazepine to decrease muscle spasm. Downward traction is applied to the posterior aspect of the mandible. The chin is then pushed posteriorly to allow the condyle to return to its fossa.

Orbital Fractures

Knowledge of the bony anatomy of the orbit is integral to the understanding of fractures at this site. The superior portion of the orbit is composed of the superior orbital rim and orbital roof, which is part of the thick frontal bone. The medial wall is formed by the ethmoid bone, which is adjacent to the nasal bones. The lateral wall is formed by the greater wing of the sphenoid and the zygoma, which are also quite thick. The floor and the inferior orbital rim are formed by the zygoma and the maxilla, which are relatively thin, and are further weakened by the groove for the infraorbital nerve.

Fractures of the floor of the orbit, sometimes known as "orbital blowout fractures," typically occur when a medium-sized, round, hard object, such as a baseball, strikes the eye (Fig. 111.3). The volume of the globe is fixed; thus, when an

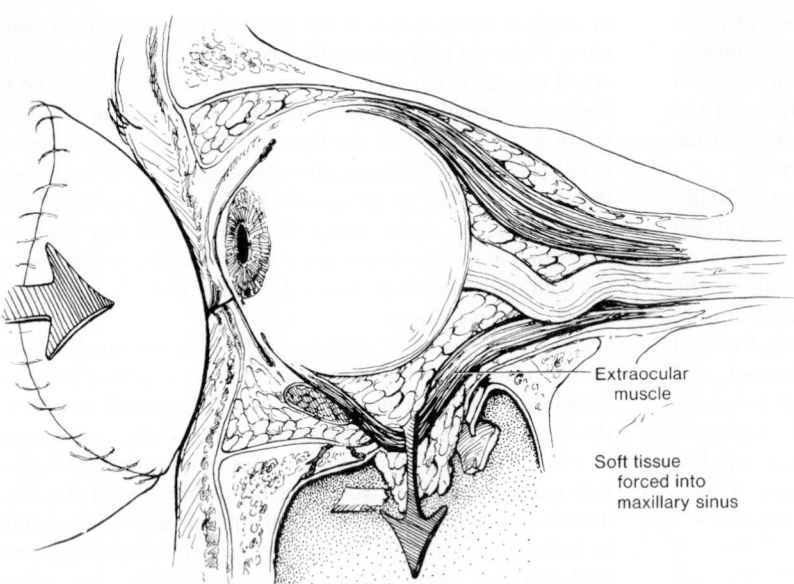

Extraocular
muscle

Soft tissue
forced into
maxillary sinus

FIGURE 111.3 Mechanism of blowout fracture. In a sagittal view, a ball is shown striking the eye, deforming it, and causing increased pressure of the intraorbital contents. The periorbital fat is forced through the floor of the orbit. Retropositioning of the eye (enophthalmos), lowering of the eye, and extraocular muscle entrapment can result.

acute increase in orbital space (an opening in the floor of the orbit) occurs, the globe may be pushed posteriorly in the orbit, producing enophthalmos, a sunken appearance to the eye. A true orbital blowout fracture denotes a fracture of the floor of the orbit, with an intact inferior orbital rim. Although these fractures are quite rare in children, they are often due to direct trauma to the zygoma rather than a compression of the globe itself. Blood and orbital fat may sink into the maxillary sinus, clouding the sinus on the radiograph (Fig. 111.4). Asymmetry in the horizontal level of the eyes (orbital dystopia) may also be present. The infraorbital nerve, the terminal branch of the maxillary division of the trigeminal nerve, exits the maxilla just below the infraorbital rim. Manifestations of injury to this nerve include decreased sensation to the cheek, upper lip, and upper gingiva on the affected side.

In children, the floor of the orbit is relatively flexible. Consequently, it may fracture in a linear pattern that snaps back to create a "trapdoor" fracture. In adults, the floor of the orbit is thick and more likely to shatter when exposed to force. If the inferior rectus muscle is entrapped in the fracture gap in the floor of the orbit, voluntary upward gaze may be limited. The presence of entrapment is one indication to operate on a blowout fracture on an urgent basis.

Studies suggest that early repair of orbital fracture and release of the entrapped muscles (within 24 to 48 hours) may help avoid muscle ischemia and fibrosis and result in better functional recovery. Corticosteroids may help decrease swelling in patients with limitation of extraocular movement.

A thorough ophthalmologic examination is warranted in all patients with orbital fractures because of the high likelihood of associated eye injuries. In particular, vision should be assessed because decreased visual acuity may be an early sign of a retrobulbar hemorrhage, or injury to the optic nerve or eye itself. A retrobulbar hemorrhage can cause compression of the central retinal artery, which can threaten vision to the affected eye if not surgically decompressed. The type of eye and orbit injuries varies on the basis of the object and mechanism involved. Typically, a low-impact mechanism with a small

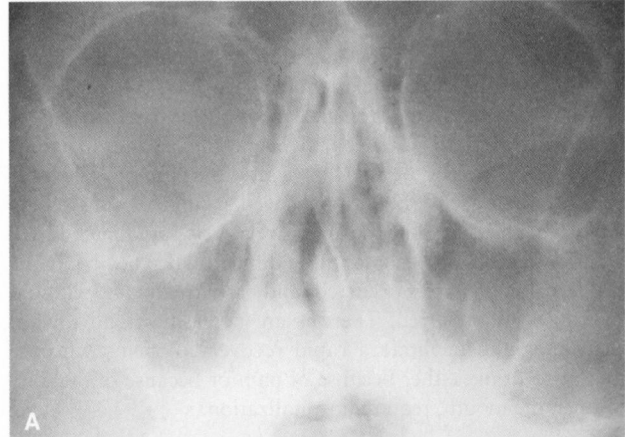

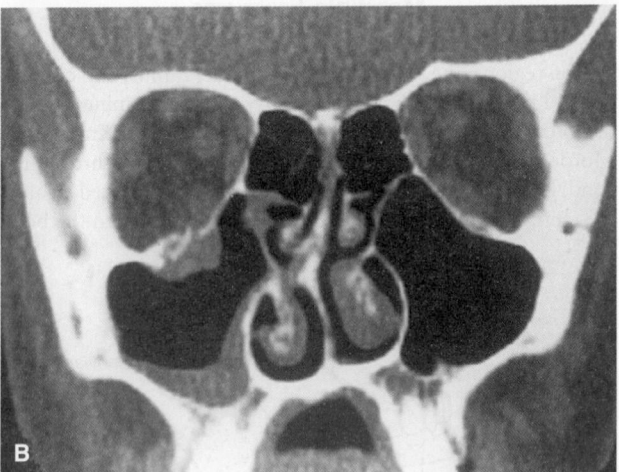

FIGURE 111.4 A: Blowout fracture. The sinus view shows teardrop configuration of the blowout fractures in the right orbit. Note associated fracture through the orbital floor and air–fluid level in the maxillary sinus. **B:** In the same patient as (**A**), computed tomography section more clearly demonstrates the multiple fragment fracture through the orbital floor. Teardrop and air–fluid level are evident in the right maxillary sinus. (Courtesy of Soroosh Mahboubi, MD.)

object will result in injuries to the eye itself, such as a corneal abrasion or hyphema. Injury to the eye from a high-speed soft object such as a tennis ball will often result in a hyphema. Hard objects striking the orbit at a high speed, such as a baseball or a fist, are likely to result in an orbital blowout fracture. High-impact mechanisms, such a those encountered when the face strikes the dashboard in a motor vehicle collision, are likely to result in complex orbital and midface fractures.

Nasal Fractures

The nasal bones are among the most commonly fractured bones of the facial skeleton because of their prominent location on the face. Nasal fractures may be difficult to detect clinically because of significant swelling associated with such injuries. Plain radiographs are needed only rarely in the emergent care of children with nasal trauma because, in most cases, they do not contribute to subsequent care and management. Most nasal injuries can be followed on an outpatient basis, and evaluation after the swelling subsides dictates the need for further intervention.

Two particular nasal injuries that deserve specific comment are the intractable nosebleed and septal hematomas. Because of the rich vascular network in the nose, supplied by branches of both the internal (anterior ethmoidal) and external (superior labial, palatine) carotid arteries, nasal hemorrhage can be difficult to stop despite usual conservative measures (e.g., elevation, compression). Treatment of persistent epistaxis may require anterior and/or posterior nasal packing with gauze or tampon, or the placement of an epistaxis balloon catheter. If a bleeding vessel can be identified, silver nitrate cauterization can be performed.

Septal hematomas arise because of hemorrhage from an artery beneath the mucoperichondrium, separating it from the septal cartilage. Because the septal cartilage is avascular and relies on the overlying mucoperichondrium for its blood supply, a hematoma may result in cartilage necrosis and eventual septal perforation. In most cases, septal hematomas require urgent incision and drainage (see Chapter 111 and Section VII).

Repair of nasal fractures should ideally be performed either within a few hours after the injury (prior to significant swelling) or after the swelling subsides (usually 4 to 7 days). Because of the significant swelling that often develops rapidly with such injuries, immediate repair is usually not possible. Patients suspected of having nasal fractures should be reevaluated within 4 to 5 days after the swelling subsides. Plain radiographs may be helpful at this time to determine whether malalignment exists. Patients with nasal deformity 4 to 5 days after injury require urgent consultation with a specialist to restore anatomic alignment.

Nasoorbital ethmoid fractures involve complete separation of the nasal bones and medial walls of the orbits from the stable frontal bone superiorly and infraorbital rim laterally. These injuries are usually the result of high-velocity trauma to the central midface. The bones are often fragmented and telescoped posteriorly into the ethmoid region. These patients display a characteristic flattened nose, with the loss of anterior projection on the lateral view of the face. Because the medial canthal tendons attach firmly to the medial walls of the orbits, lateral drift of the fracture segments results in traumatic telecanthus. Normal mean intercanthal distance is 16 mm at birth, which increases to 25 mm in a female and 27 mm in a male at

full facial growth. A significant increase in intercanthal distance or gross asymmetry in the medial canthal to facial midline distance should raise suspicion of this fracture. Traumatic telecanthus suggests the diagnosis of a nasoorbital ethmoid fracture, which unlike a nondisplaced nasal fracture, requires urgent subspecialist input.

Zygoma and Maxilla Fractures

The zygoma is composed of a body or malar eminence and the zygomatic arch and attaches to the temporal, frontal, and maxillary bones of the facial skeleton. A complete fracture of the zygoma results in fractures at each of these sites and extends through the floor of the orbit. This may result in an inferior displacement of the zygoma because of the strong inferior forces applied by the masseter muscle, which attaches to the malar eminence. Zygoma fractures often produce a flattened appearance to the cheek, with inferior displacement of the globe, and conjunctival hemorrhage. Decreased sensation along the distribution of the infraorbital nerve is also common, as zygomaticomaxillary fractures usually include the infraorbital foramen. In isolated zygomatic arch fractures, a decrease in temporal width can be appreciated when viewing the face from the front as a result of buckling of the zygomatic arch. If this buckling is severe, the mandibular condyle may be impinged, with resultant difficulty in mouth opening.

In 1901, LeFort described three fracture patterns that occurred in patients with midface trauma (Fig. 111.5). The LeFort I fracture pattern involves only the maxilla and extends through the zygomaticomaxillary region to the base of the pyriform aperture. It allows motion of a segment of alveolar bone and teeth when examined. The LeFort II pattern, also called a pyramidal fracture, is similar but extends more superiorly to the infraorbital rims and across the nasofrontal sutures. The maxilla, nasal bones, and the medial orbital wall are separated from the facial skeleton. The nose and the upper jaw are movable, whereas the zygomas are stable. The LeFort III pattern, also called craniofacial dissociation, extends across the zygomatic arch, zygomaticofrontal region, floor of the orbit, and nasofrontal sutures, effectively separating the midface from the skull base. When the nose or upper jaw is moved, the entire midface, including the zygoma, moves with it. These fractures are quite rare in children, and when they do occur, they are most often asymmetric because impact is sustained from the side rather than head on.

Patients with midface fractures typically have significant swelling over the maxilla and severe epistaxis. Particular attention to the airway is of paramount importance in these children because significant bleeding and a disruption in the normal anatomic structures may threaten the patency of the airway. Nasal manipulation should be avoided because these fractures may be associated with cribriform plate injuries and passage of a nasogastric or endotracheal tube may result in brain injury. On examination, by grasping the maxilla at the level of the central incisors, the clinician may be able to appreciate crepitus or mobility when traction is applied. Clear rhinorrhea in the setting of midface trauma may be a sign of a cerebrospinal fluid (CSF) leak and warrants neurosurgical consultation. All patients suspected of having a midface fracture require CT imaging to determine whether surgical reduction is necessary.

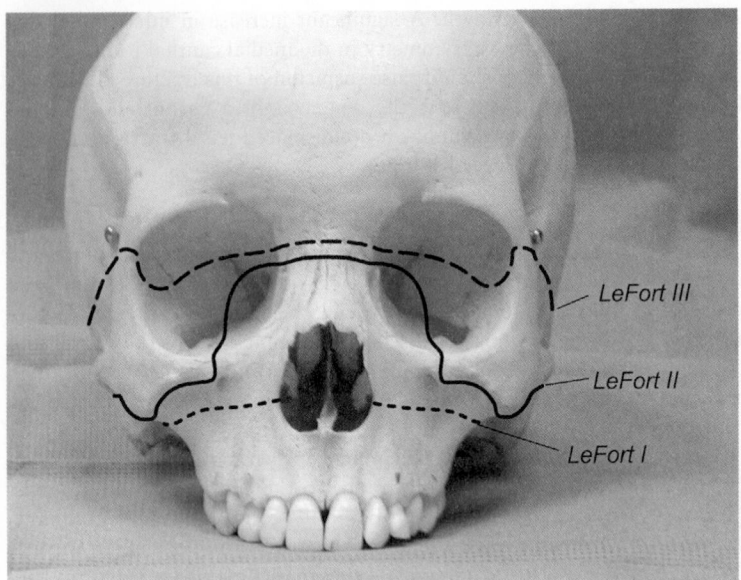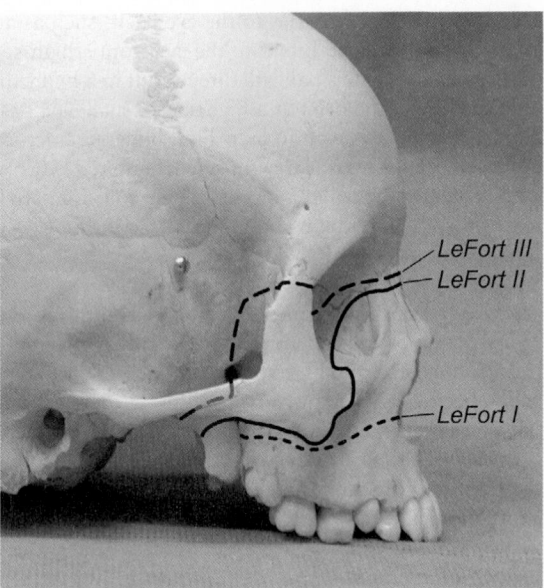

FIGURE 111.5 The LeFort classification of fractures. With type I, the maxilla is separated from its attachments. Type II (pyramidal) produces a mobile maxilla and nose. With type III (craniofacial disjunction), all attachments of the midface to the skull have been separated. Traction on the anterior maxilla produces motion up to the inferior orbital rims and zygoma. These fractures are not mutually exclusive. For example, LeFort II fracture may exist on the one side with type III on the other side.

Frontal Bone Fractures

Fractures of the frontal bone are rare in young children because the frontal sinuses do not begin to develop until 8 years of age. Injury to the frontal sinus may reveal a palpable or visible depression if the anterior wall of the sinus has been compressed. Displaced fractures of the anterior wall of the frontal sinus require surgical elevation. In patients with severe frontal sinus fractures associated with forehead lacerations, a fracture of the posterior wall of the sinus and dural tear may allow CSF to leak from the wound. Leakage of clear fluid from the wound, or clear rhinorrhea, should raise suspicion for such a leak and warrant CT imaging and neurosurgical consultation.

Soft-tissue Injuries

The approach to a child with soft-tissue injuries is discussed in the section on minor trauma (see Chapter 106). However, certain aspects of soft-tissue injuries involving the face warrant further discussion in this chapter.

Abrasions

Abrasions of the face should be evaluated for size, presence of foreign bodies, and injury to underlying structures. The severity and depth of injury may only be assessed by performing a thorough examination, which is often difficult in young children. The use of topical, local, and regional anesthetics may facilitate the examination and repair of such injuries. Deep abrasions should be irrigated to allow for optimal cleansing of the wound. Removal of debris from the wound is essential to avoid subsequent infection. Injuries on road or gravel can implant particulate matter into dermal layers. These areas require aggressive scrubbing and possible picking out of individual particles with the tip of a scalpel blade. Finally, extreme or deep wounds should be covered with sterile dressing. The use of topical antibiotic ointment on facial abrasions is controversial.

There are five general reasons to apply a dressing to a wound: protection, absorption, immobilization, compression (sometimes), and aesthetics. In most facial lacerations, the protective and aesthetic aspects of the dressing are most important. Deep abrasions should be covered with a dressing that provides controlled hydration, such as a polyurethane film, or a thicker, more absorptive dressing, such as those composed of hydrogels and hydrocolloids. These dressings help reduce pain, and studies have demonstrated that partial-thickness wounds covered with this type of dressing heal in approximately half the time it would take for an abrasion that is exposed to air or is covered with a dry dressing.

Lacerations

The goal of laceration repair is to achieve hemostasis and provide an optimal cosmetic result (Fig. 111.6, see also color plate). Although not unique to facial lacerations, cosmesis is often the primary concern among parents accompanying children with such injuries. Knowledge of the deep structures of the face, particularly the facial nerve and the lachrymal apparatus, will aid in the evaluation and management of children with deep facial lacerations. Lateral periorbital lacerations should raise suspicion of injury to the frontal branch of the facial nerve, which travels superficially along a line from just above the tragus to a point 1.5 cm above the lateral eyebrow. Lacerations in the medial periorbital region near the medial canthus should raise suspicion for lachrymal duct injury. Because 85% of tears are drained via the lower canaliculus, failure to repair a laceration to the lachrymal duct may result in excessive tearing (epiphora). If deep lacerations are present in

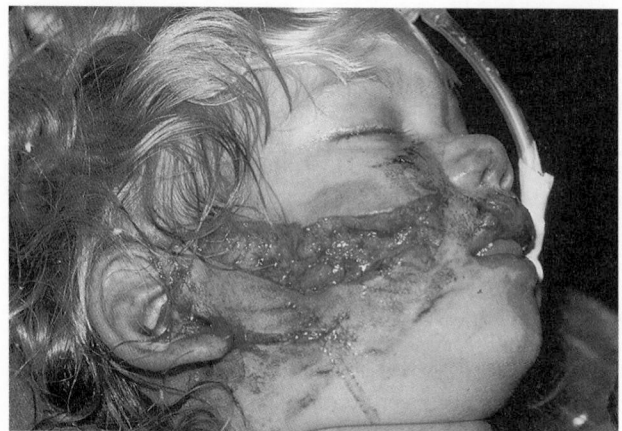

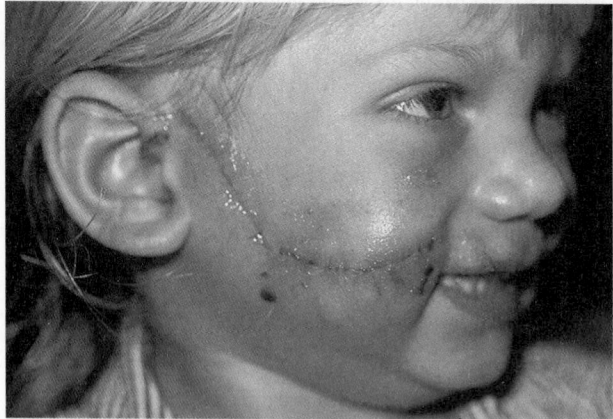

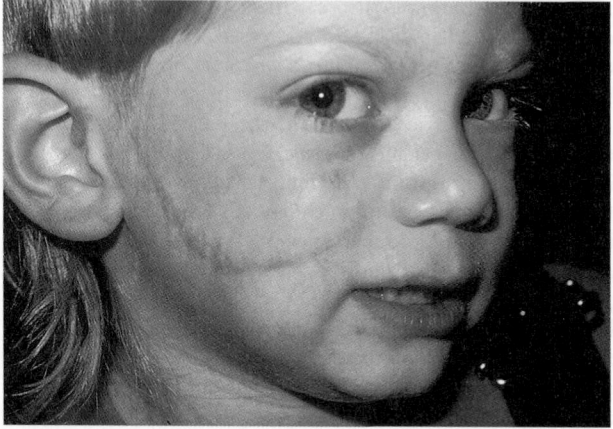

FIGURE 111.6 Photographs of a 3-year-old boy after an attack by a dog. The **top** photograph shows the child before sharp debridement, facial nerve exploration, and layered closure of his complex wound. The **middle** panel is a photograph of the child 1 week after his repair and demonstrates the precise reapproximation of the facial soft tissues. The **bottom** photograph was taken 8 months after the attack and demonstrates a nicely healed facial scar that will continue to fade and soften. (Courtesy of David W. Low, MD.)

the cheek region, the clinician must determine whether injury to the buccal branch of the facial nerve and to the parotid duct has occurred (Fig. 111.7).

Injuries to the cheek, involving the region between the mid-cheek and the tragus of the ear, should be assessed for injury to the facial nerve. When injury to the facial nerve is suspected,

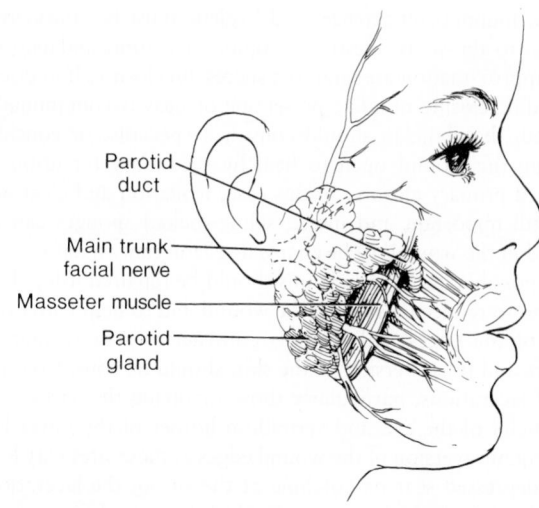

FIGURE 111.7 Deep lacerations to the cheek can injure the facial nerve, parotid gland, or parotid duct. The facial nerve becomes more superficial as it branches and proceeds distally. Distal nerve injuries can thus occur with more superficial wounds.

patients can be tested by having them move specific muscles of facial expression. This testing should take place before infiltration with local anesthetic. The frontal branch of the facial nerve can be tested by asking the patient to frown in order to look for symmetry of frontalis action. The marginal mandibular (motor) branch may course as much as 1 to 2 cm below the border of the mandible and is responsible for the depression and eversion of the lower lip. Injury to this branch results in a characteristic inward rotation of the lower lip on the affected side as a result of unopposed orbicularis tone on that side. The buccal branches are in close proximity to Stenson's (parotid) duct, usually close to a line between the tragus of the ear and the mid-upper lip. Deep lacerations in this area raise the possibility of injury to both structures.

Examination for potential injury to Stenson's duct is accomplished by grasping the commissure between the thumb and index finger and gently everting the buccal mucosa to identify Stenson's duct, which lies on a vertical line along the maxillary second premolar. With the opposite hand, gentle massage of the parotid gland is accomplished by pressing in the preauricular region. The appearance of clear fluid from Stenson's duct suggests an uninjured duct. The absence of fluid after several minutes of inspection, or bloody fluid, suggests injury to the gland or duct. In this case, inspection of the depth of the wound may reveal salivary fluid and severed ends of the duct may be identified. A sialogram can be a useful adjunct in the diagnosis of parotid duct injuries. In wounds with substantial bleeding, clamping all but the most obvious cut ends of blood vessels should be avoided for possible injury to a facial nerve branch.

Although most lacerations should be repaired within 8 to 12 hours, clean lacerations of the face can often be reapproximated up to 24 hours after the injury was sustained. Late-presenting lacerations (48 to 72 hours after the injury) can be closed after thorough sharp debridement. The risks of infection in closing such a wound must be weighed against the benefits of reducing the facial scarring that will result if the wound is allowed to heal secondarily. Factors such as mechanism of injury, immunocompetence, and hygiene must be considered. Similar to abrasions, anesthesia, copious irrigation, and tension-free approximation are vital to a successful closure. If in doubt regarding closure of a late-presenting or heavily contaminated wound, the clinician should consult a specialist or consider leaving the wound open to heal by secondary intention or delayed primary closure. In this case, irrigation and cleansing are still important and moist, saline-soaked sponges can be placed in the wound (to be changed several times a day).

If possible, facial lacerations should be repaired using deep sutures to reduce tension on the wound and to help with eversion of the edges. All wounds contract as scar formation occurs and thus eversion of the skin should be considered for facial lacerations, particularly those involving the nares, eyelids, helix of the ear, and vermillion border of the lower lip. Inadequate eversion of the wound edges at these sites may lead to a depressed scar or notching at the site of the laceration. The time after which sutures should be removed varies from approximately 5 days in the eyelids to 5 to 7 days in the face to 10 days in the nose and up to 14 days in the ear.

Repair of complex injuries to laminated structures (e.g., ear, eyelid, nose, lip) requires that each layer of the structure be reapproximated. For example, a full-thickness laceration to the nose at the nostril rim requires closure of three separate layers. The nasal lining is usually closed first with an absorbable suture material. Next, the cartilage must be repaired, also with absorbable material. Finally, the overlying skin of the nose can be reapproximated. Similarly, complex injuries of the ear, the eyelid, or the lip require layered closure to achieve the best cosmetic result. Careful attention should be paid to lip lacerations that traverse the vermillion border. Cosmetic outcome is predicated on successful alignment of tissue at this junction.

The mouth should be evaluated for lacerations of the mucosa or tongue, injury to the palate, and loose or missing teeth. Chapter 109 details specific oral injuries. Lacerations and soft-tissue injuries involving the external ear, as well as the nasal mucosa, may require plastic surgical evaluation and are described in detail in Chapter 110.

Verbal or written consent should be obtained from patients and families undergoing laceration repair and documented within the emergency department. The physician should provide a careful assessment and natural history of the injury if left untreated to heal on its own. The physician should also describe the recommended treatment, as well as alternative treatments, with its likely outcomes and possible complications. If, for instance, a dark-skinned child has sustained an abrasion or laceration to the face, the risk of pigment changes or excessive scarring in terms of hypertrophy of the scar or keloid formation is significant. Patients with lacerations resulting from dog bites and those who present for care after a delayed period of time should be warned of the high risk of infection.

Complicated facial laceration repair and laceration repair in young children may be facilitated by the use of procedural sedation. For properly selected superficial facial lacerations, tissue adhesives such as 2-octylcyanocrylate have demonstrated similar cosmetic outcome to sutures while offering the benefit of providing a painless procedure, often accomplished without the use of procedural sedation. For deep lacerations, skin closure should be performed only after tension is relieved from wound borders, usually through the use of buried absorbable

sutures. Stapling has been shown to be a fast and cosmetically acceptable alternative to suturing for simple scalp lacerations.

Regional Nerve Blocks

Local or regional anesthesia may be used to aid in the suturing of facial lacerations in children. Regional anesthesia has the distinct advantage of allowing the physician to perform a painless procedure, without distorting the anatomic structures under repair. In addition, regional blocks, in general, require fewer anesthetics. Regional nerve blockade of the face is discussed in more detail in Section VII, 12.13E to 12.13G; however, certain aspects warrant mention in this chapter.

The supraorbital nerve exits the supraorbital rim in the medial third of the eyebrow approximately 2 to 3 cm from the facial midline. Local infiltration in this region can effectively provide anesthesia to the ipsilateral hemiforehead. The infraorbital nerve exits through the infraorbital foramen, approximately 5-mm inferior to the infraorbital rim. Effective block of this nerve can provide anesthesia to the ipsilateral medial cheek and upper lip. Anesthesia of the lower lip and chin may be achieved by infiltration of the ipsilateral mental (infraoral) nerve. This nerve exists approximately 2 to 3 cm superior to the inferior border of the mandible. The supraorbital and inferior orbital nerves, as well as the mental nerve, exit the facial skeleton from foramen, which are inline with the first premolar tooth.

GUIDELINES FOR CONSULTATION

Priority must be given to the stabilization of the patient, following the airway, breathing, and circulation (ABCs) of trauma resuscitation. When a patient is stabilized, and after other associated injuries are addressed, the physician must decide whether the facial injuries warrant consultation with a subspecialist.

For the pediatric population, the parent(s) or guardian often requests a specialist consultation for problems that may not require specialist intervention, such as the repair of simple facial lacerations. Communication is of paramount importance in this scenario. Emergency physicians have the training and expertise to repair most facial lacerations in children. The provider should convey to both the child and the caregiver that he or she has the experience and procedural skills to perform the procedure and that the outcome will likely be no different if the laceration is repaired by a plastic surgeon. Injuries that require specialist consultation include (i) lacerations with evidence of injury to deep structures (a major motor nerve or a glandular duct), (ii) cases in which a substantial amount of devitalized tissue exists or actual tissue loss has occurred, (iii) wounds in which the amount of bleeding cannot be easily controlled, (iv) full-thickness defects of the ear and nose, and (v) cases in which it is unclear exactly which tissue to approximate to restore preinjury anatomy and aesthetics (e.g., lips, eyelids, nostrils, ears).

Suggested Readings

Bartlett S, Delozier JB III. Controversies in the management of pediatric facial fractures. *Clin Plast Surg* 1992;19:245–258.
Bruns TB, Robinson BS, Smith RJ, et al. A new tissue adhesive for laceration repair in children. *J Pediatr* 1998;132(6):1067–1070.

Druelinger L, Guenther M, Marchand EG, et al. Radiographic evaluation of the facial complex. *Emerg Med Clin North Am* 2000;18(3):393–410.

Eggensperger Wymann NM, Holzle A, Zachariou Z, et al. Pediatric craniofacial trauma. *J Oral Maxillofac Surg* 2008;66(1):58–64.

Ellis E, Scott K. Assessment of patients with facial fractures. *Emerg Med Clin North Am* 2000;18(3):411–448.

Flood TR, McManners J, El-Attar A, et al. Randomized prospective study of the influence of steroids on postoperative eye-opening after exploration of the orbital floor. *Br J Oral Maxillofac Surg* 1999;37(4):312–315.

Fujino T, Makino K. Entrapment mechanism and ocular injury in orbital blowout fracture. *Plast Reconstr Surg* 1980;65:571–574.

Holland AJ, Broome FX, Steinberg A, et al. Facial fractures in children. *Pediatr Emerg Care* 2001;17(3):157–160.

Jatla KK, Enzenauer RW. Orbital fractures: a review of current literature. *Curr Surg* 2004;61(1):25–29.

Khan AN, Dayan PS, Miller S, et al. Cosmetic outcome of scalp wound closure with staples in the pediatric emergency department: a prospective, randomized trial. *Pediatr Emerg Care* 2002;18(3):171–173.

Millman AL, Della Rocca RC, Spector S, et al. Steroids and orbital blowout fractures—a new systematic concept in medical management and surgical decision-making. *Adv Ophthalmic Plast Reconstr Surg* 1987;6:291–300.

Quinn J, Wells G, Sutcliffe T, et al. A randomized trial comparing octyl-cyanocrylate tissue adhesive and sutures in the management of lacerations. *JAMA* 1997;277(19):1527–1530.

Randle H, Salassa JR, Roenigk RK. Know your anatomy. Local anesthesia for cutaneous lesions of the head and neck: practical application of peripheral nerve blocks. *J Dermatol Surg Oncol* 1992;18(3):231–235.

Shaikh ZS, Worrall SF. Epidemiology of facial trauma in a sample of patients aged 1–18 years. *Injury* 2002;33(8):669–671.

Sherick DG, Buchman SR, Patel PP. Pediatric facial fractures: analysis of differences in subspecialty care. *Plast Reconstr Surg* 1998;102(1):28–31.

Stanley RB. Maxillofacial trauma. In: Cummings CW, ed. *Otolaryngology: head and neck surgery*, 3rd ed. St. Louis, MO: Mosby—Year Book, 1998:453–484.

Vyas RM, Dickinson BP, Wasson KL, et al. Pediatric facial fractures: current national incidence, distribution, and health care resource use. *J Craniofac Surg* 2008;19(2):339–349.

Zimmermann CE, Troulis MJ, Kaban LB. Pediatric facial fractures: recent advances in prevention, diagnosis and management. *Int J Oral Maxillofac Surg* 2005;34(8):823–833.

CHAPTER 112 ■ GENITOURINARY TRAUMA

CARMEN TERESA GARCIA, MD, AND VALERIE T. THOMPSON, MD

In children who sustain multiple injuries, genitourinary trauma is second in frequency only to central nervous system trauma. Approximately 10% of patients with serious multi-system trauma have urogenital injuries. Most injuries (90%) are the result of blunt trauma that involves crush injuries and acceleration/deceleration forces. Vehicular and pedestrian accidents account for a large percentage of blunt trauma. Other mechanisms of injury include falls and sports-related incidents. Penetrating injuries are less common in children than in adults. High-velocity bullet wounds produce direct tissue injury and damage to adjacent tissue because of the energy generated by the missile. Low-velocity bullet wounds and stab wounds cause injury by penetrating the tissue directly. Iatrogenic trauma has been reported after operative procedures.

Injuries to other systems are often encountered in patients sustaining genitourinary trauma. Common associated problems include head injuries, fractures (extremities, pelvis, ribs, spine, skull), spinal cord injuries, and lacerations of the liver and spleen. Simultaneous upper and lower genitourinary tract injuries are rare and are usually incompatible with survival. Isolated urologic injuries are rarely the cause of death.

The clinical approach to the injured child should strictly follow Advanced Trauma Life Support guidelines. Figure 112.1 provides an algorithm for diagnostic evaluation of pediatric patients with genitourinary trauma. Urologic management may be temporized to permit urinary drainage in the initial phases; the patient may subsequently require operative procedures.

KIDNEY

The kidney is the most commonly injured structure in the genitourinary tract. Approximately half of genitourinary injuries involve the kidney. Children are more likely than adults to sustain renal injuries. In children, the kidney is larger in proportion to the size of the abdomen than in adults. The child's kidney may retain fetal lobations, which allow for easier parenchymal disruption. The kidney has inadequate protection due to weaker abdominal musculature, a less well-ossified thoracic cage, and less developed perirenal fat and fascia than in adults. Most pediatric renal trauma is minor, requiring no intervention.

Blunt trauma accounts for more than 90% of renal injuries. Most pediatric renal trauma is sustained in motor vehicle accidents. Falls, sports-related incidents, and direct blows are also common mechanisms of injury. Penetrating trauma accounts for the remaining cases. Approximately 10% of penetrating abdominal injuries involve the kidney. Penetrating renal trauma may occur as a complication of amniocentesis or per-cutaneous manipulation.

Associated injuries often occur, with head injuries being the most common. Associated intraperitoneal injuries occur in 80% of patients with penetrating renal trauma and 20% of patients with blunt renal trauma. In general, the hospital length of stay is determined by the associated injuries and not the renal injuries.

Coincidental congenital renal anomalies and intrarenal tumors have been reported in up to 20% of injuries. More accurate recent reviews show that the incidence rate is closer to 1%. Historically, preexisting anomalies have been believed to increase the risk and severity of injury to the kidney. However, it appears that in most patients, congenital genitourinary anomalies associated with renal injury are incidental findings and do not increase morbidity. Nevertheless, a high index of suspicion should be maintained in any child who presents with gross hematuria after a relatively minor trauma. Other patients may present with an acute abdomen due to intraperitoneal rupture of a hydronephrotic kidney.

Classification

Renal injuries have been described using different classification systems based on the clinical and radiologic assessment of the patient. The Organ Injury Scaling Committee of the American Association for the Surgery of Trauma has devised an injury severity score, which represents an amalgamation of previous scales. The injury severity score was developed to facilitate clinical research. This classification system is illustrated in Fig. 112.2. Grade I injuries include contusions or subcapsular, nonexpanding hematomas. Grade II injuries include nonexpanding hematomas confined to the retroperitoneum or lacerations less than 1 cm in depth without urinary extravasation. Grade III injuries include lacerations extending more than 1 cm into the renal cortex without collecting system rupture or urinary extravasation. Grade IV injuries include lacerations extending into the collecting system or renal vascular injuries with contained hemorrhage. Grade V injuries include completely shattered kidneys or avulsions of renal hilum with devascularized kidneys.

Parenchymal contusions and hematomas are the most common renal injuries, accounting for 60% to 90% of all lesions from blunt trauma. Lacerations account for up to 10% of renal injuries and may involve disruption of the capsule, collecting system, or both.

Severe injuries, such as shattered kidney or pedicle avulsions, constitute approximately 3% of renal injuries. Pedicle injuries result from lateral displacement of the kidney with stretching of the tethered renal vessels.

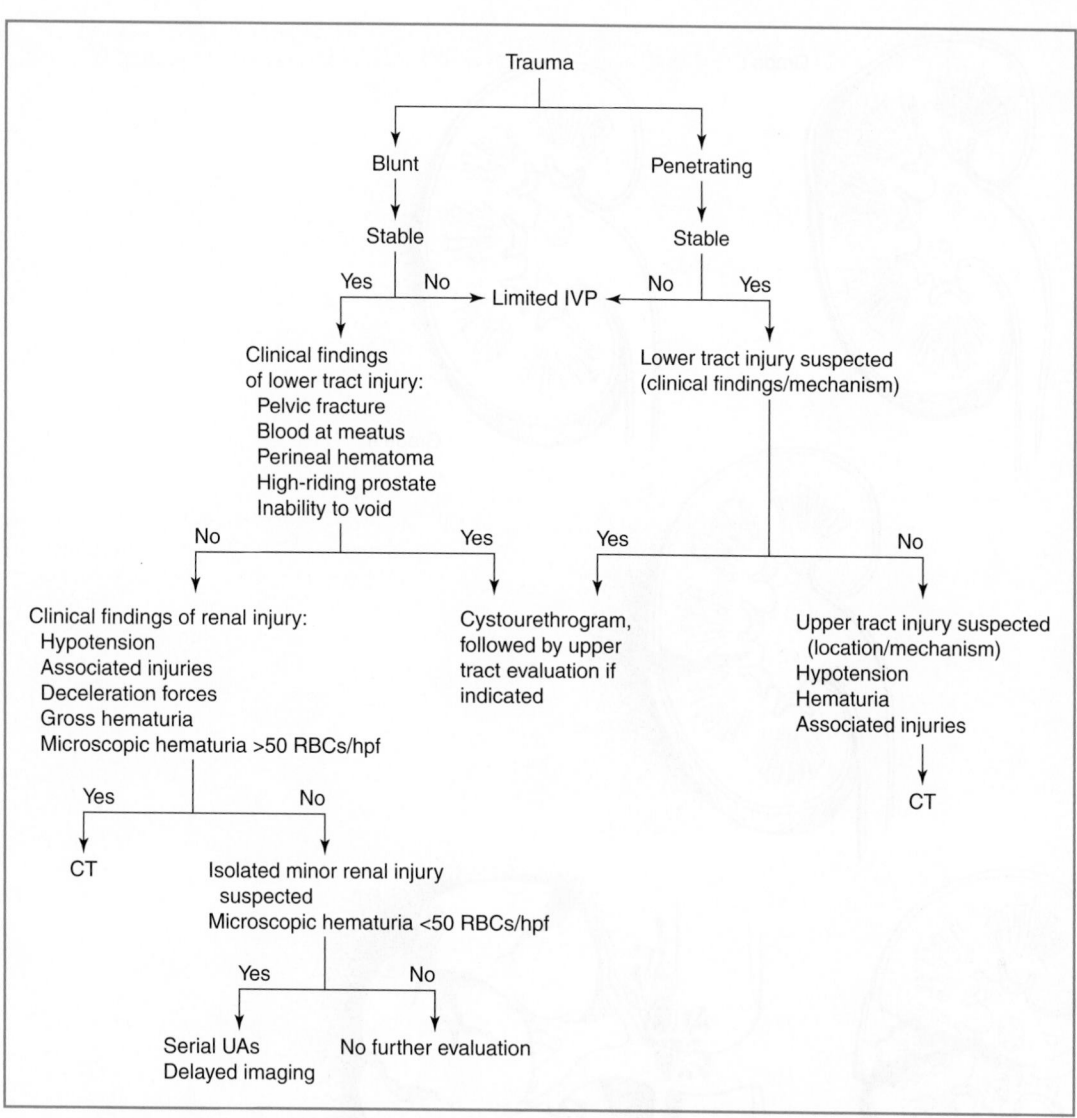

FIGURE 112.1 Algorithm for the evaluation of the pediatric patient with genitourinary trauma. IVP, intravenous pyelogram; CT, computed tomography; RBC, red blood cell; hpf, high-powered field; UAs, urinalyses.

Clinical Presentation

Children who sustain significant renal injuries usually present with localized signs such as flank tenderness, flank hematoma, or a palpable flank mass. Findings also include nonspecific signs often associated with injury to other intraabdominal organs. Generalized abdominal tenderness, rigidity of the abdominal wall, paralytic ileus, and hypovolemic shock may all be part of the clinical picture. Penetrating injuries to chest, abdomen, flank, and lumbar regions should alert the clinician to the possibility of a renal injury.

Hematuria has long been considered the cardinal marker of renal injury. Gross hematuria is a hallmark of severe injury. It should be emphasized that the degree of hematuria does not correlate with the severity of the renal lesion. Hematuria may be absent in up to 50% of patients with vascular pedicle injuries and in approximately one-third of patients with penetrating injuries.

Hematuria with abdominal symptoms has been associated with an increased risk of nonurologic intraabdominal injuries. Injuries to other organs can be seen regardless of renal injury. Some series suggest that clinically significant liver and spleen injuries are more common in children with hematuria than are renal injuries.

Diagnostic Evaluation

All injured children should undergo a thorough evaluation based on well-established trauma protocols. Assessment of the genitourinary system can be undertaken once life-threatening conditions have been identified and the child has been resuscitated. A urinalysis should be obtained in all patients with multisystem trauma or suspected isolated renal injury.

Hypotension is not a reliable indicator of significant renal injuries in children and therefore should not be used to guide management; however, most patients with multisystem trauma

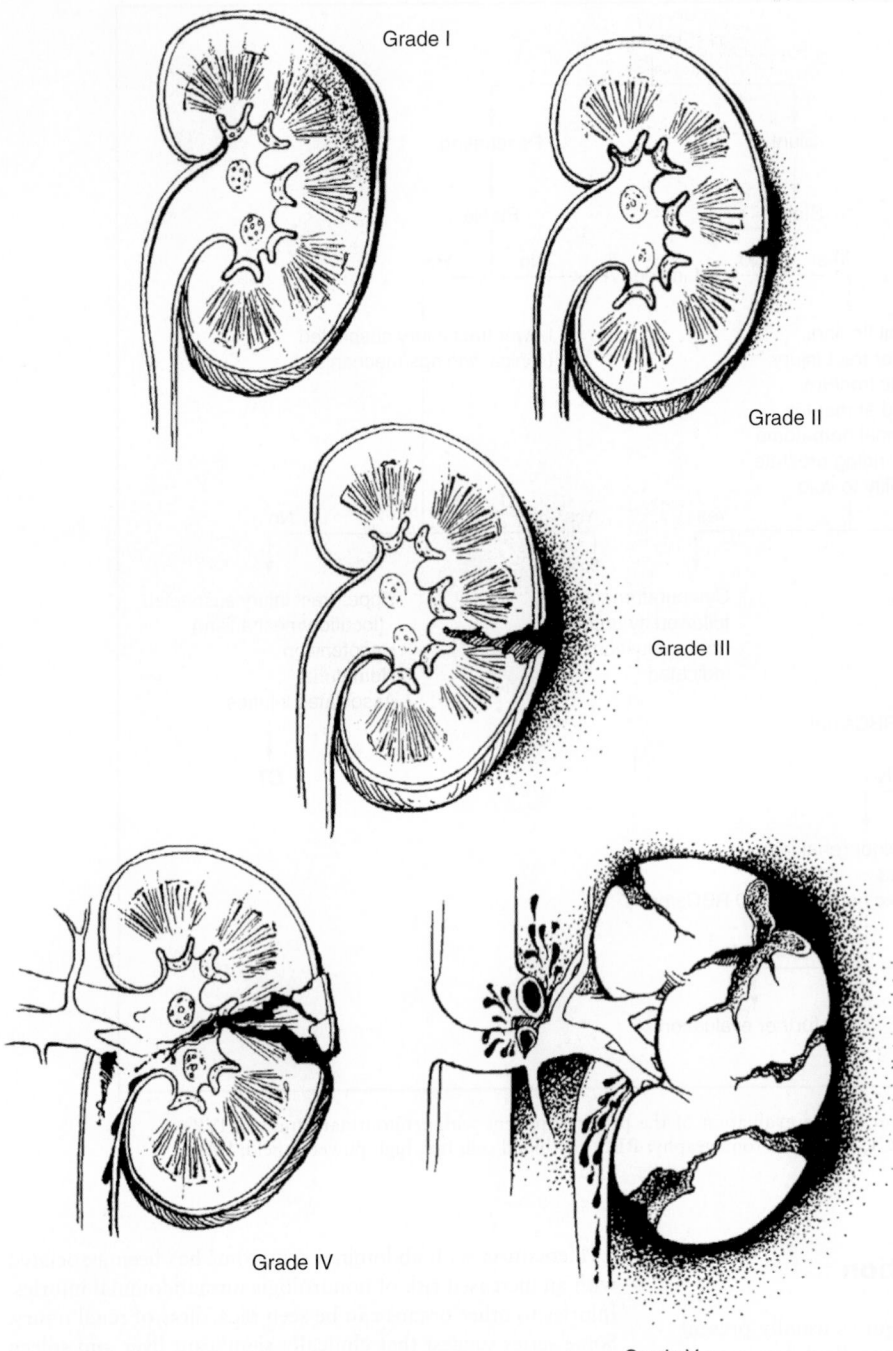

Grade I

Grade II

Grade III

Grade IV

Grade V

FIGURE 112.2 Classification of renal injuries as proposed by the Organ Injury Scaling Committee of the American Association for the Surgery of Trauma.

and hypotension undergo an abdominal computed tomographic (CT) scan to look for nonurologic injuries. Radiographic evaluation of the pediatric genitourinary tract is necessary in cases with clinical signs indicative of renal injury, gross hematuria, major associated injuries, or significant deceleration forces. Imaging all patients with blunt trauma and microscopic hematuria gives an extremely low yield. Detection of significant renal injury increases with hematuria of more than 50 red blood cells (RBCs) per high-power field (hpf). Children who present with this degree of hematuria require prompt radiographic studies. An isolated finding of microscopic hematuria of less than 50 RBCs per hpf does not alone fulfill the criteria for imaging. These patients are likely to have renal contusions and can be managed conservatively with serial urinalyses. Microscopic hematuria that persists for more than a month warrants radiographic evaluation.

Criteria regarding the imaging of children with penetrating trauma are less well established. In the adult population, radiographic evaluation is required in patients with hypotension, penetrating injuries in the vicinity of urologic organs, associated abdominal injuries, or the presence of any degree of hematuria.

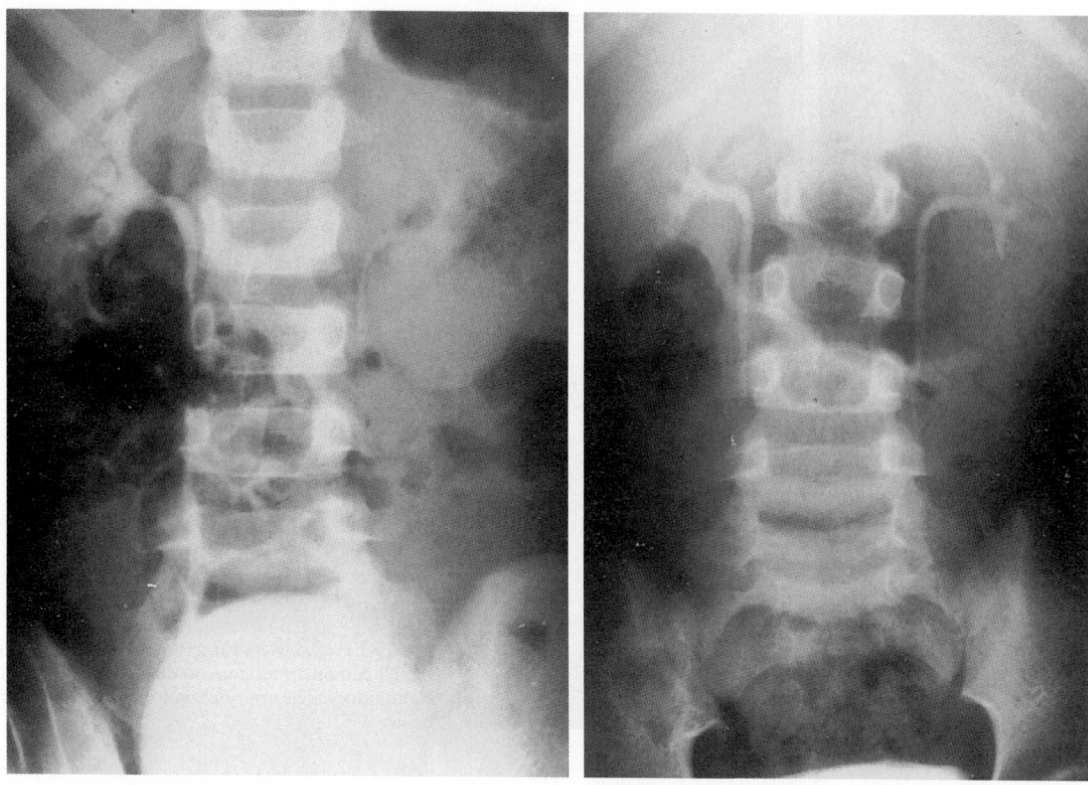

FIGURE 112.3 Renal contusion. Intravenous pyelogram (IVP) (**left panel**) shows decreased concentration of contrast material in the left kidney. Follow-up IVP (**right panel**) 1 month after the injury reveals normal renal function.

Initial evaluation of children with multisystem injuries and suspected pediatric renal trauma should include radiographs of the chest, abdomen, and pelvis. Plain radiographs may show obliterated renal and psoas shadows, scoliosis with the concavity toward the injured site, intraabdominal mass effect, or a coincident rib, spinous process, or pelvic fracture.

Traditionally, intravenous pyelogram (IVP) has been the cornerstone of evaluation in renal trauma (Fig. 112.3). The IVP is available in most institutions and provides information about the overall functional and anatomic integrity of both kidneys. It can be obtained in an unstable patient urgently in the emergency department (ED) or in the operating room before surgery. Indications of renal injury include delayed excretion of the contrast agent by the injured kidney, nonvisualization of the caliceal system, or extravasation of the contrast agent into the perinephric tissues. The presence of a normally functioning kidney contralateral to the injured kidney should be specifically noted.

Even under optimal conditions, the IVP cannot always reliably identify and stage renal trauma. The pyelogram accurately diagnoses only 5% of contusions, 50% of lacerations, and 29% of pedicle injuries. Contrast-enhanced CT is the preferred study for the evaluation of major abdominal injury, including renal injury (Fig. 112.4). CT scan has certain advantages over the IVP, the most important of which is the detection of associated injuries. In addition, CT provides three-dimensional views and imaging independent of the vascularity of the kidney. Conventional IVP should be used to evaluate major renal injuries only if CT scanning is not readily available. IVP may

also be indicated in the long-term evaluation of persistent hematuria.

CT imaging can be used to determine the degree of renal parenchymal injury, to evaluate the presence of nonviable tissue, to demonstrate extravasation and perirenal collections, and to diagnose most pedicle injuries. The diagnostic accuracy of the CT scan has been reported to be as high as 98%. Helical

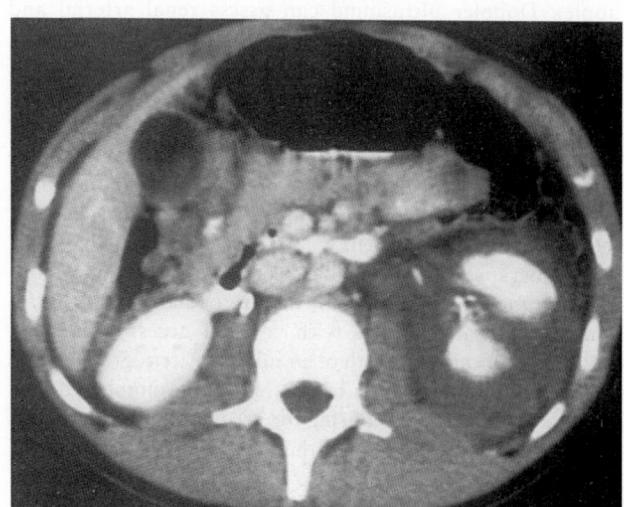

FIGURE 112.4 Renal fracture. Computed tomography section of the abdomen shows fracture of the left kidney with moderate subcapsular hematoma.

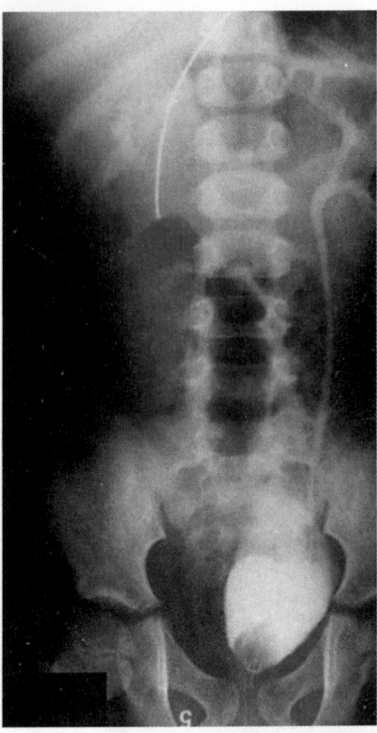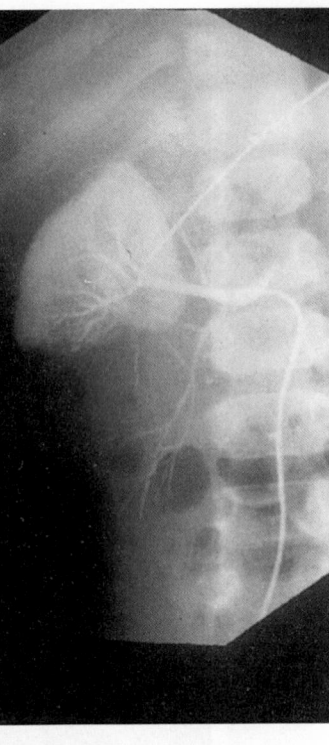

FIGURE 112.5 Renal fracture. Intravenous pyelogram (**left panel**) demonstrates nonvisualization of the lower pole of the right kidney. The arteriogram (**right panel**) confirms the diagnosis.

CT scan with immediate postcontrast and delayed imaging is the standard radiographic modality for renal trauma. CT scanning has also proven to be a useful tool for following patients after trauma.

Ultrasonography is not widely accepted for the staging of renal trauma. Its sensitivity in demonstrating renal injury is only 70% compared with CT scanning. However, ultrasound has certain advantages over CT scanning. It is readily available, can be performed at the bedside, minimizes exposure to radiation, and does not require the use of contrast material or sedation. Ultrasound can evaluate the size of the kidney and the integrity of the urinary drainage system. Pulsed-flow duplex Doppler ultrasound can assess renal arterial and venous flow and may represent the most immediate means of screening for renal pedicle injury.

Ultrasound can be particularly helpful in patients with perirenal collections who require early follow-up imaging during the hospital stay. It may be an alternative modality for the evaluation of the pregnant trauma patient. It is also often used for long-term outpatient follow-up, although its efficacy in this setting has not been proven.

Angiography (Fig. 112.5) has been largely replaced by noninvasive modalities, especially in the pediatric patients in whom technical problems with vascular access result in a higher complication rate than in adults. Arteriography does not add useful information to contrast CT scanning and may increase diagnostic delay during the preoperative workup. It is useful in patients who require therapeutic embolization of an active bleeding site.

Radionuclide imaging can assess pedicle competence, parenchymal integrity, and renal function. A nuclear scan can be obtained instead of sonography to assess change in the size of perinephric collections. Its most important role is in follow-up

evaluation of renal injury (Fig. 112.6), particularly in the setting of new-onset hypertension.

Magnetic resonance imaging (MRI) has been found to be as effective as CT scanning in staging renal injuries. However, because of cost and time restraints, its role has been limited. MRI may be indicated in carefully selected patients, such as those with either equivocal findings on the CT scan or a severe renal injury.

In conclusion, hemodynamically stable patients who present with suggestive clinical findings, gross hematuria, microscopic hematuria of more than 50 RBCs per hpf, major associated injuries, or a history of significant deceleration injury

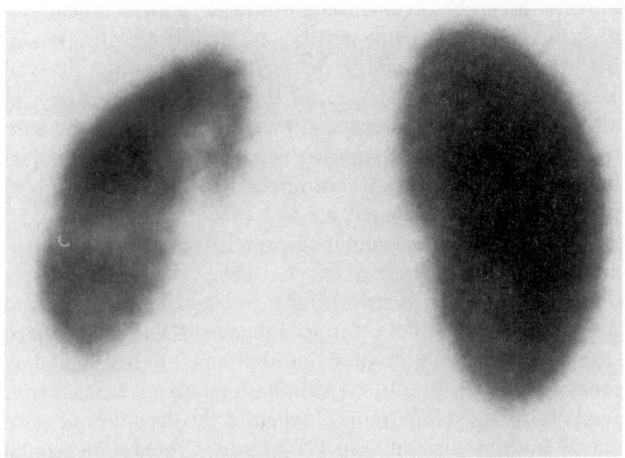

FIGURE 112.6 Follow-up renal scan of patient in Fig. 112.5 obtained 4 months after the injury. The study reveals several areas of decreased radiotracer uptake in the left kidney.

should undergo radiographic evaluation. These patients should have a CT scan. Children who remain unstable despite resuscitative measures should undergo a one-shot IVP before emergency laparotomy. This procedure is particularly important to confirm the presence of a normal contralateral kidney. Children with isolated microscopic hematuria of less than 50 RBCs per hpf do not require immediate imaging. These patients may be discharged and can be evaluated on an outpatient basis with CT, IVP, or ultrasound if hematuria persists. However, in some centers, management of these patients involves hospitalization for observation, followed by nonemergent radiographic evaluation.

Management

The principle underlying the management of pediatric renal trauma is preservation of renal tissue and function with minimal morbidity and mortality. Patients who are hemodynamically unstable or have sustained severe intraabdominal penetrating trauma require immediate surgical intervention. Management of hemodynamically stable children should proceed on the basis of staging of the traumatic lesion. Attempts should be made to manage all renal injuries conservatively.

In cases of blunt trauma, children with grade I renal injuries (contusions) can be discharged home without further imaging and followed with serial urinalyses. Patients are instructed to limit daily activity until the urinalysis is within normal limits. Outpatient radiographic evaluation is necessary if microscopic hematuria persists for more than 30 days. Grade II and III renal injuries warrant admission to the hospital for a minimum of 24 hours when the risk of bleeding is highest. Expectant treatment includes supportive care with strict bed rest, hydration, antibiotics, and serial hematocrits. Once the gross hematuria resolves, these children may be discharged home with limited activity until microscopic hematuria resolves and repeat imaging demonstrates total healing.

Management of the remaining patients (with grade IV and V injuries) evokes significant controversy. The shift from early operative intervention to a more expectant approach for most solid organ injuries has been increasingly applied to high-grade renal injuries. Advocates of early surgical exploration argue that this approach results in decreases in morbidity, hospital stay, and complications without a significant increase in the risk for nephrectomy. Opponents believe that nonoperative management of selected patients does not lead to negative consequences and may result in a higher renal salvage rate.

Nonoperative management requires time with admission to the hospital, serial examinations and hematocrits, and antibiotics. Repeat imaging should be routinely obtained at 48 hours or earlier if clinically indicated. Patients who demonstrate hemodynamic instability require surgical intervention or angiographic embolization of renal vessels. Angioembolization should be performed only in those children who have a definable segmental artery injury. Persistent urinary extravasation can be managed with percutaneous drainage or internal ureteral stenting. These procedures, as well as embolization, should be limited to institutions that can provide appropriate resources.

Operative exploration is required in 5% to 10% of cases. Absolute indications for surgery include persistent renal bleeding and expanding or pulsatile hematoma. Relative indications for exploration are urinary extravasation, nonviable tissue, segmental arterial injury, and incomplete staging. Some studies suggest that surgical intervention is more often necessary in patients with other associated nonrenal, solid organ intraabdominal injuries. Attempts to preserve the kidney are more likely to succeed in patients with grade IV injuries. Children with grade V injuries frequently require nephrectomy. In patients with vascular injuries, chances of renal salvage are improved if renal parenchyma is minimally disrupted and revascularization is achieved within a few hours of the injury. In extreme situations, such as a solitary kidney or bilateral renal injuries, surgery should be attempted even after a long delay.

Penetrating renal injuries have traditionally been managed with operative intervention. Compared with blunt trauma, far less literature is available in support of nonoperative treatment after penetrating trauma. In addition, many recommendations are extrapolated from data from adult patient populations. Careful selection of hemodynamically stable patients who can tolerate CT staging may identify a cohort of children who can be safely treated conservatively. Indications for renal exploration are similar to those for injuries caused by blunt trauma. Patients with penetrating trauma have a higher need for surgical intervention.

Complications

Short-term complications of renal trauma include delayed hemorrhage, urinary extravasation, abscess formation, and ureteral obstruction secondary to clot formation. Long-term complications include compromised renal function, hypertension, hydronephrosis, arteriovenous fistula, renal intestinal fistula, and stone formation. Children with a history of significant renal trauma require regular follow-up for at least 1 year to ensure complications are diagnosed and treated promptly.

URETER

Ureteral injuries are uncommon in children, accounting for less than 1% of all urologic trauma. These injuries can be caused by blunt, penetrating, or iatrogenic trauma.

Blunt trauma usually involves the ureteropelvic junction. Disruption of the ureter from the renal pelvis results from stretching of the ureter by sudden hyperextension of the trunk. Traditionally, this injury has been described more often in children. The degree of hyperextension necessary to cause avulsion of the ureter is believed to be fatal in adults. However, an increased number of ureteropelvic junction injuries have recently been reported in adults. In the past, many injuries in adults may have been misdiagnosed as parenchymal lacerations involving the collecting system.

Trauma to the ureter should be suspected in patients presenting with fracture of the transverse process of a lumbar vertebra. Pelvic fracture, hip fracture, lower rib fracture, splenic laceration, liver laceration, and diaphragmatic rupture have also been reported in association with ureteral injuries.

Early diagnosis of blunt ureteral injuries is critical. These injuries are often overlooked. Less than 50% of patients are diagnosed within 24 hours of presentation. The physical examination may be unremarkable. However, an enlarging flank mass in the absence of signs of retroperitoneal bleeding suggests urinary extravasation. Hematuria is an unreliable sign. The urinalysis may be normal in 30% of confirmed cases. When the diagnosis has been delayed, ureteral injury may manifest with fever, chills, lethargy, leukocytosis, pyuria, bacteriuria, flank mass or pain, fistulas, and ureteral strictures.

Avulsion of the ureter should be suspected when the IVP demonstrates extravasation of contrast material and nonfilling of the affected ureter. Contrast-enhanced CT is an appropriate alternative to the IVP. CT findings suggestive of ureteral injury include medial perirenal extravasation of contrast material, a circumrenal urinoma, and the lack of opacification of the ureter distal to the injury. Delayed images must be obtained regardless of which diagnostic modality is used. Both CT scan and IVP have been shown to have a low sensitivity for ureteral injuries, identifying only 33% of cases. Retrograde pyelogram may be a more reliable examination, but it is rarely performed in the initial evaluation of a trauma patient.

The management of complete transection of the ureter depends on the level of the injury. Important elements include debridement of devitalized tissue and a watertight, tension-free anastomosis. Ureteroureterostomy, transureteroureterostomy, or pyeloureterostomy is recommended for mid- and upper ureteral injuries. Mid- to lower ureteral injuries are best treated with ureteroneocystostomy. Placement of a ureteral stent is indicated in most cases. Conservative treatment with stent placement alone may be adequate for patients with hematomas or minor lacerations.

If the ureteral lesion is identified within 5 to 10 days of the injury, prompt repair of the ureter is indicated. If diagnosis is delayed for more than 10 days, urinary diversion above the lesion should be performed with subsequent definitive repair 4 to 6 months later. The incidence of nephrectomy is approximately 5% when the injury is detected early, but it is as high as 30% when recognition is delayed.

Penetrating injuries may occur at any point along the length of the ureter and are associated with injuries to other intraabdominal organs in up to 90% of cases. Stab wounds rarely cause ureteral injuries. However, up to 50% of patients with gunshot wounds to the abdomen have injury to the ureter. Occasionally, the ureter may be accidentally injured during pelvic operations or ureteroscopy. Most penetrating ureteral injuries are recognized intraoperatively by direct visual inspection. Intravenous or intraureteral injection of indigo carmine or methylene blue may facilitate the diagnosis. Repair of penetrating injuries to the ureter in children follows the same guidelines as those observed in adults. Injuries caused by high-velocity missiles require wide debridement to ensure an adequate anastomosis and to preserve blood supply.

BLADDER

Bladder injuries may occur after blunt or penetrating trauma. Blunt trauma secondary to motor vehicle accidents is the leading cause of bladder injuries. More than 80% of bladder injuries are associated with pelvic fractures and penetration of the bladder by a bony fragment. However, only 10% of patients with pelvic fractures sustain lower urinary tract injury. The probability of having an associated bladder injury increases proportionally with the number of fractured pubic rami. Mortality rate associated with bladder rupture may be as high as 40%. Death is usually caused by associated head injuries rather than by bladder injuries themselves.

During childhood, the bladder has a higher abdominal location, which renders the organ more susceptible to injury than in adults. The bladder can also be more easily damaged when full. The risk for this injury is especially increased in the setting of improperly fastened seat belts and lap belts. Bladder neck injuries are uncommon, but serious. Such injuries have been reported to be more common in children than in adults because of the undeveloped prostate and are often in association with a pelvic fracture. The injury may be due to longitudinal lacerations or lacerations that extend to the proximal urethra.

Bladder injuries are classified as extraperitoneal, intraperitoneal, or combined. Extraperitoneal injuries are more frequently associated with pelvic fractures of the anterior ring and may be related to either laceration or penetration from a bone spike, irrespective of bladder volume at the time of injury. In contrast, intraperitoneal injuries, which account for approximately two-thirds of major bladder injuries, are usually caused by blunt trauma, resulting in a burst mechanism to a full, distended bladder. Combined injuries are usually seen with gunshot wounds. Bladder injuries may range from contusions to rupture. Contusions are incomplete, nonperforating tears of the mucosa. Complicated injuries may involve the bladder, urethra, sacral plexus, and supporting structures of the anorectal region.

Hematuria and dysuria are symptoms commonly seen at presentation. Nearly 100% of patients with rupture of the bladder have gross hematuria. Microscopic hematuria is associated with less severe injuries such as contusions. Inability to void may be associated with large tears. Patients with intraperitoneal ruptures may develop a palpable fluid wave from extravasation of urine into the peritoneal cavity and peritoneal irritation. Elevated levels of blood urea nitrogen out of proportion to creatinine result from more rapid peritoneal reabsorption of urea.

A large, prospective series of pelvic fractures and lower genitourinary tract injury in pediatric patients found that imaging is not required if patients are stable, have a normal genitourinary examination, do not have gross hematuria, and do not have multiple associated injuries. Diagnostic evaluation is indicated in patients who sustain pelvic or lower abdominal trauma with gross hematuria, inability to void, abnormal external genitourinary examination, or multiple associated injuries. Evaluation begins with a plain radiograph to exclude a pelvic fracture. Fracture types that have been associated with bladder injury include widening of the sacroiliac joint, symphysis pubis, and fractures of the sacrum. If a pelvic fracture is not identified, the urethra can be catheterized and a cystogram is performed. Catheterization must be avoided if physical examination reveals blood at the urethral meatus or a high-riding prostate.

Conventional cystography is still considered to be the imaging "gold standard" for the evaluation of blunt bladder trauma. CT cystography has been demonstrated to have similar sensitivity, specificity, positive, and negative predictive value as conventional cystography for the presence and type of bladder injury. However, the accuracy is lower than that reported by conventional cystography for distinguishing intraperitoneal from extraperitoneal injury. It is important for the CT to have the ability to distinguish the specific type, as the management of the two may differ greatly. Sagittal and coronal multiplanar images may be helpful in identifying most sites of bladder rupture.

CT cystography does offer some advantages over plain cystography for patients undergoing CT scanning for the evaluation of other associated blunt injuries. CT scanning provides expeditious scanning of the head, chest, abdomen, and pelvis; interpretation is often less affected by overlying bone fragments from pelvic fractures and spine boards than in the plain radiographic cystogram, and the CT can detect small amounts of intra- and extraperitoneal fluid. The disadvantages of CT cystography include the much higher radiation exposure and cost than those of plain radiographs. Currently, the CT cystogram is recommended, when indicated, for patients undergoing CT scanning for other associated blunt trauma-related injuries.

Conservative management with or without urethral catheter drainage is the standard of care in patients with contusion. Extraperitoneal vesical rupture can be managed by urethral catheter or suprapubic drainage for 7 to 10 days. Treatment of extraperitoneal or intraperitoneal tears involves transperitoneal exploration and repair with the placement of a suprapubic or transurethral catheter, or transurethral catheter alone. Both have been shown to have similar outcomes and complication rates. Combined or penetrating injuries to the bladder require surgical exploration and direct closure.

Iatrogenic bladder injuries may occur during herniorrhaphy, cystoscopy, and umbilical artery cutdown. Patients with myelodysplasia who have undergone bladder augmentation may experience spontaneous bladder rupture in the presence of infection, bacteremia, or overdistension. Symptoms and signs of sepsis, as well as shoulder pain, may be encountered at presentation. Emergent exploration is indicated after a cystogram is completed.

URETHRA

Blunt trauma, due to motor vehicle accidents, high-velocity falls onto the perineum, and straddle injuries, accounts for most urethral injuries sustained during childhood. Injuries due to instrumentation and penetrating injuries, such as gunshot wounds, are less common. Urethral injuries occur primarily in males. In boys, the urethra is divided by the urogenital diaphragm into an anterior urethra (pendulous and bulbous) and a posterior urethra (membranous and prostatic) (Fig. 112.7). Anterior and posterior urethral injuries differ from each other by mechanism of injury, clinical presentation, and treatment.

Anterior urethral injuries result from direct trauma, are often isolated, and are associated with low mortality. The pendulous urethra may be damaged by blunt or penetrating forces. Bulbar injuries are commonly caused by straddle injuries, as the urethra is compressed between the symphysis pubis and a solid object. The major sign of acute anterior injury is bleeding from the urethra. Blood at the meatus has been reported in up to 90% of patients sustaining anterior urethral injuries. Other findings include hematuria, inability or difficulty voiding, and periurethral or perineal edema and ecchymosis. Perineal ecchymosis in the shape of a butterfly is typical for these injuries. Blind placement of a urethral catheter may convert a partial tear into a complete transection and therefore should be discouraged.

Diagnosis can be made by a retrograde urethrogram. A Foley catheter appropriate for the size of the patient is inserted into the urethra to the fossa navicularis without inflating the balloon. Contrast material is injected via the catheter into the

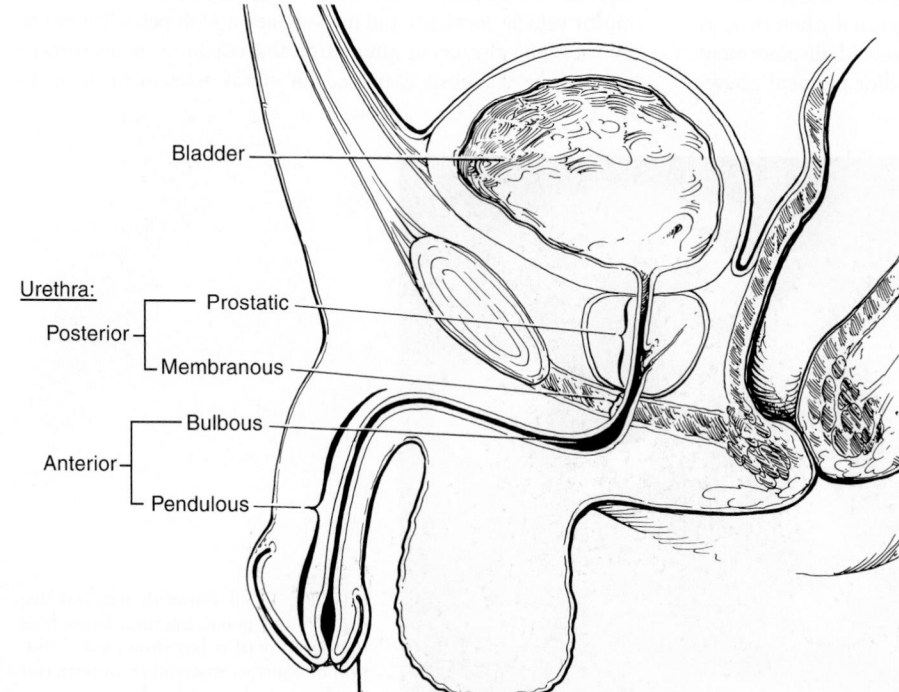

FIGURE 112.7 Sagittal section of male lower urinary tract illustrating levels of urethra.

Urethra:
Posterior — Prostatic
— Membranous
Anterior — Bulbous
— Pendulous
Bladder

urethra and images are obtained in an oblique position. If a Foley catheter is already in place, the urethrogram can still be performed via a small feeding tube passed alongside the catheter. An optional technique involves simple retrograde syringe injection through the urethral meatus. Retrograde urethrography should be performed under fluoroscopy with minimal pressure. Gross extravasation of the contrast agent at the site of the injury without visualization of the proximal urethra and bladder is diagnostic for complete rupture of the urethra. Partial rupture is represented by localized extravasation at the site of the injury, with contrast passing into the proximal urethra and bladder. If no extravasation is noted, the urinary catheter can be gently advanced into the bladder.

Anterior urethral injuries can be managed by 7 to 10 days of urethral catheterization and antibiotic therapy. More severe injuries require urinary diversion by suprapubic cystostomy.

Posterior urethral injuries occur with severe trauma to the body and are usually associated with other injuries, particularly pelvic fractures. The mortality rate with fractured pelvis has been reported to be as high as 30%. Many patients may not manifest the usual clinical signs of urethral injury. In such cases, urethral injury may be predicted by the location and displacement of associated anterior pelvic fractures, which may be valuable in making a decision to pursue further evaluation. There is a well-established association between pubic arch fractures and urethral injury, with higher risk as the number of broken rami increases. The high death rate in these patients is attributed primarily to associated injuries.

The urogenital diaphragm located between the pubic rami fixes the membranous urethra and makes it vulnerable to rupture when the pubic arch is fractured. Tears may also result from shearing of the prostatic urethra at the superior border of the urogenital diaphragm. Injuries to the prostatic urethra may extend to the bladder neck. Posterior urethral injuries in men almost uniformly occur distal to the prostate. In adults, the mature prostate, puboprostatic ligament, and bladder stabilize the prostatic urethra, making it less susceptible to trauma.

Proximal urethral injury should be suspected when there is blood at the meatus, hematuria, inability to void, displacement of the prostate on rectal examination, and/or perineal ecchy-mosis. Catheterization of the urethra is contraindicated. The diagnosis is best made by retrograde urethrography as described for anterior urethral injuries. CT scan is not adequate for diagnosing urethral injuries and is presumptive only if extravasation is detected at the bladder neck or urethra (Fig. 112.8). The IVP may demonstrate an elevation of the bladder out of the pelvis. MRI provides useful information in the determination of the need for surgical repair but is not helpful in the initial evaluation.

Initial management of posterior urethral injuries remains controversial. Therapeutic options vary from immediate exploration with primary repair to the placement of a suprapubic tube with delayed urethroplasty. Urethral rupture may also be treated by realigning the urethra over an indwelling urethral catheter. Suprapubic cystostomy and delayed repair are recommended for trauma patients who are hemodynamically unstable.

Primary realignment has become a more common treatment option. Although the incidence of urethral strictures is higher in patients undergoing primary realignment with delayed repair, impotence and urinary incontinence are more prevalent when urinary diversion is performed. Some studies suggest that long-term outcome may be determined by the location of the injury regardless of treatment method. Membranous urethral tears may have a more favorable outcome. Bladder neck injuries have the lowest rate of continence.

Penetrating wounds of the urethra demand early surgical exploration with conservative debridement and primary repair. Patients with extensive loss of urethral tissue can be managed with delayed repair and staged reconstruction.

Because the female urethra is relatively mobile and short, trauma to the urethra is uncommon. It was reported in less than 6% of cases with associated pelvic fractures in one series of women and girls. When it does occur, it is found more commonly in girls than in women. Female urethral injuries are commonly divided into avulsions and longitudinal tears. These injuries occur most often from blunt abdominal trauma in motor vehicle accidents and in association with pelvic fractures. Injuries may also occur after surgical procedures or instrumentation. The diagnosis is missed on initial assessment in up to

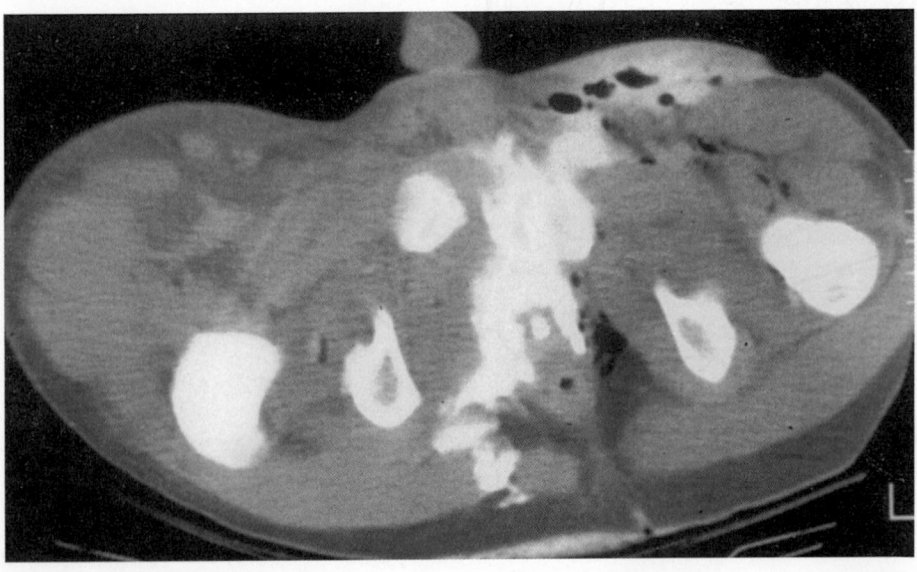

FIGURE 112.8 Posterior urethral disruption and pelvic fracture. Computed tomography of pelvis shows extravasation of contrast material from posterior urethra into the surrounding tissues.

40% of patients, emphasizing the need for careful physical examination and diagnostic evaluation. In one series, every patient with a significant urethral injury had gross hematuria or blood at the introitus and a pelvic ring fracture. Any female patient with this combination of findings should be evaluated for a urethral injury. Most serious injuries involve the vesicourethral junction and extend to the vagina. It is recommended that, whenever possible, a full speculum examination should be performed in patients in whom there is a finding of gross hematuria and pelvic ring fractures, difficulty placing a urethral catheter, and anticipated delay until the pelvic fractures is stabilized. Management of female urethral injuries relates to the location of the injury. The bladder neck and mid urethra should be repaired primarily. The distal urethra may be left open, although sutures may be required for hemostasis. Placement of a suprapubic tube and delayed repair are reserved for unstable patients, as such the placement has been associated with scarring, strictures, urethral obliteration, and fistulas. Most authors recommend some form of primary operative repair of the urethral rupture with closure of associated vaginal tears. Long-term complications of this injury include urethrovaginal fistula, vaginal stenosis, incontinence, sexual dysfunction, and urethral stricture. These patients require long-term urological follow up.

SCROTUM

Scrotal trauma may occur as a result of straddle injuries or bicycle accidents, or during sporting events. The patient may present with scrotal tenderness, edema, and ecchymosis. Potential injuries include skin or dartos ecchymoses and lacerations, intrascrotal hematomas, testicular hematomas, testicular dislocation, and testicular rupture. In addition, a testicle may torse after trauma.

When inspection of the scrotum and its contents is obscured by local swelling and pain, ultrasonography is helpful to define the extent of the injury. An intratesticular hematoma may show as an echogenic or hypoechoic testicular mass. A hematocele produces a complex extratesticular fluid collection. Sonographic findings of rupture include the presence of hematocele, mixed parenchymal echogenicity, intraparenchymal hemorrhage, and disruption of the tunica albuginea or parenchyma. If the ultrasound examination is inconclusive, radionuclide scanning may provide additional information. Both ultrasonography and nuclear scintigraphy help in the diagnosis of testicular torsion (see Chapter 124).

Patients who sustain intrascrotal hematomas, skin ecchymosis, or skin and dartos injury without evidence of injury to the testes can be managed only conservatively. Treatment consists of ice packs and scrotal support. Minor testicular injuries such as contusions or hematomas can also be treated conservatively. Large testicular hematomas may require surgical management. Delay in surgery may lead to ischemic necrosis, secondary infections, and disruption of testicular function.

Testicular dislocation may occur either as a result of an upward blow to the scrotum or, rarely, as a result of compressive displacement following severe blunt abdominal trauma. Dislocation has been described in the context of mild scrotal trauma as well.

Diagnosis of testicular dislocation can be made by thorough physical examination, including palpation of the testes,

in patients with multiple trauma, especially involving the abdomen. Examination will reveal a well-developed, but empty, scrotal sac or palpation of an abnormally located testis. Severe scrotal pain, obesity, ecchymosis, swelling, or associated pelvic injuries may make examination and diagnosis difficult. In most cases, the dislocated testis lies under the abdominal wall. Color Doppler sonography has been recommended by some to aid in the assessment but may be operator dependent. Associated injuries, such as pelvic fracture, are common. Operative repair is required if closed reduction fails.

Testicular rupture is a surgical emergency. It is characterized by a tear of the tunica albuginea and extravasation of testicular contents into the scrotal sac. Such injuries require early surgical exploration and repair to avoid the potential complications of atrophy and persistent pain. Ultrasonography has been demonstrated to be sensitive in the diagnosis of testicular rupture by informing the clinician of the integrity of the scrotal contents early. The high specificity of the ultrasonography may also provide information to guide the clinician on the necessity of surgical exploration. Testicular salvage is more likely when exploration is performed within 24 hours of the injury. Ultrasonography has shown poor accuracy, however, for the evaluation of isolated epididymal lesions. Other injuries requiring surgical management include tense hematoceles and torsion after trauma.

Superficial lacerations of the scrotum can be repaired using absorbable sutures. Local infiltration with lidocaine plus epinephrine provides adequate anesthesia. Urologic consultation should be obtained if the laceration extends through the dartos. Physical examination of the scrotal contents determines the need for debridement and primary closure. All penetrating testicular injuries require surgical exploration.

Degloving injuries of the scrotum can be seen after motor vehicle (particularly motorcycle), industrial, or farm machinery accidents. Scrotal injuries are associated with varying degrees of penile skin loss. The underlying penile and scrotal structures are usually spared. Management involves debridement and coverage of the defect by skin flaps or grafting.

PENIS

The most common cause of penile trauma in infants is iatrogenic, especially at the time of circumcision. Complications include transection of the glans, urethrocutaneous fistula, deskinning of the penile shaft, and coagulation necrosis of the entire penis from electrocautery. These injuries usually require extensive surgical repair. Penile gunshot wounds are uncommon because of the position and mobility of the penis but have the potential to significantly affect quality of life. Signs that may indicate corpora cavernosa injury include uncontrolled bleeding, expanding hematoma, blood at the meatus, or a palpable corporeal defect. Urethral injury should be ruled out by retrograde urethrography if these signs are present. These injuries require urologic evaluation to determine the need and timing of surgical management.

Blunt penile trauma from toilet seats falling on the glans or distal shaft has been described in toddlers. Significant injury to the corporal bodies or the urethra is rare and patients can be managed expectantly with warm soaks. Although the child does not commonly experience urinary retention, he may be more comfortable voiding in a tub of warm water.

Tourniquet injuries may result from bands, rings, or human hair. In the infant, strangulation with a fine hair may be difficult to recognize because of local edema. The initial diagnosis may be balanitis or paraphimosis. Local or general anesthesia may be required to expose and remove the hair. Complications include urethrocutaneous fistula or loss of the penis.

Fracture of the penis is produced by traumatic rupture of the corpus cavernosum. This injury usually occurs when the erect penis is forced against a hard surface. The patient may hear a cracking sound and develop pain, edema, and deformity of the penis shaft. The urethra is rarely involved. Most injuries require surgical treatment with evacuation of the penile hematoma, repair of the torn tunica albuginea, and a pressure dressing, but some fractures of the penis can be managed conservatively with bed rest, ice packs, and a pressure dressing.

Superficial lacerations of the penile shaft can be repaired with absorbable sutures under local anesthesia or penile block. Lacerations extending to the corporal bodies or the urethra require urologic consultation. Diagnostic evaluation includes a retrograde urethrogram to define the extent of the injury. Injuries to the corporal bodies should be repaired primarily to prevent fibrosis and impotence. Injuries to the urethra may require urinary diversion.

Zipper entrapment of the penis or foreskin is a common complaint that can be managed in the ED. Methods of emergent release have been described in relation to the zipper parts and depending on the type of zipper. The median bar of the zipper may be cut with wire cutters and thus disassembling the zipper mechanism (Fig. 112.9). This technique may sometimes prove difficult when the metal bar is sturdy and there is edema of the entrapped penile tissue within the zipper fastener, limiting access to the metal bar. Such may be the case with heavy metal zippers such as those found on jeans and dungarees, and success may depend on the strength of the operator and the availability of bone or wire cutters. Therefore, this technique may work best with plastic or lightweight zippers. Cutting the dentition of the zipper at any position, permitting unzipping of

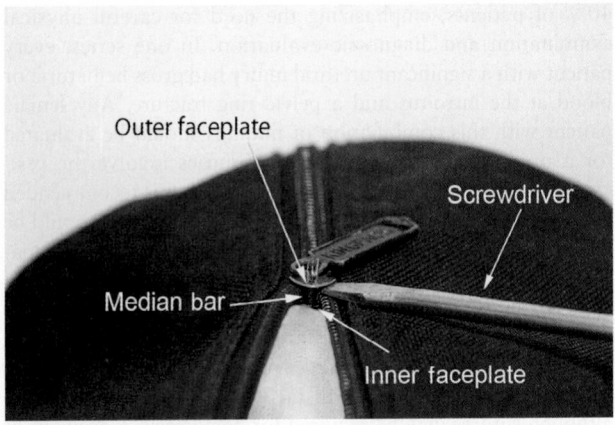

FIGURE 112.10 Screwdriver technique for the release of foreskin entrapped in the zipper. The screwdriver should be placed between the two faceplates and twisted toward the median bar.

the zipper from the rear may work best for heavy-duty metal zippers. Disengagement of the fastener by inserting a flathead screwdriver between the inner and outer faceplates and applying torque toward the median bar (Fig. 112.10) may prove helpful when it is difficult to grasp the tiny median bar with bulky cutting pliers. Elliptical incision of the entrapped foreskin or emergency circumcision can be of value when less invasive methods have failed. Regardless of technique, procedural sedation may facilitate the procedure. Edema can be treated with warm soaks.

PERINEUM

The mechanism most commonly associated with trauma to the female perineum is a straddle-type injury. These injuries may cause vulvar hematomas, which usually respond to treatment with ice packs and bed rest. Patients experiencing mild urinary retention may be more comfortable voiding in a tub of warm water. Massive or expanding hematomas may require surgical exploration and evacuation.

Superficial lacerations of the perineum can be treated conservatively at home with sitz baths. Deep lacerations may extend into the rectum or urethra and therefore require consultation by a surgeon. Rectal penetration requires a diverting colostomy. Suprapubic cystostomy or primary repair should be performed if the urethra is disrupted.

Vaginal lacerations must be suspected in patients with severe trauma to the external genitalia or penetration by foreign object. If a significant vaginal laceration is noted, endoscopy with sedation or general anesthesia is necessary for a full evaluation. The possibility of extension into the urethra, bladder, or rectum must be investigated. The vaginal laceration is debrided and repaired with fine absorbable sutures.

SEXUAL ABUSE

When common accidental situations fail to explain certain genitourinary injuries, the possibility of sexual abuse should be considered. Injuries resulting from sexual abuse include

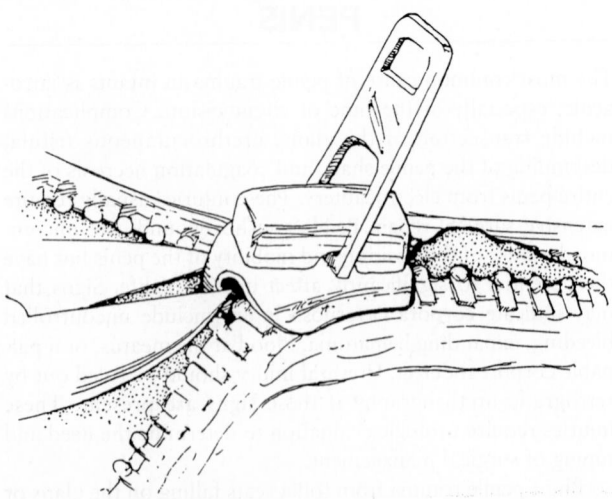

FIGURE 112.9 Penile zipper injury. A wire cutter may be used to cut the median bar of the zipper, releasing the two sides of the zipper and freeing the penis.

abrasions and hematomas in the penile shaft, vaginal lacerations, and perineal hematomas (see also Chapters 76 and 132).

Suggested Readings

Aihara R, Blansfield J, Millham FH, et al. Fracture locations Influence the likelihood of rectal and lower urinary tract injuries in patients sustaining pelvic fractures. *J Trauma* 2002;52:205–209.

Alli MO, Singh, B, Moodley J, et al. Prospective evaluation of combined suprapubic and urethral catheterization to urethral drainage alone for intraperitoneal bladder injuries. *J Trauma* 2003;55:1152–1154.

Andrich D, Day AC, Mundy AR. Proposed mechanisms of lower urinary tract injury in fractures of the pelvic ring. *BJU Int* 2007;100:567–573.

Black PC, Miller EA, Porter JR, et al. Urethral and bladder neck injury associated with pelvic fracture in 25 female patients. *J Urol* 2006;175:2140–2145.

Brandes S, Borrelli J Jr. Pelvic fracture and associated urologic injuries. *World J Surg* 2001;25:1578–1587.

Broghammer JA, Langenburg SE, Smith SJ, et al. Pediatric blunt renal trauma: its conservative management and patterns of associated injuries. *Urology* 2006;67:823–827.

Brown SL, Haas C, Dinchman KH, et al. Radiologic evaluation of pediatric blunt trauma in patients with microscopic hematuria. *World J Surg* 2001;25:1557–1560.

Buckely JC, McAninch JW. The diagnosis, management, and outcomes of pediatric renal injuries. *Urol Clin North Am* 2006;33:33–40.

Chandra RV, Dowling RJ, Ulubasoglu M, et al. Rational approach to diagnosis and management of blunt scrotal trauma. *Urology* 2007;70:230–234.

Guichard G, El Ammari J, Del Coro C, et al. Accuracy of ultrasonography in diagnosis of testicular rupture after blunt scrotal trauma. *Urology* 2008;71:52–56.

Henderson CG, Sedberry-Ross S, Pickard R, et al. Management of high grade renal trauma: 20-year experience at a pediatric level I trauma center. *J Urol* 2006;178:246–250.

Ko SF, Ng SH, Wan YL, et al. Testicular dislocation: an uncommon and easily overlooked complication of blunt abdominal trauma. *Ann Emerg Med* 2004;43:371–375.

Nguyen MM, Das S. Pediatric renal trauma. *Urology* 2002;59:762–766.

Osman Y, El-Tabey N, Mohsen T, et al. Nonoperative treatment of isolated posttraumatic intraperitoneal bladder rupture in children—is it justified? *J Urol* 2005;173:955–957.

Parry NG, Rozycki GS, Feliciano DV, et al. Traumatic rupture of the bladder: is the suprapubic tube necessary? *J Trauma* 2003;54:431–436.

Quagliano PV, Delair SM, Malhotra AK. Diagnosis of blunt bladder injury; a prospective comparative study of computed tomography cystography and conventional retrograde cystography. *J Trauma* 2006;61:410–422.

Raveenthiran V. Releasing of zipper-entrapped skin. A novel nonsurgical technique. *Pediatr Emerg Care* 2007;23:463–464.

Rogers CG, Knight V, Macura KJ, et al. High-grade renal injuries in children—is conservative management possible? *Urology* 2004;64:574–579.

Santucci RA, Langenburg, SE, Zachareas, MJ. Traumatic hematuria in children can be evaluated as in adults. *J Urol* 2004;171:822–825.

Tarman GJ, Kaplan GW, Lerman SL, et al. Lower genitourinary injury and pelvic fractures in pediatric patients. *Urology* 2002;59:123–126.

CHAPTER 113 ■ HAND TRAUMA

MICHAEL WITT, MD, MPH, AND DONALD S. BAE, MD

EPIDEMIOLOGY

Hand trauma is extremely common in the pediatric emergency department, with a broad spectrum of clinical presentations. Injuries include lacerations, soft-tissue injuries, nail bed injuries, fractures, and sprains. Understanding the epidemiology of these injuries helps the clinician identify patterns of injury as well as allows experts to modify risk factors to decrease the incidence of these injuries.

Hand injury rates follow a bimodal distribution of age, with the peaks seen in toddlers and in teenagers. Lacerations and soft-tissue injuries tend to predominate in the younger children (particularly involving the fingertips), whereas fractures are seen more frequently in older children primarily due to sports involvement. These injuries tend to occur around the home, particularly outdoors.

Fractures are most commonly seen in the little finger, especially the proximal phalanx, and fifth metacarpal. In these typically older children, sports such as football, basketball, and baseball cause the majority of injuries, though many nonathletic causes are also known, including fighting.

In cases of nonaccidental trauma, the hand is often the target. Bruises, burns, and other soft-tissue injuries are common, whereas fractures are less so. Nevertheless, during the skeletal survey of a child with suspected abuse, equal attention should be paid to the radiography of the hand.

EXAMINATION

The physical examination of the hand after trauma is perhaps the most important component of the emergency department visit. Proper treatment can only be instituted, including the need for specialist intervention, when all injuries are identified.

Every examination of the hand begins with visual inspection, particularly when compared with the opposite side. Obvious abnormalities such as edema, erythema, ecchymosis, as well as skin defects should be noted. Nail and nail bed injuries are often dramatic but may distract from other superficial or deeper trauma, such as tendon involvement. Examination of the general alignment of the hand and digits may demonstrate subtle abnormalities. Having the patient make a fist and observing any finger displacement can identify spiral phalangeal fractures. In the young, anxious, or uncooperative child, similar assessment of digital alignment may be seen with passive wrist extension, taking advantage of the tenodesis effect (Fig. 113.1).

Focused palpation of the area in question, as well as thorough examination of the other areas of the hand and wrist, is necessary. Identification of tenderness, temperature, induration, crepitance, edema, and fluctuance is critical. The ability to identify abnormalities as they relate to the different regions of the hand will help focus clinical suspicion and analysis of radiographs. Snuffbox tenderness specifically should raise suspicion of scaphoid injury.

Passive range of motion should be tested across all joints in the hand and wrist, with attention paid to discomfort and both increased and decreased range of motion. Active range of motion can be tested by isolating each joint and observing both full flexion and extension. Testing against resistance may also be helpful, particularly in cases of partial tendon injuries. When examining the fingers, recall that the flexor digitorum profundus (FDP) muscle inserts on the distal phalanx, allowing for active distal interphalangeal (DIP) flexion. Therefore, the FDP muscle should be tested by asking the patient to flex the DIP joint while holding the proximal interphalangeal (PIP) joint extended. Because FDP tendons to the digits share a common muscle belly, often individual DIP flexion is not possible. In contrast, the flexor digitorum superficialis muscle inserts into the middle phalanx of each digit; it is best tested by asking the patient to flex the PIP joint while holding the adjacent digits in full extension so as to avoid being misled by the FDP function. The thumb should be tested similarly by observing flexion of the interphalangeal joint due to the flexor pollicis longus muscle. If necessary, moving the hand from flexion to extension at the wrist can cause passive flexion of the muscles and may also identify some abnormalities (Fig. 113.2). Similarly, the extensor functions of the hand should be tested by isolating each joint.

The thumb is controlled by seven muscles. The abductor pollicis longus and abductor pollicis brevis muscles together act to abduct the thumb metacarpal and can be tested against resistance. The extensor pollicis brevis muscle acts to extend the proximal phalanx of the thumb. The extensor pollicis longus muscle acts to extend the distal phalanx and move the thumb dorsally and can be tested by placing the hand palm down on a flat surface and raising the thumb up. The thumb is flexed at both the carpometacarpal and metacarpophalangeal (MCP) joints by the flexor pollicis brevis muscle. Opposition of the thumb is the most important movement and is performed by the opponens pollicis muscle. Finally, the adductor pollicis muscle allows adduction of the thumb and gives strength during grasp movements.

The vascular examination may include the Allen test. After occluding both radial and ulnar arteries with direct pressure applied to the wrist over the palpable radial and ulnar pulses, the patient is asked to clench the fist, resulting in blanching of the skin. Upon releasing pressure over one artery, observation of color return confirms patency and function of the released artery. Digital capillary refill is tested

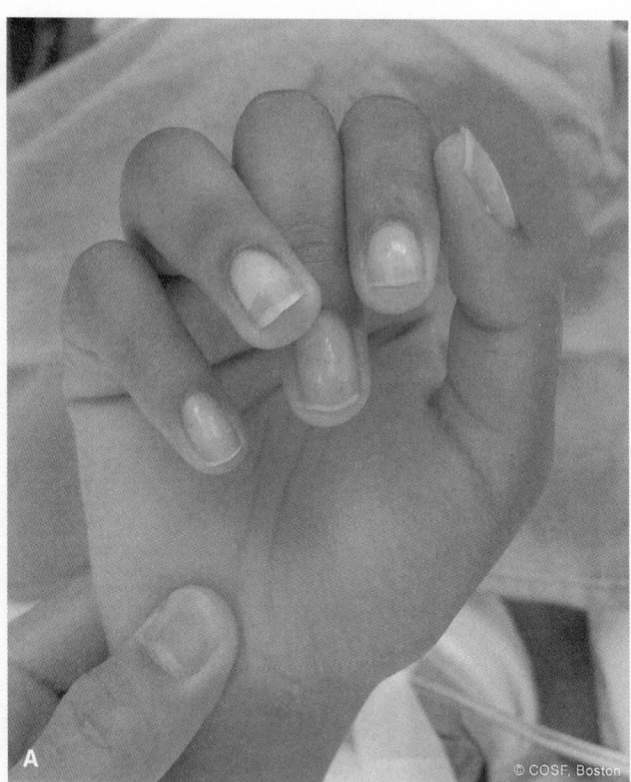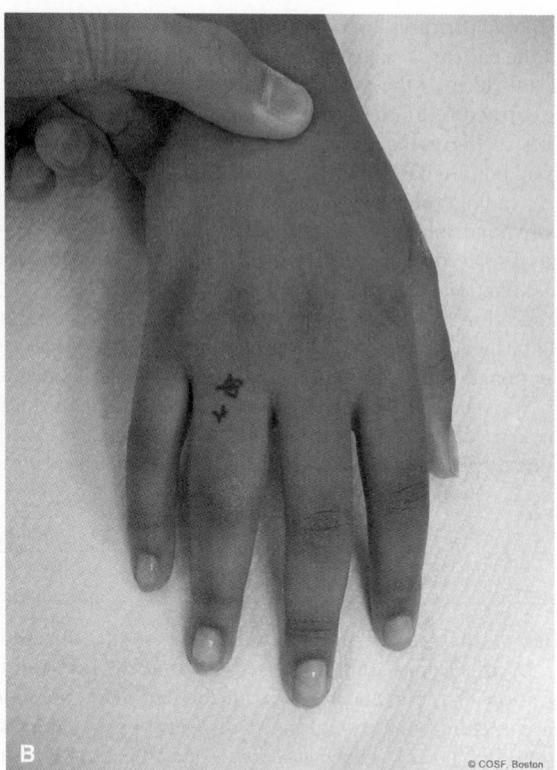

FIGURE 113.1 Abnormal tenodesis. Clinical photographs depicting abnormal rotation of the ring finger in the setting of a malrotated phalanx fracture. Note the clinical overlap of the ring finger over the long finger and increased gap between the ring finger and the small finger, with passive wrist extension (**A**) that is not clinically as apparent with the wrist in neutral position and the digits extended (**B**). (Courtesy of Children's Orthopaedic Surgery Foundation.)

by compressing the tip of the nail until blanched and then timing the return to color after releasing the pressure, generally in less than 1 to 2 seconds.

Neurologic evaluation for sensation includes light touch and pinprick, with two-point discrimination also useful in children older than 5 to 7 years who can cooperate. Motor

FIGURE 113.2 Clinical photograph of a patient with an isolated flexor digitorum profundus rupture of the long finger. Note the abnormal digital cascade and resting flexion posture of the long finger in relationship to the adjacent unaffected digits. (Courtesy of Children's Orthopaedic Surgery Foundation.)

function has effectively been tested during active range of motion, but additional attention should be paid to the ulnar innervated intrinsic muscles by asking the patient to actively abduct and adduct the fingers.

CARPALS

The incidence of carpal fractures is relatively low in children, although increasing awareness has increased its recognition. In infancy, the carpals are completely cartilaginous and are nearly immune to injury. They progressively ossify beginning with the capitate bone. The scaphoid is by far the most common fractured carpal bone, with most fractures occurring in the late childhood and adolescence. Falls are the most frequent cause.

Physical examination requires attention to edema, range of motion, and point tenderness to localize carpal injuries. Snuffbox tenderness is a useful tool for scaphoid fractures. X-ray study is obviously limited in infancy and early childhood because of the lack of ossification. As the patient ages and the carpals are progressively ossifying, comparison with the contralateral side may be of benefit. An important radiologic concept is the distance between the scaphoid and lunate bones. In a true scapholunate dissociation, this space is widened and often called the Terry Thompson sign, but in children in whom the carpals are not fully ossified, this space is naturally widened.

TRAUMA

Scaphoid fractures have different patterns depending on the age of the patient. Younger patients are more likely to fracture the distal third of the bone, whereas adolescents and adults tend to fracture at the waist. A unique fracture to young patients is the avulsion to the distal radial aspect of the scaphoid but often is not diagnosed on first presentation and is seen on radiographs 1 to 2 weeks later. Most scaphoid fractures are nondisplaced and managed with cast immobilization, though displaced fractures may require surgical reduction and internal fixation to prevent nonunion.

In addition to fractures, suspicion for ligamentous injuries should be high, particularly in late childhood and adolescence. As mentioned above, scapholunate dissociation can be identified by widened space between the two bones. Lunate dislocation is best identified with the lateral wrist radiograph, with the bone displaced from its typical midaxial location over the radius.

METACARPALS

Injuries to the metacarpals include fractures to different zones of the bones and dislocations of the MCP joint. Dislocation of the metacarpals from the carpals is possible but rare in children, although these dislocations may coexist with another injury. The metacarpals may be fractured at the base, shaft, or neck. These injuries often occur from crushing trauma in younger patients as well as from impact along the axis of the bones, such as in fighting, in older children and adolescents. Compartment syndrome in the hand can occur, particularly with multiple fractures, and thus careful physical examination and appropriate suspicion are required.

Metacarpal base fractures occur at the least common location, but most of these involve the small finger. There will be significant pain and dorsal edema, which can make accurate diagnosis challenging. Nondisplaced or minimally displaced fractures are generally managed with support via a splint or cast. Displaced fractures often require closed reduction and subsequent casting. Carpometacarpal dislocations alone or in conjunction with a fracture, however, are unstable and often require operative stabilization. Bennett fractures, or intraarticular fracture of the base of the thumb metacarpal, mandate special attention, as the thumb carpometacarpal joint is critical for full use of this digit. Similarly, Rolando fractures, comminuted fractures of the base of the thumb metacarpal, also require careful attention.

Metacarpal shaft fractures are also uncommon in the pediatric population and tend to involved the long, ring, and small fingers. They are most often spiral in nature, indicating a rotational component to the injuring force. Careful attention to the alignment of the fingers when making a fist may demonstrate subtle rotation. These injuries also result in significant edema, but significantly angulated or displaced fractures can be suspected on examination. Most nondisplaced and displaced shaft fractures can be managed with closed reduction and immobilization, though fractures with significant shortening of the length of the bone or those involved with multiple fractures may require operative repair.

The most common metacarpal fracture occurs at the neck of the bone, with the majority involving small finger (the

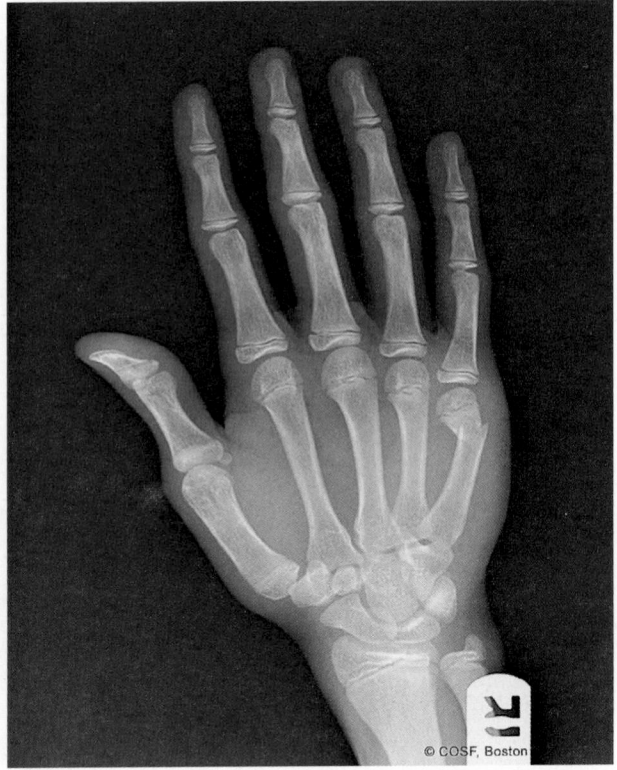

FIGURE 113.3 Anteroposterior radiograph of the hand depicting a displaced fifth metacarpal neck fracture. (Courtesy of Children's Orthopaedic Surgery Foundation.)

boxer's fracture) (Fig. 113.3). Inspection for rotational displacement of the fracture is again important, as is the evidence of skin trauma that might indicate contamination from an opponent's mouth during a fight. A considerable amount of angulation of the fracture can be tolerated without limiting ultimate hand function, with increasing tolerance in the ring and small fingers. A commonly used rule is 10–20 degrees to 30–40 degrees, indicating the progression on tolerable angulation from the index to the small finger ray. Closed reduction is often all that is needed in fractures that exceed the tolerable amount of angulation, except in unstable patients.

MCP joint dislocations are the most common dislocation among the pediatric hand injuries and most frequently involve the thumb (Fig. 113.4). Similar to dislocations of the interphalangeal joints, these dislocations occur most often with the proximal phalanx dorsal to the metacarpal and the metacarpal head palpable in the palm. In the immature patient, these dislocations on radiographs may be difficult to clarify because of the joint consisting mainly of cartilage and thus may simply seem hyperextended. Reduction attempts should maintain or exaggerate the hyperextension while putting pressure on the volar aspect of the phalangeal head toward the palm. In general, straight longitudinal traction is not recommended in an effort to avoid soft-tissue interposition and converting a reducible injury into an irreducible dislocation. If the joint is not easily relocated, specialist involvement and likely open reduction will be required because the tendons and volar plate involved may prevent reduction with inline traction.

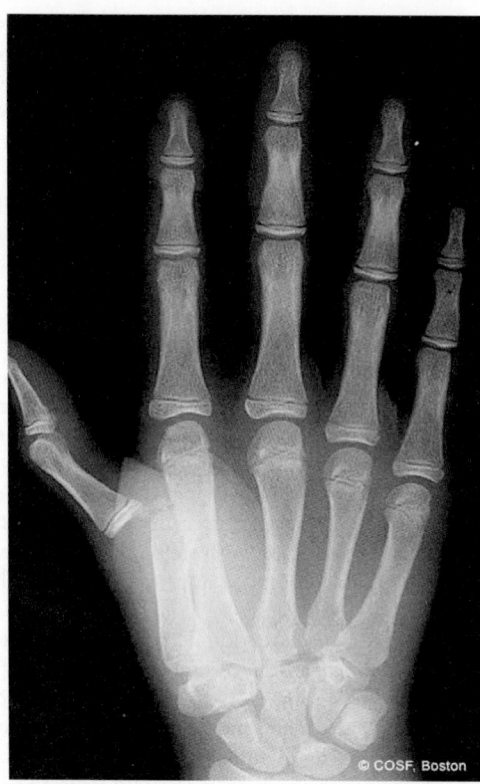

FIGURE 113.4 Anteroposterior hand radiograph depicting a dorsal complex dislocation of the thumb metacarpophalangeal joint. (Courtesy of Children's Orthopaedic Surgery Foundation.)

PHALANGES

Phalanx injuries are very common in children, as the fingers of a child are a first exploration into his or her world. Mechanisms of injury included crush, hyperextension, and "jamming" most frequently. As mentioned previously, careful examination with particular attention to rotational deformity is required. Often identifying which bone is involved in an interphalangeal joint can be challenging due to pain and edema.

Proximal phalanx injuries are some of the most common pediatric hand injuries. The base of the proximal phalanx often endures a Salter-Harris II fracture, with the little finger being most frequent. Many are managed with splinting/casting and closed reduction if necessary. Shaft fractures are also generally managed with closed reduction, though displacement or rotational deformity may require surgical stabilization. Phalangeal neck fractures can be difficult to diagnose and often oblique views on radiographs may be of assistance (Fig. 113.5). These fractures in particular require close outpatient care, as displacement and rotation may have long-term consequences on the flexion of the adjacent interphalangeal joint. Finally, condylar fractures may involve one or both condyles and long-term management may depend on the severity of the injury (Fig. 113.6). Close follow-up is also required in these injuries, as the bone may not remodel well and may require early reduction and other intervention.

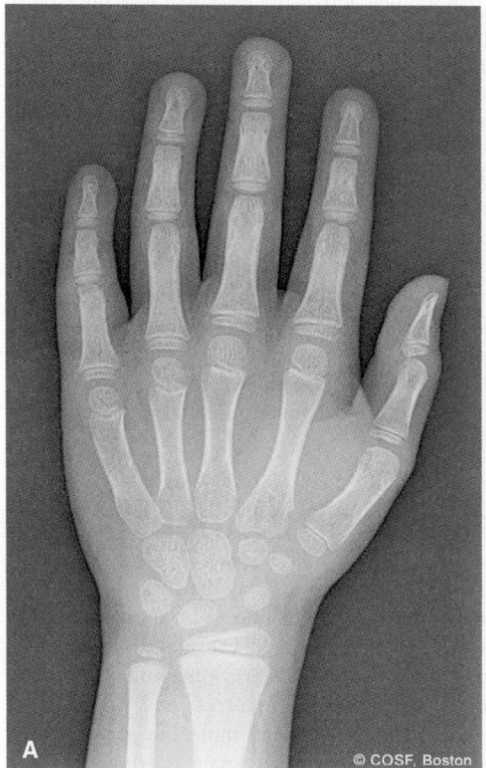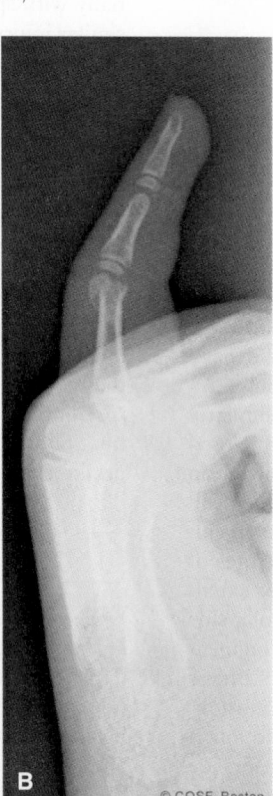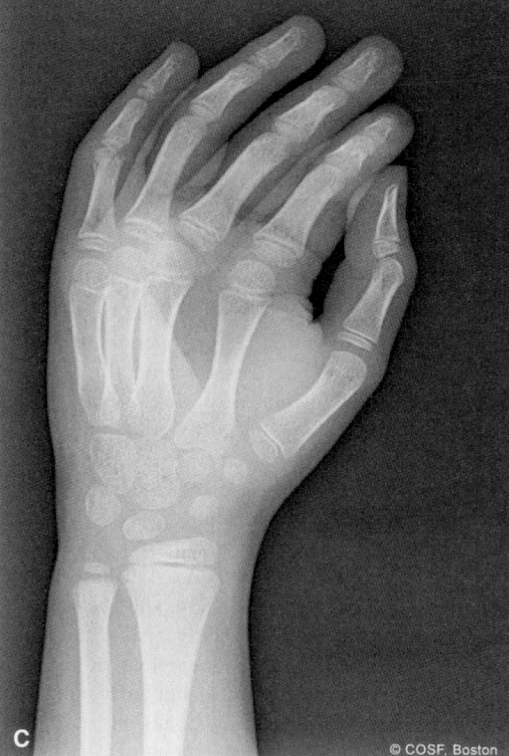

FIGURE 131.5 Radiographs of a displaced small finger proximal phalangeal neck fracture. Note the relatively subtle and benign radiographic appearance on the anteroposterior view (**A**). Fracture displacement is best seen on a dedicated lateral view (**B**) as well as on oblique projections of the small finger (**C**). (Courtesy of Children's Orthopaedic Surgery Foundation.)

TRAUMA

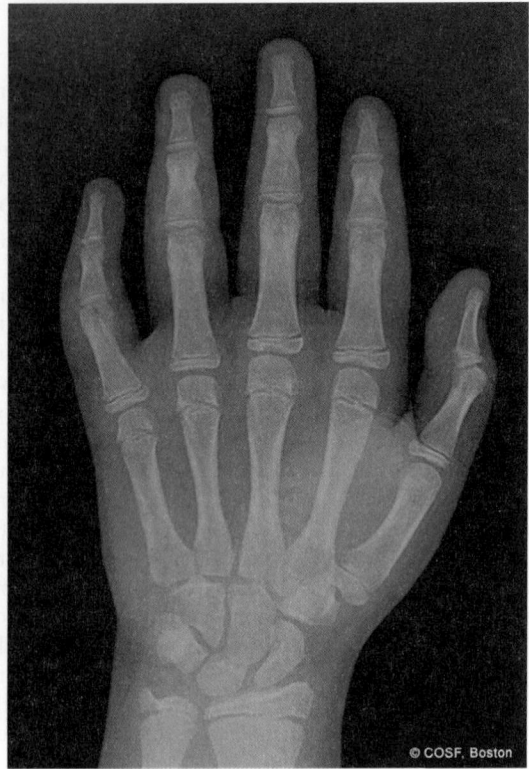

FIGURE 113.6 Anteroposterior radiograph depicting an intraarticular fracture of the head of the small finger proximal phalanx involving the radial condyle. (Courtesy of Children's Orthopaedic Surgery Foundation.)

Proximal phalanx injuries to the thumb ray are unique. In adolescents and adults, a skier's thumb or gamekeeper's thumb occurs with rupture of the ulnar collateral ligament (UCL) during stress onto the thumb away from the rest of the hand. In children, a fracture of the base of the proximal phalanx is more likely than an UCL injury, with Salter-Harris I and II fractures predominating in younger children and Salter-Harris III fractures in older children. Thumb spica splinting is appropriate for the constellation of these injuries in the emergency department. Displaced fractures require operative management.

Middle phalanx fractures are generally managed similarly to proximal phalanx injuries. Most are managed by closed management, although surgical reduction and stabilization may be required in displaced fractures. Fractures of the head of the phalanx require close management by hand surgeon because of a high rate of complications. Avulsion fractures of the middle phalanx at the insertion of the volar plate or extensor central slip are not uncommon. Avulsions on the volar side generally are from hyperextension, and generally the fragment does not reattach and frequently results in chronic stiffness and has potential for permanent loss of range of motion. Splinting is performed initially, but early range of motion is often started a week later. Small avulsions on the extensor side are generally treated similarly, though larger ones are treated with longer splinting and displaced fractures may require open reduction.

Distal phalanx injuries are very common and often associated with nail and nail bed injuries, as discussed in the following text. When associated with nail bed injuries, after the nail is removed (if necessary), the open fracture should be copiously irrigated and the nail bed repaired, followed by splinting. These should be followed by hand surgeons in case a further intervention, such as pin fixation, is required. Seymour fractures comprise a special type of injury, with a Salter-Harris I or II fracture of the distal phalanx associated with exposure of the proximal aspect of the nail and damaged germinal matrix (Fig. 113.7). The distal interphalangeal joint is often held at some flexion. Discussion with a hand surgeon is useful, as the fracture healing may be prevented by tissue present in the physis.

Lacerations in the fingers and hands that involve tendons can be serious and require attentive care. In addition to routine wound care, extensor tendon lacerations proximal to the MCP joints may be amenable to repair by the emergency physician. Extensor tendon lacerations involving the MCP joints or digits, as well as all flexor tendon lacerations, require care by a hand surgeon. In consultation with the surgeon, closure of the skin and splinting may comprise appropriate care with close follow-up.

Injuries to the extensor tendon across the distal interphalangeal joint prevent extension of that joint, commonly called mallet finger. The DIP joint rests in a somewhat flexed position. This injury occurs when the finger is "jammed" longitudinally and occurs mostly in adolescents and adults. Bony mallet fingers, on the other hand, are not a DIP issue and instead represent physeal fractures at the base of the distal phalanx. They clinically appear similar and are managed identically initially with splinting but may require surgical management. A similar injury can happen across the proximal interphalangeal joint causing a Boutonniere deformity, but the care in the emergency department is the same.

Dislocations of the MCP and interphalangeal joints are generally uncommon in younger patients, although adolescents tend to have incidence similar to adults, particularly those involved in contact sports. These dislocations most often occur with the distal bone placed dorsal to the proximal. Prompt relocation after management of pain, particularly if there is any concern of neurovascular status, is performed with inline distraction and hyperextension in the interphalangeal joints. MCP dislocation is reduced by flexing the wrist to relax the tendon and then applying dorsal pressure both in the direction of the palm and toward the fingertip. Splinting all dislocations to maintain stability is required until reevaluation.

FINGERTIP INJURIES

Fingertip injuries are very common, as the tips of the fingers are often the entry point to exploration of our surroundings. Crush injuries are the most frequent cause and can result in injuries ranging from minor lacerations and subungual hematoma to complex open fractures and tissue loss. Similarly, sharp lacerations are often simple, but particularly if the mechanism also has the force to damage the nail, complete amputations can occur. Although children often recover quite well, careful attention and care to these wounds can help reduce the risk of permanent deformity to the fingertip and nail.

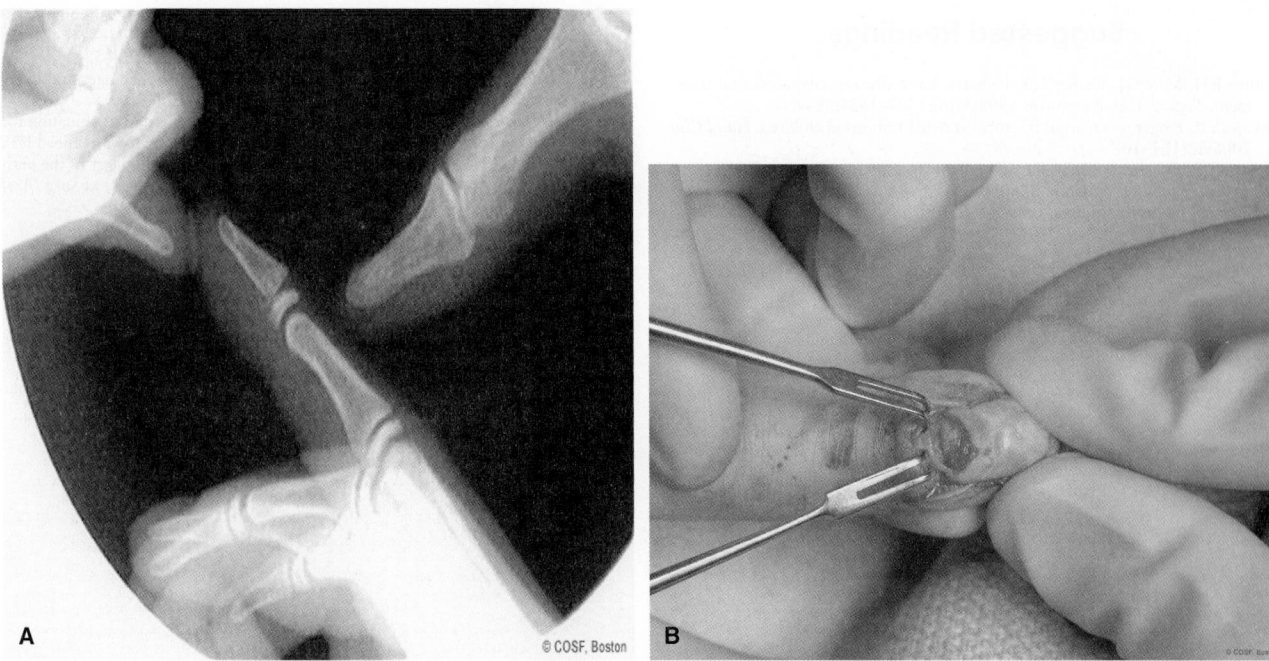

FIGURE 113.7 Seymour's fracture. **A:** Lateral radiograph depicting a displaced distal phalangeal physeal fracture in the setting of a nail bed injury. **B:** Intraoperative photograph after nail plate removal depicting the tear in the germinal matrix of the nail bed and underlying bony injury. (Courtesy of Children's Orthopaedic Surgery Foundation.)

Although the physical examination features discussed previously hold true, these injuries are often associated with significant pain and bleeding that may hamper repair efforts. Digital block of the affected digit may be required for adequate pain control. An easily removed tourniquet device is recommended if oozing from wounds precludes adequate examination and repair.

Copious irrigation is required with all wounds, with extra attention paid to open fractures. Some wound debridement may be required, though the emergency physician should hesitate before debriding the nail bed for fear of permanent effects on subsequent nail growth. When repair is complete, a nonadherent dressing should be used and splinting considered. Petrolatum-laced mesh dressings are particularly effective at optimizing healing and minimizing discomfort and damage on removal. Prophylactic antibiotics are controversial in fingertip injuries, even in open fractures. Meticulous wound care is likely most beneficial, and antibiotics should be considered in dirty wounds or those with significant devitalized tissue.

Nail bed injuries require nail removal, if not already performed traumatically, with careful wound preparation and closure of the often friable tissue with 5-0 or 6-0 absorbable suture. The nail fold must be kept open for the new nail to form and thus several placeholders are used. The salvaged nail can be placed, as can a sterile aluminum (from suture packaging), reinforced silicone sheeting, or a nonadhesive dressing. The nail should be tacked down with nonabsorbable sutures proximally and distally, though the proximal sutures should be removed early in the course at follow-up with a hand surgeon to prevent wound tracks during nail development.

Fingertip lacerations are managed similarly to lacerations in other locations with a few caveats. Wound care is performed as described above. Some literature recommends nonabsorbable suture material, though at our institution, absorbable suture is often used because the swelling and discomfort often preclude simple suture removal.

Amputations of the fingertip are not uncommon and can result in permanent deformity. When the issue of transport is concerned, the current recommendation is to transport the amputated part in saline-moistened gauze in a bag that is then kept cool in an ice–water mixture. Reimplantation has been recommended in most cases involving children if the distal piece is available and the tissues are not damaged beyond repair. Reimplantation may not be an option if the avulsed tip is too small, macerated, or grossly contaminated. If possible, the skin can be closed over the stump with sutures while taking care to protect the nail bed. Small avulsions are best cared for with local wound care and petroleum-based dressing until granulation and healing. If closure is not an option due to bone exposure, hand surgery consultation is indicated either in the emergency department or with wound care and petroleum-based dressing until seen as an outpatient.

Subungual hematomas, or the collection of blood between the nail and the nail bed, are common and generally occur with crushing injuries. Small hematomas are generally cared for without intervention, whereas hematomas involving more than 50% of the nail surface are more likely to be associated with significant nail bed injury, particularly in the setting of an associated distal phalanx fracture. Nevertheless, the literature has demonstrated that if the nail is intact and well adhered, then nail removal and nail bed reconstruction do not impart any improved outcome over simple trephination. Nail trephination can be performed with a heated paper clip, an electrocautery pen, or a large-bore needle drill rotating in a circular motion.

TRAUMA

Suggested Readings

Ablove RH, Moy OJ, Peimer CA. Pediatric hand disease. Diagnosis and treatment. *Pediatr Clin North Am* 1998;45(6):1507–1524, ix–x.

Cornwall R. Finger metacarpal fractures and dislocations in children. *Hand Clin* 2006;22(1):1–10.

Cornwall R, Ricchetti ET. Pediatric phalanx fractures: unique challenges and pitfalls. *Clin Orthop Relat Res* 2006;445:146–156.

de Alwis W. Fingertip injuries. *Emerg Med Australas.* 2006;18(3):229–237.

Kaawach W, Ecklund K, Di Canzio J, et al. Normal ranges of scapholunate distance in children 6 to 14 years old. *J Pediatr Orthop* 2001;21(4):464–467.

Light TR. Carpal injuries in children. *Hand Clin* 2000;16(4):513–522.

Papadonikolakis A, Li Z, Smith BP, et al. Fractures of the phalanges and interphalangeal joints in children. *Hand Clin* 2006;22(1):11–18.

Roser SE, Gellman H. Comparison of nail bed repair versus nail trephination for subungual hematomas in children. *J Hand Surg [Am]* 1999;24(6):1166–1170.

Zook EG, Van Beek AL, Russell RC, et al. Anatomy and physiology of the perionychium: a review of the literature and anatomic study. *J Hand Surg [Am]* 1980;5(6):528–536.

CHAPTER 114 ■ MUSCULOSKELETAL TRAUMA

DAVID BACHMAN, MD, AND STEPHEN SANTORA, MD

Orthopedic trauma currently accounts for 10% to 15% of emergency department (ED) visits in urban pediatric hospitals. The number and spectrum of musculoskeletal injuries sustained by children and adolescents appear to be on the rise since the mid-1990s, in part because of the rapid growth of organized sports. More recent reports in the medical literature have highlighted the range of injuries, many if not the majority of them orthopedic, stemming from active participation by youth in such activities as skateboarding, rollerblading, skiing, and snowboarding. The injuries associated with the use of scooters and trampolines have drawn particular attention. As the result of a number of anatomic and physiologic differences, the array of orthopedic injuries seen in pediatrics differs greatly from that seen in adult practice. An understanding of these differences allows the emergency physician to make accurate diagnosis and avoid complications. This chapter provides a set of principles and guidelines to be used in the initial evaluation, diagnosis, and treatment of common orthopedic injuries in children.

GENERAL PRINCIPLES OF PEDIATRIC ORTHOPEDICS

Structural and Physiologic Differences between the Musculoskeletal Systems of Children and Adults

The bony architecture in children includes a thick and active periosteum, a growth plate (physis), an epiphysis (secondary ossification center), and perichondrial rings (Fig. 114.1). The bones of a child are much more porous and thus more pliable than those of an adult. In contrast, because of this increased porosity, stiffness and overall bony strength are less, and the incidence of fractures is greater in children. During growth, the skeleton undergoes changes that cause different anatomic regions to be more susceptible to fracture at certain stages of development. In general, the ligaments attaching one bone to another have greater strength than the epiphyseal plates and perichondrial rings. As a result, although the number of fractures is greater, the incidence of sprains, ligamentous injuries, and dislocations is significantly lower in children.

The periosteum plays an important role in the reparative process of fracture healing. In children, the periosteum is thick and physiologically active, and is easily stripped from the bony cortex during injury. When injuries occur, the periosteum is often torn on the convex side of the fracture while remaining intact on the concave side. The intact periosteum on the concave aspect often aids the orthopedist in the reduction of the fracture fragments. Callus formation is exuberant in the young and declines with age as the physiologic activity of the periosteum decreases. Nonunions almost never occur in children.

Remodeling, although rare in adults, is expected to a degree in children. Significant remodeling can be anticipated in younger children and when the fracture occurs in the metaphysis of growing bones. Deformities occurring in the plane of motion of the adjacent joint remodel to the greatest degree. Fractures that occur in the diaphysis of long bones in adolescents, away from the plane of motion of the joint, cannot be expected to correct spontaneously with growth. The potential for remodeling with bowing fractures is particularly limited, with reduction generally recommended for cosmetically unacceptable deformities of greater than 10 degrees. In general, it is important to obtain as near an anatomic reduction of fracture fragments as possible in all age groups and not to rely on remodeling to align angulated fractures.

Fractures Unique to Children

The anatomic and physiologic differences between adults and children are reflected in a number of fractures and injuries unique to the pediatric age group, including physeal fractures, torus fractures, greenstick fractures, bowing deformities, and avulsion fractures.

Physeal Fractures

Fractures often occur at the physis (growth plate) in children. Most such fractures occur through the zone of provisional calcification, a relatively weak area of the germinal growth plate. Overall, up to 18% to 30% of pediatric fractures involve the physis. Physeal injuries are more common in adolescents than in younger children, with a peak incidence at 11 to 12 years of age. Most growth plate injuries occur in the upper limb, particularly in the radius and ulna.

Several classification systems have been described for physeal fractures. The most widely used is that of Salter and Harris, who described five types of growth plate fractures, each having specific prognostic and treatment implications (Fig. 114.2).

Salter-Harris Type I Fracture. It involves separation of the metaphysis from the epiphysis through the zone of provisional calcification. Diagnosis is often difficult if displacement is minimal. Type I fractures are generally benign, with little chance of growth disturbance if near anatomic reduction is achieved. Exceptions include type I injuries of the proximal radius, the proximal and distal femur, and the proximal tibia, all of which are subject to premature physeal closure and posttraumatic

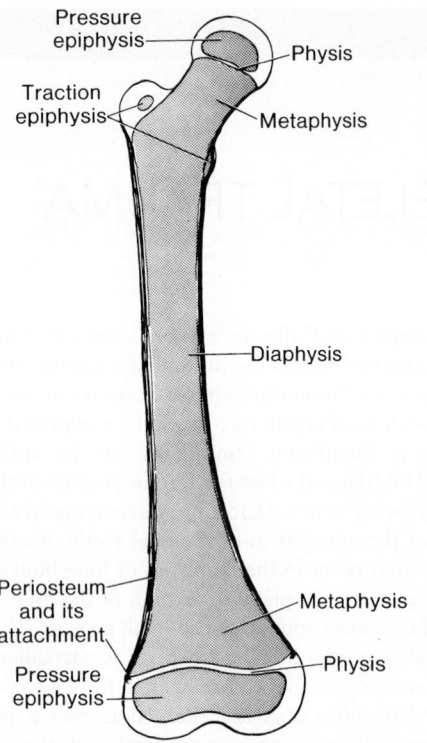

FIGURE 114.1 Diagrammatic representation of the femur in late childhood.

growth arrest. In general, when radiographic studies are negative but physical findings are suggestive of a Salter-Harris type I injury (e.g., point tenderness over a growth plate), immobilization and a follow-up examination are essential.

Salter-Harris Type II Fracture. It is the most common type of pediatric physeal fracture. It is similar to a type I fracture except that a portion of metaphyseal bone is displaced with the epiphyseal fragment.

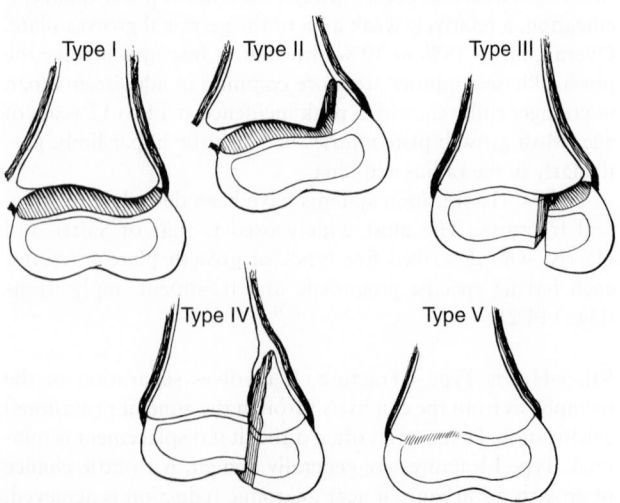

FIGURE 114.2 The Salter-Harris classification for physeal fractures. The prognosis for growth disturbance worsens from type I through type V.

The fracture line crosses the germinal growth plate as it courses toward the metaphysis. Like the type I injuries, these fractures generally carry a good prognosis.

Salter-Harris Type III and IV Fractures. These are intraarticular injuries that also involve the growth plate. Anatomic position must be reestablished to restore normal joint mechanics and prevent growth arrest. Because of the increased incidence of growth disturbance, altered joint mechanics, and functional disability following Salter-Harris type III and IV fractures, an orthopedic consultation is usually obtained for all but the most minor type III and IV injuries while the patient is in the ED.

Salter-Harris Type V Fracture. It results from axial compression of the germinal growth plate. It is often difficult to diagnose; the radiograph may be normal or may demonstrate any of the above Salter-Harris growth plate fractures. The diagnosis is often made in hindsight after a growth arrest becomes evident.

Torus Fractures

Torus (buckle) fractures are common fractures in young patients. They occur in the metaphyseal region of bone from a compressive load. The cortex of the bone buckles in a small area, resulting in a stable fracture pattern (Fig. 114.3). As the child matures, the stiffness of the metaphyseal region increases, and the incidence of this fracture pattern decreases.

Greenstick Fractures

Greenstick injuries are the most common fracture pattern in children, accounting for up to 50% of fractures before

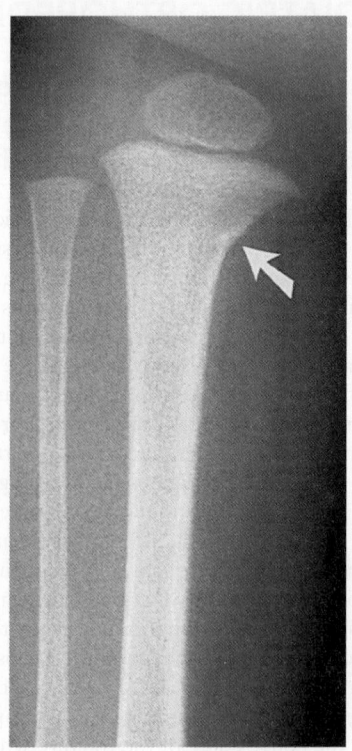

FIGURE 114.3 Torus fracture of the proximal right tibia in a 1-year-old child *(arrow)*.

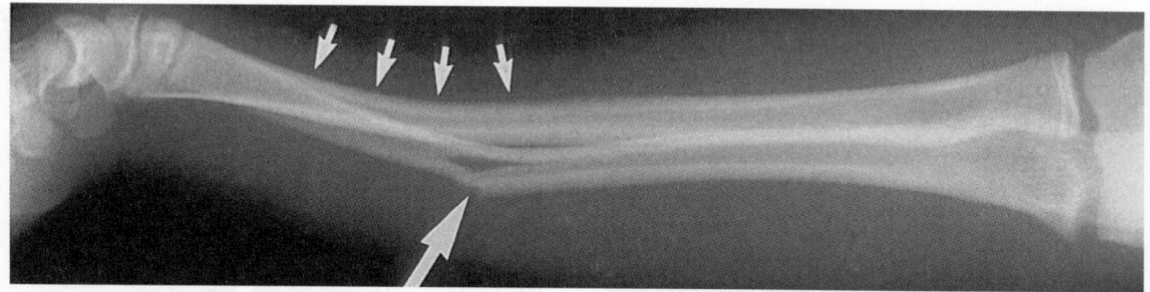

FIGURE 114.4 Greenstick fracture of the ulna *(large arrow)* and a bowing fracture *(small arrows)* of the radius. The extent of bowing can often be fully appreciated only with comparison views of the opposite extremity.

12 years of age. They are incomplete fractures that occur at the diaphyseal–metaphyseal junction and in which the cortex remains intact on one side. Angulation and rotation are common. To obtain an anatomic reduction, the fracture must often first be completed (Fig. 114.4).

Bowing Fractures

Bowing fractures occur uniquely in children. More recent evidence suggests that the force causing the deformation is longitudinal. The force stops short of creating a fracture but does cause persistent plastic deformation (bowing) of the bony structure (Fig. 114.4). Little remodeling can be expected from the injury, and both cosmetic and functional deficits are common. Anatomic reduction produces the most satisfactory result. All bowing deformities should be referred to an orthopedic surgeon.

Avulsion Fractures

Avulsion fractures are common in children. Strong muscular attachments adhere to secondary centers of ossification known as apophyses in the developing skeleton. During intense muscular contraction, fractures occur through the apophyseal plate. Most avulsion fractures occur in the pelvis and heal uneventfully. Other common sites include the tibial tubercle and the phalanges. Only infrequently do avulsion fractures require open or closed reduction. Conservative care is the mainstay of treatment.

Physical and Radiographic Examination

Approach to the Physical Examination

A systematic approach to the child with a suspected fracture is necessary to avoid overlooked injuries and undue complications. The basic principles of a history and physical examination should be followed. In all cases, it is necessary to consider the possibility of associated head and truncal injuries. Often the history is obtained from a parent or bystander who witnessed the accident. At times, no history is available. Attention to the mechanism of injury and the force causing the injury gives clues to the severity of the fracture and soft-tissue injury. The activity of the patient following the injury also helps define the likelihood and nature of orthopedic injuries. Whether the child is able to provide any details of the accident obviously depends

on the child's age, as well as the extent of associated head and internal injuries.

The physical examination should begin with careful observation of the patient's behavior. Is he or she guarding or not moving an extremity? Is there pain? How is the patient's color? Is the child interacting normally with his or her parents and the environment? After observing the child and determining the area or areas of injury, the physician can look for swelling and deformity. It is best to always begin with the extremities that do not appear to be injured. An effort should be made to gain the patient's trust by gently moving all joints and extremities that appear uninjured while trying to distract the child from the examination itself. This also allows detection of unsuspected areas of injury. Attention should then be turned to the injured extremity. Swelling, ecchymosis, deformity, and the presence of lacerations and puncture wounds should be noted. When open wounds are present, the exact location, degree of contamination, presence of fat globules, and rate of active bleeding should be documented. It is not always obvious whether there is an open fracture or simply a laceration that does not communicate with the fracture; operative exploration may ultimately be required.

While continuing to distract the child, the physician should then carefully palpate the soft tissues and bones above and below the area of injury. The point of maximal bony tenderness should next be gently defined. Evidence of increased compartment pressures should be sought both by palpation and by careful assessment of the pulses and capillary blood flow distal to the injury. However, the compartment syndrome can occur in the presence of palpable pulses (see the "Compartment Syndrome" section). If no significant deformity is discovered, joint motion both proximal and distal to the fracture should be assessed. As detailed, a sensory and motor examination as the age and overall condition of the child will permit should be performed.

Radiographic Examination

All unstable and significantly deformed fractures *must* be immobilized before the initiation of radiographic studies. By so doing, further deformity and soft-tissue injury is avoided, and patient discomfort during positioning for the radiographs is decreased. A plaster or fiberglass splint can be applied quickly and does not prevent adequate radiographic assessment of the fracture (Fig. 114.5). Unless a specific contraindication exists, pain medication, often parenteral, should also be

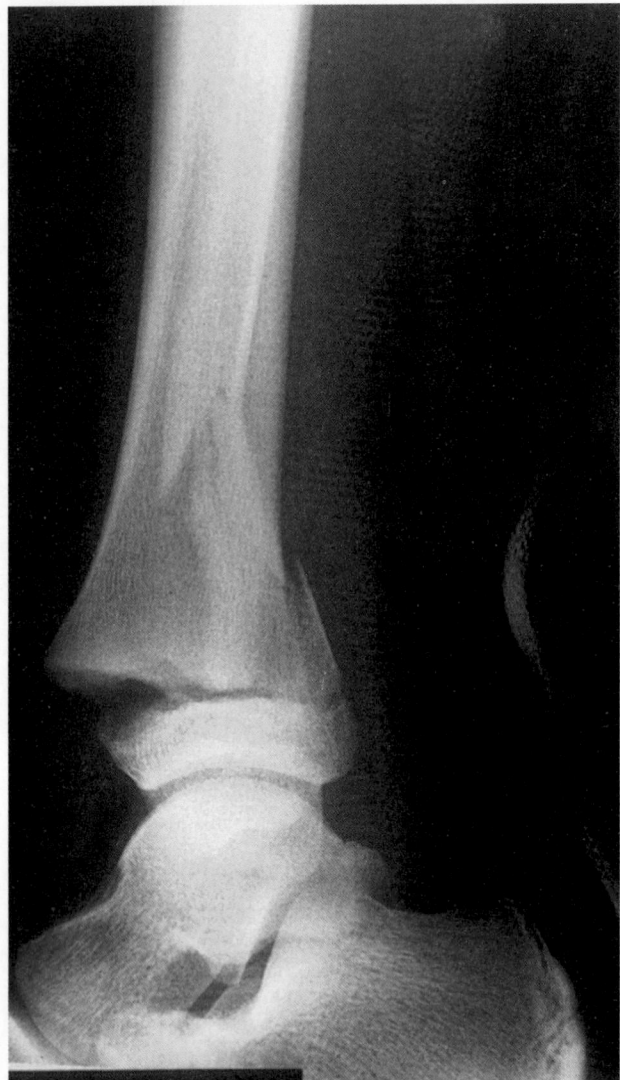

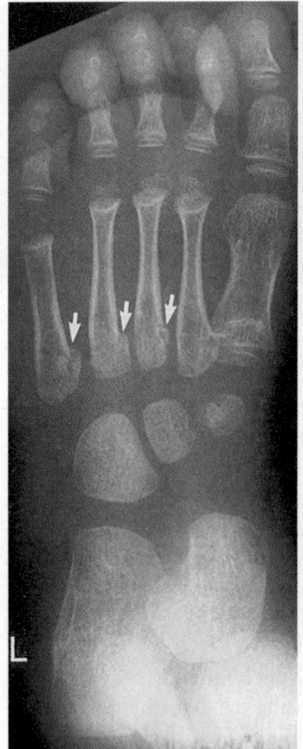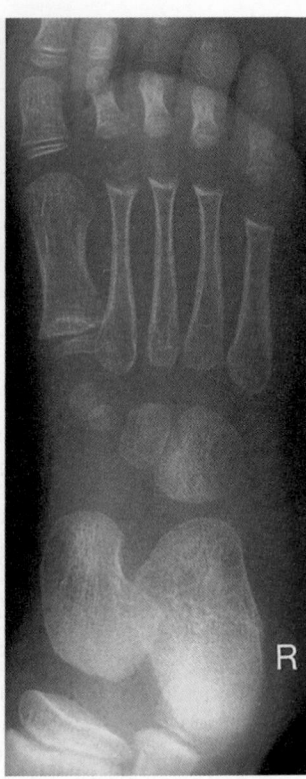

FIGURE 114.6 Radiographs of the feet of a 3-year-old child who sustained a crush injury of the left foot. The soft-tissue swelling of the left foot *(L)* is readily apparent. That the irregularities of the proximal third, fourth, and fifth left metatarsals *(arrows)* are indisputably fractures is immediately apparent when the injured foot is compared with the uninjured right foot *(R)*. A proximal second metatarsal fracture was also suspected and was better visualized on other views.

FIGURE 114.5 Lateral radiograph through a fiberglass splint showing angulated distal tibial and fibular fractures in a 13-year-old boy. Splinting before radiologic studies provides fracture stability and comfort but does not prevent adequate visualization of bony injury.

administered. Multiple studies continue to demonstrate that many children with skeletal injuries receive no or inadequate pain medication, both in the ED and on discharge. Increased emphasis of pain as a "vital sign," combined with protocolized approaches to pain management, would seem to offer a potential solution to this ongoing wave of "oligoanalgesia." No patient should be allowed to take any food or drink by mouth until all examinations and referrals are completed.

After a complete history and physical examination, the physician should be able to order specific radiologic views to identify the injury. In some instances (e.g., a toddler who is refusing to bear weight but who has no localizing signs), the history and a knowledge of the most common injuries for a given age have to guide the choice of radiographic studies. A complete examination should include the joints above and below the fracture and at least two views taken at 90 degrees to one another (generally anteroposterior and lateral views). Oblique and other additional views are necessary at times for

certain body parts (e.g., hand, ankle, foot, phalanges) and when routine views are normal but suspicions of a fracture are high. Given the degree of normal variability in bony anatomy, particularly in growing bones, comparison views are indicated on occasion (Fig. 114.6).

Although plain film radiography will no doubt remain the primary imaging technique used in fracture evaluation, other modalities, notably bone scintigraphy, computed tomography (CT), magnetic resonance imaging (MRI), and most recently, ultrasound (US) have come to play an important adjunctive role. Scintigraphy is more sensitive than plain films in certain settings, for example, when a stress fracture is suspected (Fig. 114.7). CT plays an important role in the definition of complex fractures, particularly intraarticular ones, as well as in the evaluation of spine injuries. Although seldom indicated in the acute setting, MRI has proven to be a most valuable modality in the definition of physeal and growth plate injuries, as well as in the diagnosis of avulsion and stress fractures. Its value derives from its ability to visualize cartilaginous and soft-tissue structures, as well as osseous ones, an ability of obvious value when it comes to the maturing pediatric skeleton. In the last few years, reports have begun to appear that highlight the use of US both as a diagnostic tool and as a guide during closed fracture reduction. Given the expanding role of US in the emergency setting, it seems likely that US will assume a yet to be well-defined place in acute fracture management in the years ahead.

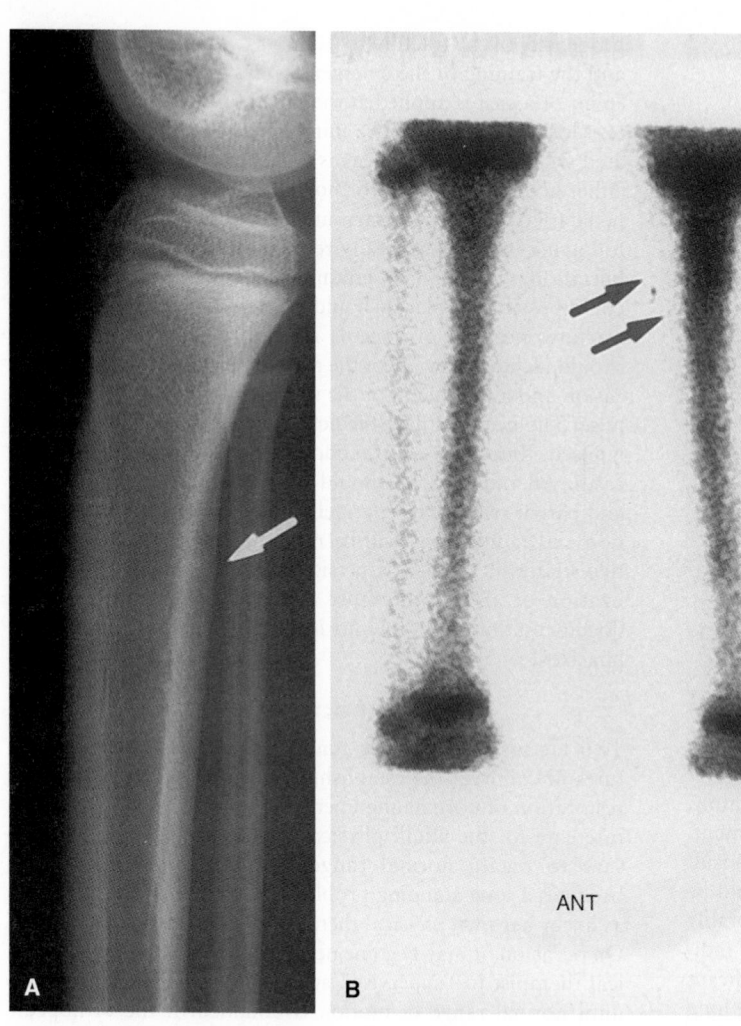

FIGURE 114.7 **A:** Routine radiographs of this 10-year-old girl revealed only a minor cortical irregularity of the posterior aspect of the proximal left tibia *(arrow)*. **B:** Bone scintigraphy was performed. The increased isotope uptake seen along the proximal left tibia *(arrows)* confirmed the clinical suspicion of a stress fracture.

Fracture Description

When obtaining an orthopedic consultation, the emergency physician must relay accurate and descriptive information to allow the orthopedist to make appropriate treatment recommendations. A clinical description should include the patient's age and gender, the mechanism of injury, the anatomic location, the status of the neurovascular structures, and the extent of associated soft-tissue injury. A careful and precise radiographic description should include the anatomic location of the fracture; the type of fracture (e.g., transverse, spiral, oblique); the amount of displacement; the degree of angulation, shortening, or malrotation; the degree of comminution; and the extent of involvement of the joint and growth plate. Accurate descriptions using appropriate terminology are helpful in assisting the orthopedist in his or her recommendations (Fig. 114.8).

Orthopedic Referral and General Principles of Acute Fracture Care

Indications for Orthopedic Referral

The indications for an orthopedic consultation vary somewhat with the ability and experience of the emergency physician and

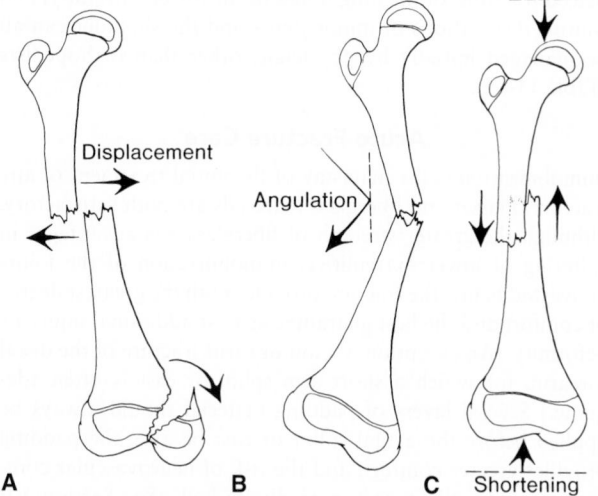

FIGURE 114.8 Diagrammatic representation of fracture deformities: displacement (**A**), angulation (**B**), and overriding with shortening (**C**).

TRAUMA

TABLE 114.1

INDICATIONS FOR ORTHOPEDIC REFERRAL

Injuries that require immediate orthopedic referral
Open fractures
Unacceptably displaced fractures
Fractures with associated neurovascular compromise
Significant growth plate or joint injuries
Complete or displaced fractures of the long bones of the
    lower extremities
Pelvic fractures (other than minor avulsions)
Spinal fractures
Dislocations of major joints other than the shoulder

Injuries that can be managed initially by emergency physician
Nondisplaced Salter-Harris type I fractures (exceptions are
    femur, proximal tibia)
Clavicular fractures
Nondisplaced upper-extremity fractures
Incomplete, nondisplaced fractures of the long bones of the
    lower extremities
Nondisplaced fractures of the hand and foot
Routine dislocations of the shoulder and minor joints
    (no fracture)

the availability and preferences of the orthopedist. Certainly, if any question exists regarding the diagnosis, treatment, complications, or follow-up of an orthopedic injury, a consultation should be obtained. An orthopedic surgeon should be called to evaluate all fractures that are open, unacceptably displaced, or causing neurovascular compromise. Other indications for immediate orthopedic referral include significant growth plate or joint involvement, many fractures of the long bones of the lower extremity, pelvic fractures (other than avulsions), spinal injuries, and dislocations of major joints other than the shoulder. In contrast, the emergency physician should be expected to provide the initial, if not the definitive, care for many pediatric fractures. Most nondisplaced Salter-Harris type I fractures; clavicular injuries; nondisplaced upper extremity, foot, and phalangeal fractures; incomplete, nondisplaced fractures of the long bones of the lower extremity; and routine dislocations of minor joints and the shoulder can all be managed initially by physicians other than orthopedists (Table 114.1).

Acute Fracture Care

Immobilization is the mainstay of the initial treatment of any fracture. Plaster and fiberglass materials are both satisfactory, although the greater strength of fiberglass has advantages in splinting of lower extremities. Immobilization of the joints above and below the fracture provides both the greatest degree of comfort and the best guarantee against additional injury or deformity. (An exception is a minor torus fracture of the distal forearm, for which a short arm splint or cast is often adequate.) Several layers of padding material should always be applied before the actual splint or cast because the padding provides greater comfort, and the risk of neurovascular compromise, if swelling occurs, is diminished. (See Section VII "Procedures," for detailed descriptions of splinting techniques.) The degree of actual or anticipated swelling, the

propensity of the fracture to lead to a compartment syndrome, and the training of the emergency physician dictate whether a splint or a cast is applied at the time of initial evaluation.

Most fractures that are initially casted should be reevaluated within 24 hours for signs of neurovascular compromise, either in the ED or by the orthopedist. Otherwise, when orthopedic follow-up is necessary, an appointment within the week following injury is generally reasonable (assuming the immobilization is adequate). Certain injuries (e.g., any fracture that could possibly displace) should be seen more promptly. Other fractures need no orthopedic referral. Discharge instructions should include a review of the need for elevation and ice application and a discussion of the signs of neurovascular compromise. The need for pain medication in children should not be ignored. Ibuprofen or oxycodone alone are adequate in most cases. All radiographs should be reviewed by a radiologist, and parents should be routinely informed that further evaluation and radiographs will be necessary despite initially negative studies if symptoms persist. The importance of immobilization of all but the most minor injuries and of careful documentation of follow-up instructions cannot be overemphasized.

Postfracture Care

Two factors influence the function regained following fractures in children: the establishment of a bony union, and the restoration of normal alignment and growth. Unlike postfracture care for the adult, physical therapy is usually not necessary to regain normal range of motion. Stiffness rarely becomes a long-standing problem for children. The child acts as his or her own physical therapist through normal activities. On occasion, it may become necessary for the parents or physical therapist to "supervise" active range-of-motion exercises until normal range of motion is obtained. If the orthopedic injury is associated with tissue loss, head injury, nerve damage, or vascular compromise, physical and occupational therapy may play a major role in reestablishing normal or near-normal function in the child.

SPECIAL CONSIDERATIONS

Open Fractures

Several considerations dictate that the emergency physician approach open fractures with special concern. Such fractures generally result from high-energy accidents, namely falls, motor vehicle collisions, and automobile–pedestrian accidents. Multiple injuries are common in such settings. The physician should not allow an open fracture to distract from the detection and orderly management of other less apparent but potentially life-threatening injuries. A complete examination is imperative.

The incidence of complications is higher with open fractures, and a complete evaluation for neurovascular compromise and for signs of compartment syndrome should be performed. In addition, the incidence of infection is increased with open fractures. Management should include cleansing the wound, applying a sterile Betadine® dressing, administering prophylactic intravenous antibiotics (e.g., broad-spectrum cephalosporins), and immobilizing the fracture. Tetanus prophylaxis should be administered according to the usual guidelines. Clearly, open fractures must be regarded as true orthopedic emergencies. Surgical debridement, irrigation, and definitive care of the wound and fracture are uniformly necessary. The patient should be given nothing by mouth, and an urgent orthopedic consultation should be obtained. The laceration over a fracture should never be closed, even if the fracture is in good alignment.

Compartment Syndrome

The compartment syndrome is a devastating fracture complication that, if left untreated, may progress to muscle necrosis and nerve palsies. It occurs when a buildup of intracompartmental pressure results in ischemia of the muscle and neurovascular tissue. The pressure initially blocks venous outflow, resulting in increased pressure in the nonelastic compartment. Eventually, the small arterioles and capillaries are occluded, and irreversible muscle and nerve damage results.

The compartment syndrome can occur in the forearm, hand, thigh, leg, or foot; the most common site is the anterior compartment of the leg. The fracture does not need to be severe; indeed, the compartments are often torn with significantly displaced fractures and thus are less subject to pressure buildup. Pain, particularly pain with passive extension, is the earliest sign of the compartment syndrome. With any fracture or blunt tissue injury presenting with pain out of proportion to the injury, the compartment syndrome must be suspected. An increasing analgesic requirement in the setting of an acute fracture should by itself prompt consideration of this diagnosis. On palpation, the muscular compartment may feel hard, swollen, and tense. Other physical signs, including pulselessness, paresthesia, pallor, and paralysis, may or may not be present. Direct measurement of compartmental pressures confirms the diagnosis. When clinical and objective signs of compartment syndrome are present, a fasciotomy should be performed as soon as possible.

In the patient with multiple injuries, it is imperative to palpate every muscular compartment to rule out impending compartment syndrome. An orthopedic consultation should be obtained in every case of suspected compartment syndrome.

Multiple Trauma

Although fractures are common in the child with multiple injuries, only rarely are they life-threatening. There is no question that orthopedic injuries are often the most obvious or that more children require operative orthopedic surgical procedures than general surgical procedures after major trauma. In contrast, it is definitely a mistake to disregard the usual tenets of trauma management and forsake an orderly and thorough evaluation of a child's respiratory, cardiovascular, and neurologic status in a rush to provide fracture care. The B of the ABCs is not for bone.

Only in a few instances is the blood loss associated with a fracture significant enough to cause signs of shock. Exceptions include extensive pelvic fractures and multiple long bone fractures (even an isolated femur fracture rarely causes hemodynamic compromise). Clearly, then, signs of significant volume loss in a child believed only to have sustained fractures should prompt an immediate search for other injuries.

In most instances, initial fracture management in the ED should consist simply of immobilization. Traction splints are extremely useful for lower-extremity fractures. The role of pneumatic antishock garments continues to be debated; their use should be considered for unstable pelvic injuries. On occasion, application of an external fixator device may help tamponade bleeding from such fractures.

Many fractures, primarily nondisplaced ones, go undetected during initial ED management. Little harm occurs as a result. In contrast, the consequences of missing a thoracic or lumbar spine fracture can obviously be much greater. Physical signs of such fractures are generally lacking, and the status of the child often precludes an assessment of pain and neurologic function. When the mechanism of injury is unknown or suggests the possibility of a spinal injury, radiographs should be ordered and careful immobilization maintained.

Child Abuse

Although the diagnostic significance of skeletal injuries in child abuse has long been recognized, only 5% to 18% of abused children sustain fractures. In contrast, a large percentage of fractures in infants younger than 1 year do not result from accidents. Careful consideration of the details of the injury, particularly from the viewpoint of the child's developmental stage, provides the first clue regarding the likelihood of abuse. Only a limited number of fracture types and patterns can be considered almost uniformly specific for child abuse (Table 114.2). The incidental discovery of rib fractures, generally posterior, on a chest radiograph should prompt consideration of abuse and raise the possibility of injuries involving the bones of the extremities. In most cases of abuse, the radiographic findings will not by themselves confirm suspicions of an intentional injury. Although spiral fractures in nonambulating children and metaphyseal-epiphyseal injuries are essentially diagnostic, transverse fractures are common and diaphyseal fractures predominate in both abused and nonabused children (Figs. 114.9 to 114.11).

As for diagnostic studies, any clinically suspected fracture should be evaluated using the radiographic views customary for the site in question. In addition, a skeletal survey must be performed routinely as part of the evaluation of all cases of

---

TABLE 114.2

FRACTURES STRONGLY SUGGESTIVE OF CHILD ABUSE

1. Fractures inconsistent with history
2. Fractures inconsistent with developmental stage of child
3. Fractures with associated injuries suggestive of abuse
4. Multiple fractures, particularly in various stages of healing
5. Multiple, complex, or depressed skull fractures
6. Epiphyseal–metaphyseal rib fractures
7. Spiral fractures of the femur or tibia in preambulating children
8. Spiral fractures of the humerus
9. Metaphyseal chip (corner) fractures
10. Avulsion fractures of clavicle and acromion process

TRAUMA

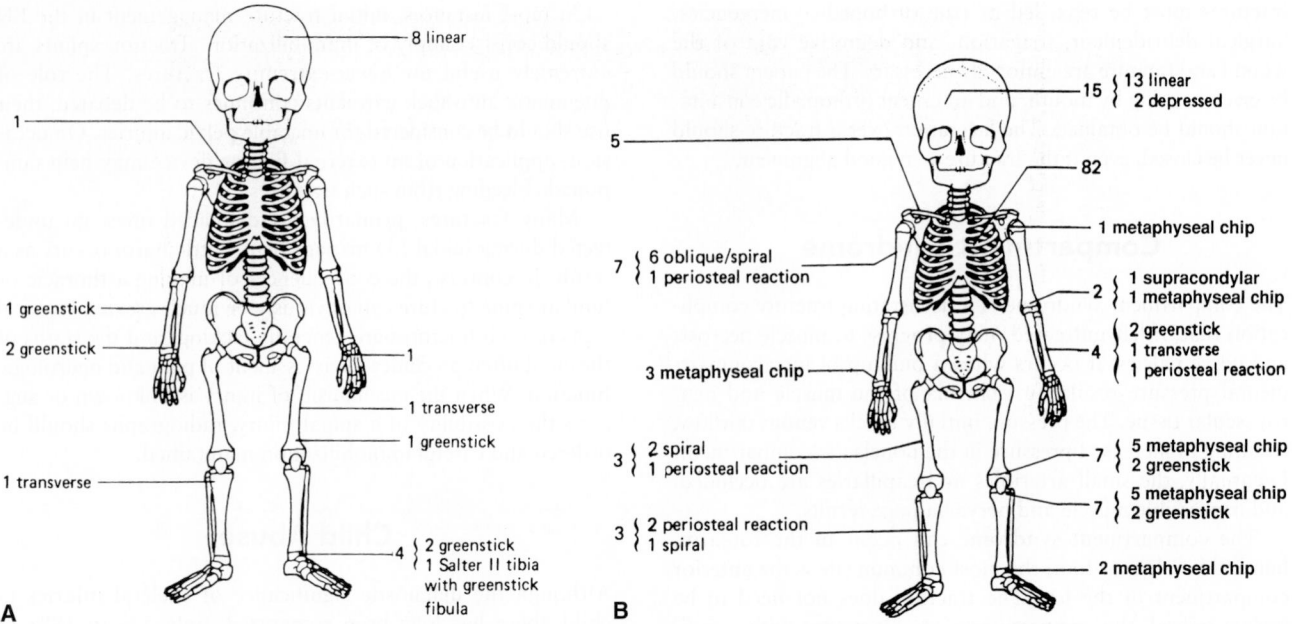

FIGURE 114.9 Comparison of the locations and types of accidental (**A**) and nonaccidental (**B**) fractures in infants younger than 18 months. (From Worlock P, Stower M, Barbor P. Patterns of fractures in accidental and nonaccidental injury in children. *BMJ* 1986;293:100–102, reprinted with permission.)

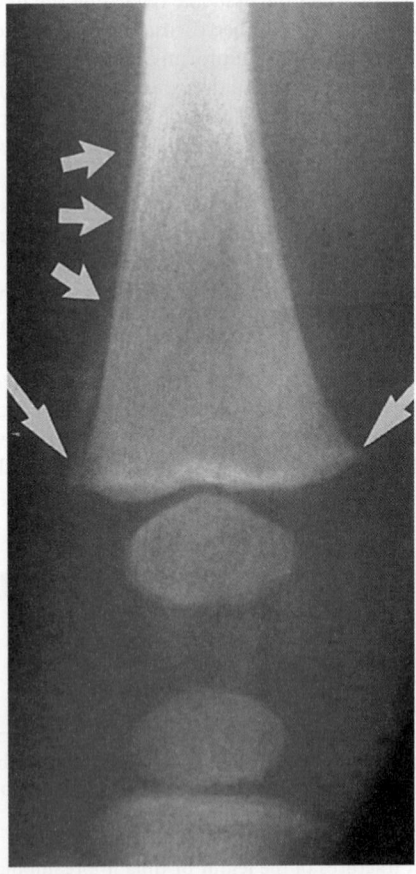

FIGURE 114.10 Radiograph of the right knee of a 3.5-month-old victim of child abuse. The metaphyseal corner fractures *(large arrows)* are considered diagnostic of abuse. Also evident is periosteal new bone formation *(small arrows)*, proof of a significant delay between injury and medical evaluation.

strongly suspected abuse in children younger than 2 years. For children 2 to 5 years of age, individual considerations determine whether a skeletal survey is needed. Skeletal surveys have little role in the evaluation of children older than 5 years. Routine radionuclide bone scans are not indicated, although this technique may be an adjunct to the detection of subtle rib and long bone shaft fractures, as well as of some spine injuries.

Pathologic Fractures

A pathologic fracture is one that occurs through abnormal bone. Many conditions, including tumors, hereditary diseases, metabolic disorders, neuromuscular diseases, and infections, can cause either generalized or localized bone weakness (Table 114.3 and Figs. 114.12 and 114.13). On occasion, the predisposing condition does not become obvious until a fracture occurs. All pathologic fractures require orthopedic consultation. The nature of the underlying disease that is identified or suspected determines the need for consultation of other specialists. In most instances, the initial treatment parallels that of a nonpathologic fracture in the same site.

INJURIES OF THE UPPER EXTREMITIES

Injuries of the Shoulder Region

For the purpose of this discussion, injuries of the shoulder region are grouped as follows: (i) clavicular fractures, (ii) scapular fractures, and (iii) shoulder dislocations.

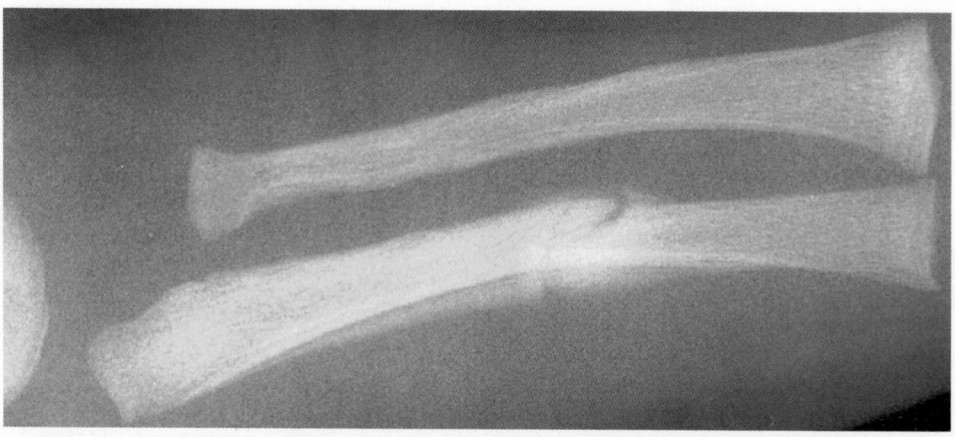

FIGURE 114.11 Radiograph of the left forearm of a 3-month-old victim of child abuse. Although the ulnar fracture is transverse and thus by itself is not diagnostic of intentional injury, both the child's age and the extent of periosteal bone formation (again establishing a significant delay between diagnosis and medical evaluation) should strongly suggest the possibility of child abuse to the examining physician.

TABLE 114.3

DIFFERENTIAL DIAGNOSIS OF PATHOLOGIC FRACTURES

Tumors and cysts—Benign
Aneurysmal bone cyst
Endochondroma
Eosinophilic granuloma
Fibrous dysplasia
Giant cell tumor
Nonossifying fibroma
Osteochondroma
Unicameral bone cyst

Tumors—Malignant
Chondrosarcoma
Ewing's sarcoma
Neuroblastoma
Osteogenic sarcoma

Hereditary diseases
Gaucher's disease
Neurofibromatosis
Osteogenesis imperfecta
Osteopetrosis
Sickle cell disease

Metabolic disorders
Copper deficiency
Cushing's syndrome
Hyperparathyroidism
Renal osteodystrophy
Rickets
Scurvy

Neuromuscular diseases (osteoporosis from disuse)
Cerebral palsy
Muscular dystrophy
Poliomyelitis
Severe head injury
Spina bifida with paraplegia
Traumatic paraplegia or quadriplegia

Infections
Osteomyelitis

Clavicular Fractures

The clavicle ranks as the most commonly fractured bone in children. More than one-half of all clavicular fractures occur in children younger than 10 years. In children younger than 2 years (excluding the newborn period), such fractures are uncommon and should provoke consideration of intentional trauma. For the sake of discussion, clavicular injuries can be divided into fractures of the shaft, the medial end, and the lateral end.

Fractures of the clavicular shaft result from direct trauma and from indirect forces transmitted by falls onto an outstretched hand. Most are greenstick injuries of the midshaft; the thick periosteum enveloping the clavicle prevents significant displacement or angulation. The diagnosis is usually self-evident. Typically, a child complains of shoulder pain and is cradling the arm on the injured side with the opposite one. Occasionally, the initial injury is unnoticed and comes to attention only when a lump appears as callus forms. Radiographs are confirmatory, although visualization of nondisplaced fractures may require several views. Despite the proximity of the brachial plexus and subclavian vessels, neurovascular injury is rare other than when a violent direct blow results in significant displacement of the fracture fragments. Medially, strong ligaments anchor the clavicle to the sternum. Eighty percent of the growth of the clavicle occurs at the medial physis. The last epiphysis in the body to close, the medial clavicular epiphysis, is rarely visible radiographically before 18 years of age. Apparent dislocations of the sternoclavicular joint are invariably epiphyseal separations in children and young adults. With such fractures, either anterior or posterior displacement can occur. The direction of displacement can often be determined by direct palpation. Radiographic visualization may be difficult; special views and/or CT scans are often required to define the degree and direction of displacement. Posterior displacement is of particular concern because compression of the mediastinal vessels and the trachea can result. If there is evidence of neurovascular or respiratory compromise, prompt orthopedic consultation and closed reduction are indicated.

TRAUMA

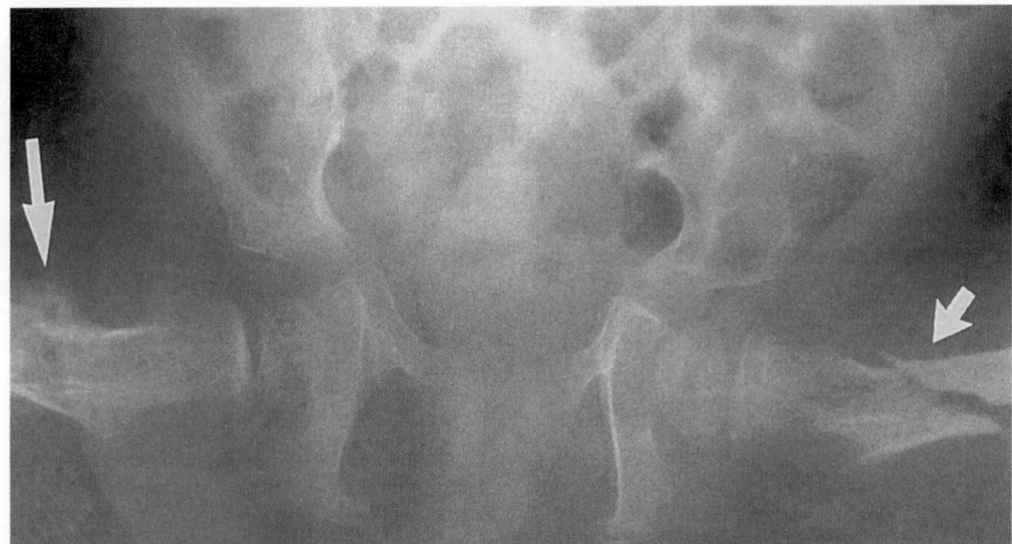

FIGURE 114.12 Radiograph of the pelvis and femur of an 18-month-old girl with osteogenesis imperfecta. There is a healing fracture of the right femur *(large arrow)*, as well as an acute fracture of the left femur *(small arrow)*.

Laterally, the coracoclavicular and acromioclavicular ligaments anchor the clavicle. Once again, fracture through the physis rather than dislocation is the rule. The usual mechanism of injury is a direct blow to the point of the shoulder. Typically, the proximal fracture fragment is displaced superiorly; the radiographic appearance suggests acromioclavicular separation. However, the periosteum remains whole inferiorly, its ligamentous connections intact. As a result, most distal clavicular fractures heal uneventfully with no loss of joint stability (Fig. 114.14).

Only infrequently is immediate orthopedic consultation necessary for a clavicular injury. Exceptions include significantly displaced (greater than 2 cm) midshaft fractures, for which closed or on occasion open reduction with fixation is desirable; posteriorly and significantly anteriorly displaced medial fractures; grossly unstable distal injuries; and all open fractures. Orthopedic referral is also indicated when there is more than 1.5 cm of clavicle shortening. Immobilization in a sling for 3 weeks followed by 3 weeks of restriction from sporting activities is adequate treatment for most shaft fractures. It

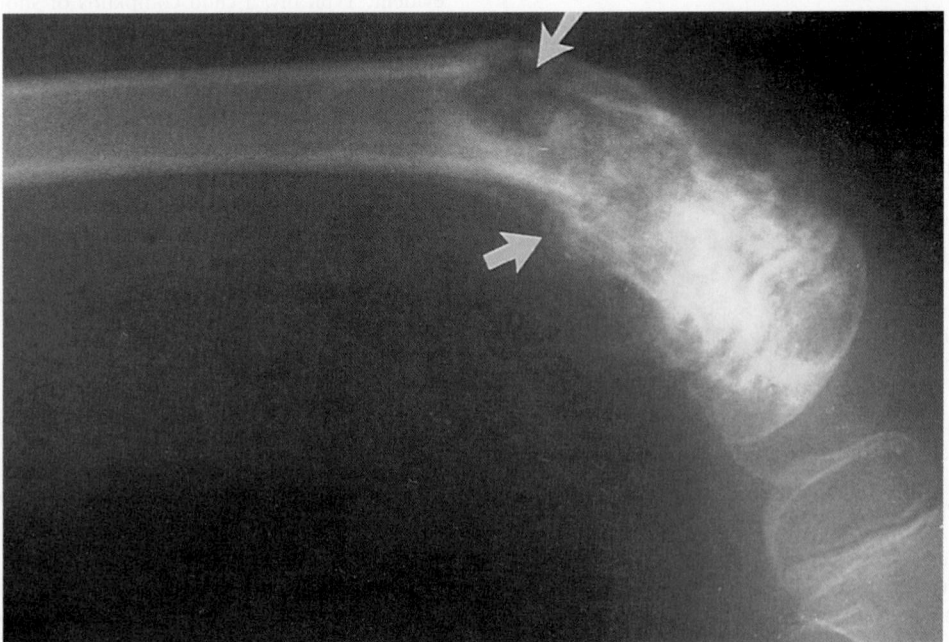

FIGURE 114.13 Radiograph of a 5-year-old girl with an osteosarcoma of the left femur showing an acute pathologic fracture *(arrows)*. Amputation was ultimately necessary.

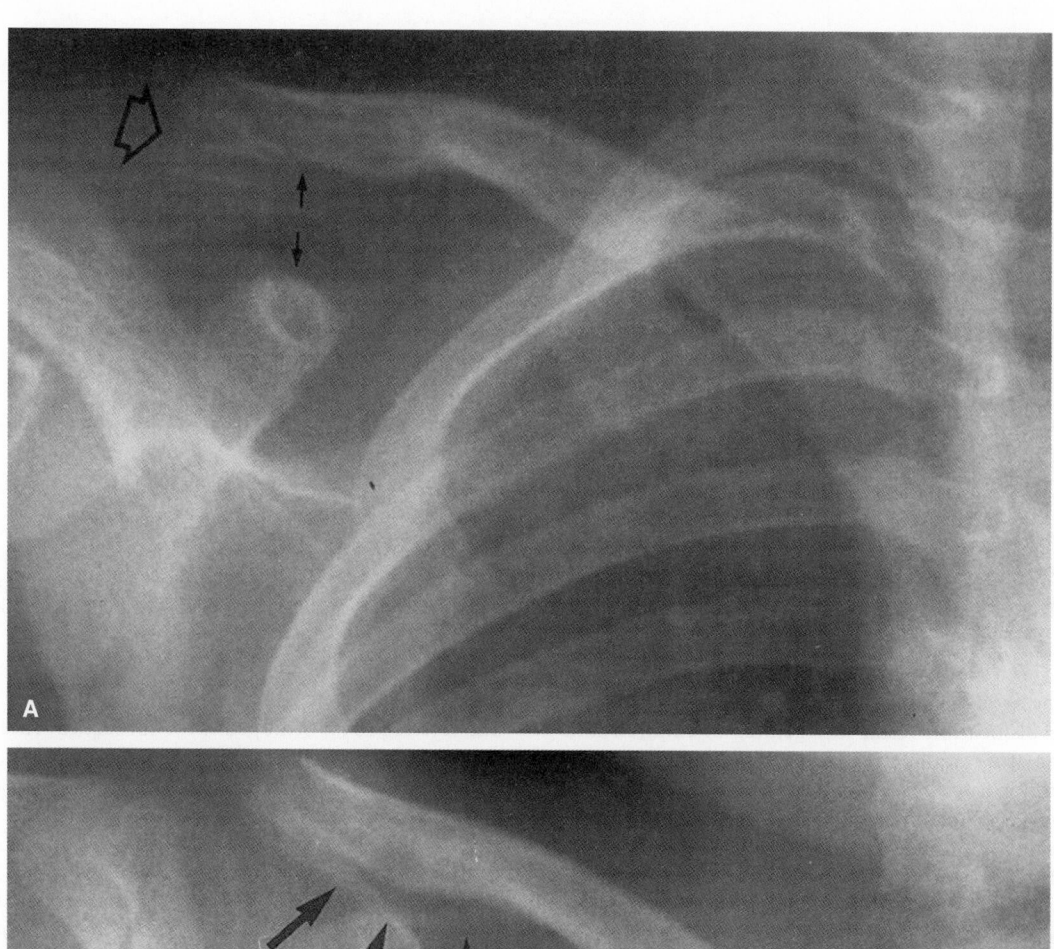

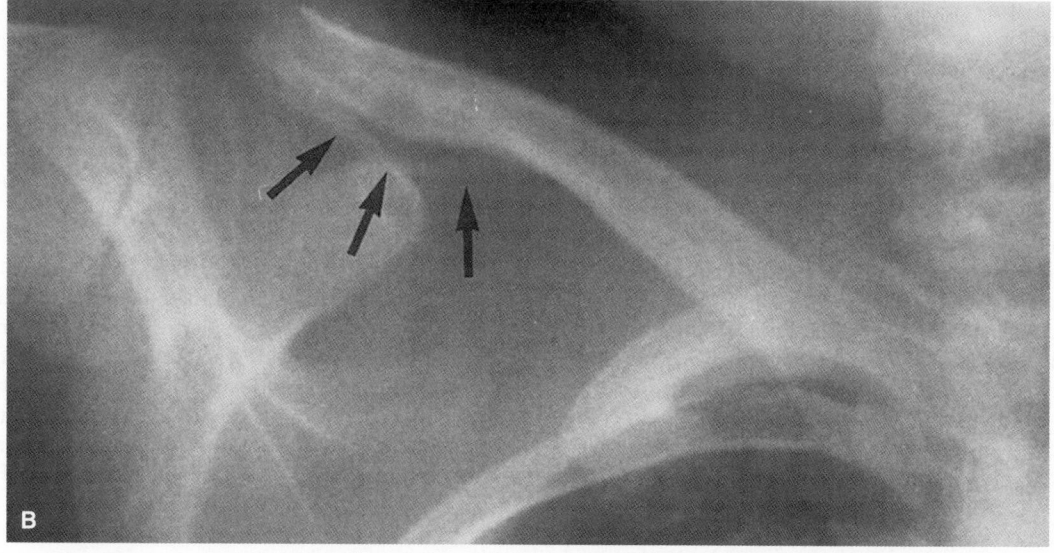

FIGURE 114.14 Radiograph of the right clavicle of a 5-year-old child. **A:** A lateral clavicular fracture *(open arrow)* and widening of the space between the clavicle and the coracoid process *(small arrows)* are evident on the initial film. **B:** The pattern of new bone formation *(arrows)* seen on the follow-up radiograph demonstrates that the periosteum and the ligaments have remained intact inferiorly.

is best to inform parents that a lump will appear as callus forms and may persist for as long as a year. With medial and distal fractures, a sling is recommended along with progressive motion as the pain subsides.

Scapular Fractures

Fractures of the scapula are unusual in adolescents and rare in children. In the isolated instances in which they do occur, the usual mechanism is a severe direct blow, such as one sustained in a fall from a height or a motor vehicle accident (Fig. 114.15). The same force that produces the scapular fracture

may result in more concerning and potentially life-threatening injuries to the chest, neck, or head. Fractures of the body and neck of the scapula are usually well visualized on plain radiographs; adequate definition of glenoid injuries may require a CT scan. Although a sling and swathe is usually the only treatment necessary, orthopedic consultation is suggested given the rarity of these injuries.

Shoulder Dislocations

Dislocations of the shoulder are unusual before physeal closure. Other than medially, the proximal humeral physis runs

TRAUMA

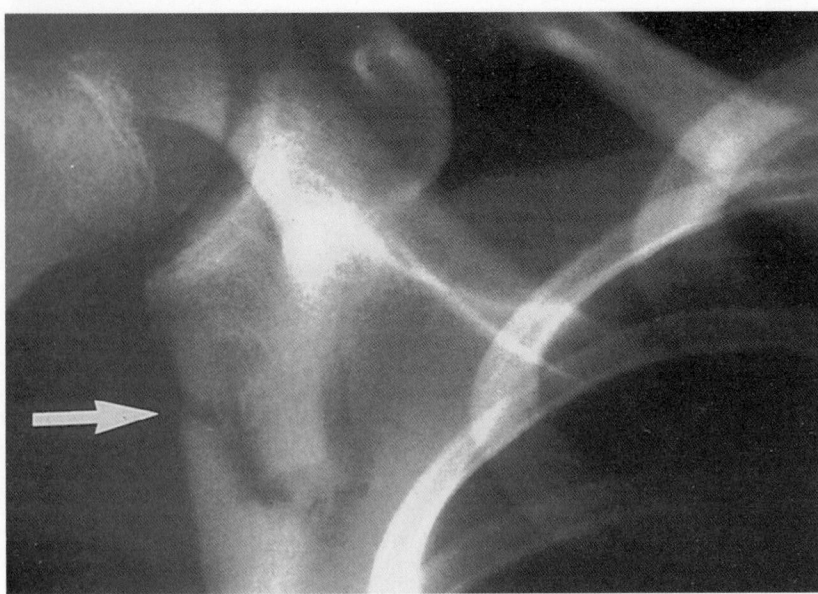

FIGURE 114.15 Radiograph of a 13-year-old boy who sustained an isolated right scapular fracture as the result of a skateboarding accident *(arrow)*.

external to the shoulder capsule, and injuries that in an adult would cause dislocation result in fractures in children and skeletally immature adolescents. Most dislocations that do occur are anterior, as is the case with adults. Findings on physical examination include swelling and deformity with loss of the usual rounded contour of the shoulder. Palpation generally reveals the displacement of the humeral head anterior to the glenoid fossa. Signs of axillary nerve injury may be present. Radiographic studies should include an axillary (Y) view in addition to the customary views of the shoulder to best define the direction of displacement. As for treatment, closed reduction of anterior dislocations can be accomplished by numerous techniques, one of which is reviewed in detail in Section VII "Procedures." Postreduction radiographs should be performed routinely in part to ensure no fracture has occurred in conjunction with the dislocation. Given their rarity, posterior dislocations merit orthopedic consultation before reduction. The rate of chronic shoulder instability and recurrent dislocation is high; even seemingly routine anterior dislocations

should be immobilized in a sling and swathe for several weeks and referred to an orthopedist for subsequent care.

Fractures of the Humerus

In this section, humeral fractures are grouped as follows: (i) proximal humeral fractures and (ii) humeral shaft fractures. Supracondylar fractures are discussed in the "Injuries of the Elbow" section.

Proximal Humeral Fractures

About 80% of the growth of the humerus occurs at the proximal humeral physis. As a result, the potential for fracture healing and remodeling with fractures that involve the proximal humeral shaft and physis is remarkable. Nonunion is unheard of and malunion is rare, other than with significantly displaced or angulated injuries in older adolescents. Before adolescence, most proximal humeral fractures are metaphyseal (Fig. 114.16),

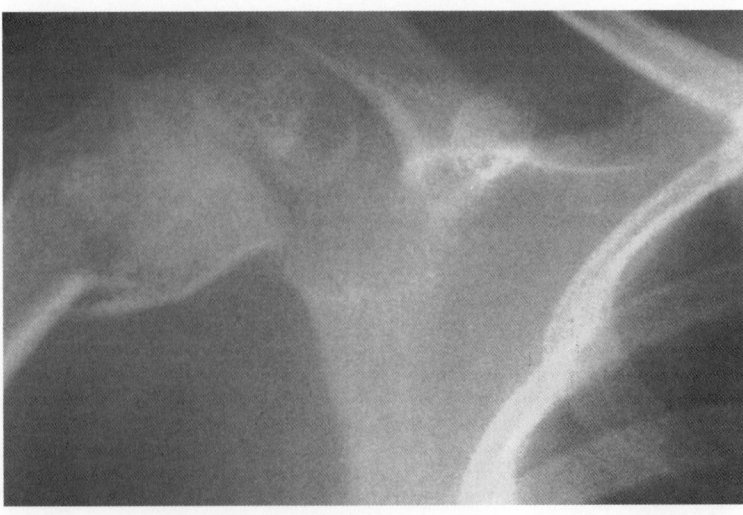

FIGURE 114.16 Impacted proximal right humeral fracture with approximately 25 degrees of angulation in a 3-year-old child. Full remodeling can be anticipated.

although Salter-Harris type I injuries are seen occasionally. With the onset of adolescence, rapid growth makes the physeal region relatively weak and thus vulnerable to injury. The incidence of proximal humeral fractures is highest in this age group; most are Salter-Harris type II injuries, and type III, IV, and V injuries are most unusual. Common mechanisms of injury include falls on an extended, adducted arm and direct blows to the shoulder.

Physical findings with proximal humeral fractures range from mild swelling to obvious deformity and shortening of the arm. Routine radiographs are generally sufficient. Care must be taken not to confuse the normal variations in the epiphyseal line with a fracture; comparison views can be useful. Conservative management is the rule. Before adolescence, as much as 50 degrees or even 70 degrees of angulation is satisfactory. In younger children, even totally displaced fractures can remodel completely. Recommendations regarding the degree of deformity acceptable in adolescents vary somewhat; 20 to 50 degrees of angulation and 50% apposition are generally tolerable. The indications for open reduction are limited. A sling and swathe for several weeks is usually the only treatment necessary. Orthopedic follow-up is recommended.

Humeral Shaft Fractures

Fractures of the humeral shaft are much less common than those involving either the proximal or distal segments. The pattern of fracture reflects the mechanism of injury; transverse fractures result from direct blows, whereas spiral fractures are caused by indirect twisting, as with a fall. When a child younger than 3 years sustains a spiral fracture of the humerus, the possibility of child abuse must be considered seriously (Fig. 114.17).

Many humeral fractures are obvious on physical examination, although only minimal swelling and tenderness may be present with buckle and greenstick injuries. Vascular injury is relatively uncommon. In contrast, evidence of radial nerve injury must always be sought, particularly with a fracture that involves the distal two thirds of the humeral shaft. Physical findings suggestive of damage to the radial nerve include loss of motor strength in the extensors of the wrist and fingers, as well as loss of sensation on the dorsum of the hand in the web space between the thumb and index finger. Of note is that, with proper fracture management, almost all cases of radial nerve palsy resolve. As for radiographs, anteroposterior and lateral views usually suffice. A prominent vascular groove in the distal humerus is a normal finding that should not be confused with a fracture.

The thick periosteal sleeve of the humeral shaft limits fracture displacement and promotes rapid healing. A sling and swathe is all that is needed for incomplete fractures. For complete or minimally displaced fractures, application of a sugar-tong splint of the upper arm, followed by a sling to support the forearm is recommended. In older children and adolescents, a hanging long arm cast is an alternative. Given the potential for overgrowth with healing, overriding of the fracture fragments by up to 2 cm is acceptable. Remodeling of as much as 40 degrees of angulation can be expected in younger children. Immediate orthopedic consultation is suggested for any completely displaced fracture, any fracture angulated more than 20 degrees in children and 10 degrees in adolescents, and any fracture with evidence of radial nerve injury. All humeral fractures should be referred for orthopedic follow-up within 5 days.

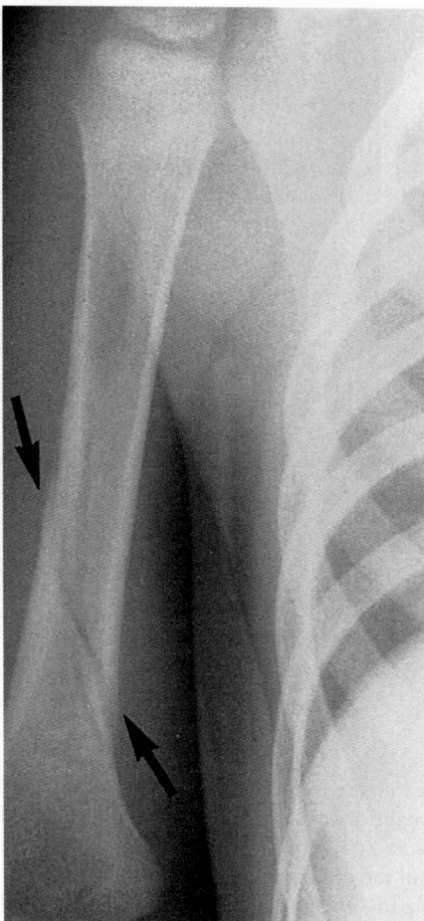

FIGURE 114.17 Spiral fracture of the right humerus in an 18-month-old girl. Although in this case the injury was accidental, spiral humeral fractures in children younger than 3 years must always evoke concerns about child abuse.

Injuries of the Elbow

Normal Anatomy and Radiographic Diagnosis

Of all the fractures encountered in the pediatric age group, those of the elbow rank as the most problematic in terms of diagnosis, treatment, and complications. In addition, they are quite common, accounting for approximately 15% of all pediatric fractures. For the emergency physician, an understanding of normal anatomy and normal radiographic findings ensures misdiagnosis and untoward outcomes are uncommon. The elbow is a complex hinge joint composed of three separate articulations, namely those between the trochlea of the humerus and the ulnar notch, the capitellum and the radial head, and the proximal radius and ulna (Fig. 114.18). To further complicate matters, there are four growth centers within the distal humerus alone, and ossification of these growth centers begins at different but predictable times (Table 114.4). The ages shown in Table 114.4 are averages; ossification begins at an earlier age in girls than in boys, and much variation exists overall. When there is confusion about what is a normal growth center and what is a fracture fragment, comparison views of the uninjured elbow can be extremely helpful.

TRAUMA

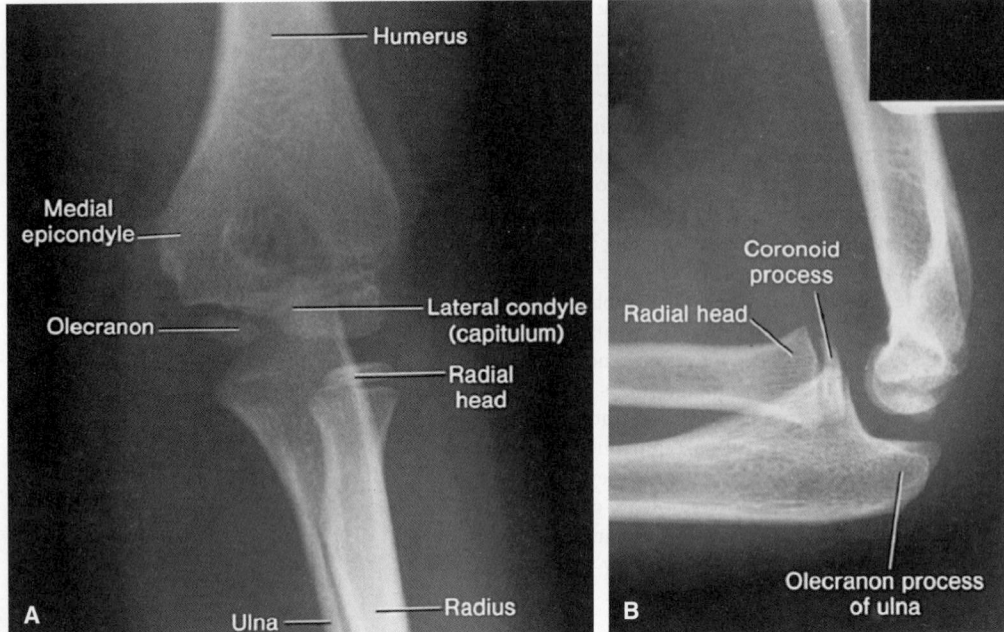

FIGURE 114.18 **A:** Anteroposterior radiograph of a normal elbow of a child. **B:** Normal lateral radiograph.

When a fracture is grossly displaced, the radiographic diagnosis is straightforward. Radiographic detection of subtle torus and nondisplaced fractures of the elbow joint is difficult. Close inspection of the radiographs for the presence of abnormalities of the fat pads and the anterior humeral line will prevent missed diagnosis in most cases. These radiographic signs are reliable only if the elbow has been properly positioned for the radiographs; the importance of a true lateral view in particular cannot be overemphasized. Of the two fat pads overlying the joint capsule along the distal humerus, only the anterior fat pad is normally visible on a lateral radiograph (Fig. 114.19). When fluid is in the joint space, as with a hemarthrosis from a fracture, these fat pads are displaced upward and outward (Fig. 114.20). If soft-tissue edema is extensive, one or both of the fat pads, although elevated, may be obscured. In the setting of known or suspected trauma, the presence of an abnormal fat pad sign should be considered a marker of an occult fracture and an indication for careful immobilization and close follow-up. Of note is that fractures of the distal humerus and of the proximal radius and ulna can produce a hemarthrosis and thus positive fat pad signs. On occasion, oblique views will reveal the fracture line. MRI studies in this setting can reveal bony

and soft-tissue injuries not evident on plain radiographs, but should not be routinely ordered given the lack of any well-defined impact on actual patient management.

Close inspection of a true lateral view of the elbow for abnormalities of the anterior humeral line is also essential. In the normal elbow, a line drawn through the anterior cortex of the humerus intersects the capitellum in its middle third

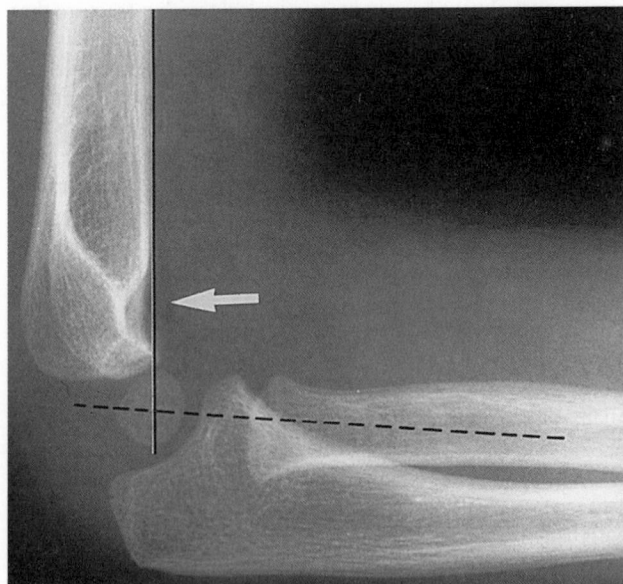

FIGURE 114.19 Normal lateral radiograph of the elbow of a 2-year-old child. The anterior fat pad is readily seen *(arrow)*; the posterior fat pad is not visible. A line drawn along the anterior cortex of the humerus intersects the capitellum in its middle third *(solid line)*. A line drawn along the axis of the radius also passes through the center of the capitellum *(dashed line)*.

TABLE 114.4

GROWTH CENTERS OF ELBOW: AVERAGE AGE FOR ONSET OF OSSIFICATION

Capitellum	11 mo
Medial epicondyle	4–6 yr
Trochlea	9–10 yr
Lateral epicondyle	10–12 yr
Radial head	5–6 yr
Olecranon	6–8 yr

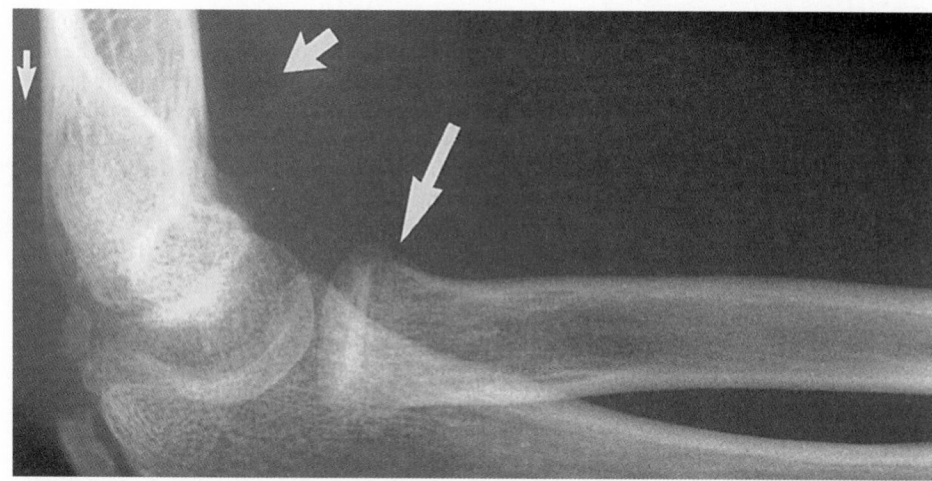

FIGURE 114.20 Lateral radiograph of the elbow of a 12-year-old girl, demonstrating marked elevations of both the anterior and posterior fat pads *(small arrows)*. A subtle radial neck fracture is also visible *(large arrow)*.

(Fig. 114.19). Because the most common mechanism of injury to the elbow is hyperextension, posterior displacement of the distal humerus is to be expected when a fracture occurs. As a result, the anterior humeral line, rather than intersecting the middle third of the capitellum, passes through its anterior third or even fails to intersect it all together (Fig. 114.21). Detection of abnormalities of the anterior humeral line in children younger than 2.5 years is complicated by the variable rates of ossification of the capitellum; once again, comparison views can be helpful in uncertain cases. In summary, errors in the management of pediatric elbow injuries can be minimized by an understanding of normal anatomy and development, careful interpretation of properly obtained radiographs, and immobilization with careful follow-up when there is even the mildest suspicion of a fracture. For the sake of discussion,

elbow injuries are divided as follows: (i) supracondylar fractures, (ii) lateral condylar fractures, (iii) medial epicondylar fractures, (iv) distal humeral physeal fractures, (v) olecranon fractures, (vi) radial head and neck fractures, (vii) elbow dislocations, and (viii) radial head subluxation.

Some of these injuries are presented diagrammatically in Figure 114.22. Fractures of the medial humeral condyle and the lateral humeral epicondyle are rare and therefore not discussed.

Supracondylar Fractures

Supracondylar fractures account for a large proportion of the fractures of the elbow in the pediatric age group. Most are sustained by children 3 to 10 years of age. A fall on the outstretched arm with hyperextension of the elbow is the most common mechanism. Accordingly, posterior angulation or displacement of the distal fracture fragment nearly always occurs (Fig. 114.23). A direct blow to the posterior aspect of the elbow can lead to anterior angulation or displacement of the

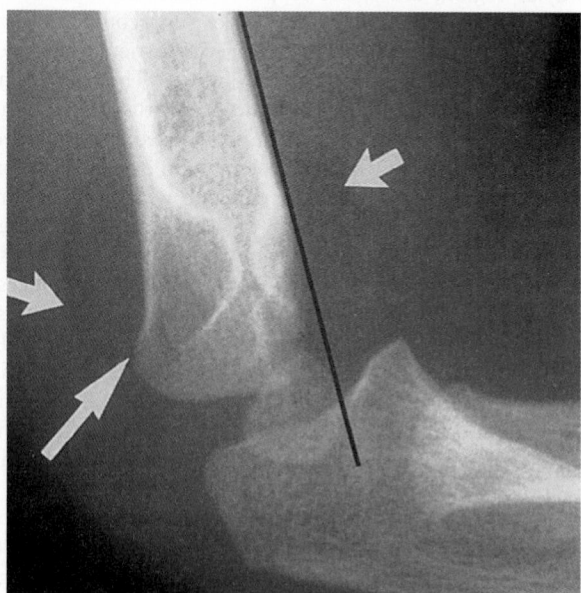

FIGURE 114.21 Lateral radiograph of the elbow of a 2-year-old girl. Once again, both the anterior and posterior fat pads are elevated *(small arrows)*. In addition, the anterior humeral line passes along the anterior edge of the capitellum rather than through its center. Mild buckling of the posterior cortex of the distal humerus can be seen *(large arrow)*.

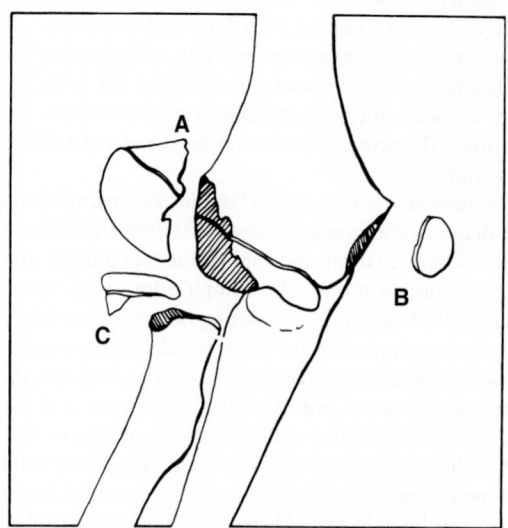

FIGURE 114.22 Common elbow fractures in children: lateral condylar fracture (**A**), medial epicondylar fracture (**B**), and radial neck fracture (**C**).

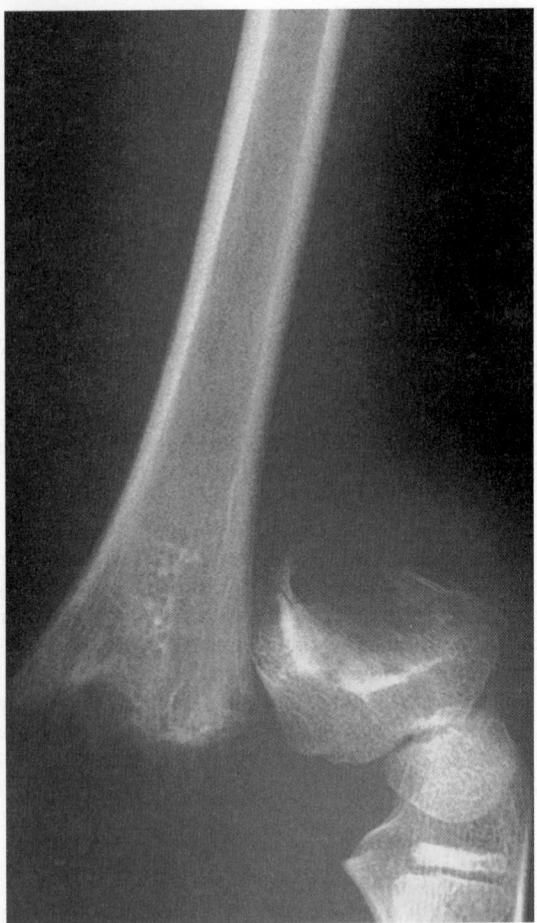

FIGURE 114.23 Displaced and rotated supracondylar fracture in an 8-year-old girl. The distal pulses were absent in this case but returned with reduction of the injury.

distal fragment, but such injuries are rare by comparison. With minimally displaced or nondisplaced fractures, recognition can be difficult. There may be only mild soft-tissue swelling. A suggestive history coupled with localized tenderness should prompt a radiologic examination. The radiographic findings may also be subtle. Close attention to the fat pads and the anterior humeral line, as detailed previously, facilitate diagnosis. At times, the actual fracture may be visualized only with an oblique view.

With more severe supracondylar injuries, the problem is not that of diagnosis (although a dislocated elbow may have a similar clinical presentation) but that of the recognition and prevention of complications. The complications associated with supracondylar fractures are multiple, ranging from immediate neurovascular compromise to long-term deformities and range-of-motion abnormalities. For the emergency physician, the first priorities are those of neurovascular assessment and fracture stabilization. The vascular examination should begin with palpation of the distal pulses and assessment of capillary refill. Use of a Doppler may allow detection of distal arterial flow when no pulse can be palpated. Absence of a pulse by itself is not extremely worrisome. Direct vascular injury is uncommon. In most instances, vasospasm or arterial compression has occurred instead, and arterial flow will resume with fracture reduction. In contrast, significant muscle ischemia can be present even when pulses and capillary refill are judged to be normal. Forearm pain, pain with passive extension of the fingers, paralysis of finger extension, and paresthesias are each worrisome and should be considered evidence of an impending compartment syndrome. Supracondylar fractures associated with ipsilateral forearm fractures are injuries at particularly high-risk for development of ischemic injury.

Neurologic deficits, usually transient, are also common with supracondylar fractures. Radial, medial, and ulnar nerve palsies all occur, as do isolated injuries of the anterior interosseous nerve (a motor branch of the median nerve). Table 114.5 outlines the innervation of these nerves and should be used as a guide to the neurologic examination. Once the neurovascular examination is completed and *before* radiographic studies, all displaced supracondylar fractures must be immobilized. It is usually best to simply splint the limb in the deformed position in which it lies. More than 20 to 30 degrees of elbow flexion will place undue tension on the neurovascular structures and should be avoided. All patients must have nothing by mouth because reduction, whether open or closed, requires general anesthesia. Frequent repeat neurovascular examinations should be performed and documented.

Minimally displaced or nondisplaced supracondylar fractures may be immobilized in a well-padded long arm posterior splint with the elbow at 90 degrees and the forearm in pronation or neutral rotation. Orthopedic referral for casting is suggested when the swelling subsides. Immobilization for a total of 3 weeks is adequate in most cases. All nonminimally displaced supracondylar fractures require immediate orthopedic referral.

Lateral Condylar Fractures

Fractures of the lateral condyle, like those of the supracondylar region, are prone to poor functional outcome if misdiagnosed or mismanaged. Unlike supracondylar fractures, lateral condyle injuries involve the articular surface; they are true Salter-Harris type IV injuries. The most commonly proposed mechanism of injury is a varus stress on the elbow, as can occur with a fall on an extended and abducted arm. The lateral ligament and the common extensor tendon remain attached to the fracture fragment, which can be partially or totally avulsed from the distal humerus (Fig. 114.24). Clinically, swelling, ecchymosis, and tenderness localized over the lateral aspect of the elbow should suggest a lateral condylar fracture. With severely displaced fractures, routine anteroposterior and lateral views usually provide adequate fracture definition. With less severe injuries, the fracture line and the degree of displacement may be evident only on oblique views. On occasion, stress views, a CT scan, or an MRI study may be needed to adequately visualize the extent of injury.

For minimally displaced and nondisplaced injuries, immobilization in a posterior splint with the elbow flexed to 90 degrees and the forearm in pronation (some authorities suggest supination instead) is satisfactory emergency management. Lateral condylar fractures as a group are inherently unstable and prone to displace despite immobilization; orthopedic follow-up within 3 to 4 days is essential. All fractures displaced more than 2 mm require reduction and often pinning.

TABLE 114.5

GUIDE TO NEUROLOGIC EXAMINATION OF DISTAL UPPER EXTREMITY

A. Motor function		
Nerve	Muscles innervated	Motor examination
Radial	Extensor carpi radialis longus	Wrist extension
Ulnar	Flexor carpi ulnaris Interosseous	Wrist flexion and adduction Finger spread
Median	Flexor carpi radialis Flexor digitorum superficialis Opponens pollicis	Wrist flexion and abduction Flexion fingers at proximal interphalangeal joint Opposition thumb to base of little finger
Anterior interosseous	Flexor digitorum profundus I and II Flexor pollicis longus	Flexion distal phalanx of index finger Flexion distal phalanx of thumb
B. Sensory function		
Nerve	Sensory innervation	
Radial	Dorsal web space between thumb and index finger	
Ulnar	Ulnar aspect palm and dorsum of hand Little finger and ulnar aspect of ring finger	
Median	Radial aspect palm of hand Thumb, index, middle, radial aspect ring finger	
Anterior interosseous	None	

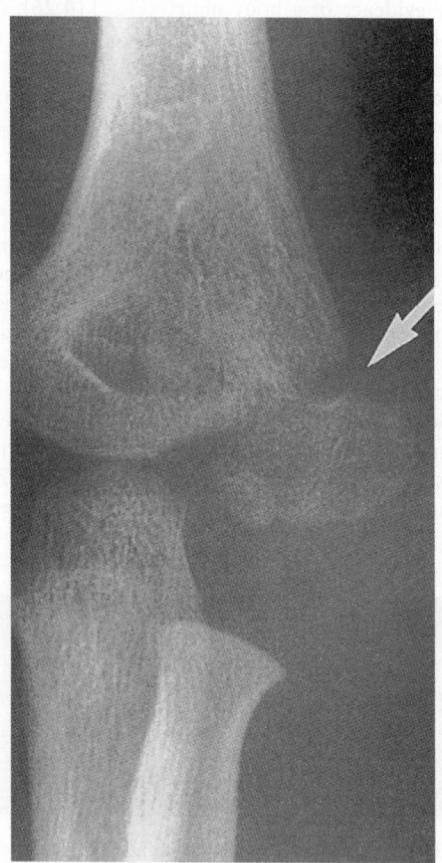

FIGURE 114.24 Lateral condylar fracture in a 2-year-old girl *(arrow)*.

Medial Epicondylar Fractures

Fractures of the medial epicondyle occur as the result of falls directly onto the elbow and falls onto the outstretched arm in which the elbow is subjected to a valgus stress. With the latter mechanism, the flexor muscles of the forearm avulse the medial epicondyle from the humerus (Fig. 114.25). Medial epicondyle injuries are particularly common with elbow dislocations. The physical findings are those that would be expected, namely swelling and tenderness localized to the medial aspect of the elbow. Valgus instability may be evident. Given its proximity, paresis of the ulnar nerve can occur. Oblique views and comparison views may be needed on occasion. The diagnosis is particularly problematic before the onset of ossification of the medial epicondyle at 4 to 6 years of age; fortunately, it is an uncommon injury in younger children. In this setting, too, MRI examination may prove useful in defining the extent of the injury. Open reduction is almost invariably necessary for displaced fractures. Nondisplaced fractures can be placed in a posterior splint with the forearm in pronation. Orthopedic follow-up is encouraged strongly, as it is with most elbow injuries.

Distal Humerus Physeal Fractures

Fractures of the entire distal humerus physis are relatively uncommon. Most such injuries take place in children younger than 2.5 years, and almost all the remainder are sustained by children younger than 7 years. Recognition is both difficult and important, especially in infants, in whom this particular injury is often the result of child abuse. The proposed mechanism in abused children is forceful twisting of the arm that shears off the distal epiphysis. In children 5 to 7 years of age,

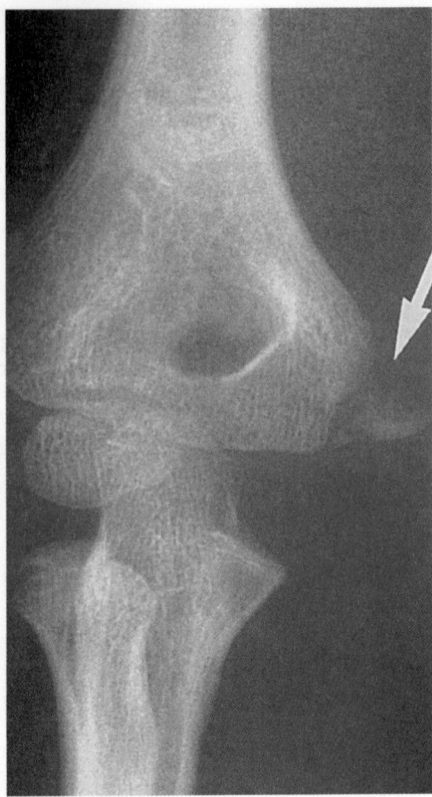

FIGURE 114.25 Displaced fracture of the medial epicondyle in an 8-year-old girl *(arrow)*. Note the extensive soft-tissue swelling.

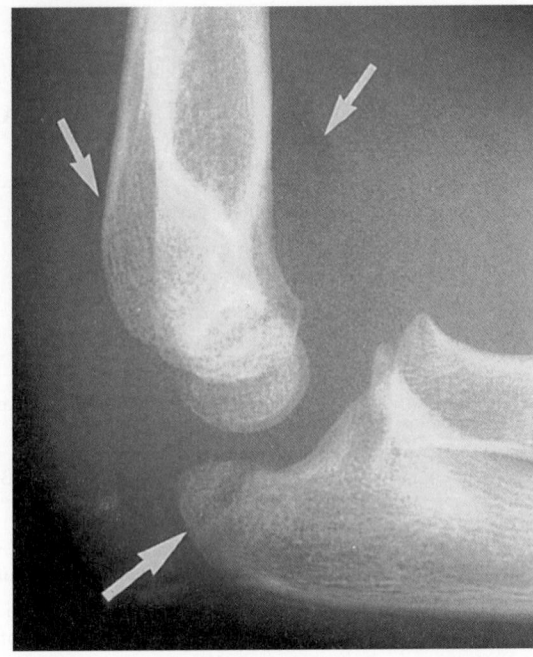

FIGURE 114.26 Nondisplaced fracture of the olecranon in an 8-year-old boy *(bottom arrow)*. Note the elevated fat pads *(top arrows)*.

a fall on an extended arm with hyperextension of the elbow usually results in a supracondylar injury but occasionally can lead to a fracture of the distal humerus physis instead.

Elbow swelling without significant deformity is the usual clinical finding. When displacement is significant, the appearance may mimic that of an elbow dislocation. The latter, however, is an injury of early adolescence. Radiographic diagnosis can be difficult, particularly in infants in whom the capitellum has not yet begun to ossify. Posteromedial displacement of the ulna and radius in relation to the humerus is the most important finding. Recognition of this displacement may necessitate comparison views. Given the difficulty in recognition and the frequent need for reduction and pinning, all suspected epiphyseal separations of the distal humerus merit immediate orthopedic referral. MRI studies may be necessary to define the extent of damage to the cartilaginous structures. In addition, the strong possibility of abuse needs to be considered seriously with this injury in children younger than 3 years.

Olecranon Fractures

Isolated fractures of the olecranon are seen only rarely. More often than not, they occur in conjunction with another injury of the elbow, in particular a fracture or dislocation of the radial head. Various mechanisms have been described, including sudden flexion of the elbow when the triceps is strongly contracted (essentially an avulsion injury) and direct trauma. Physical findings range from swelling localized to the olecranon to a marked hemarthrosis. Elbow extension may be weak or lacking altogether. Nondisplaced fractures may be some-

what difficult to discern radiographically; fat pad abnormalities are commonplace, however, and should be viewed as presumptive evidence of a bony injury (Fig. 114.26). A nondisplaced olecranon fracture can be splinted in partial extension and referred for orthopedic follow-up. Displaced fractures often require open reduction and internal fixation. Isolated olecranon fractures almost invariably heal quickly and without significant complications.

Radial Head and Neck Fractures

Falls on an outstretched, supinated arm account for most fractures of the radial head and neck. Salter-Harris type I and II and pure metaphyseal (i.e., radial neck alone) injuries are the most common. Involvement of the epiphysis (i.e., radial head), which is largely cartilage in childhood, is rare. The physical examination typically reveals localized swelling and ecchymosis. Tenderness overlying the proximal radius strongly suggests the diagnosis. Of note is that pain may be referred to the wrist and thus distract from the true injury (Fig. 114.27). As for radiographic diagnosis, oblique and comparison views can

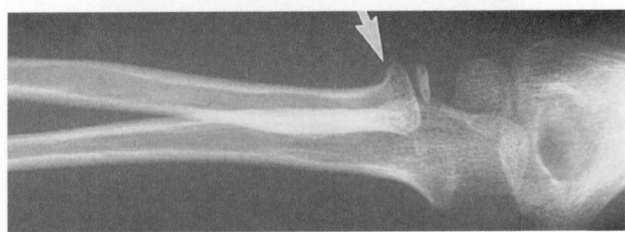

FIGURE 114.27 Buckle fracture of the radial neck in a 9-year-old girl. Wrist pain was the chief complaint. The treating physician failed to identify the proximal radial fracture, which was, however, noticed by the radiologist.

clarify the diagnosis in uncertain cases. When the metaphysis alone is injured, a hemarthrosis may be absent and the fat pads normal. Associated fractures are common. The incidence of complications, especially loss of motion and overgrowth of the radial head, is significant. For this reason, orthopedic referral is recommended for all radial head and neck fractures. Immobilization with the elbow in 90 degrees of flexion and the forearm in neutral rotation is acceptable emergency management for minimally displaced or nondisplaced fractures. Angulation of greater than 15 degrees is an indication for immediate orthopedic consultation.

Elbow Dislocations

The elbow is dislocated more often than any other major joint in children and adolescents. Nonetheless, it is an unusual injury. As discussed previously, the ligaments and tendons are relatively stronger than the neighboring bones (particularly the physeal plates) in children; injuries that would lead to dislocations in adults almost invariably result in fractures in the younger age group. It is not surprising, then, that dislocations of the elbow are accompanied by significant soft-tissue and bony damage. A fall on an extended or partially flexed arm with the forearm in supination is the usual mechanism of injury. Accordingly, the radius and ulna are displaced posteriorly and, in most cases, laterally (Fig. 114.28). The anterior capsule is torn and the medial collateral ligament typically ruptured. Fractures of the medial epicondyle, coronoid process, olecranon, and proximal radius are the most commonly associated bony injuries.

Major neurovascular compromise may accompany elbow dislocations. After reduction, patients should be evaluated carefully, placed in a posterior splint, and discharged, if neurovascularly intact, with careful instructions as to the signs of compartment syndrome. True arterial rupture is seen almost exclusively with open dislocations but has been described on occasion with closed injuries. When reduction of the dislocation fails to relieve arterial compromise, further investigation regarding the extent of vascular injury is warranted. Nerve

injury, particularly of the ulnar nerve, is even more common than vascular injury. Ulnar nerve lesions typically occur when the medial epicondyle is avulsed and then entrapped in the joint. Early recognition and appropriate treatment of such entrapment nearly always lead to complete recovery of ulnar nerve function. Median nerve entrapment is much rarer, but when it occurs, the degree of nerve damage is such that full recovery cannot be guaranteed. Moreover, recognition of median nerve injury is made difficult by the relative lack of pain and the subtlety of the initial motor and sensory deficits.

Clinical findings with dislocation of the elbow include obvious deformity and significant swelling. The forearm appears shortened. Often, the ulnar notch can be palpated posteriorly, and the humeral head can be detected as fullness in the antecubital fossa. The importance of a thorough and well-documented neurovascular examination should be obvious from the preceding discussion. Immobilization before radiographic studies is recommended to minimize the risk of further neurovascular injury. Standard radiographic views are satisfactory. They should be closely inspected for the direction of the dislocation and for the presence of associated fractures. Although most elbow dislocations can be reduced uneventfully, the risks of entrapping a fracture fragment or a nerve in the joint space during the procedure are such that immediate orthopedic consultation is recommended. Open reduction may be needed in over 50% of cases. Numerous techniques for closed reduction have been described. Whatever technique is used, hyperextension should be avoided at all times. Postreduction films are mandatory because only then will many of the associated fractures be evident. Finally, the arm should be immobilized in a posterior splint with the elbow at 90 degrees and the forearm in midpronation.

Radial Head Subluxation

Of all the injuries discussed in this section, by far the most common is radial head subluxation, otherwise known as "nursemaid's elbow" or "pulled elbow" (see Section VII, Procedures). Pathologically, radial head subluxation occurs when the annular ligament becomes partially detached from the head of the radius and slips into the radiohumeral joint where it is entrapped. The usual mechanism is that of axial traction on an extended and pronated arm. Radial head subluxation is an injury of children a few months to 5 years of age. After 5 years of age, the strength of the annular ligament is such that the injury is uncommon.

The classic history is that of a child who cries with pain and refuses to use an arm after being pulled or lifted by that same arm. With some regularity, however, the history is one of a fall. In infants, radial head subluxation can occur when an extended arm is trapped beneath the trunk as the child is rolled over. The chief complaint is typically that the child is not using the arm; concerns about a wrist or a shoulder injury are common. Children with radial head subluxation uniformly hold the arm in pronation with the elbow slightly flexed. Much more often, the degree of distress is minimal, although supination, pronation, and elbow flexion usually elicit pain. Mild tenderness may be noted with palpation of the radial head. Significant point tenderness or swelling should suggest an alternative diagnosis (e.g., a supracondylar fracture). The radiographic findings with radial head subluxation are minimal at best. Radiographs are not routinely recommended when the

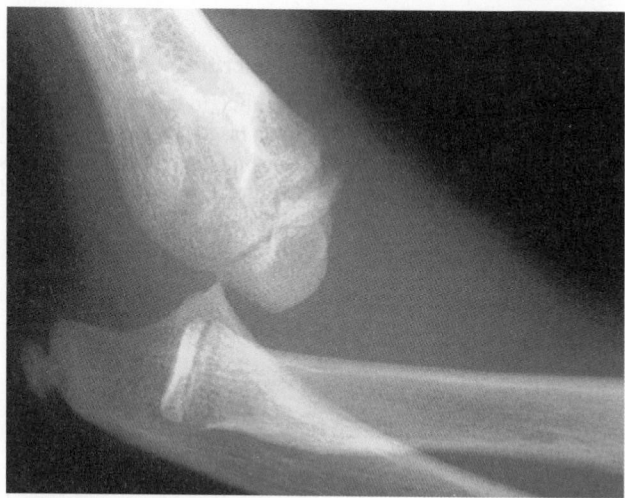

FIGURE 114.28 Elbow dislocation in an 8-year-old girl. A displaced fracture of the medial epicondyle was evident on the postreduction radiographs.

history and clinical presentation are classic. Indeed, the subluxation is often reduced when the radiology technician places the forearm in supination for the anteroposterior view.

As for treatment, various reduction techniques have been described. The most widely used is that described in Section VII "Procedures," namely, supination and flexion. If that approach is unsuccessful, either supination or pronation with elbow extension should be attempted. When reduction succeeds, the child typically uses the arm normally within 5 to 10 minutes. The delay until normal use is longer in younger children and when there has been greater than a 4- to 6-hour period between injury and treatment. When there is no evidence of recovery, the diagnosis must be reconsidered; fractures of the elbow and clavicle in particular should be excluded because the clinical presentations can be similar. With recurrent subluxations, immobilization for a few weeks in a posterior splint with the elbow at 90 degrees and the forearm supinated is suggested. Note that even when efforts at closed reduction fail, spontaneous reduction almost invariably occurs. The need for open reduction is exceedingly rare.

Fractures of the Forearm and Wrist

Children fracture the radius and ulna more often than all bones other than the clavicle. Fortunately, the incidence of neurovascular complications is low and the potential for healing with proper management high. In many instances, the emergency physician can provide the satisfactory initial, if not definitive, management for forearm injuries. However, certain types of fractures require immediate orthopedic referral, and as such they receive particular emphasis. In this section, forearm fractures are divided as follows: (i) fractures of the radial and ulnar shafts, (ii) Monteggia and Galeazzi fracture dislocations, (iii) fractures of the distal radius and ulna, and (iv) fractures of the bones of the wrist.

Fractures of the Radial and Ulnar Shafts

The usual mechanism of injury with forearm fractures, including those of the radial and ulnar shafts, is a fall on an outstretched hand. Direct blows account for some injuries, displaced and open shaft fractures in particular. Approximately three fourths of all shaft fractures involve the distal third of the shaft; most of the remainder involve the midshaft. The clinical findings generally make the diagnosis self-evident. A number of fracture patterns are seen; greenstick injuries are especially common. Standard radiographic views are sufficient other than with suspected bowing fractures when comparison views

may be necessary. The emergency physician should insist that radiographs of the forearm always include both a true lateral and a true anteroposterior view and both the elbow and the wrist. In general, isolated ulnar fractures do not occur, as is discussed further in the next section.

The periosteum and remaining intact cortex limit the degree of angulation with greenstick injuries. Keep in mind that many greenstick fractures have a significant rotational deformity and that the degree of angulation alone should not determine the need for closed reduction. It must also be remembered that the potential for remodeling decreases with the distance from the epiphysis and with the age of the child. Less angulation is therefore accepted in midshaft fractures than in more distal injuries and in adolescents than in younger children. Although it is hard to make any absolute rules, any shaft fracture angulated more than 10 degrees merits immediate orthopedic consultation, at least by telephone. This is not to say that all such fractures will require reduction. (Another simple rule is that any forearm that looks crooked should be straightened.) Dorsal angulation is usual; immobilization with the arm in supination minimizes the tendency of the forearm muscles to cause further deformity.

Complete fractures can be particularly problematic, again because significant angulation can occur. If the ends of the bones are well opposed and angulation and rotation are minimal, a well-applied sugar-tong splint is adequate initial treatment. Otherwise, immediate orthopedic referral is necessary. Closed reduction, although not always as simple as it may appear, is preferable (Fig. 114.29). In children older than 10 to 12 years, adequate alignment is often obtained only with open reduction and internal fixation.

Recognition of when a bowing fracture has occurred is crucial simply because the potential for remodeling with such injuries is minimal (Fig. 114.4). Failure to correct bowing can result in permanent loss of supination and pronation. As already mentioned, in the absence of obvious deformity, comparison views may be necessary before the true extent of bowing can be appreciated. Again, no hard and fast rules regarding indications for closed reduction are offered; however, any bowing fracture that causes obvious forearm deformity or restrictions of pronation or supination certainly merits immediate orthopedic referral.

Monteggia and Galeazzi Fracture Dislocations

In general, isolated fractures of the ulna do not occur. Instead, the same force that causes the ulnar fracture leads to a radial injury, in some instances, a dislocation of the radial head. It is this combination of an ulnar fracture and a radial head

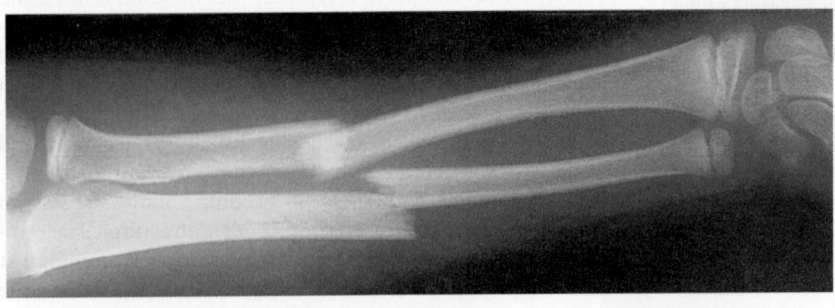

FIGURE 114.29 Complete fractures of the midshafts of the radius and ulna in a 9-year-old boy. Efforts at closed reduction failed; internal fixation was necessary.

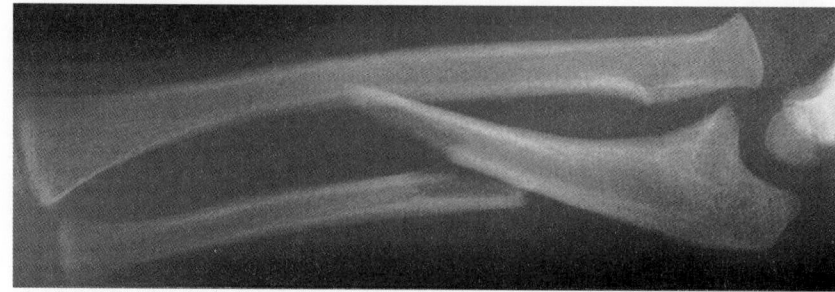

FIGURE 114.30 A Monteggia fracture in a 3-year-old boy. Note that a line drawn along the axis of the radius would fail to intersect the capitellum (compare with Fig. 114.29.)

dislocation that is known as a Monteggia fracture. Recognition is most important because failure to reduce the radial head dislocation results in permanent disability. Clues to the diagnosis on physical examination include elbow pain and swelling, which accompany signs of any ulnar fracture. Palpation may confirm the dislocation of the radial head, which may be displaced anteriorly, posteriorly, or laterally, depending on the mechanism of injury. A palsy of the posterior interosseous nerve, a motor branch of the radial nerve, may also be present.

If the radial head dislocation is to be recognized radiographically, the rule that a line drawn through the axis of the radius should pass through the center of the capitellum on all projections must be remembered (Fig. 114.30). Once again, the need for a true lateral view that includes the elbow with all forearm studies must be emphasized. Even bowing fractures of the ulna, which may require comparison views for recognition, are associated with radial head dislocation. Any suspected Monteggia injury requires immediate orthopedic referral.

The Galeazzi fracture is a radial shaft fracture, generally at the junction of the middle and distal thirds that is accompanied by disruption of the distal radioulnar joint. It is relatively rare. Physical examination reveals prominence of the distal ulna and joint instability. Radiographs are confirmatory. Once again, orthopedic consultation is necessary. The complications are few with proper management.

Fractures of the Distal Radius and Ulna

Distal radial and ulnar fractures bear special mention, not because of any undue rate of complications, but rather because of their overall frequency. Of all the fractures that occur in childhood and adolescence, those of distal forearm are by far the most common. Except for the occasional instance of nerve entrapment at the time of reduction of a complete fracture,

significant neurovascular complications are rare. Overall, the capacity for remodeling is significant. The difficulties facing the emergency physician are those of diagnosis with subtle fractures and of recognition regarding when reduction is necessary with displaced fractures.

More often than not, localized swelling and tenderness accompany distal radial fractures and can guide interpretation of the radiographic studies. However, wrist pain can be the chief complaint with more proximal injuries, for example, radial head fractures. Once again, the need for studies that include the whole forearm must be reinforced. Torus fractures are most often overlooked. Often, the location of the soft-tissue swelling on the radiographs helps highlight the position of the fracture, which may be evident on only one projection and then only as a minor irregularity in the contour of the cortex. A fracture of the ulnar styloid should also prompt a diligent search for a radial injury. Ulnar styloid fractures only rarely occur in isolation; as a rule, they are accompanied by either a torus or physeal fracture of the radius. When a torus fracture is identified, a volar splint or, if the swelling is minimal, a short arm cast for 3 to 4 weeks is recommended. A removable splint for 3 weeks was shown in one study to be as effective as casting with the additional advantage of interfering less with physical functioning and activities. Orthopedic referral is optional, and serial radiographs to document fracture healing or guide management are of limited value.

Greenstick and complete fractures are readily recognized. What must be remembered is that such fractures have a tendency to displace if not properly immobilized. The distal fragment is angulated posteriorly in most greenstick and complete fractures of the distal forearm. Angulation of greater than 10 to 15 degrees is an indication for immediate orthopedic referral (Fig. 114.31). Otherwise, immobilization with orthopedic follow-up within 3 to 5 days is adequate emergency management.

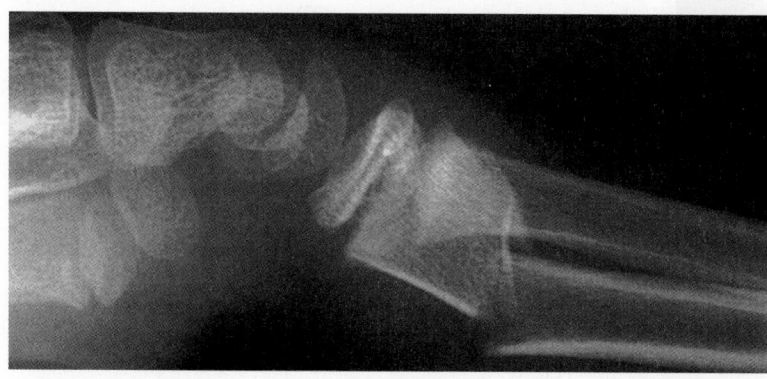

FIGURE 114.31 Complete fracture of the distal radius of a 9-year-old child demonstrating 35 degrees of posterior displacement of the distal fragment. Closed reduction was uneventful.

TRAUMA

Although there is some disagreement, immobilization with the forearm in supination is believed to decrease the likelihood of further displacement. Accordingly, either a long arm posterior splint or a well-applied sugar-tong splint are recommended with all greenstick and complete radial and ulnar fractures. Short arm volar splints should be reserved for torus injuries.

Salter-Harris type I and II injuries of the distal radial physis rarely lead to growth disturbance, which is fortunate because they are common injuries, particularly from 6 to 12 years of age. The issue again is one of recognition with these fractures. When point tenderness on the physical examination is accompanied by swelling localized to the distal radius on the radiograph, the presumptive diagnosis should be a Salter-Harris type I injury even when there is no obvious displacement of the epiphysis. Immobilization and orthopedic referral are recommended. Closed reduction is needed for all displaced physeal fractures. Of note is that the risk of growth disturbance increases with repeated and delayed manipulations.

Fractures of the Bones of the Wrist

The carpal bones are rarely fractured during childhood and adolescence. Adolescents in the later stages of skeletal maturity sustain scaphoid (navicular) fractures. Most injuries of the scaphoid in adolescence are nondisplaced fractures through the distal third of the bone (Fig. 114.32). The rate of nonunion is much lower than in adults, in whom scaphoid fractures generally involve the middle third of the bone and are more often displaced. The usual mechanism is a fall on an outstretched arm with extreme hyperextension of the wrist. Physical findings that should suggest the possibility of a scaphoid fracture include snuffbox tenderness, pain with supination against resistance, and pain with longitudinal compression of the thumb. As with adults, radiographic visualization of a nondisplaced scaphoid fracture may be difficult even with special views. If the physical signs suggest a scaphoid fracture, then immobilization in a thumb spica splint or cast for 2 weeks is recommended, regardless of the radiographic findings. At that

time, radiographs should be repeated; fractures not detectable on the initial films should now be evident. If radiographs remain normal but clinical suspicions high, a bone scan or an MRI study should be considered. Although the likelihood of complication is low, orthopedic referral is recommended once a scaphoid fracture is identified.

Injuries of the Hand and Fingers

By comparison with adults, younger children sustain relatively few bony injuries of the hand. The most commonly encountered hand injuries in the pediatric ED are crush injuries of the distal phalanx, in which lacerations and fractures often coexist. It has been stated that such injuries are often undertreated; definitive management often entails removal of the nail, repair of any nail-bed injury identified, careful immobilization, and close follow-up. (See Chapters 106 and 113 for additional discussion on the management of such crush injuries.)

A wide variety of other injuries, including an array of avulsion and physeal fractures, also occur. The types of injuries seen at a given joint reflect the underlying complex anatomy of the tendons and ligaments of the hand, a full discussion of which is beyond the scope of this chapter. However, by adhering to a few basic principles of physical and radiographic diagnosis, the emergency physician should have little difficulty in recognizing which injuries merit referral to a hand specialist.

Given the risks of permanent deformity and stiffness, all displaced fractures, particularly those extending intraarticularly, should be referred. Such fractures are generally self-evident. Before concluding that a fracture is a simple nondisplaced one and thus amenable to routine splinting, the practitioner must first assure himself or herself that there is no accompanying malrotation or joint instability. Malrotation is not always that apparent when the fingers are extended; it becomes much more obvious with finger flexion (Fig. 114.33). Joint stability must also be assessed in flexion and extension, as well as in both the lateral and anteroposterior planes. Adequate examination may be possible only after performance of a digital block. If either malrotation or joint instability is detected, consultation is again in order.

When the hand is radiographed, oblique views should be included in addition to the usual anteroposterior and lateral projections. Interpretation of the radiographs is complicated by the presence of multiple epiphyses and secondary ossification centers. It is essential to remember that the epiphyses of

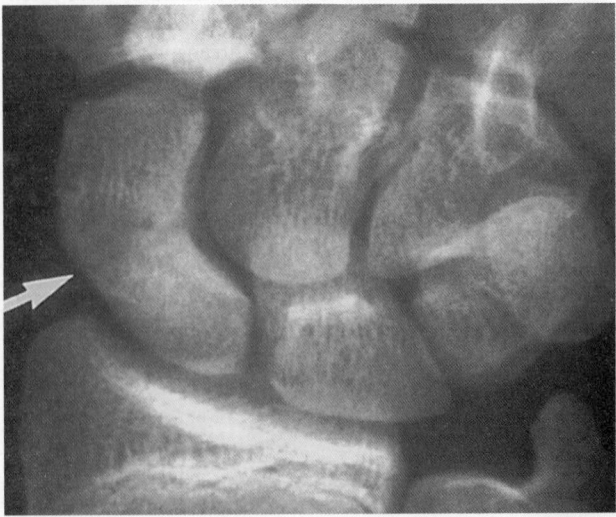

FIGURE 114.32 A scaphoid fracture in a 16-year-old boy *(arrow)*. In this case, the fracture is through the middle third of the scaphoid; fractures through the distal third are actually more common during adolescence.

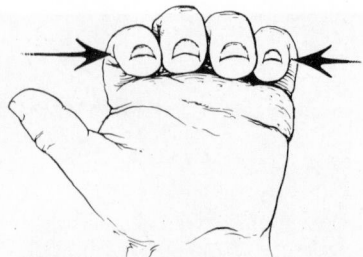

FIGURE 114.33 It is important to check for malrotation with all fractures of the metacarpals and phalanges. When flexed as shown, the fingers should all point in the same direction. If malrotation is present, overlapping will occur.

the phalanges and of the thumb metacarpal are located at the proximal ends of the bones. The growth centers of the remaining metacarpals are distal. Once again, the number of fractures missed will be minimized if close attention is paid to the physical findings and the presence of soft-tissue swelling on the radiographs. For the purposes of further discussion, hand injuries are divided into (i) metacarpal fractures and (ii) phalangeal fractures and dislocations.

Metacarpal Fractures

Perhaps the most commonly encountered metacarpal fracture in pediatrics is one of the distal fifth metacarpal in a male adolescent who has struck someone or something with a closed fist. The equivalent of a boxer's fracture in an adult, these fractures are metaphyseal rather than physeal injuries and are typically angulated. Closed reduction is usually performed if the angulation is more than 30 to 40 degrees. Salter-Harris type I and II injuries occur on occasion, primarily in the second, third, and fourth metacarpals. Nondisplaced injuries may be immobilized in a gutter splint with the wrist neutral and the metacarpal phalangeal joints at 70 degrees and then referred (Figs. 114.34 and 114.35). If they are not displaced or rotated, metacarpal shaft fractures can be managed similarly. Proximal metacarpal fractures of the second through fifth metacarpals are rarely displaced; recognition is more of an issue than management (Fig. 114.36). However, angulation is common with proximal fractures of the thumb metacarpal. Metaphyseal and Salter-Harris type II and III injuries occur and when displaced require closed reduction.

Phalangeal Fractures and Dislocations

As already mentioned, distal phalanx fractures typically accompany crush injuries of the fingertip. If only the distal tuft is fractured, anatomic closure of the laceration usually results in adequate realignment of the fracture. Displaced physeal fractures merit immediate referral (Fig. 114.37). Hyperflexion injuries of the distal phalanx, leading to so-called mallet finger deformities, are also common. In the child, Salter-Harris type I or II injuries result, whereas type III injuries are the rule in adolescents. The latter often require open reduction and internal fixation. In either case, examination reveals an extension

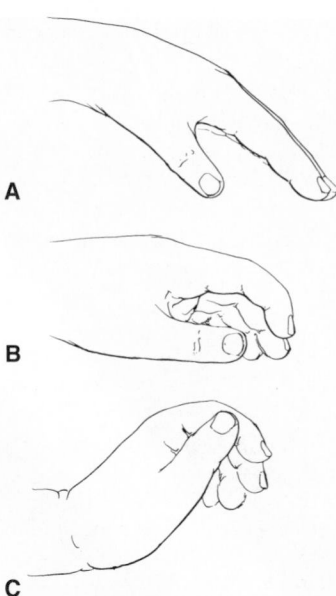

FIGURE 114.35 Splinting the hand in any of the positions shown here tends to promote joint contractures and recurrence of deformity.

lag at the distal interphalangeal joint. Recognition of the tendinous disruption is important, given that proper treatment entails 6 to 8 weeks of continuous splinting in hyperextension.

A whole range of proximal and middle phalangeal fractures occur, many of which the emergency physician can manage successfully (Fig. 114.38). Gutter splints that incorporate both the

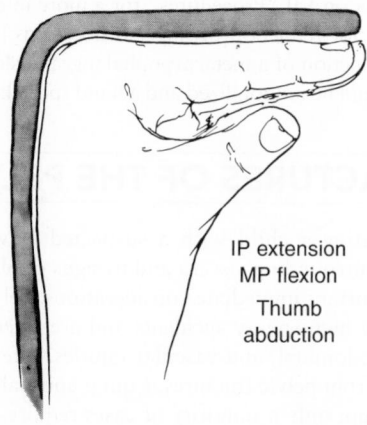

IP extension
MP flexion
Thumb
abduction

FIGURE 114.34 The hand should be splinted in this position to prevent extension contractures of the metacarpophalangeal (MP) joints and flexion contractures of the interphalangeal (IP) joints.

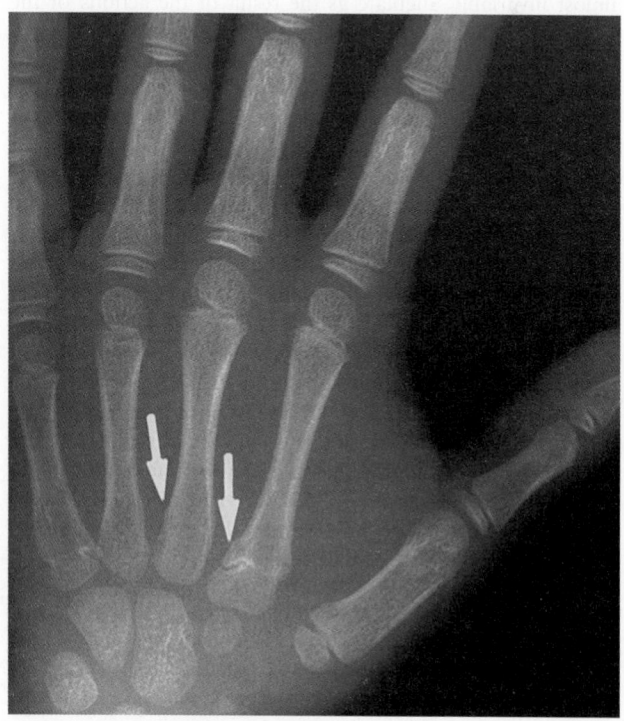

FIGURE 114.36 Radiograph of the left hand of an 8-year-old girl showing fractures of the proximal second and third metacarpals *(arrows)*. Significant displacement is unusual with proximal metacarpal fractures.

TRAUMA

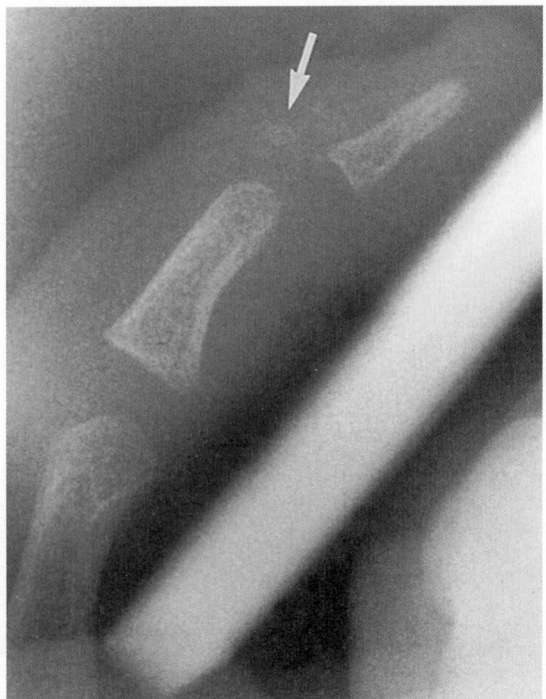

FIGURE 114.37 Displaced Salter-Harris type I fracture of the distal phalanx in an 11-month-old girl that resulted from a crush injury. The *arrow* points to the epiphysis, which is only beginning to calcify. Careful reduction is necessary if the risk of growth disturbance is to be minimized.

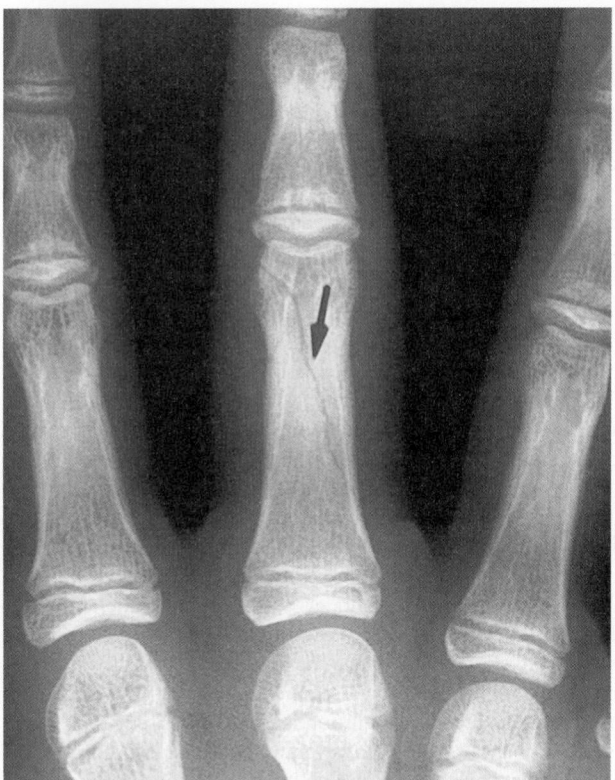

FIGURE 114.38 Oblique fracture of the proximal phalanx of the right third finger in a 12-year-old boy *(arrow)*. Before splinting such an injury, the emergency physician must first make certain that no malrotation is present.

injured and an adjacent uninjured finger are used commonly with the positioning discussed previously. Complete fractures almost invariably angulate as the result of the actions of the intrinsic muscles, the direction of angulation determined by the position of the fracture relative to the flexor and extensor tendons. Phalangeal neck fractures are of particular concern in that complete fractures can rotate by as much as 90 degrees and unicondylar fractures are prone to displacement. The radiographic findings may be subtle; the consequences of improperly evaluating such injuries are certainly substantial. In the proximal phalanx, particularly that of the fifth finger, laterally angulated Salter-Harris type II fractures are common. If the displacement is minimal, splinting with follow-up in 3 to 5 days is acceptable.

Special mention should be made of the so-called gamekeeper's or skier's thumb, an avulsion of the ulnar collateral ligament of the proximal phalanx of the thumb. Localized tenderness should raise concerns about this injury and prompt an assessment of the joint for adduction stability with the metacarpal joint extended and in 30 degrees of flexion. In the pediatric age range, this is a Salter-Harris type III injury. When there is evidence of only minor instability (firm endpoint, increased laxity of less than 30 degrees), thumb spica splinting for 3 to 6 weeks is generally sufficient. More severe injuries require operative intervention. Consultation is suggested when such injuries are suspected.

Despite the strength of the ligaments and tendons, hyperextension can lead to dislocations of the metacarpophalangeal and proximal interphalangeal joints in children. Dislocations of the proximal interphalangeal joints can usually be readily reduced (Fig. 114.39). After a digital block, the joint should be gently hyperextended and the distal bone then pushed back

into place. Radiographs, both prereduction and postreduction, should be scrutinized for fractures, and the stability of the collateral ligaments should be carefully assessed. Buddy taping for 3 weeks is adequate for routine dislocations (Fig. 114.40).

Metacarpophalangeal dislocations are particularly problematic. Although closed reduction may be successful, often the volar plate is entrapped in the joint and open reduction is therefore necessary. Such volar entrapment can be suspected when physical examination reveals puckering of the palmar skin adjacent to the affected joint. Visualization of a sesamoid bone within the joint space is pathognomonic of volar plate entrapment. (See Section VII "Procedures" for a more in-depth review of techniques for reduction of finger dislocations.) If an initial attempt at reduction of a metacarpophalangeal dislocation fails, the finger should be immobilized and a hand specialist consulted.

FRACTURES OF THE PELVIS

When evaluating a child with a suspected pelvic fracture, attention to surrounding viscera and to signs of blood loss are the most important immediate considerations. Pelvic fractures are caused by high-energy accidents and are often associated with head, abdominal, and vascular injuries. Life-threatening hemorrhage from pelvic fractures is quite unusual in the pediatric age group; only a minority of cases require transfusion. Multiple authors have questioned the role of routine screening pelvic films in pediatric trauma. In the awake, alert patient, physical examination alone has both high specificity and

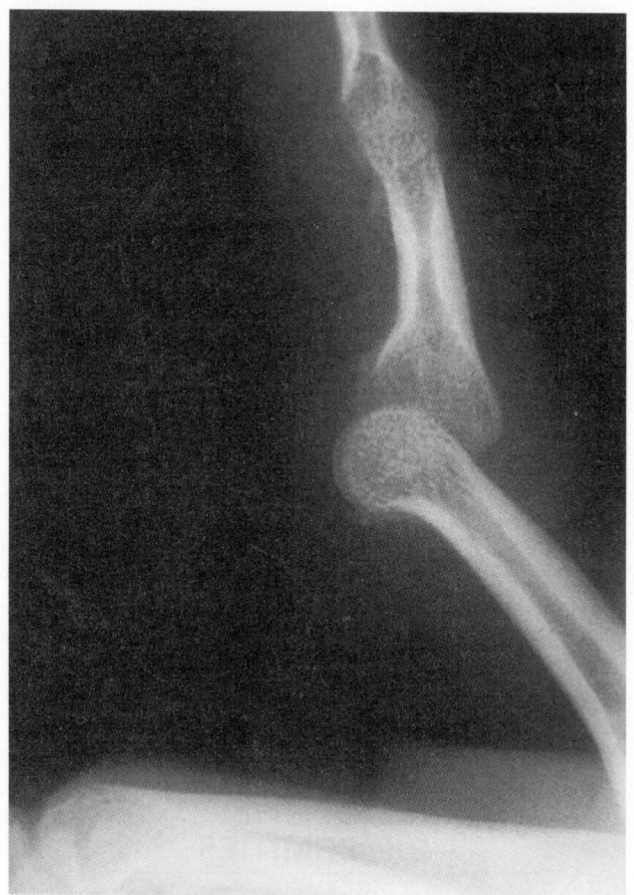

FIGURE 114.39 Dislocation of the right fourth proximal interphalangeal joint in a 15-year-old boy. Most such injuries can be readily reduced, which is not the case with metacarpophalangeal joint dislocations.

negative predictive value. When the extent of injuries is such that abdominopelvic CT scan is indicated, screening films can also be deferred as the sensitivity of CT scan for pelvic fractures is certainly higher than of a single routine radiograph. Overall, pelvic fractures in children have a favorable outcome

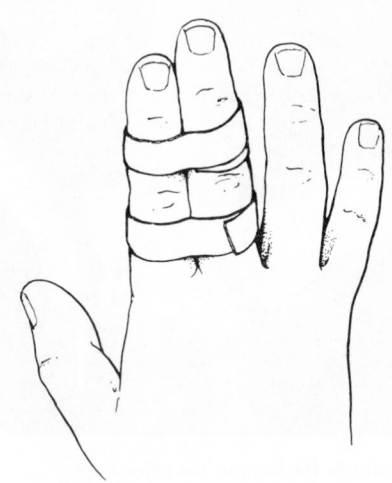

FIGURE 114.40 Buddy taping is a convenient way of splinting uncomplicated dislocations postreduction, as well as minor finger fractures.

and rarely require any more treatment than bed rest for 4 to 6 weeks. Exceptions to this rule include severely displaced sacral or sacroiliac joint dislocations and displaced acetabular fractures. An immediate orthopedic consultation is required for all pelvic fractures other than minor avulsions.

Pelvic fractures in children can be divided into three groups: (i) avulsion fractures, (ii) pelvic ring fractures, and (iii) acetabular fractures.

Avulsion Fractures

Avulsion fractures occur most commonly from sporting activities. The muscular attachments to the secondary centers of ossification (i.e., the anterior superior iliac spine, anterior inferior iliac spine, and ischial tuberosity) can be pulled off during strong, active contractions against resistance (Fig. 114.41). Localized tenderness is usually present. The diagnosis is usually readily apparent on plain film radiographs, although bone scintigraphy may be necessary to confirm the diagnosis on occasion (Fig. 114.42). Treatment is based on symptoms. Often, crutches with partial or no weight bearing for 4 to 6 weeks with slow resumption of activities are all that is required even with significantly displaced fractures. With widely separated (more than 2 cm) avulsion fractures of the ischial tuberosity, some authors recommend open reduction and fixation; others continue to advocate conservative treatment.

Pelvic Ring Fractures

Single Breaks in the Pelvic Ring

Symphysis pubis diastasis, superior and inferior pubic rami fractures, and straddle fractures are classified as single breaks in the

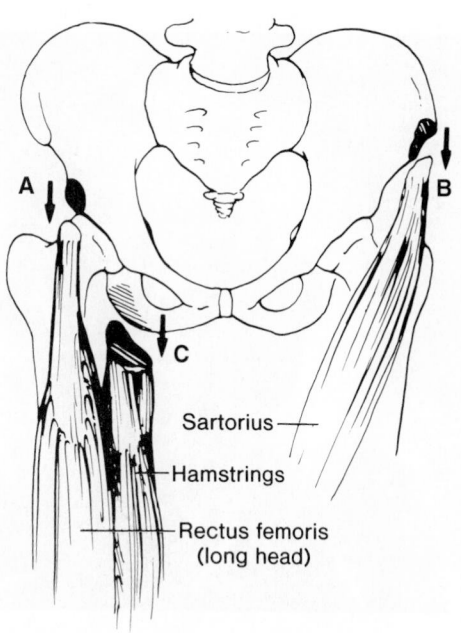

FIGURE 114.41 Common avulsion injuries of the pelvis: anterior inferior iliac spine (**A**), anterior superior iliac spine (**B**), and ischial tuberosity (**C**).

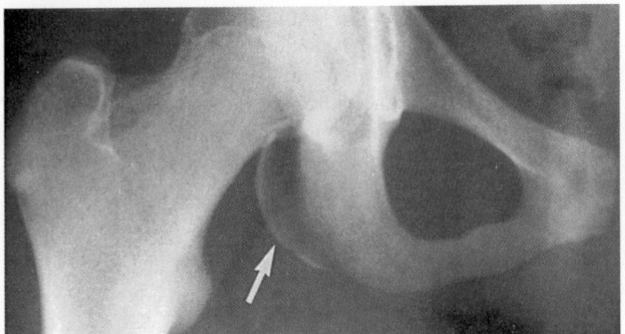

FIGURE 114.42 Avulsion fracture of the right ischial tuberosity in a 13-year-old girl *(arrow)*.

pelvic ring. These common childhood fractures often seem worse than they are. Although they are caused by high-energy accidents, they are generally stable fractures. A careful search for accompanying genitourinary and neurovascular injuries must be made. Fractures of the superior and inferior pubic rami rarely require any treatment in the child or adolescent as long as the sacroiliac joints and sacrum remain intact. One exception to this rule is a diastasis of the pubic symphysis, which is often associated with anterior disruption of the sacroiliac joint. This fracture configuration with pubic diastasis and anterior sacroiliac joint disruption is called the open book deformity. If significant displacement occurs through the symphysis pubis, closed reduction with an external fixator or a pubic plate must be considered.

Double Breaks in the Pelvic Ring

Fractures of the pubic rami or symphysis pubis associated with displaced sacroiliac joint dislocations or sacral fractures are classified as Malgaigne's fractures (Fig. 114.43). The hemipelvis is unstable and displaced cephalad. This group of fractures is associated with a high incidence of complications,

including genitourinary, abdominal, and vascular injuries. Life-threatening hemorrhage can occur from pelvic vein disruption. In severe cases of bleeding, emergent application of an external fixator or a pneumatic antishock garment in the ED with compression of the pelvis may slow bleeding by a tamponade effect. Angiographic embolization should also be considered in the face of persistent bleeding.

Initial treatment of the unstable pelvic fracture is bed rest. Special radiographic views consisting of an inlet and outlet view or CT scan assist the orthopedist in deciding whether to place the child or adolescent in traction or to undertake an open reduction and internal fixation of the posterior fracture–dislocation.

Acetabular Fractures

Fractures involving the acetabulum are rare in children. They are often associated with a dislocation of the hip joint. Attention should be directed toward obtaining an early congruent reduction and evaluating the stability of the hip. Acetabular fractures associated with major pelvic disruption should be treated like those involving double breaks in the pelvic ring. An orthopedic consultation should be obtained early and treatment of life-threatening complications initiated.

INJURIES OF THE LOWER EXTREMITIES

Injuries of the Hip and Proximal Femur

Hip dislocations and femoral neck fractures in children and adolescents are the result of high-energy accidents. The care and resuscitation of the child is paramount before addressing

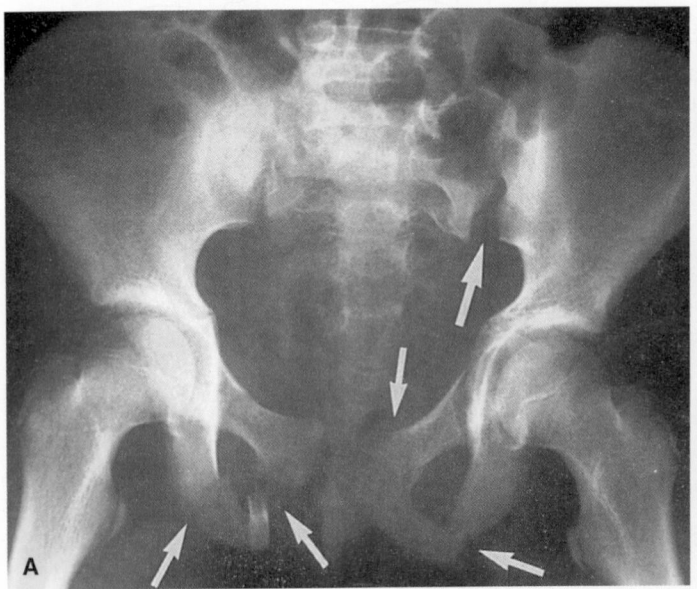

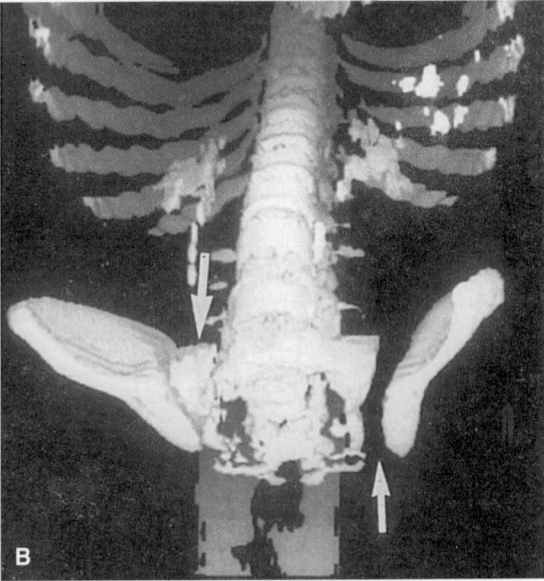

FIGURE 114.43 An unstable pelvic injury. **A:** On the plain film, multiple fractures of the pubic rami *(small arrows)* and widening of the right sacroiliac joint *(large arrow)* are apparent. **B:** On the three-dimensional reconstruction of the CT scan, the left sacroiliac fracture is even more obvious *(small arrow)*, and a right-sided sacral fracture is also seen *(large arrow)*.

the orthopedic injury. In many instances, the child can be managed in a traction splint until definitive care is given.

Injuries of the hip and proximal femur in children can be divided into five groups: (i) hip dislocation, (ii) proximal femoral physeal fractures, (iii) slipped capital femoral epiphysis (SCFE), (iv) femoral neck fractures, and (v) intertrochanteric fractures.

Hip Dislocation

Dislocation of the hip in children and adolescents is uncommon. However, it probably occurs more often than it is diagnosed because of spontaneous reduction at the time of injury. A dislocation or fracture–dislocation is rather obvious if the injured limb is shortened, externally rotated, and painful. Radiographic examinations make the diagnosis (Fig. 114.44). In evaluating suspected dislocations of the hips with spontaneous reduction, attention must be directed to the radiographic medial clear space of the hip. If a suspected dislocation with spontaneous reduction has occurred, the medial clear space is often wider than the normal contralateral side. The posterior labrum and capsule of the joint may be detached when a dislocation occurs. At the time of reduction (either spontaneous or after closed reduction), tissue may get trapped in the joint space, resulting in asymmetry of the joint space and an incongruent reduction. Further evaluation should consist of a CT scan or MRI (Fig. 114.45).

A patient presenting with a dislocated hip should undergo a closed reduction in the ED or under general anesthesia. Reduction within 6 hours of the accident is essential to decrease the incidence of osseous necrosis. The technique of closed reduction consists of hip and knee flexion to 90 degrees and axial distraction of the thigh. When closed reduction is unsuccessful or when it is suspected that tissue is trapped in the joint space, open reduction is necessary. Congruency of

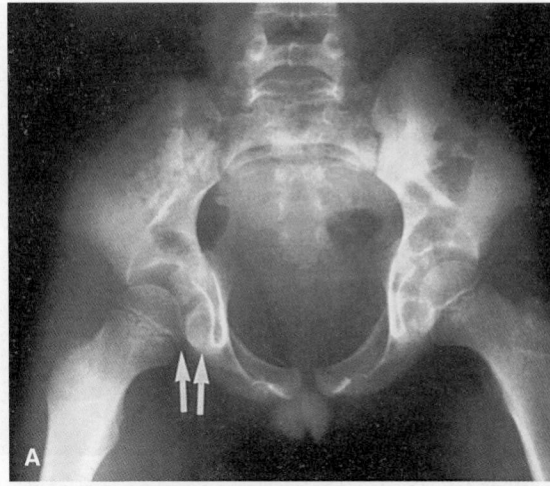
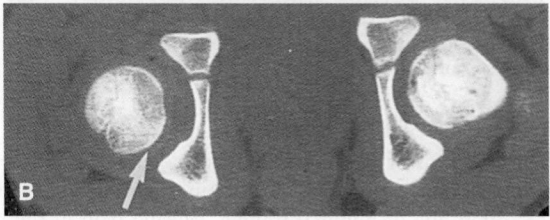

FIGURE 114.45 Radiographs taken following closed reduction of a right hip dislocation. **A:** The plain film demonstrates residual widening of the joint space *(arrows)*. **B:** Widening is also apparent with magnetic resonance imaging, as is entrapment of a portion of the posterior joint capsule. Under general anesthesia, further efforts at closed reduction were successful.

both hips is imperative to a good result. A CT scan or MRI may be needed to define the adequacy of reduction. Complications of traumatic hip dislocation in children include osseous necrosis of the femoral head, posttraumatic arthritis, and persistent instability of the hip joint.

Proximal Femoral Physeal Fractures

Proximal femoral physeal fractures occur through the zone of provisional calcification of the proximal femoral growth plate. The degree of displacement can be mild to complete (Fig. 114.46). Anatomic reduction, either by open or closed means, is essential. Unfortunately, the incidence of osseous necrosis approaches 100% in totally displaced fractures and can lead to long-term disability. In minimally displaced fractures, it may be far better to accept mild displacement than to further compromise the vascularity of the femoral head by performing a reduction.

Slipped Capital Femoral Epiphysis

Although most cases of SCFE present with chronic pain, a significant percentage present acutely. Several studies have suggested that structural weakness is present in the capital femoral physis during the onset of puberty. Others have identified a genetic or hormonal influence predisposing to SCFE. This malady occurs predominantly in children 8 to 15 years of age, with a male:female predominance of 2:1 to 4:1. Obese children and African-Americans are particularly susceptible.

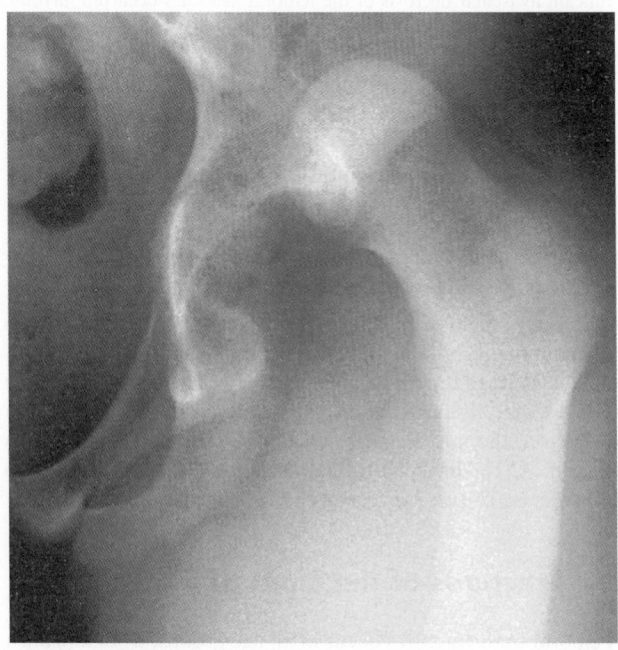

FIGURE 114.44 Dislocation of the left hip in a 9-year-old boy. If dislocation is delayed beyond 6 hours, the risk of osseous necrosis rises.

TRAUMA

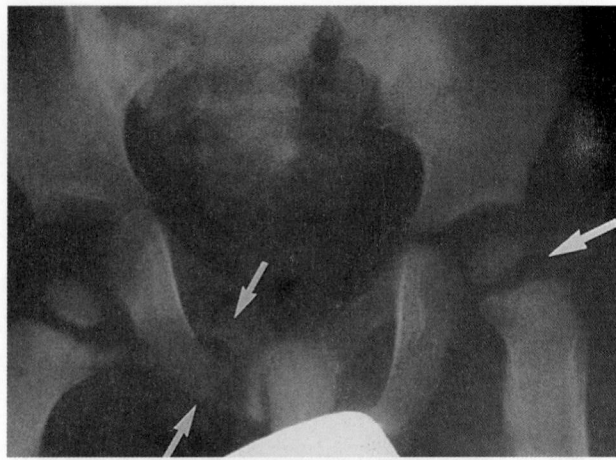

FIGURE 114.46 Displaced Salter-Harris type I fracture of the left proximal femur in a 2-year-old boy *(large arrow)*. Also seen are fractures of the right pubic rami *(small arrows)*. The pelvis is also disrupted posteriorly.

The diagnosis of SCFE should be considered in any preadolescent or adolescent complaining of hip or knee pain. The history is often one of minimal trauma, causing pain in the hip, thigh, or knee region. Vague hip or knee pain and a limp in the preceding weeks are common. The diagnosis is made by the physical and radiographic examination. Range-of-motion abnormalities of the hip, in particular limitation of internal rotation, abduction, and flexion, are almost universal. When flexing the hip from the extended position, the examiner will often note external rotation. Range of motion in all directions may be painful. The radiographic examination should include anteroposterior and frog-leg views of the pelvis. Changes on the anteroposterior film may be obscure. The slip is often seen more easily on the frog-leg view. Comparison with the normal side may assist in the diagnosis. However, 10% to 25% of slips may be bilateral (Fig. 114.47). When the diagnosis is equivocal, use of US, CT, MRI, or bone scintigraphy may be necessary.

Once diagnosis has been made, treatment should consist of strict non-weight bearing and an urgent orthopedic consultation. Prompt pinning is required to prevent further slippage. This may be performed the night of assessment or shortly thereafter, depending on the availability of anesthesia. There are those who advocate one-stage bilateral pinning as prophylaxis against contralateral disease once the diagnosis has been established.

Femoral Neck Fractures

Fractures of the femoral neck are relatively common. Initial treatment is traction and splinting followed by either closed or open reduction, depending on the position of the fracture. If the blood supply to the femoral head is damaged at the time of injury, osseous necrosis can occur. As would be expected, this complication is more likely with displaced than nondisplaced fractures. Overall, the incidence of osseous necrosis in this setting is 40% (Fig. 114.48). Stress fractures of the femoral neck are also being increasingly reported, generally in adolescents involved in repetitive activities such as long-distance running. Exercise-induced hip pain should prompt consideration of the diagnosis, which may require bone scanning or MRI study for

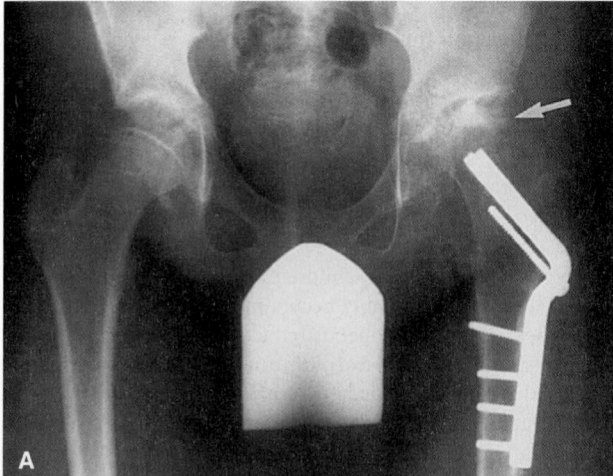

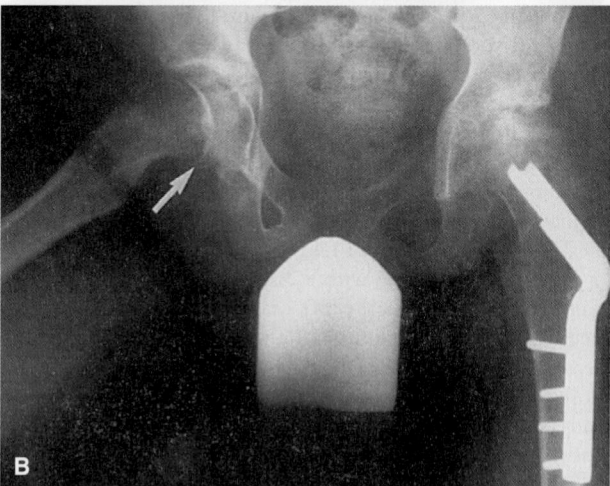

FIGURE 114.47 Radiographs of the hips of a teenager with bilateral slipped capital femoral epiphysis. **A:** Despite surgical intervention, significant avascular necrosis of the femoral head has occurred *(arrow)*. The right hip appears normal. **B:** On a simultaneous frog-leg view, however, it can be seen that the right capital femoral epiphysis has also slipped *(arrow)*.

confirmation. Early recognition is important because restriction of activity may allow healing and thus prevent progression to more complete fractures with displacement.

Intertrochanteric Fractures

Although common in adults, intertrochanteric fractures are uncommon in children and adolescents. Nondisplaced or minimally displaced fractures can be treated easily in a spica cast for 6 to 8 weeks. If significant displacement occurs, internal fixation to restore the normal anatomy may be the best approach to treatment. The incidence of complications is low in this group of patients. The rate of osseous necrosis is approximately 5%.

Fractures of the Shaft of the Femur

Femoral shaft fractures occur in all age groups, from newborn to adolescents. Each group has its specific mechanisms of injury, complications, and treatments. The following age

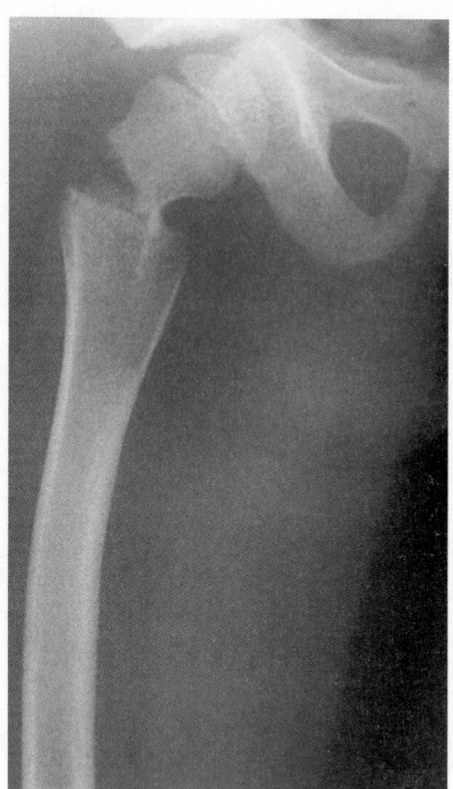

FIGURE 114.48 Fracture of the right femoral neck in a 3-year-old girl.

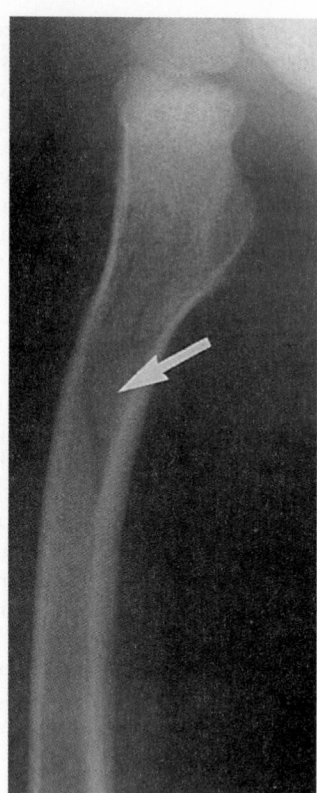

FIGURE 114.49 Spiral fracture of the right femur in a 20-month-old boy *(arrow)*. In this instance, the injury occurred as the result of a motor vehicle accident. In general, spiral femur fractures in young children should prompt consideration of child abuse.

groups are considered: (i) birth to 2 years of age, (ii) 2 to 10 years of age, and (iii) adolescents.

Birth to 2 Years of Age

Most femoral fractures in the first 2 years of life result from either a slow twisting motion or a direct blow (Fig. 114.49). A large percentage of femoral fractures in this age group are the result of intentional trauma. Overhead skin traction, once the cornerstone of the treatment, has fallen out of favor because of reports of neurovascular compromise and skin problems. Treatment options include immediate spica casting or a short period of Buck's traction followed by spica casting. Shortening and angulation are rarely problems in this age group, although rotational deformity can occur if careful alignment is not maintained during casting.

2 to 10 Years of Age

Femoral fractures in children 2 to 10 years of age are most often the result of high-energy motor vehicle or automobile–pedestrian accidents. Concomitant injuries are common. Only rarely does an isolated femur fracture cause hemodynamically significant blood loss. Neurovascular evaluation should be performed and documented at regular intervals. Initial treatment consists of traction or splinting and care of other injuries (Fig. 114.50).

Distal femoral skeletal traction for several weeks followed by spica cast application has been the cornerstone of treatment in the past. More recently, early or immediate spica casting under general anesthesia has replaced traditional methods. This has reduced the hospital stay and costs, as well as alleviated the need for the invasive intervention of the traction pin placement. Contraindications to immediate or early spica casting are shortening greater than 2.5 cm, open fractures, and major concomitant injuries. The long-term complications of femur fractures in this age group include excessive shortening or overgrowth, malrotation, and malunions of the healing femur. It is usually desirable to leave the bone fragments overlapping by 1 cm to allow for some "overgrowth" of the healing femur. Stiffness of the knee and hip has been reported following prolonged spica casting treatment but is usually not a long-term complication.

Adolescents

Femur fractures in adolescents are also caused by high-energy accidents. Once again, attention to other injuries should

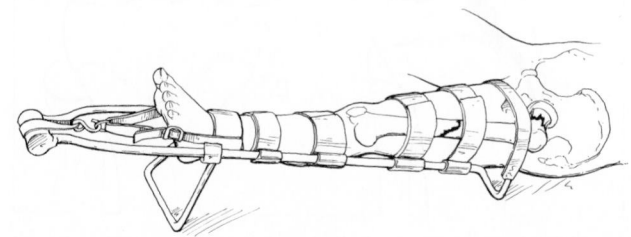

FIGURE 114.50 Use of a traction splint to stabilize femoral fractures is strongly recommended. Both adult and pediatric sizes are available.

precede treatment of the femoral fracture. Strong consideration would be given to a femoral nerve block that has been demonstrated as superior to intravenous narcotics for initial pain management. Stabilization with traction splints is adequate until an orthopedic consultation can be obtained. The management of these fractures has changed over the last several years. Closed reduction and intramedullary rodding are currently recommended to improve alignment and promote an early return to activity.

Injuries of the Knee

Although relatively uncommon, fractures about the knee arguably rank as the most serious long bone injuries in children and adolescents (Fig. 114.51). The growth centers of the distal femur and proximal tibia together account for two thirds of the length of the lower extremity. Growth arrest and deformity can occur after physeal injuries about the knee; the resultant limb-length discrepancies are hardly trivial problems. In contrast, ligamentous injuries are uncommon. For the purposes of discussion, pediatric knee injuries can be divided into the following groups: (i) ligamentous injuries and avulsion fractures, (ii) distal femoral physeal fractures, (iii) proximal tibial physeal fractures, (iv) knee dislocations, and (v) patellar fractures and dislocations.

Ligamentous Injuries and Avulsion Fractures

Compared with fractures of the epiphyses and physes about the knee, ligamentous injuries are relatively uncommon before growth plate closure. Such injuries do occur, however, both in isolation and in conjunction with fractures. Most ligamentous injuries result from direct trauma to the knee, typically when a child is struck by a motor vehicle while walking or riding a bicycle. Others occur during vigorous sporting activities when the knee is subjected to significant valgus or varus stress. The medial collateral and anterior cruciate ligaments are the ones injured most often, and injury to the latter almost invariably occurs in conjunction with an avulsion of the tibial spine. As

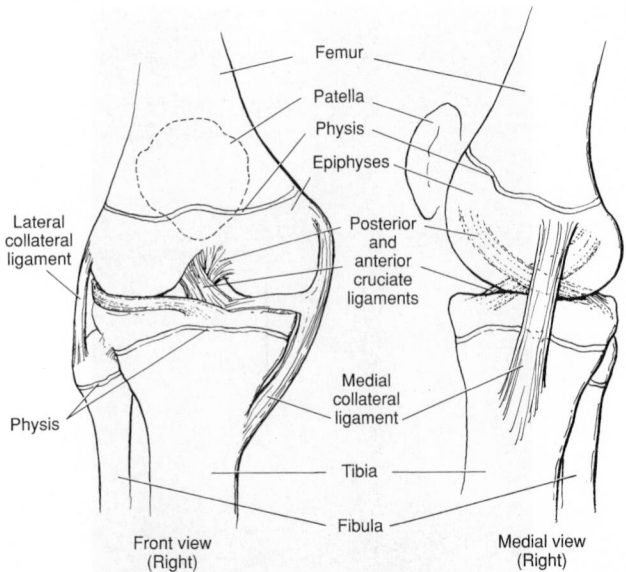

FIGURE 114.52 The ligaments of the knee. Proximally, both collateral ligaments attach to the epiphysis, whereas distally they attach to the tibia and fibula below the tibial epiphysis.

with adults, MRI studies may be necessary to define the true extent of the bony- and soft-tissue injuries.

Given the propensity for knee injuries in children younger than 14 years to result in fractures rather than ligamentous injuries, practitioners should have a low threshold for ordering radiographs. More recent studies validating the Ottawa knee rules in children provide clinicians with an evidence-based approach to imaging studies. Of the growth plates about the knee, the distal femoral physis is particularly vulnerable to injury. Both the medial and lateral collateral ligaments attach proximally to the distal femoral epiphysis. Their attachment to the tibia and fibula is distal to the epiphysis (Fig. 114.52). Given the relative strengths of the ligaments and the physeal plate, forceful valgus or varus stress results in distal femoral epiphysis separation rather than proximal tibial epiphysis injury or ligament rupture. Such injuries are discussed later in this chapter.

Avulsion of the tibial spine is the pediatric equivalent of an anterior cruciate ligament injury in an adult. The most commonly described mode of injury is hyperflexion of the knee during a fall from a bicycle. Significant pain and a refusal to bear weight are typical; a hemarthrosis is invariably present. Radiographic findings vary from minimal elevation of the anterior portion of the tibial spine (best seen on lateral views) to complete separation (Fig. 114.53). Incomplete separations can generally be managed by closed reduction with the knee held in extension. Open repair is necessary for complete avulsions and when closed manipulation does not lead to a satisfactory reduction. Arthroscopic evaluation of all tibial spine avulsions with instability on Lachman testing (see Chapter 38) has been advocated. Such an approach allows anatomic reduction of the injury with internal fixation and is believed to lead to a better long-term outcome. Immediate management in the ED should include splinting in extensions and arthrocentesis under sterile conditions when the hemarthrosis is causing severe pain.

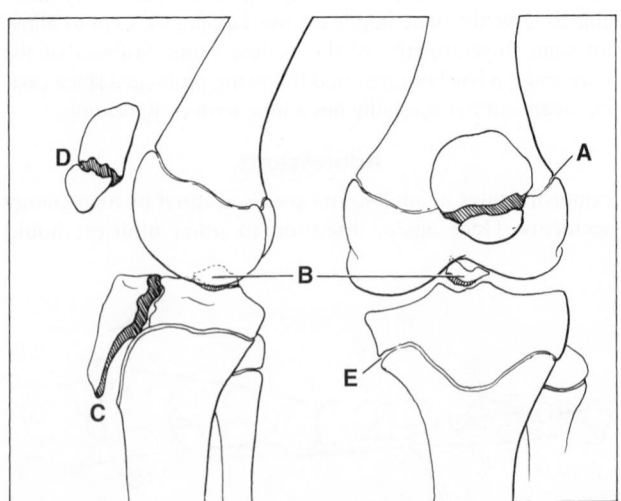

FIGURE 114.51 Common fractures of the knee in children: distal femoral physis (**A**), tibial spine (**B**), tibial tubercle (**C**), patella (**D**), and proximal tibial physis (**E**).

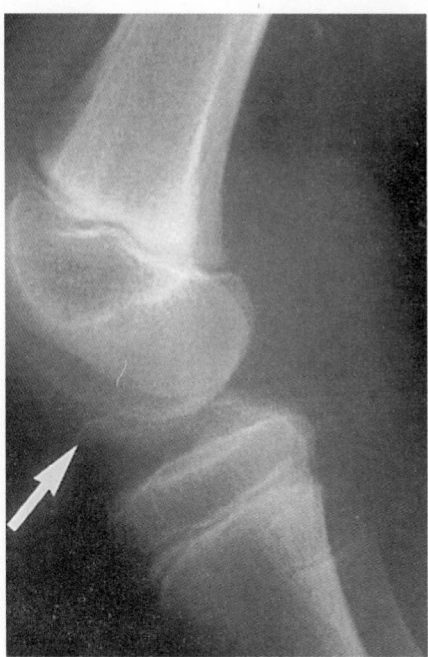

FIGURE 114.53 Avulsion fracture of the tibial spine in a 9-year-old girl. A significant hemarthrosis was present and was aspirated. In an adult, the same mechanism of injury would have resulted in a tear of the anterior cruciate ligament.

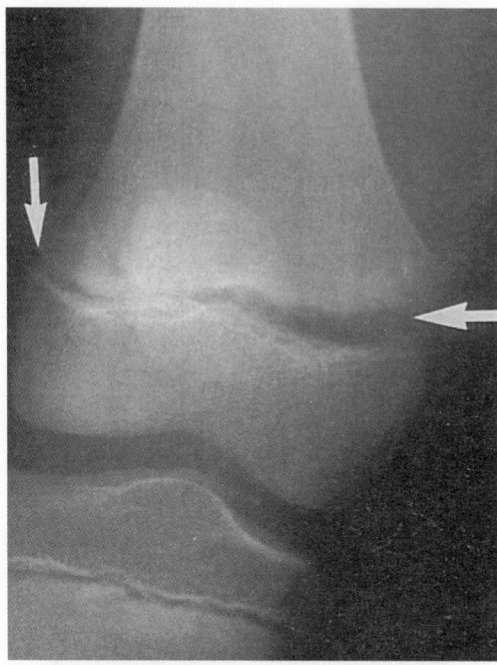

FIGURE 114.54 A Salter-Harris type II fracture of the right distal femoral physis in a 9-year-old boy. Widening of the growth plate is seen medially *(large arrow)*, and a small metaphyseal fragment has been displaced laterally *(small arrow)*. Closed reduction was successful. In an adult, the same mechanism of injury would have resulted in a medial collateral ligament sprain or tear.

Another uncommon but severe knee injury observed in adolescents is an avulsion fracture of the tibial tuberosity. This fracture occurs essentially exclusively in boys 12 to 17 years of age who are involved in vigorous sporting activities. Most such injuries occur during jumping when the quadriceps is strongly contracted. If extension is impeded, as when a basketball player jumps to shoot but is blocked, or if the contraction of the quadriceps is particularly violent, as in high-jumping, the tibial tubercle can be torn either in part or in its entirety from the proximal tibial epiphysis. The result is a Salter-Harris type III fracture. Of note is that the patient often has an antecedent history of Osgood-Schlatter's disease. Once again, the severity of the injury dictates whether closed or open management is chosen.

Distal Femoral Physeal Fractures

Historically, fractures of the distal femoral epiphysis occurred when the leg of a child was caught between the wagon and the spokes of the wheel; thus, they were known as "wagon wheel injuries" during the nineteenth century. Today these injuries are caused by high-energy sports injuries, motor vehicle accidents, and falls from a height. Overall, this injury is rare because of the undulating course of the physis and the strong perichondrial ring that surrounds it. Of all the fractures involving the growth plate, however, injuries of the distal femoral physis have the highest incidence of posttraumatic growth arrest.

These injuries are described according to the direction of displacement of the epiphysis and the corresponding Salter-Harris classification. Most common is medial or lateral displacement with a fracture of the adjacent metaphysis (a Salter-Harris type II injury) (Fig. 114.54). As already mentioned,

such injuries reflect a marked valgus or varus stress. The risk of neurovascular compromise is low, but peroneal nerve damage can accompany severe medial displacement. Even with adequate reduction, the incidence of premature growth arrest is significant. Somewhat less common is an anterior displacement of the distal epiphysis caused by hyperextension (Fig. 114.55). The risk of neurovascular compromise is high with this injury, which is the counterpart of a knee dislocation in an adult. Both compartment syndrome and direct compression of the neurovascular structures are well-recognized complications. Posterior displacement of the femoral epiphysis is uncommon but can occur as the result of a direct blow to the flexed knee. The preferred treatment of these injuries in the ED includes a thorough evaluation with splinting in place followed by prompt orthopedic consultation. Gentle closed reduction, often using general anesthesia, is usually successful. Postreduction remodeling cannot be assured because of the high rate of posttraumatic growth arrest associated with these injuries.

Proximal Tibial Physeal Fractures

Fractures of the proximal tibial physis are also rare. Hyperextension is the usual mechanism of injury. The sheer force tears the posterior periosteum and capsule of the knee, allowing a Salter-Harris fracture to occur through the growth plate. The emergency physician must recognize that the popliteal structures are tethered at this point and are therefore vulnerable to stretch or direct contusion at the time of injury. Careful, sequential neurovascular examinations are mandatory. Compartment syndrome should be considered. Closed or open

TRAUMA

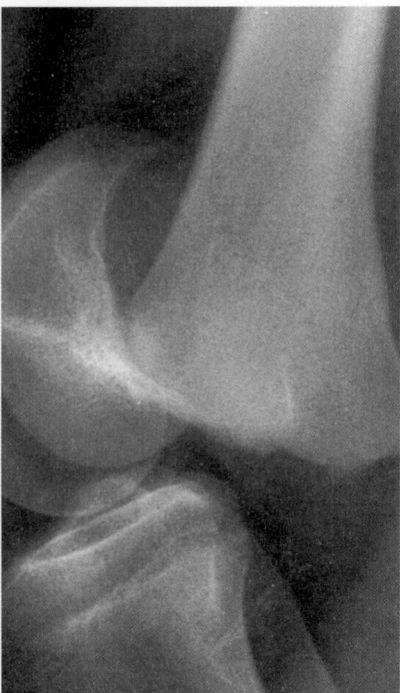

FIGURE 114.55 A Salter-Harris type I fracture of the right distal femoral physis with anterior displacement of the epiphysis in a 14-year-old boy. The injury resulted from a snowboarding accident.

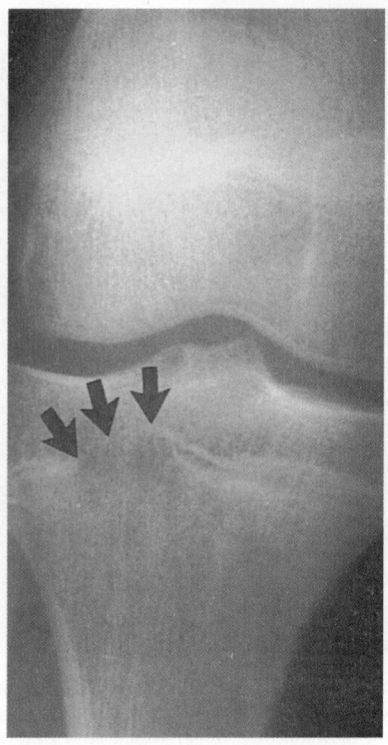

FIGURE 114.56 Although the original injury was only a Salter-Harris type I fracture of the proximal tibial physis, premature closure of the physis occurred *(arrows)*. All fractures involving the proximal tibial growth plate require orthopedic referral.

reduction will be necessary after stabilization. Complications after the injury include recurrent deformity, growth arrest, and limb length inequality (Fig. 114.56).

Knee Dislocations

Complete dislocation of the femorotibial joint, another hyperextension injury, is extremely uncommon in children. As a rule, hyperextension is much more likely to cause a distal femoral epiphyseal separation than a dislocation. Given the high likelihood of neurovascular compromise or compartment syndrome in this setting, femorotibial dislocation is considered a true emergency. A reduction maneuver may be attempted in the ED under intravenous sedation. Axial traction of the tibia with slow flexion of the knee from an extended position may lead to a reduction. Following a closed reduction, an arteriogram must be obtained to rule out an intimal tear of the popliteal artery. Definitive care of the torn ligaments resulting from this injury will ultimately be necessary.

Patellar Fractures and Dislocations

Unlike in the adult, the patella in the child is rarely fractured because of the thick covering of cartilage overlying the patella during growth and development. Fractures of the patella in adolescents are more common and present as avulsion fractures from dislocations, osteochondritis desiccans caused by overuse, symptomatic bipartite conditions, avulsion or "sleeve" fractures, and the occasional transverse displaced fracture (Fig. 114.57).

Diagnosis of a patellar fracture may be difficult. A congenitally bipartite patella can be easily confused with a fracture. In this case, an accessory ossification center is located along the superior lateral margin of the patella. The margins are smooth and rounded. A comparison view of the opposite knee may assist in the diagnosis. Sleeve fractures of the patella, in particular, can easily be misdiagnosed on radiograph. The sleeve fracture occurs when the lower half of the cartilage cap is pulled free by the patellar ligament. The visible bony portion

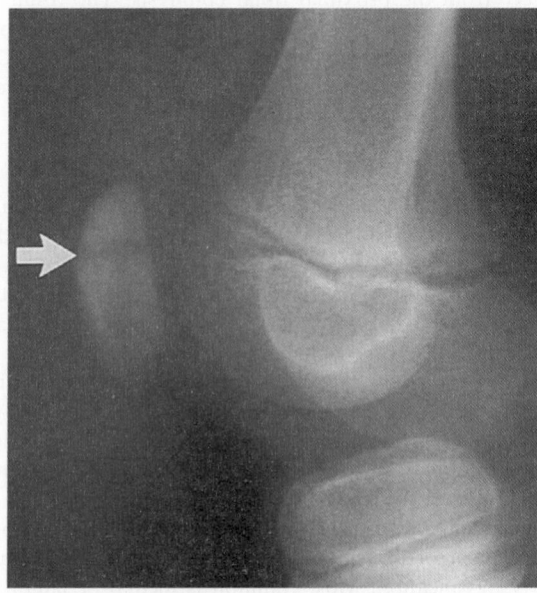

FIGURE 114.57 Transverse fracture of the patella in an 11-year-old victim of a motor vehicle accident *(arrow)*.

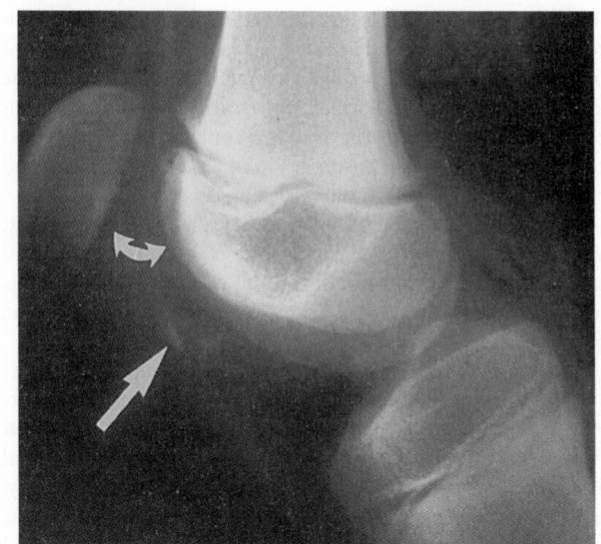

FIGURE 114.58 Radiograph demonstrating a sleeve fracture of the patella in a 10-year-old male. The inferior pole of the patella is displaced anteriorly *(curved arrow)*. The bone fragment seen *(large arrow)* was avulsed by, and remains attached to, the patellar tendon.

of the patella is displaced cephalad by the quadriceps mechanism. Often, a small fleck of bone is identified at the superior margin of the patellar ligament (Fig. 114.58). Pain usually prevents active extension of the knee.

The preferred treatment of patellar fractures parallels that of adults. Conservative care is the cornerstone of treatment in nondisplaced fractures. Cylindrical cast treatment from 4 to 6 weeks will result in union. Fractures that are displaced more than 3 to 4 mm are best treated with open reduction and internal fixation. Complications after patellar fractures include knee stiffness, quadriceps atrophy, extensor lag, and persistent pain.

Dislocation of the patella can be classified as an acute or chronic recurrent subluxation or as a dislocation. An acute traumatic dislocation of the patella results from a force displacing the patella laterally while the foot is planted. The patella may reduce spontaneously or may remain dislocated. Examination of the patient reveals an acutely swollen knee with pain to palpation noted along the medial patellar retinaculum. When reduction has already occurred, displacement of the patella laterally will usually elicit an apprehension sign. The patient may state that he or she feels like the kneecap is going to "pop out." When the patella remains dislocated, the diagnosis is readily apparent by clinical and radiographic examination. Reduction of a dislocated patella is usually accomplished easily with extension of the knee and a medial upward force on the lateral patella (see Section VII "Procedures"). Following reduction of an acutely dislocated patella, the physician must exclude the presence of an osteochondral fracture of the lateral femoral condyle or the medial patellar facet. Such fractures may be difficult to identify from a radiographic examination. Physical findings consistent with intraarticular loose bodies should suggest the diagnosis.

Chronic recurrent patella subluxation or dislocation is much less likely to result in osteochondral fractures. Predisposing factors include lateral femoral condyle hypoplasia, a loose medial

patellar retinaculum, genu valgum, external tibial torsion, and quadriceps weakness. The initial treatment of a dislocated patella should consist of a thorough examination, followed by closed reduction. Immobilization in an above-the-knee posterior splint or a commercially available knee immobilizer for 4 weeks is the appropriate ED management. Orthopedic referral is recommended.

Fractures of the Tibia and Fibula

Fractures of the tibia and fibula in children can be divided into the following groups: (i) proximal tibial metaphyseal fractures, (ii) tibial and fibular shaft fractures, and (iii) toddler's fractures.

Fractures involving the distal growth plates of the tibia and fibula are discussed with ankle injuries.

Proximal Tibial Metaphyseal Fractures

Although usually easy to manage, proximal tibial fractures can lead to two major complications, namely, compartment syndrome and progressive posttraumatic valgus deformity (Fig. 114.59). As in other settings, a careful clinical evaluation followed by direct measurement of compartment pressure is the key to the diagnosis of compartment syndrome. Progressive valgus deformity can develop after any proximal tibial injury, including greenstick and nondisplaced fractures. Deformity has been known to develop even after anatomic reduction of fracture fragments. It is speculated that stimulation of the

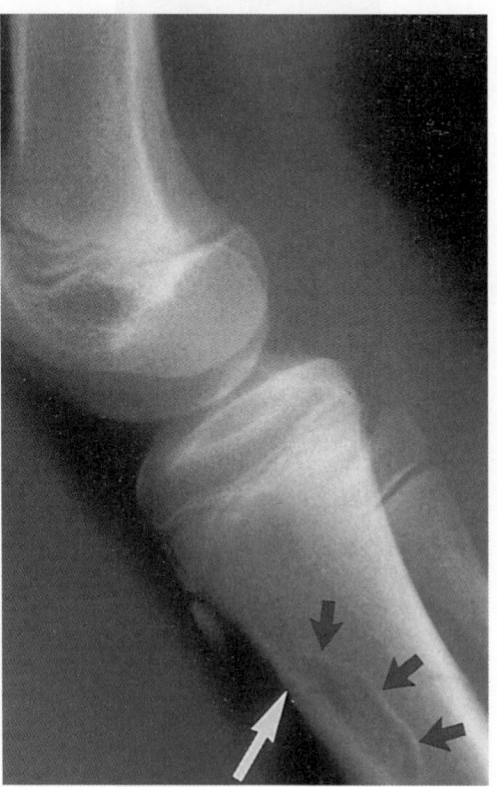

FIGURE 114.59 Nondisplaced proximal tibial metaphyseal fracture in an 11-year-old girl *(large arrow)* through a nonossifying fibroma *(small arrows)*. Orthopedic consultation is mandatory both because the fracture is pathologic and because it is located in the proximal tibia.

TRAUMA

physis from hyperemia causes asymmetric growth of the proximal tibial physis. Given the propensity for growth deformity, all fractures of the proximal tibial metaphysis should be managed by an orthopedic surgeon.

Tibial and Fibular Shaft Fractures

Fractures of the tibial and fibular shafts are the most common fractures of the lower extremity in children. The diagnosis is usually apparent by physical and radiographic examination. Most tibial and fibular fractures are stable and in acceptable alignment (Fig. 114.60). Discussion with an orthopedic consul-

tant helps decide whether any reduction is necessary. In children, these fractures rarely persist because of delayed union or nonunion. Healing time is quick, averaging 6 to 8 weeks. If the neurovascular status is normal, no signs of compartment syndrome are present, and the fracture configuration is deemed acceptable, a long leg posterior splint may be applied and orthopedic referral within the next few days arranged.

Otherwise, more immediate consultation should be sought. (Most cases of compartment syndrome result from minor closed tibial fractures; with more severe injuries, the interosseous membrane typically is torn, allowing decompression of the anterior compartment.)

The indications for open treatment of tibial and fibular shaft fractures in children include open fractures, compartment syndrome, ipsilateral femur fractures, and concomitant severe head injuries. Complications of treatment after tibial and fibular fractures include malunion, limb-length inequality, malrotation, and neurovascular deficiency.

Special consideration must be given when evaluating tibial injuries in children with paraplegia. They present with warmth and swelling over the leg or joint, which may suggest infection or inflammatory conditions rather than fractures. When identified, the fracture may be treated in a conservative manner with splints or a short 3- to 4-week period of casting.

Particular note should be made as well of the fact that the tibia and the fibula are the most common sites of stress fractures in children. Overall, the proximal third of the tibia is most often affected. The history is usually that of pain and a limp of gradual onset in a child 8 to 15 years of age. Localized swelling and tenderness are present to varying degrees. Radiographs may appear normal, show limited cortical changes, or demonstrate subperiosteal new bone formation. Bone scintigraphy confirms the diagnosis in uncertain cases (Fig. 114.7). Rest is the only treatment needed.

Toddler's Fractures

Occasionally, the emergency physician is asked to evaluate a young child with an acute gait disturbance, namely, a limp or a refusal to walk. The differential diagnosis is a broad one (see Chapter 42). One possibility that should always be considered is that of a toddler's fracture. Originally, the term *toddler's fracture* referred to an oblique nondisplaced fracture of the distal tibia in children 9 to 36 months of age. The term is now used more loosely.

In most cases, the history is that of a minor accident, such as a fall from a seemingly insignificant height or while walking or running. No history of injury may be recalled in some instances. The physical findings are often subtle and at best difficult to elicit unless a gentle, unhurried examination is performed while the child is calm. The degree of swelling is minimal; warmth and tenderness are more commonly detected but are not uniformly present. Gentle twisting of the lower leg will elicit pain on occasion.

Like the physical findings, the radiographic abnormalities are often subtle. The anteroposterior or lateral views may reveal a spiral or oblique fracture extending downward and medially through the distal third of the tibia. If a toddler's fracture is suspected clinically but the routine radiographic views are normal, an internal oblique projection should be ordered. Consideration should also be given to the possibility of a fracture elsewhere in the limb; fractures of the femur, the foot, and

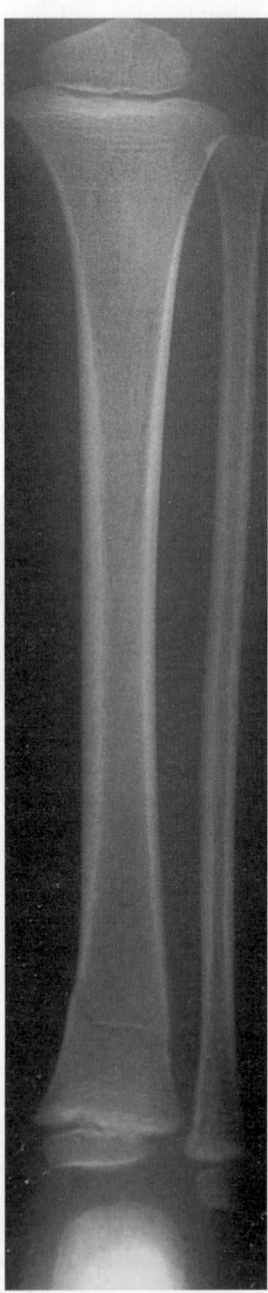

FIGURE 114.60 Nondisplaced transverse fracture of the distal tibia in a 3-year-old girl. Immobilization in a long leg posterior splint with orthopedic follow-up within 3 to 5 days would be adequate emergency treatment. The potential for growth deformity is low.

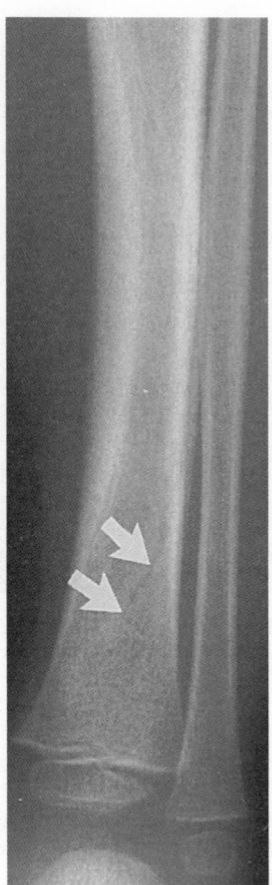

FIGURE 114.61 Toddler's fracture of the distal tibia *(arrows)*. The fracture line could not be demonstrated radiographically until 2 weeks after the onset of symptoms.

rarely, the pelvis can also present with an acute limp. If no fracture is visualized on routine radiographs, a US or a bone scan may be considered. Digital radiographs may also provide increased sensitivity compared with traditional plain films. Alternatively, if symptoms persist, it is certainly reasonable to repeat the plain films after 10 days, at which point subperiosteal new bone formation may be evident or enough sclerosis may have occurred at the fracture edges to render it visible (Fig. 114.61). Immobilization provides symptomatic relief and promotes healing, although no treatment may be necessary if the history suggests that the fracture occurred several weeks before actual diagnosis.

If a toddler's fracture is a spiral one and the caregivers can recall no specific time of injury, suspicions of child abuse may understandably arise. Notably, midshaft fractures are more common in abused children, and most toddler's fractures are distal injuries. When other circumstances or injuries suggestive of abuse are found or when spiral fractures occur in children who are not yet ambulating, the strong possibility of nonaccidental injury should obviously be seriously considered.

Injuries of the Ankle and Foot

Injuries of the ankle and foot in the pediatric age range can be divided into the following groups: (i) ankle sprains, (ii) distal

tibial and fibular fractures, (iii) hindfoot and midfoot fractures, and (iv) metatarsal and phalangeal fractures.

Ankle Sprains

Adolescents often present to the ED complaining of ankle injuries (see Chapter 36). The differential diagnosis includes ligamentous injuries; nondisplaced Salter-Harris type I fractures; osteochondral fractures of the tibia, fibula, or talus; and avulsion injuries. Once again, before growth plate fusion, physeal injuries are much more likely than ligamentous injuries. Ligamentous injuries are certainly observed in older adolescents. The most common mechanism is adduction and inversion of the foot while it is held in plantar flexion. Of the three lateral ankle ligaments, the anterior talofibular ligament is the one most commonly injured. Injury to this ligament should be suspected when palpation just anterior to the distal fibula elicits maximal tenderness. Ankle sprains are graded from I to III. In grade I injuries, ligaments are stretched but not torn. Grade II injuries include partial ligament tears without loss of stability. Complete tears of the ligamentous complex with loss of stability are present in grade III injuries. Other than with minor injuries, a three-view radiographic examination should be performed. As with adults, use of the Ottawa ankle rules, including by nursing personnel, can guide the need for radiographic studies. If the stability of a ligament is in question, stress views are recommended.

Controversy exists regarding the appropriate care of ligamentous injuries. One schema is based on the severity of the ligamentous damage. Grade I mild sprains can be treated with an elastic wrap or air splint followed by ice, elevation, and compression for 72 hours. Crutches may be used until the patient is able to walk without a limp. Grade II and grade III injuries should be immobilized either in a cast or a posterior splint. (Because posterior splints break relatively easily, use of fiberglass and/or reinforcement with a stirrup is recommended.) Crutches are used initially. Ambulation in a cast for 3 weeks aids in initial scar formation and healing. This conservative approach with more severe sprains may help prevent recurrent ankle sprains in active athletic adolescents, as may physical therapy once the injury has healed.

Distal Tibial and Fibular Fractures

Although any Salter-Harris type I through V fracture may occur in distal physes of the tibia and fibula, several specific injury patterns are described and discussed here. Fractures involving both the growth plate and the ankle joint often need open reduction and internal fixation to ensure adequate reduction of both the physis and the joint. Only minimal amounts of displacement can be accepted at the articular surface, or altered joint mechanics will develop with possible posttraumatic pain, stiffness, and arthritis.

Of the fractures of the distal fibula, a Salter-Harris type I injury is the most common. Tenderness and swelling are present over the growth plate on physical examination. Often the only radiographic finding is soft-tissue swelling overlying the distal fibula (Fig. 114.62). When suspicions of a Salter-Harris type I injury are high, a short leg cast may be applied at the time of initial evaluation. When the diagnosis is less certain, immobilization with a repeat examination in 1 week to 10 days is recommended. If tenderness persists, a presumptive diagnosis of a nondisplaced type I fracture should be made and a short leg cast, a fiberglass boot, or a posterior splint should

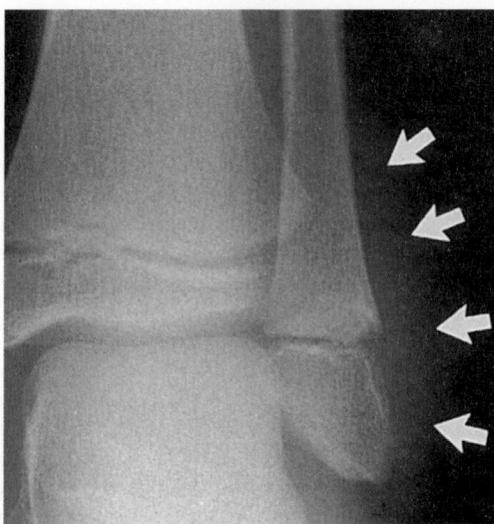

FIGURE 114.62 Radiograph of the left ankle of a 10-year-old boy notable only for soft-tissue swelling localized to the distal fibula *(arrows)*. The presumptive diagnosis must be a Salter-Harris type I injury of the fibula.

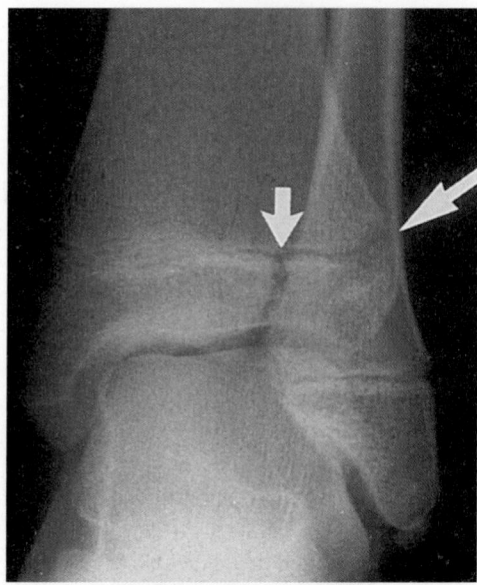

FIGURE 114.63 Classic Tillaux fracture of the distal tibia in a 14-year-old boy. The fracture line runs vertically through the epiphysis *(small arrow)* and then laterally along the physis *(large arrow)*. The lateral portion of the physis is widened.

be applied. After 10 days, repeat radiographs may reveal periosteal changes confirming the presence of a fracture. In most cases, a total of 3 weeks of immobilization is adequate.

Although type I injuries of the tibia are uncommon, type II injuries are often observed, usually in combination with a greenstick fracture of the fibula. The mechanism of injury is plantar flexion with eversion. Closed reduction and a long leg cast application usually lead to a satisfactory recovery. Growth disturbance is unusual.

The Tillaux fracture is a Salter-Harris type III injury of the ankle joint that occurs as the medial distal tibial physis begins to close in adolescents who are nearing skeletal maturity (Fig. 114.63). During external rotation of the foot, the anterior tibiofibular ligament avulses the lateral epiphysis from the medial malleolus. When displacement occurs, open reduction with internal fixation is required to ensure restoration of joint anatomy.

The triplane fracture is a complex but uncommon ankle injury that is a combination of a Salter-Harris type II fracture and a Tillaux fracture. The resultant type IV injury may appear innocuous on the anteroposterior and lateral radiographs, but the degree of growth plate damage is generally significant. Suspected triplane fractures should be evaluated by CT scan to delineate the amount of displacement at the physis and the articular surface, and to determine the number of fracture fragments (Fig. 114.64).

The treatment of physeal and ankle fractures depends on the type of fracture, the amount of displacement, and the patient's age. Nondisplaced fractures may be treated with a bulky posterior splint, crutches, and a referral to the orthopedist. Immediate orthopedic referral is otherwise necessary.

Hindfoot and Midfoot Fractures

Fractures of the foot in children are uncommon and lead to few complications. Fractures of the hindfoot, which consists of the talus and the calcaneus, are particularly uncommon. In more recent years, however, fractures of the lateral process of the talus

have become more common in the pediatric age group, primarily as the result of the increasing popularity of snowboarding. Not surprisingly, clinicians familiar with this entity commonly refer to it as the "snowboarder's fracture." When fractures of the hindfoot do occur, they are usually obvious because of swelling, pain, and occasionally, deformity. "Occult" fractures of the calcaneus have been increasingly recognized in children younger than 3 years. Pain with dorsiflexion may indicate a talar neck fracture. If suspicions of a fracture are high but routine radiographs are normal, additional views and/or bone scintigraphy may be necessary. Because calcaneal fractures generally occur as the result of a fall from a height, associated compression fractures of the spine can occur and must be considered. Treatment of hindfoot fractures are dictated by the amount of displacement. Often, a bulky posterior splint, crutches, and no weight-bearing will suffice until an orthopedic consult can be obtained. Complications include osseous necrosis of the talus and chronic pain from calcaneal fractures.

Fractures of the midfoot include the navicular; the cuboid; and the first, second, and third cuneiforms. Fractures of these bones are extremely unusual and usually form part of a more severe injury to the foot (Fig. 114.65). They can be produced by blunt trauma, in which case soft-tissue damage is usually significant and a potential for neurovascular compromise results. Occasionally, an accessory ossification center on the medial side of the navicular may be confused with a fracture.

Although well documented in the adult literature, tarsal/metatarsal fracture–dislocations have received little attention in children. These injuries present with swelling and tenderness over the dorsum of the foot. Radiographs, including anteroposterior, lateral, and oblique views, may be necessary to identify subtle abnormalities. Once again, treatment is based on the severity of the injury with reduction and stabilization necessary, if more than 2 mm of displacement is identified.

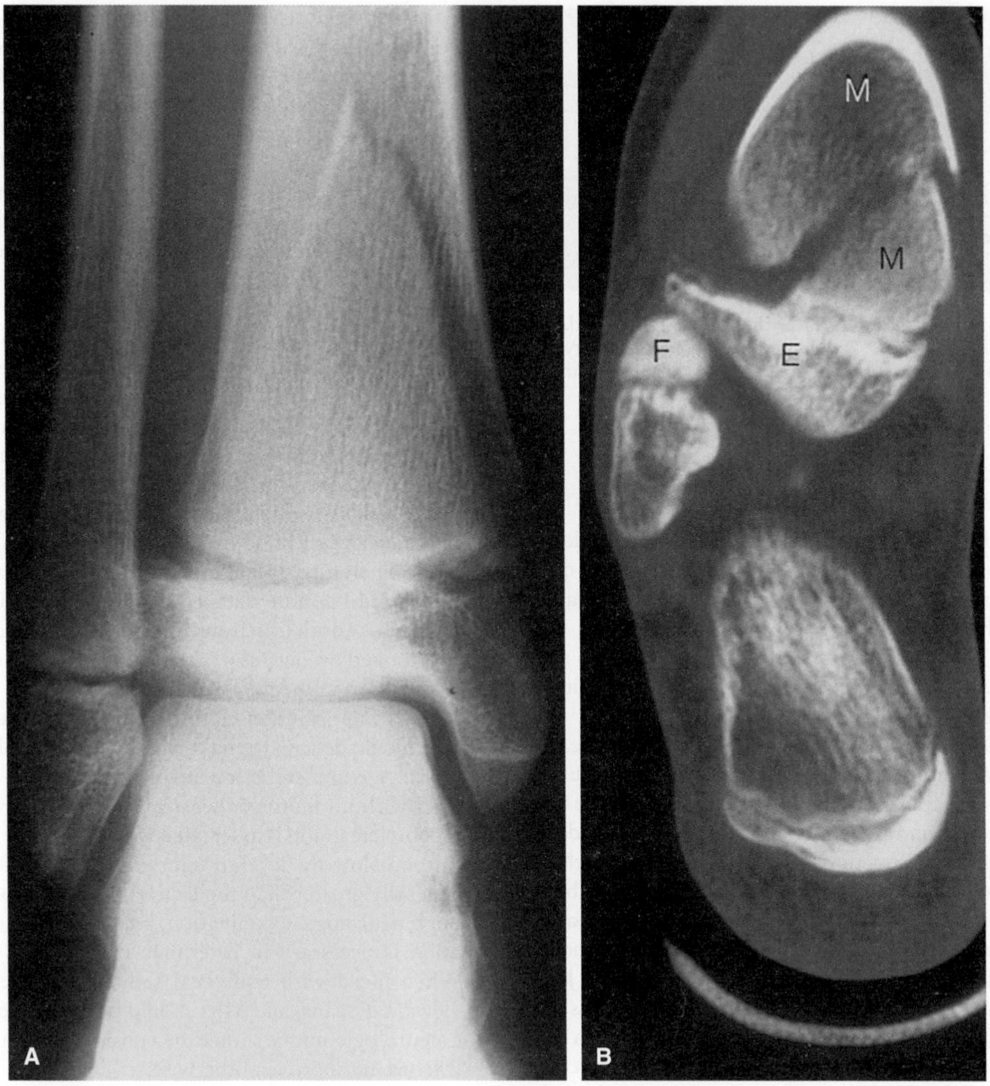

FIGURE 114.64 **A:** A triplane fracture was suspected from the plain film of the right ankle of this 11-year-old girl, although no clear epiphyseal fracture line could be seen. **B:** The coronal computed tomography scan made it possible to establish that the injury was indeed a Salter-Harris type II injury rather than the triplane fracture suspected. The fracture line runs laterally along the growth plate. E, epiphysis; F, fibula; M, tibial metaphysis.

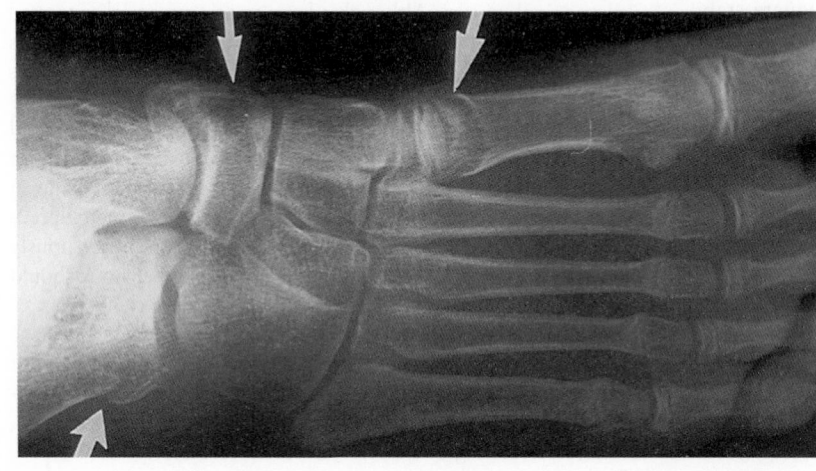

FIGURE 114.65 Radiograph of the right foot of a 13-year-old boy demonstrating fractures of the calcaneus *(small arrow)*, scaphoid *(medium arrow)*, and the first metatarsal *(large arrow)*.

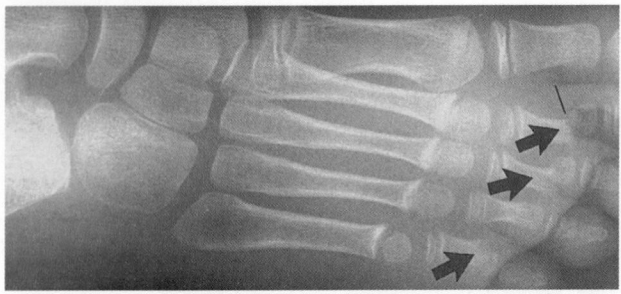

FIGURE 114.66 Displaced fractures of the right second, third, and fifth proximal phalanges in a 7-year-old girl *(arrows)*. Stability and proper healing of the fractures of the second and third toes could be guaranteed only with pinning.

Metatarsal and Phalangeal Fractures

Metatarsal and phalangeal fractures are common in children. The diagnosis is not difficult because pain, swelling, and occasionally a deformity accompany the fracture. Radiographic evaluations should include anteroposterior, lateral, and oblique views. The possibility of compartment syndrome must be kept in mind with crush injuries or multiple fractures in the midfoot or forefoot.

Two fractures that occur commonly at the base of the fifth metatarsal bear mentioning. The Jones fracture is a fracture at the diaphyseal–metaphyseal junction at the base of the fifth metatarsal. Although more common in adults, reports in adolescents can be found. This fracture has a high incidence of delayed or nonunion and should be splinted and referred to an orthopedist. An avulsion fracture of the base of the fifth metatarsal at the site of attachment of the peroneus brevis is relatively common in children. This fracture occurs more proximally than the Jones fracture and has a better prognosis. The usual treatment is 3 to 6 weeks of immobilization in a weight-bearing cast. When considering the possibility of a proximal fifth metatarsal fracture, care should be taken to distinguish a fracture fragment from the accessory ossification center found in the same location.

The care of most metatarsal and phalangeal injuries is relatively straightforward. If the fracture is nondisplaced or minimally displaced with little angulation, as is the usual case, a bulky splint can be applied and crutches prescribed. Intra-articular fractures of the big toe and significantly displaced fractures of the other toes often require pinning (Fig. 114.66). Buddy taping and hard-soled shoes provide adequate stabilization for most other phalangeal fractures.

INJURIES OF THE THORACOLUMBAR SPINE

Fortunately, injuries to the spine are rare in children and adolescents. When a child does have a spine injury, distinguishing what is normal from what is abnormal on plain radiographs can be extremely challenging. The advent of CT scans and MRI has made evaluation of spinal injuries much less problematic.

The child's spine differs from the adult's in that growth plates are present, the proportion of cartilage is higher, and the overall flexibility is greater. Because of the overall high elasticity of the pediatric spine, significant spinal cord injury can occur in the absence of radiographic signs of bony injury. By adolescence, the spine has mechanical qualities more like those of the adult, and the fracture patterns are similar. Unlike in adults, the risk of posttraumatic scoliosis after a complete spinal cord injury in children is extremely high.

In general, any child with significant head or multisystem injury should be assumed to have a spinal injury until proven otherwise. Diagnosis of a spinal injury in the child with a severe brain injury can be particularly problematic. However, certain physical findings can suggest the possibility of a coexisting spinal cord injury and should be sought routinely whenever a child with a severe head injury is examined. These findings include asymmetry of movement and reflexes between the arms and legs, absence of sacral reflexes, lax anal tone, priapism, spinal shock, autonomic hyperreflexia, diaphragmatic breathing, and urinary retention, as well as any evidence of a motor or sensory deficit level. When a child is sedated and/or paralyzed, as is often the case when a child has a severe brain injury, many of these findings will be particularly difficult to elicit. Therefore, spinal immobilization must always be maintained until a more detailed neurologic examination becomes possible. Another setting in which spinal cord injuries are overlooked on occasion is that of the lap belt complex, which is discussed in the following section.

It is important to classify spine injuries according to the neurologic deficits to make possible a determination of prognosis. A complete lesion involves the entire cord at a given level with no motor or sensory function below that level. An incomplete lesion is associated with sparing of function or sensation below the level of injury; the degree of motor deficit is generally greater than the degree of sensory loss. After a thorough neurologic examination, a complete radiographic evaluation is necessary to determine the stability of the fracture. When faced with equivocal radiographs, flexion–extension views, CT scans, and MRI should be considered. Patients with a neurologic injury should be considered to have an unstable fracture until proven otherwise.

Initial treatment in the ED must focus on maintaining the stability of the spine with a backboard and a cervical collar. Patients should not be moved unless absolutely necessary. Patients can be logrolled to inspect the spine as long as flexion, extension, or twisting movements do not occur. After stabilization of the patient and the spinal column, orthopedic and neurosurgical consultations should be obtained. Early intervention can decrease the risk of further injury to the spine in unstable, incomplete spinal injuries. Although a large multicenter trial suggested that administration of high-dose corticosteroids within 8 hours to teenagers and adults with acute spinal cord injury improves neurologic recovery, subsequent analysis of the data from this study and further investigations have not supported the initial recommendations from this group. Thus, most experts do not routinely administer corticosteroids. If a decision is made in favor of corticosteroids, according to the protocol, methylprednisolone 30 mg per kg should be administered intravenously over 15 minutes. An infusion of 5.4 mg per kg per hour should then be begun 45 minutes after the completion of the bolus.

Fractures of the spine in children and adolescents can be divided into the following groups based on the mechanism of injury and the radiographic appearance: (i) compression fractures, (ii) flexion and distraction fractures, (iii) shear fractures, and (iv) neurologic injuries without fractures.

Compression Fractures

Compression fractures result from hyperflexion producing an axial load and causing failure of the anterior vertebral body. Multiple fractures are the rule rather than the exception; the first lumbar vertebra is the most commonly injured segment (Fig. 114.67). A CT scan should be considered if there is evidence of multiple level fractures or when plain radiographs suggest the possibility of a retropulsed fragment. Compression fractures heal quickly in children and have little tendency to progress. Many children do not require hospitalization for compression fractures and can be treated with bed rest and symptomatic mobilization. Occasionally, a well-molded thoracolumbar sacral orthosis may be necessary for persistent pain or multiple areas of compression.

Flexion and Distraction Fractures

Flexion–distraction injuries are rare in the immature spine. When they do occur, the most common mechanism of injury is

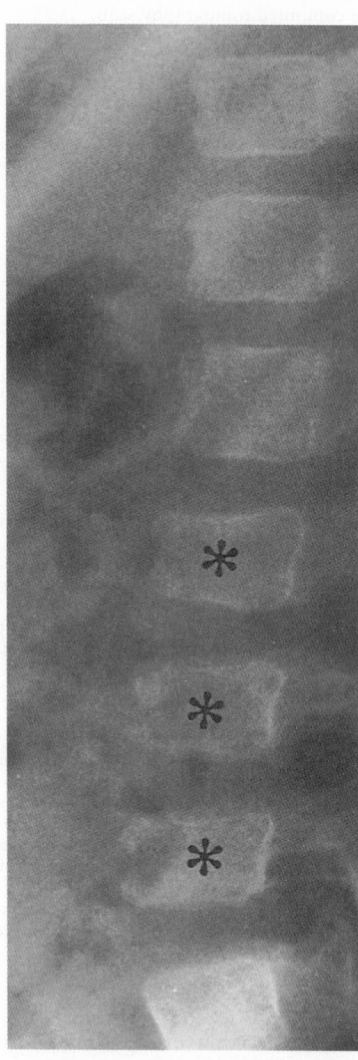

FIGURE 114.67 Compression fractures of the lumbar vertebrae in a 3-year-old boy *(asterisks)*. Multiple fractures are the rule in children.

hyperflexion over a seat belt during sudden deceleration in a motor vehicle accident. Associated intraabdominal injuries, particularly tears and transections of the duodenum, jejunum, and mesentery, are common. This combination of spinal and abdominal injuries is often referred to as either the seat belt syndrome or the lap belt complex. The tendency for lap belts to ride higher on children than the recommended position across the iliac crest combined with their relatively higher center of gravity predisposes them to both the abdominal and spinal injuries. A so-called seat belt sign, an abdominal contusion in a band corresponding to the seat belt, is often observed. Instances in which diagnosis of the spinal injury has been delayed because of the presence of the abdominal injury, as well as the reverse, have been described; the discovery of one component of the lap belt complex should obviously prompt a search for the other.

The lumbar spine is most commonly injured as the result of hyperflexion over a seat belt. Among the spinal injuries that can occur are distractions, subluxations, facet dislocations, and ligamentous ruptures, as well as fractures, including compression fractures as previously discussed. One particular fracture, the Chance fracture, merits special mention. A horizontal splitting through both the body and posterior elements of a vertebra, the Chance fracture was formerly thought to occur exclusively in adults. It is now recognized that the same fracture pattern occurs in children, almost always as a seat belt injury (and, once again, often in combination with an abdominal injury). Most Chance fractures are stable; associated neurologic injury is uncommon. Immobilization with a well-molded orthosis for several months is generally adequate treatment.

Shear Fractures

Although the cervical spine is most vulnerable to shear injuries, violent trauma can also cause such injuries in the thoracic and the lumbar spine (Fig. 114.68). Unfortunately, neurologic deficits are common in this setting. All shear fractures should be considered unstable injuries that will need stabilization procedures to avoid progressive deformity and enhance any possibility of neurologic recovery.

Neurologic Injuries Without Fractures

It is well known that the immature spine is more flexible than the spinal cord. Injuries causing hyperflexion or extension may produce damage to the cord and neurologic injury while leaving the bony, cartilaginous, and ligamentous structures intact. Termed SCIWORAs (spinal cord injury without radiographic abnormality), two thirds of such injuries occur in children younger than 8 years. Cervical and thoracic spine injuries are the most common. Both incomplete and complete neurologic deficits can occur. Any history of neurologic deficit following spinal trauma should prompt consideration of a SCIWORA. As for radiographic evaluation, MRI can best identify cord damage in the absence of a fracture. To reemphasize, in all cases of severe trauma, spinal immobilization must be maintained until the patient's condition permits a satisfactory neurologic examination.

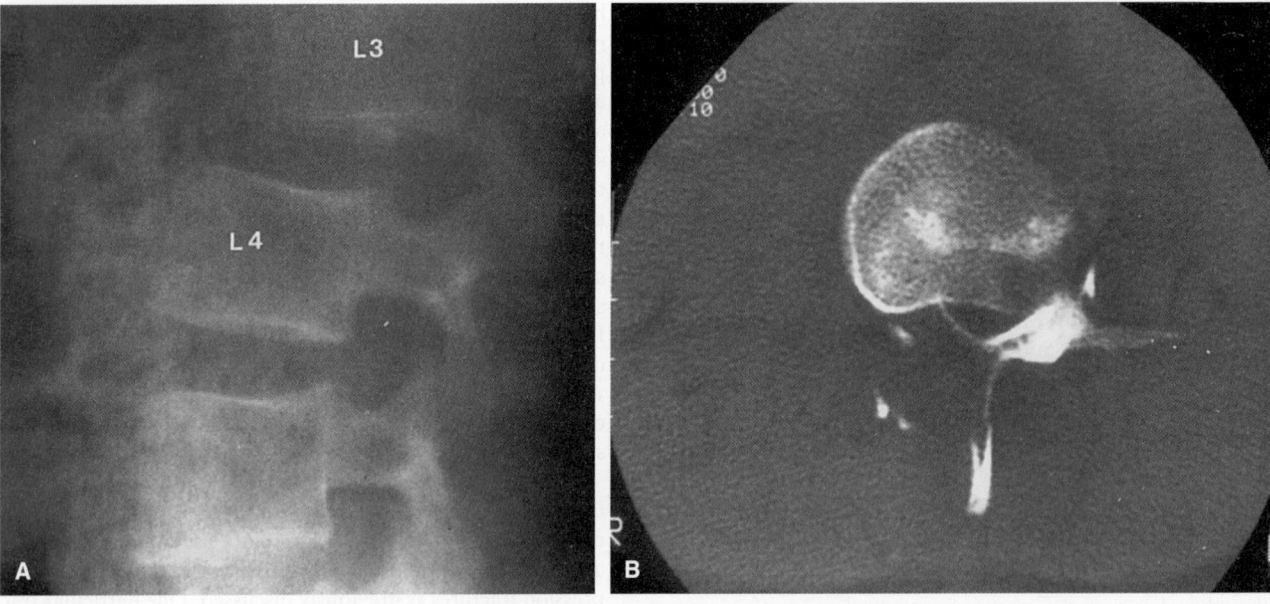

FIGURE 114.68 **A:** Fracture dislocation of the third (L3) and fourth (L4) vertebrae in a 12-year-old girl, the result of a shear injury in a motor vehicle accident. **B:** Permanent paralysis of the lower extremities resulted, as suggested by the degree of spinal canal collapse seen on the computed tomography scan.

Suggested Readings

Textbooks

Beatty JH, Kasser JR, eds. *Rockwood and Wilkins' fractures in children.* 6th ed. Philadelphia: Lippincott Williams & Wilkins, 2005.

Henretig FM, King C, eds. *Textbook of pediatric emergency procedures.* 2nd ed. Philadelphia: Lippincott Williams & Wilkins, 2008.

Swischuk LE. *Emergency imaging of the acutely ill or injured child.* 4th ed. Philadelphia: Lippincott Williams & Wilkins, 2000.

Reviews

Ecklund K. Magnetic resonance imaging of pediatric musculoskeletal trauma. *Top Magn Reson Imaging* 2002;13:203–217.

Kao SC, Smith WL. Skeletal injuries in the pediatric patient. *Radiol Clin North Am* 1997;35:727–746.

General Principles

Bae DS, Kadiyala RK, Waters PM. Acute compartment syndrome in children: contemporary diagnosis and treatment. *J Pediatr Orthop* 2001;21:680–688.

Brown JC, Klein EJ, Lewis CW, et al. Emergency department analgesia for fracture pain. *Ann Emerg Med* 2003;42:197–205.

Koller DM, Myers AV, Lorenz D, et al. Effectiveness of oxycodone, ibuprofen, or the combination in the initial management of orthopedic injury-related pain in children. *Pediatr Emerg Care* 2007;23:627–633.

Musgrave DS, Mendelson SA. Pediatric orthopedic trauma: principles in management. *Crit Care Med* 2002;30:S431–S443.

Perron AD, Miller MD, Brady WJ. Orthopedic pitfalls in the ED: pediatric growth plate injuries. *Am J Emerg Med* 2002;20:50–54.

Skaggs DL, Roy AK, Vitale MG, et al. Quality of evaluation and management of children requiring timely orthopaedic surgery before admission to a tertiary pediatric facility. *J Pediatr Orthop* 2002;22:265–267.

Turk J. Ultrasonographic findings in pediatric fractures. *J Pediatr* 2003;45:136–140.

Vorlat P, De Boeck H. Bowing fractures of the forearm in children: a long-term followup. *Clin Orthop Relat Res* 2003;413:233–237.

Worlock P, Stower M. Fracture patterns in Nottingham children. *J Pediatr Orthop* 1986;6:656–660.

Child Abuse

Caré M. Imaging in child abuse: what to expect and what to order. *Pediatr Ann* 2002;31:651–659.

Kemp AM, Dunstan F, Harrison S, et al. Patterns of skeletal fractures in child abuse. *BMJ* 2008;337:a1518.

Thomas SA, Rosenfield NS, Leventhal JM, et al. Long-bone fractures in young children: distinguishing accidental injuries from child abuse. *Pediatrics* 1991;88:471–476.

Injuries of the Shoulder Region

Pecci M, Kreher JB. Clavicle fractures. *Am Fam Physician* 2008;77:65–70.

Injuries of the Elbow

Griffith JF, Roebuck DJ, Cheng JC, et al. Acute elbow trauma in children: spectrum of injury revealed by MR imaging not apparent on radiographs. *AJR Am J Roentgenol* 2001;176:53–60.

McDonald J, Whitelaw C, Goldsmith LJ. Radial head subluxation: comparing two methods of reduction. *Acad Emerg Med* 1999;6:715–718.

Rasool MN Dislocations of the elbow in children. *J Bone Joint Surg Br* 2004;86:1050–1058.

Shrader MW. Pediatric supracondylar fractures and pediatric physeal elbow fractures. *Orthop Clin North Am* 2008;39:163–171.

Skaggs DL, Mirzayan R. The posterior fat pad sign in association with occult fracture of the elbow in children. *J Bone Joint Surg Am* 1999;81:1429–1433.

Wu J, Perron AD, Miller MD, et al. Orthopedic pitfalls in the ED: pediatric supracondylar humerus fractures. *Am J Emerg Med* 2002;20:544–550.

Fractures of the Forearm and Wrist

Memarsadeghi M, Breitenseher MJ, Schaefer-Prokop C, et al. Occult scaphoid fractures: Comparison of multidetector CT and MR imaging. *Radiology* 2007;242:169–176.

Pershad J, Monroe K, King W, et al. Can clinical parameters predict fractures in acute pediatric wrist injuries? *Acad Emerg Med* 2000;7:1152–1155.

Plint AC, Perry JJ, Correll R, et al. A randomized, controlled trial of removable splinting versus casting for wrist buckle fractures in children. *Pediatrics* 2006;117:691–697.

Waeckerle JF. A prospective study identifying the sensitivity of radiographic findings and the efficacy of clinical findings in carpal navicular fractures. *Ann Emerg Med* 1987;16:733–737.

Injuries of the Hand and Fingers

Mahabir RC, Kazemi AR, Cannon WG, et al. Pediatric hand fractures: a review. *Pediatr Emerg Care* 2001;17:153–156.

Valencia J, Leyva F, Gomez-Bajo GJ. Pediatric hand trauma. *Clin Orthop Relat Res* 2005;432:107–115.

Fractures of the Pelvis

Grisoni N, Connor S, Marsh E, et al. Pelvic fractures in a pediatric level I trauma center. *J Orthop Trauma* 2002;16:458–463.

Guillamondegui OD, Mahboubi S, Stafford PW, et al. The utility of the pelvic radiograph in the assessment of pediatric pelvic fractures. *J Trauma* 2003; 55:236–239.

Junkins EP, Nelson DS, Carroll KL, et al. A prospective evaluation of the clinical presentation of pediatric pelvic fractures. *J Trauma* 2001;51:64–68.

Injuries of the HIP and Proximal Femur

Perron AD, Miller MD, Brady WJ. Orthopedic pitfalls in the ED: slipped capital femoral epiphysis. *Am J Emerg Med* 2002;20:484–487.

Roy DR. Current concepts in Legg-Calve-Perthes disease. *Pediatr Ann* 1999;28: 748–752.

Seller K, Raab P, Wild A, et al. Risk—benefit analysis of prophylactic pinning in slipped capital femoral epiphysis. *J Pediatr Orthop* 2001;10:192–196.

Fractures of the Shaft of the Femur

Unal VS, Gulcek M, Unveren Z, et al. Blood loss evaluation in children under age 11 with femoral shaft fractures with isolated versus multiple injuries. *J Trauma* 2006;60:224–226.

Wathen JE, Gao D, Merritt G, et al. A randomized controlled trial comparing a fascia iliaca compartment nerve block to a traditional systemic analgesia for femur fractures in a pediatric emergency department. *Ann Emerg Med* 2007;50:162–171.

Yandow SM, Archibeck MJ, Stevens PM, et al. Femoral-shaft fractures in children: a comparison of immediate casting and traction. *J Pediatr Orthop* 1999;19:55–59.

Injuries of the Knee

Bulloch B, Neto G, Plint A, et al. Validation of the Ottawa knee rule in children: a multicenter study. *Ann Emerg Med* 2003;42:48–55.

Close BJ, Strouse PJ. MR of physeal fractures of the adolescent knee. *Pediatr Radiol* 2000;30:756–762.

Vaquero J, Vidal C, Cubillo A. Intra-articular traumatic disorders of the knee in children and adolescents. *Clin Orthop Relat Res* 2005;432:97–106.

Fractures of the TIbia and Fibula

Baron CM, Seekins J, Hernanz-Schulman M, et al. Utility of total lower extremity radiography investigation of nonweight bearing in the young child. *Pediatrics* 2008;121:e817–e820.

Fahr MJ, James LP, Beck JR, et al. Digital radiography in the diagnosis of toddler's fracture. *South Med J* 2003;96:234–239.

Injuries of the Ankle and Foot

Kay RM, Matthys GA. Pediatric ankle fractures: evaluation and treatment. *J Am Acad Orthop Surg* 2001;9:268–278.

Marsh JS, Daigneault JP. Ankle injuries in the pediatric population. *Curr Opin Pediatr* 2000;12:52–60.

Ribbans WJ, Natarajan R, Alavala S. Pediatric foot fractures *Clin Orthop Relat Res* 2005;432:107–115.

Injuries of the Thoracolumbar Spine

Akbarnia BA. Pediatric spine fractures. *Orthop Clin North Am* 1999;30: 521–536.

Newman KD, Bowman LM, Eichelberger MR, et al. The lap belt complex: intestinal and lumbar spine injury in children. *J Trauma* 1990;30:1133–1140.

CHAPTER 115 ■ NECK TRAUMA

GEORGE A. WOODWARD, MD, MBA

Pediatric neck injuries, fortunately, are uncommon. Many children are evaluated for cervical spine injuries secondary to trauma but few have their injuries identified. Even fewer children are evaluated for penetrating or direct blunt trauma to the neck. However, because neck injuries can be life threatening, they need to be assessed in a timely and orderly manner. It is imperative to appreciate how apparently minor or innocuous neck injuries can progress rapidly to more serious and life-threatening events. Subtle neck injuries can be easily overlooked in a patient with obvious head or chest trauma. This chapter initially discusses evaluation and management of penetrating and direct blunt injuries and then concentrates on the evaluation of the cervical spine.

When considering injuries to the neck in a child, initial management must include immediate assessment of airway, breathing, and circulation (ABCs) and treatment of abnormalities, careful not to allow an injury to progress to a more significant event. Airway abnormality may be subtle but progressive, with the precipitating injury not obvious on initial examination. Treatment should be safe and supportive and may include options within treatment categories, such as fiber-optic intubation and surgical airway placement depending on the nature and severity of the injury. Patients should be monitored closely and physically observed during their emergency department (ED) stay. A listing of common mechanisms of neck injury is given in Table 115.1.

There are several differences in neck anatomy between children and adults. The child's relatively large head and mandible and short neck make the anterior neck less accessible to direct trauma but may increase the possibility of acceleration/deceleration injuries to the cervical spine. The increased potential for acceleration/deceleration injuries is partially offset by the elasticity of the pediatric cervical spine and the child's light weight. Internal neck anatomy also differs from that of an adult and may influence the types of injuries seen. The cricoid ring is the narrowest portion of the airway and is located at the C4 level, as opposed to the adult location at C7. The arytenoids are proportionately larger, and the child's cartilage is more pliable and easily damaged.

The soft tissues and visceral components of the neck are protected by the spine posteriorly, the mandible anteriorly and superiorly, the shoulders and clavicles anteriorly and inferiorly, and the neck muscles. The head and chest of the child protrude more anteriorly than the neck and often absorb most blunt traumatic force, lessening the chance of a direct neck injury. Most injuries to the neck involve forces with relatively large masses and slow velocity, which partially account for the low incidence of serious direct trauma in this population. If the neck is hyperextended, however, the structures of the anterior neck, including the larynx, trachea, and esophagus, are more susceptible to direct trauma. The large number of vital organs and structures in the relatively small neck area enhances the potential severity of direct penetrating or blunt injuries (Table 115.2).

The neck can be divided into three anatomic zones (Figs. 115.1 to 115.3). Zone I encompasses the area between the thoracic inlet and the cricoid (the lower boundary of zone I is the thoracic inlet, the upper boundary is most often classified as the cricoid); zone II is the area between the cricoid and the angle of the mandible, the most common site of significant penetrating injuries; and zone III is the area above the angle of the mandible. Knowledge of the divisions and structures they contain is useful in the evaluation and management of neck trauma (Fig. 115.1 to 115.3). Lesions in zones I and III are often occult and difficult to diagnose by physical examination alone. Operative exploration is more difficult in zones I and III than in zone II, where injury presentation and surgical exploration are often more straightforward. The neck can also be divided into anterior and posterior elements, with the dividing line being the palpable transverse processes of the cervical spine. The posterior neck contains muscles with their individual nerve supplies and the posterior elements of the cervical spine, and the anterior neck houses most vital organs and structures. No major vascular components are contained in the posterior area of the neck. Morbidity and mortality with neck injuries result from central nervous system trauma, airway compromise, exsanguination, vascular disruption or thrombosis, venous embolism, sepsis, or mediastinitis.

PENETRATING TRAUMA

Penetrating neck trauma is uncommon in children. Penetrating trauma may be associated with extracervical injuries and may involve multiple organ systems within the neck. Most pediatric penetrating trauma is the result of a wound from a gunshot (usually low velocity), knife, broken windshield, other sharp object, or explosion (Table 115.1). The history is important in the evaluation of penetrating neck trauma. Inquiries about the mechanism of injury, time of incident, events before arrival in the ED, amount of blood loss, history of pulsatile lesions, neurologic dysfunction (including transient ischemic attack, limb paresthesias, hemiplegia, blindness, Horner's syndrome, and aphasia), and airway compromise should all be noted. In particular, knowledge of the mechanism of injury can help direct the management of both the stable and unstable patients. The mortality rate with

TABLE 115.1

COMMON MECHANISMS OF BLUNT AND
PENETRATING NECK INJURIES

Penetrating trauma	Blunt trauma
High-velocity missiles	Motor vehicle accidents, including motorcycles and all-terrain vehicles
Low-velocity missiles	Sports
Knives	Fights
Windshields	Falls
Sharp objects	Clothesline injuries
Explosions	Bicycle handlebars
Dog bites	Dog bites
Iatrogenic (intubation, endoscopy, gastric tubes)	Barotrauma (bottle cap under pressure or compressed air source)
	Nonaccidental (abuse)
	Exposures (fires, caustics)

penetrating neck trauma is between 3% and 6% with or without surgical exploration. Common causes of death include vascular, neurologic, and airway injuries.

Most gunshot wounds seen in pediatric patients involve low-velocity weapons, including handguns (90 m per second) or shotguns (300 m per second), at ranges of more than 5 m, as opposed to shotguns at close range or military-style weapons (760 m per second) (Fig. 115.4).

Unlike higher-velocity missiles, low-velocity missiles tend to be redirected when they encounter vascular or other structures. Visceral injuries may be anticipated but not completely predicted by the path of the missile. Internal injuries may be more predictable with an isolated knife wound. Low-velocity neck wounds are associated with major pathology in approximately 50% of cases compared with more than 90% with high-velocity missiles.

Vascular injury is the most common complication of penetrating trauma and is the second most common cause of death. Injuries include aneurysms, dissections, occlusions, and fistulas.

History of large blood loss, pulsatile lesion, rapidly expanding hematoma, hypovolemic shock, or neurologic deficits (paresis, visual loss or aphasia, altered level of consciousness) indicates the possibility of cervical arterial injury. Major vessels that can be injured in the neck include the common, internal, and external carotid arteries; vertebral arteries; internal and external jugular veins; and nearby innominate and subclavian vessels (Table 115.2). Injury to the vessels can be dramatic, with exsanguination, rapidly expanding hematoma causing airway compromise, acute neurologic deficits from ischemia or hypoperfusion, or venous air embolism, or it may be subtle with an initially normal examination. Approximately one-third of arterial injuries present with neurologic deficits, whereas the remaining two-thirds are often more challenging to diagnose. The symptoms and signs suggestive of vascular and other neck injuries are presented in Table 115.3. Completely transected arteries often retract and contract with minimal bleeding. Vessels that are partially severed may continue to bleed significantly with normal pulses because blood flow may not be totally interrupted. Vascular abnormalities can be assessed partially by evaluating the carotid (external), superficial temporal, and brachial pulses, although no pulses are easily accessible to evaluate for the internal carotid or vertebral arteries. Abnormal pulses suggest vascular injury, whereas normal pulses do not guarantee vascular integrity.

Auscultation of the neck is useful to identify bruits. Although a carotid bruit may be normal in children, a continuous bruit suggests a traumatic arteriovenous fistula whereas a systolic bruit suggests a partial arterial tear. Bleeding from a posterior neck wound, neurologic deficits in areas supplied by the vertebral arteries (brainstem, cerebellum), bleeding not controlled by carotid compression, a posterior bruit, or bleeding that accompanies a cervical spine transverse process fracture suggests a vertebral artery injury. Carotid artery trauma should be suspected if presentation involves an anterior triangle hematoma, Horner's syndrome (ptosis, miosis, enophthalmos, loss of sweating on the ipsilateral side of the face), transient ischemic attacks, loss of consciousness after a lucid interval, or hemiplegia. Evaluation of the chest for signs of major vessel injury, including hemothorax, widened mediastinum, and cardiac tamponade, should accompany the neck examination.

TABLE 115.2

NECK CONTENTS AND CLOSELY APPROXIMATED STRUCTURES

Musculoskeletal	Vascular	Venous	Gastrointestinal	Glandular
Cervical spine	Arterial	Jugulars: internal, external	Esophagus	Thyroid
Cervical muscles	Carotids: common, internal, external	Lymphatics	**Neurologic**	Parathyroid
Ligaments		Thoracic duct	Spinal cord	Parotid
Clavicles	Vertebral		Cranial nerves IX–XII	Submandibular
First rib	Innominate	**Airway**	Cervical nerves	
Hyoid	Subclavian	Larynx	Cervical sympathetics	
		Trachea	Brachial plexus	
		Apices of lung		

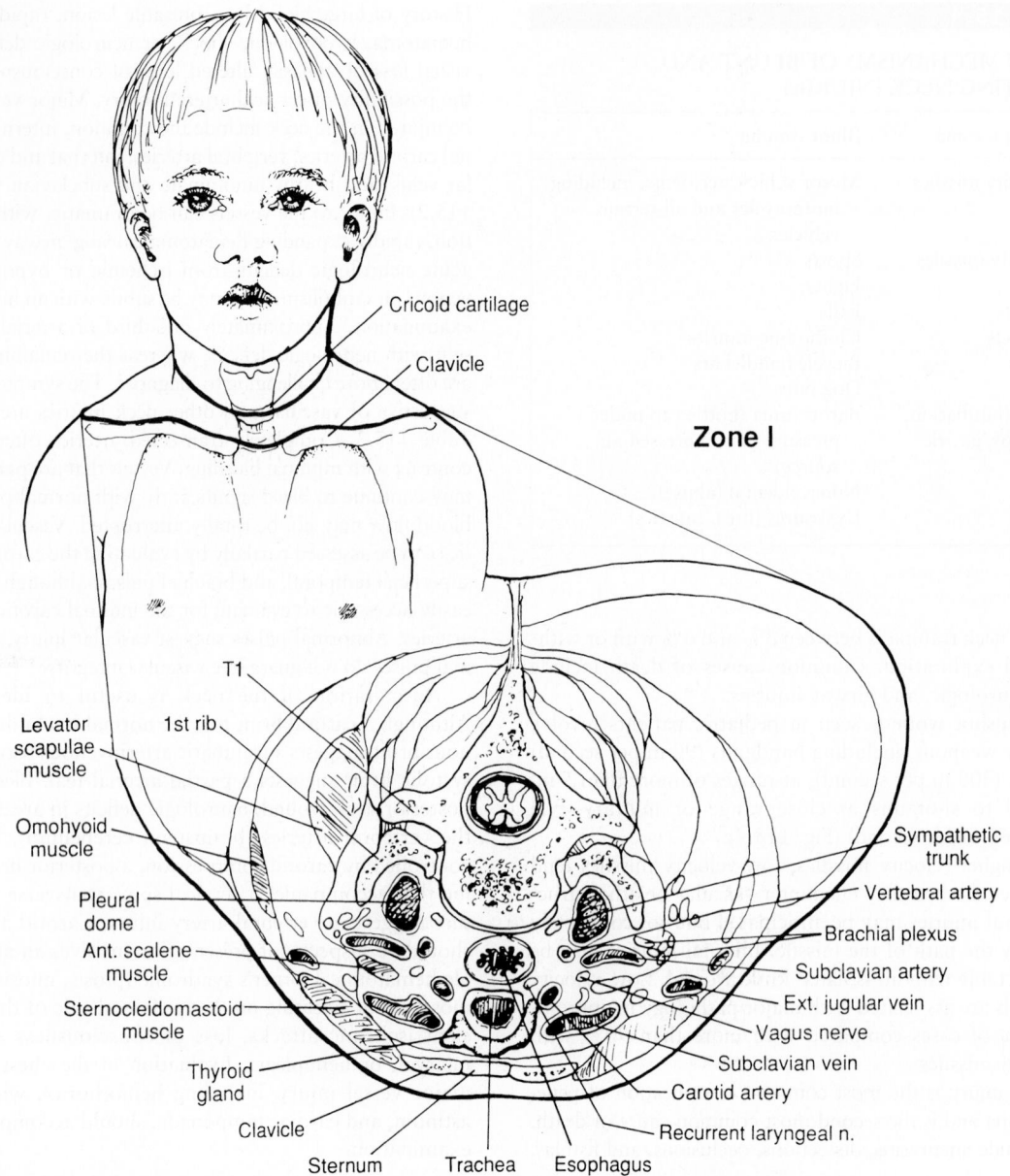

FIGURE 115.1 **A:** Anatomic neck divisions and contents of zone I. Zone I encompasses area between the thoracic inlet and the cricoid. (*continued*)

Neck vessels may be injured indirectly as a result of shock waves from a missile. These patients may have clinically unapparent vascular intimal damage that can progress to vascular thrombus or occlusion. Venous or lymphatic (thoracic duct) injuries also occur with penetrating trauma. These injuries are rarely severe and usually present as an expanding hematoma or less often with a venous air embolism. Pulmonary embolus secondary to a venous thrombus is a rare event.

Injuries to the aerodigestive tract (pharynx, larynx, trachea, and esophagus) are also seen in cases of penetrating trauma, although these relatively mobile structures are often spared. Injury may occur with rapid acceleration/deceleration events and with a direct neck blow resulting in compression of the esophagus against the cervical spinal column. The esophagus is somewhat protected in that it is usually collapsed as it courses through the neck but it may be injured by direct penetrating objects, usually a stab or gunshot wound. Penetrating injury of the larynx and trachea occur, although blunt trauma to these areas is more common and can be associated with significant morbidity and mortality (see Chapter 123). These injuries can present initially in a subtle fashion, but delays in diagnosis can lead to significant increase in observed morbidity and mortality.

Direct nervous system injury (brachial plexus, spinal cord, cervical nerves, and cervical sympathetics) is possible with penetrating neck trauma and the evaluation of the patient should assess these structures. Symptoms correspond

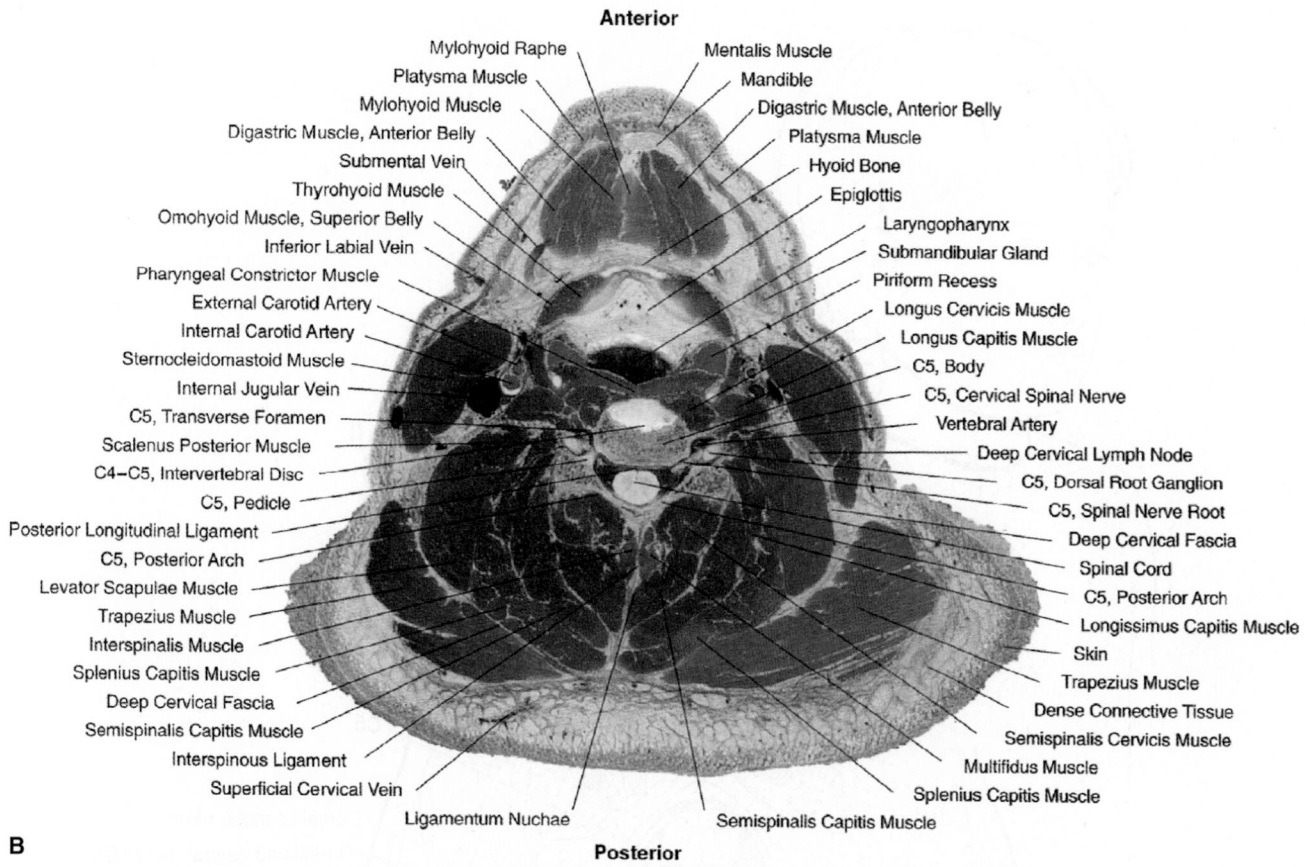

Anterior

Mylohyoid Raphe
Platysma Muscle
Mylohyoid Muscle
Digastric Muscle, Anterior Belly
Submental Vein
Thyrohyoid Muscle
Omohyoid Muscle, Superior Belly
Inferior Labial Vein
Pharyngeal Constrictor Muscle
External Carotid Artery
Internal Carotid Artery
Sternocleidomastoid Muscle
Internal Jugular Vein
C5, Transverse Foramen
Scalenus Posterior Muscle
C4–C5, Intervertebral Disc
C5, Pedicle
Posterior Longitudinal Ligament
C5, Posterior Arch
Levator Scapulae Muscle
Trapezius Muscle
Interspinalis Muscle
Splenius Capitis Muscle
Deep Cervical Fascia
Semispinalis Capitis Muscle
Interspinous Ligament
Superficial Cervical Vein
Ligamentum Nuchae

Mentalis Muscle
Mandible
Digastric Muscle, Anterior Belly
Platysma Muscle
Hyoid Bone
Epiglottis
Laryngopharynx
Submandibular Gland
Piriform Recess
Longus Cervicis Muscle
Longus Capitis Muscle
C5, Body
C5, Cervical Spinal Nerve
Vertebral Artery
Deep Cervical Lymph Node
C5, Dorsal Root Ganglion
C5, Spinal Nerve Root
Deep Cervical Fascia
Spinal Cord
C5, Posterior Arch
Longissimus Capitis Muscle
Skin
Trapezius Muscle
Dense Connective Tissue
Semispinalis Cervicis Muscle
Multifidus Muscle
Splenius Capitis Muscle
Semispinalis Capitis Muscle

B

Posterior

FIGURE 115.1 (*Continued*) **B:** Anatomic specimen demonstrating zone I relationships. (**B:** From Spitzer VM, Whitlock DG. *Atlas of the visible human male: reverse engineering of the human body.* Sodburg, MA: Jones & Bartlett, 1998. Reprinted with permission.)

to the injured structure, which may or may not require primary surgical repair (Fig. 115.5). Primary injury to the cervical cord often results from bony or foreign-body penetration or impingement or cord distraction. Secondary cord injury can occur from vascular compromise, edema, lipid peroxidation, ischemia, and ligamentous damage. When assessing neurologic findings or predicting location of the injury, it is important to remember that spinal cord and vertebral levels are not the same. In the cervical area, the cord level lies one segment higher than the corresponding vertebral level (C4 cord level lies opposite the C3 vertebral body). In the lower cervical area, a disparity of up to two levels may be present.

BLUNT TRAUMA

Blunt trauma is often the result of a motor vehicle accident, although it can also result from sports-related injuries; clothesline and handlebar injuries from bicycles, motorcycles, all-terrain vehicles, and snowmobiles; strangulation; hanging; blows from fists or feet; and the battered child syndrome (Table 115.1). Pediatric differences in exposures as well as the fact that children have a relatively short neck, mobile laryngotracheal structures, and a superior positioned

larynx protected by the mandibular arch make it less likely for children to sustain airway fractures and may impact overall severity of injury. On the other hand, the small and narrow airway increases the risk of airway-related morbidity secondary to airway edema, bleeding, swelling, and obstruction. Blunt trauma is often associated with extracervical injuries, especially maxillofacial, head, and chest injuries, but is less likely than penetrating trauma to involve multiple structures within the neck. Blunt trauma is less likely than penetrating trauma to cause vascular damage, but the incidence of aerodigestive tract injuries is increased. The airway is often injured with direct blunt trauma in part as a result of the anterior and relatively fixed position of the larynx and trachea. High-impact blunt trauma to the trachea has been associated with a mortality rate of approximately 15%, although this is likely higher when one includes patients who die at the scene. As mentioned, the anterior neck is relatively well protected by bony structures, unless the neck is extended. With neck extension, the larynx, trachea, and esophagus are exposed to direct trauma and a blunt force may crush these structures against the posterior spinal column. A tracheal tear or rupture may occur from a sudden increase in intratracheal pressure against a closed glottis, direct blunt trauma, crush, or acceleration/deceleration injury. Shearing forces can cause edema, submucosal

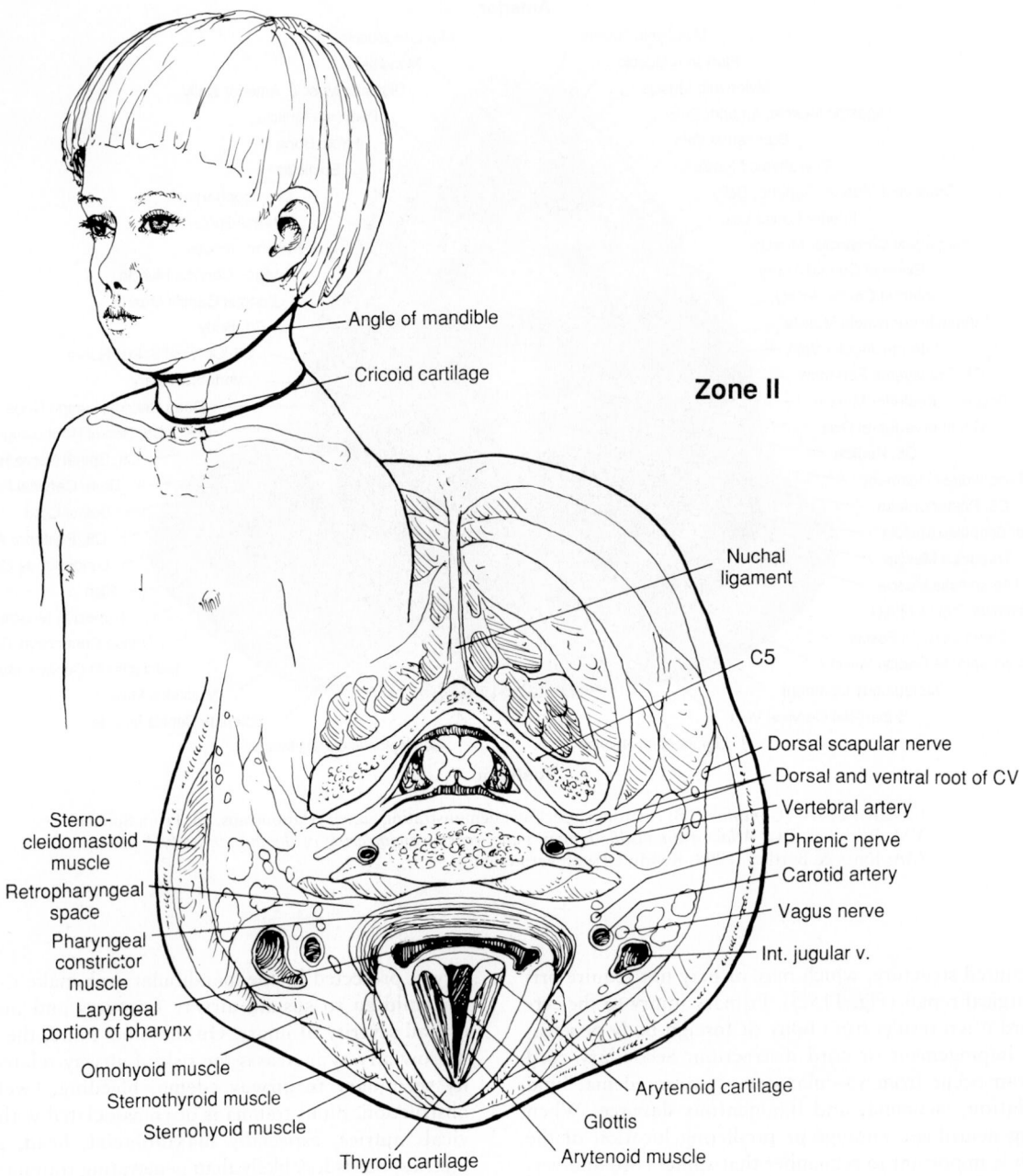

Angle of mandible

Cricoid cartilage

Zone II

Nuchal ligament

C5

Dorsal scapular nerve

Dorsal and ventral root of CV

Vertebral artery

Phrenic nerve

Carotid artery

Vagus nerve

Int. jugular v.

Sterno-cleidomastoid muscle

Retropharyngeal space

Pharyngeal constrictor muscle

Laryngeal portion of pharynx

Omohyoid muscle

Sternothyroid muscle

Sternohyoid muscle

Thyroid cartilage

Arytenoid cartilage

Glottis

Arytenoid muscle

A

FIGURE 115.2 **A:** Anatomic neck divisions and contents of zone II located between the upper boundary of zone I and the angle of the mandible. (*continued*)

hematoma, laceration, perforation, vocal cord injury, and, less commonly, partial or complete airway transection. A prime target for airway fracture is the cricoid ring, which is the only complete tracheal ring. The general triad of dyspnea, stridor, and hemoptysis suggests laryngeal injury, with injuries above the glottis often demonstrating cervical emphysema, dysphagia, hoarseness, and progressive airway obstruction whereas those below the glottis present with hemoptysis and persistent air leak, although any or all symptoms and signs listed in Table 115.3 may be present.

Approximately 85% of patients with blunt tracheal injury reportedly have subcutaneous emphysema, although the onset may be delayed (Fig. 115.6). However, airway injuries may be subtle and not apparent with initial history or physical examination. Unfortunately, these subtle injuries may progress to severe abnormalities. The same percentage of airway narrowing from edema or hematoma may lead to significantly more distress in a child than in an adult. Airway obstruction from tracheal edema has been reported as late as 48 hours after the injury. If a laryngeal injury is noted, the

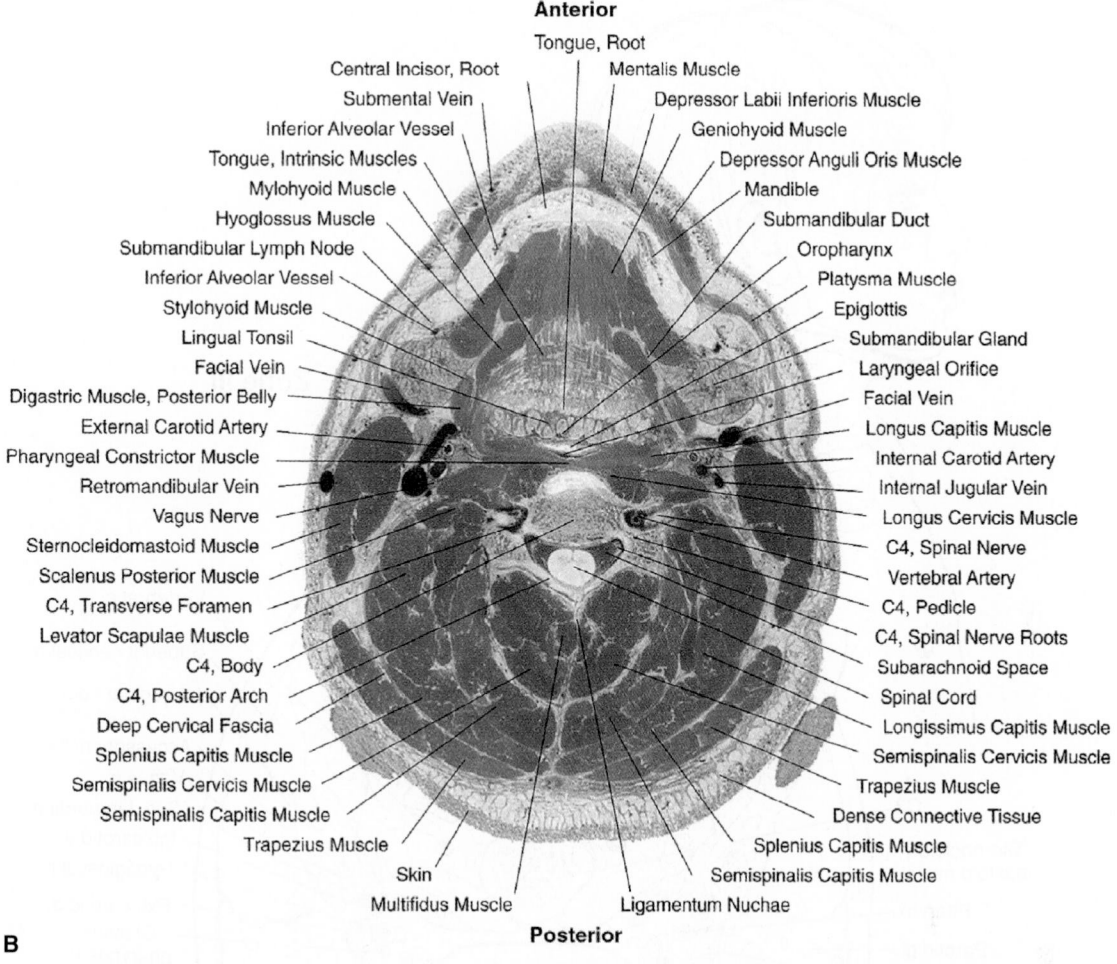

Anterior

Tongue, Root
Central Incisor, Root
Submental Vein
Inferior Alveolar Vessel
Tongue, Intrinsic Muscles
Mylohyoid Muscle
Hyoglossus Muscle
Submandibular Lymph Node
Inferior Alveolar Vessel
Stylohyoid Muscle
Lingual Tonsil
Facial Vein
Digastric Muscle, Posterior Belly
External Carotid Artery
Pharyngeal Constrictor Muscle
Retromandibular Vein
Vagus Nerve
Sternocleidomastoid Muscle
Scalenus Posterior Muscle
C4, Transverse Foramen
Levator Scapulae Muscle
C4, Body
C4, Posterior Arch
Deep Cervical Fascia
Splenius Capitis Muscle
Semispinalis Cervicis Muscle
Semispinalis Capitis Muscle
Trapezius Muscle
Skin
Multifidus Muscle

Mentalis Muscle
Depressor Labii Inferioris Muscle
Geniohyoid Muscle
Depressor Anguli Oris Muscle
Mandible
Submandibular Duct
Oropharynx
Platysma Muscle
Epiglottis
Submandibular Gland
Laryngeal Orifice
Facial Vein
Longus Capitis Muscle
Internal Carotid Artery
Internal Jugular Vein
Longus Cervicis Muscle
C4, Spinal Nerve
Vertebral Artery
C4, Pedicle
C4, Spinal Nerve Roots
Subarachnoid Space
Spinal Cord
Longissimus Capitis Muscle
Semispinalis Cervicis Muscle
Trapezius Muscle
Dense Connective Tissue
Splenius Capitis Muscle
Semispinalis Capitis Muscle
Ligamentum Nuchae

Posterior

B

FIGURE 115.2 (*Continued*) **B:** Anatomic specimen demonstrating zone II relationships. (**B:** From Spitzer VM, Whitlock DG. *Atlas of the visible human male: reverse engineering of the human body.* Sodburg, MA: Jones & Bartlett, 1998. Reprinted with permission.)

patient should be evaluated carefully for commonly associated injuries, which include cervical spine, chest, facial, pharyngoesophageal, and recurrent laryngeal nerve palsy. Airway injuries can also result from endoscopy, thermal trauma, or caustic ingestions. There are numerous reports in the literature of laryngeal and tracheal trauma secondary to intubation attempts.

As mentioned, the esophagus is mobile and is usually collapsed as it courses through the neck but may be dilated while eating. This mobility helps protect the esophagus, but its delicate mucosal walls can be damaged easily by blunt traumatic events. Iatrogenic esophageal injuries can result from endoscopy, passage of a nasogastric or orogastric tube, vigorous suctioning, and difficult intubations. Esophageal injuries can also be seen with ingested foreign bodies and caustic chemicals. The symptoms and signs associated with esophageal injury are listed in Table 115.3 and include neck tenderness and pain, dysphagia, odynophagia, drooling, crepitus, subcutaneous emphysema, hematemesis, fever, and mediastinitis (see Chapters 29, 52 and 89). The injuries, which can be subtle,

occult, and difficult to diagnose, can lead to increased morbidity and mortality if not suspected and discovered.

Isolated or concurrent hyoid bone injuries are also possible. The hyoid is mobile and fairly well protected, which explains the paucity of isolated injury. In a 1991 review by Szeremeta and Morovati, only four children 16 years or younger had been reported with an isolated hyoid fracture, three of whom sustained the injury in motor vehicle accidents. Symptoms and signs of hyoid injury include pain in the throat that worsens with swallowing or coughing, tenderness to palpation, neck crepitus, pain on head rotation, dysphagia, dyspnea, or dysphonia. As with other injuries, these symptoms and signs can be subtle initially, with progressive edema and airway obstruction.

Although vascular injuries are rare with blunt trauma, they do occur. These injuries are often unsuspected and undiagnosed on routine examination. Risk factors for injury have been reported to include Glasgow Coma Scale score of less than 8; head injury; basilar skull fracture; and facial, neck, thorax, or abdominal injury. The clinician must consider

TRAUMA

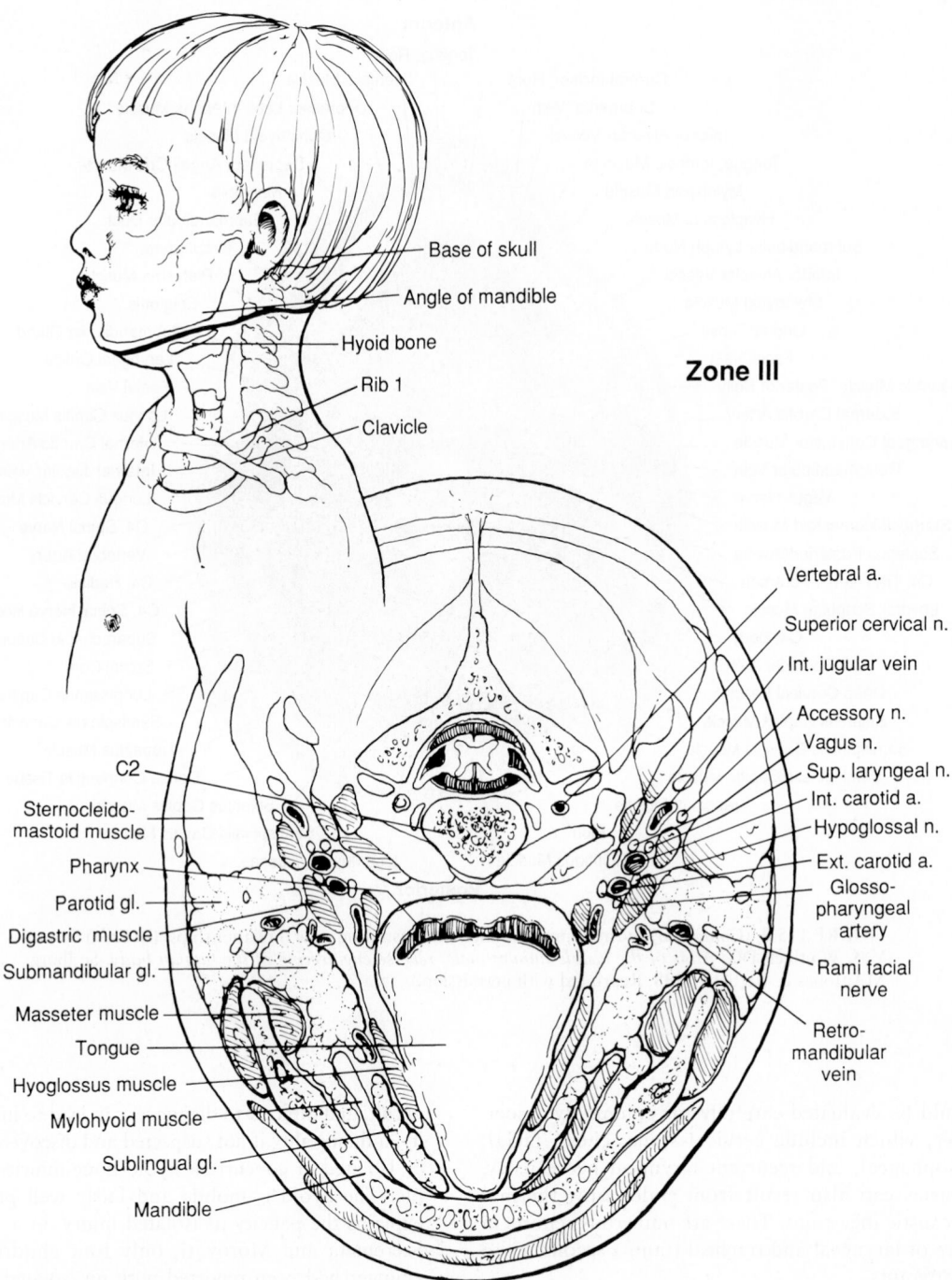

Base of skull

Angle of mandible

Hyoid bone

Rib 1

Clavicle

Zone III

Vertebral a.

Superior cervical n.

Int. jugular vein

Accessory n.

Vagus n.

Sup. laryngeal n.

Int. carotid a.

Hypoglossal n.

Ext. carotid a.

Glosso-
pharyngeal
artery

Rami facial
nerve

Retro-
mandibular
vein

C2

Sternocleido-
mastoid muscle

Pharynx

Parotid gl.

Digastric muscle

Submandibular gl.

Masseter muscle

Tongue

Hyoglossus muscle

Mylohyoid muscle

Sublingual gl.

Mandible

A

FIGURE 115.3 **A:** Anatomic neck divisions and contents of zone III. Zone III includes the area above the upper boundary of zone II. (*continued*)

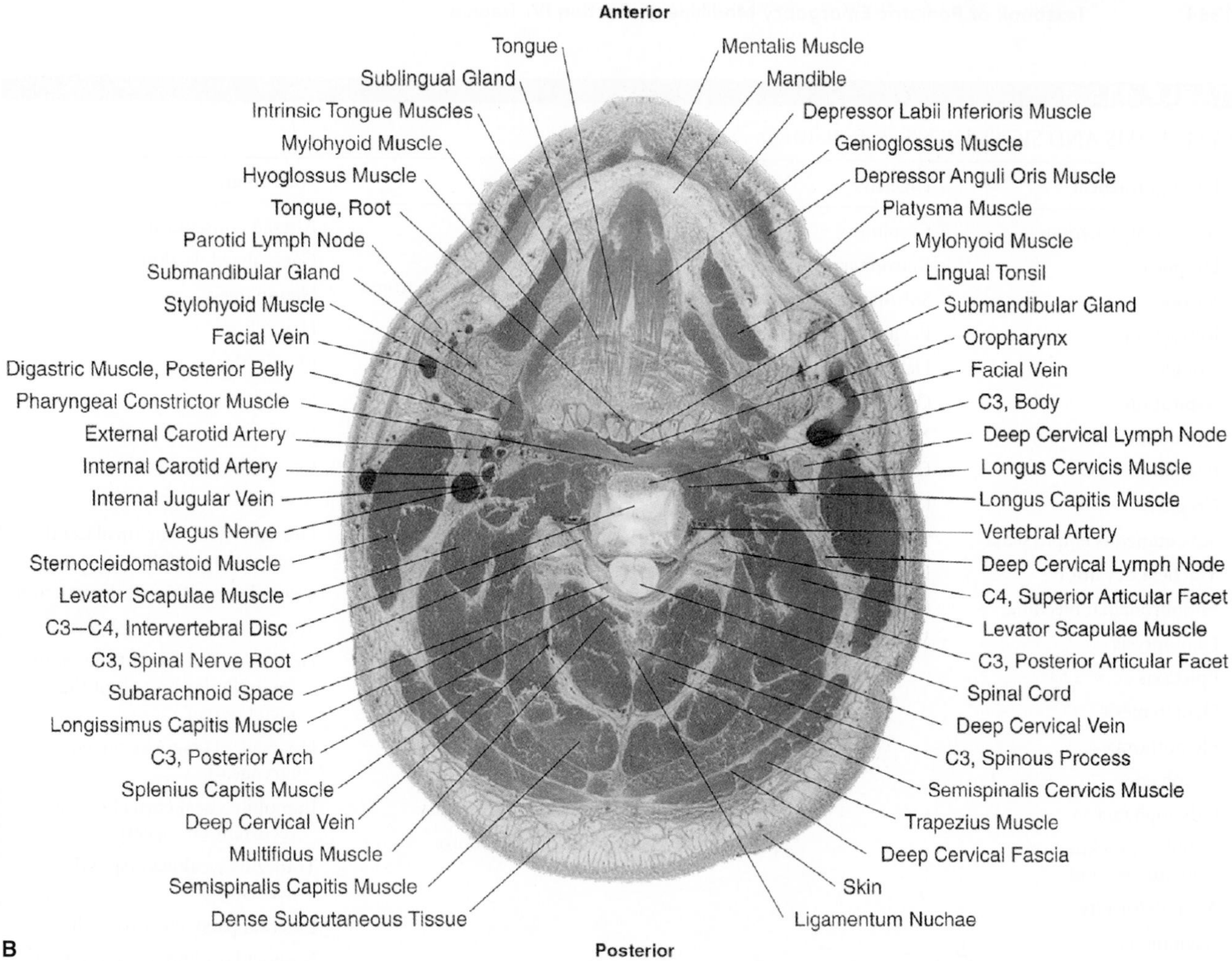

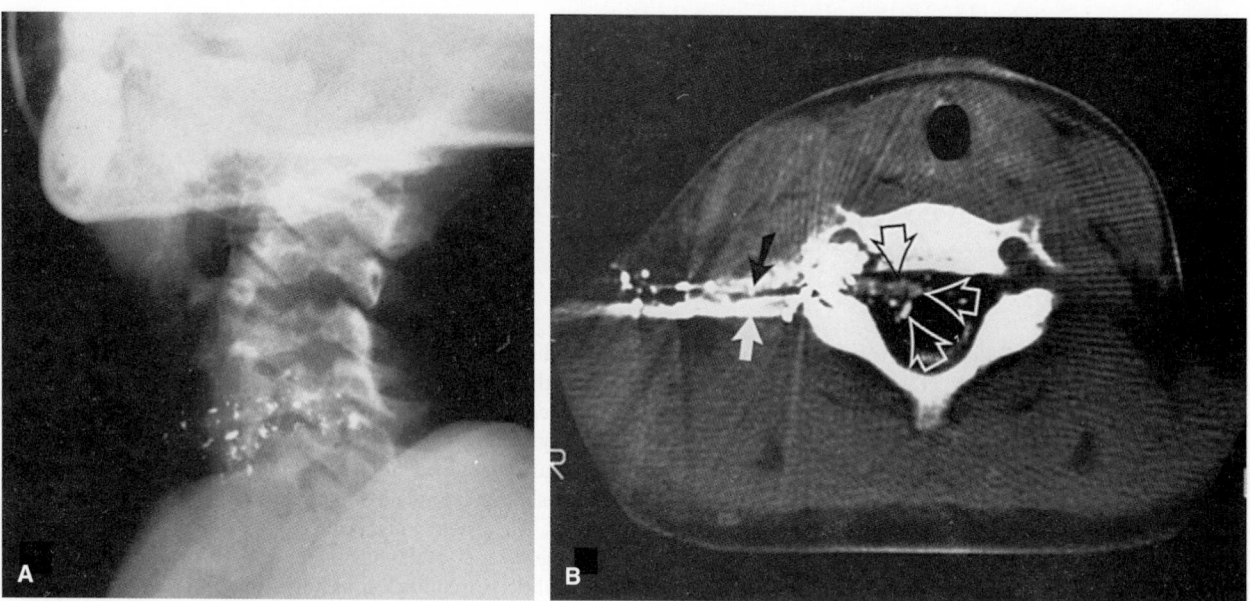

Anterior

Tongue
Sublingual Gland
Intrinsic Tongue Muscles
Mylohyoid Muscle
Hyoglossus Muscle
Tongue, Root
Parotid Lymph Node
Submandibular Gland
Stylohyoid Muscle
Facial Vein
Digastric Muscle, Posterior Belly
Pharyngeal Constrictor Muscle
External Carotid Artery
Internal Carotid Artery
Internal Jugular Vein
Vagus Nerve
Sternocleidomastoid Muscle
Levator Scapulae Muscle
C3–C4, Intervertebral Disc
C3, Spinal Nerve Root
Subarachnoid Space
Longissimus Capitis Muscle
C3, Posterior Arch
Splenius Capitis Muscle
Deep Cervical Vein
Multifidus Muscle
Semispinalis Capitis Muscle
Dense Subcutaneous Tissue

Mentalis Muscle
Mandible
Depressor Labii Inferioris Muscle
Genioglossus Muscle
Depressor Anguli Oris Muscle
Platysma Muscle
Mylohyoid Muscle
Lingual Tonsil
Submandibular Gland
Oropharynx
Facial Vein
C3, Body
Deep Cervical Lymph Node
Longus Cervicis Muscle
Longus Capitis Muscle
Vertebral Artery
Deep Cervical Lymph Node
C4, Superior Articular Facet
Levator Scapulae Muscle
C3, Posterior Articular Facet
Spinal Cord
Deep Cervical Vein
C3, Spinous Process
Semispinalis Cervicis Muscle
Trapezius Muscle
Deep Cervical Fascia
Skin
Ligamentum Nuchae

B

Posterior

FIGURE 115.3 (*Continued*) **B:** Anatomic specimen demonstrating zone III relationships. (**B:** From Spitzer VM, Whitlock DG. *Atlas of the visible human male: reverse engineering of the human body.* Sodburg, MA: Jones & Bartlett, 1998. Reprinted with permission.)

FIGURE 115.4 Gunshot wound (.22 caliber) to the neck in a 5-year-old girl. **A:** Lateral neck radiograph showing fragmentation of bullet along path. **B:** Computed tomography (CT) scan of same patient demonstrating bullet fragments in and around the spinal canal, as well as cerebrospinal fluid and contrast leak from disruption of the dura.

TRAUMA

1383

TABLE 115.3

SYMPTOMS AND SIGNS OF NECK INJURIES

Laryngotracheal	Digestive	Vascular	Neurologic
Airway obstruction	Crepitus	Vigorous bleeding, internal or external	Altered consciousness
Dyspnea	Retropharyngeal air	Expansile or pulsatile hematoma	Generalized weakness
Stridor	Subcutaneous emphysema	Bruit	Hemiparesis
Retractions	Pneumomediastinum	Absent pulsations (carotid, superficial temporal, or ophthalmic artery)	Hemiplegia
Cough	Hematemesis		Quadriplegia
Aspiration	Chest or neck pain	Unexplained hypotension	Seizures
Pneumomediastinum	Neck tenderness	Hemothorax	Bruit
Pneumothorax	Dysphagia	Cardiac tamponade	Cervicosensory deficits
Crepitus	Odynophagia	Hemiplegia	Aphasia
Subcutaneous emphysema	Saliva in wound	Hemiparesis	Horner's syndrome (ipsilateral cervical sympathetics)
Tracheal deviation	Drooling	Aphasia	Cranial nerve IX–XII dysfunction
Endobronchial bleeding	Fever	Monocular blindness	Tongue deviation (hypoglossal)
Hemoptysis	Mediastinitis	Loss of consciousness	Drooping of corner of the mouth (mandibular branch of the facial nerve)
Epistaxis		Neck asymmetry, swelling, or discoloration	
Hematemesis		Wide mediastinum	Hoarseness (vagus/recurrent laryngeal)
Hemothorax		Cranial nerve abnormality	Immobile vocal cords (vagus/recurrent laryngeal)
Dysphagia		Clavicle/first rib fracture	
Odynophagia			Trapezius weakness (spinal accessory)
Bubbling, sucking, or hissing wound			Brachial palsy (arm paresthesias)
Neck deformity			Monocular blindness (vertebral artery)
Asymmetry			Diaphragm paralysis (phrenic)
Loss of landmarks			
Flat thyroid prominence			
Laryngotracheal tenderness			
Dysphonia			
Aphonia			
Voice changes			
Hoarseness			
Drooling			
Neck pain, tenderness (with coughing or swallowing)			

subclavian or innominate vessel injuries if a fracture of the clavicle or first rib is identified. The most common vascular structure injured with blunt trauma is the common carotid artery. The vertebral arteries are rarely injured by blunt forces unless a concurrent transverse process or other fracture of the cervical spine or atlantooccipital dislocation occurs. The signs and symptoms of the vascular injury may be masked by the spinal injury. Many patients with atlantooccipital dislocation and arterial injury die in the field, but some survive and may recover with appropriate therapy. Vascular contusions with intimal damage may also be seen with blunt neck trauma.

The glandular structures in the neck, including the thyroid, parathyroid, parotid, and submandibular glands, may also be injured. Although these organs may be traumatized, they are rarely completely destroyed.

Burn management is covered in Chapter 108, but the physician should be aware of special considerations involving the neck. The airway must be evaluated and protected as indicated by the severity of the burn, realizing that initial symptoms may be subtle. Circumferential burns may become edematous and require an escharotomy for respiratory or vascular sufficiency. Escharotomy in the neck involves a vertical incision from the chin to the superior aspect of the sternal notch.

Sensory dermatomes

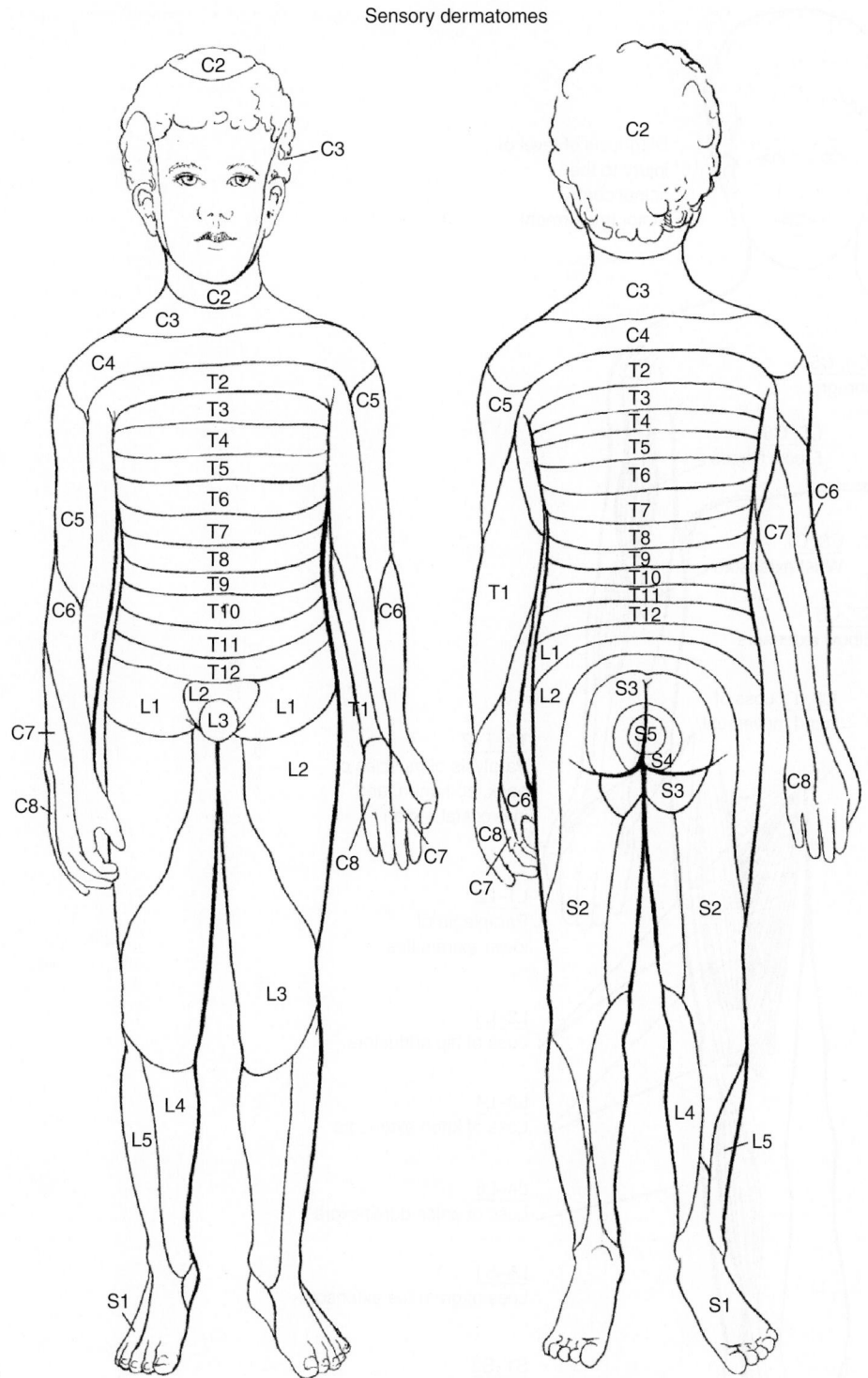

FIGURE 115.5 **A:** Sensory dermatomes. (*continued*)

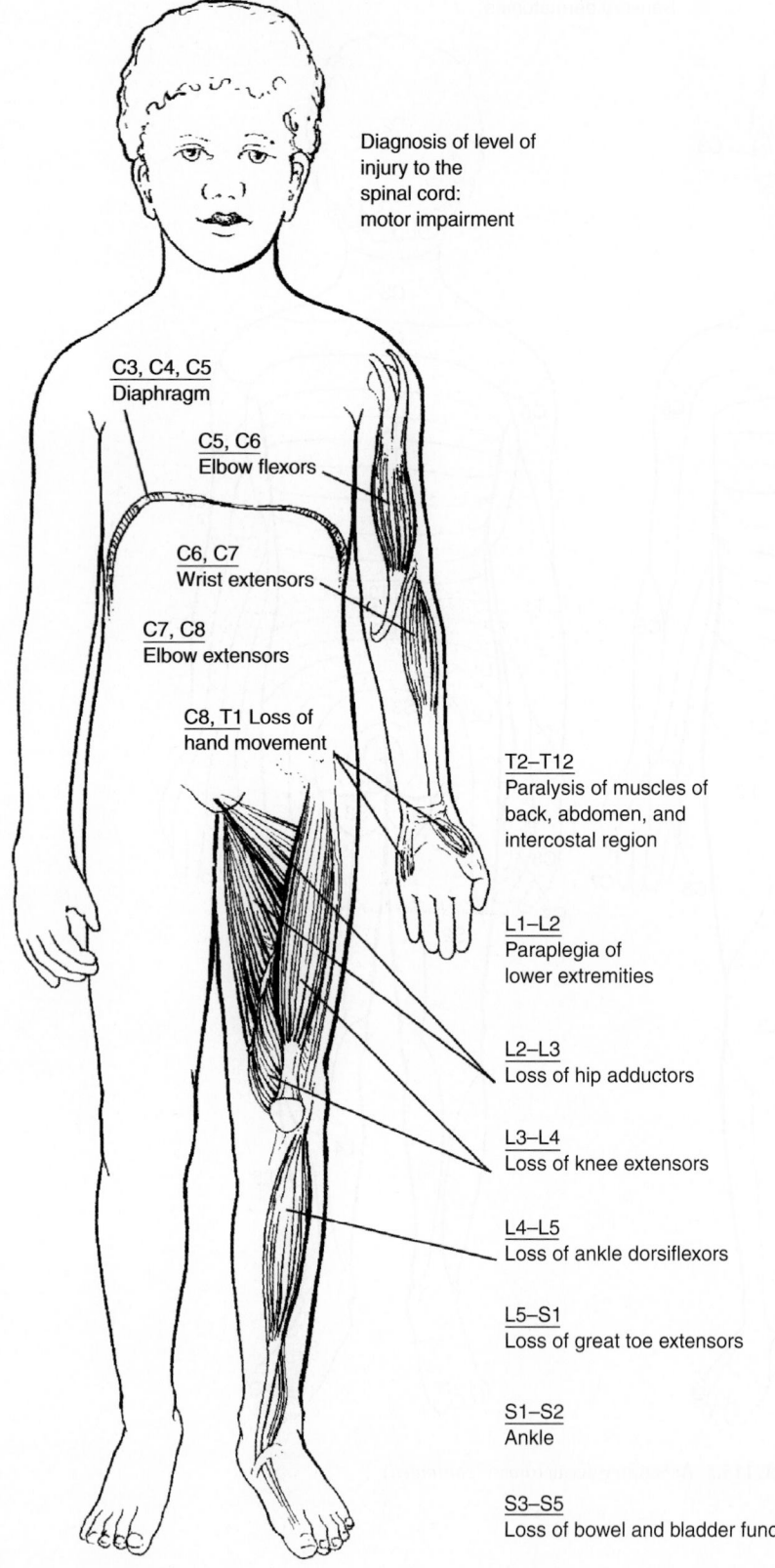

Diagnosis of level of
injury to the
spinal cord:
motor impairment

C3, C4, C5
Diaphragm

C5, C6
Elbow flexors

C6, C7
Wrist extensors

C7, C8
Elbow extensors

C8, T1 Loss of
hand movement

T2–T12
Paralysis of muscles of
back, abdomen, and
intercostal region

L1–L2
Paraplegia of
lower extremities

L2–L3
Loss of hip adductors

L3–L4
Loss of knee extensors

L4–L5
Loss of ankle dorsiflexors

L5–S1
Loss of great toe extensors

S1–S2
Ankle

S3–S5
Loss of bowel and bladder function

B

FIGURE 115.5 (*Continued*) **B:** Motor dermatomes. Knowledge of sensory and motor dermatomes can be invaluable in description of neurologic findings during initial and subsequent evaluations.

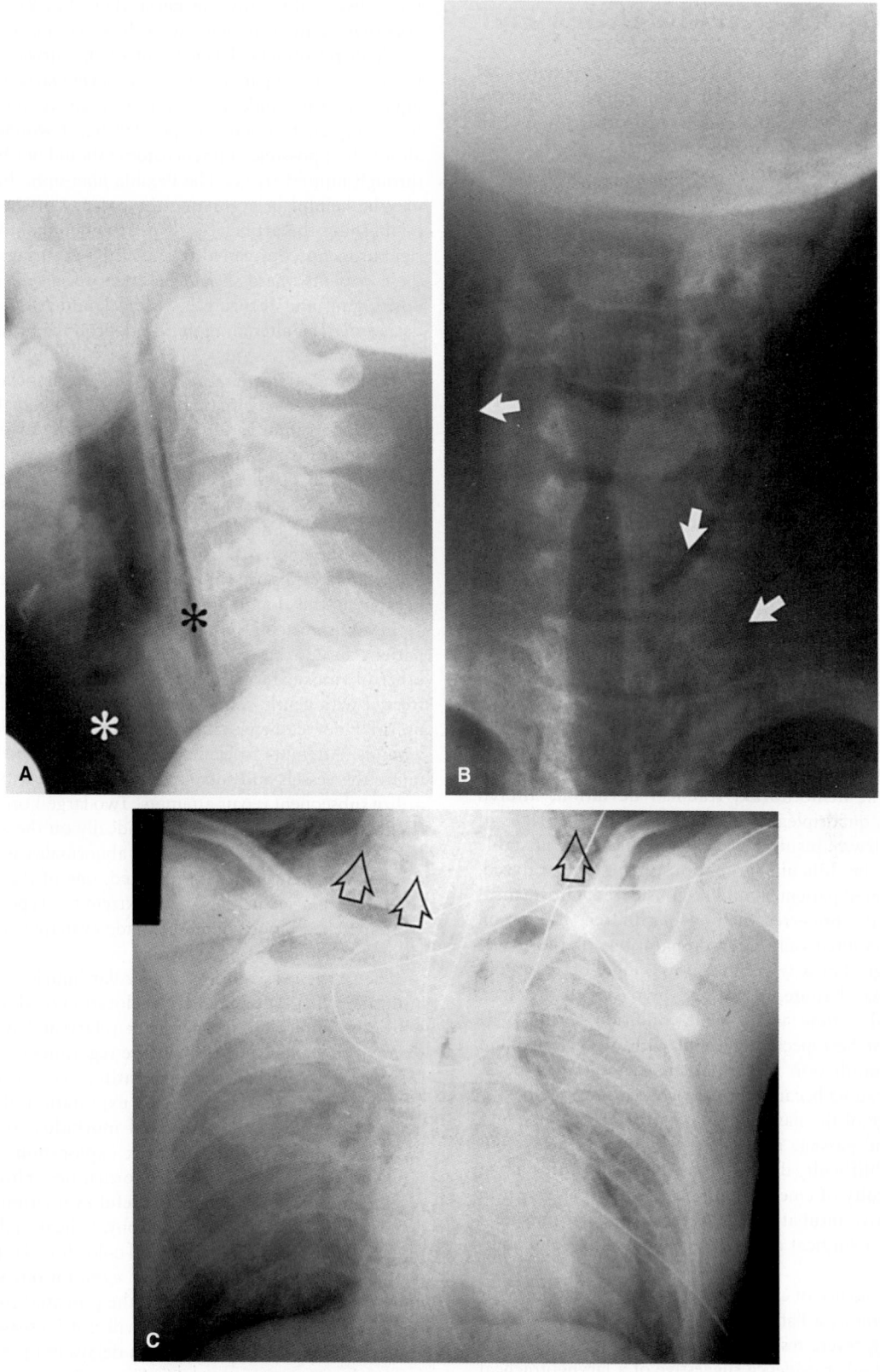

FIGURE 115.6 **A–C:** Subcutaneous emphysema of neck and chest in 11-year-old patient from baro-trauma sustained when opening carbonated beverage container with teeth.

EVALUATION AND MANAGEMENT

The goals of management are to ensure airway patency and respiratory sufficiency, control hemorrhage, maintain osseous stability, and identify and prevent progression of all injuries. Methodical and timely acquisition of historical and physical findings is mandatory. The patient must be managed with strict adherence to the ABCs, with consideration of possible rapid or gradual deterioration. Penetrating objects that are lodged in the neck on evaluation should remain in place until removed under surgical care, preferably in an operating room. All patients, other than those with minor injuries such as contusions, abrasions, or superficial lacerations (not through the platysma muscle), should receive supplemental humidified oxygen, correct airway positioning, suctioning, vigilant observation, and monitoring. The patient should be maintained in a supine or Trendelenburg position to avoid the possibility of venous air embolism. If venous air embolism is suspected because of an unexplained decrease in cardiac output and blood pressure, increase in central venous pressure, cyanosis, arrhythmias, or air in the heart on chest radiograph, the patient should be placed in the left lateral decubitus and Trendelenburg positions. A decision tree for the evaluation of direct blunt and penetrating neck trauma is presented in Fig. 115.7.

Airway assessment is the initial step in the evaluation of all patients with trauma. Any airway manipulation should be accomplished with consideration and prevention of possible cervical spine injury. Potential indications for an artificial airway with neck trauma include stridor, dyspnea, hypoxia, rapidly expanding hematoma, expanding crepitus, pneumothorax, hemothorax, tracheal deviation, altered mental status, quadriplegia, hemiparesis, and other signs of vascular or airway insufficiency. If the airway is unstable or appears to be difficult, intubation of the nonparalyzed, awake, or sedated patient should be considered. Orotracheal intubation is the preferred method in children. Intubation should be attempted only after preparation for the placement of a surgical airway, if time allows. Fiber-optic intubation via the nasal route, performed by a skilled provider, may be useful if time and patient condition permit. The physician must be especially careful with the use of blind nasotracheal intubation in the patient with blunt or penetrating neck trauma because the airway anatomy may be distorted. Passage of the nasotracheal or orotracheal tube into a false or blind passage may make subsequent airway control attempts difficult, if not impossible. Therefore, along with the difficulty of emergent surgical airway placement in children, elective intubation is not recommended outside a setting where a surgical airway can be efficiently and skillfully placed.

If there is evidence of crepitus over the larynx, laryngeal or tracheal tenderness, a flattened thyroid prominence, anterior neck deformity, severe respiratory distress, an abnormal neck radiograph, or other evidence suggestive of a laryngotracheal fracture or disruption, a tracheostomy may be preferable. Intubation should be attempted only if the airway is completely obstructed. Attempts at intubation from above may separate a tenuously attached trachea and larynx, resulting in a total loss of the airway, with the trachea commonly retracting substernally into the chest (Fig. 115.8). Attempts at cricothyrotomy in patients with direct laryngeal trauma may result in retrotracheal placement of the airway. Cricothyrotomy is helpful in patients who have severe facial or other neck injuries that preclude intubation from above. Intubation may be attempted through an open laryngeal wound if present, although, if possible, a tracheostomy should not be performed through injured tissue. The flexible fiber-optic bronchoscope may be helpful in evaluating the patency of the airway and establishing the artificial airway. If patient condition allows, rigid bronchoscopy can also be useful in securing an airway in these patients. Care should be taken to ensure correct tube positioning and securing, as usual landmarks and adjacent tissues may be altered, requiring nonroutine techniques to be considered.

Breathing abnormalities may suggest associated injuries. Missiles to the neck may also pass through or lodge in the chest. Zone I injuries of the neck can easily involve the lung apices and result in hemothorax, pneumothorax, or pneumomediastinum. Further penetration may lead to cardiac tamponade. A chest radiograph is helpful in the assessment. A report from the Eddy and the Zone I Penetrating Neck Injury Subgroup suggests that normal physical examination and chest radiographs are sufficient to obviate the need for arteriography in this population.

In addition to the usual assessment for hypovolemia, the patient should be examined for expanding hematomas or other obvious external bleeding. External bleeding should be treated with gentle compression. Navsaria et al described the use of Foley catheter tamponade for actively bleeding neck wounds. Attempts to clamp bleeding vessels in the neck can injure the vessels and surrounding structures, as well as jeopardize subsequent repair attempts. Two large-bore intravenous (IV) catheters should be inserted, ideally on the side opposite to the injury if an obvious vascular abnormality is identified. If a subclavian vein injury is suspected, one of the IV catheters should be placed in the lower extremity. Type-specific and cross-matched blood should be made available and used with volume expanders as necessary.

The subtle presentation of vascular injuries has led many authors to suggest mandatory exploration of all neck injuries when the outermost muscle layer (platysma) is penetrated. Controversy exists in the literature regarding surgical exploration with low-velocity penetrating neck trauma (Table 115.4). Proponents of mandatory exploration of penetrating neck wounds report that overall morbidity and mortality have decreased with routine neck exploration and surgical repair of vascular and other abnormalities. However, more recent literature suggests that careful evaluation with ancillary studies, including arteriography, helical multislice computed tomographic (CT) scan, and color-flow Doppler (CFD) coupled with the use of selective exploration, will identify most significant injuries and that the potential short delay in operative evaluation and repair will not increase morbidity and mortality. Others suggest that delays in operative exploration due to preoperative studies may increase morbidity and mortality. Variable results have been reported regarding the use of dynamic CT in the identification of surgically significant zone II injuries. In one study, dynamic CT was no better than esophagography in diagnosing esophageal

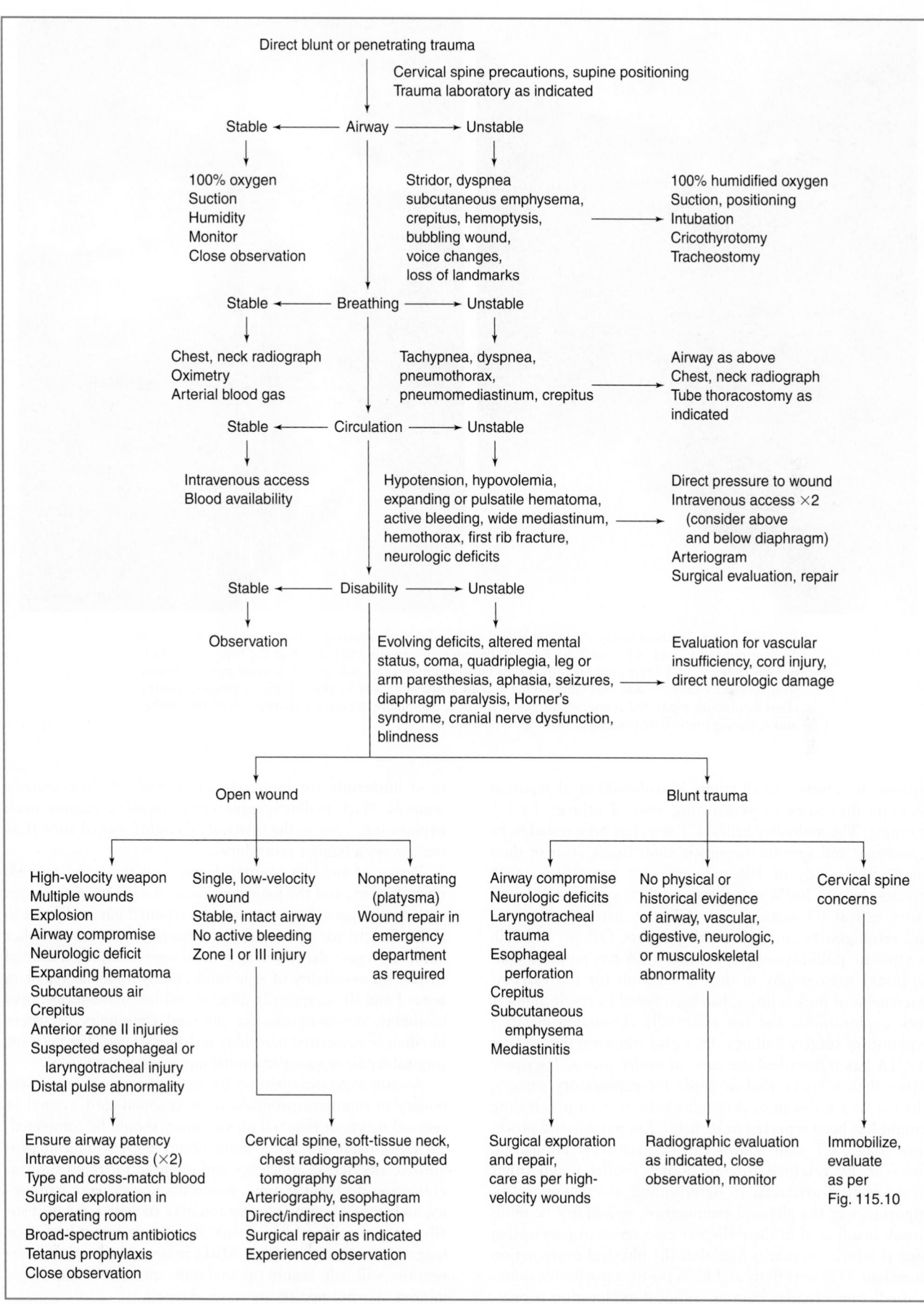

FIGURE 115.7 Evaluation of blunt and penetrating neck trauma.

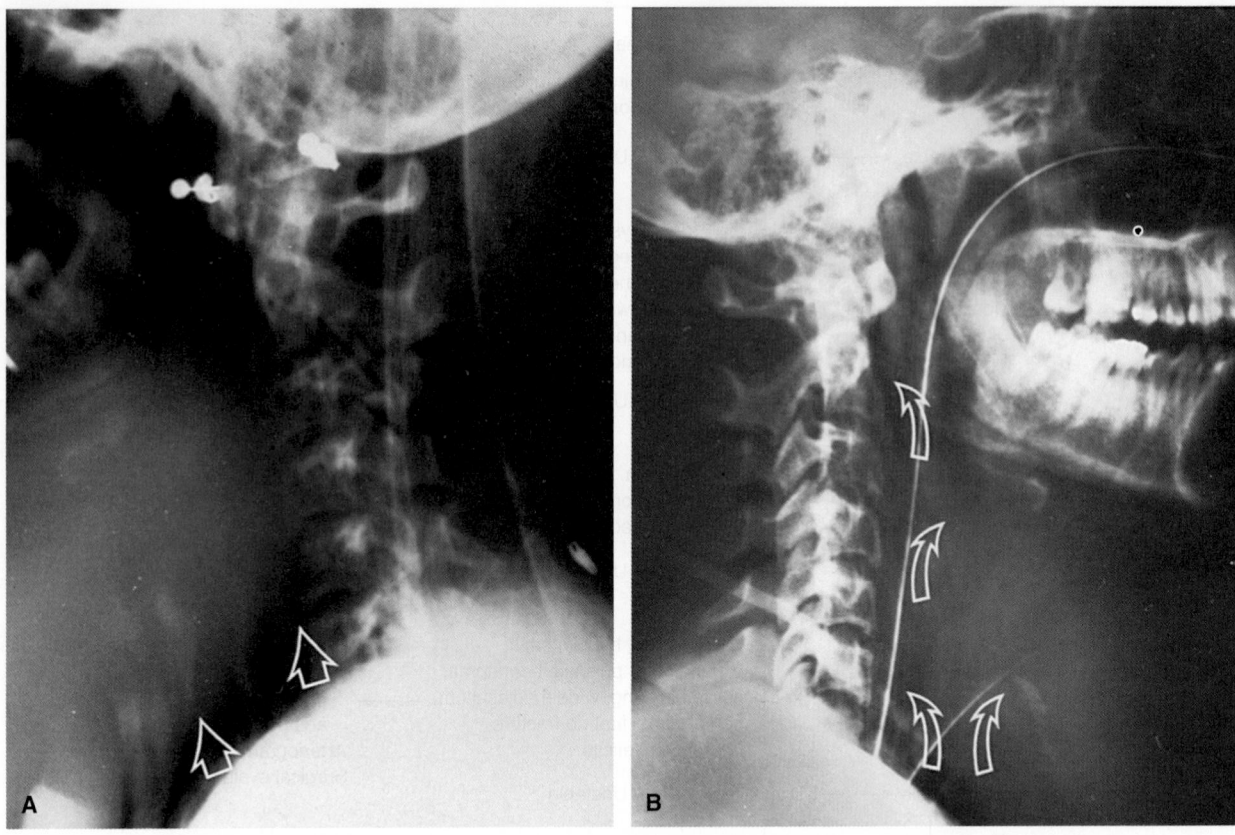

FIGURE 115.8 Tracheal injury. **A:** Initial lateral neck radiograph showing subcutaneous emphysema in 14-year-old girl kicked in the neck by a horse. Patient's airway clinically stable at the time of this radiograph (more than 1 hour after the injury). **B:** Postcricothyrotomy radiograph in same patient demonstrating significant subcutaneous emphysema and an artificial airway in place. Initial attempt at orotracheal intubation separated tenuously attached trachea, completing traumatic disruption of the trachea and requiring immediate placement of surgical airway.

injuries. In another small study, Mazolewski et al reported accurate diagnoses of penetrating zone II injuries by CT scanning. The multislice helical CT scan has been noted to be a sensitive and specific diagnostic tool. Inaba et al in their prospective study of 106 patients with penetrating neck injuries showed 100% sensitivity and 93% specificity of multislice helical CT angiography (CTA) in detecting vascular and aerodigestive injury. In stable patients, Osborn and Bell, in separate publications, report that CTA has replaced conventional angiography in their institution for the vascular assessment of neck injuries, has been noted to result in fewer neck explorations, and has essentially eliminated negative exploratory surgery findings. They also comment that the use of CTA has transcribed the zone of injury into a descriptor rather than a triage tool or guide for exploratory surgery. The use of a CT scan to determine trajectory of penetrating wound has been reported to be helpful in patient and procedure triage. CT scan images can be negatively influenced, however, by retained foreign bodies (bullets) and other injury-related artifacts. In determining assessment steps, importance of the physical examination should not be minimized. Insull et al in their 10-year case series of penetrating zone II injuries in adults note that the physical examination alone had 93% sensitivity and 87% positive predictive values in predicting vascular injuries. Surgical exploration is prac-

ticed uniformly for high-velocity or multiple low-velocity wounds. With pediatric penetrating injuries, routine neck exploration, even in the relatively straightforward zone II, is not always a benign procedure.

Repair of vascular injuries depends on the vessel injured, type of injury, and the patient's clinical status. Arterial injuries with neurologic deficits are often not repaired but are ligated to avoid the chance of reperfusion injuries to the brain. Other authors suggest that primary arterial repair may be indicated despite the possibility of reperfusion injury. Vascular repair in zones I and III is especially difficult and not without operative morbidity. Venous injuries may not need repair unless persistent bleeding or associated morbidity is demonstrated. The need for surgical repair of vascular intimal injuries is controversial.

A neurologic examination for signs of cerebral injury secondary to vascular insufficiency, direct spinal cord, cranial or cervical nerve, or brachial plexus injury should be completed. An abnormal neurologic examination result may indicate progressive vascular insufficiency and the need for rapid surgical evaluation. In blunt trauma, progressive onset pain, irritability, and signs of cord compression may suggest a spinal (usually venous) epidural hematoma. Rapid assessment by CT or magnetic resonance imaging (MRI), followed by surgical intervention, will help ensure optimal outcome. Direct neurologic injuries may not necessitate surgical repair.

TABLE 115.4

SURGICAL EXPLORATION WITH PENETRATING TRAUMA

Arguments favoring mandatory surgical exploration with penetrating trauma
Most patients have injuries to important structures
Morbidity and mortality increase with delay in surgery
Morbidity of exploration is relatively low
Negative physical examination does not preclude injury
Morbidity of missed injuries is high
Specific radiologic tests and expertise are needed for selective management
More skill is needed to observe appropriately
Length of hospitalization is similar with or without exploration

Arguments favoring selective surgical exploration with penetrating trauma
Most injuries are not secondary to high-velocity weapons
There are high negative rates of injuries with exploration in asymptomatic patients
It is unclear whether morbidity and mortality increase with delay in surgery
Zone II is involved most commonly and injuries are rarely occult
Skill is needed to explore neck
Morbidity of the more difficult zone I and III explorations is seen
Ancillary tests are helpful in zone I and III evaluation
Exploration may miss occult injuries

TABLE 115.5

INDICATIONS SUGGESTING SURGICAL EVALUATION IN PATIENTS WITH NECK TRAUMA

Unstable vital signs
Expanding or massive hematoma
Pulsatile or active bleeding
Hemorrhagic shock
Vascular deficits in the upper extremities
Abnormal distal pulses (brachial, superficial temporal, ophthalmologic, fundi)
Hematemesis, hemoptysis, epistaxis
Hemothorax
Progressive respiratory distress
Airway obstruction
Expanding subcutaneous emphysema
Bubbling or sucking wound
Pneumothorax
Progressive neurologic deficits
Hemiparesis
Horner's syndrome
Cranial or cervical nerve dysfunction
Diaphragm paralysis
Decreased sensorium
Neurologic deficits in upper extremity
Increasing dysphagia
Odynophagia or dysphonia
Hoarseness
Severe neck pain or tenderness
High-velocity wounds (rifles, explosions)
Multiple low-velocity wounds
Ancillary radiographic studies not available
Experienced observation personnel not available

Tetanus status should be assessed in all patients with penetrating trauma. The clinician should consider a broad-spectrum antibiotic for a patient with evidence of neck trauma, especially if esophageal or pharyngeal injury seems likely. Placement of a nasogastric or an orogastric tube is controversial for the patient with cervical injury because it may worsen a preexisting esophageal injury or dislodge clots in zone I of the neck. When placed, these tubes should be well lubricated, inserted gently and slowly, and withdrawn if difficulty in passage or evidence of obstruction occurs.

Superficial abrasions, lacerations, and puncture wounds are common in children. Wounds superficial to the platysma can be cleaned and sutured in the normal fashion under local anesthesia in the ED. Clean wounds can be sutured as late as 12 to 18 hours after the injury because of the excellent blood flow in the neck. In wounds beyond 12 to 18 hours postinjury, closure after 72 hours is recommended. Penetration of the external muscle layer in the neck, the platysma, is an indication for surgical referral and, in some cases, surgical exploration. When neck wounds that penetrate the platysma are evaluated, exploration in the ED is discouraged because of the risk of clot dislodgment and venous air embolism. Rapid surgical exploration and repair are indicated in patients struck by a high-velocity missile and in those with unstable vital signs, uncontrollable bleeding, rapidly expanding hematomas, progressive airway compromise, worsening neurologic symptoms, increasing subcutaneous emphysema, or bubbling wounds (Table 115.5).

Surgical evaluation may give false-negative results with esophageal tears, small vessel lacerations, pharyngeal tears, or tracheal injuries. The patient who has apparently stable vital signs, no symptoms of impaired neurologic or cardiovascular status, an intact airway, and mechanisms of injury with a low-velocity bullet or single knife wound may be managed expectantly with the use of ancillary diagnostic tests and close, experienced observation, preferably for at least 48 hours. These decisions should be made in conjunction with experienced surgical staff.

Adjuncts to the history and physical examination are given in Table 115.6. Initial evaluation should include cervical spine radiographs to detect bony or structural abnormalities, as

TABLE 115.6

ADJUNCTS TO HISTORY AND PHYSICAL EXAMINATION

Cervical spine radiographs	Xeroradiography
Soft-tissue neck radiograph	Tomography
Chest radiograph	Indirect (mirror)
Computed tomographic scan	laryngoscopy
Arteriography	Direct laryngoscopy
Doppler	Flexible bronchoscopy
Esophagram	Direct
Contrast laryngotracheography	bronchoesophagoscopy
Oculoplethysmography	Surgical exploration

TRAUMA

well as a soft-tissue lateral neck radiograph to assess for blood, edema, subcutaneous air, foreign bodies, and airway impingement or disruption. A chest radiograph should be evaluated for evidence of hemothorax or pneumothorax, mediastinal emphysema or widening, and heart size. If a serious injury is likely, these radiographs should be obtained in the ED or the patient should be accompanied to the radiology department by someone skilled in airway management. Fluoroscopy may be helpful in airway evaluation. If the patient is stable and a vascular injury is suspected, an arteriogram should be performed (Fig. 115.9). Arteriography has excellent sensitivity, specificity, and accuracy, as well as low morbidity. Some authors suggest that an arteriogram is not needed in penetrating zone II injuries if an exploration is to be performed because this can be done fairly easily without significant complications. Others suggest that, even with zone II injuries, the stable patient should receive an arteriogram before the operative procedure.

Noninvasive Doppler studies and oculoplethysmography may be useful in evaluating vascular injuries. CFD is an inexpensive, non invasive, relatively sensitive screening tool but can be limited by adjacent or overlying hematomas and pneumothoraces, as well as by the skill of the individual operator. Williams et al noted that in 4 prospective trials to evaluate penetrating neck injuries, CFD could exclude vascular injury in 77% of these cases. The collective data showed 95% sensitivity for identifying vascular injury after penetrating trauma, with specificity of 98.6%, positive predictive value of 97%, and negative predictive value of 98.6%. Contrast laryngography, tomography, and xeroradiography have been used for further evaluation; however, these methods have generally been replaced by the CT scan. The noninvasive, rapid, and safe CT scan provides excellent bone and soft-tissue detail and can be obtained easily with a stable, immobilized patient. The addition of IV contrast material allows identification and initial evaluation of the cervical vasculature. The advent of spiral CT technology allows rapid scans and illustrative coronal, sagittal, and three-dimensional reconstruction of the neck anatomy. CT may not be accurate for detection of mucosal degloving injuries, mucosal perforation in the presence of subcutaneous emphysema, endolaryngeal edema or hematoma, and partial laryngotracheal separation.

Barium or Gastrografin esophagram is helpful in evaluating the esophagus for tears or perforations, but false-negative rates of up to 50% have been reported. Evaluation can also include indirect mirror laryngoscopy to assess the larynx, vocal cord mobility, presence of mucosal edema, ecchymosis, and mucosal tears, as well as direct endoscopy to examine for tracheal, bronchial, and esophageal damage. Flexible endoscopy may be less invasive and easier to accomplish, but rigid endoscopy offers the most complete examination. Even rigid endoscopy, however, is not 100% sensitive in detecting tracheal and esophageal injuries. As mentioned, operative evaluation is mandatory for some patients and optional for others. Determinants of specific management direction include mechanism of injury, wound size and type, patient signs and symptoms, and relative stability. The clinician must maintain a high index of suspicion for potential injury to the structures contained in the neck. Consequences of missed injuries include airway obstruction, delayed hemorrhage, neurologic compro-

mise, and deep neck infection, with potentially significant morbidity and mortality.

CERVICAL SPINE EVALUATION

Cervical spine injuries are also uncommon in children, occurring in an estimated 1% to 2% of patients with multiple trauma. Traumatic brain injury has been reported to be the most common associated injury, accounting for 37% of the patients in Cirak's 2004 retrospective review of 406 patients over an 11-year period. It is estimated that 5% of all spinal injuries occur in children younger than 16 years. However, approximately 72% of spinal injuries in children younger than 8 years occur in the cervical region. Certain preexisting conditions (Down, Maroteaux-Lamy, Morquio's, Grisel, and Klippel-Feil syndromes; achondroplasia; congenital cervical stenosis; Chiari malformation; rheumatoid disease; and acute soft-tissue or bony infection or infiltration) may result in a cervical spine more predisposed to injury with minor or more significant trauma. Suspected child abuse with altered level of consciousness or neurologic deficits should alert one to the potential of cervical spine or cord injury as well. Vohra et al reported neurologic sequela in pediatric patients who underwent spinal manipulation for therapeutic purposes. Neonatal spinal injury is reported in approximately 1 in 60,000 births. These patients often have a history of cephalic forceps use during delivery and may have presenting signs that include weakness, flaccid quadriplegia, spinal shock, and apnea. These birth related injuries carry high morbidity and mortality. The clinician must assume that all children who sustain multiple trauma, have significant head or neck injuries, or have symptoms of neurologic impairment, including altered level of consciousness, have a cervical spine injury until proven otherwise. Goals in the care of these children include effectively stabilizing the primary injury that has occurred and preventing progression to a more severe or significant injury. The devastating nature of a cervical cord injury makes it imperative to not inadvertently miss a potentially unstable cervical spine injury. While attending to the basic ABCs of trauma resuscitation, the clinician should stabilize the cervical spine. Caution must be exercised when applying airway maneuvers to a child with a possible cervical spine injury. Airway interventions, however, often cannot wait until the cervical spine is "cleared." The clinician must prioritize and proceed with lifesaving airway maneuvers while minimizing motion of the potentially unstable cervical spine.

Hyperextension of the neck to facilitate intubation should be avoided. A vigorous chin lift or jaw thrust may also inadvertently hyperextend the unstable cervical spine. Gentle cricoid pressure should not cause excessive movement to the cervical spine; however, if applied vigorously, it may cause flexion of the spine. When inline neck immobilization is used to assist with airway maneuvers, the clinician should be careful to avoid applying significant traction to the spine because this pressure can also stress the unstable cervical column. Tracheal intubation in a patient with a potential cervical spine injury ideally requires at least two providers to perform the procedure safely and efficiently. Simulation models with the ability to gauge amount of cervical motion may be useful in developing, maintaining, and assessing airway skills for this subset of patients. One provider should maintain inline immobilization of the neck while

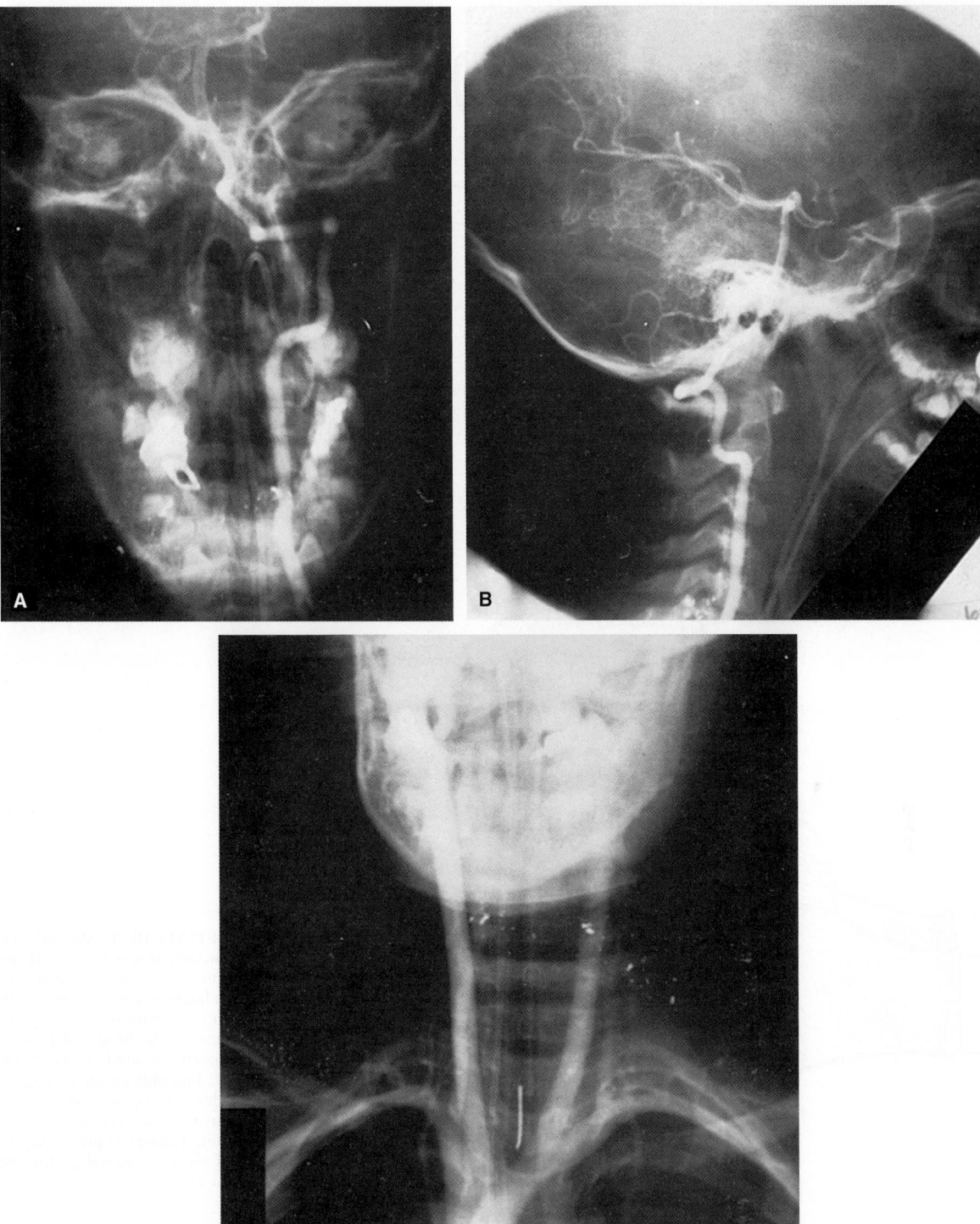

FIGURE 115.9 Angiograms in 5-year-old child shot in the neck, demonstrating normal vascular integrity.
A: Vertebral artery angiogram (anteroposterior view). **B:** Vertebral artery angiogram (lateral view).
C: Carotid angiogram.

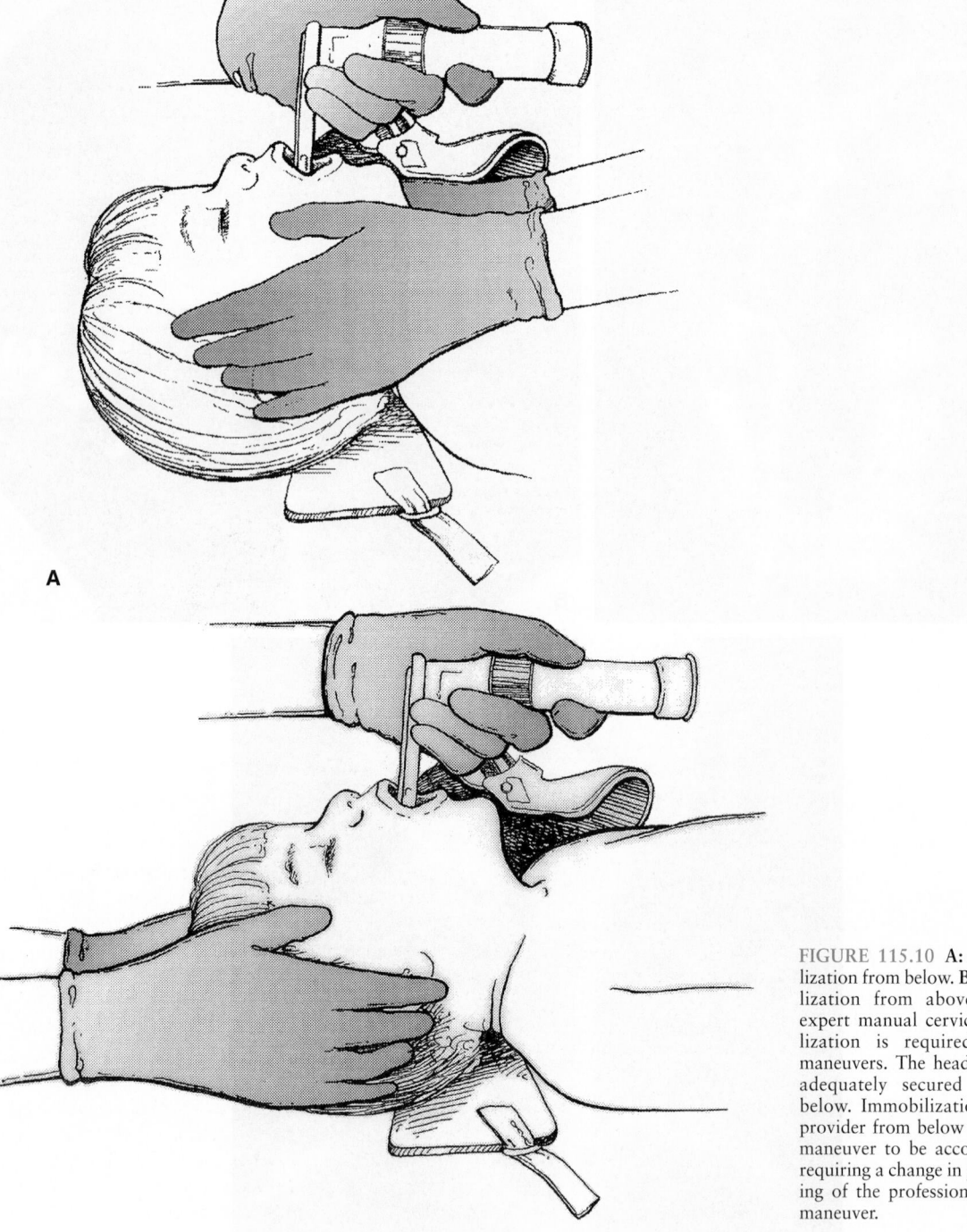

A

B

FIGURE 115.10 **A:** Manual immobilization from below. **B:** Manual immobilization from above. Adequate and expert manual cervical spine immobilization is required during airway maneuvers. The head and neck can be adequately secured from above or below. Immobilization by the second provider from below allows the airway maneuver to be accomplished without requiring a change in preferred positioning of the professional performing the maneuver.

another performs the intubation. The immobilization is often best accomplished from below, allowing the intubator as much room as possible to maneuver (Fig. 115.10). The hard cervical collar should be opened anteriorly, or removed, while this process is being performed. It is difficult to intubate a child unless the reduction in mouth opening and jaw immobilization afforded by the collar is temporarily removed, as the trachea is more anterior than in an adult. As usual, oral intubation is often

the preferred method because of the child's airway position and the usual experience of providers. Adjunctive airway techniques that do not require vigorous laryngoscopy, such as video fluoroscopy and optical stylets, may be useful in managing the airway of these patients. The collar should be resecured after the airway intervention is complete.

Several concepts should be kept in mind concerning cervical immobilization in children. It is been estimated that 3% to

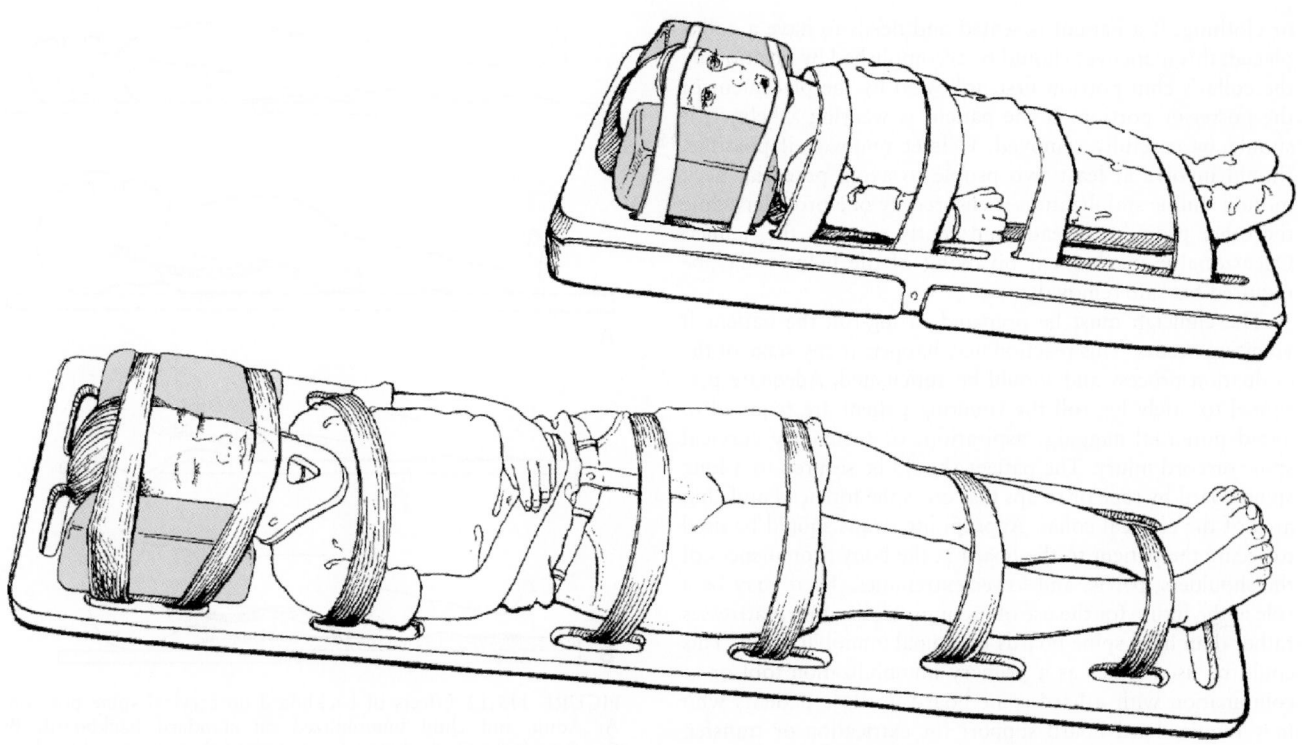

FIGURE 115.11 Cervical spine immobilization should not place the patient at an increased risk for morbidity. Securing straps should be placed around bony prominences and strap location reassessed after any movement of the patient. A neutral position of the neck should be ensured, and if necessary (younger child), a spacer can be placed underneath the child's torso and lower extremities to achieve the desired position.

25% of spinal cord injuries occur during transit or early in the course of management, although a 2001 Cochrane report noted that there are no randomized controlled studies on the effect of immobilization on mortality, neurologic injury, spinal stability, and other adverse effects. It is also important to realize that as many as 20% of spinal injuries involve noncontiguous vertebral elements, so entire spinal column immobilization is imperative. Soft cervical collars offer no protection to an unstable spine, and hard collars (Philadelphia, Stifneck) alone still allow a fair amount of flexion, extension, and lateral movement of the cervical spine. Ideal immobilization involves a hard cervical collar in conjunction with a full spine board, soft spacing devices, and securing straps (Fig. 115.11). Zhang et al noted that additional hard collars, including the C-Breeze and XTW (Deroyal Industries, Inc. Powell, TN), Miami J (Jerome Medical, Moorestown, NJ), and Aspen (International Healthcare Devices, Long Beach, CA), are effective in restricting range of motion in the cervical spine. Tescher et al report lower levels of mandibular and ocular pressures with Miami J collars, reducing the risk of occipital pressure ulcers while maintaining appropriate immobilization.

There is research suggesting that emergency medical services (EMS) protocols for selectively clearing adult cervical spines in the field are somewhat effective, but there is limited information regarding this practice in the pediatric population. For example, in the 2007 study of Armstrong et al, their prehospital cervical spine assessment protocol specifically excluded children younger than 16 years. Domeier et al in a study of more than 13,000 patients reported that prehospital protocols had a sensitivity of 92%, resulting in nonimmobilization of 8% of patients who were later evaluated for the diagnosis of spinal injury (although none developed neurologic sequela). This study included 1,200 patients who were younger than 15 years with one missed fracture. Although these are interesting data, the nuances of pediatric cervical spine evaluation, the fact that up to 75% of children with cervical spine injuries present with incomplete injuries along with the evaluation challenges encountered with variable ages and developmental status of young children, lead us to not recommend routine clinical clearance of the cervical spine by EMS in children who may have experienced potentially significant mechanisms of injury. More research may help us better understand this potential option for the prehospital care provider. An appropriately sized hard cervical collar should be chosen. The longest collar that does not hyperextend the neck is the correct choice. The choice between a one-piece collar (e.g., Stifneck) and a two-piece collar (e.g., Philadelphia) is important only in that correct fit must be ensured and the provider must understand how to apply the specific brand of collar. It is helpful to fold over the Velcro connectors on the collar before sliding it under the patient's neck to avoid Velcro attachment to the child's hair

TRAUMA

or clothing. If a patient is seated and needs to have a collar placed, this maneuver should be accomplished by positioning the collar's chin portion first, followed by the placement of the posterior portion. If the patient is wearing a helmet, it should be carefully removed. Helmet removal, if possible, should involve at least two people to avoid potential neck motion. Inline stabilization is ensured by one provider while the other provider spreads and gently removes the helmet. Occasionally, mechanical bivalving of the helmet may be required for safe removal.

The clinician must be prepared to log-roll the patient if vomiting occurs. This reaction may happen at any stage of the evaluation process and should be anticipated. Adequate personnel to safely log-roll the vomiting patient are required to avoid potential gagging, aspiration, or secondary cervical spine or cord injury. The patient should be secured to a long spine board by tape or straps that cross the forehead and chin area of the cervical collar. Appropriate straps should be used to secure the patient to the board at the bony prominences of the shoulders, pelvis, and lower extremities. There may be a role in the future for the use of vacuum stabilization mattresses rather than hard spine boards for spinal immobilization. This could be used either as a primary immobilization tool or in combination with a hard spine board in those patients who may require hard board support for extrication or transfer. Incorrect immobilization may impede respiration by obstructing chest rise or contributing to secondary spinal injury by hyperextending the neck. The securing straps should be assessed periodically to ensure adequate and safe attachment of the patient to the spine board. When a child is immobilized on a spine board, the clinician must consider that the child's head is disproportionately large compared with that of the adult. A child's head reaches 50% of postnatal growth by approximately 2 years of age, whereas chest circumference reaches 50% of postnatal growth by about 8 years of age. This disparate growth of the head and trunk causes the neck to be forced into relative kyphotic position when a child is placed on a hard spine board (Fig. 115.12). This is distinctly different from the adult patient whose neck is in 30 degrees of lordosis, the neutral position, when immobilized on a hard spine board. Suggestions have been made to allow a recess in the head area of the spine board to accommodate the child's large occiput or to place a spacing device such as a blanket underneath the torso to allow the neck to rest in a neutral position (Fig. 115.12). Figure 115.13 demonstrates how cervical spine alignment can be greatly affected and improved by this technique. As the evaluation continues, one should be aware of the consequences of prolonged hard board immobilization. These include inadequate long-term immobilization and support, pain, discomfort, pressure sores, and potential respiratory insufficiency. The spine board should be removed as soon as practical, potentially during the log-roll portion of the clinical ED assessment.

Patients often arrive in the ED with full or partial cervical spine immobilization already in place. An immediate assessment of this immobilization is imperative. Several important issues should be considered: (i) Is the patient appropriately and fully immobilized? (ii) Is the cervical collar of the correct size and type for the patient? (iii) Is the patient's neck in a neutral position? (iv) Is the patient securely strapped to a

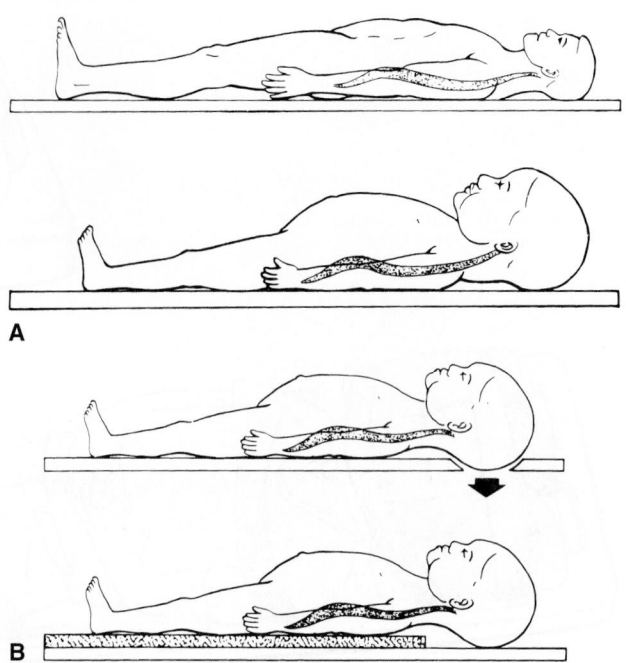

FIGURE 115.12 Effects of backboard on cervical spine position. **A:** Adult and child immobilized on standard backboard. **B:** Backboards modified with occipital recess and mattress pad to allow neutral positioning of the cervical spine in a young child. (From Herzenberg J, Hensinger R, Dedrick D, et al. Emergency transport and positioning of young children who have an injury of the cervical spine: the standard backboard may be hazardous. *J Bone Joint Surg Am* 1989;71-A:16, 21. Copyright The Journal of Bone and Joint Surgery, Inc. Reprinted with permission.)

long spine board? (v) Has there been a shift in the patient or the immobilization during the prehospital or interfacility transport that might diminish effective immobilization, cause hyperflexion or hyperextension of the cervical spine, or compromise excursion of the chest with respiration? and (vi) Does the immobilization interfere with the assessment or management of the ABCs? If these or other immobilization difficulties are identified, they should be immediately addressed.

Occasionally, the use of a semipermanent immobilization device (tongs, halo) may be indicated (Fig. 115.14). This should be accomplished after neurosurgical consultation. Attempts to rapidly reduce a cervical fracture are usually discouraged to avoid the potential for further cord injury. Frequent reassessment is necessary for the patient in cervical traction. Transport of the patient in cervical traction has the potential to further damage the injured cervical spine.

The pediatric cervical spine and its evaluation differ in many ways from the adult spine. The fulcrum of the cervical spine of an infant is at approximately C2–C3 and reaches C3–C4 by 5 to 6 years of age. At about 8 years of age, the fulcrum (C5–C6) and other characteristics of the cervical spine approximate that of an adult. The higher fulcrum of a child's spine in combination with relatively weak neck muscles and poor protective reflexes account for young children often having fractures that involve the upper cervical spine, whereas older children and adults have fractures that more often

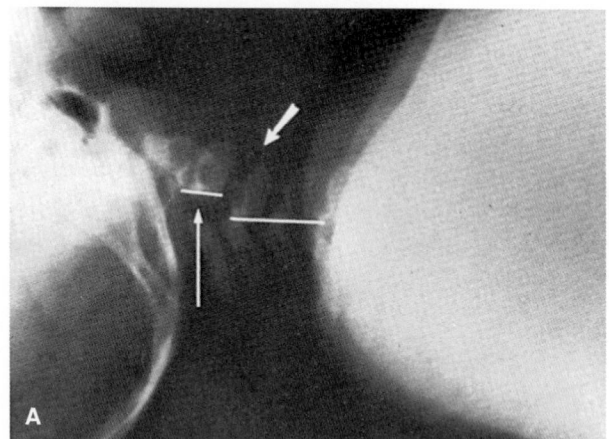

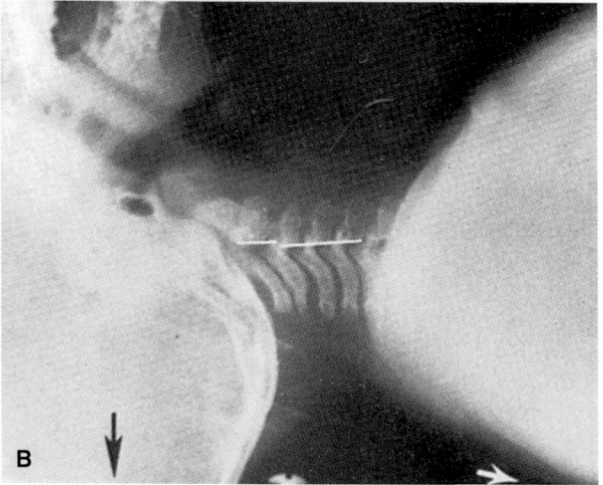

FIGURE 115.13 Effects of backboard on cervical spine position in 6-month-old child with a hangman's fracture (traumatic spondylolisthesis of posterior elements of C2) indicated by *thin arrow.* **A:** Large occiput contributes to anterior subluxation (*thick arrow*) of unstable cervical spine. **B:** Same child on backboard with occipital recess. Anterior subluxation is decreased. (From Herzenberg J, Hensiger R, Dedrick D, et al. Emergency transport and positioning of young children who have an injury of the cervical spine: the standard backboard may be hazardous. *J Bone Joint Surg Am* 1989;71-A:18. Copyright The Journal of Bone and Joint Surgery, Inc. Reprinted with permission.)

involve the lower cervical spine. Neurologic disability can occur from cervical lesions at all levels, but high cervical cord injuries are more likely to be fatal than are lower cervical cord injuries.

The large amount of cartilage present in a pediatric cervical spine not only cushions forces that are transmitted to the spine but can also make radiographic evaluation somewhat challenging. The radiolucent nature of cartilage makes the ability to appreciate soft-tissue changes on the radiograph extremely important. The pediatric cervical spine seems to have more anterior and posterior movement than its adult counterpart as a result not only of radiolucent cartilage but also of ligamentous laxity and relatively horizontal facet joints. The pediatric cervical spine also has the ability to revert to a relatively normal appearance after a significant distortion, which can hinder the radiographic search for abnormalities. It is important to

realize that any persistent distortion demonstrated on the radiographs was probably more exaggerated during the actual precipitating event. There is more room around the spinal cord within the spinal column in a young child than in an adult, which means that compressive problems such as tumors or bleeds may be slower to manifest neurologic symptoms.

Evaluation of a child with trauma begins with a focused history and complete physical examination. The history (if reliable) can be invaluable in identifying the potential for cervical spine or cord injury. The following questions should be answered: (i) Was the child involved in a high-speed motor vehicle accident? If so, was he or she restrained, and at what angle did the car(s) collide? (ii) Was there a sports injury? If so, did it involve a spearing motion? (iii) Did the child fall? If so, how high was the fall and how did the child land? A neurologic history is imperative to assess whether there was any evidence of abnormal findings such as paresthesias, paralysis, or paresis at any time after the injury. These symptoms may have been transient and may (or may not) be present at the time of the examination or volunteered by the patient during gathering of the history, yet they are important because they may suggest a cervical contusion, a concussion, or a spinal cord injury without radiographic abnormality (SCIWORA). The answers to these and other historical questions can often be obtained from the patient, parents, bystanders, and EMS personnel and can help determine the potential for cervical injury. A plethora of clues can aid in the diagnosis of a cervical cord injury (Table 115.7). The symptoms and signs may be obvious or masked by other abnormalities such as altered level of consciousness, hypovolemic shock, or concurrent head injury. Head and neck injuries may present with overlapping abnormal neurologic signs, and differentiation of causation may be difficult.

Consideration of cervical spine radiographic evaluation is the next step in assessment. Radiographic options include radiographs, CT, and MRI. MRI scans are more appropriate when evaluating the subacute or chronic stages of injury or when looking for an acute problem with cord impingement

TABLE 115.7

SYMPTOMS AND SIGNS OF CERVICAL SPINE INJURY

Abnormal motor examination (paresis, paralysis, flaccidity, ataxia, spasticity, rectal tone)	Diaphragmatic breathing without retractions
	Spinal (neurogenic) shock (hypotension with bradycardia)
Abnormal sensory examination (pain, sensation, temperature, paresthesias, anal wink)	Priapism
Altered mental status	Decreased bladder function
Neck pain	Fecal retention
Torticollis	Unexplained ileus
Limitation of motion	Autonomic hyperreflexia
Neck muscle spasm	Blood pressure variability with flushing and sweating
Abnormal or absent reflexes	Poikilothermia
Clonus without rigidity	Hypothermia or hyperthermia

TRAUMA

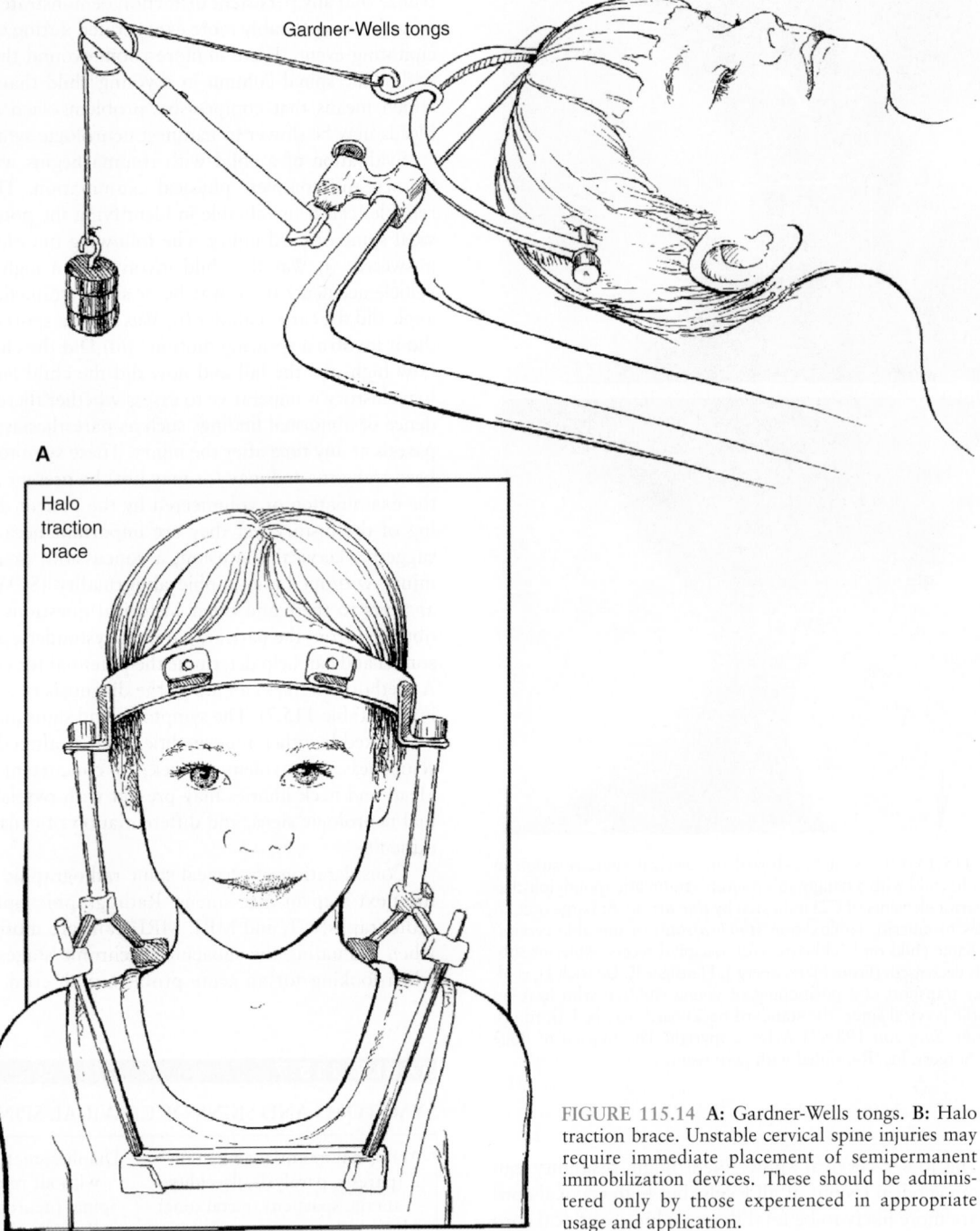

Gardner-Wells tongs

A

Halo traction brace

B

FIGURE 115.14 **A:** Gardner-Wells tongs. **B:** Halo traction brace. Unstable cervical spine injuries may require immediate placement of semipermanent immobilization devices. These should be administered only by those experienced in appropriate usage and application.

by blood or soft tissues such as tumors or intervertebral discs, instability, and ligamentous disruptions. Acute MRI evaluation is increasing in popularity in the cervical spine evaluation of patients with altered mental status. MRI does not provide images of the cortical bone well and should not be used to evaluate the cervical spine for fractures, whereas the CT scan demonstrates fractures clearly but does not offer direct evidence of ligamentous injury. A CT scan is often used as a secondary screen when adequate plain radiographs cannot be obtained or to substantiate suspected fractures. The use of the spine CT scan as an initial rapid screening tool has been sug-

gested by several authors. The detail and reconstruction provided by the CT scan promise to present greater detail to the reviewer. The issue of increased radiation exposure needs to be considered when developing institution-specific protocols. A common scenario is the use of CT to supplement viewing the C1–C2 region in young children with trauma. Several studies have demonstrated the superiority of upper cervical spine CT scan versus plain radiographs in diagnosing injuries in the region. The CT scan images soft tissue well; however, it does not demonstrate the intrathecal, ligamentous, disc, or vascular detail that can be obtained with an MRI scan.

The plain radiograph remains the preferred initial test for patients with acute trauma. Several authors have attempted to devise criteria to limit the use of cervical spine radiographs because the number of positive studies constitutes a small proportion of the total number of radiographic studies completed. The perception of unnecessary tests should be balanced against the severity of consequences that may occur with a missed cervical spine injury. The literature suggests that if the patient does not have a high-risk mechanism of injury (motor vehicle accident, fall, dive, or sports injury), is awake and alert, can have an interactive conversation (not inebriated, no altered level of consciousness, older than 4 to 5 years), does not complain of cervical spine pain, has no tenderness on palpation (especially in the midline), has normal neck mobility, has a completely normal neurologic examination without a history of abnormal neurologic symptoms or signs at any time after the injury, and has no other painful injuries (which may distract the patient and mask neck pain), the patient probably does not need radiographic evaluation of the cervical spine. The National Emergency X-Radiography Utilization Study (NEXUS) suggests the following criteria for the assessment of risk of spinal injury: (i) midline cervical tenderness, (ii) intoxication, (iii) alertness, (iv) focal neurologic deficit, and (v) distracting (painful) injury (i.e., long bone fracture, visceral injury, large laceration, degloving or crush injury, large burns, and injuries producing impairment in appreciation of other injuries). If these are negative, then the patient is believed to be at low risk for a spinal injury and may be able to forgo radiographic evaluation. NEXUS low-risk criteria have been reported to be 99.6% sensitive in detection of clinical important cervical spine injury and have a high negative predictive value for low-risk patients. Garton and Hammer's 2008 retrospective 20-year review applying NEXUS criteria to 187 eligible patients with radiographically proven cervical spine injury noted that the NEXUS criteria appeared to be more sensitive in children older than 8 years. This information, as well as the low incidence of spinal cord injuries and the presence of pediatric patients, in the studies makes the results less clear for this population, although the approach appears sound in adult patients. The provider should use clinical judgment and ancillary signs to determine whether a long bone fracture or other potentially painful injury is indeed distracting to a patient with a mechanism of injury (short fall etc.) that would suggest minor risk for a cervical spine injury. For example, if an adequate response and appreciation of painful stimuli (pinch or other effort to elicit appreciation of pain) during the physical evaluation is elicited, the provider may be more confident that the physical examination could suffice to clinically clear the patient's cervical spine. If one is unable to determine whether an injury (and associated pain) is indeed distracting, or if neck pain or appreciation of the pain may potentially have been diminished by medication for other injuries, cervical spine radiographic evaluation should be strongly considered. This approach is also being used in the out-of-hospital environment to determine initial need for immobilization. This out-of-hospital screening should not be used in the pediatric EMS population at this time, as noted above. Another screening algorithm called the Canadian C-Spine Rule evaluates high-risk factors (e.g., age, dangerous mechanism, paresthesias) and low-risk factors that would allow for safe assessment of range of motion (e.g., low-speed motor vehicle accident, delayed evaluation, delayed onset of pain, absence of midline tenderness) and ability to rotate neck 45 degrees to the right and left. This has been reported to be sensitive in alert and stable adult trauma patients. Regardless of clearing algorithm embraced, the clinician must also be sure to never "clear" the cervical spine, regardless of studies performed, in an unconscious patient in the ED.

When radiographs are obtained, a normal lateral radiograph does not "clear" the cervical spine. The sensitivity of a lateral cervical spine radiograph traditionally varies between 70% and 85%–98% in the literature. Brohi et al, in a study of 437 unconscious, intubated blunt trauma patients, reported a 53% sensitivity of adequate cross-table lateral films in identifying cervical spine fracture. When evaluating a lateral cervical spine radiograph, the clinician must ensure that C1–C7 are included as well as the C7–T1 junction. Additional films, which include an anteroposterior (AP) view of C3–C7 and an AP open-mouth (odontoid) view of C1–C2, increase the sensitivity of initial radiographic evaluation to more than 95%. Avellino and colleagues reported their experiences with radiologic misdiagnosis of pediatric cervical spine injuries found at a level 1 combined adult/pediatric regional trauma center. The most common reasons for a missed injury on initial radiologic evaluation included unfamiliarity with pediatric cervical spine anatomy, failure to recognize normal developmental variants, and suboptimal conventional film techniques. An adequate open-mouth view is often technically difficult to obtain in young children and those who are intubated. If further information is required, a CT scan of C1–C2 can be useful to augment or replace the open-mouth view. A CT scan is more expensive than a plain radiograph of C1–C2 but is easier to obtain, offers enhanced and more consistent information, and avoids the risk of missing a subtle injury in that critical area. The advent of the spiral CT scan allows this study to be completed in 1 to 2 minutes and to be reconstructed by the computer to demonstrate vivid detail of the region (Fig. 115.15). CT scan or MRI should be considered in cases where plain radiograph has identified an injury. These studies can increase the understanding regarding the severity and significance of the identified injury and potentially identify other injuries not noted on the initial screening films. Barrett et al, in 2006, reported that 36% of their patients with cervical spine injury identified from plain radiograph had a second injury identified by CT scan, and in 27% of those patients, these injuries were noncontiguous. An algorithm for considering radiographic evaluation is presented in Fig. 115.16. An approach to ordering cervical spine imaging studies is shown in Fig. 115.17.

The cervical spine has anterior (vertebral bodies, intervertebral discs, ligaments) and posterior (lamina, pedicles, neural foramen, spinous processes, ligaments) components (Fig. 115.18). The initial three-view series evaluates the anterior cervical spine well; however, it is not ideal for evaluating the posterior cervical spine. Oblique (pillar) views are helpful in imaging these posterior elements. In practice, however, oblique radiographs rarely add significant information to the initial radiographic assessment. Flexion and extension radiographs are accomplished in an awake patient by having the patient flex and extend the neck as far as possible without discomfort. As the end point involves the sensation of pain,

TRAUMA

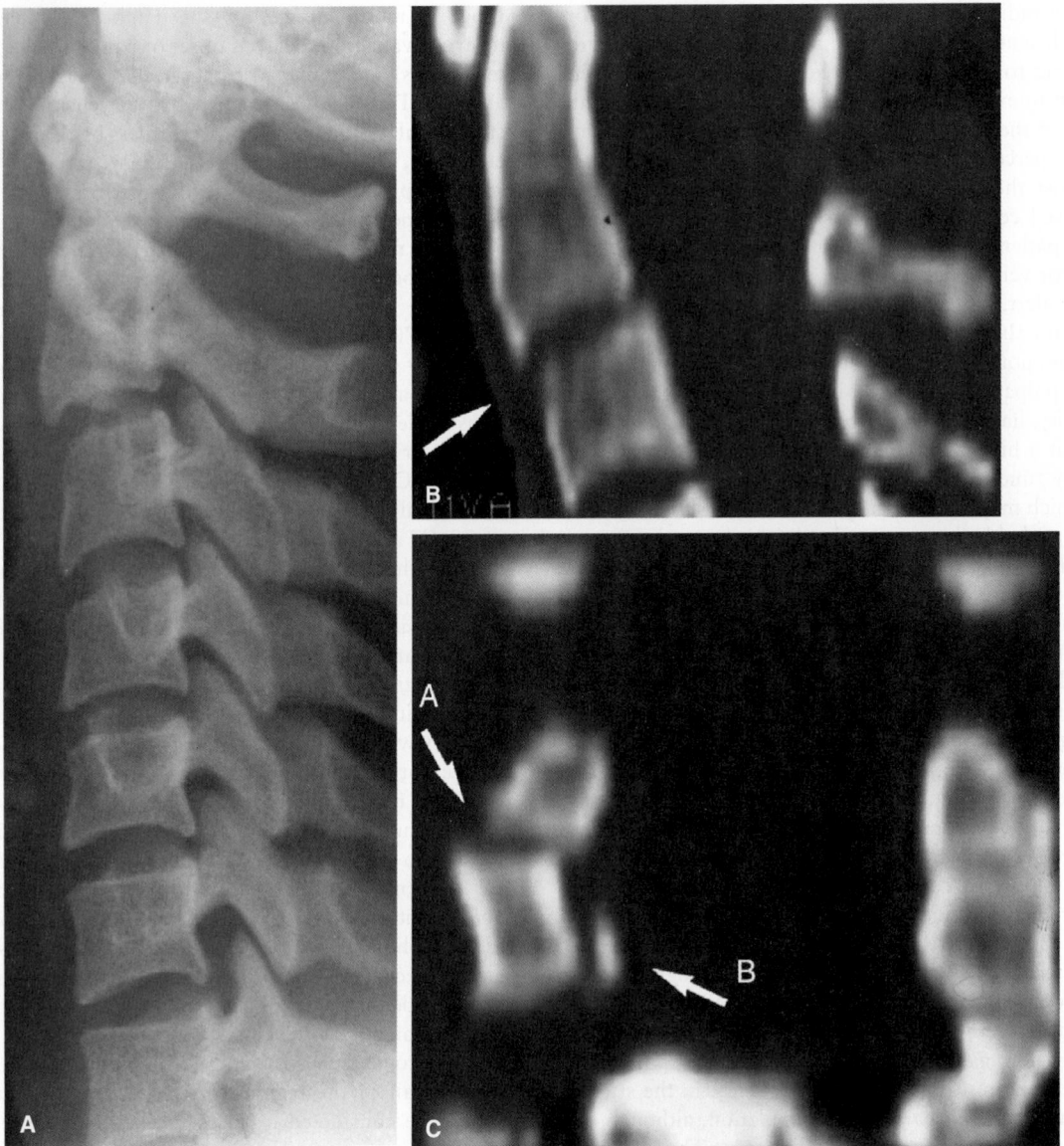

FIGURE 115.15 **A:** Apparently "normal" lateral cervical spine radiograph (16-year-old patient after motor vehicle accident). **B:** Spiral computed tomography (CT) scan demonstrating dens fracture (*arrow*). **C:** Sagittal view of spiral CT scan demonstrating dens fracture (*arrow A*) and vertebral body avulsion fracture (*arrow B*). The detail demonstrated by the spiral CT scan could help clinicians quickly identify lesions not easily visible or appreciated on conventional radiographs.

flexion/extension radiographs should not be obtained in a patient who has preexisting neck pain. Flexion and extension radiographs are believed to be of limited diagnostic use and probably should not be routinely used. Dynamic fluoroscopy could be substituted in specific instances for flexion/extension radiographs. These studies can help evaluate underlying soft-tissue or ligamentous injury that was not evident on the initial radiographs, although ligamentous injury without fracture (via radiographs and CT scan) is not a common finding. Traumatic quadriplegia has been reported during the use of this study. These radiographs are often inadequate because the neck muscles have splinted the cervical column into a

position of comfort and stability, and alignment does not change with flexion and extension. If a question remains concerning the integrity of the cervical spine following this radiographic scheme, a CT scan should be considered. Without reconstruction, a CT scan may miss a horizontal fracture or injuries obscured by artifacts from retained foreign bodies or dental work. The use of CT as a primary screening tool, as well as an adjunct to initial radiographic evaluation, is noted in the literature. Garton and Hammer noted increased sensitivity of combined plain radiograph and occiput-C3 CT (94%) compared with plain radiographs (75%) and plain radiographs coupled with flexion/extension radiographs

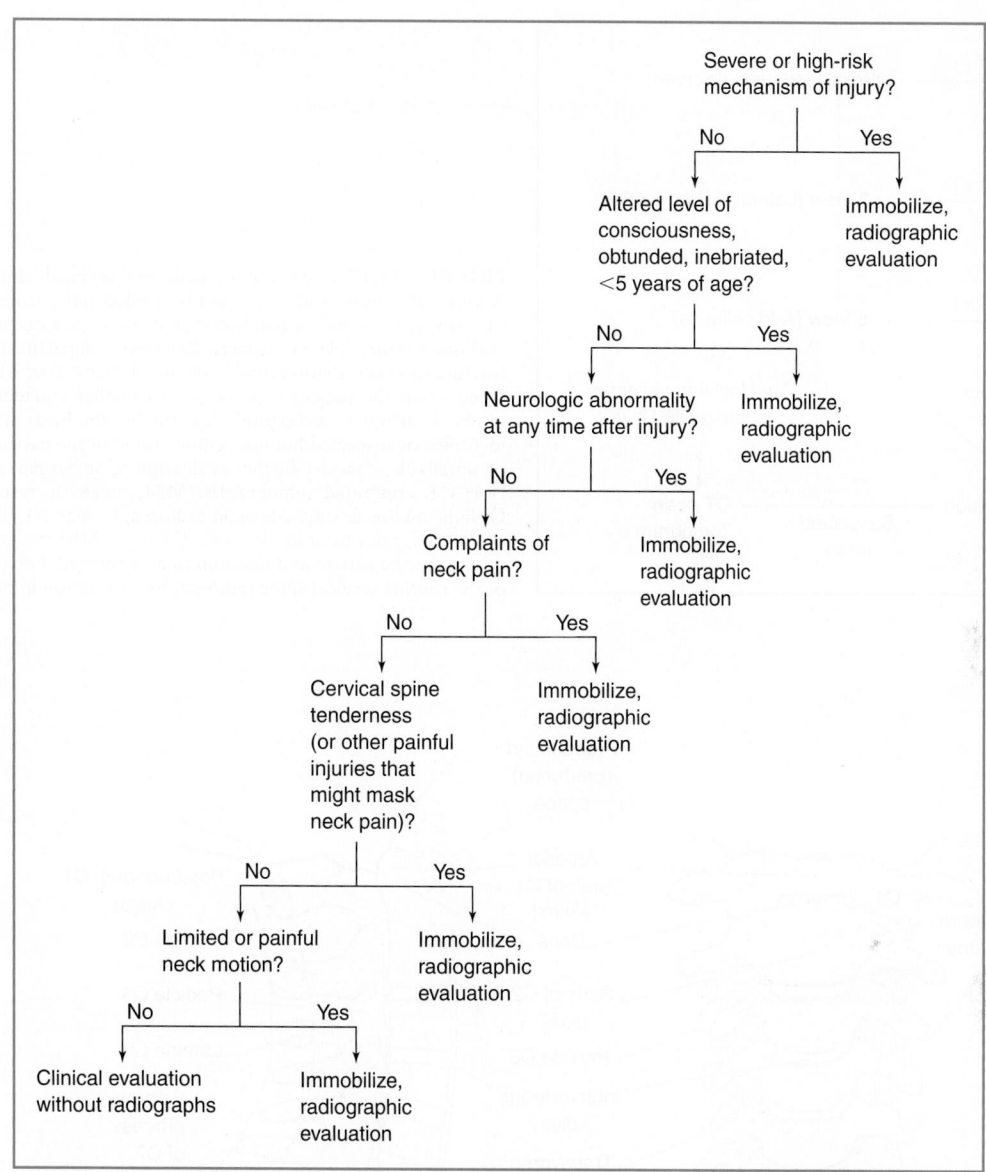

FIGURE 115.16 Decision tree for radiographic and clinical evaluation of patients with possible neck injury.

(81%) in children younger than 8 years. In children older than 8 years, the sensitivities are similar (93% to 97%), suggesting that limited use of CT may be helpful. Blackmore et al in their 1999 study reported that in adults, a CT protocol was more effective and less costly in high-risk patients (11% injury incidence), reasonably cost-effective with moderate risk of injury (4% injury incidence), but extremely costly if there is a low risk of injury (2% injury incidence). Others note that CT alone is sufficient in high-risk patients, as the combination of CT plus plain films does not markedly enhance sensitivity of injury identification. Adelgais et al noted increased radiation and radiology resource usage and no decrease in sedation usage or ED length of stay in pediatric patients using a CT screening protocol. Debate exists in the literature regarding the clearing of the cervical spine in an obtunded patient. While this should not be an ED debate, as obtunded patients should not have their cervical spine cleared in the ED, variations in practice exist. Como et al in 2007 reported that CT was sufficient to clear the cervical spine in this population, whereas Menaker et al in 2008 reported that in unreliable or obtunded adults who were admitted following a CT scan that did not demonstrate injury, the addition of MRI evaluation changed the management in 7.9% of those patients. Tomograms can also be obtained but require patient movement, are time-consuming, and are not performed easily in the acutely ill patient. An MRI should be considered to detect ligamentous, soft-tissue, or subtle cord injuries.

TRAUMA

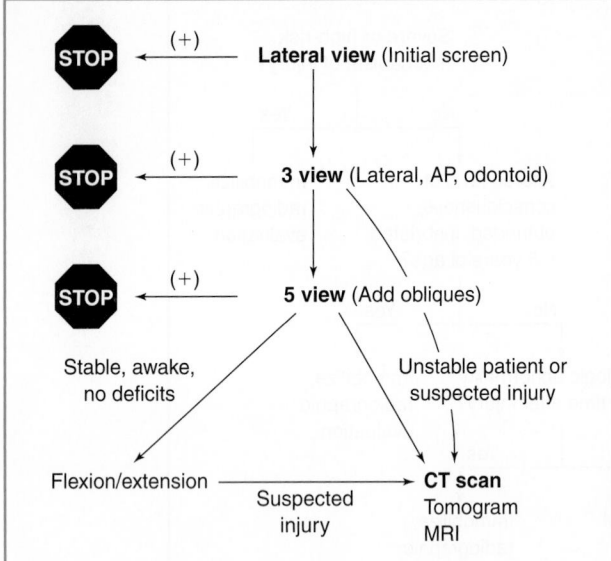

FIGURE 115.17 Approach to ordering cervical spine radiographs. Additional films or studies may not be needed in the acute CT scan images can be negatively influenced, however, by retained foreign bodies (bullets) and other injury-related artifacts. Emergency department evaluation if a fracture or other abnormality is identified, but CT or MRI may be indicated when the patient is stabilized to further elucidate the identified injury. If adequate radiographs cannot be obtained, an abnormality is identified or suspected but not demonstrated or the patient is unconscious or unreliable, consider further evaluation as suggested. AP, anteroposterior; CT, computed tomography; MRI, magnetic resonance imaging. Oblique and/or flexion/extension radiographs may also be options in the evaluation, prior to or in place of a CT or an MRI evaluation, depending on the specific patient and question to be answered, but are often not part of the routine cervical spine radiographic evaluation in pediatrics.

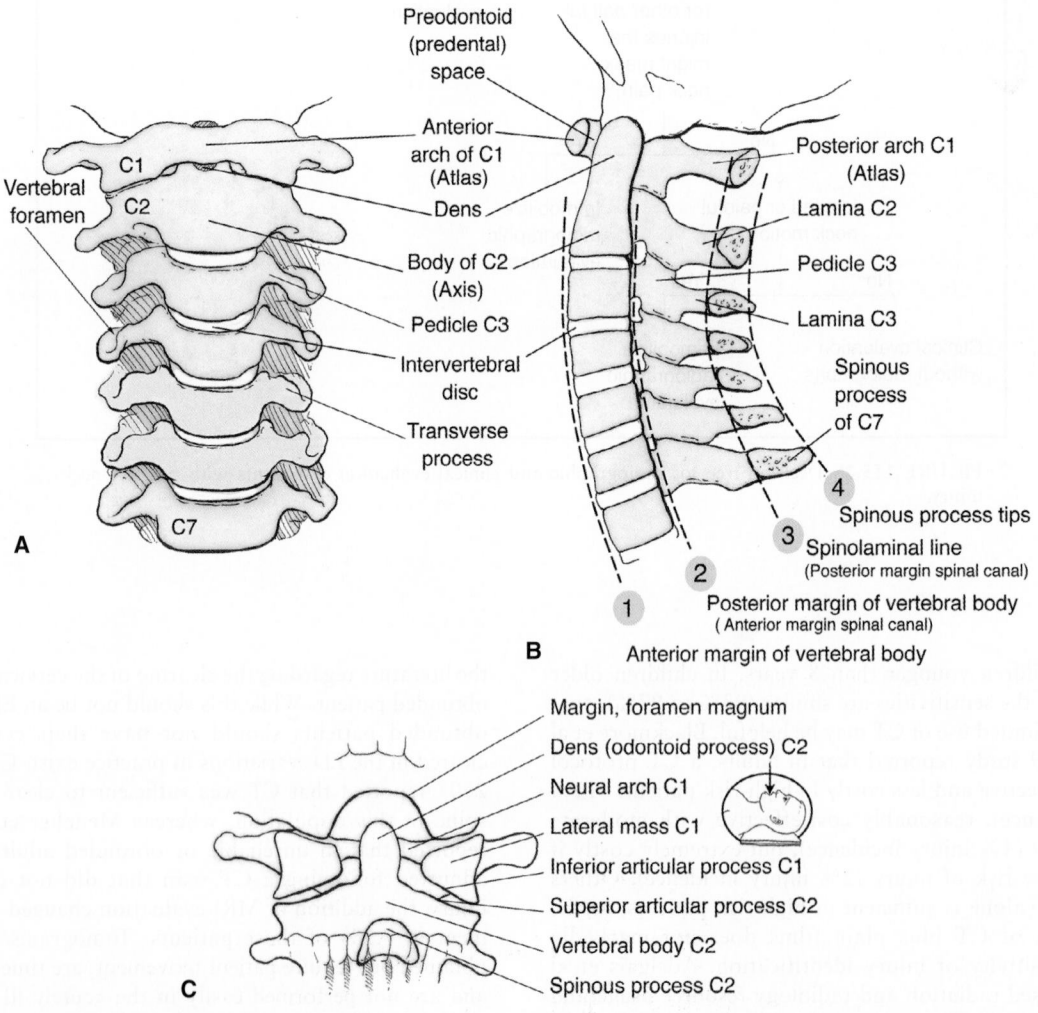

FIGURE 115.18 **A–C:** Knowledge of normal cervical spine anatomy is useful when evaluating cervical spine radiographs.

A - <u>A</u>lignment

Lordotic curves, gross malalignment,
subluxation, distraction

B - <u>B</u>ones

Fractures, anterior and posterior vertebral
columns, ossification centers

C - <u>C</u>artilage

Intervertebral disc spaces, ossification centers

S - <u>S</u>oft tissues

Prevertebral space, predental space

FIGURE 115.19 The ABCS of radiographic cervical spine interpretation.

A systematic approach should be used when evaluating radiographs of the cervical spine. The ABCS method is a useful approach (Fig. 115.19). Alignment is assessed as demonstrated in Fig. 115.20, keeping in mind that the spinal cord lies between the posterior spinal line and the spinolaminal line. These lordotic curves may not be present in children younger than 6 years, those on hard spine boards or in cervical collars, or those with cervical neck muscle spasm. Gross malalignment should be detectable with this assessment.

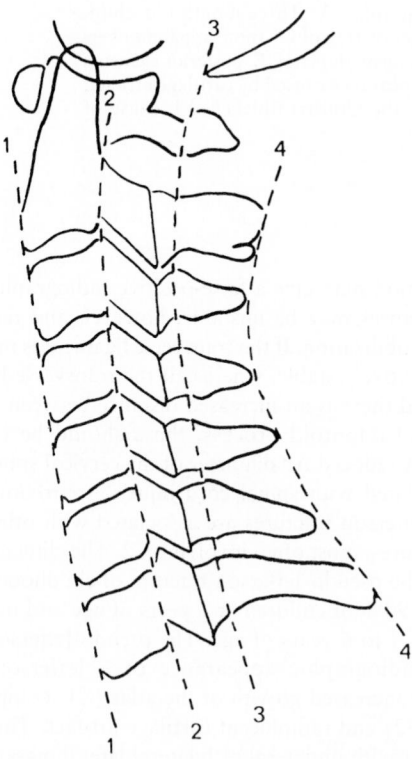

FIGURE 115.20 Four contour lines of alignment with normal cervical spine lordosis: *1*, anterior vertebral bodies; *2*, posterior vertebral bodies (anterior spinal canal); *3*, spinolaminal line (posterior spinal canal); and *4*, spinous process tips. (From Gerlock A, Kirchner S, Heller R, et al. *Advanced exercises in diagnostic radiology: the cervical spine in trauma.* Philadelphia, PA: WB Saunders, 1978:6. Reprinted with permission.)

TABLE 115.8

RADIOGRAPHIC CHARACTERISTICS OF PEDIATRIC CERVICAL SPINE

Cartilage artifact
Tapered anterior vertebrae
Apparently absent ring of C1
Atlas (C1) body not ossified at birth and may fail to close
Axis (C2) has four ossification centers
Apex of odontoid ossifies between 12 and 15 yr of age
Spinous process ossification centers
Increased mobility
Pseudosubluxation
C1 override on dens
Increased predental space (5 mm maximum)
Ligament laxity
Facet joints shallow
Growth plates (synchondrosis)
Dens ossifies between 3 and 8 yr of age (may persist into young adults)
Posterior arch of C1 ossifies at 3 yr of age
Anterior arch of C1 ossifies at 6–9 yr of age
C1 reaches adult size at 3–4 yr of age
C2 through C7 reach adult size at 5–6 yr of age
Lack of cervical lordosis
Fulcrum varies with age
Soft-tissue variability with respiration
Congenital clefts or other bony abnormalities (os odontoideum, spondylolisthesis, spina bifida, ossiculum terminale)

The bones should be evaluated for typical abnormalities, realizing that these may be subtle. Acute fractures are often irregular in location and appearance without sclerosis as compared with the more routine locations and appearance of cartilaginous growth areas. The clinician should be aware that structures that overlay the spine, including the skull and the teeth, might simulate fractures.

The next area of evaluation involves assessing the cartilage. Cartilage is radiolucent on plain radiographs. Children's spinal columns contain significant cartilage that may not only buffer a traumatic force and help prevent some injuries but can also make radiographic evaluation challenging. The cartilaginous areas include the synchondroses or growth plates and intervertebral disc spaces (Table 115.8). The growth plates may mimic fractures and may be confusing to those who are unaware of their presence. Growth centers in the anterior–superior vertebral bodies cause a sloped appearance that may appear as a compression fracture to the untrained eye. Anterior wedging can approach 3 mm and still be considered normal. Vertebral disc abnormalities may indicate specific types of injuries. A vertebral disc space that is narrowed anteriorly may indicate disc extrusion, whereas a widened space suggests a hyperextension injury with posterior ligamentous disruption.

Soft-tissue evaluation is extremely important. Abnormal soft-tissue spaces may be the only clue to the underlying ligament, cartilage, or subtle bone injury, which may not be obvious on the radiograph. The soft-tissue widening may represent blood or edema, which suggests an underlying injury. The prevertebral space at C3 should be less than one-half to two-thirds

TRAUMA

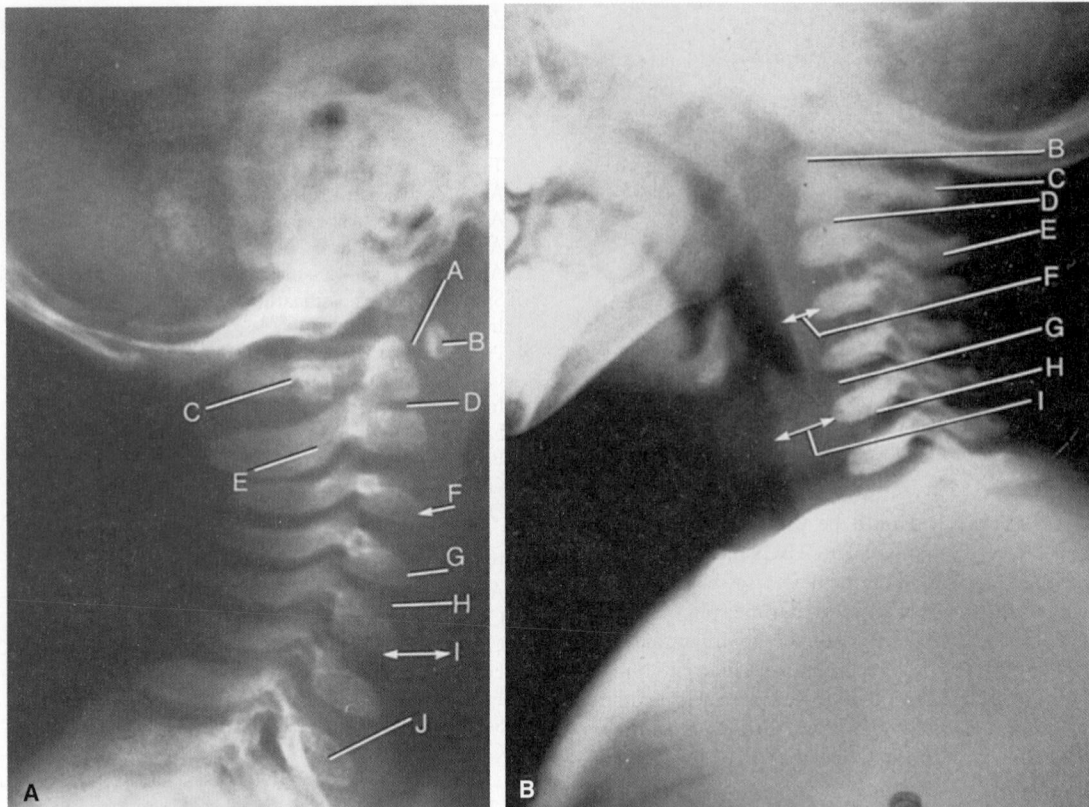

FIGURE 115.21 Normal pediatric lateral cervical spine radiographs. **A:** Three-month-old child. **B:** Twenty-month-old child. *A*, predental (predontoid) space; *B*, anterior ring of C1 (note apparent override of C1 over dens); *C*, posterior ring of C1; *D*, dens synchondrosis (growth plate); *E*, posterior elements C2; *F*, normal prevertebral space (C3 level); *G*, wedged vertebral appearance caused by cartilage artifact; *H*, intervertebral disc space; *I*, normal prevertebral space below the glottitis (thickened because of radiopaque collapsed esophagus); and *J*, vertebral body C7.

of the AP width of the adjacent vertebral body (Fig. 115.21). This space will double to approximately the width of the adjacent vertebral body below C4 (the level of the glottis) because the usually non–air-filled esophagus is present at this area. Care must be taken when evaluating the prevertebral soft-tissue space because crying, neck flexion, or the expiratory phase of respiration may produce a pseudothickening in the prevertebral space (Fig. 115.22). Soft-tissue abnormality should be reproducible on repeated radiographs if an actual underlying injury exists.

SPECIFIC INJURIES

The Jefferson fracture is a bursting fracture of the ring of C1 as a result of an axial load. The axial force compresses the ring of C1 between the occipital condyles of the skull and the lateral masses of C2. This reaction can cause an outward burst of C1, but it rarely causes immediate neurologic impairment because the fracture does not physically impinge on the spinal cord. The radiographic criterion for the diagnosis of a Jefferson fracture is lateral offset of the lateral mass of C1 of more than 1 mm from the vertebral body of C2 (Fig. 115.23).

Neck rotation may give a false-positive radiographic finding. These fractures may be unstable, however, and require adequate immobilization. If the transverse ligament is intact, these may be relatively stable, whereas if the transverse ligament is injured and there is an increased distance between the lateral masses and odontoid process, these should be considered unstable. A reduced AP diameter of the cervical spinal canal is also associated with spinal cord injury. Approximately one-third of Jefferson fractures are associated with other cervical spine fractures, most often involving C2. The clinician must be aware of the pseudo-Jefferson fracture of childhood, which is present in 90% of children at 2 years of age and usually normalizes by 4 to 6 years of age. The pseudo-Jefferson fracture has the radiographic appearance of a Jefferson fracture because of increased growth of the atlas (C1) compared with the axis (C2) and radiolucent cartilage artifact. This disorder can present with unilateral or bilateral lateral mass offset. If a Jefferson fracture is suspected by radiographic findings and mechanism of injury in children younger than 4 years, a CT scan may be necessary to further elucidate the suspected injury (Fig. 115.15).

Hangman's fracture is a traumatic spondylolisthesis of C2. This injury occurs as a result of hyperextension, which

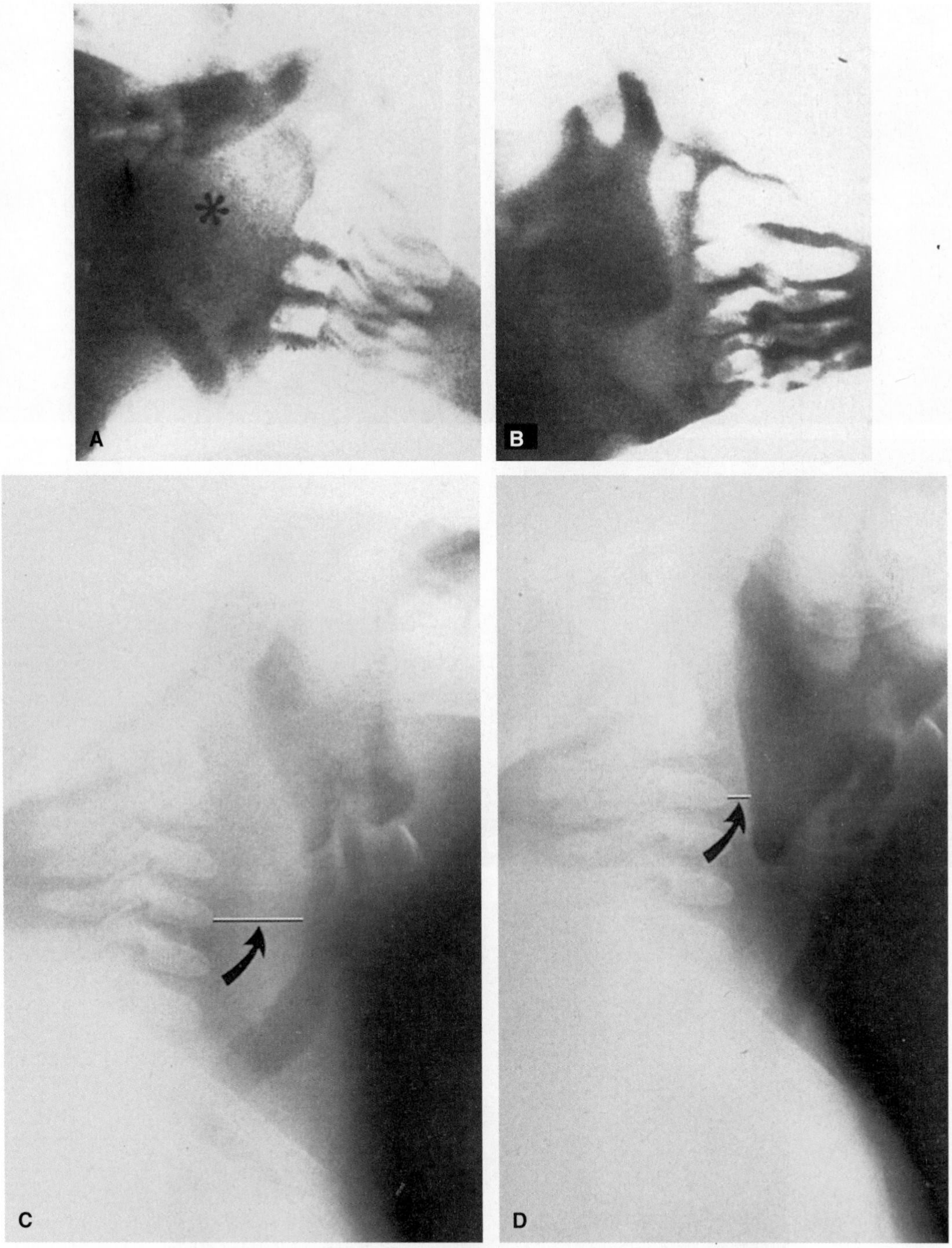

FIGURE 115.22 Effects of inspiration and positioning on prevertebral (retropharyngeal) soft tissues. A: Increased prevertebral space with expiration. B: Repeat radiograph in same patient during inspiration reveals normal prevertebral space with no suggestion of cervical spine abnormality. C: Increased soft-tissue space with expiratory phase of respiration. D: Normal soft-tissue space with inspiration in patient C. (A and B: From Harris J, Edeiken-Monroe B. *The radiology of acute cervical spine trauma*, 2nd ed. Baltimore, MD: Williams & Wilkins, 1987:6. Reprinted with permission.)

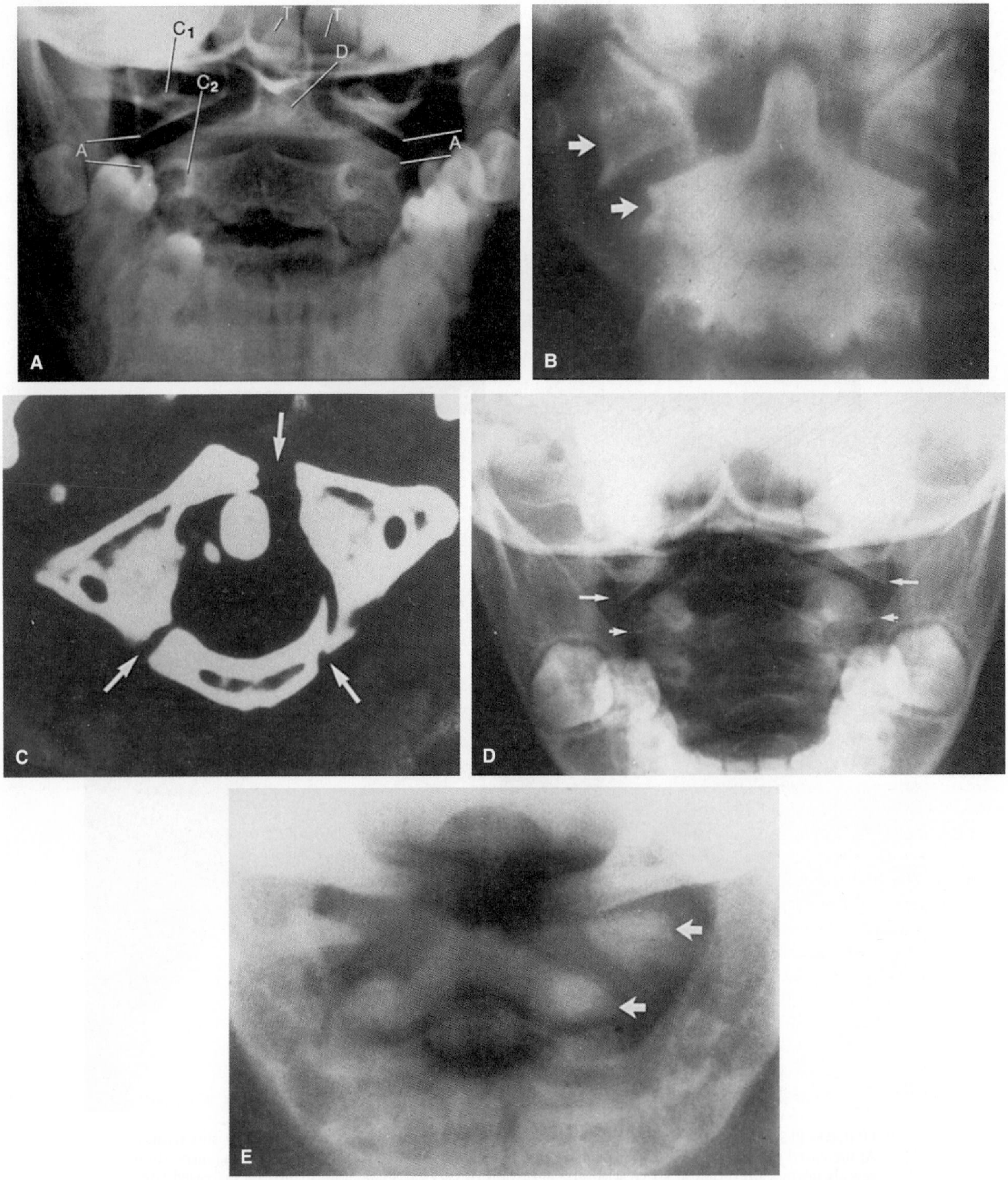

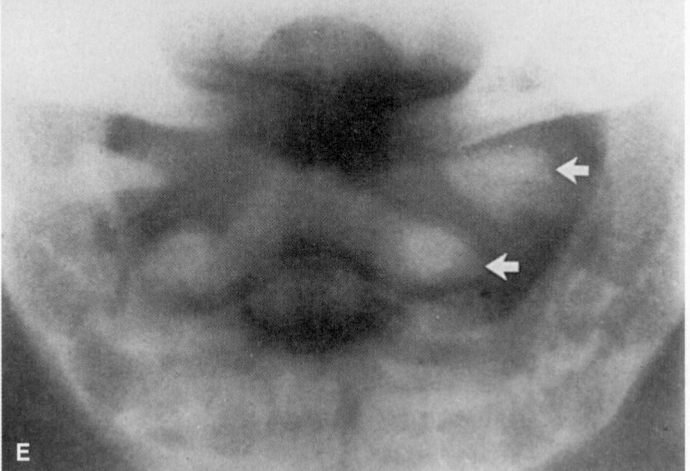

FIGURE 115.23 **A:** Normal anteroposterior (AP) (open-mouth, odontoid) view of C1 and C2. C_1, first cervical vertebra (lateral mass); C_2, second cervical vertebra; T, central incisors overlying dens (D); and A, normal relationship between lateral mass of C1 and vertebral body of C2. **B:** Jefferson fracture in AP view. Note lateral offset of C1 on C2. **C:** Jefferson fracture. Computed tomography coronal view. Note three distinct fractures and bursting nature of injury. **D:** Pseudo-Jefferson fracture of childhood in a 3-year-old child because of disparate growth of C1 and C2 and cartilage artifact. **E:** Pseudo-Jefferson fracture demonstrating marked offset of the lateral masses of C1 on C2. (**B** and **C:** From Swischuk L. *Emergency radiology of the acutely ill or injured child,* 2nd ed. Baltimore, MD: Williams & Wilkins, 1986:591. Reprinted with permission; **D:** From Aslamy W, Danielson K, Hessel S, et al. A 3-year-old boy with neck pain after motor vehicle accident. *West Med J* 1991;155:301–302. Copyright BMJ Publishing Inc. Reprinted with permission.)

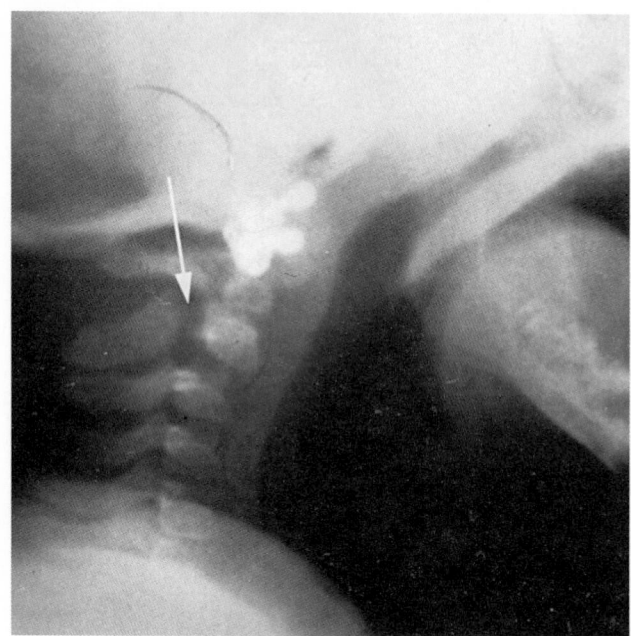

FIGURE 115.24 Hangman's fracture. A 7-week-old infant with fracture through the posterior elements of C2 as indicated by the *arrow*. (From Sumchai A, Sternback G. Hangman's fracture in a 7-week-old infant. *Ann Emerg Med* 1991;20:87. Copyright Elsevier Inc. Reprinted with permission.)

fractures the posterior elements of C2. Hyperflexion, with resultant ligamentous damage, may follow the hyperextension or may lead to anterior subluxation of C2 on C3 and subsequent damage of the cervical cord (Fig. 115.24). The subluxation associated with a hangman's fracture can sometimes be mistaken for the normal or physiologic subluxation that exists in the C2–C3 or C3–C4 region in approximately 25% of children younger than 8 years; it may also be seen in up to 16 years of age. This pseudosubluxation is caused by ligamentous laxity, relatively horizontal facet joints, weak neck muscles, and cartilage artifact. Distinguishing between a subtle hangman's fracture and pseudosubluxation can be accomplished using Swischuk's "posterior cervical line," as described in Fig. 115.25. A value of more than 1.5 to 2 mm suggests an occult hangman's fracture as the source of the anterior subluxation of C2 on C3. The increase in magnitude of the distance between the cortex of the spinous process of C2 and the posterior cervical line in a hangman's fracture is the result of anterior displacement of the skull, C1, and the anterior portion of C2 on the remainder of the lower cervical spine. Nontraumatic subluxation has also been reported at the C5/C6 and C6/C7 spinal levels, although subluxation at these lower levels should always be fully investigated for potential ligamentous injury.

Atlantoaxial (AA) subluxation is a result of movement between C1 and C2 secondary to transverse ligament rupture or a fractured dens (Fig. 115.26). Ligament instability may be precipitated by tonsillitis, cervical adenitis, pharyngitis, arthritis, or connective tissue disorders. It is also well described in patients with Down syndrome. Approximately 15% of patients with Down syndrome have radiographically demonstrated AA subluxation and therefore should be discouraged from contact sports. The presence or absence of AA subluxa-

tion in patients with Down syndrome, once believed to be a static phenomenon, may actually be transient and/or progressive. This ligament instability may progress to ligament rupture with minor trauma. Subluxation caused by a transverse ligament disruption is evidenced by a widened predental (preodontoid, atlantodental interval) space on a lateral radiograph (Fig. 115.26). Rotary subluxation can be classified as follows: type I (no displacement of C1), type II (3 to 5 mm C1 on C2 anterior displacement), type III (more than 5 mm C1 on C2 anterior displacement), and type IV (posterior displacement of C1 on C2). Normal predental measurement in children is less than 5 mm compared with less than 3 mm in adults. This space is wider in children than in adults for the same reasons as described for pseudosubluxation. *Steele's rule of three* states that the area within the ring of C1 consists of one-third odontoid, one-third spinal cord, and one-third connective tissue (Fig. 115.27). Therefore, limited space is available for dens movement or predental space widening without neurologic compromise. Neurologic symptoms are often not seen until the predental space exceeds 7 to 10 mm. A dens fracture is the cause of AA subluxation more often than ligamentous disruption in a young child because the weakest part of the musculoskeletal system in a child is the osseous component (Fig. 115.26). Several case reports describe odontoid fractures in children facing forward in car seats as a result of rapid stops. These fractures may traverse the growth plate in young children, although the clinician must be careful not to overcall fractures because of the presence of a growth plate. Neurologic damage can occur from direct spinal cord injury or secondarily from vertebral artery damage.

Cervical distraction injuries may result from rapid acceleration- or deceleration-type incidents, such as high-speed motor vehicle or pedestrian accidents (Fig. 115.28). This type of injury, although uncommon, is reported to be approximately 2.5 times more common in children than in adults. An injury that was incompatible with long-term survival, but for which initial cardiopulmonary resuscitation was successful, is shown in Fig. 115.28A. Cervical distraction injuries may be obvious or subtle on the lateral radiograph. Measurements for potential distraction injuries include the atlantooccipital and C1–C2 interspinous distances. The atlantooccipital distance should not exceed 5 mm. The C1–C2 interspinous distance should not exceed 10 mm. Sun et al noted the relationship between the C1–C2 and C2–C3 interspinous distance with regard to tectorial membrane (the stabilizing upper section of the posterior longitudinal ligament in the upper cervical spine) integrity and injury. A C1–C2:C2–C3 ratio of more than 2.5 suggests injury to the tectorial membrane and potential ligamentous instability. Sun's ratio, as well as a ratio of measurements of the basion to the posterior arch of C1 (BC) and the opisthion to the anterior arch of C1 (OA), is demonstrated in Fig. 115.29. If the BC:OA ratio is more than 1, it signifies atlantooccipital dislocation. Atlantooccipital dislocation is often fatal, but there are reports of survivors. Neurologic deficits may develop from direct spinal damage or associated carotid or vertebral artery injury. Distraction injuries may also be seen with difficult newborn deliveries. These injuries may not be visible on a plain radiograph because the pediatric cervical spine can transiently distract 2 inches before residual radiographic evidence of spinal column separation is present. However, the spinal cord can distract only 0.25 inches before permanent neurologic

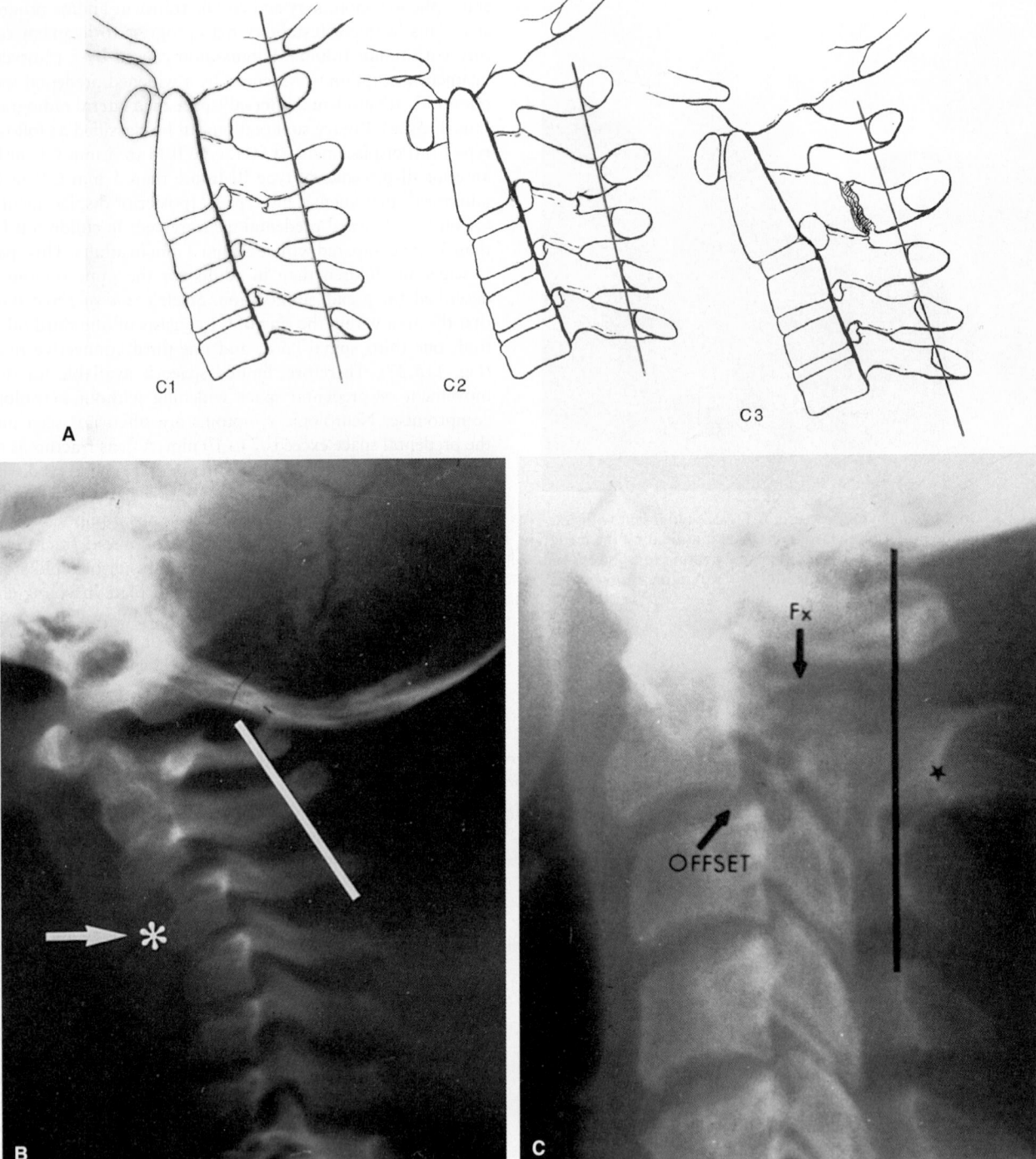

FIGURE 115.25 **A:** Posterior cervical line of Swischuk. Line is drawn from the cortex of the spinous process of C1 to the cortex of the spinous process of C3. Relationship of the line to cortex of the spinous process of C2 is noted. If the line is situated more than 2.0 mm anterior to the cortex of the spinous process of C2, underlying cervical pathology should be present. This line should be used only with anterior displacement of C2 on C3. **B:** Pseudosubluxation of C2 on C3 with normal posterior cervical line in a 2-year-old child. Note apparent widening of prevertebral soft tissue. **C:** Abnormal posterior cervical line with an underlying hangman's fracture. Actual offset is 4 mm. (**C:** From Swischuk L. *Emergency radiology of the acutely ill or injured child,* 2nd ed. Baltimore, MD: Williams & Wilkins, 1986:562–563. Reprinted with permission.)

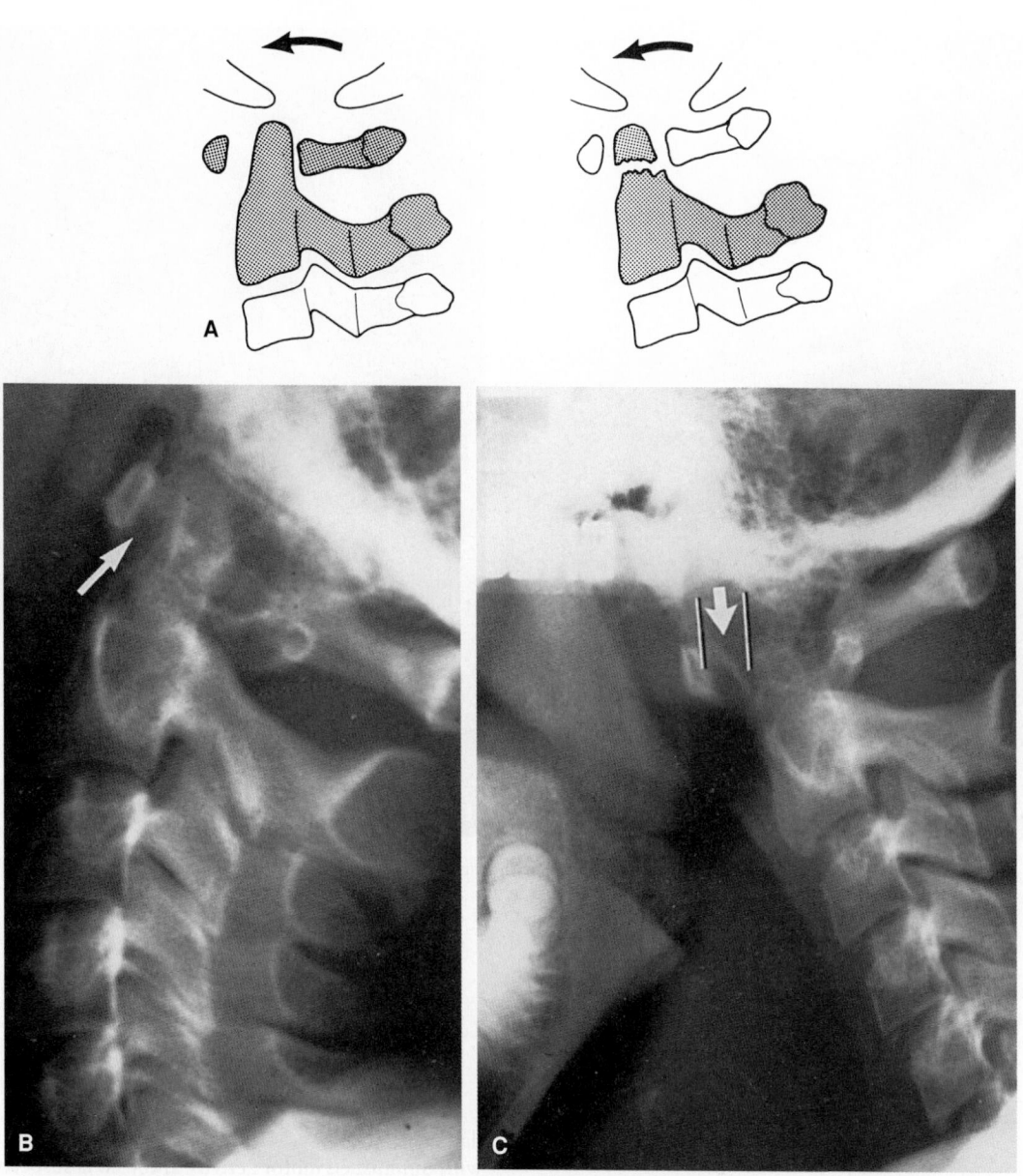

FIGURE 115.26 **A:** Diagrammatic representation of transverse ligament disruption (*left*) and dens fracture (*right*). **B:** Widened predental space on initial lateral radiograph in 15-year-old girl (actual measurement was 4 mm). **C:** Flexion radiograph in same patient demonstrating increased predental space with evidence of transverse ligament disruption. (*continued*)

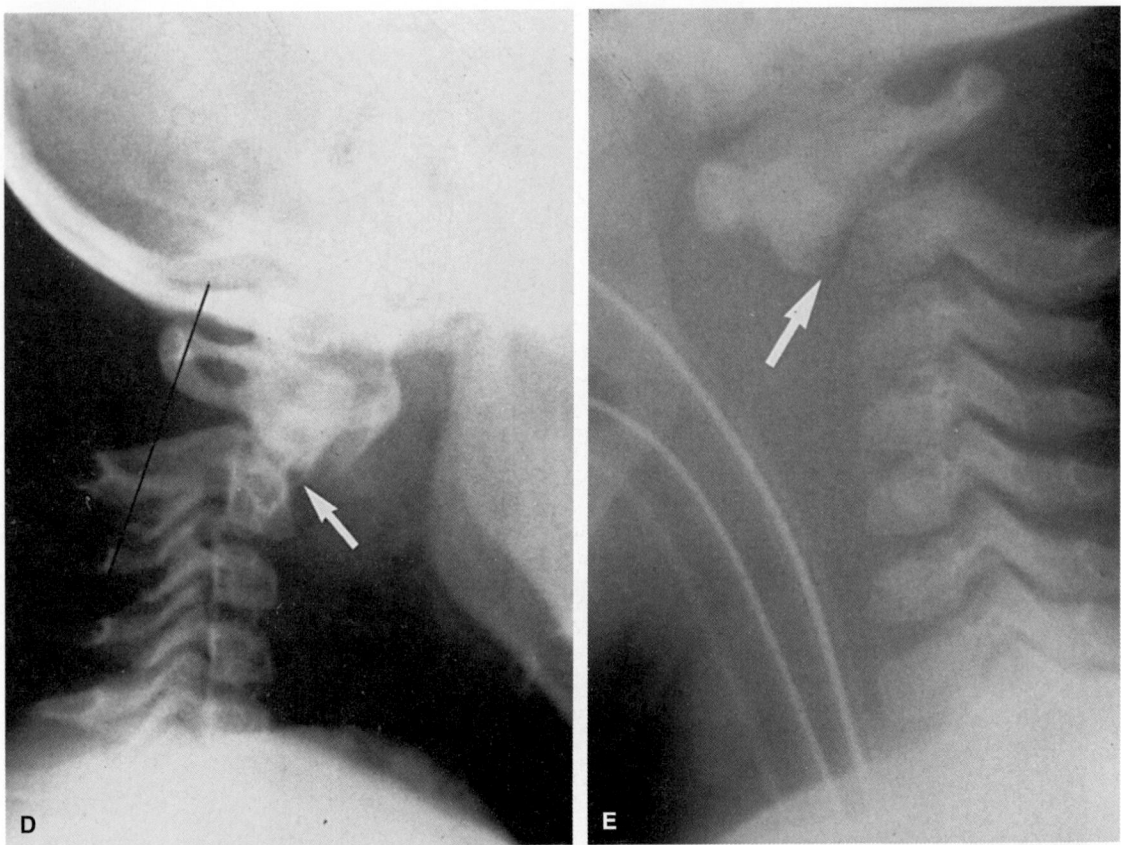

FIGURE 115.26 (*Continued*) **D:** Dens fracture with anterior subluxation of C1 and the dens on the remainder of the spinal column. *Arrow* indicates fracture. Abnormal posterior cervical *line* is also shown. **E:** Dens fracture (*arrow*) with anterior subluxation of the dens on the body of C2. (**A:** From Swischuk L. *Emergency radiology of the acutely ill or injured child,* 2nd ed. Baltimore, MD: Williams & Wilkins, 1986:572. Reprinted with permission.)

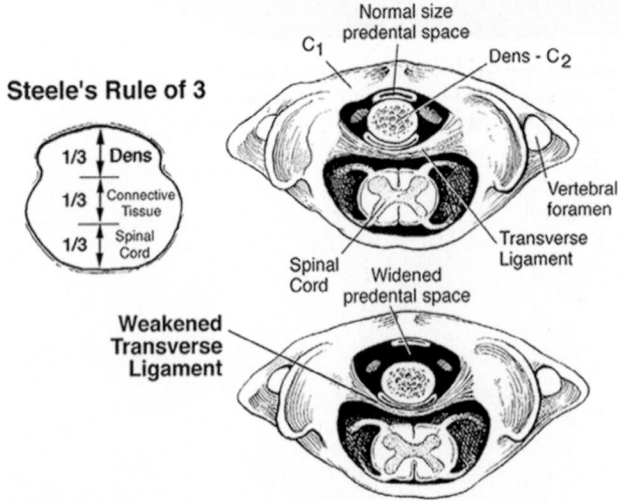

FIGURE 115.27 A cross section through the ring of C1 demonstrates Steele's rule of three. The space between the cervical cord and dens allows limited movement between C1 and C2 without immediate neurologic compromise.

damage occurs. An MRI scan is useful in evaluating an infant with diminished motor activity and who is suspected of having a distraction injury.

Vertebral compression injuries are suggested by isolated anterior wedging, teardrop fractures, or burst vertebral bodies (Fig. 115.30). The vertebral bodies should be regular, cuboid, and consistent between adjacent cervical levels (Fig. 115.30). A flexion/rotation stress can lead to anterior subluxation of one vertebral body on another with facet dislocation ("locked" or "jumped" facet) (Fig. 115.31). If the anterior displacement is less than 50% of the vertebral body width, it is consistent with a unilateral facet dislocation (Fig. 115.31). More than a 50% anterior subluxation suggests a bilateral facet dislocation (Fig. 115.31). These injuries are often accompanied by widened interspinous and interlaminar spaces, anterior soft-tissue swelling, and a narrowed disc space.

SCIWORA has been described in up to 67% of children with cervical cord injuries (Fig. 115.32). It has more recently been estimated to account for up to 25% of cervical cord injuries in children younger than 8 years. Interestingly, the 2002 NEXUS SCIWORA report, which included more than

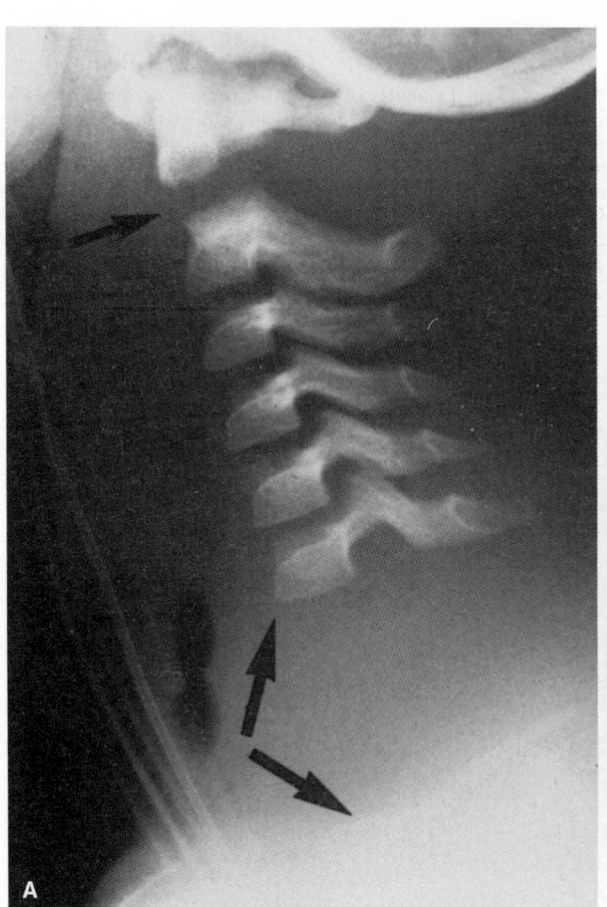

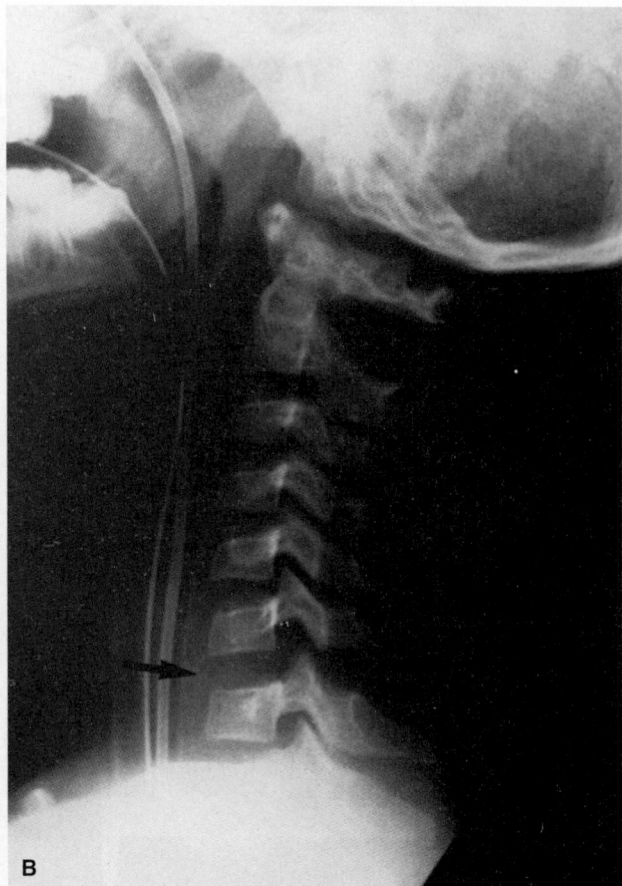

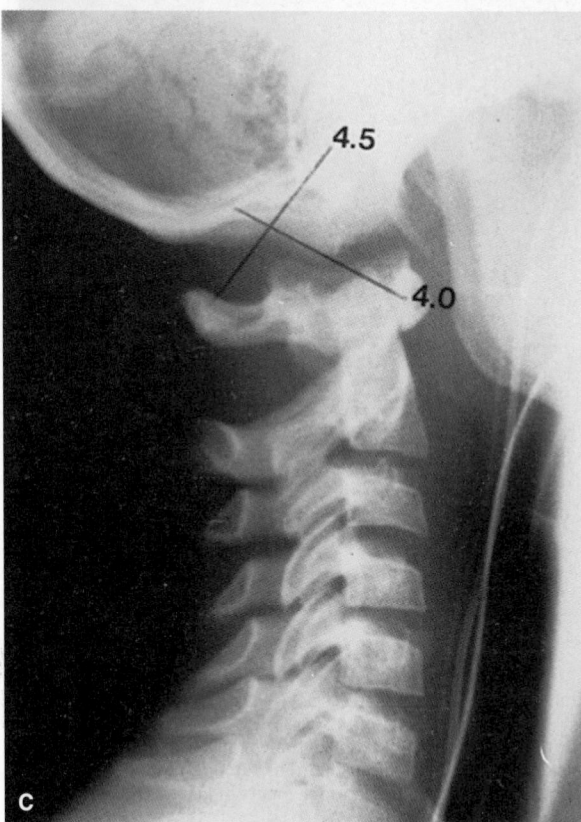

FIGURE 115.28 Distraction injuries. **A:** Dens fractures with distraction and accompanying C6–C7 distraction injury in a 3-year-old child. Injury was fatal. **B:** C6–C7 distraction injury in an 8-year-old child. **C:** BC:AO ratio is more than 1.0, suggesting atlantooccipital dislocation (see also Fig. 115.29).

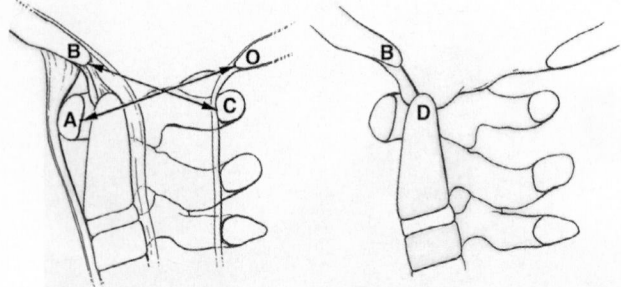

FIGURE 115.29 Examples of methods to assess occipital/C1 relationships. *A*, C1 anterior arch; *B*, basion (anterior margin of foramen magnum); *C*, anterior portion of the posterior ring of C1; *O*, opisthion (posterior margin of foramen magnum); and *D*, tip of the dens (odontoid process). These landmarks may not be easily visible on all radiographs. A BC:AO ratio of more than 0.9 to 1.0 suggests anterior dislocation or subluxation of the atlantooccipital joint. A BD distance of more than 10 to 12.5 mm should be suggestive of atlantooccipital dislocation. A C1–C2:C2–C3 ratio of more than 2.5 suggests injury to the tectorial membrane and ligamentous instability.

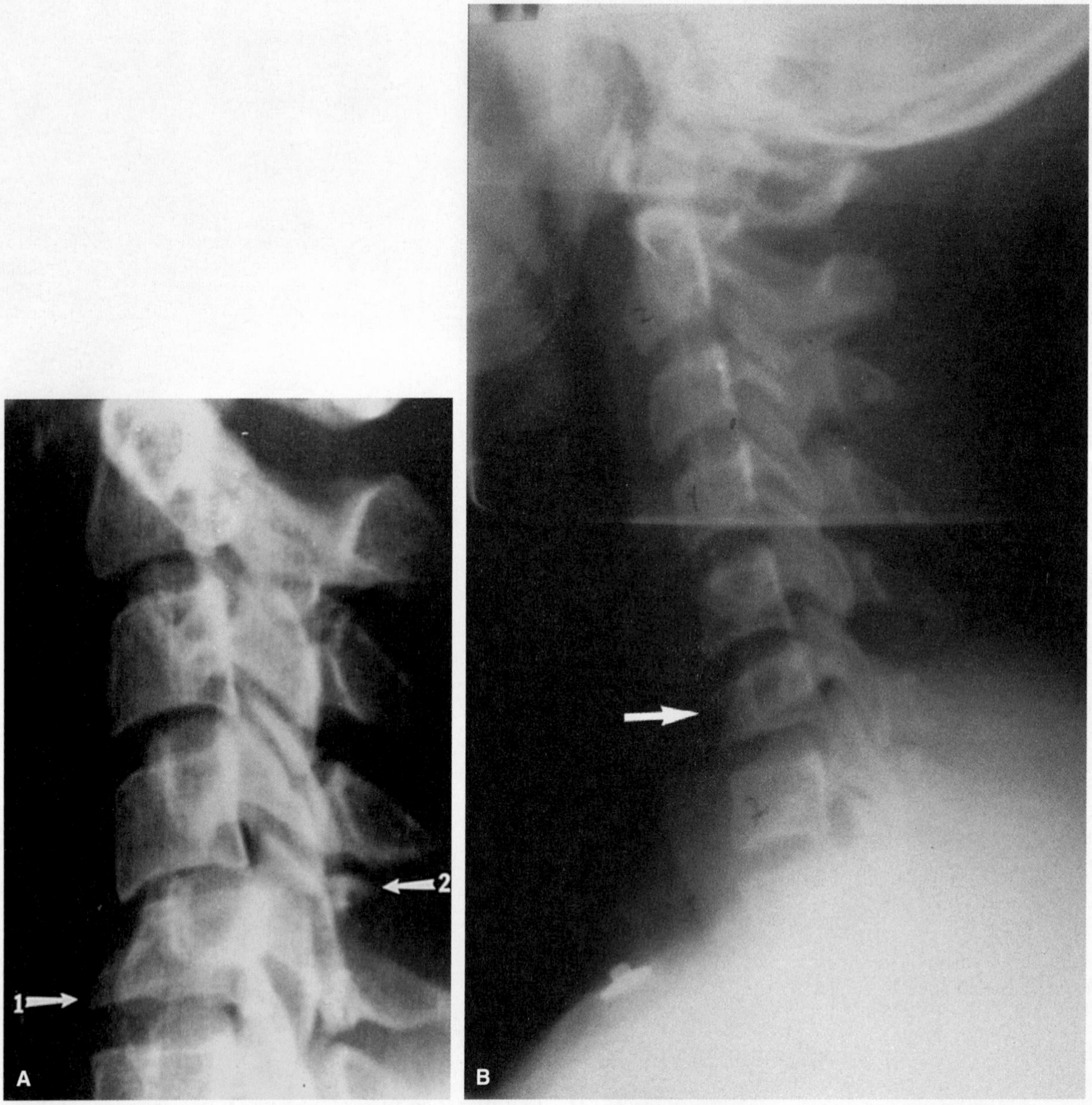

FIGURE 115.30 Examples of cervical compression injuries. **A:** Teardrop fracture. This patient sustained a whiplash injury with resultant flexion injury. A typical flexion teardrop fracture is demonstrated at (*1*). An increased interspinous distance and an associated avulsion fracture of the posterior elements of C5 are demonstrated at (*2*). **B:** Anterior C6 vertebral wedge fracture. (*continued*)

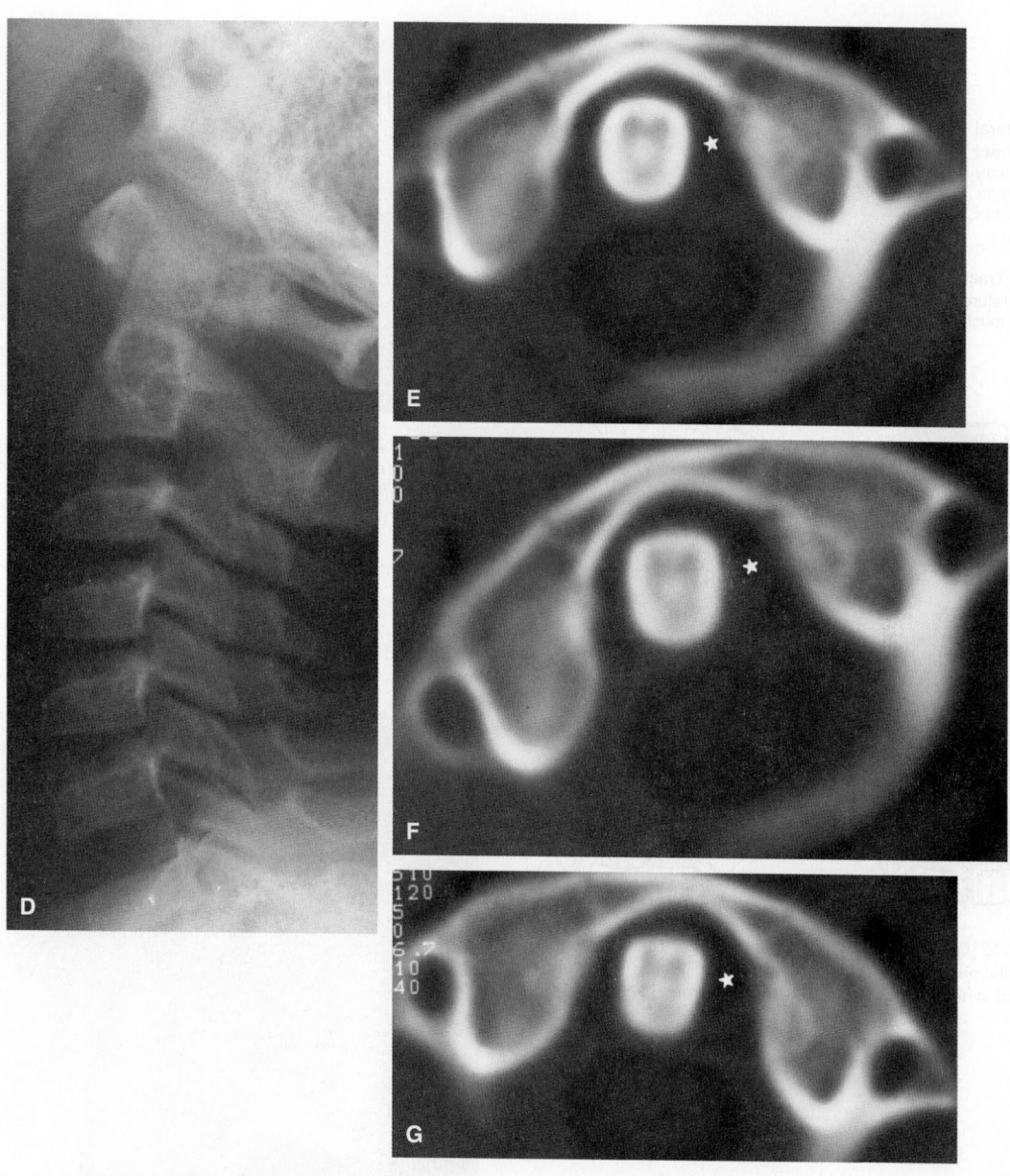

FIGURE 115.34 (*Continued*) **D–G:** CT evidence of fixed rotary subluxation in a 6-year-old child. **D:** Lateral radiograph demonstrating mild increased distance of predental space. **E:** Axial CT scan demonstrating increased distance between dens and patient's left side of C1 (asymmetry between right and left sides). **F:** Axial CT scan with patient's head turned to the right, demonstrating asymmetry between the dens and ring of C1. **G:** Axial CT scan with patient's head turned to the left, demonstrating fixed asymmetry between the dens and the ring of C1.

TABLE 115.9

METHYLPREDNISOLONE ADMINISTRATION SCHEDULE FOR BLUNT CERVICAL SPINAL CORD TRAUMA[a]

Time after injury	0–3 h	3–8 h	8 h
Initial IV dosage	30 mg/kg (over 15 min)	30 mg/kg (over 15 min)	Efficacy not demonstrated
Maintenance IV dosage	5.4 mg/kg/h	5.4 mg/kg/h	
Suggested duration	24 h	48 h	

[a]Consideration and/or potential use of methylprednisolone should be established with input from local experts. See text for discussion of methylprednisolone use in pediatrics and cervical spine trauma.

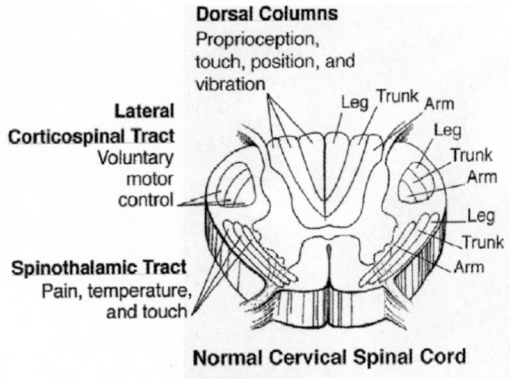

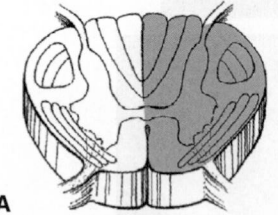
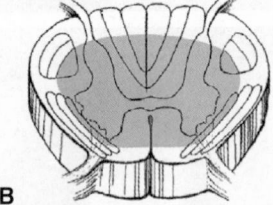

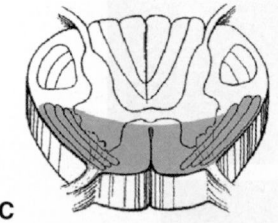
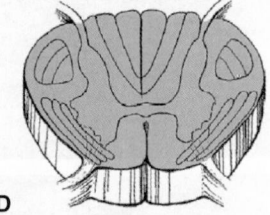

FIGURE 115.35 Graphic illustrations of a normal cervical spinal cord and specific postinjury syndromes. **A:** Brown-Sequard syndrome. **B:** Central cord syndrome. **C:** Anterior artery syndrome. **D:** Complete transection.

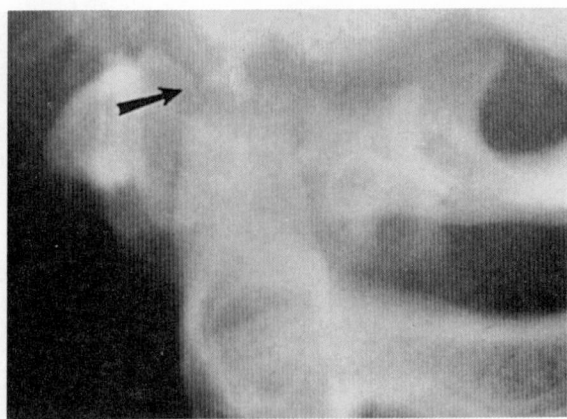

FIGURE 115.37 Normal ossiculum terminale at the tip of the dens (*arrow*). (From Swischuk L. *Emergency radiology of the acutely ill or injured child*, 2nd ed. Baltimore, MD: Williams & Wilkins, 1986:717. Reprinted with permission.)

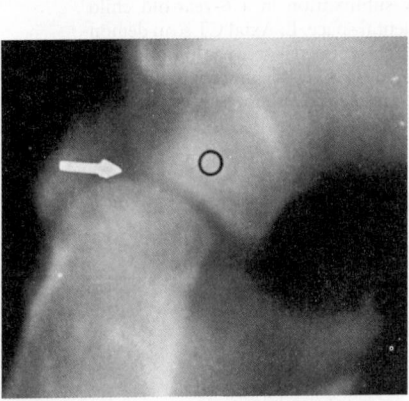

FIGURE 115.36 Example of os odontoideum. Note the hypoplastic dens and overgrown ossiculum terminale or ossiculum odontoideum (O). The *arrow* indicates posterior displacement, attesting to instability of the lesions. (From Swischuk L. *Emergency radiology of the acutely ill or injured child*, 2nd ed. Baltimore, MD: Williams & Wilkins, 1986:717. Reprinted with permission.)

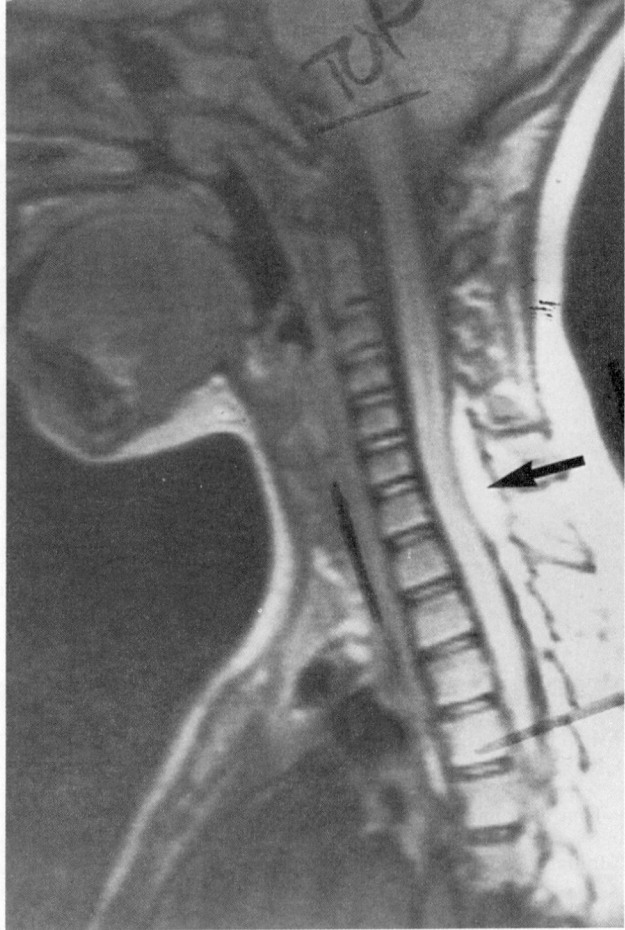

FIGURE 115.38 Magnetic resonance imaging (MRI) of cervical spine demonstrating epidural hematoma (*arrow*) from C5 to T1. Note excellent soft-tissue, intervertebral disc, and fluid detail afforded by the MRI scan.

after spinal injury in the United Kingdom and noted that steroids are not recommended by the Canadian and British spinal cord associations for acute blunt spinal cord injury. Steroid use for the pediatric patient with a clear or potential blunt cervical cord injury is not routinely indicated and should be a joint decision between the treating emergency, trauma, and neurosurgical physicians. Methylprednisolone is not recommended in conjunction with penetrating neck injuries.

Suggested Readings

Blunt and Penetrating Neck Trauma

Abujamra L, Joseph MM. Penetrating neck injuries in children: a retrospective review. *Pediatr Emerg Care* 2003;19:308–313.

Adams V, Hirsch C. Venous air embolism from head and neck wounds. *Arch Pathol Lab Med* 1989;113:498–502.

Asensio JA, Chahwan S, Forno W, et al. Penetrating esophageal injuries: multicenter study of the American Association for the Surgery of Trauma. *J Trauma-Injury Infect Crit Care* 2001;50:289–296.

Back MR, Baumgartner FJ, Klein SR. Detection and evaluation of aerodigestive tract injuries caused by cervical and transmediastinal gunshot wounds. *J Trauma* 1997;42:680–686.

Bell RB, Osborn T, Dierks EJ, et al. Management of penetrating neck injuries: a new paradigm for civilian trauma. *J Oral Maxillofac Surg* 2007;65:691–705.

Biffl WL, Moore EE, Elliott JP, et al. The devastating potential of blunt vertebral artery injuries. *Ann Surg* 2000;231:672–681.

Buchalter GM, Johnson LP, Reichman MV, et al. Penetrating trauma to the head and neck from a nail gun: a unique mechanism of injury. *Ear Nose Throat J* 2002;81:779–783.

Calkins CM, Bensard DD, Partrick DA, et al. Life-threatening dog attacks: a combination of penetrating and blunt injuries. *J Pediatr Surg* 2001;36:115–117.

Demetriades D, Charalambides K, Chahwan S, et al. Nonskeletal cervical spine injuries: epidemiology and diagnostic pitfalls. *J Trauma-Injury Infect Crit Care* 2000;48:724–727.

Demetriades D, Salim A, Brown C, et al. Neck injuries. *Curr Probl Surg* 2007; 44:13–85.

Desjardins G, Varon AJ. Airway management for penetrating neck injuries: the Miami experience. *Resuscitation* 2001;48:71–75.

Eddy VA. Is routine arteriography mandatory for penetrating injury to zone 1 of the neck? Zone 1 Penetrating Neck Injury Subgroup. *J Trauma-Injury Infect Crit Care* 2000;48:208–213.

Feldman KW, Avellino AM, Sugar NF, et al. Cervical spinal cord injury in abused children. *Pediatr Emerg Care* 2008;24:222–227.

Gee AC, Salter KD, McConnell DB, et al. Injuries to the neck. In: Flint L, Meredith J, Schwab CW, et al, eds. *Trauma contemporary principles and therapy*. Philadelphia, PA: Lippincott Williams & Wilkins, 2008:335–349.

Gold SM, Gerber ME, Shott SR, et al. Blunt laryngotracheal trauma in children. *Arch Otolaryngol Head Neck Surg* 1997;123:83–87.

Gonzalez RP, Falimirski M, Holevar MR, et al. Penetrating zone II injury: does dynamic computed tomography scan contribute to the diagnostic sensitivity of physical examination for surgically significant injury? A prospective blinded study. *J Trauma-Injury Infect Crit Care* 2003;54:61–64.

Goudy SL, Miller FB, Bumpous JM. Neck crepitance: evaluation and management of suspected upper aerodigestive tract injury. *Laryngoscope* 2002;112:791–795.

Gracias VH, Reilly PM, Philpott J, et al. Computed tomography in the evaluation of penetrating neck trauma: a preliminary study. *Arch Surg* 2001;136:1231–1235.

Graham J, Dick R, Parnell D, et al. Clothesline injury mechanism associated with all-terrain vehicle use by children. *Pediatr Emerg Care* 2006;22:45–47.

Guyot LL, Kazmierczak CD, Diaz FG. Vascular injury in neurotrauma. *Neurol Res* 2001;23:291–296.

Hanson CA, Smith JA. Penetrating neck injuries in children. *J Trauma Nurs* 2007;14:12–16; quiz 17–18.

Harrahill M. Penetrating neck trauma: a case study. *J Emerg Nurs* 2007;33:511–513.

Hersman G, Barker P, Bowley DM, et al. The management of penetrating neck injuries. *Int Surg* 2001;86:82–89.

Inaba K, Munera F, McKenney M, et al. Prospective evaluation of screening multislice helical computed tomographic angiography in the initial evaluation of penetrating neck injuries. *J Trauma* 2006;61:144–149.

Insull P, Adams D, Segar A, et al. Is exploration mandatory in penetrating zone II neck injuries? *ANZ J Surg* 2007;77:261–264.

Jurkovich GJ, Zingarelli W, Wallace J, et al. Penetrating neck trauma: diagnostic studies in the asymptomatic patient. *J Trauma* 1985;25:819–822.

Kadish H, Schunk J, Woodward GA. Blunt pediatric laryngotracheal trauma: case reports and review of the literature. *Am J Emerg Med* 1994;12:207–211.

Kim MK, Buckman R, Szeremeta W. Penetrating neck trauma in children: an urban hospital's experience. *Otolaryngol Head Neck Surg* 2000;123:439–443.

Klinkner DB, Arca MJ, Lewis BD, et al. Pediatric vascular injuries: patterns of injury, morbidity, and mortality. *J Pediatr Surg* 2007;42:178–182; discussion 182–183.

Kumar SR, Weaver FA, Yellin AE. Cervical vascular injuries: carotid and jugular venous injuries. *Surg Clin North Am* 2001;81:1331–1344.

Larsen DW. Traumatic vascular injuries and their management. *Neuroimaging Clin North Am* 2002;12:249–269.

Lee C, Woodring J, Walsh J. Carotid and vertebral artery injury in survivors of atlanto-occipital dislocation: case reports and literature review. *J Trauma* 1991;31:401–407.

Losek JD, Tecklenburg FW, White DR. Blunt laryngeal trauma in children: case report and review of initial airway management. *Pediatr Emerg Care* 2008;24:370–373.

Lupetin AR. Computed tomographic evaluation of laryngotracheal trauma. *Curr Prob Diagn Radiol* 1997;26:185–206.

Marathe US, Tran LP. Pediatric neck trauma causing massive subcutaneous emphysema. *J Trauma* 2006;61:440–443.

Markus-Rodden MM, Bojko T, Hauck LC. Traumatic tracheal laceration in a pediatric patient medically managed with high-frequency oscillatory ventilation. *Pediatr Emerg Care* 2008;24:236–237.

Marom T, Russo E, Ben-Yehuda Y, et al. Oropharyngeal injuries in children. *Pediatr Emerg Care* 2007;23:914–918.

Mazolewski PJ, Curry JD, Browder T, et al. Computer tomographic scan can be used for surgical decision making in zone II penetrating neck injuries. *J Trauma-Injury Infect Crit Care* 2001;51:315–319.

McKevitt EC, Kirkpatrick AW, Vertesi L, et al. Blunt vascular neck injuries: diagnosis and outcomes of extracranial vessel injury. *J Trauma-Injury Infect Crit Care* 2002;53:472–476.

Mezhir JJ, Glynn L, Liu DC, et al. Handlebar injuries in children: should we raise the bar of suspicion? *Am Surg* 2007;73:807–810.

Miler PR, Fabian TC, Bee TK. Blunt cerebrovascular injuries: diagnosis and treatment. *J Trauma-Injury Infect Crit Care* 2001;51:279–285.

Nason RW, Assuras GN, Gray PR, et al. Penetrating neck injuries: analysis of experience from a Canadian trauma centre. *Can J Surg* 2001;44:122–126.

Navsaria P, Thoma M, Nicol A. Foley catheter balloon tamponade for life-threatening hemorrhage in penetrating neck trauma. *World J Surg* 2006;30:1265–1268.

Phillips BJ. The penetrating neck wound: a few points. *Internet J Surg* [serial online]. 2002;3:74–77.

Rathlev NK, Medzon R, Bracken ME. Evaluation and management of neck trauma. *Emerg Med Clin North Am* 2007;25:679–694, viii.

Szeremeta W, Morovati S. Isolated hyoid bone fracture: a case report and review of the literature. *J Trauma* 1991;31:268–271.

Tallon JM, Ahmed JM, Sealy B. Airway management in penetrating neck trauma at a Canadian tertiary trauma centre. *J Can Assoc Emerg Phys*. 2007;9:101–104.

Tariq M, Kalan A, Surenthiran SS, et al. Penetrating neck injury: case report and evaluation of management. *J Laryngol Otol* 2000;114:554–556.

Verschueren DS, Bell RB, Bagheri SC, et al. Management of laryngo-tracheal injuries associated with craniomaxillofacial trauma. *J Oral Maxillofac Surg* 2006;64:203–214.

Vohra S, Johnston BC, Cramer K, Humphreys K. Adverse events associated with pediatric spinal manipulation: a systematic review. *Pediatrics* 2007;119:e275–e283. (Erratum for Vohra et al., *Pediatrics* 119(1):e275–e283. Published online July 2, 2007, accessed 11/25/2009).

Wang BS, Smith SL, Pereira KD. Pediatric head and neck trauma from all-terrain vehicle accidents. *Otolaryngol Head Neck Surg* 2007;137:201–205.

Williams EW, Cawich SO, James M, et al. Penetrating neck trauma and the aberrant subclavian artery. *West Indian Med J* 2007;56:288–293.

Zhang S, Michael M, Clowers K, Krusenklaus J. Evaluation of efficacy and 3D kinematic characteristics of cervical orthoses. *Clinical Biomechanics* 20(3):264–269.

Zonfrillo MR, Roy AD, Walsh SA. Management of pediatric penetrating oropharyngeal trauma. *Pediatr Emerg Care* 2008;24:172–175.

Cervical Spine

Adelgais KM, Grossman DC, Langer SG, et al. Use of helical computed tomography for imaging the pediatric cervical spine. *Acad Emerg Med* 2004; 11:228–236.

Anglen J, Metzler M, Bunn P, et al. Flexion and extension views are not cost-effective in a cervical spine clearance protocol for obtunded trauma patients. *J Trauma-Injury Infect Crit Care* 2002;52:54–59.

Armstrong BP, Simpson HK, Crouch R, et al. Prehospital clearance of the cervical spine: does it need to be a pain in the neck? *Emerg Med J* 2007;24:501–503.

Aslamy W, Danielson K, Hessel S, et al. A 3-year-old boy with neck pain after motor-vehicle accident. *West J Med* 1991;155:301–302.

Avellino AM, Mann FA, Grady MS, et al. The misdiagnosis of acute cervical spine injuries and fractures in infants and children: the 12-year experience of a level I pediatric and adult trauma center. *Childs Nerv Syst* 2005;21:122–127.

Baker C, Kadish H, Schunk JE. Evaluation of pediatric cervical spine injuries. *Ann Emerg Med* 2000;35:230–234.

Barba CA, Taggert J, Morgan AS. A new cervical spine clearance protocol using computed tomography. *J Trauma-Injury Infect Crit Care* 2001;51:652–656.

Barrett T, Mower W, Zucker M, Hoffman J. Injuries Missed by Limited Computed Tomographic Imaging of Patients With Cervical Spine Injuries. *Ann Emerg Med* 2006;47(2):129–133.

Bell KM, Frazier EC, Shively CM, et al. Assessing range of motion to evaluate the adverse effects of ill-fitting cervical orthoses. *Spine J* 2009;9(3):225–231.

Bivins H, Ford S, Bezmalinovic Z, et al. The effects of axial traction during oro-tracheal intubation of the trauma victim with an unstable cervical spine. *Ann Emerg Med* 1988;17:53–57.

Blackmore CC, Ramsey SD, Mann FA, et al. Cervical spine screening with CT in trauma patients: a cost-effectiveness analysis. *Radiology* 1999;212:117–125.

Bracken M, Shepard MJ, Collins W, et al. A randomized, controlled trial of methylprednisolone or naloxone in the treatment of acute spinal-cord injury: results of the second national acute spinal-cord injury study. *N Engl J Med* 1990;322:1405–1411.

Bracken M, Shepard MJ, Holford TR, et al. Administration of methylpred-nisolone for 24 or 48 hours or tirilazad mesylate for 48 hours in the treat-ment of acute spinal cord injury: results of the third national acute spinal cord injury randomized controlled trial. *JAMA* 1997;277:1597–1604.

Bracken MB. Steroids for acute spinal cord injury. *Cochrane Database Syst Rev* 2002;(3):CD001046.

Brohi K, Healy M, Fotheringham T, et al. Helical computed tomographic scan-ning for the evaluation of the cervical spine in the unconscious, intubated trauma patient. *J Trauma* 2005;58:897–901.

Brooks RA, Willett KM. Evaluation of the Oxford protocol for total spine clear-ance in the unconscious trauma patient. *J Trauma-Injury Infect Crit Care* 2001;50:862–867.

Buhs C, Cullen M, Klein M, et al. The pediatric trauma C-spine: is the "odon-toid" view necessary? *J Pediatr Surg* 2000;35:994–997.

Bulas D, Fitz C, Johnson D. Traumatic atlanto-occipital dislocation in children. *Radiology* 1993;188:155–158.

Canadian CT Head and C-Spine (CCC) Study Group. Canadian C-spine rule study for alert and stable trauma patients, part I: background and rationale. *J Can Assoc Emerg Phys* 2002;4:84–90.

Chiu WC, Haan JM, Cushing BM, et al. Ligamentous injuries of the cervical spine in unreliable blunt trauma patients: incidence, evaluation and out-come. *J Trauma-Injury Infect Crit Care* 2001;50:457–463.

Cirak B, Ziegfeld S, Knight VM, et al. Spinal injuries in children. *J Pediatr Surg* 2004;39:607–612.

Citerio G, Cormio M, Sganzerla EP. Steroids in acute spinal cord injury. An unproven standard of care. *Minerva Anestesiol* 2002;68(5):315–320.

Como J, Thompson M, Anderson J, et al. Is magnetic resonance imaging essential in cleaning the cervical spine in obtunded patients with blunt trauma? *J Trauma Injury Infect Critic Care* 2007;63(3):544–549.

Cothren CC, Moore EE, Ray CE Jr, et al. Cervical spine fracture patterns mandating screening to rule out blunt cerebrovascular injury. *Surgery* 2007;141:76–82.

Criswell JC, Parr MJ, Nolan JP. Emergency airway management in patients with cervical spine injuries. *Anaesthesia* 1994;49(10):900–903.

Curran C, Dietrich AM, Bowman MJ, et al. Pediatric cervical-spine immobiliza-tion: achieving neutral position? *J Trauma* 1995;39(4):729–732.

Daffner RH, Sciulli RL, Rodriguez A, et al. Imaging for evaluation of suspected cervical spine trauma: a 2-year analysis. *Injury* 2006;37:652–658.

d'Amato C. Pediatric spinal trauma: injuries in very young children. *Clin Orthop Relat Res* 2005;(432):34–40.

Dare AO, Dias MS, Li V. Magnetic resonance imaging correlation in pediatric spinal cord injury without radiographic abnormality. *J Neurosurg* 2002;97(1)(suppl):33–39.

Davis JW, Kaups KL, Cunningham MA. Routine evaluation of the cervical spine in head-injured patients with dynamic fluoroscopy: a reappraisal. *J Trauma-Injury Infect Crit Care* 2001;50:1044–1047.

Del Rossi G, Heffernan TP, Horodyski M, et al. The effectiveness of extrica-tion collars tested during the execution of spine-board transfer techniques. *Spine J* 2004;4:619–623.

Domeier RM, Frederiksen SM, Welch K. Prospective performance assessment of an out-of-hospital protocol for selective spine immobilization using clinical spine clearance criteria. *Ann Emerg Med* 2005;46:123–131.

Dormans JP. Evaluation of children with suspected cervical spine injury. *J Bone Joint Surg Am* 2002;84-A:124–132.

Evans D, Bethem D. Cervical spine injuries in children. *J Pediatr Orthop* 1989;9:563–568.

Fesmire F, Luten R. The pediatric cervical spine: developmental anatomy and clinical aspects. *J Emerg Med* 1989;7:133–142.

Frampton A, Eynon C. High dose methylprednisolone in the immediate man-agement of acute, blunt spinal cord injury: what is the current practice in emergency departments, spinal units, and neurosurgical units in the UK? *Emerg Med J* 2006;23:550–553.

Frank JB, Lim CK, Flynn JM, et al. The efficacy of magnetic resonance imaging in pediatric cervical spine clearance. *Spine* 2002;27(11):1176–1179.

Fuchs S, Barthel M, Flannery A, et al. Cervical spine fractures sustained by young children in forward-facing car seats. *Pediatrics* 1989;84:348–354.

Garton HJ, Hammer MR. Detection of pediatric cervical spine injury. *Neurosurgery* 2008;62(3):700–707; comments 707–708.

Goutcher CM, Lochhead V. Reduction in mouth opening with semi-rigid cervi-cal collars. *Br J Anaesth* 2005;95:344–348.

Griffen MM, Frykberg ER, Kerwin AJ, et al. Radiographic clearance of blunt cervical spine injury: plain radiograph or computed tomographic scan. *J Trauma-Injury Infect Crit Care* 2003;55:222–226.

Groopman J. The Reeve effect. *The New Yorker* November 10, 2003:83–93.

Hadley MN. Cervical spine immobilization before admission to the hospital. *Neurosurg Online* 2002;50:S7–S17.

Hadley MN. Radiographic assessment of the cervical spine in asymptomatic trauma patients. *Neurosurg Online* 2002;50:S30–S35.

Hadley MN. Management of pediatric cervical spine and spinal cord injuries. *Neurosurg Online* 2002;50:S85–S99.

Hendey GW, Wolfson AB, Mower WR, et al. Spinal cord injury without radi-ographic abnormality: results of the National Emergency X-Radiography Utilization Study in blunt cervical trauma. *J Trauma* 2002;53:1–4.

Herzenberg J, Hensinger R, Dedrick D, et al. Emergency transport and position-ing of young children who have an injury of the cervical spine: the standard backboard may be hazardous. *J Bone Joint Surg* 1989;71-A:15–22.

Hoffman JR, Mower WR, Wolfson AB, et al. Validity of a set of criteria to rule out injury to the cervical spine in patients with blunt trauma. National Emergency X-Radiography Study Group. *N Engl J Med* 2000;343:94–99.

Huerta C, Griffith R, Joyce S. Cervical spine stabilization in pediatric patients: evaluation of current techniques. *Ann Emerg Med* 1987;16:55–60.

Hugenholtz H, Cass DE, Dvorak MF, et al. High-dose methylprednisolone for acute closed spinal cord injury—only a treatment option. *Can J Neurol Sci* 2002;29:227–235.

Hurlbert RJ. The role of steroids in acute spinal cord injury: an evidence-based analysis [comment]. *Spine* 2001;26(24)(suppl):S39–S46, S55.

Insko EK, Gracias VH, Gupta R, et al. Utility of flexion and extension radiographs of the cervical spine in the acute evaluation of blunt trauma. *J Trauma-Injury Infect Crit Care* 2002;53:426–429.

Jaffe D, Binns H, Radkowski M, et al. Developing a clinical algorithm for early management of cervical spine injury in child trauma victims. *Ann Emerg Med* 1987;16:57–63.

Jagannathan J, Dumont AS, Prevedello DM, et al. Cervical spine injuries in pediatric athletes: mechanisms and management. *Neurosurg Focus* 2006;21:E6.

Kaji A, Hockberger R. Imaging of spinal cord injuries. *Emerg Med Clin North Am* 2007;25:735–750, ix.

Kerr D, Bradshaw L, Kelly AM. Implementation of the Canadian C-spine rule reduces cervical spine x-ray rate for alert patients with potential neck injury. *J Emerg Med* 2005;28:127–131.

Kerwin AJ, Frykberg ER, Schinco MA, et al. The effect of early surgical treat-ment of traumatic spine injuries on patient mortality. *J Trauma* 2007;63:1308–1313.

Knopp R, Parker J, Tashjian J, et al. Defining radiographic criteria for flexion-extension studies of the cervical spine. *Ann Emerg Med* 2001;38:31–35.

Kokoska ER, Keller MS, Rallo MC, et al. Characteristics of pediatric cervical spine injuries. *J Pediatr Surg* 2001;36(1):100–105.

Kriss VM, Kriss TC. Imaging of the cervical spine in infants. *Pediatr Emerg Care* 1996;13(1):44–49.

Kriss VM, Kriss TC. SCIWORA (spinal cord injury without radiographic abnor-mality) in infants and children. *Clin Pediatr* 1996;35(3):119–124.

Kwan I, Bunn F, Roberts I. Spinal immobilisation for trauma patients. *Cochrane Database Syst Rev* 2001;(2):CD002803.

Lanoix R, Gupta R, Leak L, et al. C-spine injury associated with gunshot wounds to the head: retrospective study and literature review. *J Trauma-Injury Infect Crit Care* 2000;49:860–863.

Lasker M, Torres-Torres M, Green R. Neonatal diagnosis of spinal cord tran-section. *Clin Pediatr* 1991;30:322–324.

Luscombe MD, Williams JL. Comparison of a long spinal board and vacuum mattress for spinal immobilisation. *Emerg Med J* 2003;20:476–478.

Lustrin SE, Karakas SP, Ortiz AO, et al. Pediatric cervical spine: normal anatomy, variants and trauma. *Radiographics* 2003;23:539–560.

Manoach S, Paladino L. Manual in-line stabilization for acute airway manage-ment of suspected cervical spine injury: historical review and current ques-tions. *Ann Emerg Med* 2007;50:236–245.

Martin B. Paediatric cervical spine injuries. *Injury* 2005;36:14–20.

Marx JA. Lateral plain films vs. helical CT for C-spine fracture: No contest. *J Watch Emerg Med* 2005;9:70–71. [Comment on: Brohi K, et al. Helical computed tomographic scanning for the evaluation of the cervical spine in the unconscious, intubated trauma patient. *J Trauma* 2005;58:897–901.]

Menaker J, Philp A, Boswell S, et al. Computed tomography alone for cervical spine clearance in the unreliable patient—are we there yet? *J Trauma* 2008;64:898–903; discussion 903–904.

Merola A, O'Brien MF, Castro BA, et al. Histologic characterization of acute spinal cord injury treated with intravenous methylprednisolone. *J Orthopaed Trauma* 2002;16(3):155–161.

Molloy S, Middleton F, Casey AT. Failure to administer methylprednisolone for acute traumatic spinal cord injury—a prospective audit of 100 patients from a regional spinal injuries unit. *Injury* 2002;33:575–578.

bone, usually as a result of frontal lobe mass lesions or swelling of the frontal lobes. The herniation may lead to distortion or compression of one or both intracranial carotid arteries, with resultant ischemia and infarction in the territories of the anterior and middle cerebral arteries.

Metabolic Derangements

Other physiologic mechanisms of secondary brain injury are also important. Hypoxia, resulting from thoracic injuries, airway obstruction, or inadequate respiratory effort, can be an important cause of brain injury. Hyperthermia increases cerebral metabolism and magnifies the severity of ischemia to an already compromised brain. Hyperglycemia also appears to contribute to cerebral injury in the compromised brain.

Excess concentrations of the neurotransmitter glutamate, released from injured neurons into the synaptic cleft, appear to contribute to brain injury through excess excitation of otherwise healthy postsynaptic neurons. Other neurotoxins such as aspartate, bradykinin, free fatty acids, and glycine may also play a role. Injured brain cells may also release various peptides that promote programmed cell death, or apoptosis, of neighboring cells. Oxidizing agents and oxygen-free radicals, released from injured neurons or elaborated as part of the brain's inflammatory response to injury, also appear to play a role in causing secondary brain injury.

Management and General Principles

Initial Resuscitation

Management of patients with head injury focuses on the prevention of secondary brain injury. Management begins with the ABCs (airway, breathing, and circulation) of resuscitation. A patient with a head injury who has altered sensorium may require assistance with the positioning of the airway or suctioning of oral and pharyngeal secretions. Cervical spine precautions must be taken during airway management. Immobilization of the cervical spine with a semirigid cervical collar or with inline manual stabilization must be maintained until the clinician is certain that no cervical spine injury has occurred.

Breathing may be impaired if neural control of respiratory function is compromised or if traumatic injuries involve the thorax. All patients with serious trauma require 100% inspired oxygen until it is certain that supplemental oxygen is not needed. Positive-pressure ventilation with a bag-valve-mask apparatus should be provided for any patient with inadequate respiratory effort. Unless there is increased ICP, the clinician should aim to achieve normocarbia (PCO$_2$ 35 to 40 mm Hg) and oxygen saturations of 100%. In cases with increased ICP, therapeutic hyperventilation may be indicated (see the following text).

Endotracheal intubation should be performed in patients making inadequate or labored respiratory effort or for patients who have a blunted gag reflex, cannot manage their oral secretions, or are comatose. Orotracheal intubation is generally safer than nasotracheal intubation, particularly if there is any concern about injuries to the midface. Care must be taken to minimize manipulation of the cervical spine.

Premedication for rapid sequence intubation begins with atropine 0.02 mg per kg (maximum dose 0.5 mg) for children younger than 8 years to lessen the vagal response to intuba-

tion. Lidocaine may also be useful at a dosage of 1 to 2 mg per kg as premedication to blunt the airway reflexes, which may increase ICP.

If possible, a sedative drug should be used, both to make the patient comfortable and to decrease the patient's responsiveness to airway manipulation. Thiopental (4 to 7 mg per kg) and etomidate (0.3 mg per kg) are both excellent choices because they decrease cerebral metabolism, thereby reducing the risk of cerebral ischemia. Thiopental must be used cautiously, however, in patients with hemodynamic instability because it may reduce vasomotor tone and cardiac contractility, thereby leading to a decrease in blood pressure. Etomidate, in contrast, tends to have little effect on systemic arterial pressure. Fentanyl (2 to 3 mcg per kg) and midazolam (0.1 mg per kg), which provide sedation and analgesia with minimal effect on cardiac contractility or vasomotor tone, could also be used. In cases in which intubation must proceed but intravenous (IV) access cannot be achieved, midazolam may be given intramuscularly (0.1 mg per kg), with onset of action in about 3 minutes. Traditional teaching has suggested that ketamine should be avoided in patients with head injuries because it can increase ICP and may in fact be beneficial. However, several recent studies have suggested that ketamine can effectively be used for the sedation of patients with head injury without leading to increased ICP and may in fact be beneficial.

For neuromuscular blockade, rocuronium (0.6 to 1.2 mg per kg IV) is commonly used because it has the fastest onset of action among the nondepolarizing agents, providing intubating conditions within 60 to 90 seconds if the high end of the dosing range is used. Succinylcholine (1 to 2 mg per kg IV) is an alternative. Succinylcholine offers the advantage of rapid action, with intubating conditions developing within 45 to 60 seconds. Because of its very short duration of action (usually about 5 minutes), succinylcholine offers the advantage of allowing ongoing clinical assessment of the neurologic status soon after intubation is complete. However, succinylcholine may cause important adverse effects, including hyperkalemia (especially in patients with prior denervating injury or neuromuscular disease) or malignant hyperthermia. For these reasons, the U.S. Food and Drug Administration has attached a "black box" warning to succinylcholine. In addition to these general risks of succinylcholine, the diffuse fasciculations caused by succinylcholine may serve to both increase resistance to venous drainage from the head and increase ICP, which could theoretically be problematic for patients with head injury.

The circulatory status of patients with isolated head trauma is generally not compromised, although the potential for other organ system trauma, with associated hemodynamic compromise, must be immediately recognized. IV access should be obtained immediately in all patients with moderate or severe head injuries.

Hypotension [systolic blood pressure less than 70 mm Hg + (age in years × 2)] should be avoided whenever possible and corrected quickly when present. The clinician should remember that the patient would only have an adequate CPP if the MAP were maintained in a normal range. Isotonic crystalloid solutions—normal saline or lactated Ringer's solution—should be given as needed to restore normal intravascular volume (see Chapter 105). Studies evaluating the role of albumin in resuscitation of hypotensive patients with

TRAUMA

traumatic brain injury have not shown benefit over isotonic crystalloid solutions. Studies comparing hypertonic saline with isotonic saline for the resuscitation of hypotensive patients with brain injury in the intensive care unit (ICU) have suggested some benefit with the use of hypertonic saline. However, the limited data currently available from prehospital or ED settings do not show a convincing benefit for hypertonic saline over isotonic solutions and thus their use is not currently recommended.

For patients with adequate intravascular volume, excess fluid administration should be avoided. Patients with a normal hemodynamic status can be managed without IV hydration for the first several hours, or with normal saline or lactated Ringer's solution, running at one-half to two-thirds the maintenance fluid rate, while evaluation and treatment of the head injuries proceeds.

Brain-specific Therapies

Once the ABCs of resuscitation have been addressed and the patient has been stabilized, attention can be given to the neurologic status. The neurologic assessment of the patient with a head injury and the criteria for deciding which patients need neuroimaging are described in detail in Chapter 37.

In any patient with signs of increased ICP on examination (i.e., a progressively deteriorating neurologic status and/or signs of impending herniation), a computed tomographic (CT) scan of the head should be performed immediately, with the goal of identifying any mass lesions that require evacuation. If a head CT scan is not available on site, emergent transfer to a facility where CT can be performed is usually the most appropriate course.

There is a long history in emergency neurotrauma care of empiric "blind" trephination (drilling of burr holes) for patients with signs of impending herniation. The goal of such therapy is to provide immediate decompression for patients who are clinically suspected of having an intracranial hematoma. As emergency CT imaging of the head has become readily available, the role for empiric trephination is very limited. In almost all cases, the benefits of the information provided by head CT scanning outweigh the costs of waiting a few extra minutes to have the scan performed, even in cases in which herniation is impending. Especially for the pediatric age group, in which most cases of increased ICP result from DBS rather than intracranial hematoma, empiric trephination is unlikely to be beneficial. Nonetheless, empiric trephination may still have a role in select patients who are too unstable to be transported to the radiology suite or in cases in which the nearest CT scanner is too far away.

When increased ICP is suspected, medical maneuvers to decrease ICP should be undertaken immediately. These maneuvers include elevation of the head of the bed to an angle of 30 degrees and maintenance of the head and neck in a midline position, both of which promote venous drainage from the head.

Sedating medications may also be used. Some sedating medications, including etomidate, barbiturates, ketamine, and midazolam, lead to lower ICP. The opiates, on the other hand, have generally been shown to cause no change or even modest increases in ICP. Propofol infusions can effectively lower ICP but are associated with a high risk of adverse effects and are therefore not recommended.

Sedation is indicated when patients are agitated or when they are coughing and choking, which may lead to dislodgement of the endotracheal tube. When sedating drugs are used, the clinician must be vigilant for hypotension. Paralytic agents should generally be reserved for situations in which sedating medications fail to adequately control the patient's behavior.

Hyperventilation lowers ICP by decreasing the volume of the intracranial vasculature. The cerebral arteriolar circulation responds to hypocarbia with reflex vasoconstriction. The therapeutic use of hyperventilation requires a delicate balance: too little ventilation leads to vasodilation and increased ICP, but too much ventilation leads to excess vasoconstriction and decreased CBF. The optimal balance for therapeutic hyperventilation appears to be achieved at a $P\text{CO}_2$ of 30 to 35 mm Hg. Arterial blood gases or end-tidal CO_2 measurements should be followed to ensure that $P\text{CO}_2$ is in the desired range.

IV mannitol (0.5 to 1 g per kg) can be administered to increase the serum osmolarity. The increased serum osmolarity draws free water into the vasculature, thereby decreasing the blood viscosity. The lower blood viscosity leads to improved CBF, which helps prevent cerebral ischemia. The autoregulatory system responds to the improved CBF and cerebral oxygenation with reflex vasoconstriction, thereby lowering intracerebral volume (and ICP) without compromising CBF. The effect of mannitol on ICP is seen within a few minutes of administration. During the ensuing hour or so, mannitol also leads to some intravascular volume depletion because of its action as an osmotic diuretic. Clinicians should be cautious when using mannitol in patients with possible hemodynamic compromise because the diuretic effect may exacerbate hypovolemia and worsen perfusion. Some clinicians advocate the use of a Foley catheter in patients receiving mannitol to prevent bladder rupture.

Hypertonic saline (typically dosed as an infusion of 0.1 to 1 mL per kg per hour of 3% saline) is an effective alternative to mannitol. As with mannitol, the hyperosmolarity of this solution leads to decreased blood viscosity and improved CBF. In contrast to mannitol, however, hypertonic saline does not have a diuretic effect. Guidelines for the care of pediatric patients with severe head injury suggest that mannitol and hypertonic saline are both reasonable alternatives for patients who require hyperosmolar therapy. There is a disagreement in the literature about the optimal use of hyperventilation and hyperosmolar therapy in the management of patients with a head injury. The clearest indication for these maneuvers is to "buy time" for several minutes in a patient with clinical signs of impending herniation. Stabilization of the patient with impending herniation with hyperventilation and/or hyperosmolar agents may allow enough time for the patient to be safely transferred to the radiology suite, for emergency head CT imaging. If an evacuable hematoma is discovered on the CT scan, these maneuvers can be used to stabilize the patient en route to the operating suite, where the increased ICP will be more definitively relieved.

It is less clear that sustained hyperventilation or repeated doses of hyperosmolar agents are useful in patients who have increased ICP but who do not have surgical mass lesions. In particular, research studies have documented a clear relationship between even mild degrees of hyperventilation ($P\text{CO}_2$ 30 to 35 mm Hg) and decreased CBF. Because the overall goal of resuscitation in patients with a head injury is to optimize CBF, prolonged hyperventilation may be counterproductive in that it may actually worsen cerebral ischemia. Therefore, hyperventilation is most useful as a transient therapy for acute changes in neurologic condition or as a second-line therapy after other methods of managing ICP have failed.

Some concern has also been raised that repeated doses of hypertonic agents may be counterproductive in the ongoing care of patients with brain swelling because the hypertonic agent can leak across the injured blood-brain barrier, with its osmotic pull serving to worsen cerebral edema. Although some experimental models of mannitol therapy have documented this phenomenon, most data from clinical studies indicate lasting improvements in CBF with repeated doses of mannitol or hypertonic saline. Therefore, many authors consider mannitol and hypertonic saline to be a useful adjunct in the management of increased ICP in patients with brain swelling.

No evidence exists that hyperventilation or a hyperosmolar agent prevents the development of brain swelling. Therefore, the prophylactic use of these therapies is not recommended.

Many studies over the years have evaluated the utility of corticosteroids in patients with a head injury. Theoretically, corticosteroids might blunt the inflammatory response to brain injury, thereby decreasing brain swelling. However, clinical researchers have been unable to show any improvement in outcome for patients with head injuries treated with corticosteroids. The use of corticosteroids for the treatment of head injury is therefore not recommended.

The potential role of intentionally induced brain hypothermia, instituted as a neuroprotective measure, has been evaluated in clinical trials. Although studies have found some modest benefit for adult patients treated with hypothermia, a multicenter randomized trial for children with severe head injury found no improvement in outcome but a possible increase in mortality among children treated with hypothermia. Thus, hypothermic therapy is not recommended.

Anticonvulsant medications are clearly indicated for patients who are having ongoing seizure activity. Short-acting benzodiazepines (lorazepam or diazepam) may be used in the short-term management of ongoing seizures, and phenytoin or fosphenytoin may be used for maintenance anticonvulsant effect.

A multicenter randomized trial showed no benefit for the use of phenytoin for seizure prophylaxis in pediatric patients with moderate to severe brain injury. Nonetheless, phenytoin (loading dose of 10 to 20 mg per kg) or fosphenytoin [loading dose of 10 to 20 mg per kg phenytoin equivalent (PE)] can be considered as an option for antiseizure prophylaxis for patients who have increased risk of early posttraumatic seizures. Younger age and lower Glasgow Coma Scale (GCS) score appear to be risk factors for seizures. Patients with parenchymal brain lesions, SAH, or subdural hemorrhage may also have some increased risk.

In recent years, researchers have designed clinical trials of novel therapies intended to block the actions of specific cytokines or neurotoxins such as bradykinin and glutamate. Other researchers have attempted to improve outcomes by infusing metabolic substrates or cytokines, such as creatine, magnesium sulfate, or nerve growth factor, that may limit brain injury or promote brain healing. To date, none of these therapies have been sufficiently proven to be recommended for routine clinical use.

Disposition

Generally, all patients with intracranial hematomas or brain injuries noted on head CT imaging should be hospitalized, no matter how mild or severe their symptoms. In addition, any patient with an abnormal neurologic examination should be hospitalized even if head CT findings are normal. More mildly symptomatic patients with a normal neurologic status and small cerebral contusions or intracranial hematomas may be candidates for observation in a ward setting.

Patients with neurologic compromise and sizable intracranial hematomas require emergency operative intervention, and they are monitored postoperatively in the ICU for the development of cerebral edema or recurrence of bleeding. Patients with neurologic compromise but no surgical lesions also need intensive care monitoring, often with the placement of a device for the measurement of ICP. In general, ICP monitors are indicated for any patient with a head injury who is comatose and whose head CT findings are abnormal. Although many different types of ICP monitors have been used, the intraventricular catheter has the advantage of being useful both for monitoring and for therapy because CSF can be drained through the catheter if needed to lower the ICP in the short term. The goal of ICU management for patients with ICP monitors is to maintain an adequate CPP, which generally entails maintaining ICP at 20 mm Hg or less. Maneuvers used to lower ICP may include CSF drainage, sedation, hyperosmolar therapy, hyperventilation, and, in some cases, decompressive craniectomy.

Well-appearing patients with head injuries who either require no head CT scan (see Chapter 37) or have no intracranial lesions on head CT imaging may be suitable for discharge to home with careful instructions.

Blunt Trauma: Specific Lesions

Concussion

Clinical Findings and Pathophysiology. Concussion is generally defined as a head injury associated with any alteration in mental status. Most clinicians use the term *concussion* to refer to mild head injuries, with no or minor depression in the level of consciousness (GCS scores of 13 to 15) and with no associated focal neurologic deficits. Concussion most commonly results from falls in infants and toddlers and from sports-related injuries in older children and adolescents.

Common symptoms of concussion include initial loss of consciousness, amnesia, confusion, headache, nausea, vomiting, and dizziness. For the most part, clinicians use the term *concussion* to describe cases of minor head trauma in which no brain imaging is performed or cases in which head CT imaging reveals no intracranial pathology.

Despite the normal CT imaging findings, patients with concussion have clearly suffered an injury to the brain. In fact, many concussed patients with normal head CT findings do in fact have subtle evidence of brain contusion or diffuse axonal injury (DAI) noted on magnetic resonance imaging (MRI) of the brain. Research studies have shown that even when there is no structural injury to the brain, there are functional disturbances, which are clearly demonstrable by imaging methodologies such as functional MRI and diffusion tensor imaging. Furthermore, researchers have found abnormalities in cerebrovascular

TRAUMA

autoregulation in some patients with concussion. Animal models of concussion have similarly shown disruptions both in CBF and in cerebral metabolism.

Patients with concussion, even if they appear normal on gross neurologic evaluation, can be demonstrated to have abnormalities on neuropsychological testing. Neuropsychological abnormalities are typically present even in seemingly minor "ding" concussions that involve no loss of consciousness and no posttraumatic amnesia.

Prognosis and Management

Most patients with concussion can be demonstrated to have persistent neuropsychological abnormalities for 5 to 7 days after a head injury. Some studies of school athletes suggest that younger players (i.e., high school students) have a higher risk for persistent cognitive deficits than college students with similar injuries. In general, patients who have amnesia at the time of initial evaluation appear to be at the highest risk for these persistent neuropsychological symptoms. Persistent complaints of amnesia or headache 24 hours after the injury have also been shown to be accurate indicators of ongoing neuropsychological dysfunction.

Patients with minor head injury who have normal head CT scans are at low risk for subsequent clinical deterioration. In general, these patients may be safely discharged to home if no other issues require inpatient care.

Numerous guidelines have been developed to help determine when patients with concussion can return to contact sports. The various proposed "return-to-play" guidelines are based on concerns that the concussed brain is especially vulnerable to repeat injury if a second head impact occurs before the brain has fully recovered from the initial concussion. A large study of NCAA football players, for instance, has shown that approximately 90% of second concussions during a given football season occur within 10 days of the initial concussion. In some respects, the concussed brain appears never to fully recover. Multiple studies have shown that patients with one or more concussions in the past, even if these prior concussions were years earlier, are at increased risk for repeated concussions.

One devastating complication of repeat head injury after concussion is the rare and poorly understood "second impact syndrome." There are several case reports in the literature of this syndrome in which patients have experienced an initial concussion during a sporting event and then have had serious neurologic deterioration and died after a second seemingly minor head impact occurred on the same day. In these cases, the initial concussion presumably led to some impairment of cerebral metabolism and cerebrovascular autoregulation that was exacerbated by the second impact. Despite the apparent rarity of this syndrome, its catastrophic nature has been one of the factors motivating the development of return-to-play guidelines.

A substantially more common outcome of repeated concussions is the progressive accumulation of subtle neuropsychological deficits. Several studies have shown persistent cognitive deficits in patients who have suffered concussions in the past, with a higher rate of abnormalities in patients who have had multiple concussions. This concern for progressive damage with repeated concussions has been a major motivation behind the dissemination of return-to-play guidelines for sports-related concussions.

The first widely accepted return-to-play guidelines were developed by the American Academy of Neurology and published in *Morbidity and Mortality Weekly Report* in 1997. These guidelines emphasized the importance of initial loss of consciousness in determining the severity of concussion. Since that time, other authors have developed alternative guidelines that depend less on loss of consciousness, which has proven to be a rare phenomenon in sports-related concussions, and more on duration of amnesia, confusion, headache, or other symptoms. Many of these later guidelines reject the classification of concussion severity on the basis of initial symptoms, because of the finding that even minor "ding" concussions can lead to neuropsychological abnormalities that persist for several days after the injury.

One widely noted set of guidelines was released by the Second International Conference on Concussion in Sports, held in Prague in 2004. These guidelines recommend a stepwise return to sports activities after concussion. The concussed athlete progresses from no-sports activity to light aerobic activity (e.g., walking) to sport-specific aerobic activities (e.g., running or skating) to noncontact training drills to full contact training drills and then finally to full game-playing activities. Each step forward is taken only if the athlete tolerates the previous step without symptoms.

Concussion guidelines emphasize the importance not only of physical rest but also of "cognitive rest," with limitations on academic work or other cognitively stressful activities, until symptoms resolve.

Acetaminophen may be used for headache, but more potent analgesics should probably be avoided so that any progression of symptoms can be detected. The warning signs of progressing intracranial injury should be reviewed with the patient before discharge, with instructions to return immediately if any of these new symptoms or signs appear.

Symptoms after a concussion generally resolve within hours to days after the injury. However, some patients develop the postconcussion syndrome, in which symptoms of confusion, amnesia, headaches, or dizziness may persist for weeks or even months after the injury. Some research in adults has indicated that a scheduled follow-up visit with a head injury clinic, involving education, neuropsychological assessment, and anticipatory guidance, reduces the likelihood of the postconcussion syndrome. Some head injury follow-up clinics for pediatric patients with concussion have been developed in recent years. Many public and private schools have developed their own programs of neuropsychological assessment and follow-up to help identify patients with persistent symptoms and to guide athletes in their decision to return to sports.

Skull Fracture

Clinical Findings and Diagnosis. Skull fractures occur in approximately 2 per 1,000 infants per year and in approximately 0.5 to 1 per 1,000 older children and adolescents. Skull fractures result mainly from falls in infants, but they may also result from child abuse, motor vehicle crashes, or other mechanisms. In older children and adolescents, skull fractures usually result from motor vehicle crashes or sports-related injuries.

Infants have a higher risk for skull fracture than older children, probably because their skulls are thinner. Many skull fractures in infants result from short distance falls; generally, about 50% of infants with skull fracture have fallen from less

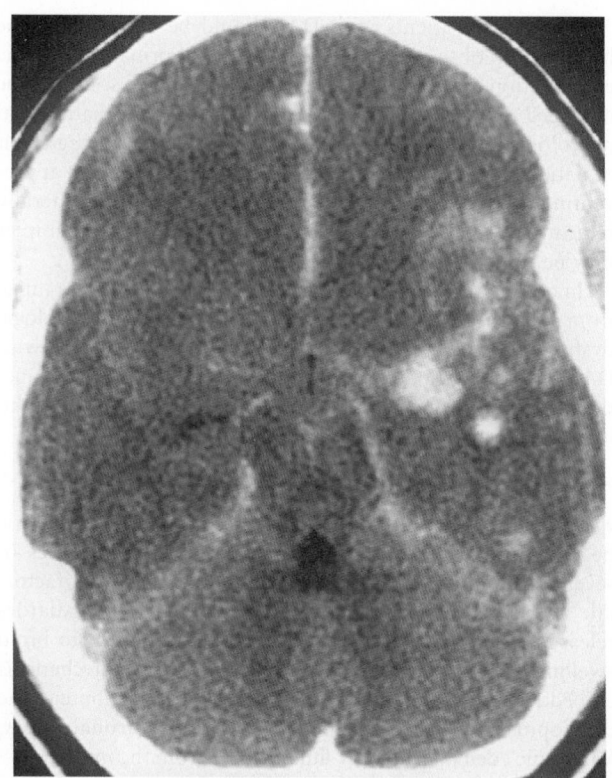

FIGURE 116.8 Cerebral contusion. This 16-year-old adolescent girl was comatose after being a passenger in a high-speed motor vehicle collision. A head computed tomographic scan shows hemorrhagic contusion of the left temporal lobe, subdural hematoma along the tentorial margins, and effacement of the sulci throughout. The patient died despite intensive medical management for increased intracranial pressure.

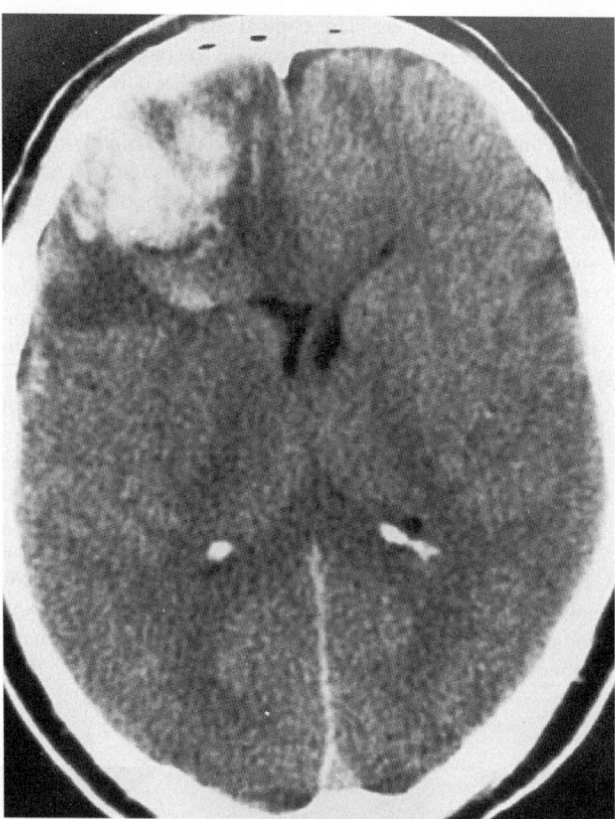

FIGURE 116.9 Intraparenchymal hemorrhage. This adolescent boy was an unrestrained passenger in a high-speed motor vehicle collision. He was comatose on presentation. A head computed tomographic scan shows a large area of intraparenchymal hemorrhage in the right frontal region. Note also the surrounding area of low-density cerebral contusion.

undergo late hemorrhage, which would manifest as a sudden increase in ICP and/or deterioration in clinical status.

Management of increased ICP for patients with cerebral contusion is similar to patients with other types of brain lesion. Hyperosmolar therapy, however, should be used with caution. Impairment of the blood-brain barrier may allow the hyperosmolar fluid to extravasate into the contused region, thereby leading to increased contusion volume.

Patients with large contusions exerting a significant mass effect may require surgical resection. Some research data indicate better outcomes for surgical versus nonsurgical management of large contusions. Nonetheless, surgical resection is typically avoided when possible because the contused tissue may actually be viable and regain function over the long term. Early decompressive craniectomy has also been used successfully in some patients with large contusions.

Operative drainage of intraparenchymal hematomas is technically difficult. Large hematomas exerting a significant mass effect require operative drainage. Smaller lesions may initially be managed nonoperatively, but with the clinician recognizing the high risk for sudden deterioration. ICP monitoring is necessary for most patients with intraparenchymal hematoma to detect early signs of a growing lesion.

The prognosis for patients with cerebral contusion varies widely, depending mainly on the patient's neurologic status on presentation and on the presence or absence of other lesions.

Patients with more significant cerebral contusion often have some residual neurologic disability. Follow-up CT scans on such patients show areas of encephalomalacia at the site of injury. Patients with brainstem or hypothalamic lesions also often have a poor prognosis. Other patients may essentially have full recovery, with no residual neurologic deficits evident. Patients with intraparenchymal hematomas usually have incurred severe brain injury, and they often have a poor outcome. However, relatively asymptomatic patients with petechial hemorrhage may have an excellent recovery.

Diffuse Axonal Injury

Pathophysiology. DAI is characterized by diffuse primary injury to the white matter tracts of the brain, often at the junction of gray and white matter or sometimes deeper at the level of the corpus callosum, brainstem, or cerebellum. Pathologically, degeneration of the axons is noted, with the presence of axonal retraction balls, microglial proliferation, and demyelination. There is usually accompanying endothelial damage to the capillaries, with some punctate areas of hemorrhage. Focal or diffuse edema may be present.

DAI results from the application of severe acceleration/deceleration or angular rotational forces to the brain, which lead to shear injuries of the axons and associated vasculature. It usually results either from motor vehicle crashes or from child abuse.

TRAUMA

Clinical manifestations. The clinical manifestations of DAI can range from symptoms of concussion to coma. Loss of consciousness is common. In one study of patients with DAI, 82% developed coma. In general, patients with more extensive DAI noted on radiographic imaging (especially if involving the brainstem) have more severe symptoms. As imaging technologies have improved, subtle signs of DAI have been noted even in patients with milder symptoms and signs of brain injury.

Diagnosis. DAI may be evident on CT scanning as small nonexpansive hemorrhagic lesions of the white matter, most typically seen at the gray–white junction of the cerebral hemispheres, or in the corpus callosum, brainstem, or cerebellum. Cerebral swelling sometimes accompanies DAI, but it need not be present for a diagnosis of DAI to be made. Slit ventricles may be seen. Intraventricular hemorrhage is sometimes noted (Fig. 116.10). Intraparenchymal hemorrhages and cerebral contusions are also commonly noted in patients with DAI.

Although some of these abnormalities may be evident on CT, advances in MRI technology such as diffusion tensor imaging have demonstrated superior sensitivity for detecting axonal hemorrhage or other forms of white matter damage that would be missed on CT.

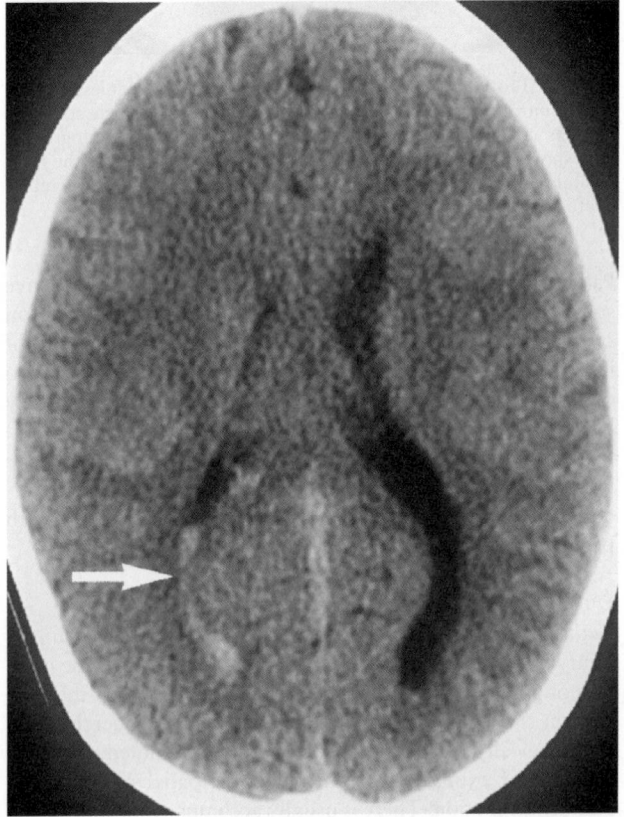

FIGURE 116.10 Intraventricular hemorrhage. This head computed tomographic (CT) scan was performed on an 8-year-old girl who was involved in a sledding accident. She presented in coma. The *arrow* indicates hemorrhage in the right lateral ventricle. Note the layering of blood inferiorly in this supine patient. Other "cuts" of the CT showed areas of punctate hemorrhage consistent with diffuse axonal injury. The patient made an excellent recovery, with minimal neurologic deficits.

Management. Patients with DAI should be admitted to the hospital for observation. Patients with a normal neurologic examination and no other lesions evident on CT scan may be managed on a general inpatient unit. Those with an abnormal neurologic status require ICU-level monitoring. Management of patients with DAI is supportive, with efforts directed at preventing secondary brain injury. ICP monitoring is generally indicated for patients who present in coma. Specific therapies may be required for the management of increased ICP.

In a large series of patients with DAI, mortality rates range from 10% to 15%. Of those who survive, persistent neurologic dysfunction occurs in 30% to 40% of patients. Children with DAI tend to have a better prognosis than adults. A good functional outcome can be expected for patients with DAI who have mild symptoms of head injury (GSC score of 13 to 15).

Diffuse Brain Swelling

Pathophysiology. DBS is a common manifestation of pediatric head trauma, occurring in approximately 40% of cases of severe head injury. The origin of DBS is probably multifactorial. Cytotoxic edema, caused by inflammatory mediators released from injured cells, is the largest contributor to brain swelling. Increased expression of aquaporins, water channels embedded in the neuronal membranes, likely contribute to the development of brain swelling in areas of neuronal injury. Vasogenic edema, caused by fluid leaking from the injured vasculature, may also contribute to a lesser extent. Cerebral vasodilation, likely reflecting disordered autoregulation in the injured brain, can also play a role in DBS. Younger children may be at higher risk for disordered autoregulation. Although some studies show increased CBF in cases of DBS, other studies suggest that abnormal vasodilation does not contribute substantially to most cases of DBS. In fact, in many cases of brain injury with DBS, the cerebral blood volume appears to be decreased below the normal level.

DBS is probably a final, common manifestation of brain injury caused by a number of different mechanisms. It can be a manifestation of primary brain injury, as when it accompanies large areas of brain contusion or DAI. In other cases, it probably represents secondary brain injury, caused by hypoxia or hypoperfusion. If left unchecked, the development of DBS can lead to a vicious cycle. That is, the presence of DBS causes an increase in ICP and then the resulting ischemia leads to the development of more DBS.

Clinical Manifestations. Most patients with DBS are comatose on initial evaluation, sometimes with associated focal neurologic deficits. Rarely, patients with DBS have less impressive symptoms with more minor neurologic deficits. These patients often experience neurologic deterioration over the ensuing several hours.

Diagnosis. DBS is diagnosed by a head CT scan when there is evidence of smaller ventricles, effacement of the sulci, or obliterated basal cisterns in the absence of other intracranial pathology that may be exerting significant mass effect (Fig. 116.11). Signs of cerebral edema per se, such as loss of gray–white differentiation, may be present. Other accompanying intracranial lesions, such as DAI, subdural hemorrhage, cerebral contusion, or SAH, are also often diagnosed. In one large study of children with DBS, 60% had no other intracranial lesions identified. It is

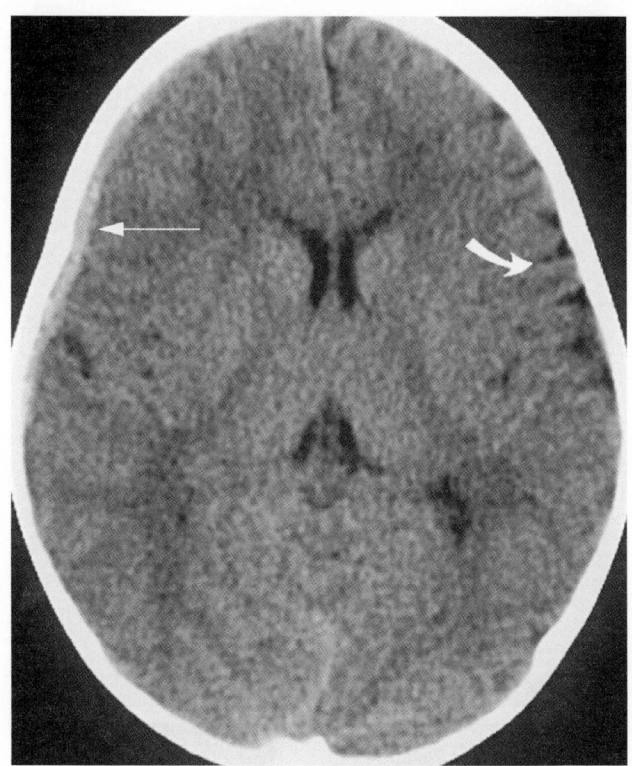

FIGURE 116.11 Brain swelling. This 1-year-old boy fell from a second-story window. The neurologic examination was normal. A head computed tomographic scan shows a small, right-sided subdural hematoma in the temporal region. Note also the effacement of the sulci on the right *(straight arrow)*, which can be compared with the normal sulci on the left *(curved arrow)*. There is also a mild shift of the midline toward the left.

likely, however, that many of these same patients would exhibit subtle evidence of DAI if more advanced imaging technologies had been used. One study found head CT scanning to have a sensitivity of 99% for detecting cases of DBS associated with increased ICP.

Management. Patients with DBS need to be admitted to the hospital. Generally, admission to the ICU is required for careful monitoring of hemodynamics, oxygenation and ventilation, and ICP. ICP monitors are indicated for any patient with DBS in coma.

Management of the patient with DBS focuses on optimizing cerebral perfusion and minimizing any stressors that may lead to worsening of the DBS. If the ICP is elevated, measures to control the ICP are required. DBS is often worse between 1 and 3 days after the occurrence of primary injury, so patients who initially have well-controlled ICP may have more serious difficulties later.

The outcome of DBS after head trauma is better for children than it is for adults. In one large study, 78% of children with DBS had a functional outcome. Patients with more severe neurologic symptoms on presentation clearly have worse outcomes, as do those with extensive areas of DAI or accompanying intracranial lesions, especially subarachnoid or intraventricular hemorrhage. Patients who experience secondary systemic insults (e.g., hypotension, hypoxia) also have a worse prognosis.

Epidural Hematoma

Pathophysiology. Most EDHs result from blunt impact to the cranium. In most EDH cases, the skull is fractured, with an associated laceration to the epidural vessels underlying the fracture site. In other cases, there is no fracture, but the deformation of the skull and associated linear deceleration from impact lead to shearing of the epidural arteries or veins. In some cases of injury to the epidural vessels, pseudoaneurysms may form.

Many patients with EDH have experienced relatively low-energy mechanisms of injury. In pediatrics, most EDH cases result from falls, although a minority of cases result from motor vehicle collisions, child abuse, or other mechanisms. About one-half of the pediatric EDH cases result from falls of 6 ft or less.

Other mechanisms of injury, such as the shaking implicated in cases of child abuse, are less likely to be associated with EDH because they do not lead to deformation of the skull. Because the low-impact falls that lead to EDH rarely involve high energy being applied to the brain itself, about 90% of EDH cases have no associated parenchymal injuries.

A small EDH may be asymptomatic. As the EDH expands, it begins to occupy an increasingly large intracranial volume. This increasing mass effect leads to an increase in ICP and, if left unchecked, may result in diffuse secondary brain injury. If the EDH continues to expand, it may ultimately lead to cerebral herniation.

If an EDH can be recognized and surgically drained before this process occurs, secondary brain injury can be prevented. In many cases, the patient has a completely normal neurologic status after the EDH is drained. If the EDH is not drained in time, however, persistent neurologic deficits may result.

Approximately 18% to 36% of patients with EDH have an arterial source of bleeding identified. In most cases, the middle meningeal artery is involved. Another 10% to 20% have bleeding from meningeal veins, the emissary veins, the diploic veins, or the dural sinuses. Finally, about 30% to 40% have no recognized source of bleeding identified and are probably oozing from small venous sites in the dura. In general, the more severe symptoms are seen in patients with arterial bleeding, an intermediate course in patients with venous sources, and the most benign course in patients with no discrete source identified. Occasionally, patients with venous or oozing EDH are first diagnosed days or even weeks after the injury.

EDH in the occipital and frontal regions or vertex may be fairly well tolerated. In contrast, bleeding in the temporal region is more likely to cause symptoms early because a temporal EDH will more quickly lead to tentorial herniation. Posterior fossa bleeding may also lead to earlier symptoms because of the potential for early compression of vital brainstem structures, as well as the potential for obstruction to CSF outflow and the development of hydrocephalus. In recent years, several cases of pediatric epidural bleeding behind the clivus as a result of ligamentous injury at the craniocervical junction have been reported, leading to cranial nerve dysfunction.

Clinical Symptoms/Signs. The classic presentation of EDH involves an initial loss of consciousness at the moment of impact, the "lucid interval" of several hours after the trauma when the patient is awake and relatively asymptomatic, and then neurologic deterioration as the enlarging hematoma begins to exert its mass effect.

In fact, however, pediatric patients with EDH rarely present with these classic symptoms. In one large series of pediatric patients with EDH, only 20% had an initial loss of consciousness and 38% were alert with normal neurologic examinations at the time of diagnosis. The most common symptoms of EDH in pediatrics are headache, vomiting, and lethargy. In addition, ataxia may be noted in cases of posterior fossa EDH. Seizures are relatively rare, occurring in less than 10% of cases.

A small number of patients with EDH may not have any symptoms of brain injury. Skull fracture may be a particularly important indicator of EDH, especially in patients with few other symptoms, because skull fracture is noted in 70% to 80% of cases of EDH. Temporal or parietal skull fractures are particularly associated with a risk of arterial bleeding.

Diagnosis. EDH can be readily diagnosed by noncontrast CT of the head. The classic appearance on CT is that of a high-density biconvex lesion subjacent to the skull (Fig. 116.12). The EDH is usually bounded by suture lines but may rarely cross these lines if diastasis of the suture has occurred. EDH is most commonly noted in the parietal, temporal, or temporoparietal region (approximately 78%) and rarely in the frontal (16%) or occipital (6%) region. The classic high-density appearance on CT indicates clotted blood. Occasionally, an adjacent or intermixed, swirled isodense lesion is noted, which represents ongoing acute bleeding that has yet to clot (Fig. 116.13).

On CT, midline shift, small ventricles, and loss of patency of the basal cisterns indicate a mass effect from the EDH. Signs of herniation may be seen. Other associated intradural hematomas or parenchymal injuries may also be present.

In more recent years, some researchers and clinicians have begun using MRI for the diagnosis of EDH. Because MRI requires a longer imaging duration and is more likely to require sedation, CT remains the preferred modality. However, MRI may occasionally be useful for regions of the brain not well imaged with CT, such as the region subjacent to the skull vertex. Some research suggests that gadolinium enhancement of the EDH indicates ongoing bleeding and an increased likelihood of expansion of the lesion.

Management. The mainstay of treatment of EDH is craniotomy, with drainage of the hematoma and repair of the lacerated epidural vessels. Patients with EDH who have depression in their level of consciousness, focal neurologic findings, pupillary abnormalities, and/or signs of increased ICP should proceed immediately to surgical intervention.

Some patients with EDH may be safely managed with observation. Conservative management is typically considered acceptable only for patients with a small EDH (generally less than 30 mL in volume and with a thickness of less than 2 cm), no focal neurologic deficits, and a normal level of consciousness. Patients with posterior fossa EDH are rarely candidates for conservative management because of the high risk of sudden deterioration resulting from medullary compression and hydrocephalus.

In virtually all cases, a neurosurgeon should be consulted immediately because children who are initially well may experience rapid neurologic deterioration in the first several

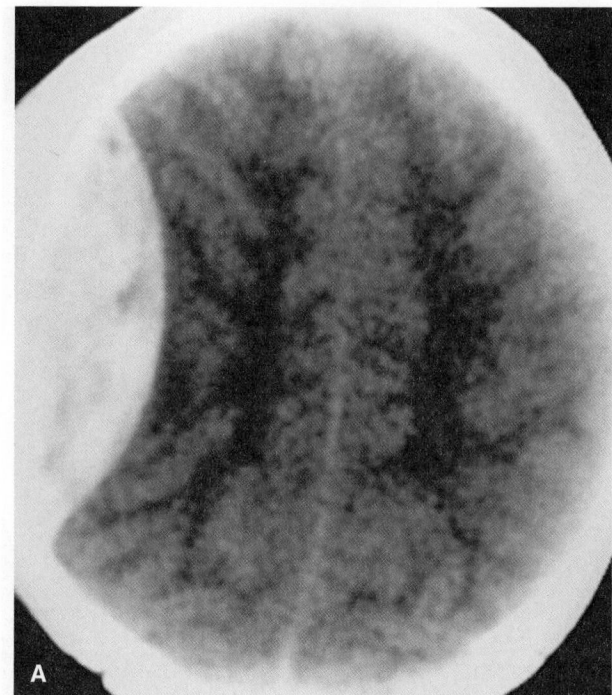

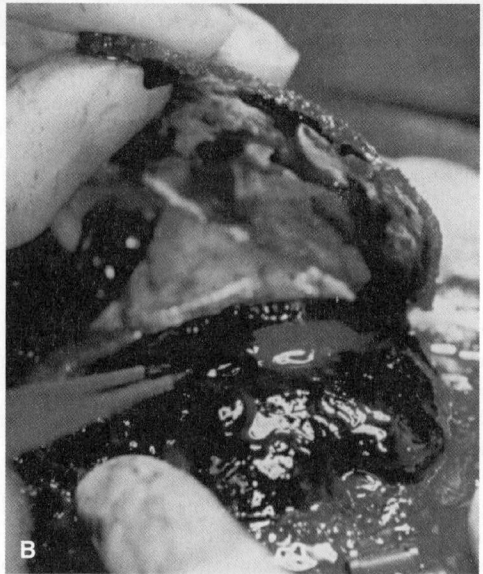

FIGURE 116.12 Epidural hematoma (EDH). This 8-year-old boy presented after a sledding accident. He had no loss of consciousness, but he complained of headache and vomiting. A head computed tomographic scan (**A**) shows the classic biconvex hyperdensity of an EDH. He proceeded to the operating room, where a large mass of clotted blood (**B**) was removed.

hours after diagnosis. In one series, 32% of patients who were initially managed conservatively ultimately required surgical drainage of the EDH. Patients who have the initial head CT performed early—especially those within 2 hours of the trauma—have a high likelihood of subsequent progression in the size of the EDH. Physicians should be especially vigilant with cases of temporal EDH because of the risk of arterial bleeding and uncal herniation associated with these lesions.

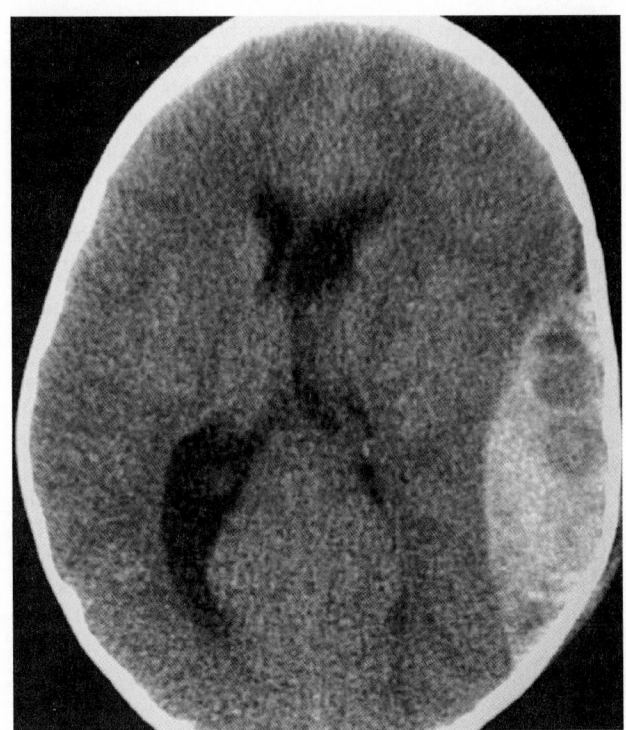

FIGURE 116.13 Epidural hematoma (EDH). This 11-month-old boy presented with progressive lethargy and vomiting after falling 2 ft off of a bed. Several hours after the injury, he became unresponsive with dilated, nonreactive pupils. This head computed tomographic scan shows a large EDH, with intermingled hypodense areas representing active bleeding. Note also the midline shift and the compression of the ipsilateral ventricle. After an emergency craniotomy, the patient made a full recovery.

Mortality rates in pediatric EDH range from 0% to 10%. Among survivors, approximately 85% have a good neurologic outcome. The most important predictor of outcome is the patient's neurologic status prior to operative intervention. Patients with coma and pupillary abnormalities are much more likely to have sustained secondary brain injury. However, even among patients who present in coma or with nonreactive pupils, a majority will have a moderate or good neurologic outcome. Minimally symptomatic patients with EDH who do not require surgery typically have a normal neurologic outcome, with no abnormalities on follow-up assessments either of neuropsychiatric outcome or of CBF.

Subdural Hematoma

Pathophysiology. SDHs result from tearing of the bridging veins that traverse the subdural space. Mechanisms of injury that are associated with shear forces being applied to these veins are especially likely to lead to SDHs. In particular, SDHs result from injuries associated with significant acceleration/deceleration forces.

In older children and adolescents, SDHs most commonly result from motor vehicle crashes. In infants, SDHs are commonly a result of the shaking impact syndrome of child abuse. Occasionally, cases of shaking impact syndrome involving SDH can be seen in older children as well. SDHs may also result from falls, especially if the fall is from a significant height. Because of the more significant forces applied to the brain in most injuries leading to SDHs, they are often associated with other intracranial lesions.

For some patients with SDH, the mass effect of the accumulating SDH is the primary cause of neurologic impairment. Many cases of SDH, however, are associated with cerebral contusions, brain ischemia, or DBS. For these patients, the SDH may be more of a marker of a high-force mechanism of injury than a cause of neurologic injury in itself. Therefore, even if the SDH is drained in a timely fashion, serious brain injury may persist.

Clinical Manifestations. SDHs are often associated both with an initial loss of consciousness and with a depressed mental status. Approximately 50% of patients with SDH present in coma. Pupillary abnormalities may also be noted, indicating impending herniation. In less severely ill patients, headaches, vomiting, lethargy, irritability, visual difficulties, or seizures may be noted. In patients with SDHs involving the posterior fossa, cerebellar signs such as ataxia or nystagmus may be noted. Some asymptomatic or minimally symptomatic patients may also be diagnosed with small SDHs.

Although most symptoms of SDH present within hours after the trauma, occasional symptoms of chronic SDH are diagnosed days or even weeks after a head trauma. In pediatrics, chronic traumatic SDH is most commonly seen in infants, usually as a consequence of child abuse. Presenting symptoms in these infants may include tense fontanel, macrocephaly, psychomotor retardation, depressed level of consciousness, seizures, vomiting, irritability, or focal neurologic deficits.

Diagnosis. On head CT scanning, acute SDH is seen as a hyperdense, crescentic collection of extraaxial fluid (Fig. 116.14). There may be areas of intermingled hypodense fluid, which represent active bleeding, sometimes termed a hyperacute SDH (Fig. 116.14). Because the subdural space is continuous around each hemisphere, subdural blood flows freely through this space, while respecting the midline and tentorial margins (Figs. 116.15 and 116.16). SDH is usually unilateral, although cases of child abuse may be associated with bilateral SDH. The CT scan should be evaluated for evidence of mass effect and associated intracranial lesions, such as brain swelling, cerebral contusions, or SAH. The density of the subdural fluid collection varies over time. With older hematomas, the collection may be almost isodense with CSF.

Management. In the early 1980s, researchers showed remarkable decreases in mortality from SDH if patients underwent timely surgical drainage. Not surprisingly, this effect was most evident in those patients with large SDHs associated with midline shift and coma. In this subgroup, the neurologic prognosis is optimized when surgery is performed within 4 hours of the trauma. It appears that early relief of the mass effect in these patients prevents secondary brain injury.

Many patients with SDH who are not so severely ill can be managed nonoperatively. Some authors have proposed nonoperative management for patients with SDH who are not comatose, who have small SDHs with no significant mass effect, and who have patent basal cisterns. Generally, even well-appearing patients with posterior fossa SDHs undergo

TRAUMA

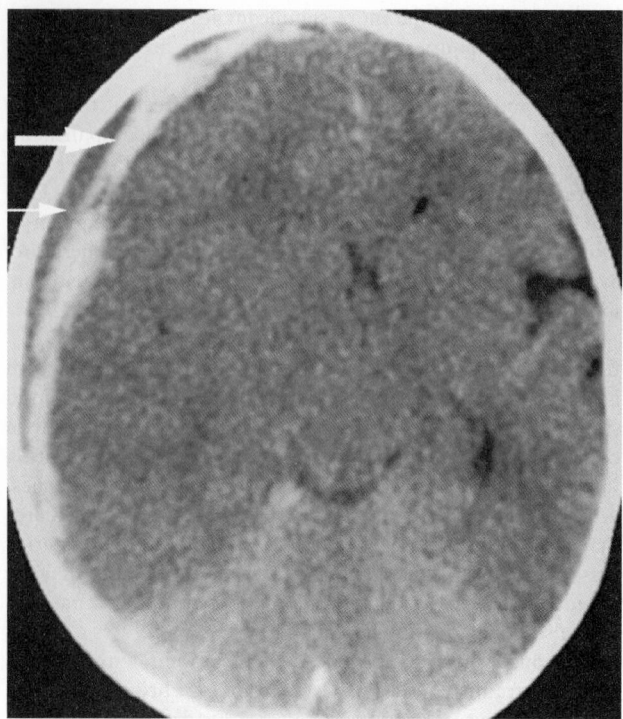

FIGURE 116.14 Subdural hematoma (SDH) and brain swelling. This 9-month-old boy reportedly became suddenly unresponsive. There was no history of trauma. On examination, he was comatose with fixed dilated pupils and extensor posturing. Massive bilateral retinal hemorrhages were seen. This head computed tomographic scan shows a right-sided SDH, with acute hyperdense *(thick arrow)* and hyperacute iso-dense *(thin arrow)* components. Midline shift to the left is noted. There is also evidence of brain swelling, with effacement of the sulci and poor gray–white differentiation. The diffuse hypodensity of the cerebral cortex can be contrasted with the normal density of the cerebellum, which appears whiter in this view. A diagnosis of child abuse was made.

surgery because of the high risk of brainstem compression. Even if a patient is a candidate for nonoperative management, immediate consultation with a neurosurgeon is essential because of the potential for rapid clinical deterioration over the first several hours of observation.

Patients with chronic SDH generally do not require craniotomy and decompression. Most centers manage these patients with a strategy of serial subdural taps or continuous external drainage. In some cases, the SDH is successfully drained in this manner and no further therapy is necessary. In most cases, eventual placement of a subduroperitoneal shunt for ongoing drainage of the lesion is necessary.

The clinician must recognize the strong association of SDH with child abuse, especially in infants with no clear mechanism of injury reported and in those patients with associated retinal hemorrhages. If the circumstances of the injury cannot be clearly explained, further evaluation for nonaccidental trauma should be pursued. Cases of SDH in which the CT findings indicate a mix of higher- and lower-density fluid collections (indicating a mix of older and newer blood) are also more suggestive of nonaccidental trauma.

Mortality rates for children with acute SDH range from 10% to 20%. Among survivors, persistent neurologic sequelae are common. Patients who present in coma or who have pupil-

lary abnormalities clearly have poorer prognoses. In addition, patients with more significant brain injury on CT or increased ICP have a worse prognosis. Even the patients who appear to be at high risk, however, may have moderate or good functional outcomes. Most patients who are managed nonoperatively do well, with few, if any, neurologic sequelae and with full resolution of the SDH. A small percentage will develop chronic SDH. Chronic SDH is seldom lethal but may be associated with ongoing neurologic problems such as seizures or developmental delay.

Subarachnoid Hemorrhage

Pathophysiology. SAH is a common complication of head trauma, especially in more severely injured patients. In one large study, SAH occurred in approximately 25% of patients who were comatose on initial evaluation.

SAH results from tearing of the small vessels of the pia mater. SAH, especially if involving the basal cisterns, can rarely indicate rupture of a dissecting traumatic arterial aneurysm. SAH generally occurs either after relatively severe blunt trauma to the head or as a result of significant shear forces.

Because the cerebral subarachnoid space is large and freely communicates with the basal cisterns and the spinal subarachnoid space, the blood in an SAH can be distributed widely. As a consequence of this wide distribution and because it is generally smaller pial vessels that bleed, SAH rarely accumulates to the extent that it causes clinically important mass effect.

SAH appears to exert its main pathophysiologic effect by causing cerebral vasospasm. SAH is associated with increased cerebrovascular resistance and, consequently, with an increased risk of cerebral ischemia or infarction. In most cases, however, even when cerebral vasospasm can be documented with imaging studies such as transcranial Doppler ultrasound, the vasospasm will not be associated with specific clinical sequelae. In general, SAH is seen in association with other intracranial injuries, especially SDH, cerebral contusion, and intraparenchymal hemorrhage. The presence of SAH may be most important as a marker for severe primary brain injury rather than as a cause of secondary injury in itself.

Because of the presence of the blood in the subarachnoid space, and probably because of associated release of inflammatory mediators from adjacent cells of the pia and arachnoid mater, SAH causes meningeal irritation and clinically mimics many of the symptoms and signs of meningitis.

Clinical Manifestations. Patients with posttraumatic SAH often have other intracranial hemorrhage or parenchymal injuries as well, so they may present with a wide range of symptoms and are those who have minimal if any symptoms and those who are comatose with signs of impending cerebral herniation. As an isolated intracranial lesion, traumatic SAH most commonly causes headache and other signs of meningeal irritation, such as nausea and vomiting, nuchal rigidity, and photophobia. Patients with isolated SAH often have a history of loss of consciousness and sometimes present with depressed mental status, or even coma. Seizures are reported in 2% to 10% of cases. Subhyaloid or preretinal hemorrhages, located just adjacent to the optic nerve head, may also be seen with SAH.

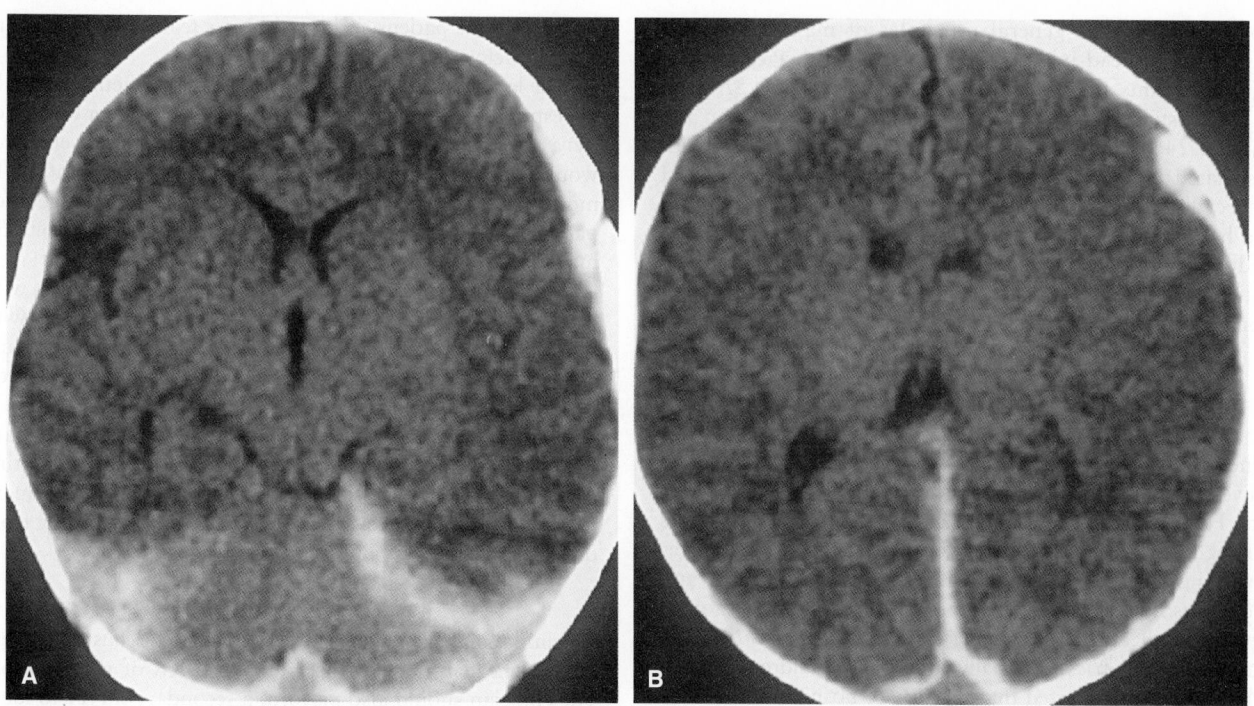

FIGURE 116.15 Subdural hematoma. This 14-day-old patient presented with a complaint of lethargy and vomiting. There was no history of trauma. This head computed tomographic scan shows subdural blood tracking along the tentorium (**A**), in the interhemispheric fissure (**B**), and in the left frontoparietal region (**A** and **B**). There is also some effacement of the sulci and loss of gray–white differentiation. Child abuse was suspected.

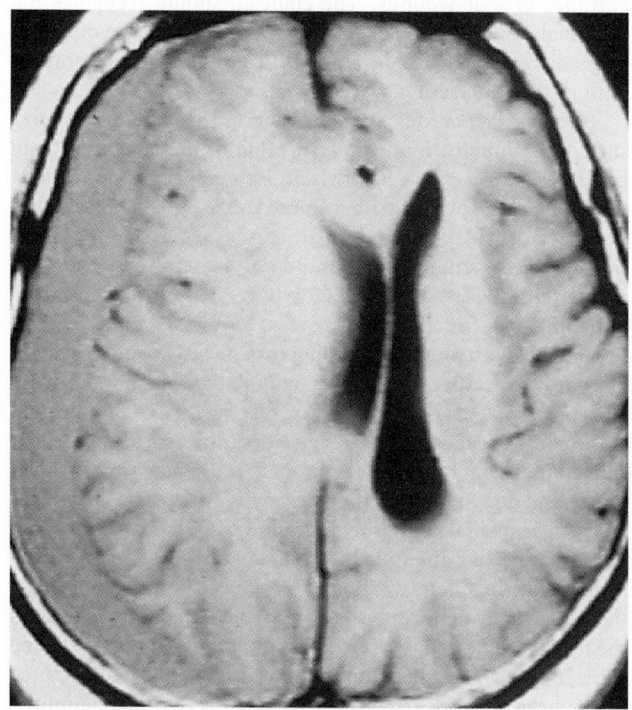

FIGURE 116.16 Subdural hematoma (SDH). This T_1-weighted magnetic resonance image shows the classic appearance of a large acute SDH, with a crescent-shaped extraaxial hematoma that covers the entire right cerebral convexity. There is significant midline shift with compression of the right lateral ventricle and enlargement of the contralateral ventricle, which probably represents obstruction to cerebrospinal fluid outflow. An emergency operative procedure was performed.

Diagnosis. SAH can usually be detected on noncontrast head CT scanning as a collection of hyperdense fluid in the CSF spaces, either in the subarachnoid space overlying the cerebral convexity or in the basal cisterns. Subarachnoid blood overlying the cerebral hemisphere can be distinguished from SDH in that the subarachnoid blood may flow into the depths of the brain sulci, fissures, and cisterns, whereas the subdural space does not penetrate into these depths. Head CT imaging has a sensitivity of only about 90% for detecting SAH, with a lower sensitivity for patients seen more than 24 hours after the SAH began. However, lumbar puncture is not recommended and may be dangerous in the setting of focal intracranial pathology or brain swelling because it may increase the risk of cerebral herniation.

Management. All patients with traumatic SAH should be admitted to the hospital for observation. In most cases, specific therapy directed at the SAH is not required. Although rare cases of traumatic SAH will result from the presence of either a preexisting cerebral aneurysm or a dissecting traumatic intracranial aneurysm, imaging studies aimed at diagnosing cerebral aneurysms are generally not indicated. Such investigations should be considered, however, when traumatic SAH is diagnosed in patients with a suggestive medical or family history, with focal neurologic findings, or with progressive or late deterioration after head injury.

Calcium channel blockers appear to be efficacious for preventing morbidity secondary to vasospasm in patients with spontaneous SAH. However, published data do not suggest a benefit from the use of calcium channel blockers in patients with traumatic SAH; thus, calcium channel blocker therapy is

TRAUMA

not indicated. The general principles of management for patients with head injuries should be followed. Prophylactic anticonvulsants are sometimes used for patients with SAH.

In one study, 24% of patients with traumatic SAH died and another 24% had a poor neurologic outcome. Patients with associated intracranial injuries and those with a larger SAH (especially if it involves both the hemispheric convexities and the basal cisterns) have the worst outcome. Posttraumatic hydrocephalus is sometimes seen as a late complication in patients with traumatic SAH. Patients with minor or no symptoms and small SAH generally do well.

Penetrating Trauma

Penetrating trauma includes injury from sharp objects, such as knives, darts, or animal bites, and from missiles, usually bullets. High-velocity penetration (as with bullets) often occurs through the skull, but lower-velocity penetrating injuries involving such objects as air gun bullets, chopsticks, and toothbrushes have occurred through the orbit or mouth. Penetrating head trauma is far less common than blunt head trauma in pediatrics, especially in younger children. Several urban hospitals reported that the rate of hospital admissions for teenagers shot in the head increased by as much as 10-fold between the 1980s and 1990s. Fortunately, surveillance data reported by the Centers for Disease Control and Prevention have shown a steady decrease in firearm injury rates since then. Nonetheless, there were about 3,000 firearm-related deaths reported in the United States in the year 2005.

Pathophysiology

Penetrating head trauma leads to brain injury by several mechanisms. First, there is direct injury along the path of the penetrating object, with laceration or contusion of neural tissue, and hemorrhage from injured vessels. For low-velocity penetrating injuries (e.g., knife wounds), this may be the primary source of brain injury.

Higher-velocity injuries (from bullets) also cause significant damage because of the shock waves created by the impact of the penetrating object. These shock waves can cause contusions or vascular injury at the sites that had no contact with the penetrating object itself.

Vascular injury may result either from direct laceration or from percussion-related damage. Dissection of an intimal flap, thrombosis of the vessel lumen, or aneurysm formation may result. Ischemia or infarction resulting from these vascular injuries may occur immediately after impact, or they may occur days or even weeks later. Occasional patients become symptomatic with rupture of an aneurysm years after the initial trauma.

Because the skull and dura are violated by the penetrating object, there is direct communication from the CSF spaces or brain to the outside world and, consequently, a risk for intracranial infection. Penetrating objects that pass through the paranasal sinuses or mastoid air cells particularly increase the risk of intracranial infection.

Clinical Manifestations

Patients with penetrating injuries sometimes may present without a clear history, either because the injury was not witnessed or because the patient and/or witnesses fear the repercussions of full disclosure.

The local signs of penetrating injury can sometimes be subtle, especially if the penetrated area is covered either by hair or by a dressing. Without careful exploration, the entrance wound might be mistaken for a superficial scalp laceration. In more obvious cases of penetrating injury, meningeal or parenchymal tissue may be visualized in the wound, or CSF may be oozing.

Signs of neurologic injury are often severe in patients with high-velocity injuries, but they may be subtler in patients with low-velocity injuries. Patients with progressively enlarging intracranial hematomas or worsening brain swelling may deteriorate quickly during the several hours after presentation.

Of course, patients with penetrating head injury may have injury to other body parts as well. Patients with penetrating head injuries sometimes develop a serious coagulopathy, manifesting either with intracranial bleeding or with bleeding from other sites of injury.

Management

The initial management of the patient who has sustained penetrating head trauma focuses on the ABCs of resuscitation. The clinician should also perform a secondary survey to identify serious injuries to other body part that might require rapid intervention. Once the ABCs and the secondary survey have been addressed, attention can be focused on the possible need for brain-specific therapies.

The patient should be examined carefully for evidence of entrance or exit wounds. The clinician should recognize the potential for multiple penetrating wounds or exit wounds in unpredicted locations because of a complicated migratory path of the penetrating object.

Bleeding lacerations should be occluded with direct pressure. Occasionally, immediate suturing of the laceration may be necessary to achieve hemostasis. Other penetrating wounds may simply be covered with a sterile gauze dressing until more definitive debridement and repair can be achieved. Any penetrating objects still in place should not be removed because of the potential for serious hemorrhage if the object is tamponading a lacerated vessel.

Patients with ongoing bleeding may have a coagulopathy. If laboratory results indicate a coagulopathy, infusion of fresh frozen plasma, cryoprecipitate, or platelets may be indicated. Although several case reports have described successful use of recombinant factor VIIa in patients with penetrating head injury and coagulopathy, this therapy is still generally considered experimental. Published data indicate that cervical spine injury is rare in patients with isolated gunshot wounds to the head. Still, the clinician should recognize the possibility that the bullet or penetrating object may have directly penetrated the neck and injured the vertebral column. Furthermore, some cases of penetrating head injury may also include a blunt force to the head or neck that might result in cervical spine injury. Cervical spine precautions should be maintained until the clinician is confident that no neck injury has occurred. In cases in which cervical spine injury cannot be excluded on the basis of clinical findings, radiographs of the cervical spine should be obtained.

Patients with penetrating head injuries generally require prophylactic antibiotic therapy. A first-generation cephalosporin such as cefazolin (30 mg per kg IV; maximum dose 2 g) is usually appropriate.

Most patients with penetrating head injuries are started on prophylactic anticonvulsant therapy [usually with phenytoin (loading dose 10 to 20 mg per kg) or fosphenytoin (loading dose 10 to 20 mg per kg PE)], especially if there is any concern about parenchymal injury or SAH.

Patients with penetrating injuries to the head require immediate head CT scanning to delineate the extent of brain injury and assess for associated intracranial hematomas, brain swelling, and/or mass effect. The head CT scan can also demonstrate the presence of intracranial foreign material.

Patients with intracranial hematomas exerting a mass effect will need an immediate operation to evacuate the hematoma. Patients with large areas of contusion exerting a significant mass effect may also require surgical resection. In addition, most patients with penetrating injuries to the head require prompt operation to debride the infected or contused brain tissue at the entry site. Traditionally, trauma surgeons have performed extensive debridement of deeper tissues along the path of the penetrating object. Many surgeons, however, have reported equally high success rates with more limited debridement. After debridement, the dura must be repaired to achieve a watertight seal.

In general, it is unnecessary to remove deeply embedded foreign material (e.g., bullets) because the risk of infection does not seem to increase when these objects are left in place. Bullets that are lodged in the ventricular system usually are removed, however, because of the potential for outflow obstruction and hydrocephalus if the bullet migrates.

All patients with penetrating head injury require hospitalization. Except in circumstances of superficial penetration with no underlying brain injury, ICU-level monitoring is indicated. Intracranial ICP monitoring is indicated for patients in coma.

Most patients with penetrating head injuries require angiography (conventional, CT, or MRI angiography) to exclude the possibility of traumatic injuries to the cerebral vasculature. Most authors recommend angiography as soon as it can be safely performed.

The prognosis after penetrating head injury depends most commonly on the level of neurologic function at the time of presentation. For patients with severe neurologic dysfunction (GCS scores in the range of 3 to 5), the likelihood of a good functional outcome is low, although occasional patients will do well. Many neurosurgeons will not operate on patients who present with an absence of neurologic function (GCS score of 3 and nonreactive pupils) because the prognosis is so dismal for this subgroup.

For patients with a better neurologic status, the prognosis is influenced by the degree of tissue damage seen on a head CT scan. Lateral-to-lateral injury paths tend to have a worse prognosis than anterior-to-posterior paths. Tracks of injury that crosses the midline or that involves the ventricles are associated with a worse prognosis. Patients with SAH also have a worse prognosis.

SPINAL CORD TRAUMA

Spinal cord injury is rare in pediatrics, occurring in approximately 2 of every 100,000 children per year. Nonetheless, spinal cord injuries, when they do occur, are associated with significant morbidity and mortality, and the consequences of missing early signs of spinal cord injury can be devastating. Furthermore, some clinical evidence suggests that prompt diagnosis and therapy for spinal cord injuries may improve the prognosis.

Anatomy

The spinal cord runs from the foramen magnum, where it extends from the base of the medulla to its distal tip in the upper lumbar region of the spine. The cord consists of an H-shaped central section of gray matter, surrounding white matter that is divided by this "H" into a ventral (motor) compartment and dorsal and lateral (sensory) compartments.

Upper motor neurons originate on one side of the cerebral cortex but then cross to the other side at the level of the medulla before entering the spinal cord. Axons from motor neurons in the left cerebral cortex, therefore, run in the right-sided white matter of the spinal cord and serve the right side of the body. Sensory neurons, in contrast, originate on one side at the level of the dorsal root ganglion and then cross immediately to the other side (at the level of the spinal nerve roots) before entering the cord. Sensory impulses from the right side of the body, therefore, run in the left-sided white matter of the spinal cord before reaching the left cerebral cortex.

The spinal cord is surrounded by three layers of meningeal tissue, which are continuous with the meninges surrounding the brain. As with the cerebral meninges, blood could potentially accumulate in the spaces between these layers of tissue, leading to spinal SDHs or EDHs.

The spinal cord runs in the vertebral canal, protected by the bones of the spinal column, with the vertebral bodies anteriorly and the vertebral arches laterally and posteriorly. Injuries to the spinal cord generally involve some injury to the surrounding spinal column. Because the spinal cord is significantly shorter than the spinal column, injuries at a certain level of the spinal column are associated with spinal cord injuries corresponding to a lower level. A low thoracic spinal column injury, for instance, may be associated with neurologic deficits corresponding to the lumbar cord.

Some unique features of the pediatric spine make spinal cord injury more likely in children. Specifically, the ligaments of the pediatric spine are especially lax, allowing more movement, or subluxation, of vertebrae on one another. In addition, the paraspinous musculature, which provides stabilization and support to the adult spine, is less developed in children. Decreased ossification of the spine, which persists throughout childhood, also makes the cervical spine more pliable. Furthermore, the facet joints between adjacent vertebral bodies are more flattened or horizontal in pediatric patients, which makes subluxation more likely.

Finally, there is excess strain on the upper cervical spine in young children because the head is a proportionately larger component of total body weight. The fulcrum of movement of the cervical spine is at the level of C2–C3 in young children, as opposed to C5–C7 in older children and adults. This feature makes the upper cervical spine especially prone to injury in young children. These "immature" features of the pediatric spine persist to around the age of 8 years. For older children,

TRAUMA

the anatomy of the spine is fairly similar to that seen in adult patients.

Pathophysiology

As with the pathophysiology of brain injury, injuries to the spinal cord can be considered to occur in two phases: primary and secondary. *Primary spinal cord injury* refers to the irreversible neural damage initiated at the time of traumatic impact. *Secondary spinal cord injury* refers to the associated pathophysiologic processes that occur hours to days later, damaging neurons not necessarily injured by the primary impact itself.

Primary injuries to the spinal cord may result from several different mechanisms. Rarely, direct transection of the cord can occur as a result of penetrating injuries to the spine or, more commonly, from bone fragments displaced after fracture or subluxation. More common are bruises or contusions of the spinal cord, which result from compression of the cord by subluxated bone or herniated intervertebral disks. Spinal cord injuries may also result from the application of shear forces to the cord, as when the spine is hyperflexed, hyperextended, or distracted during blunt trauma. The flexible spinal column of the young child makes these types of shear injuries especially common. Finally, the spinal cord can be injured if its vascular supply is disrupted, leading to ischemia and infarction of the cord, sometimes in the absence of any direct traumatic force being applied to the cord itself.

Secondary pathophysiologic changes are believed to cause much of the clinical disease noted after spinal cord injury. Proinflammatory cytokines appear to be released from injured tissue, promoting the development of more inflammation and perhaps stimulating apoptosis, which in itself leads to the release of more injurious cytokines. Much of the more recent research on acute spinal cord injury has focused on efforts to interrupt this injury cascade.

Secondary pathophysiologic changes may also result either from the local mass effect caused by SDH or EDH or from the edema associated with a contused area of cord. Secondary spinal cord injury can also be initiated or exacerbated by any systemic process that leads to hypoxia or ischemia. Areas of spinal cord that are already contused, or partially compressed by local bleeding or edema, may be especially at high risk for ischemic injury.

Clinical Manifestations

Spinal cord injuries are generally associated with significant mechanisms of injury, such as motor vehicle crashes, falls from significant heights, high-impact sports injuries (especially in football, ice hockey, and diving), or child abuse. Patients with injuries to the spinal cord often have evidence of injuries to other organ systems. In particular, there is a high association between head injuries and injuries to the cervical spine and/or spinal cord. Injuries to the thoracic or lumbar spine may also be associated with head injuries, but they are seen more often in the setting of chest or abdominal trauma. Lap belt injuries are a common cause of Chance fractures of the lumbar spine and associated spinal cord injury.

Patients with high cervical cord injuries may sometimes have abnormal vital signs, reflecting an interruption of autonomic impulses to the heart and the vasculature. These patients demonstrate bradycardia and hypotension, along with peripheral vasodilation, a syndrome known as spinal shock. They may also have abnormal or absent respiratory effort. Because most trauma patients with hypotension are hypovolemic and have a reflex tachycardia, those with bradycardia should be strongly suspected of having spinal shock.

Spinal cord injuries should also be suspected in any patient with trauma who complains of decreased motor strength or in whom focal deficits in strength or tone are noted on examination. In the acute setting, severe spinal cord injuries are usually associated with decreased or absent reflexes. Partial injuries to the cord, in contrast, may be associated with initial hypertonia and hyperreflexia. Abnormalities of bladder control and rectal tone may also be noted.

Motor deficits correspond to the spinal roots whose neural impulses are compromised by the spinal cord injury. Most typically, all motor impulses that originate from spinal nerve roots at or below the level of the spinal cord injury are affected. An understanding of the motor deficits after spinal cord injury requires knowledge of the innervation of the important muscle groups of the body. A list of the important muscle groups and the spinal roots that serve them is presented in Table 116.1.

Sensory deficits may also be noted, and these may range from paresthesias to complete loss of sensation. Because sensory impulses are carried in both the dorsal columns and the lateral compartments of the spinal cord, injuries to one of these compartments may lead to partial sensory deficits (e.g., loss of pain and temperature sense from the lateral compartment or loss of joint position sense and vibration sense from the dorsal column) but with other forms of sensation intact for the same body part. A diagram of the body's sensory dermatomes is shown in Appendix D. Often, a well-demarcated sensory "level" of the spinal cord can be identified, below which sensory impulses are absent and above which sensation is intact.

Many injuries to the spinal cord involve solely or predominantly one of the two lateral sides of the cord. Because of the distribution of sensory and motor neurons in the spinal cord, a lesion to the left spinal cord affects left-sided motor strength but right-sided sensation. This classic crossed pattern of sensory and motor deficits is known as the Brown-Sequard syndrome.

Other patterns of neurologic deficits may also be noted. Partial injuries to the spinal cord may result in partial deficits. In some cases of ventral cord injury, for instance, only motor deficits may be observed. Cases of hyperextension injury may cause more severe injury to the central or deep regions of the cord (the gray matter), while sparing the more superficial white matter. This leads to a "paradoxical" pattern of symptoms known as the central cord syndrome, in which the more distal function (served by the white matter) is spared but more proximal function (served by gray matter) is compromised. Finally, occasional patients with more minor injuries to the spinal cord report transient symptoms of paresthesias, numbness, or weakness that may have resolved by the time of evaluation.

TABLE 116.1

MAJOR MUSCLE GROUPS LISTED WITH SPINAL ROOTS AND PERIPHERAL
NERVES THAT SUPPLY THEM

Muscle	Segmental innervation	Peripheral nerve
Diaphragm	C3–C5	Phrenic nerve
Trapezius	C3–C4	Spinal accessory nerve
Deltoid	C5–C6	Axillary nerve
Supraspinatus	C5–C6	Suprascapular nerve
Biceps brachii	C5–C6	Musculocutaneous nerve
Triceps brachii	C6–C8	Radial nerve
Wrist extensors	C6–C7	Radial nerve
Finger extensors	C6–C8	Radial nerve
Wrist flexors	C6, C7–T1	Ulnar, median nerve
Intrinsic hand muscles	C8–T1	Ulnar nerve
Psoas	L1–L2	Psoas nerve
Quadriceps femoris	L2–L4	Femoral nerve
Gastrocnemius	L5–S1	Deep peroneal nerve
Urinary bladder	S2–S4	

Patients with associated head injury may be obtunded and therefore unable to report symptoms of spinal cord injury. However, even in comatose patients, asymmetric motor tone, strength, or reflexes may be noted. Abnormalities of posture or tone may be a clue to the presence of spinal cord injury in these patients. In patients with injuries at the level of C6, for instance, biceps function (with impulses from nerve root C5) is intact but triceps function (impulses from C6) is not, and the elbow is held in tonic flexion.

Patients with injury to the spinal column are at risk for spinal cord injury even if no such injury has occurred at the time of evaluation. Therefore, children with signs of spinal injury, such as pain, tenderness, decreased range of motion, or deformity of the back or neck, must be treated with the utmost caution.

Management

Care for the patient with spinal cord injury begins with the ABCs of resuscitation. This initial resuscitation must be accomplished with meticulous attention to the stabilization of the spine. For older children and adolescents, a semirigid cervical collar or manual inline stabilization should be used. For infants, a semirigid cervical collar might actually be too large and may lead to distraction or hyperextension, which could be deleterious. For some infants, therefore, it may be preferable to immobilize with sandbags on the sides of the head, without using a cervical collar. In addition, the patient should be maintained in a supine position on a backboard so that no undue manipulation of the spine occurs. Because infants have a relatively large occiput, supine positioning on a flat surface may result in flexion of the neck. Proper neutral positioning for these young patients may require that the occiput be allowed to rest at a level slightly lower than the shoulders. Any transfers of the patient from one bed to another or "log rolling" of the patient to examine the back should be done with careful attention to maintaining neutral positioning at all times.

Patients with spinal cord injury require adequate oxygenation, ventilation, and perfusion. Careful attention should be given to positioning of the airway (using the jaw-thrust maneuver rather than the chin-lift maneuver), suctioning if needed, and supplemental oxygenation. The head should never be turned in efforts to clear secretions from the oropharynx; if the patient needs to be turned, a log-roll maneuver should be used. Patients with inadequate respiratory effort require positive-pressure ventilation. Patients with coma, inadequate respiratory effort, or inadequate airway protective reflexes need intubation with mechanical ventilation. When possible, rapid sequence intubation (as previously described; also see Chapter 5) should be performed. If sedating or paralytic agents are to be used, a brief neurologic assessment (see the following text) should precede the administration of the drug if time allows.

The circulatory status of patients with spinal cord injury may be impaired if there are other organ system injuries leading to hemorrhage and hypovolemia. Fluid and blood product resuscitation should be initiated in the usual fashion (see Chapter 105), and the definitive treatment of the hemorrhagic injuries should be pursued. Rare patients with spinal cord injuries have signs of spinal shock, with bradycardia, hypotension, and peripheral vasodilation. These patients may require pressor agents to maintain adequate vascular tone. Primary α-agonists, such as norepinephrine or phenylephrine, are often first-line agents chosen in patients with spinal shock to maximize vasoconstriction with limited effect on cardiac performance.

As soon as possible after an injury, the patient's neurologic status should be recorded so that any early progression of neurologic symptoms can be noted and so that the injuries are not attributed to the emergency medical care provided. For conscious, cooperative patients, the clinician should test motor strength in all four extremities, tone in all extremities, deep tendon reflexes, and rectal tone. The sensory examination should include an assessment of light touch sensation, pain sensation (as from a pinprick), and joint position sense (of fingers and toes). For patients with depressed consciousness, an assessment of tone and reflexes may be all that is possible.

Plain radiographs of the spine should be obtained to evaluate for fractures or subluxations. However, the absence of fractures or subluxations does not eliminate the possibility of spinal cord injury. The syndrome of spinal cord injury without radiographic abnormalities (SCIWORA) is well reported in the literature. SCIWORA has also been documented in adult patients, in whom it appears to be a fairly rare phenomenon. Several series of children with spinal cord injury report that 15% to 20% of cases may be classified as SCIWORA. Children may have an especially high risk for SCIWORA because of the flexibility of the pediatric spinal column, which allows the spinal cord to withstand shear or compressive forces without necessarily causing a fracture. In some cases, the flexible and lax spinal column may sublux transiently, causing a compressive injury to the cord and then reduce back into normal position before radiographs are obtained.

In more recent years, MRI has become a mainstay for the diagnostic evaluation of patients with suspected spinal cord injury. MRI provides detailed images of the spinal cord, which cannot be well imaged by plain radiographs or CT. In cases with more severe clinical findings, spinal cord edema, hemorrhage, or even cord transaction may be seen on MRI. Increasingly, MRI has been used to document spinal cord abnormalities in cases that would be classified as SCIWORA by plain radiographs and CT. Many cases of spinal cord injury with mild or incomplete neurologic deficits are associated with normal MRI findings.

MRI should be performed as soon as possible for patients with progressive neurologic deficits who may have extraaxial mass lesions compressing the spinal cord, such as subdural or epidural hemorrhage, or a herniated intervertebral disk. In other cases, MRI may provide useful diagnostic and perhaps prognostic information, but it is less likely to alter the short-term management.

Specific therapy directed at the spinal cord focuses on the prevention of secondary cord injury. The mainstay of this therapy is careful immobilization. In all cases of spinal cord injury, a neurosurgeon should be consulted immediately. If compressive spinal cord lesions are noted, especially with incomplete but progressing neurologic injury, emergent laminectomy with surgical evacuation of the lesion may be necessary. Displaced fractures or subluxations of the spinal column require immobilization and generally some form of traction (e.g., a halo brace, skull tongs) to reduce them and maintain stability (see Chapter 115 for more details). Some patients with irreducible subluxations or unstable fractures require urgent surgery to achieve reduction. Patients with SCIWORA are often managed with long-term immobilization as well, because they are presumed to have some ligamentous instability of the spine.

High-dose corticosteroid therapy has been widely used since the mid-1980s for the management of patients with spinal cord injury. The use of corticosteroids is based primarily on the results of a multicenter prospective, randomized trial known as the National Acute Spinal Cord Injury Study II (NASCIS II). The NASCIS II trial found that a 24-hour regimen of high-dose corticosteroid therapy significantly improved the outcome for patients treated within 8 hours of injury but not in patients treated later. In more recent years, a number of authors have questioned the validity of the data from NASCIS II, pointing out that the benefit for patients treated within 8 hours was discovered only on post hoc analysis. Subsequent studies intended to replicate the results of NASCIS II have had somewhat mixed results, with one Japanese study showing some benefit to steroid administration whereas another French study showing no benefit. A subsequent trial, known as NASCIS III, found that a 48-hour regimen of high-dose steroids was better than a 24-hour regimen for patients treated 3 or more hours after the injury. In recent years, some retrospective studies have shown better outcomes for patients treated with steroids than those not treated with steroids. All studies found a higher rate of complications, including primarily gastrointestinal, pulmonary, and infectious manifestations, in patients treated with steroids than in patients treated with placebo.

Because of the lack of definitive data regarding the efficacy of steroids in spinal cord injury, most authors consider the use of steroids as an option but not a required standard of care. If steroids are used, they are probably most appropriately reserved for patients with documented motor deficits who can be treated within 8 hours of injury. As per NASCIS II, the dosing regimen is methylprednisolone at an initial IV bolus dose of 30 mg per kg, followed by an infusion of methylprednisolone at 5.4 mg per kg per hour for the subsequent 23 hours. According to the data from NASCIS III, continuation of the infusion for an additional 24 hours (total duration 48 hours) might be considered for patients for whom therapy was initiated between 3 and 8 hours after the injury.

All patients with spinal cord injury need to be admitted to the hospital for careful observation and immobilization. For patients with persistent deficits, a long-term plan for rehabilitation and ongoing medical care will need to be developed.

The prognosis after spinal cord injury depends most commonly on the severity of disease at presentation. Patients with complete loss of function below the injured level have the worst prognosis. In contrast, patients with partial injuries often have significant improvements. Although the initial neurologic status is the best predictor of long-term outcome, MRI findings may also be of prognostic value. Patients with documented transection of the cord clearly have little hope of recovery. Patients with cord hemorrhage, long segments of cord edema, or more proximal locations of cord lesions also tend to have worse prognosis. In patients with cord compression seen on MRI, the extent of cord compression also correlates well with the clinical prognosis. In contrast, patients with minor or no abnormalities on MRI generally do well.

Pediatric patients with spinal cord injuries tend to fare better than their adult counterparts. Most pediatric patients with some useful motor function at the time of presentation regain full function of the compromised motor groups. Children with no motor function distal to the site of injury usually have some permanent disability, although they still often have some improvement after their initial presentation.

Penetrating Spinal Cord Trauma

Penetrating spinal cord trauma is especially rare in pediatrics. It may occur as a result of violent injuries from stabbing or gunshot wounds. Accidental injuries may occur, most commonly from shards of glass that penetrate into the spinal column.

Wounds caused by stabbing or sharp foreign bodies usually involve penetration from the posterolateral aspects of the neck. These injuries generally lead to hemisection of the cord, with only one side of the cord affected. This predilection for unilateral injury probably reflects the fact that the posterior spinous processes and lateral transverse processes form an anatomic "gutter" through which the penetrating object is guided, thereby offering some protection to the opposite side of the cord. Bullets, in contrast, may penetrate the bones of the spinal column and cause less predictable patterns of injury.

Some cases of penetrating spinal cord injury may not be obvious on presentation. Gunshot wounds to the head, for instance, may involve migration of the bullet to the level of the spinal cord, even if the initial trajectory of the bullet might not have suggested cord involvement. Some patients with stab wounds or penetrating glass present with what appear to be innocent lacerations on the neck or back.

Plain radiographs demonstrate the presence of many radiopaque foreign bodies; in some cases, CT may be required to demonstrate less radiodense materials. In cases in which no foreign body is left in the wound, plain radiographic and CT findings may be normal. MRI is the best imaging modality for delineating injury to the cord itself.

When caring for patients with penetrating spinal cord injury, the clinician should recognize the potential for other associated injuries. Penetrating injuries of the neck, for instance, can be associated with injury to the esophagus, airway, or vasculature. Similarly, penetrating trauma to the thoracic spine may be associated with pulmonary, esophageal, or cardiovascular injury.

A neurosurgeon should be consulted in all cases of penetrating cord injury. In some cases, surgical removal of intraspinal foreign bodies, bone fragments, or expanding hematomas is indicated. Surgical repair of ongoing CSF leak from the site of injury may also be indicated. Most penetrating spinal cord injuries are not associated with instability of the spine, even in cases of gunshot wounds. Nonetheless, appropriate immobilization is recommended until spinous instability can be definitively excluded. Prophylactic antibiotic therapy is also recommended for penetrating spinal cord injury. Generally, a first-generation cephalosporin such as cefazolin (30 mg per kg IV; maximum dose 2 g) is preferred.

PERIPHERAL NERVE INJURIES

Pathophysiology

Peripheral nerve injuries in pediatrics usually involve the extremities, most commonly the hand and upper extremity. Most peripheral nerve injuries in pediatrics result from acute traumatic insults. Transection of the nerve may result either from deep soft-tissue lacerations or from severe crush injuries. Rarely, transection of a nerve may also result from a fracture, with laceration of the nerve by a displaced bony fragment.

More commonly, however, displaced fractures or dislocations lead to reversible compression injuries to the nerve. Nerve compression may also occur in the absence of acute trauma, usually because of tight anatomic compartments that exert constant pressure on the nerve (carpal tunnel syndrome is one common example).

Peripheral nerve injuries may be graded in terms of the severity of the clinical course. The mildest form of nerve injury is known as *neurapraxia*, which refers to nerve conduction impairment without structural injury to the axon itself. Neurapraxia commonly results from a situation of transient compression or ischemia, as when a patient complains that a limb has "fallen asleep." The numbness and paresthesias reflect a rapidly reversible physiologic conduction block. If biopsy of the nerve were performed in this situation, no histologic abnormalities would be expected.

More severe cases of neurapraxia may be associated with symptoms that persist for as long as several months. In these cases, histologic examination reveals focal demyelination in the injured area of the nerve, but with no injury to the axon itself. In general, as long as the axon itself is not injured, full recovery can be expected.

Axonotmesis is a more severe injury to peripheral nerve, involving injury to the axon itself, but with preservation of the surrounding connective tissue of the nerve sheath. Axonotmesis generally results from crush injuries to the nerve. Recovery of peripheral nerve function is likely to occur well, although it will progress slowly, with lengthening of the nerve axon from its proximal stump progressing at a rate of approximately 1 to 4 mm per day. Distal nerve lesions, near the target muscles or sensory regions, are associated with earlier and more complete recovery of function than do more proximal lesions.

The most severe form of nerve injury is known as neurotmesis, which involves injury both to the nerve axon and to the surrounding connective tissue. Neurotmesis usually results from direct laceration to the nerve or, rarely, from severe crush injuries. Because there is no intact nerve sheath to guide the development of the regenerating proximal nerve, spontaneous recovery of function is unlikely and surgical repair is required.

Clinical Manifestations

Significant peripheral nerve injuries are usually seen in association with other obvious signs of traumatic injury, such as a soft-tissue laceration, crush injuries to the extremity, or fracture. In some cases, however, such as with sudden stretches of the brachial plexus ("burners" or "stingers"), with repetitive microtrauma or with anatomic compressive lesions (as seen in carpal tunnel syndrome), the symptoms of peripheral nerve injury may be the primary complaint.

The cardinal symptoms of peripheral nerve injury are disturbances of sensory or motor function in the distribution of the nerve. Appropriate diagnosis of peripheral nerve injury requires an understanding of the anatomic distribution of sensory and motor functions of the major peripheral nerves. A full description of this clinical anatomy is beyond the scope of this discussion, but a summary of the motor functions of the major peripheral nerves is presented in Table 116.1.

Disturbances of sensation may include paresthesias, pain (which may be described as sharp, burning, or stabbing), or numbness. In some cases, the patient may not report a sensory deficit, but sensory abnormalities are noted on examination. A gross assessment of sensory function can be obtained simply by testing the patient's ability to recognize light touch stimuli in the distribution of the nerve in question.

TRAUMA

A more sensitive test for identifying disturbances in sensory function is two-point discrimination. Although instruments for assessing two-point discrimination are commercially available, in common practice, a paper clip is often used. The paper clip should be unfolded so that the two ends are in close proximity, with a distance of approximately 1 cm in between. The patient should then be briefly trained on an uninjured part of the body to differentiate between being touched with one or two points of the paper clip simultaneously. Once it is determined that the patient can reliably perform the task, the injured area should be assessed.

The two points must touch the skin simultaneously, and they must occur in the same axial line. If the patient is able to successfully discriminate one- and two-point stimuli, the distance between the two ends of the paper clip can be decreased successively to find the patient's threshold for discrimination. A hand with normal sensation should be able to distinguish between two points that are 2 to 5 mm apart at the fingertips, 7 to 10 mm at the base of the palm, and 7 to 12 mm on the dorsum of the hand. More proximal parts of the upper extremity may have even less sensitive discriminatory abilities.

A problem occasionally arises in trying to assess sensory function in a patient who is unresponsive or who cannot communicate with the examiner. In these cases, a test of sympathetic innervation, such as the O'Riain wrinkle test, may be useful. To perform this test, the patient's hand is immersed in a warm water bath for approximately 20 minutes. Normal digital pulps will wrinkle; fingers with disrupted sympathetic innervation will not wrinkle.

Appropriate motor testing of the peripheral nerves depends on the isolation of muscle activity that reflects the peripheral nerve in question. The clinician must be careful to recognize that a patient will compensate for a motor deficit by using other motor groups to accomplish the same task. Motor function can be assessed by examining not only active motor strength but also resting tone and, for more chronic injuries, muscle bulk.

"Burners" or "stingers" are a special form of peripheral nerve injury that result from trauma to the neck and shoulder, usually in football players after contact with another player. The injury leads to immediate onset of a burning paresthesia that radiates down the arm, often associated with ipsilateral arm weakness. The symptoms usually resolve over the course of several minutes. Although the exact pathophysiology of burners and stingers is not well understood, they appear to result from stretch of the cervical nerve roots and brachial plexus and/or compression of the nerve roots as they course through narrow cervical neural foramina. The differential diagnosis for these injuries should also include spinal cord contusion, although the characteristic involvement of a single arm, the rapid resolution of symptoms, and the absence of associated cervical spine injury help distinguish burners and stingers from spinal cord injury.

Management

Clean lacerations to a primary nerve are often repaired primarily. There is some evidence to indicate that recovery of function is better if the nerve is repaired within 48 hours of injury. Crush injuries to peripheral nerves are often repaired

secondarily, several days or weeks after the injury. For these cases, many surgeons believe that delayed repair allows better debridement of devitalized tissue and easier identification of injured nerve tissue that needs to be resected. In all cases in which transection of a peripheral nerve is suspected, prompt consultation with an appropriate surgical consultant is indicated so that a decision can be made about the appropriate timing of repair.

Injuries to peripheral nerve associated with fracture or dislocation generally improve after the orthopedic injury is reduced. If there is any question about the recovery after reduction, nerve function should be carefully followed.

For burners and stingers, no diagnostic tests are routinely necessary, but imaging of the cervical spine is appropriate if there are clinical signs to indicate possible cervical spine or spinal cord abnormalities. Patients with burners and stingers should be counseled to avoid sports activities until the symptoms have fully resolved, and they should be informed about the risk of recurrent injury. Follow-up with a sports medicine or orthopedics specialist for further diagnostic evaluation, strength training, and possible orthotics may also be helpful.

Nerve compression syndromes not associated with acute traumatic injuries, such as carpal tunnel syndrome, can generally be treated with rest and nonsteroidal antiinflammatory medications. Splinting may also be indicated for some syndromes. In all cases, appropriate follow-up should be arranged so that the patient can be referred for further interventions, if necessary.

The prognosis after peripheral nerve injury clearly depends on the severity of the injury. Compressive lesions without transection of the nerve have a better prognosis, with full recovery expected in all but the most severe or most chronic cases. With transections of the nerve, however, there is often some degree of permanent disability. In general, those lesions resulting from clean lacerations that can be repaired primarily have a somewhat better prognosis. Children, in general, have a better prognosis after peripheral nerve injury than do adults. In some cases, remarkable recoveries after severe crush injuries to the nerve have been reported.

Suggested Readings

American Association for the Surgery of Trauma, Child Neurology Society, International Society for Pediatric Neurosurgery, International Trauma Anesthesia and Critical Care Society. Guidelines for the acute medical management of severe traumatic brain injury in infants, children, and adolescents. *J Trauma* 2003;54(6)(suppl):S235–S310.

Aval SM, Durand P Jr, Shankwiler JA. Neurovascular injuries to the athlete's shoulder, part I. *J Am Acad Orthop Surg* 2007;15(4):249–256.

Balmer B, Boltshauser E, Altermatt S, et al. Conservative management of significant epidural haematomas in children [published online ahead of print November 5, 2005]. *Childs Nerv Syst* 2006;22(4):363–367.

Bourgoin A, Albanèse J, Léone M, et al. Effects of sufentanil or ketamine administered in target-controlled infusion on the cerebral hemodynamics of severely brain-injured patients. *Crit Care Med* 2005;33(5):1109–1113.

Bowman SM, Bird TM, Aitken ME, et al. Trends in hospitalizations associated with pediatric traumatic brain injuries. *Pediatrics* 2008;122(5):988–993.

Bracken MB, Shepard MJ, Holford TR, et al. Methylprednisolone or tirilazad mesylate administration after acute spinal cord injury: 1-year follow-up. Results of the Third National Acute Spinal Cord Injury Randomized Controlled Trial. *J Neurosurg* 1998;89:699–706.

Bramwell KJ, Haizlip J, Pribble C, et al. The effect of etomidate on intracranial pressure and systemic blood pressure in pediatric patients with severe traumatic brain injury. *Pediatr Emerg Care* 2006;22(2):90–93.

Centers for Disease Control and Prevention. Sports-related recurrent brain injuries—United States. *MMWR Morbid Mortal Wkly Rep* 1997;46:224–227.

Cooper DJ, Myles PS, McDermott FT, et al. Prehospital hypertonic saline resuscitation of patients with hypotension and severe traumatic brain injury: a randomized controlled trial. *JAMA* 2004;291(11):1350–1357.

De Souza M, Moncure M, Lansford T, et al. Nonoperative management of epidural hematomas and subdural hematomas: is it safe in lesions measuring one centimeter or less? *J Trauma* 2007;63(2):370–372.

Edwards P, Arango M, Balica L, et al. Final results of MRC CRASH, a randomised placebo-controlled trial of intravenous corticosteroid in adults with head injury—outcomes at 6 months. *Lancet* 2005;365(9475):1957–1959.

Erlanger D, Kaushik T, Cantu R. Symptom-based assessment of the severity of a concussion. *J Neurosurg* 2003;98:477–484.

Feldman KW, Bethel R, Shugerman RP, et al. The cause of infant and toddler subdural hemorrhage: a prospective study. *Pediatrics* 2001;108:636–646.

Guskiewicz KM, McCrea M, Marshall SW, et al. Cumulative effects associated with recurrent concussion in collegiate football players: the NCAA Concussion Study. *JAMA* 2003;290:2549–2555.

Hayashi T, Kameyama M, Imaizumi S, et al. Acute epidural hematoma of the posterior fossa—cases of acute clinical deterioration. *Am J Emerg Med* 2007;25(9):989–995.

Hendey GW, Wolfson AB, Mower WR, et al. National Emergency X-Radiography Utilization Study Group. Spinal cord injury without radiographic abnormality: results of the National Emergency X-Radiography Utilization Study in blunt cervical trauma. *J Trauma-Injury Infect Crit Care* 2002;53(1):1–4.

Hirsch W, Beck R, Behrmann C, et al. Reliability of cranial CT versus intracerebral pressure measurement for the evaluation of generalised cerebral oedema in children. *Pediatr Radiol* 2000;30:439–443.

Hosalkar HS, Matzon JL, Chang B. Nerve palsies related to pediatric upper extremity fractures. *Hand Clin* 2006;22(1):87–98.

Hutchison JS, Ward RE, Lacroix J, et al. Hypothermia therapy after traumatic brain injury in children. *N Engl J Med* 2008;358(23):2447–2456.

Inglese M, Makani S, Johnson G, et al. Diffuse axonal injury in mild traumatic brain injury: a diffusion tensor imaging study. *J Neurosurg* 2005;103(2):298–303.

Kan P, Amini A, Hansen K, et al. Outcomes after decompressive craniectomy for severe traumatic brain injury in children. *J Neurosurg* 2006;105(5)(suppl):337–342.

Kelly JD, Aliquo D, Sitler MR, et al. Association of burners with cervical canal and foraminal stenosis. *Am J Sports Med* 2000;28:214–217.

Kim TW, Lee JK, Moon KS, et al. Penetrating gunshot injuries to the brain. *J Trauma* 2007;62(6):1446–1451.

Langlois JA, Rutland-Brown W, Thomas KE. The incidence of traumatic brain injury among children in the United States: differences by race. *J Head Trauma Rehabil* 2005;20(3):229–238.

Lescot T, Degos V, Zouaoui A, et al. Opposed effects of hypertonic saline on contusions and noncontused brain tissue in patients with severe traumatic brain injury. *Crit Care Med* 2006;34(12):3029–3033.

Liao CC, Lui TN, Chen LR, et al. Spinal cord injury without radiological abnormality in preschool-aged children: correlation of magnetic resonance imaging findings with neurological outcomes. *J Neurosurg* 2005;103(1)(suppl):17–23.

Lovell MR, Pardini JE, Welling J, et al. Functional brain abnormalities are related to clinical recovery and time to return-to-play in athletes. *Neurosurgery* 2007;61(2):352–359; discussion 359–360.

Maas AI, Steyerberg EW, Butcher I, et al. Prognostic value of computerized tomography scan characteristics in traumatic brain injury: results from the IMPACT study. *J Neurotrauma* 2007;24(2):303–314.

Mannion RJ, Cross J, Bradley P, et al. Mechanism-based MRI classification of traumatic brainstem injury and its relationship to outcome. *J Neurotrauma* 2007;24(1):128–135.

Marmarou A, Signoretti S, Fatouros PP, et al. Predominance of cellular edema in traumatic brain swelling in patients with severe head injuries. *J Neurosurg* 2006;104(5):720–730.

Mastrapa TL, Fernandez LA, Alvarez MD, et al. Depressed skull fracture in ping pong: elevation with Medeva extractor [published online ahead of print May 8, 2007]. *Childs Nerv Syst* 2007;23(7):787–790.

McCrea M, Guskiewicz KM, Marshall SW. Acute effects and recovery time following concussion in collegiate football players: the NCAA Concussion Study. *JAMA* 2003;290:2556–2563.

McCrory P, Johnston K, Meeuwisse W, et al. Summary and agreement statement of the 2nd International Conference on Concussion in Sport, Prague 2004. *Br J Sports Med* 2005;39(4):196–204.

McKinley W, Santos K, Meade M, et al. Incidence and outcomes of spinal cord injury clinical syndromes. *J Spinal Cord Med* 2007;30(3):215–224.

Miyanji F, Furlan JC, Aarabi B, et al. Acute cervical traumatic spinal cord injury: MR imaging findings correlated with neurologic outcome—prospective study with 100 consecutive patients [published online ahead of print April 12, 2007]. *Radiology* 2007;243(3):820–827.

Murano T, Mohr AM, Lavery RF, et al. Civilian craniocerebral gunshot wounds: an update in predicting outcomes. *Am Surg* 2005;71(12):1009–1014.

Ng I, Lim J, Wong HB. Effects of head posture on cerebral hemodynamics: its influences on intracranial pressure, cerebral perfusion pressure, and cerebral oxygenation. *Neurosurgery* 2004;54(3):593–597; discussion 598.

Papadopoulos SM, Selden NR, Quint DJ, et al. Immediate spinal cord decompression for cervical spinal cord injury: feasibility and outcome. *J Trauma-Injury Infect Crit Care* 2002;52(2):323–332.

SAFE Study Investigators; Australian and New Zealand Intensive Care Society Clinical Trials Group; Australian Red Cross Blood Service, et al. Saline or albumin for fluid resuscitation in patients with traumatic brain injury. *N Engl J Med* 2007;357(9):874–884.

Seelig J, Becker D, Miller J, et al. Traumatic acute subdural hematoma: major mortality reduction in comatose patients treated within 4 hours. *N Engl J Med* 1981;304:1511–1518.

Tung GA, Kumar M, Richardson RC, et al. Comparison of accidental and nonaccidental traumatic head injury in children on noncontrast computed tomography. *Pediatrics* 2006;118(2):626–633.

Vignes JR, Jeelani NU, Jeelani A, et al. Growing skull fracture after minor closed-head injury. *J Pediatr* 2007;151(3):316–318.

Visocchi M, Chiaretti A, Genovese O, et al. Haemodynamic patterns in children with posttraumatic diffuse brain swelling. A preliminary study in 6 cases with neuroradiological features consistent with diffuse axonal injury [published online ahead of print February 16, 2007]. *Acta Neurochir (Wien)* 2007;149(4):347–356.

Young KD, Okada PJ, Sokolove PE, et al. A randomized, double-blinded, placebo-controlled trial of phenytoin for the prevention of early posttraumatic seizures in children with moderate to severe blunt head injury. *Ann Emerg Med* 2004;43(4):435–446.

CHAPTER 117 ■ EYE TRAUMA

ALEX V. LEVIN, MD, MHSC, FRCSC

When faced with a child who has sustained eye trauma, the pediatric emergency physician must keep in mind four important basic principles:

1. The management of life-threatening systemic illness or central nervous system trauma must always take precedence over the eye injury. Even the most serious eye injury may be acutely "neglected" if urgent lifesaving procedures are underway.
2. Ensure the structural integrity of the eyeball (i.e., rule out ruptured globe).
3. Check the vision in both the injured and uninjured eye.
4. When in doubt, and when indicated, seek ophthalmology consultation.

This chapter is designed to assist the pediatric emergency physician in the diagnosis and management of basic and uncomplicated ocular injuries, yet, it is important to recognize when ophthalmology consultation is necessary. Even with the increasing number of emergency departments (EDs) that have slit lamp biomicroscopy available to the nonophthalmologist, the ophthalmologist is more expert at using the slit lamp and has experience with a wide array of other diagnostic tools that allow viewing and recognition of intraocular injuries that can not otherwise be seen. For example, when trauma damages the retina, it often does so at the edges of the retina. This area is out of the field of view of the direct ophthalmoscope and requires indirect ophthalmoscopy to be viewed adequately. Most children who sustain high-risk blunt trauma to the eye, even in the absence of injury that can be seen on external examination, warrant a dilated retinal examination by an ophthalmologist, using the indirect ophthalmoscope. If in-house ophthalmology consultation is not readily available, it is important to identify an ophthalmologist in the community who is comfortable examining children for outpatient follow-up.

HISTORY

Certain questions help identify possible intraocular injury. What was the child's prior visual status? If the child was previously known to have poor vision in the eye, then less concern will be elicited if the same poor vision is noted after the trauma. Has the child ever had a prior eye examination, and if so, what were the results? Has the child ever had a patch over one eye for an extended period? This history would indicate that the child previously had poor vision secondary to amblyopia in the eye that was *not* patched. Has the child ever had eye muscle surgery? Children who have had strabismus are at a greater risk of developing amblyopia. Therefore, poor vision in one eye is more common. Does the patient wear glasses? If so, the glasses should be worn when visual acuity is tested. Does the patient wear contact lenses? If so, removal of the contact lenses may be necessary.

Additional questions include the following: What was the nature of the injury? How hard was the eye struck? Certain types of trauma have a particularly high risk for causing intraocular damage: significant blunt impact directly to the eyeball (e.g., fist, ball), projectiles, and sharp implements (e.g., pencil, stick). Different antibiotic coverage may be necessary for suspected contamination (e.g., *Bacillus* species) by soil or other outdoor implements. Hammering is a particularly high-risk behavior for causing intraocular foreign bodies. If an intraocular foreign body is suspected, the clinician must establish by history whether it is metallic. This may influence the choice of imaging and treatment (e.g., magnets are sometimes used by the ophthalmologist during surgical removal of a metallic intraocular foreign body).

EXAMINATION

An attempt should always be made to assess the visual acuity in the injured eye before proceeding with the rest of the eye examination. Some patients may be unable to perform this task because of eye pain, noncompliance, an inability to open swollen lids, or obtundation from accompanying head trauma. At the very least, even if the eyelids remain closed, the physician can test for light perception. By shining a bright penlight or direct ophthalmoscope in the direction of the eyeball through the closed eyelid, the physician can ask the patient to indicate whether he or she perceives the additional light on that side. Even without a patient response, a reflex contraction of the lids may be seen, indicating light perception.

If the patient is able to exhibit a greater degree of compliance, the examiner may ask the patient to count fingers that are held before the affected eye at varying distances. The maximum distance at which these fingers can be counted should be noted on the chart (e.g., counting fingers at 4 feet). If the patient cannot stand but can identify letters or numbers, a commercially available near card or any other reading material (the font isize on this page is approximately 20/60 vision) can be used to assess the quality of near vision. Very few injuries cause abnormal distance vision but normal near vision. Normal near vision usually indicates that the patient has not sustained a significant ocular injury that is impairing vision at that time. The subnormal distance vision may simply be due to uncorrected myopia or other refractive errors.

If the patient is able to comply, the examiner should try to obtain a standard visual acuity, using a distance chart. Letter charts should be used only if the child is known to be able to accurately identify all letters either by parental report or by walking up to the distance chart and identifying them at close proximity. If the child has any trouble with letters, a matching chart or a picture chart can be used (see Chapter 127).

The patient's visual acuity in each eye should be tested. The presence of bilaterally poor vision in a patient with unilateral eye trauma suggests that the cause of the poor vision is unrelated to the trauma. The eye that is not being tested should be covered well to prevent any conscious or unconscious attempt on the part of the patient to peek around the obstruction. Children will naturally try to do this if their better eye is being covered. To ensure the child is actually viewing the chart with the eye that is being tested, the examiner should stand by the chart, facing the patient, indicating which letters are to be read while observing the patient's compliance (see Chapter 127).

If a patient demonstrates poor vision in the traumatized eye, the clinician can readily establish whether this deficit is related to the trauma or uncorrected refractive error (i.e., a need for glasses). When a person looks through a pinhole and experiences improvement in performance on visual acuity testing, he or she must have an uncorrected refractive error as the cause of the initially tested poor vision. For example, if a patient comes in with a traumatized eye that is able to read only 20/400 (needs to stand at 20 feet to see what a normal person can see at 400 feet) but then improves to 20/25 by using a pinhole device, the patient has not sustained visual impairment from the ocular injury. Rather, the patient simply needs glasses. The maximum vision obtainable through a pinhole may be only 20/25 to 20/30 due to optical aberrations inherent in the pinhole test. Although commercial pinhole devices for testing vision can be used, the test can also be conducted by poking holes through opaque paper or cardboard with an 18-gauge needle. A cluster of five or six holes may be easier for the patient to use.

After visual acuity has been established, an attempt may then be made to examine the eyeball. By using a step-by-step anatomic approach, the examiner should first inspect the periorbital tissues and eyelids for the presence of ecchymosis, lacerations, and ptosis. Eye muscle movements (see Chapter 24) and the anterior surface of the eye should be evaluated next. All attempts should be made to examine these structures without touching or upsetting the child, particularly if by history or examination a ruptured globe is suspected. An upset child creates a Valsalva maneuver while crying, which may lead to extrusion of intraocular contents out of a ruptured globe. If a ruptured globe or hyphema has been ruled out, the examiner may proceed with full eye examination, including pharmacologic dilation of the pupil. Regimens for pupil dilation are suggested in Table 117.1.

TABLE 117.1

EMERGENCY DEPARTMENT OCULAR DILATING REGIMEN[a]

Phenylephrine 2.5%	For brown irides replace tropicamide with cyclopentolate 1%
Tropicamide 1%	

[a]May repeat regimen in 30 minutes if needed. Instilling proparacaine or tetracaine prior to these dilating drops will enhance the dilation effect.

A red reflex should be documented unless the vision is normal and there is no concern about a possible eye injury. By standing approximately 1 m away from the patient, the examiner should shine the largest available circle of white light from the direct ophthalmoscope onto the patient's face such that both eyes are illuminated simultaneously (see Chapter 24, Fig. 24.6). The focusing dial is then spun until the patient's face and eyes come into focus. The patient should be instructed to look at the observer. The room light should be turned out to encourage maximum physiologic pupillary dilation. The red reflex is usually orange–red or yellow–orange (see Chapter 24, Fig. 24.6); only rarely is it actually red. The absence of a red reflex (black reflex) in its entirety or in part of the pupil may indicate an obstruction within the eyeball to the passage of light, such as a corneal scar, cataract, or hemorrhage within the eyeball. A darkened reflex may also be caused by small pupils or misaligned eyes (see Chapter 24, Fig. 24.6). Rechecking the reflex after pharmacologic dilation may be helpful in these situations. A white reflex indicates white intraocular pathology such as a corneal scar, cataract, coloboma, or retinoblastoma (a malignant eye tumor). An abnormal red reflex (with the exception of a dark reflex that clears with pupil dilation) always requires ophthalmology consultation.

The emergency physician often finds the direct ophthalmoscope to be useful for the identification of possible papilledema or retinal hemorrhages in the setting of acute central nervous system injury, the latter being particularly concerning for the possibility of abusive head injury. Pupillary size should be maximized by the use of dim ambient illumination and the small white circle direct ophthalmoscope beam. Pharmacologic agents (Table 117.1) can be used to dilate the pupil and improve the view. The patient should be encouraged to fixate on a distant target. The examiner must avoid inadvertently lowering his or her head in a way that obstructs the eye that is not being examined, therefore, obstructing the fixation of that eye (Fig. 117.1A). The patient would then begin looking elsewhere, making adequate examination of the optic nerve difficult. To avoid this scenario, the examiner should sit or stand such that his or her head is at level with and parallel to the patient's head rather than leaning over (Fig. 117.1B). If the examiner is standing above the patient, the patient's head can be tilted away from the examiner such that it becomes parallel to the examiner's head when he or she leans over to look into the eye (Fig. 117.1C).

The ophthalmoscope may be used with or without the examiner's glasses (or contact lenses) in place. The examiner holds the direct ophthalmoscope approximately 30 to 60 cm from the patient while standing at his or her side, holding the instrument in the same hand and in front of the same eye that corresponds to the eye to be examined (i.e., examiner's right hand and right eye used to examine patient's right eye). The focusing dial should be set at zero, and a red reflex should be obtained. Then the examiner approaches the patient slowly until a blood vessel is seen within the red reflex. As the examiner moves closer, he or she should follow the blood vessels while turning the focusing wheel with the forefinger to keep the blood vessels in focus. The apex of any branching blood vessel points in the direction of the optic nerve head (Fig. 117.2, see also color plate). The optic nerve head (disc) is best found in this manner. When the disc is located and in focus, the examiner's forehead should be no more than 3 to 6 cm away from the patient's forehead.

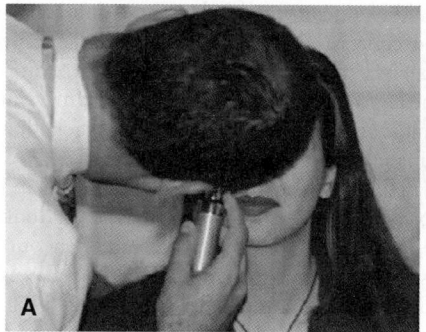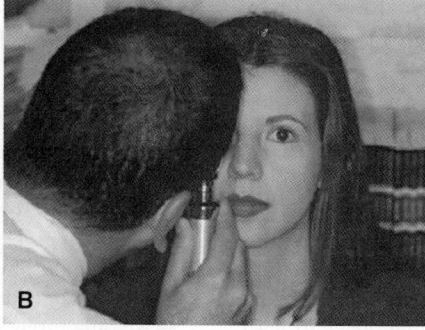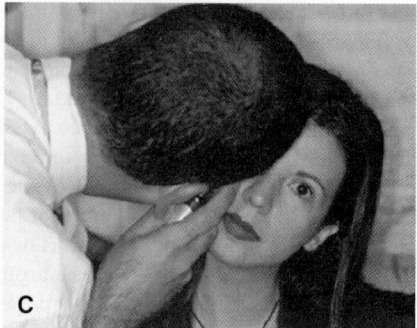

FIGURE 117.1 Use of the direct ophthalmoscope. **A:** Examiner is in incorrect position. His head is blocking patient's ability to fixate with the left eye during examination of right eye. By placing his head at level of patient's (**B**) or by tilting patient's head away (**C**), the left eye can continue to fixate.

Two common scenarios prove particularly difficult for those less familiar with direct ophthalmoscopy. If the pupil is too small relative to the light beam from the direct ophthalmoscope, not all the light will enter the pupil. Rather, some light will reflect off the iris, resulting in glare. In this situation, ensure that the smallest diameter white circle projected by the direct ophthalmoscope is being used and the pupil size is maximized by either turning off the ambient light or using pharmacologic pupil dilation. Examining infants is particularly difficult because they cannot follow the direction to fixate on one spot during the examination. If the baby is placed on an examining table or in the parent's arms in the supine position, the examiner can approach from the side as described above: lean over the child, obtain a red reflex, and then move to the usual working distance described previously. Do not chase the roving eyeball of the child. The physician should "hold his ground," staying motionless about 45 degrees away from the child's midline visual axis approximately 3 to 6 cm away from the face. Because the optic nerve head is a physiologic blind spot in the visual field, the child will eventually adopt a position to avoid the light by placing their blind spot (i.e., the optic disc) in the path of the light source, at which time the optic nerve will have come into view.

The optic nerve should be yellow–orange to pink (Fig. 117.2, see also color plate). Centrally, a white depression called the *optic cup* is apparent. Normally, this depression may be barely visible or may occupy up to 50% to 60% of the optic nerve surface area. Both optic nerves usually have symmetric cup sizes. The retinal blood vessels usually emerge from the center of the cup. In papilledema (Fig. 117.3, see also color plate), the edges of the optic nerve become indistinct and difficult to differentiate from the surrounding retina. The blood vessels may become engorged and tortuous. There may be associated hemorrhages on the optic nerve surface or immediately surrounding the disc. Yellow–white exudate may also be seen within the retina. The optic nerve cup may not be

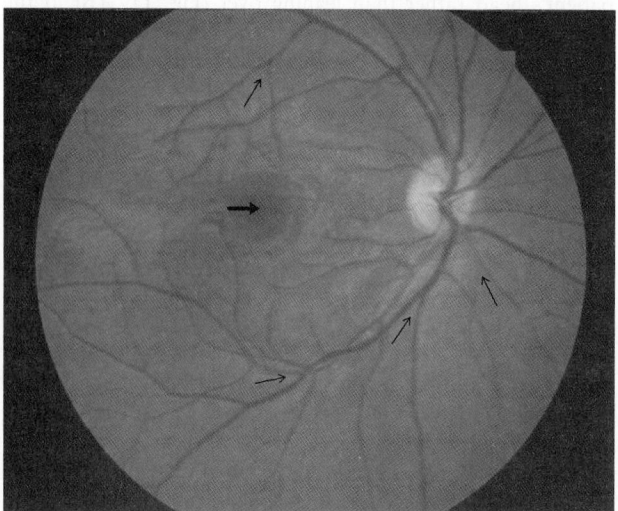

FIGURE 117.2 Normal right retina as viewed by indirect ophthalmoscope. Central dark area *(thick arrow)* represents fovea. Note that the apex of the branch point of the blood vessels *(thin arrows)* always points back toward the direction of the optic nerve head.

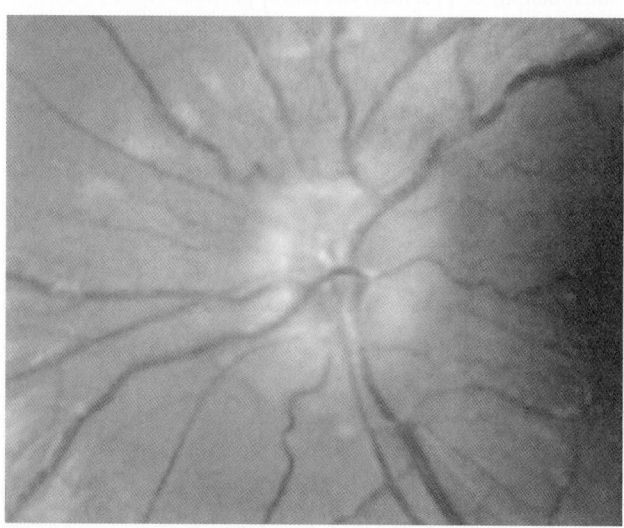

FIGURE 117.3 Papilledema. Note blurred disc margins and loss of view of blood vessels on disc.

identifiable because of swelling of the neurons. It may be difficult to focus on the optic nerve surface and the retina at the same time because of the elevation of the optic nerve. Perhaps the most important and distinguishing sign to aid in the recognition of papilledema is the disappearance of the vessels on the disc surface as they course among opaque edematous neurons. Papilledema may at times be subtle. If any question exists in the mind of the examiner that papilledema may be present, ophthalmology consultation is appropriate.

Papilledema is almost always bilateral. Presence of unilateral papilledema suggests an ipsilateral orbital trauma, such as an orbital hemorrhage, orbital tumor, or direct injury to the optic nerve. The optic nerve can be injured from blunt trauma without a penetrating orbital injury. The optic nerve can be injured even by severe blunt trauma to the frontal bone by which forces are carried to the optic foramen surrounding the optic nerve as it enters the orbit.

If the eye has been traumatized such that the patient is unable to voluntarily open the eyelids, attempts should be made to assist the patient in doing so. A warm compress may be gently applied to the eyelashes to loosen any crust or discharge that may be holding the eyelashes together. When opening the eyelids, it is essential to avoid pressure on the eyeball, which might lead to extrusion of intraocular contents via an underlying ruptured globe. By placing his or her thumbs on the supraorbital and infraorbital ridges while exerting pressure against the underlying bone, the examiner's thumbs can then be pulled away from each other such that the eyelids are separated (Fig. 117.4). Various commercially available speculums can also be used to open swollen eyelids (Fig. 117.5). A drop of topical anesthetic (e.g., tetracaine, proparacaine) should be instilled before placing a speculum or retractor. The Desmarres retractor is perhaps one of the least uncomfortable yet effective means for opening swollen lids. After instillation of a topical ophthalmic anesthetic, the

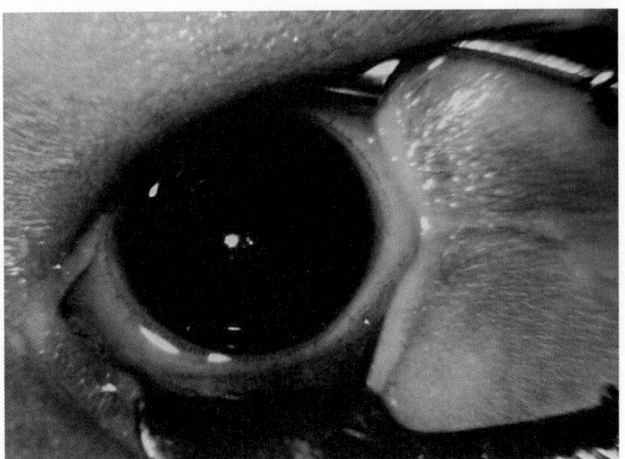

FIGURE 117.5 Commercially available eye speculum in place.

cupped end of the retractor (Fig. 117.6A) is slipped under the upper lid and gently retracted with the handle parallel to the forehead (Fig. 117.6B). A second retractor can be simultaneously applied to the lower lid to further improve exposure. Paper clips can also be bent to create a retractor (see Chapter 127, Fig. 127.3).

In the trauma setting, with enough lid swelling that precludes a readily available view of the eyeball using the techniques previously described, it is probably safer to refer the patient for an ophthalmology consultation unless the emergency physician is comfortable with the recommended techniques. Risking the use of a speculum or retractor may upset the patient and cause a struggle that could also contribute to disruption of the intraocular contents in the presence of a ruptured globe. Even the ophthalmologist may choose to abandon

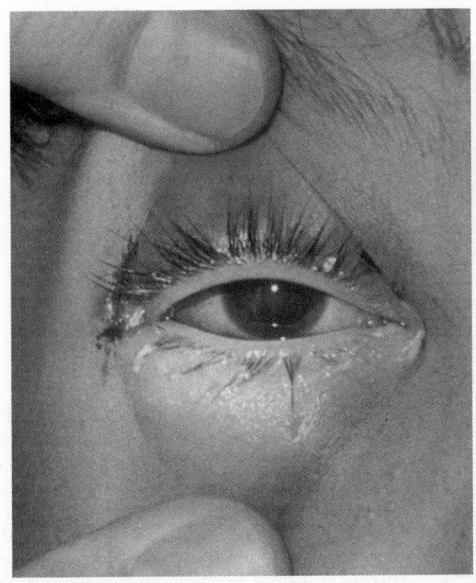

FIGURE 117.4 Opening swollen eyelids manually from the superior and inferior orbital rims.

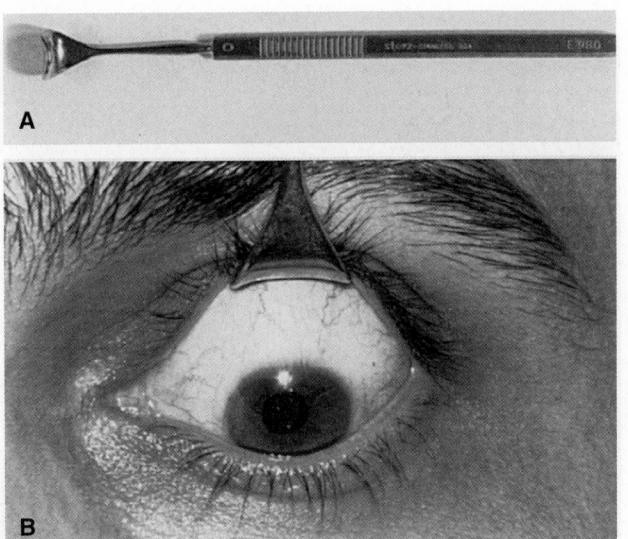

FIGURE 117.6 **A:** Desmarres retractor. **B:** Desmarres retractor in use to elevate upper lid.

TRAUMA

such attempts and proceed directly to an examination under anesthesia if the risk of ruptured globe is believed to be high.

RUPTURED GLOBE

Clinical Manifestations

Laceration or puncture of the cornea and/or sclera creates a ruptured globe. This condition can occur following trauma by projectile, sharp implement, or blunt trauma. Although severe intraocular disruption may occur, the eyeball has a remarkable ability to maintain its integrity. Immediately upon laceration, the iris or choroid (which is the extension of the iris posteriorly underneath the sclera) plugs the wound. This plug may appear as a blue, brown, or black material on the surface of the sclera (Fig. 117.7, see also color plate). At the corneoscleral junction, the iris will come forward and plug a corneal wound (Fig. 117.8). Because of this iris or choroid movement, the pupil often takes on a teardrop shape, with the narrowest segment pointing toward the rupture (Figs. 117.7 and 117.8). Hemorrhage within the anterior chamber (hyphema) often accompanies a corneal or anterior scleral laceration (Fig. 117.7). With small lacerations that are plugged by iris or choroid, the eyeball does not deflate but rather takes on a remarkably normal external appearance. Subconjunctival hemorrhage for 360 degrees may obscure an underlying scleral rupture but leave the eye fairly intact. Patients who present following trauma with this finding or with severe 360-degree conjunctival swelling without hemorrhage should be treated as if they had a ruptured globe and should be referred immediately to an ophthalmologist. The ophthalmologist can then make the assessment via intraocular examination.

Management

Although the outcome in some ruptured globes, particularly small peripheral corneal lacerations, may be good, eyeball

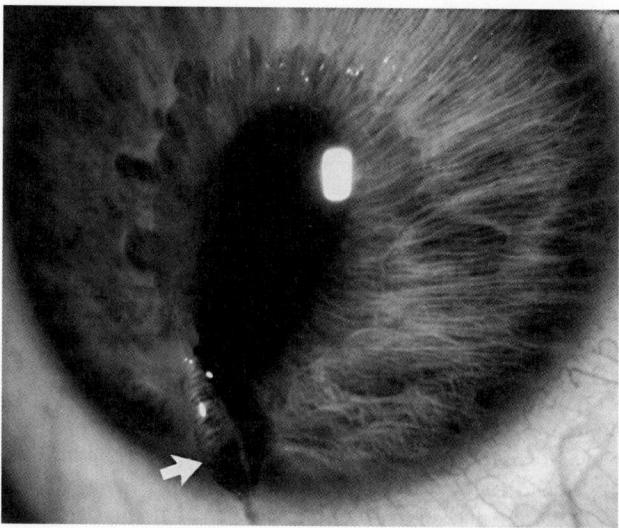

FIGURE 117.8 Corneal laceration (ruptured globe). Note iris protruding through wound *(arrow)* and teardrop-shaped pupil pointing in direction of laceration.

rupture is certainly an ominous sign that warrants emergent referral for ophthalmology consultation. Further ocular examination should be stopped immediately. No eyedrops should be instilled. A patch should never be used in this circumstance. A plastic shield should be placed over the eye such that the edges of the shield make contact with the bony prominences above and below the eyeball (Fig. 117.9). If a commercially marketed shield is not available, the clinician should cut off the bottom of a Styrofoam or plastic cup and use it as a shield, resting it against the bony prominences (Fig. 117.10). If possible, a shield can even be placed over an obviously injured eye while resuscitative efforts are ongoing to prevent further accidental injury or contamination by the medical staff.

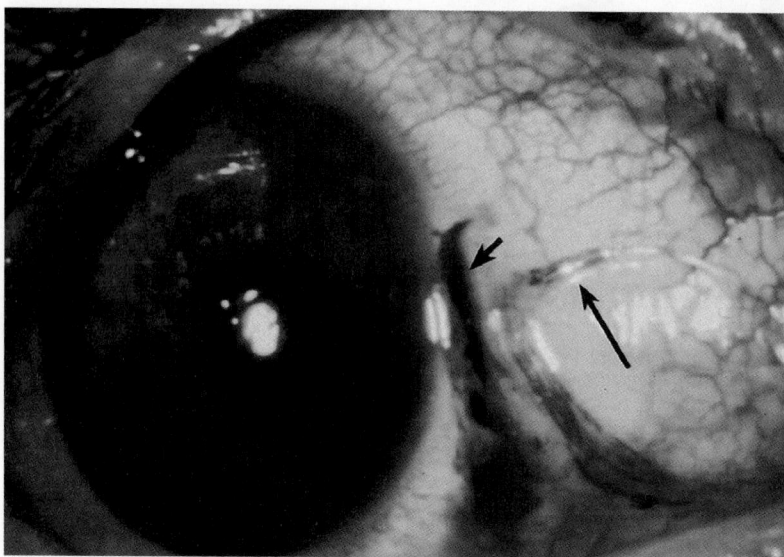

FIGURE 117.7 Ruptured globe. The scleral laceration *(short arrow)* appears as a linear brown line on the white of the eye. The pupil has a teardrop shape, the apex of which points in the direction of the rupture. The *long arrow* points to the upper border of a large conjunctival laceration. Note that the underlying sclera is intact under the conjunctival laceration. There is a diffuse hyphema in the anterior chamber, which partially obscures the pupil.

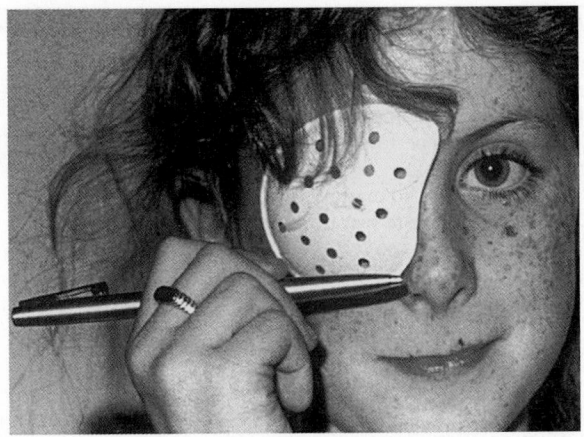

FIGURE 117.9 Patient shielded for right ruptured globe that was caused by a thrown pen.

Severe eye trauma may cause sedation or vomiting without head trauma or brain injury. Every attempt should be made to keep the child calm, even if sedation must be used. Keep in mind that crying, screaming, and Valsalva maneuvers such as vomiting can result in further extrusion of intraocular contents through the rupture. Although broad-spectrum intravenous antibiotic coverage is desirable, this treatment must be weighed against the potential aggravation of the child, which might accompany the needle puncture for catheter placement, and delay that may occur before the patient sees an ophthalmologist. Even if a ruptured globe is not seen clearly on examination, any patient who has a high-risk history, severe lid swelling, and extreme resistance to examination should be given an eye shield and referred to an ophthalmologist as if a ruptured globe was confirmed.

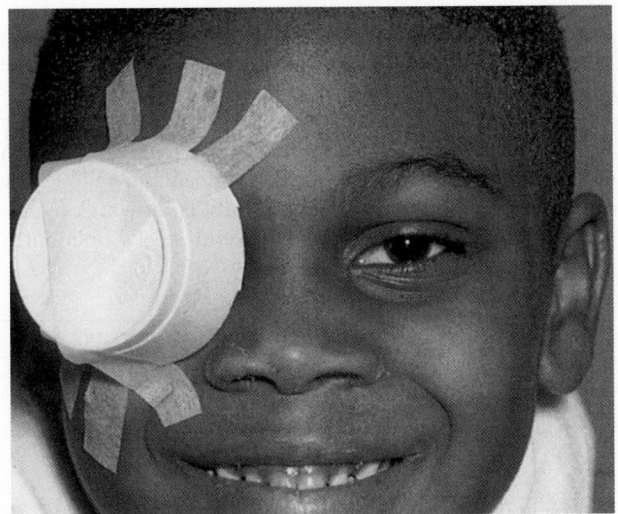

FIGURE 117.10 The bottom of a drinking cup is used as an eye shield.

BLOWOUT FRACTURE

Clinical Manifestations

The pathophysiology and diagnosis of blowout fractures are discussed in Chapter 24. Following blunt compressive eye trauma, the eyeball may be retroplaced in a manner that increases the pressure within the orbit and "blows out" one or more bones of the orbital wall. Direct blunt trauma to the orbital rims may also cause bony fractures that extend back into the orbit. Therefore, orbital fractures may occur after facial trauma with or without eyeball trauma.

The most common orbital fracture is an inferior and/or medial wall fracture. The lateral wall is the least commonly fractured. The intraocular contents often sink back into the fracture, giving an enophthalmic appearance (sunken eye). Conversely, proptosis can occur from orbital hemorrhage. Superior wall fracture (roof fractures) may be associated with pulsating proptosis as a result of communication between the orbit and intracranial cavity. Fractures of the inferior wall may be associated with numbness of the ipsilateral malar region caused by injury to the infraorbital nerve, which travels along the floor of the orbit. Palpation of the bony rim of the orbit is often remarkably normal, contrary to the common teaching about point tenderness and "step off" signs.

The hallmark sign of orbital fracture is a restriction of extraocular movement. Usually, the eye is unable to look away from the fracture site because of a tethering of intraocular muscle or other orbital tissues in the fracture (see Chapter 24, Fig. 24.4). Conversely, orbital hemorrhage at the fracture site can less commonly displace the eyeball away from the fracture and make it difficult for the eye to look in the direction of the fracture.

Management

Approximately 20% of orbital fractures are associated with eyeball injury. Therefore, ophthalmology consultation for complete dilated retinal examination and slit lamp biomicroscopy is indicated in virtually every case. Some controversy exists among ophthalmologists, otorhinolaryngologists, and craniofacial surgeons regarding the urgency for radiologic evaluation and surgical intervention in the management of orbital wall fractures. Axial (proptosis) or coronal displacement of the eyeball is an ominous finding because it may be a sign of orbital hemorrhage, which can cause compression of the optic nerve, requiring emergency surgical intervention. Some would argue that enophthalmos is also a sign that should lead to more urgent radiologic evaluation and surgical intervention. If a decision is made to proceed with radiologic imaging, the optimal test is computed tomography (CT) scan of the orbit with both axial and coronal views. The brain should be included, particularly when a roof fracture is suspected. Plain skull radiographs have little role in the management of orbital wall fractures and need not be ordered.

EYELID LACERATIONS

Clinical Manifestations

Although eyelid lacerations are usually easy to detect, the clinician must remember that the underlying eyeball might also have been lacerated or injured. Seemingly superficial lacerations of the eyelid may be associated with penetration into the orbit or intracranial cavity, particularly when the injury was caused by a pointed implement such as a tree branch or pencil. If possible, the eyelid should be everted to look for a conjunctival wound indicating that the laceration is actually a complete perforation of the eyelid. Puncture wounds of the upper lid with an implement such as a stick or pencil can result in perforation of the orbital roof and entry into the intracranial subfrontal space, with surprisingly little in the way of signs or symptoms. CT scan should be considered in all cases of full-thickness perforation of the upper lid. Likewise, it is remarkable how easily and apparently atraumatically a perforating implement can reach the orbital apex and optic nerve. Visual field defects may be the only sign, other than the small lid perforation, that the nerve has been injured. CT scan should be considered for all lid perforations.

Oblique lacerations that extend into the medial canthal area (juncture of the upper and lower lids medially) may involve the proximal portion of the nasolacrimal system (Fig. 117.11). Sometimes, the lid margin puncta, which drains tears into the system, is displaced laterally as a result of the laceration (Fig. 117.11). Lacerations in this area should usually be referred for ophthalmology consultation if any question exists regarding whether the tear drainage system is intact.

Management

Lacerations of the periorbital skin and superficial eyelid skin may be managed by standard skin closure techniques discussed elsewhere in this book. It is important that sutures not

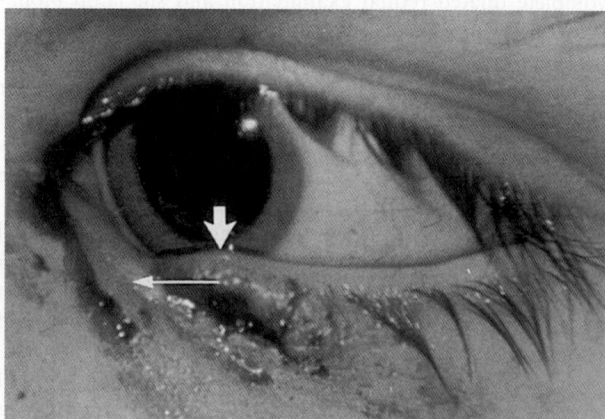

FIGURE 117.11 Lower lid laceration involving tear drainage system. *Thick arrow* indicates lower lid punctum, which has been displaced laterally. *Thin arrow* indicates normal course of canaliculus, which drains tears from the puncta to the lacrimal sac located medially.

EYELID LACERATIONS

Consult ophthalmology if laceration is associated with:
Full-thickness perforation of lid
Ptosis
Involvement of lid margin
Possible damage to tear drainage system
Tissue avulsion
Eyeball injury

grasp deep tissue within the eyelid because this may result in cicatricial eversion of the eyelid margins. Table 117.2 summarizes those findings that, when associated with eyelid lacerations, should prompt ophthalmology consultation for wound closure.

PERIORBITAL ECCHYMOSIS

Clinical Manifestations

Periorbital ecchymosis is usually a benign finding, although it may be associated with bony fracture or eyeball injury. Because of the loose connection of the eyelid skin and underlying tissues, dramatic ecchymosis can occur with mild blunt trauma. Bilateral ecchymosis may occur from midline forehead injuries. It is of forensic importance that the dating of injuries should not be made on the basis of the color of periorbital ecchymosis. Because accumulation of blood tends to be more dramatic in the eye than in other body sites, periorbital ecchymosis often looks much darker than what might be expected elsewhere for a bruise of similar age.

Management

No treatment is routinely needed for periorbital ecchymosis. Ice packs applied to the area, with the eyelids closed, can be helpful in reducing swelling.

Anticipatory guidance may be given to inform the family that the ecchymosis may persist for more than 2 weeks. An ongoing color change from purple to green and yellow may occur as the blood is resorbed and broken down. A hyperpigmented area may be left for several weeks or months thereafter.

CORNEAL AND CONJUNCTIVAL INJURY

Clinical Manifestations

The conjunctiva can be abraded or lacerated (Fig. 117.7), although the management of this problem is usually identical to that of corneal abrasion because the tissues heal so rapidly. Corneal or conjunctival abrasions may occur even from mild surface trauma. Self-inflicted abrasions may occur accidentally.

Corneal abrasion can be painful and accompanied by dramatic photophobia and resistance to opening of the eyes. Yet, some children have remarkably few symptoms. They may complain of a foreign-body sensation even though no foreign body is present. A drop of topical proparacaine 0.5% or tetracaine 0.5% may have both diagnostic and temporary therapeutic usefulness. Any patient who is made more comfortable by the instillation of either of these drops must have an ocular surface problem (conjunctiva or cornea) as the cause of pain. The child who is crying and refusing to open the eyes may be compliant and easy to examine just a few minutes after the instillation of a topical anesthetic. Onset of action is approximately 20 seconds, and duration is approximately 20 minutes.

Topical fluorescein is used as a diagnostic agent to stain the affected area. Fluorescein is available as impregnated paper strips and as a solution combined with a topical anesthetic (Fluress®, Akorn Pharmaceuticals, Lake Forest, Illinois). Considering the limited use in an ED setting, strips may be a more practical method because bacterial contamination over time is more likely with the solution. When impregnated strips are used, they must be wet before instillation. Otherwise, the strip itself may cause a corneal abrasion, thus preventing the examiner from correctly identifying the patient's problem. Topical anesthetic or saline may be used to wet the strip. The lower eyelid should be pulled down, exposing the pink inner surface (palpebral conjunctiva) against which the strip may be touched. The solution then diffuses off the strip into the area between the lower eyelid and the eyeball (inferior fornix), where it is then displaced across the ocular surface with the next blink. The clinician must avoid placing too much fluorescein because the tear film can be so oversaturated that it may be difficult to find a small abrasion.

Fluorescein, which is orange, fluoresces yellow–green when exposed to blue light. Many modern ophthalmoscopes have a blue light. The examiner can view through the peephole of the direct ophthalmoscope, spinning the focusing dial to allow the ocular surface to be in focus with the examiner 5 to 10 cm away from the patient, inspecting the cornea and conjunctiva for an area that is stained. A Wood's or Burton lamp can also be used. Some of these devices have handheld magnifying windows attached. Although the staining may not be as dramatic, white light from a direct ophthalmoscope or penlight can also be used because some blue wavelengths are incorporated in white light. Green light (red free), available on most direct ophthalmoscopes, may make identifying stained areas more difficult than white light. When a superficial abrasion may actually represent penetration into the deeper corneal tissues, a teardrop or irregular pupil may be seen. Urgent ophthalmic consultation is indicated.

If the staining pattern reveals one or more vertical linear abrasions, the examiner should suspect the presence of a retained foreign body under the upper lid. This foreign body may be viewed by upper lid eversion (Fig. 117.12). The patient should be asked to look down repeatedly throughout this procedure. With the eye in downgaze, a cotton swab should be placed against the midbody of the upper eyelid and gently rotated downward toward the eyelashes so the skin is rolled with the swab by friction. This procedure causes the eyelashes to turn out toward the examiner so they may be grasped between the examiner's thumb and forefinger. It may be necessary to grab the entire lid margin in some children. If a topical anesthetic is instilled before lid eversion, this procedure is virtually painless although some patients do not enjoy the unusual sensation. After the lashes (or margin) are grabbed, lift vertically while the cotton swab is used to apply gentle downward pressure in the opposite direction. The eyelid then flips around the cotton swab. If a foreign body is identified, it can be gently lifted away using a cotton swab or forceps. To revert the eyelid, simply

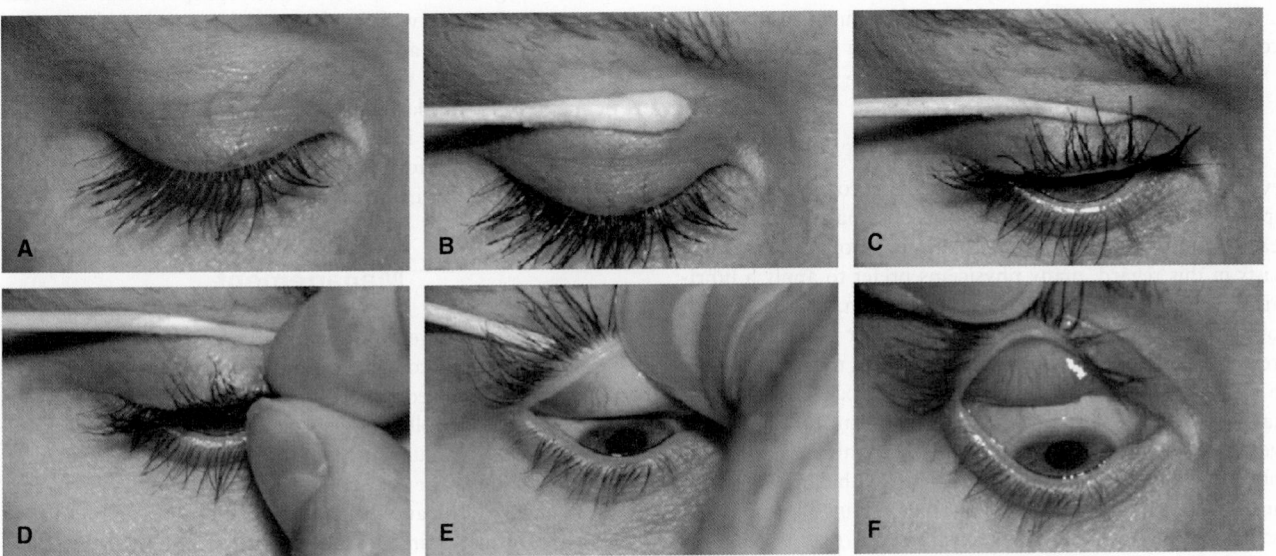

FIGURE 117.12 Upper lid eversion. Note that patient is looking down throughout procedure. In frame C, the swab is being rolled clockwise to engage skin and indirectly lift lash line. In frame E, the swab is being pushed downward as the examiner lifts the lashes upward in the opposite direction. In F, note that patient is wearing a contact lens.

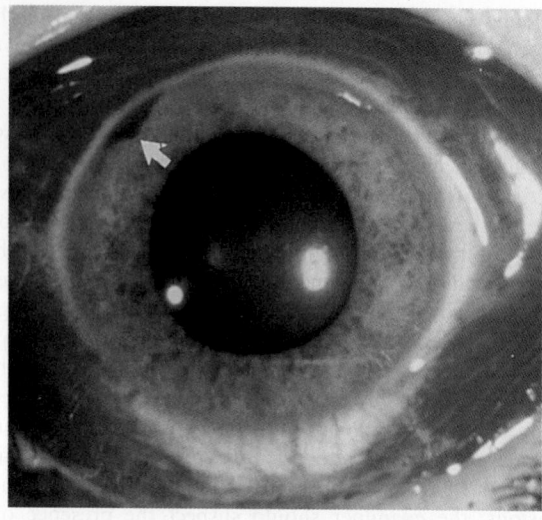

FIGURE 117.13 Subconjunctival hemorrhage extending for 360 degrees. Note the small hyphema (arrow).

have the patient look upward or the examiner can massage the lid down with his or her forefinger.

Subconjunctival hemorrhage is uncommon in children. It may result from blunt trauma, conjunctivitis, chemical irritation, and increased intrathoracic pressure (e.g., chest trauma, suffocation). Although usually focal, the lesions may be multiple or diffuse. Petechia of the surrounding periorbital skin may or may not be present if the cause is airway obstruction. Hypertension, coagulopathy, or anticoagulant medications may result in subconjunctival hemorrhage out of proportion to the injury. After blunt eyeball trauma, a 360-degree subconjunctival hemorrhage may mask an underlying ruptured globe (Fig. 117.13). No treatment is needed for isolated subconjunctival hemorrhages. They may take up to 2 weeks to resolve, turning yellowish in the process.

Chemical injuries of the cornea and conjunctiva may also occur. These injuries are discussed in Chapter 127.

Management

Several studies have suggested that patching corneal abrasions, especially in children with small abrasions, may not accelerate healing or decrease symptoms. Although some controversy exists in this regard, many physicians prefer to apply a lubricating antibiotic ointment (e.g., bacitracin, erythromycin, Polysporin®) to the ocular surface with or without a light pressure patch over the closed eyelid. If used, the patch should be worn overnight. Another alternative for pain management may be the use of topical nonsteroidal antiinflammatory agents, although this has been researched only in adults. For patients who are relatively asymptomatic with corneal or conjunctival abrasions that are small and do not involve the visual axis (i.e., not involving the central cornea over the pupil), management with antibiotic or artificial tears alone may be sufficient with no patch. For patients who are in significant pain, a drop of cyclopentolate 1% can be instilled to relieve spasm of the eye's ciliary muscle. Ointments containing

steroids or neomycin should not be used. If the patient is asymptomatic within 48 hours after patch removal (by the parents at home or by the physician), no follow-up is required. Larger corneal abrasions and those involving the visual axis should be seen on the day following trauma by an ophthalmologist. For any size of corneal abrasion, if pain or foreign-body sensation continues for more than 2 to 3 days, or if there is increasing pain and redness, the patient should be instructed to seek ophthalmologic care. A topical antibiotic ointment may be prescribed for use after patch removal two to three times daily for approximately 3 to 4 days.

Any patient with a fluorescein staining corneal defect who has a history of ocular herpes or who wears contact lenses should be referred urgently for ophthalmology consultation. Fluorescein should not be instilled while patients have their soft contact lens in place as this may result in permanent discoloration of the contact lens. Patients who wear contact lenses should never be patched for abrasions even if the contact lens has been removed. Patching an eye that often wears contact lenses may create a microenvironment that predisposes to bacterial ulceration of the cornea. The contact lenses should be removed immediately and left out until the cornea is documented by an ophthalmologist to be healed.

HYPHEMA

Clinical Manifestations

The presence of blood between the cornea and iris is a sign of severe ocular trauma. Although the entire anterior chamber may be filled with blood (8-ball hyphema), clots may also be small, requiring careful inspection for detection (Fig. 117.13). Sometimes the blood is more diffuse throughout the anterior chamber (Fig. 117.7) or may even be microscopic, requiring slit lamp examination for detection (microhyphema). The size of the hyphema is directly proportional to the incidence of secondary glaucoma and is inversely proportional to visual prognosis. Patients with hyphema are in a vulnerable period for the first 5 days after injury when spontaneous rebleeding may occur. Patients with hemoglobinopathies are also at particular risk for ocular complications of hyphema. Therefore, all patients who are in a high-risk ethnic group should receive a screening test or formal hemoglobin electrophoresis at presentation unless their status is already known.

Management

All patients who have hyphema must be seen by an ophthalmologist. Although microhyphemas and perhaps some small hyphemas may be managed in select clinical situations as outpatients with careful daily follow-up, hospital admission is often recommended. The eye trauma itself may result in some degree of physiologic sedation. The eye should be shielded, not patched (Figs. 117.9 and 117.10), and the patient should be placed on bed rest with the head elevated 45 degrees. This position helps allow blood within the anterior chamber to settle inferiorly, thus allowing clearance of the visual axis, improvement of vision, and a better view for the ophthalmologist looking into the eyeball. If an ophthalmologist is not readily available, the examining physician may recommend admission and the use of a dilating agent to paralyze the ciliary muscle within the eye but it is desirable for ophthalmology consultation to be performed at least within 24 hours. The ophthalmologist may prescribe topical steroids, but they should not be prescribed by a nonophthalmologist. In some cases, oral antifibrinolytics may be used to prevent spontaneous rebleeding, but these agents should be used only under the supervision and recommendation of an ophthalmology consultant.

TRAUMATIC IRITIS

Clinical Manifestations

Inflammation within the anterior chamber of the eye often does not present for 24 to 72 hours after blunt trauma to the eyeball. The patient may complain of eye pain, redness, photophobia, and sometimes, visual loss. The pupil on the affected side may be constricted (see Chapter 25). The ocular injection may be confined to a ring of redness surrounding the cornea (ciliary flush). Definitive recognition of traumatic iritis requires slit lamp biomicroscopy.

A beam of light projected from a light source can be seen only as it reflects from surfaces. For example, the light from a movie projector in a movie theater would not be visible unless smoke and dust were present in the air to reflect the light as it passes between the projector and the screen. Likewise, the slit beam of light projected from the slit lamp is normally visible only as it reflects off (and through) the cornea and then passes unseen through the optically clear fluid of the anterior chamber (aqueous humor), landing on the iris and lens (within the pupil), where it is again visible as it reflects from their surfaces. When white blood cells are floating within the anterior chamber fluid, along with protein that has leaked from inflamed blood vessels, the beam of light from the slit lamp then becomes visible as it passes through the aqueous humor. The white blood cells appear as small specks floating within the beam of light. Red blood cells from microhyphema can also be detected in this manner. Recognition of iritis at the slit lamp requires skill and experience. Ophthalmology consultation is recommended when the diagnosis of iritis is suspected and if the emergency physician is not expert in slit lamp examination.

Management

Traumatic iritis may be an indicator that other ocular injuries have occurred. Ophthalmology consultation should be obtained in the diagnosis and management of this condition. The ophthalmologist often recommends dilating drops and topical steroids for treatment. Because of the risks associated with the use of topical steroids, they should not be prescribed by nonophthalmologists.

TRAUMATIC VISUAL LOSS

Clinical Manifestations

Some techniques for recognizing true traumatic visual loss are discussed at the beginning of this chapter. Occasionally, the emergency physician is faced with a child who is feigning visual loss. These situations seem to be more common after motor vehicle accidents or other injuries in which legal action may be involved. Functional visual loss can also be idiopathic and transient or associated with other overt or covert stress in the child's life. In the absence of other signs of ocular or head trauma, this diagnosis should be suspected. It then becomes necessary to "trick" the child into demonstrating that he or she can actually see. Patients who are truly acutely blind should demonstrate some degree of anxiety and virtually complete inability to navigate in the new surroundings of the ED. When asked to write their names on a piece of paper, truly blind patients can do so accurately, unlike children who are functionally blind who assume they are unable to write. When a mirror is held before a truly blind eye and then tilted in the vertical and horizontal planes, the eye will not follow. Any eye that truly has enough sight to recognize its own image moves involuntarily with the motion of the mirror.

Children who are feigning visual loss but not complete blindness can be more difficult to "trick." Sometimes, by placing a drop of saline or topical anesthetic in the eye while giving the child the suggestion that these "magic drops" will cause a return of vision, the child then begins to see better. The pinhole test (discussed above) can also be used in this manner. Ophthalmology consultation is sometimes critical in discovering whether a child has truly sustained visual loss.

A rare cause of visual loss after head trauma is transient cortical visual impairment/blindness. As a result of a direct or contrecoup occipital contusion, a child may experience acute blindness despite an otherwise normal eye examination. This centrally mediated phenomenon may resolve spontaneously. Ophthalmology consultation can be useful to rule out other causes of visual loss.

A multitude of intraocular injuries, including traumatic cataract, vitreous hemorrhage, retinal bruising (commotio retinae), retinal detachment, and optic nerve injury, can result in true visual loss or blindness. Although the pediatric emergency physician is often the first to meet a child with acute traumatic visual loss, in most of these circumstances, ophthalmology consultation is then required. For the emergency physician, the best screening tests for intraocular injury are vision testing, the examination of the red reflex, and direct ophthalmoscope examination.

CHILD ABUSE

Clinical Manifestations

Virtually any eye injury can be the result of child abuse. Unusual types of ocular trauma, such as the covert instillation of noxious substances onto the conjunctiva, should also be considered in the differential diagnosis of recurrent red eyes in the absence of an apparent cause. Perhaps the most common ocular manifestation of child abuse is the finding of retinal hemorrhages associated with the abusive head injury (Fig. 117.14, see also color plate). Although these hemorrhages can be seen with the direct ophthalmoscope, ophthalmology consultation is required. Children who present to the ED before the age of 5 years with a history of head trauma or sudden unexplained cardiorespiratory arrest should have a full dilated

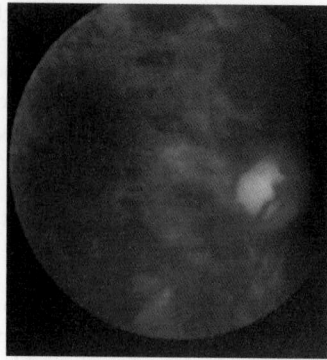

FIGURE 117.14 Retinal hemorrhages in abusive head injury.

examination conducted by an ophthalmologist to look for retinal hemorrhages that may indicate that a nonaccidental head injury has occurred. There are other cuases of retinal hemorrhage which must be differentiated based on systemic findings, laboratory evaluation where appropriate, and ophthalmology examination. The eye examination by a nonophthalmologist should not be used to decide whether or not ophthalmology consultation or neuroimaging is indicated, especially when

there are sufficient historical or clinical indicators to raise a concern about possible child abuse.

Suggested Readings

Arbour JD, Brunette I, Boisjoly HM. Should we patch corneal erosions? *Arch Ophthalmol* 1997;115:313–317.

Dutton JJ, Manson PN, Iliff N, et al. Management of blow-out fractures of the orbital floor. *Surv Ophthalmol* 1991;35:279–298.

Ehlers JP, Shah C. *Wills Eye manual: hospital office and emergency room diagnosis and treatment of eye disease*, 5th ed. Philadelphia, PA: Lippincott Williams & Wilkins, 2008.

Forbes BJ. Management of corneal abrasions and ocular trauma in children. *Pediatr Ann* 2001;30(8):465–472.

Kaiser PK. A comparison of pressure patching versus no patching for corneal abrasions due to trauma or foreign body removal. *Ophthalmology* 1995;102: 1936–1942.

Levin AV. Eye emergencies: acute management in the pediatric ambulatory setting. *Pediatr Emerg Care* 1991;7:367–377.

Levin AV. General pediatric ophthalmic procedures. In: King CK, Henretig FM, eds. *Textbook of pediatric emergency procedures*, 2nd ed. Philadelphia, PA: Lippincott Williams & Wilkins, 2008:531–544.

Levin AV. Slit lamp examination. In: King CK, Henretig FM, eds. *Textbook of pediatric emergency procedures*, 2nd ed. Philadelphia, PA: Lippincott Williams & Wilkins, 2008:545–549.

Morad Y, Kim YM, Mian M, et al. Non-ophthalmologists' accuracy in diagnosing retinal hemorrhages in the shaken baby syndrome. *J Pediatr* 2003;142: 431–434.

Riordan-Eva P, Whitcher JP. *Vaughan & Asbury's general ophthalmology*, 17th ed. New York, NY: McGraw-Hill, 2008.

CHAPTER 118 ■ THORACIC TRAUMA

HOWARD A. KADISH, MD, MBA

INTRODUCTION

Thoracic trauma in the pediatric population is relatively uncommon and only in the last two decades has it received careful scrutiny. Included in thoracic trauma are injuries to the chest wall, trachea, bronchi, lungs, heart, thoracic aorta and great vessels, esophagus, and diaphragm. The report of the National Pediatric Trauma Registry contains a detailed analysis of major thoracic trauma in children. In the United States, only 4% to 6% of children admitted to pediatric trauma centers have thoracic injuries; however, because of the severe mechanism, many patients never reach a hospital and die at the scene. In patients who do reach the hospital, most thoracic injuries do not require operative intervention other than tube thoracostomy.

When thoracic trauma occurs in isolation, the mortality rate is relatively low. The mortality rate triples when thoracic trauma occurs concurrently with head or abdominal trauma. In one study, 82% of patients with thoracic trauma had a multisystem injury, and 58% of those patients had a concomitant head injury. In the same study, children with thoracic trauma had a lower mean trauma score and a higher mean injury severity score. Mortality rates were 20 times higher for children with thoracic involvement than for those without. Another study showed that children with a pediatric trauma score of four or less had a significantly higher mortality rate than those with a score of five or greater. Most scene fatalities result from lacerations of the lung, heart, blood vessels, and bronchi. In the hospital, cardiac tamponade, injuries to the aorta and great vessels, and tension hemothorax/pneumothorax carry the greatest potential for death.

As with other types of pediatric trauma, blunt thoracic injuries are more common than penetrating. Motor vehicle–related accidents account for at least 75% of all blunt thoracic injuries. Other common mechanisms include falls, assaults, and bicycle accidents. Penetrating wounds occur in approximately 15% of children sustaining major thoracic trauma. Gunshot wounds followed by stab wounds are the most common causes of penetrating thoracic trauma, although mechanism varies with geographic location.

The most common injuries in blunt thoracic trauma include lung contusions (53%), pneumothorax or hemothorax (38%), and fractures (38%). Pneumothorax or hemothorax (64%) occur more frequently in penetrating thoracic trauma, but diaphragmatic (15%), cardiac (13%), and vascular injuries (10%) are also common.

Isolated rib fractures have a mortality rate of only 10%. The mortality rate approximates 20% in blunt thoracic trauma when only the lung or pleural space (pneumothorax or hemo-thorax) is involved. This increases to 30% if the diaphragm is injured; if the heart or great vessels are involved, it rises to 40% to 50%. In penetrating thoracic trauma, the mortality rate is less than 10% when only the pleural cavity is injured. Cardiac and vascular injuries carry a mortality rate of 50%.

PATHOPHYSIOLOGY

Children with thoracic trauma may present in respiratory or circulatory failure. Children in respiratory failure, more commonly seen than circulatory failure, may present with tachypnea, chest wall retractions, and agitation secondary to hypoxia.

Respiratory Failure

Because approximately 80% of thoracic trauma occurs as part of a multisystem injury, the most common cause of respiratory failure is neurologic compromise. If left untreated, patients will develop anoxic brain injury and a respiratory acidosis due to hypercarbia. Immediate control of the airway with positive-pressure ventilation followed by treatment of the neurologic emergency is indicated.

Airway obstruction, external compression of the pulmonary structures, direct injury to the pulmonary parenchyma, and chest wall injuries, all due to thoracic trauma, will also affect oxygenation and ventilation if left untreated.

Airway Obstruction

Blood, vomit, or foreign bodies (teeth) may obstruct the airway. Failure to remove or bypass the foreign body will lead to hypoxia and anoxic brain injury. Initial treatment includes repositioning and suctioning of the airway, along with cervical spine immobilization. If initial treatment fails, endotracheal intubation is indicated. If the endotracheal tube cannot bypass the obstruction or a foreign body cannot be extracted, a cricothyroidotomy or surgical tracheostomy should be performed.

External Compression of the Pulmonary Structures

External compression of the lungs, most commonly caused by air or blood within the pleural cavity, will cause respiratory distress. Initially patients may present with tachypnea, retractions, and hypoxia. As more lung segments are involved, ventilation is affected and the patient's carbon dioxide begins to rise. Tube thoracostomy is the treatment of choice for a pneumothorax or hemothorax.

Diaphragmatic hernia and gastric dilation can also cause respiratory distress by external compression of the lungs. Patients with a diaphragmatic hernia that compromises ventilation need prompt surgical intervention. A nasogastric or oral gastric tube helps decompress the stomach and decreases the likelihood of aspirating vomit or swallowed blood.

Pulmonary Parenchyma Injury

Aspiration of blood or vomit into the terminal bronchi and alveoli will cause a chemical pneumonitis. Direct trauma to the lung parenchyma (pulmonary contusion) will also cause a leakage of blood and fluid into the alveolar space. Both of these injuries lead to shunting of deoxygenated blood into the systemic circulation. Endotracheal intubation with positive-pressure ventilation is indicated if the patient's respiratory status worsens. Patients with a severe chemical pneumonitis or pulmonary contusion may require high inflation pressures to maintain adequate oxygenation. These patients are at risk for a pneumothorax because of high inflation pressures coupled with an already injured lung.

Although not as common as a chemical pneumonitis or pulmonary contusion, penetrating thoracic trauma may cause direct pulmonary parenchymal damage but is associated more often with a hemothorax or pneumothorax.

Chest Wall Injuries

Chest wall injuries such as rib fractures or a flail chest may cause hypoventilation, as well as hypoxia secondary to pain and inadequate air exchange. Endotracheal intubation with positive-pressure ventilation is the treatment of choice in those patients with rising carbon dioxide levels or severe hypoxia.

Circulatory Compromise

Thoracic hemorrhage, obstruction of venous return to the heart, or direct injury to the heart can cause circulatory compromise and shock.

Thoracic Hemorrhage

Laceration of the hilum of the lung, a great vessel, or the heart itself will cause a significant amount of bleeding. A patient can hemorrhage more than 50% of his or her total blood volume into the pleural cavity. The body's compensatory mechanisms for the blood loss include an increase in both heart rate and total peripheral vascular resistance. Relying solely on a decrease in systemic blood pressure to detect hemorrhage in children may be deceiving because children may lose up to 25% of their total blood volume before their systemic blood pressure is affected. Children with significant bleeding may have a normal blood pressure but be tachycardic and poorly perfused with a prolonged capillary refill time. Treatment should be initiated prior to the onset of hypotension. Therapy includes fluid resuscitation, blood transfusion, and surgical repair if the patient continues to require multiple blood transfusions.

Obstruction of Venous Return to the Heart

A tension pneumothorax or hemothorax occurs when there is progressive accumulation of air or blood within the pleural cavity, which will cause a shift of the mediastinal structures. The trachea and mediastinum are shifted to the contralateral side. Venous return to the heart is reduced because the inferior vena cava is relatively fixed in place and becomes obstructed.

Diastolic filling is reduced, and the stroke volume of the heart drops. Patients with a tension pneumothorax or hemothorax will be tachycardic, peripherally vasoconstricted, and if left untreated, will progress to shock. Initial treatment consists of needle decompression. If there is a tension pneumothorax, an immediate release of air should be noted and the patient's hemodynamic status should improve. The needle decompression is only a temporizing measure and must be followed by tube thoracostomy.

Direct Injury to the Heart

Myocardial contusion, ventricular or atrial rupture, and valvular disruption may produce cardiogenic shock. Circulatory compromise results from a decrease in cardiac output, usually from impaired in myocardial contractility. Patients may present in congestive heart failure with an enlarged liver, a gallop heard on cardiac examination, and rales with auscultation of the lungs. Echocardiography, especially transesophageal, is helpful in identifying the type of injury. Positive inotropic agents are the drugs of choice for improving myocardial contractility.

Pericardial tamponade, due to air or blood inside the pericardium, will also decrease cardiac output and cause circulatory collapse. If the patient is decompensating and a pericardial tamponade is suspected, then a pericardiocentesis should be performed. Where possible, ultrasonic confirmation and guidance are helpful.

DIFFERENCES BETWEEN CHILDREN AND ADULTS

Pediatric thoracic trauma differs from adult thoracic trauma in the mechanism of injury, type of injury, and frequency of other organ systems involved.

Falls are the most common mechanism of injury in the infant and child. Older children are often injured as pedestrians or as unrestrained passengers in motor vehicle accidents. Adolescents are more likely to be involved as occupants in motor vehicle–related accidents. Penetrating injuries secondary to violence are more common in the adolescent and young adult population.

Lung contusion is the most common pediatric thoracic injury, with intrapleural injury second. Lacerations of the heart, great vessels, and lungs are relatively uncommon, occurring in less than 10% of thoracic trauma cases. A cooperative study in adults sustaining thoracic trauma showed that 50% had a chest wall injury and that a flail chest injury occurred in 5% of those with chest wall injuries. Injuries to the lung parenchyma occurred in 26% of patients. Simple rib fractures are the most common type of thoracic injury in adults. Only 30% of pediatric patients, as compared with 50% to 75% of adults, sustain rib fractures because of increased compliance in the pediatric thoracic cage secondary to the greater cartilage content and the greater elasticity of the bones. Because of this increased compliance, kinetic energy is transferred more readily to the underlying organs. Thus, a pediatric patient may have an internal injury (lung contusion) without external evidence of trauma (rib fracture, laceration, bruising). Air and fluid within the pleural space (pneumothorax/hemothorax) more easily displace the mediastinum, compromising venous return and cardiac output in children (Fig. 118.1). Adults

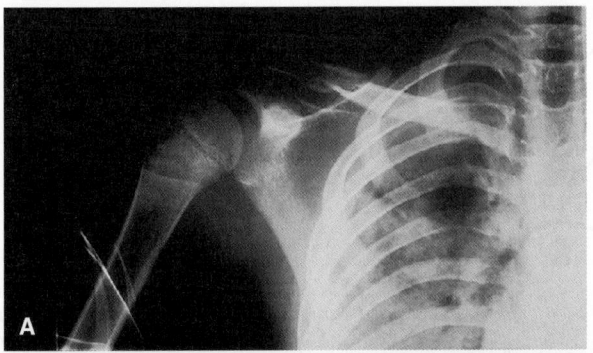

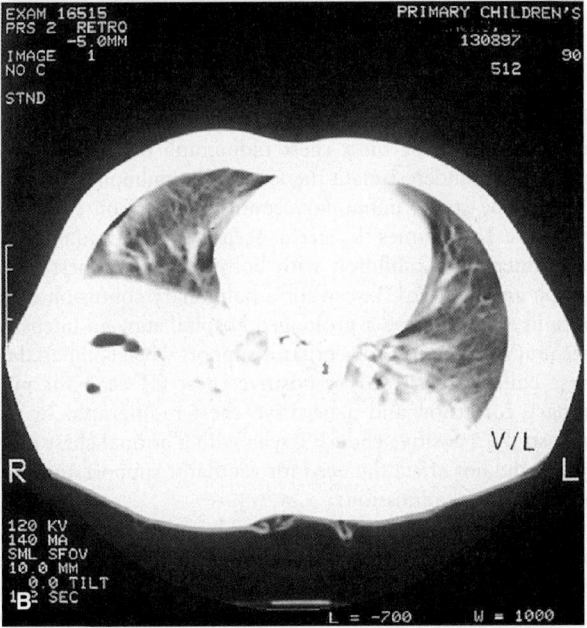

FIGURE 118.6 A 7-year-old involved in an automobile–pedestrian accident. Crepitus and decreased breath sounds were noted on the right side. Chest radiograph (**A**) shows rib fractures, clavicle fracture, and a pulmonary contusion. A pulmonary contusion and a pneumothorax are seen on the thoracic computed tomography (**B**).

laceration. Usually patients with these injuries are symptomatic (hypotension, pulse differences or deficits). In one study, all patients with a first rib fracture and injury to the great vessels exhibited physical examination abnormalities such as loss of the radial pulse on the involved side, discrepancy in blood pressure between the upper extremities, a flail chest, and/or hypotension. No patients with an isolated first rib fracture and a completely normal physical examination had an injury to a great vessel. In this and other studies, there was no correlation between level of rib fracture and associated vascular injury in the otherwise asymptomatic patient.

The pediatric patient with a rib fracture may splint and hypoventilate secondary to pain. Physical examination may reveal point tenderness, and if the pleura has been involved, crepitus. If the patient has any respiratory or circulatory compromise, a tube thoracostomy is indicated for a pneumothorax or hemothorax. The tube should be placed at a separate site from the area of the fracture. If the patient is stable, then relief of pain, monitoring the respiratory status, and further evaluation (chest radiography, thoracic CT scan) for underlying injury

is indicated. Wrapping or binding the chest wall is contraindicated because these measures may impair ventilatory function. Analgesics are helpful but should be used with caution because they may also cause respiratory depression. Epidural analgesia may be administered, especially for lower rib fracture. Intercostal nerve block is another useful modality that should be performed carefully to avoid puncturing the pleura.

Patients with rib fractures, especially more than one fracture, are usually admitted to the hospital for pain control, pulmonary physiotherapy, and observation for worsening respiratory status. Prognosis for isolated rib fractures is excellent, with most healing within 6 weeks. The chest wall will remodel leaving no permanent disability.

Sternal and Scapular Fractures

Sternal and scapular fractures are uncommon in children, secondary to the marked compliance of the chest wall (Fig. 118.7). Although a thorough evaluation for other thoracic injuries is recommended routinely because of the significant force required to fracture these bones, only rarely are vascular or brachial plexus injuries detected. In one adult study, scapular fracture alone was not a significant marker for mortality or neurovascular injury. In another adult study looking at 37 patients with sternal fractures, the authors found that only one patient had a minor blunt cardiac injury (BCI) and that this patient had an obvious abnormal EKG. They concluded that the routine use of echocardiography in the assessment of isolated sternal fractures is not indicated. In another study looking at patients with BCI, only 2% had an associated sternal fracture.

Flail Chest

Fracturing two or more ribs on the same side may result in that particular chest wall segment losing continuity with the thoracic cage causing a flail chest. Direct impact to the ribs, as in a crush injury, is the most common mechanism for a flail chest. Flail chest is uncommon in children, owing to the marked compliance of the chest wall. In published series, flail chest occurred in approximately 10% of patients as compared with less than 1% in the pediatric population. When a flail chest does occur, it is usually associated with an intrathoracic injury, most often pulmonary contusion, because of the force involved.

The pediatric patient may develop respiratory distress and failure due to a flail chest from numerous mechanisms. In the early 1900s, Bauer described the pendelluft theory, which attributes inefficient ventilation and oxygenation to a pendulum-like

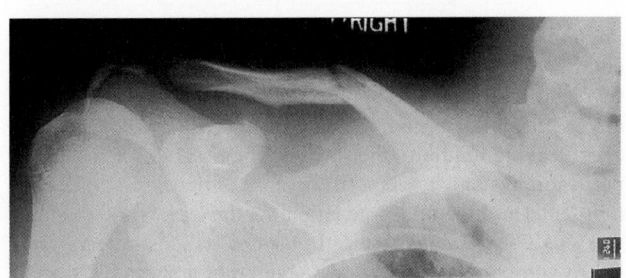

FIGURE 118.7 A 10-year-old child evaluated after a fall of more than 10 feet. The patient was asymptomatic except for shoulder pain. The only abnormalities noted were a scapular and clavicle fracture.

TRAUMA

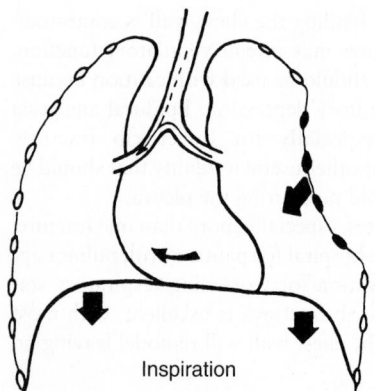
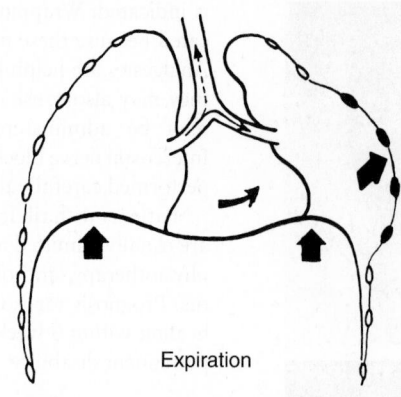

Inspiration   Expiration

FIGURE 118.8 Pathophysiologic consequence of flail chest with paradoxical motion. (From Fleisher GR, Ludwig S, Henretig FM. *Textbook of pediatric emergency medicine.* 3rd ed. Baltimore: Williams & Wilkins, Fig. 101.4, reprinted with permission.)

movement of air from the injured lung to the uninjured lung. The harder and faster a patient works to breathe, the more shifting of air from one side to the other occurs. The paradoxical movement of the chest also impairs the normal inspiratory/expiratory function of the lung (Fig. 118.8). Another mechanism for respiratory distress is the association of underlying pulmonary injury with a flail chest. Edema within the airways will alter alveolar ventilation:perfusion ratios and produce pulmonary arteriovenous shunting with hypoxemia and subsequent respiratory distress. Finally, the pain associated with rib fractures will cause voluntary and involuntary splinting. These patients are at increased risk for atelectasis and pneumonia secondary to poor pulmonary function.

The goal of treatment should be to stabilize the involved portion of the thoracic cage. At the scene of an accident, the patient can be placed with the injured side down, thus improving tidal volume and ventilation. Any patient with respiratory distress should be intubated and placed on positive-pressure ventilation. This serves two purposes. First, the patient's airway is well protected and the effectiveness of breathing is maximized. Second, the positive pressure provides optimal expansion and splinting of the injured segment. Unfortunately, high inflating pressures can cause a pneumothorax and care must be taken when delivering positive pressure to the injured child. If the patient does not need to be intubated, aggressive pulmonary physiotherapy, along with pain control, is the treatment of choice. In patients with an underlying pulmonary contusion, fluids must be carefully monitored. Fluid may leak out of the injured capillary bed, worsening the pulmonary contusion.

Pulmonary Contusions and Lacerations

Pulmonary contusion is the most common thoracic injury in children. Pulmonary contusion occurs when a blunt force, such as a crush injury, is applied to the lung parenchyma. As in any contusion or bruise, the capillary network becomes damaged, leaking fluid into the surrounding tissues. A ventilation:perfusion mismatch will occur because of the extravasation of fluid, interfering with oxygenation. As the edema and swelling worsens, the patient's respiratory status will also deteriorate. When compared with a chest radiograph, a chest CT scan is more sensitive in detecting pulmonary contusion (Figs. 118.9A and 118.9B) and often lung parenchymal injuries are noted when a few cuts of the thoracic cavity are imaged while

obtaining an abdominal CT scan. A pulmonary contusion may initially be invisible on a chest radiograph or a chest radiograph may underestimate the size of the pulmonary contusion. In one study, pulmonary contusions seen on chest CT scan were 2 to 3 times the size as seen on a chest radiograph. In another study, children with both a positive chest radiograph and a chest CT scan for a pulmonary contusion were more likely to require a prolonged hospital stay, an intensive care unit admission, and ventilator support when compared to those children with only a positive chest CT scan for pulmonary contusion and a negative chest radiograph. In the same study, a positive chest CT scan with a normal chest radiograph did not affect the need for ventilator support and prolonged hospital admission.

In one study, tachypnea, abnormal breath sounds, external thoracic wall contusion, and fracture of the bony thorax were each absent in more than 50% of patients with a pulmonary contusion. Interestingly, the chest radiograph in these patients did not dramatically worsen from time of admission. Nonetheless mild contusions require close hospital observation for worsening respiratory status and supportive care.

Patients with moderate-to-severe pulmonary contusions may be tachypneic and have an oxygen requirement secondary to shunting within the lung. If the patient can no longer maintain oxygenation, endotracheal intubation and mechanical ventilation with positive pressure is the treatment of choice. Fluid restriction is helpful to avoid exacerbation of pulmonary edema. Many of these patients will have associated injuries, making fluid restriction difficult; intensive care management with measurement of central venous and pulmonary arterial pressure may be helpful in fluid management. Double lumen endotracheal-endobronchial tubes can be used in patients with severe lung contusions refractory to normal ventilatory management.

Pulmonary lacerations usually result from penetrating trauma but can occur in rapid deceleration injuries. Rib fractures secondary to blunt trauma may also puncture the lung. Patients are usually tachypneic and have abnormal breath sounds. Large lacerations may cause hemoptysis. Chest radiograph will show pneumothorax or hemothorax. Treatment includes endotracheal intubation for those patients in respiratory distress and tube thoracostomy for pneumothorax or hemothorax. Adequate intravenous access and blood for transfusion should be available prior to chest tube placement unless the tube must be placed emergently for respiratory distress.

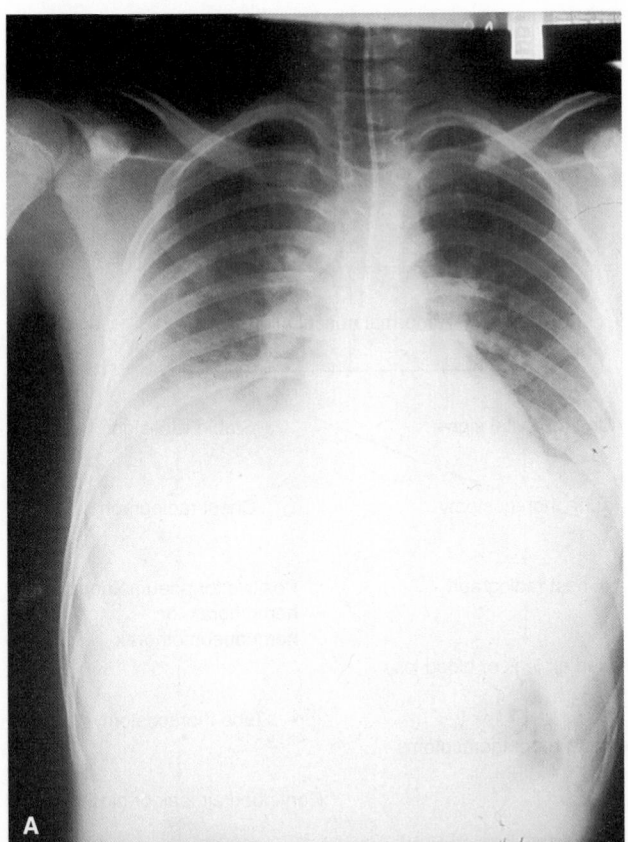

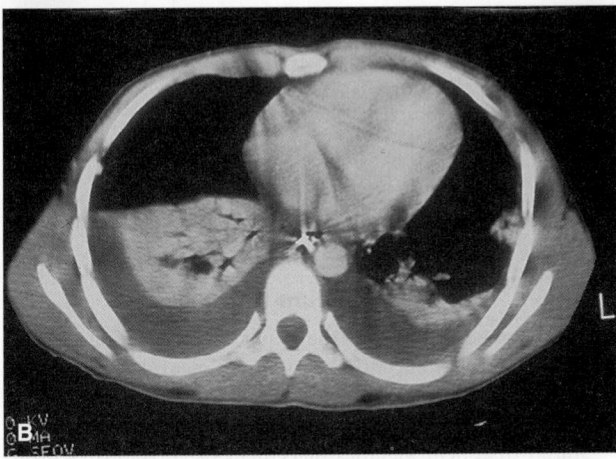

FIGURE 118.9 A 15-year-old child involved in an automobile–pedestrian accident. Vital signs were stable at the scene, but the child had decreased breath sounds bilaterally. **A:** Chest radiograph showed bilateral hemothorax and pulmonary contusions. **B:** Computed tomography confirmed and better delineated the hemothorax and pulmonary contusions.

Insertion of the chest tube can disrupt hemostasis in the chest cavity, and the patient may exsanguinate. Indications for surgery include continuous hemorrhage or air leak through the chest tube, massive hemoptysis, or air embolism.

Air embolism is usually fatal, but it should be considered when a patient deteriorates suddenly after endotracheal intubation, focal neurologic findings develop without evidence of a neurologic injury, or frothy blood is withdrawn from an

arterial puncture. Treatment includes open thoracostomy with either occlusion of the hilar structure on the affected side or direct aspiration of the air. Neither of these treatment options is very successful.

Intrapleural Injuries

In one study, intrapleural injury occurred in 40% of children with thoracic trauma. Hemopneumothorax, hemothorax, and pneumothorax were evenly distributed. Pneumothorax was associated with the lowest mortality rate (15%), whereas hemothorax had the highest (57%). Auscultation is helpful, but not 100% accurate in diagnosing a hemothorax, pneumothorax, or hemopneumothorax. A more recent report found that auscultation to detect hemothorax, pneumothorax, or hemopneumothorax had a sensitivity of 58% and a specificity of 98%. The majority of intrapleural injuries do not need surgical intervention and can be managed either by hospital observation or tube thoracostomy (Fig. 118.10).

Pneumothorax

Pneumothorax is the second most commonly encountered entity in blunt thoracic trauma and most common in penetrating thoracic trauma. Air within the pleural cavity can arise from penetration of the chest wall, disruption of the lung parenchyma, a tear of the tracheobronchial structures, or esophageal rupture.

Patients may be asymptomatic, complain of pleuritic chest pain, have tachypnea, or be in severe respiratory distress. Physical examination may be normal or may reveal diminished or absent breath sounds, crepitus, or hyperresonance to percussion on the side of the pneumothorax. In the asymptomatic or mildly symptomatic patient, a chest radiograph is helpful in diagnosing and determining the type of treatment necessary (Fig. 118.11). Plain radiographic signs of a pneumothorax may include a hyperlucent hemithorax, pleural air at the lung base, and/or an unusually well-defined heart and mediastinal outline due to pleural air rising anteriorly. If the pneumothorax is small and the patient asymptomatic, hospital observation and administration of 100% oxygen is all that is necessary. A small pneumothorax is classically described as being less than 15%, although it is common to underestimate the size of a pneumothorax on plain films, only to find a much more extensive lesion on CT scan. Tube thoracostomy is indicated in the symptomatic patient, any patient undergoing positive-pressure ventilation, or those requiring air transport. An asymptomatic patient may rapidly become symptomatic if a small, simple pneumothorax progresses to a tension pneumothorax; therefore, even asymptomatic patients with a pneumothorax should be admitted to the hospital for observation.

Tension Pneumothorax

A tension pneumothorax is the most common complicated intrapleural injury. Tension pneumothorax develops in up to 20% of children after simple pneumothorax. A tension pneumothorax occurs when there is progressive accumulation of air within the pleural cavity. A laceration to the chest wall, pulmonary parenchyma, or bronchial tree may function as a one-way valve, allowing air to enter but not leave the pleural

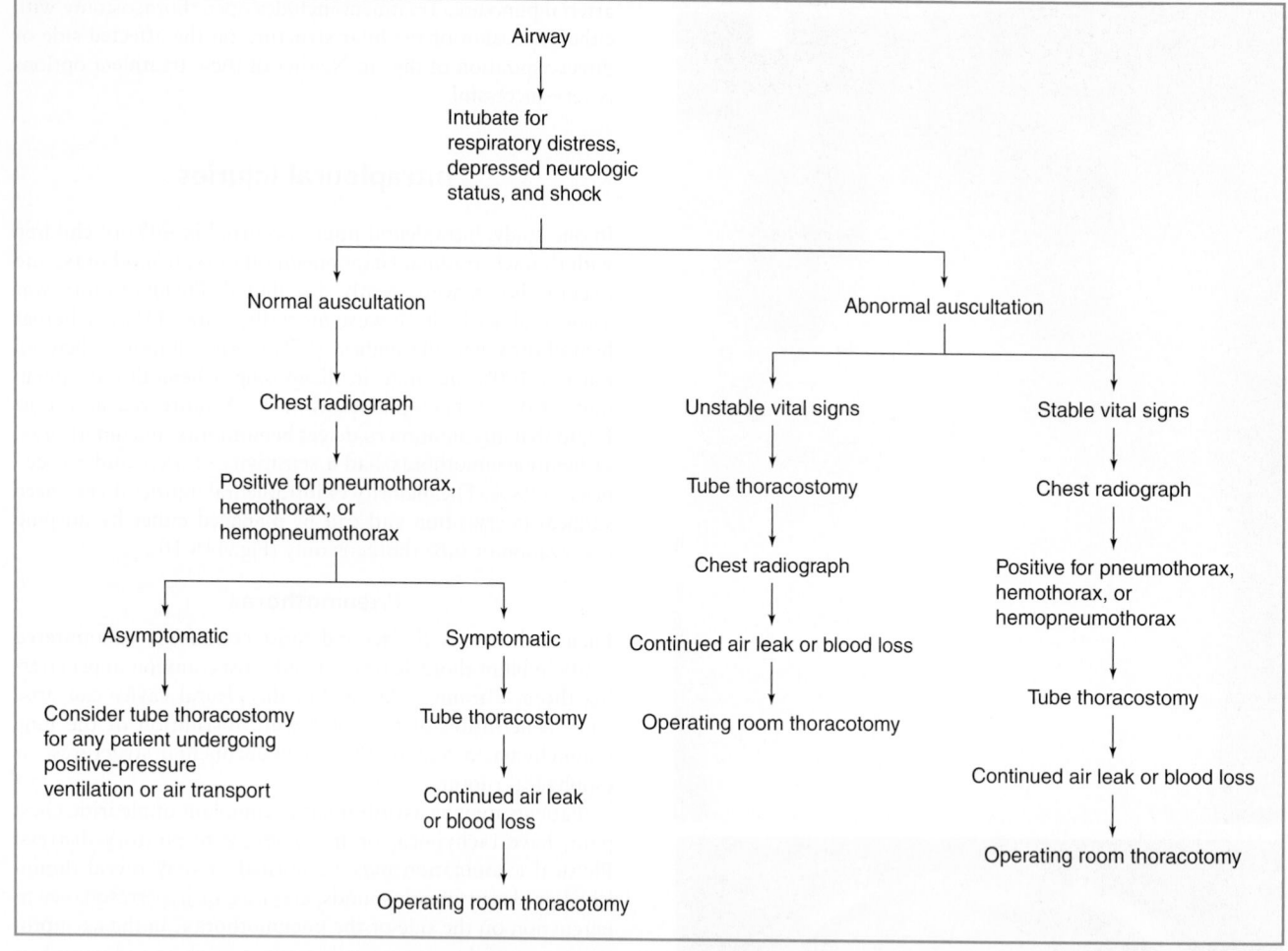

FIGURE 118.10 Algorithm for the management of intrapleural injuries.

space. The progressive accumulation of air within the pleural cavity not only collapses the ipsilateral lung, but it also compresses the contralateral lung. These patients may present in severe respiratory distress with decreased breath sounds on the side of the pneumothorax. There is also a shift of the mediastinal structures to the contralateral side (Fig. 118.12). Two thirds of the blood supply to the body is returned to the heart via the inferior vena cava. Because the inferior vena cava is relatively fixed in place and cannot shift as much as the superior vena cava, venous return to the heart is reduced and the patient may appear tachycardic, peripherally vasoconstricted, and in hypotensive shock. This underscores the importance that whenever a trauma patient suddenly deteriorates, the treating physician must return to airway and breathing, before jumping to circulation.

Initial treatment consists of needle decompression performed in the midclavicular second intercostal space of the ipsilateral side. If there is a tension pneumothorax, an immediate release of air should be noted. If positive, the needle decompression is only a temporizing measure and must be followed by tube thoracostomy. Tube thoracostomy is usually done in the midaxillary line at the level of the fifth intercostal space (nipple level). Chest x-ray is only performed after the insertion of the chest tube and should not be used to diagnose a tension pneumothorax in the symptomatic patient. If a

significant air leak continues after chest tube placement, a tracheobronchial rupture must be considered.

Open Pneumothorax

An open pneumothorax is the result of penetrating trauma. There is a direct connection between the pleural space and the outside atmosphere. As in a bronchial tear or lung parenchymal injury, air may enter but not leave the pleural space.

Initial treatment includes placement of an occlusive dressing at the wound site. This is best done when the patient is in full expiration. A chest tube should be placed immediately to prevent development of a tension pneumothorax. The chest tube should be inserted at a site different than the open wound. Larger open wounds may need surgical closure. Any patient in respiratory distress should be intubated and receive positive-pressure ventilation.

Hemothorax

Hemothorax is much more common in penetrating than blunt thoracic trauma. In blunt thoracic trauma, a hemothorax can occur from rib fractures lacerating the lung, pulmonary parenchymal injuries without rib fractures, lacerations of the internal mammary arteries or intercostal arteries, or disruption of the major vascular structures in the mediastinum or hilum. A hemothorax secondary to a major injury of the great

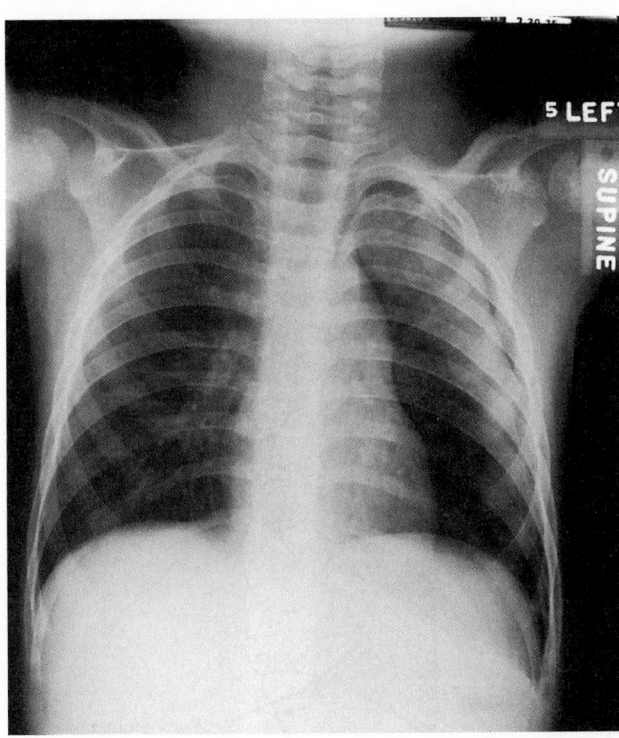

FIGURE 118.11 This 3-year-old child was an unrestrained passenger in a motor vehicle accident. The patient was tachypneic and had decreased breath sounds on the left side but was otherwise asymptomatic. Chest radiograph revealed a left pneumothorax with a pulmonary contusion.

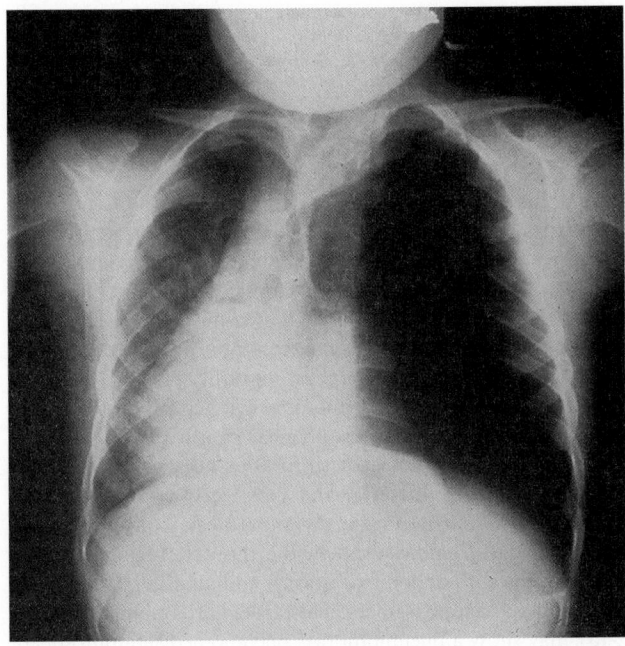

FIGURE 118.12 A 5-year-old girl fell off and was then kicked in the chest by a horse. Upon arrival of the life-flight team, the patient was found to be in both respiratory and cardiovascular distress. Chest radiograph demonstrated a left-sided tension pneumothorax. The patient was intubated, and a chest tube was placed before the patient was transported. After the intubation and chest tube insertion, both the patient's respiratory and cardiovascular status improved.

vessels usually results in death. Liver and spleen injuries can also cause a hemothorax with disruption of the diaphragm. The most common cause of a hemothorax is injury to the intercostal or internal mammary arteries, whereas injuries to the lung or great vessels causing a hemothorax are much less common, but more serious.

Patients may present in respiratory distress or in profound shock secondary to obstruction of venous return or massive blood loss. Decreased breath sounds are noted on the affected side, and there may be tracheal or mediastinal deviation. Thirty percent to 40% of the patient's blood volume may be rapidly lost in the pleural cavity. This usually occurs with major vessel lacerations. Bleeding from the intercostal or internal mammary arteries stops secondary to low systemic pressures and also when reexpansion of the lung produces effective tamponade. A chest radiograph will confirm the diagnosis. If a hemothorax is suspected clinically and the patient is in severe respiratory or circulatory distress, immediate tube thoracostomy should be performed prior to a chest radiograph.

Treatment of a major hemothorax should include aggressive airway and circulatory management, as well as evacuation of the pleural blood. Endotracheal intubation and positive-pressure ventilation should be initiated in any unstable airway. Patients should be typed and crossed for packed red blood cells and adequately volume resuscitated, preferably with two large intravenous lines in place. When time permits, O-negative blood, if type-specific blood is not available, should be at the patient's bedside prior to tube thoracostomy.

Tube thoracostomy is performed to evacuate blood within the pleural cavity, reexpand the lung, and prevent or treat any mediastinal shift. The chest tube is placed in the midaxillary line at the level of the fifth intercostal space (nipple level). This is the same location as in a pneumothorax. Many hemothoraxes may actually represent hemopneumothoraxes. After placement of a chest tube, blood should be slowly evacuated from the pleural space. Blood within the pleural cavity may tamponade a significant bleeding source within the chest and evacuating that blood may cause new bleeding to occur. Patients can exsanguinate rapidly, which is why intravenous access, adequate volume resuscitation, and blood available for transfusion should be a priority. Thoracostomy drainage needs to be closely monitored. Large ongoing blood loss from a chest tube should be collected in a system that allows autotransfusion. Thoracostomy is indicated for continued bleeding (greater than 1 to 2 mL per kg per hour), inability to expand the lung, or retained blood within the pleural cavity. Failure to adequately drain a hemothorax may result in restrictive lung disease from a fibrothorax or an empyema from the clotted material becoming infected.

Chylothorax

A chylothorax is rare in thoracic trauma and most commonly occurs secondary to iatrogenic complications. It can occur from penetrating injuries or a hyperextension injury to the spine. Disruption of the thoracic duct will lead to chyle draining into the mediastinum and pleural space. Diagnosis is confirmed when chyle is aspirated from the pleural cavity. Infection is rare because chyle is bacteriostatic, and treatment consists of tube thoracostomy, dietary manipulation, and, if all else fails, thoracic duct ligation.

TRAUMA

Tracheobronchial Injuries

Injury to the tracheobronchial tree in children occurs rarely, with an incidence of less than 1%. This injury is most commonly caused by acceleration or deceleration forces. Major vessels or pulmonary parenchyma are more likely to be injured in penetrating trauma than the tracheobronchial tree. Cervical tracheal rupture may be caused by a direct blow to the trachea or from the patient's head violently traveling forward and backward. This whiplash effect can cause a tear between two cartilaginous rings. Lower tracheobronchial injury usually occurs from a sudden increase in intrabronchial pressure. Because the child's chest wall is elastic, the trachea and main bronchi can be compressed between the chest wall and the vertebral spine. Compression of the chest with a closed glottis can cause a sudden increase in intrabronchial pressure, resulting in a tracheobronchial tear. Shear forces, traction, and crushing the airway between the chest and vertebral column may also cause a tracheobronchial injury. Approximately 80% of tracheobronchial injuries occur near the origin of the main stem bronchus.

The diagnosis of tracheobronchial injury may be difficult in the pediatric population. Mechanism of injury (fall, crush, direct blow) provides an important clue. Symptoms such as chest pain and dyspnea are common but nonspecific. Unlike the adult population, rib fractures are rare because of the elastic nature of the child's chest. Clinical signs include cyanosis, hemoptysis, tachypnea, and subcutaneous emphysema (cervical, mediastinal, or both). Pneumomediastinum and cervical emphysema are seen commonly in airway rupture (Fig. 118.13). If a pneumothorax is present with these findings, a bronchial rupture should be suspected. A continued air leak after insertion of a thoracostomy tube should also alert the physician to the possibility of a bronchial tear. Because of anatomic differences, ruptures of the bronchi occur on the right side more frequently than the left. In the absence of a pneumothorax, tracheal rupture should be suspected if a pneumomediastinum or cervical emphysema is present.

The treatment includes initial airway stabilization and then bronchoscopic evaluation of the airway. Numerous reports in the literature record a partial tracheal tear becoming complete after endotracheal intubation. Therefore, if the airway is stable and a presence of a tear is known or strongly suspected, oral tracheal intubation should be performed in the operating room under bronchoscopic guidance. This prevents further trauma to the airway, and if a complication arises, emergency surgical access to the airway is readily available. If the airway is unstable and emergent endotracheal intubation needs to be performed, efforts should be made to prepare for backup measures such as cricothyroidotomy, tracheostomy, or fiberoptic bronchoscopy. An advantage of early bronchoscopy is exact identification and location of the lesion. The best surgical results are achieved when operative exploration is performed early. In the stable patient, CT scan of the chest can also help confirm the diagnosis and identify other injuries.

Esophageal Injuries

Esophageal injury is rare in children, but presents a diagnostic challenge when it does occur. Timely and accurate diagnosis of an esophageal injury is paramount. The complications include

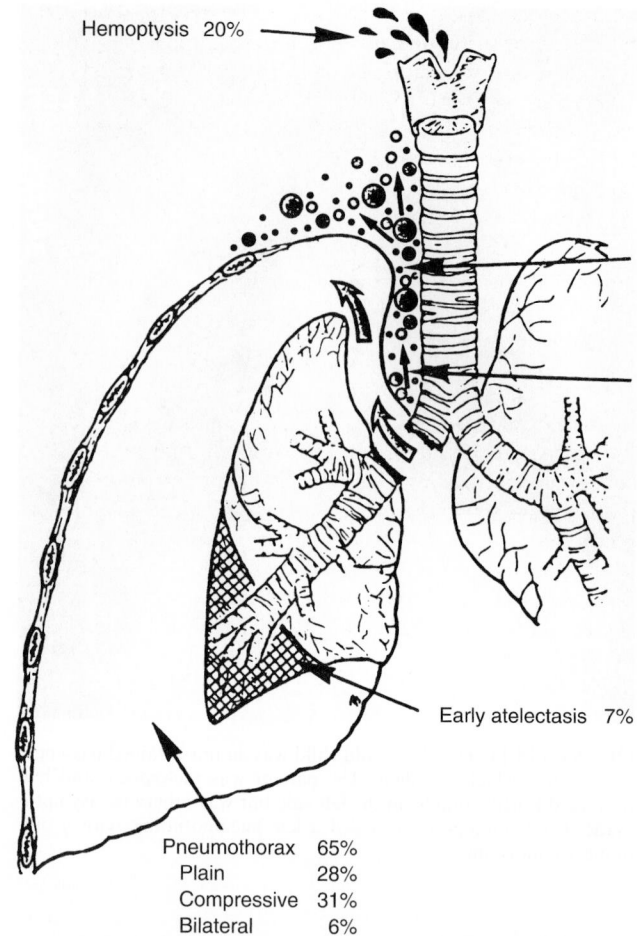

Hemoptysis 20%

Early atelectasis 7%

Pneumothorax 65%
Plain 28%
Compressive 31%
Bilateral 6%

FIGURE 118.13 Initial signs of bronchial rupture. (From Fleisher GR, Ludwig S, Henretig FM. *Textbook of pediatric emergency medicine.* 3rd ed. Baltimore: Williams & Wilkins, Fig. 101.9, reprinted with permission.)

mediastinal sepsis and death. The most common cause for esophageal perforation in the pediatric population is iatrogenic, followed by penetrating trauma (gunshot wound, stab wound). Esophageal perforation can occur in blunt trauma if there is a significant amount of chest compression. The cervical and thoracic regions are more commonly affected, with the thoracic region having the highest mortality rate (35%).

The patient's signs and symptoms will depend on the region injured. Patients with an esophageal rupture in the cervical region may complain of neck stiffness or neck pain. They may regurgitate bloody material and have cervical subcutaneous emphysema or odynophagia. A lateral neck x-ray may show retroesophageal emphysema. In the thoracic region, patients may present with abdominal spasms and guarding, chest pain, subcutaneous emphysema, tachycardia, or dyspnea. A chest x-ray may show a pneumothorax, pneumomediastinum, subcutaneous emphysema in the neck, a left pleural effusion, or an air-fluid level in the mediastinum. Perforation of the intraabdominal esophagus may cause retrosternal, epigastric, or shoulder pain.

Patients with suspected esophageal perforation should be adequately volume resuscitated, have a nasogastric tube placed, and receive antibiotics covering gram-positive, gram-negative, and anaerobic organisms. The diagnosis of an esophageal perforation can be made by either esophagography, esophagoscopy, or both. In one study, flexible esophagoscopy had a sensitivity of 100% and specificity of 96%. Depending on the expertise at each institution and the stability of the patient, these studies may be paired to lessen the chance of a misdiagnosis. Once the diagnosis is made, prompt surgical correction is mandatory. If the diagnosis is made within 24 hours, mortality rate is approximately 5%. Delayed diagnosis for more than 24 hours after injury is associated with a mortality rate of 70%.

Diaphragmatic Injuries

In the sixteenth century, diaphragmatic rupture was described by Ambrose Paré. He noted "the stomach and intestines are sometimes drawn into the thoracic cavity" after diaphragmatic injury. Diaphragmatic injuries are more common in blunt trauma. A crushing force will produce a sudden increase in the intrathoracic and intraabdominal pressure against the fixed diaphragm. Because of the flexible nature of the child's chest wall, rib fractures are rare. Even though penetrating thoracoabdominal trauma is uncommon in children, a diaphragmatic injury should be suspected in any thoracic or abdominal penetrating injury. The level of the diaphragm fluctuates greatly with respirations, and injuries of the diaphragm have been reported with penetrating wounds as high as the third rib and as low as the twelfth rib. Early reports of blunt traumatic diaphragmatic rupture were mostly left sided. Because of a greater awareness of diaphragmatic injuries, right and bilateral diaphragmatic injuries have been reported more recently. Approximately 80% of diaphragmatic injuries still occur on the left, and 20% occur on the right. The left diaphragm is relatively unprotected, whereas the liver protects the right side. Right-sided diaphragmatic injuries are associated with increased mortality rate; patients usually have a greater physiologic insult and more numerous associated injuries.

Motor vehicle accident is the most common mechanism of injury and some authors believe the direction of impact may play a role in the side and type of diaphragmatic rupture. A lateral torso impact has been shown to be three times more likely to result in a ruptured diaphragm than a frontal impact. The rupture tends to be on the same side as the impact. Right-sided diaphragmatic ruptures may be associated with right-sided impact to the passenger side of the vehicle. Associated injuries such as pulmonary contusions, hepatic or splenic lacerations, and fractures of the extremities are present in more than 75% of patients. Thoracic aortic injuries have been reported in up to 10% of adults with diaphragmatic injury and should be considered in children with diaphragmatic trauma.

Patients may present in respiratory distress and have a scaphoid abdomen, although they are more likely to be symptomatic from associated injuries than from the diaphragmatic rupture itself. The verbal child may complain of chest pain or ipsilateral shoulder pain. The presence of bowel sounds within the thoracic cavity is nonspecific because bowel sounds can be transmitted from the abdominal cavity in children. More commonly, bowel sounds are absent because of an associated ileus. A nasogastric tube may be difficult to pass in patients with a diaphragmatic injury and gastric herniation. In left-sided diaphragmatic tears, the tip of the nasogastric

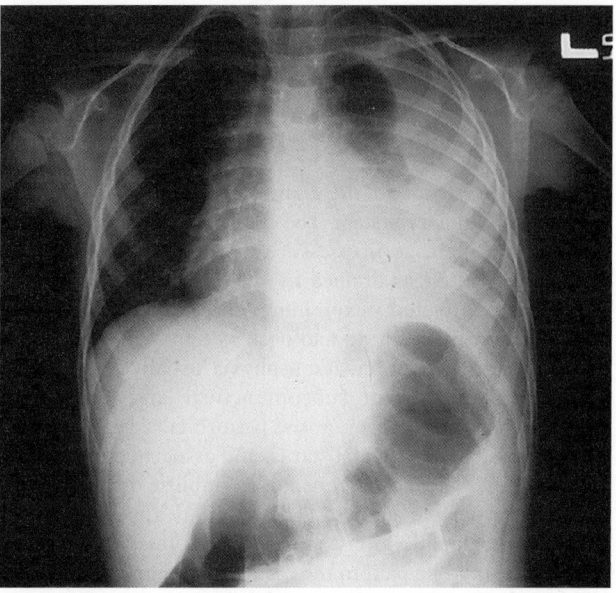

FIGURE 118.14 This 5-year-old boy was on a snowmobile when it crashed into a tree. Initially there was no respiratory distress, but upon arrival at the emergency department, the patient became tachypneic and required oxygen. Breath sounds were reportedly normal. Chest radiograph showed a left-sided diaphragmatic hernia. This injury was surgically repaired in the operating room, and the patient did well postoperatively.

tube may be seen looping into the chest. Even though the diagnosis is usually made upon initial review of the chest x-ray (Fig. 118.14), some series reported that up to 30% to 50% of initial chest x-rays were normal with a diaphragmatic injury. Right-sided diaphragmatic injury and herniation is more difficult to diagnose because the herniated organs are more likely to be solid. The chest x-ray may just show opacification of the right lung fields. This emphasizes the importance of serial evaluations and chest x-rays in patients suspected of having a diaphragmatic injury. Other diagnostic studies such as chest and abdominal CT scan with contrast or upper and lower gastrointestinal tract series can help confirm the diagnosis.

Prior to performing a tube thoracostomy for a pneumothorax or hemothorax, diaphragmatic injury should be considered to avoid injury to herniated intraabdominal organs. In patients who clinically appear to have a diaphragmatic injury (scaphoid abdomen, bowel sounds auscultated in the thoracic cavity), a finger should be inserted in the chest tube incision site and the diaphragm should be palpated before placing a chest tube.

Herniation and strangulation of bowel may result from a delayed diagnosis. Diaphragmatic defects will not spontaneously heal because of motion associated with respirations and cyclical tension. Exploratory laparotomy or laparoscopy should be performed in cases where a diaphragmatic hernia is strongly suspected.

Traumatic Asphyxia

Traumatic asphyxia results from direct compression of the chest or abdomen. The most common mechanism is a child

TRAUMA

run over by a motor vehicle or pinned underneath a heavy object. In anticipation of impending injury, the child may inspire, tensing the thoracoabdominal muscles and closing the glottis. Traumatic asphyxia also occurs in patients with asthma, seizures, persistent vomiting, and pertussis.

Positive pressure is transmitted to the mediastinum, and blood is forced out of the right atrium into the valveless venous and capillary system. The clinical manifestations occur because the increase in pressure dilates the capillary and venous system. Areas drained by the superior vena cava are particularly affected, explaining the marked difference between the patient's head and neck as opposed to the lower body. Patients with traumatic asphyxia usually present with the clinical picture of subconjunctival and upper-body petechial hemorrhages, cyanosis, periorbital edema, respiratory distress, altered mental status, and associated injuries.

The primary goal of treatment is to stabilize the patient and evaluate associated injuries. The external appearance of a child with traumatic asphyxia is quite impressive, but initial attention should be paid to the cardiopulmonary status of the child. Pulmonary contusions and hepatic injuries are commonly seen with traumatic asphyxia, and CT scan is helpful in identifying head, chest, and abdominal injuries. Because the most severe injuries cause immediate death, the prognosis is good for any patient surviving the first few hours. Cutaneous manifestations will resolve with time, and neurologic sequelae are rare. Neurologic injury usually results from hypoxia, not intracranial hemorrhage.

Aortic and Other Vascular Injuries

TRA is uncommon in children but carries a high mortality rate (75% to 95%). It is associated with sudden deceleration forces, commonly from automobile accidents, causing a sheering stress. The aortic arch remains fixed, but the descending aorta is mobile. With deceleration, bending or sheering will take place at the level of the ligamentum arteriosum, which is the most common site of aortic tears in adults and children.

TRA occurs in approximately 10% to 30% of adults sustaining severe blunt trauma but is much less common in the pediatric population. In one study, TRA occurred in only 2.1% of pediatric patients with thoracic trauma. The overall mortality rate was 93%. It is unclear why pediatric patients have a lower incidence of TRA than adults. One reason may be the mechanism of injury. In adults, most TRAs occur when the driver of an automobile forcibly strikes the steering wheel. The sudden deceleration force is isolated to the chest. Children who are passengers in a motor vehicle are less likely to strike an object that can deliver deceleration forces centrally to the chest. In children, one of the most common causes of blunt trauma is automobile-pedestrian accidents, which produce forces distributed over a much wider area.

Children are usually symptomatic from associated injuries, and TRA can easily be missed. Clinical signs may include difference in pulses between the arms or arms and legs, thoracic ecchymosis, thoracic and back tenderness, paraplegia, and anuria. Patients with paraplegia and back pain may be initially diagnosed with a spinal cord injury. Unfortunately, 50% of patients may have no signs pertaining directly to a TRA. A normal chest radiograph has been reported to have a 98%

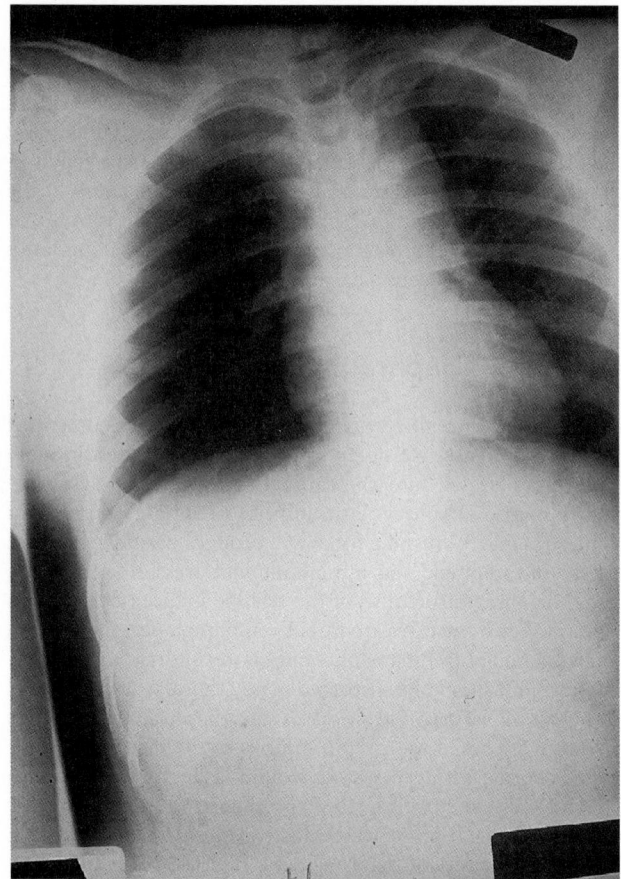

FIGURE 118.15 This 12-year-old girl was an unrestrained passenger involved in a motor vehicle accident. The patient was hypotensive at the scene and could not move her legs. In the emergency department, she had no motor or sensory function to her lower extremities and was anuric. Chest radiograph showed a widened mediastinum from traumatic rupture of the aorta.

negative predictive value in excluding aortic tear, but an abnormal radiograph is in no way diagnostic. More than 90% of patients will have an abnormal chest x-ray (Fig. 118.15). Widened mediastinum, loss of the aortic knob, left-sided pleural cap, tracheal deviation, and nasogastric tube deviation may be seen on a chest x-ray. Much has been written in the adult literature about the association of TRA with first rib fractures. More recent studies have shown that isolated first rib fractures without any other signs or symptoms do not correlate with TRA.

Early diagnosis is imperative in patients with TRA (Fig. 118.16). Morbidity and mortality increase threefold if operative intervention is delayed more than 12 hours. The gold standard for diagnosing TRA is aortography (Fig. 118.17). Thoracic CT scan is only 55% to 65% accurate but helpful in diagnosing associated injuries. In one study, transesophageal echocardiography was shown to be a highly sensitive and specific method of detecting injury to the thoracic aorta. In contrast, another study showed transesophageal echocardiography to be only 63% sensitive and 84% specific in identifying patients with a TRA. Pediatric patients were not included in either of these studies. If the patient is stable and TRA is of significant concern, aortography should be performed. Life-threatening intracranial,

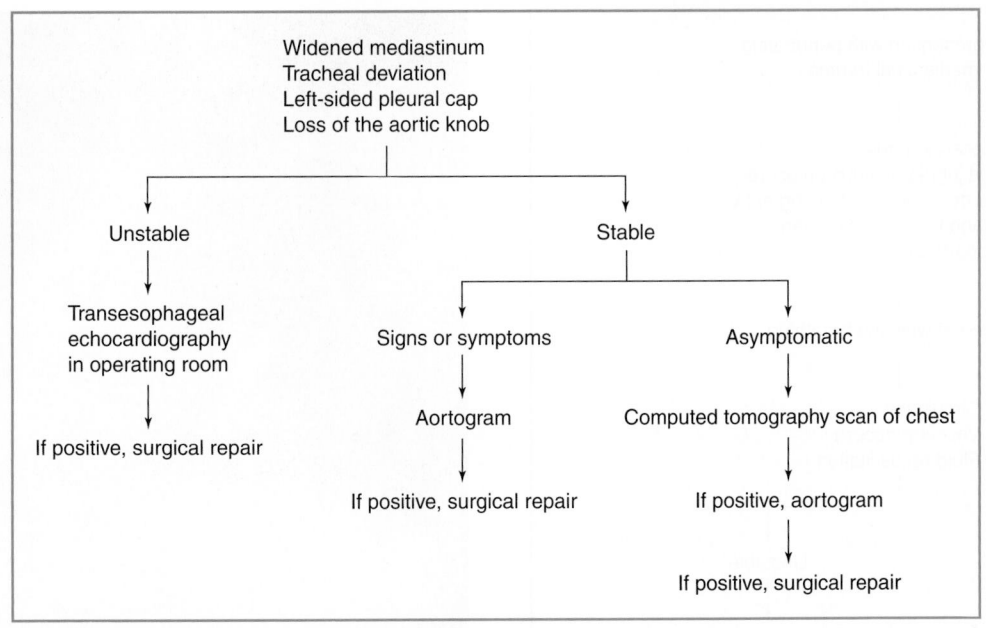

Widened mediastinum
Tracheal deviation
Left-sided pleural cap
Loss of the aortic knob

Unstable

Stable

Transesophageal
echocardiography
in operating room

Signs or symptoms

Asymptomatic

If positive, surgical repair

Aortogram

Computed tomography scan of chest

If positive, surgical repair

If positive, aortogram

If positive, surgical repair

FIGURE 118.16 Algorithm for the evaluation and diagnosis of traumatic rupture of the thoracic aorta.

thoracic, or intraabdominal injuries must first be evaluated and stabilized prior to aortography. If the patient is unstable, a transesophageal echocardiography can be performed in the operating room while the patient's other life-threatening injuries are being treated.

Pericardial Tamponade

Pericardial tamponade occurs when there is injury to the myocardium and blood accumulates in the pericardial sac. Because of the nondistensible pericardium, pressure is exerted

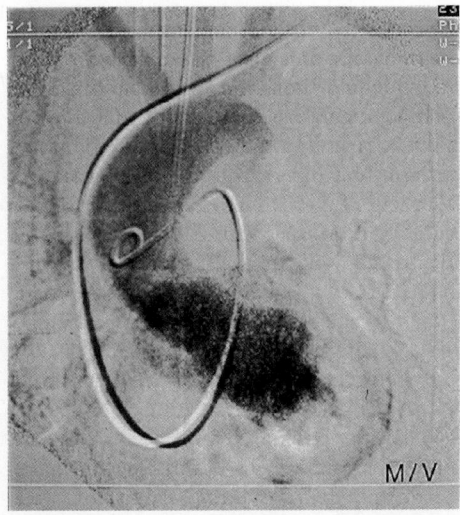

FIGURE 118.17 Emergency pulmonary angiography confirmed an aortic transection distal to the left subclavian artery with a pseudoaneurysm and narrowing of the proximal descending thoracic aorta in a 12-year-old girl.

on the heart. Cardiac output decreases secondary to a decrease in venous return and stroke volume. The body will initially try to compensate with an increase in the pulse rate and peripheral vascular resistance. As the pressure within the pericardial sac increases, the systolic blood pressure will decrease, causing a narrowing of the pulse pressure and subsequent hypotension and cardiogenic shock.

Pericardial tamponade may initially be difficult to diagnose because of associated injuries obscuring the clinical signs and symptoms. Patients may present with distant heart sounds, low blood pressure, poor perfusion, a narrow pulse pressure, or electromechanical dissociation (Fig. 118.18). Pulsus paradoxus, blood pressure falling more than 10 mm Hg during inspiration, occurs in less than one half of patients with pericardial tamponade and should not be relied on to make the diagnosis of pericardial tamponade. Chest x-ray may show an enlarged heart (Fig. 118.19) and an EKG may show low-voltage QRS waves. Neither of these tests is diagnostic for pericardial tamponade, and neither should delay treatment in the unstable patient. In the stable patient, an echocardiogram can demonstrate fluid within the pericardial sac.

In the unstable patient in whom pericardial tamponade is suspected, treatment includes control of the airway, intravascular volume resuscitation, and pericardiocentesis (Fig. 118.20). Pericardiocentesis is performed by inserting a 20-gauge spinal needle below the xiphoid process at a 45-degree angle toward the left shoulder. If time permits, an ultrasound (if available) may be performed or an EKG monitor can be attached to the spinal needle. If the needle touches the heart, a current will be noted on the EKG monitor. Blood aspirated from the pericardial sac can be differentiated from intracardiac blood because pericardial blood is defibrinated and does not clot. Even though patients may show transient improvement after removal of blood from the pericardial sac, the patient should be taken to the operating room immediately

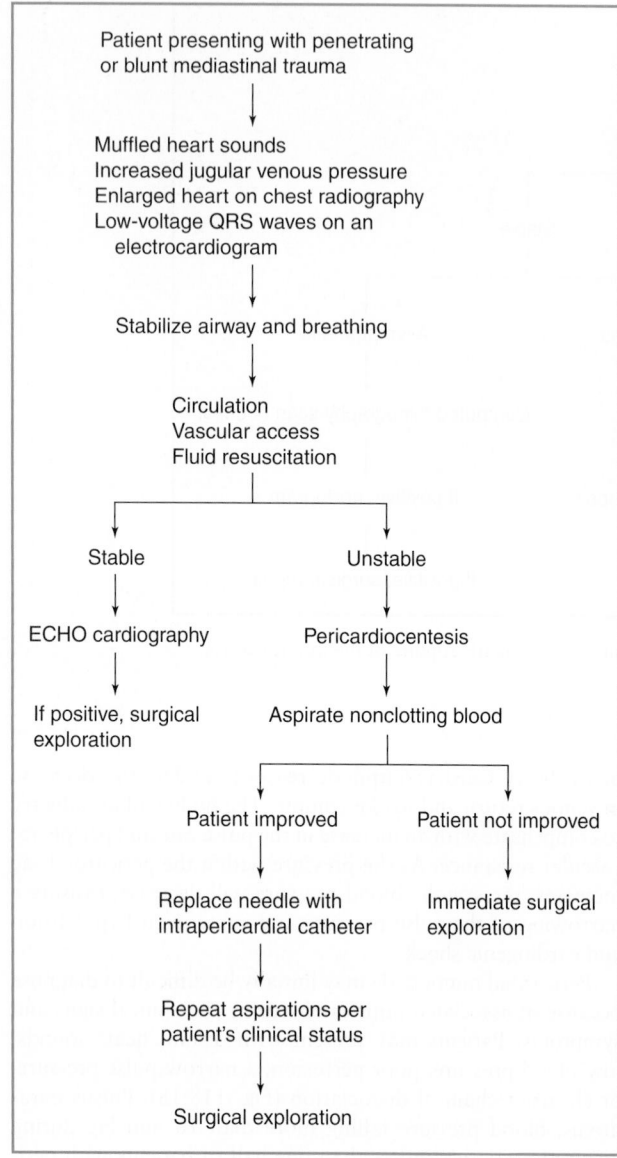

FIGURE 118.18 Algorithm for the evaluation and diagnosis of pericardial tamponade.

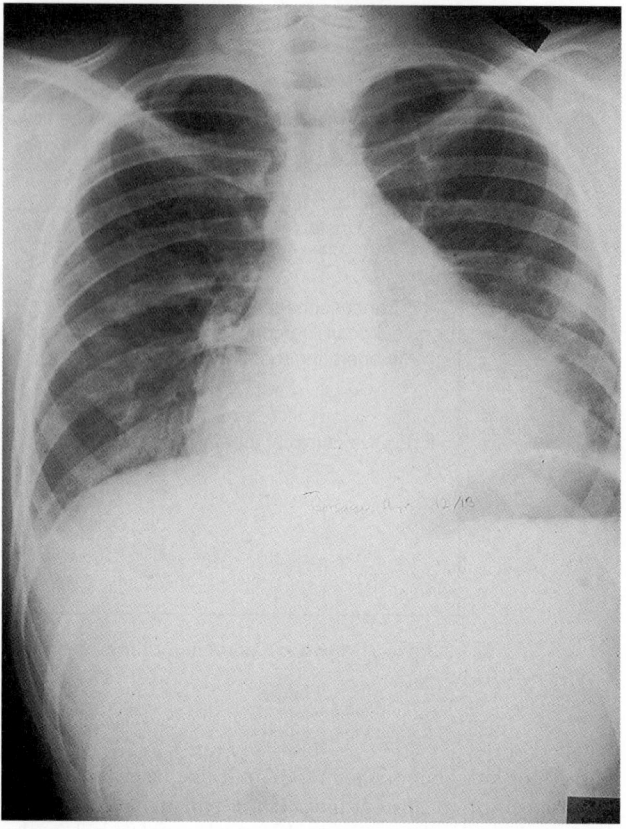

FIGURE 118.19 A 16-year-old boy had a steel bar strike him in the chest. Initially, he was hemodynamically stable but had muffled heart sounds. The patient quickly decompensated and required emergent pericardiocentesis after the chest radiograph. In the operating room, the patient was noted to have a small epicardial laceration on the surface of the heart.

BCI include arrhythmias, pump failure, congestive heart failure, and shock.

Cardiac rupture is the most common cause of death in blunt cardiac trauma. The right ventricle is the chamber most commonly ruptured because of its location directly beneath

for a pericardial window or other surgical intervention. A catheter should be placed into the pericardial sac over a wire guide for continual drainage of blood until surgical correction can be performed.

Blunt Cardiac Injuries

BCI occurs more commonly with associated injuries than in isolation and represents a spectrum of injuries. Myocardial contusion, ventricular or atrial rupture, and valvular disruption are considered BCIs. Myocardial contusion is the most common and ventricular rupture the most lethal of injuries. In one study of 1,288 patients with blunt thoracic trauma, 60 (4.6%) had a diagnosis of BCI. Other series have reported the incidence of BCI to range from 0% to 43%. Complications of

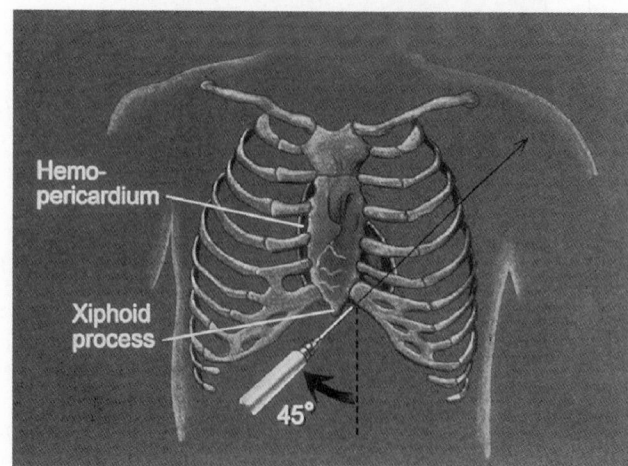

FIGURE 118.20 Pericardiocentesis is performed by inserting a 20-gauge spinal needle below the xiphoid process at a 45-degree angle toward the left shoulder.

the sternum. Septal rupture can also occur, with the condition of the patient correlating with the size of the rupture. Patients with cardiac rupture may demonstrate one or all the components of Beck's triad (jugular venous distention, low blood pressure, and muffled heart tones). Patients with valvular injury may present in congestive heart failure with a new regurgitation murmur. Coronary artery injury is rare but should be considered in patients with persistent EKG changes consistent with ischemia following blunt thoracic trauma.

Unlike adults, pediatric patients with BCI often have few presenting signs or symptoms. Approximately 70% of adults with BCI will complain of chest pain, whereas in one pediatric study less than one half of the awake patients with BCI complained of chest pain, and external evidence of thoracic injury was present in only 60% of these patients. In the same study, cardiac examination was abnormal in less than one fourth of the patients. BCI should be considered in any patient with thoracic trauma who develops a cardiac arrhythmia or a new murmur, or is in congestive heart failure.

Evaluation of suspected BCI remains controversial. In one study, all children who developed heart failure or serious cardiac arrhythmias during their hospital course initially presented to the emergency department (ED) either in shock or with a serious arrhythmia. Patients with suspected myocardial contusion can be monitored in the ED or hospital, and if no arrhythmias develop on EKG, can be safely sent home. CPK-MB ratios have a high false-positive rate and are not a helpful screening tool. Troponin I and T have low sensitivity and low predictive values in diagnosing myocardial contusion so they are not recommended as screening tools. Transesophageal echocardiography should be performed in thoracic trauma patients with an abnormal EKG, arrhythmia, or a new heart murmur. Transesophageal echocardiography has been shown to be more sensitive in detecting myocardial injury than transthoracic echocardiography.

Some general guidelines regarding patients with suspected BCI include the following:

- If a pediatric patient with suspected BCI is hemodynamically stable and has not experienced any arrhythmias, a serious life-threatening arrhythmia or pump failure is unlikely.
- Any patient with suspected BCI who is hemodynamically unstable or has arrhythmias should undergo transesophageal echocardiography and be admitted to the intensive care unit.
- All patients with suspected BCI need close follow-up.

Penetrating Thoracic Trauma

Although not as common as blunt thoracic trauma, penetrating thoracic trauma is becoming more frequent in the pediatric population. In one study, penetrating thoracic trauma occurred in 20% of pediatric patients evaluated for a thoracic injury. The most common mechanism of injury was gunshot; second was stab wounds (Fig. 118.21). Pediatric patients with blunt thoracic trauma are more likely die from associated intracranial and intraabdominal injuries. In contrast, penetrating thoracic trauma is usually a single-system disease and more than 95% of deaths are because of the thoracic wound.

The most common penetrating thoracic injuries are hemothorax and pneumothorax, almost always requiring tube thoracostomy. Intraabdominal injuries should always be suspected

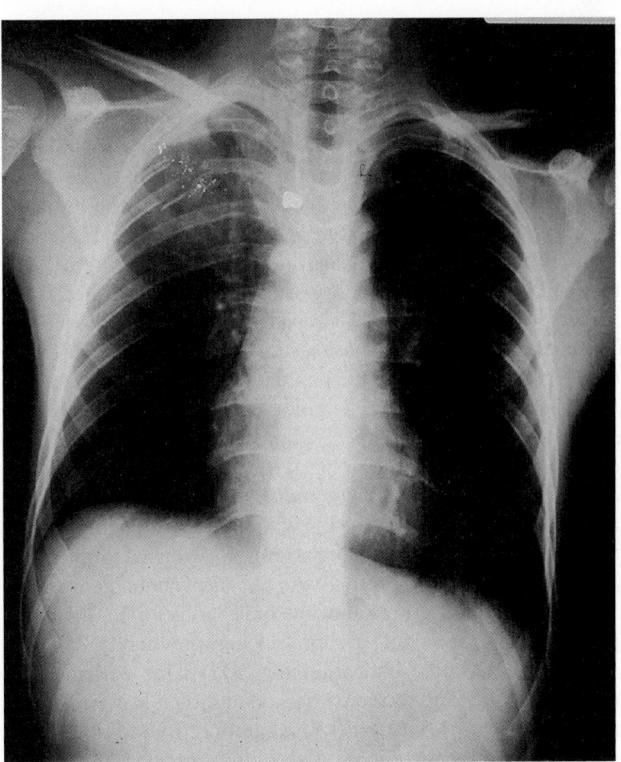

FIGURE 118.21 A 12-year-old boy playing with his father's loaded gun when it accidentally discharged. There was no cardiac or great vessel involvement, and the patient did well postoperatively.

because of the close proximity of abdominal contents to the thoracic cavity. In one study, intraabdominal injuries occurred in 20% of patients with penetrating thoracic injury. More than one half of children with penetrating thoracic injury will require operative intervention. This is higher than the 15% reported in the adult literature. It is unclear why children have this higher rate of operative intervention, but it may be because of the close proximity of the vital organs in the thoracic cavity as compared with adults.

Evaluation and treatment includes airway stabilization, fluid resuscitation, and management of the chest wound. Radiopaque markers (paper clips) may be placed by the entry and exit sites to help determine the course of the missile. Penetrating injuries near the mediastinum may be critical, especially if the patient is hemodynamically unstable. Pericardial tamponade should be considered and treated in the unstable patient. In the stable patient, transesophageal or transthoracic echocardiogram is helpful in evaluating the heart and determining if there is fluid within the pericardial sac. Diaphragmatic lacerations are difficult to diagnose and sometimes require exploratory laparotomy or laparoscopy for diagnosis and treatment.

Emergency Department Thoracostomy

Emergency department thoracostomy (EDT) is one of the most aggressive resuscitative measures for patients with thoracic trauma. With the advancement of transport systems and the regionalization of trauma centers, patients who would have died at the scene are arriving at trauma centers for evaluation and treatment. EDT allows the physician to evaluate and evacuate the pericardial sac, perform open cardiac massage, and temporarily control bleeding from the heart, hilum, or lung. Catheters can also be placed directly into the right atrium, helping with fluid resuscitation, and the thoracic aorta can be compressed, improving central circulation to the brain and heart.

Anecdotal reports have been published, suggesting EDT may be useful in the pediatric patient who has vital signs but loses them during transport or resuscitation. Other studies have shown poor outcome of EDT in pediatric blunt trauma victims. The more recent literature has reevaluated the need for EDT and tried to select a more specific population. In one study, none of the 17 pediatric patients undergoing EDT after thoracic trauma survived, although 15 of the 17 patients had blunt trauma and only 2 had isolated penetrating thoracic trauma. The authors concluded that EDT was not indicated in the blunt thoracic trauma patient arriving in the ED without any vital signs or EKG tracing. Another study of thoracic gunshot wounds in the pediatric population found no survivors in patients undergoing EDT and advocated a reappraisal of the indications for EDT among pulseless pediatric victims of thoracic gunshot wounds.

The one accepted indication for EDT is the patient with penetrating thoracic trauma who had and then lost vital signs prior to arrival or during ED resuscitation. In addition, EDT may be useful for the patient with blunt thoracic trauma who acutely deteriorates in the ED during resuscitation, but the chance of survival is dismal. Lifesaving interventions such as airway management, fluid resuscitation, and pericardiocentesis should not be delayed while waiting for EDT to be performed. The pediatric patient with vital signs, but not responding to initial treatment such as tube thoracostomy and pericardiocentesis, is a candidate for thoracostomy in the operating room, rather than the ED.

The outcome is directly dependent on the patient's status prior to arrival in the ED and mechanism of injury. In blunt thoracic trauma, essentially 100% of patients who present to the ED without vital signs have a fatal injury, regardless of whether EDT is performed. Pediatric patients who present with cardiac arrest or tamponade caused by penetrating trauma, and in whom vital signs were present either in the field or in the ED, have the best chance of survival, although small, if EDT is performed.

Suggested Readings

General

Allshouse M, Eichelberger M. Patterns of thoracic injury. In: Eichelberger M, ed. *Pediatric trauma: prevention, acute care, rehabilitation.* St. Louis, MO: Mosby–Year Book, 1993:437–448.
Balci A, Kazez A, Eren S, et al. Blunt thoracic trauma in children: review of 137 cases. *Eur J Cardiothorac Surg* 2004;26:387–392.
Bliss D, Silen M. Pediatric thoracic trauma. *Crit Care Med* 2002;30:409–415.
Cooper A. Thoracic injuries. *Semin Pediatr Surg* 1995;4:109–116.
Cooper A, Barlow B, DiScala C, et al. Mortality and truncal injury: the pediatric perspective. *J Pediatr Surg* 1994;29:33–38.
Exadaktylos AK, Sclabas G, Schmid SW, et al. Do we really need routine computed tomographic scanning in the primary evaluation of blunt chest trauma in patients with "normal" chest radiograph? *J Trauma* 2001;51:1173–1176.
Gittelman M, Gonzalez-del-Rey J, Brody A, et al. Clinical predictors for the selective use of chest radiographs in pediatric blunt trauma evaluations. *J Trauma* 2003;55:670–676.
Grisoni ER, Volsko TA. Thoracic injuries in children. *Respir Care Clin N Am* 2001;7:25–38.

Hall A, Johnson K. The imaging of paediatric thoracic trauma. *Paediatr Respir Rev* 2002;3:241–247.
Holmes JF, Sokolove PE, Brant WE, et al. A clinical decision rule for identifying children with thoracic injuries after blunt torso trauma. *Ann Emerg Med* 2002;39:492–499.
Inan M, Ayvaz S, Sut N, et al. Blunt chest trauma in childhood. *ANZ J Surg* 2007;77:682–685.
Peclet M, Newman K, Eichelberger M, et al. Patterns of injury in children. *J Pediatr Surg* 1990;25:85–91.
Peclet M, Newman K, Eichelberger M, et al. Thoracic trauma in children: an indicator of increased mortality. *J Pediatr Surg* 1990;25:961–966.
Trupka A, Waydhas C, Hallfeldt KJ. Value of thoracic computed tomography in the first assessment of severely injured patients with blunt chest trauma: results of a prospective study. *J Trauma* 1997;43:405–412.

Chest Wall Injury

Freedland M, Wilson R, Bender J, et al. The management of flail chest injury: factors affecting outcome. *J Trauma* 1990;30:1460–1468.
Garcia V, Gotschall M, Eichelberger M, et al. Rib fractures in children: a marker of severe trauma. *J Trauma* 1990;30:695–700.
Harris G, Soper R. Pediatric first rib fractures. *J Trauma* 1990;30:343–345.
Kwon A, Sorrells D, Kurkchubasche A, et al. *J Pediatr Surg* 2006;41:78–82.
Landercasper J, Cogbill T, Strutt P. Delayed diagnosis of flail chest. *Crit Care Med* 1990;18:611–613.
Sadaba JR, Oswal D, Munsch CM. Management of isolated sternal fractures: determining the risk of blunt cardiac injury. *Ann R Coll Surg Engl* 2000;82:162–166.
Schweich P, Fleisher G. Rib fractures in children. *Pediatr Emerg Care* 1985;1:187–189.
Shorr R, Crittenden M, Indeck M, et al. Blunt thoracic trauma: analysis of 515 patients. *Ann Surg* 1987;206:200–205.
Stephens N, Morgan A, Corvo P, et al. Significance of scapular fracture in the blunt-trauma patient. *Ann Emerg Med* 1995;26:439–442.
Ziegler D, Agarwal N. The morbidity and mortality of rib fractures. *J Trauma* 1994;37:975–979.

Lung Injury

Blostein P, Hodgman C. Computed tomography of the chest in blunt thoracic trauma: results of a prospective study. *J Trauma* 1997;43:13–18.
Bonadio W, Hellmich T. Post-traumatic pulmonary contusion in children. *Ann Emerg Med* 1989;18:1050–1052.
Frame S, Marshall W, Clifford T. Synchronized independent lung ventilation in the management of pediatric unilateral pulmonary contusion: case report. *J Trauma* 1989;29:395–397.
Johnson J, Cogbill T, Winga E. Determinants of outcome after pulmonary contusion. *J Trauma* 1986;26:695–697.

Pneumothorax/Hemothorax

Chen S, Markmann J, Kauder D, et al. Hemopneumothorax missed by auscultation in penetrating chest injury. *J Trauma* 1997;42:86–89.
Ma O, Mateer J. Trauma ultrasound examination versus chest radiography in the detection of hemothorax. *Ann Emerg Med* 1997;29:312–315.
Nakayama D, Ramenofsky M, Rowe M. Chest injuries in childhood. *Ann Surg* 1989;210:770–775.
Rowan KR, Kirkpatrick AW, Liu D, et al. Traumatic pneumothorax detection with thoracic US: correlation with chest radiography and CT—initial experience. *Radiology* 2002;225:210–214.
Symbas P. Cardiothoracic trauma. *Curr Probl Surg* 1991;28:742–797.

Tracheal And Bronchial Injury

Baumgartner F, Sheppard B, Virgilio C, et al. Tracheal and main bronchial disruptions after blunt chest trauma: presentation and management. *Ann Thorac Surg* 1990;50:569–574.
Gaebler C, Mueller M, Schramm W, et al. Tracheobronchial ruptures in children. *Am J Emerg Med* 1996;14:279–285.
Hancock B, Wiseman N. Tracheobronchial injuries in children. *J Pediatr Surg* 1991;26:1316–1319.
Kadish H, Schunk J, Woodward G. Blunt pediatric laryngotracheal trauma: case report and review of the literature. *Am J Emerg Med* 1994;12:207–211.
Panagiotis N, Alexander G, Richard R. Rupture of the airways from blunt trauma: treatment of complex injuries. *Ann Thorac Surg* 1992;54:177–183.
Taskinen S, Salo J, Halttunnen P. Tracheobronchial rupture due to blunt chest trauma. *Ann Thorac Surg* 1989;48:846–849.

Esophageal Injury

Backer C. Computed tomography in patients with esophageal perforation. *Chest* 1990;98:1078–1080.

Flowers J, Graham S, Ugarte M, et al. Flexible endoscopy for the diagnosis of esophageal trauma. *J Trauma* 1996;40:261–266.

Jones W, Ginsberg R. Esophageal perforation: a continuing challenge. *Ann Thorac Surg* 1992;53:534–543.

Diaphragmatic Injury

Beauchamp G, Khalfallah A, Girard R, et al. Blunt diaphragmatic rupture. *Am J Surg* 1984;148:292–296.

Boulanger B, Milzman D, Rosati C, et al. A comparison of right and left blunt traumatic diaphragmatic rupture. *J Trauma* 1993;35:255–260.

Brandt M, Luks F, Spigland N. Diaphragmatic injury in children. *J Trauma* 1992;32:298–301.

Guth A, Pachter L, Kim U. Pitfalls in the diagnosis of blunt diaphragmatic injury. *Am J Surg* 1995;170:5–9.

Murray J, Demetriades D, Cornwell E, et al. Penetrating left thoracoabdominal trauma: the incidence and clinical presentation of diaphragm injuries. *J Trauma* 1997;43:624–626.

Pagliarello G, Carter J. Traumatic injury to the diaphragm: timely diagnosis and treatment. *J Trauma* 1992;33:194–197.

Traumatic Asphyxia

Gorenstein L, Blair G, Shandling B. The prognosis of traumatic asphyxia in childhood. *J Trauma* 1986;21:753–756.

Newquist M, Sobel R. Traumatic asphyxia: an indicator of significant pulmonary injury. *Am J Emerg Med* 1990;8:212–215.

Sklar D, Baack B, McFeeley P, et al. Traumatic asphyxia in New Mexico: a five-year experience. *Am J Emerg Med* 1988;5:219–223.

Aortic and Great Vessel Injury

Dart C, Braitman H. Traumatic rupture of the thoracic aorta. *Arch Surg* 1976;111:687–690.

Eddy A, Rusch V, Fligner C, et al. The epidemiology of traumatic rupture of the thoracic aorta in children: a 13-year review. *J Trauma* 1990;30:989–992.

Lee J, Harris J, Duke J, et al. Noncorrelation between thoracic skeletal injuries and acute traumatic aortic tear. *J Trauma* 1997;43:400–404.

Saletta S, Lederman E, Fein S. Transesophageal echocardiography for the initial evaluation of the widened mediastinum in trauma patients. *J Trauma* 1995;39:137–141.

Smith M, Cassidy M, Souther S, et al. Transesophageal echocardiography in the diagnosis of traumatic rupture of the aorta. *N Engl J Med* 1995;332:356–362.

Blunt Cardiac Injury

Bertinchant J, Polge A, Mohty D, et al. Evaluation of incidence, clinical significance, and prognostic value of circulating cardiac troponin I and T elevation in hemodynamically stable patients with suspected myocardial contusion after blunt chest trauma. *J Trauma* 2000;48:924–931.

Biffl W, Moore F, Moore E, et al. Cardiac enzymes are irrelevant in the patient with suspected myocardial contusion. *Am J Surg* 1994;169:523–528.

Dowd M, Krug S. Pediatric blunt cardiac injury: epidemiology, clinical features, and diagnosis. *J Trauma* 1996;40:61–67.

Karalis D, Victor M, Davis G, et al. The role of echocardiography in blunt chest trauma: a transthoracic and transesophageal echocardiographic study. *J Trauma* 1994;36:53–58.

Maron B, Poliac L, Kaplan J, et al. Blunt impact to the chest leading to sudden death from cardiac arrest during sports activities. *N Engl J Med* 1995;333:337–342.

Maron BJ, Gohman TE, Kyle SB, et al. Clinical profile and spectrum of commotio cordis. *JAMA* 2002;287:1142–1146.

Murillo CA, Owens-Stovall SK, Kim S. Delayed cardiac tamponade after blunt chest trauma in a child. *J Trauma* 2001;52:573–575.

Penetrating Thoracic Injury

Fernandez L, Radhakrishnan J, Gordon R, et al. Thoracic BB injuries in pediatric patients. *J Trauma* 1995;38:384–389.

Inci I, Ozcelik C, Nizam O. Penetrating chest injuries in children: a review of 94 cases. *J Pediatr Surg* 1996;31:673–676.

Nance M, Sing R, Reilly P. Thoracic gunshot wounds in children under 17 years of age. *J Pediatr Surg* 1996;31:931–935.

Peterson R, Tiwary A, Kissoon N, et al. Pediatric penetrating thoracic trauma: a five-year experience. *Pediatr Emerg Care* 1994;10:129–131.

Emergency Department Thoracostomy

Beaver B, Colombani P, Buck J, et al. Efficacy of emergency room thoracostomy in pediatric trauma. *J Pediatr Surg* 1987;22:19–23.

Boyd M, Vanek V, Bourguet C. Emergency room resuscitative thoracostomy: when is it indicated? *J Trauma* 1992;33:714–721.

Durham L, Richardson R, Wall M, et al. Emergency center thoracostomy: impact of prehospital resuscitation. *J Trauma* 1992;32:775–779.

Esposito T, Jurkovich G, Rice C, et al. Reappraisal of emergency room thoracostomy in a changing environment. *J Trauma* 1991;31:881–887.

Langer J, Hoffman M, Pearl R, et al. Survival after emergency department thoracostomy in a child with blunt multisystem trauma. *Pediatr Emerg Care* 1989;5:255–261.

Lorenz H, Steinmetz B, Lieberman J. Emergency thoracostomy: survival correlates with physiologic status. *J Trauma* 1992;32:780–788.

Powell R, Gill E, Jurkovich G, et al. Resuscitative thoracostomy in children and adolescents. *Am Surg* 1988;54:188–191.

Sheikh A, Brogan T. Outcome and cost of open- and closed-chest cardiopulmonary resuscitation in pediatric cardiac arrest. *Pediatrics* 1994;93:392–398.

TRAUMA

CHAPTER 119 ■ MINOR LESIONS AND INJURIES

SARITA CHUNG, MD

A variety of minor lesions in children may prompt an emergency department (ED) visit. Most visits are the result of acute injury, infection, or combination of the two mechanisms (e.g., hair tourniquet, felon paronychia). Some formerly quiescent abnormalities (e.g., thyroglossal duct cyst, pyogenic granuloma) become clinically apparent after rapid enlargement secondary to infection or direct trauma. Alternatively, asymptomatic minor lesions (e.g., lipoma, pilomatrixoma) may be noted during the evaluation of an unrelated complaint. Regardless of the presentation, a systematic approach is necessary for proper diagnosis and subsequent management of these lesions. Although most "lumps and bumps" in children have a benign cause, the examiner should bear in mind the possibilities of associated systemic illness and future complications.

HAND AND FOOT LESIONS

Eponychia and Paronychia

Infections and/or minor trauma of the digits are the major etiologies of hand lesions in the ED. The most common infections of the digits involve the eponychium (cuticle) as a result of a breakdown of the epidermal border due to trauma such as a traumatized hangnail or, particularly in children, finger sucking or nail biting. In its initial stage, the infection consists of a superficial cellulitis that remains localized to the cuticle and is termed an *eponychia*. Symptoms include erythema and localized pain at the nail margin. With progression, pus collects in a single thin-walled pocket under the cuticle, forming an acute paronychia (Fig. 119.1A). Patients typically present with localized tenderness and have an area of fluctuance and purulence around the nail margin (Fig. 119.1B). This may progress, extending under the skin at the base of the nail, and along the nail fold. Less commonly, the pus burrows beneath the proximal nail, forming an *onychia* or subungual abscess. Causative organisms include *Staphylococcus aureus*, *Streptococcus pyogenes*, and anaerobic species. Chronic paronychia can be seen in patients repeatedly exposed to water or moist environments. Symptoms are present for weeks and are similar to those with acute paronychia. Eventually, the nail may become thickened and discolored. *Candida albicans* is the most frequent organism seen with chronic paronychia.

Treatment of a simple eponychia involves frequent warm soaks and attention to local hygiene. Topical antibacterial ointments may hasten resolution. Treatment of an acute paronychia is incision and drainage (see Section VII, Procedures). If an onychia has formed, removal of the proximal portion of nail over-

lying the abscess is essential to ensure adequate drainage and prevent destruction of the germinal matrix. When an onychia forms under the anterolateral aspect of a nail, treatment consists of elevation and excision of the overlying portion of the nail. The role of oral antibiotics after incision and drainage has not been clearly established but does represent common practice. If the infection is due to finger biting or sucking, antibiotics providing coverage against anaerobes should be considered. Oral antimicrobial therapy is definitely indicated for patients with associated lymphangitis. Oral antimicrobial therapy for methicillin-resistant *S. aureus* should be considered if there is clinical suspicion, high rate in the community or the infection is not improving. Treatment of chronic paronychia consists of topical steroids and/or antifungal agents.

A *herpetic whitlow* involving a finger is sometimes mistaken for a paronychia and is the major differential diagnostic consideration. The majority of cases are in children younger than 2 years. Clinically, this lesion is characterized by the appearance of multiple, painful, thick-walled vesicles on erythematous bases most commonly located at the pulp space of the digits but can also occur around the nail folds and lateral aspects of the digit. During the ensuing few days, vesicles begin to coalesce and their contents become pustular (Fig. 119.2). A Gram stain of pustular fluid is negative for bacteria. Tzanck prep of scrapings from the base of a lesion reveals multinucleated giant cells. Subsequently, ulceration and crusting occur. The process initially results from inoculation of herpes simplex virus into a small break in the skin. The source may be a parent with herpes labialis, or a child with herpetic gingivostomatitis or herpes labialis may inoculate his or her own finger.

If the infection is primary, fever and regional adenopathy are seen. With recurrences, these findings are usually absent. The course is usually self-limited. However, oral acyclovir may be given in the first few days of the infection to shorten the course. For the immunocompromised patient, parenteral acyclovir should be considered to prevent dissemination. A complication of herpetic whitlow is bacterial superinfection.

Felon

A *felon* consists of a deep infection of the distal pulp space of a fingertip. Felons are caused by introduction of bacteria into the pulp space, usually by punctures (which may be trivial) or splinters. Causative organisms are similar to those found in eponychial infections. A felon typically presents as an exquisitely tender and throbbing fingertip that is swollen, tense, warm, and erythematous. However, its evolution is usually relatively slow, beginning with mild pain and minimal swelling

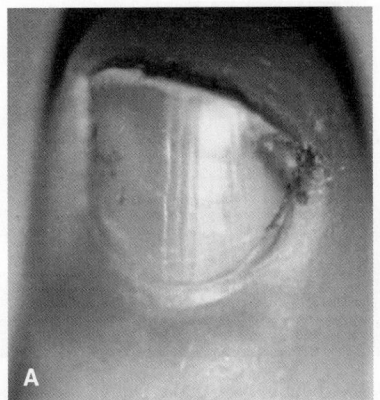

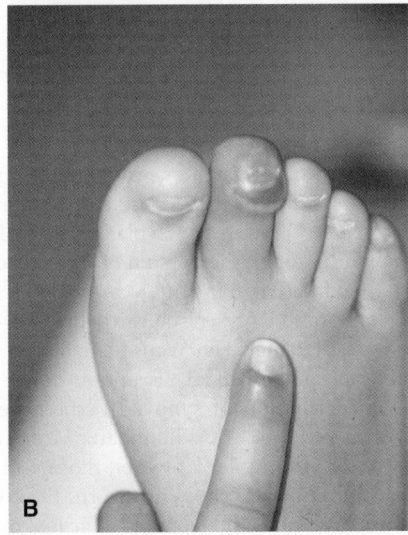

FIGURE 119.1 **A:** Small paronychia located along nail fold, noted after minor trauma. **B:** Paronychias on toe and finger.

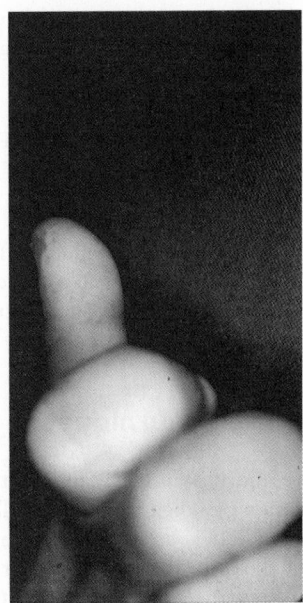

FIGURE 119.2 Herpetic whitlow of the thumb.

Subungual Hematoma

A *subungual hematoma* is a collection of blood located under a nail that arises after trauma to the nail bed, typically due to a crush injury. Because this mechanism is also a common cause of phalangeal fractures, radiographs are advisable. The patient experiences throbbing pain that worsens with increasing pressure as more blood collects. If the subungual hematoma involves more than 50% of a nail surface, is associated with a distal phalanx fracture, or the nail or its margins are disrupted, the presence of a significant nail bed injury should be suspected. Nail trephination provides drainage with relief of pressure and pain and suffices for uncomplicated subungual hematomas with intact nail margins, regardless of size of the hematoma. This procedure also reduces risk of secondary infection. The trephined opening should be large enough (larger than 3 to 4 mm) to allow for ongoing drainage without risk of closure by a new clot (see Section VII, Procedures). Sometimes producing two openings in the nail will promote more complete drainage. When the nail or its margins are disrupted and/or a displaced phalangeal fracture is present, the nail should be removed and the nail bed repaired. Antimicrobial prophylaxis for these injuries remains a source of controversy but is often prescribed by practitioners for patients with underlying fractures and those with severe soft-tissue injuries.

Subungual Foreign Body

Foreign bodies such as a wood splinter or metallic shaving become embedded under the nail and may be the source of pain and/or infection. When the foreign body is only partially embedded, the nail can be trimmed close to the nail bed, and the object's projecting end grasped with splinter forceps and gently extracted. If a portion remains or the foreign body is

that progress over a few days. This process is in part caused by the anatomy of the pulp, which consists of multiple closed spaces formed by fibrous septae that connect the volar skin to the periosteum of the distal phalanx. With progression of infection, pressure buildup within these small compartments may cause local ischemia. In some cases, organisms may spread to invade the phalanx, resulting in osteomyelitis. In others, the process may point outward to the center of the touch pad, where the septae are least dense, producing an obvious area of fluctuation. Because the deep septal attachments are distal to the distal interphalangeal (DIP) joint and flexor tendon sheath, there is less risk of spread to these structures.

Treatment consists of incision, blunt dissection, and drainage. A longitudinal incision over the area of maximal tension or fluctuance is the procedure of choice. Care should be taken to extend the incision past the DIP joint to prevent formation of a flexion contracture (see Section VII, Procedures). After drainage, a course of oral antibiotics is indicated. Close follow-up is essential to assess response to therapy and identify complications, such as septic arthritis and suppurative tenosynovitis. Patients presenting with fever, lymphangitis, or evidence of osteomyelitis should be referred to the hand service for admission, parenteral antibiotics, and definitive care.

deeply embedded from the outset, a digital block should be performed. Then the part of the nail overlying the object can be shaved down with a scalpel until the foreign body is exposed. Alternatively, the nail can be lifted and the object removed (see Section VII, Procedures). After splinter removal, the finger should be soaked in warm, soapy water, and an antibiotic ointment and protective dressing applied. Soaks should be repeated three times daily at home for the ensuing 3 to 5 days. In the unusual case of a child with multiple subungual splinters or fragments, it is best to remove the nail, clean out the foreign material, irrigate thoroughly, and then replace the nail (after trephining it to allow drainage).

Hair Tourniquet

A *hair tourniquet* injury is an entity unique to pediatrics. It involves strangulation of a digit (or occasionally the penis) by a hair or fine thread. It is seen most commonly in young infants and can be the cause of unexplained irritability or crying. The mechanism involves entwinement of the hair around an infant's digit. This may occur during a bath, during or as a result of wiggling of the toes in a sock, bootie, or mitten that inadvertently has a hair or loose thread in it. A hair shed from a parent during diapering is the probable source of penile tourniquets. As the hair or thread becomes more tightly entwined, it produces a tourniquet effect, impairing blood flow with resultant ischemic pain and distal swelling. When noted early, the hair is often visible in a crease just proximal to the swollen area. If seen later, the hair may have cut through the skin, making it difficult to visualize (Fig. 119.3). In rare cases, frank ischemic necrosis of the distal digit may be seen on presentation. Removal requires a fine-tipped forceps and the aid of a thin loupe or probe that is inserted proximally under the constricting hair. Usually the hair can be unwound from the digit intact or cut with scissors. When the hair is deeply embedded or there is any question of a remaining constricting band, a nerve block should be performed and a perpendicular incision made over the hair. To avoid damage to neurovascular structures, such an incision should be made on the lateral or ulnar aspect of a finger or toe at 3 or 9 o'clock or at 4 or 8 o'clock along the penile shaft. When the entire hair cannot be removed with certainty, plastic surgical consultation is indicated.

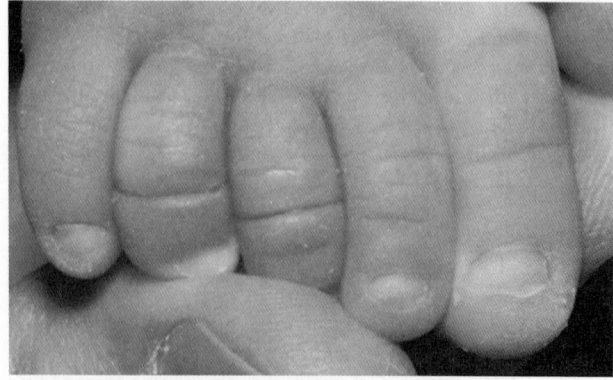

FIGURE 119.3 Hair tourniquets of third and fourth toes.

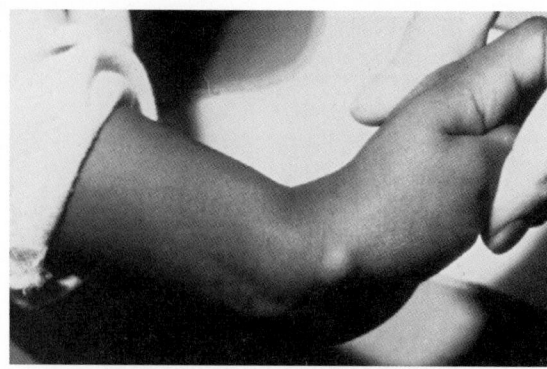

FIGURE 119.4 Ganglion cyst of the tendon sheath of flexor carpi radialis.

Ganglion

A *ganglion* is a cystic outgrowth or protrusion of the synovial lining of a tendon sheath or joint capsule. Common locations of ganglions include the dorsal or volar surface of the wrist (usually on the radial side), the dorsum of the foot, or near the malleolus of an ankle (Fig. 119.4). Occasionally, a flexor tendon sheath ganglion may present on the palmar surface of the hand at the base of a digit. The cause is believed to involve prior trauma that causes partial disruption of the synovium and subsequent herniation of synovial tissue. The cysts are soft, slightly fluctuant, and transilluminate. Most are painless or only mildly uncomfortable. However, those on the foot or ankle may cause pain when shoes are worn. Elective surgical excision with obliteration of the base is indicated only if function is impaired or the lesion is of cosmetic significance. Even then, up to 20% recur. Striking the cyst with a heavy object, an old fashion folk remedy, should be strongly discouraged because the cystic fluid may be dispersed through the surrounding soft tissue, inciting diffuse scar formation.

FACE AND SCALP LESIONS

Epidermal Inclusion Cyst

Among the most common postpubescent skin lesions is the *epidermal inclusion cyst* (EIC). These have also been termed *epithelial, sebaceous,* and *pilar cysts.* Most result from occlusion of pilosebaceous follicles, although some stem from inoculation of epidermal cells into the dermis via needlestick or other trauma. A few may arise from epidermal cells that become trapped along embryonic lines of closure. Lesions consist of firm, slow-growing, 1- to 3-cm, round nodules. Most are solitary lesions found about the scalp and face, although they also may be located on the trunk, neck, and scrotum. Histologically, these dermal and subcutaneous nodules consist of epidermally lined keratin-filled cysts. Presentation is that of a slow-growing painless lump that may provoke concerns of malignancy. At times, these cysts become acutely infected, and the patient complains of pain, erythema, and sudden increase in size. Infected cysts should be incised and drained, as well as treated with oral antibiotics before elective excision. Noninflamed cysts can be referred for elective excision that must include the entire sac to prevent recurrence.

When a patient presents with multiple large EICs, Gardner's syndrome should be suspected. This autosomal dominant disorder is characterized by multiple EICs, intestinal polyposis, desmoid tumors, and osseous lesions. Early diagnosis is especially important because of a 50% risk of malignant transformation of the intestinal polyps.

Dermoid Cyst

Dermoid cysts are congenital, subcutaneous nodules derived from ectoderm and mesoderm. There is a male predominance. They, too, are lined with epithelium, but unlike EICs, they may contain multiple adnexal structures such as hair, glands, teeth, bone, and neural tissue, as well as keratin. The cysts usually present as solitary, round, firm nodules with a rubbery or doughy consistency on palpation, a smooth surface, and normal overlying skin. Lesions tend to grow slowly, and malignant transformation is rare. Whereas some dermoids may be mobile, many are fixed to overlying skin or underlying periosteum. Occasionally, dermoids may have deeper attachments extending intracranially or intraspinally, along with an accompanying sinus. Because these cysts form along areas of embryonic fusion, common sites include the nasal bridge, midline neck, or scalp; the lateral brow (Fig. 119.5, see also color plate); anterior margin of the sternocleidomastoid; and midline scrotum or sacrum. An external ostium may or may not be visible. A small percentage of patients with dermoid cysts may have other craniofacial abnormalities. Because the sinus tract can serve as a conduit for spread of secondary infection, all midline lesions should have appropriate imaging [computed tomography (CT) and/or magnetic resonance imaging (MRI)] followed by elective excision.

Nasal Bridge Lesions

Midline nasal masses in infants and children may be acquired (e.g., EIC) or congenital, the latter stemming from improper

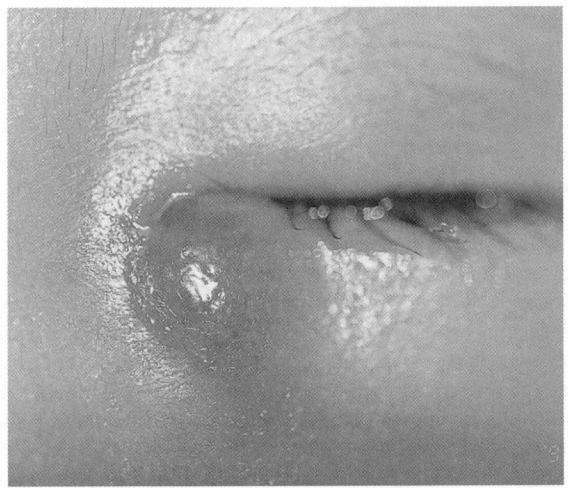

FIGURE 119.5 Dermoid cyst abscess. (From Fleisher GR, Ludwig W, Baskin MN, eds. *Atlas of pediatric emergency medicine*. Philadelphia, PA: Lippincott Williams & Wilkins, 2004. Reprinted with permission.)

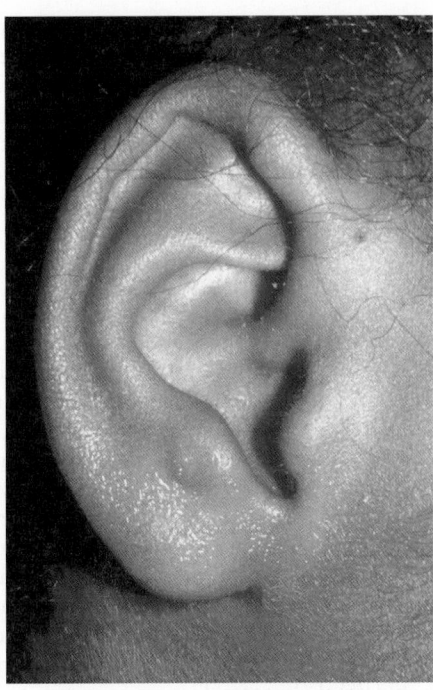

FIGURE 119.6 Preauricular surface pit. (Courtesy of David Tunkel, MD.)

embryologic development (e.g., dermoid cyst, encephalocele, glioma).

Dermoids are the most common embryologically derived midline nasal lesions (see previous discussion). Clinically, a firm, round, subcutaneous mass is seen in the midline over the dorsum of the nose. Some have an overlying dimple, which may have an extruding hair (Fig. 119.6). Its attachment may extend only to the nasal septum or may go deeper through the cribriform plate into the calvarium. Because of their proximity to the nasopharynx, these dermoids are particularly prone to secondary infection and fistula formation. Hence, prompt excision is indicated after careful MRI or CT.

Gliomas are benign growths composed of ectopic neural tissue. The lesion usually consists of a firm, gray, or red-gray nodule, ranging in size from 1 to 5 cm and can be mistaken for a hemangioma. Most are extranasal (60%), occurring on the bridge of the nose. The remainders are either solely intranasal masses (30%) or have both intranasal and extranasal elements (10%). By definition, they do not have intracranial communication. They are composed of neural and fibrous tissue, covered by nasal mucosa. There is a male predominance. To prevent possible distortion of surrounding bone and cartilage, surgical excision is the treatment of choice.

Encephaloceles consist of neural tissue that has herniated through a congenital defect in the midline of the calvarium, and thus, always have an intracranial communication. Lesions appear as soft, at times pulsatile, compressible masses that enlarge with crying or straining. Compression of the jugular veins (Furstenberg test) may also cause the mass to expand in size. Some infants with nasal encephaloceles are born with overt craniofacial deformities and a rounded swelling at the base of the nose, whereas in others, the mass is confined to the nasopharynx, and external facial features are normal. The latter may present with signs of persistent nasal obstruction. In these patients, a grapelike mass is found on nasopharyngoscopy. MRI is the modality of choice for differentiating encephaloceles from other midline nasal masses and for determining their size and extent. Neurosurgical evaluation and management is indicated for all encephaloceles.

Preauricular Lesions

Preauricular lesions, located just anterior to the tragus, may be the result of imperfect fusion of the first two branchial arches (sinus tract, pit) or may consist of first arch remnants (cutaneous tag). They may be unilateral or bilateral, single or multiple. Usually, they are seen as isolated minor anomalies, but on occasion they can be found in association with other developmental anomalies involving the first branchial arch or in infants with chromosomal disorders. Most lesions are evident shortly after birth. Some individuals simply have a surface pit or dimple, whereas in others, the overlying dimple represents the entrance to a sinus tract or blind pouch with a small cyst at its base (Fig. 119.6). The latter may contain hair and other epidermal elements. Sinuses are prone to infection and abscess formation, whereupon the child presents with sudden enlargement of a painful preauricular mass and overlying erythema. When this occurs, the patient should be treated with appropriate antimicrobial therapy before elective excision of the cyst and fistula tract. Cutaneous tags, also called *accessory auricles*, are flesh-colored pedunculated lesions that may or may not have a cartilaginous component (Fig. 119.7). Some with narrow bases may simply be tied off with silk sutures. Those with wider bases and those containing cartilage can be referred for elective excision for cosmetic reasons.

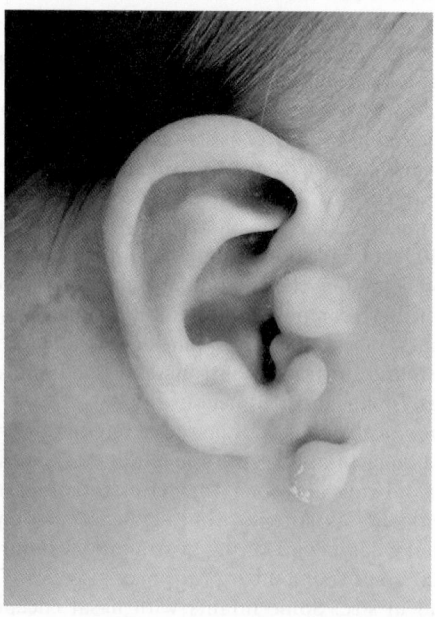

FIGURE 119.7 Multiple preauricular skin tags. (Courtesy of David Tunkel, MD.)

NECK LESIONS

Neck lesions in children may be of congenital origin or may be acquired as the result of an inflammatory process (Fig. 119.8). Although malignancy is a much rarer cause of neck masses in children, it must always be considered in the differential diagnosis. Neck masses or lesions are most conveniently divided into those occurring in the midline and those located in the lateral aspects of the neck (see Chapter 123).

Midline Neck Lesions

Submental lymphadenitis or *lymphadenopathy* occurs in the midline just beneath the chin. Nodal enlargement stems from drainage of primary infection of the lower lip, buccal floor, or anterior tongue.

Dermoid cysts (see "Face and Scalp Lesions" section) can occur throughout the midline of the neck but are usually found above the area of the hyoid. They may also be found more laterally along the anterior border of the sternocleidomastoid.

Thyroglossal duct cysts are among the more common midline neck masses in children. Approximately 40% present before 10 years of age. They are composed of an ectodermal ductal remnant that fails to regress after fetal descent of the thyroid gland. They may occur anywhere along the path of descent of the thyroid, from the foramen cecum at the base of the tongue to the sternal notch, although most are found near the level of the hyoid bone. Presentation is usually that of a painless, smooth, mobile, cystic mass that is located in the midline or just slightly off-center (Fig. 119.9). Because of its intimate association with the hyoid, the mass moves with protrusion of the tongue or swallowing. On occasion, an overlying pore is present. Some cysts go unnoticed until infection occurs, causing acute swelling, pain, and erythema of the overlying skin. Patients with asymptomatic thyroglossal duct cysts should be referred for elective surgical excision. If the thyroglossal duct cyst is infected on presentation, excision is deferred until appropriate antimicrobial therapy is completed and inflammation has subsided. If incision and drainage are required during treatment, the patient should be referred to a surgeon comfortable with thyroid anatomy. Elective excision involves removal of the cyst, the entire duct to the level of the foramen cecum, and the midportion of the hyoid bone. On rare occasions, ectopic thyroid tissue in a thyroglossal duct cyst is the patient's only functioning thyroid. Therefore, ultrasound or radioisotope scanning is recommended to confirm the presence of a normal thyroid gland before surgery.

Diffuse enlargement of the thyroid gland, or *goiter*, may be the result of infiltration, inflammation, or overstimulation of the gland. By far, the most common cause of pediatric thyroid enlargement is chronic *lymphocytic thyroiditis* (also called *Hashimoto's thyroiditis* or *autoimmune thyroiditis*). This disorder is characterized by a defect in cell-mediated immunity that results in lymphocytic infiltration of the thyroid gland. Female population is affected predominantly, and peak occurrence is during adolescence. Autoimmune thyroiditis has been associated with other autoimmune diseases such as chronic urticara and diabetes. Usual presentation is one of a slow-growing,

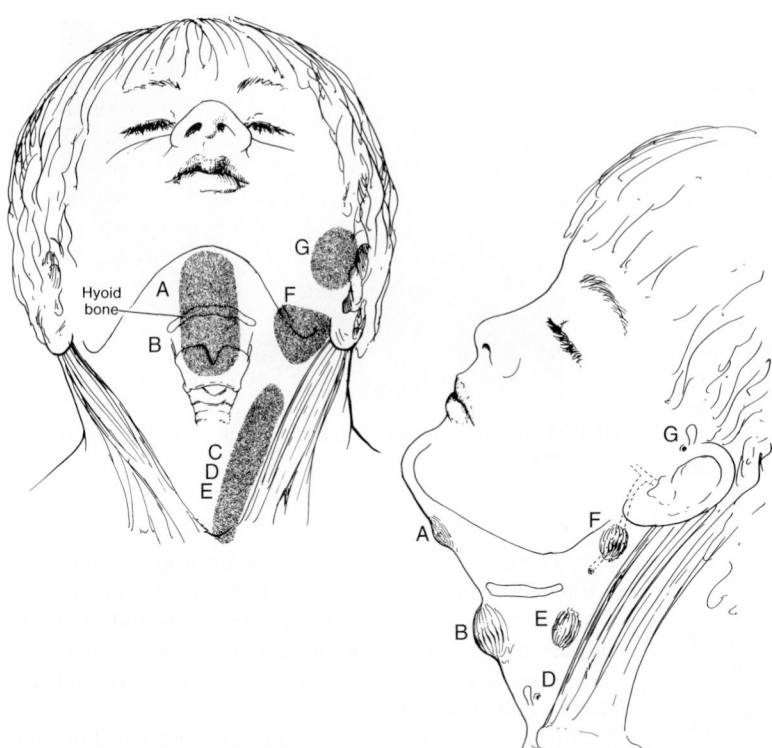

FIGURE 119.8 Head and neck congenital lesions seen in children in frontal and lateral views. The shaded areas denote the distribution in which a given lesion may be found. A, dermoid cyst; B, thyroglossal duct cyst; C, second branchial cleft appendage; D, second branchial cleft sinus; E, second branchial cleft cyst; F, first branchial pouch defect; G, preauricular sinus or appendage.

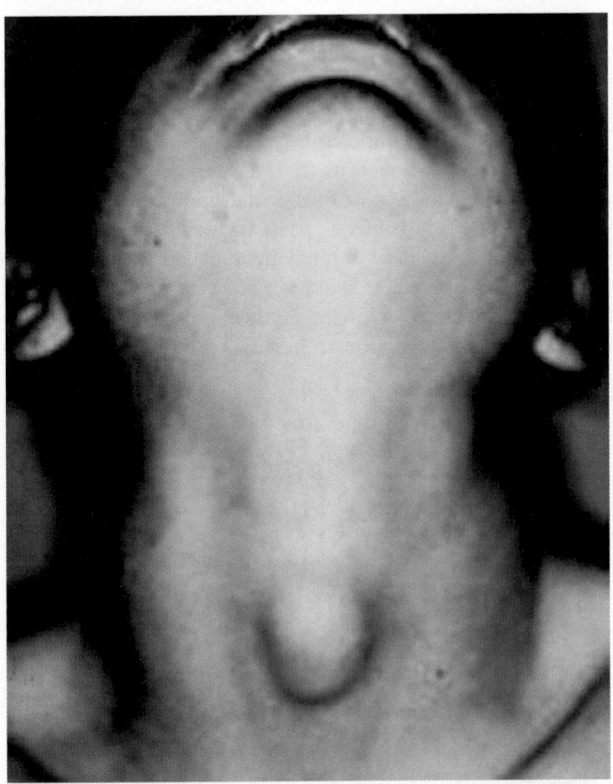

FIGURE 119.9 Thyroglossal duct cyst. (From Snell RS. *Clinical anatomy*, 7th ed. Baltimore, MD: Lippincott Williams & Wilkins; 2005:CD418. Used with permission.)

painless midline neck mass. Occasionally, a patient may complain of sore throat. Examination reveals a firm, nontender, diffusely enlarged gland in most affected children, but approximately one-third will have some lobular or nodular enlargement. Evaluation includes assessment of thyroid function and the detection of thyroid autoantibodies in the serum. Most patients with lymphocytic thyroiditis are euthyroid. When thyroid dysfunction is present, it usually takes the form of hypothyroidism. Any degree of nodularity of the gland warrants further investigation to rule out malignancy.

Inflammation of the thyroid gland secondary to infection, *acute suppurative thyroiditis*, is a rare cause of diffuse thyroid enlargement that can be associated with an underlying pyriform sinus fistula. Presentation usually follows an upper respiratory tract infection or otitis media and is characterized by abrupt appearance of a painful, tender, swollen mass in the region of the thyroid. Systemic toxicity in the form of fever and chills and severe dysphagia are often present. Flexion of the neck may alleviate pain, whereas extension worsens it. The etiologic agents include *S. aureus* and those in the oropharyngeal flora. Appropriate broad-spectrum parenteral antimicrobial therapy is usually sufficient to eradicate the infection. Abscess formation necessitates incision and drainage by a surgeon comfortable with thyroid anatomy. Evaluation with a CT or esophagography should include identification of a pyriform sinus fistula after resolution of infection to prevent recurrences.

Acute immune stimulation of the thyroid gland may also produce diffuse thyroid enlargement. In *Graves' disease*, autoantibody attachment to the thyrotropin receptor stimulates an increase in thyroid hormone synthesis and release.

Patients may initially have a history of changes of behavior, decrease in school performance, and/or increase in linear growth. On presentation, patients will have a symmetrically enlarged smooth nontender goiter and signs of thyrotoxicosis, including tachycardia, nervousness, tremor, hypertension, exophtalmos, and increased appetite. A thyroid bruit may be auscultated in half the patients. An elevated T_4 in the context of a low TSH level and presence of TSH receptor antibodies confirms the diagnosis. Consultation with a pediatric endocrinologist is indicated.

Solitary nodular thyroid masses deserve careful attention. Although most are secondary to chronic lymphocytic thyroiditis or consist of a benign adenoma, the incidence of malignant neoplasms is actually higher in children with thyroid nodules than in adults. Hence, every thyroid nodule found in a child merits a complete evaluation that may include a TSH level and ultrasound-guided biopsy.

Lateral Neck Lesions

Enlarged cervical lymph nodes constitute the most common lateral neck masses in children. Knowledge of the anatomy of the cervical lymphatics is of fundamental importance to understanding processes that cause enlargement of cervical lymph nodes. This section focuses mainly on local processes that cause nodal enlargement, but it is important to note that many systemic infections and inflammatory disorders can cause diffuse adenopathy that includes the cervical chain. Therefore, any child with a neck mass deserves a complete examination to look for the presence of generalized adenopathy and other signs of systemic disease.

Reactive cervical adenopathy refers to mild enlargement of cervical lymph nodes that accompanies a viral or bacterial upper respiratory tract infection. Involved nodes are typically located in the upper portion of the cervical chain. They are usually discrete, firm, mobile, and less than 2 cm in diameter. They may be mildly tender but have no overlying erythema, edema, or warmth. Regression within 1 to 2 weeks of resolution of the primary infection is the rule, although occasionally mild enlargement of the node may persist, if fibrosis has occurred.

Local infection of a lymph node itself is termed *acute suppurative lymphadenitis.* The involved node is solitary, typically 2 to 3 cm or larger in diameter, and extremely tender. As the infection proceeds, overlying swelling, erythema, and warmth develop and become more pronounced (Fig. 119.10). Initially the node is firm, but later it may become fluctuant. Acute suppurative lymphadenitis is most often caused by streptococcal or staphylococcal organisms. Because of the high incidence of β-lactamase production by *S. aureus,* β-lactamase stable antibiotics (dicloxacillin, cephalexin, or clindamycin) are the treatment of choice. Most patients respond to oral antimicrobial therapy and application of warm compresses. However, ultrasound may be indicated to establish if fluctance has developed, and if so, incision and drainage are recommended. Other potential causative organisms of acute, subacute, or chronic lymphadenitis include anaerobic bacteria, *Pasteurella multocida* (following animal bites), *Haemophilus influenzae, Streptococcus agalactiae, Francisella tularensis, Brucella* species, *Bartonella henselae* (cat-scratch disease), mycobacteria, and actinomycoses. Oral antimicrobial therapy for methicillin-resistant *S. aureus* should be con-

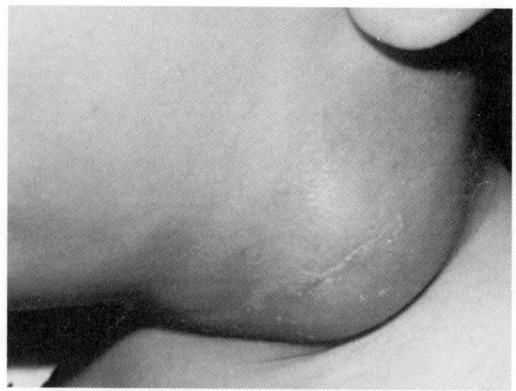

FIGURE 119.10 Suppurative lymphadenitis of an anterior cervical lymph node.

sidered if there is clinical suspicion or high rate in the community or if the infection is not improving. Kawasaki disease may also present with an acutely enlarged cervical node and should be considered when other clinical criteria are present (fever for more than 5 days, rash, conjunctivitis, extremity and oral changes, and hyperirritability).

Salivary gland infections, *sialadenitis,* and *parotitis,* may cause lateral neck or submental swelling. When the parotid gland is involved, firm indurated swelling is found extending in an arc from the preauricular area down under the ear and behind it. The degree of swelling is often sufficient to blunt the angle of the jaw, and the mass is usually mildly tender (Fig. 119.11). Patients complain of mild pain in the region of the pinna, which increases with eating. Most salivary gland infections affect the parotid gland, with involvement of the sublingual and submandibular glands being much less common. Viral agents (e.g., mumps virus, parainfluenza types 1 and 3, influenza A, Coxsackie virus A, and rarely, human immunodeficiency virus) cause most of these infections. Less commonly, parotitis is due to a bacterial agent such as *S. aureus.* In these cases, patients present with rapid gland enlargement and severe pain, and they often have high fever and signs of systemic toxicity. On examination, overlying erythema and exquisite tenderness are present, and purulent material can often be expressed

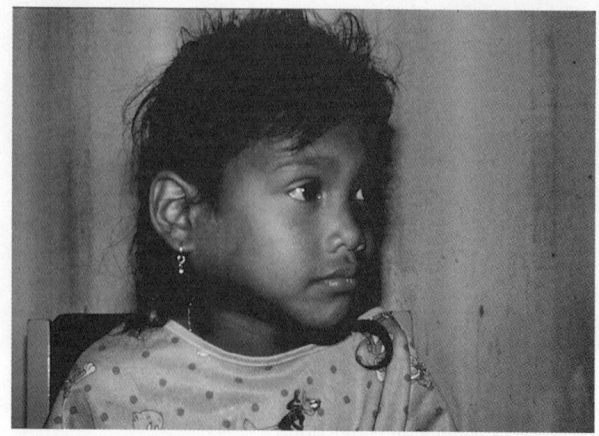

FIGURE 119.11 Parotitis.

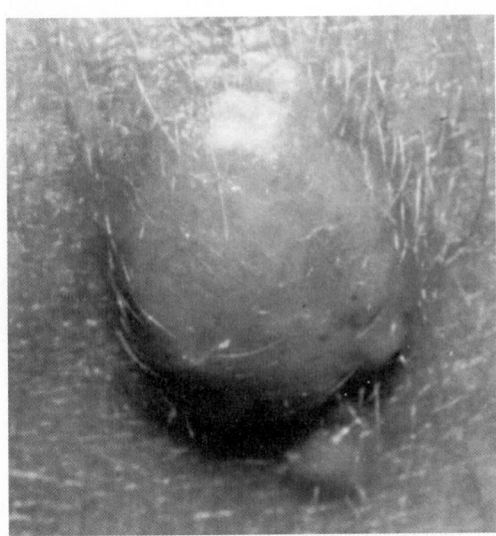

FIGURE 119.20 Yellow nodular lesion typical of juvenile xanthogranuloma.

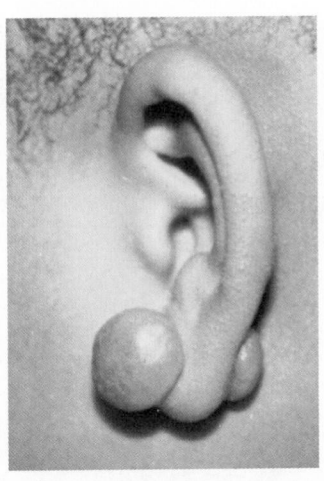

FIGURE 119.21 Large keloid that formed after ear piercing in a susceptible child.

patients may or may not have concomitant cutaneous findings. In this variant, noncutaneous lesions may involve the brain, heart, liver, spleen, and lungs. Children who have both JXG and neurofibromatosis are at a much higher risk for unusual forms of leukemia and thus should be appropriately monitored. Last, unlike children with disseminated xanthomas, there is no relationship between JXG and lipid abnormalities. All children with suspected xanthogranuloma should undergo biopsy. An ophthalmologic evaluation is necessary if JXG is confirmed, and careful observation for evidence of systemic involvement is warranted.

Neurofibroma

A neurofibroma may present as a solitary lesion in an otherwise normal patient or as a feature of neurofibromatosis type I. Cutaneous neurofibromas arise from nerve sheath cells located in the dermis. They appear as pink or flesh-colored nodules that are soft and range in size from 0.5 to 3 cm. Most do not appear until adolescence. Lesions may be confused with angiolipomas and hemangiomas; however, a distinguishing feature is the tendency of neurofibromas to be especially soft centrally and invaginate with digital pressure, described as "buttonholing." Elective excision is indicated only if the lesion is compressing a nerve, causing nerve root pain, because excision is often followed by recurrence of an even larger lesion.

Keloid/Hypertrophic Scar

Exaggerated proliferation of fibrous connective tissue in the process of cutaneous wound healing results in formation of *hypertrophic scars* and *keloids*. Wounds involving areas of skin that are thick or under high tension (shoulders, back, chest, or chin) are at greatest risk. The ear lobe is another commonly affected site. Individuals with dark skin are much more susceptible to abnormal scarring, which has its highest incidence in

adolescence and early adulthood. Hypertrophic scars remain confined to the area of original injury. They are rarely painful and tend to undergo slow regression over 6 to 12 months. In contrast, keloids extend beyond the original wound margins and rarely regress spontaneously. Initially, keloids may be painful and tender or pruritic. They have a rubbery consistency on palpation and a smooth pink surface (Fig. 119.21). Ear piercing, tattooing, and elective cosmetic procedures should be avoided in persons who have a tendency to form keloids. Severe keloids should be referred to a dermatologist or plastic surgeon for further treatment.

Lumbosacral Lesions

Pilonidal dimples, typically located in the midline in the sacrococcygeal area, are benign lesions of no clinical significance. On close inspection, there is no evidence of a central pore or opening. In contrast, pilonidal sinuses, which are found in the same area, do have a small surface opening to a tract lined by stratified squamous epithelium that extends toward, but not into, the spinal canal. In some instances, sinuses appear to be of embryonic origin, stemming from either an abnormality of midline fusion or invagination of ectodermal elements. The base of such a lesion may consist of a small cyst containing products of skin cells and epithelial appendages, including hair. In other cases, the source may be a distorted hair follicle. Pilonidal sinuses and cysts are asymptomatic until the sinus becomes obstructed and/or infected. This phenomenon is most likely to occur during adolescence or early adulthood. Male population is much more commonly affected than female population. Excess weight, hirsutism, and a sedentary lifestyle or occupation that requires prolonged sitting also appear to be predisposing factors.

Infecting organisms usually gain access through the external sinus tract. Once infection occurs, an abscess forms and tends to enlarge rapidly. Because the overlying skin is thick, expansion tends to occur deep to the skin surface, and acquired sinus tracts may form external to the postsacral facia. Patients typically complain of low back pain, increased on

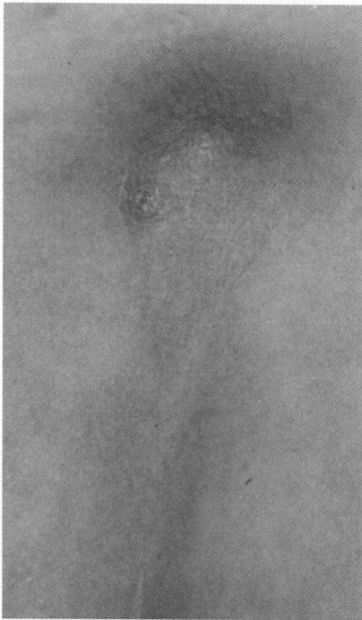

FIGURE 119.22 Infected pilonidal cyst.

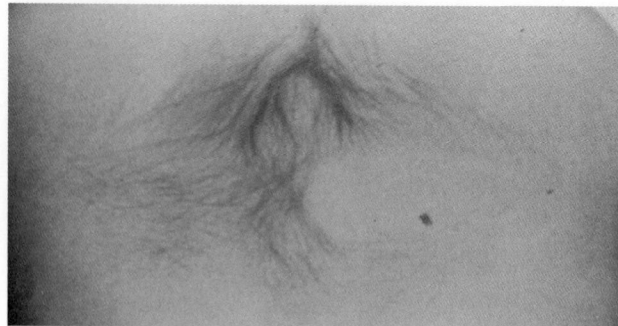

FIGURE 119.23 Lumbosacral hairy patch in a patient with diastematomyelia.

Any child found to have one of the midline cutaneous findings just described should undergo radiologic imaging to detect and delineate underlying vertebrospinal defects because early neurosurgical intervention enables substantial reduction in morbidity.

sitting, and local tenderness. On examination, a tender, indurated swelling is noted overlying the sacrococcygeal area with the original sinus at its cephalad end (Fig. 119.22). Treatment consists of incision and drainage with careful probing to break up loculations and extract any hairs present because these act as foreign bodies. Cultures grow mixed organisms, including staphylococci, anaerobes, and fecal flora. Home care includes sitz baths and oral antimicrobial therapy. Elective excision of the entire cyst and all associated sinus tracts is indicated once inflammation has resolved.

Cutaneous Manifestations of Spinal Dysraphism

A number of midline cutaneous abnormalities found in the lumbosacral area are associated with underlying vertebral or spinal cord defects that are the result of defective closure of the caudal neural tube, *occult spinal dysraphism*. Skin findings include *hairy patches* (Fig. 119.23), *skin tags*, *port-wine stains, hemangiomas,* and *congenital dermal sinuses*. The latter tend to be more cephalad than pilonidal sinuses, and their sinus tracts often extend to the spinal column. Underlying intraspinal lesions include dermoid tumors, lipomas, and diastematomyelia. In the latter condition, the lower cord is divided sagittally by an osseous or fibrocartilaginous septum, which tethers the cord at that level, impeding its normal ascent within the spinal canal as the child grows. Patients with tethering may present with lower-extremity neurologic deficits at birth or may insidiously develop symptoms later in infancy or childhood, especially during a period of rapid growth. Complaints may include back or leg pain or stiffness, buttock pain, weakness or numbness, and bowel and bladder complaints. Physical examination may reveal decreased tone and decreased deep tendon reflexes in the lower extremities.

Perineal Lesions

Urethral prolapse is a phenomenon seen primarily in obese prepubescent girls (see Chapter 90). Two-thirds or more are African American. In this condition, the urethra prolapses through the urethral meatus and is seen as a red or purplish red, friable, edematous mass overlying the anterior portion of the introitus (Fig. 119.24). It often has a doughnut shape, and close inspection reveals a central orifice. The prolapsed mucosa is usually mildly painful and tender and tends to bleed easily. Presenting complaints may include perineal pain, dysuria, and blood spotting on underwear. Urination is not impaired. The precipitating event is characterized by increased intraabdominal pressure, usually

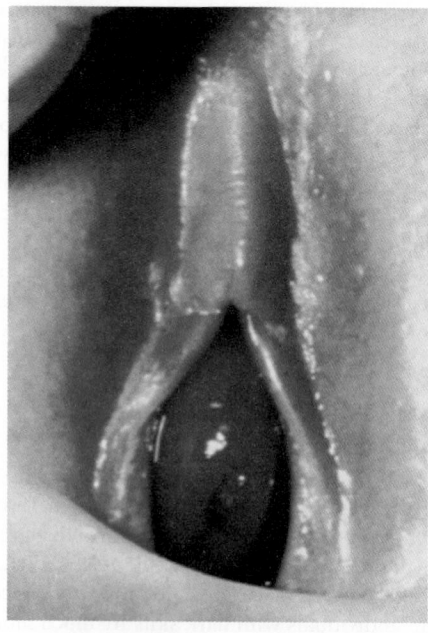

FIGURE 119.24 Typical doughnut appearance of urethral prolapse.

severe straining with constipation, a severe coughing spell, or prolonged crying. Because the red friable mass often overlies the hymenal orifice, it can be mistaken for traumatized hymenal folds, raising suspicion of sexual abuse. Correct diagnosis is made by examination under magnification after applying a topical anesthetic. This enables visualization of the central orifice and elevation of the mass to visualize the hymen. Management consists of treating the predisposing condition, oral analgesics and topical antibiotic/anesthetic creams for symptomatic relief, and twice-daily application of estrogen cream.

Hemorrhoids, internal and external, are dilated veins arising from the superior and inferior hemorrhoids veins. While very uncommon in children, incidences of hemorrhoids increase during adolescence. Development of hemorrhoids is associated with children with portal hypertension, chronic constipation, or excessive straining. Symptoms include painless bleeding (internal hemorrhoids), prolapse, pruitus, and pain secondary to vascular thrombsis. Treatment initially starts with medical management, increased fiber consumption or use of stool softeners, and topical care corticosteriods and analgesics. Refractory hemorrhoids may be managed nonoperatively with ablation or ligation. If unsuccessful, then hemorrhoidectomy should be considered. Due to the rarity of hemorrhoids in children, any presentation should prompt a careful and thorough evaluation of the underlying etiology.

Perianal skin tags are common sequelae of anal fissures and thus tend to be seen in children with a history of large, hard stools. They consist of pedunculated masses on short stalks that form during the process of healing of an anal fissure, probably in part caused by frictional forces common to this area. They are usually asymptomatic. They also can be seen in association with hypertrophic scars, another common sequela of the healing of an anal fissure. Although most patients with these lesions are otherwise normal, a small percentage have them as manifestations of perianal disease, internal fissures, and/or fistula, which may be the primary problem or one manifestation of inflammatory bowel disease. Management is directed at treating the predisposing or underlying condition. Bothersome pedunculated lesions can be tied off with silk suture.

Rectal prolapse, herniation of the rectum through the levator and then the anal orifice, is a phenomenon typically seen in children between 1 and 2 years of age (Fig. 119.25). The most common predisposing conditions, severe constipation and severe diarrhea, are characterized by repeated straining on defecation, which stretches pelvic suspensory structures, facilitating herniation. Patients with spina bifida may have prolapse as a consequence of deficits in perineal innervation with attendant atrophy of the supporting perineal muscles. Rectal prolapse may be the first presenting symptom in children with cystic fibrosis. Occasionally, an apparent rectal prolapse represents the lead end of a sigmoid intussceptens. In these cases, patients have a history of antecedent, intermittent, abdominal pain or irritability and may have vomiting, lethargy, and/or rectal bleeding as do other infants and children with intussusception. Clinically, a cylindrical mass with a central orifice and a glistening red surface is seen protruding through the anus. Acutely, the mass can be reduced with gentle pressure. Attention is then directed at identifying and treating the underlying condition to prevent recurrences. The need for operative intervention for persistent recurrences is rare and is largely limited to neurodevastated patients with intractable constipation.

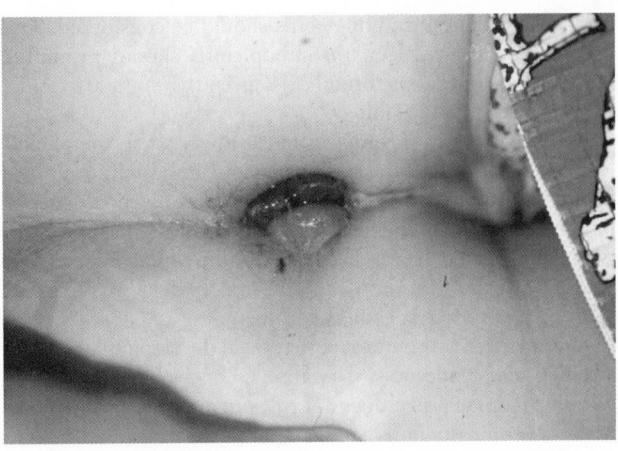

FIGURE 119.25 Rectal prolapse secondary to chronic constipation. (Courtesy of Mark Waltzman, MD.)

Acute Thromboplebitis

Because of technological advancements and treatments for diseases such as cancer and congenital heart disease, the incidence of venous thromboembolism has increased in the pediatric population. The annual incidence is 0.07 to 0.14 per 10,000 children. For hospital admissions of children, the incidence is 5.3 per 10,000, and for neonatal intensive care unit admissions, it is 0.24 per 100,000. Incidence peaks during the neonatal period and then during adolescence. Acute thrombophlebitis is increasingly recognized as a medical complication that can cause significant morbidity and mortality if not diagnosed early.

There are many medical conditions that increase the risk of thromboplebitis. In the pediatric population, one of the major causes is the presence of an indwelling central catheter. Other associated conditions that increase the risk of thromboplebitis are cancer, particularly acute lymphoblastic leukemia, chemotherapy such as asparaginase, congenital heart disease, trauma, infection, nephritic syndrome and systemic lupus erythematous.

Pathophysiology

Virchow's triad (venous stasis, endothelial injury, and hypercoagulability) illustrates the underlying mechanisms for developing thromboplebitis. Conditions that contribute to venous stasis include prolonged immobilization due to an underlying medical condition or recent surgery. Central venous lines, while crucial for many therapies, are thrombogenic as they can cause damage to the endothelium and disrupt blood flow. Hypercoagulable states include inherited thrombophilia, such as antithrombin III, protein C or S deficiency, and Factor V Leiden mutation, and acquired thrombophilia, such as infection and sepsis. Hormonal replacement and pregnancy can also contribute to increased risk of thromboplebitis.

Clinical Findings

Clinical characteristics for superficial thromboplebitis include pain, induration, and erythema along the superficial vein. Palpating a palpable cord should raise suspicion for thrombosis. If accompanied by fever or surrounding erythema or drainage, a septic thrombophlebitis should be considered. Any presence of a superficial thrombophlebitis should prompt a search for deep venous thrombosis, given that both are results of the same pathophysiology.

For deep venous thrombosis in the upper chest, initial clinical presentation can be asymptomatic. Initial clinical signs include repeated loss of patency of the central venous line, or line sepsis. Late findings include swelling of the face or neck, periorbital edema, headache, discoloration of the related limb, chylopericardium and/or chylothorax. Patient may exhibit signs of superior vena cava syndrome.

In the lower extremities, patients can develop unilateral leg swelling and tenderness. The absence of a palpable cord or negative Homans' sign does not rule out a deep venous thrombosis. Accompanying signs include inguinal and abdominal pain, discoloration of the affected leg, and prominent collateral circulation.

For clinical findings of pulmonary embolism, please see chapter "Pulmonary Emergencies."

For evaluation of thrombophlebitis, consider obtaining complete blood cell count and coagulation studies. In postpubertal girls, a urine pregnancy test is warranted. In adults, D-dimer, a marker for endogenous fibrinolysis, has been shown to be an effective screening tool in combination with a clinical prediction model in evaluating lower-extremity deep venous thrombosis. Factors used in the clinical model include immobilization, malignancy, extremity physical findings (calf circumference, leg swelling, and edema). Unfortunately, the clinical prediction model has not been validated in children and the use of D-dimer as a screening tool in children is debated. Thus, even with a negative D-dimer, one cannot exclude the diagnosis of a venous thrombosis. A persistently elevated levels of D-dimer and/or Factor VIII have been shown to predict a poor outcome in children with thrombosis.

In children with no other risk factors for venous thrombosis, or repeated episodes of venous thrombosis, consider screening for an inherited hypercoagulable state such as an antithrombin III, protein C or S deficiency, factor V Leiden mutation, antiphospholipid antibody, and lupus anticoagulant.

While venography is the gold standard for diagnosis of venous thrombosis, its use in children is limited due to its invasiveness and technical difficulties. Compression ultrasound is the imaging technique of choice for the diagnosis of venous thromboembolism in the proximal lower extremity. For evaluation of the upper chest, compression ultrasound is limited due to bony structures such as the clavicle and thoracic cage. Therefore, a combination of venography and ultrasound is recommended for evaluation of upper venous system.

Spiral CT has been shown to be accurate for diagnosis in adults, but its use in children should be limited given the radiation exposure. Currently under development, magnetic resonance venography has been shown to have high sensitivity and specificity for diagnosis of venous thrombosis in adults but has not been studied as well in children.

Management

Initial management is directed at reestablishing blood flow through the occluded vessel, resolving thrombus, and preventing embolization of the thrombus. Therapies consist of antico-agulants and thrombolytic agents. Treatment should be initiated in the ED with consultation with a hematologist.

Unfractionated heparin can be started with a loading dose of 75 units/kg and a maintenance dose of approximately 20 to 28 units/kg/hr, depending on age. Risks of unfractionated heparin include bleeding and heparin-induced thrombocytopenia.

Low-molecular-weight heparin can also be used and dosing is age-dependent. Advantages of low-molecular-weight heparin include subcutaneous administration and minimal laboratory monitoring.

Thrombolytic agents such as Recombinant tPA (alteplase) can be administered as a continuous infusion for catheter-directed thrombolysis (0.01 to 0.2 mg per kg per hour) or for systemic thrombolysis (0.1 to 0.6 mg per kg per hour for 6 hours). Use of thrombolytic agents should be reviewed in consultation with a hematologist.

Suggested Readings

Ashcraft KW. Acquired anorectal disorders. In: Ashcraft KW, Holcomb GW, Murphy JP, eds. *Pediatric surgery*, 4th ed. Philadelphia, PA: WB Saunders, 2005.

Barksdale Jr EM. Surgery. In: Zitelli BJ, Davis HW, eds. *Atlas of pediatric physical diagnosis*, 5th ed. St. Louis, MO: Mosby, 2007:623–674.

Bellinger MF. Urologic disorders. In: Zitelli BJ, Davis HW, eds. *Atlas of pediatric physical diagnosis*, 5th ed. St. Louis, MO: Mosby, 2007:535–562.

Brook I. Microbiology and management of acute suppurative thyroiditis in children. *Int J Pediatr Otorhinolaryngol* 2003;67:447–451.

Brukner AL, Frieden IJ. Hemangiomas of infancy. *J Am Acad Dermatol* 2003;48:477–493.

Canales FL, Newmeyer WL, Kilgore ES. The treatment of felons and paronychias. *Hand Clin* 1989;5:515–523.

Chi H, Lee YJ, Chiu NC, et al. Acute supportive thyroiditis in children. *Pediatr Infect Dis J* 2002;21:384–387.

Cohen BA, Davis HW, Gehris RP. Dermatology. In: Zitelli BJ, Davis HW, eds. *Atlas of pediatric physical diagnosis*, 5th ed. St. Louis, MO: Mosby, 2007:275–346.

Danielson-Cohen A, Lin SJ, Hughes CA, et al. Head and neck pilomatrixoma in children. *Arch Otolaryngol Head Neck Surg* 2001;127:1481–1483.

Davis HW, Michaels MG. Pediatric infectious disease. In: Zitelli BJ, Davis HW, eds. *Atlas of pediatric physical diagnosis*, 5th ed. St. Louis, MO: Mosby, 2007:443–508.

Derkay CS, Tunnessen WW. Picture of the month: nasal glioma. *Arch Pediatr Adolesc Med* 1994;148:954–955.

Henretig FM, King C, eds. *Textbook of pediatric emergency procedures*, 2nd ed. Baltimore, MD: Lipincott Williams & Wilkins, 2007.

Freyer DR, Kennedy R, Bostrom BC, et al. Juvenile xanthogranuloma: forms of systemic disease and their clinical implications. *J Pediatr* 1996;129:227–237.

Goldenberg NA, Bernard TJ. Venous thromboembolism in children *Pediatr Clin North Am* 2008;55:305–322.

Goldenberg NA, Knapp-Clevenger R, Manco-Johnson M. Elevated plasma factor VIII and D-dimer levels as predictors of poor outcomes of thrombosis in children. *N Engl J Med* 2004;351:1081–1088.

Guinto-Ocampo H. Incision and drainage of a felon. In: Henretig FM, King C, eds. *Textbook of pediatric emergency procedures*. Baltimore, MD: Lippincott Williams & Wilkins, 2007:1190–1094.

Johnson CF. Prolapse of the urethra: confusion of clinical and anatomic characteristics with sexual abuse. *Pediatrics* 1991;87(5):722–725.

Loiselle J, Cronan KM. Hair tourniquet removal. In: Henretig FM, King C, eds. *Textbook of pediatric emergency procedures*. Baltimore, MD: Lippincott Williams & Wilkins, 2007:1065–1069.

Male C, Kuhle S, Mitchell L. Diagnosis of venous thromboembolism in children. *Semin Thromb Hemost* 2003;29(4):377–390.

Mooney MA, Janniger CK. Pyogenic granuloma [review]. *Cutis* 1995;55:133–136.

Mulliken JB, Fishman SJ, Burrows PE. Vascular anomalies. *Curr Probl Surg* 2000;37:517–584.

Murray PJ, Davis HW. Pediatric and adolescent gynecology. In: Zitelli BJ, Davis HW, eds. *Atlas of pediatric physical diagnosis*, 5th ed. St. Louis, MO: Mosby, 2007:675–712.

Paller AS, Mancini AJ, eds. *Hurwitz clinical pediatric dermatology e-edition*, 3rd ed. Philadelphia, PA: WB Saunders, 2006.

Paller AS, Pensler JM, Tomita T. Nasal midline masses in infants and children. *Arch Dermatol* 1991;127:362–366.

Prendville JS. Diseases of the dermis and subcutaneous tissues. In: Schachner LA, Hansen RC, eds. *Pediatric dermatology*, 3rd ed. New York, NY: Churchill Livingstone, 2003.

Rahbar R, Shah P, Mulliken JB, et al. The presentation and management of nasal dermoid. *Arch Otolaryngol Head Neck Surg* 2003;129:464–471.

Raza J, Hindmarsh PC, Brook CGD. Thyrotoxicosis in children: thirty years' experience. *Acta Paediatr* 1999;88:937–941.

Sampayo EM, Henretig FM. Incision and drainage of a paronychia. In: Henretig FM, King C, eds. *Textbook of pediatric emergency procedures*. Baltimore, MD: Lippincott Williams & Wilkins, 2007:1085–1089.

Stites T, Lund DP. Common anorectal problems. *Semin Pediatr Surg* 2007: 16:71–78.

Subramaniam RM, Snyder B, Heath R et al. Diagnosis of lower limb deep venous thrombosis in emergency department patients: performance of Hamilton and Modified Wells Scores. *Ann Emerg Med* 2006:48:678–684.

Szinnzi G, Schaad UB, Heininger U. Multiple herpetic whitlow lesions in a 4-year-old girl: case report and review of the literature. *Eur J Pediatr* 2001;160:528–533.

Townsend CM Jr, Beauchamp RD, eds. *Sabiston textbook of surgery*, 18th ed. Philadelphia, PA: WB Saunders, 2008.

Roberts JR, Hedges JR, eds. *Clinical procedures in emergency medicine*, 5th ed. Philadelphia, PA: WB Saunders, 2009.

Varma R, Williams SD, Wessel HB. Neurology. In: Zitelli BJ, Davis HW, eds. *Atlas of pediatric physical diagnosis*, 5th ed. St. Louis, MO: Mosby, 2007:563–596.

Yellon RF, McBride TP, Davis HW. Otolaryngology. In: Zitelli BJ, Davis HW, eds. *Atlas of pediatric physical diagnosis*, 5th ed. St. Louis, MO: Mosby, 2007:889–938.

Young G. Diagnosis and treatment of thombosis in children: general prinicples. *Pediatr Blood Cancer* 2006;46:540–546.

CHAPTER 120 ■ APPROACH TO THE CARE OF THE TECHNOLOGY-ASSISTED CHILD

JOEL A. FEIN, MD, MPH, KATHLEEN M. CRONAN, MD, AND JILL C. POSNER, MD, MSCE

Up to almost one-fourth of the visits to a pediatric emergency department (ED) are for complaints associated with chronic illness. Many children with chronic illness have indwelling medical devices, such as cerebrospinal fluid (CSF) shunts, venous catheters, and gastrostomy tubes (G-tubes). Medical technology has enabled these children, who in the past would have required specialized inpatient or intensive care, to thrive at home. Emergency physicians must be able to diagnose and treat the common problems associated with these new technologies and recognize when it is appropriate to consult other specialists familiar with these children.

Devices most commonly found in the pediatric population include CSF shunts, tracheostomy tubes, venous catheters, and percutaneous gastrointestinal (GI), and urologic catheters. This chapter familiarizes the emergency clinician with the equipment and with the clinical manifestations and management of the problems related to these apparatuses. In addition, the clinician can advocate more effectively for the patients if he or she is aware of the emotional and social issues that may accompany these patients and families.

APPROACH TO THE CARE OF THE TECHNOLOGY-ASSISTED CHILD

The technology-assisted child who visits the ED may pose a challenge for the practitioner. Because of several factors, the evaluation of these patients may, at times, seem overwhelming. These children are often assisted by several pieces of equipment, the history can be difficult to obtain because of its inherent complexity, and a thorough physical examination may be impeded by the technology. When a common illness is superimposed on a chronic condition, the illness may appear more complex, misleading the examiner. In addition, the ED visit may have been prompted by multiple reasons. The more involved the equipment and problems, the more challenging the situation becomes.

When a technology-assisted child arrives in the ED, early contact to the primary care provider may be helpful. The primary care provider may be able to offer suggestions about the management of the child, potentially avoiding unnecessary tests and admission. In many situations, a home health nurse may accompany the patient and the family to the ED and can be a valuable source of information.

In recent years, the American College of Emergency Physicians and the American Academy of Pediatrics have provided a data form, the Emergency Information Form, for children with special health care needs that can be accessed at the time of the ED visit for patients who have subscribed to the service. This form can be located at www.aap.org/ advocacy/epcparent.htm or http://www.acep.org/patients.aspx?id=26276. A Medi-Alert bracelet provides a patient identification number that enables procurement of information about the patient. By accessing the Medi-Alert hotline, relevant medical information about the patient can be faxed rapidly to the ED for immediate use. Deriving an accurate history is imperative and greatly improves the quality of care administered.

When caring for the technology-assisted child, several important principles emerge that should be used in the acute care setting (Table 120.1).

First, *common things are common*; common pediatric illnesses may afflict these children as they do others. This point is always important to remember when evaluating a seemingly complicated child who presents with the routine signs and symptoms characteristic of typical childhood diseases. For example, a child with a CSF shunt may have vomiting caused by gastroenteritis.

Second, the presence of indwelling devices *predisposes the patient to infection*. When a child presents with symptoms associated with a specific piece of equipment, the clinician must be suspicious of infection of that equipment. For example, if a child with a tracheostomy presents with fever, cough, and increasing secretions, it is crucial to evaluate for the possibility of tracheitis. At the same time, the equipment has a tendency to become colonized with commensal organisms. Therefore, all bacterial growth does not indicate acute infection and other sources of infection should be considered.

Above all, *families should be relied on* for important information because the parents or caregivers of technology-assisted children have become sophisticated in their knowledge of specific illnesses and equipment. This information becomes crucial when an acutely ill patient presents to the ED with several forms of technology and an involved medical history. Parents are sensitive to subtle changes in their children because they provide most of the home medical care. *Families are experts* and should play an integral role in the evaluation, management, and ultimate disposition of their child in the ED setting.

Children with chronic illnesses have a higher likelihood of being admitted to the hospital, resulting in longer lengths of stay in the ED. The practitioner should realize that the families of technology-assisted children often have sufficient equipment and trained personnel available in the home setting to care for an exacerbation of a chronic problem or an unrelated acute problem. For example, family members whose child has a chronic respiratory illness often have supplemental oxygen in the home and are facile with its use. Knowing that families

TABLE 120.1

APPROACH TO THE TECHNOLOGY-DEPENDENT
CHILD IN THE EMERGENCY DEPARTMENT

Common pediatric illnesses can afflict chronically ill children
Presence of foreign bodies or hardware predisposes the
  patient to infection
Families are the experts in their children's problems—rely on
  them for important information
Consider altering the usual criteria for admission

of technology-assisted children are compliant and likely to
return to the ED if their child's degree of illness exceeds the
capabilities of the home care is reassuring. Thus, the practitioner should consider *altering the usual criteria for admission*
in this specific population.

Having a technology-assisted child in the home creates a
stressful situation for family members and other caregivers. A
visit to the ED for an acute problem exacerbates this level of
stress. These families may be more likely to question the diagnostic tests and therapies offered during the evaluation of their
child because of their level of medical knowledge, as well as the
constant illness-related anxiety that intrudes upon their lives.
The ED visit is more effective if the practitioner recognizes the
psychosocial issues associated with this population of patients.

Tracheostomy Care

Background

Advances in neonatology and pediatric critical care medicine
have enabled children to survive the complications of premature birth, congenital anomalies, and severe life-threatening
illnesses. Yet, a significant number of children are unable to be
weaned immediately from respiratory support. As home care
has become more widely recognized as an alternative to prolonged and costly hospitalization, the number of children
managed at home with tracheostomies and mechanical ventilation has increased dramatically. Consequently, these children
seek care more often in the ED when acute problems arise. To
approach these situations calmly and systematically, the emergency physician should (i) appreciate the physiologic differences in a patient with chronic respiratory insufficiency (CRI),
(ii) be familiar with the equipment used in the care, and (iii)
understand the commonly encountered complications and
their management.

Pathophysiology

In healthy people, respiration is maintained via a complex
mechanism involving the alveolocapillary network, the
diaphragm and intercostal musculature, and the central respiratory centers in the brainstem. Respiratory compromise
results when one or more components of this mechanism are
affected by disease. Chronic respiratory support may be a part
of the management plan for children with a diversity of disease
processes, including neurologic and neuromuscular disorders,
central hypoventilation syndromes, obstructive apnea, congenital facial and airway anomalies, and others. Processes such as
bronchopulmonary dysplasia once accounted for the majority

of CRI (up to 65%); however, recent epidemiologic studies
have demonstrated a shift in the proportion of CRI due to
chronic lung disease. More recent trends indicate that congenital or perinatally acquired neurologic or neuromuscular diseases are now the leading indication for chronic ventilatory
support (54% in a study by Graham et al) and chronic lung disease seems to be playing a significantly lesser role (7% in that
same study). Survival and decannulation rates depend on the
nature and severity of the underlying disease.

Equipment

The complexity of the many tubes and attachments extending
from the patient's airway can be overwhelming, especially in
the emergent situation. Familiarity with the equipment used in
caring for a patient with a tracheostomy ensures the emergency physician's adept management of these situations.
Starting from the patient's neck, each piece of equipment can
be easily identified (Fig. 120.1).

Tracheostomy Tubes. Modern tracheostomy tubes are made of
polyvinylchloride, a soft substance that conforms to the shape
of the trachea, but is rigid enough to avoid collapse. Unlike their
metal predecessors, they have little tissue reactivity, causing less
tracheal wall irritation. Several manufacturers, under sterile
conditions, package tracheostomy tubes for one-time use.
Intensivists directing the long-term airway management of their
patients may prefer one manufacturer to another, but the emergency physician does not need to know the minor differences
among the products. The emergency physician should, however,
know what types of tracheostomy tubes are stocked by the ED's
facility and how to convert from the patient's brand and size to
an available tube with suitable dimensions.

Three dimensions determine the size of a tracheostomy
tube: the inner diameter, the outer diameter, and the length.
The inner diameter refers to the same measurement used in
describing the size of an endotracheal tube, ranging from 2.5
to 10 mm. This measurement is generally imprinted on the
flanges of the tracheostomy tube and is standardized among
manufacturers. The outer diameter and length are often not

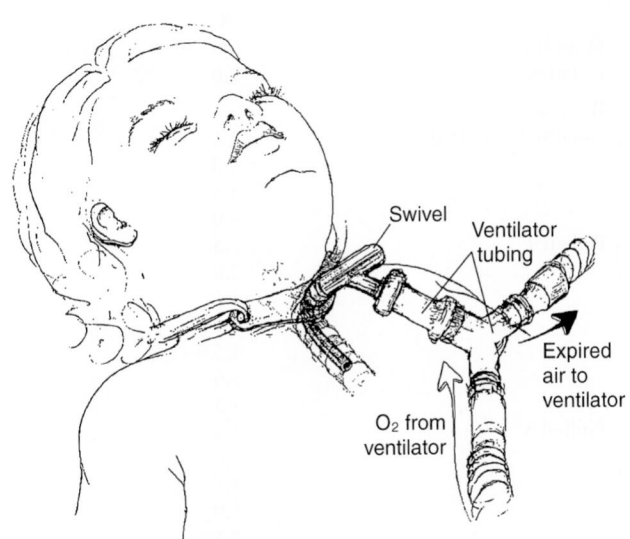

FIGURE 120.1 Tracheostomy parts.

identified on the tube and can vary considerably among manufacturers. The chart in Table 120.2 lists the dimensions of various tubes. When a tracheostomy tube change is indicated and an identical replacement is not available, this chart can be used in selecting the appropriate size tube of an available type.

A tracheostomy tube may be cuffed or uncuffed. An infant or young child may have a cuffed tracheostomy tube, especially if he or she has an airway anomaly or has developed tracheomegaly. Checking for the presence of a cuff in all patients and deflating it before removing the tube are important.

TABLE 120.2

TRACHEOSTOMY TUBE DIMENSIONS

Manufacturer	Size	Internal diameter (mm)	Outer diameter (mm)	Length (mm)
Portex				
Pediatric	3.0	3.0	5.0	36
	3.5	3.5	5.8	40
	4.0	4.0	6.5	44
	4.5	4.5	7.1	48
	5.0	5.0	7.7	50
	5.5	5.5	8.3	52
Adult	6.0	6.0	8.1	55
	7.0	7.0	9.7	75
	8.0	8.0	11.0	82
	9.0	9.0	12.1	87
	10.0	10.0	13.5	98
Shiley				
Neonatal	3.0 NEO	3.0	4.5	30
	3.5 NEO	3.5	5.2	32
	4.0 NEO	4.0	5.9	34
	4.5 NEO	4.5	6.5	36
Pediatric	3.0 PED	3.0	4.5	39
	3.5 PED	3.5	5.2	40
	4.0 PED	4.0	5.9	41
	4.5 PED	4.5	6.5	42
	5.0 PED	5.0	7.1	44
	5.5 PED	5.5	7.7	46
Long pediatric	5.0 PDL	5.0	7.1	50
	5.5 PDL	5.5	7.7	52
	6.0 PDL	6.0	8.3	54
	6.5 PDL	6.5	9.0	56
Adult with inner cannula	4	5.5	8.5	67
	6	7.0	10.0	78
	8	8.5	12.0	84
Adult with single cannula	5	5.0	7.0	58
	6	6.0	8.3	67
	7	7.0	9.6	80
	8	8.0	10.9	89
Franklin	6.0	6.0	9.3	57
Pediatric	7.0	7.0	10.0	60
Bivona				
Uncuffed or cuffed	2.5	2.5	4.0	30
	3.0	3.0	4.7	32
	3.5	3.5	5.3	34
	4.0	4.0	6.0	36
Pediatric	2.5	2.5	4.0	38
	3.0	3.0	4.7	39
	3.5	3.5	5.3	40
	4.0	4.0	6.0	41
	4.5	4.5	6.7	42
	5.0	5.0	7.3	44
	5.5	5.5	8.0	46
Phillyflex	3.5	3.5	5.3	40
	4.0	4.0	6.0	44
	4.5	4.5	6.7	48
	5.0	5.0	7.3	50
	5.5	5.5	8.0	52

Some tracheostomy tubes are fenestrated. The hole in the posterior aspect of the tube facilitates retrograde movement of air through the larynx, allowing vocalization. In addition, some tracheostomy tubes have an inner cannula that is positioned within the lumen of the tracheostomy tube (i.e., the outer cannula) so that it can be removed for cleaning while the airway is maintained by the outer cannula. Importantly, the proximal portion of the inner cannula is required to connect the tracheostomy to the manual resuscitator bag; therefore, the inner cannula must be in place when bag-valve ventilation is performed.

Swivel. A swivel is often attached to the end of the tracheostomy tube. Some unique characteristics of children make the swivel particularly useful. First, children have a natural inclination to move and explore. The swivel device accommodates movement in the ventilator-assisted child, so traction is not placed on the ventilator tubing or on the tracheostomy tube. Second, the short neck and bulky soft tissues of young children can obstruct the tracheostomy tube opening. The swivel provides additional length, so the tube opening extends beyond the soft tissues of the neck.

Heat–Moisture Exchanger. Air inspired directly into the trachea through a tracheostomy tube bypasses the important warming and humidification mechanisms provided by the natural upper airway. Therefore, a humidification system is an important component of the equipment used in a patient with a tracheostomy. A home ventilator setup includes a stationary humidification system that is used when the child is connected to the circuit. Similarly, a heat–moisture exchanger is attached to the end of the tracheostomy tube in patients who do not require the ventilator. The device is composed of a hydrophilic material that captures the patient's own heat and humidity on exhalation so that it can be inspired on inhalation. It should be placed between the tracheostomy tube and the manual resuscitator when prolonged bag-valve ventilation is performed.

Clinical Findings/Management

The approach to the ill patient with an artificial airway is the same as that for any patient who comes to the ED. The initial evaluation consists of a review of the patient's ABCDs (airway, breathing, circulation, and disability). Certainly, particular attention must be paid to the airway and breathing. An emergency physician who knows how to anticipate common problems and to recognize them early is able to institute appropriate therapy without delay.

Obstruction and Decannulation. The most life-threatening complication in a patient with an artificial airway is cannula obstruction or dislodgment. Younger children are more likely to experience accidental decannulation because of the short length of the trachea and tracheostomy tube. Some infant tubes are as short as 3 to 4 cm. In addition, the small lumen is more easily occluded by a mucous plug or by an accumulation of secretions. Infants with less developed intercostal muscles and children with neuromuscular disorders may be unable to generate an adequate cough to keep the airway clear of debris.

The presentation is similar to that of other children with respiratory compromise. The child may appear distressed with tachypnea, cyanosis, accessory muscle use, and/or nasal flaring. Alternatively, the child may be lethargic or obtunded as a result of prolonged respiratory effort or an elevated carbon dioxide level.

Any child with an artificial airway and respiratory distress is assumed to have an obstruction. The patient should be placed immediately on high-flow humidified oxygen. The physician should determine whether the tracheostomy tube appears to be in place, recognizing that a tube in the stoma does not necessarily indicate a tube in the trachea. If a cannula change was attempted before the child's arrival in the ED, a false passage into the paratracheal soft tissues may have occurred. Auscultation for the presence and symmetry of bilateral breath sounds should be performed and the quality of the patient's respiratory effort should be assessed. Immediate suctioning is appropriate in an attempt to assess tube patency and to clear the airway of secretions.

The physician should not hesitate to change the cannula. All the necessary equipment for the change should be present, including a replacement tracheostomy tube, an endotracheal tube one-half size smaller, and a bag-valve-mask ventilation circuit with oxygen flow, scissors, and tracheostomy ties. The change is best accomplished with the participation of two people; one secures the patient and removes the old tube, whereas the other inserts the new tube.

Infection. Bacterial colonization of the trachea usually occurs in a child with a tracheostomy. Common colonizing organisms include gram-positive cocci (*Staphylococcus aureus, S. epidermidis, Streptococcus pneumoniae,* α- and β-hemolytic streptococci), gram-negative bacilli (*Klebsiella, Pseudomonas, Escherichia coli, Serratia marcescens, Haemophilus influenzae*), and anaerobes (*Peptostreptococcus, Bacteroides*). These same organisms can become pathogenic, causing tracheitis or pneumonia.

A peristomal cellulitis can result from infection with skin flora. Good tracheostomy care and regular cleaning with dilute hydrogen peroxide solution can prevent most peristomal infections. Similarly, inadequate padding of the neck area beneath the tracheostomy ties can result in a contact or monilial dermatitis. Differentiating between bacterial colonization of the trachea and clinical infection can be difficult. The physician should elicit a history of any changes in the quantity, thickness, or odor of the tracheal secretions, and any systemic signs of infection or respiratory distress. Along with physical examination, there should be a determination of oxygenation by pulse oximetry. A Gram stain and bacterial culture, and a rapid viral detection assay of the tracheal secretions, may be helpful in determining the presence and cause of an infection. Leukocytosis in the tracheal secretions and a predominant organism by Gram stain may be suggestive of bacterial tracheitis; radiographic evidence of a new infiltrate indicates pneumonia.

If the child appears well and follow-up can be ensured, outpatient antibiotic therapy may be appropriate. For children with increased oxygen or ventilatory requirements, hospitalization should be considered for intravenous (IV) antibiotic therapy, aggressive pulmonary toilet, and close monitoring.

Erythema of the peristomal skin is usually caused by irritation and should be managed by increasing the frequency of the tracheostomy care at home. The additional findings of warmth, tenderness, purulent drainage, or fever may suggest the presence of a peristomal cellulitis. Depending on its severity, this condition should be treated with oral or IV antibiotics.

The skin of the neck under the ties securing the tracheostomy tube can also become inflamed. Generally, this situation can be treated by increasing the amount of padding and by keeping the area dry. An erythematous rash with satellite lesions classic for a monilial dermatitis should be treated with topical antifungal creams.

Asthma. The incidence of asthma in children with chronic lung disease has increased. Many children are maintained at home on inhaled β-agonists and inhaled steroids therapy. The usual viral and environmental triggers, such as dust, pets, and smoke, precipitate exacerbations of asthma in these children.

The presentation is similar to that of other asthmatic patients, with varying amounts of respiratory distress, wheezing, and hypoxemia. As previously mentioned, the physician must consider the possibility of cannula obstruction or dislodgment in all cases. Treatment with oxygen, bronchodilators, and steroids should be initiated promptly. Emergency clinicians should recognize, however, that children with chronic lung disease have less pulmonary reserve. Chest radiography and arterial blood gas analysis should be performed as clinically indicated. Increased ventilatory support or continuous positive airway pressure may be required to overcome fatigue and atelectasis.

Bleeding and Granuloma. The tracheal mucosa located adjacent to the stoma, the cuff, and the distal tip of the tracheostomy tube is prone to bleeding or granuloma formation. The most common reason for bleeding is inadequate humidification causing drying and friability of the tracheal mucosa. Infection or granuloma formation can also result in small amounts of bleeding. Large amounts of blood coming from the tracheostomy tube opening can signify erosion of the tube into the brachiocephalic artery. The incidence of tracheoarterial fistula formation is rare (approximately 0.7%) but commonly results in death due to massive hemoptysis and blood loss. The risk for development of this life-threatening complication is highest during the postoperative period (i.e., within 4 weeks of tube placement); it occurs with a similar incidence in patients with chronic ventilatory support.

Small amounts of bleeding from the tracheal stoma usually resolve with increased humidification of the inspired air. The persistence of minor bleeding might indicate an intratracheal granuloma, which should be evaluated by direct visualization. This procedure is best performed by an otorhinolaryngologist.

A large amount of bleeding is a surgical emergency. IV access should be obtained immediately and volume replacement should be initiated. The tracheostomy tube should not be removed because it may be the best way to ensure an airway. Frequent suctioning aids in preventing aspiration. If the site of bleeding can be identified, direct pressure should be applied to the area. Overinflating the cuff may tamponade a bleeding vessel and provide a temporary treatment until it can be ligated.

Peristomal granulomas can usually be treated with topical antibiotics. In refractory cases, cauterization with silver nitrate is indicated.

Cerebrospinal Fluid Shunts

Background

CSF shunt placement is the most common neurosurgical procedure performed in children. More than 4,400 CSF shunts were placed in 2003; that same year, CSF shunt-realted problems accounted for almost 15,000 hospital admissions and almost $300 million were charged for shunts malfunctions. CSF shunts are placed to divert CSF from the brain to another area of the body, most commonly the peritoneal cavity. The clinician evaluating a child with a CSF shunt should be aware of associated complications such as infection, obstruction, and overdrainage because certain complications can be disastrous if unrecognized and untreated. However, children with CSF shunts may often exhibit symptoms of their chronic illnesses that are unrelated to shunt malfunction.

Pathophysiology

CSF is an ultrafiltrate of plasma produced at a rate of 500 mL per day in a 70-kg adult and proportionally less in children and infants. The fluid is mainly produced by the choroid plexus and various extrachoroidal sites within the brain. CSF travels from the lateral ventricles into the third ventricle through the foramen of Monro and then again through the aqueduct of Sylvius to the fourth ventricle. The CSF then enters the subarachnoid space via the foramina of Luschka and Magendie and travels through the brain and spinal canal. CSF is reabsorbed and enters the venous system through the "one-way valves" of arachnoid villi that penetrate the dura.

Hydrocephalus can result from oversecretion, impaired absorption, or blockage of CSF pathways. *Oversecretion* can occur in some choroid plexus tumors. *Impaired absorption* can occur as a result of increased CSF protein, often a result of perinatal hemorrhage or meningitis or less commonly etiologies such as subarachnoid hemorrhage, or Guillain-Barré syndrome. Severe congestive heart failure or any other condition that raises venous pressure may impair CSF absorption as well. Impaired absorption is the cause of communicating hydrocephalus, in which flow from the lateral ventricles to the foramina of Luschka and Magendie is not obstructed. *Blockage of CSF pathways* is the most common cause of hydrocephalus in children and is often located at the narrow aqueduct of Sylvius proximal to the fourth ventricle and is referred to commonly as aqueductal stenosis. Conditions that can cause obstruction are intraventricular bleeding or scarring, tumors, or congenital malformations. Dandy-Walker cysts cause obstruction of the foramina of Luschka and Magendie and therefore may result in enlargement of all four ventricles.

Equipment

Different types of CSF shunts, which vary mostly by the location of the distal tubing and the type of reservoir or valve system, are available. The choice of CSF shunt type and the method of placement (endoscopically or nonendoscopically) depend on the individual patient's anatomy and cause of hydrocephalus and the experiences and preferences of the neurosurgeon performing the procedure. Commonly, the patient or caregiver knows the location and type of shunt and is able to provide details regarding prior shunt placement and problems. Palpation of the hardware and plain radiographs may be used

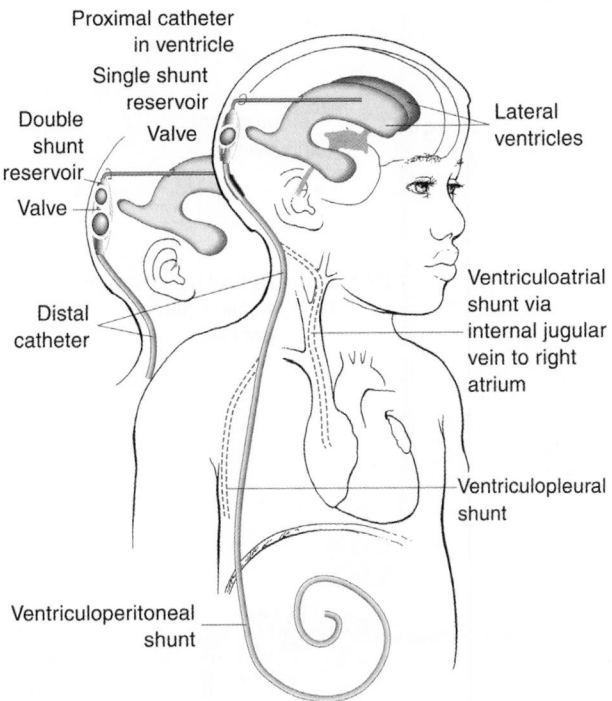

Proximal catheter
in ventricle

Single shunt
reservoir

Double
shunt
reservoir

Valve

Valve

Distal
catheter

Ventriculoperitoneal
shunt

Lateral
ventricles

Ventriculoatrial
shunt via
internal jugular
vein to right
atrium

Ventriculopleural
shunt

FIGURE 120.2 Diagram of typical ventriculoperitoneal shunt.

to acquire more information regarding the specific location of the shunt components. Most CSF shunts have the following three components: (i) proximal shunt tubing, (ii) reservoir system, and (iii) distal shunt tubing (Fig. 120.2). Occasionally, the system will not contain a reservoir and only the one-way valve can be palpated and noted on cranial radiograph.

The *proximal shunt tubing* has a fenestrated tip that is usually located in the ventricle but may also be located inside a noncommunicating cyst or in the lumbar subarachnoid space. This tip allows free passage of CSF into the shunt system. More than one proximal catheter may be present if multiple, noncommunicating areas of the brain require shunting. The *reservoir system* consists of one or two "domes" or "bubbles." Reservoirs may be placed directly over or slightly distal to the burr hole. This information is crucial when emergent access to the burr hole is needed. The *distal shunt tubing* leads from the reservoir unit to a part of the body that can accept the drained CSF, usually the peritoneum. The distal tubing may also be located in the vascular system or pleural cavity. Ventricular–atrial shunts are less commonly inserted because of the serious infectious complications that have occurred with these types of shunts but are often necessary due to severe scarring in the peritoneum from prior peritonitis either from a CSF infection or from unrelated causes. All modern shunt tubing is made of 1/8-in diameter Silastic elastomer, which causes minimal omental reaction and is resistant to cracking.

CSF shunt systems contain a one-way valve to prevent backflow of CSF into the ventricles. These valves are designed to operate at high, medium, or low pressure. Externally programmable valves, which can vary the opening pressure setting, are also available but are less commonly used in the pediatric population when compared with adults. An antisiphon device may be inserted into the distal portion of the system to

prevent overdrainage of CSF and concomitant low-pressure complications.

Clinical Findings/Management

Mechanical Malfunction. Malfunction of a CSF shunt can be caused by the obstruction of the catheter lumen or disconnection of the various components. The proximal catheter lumen is usually obstructed by choroid plexus, but floating debris or hypercellular CSF can result in the same obstruction; the distal catheter can be obstructed by the surrounding omentum or can be kinked or coiled awkwardly impeding smooth drainage. Both proximal and distal portions can be occluded by the products of infection or by migration of the catheter tip into the brain parenchyma or intraabdominal structures. Particularly in neonates, poor absorption of excess fluid in the peritoneum due to decreased surface area can create the appearance of luminal obstruction. In addition, as the child grows, the tension on the shunt system can lead to disconnection of the distal tubing.

Up to 60% of patients with CSF shunts experience a shunt malfunction in their lifetime, most commonly within the first 6 months and half within 2 years of initial shunt placement. Parental history is paramount in deciding whether a child is experiencing symptoms of shunt malfunction. The parent often notices that the child "just isn't acting right" or is less active or thinking less clearly than usual. The statement, "This is exactly how he acted the last time his shunt was obstructed," is suggestive of another malfunction, regardless of the presence or absence of the symptoms listed in the following section.

Common signs and symptoms of mechanical shunt failure include headache, visual disturbances, vomiting, lethargy, and irritability (Table 120.3). The astute parent or clinician may note mild ataxia, increased head circumference or bulging fontanel in an infant, swelling at the reservoir site, poor cognition, or abnormal behaviors. A classic sign is "sunsetting

TABLE 120.3

CONCERNING FINDINGS IN PATIENTS IN CEREBROSPINAL FLUID SHUNT MALFUNCTION

Symptoms
Fever
Headache
Altered mental status
   Irritability
   Lethargy/difficult arousal
   Confusion
Vomiting
Visual disturbances
Seizures (rare to be the only manifestation)

Signs
Papilledema
Bulging fontanel/enlarged head
Engorged head veins
Macewen's sign (cracked pot sound during percussion)
Abnormal neurologic examination
   Increased deep tendon reflexes or lower-extremity tone
   Positive Babinski's sign
   Cranial nerve palsy—lateral (sixth) or upward (fourth)
    gaze (sunsetting)
   Respiratory compromise

eyes," which is really an upgaze paresis and eyelid retraction associated with Parinaud's syndrome from pressure on the quadregeminal plate by a dilated suprapineal recess in direct communication with the third ventricle. Increased tone, hyperreflexia, or Babinski's reflex represents stretching and disruption of the corticospinal fibers originating from the motor cortex and can suggest shunt malfunction in a patient with a previously normal examination, although these symptoms are rarely present in a child without a severe alteration of consciousness and thus add little to the diagnosis. Patients with true, raised intracranial pressure (ICP), as manifest through Cushing's triad (hypertension, bradycardia, and abnormal respiratory pattern), require immediate maneuvers to decrease ICP and guide them quickly toward operative repair of the shunt. Seizures are uncommon as the sole manifestation of CSF shunt malfunction. However, seizures can occur in children who have predisposing brain lesions, and many patients with CSF shunts have epilepsy. Shunt infection must be considered in the child with symptoms of shunt malfunction, especially if the child has a history of recent shunt revision. Ronan et al reported that more than one-third of patients with shunt infection presented with symptoms of malfunction.

If the history and physical examination of the ill child with a CSF shunt suggest a possible shunt malfunction, further evaluation includes a noncontrast computed tomographic (CT) scan with comparison to the most recent prior study, if available. A plain radiograph of the skull, chest, and abdomen ("shunt series") is helpful both in assessing the integrity of the shunt connection and in identifying the components of the working system. The clinical suspicion of a shunt malfunction based on a history and physical examination may outweigh the data obtained from radiographic studies.

Much discussion and controversy surround the clinician's ability to assess CSF shunt function by "pumping" the shunt reservoirs. In a single reservoir system, this procedure involves depressing the reservoir bubble. Resistance to depression suggests distal catheter malfunction. Poor filling suggests either proximal catheter malfunction or small ventricles. The maneuver in a double-bubble shunt requires the initial depression of the proximal bubble, depression of the distal bubble to check for resistance, and subsequent release of the proximal bubble to check for poor filling. Pumping the shunt to test for obstruction is not always reliable. Piatt found that this maneuver had a positive predictive value of 21% and a negative predictive value of 78% in patients for whom the diagnosis of shunt patency or malfunction was definite. In addition, pumping of the shunt can cause entrapment of choroid plexus in the proximal shunt tubing and lead to proximal catheter obstruction where none previously existed.

If subsequent evaluation is still necessary to diagnose malfunction, a neurosurgeon should be consulted. It may be necessary to "tap" the shunt (Fig. 120.3). The patient's hair is either shaved or trimmed. The scalp is cleansed first with alcohol and then with three applications of Betadine® that are allowed to dry after each application. The shunt tap is performed by inserting a 23- or 25-gauge butterfly obliquely into the reservoir and holding the butterfly tubing perpendicular to the floor. The height that the CSF rises into the butterfly tubing, measured in centimeters, is the ICP. Normal pressure is between 5 and 10 cm; pressure of more than 20 cm is indicative of distal shunt malfunction requiring urgent revision. Slow

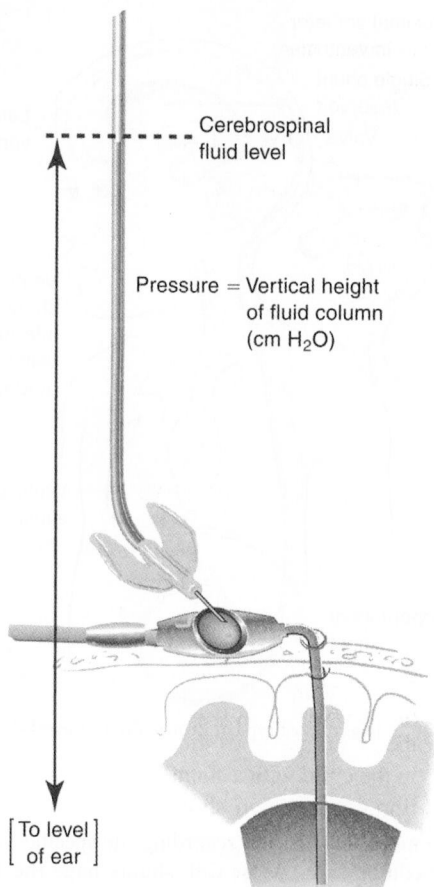

Cerebrospinal fluid level

Pressure = Vertical height of fluid column (cm H₂O)

[To level] of ear

FIGURE 120.3 Tapping the cerebrospinal fluid shunt.

or absent flow from the proximal reservoir (especially with occlusion of the distal reservoir of a double-reservoir shunt) is highly predictive proximal shunt obstruction. In this case, the physician may notice that the reservoir collapses when gentle suction is applied to the butterfly with a syringe. It is important to avoid further suctioning of this reservoir because this could lead to aspiration of debris into the proximal catheter, causing a blockage where one did not previously exist. Poor flow during the shunt tap can also indicate slit ventricles and is therefore rarely the only data required to commit a patient to an operative shunt revision.

The shunt tap can be therapeutic and diagnostic. The child with a distal shunt obstruction or partial proximal obstruction may be eligible for urgent, rather than emergent, shunt revision if symptoms of increased ICP are alleviated after the tap. However, removal of too much fluid should be avoided because abrupt fluid shifts within the cranial vault can lead to disruption of subdural vessels. It is prudent to remove just enough fluid to decrease the ICP below 20 cm and repeat the procedure if symptoms return before definitive surgical management.

The child with complete obstruction of the proximal catheter does not obtain relief of symptoms after a shunt tap because the obstruction prevents adequate aspiration of fluid from the ventricles. These children usually respond temporarily to medical management that decreases their ICP; however, it should be stressed that restoration of shunt integrity and function is the permanent treatment of shunt obstruction. This

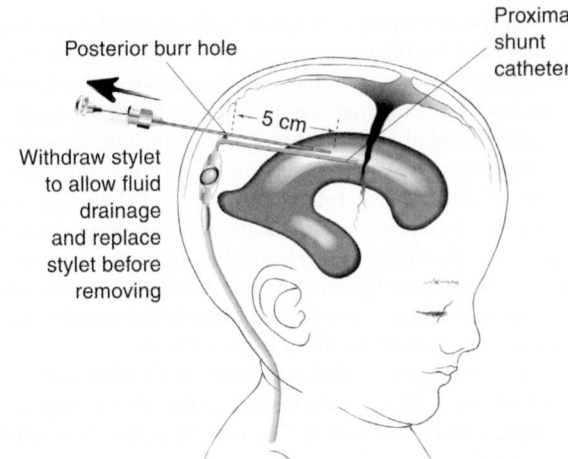

FIGURE 120.4 Burr-hole puncture.

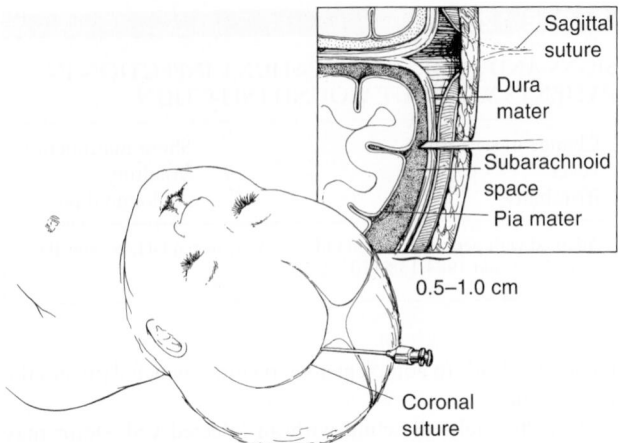

FIGURE 120.5 Ventricular tap through open fontanel.

treatment includes the administration of acetazolamide (Diamox®) 30 to 80 mg per kg per day and Decadron® 1 mg per kg per day and hyperventilation in the unstable patient. If the child is experiencing life-threatening symptoms from proximal obstruction, is unable to undergo immediate surgical repair, and is unresponsive to medical management, a burr-hole puncture procedure may be performed (Fig. 120.4) only in dire circumstances, as the procedure has attendant life-threatening risks such as disruption of intraparenchymal vessels and tissue. By nature of the procedure itself, the proximal shunt catheter is torn and urgent revision is therefore mandatory. The burr hole is best identified by direct palpation and confirmation with the skull radiographs. For example, a Rickham reservoir is located directly over the burr hole, whereas standard shunt valve/reservoir systems are usually, although not always. A 3½-in spinal needle is inserted perpendicular to the skull through the burr hole to a depth of no more than 5 cm. After the stylet is removed, fluid should drain spontaneously and should be allowed to do so until flow slows down. The patient's condition should stabilize sufficiently for transport to an operating suite or tertiary care institution.

Another method of temporarily relieving a lumen obstruction is to flush a small amount of sterile saline through the clogged tubing in an attempt to dislodge the obstruction. This method can be used for distal or proximal obstructions, with the caveat that instilling a few more milliliters into the ventricles may in fact worsen the patient's condition. In this procedure, the double-bubble reservoir that is not being used must be compressed to allow the fluid to go in only one direction.

In an infant with an open fontanel, the physician can aspirate fluid through a direct ventricular puncture (Fig. 120.5). This procedure carries as great if not greater risk of parenchymal injury as the burr-hole puncture procedure and likewise should be performed only when prompt surgery is impossible.

Infection. The reported incidence of CSF shunt infections ranges between 5% and 10% and depends on the center performing the study and the criteria used to define infection. The majority of infections are perioperative in nature. More recent advances, such as allowing fewer operating room personnel, soaking the shunt in antibiotics before insertion, and the administering prophylactic antibiotics have reduced the rate of infec-

tion. Infections generally occur within 2 months of shunt placement, with a higher incidence of infections in children younger than 4 years. Other risk factors include insertion of the shunt into a premature infant and insertion after a previous infection. The common organisms cultured from infected CSF shunts are gram-positive bacteria (Table 120.4). Staphylococci adhere well to Silastic® tubing, and these infections are often difficult to eradicate without removal of the catheter. Infections with *S. epidermidis* and *S. aureus* are common within the first few weeks after surgery. Infections that occur more than 6 months after shunt placement are more likely due to gram-negative infections such as *H. influenzae* infection, bowel erosion, or pressure necrosis from the shunt apparatus. Fungi are rare pathogens occasionally seen in premature infants.

External infection of skin and subcutaneous tissue overlying the shunt hardware can occur; however, these superficial infections may not lead to shunt infection if treated promptly. Necrosis of the area around the reservoir can occur as a result of the constant pressure in infants or nonambulatory patients. Skin breakdown leading to visualization of the shunt mechanism is, by definition, a shunt infection and must be treated accordingly.

The peritoneal portion of the shunt may become infected through the shunt mechanism or via a primary peritoneal infection. Peritoneal infection can result in loculated, cystic pools of infection around the terminal portion of tubing (pseudocysts). These infections may be indolent in their presentation, and the shunt tap from the reservoir may not show evidence of infection.

Shunt nephritis is a rare but serious complication of ventricular–atrial shunts. Renal deposition of antigen–antibody

TABLE 120.4

COMMON ORGANISMS INVOLVED IN CEREBROSPINAL FLUID SHUNT INFECTIONS

Gram positive	Gram negative
Coagulase-negative staphylococci (*Staphylococcus epidermidis*)	*Escherichia coli*
Staphylococcus aureus	*Enterococcus* species
Streptococcus species	*Haemophilus influenzae*

TABLE 120.5

SIGNS AND SYMPTOMS OF SHUNT INFECTION IN
PATIENTS WITHOUT WOUND INFECTION

Change in sensorium	Shunt malfunction
Fever	Vomiting
Irritability	Abdominal pain

Adapted with permission from Odio C, McCracken GH, Nelson JD.
Am J Dis Child 1984;138:1103–1108.

complexes leads to complement activation, which damages the
renal tissue.

Unfortunately, the child with an infected CSF shunt may
present with nonspecific signs and symptoms (Table 120.5).
Children commonly develop symptoms of shunt malfunction,
such as lethargy or irritability. Meningismus is not often present. Infection may also manifest as abdominal complaints,
such as pain or vomiting, especially when the infection
involves the distal catheter tip.

Fever is not always present in patients with shunt infections
and is uncommonly the only sign. As previously mentioned,
infection is most common within a few months of the shunting
procedure, is uncommon after 6 months, and is rare more than
1 year afterward. These rules are less applicable in patients
with gram-negative infections, which can occur later after
shunt placement. Children with gram-negative infections are
more often bacteremic, if not septic appearing.

A wound infection overlying any portion of the shunt mechanism can manifest as erythema and tenderness or swelling
along the shunt tract or over the reservoir. A reddened tract of
skin paralleling the shunt tubing from the head to chest is often
detected and is virtually diagnostic of shunt infection.

In the absence of overlying infection, aspiration of a small
amount of CSF from the shunt system should be performed to
identify the presence of a bacteriologic cause of shunt infection.
This procedure is usually performed by a neurosurgeon, if possible. The results of this procedure are sometimes helpful but
not always determinate: the white blood cell (WBC) count can
range from 0 to 2,600 if the shunt is infected, and patients
without infection can have up to 500 WBCs per mm^3. In the
absence of a positive culture result, many clinicians use more
than 50 WBCs per mm^3 in the presence of fever, shunt malfunction, and neurological or abdominal symptoms to arrive at
the diagnosis. Gram stain of the fluid may be helpful in broad-
ening antibiotic coverage if gram-negative organisms are present. However, the Gram stain should not be used to narrow
the usual antibiotic coverage until the culture and sensitivities
of the causative organisms are obtained. Most neurosurgeons
are reluctant to perform shunt taps in patients with subtle
neurologic complaints and vague infectious signs because of
the purported risk of "seeding" the shunt with skin flora. This
risk has never been clearly defined prospectively, but in a neurologically normal child, it is prudent to perform a thorough
fever workup for common infectious sources to avoid even a
small risk of causing a shunt infection.

Patients with ventriculoperitoneal shunt (VPS) who complain of abdominal pain, with or without fever, may benefit
from abdominal radiographs and ultrasound to search for a
loculated CSF collection or pseudocyst, or visceral perforation.

Various permutations of medical and surgical therapy have
been suggested for the treatment of proximal CSF shunt infections. Medical therapy alone has been found to have a relatively
low success rate compared with a combined medical–surgical
approach. Potential surgical interventions include immediate
shunt replacement or the insertion of an extraventricular
drainage (EVD) catheter, followed by delayed shunt revision.
The latter method improves the bacteriologic cure rate significantly, although it must be performed in an institution that is
facile in managing and preventing infection of EVD catheters.
Distal shunt infections are treated with antibiotics and temporary externalization of the distal shunt catheter.

Medical therapy provided in the ED for children with suspected CSF shunt infections is limited to the administration of
broad-spectrum IV antibiotics. The antibiotics should be effective against *S. epidermidis, S. aureus,* and gram-negative organisms, as well as any organisms identified from previous infections. A reasonable choice of empiric therapy is vancomycin
and cefotaxime. Therapy can be expanded to treat *Pseudomonas aeruginosa* infections in severely ill patients or those
who are unresponsive to initial therapy. Eventually, antibiotic
therapy may be narrowed on the basis of culture results of the
shunt fluid. In patients with gram-negative or fungal infections,
intrathecal antibiotics may be used; however, this procedure is
not considered appropriate in an ED setting.

Overdrainage. Occasionally, children with CSF shunts experience symptoms related to the system working too well, resulting in low ICP. "Overshunting" is more common in infants
who have had initial shunting before 6 months of age. One
consequence is the slit ventricle syndrome, in which the ventricles collapse around the proximal catheter port and block further drainage. The best means of diagnosing intracranial
hypotension is the patient's history rather than physical examination or radiographic analysis. Young infants may exhibit
sunken fontanels, microcephaly, or overriding parietal bones.
Older children may exhibit intermittent symptoms of
headache, nausea, vomiting, and lethargy. The drainage of
CSF shunts increases when the patient is upright and decreases
when supine. In contrast to the classic timing of symptoms
related to increased ICP, patients with intracranial hypotension are often worse when in the standing position or after
they are awake for several hours. Lying supine for a few hours
tends to relieve symptoms of slit ventricle syndrome. Many
patients with CSF shunts have CT scans that reveal small ventricles; however, only a small proportion of these patients have
slit ventricle syndrome. Therefore, the CT scan is best used to
differentiate between shunt malfunction and other causes of
symptoms rather than to diagnose an overdrainage problem.

Chronic or recurrent episodes of slit ventricle syndrome can
be addressed surgically by upgrading the resistance of the
valve or by insertion of an antisiphon device. Oral analgesics
may be helpful in managing mild cases.

Other Complications. Numerous other complications related
to CSF shunts deserve mention. The most common of these
complications is a benign postoperative leakage of CSF around
the proximal shunt tubing into the subgaleal space around the
reservoir. The resulting extracranial fluid collection resolves
spontaneously, so drainage of this fluid should be avoided. In
nonpostoperative patients, a new extracranial fluid collection

can suggest shunt malfunction, as the CSF takes the newest "path of least resistance."

Patients with CSF shunts have an increased risk of seizures compared with the general population. These seizures often begin years after shunt placement and are caused by epileptogenic scars. They are more common in patients with other abnormalities correlated with seizures, such as porencephalic cyst or intracranial hemorrhage.

Overdrainage can lead to shrinkage of brain tissue and concomitant subdural accumulations (hematomas or CSF effusions referred to as hygromas). Similarly, a decreased rate of head growth because of overdrainage can result in craniosynostosis in the infant.

Some important, albeit rare, complications are related to specific types of CSF shunts. The distal portions of a VPS can migrate and cause perforation of the colon or genital tract. This section of tubing can act as a fulcrum for intestinal volvulus. Ascites and abdominal cysts can form as a result of drainage of excess fluid into the peritoneum. Increased intraabdominal pressure can precipitate the formation of an inguinal hernia through a patent processus vaginalis.

Ventricular–vascular shunts can be associated with an increased risk of bacteremia. Shunt nephritis can result from complement activation and renal deposition of bacteria. Patients with ventriculoatrial shunts can experience cardiac arrhythmias or atrial perforation, usually perioperatively. Bacterial endocarditis, cardiac foreign body, and mural thrombus are rare but notable complications of vascular shunts.

After ventriculoatrial shunt, the pleural cavity is the third most common site for distal catheter placement. These can lead to pleural effusions and related complications. Often, they are placed temporarily to allow "bowel rest" after peritonitis but then revised to a standard VPS when the infectious peritoneal issues have resolved.

Avoiding Pitfalls with New Endoscopic Technology. Neurosurgeons are increasingly using endoscopic techniques in the management of pediatric hydrocephalus, particularly in obstructive hydrocephalus and the treatment of intracranial cysts. Children who have previously been shunt dependent may undergo endoscopic third ventriculostomy (ETV), which is effectively an "internal shunt" that bypasses a stenosed aqueduct of Sylvius. Parents and emergency clinicians should be cognizant that these children are still subject to the same manifestations of shunt failure; the presence of appropriate signs and symptoms of raised ICP should initiate the same evaluation and criteria for possible intervention outlined earlier in this section. It should be noted that while not subject to the myriad malfunctions that befall patients with implanted hardware such as infection, erosion, disconnection, and clogging, patients with ETVs can suffer restenosis of their fenestration site, with reports of closure as late as 8 years after the initial procedure.

Indwelling Venous Access Devices

Background

In 1973, Broviac designed the first Silastic tunneled central venous catheter (CVC). These devices provide children with relatively permanent and secure venous access during chemother-

apy, total parenteral nutrition, or prolonged IV antibiotic therapy. Pediatricians, family practitioners, and emergency physicians have increasingly been called on to access and assess these catheters. Clinicians must be familiar with the procedures for establishing patency, drawing blood, dealing with catheter occlusion or breakage, and assessing for infection. In 1983, the first totally implanted central venous access device, often referred to as a chest port, was developed and introduced.

Pathophysiology

The distal tip of tunneled venous catheters is located at the junction of the right atrium and the superior vena cava. The site of venous entry is usually the subclavian or internal jugular vein; however, access is occasionally obtained through the external jugular, cephalic, and brachiocephalic veins. The catheter is tunneled under the skin to a site in the chest away from the venous entry site and then either externalized or connected to a subcutaneous reservoir.

Equipment

Tunneled CVCs come in various types, such as Broviac, Hickman, Leonard, Raaf, Hermed, Groshong, and Corcath (Fig. 120.6). These catheters are made of Silastic elastomers

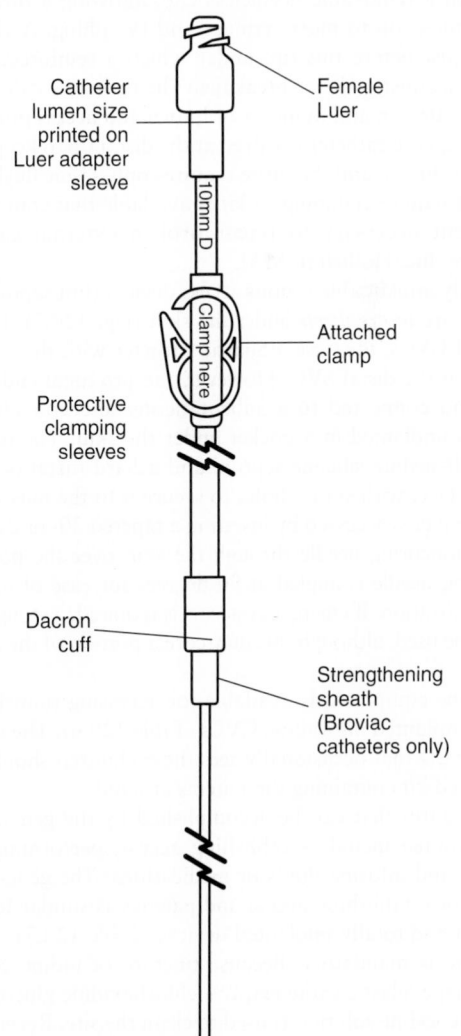

FIGURE 120.6 Partially implantable ("tunneled") venous catheter.

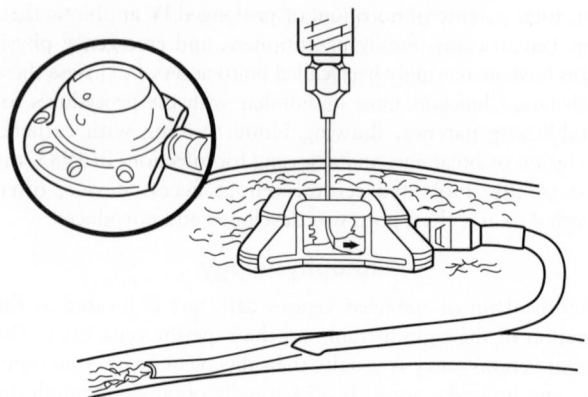

FIGURE 120.7 Totally implantable venous access device.

TABLE 120.6

EQUIPMENT NEEDED TO ACCESS CENTRAL VENOUS CATHETERS

Clamp or hemostat *without* teeth, possibly with rubber tips	Povidone-iodine ointment
T-extension tubing with clamp	Alcohol swabs
10-mL syringe of normal saline	Sterile drapes and gloves
10-mL syringe of heparin 100 U/mL	Dressing gauze and tape
(4) Injection caps	
Povidone-iodine solution with sterile gauze	Tegaderm sterile dressing (2) Tapered Huber noncoring needles, 20- and 22-gauge

and are tunneled under the skin a few centimeters before externalization. A Dacron® cuff, located around the catheter, anchors the catheter after it stimulates fibrosis of the surrounding tissue. This also serves to inhibit migration of bacteria into the catheter tract. The most proximal portion of the catheter contains a female Luer lock tip, which is usually covered with a removable needleless cap, allowing a direct and solid connection to most syringes and IV tubing. A clamp is present just before this tip, under which a reinforced sleeve protects against catheter breakage. The catheters can vary in length, diameter, and numbers of lumen and access ports. The Groshong-type catheter is valved at the distal tip to keep blood out of the lumen and therefore requires only saline flushes and does not require clamping. A kit is available that contains the equipment necessary to repair broken external catheters (Invacare, Inc, Holliston, MA).

Totally implantable venous access devices (Infusaport, Port-A-Cath) are *internalized* under the skin (Fig. 120.7). Like the tunneled CVCs, they use a Silastic catheter with the distal tip located in the distal SVC. However, the proximal end is tunneled and connected to a subcutaneous reservoir chamber, which is implanted in a pocket under the skin. The reservoir has a self-sealing silicone septum and a hard metal or plastic back surface, with suture holes to secure it to the muscle wall. The chamber is accessed by inserting a tapered 20- or 22-gauge Huber noncoring needle through the skin over the port. The noncoring needle is angled at 90 degrees for ease of insertion and stabilization. If emergency access is required, a straight needle can be used, although this may core a portion of the device's septum.

Specific equipment is available for accessing tunneled and totally implanted indwelling CVCs (Table 120.6). The medical office or ED that occasionally sees these children should have a prepared kit containing these items at hand.

Procedures that can be accomplished by the generalist or ED personnel include establishing access, performing phlebotomy, and infusing fluids or medications. The general procedure for establishing access and patency is similar for both tunneled and totally implanted devices (Table 120.7). Aseptic technique is mandatory. Because tincture of iodine solution can damage Silastic catheters, 2% chlorhexidine gluconate or povidone-iodine solution is used to clean the site. Recent studies have demonstrated lower bloodstream infection rates with the use of 2% tincture of chlorhexidine. Clamps or hemostats

with teeth can also damage the external portion of the catheter. In addition, smaller (less than 3 mL) syringes can generate too much pressure inside the catheter, causing catheter breakage. Therefore, 5- or 10-mL syringes are recommended to flush the system; never force flush against resistance. Fluid or medications should never be infused until patency is established because the risk of administering these solutions into a nonvascular space is high. To prevent air emboli from occurring, all clamps must remain closed when any part of the circuit is open. For accurate blood test results, the amount of blood that needs to be withdrawn unused is 3 mL from a tunneled CVC and 5 mL from a totally implanted CVC. Recent literature has demonstrated that compared with heparin, tissue-type plasminogen activator (tPA) is more successful in reducing the chances of clot formation in central venous hemodialysis catheter. However, further research on other types of catheters and cost analyses remain to be performed to determine if tPA should replace heparin in this regard.

When a tunneled CVC is accessed, these steps should be followed:

1. Before accessing the system, prime the intended IV circuit, including connection tubing, with saline to remove air. Clamp the IV tubing closed.
2. Clamp any external portions of central catheter on the protected area near the hub.

TABLE 120.7

TIPS FOR THE ROUTINE USE OF INDWELLING VENOUS ACCESS DEVICES

Aseptic technique
Do not use
   Clamps or hemostats with teeth
   Tincture of iodine solution
   Small (≤3 mL) syringes
Flush entire intravenous circuit before accessing system
Always close clamps when any part of the circuit is open
Do not infuse fluids or medications until patency is established
Flush the catheter with 10 mL of saline between medications
Flush cap or reservoir with heparin when procedure is complete

3. Clean the cap on the end of the system with alcohol, povidone-iodine, or chlorhexidine and allow the solution to dry.

4. Flush the system with 3 to 5 mL of saline in a 5- to 10-mL syringe and then aspirate 3 to 5 mL of blood to check patency; do not use this as a blood sample—discard. Absence of blood return may indicate the formation of fibrin sheath on internal catheter tip or malpositioning of the tip. If no blood return, consider a dye study and do not use the catheter for vesicant infusion.

5. Draw off blood needed for laboratory analysis and administer medications or fluids as needed. Flush again with saline and then either flush the device with heparin or connect the IV tubing to the needleless cap using Luer lock connections.

6. If the catheter is to be heparin locked, clamp the line prior to removal of the flush syringe; this maneuver is not necessary for the saline-flushed Groshong device.

7. If the needleless cap is removed, discard the old needleless cap and replace it with a new one using sterile technique.

The procedure differs slightly when accessing a totally implanted CVC or port. Because intact skin is penetrated, the use of a topical anesthetic cream before access should be considered when feasible. After leaving the topical anesthetic on for the manufacturer's recommended time, it should be wiped off and the skin should be cleansed with 2% chlorhexidine gluconate, alcohol, or povidone-iodine. Povidone-iodine should not be cleaned off with alcohol. Using sterile technique, a Huber needle should be inserted through the skin directly into the reservoir diaphragm and stopped when resistance is met at the back of the reservoir. The needle should be secured in place and patency should be established with aspiration and flushing. After use, the totally implanted device must be flushed using 3 to 5 mL of heparin (10 units per mL) or similar solution. When the port is not being used, patency is maintained with 3 to 5 mL of 100 units per mL flush on a monthly basis.

Complications resulting from accessing CVCs include occlusion, air embolus, catheter breakage or displacement, and infection. Although most of these complications can be avoided if care is taken to maintain aseptic technique, the clinician should be aware of their diagnosis and management.

Clinical Findings/Management

Catheter Occlusion. Difficulty drawing blood or infusing fluid through a CVC can be the result of catheter malposition or occlusion. The catheter may be positioned against a vessel wall, or fibrin or blood may clot in the lumen. In addition, various precipitates can occlude the lumen of the catheter. Waxy precipitates can result when parenteral nutrition solutions contain combinations of fat, protein, and carbohydrate, and particulate precipitates can result from the poor solubility of calcium and phosphorus. IV phenytoin (especially when administered in a glucose-containing solution) and diazepam can also get precipitated.

Children who require IV medications or fluids at home may present for short-term management of catheter occlusions. The problem is often noted only when the acute care nurse or physician cannot access the catheter during the evaluation of another problem.

Increasing the venous pressure gradient along the catheter can facilitate phlebotomy. These maneuvers include having the patient hold his or her arms above the head, cough or perform Valsalva maneuver, and placing the patient in reverse Trendelenburg position. If blood still cannot be drawn, 3 mL of saline should be used to gently irrigate the clot and aspirate it into the syringe. Two to 3 mL of fluid should be forced back and forth to avoid pushing the clot into the venous system. A number of complications can result from this maneuver. The pressure can force the clot into the bloodstream or rupture the catheter, particularly if the practitioner uses too much force or too small a syringe. Care should be taken to observe the catheter for a balloon "aneurysm," a sign of impending rupture.

Totally implanted systems are much less likely to clot than are tunneled catheters. This situation is fortunate because irrigating the clot is admittedly more difficult, if not impossible, to perform on a totally implanted system.

Specific agents may help dissolve precipitates or clots. For waxy precipitates, 70% ethanol should be used. For particulate precipitates, 0.1N hydrochloric acid (HCl) or 8.4% sodium bicarbonate should be used depending on the pH of the drugs/solutions infusing prior to the precipate formation. Fibrinolytic agents such as urokinase (0.5 to 1 mL of a 5,000 units per mL solution) or tPA (up to 2 mg, dependent on catheter size) may dissolve a blood clot, and similar to HCl, may be used up to three times if necessary. Ethanol should be used only one time per episode. Urokinase infusions may be started at the suggestion of the surgical or interventional radiology consultants, who should be involved in the treatment plan if initial attempts are unsuccessful.

Air Embolism. Failure to maintain a closed system during manipulation of indwelling venous catheters can result in embolism of air into the chambers of the heart. Passage of the embolus to the systemic or pulmonary circulation can result in severe and irreversible tissue damage.

Air embolus can cause a patient to experience sudden onset of tachypnea, tachycardia, hypotension, or loss of consciousness. Other diagnoses that should be considered in patients with these symptoms are pneumothorax, liberation of septic emboli, and direct cardiac insult. If an air embolus is suspected, the patient should be placed in the left-sided Trendelenburg position and oxygen should be administered. In addition, the indwelling catheter should be clamped and remain unused as other peripheral access is obtained.

Catheter Breakage. The family members and physicians caring for the child with a tunneled catheter may have considered the nightmare of catheter breakage and subsequent exsanguination. Although catheter breakage is a distinct possibility, most events occur during routine care rather during playtime and therefore the blood loss is easily apparent and correctable. A tunneled catheter can acquire a small hole from inadvertent needle puncture or even ordinary wear and tear. Totally implanted catheters, in contrast, are less susceptible to local events or wear and tear. However, trauma to the area can result in detachment of the proximal portion of the catheter from the implanted port.

Leakage of blood or fluid from the externalized portion of a tunneled catheter is easily noticed. Externalized catheters must be immediately clamped proximal to the break, cleaned with povidone-iodine solution, and covered with sterile dressing until repaired. Repair kits are available for each catheter size (Fig. 120.8). These kits contain a new external catheter

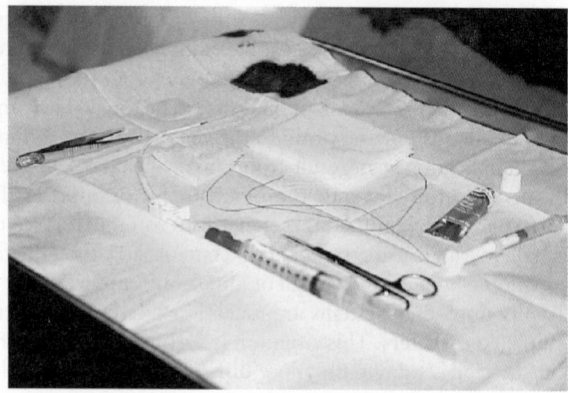

FIGURE 120.8 Repair kit for tunneled catheters.

segment with a hollow male connector that fits into a cleanly sliced proximal end. The kits also contain a syringe and needle to apply the glue to the male connector. Optimally, a person familiar with the procedure will be available within a short time of clamping the catheter. If the externalized portion is too small to clamp, hemostasis may be achieved by putting pressure on the site of venous entry. A scar is usually apparent at this site. However, if the scar is not apparent, the catheter should be palpated from the exit site on the skin to the location at which it can no longer be palpated and pressure should be applied at that site.

If an implantable catheter leaks, fluid or blood that collects subcutaneously may cause a bulge or painful swelling at the site. A broken implanted catheter must undergo prompt surgical management. The broken segment can often be easily visualized by chest radiography.

Catheter Displacement. Occasionally, the patient or caregiver inadvertently pulls on the externalized portion of a tunneled catheter. The venous portion of the catheter may eventually be displaced from the venous system. Externalized catheters are at higher risk for dislodgment within a few weeks of insertion, because the cuff is not fully anchored by fibrosis. Exsanguination after catheter dislodgment is a rare event because of the advancement of the tip inside the vein and the natural tendency toward venous hemostasis. However, children with clotting disorders are at increased risk of life-threatening blood loss after catheter displacement. Totally implanted devices are at risk of dislodgment at both ends; however, few events apart from major thoracic trauma place enough tension on the catheter to dislodge it from the vein. Migration of the venous catheter tip is rare but can lead to cardiac arrhythmias, pneumothorax, cardiac tamponade, and superior vena cava syndrome.

Detecting catheter dislodgment is easier in patients with externalized catheters. If the Dacron cuff is noted outside the skin surface, the catheter must be considered dislodged and should not be used until the tip's location can be confirmed by chest radiography. Failure to draw back free-flowing blood from the device increases the suspicion that the catheter is no longer in the central vein. In this situation, the catheter should be clamped and secured close to the skin and immediate surgical or interventional radiology consultation should be obtained. A dye study may be necessary to locate the catheter tip. For totally implanted devices, dislodgment of the catheter from the

vein should be suspected if the device no longer functions after thoracic trauma. If the catheter is disconnected from the reservoir, fluid or blood may collect subcutaneously and cause a bulge or painful swelling at the site. Prompt surgical management is required.

Catheter migration should be considered in patients with totally implanted venous catheters who experience respiratory distress or palpitations. Radiologic evaluation of catheter location should rapidly ensue, with subsequent surgical consultation if the catheter tip has migrated.

Infection. The presence of an indwelling venous catheter places a patient at higher risk for infection, which can occur at the catheter exit site, the tunnel through which the line is placed, the catheter itself, or in the patient's bloodstream. Tunneled catheters carry a higher overall risk of infection than do fully implanted devices. The presence of erythema, tenderness, or purulent drainage at any skin site related to an indwelling catheter suggests a catheter infection. Less commonly, infection can also occur at the subcutaneous pocket of a patient's fully implantable catheter. The entire dressing must be removed for these sites to be inspected. Fever is common in patients with catheter-related bacteremia or sepsis but may be absent in early, localized infection. Immunocompromised patients can exhibit rapid deterioration, and more commonly acquire fungal, gram-negative, and polymicrobial infections. Patients receiving parenteral alimentation are also at higher risk for gram-negative infections. Still, the most common pathogens in patients with indwelling catheters are gram-positive organisms such as *S epidermidis*, *S aureus*, and *S viridans*. The signs of infection may be more subtle or absent in neutropenic patients. Catheter-related bacteremia can also occur without apparent skin manifestations. It is sometimes difficult to tell if the catheter itself is infected or simply seeded the bloodstream, and many consider both to have occurred in the presence of a positive culture result. If this differentiation is necessary, it is possible to compare the extent of the colony-forming units between the peripheral and central cultures and the timing between the central and peripheral culture growth.

Blood cultures should be obtained from the catheter and, in most cases, from a peripheral vein as well. At least 1 to 2 mL of blood should be used for this purpose. More than 90% of blood cultures will yield positive results within 36 hours; gram-negative pathogens will be discovered within 24 hours after culture is obtained. Fungal cultures are appropriate in immunocompromised patients or those who have had prior invasive fungal infections. Cultures of any purulent fluid are helpful. A complete blood cell count with differential count is warranted, although a normal result should not dissuade the clinician from suspecting an invasive bacterial infection. Other blood tests, such as coagulation studies, should be considered if the patient is ill appearing.

Initial treatment consists of IV antibiotic therapy and supportive measures. Bacterial catheter infections can be eradicated without catheter removal, although infections with *S. aureus* and fungi usually necessitate catheter removal. Persistent infection, infection of the subcutaneous tunnel, critical illness, endocarditis, and thrombophlebitis are also indications for removal. Initial antibiotic therapy should include agents active against both gram-positive and gram-negative infections. Many centers use oxacillin and gentamicin as the first choice;

local antibiotic resistance patterns should determine the use of vancomycin instead of oxacillin. Ceftazidime or cefepime should be added for presumptive treatment of *Pseudomonas* infection in neutropenic patients or in those who appear to be severely ill. Local bacterial resistance patterns may alter these choices, such that centers may reserve the use of vancomycin for culture-positive resistant strains or use netilmicin in place of gentamicin. These issues should be discussed with the patient's personal physicians and the local infectious disease consultants. Persistent colonization of CVCs may respond to installation of antibiotic or ethanol into the lumen for 12 to 24 hours (antibiotic lock or ethanol lock).

Other Complications. Other complications related to indwelling catheters can occur, albeit rarely. Direct injury to the exit site can be a result of either erosion of tissue by the Dacron cuff of an externalized catheter or breakdown of the skin site from vigorous cleansing. This condition can lead to a localized infection. On physical examination, excoriation, erythema, tenderness, or purulent drainage is present at the exit site of the catheter. Select patients with a localized site infection who are afebrile and well appearing, have a normal leukocyte count, and have prearranged follow-up may be managed as outpatients with oral antibiotic therapy.

As previously mentioned, phenytoin and diazepam can interact with the silicone lining of the catheters and the administration of these medications through Silastic catheters should be avoided if possible. In addition, a large volume of saline flush should be administered between medications that are incompatible with each other, such as calcium and bicarbonate.

Enteral Feeding Tubes

Background

A stoma, derived from the Latin word for "mouth," is an opening from the GI or urinary tract to the outside of the body. A gastrostomy is a surgically or endoscopically created stoma that provides access to the stomach from the level of the skin. A jejunostomy is a surgically created stoma that brings the jejunum to the skin surface. Gastrostomy is performed most typically in children who are predicted to be unable to take adequate oral nourishment for a prolonged period. The inability to tolerate sufficient oral feedings can be related to numerous conditions, including esophageal atresia, chronic malabsorptive syndromes, significant craniofacial abnormalities, neurologic impairment, severe gastroesophageal reflux, esophageal burns, chronic systemic diseases, and rarely anorexia nervosa. Jejunostomy feedings are used when postpyloric feeding is required and carried out in such patients as those with delayed gastric emptying, recurrent aspiration pneumonia, or severe gastroesophageal reflux. Gastric feedings are much more common than jejunal feedings.

Enteral feeding via gastrostomy and jejunostomy tubes (J-tubes) has become more common in recent years. Therefore, ED physicians should become comfortable with the various types of G-tubes and jejunal tubes, the supporting types of apparatus, and the complications inherent in the use of these lifesaving enteral feeding devices.

Pathophysiology

G-tubes are inserted via percutaneous endoscopic gastrostomy (PEG), open gastrostomy, laparoscopy, or radiologic percutaneous gastrostomy. The PEG technique is the most common. It involves placing a percutaneous hole in the anterior abdominal wall. An endoscope is used to provide light at the exact site on the anterior abdominal wall as a guide for needle puncture. A long guide wire with a feeding tube is then passed through the mouth and distally until the pointed dilator is seen pushing its way through the skin of the anterior abdominal wall. In open gastrostomy, a left upper quadrant or midline incision is used to place the G-tube through the abdominal wall. The G-tube then passes through a purse string suture placed on the anterior wall of the stomach and into the lumen of the stomach at the level of the fundus. The purse string suture is then tightened around the tube to prevent gastric leakage, and the wall of the stomach around the suture is sewn to the abdominal wall where the tube makes its exit. Laparoscopic and radiologic percutaneous gastrostomies are evolving techniques of enteral tube placement.

Jejunostomy can be performed via an open technique or percutaneously. Jejunal feeding can also be accomplished by placing a jejunal tube via the gastrostomy. This method allows jejunal feeding and enables venting of gastric air.

Equipment

Gastrostomy Tubes. Several types of G-tubes are available. Most are made of polyurethane, silicone, or rubber. These devices may vary in length, the number of ports, the type of catheter tip, the number of lumens, and the manner of securing to the patient's skin (Fig. 120.9). The *mushroom* types (Button by Bard Interventional Products Division, Billerica, MA) have soft flexible tips that require an obturator or stylet to stretch the tip. These devices have a single lumen. The *balloon tip devices* (MIC-KEY, Medical Innovations Corporation, Draper, UT) have become most popular and have begun to replace the mushroom tip devices. The inflatable balloon is located at the tip, similar to a urinary Foley catheter. They are easy to secure and do not dislodge as easily. These tubes may have multiple ports and lumina. The most recent advance in G-tubes is the introduction of the low-profile G-tube, commonly referred to as buttons (Fig. 120.10). The advantage of this type of apparatus is that no long piece of tubing arises from the stoma. They may have either mushroom or balloon tips. Replacement devices need to be matched for both the size of the stoma (the external diameter of the tube) and the length of the stoma tract. These buttons have unidirectional antireflux valves that are fragile. In some centers, button devices are placed at the time of the initial gastrostomy.

Jejunal Tubes. Jejunal tubes that pass through the gastrostomy are usually small-diameter tubes (8F), an example of which is the Frederick Miller feeding tube set manufactured by Cook (Bloomington, IN). These tubes have a small mercury weight at the distal tip and are placed under fluoroscopy. Several types of surgical jejunostomy feeding tubes are available, including Malecot and MIC-KEY jejunal tubes.

Clinical Findings/Management

Patients with G-tubes or J-tubes who present with symptoms that appear to be related to the tube require a full evaluation.

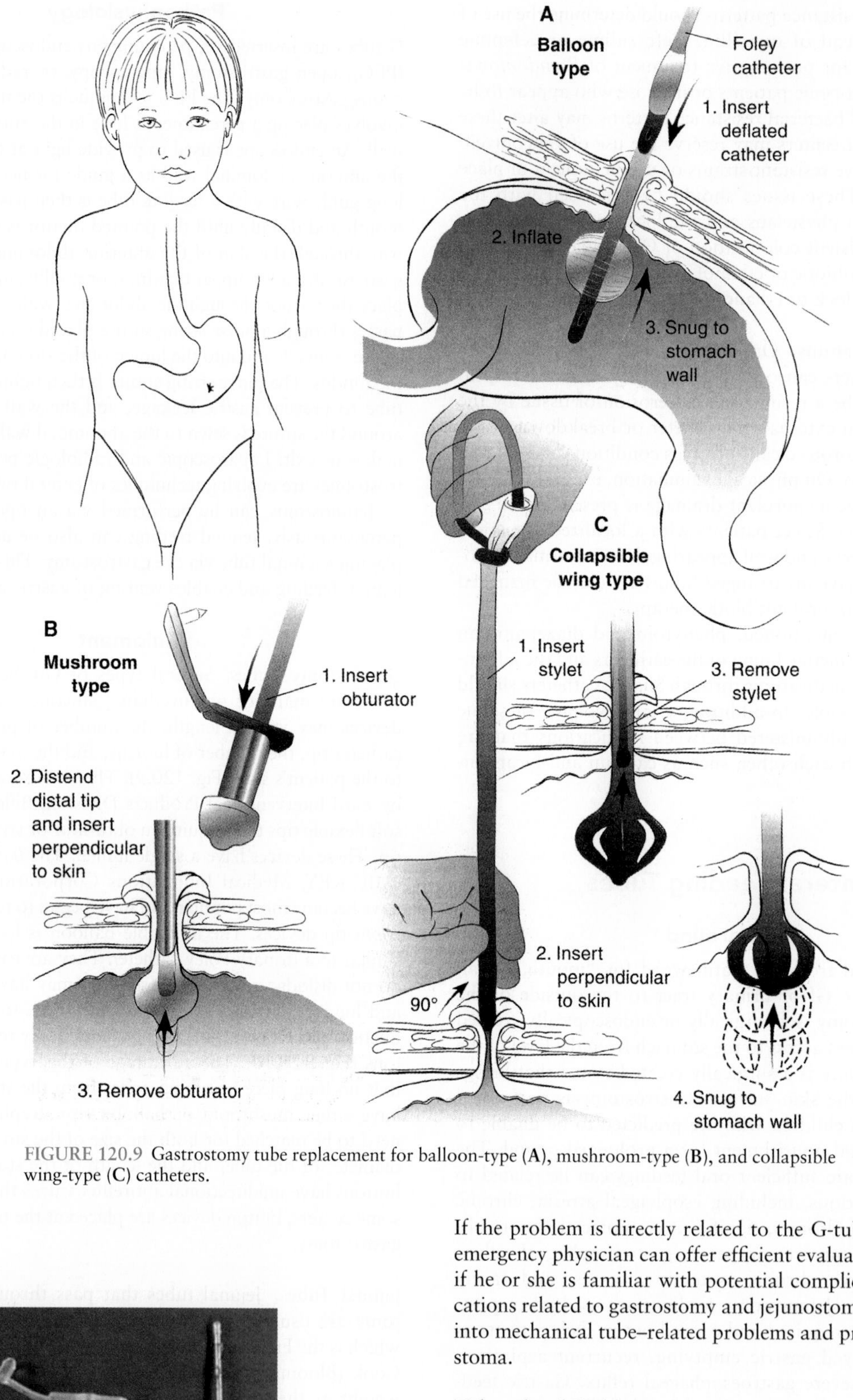

A
Balloon type

Foley catheter

1. Insert deflated catheter

2. Inflate

3. Snug to stomach wall

C
Collapsible wing type

1. Insert stylet

3. Remove stylet

2. Insert perpendicular to skin

90°

4. Snug to stomach wall

B
Mushroom type

1. Insert obturator

2. Distend distal tip and insert perpendicular to skin

3. Remove obturator

FIGURE 120.9 Gastrostomy tube replacement for balloon-type (**A**), mushroom-type (**B**), and collapsible wing-type (**C**) catheters.

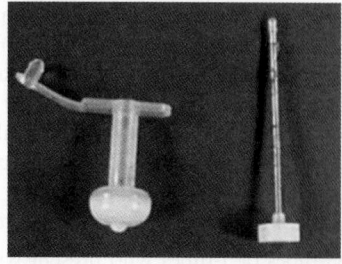

FIGURE 120.10 The button: replacement gastrostomy device.

If the problem is directly related to the G-tube or J-tube, the emergency physician can offer efficient evaluation and therapy if he or she is familiar with potential complications. Complications related to gastrostomy and jejunostomy can be divided into mechanical tube–related problems and problems with the stoma.

Tube-related Problems

Dislodgment. Dislodgment is one of the most common complications of G- and J-tubes. This situation may occur as a result of a traumatic event, such as accidental tension on the external tubing, occult balloon deflation, or rupture of the balloon leading to extrusion of the entire tube. When G-tube dislodgment precipitates an ED visit, many parents either recall the size of the tube or bring one along to the ED. If neither of these occurs, the patient's medical record usually provides the most recent tube size.

The patient with tube dislodgment may present with a benign stoma or with active bleeding secondary to trauma. If the tube size is unknown or if various tube sizes are not available, the most common temporizing method of replacement is insertion of a Foley catheter. A crucial consideration is the interval of time since the dislodgment. If hours have elapsed, the stoma may be constricted and require insertion of a smaller replacement tube.

The interval since *initial* placement of the gastrostomy is important. Perioperative displacement (within 1 month of initial placement) is treated differently than dislodgment of a tube from a mature stoma. If a G-tube dislodges, temporary replacement with a smaller Foley catheter may prevent pushing the recently fixed stomach away from the anterior abdominal wall. A series of progressively larger Foley catheters, beginning with one to two sizes smaller than the original tube, may be used to dilate the stoma if it is partially closed. A gastroenterologist or surgeon should then be consulted for definitive care. An older tube that has dislodged should be replaced urgently with the same size and type of the tube to avoid narrowing of the stoma. The physician must use caution when reinserting a G-tube because extreme force can lead to tube insertion into the peritoneal cavity through a false tract.

A jejunal tube that has dislodged needs to be replaced by the subspecialist who placed it initially. For example, a J-tube that was inserted via the gastrostomy should be replaced by the interventional radiologist under fluoroscopy. A surgical J-tube requires replacement by a surgeon.

Clogging. Clogging or obstruction of the lumen of the G-tube or J-tube can occur as a result of dried, solidified formula or twisting or kinking of the tube. Tube obstruction is discovered when the caregivers cannot infuse fluids. If formula is suspected as the cause, aspiration of the clot and gentle flushing of the lumen should be attempted. Warm water is recommended as the most effective fluid. Despite reports of the success of various carbonated drinks in this situation, their effectiveness is controversial. When the G-tube becomes clogged, insertion of a stylet is not recommended because this technique may result in perforation of the tubing beneath the skin level. Repositioning of the tube should be attempted next; if this procedure is not effective, removal and replacement are necessary. If the gastrostomy is fresh (within 1 month), the surgeon or gastroenterologist should be consulted before removal of the clogged tube. Caregivers should be reminded of the need for proper flushing with each use. If the patient has a button, the extension tubing should be removed from the button before flushing it.

Leaking. Leaking can occur directly from the lumen of the tube or from the peristomal area. Leaking from the stoma often indicates that the stoma has widened and now exceeds the size of the tube. Determining whether the leaking substance is formula, pus, or gastric fluid is important in the management. If purulent drainage is coming from the stoma, the physician needs to look further for signs of stomal cellulitis or peristomal abscess (see the next section). If formula is leaking from the lumen of the tube, the physician must assess the tube position and check the balloon. In the case of a leaking button, problems with valve patency could occur. If fluid is leaking from the stoma, the stoma may have become larger than the tube. One approach to this problem is removing the tube for a short period, thus allowing constriction of the stoma. The stoma may also have become disrupted and therefore requires surgical evaluation.

Reflux. Gastroesophageal reflux may be a complication of G-tube placement. An increase in prior reflux disease can occur when a Nissen fundoplication is not performed simultaneously. The patient may present with an increase in episodes of vomiting and symptoms of esophageal irritation after G-tube placement. Patients in this category may benefit from continuous enteral feedings. If continuous feedings are not effective in reducing symptomatic reflux, fundoplication may be indicated.

Gastric Ulceration. Gastric irritation leading to ulceration may occur as a complication of gastrostomy in several scenarios. If the tip of the G-tube is too long, it may abrade the opposite surface of the stomach mucosa, resulting in bleeding or traumatic ulceration. Similarly, the balloon may accidentally become overinflated and cause friction, especially when the stomach is empty. Balloon overdilation can occur if medications or flushes are erroneously administered via the balloon port.

A patient with gastric ulcer caused by mechanical trauma presents with symptoms similar to other ulcer patients. Common symptoms are abdominal pain, irritability, hematemesis, hematochezia, and coffee ground gastric drainage from the G-tube lumen. Saline lavage should be performed. If the fluid obtained is nonbloody, medications such as H_2-blockers, antacids, and sucralfate may be administered and upper endoscopy should be scheduled. The G-tube should be changed and the patient's symptoms should be monitored carefully.

Gastric outlet obstruction. Gastric outlet obstruction is a rare but serious complication of G-tubes. It is usually the result of the migration of the tube tip into the pyloric channel. Occasionally, the G-tube can migrate superiorly and block the esophagus. In very rare cases, the entire apparatus can migrate distally, resulting in gastric outlet obstruction. The child complains of retching or sudden onset of emesis and appears uncomfortable. The G-tube needs to be pulled back to its proper location until it is snug against the abdominal wall. If this procedure is not successful, the tube must be removed completely.

Stomal Complications
Irritant dermatitis/allergic hypersensitivity. Skin irritation around the stoma may result from chronic leakage of gastric or jejunal fluid around the tube. If the stoma widens, the leakage may become excessive, resulting in more significant dermatitis. Various brands of adhesives and cleansing solutions may result in an allergic rash around the stoma.

The peristomal skin should be thoroughly cleansed and dried before assessment. Small vesicular lesions with surrounding erythema suggest irritant dermatitis. Local treatment includes keeping the area as dry as possible and using barrier creams to protect the skin from further breakdown. Stomahesive Power (Convatec, Princeton, NJ) is useful for molding to the skin surface and keeping the area dry and free of debris. In addition, identifying and treating the cause of the leakage are important. If the leakage is caused by an enlarged stoma, surgical intervention may be required in the near future.

Hypergranulation tissue. Children with G- and J-tubes may develop hypergranulation tissue in the peristomal area, extending beyond the wound bed. Although these granulomatous lesions may be harmless, they can be distressing to caregivers. There is often drainage associated with the granulation tissue; however, this does not uniformly indicate the presence of infection. Hypergranulation tissue may begin to cause occlusion of the stoma and should be treated. Treatment options include the application of silver nitrate swabs (though this may be uncomfortable to the patient), triamcinolone cream (0.5%) twice a day, and polyurethane foam dressings.

Cellulitis. When peristomal skin surrounding the G-tube or J-tube is irritated by recurrent or intermittent exposure to drainage or other irritants, cellulitis may occur. The infection may begin as superficial skin irritation or contact dermatitis and then evolve into a deeper infection. The surrounding peristomal area may become reddened, warm, tender, and edematous. These symptoms and signs may occasionally be accompanied by systemic symptoms and fever. The patient with a G- or J-tube may become resistant to tube feedings because of the discomfort associated with manipulation of the apparatus. Once cellulitis is present, the patient requires systemic antibiotics for resolution of this infection. The common organisms, staphylococci and streptococci, usually respond to a first-generation cephalosporin. Occasionally, a peristomal abscess, heralded by a localized area of fluctuance, can complicate the cellulitis. This abscess requires incision and drainage before antibiotic administration.

Fungal infection. Recurrent moisture caused by gastric or jejunal leakage in the stomal area can predispose the patient to fungal infection. The most common causal organism is *Candida albicans*, appearing as fiery red plaques at the stoma site. Topical clotrimazole is curative in most situations. Keeping the area as dry as possible is imperative.

Gastrointestinal and Genitourinary Diversion

Background

Pediatric patients may have a GI or genitourinary diversion for one of many reasons. Congenital causes include Hirschsprung's disease, imperforate anus, cloacal exstrophy, bladder exstrophy, meningomyelocele with a neurogenic bladder, and posterior urethral valves. Acquired lesions may include ulcerative colitis, Crohn's disease, and necrotizing enterocolitis. Traumatic injuries leading to GI or genitourinary diversion include penetrating wounds and falls.

GI diversions consist primarily of colostomy and ileostomy. A colostomy brings the colon to the skin; these patients usually have semiformed stools because the absorptive and storage function of the bowel is preserved. An ileostomy brings the ileum to the skin. Since these patients do not possess large

bowel function, they consequently have a watery, frequent stooling pattern.

The major forms of chronic urinary diversions consist of ureterostomy, vesicostomy, pyelostomy, and ileal conduits. In addition, there are temporary urinary diversions that may be established by percutaneous means and maintained with a drainage catheter. Ureterostomy brings the dilated ureter to the level of the skin, whereas pyelostomy brings the dilated renal pelvis to the skin. In contrast, an ileal conduit implies that the ureters are attached to a short segment of the ileum, which is then externalized. A vesicostomy opens the bladder to the skin. Nephrostomy or cystostomy necessitates that a tube be placed into the renal pelvis or bladder via a percutaneous approach and left in place as a temporary diversion. The percutaneous nephrostomy is typically placed by the interventional radiologist. These temporary diversions are most often used to allow for minimally invasive management of stone disease. Urinary undiversion indicates that the patient has undergone a surgical procedure that internalizes the urine passage via a "neobladder" composed of the original bladder and/or a combination of large and small bowel.

In general, a stomatherapist is crucial to the physicians and families of all patients with stomal sites and appliances. However, patients continue to present to the ED with ostomy-related problems, and the emergency physician should become facile with the various types of GI and genitourinary diversions and their specific complications.

Pathophysiology

The nature of the disease and the location of the lesion(s) guide the surgeon when choosing the type of diversion to use. An ileostomy is usually performed in newborns for conditions such as meconium ileus, necrotizing enterocolitis, and intestinal atresia. It may be required in older children and adolescents because of ulcerative colitis or polyposis. The surgical method used depends on the predicted length of time required for the ostomy, as well as the location of the disease.

Colostomy in infants is required for complications of colonic atresia, high forms of imperforate anus, and Hirschsprung's disease. The level of the colostomy is related to the disease type and to anticipated future procedures. Some of the ostomy complications that occur in patients with genitourinary and GI diversions are similar. In both types of diversions, many complications relate to the actual stoma. These conditions are discussed in the previous enteral feeding section. Other complications are metabolic or mechanical in nature.

A vesicostomy is usually performed for patients with myelomeningocele, posterior urethral valves, prune belly syndrome, and spinal cord injury resulting in a neurogenic bladder. This procedure consists of bringing the dome of the bladder up to the skin below the umbilicus to serve as a vent for high bladder pressure, and it is protective of the upper urinary tract.

Ureterostomy is accomplished by bringing the ureter to the surface of the skin either in the groin (low) or in the flank (high). Most high ureterostomies are of the loop variety, in which a loop of the ureter is incised on one side and passed upward to allow the edges to be anastomosed to the skin. This path allows ureteral continuity from the kidney to the bladder, with a vent to the skin. Low ureterostomies are more common and are performed for obstructed ureters such as ectopic ureters or megaureters. To decompress an obstructed system and prevent urinary tract infection, the ureter is divided, the distal end is ligated, and the proximal edges are anastomosed to the skin.

Ileal loop conduits are created with a resected 10- to 20-cm bowel segment of the ileum and anastomosing both ureters to one end. The other end of the bowel loop is brought out to the skin. Ileal loop conduits are preferable in older children who can wear an appliance to collect the urine.

Equipment

Standard ostomies are commonly managed by placing an ostomy pouch over the stoma to collect the effluent. In young infants, sigmoid colostomies may be managed without an external pouch if the effluent is not caustic to the skin and fluid is therefore collected in the diaper. Urinary flow can also be collected in a diaper and may be preferable because some appliances do not adhere well to the skin for long periods.

Ostomy pouches for children are manufactured in various sizes. One- and two-piece configurations are available, and pouches may be soft or rigid. Supplemental adhesives are crucial to enhance adhesion, especially if the effluent is more liquidlike.

Clinical Findings/Management

Gastrointestinal Diversions. Patients with colostomies and ileostomies may present with complications that are common to both types of ostomies. Ileostomies also have metabolic complications that are specific to this type of ostomy.

Cutaneous complications. Peristomal cutaneous complications are common in patients with ostomies, and stem from the effect of chronic stool and other drainage on the peristomal skin. This chronic drainage compromises the skin integrity surrounding the stoma. The most effective management is the maintenance of a good seal between the ostomy pouch and the stoma. Contact dermatitis may occur either from leakage around the stoma or from allergy to stomal materials such as tape or pouches. Removing the offending material often successfully treats this condition. Infection with *C albicans* is fairly common because of the persistent moisture and the frequent use of prophylactic antibiotics. Treatment with antifungal agents such as clotrimazole, especially powders, is effective. The powder can be mixed with a small amount of water and painted onto the skin to enhance adherence of the pouch. Ointments and creams should be avoided in fungal infections. Skin bleeding resulting from prolonged irritation of the peristomal area is usually minor. The cellulitis that can occur if the skin excoriation worsens is treated with systemic antibiotics.

Stomal complications. Stomal stenosis is not always detectable to the parent or practitioner and may present with reduced or absent output, diarrhea, or cramping abdominal pain. When severe stenosis occurs, it usually presents as obstruction. To assess the degree of stenosis, the physician should gently examine the stoma digitally unless the stoma is too small. In this case, a catheter should be carefully passed. If abdominal obstruction is suspected, radiographs of the abdomen and urgent surgical consultation are indicated.

Prolapse of the stoma occurs in more than 20% of patients with stomas and is usually not an emergency. However, skin excoriation, bleeding, and incarceration of the bowel may occur. The situation becomes more urgent if the prolapse is associated with pain, decreased output, or a dusky stoma color that represents circulatory compromise and requires immediate surgical management. This includes easing the prolapsed contents back into the stoma using both hands. This procedure may need to be done repetitively until such time that definitive surgical repair is undertaken.

Retraction of the stoma because of excessive tension may cause the stoma to recede beneath the skin. This condition occurs more often than prolapse in patients with ileostomies. Stomal retraction makes it difficult for a pouch to adhere to the skin. Retraction can also result in cellulitis or even peritonitis, depending on the location of the detachment and the flow of the effluent. Management usually includes antibiotics and if the retraction is extensive, surgical correction is indicated.

A hernia of the peristomal contents occurs when there is a protrusion of the colon or ileum into the subcutaneous layers of skin surrounding the stoma. This complication may impede adherence of the ostomy pouch but does not usually represent an emergency. Elective surgical revision provides definitive management.

Complications specific to ileostomy. Patients with ileostomies occasionally develop metabolic derangements. In the face of large volume losses, children tend to deplete salt and water. If large fluid losses persist, the biochemical profiles of these patients are significantly altered. Determining the cause of the exceptionally high fluid losses from the ileostomy is crucial. Some possibilities are obstruction, gastroenteritis, and dietary indiscretion. Treatment is aimed at restoring normal fluid and electrolyte balance and may require hospital admission.

Patients with ileostomies are prone to acquiring urinary stones. The chemical composition of stones in this scenario is different than that in normal patients; uric acid stones constitute 60% and calcium oxalate makes up the remainder. Treatment is directed at decreasing ileostomy output and increasing urine output.

Urinary Diversions
Vesicostomy. In patients with a vesicostomy, eversion of a large portion of the bladder can occur and appear like an exstrophy. When the posterior aspect of the bladder prolapses through the stoma, the patient presents with a red mass, which may change to purple if not treated promptly. Applying an index fingertip to the bladder and gently pushing inward may manage this condition. Nonlatex gloves are required because children with urologic abnormalities are often allergic to latex. Sedatives may be required to facilitate reduction of the prolapse. A prolapsed vesicostomy should be surgically revised emergently if the manual reduction is unsuccessful.

Patients with stomal stenosis of the vesicostomy usually present with a palpable bladder, a history of unwanted urethral voiding, or with symptoms of urinary tract infection. As the bladder fails to empty at low pressures, the mean storage pressure rises and the chance for seeding bacteria into the upper urinary tract increases. These patients often have a pinpoint opening to the bladder, and the parents usually comment on how much smaller the stoma has become over time. If possible, these patients should have a catheter placed via the vesicostomy using a small (6F or 8F) catheter. If it is not possible to catheterize the vesicostomy, an attempt must be made at urethral catheterization assuming the patient has been left anatomically intact. If the vesicostomy is successfully catheterized, the catheter should be left in place until surgical revision is carried out.

Many vesicostomies are colonized with bacteria via stomal contamination. Therefore, a catheterized specimen through the stoma is sometimes unreliable. Patients with constitutional symptoms such as fever should have their urine culture carried out via vesicostomy. If no other source of fever is discovered, treatment should commence after the culture has been obtained. In an asymptomatic patient, a positive culture result may represent asymptomatic bacteriuria and is not always of concern.

Skin irritation in the area of the vesicostomy is unusual. The most important preventive measure is frequent diaper changes, even if highly absorbent diapers are used. If urine seeps onto the patient's clothes repetitively, skin breakdown may ensue. In severe cases, temporary urinary diversion with a Foley catheter while applying a barrier ointment allows time for healing.

Ureterostomy. Stenosis is the most common complication in the patient with a ureterostomy. These patients often present with fever and symptoms suggestive of pyelonephritis. The stoma should be catheterized with an 8F catheter, and urine should be sent for culture. Surgical revision of the stoma or definitive urologic reconstruction must be considered. Ureterostomy prolapse is rare.

Ileal loop conduits. Inflammation of the peristomal skin arises when the appliance fits poorly around this bud of ileum, allowing urine to seep under the protective wafer. Prolonged contact with skin causes irritation and ulceration. The use of paste to create a better seal around the bud is often all that is needed to avoid such a complication. In some cases, surgical revision is necessary, especially when the bud has retracted.

Prolapse of the ileum occurs occasionally and can be striking, especially if too long a segment was used in creating the loop initially. Prolapsed segments 20 to 30 cm long have been seen and require surgical revision. If the prolapse is minor, the clinician should perform the same gentle manual reduction technique previously described in the "Stomal Complications" section under "Gastrointestinal Diversions."

Peristomal hernia can occur when fascial defects adjacent to the ileal loop allow loops of bowel to herniate outside the abdominal wall. This condition requires urgent surgical consultation.

Stenosis of the ileal stoma may occur in these patients. Symptoms may include pain, but the usual presenting complaint for these patients is fever. This finding necessitates a workup for pyelonephritis. Stomal stenosis can also lead to the formation of urinary calculi. In this setting, surgical revision of the ileal stoma must be undertaken.

Urinary undiversions. As the child with a vesicostomy or ileal loop grows older, the social stigma of a diaper motivates many of these patients to seek urinary continence. For patients with spina bifida or exstrophy, this goal may be achieved by the use of an intestinal segment to augment bladder capacity (enterocystoplasty). In addition, a procedure to tighten the bladder neck and create resistance to leakage and creation of a channel through which the patient can perform intermittent catheterization is indicated. For all patients with spina bifida and most patients with exstrophy, continence comes at the expense of daily clean intermittent catheterization (CIC) for the rest of their lives. Careful patient and family selection is necessary for this procedure; compliance with CIC is crucial. Nevertheless, the enhanced self-esteem and improved quality of life these patients report are gratifying.

Perforation is the worst complication of intestinal augmentations to create neobladders. Most bladder perforations result from overdistension of the augmented bladder, which then diminishes perfusion to the bowel segment. In addition, the urine in these neobladders is chronically colonized secondary to the use of intermittent catheterization. Patients may present anywhere from 1 month to many years after surgery with a history of acute abdominal pain. Fever may be present within a few hours of perforation. Because many patients with spina bifida have decreased or absent abdominal sensation, peritonitis may be fairly advanced before pain is experienced. The presence of abdominal pain in a patient with a urinary diversion should prompt an immediate call to the patient's urologist. The urologic evaluation generally consists of a fluoroscopic gravity cystogram with views during filling and emptying, or a CT cystogram. Small perforations may be obscured with the full bladder and become apparent only during bladder emptying. Prophylactic antibiotics should be administered before the cystogram. Once this diagnosis is established, the patient is prepared for emergency laparotomy.

Patients may present to the ED with a sudden inability to pass a catheter into their neobladder. This situation may be because the appendiceal conduit through which they pass their catheter contains a false passage. A fluoroscopic study is warranted to delineate the passage and allow catheterization under radiographic control. The same situation is often true for patients catheterizing per urethra. In some cases, the urologists may opt to take a patient to the operating room for emergency endoscopy in order to define the obstruction point. When all else fails and the patient's bladder continues to distend, it is safest to pass a suprapubic drainage catheter into the neobladder.

Because the creation of a neobladder is an intraperitoneal operation, these patients are at risk for developing small bowel obstructions. A patient with abdominal pain and a neobladder merits radiographic evaluation.

Up to 30% of patients with a neobladder develop stones within their pouch and require either endoscopic or open surgical removal. These stones rarely cause pain by obstruction, but rather they produce foul urine that can be so irritating to the neobladder that the patient presents with a vague lower abdominal pain. These stones are calcified and show up on an abdominal radiograph. Treatment with antibiotics is palliative until surgical removal is undertaken.

The insertion of bowel segments into the urinary tract carries with it certain fluid and electrolyte complications that may not be a problem under normal circumstances. However, with GI viral infection and superimposed diarrhea and dehydration, the patient may not be able to compensate. For example, a patient with a gastric augmentation who presents with diarrhea and lethargy may have a severe, hypochloremic, hyponatremic, metabolic alkalosis. Thus, any patient with a bladder augmented with bowel who is obtunded requires careful consideration of an electrolyte disturbance as the underlying cause.

Suggested Readings

Acute Care of Chronically Ill Children

Rappo P. The care of children with chronic illness in primary care practice: implications for the pediatric generalist. *Pediatr Ann* 1997;26:687–695.

Reynolds S, Desguin B, Uyeda A, et al. Children with chronic conditions in a pediatric emergency department. *Pediatr Emerg Care* 1996;12:166–168.

Schonfeld N, McMorrow M. ED evaluation of the multiply handicapped child. *Pediatr Trauma Acute Care* 1990;3:25–26.

Tracheostomy Care

Appierto L, Cori M, Bianchi R, et al. Home care for chronic respiratory failure in children: 15 years experience. *Paediatr Anaesth* 2002;12:345–350.

Brook I. Role of anaerobic bacteria infections following tracheostomy, intubation, or the use of ventilatory tubes in children. *Ann Otol Rhinol Laryngol* 2004;113:830–834.

Fitton CM. Nursing management of the child with a tracheotomy. *Pediatr Clin North Am* 1994;41:513–523.

Graf J, Stein F. Tracheitis in pediatric patients. *Semin Pediatr Infect Dis* 2006;17(1):11–13.

Graham RJ, Fleegler WE, Robinson WM. Chronic ventilator need in the community: a 2005 pediatric census of Massachusetts. *Pediatrics* 2007;119: e1280–e1287.

Kallis JM. Replacement of a tracheostomy cannula. In: Henretig FM, King C, eds. *Textbook of pediatric emergency procedures,* 2nd ed. Baltimore, MD: Williams & Wilkins, 2007:792–798.

Katz RL. Tracheotomy care. In: Roberts JR, Hedges JR, eds. *Clinical procedures in emergency medicine,* 4th ed. Philadelphia, PA: WB Saunders, 2004.

Panitch HB, Downes JJ, Kennedy JS, et al. Guidelines for home care of children with chronic respiratory insufficiency. *Pediatr Pulmonol* 1996;21:52–56.

Pilmer SL. Prolonged mechanical ventilation in children. *Pediatr Clin North Am* 1994;41:473–512.

Posner JC. Acute care of the child with a tracheostomy. *Pediatr Emerg Care* 1999;15:49–54.

Scalise P, Prunk SR, Healy D, et al. The incidence of tracheoarterial fistula in patients with chronic tracheostomy tubes: a retrospective study of 544 patients in a long-term care facility. *Chest* 2005;128:3906–3909.

Cerebrospinal Fluid Shunts

Bondurant CP, Jiminez DF. Epidemiology of cerebrospinal fluid shunting. *Pediatr Neurosurg* 1995;23:254–259.

Borgbjerg BM, Gjerris F, Albeck MJ, et al. Frequency and causes of shunt revisions in different cerebrospinal fluid shunt types. *Acta Neurochir* 1995;136: 189–194.

Drake JM, Kestle JRW, Milner R, et al. Randomized trial of cerebrospinal fluid shunt valve design in pediatric hydrocephalus. *Neurosurgery* 1998;43: 294–303.

Ersahin Y, Mutluer S, Guzelbag E. Cerebrospinal fluid shunt infections. *J Neurosurg Sci* 1994;38:161–165.

Iskandar BJ, McLaughlin C, Mapstone TB, et al. Pitfalls in the diagnosis of ventricular shunt dysfunction: radiology reports and ventricular size. *Pediatrics* 1998;101:1031–1036.

Johnson DL, Conry J, O'Donnell R. Epileptic seizure as a sign of cerebrospinal fluid shunt malfunction. *Pediatr Neurosurg* 1996;24:223–227.

Key CB, Rothrock SG, Falk JL. Cerebrospinal fluid shunt complications: an emergency medicine perspective. *Pediatr Emerg Care* 1995;11:265–273.

Madikians A, Conway EE Jr. Cerebrospinal fluid shunt problems in pediatric patients. *Pediatr Ann* 1997;26:613–620.

McGirt MJ, Zaas A, Fuchs HE, et al. Risk factors for pediatric ventriculoperitoneal shunt infection and predictors of infectious pathogens. *Clin Infect Dis* 2003;36(7):858–862.

Naradzay JFX, Browne BJ, Rolnick MA, et al. Cerebral ventricular shunts. *J Emerg Med* 1999;17(2):311–322.

Odio C, McCracken GH Jr, Nelson JD. CSF shunt infections in pediatrics. A seven-year experience. *Am J Dis Child* 1984;138:1103–1108.

Piatt JH. Physical examination of patients with cerebrospinal fluid shunts: is there useful information in pumping the shunt? *Pediatrics* 1992;89: 470–473.

Ronan A, Hogg GG, Dlug GL. Cerebrospinal fluid shunt infections in children. *Pediatr Infect Dis J* 1995;14:782–786.

Sandberg DI. Endoscopic management of hydrocephalus in pediatric patients: a review of indications, techniques, and outcomes. *J Child Neurol* 2008;23: 550–560.

Telfeian AE, Celix JM, Sutton LN. Diagnosing ventricular shunt problems in children. *Pediatr Case Rev* 2004;4:1–15.

Villavicencio AT, Leveque JC, McGirt MJ, et al. Comparison of revision rates following endoscopically versus nonendoscopically placed ventricular shunt catheters. *Surg Neurol* 2003;59:375–380.

Walker M, Fried A, Petronio J. Diagnosis and treatment of the slit ventricle syndrome. *Neurosurg Clin North Am* 1993;4:701–714.

Duhaime AC, Wiley JF. Ventricular shunt and burr hole puncture. In: King C, Henretig FM, eds. *Textbook of pediatric emergency procedures,* 2nd ed. Philadelphia, PA: Lippincott Williams & Wilkins 2008:515–521.

Indwelling Catheters

Centers for Disease Control and Prevention. Guidelines for the prevention of intravascular catheter-related infections, 2002. *MMWR Recomm Rep* 2002;51(RR-10):1–29. http://www.cdc.gov/mmwr/preview/mmwrhtml/rr5110a1.htm. Accessed December 3, 2009.

Coulthard MG, Skinner R. Should paediatric central lines be aspirated before use? *Arch Dis Child* 2007;92:517–518.

Dyer BJ, Weiman MG, Ludwig S. Central venous catheters in the emergency department: access, utilization, and problem solving. *Pediatr Emerg Care* 1995;11:112–117.

Farr BM. Preventing vascular catheter-related infections: current controversies. *Clin Infect Dis* 2001;33:1733–1738.

Fuchs S. Accessing indwelling central lines. In: King C, Henretig FM, eds. *Textbook of pediatric emergency procedures,* 2nd ed. Philadelphia, PA: Lippincott Williams & Wilkins 2008:738–747.

Gittins NS, Hunter-Blair YL, Matthews JNS, et al. Comparison of alteplase and heparin in maintaining the patency of paediatric central venous haemodialysis lines: a randomised controlled trial. *Arch Dis Child* 2007;92:499–501.

Greene FL, Moor W, Strickland G, et al. Comparison of a totally implantable access device for chemotherapy (Port-A-Cath) and long-term percutaneous catheterization (Broviac). *South Med J* 1988;81:580–583.

Halpin DP, O'Bryne P, McEntee G, et al. Effect of a betadine connection shield on central venous catheter sepsis. *Nutrition* 1991;7:33–34.

Hartman GE, Schochat SJ. Management of septic complications associated with Silastic catheters in childhood malignancy. *J Pediatr Infect Dis* 1987;6: 1042–1047.

Mermel LA, Farr BM, Sherertz RJ, et al. Guidelines for the management of intravascular catheter-related infections. *Clin Infect Dis* 2001;32:1249–1202.

O'Grady NP, Alexander M, Dellinger EP, et al. Guidelines for the prevention of intravascular catheter-related infections. The Hospital Infection Control Practices Advisory Committee, Centers for Disease Control and Prevention. *Pediatrics* 2002;110:e51.

Onland W, Shin CE, Fustar S, et al. Ethanol-lock technique for persistent bacteremia of long-term intravascular devices in pediatric patients. *Arch Pediatr Adolesc Med* 2006;160:1049–1053.

Reynolds S, Desguin B, Uyeda A, et al. Children with chronic conditions in a pediatric emergency department. *Pediatr Emerg Care* 1996;12:166–168.

Shah SS, Downes KJ, Elliott MR, et al. How long does it take to "rule out" bacteremia in children with central venous catheters? *Pediatrics* 2008;121: 135–141.

Svoboda P, Barton R, Barbarash O, et al. Recombinant urokinase is safe and effective in restoring patency to occluded central venous access devices: a multiple-center, international trial. *Crit Care Med* 2004;32:1990–1996.

Enteral Feeding Catheters

Avitsland TL, Kristensen C, Emblem R, et al. Percutaneous endoscopic gastrostomy in children: a safe technique with major symptom relief and high parental satisfaction. *J Pediatr Gastroenterol Nutr* 2006;43:624–628.

Bumpers HL, Collure DW, Best IM, et al. Unusual complications of long-term percutaneous gastrostomy tubes. *J Gastrointest Surg* 2003;7(7):917–920.

Clevenger FW, Rodriguez D. Decision making for enteral feeding administration: the why behind where and how. *Nutr Clin Pract* 1995;10:104–113.

Crawley-Coha T. A practical guide for the management of pediatric gastrostomy tubes based on 14 years of experience. *J Wound Ostomy Continence Nurs* 2004;31:193–200.

Doede T, Faiss S, Schier F. Jejunal feeding tubes via gastrostomy in children. *Endoscopy* 2002;34(7):539–542.

Godbole P, Margabanthu G, Crabbe DC, et al. Limitations and uses of gastrojejunal feeding tubes. *Arch Dis Child* 2002;86(2):134–137.

Goldberg E, Kaye R, Yaworski J, et al. Gastrostomy tubes: facts, fallacies, fistulas, and false tracts. *Gastroenterol Nurs* 2005;28(6):485–493.

Graneto JW. Gastrostomy tube replacement. In: King C, Henretig FM, eds. *Textbook of pediatric emergency procedures,* 2nd ed. Philadelphia, PA: Lippincott Williams & Wilkins, 2008:829–834.

Kazi S, Gunasekaran TS, Berman JH, et al. Gastric mucosal injuries in children from inflatable low-profile gastrostomy tubes. *J Pediatr Gastroenterol Nutr* 1997;24:75–79.

Koulentaki M, Reynolds N, Steinke D, et al. Eight years' experience of gastrostomy tube management. *Endoscopy* 2002;34(12):941–945.

Segal D, Michaud L, Guimber D, et al. Late-onset complications of percutaneous endoscopic gastrostomy in children. *J Pediatr Gastroenterol Nutr* 2001;33(4):495–500.

Zamakhshary M, Jamal M, Blair GK, et al. Laparoscopic vs. percutaneous endoscopic gastrostomy tube insertion: a new pediatric gold standard? *J Pediatr Surg* 2005;40:859–862.

Gastrointestinal Diversion

Garvin G. Caring for children with ostomies. *Pediatr Surg Nurs* 1994;29: 645–654.

Hellman J, Lago C. Dermatologic complications in colostomy and ileostomy patients. *Int J Dermatol* 1990;29:129–133.

Walton SA, Hopkins J, Garvin G, et al. Ostomy complications in pediatrics. In: Dieckmann RA, Fiser DH, Selbst SM, eds. *Illustrated textbook of pediatric and critical care procedures.* St Louis, MO: Mosby, 1997:699–700.

Genitourinary Diversion

Barqawi A, de Valdenebro M, Furness PD III, et al. Lessons learned from stomal complications in children with cutaneous catheterizable continent stomas. *BJU Int* 2004;94:1344–1347.

Benson MC, Olsson CA. Urinary diversion. *Urol Clin North Am* 1992;19: 779–795.

Cain MP, Metcalfe PD, Rink RC. Urinary Diversion. In: Docimo S, Canning D, Khoury AE, eds. *Clinical pediatric urology.* London, England: Informa Healthcare, 2007.

Floyd S, Gray M. Managing the cutaneous vesicostomy. *J Wound Ostomy Continence Nurs* 2009;36:94–99.

Hutcheson JC, Cooper CS, Canning DA, et al. The use of vesicostomy as permanent urinary diversion in the child with myelomeningocele. *J Urol* 2001; 166(6):2351–2353.

Rapoport D, Secord S, MacNeily AE. The challenge of pediatric continent urinary diversion. *J Pediatr Surg* 2006;41:1113–1117.

CHAPTER 121 ■ ABDOMINAL EMERGENCIES

RICHARD G. BACHUR, MD

Pediatric abdominal complaints are common presentations in the emergency department (ED), mostly due to innocent gastrointestinal (GI) problems. However, ED physicians are challenged to identify those patients with more serious disorders, including surgical emergencies. The etiology of abdominal emergencies vary by age of the child, and the presentation of even common problems such as appendicitis may vary greatly based on the maturity of the child and stage of the disease. Clinicians should be aware of the variation of presentations, as well as the proper approach to diagnosis and management. Many conditions, for example, bowel obstruction, may have the same initial approach regardless of the specific etiology. Logical diagnostic schemes and prompt recognition of surgical emergencies should be the goal of the evaluation.

This chapter reviews the common, acute nontraumatic surgical conditions of the abdomen in the following categories: (i) diseases that produce peritoneal irritation; (ii) acute intestinal obstruction; (iii) chronic, partial intestinal obstruction; (iv) problems that produce rectal bleeding; (v) intraabdominal masses; (vi) abdominal wall defects; and (vii) foreign bodies of the GI tract. Nonsurgical GI emergencies are covered in Chapter 89. Chapter 107 deals with major trauma to the abdomen. Chapter 49 reviews the diagnostic approach to the child with abdominal pain.

EVALUATION

History

Once the concern of an acute abdominal process is considered, the clinician should focus on specific elements of the history: (i) presence and character of abdominal pain, (ii) history and character of emesis, (iii) bowel history, (iv) systemic symptoms, (v) associated symptoms attributable to the lower respiratory tract or urinary system, and (vi) past medical history.

Abdominal pain is a common feature of many acute surgical abdominal conditions. Unfortunately, abdominal pain can also be nonspecific and associated with many common entities such as gastroenteritis, constipation, mesenteric adenitis, nephrolithiasis, urinary tract infection, ovarian cysts, pleuritis, and pneumonias. Key elements of the history regarding pain include sudden versus gradual onset; the duration, whether it is persistent or intermittent; radiation to other areas; and whether the pain migrated. Pain that begins vaguely throughout the abdomen and then localizes to more severe, sharper pain is the classic description with appendicitis as pain transitions from a *visceral*, diffuse, and nondescript pain to a more defined, localized *peritoneal* pain. Mild intermittent pain without associated symptoms is rarely a serious condition.

Persistent pain with progressive symptoms requires a thorough evaluation for more severe conditions such as appendicitis. Sudden onset of severe pain might be seen with relatively innocent conditions such as constipation but could also represent a perforated ulcer, bowel obstruction or ischemia, renal obstruction, ovarian torsion, or ectopic pregnancy. In preverbal patients, history of irritability or "fits" of crying may be indicative of abdominal pain. Flexing the hips and crying in young infants might be indicative of abdominal pain. Paradoxical irritability, more often associated with meningeal irritation, may also be a sign of peritonitis in young infants.

Vomiting is associated with many surgical conditions. The number and frequency of the episodes along with the character of the emesis should be elicited. Specifically, questions regarding the presence or absence of bile or blood need to be determined and may substantially influence the initial management and approach to the patient. Acute onset of bilious emesis should raise concern for bowel obstructions, although some bilious emesis may also be seen with persistent emesis and ileus associated with viral gastroenteritis. Bilious emesis in a newborn infant is indicative of a surgical emergency. Bowel history should be reviewed along with the presence of blood either as fresh blood or melena. Bloody diarrhea is more likely to be seen with forms of colitis or infectious enteritis, whereas blood per rectum is more consistent with bowel ischemia, a bleeding lesion in the bowel such as a Meckel's diverticulum or polyp, or lower tract trauma. Although bloody stool may or may not be surgical in nature, it warrants a thorough assessment (see Chapters 18 and 29). In the absence of recent stool, the additional absence of flatus may suggest an ileus or obstruction. Diarrhea is not a typical feature of acute surgical processes; therefore, if the illness begins with nonbloody diarrhea, it is unlikely to represent a surgical process. However, the presence of diarrhea does not automatically exclude surgical processes because many patients with intussusception had preceding gastroenteritis. Likewise, the development of diarrhea in a child who has several days of abdominal pain may be secondary to appendiceal perforation with abscess formation.

Other systemic symptoms may help suggest the etiology of the abdominal emergency or the severity of illness. Presence of fever in the well child with abdominal pain may support viral gastroenteritis, whereas fever in the patient with concerns for acute appendicitis may suggest bowel perforation. In general, fever prior to abdominal pain is unlikely to be an acute surgical process. Distinct episodes of pain associated with profound lethargy and diaphoresis might lead to the diagnosis of intussusception. Associated weight loss, pallor, and fatigue can be seen with inflammatory bowel disease or malignancies. Associated, nonsystemic symptoms or a constellation of complaints may point toward specific etiologies of abdominal pain: cough, fever, and pleuritic pain may suggest pneumonia; fever and flank pain may be indicative of pyelonephritis; fever, dyspareunia, and vaginal discharge are seen with pelvic inflammatory disease.

Prior surgical history should always be ascertained when evaluating a patient with an acute abdomen. Abdominal complaints might indicate a complication of surgery in the immediate postoperative period, whereas more remote surgical history might indicate intestinal obstruction from adhesions.

Examination

Children vary in their ability to cooperate during the abdominal examination, and often the physician must make patient, repeated efforts to perform an adequate evaluation. A few minutes spent gaining the child's confidence will often allow a better examination. Observing the patient's ability to move in the parent's arms or bed is helpful. Patients with peritoneal signs might only get comfortable when lying still. In cases of extreme patient anxiety, watching the parents palpate the abdomen can give a general sense of tenderness and peritoneal signs. Occasionally, if an initial examination is suboptimal due to crying, repeat examinations, especially if the child falls asleep, might prove invaluable. Narcotics should not be routinely used to sedate a child for examination, but narcotics should be used to treat severe pain—knowing that subsequent examinations may be affected.

Once the child relaxes, the physical examination should follow an orderly progression: inspection and observation, abdominal palpation, auscultation, examination of nonabdominal areas, and rectal examination (Table 121.1).

The initial step of inspection should focus on the presence of distension, visible bowel loops, and asymmetry. Inspection is easily done because of the relative prominence of the child's abdomen, and thinness of the overlying muscles and subcutaneous tissue. The child should be observed in motion—for example, when moved in the parent's arms, changing position in the bed, or, in older children, when walking or hopping on command. Changes in facial expression or clutching their abdomen with motion imply significant pain. Inspection should include the oropharynx (streptococcal pharyngitis), lower chest, flanks, genitalia (testicular torsion, hernia, hematocouplos), and inguinal areas.

Palpation is the most difficult, yet most informative, aspect of physical examination. In young infants and toddlers, making the child, and hence the abdominal muscles, relax prior to the examination is important. Flexing of the hips, use of a pacifier, or providing a small sip of sugar water may change the tense abdomen of a screaming infant to an examinable abdomen. In older children, trying to engage them prior to palpation is beneficial. Ask the child to point to the place where the pain is most severe. Avoid the tender area initially, but return to palpate it last. A number of "tricks" can be used to facilitate the palpation, such as distracting the child with conversation, palpating with the head of the stethoscope in hand, and palpating while asking the child to take a deep breath. Palpation should identify any tenderness as noted by the verbal patient or change in expression or crying in the younger child. Along with tenderness, guarding and rebound should be appreciated. In addition, masses or organomegaly should be noted. Palpation should include the genitalia of males, and

TABLE 121.1

ABDOMINAL PHYSICAL FINDINGS AND THEIR MEANING

Physical findings	Meaning
Abdominal distension	Peritonitis, intestinal obstruction, ileus
Visible bowel loops	Intestinal obstruction, intussusception
Asymmetry	Appendiceal abscess tumor, constipation
Point tenderness	Appendicitis, cholecystitis
Guarding	Peritonitis, appendicitis, abscess
Rebound	Peritonitis, infarcted bowel
Rovsing's sign	Appendicitis
Palpable mass	Tumor or cyst, intussusception, chronic constipation
High-pitched bowel sounds	Intestinal obstruction
No bowel sounds	Peritonitis, infarcted bowel, ileus
Psoas sign	Appendicitis (especially retrocecal), psoas abscess retroperitoneal hematoma
Rectal examination—tenderness or bogginess on right	Appendicitis

pelvic examination should be considered in postpubertal, sexually active females. Generally, pelvic examination is not required in non–sexually active females unless specific gynecological diagnoses are probable; of note, hematocolpos does present as significant abdominal pain and possible lower abdominal mass, which can easily go unrecognized without proper examination of the genitalia.

Next, auscultate for bowel sounds. The presence of normal bowel sounds may not rule out surgical pathology, but a silent abdomen or one with high-pitched tinkles and rushes suggests the possibility of ileus or obstruction. Auscultation of the lung fields is also necessary to identify either the primary cause of pain, such as pneumonia, or associated pulmonary findings, as with pleural effusions with pancreatitis or peritonitis.

The final step in the evaluation should be a rectal examination. The important technical aspects include use of generous amounts of lubricant, slow insertion of the examiner's finger as the patient takes slow deep breaths, and the palpation of the presumed painful area last. If done carefully and gently, the rectal examination is usually well tolerated by the child. Any stool on the examiner's glove should be tested for blood.

Laboratory

Laboratory and radiographic studies vary, depending on the diagnoses that are being considered. When considering surgical diagnoses, a complete blood count (CBC) with differential is essential. As with other diagnostic workups, CBC will add information to help guide the physician toward or away from diagnoses—it will rarely make a diagnosis. A urinalysis is an important part of the evaluation of any abdominal symptoms in children: white blood cells (WBC) to suggest a urinary tract infection, blood to possibly suggest a urologic etiology such as nephrolithiasis or ureteral obstruction, and tests for glucose and ketones knowing that many patients with diabetic ketoacidosis present with abdominal pain and emesis, and finally specific gravity to help gauge hydration of the patient. Depending on the child's condition, history, physical examination, and diagnostic considerations, other tests may be ordered: serum electrolytes, blood urea nitrogen (BUN), serum amylase or lipase, liver enzymes, bilirubin, sickle cell preparation, β-HCG, erythrocyte sedimentation rate, and C-reactive protein.

An abdominal radiograph is rarely helpful for nonspecific pain in the well child, but it is very useful for consideration of obstruction, constipation, nephrolithiasis, and perforation of the bowel. An upright, lateral decubitus, or cross-table lateral radiograph should be obtained when "free air" is suspected. In evaluating possible appendicitis, look for a fecalith in the right lower quadrant. Ultrasound (US) and computed tomography (CT) have varying roles, depending on the diagnosis. Upper GI series can be done to identify upper obstructions, and dye or air enemas can be diagnostic for lower obstructions such as ileocolic intussusception.

Assessment

Once the history, physical examination, and laboratory data are available, the emergency physician must synthesize them into an overall assessment and treatment plan. The following sections detail the symptoms and signs of the common acute surgical problems in children. Initial ED management is discussed, but in all cases of presumed surgical disease, the definitive treatment requires surgical consultation. Consultation with a surgeon should be considered after the initial evaluation if the patient appears ill or serious surgical conditions are being considered; laboratory evaluation and radiologic studies should not delay surgical evaluation in such children.

DISEASES THAT PRODUCE PERITONEAL IRRITATION

The physician must perform a careful examination to elicit accurate signs of peritonitis. Tenderness is not necessarily an indication of an intraabdominal surgical problem in a child. A child with localized peritonitis may have only minimal findings, whereas a patient with a nonsurgical condition may have severe pain and generalized tenderness. The typical features of peritonitis—rigidity, involuntary guarding, and rebound—are the same in children and adults but may be more difficult to elicit or interpret in younger children and infants. Reproducible peritoneal tenderness in the same location is much more suggestive of peritonitis than deep abdominal tenderness that shifts in location with reexamination of the child. In infants and young children, irritability or screaming with any movement of the child may indicate peritonitis.

Acute Nonperforated Appendicitis

Background

Acute appendicitis is the most common, nontraumatic surgical emergency in children. There is a slight male predominance with a peak incidence of 9 to 12 years of age. Although neonatal cases have been reported, appendicitis rarely occurs in children younger than 2 years. Predictably, the diagnosis is very difficult in children younger than 5 years. The emergency physician must accurately evaluate the child and promptly consult a surgeon when the diagnosis is clear or when appendicitis cannot be safely ruled out. Such consultation is especially urgent in younger children, in whom perforation occurs more frequently and can occur within 8 to 24 hours of the onset of symptoms.

Clinical Manifestations

Usually the child with appendicitis complains initially of poorly defined and poorly localized midabdominal or periumbilical pain. Unfortunately, this symptom is common to many other intraabdominal, nonsurgical problems. In the young and, to a lesser extent, the older child, vomiting and a low-grade fever often occur soon thereafter. Characteristically, the pain then migrates to the right lower quadrant (Table 121.2).

Because the position of the appendix may vary in children, the localization of the pain and the tenderness on examination may also vary. An appendix that is located in the lateral gutter may produce flank pain and lateral abdominal tenderness; an inflamed appendix pointing toward the left lower quadrant may produce hypogastric tenderness and pain with urination

TABLE 121.2

PROGRESSION OF SYMPTOMS AND SIGNS OF APPENDICITIS

Nonperforated Appendicitis
Poorly defined midabdominal or periumbilical pain
Low-grade fever
Anorexia
Vomiting
Migration of pain to right lower quadrant
Localization depends on position of appendix
    Appendix in gutter → lateral abdominal tenderness
    Appendix pointing toward pelvis → tenderness near pubis
        may cause diarrhea or bladder irritation
    Retrocecal appendix → tenderness elicited by deep palpation
Pain on coughing, hopping, or to percussion
Rectal examination: pain on palpation of right rectal wall
WBC count: 11,000–15,000/mm^3
Urinalysis: ketosis, few WBCs

Perforated Appendix
Increasing signs of toxicity
Rigid abdomen with extreme tenderness
Absent bowel sounds
Dyspnea and grunting; tachycardia
Fever: 39–41°C (102.2–105.8°F)
WBC count: >15,000/mm^3 with shift to left
Eventual overwhelming sepsis and shock

WBC, white blood cell.

(from bladder contraction). An inflamed low-lying, pelvic appendix may not cause pain at McBurney's point, but instead may cause diarrhea from direct irritation of the sigmoid colon. Anorexia and nausea are common; vomiting is more common in younger children. In early stages, the patient may complain of pain with motion, for example, bumps in the road on the drive to the ED or walking, and as peritoneal irritation worsens, the child will prefer to lay motionless in the bed.

When obtaining the history, the physician needs to consider other causes of abdominal pain, which may appear as appendicitis but, in fact, are nonsurgical. Concurrent GI illness in other family members or friends suggests the possibility of an infectious gastroenteritis. Constipation, streptococcal pharyngitis, urinary tract infection, lower lobe pneumonia, mesenteric adenitis, and ovarian cyst are common conditions often masquerading as appendicitis. Although the presentation is generally more rapid and severe, torsion of the ovary and ectopic pregnancy should be considered in female patients with sudden onset of severe pain.

On examination, palpation is usually reliable in demonstrating focal peritoneal signs at the site of the inflamed appendix. If the appendix is in the pelvis or retrocecal area, however, typical anterior peritoneal signs may be absent. When the inflamed appendix is not close to the anterior abdominal wall, as in the case of retrocecal appendix, tenderness may be more impressive on deep palpation of the abdomen or palpation of the flank. Percussive tenderness, shake tenderness, pain with coughing, or hopping suggests peritoneal irritation. A properly performed rectal examination can contribute to the clinical impression: the examining finger should be inserted as fully as possible without touching the area of presumed tenderness and then, when the child is relaxed and taking deep breaths, the examiner can indent an area high on the right rectal wall. A sudden involuntary reaction implies localized tenderness. In a child with a history of probable appendicitis for more than 2 or 3 days, a boggy, full mass may also be in this location, suggesting an abscess.

A CBC in a child with appendicitis usually shows an elevated WBC count in the range of 11,000 to 15,000 per mm³ in the first 12 to 24 hours of the illness. As the appendix becomes more gangrenous, the WBC count rises further, and the differential demonstrates more and more neutrophils and an increasing number of bands. Urinalysis often shows ketosis. If the inflamed appendix lies over the ureter or adjacent to the bladder, a few WBCs may be found in the urine. The presence of numerous WBCs and bacteria on a freshly spun specimen may indicate an acute urinary tract infection. An abdominal radiograph may show an appendicolith (8% to 10%), localized ileus with air–fluid levels, or a gaseous loop in the right lower quadrant, or more commonly, a nonspecific bowel gas pattern. Subtle radiographic findings include a blurred psoas margins and thickened cecal wall. Rarely, pneumoperitoneum may be seen with perforated appendix.

If the clinical and laboratory diagnosis of acute appendicitis is convincing, no further studies are indicated. For patient with equivocal findings, patients should be monitored with serial examinations or have radiologic studies to aid diagnosis. CT and US have both been used for diagnosis. US has a reported sensitivity of 80% to 92% with a specificity of 86% to 98%. Technically, a noncompressible enlarged appendix is diagnostic of appendicitis, although the study must be considered unhelpful

if the appendix is not specifically identified. Focal CT has a diagnostic sensitivity of 87% to 100% with a specificity of 83% to 97%. CT can identify an enlarged appendix, focal thickening of the cecum, periappendiceal inflammation, mesenteric nodes, and fluid collections associated with perforation. Protocols using intravenous (IV) contrast plus rectal contrast or oral contrast vary by institution. In general, US has less utility in patients with a high body mass index, and CT is most interpretable in patients with adequate periappendiceal fat. US may be preferred in adolescent females as an initial study if gynecological conditions are suspected such as ovarian cyst, tuboovarian abscess, ovarian torsion, or ectopic pregnancy (see Chapter 90).

Management

The preoperative preparation of a patient with acute appendicitis should include electrolytes if the patient has been vomiting or has had poor fluid intake for more than a few hours. IV fluids should be started with the goal of rapid intravascular expansion and then correction of further fluid deficits. Protracted GI losses, as with vomiting, may lead to potassium depletion. Initial fluids should include a bolus of isotonic fluid (10 to 20 mL per kg), then changed to D5% 0.5 NS with 10 to 20 mEq per L of potassium. These fluids can then be altered, if necessary, once the serum chemistries are known.

The emergency physician must keep in mind the many variations in the way appendicitis can present. Patients with equivocal findings should be admitted for monitoring and serial examinations or have imaging studies to demonstrate a normal appendix. If the imaging studies are equivocal, the surgeon will decide to operate or continue to monitor. Patients who have a typical history for appendicitis but suddenly have diminished pain may actually represent perforation of the appendix. Such patients should be observed for several hours prior to declaring an improved condition. Even in the presence of negative imaging studies, the emergency physician should arrange close follow-up for any patient with abdominal pain. For those patients with progressive pain or persistent emesis, admission for further care and subsequent evaluation might be necessary.

Perforated Appendicitis

Ideally, once the diagnosis of appendicitis is considered seriously, the patient will have accurate diagnosis and surgery before the appendix has perforated. Unfortunately, some patients, particularly younger children and infants, may arrive for emergency care with an already perforated appendix because of a delay in seeking treatment or in making the diagnosis. Once the appendix has perforated, there are usually signs of generalized, rather than localized, peritonitis. In a young child, the omentum is thin and often incapable of walling off the inflamed appendix. As a result, perforation occurs more quickly, and secondary dissemination of the infection occurs more widely. Although the mortality from appendicitis has decreased, the incidence of perforation in children has remained the same over the last several decades.

Clinical Manifestations

Within a few hours after perforation has occurred, the child begins to develop increasing signs of peritonitis and toxicity. First, the lower abdomen and then the entire abdomen become

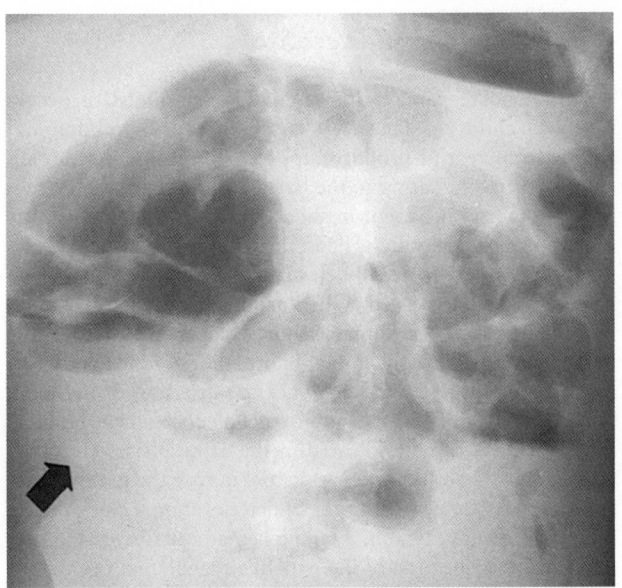

FIGURE 121.1 Perforated appendicitis with abscess and fecalith. The upright abdominal roentgenogram shows numerous dilated loops of bowel and a calcified fecalith *(arrow)*. Note that the space between the individual loops indicates the presence of intraperitoneal fluid.

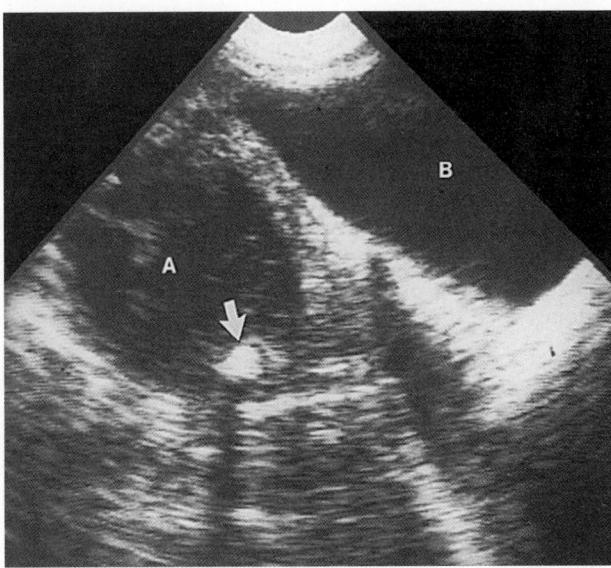

FIGURE 121.2 Perforated appendicitis with abscess and fecalith. Ultrasonography of the pelvis shows a complex mass *(A)* with a fecalith *(arrow)* producing characteristic acoustic shadowing to the right of the bladder *(B)*.

rigid with extreme tenderness. Bowel sounds are sparse to absent. Other signs include pallor, dyspnea, grunting, significant tachycardia, and higher fever [39°C to 41°C (102.2°F to 105.8°F)]. Rarely, the patient may develop septic shock (see Chapter 3) from the overwhelming infection.

Initially, the findings may be confused with those of pneumonia because the extreme abdominal pain may cause rapid shallow respirations, painful respirations associated with grunting, and decreased air entry to the lower lung fields. In young children, the findings may also be confused with meningitis because of paradoxical irritability—any motion of the child, even trying to comfort the child, may cause pain and irritability.

The laboratory findings in the child with perforated appendicitis often suggest this diagnosis. The WBC count is significantly elevated, usually greater than 15,000 per mm³, with a marked shift to left; leukopenia may be seen in perforation associated with overwhelming sepsis. The radiologic evaluation of suspected perforated appendicitis should include plain abdominal radiographs and either ultrasonography or CT. The plain film of the abdomen may show free air or evidence of peritonitis (Fig. 121.1). The US of the pelvis may show a complex mass with or without a calcified fecalith or free fluid within the abdominal cavity (Fig. 121.2). CT can better define the size and location of an associated abscess (Fig. 121.3).

Management

Initially, therapy should be directed toward proper resuscitation with assessment and management of the airway, breathing, and circulation (see Chapter 1). Extremely ill children may require endotracheal intubation to control ventilation and maximize O₂ delivery in cases of shock. Hypovolemia should be rapidly corrected with normal saline or Ringer's

lactate solution. An initial bolus of fluid starting at 20 mL per kg is given rapidly until vital signs are improved and the patient produces urine. Vasopressor therapy should be considered for patients who do not have sufficient response to 60 to 80 mL per kg of isotonic fluids. Broad-spectrum antibiotics targeting bowel flora (gram-negative enterics as well as anaerobes) should be given. Immediate surgical consultation is necessary. Placement of a bladder catheter and central venous access with measurement of central venous pressure may be necessary to monitor response to therapy. Once the emergency physician is certain that the airway can be controlled and the circulation is adequate, relief of pain can be accomplished by using narcotic agents (e.g., morphine 0.1 mg per kg). The patient's fever can usually be controlled by antipyretics or cooling blanket. A nasogastric tube should be

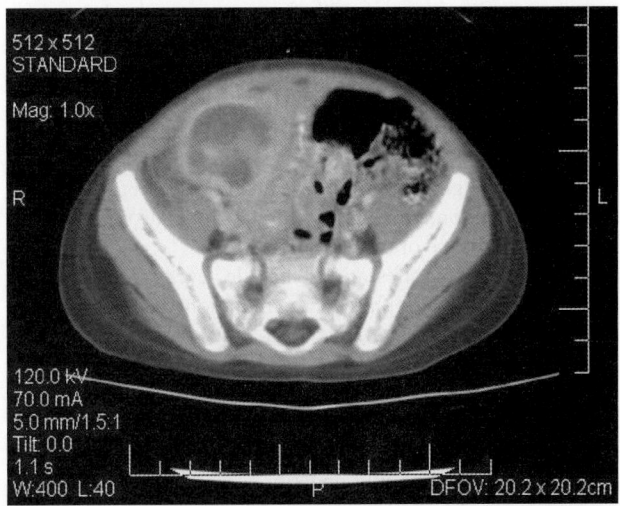

FIGURE 121.3 CT scan of perforated appendix with abscess.

placed to evacuate the contents of the stomach and to drain ongoing gastric secretions. For ill patients, blood products should be readied.

Children with perforated appendicitis can deteriorate quickly. Therefore, emergency resuscitation should be quickly followed by operative intervention. At surgery, the appendix is removed, the area is drained, and other appropriate treatments are given. For patients with minimal systemic signs, abscesses may be drained percutaneously using radiologically guided procedures—with the expectation of a delayed appendectomy.

Meckel's Diverticulitis with and without Perforation

Meckel's diverticulum is a vestige of the omphalomesenteric duct and occurs in 2% of the population. Most patients with a Meckel's diverticulum are asymptomatic or, if symptomatic, have rectal bleeding from ulceration at the junction of the ectopic gastric mucosa and the normal ileal mucosa (see the "Diseases that Produce Rectal Bleeding" section.). Classically, the bleeding is painless. Less commonly, Meckel's diverticulum presents with symptoms of diverticulitis with or without perforation. A preoperative diagnosis of an inflamed or a perforated Meckel's diverticulum is rarely made but, nevertheless, should be considered in the differential diagnosis of a perforated viscus leading to generalized peritonitis. The diagnosis is usually made in the operating room by the surgeon who finds a normal appendix, and then an exploration of the bowel finds a diseased diverticulum approximately 2 ft. from the ileocecal valve.

Primary Peritonitis

Primary peritonitis is a bacterial infection of the peritoneal cavity, usually secondary to a bloodborne or lymphborne infection. Although rare, it can occur in children with nephrosis, cirrhosis, or other etiologies of ascites, and may mimic appendicitis. Primary peritonitis is usually caused by *Streptococcus pneumoniae*, *Streptococcus pyogenes*, or gram-negative enteric organisms. Blunt trauma may lead to perforated viscus. Lacerations to the vaginal vault or rectum from instrumentation or abuse can lead to vaginal or rectal bleeding and peritonitis. Hirschspring's disease may lead to toxic megacolon and perforation. Rarely, peritonitis can spontaneously occur in girls from 5 to 10 years old in whom the cervix is open and the vaginal fluid is not yet acidic enough to retard the ascent of infection. Patients with nephritic syndromes have an increased incidence of primary peritonitis.

The clinical manifestations include fever, vomiting, and abdominal pain. The physical examination includes findings of peritoneal irritation. An elevated WBC count (greater than 15,000 per mm^3) and left shift are also seen. Often, the symptoms, signs, and laboratory findings are indistinguishable from those for perforated appendicitis; thus, the diagnosis may be made at laparotomy. If the diagnosis is suspected before surgery, the patient should undergo paracentesis. The diagnosis may be confirmed by a Gram stain showing bacteria followed by a positive culture.

Pancreatitis

Although acute pancreatitis is common in adults, it occurs rarely in children. The most common cause is abdominal trauma. Pancreatitis produces upper abdominal or periumbilical pain, often radiating to the back. Occasionally, the presentation is that of a patient in shock. Findings that support the diagnosis include paralytic ileus, distension, and ascites. Serum amylase or lipase is usually elevated. When severe, the serum calcium is also decreased. When pancreatitis occurs in a child without a history of trauma, the physician should evaluate the patient for possible congenital abnormalities of the biliary tree or pancreatic ducts, such as abnormal insertion of the main pancreatic duct or the presence of a choledochal cyst. Surgical intervention is rarely indicated in the acute phase. However, early surgical consultation is essential in case the patient deteriorates (see Chapter 89). Signs of deterioration include persistently low serum calcium, a falling hematocrit, increasing toxicity, and deterioration of the patient's coagulation profile.

ACUTE INTESTINAL OBSTRUCTION

In any child with persistent emesis, especially with bilious emesis, acute intestinal obstruction must be considered. If the obstruction is high in the intestinal tract, the abdomen does not become distended; however, with lower intestinal obstruction there is generalized distension and diffuse tenderness, usually without signs of peritoneal irritation. Only if the bowel perforates or vascular insufficiency occurs will signs of peritoneal irritation be found. If complete obstruction persists, bowel habits may change, leading to complete obstipation of both flatus and stool. All patients with suspected bowel obstruction should have radiographs of the abdomen in supine, upright, and prone cross-table lateral views. In patients with acute mechanical bowel obstruction, multiple dilated loops are usually seen. Fluid levels produced by the layering of air and intestinal contents are seen in the upright or lateral decubitus radiographs (Fig. 121.4).

Intussusception

Background

Intussusception occurs when one segment of bowel invaginates into a more distal segment. This is the leading cause of acute intestinal obstruction in infants, and it occurs most commonly between 3 and 12 months of age. The most common intussusception is ileocolic but the small bowel may intussuscept into itself. Often, it will be ileoileal at a location close to the cecum. Typically, this small bowel intussusception then prolapses through the ileocecal valve (Figs. 121.5 and 121.6). The intussusception continues through the colon a variable distance, occasionally as far as the rectum, where it can be palpated on rectal examination. Colocolic intussusceptions are rare. In infants, the lead point for the intussusception may be hypertrophied Peyer's patches. In children older than 2 years, a specific lead point such as a polyp, a Meckel's diverticulum, a duplication, or a tumor is more likely. A diarrheal illness, viral syndrome, or Henoch-Schönlein purpura may occur several days to a week before the onset of abdominal pain and obstruction.

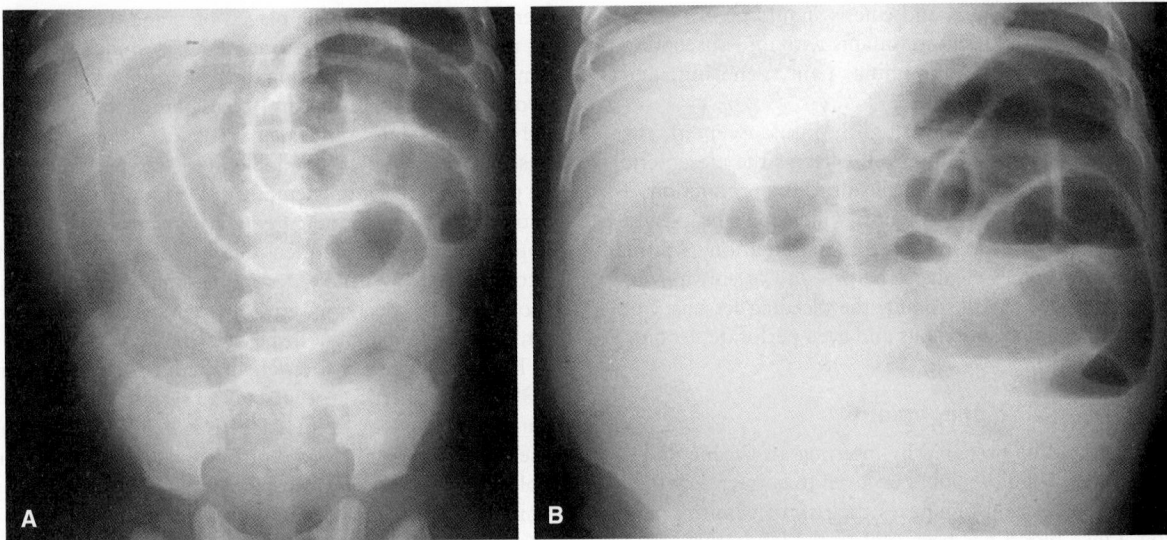

FIGURE 121.4 **A:** Small bowel obstruction. Numerous dilated small bowel loops occupy the midabdomen and have a stepladder configuration. Minimal air is seen in the rectum. **B:** Same patient as in **A.** The upright abdominal roentgenogram shows numerous dilated loops in the small bowel with differential fluid levels in one loop indicating mechanical bowel obstruction.

Clinical Manifestations

The primary manifestation of intussusception is colicky abdominal pain. This symptom may have been preceded by the symptoms and signs of a viral gastroenteritis or even an upper respiratory infection. Gradually, the child becomes more irritable and anorectic, and may vomit. The pattern of pain in a child with an intussusception is often consistent and characteristic, and the diagnosis is suggested strongly if a history of episodic pain is obtained. The child may appear to be comfortable and well between episodes. Occasionally, the infant may appear lethargic and listless. At times, patients with intussusception have been misdiagnosed as being in a postictal state or encephalopathic.

The localized portion of the intussusception leads to partial or complete obstruction and generalized abdominal distension.

In some cases, the intussuscepted mass can be palpated as an ill-defined, sausage-shaped structure if the abdomen is not too distended. This mass is most often palpable in the right upper quadrant.

When children arrive in the ED early in the course of intussusception, there is often no history of having passed a currant jelly stool, although blood may be found on rectal examination (50% to 75% of cases have occult blood). However, the absence of bloody stools should not preclude making the diagnosis of a possible intussusception. Infants and young children

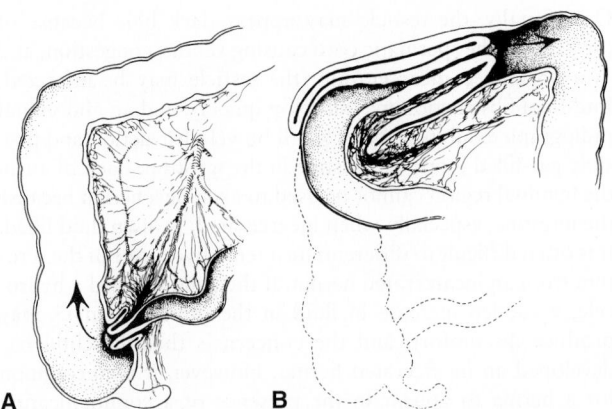

FIGURE 121.5 Ileocolic intussusception. **A:** Beginning of an intussusception in which terminal ileum prolapses through ileocecal valve. **B:** Ileocolic intussusceptum continuing through the colon. This can often be palpated as a mass in the right upper quadrant.

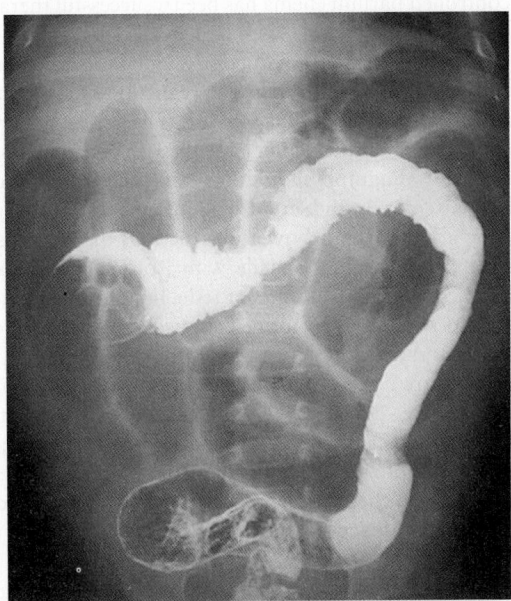

FIGURE 121.6 Ileocolic intussusception. Barium enema shows the intussusception as the filling defect within the hepatic flexure surrounded by spiral mucosal folds. Significant distended small bowel represents distal small bowel obstruction.

with colicky abdominal pain and emesis should be evaluated for intussusception. Only 20% of infants with intussusception have the triad of colicky abdominal pain, vomiting, and bloody stools.

As the bowel becomes more tightly intussuscepted, the mesenteric veins become compressed, whereas the mesenteric arterial supply remains intact. This leads to the production of the characteristic currant jelly stool, which may be passed spontaneously or found on the rectal examination. As the intussusception becomes swollen, the pressure of entrapment occludes the arteries. At this point, the bleeding lessens, but the bowel can become gangrenous and even perforate, leading to peritonitis.

Management

The patient should be prepared by inserting an IV line and a nasogastric tube. IV fluids should be given to correct dehydration. Nasogastric suction minimizes the risk of vomiting and aspiration. Once blood has been sent to the laboratory for a CBC electrolytes, and a cross-match, the patient should have radiologic studies.

Plain radiograph findings of intussusception are variable and depend primarily on the duration of the symptoms and the presence or absence of complications. In early cases, a normal gas pattern is seen. Distal colonic air cannot be interpreted as an absence of intussusception. Unless the radiograph exhibits air in the cecum, ileocolic intussusception cannot be excluded by radiograph. In the patient with symptoms longer than 6 to 12 hours, flat and upright films often show signs of intestinal obstruction, including distended bowel with air–fluid levels (Fig. 121.4). A characteristic "target" sign may be seen or more commonly a paucity of gas in the right lower quadrant. Occasionally, the actual head of the intussusception can be seen on a plain film as a soft-tissue mass. US can be used diagnostically with reported sensitivity of 98% to 100%.

In more recent years, air insufflation enema or hydrostatically controlled barium enema has been a successful therapy in up to 70% to 95% of cases with higher success rates reported with air reduction. Strict reduction guidelines must be followed to avoid perforation. The full reduction of the intussusception is confirmed only when there has been adequate reflux of barium or air into the ileum. Patients with peritonitis or free air on plain radiograph should not have an enema study or reduction attempt. In the seriously ill infant with signs of peritonitis or a frank small bowel obstruction, the diagnosis of intussusception should be made with isotonic water-soluble contrast media with no attempt at reduction. The reduction in such infants should be performed surgically. Perforation rates with enema reduction have been reported in up to 3%. Criteria that are linked to a lower reduction rate and a higher perforation rate, especially if more than one is present, are patient age younger than 3 months or older than 5 years; long duration of symptoms, especially if greater than 48 hours; passage of blood via the rectum (hematochezia); significant dehydration; and evidence of small bowel obstruction on plain radiograph.

Many children with intussusception require emergency surgery, especially if the intussusception has been of long duration or the child shows evidence of gangrenous bowel, including high fever, leukocytosis, significant distension, and general toxicity. If an enema reduction seems safe and appropriate, the operating room should be placed on standby and the operating team should be ready to commence immediate surgery if complications develop during the procedure or if unsuccessful. Preoperative preparation and resuscitation begins in the ED and continues during the enema. A general surgeon should be present or immediately available in case of perforation during the procedure. Barium enemas can lead to peritoneal contamination with barium, and air enemas can lead to massive pneumoperitoneum and sudden death unless the abdomen is decompressed (by needle decompression). Sedation has been associated with decreased rates of reduction. Delay in reduction can lead to gangrenous bowel.

The recurrence rate after enema reduction ranges from 1% to 3%. When there is a recurrence, a second attempt at reduction may be done by enema. This is usually successful in most cases, but with a third episode of intussusception, an exploratory laparotomy must be done. Recurrences are more common in older children and may be caused by a lead point such as a Meckel's diverticulum, an intestinal polyp, or an intraluminal tumor such as lymphoma. Therefore, it may be wise in an older child to operate with the first recurrence.

Incarcerated Inguinal Hernia

Incarcerated inguinal hernia is a common cause of intestinal obstruction in the infant and young child. Approximately 60% of incarcerated hernias occur during the first year of life. Incarceration occurs more often in girls than in boys, but usually involves the ovary rather than the intestine. Often, the patient or family has no previous knowledge of the presence of a congenital hernia. Incarceration does not necessarily mean that the nonreducible portion of intestine is compromised or gangrenous. However, strangulation can occur within 24 hours of a nonreduced incarcerated hernia because of progressive edema of the bowel caused by venous and lymphatic obstruction. This obstruction then leads to occlusion of the arterial supply with resulting necrosis of the bowel and perhaps perforation.

The clinical presentation of a child with an incarcerated hernia is irritability due to pain, vomiting, and occasionally abdominal distension. A firm, discrete mass can be palpated at the internal ring and may or may not extend into the scrotum. Occasionally, the testicle may appear dark blue because of pressure on the spermatic cord causing venous congestion, and in a prolonged incarceration, the testicle may be infarcted. Intestinal obstruction may develop quickly, and an abdominal radiograph exhibits signs of small bowel obstruction and possibly gas-filled loops of intestine in the scrotum. Lack of air in the inguinal region cannot be used to exclude a hernia because the intestine, especially when incarcerated, is often fluid filled. It is often difficult to differentiate a tense hydrocele in the scrotum from an incarcerated hernia. If the child has had a hydrocele, a sudden increase in fluid in the tunica vaginalis may produce discomfort, and the concern is that the child has developed an incarcerated hernia. However, it is uncommon for a hernia to appear in the presence of a communicating hydrocele because of the narrowness of the patent processus vaginalis that is associated with the hydrocele. The acute hydrocele presents only in the scrotum but may extend somewhat up into the inguinal canal. However, no mass can be felt in the area of the internal ring, indicating that no intestine is exiting from the ring.

Unless the child is extremely ill with signs of intestinal obstruction or toxic from gangrenous bowel, a manual reduction of the incarcerated hernia should be attempted. The child should be sedated with morphine 0.1 mg per kg intravenously with standard monitoring of respiratory status. The mother should then cuddle the baby until it relaxes and falls asleep. An older child may be placed in the Trendelenburg position to allow gravity to facilitate the reduction. Once the child is asleep, gentle manipulation of the incarcerated mass should be attempted. Mild pressure should be exerted at the internal ring with one hand, while the other attempts to squeeze gas or fluid out of the incarcerated bowel back into the abdominal cavity. If the reduction is unsuccessful, the child should be taken immediately to the operating room.

After the hernia has been reduced manually, the child may be admitted for observation but not immediate repair. The hernia sac and spermatic cord are edematous after a reduction, making the repair difficult. Usually, it is done 24 hours after admission. If a child has persistent emesis after a manual reduction of a hernia, consider the possibility that the bowel was incompletely reduced. Children that develop peritoneal signs after manual reduction should be evaluated for possible perforation associated with gangrenous bowel. Rarely should a child be sent home after a manual reduction unless the parents are properly informed concerning signs of recurrence or intestinal obstruction and are thoroughly reliable (see the "Inguinal Hernias and Hydroceles" section).

Incarcerated Umbilical Hernia

Incarceration of an umbilical hernia is rare. If present, there is a persistent and tender bulge in the umbilical hernia sac. If the incarceration is of short duration, a gentle effort might be made to reduce it manually, but it is often necessary to prepare the child for urgent surgery. At the time of surgery, the loop of incarcerated bowel should be inspected, rather than letting it drop back into the abdominal cavity, to be certain that there has been no vascular impairment (see the "Umbilical Hernias" section).

Malrotation of the Bowel with Volvulus

Background

Malrotation of the bowel is a congenital condition associated with abnormal fixation of the mesentery of the bowel (Fig. 121.7). Therefore, the bowel has a tendency to volvulize and obstruct at points of abnormal fixation. Although malrotation with volvulus usually occurs either in utero or during early neonatal life, malrotation can be unrecognized until childhood (25% of cases present after 1 year of age). This is an extraordinarily dangerous situation because a complete volvulus of the bowel for more than an hour or two can totally obstruct blood supply to the bowel, leading to complete necrosis of the involved segment. When a volvulus involves the midgut, the entire small bowel and ascending colon may be lost. To prevent such a catastrophe, physicians should have a high index of suspicion for malrotation in any child with signs of obstruc-

tion and be prepared to get a child with a presumed volvulus to the operating room immediately.

Clinical Manifestations

Any child with bile-stained vomiting and abdominal pain may have malrotation with volvulus. The pain is usually intense and constant. Blood may appear in the stool within a few hours and suggests the development of ischemia and possible necrosis of the bowel. Clinically, malrotation can present in several different ways: first, and most dangerous, is the sudden onset of abdominal pain with bilious vomiting with no prior history of GI problems; second is a similar abrupt onset of obstruction in a child who previously seemed to have "feeding problems" with transient episodes of bilious vomiting; and third is a child with failure to thrive because of alleged intolerance of feedings.

On physical examination, there may be only mild distension of the abdomen because the obstruction usually occurs high in the GI tract. On palpation, the physician may discern one or two prominently dilated loops of bowel. The abdomen may be diffusely tender and yet not have signs of peritonitis early in the course. On rectal examination, the presence of blood on the examining finger is an alarming sign of impending ischemia and gangrene of the bowel.

Management

The key to management is to be suspicious of malrotation and to obtain flat and upright radiographs of the abdomen immediately. The presence of loops of small bowel overriding the liver shadow is suggestive of an underlying malrotation. When complete volvulus has occurred, there may be only a few dilated loops of bowel with air–fluid levels. Distal to the volvulus, there may be little or no gas in the GI tract. A "double-bubble sign" is often present on an upright film because of partial obstruction of the duodenum causing distension of the stomach and first part of the duodenum (Fig. 121.8A).

When a child is being assessed for possible malrotation, an upper GI series is the study of choice. The ligament of Treitz is absent in the malrotation anomaly; therefore, the C-loop of the duodenum is not present, the duodenum lies to the right of the spine, and the jejunum presents a coiled spring appearance in the right upper quadrant (Figs. 121.8B and 121.9). The cecum is not fixed and usually assumes a position in the right upper quadrant. However, because of its mobility, the cecum on barium enema may be seen in its normal position in the right lower quadrant. Therefore, a barium enema is not the most reliable study to rule out malrotation. In the neonate, the cecum sometimes takes a high position, and this could give a false impression of malrotation. If a US is obtained, as with possible pyloric stenosis or intussusception, an abnormal relationship between the superior mesenteric artery and vein should lead to an upper GI series.

As in the case of a child with an unreduced intussusception, a child with a possible volvulus should be prepared for immediate surgery. The operating room and operating team should be notified. IV fluid and electrolyte replacement should begin immediately. Laboratory studies should be obtained, but they do not add to the diagnostic evaluation. A nasogastric tube should be inserted and blood cross-matched. Because this entity can present even in adulthood, every physician should understand the pathogenesis and the need for surgical therapy

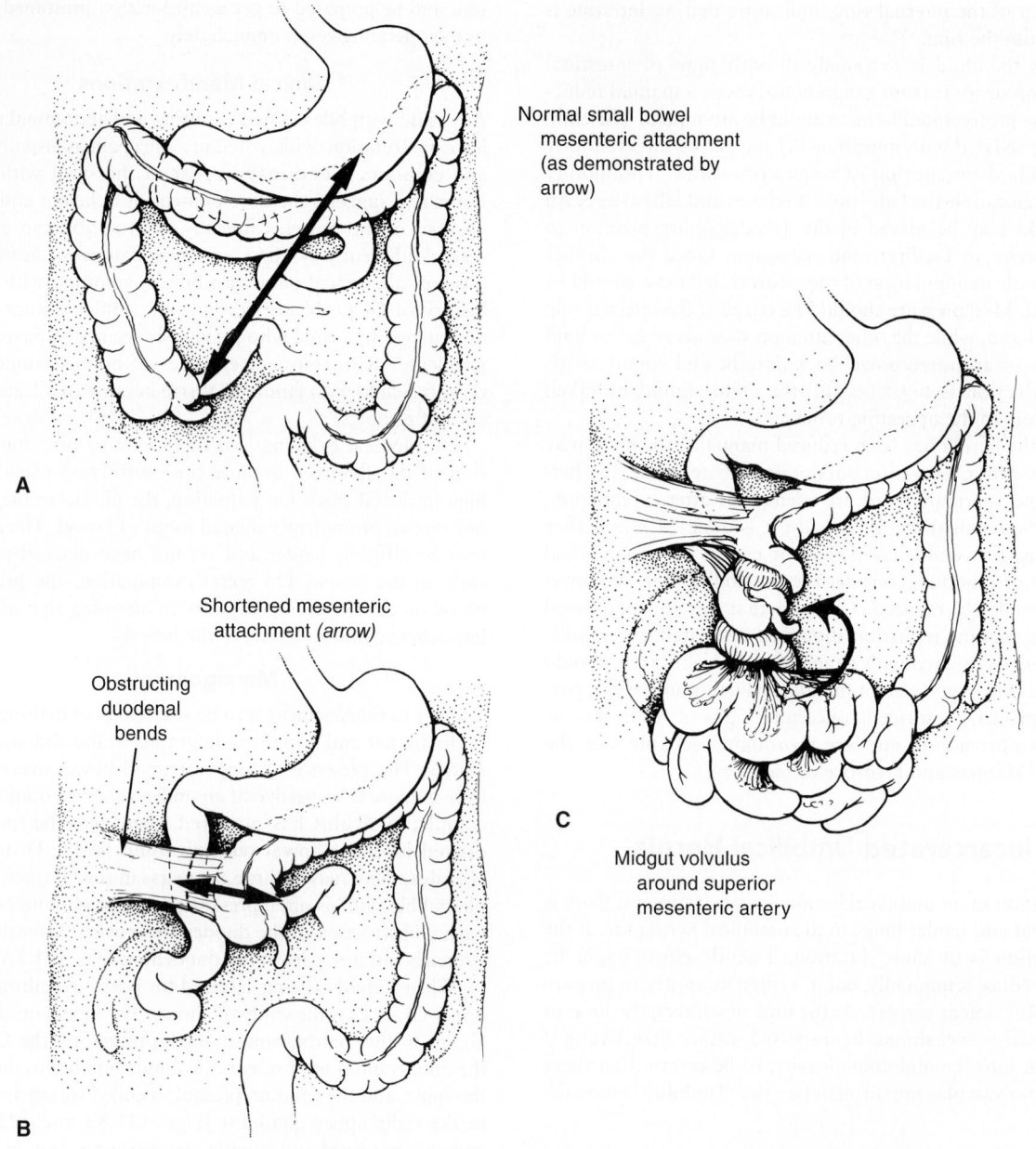

Normal small bowel
mesenteric attachment
(as demonstrated by
arrow)

A

Shortened mesenteric
attachment *(arrow)*

Obstructing
duodenal
bends

B

C

Midgut volvulus
around superior
mesenteric artery

FIGURE 121.7 Malrotation with volvulus. **A:** Normal small bowel mesenteric attachment (as demonstrated by the *arrow*). This prevents twisting of small bowel because of the broad fixation of the mesentery. **B:** Malrotation of colon with obstructing duodenal bands. **C:** Midgut volvulus around the superior mesenteric artery caused by the narrow base of the mesentery.

of malrotation. If immediate transfer to a pediatric hospital cannot be accomplished within an hour, a laparotomy should be performed without delay.

Pyloric Stenosis

Pyloric stenosis refers to an idiopathic hypertrophy of the pyloric muscle and occurs in 1 in 250 births. There is a male:female ratio of 4:1, and first born males are at higher risk. A familial incidence has been shown, particularly if the mother had hypertrophic pyloric stenosis as an infant. The age of onset is usually

2 to 5 weeks. Rarely, the onset may be late in the second month of life. The cause of the muscle hypertrophy is unknown, but the symptoms, diagnosis, and therapy are well defined. A causal relationship has been established with macrolide therapy (often used for motility), but the extent is still unknown.

Clinical Manifestations

Characteristically, the infant does well, without vomiting, for the first few weeks of life and then starts vomiting, either at the end of feedings or within 30 minutes. The infant is hungry and will eat immediately after vomiting. The vomiting becomes more prominent and eventually becomes forceful, projectile emesis.

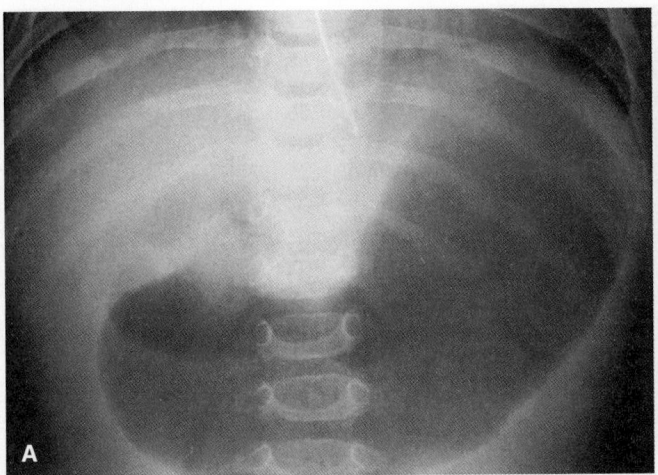
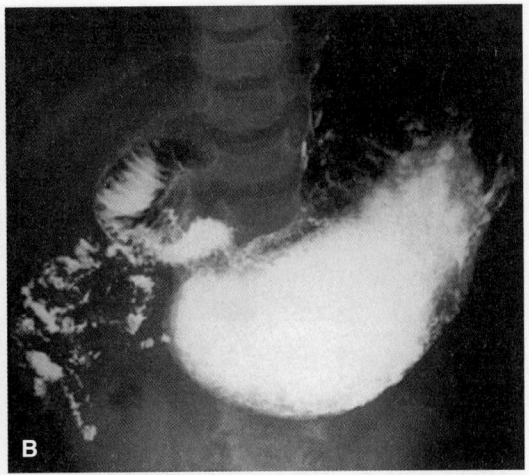

FIGURE 121.8 **A:** Malrotation of the bowel. Supine plain roentgenogram of the abdomen shows distended stomach and proximal duodenal loop. **B:** Same patient as in **A.** Upper gastrointestinal series shows dilated proximal duodenum with abrupt transition to normal caliber of small bowel. Abnormally placed ligament of Treitz. Proximal jejunum in the right abdomen.

The vomitus is always nonbilious. With protracted emesis, hematemesis can occur. Infants with pyloric stenosis may also become jaundiced with the onset of the other symptoms. The hyperbilirubinemia usually improves or abates postoperatively.

Early in the course, infants may appear perfectly active and well hydrated. In infants with protracted symptoms, moderate to severe dehydration may exist. The abdomen is soft and nondistended and if the infant is relaxed, an "olive" mass may be palpable in the midepigastrium. Sugar water can be used to help relax the infant for this part of the examination. Another

diagnostic clue is the presence of prominent gastric peristaltic waves across the abdomen. If a nasogastric tube is placed, a large volume of gastric content may be retrieved and the "olive" more easily palpated.

If the child has vomited for an extended period, he or she will show signs of growth failure. There may be loose, hanging skin and an absence of subcutaneous tissue. The infant may take on an "old man" appearance, with wrinkled skin on the face and body. Weight gain is inadequate, which may be calculated by knowing that the average child regains birth weight by 10 days of age and thereafter 15 to 30 g (0.5 to 1 oz) per day. With severe dehydration, the infant may be hypotonic and lethargic with poor feeding.

Serum electrolytes may be abnormal because of gastric losses. Accordingly, the potassium and chloride are low, and serum bicarbonate is high. This hypochloremic alkalosis may be profound with serum chlorides in the 65 to 75 mEq per L range. The patient can exhibit periods of apnea from the extreme metabolic alkalosis. When dehydration becomes severe, the patient may then develop acidosis, indicating an advanced and even more dangerous metabolic imbalance (see Chapter 100).

Management

Infants should be hospitalized and rehydrated with appropriate fluid and electrolyte replacement. Initially, IV fluids should be normal saline (lactated Ringer's solution is contraindicated) to replenish intravascular volume and supply adequate chloride. Potassium chloride should be added once urine output has been established. If hypotonic solutions are used, there is significant risk of causing hyponatremia (see Chapter 100). A volume of fluid appropriate to the patient's level of dehydration should be used.

Some pediatric surgeons will operate based on a typical history associated with a palpable pyloric mass. Commonly, US is used to confirm the diagnosis. The real-time US scanning not only increases the accuracy of the diagnosis of pyloric stenosis, but can also localize the "olive." The hypertrophic pyloric

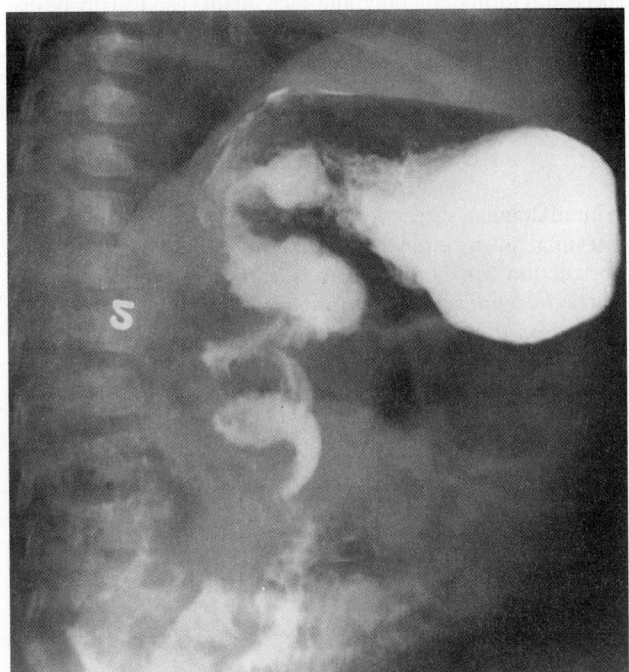

FIGURE 121.9 Malrotation. Upper gastrointestinal study showing absence of the ligament of Treitz and coiled spring appearance of jejunum.

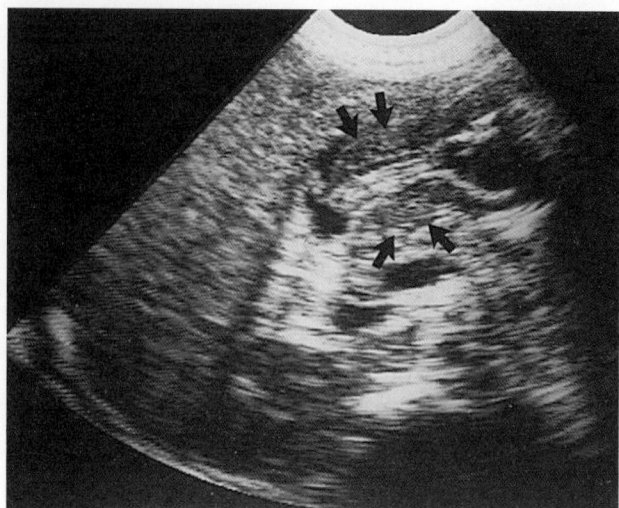

FIGURE 121.10 Hypertrophic pyloric stenosis. Ultrasonography of the abdomen shows thick pyloric muscle surrounding a centered echogenic mucosal and submucosal region *(arrows)*.

muscle is seen as a thick hypoechoic ring surrounding a central echogenic mucosal and submucosal region (Fig. 121.10). The quantitative criteria for the sonographic diagnosis of hypertrophic pyloric stenosis are 1.4 cm or longer length of the pyloric canal with 0.3 cm or greater thickness of the circular muscle.

If the US study does not show a hypertrophic pylorus, an upper GI series should then be done to eliminate gastroesophageal reflux, malrotation, and antral web as diagnostic possibilities. In general, pyloric stenosis can be identified by the presence of a "string sign" in the pyloric channel, seen best on oblique projections on the upper GI series (Fig. 121.11).

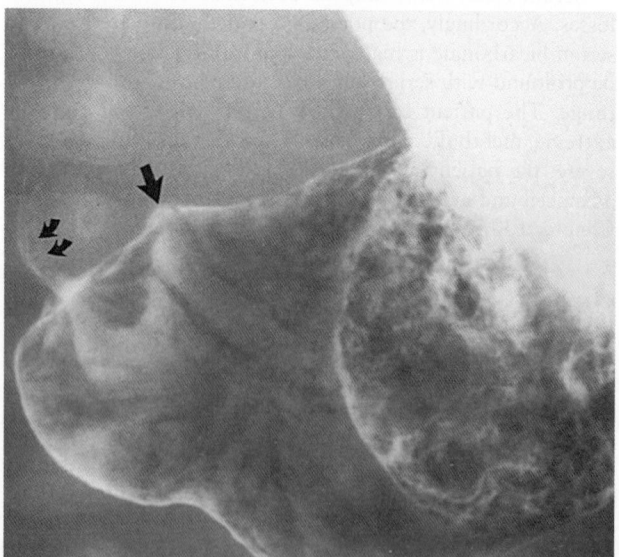

FIGURE 121.11 Pyloric stenosis. Long, narrowed, and tilting upward antropyloric canal. Parallel streaks of barium-producing typical string sign with complete obstruction *(arrows)* and eccentric lesser curvature indentation pyloric tilt *(arrow)*. The tilt is performed when the peristaltic wave meets the muscle mass.

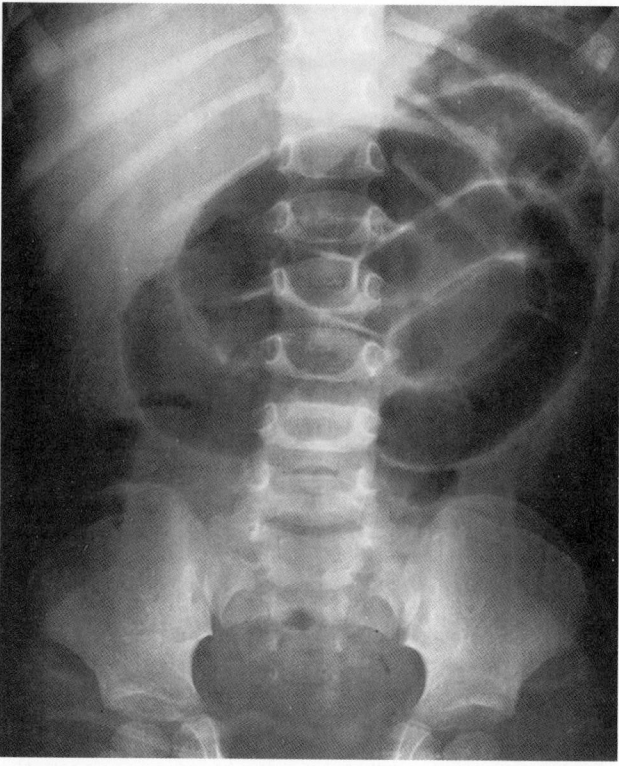

FIGURE 121.12 Dilated loops of small intestine and absence of air in lower abdomen indicating a high intestinal obstruction caused by postoperative adhesions.

To lessen the risk of vomiting and aspiration, the barium should be evacuated from the stomach after the upper GI series has been completed. Surgical pyloromyotomy is a most successful form of therapy, and such infants can usually be discharged from the hospital 2 days after surgery. Some infants will have some regurgitation postoperatively as a result of a temporary relaxation of the gastroesophageal sphincter.

Postoperative Adhesions

Prior abdominal surgery or peritonitis places a child at risk for intestinal obstruction from adhesions (Fig. 121.12). Such obstruction can occur relatively early in the postoperative course or months or even years later. The child often has the sudden onset of abdominal cramps, nausea, vomiting, and abdominal distension. Although most intestinal obstructions from adhesions do not jeopardize the perfusion of the bowel, occasionally a loop of intestine, caught under a fibrous band, can become gangrenous. All such patients need to be admitted to the hospital and evaluated by a surgeon who should direct the complete management.

CHRONIC PARTIAL INTESTINAL OBSTRUCTION

Any child with intermittent abdominal distension, nausea, anorexia, occasional vomiting, or chronic constipation or obstipation may have partial intestinal obstruction. A number of diagnostic considerations exist.

Chronic Constipation

Chronic constipation is probably one of the most common causes for abdominal pain, distension, and vomiting in children. The history, if available from a reliable parent, may attest to chronic constipation; however, occasionally, such a child is diagnosed only by palpating a large mass through the intact abdominal wall or a hard fecal mass blocking the anal outlet on rectal examination. Such children may have a history of encopresis and appear malnourished. Chapter 13 covers the diagnostic approach to the child with constipation.

These children should be disimpacted manually or managed with saline enemas and a rectal tube passed above the obstruction. For children unable to tolerate disimpaction, oral or nasogastric bowel evacuants such as polyethylene glycol electrolyte solution can be used. If the process has progressed to partial bowel obstruction, in-hospital management is necessary to clean out the bowel adequately while monitoring and hydrating the patient adequately.

Aganglionic Megacolon (Hirschsprung's Disease)

In patients with Hirschsprung's disease, the parasympathetic ganglion cells of Auerbach's plexus between the circular and longitudinal muscle layers of the colon are absent. The involved segment varies in length, from less than 1 cm to involvement of the entire colon and small bowel. The effect of this absence of ganglion cells produces spasm and abnormal motility of that segment, which results in either complete intestinal obstruction or chronic constipation.

These children have a lifelong history of constipation, so it is important to obtain an accurate account of the child's stool pattern from birth. A child with Hirschsprung's disease typically has never been able to stool properly without assistance (e.g., enemas, suppositories, anal stimulation). Normal stooling is not possible because of the failure of the aganglionic bowel and interval anal sphincter to relax. The child usually

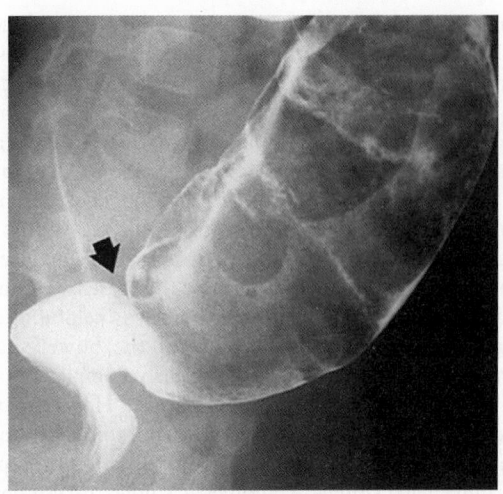

FIGURE 121.13 Hirschsprung's disease. Barium enema studies in lateral view show transition zone *(arrow)* with narrow rectum but dilated sigmoid colon.

has no history of encopresis, as one would find in chronic functional constipation. These youngsters have chronic abdominal distension and are often malnourished. Vomiting is uncommon, as are other symptoms. Complete intestinal obstruction in Hirschsprung's disease is more likely to occur in early infancy and only rarely in the older age groups. It may present with signs and symptoms of acute bowel perforation.

Table 121.3 summarizes the pertinent diagnostic features differentiating functional constipation from Hirschsprung's disease.

After flat and upright abdominal roentgenogram radiographic studies have been obtained, a properly performed barium enema with a Hirschsprung's catheter is the best initial diagnostic procedure. There should be no preparation of the bowel. Ideally, the rectum should not be stimulated by enemas or digital examination for 1 to 2 days before the procedure. The key to diagnosis is seeing a "transition zone" (Fig. 121.13) between the contracted aganglionic bowel and the

TABLE 121.3

DIFFERENTIAL DIAGNOSIS OF FUNCTIONAL CONSTIPATION AND HIRSCHSPRUNG'S DISEASE

	Functional constipation	Hirschsprung's disease
Onset	<2 yr	Birth
History	Coercive training Colicky abdominal pain Periodic volume stools	Enemas necessary No abdominal pain Episodes of intestinal obstruction
Encopresis	Present	Absent
Abdominal distension	Absent or minimal	Present
Rectal examination	Feces-packed rectum	Empty rectum
Barium examination	Dilated rectum	Narrow segment
Motility	Normal	Abnormal
Biopsy	Ganglion cells	No ganglion cells

proximal dilated ganglionated bowel. Stimulation of the rectum shortly before the study may result in decompression of the proximal bowel, with loss of definition of the transition zone. When a clear-cut transition zone is seen, it is not necessary to fill the colon with barium more than 12 to 18 in above the transition point. It is important, however, not to empty the colon of barium at the end of the study. The presence of retained barium above the transition point 24 hours later strongly suggests the diagnosis of Hirschsprung's disease.

Anorectal manometry to determine the presence or absence of relaxation of the internal anal sphincter is helpful in establishing the neurogenic dysfunction of the bowel. Barium enema studies and manometry are clearly complementary in the diagnosis of Hirschsprung's disease. However, rectal manometric studies are more reliable than radiologic methods for short aganglionic segments that are usually not apparent on barium enema studies. Manometric studies are not dependable in infants younger than 3 weeks. If the barium enema and anal manometry studies indicate Hirschsprung's disease, rectal biopsy is not necessary to confirm the diagnosis.

In children of all ages, an adequately performed suction mucosal biopsy of the rectum 2 cm or more above the dentate line can be reliable in diagnosing Hirschsprung's disease. Because of the complicated evaluation and management of this disease, referral to a pediatric surgeon is recommended.

Duplications

Duplications occur anywhere from the mouth to the anus and produce various symptoms. In the abdomen, there may be a noncommunicating cyst that gradually fills up with secretions and compresses the adjacent normal bowel, producing a palpable abdominal mass or chronic intestinal obstruction. Rarely, a marginal ulcer resulting from ectopic gastric mucosa may occur, and this produces painless bleeding. After appropriate radiographic diagnosis, surgery is indicated.

Inflammatory Bowel Disease

The older child or adolescent may develop either Crohn's disease or ulcerative colitis (see Chapter 89), and this must be included in the differential diagnosis of chronic intestinal obstruction. Usually, the child has a history of changing bowel habits, with mucus or blood in the stools, chronic abdominal pain, and weight loss. Chapter 89 covers inflammatory bowel disease in detail.

DISEASES THAT PRODUCE RECTAL BLEEDING

Rectal bleeding can be a sign of a serious condition. Blood on the outside of a formed stool is likely to originate from the distal large bowel, rectum, or anus. Blood mixed in the stool is generally from a higher source of bleeding. Blood associated with diarrhea is common with inflammatory bowel disease and infectious enteritis. A "tarry" stool suggests a source of bleeding in the proximal portion of the GI tract, and bright red

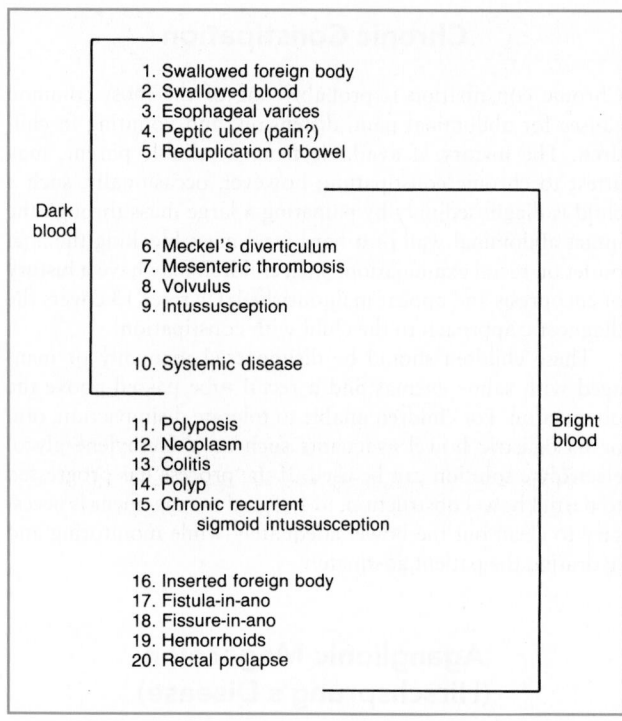

1. Swallowed foreign body
2. Swallowed blood
3. Esophageal varices
4. Peptic ulcer (pain?)
5. Reduplication of bowel

Dark blood

6. Meckel's diverticulum
7. Mesenteric thrombosis
8. Volvulus
9. Intussusception

10. Systemic disease

11. Polyposis
12. Neoplasm
13. Colitis
14. Polyp
15. Chronic recurrent sigmoid intussusception

Bright blood

16. Inserted foreign body
17. Fistula-in-ano
18. Fissure-in-ano
19. Hemorrhoids
20. Rectal prolapse

FIGURE 121.14 Causes of rectal bleeding in children.

blood suggests a more distal origin (Fig. 121.14). All patients with rectal bleeding should have a rectal examination. Those with significant hemorrhage require flexible colonoscopy. In some patients, no definite diagnosis may be reached despite extensive studies. In any patient with significant bleeding, however, surgical consultation is indicated. Chapters 29 and 89 further discuss the diagnosis and management of patients with GI bleeding.

Fissures

An anal fissure is probably the most common cause of bleeding, especially in infants. However, fissures may occur at any age. The child usually has a history of passing a large, hard stool with anal discomfort. Often, the child has a history of chronic constipation with progressive reluctance to pass stool because of the associated discomfort. If bleeding occurs, it usually involves streaking of bright red blood on the outside of the stool or red blood on the toilet tissues. The diagnosis can easily be made by inspection or anoscopic examination and appropriate measures taken to relieve the chronic constipation (see Chapter 13). Rarely does a child require hospitalization or surgery.

Juvenile Polyps

Older infants and children can develop either single or multiple retention polyps. Usually, the polyps occur in the lower portion of the colon and can often be palpated on rectal examination. Polyps bleed, but they rarely cause massive hemorrhage. They may intermittently prolapse at the anus or on

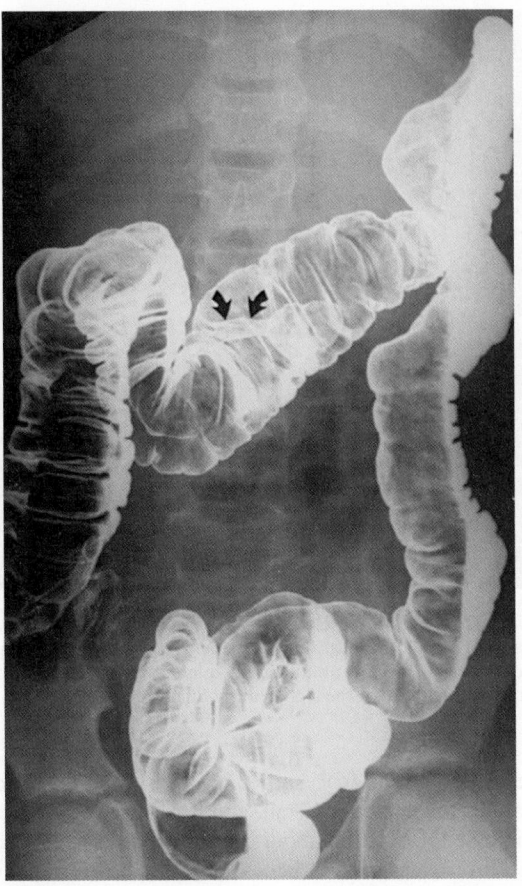

FIGURE 121.15 Juvenile polyp. Double air-contrast barium enema shows a single polyp with long stalk in transverse colon *(arrow)*.

occasion come free and be passed as a fecal mass associated with bleeding. Colonic polyps may be lead points for intussusception. Usually, however, polyps are asymptomatic except for the associated bleeding. These are not premalignant lesions, and they tend to be self-limiting (Fig. 121.15).

If a polyp can be felt on rectal examination or viewed through the sigmoidoscope, it may be safely removed. Polyps beyond the reach of the sigmoidoscope should be removed by colonoscopy.

Familial Polyposis

Families with multiple adenomatous colonic polyps are infrequently encountered. Bleeding is rare. More often, a colitis type of mucous discharge is present. Rectal examination and endoscopy reveal multiple "cobblestone" sessile polyps. These individuals are at risk for neoplasia because these are premalignant adenomatous polyps. The child should be referred to a pediatric surgeon and gastroenterologist for evaluation and long-term management.

Meckel's Diverticulum

Two percent of the population is born with a Meckel's diverticulum. This is the most common omphalomesenteric duct remnant. The diverticulum is usually located 50 to 75 cm proximal to the terminal ileum. Only 2% of persons with a Meckel's diverticulum manifest any clinical problems. The most common complication of a Meckel's diverticulum is a bleeding ulcer. Ectopic gastric mucosa in such patients is usually present in the diverticulum. The acid secretion produces ulceration at the junction of the normal ileal mucosa with the ectopic mucosa. Currant jelly stools or hemorrhage may be present. Other modes of presentation include diverticulitis, perforation with peritonitis, or intussusception as a result of the diverticulum's serving as a lead point.

Barium studies usually fail to outline a Meckel's diverticulum. The imaging modality of choice for detection of ectopic gastric mucosa in a bleeding Meckel's diverticulum is nuclear scintigraphy. A well-defined focal accumulation of radionuclide (^{99m}Tc pertechnetate) usually appears at or about the same time as activity in the stomach and gradually increases in intensity (Fig. 121.16). A duplication cyst with gastric mucosa shows the same focal accumulation of radionuclide. Preoperative differentiation between two lesions as a cause of GI bleeding is not important. The accuracy of scintigraphy in detection of ectopic gastric mucosa in Meckel's diverticula is approximately 95%. False-negative results may rarely occur in patients with rapidly bleeding Meckel's diverticula and with those diverticula that do not contain gastric mucosa.

In any child with a major rectal bleed and a negative scan, further workup, including an arteriogram if the bleeding continues to be active or colonoscopy when the bleeding is not active, is required.

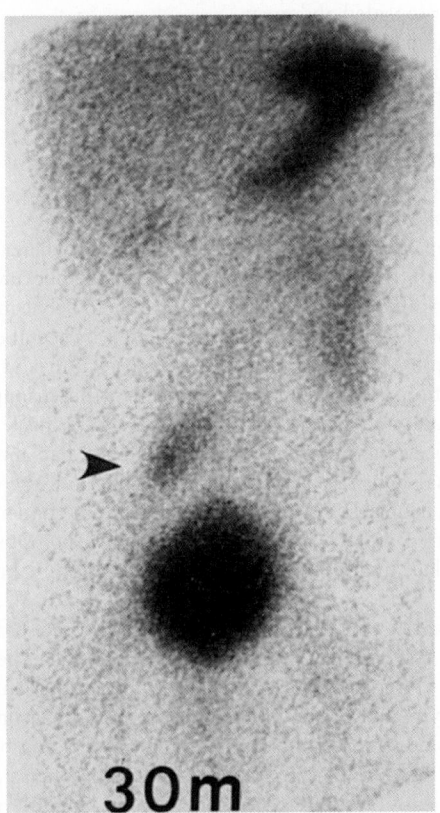

FIGURE 121.16 Meckel's diverticulum. Anterior image at 30 minutes shows an oval focal accumulation of ^{99m}Tc-pertechnetate in the right lower quadrant of the abdomen *(arrowhead)*.

Henoch-Schönlein Purpura

Henoch-Schönlein purpura (see Chapters 91 and 85) is a vasculitic disorder that can produce asymptomatic rectal bleeding or abdominal pain. Usually there is a recognizable vasculitic rash with purpura, as well as petechiae mostly of the lower extremities and buttocks. Occasionally, a child will develop a small bowel intussusception from a submucosal hemorrhage that is acting as a lead point. Other common manifestations are hematuria, arthralgias or arthritis, purpuric rash, and testicular pain.

Other Causes of Rectal Bleeding

Other causes of rectal bleeding include intestinal vascular malformations, intussusception, duplications, inflammatory bowel disease, peptic ulcer with bleeding, portal hypertension with bleeding varices, foreign bodies of the rectum, and anal fistulas. These topics are covered elsewhere in this chapter and Chapters 29 and 89.

INTRAABDOMINAL MASSES

Background

Intraabdominal masses may be benign or malignant. Children are often asymptomatic even when the tumor is large; frequently, the mass is detected by the caregiver noticing a protuberant or lopsided abdomen.

It is difficult to feel an intraabdominal mass, as well as outline its limits and its degree of mobility, if an infant or child is crying. The physician should then make an effort to palpate the intraabdominal contents carefully. These masses can be fragile and prone to rupture. Therefore, palpation of the mass should be done gently and strictly limited to as few examiners as possible.

Retroperitoneal masses tend to be fixed, whereas masses attached to the mesentery or omentum are mobile and may be shifted to different locations by the examiner. Pelvic masses are commonly fixed and often can best be felt by rectal examination. A presacral mass may narrow the rectum and produce constipation. Abdominal masses present with various characteristics and may be smooth, nodular, cystic, or firm.

Initial evaluation in the ED may include flat and upright abdominal films. If, after such an examination, the origin of the mass is unclear or suggests a neoplasm, the patient should be admitted and a workup done without delay. Observation has no place in dealing with unexplained abdominal masses in children.

Diagnostic imaging should identify the precise anatomic location and extent of the pathologic process. The general location of a mass, with or without calcification, can be confirmed by plain abdominal roentgenograms. Ultrasonography has become increasingly popular as initial imaging because it does not require GI preparation or injected contrast, yet it is diagnostically accurate. Ultrasonography can differentiate a cystic flank mass (Fig. 121.17) that could be a hydronephrotic kidney from a solid tumor such as an adrenal neuroblastoma, and thus, facilitate the proper referral of the child to either a

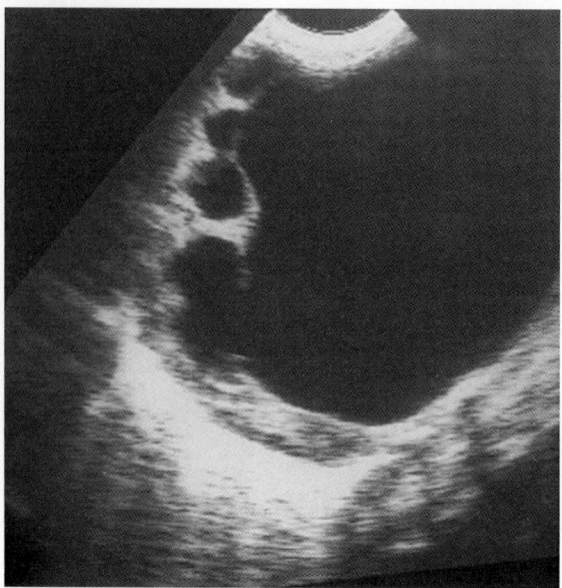

FIGURE 121.17 Ureteropelvic junction obstruction. A newborn with left flank mass. Ultrasonography of the left flank shows dilated pyelocalyceal system. The communicating dilated collecting systems are seen in the periphery of the significantly dilated renal pelvis.

urologist or a pediatric surgeon. CT is superior to other modalities for anatomic detail, and it provides anatomic and physiologic information about organs and vascular structures despite overlying gas and bones. Renal scans are superior to excretory urography for determining renal function. Angiography is indicated for an abdominal mass only if a precise knowledge of segmental vascular anatomy is required or if interventional techniques are contemplated.

Sacrococcygeal Teratoma

The presacral sacrococcygeal teratoma is the most common tumor of the caudal region in children and is more common in females than in males (4:1). Most tumors are benign and are noted at birth. Tumors in patients beyond neonatal age have a higher incidence of malignancy. Radiography shows a soft-tissue mass that arises from the ventral surface of the coccyx. Calcifications are present in 60% of presacral sacrococcygeal teratoma and are more common in benign tumors. US confirms whether presacral sacrococcygeal teratomas are cystic, solid, or mixed and can also determine impingement on the urinary tract. CT is helpful in confirming the diagnosis, particularly in older children, and demonstrates the content of a tumor, as well as its extent and bone anomalies. Tumors with more solid components are more often malignant than those with more cystic components (Fig. 121.18).

Nonmalignant Intraabdominal Masses

Fecaloma

A lower abdominal mass, particularly one on the left side, is most often related to retained stool and associated with chronic functional constipation than with Hirschsprung's

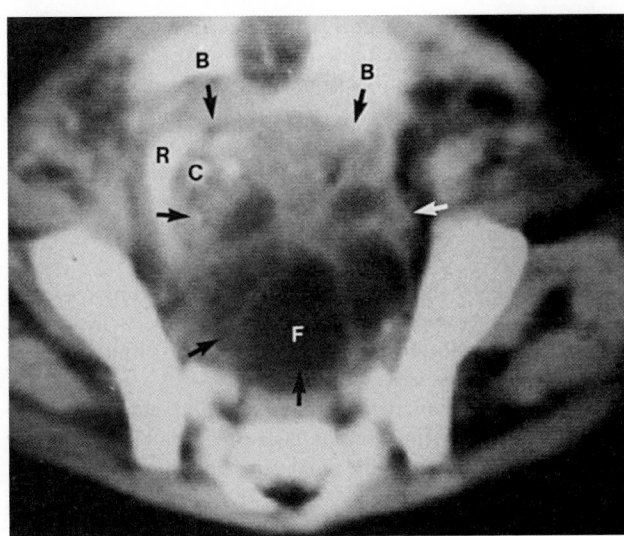

FIGURE 121.18 Presacral teratoma. Computed tomographic section of pelvis with contrast medium enhancement shows a large cystic mass *(arrows)*. The mass contains both fat and calcification, and displaces the rectum anteriorly and laterally, and the bladder anteriorly. B, bladder with Foley catheter; C, calcification; F, fat; R, rectum.

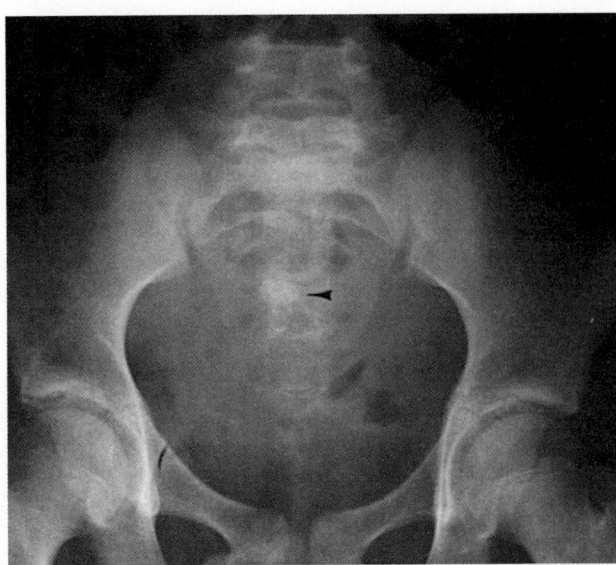

FIGURE 121.19 Ovarian dermoids. Note calcification *(arrows)* in superior aspect of a large pelvic mass in a 12-year-old girl.

disease. If a mass is found, a careful review of bowel habits is important. If an abdominal mass is a fecaloma, a large bolus of stool can usually be felt on rectal examination just inside the anus. The evaluation of the impaction, and irrigation of the upper sigmoid colon, should cause the mass to disappear. See Chapter 13 for the causes of constipation.

Ovarian Masses

Simple ovarian cysts and solid teratomas are not uncommon and may be asymptomatic even though they have reached a large size. Occasionally, the child presents with urinary complaints from the pressure on the bladder or urethra. Granulosa cell tumors of the ovary produce precocious puberty because they are hormonally active tumors. They may be malignant. The sudden onset of severe abdominal pain may indicate torsion of an ovarian mass, with resultant ovarian infarction.

Radiographs may show calcification in about half of patients with teratomas (Fig. 121.19). Because an occasional ovarian tumor is malignant in children, children with ovarian masses should be promptly evaluated and prepared for surgery (see Chapter 90).

Omental Cysts

Omental cysts are rare, are usually asymptomatic, and can fill the abdomen. It is often difficult to differentiate an omental cyst from ascites. Smaller cysts are more mobile and can be pushed freely into all quadrants of the abdomen. If a cyst volvulizes on its pedicle or has bleeding within it, it may cause abdominal pain or tenderness. Elective surgical excision is indicated.

Mesenteric Cysts

Mesenteric cysts can occur anywhere in the mesentery but are most common in the mesentery of the colon. They tend to be multilocular and are often discovered during a routine exami-

nation or after an episode of abdominal trauma with enlargement from bleeding. They are benign, but surgical therapy is indicated, both to confirm the diagnosis and to prevent complications. They can usually be removed with sparing of the bowel, or they can be marsupialized into the general peritoneal cavity where the fluid is absorbed.

Duplications

GI duplications within the abdomen can occur anywhere along the greater curvature of the stomach, the lesser curvature of the duodenum, or the mesenteric side of either the small or large intestines. They can also be pararectal, rising up out of the pelvis. Duplications that produce abdominal masses are either noncommunicating, and hence gradually enlarge, or communicating in that their secretory lining has a distal communication with the true lumen of the bowel. Except for the rare occurrence of massive rectal bleeding in a child with a communicating duplication, most duplications do not present as emergencies. Instead, they present in children either as unexplained abdominal masses or with symptoms of intermittent colic, resulting from partial obstruction of the true lumen of the adjacent bowel. The exact diagnosis is often unclear until the time of laparotomy.

Malignant Intraabdominal Masses

About 50% of the solid malignant tumors seen in children occur within the abdominal cavity. Most solid masses occur in the retroperitoneum. The most common is neuroblastoma, followed by Wilms' tumor and rhabdomyosarcoma. Other unusual tumors, such as embryonal cell carcinomas (yolk sac tumor) and lymphosarcoma, also occur in young children. Chapter 97 covers oncologic emergencies. As with most malignant tumors, early diagnosis and treatment provide the best prospects for a cure.

Neuroblastoma

Neuroblastoma most often occurs as a tumor arising from the adrenal gland, but it can develop anywhere along the sympathetic chain or in the pelvis. It can grow extensively, often crossing the midline of the abdomen and enveloping key vascular and visceral structures. The best cure rates are generally in children who are younger than 1 year at the time of diagnosis and in whom the tumor is still localized to the point of origin. In such favorable cases, the tumor can be totally excised. When widespread dissemination occurs, complete resection is unwarranted because of the risk to other vital structures.

CT with contrast enhancement demonstrates precise anatomy, as well as renal function and organ vascularity. The

CT characteristics of neuroblastoma include irregular shape, irregular margins, lack of well-defined capsules, and mixed low-density center. Neuroblastoma often displaces surrounding organs and encases vessels. Prevertebral midline extension is common. There are calcifications in at least 75% (Fig. 121.20). Ultrasonography has limitations in accurately determining tumor margins or local extension.

Wilms' Tumor

Wilms' tumor is the most common intrarenal tumor seen in children. The tumor can be massive before its discovery. Wilms' tumor should be considered in any child who has unexplained hematuria.

A solid renal mass demonstrated by US in infants and children is usually a Wilms' tumor. Because of the high frequency of tumor extension into the renal veins and inferior vena cava

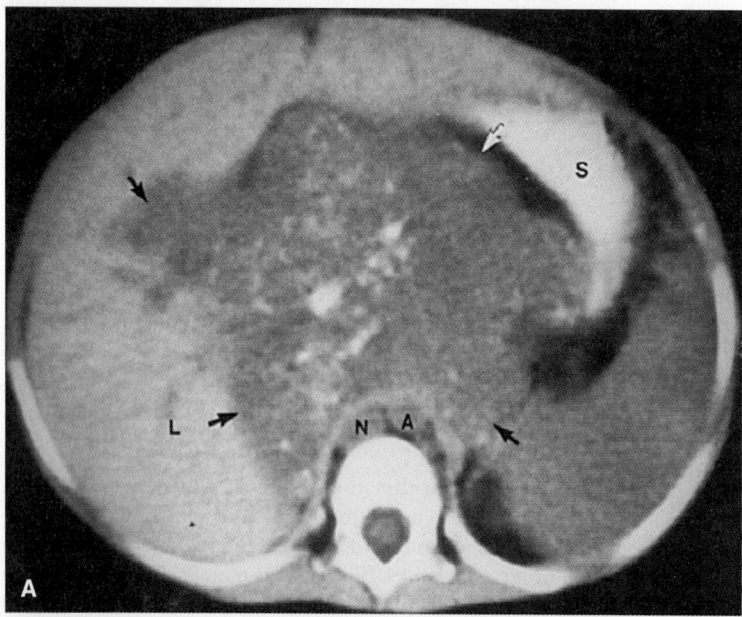

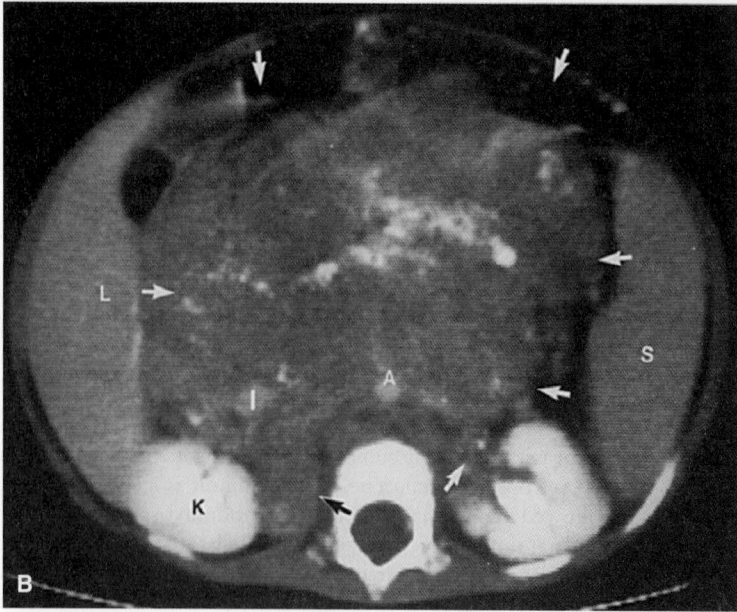

FIGURE 121.20 **A:** Celiac axis neuroblastoma. Computed tomographic (CT) section of the abdomen shows a large lobulated mass with multiple flakes of calcification displacing stomach and the liver *(white arrow)*. Note presence of retrocrural node *(black arrows)*. A, aorta; L, liver; N, node; S, stomach. **B:** Celiac axis neuroblastoma. Enhanced CT section of the abdomen at level of the kidney shows a large lobulated mass with irregular margins and calcification displacing the right kidney inferoposterior and laterally. Note encased inferior vena cava (IVC) and aorta. The IVC is displaced laterally and ventrally and to the right the superior mesenteric artery and celiac axis are completely surrounded by the mass. A, aorta; I, IVC; K, kidney; L, liver; S, spleen; *white arrows,* mass.

(IVC), these vascular structures should be examined by US. Because Wilms' tumors are usually large and expansive, the IVC often is extrinsically displaced by the tumor mass. CT with bolus contrast enhancement may be required for confirmation of equivocal invasion in a patient suspected of having Wilms' tumor. A CT scan can define the presence of an intrarenal mass and extent of tumor, visualizes vascular structures, identifies nodal involvement, defines internal hemorrhage and necrosis, evaluates the presence or absence of liver metastases, and provides some measure of renal excretory function. Also, CT can determine whether a tumor is initially nonresectable or bilateral (Fig. 121.21). Chest CT is also performed at the initial evaluation to identify pulmonary metastases. Patients with presumed Wilms' tumor require admission for coordinated approach by the surgeon and oncologists.

Rhabdomyosarcoma

Rhabdomyosarcoma can occur anywhere in the abdomen or pelvis where there is striated muscle. Tumors are particularly common in the pelvis, involving the prostate, uterus or vagina, and retroperitoneal structures, but they have also been found in the common bile duct and other unusual sites. These tumors can reach a large size before they become symptomatic, and each must be managed individually, depending on the site of origin, extent of growth, and the degree of spread. Modern selective therapy has greatly improved the survival rate of this highly malignant tumor.

Hepatomas

The most common primary GI tract neoplasm is hepatic in origin. Hepatoblastoma and hepatocellular carcinoma are the two main subgroups of liver tumors; they are clinically indistinguishable at presentation. Many are asymptomatic, but symptoms such as early satiety, weight loss, and abdominal pain may be seen especially with very large tumors. More often, the tumor is discovered after caregivers notice a change in the appearance of the abdomen. They are usually seen in older infants and young children. Increased levels of α-fetoprotein are associated

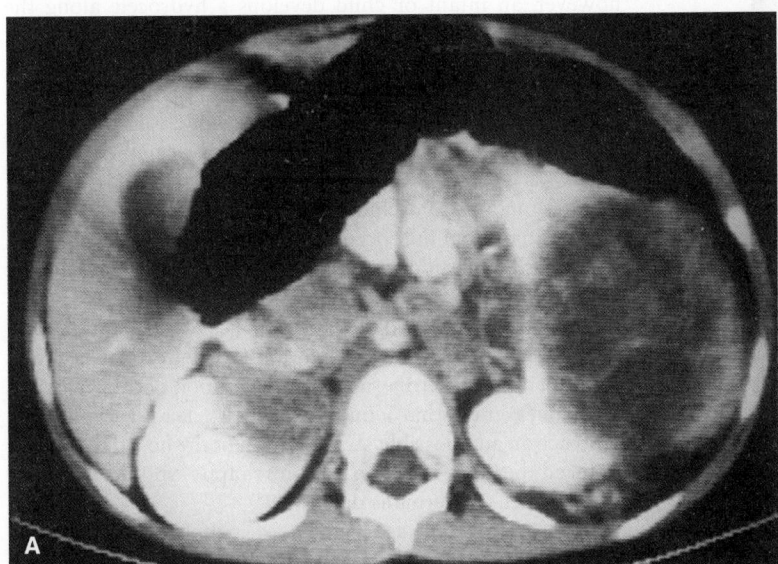

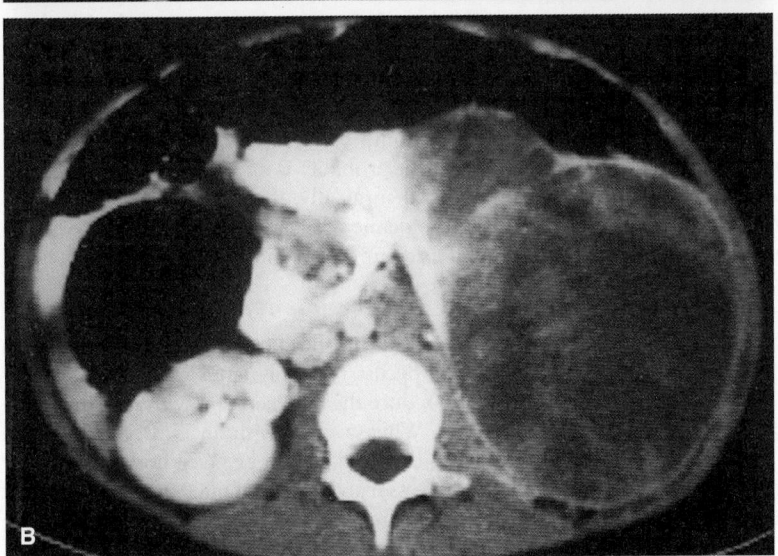

FIGURE 121.21 **A:** Bilateral Wilms' tumor. A 5-year-old girl with left flank mass. CT sections of the upper abdomen with contrast medium enhancement show a necrotic mass arising from superior aspect of the left kidney. Note a small mass in the superior medial aspect of the right kidney. **B:** Bilateral Wilms' tumor (same patient as in **A**). CT section of the abdomen with contrast medium enhancement shows extent of the large necrotic left Wilms' tumor with periaortic adenopathy.

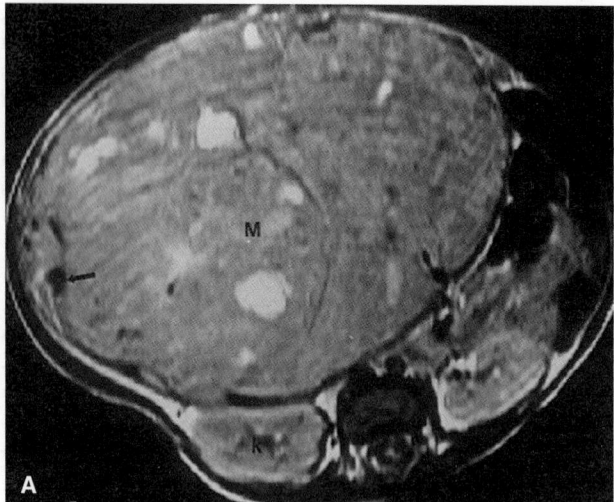

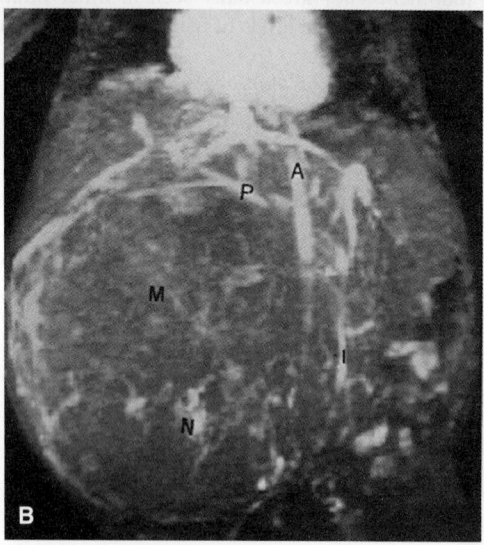

FIGURE 121.22 **A:** Hepatoblastoma in a 2-month-old boy. Axial T1 magnetic resonance imaging (MRI) shows a solid mass (M) occupying entire liver, gallbladder *(arrow)*, and right kidney (K). **B:** Coronal magnetic resonance angiography shows liver mass (M), with stretching of the hepatic vessels and multiple area of neovascularity (N). Note marked stretching and displacement of the inferior vena cava (I) with patent portal vein (P). A, aorta.

with both types. Differential diagnosis should include hemangioendothelioma, hamartoma, and renal and adrenal tumors.

Radiologic imaging is directed at diagnosis and the resectability of the tumor. CT or MRI with angiography is often required to determine surgical approach (Fig. 121.22). Long-term survival is poor unless complete resection is possible. Liver tumors commonly metastasize to the lungs, brain, and regional nodes.

ABDOMINAL WALL DEFECTS

Inguinal Hernias and Hydroceles

Indirect inguinal hernia is the most common congenital anomaly that is found in children. It is approximately 10 times more common in males than in females. There is a strong familial incidence.

Clinical Manifestations

The child with a hernia may present in different ways. The presentation is determined by the extent of obliteration of the processus vaginalis during development. A child may have a completely open hernia sac, which extends from the internal ring to the scrotum, or a segmental obliteration producing a sac that is narrow at its proximal end, creating a hydrocele of either the tunica vaginalis or the spermatic cord. The narrowing of the processus allows the abdominal fluid to seep into the distal portion of the sac. It then becomes entrapped and produces what is clinically recognized as a hydrocele. It is often difficult for this fluid to egress through the narrow patent processus vaginalis back into the abdominal cavity.

At the time of the embryologic closure of the processus vaginalis, many fetuses will have some fluid trapped around the testicle in the tunica vaginalis. This is called a physiologic hydrocele, which is a normal newborn finding. In such cases, the fluid is gradually absorbed in the first 12 months of life. If, however, an infant or child develops a hydrocele along the cord in the tunica vaginalis sometime after birth, it must be assumed the processus vaginalis is still patent and in communication with the peritoneal cavity. This patent processus vaginalis represents a hernia sac. Surgical closure of the sac and drainage of the hydrocele are then indicated on an elective basis.

Many infants and children manifest the classical bulge in the inguinal canal that occurs during straining or crying. This is caused by a loop of intestine distending into the hernia sac (or may represent the ovary in a female). Usually, the hernia sac contents reduce into the abdominal cavity when the straining ceases. If the prolapsing loop of intestine becomes entrapped in the hernia sac, an incarceration occurs. This is a true emergency that could eventually lead to intestinal obstruction and possibly strangulation of the bowel. For easily reduced hernias, elective herniorrhaphy should be done shortly after the hernia is diagnosed.

Hydroceles of the spermatic cord with associated communicating hernias are sometimes difficult to differentiate from an incarcerated hernia. If an empty hernia sac can be felt above the hydrocele, the physician can be assured that this is an asymptomatic hernia with an associated hydrocele. However, if there is fullness above the hydrocele and the mass cannot be reduced, the child should be taken to the operating room on the assumption that it probably is an incarcerated hernia that needs to be managed surgically. If there is any uncertainty, a US may be useful to define the hernia. Bowel gas in the hernia sac is not reliably present for diagnostic reasons.

Management

Fortunately, strangulation of the entrapped loop of bowel in an incarcerated hernia occurs relatively late so, contrary to adult practice, efforts to reduce the incarceration without surgery are usually warranted. When a child with an incarcerated hernia presents in the ED, the child should be given nothing to eat or drink, sedated if necessary with morphine 0.1 mg per kg, and placed in a Trendelenburg position. Often, this alone will reduce the incarceration. If it does not, bimanual reduction should be attempted. The fingers and thumb of one hand should compress the internal ring area, while an effort is made with the other hand "to milk" either gas or fluid out of the entrapped bowel back into the abdomen. This relieves the pressure and usually allows the entire loop of bowel to reduce back into the abdominal cavity. Once the incarcerated hernia is reduced, the child should be admitted or scheduled for elective surgery at the surgeon's discretion. Patients who were vomiting, had guaic-positive stools, or had difficulty reducing hernias should be admitted for serial abdominal examinations. A day or two should be allowed to pass to lessen the edema of the area, as well as to allow an easier and safer elective herniorrhaphy.

Epiploceles (Epigastric Hernias)

If a discrete mass occurs intermittently about one third of the distance from the umbilicus to the xiphoid, it is usually the result of a weakness of the linea alba through which properitoneal fat protrudes. This defect is called epiplocele. Such defects are fairly common in infants and usually close spontaneously. In older children, the mass may occasionally be tender. If it becomes excruciatingly tender, it is a sign that fat has become incarcerated in the hernia. Although there is no great urgency, these small midline defects should be repaired surgically when they become symptomatic.

Umbilical Hernias

Umbilical hernias are common in small infants, particularly in African Americans. Fortunately, most of the hernias tend to close spontaneously, and only rarely does incarceration occur. Umbilical hernias can be large and unsightly, and families need reassurance that watchful waiting is the best course. However, if the umbilical hernia fails to close by the age of 5 to 6 years, surgical repair is indicated. Umbilical hernias may be repaired earlier if there is a large ring that shows no signs of diminishing in size over 1 to 2 years, if there is a thinning of the umbilical skin, or if an incarceration has occurred. Hernias that have a supraumbilical component tend not to close spontaneously and may be operated on at an earlier time of life.

Other Umbilical Defects

Omphalomesenteric duct remnants may persist in either of two forms. When the duct is patent from the ileum to the umbilicus, there is a release of small bowel contents via an opening in the umbilicus. A second form involves a remnant of the omphalomesenteric duct that contains a secreting mucosal patch that is attached to an opening in the center of the umbilicus. Passage of a sterile blunt probe or instillation of contrast dye under fluoroscopy via the umbilical opening will usually confirm either of these conditions. Once identified, these remnants must be excised surgically. In contrast, some infants present with umbilical granuloma in which an excessive amount of granulation tissue has built up after separation of the umbilical cord. In these patients, no opening in the gran-

ulation tissue can be seen or felt by means of a probe. These granulomas are usually best treated by application of silver nitrate to the granulation tissue. After each treatment, the area should be rinsed thoroughly to prevent burning of adjacent skin. If the granuloma is allowed to persist, it will eventually epithelialize and become an umbilical papilloma (Fig. 121.23).

If the urachus persists after birth, it can form a urinary fistula that drains at the umbilicus. This problem is ordinarily noted in the newborn period. Older infants or children may present with drainage at the umbilicus caused by persistence of part of the urachus, even though connection with the bladder may be obliterated. These urachal remnants also require surgical excision.

FOREIGN BODIES OF THE GASTROINTESTINAL TRACT

When a child ingests a foreign body, it causes great concern to the family. Most swallowed foreign bodies move through the GI tract without complication. Occasionally, a foreign body lodges in the esophagus, necessitating removal. Plain film roentgenograms for suspected foreign body should focus on the suspected area initially but then expanded to locate the object. Foreign bodies lodged in the esophagus should be removed promptly to prevent complications such as edema, ulceration, aspiration, pneumonia, or perforation. If initial radiographic studies identify a smooth, small object, such as a coin, a period of conservative observation may allow the foreign body to move into the stomach. If the history of radiographic appearance suggests a battery, emergency endoscopy and removal should be performed. Esophageal foreign bodies in the esophagus greater than 24 hours require removal. Patients with esophageal foreign bodies require follow-up radiographs to show movement into the stomach or evidence of successful passage (by identification in stool).

Foreign bodies that reach the stomach, whether pointed or sharp edged, usually pass completely through the intestinal tract and are evacuated. Cathartics and other efforts to hurry their transit are unnecessary. Whether all GI tract foreign bodies should be followed until evacuation is not clear. Persistent emesis may represent pyloric obstruction.

Occasionally, a long, thin foreign body such as a bobby pin may not be able to traverse the turn where the duodenum joins the jejunum at the ligament of Treitz. If a foreign body is trapped in this area, perforation with local or generalized peritonitis may occur. When entrapment occurs anywhere beyond the pylorus, surgical removal is indicated either to prevent or to treat local perforation. Occasionally, objects such as straight pins, toothpicks, and broom straws become entrapped in the appendix. When this occurs, the appendix should be removed. Special consideration should be given to magnets; when two magnets attract across a loop of bowel, the compressed bowel may necrose. Coins may remain in the child's stomach for considerable time, and if they do not become embedded in the gastric mucosa, they eventually pass, even after several weeks. Objects stuck in the pylorus may cause vomiting and should be removed. With the aid of modern flexible endoscopic equipment, foreign bodies in the stomach can usually be removed with ease. Chapter 123 covers pharyngeal foreign bodies.

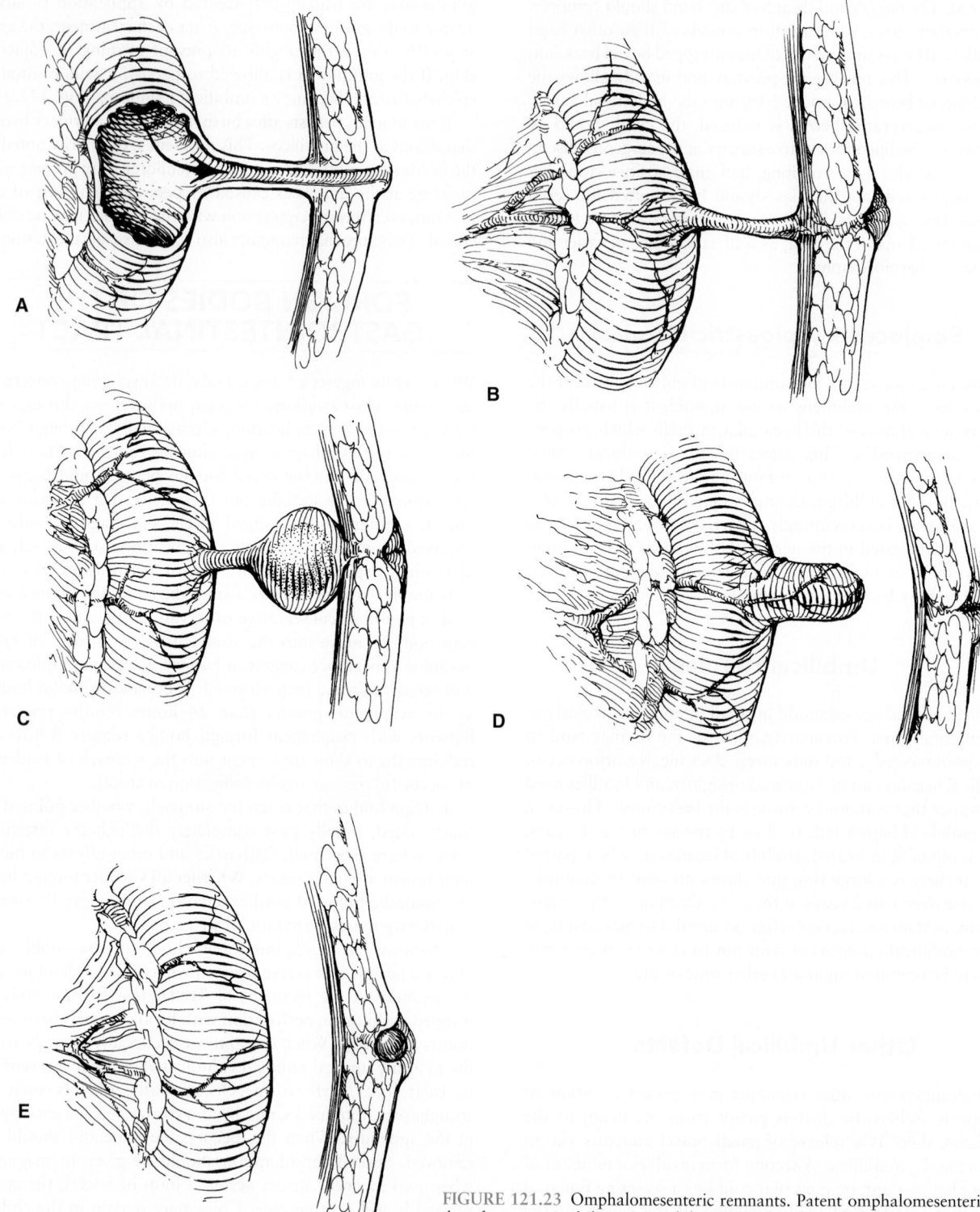

FIGURE 121.23 Omphalomesenteric remnants. Patent omphalomesenteric duct from terminal ileum to umbilicus (**A**); closed omphalomesenteric duct with mucosal patch at umbilicus (**B**); omphalomesenteric cyst below umbilicus (**C**); Meckel's diverticulum (**D**); and umbilical granuloma (**E**).

Suggested Readings

Appendicitis

Alloo J, Gerstle T, Shilyansky J, et al. Appendicitis in children less than 3 years of age: a 28-year review. *Pediatr Surg Int* 2004;19:777–779.

Becker T, Kharbanda A, Bachur R. Atypical clinical features of pediatric appendicitis. *Acad Emerg Med* 2007;14:124–129.

Bundy DG, Byerley JS, Liles EA, et al. Does this child have appendicitis? *JAMA* 2007;298:438–451.

Callahan MJ, Rodriguez DP, Taylor GA. CT of appendicitis in children. *Radiology* 2002;224:325–332.

Friday JH. Update on appendicitis: diagnosis and presurgical management. *Curr Opin Pediatr* 2006;18:234–238.

Garcia Pena BM, Cook EF, Mandl KD. Selective imaging strategies for the diagnosis of appendicitis in children. *Pediatrics* 2004;113:24–28.

Kaiser S, Finnbogason T, Jorulf HK, et al. Suspected appendicitis in children: diagnosis with contrast-enhanced versus nonenhanced helical CT. *Radiology* 2004;231:427-433.

Kaiser S, Frenckner B, Jorulf HK. Suspected appendicitis in children: US and CT—a prospective randomized study. *Radiology* 2002;223:633–638.

Meier DE, Guzzetta PC, Barber RG, et al. Perforated appendicitis in children: is there a best treatment? *J Pediatr Surg* 2003;38:1520–1524.

Morrow SE, Newman KD. Current management of appendicitis. *Semin Pediatr Surg* 2007;16:34–40.

Newman K, Ponsky T, Kittle K, et al. Appendicitis 2000: variability in practice, outcomes, and resource utilization at thirty pediatric hospitals. *J Pediatr Surg* 2003;38:372–379; discussion 372–379.

Samuel M. Pediatric appendicitis score. *J Pediatr Surg* 2002;37:877–881.

Sivit CJ, Applegate KE, Stallion A, et al. Imaging evaluation of suspected appendicitis in a pediatric population: effectiveness of sonography versus CT. *AJR Am J Roentgenol* 2000;175:977–980.

Vernon AH, Georgeson KE, Harmon CM. Pediatric laparoscopic appendectomy for acute appendicitis. *Surg Endosc* 2004;18:75–79.

Ziegler MM. The diagnosis of appendicitis: an evolving paradigm. *Pediatrics* 2004;113:130–132.

Intussusception

Bajaj L, Roback MG. Postreduction management of intussusception in a children's hospital emergency department. *Pediatrics* 2003;112:1302–1307.

D'Agostino J. Common abdominal emergencies in children. *Emerg Med Clin North Am* 2002;20:139–153.

Harrington L, Connolly B, Hu X, et al. Ultrasonographic and clinical predictors of intussusception. *J Pediatr* 1998;132:836–839.

Kaiser AD, Applegate KE, Ladd AP. Current success in the treatment of intussusception in children. *Surgery* 2007;142:469–475; discussion 475–467.

Lui KW, Wong HF, Cheung YC, et al. Air enema for diagnosis and reduction of intussusception in children: clinical experience and fluoroscopy time correlation. *J Pediatr Surg* 2001;36:479–481.

Ramachandran P, Gupta A, Vincent P, Sridharan S. Air enema for intussusception: is predicting the outcome important? *Pediatr Surg Int* 2008;24:311–313.

Sohoni A, Wang NE, Dannenberg B. Tension pneumoperitoneum after intussusception pneumoreduction. *Pediatr Emerg Care* 2007;23:563–564.

Waseem M, Rosenberg HK. Intussusception. *Pediatr Emerg Care* 2008;24:793–800.

Malrotation

D'Agostino J. Common abdominal emergencies in children. *Emerg Med Clin North Am* 2002;20:139–153.

Gauderer MW. Acute abdomen. When to operate immediately and when to observe. *Semin Pediatr Surg* 1997;6:74–80.

Hajivassiliou CA. Intestinal obstruction in neonatal/pediatric surgery. *Semin Pediatr Surg* 2003;12:241–253.

Spigland N, Brandt ML, Yazbeck S. Malrotation presenting beyond the neonatal period. *J Pediatr Surg* 1990;25:1139–1142.

Hernias

Brandt ML. Pediatric hernias. *Surg Clin North Am* 2008;88:27–43, vii-viii.

Chen LE, Zamakhshary M, Foglia RP, et al. Impact of wait time on outcome for inguinal hernia repair in infants. *Pediatr Surg Int* 2009;25:223–227.

Erez I, Rathause V, Vacian I, et al. Preoperative ultrasound and intraoperative findings of inguinal hernias in children: a prospective study of 642 children. *J Pediatr Surg* 2002;37:865–868.

Gill FT. Umbilical hernia, inguinal hernias, and hydroceles in children: diagnostic clues for optimal patient management. *J Pediatr Health Care* 1998;12:231–235.

Graf JL, Caty MG, Martin DJ, et al. Pediatric hernias. *Semin Ultrasound CT MR* 2002;23:197–200.

McCollough M, Sharieff GQ. Abdominal pain in children. *Pediatr Clin North Am* 2006;53:107–137, vi.

Myers JB, Lovell MA, Lee RS, et al. Torsion of an indirect hernia sac causing acute scrotum. *J Pediatr Surg* 2004;39:122–123.

Sheldon CA. The pediatric genitourinary examination. Inguinal, urethral, and genital diseases. *Pediatr Clin North Am* 2001;48:1339–1380.

Intraabdominal Masses

Golden CB, Feusner JH. Malignant abdominal masses in children: quick guide to evaluation and diagnosis. *Pediatr Clin North Am* 2002;49:1369–1392, viii.

Islam S, Yamout SZ, Gosche JR. Management and outcomes of ovarian masses in children and adolescents. *Am Surg* 2008;74:1062–1065.

Waldhausen JH, Tapper D, Sawin RS. Minimally invasive surgery and clinical decision-making for pediatric malignancy. *Surg Endosc* 2000;14:250–253.

Foreign Bodies In The Gastrointestinal Tract

Dokler ML, Bradshaw J, Mollitt DL, et al. Selective management of pediatric esophageal foreign bodies. *Am Surg* 1995;61:132–134.

Kay M, Wyllie R. Pediatric foreign bodies and their management. *Curr Gastroenterol Rep* 2005;7:212–218.

Macpherson RI, Hill JG, Othersen HB, et al. Esophageal foreign bodies in children: diagnosis, treatment, and complications. *AJR Am J Roentgenol* 1996;166:919–924.

Wildhaber BE, Le Coultre C, Genin B. Ingestion of magnets: innocent in solitude, harmful in groups. *J Pediatr Surg* 2005;40:e33–e35.

CHAPTER 122 ■ DENTAL EMERGENCIES

LINDA P. NELSON, DMD, MSCD, AND STEPHEN SHUSTERMAN, DMD

Nontraumatic orofacial emergencies can appear suddenly and are frightening for children and their families. The major task in evaluating a child with a nontraumatic orofacial emergency is to identify the cause of the problem. In cases of facial swellings, the first step in treatment is determining whether a tooth is the causative agent. In cases of postextraction complications, historical information suggesting a preextraction infection, fractured tooth, or overlying chronic systemic problem may be elicited. Therefore, initial assessments must be performed in the same manner as traumatic orofacial emergencies (see Chapter 109).

POSTEXTRACTION COMPLICATIONS

Hemorrhage

It is expected that any extraction site may ooze for 8 to 12 hours and perhaps longer for a permanent site. However, it is important to check the history for any prior bleeding episodes to rule out a systemic hematologic abnormality. If there is a concern for abnormally prolonged bleeding, a complete blood cell count and coagulation profile would be indicated.

Emergency treatment may include the following steps:

1. Apply pressure, using folded gauze sponges that are placed over the socket with biting pressure applied directly on the site for 30 minutes. If unsuccessful, proceed to step 2.
2. Physically close the socket by suturing. Administer local anesthesia (2% lidocaine with 1:100,000 epinephrine infiltration), and approximate the extraction site with the appropriate sutures. Alternatively, the socket may be packed with Gelfoam®.

A possible home remedy before coming to the emergency department (ED) might include the use of a tea bag. A tea bag is dipped in hot water and allowed to cool, then placed over the socket with pressure. The tannic acid in the tea bag may initiate or accelerate coagulation.

Infection

Postextraction infection is rare in children. If it occurs, it may present as localized swelling or edema surrounded by an erythematous zone. A purulent exudate may be evident from the socket. Emergency treatment includes the application of moist heat, oral saline rinses (if the age is appropriate), and antibiotic therapy. Amoxicillin or Augmentin© (amoxicillin with clavulanate potassium) is the drug of choice. (See the "Dentoalveolar Abscess" section for dose and duration.)

Alveolar Osteitis

Alveolar osteitis, or *dry socket*, is a painful postoperative condition produced by a disintegration of the clot in the tooth socket. This condition usually is seen in adults and only rarely in children younger than 12 years. It generally occurs approximately 72 hours after mandibular extractions and is painful. Emergency dental treatment is variable, but the immediate goal is relief of pain. Under local anesthesia, the socket may be debrided and then packed with ¼-in. iodoform gauze or BIPP (bismuth, iodoform, paraffin) paste. Oral analgesic and antiinflammatory (NSAID) medications should be prescribed for pain. Since it is an osteitis, antibiotics should only be used if there is evidence of infection.

ORAL INFECTIONS

In a retrospective analysis of pediatric dental patients presenting to the ED and dental clinics, toothaches, pain, and facial swellings accounted for 44% of the chief complaints. This is consistent with other studies. It is important to remember that the infant or small child who may be in pain often cannot localize the discomfort. It may be the first opportunity for many children to receive dental care. A complete history from the parents and a thorough oral examination are mandatory. Figure 122.1 shows a diagram of the normal tooth.

Odontalgia—Simple Toothache

The child with a simple toothache often complains of diffuse mouth pain and may not be able to identify a specific tooth. Children often cannot distinguish between tooth pain and soft-tissue pain from a lesion such as an aphthous ulcer. A careful intraoral examination should be preformed to identify the true source of the discomfort. The emergency physician may note a grossly carious tooth or large restoration. Swelling or inflammation in the surrounding soft tissue may be present. The tooth may be sensitive to percussion and may exhibit excessive mobility. A dental consultation is necessary, especially if swelling is noted. In the case of swelling, the tooth may be opened for drainage to relieve the pressure, in a manner similar to the management of any abscess.

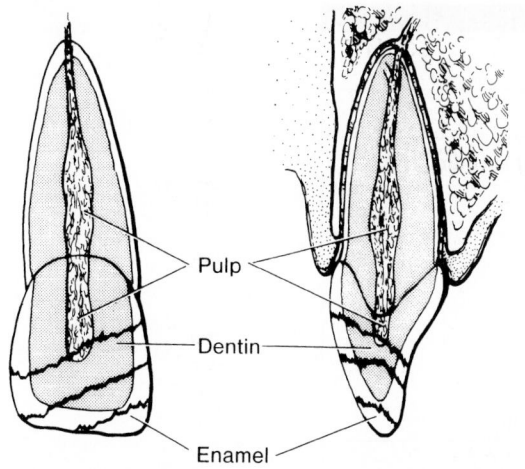

FIGURE 122.1 The anatomy of a tooth that should be considered during a traumatic injury. Enamel fracture, no emergency treatment; dentin fracture, emergency treatment as soon as convenient; and pulpal fracture, emergency treatment as soon as possible.

Dentoalveolar Abscess

Dental abscesses are common in children because of the morphologic characteristic of the primary tooth and immature permanent tooth. In the dentoalveolar abscess, the causative factors are gross or recurrent decay, trauma, or perhaps, chronic irritation from a large restoration. If there is an acute pulpitis, there may be severe pain and swelling, but other symptoms, such as mobility or purulence, may not be present. Establishing drainage through the tooth or soft tissue is key to relief of the symptoms, but antibiotics and/or analgesics may also be necessary. If the infection is long standing, suppuration is usually confined to the bone around the tooth. The swelling can perforate the thin buccal bony plate adjacent to the root of the involved tooth and spread into the subperiosteal area and then to the surrounding soft tissues. In a child, the dentoalveolar abscess usually perforates the buccal plate of bone because of the position of the tooth and the thinness of the overlying bone. If it does not drain intraorally, the infection can spread rapidly through the fascial planes of the face or neck.

The following are clinical manifestations of a dentoalveolar abscess in a child:

- Pain: The tooth may be painful to percussion or may exhibit spontaneous painful episodes.
- Mobility: The tooth may have a more than the normal degree of movement in the socket when palpated.
- Swelling: The soft tissues surrounding the tooth may be edematous and erythematous.
- Temperature elevation: The child may be febrile [temperature higher than 37.5°C (99.5°F)], have general malaise, and have a decrease in appetite.
- Fistulous tracts: These appear clinically as a pustule-like lesion on the gingiva (rarely on the face) when the infection has been present for a long time.

- Extrusion: The tooth may become extruded because of the presence of fluid in the periradicular space.
- Lymphadenopathy: Major lymph node enlargement can occur at any time during the infective process.

The first step in treating a perioral abscess is to determine whether a tooth is the causative agent. This can be accomplished by clinical examination and available radiographs. Corroboration of dental origin can be established by reviewing intraoral radiographs with a dentist. A computed tomography (CT) scan with contrast will enhance the visualization of a dental abscess. If the child is febrile, a blood culture should be obtained, although it may not yield a definitive microorganism. The location and extent of any swelling and/or fistulous tracts, whether intraorally or extraorally, should be noted.

It is important that the treatment of choice for a localized dentoalveolar abscess is local in its focus (e.g., drainage, moist heat). In cases of facial cellulitis with lymphadenopathy caused by acute dentoalveolar abscess, the antibiotic of choice is Augmentin® (amoxicillin with clavulanate potassium), or alternatively clindamycin if there is a known allergy to penicillin derivatives. The initial dose of Augmentin® is 25 mg of amoxicillin/kg/dose orally three times a day, rounding to the nearest 250 mg increment in older children.

Penicillin-sensitive streptococci and anaerobic organisms predominate as the cause of acute dentoalveolar abscesses. If there is facial cellulitis over the maxilla extending toward the inferior border of the orbital rim or if there is mandibular cellulitis, which might be a potential cause of airway compromise, the child may be admitted to the hospital where intravenous antibiotic therapy can be managed. Treatment for facial cellulitis is covered in Chapter 92.

Other factors to consider in determining the need for hospital admission include the child's ability to take fluids and the likelihood of the parent's cooperation for follow-up dental care. Obviously, if the child has signs of sepsis, a hospital admission is indicated. In addition to antibiotics, warm oral saline rinses should be used. Heat should be applied extraorally. There is some concern that extraoral heat will cause the abscess to point extraorally and thus produce an exterior fistula. This has not proven true in our experience. Mild analgesic therapy such as acetaminophen is usually sufficient. Dental consultation should be obtained to vent the offending tooth, to establish drainage, to incise a fluctuant mass, or to remove the tooth.

As with infection elsewhere in the body, the basic surgical principles of treatment must be used to establish drainage and remove the cause. An abscessed primary tooth must be vigorously treated because such infections can affect the developing unerupted permanent tooth bud. A facial cellulitis can have severe systemic consequences, including cavernous sinus thrombosis, airway obstruction, meningitis, orbital cellulitis, and septicemia.

In some cases, there may be a need for additional consultation with infectious disease experts, especially in a situation in which systemic disorders render the child more susceptible to infection.

TABLE 122.1

ERUPTION SCHEDULE FOR SPECIFIC TEETH

A. Primary teeth				
	Age at eruption (mo)		Age at shedding (yr)	
	Lower	Upper	Lower	Upper
Central incisor	6	7½	6	7½
Lateral incisor	7	9	7	8
Cuspid	16	18	9½	11½
First molar	12	14	10	10½
Second molar	20	24	11	10½
Incisors	Range ±2 mo			
Molars	Range ±4 mo		Range ±6 mo	

B. Permanent teeth[a]		
	Age (yr)	
	Lower	Upper
Central incisors	6–7	7–8
Lateral incisors	7–8	8–9
Cuspids	9–10	11–12
First bicuspids	10–12	10–11
Second bicuspids	11–12	10–12
First molars	6–7	6–7
Second molars	11–13	12–13
Third molars	17–21	17–21

[a]The lower teeth erupt before the corresponding upper teeth. The teeth usually erupt earlier in girls than in boys.
(Modified with permission from Massler M, Schour I. *Atlas of the mouth and adjacent parts in health and disease.* Chicago, IL: The Bureau of Public Relations Council on Dental Health, American Dental Association, 1946.)

Pericoronitis

Pericoronitis is a localized infection surrounding an erupting tooth. It is usually associated with erupting molars in the adolescent patient, although a mild form may be associated with the eruption of the first permanent molar at age 6 (Table 122.1). Symptoms usually include pain distal to the last erupted tooth in the dental arch, along with erythema and edema localized to the gingiva in the retromolar area. Lymphadenopathy, trismus, and dysphagia may accompany these symptoms. An elevated body temperature is an occasional finding. It is not unusual to see or palpate the cusps of the erupting tooth. The patient may complain of an inability to completely close his or her mouth because of the edematous gingiva. Otalgia is an uncommon complaint.

Emergency treatment includes local curettage, oral rinses, heat, and scrupulous oral hygiene. Amoxicillin or Augmentin® may be necessary (for dose, see "Dentoalveolar Abscess" section) when there are systemic symptoms of infection or facial swelling.

Primary Herpetic Gingivostomatitis or Herpes Simplex Virus Type 1

Primary herpetic gingivostomatitis, or herpes simplex virus type 1, is a communicable childhood disease that is not a true dental emergency but is a common cause of ED visits. The child is usually an infant or toddler who stops eating, drinking, or talking and is extremely irritable. The child usually has had an elevated temperature for 3 to 5 days before any clinical oral findings. A higher incidence of primary herpes has been noted after other viral illnesses. Older children may complain of headaches, malaise, nausea, regional lymphadenopathy, and/or bleeding gums. The physical examination reveals fiery red marginal gingiva with areas of spontaneous hemorrhage. Within 1 or 2 days, yellowish, fluid-filled vesicles develop on the mucosa, palate, lips, or tongue and coalesce. The vesicles may coalesce or rupture spontaneously, leaving extremely painful ulcers, covered by a yellow or gray membrane and surrounded by an erythematous zone. Ulcers, especially on the lips, may become encrusted, as seen in Fig. 122.2.

If necessary, a definitive diagnosis can be made by isolation of the herpes simplex virus in tissue culture (although this is rarely indicated). Emergency treatment includes reassuring the parent and rehydrating the patient. The disease, like recurrent herpes labialis, is self-limiting, with a duration of 7 to 14 days. Dehydration and weight loss are the major concerns; therefore, high-calorie and high-protein shakes, ice cream, and liberal quantities of clear fluids should be encouraged. The young child with extensive lesions may require hospitalization for intravenous hydration.

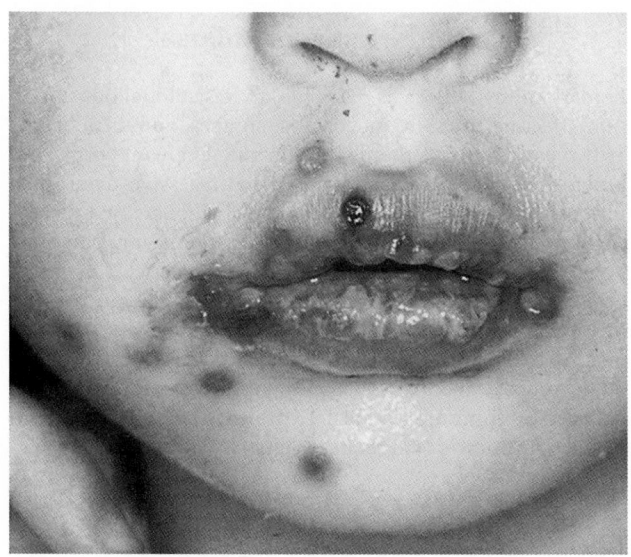

FIGURE 122.2 A child with typical crusted extraoral lesions of late primary gingivostomatitis.

Viscous lidocaine rinses and "magic mouthwash," Maalox® and Benadryl® with or without lidocaine combinations, may be helpful but may be unrealistic for children in this age range. The unpleasant taste sometimes makes administration difficult, therefore negating any benefit that the child may receive. If using lidocaine do not exceed 3 mg/kg/dose and do not give any more frequently than every 3 hours.

Secondary infection, although rare, is of concern for those children who may be immunosuppressed, and in those cases, antibiotic therapy may be indicated.

Acute Necrotizing Ulcerative Gingivitis, Vincent's Disease, Trench Mouth

Acute necrotizing ulcerative gingivitis (ANUG), Vincent's disease, or trench mouth is characterized by increases in the fusiform bacillus and *Borrelia vincentii*, a spirochete, which usually coexist in a symbiotic relationship with other oral flora. Adolescents complain of soreness and point tenderness at the gingiva and often tell the physician that they feel as if

they "cannot remove a piece of food that is painfully stuck between their teeth" (a wedging sensation). They may also complain of a metallic taste in their mouth and bleeding gums. Upon examination, the breath has an obvious fetid odor. The gingivae are hyperemic, and the usually triangular gingiva between the teeth is missing or "punched out" (Fig. 122.3). Intense pain is produced with probing, and a gray, necrotic pseudomembrane may cover some areas of gingiva.

It is extremely rare to find ANUG in a young child, but a mistaken diagnosis is often made by physicians, confusing this disease with primary herpetic gingivostomatitis. Primary herpes is usually seen in infants and toddlers, and ANUG is characteristically seen in adolescents and young adults (ages 15 to 35 years). Emotional stress has been linked to the onset of the disease process, as have malnutrition, severe dehydration, poor oral hygiene, immunodeficiency disorders, especially acquired immunodeficiency syndrome (AIDS), and infectious mononucleosis. The adolescent should be advised to maintain better oral hygiene, rest and reduce stress, and use oral rinses such as Peridex® (0.12% chlorhexidine). Hydrogen peroxide, diluted 1:1 with warm water, may alternatively be used as often as possible throughout the acute phase. Because of the rapidity of tissue destruction and sensitivity of the organisms, as well as risk of secondary infection, penicillin, metronidazole, tetracycline, or erythromycin should be prescribed for the first week, especially in the presence of fever or lymphadenopathy. When the acute phase is over, the patient should be sent to the dentist for a thorough debridement of the area. If the patient is resistant to therapy, a thorough workup of the underlying causes of immunosuppression is indicated, because of the relationship of ANUG and immunosuppression.

ORAL AND PERIORAL PATHOLOGY PRESENTING AS DENTAL EMERGENCIES

Aphthous Stomatitis

Aphthous stomatitis is the most common disease of the oral mucosa and may affect 20% or more of the population. These painful, shallow, circular ulcerations are distinctive because of their size (2 to 4 mm), distribution, and recurrence. Clinically,

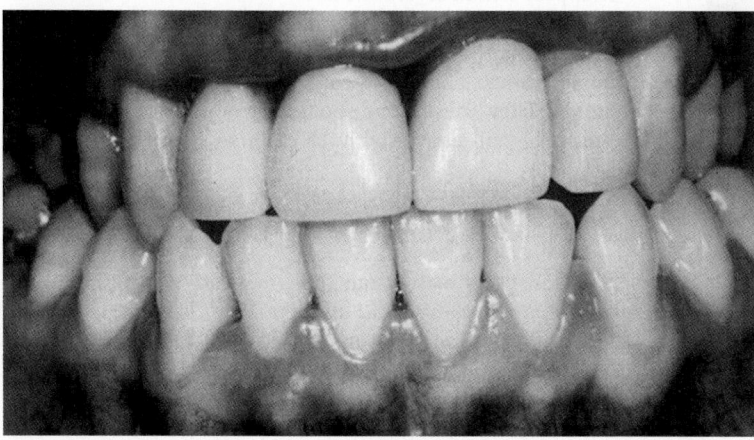

FIGURE 122.3 A child with typical "punched out" gingiva—pathognomonic for acute necrotizing ulcerative gingivitis. (Courtesy of Dr. Mark Snyder.)

the floor of the ulceration is yellowish, with a sharply defined red margin. Aphthae affect only nonkeratinized areas of the mouth, such as the tongue, cheek, or vestibule. If the hard palate or gingival margins are affected, it is unlikely to be aphthae. Recurrent aphthae often start in childhood or adolescence. In young children, there is a syndrome of recurring aphthous ulcers and periodic fevers. They peak in early adult life and then seem to spontaneously resolve. Recurrent aphthae usually occur during periods of anxiety, such as during final examinations at school or during domestic disturbances. The ulcerations may appear singly or in clusters. They are usually painful and tender, have a clinical course of 10 to 14 days, and often cause difficulties with eating. Treatment is largely empirical and also usually unsatisfactory. Drugs used in the management of aphthae have included topical local analgesics, such as lidocaine gel or benzocaine oral emollient (Orabase® with benzocaine), which allow the patient to eat in some degree of comfort. Due to the risk of methemoglobinemia secondary to benzocaine toxicity, Orabase® should not be used for more than 2 days in children < 2 years of age. Bland nonacidic diets to avoid further irritation may be the best recommendation.

Erythema Multiforme

Erythema multiforme is primarily a dermatologic disease characterized by macular, papular, vesicular, or bullous lesions on the skin or oral mucosa (Fig. 122.4). The lips may appear crusted, as in primary herpes. Lesions arise from an erythematous area that enlarges and develops a central vesicle or "target lesion." Oral lesions arise at about the same time as skin lesions and are also variable in their clinical appearance, producing painful, bleeding, crusting erosions. These symptoms may occur as an acute drug reaction but can be precipitated by herpes simplex. Stevens–Johnson syndrome is a more disseminated form of erythema multiforme in which conjunctival and genital lesions are seen concomitant with the oral and cutaneous lesions (see Chapter 99). Identifying and eliminating the precipitating drug is the first step in treatment. Immediate care may include caloric and fluid support. Steroids may be of help in severe cases.

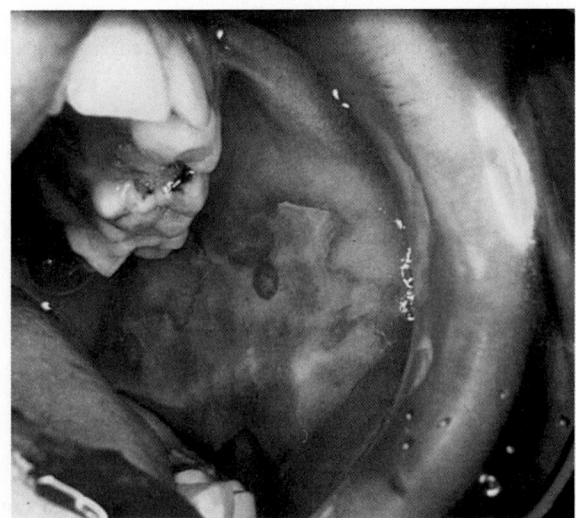

FIGURE 122.4 Intraoral view of erythema multiforme.

Epidermolysis Bullosa

Epidermolysis bullosa is a hereditary vesiculobullous condition affecting the skin, mucous membranes, and teeth. There are several forms of the disease. In the dominant form, oral bullae have been documented. In the recessive dystrophic form, the teeth have hypoplastic enamel, an increased susceptibility to dental caries, and delayed eruption. Oral mucosal involvement appears soon after birth with vesicles from the negative pressure of the sucking reflex. The labial mucosa and lips can appear scarred and taut. Even routine dental management such as toothbrushing may cause the eruption of bullae on the mucosa and lips. Emergency visits may result from pain or bleeding from oral lesions. Treatment should palliate pain and support nutritional requirements.

Pyogenic Granuloma

Pyogenic granulomas develop as granulation tissue in response to an irritant or trauma. Clinically, they are red, elevated, and usually ulcerated. Initial growth is rapid. Pyogenic granulomas are most common on the gingivae and may remain static for a time before becoming fibrotic. Treatment consists of simple excision, but recurrence is common unless the causative agent (calculus or foreign body) is removed.

Neonatal Cysts

Epstein's pearls are keratin-filled cystic lesions located along the midpalatine raphe in the newborn. They appear as round or ovoid, white, raised nodules. Often, only a few can be visualized, but sometimes there are too many to count. They are believed to arise from embryologically trapped epithelium. They are present in about 80% of neonates and should be considered a variation of normal. No treatment is necessary because they disappear within several weeks.

Bohn's nodules are remnants of the dental lamina that appear as cysts on the buccal or lingual aspect of the maxillary and mandibular dental ridges in the newborn. They may appear in the palate but are far removed from the midpalatine raphe. Although similar in shape and color, they are located differently and should not be confused with Epstein's pearls. No treatment is necessary because they, too, are normal and disappear within several weeks.

Dental lamina cysts are multiple, or occasionally solitary, nodules on the alveolar ridge of newborn (Fig. 122.5) or young infants. They represent trapped remnants of the dental lamina. They are soft and spongy, asymptomatic, and tend to disappear with time or with the eruption of teeth.

Eruption Cysts

Eruption cysts arise from the preeruptive dental sac and appear as a swelling of the alveolar ridge. They are associated with the eruption of primary (Fig. 122.6) and permanent teeth. Occasionally, they fill with blood and may be termed *eruption hematomas* (Fig. 122.7). Treatment is unnecessary because the erupting tooth usually emerges within several

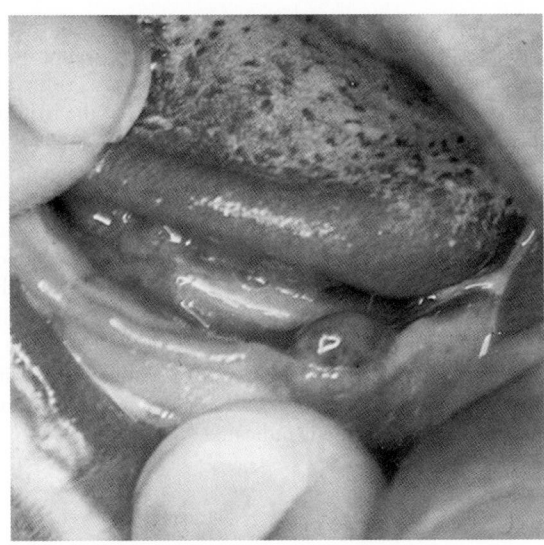

FIGURE 122.5 Dental lamina cyst in a neonate.

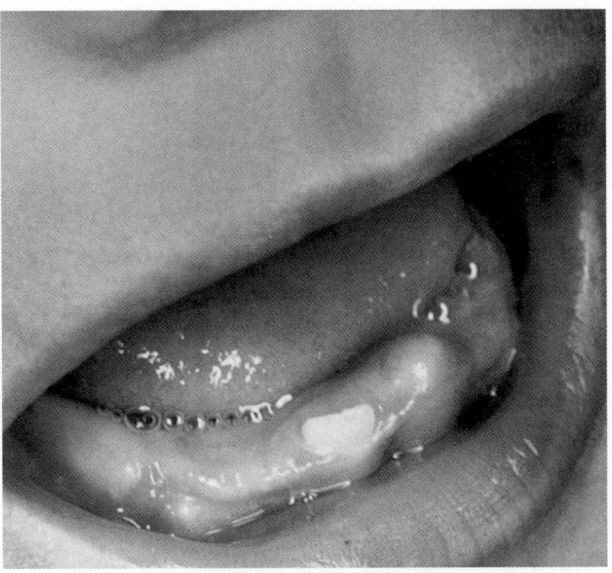

FIGURE 122.6 An eruption cyst associated with an erupting primary central incisor.

days. If treatment is necessary because of the size of the lesion, excision of the overlying soft tissue to expose the erupting tooth eliminates the problem.

Riga-Fede Disease/Natal or Neonatal Teeth

Riga-Fede disease is a condition observed in infants with natal or neonatal teeth. It is characterized by ulcerations on the ventral surface of the tongue from irritation caused by the incisal edges of lower incisors during nursing or suckling. Treatment should be avoided, but the incisal edge of the erupting teeth can be smoothed off in the dental office if there is bleeding and pain associated with the lesion. In very severe cases, extraction may be necessary if the natal or neonatal teeth interferes with feeding. Natal or neonatal teeth in general should be removed only when they interfere with feeding or represent a danger of aspiration.

Orofacial Neoplasms

Orofacial neoplasms in children are rare. Some benign and malignant neoplasms may result in emergency visits and, therefore, are included. Identification is central to the triage process.

The oral papilloma is a benign epithelial neoplasm that is an exophytic elevation of the surface epithelium with small fingerlike projections from its surface. These lesions, which rarely become malignant, constitute about 8% of all oral neoplasms in children. Slightly more than one-third of the lesions occur on the tongue and (in decreasing order of frequency) palate, buccal mucosa, gingiva, and lip. If spontaneous involution does not occur, the usual treatment is surgical removal.

The fibroma is a common smooth-surfaced lesion with a sessile base. Its consistency varies from soft to firm, and its size ranges from a few millimeters to a centimeter or more in diameter. It may become whitened secondary to the overlying

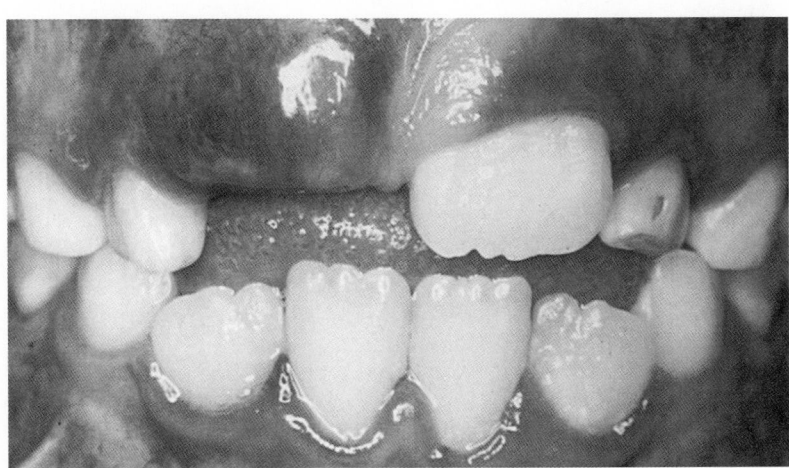

FIGURE 122.7 Erupting hematoma over erupting maxillary permanent central incisor.

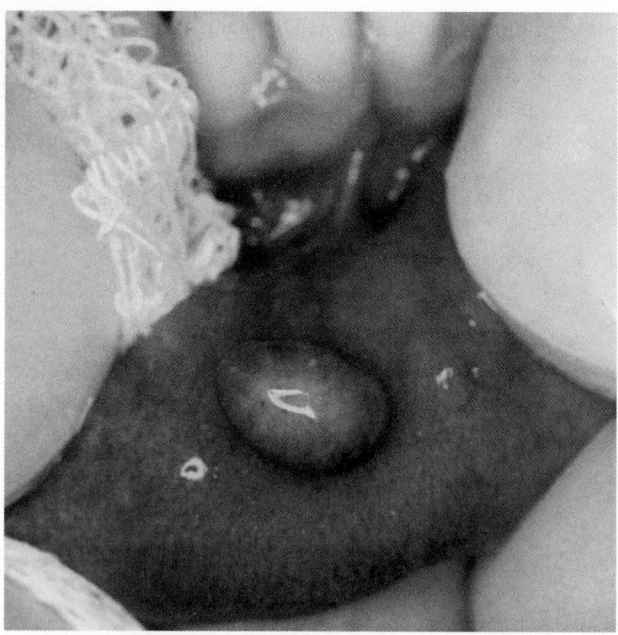

FIGURE 122.8 Mucocele associated with minor salivary gland of the lower lip.

hyperkeratosis caused by trauma. Fibromas occur during the first and second decades of life and are usually found on the palate, tongue, cheek, and lip. Surgical removal is sometimes indicated, and recurrence is rare if the source of the irritation is removed.

The mucocele appears as a soft, raised, fluid-filled, and well-delineated nodule, most commonly on the lower lip or the mucosal lining of the lower lip (Fig. 122.8). Superficial lesions appear translucent and are bluish, whereas deep-seated lesions have a normal color. A mucocele in the floor of the mouth is termed a *ranula* and is seen as a dome-shaped, fluid-filled lesion. Mucoceles are believed to result from severance or obstruction of a salivary gland duct, with pooling of mucin in the lamina propria. Complete excision of the mucocele or marsupialization of the ranula is indicated.

Suggested Readings

Cawson R, Binnie W, Barrett A, et al. *Oral disease*, 3rd ed. Edinburgh, United Kingdom: Mosby, 2001.
Kaban L, Troulis M. *Pediatric oral and maxillofacial surgery.* Philadelphia, PA: WB Saunders, 2004.

CHAPTER 123 ■ OTOLARYNGOLOGIC EMERGENCIES

LISA M. ELDEN, MD, CM, AND WILLIAM P. POTSIC, MD, MMM

The ear, nose, and throat are common sites for infection and neoplasms and may be the sources of acute pain. Although the diseases prompting the emergency department (ED) visit may be distressing to the patient and cause considerable anxiety for the parents, they are rarely life threatening. This chapter includes discussion of disorders of the ear, nose, nasal sinuses, oral cavity, pharynx, esophagus, larynx, trachea, and neck.

EAR

Methods of Examination

The equipment necessary to properly evaluate the head and neck in an ED should include an otoscope with a pneumatic insufflator, wax loop (curette), illuminated headlight, and otologic forceps.

Examination of the ear begins by inspection of the auricle and surrounding areas. The external meatus should be visualized directly with a bright light after it is fully opened by pulling the pinna posteriorly and superiorly. The tragus may be displaced forward by traction on the skin in front of the ear with the examiner's other hand (Fig. 123.1). The ear canal can then be examined with a pneumatic otoscope, using the largest speculum that will fit in the meatus without discomfort. Wax or debris occluding the ear canal should be removed with a curette or by repeated irrigation with body temperature water (see Procedure 5.3 in Section VII). Irrigation of the canal should not be performed if a ventilating tube is in place or if a perforation of the tympanic membrane (TM) is suspected.

The TM should be evaluated for its appearance, and part of the middle ear contents can usually be seen if the eardrum is translucent (Fig. 123.2). Mobility should be evaluated with the pneumatic otoscope because the accuracy of diagnosing middle ear pathology increases greatly when mobility is assessed by pneumatic otoscopy compared with observation alone. Pneumatic otoscopy is performed by applying positive and negative pressure to the TM, with the pneumatic otoscope fitted snugly into the ear canal. The pressure applied to the ear can be varied by squeezing a rubber bulb (see Procedure 5.1 in Section VII). Middle ear effusion is more likely to be present if the TM fails to move with this technique. The use of tympanometry may be helpful in instances when the clinician cannot assess mobility with a pneumatic otoscope. The test is most useful in excluding the disease because the presence of a normal type A tympanogram (peaked curve at zero pressure) is 90% to 95% sensitive and specific in predicting absence of middle ear effusion. Alternatively, a B type tympanogram (flat tracing), which occurs when there is absence of TM move-

ment, is less accurate in predicting the presence of fluid in the ear with a sensitivity of 81% and specificity of 74%.

The ear of a neonate requires special attention to perform an adequate otologic examination. The ear canal itself is narrow and collapsible. Often, only the otoscopic speculum can be inserted, as positive pressure from the pneumatic bulb is used to distend the canal ahead of the advancing speculum. The canal may be filled with vernix caseosa, which must be removed or irrigated out of the canal to permit visualization of the TM. The neonate's TM lies at a more oblique angle to the ear canal (compared with older children) and may make recognition of the TM and its landmarks more difficult. Amniotic fluid may be present in the middle ear cavity for days to weeks after birth and should not be confused with middle ear infection unless other symptoms such as fever and irritability are present.

In older children, crude hearing acuity can be tested with a ticking watch or a 512-Hz tuning fork. The sound should be heard equally in each ear. However, this does not rule out a symmetric bilateral hearing deficit. If the tuning fork is applied to the forehead, it should be heard equally in both ears. If it is heard only in one ear, it signifies either a conductive loss in the ear that hears the tone or a sensorineural hearing loss (SNHL) in the opposite ear. Audiometry (behavioral) is required for an accurate evaluation of hearing at all frequencies. Auditory brainstem response testing is helpful for a child who cannot cooperate with behavioral testing.

Infections

Acute Otitis Media

Apart from viral infections of the upper respiratory tract, acute otitis media (AOM) is the most common head and neck infection in children and is the second most common diagnosis made in the ED. It may occur as an isolated infection or as a complication of an upper respiratory tract infection. Risk factors that make children more susceptible to recurrent AOM include the presence of otitis media with effusion (OME), which is noninfected fluid in the middle ear (also called serous otitis media or secretory otitis media), day care attendance, exposure to secondhand smoke, and immunodeficiency states.

The more common organisms causing acute otitis at all ages are *Streptococcus pneumoniae*, *Haemophilus influenzae*, and *Moraxella catarrhalis*, and less commonly, group A β-hemolytic streptococci and various upper respiratory viruses. Gram-negative organisms may occur in hospitalized patients who are younger than 8 weeks or immunosuppressed.

Clinical Manifestations. Over the last decade, The American Academy of Pediatrics (AAP) and the Joint Committee of

1545

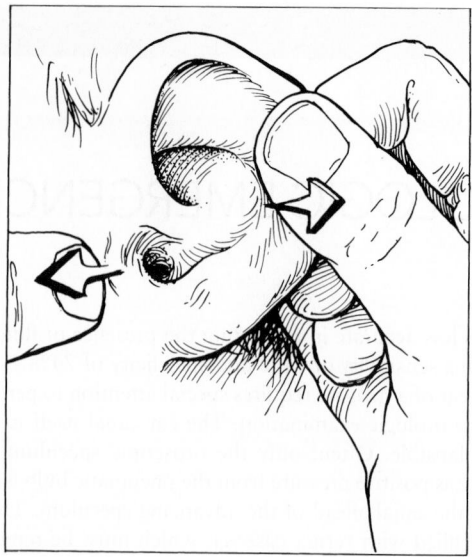

FIGURE 123.1 The external meatus is opened by pulling the auricle in the posterior superior direction and placing traction on the skin immediately in front of the tragus.

American Academy of Family Practitioners (AAFP) have developed guidelines to improve accuracy of diagnosis of AOM. Based on the best available evidence in the literature, three components should be present to diagnose AOM.

1. History of acute onset of symptoms within 48 hours of presentation.
2. Presence of middle ear effusion confirmed by pneumatic otoscopy (or tympanometry).
3. Signs of middle ear inflammation.

AOM should be suspected in any child who is irritable or lethargic, has a low-grade fever, and has localized pain in the ear. The pain develops rapidly and is often severe. Spontaneous perforation of the TM with serosanguineous drainage may occur in less than 1 hour after the onset of pain. On examination, the TM is hyperemic and mobility is decreased. The strongest predictor of AOM is the presence of a bulging TM that obliterates normal landmarks, whereas redness is least helpful in predicting the disease. Infection with *Mycoplasma pneumoniae* and other bacteria may cause blebs on the lateral surface of the drum. The vesicles of bullous myringitis are filled with clear fluid and are painful. The appearance of the TM in AOM secondary to bacterial pathogens does not differ significantly from AOM of viral etiology.

Complications.   The following complications of AOM may be encountered in the ED:

1. The purulent exudate that fills the middle ear space causes a conductive hearing loss. The congealed exudate may organize and stimulate hyalinization and calcification, leading to myringosclerosis (white patches within the TM) and sometimes tympanosclerosis (white deposits in the middle ear).
2. Spontaneous perforation of the TM usually produces a small hole that heals rapidly; however, large perforations may occur that do not heal even after the infection has cleared.
3. Ossicular necrosis may also occur in children who have had AOM or OME and can cause a persistent conductive hearing loss. The distal tip of the incus is most susceptible to erosion that can cause eventual disconnection of the incus from the stapes, resulting in conductive hearing loss.
4. As the TM heals after a perforation, skin from the lateral surface of the TM may be trapped in the middle ear to form

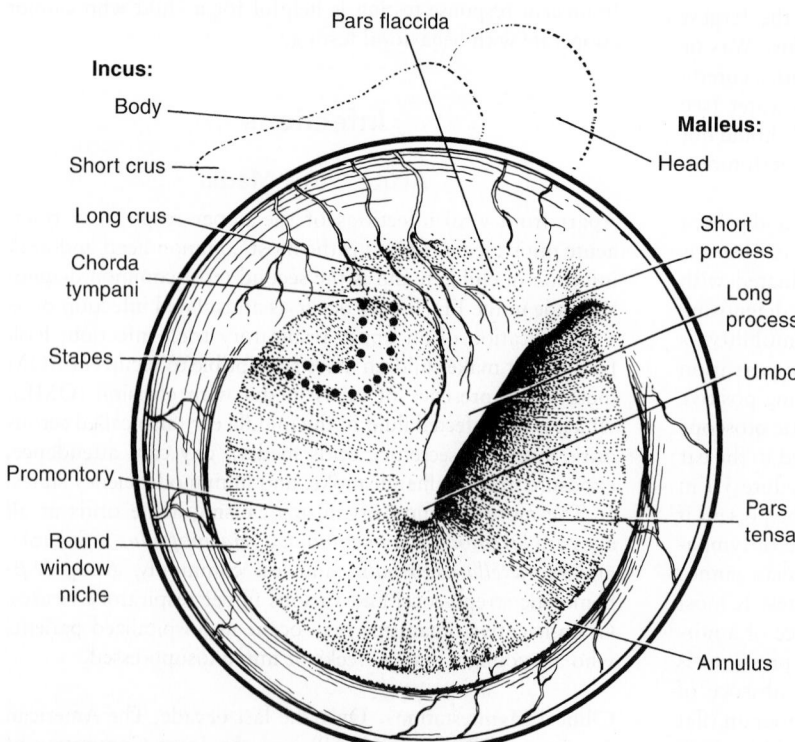

FIGURE 123.2 Right tympanic membrane.

a cyst (cholesteatoma) that can expand and destroy the structures of the middle ear and surrounding bone.

5. Facial nerve paralysis may occur suddenly during AOM. The nerve paralysis may be partial or complete when the child is first examined. The facial nerve usually recovers complete function if appropriate systemic [intravenous (IV) followed by oral] antibiotic therapy is administered and a wide myringotomy with or without tube placement for drainage is carried out as soon as possible.

6. AOM may cause inflammation in the inner ear (serous labyrinthitis). This causes mild to moderate vertigo without a sensorineural hearing loss.

7. Bacterial invasion of the inner ear (suppurative labyrinthitis) causes severe sensorineural hearing loss and severe vertigo that is usually associated with nausea and vomiting. Early treatment with IV antibiotics and wide myringotomy with tube placement may prevent permanent inner ear damage.

8. Suppurative mastoiditis (acute coalescent mastoid osteomyelitis) may develop, causing destruction of the mastoid air cell system. Temporal bone computed tomographic (CT) scans are helpful in differentiating otitis media from mastoiditis. Patients with otitis media or mastoiditis have opacified mastoid air cells when disease is present, but those with mastoiditis also have radiographic evidence of erosion of the mastoid air cells creating larger opacified spaces. As the infection spreads to the postauricular tissues, subperiosteal collection of purulent material displaces the auricle laterally and downward from its normal position. The pus may extend through air cells to the medial portion of the temporal bone, causing sixth cranial nerve paralysis, deep retroorbital pain, and otorrhea (Gradenigo's syndrome). Pus may also break through the mastoid tip and extend into the upper neck (Bezold abscess).

9. The most common intracranial problem associated with AOM is meningitis, which may cause severe sensorineural deafness and irreversible vestibular damage. Less commonly associated problems are cerebritis, epidural abscess, brain abscess, lateral sinus thrombosis, and otitic hydrocephalus. The child with overt or impending intracranial complications should be stabilized, be given IV antibiotics, and have a CT scan with contrast or magnetic resonance imaging (MRI) scan performed.

Children who are younger than 6 years with SNHL who have cochlear implants are 30 times more likely to develop pneumococcal meningitis than are age-matched cohorts without SNHL. This increased risk of meningitis may be caused by the presence of the implant that can act as a pathway for spread of infection into the meninges in children who develop ear infections or because other inner ear malformations coexist in these patients that may allow bacteria to spread to the brain. However, the majority of meningitis in children is a result of bloodborne bacterial seeding of cerebrospinal fluid. The Centers for Disease Control and Prevention recommends that age-appropriate pneumococcal vaccinations be given to all children to prevent the occurrence of meningitis.

Management. Antibiotics prescribed for AOM account for 25% to 50% of all outpatient antibiotics and are partly responsible for the global finding that bacteria, especially *S. pneumoniae*, *H. influenzae*, and *M. catarrhalis*, are becoming increasingly resistant to these medications. As such, expert panels and various medical societies have been forced to examine the benefits and choice of antibiotics used for this disease. The AAP/AAFP guidelines stress the need to improve accuracy of diagnosis to use antibiotics judiciously in treating AOM. Using the best available literature, including randomized clinical trials and cohort studies of patients with suspected AOM treated with antibiotics versus those treated with observation, the AAP/AAFP panel concluded that 80% of children who were not treated with antibiotics had spontaneous resolution of symptoms within a 2- to 7-day onset of symptoms. With this information, the panel suggested that a period of observation might be appropriate for otherwise healthy patients with AOM. However, very young children, those with immune, genetic, or craniofacial anomalies, known or underlying OME, or recent AOM in the previous 30 days should not be considered candidates for this option because they are more likely to suffer adverse consequences from observation alone. The panel also specified that the observation option must be used only if there is a high probability that the parent will be compliant in returning for evaluation if symptoms of AOM persist over the next 72 hours. Specifically, any patient younger than 6 months should be treated with antibiotic even when the diagnosis of AOM is uncertain. The observation option is recommended for children 6 months to 2 years of age whose baseline health is good, who are not seriously ill at presentation, and who have an uncertain diagnosis. The option of observation is available for children older than 2 years, with nonsevere illness at presentation with or without a certain diagnosis (Table 123.1). In prospective studies, 25% of those children did eventually require antibiotic upon follow-up within 48 to 72 hours. With regard to follow-up, the guideline suggests that the observed patients be contacted or seen within 72 hours so that they may be treated if symptoms persist. Other authors have advocated writing a "safety net prescription" to be given to parents of children who are observed at the time of the initial assessment with instructions to fill it if symptoms persist. Children with persistent OME lasting longer than 6 to 8 weeks, complications of middle ear disease, or recurrent bouts of AOM (five episodes in 6 months) should be referred to an otolaryngologist for evaluation for possible surgical treatment (myringotomy and tube placement)

To effectively treat AOM, the most important pathogen to address is *S. pneumoniae* because it is less likely to resolve spontaneously without treatment compared with *H. influenzae* and *M. catarrhalis*. Although a large number of species exist that are resistant to amoxicillin and cephalosporins, evidence from the literature and guidelines suggest that no antibiotic outperforms amoxicillin as the first-line drug to treat AOM in patients who are not allergic to penicillin. Higher dose amoxicillin (80 mg per kg per day) in two divided doses for 5 to 10 days) has been shown to be more effective than standard dosing (40 mg per kg per day) in that it overcomes the minimum inhibitory concentrations of penicillin to kill intermediate and some highly resistant strains of *S. pneumoniae*. Initial therapy in uncomplicated AOM in patients who have type 1 allergy (anaphylaxis or history of hives) to penicillin or cephalosporins should be treated with one of the following antibiotics: azithromycin, clarithromycin, or erythromycin.

In general, if symptoms persist after a child has taken first-line antibiotic for 48 to 72 hours, then the child should be

OPTIONS FOR THE TREATMENT OF ACUTE OTITIS MEDIA
(AAP/AAFP) GUIDELINES

Child age	Certain diagnosis	Uncertain diagnosis
Younger than 6 mo	Antibiotics	Antibiotics
6 mo–2 yr	Antibiotics	Antibiotics if severe illness; observe if nonsevere illness[a]
2 yr or older	Antibiotics if severe illness; observe if nonsevere illness[a]	Observe

[a]Nonsevere illness: fever <39°C and/or mild otalgia; severe illness: fever >39°C and/or moderate to severe otalgia

reevaluated by the health care provider (either by phone or in the office). Antibiotics should then be prescribed to cover β-lactam producing organisms. Specifically, amoxicillin-clavulanate (90 mg per kg per day in twice a day dosing) or the modified extra strength version of that antibiotic is appropriate for those who have a history of gastrointestinal intolerance. Other options include oral cefdinir, cefuroxime, cefpodoxime and, less commonly, ceftriaxone in IV or intramuscular dosing.

Pain should be controlled with acetaminophen or ibuprofen. Codeine should be limited for use in those with severe pain. Topical benzocaine (Auralgan or Americaine Otic) provides additional, but brief, relief for some children (30 to 60 minutes) but should not be used in patients who have TM perforations or ear tubes. Antihistamines, decongestants, and corticosteroids have shown only minimal benefit and are not recommended.

External Otitis

External otitis is usually caused by water trapped in the ear canal after swimming and is often called swimmer's ear. Ear canal trauma or foreign bodies may also contribute to the development of external otitis.

Otitis externa (OE) may be localized or diffuse. Localized external otitis is the result of an abscessed hair follicle in the outer two-thirds of the ear canal. These abscesses are most often caused by *Staphylococcus aureus*.

Diffuse external otitis is caused by *Pseudomonas aeruginosa,* staphylococci (including methicillin-resistant staphylococci), fungi, or a mixture of gram-negative and gram-positive organisms. Viral external otitis is usually caused by herpes simplex or herpes zoster virus.

Clinical Manifestations. External otitis usually begins with itching and fullness that progress to severe pain. The pain is worsened by chewing or by touching the ear. The external canal is red, edematous, and narrowed. The diagnosis of external otitis is usually readily made by external inspection and otoscopy. Otoscopy may be painful, and visualization of the eardrum may be impossible because of edema of the canal walls. A foul-smelling, purulent discharge is usually present. Surrounding cellulitis and regional cervical adenitis may also be present. Malignant external otitis occurs rarely in debilitated patients who have diabetes or who are immunosuppressed. It may cause extensive tissue necrosis and can be rapidly fatal if not treated immediately with antibiotics and may require surgical debridement.

Management. If the abscess in localized external otitis is about to drain spontaneously, it should be opened where it is pointing with an 18-gauge needle or a no. 11 scalpel blade. Drainage results in immediate relief of pain. Antibiotic therapy with an antistaphylococcal antibiotic (e.g., erythromycin, dicloxacillin, clindamycin, or cephalosporin) should be administered for 10 days. Clindamycin or trimethoprim-sulfamethoxazole should be considered in regions where methicillin-resistant *S. aureus* (MRSA) is more prevalent. The treatment of diffuse external otitis comprises antibiotic eardrops containing either ciprofloxacin with or without steroids or a combination drop with neomycin, polymyxin, and hydrocortisone (four drops, three times daily) in the affected ear for 10 days. Before the drops are started, the pus and debris should be cleaned from the ear canal with gentle suction, a curette, or cotton-tipped applicators. If the meatus is so swollen that drops cannot enter the external canal, a wick of gauze or Merocel sponge should be gently advanced into the ear canal with a forceps (Fig. 123.3) to facilitate instillation of the topical medicine. The wick should be left in place for 24 to 48 hours, by which time the canal swelling should resolve to permit entrance of the drops. Broad-spectrum systemic antibiotics should be used if cellulitis or regional cervical adenitis is present. No water should be allowed to enter the ear canal during the 10 days of therapy. If OE becomes recurrent or fails to improve after a course of therapy, the discharge should be cultured for fungal and routine bacteria.

Chronic Suppurative Otitis Media

Chronic suppurative otitis media (CSOM) is a persistent perforation of the TM of more than 3 months' duration; the perforation may be acquired (from AOM or trauma) or iatrogenic (by tympanostomy tube) and may or may not be associated with active infection. When infection is present, the causative organism is usually *P. aeruginosa* or *S. aureus,* and it presents with a profuse, foul-smelling discharge. Perforation may be associated with a cholesteatoma (white skin-lined cyst) that can destroy the structures of the ear as it expands.

Clinical Manifestations. COM is usually diagnosed by otoscopy. A perforation of the eardrum is readily seen and the white, pearly, flaky debris from a cholesteatoma may also be present.

Management. Dry perforations require no active treatment. When otorrhea is noted, antibiotic-containing eardrops (four to five drops, three times daily) should be placed in the ear

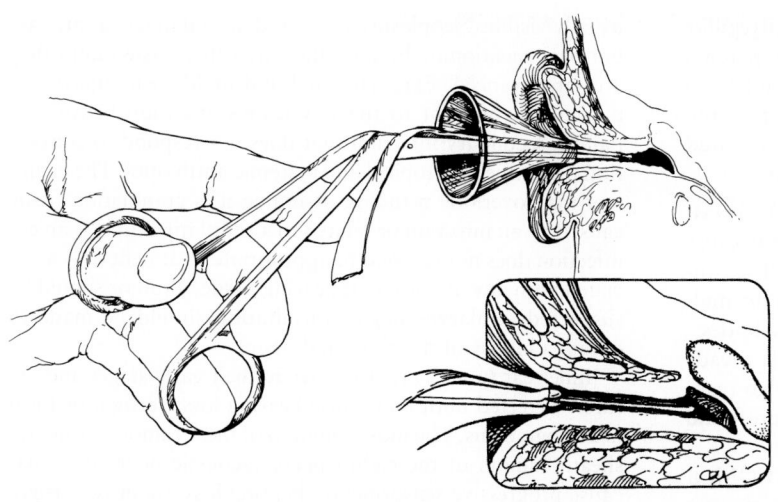

FIGURE 123.3 Gauze wick (¼ × 1½ in) being placed in ear canal to facilitate topical treatment of otitis externa.

canal. Ototoxicity manifested by either SNHL or dizziness has been reported with certain antibiotic drops but is less likely to occur when profuse otorrhea is present. The U.S. Food and Drug Administration has approved flouroquinolones with or without steroids (Ciprodex® and Floxin®, with or without steroids, respectively) in children who have otorrhea and who also have tubes or other openings into the middle ear to lower the risk of ototoxicity. Aerobic, anaerobic, and fungal cultures should be obtained in children who fail a 10-day course of drops. Clotrimazole drops have been shown to be beneficial in clearing fungal infections caused by *Aspergillus* or *Candida* species. Systemic antibiotics are of limited value unless regional cellulitis or cervical adenitis is present but may shorten the course of otorrhea in some instances. In those cases, an anti-staphylococcal antibiotic (e.g., erythromycin, dicloxacillin, clindamycin, or cephalosporin) should be administered for 10 days. Cultures are sometimes helpful in recalcitrant cases to identify less common pathogens including fungi (*Aspergillus* or *Candida* species) or MRSA. Chronic perforation and cholesteatoma require surgical correction. All cases should be referred to an otolaryngologist for definitive management.

The complications of COM with infection are the same as those that occur in AOM, including intracranial spread of the infectious process. In addition, with repeated infection, a progressive high-frequency sensorineural hearing loss may develop.

Infection of the Pinna

The pinna may become infected in a fashion similar to skin surfaces anywhere else on the body (see Chapter 92). Preauricular cysts and sinuses may occasionally be infected with *S. aureus* and should be treated with antistaphylococcal penicillin, clindamycin, or cephalosporin for 10 days. If an abscess forms, it should be drained surgically. Infected preauricular sinuses/cysts require surgical excision once the acute infection has been treated. Perichondritis requires immediate antipseudomonal and antistaphylococcal antibiotic treatment.

Sudden Hearing Loss

Sudden hearing loss is not a common complaint in the ED, but it requires prompt attention, especially if the loss is determined to be sensorineural. Sudden conductive losses almost never occur without a known antecedent such as head trauma, ear infection, or wax occlusion of the ear canal. History and otoscopy can usually establish the cause of the conductive hearing loss. However, the cause of sensorineural sudden hearing loss is obscure when the history is unrevealing and otoscopy findings are normal. Tuning fork testing helps confirm the presence of a sensorineural hearing loss.

Sudden sensorineural hearing loss that occurs after an airplane trip, scuba diving, straining, or head trauma is highly suggestive of a perilymph fistula. A perilymph fistula occurs when inner ear fluid leaks out into the middle ear through a rupture in the round window or stapes footplate (oval window). The leaking fluid causes a fluctuating sensorineural loss and vertigo. Urgent surgical exploration of the middle ear is required for repair.

Sudden sensorineural deafness may occur without a history suggestive of a fistula and without otoscopic abnormalities. This is often secondary to concussive middle ear injury or a viral infection of the cochlear labyrinth. Measles, mumps, and cytomegalic viral illnesses are common causes of sudden sensorineural deafness. Other viruses may also injure the cochlea. There may be no systemic symptoms or signs of such a viral infection. These patients may have partial or complete recovery of hearing that usually improves over several weeks. Lyme disease has also been found to be a cause of sensorineural hearing loss.

There is no proven effective treatment of sudden hearing loss. Aspirin has been recommended (in older children) both to decrease platelet aggregation and to maintain patency of the cochlear blood vessels, and corticosteroids have been recommended by some authors who believe that the etiology of some cases is autoimmune. Other treatments have been proposed (e.g., cyclophosphamide, hyperbaric oxygen, inhaled CO_2), but these therapies are of uncertain efficacy. Antivertigo medications may be prescribed for patients experiencing dizziness. All patients with a sudden sensorineural hearing loss should be referred to an otolaryngologist.

Vertigo

Sudden vertigo is a disturbing and sometimes confusing symptom. Vertigo caused by middle ear pathology is often accompanied by nausea, vomiting, imbalance, and irregular gait. A child may be brought to the ED because the parents think he or she is having a seizure. Vertigo may result from dysfunction of any part of the vestibular system (from the labyrinth to the vestibular cortex). Vertigo may be associated with a number of conditions affecting the middle ear:

1. Serous labyrinthitis may develop in a child with OME, AOM, or COM. Pressure and infection in the middle ear may cause inner ear inflammation and vestibular dysfunction. The conductive hearing loss and the dizziness resolve when the middle ear pressure is normalized or the inflammation subsides.

2. Suppurative labyrinthitis may occur when bacteria invade the inner ear. This condition results in severe vertigo (usually with associated nausea and vomiting) and profound sensorineural hearing loss.

3. When a cholesteatoma arises in association with COM, it may invade the bony wall of the labyrinth. Pneumatic otoscopy may produce the sensation of vertigo by transmitting the pressure directly to the inner ear.

4. A common cause of sudden vertigo is vestibular neuronitis. The origin of this entity is uncertain, and the vertigo resolves spontaneously over several weeks. It may be associated with a minor upper respiratory tract infection.

5. Trauma can be associated with vertigo in several ways. Perilymph fistulae, which occur most often after barotrauma, blunt head trauma, or straining, produce vertigo that fluctuates in severity. However, labyrinthine concussion or hemorrhage (hemorrhagic labyrinthitis) caused by blunt or direct trauma to the head can also result in vertigo. Cerebral injuries involving the temporal lobe (with or without temporal bone fracture) are more likely to cause vertigo. In most instances, the child can compensate for complete vestibular loss in several weeks as long as only one ear is affected and he or she has normal cerebellar and visual functions.

6. Measles and mumps may also infect the inner ear and cause vertigo.

7. Meniere's disease (endolymphatic hydrops) is rare in children. Its origin is unknown. The symptoms are intermittent vertigo, tinnitus, a feeling of fullness in the ear, and fluctuating hearing that lasts several hours and then usually passes.

8. Miscellaneous causes of sudden vertigo in children include benign paroxysmal vertigo of childhood and retrolabyrinthine lesions such as tumors, demyelinating diseases, and temporal lobe seizures. Migraine headaches may also present with episodes of vertigo.

The emergency physician should be reminded that vertigo is only a symptom of an underlying disease. Emergency treatment should consist of searching for the underlying disease, as well as providing symptomatic relief. Vertigo is rarely associated with a life-threatening illness, but CT or MRI scans of the head should be considered in more severe cases to look for intracranial sources of the vertigo. Because sensorineural hearing loss usually accompanies serious causes of vertigo, its absence can provide some level of confidence that no life-threatening disease is present. (See Chapter 20 for further discussion.)

Neoplasms

Neoplasms of the external ear are as varied as the tissue types of the auricle and are not difficult to diagnose because they are usually visible. Neoplasms of the middle and inner ear are rare but bear mentioning because they are often missed until they are far advanced. External canal and middle ear tumors are most often brought to the physician's attention because of painful secondary infection that does not respond to conventional treatment of topical and systemic antibiotics. The examiner may overlook a tumor, assuming it is granulation tissue caused by an infection or related to a ventilating tube. If an ear infection does not respond to appropriate treatment or is associated with any abnormal-appearing tissue, a tumor should be suspected; otolaryngologic consultation should be made to obtain a biopsy of the abnormal tissue.

Inner ear tumors are deceptive in their early stages and are rarely detected until they cause hearing loss, vertigo, or focal neurologic signs. The most common of these tumors are neural sheath tumors of the eighth nerve (acoustic neuromas) that cause progressive sensorineural hearing loss, tinnitus, vertigo, and fifth nerve anesthesia. These tumors are more likely to occur in children who are in their teens or who have neurofibromatosis type 2.

Facial Nerve Paralysis

Facial nerve paralysis is a frightening occurrence in children. Bell's palsy (idiopathic facial paralysis) is the most common cause of facial paralysis. (See Chapter 83 for management of this presumed viral infection.) A child presenting with facial paralysis must have a careful examination to detect any other treatable cause for the nerve dysfunction. Facial paralysis secondary to AOM requires a course of systemic (24 to 48 hours of IV followed by oral) antibiotics and an urgent wide-field myringotomy and tube for drainage. Temporal bone fractures, facial trauma, and neoplasms of the middle ear and parotid area can also present with facial nerve paralysis. A child with a facial nerve paralysis should be referred to an otolaryngologist for a complete evaluation of the head and neck, audiogram, and radiographic imaging.

The most common infectious cause of facial nerve paralysis in children is Lyme disease. It has been reported to be bilateral in 28% of patients. The treatment is doxycycline in adults, but amoxicillin is also effective in children. The majority of cases resolve within 6 months after treatment has been started.

Other less common causes of facial nerve paralysis include herpes zoster virus, herpes simplex virus, Epstein-Barr virus, *M. pneumoniae*, and, less often, cat-scratch disease. Acyclovir has been used with some success in cases of herpes virus infections. Facial nerve paralysis has also been associated with inflammatory disease, including Kawasaki's disease, Wegener's granulomatosis, and Melkersson-Rosenthal syndrome.

NOSE AND PARANASAL SINUSES

Methods of Examination

The external nose and anterior portion of the nasal cavities can be examined by direct visual inspection. A nasal speculum and directed light source are necessary to permit good visualization of the anterior septum and inferior and middle turbinates. In younger children, the examiner's thumb can elevate the mobile nasal tip to allow adequate inspection of the anterior nasal structures. Vasoconstrictors such as 0.25% phenylephrine or 0.05% oxymetazoline (two or three drops) can be applied to the nose to shrink the mucosa and allow a more complete examination. The posterior nasal structures and nasopharynx can be seen with the aid of a flexible fiber-optic endoscope placed in the nose or the posterior oropharynx (see Procedure 7.5 in Section VII). Patency of the nasal cavities in the neonate can be assessed by the passage of small rubber catheters through the nose and into the pharynx. Palpation is also important in the evaluation of nasal and facial trauma. Tenderness to palpation over the sinuses is a common sign of acute sinusitis.

A careful examination of adjacent areas is important when evaluating a child with sinus disease. Dental pathology may be a possible cause of a bacterial maxillary sinusitis. An examination of the orbit with assessment of visual acuity and ocular mobility should be performed to detect possible orbital complications of sinus disease.

Radiographs are very helpful in evaluating diseases of the nose and sinuses. Plain films (sinus or facial series) can be used as screening devices to evaluate a mass or fluid in a sinus, but CT scans are indicated for more precise and detailed evaluation of sinusitis or tumors of this area. (See the following text.)

Infections

The common cold/upper respiratory tract infection accounts for the majority of infections of the nose and paranasal sinuses. The symptom complex of fever, nasal congestion/rhinorrhea, and headache is most often caused by a viral agent. Physical examination often reveals swollen, erythematous, nasal turbinates. The rhinorrhea can be clear or white. Facial tenderness is usually absent. Viral rhinitis requires a little more than supportive care with hydration, rest, and antipyretics. Topical decongestants should be avoided and their use limited to 3- to 5-day duration because of their tendency to cause rebound congestion as their vasoconstricting effect on the nasal mucosa wears off.

Bacterial infection of the nose and paranasal sinuses is a more serious condition that requires careful examination and prompt treatment. Bacterial rhinosinusitis should be suspected when cough, halitosis, low-grade fever, and purulent rhinorrhea are present. A bacterial infection is more likely to be present when the nasal discharge lasts more than 7 days and the discharge is thick yellow to yellowish green, especially if it is localized in the nasopharynx or middle meatus of the nose. Tenderness over the face may indicate clinical involvement of one or more of the paranasal sinuses, but direct rhinoscopy with an otoscope is more helpful in locating the source of infection. The AAP developed guidelines in 2001 with recommendations that sinus radiographs (plain or CT) should not be used as a routine clinical adjunct to diagnose acute rhinosinusitis in children 6 years or younger because clinical history predicts outcome of imaging studies with 88% accuracy in that age group. They may be considered in older children, but false-positive rates of CT scans are high unless any of the following findings are present: mucosal thickening greater than 4 mm, an air–fluid level, or complete opacification of the sinus. A sinus CT scan should be obtained when the child is severely ill or when complications of disease are suspected in the orbit

or brain. Nasal culture should not be obtained unless taken directly from the middle meatus or sinus. Because the most common organisms responsible for bacterial rhinosinusitis are *S. pneumoniae*, nontypeable *H. influenzae*, and *M. catarralis*, amoxicillin (80 mg per kg per day) for 10 days is the treatment of choice. Short courses of saline, humidified air and nasal steroids should be used to help promote drainage.

Complications of acute sinusitis, such as orbital cellulites/abscess, facial cellulitis/abscess, meningitis, or intracranial abscesses require admission to the hospital for appropriate IV antimicrobial therapy and possible operative intervention. Otolaryngologic consultation should be obtained in the evaluation of these patients with complicated acute sinusitis because surgical drainage may be needed. Intracranial complications of sinusitis should be suspected in those who also have sinusitis with changes in mental status, fever, headache, and vomiting. Adolescent boys are more likely to have intracranial complications involving the frontal sinus because the frontal bone and sinuses are developing, and because there is an increase rate of growth of diploic bone at that time. CT of sinuses and brain with contrast are usually necessary to avoid missing complications of frontal sinuses in severely ill children.

The sinus mucocele is a late complication that can flare up, causing a child to present to the ED with acute symptoms. Mucoceles are expansile cystic lesions that occur secondary to a long-standing blockage of a sinus ostium. Although the lesion evolves over several months or even years, the child usually presents with the sudden onset of signs and symptoms usually related to an acute infection of the mucocele. These include pain and swelling secondary to osteomyelitis of the frontal bone, inferior and lateral displacement of the globe with proptosis, limitation of ocular mobility, and chronic nasal/postnasal discharge. Radiographs (plain films and CT) are often needed to determine the presence and extent of a mucocele. The patient should be referred to the otolaryngology service for appropriate IV antimicrobial therapy and surgical drainage.

Underlying conditions should be suspected if rhinosinusitis persists after a prolonged course of antibiotics. The presence of foreign bodies, choanal atresia, neoplasms, septal deviation, dental disease, adenoid hypertrophy, allergic polyps, or immunodeficiency states may all be associated with recurrent or persistent rhinosinusitis.

Chronic Nasal Obstruction

Obstruction to the normal passage of air can occur with various conditions and gives the sensation of a blocked or "stuffy" nose. Temporary partial obstruction of one nasal cavity at a time occurs normally in the nasal respiratory cycle. However, prolonged blockage is not physiologic, and the physician should search for a cause.

Although most instances of nasal obstruction cause only mild feelings of discomfort, some children may present with a history of obstructive apnea (Pickwickian syndrome—see the "Adenotonsillar Hypertrophy" section) and even cor pulmonale. Nasal trauma or a foreign body may be a cause of the obstruction. A careful examination of the nasal cavities and pharynx is necessary to determine the cause of the obstruction. Septal deviation, and turbinate hypertrophy related to allergy and/or infection are common causes.

Adenoid hypertrophy, nasal tumor nasopharyngeal tumor (lymphoma, rhabdomyosarcoma), and choanal atresia (unilateral or bilateral) can all present with nasal obstruction. Flexible fiber-optic examination (see Procedure 7.5 in Section VII) and radiographs (usually CT scan) of the nose and nasopharynx may be useful in the evaluation of the blocked nasal airway. If the source of the obstruction is not apparent after these maneuvers, referral should be made to an otolaryngologist to perform a complete examination of the nose and nasopharynx.

Epistaxis

Epistaxis is relatively common in children, and may cause significant anxiety in both the child and the parent. Although bleeding occasionally occurs secondary to the mucosal maceration caused by upper respiratory tract infections, nose picking accounts for most cases of recurrent epistaxis. (A more complete discussion on the differential diagnosis is presented in Chapter 22.) The usual site of bleeding is the anterior nasal septum, Kiesselbach's or Little's area (Fig. 123.4).

It is important to obtain information regarding the site of bleeding (one or both sides of the nose), frequency, and presence of bleeding from other places, history of trauma, and family history of bleeding in order to properly manage a patient with epistaxis. Figure 123.5 presents an algorithm for the management of epistaxis. A careful examination of the nose should be performed to identify the site and cause of the bleeding. Good lighting, suction, and material for cauterization and packing should be readily available (see Procedure 7.1 in Section VII). Topical vasoconstrictors such as phenylephrine (0.25%), oxymetazoline (0.05%), or epinephrine (1:1,000) on a cotton pledget can be placed in the nose to shrink the nasal mucosa, allowing better visualization of the nasal cavity; vasoconstrictors may slow or even stop the bleeding. Applying pressure for 10 to 20 minutes by squeezing the nostrils together is usually sufficient to stop most epistaxis. Occasionally, a roll of cotton placed under the upper lip will stop bleeding by compression of the labial artery. If pressure is not successful, cauterization with silver nitrate sticks or packing of the nose is performed (see Procedures 7.1

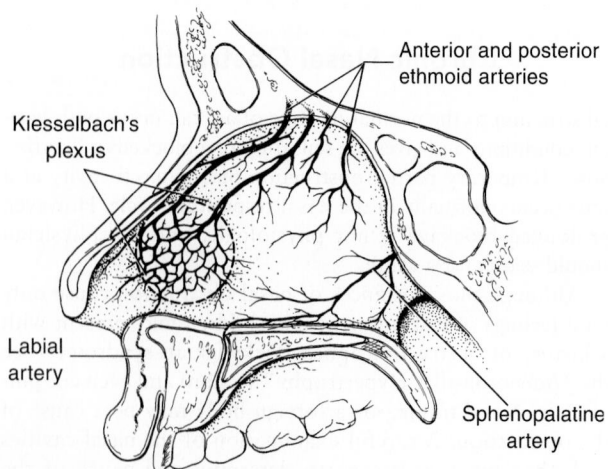

FIGURE 123.4 Vascular supply of nasal septum. Note confluence of vessels that forms Kiesselbach's plexus.

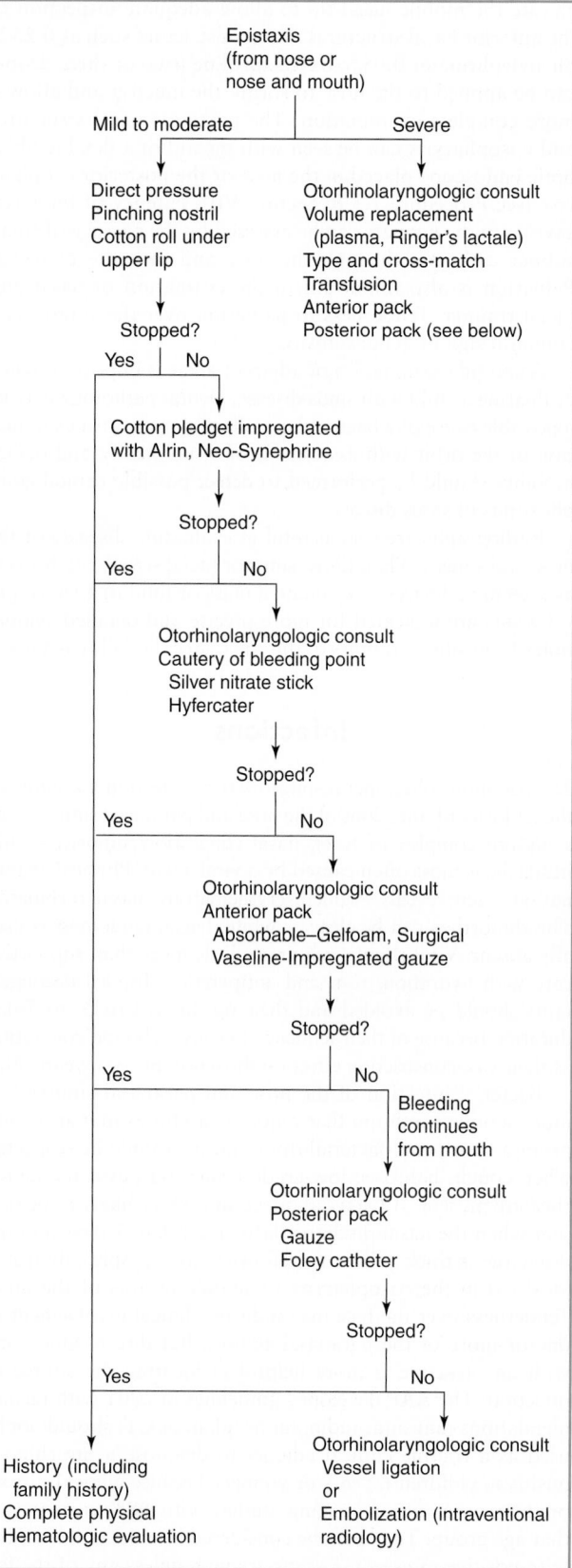

FIGURE 123.5 Algorithm for the management of epistaxis.

and 7.2 in Section VII). Absorbable packing such as oxycellu-lose (Surgicel®) or gelatin (Gelfoam®) is usually adequate for most epistaxis and is advantageous because it does not need to be removed. Micofibrillar collagen (Avitene©, Davol) is a foam/gel that could be used to prohibit further bleeding but is less helpful when the nose is actively bleeding.

Further treatment should also be directed toward prevent-ing the child from continuing to traumatize his or her nose, which could result in further bleeding. Using a vaporizer to increase the humidity in the child's room and applying petro-leum jelly to the anterior septal areas twice daily can aid in healing the irritated nasal mucosa and preventing recurrent epistaxis. Fingernails should be cut short.

Otolaryngologists should be called to assist in diagnosis and management of children who have severe or recurrent episodes of epistaxis. Epistaxis that does not stop with simple pressure or oxycellulose or gelatin packing may require a more substantial anterior nasal pack of petroleum jelly-impregnated gauze. A posterior nasal pack (using gauze or a Foley catheter) may be necessary in managing severe epistaxis that originates in the posterior nasal cavity or nasopharynx (see Procedure 7.2 in Section VII).

If the epistaxis recurs despite these treatments, an otolaryn-gologist should be consulted to look for other causes for the epistaxis. Nasal septal deviation or perforation, sinusitis, tumor (nasal, nasopharyngeal, or sinus), Rendu-Osler-Weber disease (hereditary hemorrhagic telangiectasia), and nasal for-eign body can all present with epistaxis. Blood dyscrasias such as hemophilia, idiopathic thrombocytopenia purpura, von Willebrand's disease, and those hematologic conditions that are associated with leukemia or the administration of chemothera-peutic agents may lead to severe epistaxis. Treatment consists of correcting the underlying hematologic problem in addition to the previously described local measures. Recurrent or severe bleeding may require more extensive cauterization of the ves-sels on the septum or ligation or embolization of the regional blood vessels, including the maxillary and ethmoid vessels.

Neoplasms

Neoplasms of the nose and sinuses are uncommon in children. They may present as mass lesions or as chronic/recurrent rhi-nosinusitis. When a neoplasm is suspected, the child should be referred to an otolaryngologist for a complete evaluation of the nose and sinuses and appropriate radiographic imaging, which is a prerequisite to the proper treatment of these lesions.

Hemangiomas are the most common benign neoplasms of the head and neck in children and often occur on the skin near or on the nose. Because hemangiomas often go through a period of rapid growth for the first 12 to 18 months of life before they begin to involute, a period of observation is recommended before corticosteroids or surgical excision is considered. Recurrent bleeding, thrombocytopenia, skin breakdown, obstruction to vision, respiratory distress, and cardiac failure are some indications for early intervention. Papillomas are viral-induced verrucous growths that are the most common neo-plasms of the aerodigestive tract. When they appear in the nose, they are most often found on the nasal septum. Simple excision or fulguration is the preferred treatment of these lesions. In addition to these conditions, there are various benign and malignant mass lesions of the nose. Early consultation with an otolaryngologist should be obtained for any tumor of the nose, especially one with recent changes in size or character.

ORAL CAVITY, PHARYNX, AND ESOPHAGUS

Methods of Examination

The oral cavity and oropharynx are directly visible with the aid of a tongue blade. A headlight or brightly lighted flashlight is required for this examination. The tongue should be dis-placed down and forward with the tongue blade placed on the anterior two-thirds of the tongue to avoid gagging. The exam-ination of the nasopharynx, hypopharynx, and esophagus requires special instrumentation. The nasopharynx and hypopharynx can be examined with a flexible nasopharyngo-scope. Nasopharyngoscopy requires special skills and may be best left to the otolaryngology consultant (see Procedure 7.5 in Section VII). Examination of the esophagus requires direct visualization with an esophagoscope under general anesthesia. Palpation of the hypopharynx and nasopharynx should not be performed because it is uncomfortable to the child and poten-tially dangerous.

Radiography contributes minimally to the examination of the oral cavity and oropharynx because these areas are visible by direct examination. The lateral neck radiograph is useful to evaluate the presence of abnormal tissue or masses in the nasopharynx and hypopharynx because air–tissue interfaces are present. Barium esophagrams may be helpful in diagnosing esophageal strictures or fistulas, and they are helpful in defin-ing areas of external compression caused by extrinsic masses or congenital vascular anomalies.

Infections

Stomatitis

The most common infectious lesion of the oral cavity is the aphthous ulcer. The ulcers are often recurrent, may appear as a single lesion or a confluence of many lesions, and can cause severe stomatitis. The exact cause of aphthous ulcerations is unknown, but it is believed to be infectious.

Herpes simplex virus can cause severe gingivostomatitis, whereas the pharynx is relatively spared. In contrast, coxsack-ievirus infection (herpangina) causes severe ulcerative lesions of the pharynx but not the anterior mouth. These viral infections cause severe oral pain and inability to eat. They are self-limited and require only symptomatic relief (see Chapters 84 and 124).

Candida albicans oral infection (thrush) usually appears as white patches with surrounding inflammation on the oral mucosa. It often occurs in newborns, immunosuppressed patients, and patients receiving antibiotic therapy. Nystatin is an effective treatment. The dosage is 100,000 to 200,000 units (1 to 2 mL) four times per day for 5 to 10 days.

Acute necrotizing ulcerative gingivitis (trench mouth) causes painful, bleeding gums. Vigorous brushing of the teeth and gums with a soft brush promotes rapid healing. Antibiotics are of limited value.

Pharyngitis/Tonsillitis

Pharyngitis/tonsillitis (pharyngotonsillitis) may be caused by viral or bacterial organisms. Differentiating viral pharyngotonsillitis including mononucleosis from an infection of bacterial origin is difficult on clinical grounds. A child is more likely to have a bacterial pharyngotonsillitis if three of four indicators are present: red tonsils with exudate, cervical lymphadenopathy, fever greater than 101°F, and absence of cough. Rapid strep tests are quick (5 to 10 minutes) and may be helpful in confirming the diagnosis but may miss up to one-third of infections. If this test result is negative and bacterial infection is still suspected, then a routine throat culture may be helpful, but the results are not available for 24 to 48 hours. Bacterial pharyngotonsillitis should be treated with a 10-day course of penicillin or amoxicillin. Patients with repeated debilitating bouts of pharyngotonsillitis (five to seven in a 1-year period or several per year for several years) or complications including peritonsillar abscess should be referred to an otolaryngologist for consideration for tonsillectomy and adenoidectomy.

Pharyngeal infections may spread to the peritonsillar area, causing cellulitis. The affected tonsil bulges forward and medially to touch the uvula. If pus localizes in the peritonsillar space, a peritonsillar abscess is formed. The peritonsillar abscess causes trismus. Suspected abscess formation requires immediate consultation with an otolaryngology specialist. Short-term treatment of peritonsillar abscess requires systemic (24 to 48 hours of IV followed by oral) antibiotics and needle aspiration or incisional drainage (if possible) of the abscess. Occasionally, a "hot" or quinsy tonsillectomy may be required to treat the acute infection. Later, elective tonsillectomy is indicated if there is a previous history of tonsillar or peritonsillar infections.

Retropharyngeal and Parapharyngeal Infections

Retropharyngeal and parapharyngeal lymph nodes may also become infected during an episode of pharyngitis and progress to abscess formation. Retropharyngeal abscess is usually easily seen on the lateral neck radiograph and confirmed by CT of the neck with contrast. Abscess is more likely present when the soft-tissue mass (lymph nodes) has a hypolucent core that has complete rim enhancement (Fig. 123.6). Peritonsillar, retropharyngeal, and parapharyngeal abscesses must be treated with IV antibiotics, and 60% to 80% require surgical drainage. (See also "Infections" under the "Neck and Associated Structures" section.)

Other unusual infections that may occur in the oral cavity include actinomycosis, mucormycosis, and syphilis. Infections due to actinomycosis may cause oral–cervical fistulas, whereas infections due to *Mucor* cause necrosis of the palate. Syphilis is visible in many ways (e.g., ulceration or raised lesion) and has no one characteristic appearance.

Adenotonsillar Hypertrophy

Lymphoid hyperplasia (enlarged tonsils and adenoids) can cause airway obstruction that can range from mild snoring to severe sleep apnea with right-sided heart strain. Young children with obstructive sleep apnea most often weigh in the lower 25th percentile and some have failure to thrive. Alternatively, older children with severe obstructive sleep apnea are often obese and present with daytime somnolence (Pickwickian syndrome). If significant oxygen desaturation with or without bradycardia is present, or signs of right-sided heart strain or daytime somnolence are present, a tonsillectomy and adenoidectomy may be required urgently.

Neoplasms

Benign and malignant neoplasms occur in the oral cavity, pharynx, hypopharynx, and esophagus. Benign neoplasms in the oral cavity may rise from the mucosa or underlying tissues. Minor salivary gland tumors, hemangiomas, lymphangiomas,

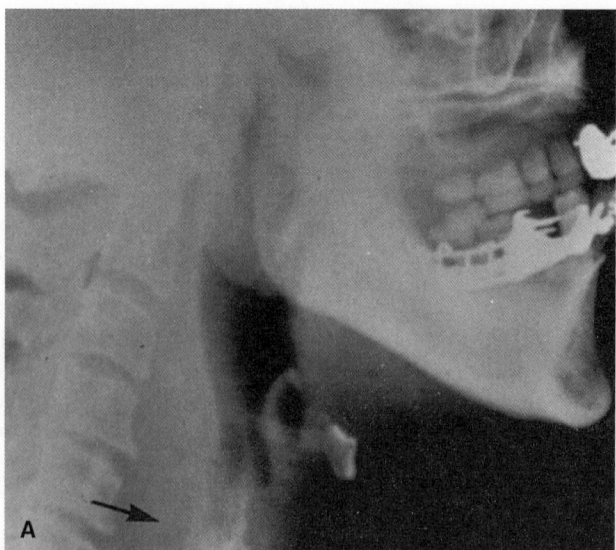
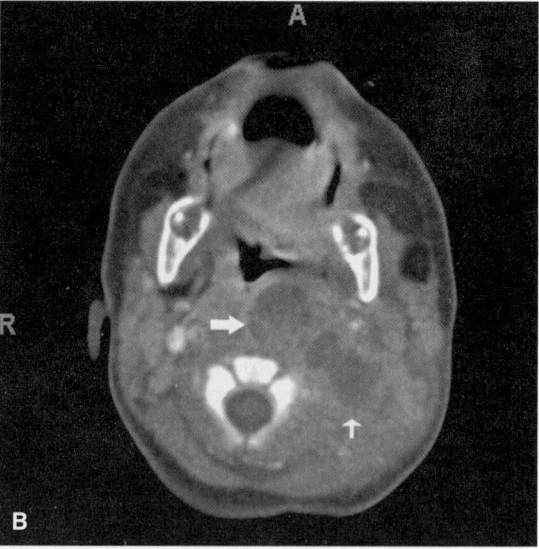

FIGURE 123.6 **A:** A lateral neck radiograph demonstrating retropharyngeal abscess *(arrow)*. **B:** A computed tomographic scan of neck with contrast demonstrating a retropharyngeal abscess *(large arrow)* and smaller, contiguous parapharyngeal abscess *(small arrow)*.

pyogenic granulomas, and neurofibromas are found in the oral cavity, but they rarely require emergency intervention.

Nasopharyngeal angiofibromas occur in pubescent males, and most often present with unilateral bleeding and nasal obstruction. They may appear in the ED with massive epistaxis. Posterior packing is usually required to control the hemorrhage that may be life threatening (see Procedure 7.2 in Section VII).

Malignant neoplasms are rare but can occur throughout the oral cavity, pharynx, and esophagus. Rhabdomyosarcoma, lymphoma, and squamous cell carcinoma (lymphoepithelioma) are the most common lesions and are rarely seen as emergencies unless there is extensive hemorrhage or a compromised airway.

Biopsy of oral, pharyngeal, and esophageal tumors is best done in the operating room, where adequate exposure and control of hemorrhage is most effectively obtained.

LARYNX AND TRACHEA

Methods of Examination

Examination of the larynx is often difficult in young children. Commonly, however, the tip of the epiglottis may be visualized when the tongue is protruded during the examination of the oropharynx. Examination of the larynx can be performed with a flexible fiber-optic endoscope. Vocal cord mobility, the structures of the larynx, and the presence of laryngeal masses can usually be assessed in this manner (see Procedure 7.5 in Section VII). The otolaryngologist may need to be consulted to perform this examination for the child presenting in the ED with symptoms related to the larynx.

Lateral and anteroposterior plain radiographs of the neck can provide significant information about the larynx and upper trachea. Although xeroradiographs offer more precise detail of the airway by virtue of their property of edge enhancement, the extra radiation exposure inherent in this study makes this a less desirable imaging modality. CT and MRI scans are useful in examining the fine detail of laryngeal and tracheal structures, but the sedation may be required to keep the child still for these examinations, restricting their use to specific situations. Fluoroscopic examination of the larynx is another method used to evaluate the movements of the vocal cords during phonation and respiration. Vocal cord paralysis and laryngomalacia can often be identified in this manner. Contrast studies can also be used in the evaluation of laryngeal function. A barium swallow is useful in detecting aspiration associated with vocal cord paralysis, posterior laryngeal cleft, extrinsic masses such as vascular webs, or tracheoesophageal fistula.

Infections

Viral laryngitis usually occurs along with a common upper respiratory tract infection, resulting in vocal cord edema manifested by a hoarse, raspy voice. Airway obstruction is rare in viral laryngitis. Symptomatic treatment with humidification, antipyretics, analgesics, throat gargles, and voice rest is recommended while the disease runs its natural course. When the viral infection involves the subglottic space, a more serious clinical problem appears. Laryngotracheobronchitis (croup) is a common and potentially life-threatening infection occurring in early childhood. The diagnosis and management of croup is discussed in Chapters 72 and 92.

Bacterial laryngotracheobronchitis does occur but is not nearly as common as its viral counterpart. Children aged 3 to 6 years are more commonly affected by bacterial tracheitis than by the infection of viral origin that usually appears in children younger than 3 years. It may be difficult to distinguish bacterial laryngitis on clinical grounds from a similar infection of viral origin. Etiologic agents responsible for bacterial laryngitis include staphylococci, streptococcus, and *H. influenzae*. Severe airway obstruction is a common symptom of bacterial laryngotracheobronchitis. This is caused by thick, inspissated secretions that fill the trachea and are difficult for the child to clear. In addition to the treatment measures recommended for viral laryngitis, patients should be prescribed antimicrobial agents and may require observation in the hospital if airway symptoms are severe. The otolaryngologist is usually required to perform a direct laryngoscopy and bronchoscopy to confirm the diagnosis and to aspirate the thick secretions for therapeutic and diagnostic purposes.

Diphtheria may involve the larynx, as well as other areas of the upper aerodigestive tract. The diagnosis is suspected by the presence of a membrane covering the pharynx and larynx that leaves a raw, bleeding surface when it is removed. The diphtheria membrane can obstruct the laryngeal airway to cause respiratory distress. Endoscopic removal of the membrane and/or tracheostomy may be required, in addition to antimicrobial therapy.

Bacterial infection of the supraglottic larynx can cause a symptom complex with potentially life-threatening airway obstruction. Epiglottitis (more appropriately called supraglottitis) is an infection of the supraglottic larynx that is caused most often by *H. influenzae* type b. Although the *H. influenzae* type b vaccine is generally effective (with reported overall efficacy of 98%), vaccine failures do occur. Up to 27% of reported cases of epiglottitis occur in children who have been vaccinated. Other bacteria that can cause epiglottis include *S. pneumoniae* and group A, B, or C streptococci. The diagnosis and management of epiglottitis are discussed in Chapters 72 and 92.

Neoplasms

Neoplasms of the larynx and trachea are uncommon in children. The otolaryngologist should be consulted to assist the emergency physician in the management of these patients.

The most common neoplasm of the larynx in children is the laryngeal papilloma. This is believed to be a viral-induced neoplasm (human papillomavirus, HPV) that has a predilection for the upper aerodigestive tract and the larynx in particular. The disease is most often transmitted from the mother to the infant at birth, but symptoms do not usually become apparent until the child is between 2 and 5 years of age. The child presents with persistent or worsening hoarseness and, occasionally, airway obstruction. Vaccination with HPV vaccine Gardasil® has been recommended for use in teenage women and has been shown to prevent cervical HPV infections that can later be transmitted to their offspring during pregnancy or childbirth.

If papillomas are suspected as the source of hoarseness in a child, the otolaryngologist should be consulted to perform the

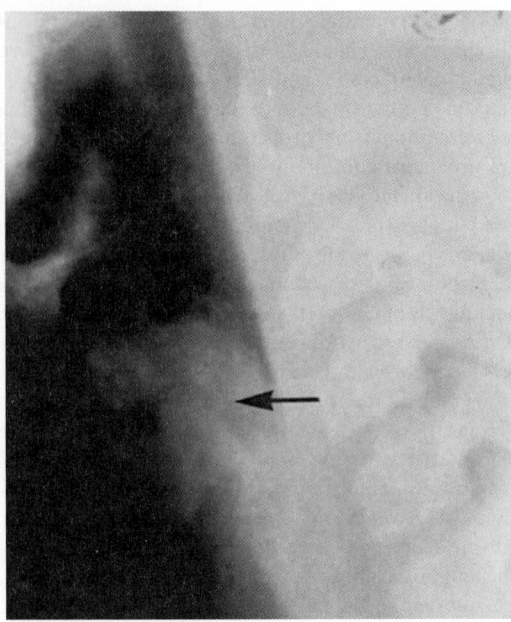

FIGURE 123.7 Lateral neck radiograph demonstrating soft-tissue density *(arrow)* at the level of larynx. Direct laryngoscopy revealed this to be papilloma.

indirect or direct laryngoscopy required to confirm the diagnosis. A lateral neck radiograph may demonstrate a soft-tissue mass in the area of the larynx (Fig. 123.7). The course of the disease is characterized by multiple cycles of growth and regression until a spontaneous remission occurs, usually around puberty. The otolaryngologist's goal in managing these patients is to maintain an adequate voice and unobstructed airway by frequent repeated excision (with cup forceps, carbon dioxide laser, or microdissectors) of the papillomas. A tracheostomy may be required in cases of severe airway obstruction. Hemangiomas may occur in the larynx, primarily in the subglottic area. As with most juvenile hemangiomas, these lesions present in the second to sixth months of life and can enlarge over several months to cause significant airway obstruction. Episodes of stridor may be precipitated by an upper respiratory tract infection. Of children with subglottic hemangiomas, 50% have other cutaneous lesions. The presence of cutaneous hemangiomas in an infant with stridor should suggest to the emergency physician the possibility of a subglottic hemangioma; however, only 1% of patients with cutaneous hemangiomas have airway lesions. Hemangiomas may appear as posterior subglottic masses on lateral neck radiographs, but the diagnosis must be confirmed by laryngoscopy performed by an otolaryngologist. Because most hemangiomas of infancy tend to involute after an initial period of rapid growth during the first 1 to 2 years of life, close observation is the only treatment required for those lesions that are causing minimal symptoms. If there is severe, persistent, or recurrent respiratory distress, intervention is indicated. Systemic corticosteroids, direct surgical excision, and tracheostomy are some of the modes of treatment presently being advocated. The carbon dioxide laser has been used as another method to vaporize hemangiomas but is used less frequently because it has been associated with increased scarring leading to subglottic stenosis.

Malignant neoplasms of the larynx are uncommon. They include rhabdomyosarcoma, chondrosarcoma, and lymphoma.

These tumors are seen with varying degrees of hoarseness and respiratory obstruction. If a laryngeal malignancy is suspected, the otolaryngologist should be asked to perform indirect or direct laryngoscopy to confirm the laryngeal problem and obtain tissue for histologic identification of the tumor.

Stridor

The differential diagnosis and emergency management of a child presenting with stridor is discussed in detail in Chapter 72.

NECK AND ASSOCIATED STRUCTURES

Methods of Examination

Visual inspection and palpation provide the basis for examination of the neck and its enclosed structures. The head should be erect during the examination, with the normal prominence of the sternocleidomastoid muscle on each side. Anterior projection of the thyroid cartilage or "Adam's apple" is seen in postpubescent males. Palpation of the neck is performed to assess the normal structures in the neck and to detect the presence and nature of any cervical masses. Examination of the two sides is done simultaneously so that they can be compared with one another. The examiner should be able to grasp the thyroid cartilage and move it gently from side to side without any discomfort to the patient. Immobility or significant pain may indicate the presence of laryngeal pathology. Crepitance of the neck indicates free air in the tissue planes of the neck from perforation of a hollow viscous. Passive and active range of motion of the neck should be complete in all directions. Restriction in movement may be caused by tender cervical adenopathy, cervical spine disease, spasm or fibrosis of the sternocleidomastoid muscle, or meningeal irritation (Brudzinski's sign). Arterial pulses of equal strength should be palpable in the carotid artery on each side of the neck. The carotids can also be auscultated for evidence of bruits.

Radiographs are often invaluable in the examination of the neck. Plain anteroposterior and lateral views provide significant information in the evaluation of cervical problems. The presence of masses projecting into and compromising the airway can be detected. Air between the muscle planes of the neck indicates a perforation of a hollow viscus such as the pharynx, esophagus, larynx, trachea, or pulmonary alveolus. CTs and MRIs of the neck obtained with contrast are often helpful in determining the cause of a neck mass.

Infections

Cervical adenitis is the most common cause of a neck mass in a child. The lymphatic system of the neck drains the internal cavities of the head and neck (ear, nose, mouth, pharynx, sinuses, and larynx), as well as the skin and associated adnexal structures of the face and scalp. Regional cervical lymph nodes respond when there is a primary infection in any area of the head and neck. Because certain groups of nodes drain into specific sites in the head and neck, the location of the swollen and infected lymph node can often help the practitioner to identify the area of the primary infection. Infraauricular nodes most often drain during ear infections, jugulodigastric nodes usually swell during pharyngeal infections (e.g., tonsillitis), and posterior neck nodes swell during nasopharyngeal infections (e.g., adenoiditis).

Cervical adenitis does not usually occur following a brief, uncomplicated viral infection of the upper respiratory tract. Instead, these tender and enlarged nodes occur more often as a result of bacterial infection of the head and neck. Infections of the ear and throat are the most common source. Because *Streptococcus* species are the causative agents in the majority of bacterial infections of the head and neck, the infected lymph nodes usually contain the same organisms. Treatment with amoxicillin or penicillin usually clears the primary infection and causes regression of the enlarged lymph nodes. Culture of the nasopharynx, throat, or aspirate of the cervical node can assist the physician in the choice of antimicrobial agents.

Although most children respond to oral antibiotics, a small group of children develop nodes that progress to suppurative cervical adenitis that usually requires hospitalization. A recent study of children hospitalized with cervical adenitis has shown a predominance of *S. aureus* as the causative agent (63% of positive cultures were *S. aureus* and 22% were group A streptococci, respectively). Of the staphylococcal infections, 27% were MRSA and all of these were sensitive to clindamycin and trimethoprim-sulfamethoxazole, 63% were sensitive to ciprofloxacin, and 25% to erythromycin. Of the methicillin-sensitive *S. aureus* isolates, 100%, 86%, and 82% were sensitive to trimethoprim-sulfamethoxazole, clindamycin, and ciprofloxacin, respectively. The high incidence of staphylococci in these hospitalized patients may occur because they have not responded to oral antimicrobials effective against the more commonly occurring *Streptococcus* species. Therefore, if cervical adenitis has not responded to the primary antimicrobial treatment, agents should be added that are effective against *S. aureus* (as well as other *Streptococcus* species).

A child who has demonstrated rapid enlargement of cervical nodes, poor response to oral antimicrobials, cellulitis of the overlying skin, abscess formation, or signs of toxicity (high fever, malaise, dehydration) should be admitted to the hospital for treatment with IV fluids and antimicrobials. Surgical consultation should be obtained in the management of these complicated cases in which needle aspiration, incision and drainage, or biopsy (for possible neoplasm) may be required.

Retropharyngeal or parapharyngeal nodes are commonly involved with inflammatory processes that originate in the pharynx. Sore throat, dysphagia, and stiff neck are some of the symptoms that can significantly accompany enlarged pharyngeal nodes. Retropharyngeal nodes can sometimes be seen overlying the cervical spine during examination of the oropharynx. They also can cause widening of the retropharyngeal soft tissues on lateral neck radiographs. Parapharyngeal nodes are seldom detected clinically unless they enlarge sufficiently to deviate the tonsil and pharyngeal wall medially. Treatment of enlarged pharyngeal nodes consists of IV antimicrobials (usually β-lactamase–resistant penicillin) and observation of the child's airway. Biopsy of the mass is indicated if resolution does not occur with treatment or if a malignancy is suspected.

A collection of purulent material within the tissues of the neck, a neck abscess, requires prompt and specific treatment.

The most common cause of a neck abscess is breakdown or necrosis of an infected lymph node. Purulent material may be located within a single node or may accumulate between several adjacent nodes. Once the process of cervical adenitis has progressed to the point of abscess formation, treatment involves evacuation of the infected material and the prevention of further spread of the infection. The child is hospitalized, and IV antimicrobials are administered that are effective against *S. aureus* and *Streptococcus* species (with antistaphylococcal and β-lactamase–resistant activity). Otolaryngologic consultation is obtained to perform a needle aspiration or incision and drainage to evacuate and culture the infected material. Less common causes of cervical adenitis include cat-scratch fever, atypical *Mycobacterium* tuberculosis, and tuberculosis.

Deep neck abscesses are uncommon in children but can be dangerous when they occur. Parapharyngeal abscess occurs when purulent material collects in the parapharyngeal space lateral to the pharyngeal constrictors and medial to the vascular compartment of the neck. Necrosis of parapharyngeal lymph nodes and lateral extension of a peritonsillar abscess are the two main sources of this infection in children. The child with a parapharyngeal abscess presents with a stiff neck, high fever, malaise, dehydration, and other signs of toxicity. The child usually has dysphagia and may not be able to swallow his or her own saliva. Physical examination reveals diffuse swelling and tenderness of one side of the neck, but fluctuance is seldom appreciated. Intraoral examination may demonstrate medial displacement of the lateral pharyngeal wall and tonsil. Lateral neck radiographs are usually not helpful in evaluating this disease process. CT or MRI scans with contrast provide the best evaluation of suspected deep neck abscesses (Fig. 123.8). If left to progress, the parapharyngeal abscess can involve the adjacent vascular structures in the neck, descend

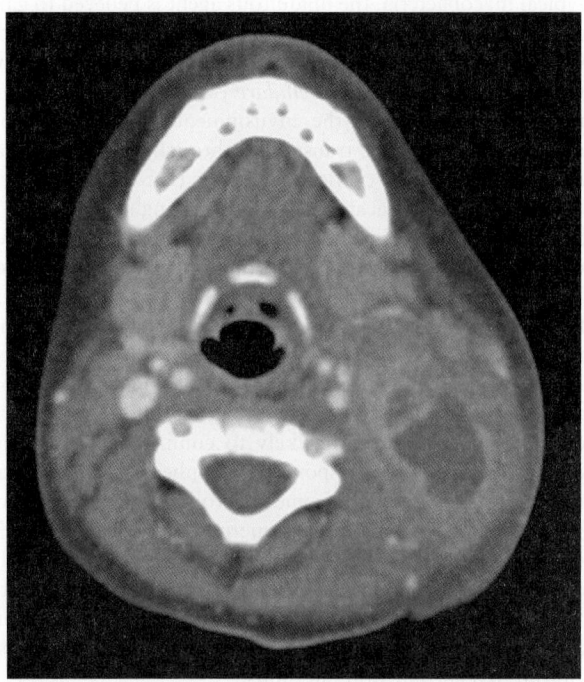

Figure 123.8 Computed tomographic scan with contrast demonstrating left lateral neck abscess/necrotic lymph nodes from cervical adenitis.

into the mediastinum, or spontaneously rupture into the pharynx, causing aspiration of purulent material.

Otolaryngologic consultation should be obtained to assist the emergency physician in the evaluation of a patient with a parapharyngeal abscess. Appropriate treatment consists of hospitalization, IV fluids, antimicrobials effective against *S. aureus* and *Streptococcus* species (antistaphylococcal and β-lactamase–resistant penicillins, clindamycin, cephalosporins), and external drainage of the abscess. Occasionally, infections may be polymicrobial in nature and include anaerobic bacteria from the oral cavity and, less often, gram-negative organisms.

Retropharyngeal abscess occurs as a result of the necrosis of retropharyngeal lymph nodes or secondary to perforation of the pharynx or esophagus. Purulent material collects between the retropharyngeal and prevertebral layers of the cervical fascia, also called the danger space. This potential space extends from the base of the skull to the mediastinum, thus allowing extensive spread of the infection. A child presents with symptoms similar to those associated with parapharyngeal abscess. Lateral neck radiographs demonstrate widening and bulging of the retropharyngeal space, but these radiographs have a high false-positive rate and are best used as screening tests (Fig. 123.6). CT scanning with IV contrast is most useful to diagnose the presence of a retropharyngeal infection but is less helpful in differentiating a drainable abscess from cellulitis. Treatment consists of hospitalization, IV fluids, and antimicrobials effective against *S. aureus* and *Streptococcus* species. Drainage of the abscess (either intraoral or through the external neck) is necessary in 60% to 70% of cases and should be done if the child has signs of airway compromise, has findings of a large hypolucent mass with thick enhancing capsule on CT radiographs, or has failed to respond to IV antibiotic therapy after 48 to 72 hours.

Nontubercular mycobacterial (NTM) infection is a common cause of chronic cervical adenitis in children. Also called atypical mycobacteria, the ubiquitous agent is believed to gain access to the cervical lymph nodes through oral mucosal or skin breaks (e.g., teething, minor trauma). Most cultures grow *Mycobacterium avium intracellulare* (MAI). These organisms are commonly found in the environment in dirt, dust, and water. They can also be transmitted through food. The usual presentation of NTM cervical adenitis is that of a nontender, slightly fluctuant cervical mass with overlying skin that has a characteristic violaceous hue. By history, the mass may have been present for weeks, so it is important to rule out other causes of persistent lymphadenopathy such as lymphoma or other malignancies. Chest radiographs are usually normal and purified protein derivative test results are most often reported as negative or intermediate in their response. Fine needle aspiration to collect specimens for cytology or culture/smears for acid-fast bacteria are more likely to confirm the diagnosis. NTM infections do not respond to antitubercular antibiotics. Long courses (months) of some macrolides (clarithromycin) with or without rifabutin are sometimes effective, especially when surgical treatment has not been thoroughly effective. In general, the child should be referred to an otolaryngologist to consider surgical biopsy and excision or curettage to cure this condition. Incision and drainage are discouraged because these can lead to a chronic draining sinus.

Salivary gland infections should be considered in the differential diagnosis of a cervical mass suspected to be infectious in origin. Both viral and bacterial agents can be responsible for the infection, with the former being more common. Mumps (endemic parotitis) is the most common salivary infection in children. Although the parotid gland is involved in more than 85% of the cases, the submandibular gland may also be involved with the viral infection. The infection appears with acute painful swelling of the involved gland or glands. There is erythema around the intraoral orifice of the salivary duct, and the saliva expressed is generally clear. Treatment is supportive, with clear fluids, antipyretics, and analgesics as necessary.

Bacterial infections of the salivary glands are seen with signs and symptoms similar to those associated with cervical lymphadenitis. Neonatal parotitis and, less commonly, submandibular sialadenitis usually occur in a 3- to 4-week-old child after a systemic illness has caused dehydration. The affected gland is swollen and abscess formation may occur. Purulent material may be expressed from either Stenson's or Wharton's duct by massage of the affected salivary gland. Otolaryngologic consultation should be obtained. The child is hospitalized for treatment with IV antimicrobials effective against *S. aureus* (antistaphylococcal penicillin) and surgical drainage of any collection of purulent material. Recurrent or chronic infections of the salivary glands are usually related to some predisposing factors such as stones, ductal stenosis, or secretory immunodeficiency. Management should include the detection and correction of these conditions.

Neoplasms

Neoplasms of the neck, both primary and metastatic, occur in children. If a cervical neoplasm is suspected, an otolaryngologist should be consulted to perform a complete examination of the head and neck, including endoscopy of the nasopharynx, larynx, and hypopharynx.

The hemangioma is the most common neoplasm of the head and neck in children. Although they are more common on the skin of the face and scalp, lesions can occur on the skin of the neck and involve deeper structures such as the parotid gland. The diagnosis of cutaneous hemangiomas of the cervical skin is usually obvious on physical inspection; the lesions are red to reddish purple, flat or raised, blanch with pressure, and increase in size with crying or straining. Deep-seated lesions without cutaneous manifestations may require special diagnostic aids such as CT or MRI scans and, rarely, biopsy to confirm the diagnosis.

These juvenile hemangiomas demonstrate a cycle of rapid growth for the first 12 to 18 months of life. Slow regression and even total disappearance occurs over the next year or two. Because of this natural history, once the diagnosis of hemangioma is made, the preferred treatment is close observation. Lesions that grow rapidly to produce complications such as airway obstruction, skin necrosis, hemorrhage, high-output cardiac failure, or thrombocytopenia require more active intervention. The child should be admitted and otolaryngologic consultation obtained. Treatment modalities presently advocated include systemic corticosteroids, cryotherapy, CO_2 laser excision, interferon, sclerosing agents, and surgical excision.

Lymphangiomas are uncommon benign lesions of the neck. Cystic hygroma is the most common type of lymphangioma found in the neck. These lesions consist of multiple cystic spaces filled with lymph and, occasionally, blood. They appear most commonly as large lateral neck masses in neonates. The diagnosis is often obvious on physical examination of a large cystic lesion that transilluminates. The natural history of these lesions is usually one of progressive growth and enlargement. Lymphangiomas can fluctuate in size secondary to a concurrent infection of the head and neck or hemorrhage into a cyst. Small, stable, asymptomatic lesions can be managed by close observation. Surgical excision has been the treatment of choice for large symptomatic lesions, with several staged procedures often being required. Aspiration of a large cyst (or cysts) can temporarily decompress a lesion, and use of sclerosing agents introduced by needle under radiographic guidance has been useful in controlling symptoms in those who have disease that is difficult to excise. Large cystic hygromas may cause feeding difficulties or respiratory distress in the newborn and may necessitate early surgical intervention, which can include tracheostomy and gastrostomy.

Less common benign neoplasms of the neck in children include teratomas, paragangliomas (carotid body tumors, glomus tumors), neural sheath tumors (neurofibromas, neurolemmomas), and thyroid and salivary gland neoplasms.

The sternocleidomastoid "tumor" of infancy is an unusual lesion that appears as a discrete mass within the substance of the sternocleidomastoid muscle in a child 4 to 8 weeks old. The cause of this localized area of fibrosis is unknown. The lesion usually resolves with range-of-motion exercises. Surgical intervention is indicated in those cases in which the fibrosis progresses to cause persistent torticollis (see the "Neck Stiffness" section in Chapter 46), or if there is suspicion of a malignancy.

The most common malignant neoplasm of the neck in children is lymphoma, being almost equally divided into Hodgkin's and non-Hodgkin's types. The disease may be localized in the neck or be a part of a more generalized disorder. Physical examination often reveals multiple firm, rubbery, unilateral, or bilateral nodes. If the diagnosis of lymphoma is suspected, otolaryngologic consultation should be obtained for a careful examination of the oral cavity, pharynx, and paranasal sinuses to look for a primary or associated lesion. This not only aids in the evaluation of the extent of the lymphoma but may also locate a site from which a biopsy can be obtained without the morbidity of a neck exploration.

Cervical lymph nodes may appear as neoplasm metastatic from a nonlymphogenous primary tumor. Thyroid carcinoma, squamous carcinoma (lymphoepithelioma) of the nasopharynx, and malignant melanoma may all be seen first with enlarged cervical lymph nodes. These nodes tend to be hard, singular, and may be fixed to underlying structures. Otolaryngologic consultation should be obtained for a complete examination of the head and neck to search for a primary lesion. Biopsy of the node is usually required for diagnosis.

Rhabdomyosarcoma is the most common soft-tissue sarcoma of the head and neck in children, and its frequency of occurrence in the neck is second only to that in the orbit. The child usually presents with a history of rapid enlargement of a painless neck mass. The mass itself is hard, often diffuse, and poorly mobile. Although the diagnosis of rhabdomyosarcoma may be suspected from the history and physical examination, biopsy is always required for confirmation.

Many other malignant neoplasms can also occur in the neck. These include soft-tissue sarcomas other than rhabdomyosarcoma, malignant fibrous histiocytoma, and neuroblastoma.

Neck Mass

The differential diagnosis and ED management of the child with a neck mass are presented in detail in Chapter 44.

Torticollis (Wryneck)

The differential diagnosis and ED management of the child with torticollis or stiff neck are presented in detail in Chapter 45. For further details, see Chapters 111 and 110.

Suggested Readings

Albright JT, Pransky SM. Nontuberculous mycobacterial infections of the head and neck. *Pediatr Clin North Am* 2003;50(2):503–514.

American Academy of Pediatrics Subcommittee on Management of Acute Otitis Media. Diagnosis and management of acute otitis media. *Pediatrics* 2004; 113:1451–1465.

American Academy of Pediatrics Subcommittee on Management of Sinusitis and Committee on Quality Improvement. Clinical practice guideline: management of sinusitis. *Pediatrics* 2001;108(3):798–808.

Centers for Disease Control and Prevention, Advisory Committee on Immunization Practices. Pneumococcal vaccination for cochlear implant candidates and recipients: updated recommendations of the Advisory Committee on Immunization Practices. *MMWR Morbid Mortal Wkly Rep* 2003;52(31):739–740.

Chatrath P, Black M, Jani P, et al. A review of the current management of infantile subglottic haemangioma, including a comparison of CO_2, laser therapy versus tracheostomy. *Int J Pediatr Otorhinolaryngol* 2002;64:143–157.

DeSutter AI, DeMeyere MJ, Christiaens TC, et al. Does amoxicillin improve outcomes in patients with purulent rhinorrhea? A pragmatic randomized double-blind controlled trial in family practice. *J Fam Pract* 2002;51(4):317–323.

Dotevall L, Hagberg L. Successful oral doxycycline treatment of Lyme disease associated facial palsy and meningitis. *Clin Infect Dis* 1999;28(3):569–574.

Elden L, Tom LWC. Pediatric perspectives of rhinosinusitis. In: *Rhinosinusitis.* Thaler ER, Kennedy DW, eds. New York, NY: Springer, 2008:205–222.

Eppes SC. Diagnosis, treatment and prevention of Lyme disease in children. *Paediatr Drugs* 2003;5(6):363–372.

Guss J, Kazahaya K. Antibiotic-resistant *Staphylococcus aureus* in community-acquired pediatric neck abscesses. *Int J Pediatr Otorhinolaryngol* 2007;71 (6):943–948.

Jose J, Coatesworth AP, Anthony R, et al. Life threatening complications after partially treated mastoiditis. *BMJ* 2003;327(7405):41–42.

Marchetti F, Ronfani L, Nibali SC, et al. Delayed prescription may reduce the use of antibiotics for acute otitis media. *Arch Pediatr Adolesc Med* 2005;159:679–684.

McEwan J, Wijayasingham G, Clarke RW, et al. Paediatric acute epiglottitis: not a disappearing entity. *Int J Pediatr Otorhinolaryngol* 2003;67:317–321.

Ong YK, Tan HK. Suppurative intracranial complications of sinusitis in children. *Int J Pediatr Otorhinolaryngol* 2002;66(1):49.

Piglansky L, Leibovitz E, Raiz S, et al. Bacteriologic and clinical efficacy of high dose amoxicillin for therapy of acute otitis media. *Pediatr Infect Dis J* 2003; 22(5):405–413.

Reefhuis J, Honein MA, Whitney CG, et al. Risk of bacterial meningitis in children with cochlear implantation. *N Engl J Med* 2003;349(5):435–445.

Ruohola A, Heikkinen T, Meurman O, et al. Antibiotic treatment of acute otorrhea through tympanostomy tube: randomized double-blinded placebo controlled study with daily follow-up. *Pediatrics* 2003;111(5, pt 1):1061–1067.

Shah MB, Haddad J. Nontuberculous mycobacteria-induced parotid lymphadenitis successfully limited with clarithromycin and rifabutin. *Laryngoscope* 2004;114(8):1435–1437.

Weber SM, Grundfast KM. Modern management of acute otitis media. *Pediatr Clin North Am* 2003;50(2):399–411.

CHAPTER 124 ■ UROLOGIC EMERGENCIES

HOWARD M. SNYDER III, MD

Early in their lives, children become familiar with the act of voiding and the appearance of their genitals. Disturbances of either are a great source of concern to them and their parents. This may result in an anxious trip to the emergency department (ED), requiring the emergency physician to be familiar with the problems discussed in the chapter on scrotal pain (see also Chapter 57). This chapter discusses (i) penile problems, (ii) testicular problems, and (iii) urinary tract infections (UTIs). Renal trauma is covered in Chapters 100 and 112.

PENILE PROBLEMS

Penile Care in the Uncircumcised Male Infant

Although the data of Wiswell and Roscelli suggest that the presence of the foreskin may make ascending urinary infection an increased risk in newborn males, the overall low incidence of problems associated with the foreskin and the lack of benefits from its removal led us to continue to discourage routine circumcision. This view is common and increasing numbers of uncircumcised children are seen in EDs. Surprisingly, few physicians know how to care for uncircumcised boys. It is important to realize that, in male infants, adhesions between the glans and the foreskin are normal (Fig. 124.1). The foreskin is not normally retractable in this age group. No effort should be made to strip the foreskin back in infants because that not only produces undue pain for the child but also may result in a raw surface with consequent inflammation and scarring. Between ages 2 and 4, lysis of the adhesions is spontaneous in 90% of children. It is rare for the male infant to have any adverse hygienic consequence from leaving the foreskin in place until spontaneous lysis of the adhesions takes place. The small, whitish lumps that may be seen and felt beneath the foreskin represent only desquamated epithelium and need not be removed. When toilet training has occurred, it is wise to teach a boy to retract the foreskin enough to expose the meatus when he voids. Not only does this facilitate better aiming, but it also avoids leaving the inner foreskin wet with urine. Ammoniacal irritation can lead to inflammatory adhesions and may create a portal of entry for a bacterial balanoposthitis. When a boy is able to retract his foreskin, usually between 4 and 6 years of age but sometimes later, he may be taught to withdraw the foreskin and perform normal hygiene as part of bathing.

Phimosis and Paraphimosis

Phimosis exists when tightness of the distal foreskin precludes its being withdrawn to expose the glans. Although inflamma-

tion of the foreskin from severe chronic ammoniacal rash or infection may lead to scarring and a true phimosis, this is uncommon in children. More often, normal penile adhesions are confused with phimosis.

In the uncircumcised male infant, if the foreskin is retracted behind the glans and left in that position, venous congestion and edema of the foreskin results, making it difficult to reduce the foreskin to a normal position. This condition of a swollen, retracted foreskin is called *paraphimosis* (Fig. 124.2). The application of ice and steady local manual compression usually reduces the edema and permits manual reduction of the paraphimosis. Topical anesthetic cream or a local anesthetic penile block of the dorsal nerve of the penis at the base of the shaft will reduce the discomfort experienced by the child during compression of the edematous foreskin. Once a portion of the edema has been reduced, pressure on glans (like turning a sock inside out) usually permits reduction of the foreskin back to its normal position (Fig. 124.3). If manual reduction fails, a surgical division of the foreskin to permit reduction is indicated (Fig. 124.4). This may usually be accomplished with sedation and local anesthetic. If surgical reduction of the foreskin is required, it should be followed a few weeks later by a circumcision. Education in the care of the uncircumcised boy will reduce the incidence of this condition.

Balanoposthitis

Balanoposthitis is an infection of the foreskin that may extend onto the glans (Fig. 124.5A). It is a form of cellulitis and has its origin from a break in the penile skin, commonly associated with ammoniacal dermatitis. It may be the result of local trauma or may, in the older boy, be associated with poor penile hygiene. Scarring after the inflammatory reaction may lead to true phimosis. The acute infection is dealt adequately by warm soaks and the administration of an appropriate antibiotic, usually ampicillin (50 to 100 mg per kg every 24 hours in four divided doses) (Fig. 124.5B). It is unusual for a child to be unable to void as a result of this condition, although he may be more comfortable voiding while in a tub of warm water. After resolution of the acute infection, the youngster should be examined again, and, if true phimosis is present, a circumcision is advisable. One episode of balanoposthitis with a normal retractable foreskin does not indicate a need for a circumcision. However, if a child has recurrent infections, a circumcision is in order.

Penile Swelling

Although most penile swellings are painful and the result of either infection, as described previously, or trauma, to be

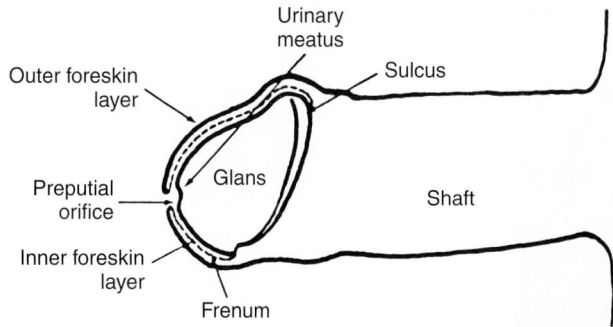

FIGURE 124.1 Anatomy of normal uncircumcised male. Adhesions between inner foreskin layer and glans are normal in newborns and prevent retraction of the foreskin. (From Wallerstein E. *Circumcision: an American health fallacy*. New York: Springer, 1980:201. Reprinted with permission.)

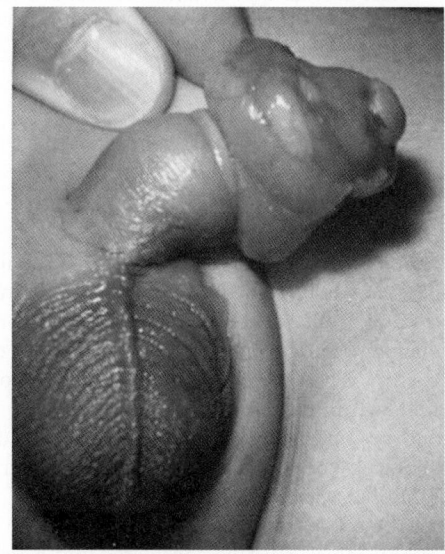

FIGURE 124.2 Paraphimosis—a foreskin that is left in a retracted position leads to venous congestion and edema of the foreskin.

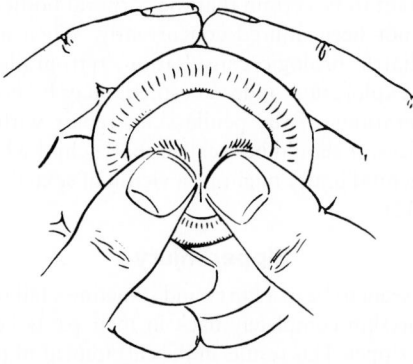

FIGURE 124.3 Manual reduction of paraphimosis. After a local anesthetic block of the dorsal nerve of the penis, the foreskin is manually compressed to reduce edema. The foreskin can be reduced by pressure on glans—like turning a sock inside out. (From Klauber GT, Sant GR. Disorders of the male external genitalia. In: Kelalis PP, King LR, Belman AB, eds. *Clinical pediatric urology*, 2nd ed. Philadelphia, PA: WB Saunders, 1985:287. Reprinted with permission.)

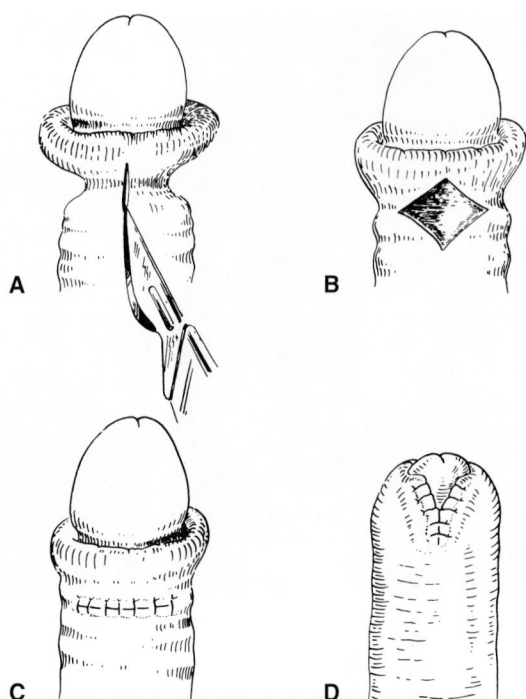

FIGURE 124.4 Surgical correction of phimosis. **A:** Constricting foreskin is incised vertically on dorsum. **B:** The incision opens laterally, relieving constriction. **C:** Incision is closed transversely with chromic catgut sutures. **D:** Foreskin can now be reduced. (From Klauber GT, Sant GR. Disorders of the male external genitalia. In: Kelalis PP, King LR, Belman AB, eds. *Clinical pediatric urology*, 2nd ed. Philadelphia, PA: WB Saunders, 1985:827. Reprinted with permission.)

described later, occasionally a child has isolated penile edema that is either nontender or minimally tender. This may result from an insect bite, with local edema secondary to histamine release. A history of a bite or the finding of a small punctate lesion may give the clue to diagnosis. Painless penile edema may be present with a generalized allergic reaction or as part of the manifestation of a general edematous state secondary to renal, cardiac, or hepatic problems. Here, the diagnosis is suggested by evidence of dysfunction in these organ systems on general examination. It is also important to remember that penile swelling may be caused by a strangulation injury (see "Strangulation" section).

Priapism

Prolonged, painful penile erection unaccompanied by sexual stimulation is called *priapism*. In the pediatric age group, this entity may be caused by trauma or leukemic infiltration, but it is most often seen in African American male persons with sickle cell disease. A sickling crisis that involves the corporal bodies does not necessarily need to be related to symptomatic sickling elsewhere in the body. Sickling of the erythrocytes produces sludging and stasis in the erectile tissue of the corporal bodies. This stasis leads to further hypoxia, acidosis, and more sickling. The thick, dark sludge that is formed prevents detumescence of the erectile tissue and thus causes priapism.

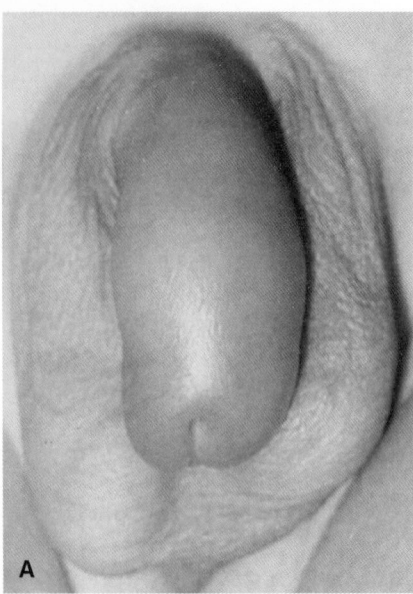
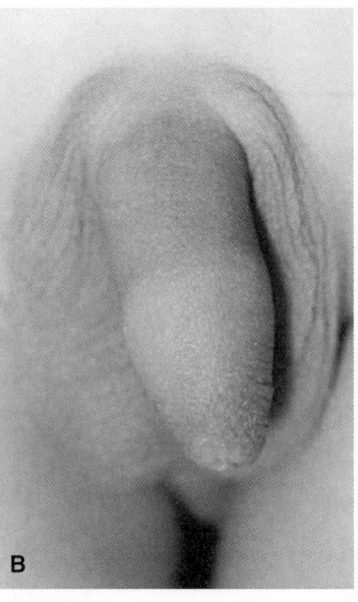

FIGURE 124.5 **A:** Balanoposthitis—cellulitis of normal foreskin with erythema, edema, and tenderness. **B:** Normal foreskin after treatment of balanoposthitis with antibiotics and warm soaks.

Pain results from ischemia. It is speculated that an inflammatory reaction to this material may lead to fibrosis of the erectile tissue. Impotence may result.

Although recommendations for treating priapism have ranged from ice or hot packs, estrogens, and spinal anesthesia to radiation therapy, the best treatment for priapism associated with sickle cell diseases now appears to be hydration and irrigation of the corporal bodies with saline in combination with vasoactive substances. This is best performed with urologic consultation. Although priapism has been documented to lead to impotence in some cases, impotence is rare in priapism related to sickle cell disease, unless the patient has been subjected to a surgical procedure. It may be that the more difficult cases are the ones most likely to come to surgical treatment, and impotence thus may reflect more the basic disease, rather than the type of treatment.

Meatal Stenosis

Meatal stenosis is a problem almost exclusively of circumcised male persons and follows an inflammatory reaction around the meatus, usually the result of the lower edge of the meatus rubbing against a wet diaper, with inflammation of the meatus resulting from mechanical and ammoniacal chemical dermatitis. Meatal stenosis is rare in the boy who has a circumcision after becoming continent. Appearances are often deceiving. The meatus may appear to be stenotic but may be functioning adequately. Significant meatal stenosis causes spraying of the urinary stream or, more commonly, dorsal deflection of the stream. Surgical treatment of the meatus is warranted only if these symptoms are present. Meatal stenosis is not a cause of frequency, enuresis, or UTI. When it is indicated, we perform a meatotomy in our office after application of topical penile anesthesia with EMLA Cream. A general anesthetic is usually neither necessary nor indicated.

Penile Trauma

Direct Injury

The most common cause of direct injury to the penis comes from a toilet seat's falling on the penis of a little boy who is learning to stand at the toilet to void. Although the resulting penile edema may be notable, significant injury to the corporal bodies or urethra is rare. Although parents may be concerned that the child will be unable to void, this generally is not a problem, but the child may be more comfortable voiding in a tub of warm water. The only treatment required is warm soaks and expectant observation.

After blunt or sharp trauma, if blood is seen at the urethral meatus, urethral injury must be considered and a retrograde urethrogram performed. Pediatric urologic consultation is appropriate, as is follow-up for possible stricture formation (see Chapter 112).

If a child is seen for a laceration of the shaft of the penis, it is important to be certain that the corporal bodies and urethra have not been injured concurrently. When a question exists, pediatric urologic consultation, retrograde urethrogram, and exploration under anesthetic may be needed. For simple lacerations of the penile skin, repair with chromic catgut suffices. It should be recalled that a child who has any form of a genital injury might be a victim of sexual abuse (see Chapter 132).

Zipper Injury

Boys often seem to be in a hurry and sometimes fail to get their penis or foreskin completely back in their pants before they pull up the zipper. This results in the entrapment of penile skin or foreskin in the teeth of the zipper. The teeth may be so engaged that it is impossible to simply unzip the zipper. Often, the problem may be dealt with simply, as shown in Fig. 124.6. The median bar of the zipper may be cut with a pair of wire cutters, which will permit the two halves of the zipper to fall

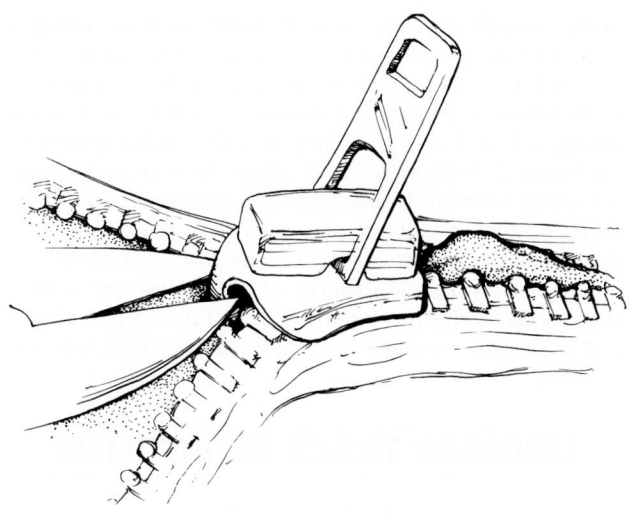

FIGURE 124.6 Penile zipper injury. A wire cutter may be used to cut the median bar of the zipper, releasing the two sides of the zipper and freeing the penis.

apart, releasing the entrapped skin. Mineral oil has also been used quite effectively to allow the tissue to slide free of the metal zipper. Local infiltration of lidocaine (Xylocaine®) or application of anesthetic cream makes this procedure less traumatic to the child. Only rarely is a general anesthetic required. After the zipper is removed, the penis may become edematous, but generally nothing more than warm soaks is required for further treatment.

Strangulation

The penis may be encircled by a constricting ring formed by a hair, fiber, or thread, just as occurs with digits. Many times, the cause of the problem is not immediately evident because local edema may hide the ring of hair. The edema is produced by venous engorgement, which takes place early, after the development of this type of constriction around the penis. Once the source of the problem has been identified, therapy requires the division of the hair and the release of the constriction. This may require a general anesthetic. Pediatric urologic consultation is advisable. A urethrocutaneous fistula, or even loss of the penis, has been reported but is rare. How the hair comes to encircle the penis is generally unknown, but it should be remembered that such constriction occasionally has been reported as a form of sexual abuse.

TESTICULAR PROBLEMS

Background

Primordial germ cells have their origin in the entoderm of the yolk sac. By the fifth week of intrauterine life, they have reached the ventromedial portion of the urogenital ridge, the portion destined to form the testes. A mesodermal cord, the gubernaculum, becomes attached to the bottom of the testis at the epididymis and runs to the bottom of the scrotum. With rapid growth of the trunk, the testes lie adjacent to the internal

ring by the third month of gestation. The testes remain at this location until the seventh month when, preceded by a fold of peritoneum (the processus vaginalis), the testes move down the inguinal canal and reach their final scrotal position shortly before birth. This fact accounts for the higher incidence of undescended testis in premature boys.

The gubernaculum appears to have an important role in testicular descent, although the exact nature of that role remains incompletely understood. Acute conditions involving the testes are discussed in Chapter 57.

Retractile Testis

In the physical examination of the child in the ED, an empty scrotum on one or both sides is a common finding. Although the testis may be found to be truly undescended, more often it is merely a retractile testis. In a boy with a retractile testis, the active cremaster muscle attached to the small prepubertal gonad is able to draw the testis up into a position near the pubic tubercle. There is no evidence that this causes any harm to the gonad. When the testis enlarges at puberty, it will assume a scrotal position permanently because the cremaster is no longer able to draw it out of its more normal position. The diagnosis of a retractile testis is made when one is easily able to milk the testis down into a position in a dependent portion of the scrotum where the testis stays, at least briefly, after overstretch of the cremaster muscle. In an obese youngster, it may be difficult to grasp the testis to pull it down. It is worthwhile putting a youngster in a "catcher's position," in which the testis is pushed down to where it can be grasped and drawn into the scrotum. If the testis can be pulled into the scrotum but, regardless of how much the cremaster is overstretched, the testis "pops up" when released, this is a low form of a true undescended testis and not a retractile testis. This is a common diagnostic difficulty, and pediatric urologic consultation should be sought if the situation is questionable.

Undescended Testis

True undescended testes are seen in 4% of newborn males. That instance decreases to 1.6% by 1 year of age, indicating that some undescended testes do descend after birth. Spontaneous descent rarely occurs after 6 months of age. Although it may be appropriate to continue for a few months to observe an infant who has an undescended testis, the child older than 6 months should have urologic consultation.

Testicular malignancy and infertility are increased in the male infant with an uncorrected undescended testis. By electron microscopy, it is possible to demonstrate degenerative changes in the undescended testis by 1 year of age. Early referral to a urologist for orchiopexy (before age 2 and preferably near age 1) appears advisable because data are now accumulating that indicate early surgery may decrease the incidence of both testicular malignancy and infertility.

Usually, an undescended testis is asymptomatic. However, in a position against the abdominal wall, it may be more subject to trauma than when freely mobile in the scrotum. The undescended testis is also malfixed and may undergo torsion more easily than a normally descended one. The boy who presents with an acutely tender groin mass with an ipsilateral empty scrotum may have torsion of his undescended testis. The physician must consider the differential diagnosis of an incarcerated inguinal hernia or acute hydrocele of the cord. Prompt surgical treatment is required.

Varicocele

Varicoceles are abnormal dilations of the cremasteric and pampiniform venous plexuses surrounding the spermatic cord (Fig. 124.7). They generally present as an asymptomatic scrotal swelling about the time of puberty and are rare in the prepubertal boy. Almost all are of congenital origin and affect the left testis. The anatomic problem is a defect in the valves of the left spermatic vein that, on the left, drains directly into the left renal vein. A higher left renal vein pressure may also play a role. Why varicoceles are often not noted until boys approach puberty is unclear, but they are common in that age group, affecting about 15% of adolescent boys. If the varicocele does not disappear when the child lies down, it suggests a varicocele secondary to obstruction of the left renal vein, and a renal and bladder ultrasound is appropriate. Varicoceles are rarely symptomatic; a heavy or tugging sensation is occasionally reported.

Approximately 15% of these boys with a varicocele will have an adult problem with infertility, although the exact mechanism of injury to the spermatogenic elements remains to be defined. Thus, periodic examination of these boys as they progress through pubertal change is recommended. As

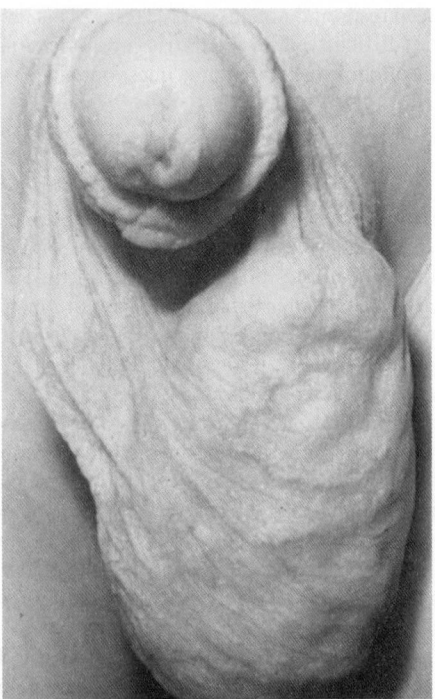

FIGURE 124.7 Varicocele—abnormal dilation of cremasteric and pampiniform venous plexuses surrounding the spermatic cord, giving the scrotum the appearance of a "bag of worms."

in the postpubertal testis, more than 80% of testis volume is a result of the spermatogenic elements; testis size is generally accepted as an indication of the effect of the varicocele on testis function. Although testicular asymmetry is common during pubertal change, a progressively smaller ipsilateral testis over 2 years or more of follow-up is an appropriate indication for surgical or radiographic treatment of the varicocele. "Catch-up" enlargement may occur after treatment of the varicocele. In our experience, any form of treatment is needed in only a small minority of cases. However, controversy exists on this point and long-term follow-up of adolescent boys with a varicocele is insufficient to permit firm conclusions.

URINARY TRACT INFECTIONS

Background

UTI ranks behind upper respiratory tract problems as the second most common form of bacterial infection in children. Between 1% and 2% of infants and children have bacteriuria at any given time, and 5% of all girls have UTI during their school years. Most UTIs result from fecal bacteria on the perineal skin ascending the urethra. The short female urethra, with resultant ease of bacterial contamination of the bladder, accounts for the higher incidence of UTIs in girls. The uncircumcised male infant younger than 6 months also appears to be at increased risk of ascending urinary infection because foreskin bacterial colonization may lead to increased meatal contamination. However, because the absolute risk of UTI in male infants is in the order of 1%, it is questionable to suggest the risk of UTI is an indication for routine circumcision.

It is now recognized that the major risk factor in the development of UTI is the physical nature of the uroepithelium lining the urethra and bladder. In some children and adults, adherence factors in the mucosa lead to recurrent episodes of symptomatic infection. In addition, some bacteria (piliated ones) have increased adherence characteristics that add to the risk of invasive infection. Because voiding dysfunction may also contribute to recurrent infection, this is another reason to consider pediatric urologic consultations, especially in the older child who persists with wetting after appropriate treatment of infection.

A UTI may be defined as the multiplication of bacteria in the urinary tract. Normally, urine from the bladder and upper urinary tract should be sterile. The concept of "significant bacteriuria" (10^5 or more organisms per milliliter of one colony type) in a cleanly voided midstream specimen is based on the statistical likelihood that this colony count is associated with the actual presence of bacteria in the bladder. A colony count of 10^5 or more organisms per milliliter of a single type suggests infected urine, with an 80% confidence level. Reliability can be increased to 95% if a second culture confirms the presence of the same bacteria type with identical antibiotic sensitivity; 10^4 to 10^5 bacteria per milliliter is an equivocal result and requires repeat culture. Less than 10^4 organisms per milliliter or the presence of several different organisms suggests no infection or contamination of the specimen (see Chapter 84).

Clinical Manifestations

Particularly in the infant, UTIs may produce nonspecific findings. The urine may be cloudy or have a foul odor. There may be a history of unexplained fevers, general irritability, or failure to thrive and gain weight normally. Gastrointestinal (GI) symptoms are common, and many times, the youngster with a UTI is believed to have gastroenteritis or a food allergy. A high index of suspicion is required. If a urine culture is not obtained, the source of the child's problem will be missed.

In the older child, symptoms may point more directly at the urinary tract. Frequency, urgency, and dysuria are produced by inflammation of the bladder and urethra. A previously toilet-trained child may begin to have "accidents." Particularly in girls, hematuria may be seen. Although symptoms do not provide a completely reliable way of differentiating cystitis from pyelonephritis, the presence of systemic findings such as a high fever and malaise or abdominal/flank pain suggests renal involvement. A UTI, especially when chronic, may also have few or no symptoms. It is important to emphasize that in children, anything that irritates the urethral meatus may produce dysuria and, occasionally, urgency and frequency (see Chapter 53). The source of the irritation may be a tight or moist bathing suit, underwear, or an ammoniacal rash. Bubble bath or other soap in contact with the urethral meatus may not only produce these symptoms but also, by producing inflammation, contribute to the ascent of bacteria up the urethra and to the development of true infection. To avoid being confused by a noninfectious cause of symptoms, it is important that UTIs be proven by urine culture and not diagnosed by history and urinalysis alone.

Escherichia coli is the most commonly isolated organism responsible for UTI in children, constituting 80% to 90% of the total. This is because of the prevalence of the organism in GI tract flora, as well as its short mean generation time, which enables it to multiply rapidly once it has entered the bladder. The other organisms commonly found can be seen in Table 124.1.

Management

The first step in management is to make an accurate diagnosis. The presence of pyuria does not provide an accurate criterion for the diagnosis of UTI. At least 20% of children with pyuria do not demonstrate significant bacteriuria. In any febrile illness, mobilization of the peripheral leukocyte pool may be adequate to produce the presence of white blood cells in the urine. Conversely, a child with bacteriuria occasionally does not demonstrate pyuria. Bacteria demonstrated by Gram stain of an unspun urine specimen are more reliably indicative of a UTI. However, it is difficult to determine whether one type of bacteria or several different contaminants are present. Thus, culture of the urine must continue to be the benchmark for the diagnosis of a UTI in children. Obtaining an adequate urine specimen for bacterial culture is the most critical step in diagnosing UTI. A cleanly voided specimen obtained as a midstream catch after washing of the periurethral area is the preferred technique in the toilet-trained child. Simple soap and water washing of the periurethral area is preferred because antimicrobial soaps or solutions may become mixed with a voided specimen and lead to a false-negative result.

In the infant, obtaining an adequate urine specimen is more difficult. Specimens collected in a plastic bag (U-bag) attached to the perineum are rapidly contaminated by perineal bacterial skin flora. If a culture from a bag is sterile, it is acceptable. However, the demonstration of bacterial growth must be confirmed by some other means before a bona fide UTI can be presumed to be present. The most reliable way to obtain a confirming specimen of urine is by urethral catheterization or suprapubic aspiration of urine from the bladder, a procedure that is not dangerous and that has a reliability approaching 100%. The procedure for performing suprapubic aspiration is covered in Section VII. If it is essential that the first specimen be the definitive one for diagnosis of UTI, as in the infant undergoing septic workup, the primary use of these techniques is justified. When symptoms strongly suggest the possibility of a UTI, beginning antibiotic therapy as soon as an adequate urine specimen for culture has been obtained is recommended. The matter of just 1 or 2 days before the institution of antibiotics may make a difference in the degree of eventual pyelonephritic scarring. If the urine culture turns out to be negative for UTI, the antibiotics may be stopped. Table 124.2 lists the most commonly used outpatient antibiotics for UTIs.

Although any of these antibiotic choices is acceptable in the initial therapy of a UTI, sulfamethoxazole–trimethoprim has become most commonly used in recent years because of its acceptance by children and its high efficacy. Nitrofurantoin, although effective, can produce GI upset (lessened by taking with meals) and is less well-tolerated by most children. Also poor serum levels make it a poor choice in the treatment of pyelonephritis. Methenamine mandelate is not useful unless there is urinary stasis and acid urine and accordingly has little role in most childhood UTIs. Tetracycline is not recommended for the child younger than 10 years because of its potential for discoloration of the teeth. When the organism causing UTI is sensitive to the antibiotic selected, the urine is usually sterilized rapidly. It is advisable to repeat a culture 48 hours after starting an antibiotic. The continued presence of infection suggests inaccuracy of the sensitivity, noncompliance, or obstruction.

If a child is sufficiently toxic to warrant hospitalization, the intravenous administration of antibiotics is appropriate. The drug of choice while cultures are pending is ampicillin or cephalosporin, usually combined with an aminoglycoside.

More recently, the duration of therapy has been a subject of debate. For uncomplicated cystitis, 1 to 3 days of therapy is usually adequate. For children with a febrile UTI or who have not been radiographically evaluated or for any child with a congenital anomaly, a 10-day course of antibiotics continues to be recommended.

TABLE 124.1

BACTERIA COMMONLY CAUSING URINARY TRACT INFECTIONS

Escherichia coli	*Proteus* species
Klebsiella pneumoniae	*Pseudomonas aeruginosa*
Streptococcus faecalis	*Staphylococcus epidermidis*
(enterococcus)	

TABLE 124.2

ANTIBIOTIC AGENTS FOR URINARY TRACT INFECTIONS

Drug	Oral dosage	Number of doses
Sulfamethoxazole–trimethoprim	1 mL suspension/kg/day	2
Sulfisoxazole	120 mg/kg/day	4
Nitrofurantoin	5–7 mg/kg/day	4
Amoxicillin	50–100 mg/kg/day	3
Cephalexin	50–100 mg/kg/day	4

Other factors in the treatment of UTI involve high fluid intake with regular and frequent voidings to promote bladder washout of bacteria. If the child has a history of wetting, infrequent voiding, or frequent urge episodes, the possibility of dysfunctional voiding, which can contribute to recurrent infections, should be considered and appropriate consultation obtained. Avoiding constipation helps ensure better bladder emptying. Constipation is being recognized increasingly as a factor that contributes to UTI. Good perineal hygiene, including wiping from front to back after a bowel movement, is important. Eliminating pinworms prevents a source of inflammation, excoriation, and secondary increase in perineal skin flora. Bubble bath, by producing inflammation at the meatus, may promote the ascent of bacteria and should be avoided. Acidification of the urine with oral vitamin C or juices high in citric acid content may be useful to produce an acid urine in which bacteria multiply less rapidly.

Urologic Follow-up and Radiographic Investigation

A suppressive dose of antibiotics should be begun after the acute phase of full-dose treatment. It is customary to use one-third to one-half the dose of antibiotic used for acute treatment, usually administered in a once-per-day evening dose. Suppressive antibiotics reduce the likelihood of recurrent infection, pending urologic consultation and radiographic investigation.

The routine radiographic evaluation of a UTI is by means of a voiding cystourethrogram (VCUG), followed by an ultrasound examination of the kidneys and bladder. These studies are usually performed about 2 to 4 weeks after the acute treatment of a UTI; however, failure of a child to respond promptly to appropriate antibiotic therapy should lead to the urgent performance of an ultrasound examination to rule out urinary obstruction. The cystogram must include a voiding phase or else significant pathology may be missed, particularly vesicoureteral reflux, which may be evident only on voiding films. In the usual child with a UTI, cystoscopy contributes little to the initial investigation; therefore, it is not recommended.

Any child with a history of a febrile UTI and all boys should be investigated after their first UTI. In girls without a febrile UTI, the usual recommendations have been to wait until a second infection before recommending urographic investigation. However, Kunin's data demonstrate that after one UTI there is an 80% likelihood of a second episode of bacteriuria and that half of these children will be asymptomatic. Thus, it appears justified to perform radiographic studies after a first documented infection in girls, as well as boys, or at the least to follow girls who have recovered from a first UTI, with repeat cultures at regular intervals.

In approximately 50% of infants and 30% of older children, an anatomic abnormality is found in association with a UTI. The most common finding is vesicoureteral reflux. Reflux permits infected urine to ascend to the kidney, where pyelonephritic damage may occur. With linear growth of the child, many milder cases of reflux may spontaneously resolve, leaving surgical management primarily for the more severe cases. These decisions are best made in consultation with a pediatric urologist.

As for the child who has no abnormality demonstrated by ultrasound and VCUG, the parents can be reassured that although the child may have a symptomatic problem from cystitis, there is little likelihood of renal damage. Occasionally, if a child has frequent episodes of symptomatic cystitis, suppressive antibiotics are justified to reduce the morbidity of these infections. The primary factor responsible for the development of urinary infection appears to be an adherent uroepithelium, which leads bacteria that ascend the urethra to stick to the bladder lining and become invasive. Like adults, children who have such bladder lining may experience several UTIs per year. Surgical manipulation, such as urethral dilation, does nothing to change the basic bladder problem and is no longer performed. When infections recur in rapid sequence, this may indicate the colonization of the GI bacterial flora by organisms with increased adherence characteristics. Fortunately, during 3 to 6 months of suppressive antibiotic therapy, these organisms tend to modulate to less adherent bacteria. It should also be borne in mind that children with dysfunctional voiding patterns also tend to be troubled with frequent UTIs. Thus, if a child has an abnormal voiding pattern when uninfected (wetting, infrequent voiding), a pediatric urologic assessment is in order.

ACUTE URINARY RETENTION

A patient with acute urinary retention is unable to empty the bladder even though it is full. In children, as in adults, the cause may be a urethral obstruction. Congenital lesions, such as urethral valves, or acquired lesions, such as posttraumatic strictures, may lead to urinary retention. In such cases, a careful history often elicits symptoms of a weak stream or difficulty initiating the stream. Children who have any form of urethral irritation and dysuria may voluntarily retain urine. That is a different situation and needs to be separated carefully from organic obstruction causing retention. For the child with voluntary retention, gentle massage of the lower abdomen, combined with a soak in a warm tub, usually leads to spontaneous evacuation of the bladder. Rarely does a child's bladder become so distended, as after an outpatient surgical general anesthetic, that the child is unable to void. A simple one-time emptying of the bladder by catheterization with a feeding tube usually corrects the problem. It should be remembered that a child is able to hold urine voluntarily for longer periods than would be suspected; up to 12 hours is not unusual. Unless the child has a history suggestive of an organic obstruction or has a palpably enlarged bladder that cannot be emptied by massage and warm tub soaks, instrumenting the child's urethra should not be considered. Urologic consultation would be advisable before undertaking such maneuvers.

Suggested Readings

General

Brown MR, Cartwright PC, Snow BW. Common office problems in pediatric urology and gynecology. *Pediatr Clin North Am* 1997;44:1091–1115.

Middleton RG, Matlack ME, Nixon GW, et al. Genitourinary injuries in children. In: Mayer TA, ed. *Emergency management of pediatric trauma.* Philadelphia, PA: WB Saunders, 1985:341–352.

Shalaby-Rana E, Lowe LH, Blask AN. Imaging in pediatric urology. *Pediatr Clin North Am* 1997;44:1065–1089.

Penile Problems

Boran P, Tokuc G, Yegin Z. Methemoglobinemia due to application of prilocaine during circumcision and the effect of ascorbic acid. *J Pediatr Urol* 2008;4: 475–476.

Brown-Trask B, Van Sell S, Carter S, et al. Circumcision care. *RN* 2009;72:22–28.

Docimo SG, Canning D, Khoury A, eds. *The Kelalis-King-Belman textbook of clinical pediatric urology,* 5th ed. London, England: Informa Healthcare, 2007.

El-Bahnasawy MS, El-Sherbiny MT. Paediatric penile trauma. *BJU Int* 2002;90: 92–96.

McHardy P, McDonnell C, Lorenzo AJ, et al. Management of priapism in a child with sickle cell anemia; successful outcome using epidural analgesia. *Can J Anaesth* 2007;54:642–645.

Mydlo JH, Harris CF, Brown JG. Blunt, penetrating and ischemic injuries to the penis. *J Urol* 2002;168:1433–1435.

Nakagawa T, Toguri AG. Penile zipper injury. *Med Princ Pract* 2006;15:303–304.

Nolan VG, Wyszynski DF, Farrer LA, et al. Hemolysis-associated priapism in sickle cell disease. *Blood* 2005;106:3264–3267.

Prais D, Shoov-Furman R, Amir J. Is ritual circumcision a risk factor for neonatal urinary tract infections? *Arch Dis Child* 2009;94:191–194.

Rogers ZR. Priapism in sickle cell disease. *Hematol Oncol Clin North Am* 2005;19:917–928.

Towbin R, Hurh P, Baskin K, et al. Priapism in children: treatment with embolotherapy. *Pediatr Radiol* 2007;37:483–487.

Wallerstein E. *Circumcision: an American health fallacy.* New York, NY: Springer, 1980.

Wiswell TE, Roscelli JD. Corroborative evidence for the decreased incidence of urinary tract infections in circumcised male infants. *Pediatrics* 1986;78:96–99.

Zampieri N, Pianezzola E, Zampieri C. Male circumcision through the ages: the role of tradition. *Acta Paediatr* 2008;97:1305–1307.

Testicular Problems

Barthold JS. Undescended testis: current theories of etiology. *Curr Opin Urol* 2008;18:395–400.

Bierich JR, Giarola A, eds. *Cryptorchidism.* London, England: Academic Press, 1979.

Fonkalsrud EW, Mengel W. *The undescended testis.* Chicago, IL: Year Book, 1981.

Foresta C, Zuccarello D, Garolla A, et al. Role of hormones, genes, and environment in human cryptorchidism. *Endocr Rev* 2008;29:560–580.

Hughes IA, Acerini CL. Factors controlling testis descent. *Eur J Endocrinol* 2008;159(suppl 1):S75–S82.

Hutson JM, Clarke MC. Current management of the undescended testicle. *Semin Pediatr Surg* 2007;16:64–70.

Kass EJ, Lundak B. The acute scrotum. *Pediatr Clin North Am* 1997;44: 1251–1266.

Main KM, Skakkebaek NE, Toppari J. Cryptorchidism as part of the testicular dysgenesis syndrome: the environmental connection. *Endocr Dev* 2009;14: 167–173.

Oster J. Varicocele in children and adolescents: an investigation of the incidence among Danish school children. *Scand J Urol Nephrol* 1971;5:27–32.

Scorer CG, Farrington GH. *Congenital deformities of the testis and epididymis.* London, England: Butterworth, 1971.

Skoog JS. Benign and malignant pediatric scrotal masses. *Pediatr Clin North Am* 1997;44:1229–1250.

Urinary Tract Infections

Downs SM. Technical report: urinary tract infections in febrile infants and young children: the Urinary Tract Subcommittee of the American Academy of Pediatrics Committee on Quality Improvement. *Pediatrics* 1999;103:e54.

Feld LG, Waz WR, Perez LM, et al. Hematuria: an integrated medical and surgical approach. *Pediatr Clin North Am* 1997;44:1191–1210.

Keren R. Imaging and treatment strategies for children after first urinary tract infection. *Curr Opin Pediatr* 2007;19:705–710.

Rushton HG. Urinary tract infections in children: epidemiology, evaluation and management. *Pediatr Clin North Am* 1997;44:1133–1169.

Shaikh N, Morone NE, Bost JE, et al. Prevalence of urinary tract infections in childhood. *Pediatr Infect Dis J* 2008;27:302–308.

Stahl GE, Topf P, Fleisher GR, et al. Single-dose treatment of uncomplicated urinary tract infections in children. *Ann Emerg Med* 1984;13:705–708.

CHAPTER 125 ■ ORTHOPEDIC EMERGENCIES

MARK D. JOFFE, MD, AND JOHN M. LOISELLE, MD

ORTHOPEDIC CONDITIONS

Orthopedic emergencies usually result from trauma (see Chapter 114). Nontraumatic orthopedic problems are often a clinical challenge because they may present as suspected injuries. Physicians must not be misled by the virtually ubiquitous history of injury in active young children. The nontraumatic orthopedic conditions described in this chapter are especially important to consider when a reported injury mechanism is minor or onset of symptoms is delayed. Evaluation of children with complaints such as limp (see Chapter 42), joint pain (see Chapter 56), and back pain (see Chapter 50), to name a few, requires consideration of both traumatic and nontraumatic causes. Children involved in competitive athletics train more intensively and at younger ages than in previous years, resulting in overuse syndromes. With knowledge and appropriate suspicion, physicians caring for children can identify nontraumatic orthopedic problems, begin treatment, and make intelligent recommendations about referral.

Osteomyelitis

Background

Osteomyelitis is an inflammation of the bone and bone marrow, most commonly of infectious origin. Infection is confirmed by the presence of two of the following: pus on an aspirate of the bone, clinical findings consistent with the diagnosis, positive blood or bone aspirate cultures, and consistent findings on medical imaging. Osteomyelitis is more common in boys with the highest incidence found among infants and preschool age children. Age and underlying disorders are associated with an increased risk for contracting osteomyelitis, as well as for the particular pathogens involved.

Pathophysiology

Infection occurs by one of three routes: hematogenous, direct spread, or inoculation through a penetrating wound. Hematogenous spread is the most common route of infection in children. A transient bacteremia is believed to be the initiating event in the infection. Bacteria enter the bone at the level of the metaphysis where the predominant vascular supply is located. The sluggish blood flow within the microvasculature of the marrow predisposes to infection. Local trauma has been suggested as a possible cause of microthrombotic events further predisposing bone to infection. This is supported by an association of trauma with the occurrence of osteomyelitis and the preponderance of infections occurring within the long bones,

especially those of the lower extremities. In sickle cell patients, microinfarcts within the more tenuously supplied area of the diaphysis may explain the increased occurrence in this region of the bone. As infection progresses, pressure increases and organisms penetrate up through the cortex to the subperiosteal space. If left untreated, the infection may spread along this space or rupture through the periosteum into the surrounding soft tissue.

Differences in the underlying bony structure in the neonate and young infant predispose them to a higher incidence of multifocal osteomyelitis and concomitant septic arthritis. The thin cortex allows easier penetration to the subperiosteal space. The periosteum is less adherent in these ages and less effective in limiting the spread of infection. Transphyseal vessels, which are present through the first 18 months of life, allow bacteria to gain access to the adjoining epiphysis and joint space.

A less common source of osteomyelitis in children is penetration of the periosteum by adjacent infections. Inoculation of the bone from stepping on a nail, surgical instrumentation, or intraosseous needle placement provides a third means for infection to gain entrance to the bone.

Inadequately treated infections can progress to a chronic osteomyelitis and may result in potentially deleterious effects on growth. There have also been reported cases of chronic recurrent multifocal osteomyelitis (CRMO), which is an autoinflammatory disorder characterized by bone pain and fever. Its course is one of exacerbations and remissions. The etiology of this condition is still unknown. Cultures of bone are sterile and radiographs may show lytic lesions. The presentation may mimic acute bacterial osteomyelitis, which must be ruled out and CRMO is a diagnosis of exclusion.

Clinical Findings

Physical signs of osteomyelitis are age dependent. The older child is more likely to have localized infection and is more capable of expressing or identifying a site of localized pain and point tenderness. The neonate or young infant may present with a pseudoparalysis of the affected limb. Another common, although nonspecific, finding in this age group is paradoxical irritability in which the infant exhibits pain or distress upon handling and is more comfortable when left alone.

Fever and pain are highly sensitive findings but are not universally present. Fever is described in up to 90% of children with osteomyelitis upon presentation and may be quite elevated. Pain is expressed through limp, refusal to bear weight, or a decreased range of motion when a limb is involved. Erythema and swelling are less frequent but can also be observed at the site, and usually suggest more advanced periosteal involvement.

Diagnosis

The diagnosis of osteomyelitis in the child can be challenging and misdiagnoses are common. Several injuries and illnesses with overlapping clinical, laboratory, and radiologic findings can mimic osteomyelitis. In addition to clinical findings, the diagnosis of osteomyelitis depends on culture results. Blood cultures and bone aspirates should be obtained in suspected cases of osteomyelitis before the initiation of antibiotics. Isolation of the causative organism is important not only in diagnosis, but also in antibiotic selection and the possibility of eventual outpatient therapy. Reports of positive blood cultures in the setting of osteomyelitis range from 30% to 57%. An organism is recovered from a bone aspirate in 51% to 90% of cases. The combination will identify a pathogen in 75% to 80% of cases. Bone aspirates may remain positive for several days after antibiotic use, whereas blood cultures are often sterile within 24 hours of the initiation of antibiotics.

Laboratory tests vary in sensitivity. The white blood cell (WBC) count rises in only one-third of the cases of osteomyelitis, whereas both the erythrocyte sedimentation rate (ESR) and C-reactive protein (CRP) are elevated in more than 90% of the cases. The latter tests are useful in diagnosis and in monitoring the response to therapy. The CRP peaks at 2 days and returns to normal following 7 to 10 days of appropriate therapy. The ESR may remain elevated for several weeks despite adequate treatment.

The plain radiograph is the initial imaging study of choice. It is useful both in detecting early signs of osteomyelitis and excluding other diagnostic possibilities. The earliest radiograph changes suggestive of osteomyelitis include deep soft-tissue swelling with elevation of the muscle planes from the adjacent bone (Fig. 125.1). These may be seen as early as 3 to 4 days after the onset of symptoms. Lytic bone changes are not detectable until 10 to 14 days. Periosteal elevation, when present, is not generally visible until 10 to 21 days after infection (Fig. 125.1). A negative radiograph in the first 10 days of illness does not rule out osteomyelitis. When suspicion remains high in the setting of a negative radiograph, further imaging studies should be obtained. The triple-phase technetium bone scan has a reported sensitivity and specificity of more than 90%, and will detect osteomyelitis within 24 to 48 hours of symptom onset. The bone scan can localize the site of infection and differentiate soft-tissue infection from bony involvement. It is the test of choice when osteomyelitis is suspected but a specific site of concern can not be identified by physical examination or when multiple foci of infection are possible. Magnetic resonance imaging (MRI) is also highly sensitive in detecting osteomyelitis and does not expose the child to ionizing radiation. In addition, MRI provides a higher degree of detail than the bone scan (Fig. 125.2). This is useful in detecting suspected complications of osteomyelitis such as a subperiosteal abscess or bone sequestrum. Many orthopedic surgeons prefer this high degree of resolution to guide a bone aspirate or biopsy. Both imaging studies commonly require sedation of the young child, but the bone scan is not as affected by small movements. A bone aspirate preceding a bone scan or MRI will not alter the results and should not be delayed because of this concern.

Microbiology

Organisms responsible for osteomyelitis differ according to the age of the patient, the route of infection, and any underlying

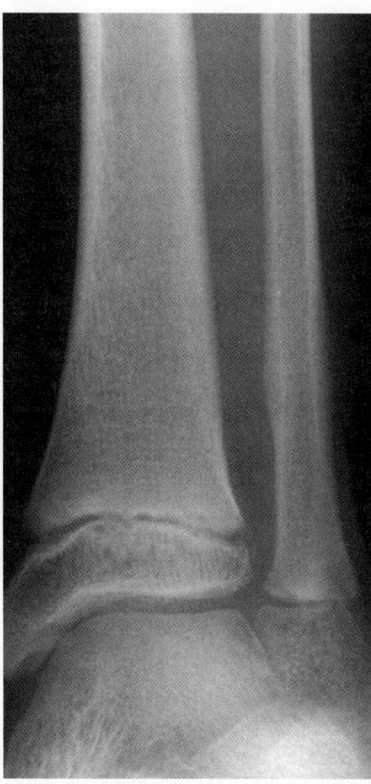

FIGURE 125.1 Periosteal activity in distal fibula in child with *Staphylococcus aureus* osteomyelitis; day 20 of illness.

medical problems. *Staphylococcus aureus* is the most common pathogen across all age groups accounting for 70% to 90% of cases. The incidence of community-acquired methicillin-resistant *S. aureus* (CA-MRSA) has increased dramatically in most areas of the United States. Some studies have found over 50% of cases due to MRSA. Osteomyelitis due to MRSA has been associated with longer duration of fever, extended hospitalization and increased frequency of complications. This may be a result of the high prevalence of certain genes encoding for virulence factors such as Panton-Valentine leukocidin (PVL). Group A β-hemolytic streptococcus is the second most common organism isolated in childhood osteomyelitis and accounts for 10% of cases outside of the neonatal period. A high prevalence is found in association with recent varicella infections. *Kingella kingae* has been sporadically reported in the toddler and preschool age group. It is a gram negative organism and therefore resistant to vancomycin and clindamycin, but sensitive to cephalosporins and β-lactam antibiotics. Bacterial isolates from neonates younger than 2 months include *S. aureus*, group B streptococcus, and *Escherichia coli*, and antibiotic coverage should reflect this.

Certain groups are at risk for particular organisms. Patients with sickle cell disease have a high incidence of osteomyelitis caused by salmonella. *Pseudomonas aeruginosa* is a common organism found in osteomyelitis of the foot, often resulting from a nail penetrating a sneaker.

Management

Initial therapy for osteomyelitis includes intravenous antibiotics. Empiric antibiotic coverage should be based on the predominant

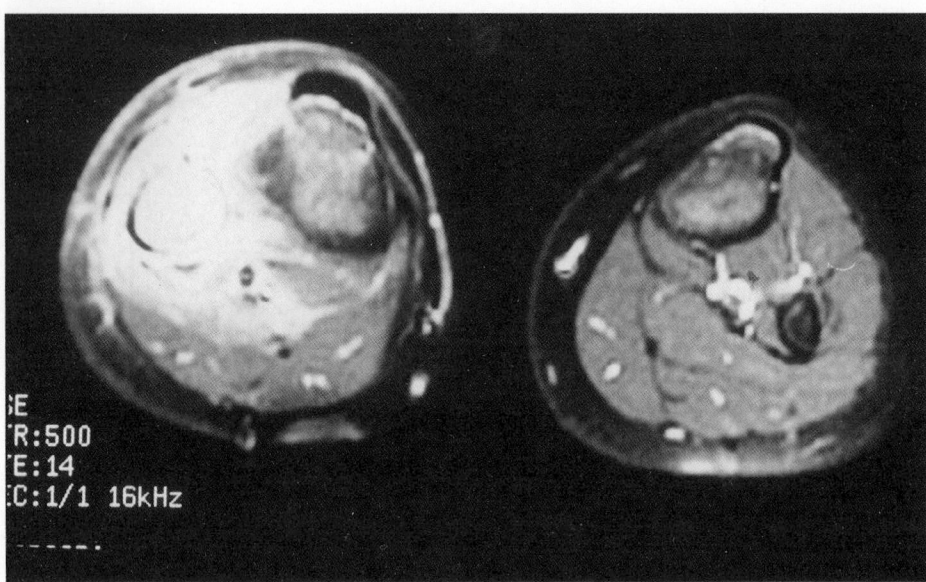

FIGURE 125.2 Magnetic resonance imaging of osteomyelitis of the proximal right fibula.

organisms in each age group, local sensitivity patterns, the mechanism of infection, and Gram stain results. Clindamycin is the treatment of choice for osteomyelitis outside of the neonatal age range when MRSA is suspected. Vancomycin may be indicated for empiric treatment when the incidence of clindamycin resistance in the community is high. Definitive treatment is ultimately based on the identification and sensitivity of recovered isolates. A third-generation cephalosporin or the addition of an aminoglycoside is indicated in the neonatal age group.

Suggested agents are listed in Table 125.1. Early aggressive antibiotic therapy frequently prevents the need for surgical intervention.

Septic Arthritis

Background

The presence of bacterial pathogens within the articular capsule presents a true surgical emergency. Delay in the identification and treatment of an infected joint in a child can result in severe and permanent sequelae. The urgency associated with this diagnosis has given rise to the maxim, "The sun should never rise or set on a septic hip." In many cases, the pediatric emergency physician will be the initial point of contact, and must maintain a high index of suspicion to recognize and appropriately treat these patients at the time of the first visit.

Pathophysiology

Bacteria gain entry to the joint space through one of three means. The highly vascular synovium is most commonly infected through hematogenous seeding. The role of local injury in predisposing joints to infection by this means is unclear. Organisms from adjacent areas of infection may invade the joint, or direct inoculation can occur through penetrating injuries. Infection secondary to penetrating objects may be delayed from the actual time of injury. External wounds may be small or healed at the time of presentation. Undetected penetration of the knee joint by a sewing needle in a crawling infant may give rise to a septic knee. A metatarsal joint infection may be the result of a nail puncture wound to the foot that occurred several weeks earlier.

TABLE 125.1

INITIAL ANTIBIOTIC THERAPY: OSTEOMYELITIS[a]

Age	Pathogens	Antibiotics
Neonate <2 mo	*Staphylococcus aureus*, group B streptococcus, gram-negative bacilli	Vancomycin and cefotaxime
>2 mo–5 yr	*S. aureus*, group A streptococcus, *Streptococcus pneumoniae*, *Kingella kingae*	Clindamycin[b,c]
>5 yr	*S. aureus*, group A streptococcus, *S. pneumoniae*	Clindamycin[c]
Special Cases		
Sickle cell disease	Salmonella, *S. aureus*	Clindamycin and ceftriaxone
Foot puncture wound	*Pseudomonas aeruginosa*, *S. aureus*	Cefepime or piperacillin/tazobactam

[a]Coverage modified on the basis of culture results and sensitivities.
[b]Add ceftriaxone for Gram stain negative for gram-positive cocci or culture positive for *Kingella kingae*.
[c]Vancomycin if high incidence of clindamycin resistance in community.

Eighty to 90% of septic joints occur in the lower extremities. The knee and hip are most commonly afflicted. The same distribution is found in the preambulatory child. Infections involve only a single joint in greater than 90% of cases. Multifocal infections are more common in neonates.

Once established within the joint, bacteria release endotoxins that stimulate the production of proteolytic enzymes by neutrophils and synovial cells. These enzymes directly damage the intraarticular cartilage. Pressure elevation within the minimally distensible joint capsule can compromise vascular flow, resulting in ischemic injury to the bone. This is a particular concern in the hip, where avascular necrosis of the femoral head is a well-described complication of septic arthritis. Prognosis is worse in children younger than 1 year, with involvement of the hip joint, with delay to the initiation of therapy, and with infection by *S. aureus*.

Clinical Findings

Pain is the most common presenting complaint in the child with a septic joint. The child may express this in many ways. The older child is better able to localize the area of discomfort. Because of the predominance of septic arthritis in the lower extremities, the younger child often presents with a limp, abnormal gait, or inability to bear weight. Referred pain from the hip may manifest as groin, thigh or knee pain.

Range of motion around the affected joint is dramatically reduced. Any degree of movement causes great distress and is vigorously resisted. Many clinicians rely on this aspect of the evaluation more than any other in differentiating infection from alternative causes of joint pain.

Clinical signs are more subtle in the neonate or young infant with a septic joint. Nonspecific findings such as septic appearance, irritability, and pseudoparalysis of a limb are common presenting findings in these ages. Parents may note excessive irritability associated with diaper changes in the infant with a septic hip. The child with a septic hip will typically hold the lower extremity in abduction and external rotation in order to decrease intracapsular pressure by maximizing the volume of joint space (Fig. 125.3). A high degree of suspi-

cion, close observation, and isolated manipulation of each extremity will help locate the particular area of involvement.

The skin surface should be closely evaluated for local signs of injury. Most involved joints will have obvious erythema, warmth, and swelling. The exception is the hip joint because of its deep-seated location. Swelling may be less obvious in the pudgy infant. Fever is a commonly associated sign but is absent in up to one-third of patients.

Diagnosis

The diagnosis of septic arthritis is confirmed by the identification of purulent fluid within the joint space. Arthrocentesis is a mandatory procedure in all suspected causes of septic arthritis. The decision to perform this procedure is based on the degree of clinical suspicion in combination with results of laboratory tests and imaging studies. None of these in isolation are 100% sensitive in detecting or excluding septic arthritis from other conditions. A sample of synovial fluid is often the only means of discriminating septic arthritis from less serious inflammatory processes.

The mean peripheral WBC count is elevated in children with septic arthritis, however, more than half of the patients will have a WBC count less than 15,000 per mm^3. The ESR and CRP are more sensitive markers and are elevated in 90% to 95% of patients.

Plain radiographs may demonstrate signs of an effusion ranging from subtle blurring or displacement of fascial planes to complete dislocation of the joint. The main role of the radiograph in the evaluation is to exclude fractures or other bony abnormalities that may mimic septic arthritis. Ultrasound is most useful in evaluating the hip. It is much more sensitive than the radiograph in detecting a joint effusion. Some have suggested that the absence of an effusion on an ultrasound scan effectively excludes the diagnosis of septic arthritis. The ultrasound cannot, however, distinguish between infected and sterile inflammatory effusions. Ultrasound guidance is useful in performance of a needle aspiration of the hip joint.

The bone scan localizes areas of inflammation and is unaffected by prior arthrocentesis. It cannot differentiate infection from other causes of inflammation. A bone scan may be helpful in excluding osteomyelitis. Inflammation is found symmetrically across a joint in septic arthritis, whereas in osteomyelitis it is limited to one side. The reliability of a bone scan in differentiating joint from bone involvement decreases in the neonatal age group.

The isolation of a bacterial pathogen is important in diagnosis and in directing subsequent management. Cultures of joint fluid and blood should be performed on all patients with a possible septic joint. The yield of organisms can be increased by directly inoculating joint fluid into a blood culture bottle. When indicated, cultures from additional sites should be obtained to increase the potential isolation of a pathogen. Cultures of the joint fluid demonstrate the highest yield and are positive in 50% to 80% of cases. Blood cultures identify an organism in 15% to 46% of patients with septic arthritis and are positive in many cases in which the organism is not isolated from the joint fluid. Cervical or urethral cultures in sexually active adolescents with septic arthritis may identify *Neisseria gonorrhoeae* as the responsible organism. In 20% of cases, a causative organism is not recovered. Improvement in polymerase chain reaction (PCR) techniques may increase the ability to identify pathogens.

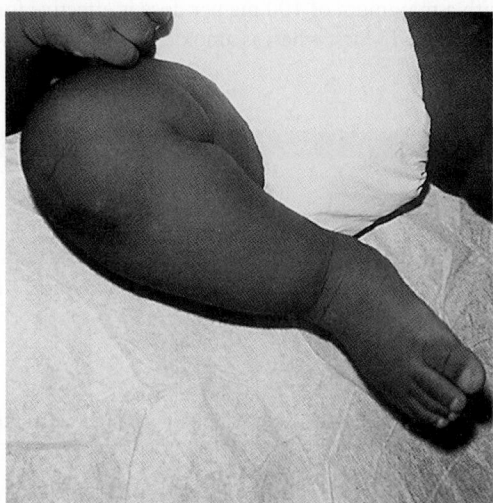

FIGURE 125.3 Five-month-old infant with septic arthritis of the right hip. Hip joint is held in flexion, abduction, and external rotation.

A Gram stain should be performed on joint fluid, and it occasionally provides additional assistance in identifying both the presence of an infection and the infecting organism. Although elevation of the WBC count more than 100,000 per mm^3 in the synovial fluid is considered strong evidence of infection, the actual counts are often much lower. Presence of purulent fluid, a positive Gram stain, and a highly elevated WBC count with a left shift in the synovial fluid are often used as indications for operative intervention when there is a concern of a septic hip.

Microbiology

With a few exceptions, bacteria found in septic arthritis are the same as those in osteomyelitis. *S. aureus* is the most common reported isolate in all age groups. Prior to the introduction of the Hib vaccine, *Haemophilus influenzae* type b was the leading cause of septic arthritis in the 6-month-old to 5-year-old age group. Through immunization, this organism has now been essentially eliminated and surpassed in frequency by group A streptococcus and Streptococcus pneumoniae. *S. aureus* is also the predominant pathogen in neonatal patients. Gram-negative coliforms and Group B β-hemolytic streptococcus are also found in this age group. *N. gonorrhoeae* is found in the neonatal ages and is a frequent pathogen in sexually active teenagers. *K. kingae* is a fastidious gram-negative rod, susceptible to beta lactam antimicrobials, which has recently been isolated as a pathogen in numerous childhood bone and joint infections. It is found most commonly in children younger than 36 months. *Neisseria meningitidis* is a rare but reported cause of septic arthritis in children.

Management

The management of septic arthritis consists of parenteral administration of antibiotics (Table 125.2) and joint immobilization. Joint irrigation should be performed in selected cases. Empiric antibiotic therapy is dictated by the common organisms in the age group, local sensitivities and by results of the synovial fluid Gram stain. Vancomycin or clindamycin is indicated depending on the incidence of clindamycin-resistant MRSA in the community. Gram-negative coverage should be added in neonates and adolescents. A third-generation cephalosporin should be added in patients with sickle cell disease because of susceptibility to salmonella infection.

Surgical intervention for joint irrigation is generally indicated for all cases involving the hip joint; infections in which large amounts of fibrin, debris, or loculations are found within the joint space; or when the patient fails to improve following several days of intravenous antibiotic therapy. Expeditious and aggressive management limits but does not eliminate potential sequelae of septic arthritis.

Lyme Arthritis

Lyme disease is a common cause of infectious arthritis in certain geographic locations within the United States. The infection is caused by the spirochete *Borrelia burgdorferi*. Arthritis is a manifestation of late disease and can occur 1 to 12 months following inoculation. Lyme arthritis is most often a monoarticular infection of the knee. If left untreated, symptoms can be episodic, lasting several days followed by several weeks to months without symptoms. Clinical and laboratory findings are similar to those for septic arthritis. Joint swelling is marked and out of proportion to the degree of pain. Fever is often absent and is generally low grade when present. Pain and limitation of movement of the affected joint is less than in septic arthritis, and patients are often able to ambulate despite the swelling. Infection can occur without a preceding history of a tick bite or the classic skin manifestations of erythema migrans. Extraarticular manifestations such as facial palsy or meningitis are rare but are helpful in the diagnosis when present. The ESR and CRP are elevated. The mean leukocyte count in synovial fluid is usually 10,000 to 25,000 cells per mm^3 but can exceed 50,000 cells per mm^3 with a neutrophil predominance. Routine cultures of synovial fluid are negative. Diagnostic testing for Lyme arthritis is indicated in endemic areas and should include serum enzyme-linked immunosorbent assay. Positive results should be confirmed by a Western immunoblot for IgG antibodies to *B. burgdorferi*. An IgM immunoblot assay is not necessary in late disease and may result in false-positive results. Negative serum IgG serology virtually excludes Lyme as the cause of arthritis. Treatment for Lyme arthritis consists of a 4-week course of oral antibiotics. Doxycycline in a dose of 4 mg per kg per day divided twice daily with a maximum of 100 mg per dose is effective for children older than 8 years, whereas amoxicillin (50 mg per kg per

TABLE 125.2

INITIAL ANTIBIOTIC THERAPY: SEPTIC ARTHRITIS[a]

Age	Pathogens	Antibiotics
Neonate <2 mo	*Staphylococcus aureus*, group B streptococcus, gram-negative bacilli	Vancomycin and cefotaxime
>2 mo–5 yr	*S. aureus*, group A streptococcus, *Streptococcus pneumoniae*, *Kingella kingae*	Clindamycin[b,c]
>5 yr	*S. aureus*, group A streptococcus	Clindamycin[c]
Adolescent	*S. aureus*, group A streptococcus, *Neisseria gonorrhoeae*	Clindamycin and ceftriaxone[d]

[a]Common pathogens and empiric antibiotic coverage by age.
[b]Add ceftriaxone for Gram stain negative for gram positive cocci or culture positive for *K. kingae*.
[c]Vancomycin, if high incidence of clindamycin resistance in community.
[d]Empiric treatment in sexually active adolescent.

day in three divided doses with a maximum of 1.5 g per day) is sufficient in younger children. Serum antibody titers remain elevated even after adequate antibiotic treatment and should not be used as a measure of success of treatment. Persistent or recurrent joint swelling may occur two months beyond the initiation of treatment. Although this may represent a local autoimmune response, experts recommend retreatment with a second 4-week course of oral antibiotics or a 2- to 4-week course of parenteral ceftriaxone.

Transient Synovitis

Background

Transient or toxic synovitis is a benign, self-limiting inflammatory condition of the hip. It afflicts males more frequently than females and is the most common cause of acute hip pain in children 3 to 10 years of age. The underlying cause is unknown, although a postinfectious inflammatory response has been suggested. Its presentation can mimic that of septic arthritis of the hip (Fig. 125.4), a distinction that is as crucial in management as it is difficult in diagnosis.

Clinical Findings

The onset of symptoms is abrupt with unilateral hip pain and limp. Fever is rare, occurring in less than 10% of cases, and when present, is usually low grade. Although patients complain of discomfort with movement of the limb, it is generally possible to gently maneuver the hip through a full range of motion. This contrasts with the septic hip in which pain and spasm are more extreme, and patients resist a full range of motion. Additional signs of systemic illness are absent and, despite the title, the child is nontoxic appearing.

Laboratory

Laboratory tests are generally useful only in attempting to distinguish transient synovitis from more serious conditions. The WBC count, ESR, and CRP are generally normal or only slightly elevated. The mean WBC count, ESR, and CRP are significantly lower than in septic arthritis; however, sufficient

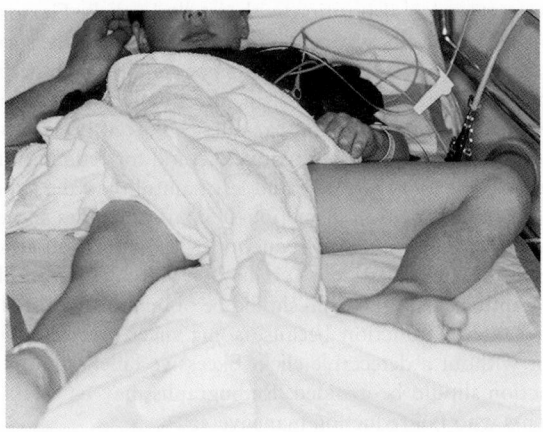

FIGURE 125.4 Seven-year-old child with transient synovitis of the left hip. Hip joint is held in same position of comfort as in septic arthritis.

overlap exists between values in transient synovitis and septic arthritis such that they do not reliably distinguish between the two conditions in individual patients.

Radiographs may demonstrate an effusion but principally serve to exclude pathologic osseous conditions. Ultrasound is more sensitive than plain films at detecting joint effusions, although accuracy declines in patients younger than 1 year of age. Reports of an effusion of the hip by ultrasound in transient synovitis vary from 50% to 95%. The clinician must use a combination of clinical, laboratory, and radiographic findings to determine which patients require further evaluation with needle aspiration of the hip. Although patients often report relief of pain following aspiration, the procedure is unnecessary except to exclude the presence of a bacterial infection. Synovial fluid, when obtained, is sterile. The synovial fluid WBC count is typically less than 50,000 cells per mm³.

Management and Prognosis

Treatment occurs on an outpatient basis, and emphasizes rest and analgesics. Traction is of unproven benefit and is potentially harmful. Nonsteroidal antiinflammatory medications are the first-line therapy for pain. Pain duration is typically 3 to 4 days but may last as long as 2 weeks. Exacerbations can occur if activity is resumed too early.

There is no evidence of serious sequelae resulting from transient synovitis. The relationship between transient synovitis and the subsequent development of Legg-Calvé-Perthes disease (LCPD) is unclear. Studies have been unable to demonstrate cause and effect. Some suggest that these patients are at increased risk for developing LCPD, whereas others believe only that the clinical presentations are similar. Recurrences of transient synovitis can occur up to several years later and are not associated with worse outcomes.

Penetrating Intraarticular Wounds

Penetrating intraarticular wounds are not specific to children, but they are injuries that the pediatric emergency physician must recognize and treat on an urgent basis in order to prevent serious and potentially permanent sequelae. Knees are the most commonly injured joints. Motor vehicle accidents are the cause in the overwhelming number of cases. A penetrating joint injury commonly missed in the emergency department is the closed fist injury in which the patient strikes an opponent in the mouth. A tooth can disrupt the capsule of the metacarpophalangeal joint and introduce oral bacteria. Failure to recognize this injury can result in septic arthritis, osteomyelitis, and permanent joint damage.

An open joint may be detectable on direct visualization or by palpation through a periarticular laceration. Injuries that extend below the skin surface adjacent to a joint effusion should raise a high level of suspicion that the joint space has been violated. The presence of air in the joint on radiograph is diagnostic for joint penetration (Fig. 125.5). In less obvious cases, disruption of the joint capsule can be demonstrated by the saline load test. Arthrocentesis is performed through an uninjured site on the skin surface, and saline is injected. Extravasation of saline from the joint into the wound is diagnostic for penetrating injury. A volume of 60 mL of saline is generally adequate to evaluate knee joint integrity, 20 mL for

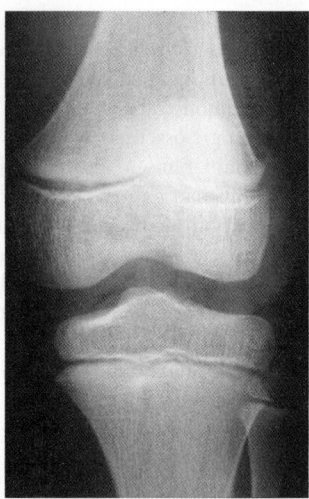

FIGURE 125.5 Intraarticular air in knee joint following penetrating injury sustained from fall on edge of stone.

elbow or ankle joints, and 1 to 2 mL for finger joints. The addition of a small amount (<0.1mL) of methylene blue to the saline may improve visualization of extravasated fluid. Voit et al. found that clinical evaluation had poor sensitivity in identifying penetrating wounds compared with saline injection. Other studies have shown that the saline load test may also miss a significant number of joint disruptions. If a question still remains regarding the integrity of the joint after such testing, then further imaging studies or surgical exploration is necessary.

The treatment of an open joint wound is similar to that of an open fracture. Open wounds of the joint are considered contaminated and broad-spectrum antibiotics should be administered. Surgical intervention consists of vigorous irrigation and debridement, often in the operating room. Attention should be given to appropriate tetanus prophylaxis, splinting, wound dressing, and pain control while the patient remains in the emergency department.

The prognosis of penetrating intraarticular wounds is dependent on the degree of overlying soft-tissue injury and the extent of intraarticular damage. Infectious complications are the most common. Septic arthritis with a variety of both gram-positive and gram-negative organisms is an early and common outcome of inadequate early intervention. Delayed synovitis, often necessitating synovectomy, has been described after unidentified penetration of small foreign bodies.

Annular Ligament Displacement (Radial Head Subluxation)

"Nursemaid's elbow" is the most common joint injury in pediatric patients, usually occurring in children between 6 months and 5 years of age. The term annular ligament displacement (ALD) is replacing radial head subluxation for this entity because it is more anatomically correct. Displacement of the annular ligament occurs as a result of traction on a pronated hand or wrist, causing the ligament to slide overtop of the radial head and become interposed between the radius and capitellum. Except for a very slight increase in the distance

between the radial head and capitellum that can be seen on ultrasound, the relationship between radial head and capitellum remains essentially unchanged, and radiographs are normal in patients with ALD. The radial head is not abnormal and the annular ligament does not always tear when this injury occurs. The left elbow is more often affected because adult caregivers tend to hold the child's left hand with their dominant right hand.

In up to half of the cases, a history of traction on the arm is not obtained, which may suggest another mechanism for this injury or perhaps caregivers who are reluctant to volunteer self-incriminating information. Astute clinicians should suspect this injury even in the absence of the typical history.

ALD can be strongly suspected from across the examining room. The child generally holds the arm slightly flexed and against his or her body. When left alone, the child does not appear to be in significant pain. Parents may report a problem with the wrist or shoulder because, in their attempts to assess these joints, inadvertent movement of the elbow causes pain. Physicians can be similarly fooled, especially when a classic history is not obtained.

Evaluation and Management

The young child must be approached in a slow and nonthreatening manner. Examination that does not move the elbow joint at all is necessary to exclude point tenderness of the clavicle, humerus, radius, and ulna that may suggest a fracture. True tenderness and swelling at the elbow are usually absent. When disuse of the elbow is present without significant pain or bony tenderness, the clinician should perform the reduction maneuver to confirm the diagnosis of radial head subluxation. Radiographs of the elbow are unnecessary unless the physician suspects another injury. Swelling and localized tenderness of the distal humerus are usually apparent with supracondylar fractures, the next most common elbow injury in this age group.

Reduction of a displaced annular ligament is one of the most gratifying procedures for physicians and parents alike. Nonmedical caregivers have been instructed by telephone to reduce recurrent ALDs. Several effective reduction maneuvers have been described. In performing the traditional supination–flexion maneuver, the clinician holds the elbow with his or her thumb over the radial head (Fig. 125.6). In the majority of patients, full supination of the affected arm rotates the flared aspect of the radial head, snapping the annular ligament back to its original position with a telltale click. Flexion or extension of the elbow after supination may add to the success rate. If no click is felt, a second attempt can be made, perhaps exerting mild traction to disengage the annular ligament from between the radial head and capitellum. Forced pronation or pronation–flexion is an alternative method for reduction that appears to be more effective and less painful than the supination–flexion maneuver. Pronation–flexion sometimes succeeds after the initial attempt at reduction with supination–flexion has failed. After an attempt at reduction that does not result in a perceptible click, the child should be observed and tested for return of arm function because some successful reductions occur without a detectable click. Excessive failed attempts at reduction should be avoided. Radiographs may be useful for patients who fail reduction maneuvers.

Return of function after successful reduction is usually prompt, but not immediate. Toys, bottles, or interesting objects can be used to encourage the child to use the affected

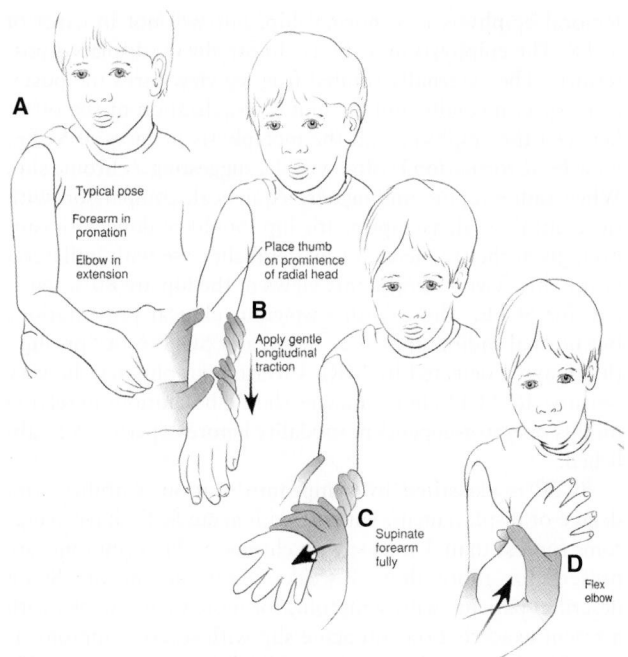

FIGURE 125.6 **A–D:** Supination–flexion maneuver for reduction of radial head subluxation (nursemaid's elbow).

arm. Voluntary use of the arm will return in less than 15 minutes in almost 90% of patients. Younger children generally take longer to begin reusing the arm. Longer duration of subluxation does not appear to be associated with delayed return of function. Many clinicians relate experiences with "failed" reductions in children whose arms are better the following morning. If disuse of the arm persists and radiographs are normal, a sling should be placed and the child should be seen in follow-up by an orthopedist.

Recurrent ALDs are common, occurring in a quarter to one-third of cases. Caregivers should be counseled to lift the child from the axillae, avoiding traction on the distal extremities.

Shoulder (Glenohumeral) Subluxation/Dislocation

Shoulder dislocation is extremely uncommon in young children. Shoulder dystocia at delivery can lead to displaced Salter I fractures that look like dislocations because the unossified proximal humeral epiphysis remaining in the glenoid fossa is not visible radiographically. True dislocations become more common in adolescence, and their management is described in Chapter 135. Intraarticular lidocaine injection is an alternative to intravenous narcotic/benzodiazepine as analgesia for reduction of shoulder dislocations that has a lower complication rate and requires less time in the emergency department.

Glenohumeral subluxation/dislocation will be recurrent in about half of all the cases managed nonoperatively, especially if the anterior glenoid rim is avulsed (Bankhart lesion). Patients may report functional impairments from a shoulder that "pops out" and reduces spontaneously. Some disturbed individuals intentionally dislocate their shoulder. Arthroscopic surgery can

stabilize the shoulder, reducing the likelihood of recurrent dislocation. Data are insufficient and opinion is divided on whether surgical intervention is indicated after the first shoulder dislocation or better reserved for cases that are recurrent.

Slipped Capital Femoral Epiphysis

Background

Slipped capital femoral epiphysis (SCFE) is the most common hip disorder in adolescent patients and should be familiar to all who care for children in this age group. It is twice as common in males as females, and more common in African–American patients. Over 80% of patients with SCFE have body mass index above the 95th percentile, but clinicians must also consider SCFE in patients who are not obese to avoid delayed diagnosis. As expected, increasing rates of childhood obesity have been associated with increase in the incidences of SCFE. Cases of SCFE are usually sporadic, but some familial tendency has been noted. Most children with SCFE are early adolescents in their growth spurt. Boys are most commonly affected between 13 and 15 years of age, and girls between 11 and 13 years of age because of their earlier pubertal development. SCFE onset after menarche is extremely rare.

Slippage of capital femoral epiphysis is almost always posterior and inferior relative to the proximal femoral metaphysis, however, displacement anteriorly or superiorly has been reported. The epiphysis maintains a normal relationship with the acetabulum. The left hip is affected more often than the right. Although symptoms are usually unilateral, plain radiographs document bilateral slippage in about 25% of cases, computed tomographic (CT) scans and MRI in up to 50%.

Pathophysiology

The pathogenesis and biomechanics of SCFE have been the subject of some research and much reasoned speculation. The perichondrium is primarily responsible for the strength of the proximal femoral physis. SCFE differs from a displaced Salter I fracture in that the perichondrium remains intact in most cases of SCFE and is disrupted with acute Salter I fractures. Collagenous bridges that traverse the physeal cartilage and the undulating convexity of the physis toward the epiphysis contribute to the shear strength of the physis. Children with more vertically inclined physeal angles have greater shear stress across their proximal femoral physes and therefore are at greater risk for SCFE. Although it takes an enormous shearing force to produce acute slippage of an initially normal hip joint, the viscoelasticity of the physeal cartilage allows for gradual slippage. Most children with acute presentations will have radiographic evidence of chronic slippage. A so-called "preslip" may be diagnosed in a symptomatic child with normal radiographs. MRI will usually document physeal widening posteromedially on T1-weighted images.

Most patients with SCFE do not have identifiable endocrinologic problems. However, several hormonal abnormalities have been associated with increased risk. Elevated growth hormone and somatomedin, hypogonadism, hypothyroidism, and secondary hyperparathyroidism from renal failure (renal osteodystrophy) have been associated with SCFE. Short children receiving exogenous growth hormone therapy and tall, thin, rapidly growing children with high levels of endogenous growth hormone are both at increased risk. Children outside the usual age range for SCFE, and those with other signs and symptoms that suggest possible endocrine abnormalities, should be referred for endocrine evaluation.

Clinical Presentation

Pain and/or limp are the most common chief complaints in patients with SCFE. Physicians may be misled when the pain is referred to the thigh, knee, or groin. It is often dull, vague, intermittent, and chronic in nature. The average duration of symptoms prior to diagnosis of SCFE is 2 months and slip severity is correlated with delay in diagnosis. A history of trivial injury is sometimes obtained, perhaps causing the additional slippage that precipitates a medical evaluation. Acute onset of severe symptoms suggests acute or acute-on-chronic slippage, sometimes referred to as "unstable" SCFE. These patients are often unable to bear weight and may be in significant pain. Major trauma can cause SCFE, but these presentations are rare.

Examination findings in patients with SCFE include a resting position with hip flexion and some external rotation. Range of motion of the hip, especially full flexion, medial rotation, and abduction, is decreased and painful. Hip flexion will often be associated with obligate external rotation. Patients with significant displacement may have evidence of limb shortening. Occasionally, there is tenderness of the hip anteriorly. Patients with more acute presentations should not be forced to walk as part of the evaluation. Testing for full range of motion is unnecessary once a decision to obtain radiographs has already been reached.

Diagnosis

It is important for emergency physicians to have skill in interpreting plain radiographs for SCFE. Radiographs of the hip should include two views because SCFE is inapparent in one-third of cases in which a single anteroposterior (AP) view is obtained (Fig. 125.7). On the AP view, widening of the physis is usually seen, even if the displacement is inapparent. A line drawn along the lateral aspect of the femoral neck on the AP view (Klein's line) should intersect a small portion of the

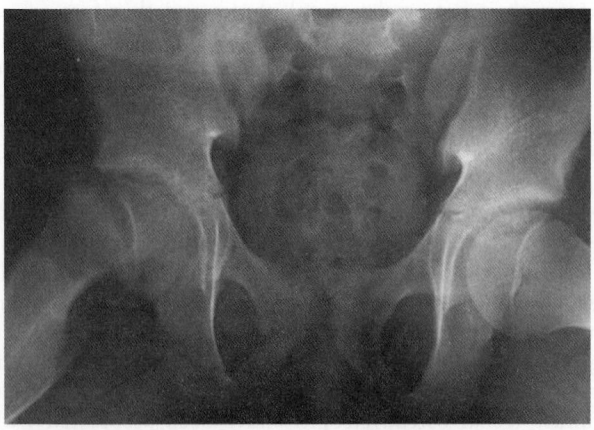

FIGURE 125.7 Slipped capital femoral epiphysis of right hip. Epiphysis is displaced medially on the frog view.

femoral epiphysis in a normal hip, but will not in cases of SCFE. The epiphysis in SCFE is almost always displaced posteriorly. The externally rotated frog-leg view turns the posterior aspect medially and facilitates visualization of the offset between the epiphysis and the metaphysis in cases of SCFE. New bone formation is often visible, suggesting a chronic slip. When radiographic findings are equivocal, comparison with the contralateral, asymptomatic hip should be done with caution, given the frequency of bilateral slippage with unilateral symptoms. Two radiographic views of the hip are 80% sensitive for SCFE. Those with suspicious clinical presentations but normal radiographs may have early SCFE or a "preslip" that may be detected by MRI. Ultrasonography may be very sensitive for SCFE, but clinicians should be cautious in relying on this operator-dependent modality before expertise is established.

SCFE is classified by symptom duration, stability, and degree of displacement. Patients with acute SCFE have symptoms for less than 3 weeks; with chronic SCFE, symptoms are present for more than 3 weeks. Acute-on-chronic SCFE describes patients with symptoms for more than 3 weeks with a recent exacerbation. An acute slip with severe symptoms is unstable. Acute or chronic slips with mild symptoms are stable and have a more favorable prognosis. The degree of slippage is expressed with a grading system: grade I or preslip with possible widening of the physis but no displacement, grade II with displacement less than one-third of the width of the metaphysis, grade III with displacement of one-third to half of the metaphyseal width, and grade IV with displacement of greater than half the metaphyseal width.

Management

Children with SCFE who present with severe symptoms and/or acute onset should be admitted and promptly evaluated by an orthopedic surgeon. Those with milder symptoms may be sent home on crutches, assuming timely orthopedic follow-up has been arranged. Treatment of SCFE is primarily surgical. Screws are usually placed through the femoral neck into the epiphysis. Reduction of the displacement is not performed because there is some evidence that it may increase the likelihood of avascular necrosis of the femoral head and chondrolysis. Chondrolysis is the most common complication of SCFE, occurring in about 8% of patients. Pain and persistent decreased range of motion after pinning are the usual presenting symptoms. If the pins extend into the joint space, the risk of chondrolysis is increased. Two-thirds of patients with chondrolysis have a progressive course. Ankylosis may ensue, leading to long-term disability. Some pediatric orthopedists advocate prophylactic pinning of the contralateral hip after unilateral SCFE if the risk for subsequent slippage is high. Younger chronological age (girls younger than 10 years, boys younger than 12 years) is a very significant predictor for development of a contralateral slip.

Legg-Calvé-Perthes Disease

LCPD is a hip disorder that affects about 1 in 1,200 children and generally has onset between the ages of 4 and 9 years. Males outnumber females by a ratio of 4:1. Most children with LCPD are short, with average or above-average weight, and often have delayed skeletal maturation.

LCPD, or osteonecrosis of the capital femoral epiphysis, is the result of ischemia. LCPD can be simulated in experimental animals by embolizing the blood supply to the femoral head. The theory that LCPD is the result of a variety of clotting abnormalities has gained support in recent years. Thrombotic venous occlusion in the proximal femur may increase intramedullary pressure and lead to ischemia. Patients may remain asymptomatic despite varying degrees of necrosis and resorption of the femoral head. Some children recover completely without developing symptoms. Symptoms usually begin when routine trauma causes stress fracture of the abnormal subchondral bone. Rarefaction of the femoral head with subluxation and deformity may ensue. The process of reossification and remodeling takes 2 to 4 years.

The onset of symptoms in LCPD is usually insidious. Presentation as an acute emergency is rare. Mild hip pain and limp have usually been present for weeks to months before diagnosis. Pain is often referred in the distribution of the obturator nerve to the knee, anteromedial thigh, or groin. Physical findings include decreased hip abduction and internal rotation. Thigh muscle atrophy, and in advanced cases, limb shortening may also be noted.

The sequence of radiographic changes in LCPD has been described in detail (Fig. 125.8). Gadolinium subtraction MRI may offer radiographic evidence of disease during the first 3 to 6 months of symptoms when plain radiographs are normal. At diagnosis, most patients have widening of the articular cartilage with a small, dense proximal femoral epiphysis. Subchondral fracture may be visible. Irregularity and flattening of the epiphysis develops over time. The differential diagnosis includes various bone tumors and skeletal dysplasias. As the disease progresses, anterolateral subluxation may be quantitated radiographically.

Management of LCPD requires a pediatric orthopedist who will follow and treat the child through the various stages of the disease. Prompt referral may influence long-term prognosis. Older children, obese children, girls, and those with more severe disturbance of the epiphysis on radiographs have a poorer prognosis.

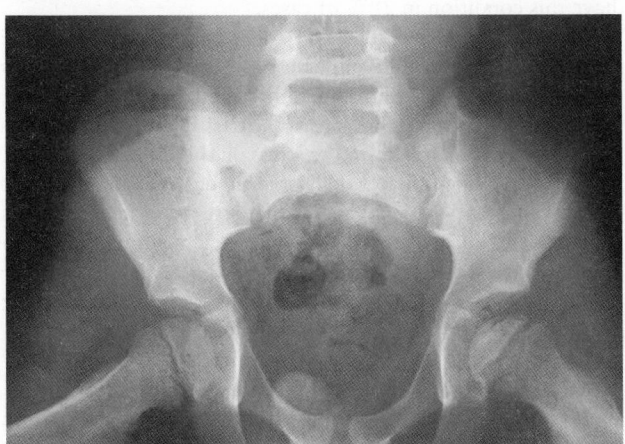

FIGURE 125.8 Legg-Calvé-Perthes disease of left hip. Epiphysis is narrowed and radiodense. A subchondral fracture is also visible.

Discitis (Diskitis)

Background

Discitis is an uncommon and poorly understood inflammatory condition involving the intervertebral disc space. Vertebral osteomyelitis with involvement of the disc space is a distinct diagnostic entity with different epidemiology and pathophysiology from discitis. The mean age of patients with discitis is less than children with vertebral osteomyelitis. No gender or racial predilection has been noted. The involved disc space is usually lumbar or lower thoracic. Most authorities believe discitis results from infection. A history of trauma is obtained in some patients with discitis, but whether the injury plays a role or is a "red herring" is unclear. The vascular anatomy of the disc space supports the notion that organisms reach the disc space via the hematogenous route. In children, the blood supply of the disc space comes from adjacent vertebral body end plates. These vascular connections are absent in older adolescents and adults, and may be the reason discitis is so rare in this age group. Discitis can also be a complication of lumbar puncture.

Bacteria are cultured from a minority of children with discitis. *S. aureus* is the predominant isolate from disc space aspirates and occasionally blood, but other organisms including anaerobes have also been recovered.

Diagnosis

Children with discitis are a diagnostic challenge for clinicians. The condition is uncommon and symptoms are often nonspecific and vague, especially in the younger child. They usually have been present for more than 1 week at the time of diagnosis. Back pain is not always described. Limp, refusal to walk, leg pain, hip pain, and abdominal pain are common presenting complaints. Unlike vertebral osteomyelitis, which is usually associated with fever, only about a quarter of patients with discitis are febrile. Irritability may also be reported.

Physical findings suggesting discitis will be missed if this entity is not considered because careful examination of the spine is not performed routinely by most clinicians. Many children assume a recumbent position of comfort from which they do not want to be moved. Decreased range of motion of the spine and paravertebral muscle spasm are usually present. There is often a change in the lumbar lordosis, which may be decreased or increased. Tenderness to palpation of the disc space can usually be demonstrated. Range of motion of the hips is essentially normal, but inadvertent movement of the lumbar spine during hip examination may cause pain that is misinterpreted to suggest hip pathology. Straight leg raise may be limited by muscle spasm in the hamstrings. Neurologic assessment of the lower extremities is generally normal, but there are reports of discitis with neurologic involvement. Abnormalities in strength, sensation, and/or deep tendon reflexes suggest a spinal cord lesion, tumor, epidural abscess, or herniation of the disc (rare). Signs of discitis may vary, depending on the location of the inflamed disc. Patients with lesions of the upper spine may have meningismus. Imaging studies can be useful in the diagnosis of discitis. Plain radiographs may be normal initially, but intervertebral disc space narrowing develops

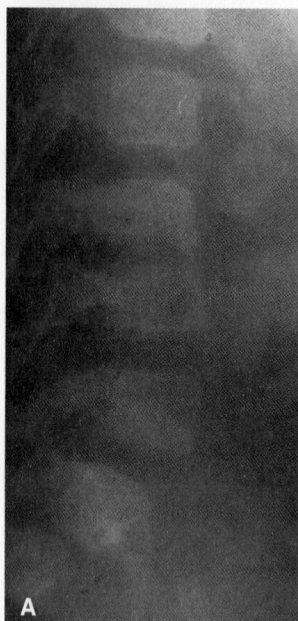
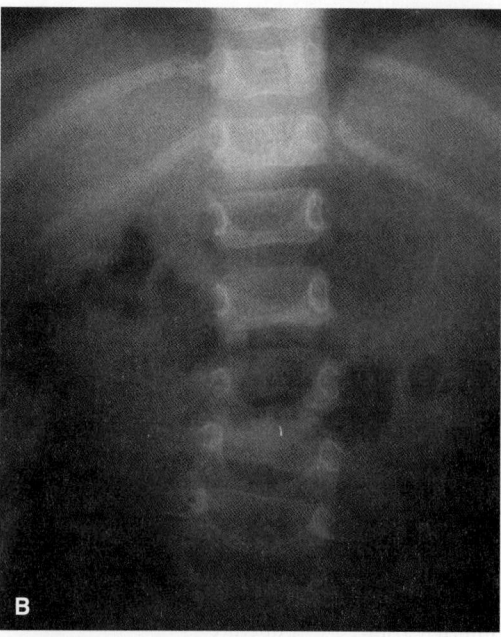

FIGURE 125.9 Discitis. L3–L4 intervertebral disc space is narrowed. Anteroposterior (**A**) and lateral (**B**) views.

after 2 to 3 weeks of illness (Fig. 125.9). At the time of diagnosis, 76% of children with discitis will have abnormal radiographs. MRI is 90% sensitive for discitis, and bone scan is perhaps the most sensitive imaging modality, especially early in the course of this disease. Increased uptake at the level of the involved disc can confirm the diagnosis. CT scanning can demonstrate the degree of bony erosion of the vertebral end plates and paravertebral soft-tissue involvement.

Laboratory testing plays a minor role. Elevation of the WBC count is sometimes noted at the time of diagnosis. ESRs of 40 to 60 mm per hour are usually noted in patients presenting with discitis and decrease with resolution of the disease. Skin testing for tuberculosis, as well as serologic testing for brucellosis and salmonellosis, are often performed but not routinely recommended. Discitis can usually be diagnosed and treated without biopsy or aspiration of the involved disc space. If the presentation is atypical, signs and symptoms severe, or response to therapy unsatisfactory, obtaining a guided-needle aspiration can be helpful.

Management

Discitis is a self-limited disease and need not be treated aggressively. Virtually all children in reported series return to normal function in a few months. Resting the spine usually results in improved symptoms in days to weeks. Immobilization with plaster has not been shown to improve outcome over bed rest alone, but therapeutic decisions should be individualized with input from an orthopedist.

Although there are no data to suggest that they speed recovery or improve outcome, antistaphylococcal antibiotics seem prudent, given the frequency of documented staphylococcal infection. When cultures demonstrate particular organisms with known antimicrobial susceptibilities, antibiotic therapy can be individualized.

SPONDYLOLYSIS AND SPONDYLOLISTHESIS

Spondylolysis, with or without spondylolisthesis, occurs in 2% to 5% of children, but the majority are asymptomatic. Most children presenting with low back pain will not receive a definitive diagnosis, but of those that do, spondylolysis is the most common condition identified. Adolescents involved in sports are at highest risk.

Spondylolysis is a defect in the pars interarticularis of the vertebral body. Spondylolisthesis is displacement of the vertebral bodies, usually involving L5 slipping anteriorly on S1. Spondylolisthesis may result from structural abnormalities of the vertebral bodies (dysplastic type) or acquired defects of the pars interarticularis (isthmic type) that allow slippage. There is a genetic predisposition to spondylolysis and spondylolisthesis. Parents of children with spondylolisthesis are found to have this condition in 28% of cases.

The cause of the defect of the pars interarticularis in spondylolysis is not fully understood. Repeated stress, such as occurs in gymnasts with frequent hyperextension of the spine, causes stress fracture. One side of the pars interarticularis fractures overtly, which adds to the stress on the contralateral side. Fracture becomes bilateral. Displacement may or may not occur. Children who play sports that stress the spine, such as gymnastics, football, rowing, diving, weight lifting, and high jumping, are at particular risk.

Patients who develop symptoms generally present during the adolescent growth spurt. Back pain usually has an insidious onset and worsens with activity, improves with rest. Over time, there may be pain in the buttocks and posterior thighs. Symptoms radiating down the legs suggest significant nerve root irritation. Parents may describe an increase in the lumbar lordosis or a change in the child's gait.

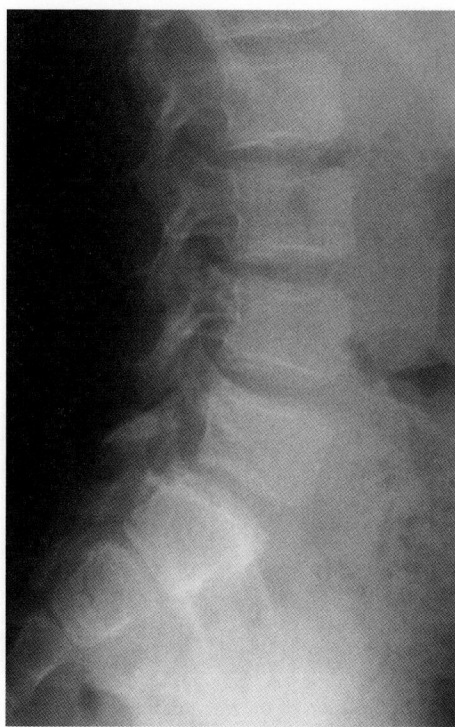

FIGURE 125.10 Spondylolisthesis with slippage of L5 anteriorly on S1.

Physical examination in the prone position shows tenderness with hyperextension of the lumbar spine and with deep palpation. The hamstrings are usually tight, with decreased range of motion on straight leg raise and flexion of the trunk. Children seldom have motor (10%), sensory (15%), or reflex (10%) deficits in the legs.

Plain radiographs should include AP, lateral, and oblique views. The "scotty dog" of the oblique view will have a collar on the neck if spondylolysis is present. Spondylolisthesis can be diagnosed on the lateral view, and the degree of displacement can be quantitated relative to the width of the vertebral body (Fig. 125.10). A bone scan or MRI in children with chronic back pain and normal plain radiographs can identify spondylolysis in its early stages, when conservative therapy can result in bony union.

Treatment varies, depending on symptoms and degree of displacement, if any. Most cases of asymptomatic spondylolysis and spondylolisthesis with mild displacement will not progress. Children with displacement greater than 25% should avoid rough sports. Symptomatic children with displacement may benefit from immobilization. Decisions about treatment should be made in consultation with an orthopedic surgeon.

OVERUSE SYNDROMES

Overuse syndromes is a general term that encompasses various injuries that result from excessive and repetitive forces on susceptible structures. Children are at unique risk for such injuries, which are particularly common in adolescent athletes. There is an increased susceptibility during the growth spurt when skeletal growth exceeds the growth of the muscle—tendon unit. This results in increased stress at the apophysis, the musculotendinous origin, or insertion. In children, cartilage is interposed between the tendon and bone, and is most prone to injury from repetitive forces. Repetitive tensile forces at these sites result in chronic irritation and microfractures or avulsions of the apophysis. If allowed to progress, there is evidence that the repetitive microtrauma may weaken the bone and predispose to major avulsion fractures. Underlying anatomic variations, poor quality sporting equipment and unforgiving playing surfaces may predispose young athletes to overuse injuries. Traction apophysitis is unique to the growing child. By adulthood, the tendon has fused to the bone. Repetitive forces then cause tendinitis rather than apophysitis. The late childhood and early teenage years coincide with increased participation in organized sporting activities. There is a tendency in high-intensity programs to overtrain young athletes, and at times, to encourage them to work through or ignore the early warning signs of pain.

General therapy for these injuries must emphasize several points. Rest is crucial for the specific area involved until pain has completely resolved. The athlete should be actively encouraged to use alternative activities to maintain conditioning during this time. The role of inflammation in overuse injuries is controversial, but the application of ice and use of antiinflammatory agents is generally recommended. Directed stretching exercises reduce tension on affected areas. Biomechanics should be assessed and corrected when necessary. When returning to full activity, an appropriate training regimen should emphasize a slow gradual buildup in intensity and duration and should include explicit limits. The sudden increase in intensity and duration of training that occurs with a change of sporting seasons is a major culprit in overuse injuries.

Numerous overuse syndromes have acquired popular eponyms. Among the most common overuse syndromes in children are Osgood-Schlatter disease, Little Leaguer's elbow, and Sever's disease.

Osgood-Schlatter Disease

Osgood-Schlatter disease is an apophysitis of the tibial tubercle. Repetitive stress imposed by the patellar tendon on its site of insertion results in a series of microavulsions of the secondary ossification center and underlying cartilage. The condition is most common in running and jumping athletes between the ages of 11 and 15 years, and has been associated with tibial torsion. Boys are most commonly affected, but the rising incidence among girls may be because of increased participation in previously male-dominated sports. Cases are bilateral in a quarter of cases, although symptoms are commonly asymmetric.

The physical examination is notable for localized tenderness at the tibial tubercle. Any action that applies tension to the patellar tendon elicits pain. Placing the patient prone and flexing the knee so the heel contacts the buttocks will typically trigger pain at the tibial tubercle. Additional maneuvers likely to cause pain include forced extension of the knee, jumping, squatting, or direct pressure as when kneeling. In advanced cases, callus formation occurs, resulting in further prominence of the tubercle. Some experts have suggested a relationship

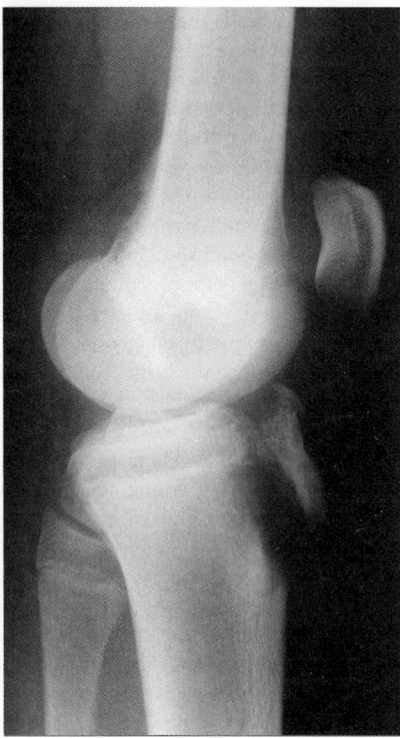

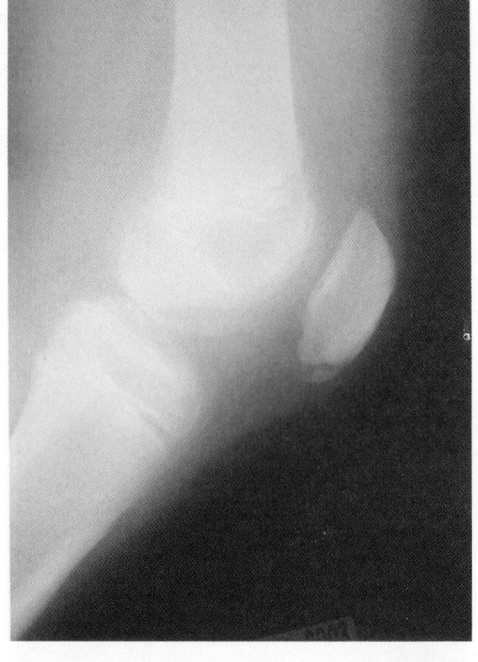

FIGURE 125.12 Avulsion of the inferior pole of the patella in a 10-year-old child with Sinding-Larsen-Johansson disease.

FIGURE 125.11 Acute tibial tubercle avulsion fracture in child with history of Osgood-Schlatter disease.

between Osgood-Schlatter disease and acute avulsion fractures of the tibial tubercle (Fig. 125.11). The diagnosis is based on the clinical features. Radiographs are not necessary in typical cases, although some orthopedic surgeons recommend imaging in unilateral cases to rule out bony disorders that may mimic Osgood-Schlatter disease. In the early stages of the disease, radiographs are normal. Fragmentation of the tibial tubercle can be a normal finding in the adolescent and must be correlated with clinical findings. In advanced stages of the disease, avulsions from the secondary site of ossification may form ossicles that are visible on a lateral radiograph of the knee.

Management consists first and foremost of avoiding activities that place stress on the tibial tubercle. This is perhaps the most difficult instruction to enforce in young athletes. A brief period of immobilization or non–weight bearing is recommended by some as a means of ensuring compliance. Application of ice will reduce pain and swelling. Nonsteroidal antiinflammatory medications are commonly recommended. Activity may be resumed when the patient is free of pain. Flexibility exercises concentrate on stretching the quadriceps and hamstrings to alleviate stress on the tubercle and avoid recurrences. A neoprene sleeve on the knee will reduce patellar mobility and reduce forces on the tubercle. Over 90% of cases resolve within 12 to24 months with conservative treatment.

Sinding-Larsen-Johansson Disease

The tension in the infrapatellar tendon that causes Osgood-Schlatter disease is also transmitted proximally to the inferior pole of the patella. A traction apophysitis at this site results in pain and localized tenderness, and is known as Sinding-Larsen-Johansson disease. The predisposing factors for this injury are the same as those for Osgood-Schlatter disease, and include running and jumping acitvities. Sinding-Larsen-Johansson disease and Osgood-Schlatter disease can occur simultaneously. Provocative maneuvers that produce discomfort in Osgood-Schlatter disease produce pain at the distal patella. Radiographs are nonspecific but may show fragmentation or a small avulsion at the distal pole of the patella (Fig. 125.12), which must be differentiated from an acute sleeve fracture of the patella or a bipartite patella. Treatment emphasizes rest, application of ice, stretching exercises and oral anti-nflammatory agents. Resolution occurs over a period of 12 to 18 months.

Little Leaguer's Elbow

Little Leaguer's elbow refers to a group of disorders resulting from repetitive valgus stress applied to the skeletally underdeveloped elbow. The cause of these injuries is multifactorial and includes the number of pitches thrown per outing, the number of outings, type of pitches thrown, throwing technique, and degree of skeletal maturity. Valgus force places tension on the medial collateral ligaments, which is translated to the medial epicondyle. A medial epicondylitis or apophysitis is the most commonly resulting lesion. An avulsion fracture of the medial epicondyle may result from an acute valgus force once the site has become weakened from repetitive microtrauma. As expected, Little Leaguer's elbow occurs most commonly in boys aged 9 to 12 years.

Patients complain primarily of elbow pain that is exacerbated by throwing. Athletes report progressive drop off in throwing distance. Tenderness is localized over the medial elbow. Applying a valgus stress to the partially flexed elbow will reproduce the pain. Flexion of the wrist or fingers against resistance will also elicit pain. In advanced cases, extension of the elbow becomes limited.

Radiographs may reveal nonspecific changes such as an irregular or widened medial epicondylar physis, but in general an apophysitis is not visible. An avulsion fracture may appear as a bony fragment separated from the medial epicondyle. Comparison views of the nonthrowing elbow may confirm asymmetric changes.

Treatment emphasizes rest for a period of at least 1 month, application of ice, and return to activity only after all pain is gone. Once activity is resumed, the athlete must concentrate on limiting the total amount of pitching, as well as minimizing stress on the medial epicondyle by employing an overhand rather than sidearm pitching motion. Routine stretching and range of motion exercises will reduce the risk of recurrence. Displacement of an avulsion fragment may require surgical repair to restore full elbow function.

Sever's Disease

Sever's disease is a calcaneal apophysitis occurring at the insertion of the Achilles' tendon at the posterior aspect of the calcaneus. It afflicts predominantly runners, jumpers, and soccer players. Sever's disease is often bilateral, is more common in males, and has its peak incidence between 10 and 12 years of age.

Localized tenderness occurs at the insertion of the Achilles' tendon on the calcaneus. A maneuver such as hanging the heels over the edge of a step, climbing steps, or hopping applies tension to the Achilles' tendon and exacerbates the pain. Patients are often found to have a tight gastrocnemius-soleus muscle complex and limited dorsiflexion of the foot. Radiographs of the site are usually normal and are unhelpful, except to exclude bony injuries such as stress fractures.

Management includes rest, ice, and antiinflammatory medications. Heel padding or lifts may be helpful in relieving tension in the area. Flexibility exercises should concentrate on both the hamstrings and the calf muscles. When therapy is initiated early in the disease, most patients are able to return to normal activity by 2 months.

Bursitis

Bursa sacs are both the shock absorbers and the ball bearings of the musculoskeletal system. They disperse forces from blows on bony prominences and reduce friction where tendons or ligaments are in frequent motion.

Trauma, either in a single blow or by repetitive forces, can inflame the bursa, which responds with increased production of synovial fluid. The bursa sac subsequently swells and a cycle of swelling, irritation, and inflammation ensues. Bursitis is most commonly an overuse syndrome seen in adults and adolescents, and is less common in young children.

Injury or cellulitis of the skin overlying a bursa sac can predispose to infection. Aspiration and culture are necessary for definitive diagnosis. The organisms found in septic bursitis are the same as those in septic arthritis, with *S. aureus* accounting for more than 90% of cases. There is no consensus on the need for parenteral versus oral antibiotics. The prepatella bursa and olecranon bursa are most commonly infected.

Bursae are located throughout the body, but bursitis occurs only in a few. Prepatella bursitis, commonly called "housemaid's knee" results from frequent or prolonged kneeling. Pes anserinus bursitis occurs on the lateral aspect of the knee where the tendons of the hamstring muscles overlie the tibia. Retrocalcaneal bursitis occurs between the calcaneus and Achilles' tendon, and is often caused by direct pressure from ill-fitting footwear or high-heeled shoes. Olecranon bursitis most often results from a single direct blow to the elbow. Shoulder or subacromial bursitis is often associated with calcifications and produces severe pain with abduction. Other commonly affected bursae include the inferior calcaneal bursa and the trochanteric bursa.

An unusual form of bursitis is known as a popliteal or Baker's cyst. This occurs in the bursa that cushions the tendons of the gastrocnemius and semimembranous muscles from the distal femur. The presence of this condition in adults is highly suggestive of intraarticular knee damage. In children with a Baker's cyst, there is frequently a congenitally wide opening joining the bursa sac with the knee joint itself. One-way flow of synovial fluid into the bursa produces swelling just below the popliteal fossa on the medial side. Patients with chronic inflammatory conditions of the knee, such as juvenile rheumatoid arthritis, are at increased risk of developing popliteal cysts. The swelling limits full flexion of the knee and produces the sensation of tension with extension. An arthrogram or bursagram may outline the cyst, document the articular connection, and detect ruptures of the cyst. Ultrasound is a useful noninvasive diagnostic modality. MRI is more accurate than ultrasound but not as essential in children, given the lower incidence of accompanying intraarticular injury.

Bursa inflammation produces swelling and localized pain with direct palpation. Any movement of the tendons overlying the site will reproduce the pain.

Conservative therapy consisting of restricted activity, frequent application of ice, and regular use of nonsteroidal antiinflammatory medications is successful in most cases. Resistant cases respond well to aspiration of synovial fluid and injection of corticosteroids. Frequently recurring cases may require surgical removal of the bursa sac. A new bursa will be generated.

Osteochondritis Dissecans

Background

Osteochondritis dissecans is an acquired lesion involving separation of an osteochondral fragment from underlying healthy bone. Various articular lesions are often lumped together under this term, including acute osteochondral fractures and epiphyseal dysplasias. This results in confounding descriptions of the natural course and outcome of the true condition. Adults are often diagnosed with osteochondritis dissecans; however, it remains primarily a condition of the adolescent age group, with the highest incidence occurring among male athletes between 12 and 16 years of age. The term "juvenile osteochondritis dissecans" (JOCD) refers to lesions that occur prior to the closure of the growth plates, whereas "adult osteochondritis disse-cans" presents after the closure of the growth plate. This dis-tinction has important implications for prognosis and treat-ment because the likelihood of spontaneous healing is significantly greater in JOCD. The primary sites of osteochon-dritis dissecans include the medial femoral condyle in the knee, the posteromedial aspect of the talus in the ankle, and the capitellum in the elbow. It is less frequently reported in the hip, foot, and wrist. Involvement of multiple sites is rare, although some series report bilateral knee lesions in up to 30% of cases.

Pathophysiology

The underlying cause of osteochondritis dissecans remains controversial and may differ based on the anatomic location of the lesion. Trauma, vascular insult, genetic predisposition, and abnormalities of ossification have all been proposed as possible etiologies. The greatest evidence supports repetitive trauma as the sole or major contributory cause of the pathol-ogy. Overuse injury is most clearly associated with osteo-chondritis dissecans of the capitellum, where the majority of cases occur in Little League pitchers. Higher incidences of osteochondritis dissecans of the knee and ankle are seen in participants of activities that place increased stress on these areas, such as distance running, ballet, and basketball. Focal necrosis is suspected to follow the initial insult. Spontaneous resolution may occur at this point, or the lesion may progress with the subchondral bone undergoing various degrees of sep-aration from the underlying epiphysis. In advanced stages, complete separation of the osteochondral fragment results in a free-floating body within the joint, which can disrupt nor-mal mechanical function.

When the disease occurs in the second decade of life, long-term outcome is generally good. Progression to osteoarthritis or other degenerative joint diseases is rare. A worse prognosis is associated with a diagnosis after skeletal maturity, a larger lesion, and complete separation of the fragment.

Clinical Findings

Symptoms develop gradually over several months. Joint pain and stiffness typically occur following strenuous exercise and improve over several hours with rest. Swelling may occasion-ally be present with activity.

When a free body is present, patients describe intermittent, abrupt locking of the joint. Locking in the knee or elbow pre-vents full extension of the extremity. This is in contradistinction to buckling, stiffness, or pain with extended range of motion.

The physical examination of the joint is frequently normal. Occasionally, a small effusion may be detectable. Lesions in the medial femoral condyle may be directly palpated and pain elicited when the knee is held in 90 degrees of flexion. The typi-cal location of a lesion in the talus is not accessible on examina-tion. Osteochondritis dissecans in the femoral condyle may give rise to an abnormal gait with external rotation of the affected limb.

Wilson described a clinical test for osteochondritis disse-cans of the knee. Wilson's sign is elicited by flexing the affected knee to 90 degrees. The tibia is held in internal rotation while the leg is slowly extended. In a positive test, pain occurs at approximately 30 degrees of flexion as the tibial spine contacts the classic location of osteochondritis dissecans in the femur. External rotation of the tibia relieves the pain. Wilson's sign has demonstrated low sensitivity in validation studies but,

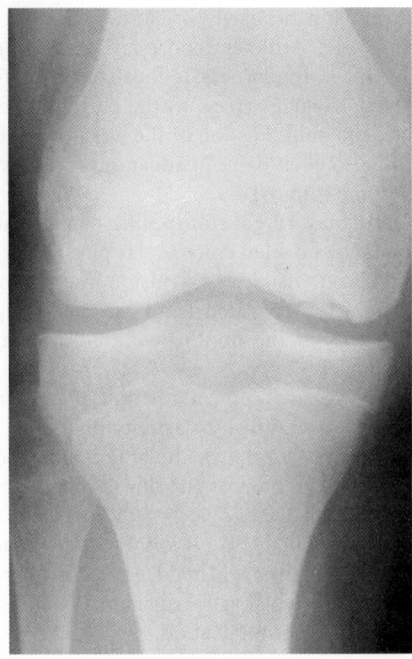

FIGURE 125.13 Osteochondritis dissecans of the medial femoral condyle. Crescentic lesion with radiolucent margin in a 14-year-old girl.

when present, is considered specific for a medial femoral condyle lesion. Conversion from a positive sign to a negative sign over time correlates with clinical healing.

Diagnosis

Plain films of the joint should be obtained, and are often diag-nostic when osteochondritis dissecans is suspected (Fig. 125.13). Radiographs reveal a crescentic-shaped defect within the subchondral bone. The avascular segment of subchondral bone may have increased density. A radiolucent line may demar-cate the separation from the remainder of the epiphysis. A free body often includes a portion of dead subchondral bone, which appears as a radiodense object within the joint space. In addi-tion to the standard AP and lateral views of the knee, tunnel and sunrise views are useful in detecting lesions within the femoral condyle. Lateral, AP, and mortis views of the ankle are adequate when a lesion of the talus is suspected, and AP and lateral views of the elbow are indicated for lesions in the capitellum.

Early lesions may not be detected on plain films, and alter-nate imaging modalities may improve overall sensitivity. When correlated with arthroscopic or surgical findings, MRI has been shown to have excellent ability to detect osteochondritis dissecans and accurately define the extent and stage of the lesion. Osteochondritis dissecans lesions are staged according to the degree of separation from the underlying bone. Stage three or four lesions by MRI have significant separation and are considered unstable. Most orthopedic surgeons consider MRI useful in distinguishing JOCD from other pathologic conditions, guiding therapy and monitoring healing.

Management

The management of osteochondritis dissecans depends on the age and skeletal maturity of the patient, the location of the lesion, and the stage of the lesion. Conservative therapy consist-ing of restricted activity and relief of stress on the involved joint is the first line of treatment in children who have not reached skeletal maturity and for those diagnosed at an early stage of the disease. Immobilization in a cast or non–weight bearing for lower-extremity lesions is unnecessary but occasionally employed to enforce rest. Early return to sports may increase the risk of arthritis or further joint disease. Patients should be followed closely by an orthopedic surgeon both for resolution of clinical symptoms and evidence of healing on serial radiographs or MRIs. Most stable lesions occurring in patients prior to physeal closure go on to heal; however, a few will progress to separation. Lesions occurring in adults generally do not heal without surgery. Surgical intervention is generally recommended when lesions fail to improve clinically or radiographically after 6 months of rest. The presence of an unstable or free-floating fragment is also considered an indication for surgery. Most corrective surgical procedures can now be performed arthroscopically. Fine transarticular or retroarticular drilling through the subchondral fragment into healthy bone appears to stimulate revascularization and promote healing. Fragments are replaced whenever possible. Loose fragments and larger free bodies may be reduced and fixed in place with the use of screws or Kirschner wires. When free bodies must be removed from the joint space, the resulting defects may be repaired with the use of a bone graft or through stimulation of fibrocartilage or scar tissue formation to restore congruity to the articular surface.

Chondromalacia Patellae

Chondromalacia patellae is a pathologic diagnosis referring to damage of the articular cartilage of the patella. Specific changes include softening, fissures, and erosions. Patellofemoral pain syndrome, a term often used interchangeably with chondromalacia patellae, more accurately describes a constellation of symptoms, principally anterior knee pain arising from the patellofemoral joint. Whether the two conditions are actually related is the subject of debate. They share a number of symptoms and precipitating factors. Patellofemoral pain syndrome may represent the early end of the spectrum of injury, which ultimately may or may not progress to true pathologic changes within the cartilage.

Patellofemoral pain syndrome and chondromalacia patellae are first seen in early adolescents. The rise in incidence tends to parallel the growth spurt. A number of underlying causes or associated factors have been identified. Malalignment of the patella and an abnormal tracking of the patella over the femoral condyles appear to be the major contributors to patellofemoral disorders. The quadriceps or Q angle is the angle between a line from the center of the tibial tubercle to the center of the patella and a second line from the center of the patella to the anterior superior iliac spine. A Q angle greater than 20 degrees has been found in a significant number of affected individuals and results in disproportionate lateral traction applied to the patella during extension. The wider pelvic bones in females result in a generally wider Q angle, which may account for the higher proportion of patellofemoral problems in females. Another contributing anatomic factor is a relative strength imbalance of the four muscles composing the quadriceps. A shallow femoral intracondylar sulcus has also been associated with the disorder.

Chondromalacia patellae and patellofemoral pain syndrome are often classified as overuse syndromes because individuals exposed to repetitive trauma are at higher risk for these disorders. Runners are particularly predisposed to develop these conditions. Poor training regimens, rapid increases in duration or intensity of training, hard or uneven running surfaces, and inadequate shoes have been blamed.

Symptoms consist mainly of anterior knee pain often described as arising from beneath or on the sides of the patella. Pain is usually of gradual onset and is exacerbated by exercise. Activities that involve loading of the knee when it is in flexion, such as climbing steps, are particularly painful.

The physical examination is notable for tenderness along the patellar margins or the posterior surface, which is accessible when the patella is manually displaced medially or laterally. Pain, and occasionally crepitus, are elicited with flexion and extension of the knee, or tightening the quadriceps while compressing the patella against the femoral condyles. Range of motion is not limited, and swelling is rare. The presence of an effusion is suggestive of significant cartilaginous damage. Provocative tests that reproduce the pain include climbing steps, squatting, or knee extension against resistance.

Radiographs are generally insensitive but may show changes to the patella in advanced cases. Radiographs may also be obtained to more accurately measure the intracondylar sulcus or Q angle, or to rule out alternative diagnoses. MRI, with sensitivity greater than 80%, is considered the best non-invasive diagnostic modality for chondromalacia patellae. True confirmation of lesions requires arthroscopy.

Treatment is conservative. More than 90% of cases of patellofemoral pain syndrome resolve after instituting a program of rest, antiinflammatory medications, and ice followed by physical therapy. Exercises that begin once the initial pain has resolved emphasize strengthening of the quadriceps muscles. Recommended exercise regimens include isometric contractions of the quadriceps with the knee in extension, straight leg raises, and knee extensions, first without and then with weights. Training routines for athletes may need modification and should emphasize soft, even running surfaces; proper biomechanics; and shoes with appropriate cushioning and support. Surgery is recommended only as a last resort in the most recalcitrant cases because results have been generally less than satisfactory. Surgery is directed at either correcting unequal tension applied to the patella or removing loose or nonviable cartilage from the posterior patellar surface.

COMPARTMENT SYNDROME

Compartment syndrome refers to vascular insufficiency caused by elevated tissue pressures that usually occurs after an injury involving hemorrhage or edema within an enclosed fascial compartment. Tight circumferential bandages or casts can also limit expansion of swollen tissues and result in elevation of tissue pressures. Fluid extravasation from intravenous or intraosseous lines, especially pressure-driven extravasation, may significantly elevate compartment pressures. Direct injury to an artery is less common as the cause of vascular insufficiency after injury but is also considered as compartment syndrome.

Abdominal compartment syndrome is a life-threatening condition in which intraabdominal pressure elevation compromises blood flow to the intestine and kidneys, impairs ventilation, and reduces cardiac output by compressing the inferior vena cava thereby reducing venous return to the heart. The most frequent causes of abdominal compartment syndrome are trauma, burns, pancreatitis and intestinal obstruction.

When compartment pressures approach the perfusion pressure of muscle, which is approximately 30 mm Hg, arterial inflow is reduced and veins and capillaries are collapsed. Ischemia of muscle leads to further swelling, and a positive feedback loop of ischemia—edema can further elevate tissue pressures and lead to complete cessation of perfusion. Muscle necrosis is irreversible after 6 to 8 hours of tissue anoxia. Fibrosis develops and ischemic contracture results in permanent disability. The emergency physician must identify patients at risk for compartment syndromes, and consult with an orthopedist who can monitor tissue pressures and treat compartment syndromes before irreversible injury occurs.

Knowledge of the common pediatric injuries that are associated with compartment syndromes can raise the clinician's index of suspicion appropriately. Displaced supracondylar fractures may injure the anterior interosseous artery and the flexor compartment of the forearm causing a compartment syndrome that leads to the classic Volkmann's contracture. Though controversial, some have suggested that delayed reduction is a risk factor for compartment syndrome after supracondylar fracture. Forearm fractures may also cause compartment syndromes, affecting either the flexor or extensor musculature. Fractures of the tibia and/or fibula can lead to compartment syndrome of the lower leg. Fractures that are open are at greater risk for the development of a compartment syndrome, perhaps because they result from higher-energy mechanisms. Compartment syndromes may occur from crush injuries and other soft-tissue trauma that does not necessarily involve a fracture. Poisonous snakebites, especially pit vipers, and deep tissue infections such as myositis or fasciitis may also lead to dangerous elevations of compartment pressures.

The "five Ps" of compartment syndrome is a mnemonic that can be misleading. One "P," pain, is often the only early symptom or sign of vascular insufficiency. The astute clinician will have consulted an orthopedic surgeon and suspected compartment syndrome before paresthesia, pallor, paralysis, and pulselessness are present.

Pain, the hallmark of compartment syndromes, is a symptom in almost all significant injuries. Distinguishing the pain from the injury itself from that related to the vascular insufficiency is difficult. Pain that increases over time or seems out of proportion to the injury itself suggests muscle ischemia. Full extension of the fingers or toes stretches ischemic muscles and exacerbates the pain in compartment syndromes, making this part of the examination especially important in patients at risk for compartment syndromes.

Paresthesia may be noted in the distribution of the nerves that traverse the ischemic compartment. When the flexor compartment of the forearm is involved, the median nerve is usually affected. Over time, paresthesias may progress to complete anesthesia, and pain may decrease.

Pallor from decreased perfusion may be noted distally. Sluggish circulation may cause cyanosis. Paralysis is a late finding and is probably the least sensitive marker for compartment syndrome. Pulselessness is a useful finding if present, but some physicians are falsely reassured when distal pulses are palpable. Collateral circulation can preserve pulses in larger vessels but the ischemia in compartment syndromes results from vascular occlusion of small vessels.

Treatment of a compartment syndrome should begin from the moment it is suspected. All circumferential bandages should be removed. If symptoms persist, measurement of compartment pressures should be obtained. Reduction of displaced fractures can improve blood flow to affected compartments. Fasciotomy in the operating room is indicated if compartment pressures remain high.

COMPLEX REGIONAL PAIN SYNDROME TYPE 1 (REFLEX SYMPATHETIC DYSTROPHY)

Complex regional pain syndrome type 1 (CRPS1), formerly known as reflex sympathetic dystrophy (RSD) or reflex neurovascular dystrophy (RND), is a poorly understood disorder characterized by pain, abnormal sensation, and circulatory irregularities. Over time, atrophic changes of the extremity may develop. Initially thought to be primarily an adult disease, CRPS1 is increasingly being recognized in children. There are often delays in diagnosing children with CRPS1. Emergency physicians can play a valuable role by considering CRPS1 in children with pain and making appropriate referrals for a prompt, definitive diagnosis. In many patients symptoms of CRPS1 will eventually resolve, but early treatment may prevent prolonged disability.

Children with CRPS1 as young as 3 years have been described. The average age of children with CRPS1 is approximately 12 years, girls outnumbering boys by as much as 6:1. Most cases in children involve the lower extremity. CRPS1 usually follows minor trauma, but some cases develop without an identified precipitant.

The pathophysiology of CRPS1 is not well-understood. Early theories suggested abnormal synapses develop between sensory afferent nerves and sympathetic afferents after an injury. "Sympathetic" dystrophy is probably a misnomer, and nomenclature has changed because local epinephrine and norepinephrine levels are lower, not higher, than normal, and vasodilation, not sympathetic vasoconstriction, may predominate. Current theories include regional sensitization of the central and perhaps peripheral nervous system from an initial injury. Experimental evidence suggests involvement of glutamate and NMDA (N-methyl-D-aspartic acid) receptors in this process. The role of cytokines in the development and maintenance of sensitization is also under investigation. Patients with other dysautonomic conditions, including gastrointestinal dysmotility, migraine, cyclic vomiting and chronic fatigue, may also have CRPS1. Most of these patients meet criteria for maternally inherited mitochondrial disease, the significance of which has yet to be elucidated.

Pain is usually the presenting complaint with CRPS1. The pain is continuous, often burning in quality, with exacerbations but no complete remissions. Abnormal sensitivity is distinctive, with severe pain provoked by normally nontender touching (allodynia). The extremity is usually swollen and cool to the touch, although warmth has also been reported (Fig. 125.14). Dusky discoloration of the skin with hyperhidrosis or anhydrosis may be present. The arm or leg is not used, and atrophic muscle, skin, and bony changes develop in some patients over time. There is some evidence that demineralization of bone occurs more rapidly than would be expected from disuse alone.

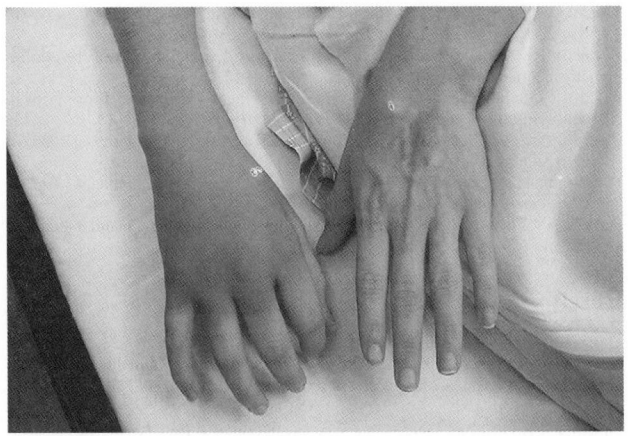

FIGURE 125.14 Reflex sympathetic dystrophy in a 10-year-old girl after a minor wrist injury.

Psychiatric and personality problems have been suspected in many patients with CRPS1, but controlled prospective studies are lacking. Factitious illness or conversion reactions are often considered because symptoms are out of proportion to the inciting injury.

The characteristic history and physical examination, including pain, loss of function, and evidence of autonomic dysfunction, allow for a clinical diagnosis of CRPS1 in most cases. Radiographs in children may not demonstrate the osteoporosis described in adults, especially early after the onset of symptoms. Radionuclide bone scans generally show increased blood flow and periarticular uptake in adults, but in children with CRPS1 the blood flow and osseous uptake is more often reduced. Thermography may document decreased temperature in the affected extremity. Treatment of CRPS1 focuses on early mobilization of the extremity through physical therapy to avoid atrophic changes. Physiotherapy may initially exacerbate symptoms, but experienced clinicians believe it both prevents atrophy and decreases the duration of pain. The knee-jerk response to splint for comfort may be counterproductive with CRPS1. Referral to a pediatric pain program is advisable if symptoms persist. Sympathetic block with local anesthetic is commonly performed in patients with CRPS1 but evidence of its effectiveness is lacking. There are case reports of successful treatment of CRPS1 with intravenous regional block using guanethidine, transcutaneous nerve stimulation, and sympathectomy.

Suggested Readings

Osteomyelitis

Bocchini CE, Hulten KG, Mason EO, et al. Panton-Valentine leukocidin genes are associated with enhanced inflammatory response and local disease in acute hematogenous *Staphylococcus aureus* osteomyelitis in children. *Pediatrics* 2006;117:433–440.

Chun CS. Chronic recurrent multifocal osteomyelitis of the spine and mandible: case report and review of the literature. *Pediatrics* 2004;113:e380–e384.

Ekopimo OI, Imoisili M, Pikis A. Group A β-hemolytic streptococcal osteomyelitis in children. *Pediatrics* 2003;112:e22–e26.

El-Shanti HI, Ferguson PJ. Chronic recurrent multifocal osteomyelitis: a concise review and genetic update. *Clin Orthop Relat Res* 2007;462:11–19.

Frank G, Mahoney HM, Eppes SC. Musculoskeletal infections in children. *Pediatr Clin North Am* 2005;52:1083–1106.

Gutierrez K. Bone and joint infections in children. *Pediatr Clin North Am* 2005;52:779–794.

Jacobs RF, McCarthy RE, Elser JM. Pseudomonas osteochondritis complicating puncture wounds of the foot in children: a 10-year evaluation. *J Infect Dis* 1989;160:657–661.

Jurik AG. Chronic recurrent multifocal osteomyelitis. *Semin Musculoskelet Radiol* 2004;8:243–253.

Martinez-Aguilar G, Avalos-Mishaan A, Hulten K, et al. Community-acquired, methicillin-resistant and methicillin-susceptible Staphylococcus aureus musculoskeletal infections in children. *Pediatr Infect Dis J* 2004;23:701–706.

Oudjhane K, Azouz ME. Imaging of osteomyelitis in children. *Radiol Clin North Am* 2001;39:251–266.

Saavedra-Lozano J, Mejias A, Ahmad N, et al. Changing trends in acute osteomyelitis in children: impact of methicillin-resistant Staphylococcus aureus infections. *J Pediatr Orthop* 2008;28:569–575.

Sonnen GM, Henry NK. Pediatric bone and joint infections. *Pediatr Clin North Am* 1996;43:933–947.

Tuson CE, Hoffman EB, Mann MD. Isotope bone scanning for acute osteomyelitis and septic arthritis in children. *J Bone Joint Surg Br* 1994;76:306–310.

Unkila-Kallio L, Kallio MJT, Eskola J, et al. Serum C-reactive protein, erythrocyte sedimentation rate, and white blood cell count in acute hematogenous osteomyelitis of children. *Pediatrics* 1994;93:59–62.

Vazquez M. Osteomyelitis in children. *Curr Opin Pediatr* 2002;14:112–115.

Wong M, Isaacs D, Howman-Giles R, et al. Clinical and diagnostic features of osteomyelitis occurring in the first three months of life. *Pediatr Infect Dis J* 1995;14:1047–1053.

Septic Arthritis

Arnold SR, Elias D, Buckingham SC, et al. Changing patterns of acute hematogenous osteomyelitis and septic arthritis: emergence of community-associated methicillin-resistant Staphylococcus aureus. *J Pediatr Orthop* 2006;26:703–708.

Kallio MJT, Unkila-Kallio L, Aalto K, et al. Serum C-reactive protein, erythrocyte sedimentation rate and white blood cell count in septic arthritis of children. *Pediatr Infect Dis J* 1997;16:411–413.

Kocher MS, Lee B, Dolan M, et al. Pediatric orthopedic infections: early detection and treatment. *Pediatr Ann* 2006;35:112–122.

Lundy DW, Kehl DK. Increasing prevalence of *Kingella kingae* in osteoarticular infections in young children. *J Pediatr Orthop* 1998;18:262–267.

Moumile K, Merckx J, Pouliquen JC, et al. Bacterial aetiology of acute osteoarticular infections in children. *Acta Pediatr* 2005;94:419–422.

Yagupsky P, Bar-Ziv Y, Howard CB, et al. Epidemiology, etiology, and clinical features of septic arthritis in children younger than 24 months. *Arch Pediatr Adolesc Med* 1995;149:537–540.

Lyme Arthritis

Bachman DT, Srivastava G. Emergency department presentations of Lyme disease in children. *Pediatr Emerg Care* 1998;14:356–361.

Puius YA, Kalish RA. Lyme arthritis: pathogenesis, clinical presentation, and management. *Infect Dis Clin North Am* 2008;22:289–300.

Rose CD, Fawcett PT, Eppes SC, et al. Pediatric Lyme arthritis: clinical spectrum and outcome. *J Pediatr Orthop* 1994;14:238–241.

Shapiro ED, Gerber MA. Lyme disease: fact versus fiction. *Pediatr Ann* 2002;31:170–177.

Willis AA, Widmann RF, Flynn JM, et al. Lyme arthritis presenting as acute septic arthritis in children. *J Pediatr Orthop* 2003;23:114–118.

Wormser GP, Dattwyler RJ, Shapiro ED, et al. The clinical assessment, treatment, and prevention of Lyme disease, human granulocytic anaplasmosis, and babesiosis: clinical practice guidelines by the Infectious Diseases Society of America. *Clin Infect Dis* 2006;43:1089–1134.

Transient Synovitis

Caird MS, Flynn JM, Leung YL, et al. Factors distinguishing septic arthritis from transient synovitis of the hip in children. A prospective study. *J Bone Joint Surg Am* 2006;88:1251–1257.

Del Becarro MA, Champoux AN, Bockers T, et al. Septic arthritis versus transient synovitis of the hip: the value of screening laboratory tests. *Ann Emerg Med* 1992;21:1418–1422.

Fink AM, Berman L, Edwards D, et al. The irritable hip: immediate ultrasound guided aspiration and prevention of hospital admission. *Arch Dis Child* 1995;72:110–114.

Kocher MS, Zurakowski D, Kasser JR. Differentiating between septic arthritis and transient synovitis of the hip in children: an evidence-based clinical prediction algorithm. *J Bone Joint Surg Am* 1999;81:1662–1670.

Mukamel M, Litmanovitch M, Yosipovich Z, et al. Legg-Calvé-Perthes disease following transient synovitis. How often? *Clin Pediatr(Phila)* 1985;24:629–631.

Zawin JK, Hoffer FA, Rand FF, et al. Joint effusion in children with an irritable hip: US diagnosis and aspiration. *Radiology* 1993;187:459–463.

Penetrating Intraarticular Injuries

Collins DN, Temple SD. Open joint injuries: classification and treatment. *Clin Orthop Relat Res* 1989;243:48–56.

Tornetta P, Boes MT, Schepsis AA, et al. How effective is a saline arthrogram for wounds around the knee? *Clin Orthop Relat Res* 2008;466:432–435.

Voit GA, Irvine G, Beals RK. Saline load test for penetration of periarticular lacerations. *J Bone Joint Surg Br* 1996;78:732–733.

Radial Head Subluxation

Kaplan RE, Lillis KA. Annular ligament displacement. *Pediatrics* 2002;110: 171–174.

McDonald J, Whitelaw C, Goldsmith LJ. Radial head subluxation-comparing two methods of reduction. *Acad Emerg Med* 2000;7:207–208.

Green DA, Linares MY, Garcia Pena BM, et al. Randomized comparison of pain perception during radial head subluxation reduction using supination-flexion or forced pronation. *Pediatr Emerg Care* 2006;22:235–238.

Schunk JE. Radial head subluxation: epidemiology and treatment of 87 episodes. *Ann Emerg Med* 1990;19:1019–1023.

Slipped Capital Femoral Epiphysis

Futami T, Suzuki S, Seto Y, et al. Sequential magnetic resonance imaging in slipped capital femoral epiphysis: assessment of preslip in contralateral hip. *J Pediatr Orthop* 2001;10:298–303.

Kocher MS, Bishop J. Delay in diagnosis of slipped capital femoral epiphysis. *Pediatrics* 2004;113:e322–e325.

Manoff EM, Banffy MB, Winell JJ. Relationship between Body Mass Index and slipped capital femoral epiphysis. *J Pediatr Orthop* 2005;25:744–746.

Mooney JF 3rd, Sanders JO, Browne RH, et al. Management of unstable/acute slipped capital femoral epiphysis: results of a survey of the POSNA membership. *J Pediatr Orthop* 2005;25:162–166.

Riad J, Bajelidze G, Gabos PG. Bilateral slipped capital femoral epiphysis: predictive factors for contralateral slip. *J Pediatr Orthop* 2007;27:411–414.

Legg-Calvé-Perthes Disease

Frick SL. Evaluation of the child who has hip pain. *Orthop Clin North Am* 2006;37:133–140.

Glueck CJ, Freiberg RA, Wang P. Role of thrombosis in osteonecrosis. *Curr Hematol Rep* 2003;2:417–422.

Wall E. Legg-Calvé-Perthes disease. *Curr Opin Pediatr* 1999;11:76–79.

Wingstrand H. Significance of synovitis in Legg-Calvé-Perthes disease. *J Pediatr Orthop* 1999;8:156–160.

Discitis

Fernandez M, Carrol CL, Baker CJ. Discitis and vertebral osteomyelitis in children: an 18 year review. *Pediatrics* 2000;105:1299–1304.

Early SD, Kay RM, Tolo VT. Childhood diskitis. *J Am Acad Orthop Surg* 2003;11:413–420.

Nussinovitch M, Sokolover N, Bolovitz B, et al. Neurologic abnormalities in children presenting with diskitis. *Arch Pediatr Adolesc Med* 2002;156:1052–1054.

Spondylolysis and Spondylolisthesis

Akiyoshi V, Sasidhar B, Ashok EN. MRI signal changes of the pedicle as an indicator for early diagnosis of spondylolysis in children and adolescents: a clinical and biomechanical study. *Spine* 2006;31:206–211.

Beutler WJ, Fredrickson BE, Sweeney CA, et al. The natural history of spondylolysis and spondylolisthesis: 45-year follow-up evaluation. *Spine* 2003;28: 1027–1035.

Logroscino G, Mazza O, Aulisa G, et al. Spondylolysis and spondylolisthesis in the pediatric and adolescent population. *Childs Nerv Syst* 2001;17:644–655.

Overuse Syndromes

Duri ZA, Patel DV, Aichroth PM. The immature athlete. *Clin Sports Med* 2002;21:461–482.

Dyment PG, ed. *Sports medicine: health care for young athletes*. Elk Grove Village, IL: American Academy of Pediatrics, 1991.

Gerbino PG. Elbow disorders in throwing athletes. *Orthop Clin North Am* 2003;34:417–426.

Gill TJ, Micheli LJ. The immature athlete: common injuries and overuse syndromes of the elbow and wrist. *Clin Sports Med* 1996;15:401–423.

Gomez JE. Upper extremity injuries in youth sports. *Pediatr Clin North Am* 2002;49:593–626.

Hogan KA, Gross RH. Overuse injuries in pediatric athletes. *Orthop Clin North Am* 2003;34:405–415.

Kennedy JG, Knowles B, Dolan M, et al. Foot and ankle injuries in the adolescent runner. *Curr Opin Pediatr* 2005;17:34–42.

Micheli LJ, Ireland ML. Prevention and management of calcaneal apophysitis in children: an overuse syndrome. *J Pediatr Orthop* 1987;7:34–38.

Purushottam AG, Scher DM, Khakharia S, et al. Osgood Schlatter syndrome. *Curr Opin Pediatr* 2007;19:44–50.

Saperstein AL, Nicholas SJ. Pediatric and adolescent sports medicine. *Pediatr Clin North Am* 1996;43:1013–1033.

Soprano JV, Fuchs SM. Common overuse injuries in the pediatric and adolescent athlete. *Clin Pediatr Emerg Med* 2007;8:7–14.

Bursitis

Harwell JI, Fisher D. Pediatric septic bursitis: case report of retrocalcaneal infection and review of the literature. *Clin Infect Dis* 2001;32:e102–e104.

Lang IM. MRI appearance of popliteal cysts in childhood. *Pediatr Radiol* 1997;27:130–132.

Raddatz DA, Hoffman GS, Franck WA. Septic bursitis: presentation, treatment, and prognosis. *J Rheumatol* 1987;14:1160–1163.

Southmayd W, Hoffman M. *Sports health: the complete book of athletic injuries.* New York: Quick Fox, 1981.

Szer IS, Klein-Gitelman M, DeNardo BA, et al. Ultrasonography in the study of prevalence and clinical evolution of popliteal cysts in children with knee effusions. *J Rheumatol* 1992;19(3):458–462.

Osteochondritis Dissecans

Bradley J, Dandy DJ. Osteochondritis dissecans and other lesions of the femoral condyles. *J Bone Joint Surg Br* 1989;71:518–522.

Conrad JM, Stanitski CL. Osteochondritis dissecans: Wilson's sign revisited. *Am J Sports Med* 2003;31:777–778.

Letts M, Davidson D, Ahmer A. Osteochondritis dissecans of the talus in children. *J Pediatr Orthop* 2003;23:617–625.

Pill SG, Ganley TJ, Milam RA, et al. Role of magnetic resonance imaging and clinical criteria in predicting successful nonoperative treatment of osteochondritis dissecans in children. *J Pediatr Orthop* 2003;23:102–108.

Robertson W, Kelly BT, Green DW. Osteochondritis dissecans of the knee in children. *Curr Opin Pediatr* 2003;15:38–44.

Wall E, Von Stein D. Juvenile osteochondritis dissecans. *Orthop Clin North Am* 2003;34:341–353.

Chondromalacia Patellae

Davidson K. Patellofemoral pain syndrome. *Am Fam Physician* 1993;48: 1254–1262.

Dyment PG, ed. *Sports medicine: health care for young athletes.* Elk Grove Village, IL: American Academy of Pediatrics, 1991.

Tria AJ, Palumbo RC, Alicea JA. Conservative care for patellofemoral pain. *Orthop Clin North Am* 1992;23:522–526.

Compartment Syndrome

Grottkau BE, Epps HR, Di Scala C. Compartment syndrome in children and adolescents. *J Pediatr Surg* 2005;40:678–82.

Bae DS, Kadiyala RK, Waters PM. Acute compartment syndrome in children: contemporary diagnosis, treatment and outcome. *J Pediatr Orthop* 2001;21: 680–688.

Ramachandran M, Skaggs DL, Crawford HA, et al. Delaying treatment of supracondylar fractures in children: has the pendulum swung too far? *J Bone Joint Surg Br* 2008;90:1228–1233.

Sharrard WJW. *Paediatric orthopaedics and fractures.* London: Blackwell Scientific, 1993.

Reflex Sympathetic Dystrophy

Cimaz R, Matucci-Cerinia M, Zulian F, et al. Reflex sympathetic dystrophy in children. *J Child Neurol* 1999;14:363–367.

Cepeda MS, Carr DB, Lau J. Local anesthetic sympatheric blockade for complex regional pain syndrome. *Cochrane Database Syst Rev* 2005:19:CD004598.

Lloyd-Thomas AR, Lauder G. Reflex sympathetic dystrophy in children. *BMJ* 1995;310:1648–1649.

Tan EC, Zijlstra B, Essink ML, et al. Complex regional pain syndrome type 1 in children. *Acta Paediatr* 2008; 97:875–879.

Wilder RT, Berde CB, Wolohan M, et al. Reflex sympathetic dystrophy in children. Clinical characteristics and follow-up of seventy patients. *J Bone Joint Surg Am* 1992;74:910–919.

CHAPTER 126 ■ NEUROSURGICAL EMERGENCIES, NONTRAUMATIC

DANIEL S. TSZE, MD, MPH, AND DALE W. STEELE, MD

Patients with nontraumatic neurosurgical emergencies present to the emergency department (ED) with a variety of signs and symptoms, including headache, vomiting, seizures, changes in mental status, weakness, and coma. Although headache and vomiting are commonly associated with many benign self-limiting conditions, a high index of suspicion for more serious pathology is required. Because the most urgent problems are related to the onset of increased intracranial pressure (ICP), this chapter opens with a general discussion of ICP, followed by descriptions of the common congenital, infectious, vascular, and neoplastic conditions that may present as neurosurgical emergencies.

INCREASED INTRACRANIAL PRESSURE

Pathophysiology

The functions of the buffering systems that maintain ICP at normal levels have been detailed in Chapter 116. The cranium contains three components: brain tissue predominantly, cerebrospinal fluid (CSF), and blood. An abnormal increase in volume of any of these components (by means of edema or mass lesion, increased production or diminished absorption of CSF, or increased blood flow) may result in elevated ICP. This closed space has limited capacity to compensate for increased volume. ICP levels normally rise and fall over the course of the day. ICP is at its peak during sleep because the horizontal posture and the relative hypoventilation that increases arterial P_{CO_2} result in increased cerebral blood flow. This is especially true during rapid eye movement sleep, which usually occurs just before awakening. Headaches that awaken a child during the night or that occur on awakening may be caused by ICP waves elevated beyond the normal nighttime peaks. With the improved ventilation and the assumption of upright posture on arising, P_{CO_2} is lowered and cerebral vasodilation is lessened. If vomiting occurs, the accompanying hyperventilation also decreases cerebral blood flow. As a result, the severity of the headache may then lessen significantly in the awakened child.

Clinical Manifestations

A careful history must be taken with respect to the timing and severity of headaches, vomiting, changes in behavior, visual changes, and episodic decreases in level of consciousness (Table 126.1). Nighttime and morning headaches that improve on arising are always ominous, as is recurrent vomiting without fever, abdominal pain, or diarrhea. Most children presenting to the ED with headache will have common diagnoses, including viral infections, migraine, and sinusitis, and do not require routine neuroimaging. The need for further evaluation will depend on the age of the child and the clinical examination. For example, children younger than 7 years of age do not have frontal sinuses, thus ruling out the possibility of frontal headache caused by sinusitis. Conversely, frontal sinusitis in adolescent boys has a significant rate of intracranial complications, especially subdural and epidural abscesses.

The clinical examination can help confirm the presence of intracranial hypertension, but a normal examination cannot reliably exclude it. Fundoscopy will identify papilledema but it is possible to have ICP without papilledema. Visual fields and visual acuity should be checked. Cranial sutures may split in infants and young children with chronic elevation of ICP, resulting in a hyperresonant note when the skull is percussed, a "cracked pot" sound known as Macewen sign. Cranial nerve palsy may occur, usually affecting the third and sixth nerves, resulting in dilated pupil, diplopia, and strabismus. When the fourth nerve is affected, the child may exhibit a "cock robin" head tilt. Cerebellar herniation may also cause head tilt; if bilateral, the neck may be held in an extended position.

The possibility of cerebral herniation should be considered and aggressively treated in the presence of an evolving pattern of diminishing level of consciousness, unexplained bradycardia, pupillary changes, or abnormal or asymmetric posturing with stimuli. Spontaneous posturing should not be confused with seizure activity. Cushing's triad (hypertension, bradycardia, and irregular respirations) is a near terminal event, with bradycardia usually the first and most sensitive indicator.

Management

The emergency treatment of increased ICP depends on the patient's clinical state and the cause of the intracranial hypertension (Table 126.2). The first priority in all patients is to follow the ABCs (airway, breathing, and circulation) of resuscitation and to prevent hypoxemia, hypercarbia, and systemic hypotension with oxygenation, ventilation, and appropriate fluid therapy. Seizures should be treated aggressively and, if possible, prevented because ICP spikes during seizures will aggravate intracranial hypertension.

Sedative agents given without controlled ventilation may result in hypercarbia, causing an increase in cerebral blood volume and, consequently, in ICP. Therefore, it is often prudent to

SIGNS AND SYMPTOMS OF ELEVATED
INTRACRANIAL PRESSURE

Symptoms	Signs
Headache	Papilledema/retinal hemorrhage
Nocturnal, episodic severe	Cranial nerve palsies/ sunset sign
Vomiting	Meningismus
Stiff neck	Head tilt
Double vision	Bulging fontanel/prominent scalp veins
Transient visual loss	Macewen (cracked pot) sign
Gait difficulties	Decorticate/decerebrate posturing
Behavioral changes	Coma
Irritability/screaming episodes	Progressive hemiparesis
	Bradycardia

Modified from Bruce DA. Neurosurgical emergencies. In: Fleisher GR, Ludwig S, eds. *Textbook of pediatric emergency medicine*, 3rd ed. Baltimore: Williams & Wilkins, 1993:1410.

perform tracheal intubation using an rapid sequence intubation (RSI) technique to blunt increases in ICP (see Chapter 5) before CT scan or interfacility transport.

Hyperventilation is only recommended for acute herniation. The effects of hyperventilation are transient and not recommended for prophylactic treatment of increased ICP. Hyperventilation decreases cerebral blood flow leading to cerebral ischemia, depletion of brain tissue interstitial bicarbonate buffering capacity leading to a loss of local vasoconstrictor effects, and a possible rebound phase of increased ICP as the CSF pH equilibrates. Mild hyperventilation (PCO_2 30 to 35 mm Hg) may be implemented to allow time for more definitive treatments. More extreme reductions in PCO_2 and routine chronic

TREATMENT OF INCREASED INTRACRANIAL
PRESSURE

Prevent hypoxia and hypercarbia
  Tracheal intubation/controlled ventilation
  Seizure treatment and prophylaxis
Maintain adequate cerebral perfusion pressure and cerebral
  perfusion
  Treatment of shock
  Limitation of excessive hyperventilation
Decrease cerebral blood volume
  Acute hyperventilation
Decrease brain tissue volume
  Mannitol/hypertonic saline
  Dexamethasone for vasogenic edema
Decrease cerebrospinal fluid (CSF) volume
  CSF drainage
  Acetazolamide
Removal of mass lesion
  Surgical removal/decompression

hyperventilation (to PCO_2 of 20 to 25 mm Hg) will result in brain hypoperfusion and have a detrimental effect on outcome. Continuous, portable capnometry may be useful to avoid excessive hyperventilation during transport or diagnostic imaging.

The head of the bed should be elevated to 30 degrees to promote displacement of CSF from the intracranial compartment to the spinal compartment, and the head maintained in a neutral position to minimize venous outflow resistance. A ventriculostomy catheter may be used to measure ICP, direct medical therapy, and allow drainage of CSF. CSF volume may also be reduced by drainage from a shunt reservoir or by a ventricular tap via an open fontanel, a split suture, or a burr hole. Hyperosmolar therapy is used to acutely decrease ICP in the deteriorating patient. Mannitol is most commonly used, lowering ICP in 1 to 5 minutes with a peak effect in 20 to 60 minutes. Mannitol is relatively contraindicated in hypovolemic patients because of its diuretic effects. Hypertonic saline reduces ICP while augmenting intravascular volume and thus has a clear advantage over mannitol in hypovolemic or hypotensive patients. Dexamethasone is useful in treating vasogenic brain edema associated with tumor and abscess, but onset of this effect is slow, with ICP decreasing over the course of 2 to 5 days. Steroids have been shown to have no benefit or a detrimental effect in other neurosurgical disorders, such as traumatic brain injury and spontaneous intracerebral hemorrhage.

HYDROCEPHALUS

Hydrocephalus is characterized by dilated cerebral ventricles that contain an excessive amount of CSF, resulting from imbalance between production and absorption. Production occurs in the choroid plexus, almost always remains stable, and is only rarely excessive. In noncommunicating hydrocephalus, CSF in the ventricular system is blocked from communicating with CSF in the subarachnoid spaces and basal cisterns by a congenital or acquired defect. In communicating hydrocephalus, the block in absorption is on the meningeal surfaces, outside the ventricular system. Congenital hydrocephalus may result from aqueductal stenosis or in association with Dandy-Walker or Arnold-Chiari malformations. Acquired hydrocephalus may follow bacterial meningitis, obstruction by tumor, or result from the inflammatory response to subarachnoid or intracranial hemorrhage.

Previously Undiagnosed Hydrocephalus

Children with undiagnosed hydrocephalus rarely present first to the ED, but hydrocephalus must be considered in infants with increasing head circumference, bulging fontanel, dilated scalp veins, lower extremity spasticity, and other signs and symptoms of increased ICP (Table 126.1).

Management

Noncontrast head CT demonstrates enlarged ventricles. The urgency of ventricular drainage depends on the child's condition. Ventricular puncture through an open fontanel or coronal suture may be lifesaving in a child with evidence of herniation. Endoscopic third ventriculostomy and other endoscopic techniques have been increasingly utilized for treating selected patients with hydrocephalus, avoiding the need for an indwelling shunt.

Previously Shunted Hydrocephalus

CSF shunts allow diversion of CSF into another area of the body outside the brain. Unfortunately, placement of shunts may be accompanied by numerous complications.

Pathophysiology

Many different types of shunts are in use; therefore, emergency physicians must become familiar with those commonly used in their area. All shunts share three common features: a radiopaque ventricular catheter; a one-way valve; and distal tubing that is palpable subcutaneously and most commonly enters the peritoneal cavity, or rarely into the right atrium or pleural cavity. Many shunts also include a pumping mechanism and a reservoir, which enables percutaneous sampling of CSF without damage to the shunt. Some shunts are programmable, allowing noninvasive adjustments in valve pressure to treat both under- and over-drainage.

Shunt-related problems include obstruction, infection, mechanical failure, overdrainage, loculation of the ventricles, and abdominal complications. The risk for shunt failure is greatest in the first months after placement. Up to 40% of shunts fail during the first year after placement, and 80% require revision by 10 years. Approximately 80% of obstructions occur at the proximal (ventricular) end of the shunt tip as a result of occlusion by tissue or migration of the shunt tip into the brain parenchyma. Shunt infections are most common in the early postoperative period. Mechanical failures include fracture of the distal tubing, disconnection of shunt components, or migration or misplacement of either the ventricular or the distal end of the catheter. Overdrainage implies a properly functioning shunt that removes more fluid than necessary. Rarely, over-drainage can acutely cause extra-axial fluid accumulation or subdural hematoma. Noncommunicating loculations may form so that a single shunt does not drain the entire ventricular system. The most common abdominal complication is pseudocyst formation around the catheter. Pseudocysts are often associated with low-grade shunt infection and can be seen on abdominal ultrasound or CT. Severe constipation may cause reversible ventriculoperitoneal shunt failure due to increased intra-abdominal pressure. Other intra-abdominal complications include ascites and bowel or bladder perforation.

Shunt Malfunction

Clinical Manifestations

Patients with shunt malfunction commonly present with manifestations of increased ICP (Table 126.1), and presentation may differ by age. Uncommon, but relatively specific signs are nonlocalizing sixth nerve palsy, intermittent downward gaze (sunset sign), and swelling from CSF tracking along the shunt tract. The fontanel may be full and tense, even when the infant is upright. Papilledema is uncommon in acute shunt malfunction. Although seizures are common in patients with shunts, one series found that only 2.9% of ED visits by patients with

shunts for isolated seizures culminated in shunt revision. A history of onset or worsening of symptoms with upright posture suggests overdrainage. Parents, particularly those who have witnessed prior episodes of shunt malfunction, are perceptive to the subtle and often intermittent symptoms that herald shunt malfunction.

Shunts should not be routinely pumped as this test lacks sensitivity, and because the negative pressure generated in a small ventricle may occasionally result in obstruction. However, if the ventricular catheter is shown on CT scan to be in the center of a dilated ventricle and the shunt umbilicates on depression with slow refill, shunt obstruction is likely.

Management

If the history or physical examination suggests shunt malfunction, early neurosurgical consultation is strongly recommended. A plain radiographic "shunt series" should be done, consisting of anteroposterior and lateral views of the skull, neck, thorax, and abdomen. These radiographs allow the type, location, connections, and intactness of the system to be evaluated.

A noncontrast head CT should also be done and compared, if possible, with previous scans taken when the shunt was functioning. In some patients, ventriculomegaly may persist despite a functioning shunt. Conversely, some patients have increased ICP despite small or unchanged ventricles. Rapid-sequence (quick-brain) MRI avoids radiation exposure and may be used to visualize ventricular catheters and ventricular size. Although CT and shunt series are useful, a normal result for either should still be scrutinized. Several series have shown that as many as 8.4% of patients with shunt malfunction were identified by an abnormal shunt series, while having a normal CT scan. Another series demonstrated that out of 267 patients with both normal head CT and shunt series, 14 (5.2%) patients were subsequently diagnosed with shunt malfunction. If there is persistent concern for shunt malfunction, a radionucleotide shuntogram may be done to further assess the patency of both the proximal and distal shunt catheters, as well as the integrity of the valve mechanism.

Shunt tap, performed selectively by the neurosurgical consultant, may be useful in patients in whom shunt function is questionable. Assuming the ventricular end is patent, the pressure in the system can be estimated by the level to which CSF rises when the butterfly tubing is held erect. Poor flow of CSF on shunt tap is highly predictive of proximal catheter obstruction, but both distal and proximal obstruction may still be present despite good CSF return. In patients with distal shunt obstruction, the need for emergency shunt revision is less because the ICP can be controlled by withdrawing CSF until a pressure of approximately 10 cm of water is reached.

The urgency of shunt revision depends on the patient's status. Patients with proximal obstructions may worsen quickly, and if the child suddenly deteriorates, CSF cannot be quickly withdrawn from the shunt reservoir to relieve pressure. In this instance, the ventricle must be tapped through the fontanel if open, through the sutures if they are split, or through the shunt burr hole. This latter maneuver usually damages the shunt and is only a temporizing measure to lower the ICP before definitive shunt revision. Acetazolamide is sometimes used to reduce CSF production in the chronic medical management of hydrocephalus. However, acetazolamide may cause transient, paradoxical increases in ICP and should be avoided in patients with rapidly progressive hydrocephalus and signs of increased ICP.

Shunt Infection

Pathophysiology

The incidence of shunt infection is greatest in the first 8 weeks after surgery, with 90% of infections occurring in the first 6 months. *Staphylococcus aureus* infections are most common in the early postoperative period and gram-negative infections are more common after 6 months. However, approximately 75% of infections are caused by low virulence *Staphylococcus epidermidis*. These organisms secrete an extracellular polysaccharide "slime" substance that coats the shunt, making the enclosed colonies of organisms highly resistant to phagocytosis and systemic antibiotics.

Clinical Manifestations

In the immediate postoperative period, erythema and warmth along the course of the shunt are highly predictive of early wound infection. Infections are associated with fever in only 42% of patients which, if present, may be low grade and intermittent. Signs of obstruction may be present, but infection can and often does occur in the setting of a functioning shunt. When present, abdominal pain, peritoneal signs, and meningeal signs are strongly associated with infection. A rare presentation of shunt infection is glomerulonephritis, most commonly seen in association with ventriculoatrial shunts.

Management

The diagnosis of shunt infection requires CSF obtained from the shunt. However, there is some, albeit small, risk that tapping the shunt may cause an infection. Thus, shunt tap is not indicated in all children with a shunt who present with fever. A diligent search for alternative explanations of fever should be undertaken. Urinary tract infections are a particularly common cause of fever in children with myelomeningocele. Debilitated patients with severe developmental delay are at risk for pneumonia. Fever without localizing signs in patients whose current shunt was placed or revised years ago, and who lack signs and symptoms of shunt malfunction, may be appropriately managed with close follow-up or observation without shunt tap.

In patients with noncommunicating hydrocephalus, if the shunt tap is negative but a CNS infection is clinically suspected, a lumbar puncture is required because ventriculitis may not accompany meningitis. A false-negative shunt tap may also occur when children are on chronic antibiotics (e.g., child with myelomeningocele on antibiotics for urinary tract infection prophylaxis) or if the focus of infection is distal and below a one-way valve. In the latter case, identifying the infection may require exteriorizing of the shunt so that the intra-abdominal portion may be cultured.

CSF obtained from the shunt tap is sent for Gram stain, cell count, glucose, protein, and culture. If the CSF contains more than 100 cells per mm^3, cultures are positive in about 90% of patients. However, most infected shunts have only modest pleocytosis (less than 200 white blood cells per mm^3), slight

decrease in glucose, and modest protein elevation. Blood cultures are infrequently positive.

If shunt infection is presumed, empiric treatment with broad-spectrum antibiotics is begun until specific organisms are identified and sensitivities are available. Patients may require either externalization of the abdominal catheter or complete removal of the shunt and a period of external drainage followed by placement of a new shunt into a different anatomic location.

STROKE

Stroke denotes a sudden onset of a persistent focal neurologic deficit, resulting from interruption of blood flow to a localized area of the brain. Pediatric stroke has a wide range of causes and risk factors distinct from those in adults, thus limiting comparison to stroke in adults. Strokes can be categorized into hemorrhagic or ischemic. Unlike the adult population, in which ischemic episodes account for 80% to 85% of strokes, approximately 55% of strokes in children are ischemic. Stroke is often undiagnosed or diagnosed late in its course. The ED physician must have a high index of suspicion for this condition.

Pathophysiology

Hemorrhagic strokes refer to spontaneous intraparenchymal hemorrhage and nontraumatic subarachnoid hemorrhage (causes of hemorrhagic stroke are listed in Table 126.3). Intraparenchymal hemorrhages are the result of bleeding from a ruptured blood vessel within the brain parenchyma and can result in progressive surrounding edema and focal mass effect. They are most often the result of anteriovenous malformation (up to 50%), followed by hematologic abnormality and hemorrhage into brain tumors. Congenital or acquired disorders, such as sickle cell disease, severe factor VIII deficiency, or severe thrombocytopenia, have been reported to be the major risk factor in 10% to 30% of hemorrhagic stroke in most series and may result in spontaneous intracranial bleeding with minimal or no preceding head trauma.

TABLE 126.3

CAUSES OF HEMORRHAGIC STROKE

Secondary hemorrhage into ischemic brain
Arteriovenous malformations
Vascular malformations
  Sickle cell disease
  Saccular (berry) aneurysms
Hemorrhage into intracranial tumor
Coagulopathy
  Hemorrhagic disease of the newborn (vitamin K deficiency)
  Clotting factor deficiency (VIII, IX, XI)
  Thrombocytopenia
Arterial hypertension
  Renal vascular or parenchymal disease
  Coarctation of the aorta
  Pheochromocytoma
  Illicit drugs with sympathomimetic effect
  Amphetamines, cocaine

TABLE 126.4

CAUSES OF ISCHEMIC STROKE

Cardioembolic
    Left atrial myxoma
    Cyanotic congenital heart disease
    Right-to-left shunts (e.g., patent foramen ovale)
    Congenital or acquired valvular defects
    Contractile dysfunction
    Rhythm disturbance
Vascular disease
    Sickle cell disease
    Arterial dissection
    Homocystinuria
    Vasculitis
    Moyamoya
    Migraine
Thrombotic (arterial and sinovenous)
    Hypercoagulable state, congenital or acquired protein C, S,
        antithrombin III deficiencies, factor V Leiden, prothrom-
        bin 20 210A mutation, oral contraceptives, anticardiolipin
        antibodies
    Hyperviscosity (polycythemia, dehydration)
Genetic/metabolic

Nontraumatic subarachnoid hemorrhages are most often because of intracranial aneurysms. Ruptured aneurysms account for 10% of intracranial hemorrhage in children. About 5% of children with intracranial aneurysms will have more than one aneurysm. Congenital ruptured aneurysms may rarely occur as early as the first week of life. Bleeding occurs from an aneurysm located at branching points of the major arteries coursing through the subarachnoid space at the base of the brain. The incidence of aneurysm is increased in various congenital and hereditary conditions, including coarctation of the aorta, autosomal-dominant polycystic kidney disease, fibromuscular dysplasia, Ehlers-Danlos type IV, neurofibromatosis type 1, and Marfan syndrome.

Ischemic strokes include both arterial ischemic strokes (AIS) and cerebral venous sinus thrombosis (CVST). Ischemic injury to the brain occurs as a result of embolism from the heart or proximal circulation or from thrombosis in the arterial or sinovenous system. Almost half of all children with an ischemic stroke have a known risk factor. The most common risk factor (in about 25% of patients) is congenital heart disease. At least two-thirds of children will have one or more risk factors identified after an extensive workup (Table 126.4).

Clinical Manifestations

The diagnosis of stroke in children is often delayed by the failure to consider it, as signs and symptoms can be subtle and nonspecific. There are some generalizations that can be made as to how strokes present in children. Ischemic strokes most often present as a focal neurologic deficit. Hemiplegia is the most common focal manifestation, occurring in up to 94% of cases. Hemorrhagic strokes, on the other hand, most commonly present with headache or altered level of consciousness and are more likely to cause vomiting than ischemic strokes. Seizures are common, occurring in up to 50% of children with strokes.

There are significant differences in clinical presentation based on the age of the child: the younger the child, the more nonspecific his or her symptoms may be. Perinatal strokes may present with focal seizures or lethargy. Similarly, infants in the first year of life may present with apnea or hypotonia. In arterial dissection, patients may complain of sudden ipsilateral pain in the head, neck, or eye. There may be an associated Horner syndrome if the cervical sympathetic chain is involved. A bruit may be heard over the involved carotid. A posterior circulation stroke may result in vertebrobasilar insufficiency and cranial neuropathy, difficulties with balance and coordination, and tremor. After a subarachnoid hemorrhage (SAH), neck stiffness may be followed by lower back pain and radicular leg pain which may subsequently predominate as CSF circulates.

Management

The management of stroke in children is understudied and largely extrapolated from the adult literature and can be categorized into general supportive measures applicable to all types of strokes, diagnostic modalities, and stroke-specific treatment. It is prudent to have a stroke protocol in place.

General supportive measures include correction of hypoxemia, control of fever, normalization of serum glucose, and treatment of increased ICP. Judicious control of severe systemic hypertension is recommended. However, rapid reduction of blood pressure has been associated with worse neurological outcomes and larger infarcts in adults. There is no evidence to support prophylactic anticonvulsants in the absence of clinical or subclinical seizures in children with AIS, but they should be considered in children with hemorrhagic stroke and CVST.

The next priority is to exclude an acute intraparenchymal bleed or SAH. Non-contrast head CT is readily obtained, quickly completed, and sensitive for acute hemorrhage although the adult literature suggests that a lumbar puncture is still needed to exclude SAH not seen on CT. MRI is as good as CT for identifying hyperacute hemorrhage (less than 6 hours).

In ischemic stroke, CT may reveal low-density lesions within vascular territories in AIS and evidence of CVST. However, CT is usually normal within the first 12 hours after the onset of symptoms. CT angiography (CTA) may be used to identify arterial dissection. However, CTA requires larger radiation doses than standard CT. The contrast required may also limit the volume of contrast that can be safely administered for subsequent, more definitive delineation by catheter angiography (CA).

MRI should be performed if a hemorrhagic stroke is not found on CT. MRI is sensitive for ischemic stroke, even within a few hours of symptom onset. Magnetic resonance angiography (MRA) will yield further information about blood flow and vessel patency, and magnetic resonance venography (MRV) will more reliably identify CVST.

CA yields the most precise detail of vascular anatomy and affords the option of endovascular therapy. It will also identify specific signs of vasculitis or dissection and abnormalities in medium or smaller arteries, which MRA may miss. However, CA is an invasive procedure, less commonly performed in children, and has a similar diagnostic yield as MRI when combined with MRV and MRA. Other investigations to consider include ultrasound of the extracranial carotid circulation and echocardiography.

Once the type of stroke is identified, specific treatment is tailored to the etiology. In hemorrhagic stroke, coagulation defects should be corrected (see Chapter 91). Emergent splenectomy is indicated for intraparenchymal bleeding associated with idiopathic thrombocytopenic purpura. Recombinant factor VIIa is a promising therapy which promotes hemostasis and may stabilize intracerebral hematoma and reduce hemorrhage volume and improve clinical outcome.

Surgical management of hemorrhagic strokes is controversial. However, evacuation of a rapidly expanding hematoma causing cerebral herniation may be of benefit.

The goal of medical management of ischemic stroke is to preserve neurologic function and prevent recurrent stroke. Treatment may include short-term anticoagulation with low–molecular-weight heparin (LMWH) or unfractionated heparin. Although LMWH has reproducible pharmacokinetics and requires fewer monitoring tests, its effects cannot be completely reversed within minutes as it could be in someone who received unfractionated heparin. The loading dose of heparin is 75 units per kg intravenously over 10 minutes, followed by 20 units per kg for children older than 1 year of age, or 28 units per kg for children younger than 1 year of age titrated to a target partial thromboplastin time of 60 to 85 seconds. Alternatively, LMWH (enoxaparin 1 mg per kg subcutaneously for children more than 2 months of age, or 1.5 mg per kg for infants less than 2 months of age) may be given. It is prudent to start anticoagulation in children because the likelihood of a child having an underlying condition that would benefit from anticoagulation is high. Anticoagulation is also often used in children with arterial dissection, dural sinus thrombosis, or hypercoagulable disorders; in those at high risk of embolism; or in response to progressive deterioration during the initial evaluation of a new cerebral infarction.

The decision to use thrombolytic therapy in children with ischemic strokes must be made in a guarded and judicious manner. Although there have been anecdotal reports of successful endovascular thrombolysis in children, there are also reports of a high complication rate in children with systemic thromboses who receive tissue-type plasminogen activator (tPA) despite successful lysis of said thromboses. Published guidelines suggest that tPA may be considered in a select group of children with CVST, and that it would be most prudent to consider the same guidelines used in adults: administration of intravenous tPA within 3 hours of stroke onset and intra-arterial tPA within 6 hours of stroke onset for anterior circulation strokes. Delayed administration may lead to an unacceptable rate of intracerebral hemorrhage in children, as has been demonstrated in adults. Whether adult guidelines can be readily applied to older adolescents nearing adulthood is unclear, but there is as of yet little evidence to support the use of tPA in children outside of a clinical trial.

Rates of stroke in children with sickle cell disease (SSD) are much higher than in the rest of the pediatric population, and the management in this context requires specific considerations. In addition to supportive measures, ischemic strokes should be treated with hydration and simple or partial exchange transfusion to achieve a hemoglobin SS fraction of less than 30% and a hemoglobin level below 10 g per dL to avoid hyperviscosity. Evaluation for a structural vascular lesion in children with sickle cell disease and a hemorrhagic

stroke is reasonable. Aneurysm is often present in adolescents with SCD and an SAH, and there is potential for rebleeding in these individuals. Evaluation with CA should be deferred until after reduction of the percentage of sickle hemoglobin because of concerns that CA might facilitate sickling.

CENTRAL NERVOUS SYSTEM INFECTIONS

Infection of the CNS, including subdural empyema, brain abscess, bacterial and viral meningitis, and viral encephalitis, are often associated with some degree of increased ICP. Acute hydrocephalus may complicate tuberculous, fungal, amebic, and rarely bacterial meningitis. Subdural empyema and epidural abscess may occur as a complication of parameningeal infections (e.g., sinusitis, orbital cellulitis, or mastoiditis) and are true neurosurgical emergencies, often progressing to death if not recognized early. Children with CNS infectious processes may present with fever, evidence of meningeal irritation, seizures, increased ICP, focal neurologic findings, and herniation.

Management

Supportive care and antibiotics are the first priority in treatment of suspected meningitis. Lumbar puncture should be deferred in patients with cardiorespiratory instability, signs of impending herniation, papilledema, or focal neurologic deficits. A CT may identify acute brain edema or other signs of increased ICP, but a normal CT scan does not eliminate the possibility that ICP is increased. Normal CT scans have been seen in patients with fatal herniation. MRI may be more sensitive than CT for identifying potential complications of meningitis, such as infarction, ventriculitis, and venous sinus thrombosis. If a subdural empyema or brain abscess is suspected, a contrast-enhanced CT may be helpful. However, MRI is more sensitive for identifying this intracranial complication, particularly the early cerebritis phase of brain abscess and those located in the brain stem or posterior fossa.

Subdural empyema requires immediate surgical drainage. For brain abscess, closed-needle drainage with stereotactic CT guidance permits precise targeting of small lesions. This technique allows rapid relief of mass effect by removing purulent material and provides a specimen for culture and sensitivity testing to guide subsequent antibiotic therapy. The use of corticosteroids for treatment of brain abscess is controversial because of concerns related to decreasing antibiotic penetration and inhibition of leukocyte migration and host defense mechanisms. However, steroids may be selectively used to control life-threatening intracranial hypertension due to mass effect and edema.

BRAIN TUMORS

Brain tumors account for nearly 20% of all cancers in children, second only to leukemia. Early signs and symptoms are often attributed to benign causes resulting in delayed diagnosis.

Pathophysiology

The most common pediatric brain tumors are gliomas, primarily astrocytomas. The majority are infratentorial and arise in the posterior fossa. The clinical features can be either generalized, resulting from elevated ICP due to mass effect, edema, or obstructive hydrocephalus; or focal, resulting from mass effect on specialized brain regions.

Clinical Manifestation

Early signs and symptoms are often nonspecific, and neurologic abnormalities may be subtle. Behavioral symptoms account for up to one-fifth of initial symptoms in children. Isolated persisting vomiting and vomiting on awaking, due to position change, is ominous. Headaches associated with intracranial mass lesions may be nonspecific but are usually of recent onset. Other predictors of surgical space-occupying lesions include absence of a family history of migraine; sleep-related headache (headache either wakes child from sleep or is present immediately on awakening); confusion; and an abnormal neurologic examination.

Physical examination should include fundoscopy to look for papilledema, cranial nerve examination for palsy, and search for focal motor deficits and ataxia. Acute symptoms may result from seizure, acute intracranial hypertension with pressure waves, or acute obstructive hydrocephalus or hemorrhage into tumor.

Management

Most children who require emergent management for tumor-related obstructive hydrocephalus, mass effect, and hemorrhage are recognized using noncontrast CT. In the stable patient who does not require sedation, when local resources permit, one may consider obtaining an MRI as the first-line imaging study. MRI is more sensitive than CT in identifying small brain tumors, particularly in the posterior fossa and is useful for identifying other potential pathologies that may be responsible for the presenting symptoms, including hyperacute hemorrhages. MRI will eventually be necessary for definitive management. Dexamethasone may be useful in treating increased ICP before surgery.

SPINAL CORD COMPRESSION

Nontraumatic acute spinal cord compression is relatively uncommon but will result in devastating sequelae if not considered early and diagnosed promptly. In children, it occurs most frequently with paravertebral neoplasms. Back pain in a child with known cancer should raise concern for cord compression until proven otherwise.

Pathophysiology

Spinal cord compression may be caused by paravertebral neoplasms or vertebral metastases; spinal epidural or, rarely, sub-dural, abscesses; epidural hematoma; central disc herniation; or congenital tethered cord. Spinal epidural abscesses (SEA) occur most frequently in children younger than 2 or older than 12 years of age. SEA is most frequently caused by seeding in the epidural space following hematogenous spread from a distant infectious focus including cellulitis, tonsillitis, and pneumonia, or in association with IV drug abuse.

Clinical Manifestations

Back pain in children commonly signals an important diagnosis. A history of localized or radicular back pain or refusal to walk mandates a careful evaluation. Radicular pain may misdirect the clinician depending on the nerves involved, manifesting instead as hip, extremity, or abdominal pain. The back pain of SEA in older children may be excruciating, causing them to lie absolutely still. Younger children may present with a nonspecific reluctance to lie prone. A history of change in gait or difficulty with bowel or bladder control should be sought. The level of maximal spinal tenderness is usually the site of pathology. Deep tendon reflexes, Babinski reflex, motor strength, sensation, and anal sphincter tone should be assessed.

Management

Blood cultures may help guide antibiotic therapy during hospitalization. If SEA is suspected, a lumbar puncture should not be performed, as it does not significantly contribute to the diagnosis and may spread bacteria into the subdural or subarachnoid space. Plain radiographs of the spine may show evidence of osteomyelitis or vertebral abnormalities but will miss significant pathology. Therefore, emergent MRI should be carried out to identify the cause and degree of spinal compression. The entire spine should be imaged as metastases or abscesses may be seen in multiple places.

Tumor-related cord compression with neurologic deficits mandates immediate treatment. Prompt initiation of high-dose corticosteroid therapy is indicated. Additional treatment options include decompressive surgery, radiation therapy, and chemotherapy. Abscess formation, subdural or epidural hemorrhage, and symptoms related to cord tethering are usually indications for surgical intervention.

Suggested Readings

Increased Intracranial Pressure

Herrmann BW, Chung JC, Eisenbeis JF, et al. Intracranial complications of pediatric frontal rhinosinusitis. *Am J Rhinol* 2006;20(3):320–324.
Rangel-Castilla L, Gopinath S, Robertson CS. Management of intracranial hypertension. *Neurol Clin* 2008;26(2):521–541.

Previously Shunted Hydrocephalus

Anderson CM, Sorrells DL, Kerby JD. Intraabdominal pseudocysts as a complication of ventriculoperitoneal shunts. *J Am Coll Surg* 2003;196(2):297–300.
Ashley WW Jr, McKinstry RC, Leonard JR, et al. Use of rapid-sequence magnetic resonance imaging for evaluation of hydrocephalus in children. *J Neurosurg (Pediatrics 2)* 2005;103:124–130.
Barnes NP, Jones SJ, Hayward WJ, et al. Ventriculoperitoneal shunt block: what are the best clinical indicators? *Arch Dis Child* 2002;87:198–201.

Browd SR, Ragel BT, Gottfried ON, et al. Failure of cerebrospinal fluid shunts: part I: obstruction and mechanical failure. *Pediatr Neurol* 2006;34(2): 83–92.

Browd SR, Ragel BT, Gottfried ON, et al. Failure of cerebrospinal fluid shunts: part II: overdrainage, loculation, and abdominal complications. *Pediatr Neurol* 2006;34(3):171–176.

Duhaime A, Wiley JF. Ventricular shunt and burr hole puncture. In: Henretig FM, King C, eds. *Textbook of pediatric emergency procedures.* Baltimore: Williams & Wilkins, 2008:515–521.

Iskandar BJ, Sansone JM, Bedow J, et al. The use of quick-brain magnetic resonance imaging in the evaluation of shunt-treated hydrocephalus. *J Neurosurg* 2004;101(2):147–151.

Kim TY, Stewart G, Voth M, et al. Signs and symptoms of cerebrospinal fluid shunt malfunction in the pediatric emergency department. *Pediatr Emerg Care* 2006;22(1):28–34.

Lee P, DiPatri AJ. Evaluation of suspected cerebrospinal fluid shunt complications in children. *Clin Pediatr Emerg Med* 2008;9:76–82.

Martinez-Lage JF, Martos-Tello JM, Ros-de-San Pedro J, et al. Severe constipation: an under-appreciated cause of VP shunt malfunction: a case-based update. *Childs Nerv Syst* 2008;24:431–435.

May CH, Aurisch R, Kornrumpf D, et al. Evaluation of shunt function in hydrocephalic patients with the radionuclide 99mTc-pertechnetate. *Childs Nerv Syst* 1999;15:239–244.

Piatt JH, Garton HJ. Clinical diagnosis of ventriculoperitoneal shunt failure among children with hydrocephalus. *Pediatr Emerg Care* 2008;24(4):201–210.

Pitetti R. Emergency department evaluation of ventricular shunt malfunction: Is the shunt series really necessary? *Pediatr Emerg Care* 2007;23(3):137–141.

Poca MA, Sahuquillo J. Short-term medical management of hydrocephalus. *Expert Opin Pharmacother* 2005;6(9):1525–1538.

Rocue BG, Lapsiwala S, Iskandar BJ. Ventricular shunt tap as a predictor of proximal shunt malfunction in children: a prospective study. *J Neurosurg Pediatr* 2008;1(6):439–443.

Sandberg DI. Endoscopic management of hydrocephalus in pediatric patients: a review of indications, techniques, and outcomes. *J Child Neurol* 2008;23(5): 550–560.

Zorc JJ, Krugman SD, Ogborn J, et al. Radiographic evaluation for suspected cerebrospinal fluid shunt obstruction. *Pediatr Emerg Care* 2002;18(5):337–340.

Shunt Infection

Duhaime A. Evaluation and management of shunt infections in children with hydrocephalus. *Clin Pediatr* 2006;45:705–713.

Schreffler RT, Schreffler AJ, Wittler RR. Treatment of cerebrospinal fluid shunt infections: a decision analysis. *Pediatr Infect Dis J* 2002;21(7):632–636.

Scribano PV, Pool S, Smally AJ. Comparison of ventriculoperitoneal shunt tap and lumbar puncture in a child with meningitis. *Pediatr Emerg Care* 2002;18(4):E1–E3.

Hemorrhagic and Ischemic Stroke

Bernard TJ, Goldenberg NA, Armstrong-Wells J, et al. Treatment of childhood arterial ischemic stroke. *Ann Neurol* 2008;63:679–696.

Calder K, Kokorowski P, Tran T, et al. Emergency department presentation of pediatric stroke. *Pediatr Emerg Care* 2003;19(5):320–328.

Edlow JA, Panagos PD, Godwin SA, et al. Clinical policy: critical issues in the evaluation and management of adult patients presenting to the emergency department with acute headache. *Ann Emerg Med* 2008;52(4):407–436.

Gabis LV, Yangala R, Lenn NJ. Time lag to diagnosis of stroke in children. *Pediatrics* 2002;110(5):924–928.

Huang J, McGirt MG, Gailloud P, et al. Intracranial aneurysms in the pediatric population: case series and literature review. *Surg Neurol* 2005;63:424–432.

Jordan LC, Hillis AE. Hemorrhagic stroke in children. *Pediatr Neurol* 2007; 36:73–80.

Kidwell CS, Chalela JA, Saver JL, et al. Comparison of MRI and CT for detection of acute intracerebral hemorrhage. *JAMA* 2004;292(15):1823–1830.

Kirton A, Wong JH, Mah J, et al. Successful endovascular therapy for acute basilar thrombosis in an adolescent. *Pediatrics* 2003;112(3, pt 1):e248–e251.

Liu AC, Segaren N, Cox TS, et al. Is there a role for magnetic resonance imaging in the evaluation of non-traumatic intraparenchymal haemorrhage in children? *Pediatr Radiol* 2006;36:940–946.

Mendelow AD, Gregson BA, Fernandes HM, et al. Early surgery versus initial conservative treatment in patients with spontaneous supratentorial intracerebral haematomas in the International Surgical Trial in Intracerebral Haemorrhage (STITCH): a randomized trial. *Lancet* 2005;365:387–397.

Roach ES, Golomb MR, Adams R, et al. Management of stroke in infants and children: a scientific statement from a Special Writing Group of the American Heart Association Stroke Council and the Council on Cardiovascular Disease in the Young. *Stroke* 2008;39:2644–2691.

Central Nervous System Infections

Foerster BR, Thurnher MM, Malani PN, et al. Intracranial infections: clinical and imaging characteristics. *Acta Radiol* 2007;48:875–893.

Hakan T, Ceran N, Erdem I, et al. Bacterial brain abscesses: an evaluation of 96 cases. *J Infect* 2006;52(5):359–366.

Oliver WJ, Shope TC, Kuhns LR. Fatal lumbar puncture: fact versus fiction—an approach to a clinical dilemma. *Pediatrics* 2003;112(3, pt 1):e174–e176.

Brain Tumors

Dobrovoljac M, Hengartner H, Boltshauser E, et al. Delay in the diagnosis of paediatric brain tumours. *Eur J Pediatr* 2002;161(12):663–667.

Hutter A, Schwetye KE, Bierhals AJ, et al. Brain neoplasms: epidemiology, diagnosis, and prospects for cost-effective imaging. *Neuroimaging Clin N Am* 2003;13:237–250.

Kukal K, Dobrovoljac M, Boltshauser E, et al. Does diagnostic delay result in decreased survival in paediatric brain tumours? *Eur J Pediatr* 2009;168: 303–310.

Squires RH Jr. Intracranial tumors: vomiting as a presenting sign. A gastroenterologist's perspective. *Clin Pediatr (Phila)* 1989;28(8):351.

Spinal Cord Compression

Jacobsen FS, Sullivan B. Spinal epidural abscesses in children. *Orthopedics* 1994;17(12):1131–1138.

Pollono D, Tomarchia S, Drut R, et al. Spinal cord compression: a review of 70 pediatric patients. *Pediatr Hematol Oncol* 2003;20(6):457–466.

Reihsaus E, Waldbaur H, Seeling W. Spinal epidural abscess: a meta-analysis of 915 patients. *Neurosurg Rev* 2000;232:175–204.

Spinazze S, Caraceni A, Schrijvers D. Epidural spinal cord compression. *Clin Rev Oncol Hematol* 2005;56:397–406.

CHAPTER 127 ■ OPHTHALMIC EMERGENCIES

ALEX V. LEVIN, MD, MHSC, FRCSC

Many ocular disorders in children may be seen first by the pediatric emergency physician. Although ophthalmology consultation is necessary in some cases, some problems can and should be treated by the emergency physician. This chapter provides the emergency physician with a basic foundation for the diagnosis and treatment of common pediatric eye emergencies.

EXAMINATION

Many children regard eye examinations and eye drops with the same fear that they harbor for injections. Therefore, it is important to gather as much information as possible before touching the patient or instilling eye drops. This can be accomplished by turning the initial parts of the eye examination into a game, using toys and distracting stimuli, and exploiting the full potential of the direct ophthalmoscope, the main instrument for ophthalmic examination available to the pediatric emergency physician.

A detailed history can be a valuable tool in focusing the examination and making a diagnosis. Questions regarding unilaterality/bilaterality, acute/chronic onset of symptoms, and prior ophthalmic care are particularly helpful. Perhaps the child is known to have an eye with poor vision. Even if the parent does not know that this is the case, a history of having one eye patched for a visual problem suggests that the unpatched eye had amblyopia. If a child has previously passed his or her visual screening examination at school, this does not necessarily imply that the vision was normal because false-negative tests are well known to occur. The child may also be unaware of having poor vision in one eye because the pediatric brain is able to suppress recognition of the blurred image and focus solely on the clear image, allowing the child to proceed with normal activity unaware of the unilateral visual deficit.

The examiner starts the evaluation either by testing visual acuity in children who are readily verbal and interactive, or by using other techniques in children who need to be "warmed up." In the latter case, it is often useful to start with assessment of the extraocular muscle movements. This procedure is discussed in Chapter 23. By using a toy or another interesting hand-held object, the physician can distract the child to look in the direction in which the object is placed. Both eyes should move equally, quantitatively and qualitatively, in all directions. The examiner should test up, down, left, and right gaze.

The examiner can use the direct ophthalmoscope as a tool to accomplish several tasks without touching the child. The direct ophthalmoscope light may be useful as a fixation target in testing eye movements. It can also be used to assess whether the eyes are aligned (Hirschberg light reflex test, see Chapter 23) and to test for a red reflex (see Chapter 117). In addition,

the ophthalmoscope can be used as a simple hand-held magnifier by viewing through the ophthalmoscope and dialing the focusing wheel in the direction of the black or green numbers. This allows the eyeball to come into focus regardless of the distance between the examiner and the patient. The closer one gets, the higher the black or green number needed on the focusing wheel, and the greater the magnification. The examiner can perform this maneuver with or without his/her own glasses on.

Visual acuity testing is usually performed at a distance of 20 ft or 10 ft. Most standard wall charts are calibrated to be read at 20 ft. If space does not permit this distance to be used, the patient can be placed 10 ft from the chart and the results interpreted with an adjustment for this distance. For example, the line marked 20/60 on the chart (a line that a person with normal sight can see at 60 ft, but a person with that visual acuity would need to stand at 20 ft to see) becomes a 20/30 line at a distance of 10 ft. In some centers or with some vision charts, the metric system is used with 20 ft being equivalent to 6 m. As examples, vision of 20/20 is written as 6/6, 20/30 as 6/9, and 20/200 as 6/60.

Chart selection is important when trying to obtain an accurate visual acuity. Letter charts should be used only for patients who can clearly recognize the alphabet. If there is any question by parental report, a number or picture chart (Fig. 127.1) should be used. The patient may be asked to walk right up to the chart to identify the letters, numbers, or pictures. If the patient can perform this task, the chart may then be used for distance testing. Some children give remarkably unique interpretations of the pictures (e.g., calling the birthday cake a bag of French fries). When using picture charts that have colored figures, the examiner should avoid using those figures that are yellow because the bright illumination of the emergency department (ED) lessens the contrast between these figures and the white chart background, thus making recognition more difficult. The "tumbling E" chart is not recommended in young children as it may be too complex for their developmental level and requires some sense of handedness, which is not developed until an age when they should easily be able to perform the other tests. This chart is more useful for older non–English-speaking children and illiterate adults. It is sometimes referred to as the "illiterate E" test.

A useful option for children who are not "in the mood" to verbalize their responses or are very shy is the use of matching acuity chart systems. The two most common are the Sheridan Gardiner (Keeler Instruments, Inc., Broomal, PA) and HOTV (Precision Vision, La Salle, IL). In both situations, the child is holding a card that has all of the letters that are on the posted or hand-held chart 10- or 20-ft away. The child need not know letters but can identify them as shapes. For example, the H can be called a little ladder and the O a circle. Instead of verbally

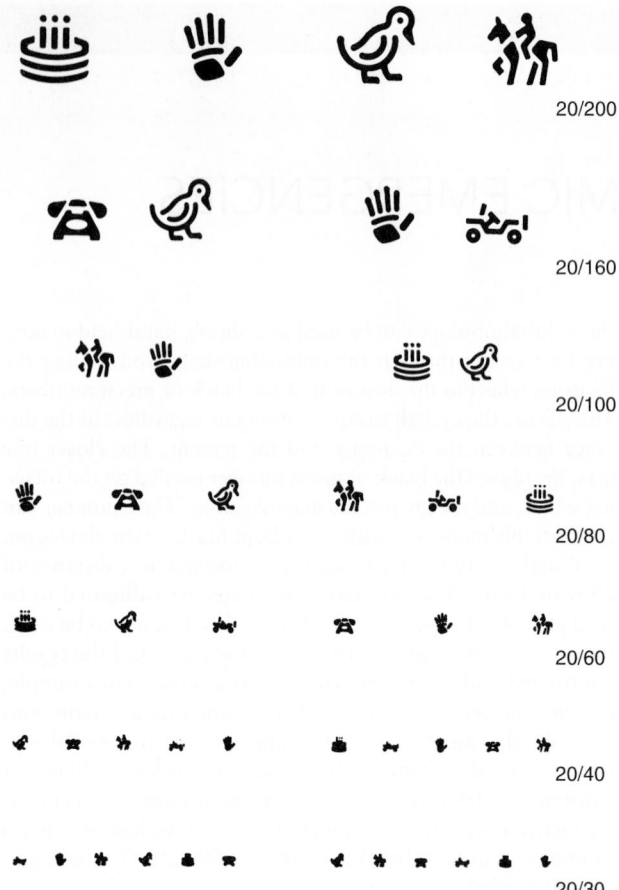

FIGURE 127.1 Picture visual acuity chart.

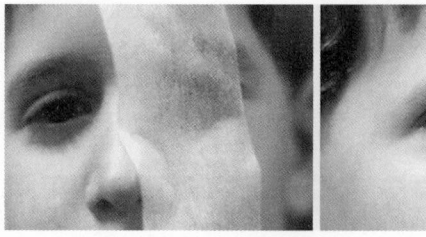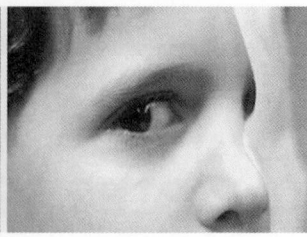

FIGURE 127.2 A broad piece of tape can be used to obstruct the vision of the eye not being tested. If the tape is not adherent to the bridge of the nose, the child can peek out by turning the face to the side (**right frame**).

responding, the child points to the matching shape (letter) on the card he/she or his/her parent is holding. EDs can even make their own hand-held card to match whatever wall chart they have posted to accommodate to children in this younger age range where matching is more easily accomplished than verbal response.

When using any visual acuity chart, it is not necessary to start with the largest symbol and have the patient read every symbol on every line thereafter. Doing so risks losing the child's attention. Rather, one can start with the 20/20 line and then go to larger lines if the child is having trouble. The child needs to recognize only a few letters on each line. Minor errors such as the substitution of the letter F for the letter P, or the letter C for the letter O, may be tolerated.

It is almost an instinct for young children to use their better eye and suppress the vision in their lesser eye. Therefore, if the good eye is covered inadequately, the patient will naturally try to read the chart with what the examiner thought was the covered eye. Children should never be allowed to cover their eye with their own hand because the small cracks between the fingers can actually allow vision out of the "covered" eye and even improve that vision by the pinhole effect (see Chapter 117). Children may also look around commercially available occluders for the same reasons. Perhaps the best way to obstruct the vision in the eye not being tested is to use a broad piece of tape, ensuring the tape also covers the depression at the bridge of the nose (Fig. 127.2). To help ensure the patient

is not "cheating," the examiner should stand by the chart indicating the letters or pictures while looking back at the child.

Any child who shows a reduced visual acuity should be offered the pinhole test. If the patient is unable to identify any object or picture on the chart, the examiner should at least try to determine whether vision is present. After external examination and visual acuity are completed, the examiner can then proceed with other procedures as indicated, such as upper lid eversion and dilating the pupil. These techniques, along with the proper methods of examining the retina and optic nerve using the direct ophthalmoscope, are discussed in Chapter 117.

One circumstance that may present an obstacle to proper examination of the eye is the situation in which the eyelids are swollen or the patient refuses to voluntarily open the eyelids. The techniques described in Chapter 117 for opening the traumatized eye may be useful. Commercially available speculums, when used in association with a topical anesthetic, are a painless and efficient way of opening the eyelids (see Chapter 117, Fig. 117.5). If these are not available, either a Desmarres retractor (see Chapter 117, Fig. 117.6) can be used or a similar device can be fashioned out of paper clips (Fig. 127.3). These types of single-blade retractors are most helpful when used on the upper eyelid (see Chapter 117, Fig. 117.6). A retractor can also can be applied simultaneously to the lower eyelids, although this often requires an extra assistant if there is a problem holding the child still while the eyelids are retracted. When paper clips are used, it is important to inspect the paper clip after bending. Some paper clips have a coating that may become fragmented, potentially causing particles that could be dispersed to the conjunctiva or cornea as tiny foreign bodies. Eyelid speculums and retractors should be sterilized between patients. Paper clip speculums are designed for single usage and may be prepared by cleansing with an alcohol swab.

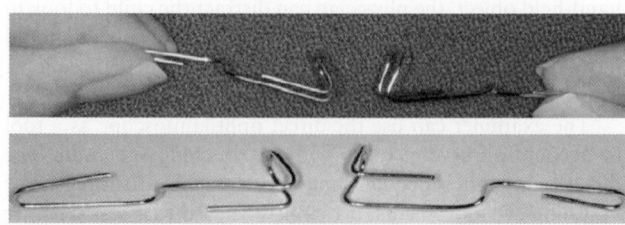

FIGURE 127.3 Paper clips can be bent into a retractor to open the eyelids.

In infants, the eyelids may be separated by using cotton swabs. The swabs should be placed at the midbody of the upper and lower eyelids. As they are separated, pressure should be applied down against the eyelid and the swab should be rotated inward toward the eyelashes. This will keep the eyelids in place so they do not spontaneously evert and further obstruct the examiner's view. When long cotton swabs are used, the stick should be grasped close to the patient to prevent breakage when pressure is applied. The cotton swab technique should not be used in patients being evaluated for eye trauma because pressure on the eyeball from this technique could cause further injury (see Chapter 117).

COMMON EYE EMERGENCIES

The pediatric emergency physician is called on to care for a number of eye problems. The reader is referred to other sections of this book for discussions of eye injuries (see Chapter 117), red eye (see Chapter 23), disorders of the eye muscle movement and strabismus (see Chapter 24), iritis (see Chapters 23 and 117), and unequal pupils (see Chapter 25).

Periorbital and Orbital Cellulitis

Clinical Manifestations

The primary concern when making the diagnosis of periorbital cellulitis (preseptal cellulitis) is to rule out the possibility of orbital cellulitis. The cardinal signs of orbital cellulitis include decreased eye movement, proptosis, decreased vision, and papilledema (or other signs of optic nerve involvement such as decreased color vision, visual field defects, or Marcus Gunn pupil). Both orbital and periorbital infection may be associated with fever, pain, swollen eyelids, and red eye. If orbital cellulitis is suspected, computed tomography (CT) scanning of the orbit is indicated, keeping in mind that a CT scan taken in the first 24 to 48 hours of infection can appear normal. Clinical examination is therefore very important. Ophthalmology consultation is indicated in all cases of suspected or proven orbital cellulitis. Surgical intervention may be required. Otorhinolaryngology consultation should also be considered when orbital cellulitis is secondary to contiguous sinus infection.

Historical and clinical information can also be helpful in establishing the probable bacterial etiology of the infection. Infection secondary to a bug bite or other skin wound that may have served as a route of entry for local bacteria is more often caused by staphylococci or streptococci. The bluish hue of the periorbital skin that is sometimes attributed to *Haemophilus influenzae* is not a specific or sensitive indicator. In fact, since the introduction of the *H. influenzae* type b vaccine in 1985, the incidence of this pathogen as a cause for periorbital or orbital cellulitis has dropped substantially. It is now an uncommon cause.

One must rule out other conditions that can mimic a periorbital cellulitis. Insect bites and allergic reactions can cause dramatic acute periorbital swelling. These conditions are not usually associated with fever. Often, close inspection of the skin with magnification (using the direct ophthalmoscope) can localize the site of an insect bite. Allergic swelling is often bilateral, whereas periorbital cellulitis is rarely bilateral. Underlying sinusitis can also cause periorbital swelling. Some

authors have argued that CT scan evaluation of the sinuses is indicated in all cases of presumed periorbital cellulitis but this is not common practice in many centers. Severe conjunctivitis, especially adenoviral infection and neonatal gonorrhea conjunctivitis, can also result in significant lid swelling. The presence of conjunctival discharge is helpful in making these diagnoses. Contiguous spread of conjunctival infections to the periorbital tissues can occur, and one must be careful about falsely eliminating the diagnosis of periorbital infection based on the presence of conjunctivitis.

Management

There is some controversy about the appropriate route of antibiotic administration in periorbital cellulitis. When *H. influenzae* was more common with the risk of hematogenous spread, it seemed prudent to use intravenous (IV) antibiotics. Clinicians have generally become more liberal with oral antibiotic treatment now that the risk of *H. influenzae* has declined. In otherwise well children who are beyond infancy and have mild periorbital cellulitis and no systemic signs or symptoms, particularly when the cause of the cellulitis is believed to be a skin wound, intramuscular and/or oral antibiotics may be tried. The patient should be seen again (or with telephone follow-up) within 24 to 48 hours, at which time improvement should be documented. If no improvement occurs, the patient could then be admitted for IV antibiotics. Clinical scales are available for assessing the patient's status and response to treatment. Periorbital cellulitis is a potentially fatal disease because complications such as meningitis may develop if inadequately treated. All cases of orbital cellulitis must be treated with IV antibiotics.

The choice of antibiotics should reflect the probable causative organism. Antibiotic coverage that would be used for presumed sepsis in an immunocompetent host with an unknown organism is usually appropriate. Before starting IV antibiotics, blood culture should be obtained. Other systemic cultures (e.g., cerebrospinal fluid, urine) may be indicated if signs of systemic toxicity are present. Percutaneous aspiration from the area of cellulitis is not recommended. Conjunctival cultures do not necessarily identify the causative agent of the cellulitis, but it may be reasonable to treat a predominant organism, particularly if purulent conjunctivitis is present. The patient should be monitored daily for signs of orbital cellulitis if there is no improvement.

Chalazions and Styes

Clinical Manifestations

Chalazion (internal hordeolum) and stye (external hordeolum) represent blocked glands within the eyelids. Both may present acutely with localized lid swelling, erythema, and tenderness. Styes are associated with swelling and purulent drainage at or near the lid margin (Fig. 127.4, see also color plate). More than one lesion may occur simultaneously, and more than one lid may be involved. Acute chalazion causes swelling and redness in the body of the eyelid and may be associated with drainage on the conjunctival surface of the eyelid with or without a red eye. They may also point and drain via the skin (Fig. 127.5, see also color plate). A chalazion may enter a chronic phase in which there is a nontender, noninflamed, mobile pea-size nodule within the body of the eyelid (Fig. 127.6). History

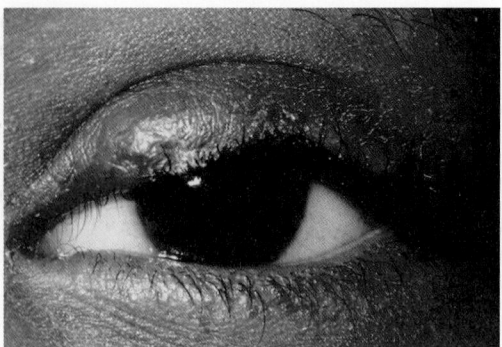

FIGURE 127.4 Acute sty (external hordeolum).

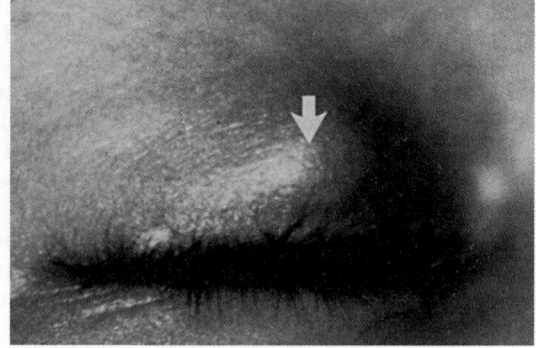

FIGURE 127.6 Chronic chalazion *(arrow)* within upper lid.

can be helpful in establishing these diagnoses because patients often have had recurrent lesions in the same or other eyelids.

Management

The treatment for both chalazion and stye is essentially the same. Eyelash scrubs with baby shampoo once or twice daily are helpful in mechanically establishing drainage. Baby shampoo is applied to a washcloth and then used to gently scrub the base of the eyelashes while the eyelids are shut. Some authors prefer cotton swabs for this procedure but this raises the risk of a swab injuring the eye if the swab slips between the lids. Warm compresses over closed eyelids are also sometimes recommended, but rarely tolerated well by younger children. Optimally, warm compresses should be applied four times daily for 10 to 20 minutes at each sitting. This is very difficult to accomplish. Antibiotics probably play a minimal role in the treatment of stye and chalazion. If desired, a topical antibiotic ointment with coverage for coagulase-negative staphylococcal species (Table 127.1) can be given twice daily following eyelash scrubs. If medical treatment has failed to cause adequate resolution after at least 4 weeks, surgery can be offered either for cosmesis or for uncomfortable lesions. In severe recurrent cases, particularly when associated with red eye or facial rosacea, oral erythromycin or tetracycline (only for patients older than 8 years) may be tried, although at this stage ophthalmic consultation should be obtained.

Chemical Injury

Clinical Manifestations

When the child has a clear history of a noxious substance coming in contact with the ocular surface, it is important to determine whether this substance is an acid or an alkali. Alkali injuries tend to be much more severe as they can cause aggressive tissue necrosis. It is also important to determine whether particulate matter may have been deposited on the ocular surface. Smoke can also cause chemical conjunctivitis, particularly in house fires when chemicals are liberated into the air from the burning of

TABLE 127.1

PEDIATRIC EMERGENCY DEPARTMENT
OPHTHALMIC DRUG GUIDELINES

Use	Avoid
Dilating drops	
Phenylephrine 2.5%	Scopolamine
Tropicamide 1%	Atropine
Cyclopentolate 1%	Homatropine
	Cyclopentolate 2%
Antibiotics	
Bacitracin ointment	Neomycin
Erythromycin ointment	Sulfacetamide
Polysporin drops or ointment	Aminoglycosides
Polytrim (trimethoprim/	(except neonate)
polymyxin B) drops	Quinolones
Lubricants	
Artificial tear drops or ointment	
Vasoconstrictors/antihistamines	
(e.g., naphazoline/antazoline)	
Diagnostic agents	
Topical fluorescein	
Anesthetic agents	
Proparacaine, tetracaine	Cocaine
(DO NOT PRESCRIBE)	

AVOID ALL ANTIVIRALS, MIOTICS (see Chapter 26),
STEROIDS,[a] and ANTIGLAUCOMA AGENTS.

[a]Including steroid-containing preparations, such as combination antibiotic-steroids.

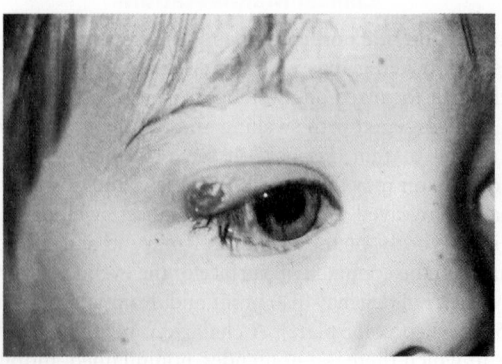

FIGURE 127.5 Chalazion draining spontaneously via skin.

plastics and other substances. Foreign bodies due to ashes and other particulate matter in the smoke are not uncommon.

The examiner must also assess the degree of exposure. If a child has no symptoms (pain, photophobia) or signs (red eye, epiphora, conjunctival swelling) and a weak history of actually getting the chemical into the eye, it may be acceptable to avoid lavage.

Management

Chemical injury to the eyeball is a true ocular emergency. Immediate intervention by ED personnel is essential to improving the patient's prognosis. Any patient with sufficient history should be immediately placed in the supine position, even if some level of restraint is needed, so ocular lavage may be started. Ocular lavage can often be frightening to a child. If sedation can be administered promptly, it may be helpful. The physician should never wait for the effects of sedation before proceeding with lavage. Although a drop of topical anesthetic can make this procedure more comfortable, the physician should not wait for this to become available if it is not immediately handy. Usually, the irrigating solution itself will induce cold anesthesia. If a speculum, Desmarres retractor, or paper clip is readily available (see above), this may be used to help obtain optimal exposure of the ocular surface. Commercially available irrigation lenses achieve similar results but often at greater monetary cost. Again, the physician should not wait for these to become available.

Virtually any IV solution can be used for ocular lavage, although normal saline solution or Ringer's lactate is perhaps preferable (although there is some controversy). A standard IV bag and tubing set is used without a needle on the end. Rather, the solution is allowed to flow, with the system at its maximum flow rate, across the surface of the open eye from medial to lateral. If both eyes have been exposed, they should both be lavaged simultaneously with two separate setups. Lavage should be continued until the involved eye(s) has received either 2 L of fluid or until approximately 20 minutes has elapsed. Lid eversion should be performed (see Chapter 117, Fig. 117.12), and lavage should be continued with the lid in this position so that the conjunctiva under the upper lid may also be cleansed. Mechanical debridement should be limited to the removal of visible particles from the ocular surface.

It is useful to have a strip of standard litmus paper available in the ED. The litmus paper is touched against the surface of each conjunctiva before beginning lavage. The pH is noted and the lavage is continued if, after the required minimum time/volume, the pH has not become normal (6.5 to 7.5) and equal between the two eyes. The end point of equality should only be used if one eye has not been exposed to chemical injuries. The conjunctiva under the upper lid may also be tested separately because noxious material can be harbored in the recess above the eye under the lid.

Ophthalmology consultation is usually indicated in cases of significant chemical injury. The consultant should be notified while lavage is ongoing. Do not delay lavage while awaiting the arrival of the ophthalmologist. In cases of minor exposure to substances that are clearly not alkaline or strongly acidic, and when the eye is not injected, an ophthalmology consultation may be deferred or may not be necessary, but emergency physicians must be cautious about the absence of conjunctival injection because alkali burns can cause blanching of the conjunctiva, which is a poor prognostic sign.

Conjunctivitis

Clinical Manifestations

Chapter 23 provides an approach for eliminating other causes of red eyes from the differential diagnosis. Table 127.2 is designed to give some additional help in differentiating causes

---

TABLE 127.2

DIFFERENTIAL DIAGNOSIS OF CONJUNCTIVITIS

	Bacterial	Viral (nonherpes)	Herpetic	Chlamydial	Allergic
Discharge—purulent	+++	±	—	±	—
Discharge—clear	—	+++	+++	±	+++
Swollen lids	++	+ to +++	+ to ++	+	+ to +++
Acute onset	++	++	+++	Chronic	+++ unless seasonal
Red eye	+++	+ to +++	Focally or diffuse +++	++	+
Cornea-staining with fluorescein	Nonspecific	Nonspecific	Dendrite	—	—
White cornea infiltrates	—	—	Possible	Multiple peripheral	—
Unilateral or bilateral	Uni/bi	Uni/bi	Uni	Usually bi	Usually bi
Contact history	+	+++	—	?STD	—
Preauricular node	++	+++	Usually—	±	—
Other associations	Otitis media? (*H. influenzae*)	Otitis media? Malaise, fever, pharyngitis	Prior or current skin lesions Recurrent	Genital discharge	Chemosis if acute

STD, sexually transmitted disease.
Adapted from Levin AV. Ophthalmology. In: Kropt SP, ed. *The HSC handbook of pediatrics.* 9th ed. Toronto: Mosby, 1997.

of conjunctivitis. The patient's age is often useful in determining a diagnosis. Neonates presenting in the first 3 days of life can have a chemical conjunctivitis caused by silver nitrate used for ocular prophylaxis perinatally. Almost all hospitals should have now discontinued this practice, and instead should be using erythromycin ointment or dilute betadine solutions. No prophylaxis is completely effective in eliminating subsequent gonorrheal or chlamydial conjunctivitis in the neonatal period. These two forms of conjunctivitis, as well as bacterial conjunctivitis often secondary to enteric organisms, can be difficult to distinguish clinically. Each can present as either a mild purulent form or more severe acute purulent conjunctivitis. A dramatically hyperacute conjunctivitis with significant lid swelling and copious purulent ocular discharge is more characteristic of gonorrhea (Fig. 127.7, see also color plate). In view of the risk of spontaneous corneal perforation associated with gonorrhea conjunctivitis, infants should be presumed to have this infection until proven otherwise. Immediate Gram stain should be performed looking for gram-negative diplococci. If present, treatment for gonorrheal conjunctivitis should be started emergently while awaiting culture results.

In this age group, chlamydia studies may also be useful. Conjunctival scrapings are useful to look for inclusion bodies of chlamydial conjunctivitis. However, the sensitivity of this test depends on sampling, and the techniques may not be readily available or properly performed. Other methods to detect chlamydia must always be used. Although rapid slide methods are approved for conjunctival samples, chlamydia cultures are preferred because they increase diagnostic sensitivity. Even if chlamydia is detected by Giemsa staining, this does not rule out the presence of concomitant gonorrheal infection.

In children beyond the neonatal period, a wide range of organisms, both viral and bacterial, as well as chlamydia, can cause conjunctivitis. Clinically, these entities may be indistinguishable. In general, purulence is more characteristic of bacterial infections, whereas clear serous discharge is more characteristic of viral infection. Although both viral and bacterial

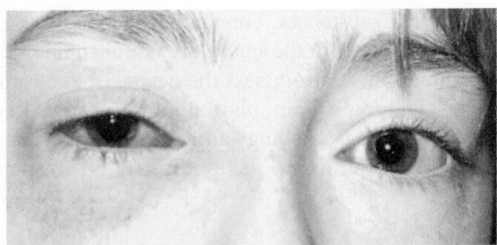

FIGURE 127.8 Patient with right epidemic keratoconjunctivitis infection. Note the lid swelling, red eye, and absence of purulent discharge. Patient also has right preauricular adenopathy (not visible). Note the early injection of left eye, representing sequential involvement.

conjunctivitis may be unilateral or bilateral, a history of multiple infected contacts argues in favor of a viral etiology. Likewise, dramatic lid swelling associated with preauricular adenopathy, mucoid or serous discharge, and perhaps an uncomfortable, sandy, foreign-body sensation is strongly suggestive of epidemic keratoconjunctivitis secondary to adenovirus. This fulminant viral infection is usually easy to recognize (Fig. 127.8, see also color plate). Rapid tests for adenovirus are now available. Infectious conjunctivitis may present as a unilateral or bilateral disease, but consecutive involvement of one eye and then the other is particularly suggestive. Viral culturing is rarely necessary. Bacterial cultures should be considered in cases of purulent conjunctivitis, particularly when antibiotic treatment is going to be instituted.

Non seasonal acute allergic conjunctivitis is usually a hyperacute conjunctival injection associated with tearing and a blister-like swelling of the conjunctiva (chemosis) (Fig. 127.9). Itching is often a prominent symptom, although this may also be a symptom of blepharitis (see Chapter 23). Conjunctival smears stained with Gram or Wright methods may reveal abundant eosinophils.

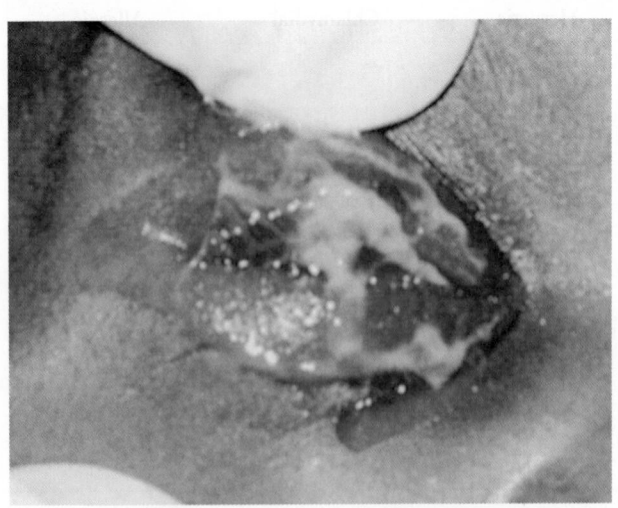

FIGURE 127.7 Neonatal gonorrheal conjunctivitis. Note the dramatic lid swelling and severe purulent discharge.

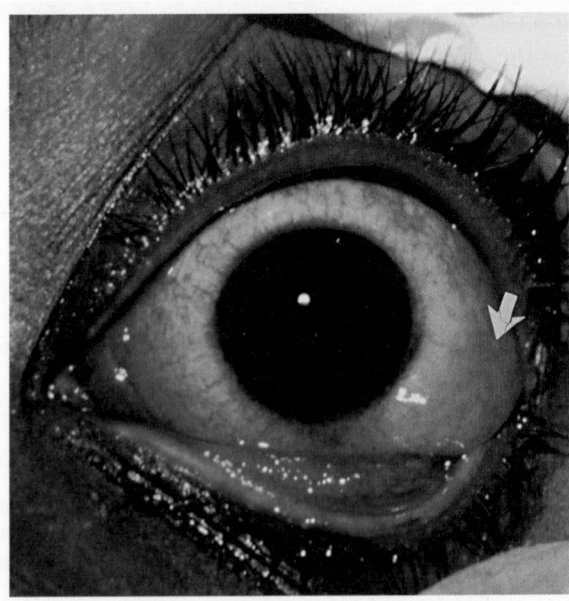

FIGURE 127.9 Non seasonal acute allergic conjunctivitis. Acutely swollen conjunctiva (chemosis) is indicated (arrow).

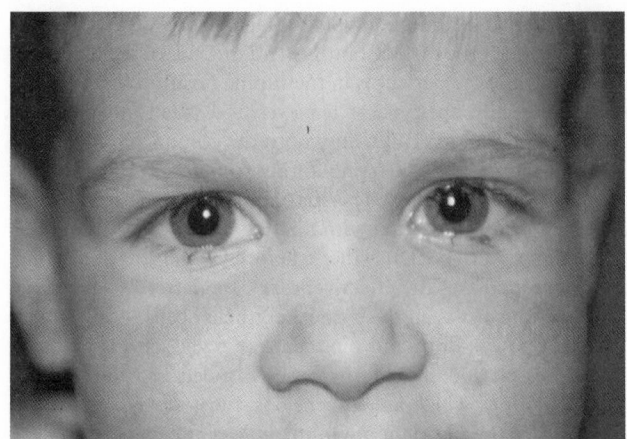

FIGURE 127.10 Left nasolacrimal duct obstruction. Note discharge on medial lower lid and wet lower lid lashes. The conjunctiva is non-inflamed (no "red eye") indicating that the child does not have conjunctivitis.

Nasolacrimal duct obstruction is often confused with conjunctivitis because discharge may be present, but the conjunctiva is rarely inflamed (i.e., no "red eye"), indicating the absence of true conjunctivitis (Fig. 127.10, see also color plate). The discharge is mostly mucus that has precipitated out of the tear film because of stagnation of tear flow. Patients are usually younger than 1 year, with a history of symptoms dating back to the first weeks of life. The discharge is usually worse on waking. Crusts may form on the lashes (Fig. 127.10). Chronic skin changes of the lower lid will develop over time. Tearing may become more prominent after the first few months of life. Older children often have epiphora without discharge. The diagnosis can be confirmed by placing pressure on the lacrimal sac, which lies under the skin against the lacrimal bone between the medial canthus and bridge of the nose. This maneuver may cause an increase in the amount of discharge as it is forced out of the sac back onto the surface of the eye via the medial upper and lower lid margin puncta.

Management

Until proven otherwise, and in the presence of gram-negative diplococci, neonatal purulent conjunctivitis should be treated as gonorrheal conjunctivitis, pending the results of cultures. The patient should be admitted for parenteral antibiotic therapy with cephalosporin (ceftriaxone 25 to 50 mg per kg, maximum 125 mg, intramuscularly or intravenously as single dose, or cefotaxime 100 mg per kg intramuscularly or intravenously as single dose), particularly in areas where penicillinase-producing strains are common. Ophthalmology consultation is indicated. Saline ocular lavage on an hourly basis may be helpful in decreasing the amount of organisms having access to the cornea. Topical erythromycin ointment is helpful because it will also treat chlamydia, but topical treatment alone is insufficient for either organism. If chlamydia is laboratory proven, then the child must also receive a 14- to 21-day course of oral erythromycin. This is necessary to eradicate carriage of chlamydia in the nasopharynx, which can subsequently lead to pneumonitis. The mother and father should also be tested for any sexually transmitted disease found in the child. The child

should be tested for other sexually transmitted diseases. Consideration of possible covert sexual abuse should be given for postneonatal, prepubertal children with gonorrhea or chlamydia conjunctivitis, although there is evidence that nonsexual transmission to these sites may occur (unlike infection of the vagina, urethra, anus, or throat).

Any of the topical antibiotics suggested in Table 127.1 would be appropriate for empiric coverage in treating a presumed bacterial conjunctivitis other than gonorrhea while awaiting culture results. Gram stain can be helpful when narrowing down the possible causes, particularly when sheets of one predominant type of organism are seen. In the first 3 months of life, topical aminoglycosides might be a reasonable choice because gram-negative and enteric organisms are more common. In older children, without strong evidence to suspect such organisms, aminoglycosides should be avoided because they may be toxic to the corneal epithelium and may select for resistant organisms.

If the patient clearly has a viral conjunctivitis, antibiotic treatment is probably not needed. Some physicians use antibiotics to "prevent secondary infection." This is not a clinically significant problem in immunocompetent children. Rather, these patients are best soothed with cool compresses and over-the-counter artificial tear preparations. Depending on the virus, symptoms may last for up to 2 to 3 weeks. Patients with symptoms that appear to be getting worse or persisting for longer than 1 week may benefit from ophthalmology consultation.

Allergic conjunctivitis is soothed by topical lubricants and cool compresses. The combination vasoconstrictor/antihistamine preparations listed in Table 127.1 may also be prescribed. Patients with recurrent allergic conjunctivitis, atopy, or asthma may benefit from long-term or seasonal topical mast cell stabilizers. A host of antiallergy eye drops are now available, the review of which is well beyond the scope of this chapter. Ophthalmology consultation may be useful, especially when symptom relief is not obtained or pain and red eye are present. Steroids should not be used without ophthalmology consultation.

Any patient with a history of herpetic ocular infection, should be referred immediately for ophthalmology consultation. Herpetic corneal infection is usually painful. Patients may or may not have a history of skin lesions. Characteristic fluorescein dendritic staining patterns can be seen on the cornea or conjunctiva (Fig. 127.11, see also color plate). Even if there is no staining

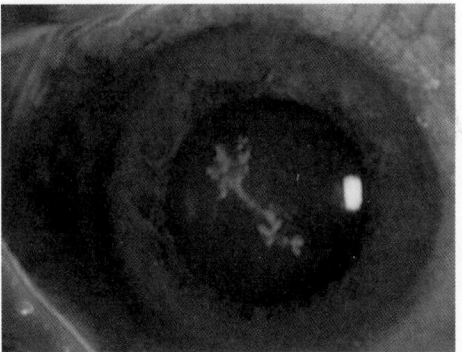

FIGURE 127.11 Fluorescein staining pattern of herpes simplex virus corneal infection. Eye is illuminated with blue light to demonstrate yellow/green branching fluorescein staining pattern of herpetic dendrite.

but a history of herpetic (varicella-zoster or simplex) corneal infection, urgent ophthalmology consultation is essential. Skin lesions on the lids without any conjunctival injection do not require ophthalmology consultation.

Any patient who wears contact lenses and has conjunctivitis, should be referred immediately for ophthalmology consultation.

DRUGS

Table 127.1 is designed to give emergency physicians some guidelines regarding the prescription and use of ophthalmic medications. Those drugs that should be avoided are listed because of problems with ocular toxicity, systemic toxicity, undesirable selection of resistant organisms, or the need for ophthalmology consultation and management regarding the problem that those drugs are designed to treat. In addition, emergency physicians are advised to follow these guidelines:

1. No topical drugs should be prescribed to patients who wear contact lenses without the supervision and consultation of an ophthalmologist.
2. Topical anesthetics must never be prescribed for outpatient use. These are strictly diagnostic agents. Prolonged use of topical anesthetics may result in corneal ulceration.
3. Steroids should never be prescribed by the emergency physician. Inappropriate use of steroids may lead to glaucoma, cataract, increased severity of corneal viral infection, or rebound symptoms when the drug is discontinued.

Instillation of eye drops can sometimes be difficult because of swollen eyelids or noncompliance from the patient. Some of the drop is often expelled upon blinking after drop instillation. This is not an indication for repeat instillation because only approximately 20% of an eye drop is actually absorbed for use. Ophthalmic solutions are designed for a one-drop dose. Drops are most efficiently delivered by pulling down the lower eyelid and placing the drop in the inferior fornix. In patients who are extremely resistant, forced eyelid opening is needed to expose just a small strip of palpebral conjunctiva. The eyeball itself does not need to be visualized. The same techniques described previously and in Chapter 117 for opening the eyelids may be used for the administration of eye drops in the ED.

An alternative technique involves placing the eye drop in the sulcus between the medial canthus and the side of the bridge of the nose while the patient is in the supine position. Every child must eventually open his or her eyes and when this happens the eye drop will naturally flow onto the conjunctiva.

Topical anesthetics do sting for approximately 10 to 20 seconds before taking effect. This may still be more desirable than the severe sting associated with dilating drops. In addition, the placement of a topical anesthetic before instillation of dilating eye drops increases the effectiveness of the latter by loosening gap junctions between the corneal epithelial cells.

When an eye drop and ointment are to be used simultaneously, the solution should always be instilled before the ointment. Solutions which are suspensions, must always be shaken very well before instillation. Ophthalmic ointments are applied by placing a strip of ointment along the conjunctiva of the lower lid without touching the tip of the applicator to the eye. When treating stye or chalazion located within the eyelid, ointment can be placed on the lashes or conjunctiva. Some parents find ointments harder to instill. Blepharitis, styes, and chalazion are more effectively treated by ointment as the site of action is the lid margin. Ointment antibiotic doses are usually twice daily whereas drops are usually four times daily. Ointments last longer and can give coverage while the child is sleeping. The choice of ointment versus drops may be come a matter of parental preference.

Suggested Readings

Ehlers JP, Shah C. *Wills Eye manual: office and emergency room diagnosis and treatment of eye disease.* 5th ed. Philadelphia: Lippincott Williams & Wilkins, 2008.

Lessner A, Stern GA. Preseptal and orbital cellulitis. *Infect Clin North Am* 1992;6:933–952.

Levin AV. Eye emergencies: acute management in the pediatric ambulatory care setting. *Pediatr Emerg Care* 1991;5:367–377.

Sadow KB, Chamberlain JM. Blood cultures in the evaluation of children with cellulitis. *Pediatrics* 1998;101:e4.

Simon JW, Kaw P. Commonly missed diagnoses in the childhood eye examination. *Am Fam Physician* 2001;64(4):623–628.

Teoh DL, Reynolds S. Diagnosis and management of pediatric conjunctivitis. *Pediatr Emerg Care* 2003;19(1):48–55.

Vu BLL, Dick PT, Levin AV, et al. Development of a clinical severity score for preseptal cellulitis in children. *Pediatr Emerg Care* 2003;19(5):302–307.

Wagoner MD. Chemical injuries of the eye: current concepts in pathophysiology and therapy. *Surv Ophthalmol* 1997;41(4):275–313.

CHAPTER 128 ■ THORACIC EMERGENCIES

JOY L. COLLINS, MD, FAAP, AND MICHAEL L. NANCE, MD

INTRODUCTION

Thoracic emergencies in children often result in life-threatening alterations in cardiorespiratory physiology. A rapid, yet organized, approach to the child with a thoracic emergency is essential. The purpose of this chapter is to describe nontraumatic surgical diseases of the thorax and guide the evaluating health care provider in the diagnosis and treatment of these conditions. Congenital abnormalities that are usually diagnosed at birth are not included. Thoracic trauma is discussed in Chapter 118.

This chapter reviews the pathophysiology and clinical manifestations of thoracic emergencies, as well as the general principles of physical and laboratory assessment. Subsequent sections cover specific entities within the following categories: (i) airway obstruction, (ii) violations of the pleural space, (iii) circulatory impairment, (iv) intrinsic pulmonary lesions, (v) mediastinal tumors, (vi) diaphragmatic defects, and (vii) chest wall tumors.

Pathophysiology

Thoracic conditions of surgical significance frequently present as a result of a mechanical or infectious complication of an anatomic abnormality. These anatomic distinctions may be grouped into conditions resulting in airway compromise, violations of the pleural space, intrinsic lesions of the lung, mediastinal masses, and diaphragmatic defects.

Within each category, it is particularly useful to consider *fluid pressure* changes and that fluids, including air, move in the body down pressure gradients. During inspiration, the pressure within the thoracic cavity is negative with respect to atmospheric pressure, thereby allowing air to be drawn through the oropharynx, the trachea, and into the lungs and alveoli. Any barriers to this pressure gradient, such as accumulation of air or fluid around the lungs in the pleural space, need to be corrected if limiting lung expansion. Obstructions to flow caused by masses compressing the airway or esophagus also impact the necessary pressure gradient.

Infectious problems requiring surgical care usually evolve in the setting of an underlying *anatomic abnormality*. Examples include congenital lung lesions such as infected bronchogenic cyst or pulmonary sequestration, or an H-type tracheoesophageal fistula producing aspiration pneumonia. An exception to this rule is empyema, the accumulation of infected pleural fluid, often a complication of severe pneumonia in childhood. The pathophysiology of this condition and its predilection for younger children remain poorly understood.

In patients with thoracic masses in which there is no compressive effect, or in those in which the anatomically urgent issue has been addressed, it is important to remember that some of these entities will require further evaluation or biopsy. Appropriate referral of such patients is imperative.

The emergency physician evaluating the child with a thoracic problem must attempt to determine whether the patient has evidence of airway compromise, circulatory compromise, or components of both.

Airway Compromise

Airway compromise can occur anywhere in the respiratory tract from the nose to the alveolus. Obstructive emergencies relating to the oropharynx, larynx, and proximal trachea are discussed in Chapters 110 and 123.

Compromise of the more distal tracheobronchial tree may be caused by lesions in the lumen, in the wall, or extremities to the bronchus. Intrinsic bronchial obstructions may result from compression by a tumor within the bronchial lumen (e.g., carcinoid tumor), foreign body, or a mucous plug. Obstruction from lesions in the wall of the bronchus includes collapse from tracheomalacia and stenosis after tracheostomy. Extrinsic lesions (e.g., bronchogenic cyst or inflamed lymph nodes) may be symptomatic by producing impingement on a bronchus. Table 128.1 lists intraluminal, mural, and extrinsic conditions that produce airway obstruction.

The anatomic level of the obstruction correlates with its effects: an obstruction of the distal tracheobronchial tree may lead to segmental lung overdistension or segmental infection. An obstruction of the proximal trachea affects both lungs, with a much greater likelihood of catastrophe for the patient. Similarly, greater degrees of obstruction, as a rule, lead to greater effects on gas exchange and severity. Infection commonly follows obstruction of bronchial drainage because the clearance of bacteria or inhaled foreign materials by the mucociliary elevator is prevented.

Circulatory Impairment

Hemorrhage has somewhat different effects on the circulation in children than in adults. The ability of the child to support blood pressure in the face of significant blood loss has particular implications in the chest. Significant blood loss may go unrecognized in the large volume of the chest. It is important to recognize the early signs of shock (monitor pulse/pressure, increased pulse, cool extremities, prolonged capillary refill) before significant decreases in blood pressure occur because this may represent a loss of 30% to 40% or more of the blood

TABLE 128.1

TRACHEOBRONCHIAL CONDITIONS ASSOCIATED
WITH AIRWAY COMPROMISE

Intraluminal
Foreign bodies
Aspiration (esophageal reflux, tracheoesophageal fistula,
   bronchial fistula, biliary fistula, or esophageal fistula)
Mucous plugs (cystic fibrosis)
Granuloma (chronic intubation, tuberculosis)
Hemoptysis (vascular malformations, cystic fibrosis,
   tuberculosis, sarcoidosis, hemosiderosis, lupus)
Acute infection (tracheitis)

Mural
Tracheomalacia
Lobar emphysema
Bronchial atresia
Bronchial tumors

Extrinsic
Lymphadenopathy
Bronchogenic cyst
Cystic hygroma
Esophageal duplication
Mediastinal tumors

volume. Fortunately, nontraumatic causes of intrathoracic
major blood loss are rare in children.

Collections of fluid in the pleural space and mediastinum,
whether the result of bleeding or other causes, may produce
obstruction of the venous return by *tension physiology*: a
child's mediastinum is mobile, and kinking of the great veins
[e.g., inferior vena cava (IVC) and superior vena cava (SVC)]
occurs much more easily than in adults. In a patient who requires
positive-pressure ventilation, the positive inspiratory pressure
inside the chest may be greater than the venous pressure returning blood to the heart. Thus, major intrathoracic bleeding may
produce more than one difficulty: the central venous pressure
and systolic arterial pressure are decreased because of loss of
blood volume, and in addition, the pressure inside the chest of a
ventilated patient may collapse the veins, returning blood to the
heart. Both problems require rapid administration of volume to
the patient.

Rarely, the heart itself can be obstructed by primary tumors
such as rhabdomyosarcoma or metastatic Wilms' tumor. Tamponade of the heart can be caused by pericardial effusion,
hemopericardium, or, more rarely, by pneumopericardium or
pneumomediastinum. These topics are addressed in Chapter 84.

Clinical Manifestations

Physical Examination

Evaluation of the child with a thoracic emergency requires a
calm, orderly assessment of airway, breathing, and circulation
(ABCs). In assessing the airway, the physician must evaluate the
adequacy of air movement and gas exchange. Pulse oximetry
should be performed upon the patient's arrival. Anxiety or confusion in a patient with a thoracic emergency may be evidence
of hypoxemia. Increased work of breathing may indicate partial
airway obstruction and can be evaluated by assessing the use of
intercostal, subcostal, and supraclavicular accessory muscles.

Prolonged use of these accessory muscles may result in the most
common cause of cardiac arrest in children—respiratory arrest.

Breathing is best evaluated by palpation and auscultation of
the chest. The trachea should be palpated to ensure it is midline.
Any lateralization of the trachea is suggestive of either unilateral
volume loss or a lateral space-occupying process, such as a
pneumothorax, pleural effusion, or mass. The neck and chest
should be palpated for signs of subcutaneous emphysema, suggestive of a pneumothorax or airway injury with an air leak.
Finally, breath sounds should be assessed via auscultation for
symmetry and adequacy of inspiratory and expiratory airflow.

Evaluation of the cardiovascular system should include an
assessment of the patient's pulse for quality, rate, and regularity. The peripheral skin should be assessed for color, temperature, and capillary refill. Signs of poor perfusion often precede
that of pressure instability. The neck should be assessed for
signs of jugular venous distension. Finally, the heart should be
examined for signs of displacement of the point of maximal
impulse; shift or alteration in the heart tones; or new murmurs,
gallops, or friction rubs.

Laboratory Studies

The most important study when evaluating any patient with a
thoracic emergency is a good quality chest radiograph. The
radiographs of the chest in the posteroanterior (PA) and lateral
views should be performed in an upright position (unless contraindicated by the patient's condition). The width of the mediastinum and the degree of mediastinal shift are much better seen
in the upright chest radiograph. Moreover, abnormalities in the
lung, pleural cavity, and diaphragm are also best appreciated in
this view. When a pulmonary effusion exists, lateral decubitus
anteroposterior views of the chest can be obtained to determine
whether the effusion layers freely or is loculated.

In interpreting the chest radiograph, the physician should
distinguish between a diffuse pulmonary problem and a focal
lesion. Hyperaeration of one portion of the lung suggests air
trapping in the involved lobe. Hyperaeration of the entire lung
field on one side is usually the result of compensatory enlargement of the lung because of atelectasis and loss of lung volume
on the opposite side.

Other studies that should be considered in a patient with a
thoracic emergency include a complete blood cell (CBC) count,
blood urea nitrogen, serum glucose, electrolytes, CO_2 concentration, and arterial blood gas or measurement of oxygen saturation. Depending on the patient's specific problem, a cross-match,
blood cultures, and an assessment of any sputum by Gram stain
and bacteriologic culture may be helpful. Clinical evidence of a
bleeding problem, but not need for operation alone, mandates
evaluation of platelet count, prothrombin time, and partial
thromboplastin time. Other diagnostic studies, such as pulmonary function tests, barium contrast studies, echocardiography, computed tomographic (CT) scans, and magnetic resonance
imaging (MRI), can be used as indicated.

AIRWAY OBSTRUCTION

Tracheal Obstruction

Tracheal obstruction may be produced by stenosis or lesions
within the lumen of the trachea (Fig. 128.1), in the wall of the
trachea, or by extrinsic compression. One of the most common

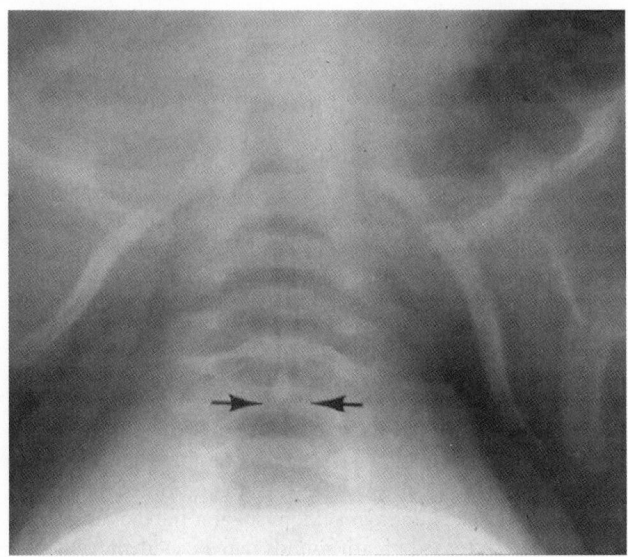

FIGURE 128.1 Foreign body (glass) oriented in an anteroposterior (AP) position in the trachea as evidenced on AP radiograph.

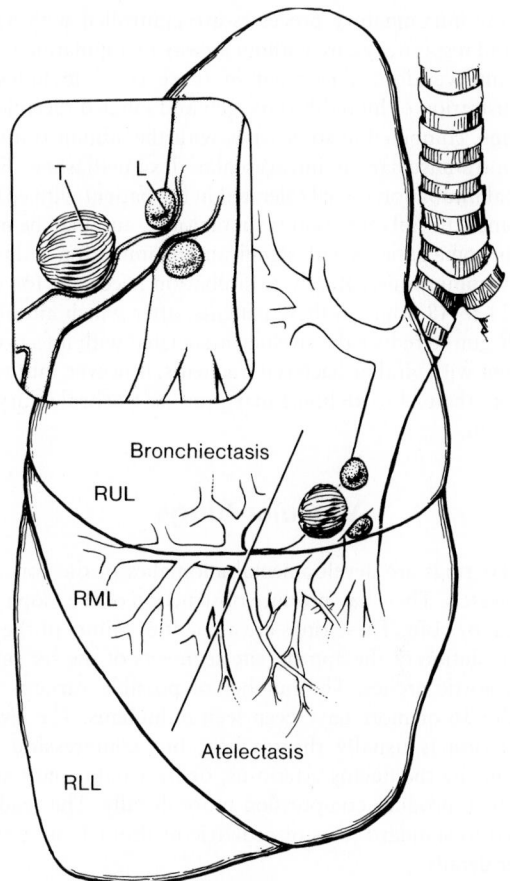

FIGURE 128.2 Acute and chronic obstruction of a bronchus owing to tumor or cyst (T) or lymph nodes (L). When the obstruction is acute, there may be bronchiectasis caused by recurrent pneumonia. The right middle lobe as shown here is particularly prone to bronchial obstruction caused by pressure from encircling lymph nodes. RUL, right upper lobe, RML, right middle lobe, RLL, right lower lobe.

causes of intrinsic obstruction in children is an aspirated foreign body. Other causes include congenital anomalies such as subglottic stenosis, laryngomalacia, and vocal cord paralysis; acquired subglottic stenosis after tracheostomy or prolonged intubation; viral or bacterial tracheitis or any process that causes significant mucosal edema, particularly in an infant with small baseline airway diameter; or more rarely, a space-occupying lesion such as a hemangioma. Tracheomalacia, sometimes complicating lung disease of prematurity, is characterized by a floppy trachea that collapses during expiration when the intrathoracic trachea is compressed by the positive intrathoracic pressure. Laryngomalacia, or tracheomalacia outside the thoracic inlet, may produce obstruction during inspiration when the negative intraluminal pressure transmitted from the chest causes the floppy wall to collapse. Tracheomalacia often occurs in infants born with tracheoesophageal fistula. Extrinsic compression may occur both from mass lesions (Table 128.1) and as a result of anomalous arteries.

Clinical Findings

Tracheal compromise produces symptoms that vary from mild to severe, depending on the degree of obstruction present. When symptoms are mild, the underlying cause may not be evident. Occasional episodes of respiratory infection that are believed to result from croup or bronchitis may be the only symptom. Stridor, wheezing, or cough occurs in patients with more significant obstruction, and a history of previous hospitalizations for treatment with mist tent, antibiotics, and chest percussion may be obtained.

Severe tracheal compromise is usually manifested by a history of stridor at rest. Progressive cyanosis and apneic episodes may occur. On examination, a child with obstruction caused by extrinsic compression often has wheezing or stridor throughout the respiratory cycle. In contrast, a patient with the floppy trachea of tracheomalacia often wheezes only during expiration.

Radiographic evaluation of the stable patient should begin with PA and lateral chest radiographs, ideally obtained at full inspiration and again at full expiration. Lateral radiographs of the neck may be useful in showing an edematous epiglottis in patients with suspected epiglottitis. Mass lesions will require cross-section imaging (e.g., CT) for evaluation. Bronchoscopy is often indicated to evaluate obstructive lesions, whether in the lumen, the wall, or extrinsic to the wall of the trachea (Fig. 128.2).

Management

If the patient has a life-threatening airway obstruction, he or she should receive airway management as outlined in Chapters 1 and 5. A coordinated effort between the emergency department (ED) physician, the surgeon, and the anesthesiologist or critical care physician may be necessary to establish an airway by endotracheal intubation, bronchoscopy, or tracheostomy. Intubation of the airway to within a short distance of the carina supports most patients with lesions extrinsic to the trachea or in the tracheal wall with a critical obstruction. Such a patient requires admission to an intensive care or other unit with ventilator capability. Lesions within the lumen will likely require endoscopic management in an operating room, and early involvement of an experienced surgeon is recommended.

Many inflammatory processes are controlled with antibiotics and respiratory care without airway manipulation or surgical intervention. Treatment in these cases includes the administration of humidified oxygen and inhaled racemic epinephrine, combined in some cases with the administration of oral, intramuscular, or intravascular dexamethasone. Endotracheal intubation is well tolerated in the patient with epiglottitis, since the inflammation is supraglottic, and may be necessary for some patients with significant inflammation and upper airway compromise. Rarely is intubation necessary for more than 24 to 48 hours in these patients, after which antibiotics have begun to reduce the swelling associated with infection. In a patient with viral or bacterial tracheitis, however, intubation for more than 24 to 48 hours may produce tracheal injury and ulceration.

Vascular Rings

Vascular rings are developmental anomalies of the aorta and great vessels. They may produce obstruction of the esophagus, trachea, or both. These rings are a result of failure of the normal involution of the appropriate segments of the six embryologic aortic arches. The number of possible variants is at least 36; 16 or more have been seen in humans. The level of obstruction is usually the trachea, but compression of a bronchus by the ductus arteriosus, or by a pulmonary artery sling, may produce compression more distally. The reader is referred to standard texts of pediatric or thoracic surgery for further details.

Clinical Findings

Vascular rings may be asymptomatic in infancy but lead to significant airway obstruction in childhood. The wide variety of anomalies produces varying degrees of symptoms. Vascular rings should be suspected in infants with stridor, dysphagia, failure to thrive associated with difficult feeding, or recurrent pneumonia. Esophageal obstruction can produce difficulty swallowing, coined *dysphagia lusoria* by Bayford in 1794. A patient with esophageal compression may also have respiratory symptoms from compression on the trachea from a distended esophageal pouch. This may lead to reflex apnea during feeding, and eventually tracheomalacia in a more chronic setting. Often, diagnosis is delayed by failure to consider these anatomic obstructions. In a patient presenting with an acute airway obstruction or other medical problems requiring intubation and nasogastric tube placement, detection of a vascular ring can be more difficult because of the presence of these tubes. Chest radiographs may be supplemented by various diagnostic tests: contrast esophagography, angiography, echocardiography, MRI, and digital subtraction angiography are needed in some combination to define the anatomy.

Management

Although some patients with constricting anomalies improve as they grow, most will require surgical correction. Surgical treatment is usually indicated to relieve the obstruction, with predictable and immediate resolution of symptoms. This is accomplished by dividing the vascular ring and preserving the blood supply to the aortic branches. This is usually accomplished by a left thoracotomy.

BRONCHIAL LESIONS

Bronchial Atresia

Congenital bronchial atresia is a rare anomaly characterized by a bronchocele caused by a mucus-filled, blindly terminating segmental or lobar bronchus, with resulting hyperinflation of the distal obstructed segment of lung. Hyperaeration is believed to result from communication with the normally aerated lung via the pores of Kohn and the channels of Lambert.

Clinical Findings

Neonates and infants with the lesion are usually seen for respiratory distress. In older patients, a history of episodic upper respiratory infection and wheezing may be elicited. Some older patients may complain of dyspnea on exertion or unilateral chest pain. Physical findings seldom suggest the diagnosis, but unilaterally decreased breath sounds may be evident.

Management

Often, the diagnosis is suggested by chest radiograph, but chest CT scan may be necessary to help more closely define the anatomy. Bronchoscopy is the most efficient way to identify the atretic opening to the involved bronchus. Bronchography has been used in the past, but high-resolution CT scan can often provide the same anatomic information noninvasively. Complete atresia of a main stem or lobar bronchus may lead to infectious complications or compression symptoms from overdistention of the affected lobe. This may require surgical management, such as lobectomy.

Right Middle Lobe Syndrome

Right middle lobe syndrome is the recurrence or persistence of atelectasis or pneumonitis of the right middle lobe, sometimes associated with bronchiectasis. It has been described in all age groups, in both the right middle and lower lobes concomitantly, and has also been observed in the lingula segment. This process can be caused by extraluminal or intraluminal obstruction, or by nonobstructive causes. The right middle lobe is anatomically predisposed to compression of its bronchus by the lymph nodes in the vicinity that encircle it. Previously, especially in the era before antituberculous chemotherapy, this resulted in compression of the right middle lobe bronchus alone, eventually leading to bronchiectasis. Because the right middle and lower lobes are favored sites for aspirated material (Fig. 128.3), recurrent inflammation caused by pneumonia can lead to chronic atelectasis and adenopathy. A similar situation can be seen with intraluminal tumors and other space-occupying lesions. Nonobstructive causes such as asthma can result in prolonged atelectasis, which promotes recurrent infection and eventual bronchiectasis.

Clinical Presentation

Middle lobe syndrome may present as symptomatic or asymptomatic atelectasis of the right middle lobe on chest radiograph and may be recurrent or persistent. It may also present as bronchiectasis or pneumonitis of the affected area. Recurrent episodes of pneumonia and associated atelectasis in

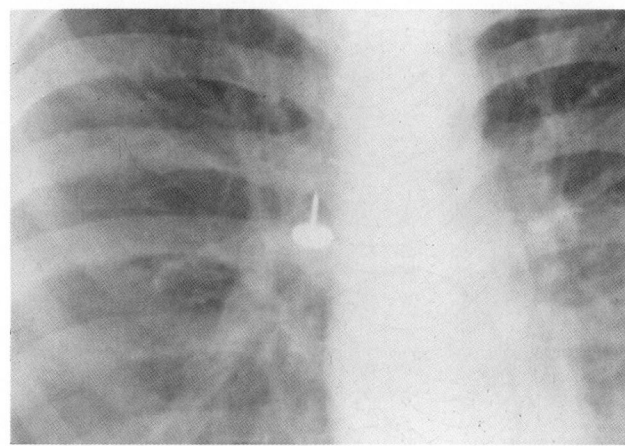

FIGURE 128.3 Foreign body (thumb tack) in the right main stem bronchus.

the lingula or right middle (and often lower) lobes occur in these patients and are not responsive to chest percussion, postural drainage, or antibiotic treatment. Radiographic findings reveal right middle lobe collapse or atelectasis. The mechanical compression of the bronchus leads to a sequestered infection that may require resection of the right middle or right middle and lower lobes for resolution.

Management

Although the need for resection is far less common than in the past, acute pneumonia in these anatomic locations should prompt a discussion of previous pneumonias and treatment. There are some data suggesting a beneficial role for fiber-optic bronchoscopy and bronchoalveolar lavage in some patients, which may restore patency of the bronchus and allow better postural drainage and enhance antibiotic effectiveness. Those patients with obstructing lesions, bronchiectasis, bronchial stenosis, or failure to respond to medical management should be considered candidates for lobectomy.

ESOPHAGUS-RELATED CAUSES OF AIRWAY DIFFICULTIES

Tracheoesophageal Fistula

Tracheoesophageal fistula (TEF) occurs in children both as a congenital lesion and, rarely, as an acquired problem after suppuration of mediastinal nodes. The congenital fistula is accompanied by atresia of the esophagus in more than 85% of patients and generally presents in the immediate perinatal period with feeding intolerance and inability to handle secretions. These patients with esophageal atresia undergo repair shortly after diagnosis, typically via a right thoracotomy. More recently, surgeons who are adept at minimally invasive techniques will perform thoracoscopic repair in select patients. Approximately 3% of all patients with TEF have "H-type" fistula, in which both the trachea and the esophagus are intact and patent but are connected by a fistula that is frequently in the cervical region or high in the thorax (Fig. 128.4). Because there is no accompanying esophageal atresia, these patients are more likely to present

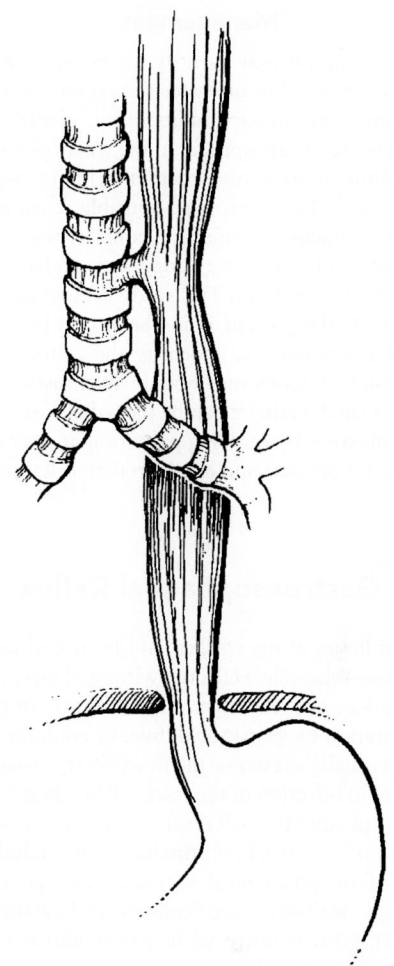

FIGURE 128.4 H-type tracheoesophageal fistula.

to the ED later in infancy or childhood for symptoms of recurrent respiratory distress or pulmonary aspiration.

It is this "H-type" fistula that is most likely to be seen in patients presenting to the ED and is therefore the type that we will discuss primarily in this chapter. The acquired form is usually in the distal trachea or proximal bronchial tree and is extremely uncommon.

Clinical Findings

H-type fistulae are notoriously difficult to diagnose. Children generally develop recurrent pulmonary infections with no obvious source. The characteristic history of choking or gagging when swallowing that accompanies esophageal atresia with TEF may not be present, but parents may describe excessive secretions or noisy breathing after feeds.

Mention should be made of the fact that children in whom the more common esophageal atresia with repaired distal TEF may present to the ED with wheezing, stridor, and other respiratory symptoms because of potential tracheomalacia and an increased susceptibility to respiratory compromise with viral illnesses. These children are also at high risk for esophageal food bolus obstruction or esophageal foreign bodies, with the site of retention being a stricture or relative narrowing at the site of anastomosis.

Management

Contrast esophagram may identify an H-type TEF. Most of these fistulae are small in diameter (less than 1 cm) and short (also less than 1 cm), making radiographic identification difficult. Even when contrast appears in the tracheobronchial tree, it may be difficult to know whether primary aspiration of orally administered contrast is responsible. Placing a feeding tube in the esophagus and injecting contrast while pulling the tube back up from the lower esophagus under fluoroscopic observation may be helpful. This study is most accurate when performed with the patient is in the prone position. High-resolution CT scanning may identify the anatomy. Bronchoscopy and esophagoscopy may both be diagnostic and may aid the repair if a small catheter can be passed across the fistula to aid its identification by enabling palpation at operation. Most such fistulae are cervical and can be repaired without a thoracotomy.

Gastroesophageal Reflux

The mucosal lining of the trachea and bronchial tree tolerates periodic soilage relatively well; even witnessed aspiration of gastric contents does not reliably produce infection or pneumonia. Ongoing irritation by gastric acid, bile, or contaminated secretions will eventually overcome the mucociliary elevator and the other barriers to infection of the tracheobronchial mucosa, and bronchitis or pneumonia will result. Common causes of repetitive soilage of the tracheobronchial tree include primary aspiration of oropharyngeal secretions, often in children with impaired swallowing mechanisms, and gastroesophageal reflux (GER). GER is universal in babies and is usually outgrown without the need for intervention. In patients with neurological impairment or in patients with significant cardiac or pulmonary disease, however, GER may require medical or surgical treatment.

Clinical Presentation

GER often presents with symptoms of spitting up or vomiting after eating. Aspiration may lead to presentation with recurrent pneumonia. Complications that follow prolonged GER include failure to thrive because of inadequate nutrition, esophagitis, esophageal ulceration, and esophageal stricture (Fig. 128.5). Some patients present with an acute life-threatening event (ALTE) in which laryngospasm or bronchospasm precipitated by aspiration of gastric contents produces profound hypoxia and even respiratory or cardiac arrest. GER is common in patients with an anatomic abnormality or a history of surgery around or near the esophagus or gastroesophageal junction, as in patients who have undergone TEF repair or repair of congenital diaphragmatic hernia (CDH).

Management

Management of GER begins with establishing the diagnosis. If this is evident clinically and the child responds to medical management, no further evaluation may be needed. Recalcitrant GER may be an indication for an upper gastrointestinal contrast study (UGI series) to establish that there is no anatomic obstruction to gastric emptying such as pyloric stenosis, malrotation, a duodenal web or annular pancreas. Recording the

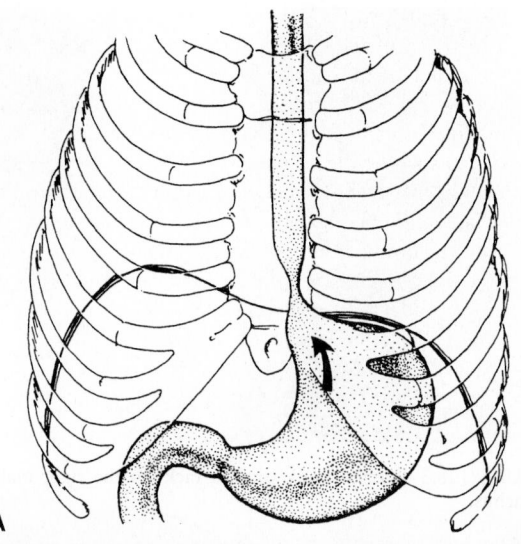

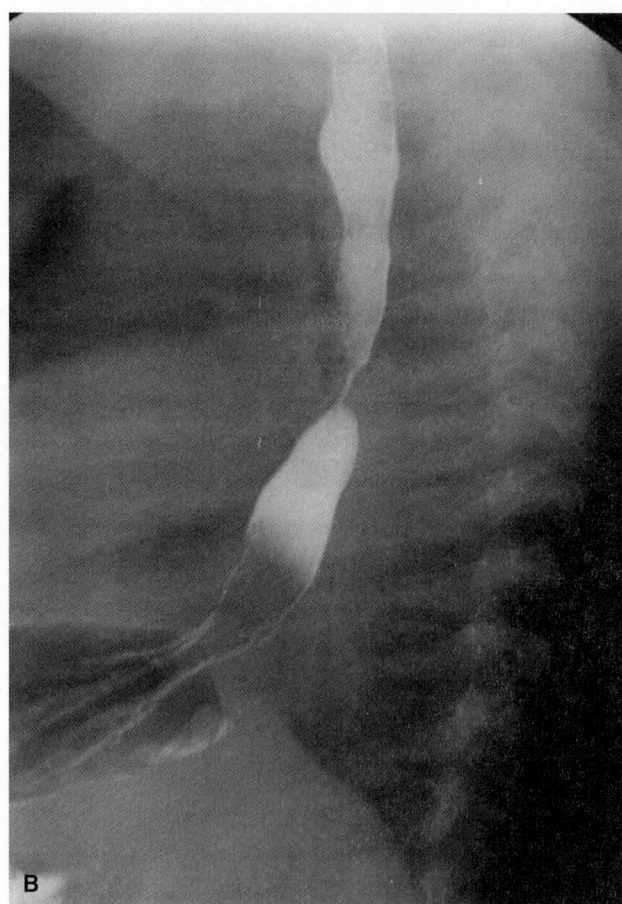

FIGURE 128.5 A: Distal esophageal stricture caused by prolonged reflux esophagitis. Note the loss of the normal angle between the esophagus and the stomach. **B:** Esophageal stricture. Lateral barium esophagram shows narrowing of midesophagus in an infant with gastroesophageal reflux.

esophageal pH over a 12- to 24-hour period with a pH probe will help quantify the severity of the problem. Scintigraphy for the evaluation of GER may also be useful, as it identifies GER and aspiration of gastric contents into the tracheobronchial tree and quantifies the efficacy of gastric emptying.

GER is managed by a three-tiered approach. Initially, elevating the head of the bed, thickening the feeds, and decreasing the volume of individual feeds are useful to allow gravity and mechanical effects to help. If these measures are ineffective, medical management of this problem includes efforts to decrease gastric acidity and to improve motility. The most common agents to neutralize or decrease acid production include antacids, H_2-receptor antagonists such as ranitidine, and proton pump inhibiting drugs (e.g., omeprazole, lansoprazole). Many clinicians add prokinetic medications such as metoclopramide to improve the gastric motility, however, reports of irreversible tardive dyskinesia and movement disorders are decreasing the use of metoclopramide in favor of low dose erythromycin. Concerns regarding the association between the prokinetic drug, cisapride, and drug interactions leading to ventricular tachycardia have led to virtual cessation of its use. Indications for surgical management of GER include failure of medical management or the occurrence of complications, such as esophageal stricture or repeated ALTEs without other evident cause. Also, patients who have an anatomic reason for reflux, such as a hiatal hernia or a neurologic or other condition that severely impedes the ability to protect their airway, should be considered for surgical treatment of significant GER. Presently, the favored operative treatment in North America is fundoplication: wrapping the fundus of the stomach either partially (a Thal operation if anterior to the esophagus or Toupet operation if posterior) or completely (the Nissen operation) around the esophagus just above the gastroesophageal junction. All of these procedures may be performed laparoscopically in appropriate patients.

Esophageal Web

Rarely, a patient presents with reflux that is caused by an esophageal web (Fig. 128.6). The membranous, congenital narrowing of unclear origin can usually allow liquids to pass, and symptoms often do not arise until the child begins to eat solid food. Recurrent aspiration pneumonia may also develop. Rarely, it can present with associated anemia, in the form of Plummer-Vinson syndrome. An esophagram is usually diagnostic. Often, a thin, membranous web may be split by esophageal dilators, cautery, or a hydraulic balloon placed endoscopically across the stenosis. If this approach is unsuccessful because the lumen is too small to transmit the dilator or the tissue is unyielding, segmental esophageal resection may be necessary via thoracotomy.

CIRCULATORY IMPAIRMENT

Thoracic emergencies leading to shock are often due to a decrease in cardiac preload or filling pressure. Preload may be reduced by tension pneumothorax causing kinking of the great veins returning blood to the heart in the child's mobile mediastinum; by massive intraabdominal hemorrhage compressing the IVC; by a cardiac tumor obstructing one of the atria; or by tamponade of the heart from mediastinal pressure caused by blood, pericardial fluid, or air. The causes, presentation, and management of cardiogenic shock are reviewed in detail in Chapter 3. Shock as a result of trauma is reviewed in Chapters 3, 104, and 118.

Clinical Findings

Findings are dependent on the type of shock and the primary lesion. Whether caused by tension pneumothorax, intracardiac tumor, or tamponade, hypovolemic (or decreased preload) shock is accompanied by tachycardia. Usually blood pressure is maintained until upwards of 30% to 40% of the blood volume is lost; predicting the onset of hypotension with tension pneumothorax or a compressive phenomena is difficult. Characteristically, the extremities are cold and poorly perfused as peripheral vasoconstriction compensates for the loss of central venous pressure. Tamponade is accompanied by muffled heart tones, often difficult to recognize in a noisy ED, especially in the setting of trauma. Distended neck veins are often present. Once tamponade has reached a critical compression pressure, it often does not respond to intravenous (IV) fluid. Pulsus paradoxus may not accompany acute tamponade.

Clinical findings suggestive of cardiogenic shock are discussed in Chapter 3. Septic and neurogenic shocks are "warm shock" in which the extremities are well perfused because of loss of vascular tone; tachycardia is commonly typically present. Fever in septic shock, as well as flaccid extremities with loss of bladder control and rectal tone in neurogenic shock, may aid the different ED diagnosis.

Management

IV support with two large-gauge peripheral catheters, electrocardiogram monitoring, pulse oximetry, and oxygen supplementation are indicated for any type of circulatory collapse. Stable patients should undergo a chest radiograph immediately. Afterward, management is directed to relieving the condition suspected of causing the shock.

If acute cardiac tamponade is suspected, emergency pericardiocentesis is indicated (see Section VII, Procedures). If the patient is not improved by pericardiocentesis, the pericardium may be filled with clotted blood not amenable to drainage. In this circumstance, pericardial drainage will require a larger

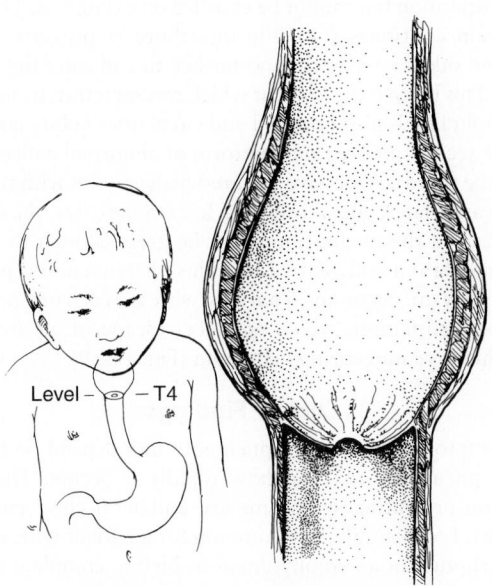

FIGURE 128.6 A child with chronic partial obstruction of the esophagus caused by a congenital web. Similar bulbous enlargement of the proximal esophagus can occur with any type of stricture and results in pressure on the trachea and recurrent regurgitation with aspiration. T4, 4th thoracic vertebrae.

Level — — T4

opening in the pericardium. In a patient with shock and incipient cardiac arrest, a vertical subxiphoid incision should be made in the ED (i.e., pericardial window). After opening the linea alba, the pericardium can be opened widely enough to digitally extract hematoma from the pericardium.

PLEURAL DISEASES

The lung is covered by the densely adherent visceral pleura, which moves smoothly over the parietal pleura of the chest wall because of a thin film, and the friction created by apposition of the pleural layers (like two plates of glass held together by a film of water) contributes to the full expansion of the lung mechanically. When air, excess fluid, or purulent material comes between the two layers of the pleura, the lung may collapse or become significantly compressed and consideration needs to be given to drainage of the pleural space.

Pneumothorax

A pneumothorax is a collection of air in the pleural space. It can occur for short- or long-term duration and can be static or accumulate progressively. Because atmospheric pressure is greater than intrapleural pressure, any mechanism that allows even momentary communication between the atmosphere outside the chest wall or within the tracheobronchial tree can result in a rapid shift of air into the pleural space. A pneumothorax may occur spontaneously, or it may be the result of trauma or a therapeutic intervention. Spontaneous pneumothorax can occur in children with no known underlying condition or as a result of a congenital bleb, pneumatocele, congenital cystic adenomatoid malformation, or other such structural abnormality. Such a process can lead to a small pneumothorax or complete collapse of the involved lung (Fig. 128.7). In patients with cystic fibrosis, spontaneous pneumothorax is the second most common pulmonary complication and usually occurs in teenage or young adult patients with far advanced, diffuse disease. Another group of children with a high incidence of spontaneous pneumothorax are those with pulmonary metastases, such as patients with osteogenic sarcoma. Children with staphylococcal pneumonia are especially prone to develop unilateral or bilateral pneumothorax. Iatrogenic causes of pneumothorax include thoracentesis or central venous catheter insertion, bronchoscopy, aggressive mechanical ventilation ("barotrauma"), or cardiopulmonary resuscitation. Penetrating and blunt trauma to the chest may cause injuries to the lung, pleura, esophagus, trachea, and bronchi, all of which can result in pneumothorax. A more detailed discussion of trauma-related causes of pneumothorax can be found in Chapter 107.

Two special forms of pneumothorax require emphasis because these conditions may result in the death of the patient if not recognized early and attended to rapidly. The first is a tension pneumothorax, which results not only in a complete collapse of the ipsilateral lung but also in progressive pressure across the mediastinum (Fig. 128.8). This pressure impedes ventilation of the contralateral lung resulting in further compromise. Tension pneumothorax results for air accumulating in the pleural space with each inspiration. Whether the entry site of air into the pleural space is through the chest wall, a torn bronchus,

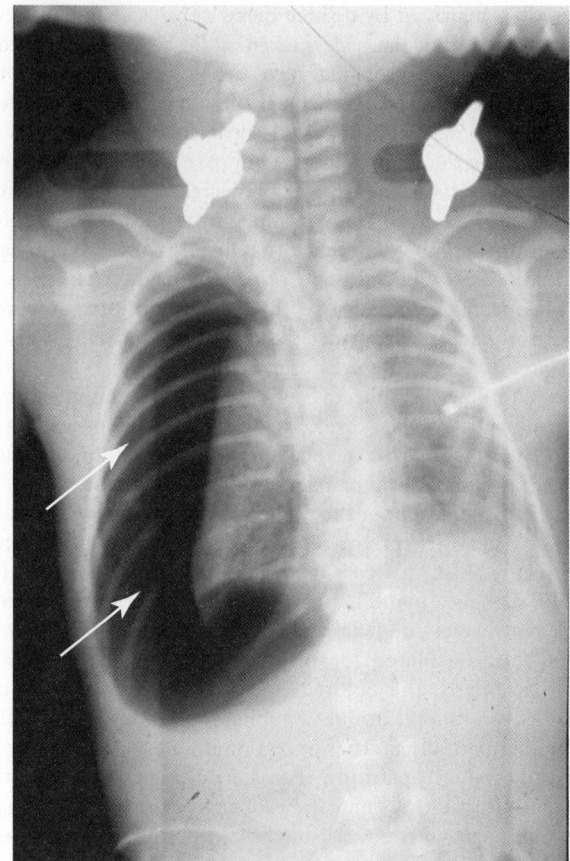

FIGURE 128.7 Large pneumothorax involving the entire thorax. Atelectatic lung border is marked by *arrows*.

or an injured lung, the physiologic result is that of a one-way valve, whereby air continues to accumulate in the pleural cavity with inspiration but cannot be expelled on expiration. This phenomenon continues until the intrathoracic pressure on the involved side is so high that no further air can enter the pleural space. This is often the point at which venous return from below the diaphragm is also impeded and circulatory failure ensues.

The second life-threatening form of abnormal collection of air in the thorax is massive pneumomediastinum with or without an associated pneumothorax. In extreme cases, the tension produced in the mediastinum can be great enough to impair both circulation and ventilation. This phenomenon is particularly likely to occur in a patient who is receiving positive-pressure ventilation, which enhances escape of air from the bronchial tree into the mediastinum (Fig. 128.9).

Clinical Findings

The symptoms and signs of pneumothorax depend on the size of the pneumothorax and how rapidly it occurs. The most common presenting symptoms are unilateral chest pain and dyspnea. For example, it is common for a patient with spontaneous rupture of an emphysematous bleb to complain of sudden acute pain on the involved side of the chest followed by tachypnea, pain at the tip of the ipsilateral shoulder, and a sense of shortness of breath. Such patients usually have a small to moderate pneumothorax (less than 20% of the lung volume), often with no accompanying hypoxia. Decreased breath

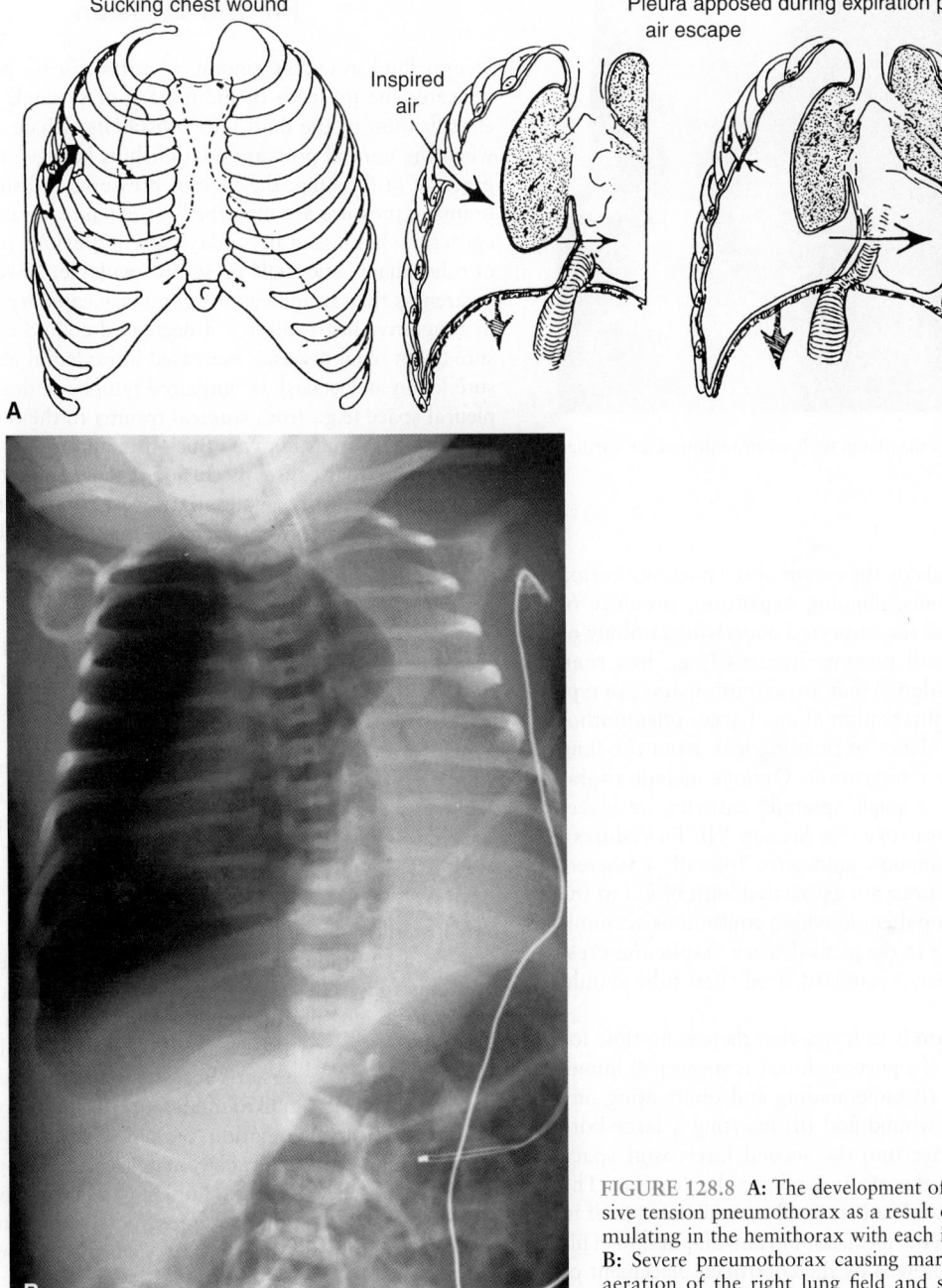

Sucking chest wound

Inspired air

Pleura apposed during expiration preventing air escape

A

B

FIGURE 128.8 **A:** The development of a progressive tension pneumothorax as a result of air accumulating in the hemithorax with each inspiration. **B:** Severe pneumothorax causing marked hyperaeration of the right lung field and shift of the mediastinum to the left side.

sounds may be heard on the ipsilateral side, and a chest radiograph will usually demonstrate the pneumothorax, particularly if taken at end expiration.

In general, a patient with a pneumothorax of 50% or more of the lung volume will to exhibit signs and symptoms of ventilatory impairment: dyspnea, tachypnea, pain, splinting on the involved side, agitation, increased pulse rate, diminished breath sounds, and increased resonance to percussion on the involved side and, possibly, displacement of the trachea and heart away from the involved side. Severe dyspnea should alert the physician to the possibility of a very large or possible tension pneumothorax. A child with existing underlying lung disease may display more severe symptoms and hypoxemia with a small or moderate pneumothorax.

Management

The essential components of management involve confirmation that a pneumothorax exists and reexpansion of the lung. If the patient's condition is not severe, an immediate upright PA and a lateral chest radiograph should be taken. These radiographs are important to determine not only the site and extent of the pneumothorax but also any complicating features such as tumor, fluid within the pleural space, or abnormalities of the lungs, diaphragm, or mediastinum.

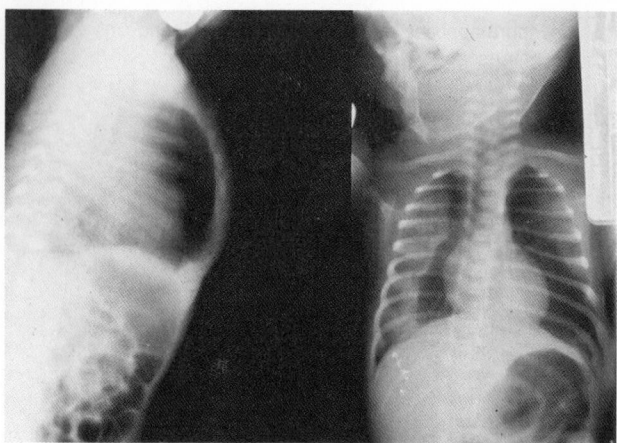

FIGURE 128.9 Pneumomediastinum with accentuation of the cardiac silhouette.

Management depends on the extent of the pneumothorax, the severity of symptoms, ongoing expansion, presence of tension, physiology, and the suspected underlying etiology or clinical condition. Small pneumothoraces (e.g., less than 15% to 20% of lung volume) that are asymptomatic can typically be followed by observation alone. Larger pneumothoraces or those with evidence of ongoing leak from the lung surface usually require intervention. Options include thoracentesis, placement of a small "pigtail" catheter, or placement of a standard chest tube (see Section VII, Procedures). In the ED, the percutaneous, guidewire "pigtail" catheters are ideal for pneumothorax not associated with blood in the chest or empyema. In a patient in whom continuous accumulation of air takes place in the pleural space despite the presence of a pigtail catheter, a standard-sized chest tube should be placed.

If the child's condition is so severe that there is no time for a chest radiograph and if a pneumothorax is suspected, immediate therapy includes (i) tamponading and obliterating any sucking or open chest wound and (ii) inserting a large-bore (14-gauge) angiocatheter into the second intercostal space anteriorly to evacuate the air and relieve the tension. The insertion of the needle and catheter will immediately result in release of the tension on the mediastinum and diaphragm. This maneuver should be followed by the controlled placement of an appropriate-sized chest tube. Depending on the suspected etiology, further studies may be needed.

Many infants can be effectively managed in this way if the amount of air present in the pleural space is small. However, these temporary catheter devices are small gauge and thus tend to easily develop fibrin plugs. Therefore, in any infant or older child who requires a tube within the pleura for more than 24 hours, it is best to proceed with a standard chest tube insertion. Patients with a pneumothorax should be admitted to the hospital, even if no chest tube is believed necessary, to monitor for signs of clinical deterioration (e.g., hypoxia) and to repeat a chest radiograph to ensure no progression of the process.

A surgical consultation is generally warranted for any patient with a pneumothorax, particularly if there is evidence of a continuing air leak or the mechanism was traumatic, or due to an underlying anatomic abnormality.

Pleural Effusion

Pleural fluid in excess amount is not a disease per se, but it indicates the presence of pulmonary or systemic illness. The classification of the fluid into *transudate*, which accumulates when the normal pressure relationships between the capillary pressure in the lung, the pleural pressure, and the lymphatic drainage pressure are disturbed, or *exudate*, an inflammatory collection, has less utility today than in previous years because of other diagnostic tools presently available. Nevertheless, an awareness that an increased pulmonary capillary pressure (as in congestive heart failure), a decreased colloid osmotic pressure (as in renal disease), increased intrapleural negative pressure (as in atelectasis), or impaired lymphatic drainage of the pleural space (e.g., from surgical trauma to the thoracic duct) may result in transudative effusion is important. In children, the inflammatory cause of effusion is most commonly a result of pneumonia, with accumulation of infected fluid in the pleural space, or empyema. The accumulation of blood in the pleural space because of trauma is discussed in Chapter 107. Hemothorax may also result from nontraumatic conditions. Necrotizing pulmonary infections, tuberculosis, pulmonary arteriovenous (AV) malformation, torn pleural adhesions with spontaneous pneumothorax, hemophilia, thrombocytopenia, and systemic anticoagulation, and pleural tumors have all been reported to cause hemothorax. Chylothorax, or the accumulation of lymphatic fluid in the pleural space, has increased in frequency as thoracic, especially complex cardiac, surgical operations have become more common in children.

Clinical Findings

Small, sterile collections, as well as large, chronic collections, may be asymptomatic. Acute collections produce symptoms by compressive effects on the lung, with resultant atelectasis, and right-to-left shunting, with resultant hypoxia and hypercapnia. Respiratory distress may follow, marked by dyspnea, tachypnea, increased use of accessory muscles of respiration, and even cyanosis. Small to moderate effusions may not be evident on physical examination, with most effusions detected by chest radiograph. Bilateral decubitus chest radiographs help define the presence of pleural fluid in patients in whom it is difficult to see because of the concurrent parenchymal disease. This examination also demonstrates whether the fluid is free to move about in the chest.

Management

If the presence of a significant effusion is evident by examination and radiograph, no further radiographic studies may be needed. A CT scan or an ultrasound examination of the chest helps determine whether opacity seen on a chest radiograph is due to parenchymal disease or due to pleural fluid. All patients should have a CBC count with differential and blood culture. Analysis of the pleural fluid itself (including cultures) may be a useful diagnostic test. The technique for thoracentesis is given in Section VII.

Aspirated fluid should be sent for cell count, differential, Gram stain, acid-fast bacillus (AFB) stain, total protein, lactate dehydrogenase (LDH), protein, specific gravity, and a complete set of cultures (aerobic, anaerobic, AFB, and

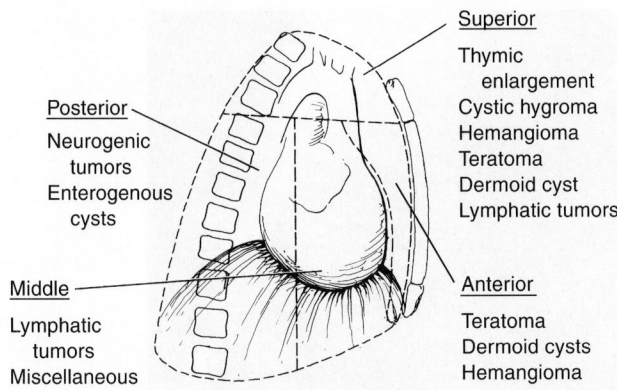

FIGURE 128.14 Mediastinal tumors in children. Differential diagnosis is based on anatomic location within the mediastinum.

with the likelihood of malignancy increasing with age of the patient. More than 90% of the asymptomatic masses are benign. The mediastinum is commonly divided into anterior, superior, middle, and posterior compartments (Fig. 128.14). The superior mediastinal compartment contains germ cell tumors of the thymus, thymomas, and lymphangiomas. The anterior compartment contains thymic tumors, lymphangiomas, as well as lymphomas and teratomas. Bronchogenic cysts in the area of the hilum are located in the middle mediastinum. Most neurogenic tumors, such as neuroblastomas and ganglioneuromas, as well as esophageal cysts, are found in the posterior compartment. Neurogenic tumors are the most common cause of mediastinal masses, with lymphomas and germ cell tumors being second and third in frequency. Infection is an uncommon cause of mediastinal node enlargement but, when present, is largely caused by histoplasmosis. Thymic enlargement may mimic an anterior mediastinal mass.

Clinical Presentation

Mediastinal masses usually present with chest pain or respiratory symptoms as a result of airway obstruction or erosion. Patients may present with cough, wheezing, recurrent respiratory infections, bronchitis, atelectasis, and hemoptysis. Dysphagia and hematemesis may occur with compression of the esophagus. SVC syndrome is a rare complication, usually in association with a rapidly growing tumor. If the recurrent laryngeal nerve is compressed as a result of the mass, hoarseness and inspiratory stridor may result. Spinal cord compression and vertebral erosion can be seen with a posterior mediastinal tumor.

Management

Children with tumors of the anterior or superior mediastinum should be admitted to a hospital to undergo urgent evaluation because these tumors may pose an immediate threat to life. CT scan or MRI of the chest is generally needed to supplement plain radiographs in order to further define the location and extent of the mass, as well as potentially provide details that may help establish the diagnosis.

When biopsy of a large mediastinal mass is necessary, the logistics of biopsy require careful, thoughtful evaluation, ideally involving the pediatrician, surgeon, oncologist, and anesthesiologist. Airway compression by large mediastinal masses

may be critical. Endotracheal intubation and delivery of general anesthesia may decrease negative intrathoracic pressure leading to occlusion of the thoracic trachea by the tumor. This situation can be challenging to manage; passage of a rigid bronchoscope may be necessary to stent the trachea open to allow gas exchange. CT scan should be used to evaluate large mediastinal masses in order to assess the likelihood of tracheal compression. MRI may be a better diagnostic modality for posterior mediastinal masses because many of them are neurogenic in origin and may have extension into the spinal canal. If tracheal compression is present, consideration should be given to the feasibility of biopsy under local anesthesia. An echocardiogram should be obtained prior to surgery in order to assess the extent of mediastinal shift and the degree of atrial or ventricular compression by the mass. The anesthesiologist should be apprised of the nature of the tumor, and a bronchoscope should be at hand if a general anesthetic is needed. Tissue may be obtained in numerous ways, with the location of the tumor dictating the approach: (i) with a mediastinoscope, inserted via an incision above the sternal notch and passed behind the sternum; (ii) a video-assisted thoracic surgery (thoracoscopy); (iii) a thoracotomy, usually limited, or (iv) through a high, anterior interspace approach (Chamberlain procedure). In some cases, mediastinal masses can be accurately diagnosed by biopsy of supraclavicular or other extrathoracic adenopathy.

DIAPHRAGMATIC PROBLEMS

Congenital Diaphragmatic Hernia

CDH is the presence of intestinal viscera in the chest through a defect in the diaphragm not caused by trauma. Nearly 90% of CDHs occur on the left side through the foramen of Bochdalek. Herniation may also occur through the foramen of Morgagni, which lies just posterior to the sternum comprising 2% or 3% of all diaphragmatic hernias. CDH may be associated with a variety of genetic conditions, including Cornelia de Lange, Fryns, and Beckwith-Wiedemann syndromes. Traumatic diaphragmatic rupture may occur through any portion of the diaphragm and may present in a delayed time frame. Information in this chapter focuses on diaphragmatic hernias diagnosed in stable older babies and children who are more likely to present to the ED than those in whom the diagnosis is made in the perinatal period.

Pathophysiology

Most babies with CDH become symptomatic as newborns when profound respiratory compromise leads to diagnosis. Until recent years, it was believed that the respiratory difficulties of babies with CDH were caused by mechanical compression of the lung by the intestinal viscera extruded through the diaphragmatic opening into the chest. It has become clear that the situation is more complex. Pulmonary hypertension, surfactant deficiency, and a vicious cycle of hypoxia, acidosis, and intrapulmonary shunting lead to the death of a significant number of newborns with this diagnosis. CDH may also be identified after the neonatal period. Older infants and children are less likely to present with this form of respiratory distress but may present with features of bowel obstruction, visceral

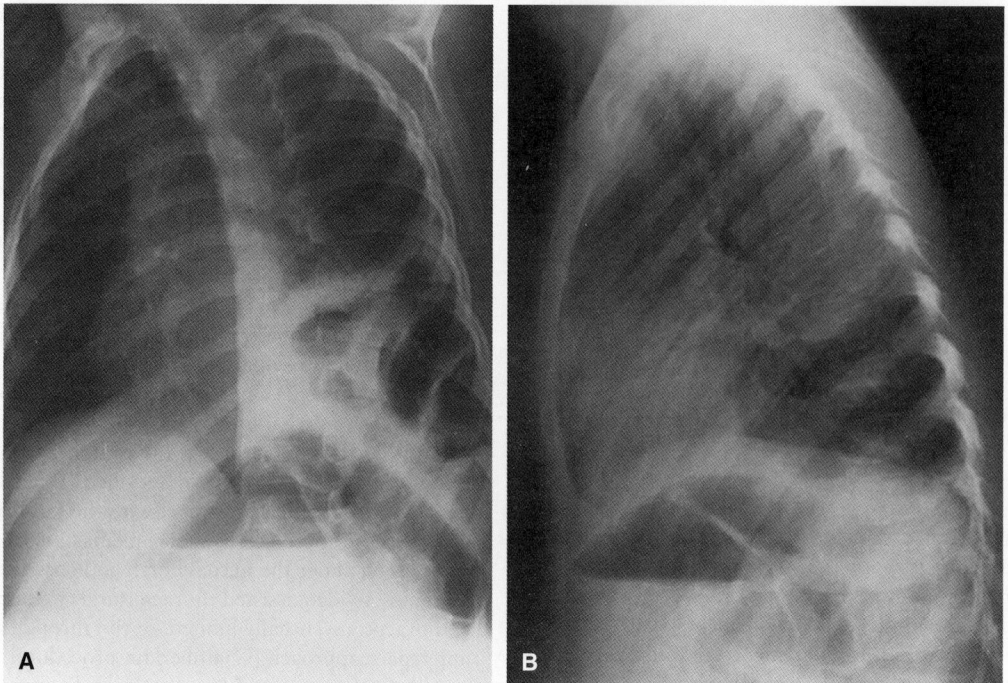

FIGURE 128.15 A 4-year-old boy admitted with 1-day history of recurrent severe upper abdominal colicky pain with dyspnea and decreased breath sounds in the left base. Posteroanterior (**A**) and lateral (**B**) chest films demonstrate multiple bowel loops in the lower, posterior, left side of chest, indicative of a foramen of Bochdalek hernia that was subsequently repaired without difficulty.

ischemia, or pleural inflammation arising from sudden shift of abdominal viscera into the chest.

Clinical Presentation

When found in older babies and children, identification is usually by a chest radiograph obtained for nonspecific symptoms such as fever, cough, chest or abdominal pain, or vomiting. The presence of loops of intestine above the diaphragm may be seen on the chest radiograph, and the stomach may be confirmed to be in the chest by the passage of a nasogastric tube that demonstrates its tip in the thorax. Loops of intrathoracic intestine on the chest radiograph may suggest pneumonia with pneumatocele formation (Fig. 128.15). A gastrointestinal contrast study or preferably a chest and abdominal CT scan may provide clarity if the diagnosis is uncertain. Potential intestinal or visceral ischemia caused by obstruction and strangulation is one of the reasons operative repair is undertaken.

Management

In the stable patient, surgical repair should be undertaken soon after the diagnosis is made but may be elective in the asymptomatic patient. Because diagnosis may be made incidentally during evaluation for a condition such as pneumonia, which would increase the risk of elective operation, the timing of surgery must be tailored to the individual situation. Certainly, the pediatric surgeon should be consulted as soon as the diagnosis is suspected. If a patient is symptomatic from an acute ischemia of the herniated viscera, an urgent operation may be required. Usually, a transverse or subcostal abdominal incision is used because it permits reduction or resection of compromised intestine or other abdominal viscera and allows

for correction of the malrotation that usually accompanies this condition. In selected patients, thoracoscopic repair has been performed safely and effectively.

Foramen of Morgagni Hernias

Frequently asymptomatic or presenting with vague symptoms of abdominal discomfort, a Morgagni diaphragmatic hernia results from a defect in the anterior diaphragm just behind the sternum. Substernal or epigastric pain and bowel obstruction resulting from the narrow neck of the sac may occur spontaneously or be precipitated by any condition that increases intraabdominal pressure (Fig. 128.16).

Clinical Findings/Management

A lateral chest radiograph should clarify the abnormality as anterior and demonstrate that the herniation is not through the esophageal hiatus. A contrast enema or a CT scan in stable patients should be considered if doubt persists. Surgical repair, indicated to prevent incarceration of bowel even in asymptomatic patients, may be performed laparoscopically or through an upper abdominal incision.

Diaphragmatic Eventration

Eventration is an abnormal elevation of the diaphragm and may present to the emergency physician as an unexpected finding on a chest radiograph obtained for another reason. Eventration may be congenital or acquired. Acquired diaphragmatic even-

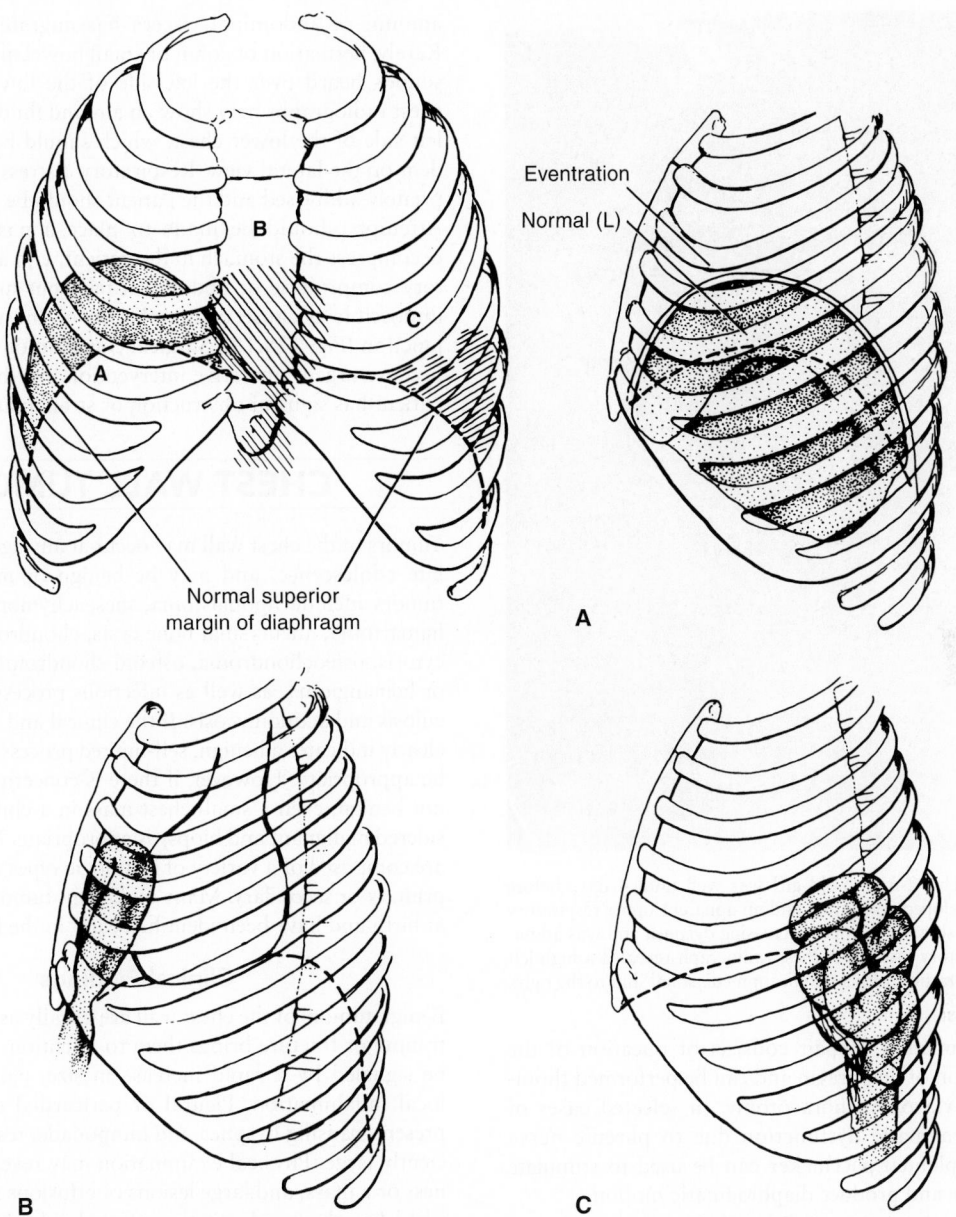

FIGURE 128.16 Diaphragmatic defects in infants and children. The nature of these defects are often better appreciated on a lateral view of the chest. Eventration of the diaphragm (**A**); foramen of Morgagni hernia (**B**); and left foramen of Bochdalek hernia (**C**).

tration is commonly the result of a phrenic nerve paralysis, which may be caused by birth, operative, or other trauma. Neoplastic or inflammatory processes near the phrenic nerve can also lead to eventration.

Diaphragmatic eventration occurs most commonly on the left side but may be bilateral. The affected hemidiaphragm moves paradoxically during inspiration and expiration, with compromise of pulmonary mechanics and function. A large enough congenital eventration may affect prenatal and postnatal lung development, potentially resulting in pulmonary hypoplasia.

Clinical Findings

Patients with eventration may be asymptomatic but potentially will exhibit respiratory distress as a result of alveolar hypoventi-

lation and paradoxical diaphragmatic movement. This frequently manifests as tachypnea, pallor, and feeding difficulties. Physical examination findings of nonaerated lung, including absent breath sounds and dullness to percussion, should be investigated by chest radiograph. Chest radiographs usually confirm the presence of an elevated hemidiaphragm (Fig. 128.17). This study may be confirmed by fluoroscopy or ultrasonography, which will demonstrate paradoxical motion of the hemidiaphragm and mediastinal shift with inspiration and expiration.

Management

Small degrees of eventrations that are incidentally identified and asymptomatic may be observed. The need for repair is based on the severity of the eventration and the degree of

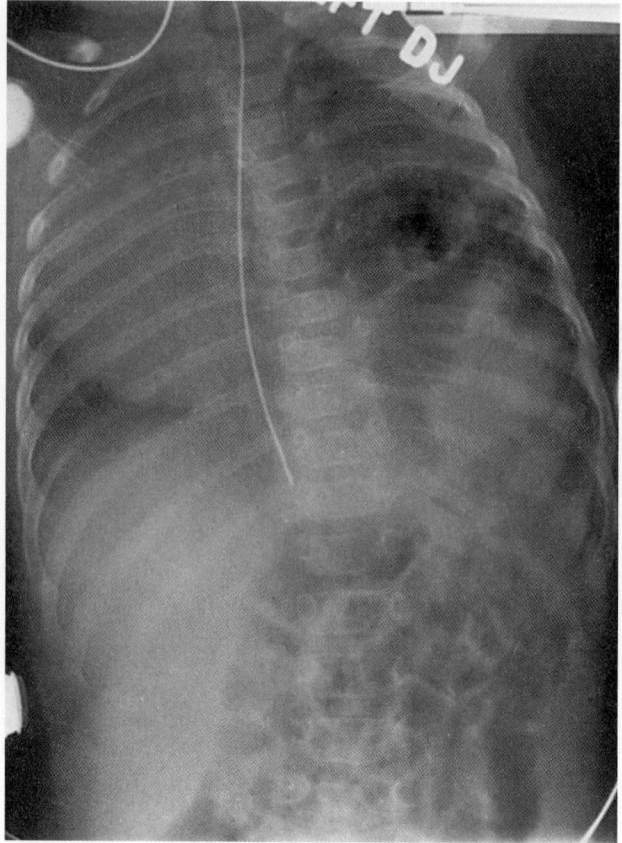

FIGURE 128.17 This 2-month-old girl was well until 4 days before admission. She developed congestion and an apparent upper respiratory tract infection. She slowly developed increasing dyspnea and was admitted in acute respiratory distress. A chest radiograph revealed a high left diaphragmatic eventration with a significant mediastinal shift to the right.

pulmonary dysfunction. Repair consists of plication of the attenuated portion of diaphragm and can be performed thoracoscopically or via open thoracotomy. In selected cases of acquired diaphragmatic dysfunction due to phrenic nerve paralysis, an implanted pacemaker can be used to stimulate the phrenic nerve and produce diaphragmatic motion.

Paraesophageal Hernia

A paraesophageal hernia is a form of hiatal hernia in which the stomach and potentially other intraabdominal organs protrude through the esophageal hiatus. It is uncommon in children and may be congenital and/or associated with other anomalies. A paraesophageal hernia typically presents with symptoms of respiratory distress, vomiting, and failure to thrive. Symptoms of upper abdominal pain, tachypnea, and tachycardia may accompany the condition, as the herniated stomach distends with swallowed air inside the chest. Such symptoms may also be indicative of gastric volvulus, strangulation, and necrosis, although these findings are uncommon in children with paraesophageal hernia.

Clinical Findings/Management

Physical examination may reveal decreased breath sounds and dullness to percussion over the left side of chest if a significant

amount of abdominal viscera has migrated into the chest. Rarely, herniation of colon or small bowel may result in bowel sounds heard over the left side of the lower chest. Upright chest radiographs may show an air- and fluid-filled mass in the left side of the lower chest, which should be particularly evident on the lateral view. Respiratory distress should be appropriately addressed and the patient should be fluid resuscitated. Attempts should be made to place a nasogastric tube to decompress the stomach in the patient with associated respiratory compromise or abdominal pain but may be difficult or impossible because of angulation of the gastroesophageal junction (Fig. 128.18). Surgical consultation should be sought because urgent operative intervention may be necessary if the patient has signs of obstruction or strangulation.

CHEST WALL TUMORS

Tumors of the chest wall may occur at any age, from infancy to late adolescence, and may be benign or malignant. Benign tumors include lipoblastoma, mesenchymoma, mesenchymal hamartoma, aneurysmal bone cysts, chondroma, lipoid histiocytosis, osteochondroma, osteoid chondroma, lymphangioma, or hemangioma, as well as infectious processes such as tuberculosis and actinomycosis. If the clinical and radiologic picture clearly indicates a benign, self-limited process, observation may be appropriate. However, if there is concern that the lesion is not benign, even a small chest mass in a child should be considered malignant and biopsy is appropriate. Malignant tumors are composed of a variety of histologic types and may be either primary or secondary. Many malignant tumors may be present at birth and have been identified early in the first year of life.

Clinical Findings

Benign tumors of the chest wall are usually asymptomatic until trauma or fracture brings them to attention. Malignancy may be signaled by a rapid increase in size, pain, tenderness, or local inflammation. Pleural or pericardial effusions may be present, causing dyspnea and tamponade, respectively, if sufficiently large. Physical examination may reveal chest wall fullness or a mass, and large lesions or effusions may cause diminished breath sounds on the affected side. Chest radiographs may show pleural effusion and a peripheral mass, the depth and extent of which are better demonstrated by a CT scan.

The site of the lesion may suggest certain diagnoses (Fig. 128.19). Ewing's tumor typically involves the lateral aspects of the ribs. Chondrosarcoma typically involves the costal cartilages between the sternum and the distal rib end. The sternum is a favored site for anaplastic sarcomas. These last two tumors may extend intrathoracically and outside the bony thorax.

Management

Initial management of patients presenting with respiratory distress includes supplemental oxygen administration, evaluation for pleural and pericardial effusions with aspiration or tube thoracostomy drainage if present, and pain management if clinically indicated. Radiographic evaluation should include a CT scan of the pertinent area, bone scans of the entire body, and a metastatic bone survey. Multimodal, coordinated treatment involving surgery, chemotherapy, and radiotherapy is frequently required. Initial biopsy should be performed by a

TABLE 129.1

ADVERSE EFFECTS OF IMMUNOSUPPRESSIVE AGENTS[a]

Adverse effect	Cyclosporine	Tacrolimus	Azathioprine	Mycophenolate	Steroids	Sirolimus
Systemic increased risk of infection	+	+	+	+	+	+
Increased risk of malignancy	+	+	+	+	−	−
Hyperglycemia/posttransplant diabetes mellitus	+	+	−	−	+	−
Bone marrow suppression	−	−	+	+	−	+
Nephrotoxicity	+	+	−	−	−	−
Hyperkalemia, hypomagnesemia	+	+	−	−	−	−
Hypertension	+	+	−	−	+	−
Hyperlipidemia	−	−	−	−	+	+
Anaphylaxis/hypersensitivity	+	+	+/−	−	−	−
Dermatologic						
Hirsutism	+	−	−	−	+/−	−
Rash	−	−	+	+	+	+
Gastrointestinal						
Gingival hypertrophy	+	−	−	−	−	−
Abdominal pain	+	+	−	+	+	−
Gastritis	−	+	−	+	+	−
Diarrhea, nausea, emesis	−	+	+	+	−	−
Hepatotoxicity	+	+	+	−	−	−
Pancreatitis	+/−	+/−	+	+/−	+	−
Neurologic						
Headache	+	+	−	−	+	−
Tremor	+	+	−	−	−	−
Seizures	+	+	−	−	−	−

[a]Does not include adverse effects rarely encountered with a medication.
+/− Small case series indicate potential adverse effect.

GENERAL PRINCIPLES OF TRANSPLANT MEDICINE

Solid organ transplantation is a complex undertaking considered only for children with life-threatening primary or secondary disease of vital organs. The evaluation of a candidate for pediatric transplantation is a complex process, with wide and variable indications for each organ type. Despite the variation and complexity of the different types of organ transplants, there are many similarities in the postoperative monitoring and management of graft recipients. The ultimate goal of any organ transplantation is to restore normal quality of life, and to that end, various general principles hold across all organ transplant fields.

The general principles of management include (i) monitoring of graft function; (ii) surveillance for infectious complications; (iii) monitoring for long-term adverse effects of immunosuppression; and (iv) maintenance of standard well child care (including modified immunization schedule, growth and nutrition, and psychosocial issues). ED evaluations are directed by the acute problems that may arise from surgical or medical complications and that may manifest as fever, graft dysfunction, pain, or drug toxicity. To evaluate the common complaints of the transplant recipient, it is helpful to review the immunosuppression medications that both sustain the graft and health of the recipient and precipitate many of the complications of transplantation. Table 129.1 summarizes typical adverse effects of the most commonly used medications. Table 129.2 indicates drug interactions that frequently precipitate toxicities. Each medication is discussed in further detail in the next section.

IMMUNOSUPPRESSIVE MEDICATIONS

Corticosteroid

Corticosteroid therapy is used for induction of immunosuppression, with dosing often beginning in the operating room. Steroid therapy is effective for both treatment and prevention of acute rejection. Although for many years, long-term, low-dose steroid dosing was believed to be necessary for most transplant recipients, there is growing evidence that this therapy is not required for many heart and liver recipients. Corticosteroid therapy decreases inflammatory response by preventing the chemotaxis and recruitment of mediating lymphocytes, and it can also be lympholytic at higher doses. Intravenous methylprednisolone (Solumedrol®) is used in the immediate perioperative period with a transition to oral prednisone. It is also used for treatment of acute rejection and is extremely effective. Reasonably common acute adverse effects include hypertension, hyperglycemia (sometimes requiring insulin), psychosis, and joint pain (Table 129.1). Chronic adverse effects include those listed in this section, plus the Cushing's syndrome, bone demineralization, linear growth delay/arrest, adrenal suppression, and cataracts, as well as others.

TABLE 129.2

MEDICATIONS THAT ALTER IMMUNOSUPPRESSANT MEDICATION METABOLISM

Drug	Agents that increase blood concentrations (decrease metabolism)	Agents that decrease blood concentrations (increase metabolism)
Calcineurin inhibitors (cyclosporine and tacrolimus)	Diltiazem Nicardipine Nifedipine Verapamil Fluconazole/ketoconazole Voriconazole Clotrimazole Clarithromycin/erythromycin Azithromycin Metoclopramide Amiodarone Methylprednisolone Omeprazole Nefazodone	Carbamazepine Phenobarbital Phenytoin/fosphenytoin Rifabutin Rifampin Rifapentine St. John's Wort Probucol Terbinafine
Azathioprine	Allopurinol Methotrexate Angiotensin converting enzyme inhibitors	Antacids Cholestyramine Iron preparations
Mycophenolate	Probenecid Tacrolimus	Antacids Cholestyramine Iron preparations
Sirolimus	Diltiazem Nicardipine Nifedipine Verapamil Fluconazole/ketoconazole Voriconazole Clotrimazole Clarithromycin/erythromycin Azithromycin Metoclopramide Amiodarone Methylprednisolone Omeprazole Cyclosporine	Carbamazepine Phenobarbital Phenytoin/Fosphenytoin Fosphenytoin Rifabutin Rifampin Rifapentine St. John's Wort

Tacrolimus (Prograf®, FK506)

Tacrolimus is a macrolide immunosuppressant in the category of calcineurin inhibitors produced by the fungus *Streptomyces tsukubaensis*. A potent immunosuppressive, tacrolimus is effective as treatment for acute and chronic rejection, as well as for maintenance prophylactic immunosuppression, either alone or in combination with adjuvant drugs. Tacrolimus is dosed orally every 12 hours, with monitoring of trough levels to adjust dosing daily in the perioperative period. Once the therapeutic dose is established, levels may be checked as infrequently as every 3 months for a stable liver recipient (or thoracic transplant recipient) for as long as 2 years posttransplantation. Common side effects include hyperglycemia (sometimes requiring insulin), hypertension, headache, increased creatinine, and renal electrolyte wasting (particularly magnesium and potassium). Less common adverse effects include dermatologic diseases, such as eczema, common warts (the severity of which can range from mild to disfiguring), and neurotoxicity (seizures) (Table 129.1).

All immunosuppression leaves the recipient more prone to infections and posttransplant lymphoproliferative disease (PTLD). PTLD is a special problem in infant recipients who are more commonly Epstein-Barr virus (EBV) naive. Tacrolimus is erratically absorbed orally; food and various other medications, particularly anticonvulsants, macrolide antibiotics, fluconazole, and related drugs, will alter absorption (Table 129.2). Target levels for tacrolimus will vary depending on the organ received, the time elapsed from transplant, history of rejection, current infections, and renal function. It is important to note that immunosuppression and toxicities (particularly nephrotoxicity) are synergistic with cyclosporine and ibuprofen, among others (Table 129.2).

Cyclosporine (Neoral®, SangCya®, Sandimmune®)

Cyclosporine is a cyclic, 11 amino acid polypeptide produced by fungi. Cyclosporine is quite effective for prophylaxis for rejection but is less effective as treatment for acute or chronic rejection. This agent was essentially the only immunosuppressive drug available for many years, and it is still widely used as a primary agent or in combination with other medications. Oral dosing is every 8 hours for infants and toddlers, and twice daily for older children and adults. Morning trough levels or area-under-the-curve levels are monitored to optimize dosing. The original form of cyclosporine required bile micelle formation for absorption, which may be a problem for liver recipients with acute or chronic rejection or other causes of cholestasis, but the Neoral/SangCya® brands form do not. In fact, these are better absorbed in the face of the cholestasis of rejection. Regardless of the brand chosen, it is important not to interchange one for another. Adverse effects are similar to those of tacrolimus, with hypertension, renal injury, infection, skin problems, PTLD, and seizures (Table 129.1). In addition, there is frequent hirsutism and gingival hyperplasia. As with tacrolimus, target levels vary depending on the organ, time from transplant, and status of the patient.

Azathioprine (Imuran®)

Azathioprine is used as an adjuvant immunosuppressive therapy in combination with a calcineurin inhibitor and/or corticosteroid therapy. Azathioprine is rapidly converted to 6-mercaptopurine, the active form of the drug, which acts as a lymphocytic antiproliferative by inhibition of purine synthesis. The most common adverse effect is myelosuppression. Indeed, the level of myelosuppression can be used to monitor dosing and compliance; however, active metabolite levels can now be measured directly. Dosing should be adjusted in renal failure due to renal metabolism and clearance. Idiosyncratic reactions include drug fever, hepatotoxicity, and pancreatitis. Increased risk of infection and late neoplasm have been attributed to long-term use of azathioprine.

Mycophenolate Mofetil (CellCept®, MMF)

Mycophenolate mofetil (MMF) is an ester of mycophenolic acid (MPA), which is the active metabolite, and has lymphocytic antiproliferative properties. The drug is administered orally on a bid or tid basis, and levels are generally not monitored. The drug is rapidly metabolized to MPA, which is a potent selective competitive inhibitor of inosine monophosphate dehydrogenase and, therefore, inhibits synthesis of the purine nucleotide guanosine. T and B lymphocytes are dependent for proliferation on de novo purine synthesis, whereas other cell types can use alternate salvage pathways. The drug, therefore, selectively inhibits proliferation of B and T lymphocytes and also inhibits antibody formation by B cells. Mycophenolate is effective as treatment for acute rejection and is used mainly as a short-term adjuvant immunosuppressive therapy. Common adverse effects are primarily gastrointestinal (GI) symptoms, including diarrhea and cramping. Other effects include vomiting, anorexia, leukopenia, infection, and PTLD (Table 129.1).

Sirolimus (Rapamune®)

Sirolimus is a newer immunosuppressive medication used primarily in adults but with growing indications in children. Sirolimus inhibits T-lymphocyte activation and proliferation in response to antigenic and cytokine stimulation. Its mechanism differs from the calcineurin inhibitors, and its toxicity profile is different. Sirolimus can be used as a single agent or in combination with calcineurin inhibitors. Reports of serious complications with sirolimus as a primary agent in liver (hepatic vascular thrombosis) and lung (bronchial anastomotic breakdown) recipients have limited its use in the perioperative period. However, it has been very effective for long-term maintenance, especially in children with renal injury from calcineurin inhibitors. Sirolimus is dosed once daily and has excellent absorption and biliary excretion. Common adverse effects (primarily reported in adults) include edema, hypertension, hyperlipidemia, and hypercholesterolemia, with many other effects reported. Side effects seen in the pediatric population include nephrotoxicity (typically dose-related and short-lived) and marrow suppression.

Lympholytic Agents: OKT3 and Antithymocyte Globulin (ATG)

OKT3 is a mouse antibody against the CD3 antigen of human T cells. It is available only for IV use. Levels of OKT3, human anti-OKT3 antibodies, and T-cell subtype counts are monitored. OKT3 is used for treatment of acute rejection that is steroid resistant or for induction of immunosuppression for patients with hepatorenal syndrome who cannot tolerate tacrolimus or cyclosporine in the perioperative period. Common side effects are attributable to a cytokine release syndrome (CRS) associated with the first few doses of OKT3; hyperpyrexia is most common. The first dose is typically administered in the intensive care unit for monitoring and rapid response to the CRS should it occur. OKT3 is administered after appropriately timed premedication with steroids, acetaminophen, and antihistamine. CRS can be severe and can progress rapidly to life-threatening shock, with cardiovascular collapse and pulmonary edema. Resuscitation equipment and medications should be available, and fluid overload and/or pulmonary edema should be treated prior to administration. Cerebral edema (and herniation) may occur. Use of OKT3 is associated with increased risk for bacterial and viral sepsis and development of PTLD. Aseptic meningitis is also associated with OKT3 use, with typical manifestations and cerebrospinal fluid findings; seizure risk is also increased. Treatment with OKT3 imparts increased risk for viral infections and PTLD, even after the treatment course is completed.

Other antilymphocyte antibodies, such as antithymocyte globulin (ATG), are available with various modifications designed to reduce CRS and improve efficiency of induction, particularly useful in renal transplantation. Monoclonal preparations arising from nonhuman hosts (e.g., rabbit ATG, horse ATG) carry with them a risk of serum sickness, which can occur 2 or 3 weeks after treatment. Symptoms of malaise, fever, skin rash, and joint pain may implicate this diagnosis.

COMPLICATIONS RELATED TO IMMUNOSUPPRESSION

Although immunosuppression puts patients at greater risk for infectious complications and this likely accounts for the majority of ED visits in transplant recipients, there are certain drug-related side effects that may commonly be encountered in

TABLE 129.3

OVERVIEW OF COMPLICATIONS OF SOLID ORGAN TRANSPLANTATION

Organ	Vascular	Surgical	Immunosuppression	Graft function and rejection	Common presentation of rejection
Kidney	Bleeding Renal artery stenosis Vascular thrombosis	Urinary leak Ureteral obstruction	Infection Cosmetic changes Hypertension Nephrotoxicity PTLD noncompliance	Hyper acute rejection Rejection Drug toxicity Recurrent disease	Nonspecific: fever, abdominal pain Specific: uremia
Liver	Bleeding Hepatic artery thrombosis Portal vein thrombosis	Biliary leak Biliary obstruction/ stricture	Infection Cosmetic changes Hypertension Nephrotoxicity Hepatotoxicity PTLD Noncompliance	Primary nonfunction Rejection Recurrent disease	Nonspecific: fever, itching, abdominal pain, anorexia Specific: cholestasis, pleural effusion
Heart	Bleeding Pulmonary artery hypertension[a] Pulmonary venous obstruction[a]	Pulmonary artery hypertension Pulmonary venous obstruction	Infection Cosmetic changes Hypertension Nephrotoxicity Hepatotoxicity PTLD Noncompliance	Primary graft failure Acute rejection Chronic (vascular) rejection Arrhythmia Hypotension	Nonspecific: fever, malaise, abdominal pain, cough, weakness Specific: ventricular failure/CHF, low cardiac output, arrhythmia, pericar- dial effusion
Lung	Bleeding	Dehiscense, tracheal obstruction, diaphragmatic paralysis	Infection Cosmetic changes Hypertension Nephrotoxicity Hepatotoxicity PTLD Noncompliance	Graft failure Obliterative Bronchiolitis (rejection)	Nonspecific: fever, cough, malaise Specific: hypoxia, chest radiograph findings, pulmonary function test deterioration

PTLD, posttransplant lymphoproliferative disease; CHF, congestive heart failure.
[a]Typically as a result of pretransplant diagnosis and/or prior surgeries.

an urgent care setting (Table 129.3). Patients receiving calcineurin inhibitors are at risk for nephrotoxicity. Patients who have had low cardiac output for long periods prior to transplantation may also be at increased risk. Renal dysfunction may be manifest by edema and decreased urine output and may follow a course of antibiotics, use of nonsteroidal antiinflammatory drugs (NSAIDs), or a diarrheal illness resulting in dehydration. Patients should be closely evaluated and immediate drug levels obtained and followed. Calcineurin inhibitors should not be subsequently administered until drug levels are determined and the etiology of renal insufficiency is explained. Renal failure is a possible temporary or permanent outcome of an acute insult on an overlay of chronic calcineurin inhibitor exposure. Although relatively few patients progress to requiring chronic dialysis, this is a potential end point for these patients.

Patients receiving calcineurin inhibitors, especially in conjunction with steroids, are at risk for systemic hypertension. It is notable that about two-thirds of postcardiac transplantation patients have hypertension, and most require some antihypertensive therapy. Typical medications used to control hypertension are calcium channel blockers (especially amlodipine) and angiotensin-converting enzyme inhibitors. The latter class of

drugs may also contribute to renal toxicity; therefore, renal function must be closely monitored.

INFECTION PROPHYLAXIS

One important complication related to immunosuppression in transplant patients is that it places the patient at increased risk for developing infections, both conventional and opportunistic (Table 129.3). The child's susceptibility to infection will vary, depending on the level of immunosuppression used, his or her overall health at the time of transplant, and exposures and immunities prior to transplant. Young children and infants who have had little infectious exposure and have few immunizations are at particular risk for early viral infections posttransplant. The most common viral infections posttransplant include cytomegalovirus (CMV), EBV, herpes simplex virus (HSV), and varicella-zoster virus. Patients who have complicated postoperative courses in which there are bile leaks or collections, or complications that necessitate multiple abdominal surgeries and long-term antibiotic use, are at high risk for fungal infections. Most viral and fungal infections begin to appear approximately 1 month posttransplant, whereas the risk of bacterial infection is highest in the first few postoperative days. Most transplant programs employ protocol use of perioperative prophylactic antibiotics, as well as antifungal and antiviral therapy. The regimen varies slightly with the age and exposure history of the patients.

Given that both primary and reactivated CMV infections can be serious threats to transplant recipients, antiviral therapy is an important part of the posttransplant regimen. Prophylactic therapy for CMV infections may include CMV hyperimmunoglobulin (CMV-IG), oral acyclovir, and IV or oral ganciclovir or valganciclovir for the first 3 to 6 months after the transplant and during treatment with monoclonal or polyclonal antibodies. The risk is particularly high in CMV-negative recipients who have received CMV-positive allografts. CMV infections may be asymptomatic or may present with symptoms such as fever, leukopenia, pulmonary disease, hepatic dysfunction, intestinal bleeding, or diarrhea. Some programs monitor the presence of CMV antigen in the blood and treat intermittently with IV ganciclovir.

Pneumocystis jiroveci can also be an important pathogen posttransplant. Prophylactic regimens may include sulfamethoxazole–trimethoprim as a single dose (at half the therapeutic dose) daily or as a full dose (10 mg per kg per day trimethoprim), in two divided doses three times per week. Other regimens include monthly IV pentamidine and monthly aerosolized pentamidine. Sulfamethoxazole–trimethoprim may also serve as a urinary tract infection suppressant in renal transplant recipients. These patients are also at increased risk for oral and esophageal candidiasis because of steroid and antibiotic treatment. Therefore, oral nystatin is given for 6 to 12 months after the transplant.

IMMUNIZATIONS IN THE SOLID ORGAN TRANSPLANT RECIPIENT

Ideally, every solid organ transplant recipient would receive all standard childhood immunizations prior to transplantation. In reality, many young infants undergo transplantation before completing childhood immunizations and, more distressingly, immunizations are often withheld from children with chronic diseases on the basis of misunderstanding the necessity to continue immunizations by parents and primary care providers. Although infants and children with chronic disease may have reduced efficacy from immunization, failure to provide immunization has still lower protection. When evaluating a febrile transplant patient, careful consideration should be given to immunization status.

Following initial recovery from the transplantation procedure and any perioperative complications, a standard immunization schedule (with catch up as necessary) should be implemented as per the Advisory Committee on Immunization Practices (ACIP) and American Academy of Pediatrics (AAP) recommendations, with modifications only for live virus immunizations. It is generally accepted that inactivated virus immunizations are safe in the immunocompromised patient, although reduced rates of seroconversion may be expected, especially for children with higher degrees of immunosuppression. Patients often receive relatively more immunosuppression during the first year after transplant and, from a practical perspective, routine immunizations may be more effective if resumed thereafter. Attenuated live virus immunizations have been the subject of greater con-

troversy; the standard recommendation is that immunocompromised individuals should not receive live virus immunization. Retrospective studies from centers administering live virus immunizations (MMR and Varivax®, in particular) to selected liver transplant recipients on maintenance immunosuppression have shown no evidence of infectious complications and a reduced but still significant rate of serologic protection.

GENERAL PRINCIPLES OF MANAGEMENT

Hospitalizations in the first 6 months after transplant are common. For example, 60% of recipients of cadaver donor renal allografts and 50% of living donor recipients are hospitalized in the first 6 months after transplant. The most common causes for hospitalization include treatment of acute rejection, viral and bacterial infections, and treatment of hypertension (Table 129.3). These are also the most likely reasons for presentation to the ED. The encounter in the ED with the renal, liver, or heart transplant recipient need not provoke a sense of uneasiness in the physician if the following pertinent principles of evaluation and treatment are applied:

1. If the transplant patient is critically ill or hemodynamically unstable, the patient should be stabilized by using the same lifesaving interventions used for any critically ill individual with attention to the ABCs of resuscitation. The primary focus should be on the patient and not on graft survival. A critically ill transplant patient should be stabilized and then transported to a transplant center.

2. The transplant center should be regarded as a valuable source of information and assistance. The transplant center should be contacted early in the ED evaluation. No changes in immunosuppressive medication should be undertaken independent of input from the transplant center unless the medication is determined to be the cause of the life-threatening event (i.e. anaphylaxis).

3. All symptoms require thorough evaluation because a patient receiving immunosuppressive medications may have blunted or atypical presentations of severe disease, particularly when infection is involved. Abdominal pain may represent a surgical emergency even when mild in nature. Steroid therapy may blunt the inflammatory response in a transplant patient such that visceral perforation, urine or bile leak, or infectious peritonitis may not be accompanied by classic peritoneal signs. Therefore, all complaints warrant full investigation.

4. Conditions that impair the patient's ability to take or absorb medications (e.g., vomiting, diarrhea) necessitate hospital admission for parenteral administration of the immunosuppressive medications and careful monitoring. Simple conditions, such as gastritis with vomiting or gastroenteritis with diarrhea, may lead to significantly diminished cyclosporine levels and the potential for rejection and graft loss.

5. Fever in the immunocompromised patient requires aggressive investigation because it could be a manifestation of a wide spectrum of disease from severe opportunistic infection to acute graft rejection. If the patient is obviously septic or meningitic, blood cultures should be drawn and broad-spectrum antibiotics administered expeditiously. Headache, seizures, or neurologic changes in the setting of

a fever are indications for a lumbar puncture with cerebrospinal fluid cell count, as well as comprehensive stains and culture for bacteria, viruses, fungi, and acid-fast organisms, to be performed as part of the primary evaluation.

6. Renal or liver allograft dysfunction may be secondary to causes other than rejection. Problems such as bile duct or ureter obstruction, infection, drug toxicity, and rejection may mimic each other but require different therapy. In addition, volume depletion can significantly increase the serum creatinine level in renal transplant recipients. Therefore, these patients must be fully evaluated in a transplant center where they may have prompt immunosuppressive drug levels, graft-specific imaging studies, and possibly graft biopsy before antirejection therapy is initiated.

7. Cyclosporine and tacrolimus have several drug interactions (Table 129.2) that alter patients' metabolism and may lead to dangerously high or low levels. Numerous medications, such as NSAIDs, can also act synergistically with these agents to increase their nephrotoxic effects. Careful attention should be paid to potential drug interactions and to the levels of cyclosporine or tacrolimus in all transplant patients.

APPROACH TO FEVER

Fever is the most common reason for the pediatric transplant recipient to seek evaluation in an ED. A fever in a transplant patient may be a manifestation of any number of infections or processes from acute graft rejection to systemic sepsis. Assessing these patients is challenging because their immunosuppression may mask many of the typical physical findings associated with their disease process (e.g., peritoneal signs).

Patient assessment should include (i) a careful physical examination that includes examination of all wounds; (ii) pulse oximetry and chest radiograph if the patient has cough, dyspnea, tachypnea, or other signs of hypoxia; (iii) a screen of graft function (liver function tests and creatinine level analysis), in addition to other routine laboratory tests such as complete blood cell count, differential prothrombin time/partial thromboplastin time, and possibly disseminated intravascular coagulation panel, if the patient appears septic; and (iv) a blood culture for bacterial and viral pathogens, blood buffy coat CMV antigen assay by rapid assay technique, urine for urinalysis, rapid CMV assay, and viral culture of the urine and a standard urine culture if the child has a fever or appears ill. Because some patients may have a central venous catheter, line sepsis should always be considered in the differential diagnosis.

If the patient appears well, has normal laboratory evaluation and chest radiograph (if presenting with respiratory symptoms), and has an obvious minor source of infection, such as otitis media or an upper respiratory tract infection, the patient may be sent home with appropriate therapy. As previously mentioned, the transplant center should always be notified at the time of the visit that the patient had been evaluated and what the diagnosis was. Close outpatient follow-up is mandatory within 48 hours.

In the liver transplant patient, elevated levels of liver aminotransferases may be a sign of rejection, arterial or venous thrombosis of the graft, or even biliary stricture and obstruction with resultant cholangitis. The initial study required in this case is an ultrasound examination with Doppler flow study to view arterial and venous blood flow to the graft and to assess

the biliary tree for evidence of dilation, which suggests obstruction. If obstruction is suspected from the ultrasound evaluation, percutaneous transhepatic cholangiography (PTC) is usually necessary to image the biliary tree and biliary–enteric anastomosis. Prior to the PTC, the patient is given broad-spectrum antibiotic coverage for the common biliary pathogens (e.g., gram-negative enteric organisms). Ampicillin (200 mg per kg per day) and cefotaxime (100 mg per kg per day) are usually adequate. If the ultrasound evaluation is otherwise abnormal (i.e., demonstrating a fluid collection), the situation could require surgical revision of the biliary anastomosis or biliary stent placement either by the interventional radiologists or by open procedure by the transplant surgeons.

If the ultrasound evaluation is normal and no source for the fever or increased liver function tests is found, the patient requires admission and liver biopsy to rule out rejection or viral infection. In the renal transplant recipient, particular attention should be paid to the graft site because fever, tenderness over the transplanted kidney, poorly controlled hypertension, diminished urinary output, and recent weight gain may all be signs of rejection. A rise in the blood urea nitrogen and creatinine levels also suggests rejection. However, ascending urinary tract infection, infected perinephric collections (lymphocele, seroma, and urinoma), ureteral stenosis or obstruction, and renal vascular thrombosis may also present with similar findings. These emergencies require in-hospital workup, beginning with urine culture, blood culture, Doppler and conventional ultrasound, nuclear renal scan, antegrade or retrograde pyelogram when indicated, and possible renal biopsy.

INFECTION

In general, the onset and type of infection and the responsible agent is related to the intensity and type of immunosuppression, as well as the time since the transplant procedure. In the first few weeks after transplant, the most common infections are urinary tract infection and wound infection with bacterial pathogens. After this period, the incidence of opportunistic infections increases.

Pneumocystis jiroveci Pneumonia

P. jiroveci pneumonia (PCP) is most common within the second to sixth month after transplant. In most cases, a patient with PCP presents with dry cough, dyspnea, diffuse interstitial infiltrates, and hypoxemia. Suspicion of infection with this pathogen necessitates a diagnostic intervention such as bronchoscopy with a bronchoalveolar lavage as soon as possible. The isolation of pneumocysts on the silver stain of the lavage fluid confirms the diagnosis. Infection is treated with IV sulfamethoxazole–trimethoprim (20 mg per kg per day of trimethoprim given IV in four divided doses) or pentamidine (4 mg per kg given IV in a single daily dose).

CMV Infection

CMV infection is the single most important infection in the transplant recipient. CMV infection in an immunocompetent host is usually asymptomatic, whereas in a transplant patient, it may be devastating. CMV causes a syndrome characterized by anorexia, malaise, myalgias, and arthralgias, usually heralded by the initial presentation of fever. These symptoms may be accompanied by an atypical leukocytosis and usually occur within 2 to 3 months of transplant but may occur at any time. In approximately one-third of febrile patients with CMV infection, pulmonary disease develops and may rapidly progress to adult respiratory distress syndrome and death. The risk of succumbing from disseminated CMV disease, prior to the availability of ganciclovir, is 4%, 14%, and 19% in patients after kidney, heart, and heart-lung transplantation, respectively. CMV may also cause localized disease, which in transplant patients may localize to the renal or hepatic graft (causing a picture of hepatitis) and mimic rejection. Another specific site of CMV involvement is the mucosal lining of the GI tract where the virus may cause ulceration and massive GI tract hemorrhage. The effects of the organ-specific infection are amplified by several of the systemic effects of the virus, including thrombocytopenia and leukopenia caused by bone marrow suppression, and impairment in alveolar macrophage function and cell-mediated immunity, which predispose the patient to further opportunistic infections by other viral agents or *Pneumocystis*. Diagnosis of CMV is made by culture, serology, or antigen detection, and therefore, cannot be determined in the ED. However, blood samples can be sent for early antigen detection and culture if CMV is suspected. The transplant physicians can determine by weighing the patient's presentation and risk factors whether preemptive treatment is indicated in any particular patient in the ED. Treatment of active CMV includes lowering of the immunosuppression and administering IV ganciclovir (5 to 10 mg per kg per 24 hours in two divided doses). CMV disease may represent (i) a primary infection in a CMV-nonimmune recipient who acquires the infection from the allograft or transfusion of CMV-positive blood products, (ii) reactivation of latent virus as a consequence of immunosuppression (most recipients in this situation show some evidence of CMV infection, although only 20% become symptomatic), and (iii) superinfection of a CMV-immune patient with a strain of CMV of donor or environmental origin. The course of CMV infection is influenced by the type and intensity of immunosuppression the patient has received. Azathioprine and particularly OKT3 and Antithymocyte globulin (ATG) have the highest risk of reactivating CMV disease.

Epstein-Barr Virus and Posttransplant Lymphoproliferative Disease

EBV is a ubiquitous virus and, similar to CMV, is associated with hepatitis as well as a more systemic illness. Acute EBV infection presents as a mononucleosis-like syndrome with diffuse B-cell hyperplasia. However, of particular concern with EBV infection is the risk of PTLD. PTLD refers to a range of lymphoproliferative disorders—resulting from EBV activation of lymphocytes—that are under the influence of immunosuppression. This can present anytime from 1 month after transplant to many years after transplantation. The clinical presentation of PTLD is highly variable and may include fever, lymphadenopathy, sinusitis, upper airway obstruction from tonsillar enlargement, splenomegaly, GI bleeding from necrotic intestinal lymph nodes, or intestinal obstruction or perforation. This disorder is most common in children who are not immune to EBV at the time of transplant and thus develop EBV infection. The overall incidence in pediatric renal transplant recipients is less than 1%, but the risk increases with increasing exposure to immunosuppressive medications such as OKT3 and tacrolimus-based immunosuppression.

The diagnosis of PTLD is rarely made in the ED. It usually requires a combination of analysis of tissues (lymph node, tonsil, liver) for evidence of EBV-transformed B cells and quantitative EBV polymerase chain reaction (PCR) from blood confirming viral replication. However, blood can be sent from the ED for EBV PCR if this condition is suspected. Specific T-cell studies are used to determine the clonality of the lymphoproliferation and thereby to determine the appropriate therapy, which can range from reduction of immunosuppression and antiviral therapy to cytotoxic chemotherapeutic agents, such as cyclophosphamide and anti-CD20 antibody therapy. In many cases, the PTLD responds to discontinuation of immunosuppressive medications without ensuing allograft rejection.

Herpes Simplex Virus

Reactivation of latent HSV infection is common in transplant recipients. Patients presenting with an oral or genital lesion resembling herpes should have a scraping for immunofluorescence performed on the lesion. If HBV is present, oral acyclovir is used for minor lesions without systemic symptoms. Extensive lesions, fever, or other systemic symptoms require IV acyclovir treatment (750 to 1,500 mg per square meter per 24 hours given IV in three divided doses) to prevent disseminated herpes infection.

Varicella

Varicella is a highly contagious pathogen that is common among school children. In a transplant patient who is immunocompromised, it may become a disseminated disease spreading to the liver, lungs, and central nervous system (CNS). If a patient has been exposed only to varicella (household contact or played in the same room with an infected individual), the patient should receive varicella-zoster immunoglobulin (VariZIG). VariZIG (125 units or one vial per 10 mg) should be given within 96 hours of exposure, but the sooner it is administered, the more efficacious it will be. VariZIG has been on a patient specific allocation for approximately 3 years in the United States, requiring registration of the patient and a drop shipment to the institution that arrives within 24 hours. Thus it is imperative to request the drug as soon as the diagnosis is made. If the transplant patient is diagnosed with varicella, he or she should be admitted to the hospital for IV acyclovir therapy (1,500 mg per square meter per 24 hours in three divided doses) and a sharp reduction in steroid dosage. Herpes zoster may occur in as many as 5% to 10% of adult transplant patients, representing reactivation of old varicella infection, although it rarely disseminates. Acyclovir may hasten resolution of lesions, but no change in immunosuppressive regimen is usually needed.

Adenovirus

This viral infection occurs in up to 7% of pediatric transplant patients and should be considered when the patient presents with high fever and liver and/or pulmonary dysfunction with or without diarrhea. A nasopharyngeal swab and stool for viral culture should be sent to screen for the virus in the febrile posttransplant patient.

Other Viral Pathogens

Recently, other viruses have been identified as pathogens in transplant patients. Human herpesvirus-6 (HHV-6) and human herpesvirus-7 (HHV-7) are causative agents of severe disease in stem cell transplantation. In solid organ recipients, the most common clinical manifestation is a nonspecific febrile syndrome. Other symptomatic infections are rare and may include hepatitis, colitis and nonspecific neurologic sequelae. In adult liver transplant patients, active infection with HHV-6 or HHV-7 may increase the risk of developing severe CMV disease and invasive fungal infections. Risk factors for infection with HHV-6 include antirejection therapy with OKT-3 or antithymocyte globulin. The role of HHV-6 or HHV-7 in solid organ rejection is still unclear.

Fungal and Nocardial Infections

Fungal infections in the posttransplant patient can have various clinical presentations. They may present as a subacute respiratory illness with local or disseminated findings on chest radiograph. Alternatively, the patient may have a systemic illness with nonspecific symptoms of malaise and fever that may be acute or chronic. Fungal infections may also present with metastatic disease. Examples are the 20% to 30% of patients with cryptococcal infection who demonstrate skin lesions weeks or months before the development of CNS lesions and the 10% to 15% of patients with disseminated *Candida* infection who have skin lesions early on in its course. Similarly, *Nocardia* and *Mucor* species may show early skin lesions before evidence of more serious deep-seated infection presents itself. Another common fungal infection is candidal esophagitis, which may present with dysphagia or odynophagia. CMV and HSV infection of the esophagus may also occur with similar symptoms.

Fungal infections generally do not occur in the first month after transplant but rather in the subsequent months. Between the first and sixth months, *Candida* species are the major fungal pathogens. Infections with *Aspergillus* are less common but are associated with high mortality. Fungal infection of the CNS may be difficult to assess because the classic signs of CNS infection, such as meningismus, are often absent in immunosuppressed patients. The common presentation of headache, often without fever, may be the only indication that a CNS infection exists and warrants thorough neurological evaluation, lumbar puncture with fungal stains and cultures, and possibly an imaging study of the brain, preferably magnetic resonance imaging. Acute or subacute meningitis is most commonly caused by *Listeria monocytogenes,* whereas chronic meningitis is most often caused by *Cryptococcus neoformans* and focal brain abscess is often indicative of *Aspergillus* infection.

GASTROINTESTINAL EMERGENCIES

Transplanted patients may develop GI complications that are secondary to many different causes, ranging from infection to postsurgical complications to dehydration of any cause. Perforation and bleeding may occur secondary to necrotic lymph nodes from PTLD or because of small bowel ulcerations from CMV infection. Intussusception or luminal obstruction may occur secondary to enlarged lymph nodes from PTLD, and peritonitis may be caused by any of the aforementioned conditions, including bile leak from an anastomotic breakdown or bile duct ischemia, particularly in the early posttransplant period. Severe variceal bleeding is also seen in the liver transplant patient with portal venous thrombosis and consequent prehepatic portal hypertension. Dehydration should be promptly addressed as it may lead to renal toxicity of immunosuppressive medications. In such instances, the medication should be held and a medication level checked, if possible. Interpretation will depend on the timing of the last dose given. Pancreatitis may be seen as a complication of taking azathioprine. Tacrolimus toxicity can produce complaints of severe epigastric pain or diffuse abdominal pain. Mycophenolate can cause gastritis, esophagitis, and diarrhea. In addition to viral involvement of the GI tract, infectious processes that are most common in transplant recipients include *Clostridium difficile* colitis and candidal esophagitis.

The approach to these patients in the ED is the same as for the nonimmunocompromised patient: (i) stabilize with fluid resuscitation or blood products if necessary, (ii) nasogastric intubation if evidence of upper GI bleeding or obstruction, and (iii) frequent monitoring of vital signs while transfer to the transplant center is arranged.

MISCELLANEOUS EMERGENCIES

Transplant recipients may also experience many of the usual childhood emergencies, including hydroceles and herniae. Scrotal edema on the side of the renal transplant is a common finding; it is generally self-limiting and not a problem. Other possible complications include deep venous thrombosis on the side of the transplanted kidney, which is confirmed by noninvasive venous imaging and managed with anticoagulant therapy. Less common complications are suture-line disruption with subsequent "blow out" or aneurysmal rupture at the anastomotic site in both liver and renal transplants.

Careful attention should be paid to a transplant recipient with a headache. In addition to usual causes of headaches, meningitis, pseudotumor cerebri, malignancy, and malignant hypertension must be considered. In a patient with papilledema, the most likely cause is pseudotumor cerebri, which is a complication of steroid treatment and may be related to changes in steroid dose.

CONCLUSION

Emergencies in the pediatric transplant patient are common, consequent to the complex nature of the procedures and the depressed state of the immune system. With the ever-increasing number of organ transplants being performed each year in children, more of these patients are likely to be seen in the ED. Therefore, a working knowledge of the nature of these procedures and the common emergency situations that may arise in this patient group is essential to proper assessment and management of these patients' problems.

Suggested Readings

Alonso MH, Ryckman FC. Current concepts in pediatric liver transplant. *Semin Liver Dis* 1998;18:295–307.

Ascher NL, Stock PG, Bumgardner GL, et al. Infection and rejection of primary hepatic transplant in 93 consecutive patients treated with triple immuno-suppressive therapy. *Surg Gynecol Obstet* 1988;167:474–484.

Badley AD, Seaberg EC, Porayko MK, et al. Prophylaxis of cytomegalovirus infection in liver transplantation: a randomized trial comparing a combination of ganciclovir and acyclovir to acyclovir. *Transplantation* 1997;64(1):66–73.

Bartosh SM, Alonso EM, Whitington PF. Renal outcomes in pediatric liver transplantation. *Clin Transplant* 1997;11:354–360.

Bock GH, Sullivan EK, Miller D, et al. Cytomegalovirus infections following renal transplantation—effects on antiviral prophylaxis: a report of the North American Pediatric Renal Transplant Cooperative Study. *Pediatr Nephrol* 1997;11(6):665–671.

Breinig MK, Zitelli B, Starzl TE, et al. Epstein-Barr virus, cytomegalovirus, and other viral infections in children after liver transplantation. *J Infect Dis* 1987;156(2):273–279.

Cames B, Rahier J, Burtomboy G, et al. Acute adenovirus hepatitis in liver transplant recipients. *J Pediatr* 1992;120(1):33–37.

Cao S, Cox KL, Berquist W, et al. Long-term outcomes in pediatric liver recipients: comparison between cyclosporin A and tacrolimus. *Pediatr Transplant* 1999;3(1):22–26.

Crandall WV, Norlin C, Bullock EA, et al. Etiology and outcome of outpatient fevers in pediatric heart transplant patients. *Clin Pediatr (Phila)* 1996;35(9):437–442.

Cronin DC II, Faust TW, Brady L, et al. Modern immunosuppression. *Clin Liver Dis* 2000;4(3):619–655, ix.

Duvoux C, Pageaux GP, Vanlemmens C, et al. Risk factors for lymphoproliferative disorders after liver transplantation in adults: an analysis of 480 patients. *Transplantation* 2002;74(8):1103–1109.

George DL, Arnow PM, Fox A, et al. Bacterial infection as a complication of liver transplantation: epidemiology and risk factors. *Rev Infect Dis* 1991;13:387–396.

George DL, Arnow PM, Fox A, et al. Patterns of infection after pediatric liver transplantation. *Am J Dis Child* 1992;146:924–929.

Goldstein G, Kremer AB, Barnes L, et al. OKT3 monoclonal antibody reversal of renal and hepatic rejection in pediatric patients. *J Pediatr* 1987;111(6, pt 2):1046–1050.

Guthery SL, Heubi JE, Bucuvalas JC, et al. Determination of risk factors for Epstein-Barr virus-associated posttransplant lymphoproliferative disorder in pediatric liver transplant recipients using objective case ascertainment. *Transplantation* 2003;75(7):987–993.

Hamburger J, Vaysse J, Crosnier J, et al. Renal homotransplantation in man after radiation of the recipient. *Am J Med* 1962;32:854–871.

Holmes RD, Sokol RJ. Epstein-Barr virus and post-transplant lymphoproliferative disease. *Pediatr Transplant* 2002;6(6):456–464.

Hughes WT, Rivera GK, Schell MJ, et al. Successful intermittent chemoprophylaxis for *Pneumocystis jiroveci* pneumonitis. *N Engl J Med* 1987;316(26):1627–1632.

Jan D, Laurent J, Lacaille F, et al. Liver transplantation in children with inherited metabolic disorders. *Transplant Proc* 1995;27(2):1706–1707.

Kirk AJB, Omar I, Bateman DN, et al. Cyclosporine-associated hypertension in cardiopulmonary transplantation. *Transplantation* 1989;48:428–430.

Kuss R, Legrain M, Mathe G, et al. Homologous human kidney transplantation: experience with six patients. *Postgrad Med J* 1962;38:528–531.

Lawless S, Demetrius E, Thompson A, et al. Mechanisms of hypertension during and after orthotopic liver transplantation in children. *J Pediatr* 1989;115:372–379.

Lumbreras C, Cuervas-Mons V, Jara P, et al. Randomized trial of fluconazole versus nystatin for the prophylaxis of *Candida* infection following liver transplantation. *J Infect Dis* 1996;174(3):583–588.

Lynfield R, Herrin JT, Rubin RH. Varicella in pediatric renal transplant recipients. *Pediatrics* 1992;90(2, pt 1):216–220.

Mazzaferro V, Esquivel CO, Makowka L, et al. Hepatic artery thrombosis after pediatric liver transplantation—a medical or surgical event? *Transplantation* 1989;47:971–977.

McDiarmid SV. Management of the pediatric liver transplant patient. *Liver Transpl* 2001;7(11)(suppl 1):S77–S86.

McDiarmid SV. Renal function in pediatric liver transplant patients. *Kidney Int Suppl* 1996;53:S77–S84.

McDiarmid SV. The use of tacrolimus in pediatric liver transplantation. *J Pediatr Gastroenterol Nutr* 1998;26(1):90–102.

Michaels MG, Green M, Wald ER, et al. Adenovirus infection in pediatric liver transplant recipients. *J Infect Dis* 1992;165(1):170–174.

Murray JE, Merrill JP, Dammin GJ. Study of transplantation immunity after total body irradiation: clinical and experimental investigation. *Surgery* 1960;48:272–284.

Murray JE, Merrill JP, Harrison JH, et al. Prolonged survival of human-kidney homografts by immunosuppressive drug therapy. *N Engl J Med* 1963;268:1315–1323.

Neuhaus P, Bechstein O, Blumhardt G, et al. Comparison of quadruple immuno-suppression after liver transplantation with ATG or IL-2 receptor antibody. *Transplantation* 1993;55:1320–1327.

Paya CV. Prevention of fungal infection in transplantation. *Transpl Infect Dis* 2002;4(suppl 3):46–51.

Paya CV, Hermans PE, Smith TF, et al. Efficacy of ganciclovir in liver and kidney transplant recipients with severe cytomegalovirus infection. *Transplantation* 1988;46(2):229–234.

Paya CV, Hermans PE, Washington JA II, et al. Incidence, distribution, and outcome of episodes of infection in 100 orthotopic liver transplantations. *Mayo Clin Proc* 1989;64(5):555–564.

Post DJ, Douglas DD, Mulligan DC. Immunosuppression in liver transplantation. *Liver Transpl* 2005;11(11):1307–1314.

Rand EB, McCarthy CA, Whitington PF. Measles vaccination following orthotopic liver transplantation. *J Pediatr* 1993;123:87–89.

Rothwell WS, Gloor JM, Morgenstern BZ, et al. Disseminated varicella infection in pediatric renal transplant recipients treated with mycophenolate mofetil. *Transplantation* 1999;68(1):158–161.

Serinet MO, Jacquemin E, Habes D, et al. Anti-CD20 monoclonal antibody (Rituximab) treatment for Epstein-Barr virus-associated, B-cell lymphoproliferative disease in pediatric liver transplant recipients. *J Pediatr Gastroenterol Nutr* 2002;34(4):389–393.

Shapiro R, Scantlebury VP, Jordan ML, et al. A pilot trial of tacrolimus, sirolimus, and steroids in renal transplant recipients. *Transplant Proc* 2002;34(5):1651–1652.

Sindhi R, Webber S, Venkataramanan R, et al. Sirolimus for rescue and primary immunosuppression in transplanted children receiving tacrolimus. *Transplantation* 2001;72(5):851–855.

Smets F, Vajro P, Cornu G, et al. Indications and results of chemotherapy in children with posttransplant lymphoproliferative disease after liver transplantation. *Transplantation* 2000;69(5):982–984.

Starzl TE. The saga of liver replacement, with particular reference to the reciprocal influence of liver and kidney transplantation (1955–1967). *J Am Coll Surg* 2002;195(5):587–610.

Stratta RJ, Shaeffer MS, Markin RS, et al. Cytomegalovirus infection and disease after liver transplantation: an overview. *Dig Dis Sci* 1992;37:673–688.

Studies of Pediatric Liver Transplantation (SPLIT): Year 2000 outcomes. *Transplantation* 2001;72(3):463–476.

Webber SA. The current state of, and future prospects for, cardiac transplantation in children. *Cardiol Young* 2003;13(1):64–83.

Yoshikawa, T. Human herpesvirus-6 and -7 infections in transplantation. *Pediatr Transplant* 2003;7:11–17.

Younes BS, Ament ME, McDiarmid SV, et al. The involvement of the gastrointestinal tract in posttransplant lymphoproliferative disease in pediatric liver transplantation. *J Pediatr Gastroenterol Nutr* 1999;28(4):380–385.

Zitelli BJ, Gartner JC, Malatack JJ, et al. Pediatric liver transplantation: patient evaluation and selection, infectious complications, and life-style after transplantation. *Transplant Proc* 1987;19(4):3309–3316.

CHAPTER 130 ■ ADOLESCENT EMERGENCIES

MONIKA GOYAL, MD, CYNTHIA J. MOLLEN, MD, MSCE, AND JANE M. LAVELLE, MD

OVERVIEW

Adolescence is a cultural construct that can be defined as the transition from the dependent state of childhood to the independence of adulthood. This process usually begins with the changes in physical growth caused by activation of the hypothalamic-pituitary-gonadal axis, termed puberty, which commonly occurs between the ages of 8 and 11 years in girls and 9 to 12 years in boys. As discussed in more detail in this chapter, many physiologic, psychological, and environmental factors can delay the onset of puberty; therefore, adolescence may begin with changes in cognitive processes or relationships with peers and family members. At the other end of this transition process, an individual may not achieve true independence until well into the third or fourth decade of life. Because an end point is difficult to define, individuals are usually categorized as adolescents through age 21 years, although some pediatric facilities only care for adolescents without chronic illnesses until their 19th birthday. For many reasons, it is not unusual for individuals with special health and emotional needs to seek health care in pediatric settings well after they have achieved independent adult status.

Although the physical, psychological, and social changes associated with adolescence are well defined, the process is extraordinarily unique for each individual. There are many pathways by which biological, emotional, and environmental conditions can affect the rapidly changing adolescent. Surprisingly, although many adolescents struggle with the transition to independence from parents and childhood caregivers, for most adolescents these transitions occur smoothly with relatively little emotional distress or physical ailment. This may not be true for their parents or caregivers. Because optimal emergency care of adolescents is based on an understanding of the patient's developmental processes, a brief overview of the principles of adolescent development is presented, followed by a summary of health problems and patterns of emergency department (ED) use by adolescents.

The developmental tasks of early adolescence include establishing autonomy from parents or caregivers, moving from concrete to abstract thought and decision-making processes, and adopting a peer group identity. During the middle phase of adolescence, the struggle toward establishing an individual identity occurs, as one becomes aware of him- or herself as a sexual being and progressively longer-lasting intimate relationships evolve. Relationships with peers and adults change rapidly during middle adolescence. Family and social roles may become strained, and frameworks for moral decision making may develop at what may seem in opposition to traditional value systems. In the third phase of adolescent psychosocial development, individuals may strive to accept a sexual identity, establish meaningful interpersonal relationships, and work toward long-term life goals. It is not surprising that with so many somatic, psychological, and social changes occurring simultaneously, presentation for emergency medical attention is likely. Although the vast majority of adolescents cope well with their development and have only occasional episodic need for emergency medical services, up to one-fifth of teenagers have serious behavioral or medical problems, including conditions that can cause serious injury and threaten their lives. It is of paramount importance to approach each teenager and young adult on an individual basis. A standard approach based on chronologic age or physical appearance is never indicated or prudent. It is important to note that as teenagers develop a growing sense of self-awareness, the ways that their physical development differs from their peers can have significant impact on their identity and behavior. In particular, the physical development of individuals with chronic physical or emotional health conditions provides little insight into their psychosocial development.

The health care needs of adolescents are reflected by the chief causes of their mortality and morbidity. Since the 1980s, although there has been a gradual decrease in the adolescent death rate, it still remains high. The death rate for adolescents is 80 per 100,000 with a male:female ratio of 2:1. The root cause of the majority of adolescent deaths can be attributed to the "social morbidities" (substance abuse, sexually transmitted diseases, accidents, homicides, suicides, mental health disorders, and eating disorders).

Of all deaths of individuals between 15 and 24 years of age in the United States, three-fourths are the result of motor vehicle crashes, other unintentional injuries, homicide, and suicide. The leading causes of these unintentional injuries include motor vehicles, drowning, poisoning, firearms, fires, and falls. Homicide, the second leading cause of death, accounts for almost 15% of all deaths in the adolescent age group, the majority of which are caused by firearms; suicide accounts for more than 10%. Surveys of teens have revealed some insight about the extent they are at risk for some of these health problems. Results from the 2007 National Youth Risk Behavior Survey, which surveys a nationally representative sample of high school students, indicates that more than 10% of teens reported never or rarely wearing a seat belt and almost 30% reported traveling in a car driven by someone who had been drinking. Moreover, 18% reported carrying a weapon. Substance abuse is also a major contributor as 75% reported drinking alcohol, 20% smoked cigarettes, almost 40% smoked marijuana, and 7% had tried cocaine at least once.

More recent trends and changes in American family life, including increased incidence of unwed teenage pregnancy, high divorce rate, the deterioration of public education in some segments of our society, and unemployment, undoubtedly contribute to the health care problems of adolescents. These findings indicate that adolescent death and injury are not random events but have an epidemic cause that may be altered by timely, appropriate interventions.

Another important influence on the overall health of adolescents is their lack of access to the health care system. The National Health Interview Survey revealed that one in seven adolescents has no health insurance; overall, 16- to 24-year olds comprise the highest portion of uninsured individuals. Adolescents from poor, nonwhite families that are headed by one adult are most likely to be uninsured, contributing to ethnic disparities in health care access and overall health status. Other populations that may have limited access to coordinated health care for other reasons include youth who develop a minority sexual identity or those who have been displaced or abused. As a whole, 10% of adolescents have no regular source of health care, and 18% identify local EDs, outpatient clinics, and city clinics as their only source of health care. When adolescents do have a regular physician, it is usually a family practitioner; the remaining are cared for by internists or pediatricians. Unfortunately, studies indicate that most of these primary care physicians perceive themselves to be deficient in experience, knowledge, and training in the care of adolescents.

Adolescents account for approximately 10% to 15% of all ED visits; of these, 13% require acute hospitalization. In one report, 78% of these visits were triaged to the acute and urgent categories. A more recent survey of hospital discharges revealed that more than one-half of all discharges in patients 15 to 24 years of age were a result of pregnancy and its complications, poisoning (substance abuse and suicide gestures/attempts), and trauma (including physical and sexual abuse). Other reasons for ED visits include minor trauma, sexually transmitted infections (STIs), mental health disorders not associated with suicide, and routine visits for acute and chronic illness. There are multiple reasons contributing to an adolescent's choice to seek care in an ED setting. Inexperience, denial, and fear may delay the recognition of disease symptoms and the timely seeking of medical care. The anonymous setting of the ED is often preferred because they can be treated in certain instances without parental consent and are rarely, if ever, refused. Although the adolescent's acute health care needs may be well served this way, proper follow-up, patient education, and recognition of chronic problems may be less than adequate.

Just as children are not just small adults, adolescents are not just large children. Adolescents are prone to a distinct group of diseases and have special medical needs that are much different from those confronted by younger children or adults. Tolmas eloquently listed some important considerations for medical professionals preparing to care for this group of patients: "a knowledge of the growth and developmental tasks that young people address, a personal interest, respect for confidentiality, honesty and pragmatism in all aspects of behavior and conversation, and a genuine attempt to keep from projecting one's own moral code." This chapter addresses these considerations by first briefly reviewing some special considerations in the history and physical examination of adolescents, then, in following sections, focusing on legal rights of adolescents in obtaining health care, adolescents with special health care needs, pregnancy, rape and sexual abuse, and interpersonal violence.

GENERAL CONSIDERATIONS FOR THE HISTORY AND PHYSICAL EXAMINATION

While evaluating the history, it is important to assess the developmental age of the adolescent and not to simply treat the adolescent with a standard approach or strictly on the basis of his or her physical appearance. As for all patients, listening to the adolescent's fears and concerns is extremely important. Taking a moment to establish rapport and eye contact, while demonstrating patience and a caring demeanor, aids in conducting a successful interview. Medical staff may grossly underestimate an adolescent patient's concerns regarding health, because more than 50% of adolescents worry about their health. Teens may avoid seeking appropriate care for social or psychiatric concerns, and psychosocial strain occurring within this period of immense change is often translated into somatic complaints. The reason for the visit is thus often intentionally or unintentionally disguised and presented in conventional or acceptable, nonspecific medical complaints because of the adolescent's fears, embarrassment, or lack of insight. The clinician must always be alert to the possibility of a "hidden agenda," of which the adolescent and his or her family may not be completely aware.

Because nonspecific somatic complaints can be related to pregnancy; sexual, emotional, or physical abuse; mental health disorders; or substance abuse, at some point during the patient evaluation the adolescent should be interviewed without the presence of the parent or other caregiver. The physician must always ensure the patient that confidentiality will be maintained and that openness and honesty between patient and physician is a prerequisite for good medical care.

General questions about the adolescent's home and school life are helpful in assessing overall "wellness" of the teen. Table 130.1 lists the components of the psychosocial interview—Home, Education/Employment, Activities, Drugs, Sexuality, and Suicide (HEADSS)—providing a framework to identify health risk behaviors. Reviewing components of this list may well be pertinent to the chief complaint that brings the teen to the ED. It is important for the adolescent patient to understand the relevance of personal questions to foster both respect and trust. Adolescents who believe that they must keep behaviors, thoughts, or personal identity concerns secret from adult caregivers may be more willing to disclose to an acute care provider who they may see only once. In some EDs, a computer-based survey may be a more comfortable way for adolescents to express their concerns. Once information pertinent to the adolescent's physical and emotional health has been disclosed, it is imperative that a plan for disclosure to the appropriate supportive adults be discussed.

A brief sexual history must be taken for almost every complaint (see Chapters 90 and 93). Interviewers obtain more reliable information if questions are asked in a matter-of-fact but nonleading and open-ended fashion. Adolescents give the "proper" or perceived "desired" answer to such questions to

TABLE 130.1

THE PSYCHOSOCIAL INTERVIEW

Home	Activities	Sexuality
Where and with whom do you live?	What do you do for fun?	Have you ever had sex with someone?
Who is your legal guardian?	Do you have a best friend?	Do you have sex with men or women?
How do you get along with everyone at home?	Group of friends?	How many partners have you had?
Do you feel safe at home?	Who do you talk to about problems?	Are you using birth control?
Education/employment	Have you ever been in trouble with the police?	Have you ever been pregnant?
What school do you attend?	**Drugs**	Do you use condoms every time?
What grade are you in?	Do your friends smoke, drink, or use drugs?	Did anyone ever hurt/scare you?
How are you doing?	Did you ever smoke?	**Suicide**
Did you ever repeat a grade?	Do you drink? How often? How much?	Do you ever feel down?
Are you in a special class/program?		What do you do to feel better?
Do you have a job?		Did you ever feel like hurting yourself?

From Ehrman WG, Matson SC. Approach to assessing adolescents on serious or sensitive issues. *Pediatr Clin North Am* 1998;45:189–204.

gain the provider's acceptance and sympathy; alternatively, they could withhold information for fear of judgment or stigmatization. It is relevant here to note that there are reliable and unreliable personal historians, and it is extraordinarily difficult for the acute care provider to distinguish between the two. Therefore, it is prudent to obtain noninvasive (urine-based) testing for prevalent bacterial sexually transmitted infections (STIs), regardless of personal history. The decision to pursue more invasive examinations, such as speculum or bimanual examinations, should be made after careful consideration of the history, physical examination, and potential sequelae of suspected infections and procedures. Just as a delay in treatment of pelvic inflammatory disease can lead to infertility and chronic pain, a rushed judgment to perform a full pelvic examination on a virginal adolescent can have equally as devastating emotional, and possibly social, sequelae, not the least of which may be a lifelong mistrust of health care providers.

Phenotypic changes associated with puberty were defined and standardized by Tanner in the mid-20th century, using largely Caucasian subjects. In the last two decades, there has been a growing recognition that the timing and progression of physical development can be dramatically affected by genetic, cultural, social, and psychological factors. Thus, the staging of pubertal development is now referred to as sexual maturity rating (SMR), reflective of a broader basis and range of what is accepted as normal. Figures 130.1, 130.2, and 130.3 illustrate the progression of breast and pubic hair development, and Figs. 130.4 and 130.5 are the currently accepted SMR growth charts that reflect growth curves for "early" and "late" bloomers, as well as "normal." Abnormal progression is a sign of underlying pathology, which may be the product of organic disease, social distress, emotional problems, or any combination of these. Abnormal progression almost always requires a thorough evaluation and close follow-up. Therefore, maturity rating becomes important in the evaluation of many adolescent complaints.

LEGAL ISSUES

When caring for a minor patient, it is important for the health care provider to have a basic understanding of the legal and

ethical issues that may arise. Each state has individual provisions; however, the following general discussion applies to most situations.

Consent

There are many exceptions to the requirement that a parent or legal guardian must consent to medical care for a minor before care can be provided. In the emergency setting, it is often

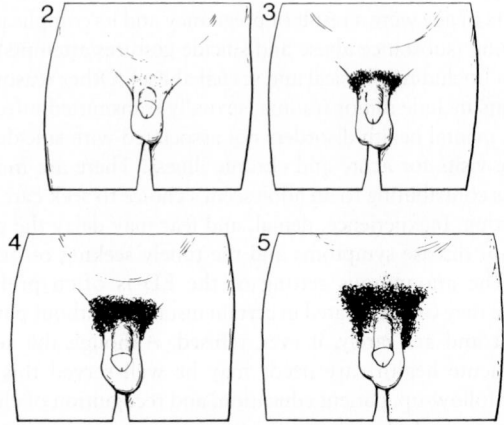

FIGURE 130.1 Stages of pubic hair growth and development of the external genitalia in boys. Numbers in left-hand corner refer to staging according to Tanner. Description of stages of pubic hair: 1, no pubic hair (not shown); 2, long, downy pigmented hair at and lateral to the base of the penis; 3, dark, coarse, curled hair at and lateral to the base of the penis; 4, abundant adult-type sexual hair limited to the pubic region with no extension to the thighs; 5, sexual hair is adult type in quantity and distribution with spread to the medial aspects of the thighs. Description of genitalia stages: 1, prepubertal; 2, enlargement of the testes and scrotum, with pigmentation and thinning of the scrotum; 3, lengthening of the penis, further enlargement of the testes and scrotum; 4, increase in width and length of the penis, further enlargement of the testes and scrotum, increased pigmentation of the scrotum; 5, adult size and shape of genitals. (Modified from Marshall WA, Tanner JM. Variations in patterns of pubertal changes in girls. *Arch Dis Child* 1969;44:291–303; and Root AW. Endocrinology of puberty. I. Normal sexual maturation. *J Pediatr* 1973;83:1–19.)

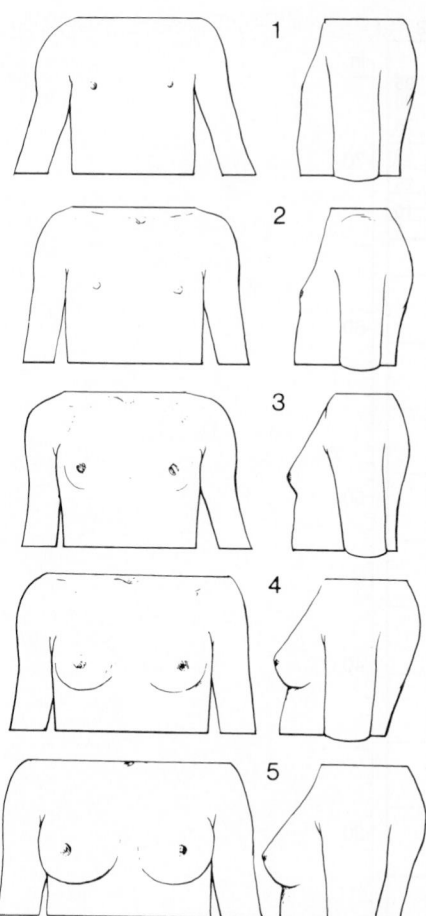

FIGURE 130.2 Stages of breast development in girls. Numbers refer to staging according to Marshall and Tanner. Description of stages: 1, no breast development; 2, breast budding widening of areola and elevation on mound of subareolar tissue, erect papilla; 3, continued enlargement of breast and widening of areola without separation of their contours; 4, areola and papilla project above the plane of enlarging breast; 5, mature breast, areola and breast in same plane, erect papilla. (Modified from Marshall WA, Tanner JM. Variations in patterns of pubertal changes in girls. *Arch Dis Child* 1969;44:291–303; and Root AW. Endocrinology of puberty. I. Normal sexual maturation. *J Pediatr* 1973;83:1–19.)

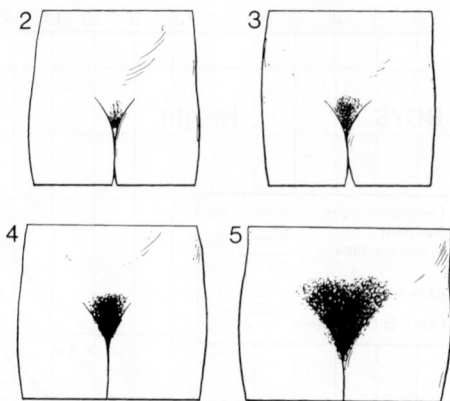

FIGURE 130.3 Stages of pubic hair growth in girls. Numbers in left-hand corner refer to staging according to Marshall and Tanner. Description of stages: 1, no pubic hair (not shown); 2, long, pigmented hair over mons veneris or labia majora; 3, dark, coarse, curled hair spread sparsely over the mons veneris; 4, abundant, adult-type sexual hair limited to the mons veneris; 5, sexual hair is adult type in quantity and distribution with spread to the medial aspect of the thighs. (Modified from Marshall WA, Tanner JM. Variations in patterns of pubertal changes in girls. *Arch Dis Child* 1969;44:291–303; and Root AW. Endocrinology of puberty. I. Normal sexual maturation. *J Pediatr* 1973;83:1–19.)

trine states that a minor may consent to medical care if (i) he or she understands the nature of the proposed treatment and its risks, (ii) the physician believes the patient can give the same informed consent as an adult patient, and (iii) the treatment proposed does not involve very serious risks. It is generally applied to adolescents who are at least 14 years old. There have been no cases in over 30 years in which a parent has successfully sued a treating physician for nonnegligent care of an adolescent without the parent's knowledge. This doctrine must be applied carefully, however, taking each case on an individual basis. As discussed previously, some 14-year olds will be very mature and able to understand the risks and benefits of treatment, whereas some older adolescents may not have the maturity to consent. When obtaining consent from a minor patient, the physician should document the information that led to the judgment that the patient is "mature" in the medical record.

Confidentiality

The practice of confidentiality encourages the adolescent patient to provide an honest history and to begin to take control of his or her own health care. Furthermore, some amount of confidentiality is required by law. In 1996, the Health Insurance Portability and Accountability Act (HIPAA) was passed, which delineates strict guidelines protecting the disclosure of patient information. In general, if a minor is able to legally consent to medical care, then that minor also controls disclosure of information related to that service. Importantly, HIPAA regulations do not overrule state laws that authorize a health care provider to disclose a minor's health information to a parent or guardian. As of this writing, the U.S. Department of Health and Human Services has not issued a final rule related to proposed changes in HIPAA that may affect health care provision to minors.

A private interview with the adolescent patient should be a routine part of the health care provider's approach to all

appropriate to initiate care prior to the arrival of the parent. In addition, there are situations where the minor may be legally able to provide informed consent. Such provisions vary by state, but services covered generally include contraceptive services, pregnancy-related care, diagnosis and treatment of STIs or other reportable diseases, including HIV (human immunodeficiency virus), examination and treatment related to sexual assault, and counseling for alcohol and drug problems. In addition, some mental health services may be included. Finally, minors who have achieved a certain status can consent for care; although the specifics vary by state, they usually include having graduated from high school or having served in the armed services, as well as married minors, minors who have been pregnant or given birth, and minors living independently from their parents.

In addition to specific legal statutes, over the years the "Mature Minor Doctrine" has developed under the common law and has been written into statute in some states. This doc-

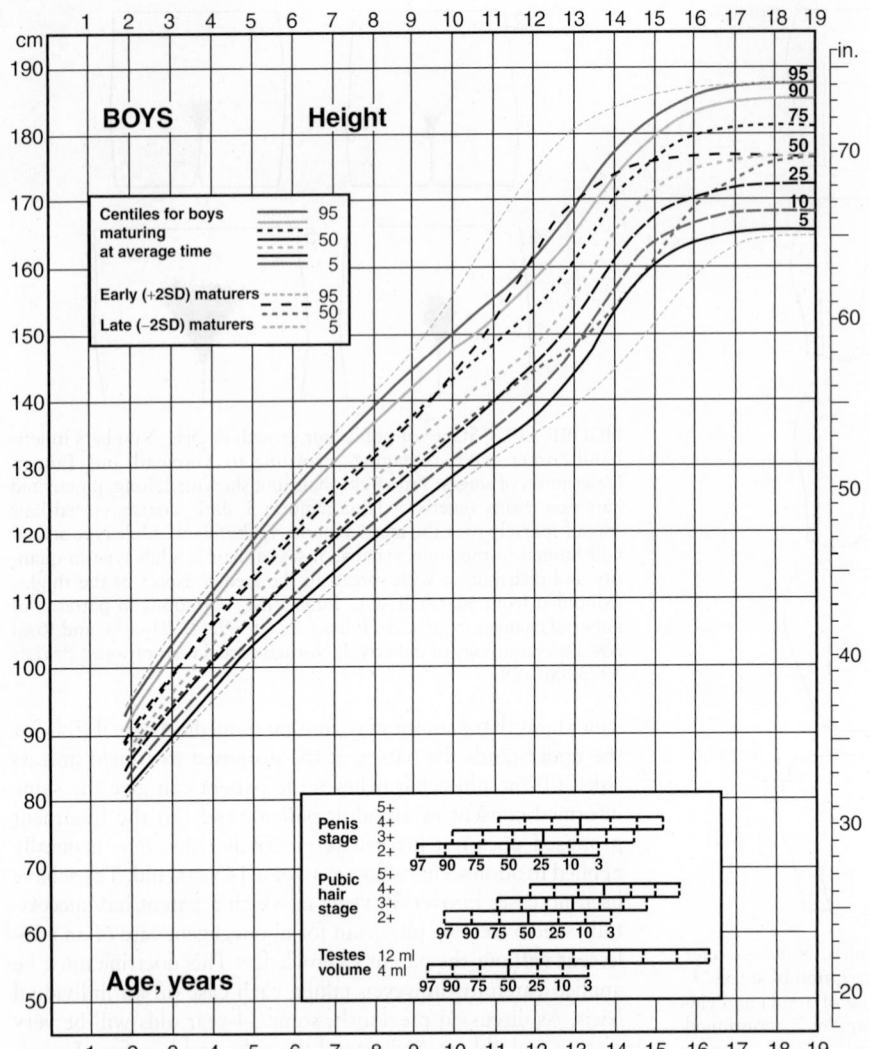

FIGURE 130.4 The currently accepted sexual maturity rating growth chart for boys that reflects growth curves for "early" and "late" bloomers, as well as "normal."

adolescent patients. Confidentiality is best defined at the start of the interview in front of the patient and parent/guardian. The limits of confidentiality, based on local mandated reporter statute, should also be defined at the outset. These limits may include clinical evidence or suspicion of physical abuse, suicidal ideation or intent, and homicidal intent; some states may include the diagnosis of pregnancy or sexually transmitted infections under their definition of "abuse." Thus, confidentiality is not unqualified, and it is critical to maintain up-to-date knowledge of the laws of the state in which one practices. If a teen is in imminent danger, he or she should be informed of the need to disclose this important information to a responsible, caring adult either alone or with the clinician's assistance. The primary physician, social work counselor if available, and appropriate child protective or mental health agency should always be involved to ensure necessary follow-up and community-based services.

Documentation and Payment

Both the release of medical records to a parent or guardian and a bill for services sent to the guardian can effectively breach the adolescent's confidentiality. It may not be necessary to document everything that is learned during an interview with a patient, particularly if it does not directly relate to the patient's chief complaint. In addition, it is advisable to be familiar with the billing procedures and codes of your particular environment so that you can discuss with the patient the likelihood of a parent learning about a health care visit when a bill arrives.

SPECIFIC ISSUES

Patients With Special Health Care Needs

The prevalence of chronic health conditions in adolescents and adults has dramatically increased over the last several decades. The adolescent with special health care needs may face problems as he or she struggles to establish a personal identity and cope with the rigors of chronic illness in family and health care settings that stress compliance and may overemphasize short-term physical health. As individuals with chronic health conditions age to adulthood, they and their families often find that different systems and supports exist once they cross the threshold of their 21st birthday. The new systems may be seen in a

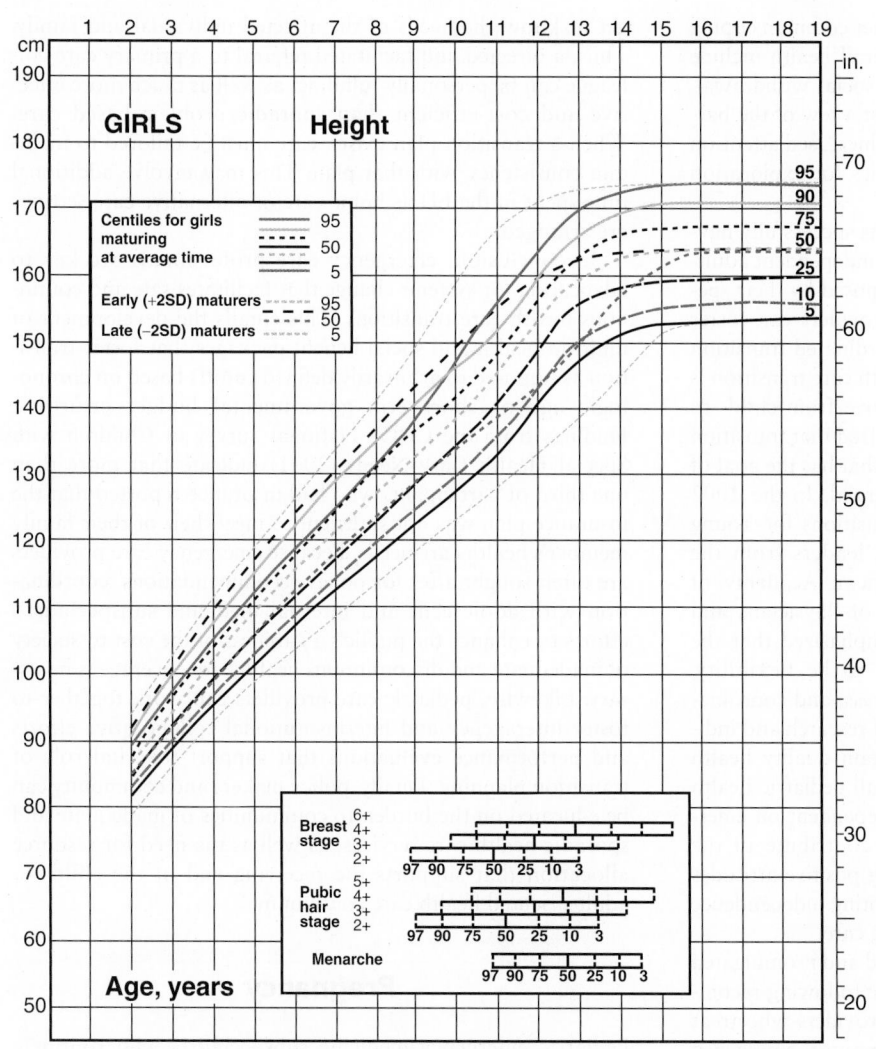

PSYCHOSOCIAL EMERGENCIES

FIGURE 130.5 The currently accepted sexual maturity rating growth chart for girls that reflects growth curves for "early" and "late" bloomers, as well as "normal."

negative light by the patient and the family, due in part to increasing expectations of personal responsibility, facilities that seem less attractive and receptive, and the grief experienced by young adults and their families as they face the loss of lifelong child-oriented care providers and support systems. Interest and research toward understanding how to provide effective and compassionate care to adolescents with chronic health conditions, as well as to promote safe and continuous health care transition, has been a growing focal point in the health literature for the last 20 years. This section focuses on the role of emergency care providers in meeting these goals by first describing the nature of the problem. This is followed by a discussion of developmental and behavioral needs of affected adolescents and of the necessity of coordinated transition planning as it relates to emergency care.

Stein and Silver estimated that 14.8% (10.3 million) of all children in the United States have chronic health conditions. Children with special health care needs are typically defined as those who have, or are at increased risk for, a chronic physical, developmental, behavioral, or emotional condition and who also require health or related services of a type or amount beyond that required by children generally. Adolescents with special health care needs can exhibit a number of developmen-

tal and behavioral sequelae of their functional limitations and increased dependence on family members and health care systems. Because physical growth and pubertal development are often affected, they must struggle with developing a healthy body image at a time when biological, psychological, and societal forces emphasize the importance of being "normal." Furthermore, increased health risks of pregnancy or STI, and limitations of reproductive function and capacity, often interfere with normal risk taking and developing age-appropriate gender roles. Frequent time spent in hospitals or recuperating from acute exacerbations at home limits peer group activities and further curtail opportunities to learn expectations of social behavior. The struggle for autonomy and transition from dependence to independence is almost always affected by special health care needs. Although the duration and intensity of parental and professional supervision may be significantly increased, there is often little else to prevent affected youth from developing behaviors that are counterproductive to health, but may foster a short-term sense of independence or temporarily soothe discordant emotions. There are numerous reports in the adolescent health literature reporting rates of substance abuse and sexually transmitted infections in populations with special health care needs that approach and surpass rates in their nonaffected counterparts. Other common coping behaviors that can contribute to poor overall health include poor adherence with treatment regimens, social withdrawal, and developmental regression. This lists just a few of the barriers faced by this population that demand increased attention to ensuring adequate time and opportunities for exploration and personal growth.

There is no doubt that most young adults successfully navigate adolescence and achieve some level of independent adulthood in spite of the additional burdens imposed by their special health care needs. Emergency care providers can foster success by supporting continuous and coordinated transition to adult roles and health care systems. Health care transition is defined as the purposeful and planned move from child- to adult-oriented care. It has long been recognized that transition is a complex and dynamic lifelong process that has the goal of maximizing lifelong functioning and potential. In the 2002 Consensus Statement on Health Care Transitions for Young Adults with Special Health Care Needs, leaders from the American Academy of Pediatrics, American Academy of Family Physicians, the American College of Physicians and American Society of Internal Medicine emphasized that the core components of effective transition to be flexibility, responsiveness, continuity, comprehensiveness, and coordination. This statement summarized decades of research and indicates that transition is necessary to maintain quality health care, and therefore, must be a priority for all pediatric health care providers. Although not specifically dependent on emergency care providers, any provider can contribute in the process of successful transition by fostering positive attitudes about adult-oriented health care and promoting independence in the young adult patient and coordinating care.

Based on the medical home model created and promulgated by the American Academy of Pediatrics, the following recommendations are made to emergency care providers who treat youth with special care needs. First and foremost, emergency care professionals should maintain a future orientation by proactively asking adolescents about transition plans in regard to work, school, and goals for independence. Asking in this way is usually perceived as supportive. A future-oriented approach can also be emphasized by clearly establishing decision-making roles of the patient and supportive family members. This also fosters a sense that personal independence is a reasonable and desirable objective. Every adolescent and young adult with special care needs should have a primary care provider (PCP) who takes responsibility for coordinating subspecialty care and supports a comprehensive transition plan. Once the patient has been medically stabilized, a member of the emergency care team should attempt to communicate with the PCP. In addition, the patient may possess a portable medical summary and transition plan that can be relied on in determining optimal treatment options and dispositional planning. Researchers from the Centers for Disease Control and Prevention (CDC) reported in 2001 that 1 in 11 (9.3%) children with special health care needs relied on the emergency room as their usual source of care. This proportion surpasses 1 in 10 in many regions of the country, including the upper midwest, west, and southeastern United States. In the absence of an identifiable PCP, there is an opportunity to emphasize the necessity of establishing a medical home and transition plan. Often, emergency care providers establish relationships and

get to know the needs of the affected individual and family. Thus, a directed and facilitated referral to a primary care colleague can be personally fulfilling, as well as much more effective and cost-efficient than sporadic problem-based care. When a transition plan exists, care must be tailored to maintain consistency with that plan. This may involve additional time spent in the ED as home care or alternative care settings are arranged.

In conclusion, emergency care professionals are key to advocating for systems change that facilitates safe and continuous health care transitions. This entails the development of uniform health and social benefit packages that foster transition as opposed to arbitrarily defined cutoffs based on chronologic age or short-term governmental budget priorities. Findings from the CDC's National Survey of Children with Special Health Care Needs (2001) indicate that more than one-third of participants who had insurance reported that the insurance plan was not sufficient to meet their or their family member's health care needs. Because emergency care providers are often sought after for policy recommendations, coordination with adolescent and internal medicine subspecialist's efforts to enhance the public's awareness of the cost to society of inadequate and discontinuous health care coverage is necessary. Likewise, pediatric care providers can work together to foster interagency and interinstitutional collaborative efforts and performance evaluations that support the vital role of transition planning. Finally, policy makers and community can be educated on the burden to communities of inadequate and sporadic health care services, as well as the need for resource allocation that supports the receiving end of the child- to adult-oriented health care continuum.

Pregnancy

Pediatric emergency medicine subspecialists who routinely care for adolescents will frequently evaluate patients for the diagnosis of potential pregnancy and for complications of early pregnancy. Therefore, it is important to possess the necessary knowledge and skills to care for sexually active teenagers and to identify and access appropriate resources to ensure adequate treatment and follow-up. Twenty percent of sexually active teenagers become pregnant yearly, accounting for approximately 750,000 pregnancies. Although many pregnant teenage women may not have intended to become pregnant, several qualitative and quantitative studies report that many of these young women may have desired pregnancy for various reasons. More than one-half (56%) of teenage pregnancies result in a live birth, whereas 30% end in therapeutic abortion, and 14% end in spontaneous abortion.

Clinical Manifestations

The symptoms of pregnancy in teenagers are variable. It should be considered in the differential diagnosis for almost every chief complaint of the postpubertal adolescent girl. In a retrospective review of adolescents found to be pregnant during a visit to a pediatric emergency department (PED), only 8% mentioned pregnancy as part of their chief complaint in triage. Physicians elicited concern for possible pregnancy in only 36% of cases, and 10% of the patients denied sexual activity. Silber and Sadaat noted that the diagnosis of pregnancy was missed in 14% of these teens on their initial visit. Causey and colleagues retrospectively compared adolescents presenting to a general emergency department (GED) who were diagnosed with pregnancy with those in whom the diagnosis was not made during an ED visit but subsequently went on to have a child. They found that 43% presented during the first trimester, 25% in the second trimester, and 33% in the third trimester. Of the 100 patients in whom the diagnosis was not made, one-third of these patients had complaints that were suspicious for pregnancy.

The most common presenting complaint associated with early pregnancy is a missed or abnormal menstrual period. However, the menstrual history is particularly unreliable in teenage women secondary to anovulatory cycles. As many as two-thirds of pregnant teens report a missed period. Other symptoms commonly associated with pregnancy include fatigue, dizziness, breast tenderness, weight gain, nausea, syncope, and morning sickness. Many adolescents report nonspecific complaints related to the gastrointestinal or genitourinary tracts. In the previously described PED study, 77% of pregnant patients complained of gastrointestinal symptoms. Similarly, in the GED study, 91% of patients diagnosed with pregnancy had abdominal or genitourinary complaints. Less commonly, the presenting symptom is associated with complications of early pregnancy, including vaginal bleeding, hyperemesis, hypertension, headache, hyperglycemia, vaginal discharge, or dysuria.

Thus, it is important to consider performing a pregnancy test in peri- and postmenarcheal teenage women. Even if a positive pregnancy test is unrelated to the presenting symptoms, there are several advantages to the patient in identifying pregnancy as early as possible. These include earlier initiation of pregnancy precautions and prenatal care if childbirth is desired, earlier detection of life-threatening complications such as ectopic pregnancy, opportunity for consideration of options such as therapeutic abortion or adoption, and increased time for counseling, regardless of the patient's ultimate choice.

Pregnancy Testing

Urine pregnancy tests use the enzyme-linked immunosorbent assay (ELISA) technique, using a highly specific monoclonal antibody directed against the β-subunit of human chorionic gonadotropin (β-hCG). Following implantation, the trophoblast begins to secrete β-hCG 9 to 11 days following ovulation. Concentration of this hormone doubles approximately every 1 to 3 days, reaching about 100 mIU per mL at the time of the first missed menses. Levels rise rapidly during the early stages of pregnancy, roughly doubling every 2 to 3 days until 6 to 8 weeks' gestation, and then fall gradually and level off by 20 weeks' gestation. Available urine pregnancy kits are qualitative and detect levels of 5 to 50 mIU per mL, which allows the diagnosis of pregnancy to be made 7 days after implantation (10 to 14 days following conception), with a sensitivity of 98%; this timing usually coincides with a missed menses. These tests can be performed in less than 5 minutes and have a false-negative rate of less than 1%. The most common cause of a false-negative test is very early pregnancy, with a β-hCG level below the test's detectable range. Therefore, if pregnancy is suspected, repeat testing should be done in 1 week. Urine pregnancy tests using ELISA are specific to the β-subunit of β-hCG, and generally do not cross-react with structurally similar proteins such as Follicle Stimulating Hormone (FSH) and Leutenizing Hormone (LH). Conditions other than pregnancy that can lead to β-hCG production and a false-positive pregnancy test include choriocarcinoma, embryonal cell carcinoma of the ovary, and neuroendocrine tumors of the lung, adrenal, and liver, and a recent pregnancy loss usually within the last month.

An alternative test is the quantitative β-hCG level, measured on serum samples, employing radioimmunoassay. Quantitative β-hCG testing is expensive and time-consuming and offers no advantage over urine tests in making the diagnosis of uncomplicated pregnancy. However, this test is helpful when complications of pregnancy are suspected. Levels of β-hCG that are abnormally elevated for gestational age may indicate multiple gestation or molar pregnancy. Abnormally low levels, or levels that fail to increase appropriately in the first 8 weeks, may indicate spontaneous abortion or ectopic pregnancy. After delivery or fetal loss beyond the first trimester, the β-hCG level decreases rapidly over 2 weeks, and may be undetectable by urine or serum test by 3 to 4 weeks. Following first trimester loss when the serum concentrations are much higher, β-hCG may be detected for 8 weeks.

Evaluation

Once the diagnosis of pregnancy has been determined, goals of the ED evaluation include (i) dating the pregnancy, (ii) recognizing symptoms that require immediate referral for obstetric or gynecologic evaluation, (iii) identifying and treating presenting and potential nonsurgical complications, (iv) assessing chronic medical conditions, (v) providing appropriate counseling, and (vi) securing appropriate and timely follow-up.

The Nagele rule can be used to establish the estimated date of confinement if the date of the last menstrual period is known and the teen has regular periods. To use this rule, add 7 days to the first day of the last menstrual period, subtract 3 months, and add 1 year. A bimanual examination is indicated to determine uterine size and to assess the integrity of the cervical os. The uterus is enlarged to the size of an orange at 8 weeks' gestation, and at 12 weeks is palpable just above the pelvic brim. The fundus reaches the umbilicus by 20 weeks.

Key components of the history, physical examination, and laboratory examination for all teenagers diagnosed with pregnancy are reviewed in Table 130.2. In the ED, it is imperative to recognize those patients who are immediately at risk for life-threatening complications and require acute resuscitation and emergent evaluation by a surgical subspecialist. Figure 130.6 describes an overall approach to teens with possible pregnancy. It is imperative that both the medical and psychosocial aspects of the diagnosis be addressed.

Pregnant patients who present with vaginal bleeding, with or without abdominal pain, represent a high-risk group. First-trimester vaginal bleeding occurs in 20% to 25% of patients. Common etiologies include ectopic pregnancy, spontaneous and incomplete abortion, missed or threatened abortion, STI, and trauma. The initial laboratory workup should always include a complete blood count, both to assess the amount of blood loss and to provide a baseline if bleeding continues. A urinalysis can detect the presence of white blood cells, bacteria, glucose, or protein. Other laboratory screening tests that are rarely indicated during an ED evaluation include Papanicolaou smear, syphilis serology, HIV testing, rubella

TABLE 130.2

EVALUATION OF THE TEEN WITH
SUSPECTED PREGNANCY

History
Date of last menstrual period (date of conception)
Contraceptive use
Previous sexually transmitted disease
Previous upper genital tract infection or surgery
Gravity, parity, previous abortion
History of previous ectopic pregnancy
Lower abdominal pain
Vaginal bleeding, discharge, dysuria
Vomiting, diarrhea
Past medical history
Medications
Allergy

Physical examination
Vital signs
Abdominal examination/fundal height
Pelvic examination/uterine size (first trimester)

Laboratory tests
Urine β-hCG
Baseline serum quantitative β-hCG (if uterine size discordant
  with dates)
Urinalysis
CBC, RPR
Testing for *Neisseria gonorrheae* and *Chlamydia trachomatis*
Wet mount (*Trichomonas vaginalis*, presence of WBCs)
Pelvic/transvaginal ultrasound

hCG, human chorionic gonadotropin; CBC, complete blood count;
RPR, rapid plasma reagent, WBCs, white blood cells.

serology, and hepatitis B serology. If unknown, Rh determination is indicated if there is uterine bleeding. It is important to note that Rh-negative teens with pregnancies greater than 8 weeks' gestation should receive Rh immunoglobulin if there is risk of fetal or placental blood loss.

Ectopic pregnancy is the leading cause of maternal mortality in the United States during the first half of pregnancy; therefore, timely recognition and treatment is imperative. The prevalence of ectopic pregnancy among women presenting to an ED with first trimester bleeding and/or pain ranges from 6% to 16%. The CDC has reported that the overall mortality from ectopic pregnancy fell from 35.5 to 5.4 deaths per 10,000 ectopic pregnancies from 1970 to 1988, attributed to improvements in earlier diagnosis and treatment. Although the overall incidence of ectopic pregnancy in teenagers is low, this group has the highest mortality rate, largely due to a tendency to delay seeking care. Risk factors for ectopic pregnancy include prior ectopic pregnancy, tubal abnormalities, prior upper genital tract infection, and assisted reproduction. The use of intrauterine devices does not increase the risk of ectopic pregnancies. Their use has been associated with ectopic pregnancies because they are effective in preventing intrauterine pregnancies. In the rare occasion that implantation does occur, it is more likely to be in an ectopic location.

The diagnosis of ectopic pregnancy must be considered in any patient with vaginal bleeding and/or abdominal pain. Patients can present with a wide spectrum of symptoms, including abnormal vaginal bleeding; intermittent crampy,

lower abdominal pain; or acute abdominal pain associated with shock (with or without vaginal blood loss). Fortunately, with the development of sensitive urine pregnancy tests, most patients with ectopic pregnancy present before rupture has occurred. The approach to these more stable patients includes subspecialty consultation, quantitative serum β-hCG levels, serum progesterone levels, abdominal and/or transvaginal ultrasound, and close follow-up. In a normal singleton pregnancy, serial serum β-hCG levels should increase by 67% every 48 hours during the first month of pregnancy. Levels that do not rise or rise more slowly than expected are indicative of an abnormal pregnancy (usually an ectopic pregnancy or a pregnancy that is destined to spontaneously abort). Serum progesterone levels may play some role in the diagnosis of normal versus abnormal pregnancy. A progesterone level greater than 25 ng per dL is seen in 95% of normal pregnancies; a level less than 5 ng per dL suggests an abnormal pregnancy. Ultrasound is used to visualize the uterine cavity to assess for the presence of a gestational sac. When the β-hCG level reaches the discriminatory zone (a level that varies based on local transvaginal ultrasound expertise), a gestational sac should be visible within the uterus. If no sac is seen, the pregnancy is presumed to be ectopic.

Therapeutic options at this point include curettage or medical termination with methotrexate or etoposide therapy, both chemotherapeutic agents. For patients undergoing curettage, the diagnosis of ectopic pregnancy can be confirmed by a lack of villi on pathologic specimens or by a fall in β-hCG levels 12 to 24 hours after the procedure. Emergency laparoscopy is indicated for patients in whom there is concern about hemodynamic stability or correct diagnosis, or in those with gestational sacs greater than 4 cm or hCG levels greater than 10,000 mIU per ng. Conservative medical management may be appropriate in adolescents who are stable; have no evidence of any bleeding; and have a hemoglobin of greater than 8 g per dL and a gestational sac less than 4 cm, without immunocompromise, bleeding diathesis, liver, or renal disease, providing that close follow-up can be secured. As many as 83% of patients meeting these criteria may experience spontaneous abortion and resorption. Methotrexate given as a single 50 mg per m² intramuscular shot results in successful involution of the pregnancy in 95% of cases. Slaughter and Grimes demonstrated a 92% cure rate in outpatient candidates using methotrexate therapy, with only 5% to 16% requiring a second dose. Lipscomb demonstrated a success rate of 94% when hCG levels were less than 10,000 mIU per ng. The side effects of this therapy are generally mild and self-limited. However, tubal rupture has been reported in 3% to 4% of cases. Thus, thorough discharge instructions along with close follow-up are very important.

Although less common, those presenting with an acutely ruptured ectopic pregnancy have an immediate life-threatening condition. These patients usually have a history of abnormal vaginal bleeding and intermittent pelvic pain. On physical examination, vital signs may reflect compensated or uncompensated shock, the abdomen is tender, the uterus is tender and may be slightly enlarged, and an adnexal mass may or may not be palpated after rupture has occurred. These patients require immediate subspecialty consultation with either gynecology or pediatric surgery, depending on the care setting. They should have continuous vital sign monitoring, fluid resuscitation with normal saline, and packed red blood cells as needed. Serial

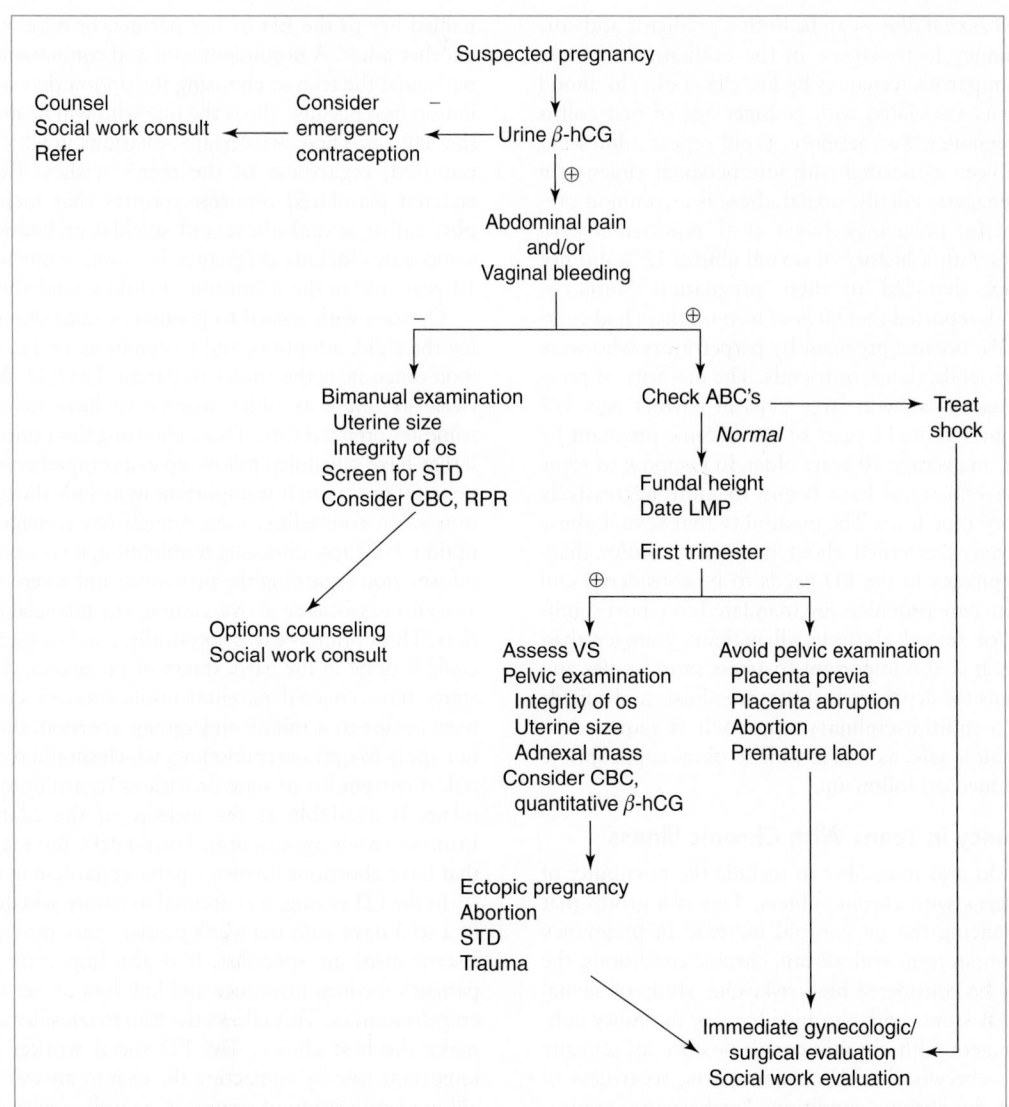

FIGURE 130.6 General approach to the pregnant teen. (From Mollen CJ, Pletcher J, Lavelle J. Emergency department management of teen pregnancy. *Clin Pediatr Emerg Med* 2002;4:61.). hCG, human chorionic gonadotropin; ABCs, airway breathing circulation: LMP, last menstrual period; VS, vital sign; STD, sexually transmitted disease; CBC, complete blood count; RPR, rapid plasma reagent.

hemoglobin determination, coagulation profile, Rh screening, and type and cross are important components of the laboratory evaluation. Emergency surgical evaluation is the treatment of choice. Ultrasound is contraindicated in the unstable patient and may delay surgical intervention.

Spontaneous abortion is another cause of vaginal bleeding in the pregnant teenager, which can be septic, threatened (or missed), inevitable, or complete. Spontaneous miscarriage is very common in early pregnancy, up to one-half of all fertilized ova that implant into the endometrium are lost. Most spontaneous abortions occur during the first trimester, although a small number occur after 20 weeks' gestation. Vaginal bleeding can indicate threatened abortion, when the patient's external cervical os is closed, or an inevitable abortion, when the external os is open. If products of conception are found in the vaginal vault of a patient with an inevitable abortion, the abortion is incomplete. Uterine curettage or

vacuum aspiration may be indicated if bleeding is heavy and life-threatening, or if the patient desires to discontinue the pregnancy. The diagnosis of a complete abortion is made if an intact gestational sac is present following uterine curettage, or if there is reversion to a negative β-hCG.

Sexually transmitted infections should be considered in all pregnant teens. Screening for *Chlamydia trachomatis* and *Neisseria gonorrhoeae* can be accomplished using polymerase chain reaction (PCR) or ligase chain reaction (LCR) technology on a dirty urine specimen. A blind high vaginal swab for wet mount and Gram stain can be used to identify the presence of trichomonads and white blood cells. Trichomoniasis also is best detected by performing rapid antigen or PCR testing on a vaginal swab. When vaginal blood is present, a speculum examination is necessary to identify the site of bleeding. A bimanual examination detects the presence of upper genital tenderness, uterine size and presence of abnormal mass or fullness.

Physical and sexual abuse can be both a predictor and correlate of pregnancy in teenagers. In the evaluation of more than 1,000 primiparous teenagers by Fiscella et al., childhood sexual abuse was associated with younger age of first coitus and of first pregnancy. Furthermore, rapid repeat adolescent pregnancy has been associated with interpersonal violence in low-income teenagers. Finally, sexual abuse is a common precipitating event for pregnancy. Boyer et al. reported that of 295 adolescents with a history of sexual abuse, 12% did not consent to sex that led to their pregnancy. Similarly, Gershenson et al. reported that 60% of teen mothers had coercive sex and 23% became pregnant by perpetrators who were most often boyfriends, dates, or friends. The majority of pregnancies were associated with large gaps in partner age. For example, teen girls 11 to 12 years of age became pregnant by boys who were on average 10 years older. In response to some of this data, several states have begun to more aggressively enforce statutory rape laws. The possibility that sexual abuse may exist in teens concerned about pregnancy and/or diagnosed with pregnancy in the ED needs to be considered and explored. Health care providers are mandated to report significant concern for sexual abuse in all patients younger than 18 years of age. It is also important to assess safety issues and screen these teens for depression, substance abuse, and suicide risk. Usually, a multidisciplinary approach is required to ensure the patient is safe, as well as able to obtain appropriate counseling and medical follow-up.

Pregnancy in Teens With Chronic Illness

Physicians should also remember to include the possibility of pregnancy in teens with chronic illness. This is a group that may be experiencing the most rapid increase in pregnancy rates. In addition, in teens with certain chronic conditions, the pregnancy may be considered high risk. One study of sexual behaviors in adolescents with chronic illness or disability indicates that teenagers with chronic conditions are as sexually active as their otherwise healthy counterparts, regardless of the visibility of the chronic condition. Furthermore, contraception may be less effective in teenagers with chronic illness for multiple reasons.

Counseling and Legal Issues

Counseling the teen regarding the options for pregnancy may be the most important part of the visit. In the changing, demanding environment of the ED, it is important to secure a quiet, focused time. This is best done using a multidisciplinary team comprised of physicians, nurses, and social workers. The social worker plays a crucial role in providing continuous support, identifying important social and mental health concerns and important outpatient resources, and providing ongoing dialog throughout the ED visit.

Confidentiality should be maintained throughout the visit to encourage autonomy, protect privacy, promote necessary medical follow-up, and guard the teen from any physical harm or humiliation that may result from disclosing pregnancy status to family member. The results of the test are best initially shared with the adolescent alone. At this time, the practitioner has the opportunity to encourage the teen to share the information with a trusted adult friend who can offer support and assistance to the teen in necessary follow-up. The teen may choose to share this information with those that have accom-

panied her to the ED or her partner, or may want to contact another adult. A nonjudgmental and compassionate approach will assist the teen in choosing the option that suits her life situation best because she is the one who will be most affected by that choice. There are certain situations in which disclosure is required, regardless of the teen's wishes. Every state has enacted mandated reporter statutes that include suspected physical or sexual abuse and suicidal or homicidal ideation; some states include pregnancy in young women younger than 13 years old in the definition of child sexual abuse.

Options with regard to pregnancy outcome include parenting the child, adoption, and termination. By far, the most common outcome is the choice to parent the child. Adolescents are twice as likely as older women to have no or only third-trimester prenatal care. Those choosing this option will fare best if they have scheduled follow-up in a comprehensive, teen-based prenatal program. It is important to include the option of adoption when counseling, even though few teenagers choose this option. For those choosing termination, it is essential to provide information regarding the procedure and where it can be done, as well as assistance in overcoming any financial and social barriers. This option is easier physically, psychologically, and financially if done in the early stages of pregnancy. Although many states have enacted parental notification or consent requirements prior to a minor undergoing abortion, these statutes do not apply to options counseling, which should remain confidential. A current list of state provisions regarding specific requirements is available at the website of the Alan Guttmacher Institute (www.agi-usa.org). Fortunately, the majority of teens that have abortions involve a parent/guardian in this process.

In the ED setting, it is optimal to ensure scheduled follow-up in 2 to 3 days with the teen's primary care provider or an adolescent medicine specialist. It is also important to review the patient's medical insurance and link him or her to eligible coverage/resources. This allows the teen to consider all options and make the best choice. The ED social worker also plays an important role by contacting the teen to answer questions and aid in identification of resources, as well as ensuring follow-up. Forman et al. prospectively followed 96 diagnosed teen pregnancies and found that the time to referral appointment was significantly shorter for patients who planned to terminate their pregnancy, compared with those who planned to continue it. The need to arrange close follow-up and to facilitate connection to care following the ED visit should not be underestimated.

Adolescents With Negative Pregnancy Tests

Those teens that present with concern for possible pregnancy, but whose pregnancy tests are negative, represent a group at higher risk for future pregnancy and STI acquisition. Intervention in the ED should include evaluation for STIs, as well as counseling regarding effective birth control and emergency contraception (EC). These patients benefit from a social work evaluation with focus on the teen's home environment, need for mental health services, medical insurance, and access to health care. Approximately, one-third of adolescents presenting to a clinic setting requesting a pregnancy test are pregnant. Almost three in every five teens had a negative pregnancy test result at a clinic before ever becoming pregnant. Further, at least one-half of these teens are not using effective birth control. The majority feel positive or ambivalent with regard to becoming pregnant, 15% may actively try to conceive, and 50% believe their partner wants them to become pregnant. Overall, 56% of teens who initially test negative will become pregnant over the following 18 months. Obviously, pregnancy prevention requires a comprehensive, longitudinal program; however, education can begin during the ED visit and an effort can be made to link the teen with an effective health care program.

Emergency Contraception

More recently, the U.S. Food and Drug Administration (FDA) declared that using a combination of ethinyl estradiol and levonorgestrel, or levonorgestrel alone, to be safe and effective forms of emergency contraceptive. In 1998, Preven was approved by the FDA and includes a pregnancy test, four Ovral® tablets (each containing 0.05 mg ethinyl estradiol and 0.5 mg norgestrel), two tablets to be taken 12 hours apart, along with instructions. In 1999, a dedicated progestin-only product (Plan B®) was approved, which includes two tablets of 1.5 mg norgestrel. Initial labeling indicated the tablets to be taken 12 hours apart, but recently that was changed to give both tablets at once and now has been updated to give one 1.5 mg tablet × 1 dose. Both regimens should be given within 120 hours of unprotected intercourse. Two years ago, the FDA approved the nonprescription sale of Plan B to anyone older than 17 years.

There are very few side effects to the use of emergency contraception. Nausea, less commonly seen in patients using the progestin-only method, can be relieved by prescribing an antiemetic 1 hour prior to each dose. Ninety-eight percent of women will have withdrawal bleeding by 3 weeks; if this does not occur, a follow-up pregnancy test is required. Contraindications for the combined method are the same as those for combined oral contraceptive use. Contraindications for the progestin-only method include pregnancy, undiagnosed vaginal bleeding, and allergy. Pregnancy is considered a contraindication simply because if pregnant, the medication will not work, not because its use will impose any risk to the fetus. Use of the combined regimen results in approximately 75% reduction of pregnancy. The use of the progestin-only method results in an 89% reduction. The mechanism of action is presumed to be delay or inhibition in ovulation, or decrease in tubal motility.

Employing a telephone survey, Delbanco et al. found that only 23% of teens were aware that anything could be done to prevent pregnancy after unprotected sex. Of those teens who did have some knowledge of it, 32% did not know that a prescription was required and 78% underestimated the length of time after unprotected sex that this method would be effective. However, after hearing about this option, two-thirds of the teens stated they would likely use them. Todd and colleagues found that almost one-third of women younger than 18 years of age, presenting to an urban ED, had an unintended pregnancy risk, thus the option of EC may be underutilized. Providers should document the date of the last menstrual period, the time/times of intercourse, use of other methods of contraception, symptoms of pregnancy, any contraindications that the patient may have for this therapy, and the results of a urine pregnancy test. Knowledge regarding this safe and effective method of pregnancy prevention is important to health providers routinely caring for adolescents.

Delivery

Patients presenting to the ED in active labor should be transferred to the obstetrical unit as soon as possible. However, even in a PED, patients have presented when the newborn is crowning, making transfer impossible. Fortunately, the majority of deliveries occur spontaneously, and the primary role of the clinician is to control the process. However, a subspecialist should be called to the ED to deliver the newborn whenever possible.

All EDs should have the necessary equipment for this procedure, which includes surgical scissors, three hemostats, a cord clamp, a bulb syringe, sterile sponges, sterile towels, a basin, and povidine–iodine solution. Warm blankets, a warmed isolette, and neonatal resuscitation equipment are also needed. If possible, document date of the last menstrual period, the estimated date of conception, prenatal care, significant health problems, current medications, the time the contractions began and the interval between them, and whether membranes have ruptured. Examine the perineum for bleeding, prolapsed cord, crowning, or fetal parts. If there is significant vaginal bleeding, avoid cervical examination so as not to precipitate bleeding if the patient has a placenta previa. If there is no significant bleeding, cleanse the vaginal area, and using a sterile gloved hand, assess degree of cervical dilation and effacement. When there is complete cervical dilation (10 cm) and effacement (thin, flat cervix), and the head is at the perineum, delivery is imminent. As the head advances place one hand on the suboccipital area of the infant's head to control the speed of delivery, with the other hand apply moderate upward pressure to the fetal chin to decrease perineal injury. Gently suction the nose and mouth of the infant. Check for the presence of a nuchal cord, and gently slip it over the infant's head. If this is not possible, the cord should be clamped in two places and cut in between these clamps to avoid anoxia. Gentle downward traction of the head assists delivery of the anterior shoulder followed by upward traction to deliver the posterior shoulder. Control the remainder of the delivery, then hold the infant with the head down at a 15-degree angle for approximately 1 minute, allowing for secretion drainage and a small blood transfusion from the placenta. The umbilical cord is then clamped and cut, and the infant can be handed off to another clinician. The placenta usually spontaneously delivers within 5 to 30 minutes; palpate the uterus afterward to stimulate contractions and reduce blood loss. The mother should be transferred to an obstetrical unit as soon as possible.

Rape/Sexual Assault

Rape is defined as genital contact without consent, through use or threat of use of force or fraud, or when the victim is unable to give consent because of physical or mental disability. Statutory rape is intercourse with a female younger than the age of consent, which is considered to be 16 years in most states. The term *incest* applies to the situation in which the assailant and victim are related, and therefore, could not legally marry or have a functional situation simulating this relationship. *Sexual abuse* or *molestation,* a broader term, is involvement of the adolescent in activities that he or she does not fully comprehend. These include exhibitionism, fondling, oral–genital contact, and rectal or vaginal penetration. Incest is probably the most common form of adolescent abuse, and is the most underreported and difficult to prove.

Females of ages 12 to 24 years are at the greatest risk for experiencing a rape or sexual assault. More than one-half of all rapes of women occur before age 18 years; 22% occur before age 12 years. Fewer than one-half (48%) of all rapes and sexual assaults are reported to the police; these represent the tip of the iceberg. According to the 2007 Youth Risk Behavior Surveillance System (YRBSS), 7.8% of students had been forced to have sexual intercourse. Female students (11.3%) were significantly more likely than male students (4.5%) to have been forced to have sexual intercourse. Black students (10.5%) were more likely than white students (7.0%) to have been forced to have sexual intercourse. According to the 2000 National Crime Victimization Survey, 62% of rape and sexual assault victims knew the perpetrator. More than 40% of rapes and sexual assaults came at the hands of a person the female victim called a friend or acquaintance.

Due to the magnitude of this problem in the pediatric age group, the pediatric emergency physician should develop skills in treating these patients. In many cities, Sexual Assault Response Teams have been developed to provide comprehensive and consistent care to these patients. Physicians practicing in a particular area must be knowledgeable of the state laws regarding the care of adolescents.

Clinical Manifestations

Adolescent victims present in one of the following two ways: (i) following an acute event with an unknown perpetrator, or (ii) after acute stress when an incestuous relationship is revealed. All patients who have been assaulted within the previous 72 hours or those with symptoms should be evaluated on an emergency basis. Asymptomatic patients with ongoing chronic abuse (not occurring in the preceding 72 hours) can be scheduled in special outpatient clinics designed to care for this particular group. These patients benefit from a multidisciplinary approach, including physicians, social workers, nurses, and psychologists, to provide optimal care. SANE (sexual assault nurse examiner) programs have been very successful in providing standardized evaluation and evidence collection in these patients. The aim of the acute intervention is to obtain the details of the incident, perform a complete medical evaluation, collect medicolegal evidence, and provide appropriate medical and psychological follow-up. The acute intervention is not intended to ascertain whether a crime was committed. All suspected cases of abuse/rape must be reported to the police.

Evaluation and Management

Consent for interview, examination, and collection of evidence should be obtained from the victim. Accurate and thorough records are of the utmost importance. The victim should be given control of the situation and has the right to terminate the process at any point. A supportive female or male, or ideally an experienced rape counselor/nurse, should be present throughout the interview and examination. The patient should be placed in a secluded, quiet room as soon as possible after arrival.

The history should include the details of the event, including time and place; the details of the sexual acts (including whether oral, rectal, or vaginal penetration occurred); whether ejaculation occurred; the force or threat that was used by the assailant; the name and relationship of the perpetrator; and the associated use of alcohol, drugs, or weapons. Hygiene, including bathing, douche, or change of clothes after the event, should be recorded. Medical history, including menstrual his-

tory, sexual activity, previous history of STIs, birth control use, last intercourse, previous obstetric and gynecologic history, and history of health problems, should be documented.

As many as 46% of victims have nongenital injuries, with as many as 15% of them requiring therapy and follow-up. Up to 80% of victims have minor genital injuries, most of which are external and involve the posterior fourchette. These observations emphasize the need for a complete, careful examination. However, the presence of a normal examination does not imply that assault did not occur. Photographs should be taken with the victim's consent, whenever possible. However, the taking of photographs does not preclude careful, descriptive documentation of existing injuries on the patient's chart.

The physician should explain the parts of the examination before performing them to allow the patient to assume control and to alleviate as much anxiety as possible. A chaperone should always be present. A complete physical examination to assess for bruises, scratches, and SMR is needed. To prevent cross-contamination, the examiner should wear gloves and change them as often as needed.

There are a few general rules to consider when collecting forensic evidence. When in doubt, always collect the specimen for evaluation. Always air-dry the swabs used to collect the evidence. Place specimens in glass or paper containers for transfer. Do not lick the envelopes, and be careful when touching items that may have fingerprints. Core evidence includes cotton Q-tip swabs from the oral cavity, the vaginal vault, and the anus.

A description of the patient's general appearance and emotional status, as well as a description of clothing condition, begins the physical examination. The patient should undress while standing on a clean sheet. Each article of clothing is then placed in a separate, labeled, paper bag. The sheet that the patient stood on is also submitted as evidence. Describe all injuries, noting size, location, and color.

Comb the patient's hair over a clean sheet of paper to collect any debris/assailant hair, fold the paper, and place it in a labeled envelope. If there is history or evidence of oral trauma, a swab from the gum line and buccal mucosa can also be evaluated for the presence of sperm. Next, the victim should be asked to chew on a piece of filter paper or a cotton ball to obtain a sample of saliva. Eighty percent of people secrete blood group antigens in their saliva, sweat, and other body fluids.

Stains on the skin should be swabbed with saline-moistened swabs and stored in dry, labeled test tubes. These should be air-dried and placed in labeled glass tubes. The use of a blue light source may aid in identifying areas that should be swabbed and sent for forensic analysis. Debris under the fingernails should be removed with a wooden curette and placed in a labeled envelope. A careful external examination is paramount, and then the hymen and the posterior fourchette should be carefully inspected for areas of laceration. Matted pubic hair should be removed, and the remaining pubic hair gently combed into a labeled envelope.

The decision to perform and how to perform a speculum examination should be given careful thought. Although speculum examinations are almost never indicated on prepubertal females after assault, they are more commonly conducted in adolescents. However, the examination should always be preceded by clear and precise instructions about what the process will entail, as this may be the first time an adolescent female has an internal examination. Moreover, the decision to perform a speculum examination becomes even more difficult if the patient is developmentally delayed. Given that the patient has already experienced significant trauma by virtue of being a victim of sexual assault, it may be necessary to perform the examination with the patient sedated to avoid any additional emotional or psychological trauma.

A speculum examination is indicated to assess for the presence of vaginal and cervical trauma. Avoid lubricants because they affect both sperm motility and culture results. If secretions are present in the posterior fornix, aspirate it and place it in a sterile container for sperm and acid phosphatase detection. Cotton swabbings taken from the posterior fornix should be used to make slides for detection of motile sperm, acid phosphatase, and blood group antigens. Vaginal swabs for wet mount and Gram stain should also be obtained. The remainder of the pelvic examination is completed in the usual manner. The rectum should be carefully examined. Some centers use colposcopy to identify and photograph genital injury.

Between 4% and 30% of rape victims contract STIs as a result of the victimization. Studies have shown that 2% to 12% of adolescents at the initial visit have gonorrhea, and 1.5% to 10% have chlamydia. On follow-up visit, 1% to 3% have positive cultures. The risk of *Trichomonas* and bacterial vaginosis range from 5% to 25%. Therefore, evaluation for STIs and prophylactic treatment is indicated (Table 130.3). The risk of human papillomavirus is unknown; however, the proportion of patients having abnormal Papanicolaou smears ranges from 3% to 27%. The risk of herpes simplex virus, syphilis, and HIV is low. Laboratory evaluation includes culture/LCR for chlamydia and gonorrhea, and vaginal specimens for trichomoniasis. Serum is sent for blood type, DNA identification, drug testing, syphilis, hepatitis B if the patient is not fully immunized, and HIV testing. Urine and serum for drug evaluation should be considered.

Follow-up of the patient 7 days after the initial examination is recommended by the CDC for repeat urine or vaginal

TABLE 130.3

PROPHYLAXIS OF ADOLESCENTS FOLLOWING SEXUAL ASSAULT

Chlamydia trachomatis	Azithromycin 1 g po once Doxycycline 100 mg po bid for 7 days
Neisseria gonorrhoeae	Ceftriaxone 125 mg IM/IV once
Trichomonas	Metronidazole 2 g po once Cefixime 400 mg po once Metronidazole 500 mg po for 7 days
Hepatitis B	Give vaccine if patient not fully immunized
HIV	Consider prophylaxis
Emergency contraception	

bid, twice a day; HIV, human immunodeficiency virus; IM, intramuscular; IV, intravenous; po, orally.
From Centers for Disease Control and Prevention. Sexually transmitted treatment guidelines 2002. *MMWR Morbid Mortal Wkly Rep* 2002;51(RR-6):1–77.

specimens for gonorrhea, chlamydia, and *Trichomonas*. A test for syphilis should be repeated at 6 to 8 weeks. Testing for HIV is done again at 3 to 6 months after the incident, and if negative, again at 1 year. The risk of transmission after a single sexual assault is very low. Prophylaxis may be considered for patients presenting within 48 hours of the assault.

All patients should have a pregnancy test performed. Pregnancy occurs as a result of rape in 1% of victims. If the patient is not at risk for early pregnancy, a protocol for pregnancy prevention may be followed. This treatment should be given within 120 hours of the event.

A list of the comprehensive list of the evidence collected should be included in the patient's medical record. All specimens should be labeled carefully with the patient's name, medical record number, date and time of evidence collection, the location from which the evidence was collected, and the examiner's name and signature. Transfer of custody must be documented with the name of the person receiving the evidence and the date and the time of transfer.

Finally, all patients should have scheduled medical and psychological follow-up before discharge from the ED.

Interpersonal Violence: Detection and Intervention

Interpersonal violence has reached epidemic proportions in the United States, and adolescents are at particularly high risk for violence-related injuries. Homicide is the second leading cause of death for 15- to 19-year olds, and the CDC estimates the ratio of nonfatal injuries from physical assaults to homicides as 90:1. According to the 2007 YRBSS, 35% reported being in a fight in the last year and 18% reported carrying a weapon. Violence is not limited to the inner city; one study reported that 89% of students in a suburban middle school knew someone who had been robbed, beaten, stabbed, shot, or murdered, and 57% had witnessed such an event. In addition to physical injuries, youth involved in interpersonal violence are at risk for posttraumatic stress disorder, major depression, and substance abuse.

Multiple studies have helped refine the risk factors for violent injury; knowledge of these risk factors can assist the clinician in obtaining an appropriate screening history. Several key risk factors include a prior history of fighting, failing in school or having dropped out of school, and substance use. Other risk factors include weapon carrying, witnessing violence (in the home, in the community, through the media), lack of school "connectedness," depression, and quick temper. Although few studies have described effective screening tools for interpersonal violence, the emergency medicine physician can roughly gauge a youth's risk for future violent injury by inquiring about the risk factors described previously. Any adolescent being treated for a violent injury should be screened for future risk, with social work and community referrals available as needed. In the hectic environment of the ED, it is not always feasible to provide appropriate counseling for risk reduction; instead, knowledge of available community resources and linking the patient back to the PCP are key interventions.

More specifically, the American Academy of Pediatrics Task Force on Adolescent Assault Victim Needs outlines appropriate care for the victims of interpersonal violence. After stabilizing and treating the patient's injuries, the guidelines recommend providing a thorough social work evaluation and determining appropriate follow-up, notifying the police when appropriate, and providing support for the patient's family and friends. In addition, the emergency physician should assess the risk of retaliation, both for the safety of the patient and the safety of the others involved in the incident, and be prepared to intervene if retaliation seems imminent (through the police or community resources).

CONCLUSION

The care of adolescents is both challenging and rewarding. They present to the ED with a wide spectrum of diseases and often require gynecologic evaluation and referral, crisis intervention, and medical or psychological follow-up. Thus, the ED should design an organized approach to the care of the adolescent patient.

Suggested Readings

Growth (Weight and Height Velocity) Standards

Tanner JM, Davies PS. Clinical longitudinal standards for height and height velocity for North American children. *J Pediatr* 1985;107:317.

Pubertal Delay

Fenichel P. Delayed puberty. *Endocr Dev* 2004;7:106–28.
Hoffman B, Bradshaw KD. Delayed puberty and amennorhea. *Hor Res* 2003;60(suppl 3):35–48.

Confidentiality/Consent/legal Issues

American Academy of Pediatrics Committee on Adolescence. Achieving quality health services for adolescents. *Pediatrics* 2008;121:1263–1270.
American Psychiatric Association. *Diagnostic and statistical manual of mental disorders, fourth edition, text revision (DSM-IV-TR®).* Washington, DC: American Psychiatric Association, 2000.
English A. Sexual and reproductive health care for adolescents: legal rights and policy challenges. *Adolesc Med* 2007;18:571–581.
Ford CA, English A. Limiting confidentiality of adolescent health services: what are the risks? *JAMA* 2002;288:752–753.
Ford C, English A, Sigman G. Confidential health care for adolescents: a position paper of the Society for Adolescent Medicine. *J Adolesc Health* 2004; 35:160–167.
Grupp-Phelan J, Harman JS, Kelleher KJ. Trends in mental health and chronic condition visits by children presenting for care at U.S. emergency departments. *Public Health Rep* 2007;122:55–61.
Jacobstein CR, Baren JM. Emergency department treatment of minors. *Emerg Med Clin North Am* 1999;17:341–351.
Lehrer JA, Pantell R, Tebb K, et al. Forgone health care among U.S. adolescents: associations between risk characteristics and confidentiality concern. *J Adol Health* 2007;40:218–226.
Lerand SJ. Teach the teacher: adolescent confidentiality and minor's consent. *J Pediatr Adolesc Gynecol* 2007;20:377–380.
Luo X, Liu G, Frush K, et al. Children's health insurance status and emergency department utilization in the United States. *Pediatrics* 2003;112:314–319.
National Center for Health Statistics. *Advance report of final mortality statistics, 2005.* Hyattsville, MD: Department of Health and Human Services, Public Health Service, Centers for Disease Control, 2007.
National Center for Health Statistics. Health insurance coverage: early release of estimates from the National Health Interview Survey, January-June 2008. *Centers for Disease Control and Prevention,* 2008.
Newacheck PW, Park MJ, Brindis CD, et al. Trends in private and public health insurance for adolescents. *JAMA* 2004;291:1231–1237.
Sigman GS, O'Connor C. Exploration for physicians of the mature minor doctrine. *J Pediatr* 1991;119:520–525.

United States Department of Health and Human Services, Health Resources and Services Administration, Maternal and Child Health Bureau. *Child Health USA 2004.* Rockville, MD: U.S. Department of Health and Human Services, 2004.
Viner RM. Do adolescent inpatient wards make a difference? Findings from a national young patient survey. *Pediatrics* 2007;120:749–755.
Wilson KM, Klein JD. Adolescents who use the emergency department as their usual source of care. *Arch Pediatr Adolesc Med* 2000;154:361–365.
Ziv A, Boulet JR, Slap GB. Emergency department utilization by adolescents in the United States. *Pediatrics* 1998;10:987–994.

Patients with Special Health Care Needs

American Academy of Pediatrics, Committee on Children with Disabilities. General principles in the care of children and adolescents with genetic disorders and other chronic health conditions. *Pediatrics* 1997;99:643.
American Academy of Pediatrics, Council on Children with Disabilities. Sexuality of children and adolescents with developmental disabilities. *Pediatrics* 2006;118:398–403.
Britto MT, Garrett JM, Dugliss MAJ, et al. Risky behavior in teens with cystic fibrosis or sickle cell disease: a multicenter study. *Pediatrics* 1998;101: 250.
Centers for Disease Control and Prevention, National Center for Health Statistics. State and Local Area Integrated Telephone Survey, National Survey of Children with Special Health Care Needs, 2001. Available at: http://www.mchb.hrsa.gov/chscn.
Kyngas HA, Kroll T, Duffy ME. Compliance in adolescents with chronic diseases: a review. *J Adolesc Health* 2000;26:379.
Rew L. Sexual health of adolescents with chronic health conditions. *Adol Med.* 2007;18:519–29.

Pregnancy

American Academy of Pediatrics. *Red Book: 2009 Report of the Committee on Infectious Diseases,* 28th ed. Elk Grove Village, IL: American Academy of Pediatrics, 2009.
American Academy of Pediatrics, Committee on Adolescence. Emergency contraception. *Pediatrics* 2005;116:1026–1035.
American College of Obstetricians and Gynecologists. ACOG practice bulletin. Emergency oral contraception. Number 25, March 2001. (replace practice pattern number 3, December 1996). American College of Obstetricians and Gynecologists. *Int J Gynaecol Obstet* 2002;78:191–198.
Bastian LA, Nanda K, Hasselblad V, et al. Diagnostic efficacy of home pregnancy kits: a meta-analysis. *Arch Fam Med* 1998;7:465.
Centers for Disease Control and Prevention. Sexually transmitted treatment guidelines 2006. *MMWR Morb Mortal Wkly Rep* 2006;55(RR-11):1–98.
Chande VT. Obstetrical procedures for adolescents. In: Henretig FM, King C, eds. *Textbook of pediatric emergency medicine procedures.* Baltimore, MD: Lippincott Williams & Wilkins, 2008:911.
English A. Understanding legal aspects of care. In: Neinstein LS, ed. *Adolescent health care: a practical guide,* 4th ed. Philadelphia, PA: Lippincott Williams & Wilkins, 2002:186.
Harner HM. Childhood sexual abuse, teenage pregnancy, and partnering with adult men: exploring the relationship. *J Psychosoc Nurs Ment Health Serv* 2005;43:20–28.
Jacoby M, Gorenflo D, Black E, et al. Rapid repeat pregnancy and experiences of interpersonal violence among low-income adolescents. *Am J Prev Med* 1999;16(4):318.
Lozeau AM, Potter B. Diagnosis and management of ectopic pregnancy. *Am Fam Phys* 2005;72:1707–1714.
Menon S, Sammel MD, Vichnin M, et al. Risk factors for ectopic pregnancy: a comparison between adults and adolescent women. *J Pediatr Adolesc Gynecol* 2007;20:181–185.
Mollen CJ, Pletcher J, Lavelle J. Emergency department management of teen pregnancy. *Clin Pediatr Emerg Med* 2002;4:58–68.
Neinstein LS, Farmer M. Teenage pregnancy. In: Neinstein LS, ed. *Adolescent health care: a practical guide,* 4th ed. Philadelphia, PA: Lippincott Williams & Wilkins, 2002:810.
Neinstein LS, Nelson AL. Ectopic pregnancy. In: Neinstein LS, ed. *Adolescent health care: a practical guide,* 4th ed. Philadelphia, PA: Lippincott Williams & Wilkins, 2002:1029.
Tay JI, Moore J, Walker JJ. Ectopic pregnancy. *West J Med* 2000;173:131.
Thomas BJ, Pierpoint T, Taylor-Robinson D, et al. Sensitivity of the ligase chain reaction assay for detecting *Chlamydia trachomatis* in vaginal swabs from women who are infected at other sites. *Sex Transm Infect* 1998;74(2):140.
Todd CS, Mountvarner G, Lichenstein R. Unintended pregnancy risk in an emergency department population. *Contraception* 2005;71:35–39.
Weinstock H, Berman S, Cates W Jr. Sexually transmitted diseases among American youth: incidence and prevalence estimates, 2000. *Perspect Sex Reprod Health* 2004;36(1):6–10.
Zabin LR, Emerson M, Ringers PA, et al. Adolescents with negative pregnancy test results: an accessible at-risk group. *JAMA* 1996;275:113.

Sexual Assault

Administration on Children, Youth, and Families, U.S. Department of Health and Human Services. *Child maltreatment 2000.* Washington, DC: U.S. Government Printing Office, 2002. Available at: http://www.acf.hhs.gov/programs/cb/publications/cm00/index.htm.

American Academy of Pediatrics: Committee on Adolescence. Care of the adolescent sexual assault victim. *Pediatrics* 2001;107:1476–1479.

American College of Emergency Physicians. *Evaluation and management of the sexually assaulted and sexually abused patient.* Dallas, TX: American College of Emergency Physicians, 1999. Available at: http://www.acep.org/workarea/downloadasset.aspx?id=8984.

Banyard VL, Cross C. Consequences of teen dating violence: understanding intervening variables in ecological context. *Viol Against Women* 2008;14:998–1013.

Bechtel K, Carroll M. Medical and forensic evaluation of the adolescent after sexual assault. *Clin Pediatr Emerg Med* 2002;4:37–46.

Bechtel K, Ryan E, Gallagher D. Impact of sexual assault nurse examiners on the evaluation of sexual assault in a pediatric emergency department. *Pediatr Emerg Care* 2008:24;442–447.

Centers for Disease Control and Prevention. Youth Risk Behavior Surveillance—United States, 2007. *MMWR Morb Mortal Wkly Rep* 2008;57(SS-4):1–131.

DeLago C, Deblinger E, Schroeder C, et al. Girls who disclose sexual abuse: urogenital symptoms and signs after genital contact. *Pediatrics* 2008;122:e281–e286.

Violence

American Academy of Pediatrics, Task Force on Adolescent Assault Victim Needs. Adolescent assault victim needs: a review of issues and a model protocol. *Pediatrics* 1996;98(5):991–1001.

American Medical Association, Council on Scientific Affairs. Adolescents as victims of family violence. *JAMA* 1993;270:1850–1856.

Baren JM, Mace SE, Hendry PL. Children's mental health emergencies—part 3: special situations: child maltreatment, violence, and response to disasters. *Ped Emer Care* 2008:24;569–577.

Centers for Disease Control and Prevention. Youth Risk Behavior Surveillance—United States, 2007. *MMWR Morb Mortal Wkly Rep* 2008;57(SS-4):1–136.

Copelan RI, Messer MA, Ashley DJ. Adolescent violence screening in the ED. *Am J Emer Med* 2006;24;582–594.

Cunningham R, Walton M, Trowbridge M, et al. Correlates of violent behavior among adolescents presenting to an urban emergency department. *J Pediatr* 2006;149;770–776.

Johnson SB, Bradshaw CP, Wright JL, et al. Characterizing the teachable moment: is an emergency department visit a teachable moment for intervention among assault-injured youth and their parents? *Pediatr Emerg Care* 2007;23;553–559.

Martin JA, Kung HC, Mathews TJ, et al. Annual summary of vital statistics: 2006. *Pediatrics* 2008;121:788–801.

Saluja G, Marquez V, Cheng TL, et al. Adolescents as victims of familial violence: a hospital based surveillance. *Int J Inj Contr Saf Promot* 2007:14;19–23.

PSYCHOSOCIAL EMERGENCIES

CHAPTER 131 ■ BEHAVIORAL EMERGENCIES

MIRNA M. FARAH, MD, AND JOSEPH ZORC, MD, MSCE

This chapter reviews a number of conditions with prominent behavioral and somatic symptoms that may cause an infant or child to be brought to the emergency department (ED) (Table 131.1). Although these conditions rarely require emergency intervention, the associated symptoms, such as stereotyped movements or cyanosis, may mimic other disorders with important physiologic consequences. The conditions reviewed in this chapter are heterogeneous; age of onset, symptoms, and prognosis vary widely. Some are part of normal childhood development, and others likely have an organic or genetic basis. All these conditions, however, have prominent behavioral features as part of the history that are the key to diagnosis. Familiarity with these disorders aids the emergency practitioner in an appropriate evaluation followed by reassurance of the family and referral, if necessary, to a source for ongoing care that is the basis for treatment.

GENERAL APPROACH

Diagnosis of these disorders depends on obtaining a history of symptoms associated with the child's other activity at the time. Organic conditions such as seizures (see Chapter 69) or syncope (see Chapter 73) are involuntary and usually unrelated to other behaviors. Gathering the necessary information requires a careful history because the child's caregiver may not recognize the behavioral nature of the event and emotional response may cloud recall. The clinician should review the episode chronologically in detail; key data include any precipitating events (e.g., breath-holding attacks, hyperventilation); the child's level of consciousness before, during, and after the episode (sleep disturbances); and any history of similar symptoms in the child or family members (tics). Having the caregiver act out the episode to demonstrate it and allow for measurement of duration may be useful. Social history and assessment of family dynamics (see Chapter 133) may further strengthen the diagnosis of some of these disorders.

Further evaluation beyond a careful history and physical examination is generally unnecessary for these conditions. The clinical picture may be specific enough to lead to the correct diagnosis. Laboratory values are generally normal or merely document the degree of symptoms (e.g., cyanosis) that has occurred. If the history is unclear or ambiguous, further investigation or referral may be warranted to rule out an important diagnosis, as discussed in the appropriate chapter of this text. As in all uncertain clinical scenarios, the degree of evaluation should reflect the seriousness of potential diagnoses, in accordance with the maxim primum non nocere (above all, do no harm).

Management of these disorders generally requires referral to a physician with an ongoing relationship with the patient, the child's medical home. For some of the conditions that are part of normal development (e.g., night terrors), reassurance may be all that is necessary. Nevertheless, the emergency practitioner may play an important role in this process because he or she may have the best opportunity to obtain important historical information that may be forgotten by the time of a later evaluation. The effect that a correct initial diagnosis may have on preventing unnecessary tests and reducing further anxiety should not be underestimated.

BREATH-HOLDING SPELLS

Background

Breath-holding spells in young children have been described since antiquity; accounts of this condition can be found in the works of Hippocrates, Rousseau, and Dickens, among others. In the modern medical literature, Lombroso and Lerman characterized the clinical syndrome in a group of 225 children with breath-holding spells. These patients were identified in a prospective study of almost 5,000 children, suggesting an incidence of 4.6%. The physicians described episodes of apnea and color change followed by loss of consciousness and postural tone that appeared to be triggered by an inciting event such as pain, fright, or agitation. Breath-holding children were categorized as cyanotic (62%), pallid (19%), or indeterminate (19%), on the basis of the type of color change. These subgroups appeared to have distinctly different clinical features. Cyanotic breath-holding spells were usually preceded by vigorous crying; pallid spells were sudden and more likely to be followed by convulsive activity.

Pathophysiology

Although the cause of breath-holding spells remains unclear, research has refined the understanding of this condition. The diagnostic term itself is a misnomer. *Breath-holding* would suggest voluntarily "waiting to exhale"; however, most episodes appear to be involuntary and to occur at the end of expiration. Studies of breath-holding children have reported associations with autonomic dysfunction and anemia, as well as an apparent familial predisposition. The clinical difference observed between pallid and cyanotic spells may have a basis in pathophysiology; pallid breath-holding spells can be reproduced by a vagal stimulus and are associated with subtle differences in autonomic function. These findings suggest a similarity to vasovagal syncope or neurally mediated hypotension

TABLE 131.1

BEHAVIOR-RELATED PROBLEMS PRESENTING WITH
SOMATIC SYMPTOMS

Cyanosis
Cyanotic breath-holding spells

Syncope
Cyanotic or pallid breath-holding spells

Motor Activity
Tic disorders and Tourette's syndrome
Paroxysmal choreoathetosis
Benign paroxysmal torticollis
Opsoclonus and myoclonus
Spasmus nutans
Gratification disorder (infantile masturbation)

Hyperventilation Syndrome

Sleep-Related Disorders

as described in adults, although further confirmatory research
is needed.

Diagnosis

The diagnosis of breath-holding spells is based on the clinical
history. Initial presentation usually occurs within the first
2 years of life and is not associated with other physical, developmental, or behavioral disorders. The typical episode begins
with an inciting stimulus such as anger, frustration, fear, or
pain. The child begins to cry, either briefly or for a prolonged
period, and then suddenly stops in full expiration with mouth
wide open. The spell may resolve at this point or proceed to
color change followed by loss of consciousness. The child then
becomes limp but soon may progress to an opisthotonic posture. Return to consciousness usually occurs within 1 minute.
Severe breath-holding episodes may be associated with body
jerks or incontinence and a transient recovery period of several
minutes.

When a child is evaluated after a breath-holding spell, the
clinician should expect to find normal findings in physical
examination. Laboratory test results are also usually normal
and add little to the evaluation. Some physicians suggest measuring hemoglobin level because anemia has been associated
with breath-holding spells. Electroencephalogram (EEG) performed during a spell reflects hypoxemia but returns to normal
afterward. Thus EEG is not recommended as a diagnostic test.

The differential diagnosis of breath-holding spells includes
seizure disorders (see Chapter 69), structural cardiac disease
(e.g., tetralogy of Fallot), arrhythmia (e.g., long QT syndrome;
see Chapter 84), syncope (see Chapter 73), and apnea (see
Chapter 9) secondary to infection, brain tumor, injury, or congenital causes. A characteristic history in a healthy child with
normal physical examination findings should be sufficient to
make the diagnosis. The key elements of the history are identifying the precipitating event (which may include minor
trauma) and determining that the color change preceded any
motor activity (unlike most seizures). In uncertain cases
involving syncope, an electrocardiogram (EKG) is advisable to
measure the QT interval corrected for heart rate.

Management

Once the diagnosis has been made, parents should be reassured
that there is no evidence of long-term sequelae from typical
childhood breath-holding spells. The relationship between the
inciting event and the spell should be explained, as well as the
possibility of recurrence. Frequency of recurrence varies from
daily to yearly, but most breath-holding children stop having
spells by school age. Inciting events such as pain and frustration are to be expected in healthy children, and overzealous
attempts at prevention may impair the exploratory behavior
and appropriate limit setting that is part of normal development. If a spell recurs, parents should be instructed to clear the
airway and place the child in a lateral, supine position away
from other objects. In severe cases, referral to a specialist is
indicated because treatment with atropine, scopolamine, other
medications, or a cardiac pacemaker has been helpful in
selected cases. A randomized trial found a reduced frequency of
spells in children treated with iron, although the efficacy of this
treatment in nonanemic children remains unclear.

TICS AND MOVEMENT DISORDERS

Tics are involuntary, rapid, repetitive movements or vocalizations that may present throughout childhood and be confused
with seizures or other disorders. Tic disorders affect 2% to 5%
of school-aged children and range from mild, self-limited symptoms to the chronic Gilles de la Tourette's syndrome, which can
be severe and debilitating. Boys are affected with tics three times
as commonly as girls, and familial predisposition has been well
documented. Attention deficit/hyperactivity disorder (ADHD)
and obsessive-compulsive disorder are more common in children with tics. A recent area of research interest has been a
hypothesized increase in tics and obsessive-compulsive symptoms following group A streptococcal infections known as
PANDAS (pediatric autoimmune neuropsychiatric disorders
associated with streptococcal infections). A recent large cohort
study suggests that this association, if present, accounts for a
small subset of these symptoms among selected children.

Diagnosis of tic disorders relies on obtaining a history of
stereotypical, involuntary motor activity that most often
involves the muscles of the head and neck. Eye movements,
head twitches, and shoulder shrugs are common, although
complex movements and vocalizations may also occur. Unlike
partial seizures, tics are nonrhythmic and partially suppressible, which may result in their being absent at the time of an
evaluation. Tics tend to increase at times of anxiety, stress, and
fatigue and decrease during sleep or relaxation. Tics may be
precipitated by medications, especially stimulants such as
methylphenidate. The differential diagnosis of tic disorders
includes chronic diseases affecting the central nervous system,
such as Wilson's disease, Sydenham's chorea, and metabolic
disorders. A toxic cause should be considered because adverse
reactions to many medications, including neuroleptics, metoclopramide, and antihistamines, can present with dystonic
symptoms simulating tics.

ED evaluation and management of tics should be limited
to establishing the diagnosis by history and ruling out other
conditions. Physical examination finding is usually normal.

Laboratory tests, imaging studies, and EEG results are also usually normal and generally unnecessary. The emergency practitioner should reassure the family that tics are not harmful and should encourage further discussion with a continuing care provider. Mild tics in young children often resolve spontaneously; more severe tics may require referral to a neurologist or psychiatrist for consideration of pharmacologic treatment.

Other movement disorders of childhood are listed in Table 131.1. Disorders of paroxysmal choreoathetosis are usually chronic and familial. Opsoclonus–myoclonus is a syndrome of chaotic, irregular eye movements that is associated with neuroblastoma in more than 50% of affected patients. *Spasmus nutans* is a condition involving head tilt, nodding, and nystagmus that presents in infancy and is associated with optic glioma in some cases. Benign paroxysmal torticollis presents in infancy with recurring episodes lasting minutes to days and must be differentiated from posterior fossa tumors and other conditions. Gratification disorder is a condition of stereotyped self-stimulatory movements in young children that may resemble epilepsy but can be interrupted with distraction.

HYPERVENTILATION SYNDROME

Background

Hyperventilation is defined as ventilation in excess of that required to maintain normal arterial blood partial pressure of oxygen (PaO_2) and partial pressure of carbon dioxide ($PaCO_2$). This causes the elimination of more carbon dioxide than is produced, resulting in respiratory alkalosis and an elevated blood pH. Hyperventilation may be produced by an increase in either frequency or depth of respiration. The pathophysiology of the hyperventilation syndrome contains two components: (i) physiologic derangement produced by hyperventilation and (ii) underlying psychiatric disturbance most often including anxiety and panic.

Clinical Manifestations

Onset is typically around 13 to 14 years of age. Girls are affected twice as often as boys. Patients almost always report that their symptoms occur in "spells" or "attacks" lasting a few minutes to several hours each. In the ED, patients can present with various combinations of symptoms, including dyspnea, tachypnea, breathlessness, chest tightness and pain, palpitations, anxiety, panic and a feeling of impending doom, paresthesias, coldness of the extremities, tetany, trembling, blurred vision, light headedness, syncope, or seizure. Physical examination may reveal obvious hyperventilation, or more commonly, periodic deep-sighing respirations.

EKG changes, such as ST-segment depression and flattening and inversion of T waves, both in the resting and exercise EKG, have been reported in adults who hyperventilate. However, unlike in ischemia, these changes occur early in exercise and disappear as exercise continues.

Differential Diagnosis

The manifestations of hyperventilation syndrome are variable and can initially seem worrisome. Organic disorders that require serious consideration in the differential diagnosis include asthma, metabolic acidosis (e.g., diabetic ketoacidosis), hyperammonemia, hypocalcemia, drug intoxication (including salicylism), hypercapnia, cirrhosis, organic central nervous system disorders, fever, and the response to severe pain. A few paroxysmal disorders, such as hypotensive syncope, Stokes–Adams attacks, epilepsy, and migraine, should be ruled out. However, many of the previous organic disorders can be excluded on the basis of careful history and physical examination. A clinical problem is that hyperventilation syndrome and asthma often coincide, leading to a vicious circle—that is, asthma symptoms increase anxiety, which may induce hyperventilation.

Elements of history that suggest the diagnosis of hyperventilation syndrome include lack of nocturnal symptoms; sudden occurrence, sometimes at rest without typical trigger factors; chronicity or variable duration of symptoms; lack of response to adequate pharmacotherapy (e.g., for asthma); reference to breathlessness; expression of anxiety; and finally, normal results of a diagnostic workup. Intensive efforts should be made to diagnose functional symptoms at an early stage because this will prevent stigmatization and fixation of symptoms and disease and will also prevent children from undergoing unnecessary and potentially harmful therapies. Assessing whether voluntary hyperventilation reproduces the patient's symptoms is also helpful. This provocation test is currently the best diagnostic method and is accomplished by asking the patient to hyperventilate for at least 3 minutes, enough to bring the $PaCO_2$ to less than 50% of baseline. Termination of symptoms on rebreathing into a paper bag is another suggestive finding. When the syndrome is recognized, extensive laboratory evaluation is rarely required in the pediatric population and may add to the child's anxiety. However, as in many clinical situations that result in a diagnosis with psychological or psychiatric implications, the emergency physician may rarely elect to order laboratory data to support the diagnosis. The specific tests obtained should be determined by the patient's symptoms but will usually be selected from among chest radiograph, EKG, serum calcium and electrolytes, and blood gas determinations.

Treatment

The therapeutic approach to hyperventilation syndrome has several stages and/or degrees of intervention:

1. Psychological counseling: "Reassurance" by physicians, family, and professionals is the most prominent instrument to reduce or diminish observed respiratory symptoms in the absence of significant organic abnormality. Reassurance measures may include the demonstration of normal diagnostic results to patients and parents. Children and adolescents need to be reassured in specific terms relevant to their fears. Child life specialists or social workers are most helpful in this treatment. Counseling and supportive therapy are necessary to discover the sources of the psychological disturbance experienced by the child. These efforts should start in the ED, but psychiatric consultation and/or referral is often required.
2. Physiotherapy: The classic remedy for hyperventilation is relaxation and breathing into a paper bag. The patient rebreathes his or her own expired air and thus inhales air

enriched with CO_2. Most experts recommend that the patient understand the mechanism by which the symptoms are produced. For adolescents, in particular, emphasizing that the patient has control over the production of symptoms is important. This understanding is often accomplished by voluntary overbreathing and attribution of cause of symptoms to hyperventilation. Relaxation techniques such as self-hypnosis may positively influence the pathological breathing pattern and slow down the respiratory rate. Relaxation may also diminish the underlying anxiety. Parents and others should also avoid reinforcing the patient's symptoms through attention.

3. Pharmacotherapy: A major goal is to avoid or reduce the use of pharmacotherapy, limiting it to patients who fail to respond to education and counseling. Propranolol and anxiolytics have been used successfully in children to interrupt these spells. The prognosis of hyperventilation syndrome in children and adolescents is worrisome, with 40% of patients showing persistent symptoms into adulthood.

SLEEP DISTURBANCES

Background

Childhood sleep disturbances are common, occurring in 20% to 30% of children between the ages of 1 and 8 years. They are often a clue to underlying emotional or family stresses during certain childhood developmental stages. The predominant sleep disturbances include resistance to being put down for the night, frequent nighttime awakenings in infancy, and parasomnias in school-aged children. Anticipatory guidance on the part of the primary care physician can minimize the impact of these disturbances.

Clinical Manifestations and Management

Parasomnias

Parasomnias are physical phenomena during sleep that do not usually result in excessive daytime sleepiness. They can be subdivided into four groups: arousal disorders, sleep–wake disorders, rapid eye movement (REM) sleep disorders, and other parasomnias, such as sleep enuresis and sleep bruxism.

Arousal Disorders. Arousal disorders tend to occur during the first third of the night, in the transition from deep non-REM to light non-REM sleep. A positive family history is often present. The disorders are paroxysmal, often associated with activation of the autonomic nervous system and skeletal muscles, unresponsiveness to the environment, and amnesia for events. Most of these episodes last 2 to 10 minutes, followed by a rapid return to sleep. Intercurrent illnesses, medications, physical or mental fatigue, sleep deprivation, and emotional distress can trigger these parasomnias in susceptible individuals.

Confusional arousals are brief episodes of confused state seen most commonly in children younger than 5 years. The brain is only partially awakened during these episodes. They consist of disorientation in time and space, slow speech and mentation, and bizarre behavior, such as placing a piece of cloth in the refrigerator. Children do not express fear or panic and spontaneously return to sleep with no recollection of the event the following morning. These episodes are benign and gradually decrease in frequency with age.

Pavor nocturnus (night terrors) are dramatic events which may occur at any age and seen in as many as 20% of children between 5 and 7 years of age. The child abruptly awakens 15 to 90 minutes after sleep onset, with a piercing scream or cry, sits up in bed with wide-open eyes, extreme anxiety, and autonomic phenomena (sweating, flushing, and rapid heartbeat and breathing). The child appears confused, is not able to recognize the parents, and is inconsolable for 10 to 15 minutes. Then he or she relaxes and falls back to a quiet sleep with no recollection of the event in the morning. Night terrors usually occur so rarely that treatment is not necessary. Their frequency decreases with age.

Somnambulism (sleepwalking) appears in children 4 to 6 years of age. The child sits up suddenly with eyes glassy and staring and may then arise and walk around clumsily toward a light or a noise. During sleepwalking, children often appear confused, and many attempt to vocalize inappropriate answers to questions. Other bizarre behaviors include urinating in closets, ambulating outside, or climbing out of a window. The episodes usually last less than 15 minutes, and when the child is returned to bed, he or she will fall asleep uneventfully. Temporal lobe epilepsy may be difficult to distinguish from somnambulism but can be differentiated by adequate sleep EEG studies. Unlike in adults, somnambulism in children is benign and self-limited, but there is a high potential for harm. Management consists of "sleep-proofing" the home: windows and doors should be locked, and gates placed across stairs. A bell could be placed on the child's door to alert the caregivers of these events. Parents can be reassured that most children outgrow sleepwalking over several years.

Sleep–Wake Transition Disorders. Sleep–wake transition disorders occur in the transition from wakefulness to sleep, from sleep to wakefulness, or in sleep-stage transitions.

Rhythmic movement disorder starts at around 8 months of age and generally stops by age 4. Boys outnumber girls 3:1. The usual pattern is body rocking followed by head rolling or banging against the crib sides immediately before sleep onset and throughout light sleep, lasting several minutes to an hour. Head banging is typically not associated with crying. No significant injuries are incurred, although callus formation and contusions may be observed. Management consists of reassurance and advice to pad the crib.

Somniloquy (sleep talking) appears in school-aged children. The speech can be spontaneous or induced by conversation from another person. Sleep talking may be vivid and revealing but is also usually outgrown with time.

Nocturnal leg cramps and *restless leg syndrome* may prevent children from initiating or returning to sleep. Patients feel the need to frequently toss, turn, and kick to relieve their leg discomfort. Children with restless leg syndrome may be misdiagnosed with growing pains or ADHD. Restless leg syndrome may be associated with sleep apnea. Symptoms can improve with dopaminergic agents and benzodiazepines.

REM Sleep Disorders. REM sleep disorders often occur during the last part of the night when REM sleep predominates.

Nightmares are unpleasant dreams from which the child is usually awake and responsive by the time the parents arrive, and for which substantial recall can occur. Approximately 10% to 50% of children between the ages of 3 and 6 years experience nightmares, but this frequency decreases over time. The child who just had a nightmare should be reassured with embraces and soothing words, and the parent should stay until the child is calm. Parents of children with occasional nightmares should be reassured about the benign nature of these episodes. Frequent nightmares may be a sign of distress that merits a psychological evaluation. Certain medications can trigger nightmares, such as L-DOPA, β-blockers, and withdrawal from REM-suppressing drugs.

Other Parasomnias. *Bruxism* (clenching and grinding of teeth during sleep) occurs in 50% of healthy infants at the time of tooth eruption, but it also occurs in children 10 to 20 years of age due to stress. Bruxism can also be caused by dental malocclusion and neurologic conditions. For persistent nightly bruxism, tooth guards can protect the teeth and reduce potential damage to the temporomandibular joint. Relaxation exercises such as self-hypnosis to relax the body at bedtime can be helpful for older children.

Primary nocturnal enuresis is defined as enuresis occurring in a child older than 3 years, who is otherwise well and has never been dry at night, although he or she can stay dry all day. This condition is the most common non-REM disorder, with an incidence ranging from 5% to 17% of all children between 3 and 15 years of age. The enuretic episode typically occurs during the first cycle of the night. It is characterized by tachycardia, tachypnea, penile erection in boys, increased intravesical pressure, and spontaneous bladder contraction. The differential diagnosis includes organic problems such as diabetes mellitus, diabetes insipidus, and urinary tract infection, although these symptoms would be rare if the definition just given is adhered to. The sleep quality of children with nocturnal enuresis is poor due in part to the fear or anxiety of bedwetting during sleep. So, active treatment should be started as soon as the enuretic child is ready and wants to be dry during sleep. Treatment starts with conditioning modalities. Medications, such as imipramine, that have both anticholinergic effects on the bladder and stimulant effects on sleep-stage patterns, or antidiuretic hormones are considered a last resort and should be prescribed only in severe cases, under the supervision of the primary care physician.

Dyssomnias

Dyssomnias are primary disorders of sleep excess or insomnia.

Narcolepsy is a rare syndrome characterized by excessive daytime sleepiness. Onset is gradual, often between 15 and 35 years of age with a strong genetic predisposition. The two most important symptoms of narcolepsy are daytime sleepiness (that is irresistible and that cannot be fully relieved by any amount of sleep) and cataplexy (sudden loss of muscle tone with preservation of consciousness, triggered by strong emotions such as laughter, crying, anger, or fear). Other complaints include attacks of daytime sleep (short, 10- to 20-minute naps after which children feel refreshed, then feel sleepy again within 2 to 3 hours), sleep paralysis (inability to move during the onset of sleep or on awakening), hypnagogic hallucinations (vivid imagery at the onset of sleep or awakening), and disturbed nighttime sleep. The occurrence of REM sleep at the onset of sleep is the most characteristic and striking abnormality observed in narcolepsy. Management includes a regular schedule of naps and adherence to a consistent sleep schedule. Short-acting stimulant drugs, such as a low dosage of dextroamphetamine or methylphenidate for daytime sleepiness, and sodium oxybate, tricyclic antidepressants, or serotonin reuptake inhibitors are recommended for cataplexy, sleep paralysis, and hypnagogic hallucinations. Issues to be addressed with adolescents are driving, poor school performance, and difficult peer interactions. The degree of sleepiness rarely lessens, but cataplexy, sleep paralysis, and hypnagogic hallucinations improve or disappear with age in one-third of patients.

Obstructive sleep apnea syndrome affects 1% to 3% of all children and peaks between 2 and 6 years of age. It is caused by upper airway obstruction, resulting in frequent apneic spells during sleep, hypoxia, hypercarbia, frequent arousals, and sleep fragmentation. This leads to neurocognitive disruption and decreased stages 3 and 4 of non-REM sleep. Children may present with loud snoring, excess daytime somnolence, morning headaches, hypertension, cardiac arrhythmias, cor pulmonale, failure to thrive, enuresis, anoxic seizures, aggressiveness, decreased attention span, and poor school performance. Predisposing risk factors to obstructive sleep apnea include obesity, craniofacial abnormalities, and hypotonia. An overnight polysomnogram is the gold standard for confirming the presence and severity of obstructive sleep apnea. Management involves otolaryngologic or pediatric sleep medicine consultation for thorough airway evaluation and appropriate measures to relieve obstruction, maintenance of continuous positive airway pressure, and initiation of weight loss in obese children. However, the most common and effective treatment for obstructive sleep apnea is tonsillectomy and adenoidectomy, after which symptoms resolve in 70% to 80% of the cases.

Suggested Readings

General Approach

DiMario FJ. Paroxysmal nonepileptic events of childhood. *Semin Pediatr Neurol* 2006;13:208–221.

Breath-Holding Spells

DiMario FJ. Prospective study of children with cyanotic and pallid breath-holding spells. *Pediatrics* 2001;107:265–269.
Lombroso CT, Lerman P. Breathholding spells (cyanotic and pallid infantile syncope). *Pediatrics* 1967;39:563–581.

Tics and Movement Disorders

Kurlan R, Johnson D, Kaplan EL, et al. Streptococcal infection and exacerbations of childhood tics and obsessive-compulsive symptoms: a prospective blinded cohort study. *Pediatrics* 2008;121:1188–1197.
McMahon WM, Filloux FM, Ashworth JC, et al. Movement disorders in children and adolescents. *Neurol Clin Am* 2002;20:1101–1124.

Hyperventilation

Niggemann B. Functional symptoms confused with allergic disorders in children and adolescents. *Pediatr Allergy Immunol* 2002;13:312–318.

Weinberger M, Abu-Hasan M. Pseudoasthma: when cough, wheezing, and dyspnea are not asthma. *Pediatrics* 2007;120(4):855–864.

Sleep Disorders

American Sleep Disorders Association. *International classification of sleep disorders: diagnostic and coding manual.* Lawrence, KS: Allen Press, 1990.

Goldstein NA, Pugazhendhi V, Rao SM, et al. Clinical assessment of pediatric obstructive sleep apnea. *Pediatrics* 2004;114(1):33–43.

Gozmen S, Keskin S, Akil I. Enuresis nocturna and sleep quality. *Pediatr Nephrol* 2008;23(8):1293–1296.

Moore M, Allison D, Rosen CL. A review of pediatric nonrespiratory sleep disorders. *Chest* 2006;130(4):1252–1262.

Trenkwalder C, Benes H, Poewe W, et al. Efficacy of rotigotine for treatment of moderate-to-severe restless legs syndrome: a randomised, double-blind, placebo-controlled trial. *Lancet Neurol* 2008;7(7):595–604.

Ward T, Mason TB II. Sleep disorders in children. *Nurs Clin North Am* 2002; 37(4):693–706.

Xyrem International Study Group. A double-blind, placebo-controlled study demonstrates sodium oxybate is effective for the treatment of excessive daytime sleepiness in narcolepsy. *J Clin Sleep Med* 2005;1(4):391–397.

CHAPTER 132 ■ CHILD ABUSE

JOANNE N. WOOD, MD, MSHP, AND STEPHEN LUDWIG, MD

Child abuse is the single diagnostic term used to describe a range of behaviors, from somewhat harsh discipline to intentional repetitive torture. This phenomenon is complex and results from a combination of individual, familial, and societal factors. The common final pathway for these factors is parental behavior destructive to the process of normal growth, development, and well-being of the child. Abuse may be subdivided into four broad categories: (i) physical abuse, (ii) sexual abuse, (iii) neglect, and (iv) emotional abuse. Each form of abuse has individual characteristics of family dynamics and clinical manifestations and requires skillful physician management.

The task of the emergency physician is difficult. The physician must first maintain an open mind to the possibility that abuse not just occurs but also occurs commonly. Thus, abuse should be included in the differential diagnosis of any injury or any physical or psychological complaint that does not have an obvious etiology. Second, the physician must identify signs and symptoms of suspected abuse. Next, the potential family crisis must be managed to protect the child, yet maintain the abusive parents' motivation for help. Finally, the legal requirements for reporting abuse to the proper social service or police authority should be thoroughly understood.

The demands of managing a case of child abuse may be lessened by sharing the responsibility with other health care professionals. The skills of physician colleagues, as well as nursing and social work staff, are invaluable. The child abuse field has been a model for multidisciplinary collaboration, which is most productive if begun in the initial phases of case management in the emergency department (ED). Establishing an institutional or departmental protocol for the management of abuse cases is also essential. This protocol relieves the emergency physician from having to reconstruct a complete management plan for each new case. Having a standard protocol to follow allows the physician more time to concentrate on the individual needs of the patient and parents.

To the unfamiliar observer, the easy solution to all abuse cases is to "take away the child and put the parents in jail." This commonly held treatment philosophy would be practiced more if it were truly a panacea. However, the alternative forms of child care (i.e., institutional care, foster care, extended family care) are each fraught with their own hazard. With the use of well-organized community services, abusive behavior can be controlled while the child and family receive therapy. In some cases, however, removal of the child and establishing data on which to effect the removal will be the main focus of the ED visit.

There may be support for the notion that parents who bring their abused child to the ED are motivated to seek help for their child and for themselves. Most parents feel remorse about their abusive behavior. The severity of injuries inflicted is often overestimated as a result of parental guilt. The emergency physician must neither overlook nor mismanage the opportunity to identify abuse early and help control the parents' behavior. Sharp focus must be maintained on the dual goals of case management—protect the child and use the crisis to strengthen and preserve family life. When these dual goals are in conflict, it is the former that must take priority.

PHYSICAL ABUSE

Background

Physical abuse is the most often reported form of child abuse. Definitions of physical abuse vary from state to state. Operationally, the definitions vary from institution to institution and indeed from person to person. Even the definition of physical abuse is a definition in transition. Over the past century, many advances in the "rights of the children" have been made. For example, the enactment of child labor and compulsory education laws has been an important step forward. As the history of abuse is traced through the centuries, the forms and definitions of abuse have changed. Definitions currently used are likely to continue to change with time. The present widespread medical interest in abuse was stimulated by C. Henry Kempe with the introduction of the term *battered child syndrome* in 1962. It was only as recently as 1968 that the last of the 50 states enacted child abuse legislation. Many states are now using their second or third generation of child abuse laws.

The Child Abuse Prevention and Treatment Act (CAPTA), as amended and reauthorized in June 2003 by the Keeping Children and Families Safe Act of 2003 (Pub L No. 108-36), defines child abuse and neglect as, at a minimum, any recent act or failure to act.

■ Resulting in imminent risk of serious harm, death, serious physical or emotional harm, sexual abuse, or exploitation
■ Of a child (a person younger than age 18, unless the child protection law of the state in which the child resides specifies a younger age for cases not involving sexual abuse)
■ By a parent or caregiver (including any employee of a residential facility or any staff person providing out-of-home care) who is responsible for the child's welfare.

There are four major types of child maltreatment: (i) physical abuse, (ii) child neglect, (iii) sexual abuse, and (iv) emotional abuse. Physical abuse is the infliction of physical injury as a result of punching, beating, kicking, biting, burning, shaking, or otherwise harming a child. The parent or caregiver may not have intended to hurt the child but rather the injury may have resulted from overdiscipline or physical punishment.

The true incidence of abuse is elusive. Many cases of abuse occur in the privacy of the home and are never recognized or reported. The federal government has collected three national incidence studies in 1979–1980, 1986–1987, and 1993–1995. A fourth cycle of data is being collected and a report is pending. These data are shown in Fig. 132.1. The National Center for Child Abuse and Neglect (NCANDS) also collects data through voluntary reporting by state child protective services (CPA) agencies. These data sources all underestimate the incidence of abuse. There are about 3 million reports and 1 million substantiated cases per year or an incidence of 42 per 1,000 children. The breakdown in the forms of abuse is shown by type and age in Fig. 132.2.

Homicide is now the fifth leading cause of death in children aged 1 to 4 years and the fourth leading cause of death in

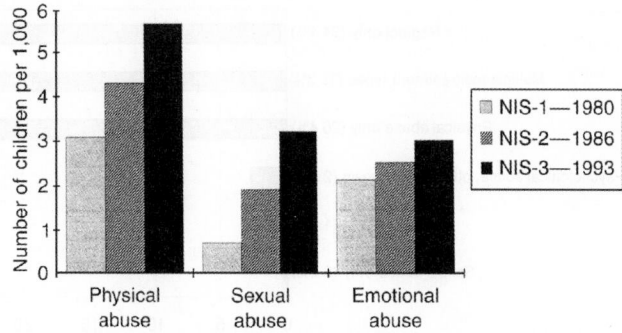

FIGURE 132.1 Incidence of child abuse per 1,000 children by abuse type determined by three national incidence studies. (From the U.S. Department of Human Services. Reprinted with permission.)

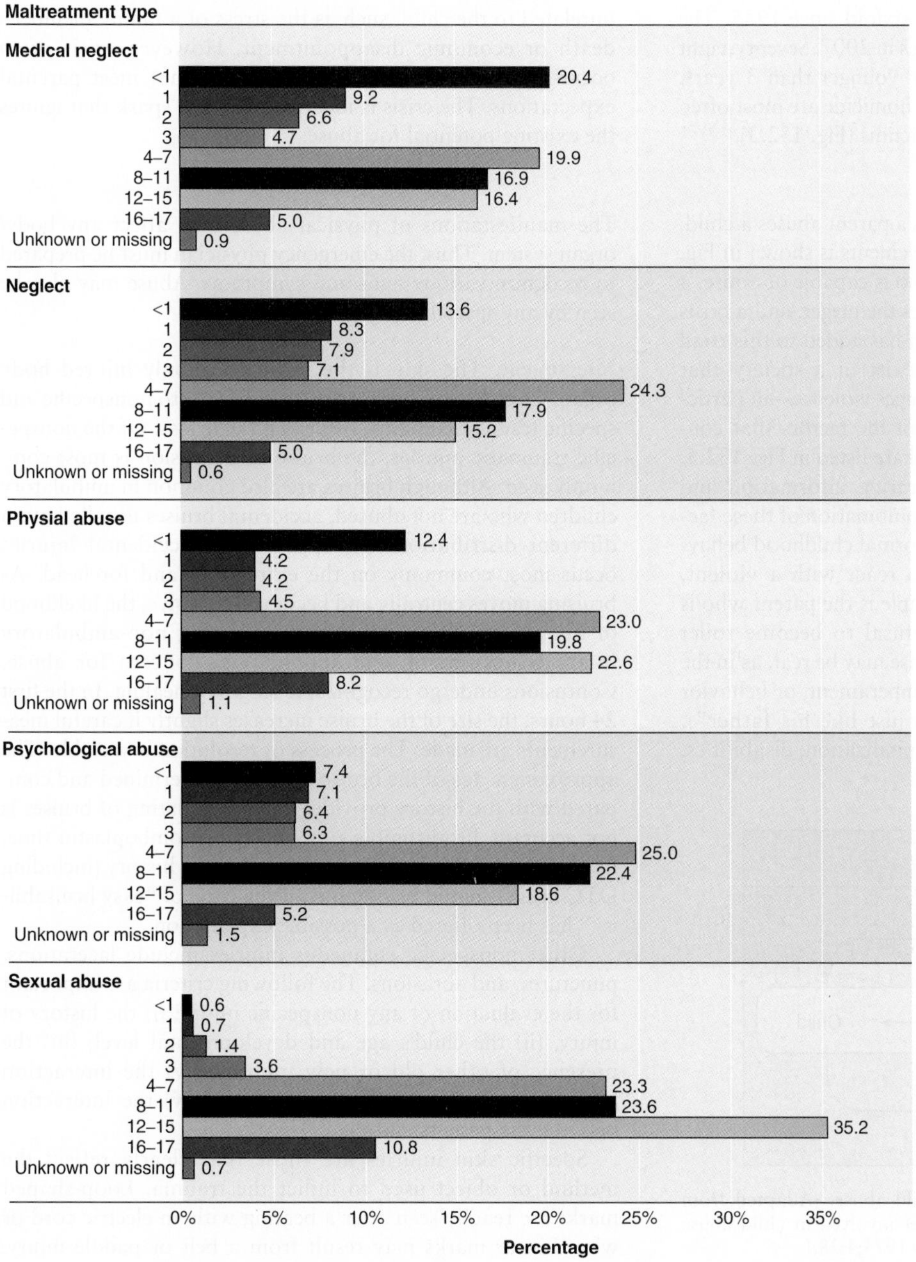

Maltreatment type

Medical neglect

Age	Percentage
<1	20.4
1	9.2
2	6.6
3	4.7
4–7	19.9
8–11	16.9
12–15	16.4
16–17	5.0
Unknown or missing	0.9

Neglect

Age	Percentage
<1	13.6
1	8.3
2	7.9
3	7.1
4–7	24.3
8–11	17.9
12–15	15.2
16–17	5.0
Unknown or missing	0.6

Physial abuse

Age	Percentage
<1	12.4
1	4.2
2	4.2
3	4.5
4–7	23.0
8–11	19.8
12–15	22.6
16–17	8.2
Unknown or missing	1.1

Psychological abuse

Age	Percentage
<1	7.4
1	7.1
2	6.4
3	6.3
4–7	25.0
8–11	22.4
12–15	18.6
16–17	5.2
Unknown or missing	1.5

Sexual abuse

Age	Percentage
<1	0.6
1	0.7
2	1.4
3	3.6
4–7	23.3
8–11	23.6
12–15	35.2
16–17	10.8
Unknown or missing	0.7

0%   5%   10%   15%   20%   25%   30%   35%

Percentage

FIGURE 132.2 This bar chart displays the medical neglect, neglect, physical abuse, psychological abuse, and sexual abuse maltreatment types by age within each maltreatment type. The percentage of victims for each age group within each maltreatment type is shown. (From U.S. Department of Health and Human Services, Administration for Children & Families, Administration on Children, Youth & Families, Children's Bureau. *Statistics & research, child maltreatment 2007.*)

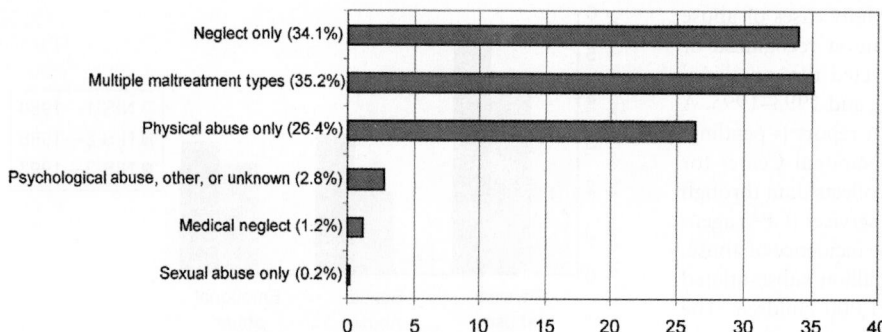

FIGURE 132.3 Causes of child abuse and neglect fatalities by maltreatment type in 2007 data from the National Center for Child Abuse and Neglect. (From U.S. Department of Health and Human Services, Administration for Children & Families, Child Welfare Information Gateway. *Child abuse and neglect fatalities: statistics and intervention.*)

children aged 5 to 14 years. There are 2,000 to 5,000 deaths annually or an incidence of 5.4 per 100,000 children 4 years and younger. The incidence of child homicide has steadily increased. According to a review by the Centers for Disease Control and Prevention (CDC), the rate of homicide in the 1- to 4-year-old age group has increased sixfold since 1925. The NCANDS reported 1,760 child fatalities in 2007. Seventy-eight percent of deaths occurred in children younger than 3 years. The perpetrators in these cases of child homicide are most often adults who are known by their child victims (Fig. 132.3).

Dynamics

Many factors contribute to the reasons a parent abuses a child. Helfer's formulation of the necessary elements is shown in Fig. 132.4. The factors include a parent who is capable of abuse, a child who actively or passively becomes the target, and a crisis that triggers the angry response. Green has added to this triad the concept that the process must exist in a society that unknowingly condones or even encourages violence—in particular, violence against children. Some of the factors that contribute to the parents' abusive potential are listed in Fig. 132.5.

Stress and lack of specific child-rearing information and experience play dominant roles. The combination of these factors causes many parents to misread normal childhood behavior as defiant or provocative and to react with a violent, destructive response. The typical example is the parent who is angered by the 1-year-old child's refusal to become toilet trained. The child's contribution to abuse may be real, as in the case of negative behavior, disparate temperament, or behavior imagined by the parent (e.g., "He's just like his father"). Children with prolonged neonatal hospitalization, disabilities,

or developmental delays are at increased risk. Living situations in which nonbiological parents are present are also high risk. For example, the adopted child or the child living with a parent's significant other may be the target of abusive behavior. The crisis that initiates abuse varies tremendously. It may be unrelated to the child, such as the stress of a family member's death or economic disappointment. However, crisis often occurs because the child's behavior does not meet parental expectations. The crisis is identifiable as the spark that ignites the existing potential for abuse.

Manifestations

The manifestations of physical abuse may affect any body/ organ system. Thus, the emergency physician must be prepared to recognize various signs and symptoms. Abuse may also be seen by any specialist physician.

Integument. The skin is the most commonly injured body organ. Cutaneous injuries may be divided into nonspecific and specific traumatic lesions, burns, and hair loss. Of the nonspecific traumatic injuries, the bruise or contusion is most commonly seen. Although bruises are also common in ambulatory children who are not abused, accidental bruises usually have a different distribution and appearance. Accidental injuries occur most commonly on the extremities and forehead. As bruising moves centrally and becomes extensive, the likelihood of abuse rises. Also, bruising in a young non-ambulatory infant is uncommon and should raise concern for abuse. Contusions undergo recognizable stages of healing. In the first 24 hours, the size of the bruise increases slightly if careful measurements are made. The process of resolution is variable. The approximate age of the bruise should be determined and compared with the history provided but exact dating of bruises is not accurate. Prothrombin time, partial thromboplastin time, bleeding time, platelet count and medication history (including OTC drugs) should be obtained if the issue of "easy bruisability" has been offered as a possible explanation.

Other nonspecific cutaneous injuries include lacerations, punctures, and abrasions. The following criteria are important for the evaluation of any nonspecific injury: (i) the history of injury, (ii) the child's age and developmental level, (iii) the presence of other old or new injuries, (iv) the interaction between the parents and the child, and (v) the interaction between the parents and the ED staff.

Specific skin injuries are those that clearly reflect the method or object used to inflict the trauma. Loop-shaped marks are readily seen after a beating with an electric cord or wire. Linear marks may result from a belt or paddle injury.

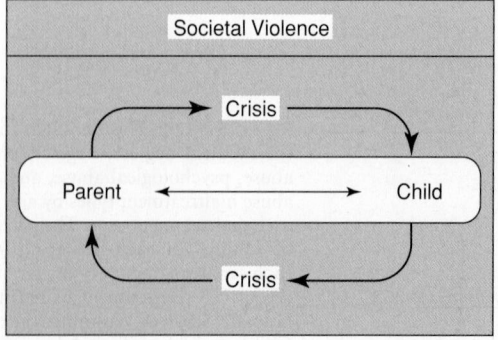

FIGURE 132.4 Essential elements of child abuse. (Adapted from Helfer RE. Why most physicians don't get involved in child abuse cases and what to do about it. *Child Today* 1975;4:28.)

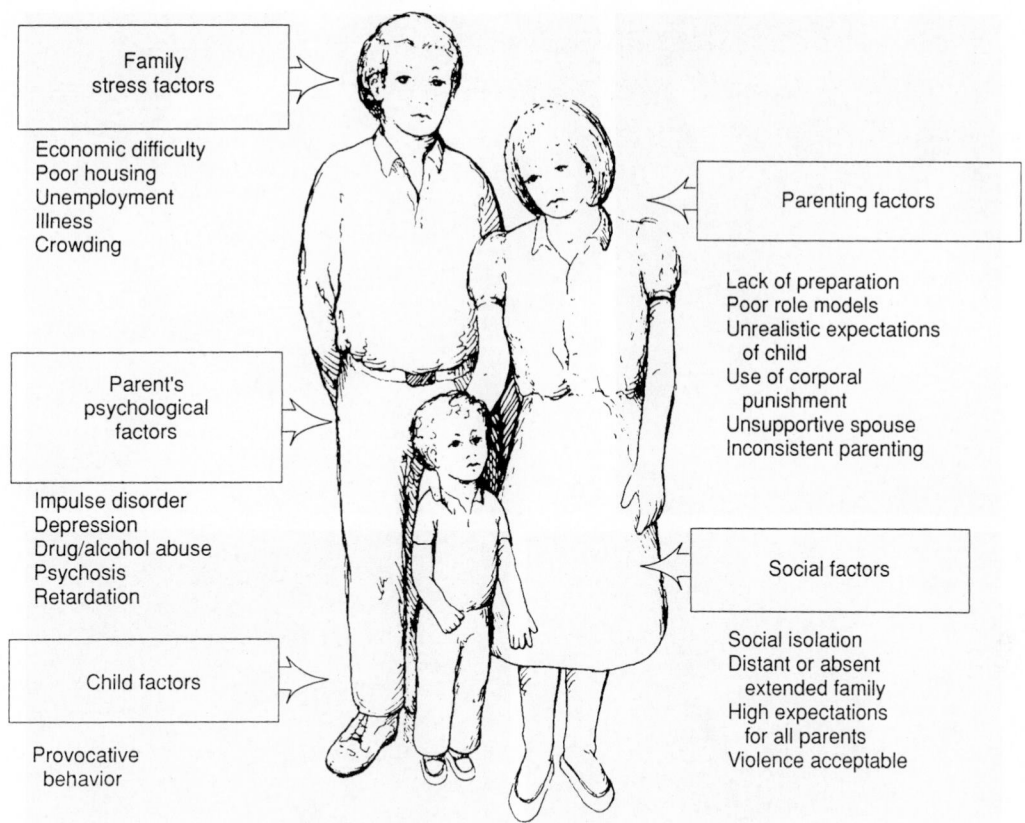

FIGURE 132.5 Risk factors that contribute to abuse and neglect.

Rope burns result in circumferential marks on the wrists, ankles, or around the neck when a child has been bound. Another common specific integument lesion is a handprint on the side of the face or symmetrically on the upper arms. The lesion produced by a slap leaves ecchymotic areas in the location of the interphalangeal spaces. Human bites appear as circular lesions 1 to 2 in. in diameter. Forensic dentistry can match the skin lesion with the dentition of the alleged perpetrator. Some specific skin lesions are shown in Fig. 132.6.

Burns of the skin may be caused by abuse or neglect. Burns account for 5% of cases of physical abuse. In particular, tap water scald burns that occur in an immersion pattern (Fig. 132.7A) are often the result of intentional trauma. Immersion burns are likely to be inflicted by an abusive parent when they occur on a child who is being toilet trained. Other indications of abuse are (i) a delay in seeking treatment, (ii) a history of the child being unsupervised, and (iii) the child being brought to the hospital by the parent who was not present at the time the burn occurred.

In attempting to match the physical findings of the burn with the available history, several factors must be appreciated. The extent of the burn depends on the temperature of the water, duration of exposure, thickness of the skin involved, and presence or absence of clothing. Water temperature 54°C (130°F) or greater causes a full-thickness burn with less than a 30-second exposure. Because palms and soles are thick, they are often spared. Clothing tends to keep the hot water in contact with the skin and causes more severe burns. Burns presumably caused by falling or thrown fluids should produce a droplet or splash pattern. When the child has several small bullous lesions, the main differential diagnosis is a second-degree burn versus bullous impetigo caused by bacterial infection. This differentiation is easily made by Gram stain and culture of a bulla.

Other burns may occur through contact with a hot solid rather than a hot fluid. Cigarette burns are the most common. If the history given is of a child brushing against a cigarette or of hot ashes falling on the child, the resulting injury should be a nonspecific first- or second-degree burn. When a cigarette is extinguished on the child's skin, the injury is a burn that is 8 to 10 mm in diameter and indurated at its margin. A healed cigarette burn is indistinguishable from any other circular skin lesion such as impetigo, abscess, or vesicles. Burns from radiators, hot plates, cigarette lighters (Fig. 132.7B), curling irons, or standard irons imprint the shape of the hot object. More recently, there have been reports of children burned by microwave ovens.

The final category of integumental injury is injury to the hair. Traction alopecia is seen when a parent pulls the child by the hair. The scalp is usually clear, differentiating this lesion from tinea capitis, seborrhea, and scalp eczema. Alopecia areata produces a lesion in which the hair is uniformly absent. In the case of traction or traumatic alopecia, patches of broken hair remain.

Skeletal System. The skeletal system is also commonly traumatized when children are physically abused. As previously

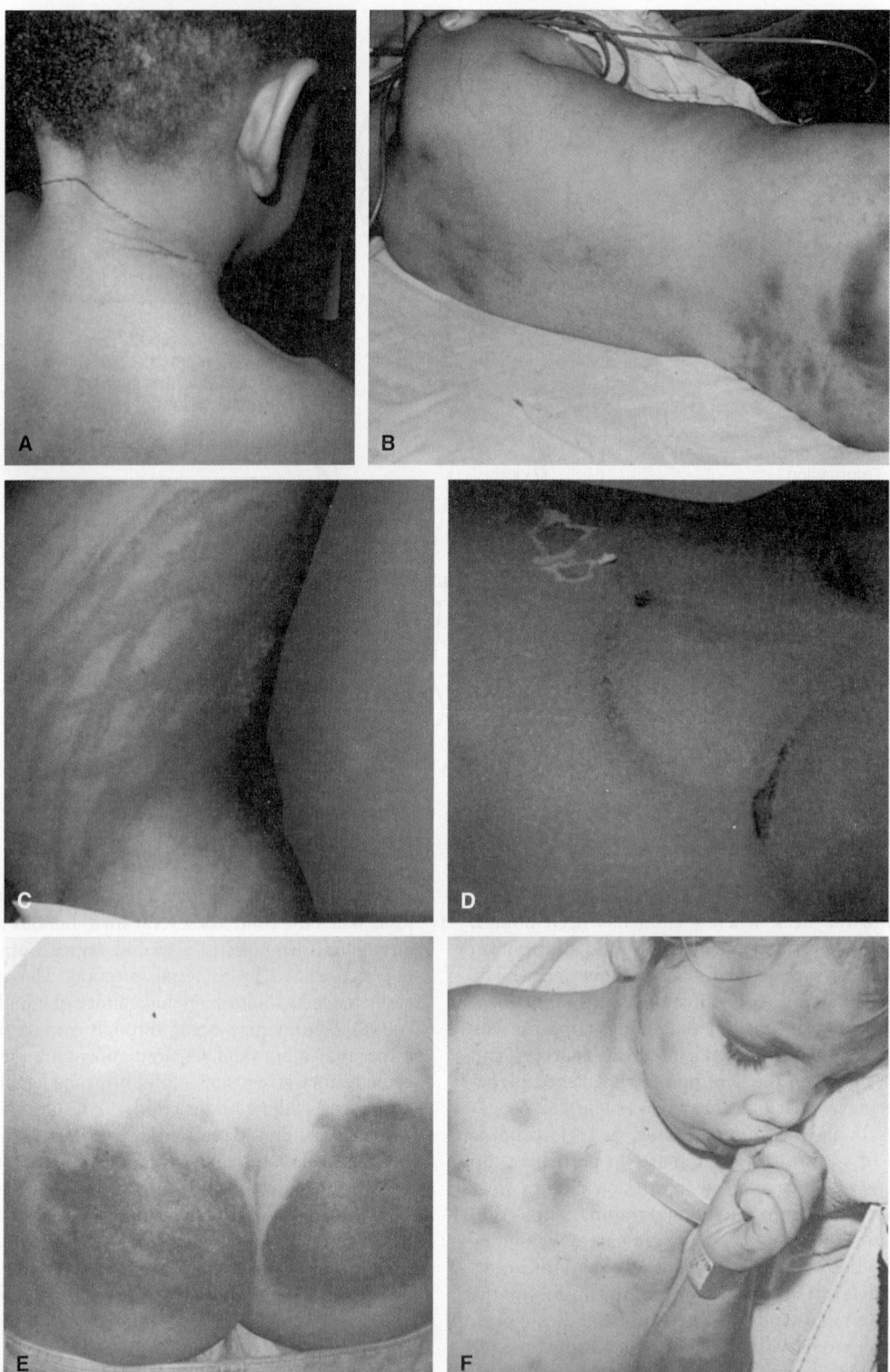

FIGURE 132.6 Cutaneous manifestations of child abuse. **A:** Strangulation mark. **B:** Bruises at various stages of healing. **C:** Linear loop-shaped marks. **D:** Multiple loop-shaped marks. **E:** Buttocks bruises as a cause of myoglobinuria. **F:** Multiple bruises in a central pattern.

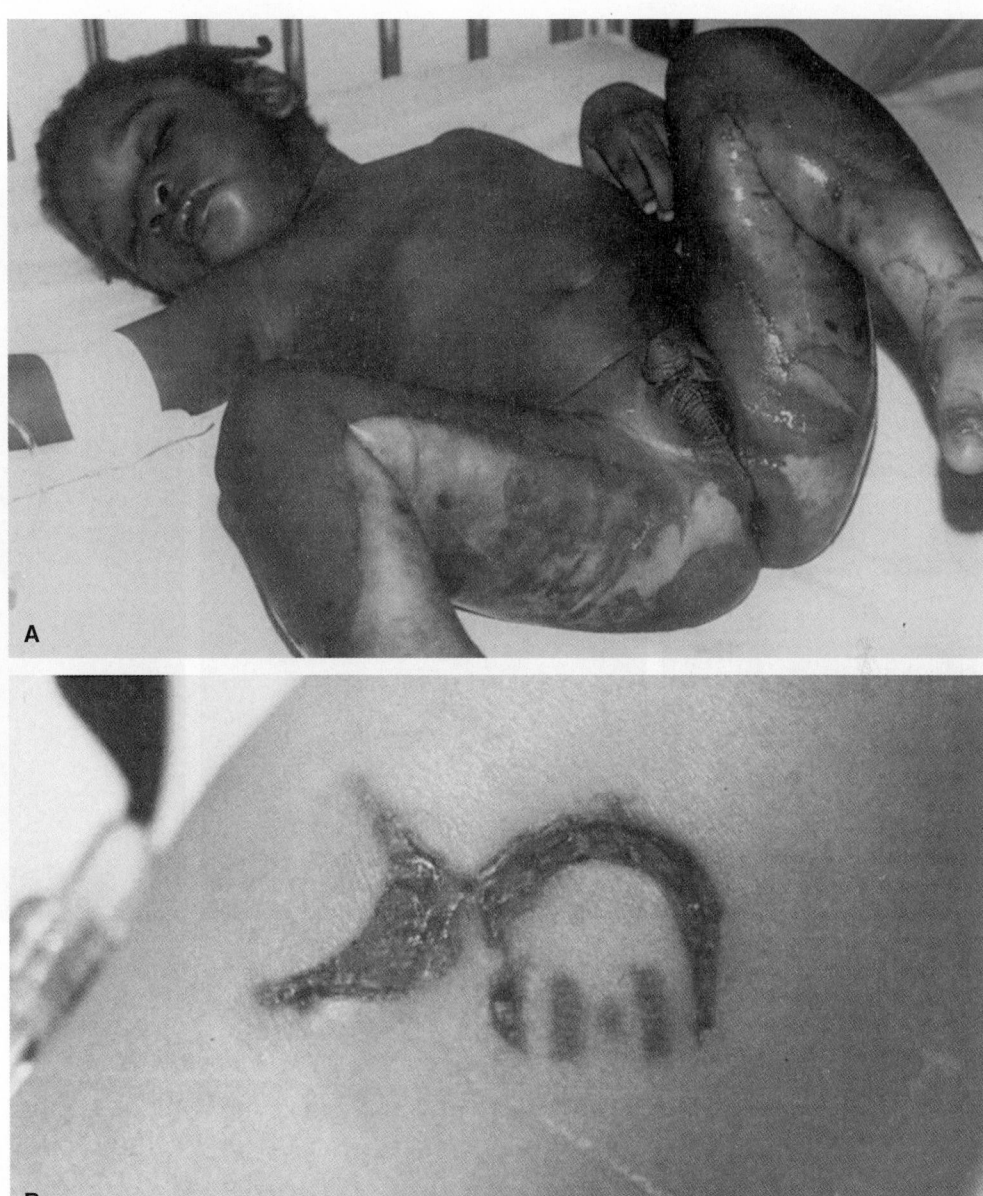

FIGURE 132.7 **A:** Hot water burn in an immersion pattern. **B:** Pattern burn from cigarette lighter.

mentioned, matching the history of injury with the physical findings is important. Considering the mobility and strength of the child is also important in identifying suspicious injuries. The radiologist needs to review the patient's past radiographs to identify the child with multiple visits to the hospital for the treatment of fractures. When suspicion of abuse is high, a radiographic skeletal survey should be obtained to ascertain the condition of the entire skeletal system. It may be helpful to repeat a skeletal survey 2 weeks after a suspected injury, as healing may make the injuries more apparent.

Support for the use of radioisotope scans and magnetic resonance imaging (MRI) as a more sensitive and immediate way of demonstrating bone injury is increasing. However, radionuclide scans and MRIs are still second-line studies. Some of the indications for a radiographic skeletal survey or bone scans are listed in the "Management" section of this chapter. A skeletal survey is often performed on a young child with one obvious fracture and then reveals multiple healing old fractures. The skeletal survey is the preferred radiographic study because it provides information on the type, location, and age of fractures, as well as presence or absence of bone diseases.

Bone injuries may be of several types, including simple transverse fractures, impacted fractures, spiral fractures, metaphyseal fractures, or subperiosteal hematomas. Radiographs of some of these injuries are shown in Fig. 132.8. To explain a transverse fracture, the history should be that of direct force applied to the bone. Differentiating the true cause of this type of fracture is often difficult. The impacted fracture should have an accompanying history of force along the long axis of the bone, such as the child's falling on his or her outstretched hand. In the case of a spiral fracture, a history of twisting or torque during the traumatic event should be present. Metaphyseal chip fractures

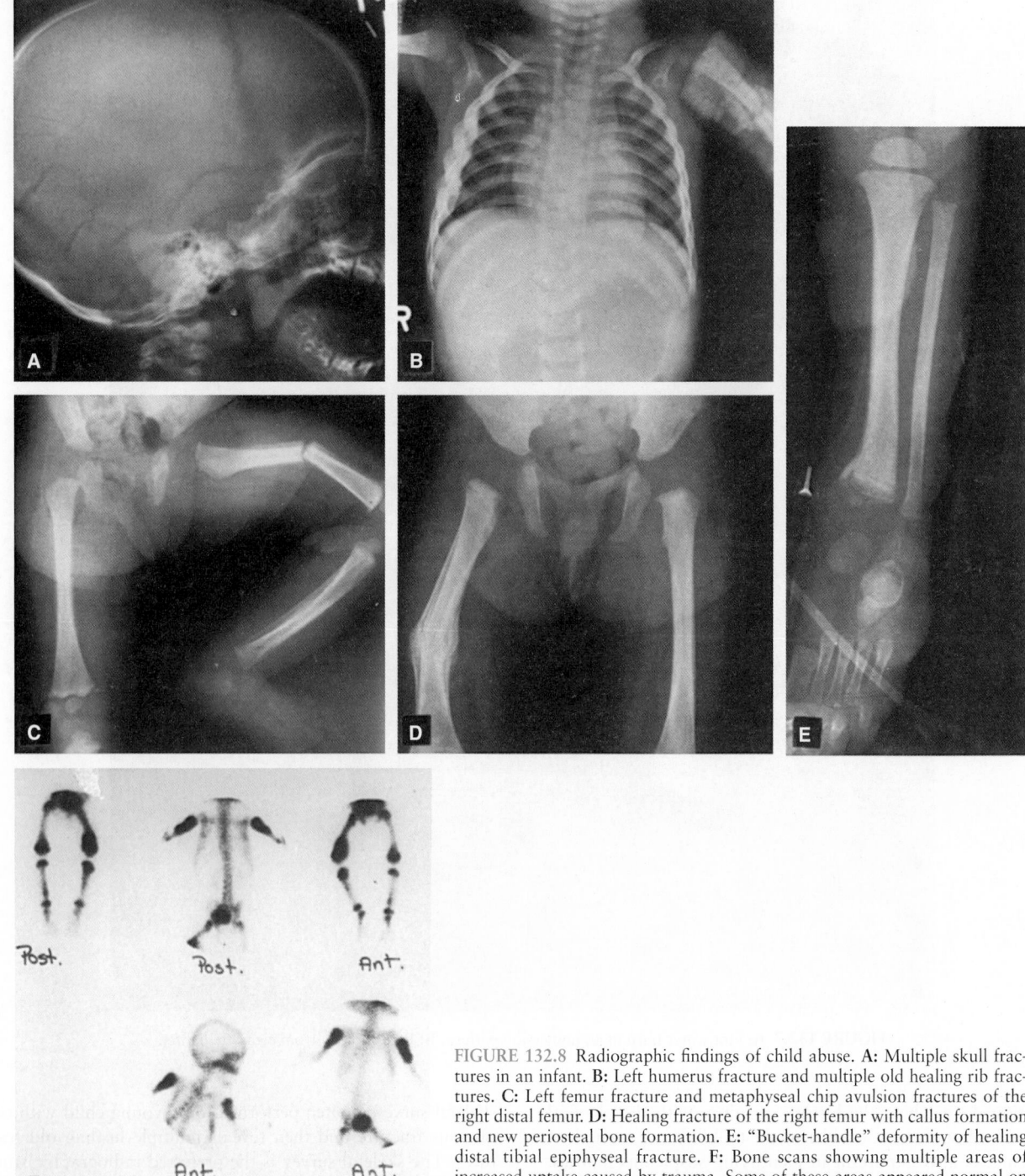

FIGURE 132.8 Radiographic findings of child abuse. **A:** Multiple skull fractures in an infant. **B:** Left humerus fracture and multiple old healing rib fractures. **C:** Left femur fracture and metaphyseal chip avulsion fractures of the right distal femur. **D:** Healing fracture of the right femur with callus formation and new periosteal bone formation. **E:** "Bucket-handle" deformity of healing distal tibial epiphyseal fracture. **F:** Bone scans showing multiple areas of increased uptake caused by trauma. Some of these areas appeared normal on the original radiographs. Ant., anterior; Post., posterior.

occur when the extremity is pulled or yanked. It is hypothesized that the periosteum is most tightly adhered at the metaphysis, causing small bone fragments to avulse. Metaphyseal chip fractures are almost exclusively caused by abuse. Subperiosteal hematomas produce a characteristic radiograph. The elevation of the periosteum is seen as a linear opacification running parallel to the bone surface. Subperiosteal hematomas are produced by direct trauma to the bone.

However, in up to 10% of small and premature infants, symmetric periosteal elevation that is not caused by abuse may occur along the tibia or humerus. The reason for this finding is unknown, but it should not be confused with abuse.

The location of the fracture is important in the identification of abuse. The fracture of a clavicle or the dislocation of a radial head is a common noninflicted injury. However, when the femur and/or ribs of a young child are fractured, the suspicion of abuse increases. Anderson reported on a series of children with femur fractures. Of 24 children who were younger than 2 years, abuse was proved in 19 cases. In two-thirds of these children, the fracture was the only sign of abuse.

Feldman and Brewer reported on a series of children with rib fractures and noted an obvious history of trauma—for example, motor vehicle accident, an obvious bone disease such as osteogenesis imperfecta, or child abuse.

Feldman and Brewer also report examining several children who received external cardiac compression and finding that none of them had sustained rib fractures as a result of their cardiopulmonary resuscitation. In a confirmatory report, Schweich and Fleisher found that when the parents could not provide a history for rib fractures, the cause was abuse. The mean age of the group of children who had inflicted trauma was 3 months, whereas the group having accidental rib fractures had a mean age of 8.5 years. Abusive rib fractures are frequently posterior in location and are thought to result from anterior-posterior compression of the thorax rather than blunt trauma in most cases. The history of injury must be matched with the physical finding.

Other uncommon and therefore suspicious fractures are located in the vertebrae, sternum, pelvis, or scapulae. Uncommon fractures need to be carefully evaluated unless a clear history of significant trauma, such as an automobile injury, is reported.

The age of a fracture may be estimated from the amount of callus formation and bone remodeling seen on the radiograph. Table 132.1 lists fracture landmarks by date. Dating of fractures is not an exact science because many confounding variables, such as the child's age, location of the fracture, and nutritional status, must be considered. Nonetheless, the child who presents with an acute fracture and has a second fracture with a callus stands out as having sustained more than one episode of trauma. The usual long-bone fracture may take 8 to 10 days to form callus and several months to heal completely. In the acute stages of injury, soft-tissue swelling should be seen for 2 to 5 days. Soft-tissue swelling may be clearly seen on standard radiographs. Skull fractures or fractures of other flat bones cannot be dated in the same way. Caution should also be exercised in dating metaphyseal fractures as some metaphyseal fractures will not develop much callus or exhibit the classic stages of healing.

TABLE 132.1

DATING FRACTURES

0–10 days
Soft-tissue edema
Joint fluid
Visible fracture fragments
Visible fracture lines

10 days–8 wk
Periosteal new bone (layered)
Callus (first subtle and then heavy)
Bone resorption along fracture line makes fracture line more visible
Metaphyseal fragments often more visible

≥8 wk
Periosteal new bone matures, becomes thicker
Callus formation becomes more dense and smoother
Metaphyseal fragments are incorporated into metaphyseal callus and become smoother
Fracture line less visible and then invisible
Deformities and cortical bumps persist

When a young child sustains multiple fractures, the differential diagnosis must be widened beyond accidental trauma and abuse to include osteogenesis imperfecta, infantile cortical hyperostosis, scurvy, syphilis, osteoid osteoma, neoplasms, rickets, hypophosphatasia, and osteomyelitis. Table 132.2 details the distinction between child abuse and osteogenesis imperfecta. The other conditions are much more rare than abuse and can be ruled out both by the appearance of the bone on the radiograph and by the levels of calcium, phosphorus, and alkaline phosphatase in the serum.

Central Nervous System. Injuries to the central nervous system (CNS) are the main cause of child abuse deaths. These injuries may be subdivided into two categories: direct trauma

TABLE 132.2

OSTEOGENESIS IMPERFECTA VERSUS CHILD ABUSE

Finding	Osteogenesis imperfecta	Child abuse
Incidence	Rare	Common
Positive family history	Common	Common
Blue sclerae	Common	Rare*
Abnormal teeth	Common	Rare
Hearing impairment	Common	Uncommon
Osteoporosis	Common	Rare
Abnormal fracture healing	Common	Rare
Wormian bones	Common	Rare
Joint laxity	Common	Rare
Short stature	Common	Occasional
Fracture recurrence in protected environment	Common	Rare
In utero fracture	Occasional	Rare
Biochemical studies	Abnormal	Normal

*Light blue sclera can be a normal finding in young infants.

and shaking injuries. Direct trauma is inflicted either by striking the child with an object or by dropping or throwing the child against a wall or onto the floor. The extent of the resulting trauma depends on the amount of force used, the surface contacted, and the child's age. The child may be brought to the ED with a small subgaleal hematoma or in coma. Injuries may vary from scalp contusions to intracerebral hematomas.

A history of a young infant falling off a bed or dressing table is often presented. The precise extent of injury from this type of fall is unknown, but several reports suggest that even uncomplicated skull fractures are as uncommon as 1% to 2% of cases. If the injury is more severe and the only history is of a fall from less than 8 to 10 feet, abuse should be suspected. Another scenario is that of a child who sustained trauma 1 week before the ED visit. The visit is prompted by the parent's noticing a soft spot on the child's cranium. This sequence may occur when the initial scalp hematoma so rapidly expanded that it had a bony consistency. Only with degradation and softening of the mass does the parent now perceive the hematoma. Although a delay in seeking treatment is a well-recognized red flag for child abuse injuries, this case provides a plausible exception. In all children younger than 1 year who have a history of head trauma, skull radiographs are recommended. Infants tend to sustain skull fracture more easily and are more vulnerable to serious sequelae. If a fracture does exist and abuse is suspected, a skeletal survey and further head imaging with a CT and/or MRI should also be obtained. For the diagnostic methods to be used for more serious head injuries, refer to Chapter 116.

Shaking injuries characteristically cause serious CNS damage without evidence of external trauma. The infant's relatively large head size and weak neck muscles are predisposing factors for whiplash injury. Whether the injury is caused by shaking alone or shaking followed by an impact is controversial (Fig. 132.9). There are some parent defense experts who have attempted to discredit this form of injury, but it remains one of the most important and lethal forms of abuse. In most fatal cases, minor bruising to the scalp is apparent, although such scalp injuries may not be apparent until the scalp is reflected during the autopsy.

The shearing and contusive forces that result from shaking the infant produce this type of injury. Specific lesions that occur include hematomas, subarachnoid hemorrhages, or brain contusions, particularly in the frontal and occipital lobes. The child may present with lethargy and a "septic" appearance, with seizures, or in a coma. The physical examination is often otherwise unremarkable except for retinal hemorrhages (Fig. 132.10A). Occasionally, bruises on the upper arms or shoulders indicate the sites where the child has been grasped. Lumbar puncture may produce grossly bloody, xanthochromic or normal spinal fluid. If computed tomography is available, it shows the characteristic findings of occipital contusion and intrahemispheric blood (Fig. 132.10B). This form of abusive behavior by the parent is usually triggered by the infant's persistent crying. Excessively rough forms of play and misguided resuscitative efforts have been cited as alternative explanations for head injuries by caregivers but there is not any data to support the claims that these activities can result in the types of injuries seen in abusive head trauma. Imaging the CNS has been advocated for all children under 2 years of age who have signs of physical abuse, as there may be occult or old injury independent of neurologic signs and symptoms.

Gastrointestinal System. Gastrointestinal (GI) injuries are relatively uncommon abuse manifestations but, similar to CNS injuries, account for a significant percentage of fatal injuries. Of all GI injuries, mouth trauma is perhaps the most common.

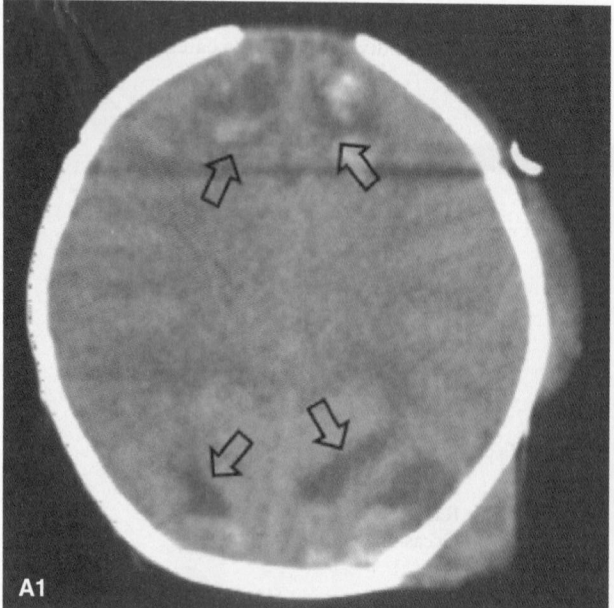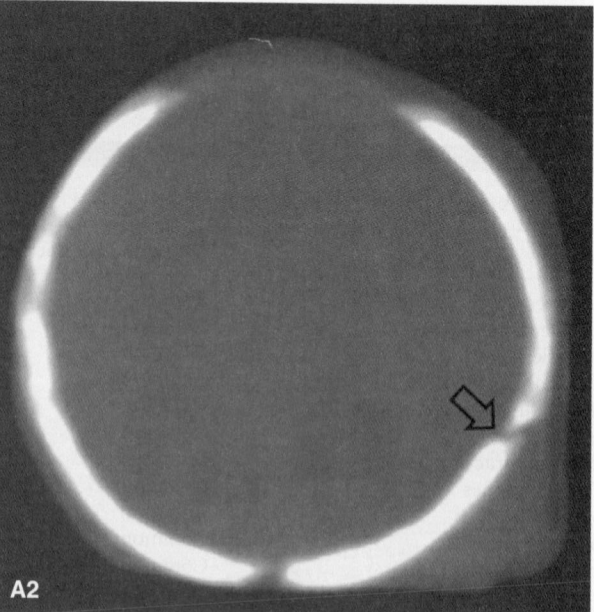

FIGURE 132.9 **A:** Six-week-old infant examined by computed tomography (CT) without contrast. **A1:** Axial CT shows focal areas of increased and decreased density in the anterior and posterior parasagittal regions *(arrows)*. Scalp swelling is present on the left. **A2:** Axial bone window shows fracture of the right parietal bone *(arrow)*. *(continued)*

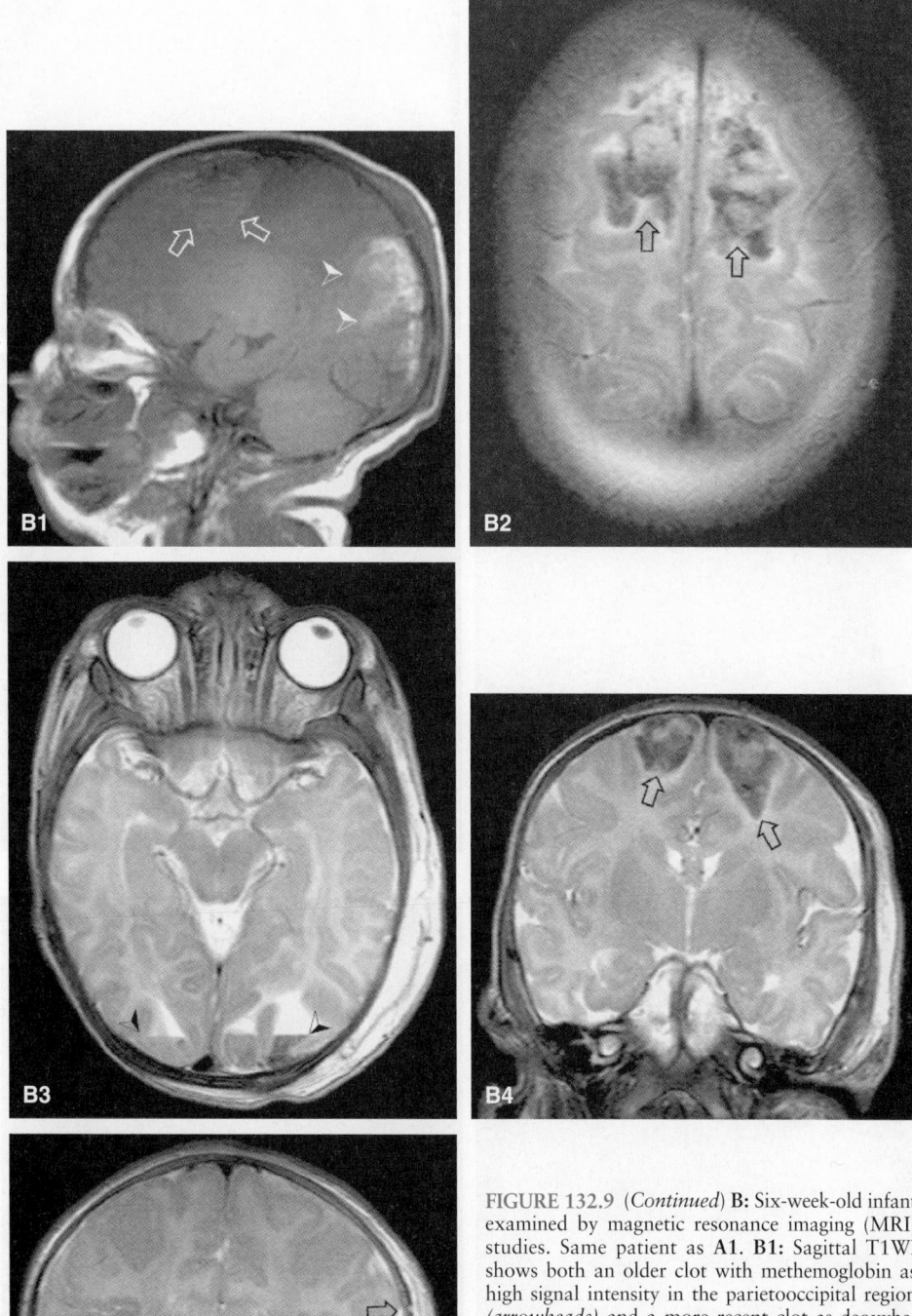

FIGURE 132.9 (*Continued*) **B:** Six-week-old infant examined by magnetic resonance imaging (MRI) studies. Same patient as **A1. B1:** Sagittal T1WI shows both an older clot with methemoglobin as high signal intensity in the parietooccipital region (*arrowheads*) and a more recent clot as deoxyhemoglobin in the frontal region (*arrows*). **B2:** Axial T2WI shows the frontal parasagittal hemorrhagic areas of injury (*arrows*). **B3:** Axial T2WI shows the posterior, parietooccipital older areas of injury as areas of bleeding with blood fluid levels (*arrowheads*). **B4:** Coronal T2WI through the frontal region shows bilateral parasagittal hemorrhagic changes (*arrows*). **B5:** Coronal T2WI at the site of fracture (*arrow*) shows overlying scalp swelling and bleeding. (Courtesy of Robert A. Zimmerman, MD.) (*continued*)

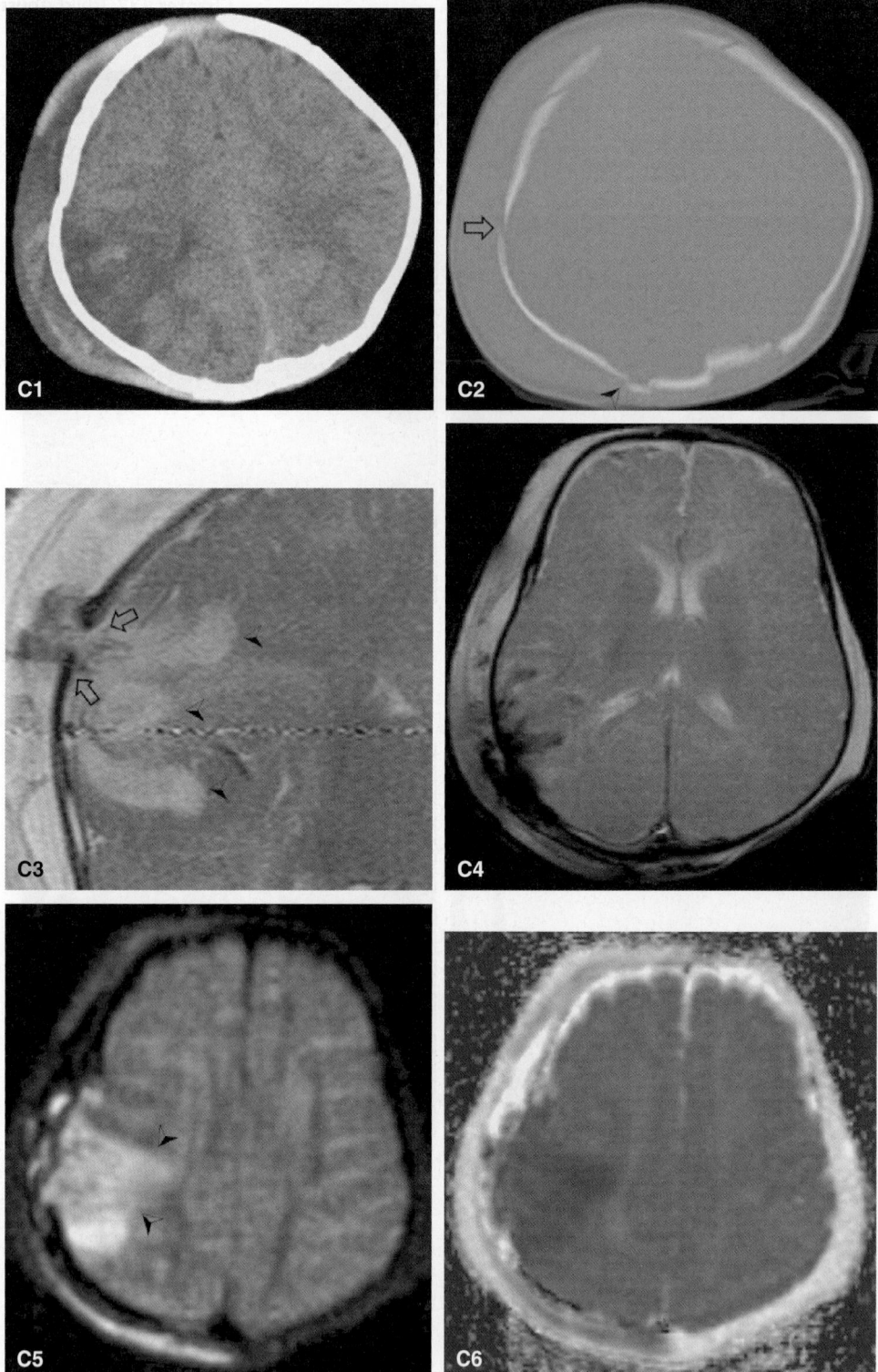

FIGURE 132.9 (*Continued*) **C:** Five-month-old male infant examined by CT and MRI on the day of admission. Parts **C1** and **C2**, axial CTs without contrast; parts **C3–C6**, MRI images. **C1:** Axial CT, brain windows, shows hemorrhage within the soft tissues of the scalp; underlying hypodensity and hyperdensity within the brain in the right parietal region consistent with contusional change. **C2:** Axial bone window at the same level as **C1** shows a fracture of the right parietal bone *(arrow)* and an additional area of fracture posteriorly at the lambdoid suture *(arrowhead)*. **C3:** Coronal T2WI demonstrates separation of the bone at the site of fracture *(arrow)* and underlying brain swelling involving the cortex, consistent with contusion *(arrowheads)*. Abnormality is present at the site of the fracture in the extracalvarial soft tissues, consistent with hemorrhage and/or herniation of brain tissue through the fracture. **C4:** Axial two-dimensional FLASH susceptibility gradient echo scan demonstrates extensive intraparenchymal and soft-tissue scalp areas of signal loss consistent with bleeding. **C5:** Axial diffusion imaging through the site of contusion shows restricted motion of water consistent with cytotoxic edema *(arrowheads)*. **C6:** Axial apparent diffusion coefficient (ADC) map at the site of the restricted motion of water shows hypointensity consistent with cytotoxic edema. (Courtesy of Robert A. Zimmerman, MD.) (*continued*)

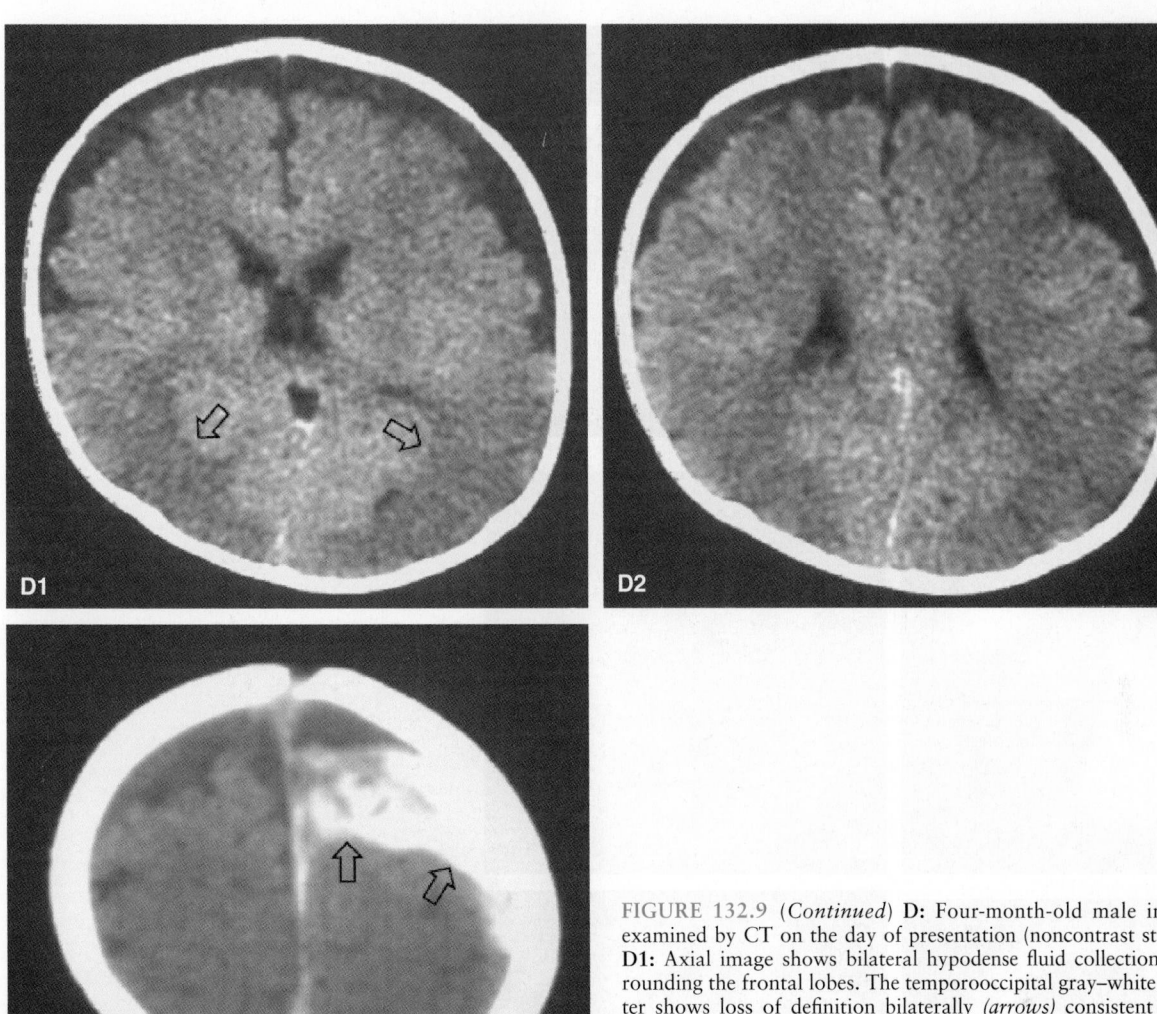

FIGURE 132.9 (*Continued*) **D:** Four-month-old male infant examined by CT on the day of presentation (noncontrast study). **D1:** Axial image shows bilateral hypodense fluid collection surrounding the frontal lobes. The temporooccipital gray–white matter shows loss of definition bilaterally *(arrows)* consistent with injury. **D2:** Axial CT at a higher level in the brain shows the same findings as in **A. D3:** Still higher axial CT shows extensive subdural hemorrhage on the left side covering the frontal lobe *(arrows)* and extending into the midline along the falx cerebri. (Courtesy of Robert A. Zimmerman, MD.) (*continued*)

Small infants may sustain a tear of the frenulum resulting from "bottle jamming." In older children, dental trauma may be a sign of abuse.

Other GI system manifestations are more medically serious and generally result from blunt trauma to the abdominal contents. Rupture of the spleen or laceration of the liver causes the child to present with elevated levels of liver enzymes, with an acute abdomen, or in shock, with no external source of bleeding and with absent or only minor bruising of the abdominal wall as shown in figure 132.11. The identification and management of these emergencies are covered in Section IV. A less acute presentation is the afebrile child with persistent bilious vomiting from a duodenal hematoma with small-bowel obstruction. Documenting an elevated serum amylase or lipase level or increased liver enzyme levels is important in providing tangible evidence of abdominal trauma in cases that lack any radiographic finding or abdominal wall bruising. Due to the recognition that abusive abdominal injuries may be occult at the time of presentation for medical care, some experts advocate screening all victims of suspected child abuse for occult abdominal trauma. Recommended screening tests include liver enzyme tests, amylase and lipase and urine analysis. Elevation of the serum amylase level may also identify those cases that should be followed for possible development of a pancreatic pseudocyst. See Chapter 107 for more detailed information on abdominal trauma.

Cardiopulmonary System. Abuse may be manifested in cardiac or pulmonary trauma, with no injuries that are characteristically induced by abuse. Pulmonary contusion, pneumothorax, hemothorax, cardiac tamponade, and myocardial contusion may all occur occasionally. Specifics of identification and management of these problems are covered in Chapter 118. Measurement of cardiac enzymes may help identify cardiac trauma.

Genitourinary Systems. Common genitourinary complaints, such as hematuria, dysuria, urgency, frequency, and enuresis, may be the initial signs of abuse. These problems may result

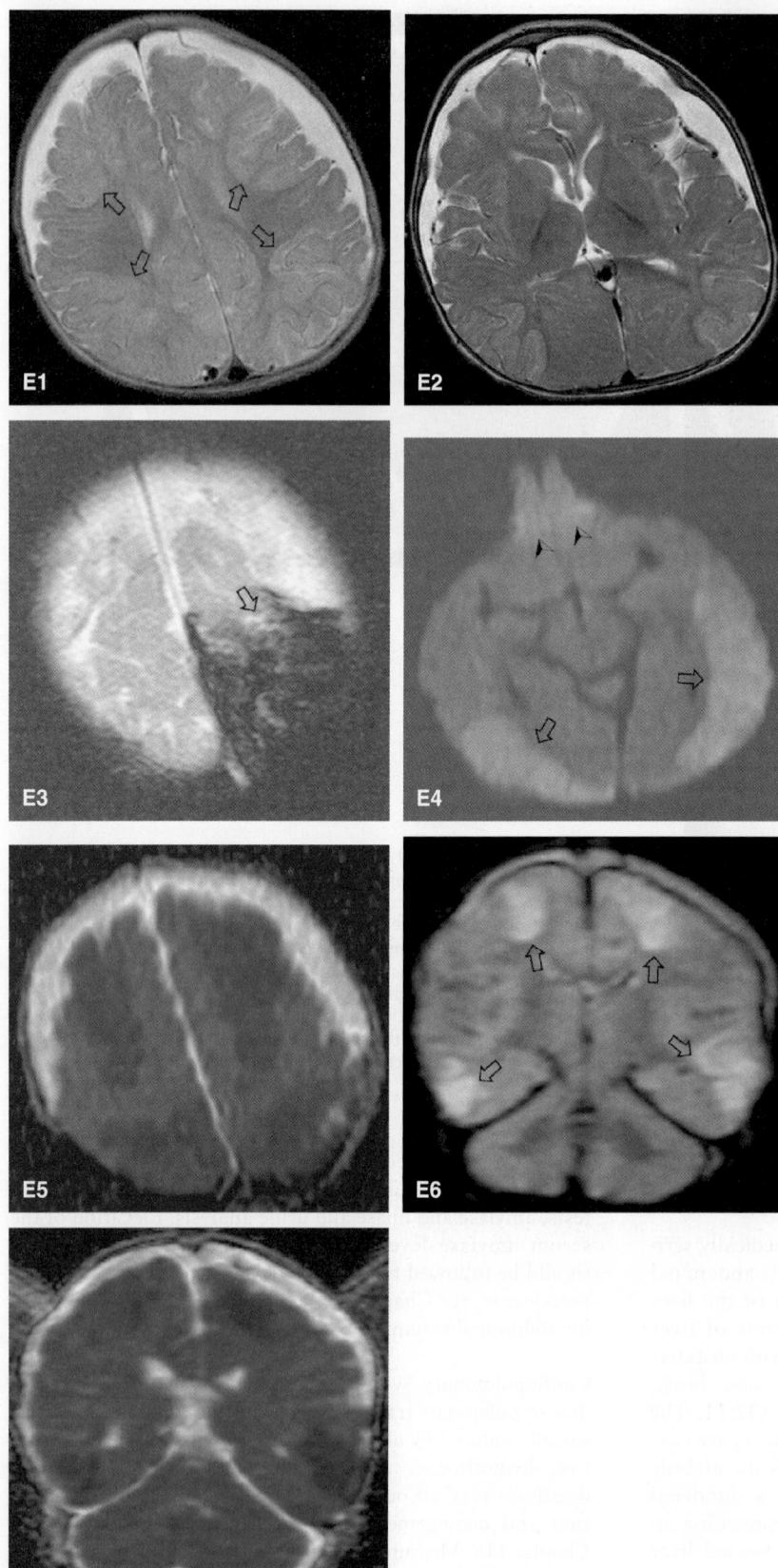

FIGURE 132.9 (*Continued*) **E:** Four-month-old male infant (same as **D**) examined on the day of presentation. **E1:** Axial T2WI shows bilateral subdural fluid collection surrounding the frontal lobes. There is abnormal subtle increased T2 signal intensity in the cortex both anteriorly and posteriorly within the brain *(arrows)*. There is sparing of the rolandic region. **E2:** Axial T2WI at a lower level shows the same findings. **E3:** Axial T2WI gradient echo susceptibility scan shows extensive area of hemorrhage in the subdural space overlying the left parietal region *(arrow)*. **E4:** Axial diffusion weighted image shows bilateral temporooccipital areas of restricted diffusion consistent with cytotoxic edema *(arrows)*. Note anteriorly in the region of the gyrus rectus that there is also bilateral cytotoxic edema *(arrowheads)*. **E5:** Axial ADC map at a higher level in the brain shows the hypointense signal in the bilateral parasagittal watershed region frontally, consistent with cytotoxic edema, as well as posteriorly in the bilateral parietal region. **E6:** Coronal diffusion weighted image shows bilateral parasagittal posterior frontal areas of cytotoxic edema and bilateral temporal watershed areas *(arrows)*. **E7:** Coronal ADC map of these injuries shows hypointense signal at the site of cytotoxic edema. (Courtesy of Robert A. Zimmerman, MD.)

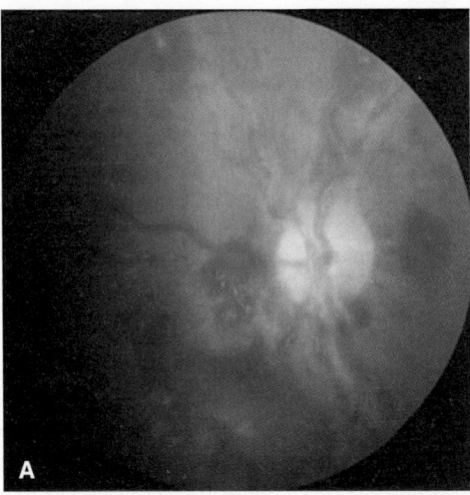

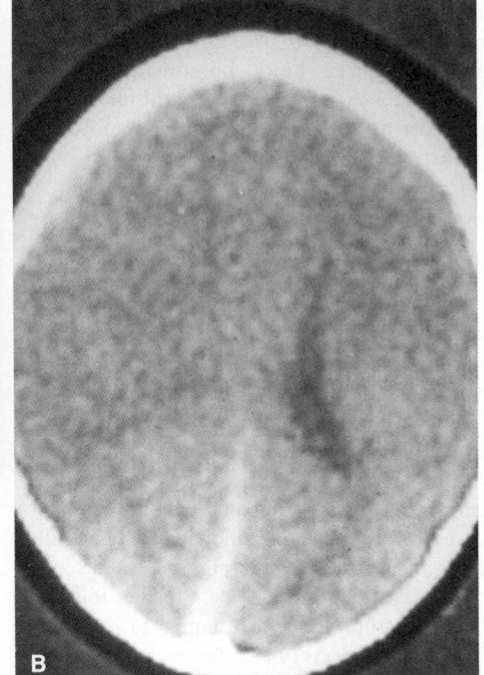

FIGURE 132.10 Manifestations of abusive head trauma. **A:** Retinal hemorrhages as seen on fundoscopic examination. **B:** Computed tomography showing intrahemispheric subdural bleeding and right cortical brain swelling.

from direct trauma, sexually transmitted infections (SITs), or emotional abuse. Some aspects of genitourinary manifestation are covered subsequently in the "Sexual Abuse" section. As for direct trauma, any part of the genitourinary system may be involved, from the renal parenchyma to the urethral meatus. Penile trauma that does not have an adequate explanation may be an alerting sign of abuse. Traumatic hematuria is managed as described in Chapter 112.

A life-threatening renal manifestation may be the occurrence of rhabdomyolysis and myoglobinuria. With extensive deep soft-tissue and muscle trauma, myoglobin may be liberated in quantities sufficient to cause acute renal failure. Such children have dark or tea-colored urine that tests positive for blood with urine dipstick but has no visible red blood cells on microscopic examination. Serum myoglobin levels confirm the diagnosis, and the serum creatine phosphokinase

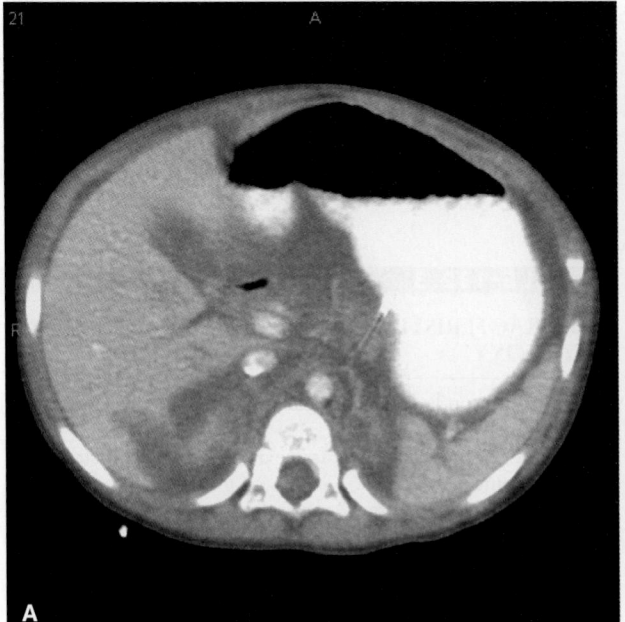

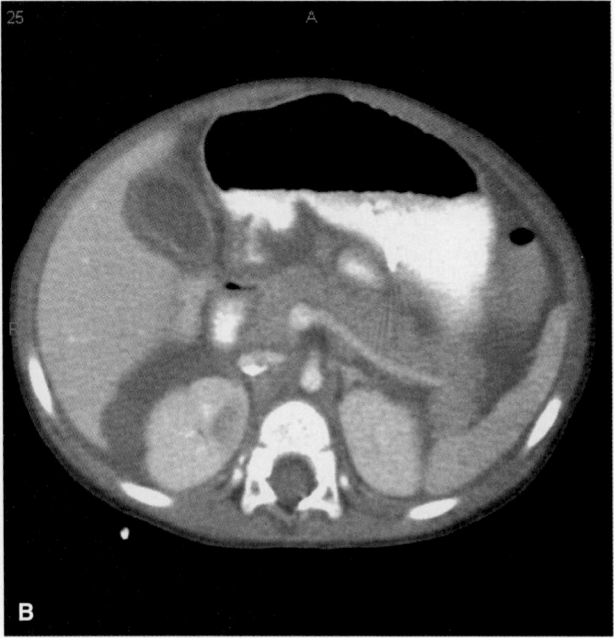

FIGURE 132.11 **A:** Abuse victim with computed tomographic (CT) scan evidence of injury to the liver and spleen. **B:** CT scan showing injury to the kidney and pancreas.

can reach extremely high values. Before using hypertonic intravenous contrast materials in the child with heme-positive urine, myoglobinuria should be considered and ruled out. The patient with possible myoglobinuria and acute renal failure must not be given potassium-containing intravenous solutions.

Sensory. The sensory organs are vulnerable to physical abuse, including ocular, nasal, and otic injuries. The eye may sustain several different forms of injury, including periorbital ecchymosis, corneal abrasion, subconjunctival hemorrhage, hyphema, dislocated lens, retinal hemorrhages, or detached retina. Each lesion is discussed in Chapters 110, 111 and 117. A careful history of injury is important when treating any of these conditions. Injury to the nose may result in simple hemorrhage or fracture and dislocation.

A direct blow to the ear may also cause ecchymosis, hemo-tympanum and perforation of the tympanic membrane (Fig. 132.12). In such cases, hemotympanum following basilar skull fracture should also be considered. The presence of discoloration behind the ear (Battle's sign) may be a further indication of a basilar skull fracture. Refer to Chapter 116, which deals specifically with these aspects of emergency care.

Unusual Manifestations. Rarely, the emergency physician is confronted by one of the unusual abuse manifestations. Cases of toxic and nontoxic ingestions, electrolyte disorders such as hyponatremia and hypernatremia, foreign bodies,

bathtub drowning, strangulation, and multiple serious infections may be the result of abuse. In these situations, the parent actively abuses the child by feeding, instilling, or injecting harmful substances or objects into the child's body. Some children with a toxic ingestion reveal that their parents forced them to ingest the substance. The most common toxic ingestants of this type are alcoholic beverages that are given to or forced on the child to either quiet the child or demonstrate "manly" qualities. Other drugs may be used to poison the child. Most recent reports are of cocaine ingestions and passive inhalation of "crack" cocaine that has been vaporized (see Chapter 102).

Several cases have been reported in which parents have placed their children on high-salt, water-only, or pepper diets as a form of punishment. Such children may present with signs of hypernatremia or hyponatremia, possibly with seizures. Foreign bodies have been found in every orifice, as well as under the skin and in fingernail beds. There have been case reports of children who were smothered and present to the ED with florid pulmonary edema. Several cases of Munchausen syndrome by proxy (also referred to as pediatric condition falsification and child abuse in a medical setting) have been reported in which a parent has inflicted illness on the child rather than feigning or inducing illness (Table 132.3). Cases of fictitious fever, hematuria, and even sepsis have resulted from this form of abuse. Although rare, the unusual manifestations of abuse should be considered when more common causes of these problems could not be identified.

Management

The management of a child abuse case is difficult unless the emergency physician has a previously prepared, well-structured protocol. If reports of abuse are not a daily occurrence, an institutional policy serves as an important guide to the mechanics of management. Consultants from different disciplines, such as nursing and social work, provide invaluable assistance. A multidisciplinary approach simplifies the initial decision making and subsequent case management. The steps in the protocol are shown in Fig. 132.13.

Suspect Abuse. The first step is to decide whether a reasonable likelihood of abuse exists. Many shades of suspicion make the term *abuse* imprecise. Although every traumatic

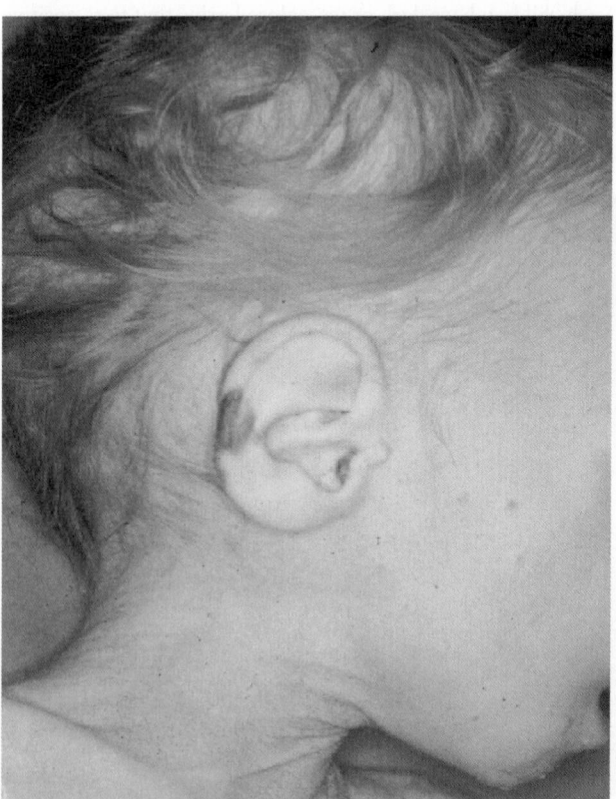

FIGURE 132.12 Ecchymosis on the internal surface of the pinna may result from "boxing" the ear, crushing it against the skull.

TABLE 132.3

CHARACTERISTICS OF MUNCHAUSEN SYNDROME BY PROXY

Difficult to understand medical situation, often with recurrent episodes
Failure of other centers to arrive at diagnosis—"doctor shopping"
Unsupportive or "absent" marital relationship
Compliant, cooperative, overinvolved mother
Medical knowledge in parent's background
Findings abort with surveillance of child
Findings correlate to the presence of parent
Extensive medical care in parent's medical history

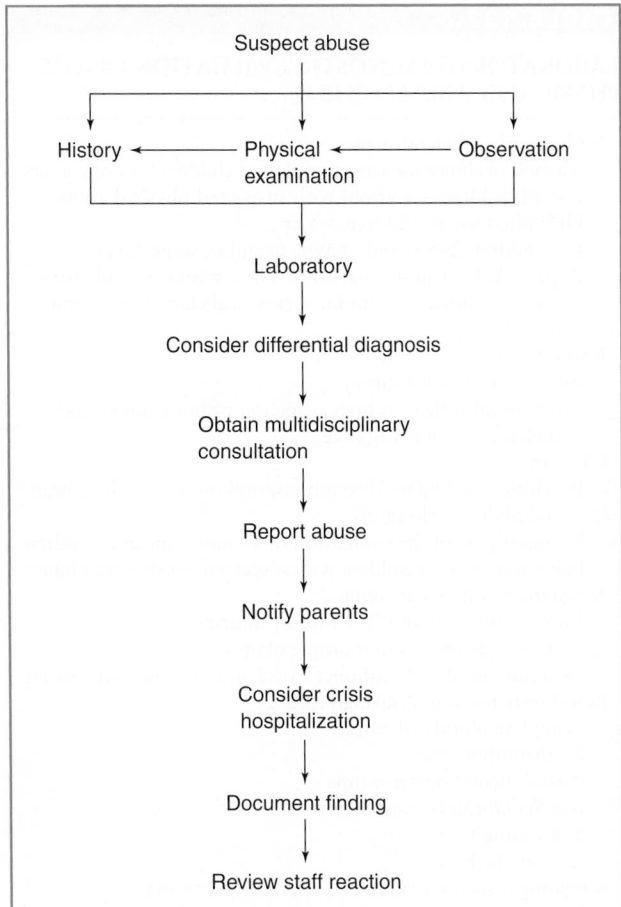

FIGURE 132.13 Procedure for emergency department management of suspected physical abuse.

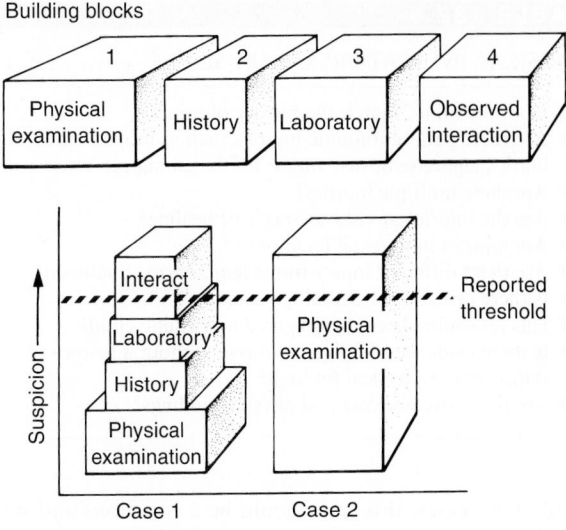

FIGURE 132.14 Building a level of suspicion.

As with the history, the physical examination must be thorough. The signs of physical abuse are detailed in the "Clinical Manifestations" section. A thorough examination serves as a means to uncover these findings. Although the clinician may be tempted to merely glance at a small contusion on a child's face, such a cursory examination fails to reveal possible linear and loop-shaped marks on the upper thighs and buttocks. Table 132.5 lists some of the important physical examination features that are indicators of abuse.

After completion of the history and physical examination, the next step is to compare them. Does the stated history match the physical findings? Does the history make sense? Does the history correlate with the developmental level of the child? Answers to these important questions may add further elements of suspicion.

This step of comparing history and physical examination is completed subconsciously by most practitioners. Physicians often attempt to match the patient's degree of symptoms with the presence or absence of physical findings, particularly in patients with psychosomatic complaints. In

injury should be suspected as abuse, the physician has the onerous task of deciding how much suspicion is necessary to take some action (i.e., report). To establish the level of suspicion, data are gathered by obtaining a complete history, performing a thorough physical examination, comparing the history and physical examination, observing interactions, and obtaining laboratory studies and/or radiographs. Then, the physician can formulate a differential diagnosis and assign a rank to abuse. Indications of abuse in the history and physical examination and observational data must be used as building blocks that are added until they achieve a certain threshold of suspicion. As demonstrated in Fig. 132.14, when the threshold is reached, a report of suspected abuse must follow. In the example of case 1, the building blocks must be used to build a level of suspicion; in case 2, the physical injury is sufficient to make the diagnosis.

A highly detailed history is always important. As in many other medical situations, this process is initiated by asking some general, open-ended questions about "what happened." If the child has sufficient verbal skills, the first questions are directed at him or her. General inquiries must then be followed with specific requests for information; however, a harsh interrogation only alienates the family. Some specific historical indications are listed in Table 132.4.

TABLE 132.4

HISTORICAL INDICATORS OF ABUSE

- Is the history one of inflicted injury?
- Is there an absence of history, a "magical" injury?
- Could the injury have been avoided by better care and supervision?
- Are there inconsistencies or changes in the history?
- Is there a history of repeated injury or hospitalization?
- Was there a delay in seeking medical care?
- Does the history over- or underestimate the injury?
- Is there a medical history of prematurity, failure to thrive, and/or failure to receive adequate medical care, such as immunization?
- Is this a high-risk history (e.g., fall down stairs, dropped baby)?

TABLE 132.5

PHYSICAL INDICATORS OF ABUSE

- Does the injury match the history of injury?
- Are there pathognomonic injuries such as looped wire marks, cigarette burns, and/or bottle jamming?
- Are there multiple injuries?
- Are the injuries at various stages of healing?
- Are injuries in unusual locations?
- Are there different injury forms (e.g., burns, fractures)?
- Is there evidence of overall poor care?
- Has poisoning been documented in a young child?
- Is there evidence of failure to thrive without a history of symptoms or physical findings?
- Are there any unexplained physical findings?

child abuse cases, this step should be a conscious and well-defined step because it is vital to establishing suspicion. In some cases, a lack of consistency is obvious, such as a parent's claim that burns on the child's buttocks occurred when the child inserted his or her finger into an electric socket. Other situations may be less clear, such as the injury being attributed to hot plastic seat covers on an automobile. Although the latter explanation has in fact been reported as a case of accidental injury, it rarely explains burns on the buttocks.

Laboratory data and radiographs are another source of indicators of abuse. The laboratory studies used are few and, for the most part, document the obvious or rule out other disease states. Biochemical, hematologic, and urinary studies that are used appear in Table 132.6, along with their indications. Radiographs document a specific bony or soft-tissue injury. They may provide a comprehensive and longitudinal record of osseous injury at any site in the skeletal system. Indications for performing a skeletal survey include (i) any child younger than 2 years presenting for an injury suspicious for abuse (ii) any child with severe or extensive fractures, (iii) any child who has a history of more than one fracture, (iv) a history in the child or the family of "soft" or easily broken bones, and (v) anytime there is suspicion. Due to the high risk of occult head injury, head imaging with CT and/or MRI is also recommended in children younger than 1 to 2 years presenting with abusive injuries.

During the time occupied by the history, physical examination, and performance of laboratory studies, the physician should be cognizant of the interactions among family members and among the parents, the child, and the ED staff. Such awareness often uncovers subtle indicators of abuse. The observation of parents arguing vehemently on the way to the radiology department may be a clue. The parent who appears to be distant from both the child and the physician is also a suspect. Although the parent who is intoxicated or incoherent never fails to gain staff attention, such individuals are in the minority of abusive parents. Observation of the child is also important. All abused children are not withdrawn, passive, and depressed. On the contrary, some are competent, outgoing, or "pseudomature."

The observed state of the child depends on several factors: (i) the length, frequency, and severity of abuse; (ii) the child's developmental level and age; and (iii) the amount of positive

TABLE 132.6

LABORATORY/DIAGNOSTIC EVALUATION OF THE PHYSICALLY ABUSED CHILD

Radiographic skeletal survey
    Method of choice for screening abused children for bony injury
    For all children <2 yr old with suspected physical abuse
    Of limited use in children >5 yr
    For children 2–5 yr old, maybe useful in some cases
    Repeat skeletal survey performed in 2 weeks may identify fractures missed on initial survey and clarify indeterminate findings.
Radionuclide bone scan
    Adjunct to skeletal survey
    Most useful if there is high suspicion of bony injury and skeletal survey is negative
CT scan
    Provides sliced views through internal organs, such as brain and abdominal organs
    Essential part of the evaluation of seriously injured children
    Initial test used for children with suspected abusive head injury
Magnetic resonance imaging
    More sensitive than CT for many injuries
    Can provide images in multiple planes
    Generally used as an adjunct to CT in the acute care setting
Blood tests for easy bruising/bleeding
    Complete blood cell count
    Prothrombin time
    Partial thromboplastin time
    von Willabrand's panel
    ± Bleeding time
    Clotting factors
Screening tests for evidence of abdominal trauma
    Liver
        Alanine aminotransferase
        Aspartate aminotransferase
    Pancreas
        Amylase
        Lipase
    Kidney
        Urinalysis
Toxicology screens
    For children with unexplained neurologic symptoms or symptoms compatible with ingestion
    Variance among laboratories in drugs tested in "tox screen"
    Screening of urine *and* blood and/or gastric contents
    Consideration of blood alcohol levels for children with altered mental status

CT, computed tomography.
Adapted from U.S. Department of Health and Human Services. *A nation's shame: fatal child abuse and neglect in the United States: a report of the U.S. Advisory Board on Child Abuse and Neglect: fifth report.* Washington, DC: U.S. Department of Health and Human Services, April 1995.

interaction the child's parents and extended family have had between abusive episodes. Physicians are often surprised that the child does not immediately state the nature and extent of the abuse and ask for asylum. Such statements by children are actually rare and occur mainly in adolescent patients. Children are loyal to their parents. Abusive parents may be only episodically abusive and at other times nurturing and loving. Young children may have no framework for comparison and may accept the abuse as the norm. Somewhat older children may understand and dislike the abuse but may fear the consequence of reporting it even more. In the child's mind, it may be better to live with the pain of abuse than to face the unknown of institutional or foster placement.

The final step in establishing a threshold level of suspicion is to review the differential diagnosis. At this point in the management scheme, the physician must add up the indicators and arrive at a judgment. If the process does not lead to a clear determination, most state laws imply that reporting suspected abuse is more prudent than not. Physicians are asked to report suspected, not proven, abuse. The major differentiation is between accidental and nonaccidental trauma. The other elements of the differential diagnosis are all uncommon diseases, including (i) bone diseases such as osteogenesis imperfecta, osteoid osteoma, and hypophosphatasia; (ii) hematologic disorders such as idiopathic thrombocytopenic purpura and hemophilia; (iii) neoplasms; (iv) metabolic disorders such as rickets or scurvy; (v) infections such as syphilis or osteomyelitis; and (vi) syndromes in which pain sensation is absent, such as spina bifida or congenital indifference to pain. These diseases occur with much less frequency than abuse but deserve consideration. Simple laboratory and radiographic studies will confirm or deny these diagnoses.

A special note should be made concerning the child younger than 12 months who is brought to the hospital deceased. In this situation, the central differential diagnosis exists between sudden infant death syndrome (SIDS) and child abuse. Other rare causes of sudden death include hypoglycemia, medium-chain fatty acid defects, mitochondrial defects, intoxication, and smothering. Victims of SIDS may appear to have bruising as a postmortem change. Clearly, their parents have no adequate explanation for the death. In this situation, the presumption should always be SIDS. Most localities require an autopsy to be performed. If not required, the physician should insist on a postmortem examination and wait for the autopsy to ultimately make the differentiation. Interrogating parents in cases of SIDS about the possibility of abuse can produce unnecessary psychological harm. With the death of a child, supportive ED treatment becomes paramount and suspicions of abuse can be pursued by the medical examiner and law enforcement personnel if warranted. If two or three SIDS deaths have occurred in the immediate family, the level of suspicion for abuse should be elevated.

Multidisciplinary Consultation. If consultation with a nurse, social worker, or physician with more extensive experience in the management of child abuse is available, it should be obtained. The advantages of consultations are many. They allow for (i) information sharing, (ii) joint decision making, (iii) planning, and (iv) mutual support. Planning an approach to the family and subsequent case management is useful. This brief consultation enables the physician to be more secure in making decisions about matters that are generally unfamiliar and often value laden. Joint interviewing is not only time efficient but also gives the family a uniform approach from the professional staff.

Reporting. Once the suspicion of abuse has been established and consultations obtained, the next step is reporting. Although laws vary from state to state, most have common elements. The emergency physician should become familiar with his or her current state law. The definition of abuse is central to each reporting law. A stated age defines a child. The laws also specify who must report (mandated reporters) and who may report (nonmandated reporters). For most mandated reports, the law requires a specific penalty (as well as malpractice liability) for failure to report and provides protection from liability if the report of suspected abuse turns out to be unfounded once investigated. Finally, the law dictates to whom and how the report should be made. Generally, reports are made to child protective services (CPS) agencies, to police departments, or to some combination of law enforcement and social work personnel. Many states now have statewide central registries for receiving reports.

Notifying the Parents and Managing Their Reactions. An important, but often avoided, step in case management is notification of the parents. This step is often forgotten because it is a difficult interpersonal task; nonetheless, it must be done. Nothing makes parents more resistant to change than completing a "routine" ED visit, only to later receive notification that the physician has filed a suspected child abuse report. Some specific guidelines are helpful in avoiding this breech of trust. The overall approach to the parents must be based on concern for the child. Concern for the child, not accusation, should be stressed. The physician should not confront the parents or attempt to seek an admission of guilt. Often, the parent in the ED may not be the abusive parent and may know as little about the episode as the hospital staff. The physician should explain the requirement for a mandated reporter to report all suspected cases. However, stating the requirement should not be used as an excuse. The desire to report should also be stated.

In many states, the reporter is required to report all injuries that are not fully explained. This requirement may also be stated to the parent. Using the words *child abuse report* is important. This situation is not a time to "soft pedal." However, child abuse does represent a range of behaviors, from the parent who overvigorously disciplines to the parent who sadistically tortures. Parents often have not seen themselves as abusers, and an explanation of the range of abuse is helpful in demonstrating how a child abuse report applies to them. Parents are fearful of what a child abuse report means and of what will happen. Therefore, the consequences of the report should be explained (e.g., "a social worker will call and come visit you in 1 or 2 days"). The physician's natural fear is that the parent will have a dramatic and hostile reaction.

The emergency physician can expect a wide variety of reactions, from hostility to appreciation. To minimize the angry reactions, the physician should stress the focus as being concern for the child. This perspective puts the physician on common ground with the parent. An angry reaction is more likely if guilt or fear is increased. This reaction may be seen as a feedback relationship. Stoking the fire by increasing the parent's guilt or fear results in a flare of angry emotion directed at the staff, the child, or the other spouse. Figure 132.15 illustrates this relationship.

Although the child does not need to be formally notified, the child may often be aware of what is happening and may even ask some pointed questions. The physician may want to discuss

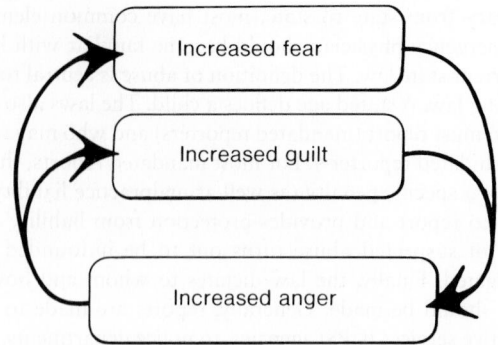

FIGURE 132.15 The cycle of fear, guilt, and anger.

the report with the child. The physician should stress the outcomes of protection and help for the child and the family. The ED staff should never be accusatory or belittling of the parent.

Crisis Hospitalization. In some cases of abuse, the family crisis is at such an acute level that hospitalization is necessary. The physician must ask, "Is the home safe?" If the child's environment poses a potential danger, the child should be admitted, no matter what the extent of injury. Some state laws have included protective custody sections that allow physicians to have virtual police powers in detaining a child for protection. In other states, the physician may need to obtain parental consent for admission.

This task is also difficult. As with reporting, the approach to the parents must be honest and nonaccusatory. The reasons for admission are to observe the child and allow time to evaluate the possibility of such an injury happening again. The focus must be the physician's concern for the child's health. In hospitalizing the child, the physician also makes a statement about the seriousness of the situation and the depth of his or her concern. Most hospitals do not have the resources to hospitalize every abused child, and it is not necessary or advisable to do so in every case. Factors that favor sending the child home are (i) a concerned relative or neighbor available to support the family, (ii) a solution to the inciting crisis, (iii) parental acceptance of responsibility, (iv) prompt (less than 24 hours) CPS or police response, (v) a first episode or minor degree of abuse, and (vi) an alternative environment (e.g., grandmother's house) (vii) older, less vulnerable child. If the physician is unable to hospitalize the child and has lingering doubts, a specific agreed-upon return appointment for the next day may be a solution. If the family is unable to keep the appointment, there should be a grave concern and emergency CPS or police involvement should be requested.

Documentation. Throughout each step of case management, documentation is important. The record of this visit is both a medical and a legal document. A precise description of the injuries enhances the document's value, and small sketches are also helpful. Photographs are invaluable in documenting extensive injuries. Photographs may be used in court to illustrate, for a judge or jury, injuries that would be difficult for most witnesses to describe. Even if the photographs are not admissible in court, they refresh the mem-

ory of the physician for testimony. Often, court proceedings may not take place for several months after the ED visit. If photographs are taken, their quality must be good. Poor-quality photographs can damage a case by failing to show all the pertinent findings.

Written descriptions of an injury are adequate for less extensive trauma, but as much detail as possible should be included. The record of the history should be as factual as possible; conclusions or impressions should not be listed. For example, rather than recording "the child looked fearful," describing the physical components or behaviors that prompted that judgment, under standard courtroom procedure, is more appropriate. Direct quotes from the child or parents should be included because quotes from another person are generally considered hearsay and are disallowed. When such quotes are included in the text of a business (medical) record, they may become more acceptable. General legibility and, in particular, a clearly written signature are always important record requirements. At the time of the ED visit, detailed record keeping seems to be a burden and waste of time. When a case record requires review before court testimony, good documentation is a necessity. Upon completion of the record, the physician should read it again as if he or she was the defendant's attorney.

Staff Reactions. Child abuse triggers many emotions in the physician and in the ED staff. Sadness and pity for the child and, often, anger for the parents are exhibited. The staff may have a general feeling of disbelief, "How can this happen?" The case management plan previously described requires that each ED staff member be professional and in control of these emotions. The offhand comment of a clerk or the whispering among nurses can undermine the work being done with the family. If a staff member is too upset by abuse, he or she should be relieved of the responsibility of working in such situations. Physicians or nurses who openly attack the family or who are blatantly accusatory should not be involved in these types of cases. Only after having experience with large numbers of cases can an ED staff member develop an appreciation of abuse as a negative but understandable human response. With such a perspective, the physician can become less angry and more zealous in attempting to provide constructive case management.

If problems relating to the staff reaction exist, as they often will, several corrective actions should be taken. At times, a brief meeting of the involved staff members can be called after the family has been discharged from the ED. This meeting allows staff members an immediate opportunity to ventilate their feelings. In-service education serves the same purpose, providing a forum for staff members to discuss their personal feelings about abuse, as well as their past experiences. ED staff members are always involved in the negative aspects of identifying and reporting abuse, but they never see the long-term treatment and rehabilitation phase. If a therapist, or better yet a family member, can present this side of abuse to the staff, it engenders more positive attitudes. Without learning about the successes, the staff often displaces this anger, charging "incompetence" of the CPS agency or "leniency" of a family court judge. Scapegoating should be put into the proper perspective. Again, in-service education and case reviews are useful. The integrity of the entire treatment team, both in the hospital and in the community, must be maintained to accomplish the difficult goals of protecting the child and preserving family life.

SEXUAL ABUSE

During the last 30 years, sexual abuse has been increasingly recognized as an important pediatric medical problem. According to the NCANDS, CPS agencies have determined more than 78,000 children in the United States to be victims of sexual abuse in 2006. Research studies, however, suggest that only a small percentage of sexual abuse cases are reported to CPS agencies. Experts estimate that each year, 1% of children become victims of sexual abuse. In addition to leading to increased recognition of the magnitude of the problem, recent research has also led to the development of improved medical guidelines for the identification, evaluation, and treatment of sexual abuse. Prompt diagnosis, humane emergency management, and referral to long-term treatment resources are the goals of the emergency physician. Working in a multidisciplinary fashion with nursing and social work staff is important. As with the physically abused, the sexually abused child engenders a great deal of emotion from the health care professionals in the ED.

Background

The term *sexual abuse* often conjures up images of a violent, forced sexual attack and rape. Many people think of the psychopathic criminal luring children on their way home from school by offering them gifts, but such stereotypes are the exception. Commonly, a relationship exists between the perpetrator and the victim. The misuse of that relationship is central to the sexual abuse of the child. The relationship may be a familial one, such as father–daughter. In more than half of the cases of sexual abuse identified by CPS agencies in 2006, the perpetrator was a relative. The relationship may also be a household relationship, such as mother's live-in paramour and the child, or a more casual relationship, such as that with a neighbor, teacher, or friend of the family. Many experts believe that sexual abuse is the most underreported form of child maltreatment because of the secrecy or "conspiracy of silence" that so often characterizes these cases. Most often, no overt violence is perpetrated, although harsh threats of violence as a consequence of the child's revealing the act to another person may be issued.

The definition of sexual abuse varies from state to state, but federal law under CAPTA provides a minimum definition of sexual abuse that applies to all states. CAPTA defines *sexual abuse* as

- "The employment, use, persuasion, inducement, enticement, or coercion of any child to engage in, or assist any other person to engage in, any sexually explicit conduct or any simulation of such conduct for the purpose of producing any visual depiction of such conduct;
- Or rape, and in cases of caregiver or interfamilial relationships, statutory rape, molestation, prostitution, or other form of sexual exploitation of children, or incest with children."

Sexual abuse encompasses a wide range of inappropriate sexual activities, including fondling a child's genitals, inter-

course, incest, rape, sodomy, exhibitionism, and commercial exploitation through prostitution or the production of pornographic materials. Emergency physicians should become familiar with the specific laws governing sexual abuse in their area. For example, in the commonwealth of Pennsylvania, statutory rape occurs when a person engages in sexual intercourse with a complainant younger than 16 years and that person is 4 or more years older than the complainant and the complainant and the person are not married to each other. In Nebraska, however, first-degree sexual assault occurs when a person 19 years or older sexually penetrates a person younger than 16 years. Some state laws define specific acts of sexual abuse such as rape, incest, statutory sexual abuse, and involuntary deviate sexual abuse, but other state laws refer to sexual abuse in more general terms.

Clinical Manifestations

Child sexual abuse victims usually come to medical attention due to one of the following five reasons: (i) a disclosure of inappropriate sexual contact, (ii) anogenital complaints, (iii) nongenital physical complaints, or (iv) inappropriate sexualized behaviors or (v) nonspecific behavioral complaints (Table 132.7).

Disclosure of Sexual Abuse. The majority of child victims of sexual abuse present for care after making a disclosure. Children frequently do not disclose that they have been sexually abused immediately after the event but may wait days, months, or even years before telling anyone and presenting for medical care. Even when a child does disclose, he or she may not fully disclose the extent of the abuse. When a child makes

PSYCHOSOCIAL EMERGENCIES

TABLE 132.7

PRESENTATIONS FOR EVALUATION OF SEXUAL ABUSE

Disclosure	
Child discloses history of inappropriate sexual contact	
Physical complaints	
Anogenital	**General**
Anogenital injury	Abdominal pain
Bruises	Anorexia
Lacerations	Dysuria
Bleeding	Encoporesis
Pain	
Sexually transmitted disease	
Pregnancy	
Behavioral complaints	
Inappropriate sexual behaviors	**Nonspecific behavioral complaints**
Compulsive masturbation	Excessive fears, phobias
Inappropriate knowledge of adult sexual behavior	Refusal to sleep alone, nightmares
Excessive sexual curiosity, sexual acting out	Runaways
	Any abrupt change in behavior

a disclosure and offers the specifics of an encounter, a report to CPS should be made. Reports of suspected sexual abuse are often based on history alone. Children do not usually make up allegations of sexual abuse. Most children who are not abused are not knowledgeable in the details of sexual encounters. The detail of the disclosure varies with the child's age and language development, but even children of 3 or 4 years of age may be able to make statements about someone touching their genitals.

Genital Complaints. Child victims of sexual abuse may present with genital complaints resulting from trauma, infection, or pregnancy. A physical injury such as a laceration, abrasion, or bruising to the genitalia or anus of a child should elicit a suspicion of sexual abuse and be evaluated. Accidental straddle injuries can produce external genital trauma and are the most common form of accidental genital injury to young girls. Straddle injuries, however, rarely produce hymenal injury and do not cause vaginal injury. The premenstrual child who presents with vaginal hemorrhage may be bleeding from a vaginal laceration that is not visible on external examination. Prompt surgical or gynecologic consultation should be obtained to identify and treat unseen sites of trauma. In males, accidental penile trauma may occur from zipper accidents or from a toilet seat that falls. Beyond these common accidental situations, the emergency physician should scrutinize the history given and consider sexual abuse.

The presence of an STI in a prepubertal child raises suspicion for sexual abuse. While some STIs should be considered as evidence of sexual abuse, other STIs may frequently be transmitted through nonsexual modes. On the basis of an understanding of disease transmission, the American Academy of Pediatrics (AAP) and the CDC have placed these infections into four categories. The first category includes those infections that are virtually always transmitted through sexual contact (Table 132.8). In this category, syphilis, *Neisseria gonorrhoeae* infection, and *Chlamydia trachomatis* infection are considered diagnostic for sexual abuse in prepubertal children if perinatal acquisition and rare nonsexual vertical transmission have been excluded. In the absence of perinatal or transfusion-related transmission, human immunodeficiency virus (HIV) infection is also considered diagnostic for sexual abuse. In the second category is *Trichomonas vaginalis* infec-

tion, which to the best of clinical knowledge is usually transmitted sexually and should be considered highly suspicious for abuse. Category 3 includes condyloma accuminata (anogenital warts) and herpes simplex, which are suspicious for abuse but may be transmitted by nonsexual contact. Although the CDC and the AAP categorize condyloma accuminata as suspicious for abuse and recommend making a report of suspected sexual abuse to CPS, recent literature suggests that the majority of cases of anogenital warts in children likely result from nonsexual transmission of the human papillomavirus (HPV). Thus, although sexual abuse must be considered during the evaluation of child with genital warts, in the absence of a disclosure or other concerning findings, a report to CPS may not be warranted in a young child infected with HPV. Category 4 includes bacterial vaginosis, which is not considered indicative of sexual abuse. Although not included in the AAP categories, scabies and lice can also be transmitted non-sexually and should be considered inconclusive findings.

The pregnant adolescent may be a victim of sexual abuse. The physician should try to obtain a specific history of conception. Often, the focus of case management centers on how the adolescent plans to notify her parents or whether she considers abortion or adoption as an option. If the issue of paternity is not pursued, sexual abuse escapes detection.

Nongenital Physical Complaints. In addition to presenting with genital concerns, child victims of sexual abuse may be brought for medical evaluation of a broad range of nonspecific physical complaints. Sexual abuse may be related to cases that present with headache; pain in the abdomen and thighs; dysuria; pain on defecation; hematuria; or hematochezia. For example, gonorrhea can present with vaginal discharge but may also appear in cases of less well-defined symptoms such as vaginal pain, itching, urinary frequency, or enuresis. Abuse may manifest as a change in habits, such as urinary frequency, enuresis, constipation, or encopresis; other complaints may include a chronic sore throat. The cause of each of these complaints may be any number of things. For example, in studying a group of children with enuresis, sexual abuse is an uncommon cause of the complaint. Nonetheless, sexually abused children are regularly brought to EDs with nonspecific complaints. If sexual abuse is not considered, it goes unnoticed.

TABLE 132.8

SEXUALLY TRANSMITTED INFECTIONS AND LEVEL OF CONCERN FOR SEXUAL ABUSE

Diagnostic for Sexual Abuse in Most Cases[*]	Highly Concerning for Sexual Abuse[*]	Concerning for Sexual Abuse	Inconclusive: Non-Sexual Transmission Possible
Neisseria gonorrhoeae *Chlamydia trachomatis* Syphilis HIV	*Trichomonas vaginalis*	Genital herpes simplex virus (HSV)[**] Anogenital *Condyloma accuminata*[***]	Pediculosis pubis Scabies Bacterial vaginosis

[*]In the absence of clear alternative mechanism for transmission of infection, a report should be made to child protective services (CPS). Perinatal transmission and non-sexual transmission (although rare) should be considered for *Neisseria, Chlamydia,* and syphilis. Perinatal or transfusion related transmission should be considered for HIV.
[**]In the absence of a history of autoinoculation from a non-genital HSV infection a report to CPS is recommended.
[***]Although the AAP guidelines recommend reporting cases of anogenital warts to CPS, recent research suggests that the majority of cases in children result from nonsexual transmission. If a thorough evaluation reveals no other findings concerning for sexual abuse, a report to CPS may not be indicated.

TABLE 132.9

SEXUAL PLAY

Normal	Needs further assessment
Discreet, private	No regard for privacy
Mutual consent	One child does not freely consent
No power imbalance	Power imbalance
No threats or violence	Actual or implied threats or violence
Infrequent	Frequent, compulsive
Age-appropriate language and sexual knowledge	Language beyond age-appropriate level of sexual knowledge
Does not result in injury	Causes injury
Basic, rudimentary sexual activity	Explicit, graphic, and detailed sexual activity; attempted or actual penetration of genital orifices

Adapted from Haka-Ikse K, Mian M. Sexuality in children. *Pediatr Rev* 1993;14:401–407.

Behavioral Manifestations. Some children manifest behaviors in their play or in their conversation that indicate that they have been exposed to sexual experiences and perhaps abused. These signs are less specific than a clearly stated history, but they are significant enough to require evaluation. All children manifest sexual curiosity and may engage in some form of masturbation, but when either behavior appears in excess, it deserves investigation because sexual abuse may be the cause. For example, children who want to fondle their parents' genitals as an expression of affection are cause for concern. Tables 132.9 and 132.10 help differentiate normal play and masturbation from more worrisome sexually inappropriate behaviors. These behaviors are usually learned. Although, inappropriate sexual behaviors should trigger a suspicion and evaluation for abuse, they are not by themselves diagnostic for abuse. Children may be exposed to sexual material through many routes, including television and the Internet.

TABLE 132.10

MASTURBATION

Normal	Needs further assessment
Occasional	Frequent, compulsive
Discreet, private	No regard for privacy
Not preferred over other activity or play	Often preferred over other activity or play
No physical symptoms or signs	Produces genital discomfort, irritation, or physical signs
External stimulation of genitalia only	Involves penetration of the genital orifices; includes bizarre practices or rituals

Adapted from Haka-Ikse K, Mian M. Sexuality in children. *Pediatr Rev* 1993;14:401–407.

Sexually abused children may also exhibit relatively minor unexplained behavioral changes, such as the recent episodes of nightmares or phobias, or major changes, such as school truancy and adolescent runaways. Children who bear no physical evidence of their abuse and in whom no physical symptoms develop may express themselves behaviorally. Many children demonstrate change in one or more of the important spheres of their life: at home, in school, or with peers. A sudden change in school performance unexplained by the teacher, social withdrawal, and isolation may also be nonspecific behavioral manifestations of sexual abuse. Thus, sexual abuse should be considered in the differential diagnosis of a child with nonspecific behavior changes.

Management

The primary goals in case management of most sexually abused child are the following: (i) identify and report the abuse, (ii) test for and provide prophylaxis and or treatment of STIs if indicated, (iii) test for and provide prophylaxis for pregnancy if appropriate, (iv) collect forensic evidence if appropriate, and (v) provide referral for psychological evaluation and treatment. A minority of pediatric sexual abuse victims will also have traumatic injuries requiring medical treatment. Care should be taken to avoid causing *secondary abuse phenomenon* while completing these goals. *Secondary abuse phenomenon* refers to the physical examination that is so overzealous that it assumes a rape-like quality in the mind of the child. Also to be avoided are parental or staff reactions that make the child feel responsible or blamed for the abuse. To allow long-term sexual assault evaluations to be performed in a less stressful environment, many ED centers have moved to performing a screening function. Children who have been abused within the past 72 hours or have acute symptoms (e.g., bleeding, signs of sexually transmitted disease) need immediate evaluation because forensic evidence may be collected or they may require urgent medical treatment. Children who were abused more than 72 hours ago and do not have any acute symptoms may be referred to a sexual assault center for a nonemergent evaluation. In places where no center is functioning, evaluations must be done in the ED. The following sections offer management techniques to identify suspected sexual abuse and gather enough documentation for legal purposes in a manner that is humane for the child and supportive for the family. Chapter 130 details the management of adolescent rape victims.

Interviewing the Parent. Parents may present the problem of sexual abuse either directly or indirectly. For the parent who is direct (i.e., "My child's been abused"), it is important to provide a controlled, quiet environment because he or she may be upset and angry. With such parents, the interviewer's tasks are calming, limiting, and clarifying. If possible, the parent should be interviewed without the child present. In an example of the indirect presentation, the parent brings the child for complaints such as those detailed in the sections on nonspecific physical or behavioral manifestations. With this parent, the task of the interviewer is to bring the possibility of sexual abuse into the open. Once the topic is nominally broached, it may become apparent that the parent has already considered sexual abuse. With both types of parents, exploring their concerns and their information in detail is important. Most of the parents bringing their child to the ED initiate their visit on the basis of a real observation or a strong feeling that something has happened to their child. The emergency physician must help clarify what the initiating cause may have been. In some cases, the parent may have responded to anxiety that their child may have been abused and can provide no substantive cause for their concern. In some of the latter cases, a follow-up visit to a sexual abuse center may be needed for the parents to again explore the motivation for their anxiety before their concerns can be put to rest. During the parental interview, information regarding the child's medical history and relevant signs and symptoms should be obtained.

Interviewing the Child. In most cases of child sexual abuse, the key to making the diagnosis rests with the history. Beyond standard history taking from the parents, the emergency physician should obtain a history from the child. This task may difficult for several reasons: (i) the child's level of language development, (ii) the child's level of psychosexual development, (iii) the desire not to contaminate what may be important evidence, (iv) the apprehension of the child and the parent, and (v) the awkwardness and apprehension felt by the interviewer in discussing sexual matters with a child. If possible, the child should be interviewed without the parent or caregiver present. A third party (e.g., a nurse or social worker) should be present. An initial discussion of topics, other than the alleged abuse, may comfort the child and encourages him or her to talk to the interviewer. Information about school, peers, and family adjustment is important in looking for nonspecific behavioral manifestations, and this preliminary conversation also helps evaluate the child's developmental level. Table 132.11 briefly outlines normal sexual developmental stages and appropriate interviewing techniques for each level.

On focusing the conversation on the abuse, one technique may be to ask the child why his or her parents brought him or her to the hospital. More specific questions may be necessary in some cases. One approach is for the physician to explain that sometimes he or she cares for children who have been hurt or touched by someone in a way that they did not like. The physician can then ask the child if anyone has hurt or touched him or her in a way that he or she did not like. Care should be taken to use open-ended questions and avoid leading questions. New words should not be introduced into the child's vocabulary. The physician may establish common vocabulary by asking the child the term used for his or her genitalia. Children offer a rich variety of terms and may have no understanding of the words "vagina" and "penis." In eliciting and using common language, the physician gets to the point of the interview more easily.

Children younger than 3 years are often not able to be interviewed. Techniques using anatomically correct dolls may be useful in preverbal children (Table 132.11). These dolls allow the child to play out the episode. Similarly, some children may choose to draw a picture that tells the story or that may be used by the interviewer to initiate the interview. These techniques are usually only employed by professionals with specific training in interviewing young children and may not be appropriate in the ED setting.

Emotional Support. Throughout the interview and in all contacts with the child, the rightness of his or her decision to discuss the abuse should be stressed. A child experiences conflict about revealing a secret, especially a long-standing secret. The patient may also feel conflict in sensing that his or her actions may be provoking a great deal of emotional turmoil. Often, the child has a relationship with the perpetrator and realizes that this admission may alter or end the relationship. At times, the child is aware or is made aware of getting the perpetrator "in trouble." Reaffirm the importance of what the child has revealed and focus the wrongdoing on the perpetrator. The child may have been threatened not to tell. Thus, bringing the nature of the threats into the open and offering protection to the child are important concerns. Finally, many children have fears about the abuse. Common fears are shown in Table 132.11. The physician may anticipate and address these fears on the basis of the child's development.

Physical Examination. A complete physical examination should be conducted with the knowledge that in many cases, the examination including the genital examination will be normal. Research by Kellogg, Heger, and other experts has repeatedly shown that the majority of pediatric sexual abuse cases do not have physical evidence of abuse on examination. In some cases, the sexual abuse may have involved fondling, labial coitus, or other forms of inappropriate touching that did not cause genital trauma. Even when vaginal penetration occurs, the physical examination may be normal as evidenced by Kellogg's study of pregnant sexually abused adolescents. Despite being pregnant, 86% of the adolescents had normal or nonspecific findings at the time of their examination. In some cases, the child may have sustained trauma that healed by the time of his or her medical evaluation. Many injuries to the hymen can heal rapidly and completely as evidenced by several research studies including the work of McCann and Heppenstall-Heger. Similarly, research has shown that the majority of children who disclose a history of anal penetration have normal physical examinations.

The examination should be conducted in a standard fashion, with all parts of the body examined. The child should be evaluated for signs of physical abuse or neglect. Other physical findings to note carefully are any contusions, abrasions, or lacerations in nongenital areas. Common sites for these signs of trauma are the upper thighs, buttocks, and upper arms. Figure 132.16 shows some of the visible findings of child sexual abuse. The oropharynx should also be carefully examined, especially if the child discloses a history of oral penetration. The genital examination may be a point of significant trauma for the child and care should be taken to minimize the child's anxiety. Young children may prefer to be examined while sitting in their parent's lap. In examining the genitalia of young girls, two positions are recommended. One is a frog-leg posture, which can be done with the child supine on the examination table or in an adult's lap. Alternatively, the child can lie prone with knees tucked under the thorax (i.e., the knee–chest position).

The external genitalia should be inspected for any signs of trauma or infection. In females, the labia majora and minora, clitoris, urethra, periurethral tissue, hymen, fossa navicularis, posterior fourchette, perineum, should all be examined. In particular, the rim of the hymenal opening should be examined for any notches, transections, or lacerations. In postpubertal girls with redundant hymenal tissue, examinations in different positions or the use of a dampened cotton swab or other techniques may be needed to fully visualize the hymenal rim. In

TABLE 132.11

DEVELOPMENTAL ISSUES IN MANAGING THE SEXUALLY ABUSED CHILD[a]

Age	Developmental issues	Fears	Techniques
0 to approximately 3 yr	*General* Depend on protection of adult Little or no ability to label time or sequence events Language only partially intelligible May not be able to identify body parts Toilet training in process *Sexual* Normal self-exploration of genital area is pleasurable Confused if this behavior is labeled "wrong" or "dirty" If sexual abuse is not painful, it may be accepted By age 3, curious about genitals of others	Terrified of painful assault Terrified of losing protection of adult	May not be able to be interviewed Consider having parent present during interview Use dolls to[a]: Point to body parts Do actions
Preschool, 3–6 yr	Language skills better Able to sequence events Gender differentiation established Cannot tell time but can have established time concepts, "before or after" Sexually curious Younger children exhibit bodies Modesty develops Vocabulary of sex parts and body functions After abuse, there may be masturbation and/or sexual play	Confused over incident Frightened by parents' anxiety and anger Feel they are "bad" for causing parents to be upset Behavior changes and phobias may develop (e.g., fear of dark, fear of strangers)	Ask children to draw pictures[a] Use doll or puppet play to note response[a]
School age	*General and sexual* Sexual interest increases but usually more curious than erotic Discomfort discussing their bodies, especially outside family Extremely modest with strangers and often with parents Abusive incident may have been pleasurable and nontraumatic	Abuse is perceived as sexual, may feel "sex is wrong" Often have been threatened by adult perpetrator Guilt about what they did vs. guilt over getting adult and family into trouble Fear about their bodies, feel "dirty" or "different" after incident	Use same-sex interviewer Do not assume correct knowledge of body; a physically mature 10-yr-old child is not necessarily emotionally mature or well informed Give reassurance of their nonresponsibility for the abuse Give praise for having reported incident Encourage child to talk about parents' reaction Mobilize family to support victim
Adolescent	Strong urge to conform and be "normal" Knows what is and is not socially acceptable Developing body image and self-esteem is very fragile Conflict between the need to assert independence, and the need for adult protection and approval	Forcible nature of sex is terrifying even to a sexually active adolescent Grief over loss of virginity Feeling that he or she is dirty or abnormal Fear of unavoidable further encounters with perpetrator Fear that a homosexual encounter may have lifelong consequences	Stress the normality of the victim—not branded for life Use charts or models Victims need to know that you have seen others with similar experiences who have recovered well Mobilize active family support Be available—give victim your phone number at work or social worker's phone number Victim advocate groups very helpful

[a]These techniques are usually only employed by professionals with specific training in interviewing young children and may not be appropriate in the emergency department setting.
Adapted from J. Michaelson, J. Paradise, S. Ludwig, unpublished data, 1983.

PSYCHOSOCIAL EMERGENCIES

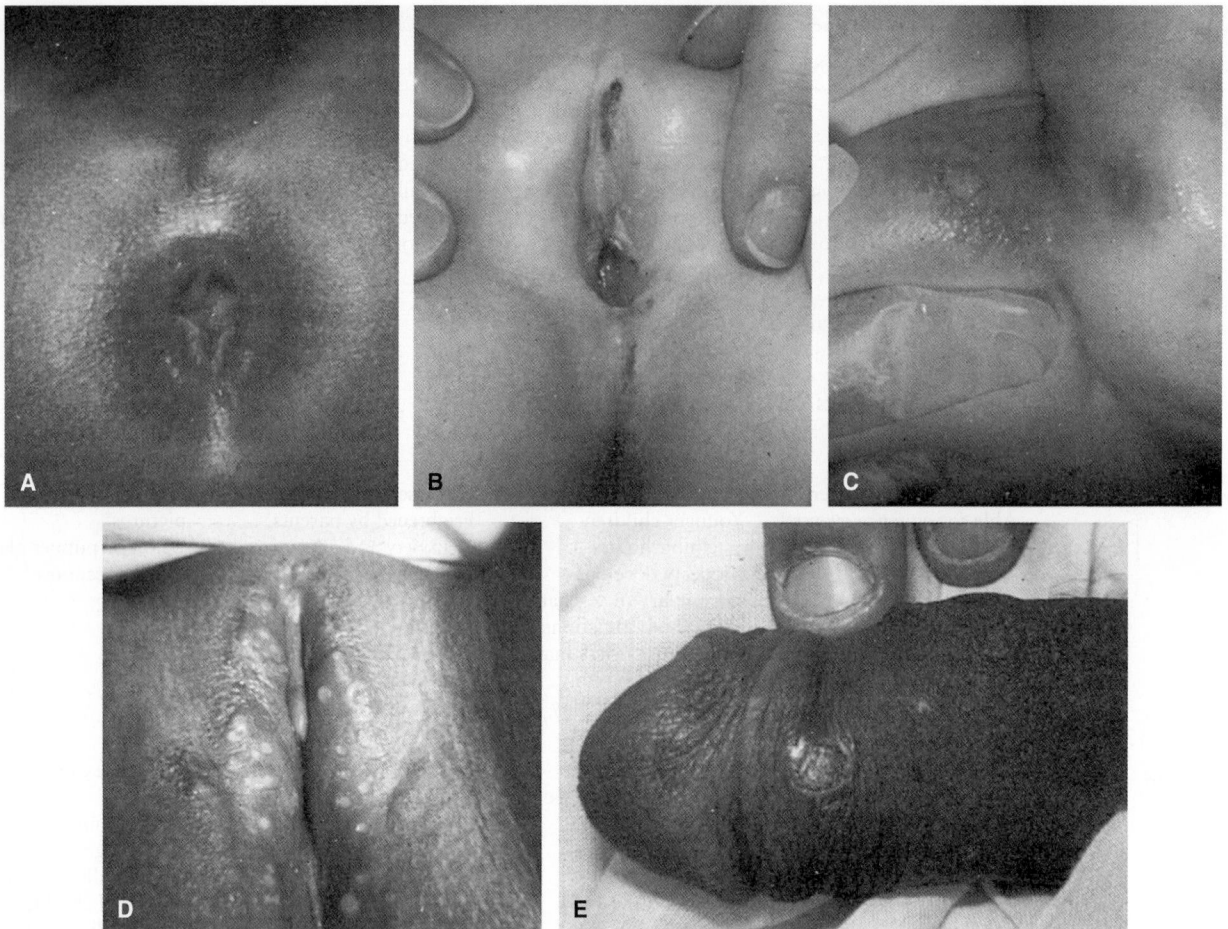

FIGURE 132.16 Physical signs of child sexual abuse. **A:** Rectal dilation and multiple lacerations after sodomy. **B:** Multiple vaginal and paraclitoral lacerations. **C:** Herpes simplex virus infection in perirectal area. **D:** Herpes virus vaginitis. **E:** Syphilis in a sexually abused adolescent.

prepubertal females, the hymen is sensitive and the examiner should avoid touching it if possible. Attempts to measure the size of the hymenal opening are unreliable and are not recommended as part of the examination. The location of any hymenal findings can be described using a clock face. In males, the penis and scrotum should be inspected. The perineum and perianal tissue should be examined in both genders even if the child did not disclose anal penetration. Any lesions, bruises, lacerations, scars, bleeding, discharge, or other findings should be documented. Figure 132.16 shows some of the visible findings of child sexual abuse. The child's tanner staging should be noted as part of the examination.

Only the external genitalia need be examined unless there is concern for internal injury. Speculum or digital examination is not necessary in most cases and should not be performed on prepubertal children unless under anesthesia. If even minimal vaginal bleeding appears to be coming from a more internal source, exploration and possible surgical repair are best done under general anesthesia in the operating room. Digital rectal evaluation is also not necessary.

If the physical examination proves too traumatic for the child, the physician is faced with a significant dilemma. The choices are to further traumatize the child or to perform an incomplete examination and collect inadequate evidence. As

with all dilemmas, the best choice is not obvious. Physically or psychologically traumatizing the child should be avoided. Often, no physical evidence is present and the history, if detailed enough, may be sufficient. The guiding principle should be primum non nocere (first do no harm).

Evidence Collection. In cases of acute sexual assault presenting within 72 hours, the physician should consider collecting forensic evidence, including clothing, debris, body swabs, genital swabs, and oral swabs, but recognize that no evidence will be recovered in most cases. Although forensic evidence collection should be considered in up to 72 hours after a sexual assault, research studies by Christian and Young have suggested that forensic evidence is unlikely to be recovered from a child's body after 24 hours. Research by Palusci has suggested that bathing and age less than 10 years are associated with a lower likelihood of forensic evidence recovery. Forensic evidence may be recovered from clothing and bed linens even after 24 hours, however, and these items should be collected in the ED if available. The type of evidence to be collected, the collection methods used, and the procedures for processing the results vary by locale. Whatever the specifics of a particular jurisdiction, some general principles should be followed. Establishing a standard protocol is important so

TABLE 132.12

FORENSIC EVIDENCE COLLECTION KIT

Use a standardized forensic evidence kit that meets the requirements of the police authority in your location. The exact content of the kit may vary based on the jurisdiction but in general most kits will include the following items:

- Container in which most of the evidence will be placed
- Form for obtaining authorization to collect and release evidence and information to law enforcement
- Checklists to guide history taking, physical examination, and specimen collection
- Evidence seals
- Form for documenting chain of custody
- Labels for identifying information and evidence
- Paper bags to hold clothing and other bulky items that do not fit in container*
- Envelopes or other containers for collection of debris, nail scrapings, hair, etc.
- Several cotton swabs for collection of specimens plus or minus glass slides**
- Tubes or containers for collection of secretions
- Blood sample tubes for blood typing and DNA analysis.
- Combs for scalp and/or pubic hair combings
- Instrument for obtaining nail scrapings and/or cuttings
- Gauze or swabs for saliva sample

Other items that may be needed but that are not necessarily in the kit include:

- Camera or colposcope for photographic documentation
- Alternate light source

*Plastic bags should not be used for evidence collection because they retain moisture which can lead to degradation of evidence.
**Slides may be included if the forensic laboratory prefers that the swabs be made into slides at the hospital. Other forensic laboratories may prefer that the swabs be placed in envelopes or containers without slides being made.

that each new case does not force the emergency physician to reformulate the entire process (Table 132.13). The ED should have on hand standard forensic evidence collection kits containing the necessary tubes, swabs, and supplies (Table 132.12). The patient should be instructed not to wash, change clothes, urinate, defecate, smoke, drink, or eat until initially evaluated by the physician, unless medically necessary. Evidence collection should be performed with another health care professional present. Evidence should be collected before obtaining specimens for STI testing. A standard for labeling the specimens should be established, including the patient's name, date of birth, and medical record number. Finally, the protocol should include a procedure for a specified person to give the specimens to law enforcement agency or to take the specimens to a specified safe storage area so that the chain of evidence is maintained. This detail becomes important in the court proceedings against the perpetrator.

Consider a Differential Diagnosis. In any consideration of abuse, the physician must always consider the question, "What else could it be?" There may be plausible explanations for physical findings such as straddle injuries causing accidental injuries to the genitals. Other important alternatives to consider are (i) infections caused by *Streptococcus*, *Haemophilus influenzae*, and *Monilia*; (ii) congenital anomalies such as

hydrometrocolpos, hemangioma, and perineal groove; (iii) foreign bodies of the rectum and vagina; and (iv) dermatologic conditions such as lichen sclerosus et atrophicus, diaper dermatitis, and contact dermatitis and other conditions such as a prolapsed urethra, which appears as a hemorrhagic mass covering the upper vaginal area (Table 132.14).

Documentation. Careful record keeping cannot be stressed too strongly. As with the collection and processing of evidence, ED records can make or break a case. The Children's Hospital of Philadelphia has developed a separate form that guides the examining physician to include all pertinent information (Fig. 132.17). The aspects of record keeping mentioned in the "Physical Abuse" section apply. In particular, what the child said in his or her own words should be carefully recorded. Quotations should be used if possible. Good records not only help the police and lawyers involved but also help the physician review the case before a hearing that may not take place months or even years. In some jurisdictions, legal provisions allow videotaping patient interviews. This tool is particularly helpful to the victim in that he or she may not have to repeat the history so many times. It may also be helpful to the physician by serving as another form of documentation. Photographs should be taken of physical examination findings. If photographs are not possible, the physician should draw diagrams of the findings.

Diagnosis. The diagnosis of sexual abuse should be based on a composite of the history, physical examination, and laboratory findings. In the majority of cases, however, no physical examination or laboratory findings are present and reports to CPS are made based solely on the child's statements. In some cases, the diagnosis may be unclear but a report to CPS may be indicated because of a reasonable suspicion of sexual abuse. Many pediatric centers rely on a classification scale for the assessment of suspected sexual abuse cases developed by Adams et al. The classification scale (Table 132.15) was most recently revised in 2007 and incorporates physical and laboratory findings. When using the classification scale to guide the interpretation of findings, the emergency physician must remember that in the vast majority of child sexual abuse cases, there are not any physical or laboratory findings present and a diagnosis may be made on the basis of the child's disclosure. A guideline for assessing the overall level of concern and making the decision to report sexual abuse has been developed by the AAP and is provided in Table 132.16.

Reporting. The laws governing which cases should be reported to the CPS or the police or both vary by jurisdiction. In most jurisdictions, sexual abuse is a criminal offense. Thus, all cases are reported to the police department. When a caregiver is responsible for the abuse, a civil report to the CPS agency is also required. ED protocols for reporting to CPS and police should be developed according to local guidelines and included in an ED sexual assault procedure. In the event of a criminal (police) report, a civil (child abuse) report, or both, the parent should be informed that such reports are being made. The physician or social worker must spell out the practical consequences of the reports for the parent.

Preparing the Parent. Beyond notifying the parent about reporting the sexual abuse, additional preparation must be

TABLE 132.13

GUIDELINES FOR FORENSIC EVIDENCE COLLECTION

General

1. Obtain consent to collect forensic evidence in adolescent sexual assault cases. In cases of child sexual abuse, consent is not needed
2. Instruct patient to not wash, change clothes, urinate, defecate, smoke, drink, or eat until evaluated by examiners, unless medically necessary
3. Wash your hands and wear gloves
4. Use photographs to document physical findings
   a. The first photograph should be that of the child's ID label with full name, date of birth, and medical record number.
   b. Take as many photographs as needed to document injuries.
   c. Document each injury separately with ruler/color guide in photographs.
5. Use anatomical diagrams to document findings including location, size, and appearance.

Initial debris and clothing collection

1. **Debris collection:** Carefully inspect patient's head, hands, and other exposed skin surfaces, as well as outer surface of clothing, for any loose debris including hairs, grass, leaves, fibers, threads, etc. Using one piece of clean white copy paper carefully remove the loose material and place it inside the unfolded paper. Refold paper to retain material; indicate location on patient's body or clothing from which material was collected. Repeat as necessary. Place sealed paper folds into envelope marked "Miscellaneous," seal, and label envelope as indicated.
2. **Clothing collection:** Spread clean sheet on floor, place large paper sheet from "Foreign Material" envelope in the middle of the cloth sheet. Have patient stand in the middle of the sheet and remove clothing one piece at a time, careful not to shake the clothing. If parents or the nurse is helping patient, advise them to not stand on the sheet with the patient. Ask the patient to remove one article of clothing at a time. If the article of clothing has wet stains of potential biological material (blood, saliva, semen, etc.), lay flat to dry. Place each article of clothing in a separate paper bag, labeled with patient identification sticker, date, time, and forensic examiner's initials.
   a. Underpants and/or diapers should be collected even if they are not the pair worn during or immediately after the incident. Vaginal secretions may accumulate, even if the patient has bathed or showered.
   b. Collect all clothing if worn during assault or immediately after. If patient is not wearing the same underwear from the assault, the examiner should inquire about the location of the garment and instruct patient or family to save the garment for police/SVU (ideally unlaundered in a paper bag).

Physical examination evidence collection

1. **Skin surface assessment:** Carefully perform a visual inspection of the patient's external skin surfaces. Locate, describe, and photograph any evidence of trauma or adherent foreign matter.
   a. If areas of dried secretions are noted on external skin surfaces, document findings on anatomical diagrams.
2. **Secretions collection:** Prior to any swabs or evidence collection, an alternative light source should be utilized in a dark room over the patient's entire body. If there is a pos-

itive (fluorescent specimen), a sterile swab moistened with sterile water should be used to swab area. Allow to air dry. Place in "Debris or Miscellaneous" envelope—noting where specimens were collected.
   a. Use extra swabs to collect specimens if needed. Be sure to label the "Debris or Miscellaneous" envelopes carefully to what evidence is inside and where it was obtained.
3. **Bite mark evidence:** Document location of bite mark(s) on anatomical diagram form and, where possible, photograph the bite mark with and without scale. Use a lightly moistened swab to gently rub inside the parameters of the bite mark in order to collect any dried saliva left by the offender. Do not moisten the second swab, again gently rub the inside parameters of the bite mark with the second dry swab.
4. **Examination of hands:** Carefully inspect dorsal and palmar surface of hands for any signs of trauma. Document all findings on anatomical diagram. Swab only fingernails if there are dried secretions, if so, follow directions for dried secretions.
5. **Oral swabs:** Open the swab packet from the envelope marked "Oral Swabs," grasp both swabs together by the shaft, and swab the area between the patient's cheek and gum, and behind the back molars on both the upper and lower jaws.
   a. Mucosal membranes swabs do not need to be moistened.
6. **Genital inspection:** Carefully inspect entire external genital area for signs of trauma. Use colposcope or other light source to examine for injuries. Document findings, including size, shape, color and location, on anatomical diagrams of genitalia.
7. **Pubic hair combings:** Remove paper fold from envelope marked "Pubic Hair Combings." Ask patient to sit on unfolded paper so that the paper protrudes between the thighs; comb downward on pubic hair to dislodge any debris or loose hairs onto the paper. Place comb on paper and fold paper to retain debris; place paper in the envelope marked "Pubic Hair Combings," seal, and label as indicated.
8. **Perianal swabs:** Carefully evaluate the anus and buttocks for signs of injury. Document positive findings on gender-appropriate anatomical diagrams. Using two moistened swabs simultaneously, gently rub swabs on anal folds and anal opening. Dry completely and place in the envelope marked "Perianal Swabs."
9. **Rectal swabs:** After external anal swabs have been collected, the anal area should be cleansed by wiping carefully with a moistened gauze pad. Simultaneously insert two sterile cotton swabs approximately 2 cm into the rectum and swab rectal walls. Remove swabs, avoiding contact with the external anal tissue. Dry completely and place in the envelope marked "Rectal Swabs."
10. **External genital swabs:** Use swabs in external genital envelope. For male patients, wipe the surface of the glans and the shaft; for female patients, wipe the inner surfaces of the labia minora with a downward motion. After drying, place in a marked envelope.
11. **Vaginal swabs:** Using two swabs simultaneously, collect secretions from the vagina near the vaginal fornix (area below the cervix). (This step may be performed with a speculum in place in postpubertal children, or by blind sweep without the use of a speculum.)

(continued)

TABLE 132.13

CONTINUED

12. **Cervix swabs:** Using two swabs simultaneously, collect secretions from cervical os. This step should be performed only with the use of a speculum to ensure visualization of the cervix and thus should not be performed in prepubertal children unless under anesthesia. Dry completely and place in envelope marked "Cervix Swabs."
    a. If using a speculum for cervical examination, after evidence is collected, use the Aptima Cervical Swab to obtain specimen for STIs.
13. All tampons, pads, pantyliners should be collected and dried. Once dry, place in the "Miscellaneous" envelope.
14. All evidence should be dry before packaging. To dry swabs, place swabs in swab drying machine, with cotton tip pointing upward to promote drying.
15. Do not allow cotton tip of swabs to contact other objects or surfaces during drying process. (Use the test tube rack not allowing it to touch any other swabs.)

16. After drying, swabs should be placed in swab boxes and then into the envelopes provided for each specimen. (If additional specimens were collected and no swab box or evidence envelope is available for packaging, dried swabs may be placed in a plain envelope.)
17. All envelopes and boxes should be labeled with patient's name, case number, date, and name of the examiner.
18. Seal enveloped: Do not lick envelopes to seal them. Use a clean gauze or cotton and wet with sterile water to moisten adhesive on collection envelopes.
19. All envelopes containing evidence specimens should be placed inside the evidence kit box. The sealed bag containing underpants may be placed inside evidence kit box if space permits; all other clothing bags should remain outside of evidence box. Each item collected must be noted on the evidence receipt form.

Adapted from *Forensic Exam Checklist*, Children's Hospital of Philadelphia, Philadelphia, PA.

given. Many workers believe that, for the young child, the parental reaction to sexual abuse may have as important a role as the abuse itself in producing subsequent manifestations. Long-term follow-up studies of sexually abused children performed by a case–control methodology show that sexually abused children are at long-term risk for various psychological and behavioral consequences. Parents need to be aware of this

TABLE 132.14

DIFFERENTIAL DIAGNOSIS OF ANOGENITAL ERYTHEMA, EXCORIATION, AND PRURITUS

Local irritation
Sexual abuse
Poor hygiene
Tight/poorly ventilated underwear
Chemical
Sandbox vaginitis

Infection
Sexually transmitted disease
Nonspecific vaginitis
Pinworms
Scabies
Candidal infection
Perianal streptococcal cellulitis

Dermatologic
Atopic dermatitis
Contact dermatitis
Seborrheic dermatitis
Diaper dermatitis/candidal infection
Psoriasis
Lichen sclerosus/balanitis xerotic obliterans

Systemic
Crohn's disease
Kawasaki's syndrome
Stevens-Johnson syndrome

correlation. Social worker consultation and collaboration for this aspect of case management are essential.

The first step is to focus the parent's attention on the child. Especially in situations of father–daughter incest or surrogate father–daughter incest, the maternal reaction may initially be more self-centered. In directing the parent's attention to the child, the physician returns the parent to a more comfortable traditional role and raises many important issues to which the parent must attend. The physician should review with the parent that manifestations of sexual abuse may be physical and/or psychological. The physical manifestation may seem minor to the physician, but parents must be specifically told that whatever the injury, it can be repaired with no impairment of the victim's sexual functions as an adult.

Parents must be told that the psychological outcome, in part, relates to their reactions to the situation. Their role must be to provide comfort, support, and reassurance to the child. Methods of supporting the child have been raised previously in this section. These techniques must be used by the parents. Unfortunately, parental anger and blame may sometimes be displaced onto the child. All attempts to place responsibility or blame on the victim need to be eliminated. The ultimate responsibility is that of the perpetrator, no matter what the behavior of the child.

Some parents may focus their anger clearly on the perpetrator but want to "take the law into their own hands." Parents should be cautioned about leaving the ED to find and confront the perpetrator. This action is a police responsibility. The parental role is to provide safety for the child. Parental ire can be modified by pointing out that a parent's arrest for assault of the perpetrator will not benefit the child.

Yet, another common parental reaction is the desire to institute several lifestyle changes. Parents may want to change their place of residence, change the child's school, or quit their jobs to be able to guard the child 24 hours per day. The ED staff should stress that returning to as normal a lifestyle as possible is best for the child. Change is always difficult for children, and

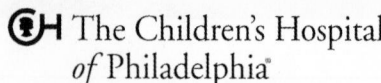

The Children's Hospital
of Philadelphia®

ED-5490
Rev. 7/07

SEXUAL ASSAULT EVALUATION

(Page 1 of 4)

(PATIENT LABEL)

Attending M.D. _____ Brought in by _____

CHOP S.W. _____ _____

Referred by _____ Contact Phone _____

History of Assault/Abuse

History provided by _____ Child Interviewed by _____

Alleged Perpetrator(s) (if known):

Name/Nickname _____ Age _____ Sex _____

Relationship to child _____ Time elapsed since last
contact (if known): _____

Hx: (to be patient's own words whenever possible)

_____

_____

_____

_____

_____

_____

_____

_____

_____

_____

_____

_____

_____

_____

_____

_____

_____

_____

_____

_____

_____

_____

_____

For **Recent Assault:** (within 72 hours) has patient:

Eaten / rinsed Mouth? _____ Bathed? _____ Urinated? _____ Defecated? _____

Initials _____

ATTENDING / TEACHING PHYSICIAN

Date: _____ Time: _____

_____

_____

_____

_____

_____

_____

_____

_____

_____

_____

_____

_____

_____

_____

_____

_____

_____

_____

_____

_____

_____

_____

_____

_____

_____

_____

_____

_____

Initials _____

AEL 7/2007

FIGURE 132.17 Sexual assault checklist. (Courtesy of The Children's Hospital of Philadelphia, Philadelphia, PA.) (*continued*)

CH The Children's Hospital
of Philadelphia®

ED-5490
Rev. 7/07

SEXUAL ASSAULT EVALUATION

(PATIENT LABEL)   **(Page 2 of 4)**

	ATTENDING / TEACHING PHYSICIAN
PMH:	

Date: _____   Time: _____

Age at menarche_____   LMP_____   Tampon use?_____   Contraception used_____

ROS: (D/C, bleeding, dysuria, pain, UTIs, change in bowel or urinary habits, behavioral changes)

Are you having pain now?   Yes _____   No _____

Physical Examination: Wt._____   Ht._____   P_____   BP_____

General description:

General Examination: (if abnormal, please describe and include any bruising or skin injury.)

PE:	NORMAL	ABNORMAL	SIGNIFICANT FINDINGS
(1) Head / Face			
(2) Ears			
(3) Eyes			
(4) Throat			
(5) Neck			
(6) Chest			
(7) Heart			
(8) Abdomen			
(9) Extremities			
(10) Skin			
(11) Neuro			

Initials _____   Initials _____

FIGURE 132.17 (*Continued*)

PSYCHOSOCIAL EMERGENCIES

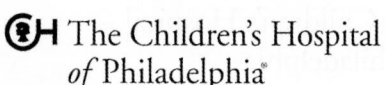

ED-5490
Rev. 7/07

SEXUAL ASSAULT EVALUATION

(Page 3 of 4)   (PATIENT LABEL)

Genital / Pelvic Examination	**ATTENDING / TEACHING PHYSICIAN**

Colposcope used?_____   Hand held magnifier used?_____

Position Examined: Frog Leg Supine_____   Knee Chest Prone_____   Lateral decub_____

Other _____

ATTENDING / TEACHING PHYSICIAN

Date: _____   Time: _____

_____

_____

FEMALE:

Tanner: Breasts _____

Pubic Hair _____

External Exam (Vulva, Hymen, Vagina)

_____

_____

_____

_____

Anus_____

Pelvic (post pubertal)

Cervix_____

Adnexa_____

MALE:

Tanner: Genitals _____

Pubic Hair _____

Penis _____

Scrotum _____

Anus_____

_____

_____

_____

_____

_____

_____

_____

_____

_____

_____

_____

_____

_____

_____

Initials _____

_____

Initials _____

_____

_____

_____

_____

_____

_____

_____

_____

_____

_____

_____

_____

_____

_____

_____

_____

_____

_____

_____

_____

_____

_____

_____

_____

Initials _____

FIGURE 132.17 (*Continued*)

⊕H The Children's Hospital
of Philadelphia®

ED-5490
Rev. 7/07

SEXUAL ASSAULT EVALUATION

(PATIENT LABEL)

(Page 4 of 4)

Laboratory (check if done):

_____ Urine aptima GC / chlamydia

_____ Vaginal aptima GC / chlamydia

_____ GC culture body site_____

_____ Routine vaginal culture

_____ Gram stain_____

             location

_____ Trichomonas

_____ HIV (with consent)

_____ RPR

_____ Hepatitis C Ab / PCR

_____ Urine / serum pregnancy test

_____ UA

_____ Urine Culture

_____ Stool hematest

_____ Other (specify)_____

ATTENDING / TEACHING PHYSICIAN

Date: Time:

Photographs? Yes_____   No_____   Camera?_____

Forensic Evidence Kit: completed? Yes_____   No_____   N/A_____

2 air dried swabs for sperm/acid phosphatase from:

labia_____ vagina/cervix_____ rectum_____ mouth_____ other_____

_____ Saliva sample

_____ Blood sample in red top tube

_____ Clothing (list)_____

_____ Other (hair, foreign objects, etc.)_____

Specimens given to:_____ Time_____ Date_____

Impression:

_____

_____

_____

_____

_____

Plan/Recommendations:

_____

_____

_____

_____

_____

Name of CHOP S.W. notified_____

Child Protective Services notified?_____
                    State/County

Contact Person's name and time of call: _____

Police notified?_____
            State/County

Resident/Fellow M.D. Signature _____

Printed name _____

Date / Time _____

Attending M.D. Signature

_____

Printed name

Date / Time

FIGURE 132.17 *(Continued)*

TABLE 132.15

APPROACH TO INTERPRETING PHYSICAL AND LABORATORY FINDINGS IN SUSPECTED CHILD SEXUAL ABUSE: DECEMBER 2006

A Product of an ongoing collaborative process by child maltreatment physician specialists, under the leadership of Joyce A. Adams, MD (Numbering of findings is for ease of reference only and does not imply increasing significance)

Findings documented in newborns or commonly seen in non-abused children: (The presence of these findings generally neither confirms nor discounts a child's clear disclosure of sexual abuse)

Normal Variants	Findings commonly caused by other medical conditions
1. Periurethral or vestibular bands 2. Intravaginal ridges or columns 3. Hymenal bumps or mounds 4. Hymenal tags or septal remnants 5. Linea vestibularis (midline avascular area) 6. Hymenal notch/cleft in the anterior (superior) half of the hymenal rim (prepubertal girls), on or above the 3 o'clock - 9 o'clock line, patient supine 7. Shallow/superficial notch or cleft in inferior rim of hymen (below 3 o'clock - 9 o'clock line) 8. External hymenal ridge 9. Congenital variants in appearance of hymen, including: crescentic, annular, redundant, septate, cribiform, microperforate, imperforate 10. Diastasis ani (smooth area) 11. Perianal skin tag 12. Hyperpigmentation of the skin of labia minora or perianal tissues in children of color, such as Mexican–American and African–American children 13. Dilation of the urethral opening with application of labial traction 14. 'Thickened hymen' (may be due to estrogen effect, folded edge of hymen, swelling from infection, or swelling from trauma. The latter is difficult to assess unless follow-up examination is done)	15. Erythema (redness) of the vestibule, penis, scrotum or perianal tissues. (May be due to irritants, infection or trauma*) 16. Increased vascularity ('Dilatation of existing blood vessels") of vestibule and hymen. (May be due to local irritants, or normal pattern in non estrogenized state) 17. Labial adhesions. (May be due to irritation or rubbing) 18. Vaginal discharge. (Many infectious and noninfectious causes, cultures must be taken to confirm if it is caused by sexually transmitted organisms or other infections) 19. Friability of the posterior fourchette or commisure. (May be due to irritation, infection, or may be caused by examiner's traction on the labia majora) 20. Excoriations/bleeding/vascular lesions. (These findings can be due to conditions such as lichen sclerosus, eczema or seborrhea, vaginal/perianal Group A Streptococcus, urethral prolapse, hemangiomas) 21. Perineal groove (failure of midline fusion), partial or complete 22. Anal fissures (Usually due to constipation, perianal irritation) 23. Venous congestion or venous pooling in the perianal area. (Usually due to positioning of child, also seen with constipation) 24. Flattened anal folds. (May be due to relaxation of the external sphincter or to swelling of the perianal tissues due to infection or trauma*) 25. Partial or complete anal dilatation to less than 2 cm (anterior–posterior dimension), with or without stool visible. (May be a normal reflex, or have other causes, such as severe constipation or encopresis, sedation, anesthesia, neuromuscular conditions)

Indeterminate findings: Insufficient or conflicting data from research studies: (May require additional studies/evaluation to determine significance. These physical/laboratory findings may support a child's clear disclosure of sexual abuse, if one is given, but should be interpreted with caution if the child gives no disclosure. In some cases, a report to Child Protective Services may be indicated to further evaluate possible sexual abuse.

Physical examination findings	Lesions with etiology confirmed: Indeterminate specificity for sexual transmission (Report to protective services recommended by AAP Guidelines unless perinatal or horizontal transmission is considered likely)
26. Deep notches or clefts in the posterior/inferior rim of hymen in pre-pubertal girls, located between 4 and 8 o'clock, in contrast to transections (see 41) 27. Deep notches or complete clefts in the hymen at 3 or 9 o'clock in adolescent girls 28. Smooth, noninterrupted rim of hymen between 4 and 8 o'clock, which appears to be less than 1 mm wide, when examined in the prone knee–chest position, or using water to 'float' the edge of the hymen when the child is in the supine position. 29. Wart-like lesions in the genital or anal area. (Biopsy and viral typing may be indicated in some cases if appearance is not typical of Condyloma accuminata) 30. Vesicular lesions or ulcers in the genital or anal area (viral and/or bacterial cultures, or nucleic acid amplification tests may be needed for diagnosis) 31. Marked, immediate anal dilation to an AP diameter of 2 cm or more, in the absence of other predisposing factors	32. Genital or anal Condyloma accuminata in a child, in the absence of other indicators of abuse. 33. Herpes Type 1 or 2 in the genital or anal area in a child with no other indicators of sexual abuse.

(continued)

TABLE 132.15

CONTINUED

Findings Diagnostic of Trauma and/or Sexual Contact (The following findings support a disclosure of sexual abuse, if one is given, and are highly suggestive of abuse even in the absence of a disclosure, unless the child and/or caretaker provide a clear, timely, plausible description of accidental injury. It is recommended that diagnostic quality photo-documentation of the examination findings be obtained and reviewed by an experienced medical provider, before concluding that they represent acute or healed trauma. Follow-up examinations are also recommended.)

Acute trauma to external genital/ anal tissues	Residual (healing) injuries (These findings are difficult to assess unless an acute injury was previously documented at the same location)
34. Acute lacerations or extensive bruising of labia, penis, scrotum, perianal tissues, or perineum (May be from unwitnessed accidental trauma, or from physical or sexual abuse) 35. Fresh laceration of the posterior fourchette, not involving the hymen (Must be differentiated from dehisced labial adhesion or failure of midline fusion. May also be caused by accidental injury or consensual sexual intercourse in adolescents)	36. Perianal scar (Rare, may be due to other medical conditions such as Crohn's disease, accidental injuries, or previous medical procedures) 37. Scar of posterior fourchette or fossa. (Pale areas in the midline may also be due to linea vestibularis or labial adhesions)
Injuries indicative of blunt force penetrating trauma (or from abdominal/pelvic compression injury if such history is given)	**Presence of infection confirms mucosal contact with infected and infective bodily secretions, contact most likely to have been sexual in nature**
38. Laceration (tear, partial or complete) of the hymen, acute. 39. Ecchymosis (bruising) on the hymen (in the absence of a known infectious process or coagulopathy). 40. Perianal lacerations extending deep to the external anal sphincter (not to be confused with partial failure of midline fusion) 41. Hymenal transection (healed). An area between 4 and 8 o'clock on the rim of the hymen where it appears to have been torn through, to or nearly to the base, so there appears to be virtually no hymenal tissue remaining at that location. This must be confirmed using additional examination techniques such as a swab, prone knee-chest position or Foley catheter balloon (in adolescents), or prone-knee chest position or water to float the edge of the hymen (in prepubertal girls). This finding has also been referred to as a 'complete cleft' in sexually active adolescents and young adult women. 42. Missing segment of hymenal tissue. Area in the posterior (inferior) half of the hymen, wider than a transection, with an absence of hymenal tissue extending to the base of the hymen, which is confirmed using additional positions/methods as described above.	43. Positive confirmed culture for gonorrhea, from genital area, anus, and throat, in a child outside the neonatal period. 44. Confirmed diagnosis of syphilis, if perinatal transmission is ruled out. 45. Trichomonas vaginalis infection in a child older than 1 year of age, with organisms identified by culture or in vaginal secretions by wet-mount examination by an experienced technician or clinician. 46. Positive culture from genital or anal tissues for Chlamydia, if child is older than 3 years at time of diagnosis, and specimen was tested using cell culture or comparable method approved by the Centers for Disease Control. 47. Positive serology for HIV, if perinatal transmission, transmission from blood products, and needle contamination has been ruled out. **Diagnostic of sexual contact** 48. Pregnancy 49. Sperm identified in specimens taken directly from a child's body.

*Follow-up examination is necessary before attributing these findings to trauma
Reprinted with minor adaptations from Adams JA, Kaplan RA, Starling SP, et al. Guidelines for medical care of children who may have been sexually abused. *J Pediatr Adolesc Gynecol*; 20:163–172, 2007, with permission from Elsevier.

the stress of entering a new school or meeting a new set of friends is a burden the sexual abuse victim does not need. Parents should be cautioned about limiting the amount of open conversation with friends and relatives that the child may overhear. The victim's desire to discuss the abuse should regulate how much abuse-related conversation should take place between family members. Some children may want repeated reassurances about their parents' approval and about their future safety. Other children may want to let the episode be forgotten and return to school and play. If the sexual abuse triggers disruption and chaos in the parents' life and disap-

proval of the child, it will surely have psychological ramifications. The best prognosis results if the parents can show their concern in a way that ensures the child of approval, protection, and resumption of a normal lifestyle.

Hospitalization

Two indications for hospitalizing the sexually abused child are (i) severe injury requiring treatment and (ii) an unsafe home. Outpatient management of sexual abuse victims is always preferable. The rationale is to avoid victimizing the child twice. Children who are hospitalized because the home is

TABLE 132.16

GUIDELINES FOR MAKING THE DECISION TO REPORT SEXUAL ABUSE OF CHILDREN

Data Available				Response	
History	Behavioral Symptoms	Physical Examination	Diagnostic Tests	Level of Concern About Sexual Abuse	Report Decision
Clear statement	Present or absent	Normal or abnormal	Positive or negative	High	Report
None or vague	Present or absent	Normal or nonspecific	Positive for *C trachomatis*, gonorrhea, *T vaginalis*, syphilis, or herpes*	High	Report
None or vague	Present or absent	Concerning or diagnostic findings	Negative or positive	High†	Report
Vague or history by parent only	Present or absent	Normal or nonspecific	Negative	Indeterminate	Refer when possible
None	Present	Normal or nonspecific	Negative	Indeterminate	Possible report, ‡refer, or follow

*If nonsexual transmission is unlikely or excluded.
†Confirmed with various examination techniques and /or peer review with expert consultant.
‡If behaviors are rare / unusual in normal children.
Reproduced with permission from *Pediatrics,* Vol, 116(2), 506-512, Copyright 2005 by the AAP.

unsafe may believe that they are being sent away for their wrongdoing. Another message hospitalization may transmit is that the parent is incapable of providing protection. Both of these messages are harmful to the child's psychological adjustment. If an adult in the home has been the intrafamilial perpetrator, CPS should remove the perpetrator from the home so that the child may return.

Treatment. Whether the child is hospitalized or discharged from the ED, three additional issues should be considered: (i) STI testing (ii) STI prophylaxis, and (iii) pregnancy prevention. SITs are identified in approximately 1 in 20 sexually abused children. All children who have symptoms of a possible STI should be tested and treated. All asymptomatic postpubertal children should also be tested for STIs. The rate of asymptomatic STIs in prepubertal children is lower and the decision to screen for STIs should be made on a case-by-case basis. The presence of any of the following risk factors for STIs may indicate a need for testing: (i) high prevalence of an STI in the community, (ii) presence of an STI in a family member or close contact, (iii) suspected perpetrator has a known STI, (iv) suspected perpetrator is at high risk for an STI, and (v) there is evidence of penetration or ejaculation. STI testing should also be performed at the patient's or family's request. When STI screening is indicated in prepubertal children, testing for *N. gonorrhoeae* and *C. trachomatis* infection is performed. Testing can be expanded to also include syphilis, hepatitis B, *T. vaginalis* infection (Table 132.17). Hepatitis C testing is not included in CDC guidelines for STI testing in victims of sexual assault, but some centers do send hepatitis C PCR and antibody because hepatitis C can be transmitted via sexual con-

tact. HIV testing is already an issue on the minds of most parents of sexual abuse victims. Transmission of HIV during child sexual abuse contacts is uncommon but has been reported. Testing for HIV may depend on the nature and extent of sexual contact, regional rates of HIV infection, ability to test the alleged perpetrator, and parental desires for testing. See Chapter 85 for more on HIV infections. Routine screening for HPV and herpes simple virus (HSV) in the absence of lesions is not indicated in prepubertal children. Genital warts from HPV can often be diagnosed on the basis of clinical appearance. If any vesicular lesions suspicious for HSV are present, testing should be performed to confirm the presence of the virus and to distinguish type 1 form type 2.

Antimicrobial prophylaxis for STIs should be offered to postpubertal victims of sexual assault who present within 72 hours. Specimens for STI testing should be obtained before providing prophylaxis. Recommended prophylaxis regimens for adolescents are shown in Chapter 94 and for preadolescents in Table 132.18. Routine antimicrobial prophylaxis is not indicated in prepubertal children unless the history or examination suggests that the child is at an increased risk of having an STI. All children who receive prophylaxis should have testing performed for STIs first. HIV prophylaxis should also be considered for sexual assault victims presenting within 72 hours. The efficacy of the HIV postexposure prophylaxis in children has not been established and the decision to start HIV prophylaxis must be made on a case-by-case basis. The AAP and the CDC recommend that physicians consider the following factors: (i) local HIV/AIDS epidemiology, (ii) risk of HIV infection in alleged perpetrator, and (iii) risk of HIV transmission based on circumstances of abuse. If the physician determines

TABLE 132.17

STI TESTING IN SUSPECTED VICTIMS OF CHILD SEXUAL ABUSE

Specimen Source	Infections	Recommended Test
Vaginal	*Neisseria gonorrhoeae*	Culture*
	Chlamydia trachomatis	Culture*
	Trichomonas vaginalis	Wet mount and culture
	Bacterial vaginosis	Wet mount and culture
Urethral (male)**	*Neisseria gonorrhoeae*	Culture*
	Chlamydia trachomatis	Culture*
Rectal	*Neisseria gonorrhoeae*	Culture
	Chlamydia trachomatis	Culture
Throat	*Neisseria gonorrhoeae*	Culture
Serum	Syphilis	Serologic tests at time of presentation and 6, 12, and 24 weeks after last episode of sexual abuse.
	HIV	Serologic tests at time of presentation and 6, 12, and 24 weeks after last episode of sexual abuse. Serologic testing of alleged perpetrator if available.
	Hepatitis B virus	Hepatitis B surface antibody if child did not complete 3 dose series of Hepatitis B vaccine. If concern for Hepatitis B infection and initial test is negative, test can be repeated at 6, 12, and 24 weeks.
Lesion Specimen	Human papilloma virus	Biopsy of wart
	Herpes simplex virus	Culture. PCR is more sensitive than culture and should be performed if the lesion has crusted.
	Syphilis (chancre)	Darkfield examination of ulcer exudate

*Initial studies in prepubertal children have suggested that nucleic acid amplifications tests (NAATs) performed on urine or vaginal specimens for *C trachomatis* and *N gonorrhoeae* are sensitive and specific and may be an alternative to cultures. According to the 2006 CDC guidelines and the 2009 AAP Red Book recommendations, however, the evidence to support the use of NAATS in children is currently insufficient. The CDC and AAP state that NAATs might be used if culture is not available and if confirmation with a second FDA approved NAAT targeting a different sequence was performed. The CDC recommends using culture or FDA approved NAATs in adolescents.
** If urethral discharge is present a meatal discharge specimen can be performed instead.
Data included in table from following sources:
American Academy of Pediatrics. *Sexual Victimization and STIs*. Pickering LK, ed. *Red Book:2009 Report of the Committee on Infectious Diseases*. 28th ed. Elk Grove Village, IL: American Academy of Pediatrics; 2009: 167–172
Black CM, Driebe EM, Howard LA, et al. Multicenter Study of Nucleic Acid Amplification Tests for Detection of Chlamydia trachomatis and Neisseria gonorrhoeae in Children Being Evaluated for Sexual Abuse. *Pediatr Infect Dis J*. Jul 2009;28(7):608–613.
Centers for Disease Control and Prevention. Sexually Transmitted Diseases Treatment Guidelines – 2006/ MMWR 2006;55(No. RR-11):80–85.

the child may be at risk of HIV transmission, he or she should consult with a specialist in HIV prophylaxis. The risks and unknown efficacy of postexposure prophylaxis should be discussed with the child's caregiver. If HIV prophylaxis is started, a 3- to 7-day supply should be given and the child should be seen in follow-up visits. A prescription for the remainder of the HIV prophylaxis can then be given.

Pregnancy prophylaxis should be considered if the child has reached menarche and presents within 72 hours of genital–genital contact. For pregnancy prophylaxis, one 1.5 mg or two 0.75 mg of levonorgestrel tablets are taken. Documenting that the patient does not have an existing pregnancy is important. Antiemetic therapy may be considered and offered to children provided with pregnancy prophylaxis and antimicrobial prophylaxis because of the risk of nausea and emesis, although now considerably less with levonorgestrel-based prophylaxis.

Children with physical injuries on examination in the ED should be referred from medical follow-up in 2 weeks. In some cases, particularly if there are new symptoms, repeat evaluation for STIs may be indicated even if the initial STI screening finding was negative. In addition, if there is a concern for hepatitis B, syphilis, or HIV infection with negative baseline testing, repeat testing should be performed at 6, 12, and 24 weeks after the last exposure. Recommendations for treating identified STIs in children are included in Table 132.19. See chapter 85 for information on STI treatment in adolescents.

Psychosocial Referral and Follow-up. All sexually abused children need some form of referral and careful follow-up care. Referral may initially be to the hospital social worker for monitoring of the child's symptoms and the family's ability to cope with this stress. In some locales, volunteer self-help groups organized for women who have been raped may provide support to the child victim and parent. Referral for more in-depth mental health counseling depends on the (i) symptoms manifested by the child, (ii) state of family organization, (iii) length of time the abuse has occurred, and (iv) the child's age. In general, the older the child and the longer the abuse has occurred, the more likely he or she may have or may develop a serious mental health problem. All children should be referred to mental health services.

PSYCHOSOCIAL EMERGENCIES

STI PROPHYLAXIS AFTER SEXUAL VICTIMIZATION OF PREADOLESCENT CHILDREN

Weight <100 lb (<45 kg)		Weight ≥100 lb (≥45 kg)
	For prevention of gonorrhea	
1. Ceftriaxone, 125 mg, intra-muscularly, in a single dose		1A. Ceftriaxone, 125 mg, intramuscularly, in a single dose **OR** 1B. Cefixime, 400 mg, orally, in a single dose
	For prevention of *Chlamydia trachomatis* infection	
PLUS 2A. Azithromycin, 20 mg/kg (maximum 1 g), orally, in a single dose **OR** 2B. Erythromycin base or ethylsuccinate, 50 mg/kg per day, divided into 4 doses for 14 days		**PLUS** 2A. Azithromycin, 1 g, orally, in a single dose **OR** 2B. Doxycycline, 100 mg, twice daily, for 7 days (if at least 8 years of age)
	For prevention of hepatitis B virus infection	
PLUS 3. Begin or complete hepatitis B virus immunization if not fully immunized		**PLUS** 3. Begin or complete hepatitis B virus immunization if not fully immunized
	For prevention of trichomoniasis and bacterial vaginosis	
PLUS 4. Consider adding prophylaxis for trichomoniasis and bacterial vaginosis (metronidazole, 15 mg/kg per day, orally, in 3 divided doses for 7 days; maximum 2 g)		**PLUS** 4. Consider adding prophylaxis against trichomoniasis and bacterial vaginosis (metronidazole, 2 g, orally, in a single dose)

*See text for discussion of prophylaxis for human immunodeficiency virus infection in children after sexual abuse or assault.
Reproduced with permission from the American Academy of Pediatrics. Prophylaxis After Sexual Victimization of Preadolescent Children. Sexual Victimization and STIs. Pickering LK, ed. Red Book: 2006 Report of the Committee on Infectious Diseases. 26th ed. Elk Grove Village, IL: American Academy of Pediatrics; 170.

Follow-up health care visits should be arranged with an informed and sympathetic practitioner who can continue the humane and supportive care initiated in the ED.

Suspected Sexual Abuse in the Setting of Parental Conflicts

In some cases, children will present for evaluation when one parent suspects another parent of sexually abusing the child in the setting of parental divorce. These cases can be challenging, especially if the physician is concerned that the allegations of sexual abuse may be related to a custody dispute or conflict between the parents. The physician, however, cannot ignore concerns of sexual abuse in theses cases and must perform a thorough evaluation. If the child makes a disclosure of sexual abuse or the evaluation is concerning for sexual abuse, the physician is obligated to make a report to the CPS agency. If the evaluation does not support a history of sexual abuse but a parent continues to express concern, the ED physician may need to refer the family for further evaluation by a pediatric child abuse expert and or mental health expert.

NEGLECT

Child neglect is by far the most prevalent form of child abuse. When neglect is blatant, it is easily recognized and reported.

More often, neglect is not obvious and goes undetected for long periods. Although the manifestations of neglect are less dramatic than those of physical abuse, the long-term effects may be more destructive to the child. The indolent nature of child neglect makes it a serious public health problem. For ED staff members, neglect cases are difficult because they require that certain value judgments be made. The balance between supporting the independent rights of the child and maintaining the privacy and sanctity of family rights is delicate. With neglected children, the questions are as follows: (i) How much should the family be doing? (ii) How much are they capable of doing? (iii) How much support from the community or society do they require? and (iv) How much support or help are they willing to accept on behalf of their child? As with the other forms of child abuse, the management of child neglect cases is made easier by working with a multidisciplinary team. In the ED, the team would generally consist of the physician, nurse, and social worker. Particularly in situations in which the line between adequate child care and neglect needs to be drawn, the diversity of personal and professional opinions adds credibility to decision making and lessens the burden on the single practitioner.

Background

The definition of child neglect is difficult because no societal standards for child care are explicitly stated. This vagueness creates a situation in which parents and professionals are left

TABLE 132.19

TREATMENT OF SEXUALLY TRANSMITTED INFECTIONS IN CHILDREN

Infection	Recommended Treatment
Chlamydia trachomatis (vulvovaginitis and urethritis)	*Children <45 kg:* Erythromycin base or ethylsuccinate 50 mg/kg/day orally divided into 4 doses daily (maximum 2 g/day) for 14 days *Children >45 kg but <8 years old.:* Azithromycin 1g orally in single dose *Children >8 years old:* Azithromycin 1 g orally in single dose OR Doxycycline 100 mg orally twice a day for 7 days
Neisseria gonorrhoeae (vulvovaginitis, urethritis, cervicitis, pharyngitis, & proctitis)	*Children <45 kg:* Ceftriaxone, 125 mg, in a single dose
Treponema vaginalis	*Children <45 kg:* Metronidazole, 15 mg/kg per day, orally, in 3 divided doses (maximum 2 g/day) for 7 days
Bacterial vaginosis	*Children <45 kg:* Metronidazole, 15 mg/kg per day, orally, in 2 divided doses (maximum 1 g/day) for 7 days
HSV—primary infection	*Children <45 kg:* Acyclovir, 80 mg/kg per day, orally, in 3–4 divided doses (maximum 1.2 g/day) for 7–10 days
Treponema pallidum	Treatment regimen depends on syphilis stage. See Chapter 85.3, Table 85.3 for details.
Human papillomavirus (external anogenital warts)	*Children <45 kg:* Patient-applied: Podofilox 0.5% solution or gel* OR Imiquimod 5% cream* Provider-administered: Cryotherapy OR Podophyllin resin 10%–25%* OR Trichloroacetic acid OR Bichloroacetic acid OR Surgical removal

*Contraindicated in pregnancy.
Based on data from the following sources:
Centers for Disease Control and Prevention. Sexually Transmitted Diseases Treatment Guidelines – 2006/ MMWR 2006;55(No. RR-11):1–94.
Prophylaxis After Sexual Victimization of Preadolescent Children. Sexual Victimization and STIs. Pickering LK, ed. Red Book: 2006 Report of the Committee on Infectious Diseases. 26th ed. Elk Grove Village, IL: American Academy of Pediatrics; 2006:172–177.

PSYCHOSOCIAL EMERGENCIES

to define their own standards, which may produce many problems. Defining *abandonment* (the ultimate neglect) is an excellent example of the difficulties encountered in setting standards. No societal norm is established for either the age of the child left alone or the duration of time. Thus, if a parent leaves a 3-year-old child unattended in a home for several hours, most neighbors and professionals would consider that neglect. But what if the child was 10 years old and the parent was gone for 20 minutes? Then the situation becomes less clear.

Many states have tried to partially define the condition by making it depend on a physical manifestation in the child. Thus, the child left alone who stays out of trouble is not neglected; the one who burns himself or herself and cries to the point that the neighbors become aware is neglected. The NCANDS uses the following definition: child neglect is charac-

terized by failure to provide for the child's basic needs. Neglect can be physical, educational, or emotional. Physical neglect includes refusal of or delay in seeking health care, abandonment, expulsion from the home or refusal to allow a runaway to return home, and inadequate supervision. Educational neglect includes the allowance of long-term truancy, failure to enroll a child of mandatory school age in school, and failure to attend to a special educational need. Emotional neglect includes actions such as significant inattention to the child's needs for affection, refusal of or failure to provide needed psychological care, spouse abuse in the child's presence, and permission for drug or alcohol use by the child. The assessment of child neglect requires consideration of cultural values and standards of care, as well as recognition that the failure to provide the necessities of life may be related to poverty.

Other apparent societal conflicts are inherent in defining neglect. One conflict centers on the relationship between neglect and poverty. This situation relates to the questions asked previously and the issue of what the family should be doing versus what they are financially capable of doing. Certainly, at times, poverty may be coincident with neglect, but the issues are distinctly separate. Most poor families find a way to provide the material essentials and, more important, the emotional essentials for their children. The contrasting example is that of families who are in the middle or upper socioeconomic scale and who could provide for their children but are neglectful. Another conflict is based on the failure to recognize the evils of excess. The child who is underfed and wasted is promptly labeled *failure to thrive*. The child who is overfed to the point of obesity may face as many serious consequences. The child who is developmentally delayed from understimulation may be labeled *neglected*. The child who has psychosomatic illness from being stressed to overachieve also deserves identification and help. The term *neglect* generally refers to underprovision on the part of the parent. Overprovision may be as deleterious, which presents a serious conflict to the definition of neglect. The true incidence of neglect is not ascertainable.

Dynamics

The dynamics of child neglect have been explained by several different theorists. Some theories are based on purely individual dynamics and point to the immature, overwhelmed, overstressed parent who responds by withdrawal. Polansky has well documented and labeled this condition as the "apathy futility syndrome." Theories that have a more social orientation point to societal pressures and the existence of poverty. David Gil considers all children existing on a welfare stipend as neglected and recommends a change in the distribution of societal resources as a solution. Most theories would support the notion that the neglectful parent does not see himself or herself as such. Most parents are caught up in a neglectful lifestyle that is self-perpetuating. Most neglect is not purposeful, it just happens. Studies have clearly shown that women who fail to seek prenatal care are also likely to not obtain health care for their children. In the parents' view, it is a pattern of living that seems to be the norm. This facet of the dynamics of neglect is important to the ED management.

Manifestations

The manifestations of neglect are countless. The manifestation may be tangible, such as the weight loss of a child whose diet has been inadequate, or intangible, such as the psychological effects of unsatisfactory relationships. A categorization of neglect can be made by looking at the standard functions of the family and then considering the failure to fulfill these functions. A family must (i) provide and distribute material goods—food, clothing, and shelter; (ii) ensure health; (iii) promote safety; (iv) socialize and educate; and (v) provide emotional support, security, and love. The manifestations of neglect may occur in one or more of these functional areas. The most commonly reported manifestations are (i) nonorganic failure to thrive—a lack of food and feeding skills; (ii) medical neglect—a failure to provide needed health care; (iii) abandonment—total neglect, generally viewed as a lack of supervision and as a safety hazard; and (iv) truancy and school avoidance.

Failure to Thrive. The term *failure to thrive* has been used as a diagnostic term to group several diseases and disorders that result in growth failure. Growth failure is generally measured in weight, length, and head circumference as compared with standard growth curves for these parameters. Growth failure may be defined as measurements that fall below 2 SD for age or patterns that cross percentile lines (i.e., move 2 SD) and do not follow the normal lines of growth. Patients diagnosed as failure to thrive may be subcategorized into three groups: (i) organic, (ii) nonorganic, and (iii) mixed group. *Organic* refers to children whose failure to thrive is based on a physical cause such as congenital heart disease, renal disease, or a genetic abnormality. *Nonorganic* refers to the group whose growth failure is environmentally related. When these children are hospitalized and fed standard diets, they grow rapidly and thrive. The group of patients with nonorganic failure to thrive include a substantial number of neglected children who may be brought to the ED for care. The mixed group refers to patients who have a combination of physical and environmental factors. An example might be a physical condition that so overstresses a family that they cannot function; thus, they neglect the child in some aspect of the feeding process.

In recognizing the patients with nonorganic failure to thrive, the following factors are suggestive:

- *History:* (i) an idealized feeding history; (ii) a chief complaint and history that do not identify the child's growth pattern as a problem; (iii) no description of losses such as vomiting or diarrhea; and (iv) failure to give a history of a schedule or scheduled pattern of feeding (e.g., baby eats about every 4 hours).
- *Physical examination:* (i) measurements in which weight is more depressed than length, which is more depressed than head circumference; (ii) other signs of neglect such as poor hygiene, diaper rash, and flat and balding occiput; (iii) dull, apathetic facies; (iv) body posture of an understimulated child; (v) excessive oral self-stimulation; and (vi) developmental delay, particularly in the social adaptive and language areas.
- *Parental observation:* the parent who (i) has an uninterested attitude; (ii) does not respond to child's needs (e.g., react to crying); (iii) lacks concern about health issues; and (iv) appears to be a drug or alcohol abuser.

These factors are shown in Fig. 132.18.

Medical Neglect. The differentiation between medical neglect and noncompliance is often difficult. The key to differentiating them is to ask, "Has identifiable harm come to the child?" If a parent fails to complete a course of therapy prescribed by a physician, noncompliance exists. However, if the failure to give medication results in further illness in the child, medical neglect exists. The manifestations of medical neglect can be documented and reported as such. Noncompliance merely results in a worsening doctor–patient relationship. Proving that the failure to give medication, attend follow-up appointments, or obtain a procedure directly resulted in damage to the child's health may be difficult. Intervening variables, such as the complexity of the disease (e.g., the exacerbations of an asthma attack), or the proven efficacy of the treatment often exist. The ED is often the central place for identifying the manifestations of medical neglect. Good documentation of prescribed treatments and good communication with the source of the child's ongoing health care are important.

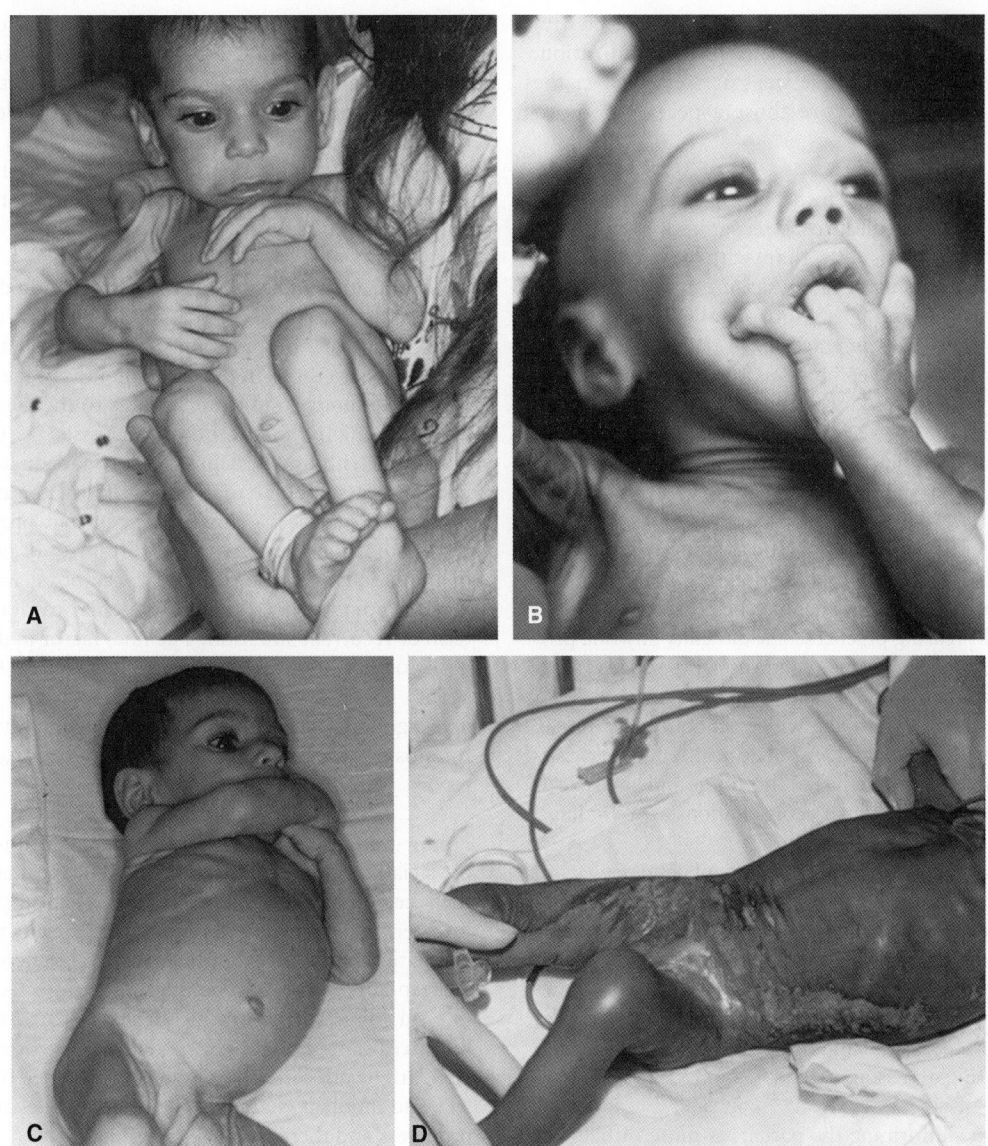

FIGURE 132.18 Physical signs of failure to thrive. **A:** Dull, apathetic eyes that avoid eye contact. **B:** Oral self-stimulatory behavior. **C:** Wasted extremities and protuberant abdomen. **D:** Severe diaper rash as a sign of overall neglect.

Abandonment. Local jurisdictions may dictate the length of time a child must be without supervision before he or she is declared legally abandoned. These cases often come to the ED as the result of a neighbor's call or the initiative of a relative who is aware of the neglect. At times, the situation may become apparent as the ED attempts to obtain permission to treat a child and has difficulty locating a parent or responsible adult. Manifestations of abandonment include (i) physical findings such as excessively dirty diapers, poor hygiene, or hoarse cry; (ii) excessive hunger documented by unusual intake; and (iii) dehydration as documented by urine-specific gravity or blood urea nitrogen. Other manifestations may relate to a lack of supervision and protection and may include burns, ingestions, or repeated accidents. Children with these manifestations may be brought to the ED for treatment. Good case management results in their identification.

Truancy. Truancy as a manifestation of neglect may be less commonly recognized in the ED. The section on school avoidance (see Chapter 133) details many of the aspects of this complex psychosocial emergency. The emergency physician may recognize truancy as a neglect problem when the truant child presents with multiple somatic complaints. As the complaints are explored and no organic basis is found, the parent may be instructed to return the child to school. A failure to comply with this aspect of treatment constitutes medical neglect. For the child who makes frequent visits to the ED, neglect needs to be considered.

Management

The management of cases of child neglect follows the principles detailed in the "Physical Abuse" section. The steps are to (i) suspect and recognize neglect manifestations, (ii) obtain multidisciplinary consultation, (iii) report the neglect, (iv) inform the parents, (v) determine the need for hospitalization, and (vi) arrange follow-up. These steps are reviewed in the following sections to underscore those aspects unique to neglect.

Suspect Neglect. As with other forms of abuse, the open mind of the physician allows neglect to be recognized. Because the manifestations are more subtle than with physical abuse, recognition is more difficult. The physician can overcome this difficulty by only obtaining a more detailed history and observing the parent–child interaction. In-depth social work evaluation can often uncover previous reports of neglect or involvement with child welfare agencies. Piling the building blocks of suspicion to the height of a threshold point may be more difficult because the size of each block may be smaller and less dramatic than that in physical abuse.

Multidisciplinary Consultation. Because much of defining neglect is value laden, using a multidisciplinary consultation is vital. Such consultation can broaden perspectives on "normal" lifestyles and child-rearing practices. The difficulty any one professional feels in making a value judgment can be shared by a group. The multidisciplinary consultation may be made with someone outside the ED. Speaking with a schoolteacher, nurse, or counselor may be informative. A public health nurse or visiting nurse may have worked in the family's home and have excellent insights. Any multidisciplinary consultations are of value.

Reporting. Most states provide that reports of child neglect go to the CPS agency. Some states have joint police and social work (CPS) reporting. Criminal charges under the rubric of "endangering the welfare of another" may be brought against some neglectful parents. However, most neglect cases come under the supervision of CPS. Police involvement becomes almost essential in cases of abandonment, and police have special skills in locating a missing parent.

Informing Parents. Informing the parents is more difficult in cases of neglect. Responses may be either active or passive. The term *neglect* often triggers an active and angry response. This reaction occurs because neglectful parents believe they are trying to parent as best as they can. Their perceptions of the neglect are different from those of the ED staff. This difference invariably creates conflict and evokes guilt and anger. When informing the parents, the focus should be on the child. The physician may need to verbally recognize the positive efforts of the parent. Nonetheless, if the result in the child is inadequate, action needs to be taken to help the child. Taking this approach often directs the parents' energy toward the child and sufficiently quiets emotional reactions.

The passive response may be equally disquieting to the physician. It may be seen in parents who are overwhelmed, have inadequate personalities, or are depressed, intoxicated, or mentally retarded. Separating these parental problems from each other may be difficult. The physician may incorrectly assume the parent does not care what happens to the child because of the lack of response. With extremely passive parents, even engaging them in conversations may be difficult. Approaching the withdrawn parent with simple questions that do not directly relate to the neglect may be helpful. Often, by initiating a neutral conversation, the physician can learn about the parental problem. Asking the parent to perform a task that requires reading or writing may also be instructive. When informing the parent of the neglect report does not trigger active resistance, the physician may be left with an uneasy feeling that the communication was not clearly understood. However, repeat explanations may not stimulate more parental response.

Hospitalization. The need for hospitalization depends on several factors. Certainly, if the child's physical condition warrants treatment, hospitalization is indicated. For example, a child failing to thrive in the first 6 months of life should be hospitalized. Another indication relates to the degree of parental dysfunction. If the parents are assessed as being so overwhelmed, withdrawn, depressed, or inadequate that they are unable to assume parental responsibility, the child should be protected regardless of his or her current physical status. A third indication stems from the chronicity of neglect. Because of the indolent nature of neglect, the physician may need to make a point of hospitalizing the child to dramatize a long-term or recurrent situation. The final factor in determining the need for hospitalization is the time required for community agency response. If the report of neglect triggers an immediate investigation and institution of therapeutic services, the need for hospitalization is diminished. The response to neglect reports varies by community.

Follow-up. In cases of neglect, arranging follow-up care by a physician or clinic is important. Often, the step of informing the receiving physician is overlooked. The staff providing the long-term care is expected to have the capacity to closely monitor patients and to become aggressive about correcting failure to keep appointments. The treatment of neglected children is often a long and frustrating process. Thus, special referral resources should be sought. Attempts to provide treatment in standard health care facilities may be doomed because the passive and indolent character of neglect may escape health care providers and thereby injure the child.

EMOTIONAL ABUSE

Emotional abuse is the form of child abuse that most seriously and most often affects children. With every episode of physical or sexual abuse, a negative psychological message is being inflicted. The child is told, "You are bad!!" and often comes to believe this statement. When the bruises, burns, and broken bones are healed, psychological injury may remain untreated. The neglected child also feels devalued and unloved. Emotional abuse always accompanies other forms of abuse and at times is inflicted independently.

Yet, this form of abuse is the least well understood. Furthermore, a report of suspected abuse is rarely based solely on emotional abuse. Gathering enough objective data to prove that emotional abuse has occurred is difficult. Courts and legal authorities remain unconvinced that a given parental behavior or set of behaviors can be shown to be responsible for effects in the child. Emotional abuse rarely results in a psychosocial emergency. More often, similar to neglect, it is a long-term impediment to normal growth and development.

Background

Emotional abuse has been defined in many different ways. The NCANDS defines it simply: "Child abuse which results in impaired psychological growth and development. Frequently occurs as verbal abuse or excessive demands on a child's performance and results in a negative self-image on the part of the child and disturbed child behavior." The Pennsylvania Child Abuse Law provides for reporting a serious mental injury, which is defined as a psychological condition determined by a psychologist, psychiatrist, or pediatrician, and caused by the acts or omissions of a parent or person responsible for the child's welfare, which: (i) renders the child chronically and severely anxious, agitated, depressed, socially withdrawn, or in reasonable fear of his or her life; (ii) makes it extremely likely that the child will be chronically and severely anxious, agitated, depressed, socially withdrawn, or be in reasonable fear that his or her life is threatened; or (iii) seriously interferes with the child's ability to accomplish age-appropriate developmental milestones or school or community tasks or peer relations.

The Pennsylvania law identifies some of the potential manifestations of emotional abuse but does not define the difficult issue of a child's behavior as "caused by" an act or omission on the part of the parent. The issue of causality hampers the reporting of emotional abuse. The incidence of emotional abuse is unknown, and reasonable estimates of its frequency are not available. Although neglect is reported most often, emotional abuse is the most common form of abuse because it occurs along with all other forms of abuse and neglect, as well as independently.

Dynamics

Emotional abuse occurs when a parent attacks, belittles, humiliates, or devalues a child. Such behavior is not the infrequent reaction of a normal angry parent, but it is an often-repeated message to the child. An emotionally abusive parent appears to be determined to verbally destroy his or her child. The reasons for this behavior are many. The dynamics responsible for physical abuse may be operative for emotional abuse. Often, poor parental self-image is a strong component. The child either threatens the parent or reflects unwanted parental characteristics. In either case, the parent is unable to withstand the stress and attacks the child. When there are many children in a family, a parent may scapegoat the one child with whom he or she most identifies. At times, the child may be identified with another family member, such as an estranged father or a grandparent.

Helfer capsulized the intergenerational nature of emotional and physical abuse in his "World of Abnormal Rearing" formulation (Fig. 132.19). The child who is told repeatedly that he or she is "bad" and "worthless" eventually accepts it. Once the belief that "I'm no damn good" exists, the child's behavior matches the expectation. Ultimately, the poor self-image is reflected in the inability to choose friends or a mate and to accept help. The cycle is completed with poor parenting and emotional abuse of the next generation of children. The intergenerational potential for emotional abuse makes it a serious public health problem.

Manifestations

Emotional abuse manifests in many forms, including children who are excessively withdrawn and passive and those who are

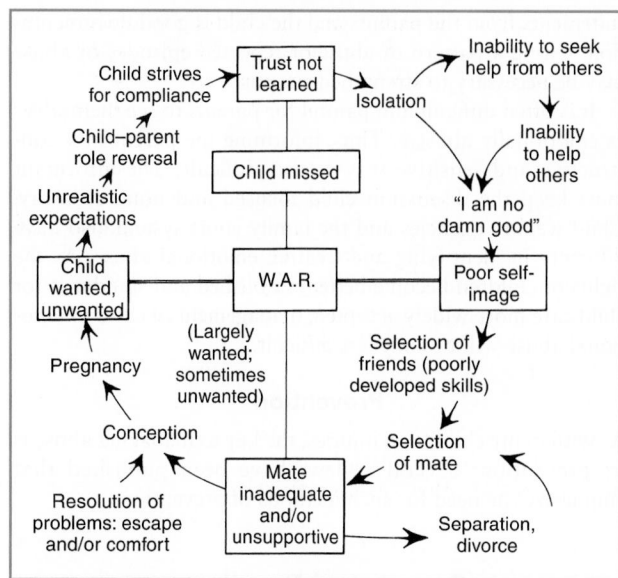

FIGURE 132.19 World of Abnormal Rearing (W.A.R.). (Adapted from R.E. Helfer.)

aggressive and act out. The manifestations are so varied that it is difficult to identify any constant characteristics of the emotionally abused child. To identify emotional abuse, the physician must witness family interactions on repeated occasions; however, the emergency physician does not often have the opportunity for such comprehensive evaluation.

Rarely, more direct presentations of emotional abuse may be seen in the ED. Some children may seek hospital asylum because of excessive fear of their parents. Adolescent "runaways" may include a subset of children who are emotionally abused (see Chapters 130, 131, and 133). Developmental delay may be recognized in the ED, but the cause of the delay can rarely be identified. Finally, children with drug or alcohol abuse may be in a high-risk group for prior emotional abuse. The effects of emotional abuse closely parallel the findings in children with substance abuse (e.g., poor self-image, difficulty in establishing relationships).

Another group of emotionally abused children frequently seen in the ED are youngsters caught in the conflict between estranged parents. These victims have been called "yo-yo" children because they are pulled between arguing parents. Sometimes the children are virtually kidnapped by one parent. These presentations to the ED are based on one parent's attempt to document the poor parenting or neglect of the other. The misuse of the child as a pawn in the marital dispute constitutes emotional abuse. Despite the credibility and motivation of the parent in the ED, emotional abuse should be reported to remove the child from the middle.

Management

The management principles for emotional abuse are the same as those for other forms of abuse. To substantiate emotional abuse, documentation of behavior must be precise. The physician, nurse, and social worker must record observed interactions in behavioral terms using a minimum of subjective assessments and personal conclusions. Recording significant

PSYCHOSOCIAL EMERGENCIES

statements from the parents and the child is good documentation. Citing a pattern of abuse or repeated episodes of abuse may be necessary to strengthen a report.

It is often difficult and painful for parents to see themselves as emotionally abusive. Thus, informing the parent in a constructive and sensitive way is also difficult. The informant must keep the discussion child focused and nonaccusatory. Child welfare agencies and the family court system also have difficulty in identifying and treating emotional abuse. As the rights of children become better established and standards for child care more widely accepted, management of cases of emotional abuse will become less difficult.

Prevention

As with many childhood injuries, the key to managing abuse is its prevention. Several reviews have been published that emphasize the need for such methods of prevention.

Suggested Readings

General

AAP. Diagnostic imaging of child abuse. *Pediatrics* 2000;105:1345–1348.

Carty H, Pierce A. Non-accidental injury: a retrospective analysis of a large cohort. *Eur Radiol* 2002;12:2919–2925.

Centers for Disease Control and Prevention. Nonfatal maltreatment of infants—United States, October 2005–September 2005. In: *MMWR Morb Mortal Wkly Rep* 2008;57(13):336–339.

Durfee M, Parra JM, Alexander R. Child fatality review teams. *Pediatr Clin North Am* 2009;56:379–387.

Flaherty EG, Sege RD, Griffith J, et al. From suspicion of physical child abuse to reporting: primary care clinician decision-making. *Pediatrics* 2008;122: 611–619.

Green FC. Child abuse and neglect: a priority problem for the private physician. *Pediatr Clin North Am* 1975;22:329.

Guenther E, Olsen C, Keenan H, et al. Randomized prospective study to evaluate child abuse documentation in the emergency department. *Acad Emerg Med* 2009;16:249–257.

Jones R, Flaherty EG, Binns HJ, et al. Clinicians' description of factors influencing their reporting of suspected child abuse: report of the child abuse reporting experience study research group. *Pediatrics* 2008;122:259–266.

Kellogg ND; American Academy of Pediatrics Committee on Child Abuse and Neglect. Evaluation of suspected child physical abuse. *Pediatrics* 2007;119: 1232–1241.

Kempe CH, Silverman FH, Steele BF, et al. The battered child syndrome. *JAMA* 1962;181:17.

Kleinman PK. *Diagnostic imaging of child abuse,* 2nd ed. Baltimore, MD: Williams & Wilkins, 1998.

Ludwig S. A multidisciplinary approach to child abuse. *Nurs Clin North Am* 1981;16:161.

Ludwig S, Kornberg AE. *Child abuse: a medical reference.* New York, NY: Churchill-Livingstone, 1992.

Reece RM, Christian C, eds. *Child abuse: medical diagnosis and management,* 3rd ed. Elk Grove Village, IL: AAP Press, 2009.

Sedlak AJ, Broadhurst DD. *Third national incidence study of child abuse and neglect: final report (NIS-3).* Washington, DC: U.S. Department of Health and Human Services Administration for Children and Families, Administration on Children, Youth and Families, National Center on Child Abuse and Neglect, 1996.

Smith JR, Brooks-Gunn J. Correlates and consequences of harsh discipline for young children. *Arch Pediatr Adolesc Med* 1997;151:777–786.

Straus MA, Sugarman DB, Giles-Sims J. Spanking by parents and subsequent antisocial behavior of children. *Arch Pediatr Adolesc Med* 1997;151:761–767.

Teicher MH. Scars that won't heal: the neurobiology of child abuse. *Sci Am* 2002;286:68–75.

Trokel M, Griffith J, Sege R. Variation in the diagnosis of child abuse in severely injured infants. *Pediatrics* 2006;117:722–728.

U.S. Department of Health and Human Services. *A nation's shame: fatal child abuse and neglect in the United States: a report of the U.S. Advisory Board on Child Abuse and Neglect: fifth report.* Washington, DC: U.S. Department of Health and Human Services, April 1995.

U.S. Department of Health and Human Services, National Center on Child Abuse and Neglect. *Child maltreatment 1995: reports from the states to the National Child Abuse and Neglect Data System.* Washington, DC: U.S. Government

Printing Office, 1997. http://www.acf.hhs.gov/programs/cb/publications/ncands/index.htm.

U.S. Department of Health and Human Services, National Center on Child Abuse and Neglect. *Child maltreatment 2001: reports from the states to the National Child Abuse and Neglect Data System.* Washington, DC: U.S. Government Printing Office, 2003. http://www.acf.hhs.gov/programs/cb/publications/cm01/index.htm.

U.S. Department of Health and Human Services, National Center on Child Abuse and Neglect. *Child maltreatment 2002: reports from the states to the National Child Abuse and Neglect Data System.* Washington, DC: U.S. Government Printing Office, 2004. http://www.acf.hhs.gov/programs/cb/publications/cm02/index.htm

U.S. Department of Health and Human Services, Administration for Children & Families, Administration on Children, Youth & Families, Children's Bureau. *Statistics & Research, Child Maltreatment 2007.* http://www.acf.hhs.gov/programs/cb/pubs/cm07/figure3_5.htm.

U.S. Department of Health and Human Services, Administration for Children & Families, Child Welfare Information Gateway. *Child abuse and neglect fatalities: statistics and interventions.* http://www.childwelfare.gov/pubs/factsheets/fatality.cfm.

Physical Abuse

Cutaneous Injury

Angel C, Shu T, French D, et al. Genital and perineal burns in children: 10 years of experience at a major burn center. *J Pediatr Surg* 2002;37:99–103.

Banco L, Lapidus G, Zavoski R, et al. Burn injuries among children in an urban emergency department. *Pediatr Emerg Care* 1994;10:98–101.

Bariciak ED, Plint AC, Gaboury I, et al. Dating of bruises in children: an assessment of physician accuracy. *Pediatrics* 2003;112:804–807.

Dailey JC, Bowers CM. Aging of bite marks: a literature review. *J Forensic Sci* 1997;42:792–795.

Gilliland MGF, Folberg R. Shaken babies—some have no impact injuries. *J Forensic Sci* 1996;41:114–116.

Greenbaum AR, Donne J, Wilson D, et al. Intentional burn injury: an evidence-based, clinical and forensic review. *Burns* 2004;30:628–642.

Hicks Ra, Stolfi A. Skeletal surveys in children with burns caused by child abuse. *Pediatr Emerg Care* 2007;23:308–313.

Joffe M, Ludwig S. Stairway injuries in children. *Pediatrics* 1988;82:457–472.

Labbé J, Caouette G. Recent skin injuries in normal children. *Pediatrics* 2001;108:271–276.

Maguire S, Mann MK, Sibert J, et al. Are there patterns of bruising in childhood which are diagnostic or suggestive of abuse? A systematic review. *Arch Dis Child* 2005;90:182–186.

Maguire S, Mann MK, Sibert J, et al. Can you age bruises accurately in children? A systematic review. *Arch Dis Child* 2005;90:187–189.

Ng CS, Hall CM, Shaw DG. The range of visceral manifestations of non-accidental injury. *Arch Dis Child* 1997;77:167–174.

Schwengel D, Ludwig S. Rhabdomyolysis and myoglobinuria as manifestations of child abuse. *Pediatr Emerg Care* 1985;1:194.

Sugar NF, Taylor JA, Feldman KW. Bruises in infants and toddlers: those who don't cruise rarely bruise. *Arch Pediatr Adolesc Med* 1999;153:399–403.

Head Trauma

Barr RG, Trent RB, Cross J. Age-related incidence curve of hospitalized shaken baby syndrome cases: convergent evidence for crying as a trigger to shaking. *Child Abuse Negl* 2006;30:7–16.

Bechtel K, Stoessel K, Leventhal JM, et al. Characteristics that distinguish accidental from abusive injury in hospitalized young children with head trauma. *Pediatrics* 2004;114:165–168.

Biron D, Shelton D. Perpetrator accounts in infant abusive head trauma brought about by a shaking event. *Child Abuse Negl* 2005;29:1347–1358.

Block RW. Follow-up skeletal surveys prove to be valuable in evaluation of child physical abuse. *Child Abuse Negl* 2005;29:1073–1074.

Bonnier C, Nassogne MC, Saint-Martin C, et al. Neuroimaging of intraparenchymal lesions predicts outcome in shaken baby syndrome. *Pediatrics* 2003;112:808–814.

Chiesa A, Duhaime AC. Abusive head trauma. *Pediatr Clin North Am* 2009;56: 317–331.

Duhaime AC, Alario AJ, Lewander WJ, et al. Head injury in very young children: mechanisms, injury types, and ophthalmologic findings in 100 hospitalized patients younger than 2 years of age. *Pediatrics* 1992;90:179–185.

Duhaime AC, Christian CW, Rorke LB, et al. Nonaccidental head injury in infants—the "shaken-baby syndrome." *N Engl J Med* 1998;338(25):1822–1829.

Feldman KW, Bethel R, Shugerman RP, et al. The cause of infant and toddler subdural hemorrhage: a prospective study. *Pediatrics* 2001;108:636–646.

Hettler J, Greenes DS. Can the initial history predict whether a child with a head injury has been abused? *Pediatrics* 2003;11:602–607.

Hymel KP, Rumack CM, Hay TC, et al. Comparison of intracranial computed tomographic (CT) findings in pediatric abusive and accidental head trauma. *Pediatr Radiol* 1997;27(9):743–747.

Ichord RN, Naim M, Pollock AN, et al. Hypoxic-ischemic injury complicates inflicted and accidental traumatic brain injury in young children: the role of diffusion-weighted imaging. *J Neurotrauma* 2007;24:106–118.

Jenny C, Hymel KP, Ritzen A, et al. Analysis of missed cases of abusive head trauma. *JAMA* 1999;281:621–626.

Kapoor S, Schiffman J, Tang R, et al. The significance of white-centered retinal hemorrhages in the shaken baby syndrome. *Pediatr Emerg Care* 1997;13(3): 183–185.

Laskey AL, Holsti M, Runyan DK, et al. Occult head trauma in young suspected victims of physical abuse. *J Pediatr* 2004;144:719–722.

Levin AV. Retinal hemorrhages: advances in understanding. *Pediatr Clin North Am* 2009;56:333–344.

Minns RA, Brown JK. Shaking and other non-accidental head injuries in children. *Arch Pediatr Adolesc Med* 2007;161:108–109.

Nichols JS, Elger C, Hemminger L, et al. Magnetic resonance imaging: utilization in the management of central nervous system trauma. *J Trauma* 1997;42:520–524.

Odom A, Christ E, Kerr N, et al. Prevalence of retinal hemorrhages in pediatric patients after in-hospital cardiopulmonary resuscitation: a prospective study. *Pediatrics* 1997;99(6):e3.

Reece RM, Nicholson CE, eds. *Inflicted childhood neurotrauma.* Elk Grove Village, IL: American Academy of Pediatrics, 2003.

Rubin DM, Christian CW, Bilaniuk LT, et al. Occult head injury in high-risk abused children. *Pediatrics* 2003;111:1382–1386.

Salehi-Had H, Brandt JD, Rosas AJ, et al. Findings in older children with abusive head injury: does shaken-child syndrome exist? *Pediatrics* 2006;117: e1039–e1044.

Shah M, Vavilala MS, Feldman KW, et al. Motor vehicle crash brain injury in infants and toddlers: a suitable model for inflicted head injury? *Child Abuse Negl* 2005;29:953–967.

Thackeray JD. Frena tears and abusive head injury. *Pediatr Emerg Care* 2007; 23:735–737.

Zimmerman RA, Bilaniuk LT. Pediatric head trauma. *Neuroimaging Clin N Am* 1994;4:349–366.

Fracture

American College of Radiology. *ACR practice guideline for skeletal surveys in children.* Reston, VA: American College of Radiology, 2006.

Anderson WA. The Significance of Femoral Fractures in Children. *Ann Emerg Med* 1982;11(4):174–177.

Barsness C, Cha E, Bensard D, et al. The positive predictive value of rib fractures as an indicator of nonaccidental trauma in children. *J Trauma* 2003;54: 1107–1110.

Belfer RA, Klein BL, Orr L. Use of the skeletal survey in the evaluation of child maltreatment. *Am J Emerg Med* 2001;19:122–124.

Bulloch B, Schubert CJ, Brophy PD, et al. Cause and clinical characteristics of rib fractures in infants. *Pediatrics* 2000;105:e48.

Feldman KW, Brewer DK. Child abuse, cardiopulmonary resuscitation, and rib fractures. *Pediatrics* 1984;73:339.

Harris VJ, Lorand MA, Fitzpatrick JJ, et al. *Radiographic atlas of child abuse: a case studies approach.* New York, NY: Igaku-Shoin, 1996.

Jenny C. Committee on Child Abuse and Neglect. Evaluating infants and young children with multiple fractures. *Pediatrics* 2006;118:1299–1303.

Kemp AM, Butler A, Morris S, et al. Which radiological investigations should be performed to identify fractures in suspected child abuse? *Clin Radiol* 2006;61:723–736.

Kleinman PK, Schlesinger AE. Mechanical factors associated with posterior rib fractures: laboratory and case studies. *Pediatr Radiol* 1997;27:87–91.

Lane WG, Rubin DM, Monteith R, et al. Racial differences in the evaluation of pediatric fractures for physical abuse. *JAMA* 2002;288:1603–1609.

Leventhal JM, Martin KD, Asnes AG. Incidence of fractures attributable to abuse in young hospitalized children: results from analysis of a United States database. *Pediatrics* 2008;122:599–604.

Schweich P, Fleisher G. Rib fractures in children. *Pediatr Emerg Care* 1985;1(4): 187–189.

Spevak MR, Kleinman PK, Belanger PL, et al. Cardiopulmonary resuscitation and rib fractures in infants. *JAMA* 1994;272(8):617–618.

Swischuk LE. Radiographic signs of skeletal trauma. In: Ludwig S, Kornberg A, eds. *Child abuse: a medical reference,* 2nd ed. New York, NY: Churchill-Livingstone, 1992.

Williams RL, Connolly PT. In children undergoing chest radiography what is the specificity of rib fractures for non-accidental injury? *Arch Dis Child* 2004; 89:490–492.

Abdominal Trauma

Arkovitz MS, Johnson N, Garcia VF. Pancreatic trauma in children: mechanisms of injury. *J Trauma* 1997;42(1):49–53.

Cameron CM, Lazoritz S, Calhoun AD. Blunt abdominal injury: simultaneously occurring liver and pancreatic injury in child abuse. *Pediatr Emerg Care* 1997;13:334–336.

Coant PN, Kornberg AE, Brody AS, et al. Markers for occult liver injury in cases of physical abuse in children. *Pediatrics* 1992;89(2):274–278.

Slosberg E, Ludwig S, Duckett J, et al. Penile trauma as a sign of child abuse. *Am J Dis Child* 1978;132:719.

Trokel M, DiScala C, Terrin NC, et al. Blunt abdominal injury in the young pediatric patient: child abuse and patient outcomes. *Child Maltreat* 2004; 9:111–117.

Wood J, Rubin DM, Nance ML, et al. Distinguishing inflicted versus accidental abdominal injuries in young children. *J Trauma* 2005;59:1203–1208.

Fatality

Brewster A, Nelson J, Hymel K, et al. Victim, perpetrator, family and incident characteristics of 32 infant maltreatment deaths in the United States Air Force. *Child Abuse Negl* 1998;22:91–101.

Hodge D, Ludwig S. Child homicide: emergency department recognition. *Pediatr Emerg Care* 1985;1:3.

Nashelsky MB, Dix JD. The time interval between lethal infant shaking and onset of symptoms: a review of the shaken baby syndrome literature. *Am J Forensic Med Pathol* 1995;16(2):154–157.

Wyatt JP, McLeod L, Beard D, et al. Timing of paediatric deaths after trauma. *BMJ* 1997;314(7084):868.

Other

Ayoub CC, Schreier HA, Alexander R. Munchausen by proxy. *Child Maltreat* 2002;7:103–165.

Bryk M, Siegel PT. My mother caused my illness: the story of a survivor of Munchausen by proxy syndrome. *Pediatrics* 1997;100:1–7.

da Fonseca MA, Feigal RJ, ten Bensel RW. Dental aspects of 1248 cases of child maltreatment on file at a major county hospital. *Pediatr Dent* 1992;14: 152–157.

Finkel MA, Ricci LR. Documentation and preservation of visual evidence in child abuse. *Child Maltreat* 1997;2:322–330.

Leavitt EB, Pincus RL, Bukachevsky R. Otolaryngologic manifestations of child abuse. *Arch Otolaryngol Head Neck Surg* 1992;118:629–631.

Ludwig S. The treatment of child abuse and violence. *Ann Nestle [Fr]* 2004;62: 25–31.

Rubin D, McMillan CO, Helfaer M, et al. Experience and reason—briefly recorded. Pulmonary edema associated with child abuse: case reports and review of the literature. *Pediatrics* 2001;108:769–775.

Southall DR, Plunkett MCB, Banks MW, et al. Covert video recordings of life-threatening child abuse: lessons for child protection. *Pediatrics* 1997;100: 735–760.

Sexual Abuse

Adams JA. In training: medical evaluation of suspected child sexual abuse. *J Pediatr Adolsc Gynecol* 2004;17:191–197.

Adams JA. Guidelines for medical care of children evaluated for suspected sexual abuse: an update for 2008. *Curr Opin Obstet Gynecol* 2008;20(5): 435–441.

Adams JA, Harper K, Knudson S, et al. Examination findings in legally confirmed child sexual abuse: it's normal to be normal. *Pediatrics* 1994;94:310–317.

Adams JA, Kaplan RA, Starling SP, et al. Guidelines for medical care of children who may have been sexually abused. *J Pediatr Adolesc Gynecol* 2007;20: 163–172.

American Academy of Pediatrics. Sexual victimization and STIs. In: Pickering LK, ed. *Red Book: 2009 Report of the Committee on Infectious Diseases,* 26th ed. Elk Grove Village, IL: American Academy of Pediatrics, 2009:167–172.

Bernet W. Practice parameters for the forensic evaluation of children and adolescents who may have been physically or sexually abused. American Academy of Child and Adolescent Psychiatry. *J Am Acad Child Adolesc Psychiatry* 1997;10(suppl):37S–56S.

Black CM, Driebe EM, Howard LA, et al. Multicenter Study of nucleic acid amplification tests for detection of *Chlamydia trachomatis* and *Neisseria gonorrhoeae* in children being evaluated for sexual abuse. *Pediatr Infect Dis J.* 2009;28(7):608–613.

Centers for Disease Control and Prevention. Sexually transmitted diseases treatment guidelines, 2006. *MMWR Morb Mortal Wkly Rep* 2006;55(RR-11): 1–94.

Child Welfare Information Gateway. Definitions of child abuse and neglect. www.childwelfare.gov/systemwide/laws_policies/statutes/define.cfm. Published 2007.

Committee on Child Abuse and Neglect, American Academy of Pediatrics. Gonorrhea in prepubertal children. *Pediatrics* 1998;101:134–135.

DeJong AR, Rose M. Legal proof of child sexual abuse in the absence of physical evidence. *Pediatrics* 1991;88(3):506–511.

Dubow SR, Giardino AP, Christian CW, et al. Do pediatric chief residents recognize details of prepubertal female genital anatomy: a national survey. *Child Abuse Negl* 2005;29:195–205. Accessed 12/20/2009

Finkel M, Giardino A, eds. *Medical evaluation of child sexual abuse: a practical guide,* 2nd ed. Thousand Oaks, CA; Sage, 2002.

Haka-Ikse K, Mian M. Sexuality in children. *Pediatr Rev* 1993;14:401–407.

Heger A, Ticson L, Velasquez O, et al. Children referred for possible sexual abuse: medical findings in 2384 children. *Child Abuse Negl* 2002;26:645–659.

Hymel KP, Jenny C. Child sexual abuse. *Pediatr Rev* 1996;17(7):236–249.

Heppenstall-Heger A, McConnell G, Ticson L, et al. Healing patterns in anogenital injuries: a longitudinal study of injuries associated with sexual abuse, accidental injuries, or genital surgery in the preadolescent child. *Pediatrics* 2003;112:829–837.

Jones V, Smith SJ, Omar HA. Nonsexual transmission of anogenital warts in children: a retrospective analysis. *Sci World J* 2007;7:1896–1899.

Kamarashev JA, Vassileva SG. Dermatologic diseases of the vulva. *Clin Dermatol* 1997;15:53–65.

Kellogg N, Baillargeon J, Lukefahr J, et al. Menard. Comparison of nucleic acid amplification tests and culture techniques in the detection of *Neisseria gonorrhoeae* and *Chlamydia trachomatis* in victims of suspected child sexual abuse. *J Pediatr Adolesc Gynecol* 2004;17(5):331–339.

Kellogg N, The Committee on Child Abuse and Neglect. The evaluation of sexual abuse in children. *Pediatrics* 2005;116(2):506–512.

McCann J, Miyamoto S, Boyle C, et al. Healing of hymenal injuries in prepubertal and adolescent girls: a descriptive. *Pediatrics* 2007;119:e1094–e1106.

Palusci VJ, Cox, EO, Shatz, EM, Schultze JM. Urgent medical assessment after child sexual abuse. *Child Abuse Negl* 2006;30(4):367–380.

Paradise JE, Rostain AL, Nathanson M. Substantiation of sexual abuse charges when parents dispute custody or visitation. *Pediatrics* 1988;81:835–839.

Sinclair KA, Woods CR, Kirse DJ, et al. Anogenital and respiratory tract human papillomavirus infections among children: age, gender, and potential transmission through sexual abuse. *Pediatrics* 2005;116:815–825.

U.S. Department of Health and Human Services, Administration on Children, Youth and Families. *Child maltreatment 2006.* Washington, DC: U.S. Government Printing Office, 2008.

Young KL, Jones JG, Worthington T, et al. Forensic evidence in sexually abused children. *Arch Pediatr Adolesc Med* 2006;260:585–588.

Neglect

Adedoyin A, Gottlieb B. Evaluation of failure to thrive: diagnostic yield of testing for renal tubular acidosis. *Pediatrics* 2003;112:463–466.

Bailey E. Child abuse and neglect: a system that still needs pediatric leadership. *Pediatrics* 2008;122:654–655.

Block RW, Krebs NF, AAP Committee on Child Abuse and Neglect and the Committee on Nutrition. Failure to thrive as a manifestation of child neglect. *Pediatrics* 2005;116:1234–1237.

Dubowitz H. Tackling child neglect: a role for pediatricians. *Pediatr Clin North Am* 2009;56:363–378.

Frank DA, Silva M, Needlman R. Failure to thrive: mystery, myth, and method. *Contemp Pediatr* 1993;10:114–133.

Harrington D, Black MM, Starr RH Jr, et al. Child neglect: relation to child temperament and family context. *Am J Orthopsychiatry* 1998;68:108–116.

Homer C, Ludwig S. Categorization of etiology of failure to thrive. *Am J Dis Child* 1981;135:848.

Hymel KP, AAP Committee on Child Abuse & Neglect. When is lack of supervision neglect? *Pediatrics* 2006;118:1296–1298.

Ludwig S. Failure to thrive/starvation. In: Ludwig S, Kornberg A, eds. *Child abuse: a medical reference,* 2nd ed. New York, NY: Churchill-Livingstone, 1992;303–319.

Margolin L. Fatal child neglect. *Child Welfare* 1990;69:309–319.

Polansky NA, Chalmers MA, Buttenwieser E, et al. *Damaged parents: an anatomy of child neglect.* Chicago, IL: University of Chicago Press, 1981.

Schwartz ID. Failure to thrive: an old nemesis in the new millennium. *Pediatr Rev* 2000;21:257–264.

Straus MA, Kantor GK. Definition and measurement of neglectful behavior: some principles and guidelines. *Child Abuse Negl* 2005;29:19–29.

Psychological/Emotional Abuse

Jellen LK, McCarroll JE, Thayer LE. Child emotional maltreatment: a 2-year study of US Army cases. *Child Abuse Negl* 2001;25:623–639.

Kilpatrick KL, Litt M, Williams LM. Post-traumatic stress disorder in child witnesses to domestic violence. *Am J Orthopsychiatry* 1997;67:639–644.

Ludwig S, Rostain A. Family function & dysfunction. In: Carey WB, Crocker AC, eds. *Developmental-behavioral pediatrics,* 4th ed. Philadelphia, PA: Saunders-Elsevier, 2009;103–118.

Shipman K, Taussig H. Mental health treatment of child abuse and neglect: the promise of evidence-based practice. *Pediatr Clin North Am* 2009;56:417–428.

Stirling Jr J, AAP Committee on Child Abuse & Neglect & Section on Adoption & Foster Care, Amaya-Jackson L. Understanding the behavioral and emotional consequences of child abuse. *Pediatrics* 2008;122:667–673.

van der Kolk BA. The psychobiology of posttraumatic stress disorder. *J Clin Psychol* 1997;58:16–24.

Widom C. The cycle of violence. *Science* 1989;244:160–164.

Prevention

Dubowitz H. Preventing child neglect and physical abuse: a role for pediatricians. *Pediatr Rev* 2002;23:191–195.

Rubin D, Lane W, Ludwig S. Child abuse prevention. *Curr Opin Pediatr* 2001;13:388–401.

Toomey S, Bernstein H. Child abuse and neglect: prevention and intervention. *Curr Opin Pediatr* 2001;13:211–215.

CHAPTER 133 ■ PSYCHIATRIC EMERGENCIES

EMILY R. KATZ, MD, LAURA L. CHAPMAN, MD, AND THOMAS H. CHUN, MD

The emergency department (ED) is frequently the setting for the initial evaluation of various emotional and psychiatric difficulties of children and their families. As such, ED physicians must be proficient in psychiatric diagnosis, crisis intervention, and disposition planning, regardless of whether a mental health professional is consulted to evaluate the patient. Even when a consultant is involved, the ED physician still shares responsibility for the patient's care and disposition. As in any other situation involving a consultant, it is critical that the ED physician and the consultant agree on a treatment plan, both from a patient care perspective and from a medicolegal standpoint.

CRISIS AND CRISIS INTERVENTION

Psychiatric emergencies are best understood as crisis situations. Crisis involves the acute development of circumstances or events that render the usual coping and adaptive patterns of an individual or social unit inadequate. A useful conceptual approach to these crises is "Why now?" (i.e., what in the person's behavior or their overall situation has become unmanageable). It is at this point that patients and/or families seek professional help and the patient may be brought to the ED.

Psychiatric emergencies during childhood may be defined as crises in which the adults around the child are no longer able to help the child control his or her emotions and can no longer provide adequate support and control of the child's emotional reactions and behavior. Therefore, comprehensive assessment and treatment of psychiatric emergencies in children must involve the participation of the child's family.

Requirements of the ED

The ability to respond effectively to psychiatric emergencies of children and families requires special capacities of the ED and its staff. The safety of patients and the ED staff is of paramount importance. Ensuring safety includes not only the physical characteristics of the patient room but also the access to medical and hospital security personnel, as well as appropriate safety procedures and policies.

It is vitally important to ensure patients do not bring weapons or other dangerous objects into the ED. Procedures to achieve this end may include use of metal detectors or a physical search of the patient and their belongings for such objects. Some EDs use a protocol whereby all patients must wear a hospital gown and slippers while in the ED. This separates the patient from their belongings and can facilitate a search for harmful objects. Such a policy may also theoretically reduce the risk of patient elopement.

A safe and adequate physical space is an absolute requirement of the ED. Patients should be under constant supervision by ED personnel—by either by the medical staff or the security staff. ED staff must always be able see the patient, either by direct visualization of the patient or by continuous video monitoring. At the minimum, the room in which patients are medically evaluated must be free of objects with which the patient can harm him- or herself. This includes not only sharp objects but also objects with which they could strangle themselves (e.g., medical tubing, electrical or equipment cords). Such objects should be either inaccessible to the patient (e.g., in locked cabinets) or physically removed from the room. Ideally, the ED should have a separate holding or observation area for patients recovering from overdoses or being stabilized with psychotropic medication, where they can be observed and evaluated regularly.

The optimal setting for a psychiatric evaluation would have the following characteristics. It would be a quiet, low-stimulus environment in which interruptions are uncommon and privacy and confidentiality are assured. A specific area for psychiatric emergencies distinct from the main ED may be calming and may enable a mood of concern and deliberation. Examination rooms should have seats for each family member and the clinician. This area should be adequately staffed by medical and security personnel and have rapid access to additional personnel. There should also be the capacity for using restraints, if necessary.

Clinicians in the ED should have a preexisting relationship with a mental health team that is committed to providing child psychiatric consultation at all times. The emergency physician and the consultant need to collaborate in the care of these patients. The ED should also have relationships with various psychiatric inpatient units so that hospitalization, when needed, can be arranged efficiently. The staff should be thoroughly familiar with the procedures for psychiatric hospitalization, including the specific legal requirements for involuntary commitment. In certain situations, such as children recovering from medically serious suicide attempts, medical hospitalization may be necessary. The hospital should have specific guidelines or protocols for the management of psychiatric patients on medical floors.

Finally, the ED should have relationships with other social agencies and an awareness of relevant laws. The police should be aware of which children to bring to the ED for psychiatric assessment and should be prepared to remain in the ED until adequate security has been arranged. Relationships should be developed with mental health base service units, temporary shelters, and other crisis intervention centers, ensuring effective referrals when necessary. Staff should be aware of child protection laws and the procedures for emergency intervention in situations of abuse and neglect.

CHILDHOOD/ADOLESCENT PSYCHIATRIC
EMERGENCIES: EMERGENCY PHYSICIAN
RESPONSIBILITIES

Rapidly identify crisis situation
Assess nature and degree of child and family stress
Acute medical management
Acute psychiatric management
Develop specific crisis interventions
Psychiatric consultation
Independent disposition planning

Physician Responsibilities and Skills

The responsibilities of the emergency physician with psychiatric emergencies are shown in Table 133.1. The physician needs to handle the family's anxiety and uncertainty by approaching the family crisis calmly and systematically. In doing so, the physician establishes the leadership and authority that enables the family to discuss its problems freely and to consider and act on recommendations. Another important skill of the emergency physician involves the ability to obtain and assess relevant information about the child, the family, and their community supports. This topic is covered subsequently in the "Evaluation of Psychiatric Emergencies" section.

Family Responsibilities

A childhood psychiatric emergency implies a limitation of effective interaction between the child and his or her caregivers. The emergency physician must establish who the child's actual caregivers are and try to involve as many of them as possible in the ED. When evaluating the child, the caregivers, and their relationships with each other, the emergency physician should assess the degree to which the parents (or other caregivers) are meeting the following responsibilities:

1. Ensure the physical and emotional safety of the child. Parents need to protect the child as much as possible from external danger (e.g., getting lost, walking into traffic, going off with strange adults) and internal family danger (e.g., neglect, physical and emotional abuse, sexual abuse).
2. Provide support and nurturance, especially to younger children, such that an emotional bond is established between the child and parent.
3. Provide enough socialization to set limits on the child's behavior.
4. Promote the child's efforts in age-appropriate tasks, including consistent school attendance and performance, learning to relate to peers, and assuming greater autonomy within the family as the child grows older.
5. Assist the child in coping with unexpected failures and losses, including academic disappointment, family disruption, and disability resulting from physical illness.

By keeping these family responsibilities in mind, the emergency physician can assess families in crisis, determining which functions are being met and which need to be supported.

Working with Strengths

The emergency physician working with a family in crisis must look for problem areas, as well as areas of competence in both the child and the family. These areas of strength form the basis for a successful treatment plan that enables the family to master the crisis. Typically, families in crisis do not use their existing abilities enough as they pursue a narrow range of responses to the problem at hand. Once a family's assets are recognized, these skills enable the parents to be more confident and competent in dealing with their child. The emergency physician should help the family recognize its capabilities at a time when confidence is at its lowest level.

EVALUATION OF PSYCHIATRIC EMERGENCIES

The evaluation of acute psychosocial emergencies can be divided into five sections (Table 133.2). Orienting data and relevant history indicates the general living situation and previous psychosocial adaptation of the child or adolescent patient. It also provides a complete description of the current crisis, including apparent precipitants. Medical history and physical evaluation determine the child's current physical status. The mental status examination of the child provides information about the patient's current psychological well-being. A family evaluation, using both history and observation of the family's behavior during the ED visit, enables the physician to determine the family's ability to respond to the child's distress. By integrating these sources of information, the emergency physician is well equipped to understand the crisis and to pursue appropriate treatment alternatives.

Orienting Data and Relevant History

Psychosocial orienting data, as shown in Table 133.3, provide information that enables the physician to appreciate the basic living situation of the child and family. This information can be quickly obtained and includes the child's age, gender, and race; the child's grade in school and the type of classroom setting; and the address and type of neighborhood where the family lives. Family composition includes who lives at home, what their relationships are to each other and to the identified patient, and who are the primary and secondary caregivers.

CHILDHOOD/ADOLESCENT PSYCHIATRIC
EMERGENCIES: CATEGORIES OF NECESSARY
INFORMATION

1. Orienting data
2. Relevant history
3. Medical history and physical examination
4. Mental status of the child
5. Family evaluation

TABLE 133.3

CHILDHOOD/ADOLESCENT PSYCHIATRIC EMERGENCIES: ORIENTING DATA

Age of child, gender, race
Grade in school, name of school, classroom setting
Family address, type of neighborhood, parental occupations
Family composition
  One- or two-parent family; approximate ages of parents
  Siblings of patient and their ages
  Other family members, if any, living in the home
  Other significant relatives and caregivers

Relevant history, as shown in Table 133.4, builds on identifying information to provide a more complete description of the problem at hand. Historical information should include a thorough understanding of the current crisis and its apparent precipitants, as well as similar problems in the past and previous psychiatric involvement for either child or family. The recent school performance of the child and the adequacy of his or her relationships with peers and family members should also be determined.

The history of the current crisis should be obtained directly by asking family members in turn to give their account. Usually, beginning with the parents and other adults in the room is easiest. The physician must also obtain the child's version of the current difficulties. If the family does not provide a coherent history, the physician should guide the interview by interrupting respectfully and asking relevant questions. The physician can ensure a more complete understanding of the problem by periodically summarizing what family members have said and then checking for accuracy. When accounts and opinions differ among family members, this disparity should be made explicit. When important issues such as suicidal thinking and severe depression are not brought up, the physician should inquire about them directly. This inquiry often reassures the family that its distress is understood and enables the emergency physician to have all the relevant information needed for assessment.

Medical History and Physical Examination

"Medical clearance" of psychiatric patients is one of the prime reasons why children with psychiatric emergencies are sent to an ED. There are several major objectives of this medical evaluation. First and foremost is to determine whether a patient has an unstable medical condition or acute injuries requiring immediate treatment. Many psychiatric facilities do not have

TABLE 133.4

CHILDHOOD/ADOLESCENT PSYCHIATRIC EMERGENCIES: RELEVANT HISTORY

History of presenting crisis and apparent precipitants
Past episodes or other major psychosocial problems
Psychiatric treatment, past or current, for child or family member
School performance of child
Child's relationships with siblings and peers

the capacity to care for acute medical problems. Such problems must thus be stabilized and/or treated before the patient can be safely transferred to the psychiatric facility. The second aim is to evaluate the patient for possible medical causes of their psychiatric symptoms. Many medical conditions, as well as acute intoxications, can mimic psychiatric disorders (Table 133.5). Failing to diagnose an underlying medical condition may result in significant morbidity to the patient. It is important to note that psychiatrically ill children may also have concomitant medical problems and, in fact, are at greater risk for presenting with emergent medical conditions such as injuries and ingestions than are nonpsychiatrically ill children.

The emergency physician must obtain a thorough medical history of the child, including current medication and possible medicines available to the child, followed by a complete physical examination, including assessment of neurologic functioning. There is no "standard" set of laboratory evaluations that must be obtained to "clear" a psychiatric patient. Many psychiatric patients, particularly those with preexisting psychiatric diagnoses, can be medically cleared by history and physical examination alone. Patients with new onset of or acute change in psychiatric symptoms, especially psychosis or alterations in mental status, must be carefully evaluated for possible underlying medical conditions. These patients frequently require at least some laboratory evaluation. In addition, some inpatient psychiatry facilities require baseline laboratory data before accepting a transfer.

Toxicologic screens and pregnancy tests in women of childbearing age are the most frequently obtained laboratory tests. Table 133.6 lists laboratory evaluations that may be considered for psychiatric patients.

Mental Status of the Child

Evaluation of the child's mental status takes place throughout the entire ED visit. The mental status examination provides a psychological profile of the child at the same time that it assists in determination of a psychiatric diagnosis. Generally, the physician does not need to perform a formal mental status examination of the child because most of the relevant data emerge from history, the physical examination, and the interactions that the child has with family members and with the physician during the emergency assessment. However, the emergency physician should have a systematic and thorough understanding of the mental status examination and should follow up areas of concern with more specific questions. Table 133.7 lists the major categories of the mental status examination. These categories are described as they apply to emergency psychiatric assessment.

Orientation

The level of consciousness and orientation of the child is the first area of assessment. The child not under the influence of drugs or with severe medical illness should be oriented in all spheres: person, place, time, and situation.

Appearance

The physical appearance of the child reveals important information about both the way the child feels about and cares for him- or herself and the supervising care by the family. The examiner

TABLE 133.5

MEDICAL CONDITIONS THAT MAY MANIFEST WITH NEUROPSYCHIATRIC SYMPTOMS

Neurological
Cerebrovascular disorder (hemorrhage, infarction)
Head trauma (concussion, posttraumatic hematoma)
Epilepsy (especially complex partial seizures)
Narcolepsy
Brain neoplasms (primary or metastatic)
Normal-pressure hydrocephalus
Parkinson's disease
Multiple sclerosis
Huntington's disease
Dementia of the Alzheimer's type
Metachromatic leukodystrophy
Migraine

Endocrine
Hypothyroidism
Hyperthyroidism
Hypoadrenalism
Hyperadrenalism
Hypoparathyroidism
Hyperparathyroidism
Hypoglycemia
Hyperglycemia
Diabetes mellitus
Panhypopituitarism
Pheochromocytoma
Gonadotropic hormonal disturbances
Pregnancy

Metabolic and systemic
Fluid and electrolyte disturbances (e.g., syndrome of
  inappropriate antidiuretic hormone secretion)
Hepatic encephalopathy
Uremia
Porphyria
Hepatolenticular degeneration (Wilson's disease)
Hypoxemia (chronic pulmonary disease)
Hypotension
Hypertensive encephalopathy

Toxic
Intoxication or withdrawal associated with drug or
  alcohol abuse
Adverse effects of prescribed and over-the-counter
  medications
Environmental toxins (volatile hydrocarbons, heavy metals,
  carbon monoxide, organophosphates)

Nutritional
Vitamin B_{12} deficiency (pernicious anemia)
Nicotinic acid deficiency (pellagra)
Folate deficiency (megaloblastic anemia)
Thiamine deficiency (Wernicke–Korsakoff syndrome)
Trace metal deficiency (zinc, magnesium)
Nonspecific malnutrition and dehydration

Infectious
AIDS
Neurosyphilis
Viral meningitides and encephalitides (e.g., herpes simplex)
Brain abscess
Viral hepatitis
Infectious mononucleosis
Tuberculosis
Systemic bacterial infections (especially pneumonia)
  and viremia
Streptococcal infections
Pediatric infection-triggered, autoimmune neuropsychiatric
  disorders

Autoimmune
Systemic lupus erythematosus

Neoplastic
Central nervous system primary and metastatic tumors
Endocrine tumors
Pancreatic carcinoma
Paraneoplastic syndromes

AIDS, acquired immunodeficiency syndrome.
From Sadock BJ, Sadock VA, eds. *Kaplan & Sadock's synopsis of psychiatry*. 9th ed. Philadelphia, PA: Lippincott Williams & Wilkins, 2003:2.

TABLE 133.6

SCREENING TESTS FOR MEDICAL ILLNESS

1. Complete blood cell count with differential
2. Complete blood chemistries (including measurements of
   electrolytes, glucose, calcium, and magnesium levels and
   tests of hepatic and renal function)
3. Thyroid function tests
4. Pregnancy test
5. Urinalysis
6. Urine and serum toxicology screen
7. EKG
8. Plasma levels of any drugs being taken, if appropriate
9. Head CT (if clinically indicated)
10. Lumbar puncture (if clinically indicated)

EKG, electrocardiogram; CT, computed tomography.
Adapted from Sadock BJ, Sadock VA, eds. *Kaplan & Sadock's synopsis of psychiatry*. 9th ed. Philadelphia, PA: Lippincott Williams & Wilkins, 2003:24.

TABLE 133.7

CHILDHOOD/ADOLESCENT PSYCHIATRIC
EMERGENCIES: CHILD MENTAL STATUS
EXAMINATION

Orientation
Appearance
Memory
Cognition
Behavior
Relating ability
Speech
Affect
Thought content and process
Insight and judgment
Synthesis of evaluation

should carefully observe factors such as physical size, personal hygiene, choice of clothes, neatness, grooming, posture, and gait.

Memory

The child's memory can be evaluated while listening to the history and through direct questioning. Impairment of memory in a child is a strong indication that his or her emotional and behavioral disturbance may have an underlying medical cause.

Cognition

Intelligence, fund of knowledge, and the ability to think and reason are evaluated while talking with the child. Intelligence and fund of knowledge only need to be categorized as adequate or inadequate for the child's age.

Behavior

The child's behavior can be observed throughout the visit. Activity level may be at the appropriate age level and goal directed, too rapid and random (hyperactive), or too slow and diffuse (psychomotor retarded). The child may appear well focused or may be distractible. Behavioral tendencies are revealed in the child's talking with the examiner and in interactions with various family members. Psychotic youngsters may act in a bizarre, disorganized manner or seem completely disconnected from the world around them. Nonpsychotic children, when aggressive, tend to be more oppositional and defiant than psychotic children. The child's ability to control his or her behavior in response to the examiner's or family's request should be carefully noted.

Relating Ability

The child's capacity to relate to the examiner is a key element in the mental status evaluation. In a sense, the examiner is a window to the outside world, and the degree to which a positive relationship can develop during the assessment suggests the child's current capacity for forming relationships in general. The examiner should be concerned with what occurs at any moment during the evaluation and, even more important, how the interaction evolves during the course of the visit. The following questions should be considered: (i) to what degree does the child offer eye contact and speak spontaneously; (ii) how trusting does the child appear to be and to what degree does the child appear to desire the examiner's approval; and (iii) in contrast, is the child too friendly and open, suggesting extreme neediness? The child's cooperativeness and tendency to alter his or her mood in response to the examiner's encouragement are important components of his or her capacity to relate.

Speech

Speech includes elements such as spontaneity, coherence, articulation, and vocabulary. As such, the category of speech overlaps with the capacity to relate, the quality of thought processes, and the level of intelligence. Rapid speech that is difficult or impossible to interrupt may be a sign of mania or ingestion (e.g., a stimulant). Poor vocabulary and articulation may suggest mental retardation, psychosocial deprivation, specific language disabilities, or combinations of these.

Affect

The child's affect, as the external manifestation of predominant feeling states, is assessed informally during the course of the interview. Fluctuations of affect according to changes in content and interactions should be carefully observed, with more serious concern raised by children whose affect does not change as different subjects are discussed. Depressed children may show both sad and angry affect, which suggests the way in which the child sees both self and the external world. Some angry children express their anger directly, even in the form of rage. Other children become so well defended that their affect appears flat and constricted. Frankly psychotic children, in addition to blunted affect, show an inappropriate response to internal and external events, such as smiling while serious topics are discussed. Manic children may have either an irritable or elated affect.

Thoughts

Thoughts include both thought processes and thought content. The evaluation of the preceding categories necessarily yields much information on thinking. Thought process involves the coherence and goal directedness of verbal communication. Evasiveness and guardedness must be distinguished from the looseness of associations of the psychotic child or adolescent. Loose associations have no logical coherence or connection with previous statements. Flight of ideas, as found in bipolar disorder, involves rapid shifting from one topic to another, often triggered by the patient's ongoing monologue. Thought content involves the major themes that emerge as the child talks spontaneously and responsively to the examiner. If themes of violence and insecurity are evident, are other more hopeful and positive themes also present? Such information can often be obtained by eliciting fantasy material, such as three wishes, personal goals, and views of the future. Self-concept, when low, may become apparent as persistent themes and fantasies are pursued. Thorough screening also involves determining the possible presence of psychotic phenomena (hallucinations, delusions, grandiosity, and ideas of reference) and present or past tendencies toward suicide or homicide.

Insight and Judgment

Insight involves the degree of recognition and acknowledgment of current problems by the child. A child with a high degree of insight can also identify possible precipitating factors. Judgment involves the child's ability to think before acting. Over the course of the interview in the ED, the examiner can assess these elements informally.

Synthesis

After the component parts of the mental status examination have been determined, the physician should integrate them into a comprehensive picture of the child. For example, a 14-year-old boy presents to the ED fully alert and oriented, but disheveled and malnourished. His cognitive abilities appear to be intact, but his actions are slow and labored. The child's thinking shows no evidence of incoherence, but themes of disappointment emerge from the conversation. The boy relates to the physician in a withdrawn manner and appears to be preoccupied. The data from this mental status examination suggest that the adolescent described is depressed. This impression should then be integrated with historical, medical, and family information as the examiner plans appropriate treatment.

Family Evaluation

To assess families, the physician needs to have an organized framework to guide the evaluation process (Table 133.8). The goal of a family evaluation for childhood psychiatric emergencies is to determine the methods that the family uses to help its members when distressed, the adequacy of these efforts, and the possibilities for new alternatives that will help the family cope successfully with the current crisis. In obtaining the history from the family and proceeding with the assessment, the emergency physician should keep in mind these specific aspects of family functioning so that he or she can evaluate the family systematically during the ED visit. When conducting the interview with child and family, the emergency physician is encouraged to remember that, despite the disruption caused by the crisis, families know their child the best. When the physician approaches parents as partners, the likelihood of an effective collaboration between parents and medical staff is maximized.

Family Mental Status

Just as it is important to know the child's mental status, the emergency physician must also determine the mental status of the rest of the family. This task can be accomplished as the physician observes the family members and listens to their presentation of the history. The history should be coherent and logical and should follow a temporal sequence. Families that do not present an organized history may have serious difficulties resolving crises. Family members under the influence of drugs or alcohol may not be fully alert and oriented. Their history may not be clear. Depressed parents appear withdrawn and downcast. They may be so preoccupied with their depression that they do not focus effectively on the child's problem or they may describe the problem in extremely hopeless terms.

Although anxiety, distress, and even anger may be appropriate responses to a psychiatric emergency, parents should be able to use the physician's support to control these responses so that the crisis can be approached systematically. When this

TABLE 133.8

CHILDHOOD/ADOLESCENT PSYCHIATRIC EMERGENCIES: FAMILY ASSESSMENT

Signs of Competence and Strength
Level of concern
Verbal communication
Problem-solving ability

Relationships
Parents and child
Parents or caregivers
Parents and physician

Danger Signs with Parents/Caregivers
Psychosis
Intoxication/drug abuse
Depression
Violence
History of abuse (physical, emotional, sexual) and/or neglect

cooperation does not occur, the emergency physician should consider psychiatric consultation. Other indications for psychiatric consultation include the presence of psychosis or other severe psychiatric disturbance in a parent or caregiver. When the family presents a disorganized history, the physician can indicate that he or she is confused and ask for clarification. The physician can also suggest that only one person talk at a time and can repeat the history given and ask the family to confirm it. When these attempts to provide structure to the family fail, psychiatric consultation is needed.

Conflict Resolution Versus Conflict Avoidance

All families have disagreements among their members. In some families, disagreements are acknowledged and confronted directly, whereas in others, potential conflict is consistently avoided. Other families disagree openly but are unable to reach a constructive resolution. The capacity of the family for conflict resolution is an important area for the emergency physician to assess because unresolved disagreements typically lead to chronic hostility, undermining of relationships, and ineffective parenting.

Families that are unable to resolve conflict often have significant marital problems. The parents, unable to deal effectively with each other, instead become overinvolved with one of the children. The child may have a chronic illness, may be either the oldest or the youngest, or may be chosen for another reason. The child gets caught in the marital struggle of the parents, in part through their efforts and in part through his or her own desire to remain close to the parents and keep them together. This child often develops physical and psychiatric symptoms and may present to the ED with the family.

The emergency physician may observe several possible patterns of conflict avoidance. The parents may agree that the only problem in the family is the child and that, if it were not for him or her, everything would be fine. However, the physician notes that the parents do not look at each other or talk to each other. Their one common ground of agreement is the scapegoated child and his or her symptoms. In a related pattern, the parents suppress all conflict by focusing excessive concern on the symptomatic child, who is seen as vulnerable and weak. This reaction often occurs in families with a child with psychosomatic symptoms, where the child is overprotected and his or her symptoms are typically exacerbated by family conflict. The third pattern involves parental focusing on the child and his or her symptoms as the battleground for overt parental and spousal disagreements. The parents deny the existence of any disagreements except those related to the identified patient, about whom they disagree openly and angrily.

Using Social Support

Some families come to the ED feeling isolated, overwhelmed, and exhausted. Often, such families have not used all the family and community resources available to them. Effective crisis intervention for psychiatric emergencies involves not only emergency treatment but also effective disposition planning for the family. The ED staff should determine what community resources are available, or potentially available, to the family. The parents should be asked about relatives or neighbors who might be able to help them.

AGITATED OR VIOLENT BEHAVIOR AND THE USE OF RESTRAINT

Background

Agitated or violent behavior is a frequent reason that children and adolescents are brought to the ED for evaluation. Such behavior may be especially problematic for the ED physician in that it may interfere with the physician–patient relationship and impair the physician's ability to fully assess and treat the patient. ED physicians may need to rapidly decide on a treatment strategy with little or no input from the patient. Differentiating among the varied possible causes is critical in successfully selecting the least restrictive yet efficacious treatment strategy, while minimizing the potential for adverse effects to the patients.

Clinical Manifestations

Agitation may manifest in a wide variety of behaviors, depending on the patient's age and developmental and physical state. Signs and symptoms may include catatonic withdrawal, restlessness, hyperactive motor activity, confusion or disorientation, uncontrollable crying, verbal threats, and overt physical violence toward oneself, others, or physical property.

It is important to remember that agitated or violent behavior may be situation dependent. Once removed from that situation, the child's or adolescent's behavior may significantly improve. In fact, the behavior may appear to be normal by the time he or she arrives at the ED. It is potentially a grave mistake to equate the lack of significant symptoms in the ED with the absence of a significant problem. The problematic behavior may easily reoccur if the patient is returned to the same situation without any appropriate intervention(s).

Assessment

Agitation or violence is not a diagnosis unto itself. Such behavior is the final common pathway for various psychological, medical, and toxicological disturbances. An agitated or violent patient may be experiencing dysfunction in one or more of these areas. The ED physician's assessment should thus focus on differentiating among the many possible causes.

Paramount in evaluating these patients is assessing their potential for violence, both imminently in the ED and in the future should they be discharged. Table 133.9 lists signs and symptoms commonly used in assessing and predicting violent behavior. Table 133.10 lists other commonly cited predictors of dangerousness to others. Patients should be asked if they currently have any violent or homicidal thoughts. Do they have any specific plans or thoughts on how they would hurt someone? Do they have access to firearms or other weapons? No single sign, symptom, or set of criteria successfully identifies all patients with significant risks for violence. When there is a concern for such violence, prompt psychiatric evaluation should be obtained. Appropriate safety measures should be undertaken in the ED, including searching the patient for weapons or potential

TABLE 133.9

ASSESSING AND PREDICTING VIOLENT BEHAVIOR

Signs of impending violence
  Recent acts of violence, including property violence
  Verbal or physical threats (menacing)
  Carrying weapons or other objects that may be used as weapons (e.g., forks, ashtrays)
  Progressive psychomotor agitation
  Alcohol or other substance intoxication
  Paranoid features in a psychotic patient
  Command violent auditory hallucinations—some but not all patients are at high risk
  Brain diseases, global or with frontal lobe findings; less commonly with temporal lobe findings (controversial)
  Catatonic excitement
  Certain manic episodes
  Certain agitated depressive episodes
    Personality disorders (rage, violence, or impulse dyscontrol)
Assess the risk for violence
  Consider violent ideation, wish, intention, plan, availability of means, implementation of plan, wish for help
  Consider demographics—gender (male), age (15–24), socioeconomic status (low), social supports (few)
  Consider the patient's history—violence, nonviolent antisocial acts, impulse dyscontrol (e.g., gambling, substance abuse, suicide or self-injury, psychosis)
  Consider overt stressors (e.g., marital conflict, real or symbolic loss)

From Sadock BJ, Sadock VA, eds. *Kaplan & Sadock's synopsis of psychiatry.* 9th ed. Philadelphia, PA: Lippincott Williams & Wilkins, 2003.

TABLE 133.10

PREDICTORS OF DANGEROUSNESS TO OTHERS

High degree of intent to harm
Presence of a victim
Frequent and open threats
Concrete plan
Access to instruments of violence
History of loss of control
Chronic anger, hostility, or resentment
Enjoyment in watching or inflicting harm
Lack of compassion
Self-view as victim
Resentful of authority
Childhood brutality or deprivation
Decreased warmth and affection in home
Early loss of parent
Fire setting, bed-wetting, and cruelty to animals
Prior violent acts
Reckless driving

From Sadock BJ, Sadock VA, eds. *Kaplan & Sadock's synopsis of psychiatry.* 9th ed. Philadelphia, PA: Lippincott Williams & Wilkins, 2003.

weapons and placing the patient in a room where he or she does not have access to items that could be used as a weapon and where he or she can be constantly observed by ED or security personnel.

In the rare event that an ED physician is the sole person evaluating and managing a truly homicidal patient, the ED physician has a duty to both warn the potential victim and to take actions to protect the potential victim from harm, that is, by psychiatrically hospitalizing the patient. This duty was established in the landmark case of *Tarasoff versus the University of California* and has withstood numerous court challenges. This duty to warn and protect the potential victim supersedes the physician's duty to maintain patient confidentiality.

Management

Verbal De-escalate

The importance and impact of verbal de-escalation strategies should not be overlooked. Several studies have shown that when hospital staff is trained in verbal restraint techniques, the result is a significant decrease in the need for and use of chemical and physical restraint in the care of psychiatric patients. Ideally, all ED staff participating in the care of psychiatric patients should have training in verbal de-escalation techniques (see Table 133.11). Various verbal de-escalation programs have been described in the psychiatric literature. Some of these programs have developed training manuals, which are readily available for purchase. Other programs offer courses in verbal de-escalation.

All verbal de-escalation techniques share common features. The agitated patient should be approached with a calm, non-

TABLE 133.11

VERBAL DE-ESCALATION/CALMING TECHNIQUES

Clearly introduce yourself
Use simplified language, a soft voice, and slow movements
Explain what will happen in the ED
Reduce environmental stimulation, if possible (less noise or light, fewer people)
Remove access to breakable objects/equipment
Allow room for pacing, if possible
Offer food or drink, which is inherently calming
Reassure child that you are there to keep him or her safe, that this is your job
Listen and empathize (a treatment cornerstone)
Tell child how you plan to honor his or her reasonable requests
Clarify the child's goal and then try to link his or her cooperation to that goal
Find things for the child to control, like choice of drinks
Engage available consultants: security, social work, psychiatry
Offer distracting toys/sensory modalities
Remain engaged; perceived ignoring may encourage escalations
Remember not to take their anger personally

ED, emergency department.
From Hilt RJ, Woodward TA. Agitation treatment for pediatric emergency patients. *J Am Acad Child Adolesc Psychiatry* 2008;47(2): 132–138.

judgmental manner. Asking the patient to verbalize what is on his or her mind and being an empathetic listener may be all that is needed to calm him or her. The simple act of listening can have a powerful effect. The patient should be reassured that the ED staff is there to help and work with the patient. Discussing what the patient can expect (e.g., what will happen while they are in the ED, how long he or she will be there, who will be working on him or her) provides structure, which will reassure the patient and alleviate much of his or her agitation.

Patients should be given as much autonomy as possible. This can be achieved by presenting them with as many reasonable treatment options as possible and allowing them to choose among the options. By promoting the patient's autonomy, patients often feel empowered and, in feeling so, are better able to control themselves. That said, it is equally important to set clear limits with the patient. Setting limits are for the safety of all involved. Limit setting may include discussing what is acceptable and unacceptable behavior and what are the consequences of the patient's behavior. With few exceptions, one should avoid "bargaining" with patients because this often encourages testing of limits. It is imperative that the limits and consequences for patient behavior are discussed and applied in a nonpunitive manner. Feeling threatened or punished may exacerbate a patient's agitation and/or behavior.

Restraints

Physical and chemical restraint may be necessary to contain the patient's violent behavior toward self, others, or medical staff. However, controversy exists regarding in what situations and when restraint is indicated. While the use of restraints can prevent significant and potentially life-threatening violent outbursts and can help an out-of-control patient calm down, restraints can also be physically harmful to the patient and traumatizing to the patient, the family, and the staff who witness it.

It is important to be cognizant that restraint has the potential to harm patients. Adverse reactions to chemical restraint, physical harm and death due to physical restraint, as well as psychological harm [e.g., feelings of shame and/or of being personally violated, frank symptoms of posttraumatic stress disorder (PTSD)] have all been reported. Both the Centers for Medicare & Medicaid Services (CMS) and the Joint Commission for the Accreditation of Healthcare Organizations (JCAHO) mandate that health-care institutions monitor their use of restraints, as well as develop and maintain protocols in which patients are treated in the least restrictive manner possible. ED physicians and staff thus need to be familiar with their institution's restraint policies, practices, and guidelines.

Chemical Restraint. CMS defines chemical restraint as "a medication used to control behavior or to restrict a patient's freedom of movement and not standard treatment for the patient's medical or psychiatric condition." Although such medications are extensively used and there are numerous published studies of their use in the adult ED and psychiatric settings, there is scant literature on their use in pediatric populations. In addition, as is the case with many medications and pediatric populations, these medications have not been approved by the U.S. Food and Drug Administration (FDA) for the purpose of chemical restraint in children and adolescents. Any medication(s) used for chemical restraint is thus an "off-label" use of the medication(s). Although there are published studies of using the oral forms of the newer, atypical antipsychotics in children and adolescents, there are no published studies of the parental forms of these medications used in this population. These limitations aside, it is widely held by experienced psychiatric and pediatric emergency physicians that these medications are both safe and efficacious. Adverse reactions to these medications in the acute setting are rare and usually easily managed should they arise.

Table 133.12 lists medications that are commonly used for chemical restraint and the appropriate initial dose of these medications. When using these medications, it is acceptable to round the dose to the nearest half or whole milligram or the nearest whole pill dose. Alternatively, for patients already on psychiatric medications, their current dose or an increased dose of one of their medications may be appropriate.

The choice of medication(s) for chemical restraint should be based on the level of the patient's agitation or dangerousness. For mild agitation, antihistamines, such as diphenhydramine and hydroxyzine, or benzodiazepines are the first line of treatment. For moderate agitation, possible medications include benzodiazepines, antipsychotics, and atypical antipsychotics. The ED physician should choose between these different agents on the basis of the degree of agitation, the patient's willingness to take oral medications, and the medication side effect profile. The newer, atypical antipsychotics may have fewer adverse effects than traditional antipsychotics [e.g., extrapyramidal symptoms (EPS), dystonic reactions, neurolep-

tic malignant syndrome]. However, their use in the ED may be limited in that ziprasidone and olanzapine are the only atypical antipsychotics that have a parenteral form, and there is only limited experience using these medications in pediatric populations. The rapidly dissolving oral forms of olanzapine and risperidone may be an acceptable alternative to physicians and patients.

For patients with severe agitation, *rapid tranquilization* is the strategy favored by most experts. In this approach, a dose of a benzodiazepine and an antipsychotic are given simultaneously. These medications can be given orally but almost always will need to be given parenterally. If needed, subsequent doses can be given 60 and 120 minutes after the initial dose. This approach is more effective than medication alone and results in the use of less total medication. A variation of this approach is to give a dose of one of these medications and reassess the patient 30 minutes later. If the patient's agitation has not sufficiently resolved, a dose of the other medication is given. The patient is reassessed every 30 minutes and redosed with the appropriate medication if needed.

Both haloperidol and the atypical antipsychotics, ziprasidone to the largest degree, may cause QTc prolongation. As such, patients receiving these medications should be closely monitored. There is no consensus regarding the prophylactic use of benztropine [1 mg oral (PO)/intramuscular (IM)] or other anticholinergic agents in patients receiving antipsychotics. Some experts favor giving such medications to all patients receiving

TABLE 133.12

CHEMICAL RESTRAINT MEDICATIONS

Medication	Initial dose[a]	Onset of action (min)	Half-life, $t_{1/2}$ (h)	Comments/adverse effect
Diphenhydramine	1.25 mg/kg[b] Teen: 50 mg	5–15 (IM/IV) 20–30 (PO)	2–8 2–8	Paradoxical reaction[a]
Hydroxyzine	1.25 mg/kg[b] Teen: 50 mg	5–15 (IM/IV) 20–30 (PO)	7–10 7–10	Paradoxical reaction[a] Paradoxical reaction[a]
Lorazepam	0.05–0.1 mg/kg[b] Teen: 2–4 mg	5–15 (IM/IV) 20–30 (PO)	12 12	Paradoxical reaction[a]; respiratory depression
Midazolam	0.05–0.15 mg/kg[b] Teen: 2–4 mg	5–15 (IM/IV) 20–30 (PO)	3–4 3–6	Paradoxical reaction[a]; respiratory depression
Haloperidol[c]	0.1 mg/kg[b] Teen: 2–5 mg	15–30 (IM) 30–60 (PO)	21 21	EPS/NMS Transient hypotension, may prolong QTc[d]
Risperidone[e,f]	<12 yr: 0.5mg Teen: 1mg	45–60 (PO) 45–60 (PO)	20 20	EPS/NMS may prolong QTc[d]
Olanzapine[e]	<12 yr: 2.5 mg Teen: 5–10 mg	30–60 (IM) 45–60 (PO)	30 30	EPS/NMS may prolong QTc[d]
Quetiapine	25 mg	45–60 (PO)	6	EPS/NMS may prolong QTc[d]
Ziprasidone	<12 yr: 5 mg Teen: 10–20 mg	30–60 (IM) 60 (PO)	2–5 7	EPS/NMS may prolong QTc[d]

IM, intramuscular; IV, intravenous; PO, oral; EPS, extrapyramidal symptoms; NMS, neuroleptic malignant syndrome.
[a]A paradoxical reaction, such as behavioral disinhibition, agitation, hyperexcitability, and insomnia may occur.
[b]Round dose to nearest milligram or half milligram.
[c]Although not U.S. Food and Drug Administration approved, haloperidol lactate has been used IV (with dosage usually approximated at PO dose × 0.625).
[d]Relative risk for QTc prolongation: ziprasidone > quetiapine > risperidone, olanzapine, haloperidol.
[e]Rapidly disintegrating oral tablet available.
[f]Liquid formulation available.

antipsychotics, for the prevention of EPS. Others prefer to use these medications only if and when EPS develop.

Neuroleptic malignant syndrome (NMS) is a rare complication of antipsychotic use. It is more commonly seen in young, muscular males, although it may occur in patients of any age, gender, and body habitus. Preexisting dehydration and chronic antipsychotic use are other risk factors for developing NMS. Because there is no test that absolutely confirms it, NMS can be vexing to diagnose. In addition, the clinical picture of fever, altered mental status, and autonomic hyperactivity may be difficult to differentiate from meningoencephalitis, intracranial injury, various toxins, serotonin syndrome, or an underlying psychiatric condition. It should be strongly considered in any agitated patient whose conditions worsen or do not resolve when given antipsychotic medication.

Two antipsychotics, thioridazine and droperidol, currently carry FDA "black box" warnings against their use because they may cause fatal arrhythmias. Thioridazine has been largely replaced by newer agents with more favorable side effect profiles. Droperidol is a high-potency butyrophenone (typical) antipsychotic that has been widely used in the ED setting for agitated patients. There is a wealth of literature supporting droperidol's efficacy, as well as numerous papers citing its safety. Currently, the safety record of droperidol and the issue of whether the FDA's black box warning is justified remain unresolved and is being hotly debated.

Physical Restraint. Any device that restricts a patient's mobility is a physical restraint. Theoretically, a bed rail is a form of restraint. In the treatment of agitated patients, however, physical restraints specifically refer to devices (e.g., leather restraints) with the express purpose of restraining a patient's limbs. Only such approved devices should be used for physical restraint. "Soft restraints" or other makeshift devices should not be used.

Physical restraints are not without risks. In 1999, the *Hartford Courant* reported that in the previous 10 years in the United States, 142 people had died during or shortly after being physically restrained. A disproportionate number of deaths were in children. In response to these concerns, the JCAHO Board of Commissioners analyzed a number of these cases. They identified several risk factors associated with patient deaths.

Asphyxiation was associated with excess weight being placed on the back of prone patients, a towel or sheet being placed over the patient's head to protect against spitting or biting, and airway obstruction due to placing the patient's arm across the neck area. A minimum of five trained staff are needed to restrain a patient, one to control each limb and one for the patient's head. For extremely violent or agitated patients, the prone position, although more restrictive, is safer for both the patient and the care provider. Physically restrained patients need constant observation by medically trained personnel because the patient may medically decompensate. JCAHO standards were developed in response to the previously mentioned analysis. They mandate documentation of patient's vital signs and observation, assessment of behavioral status, and offering of food, water, and access to bathroom facilities at regular intervals. These standards also mandate a face-to-face evaluation of the patient by the physician ordering the restraint within 1 hour of the patient being placed in restraints. Orders for restraint can

be renewed, but each order cannot exceed 1 hour for children younger than 9 years, 2 hours for children and adolescents between 9 and 17 years, or 4 hours for adults.

Once a patient has calmed down and follows instructions, consideration should be given to removing the restraints. Restraints should be removed in an organized manner, taking into account the severity of the patient's agitation. The same number of personnel needed to place the restraints should be present when the restraints are removed, in case the restraints need to be reapplied. There is no consensus as to the optimal method for removing restraints. Some remove all restraints once the patient is judged to be safe. Others prefer a stepwise approach, releasing an arm first, then the opposite leg, and finally the remaining limbs. Between each step, the patient is informed that if they remain under control, the removal process will continue. Patients should not be left with only one limb restrained. They have too much mobility and could injure themselves or others if they become combative.

SUICIDE ATTEMPTS

Background

Suicidal behavior involves thoughts or actions that may lead to self-inflicted death or serious injury. A distinction is made between suicidal ideation and suicidal attempts in which deliberate attempts to take one's life occurred.

The increasing trend toward suicidal behavior by children and adolescents is alarming. Table 133.13 provides information on the nature and scope of this problem.

TABLE 133.13

CHILDHOOD AND ADOLESCENT SUICIDE: NATURE OF THE PROBLEM

Adolescent Suicide
Now epidemic
44% rise in suicide rate, adolescents ages 15–19 yr, since 1970
4,000 completed adolescent and young adult suicides, 2000
Estimated 400,000 adolescent attempts, 2000 (1:50–1:100 attempts succeed)
Suicide is the third leading cause of death, ages 15–24 yr (after accidents, homicides)

Childhood Suicide
Serious problem
Younger children attempt suicide as a result of depression and/or poor judgment
Increase in attempted and completed suicides, children ages 6 yr and older
Suicide attempts via ingestions (children ages 5–14 yr) five times more common than all forms of meningitis

Additional Data
Girls *attempt* at least three times more often than boys
Boys *succeed* at least two times more often than girls
80% of attempts are pill ingestions
More lethal means—gun, knife, jumping, running into car—more common with boys
Many car "accidents" are not accidents

Suicide can be seen as the final common pathway for various situations in which the child experiences a pervasive sense of helplessness, with a perceived absence of alternative solutions. To the distressed child, suicide appears to be the only solution to his or her problems and also to the family's problems. Most suicide attempts occur in depressed children. Others occur with children experiencing major losses, such as serious illness or death in the family. Still others occur in children with depression in association with problems of impulsivity. A small but significant percentage of suicide attempts occur in psychotic children and adolescents. Table 133.14 outlines the potential sources of adolescent suicide attempts.

A factor that complicates the discussion of suicide in children is their differing conceptions of death at various ages. Up to age 5, death is seen as a reversible process in which the activities of life still occur. From 5 to 9 years, the irreversibility of death is beginning to be understood, but death is personified rather than seen as an independent event. It is not until about age 9 that death is seen as irreversible in the adult sense of being both final and inevitable. Even then, however, the child may imagine his or her own death as being reversible. Under such circumstances, a suicide attempt may have a different meaning than for an adult, where suicide corresponds to a definite end of one's life.

TABLE 133.14

POTENTIAL SOURCES OF ADOLESCENT
SUICIDE ATTEMPTS

Developmental stress—identity crisis
   Dependence/independence
   Accepting disappointments/limitations
   Planning for future
Body changes and self-image
   Physical growth
   Onset of puberty
   Awareness of sexuality/need to look attractive
Peer pressures
   Friendships and competition with peers of same gender
   Dating, romantic involvements, dealing with sexuality
   Rejection by special person or peer group
School pressures
   Academic competition
   Personal need to succeed
   Meeting parental expectations
Family pressures
   Parent–child expectations/problems
   Parental impairment (medical, psychiatric, drug
    or alcohol)
   Parental conflict or divorce
   Financial/job-related crises
Societal influences
   Mobility and social isolation
   Romanticizing of violence and suicide
   Lack of confidence in secure future
Adolescent depression
   Physiologic vulnerability
   Situational stresses
   Homosexuality or other minority sexual identity

TABLE 133.15

CHARACTERISTICS ASSOCIATED WITH CHILDHOOD
AND ADOLESCENT SUICIDE ATTEMPTS

Positive family history
Hopelessness
Low self-esteem
Active desire to die
Depression
Anger/desire for revenge

Clinical Manifestations

In school-aged children, certain risk factors have been identified that distinguish children with suicidal behavior from other children with emotional problems (Table 133.15). Suicidal children are likely to be depressed and hopeless. Self-esteem is low, and they see themselves as worthless. The want to die is present, as are preoccupations with death. The family history may include past episodes of parental depression and suicidal behavior. Suicidal children tend to view death as temporary and pleasant rather than irreversible.

Adolescent suicide attempts are usually not simply impulsive acts. Before the suicide attempt, preceding family problems often have been present. These problems include a parent or close relative attempting suicide, many residential and environmental changes, and unexpected separations from meaningful relationships (divorce, separation, or death). With the onset of adolescence, an escalation phase occurs in which frustration results from the teenager's desire for autonomy and the belief that his or her parents do not understand. The teenager withdraws or rebels, becoming alienated from his or her parents at a time when they are still needed. The scene is then set for the final stage, in which some precipitating event leads to the suicide attempt.

Table 133.16 indicates the high-risk situations for suicidal behavior in which direct questioning about suicide should occur. The first two situations immediately alert the physician to the danger of suicidal behavior. The other situations involve a different chief complaint, masking possible suicidal ideation

TABLE 133.16

CHILDHOOD AND ADOLESCENT SUICIDE: HIGH-RISK
SITUATIONS FOR SUICIDE ATTEMPTS

Suicide attempt just made
Suicidal threat made
"Accidental" ingestion
Child complains of depression
Psychotic child
Significant withdrawal by child
History of aggressive or violent behavior
History of substance abuse
History of previous suicide attempt(s)
Medical concerns, but child appears depressed
Highly lethal method of suicide attempt
Availability of or access to firearms

TABLE 133.17

ASSESSING CHILDHOOD/ADOLESCENT SUICIDE
ATTEMPTS: FOUR MAJOR DIMENSIONS

Medical lethality
Suicidal intent
Impulsivity
Strengths/supports

or behavior. All accidental ingestions should be screened for
the possibility of a suicide attempt. Overtly depressed children
are at risk for suicide, as are depressed children who present
with somatic complaints. Children who have acted violently
are also at risk because violence can be turned inward.
Psychotic children present a special problem and may present
with inadvertent suicide attempts as the result of impaired
judgment, hallucinations, and delusions of persecution. The
isolated, withdrawn child may harbor suicidal thoughts that
are uncovered only by direct questioning.

Assessment

The emergency physician should specifically ask about suicidal
thinking in all high-risk children. The dichotomy sometimes
drawn between suicide "attempts" and suicide "gestures" is ill
conceived. All suicidal behavior should be regarded as suicide
attempts, which are best evaluated by appreciating the medical
lethality of the act, the suicidal intent of the child, the impulsivity of the act, and the strengths and supports within the
family (Table 133.17). The lethality of a suicide attempt by
itself may be misleading because suicidal children may miscal-
culate, causing at times more harm than was intended and at
other times less harm than was intended. As an example, the
child who takes 10 tablets of his mother's tricyclic antidepressant (TCA) medication could make a fatal miscalculation
because TCAs can cause fatal arrhythmias in children. In contrast, a child who takes 10 aspirins may be far more suicidal
than the lethality of his or her ingestion would suggest. In general, more violent methods of attempted suicide (e.g., hanging,
shooting, jumping) usually reflect greater suicidal intent (Table
133.18). However, the physician cannot conclude that
attempts with low lethality are not serious attempts until he or

TABLE 133.18

CHILD AND ADOLESCENT SUICIDE: ASSESSING
MEDICAL LETHALITY

Vital signs
Level of consciousness
Evidence of drug/alcohol intoxication (e.g., pupils, smell
    on breath)
Need for emesis, lavage, or catharsis
Acute medical complications (cardiac, respiratory, renal,
    neurologic)
Indications for medical hospitalization, including
    intensive care
Residual abnormalities

TABLE 133.19

CHILDHOOD AND ADOLESCENT SUICIDE:
ASSESSING SUICIDE INTENT

Circumstances of Suicide Attempt
Nature of suicide attempt (e.g. ingestion vs. violent means)
Use of multiple methods
Method used to extreme (all vs. some pills ingested)
Suicide note written
Secrecy of attempt (attempt concealed vs. revealed)
Premeditation (long planned vs. impulsive attempt)
History of prior attempts

Child Self-report
Premeditation of attempt
Anticipation of death
Desire for death
Attempt to conceal attempt
Nature of precipitating stresses

Child's Mental Status
Orientation/cognitive intactness
Presence/absence of psychosis
Manner of relating to physician
Current suicidality
    Response to being saved/being unsuccessful in attempt
    Active plan for another attempt
    Readiness to discuss stresses
    Readiness to accept external and family support
Nature of orientation toward future

she has specifically asked about and assessed the child's suicidal intent, that is, just how seriously the child wanted to end
his or her life (Table 133.19). These questions should be asked
of the child without the parents in the room.

In addition to asking directly about suicidal intent ("When
you took those pills, what did you think would happen? What
did you hope would happen?"), the physician should gather as
much information as possible about the attempt itself to help
infer the degree of suicidal intent on the part of the child. Did
the child take all the pills that were available? Did he or she
expect to wake up? Did he or she tell anyone after taking the
pills? Did he or she leave a suicide note? Now that he or she is
awake, is the child pleased or displeased to be alive? Does he
or she intend to try again?

Children who threaten suicide without making an actual
attempt should also be questioned carefully about suicidal
intent. How long has the child considered suicide; what methods
are planned; when will this take place? Has the child ever made
previous attempts? How about other family members? Psychotic
and depressed children, especially when the parents appear
unable to supervise the child, should elicit particular concern.

Assessment of the child's level of impulsivity is also important (Table 133.20). Does the attempt appear to have been
impulsive rather than planned? Is there a history of prior
impulsive behaviors? Is there evidence of impulsivity during
the ED interview?

The physician should ask the child and family about possible precipitating events to determine what changes in the environment may be needed. The strengths of the family should be
assessed to determine whether sufficient social support exists
to allow for outpatient management (Table 133.21).

TABLE 133.20

CHILDHOOD AND ADOLESCENT SUICIDE: ASSESSING IMPULSIVITY

Evidence of impulsive suicide attempt
History of prior impulsive behaviors
Evidence of impulsivity during interview

Management

Evaluation for Hospitalization

No universally agreed-on criteria have been established for when to hospitalize a child with suicidal behavior and when to manage him or her on an outpatient basis. Garfinkel and Golombek identified seven areas to assess to determine whether hospitalization is indicated (Table 133.22).

Social set involves the degree of privacy that the child arranged at the time of the attempt. Did he or she tell anyone before or after the attempt, or were pains taken to set up a situation in which detection was unlikely? Intent may be reflected in a suicide note left by the child, by the degree of detail of the suicide plans, and by direct questioning of the child regarding his or her suicidal intent at the time of the attempt and at the time of examination. The choice of method also helps in the assessment of the suicide attempter. Was a method with high lethality used or desired? Did the child understand the likely outcome of the method used? The history reveals both the presence of past suicide attempts by the child and past attempts by other family members. The evaluation of the stressful precipitating events is important in planning disposition, as is the mental status of the child at present and in comparison with the past. Finally, the degree of support expected from within the family and outside the immediate family (extended family, neighbors, peers, and teachers) must

TABLE 133.21

CHILDHOOD AND ADOLESCENT SUICIDE: ASSESSING STRENGTHS AND SUPPORTS

Strengths and Assets of Child
Ability to relate to physician
Ability to rely on parents in crisis
Ability to acknowledge problem
Positive orientation toward future

Strengths and Assets of Family
Commitment to child
Ability to unite during crisis
Problem-solving abilities
Capacity to supervise child (support *and* limits)
Ability to use external supports

Nature of External Supports
Outpatient psychiatrist/family physician
Extended family
Neighbors/other significant adults
Religious community
Self-help groups

TABLE 133.22

AREAS TO ASSESS FOLLOWING A SUICIDE ATTEMPT

Social set
Intent
Method
History
Stress
Mental status
Support

be assessed. To what degree can the family unconditionally commit itself to support the child's safety and well-being? Are there resources present for the family and larger network to implement this commitment? The decision to hospitalize the child is made when the child's safety is still in doubt after these questions have been answered.

In general, any suicide attempt deserves a thorough assessment by the emergency physician and a complete psychiatric consultation. Hospitalization should be used in the circumstances listed in Table 133.23. These are as follows: (i) the physician has had difficulty in gaining the cooperation of the child and the family, (ii) the child has made a serious suicide attempt, (iii) the child is continuing to be actively suicidal, (iv) the child is unwilling/unable to provide a no-suicide commitment to the parents, (v) the child is psychotic, (vi) the family appears unable to provide necessary supervision and support to the child, and (vii) the child and family deny the significance of a serious suicide attempt.

Initiating Treatment

The critical goal in dealing with suicidal behavior in a child is to create a context for living—an immediate response to the crisis that increases the likelihood that the child remains alive. The emergency physician creates a context for living through his or her thorough assessment of child and family, the eventual disposition, and the encouragement of family and child to increase communication and develop alternative solutions to problems that have arisen.

Parents should be encouraged to tell the child that they want him or her to live and that suicidal behavior is forbidden. Parents can be tender in expressing their love for the child, but they need to be firm in establishing the rule that self-destructive

TABLE 133.23

INDICATIONS FOR PSYCHIATRIC HOSPITALIZATION FOLLOWING CHILDHOOD/ADOLESCENT SUICIDE ATTEMPT

1. Failure of rapport among physician, child, and family
2. Serious suicide attempt (lethality and intent)
3. Continuing active suicidality
4. Inability to provide no suicide commitment to parents
5. Psychosis of child
6. Divisive/disturbed family, incapable of support and supervision
7. Denial of significance of suicide attempt

behavior is an unacceptable response to problems. The child should also be told that he or she has a responsibility to him- or herself and the family to keep him- or herself alive. The emergency physician may need to remind tentative parents that, regardless of whether hospitalization is used, they still have primary responsibility for their child.

A critical moment occurs when the parents, guided by the emergency physician, ask the child to make a no-suicide commitment, also known as a *safety contract*. This commitment signifies the child's promise to the parents that he or she will not try to harm him- or herself again, no matter how upset he or she is. Instead, the child will seek out the parents or another responsible adult for assistance. The emergency physician should recognize the common tendency toward denial by the child in the ED after the actual suicide attempt. As a result of this denial, or in an effort to simply appease the parents, the child may make an insincere no-suicide commitment. Therefore, when this commitment is being made, parents and child should discuss it carefully and thoughtfully, so that the parents and ED physician can determine the real intentions of the child and convey the urgency of the no-suicide commitment. While there are no well-controlled studies to support to contention that a no-suicide commitment is protective against future suicidal or self-injurious acts, it can still be diagnostically and therapeutically useful to discuss this concept. When a child and his or her parents are able to agree on a contract for safety, it can help foster a sense of collaborative problem solving and open communication. Alternatively, if an earnest contract for safety cannot be established, this failure alone is often sufficient indication for inpatient admission.

If inpatient treatment is required, the child and family should be informed about how the hospital operates and what to expect. The goals of the hospitalization should be discussed and the active role of the family in the treatment emphasized. In many states, voluntary consent forms need to be signed. In instances in which the child or parents do not agree to hospitalization, involuntary commitment may need to be used, although every effort should be made to enlist the concurrence of the parents first. When possible, the child and family should be accompanied to the psychiatric hospital by the consultant psychiatrist or an involved social worker so that the transition to the psychiatric facility is made smoother.

Outpatient management of suicidal behavior becomes feasible when (i) the child and family are cooperative and engageable,

TABLE 133.24

PREVENTION OF CHILDHOOD AND ADOLESCENT SUICIDE: GUIDELINES FOR PARENTS

Understand nature of parent–child dilemma during adolescence
Maintain physical contact—be around, combat tendency toward isolation
Maintain emotional contact—stay involved, show positive regard
Listen to child before responding—promote safety in talking
Respond to child once child has finished—take child seriously, do not dismiss or attack
Encourage choices by adolescent
Acknowledge child and provide respect

TABLE 133.25

PREVENTION OF CHILDHOOD AND ADOLESCENT SUICIDE: WARNING SIGNS FOR PARENTS

Withdrawal (peers, parents, siblings)
Somatic complaints
Irritability
Crying
Diminished school performance
Sad or anxious appearance
Significant loss (rejection by peer group, breakup of romance, poor grades, failure to achieve important goal)
Major event or change within family
Casual mention of suicide or being "better off dead"
Explicit suicide threat
Minor, seemingly unimportant suicide "gestures"
Apparent "accidents"
Other unusual behavior pattern—housebound behavior, breaking curfew, running away, drug or alcohol abuse, bizarre or antisocial actions

(ii) the attempt is determined not to have been too serious in terms of intent and medical lethality, (iii) the child is not actively suicidal or psychotic at the time of the evaluation, (iv) the child provides an earnest no-suicide commitment, and (v) the family can take responsibility for the child until formal psychiatric treatment is begun the next work day and appears capable of managing the child within the home setting as mental health treatment is provided. Before sending a family home, the psychiatrist or emergency physician should have the family formulate a concrete plan concerning how it will manage the child. The expectations and responsibilities of each family member, including the suicidal child, should be spelled out.

Outpatient psychotherapy can begin immediately with emergencies that occur during the workday. When outpatient treatment cannot begin until the next day, the physician should give the family a therapist's name or the name of the "intake person" at the mental health agency. This information personalizes the agency and increases the chances that the family will follow through. The family should be instructed to use the physician's name as the source of referral and should be reassured that the physician will contact the agency before the family's call. At least one parent and the child, if an adolescent, should be asked to sign a release of confidentiality to authorize communication between the physician and the mental health agency. This release also enables the agency or the psychiatrist to contact the family if the family fails to follow through in making an appointment to be seen. Any discussion of suicide must contain careful consideration of prevention. Parents should be given guidelines for the prevention of suicide (Table 133.24) and instruction in the early warning signs (Table 133.25).

DEPRESSION

Background

Depression can refer to the symptom of feeling sad, but most appropriately, it describes a symptom complex or syndrome that includes cognitive and physiologic components in addition to mood symptoms. Depression involves a pervasive inflexibility of sad mood, accompanied frequently by self-deprecation and suicidal ideation. Depression also implies a change in functioning from an earlier state of relatively good adjustment, rather than a temperamental or personality type. The depressed child typically experiences a profound sense of helplessness, feeling unable to improve an unsatisfactory situation.

Data on the incidence of depression in children and adolescents vary. In one suburban Boston study of high school students who were aged 11 to 15 years, 33% of these early adolescents were believed to have moderate to severe symptoms of depression. Other estimates put the incidence of depression in children and adolescents in the 20% range. The incidence of depression is higher in children with school problems (including learning disabilities and attention-deficit/hyperactivity disorder (ADHD)) and in children with significant medical problems. Because most children with depression come to the ED with another chief complaint (e.g., somatic symptoms, school problems, behavior problems), the physician must keep in mind the possibility of depression in all children seen with recurrent or vague somatic complaints.

Considerable evidence suggests that a genetic predisposition exists for depression, particularly severe depression. Depressive episodes may be triggered by environmental events of significance to the child.

Clinical Manifestations

Depression appears differently at different stages of development. In infancy, depression is usually the result of loss of mother and/or lack of nurturance and is seen as a global interference of normal growth and physiologic functioning. Thus, some of the manifestations of depression in infancy include apathy and listlessness, staring, hypoactivity, poor feeding and weight loss, and increased susceptibility to infection.

In school-aged children, depression can appear as part of a syndrome or may be masked by other symptoms. Petti described the two key features in childhood depression as dysphoric mood and self-deprecatory ideation. Dysphoric mood is manifested by looking or feeling sad and forlorn, being moody and irritable, and crying easily. Self-deprecatory thoughts are reflected by low self-esteem, feelings of worthlessness, and suicidal ideation. Depression in this age can also appear as other common symptoms, including irritability, multiple somatic complaints, school avoidance or underachievement (including learning disabled children or children with ADHD), angry outbursts, runaway behavior, phobias, and fire setting.

Depression during adolescence is more similar to adult-onset depression. The major symptom is a sad, unhappy or irritable mood, and/or a pervasive loss of interest and pleasure. Other symptoms may include a change in appetite, change in a sleep behavior, and psychomotor retardation or agitation. Also present in many depressed teenagers are loss of energy, feelings of worthlessness or excessive guilt, decreased ability to concentrate, indecisiveness, and recurrent thoughts of death or suicide. Depressed teenagers can also present with somatic complaints, academic problems, promiscuity, drug or alcohol use, aggressive behavior, and stealing. Many teenagers with behaviors such as these are unaware of their depression

because it is not on the surface. Others simply deny the painful depressive affect. In talking with these patients about their lives at home, at school, and with peers, the underlying depression usually becomes apparent.

As with all children presenting with psychiatric symptoms, especially those that are acute in onset or significantly changed in severity or character, a medical evaluation in indicated to rule out potential medical causes of their symptoms or concurrent medical illness, to assess for physical or laboratory signs of self-injurious/suicidal behaviors and, when indicated, to screen to side effects of prescribed medications (e.g., renal dysfunction in a child on lithium). See Table 133.5 and the section on medical history and physical examination for additional information.

Management

The three major goals in the management of depression involve (i) determining suicidal potential, (ii) uncovering acute precipitants, and (iii) making an appropriate disposition.

The emergency treatment of depression can usefully be thought of as the prevention of suicide attempts. The task of the physician is to carefully determine whether any suicide attempts have been made and whether suicidal ideation is present. The physician should not be hesitant to ask the child about suicidal deeds, thoughts, or wishes. Such questions represent a positive confrontation of the problem of depression and are unlikely to catalyze a subsequent suicide attempt. In fact, questions about suicide may actually provide a sense of relief for the depressed child.

The physician should attempt to determine possible acute precipitants of the current depression to guide subsequent recommendations. The duration of the depression should be determined, as well as the family response. Assessing overall adjustment at home, in school, and with peers is important, as well as looking for the strengths of child and family for use in the treatment plan.

When suicidal ideation is present, the emergency physician should request psychiatric consultation. A decision can then be jointly made regarding outpatient or inpatient treatment. Whether suicide is an imminent danger, the task of the physician is to create a sense of hope that things will improve. To achieve this goal, the physician must form a solid doctor–patient relationship with child and family. Outpatient management can be used when adequate social support is present. The parents must first acknowledge the existence of depression in the child and then come to understand that the solution involves a strong commitment on their part, including, at times, their participation in family therapy.

Although fluoxetine is the only psychotropic medication approved by the FDA for depression management in children and adolescents, it and other medications are commonly being used in the treatment of childhood and adolescent depression. As an acute intervention, however, the emergency physician should not prescribe antidepressant medication because its desired mood-elevating effects generally require up to 1 month to take effect, and the act of prescribing medication in the ED may decrease the likelihood of successful referral for follow-up mental health treatment.

The emergency physician should be familiar with commonly used antidepressants, which are used in the treatment of depression. In more recent years, the selective serotonin reuptake inhibitors (SSRIs) have displaced TCAs as first-line medications. Advantages of SSRIs over TCAs include a decreased likelihood of cardiotoxicity, the absence of anticholinergic side effects, and the relative safety of these medications when used in overdose. Another commonly prescribed antidepressant is bupropion, which is chemically distinct from other agents and primarily acts on the dopaminergic system. A side effect of potential concern with bupropion involves seizures. Newer mixed mechanism agents such as duloxetine, venlafaxine, and mirtazapine are also being used in children and adolescents.

Currently, a hotly debated topic is the safety of antidepressants in the treatment of adolescents. In 2003, the British counterpart of the FDA banned the use of SSRIs in children and adolescents, citing cases where patients' symptoms, including suicidality, worsened while on these medications. In December 2004, the FDA mandated a "Black Box" warning label on all antidepressants. The labels warn about possible increase risk of suicidality with these drugs and about the need to monitor patients for the worsening of depression and the emergence of suicidal ideation. The FDA has not yet taken a position on whether antidepressants cause the emergence of suicidal thinking and behavior. The agency advises that children and adolescents on antidepressants should be closely monitored, particularly after starting or increasing the dose of medication.

PSYCHOSIS

Background

Psychosis is the term used to describe severe disturbances in a patient's mental functioning. It is manifested by significant aberrations in cognition, perception, mood, impulses, and reality testing. Behavior may also become extremely agitated and potentially violent or excessively withdrawn to the point where the patient does not recognize and attend to his or her physical needs. Psychotic patients are actively attempting to regain control over their mental capacities and are trying to understand and deal with highly unusual thoughts, perceptions, and impulses. Their subjective experience is often one of helplessness and extreme anxiety.

Psychosis in children and adolescents can be divided into two groups based on cause: medically based psychosis and psychiatrically based psychosis. Psychiatrically based psychosis in children and adolescents has three major causes: (i) adult-type schizophrenia with onset in adolescence, (ii) brief psychotic episode, and (iii) bipolar or depressive illness with onset in late childhood or adolescence. Emergency management of psychosis due to a medical condition and the three major types of psychiatrically based psychosis are described in the following sections.

Misdiagnosing children and adolescents with psychosis is a significant problem. Werry and Thomsen each described groups of patients initially diagnosed as psychotic, who ultimately were found to have bipolar disorder and personality disorders. In addition, there are numerous case reports of patients with medical causes of their symptoms, who suffered morbidity because of inaccurate diagnosis and inappropriate treatment. Developmental and cultural factors contribute to the difficulty in accurately diagnosing psychosis. Hallucinations can be seen in various normal developmental conditions and may be difficult to differentiate from those of true psychosis. In addition, cultural and religious beliefs, taken out of context or inadvertent clinician biases, may be misconstrued as psychotic symptoms. For these reasons, patients with new onset of or sudden change in psychotic symptoms need to be carefully evaluated for underlying medical conditions and thoroughly evaluated by a psychiatrist.

Psychosis due to a Medical Condition

Differentiation of psychosis secondary to a medical condition as a separate class does not imply that psychiatrically based psychosis is completely independent of brain processes. On the contrary, all psychosis is assumed to be associated with aberrant brain function. The term *psychosis due to a medical condition* merely implies that the cause of the aberrations in mental functioning is known, and resolution of the psychosis depends on improvement in the underlying medical problem(s). Psychiatrically based psychoses, in contrast, are those in which specific medical causes have not yet been determined (Table 133.26). The causes of medically based psychoses can be acute or chronic illnesses, trauma, or intoxications with an exogenous substance (Tables 133.27 through 133.29).

Clinical Manifestations

The child or adolescent with psychosis due to a medical condition often presents to the ED in an agitated and confused state. The child's orientation to time and place is often disturbed, and he or she may be highly distractible, with significant disturbance of recent memory. Evidence of bizarre and distorted thoughts is apparent, and disconnected ideas may be juxtaposed. The child may also have significant difficulty controlling behavior and may persist in activities without regard for personal safety. The child may get up to leave the room without saying where he or she is going or why he or she needs to leave. Intellectual functioning may also be impaired, and the child may be unable to concentrate on simple reading or arithmetic tasks.

The child with psychosis due to a medical condition may experience visual hallucinations, which may be frightening in nature. Tactile hallucinations may be present. Auditory hallucinations, more common in psychiatric illness, are less common in medically based psychoses. As a result of impaired reality testing, children and adolescents with psychosis due to a medical condition are often extremely difficult to control and may strike out at family or staff when attempts are made to control their behavior.

An accurate and thorough history is essential in the evaluation of any child or adolescent for psychosis and is also helpful in appreciating its underlying cause. A complete medical history helps determine whether the psychosis is a concomitant feature of an already existing chronic illness (e.g., lupus cerebritis), a result of medication prescribed to treat an ongoing disease (e.g., steroids for lupus erythematosus), or a result of drug ingestion (e.g., amphetamine psychosis). Typically, an acute intoxication or drug ingestion causes the acute onset of psychosis and represents an abrupt change from the child's previous psychological functioning. The possibility of alcohol use must also be considered in the cause of psychosis, and the

TABLE 133.26

MEDICALLY VERSUS PSYCHIATRICALLY BASED PSYCHOSIS: MAJOR DIFFERENTIATING FEATURES

Assessment feature	Medically based psychosis	Psychiatrically based psychosis
History		
Nature of onset	Acute	Insidious
Preillness history	Prior illness/drug use	Prior psychiatric history (self or family)
Medical Evaluation		
Vital signs	May be impaired	Usually normal
Level of consciousness	May be impaired	Normal
Pathologic autonomic signs	May be present	Normal
Laboratory studies	May be abnormal	Normal
Mental Status Evaluation		
Orientation	May be impaired	Intact
Recent memory	May be impaired	Intact
Cognitive/intellectual functioning	May be impaired	Intact
Nature of hallucinations	Usually not auditory (e.g., visual, tactile)	Auditory
Response to support and medication	Often dramatic	Often limited

history should explore the possibility of trauma. No specific features of the mental status examination differentiate the various causes of psychosis.

The physical examination is often extremely helpful in both differentiating medically based from psychiatrically based psychosis and determining the underlying cause of an acute psychosis. Fever is likely to be present in infections, and tachycardia is often associated with chronic illness or intoxication. The general physical examination gives indications of pulmonary, cardiac, liver, or autoimmune disease, and the neurologic examination assists in the diagnosis of central nervous system (CNS) disease. Abnormalities of reflexes or of motor, sensory, or coordination systems always require complete neurologic evaluation. Signs of increased intracranial pressure may be indicative of a cerebral vascular accident, CNS tumor, or cerebral edema. Signs of autonomic dysfunction, such as pupillary abnormalities, are often indicative of acute intoxication.

In instances of suspected psychosis due to a medical condition, laboratory evaluation should include a complete blood cell count, urinalysis, serum electrolytes, calcium, blood urea nitrogen, blood glucose, and complete drug and alcohol screens. Serum and urine should be obtained for toxicology screening. Other laboratory and radiologic studies depend on abnormalities noted in the history and physical examination. If CNS disease is suspected, CNS imaging studies and a lumbar

TABLE 133.27

CAUSES OF MEDICALLY BASED PSYCHOSIS

Medical conditions (acute and chronic)
Trauma (acute and chronic)
Prescribed medications (toxicity/side effects/withdrawal)
Drug intoxications
    Accidental, including misuse of proprietary medication
    Drug abuse/experimentation
    Alcohol abuse (alone or with drugs)
    Deliberate suicide attempt

TABLE 133.28

MEDICAL CONDITIONS THAT MAY LEAD TO PSYCHOSIS

Central Nervous System Lesions
Tumors
Brain abscess
Cerebral hemorrhage
Meningitis or encephalitis
Temporal lobe epilepsy

Cerebral Hypoxia
Pulmonary insufficiency
Severe anemia
Cardiac failure
Carbon monoxide poisoning

Metabolic and Endocrine Disorders
Electrolyte imbalance
Hypoglycemia
Hypocalcemia
Thyroid disease (hyper and hypo)
Adrenal disease (hyper and hypo)
Uremia
Hepatic failure
Diabetes mellitus
Porphyria

Rheumatic Diseases
Systemic lupus erythematosus
Polyarteritis nodosa

Infections
Malaria
Typhoid fever
Subacute bacterial endocarditis

Miscellaneous Conditions
Wilson's disease
Reye's syndrome

EXOGENOUS SUBSTANCES THAT CAUSE PSYCHOSIS
FOLLOWING INGESTION OF SIGNIFICANT
QUANTITY

Alcohol
Barbiturates
Antipsychotics (e.g., phenothiazines)
Amphetamines
Hallucinogens—Lysergic acid diethylamide (LSD) peyote,
    mescaline
Marijuana
Phencyclidine (PCP)
Quaalude
Anticholinergic compounds
Heavy metals
Cocaine and crack
Corticosteroids
Reserpine
Opiates (e.g., heroin, methadone)

puncture may be necessary. Liver function studies, thyroid
studies, and other specialized and specific laboratory tests may
be obtained as required.

Brief Psychotic Episode

Brief psychotic episode, a relatively uncommon psychiatrically
based psychosis, involves a time-limited loss of reality, caused
by the accumulated effects of externally imposed traumatic
events. Although vulnerability may vary from child to child,
children and teenagers can develop acute psychotic symptoms
in response to trauma. The diagnosis of reactive psychosis can
be made partly by history, but only after a complete medical
and psychiatric evaluation has eliminated medically based and
other psychiatrically based psychoses. The acuteness of the
clinical presentation and its precipitating events differentiates
brief psychotic episode from PTSD.

Clinical Manifestations

The clinical picture of brief psychotic episode varies, in some
instances resembling schizophrenia and in others a less-defined
disorganized state characterized by loss of contact with reality,
panic, and specific hallucinations (usually auditory or visual).

Different traumatic experiences, including physical or sexual abuse, rape, homelessness, and running away, may elicit a
reactive psychosis. All such situations impose stress on the
child and may also disrupt usual patterns of living. Confronted
with a new environment and a new reality, the child's familiar
cues are absent and confusion or frank psychosis may occur.

Schizophrenia

Schizophrenia often has its onset in adolescence and occurs in
approximately 0.5% of the population. This disorder is
equally common in male and female patients, although the age
of first diagnosis tends to be earlier in male patients. It is more
prevalent among family members of known individuals with
the disease.

ACUTE SCHIZOPHRENIA IN ADOLESCENCE:
MOST COMMON FEATURES

Flat affect
(Patient uninvolved and without emotion)
Auditory hallucinations
(Physician: "Have you been hearing voices even when no one
    is there?")
Thoughts spoken aloud
(Physician: "Can other people read your mind? Can you read
    their minds?")
Delusions of external control
(Physician: "Is anyone trying to kill you? . . . trying to control
    your mind or your body?")

Clinical Manifestations

Symptoms of schizophrenia involve impairment of basic psychological processes, including perception, thinking, affect,
capacity to relate, and behavior (Table 133.30). Impaired
thought content includes delusions (strongly held beliefs
involving the self with no basis in reality), such as delusions of
persecution and external control. For example, an adolescent
with schizophrenia may think that others can read and insert
thoughts into his or her mind. Significantly illogical thinking
occurs. Speech is often characterized by loose associations, in
which ideas shift from one subject to another entirely unrelated subject without the speaker recognizing that the topics
are not connected. Auditory hallucinations are common and
may include direct commands for suicide or violence to others.
Typically, but not always, the voices talk to the patient in the
third person, with a highly critical and demeaning message.
Affect may be blunted and flat or inappropriate and bizarre.
Sudden and unpredictable changes in mood may occur. These
teenagers may appear extremely agitated or may be withdrawn, speaking only in monosyllables and describing only
concrete objects. Schizophrenic patients typically have significant distortions of their identity and their abilities and demonstrate behavior that is not goal directed.

The history often reveals a prodromal phase that includes
social withdrawal, peculiar behavior, failure to look after one's
appearance, and significant reduction in performance in
school or work. This phase is followed by an acute phase in
which the previously described symptoms develop, sometimes
as a result of an acutely stressful event. The overall course of
schizophrenia is often chronic and associated with remissions
and exacerbations. Exacerbations often occur when treatment,
including medication, is suspended. However, other individuals experience a schizophrenic-like acute psychosis and recover
completely with appropriate treatment, experiencing no further deterioration.

Management

Psychosis due to a Medical Condition

Management of these children and adolescents involve several
steps (Table 133.31). First and foremost is diagnosing the
underlying cause. Medical treatment is then pursued as

TABLE 133.31

GUIDELINES FOR MANAGEMENT OF ACUTE
ADOLESCENT PSYCHOSIS

Diagnose underlying cause.
Request immediate psychiatric consultation.
Use medical hospitalization, if clinically indicated, with
  medically based psychosis.
Request psychiatric consultation with psychotic drug
  intoxications, either immediately or when mental
  status stabilizes.
Use quiet room, family and friends, and constant medical
  supervision.
Use restraints, if necessary.
Recognize clinical variations of extrapyramidal reactions to
  antipsychotic medications.

indicated for the specific medical condition. Any child with
psychosis in which underlying medical condition is suspected
should be admitted to a medical inpatient unit for diagnostic
evaluation and treatment. This treatment is especially important because psychosis may be a transitory condition in a child
or adolescent whose illness or intoxication is progressive and
life-threatening.

Other important components of the management of a
psychotic child involve controlling the child's behavior, preventing injury to him- or herself or others, and alleviating
the child's fear and anxiety. This goal should be attempted
first through supportive statements indicating the physician's appreciation of the child's condition and his or her
distress. Specific instructions to the child (e.g., "Try to relax
and look at your mother") may also be effective. Often, such
interventions calm the child, but because the child is distractible and anxious, instructions may need to be repeated
frequently.

Brief Psychotic Episode

The emergency physician should appreciate that most children
who present with brief psychotic episode do not have a permanent psychiatric disorder. The emergency management is similar
to that of other psychotic states. Physical and emotional protection of the child is the first priority. The child should be given
support and time to reconstitute. Efforts to avoid antipsychotic
medication should be made in the beginning, but, when necessary, low-dose antipsychotic medication can be used. When the
parents or other caregivers are not implicated in the traumatic
events, emergency staff members should encourage their active
involvement with the child. When the parents are implicated in
the trauma or when the facts are unclear, immediate investigation should take place and contact made with appropriate child
protection authorities, if indicated.

After emergency treatment, the prognosis of the child
depends in large measure on the restoration—or creation—of
a safe and dependable family support system. Referral for outpatient family therapy should be made unless the child
requires psychiatric hospitalization for further evaluation or
treatment. In the absence of adequate family support, some of
these children may eventually require foster placement, residential treatment, or other placements.

Schizophrenia

The management of an acute schizophrenic episode should
always take place in collaboration with psychiatric consultation. Patients with suicidal or homicidal ideation should
receive psychiatric hospitalization. Psychotic patients from
disorganized home environments should also be hospitalized
for initial treatment. In general, the approach to the psychotic
patient in the ED depends on the condition of the patient and
the anticipated site of the ongoing treatment. For agitation and
dangerous thoughts or behaviors, approaches include reassurance and a quiet setting, psychotropic medication, and/or
physical restraint. Antipsychotic medication is discussed in the
next paragraph. The patient's vital signs, general condition,
and possible side effects should be monitored frequently. If the
patient does not respond to medication, inpatient psychiatric
hospitalization is necessary. If significant improvement occurs,
suicidality and homicidality are absent, and side effects do not
occur, the patient can be considered for discharge to outpatient
psychiatric treatment with careful follow up, as long as the
parents or caregivers are well organized, appreciate the child's
condition, and feel capable of managing the child at home.

Commonly used antipsychotic medications, their trade names,
relative potency, and usual dosage ranges are listed in Table
133.32. Long-standing antipsychotic medications, now referred
to as *typical antipsychotics*, exert their influence primarily on
dopaminergic neurons. A new class of antipsychotic medications,
called *atypical antipsychotics*, has emerged. These medications
affect multiple neurotransmitter systems, most frequently
dopamine and serotonin. In this growing class are risperidone
(Risperdal), clozapine (Clozaril), olanzapine (Zyprexa), aripipra-
zole (Abilify), quetiapine (Seroquel), and ziprasidone (Geodon).
Clinical advantages offered by this new class of medications
include clinical effects on the "positive symptoms" of schizophrenia (e.g., an improvement in the ability of the individual to relate
to the environment and to others, not just a positive effect on hallucinations and delusions) and a decreased likelihood of EPS and
long-term tardive dyskinesia.

The major side effects of typical antipsychotic medications
are EPS, including acute dystonic reactions (abnormal muscle
tone or posturing), akathisia (motor restlessness), and parkin-
sonian effects (rigidity, tremor, slowed movement, and loss of
balance). Acute dystonic reactions are best treated by PO, intravenous, or IM administration of diphenhydramine (25 to 50 mg)
or PO or IM administration of benztropine (1 to 2 mg per day).

MANIA/BIPOLAR DISORDER

Childhood and adolescent bipolar disorder is one of the most
active areas of research in child and adolescent psychiatry. It is
now generally accepted that the clinical presentation of mania
in childhood may be atypical by adult standards. In contrast,
symptoms of bipolar disorder in adolescents are similar to
those in adults. Between 20% and 40% of adolescents initially
diagnosed with major depressive disorder develop bipolar disorder within 5 years.

Clinical Manifestations

Unlike adults, mania in childhood is not typically characterized by euphoric mood. Irritable mood is much more common.

TABLE 133.32

ANTIPSYCHOTIC MEDICATIONS

Generic name	Brand name	Estimated equivalent dosage (mg)	Total daily dosage
Phenothiazines			
Chlorpromazine	Thorazine	100	50–1,000
Trifluoperazine	Stelazine	5	5–30
Fluphenazine	Prolixin	2	1–20
Butyrophenone			
Haloperidol	Haldol	2	2–40
Atypical Antipsychotics			
Clozapine	Clozaril	75	300–450
Risperidone	Risperdal		1–6
Olanzapine	Zyprexa		2.5–20
Quetiapine	Seroquel		150–400
Ziprasidone	Geodon		20–200
Aripiprazole	Abilify		10–30

Children often have remarkable shifts in mood, involving sudden changes from depressed to irritable or happy, and then back to irritable or depressed. This emotional lability can be disorienting to parents, who cannot understand why the child changes so much and so dramatically, possibly even several times the same day. Unlike the older adolescent, the child often does not have a clear recovery from identified episodes but rather may continue to present in at least a mildly unstable way with irritability and anger for much of the time. Explosive, disorganized behavior may also be seen. True psychotic features are rare in childhood bipolar disorder. The course of childhood bipolar disorder tends to be chronic and continuous, rather than episodic. Approximately 90% of children with bipolar disorder have concurrent symptoms of ADHD, which may, in fact, present before the onset of the mood instability.

Symptoms of bipolar disorder in adolescents are often similar to the adult form, but atypical presentations are also common. Psychotic symptoms, suicide attempts, inappropriate sexual behavior, and a "stormy" first year of illness may be typical of adolescent mania. However, when compared with adults, adolescents may have a more prolonged early course and be less responsive to treatment.

The adolescent with mania has a distinct period of predominantly elevated, expansive, and/or irritable mood (Table 133.33). The patient has a significant decrease in need for sleep, high distractibility, hyperactivity and pressured speech, and emotional lability. These patients also exhibit what is called *flight of ideas*—a nearly continuous flow of accelerated speech with abrupt changes from topic to topic, usually based on understandable associations, distractions, or plays on words. Unlike the loose associations of the schizophrenic patient, the flight of ideas of a manic patient retains logical connection from one idea to the next but moves quickly from one topic to another. The manic patient may at times have a remarkably inflated self-esteem, with uncritical self-confidence and significant grandiosity. This grandiosity may also include delusional ideas. The individual may be aggressive and combative. He or she may go on buying sprees or pursue other reckless behaviors or be hypersexual. Manic patients usually have a history of previous depressive episodes, but an acute manic episode in adolescence may be the initial presentation of the disorder. A family history of psychiatric disturbance usually exists in patients with manic–depressive disorder. Typically, manic patients report feeling extremely well, and they are brought to the ED against their will.

Sometimes, patients will present with symptoms of both mania and depression. In these instances, referred to as *mixed episodes*, the mania is usually primarily characterized by irritability. Mixed episodes are particularly dangerous, as patients are at significantly increased risk for suicidal behaviors.

The differentiation of mania and schizophrenia in an initial episode of psychosis in adolescence may at times be difficult. Hyperactivity, distractibility, and expansive and euphoric mood are often helpful in identifying manic individuals. Both groups may have auditory hallucinations and delusions, but someone listening to the speech of the manic adolescent should recognize the flight of ideas and their connection with each other.

Children presenting with symptoms suggestive of mania should receive a thorough medical evaluation to rule out any potential medical causes of their symptoms (Table 133.5). Special attention should be paid to the possibility of toxic ingestions or drug-induced symptoms. For example, steroids

TABLE 133.33

ACUTE MANIA IN ADOLESCENCE: MOST COMMON FEATURES

Pressured speech
Grandiosity
Apparent "high" (euphoria)
Rapid shifts of emotion
Euphoria
Anxiety/irritability
Combativeness/panic
Hypersexuality

at doses commonly used in patients undergoing chemotherapy or treatment for chronic diseases such as inflammatory bowel disease are a common culprit of iatrogenically induced mania. Patients with mania should also be assessed for potential medical sequelae of behaviors that they engaged in as a result of their impaired judgment, for example, exposure to sexually transmitted diseases (STDs), emergency contraception, occult head trauma. Laboratory and imaging work-up should be based on history and clinical findings.

Management

Psychiatric consultation should be obtained whenever a new diagnosis of bipolar disorder is being considered, a manic/mixed episode is present, or if the patient is engaging in any unsafe behaviors. In younger children, especially those who are not floridly manic, outpatient management—usually with the combination of mood-stabilizing medications and intensive behavioral treatment—may be sufficient. However, inpatient hospitalization is often required to maintain the patient's safety while effective treatments are being initiated. Patients who are manic can have severely impaired insight and judgment. This can lead them to engage in dangerous behaviors that can have lifelong consequences or even lead to the death of themselves or others, such as unprotected sex with multiple partners, unsafe driving, engaging in felony-level criminal offenses. Involuntary commitment may be necessary.

Initial emergency treatment of the agitated manic patient may require the use of restraints and the acute administration of antipsychotic agents, in doses equivalent to those used for schizophrenic patients.

AUTISM AND OTHER PERVASIVE DEVELOPMENTAL DISORDERS OF CHILDHOOD

Because of the subacute nature of presentations and the chronicity of their course, it is unusual for children with either infantile autism or other pervasive developmental disorders (PDDs) to present to an ED undiagnosed. However, children with these disorders may present in the ED for the treatment of intercurrent illnesses or an acute exacerbation of the child's behavior. Given the limited verbal skills of many of these children, they are often unable to effectively communicate what is causing them distress. As a result, these children can exhibit behavioral or mood in response to a wide variety of stressors or physical symptoms (as seemingly minor as constipation or a sore throat or as potentially life-threatening as a septic joint). Therefore, the ED clinician should obtain a thorough history from caregivers and maintain a high suspicion for a medical etiology of the patient's altered behavior.

Autism

According to the *Diagnostic and Statistical Manual*, fourth edition (*DSM-IV*), autism is a specific type of PDDs of childhood. The major differentiating feature between autism and other forms of PDDs is the age of onset. Autism always has an onset

before 30 months of age. Children with autism have a generalized lack of responsiveness to other people and a failure to develop normal attachment behavior. They do not develop relationships and instead play alone, often showing stereotyped behavior and using objects in bizarre, inappropriate ways. The autistic child becomes extremely upset if objects in his or her environment are disturbed or changed. Language development is impaired or absent. Only 30% of autistic children have an IQ higher than 70. Some autistic children have underlying illnesses, such as maternal rubella syndrome or previous encephalitis or meningitis, but in many cases, the cause is unknown. Many autistic children have coexisting seizure disorders. The course of infantile autism is generally chronic, with two-thirds of all autistic children remaining severely disabled throughout life.

A comprehensive educational and socialization program with psychiatric monitoring is essential for autistic children. If an autistic child seen in the ED is not participating in such a program, outpatient psychiatric referral is indicated. Medication management of autism at times may involve careful use of psychotropic medication, including antipsychotics, antidepressants, and α-adrenergic agents. Such psychotropic strategies should be used only in conjunction with ongoing psychiatric treatment. Clear justification must be present for psychotropic medication use, not just the diagnosis of autism. In general, acute psychiatric hospitalization is rarely necessary with autism. In instances of extremely disturbing behavior or acute agitation, sedation with either diphenhydramine or risperidone may be helpful. Alternatively, if a child is already prescribed a standing medication for aggressive behaviors, treating the child additional dose of that medication can be considered. Children with autism or related disorders are often exquisitely sensitive to medications and their side effects, so the use of medications to control agitation should be avoided or minimized whenever possible. General calming interventions and behavioral techniques that are used by caregivers in the school or home setting should be employed to help the child remain safe and calm while in the ED. Child life specialists, when available, should be consulted. If the parents are distressed by their child's immediate behavior and the child is receiving psychiatric treatment, phone contact with the psychiatrist may be helpful to both the emergency physician and the family. In the absence of ongoing care, a psychiatric consultation should be requested.

Other Pervasive Developmental Disorders

Pervasive developmental disorder of childhood is a generic term that includes other developmental impairments in which an incapacity to form reciprocal relationships with others results in severe, sustained impairment of attachment and social relationships. Other features may include extreme anxiety and severe emotional reactions to minor difficulties, with inappropriate affect and extreme mood lability. Abnormalities of speech, hypersensitivity to sensory stimuli, peculiar posturing, and self-mutilation may also occur. PDD other than autism has onset after 30 months and before 12 years of age.

The term PDD incompletely incorporates entities such as childhood schizophrenia, symbiotic psychosis, and atypical psychosis, as well as other recently added conditions. One type of PDD with which the emergency physician should be familiar is

Asperger's syndrome. Children with this disorder typically have normal or above-average intelligence, with a well-developed capacity for speech and language. The impairment is in the capacity to form reciprocal relationships, and emotional rigidity, idiosyncratic thinking, and intense pursuit of a narrow range of interests may be present. Children with Asperger's syndrome may be confusing to the emergency physician because they present as higher functioning than other children with PDD and are not psychotic, yet they may appear to be significantly strange.

All children with PDD, including children with autism, require comprehensive psychiatric and educational treatment. Parents of children with autism and PDD should be given appropriate referrals because children who receive services early in their development are believed to have an improved prognosis. When necessary, the same acute pharmacologic approaches for children with autism are also relevant for other PDDs. Low-dose antipsychotic medication may also be used. With the acute exacerbation of a child with PDD, psychiatric hospitalization may be necessary, both to provide assistance to the parents and to develop or modify a comprehensive treatment program. Families with acute concerns about their child's behavior should receive psychiatric consultation.

POSTTRAUMATIC STRESS DISORDERS

PTSD can occur in childhood and adolescence, typically based on the experience of severe trauma during earlier years. Children may be more sensitive to the effects of trauma than are adults and thus may have higher rates of PTSD. Either the reemergence of the old trauma, the emergence of a new similar one, or the recollection of the original trauma can activate a PTSD. A summary of the official *DSM-IV* description of PTSD is helpful in understanding this concept.

The person has been exposed to a traumatic event in which the person experienced, witnessed, or was confronted with an event that involved actual or threatened death or serious injury, or a threat to the physical integrity of self or others. The person's response involved intense fear, helplessness or horror, or, in children, disorganized or agitated behavior. In addition, the traumatic event is persistently reexperienced in one or more ways, there is persistent avoidance of stimuli associated with the trauma and numbing of general responsiveness, and there are persistent symptoms of increased arousal.

Highly stressful situations that may precipitate severe emotional reactions by the child and PTSD include physical beatings and other violence, repeated threats and belittling by adults, long-standing hunger and poverty, sexual abuse, and rape. PTSD symptomatology has also been reported following bone marrow transplant, severe burns or injuries, or motor vehicle accidents. In some cases, a separate dissociative reaction may occur instead (see the next section). With the child, PTSD probably emerges through a combination of traumatic events, along with a silent or nonaccepting environment that fails to provide the child with adequate protection and support.

Symptomatically, the child may persistently reexperience the traumatic event in many ways, including recurrent and distressing recollections of the event, which may be observed through repetitive play by young children in which themes or aspects of the trauma are expressed. Recurrent and distressing

dreams of the event may also occur. Hallucinations and flashbacks may follow the child's sudden reliving of the experience. In addition, events that symbolize or resemble some aspect of the traumatic event may produce intense anxiety and distress; the connection between precipitating event and distress is not always evident to parents or child.

Other PTSD symptoms experienced by children include generalized numbing of responsiveness to events and people. Stimuli associated with the trauma may be consistently avoided. The emergency physician should also be alert for signs of increased arousal—anxiety and agitation, difficulty falling asleep, irritability or anger, suspiciousness, difficulty concentrating—and various physiologic complaints in response to events that resemble or symbolize the traumatic event.

The key task for the emergency physician is to recognize PTSD in the differential diagnosis of an agitated, confused, or even psychotic child or adolescent. A careful history usually provides clues to this diagnosis. Supportive management in the ED, including using family and friends, is often sufficient. Low-dose antipsychotic medication should be reserved for children who are frankly psychotic and who do not respond to reality-based support. Often, an antihistamine or anxiolytic medication may suffice.

The ED physician may also have an important role in the prevention of PTSD. When patients are being treated for an acute traumatic episode, the ED should have forethought. The PTSD may be a consequence and attempt to refer a patient for mental health counseling.

When parents dismiss or doubt the child's symptoms or worries, the emergency physician can encourage the parents to respond supportively to their child. When the physician suspects parental abuse, this concern must be addressed directly with the family and with appropriate authorities brought in, if justified. Many children with PTSD benefit significantly from individual and family therapy. If child and family are not already in treatment, a referral is appropriate.

DISSOCIATIVE DISORDERS

Some children develop a dissociative disorder in response to extreme trauma. In a dissociative disorder, the child separates the usually integrated functions of identity, memory, and consciousness. As a result, the child's affect appears split off from the rest of the person. Specific symptoms vary, but in most cases, the child appears distant, even weird, but is not psychotic. Dissociative disorders occur most commonly in female patients, with sexual abuse a common original trauma.

The function of dissociative reactions is believed to decrease the child's awareness of emotional pain caused by the trauma. The process of splitting off the affect from the body may help a severely traumatized child deal with and survive the assault. This response probably begins at the time of the trauma, especially if it occurs repeatedly, and is then continued afterward as a form of coping. However, a consequence is that the child may continue to split off full emotional responsiveness to daily experiences, creating a profound isolation. This process may continue into adulthood.

The emergency physician may encounter a child with depersonalization, a feeling of detachment from one's self or a feeling of being an automaton or in a dream. Another dissociative response is psychogenic amnesia, the sudden inability to recall important personal information (or even know one's own identity). Some runaway adolescents may present with a psychogenic fugue, another dissociative disorder. In a fugue state, the individual leaves home unexpectedly with no apparent justification and may at times assume a partial or complete new identity.

The most extreme form of dissociative disorder is dissociative identity disorder (formerly *multiple personality disorder*). In this condition, the child has two or more personalities and appears puzzling to parents, teachers, and physicians. At least two of these personalities recurrently take full control of the child's behavior, with the child unaware of the process. Children with this disorder are aptly described as erratic, inconsistent, and even mercurial.

The emergency physician should consider the possibility of dissociative disorders in all children and adolescents who present in a confused and confusing way. None of these children are psychotic; in fact, an entirely different emotional process is operating. A thorough history is most rewarding and may reveal a female patient with repeated sexual abuse who often appears far off into her own world. Psychiatric referral is appropriate for patients with dissociative disorders. The emergency physician should also determine any possible ongoing abuse before releasing the child to the family.

Panic Attacks

It is not uncommon for children experiencing panic attacks to present to the ED for medical attention. After ruling out any medical cause for the child's symptoms, the ED physician should educate the patient and their family about the nature of panic attacks and explain that no additional medical testing or observation is indicated at this time. Benzodiazepines should be avoided when possible, so as to help the patient and their family recognize that the symptoms of a panic attack are time limited and self-resolving. The patient and their family should be receive brief bedside teaching about basic anxiety management techniques and the appropriate level of response should symptoms recur, for example, when to forego versus when to seek medical attention. It can sometimes be helpful and instructive to ask the patient to practice deep breathing or relaxation techniques while they are connected to a cardiorespiratory monitor, so they can receive immediate feedback on how anxiety level and physical signs/symptoms are related. If the panic attacks are frequent, cause significant distress, or are leading the patient/family to repeatedly seek medical care, use of antianxiety medication and referral to an outpatient mental health provider is indicated. If left untreated, panic attacks can blossom into life-long and severely impairing anxiety disorders. However, with appropriate and early treatment, future panic attacks and their sequelae can be prevented.

SCHOOL REFUSAL

Background

School refusal, also called *school avoidance* and *school phobia*, entails a child's not attending school and expressing somatic complaints that keep him or her at home. Usually, some somatic complaint is the justification for school absence. School refusal involves the knowledge and complicity of the family. A parent, usually the mother, is aware of the child's school absence and has endorsed his or her being home, in part because the parent may consider the child to be physically ill. Children with school refusal often meet criteria for what psychiatrists would refer to as a *somataform disorder* or what medical specialists might refer to as a *functional syndrome*. In some circumstances, they may even present with neurological symptoms suggestive of a conversion disorder. Therefore, the ED evaluation and management recommendations discussed below can be applied to these children as well.

School refusal is an important condition with which the emergency physician should be familiar. Usually, it is not the initial complaint. Typically, one or more physical complaints bring the child to the ED, and information about school attendance is not offered. The physician must maintain an "index of suspicion" in a child with recurring complaints for which no medical cause is apparent.

Clinical Manifestations

Certain school attendance patterns are suggestive of but not necessary for the diagnosis of school refusal. More absences occur in the fall, when school begins, than in the spring. The child often exhibits a reluctance to return to school after weekends and holidays. There may be a lessening of somatic complaints on weekends and over the summer. Similar sporadic attendance patterns may often be elicited at some other time in the child's past. In other instances, however, school refusal may develop in a child who has previously given no cause for concern.

Schmitt formulated a diagnostic triad of the clinical manifestations of school refusal: (i) vague physical symptoms; (ii) normal physical and laboratory findings; and (iii) poor school attendance. The child may have one or more complaints. Schmitt also pointed out that many of the symptoms are reflective of depression and anxiety. This finding is consistent with the fact that many children with school refusal are also depressed. Other psychiatric conditions that may be comorbid with school refusal are specific phobias, other anxiety disorders, conduct disorder, substance abuse, or family psychopathology.

Characteristics of families with school refusal have been noted. An illness orientation is revealed by physical complaints in other family members and frequent somatic references in verbal communication. The closeness between the mother and child may be manifested by the mother's frequent use of "we" when talking about the child. Active undermining by the parents may at times be observed.

Management

The major responsibility of the emergency physician is the detection of school refusal. Although the emergency physician cannot guide the entire treatment of school refusal, he or she can get the process going. The physical examination should be done in the presence of the parents in a thorough manner, with the physician emphasizing the absence of physical findings. Appropriate, but not excessive, laboratory work should be performed, and medication should not be prescribed. After acknowledging the genuineness of the child's symptom so that there is no misunderstanding that the child is "faking it," the physician should provide a firm and unequivocal statement to the family that the child has no serious illness. He or she should then ensure that the family understands what has been said and accepts it. In this way, misunderstandings or disagreements can be confronted directly, thereby decreasing the likelihood of subsequent "doctor-shopping" by the family. The emphasis is then placed on the child's learning to function despite his or her symptoms.

Once school refusal is recognized and the possibility of medical diseases are ruled out, the principal goals in the treatment of school refusal are (i) getting the child back to school as soon as possible, (ii) ensuring continuity of medical care, and (iii) referring the patient and family to a mental health professional to address underlying individual and family issues that contributed to the development of the problem.

It may be helpful for the parents rather than the physician to tell the child that he or she needs to return to school. In this way, the family takes responsibility for the resolution of the problem from the beginning of the intervention. The parents should be encouraged to work closely together to achieve their desired goal.

CONDUCT DISORDERS

Background

A child with a disorder of conduct engages in repetitive, socially unacceptable behavior, without evidence of medical or other psychiatric disorder. The diagnosis of conduct disorder implies a continuing pattern of disruptive or deviant behavior, rather than isolated antisocial acts. This may involve behavior this is violent and aggressive (e.g., vandalism, mugging, assault, rape) or behavior that is socially unacceptable but nonaggressive (e.g., truancy, running away, lying, stealing, substance abuse). Therefore, a disorder of conduct involves more serious behavior than ordinary mischief and pranks of children and adolescents. Because violent and other unacceptable behaviors may be performed by children with medical illnesses and intoxications, these causes must be ruled out before the diagnosis of conduct disorder can be made. Similarly, because children with psychosis and depression can also behave in socially unacceptable ways, these serious psychiatric disorders must also be considered and eliminated before diagnosing a conduct disorder (see Chapter 19). However, even with primary medical and psychiatric causes of socially unacceptable behavior ruled out, some youth with conduct disorder may have ill-defined physiologic predispositions that contribute to its emergence.

Society disagrees about whether to regard children and adolescents with conduct disorders as psychiatrically impaired and needing treatment, or as delinquent and needing detention or incarceration. No consistent agreement exists about the appropriate criteria for taking such children to an ED as opposed to a juvenile center. In actual practice, certain factors probably influence the choice of disposition, such as age (younger children are more likely to receive medical evaluation), socioeconomic level (children belonging to middle- and upper-level income family are more likely to be taken to an ED), race (Caucasian children are more likely to be taken to an ED than are African American or other minority children), and nature of the infraction (children with aggressive acts directed outside the family are more likely to be taken to a detention center). Aggressive children should always undergo an emergency medical and psychiatric evaluation any time intoxication, an underlying medical condition, or other psychiatric disorder is suspected.

Clinical Manifestations

Children with conduct disorders typically have poor adjustment at home and in the community. Peer relationships are superficial, based more on what the child can get from the other person than on a sense of empathy. The child thinks primarily about him- or herself, trying to manipulate situations to personal advantage without significant concern for the feelings and needs of others. The child with a conduct disorder is unlikely to extend him- or herself for others when no immediate advantage can be gained. When the child is apprehended, little sense of remorse or guilt is exhibited, but rather a sense of anger at being detected and detained. Such children rarely accept responsibility for their own actions and instead tend to blame others for their mistakes.

School attendance of children with a conduct disorder is often sporadic, and academic performance is often poor. This may be caused by various factors, including lack of interest and discipline, but may also be caused by specific learning disabilities and a concurrent ADHD, diagnoses that are remediable but often missed.

The child or adolescent with a conduct disorder shows low frustration tolerance, irritability, and temper outbursts. He or she may be reckless in behavior and project an image of "toughness." Smoking, drinking, drug use, and precocious sexual activity may all occur. In addition to possible legal difficulties, the child may have other problems, including school suspensions, drug dependence, STD, pregnancy, and physical injury from accidents and fights.

The presence of a conduct disorder implies a failure of the child's environment to instill familial and societal values, and to implement their rules effectively. As a result, the child comes to believe that he or she can act as he or she chooses and does not develop control of impulses. The specific pattern of inadequate limit setting varies, but families share an inconsistency in enforcing rules and do not hold the child accountable for his or her behavior. In some families, discipline may fluctuate from being perfunctory at times to being harsh and even physically abusive at other times. Parental role models may show poor impulse control themselves and disregard societal norms.

In addition to inconsistent limit setting, parental separations and divorce, mental illness, and alcohol or drug abuse may also be factors. Parental criminality and incarceration occur in some families. Families with aggressive and impulsive children often do not know how to effectively use social service resources and may consider themselves helpless in controlling their child and in dealing with the world at large.

When brought to the ED, children with a conduct disorder have variable presentations. For example, the child or adolescent may be angry, hostile, uncooperative, and even violent, refusing to answer questions directed to him or her, but quick to interrupt to defend him- or herself when others speak. Alternatively, the child may present with a superficially smooth and pleasant facade, hoping to persuade the physician and authorities of his or her innocence. Often, once the child realizes that he or she will not be permitted to act out or manipulate in the ED, he or she may settle down and cooperate more fully. At other times, the child maintains an essentially impenetrable persona.

Management

The goals for managing aggressive and disruptive children in the ED are to (i) ensure the safety of the child, family, and staff; (ii) rule out possible medical conditions and severe psychiatric disorders before making the diagnosis of conduct disorder; and (iii) gather sufficient information to make an appropriate disposition.

The safety of the child and staff and control of the child's unacceptable behavior must be achieved in the ED. In many instances, the disruptive behavior occurred and ended before the child's coming to the ED and gaining the child's cooperation is not a problem. In other instances, however, the child may remain combative and aggressive in the ED. Dealing with such a problem requires the presence of adequate security staff and a quiet space where attempts to control the patient do not disrupt the remainder of the ED. The patient should be told firmly that he or she is in the hospital for medical and psychiatric evaluation and will not be permitted to harm him- or herself or others. The child should be informed of the need to cooperate with the staff and control his or her behavior. The child's parents, if present, should be asked to assist in controlling the child. The child can be reassured that he or she will get a chance to tell his or her side of the story completely. These interventions are usually sufficient to gain the child's cooperation.

The history and physical examination assist in ruling out medical conditions and intoxications. The presence of ongoing medical conditions should be specifically asked about, as should any recent alcohol use or drug ingestion because substance abuse is common. As indicated, specimens for toxicologic screening should be obtained. Epilepsy can be ruled out as the cause of the abnormal behavior in the presence of a normal neurologic examination and the absence of an aura, abnormal neurologic signs, or postictal phenomena.

Children with medical conditions and acute intoxications are best managed through medical hospitalization. The presence of psychosis or depression requires psychiatric consultation and possible psychiatric hospitalization. Psychiatric consultation should be obtained for children with presumptive conduct disorder and no underlying medical condition. Less severe and complicated cases can be managed through referral for outpatient therapy. More severe cases may require more intensive community-based services, such as partial hospitalization or even psychiatric hospitalization, which should be considered in cases of severe, chronic conduct disorders, especially when the child's behaviors are escalating and treatment to date has been ineffective. For intervention to be effective with such children, the family must be willing to participate actively, with the goal of altering persistent patterns of disturbed behavior.

Involuntary hospitalization may be necessary when the child's condition continues to pose a threat to him- or herself or others or when overt homicidal or suicidal ideation is present. When the child is not suicidal or homicidal and refuses to make a commitment to work in psychotherapy and when the family does not support the proposed psychiatric hospitalization, problematic behaviors are more likely to continue and the child may eventually enter the juvenile justice system.

FIRE SETTING

Virtually all children in our society develop a fascination with fire and may experiment with it at a relatively early age. For most children, this experimentation is transient and consists mainly of playing with matches or lighting small fires. However, some children may persist with fire-setting behavior, actually planning to set larger fires that are destructive to both people and property. At this point, the child is demonstrating evidence of a significant psychiatric disorder and requires intensive treatment. The exact incidence of fire setting is unknown, but serious repetitive fire setting is believed to be uncommon in children and adolescents. In general, fire setting is a symptom of serious underlying emotional difficulty and is often associated with other disturbances of behavior and impulse control. Fire setting is also associated with significant anger and aggressiveness on the part of the child. The background of fire-setting children is likely to be highly unstable. These children may have had multiple contacts with social agencies in the past, and some may have been placed outside the home in foster homes or institutions. Although the exact percentage of fire setters with underlying ADHD is unknown, many of these children are described as having been hyperactive, with significant learning problems and long-standing truancy from school.

Management

The clinical manifestations of fire setters in the ED are similar to those of other children with conduct disorders as previously described. Effective ED evaluation should always consider psychiatric hospitalization. As psychiatric hospitalization is arranged, the facility must be informed about the child's previous fire-setting behavior so that appropriate behavior monitoring and safety measures can be employed during the admission.

ATTENTION-DEFICIT/ HYPERACTIVITY DISORDER

Background

ADHD refers to a syndrome found in school-aged children, characterized by a pervasive difficulty in maintaining attention and goal-directed behavior. ADHD has an incidence of between 5% and 10% of school-aged children, occurring two to five times more often in boys than in girls. It is presumed to have an underlying neurologic cause. It is the most common cause of chronic behavioral problems for school-aged children.

The emergency physician should be familiar with ADHD because many children so affected become depressed and may make suicide attempts. ADHD is also common in children with bipolar disorder and may in fact initially mask the bipolar disorder. During adolescence, ADHD may itself be masked by antisocial behavior. Because identification and treatment can produce significant improvements in the clinical picture, the diagnosis of ADHD should not be missed.

Clinical Manifestations

Although some children with attentional problems present without hyperactivity, most children have hyperactivity in association with inattention and impulsivity and, therefore, fit within the full ADHD umbrella. Wender described the various possible components of the ADHD picture. Attentional difficulties occur both at home and in school and are often more severe in school. Rather than persisting in schoolwork and other tasks, the child often appears not to be listening to the teacher, and discipline may be a problem.

Impulsivity is another essential characteristic of ADHD. The child has difficulty with self-control, exhibiting behaviors that get him or her in trouble with parents, siblings, teachers, and peers. At home, the child typically has outbursts and temper tantrums, and enforcement of discipline may be difficult. Lack of self-control may also manifest through stealing, lying, playing with matches, and other forms of acting out.

ADHD symptoms tend to be worse in a group situation than at home or in one-to-one interactions. This characteristic at times creates difficulty in the diagnosis of ADHD because the telltale signs are least likely to occur during an individual assessment by the physician.

The child with ADHD may be labile, with fluctuations in mood and a tendency toward overreaction and temper tantrums, but such responses are not always extreme. Appreciating the low self-esteem and possible depression that may be present in these children as a result of academic failure, conflicts at home, and peer and sibling rejection is important. In acute situations, the depression may find expression as suicide attempts or violent behavior. ADHD children are a high-risk group for self-destructive behavior. The physician often perceives the child's sense of sadness beyond a cocky bravado that masks feelings of frustration and inadequacy.

Family problems are typically found in the families of ADHD children, if only as a consequence of the child's impulsivity and challenging behaviors. The child may provoke the parents, interrupt family members, and fail to learn consistently from experience. The child is often difficult to discipline effectively. Conflicts with siblings may occur.

Management

The principal responsibility of the emergency physician is to recognize the possibility of ADHD in children who present with other problems—including depression, mood instability, and conduct disorder—and consider the diagnosis. The physician is then in a position to clarify the meaning of this disorder with the family, as well as to restore hope for the child's improved behavior and adaptation by making a psychiatric referral when indicated. The history is the most reliable diagnostic indicator. Once a presumptive diagnosis is made, appropriate referral and treatment can follow.

Psychostimulant medication is often helpful in alleviating the symptoms of ADHD. Although psychostimulant medication should not be prescribed in the ED, the emergency physician should have a familiarity with the commonly used drugs, including stimulants, such as methylphenidate and D-amphetamine, and their long-acting forms. Tricyclic antidepressants, bupropion, modafinil, and α-adrenergic agents have also been successfully used in the treatment of ADHD but constitute a second line of medication and are not approved by the FDA for this purpose. Atomoxetine is a noradrenergic reuptake inhibitor that is FDA approved for the treatment of ADHD. In general, response rates to the stimulant medications are higher than 75%. The principal short-term side effects of the stimulants are appetite suppression and insomnia. The principal concerns of long-term use of stimulants are suppression of weight gain and linear growth. However, rebound growth appears to occur when the medication is discontinued. Recently, cardiac dysrhythmias and sudden death secondary to the use of stimulants has come under greater scrutiny and is the subject of ongoing research.

ATTACHMENT DISORDERS OF INFANCY

Occasionally, infants will be seen in the ED who are withdrawn and apathetic. These infants demonstrate severe disturbances of attachment with their primary caregivers, often have feeding disturbances, and may fail to thrive. The most significant disability of these children is a dramatic failure of social development. They do not track with their eyes, and they rarely smile. They do not interact with caregivers in age-appropriate fashion, and facial responsiveness may be entirely absent. The child may be noted to be weak, may have poor muscle tone, and may emit a feeble cry. The child demonstrates little spontaneous activity, sleeps excessively, and has a generalized lack of interest in the environment.

The cause of attachment disorders in infants is a continuing lack of adequate caregiving. Features that interfere with maternal–infant bonding are often noted in the history. These may include significant maternal depression and isolation, other maternal incapacitation including substance abuse, maternal indifference toward the infant, history of prolonged separation between mother and infant following birth because of perinatal difficulties, and actual physical abuse. Infants who are temperamentally placid, those who make their needs known quietly, often have more difficulties in the presence of maternal depression or maternal preoccupation than more active and responsive infants.

Underlying chronic illness may also lead to the development of social withdrawal and apathy. Also, children with physical problems in infancy may be more difficult to care for, thus parental reactions to the child's illness may interfere with attachment. Children with mental retardation, although they develop slowly, do not generally demonstrate the profound apathy of the child with an attachment disorder. Furthermore, children with mental retardation receive generally adequate caregiving and do not fail to thrive.

Management

Children with attachment disorders require complete medical evaluation, along with careful assessment of their environment. Such children are often seen in the ED for minor physical complaints and may not be receiving regular pediatric care. Thus, the emergency physician must recognize attachment disorders and make effective referrals for ongoing health care for child and family. When parental apathy accompanies severe failure to thrive, hospitalization may be necessary to initiate needed changes and to plan continuing treatment. The physician should recognize that attachment disorders and the associated failure to thrive are often reversible once adequate caregiving is instituted and maintained. If the physician suspects that the child's problems are a result of actual abuse or neglect, this belief should be reported to the appropriate agencies. (Child neglect is discussed in detail in Chapter 132.)

Suggested Readings

General

American Psychiatric Association. *Diagnostic and statistical manual of mental disorders*, 4th ed., text rev. (DSM-IV-TR). Washington, DC: American Psychiatric Association Press, 2000.

Dubin W, Weiss K. *Handbook of psychiatric emergencies*. Torrance, CA: Homestead School, 1997.

Green WH. *Child and adolescent clinical psychopharmacology*, 3rd ed. Philadelphia, PA: Lippincott Williams & Wilkins, 2001.

McClellan JM, Werry JS. Evidence-based treatments in child and adolescent psychiatry: an inventory. *J Am Acad Child Adolesc Psychiatry* 2003;42:1388–1400.

McDaniel KD. Pharmacologic treatment of psychiatric and neurodevelopmental disorders in children and adolescents (3 parts). *Clin Pediatr* 1986;25:65–71, 143–146, 198–204.

Riddle MA. *Child and adolescent psychiatric clinics of North America: pediatric psychopharmacology I*, vol. 4. Philadelphia, PA: WB Saunders, 1995.

Riddle MA. *Child and adolescent psychiatric clinics of North America: pediatric psychopharmacology II*, vol. 4. Philadelphia, PA: WB Saunders, 1995.

Riddle MA, Kastelic EA, Frosch E. Pediatric psychopharmacology. *J Child Psychol Psychiatry* 2001;42:73–90.

Volkmar FR, Tsatsanis KD. Childhood schizophrenia. In: Lewis M, ed. *Child and adolescent psychiatry: a comprehensive textbook*. Philadelphia, PA: Lippincott Williams & Wilkins, 2002.

Agitated or Violent Behavior and the Use of Restraint

Allen MH. Managing the agitated psychotic patient: a reappraisal of the evidence. *J Clin Psychiatry* 2000;61(suppl 14):11–20.

Binder RL, McNiel DE. Contemporary practices in managing acutely violent patients in 20 psychiatric emergency rooms. *Psychiatr Serv* 1999;50:1553–1554.

Busch AB, Shore MF. Seclusion and restraint: a review of the recent literature. *Harv Rev Psychiatry* 2000;8:261–270.

Currier GW. Atypical antipsychotic medications in the psychiatric emergency service. *J Clin Psychiatry* 2000;61(suppl 14):21–26.

Currier GW, Allen MH. Physical and chemical restraint in the psychiatric emergency service. *Psychiatr Serv* 2000;51:717–719.

Dorfman DH. The use of physical and chemical restraints in the pediatric emergency department. *Pediatr Emerg Care* 2000;16:355–360.

Hilt RJ, Woodward TA. Agitation treatment for pediatric emergency patients. *J Am Acad Child Adolesc Psychiatry* 2008;47(2):132–138.

Practice parameter for the prevention and management of aggressive behavior in child and adolescent psychiatric institutions, with special reference to seclusion and restraint. *J Am Acad Child Adolesc Psychiatry* 2002;41(2)(suppl):4S–25S.

Sachdev P, Mason C, Hadzi-Pavlovic D. Case-control study of neuroleptic malignant syndrome. *Am J Psychiatry* 1997;154:1156–1158.

Sorrentino A. Chemical restraints for the agitated, violent, or psychotic pediatric patient in the emergency department: controversies and recommendations. *Curr Opin Pediatr* 2004;16:201–5.

Yildiz A, Sachs GS, Turgay A. Pharmacological management of agitation in emergency settings. *Emerg Med J* 2003;20:339–346.

Suicide

Brown LK, Overholser J, Spirito A, et al. The correlates of planning in adolescent suicide attempts. *J Am Acad Child Adolesc Psychiatry* 1991;30:95–99.

Garfinkel BD, Golombek H. Suicide and depression in childhood and adolescence. *Can Med Assoc J* 1974;110(11):1278–1281.

Henden H. Psychodynamics of suicide, with particular reference to the young. *Am J Psychiatry* 1991;148:1150–1158.

Lewinsohn PM, Rohde P, Seeley JR. Psychosocial risk factors for future adolescent suicide attempts. *J Consult Clin Psychol* 1994;62:297–305.

Masters KJ, Bellonci C, Bernet W, et al. Practice parameter for the prevention and management of aggressive behavior in child and adolescent psychiatric institutions, with special reference to seclusion and restraint. *J Am Acad Child Adolesc Psychiatry* 2002;41(2)(suppl):4S–25S.

Pfeffer CR. Childhood suicidal behavior: a developmental perspective. *Psychiatr Clin North Am* 1997;20:551–562.

Safren SA, Heimberg RG. Depression, hopelessness, suicidality, and related factors in sexual minority and heterosexual adolescents. *J Consult Clin Psychol* 1999;67:859–866.

Depression and Bipolar Disorder

Birmaher B, Ryan N, Williamson D, et al. Childhood and adolescent depression: a review of the past 10 years, part I. *J Am Acad Child Adolesc Psychiatry* 1996;35(11):1427–1439.

Garrison CZ, Jackson KL, Marsteller F, et al. A longitudinal study of depressive symptomatology in young adolescents. *J Am Acad Child Adolesc Psychiatry* 1990;29:581–585.

Geller B, Fox LW, Clark KA. Rate and predictors of prepubertal bipolarity during follow-up of 6- to 12-year old depressed children. *J Am Acad Child Adolesc Psychiatry* 1994;33:461–468.

Geller B, Luby J. Child and adolescent bipolar disorder: a review of the past 10 years. *J Am Acad Child Adolesc Psychiatry* 1997;36:1168–1176.

Kessler RC, Walters EE. Epidemiology of DSM-III-R major depression and minor depression among adolescents and young adults in the National Comorbidity Survey. *Depress Anxiety* 1998;7:3–14.

Practice parameters for the assessment and treatment of children and adolescents with depressive disorders: AACAP. *J Am Acad Child Adolesc Psychiatry* 2007;46(11):1503–1526.

Rao U, Ryan ND, Birmaher B, et al. Unipolar depression in adolescents: clinical outcome in adulthood. *J Am Acad Child Adolesc Psychiatry* 1995;34:566–578.

Strober M, Schmidt-Lackner S, Freeman R, et al. Recovery and relapse in adolescents with bipolar affective illness: a five-year naturalistic, prospective follow-up. *J Am Acad Child Adolesc Psychiatry* 1995;34:724–731.

Weller EB, Weller RA, Fristad MA. Bipolar disorder in children: misdiagnosis, underdiagnosis, and future directions. *J Am Acad Child Adolesc Psychiatry* 1995;34:709–714.

Psychosis

Kilgus MD, Pumariega AJ, Cuffe SP. Influence of race on diagnosis of adolescent psychiatry inpatients. *J Am Acad Child Adolesc Psychiatry* 1995;34:67–72.

Masters KJ, Bellonci C, Bernet W, et al. Practice parameter for the prevention and management of aggressive behavior in child and adolescent psychiatric institutions, with special reference to seclusion and restraint. *J Am Acad Child Adolesc Psychiatry* 2002;41(2)(suppl):4S–25S.

Thomsen PS. Schizophrenia with childhood and adolescent onset: a nationwide register-based study. *Acta Psychiatr Scand* 1996;94:187–193.

Volkmar FR. Childhood and adolescent psychosis: a review of the past 10 years. *J Am Acad Child Adolesc Psychiatry* 1996;35:843–851.

Werry JS, McClellan JM, Chard L. Childhood and adolescent schizophrenic, bipolar, and schizoaffective disorders: a clinical and outcome study. *J Am Acad Child Adolesc Psychiatry* 1991;30:457–465.

Autism and Other Pervasive Developmental Disorders of Childhood

Masters KJ, Bellonci C, Bernet W, et al. Practice parameter for the prevention and management of aggressive behavior in child and adolescent psychiatric institutions, with special reference to seclusion and restraint. *J Am Acad Child Adolesc Psychiatry* 2002;41(2)(suppl):4S–25S.

Tsai LY. Autistic disorder and other pervasive developmental disorders. In: Wiener JM, Dulcan MK, eds. *Textbook of child and adolescent psychiatry*, 3rd ed. Arlington, VA: American Psychiatric Publishing, 2004;261–350.

Tsai LY. *Taking the mystery out of medication in autism/Asperger syndromes*. Arlington, TX: Future Horizons, 2001.

Posttraumatic Stress Disorder

Nader K, Pynoos R, Fairbanks L, et al. Children's PTSD reactions one year after a sniper attack at their school. *Am J Psychiatry* 1990;147:1526–1530.

PSYCHOSOCIAL EMERGENCIES

Pfefferbaum B. Posttraumatic stress disorder in children: a review of the past 10 years. *J Am Acad Child Adolesc Psychiatry* 1997;36:1503–1511.

Terr L. Childhood traumas: an outline and overview. *Am J Psychiatry* 1991;148:10–20.

Ursano RJ. Post-traumatic stress disorder. *N Engl J Med* 2002;346:130–132.

Dissociative Disorders

Chu J, Dill D. Dissociative symptoms in relation to childhood physical and sexual abuse. *Am J Psychiatry* 1990;147:887–892.

Deel P, Eisenhower J. Adolescent multiple personality disorders: a preliminary study of 11 cases. *J Am Acad Child Adolesc Psychiatry* 1990;29:359–366.

School Refusal

Bernstein G, Svingen PH, Garfield BD. School phobia: patterns of family functioning. *J Am Acad Child Adolesc Psychiatry* 1990;29:24–30.

King NJ, Bernstein GA. School refusal in children and adolescents: a review of the past 10 years. *J Am Acad Child Adolesc Psychiatry* 2001;40:197–205.

Last C, Strauss C. School refusal in anxiety-disordered children and adolescents. *J Am Acad Child Adolesc Psychiatry* 1990;29:31–35.

Steiner H. Practice parameters for the assessment and treatment of children and adolescents with conduct disorder. *J Am Acad Child Adolesc Psychiatry* 1997;36(suppl):122S–139S.

Conduct Disorders

Boyle M, Offord D. Primary prevention of conduct disorders: issues and prospects. *J Am Acad Child Adolesc Psychiatry* 1990;29:227–233.

Coccaro E, Kavoussi R. Fluoxetine and impulsive aggressive behavior in personality-disordered subjects. *Arch Gen Psychiatry* 1997;54:1081–1089.

Cox-Jones C, Lubetsky MJ, Fultz SA, et al. Inpatient psychiatric treatment of a young recidivist firesetter. *J Am Acad Child Adolesc Psychiatry* 1990;29: 936–941.

Farrington DP, Loeber R. Epidemiology of juvenile violence. *Child Adolesc Psychiatr Clin N Am* 2000;9:733–748.

Klein RG, Abikoff H, Klass E, et al. Clinical efficacy of methylphenidate in conduct disorder with and without attention deficit hyperactivity disorder. *Arch Gen Psychiatry* 1997;54:1073–1080.

Loeber R, Burke JD, Lahey BB, et al. Oppositional defiant disorder and conduct disorder: a review of the last 10 years, part I. *J Am Acad Child Adolesc Psychiatry* 2000;39:1468–1484.

Prothrow-Stith D. *Deadly consequences: how violence is destroying our teenage population and a plan to begin solving the problem.* New York, NY: Harper Perennial, 1993.

Rey J, Plapp J. Quality of perceived parenting in oppositional and conduct disordered adolescents. *J Am Acad Child Adolesc Psychiatry* 1990;29: 382–385.

Attention-Deficit/Hyperactivity Disorders

Barkley RA. *Taking charge of ADHD: the complete authoritative guide for parents.* New York, NY: Guilford Press, 1995.

Cantwell DP. Attention deficit disorder: a review of the past 10 years. *J Am Acad Child Adolesc Psychiatry* 1996;35:978–987.

Greenhill LL, Halperin JM, Abikoff H. Stimulant medications. *J Am Acad Child Adolesc Psychiatry* 1999;38:503–512.

National Institutes of Health Consensus Development Conference Statement: diagnosis and treatment of attention-deficit/hyperactivity disorder (ADHD). *J Am Acad Child Adolesc Psychiatry* 2000;39:182–193.

Pliszka S; AACAP Work Group on Quality Issues. Practice parameter for the assessment and treatment of children and adolescents with attention-deficit/hyperactivity disorder. *J Am Acad Child Adolesc Psychiatry* 2007; 46(7):894–921.

Scahill L, Schwab-Stone M. Epidemiology of ADHD in school-age children. *Child Adolesc Psychiatr Clin N Am* 2000;9:541–555.

Silver LB. *Attention-deficit hyperactivity disorder: a clinical guide to diagnosis and treatment.* Washington, DC: American Psychiatric Association Press, 1992.

Infancy

Campbell M, Schopler E, Cueva J, et al. Treatment of autistic disorder. *J Am Acad Child Adolesc Psychiatry* 1996;35:134–143.

Goldberg C. Outcome in autism and autistic-like conditions. *J Am Acad Child Adolesc Psychiatry* 1991;30:375–382.

Rogers S, DiLalla D. Age of symptom onset in young children with pervasive developmental disorders. *J Am Acad Child Adolesc Psychiatry* 1990;29: 863–872.

CHAPTER 134 ■ ULTRASOUND

JASON LEVY, MD

INTRODUCTION

Emergency bedside ultrasound has been used in the emergency department (ED) for more than two decades. Its beginnings are rooted in the general ED adult population, which now has well-established, evidence-based applications, such as the focused assessment with sonography in trauma (FAST) or evaluation for abdominal aortic aneurysm. It is now a required component of emergency medicine residencies and is considered as core content by the American Board of Emergency Medicine and the American College of Emergency Physicians (ACEP).

Traditionally, ultrasound performed by imaging specialists involves comprehensive examinations in which entire anatomic areas are evaluated. In contrast, emergency bedside ultrasound is intended to answer a focused, limited clinical question (e.g., "Is there cardiac activity or not?") or assist in a specific procedure. As such, each examination type listed below will be presented with this type of question in mind.

Pediatric emergency medicine has been later to adopt bedside ultrasound into everyday clinical practice. In recent years, however, it has gained more widespread acceptance as the body of literature has expanded and training has become more accessible. Besides the obvious advantage of being conducted directly at the patient's bedside, emergency ultrasound offers several other benefits to the pediatric patient. It is generally pain free and does not require sedation to complete; it is readily available; and it does not expose the patient to ionizing radiation. Furthermore, published data support its use with respect to improved patient care and patient satisfaction with decreased ED lengths of stay. Although a substantial amount of pediatric-specific research exists, its growing use will necessitate further investigation to determine which adult applications can be adopted in children. Innovative development of sound bedside ultrasound examinations specific to the pediatric patient will also be required.

ADMINISTRATIVE ASPECTS

Starting an Ultrasound Program

The process of implementing an ultrasound program requires ED leadership, a partnership with hospital leadership in clinical care, and support for an appropriate credentialing and quality assurance protocol. Appointment or recruitment of a point person who either is already well trained in bedside ultrasound or is prepared to undertake additional ultrasound training is a first step. Responsibilities of the lead person are to develop the skills necessary to conduct the evaluation and teach other clinicians and to work to set the standards by which to judge competencies as the program grows.

Second, starting a program is best done in concert with hospital leadership, including radiology and surgery and with the hospital physician–credentialing committee leaders. Whenever possible, evidence-based data should be employed to justify implementation of specific bedside ultrasound examinations. There must be a consensus that this will improve patient outcomes and will be of high quality.

Third, the program requires an ultrasound system designed for the purposes of ED usage, which should be immediately available. Staff and trainees must be able to put what they have learned into use, and only those who perform ultrasound scans routinely will gain sufficient facility to incorporate it into their everyday practice. There are now many companies that recognize the need for ED-specific machines and have numerous quality products that cater to this niche.

Although some standards for training in ultrasound have been published, there is still debate among different governing bodies as to minimal requirements. Guidelines from the American College of Radiology and the American Institute of Ultrasound in Medicine are geared toward comprehensive, diagnostic examinations and are not applicable to emergency bedside ultrasound. ACEP has published consensus guidelines based on expert opinion and previous published data that have now become the current standard for emergency medicine. In general, programs should establish a minimum number of didactic hours, a minimum number of overall ultrasound examinations, and a minimum number of examinations to look for a specific finding. These requirements will form the basis of the credentialing process for staff physicians.

Equipment Considerations

Most important, the anticipated type of ultrasound scans should guide the purchasing of all equipment. If a machine were being purchased only for vascular access, then one with a high-quality cardiac application would not be justified. There are ultrasound systems that are tailored to the practice of emergency medicine, and the technology is ever advancing. All machines should be portable and maneuverable enough to fit into the cramped spaces of an ED. A cart-based system is ideal for ease of movement, changing of probes, storage space, and housing considerations. A device's ease of use is important, as the more complicated systems may intimidate novice users and be a roadblock to gaining experience. Other factors to consider when buying a system include durability, image quality, storage capability, power supply (battery option), boot-up times, and service plans.

There are numerous types of transducers (probes) from which to choose. Transducers are generally classified based on frequency, with low-frequency probes for improved penetration (but poorer image quality) and high-frequency probes for better image resolution (but weaker penetration into deep tissue). Transducers should be purchased based on the anticipated type of ultrasound examinations. For example, if a significant percentage of patients present with pregnancy-related complaints, an endocavitary probe would be warranted. The footprint of the probe should also be considered. The footprint is that portion of the probe that comes into contact with the skin and sends out the ultrasonic waves. Probes with a large footprint can give a wider field of view but are difficult to fit into the small intercostals spaces of infants and children. Generally speaking, at least two probes should be considered essential when purchasing an ultrasound machine, a low-frequency probe that can be used for abdominal and cardiac examinations, and a high-frequency linear probe that can be used for procedural applications (Fig. 134.1).

ULTRASOUND BASICS

Ultrasound Physics

This section will review the basic principles to help lead to a higher comfort level with machine operation and to greater facility with image acquisition and interpretation.

Ultrasound refers to sound waves that have a frequency greater than 20,000 Hz (the upper range of audible sound). Frequencies used in diagnostic and procedural ultrasound generally range from 2 to 15 MHz. The general principle of diagnostic ultrasound is the pulse–echo effect. Sound waves

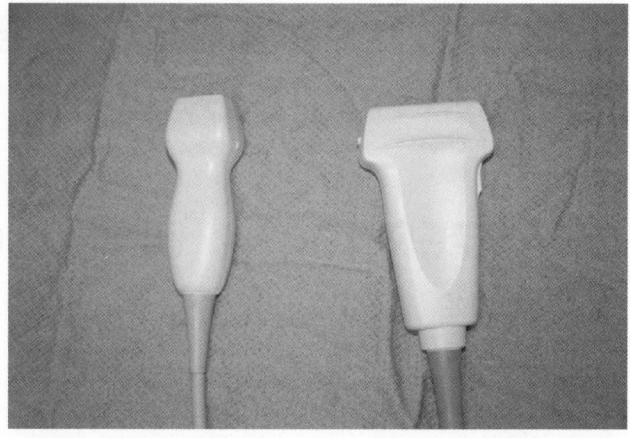

FIGURE 134.1 On the left is a low-frequency phased array probe commonly used in cardiac or abdominal applications. On the right is a high frequency linear probe used for procedures and identifying superficial structures.

are generated from the transducer and sent into a medium (the body). The transducer then "listens" for the return, or echo, of that sound. The emitted sound wave encounters the body tissues, with different densities at different distances from the surface of the skin. Some of the wave is reflected back to the transducer footprint. Once the transducer "hears" a returning echo, the ultrasound system calculates the distance of an object from the transducer on the basis of the time it took the echo to return. The intensity of the returning sound wave determines the grayscale assignment on the image. For example, fluid does not reflect sound waves at all, leading a fluid-filled bladder to appear black or anechoic (i.e., the transducer did not "hear" any sound waves reflected back). The diaphragm is highly reflective and appears bright on the screen (Fig. 134.2). The overall ultrasound image consists of all the pixels on the screen that are generated in this fashion.

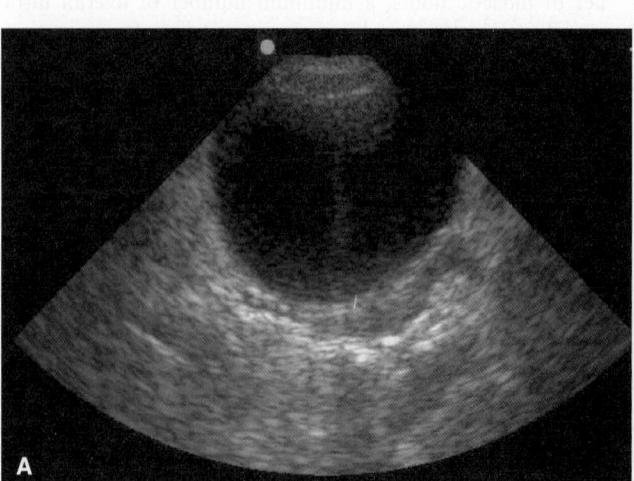 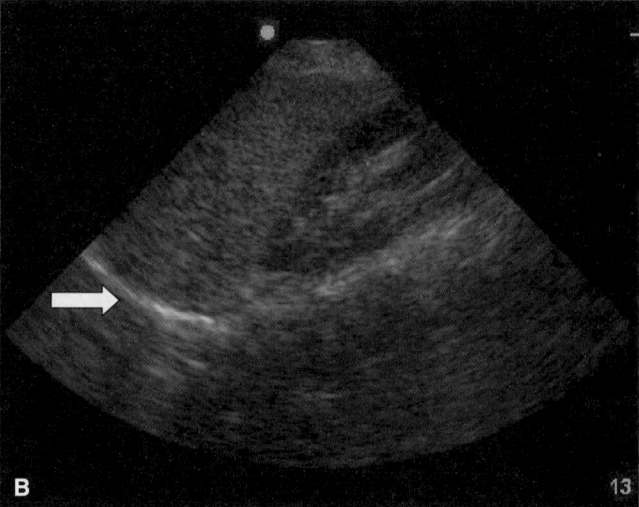

FIGURE 134.2 **A:** A full bladder. Note that fluid is anechoic *(black)*. **B:** Morison's pouch. Note the bright reflection of the diaphragm just superior to the liver *(arrow)*.

Basic Controls

Ultrasound machines, at first glance, can appear complicated with the presence of multiple buttons and knobs, and it remains important to gain an understanding of the equipment to avoid being overwhelmed or disheartened. The good news is that the controls simply allow one to adjust and optimize the image on the basis of the basic principles of the ultrasound image.

Gain refers to the intensity of the returning echoes on the display screen. Adjusting the gain essentially changes the brightness without improving the quality of the image. *Depth* of the image can be adjusted as well. For superficial structures, decreasing the depth allows for higher image quality, increasing the size on the screen of the structure under scrutiny and reducing wasted space on the screen. Increasing the depth allows for visualization of deeper structures (i.e., farther away from the skin and transducer). *Zoom* allows the sonographer to magnify a section on the display screen. This can be especially useful when attempting to focus on smaller, deeper structures, such as foreign bodies. Finally, the *freeze* button allows the sonographer to hold an image. On most machines, several seconds of memory are saved when the freeze function is used, and the image can be toggled forward and backward to find a desired image.

Other control panel functions on ultrasound machines vary widely but often include color flow, Doppler, motion-mode (m-mode), focus, and tissue harmonics. As the practitioner gains more and more experience, these machine capabilities will become more familiar and will allow for more advanced applications of emergency bedside ultrasound.

General Scanning Techniques

One of the greatest advantages of ultrasound is that it is dynamic, with the ability to capture images in multiple imaging planes and different orientations. However, because this may lead to confusion in interpretation, standard and consistent orientation should be used whenever possible.

The standard ultrasound examination is performed with the sonologist and machine on the right-hand side of the patient's bed. The probe should be held in the right hand and ultrasound system adjustments made with the left hand during scanning.

All transducers have some marking that correlate with a dot (or some other identifier) on the monitor screen (Fig. 134.3). By convention, the transducer marker is always placed on the patient's right-hand side in transverse views and on the cephalad side in sagittal views and the dot on the screen is located at top, left side of the monitor (with the exception of cardiac scanning). Adhering to this principle allows for uniformity of images and makes interpretation and review more seamless. Objects that are closer to the probe marker appear closer to the dot on the monitor and vice versa.

Most ultrasound imaging is performed in B-mode (brightness), which is the standard, 2-D representation of the reflected ultrasound waves. As mentioned above, each pixel represents the intensity of echo (black, no echo; white, very echogenic) and distance from the probe (determined by time of a returning sound wave). M-mode (motion) creates a single

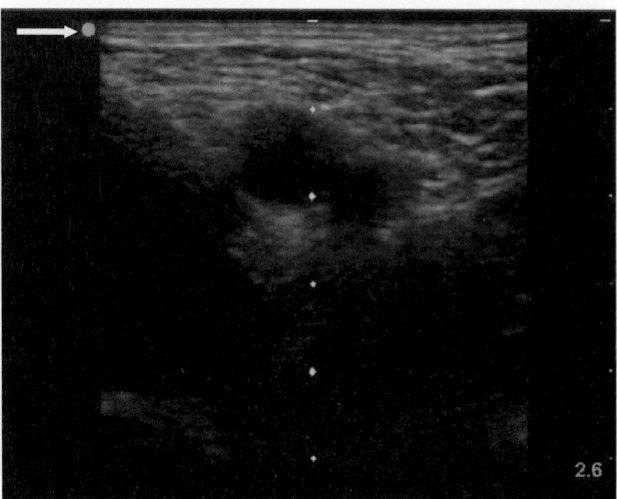

FIGURE 134.3 Image of femoral anatomy. Note the marker on the screen *(arrow)* is a large at upper left dot. By convention, the marker should always be on the left, upper side of the monitor.

line of a sound wave through an object of interest and then displays the grayscale image along that vertical scanning line with respect to time on the horizontal access. M-mode is useful to document movement of a structure, such as cardiac valves or the fetal heart.

Finally, Doppler senses the movement of the ultrasound waves as they encounter a moving medium, represented by either color changes or audible sound generated by the ultrasound machine. Doppler ultrasound is especially useful when identifying vessels, discerning between arterial and venous flow or possible vessel obstruction.

DIAGNOSTIC EXAMINATIONS

Focused Assessment with Sonography in Trauma

Introduction

The use of sonography in trauma was one of the very first applications of emergency bedside ultrasound, and many now consider it a standard part of the evaluation of the injured patient. The basic sonographic question when performing the FAST examination is: "Is there free fluid in the peritoneum or pericardium?" Initially, the FAST scan was meant to detect peritoneal blood in patients with blunt or penetrating abdominal injuries. The FAST scan has evolved to include a view of the pericardial space and, in some cases, the pleural space (referred to as the *enhanced FAST* or *eFAST*). The overarching principle of the examination is that hemoperitoneum or hemopericardium is an indication of organ injury in the setting of blunt or penetrating torso trauma. Blood in the abdomen or thorax will appear hypoechoic or anechoic (dark) against the hyperechoic (bright) background of the internal organs (Fig. 134.4). Thus, the detection of peritoneal or pericardial fluid by sonography may be evidence of injury to the abdominal organs or heart, respectively.

PROCEDURES

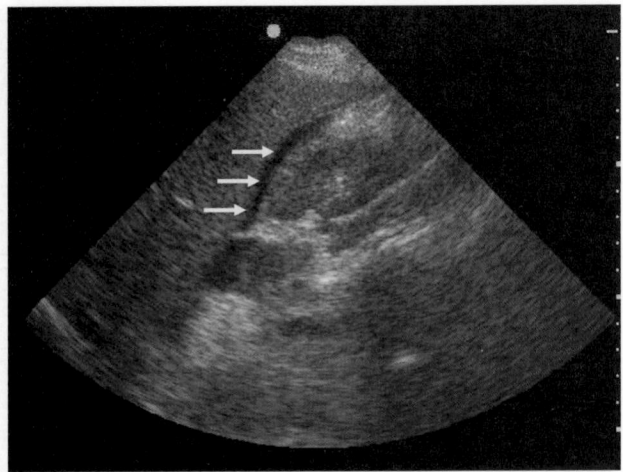

FIGURE 134.4 A positive FAST examination. Note the anechoic stripe of fluid *(arrows)* in Morison's pouch, between the liver and kidney. FAST indicates focused assessment with sonography in trauma.

Although computed tomography (CT) remains the study of choice for the stable pediatric patient with suspected intraabdominal injury, the FAST scan has several distinct advantages. First, it can be performed immediately at the bedside and is interpreted by the person performing the test, who is privy to the clinical context. Second, there is no exposure to the ionizing radiation of CT. Sedation, which may be required for CT scan, is not required. The FAST scan can be repeated with serial examinations as the patient condition changes. Last, for unstable patients, CT is often not a viable option and the FAST scan can frequently provide valuable information that may guide therapeutic or operative interventions.

Research pertaining to the FAST scan has been plentiful, mainly focused in the adult population, with several pediatric studies. Published data indicate that the sensitivity of FAST scan in children is not as robust as in adults but indicate that specificity remains very high. Thus, a positive FAST scan should always prompt either further investigation or therapeu-

tic intervention. A negative FAST scan does not necessarily obviate the need for CT scan but still be valuable in patients with a low pretest probability of intraabdominal injury.

Anatomy

When supine, there are several dependent areas of the peritoneal cavity where blood or fluid has a tendency to accumulate. The hepatorenal recess, also known as *Morison's pouch*, is the space located between the liver and right kidney. In a normal person, this is a potential space and, thus, fluid is not usually found here. The splenorenal recess is the space located between the spleen and left kidney. Again, no fluid should be seen here in the healthy person. The rectovesical pouch (male patients) and the pouch of Douglas (female patients) are formed by the space between the rectum and bladder or uterus, respectively. These potential spaces form the basis of the FAST abdominal views (Fig. 134.5).

In the supine patient, free fluid from the right upper quadrant will tend to collect in Morison's pouch first, but free fluid from the left upper quadrant will often accumulate in the left subphrenic space initially (i.e., not the splenorenal recess). The amount of intraperitoneal fluid needed for detection by ultrasound has been reported to be as little as 100 mL in adults and will depend on the source of the bleeding and patient positioning.

Technique (Also See Chapter 135 Procedure 13.2)

Probe selection is the first step. Any low-frequency (2–5 MHz) probe should be chosen for adequate penetration. Most commonly, a large footprint (the transducer head) curvilinear probe is used. In pediatric trauma, however, the smaller head of a phased array probe or microconvex probe may be more useful to obtain images in the small intercostals spaces.

There are 4 views of the FAST examination: (i) hepatorenal recess or Morison's pouch, (ii) splenorenal recess, (iii) pelvic/bladder view, and (iv) subcostal pericardial view (Fig. 134.6). Many are now also incorporating views of the thorax to assess for hemothorax or pneumothorax, referred to as the enhanced FAST or eFAST. The sonographer should perform the FAST

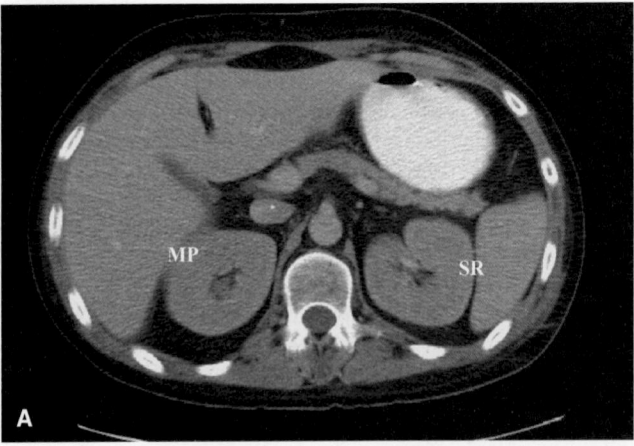
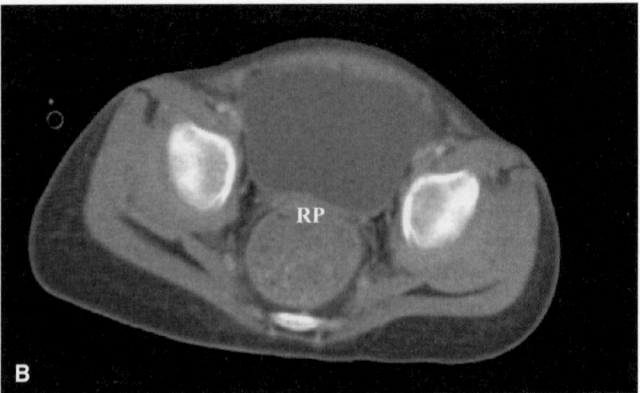

FIGURE 134.5 **A:** Computed tomography cross-sectional view of abdominal anatomy. Note the dependent areas of Morison's pouch (MP) and the splenorenal recess (SR). **B:** Pelvic anatomy. Note the dependent rectovesical pouch (RP) between the posterior wall of the bladder and stool-filled rectum.

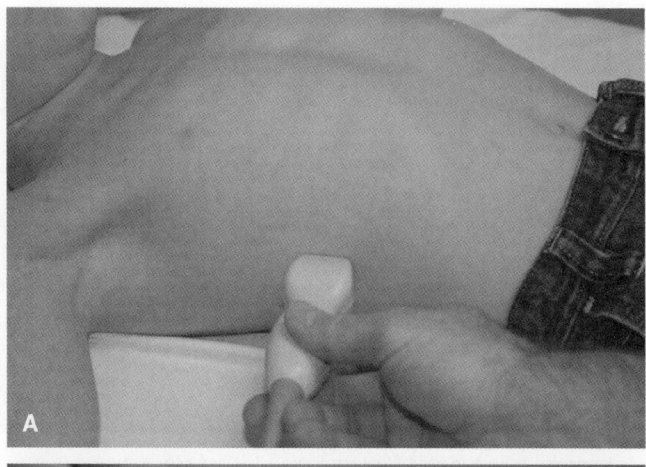

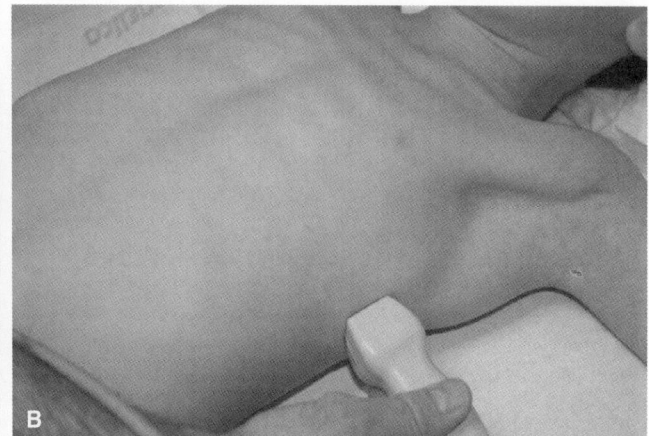

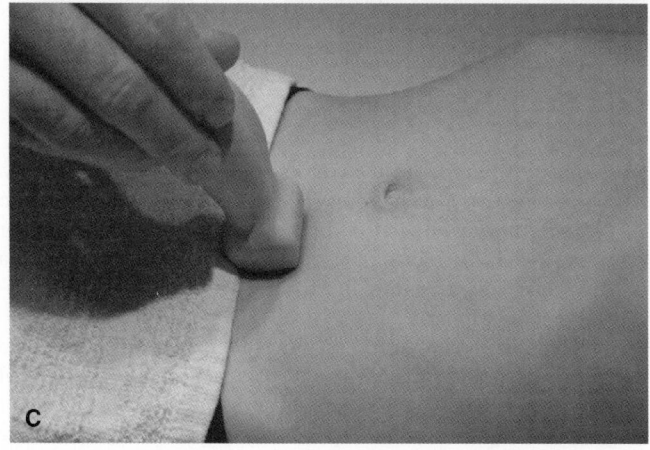

FIGURE 134.6 Probe positions for the abdominal FAST scan. **A:** Morison's pouch, **(B)** splenorenal recess, and **(C)** pelvis. FAST indicates focused assessment with sonography in trauma.

examination in a systematic manner in a standard sequence. This will allow greater focus on image acquisition and optimization as the examination order becomes routine.

A view of Morison's pouch can be obtained by placing the probe coronally (marker toward the patient's head) in the anterior axillary line between the seventh and ninth ribs on the patient's right-hand side. If rib shadows prevent optimal images, the probe can be rotated slightly in a counterclockwise fashion such that the head is oriented in between and parallel to the ribs. Once the hepatorenal recess comes into view, the probe can be moved superiorly toward the head and inferiorly toward the feet to visualize Morison's pouch completely, as well as the inferior portions of the liver and kidney (Fig. 134.7). As mentioned earlier, blood will tend to accumulate in these dependent portions of the peritoneal cavity initially.

The splenorenal recess is a more difficult view to obtain. Because the left kidney sits more superior and posterior than the right kidney, starting position for the probe is the coronal plane (marker to the patient's head) between the fifth and seventh ribs in the posterior axillary line on the left. Rotation of the probe slightly should help avoid rib shadows. In this view, blood will frequently accumulate between the spleen and diaphragm, so it is important to visualize the superior portion of the spleen in addition to the splenorenal junction (Fig. 134.8).

The pelvic view is obtained by placing the probe transversely (marker to the patient's right), just above the symphysis pubis and angling the probe inferiorly toward the feet. A full bladder will appear as a large anechoic structure and free fluid will be seen either posterior to or superior to the bladder wall (Fig. 134.9). For this reason, a sagittal view visualizing the superior bladder wall is always necessary for a complete examination.

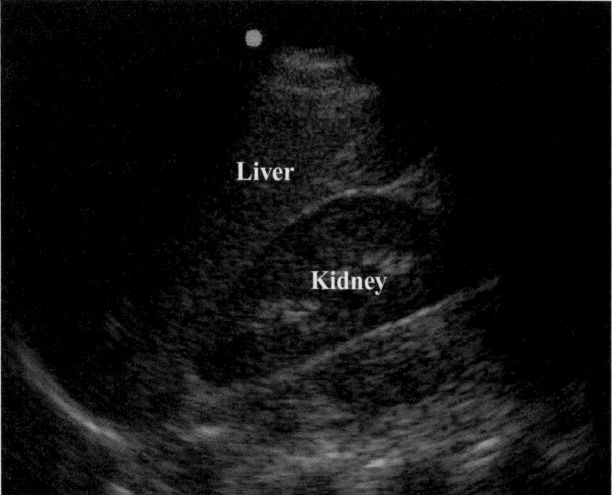

FIGURE 134.7 Normal view of Morison's pouch. In a positive study, there would be an anechoic *(dark)* stripe between the liver and kidney (see Figure 134.4).

PROCEDURES

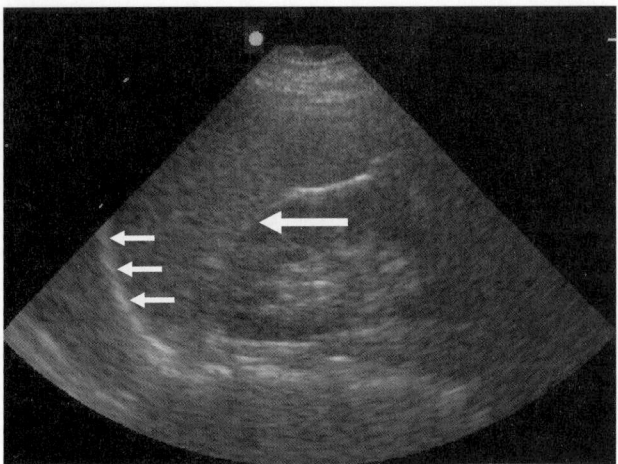

FIGURE 134.8 Normal view of splenorenal junction. Fluid may accumulate between the spleen and the kidney *(single arrow)* or between the spleen and the diaphragm *(multiple arrows)*.

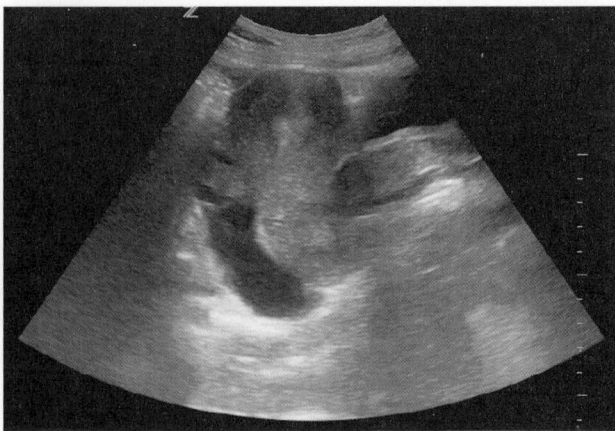

FIGURE 134.9 Positive FAST pelvic view. FAST indicates focused assessment with sonography in trauma.

Finally, the subcostal or subxiphoid view of the heart is obtained. It is important to remember that the heart sits slightly rotated in the thorax, with the right ventricle most anterior and the left ventricle posterior and toward the patient's left hip. The transducer should lie almost parallel to the abdomen, just below the xiphoid process, with the marker to the patient's right-hand side and angled toward the left shoulder (Fig. 134.10). The probe can be slid rightward along the inferior portion of the rib to avoid the acoustic artifacts caused by air in the stomach, using the liver as an acoustic window instead. The normal pericardium is seen as a hyperechoic (bright) line surrounding the heart. Pericardial fluid will appear as an anechoic collection between the myocardium and bright pericardium (Fig. 134.11). A more detailed description of bedside echocardiography is discussed in the next section.

Pitfalls

For the Morison's pouch and splenorenal recess views, the most common difficulty arises from rib shadows. The probe can be rotated about 20 degrees such that the orientation of

the head is parallel to the course of the rib above and below. The probe can also be moved either anterior or posterior to optimize images. It is also important to recognize the inferior vena cava in the right upper quadrant scan. The inferior vena cava can mimic free fluid in Morison's pouch for the inexperienced sonographer.

The splenorenal recess is more difficult to visualize than Morison's pouch because of the relative superior position of the left kidney and smaller spleen size. Often, the probe is not positioned posterior or cephalad enough to visualize these structures.

A frequent pitfall with the pelvic view is the inability to visualize the bladder. Sometimes the bladder is empty (i.e., when a Foley catheter has been placed). More often, the probe is positioned too superior and should be slid and/or angled toward the feet. Less commonly, the bladder is off of midline to the right or left.

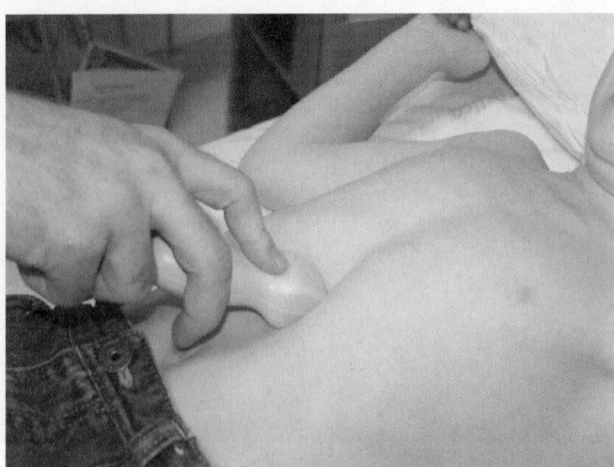

FIGURE 134.10 Probe position for the FAST subxiphoid cardiac view. FAST indicates focused assessment with sonography in trauma.

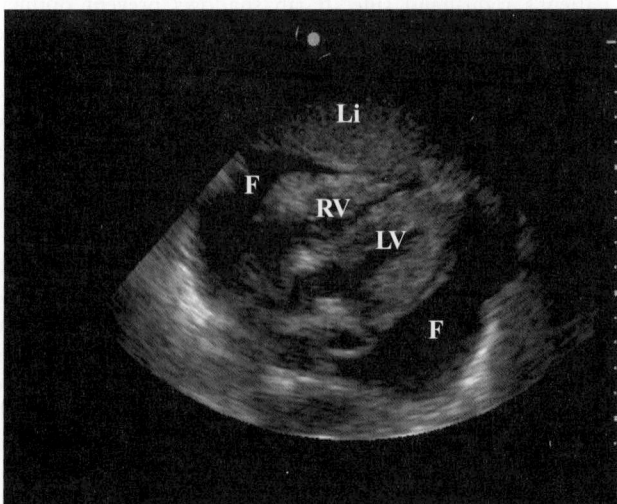

FIGURE 134.11 Pericardial effusion: An anechoic fluid collection *(F)* surrounds the myocardium. Note the liver *(Li)*, right ventricle *(RV)*, and left ventricle *(LV)*.

There are several reasons why a sonographer may not view the heart during the cardiac examination. First, the depth has not been adjusted from the abdominal scans. The abdominal organs lie relatively closer to the skin than the heart does to the subxiphoid process, and thus, the heart will often be deeper than the maximal depth set on the monitor. By increasing the depth prior to the cardiac scan, the heart will come into view easily. Second, the angle of the probe may be too steep. Remember that from the subcostal position, the heart lies superiorly and the head of the transducer must be pointed in that direction. Third, air from the stomach can scatter the ultrasound beams, rendering the image unreadable. The probe should be slid to the patient's right, away from the stomach, thereby using the liver as an acoustic window instead.

Cardiac

Introduction

Cardiac ultrasound as part of the FAST examination was one of the first applications of bedside ultrasound. Subsequent to its use in trauma, however, more focused cardiac examinations have become frequent. The basic questions asked when performing focused bedside echocardiography are: (i) "Is the heart beating?" and (ii) "Is there a pericardial effusion?" As such, the two most common indications for bedside cardiac ultrasound are (i) assessing for pericardial effusions and (ii) evaluating for cardiac activity in patients with cardiac arrest or pulseless electrical activity (PEA). Although these scenarios are much less common than in the adult patient, their relative clinical importance makes cardiac ultrasound an invaluable tool when examining pediatric patients with these conditions. Evaluating global cardiac function and overall volume status can also have an immediate impact on patient care. These echocardiographic skills, however, are much more difficult to acquire and necessitate more extensive, cardiac-focused training. As such, practitioners should know their limits and use ultrasound accordingly. The purpose of focused echocardiography is to provide the clinician with immediate bedside information and is not meant to replace comprehensive, formal echocardiograms.

Much of the early research regarding emergency physician–performed echocardiography centered on the identification of pericardial effusion and cardiac activity in the pulseless patient. Numerous studies of adult patients have shown that emergency physicians can accurately identify pericardial effusions in the setting of both traumatic and nontraumatic etiologies. In penetrating chest trauma, early identification of pericardial effusion has been shown to dramatically improve patient outcomes. Although case reports exist, there have been no prospective studies evaluating the use of bedside ultrasound to identify pericardial effusions in the pediatric emergency department.

In adult patients with cardiac arrest, the use of ultrasound has been shown to be valuable. Patients with PEA who have cardiac activity demonstrated on bedside ultrasound are more likely to survive when compared with patients with cardiac standstill. Because cardiac arrest is such a rare event in children, prospective studies have not been performed and single-institution protocols may not be practical in pediatric patients. Studies of adults indicate that emergency bedside ultrasound may be valuable in guiding resuscitative efforts or identifying life-threatening causes of PEA such as cardiac tamponade.

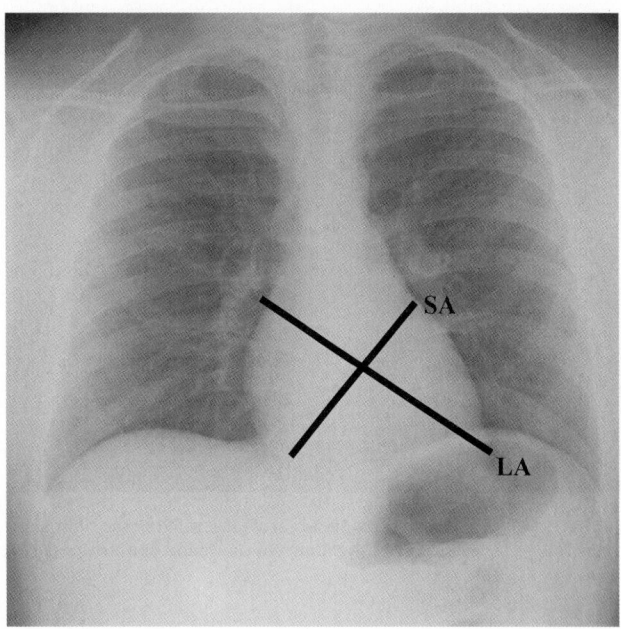

FIGURE 134.12 Ultrasound axes of the heart. Long axis *(LA)* and short axis *(SA)*.

Anatomy

The standard terminology used in other ultrasound examinations is less useful when discussing cardiac ultrasound due to the position of the heart in the thorax. Instead, standard views are along two different cardiac planes. The cardiac long axis views the heart along its plane from the atria to apex. The short axis cuts across the heart from anterior to posterior, along the plane from the right hip to the left shoulder (Fig. 134.12). These axes form the basis for the standard cardiac views used in emergency bedside echocardiography.

Technique (See Also Chapter 135, Procedure 13.4)

The subcostal or subxiphoid view is the same view as obtained when performing the FAST examination. A low-frequency (2–5 MHz) curvilinear or phased array probe should be chosen. Phased array probes (Fig. 134.1) are more ideal for moving structures such as the heart. Furthermore, smaller footprint probes may prove useful when attempting cardiac views in between rib spaces of pediatric patients.

Some controversy still exists in emergency medicine as to the direction of the probe marker and location of the marker indicator on the monitor. This author has found that for the novice sonographer, keeping the "dot" on the left side of the screen and marker toward the patient's right for the subcostal four-chamber view maintains consistency and convention. Classic echocardiography dictates the opposite approach, with the probe marker directed leftward and the marker indicator on the right side of the machine. In both instances, the same image orientation will appear on the screen.

Recall that the heart lies obliquely in the chest, with the apex pointed toward the left hip. The subcostal four-chamber view cuts across the heart from its atria to apex and is thus considered a long-axis image. The transducer should lie almost parallel to the abdomen, just below the xiphoid process and the head of the

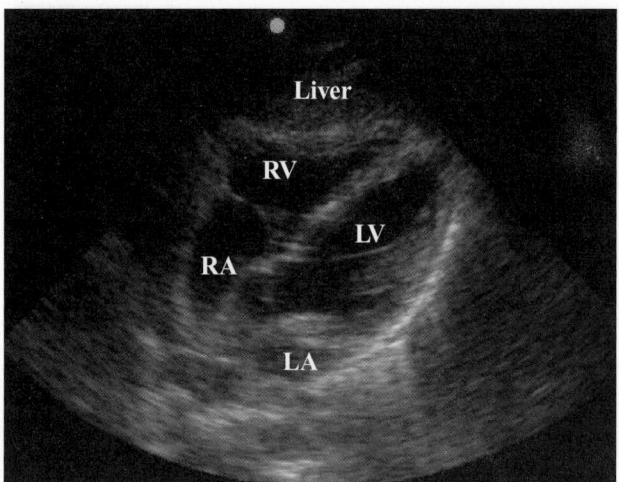

FIGURE 134.13 Normal subxiphoid cardiac view. Note the right ventricle *(RV)*, left ventricle *(LV)*, right atrium *(RA)*, and left atrium *(LA)*.

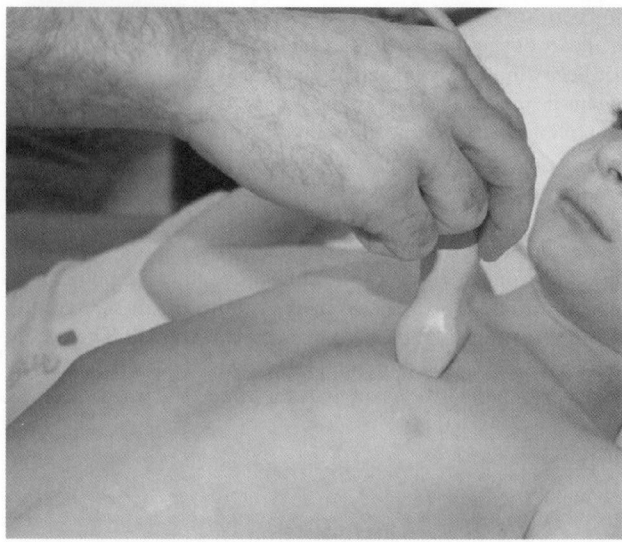

FIGURE 134.14 Probe position for the parasternal long cardiac view.

probe angled toward the left shoulder (Fig. 134.10). The probe can be slid rightward along the inferior portion of the last rib to avoid the acoustic artifacts caused by air in the stomach, using the liver as an acoustic window instead. As the ultrasound wave moves toward the left shoulder from the subxiphoid space, it will encounter the liver first, then right ventricle and right atrium, followed by the left ventricle and left atrium. The image obtained will correlate such that the liver is at the top of the screen and the left ventricle is near the bottom of the screen (Fig. 134.13). Normally, the bright white pericardium abuts the gray myocardium. When a pericardial effusion is present, a hypoechoic (dark) stripe will appear between the two (Fig. 134.11).

The left parasternal long view is obtained by placing the probe in the third or fourth intercostal space, immediately left of the sternum, with the marker pointed toward the left hip. Unlike the subcostal view in which the probe can lie almost flat, it should be perpendicular to the chest wall in the parasternal long view (Fig. 134.14). The image acquired should cut across the long axis of the heart, from the atria (right shoulder) to apex (left hip). This view can be quite useful in obese patients in whom the subcostal view is often difficult to obtain. Just as in the subcostal view, the right ventricle is the first cardiac structure encountered by the sound wave as it lies most anterior and closest to the probe (Fig. 134.15).

The subcostal and parasternal long views are the most useful when assessing for cardiac activity or pericardial effusions. Other cardiac windows include the parasternal short view and apical four-chamber view. While these can provide further information about global cardiac function and potential valvular pathology, they are beyond the scope of this chapter.

Pitfalls

There are several reasons why a sonographer may not see the heart during the cardiac examination. In the subcostal view, the heart often lies deeper than the depth set on the screen. To avoid this, the depth should be set to its maximum level and once the heart is located, the depth should be changed accordingly to optimize and center the image. In addition, the angle of the probe in the subcostal view may be too steep. Remember

that from the subxiphoid position, the heart lies superiorly, and thus the head of the transducer must be pointed in that direction, toward the left shoulder. In the subxiphoid view, air from the stomach can scatter the ultrasound beams, rendering the image useless. Slide the probe to the patient's right, away from the stomach, thereby using the liver as an acoustic window instead. In the parasternal view, rib shadows are often encountered. The probe may be shifted to the patient's left, be rotated, or be angled obliquely to better fit the transducer footprint in between adjacent ribs.

First Trimester Ultrasound

Introduction

Abdominal pain in the pregnant adolescent female is a common presenting complaint to many pediatric EDs. The differential

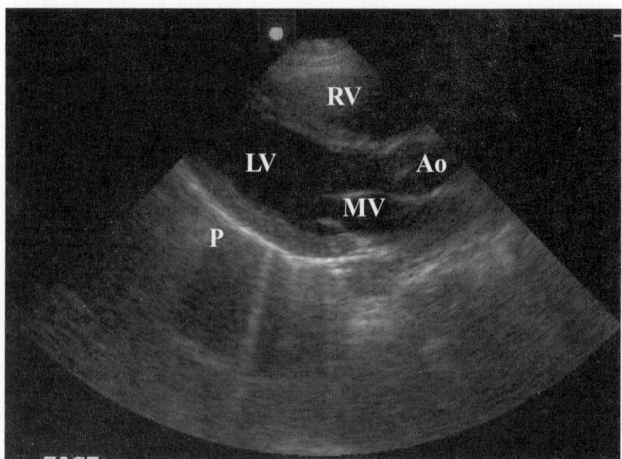

FIGURE 134.15 Normal parasternal long cardiac view. Note the right ventricle *(RV)*, left ventricle *(LV)*, mitral valve *(MV)*, aortic root *(Ao)*, and pericardium *(P)*. Fluid will accumulate just above the pericardium in a pericardial effusion.

diagnosis is broad, ranging from benign self-limited conditions to a spectrum of life-threatening and organ-threatening conditions. Ectopic pregnancy must be identified and treated rapidly. It is the leading cause of maternal mortality in the United States and has a reported prevalence as high as 8% for any pregnant patient presenting to the ED.

Multiple studies have shown emergency bedside ultrasound to be valuable in the evaluation of first-trimester pregnant women who present with vaginal bleeding or abdominal pain, specifically in *ruling in* those patients with normal intrauterine pregnancy (IUP) and, thus, ruling out ectopic pregnancy. Studies have demonstrated excellent sensitivity and specificity not only for identifying IUP by bedside ultrasound but also in shortening the time to definitive therapy and ED length of stay.

The basic question that needs to be answered in a first-trimester ultrasound is: "Is there an intrauterine pregnancy?" By visualizing an IUP, an ectopic pregnancy may be ruled out in most cases. In other words, finding the ectopic pregnancy is not the goal and is, in fact, much more difficult. In patients with increased risk of heterotopic pregnancies, confirming an IUP does not obviate the need to search for an ectopic pregnancy when there is any clinical suspicion. This subset of pregnant patients should always have a formal comprehensive ultrasound performed by the radiology or gynecology service.

The value of bedside ultrasound in the nonpregnant woman with abdominal pain is less clear. Conditions such as ovarian cysts, ovarian torsion, and tuboovarian abscesses require a greater amount of sonographic skill, and it is not yet clear that emergency physicians will identify these conditions with adequate reproducible accuracy.

Anatomy

The important anatomical consideration to remember is that the bladder lies anterior to the uterus. This relationship allows a full bladder to be used as an acoustic window to visualize the uterus. An empty bladder makes the transabdominal approach much more difficult. When the bladder is empty, the uterus will often lie more anterior and superior, making the transvaginal approach less difficult.

Technique

Before undergoing sonography for evaluation of the pregnant woman, one must consider that a pregnancy of less than 5 weeks' gestational age (3 weeks postconception) may not be visible. Either a transabdominal or transvaginal approach can be used. A low-frequency curvilinear or phased array probe should be used for the transabdominal approach. Ideally, transabdominal sonography should be performed through a distended urinary bladder, which serves as an acoustic window. This may not be practical in a busy ED. A pregnancy of 5 to 6 weeks' gestation can usually be seen. The probe should be positioned longitudinally just above the pubic symphysis and directed through the bladder to visualize a longitudinal view of the uterus, cervix, and the pouch of Douglas, with cephalad structures on the left side of the monitor (Fig. 134.16). In the nonpregnant woman, the endometrial stripe will be visualized without any uterine contents. The ovaries can often be visualized by sliding the probe laterally and directing the beam toward the opposite side. Transverse

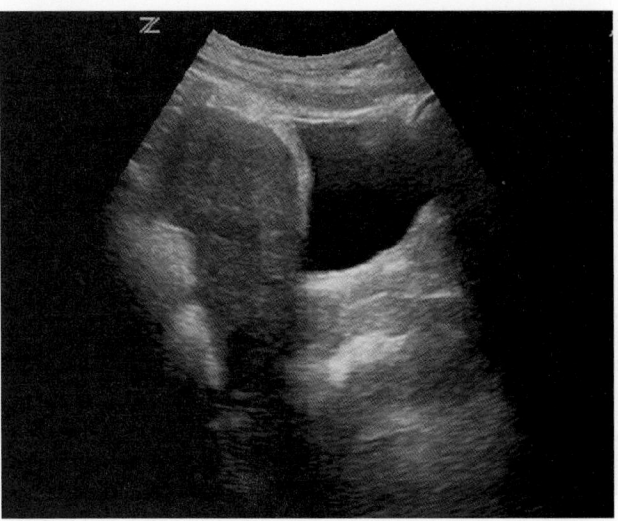

FIGURE 134.16 Normal transabdominal view of the female pelvis.

images should also be obtained and may allow for visualization of the uterus and adjacent adnexa in the same image.

An endocavitary probe should be used for the transvaginal approach. Although the transvaginal transducer is of higher frequency and produces sharper images, the field of view is more limited. The bladder should be emptied before performing the scan. After the probe is cleaned and covered, it is inserted into the vaginal canal with the marker facing up (to the sky). It often helps to have the anxious patients insert the probe into the vaginal canal themselves. A standard transvaginal longitudinal view is obtained (Fig. 134.16). Once the longitudinal view is obtained, the probe should be rotated such that the marker is to the patient's right-hand side, to obtain a transverse view. With each planar view, it is important to fan the probe along the scanning plane axes to visualize the entire body of the uterus. One with greater sonographic skill may be able to also view the fallopian tubes and ovaries, but it is important to emphasize again that the purpose of the examination is to determine whether there is an IUP or not.

In normal pregnancy, the earliest sonographic finding of an IUP is the gestational sac, which appears as a round fluid collection within the uterus (Fig. 134.17). In transabdominal scanning, the gestational sac can be seen at 5 to 6 weeks' gestational age. Transvaginal scanning can reliably detect this finding about 7 to 10 days earlier. Visualization of the gestational sac alone is not adequate in confirming an IUP. The yolk sac can be seen inside the gestational sac at approximately 6 to 7 weeks' gestational age (5 to 6 weeks by transvaginal scanning), and most authors consider this as definitive evidence of IUP. A normal embryo will appear at the margin of the yolk sac at about 6.5 to 7.5 weeks' gestational age, and cardiac activity can be detected shortly thereafter (Fig. 134.18).

In the pregnant woman, the standard for confirming an IUP for emergency physician–performed bedside ultrasound requires visualization of an intrauterine yolk sac, fetal pole, or intrauterine fetal heartbeat. Visualizing only the gestational sac is not adequate as this can be the result of hormonal stimulation from an ectopic pregnancy. When a fetal heartbeat can be seen, it should be documented with m-mode.

PROCEDURES

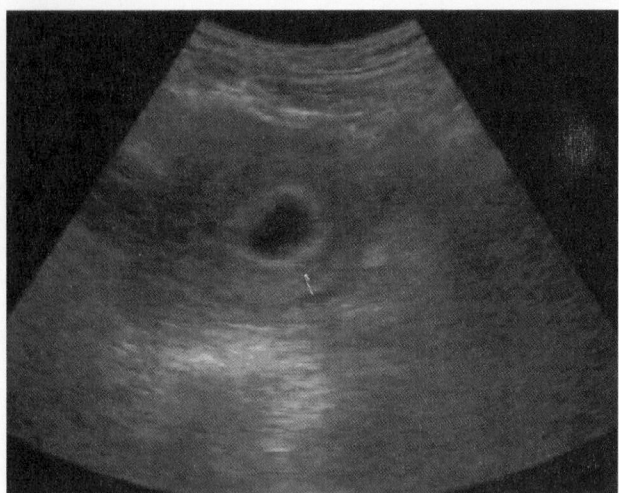

FIGURE 134.17 Normal intrauterine pregnancy with gestational sac within the uterus.

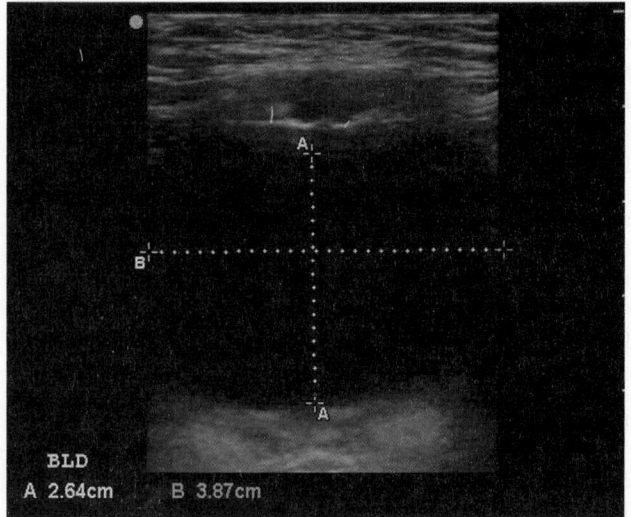

FIGURE 134.19 Full bladder measured in two different planes.

In an ectopic pregnancy, an adnexal mass or free fluid in the pelvis can sometimes be seen. Again, visualization of the ectopic pregnancy, however, should not be the goal of the emergency physician. Several protocols have been developed, addressing the use of bedside pelvic sonography in the pregnant woman. In general, if an IUP is not seen in a woman with a positive urine β-human chorionic gonadotropin (β-hCG), gynecology consultation should be arranged and a formal ultrasound conducted. A low serum-hCG level, implying an early IUP, may prompt the practitioner to arrange outpatient follow-up instead, with ectopic precautions taken.

Bladder Ultrasound

Introduction

Bladder ultrasound is performed for a variety of reasons. For the child who has not voided for a prolonged period, simply assessing bladder size can inform the practitioner whether a

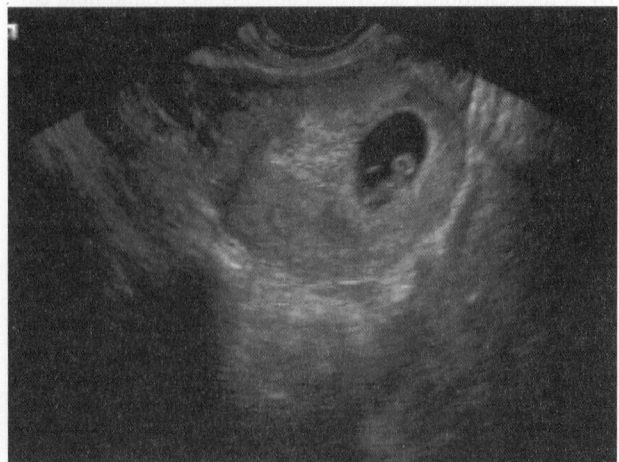

FIGURE 134.18 Normal intrauterine pregnancy with gestational sac and embryo.

problem exists and where (anatomically) it is located. More commonly, bladder ultrasound is performed prior to bladder catheterization or suprapubic aspiration to assess volume of urine and thereby improve success rates of the procedure. It may be used dynamically as well to guide needle placement during suprapubic aspiration.

Numerous studies have been conducted using ultrasound prior to both bladder catheterization and needle aspiration. Authors have found that use of ultrasound leads to increased success rates and can reliably predict successful and unsuccessful catheterizations. Similarly, ultrasound use has been shown to increase success rates of suprapubic aspiration and decrease number of needle passes when used dynamically.

Technique (See Chapter 135, Procedure 13.3)

The same approach as the pelvic view of the FAST examination should be taken when performing a bladder ultrasound. A high-frequency linear probe or low-frequency abdominal probe may be used. A full bladder will appear as a well-circumscribed, fluid-filled (anechoic) structure within the pelvis (Fig. 134.2). Once the bladder is identified, it should be measured in at least two planes (Fig. 134.19). Although studies differ with respect to exact measurements, generally speaking, if the wall-to-wall distance measures more than 2 cm in both planes, catheterization or suprapubic aspiration will likely be successful.

PROCEDURAL APPLICATIONS

Bedside ultrasound for diagnostic purposes can direct care and decision making. By contrast, use of bedside ultrasound for procedures is aimed at improving patient care. The pediatric ED is replete with opportunities in which bedside ultrasound can not only improve success rates of the procedure itself but also augment patient safety by reducing complications. It can be the driving force behind both implementing an emergency ultrasound program and compelling staff to acquire ultrasound skills.

Central Vascular Cannulation

Introduction

Utilization of ultrasound for vascular access is not a new application. Interventional radiologists and anesthesiologists have used sonography to aid in vessel cannulation for decades. More recently, it has become the standard of care for cannulating the internal jugular vein in adults in the ED. Moreover, the Agency for Healthcare Research and Quality has stated that ultrasound for central venous access is a clear opportunity for safety improvement and listed it as one of the "top 11 highly proven" patient safety practices that are not routinely practiced. This use of ultrasound represents a unique opportunity for the pediatric emergency medicine physician to reduce morbidity associated with line placement and may soon represent the standard of care for all central venous cannulation.

The literature supporting ultrasound use for central line placement is vast. In the ED setting, bedside ultrasound has been shown to increase success rates and decrease the number of procedural complications in adults. Similar reports exist in the pediatric population but not in the acute care setting. The overwhelming evidence in the adult population, however, along with the generalizability of the procedure, suggests that ultrasound is a necessary skill for the practitioner who places central venous lines in children. Given the relative infrequency of attaining central access in children when compared with adults, multiinstitutional studies may be needed to confirm the utility of ultrasound in the pediatric population.

Technique (See Chapter 135, Procedure 13.1)

A high-frequency linear probe should be used. Relevant anatomy for the particular site chosen (femoral, internal jugular) should be reviewed. It is also advisable to survey and confirm the target vessels with ultrasound before the procedure begins. Preprocedure steps are important to maximize success and include adjusting the height of the bed and positioning of the patient, positioning of the ultrasound machine, and having equipment and extra personnel ready for assistance. Aseptic technique should be used with sterile probe covers and sterile gel (if probe covers are unavailable, a sterile glove will suffice).

Either a static or dynamic approach may be used. In the static approach, the vasculature and surrounding anatomy are identified by ultrasound prior to vessel cannulation. The position of the vein should be marked on the skin at two points. The machine is then set aside and the procedure continues using the landmarks identified under ultrasound but without active ultrasound assistance. Data have shown that this method does improve success rates, although complications are less reduced when compared with the dynamic method.

The dynamic method uses ultrasound in real time to visualize the needle puncturing the vein. When using ultrasound dynamically, a one- or two-person approach can be used. The author feels that, for femoral vein catheterization, the ultrasound machine should be positioned across the bed from the side chosen. For example, when attempting to cannulate the right femoral vein, the machine should be situated across the bed, on the patient's left. This enables the proceduralists to maintain a direct line of site with both the patient and the image on the screen without having to turn their head, making the process more fluid. The marker on the transducer should face in the same direction as the marker on the screen. In other words, if the marker is on the left side of the screen (the standard convention), the probe marker should face to the *proceduralist's* left. This becomes useful when repositioning the needle; when the needle is moved toward the left of the probe, it moves toward the left side of the screen.

The vascular bundle should be identified in cross section. Color flow, Doppler, and compressibility can aid in the identification of the medially located femoral vein (Fig. 134.20, see also color plate). Ultrasound scanning during a Valsalva maneuver may make the vein larger and easier to visualize. Once the vein is identified, the sonographer should attempt to center the vein the screen. Some probes have an electronic guide that can be placed directly in the center of the image and that represents a marked point on the probe. Once the vein is positioned appropriately in the center of the screen, the finder needle can be inserted, lining up with the center of the probe. When viewed in cross section, the needle may appear as a single bright dot, with or without artifact, or not at all (Fig. 134.21). When the needle encounters the vein, tenting of the vessel wall will be seen and will "pop" back once the needle tip punctures the vessel wall. At this point, blood should be aspirated and the ultrasound probe can be laid aside as the procedure is continued in normal fashion.

The two-person technique may be easier for the more inexperienced ultrasound user. In this situation, one person is responsible for holding the probe and keeping the vein centered on the screen. The proceduralist can thus focus his attention solely at the site of puncture on the patient, without having to look away at the screen. The more experienced ultrasonographer should be the one holding the probe and centering the vein on the screen.

For internal jugular vein catheter placement, the same principles apply. Here, the machine may be placed on the same side of the procedure as this creates the most direct line of site. Once again, the vein should be identified, placed in the center of the screen, and cannulated under ultrasound guidance. Although ultrasound-guided catheter placement of the subclavian vein has been described in the literature, it is much more difficult due to the shadows created by the clavicle and should only be undertaken by the experienced sonographer.

The long-axis approach is more difficult and requires much finer movements of the transducer. Again, the short-axis approach has been shown to be more successful for the novice user and should be the method of choice for most users. For the experienced sonographer, however, the long-axis view offers the advantage of visualizing the vein (and thus needle and catheter) along its entire course of cannulation (Fig. 134.22). In general, the long axis technique should be reserved for peripheral access.

Pitfalls

While ultrasound can certainly enhance placement of a central venous catheter, there are certain caveats one must keep in mind. First, the depth of the vessel and distance the needle must travel to hit the vessel calculated should be noted. Remember that when the needle is inserted into the skin, it is traveling along the hypotenuse of a right triangle, and the distance it must traverse before hitting the vein should be calculated. This concept becomes important when the angle of

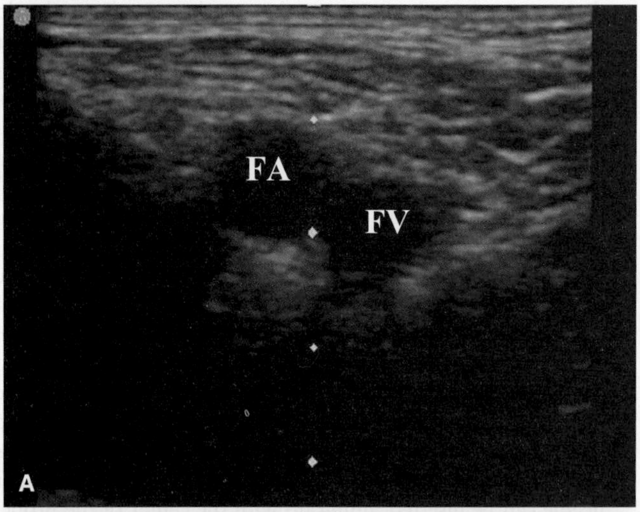

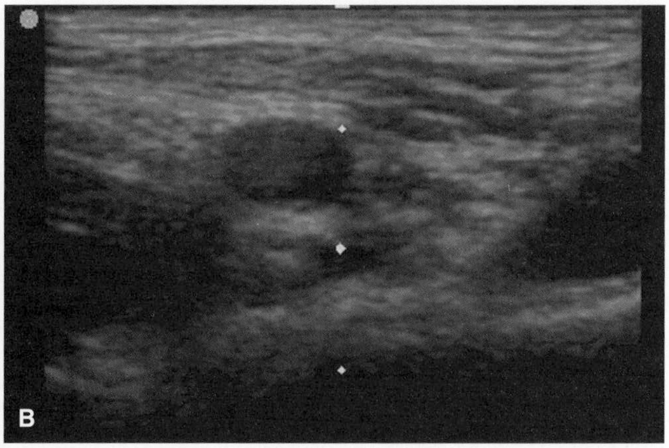

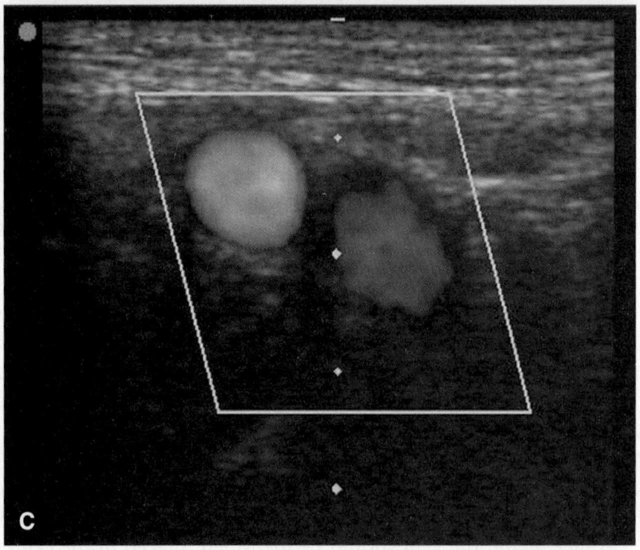

FIGURE 134.20 Femoral vascular anatomy. **A:** Femoral artery *(FA)* and femoral vein *(FV)*. **B:** During compression, the vein collapses and is not visible, whereas the artery remains patent and visible by ultrasound. **C:** The femoral artery will pulsate, whereas the vein will have low constant flow or no flow depending on the sensitivity settings of the color Doppler.

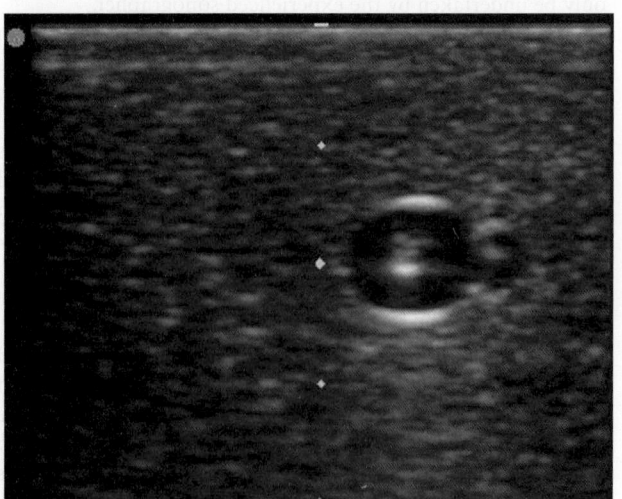

FIGURE 134.21 Transverse-axis image of a needle within a "vessel" of an ultrasound phantom model.

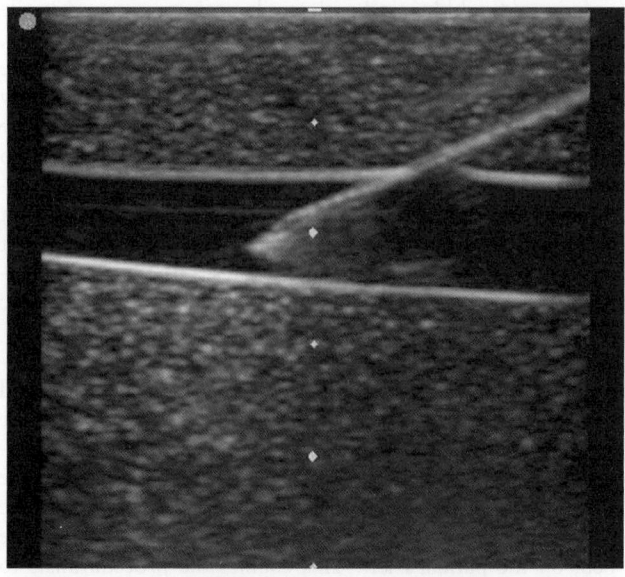

FIGURE 134.22 Long-axis image of a needle entering a vessel. Note that the entire course of the needle can be followed.

insertion is, closer to parallel to the skin surface increasing the distance the needle must travel before puncturing the vein.

Puncturing the skin either too close or too far from the transducer may be problematic. If the needle is inserted too close to the transducer, it will pass under the probe (i.e., through the plane of sound waves) before encountering the vessel. The point at which the needle contacts the vessel will not be visualized unless the probe is repositioned. If the needle is inserted into the skin too far from the transducer, it will encounter the vessel before being visualized. In the short-axis view, the transducer should always be repositioned such that the plane of ultrasound waves follows the tip of the needle. In the long-axis view, the opposite is true. As long as the transducer is correctly centered over the target vessel, the needle should be repositioned to follow the ultrasound waves. In other words, the transducer should never be repositioned to find the needle in the longitudinal view, as this may lead to cannulation of the wrong vessel (and potentially an artery).

Using ultrasound statically should be performed always *after* the patient has been positioned. Repositioning the patient after identification can lead to changed anatomic relationships and may result in failed attempts at catheterization.

The proceduralists must pay attention to both the ultrasound image on the screen and the site of the procedure. All too often, the inexperienced sonographer will focus too heavily on the screen and a flash of blood in the hub will go unnoticed. A slow and methodical approach, along with experience, can help minimize this occurrence.

Peripheral Venous Cannulation

Introduction

Peripheral intravenous catheter placement can be difficult in children as well. Multiple attempts are sometimes needed for successful placement. Ultrasound has been shown to improve. success rates of placement of peripheral catheters in adult patients who are difficult to access and to reduce failure rates when used in children. The most common anatomical sites attempted under ultrasound guidance are the brachial, cephalic, and basilic veins of the upper arm. In obese older children, ultrasound can be useful to locate the antecubital veins when palpation proves difficult.

Technique

Cannulation of the peripheral veins uses the same principles as central venous catheter placement. The desired vein for cannulation should be identified in cross section once the relevant anatomy has been reviewed. Color flow, Doppler, and compressibility should again be noted, although in smaller veins, velocity of blood flow may not be adequate to generate a color change or Doppler signal. The vein image should be centered on the screen, and catheter placement should proceed in the same fashion as central venous catheter placement.

Pitfalls

Several additional pitfalls must be considered when placing an ultrasound-guided peripheral catheter. Standard intravenous catheters are usually not long enough to reach the deeper veins of the upper arm. Long catheters are available and should be used, but even these catheters may fall out when the patient's

arm is moved because of excessive subcutaneous tissue. Second, peripheral veins are much easier to compress than central veins, and it is not uncommon for the inexperienced sonographer to apply too much pressure with the probe during the procedure, thereby compressing the vein. Third, the angle of insertion of a peripheral catheter may be shallower than that of a central catheter. One must avoid the temptation to take a steeper approach when using ultrasound guidance as this often leads to inability to advance the catheter over the needle.

Abscess Identification and Drainage

Introduction

Soft-tissue infection is not an uncommon presentation to the pediatric ED. The decision to incise and drain is often straightforward based on physical examination findings. Clinical findings are sometimes ambiguous, where an abscess may be present when only cellulitis is suspected clinically. Ultrasound has been shown to be accurate not only in correctly diagnosing abscesses but also in appropriately guiding management plans when it is unclear whether a skin infection represents an indurated cellulitis versus a fluid-filled abscess. Moreover, ultrasound can identify blood vessels that may lie near or deep to the abscess. Knowledge of important anatomical structures in close proximity allow the practitioner to proceed with caution when incising, thereby maximizing patient safety.

Technique

A high-frequency linear probe should be used. The probe should be placed directly over the site of interest to look for areas for drainage and to evaluate for nearby vascular structures. Skin infections may appear in multiple, different stages. Some are filled with thin, hypoechoic pus and are clearly ripe for drainage (Fig. 134.23), while others have a "cobblestone" appearance and need more time to coalesce (Fig. 134.24). It is advisable to conduct ultrasound with color flow over the area of interest in instances when clinically a vascular structure such as an arteriovenous malformation is possible. Once a drainable collection is identified and important surrounding structures are noted, incision and drainage may proceed in normal fashion.

Pitfalls

Some soft-tissue infections progress in stages, and in the pre-abscess phase, it may be difficult to determine if there is a drainable collection of thick pus, even with the aid of ultrasound. Abscesses are not always hypoechoic or anechoic, and clinical examination should help guide decision making when ultrasound is inconclusive.

Hematomas, inflamed lymph nodes, and vascular malformations may appear similar to abscesses on ultrasound imaging. Color flow will differentiate abscesses from vascular malformations. Lymph nodes will appear more homogenous with smoother borders and a rounded appearance (Fig. 134.25). Discerning a recent hematoma from the thick pus of an abscess can be difficult and clinical context becomes important. The experienced sonographer may notice a slightly more homogeneous appearance and the noninflamed epidermis of a hematoma.

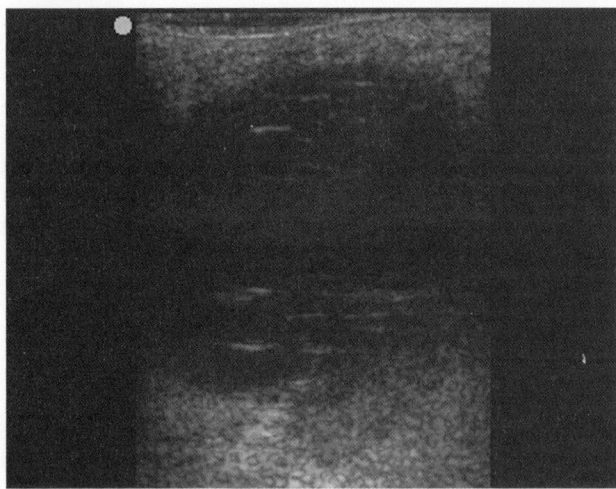

FIGURE 134.23 Pus-filled abscess.

Foreign Body Identification and Removal

Introduction

Ultrasound may be used to both identify subcutaneous foreign bodies and aid in their removal. Literature has demonstrated that physical examination can be unreliable for foreign body detection and that adjunct imaging is often required. There are numerous types of materials that will not be apparent by radiography, and ultrasound may help not only in locating these radiolucent foreign bodies but also in pinpointing a more exact location by imaging in multiple different planes.

The use of ultrasound for detection of soft-tissue foreign bodies is well established, especially when the suspicion of a radiolucent foreign body is high. Studies have demonstrated similar rates of accuracy between emergency medicine physi-

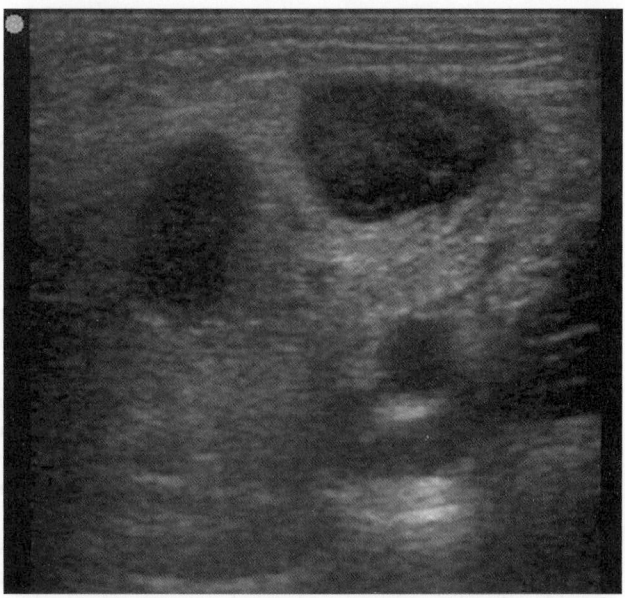

FIGURE 134.25 Inguinal lymphadenitis.

cians and more experienced personnel, as well as greater sensitivity in foreign body detection in children when using ultrasound in combination with radiography.

Technique

A high-frequency linear transducer should be used. The operator should scan over the area of interest. A foreign body may appear hyperechoic or isoechoic but with a shadow cast distal to the object (Fig. 134.26). Once the foreign body is located, the area may be marked with a pen and removal may proceed under normal fashion. Alternatively, ultrasound may be used to guide the procedure.

When ultrasound is used to guide foreign body removal, a long-axis approach should be used. The object should be identified along its long axis and the needle (for local anesthesia)

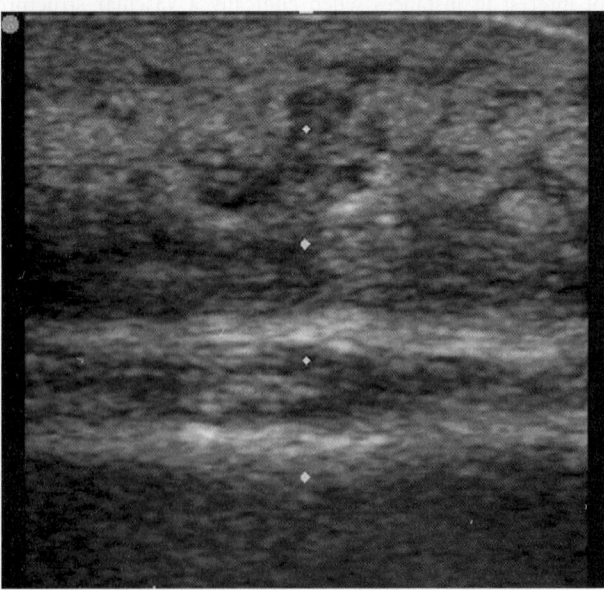

FIGURE 134.24 Ultrasound of inflamed skin with "cobblestone" appearance.

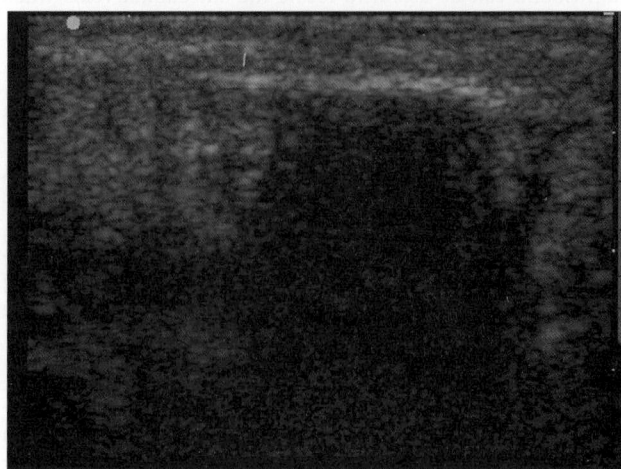

FIGURE 134.26 Bedside ultrasound was able to identify this toothpick in the foot of a pediatric patient, not identified by radiography. The hyperechoic toothpick is more obvious due to distal shadowing artifact.

inserted along that same line toward one tip of the embedded material. Once the tip of the needle comes in close contact with the tip of the object, anesthetic should be injected. This will not only anesthetize the area but also allow for better visualization of the object as it will now be surrounded by anechoic fluid. After local anesthetic is injected, forceps should be inserted along the same track and axis under ultrasound guidance. Once the object is encountered, the forceps jaws are opened slightly and the foreign body may be grasped and pulled out along the same track.

Using ultrasound dynamically to remove a foreign body is technically challenging. It requires a moderate amount of ultrasound experience and dexterity. The novice user may have greater success in identifying the foreign body statically in multiple planes, marking the site and attempting removal in standard fashion.

Suggested Readings

Review Articles

Chen L, Baker MD. Novel applications of ultrasound in pediatric emergency medicine. *Pediatr Emerg Care* 2007;23(2):115–126.
Levy JA, Noble VE. Bedside ultrasound in pediatric emergency medicine. *Pediatrics* 2008;121(5):e1404–e1412.

Cardiac

Pershad J, Myers S, Plouman C. Bedside limited echocardiography by the emergency physician is accurate during evaluation of the critically ill patient. *Pediatrics* 2004;114(6):e667–e671.

Abscess

Squire BT, Fox JC, Anderson C. ABSCESS: applied bedside sonography for convenient evaluation of superficial soft tissue infections. *Acad Emerg Med* 2005;12(7):601–606.

Trauma

Holmes JF, Gladman A, Chang CH. Performance of abdominal ultrasonography in pediatric blunt trauma patients: a meta-analysis. *J Pediatr Surg* 2007;42: 1588–1594.
Melniker LA, Leibner E, McKenney MG, et al. Randomized controlled clinical trial of point-of-care, limited ultrasonography for trauma in the emergency department: the first sonography outcomes assessment program trial. *Ann Emerg Med* 2006;48(3):227–235.

Central Venous Access

Leung J, Duffy M, Finckh A. Real-time ultrasonographically-guided internal jugular vein catheterization in the emergency department increases success rates and reduces complications: a randomized, prospective study. *Ann Emerg Med* 2006;48(5):540–547.

ACEP Guidelines

American College of Emergency Physicians. Emergency ultrasound guidelines. *Ann Emerg Med* 2009;53(4):550–570.

PROCEDURES

CHAPTER 135 ■ ILLUSTRATED TECHNIQUES OF PEDIATRIC EMERGENCY PROCEDURES

LYNN BABCOCK CIMPELLO, MD, ROBERT JAY DEUTSCH, MD, MPH, FAAP,
CINNAMON DIXON, DO, JAVIER A. GONZALEZ DEL REY, MD,
DEE HODGE III, MD, DAVID M. JAFFE, MD, LISA L. LEWIS, MD,
MATTHEW MITTIGA, MD, JOHN M. LOISELLE, MD,
CONSTANCE M. MCANENEY, MD, MS, AND RICHARD M. RUDDY, MD

1.0. PREPARATION OF THE CHILD

Proper preparation of the child and family is important to effectively perform diagnostic and therapeutic procedures on children in the emergency department (ED). Even a relatively short procedure may be very prolonged or difficult to complete without the best preparation possible. The ED staff should be prepared to team up and assist in the procedure to minimize delay, by having the necessary equipment available in the ED, and by providing the needed support. The medical team should consider whether the ED is the appropriate location and environment in which to care for the consequences and complications of a procedure, particularly one in a high-risk patient or where the length of the procedure depletes resources or would suggest doing it more safely in the operating suite. Delay in care for other potentially ill or injured children must be minimized.

Except when the procedure is immediately necessary for a life-threatening emergency, approval and support for the procedure should be obtained from the child and parents beforehand. An informative, efficient discussion of risks and benefits of the procedure for a particular child almost always reassures the parents of the need for the procedure. Written consent may not be necessary for all simple procedures, but it is key for the ED to have standards around which procedures require this to be completed, what defines the emergency to forgo the written consent, and under what conditions the minor should also assent. During the advanced life support of resuscitation or other life-threatening situation, the ED staff should provide a professional staff member to privately prepare the family for the ensuing issues and questions.

The child's developmental maturity should be assessed to determine how capable the child is of understanding and cooperating in the performance of the procedure. Substantial variations in developmental age also affect the fears of children. Specifically, the parents need to understand the risk–benefit ratio of the procedure being performed, the need for it to be done safely and with the best success. This may require tools such as guided imagery or forms of hypnosis such as performed by child life specialists, the need for pharmacologic sedation, and the need for the use of various well-known physical or mechanical restraints to minimize discomfort and maximize safety and efficiency. The parents should be made aware of possible complications, the effects of sedation and of equipment that will be attached to their child, and any discomfort subsequent to the procedure. The assurance that restraint may minimize repeated discomfort cannot be overemphasized. It needs to be emphasized that the ED staff and clinician should be prepared to set up and perform the procedure with a positive attitude.

Lastly, prior to starting a procedure on any patient the use of a team time-out prior to starting needs to part of the culture of performing procedures to maximize safety. The use of a check list followed by a time-out to make sure that the right procedure is being done on the right patient, on the right anatomic location.

1.1. RESTRAINTS

Indications

Restraint should be considered in the performance of all procedures in which patients may be unmanageable; it is possible that they may directly hurt themselves or may indirectly delay important treatment. Physical restraints are usually more effective than human restraints and may be necessary in a proportion of infants, toddlers, and preschool children. In conjunction with restraint, standard methods of pharmacologic sedation and local anesthetic are often indicated. Clearly, the use of anxiety-reducing methods by trained staff, as well as the continued calm presence of the parents, may be of great benefit to the child.

Complications

1. Bruising, edema
2. Vascular compromise (too tight a restraint or restraint for excessive time)
3. Mistrust and future medical procedure fears (if not discussed truthfully or if highly traumatized)
4. Airway compromise or musculoskeletal injury (rare except in high-risk patients or with unsafe restraint practice)

Procedure

Papoose

Figure 1.1A represents the example of the papoose, which is commonly used for restraint during repair of lacerations and other wounds. It is used to expose the head, face, and extremities with minimal discomfort to the child. In recent years, with child life presence many centers have narrowed the use of this tool a good deal. After explaining the procedure to the family, open the papoose across the ED stretcher. Place the child supine on the papoose and expose the body area necessary for treatment. Beginning with the midabdominal restraints, cover the child across the midline with the Velcro-lined sides (Fig. 1.1A). Better exposure of the extremities, such as the hand, is obtained by flexion of the area under the harness (Fig. 1.1B). Before starting a wound repair or other procedure, reassess for the safety and adequacy of the immobilization of the child and correct it if necessary.

Mummy Wraps

The mummy wrap is an alternative restraint to use for treating emergency problems of the head, especially minor trauma. By slight variation, it also provides access to the distal extremities. Prepare the patient and family for the procedures. Fold a bedsheet on itself so the width measures from the axillae to the heel of the child. Stand the child on the bed and place the bedsheet behind his/her back, under the axilla, and in front of the arms as in Figure 1.1C, with the short end of the sheet tucked behind one

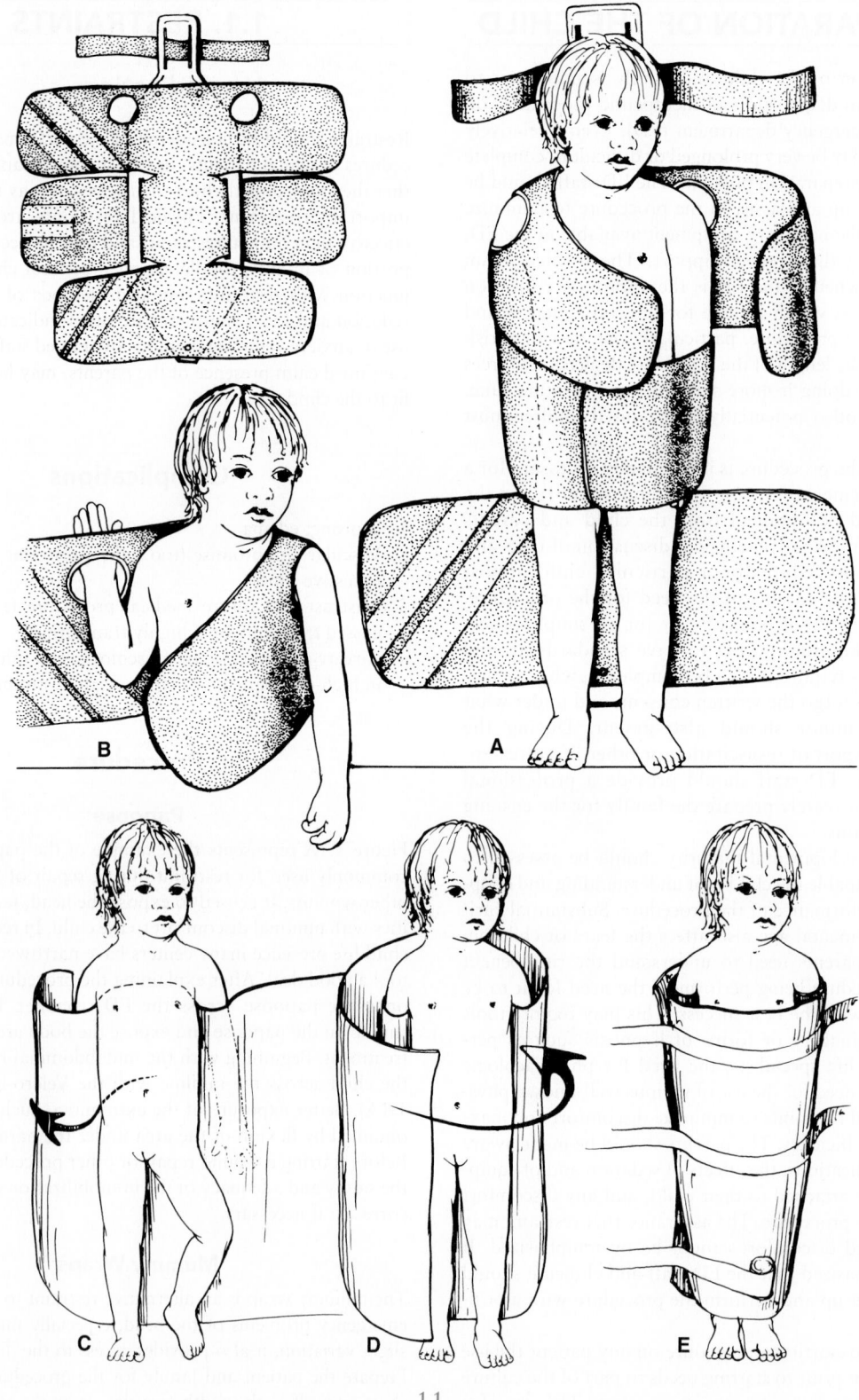

1.1

arm around the child's back. With the child standing, wrap the long end of the sheet on the child's other side, around the back to the front and across the trunk again, finishing behind the child, as in Figure 1.1D. Lay the child supine or prone to best expose the injury to be treated. Extend several lengths of 2- or 3-in wide

adhesive tape across the patient, attaching it to the sides of the stretcher to firmly hold the child's trunk in place (Fig. 1.1E). In some settings, using the mummy wrap inside of a papoose without the need for adhesive tape is an excellent alternative. An injured extremity can be left out of the wrap for better exposure.

Head Box

A head box can be placed behind the head and along the sides to help keep the child's head midline when supine. It will fit under the papoose, and the side should fit snugly (not tightly) on the lateral aspect of the child's head. It is of great value when repairing facial lacerations in young infants. Be careful that the head box is not excessively tight.

Restraint by Personnel

Many physical methods can be used to restrain children for simple emergency procedures. Often, a single assistant can grasp and immobilize a child. The specific positioning for procedures is illustrated with individual procedures. The assistant's hold must be firm enough to prevent movement that would make the procedure more difficult to perform or more likely to induce complications. Though uncommon, the use of excessive force may cause superficial or more serious injury.

2.1. EXTERNAL JUGULAR VENIPUNCTURE

Indications

Venous blood sampling in infants generally younger than 2 years of age with inadequate peripheral veins on the extremities or during resuscitation measures at any age

Complications

1. Hematoma
2. Pneumothorax (apical)
3. Infection

Equipment

Butterfly (21 to 23 gauge); 5- to 10-mL syringe; povidone–iodine or chlorhexidine solution; 70% alcohol; sterile gauze

Procedure

Place the infant on the examining table in the supine position with the infant's shoulders 7 to 10 cm from the end of the table. Have the assistant lean over the patient to stabilize the trunk. The assistant then holds the shoulder ipsilateral to the external jugular vein to be punctured with one hand and places the other hand over the ipsilateral zygoma and forehead, turning the head toward the contralateral shoulder and dropping the head 15 to 20 degrees over the table top.

Attach the butterfly to the syringe and check for patency. Cleanse the skin over the vein circumferentially with the povidone–iodine or chlorhexidine solution. After drying, povidine–iodine may be wiped off with alcohol and them the skin dried with sterile gauze. If the vein is not easily visualized in this position, it may be necessary to stimulate the infant to Valsalva or to cry to improve filling and visualization of the blood vessel. Align the butterfly needle parallel to the vessel as

shown in Figure 2.1, and pierce the skin near the white circle shown overlying or just next to the vein approximately one half to two thirds of the distance between the angle of the jaw and the clavicle. The puncture often improves venous engorgement by stimulating the infant to cry. Then with constant suction on the syringe, advance the needle (Fig. 2.1, *dotted line*) until the external jugular vein is entered, keeping the needle steady with the heel of the hand on the infant's head. After withdrawing an adequate blood sample, relieve the suction on the syringe and withdraw the needle. Apply sterile dry gauze immediately. The assistant should bring the infant to the upright position and compress the venipuncture site for 5 minutes.

2.2. RADIAL ARTERIAL PUNCTURE

Indications

Procurement of blood samples, especially for arterial blood gas analysis

Complications

1. Arterial occlusion by thrombosis/hematoma
2. Infection—thrombophlebitis
3. Ischemia (especially if the ulnar collateral circulation is insufficient)
4. Hematoma—from hemostatic problems or inadequate pressure afterwards

Equipment

Butterfly (23 to 25 gauge); 1- to 3-mL syringe or standard blood sample collecting system; heparin flush (10 U per mL); povidone–iodine or chlorhexidine solution; 70% alcohol; sterile gauze

Procedure

Prepare the equipment—attach the butterfly to the syringe and flush the system with the heparin solution and empty it. Assess the adequacy of both radial and ulnar arterial flow by palpation before the puncture (i.e., Allen test). Have the assistant firmly restrain the infant or child by holding the arm just proximal to the wrist in supination and hyperextending the hand approximately 20 to 30 degrees.

Cleanse the skin overlying the radial artery with povidone–iodine or chlorhexidine solution followed by 70% alcohol and then dry with sterile gauze. Using gentle pressure with the gloved palpating fingers, locate the vessel. Hold the needle as shown in Figure 2.2 and pierce the skin between index and middle fingers of the palpating hand, directing the needle at 30 to 60 degrees from the horizontal plane. When the needle enters the radial artery, blood begins to flow into the tubing. It will freely flow into a glass syringe, but slight suction is needed to fill plastic syringes. If the initial thrust is unsuccessful, attempt to enter the artery from a different angle, either medially or laterally as determined by careful palpation. To reduce the likelihood of vessel injury and to obtain a more reliable

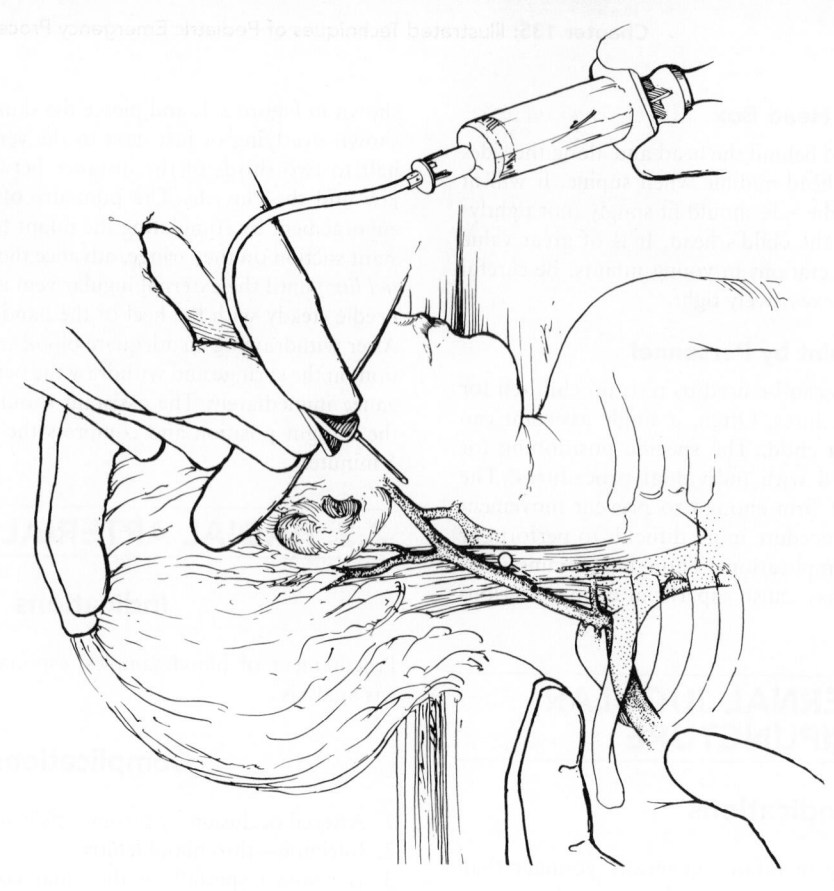

2.1

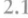

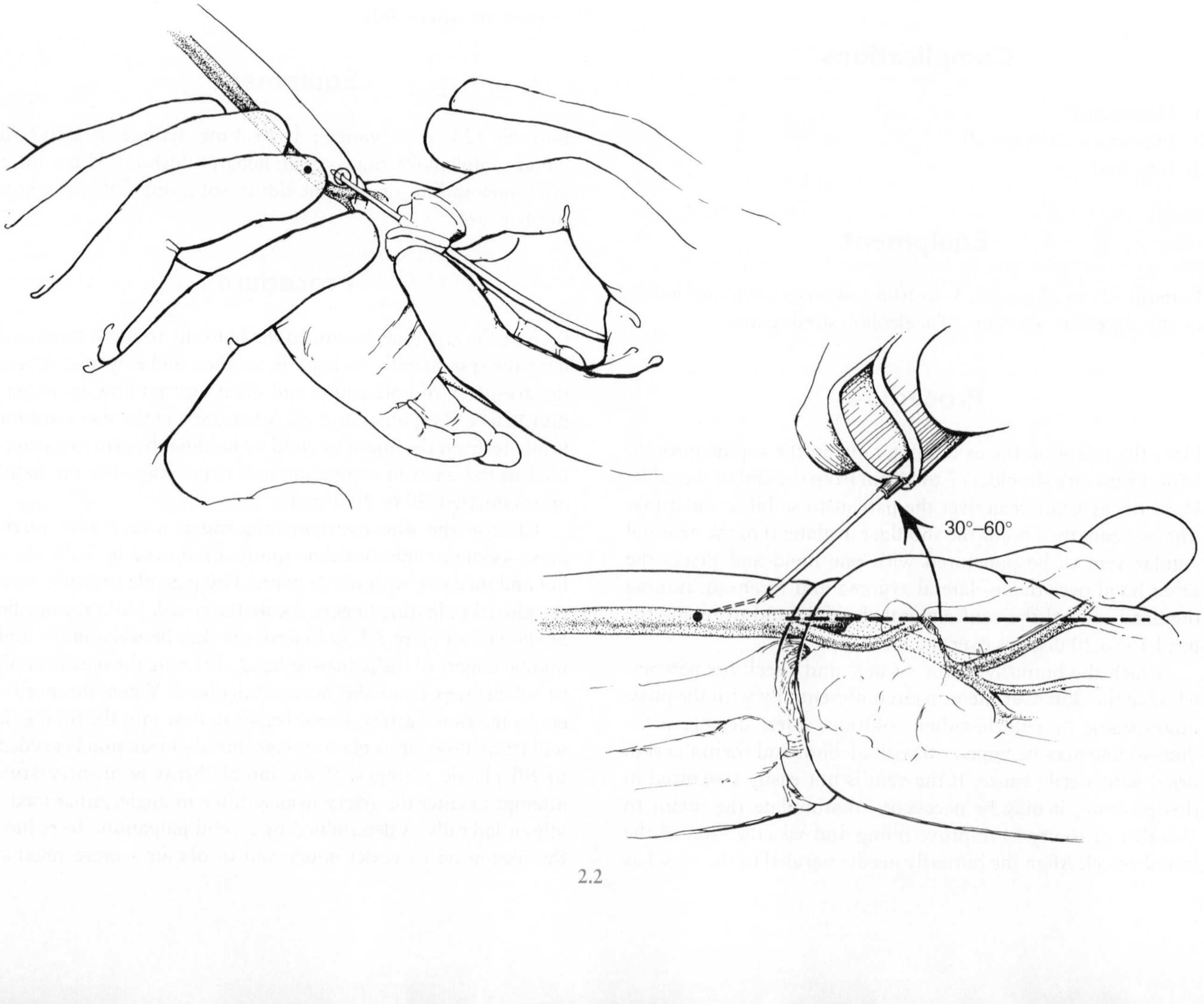

30°–60°

2.2

blood gas analysis, every effort should be made to minimize the number of punctures.

After obtaining the specimen, quickly remove the needle and apply pressure to the puncture site for 5 minutes. Any air bubbles must be immediately removed from the sample to achieve accurate results.

2.3. FEMORAL ARTERY/VEIN PUNCTURE

Indications

1. Arterial or venous blood sampling during acute resuscitations
2. Venous blood sampling in infants with inadequate peripheral veins

Contraindications

Avoid femoral punctures in children who have coagulation defects, hypercoagulable states, or cardiac shunts.

Complications

1. Hematoma of femoral triangle
2. Thrombosis—femoral artery or vein
3. Superficial infection
4. Osteomyelitis/arthritis—proximal femur, hip joint

Equipment

Butterfly needle (1-in, 21- to 23-gauge needle in a child 2 to 3 years of age or older); syringe on 1.5-in, 19- or 21-gauge needle when child is 9 to 10 years of age or older; 5- to 10-mL syringe; povidone–iodine or chlorhexidine solution; 70% alcohol; sterile gauze; blood sample containers

Procedure

Have the assistant restrain the infant. This can be done using one of the two methods. The first method is illustrated in Figure 2.3A, whereby the trunk and contralateral leg are restrained by the assistant and the ipsilateral leg is restrained by the operator. The second method is diagrammed with the illustration for suprapubic bladder aspiration (see Procedure 11.2), in which the assistant leans over the infant with arms pressing on the infant's arms above and holding the distal thighs below in the frog-leg position.

Gently flex the knee and externally rotate the hip to identify the landmarks of the femoral triangle. Locate the inguinal ligament, and gently palpate midway between the anterior superior iliac spine and pubic symphysis. The femoral artery lies halfway between the two landmarks; the vein lies 0.5 to 1 cm medially (Fig. 2.3B). The empty space between flexor and extensor muscles of the medial thigh will also reveal the location of the vessels.

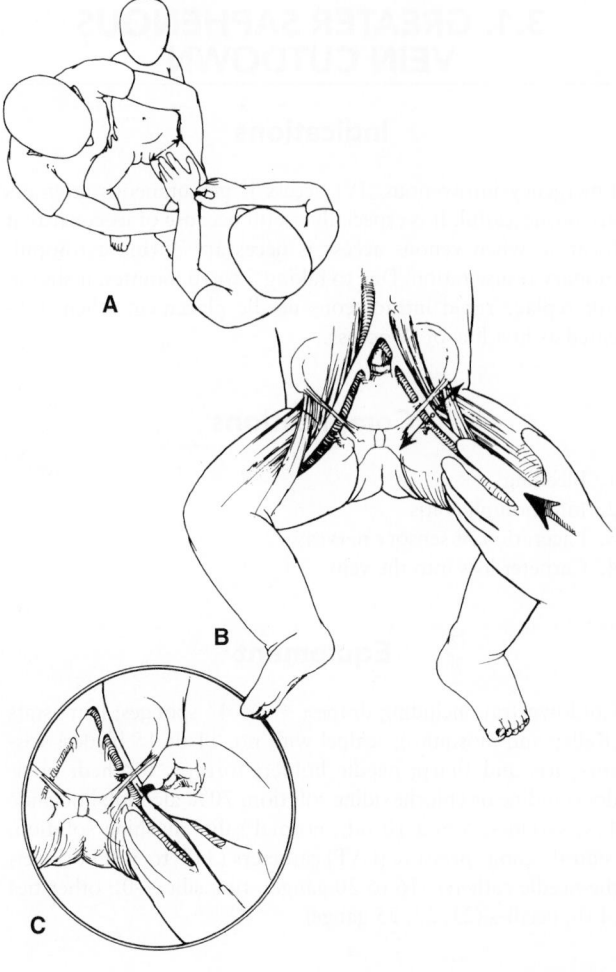

2.3

Cleanse the femoral triangle circumferentially with povidone–iodine or chlorhexidine solution several times, and then wipe the dried povidone–iodine off with 70% alcohol and dry with sterile gauze. With the palpating index finger, relocate the femoral artery approximately 2 cm below the inguinal ligament. Use the palm of this hand to control the movement of the child's leg. Minimize the infant's agitation and movement because this will make the abdominal musculature taut and the transmitted pulse difficult to palpate.

Direct the needle 60 to 75 degrees from the horizontal, just cephalad on the leg to the palpating finger, as shown in Figure 2.3C. Puncture the skin over the pulsatile femoral artery or 0.5 cm medially for the vein, whichever is desired. Apply constant suction to the syringe as the needle is advanced into the thigh to ensure blood is obtained on entering the vessel. The assistant should work to avoid uncontrolled leg movements by the infant because this makes it possible to lose alignment of the needle and vessels. If unsuccessful, withdraw the needle to just below the skin surface and reattempt vessel puncture after shifting the medial or lateral alignment of the needle tip. After obtaining the sample, stop suction on the syringe. Concomitant with needle withdrawal, the assistant should provide constant pressure on the puncture site for 5 minutes with sterile gauze.

PROCEDURES

3.1. GREATER SAPHENOUS VEIN CUTDOWN

Indications

Emergency intravenous (IV) access if percutaneous attempts are unsuccessful. It is especially useful because of its consistent location when venous access is necessary during cardiopulmonary resuscitation. Due to taking 5 to 10 minutes, it should not replace rapid intraosseous needle placement when indicated as first line of IV access.

Complications

1. Bleeding
2. Infection/phlebitis
3. Laceration of sensory nerves
4. Catheter loss into the vein

Equipment

Cutdown tray including drapes; 4″ × 4″ sponges; hemostats (Kelley and mosquito); scalpel with no. 11 or 15 blades; scissors, iris and sharp; needle holder; forceps, toothed; povidone–iodine or chlorhexidine solution; 70% alcohol; lidocaine 1%; syringes, 5 and 10 mL; normal saline flushing solution; central venous pressure (CVP) catheters (3.0F to 5.0F) or over-the-needle catheter (16 to 20 gauge); ties, silk (3-0); other ties (4-0); needles (21, 22, 25 gauge)

Procedure

Prepare the catheter by attaching it distally to a stopcock and 10-mL syringe. Fill the catheter system with routine flushing solution. Prepare the child for the procedure. Place the patient supine and externally rotate the leg and ankle. Restrain the patient's foot while allowing proper exposure of the area.

Palpate the medial malleolus of the tibia and anterior tibial tendon between which the saphenous vein lies. Cleanse the ankle with povidone–iodine or chlorhexidine solution followed by 70% alcohol and dry with sterile gauze. Using sterile technique, drape the area with sterile towels, leaving a rectangular 5 ×8 -cm^2 field exposed over the ankle. Inject 1% lidocaine to achieve local anesthesia at the incision site.

After relocating the landmarks, make a 2-cm transverse incision with a no. 15 scalpel blade just proximal and anterior to the bony prominence of the medial malleolus, as shown by the dotted lines in Figure 3.1. In infants <1 year, a 1-cm incision may be sufficient. Do not use a proximal tourniquet because it may increase capillary bleeding and obscure the field.

With a curved hemostat, spread the subcutaneous tissue proximal from distal along the course of the vein. The vein can be located by lifting up the tissue directly on top of the fascia. Just anterior to the vein is a sensory nerve, which will be spared if the vein is separated well from the surrounding tissue. Isolate the vein and pass two 3-0 or 4-0 silk ties under-

neath it. Tie the distal suture, as shown in Figure 3.1A, and hold the suture with a clamp distally. Then loosely knot the proximal tie.

As shown in Figure 3.1B, incise the vein after applying traction to it by exerting tension on the distal ligature. Use a no. 11 scalpel blade and insert its sharp point at 45 degrees from the horizontal to produce a vein wall flap halfway through the vein. Figure 3.1C shows the procedure in small veins and how grasping the vein on either side flattens it out. This method exposes the lateral vein surface and makes it easier to incise the 45-degree flap. Often it is helpful to make a hook to hold the proximal vein flap. This is accomplished by using a hemostat to bend the tip of a 22-gauge needle into a curved hook. Lift the top of the vein flap with it to expose the venotomy opening. Next, as in Figure 3.1D, hold the vein flap open with the curved hook and insert the beveled catheter through the vein opening and up the leg. Figure 3.1E shows the technique for advancing the catheter once patency is confirmed. Running IV fluids while advancing the catheter dilates the vein and facilitates passage of the remaining 15-cm length of catheter. At this point, secure the proximal tie around both the vein and the indwelling catheter, and distal to the cutdown site, suture the catheter to the skin. The incision may be closed with several sutures. Apply a sterile dressing.

Alternative

Rather than making an incision in the vein, the emergency physician may choose to insert an "over-the-needle" catheter into the vessel after it has been exposed. This may be done without tying off the distal end of the vein. The technique is similar to that of percutaneous venipuncture, except the vein is under direct visualization. After the catheter has been advanced and patency confirmed, secure the catheter and close the incision as previously described. If the vein is not ligated, disconnect the distal tie. This may assist in reuse of the vein if the patient may require it later. In most instances where the vein may have not been tied off, future attempts for IV placement will not be tried unless it is well documented.

3.2. CENTRAL VENOUS CATHETER: PERCUTANEOUS SELDINGER TECHNIQUE—FEMORAL

Indications

Emergency access to central venous circulation. See Procedure 13.1 for ultrasound guidance. The femoral vein is more accessible than the external or internal jugular vein during resuscitation but should be avoided when possible interruption of the inferior vena cava exists, such as in trauma or severe abdominal catastrophe.

Complications

1. Arterial or venous laceration
2. Infection (especially if placed in emergency without reliable use of infection control technique)
3. Catheter fragment in circulation

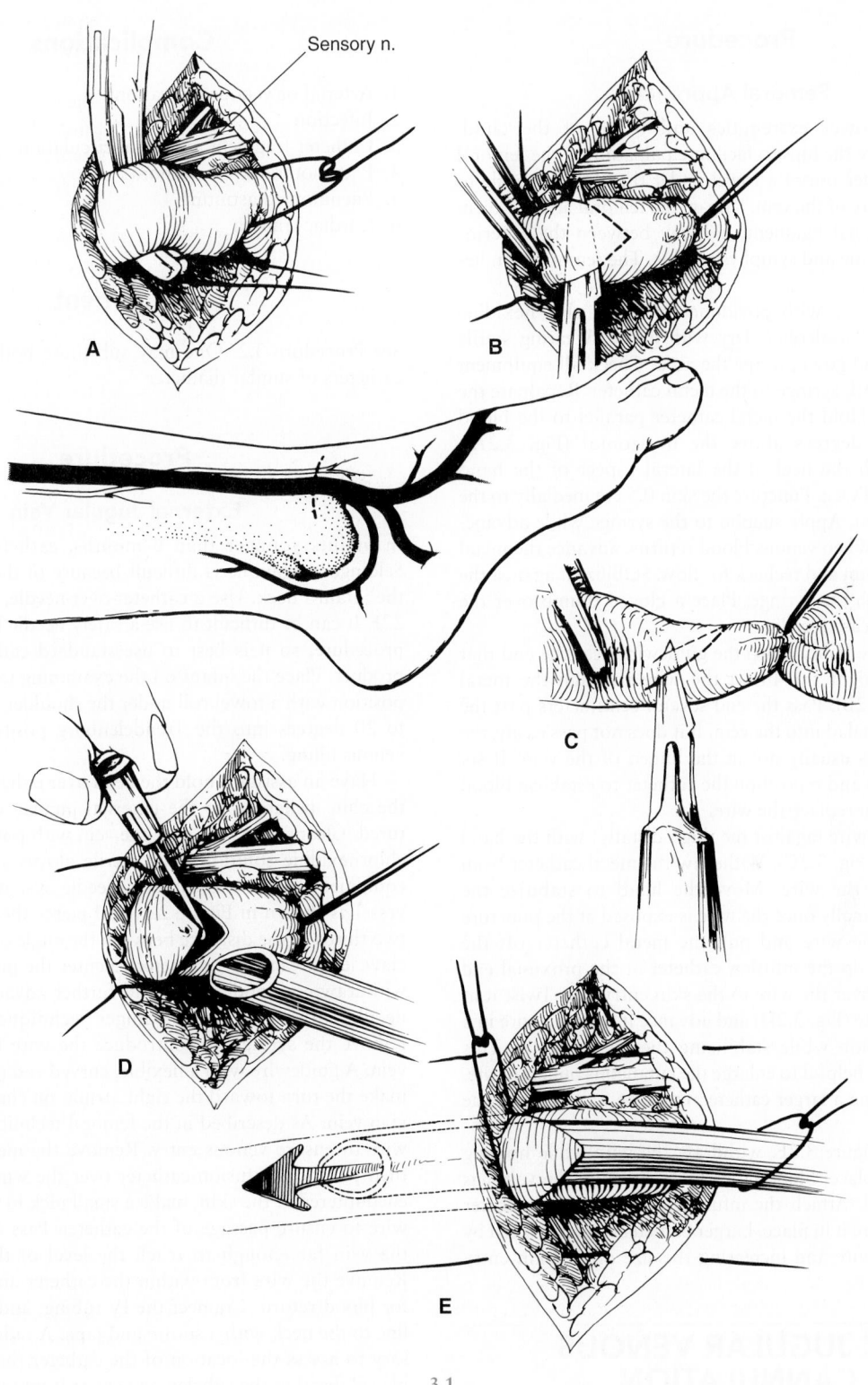

Sensory n.

A

B

C

D

E

3.1

Equipment

Commercial tray (i.e., Abbott®, Arrow®, Cooke®, Viggo-Spectramed®), with metal catheter; guidewire; 3F, 20-gauge (younger than 2 years of age) or 4F, 18-gauge (2 to 7 years old) or 5F, 16-gauge (older than 8 years of age) infusion catheter; sterile drapes and gloves; 5- to 10-mL syringe; T-connector; three-way stopcock; infusion fluid; povidone–iodine or chlorhexidine solution; 70% alcohol; sterile gauze pads; use larger set in trauma patients

Procedure

Femoral Approach

Restrain the lower extremities and trunk of the child. Externally rotate the hips to facilitate palpation of the femoral triangle. Consider use of a towel under the gluteal muscle to improve exposure of the vein. Palpate the femoral artery 1.5 cm below the inguinal ligament, halfway between the anterior superior iliac spine and symphysis pubis. The femoral vein lies 0.5 cm medially.

Cleanse the site with povidone–iodine or chlorhexidine solution and 70% alcohol. Dry with gauze. Wearing sterile gloves, mask and gown, drape the area. Check all equipment and attach a 5-mL syringe to the metal catheter. Repalpate the femoral artery. Hold the metal catheter parallel to the blood vessel and 30 degrees above the horizontal (Fig. 3.2A). Stabilize it with the heel of the lateral aspect of the hand against the child's leg. Puncture the skin 0.5 cm medially to the arterial pulsation. Apply suction to the syringe while advancing the needle. When venous blood returns, advance the metal catheter 1 to 2 mm and recheck for flow. Stabilize it against the thigh and detach the syringe. Place a gloved thumb over the catheter to decrease bleeding.

Using the free hand, grasp the guidewire near the end that has a soft, straight tip. Insert the wire through the metal catheter (Fig. 3.2B). Pass the end several centimeters past the catheter tip cephalad into the vein. If it does not pass easily, the metal catheter is usually not in the lumen of the vein. If so, remove the wire and reposition the catheter to establish blood flow again. Then replace the wire.

Stabilize the wire (against the thigh distally) with the hand that inserted it (Fig. 3.2C). Withdraw the metal catheter from the vein along the wire. Move the hand to stabilize the guidewire proximally once the wire is exposed at the puncture site. Support the wire and pull the metal catheter off the guidewire. Pick up the infusion catheter at the proximal end and advance it over the wire to the skin entry site. Twist it at the skin entry site (Fig. 3.2D) and advance it over the wire in a cephalad direction while stabilizing the wire distally. This rotary motion is helpful to enlarge the cutaneous puncture site. When introducing a larger catheter, make an incision over the wire.

Last, as in Figure 3.2E, withdraw the wire while holding the catheter in place; blood flows immediately if the vein has been cannulated. Attach the infusion system to the catheter and tape or suture it in place. Larger catheters can be placed by reinserting the wire and increasing the size of the skin entry site.

3.3. JUGULAR VENOUS CANNULATION

Indications

Emergency central vein access. The internal or external jugular veins are preferred entry sites particularly when abdominal trauma with possible vena cava injury is present. This is a relative contraindication to femoral vein cannulation. The main delay in early access to the jugular vein is the need to stabilize the airway or maintain protection of the C-spine.

Complications

1. Arterial or venous lacerations
2. Infection
3. Catheter fragment in central circulation
4. Pneumothorax, hemothorax
5. Pneumomediastinum
6. Cardiac trauma

Equipment

See Procedure 3.2. One may substitute both over-the-needle catheters of similar diameter

Procedure

External Jugular Vein

In infants younger than 6 months, catheterization by the Seldinger technique is difficult because of the short length of the infant's neck. Use a catheter-over-needle, usually a 20F or 22F. It can be difficult to use a safety needle IV set up for this procedure, so it is best to use standard catheter-over-needle product. Place the infant on the examining table in the supine position with a towel roll under the shoulder or tilt the bed 15 to 20 degrees into the Trendelenburg position to maximize venous filling.

Have an assistant hold the head over either the forehead or the chin ipsilateral to the external jugular vein to be punctured. Cleanse the skin over the vein with povidone–iodine or chlorhexidine solution. Don sterile gloves and assemble the equipment. Align the catheter–needle system parallel to the vessel as shown in Figure 2.1, and pierce the skin one half to two thirds of the distance between the angle of the jaw and the clavicle. Advance the catheter to enter the jugular vein. After withdrawing blood, proceed to further advance the over-the-needle catheter. If the Seldinger technique is being used, remove the syringe and introduce the wire to cannulate the vein. A guidewire with a flexible, curved end (J-wire) may help make the turn toward the right atrium on entry of the subclavian vein. As described in the femoral technique, pass enough wire to ensure venous entry. Remove the metal catheter and then place the infusion catheter over the wire. If difficulty is encountered at the skin, make a small nick in the skin over the wire to ensure passage of the catheter. Pass the catheter into the vein far enough to reach the level of the right atrium. Remove the wire from within the catheter and check the line for blood return. Connect the IV tubing, and then secure the line to the neck with a suture and tape. A radiograph is necessary to assess the location of the catheter (because it may be placed distal in the subclavian vein or if into the ventricle).

Internal Jugular Vein

Position the infant or child in 15 to 20 degrees of Trendelenburg with the head turned over the bed or table edge. Mild hyperextension of the neck tenses the sternocleidomastoid muscle to localize the landmarks. The medial approach uses the apex of the triangle formed by the sternal and clavicular heads of the sternomastoid muscle as the entry site (Fig. 3.3). Using a needle attached to a tuberculin syringe, advance it at a 45-degree angle

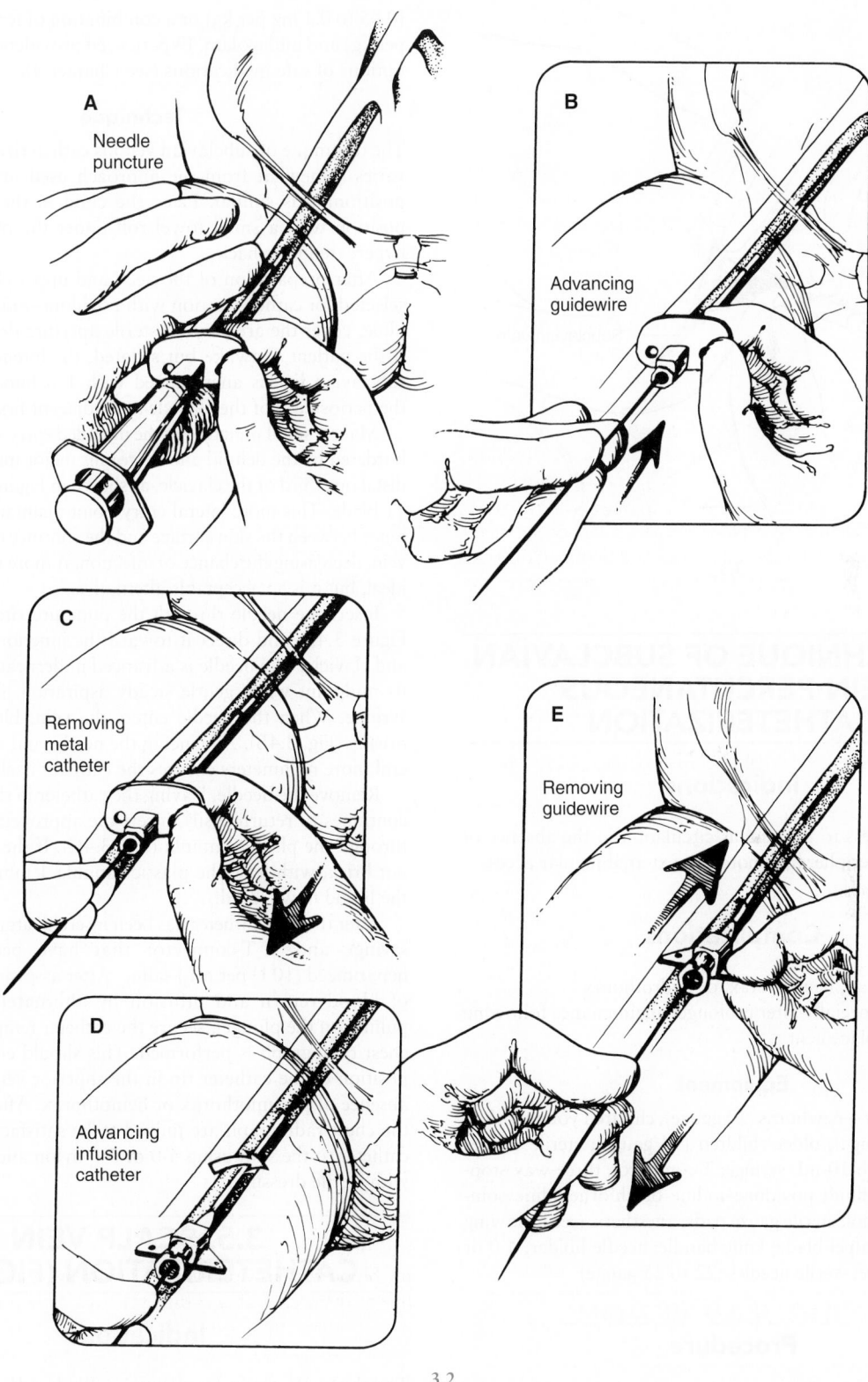

A
Needle
puncture

B
Advancing
guidewire

C
Removing
metal
catheter

E
Removing
guidewire

D
Advancing
infusion
catheter

3.2

to the skin in the caudal direction. Aim toward the ipsilateral nipple. Aspirate on the syringe as advancing; the vein should be entered at a depth of 1 to 2 cm. If this fails, withdraw the needle slowly with constant traction on the plunger of the syringe. If blood return does not signify venous entry, reattempt cannulation by advancing the needle slightly lateral to the initial attempt

(do not advance the needle more medial to the ipsilateral nipple line). After obtaining blood flow, introduce the guidewire and then the catheter, as previously described. Check for blood return, and secure the line with suture and tape. A radiograph of the chest should be taken to check for line position and assess for pneumothorax.

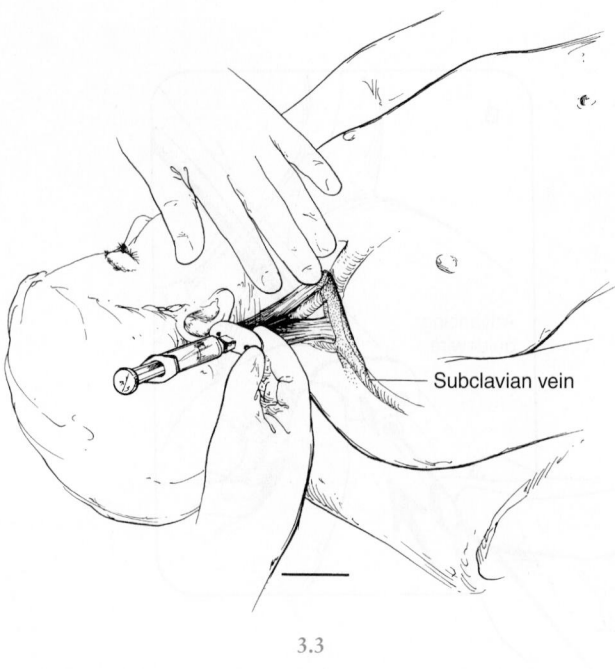

Subclavian vein

3.3

3.4. TECHNIQUE OF SUBCLAVIAN VEIN PERCUTANEOUS CATHETERIZATION

Indications

Emergency access to the venous circulation in the absence of percutaneous peripheral, femoral, or external jugular access

Complications

1. Pneumothorax, hemothorax, or hydrothorax
2. Infection, especially after prolonged maintenance following emergency placement

Equipment

Venous catheter—newborns (20 gauge), children younger than 9 years (18 gauge), older children (14 gauge); sterile drapes and gloves; 5- to 10-mL syringe; T-connector, three-way stopcock; infusion fluid; povidone–iodine or chlorhexidine solution; 70% alcohol; sterile gauze pads; anesthetic (see following text); no. 11 scalpel blade; knife handle; needle holder; 4-0 or 5-0 nylon suture; sterile needles (22 to 25 gauge)

Procedure

Anesthesia

Except in premature infants or obtunded children, adequate restraint in the Trendelenburg position can be difficult without pharmacologic sedation or general anesthesia; this requirement precludes the insertion of a subclavian line in many situations. However, in children older than 6 years of age who are stable and cooperative, the procedure can be done with a local anesthetic of 1% lidocaine and/or sedation with IV midazolam

(0.05 to 0.1 mg per kg) or a combination of fentanyl (1 to 2 μg per kg) and midazolam. Experienced providers may have other options of safe medications (see Chapter 4).

Technique

The technique of subclavian venous catheterization in children varies somewhat from the approach used in adults, but the positioning is similar. Place the child in the Trendelenburg position with a small towel roll under the thoracic spine to hyperextend the back.

After preparation of the neck and upper chest on the side selected for catheterization with povidone–iodine or chlorhexidine, cover the area with a sterile aperture drape and towels. If the patient is awake but sedated, the intended tract of the subclavian line is anesthetized with 1% lidocaine, including the periosteum of the clavicle and adjacent first rib.

Make a small puncture at the intended entry site, a depression bordered by the deltoid and pectoralis major muscles, under the distal one third of the clavicle, as shown in Figure 3.4A; use a no. 11 blade. This more lateral entry point maintains a greater distance between the skin surface and the entrance to the subclavian vein, decreasing the chance of infection. A more medial site is less ideal, but it is an acceptable alternative.

Insert the needle through the puncture site as depicted in Figure 3.4A, and direct it toward the junction of the first rib and clavicle. The needle is advanced underneath the clavicle at its midpoint while gentle steady aspiration is applied to the syringe. When the needle enters the vein, blood flows back briskly (Fig. 3.4B). Advancing the needle and catheter for several more millimeters ensures the catheter itself is in the vein.

Remove the needle, leaving the catheter in the vein. If blood continues to return easily, insert the appropriate size catheter through the plastic cannula (Fig. 3.4C). If the blood return is not brisk, withdraw the plastic cannula 1 mm at a time until the blood flows rapidly.

After the long catheter has been inserted, attach it to a 10-mL syringe and a T-connector that have been filled with heparinized (10 U per mL) saline. After assessing for adequacy of blood return and infusion by alternately pushing and pulling on the plunger, secure the catheter temporarily while a chest radiograph is performed. This should confirm both the position of the catheter tip in the superior vena cava and the absence of pneumothorax or hemothorax. After the results of the chest radiograph are judged to be satisfactory, suture the catheter to the skin using 4-0 or 5-0 nylon and cover the area with sterile dressing.

3.5. SCALP VEIN CATHETERIZATION (FIG. 3.5)

Indications

To achieve IV access for delivering fluid and/or medication in an infant usually younger than 1 year of age, when peripheral extremity veins are unavailable

COMPLICATIONS

1. Inadvertent arterial puncture
2. Ecchymoses and hematoma of the scalp

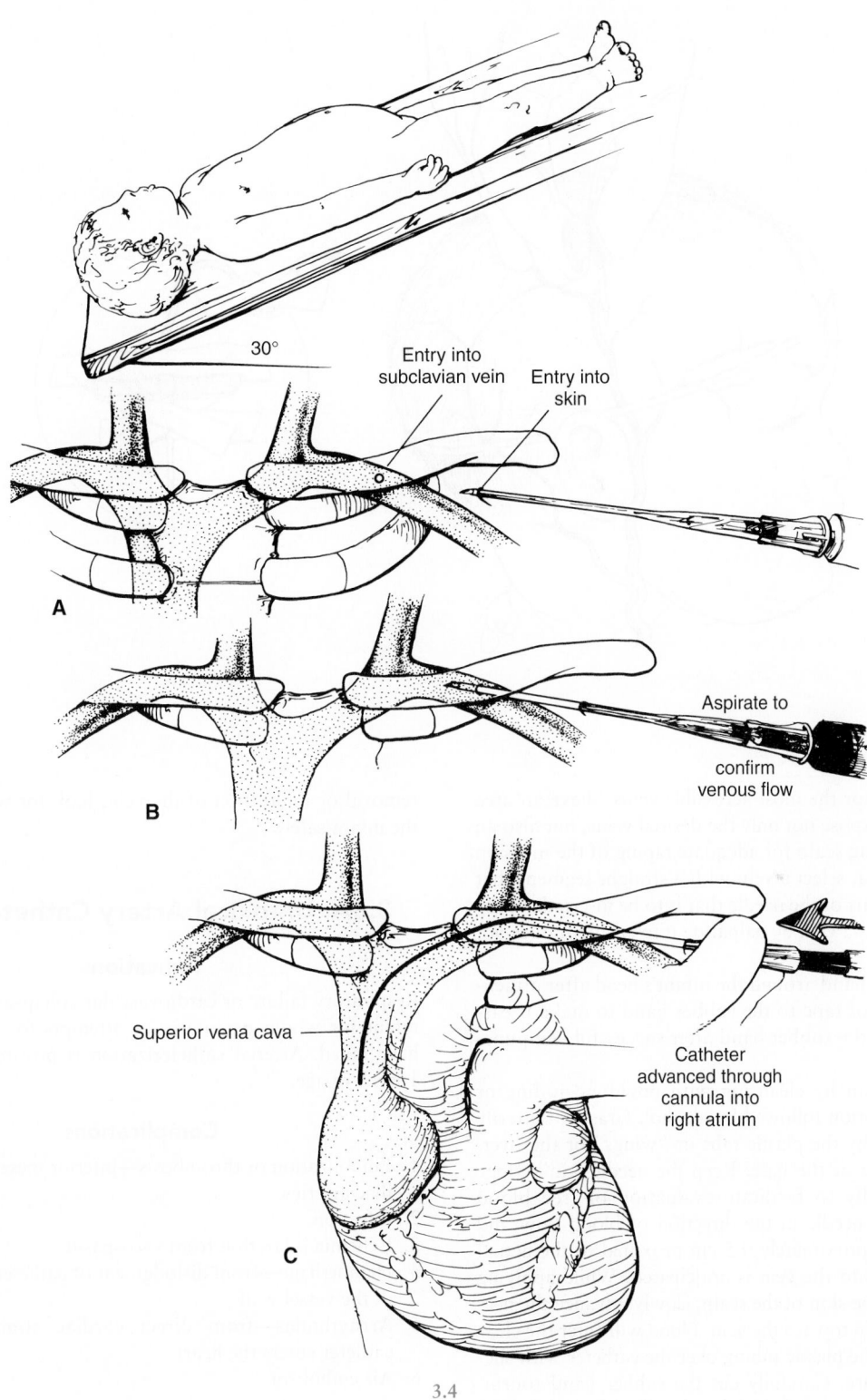

30°

Entry into
subclavian vein

Entry into
skin

A

Aspirate to

confirm
venous flow

B

Superior vena cava

Catheter
advanced through
cannula into
right atrium

C

3.4

EQUIPMENT

Butterfly scalp vein needle no. 23, 25, or 27, or an over-the-needle catheter, 22 or 24 gauge; rubber band with tape; flush solution; 3-mL syringe; tincture of benzoin; tape; razor blade; povidone–iodine or chlorhexidine solution; 70% alcohol; sterile gauze

PROCEDURE

The infant younger than 1 year of age has several easily accessible scalp veins. These include the frontal, supraorbital, posterior facial, superficial temporal, and posterior auricular veins and their tributaries. Restrain the patient in a supine position and have an assistant stabilize the infant's head.

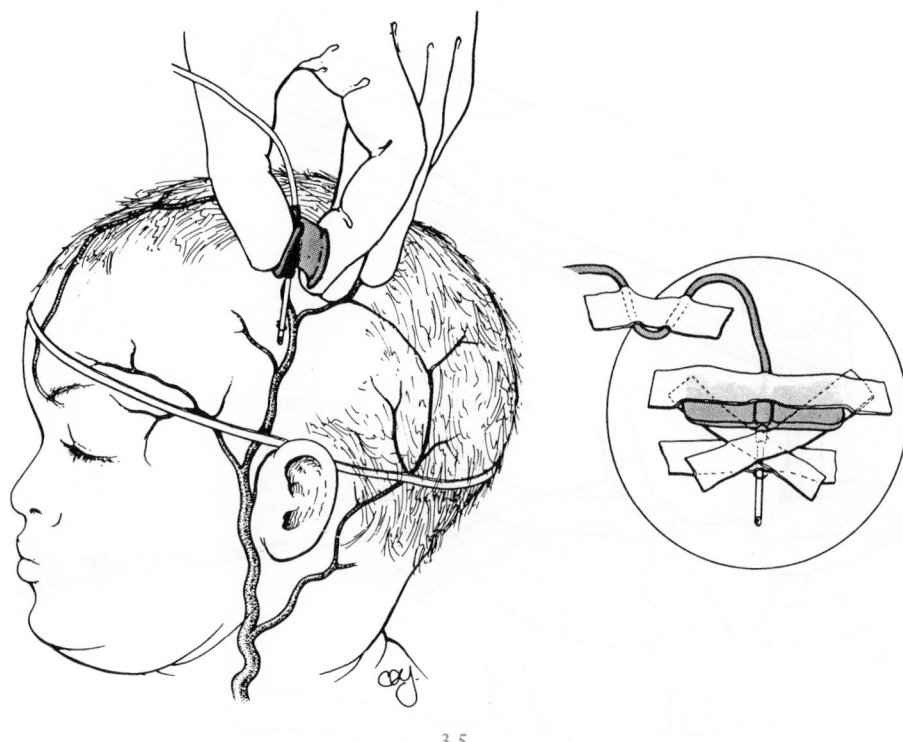

3.5

After assessment for the most accessible veins, shave an area large enough to expose not only the desired veins, but also an area of surrounding scalp for adequate taping of the infusion needle. In this area, select a vein with a straight segment that is as long as the part of the needle that is to be inserted. Verify the chosen vessel is a vein by palpating it to ensure it does not pulsate.

Place a rubber band around the infant's head after attaching a small piece of tape to the rubber band to make it easier to lift and cut the rubber band after successful venipuncture.

Prepare the skin by cleansing with povidone–iodine or chlorhexidine solution followed by alcohol. Grasp a butterfly scalp vein needle by the plastic tabs or "wings" or the over-the-needle catheter at the base. Keep the needle and syringe unattached initially to facilitate evaluation of free blood return. Insert the needle in the direction of blood flow and pierce the skin approximately 0.5 cm proximal to the actual site where entry into the vein is anticipated. While applying mild traction on the skin of the scalp, slowly advance the needle through the skin toward the vein. Blood will enter the clear plastic tubing or the plastic tubing over the catheter with successful venipuncture. Carefully cut the rubber band tourniquet, attach the syringe filled with saline flush solution, and slowly inject 0.5 mL of flush. If the needle is satisfactorily inserted into the lumen of the vein, the solution will flow easily. Thread the catheter over the needle further into the vein continuing to assess for flow. Appearance of a skin wheal indicates that the vein has not been satisfactorily cannulated, and another attempt must be made.

After successful catheterization, carefully tape the scalp vein needle as shown in the diagram. To prevent accidental removal or infiltration of the vein, look for ways to position the infant safely.

3.6A. Umbilical Artery Catheterization

Indications

Respiratory failure or cardiovascular collapse in the newborn infant for whom percutaneous attempts for vascular access have failed. Arterial catheterization is possible until around 1 week of age.

Complications

1. Embolization or thrombosis—inferior mesenteric, renal, or iliac arteries
2. Infection
3. Ischemia/infarction from vasospasm
4. Hemorrhage—from dislodgment of catheter or perforation of the vessel wall
5. Arrhythmias—from direct cardiac stimulation if the catheter enters the heart
6. Air embolism

Equipment

3-0 or 4-0 silk suture on straight or curved needle; antiseptic solution (povidone–iodine); sterile gauze pads; drapes and gloves; hemostats (four pairs), curved non-tooted iris forceps (4 in) or metal dilator and iris scissors; needle holder, sterile scalpel and no. 11 or 15 blade; 22-gauge needle; 10-mL syringe filled with normal saline; T-connector (optional); three-way stopcock; nonthrombogenic umbilical catheter, 3.5,

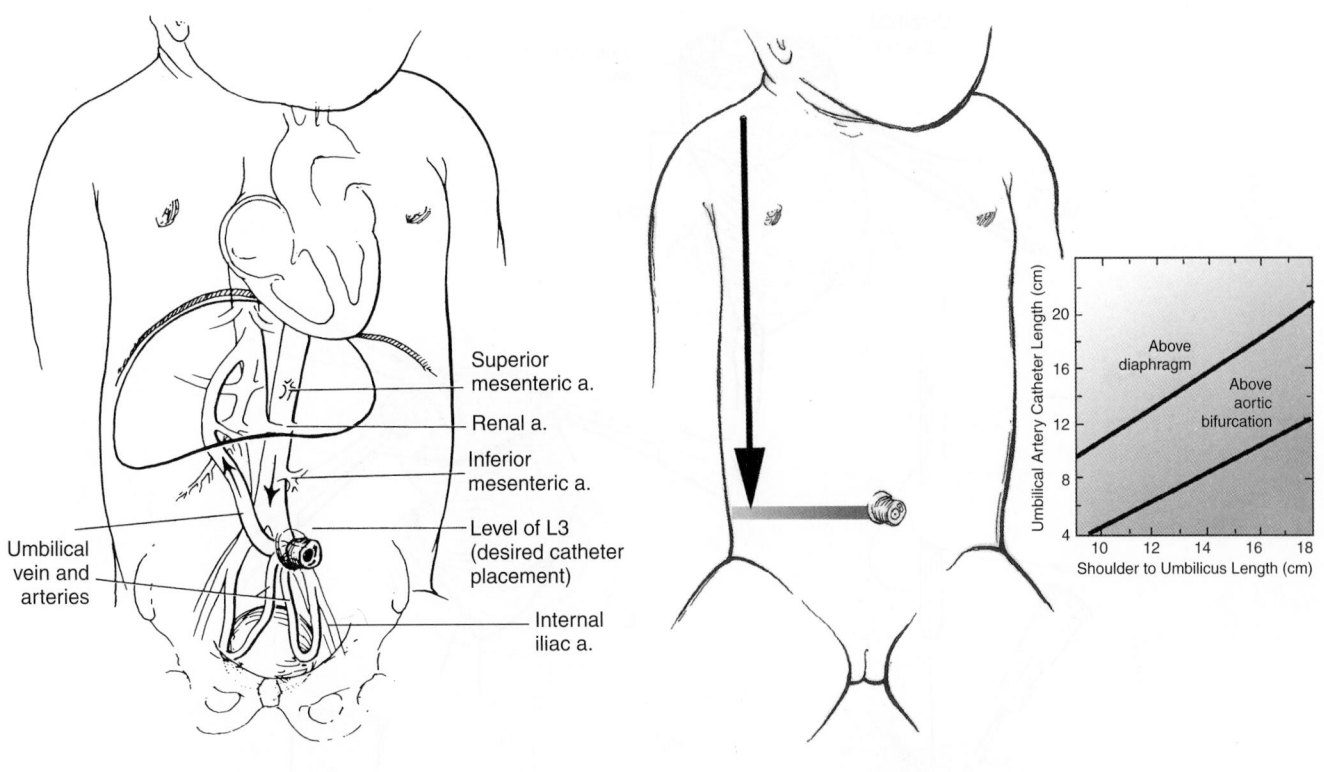

Superior mesenteric a.

Renal a.

Inferior mesenteric a.

Level of L3 (desired catheter placement)

Internal iliac a.

Umbilical vein and arteries

3.6A

4 Fr (premature babies) or, 5F (full-term); infusion solution, often normal saline, containing heparin (1 U per mL)

Procedure

Initiate therapy for any cardiorespiratory disturbances before beginning procedure. During the catheterization, monitor the cardiac rate and keep the infant under a radiant heater to maintain normothermia. Figure 3.6A shows the pertinent anatomy.

Place the infant supine in the frog-leg position and restrain him/her as necessary. Gauze pads may be wrapped around the ankles and wrists and either pinned or taped securely to the bed/sheet. Wearing mask, gown, and gloves, hold the sterile umbilical catheter over the infant to measure the vertical distance from the lateral aspect of the clavicle to the umbilicus. The catheter will be advanced into the artery 60% of this distance, beginning at the skin surface so its tip will reach the bifurcation of the aorta, the subdiaphragmatic location. For catheters that may need to be longer, use the nomogram, Figure 3.6A, to establish the length to place it. These amounts do not account for the length of catheter that is within the umbilical stump from the abdominal wall. Mark the catheter appropriately and attach it to the T-connector, stopcock, and syringe. Flush it, leaving it full of fluid. While lifting the umbilical cord with gauze in one hand, scrub the lower umbilical cord and abdomen from the xiphoid process to the symphysis pubis with povidone–iodine solution. Drape the infant on both sides by folding two drapes into triangles or use an aperture drape; cover the area below the umbilicus with a third square drape.

At the base of the umbilical stump, suture a 3-0 or 4-0 silk tie around the cord to make a purse string, but leave the knot untied. While holding the gauze on the nonsterile distal umbilicus, sever the cord 1.5 to 2 cm above the abdominal wall with the scalpel as shown in Figure 3.6B, part A. Remove the cut umbilicus and gauze from the sterile area. Bleeding is usually minimal, stopping with gentle pressure or wiping; rarely, the purse string must be tightened.

Locate the umbilical vessels, usually two thick, white-walled arteries on one side, and a larger vein on the other. If the arteries in the stump are tortuous, cut it closer to the abdominal wall to facilitate cannulation.

Attach two clamps on opposite sides of the umbilicus, being careful to grasp a fibrous portion of the cord and not just Wharton's jelly or an artery. Evert the clamps to immobilize and expose the cord, and use the small curved forceps, as in Figure 3.6B, part B, to enter and then stretch the lumen of the artery. Gentle, repetitive stretching is most effective with a solid metal dilator. An attempt at catheter placement should be undertaken when the artery remains dilated to a diameter that is greater than that of the catheter for the depth of 1 cm.

To insert the catheter, hold the distal end near the tip as in Figure 3.6B, part C, and place it in the arterial lumen between the prongs of the forceps that are holding open the artery. An alternative method, pictured in Figure 3.6B, part C, shows the inner wall of the vessel held with a 22-gauge needle (bent in the shape of a hook by a hemostat), allowing the vessel to be entered directly. Pass the catheter under gentle, constant tension to overcome the resistance encountered at the points where the artery turns (just below the skin surface and where the arteries turn upward toward the iliacs; see Fig. 3.6A). Blood should flow readily after the second bend when the iliac artery is entered.

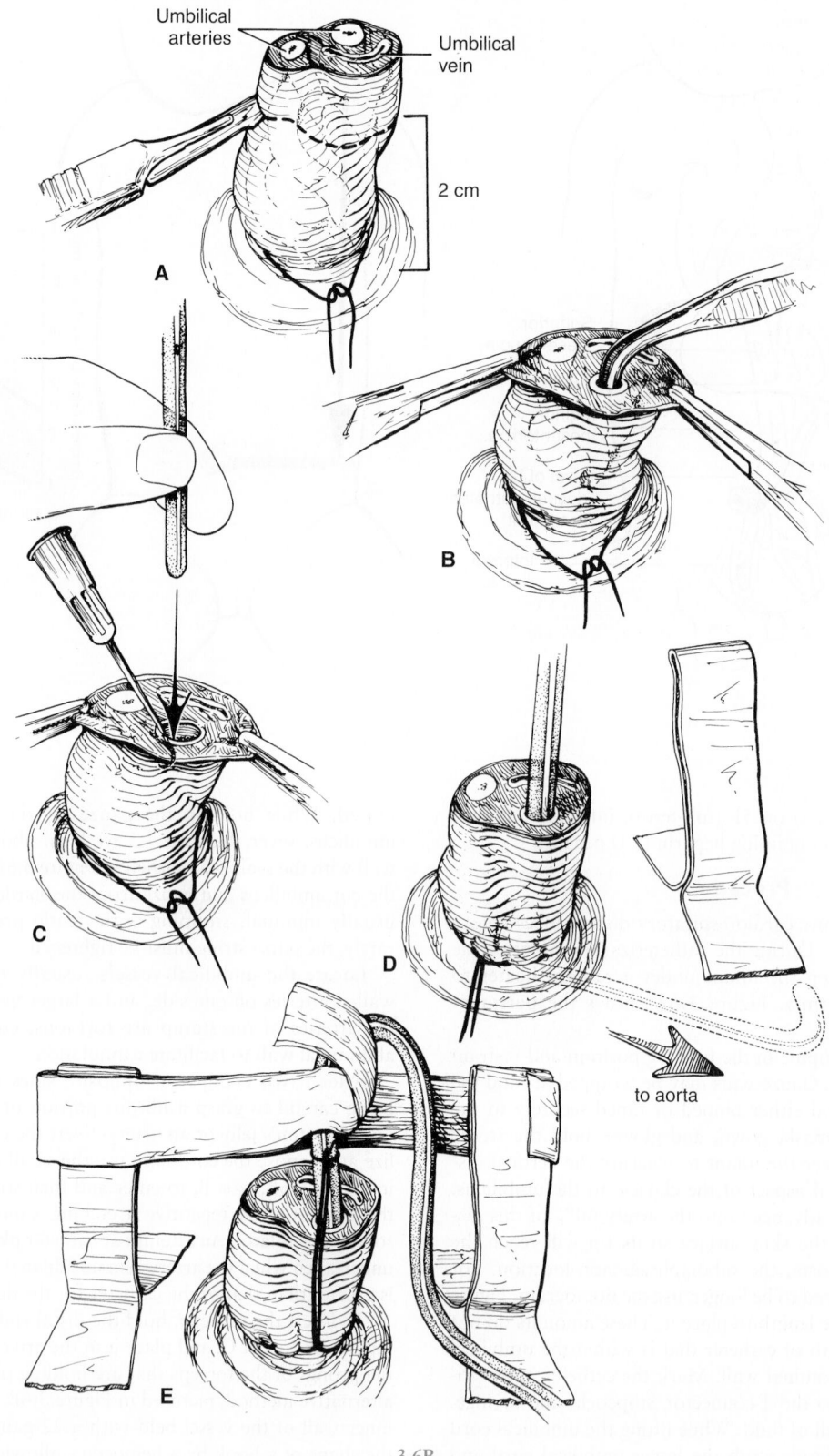

Umbilical
arteries

Umbilical
vein

2 cm

A

B

C

D

to aorta

E

3.6B

As shown in Figure 3.6B, part D, advance the catheter as far as the mark made on it at the outset; confirm blood flow at the final point. Turn the handle of the stopcock toward the infant. Then, tighten and knot the purse string, leaving both ends of the suture long. Approximately 5 cm from the knot at the base of the cord, make a square knot and then loop and tie the suture around the catheter to help secure it in place, as shown in Figure 3.6B, part E. An alternative is to suture in a purse string circumferentially around the umbilical cord. Then tie the knot around the catheter to assist in maintaining it securely. Also place tape on the abdominal wall as shown in the figure. Verify with an abdominal radiograph that the tip of the catheter lies below the level of third lumbar vertebral body, or withdraw it to this position manually if the tip is higher on radiograph.

Infuse solutions containing heparin (1 U per mL) unless contraindicated for bleeding diathesis.

3.6B. Umbilical Vein Catheterization

Indications

To gain vascular access rapidly in a newborn with respiratory failure or cardiovascular collapse. Venous catheterization is possible until around 2 weeks of age.

Complications

1. Infection
2. Embolization or thrombosis
3. Vessel perforation
4. Hemorrhage
5. Air embolus

Equipment

Umbilical tape or 3-0 silk suture on straight or curved needle, antiseptic solution (povidone–iodine), sterile gauze pad, drapes, mask, gown, gloves, small curved hemostat

Sterile scalpel and no. 11 or 15 blade, iris scissors, 5F umbilical catheter three-way stopcock, 10-mL syringe with normal saline, infusing solution

Procedure

The umbilical vein is preferred for vascular access during neonatal resuscitation because the vessel is readily located and cannulated. Catheterizing the umbilical vein is generally much easier than catheterizing the umbilical artery.

Place the newborn supine and restrain the extremities as necessary. The newborn should be on a radiant warmer bed, and the heart rate and pulse oximetry ideally should be monitored throughout the procedure. Prepare the equipment. Attach a 5F umbilical catheter to a three-way stopcock and a saline-filled syringe. Prime the catheter with normal saline. Wearing mask, gown and sterile gloves, cleanse the umbilical cord and the abdomen from the xiphoid process to the pubic symphysis with povidone–iodine solution. At the base of the umbilical cord, loosely tie umbilical tape or insert 3-0 silk suture around the cord to make a purse string. Cut the cord 1 to 2 cm from the abdominal wall. Locate the vein orifice and remove any visible solid clot with fine forceps.

Gently grasp the umbilical vein catheter about 2 cm from the tip with either a small clamp or your gloved fingers (Fig. 3.6C). Introduce the catheter tip into the umbilical vein. Apply gentle pressure and advance the catheter through the venous lumen. The catheter is inserted until blood flows freely. This generally occurs when the catheter tip is just beyond the junction of the umbilicus and the abdominal wall. The catheter is inserted a short distance further to avoid infusing fluids directly into the liver. Take the vertical lateral clavicle to umbilicus measure and 0.6 times this is the distance to insert it to be above the level of the diaphragm. When placing it higher, it is important to confirm location with an x-ray.

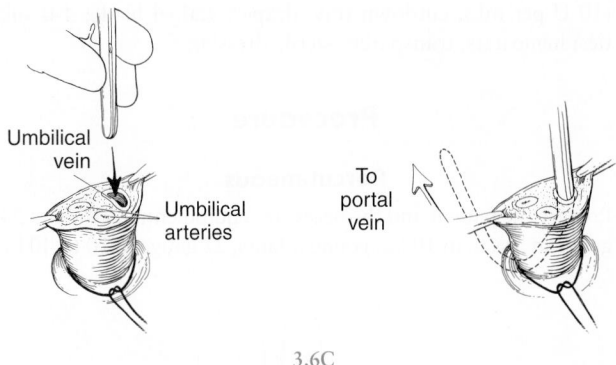

3.6C

When good blood flow has returned, tighten the umbilical tape or the purse string suture. Tape the catheter in place to further secure it. The umbilical vein catheter is usually withdrawn at the end of resuscitation to minimize the danger of infection or portal vein thrombosis; therefore, it is generally not necessary to suture this line in place.

3.7. RADIAL ARTERY CATHETERIZATION

Percutaneous and cutdown techniques

Indications

Percutaneous

1. Frequent blood gas determinations
2. Continuous blood pressure monitoring in cardiovascular collapse/shock syndromes and major surgical procedures

Cutdown

1. Infants weighing less than 5 kg
2. Emergency arterial access if percutaneous attempts are unsuccessful

Complications

1. Hemorrhage
2. Embolization or thrombosis
3. Ischemia and/or infarction of hand
4. Infection

Caution

No medications or hyperosmolar solutions should be administered through peripheral arterial catheters.

Equipment

Arm board; 1- and 2-in tape; 1% lidocaine solution in a 3-mL syringe with a 25-gauge needle; 18- or 19-gauge sterile needle; povidone–iodine or chlorhexidine solution; 70% alcohol; gauze pads; catheter (20- to 24-gauge catheter over needle); T-connector, 5- or 10-mL syringe with heparin flush solution

PROCEDURES

(10 U per mL); cutdown tray; drapes; scalpel blade; 4-0 silk ties; hemostats, transparent sterile dressing

Procedure

Percutaneous

Prepare the patient and the necessary equipment. Consider a 24 gauge in less than 10 kg, young infants, 22 gauge in 10 to 40 kg and 20 gauge in more than 40 kg. Secure the child's hand and forearm to an arm board with the wrist in moderate extension using a gauze roll under the wrist. Cleanse the wrist with antiseptic solution several times and allow to dry followed by 70% alcohol and dry with sterile gauze. Locate the radial artery by palpating distally over the distal volar forearm as shown in Figure 3.7. Then, assess collateral circulation by palpation of the ulnar pulse and performance of the Allen test. After infiltration at the intended puncture site with lidocaine, make a

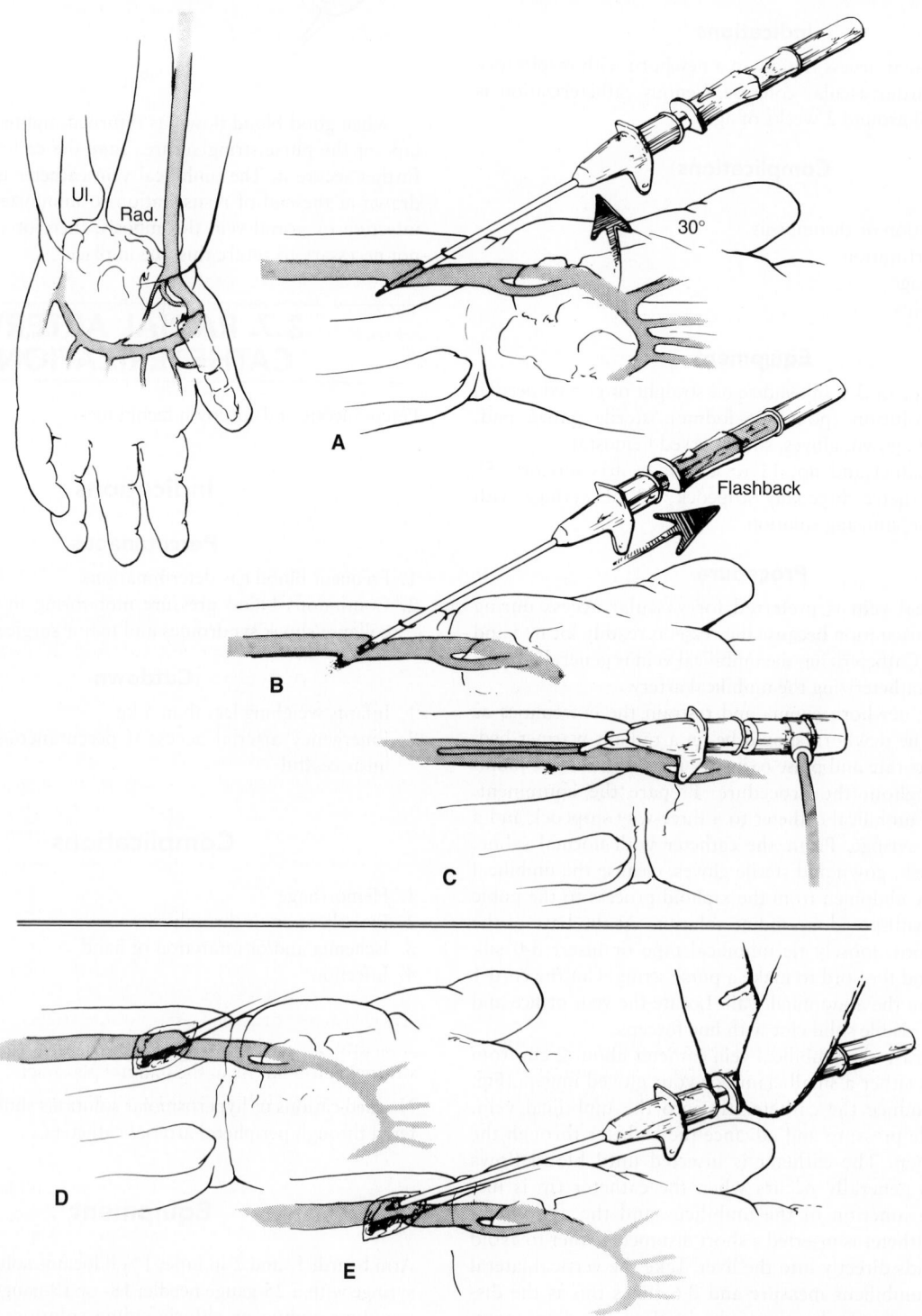

puncture wound with the sterile needle of the skin over the radial artery 0.5 to 1 cm proximal to the distal wrist crease.

Remove the syringe from the over-the-needle catheter system. Again, palpate the radial artery proximally to the previous puncture site while advancing the catheter through the site. After puncturing the artery and obtaining blood flow, advance the needle 1 to 2 mm farther, and then hold the needle steady and slowly advance the catheter into the vessel.

If blood flow never occurs or stops spontaneously, the needle tip may have penetrated the posterior wall of the vessel, as shown in Figure 3.7A. Remove the needle, holding the catheter steady, and begin pulling back the catheter 1 mm at a time until a sudden flash of arterial blood is identified (Fig. 3.7B). Then, advance the catheter forward into the artery. If no blood returns, make another attempt starting over again with new equipment as previously described.

If blood flow is satisfactory in the position shown in Figure 3.7C, attach the connecting tubing to the catheter with a T-connector, stopcock, and syringe, and recheck arterial flow. The catheter should be securely taped or sewn to the forearm to prevent dislodgment. Use of a transparent sterile dressing is recommended to enhance visibility and security.

Cutdown (Figs. 3.7D and 3.7E)

After preparing the equipment and the patient, the wrist is restrained, cleansed, and anesthetized as before. Wearing sterile gloves, drape the area. Make a 1-cm transverse skin incision proximal to the crease closest to the wrist joint (Fig. 3.7D). By carefully spreading the subcutaneous tissue along the incision line, visualize the artery with care to avoid cutting the adjacent veins.

The best approach is to directly puncture the exposed artery with the over-the-needle catheter setup, as shown in Figure 3.7E. A 4-0 silk tie is placed distally to the entry site and pulled to give back traction on the artery. This secures and accentuates it, usually enabling easy puncture and threading of the catheter. Attach the syringe and stopcock system, and check for patency.

The system is secured by suturing the catheter to the skin distal to the incision. Closure of the incision should be accomplished with several 4-0 skin sutures, and a dressing should be applied to stabilize and protect the system.

3.8. INTRAOSSEOUS INFUSION

Indications

This emergency intravascular access is a rapidly placed alternative if percutaneous attempts after 1 to 2 minutes are unsuccessful for life-threatening therapies. This method is especially useful in children up to 6 years of age with circulatory collapse and/or cardiac arrest but can be used at any age. In most instances, the goal is to remove the needle in 3 to 4 hours.

Complications

1. Extravasation of fluids or medications into subcutaneous tissue

2. Subcutaneous abscess, osteomyelitis, and bacteremia
3. Epiphyseal injury and fracture
4. Fat embolus

Equipment

Povidone–iodine solution; sterile gauze; gloves; drapes; 1% lidocaine; 3- to 5-mL syringe; 18- or 20-gauge intraosseous infusion needle; or IO devices (EZ-IO (Vidacare) or bone injection gun (WaisMed). Alternatives: bone marrow aspiration needle; 20-gauge lumbar puncture (LP) spinal needle; saline flush solution; IV fluids and tubing

Procedure

The preferred locations are the proximal tibia or distal femur for both ease of access and safety. The distal tibia may be used in children 3 to 4 years of age or older. By aseptic technique, prepare the selected site; then inject the skin to the periosteum with 1% lidocaine for anesthesia in the awake patient. The site for penetration of the proximal tibia is the flat, medial surface of the proximal shaft (tibial plateau) 1 to 2 cm below the tibial tuberosity (Fig. 3.8A). Alternatively, use the lower third of the femur in the midline approximately 3 cm above the lateral condyle (Fig. 3.8B). In the absence of an intraosseous needle, use a spinal needle with bevel or a bone marrow sampling needle. The distal tibia site is 1 to 2 cm proximal to the medial malleolus of the tibia (Fig. 3.8C).

After penetrating the skin with the needle, direct it at a slight angle 10 to 15 degrees from vertical and away from the growth plate of the long bone (caudad for the tibia insertion; cephalad for the femur insertion). Apply downward pressure with a "to-and-fro" rotary motion to advance the needle. When the needle passes through the cortex of the bone into the marrow cavity, resistance will suddenly decrease (a "trap door effect"). Now the needle should stand without support. Remove the stylet and connect a 5-mL syringe to the needle. Confirm proper placement by aspiration of bone marrow; then flush the needle with heparinized saline and connect it to conventional IV infusion tubing. Observe the site for extravasation of fluid, which is an indication that either the placement is too superficial or the bone has been pierced through both sides. Restrain the leg and maintain a clean infusion site while the needle is in place.

Use of an EZ-IO for placement involves all the same preparation. Use the 15 mm size for patients under 40 kg and 25 mm for those over 40 kg. After marking of the spot to place the IO, aim the needle away from the growth plate with pressure against the skin and pull the trigger. The needle will pass into the bone and stop xx after entry to insure not advancing too far. As in the manual placement, it is important to maintain a steady pressure to guide it directly into the bone.

3.9. AXILLARY VEIN CATHETERIZATION

Indications

For difficult peripheral or central venous access in emergency conditions

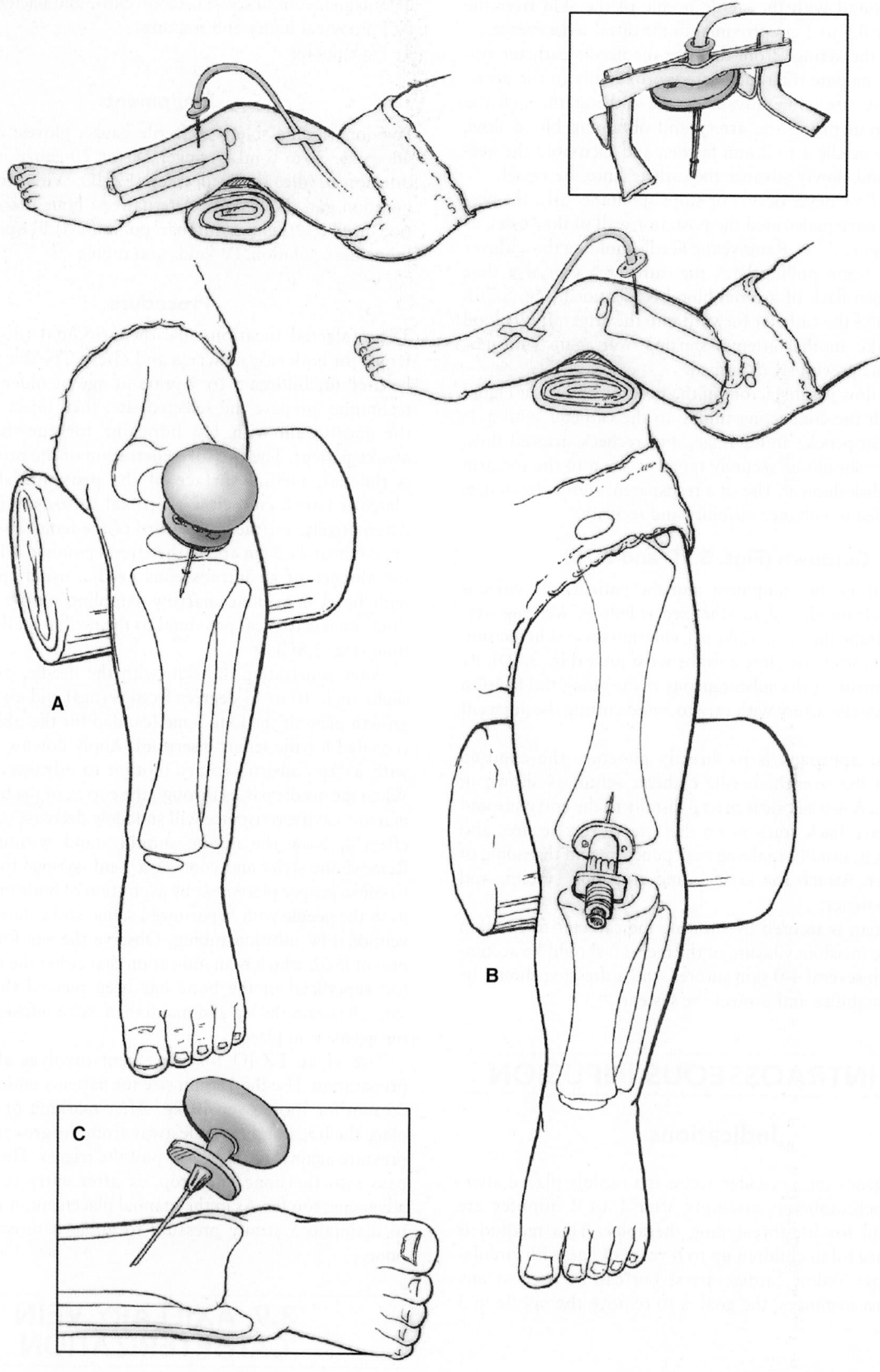

3.8

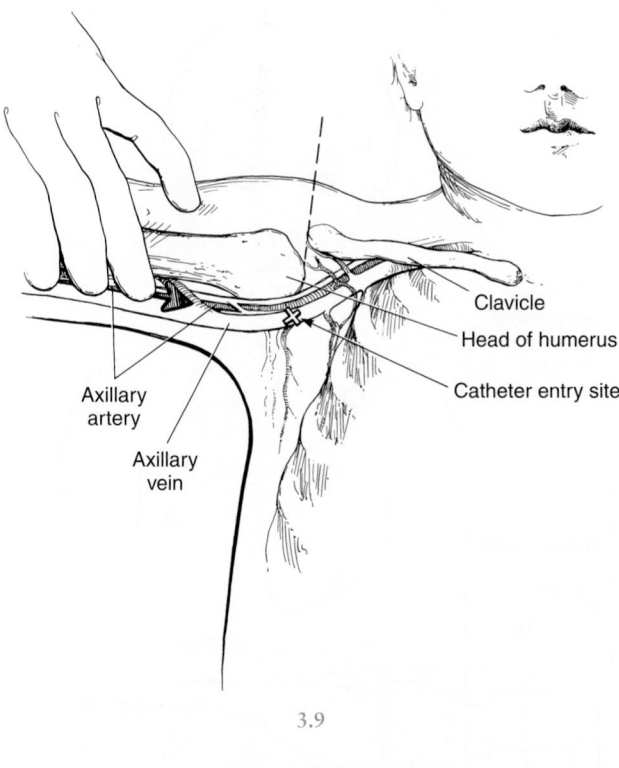

Axillary artery

Axillary vein

Clavicle

Head of humerus

Catheter entry site

3.9

Complications

1. Pneumothorax
2. Hematoma
3. Injury to axillary artery, median, or ulnar nerve
4. Thrombosis
5. Infection

Procedure

Use a catheter over needle (peripheral) or Seldinger technique (central) to access the vein.

Prepare the patient for the procedure, preferably placing him/her in the Trendelenburg position. Abduct the arm 90 to 130 degrees to maximize exposure. Palpate the course of the axillary artery (usually the vein is not visible, except in neonates). Prepare the site with povidone–iodine solution. Puncture the skin and enter the vein distal to the humeral head (Fig. 3.9) just inferior and anterior to the axillary artery. Be sure to be parallel to the palpated course of the axillary artery. After entering the vein, advance the catheter or place the wire through the needle as indicated. After securing the catheter, check again for flow. In use for peripheral venous placement, short catheters occasionally have flow problems with arm positioning. Apply a transparent clean dressing.

3.10. ACCESSING CENTRAL VENOUS CATHETERS

Types

1. Central venous access catheters—include brands such as Arrow, Broviac®, Hickman®, Bard®, Corcath®, Leonard®,

Raaf®, and Hemed®. The access to central circulation is via cephalic, external jugular, internal jugular, brachiocephalic subclavian, or saphenous veins. Peripherally inserted central lines—PICC

2. Implanted venous access catheters—Port-A-Cath, Infuse-A-Port, and Mediport and Babyport. These devices are subcutaneous chambers attached to an IV catheter, which are surgically implanted.

Indications

1. IV fluid administration
2. Medication administration
3. Phlebotomy

Equipment

Central Venous Catheters

1. Sterile gloves, mask, and eyewear
2. Povidone–iodine solution
3. Sterile drapes
4. Catheter clamp or hemostat without teeth
5. Three needles (18-, 19-, or 20-gauge)
6. 10-mL syringe with normal saline flush
7. 5-mL syringe with heparin (100 U per mL)
8. Two sterile 10-mL syringes (for phlebotomy)
9. Fluids and/or medications to be administered
10. 4 × 4 gauze pads

Implantable Venous Access Catheters

1. Sterile gloves, mask, and eyewear
2. Povidone–iodine solution
3. Sterile drapes
4. Two Huber needles (19-, 20-, or 22-gauge) with 90-degree bend or standard 19-gauge needle in an emergency
5. Extension tubing with clamp or stopcock
6. 10-mL syringe with normal saline flush
7. 5-mL syringe with heparin solution (100 U per mL)
8. 4 × 4 gauze pads
9. Silk tape
10. Fluids and/or medications to be administered

Complications

1. Line sepsis
2. Air embolus
3. Perforation of catheter
4. Embolization of thrombi while flushing
5. Catheter displacement
6. Cardiac arrhythmias
7. Infusion of medications that interact with silicone, i.e., phenytoin, diazepam
8. Infusion of incompatible medications.

Procedure

Central Venous Catheters

Sterile technique should be maintained at all times. Clamp catheter (clamp will be on catheter or a hemostat without teeth

PROCEDURES

can be used). Remove cap. Place a 10-mL syringe with normal saline flush, unclamp, and inject 5 mL; then withdraw from the central catheter to ensure patency. Clamp catheter. Bolus medication or venous fluids should be attached to end of catheter. Unclamp and open solutions to infuse.

If a blood specimen needs to be drawn, clamp catheter. Place a 10-mL syringe on the end of the catheter. Unclamp and withdraw approximate dead space solution (5 to 10 mL). Clamp. Place a separate 10-mL syringe and withdraw the desired amount of blood sample. Clamp. When blood drawing is completed, flush with normal saline and then heparin. In small infants or when sampling may be frequent, consider reinfusing the initial blood sample to clear the line to the patient prior to the saline flush and heparin. After completion, clamp and replace the cap.

If difficulty occurs with blood flow from catheter, this may be secondary to catheter placement, clot, or malfunction. Certain maneuvers that may aid in blood flow include placement of the patient in reverse Trendelenburg position, placing slight tension on the catheter, holding patient's arms over head, or use of a Valsalva maneuver. Withdrawing with force will only collapse the tubing. If the aforementioned maneuvers are not successful, gently flush catheter with 3 to 5 mL of heparin solution (100 U per mL). If this attempt fails, streptokinase or urokinase may be used, which is detailed to follow.

Implantable Venous Access Catheters (Fig. 3.10)

Sterile technique should be maintained at all times. Palpate the circular reservoir. Prepare the overlying skin with povidone–iodine solution. If have time, consider placement of topical anesthetic 30 to 40 minutes before access is desired. Connect the Huber needle to extension tubing at one end, and syringe with normal saline at other end. Tubing should be purged with normal saline and the clamp closed. Insert the Huber needle slowly through the skin into the septum of the circular reservoir until the back of the reservoir is reached. Unclamp and slowly inject saline. Watch for local infiltration, which may occur if the needle is not properly placed. Gently withdraw the plunger of the syringe to ensure placement. Lack of blood return is not an absolute contraindication for use. Blood drawing is accomplished through extension tubing after clearing the line of dead space solution. Medications or IV fluids may be attached. Remember that normal saline flush should be administered between medications. Flush with 5 mL of heparinized solution when medication or venous fluid administration is complete or blood drawing is accomplished. Remove the Huber needle.

Nonpatent Catheters—Use of Fibrinolytics

When central venous catheters or implantable catheters are not readily accessed, the most common reason is a clot being present. In the absence of central nervous system (CNS) or respiratory distress, the clinician should consider use of a fibrinolytic to assist in clot dissolution.

Urokinase (5,000 U per mL) or Streptokinase (10,000 U per 3 mL)

For 3F or 4F catheter, inject 0.5 mL into the catheter. Use 1 mL for larger size. The volume should approximate the catheter lumen priming volume. Allow to stand within the catheter for 20 minutes. Then, attempt to withdraw blood or dot with

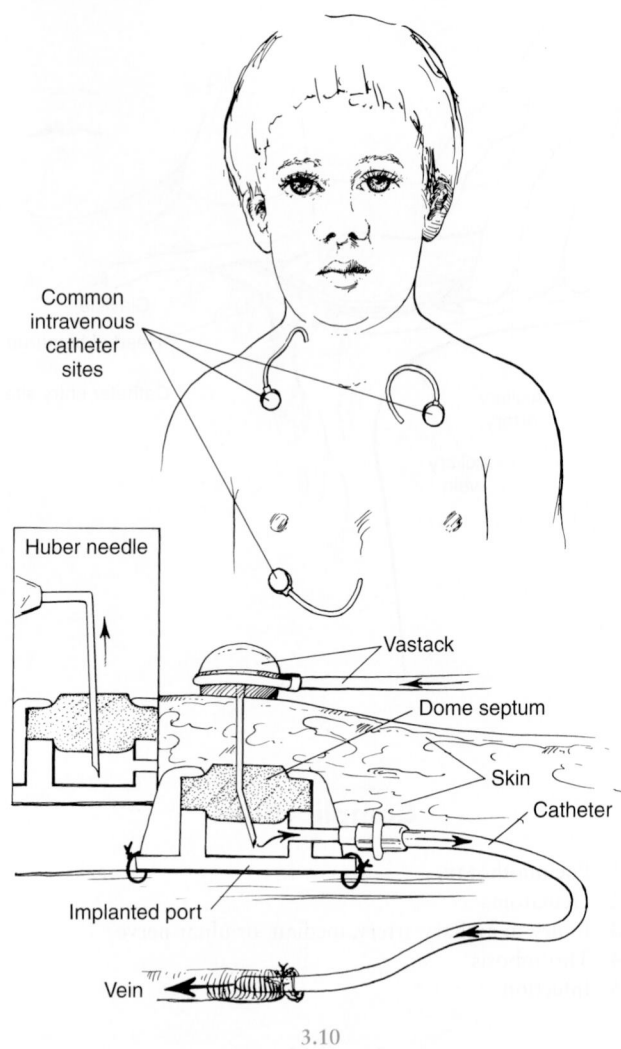

Common intravenous catheter sites

Huber needle

Vastack

Dome septum

Skin

Catheter

Implanted port

Vein

3.10

a 5- to 10-mL syringe. If this is unsuccessful, consider repeating one more time.

For more complex problems, including consideration of other precipitants, refer to the staff caring for the catheter or other texts. Because urokinase is biological, be sure to weigh the risk of its use in children at risk.

4.1. LUMBAR PUNCTURE

Indications

To obtain cerebrospinal fluid (CSF) for the diagnosis of meningitis, meningoencephalitis, subarachnoid hemorrhage, and other neurologic syndromes

Complications

1. Headache (uncommon in children younger than 10 years of age)
2. Apnea (central or obstructive)
3. Local back pain—occasionally with short-lived referred limp

4. Spinal cord bleeding—especially in the presence of bleeding diathesis
5. Infection
6. Subarachnoid epidermal cyst—secondary to foreign-body reaction
7. Ocular muscle palsy (transient)
8. Epidural CSF leak—asymptomatic to cauda equina syndrome
9. Brainstem herniation—in the presence of symptomatic intracranial hypertension

Equipment

Commercial trays; CSF manometers; spinal needle—22 gauge; 3.75 cm (1.5 in) for younger than 1 year old, 6.25 cm (2.5 in) for 1 year to middle childhood, and 8.75 cm (3.5 in) for older children and adolescents; povidone–iodine solution; consider EMLA® or Zylocaine® cream

Procedure

Lateral Decubitus Position

Restrain the patient in the lateral decubitus position. Maximally flex the spine without compromising the upper airway. Often, in infants younger than 3 months, the patient's hands can be held down between the flexed knees with one of the assistant's hands. The other hand can flex the neck at the appropriate time.

The spinal cord ends at approximately the level of the L1 and L2 vertebral bodies. Caudal to L2, only the filum terminale is present. The desired sites for LP are the interspaces between the posterior elements of L3 and L4 or L4 and L5. Locate these spaces by palpating the iliac crest (Fig. 4.1B, parts A and D). Follow an imaginary "plumb line" from the iliac crest to the spine. The interspace encountered is L4–L5. Use it or the one cephalad to it.

Use sterile technique for the LP. Cleanse the skin with povidone–iodine solution after donning sterile gloves. Using sponges, begin at the intended puncture site and sponge in widening circles until an area 10 cm in diameter has been cleansed. Repeat this three times. Drape the child beneath his/her flank and over the back with the spine accessible to view (as in Fig. 4.1A). Allow the solution to dry.

Use local anesthesia in children—this includes placement of EMLA® or ELA-Max® cream 45 to 60 minutes before LP when time is available. Alternatively, anesthetize the site by injecting 1% lidocaine intradermally to raise a wheal, then advance the needle into desired interspace, injecting anesthetic and being careful not to inject it into a blood vessel or spinal canal.

Check the spinal needle and ensure the stylet is secure. Grasp the spinal needle firmly with the bevel facing "up" toward the ceiling, making the bevel parallel to the direction of the fibers of the ligamentum flavum. Recheck the patient's position to ensure the needle's trajectory is midsagittal to his/her back. Insert the needle into the skin over the selected interspace in the midline sagittal plane. Two methods of stabilizing and guiding the needle are shown (Fig. 4.1B, parts B and D). Insert the needle slowly, aiming slightly cephalad toward the umbilicus. When the ligamentum flavum and then the dura are punctured, a "pop" and decreased resistance are felt. Remove the stylet and check for flow of spinal fluid. If no fluid is obtained, reinsert the stylet, advance the needle slowly, and check frequently for the appearance of CSF. An alternative to keeping the stylet in during the procedure is to remove it after the needle is inserted into the skin. Introducing the needle without a stylet from the start increases the risk of a small bit of epidermis entering the spinal needle and either blocking it from CSF drainage or being unintentionally introduced into the CSF space, where a epidermoid cyst may be produced. When CSF flows, attach the manometer to the needle's hub if you are to obtain an opening pressure reading. Collect 1 mL of CSF in each of the three sterile tubes. Send the CSF for routine culture, glucose and protein determination, and cell count. Collect additional tubes as indicated. After collecting CSF, a closing pressure can be obtained. Reinsert the stylet and then remove the spinal needle with one quick motion. Cleanse the back and cover the puncture site.

Sitting Position

Restrain the infant in the seated position with maximal spinal flexion (Fig. 4.1B, part C). Have the assistant hold the infant's hands between his/her flexed legs with one hand and flex the infant's head with the other hand.

Place drapes underneath the child's buttocks and on the shoulders with an opening near the intended spinal puncture site. Choose the interspace as noted earlier and follow the procedure as outlined for the lateral position. Insert the needle so it runs parallel to the spinal cord (Fig. 4.1B, part D).

4.2. EVALUATION OF VENTRICULOPERITONEAL SHUNT

Indications

To evaluate the role of shunt malfunction as the cause of signs and symptoms, including vomiting, drowsiness, headache, seizures, bradycardia, coma, focal neurologic findings, or swelling around the shunt site

Complications

1. Proximal shunt dysfunction—Repetitive pumping of a functioning shunt may lead to blockage of the proximal

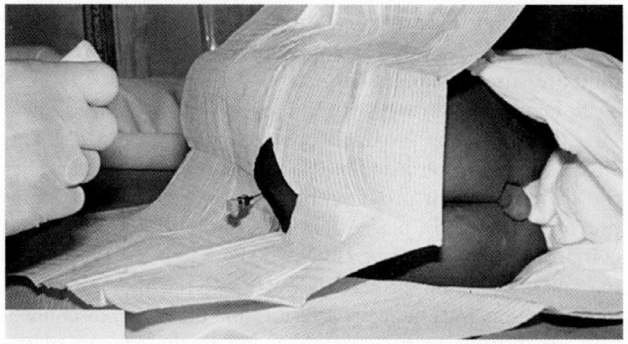

4.1A

PROCEDURES

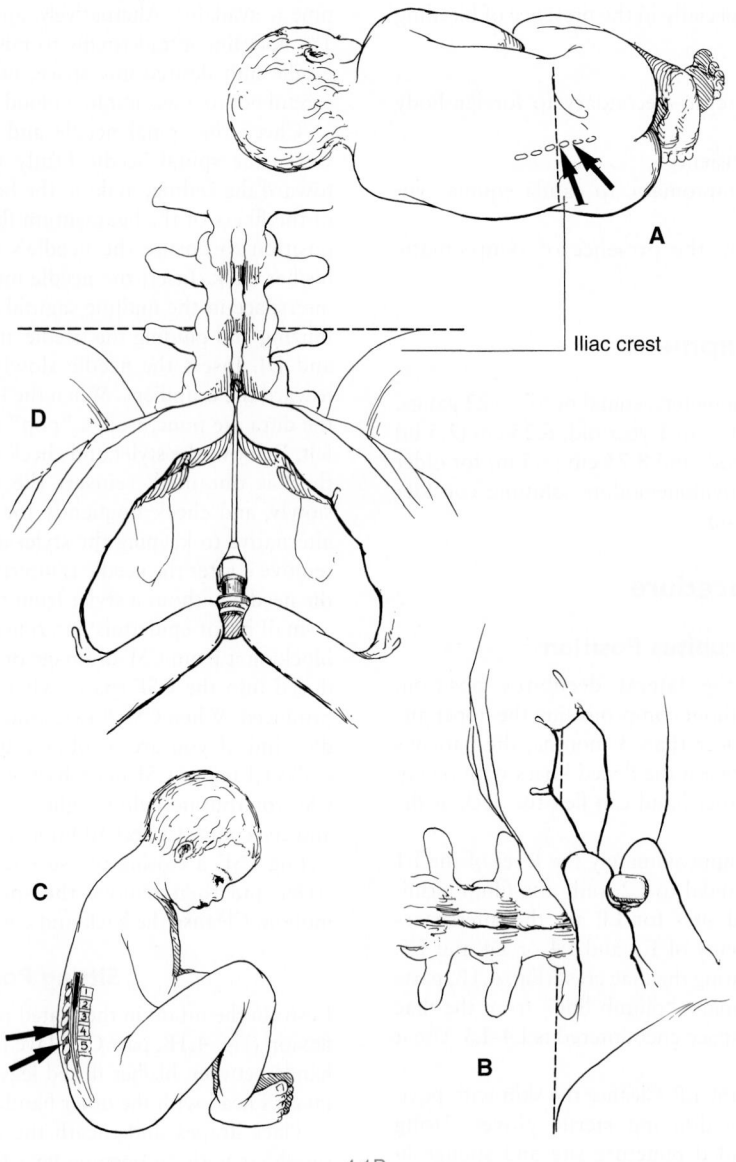

Iliac crest

4.1B

shunt with tissue from the choroid plexus or blood from irritation of the ventricular wall.

2. CSF leakage—If a complete blockage occurs distally, some patients develop a CSF collection in the subgaleal space that may be exacerbated by vigorous pumping.

Procedure

Figures 4.2 and 4.3 show two types of common permanent ventricular drainage systems. Figure 4.2 is a "double-bubble" ventriculoperitoneal shunt. Its distal end, located in the abdominal cavity, has a one-way valve. The shunt tubing travels from the lateral ventricle, through the skull, to the subcutaneous space of the scalp where a right angle is made. At this point, it connects to a double-bubble rubber reservoir that lies posterior and superior to the ear in the parietooccipital area of the skull. Finally, it continues subcutaneously, as shown, to the

abdominal cavity, where the CSF drains, if the system functions properly, and is absorbed by the peritoneum.

To check the function and patency of the system, place the child in a comfortable position during the physical examination. Locate the tubing and trace its entire course to look for disconnections, fluid accumulations, or short tubing length at the distal end. This should not cause pain, as it involves only mild pressure on skin surface.

In Figure 4.2, three maneuvers to assess patency are shown. First, compress the proximal bubble as in Figure 4.2A. This ensures filling of the distal bubble for the next step and empties the chamber to test proximal blockage later. While still compressing proximally, place a finger over the distal bubble and compress it as in Figure 4.2B. Normally, there is no resistance to emptying of fluid through the valve into the abdominal cavity. Undue pressure suggests a distal tube blockage, disconnection, or insufficient tube length owing to the growth of the child. Finally, release the proximal bubble as in Figure 4.2C.

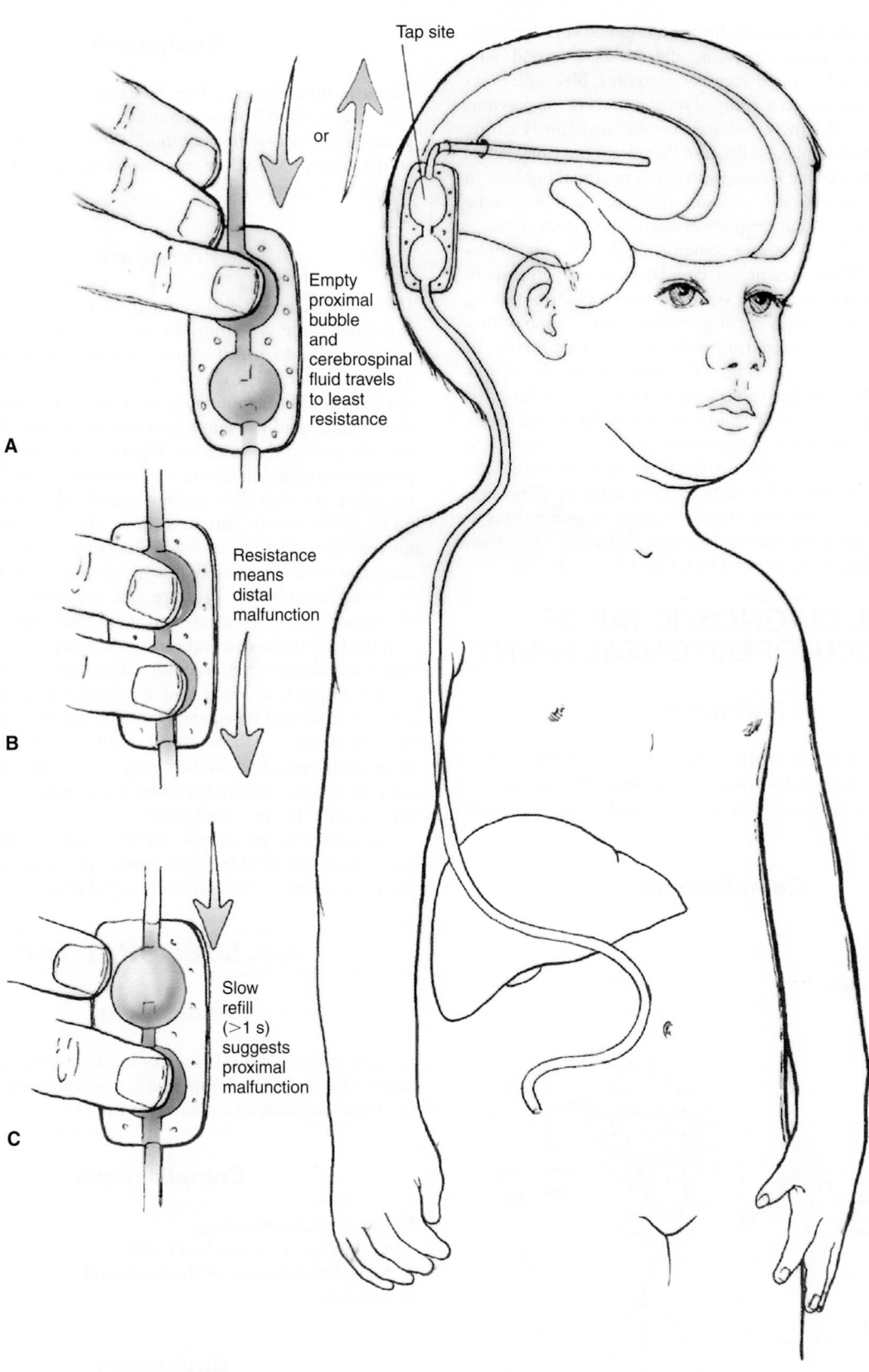

Tap site

A Empty proximal bubble and cerebrospinal fluid travels to least resistance

or

B Resistance means distal malfunction

C Slow refill (>1 s) suggests proximal malfunction

4.2

Now the negative pressure in this bubble should suck fluid into it from the ventricular cavity, usually within 1 second. Any longer delay in filling often suggests a proximal blockage; however, if the shunt has been pumped several times in the previous hours, it may fill slowly because the proximal tip is sitting against the choroid plexus. Because there is no proximal valve, when the distal bubble is compressed, the proximal bubble can be repeatedly depressed to measure resistance to filling of the proximal shunt without draining excessive fluid from above.

Figure 4.3 shows the very common single-reservoir, single-pump shunt. When present, the circular chamber perpendicular to the shunt entering the skull is a reservoir for obtaining specimens. More distally a compressible rubber pump with a pressure valve is connected on each end to plastic tubing. In most, there is a valve often near the reservoir, which controls flow. It may be an in-line valve as part of the distal catheter. To pump this type, compress and release the distal soft tube, checking for refill. Each compression will test distal patency, whereas the release verifies proximal patency. Generally, the release is immediate in this shunt, so any delay of filling suggests blockage or choroid collapse. Because the connections of the pump to the shunt tubing are purse strings on either end, this system can disconnect and leak CSF subcutaneously.

4.3. DIAGNOSTIC TAP OF VENTRICULOPERITONEAL SHUNT

Indications

1. Reduction of intracranial pressure in a child with acute symptomatic hydrocephalus typically from shunt obstruction
2. Diagnostic evaluation of possible ventricular or shunt infection

Complications

1. Infection
2. CSF leak
3. Local hematoma

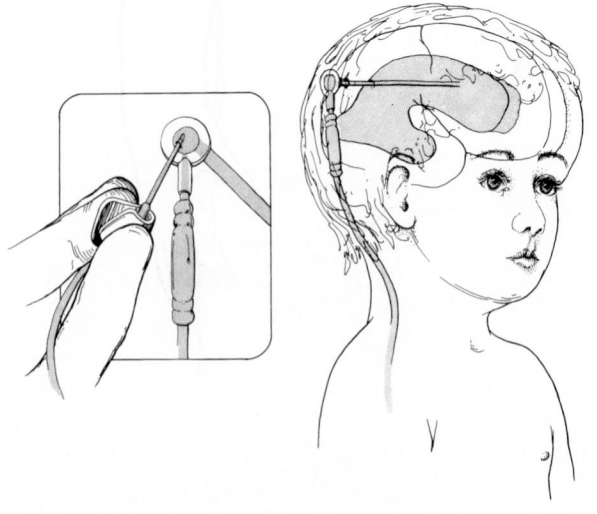

Equipment

Butterfly infusion set, 23 or 25 gauge; 5- to 10-mL syringe; sterile collection tubes; manometer; sterile gloves, sterile gauze; povidone–iodine solution; 70% alcohol; razor blade; sterile drape; EMLA® or anesthetic cream; 1% lidocaine with needle and syringe

Procedure

Locate the reservoir and pump(s), and assess the function of the shunt if the symptoms are suggestive of blockage. When time permits 45 to 60 minutes to procedure, consider the application anesthetic cream to skin over the tap site. Restrain the patient in the supine position with the face turned toward the shoulder and the shunt reservoir facing up; shave the hair directly around the reservoir. Wash the site several times with povidone–iodine solution in a circumferential fashion; clean it off when dry with 70% alcohol and dry the area with sterile gauze. Don sterile gloves. Palpate the reservoir with one gloved finger (Figs. 4.2 and 4.3). Puncture the skin and quickly enter the reservoir. If distal obstruction is present, the fluid will be under considerable pressure and will flow readily. Attach the manometer immediately and standardize the zero mark on it at the level of the cerebral ventricles. Samples of CSF are collected aseptically into sterile tubes. Use slight negative pressure on the syringe to enhance flow if proximal obstruction or viscous infected fluid is evident. Drainage may be continued until the CSF pressure is between 10 to 20 mL (cm H_2O). Refrain from applying suction on the syringe to minimize the chance of choroid plexus entering the shunt if the ventricle were to collapse around the proximal shunt.

Figure 4.3 shows a single reservoir system being tapped. In general, on the double-bubble setup, puncture the proximal bubble in a similar fashion as described earlier.

4.4. SUBDURAL TAP

Indications

Evacuations of subdural blood or fluid in young infants, when such collections cause symptoms (i.e., seizures, unilateral paresis) from increased intracranial pressure

Complications

1. Intracranial hemorrhage
2. Contusion of the cerebral cortex
3. Subgaleal collection of fluid or blood
4. Infection

Equipment

Subdural or spinal needle (19 or 20 gauge); 10-mL syringe; razor blade; povidone–iodine solution; 70% alcohol; sterile gauze; 1% lidocaine with epinephrine; 22- and 25-gauge needles (Fig. 4.4); strongly consider pharmacologic sedation

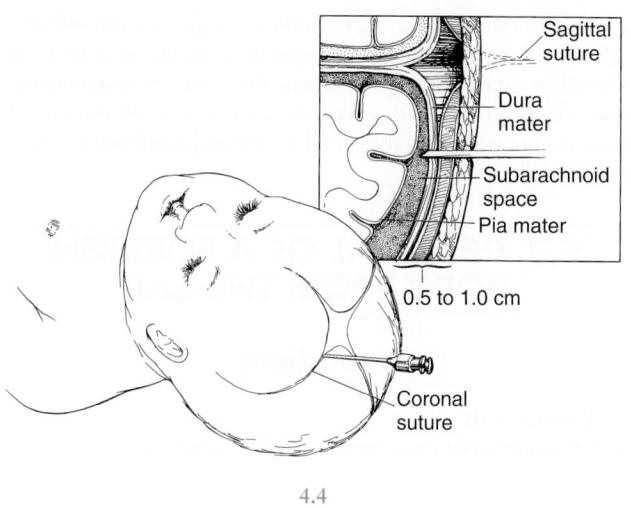

4.4

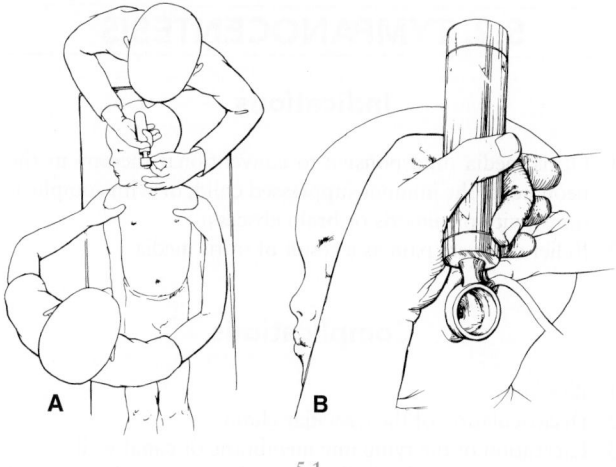

5.1

Procedure

Prepare the infant for the procedure in the supine position after performing the appropriate measures for resuscitation and stabilization. Have an assistant restrain the patient in a mummy wrap or by leaning over the infant with his/her arms firmly pinned at the side. The head should be face up. Continuous monitoring of the cardiorespiratory status is essential.

Shave the scalp widely in an area around the lateral boundaries of the anterior fontanel (the anterior two thirds of the head). Prepare the site(s) with povidone–iodine solution and 70% alcohol, and then dry with sterile gauze. Wearing sterile gloves, palpate the coronal suture at the lateral aspect of the anterior fontanel. If the fontanel opening is extremely small, move several millimeters farther laterally in the coronal suture. Inject local anesthetic (i.e., 1% lidocaine with epinephrine) in the conscious child.

Grasp a 19- or 20-gauge subdural or spinal needle by the hub and check its patency. Hold it between the thumb and index finger, and rest the heel of the hand against the infant's scalp. Puncture the skin at a right angle to surface, stretching it slightly to obtain a Z-track. Advance the needle through the puncture site between the edges of the coronal suture until the feeling of resistance lessens. Then, remove the stylet to allow fluid or blood to drain; 10 to 15 mL can be safely evacuated from each side. Normally, the needle is not advanced more than 5 to 8 mm below the scalp's surface. Some infants may require bilateral taps.

5.1. PNEUMATIC OTOSCOPIC EXAMINATION

Indications

Evaluation of middle ear

Complications

Pain or bleeding from contusion or laceration of the external canal

Procedure

To safely and accurately evaluate the middle ear structures in infants, the lack of movement while performing the examination is critical. In many infants, this requires appropriate restraint. Many young children fear the approach of a physician, particularly to examine their ears. Usually a parent can provide proper immobilization. Place the infant supine on the examination table, and ask a parent to hold the arms firmly against the trunk (Fig. 5.1A) or against the head, grasping them just above the elbow. When assisting, the parent may hold his/her hand across the forehead against his/her own chest to minimize movement. Hold the otoscope as shown in Figure 5.1B, grasping it between the thumb and index finger of the dominant hand. The heel of the hand should rest against the anterior portion of the infant's head to maintain constant, firm pressure against the temporal skull while bringing the infant's head horizontal to the table. This assists the operator in ensuring the otoscope will move in conjunction with the child if he/she is not still during the procedure.

Once the infant is restrained, use the other hand to grasp the upper portion of the helix, stretching it superiorly and posteriorly in the child to straighten the external canal. In young infants, pull the helix inferiorly and posteriorly to best visualize the tympanic membrane. Simultaneously, observe the entrance to the auditory canal through the otoscope and flex the thumb to direct the speculum down the canal entrance. Then, straightening of the external canal is performed under direct visualization. The removal of cerumen obscuring the field may be necessary (see Procedure 5.3). Observe the tympanic membrane for color, contour, and presence of the bony and vascular landmarks (see the "Otitis Media" section in Chapter 54).

For evaluation of the compliance of the tympanic membrane, a tight seal is required between the auditory canal and the speculum. If the diameter of the speculum is found to be less than that of the canal, replace it with one of a larger size. Reenter the canal to one third to one half of its depth, establish a seal, and lightly squeeze the bulb while observing the tympanic membrane.

PROCEDURES

5.2. TYMPANOCENTESIS

Indications

1. Otitis media unresponsive to conventional therapy in the neonate, in the immunosuppressed child, or with complications (with meningitis or brain abscess)
2. Relief of severe pain as a result of otitis media

Complications

1. Bleeding
2. Disarticulation of the ossicular chain
3. Laceration of the tympanic membrane or canal wall
4. Contamination of middle ear by bacteria in the external canal

Procedure

After full explanation of the procedure to the parents and patient, obtain consent including the use of pharmacologic sedation to reduce anxiety and movement. Prepare all equipment, include child life assistance if available and restrain the child securely in a supine position. Use the mummy or papoose restraint, or ask an assistant to restrain the trunk. Have the child's head held in the horizontal plane by an assistant. Visualize the external canal and clean any wax or debris from it. When available, use of operating head otoscope improves visualization of landmarks. Sterilize the ear canal by filling it with 70% alcohol or povidone–iodine solution for 60 seconds, and then drain out excess solution by placing the ear down. Again restrain the child's head in the horizontal plane, and visualize the tympanic membrane with an otoscope fitted with an operating head. Insert the aspiration set (a 22-gauge, 8- to 10-cm spinal needle bent 30 degrees 4 to 5 cm from the tip and attached to a 1-mL tuberculin syringe) into the otoscope, through the speculum as shown in Figure 5.2A. Pierce the

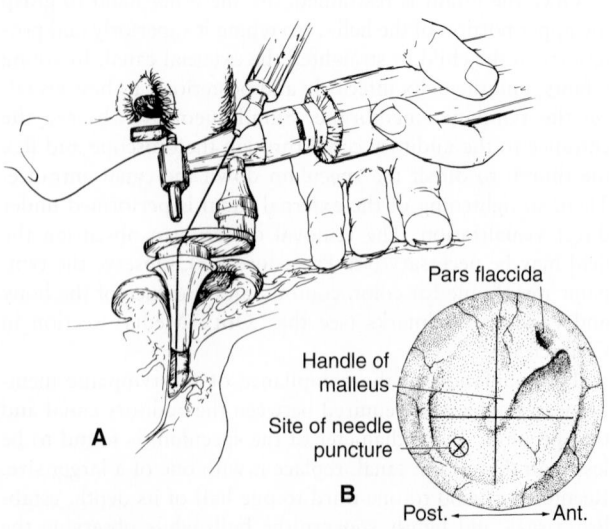

Pars flaccida

Handle of malleus

Site of needle puncture

A

B

Post. ◀——————▶ Ant.

eardrum as shown (Fig. 5.2B) in the inferoposterior quadrant. After entering the middle ear, aspirate with the syringe. Care should be taken not to contaminate the needle by touching the ear canal or otoscopic speculum. If only a small amount of fluid is obtained, flush the spinal needle with nonbacteriostatic normal saline.

5.3. REMOVAL OF A FOREIGN BODY FROM THE EAR

Indications

1. Foreign body
2. Obstruction of the external canal by cerumen

Complications

1. Laceration of the canal wall
2. Perforation of the tympanic membrane
3. Ossicular disruption

Procedure

Three methods are available for removal of a foreign body; all require cooperation from, or restraint of, the child. Other options include pharmacologic sedation to assist the operator. Because the material may not be emergent to remove and may be difficult in this setting, it is often ideal not to go to extreme measures where there may be local trauma or unnecessary anxiety/pain and to refer to an ear, nose, and throat specialist for more elective removal. Because a minor laceration of the ear canal is often unavoidable, the parents should be aware of this complication before the physician undertakes the use of a curette or forceps. After removal of foreign body or cerumen by any method, it is important to visualize the eardrum and document its condition.

Curette (Fig. 5.3A)

Visualize the foreign body with a speculum, preferably using an operating head otoscope. Then, slowly advance the curette just beyond the foreign body as shown. While applying pressure to the foreign body, slowly withdraw the curette until the foreign body is removed.

Forceps (Fig. 5.3B)

Visualize the foreign body with a speculum and look for a protruding edge of the foreign material. Carefully guide the forceps in the closed position under direct visualization through the speculum. Just a few millimeters from the edge of the foreign body, open the forceps and grasp the edge gently. Withdraw the forceps, visualizing the foreign body simultaneously to minimize the chance of a complication.

Irrigation (Fig. 5.3C)

Straighten the ear canal and visualize the foreign body directly with a speculum, ensuring the tympanic membrane is intact. If the foreign body is spongy or could be expansile when wet, such as a bean or other food material, do not use this method.

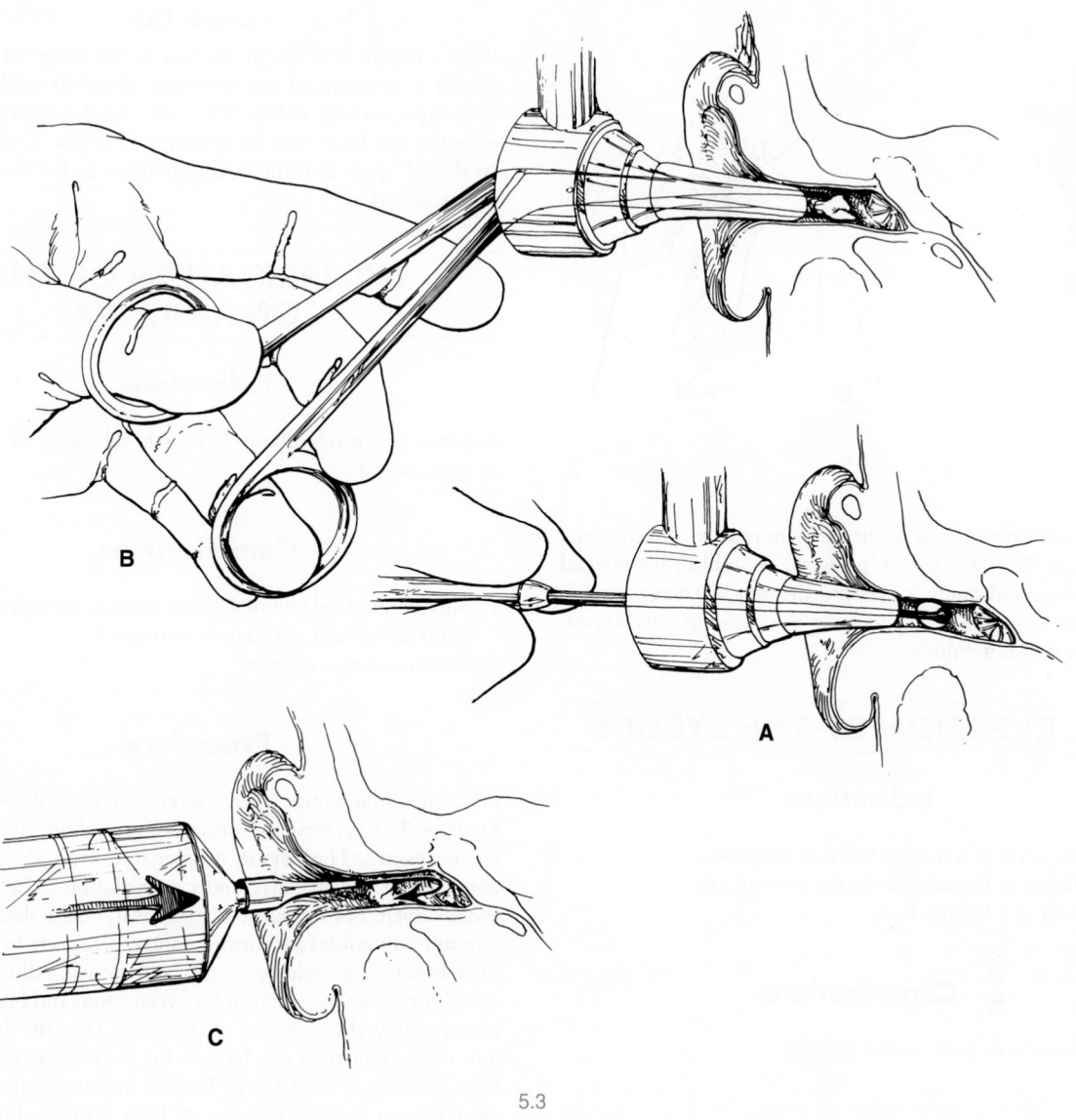

5.3

Do not attempt to remove a disc battery with irrigation. Remove the speculum and irrigate the ear canal by injecting a constant stream of water at body temperature. Use a 20- to 50-mL syringe attached to a flexible IV catheter tip (i.e., a cut section of tubing from a butterfly needle). Repeated irrigation may be necessary to provide complete emptying.

5.4. ASPIRATION OF AN AURICULAR HEMATOMA

Indications

Traumatic auricular hematoma or seroma

Complications

1. Recurrent hematoma or seroma
2. Infection (abscess)

Procedure

Restrain the child in a standard method. Palpate the hematoma to find the most fluctuant portion. Cleanse the skin over the hematoma with povidone–iodine solution and dry with sterile gauze. Topical anesthesia may be provided with EMLA® or topical lidocaine directly applied 30 to 45 minutes before aspiration on the hematoma. In very anxious children or those requiring longer procedure, consider the use of pharmacologic sedation prior to the procedure.

Use a 10- or 20-mL syringe with an 18-gauge straight needle. While stabilizing the syringe against the scalp with the nondominant gloved hand, puncture the most fluctuant portion of the hematoma with the needle (Figs. 5.4A and 5.4B). Maintain negative pressure on the syringe with one hand, while "milking" the hematoma with the thumb and index finger of the other. Withdraw the needle after emptying the hematoma, but continue to maintain pressure on the auricle between the thumb and the finger to tamponade any ongoing bleeding for 3 to 5 minutes. If blood clots are difficult to

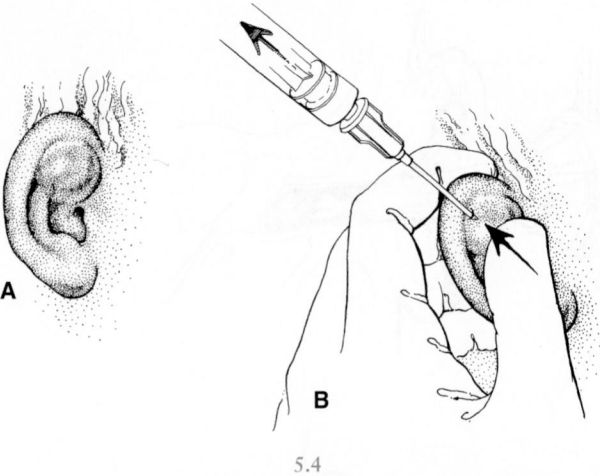

5.4

remove, consider use of a curved hemostat to improve the evacuation. With wet cotton pledgets, reestablish the normal ear contours and apply a pressure dressing. Arrange for follow-up in 12 to 24 hours to have the dressing unwrapped, check the ear, and redress.

6.1. EVERSION OF THE EYELIDS

Indications

1. Identification of a foreign body or infection
2. Instillation of medications to the conjunctiva
3. Removal of a foreign body

Complications

Mild contusion or ecchymoses (rarely)

Procedure

Have an assistant restrain the infant on the examination table in the supine position with the arms wrapped around the head. Alternatively, small infants can sit on the lap of a parent who then holds the infant's head still. Older cooperative patients may sit up for the procedure.

Upper Lid

Upper lid eversion is the more difficult, normally requiring cooperation or restraint, because the examiner needs to use both hands. After restraint, grasp the eyelash and distal upper lid between the index finger and the thumb. Ask the child to look down at the floor if he/she will cooperate. Draw the eyelid downward as shown in Figure 6.1A. Place a clean cotton swab across the superior tarsal margin, as shown in Figure 6.1B. In one motion, move the swab slightly downward and pull the eyelid slightly upward. This maneuver should bend the eyelid slightly upward and backward and expose the palpebral surface, as shown in Figure 6.1C. To restore the lid to its usual position, lift the swab slightly while maintaining pressure along the upper lid margin, and turn the thumb and index finger downward.

Lower Lid

Place a thumb or finger at the base of the lower lid and gently retract it in a caudal and posterior direction while the child looks upward (Fig. 6.1D). While the eyelid is everted, removal of a foreign body can be accomplished. Use a clean cotton swab and apply it to the foreign body to flick it from the conjunctival surface.

6.2. IRRIGATION OF THE CONJUNCTIVA

Indications

Presence of a foreign body or caustic substance on the cornea or conjunctiva

Complications

1. Subconjunctival hemorrhage or corneal abrasion (rare) in a child who is not adequately restrained
2. Conjunctival erythema

Procedure

Place the child supine over a large sink or pail, as shown in Figure 6.2. To restrain an uncooperative child, two assistants are necessary. The person holding the head should wear a gown and may use gauze under each thumb to help keep the eyelids open. For foreign-body removal, where delay of a few minutes will not lead to further injury, place one to two drops of ophthalmic anesthetic on the conjunctiva. Allow bacteriostatic normal saline solution (between room and body temperature) to flow through a set of IV tubing. Drip the fluid rapidly into the conjunctival sac. Irrigate for a minimum of 5 minutes for acid using at least 1 liter. Irrigate for 20 minutes for alkali or unknown substances using at least 2 liters. Tap water at room temperature is an acceptable alternative for irrigation fluid, especially if it can be done immediately, such as in a home or office setting.

After irrigation, the eye should be carefully examined for corneal and conjunctival integrity, including staining with fluorescein dye.

6.3. EYELID RETRACTION

Indications

1. Identification and removal of a foreign body
2. Enable examination of the anterior surface of the eye, cul de sac, and palpebral conjunctiva, especially in the uncooperative patient or when concern for traumatic rupture of the globe exists

Complications

1. Contusion of lid/globe
2. Corneal abrasion

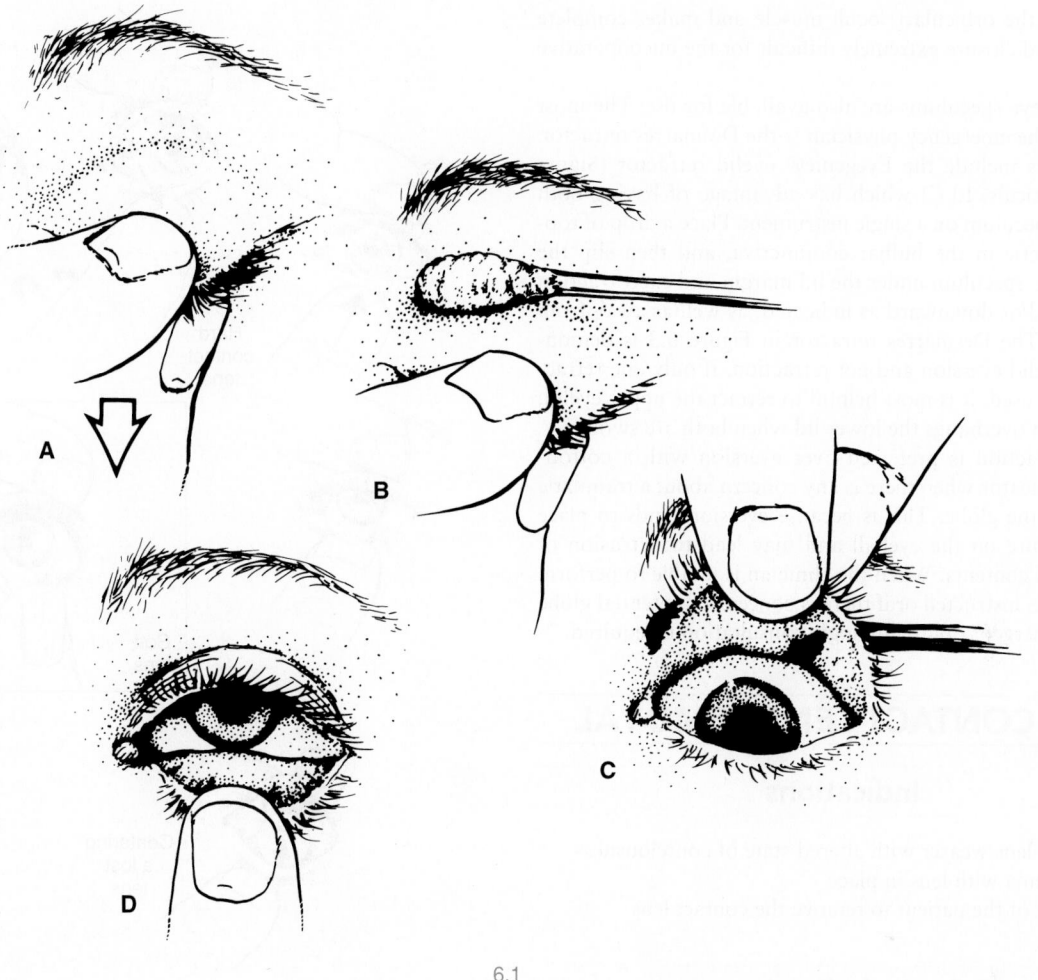

6.1

Procedure (Fig. 6.3)

As in all emergency procedures, universal blood and body fluid precautions (e.g., use of gloves) are a consideration. Place one finger on the orbital rim and gently but firmly roll the finger to gather the elastic tissue at the lid either upward (for the superior orbital rim) or downward (inferior rim). This maneuver

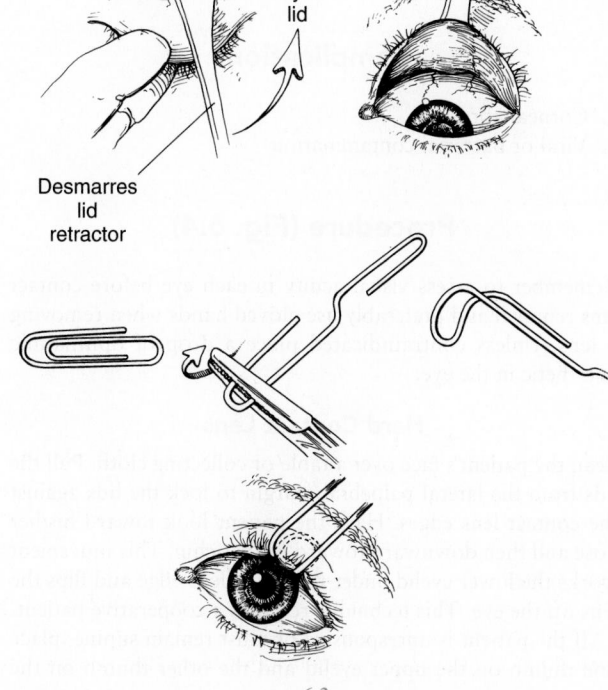

Everting eye lid

Desmarres lid retractor

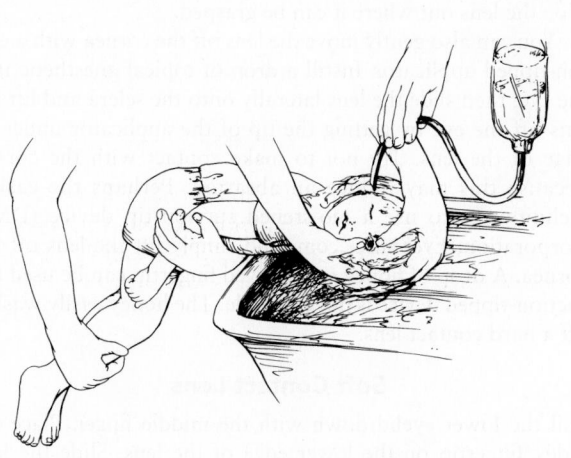

6.2

6.3

overcomes the orbicularis oculi muscle and makes complete forced eyelid closure extremely difficult for the uncooperative patient.

Several eye speculums are also available for use. The most useful for the emergency physician is the Desmarres retractor. Alternatives include the Eyegenie® eyelid retractor (Sigma Pharmaceuticals, LLC) which has advantage of having both ends of a speculum on a single instrument. Place a drop of topical anesthetic in the bulbar conjunctiva, and then slip the blade of the speculum under the lid margin and exert traction upward and/or downward as indicated, as well as away from the globe. The Desmarres retractor in Figure 6.3 is demonstrating eyelid eversion and not retraction. If only one retractor is to be used, it is most helpful to retract the upper eyelid, which often overhangs the lower lid when both are swollen.

Lid retraction is preferred over eversion with a cotton-tipped applicator when there is any concern about a traumatic rupture of the globe. This is because eversion tends to place some pressure on the eyeball and may lead to extrusion of intraorbital contents. When the clinician is unable to perform this easily as instructed or if there is concern of potential globe rupture, emergent ophthalmologic consultation is required.

6.4. CONTACT LENS REMOVAL

Indications

1. Contact lens wearer with altered state of consciousness
2. Eye trauma with lens in place
3. Inability of the patient to remove the contact lens

Contraindications

Possible corneal perforation—suction cup technique preferred in this instance

Complications

1. Corneal abrasion
2. Viral or bacterial contamination

Procedure (Fig. 6.4)

Remember to assess visual acuity in each eye before contact lens removal and preferably use gloved hands when removing a lens. Unless contraindicated place a drop of ophthalmic anesthetic in the eye.

Hard Contact Lens

Lean the patient's face over a table or collecting cloth. Pull the lids from the lateral palpebral margin to lock the lids against the contact lens edges. Have the patient look toward his/her nose and then downward toward his/her chin. This movement works the lower eyelid under the lower lens edge and flips the lens off the eye. This technique requires a cooperative patient.

If the patient is unresponsive or must remain supine, place one thumb on the upper eyelid and the other thumb on the

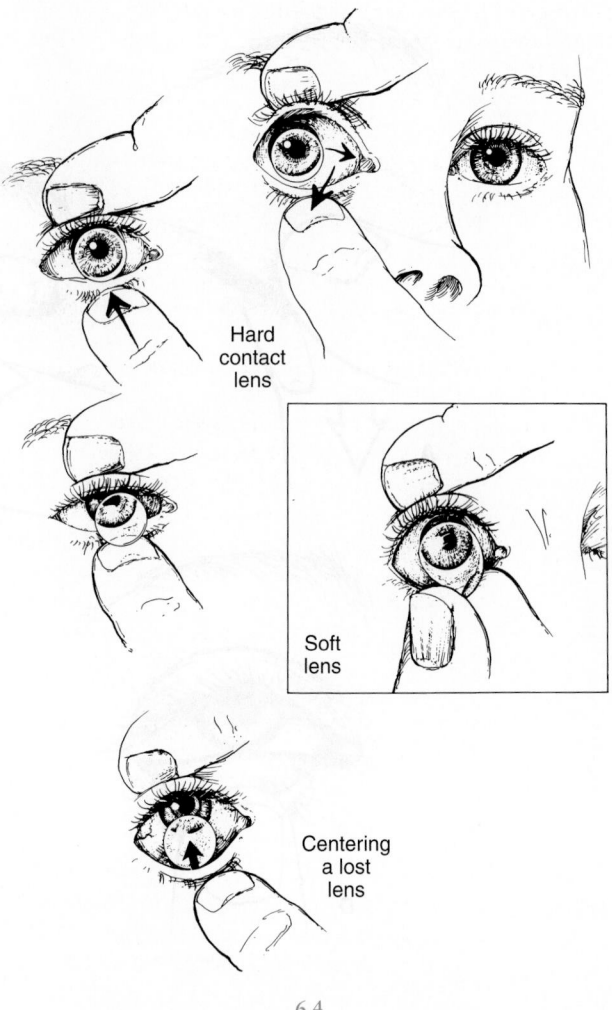

Hard
contact
lens

Soft
lens

Centering
a lost
lens

6.4

lower eyelid near the lid margins. With the lens centered over the cornea, open the eyelids until the lid margins are beyond the edges of the lens. Then press both eyelids gently but firmly on the globe and move the lids so they barely touch the edges of the lens. Press slightly harder on the lower lid to move it further under the bottom edge of the lens. As the lower lens edge begins to tip away from the eye, move the lids together and slide the lens out where it can be grasped.

You can also gently move the lens off the cornea with a cotton-tipped applicator. Instill a drop of topical anesthetic into the eye, then slide the lens laterally onto the sclera and lift the lens off the eye by getting the tip of the applicator under an edge of the lens. Try not to make contact with the cornea because this may induce an abrasion. Perhaps the easiest technique is to use a moistened suction-tip device (DMV Corporation; EyeSource.com) and simply lift the lens off the cornea. A drop of honey on a gloved fingertip can be used if a suction-tipped device is not available. The honey easily washes off a hard contact lens.

Soft Contact Lens

Pull the lower eyelid down with the middle finger. Place the index fingertip on the lower edge of the lens. Slide the lens down onto the sclera and pinch the lens slightly between the thumb and index finger. This folds the lens and allows removal from the eye.

"Lost" Contact Lens

Patients may be uncertain whether their lens is hidden under a lid, remains on the cornea, or is truly off the eye. As with all other eye examinations, begin the evaluation with an assessment of visual acuity. Then inspect the eye for the contact lens. Although transparent, lenses are usually seen easily as a fine line on the sclera several millimeters peripheral to the limbus. If the lens is not evident on initial inspection, evert the eyelids as discussed in Procedure 6.1. If the lens is still not visible, place a drop of topical anesthetic in the eye. Then, with the patient looking toward his/her chin, sweep over the upper fornix gently with a moistened cotton-tipped applicator. If the lens remains elusive and the patient is insistent that it is still in the eye, a fluorescein examination may be performed after explaining that the dye will permanently stain a soft contact lens. If the contact lens is still not found, reassure the patient that a thorough examination has not located the missing lens. Be sure to check that the patient has not inadvertently placed one contact over the other in the same eye.

7.1. NASAL CAUTERIZATION

Indications

Epistaxis recalcitrant to conservative management with the application of a topical vasoconstrictor and manual pressure

Contraindications

Bleeding diathesis (e.g., hemophilia, thrombocytopenia)
Prior nasal cauterization within the past 4 to 6 weeks

Complications

1. Septal perforation
2. Staining of the external nose or upper lip with the use of silver nitrate
3. Thermal damage to the anterior nares or inferior turbinate with the use of electrocautery
4. Secondary bacterial infection of the cauterized area

Procedure

The patient should be sitting or lying in a supine position and, if necessary, manually restrained; distraction techniques, anxiolysis, or procedural sedation may be useful for the apprehensive patient. Care should be taken with patient positioning as well as with medication administration as brisk epistaxis may result in airway compromise in the supine or sedated patient. Topical anesthesia and vasoconstriction of the nasal mucosa can be achieved with the use of an atomizer or cotton pledgets soaked with the desired agents (Table 7.1). This will allow better visualization of the interior of the nose and may slow or

TABLE 7.1

EQUIPMENT—OTORHINOLARYNGOLOGIC PROCEDURES

Directed light source (e.g., headlight, flashlight)
Frazier section tip
Nasal speculum
Bayonet forceps
Topical vasoconstrictor [phenylephrine (0.25%, 0.5%), epinephrine (1:1,000), cocaine (3% to 5% solution)]
Topical anesthetics [cocaine (3% to 5% solution), lidocaine (4%), ethyl chloride]
Absorbable gelatin sponge (Gelfoam)
Oxycel gauze (Surgicel)
Silver nitrate sticks
Expandable sponge nasal pack (Merocel, Rhino-Rocket)
Vaseline gauze (0.5 × 72 in)
Gauze (4 × 4) to make posterior pack
Suture (0-silk) 18 in length
Foley catheter (12 or 14 gauge with 30-mL balloon)
Red rubber catheters
Cuff (made of 1-in length of suction tubing)
Syringe (50 mL)
Sterile saline solution
Hoffman clamp (for Foley catheter)
Scalpel blade, no. 15
Alligator forceps

even stop the bleeding. In addition, the topical anesthetic will aid in minimizing the pain associated with instrumentation of the nose. Prior to topical medication application, the patient should gently blow their nose to clear mucous, blood, and clot that may be present.

Insert the nasal speculum into the nose and open the blades widely, using a headlight or directed light source (i.e., flashlight or penlight) to illuminate the interior of the nose. Most epistaxis originates from Kiesselbach's plexus in Little's area (the anterior septum), and this area should be examined first. Suction any remaining clots or fresh blood gently with a Frazier suction tip on low-pressure wall suction to expose the source of hemorrhage. Once the site of bleeding is located, apply the tip of a silver nitrate stick to it and roll it over the bleeding area for 5 to 10 seconds (Fig. 7.1). Two or three sticks are often required to control an episode of epistaxis. Once the bleeding has stopped, petroleum jelly (Vaseline®) or oxidized cellulose gauze (Surgicel®) may be placed on the septum to stabilize the clot and protect the area from further trauma.

If electrocautery is available, it can be used in place of the silver nitrate sticks, but certain precautions must be taken. Although topical anesthesia is often effective for the application of silver nitrate sticks, injected local anesthesia with bilateral application is required before the use of electric current. If unilateral anesthesia is performed, the electric current may be transmitted through the septum causing significant discomfort to the non-anesthetized side. Also, the electrocautery must be properly grounded electrically and have a manual setting so that low voltage can be used. A conservative amount of cauterization is recommended to avoid septal perforation.

With either method of cauterization, refrain from cauterizing both sides of the nasal septum during the same treatment.

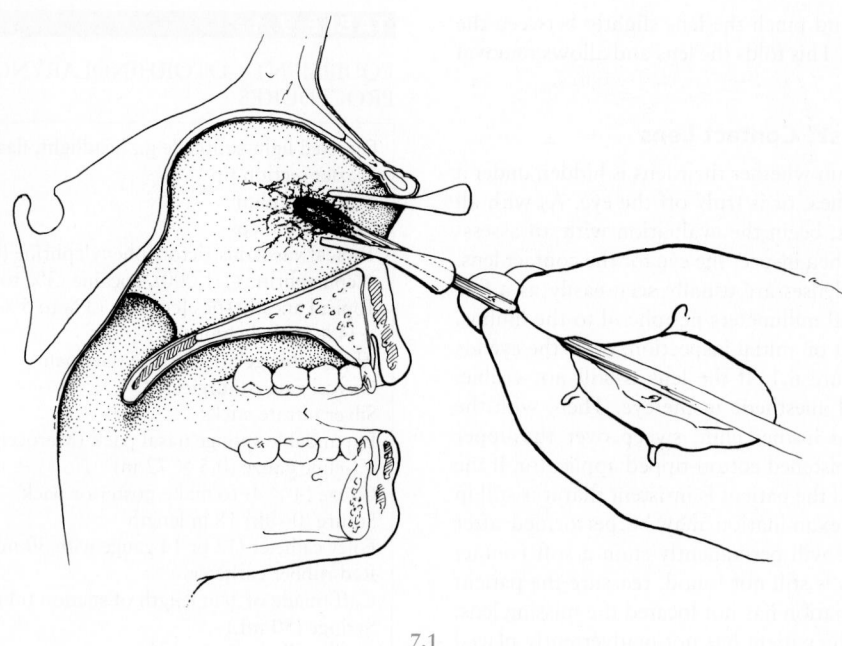

7.1

Vigorous bilateral cauterization may deprive the underlying septal cartilage of its blood supply leading to a septal perforation.

7.2. NASAL PACKING—ANTERIOR AND POSTERIOR

Indications

Epistaxis recalcitrant to or not amenable to medical management or cauterization

1. Bacterial rhinosinusitis
2. Toxic shock syndrome
3. Nasal alar or columellar necrosis
4. Septal ulceration or perforation
5. Synechiae formation
6. Hypoxemia or respiratory distress from sedation and nasal airway obstruction

Procedure

Anterior Pack (Fig. 7.2A)

Anterior packing can be performed using a variety of commercially available nasal tampons or as classically described using petroleum jelly or antibiotic ointment impregnated gauze. Prior to insertion of packing, consider the use of an anxiolytic/amnestic or procedural sedation to minimize the pain and emotional trauma associated with the packing procedure in a pediatric patient. Prepare the patient in the same manner as for cauterization, including the careful visualization of the nasal cavity and suctioning of active bleeding. Mild anterior nasal bleeding can often be stopped with a small pack created out of absorbable (gelatin foam, oxidized cellulose, or thrombin-gelatin) material. Although this type of material does not

apply a lot of pressure to a bleeding site, it facilitates clotting, protects the nasal mucosa, and does not require removal.

Nasal Tampons and Inflatable Devices. There are several commercially available products that all function by expansion when placed into the nasal cavity thereby tamponading the site of bleeding. A nasal tampon, such as Merocel®, is inserted in a dry, compressed state along the floor of the nasal cavity. When it contacts nasal secretions, blood, or added sterile saline, the tampon expands to fill the nasal cavity and applies direct pressure to the walls of the nasal cavity. The Rhino Rocket® represents a compressed foam polymer tampon made of polyvinyl alcohol and a delivery device to aid insertion. The nasal tampon comes loaded in a slim, syringe-like applicator, which is placed on the floor of the nose at the entrance or just inside the nose. The tampon is expelled into the nose from the applicator expanding as it contacts blood and nasal fluid. The retention strings should be secured to the side of the face. The Rapid Rhino® is a carboxymethylcellulose pack with an inflatable balloon that secures it in the nasal cavity after insertion. It facilitates platelet aggregation and also forms a gel-like lubricant over its surface easing insertion and removal.

Classic Anterior Pack with Ribbon Gauze. Using bayonet forceps, grasp a length of petroleum-jelly-impregnated gauze approximately 5 to 7 cm from its end, and insert it straight back along the floor of the nose for 3 to 4 cm. The end of the gauze should protrude from the nostril by 2 to 3 cm to prevent it from falling into the nasopharynx and causing the child to gag. Withdraw the bayonet forceps and grasp the gauze again approximately 7 cm from where it is now exiting the nose. This portion of the gauze should then be placed into the nose on top of the initial layer. Repeat the process until the nasal cavity is filled with layers of gauze from bottom to top. Any free end of gauze should be directed anteriorly so that it does not fall into

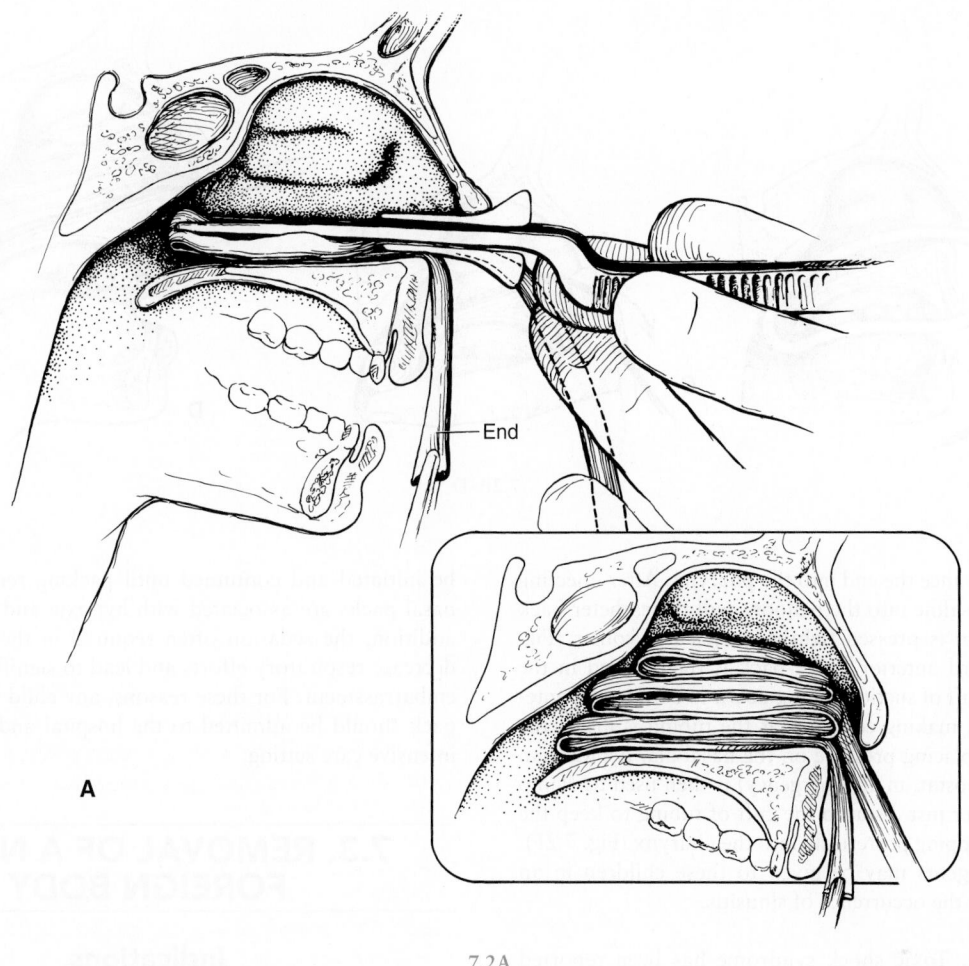

A

7.2A

the posterior nasopharynx and lead to gagging. A small piece of tape can be used to cover the nostril and prevent the child from disturbing the pack. Because the nasal pack causes stasis of the nasal secretions, oral antimicrobial drugs may be considered to prevent the occurrence of sinusitis. Nonresorbable anterior packs should be removed in 3 to 5 days.

Posterior Pack

If an anterior pack is not sufficient to stop an episode of epistaxis, a posterior pack may be required. The placement of posterior packs is extremely uncomfortable; therefore, procedural sedation is strongly recommended. Posterior packs can consist of a double-balloon catheter, 4″ × 4″ gauze, or a Foley catheter.

The double-balloon catheter has a distal, spherical, small balloon and a proximal, oblong, large balloon. The catheter should be lubricated and then inserted until the tip is in the pharynx beyond the choana. The distal, smaller balloon is then inflated with saline or water, and the catheter is pulled anteriorly to occlude the choana. The proximal, larger balloon is then inflated within the nasal cavity providing direct pressure. The portion of the catheter that is protruding from the nose should be padded with a gauze bolster to prevent pressure necrosis of the ala and columella as well as slippage of the catheter posteriorly.

To make the gauze pack, roll up a 4 × 4 gauze sponge until it is approximately 2 to 5 cm long and 2 cm in diameter; three

no. 0 silk sutures (50 cm in length) are knotted around the middle of this roll. Next, thread a red rubber catheter into the nose and bring the end out the mouth by grasping it with a hemostat when it appears in the posterior oropharynx. Tie two of the silk sutures to the end of the catheter, as shown in Figure 7.2B, but hold the third with a hemostat. As the catheter is withdrawn from the nose, guide the pack into the mouth and then up into the nasopharynx (Figs. 7.2C and 7.2D). The pack is held in position by the two silk sutures, which pull the pack up against the vomer (posterior nasal septum). Tie these sutures together after placing an anterior gauze pack as previously described. The third silk suture, which is protruding from the child's mouth, is taped to the cheek to prevent aspiration of the pack if the nasal ties should loosen.

An alternative is to use two red rubber catheters and insert one through each nare. On completion, the sutures on each side can be loosely tied in front of the septum. An anterior pack is still used at the site of bleeding.

To place a posterior pack using a Foley catheter, make a plastic cuff by cutting a 2- to 3-cm length of clear plastic tubing (e.g., suction tubing) and pass it over a 12- or 14-gauge Foley catheter that has a 30-mL balloon. The cuff serves to hold the catheter in place outside the nose. Slide the cuff up to the bifurcation of the catheter; the distal tip of the Foley catheter beyond the balloon should be cut off. Test the inflation of the balloon by injecting saline. Place the catheter into

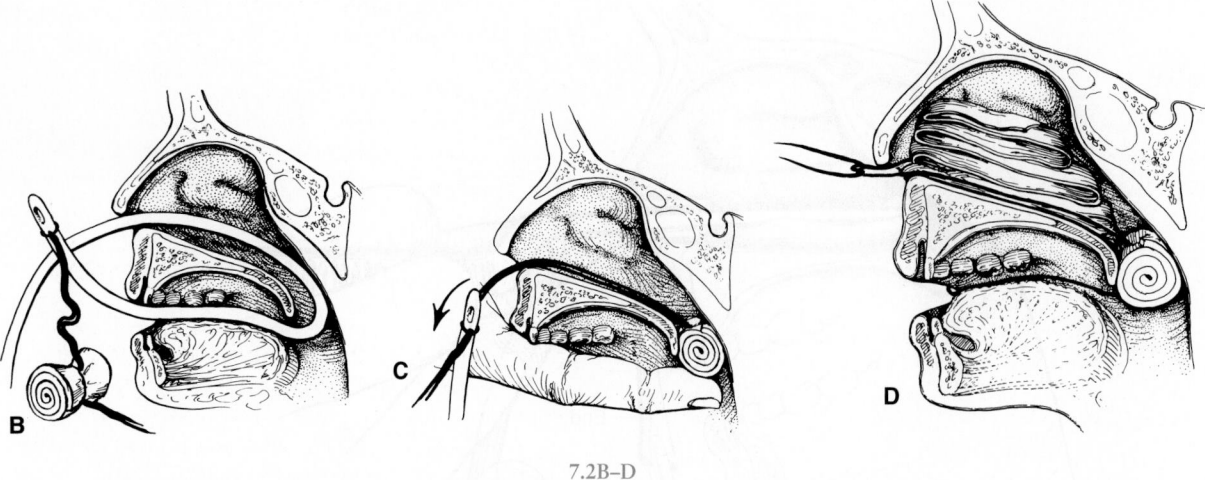

7.2B–D

the nose and advance the end into the pharynx. After injecting 10 to 15 mL of saline into the balloon, pull the catheter back until the balloon is pressed tightly against the vomer (Fig. 7.2E). A standard anterior gauze pack is then placed in the nose. Slide the cuff of suction tubing down to contact the anterior gauze pack, making certain that the tubing is inside the nostril and not placing pressure on the nasal ala. A Hoffman clamp (or a hemostat, in an emergency) is then used to clamp the Foley catheter just distal to the cuff of tubing to keep the catheter from slipping posteriorly into the pharynx (Fig. 7.2F). Antimicrobial agents may be given to these children in an effort to prevent the occurrence of sinusitis.

Important Note. Toxic shock syndrome has been reported with nasal packing. If a nasal pack is left in place, it is recommended that an oral antibiotic, such as amoxicillin-clavulanate,

be initiated and continued until packing removal. Posterior nasal packs are associated with hypoxia and hypercapnia. In addition, the sedation often required in these patients may decrease respiratory efforts and lead to significant respiratory embarrassment. For these reasons, any child with a posterior pack should be admitted to the hospital and observed in an intensive care setting.

7.3. REMOVAL OF A NASAL FOREIGN BODY

Indications

Presence of a nasal foreign body

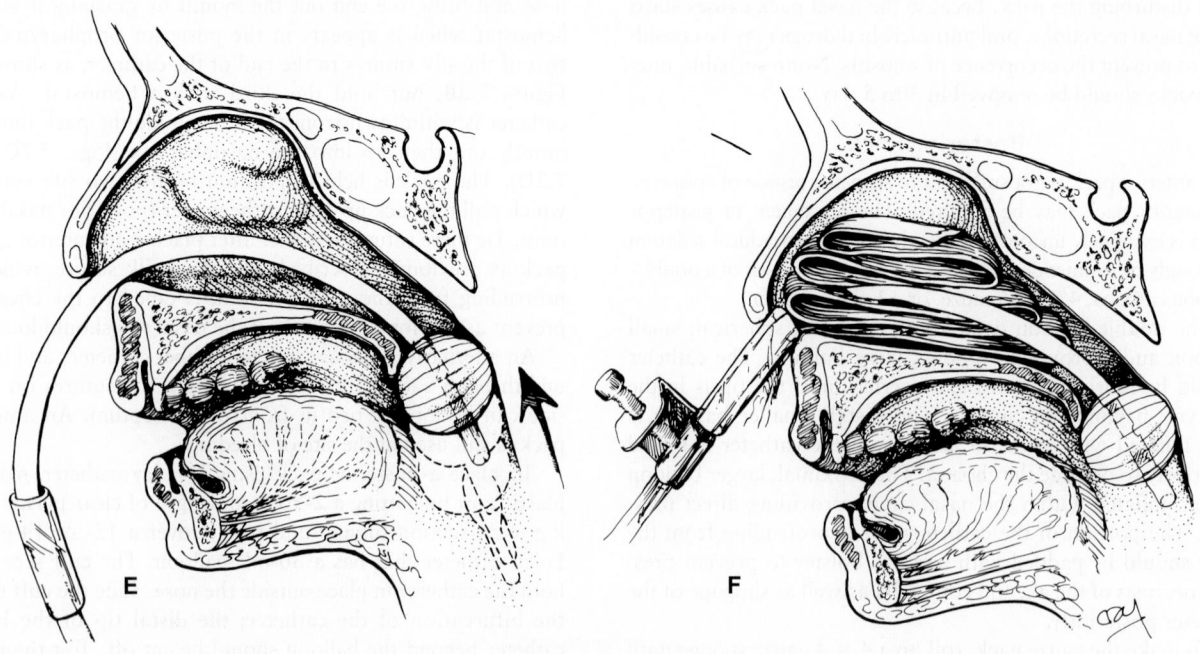

7.2E–F

Complications

1. Rhinosinusitis
2. Mucosal laceration
3. Epistaxis
4. Aspiration
5. Incomplete removal of the foreign body

Procedure

Preparation for the procedure to minimize the pain or anxiety and maximize visualization is the key to success. The patient must be still during instrumentation of the nose to prevent injury to the internal nasal structures. In most instances, it is useful to apply topical vasoconstrictor–anesthetic agent (neosynephrine 0.25%) to shrink the nasal membranes. The child should be supine and restrained. Then, visualize the interior of the nose with a nasal speculum and a headlight or directed light, as shown in Figure 7.3A. Purulent secretions should be gently removed by use of Frazier suction tip until the foreign body is clearly seen. The parent's kiss method of removal may be attempted and has demonstrated success in over 60% of children in some studies. The child is best held in another caregiver's lap and the parent explains that he/she is going to kiss the child. With one finger occluding the nares that is unaffected, the parent covers the child's mouth with his/hers and instills a short puff of air into the child's mouth to expel the foreign body.

If that fails or is felt to not be an option, attempt to extract the object with suction, a hook, or alligator forceps as determined by the size, nature, and position of the object. In some instances, procedural sedation may be necessary to enhance the removal of the foreign body. Figure 7.3B shows a hook being placed around a round foreign body. Do not push the foreign body into the posterior nasopharynx because it may be aspirated by the struggling child. The use of irrigation is *not recommended* because the foreign body may slip posteriorly and be aspirated, or hygroscopic foreign bodies (i.e., sponges) may swell and become lodged in the nose. The use of cyanoacrylate has been effective but requires the glue to directly be in contact with the foreign body for up to 30 seconds against a wooden stick; contact to the mucosa can adhere the stick with the intraluminal mucosa. After the foreign body has been removed, oral antimicrobial agents may be used to prevent an infection in the traumatized area.

7.4. DRAINAGE OF SEPTAL HEMATOMA/ABSCESS

Indications

Presence of a nasal septal hematoma or abscess

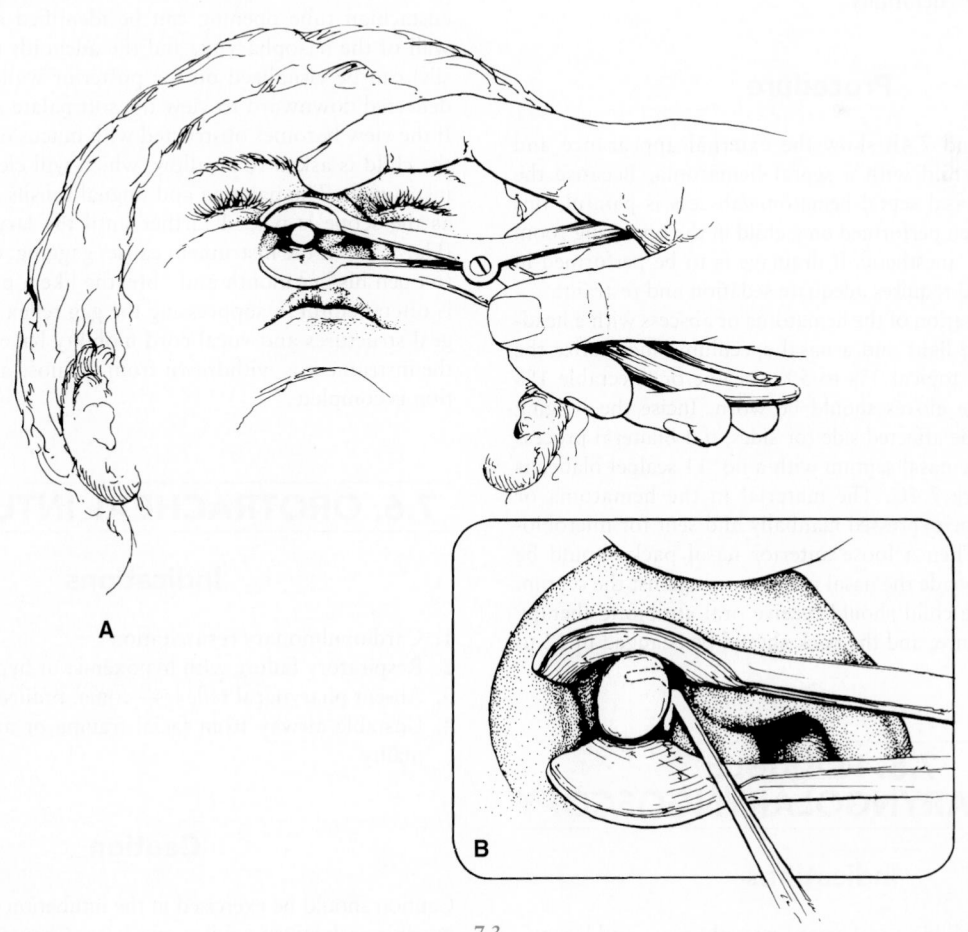

A

B

7.3

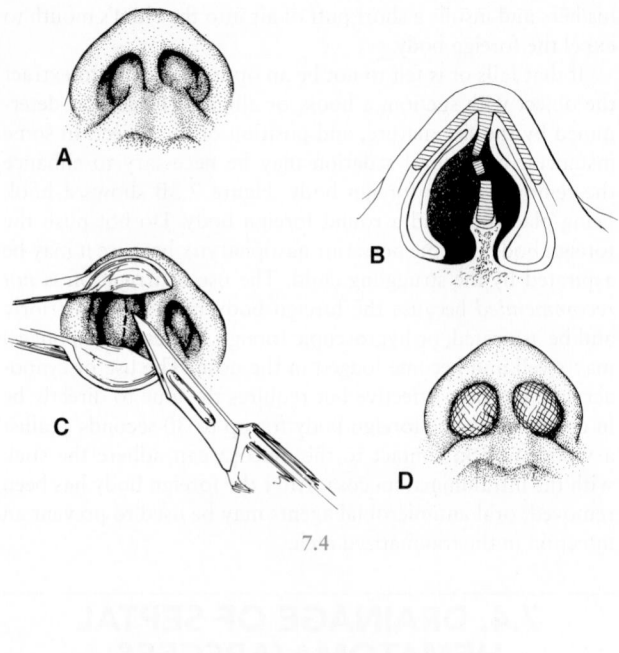

7.4

Complications

1. Perichondritis
2. Septal abscess
3. Septal perforation
4. "Saddle nose" deformity

Procedure

Figures 7.4A and 7.4B show the external appearance and anatomy in a child with a septal hematoma. Because the drainage of a nasal septal hematoma/abscess is painful, this procedure is often performed on a child in the operating room under a general anesthetic. If drainage is to be performed in the ED, the child requires adequate sedation and restraint.

After visualization of the hematoma or abscess with a headlight or directed light and a nasal speculum, anesthetize the membrane with topical 3% to 5% cocaine or injectable 1% lidocaine. Sterile gloves should be worn. Incise the bulging membrane on the affected side (or sides, if a bilateral process is present) of the nasal septum with a no. 11 scalpel blade, as shown in Figure 7.4C. The material in the hematoma or abscess should be expressed manually and sent for microbiologic culture. Then a loose anterior nasal pack should be placed to tamponade the nasal membranes against the septum (Fig. 7.4D). The child should receive oral antibiotic therapy after the procedure, and the pack should be changed in 12 to 24 hours.

7.5. FLEXIBLE NASOPHARYNGOLARYNGOSCOPY

Indications

To evaluate the child's nasal cavity, nasopharynx, and larynx

Complications

1. Epistaxis
2. Edema of nasal airway
3. Laryngospasm
4. Aspiration

Procedure

The child is usually seated (on the parent's lap, if necessary). Consider an anxiolytic/amnestic, such as midazolam, in the apprehensive patient. The anterior nasal cavity is inspected to detect any nasal septal deformity or enlarged turbinate, and any blood or excess mucus is removed. Topical anesthesia is achieved by spraying 2% to 4% lidocaine solution into the more accessible of the two nasal cavities. Vasoconstriction with oxymetazoline nasal spray prior to the procedure may prevent bleeding and reduce edema optimizing the operator's view of the nasal cavity. If an atomizer is not available, a cotton pledget soaked with lidocaine and oxymetazoline is placed along the floor of the nose and left in place for 10 to 15 minutes.

The examiner sits opposite the child and inserts the tip of the flexible nasopharyngoscope with his/her left hand as the right hand controls the flex of the tip. The instrument is advanced along the floor of the nose through the inferior meatus until the nasopharynx is visualized (Fig. 7.5A). The eustachian tube opening can be identified along the lateral wall of the nasopharynx, and the adenoids (pharyngeal tonsils) can be visualized on the posterior wall. The tip is then deflected downward to view the soft palate and oropharynx. If the view becomes obstructed with mucus or the tip fogs up, the child is asked to swallow, which will clear the tip of the instrument. The palatine and lingual tonsils can be inspected as the scope is passed farther until the larynx is visualized (Fig. 7.5B). If the instrument causes gagging, the child is asked to open his/her mouth and "breathe like a puppy dog." This is often helpful in suppressing the gag reflex. After the laryngeal structures and vocal cord mobility have been evaluated, the instrument is withdrawn from the nose and the examination is complete.

7.6. OROTRACHEAL INTUBATION

Indications

1. Cardiopulmonary resuscitation
2. Respiratory failure with hypoxemia or hypercarbia
3. Absent pharyngeal reflexes—coma, brainstem dysfunction
4. Unstable airway from facial trauma or an airway abnormality

Caution

Caution should be exercised in the intubation of the child with possible neck injury, a full stomach (see Chapters 1, 5, and 104),

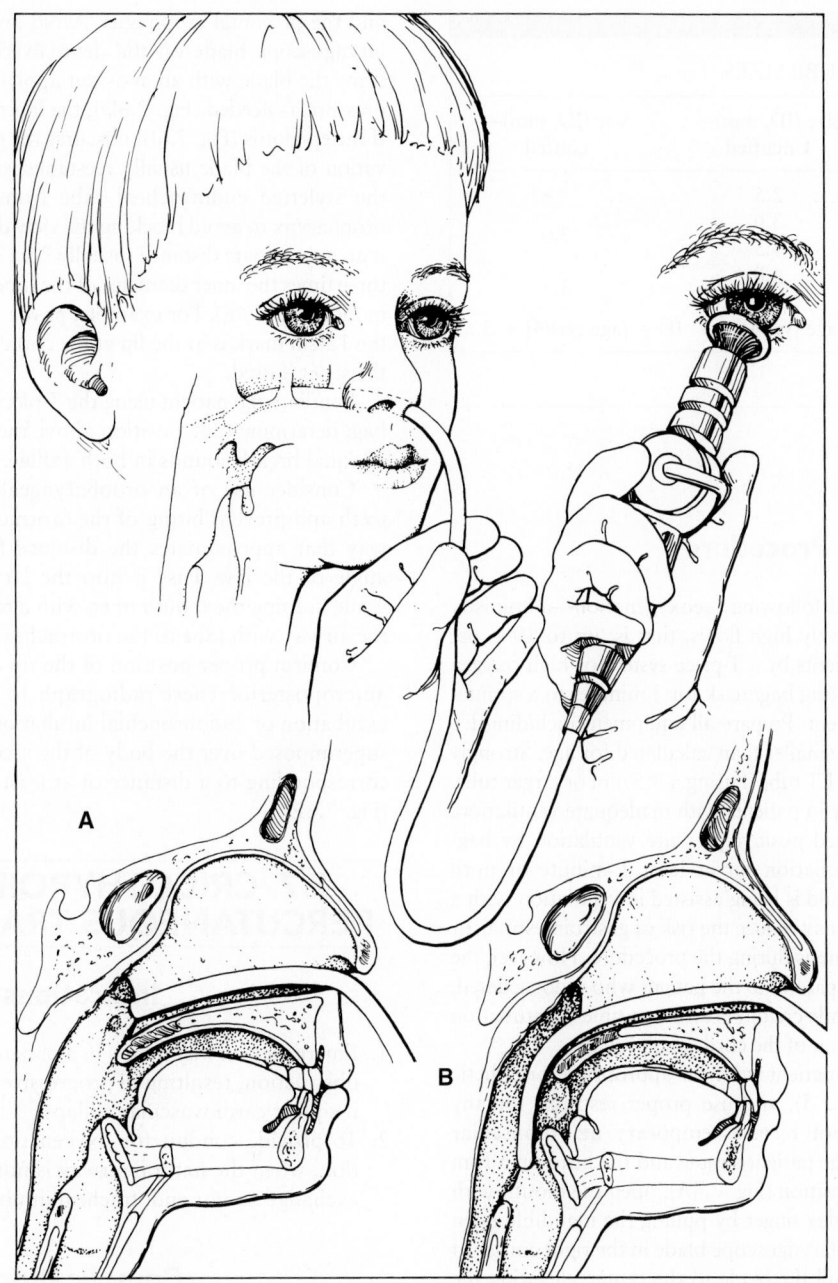

7.5

temporomandibular ankylosis or a hypoplastic mandible (see Chapter 5), or a defect in blood coagulation.

Complications

1. Hypoxemia or cardiac arrest
2. Bronchial intubation with secondary contralateral atelectasis or ipsilateral pneumothorax
3. Vomiting and/or aspiration secondary to a full stomach
4. Dislodgment of teeth
5. Laceration of the lips and gums
6. Laryngeal trauma
7. Esophageal intubation

Equipment

Resuscitator with mask and oxygen source; oropharyngeal airways (Guedel 00, 0, 1, 2, 3, 4); uncuffed orotracheal tubes, 2.5- to 8-mm inner diameter (ID), cuffed tubes 3.5- to 8-mm ID (all with 15-mm male connector) (Table 7.6A); laryngoscope handle and several blades (Table 7.6B), extra batteries and bulbs; stylet—infant and adult, Teflon coated; Magill forceps—child and adult; suction equipment—central or portable suction source; Yankauer tonsil aspirator (replace tip by thick-walled rubber tubing); disposable sterile plastic suction catheters (5F, 8F, 10F, 14F)

TABLE 7.6A

ENDOTRACHEAL TUBE SIZES

Age	Size (ID, mm)—Uncuffed	Size (ID, mm)—Cuffed
Premature	2.5	—
Term to 3 mo	3.0	3.0
3–7 mo	3.5	
7–15 mo	4.0	3.5
15–24 mo	4.5	
2–15 yr	ID = [age (yr)/4] + 4	ID = [age (yr)/4] + 3.5

ID, inner diameter.

Procedure

Intubation is performed following preoxygenation—administer 100% oxygen at relatively high flows, that is, up to 10 L per minute in pediatric patients by a T-piece system or high oxygen concentration, self-inflating bag/mask for 3 minutes to a spontaneously ventilating patient. Prepare all equipment including ET tubes ½ size larger and smaller than calculated for age. Strongly consider use of a cuffed ET tube if using a 3.5 mm or larger tube. During resuscitations or in patients with inadequate ventilation, use assisted or controlled positive-pressure ventilation by bag-valve-mask before intubation for at least 1 minute or until cyanosis clears. If the child is being assisted in ventilation with a BVM, cricoid pressure may reduce the risk of gastrointestinal air increasing the risk of emesis during the procedure. However, the evidence is weak and is painful to the patient who is not sedated. Some operators find gentle cricoid pressure at time of intubation improves the visualization of the cords and airway.

Prepare the awake patient with an appropriate anesthetic (see Chapters 1, 4, and 5), and use proper restraint for any patient who should not receive temporary neuromuscular blockade. Then, with the patient supine and the head on a firm pad in the "sniffing" position (Fig. 7.6A), open the mouth with the right thumb and index finger by pulling the mandible open and forward. Insert the laryngoscope blade in the right corner of the mouth, and then pull the blade to the center, elevating the tongue and clearing the lower lip from between the teeth and the blade (Fig. 7.6B). Advance the blade under direct visualization into the hypopharynx (Fig. 7.6C). Elevate the mandibular tissue block by exerting force along the axis of the laryngoscope handle to expose the posterior pharyngeal wall

TABLE 7.6B

LARYNGOSCOPE BLADES

Age	Name and size
Premature	Miller 0
Term to 1 yr	Wis-Hipple 1 or Miller 1
1 to 1.5 yr	Wis-Hipple 1½
1.5 to 12 yr	Miller or Flagg 2
13 yr +	Macintosh 3

and the proximal esophagus. Avoid any direct pressure of the laryngoscope blade on the dentoalveolar ridge. Slowly withdraw the blade with an assistant applying simultaneous cricoid pressure as needed (Fig. 7.6D); the larynx will ascend into view. If the epiglottis (Fig. 7.6B) obscures the glottic chink, further elevation of the blade usually reestablishes a good view. Advance the styletted endotracheal tube from the right side of the oropharynx to avoid blocking the view during tube passage. Pass it an appropriate distance (usually 2 to 3 cm) into the trachea or three times the inner diameter of the tube in centimeters from the mouth (Fig. 7.6E). For example, pass a 4F endotracheal tube so the 12-cm mark is at the lip at the corner of the mouth. Remove the stylet if used.

Ventilate the patient using the T-piece system or self-inflating bag; determine tube position above the carina by auscultation of equal breath sounds in both axillae.

Consider use of an oropharyngeal airway to protect the teeth and prevent biting of the orotracheal tube. Pick the airway that approximates the distance from the mouth to the angle of the jaw. Pass it into the larynx curved downward while keeping the mouth open with a tongue depressor. Secure the airway with tape to the orotracheal tube and child's skin.

Confirm proper position of the tip of the tube by portable anteroposterior chest radiograph to help avoid accidental extubation or endobronchial intubation. Aim for the tip to be superimposed over the body of the second thoracic vertebrae, corresponding to a distance of at least 2 cm above the carina (Fig. 7.6E).

7.7. CRICOTHYROIDOTOMY/ PERCUTANEOUS TRACHEOTOMY

Indications

1. Emergency airway access in a patient with an upper airway obstruction, resulting in progressive cyanosis, acidosis, and incipient cardiovascular collapse
2. To provide conduit for oxygenation and, ideally, ventilation, when the natural airway is not accessible for safe gas exchange and/or endotracheal intubation

Complications

1. Bleeding or hemorrhage
2. Subcutaneous and/or mediastinal emphysema
3. Perforation of the posterior wall of the trachea
4. Malposition of the catheter or cannula outside the trachea
5. Barotrauma—when complete proximal airway obstruction is present
6. Pneumothorax and/or pneumomediastinum
7. Infection—periosteal or mediastinal
8. Vocal cord injury and/or voice changes
9. Injury to great vessels, cricothyroid muscle or cricoid cartilage
10. Subglottic stenosis/edema
11. Specific complications with needle cricothyroidotomy:
    a. Kinking and obstruction of the soft IV cannula
    b. Ineffective ventilation with rapid development of severe respiratory acidosis

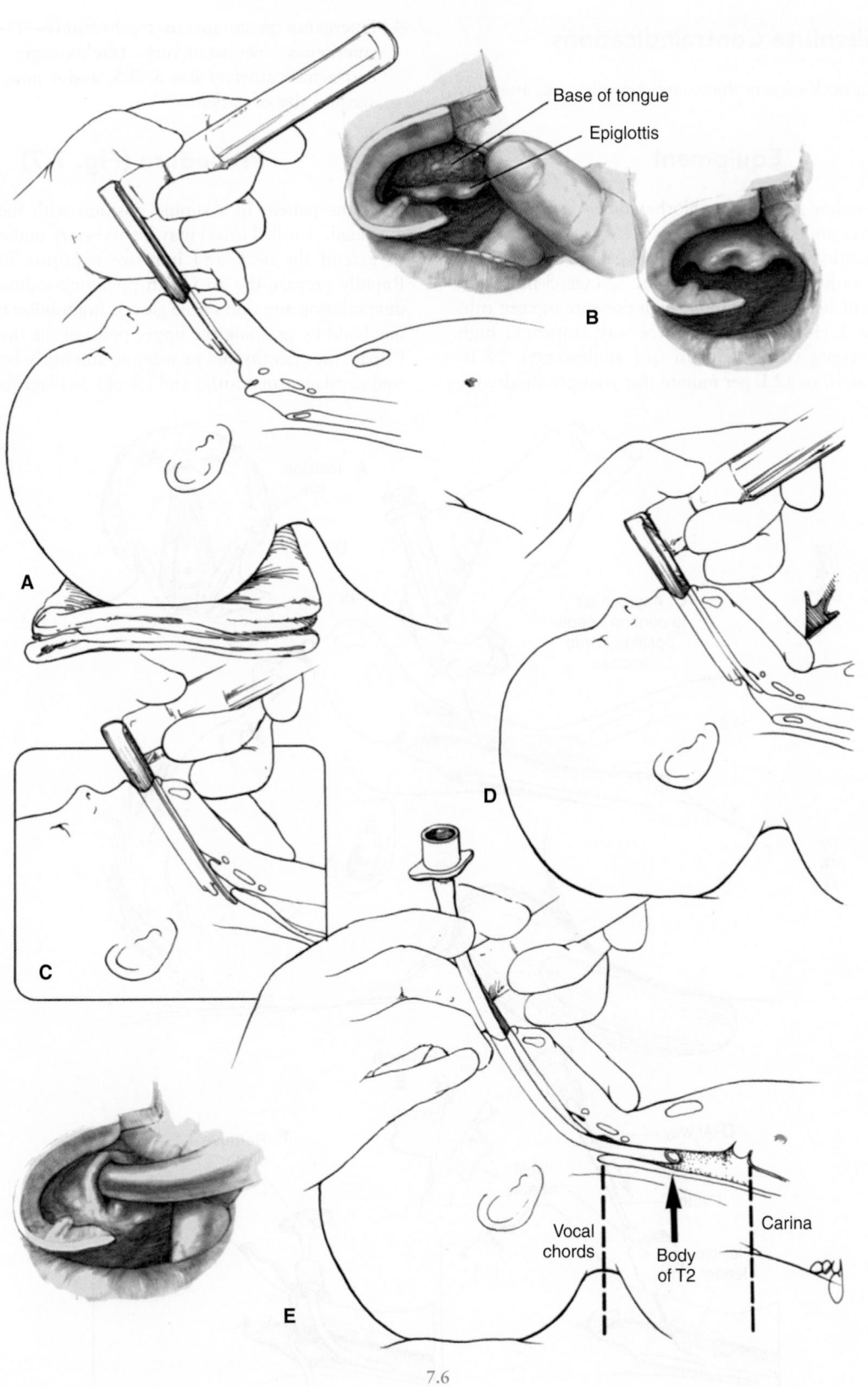

Base of tongue
Epiglottis

A

B

C

D

E

Vocal
chords

Body
of T2

Carina

7.6

Absolute Contraindications

1. Prior major neck surgery that completely obscures anatomy

Equipment

1. Povidone–iodine solution or chlorhexidine
2. Sterile gloves and sterile gauze
3. Needle cricothyroidotomy—16- to 18-gauge, 8.5-cm over-the-needle catheter attached to a 5-mL syringe; 3-mm pediatric endotracheal tube adaptor; high pressure oxygen tubing with a Y-H–connector or three-way stopcock; high pressure oxygen source—50 psi (for adolescents), 25 to 35 psi set at 10 to 12 L per minute (for younger children)

4. Emergency percutaneous tracheotomy—11-blade scalpel, emergency percutaneous tracheotomy device (i.e., Pertrach® catheter) size 3, 3.5, and 4 mm, depending on age and size of patient

Procedure (Fig. 7.7)

Place the patient in a supine position with the neck slightly extended. A rolled towel may be necessary under the shoulders to extend the neck and improve exposure of the trachea. Rapidly prepare the area with povidone–iodine or chlorhexidine solution and don sterile gloves. Immobilize the larynx with one hand by grasping the upper poles of the thyroid cartilage. Palpate the cricothyroid membrane anteriorly between the thyroid cartilage (superiorly) and cricoid cartilage (inferiorly).

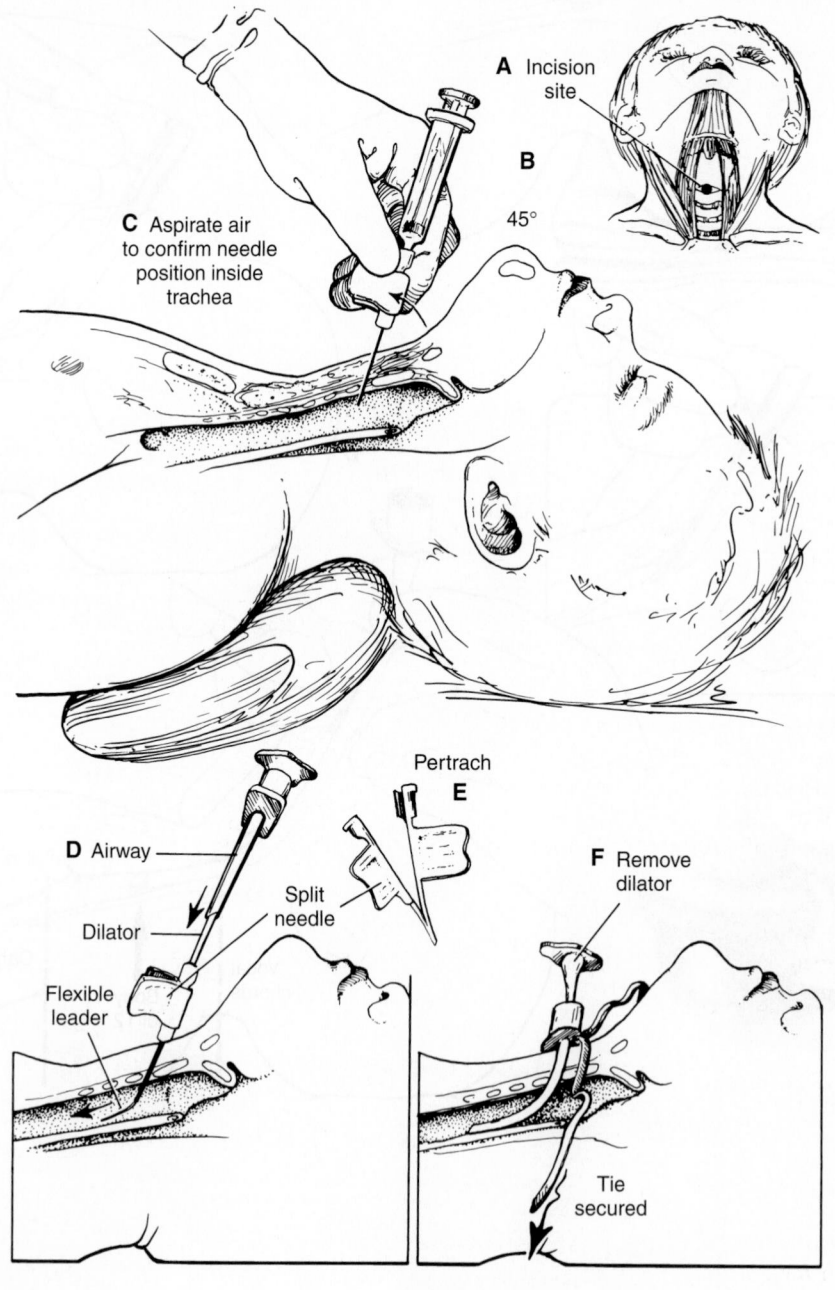

A Incision site

B

45°

C Aspirate air to confirm needle position inside trachea

D Airway

Dilator

Flexible leader

Split needle

Pertrach

E

F Remove dilator

Tie secured

Needle Cricothyroidotomy

When performing a needle cricothyroidotomy, make a small puncture in the skin first with a 16- to 18-gauge needle (with attached syringe) over the center of the cricothyroid membrane. Then, at a 45-degree angle caudad, insert the IV cannula downward through the cricothyroid membrane until a pop is felt. As the cannula is advanced, aspirate continuously. When the pop is felt, there will be an immediate return of air in the syringe. Slide the IV plastic cannula off the needle and into the trachea. Take the syringe, attach it to the IV cannula, and aspirate to confirm successful aspiration of air. Remove syringe and attach the catheter needle hub to a 3-mm pediatric endotracheal tube adaptor. Then, connect this adaptor to high pressure oxygen tubing with a preprepared Y-connector. Set the oxygen flow meter at 50 psi (50 L per minute) for adolescents and at 25 to 35 psi (10 to 12 L per minute) for younger children. Apply intermittent occlusion of the open end of the Y-connector for 1 second, and then release the open end of the Y-connector for 4 seconds. Listen for breath sounds with each delivery of oxygen. Manually guard the plastic cannula to prevent it from kinking, and prepare for more definitive airway access from above, if possible.

Percutaneous Tracheotomy

When inserting an emergent pediatric percutaneous tracheotomy, make a 1-cm vertical and midline incision over the cricothyroid membrane using the 11-blade scalpel. Using an emergency pediatric percutaneous tracheotomy device, (i.e., Pertrach® device), insert the prepared splittable needle (already attached to a syringe), through the incision site at a 45-degree downward (caudal) angle. Within a few millimeters, the give of a "pop" will be felt as the needle bevel enters the trachea. Aspirate air, confirming the position within the tracheal lumen. Oscillate the tip of the intratracheal needle from side to side to confirm that it has not punctured the posterior wall of the trachea. Remove the syringe while stabilizing the splittable needle. Angle the splittable needle acutely toward the carina. Then, lubricate the leader and overlying endotracheal tube, and insert the leader through the needle beyond the needle bevel down toward the carina as far as possible. (If the needle bevel is outside the trachea, the leader will not thread.) Squeeze the flanges of the needle together and pull apart the flanges of the splittable needle. Keep the leader stable when performing this step. With steady pressure, advance the remainder of the leader, the dilator, and the tracheostomy tube directly into the trachea. Remove the leader and dilator, and attach the tracheostomy tube to a bag-valve-mask and ventilate the patient. Observe for chest wall excursion, auscultate for breath sounds, and then secure the tracheostomy tube in place with ties snugly fitted around the neck.

7.8. REPLACEMENT OF A TRACHEOSTOMY CANNULA

Indications

1. Relief of obstruction of a tracheostomy tube (i.e., secretions, mucous plug, or foreign body)
2. Accidental decannulation

Complications

1. Respiratory distress—hypoxemia and hypercarbia
2. Creation of a false tracheal passage, leading to pneumomediastinum and pneumothorax

Procedure

Replacement of an Obstructed Tracheostomy Cannula

The child with a tracheostomy who develops tachypnea, cyanosis, decreased breath sounds, or severe retractions should be assumed to have a mechanical obstruction of his/her cannula until proven otherwise. Have an assistant obtain a scissors, a new cannula (often available from the parents), or an endotracheal tube of the same diameter or one size smaller than the obstructed tube. Ventilate the child with 100% oxygen. Place a small, folded towel under the child's shoulder, and extend the head and neck. This maneuver exposes the tracheostomy site and eliminates redundancy or flaccidity of those tissues, which lie between the trachea and the anterior surface of the neck. The trachea is thereby forced closer to the plane of the skin. An attempt should be made to pass a suction catheter. If the catheter passes, apply suction at 80 to 120 cm of water and withdraw over 3 to 5 seconds. Immediately reventilate with 100% oxygen. *If the suction catheter will not pass through the tracheal cannula, the cannula must be changed immediately.* Carefully cut the strings that secure the cannula with bandage scissors so as not to lacerate the child's neck. Remove the tube, observe the tract of the tracheocutaneous fistula, and introduce the new cannula, preferably with internal obturator in place so the tip follows the course of the tracheocutaneous fistula (Fig. 7.8A). Press the flanges of the tracheostomy tube against the child's neck, and attach a swivel connector and resuscitator to the system. Remove the obturator if used, ventilate the child, and check for symmetric breath sounds by auscultation. Insert a hemostat through a flange hole on the lateral aspect of the cannula and pull the tracheostomy twill (cloth tape) through so two equal lengths of twill are left that are long enough to go around the neck to knot through the opposite flange hole. Before securing the knot, apply adhesive-backed foam, if available, to the string crossing the back of the neck. With the neck flexed, tie the string snugly. If the cannula is properly secured, an index finger should fit snugly under the strings while the head is flexed. Obtain a chest radiograph to ensure proper placement and to assess for pulmonary parenchymal change.

If a tracheostomy cannula is not immediately available, a standard endotracheal tube of the same diameter can be used instead. Care must be taken not to advance this longer tube beyond the carina by measuring it against the tracheostomy removed to estimate distance. The chest should be auscultated for equal breath sounds bilaterally and, in addition, position of the distal tip should be confirmed by a chest radiograph. Because this is temporary, obtain the correct size tracheostomy tube to change the endotracheal tube as soon as possible.

Replacement of a Dislodged Cannula

When a tracheal cannula is dislodged from the stoma of a child totally dependent on that cannula, it must be replaced

PROCEDURES

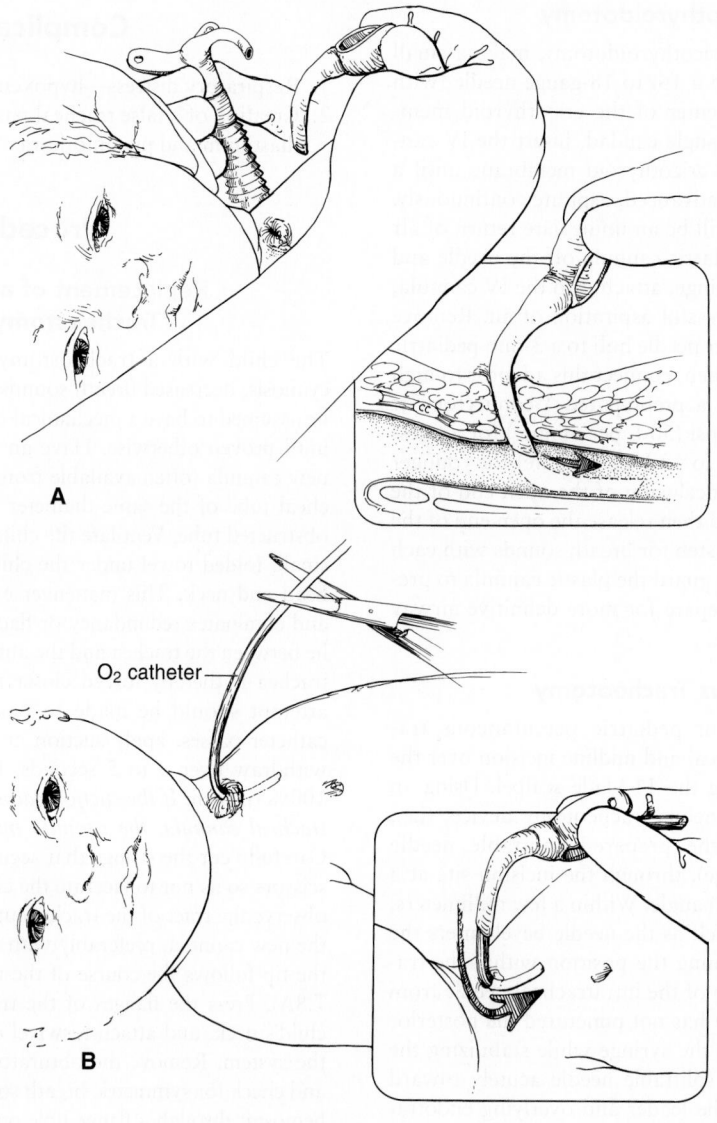

A

O$_2$ catheter

B

7.8

immediately. Time may not allow for acquiring a clean tube. Cut the strings and replace the dislodged cannula. Hold it firmly in place until it can be secured or until a clean cannula is made available. Occasionally, the tracheocutaneous stomal tract will constrict so the cannula cannot be replaced. Several options are then available. First, place a smaller tracheal cannula or endotracheal tube to allow oxygenation and ventilation. Second, electively dilate the stoma and replace the appropriate size tube. Alternatively, as in Figure 7.8B, pass a smaller oxygen catheter (10F or 14F). If the child is cyanotic, connect the catheter to an oxygen hose and run oxygen at a minimal flow rate of 1 L per minute (2 to 3 L per minute if older than 3 years of age.). If the child is not cyanotic, move directly toward passing a tracheostomy cannula over the oxygen catheter into the stoma. The oxygen catheter will serve as a stylet and guideline to keep the tracheostomy cannula from being forced into a false passage. If the cannula cannot be advanced, it may be necessary to oxygenate and ventilate the child with a resuscitator, and mask through the upper airway while an assistant covers the stoma with a gloved finger. If the upper airway is obstructed, place a small endotracheal tube (size 3.5 to 4.5) through the stoma, hold it in place, and use it to oxygenate the patient. Efforts to

place a more appropriate size airway can then be reasonably made, using the surgical approach if other efforts fail.

Important Note

Remember that cardiopulmonary failure or respiratory distress often means obstruction of the tracheostomy. First, if unable to ventilate or suction, remove. Second, try to cannulate. Third, remember in some patients, an ET tube can be passed through the mouth or tracheostomy stoma. Last, remember to try the other procedures (e.g., oxygen catheter).

8.1. INSERTION OF A CHEST TUBE

Indications

1. Evacuation of a pneumothorax
2. Drainage of a hemopneumothorax, symptomatic empyema, or large pleural effusion
3. Esophageal rupture with gastric leakage into the pleural space

Complications

1. Bleeding (local and/or perforation of major vessels)
2. Pulmonary contusion
3. Pneumothorax or hemothorax
4. Infection (at insertion site, pneumonia, or empyema)
5. Bronchopleural fistula or pleurocutaneous air leak
6. Laceration or perforation of visceral organs (heart, lungs, diaphragm, spleen, liver, or other intraabdominal organs)
7. Subcutaneous emphysema
8. Reexpansion pulmonary edema
9. Intercostal neuralgia/neuritis

Contraindications

Absolute

1. Lung is completely adherent to chest wall throughout hemothorax

Relative

1. Risk of bleeding with patient treated with anticoagulants
2. Coagulopathies and platelet dysfunctions

Equipment

1. Povidone–iodine solution or chlorhexidine
2. Sterile gown, mask, hat, gloves, gauze and drapes
3. 11-blade scalpel; 5- to 10-mL syringe; needle (18- to 25-gauge) for anesthetic; 1% lidocaine
4. Needle driver; curved Kelly clamps or artery forceps; scissors; strong, non-absorbable suture
5. Age/size-appropriate thoracostomy tube (as designated in Table 8.1)
6. Pleural drainage system (e.g., Pleur-evac)

Procedure

Identify the side(s) with the hemothorax or pneumothorax by physical examination and chest radiograph, if time allows. Initiate treatment of cardiorespiratory disturbances before beginning the procedure. If abdominal distension is present, especially from a dilated stomach, pass a large-bore nasogastric tube to reduce diaphragmatic elevation.

Figure 8.1A shows the anatomy of a child with a right-sided pneumothorax from an anterior view, and the preferred sight of entry into the thorax between the anterior axillary and midaxillary lines at the level of the nipple (fifth intercostal space). Restrain the child, if necessary; minimize any respiratory compromise. Consider use of pharmacologic sedation. Generally, a young or seriously ill child should be supine, but an older, cooperative patient may sit. Locate the landmarks and cleanse the site with povidone–iodine or chlorhexidine solution. Prior to starting, mark the side affected and use your institution's "hold point" method to ensure correct side tube placement. Using aseptic technique with sterile gown, gloves and mask, create a sterile field. Infiltrate the skin, subcutaneous tissue, intercostal muscles and periosteum of the rib with a local anesthetic (1% lidocaine). Make a skin incision parallel to the rib and at least one intercostal space below the rib over which the catheter will pass. This spot provides an oblique trajectory for the chest tube, which helps maintain an airtight seal when the tube is in position and after its removal.

Figure 8.1B shows a 1.5- to 2-cm transverse skin incision made with a no. 15 scalpel blade. Using a curved hemostat or Kelly clamp, bluntly dissect through the muscle and fascial layers to the upper surface of the chosen rib. Determine the proper position by palpation of the rib with the tip of the instrument. Then, slide the tip over the superior rib margin, puncturing the intercostal muscles and pleura well below the neurovascular bundle of the adjacent cephalad rib, as shown in Figure 8.1C. Control the instrument so the tip does not enter more than 1 cm into the thoracic cavity. Spread the tips of the instrument widely to provide an opening through the intercostal muscles and pleura that is at least 1.5 to 2 cm in diameter. At this point, any fluid or air under pressure in the pleural space may surge out. Use your gloved finger to explore the tract and remove the curved hemostat, exploring the pleura to ensure lung falls away from pleural wall and to clear adhesions or clots.

As shown in Figure 8.1D, grasp the chest tube between the tips of the curved hemostat or clamp. In general, the smaller thoracic cavity in children as compared with that of adults makes the use of a trocar more risky. Then, advance the instrument through the incision and previously dissected tract to the pleural space. When the tube tip has entered this cavity, open the hemostat and advance the catheter posteriorly, in the apical direction, until it meets some resistance. The tip will most likely be at the apex of the hemithorax. Approximate the incision with several nylon sutures, some of which should encircle the tube to secure it in place. Sterile ointment and a sterile occlusive dressing should be applied to the wound. Further taping will help prevent dislodgment. After the tube has been attached to a drainage set (e.g., a Pleur-evac), obtain an upright or decubitus chest radiograph immediately.

8.2. THORACENTESIS

Indications

Diagnostic or therapeutic drainage of a pleural effusion

Complications

1. Pneumothorax or hemothorax
2. Pulmonary contusion or lung laceration
3. Hepatic or splenic trauma

TABLE 8.1

CHEST TUBE SIZES BY AGE

Age	Size (F)
Newborn	10–12
6 mo	10–12
1 yr	16–20
4 yr	20–28
10 yr	28–32
>14 yr	28–32

PROCEDURES

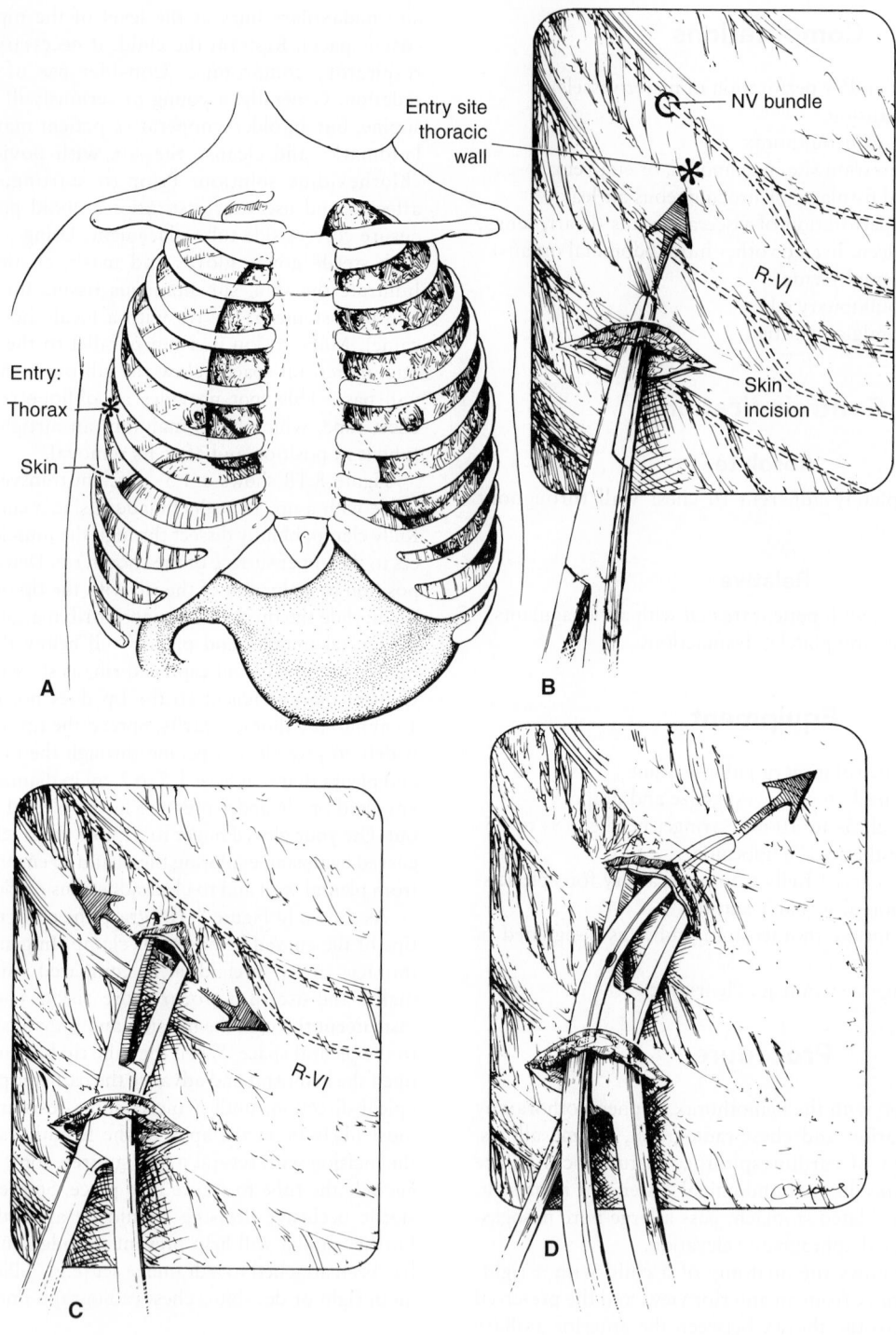

8.1

Equipment

1. Povidone–iodine solution or chlorhexidine
2. Sterile gown, mask, hat, gloves, and gauze
3. 5-mL syringe, 22-gauge needle, 1%. lidocaine
4. Over-the-needle catheter, no. 16 to 20, or 4-0 to 5-0 central line catheter tray, or pigtail thoracentesis catheter
5. Stopcock, T-connector, 20- to 50-mL syringe

Procedure

To confirm the presence of a free pleural effusion and the side involved, obtain erect and decubitus chest radiographs before the procedure. Prepare the equipment and the patient. Some children may do better with mild sedation if they are not having respiratory distress because restraint is difficult. Figure 8.2 shows the position useful in most toddlers and older children.

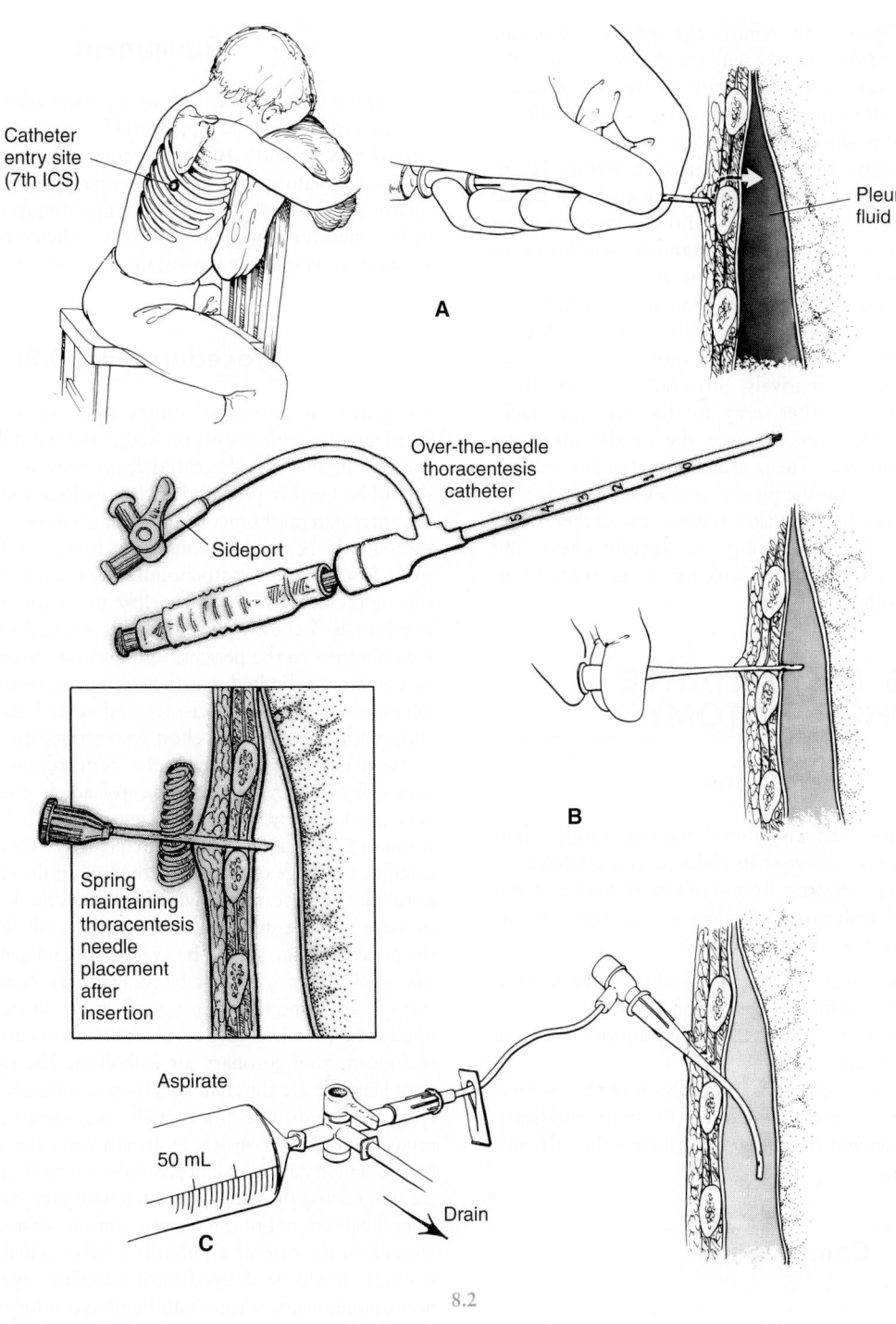

Catheter entry site (7th ICS)

Pleural fluid

A

Over-the-needle thoracentesis catheter

Sideport

B

Spring maintaining thoracentesis needle placement after insertion

Aspirate

50 mL

Drain

C

8.2

Place the child in the sitting position with the arms and head supported on a pillow. With the arm on the involved side elevated, the lower tip of the scapula lies just above the seventh intercostal space in the posterior axillary line. Significant amounts of free fluid in the thoracic cavity will usually be present at this point. Prior to starting the procedure, complete your institution's "hold point" procedure for the correct location/ side. After donning sterile gloves, scrub the area of the intended puncture with antiseptic solution. Then, anesthetize the site with 1% lidocaine from the skin to the periosteum of the rib.

Figure 8.2A shows the use of an over-the-needle catheter device. Advance the needle through the skin at a right angle to the chest wall at the point marked in Figure 8.2. Direct the needle against the upper rib surface and then draw it back slightly. Next, lift up the catheter system gently and slowly advance it so the needle slides over the top surface of the rib. Maintain continuous suction on the syringe while entering the pleural cavity; a decrease in the resistance to advancement of the needle and flow of fluid signals penetration of the parietal pleura. Advance the catheter slightly further, holding the needle steady.

As shown in Figure 8.2B, remove the syringe and needle and cover the hub of the catheter with the thumb. Because the catheter is soft, it can be advanced further into the thoracic cavity with little risk of puncturing the lung. Aim caudally to achieve an optimal position for evacuation of fluid.

As shown in Figure 8.2C, quickly attach a syringe (20 to 50 mL), stopcock, and T-connector to the catheter tip to minimize any leakage of air into the thorax. Increments of up to 50 mL can be removed for diagnostic studies or to provide symptomatic relief. If suction becomes difficult, reposition the catheter to maximize drainage. If insufficient fluid is obtained using a large-bore catheter, insert a longer through-the-needle catheter deeper into the thorax to improve emptying. Alternatively, introduce a needle from the central catheter or other setup for the Seldinger technique. Introduce the wire through the needle after the pleural space is entered. Then, after removing the needle, advance the catheter into the pleural space over the wire. At the end of the procedure, quickly remove the catheter and apply a sterile occlusive dressing. An upright chest film should be obtained afterward to look for the presence of an iatrogenic pneumothorax.

8.3. RESUSCITATIVE THORACOTOMY

Indications

In penetrating chest and abdominal trauma, rarely blunt trauma or other cause of arrest in children and adolescents. Best outcome with penetrating from stabbing and not gunshot and in the patients with progressive loss of vital signs or cardiac arrest for but a few minutes.

1. To provide access to the pericardium and heart for relief of tamponade and to institute open cardiac massage
2. To obtain control of any active bleeding injuries from the lung, hilum, or heart
3. To provide direct compression or occlusion of the thoracic aorta to improve central circulation of the brain and heart
4. To provide placement of large-bore catheters directly into the right atrium

Complications

1. Bleeding
2. Intrathoracic or chest wall infection
3. Delayed pericardial effusion

Relative Contraindications

1. Any patient with absence of vital signs at the prehospital scene and on arrival to the ED, following cardiopulmonary resuscitation for more than five minutes
2. Any patient with no signs of life, or asystole, on arrival to the ED, following blunt thoracic trauma
3. Any patient with head or thoracic injury, as part of a severe multisystem trauma

Equipment

A complete thoracotomy tray with rib spreaders; large vascular clamps and an aortic clamp; toothed forceps and artery forceps; curved scissors; and a 10-blade scalpel and preprepared 3-0 cardiovascular suture with cardiovascular pledgets; internal defibrillator paddles; 4-0 and 3-0 silk suture on tapered needle; sterile IV connector tubing; an 8 Fr Foley catheter; povidone–iodine solution; gloves, sterile gowns, masks, and drapes

Procedure (Fig. 8.3)

The patient is positioned supine with side of operation elevated slightly with towels or wedge-shaped pillow. The entire chest from sheet to sheet and from neck to lower abdomen should be quickly prepared with povidone–iodine solution. A left anterolateral thoracotomy incision (most common incision site) should be made through the fourth or fifth intercostal space from anterior costochondral junction to midaxillary line cutting the intercostal muscle close to the top of the respective inferior rib. A chest wall retractor is inserted and opened, providing access to the pericardium and the descending aorta. If access remains limited, cut the sternum across to the opposite interspace using heavy scissors and spread the right anterior chest with another set of chest wall retractors.

Next is the inspection of the pericardium, followed by a pericardiotomy, if pericardial tamponade is present. Perform a pericardiotomy by making a longitudinal cut through the pericardium 1 cm anterior to the phrenic nerve. This is best done by catching one edge of the pericardium with the scissors and then grasping the pericardium with forceps so the longitudinal incision can be made superiorly and inferiorly. All blood and clots in the pericardial sac should be evacuated, and gentle digital pressure applied to any cardiac bleeding points. Next step is a thorough heart inspection, during which the heart should not be lifted if there is a left-sided cardiac perforation because of the risk of sudden, fatal coronary air embolism. The right atrium and right ventricle are the chambers most commonly injured by penetrating wounds. Use of a partially occluding vascular clamp is preferred for major vessels or atrial bleeds. For temporary control of hemorrhaging wounds, a Foley catheter can be inserted in the wound and the balloon inflated with tube clamped so as not to pull balloon out of the wound, thus increasing the size of the wound. In the case of a pulsatile cardiac activity, repair of the wounds should be delayed until adequate resuscitation; for a non-beating heart, sutures can be placed prior to resuscitation. Atrial and ventricular wounds can be temporarily controlled with 3.0 non absorbable mattress sutures or a stapling device.

After the heart has been repaired, or if perforation of the heart has not occurred, internal cardiac massage may be done using the palms and proximal fingers of two hands proceeding from the apex to base of the heart. Avoid compressions between the thumb and the hand because these may cause perforation. Internal defibrillation may be necessary in the event of ventricular tachycardia, ventricular fibrillation, or to restore adequate cardiac output. With defibrillation, internal paddles are used and energy settings are reduced.

If bleeding is occurring from a major portion of the lung or parenchyma, it may be tamponaded or clamped with a

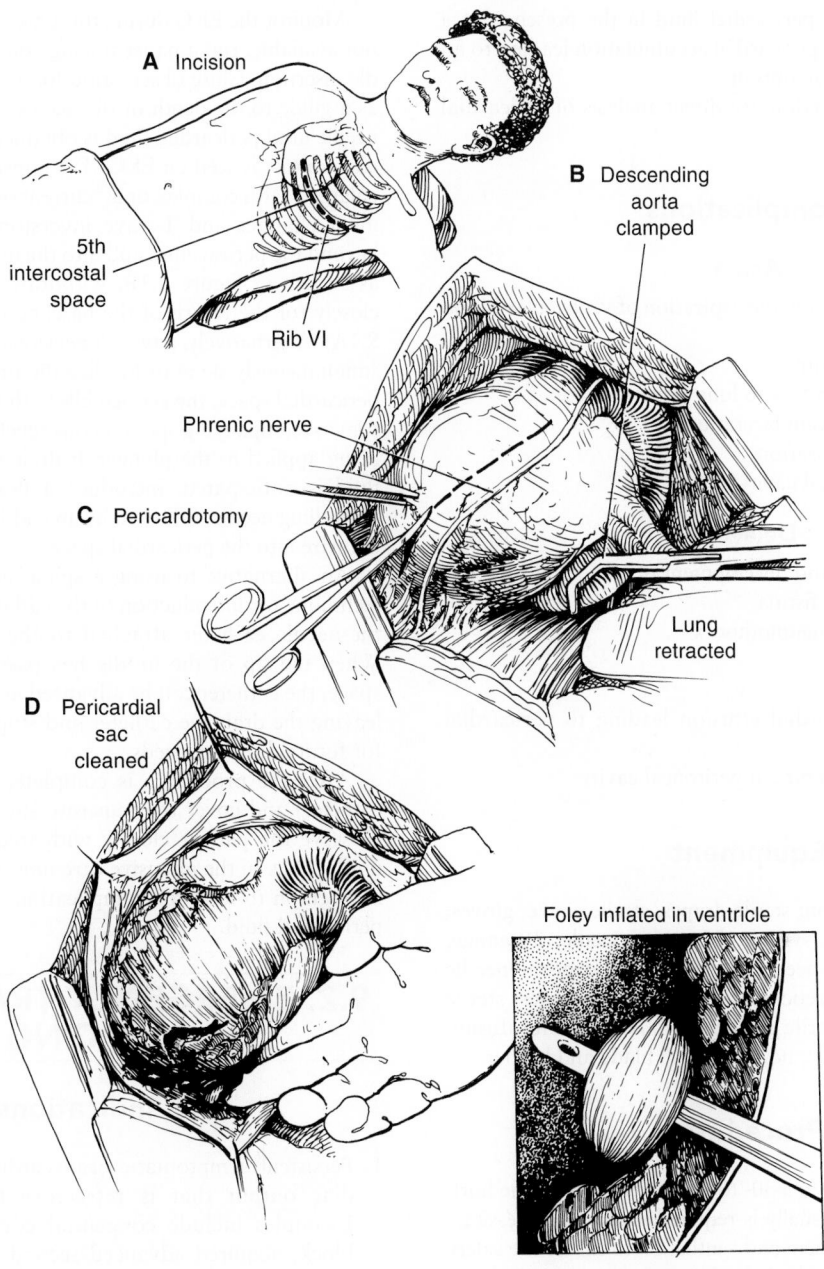

A Incision

5th intercostal space

Rib VI

B Descending aorta clamped

Phrenic nerve

C Pericardotomy

Lung retracted

D Pericardial sac cleaned

Foley inflated in ventricle

8.3

PROCEDURES

Satinsky clamp. Likewise, if bleeding is occurring from the hilum of the lung, a large, curved vascular clamp should be placed across the hilum of the lung to secure hemostasis.

Cross-clamping of the descending thoracic aorta is an adjunctive measure to maintain proximal arterial pressure, thus increasing brain and heart perfusion, and decreasing subdiaphragmatic hemorrhage. In this case, the left lung is elevated anteriorly and superiorly by an assistant on the right of the patient. The operator on the left side of the patient should spread a DeBakey aortic clamp medial and lateral to the mid-descending aorta. The operator passes his/her finger around the descending aorta, and then applies the clamp to the descending aorta under direct visualization, with care to avoid avulsion to other aortic branches.

Once hemorrhage has been controlled and adequate resuscitative measures applied, the patient is moved to the operating room where definitive hemostasis is secured and all clots/debris are lavaged from the pericardial and pleural cavities. Finally, the chest will be closed after placement of appropriate chest and pericardial tubes.

9.1. PERICARDIOCENTESIS

Indications

1. Emergent removal of intrapericardial fluid in the treatment of cardiac tamponade

2. Elective removal of pericardial fluid in the presence of a chronic or recurrent pericardial accumulation leading to an impairment of cardiac output
3. As a diagnostic procedure for direct analysis of pericardial fluid

Complications

Acute

1. Myocardial penetration and aspiration of ventricular blood
2. Cardiac arrhythmias
3. New hemopericardium
4. Pneumothorax secondary to lung puncture
5. Coronary artery or vein laceration
6. Diaphragmatic perforation
7. Puncture of peritoneal cavity

Delayed

1. Pericardial leakage and development of a cutaneous fistula
2. Pericardioperitoneal fistula
3. Slowly developing pneumothorax
4. Pneumopericardium
5. Local infection
6. Hemorrhagic pericardial effusion leading to pericardial tamponade
7. Peritonitis from puncture of peritoneal cavity

Equipment

Povidone–iodine solution; sterile drapes, sterile gauze, gloves; 1% lidocaine, 3–5 mL syringe; 22-gauge needle; 20-gauge, 2.5-in or 3.5-in spinal needle or long (6 in) over-the-needle catheter; three-way stopcock; 20- and 50-mL syringes; sterile alligator clip; flexible sterile guidewire (0.018 in); soft infusion catheter (18 or 20 gauge); no. 15 scalpel blade and holder

Procedure

Position the child supine at a 30- to 45-degree angle to the horizontal plane. Sedation usually is required, and may necessitate capable airway management and ventilation to ensure the safety of the child. Attach the limb leads of an electrocardiogram (EKG) monitor. Clean and sterilize the precordium with povidone–iodine solution, and donning sterile gloves, drape the area with sterile towels. Infiltrate the area 1 to 2 cm below and to patient's left of the xiphoid process with 1% lidocaine; penetrate through the muscle layer to achieve satisfactory local anesthesia. Attach the spinal needle to a stopcock and a 20- to 50-mL syringe. Connect the "V" lead of the EKG to the hub of the needle with a sterile clip (alligator type) after checking that the lead is grounded. Turn the EKG recorder on to the "V" lead position.

Before inserting the needle, make a 2-mm incision 1 to 2 cm below and slightly to the patient's left of the xiphoid to facilitate penetration of the skin. Holding the needle perpendicular to the skin, advance it through this incision. Once below the skin, angle the needle at approximately 45 degrees up from the abdominal surface, pointing cephalad and toward the tip of the left scapula. Slowly advance, maintaining a slightly negative pressure on the syringe.

Monitor the EKG during this procedure. If an oscilloscope is not available, run a paper tracing continuously during the needle insertion. Close observation for a change in the EKG serves as a guide to the depth of the needle penetration. Advance the needle until pericardial fluid is obtained or evidence of myocardial contact is seen on EKG. The appearance of a widened and enlarged QRS complex or a "current of injury" pattern (ST segment changes and T-wave inversion) indicates penetration beyond the pericardium and into the myocardium. If this occurs as shown in Figure 9.1B, withdraw the needle and observe closely for the return of the baseline pattern of the EKG (Fig. 9.1A). Alternatively, a two-dimensional echocardiogram can be simultaneously done to localize the drainage site. Once in the pericardial space, the syringe fills with the pericardial fluid with some accompanying spontaneous relief of the negative pressure being applied to the plunger. If drainage of a large volume of fluid is anticipated, introduce a flexible wire through the indwelling needle, followed by an end-hole catheter passed over the wire into the pericardial space.

An alternative to using a spinal needle and the Seldinger technique for introduction of the catheter is to use a long over-the-needle catheter attached to the syringe and stopcock. When the tip of the needle has passed into the pericardial space, the catheter can be advanced and the needle withdrawn leaving the drainage catheter and stopcock assembly in place for future drainage needs.

After the procedure is complete, remove the needle (or catheter) and cover the puncture site with a sterile dressing. Observe the patient closely with frequent vital sign checks, until stable, in the intensive care unit. Obtain an upright chest radiograph to look for complications or a reaccumulation of pericardial fluid.

9.2. EMERGENCY TRANSVENOUS PACING

Indications

1. Persistent symptomatic bradycardia with inadequate cardiac output that is refractory to medical treatment. Examples include congenital complete atrioventricular block, acquired advanced second degree or third degree atrioventricular block, sinus bradycardia or sinus node dysfunction leading to symptomatic age-inappropriate bradycardia, and junctional or idioventricular rhythms.
2. Overdrive suppression of atrial or ventricular tachyarrhythmias refractory to other treatment modalities.

Contraindications

Congenital heart disease or surgery precluding transvenous access to the cardiac chambers

Complications

Acute

1. Perforation of vessel, heart, and/or contiguous structures (e.g., pneumothorax)

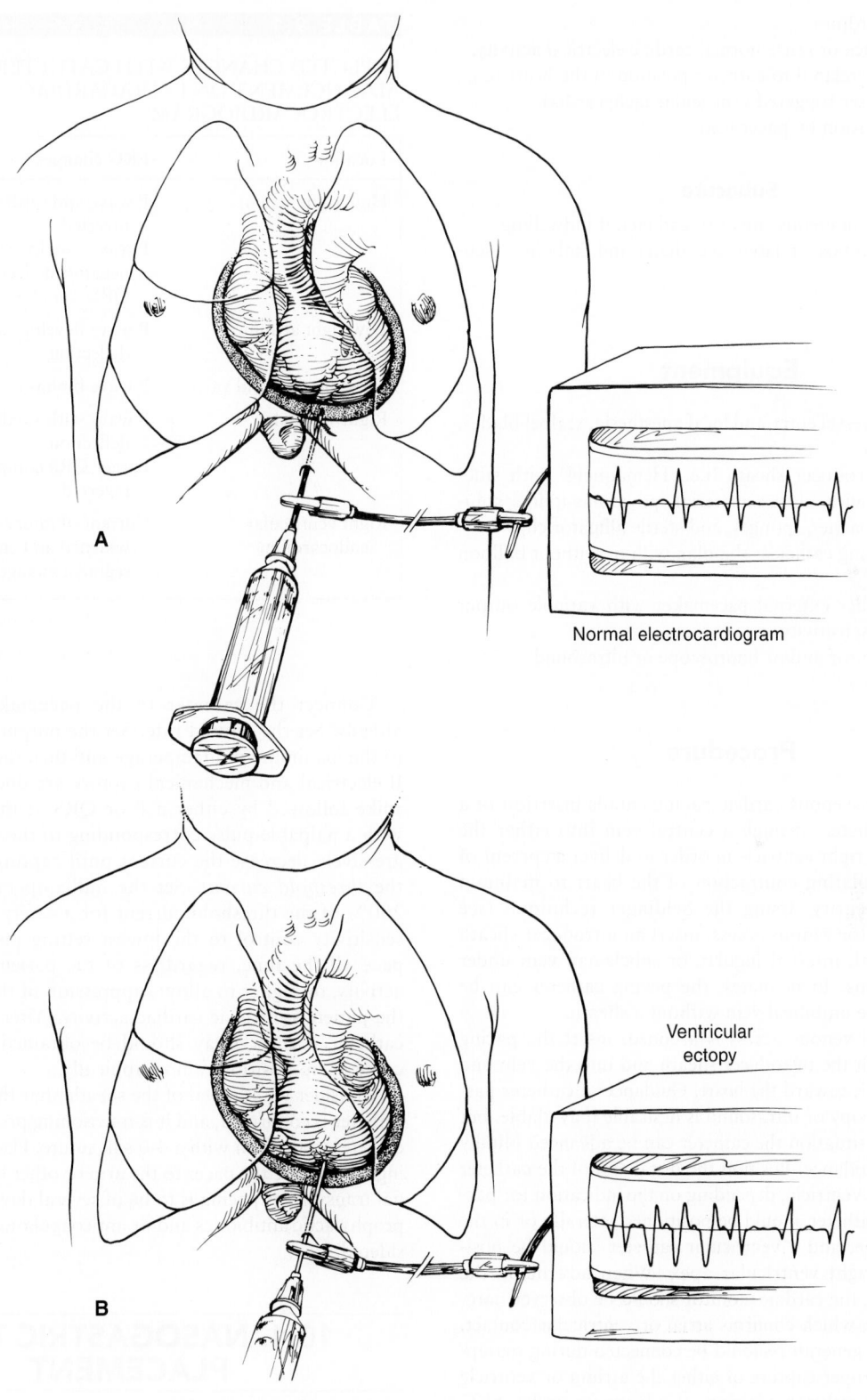

Normal electrocardiogram

Ventricular ectopy

9.1

2. Hemopericardium
3. Failure to pace or sense normal cardiac electrical activity.
4. Arrhythmias related to catheter position in the heart (e.g., pacing catheter triggered ventricular tachycardia)
5. Venous occlusion by pacer lead

Subacute

1. Infection of cutaneous site or of catheter, if indwelling
2. Venous thrombosis related to catheter and embolic vascular events

Equipment

1. Needles for vessel entry and local anesthesia, scalpel blades, 1% lidocaine
2. Catheter introducer sheath (i.e., Hemaquet® with side-port), guidewire, suture material, povidone–iodine solution, sterile barrier, sponges, and sterile alligator clip
3. 3F to 5F pacing catheter—bipolar, with or without balloon tip
4. Single chamber external pacemaker with variable output current and sensitivity
5. Cardiac monitor and/or fluoroscope or ultrasound

Procedure

Temporary transvenous cardiac pacing entails insertion of a pacemaker catheter through a central vein into either the right atrium or right ventricle in order to deliver a current of electricity stimulating contraction of the heart to maintain circulatory integrity. Using the Seldinger technique (see Procedure 3.2) for venous access, insert an introducer sheath into the femoral, internal jugular, or subclavian vein under sterile conditions. In neonates, the pacing catheter can be inserted into the umbilical vein without a sheath.

After central venous access is attained, insert the pacing catheter through the introducer sheath and into the vein and *gently* advance it toward the heart. Guidance of catheter passage by fluoroscopy or ultrasound is desirable if available, but in an emergent situation the catheter can be advanced blindly or with EKG guidance. Position the distal end of the catheter in the atrium or ventricle, depending on the indication for pacing. An atrial catheter should be positioned laterally or in the atrial appendage, and a ventricular catheter should be positioned in the right ventricular apex. When advancing the catheter blindly, the cardiac monitor should be observed carefully for ectopy, which confirms atrial or ventricular contact. The pacemaker generator should be connected during manipulation, with proper capture of either the atrium or ventricle confirming the catheter position. If advancing under EKG guidance, the negative pole of the bipolar pacing electrode should be connected to a surface precordial lead with an alligator clip. The pacing electrode should be advanced and as the electrode traverses the right atrium and comes into contact with the right ventricle predictable EKG changes should be observed consistent with those expected on an intracardiac EKG (Table 9.1).

TABLE 9.1

EXPECTED CHANGES WITH CATHETER ADVANCEMENT ON INTRACARDIAC ELECTROCARDIOGRAM

Location	EKG changes
High right atrium	P wave and QRS complex inverted
	P wave usually with larger negative deflection than the QRS complex
Low right atrium	P wave develops a positive deflection
Crossing tricuspid valve	P wave biphasic
Right ventricle	P wave with small positive deflection
	Larger QRS complex deep and inverted
Right ventricular endocardium	Current of injury pattern—widened and enlarged QRS, ST segment changes

Connect the catheter to the pacemaker if not done already. Set the desired rate. Set the output current control to the maximum milliamperage and turn the pacemaker on. If electrical and mechanical capture are documented (pacer spike followed by either a P or QRS at the set rate along with a palpable pulse corresponding to the QRS), then progressively decrease the current until capture is lost. This is the *threshold current*. Set the milliamperage at 150% to 200% of the threshold current for a safety margin. Set the sensitivity control to the lowest setting (asynchronous) to pace all the time, regardless of the patient's own cardiac activity, or higher to allow suppression of the pacemaker by the patient's intrinsic cardiac activity. After insertion of the catheter, a chest x-ray should be obtained to confirm the catheter tip position radiographically.

Consider withdrawal of the sheath after the position of the catheter is confirmed, and it is functioning properly. Secure the catheter to the skin with a 4-0 silk suture. Place a sterile dressing, and secure the pacer to the arm or other location. If external transvenous pacing is to be of several days' duration, then prophylactic antibiotics and/or anticoagulation should be considered.

10.1. NASOGASTRIC TUBE PLACEMENT

Indications

1. Decompression of the stomach and proximal bowel for obstruction or trauma
2. Gastric lavage in the child with upper gastrointestinal (GI) bleeding or an ingestion/overdose
3. Administration of medication or nutrition

Complications

1. Tracheal intubation
2. Nasal, pharyngeal or esophageal trauma or laceration
3. Reflux or vomiting leading to aspiration
4. Direct airway instillation of tube contents—medications, food, etc.

Procedure

Choose the largest size tube feasible to perform the indicated task, without causing undue discomfort to the child. In general, choose an 8F tube in the newborn, and around a 12F by the age of 1 year. A teenager will usually tolerate an 18F. In between, pick the size accordingly. In an adolescent overdose, the use of a 28F to 40F tube will assist in the efficient drainage of pill fragments from the GI tract, but its use has become very uncommon in the management of overdoses. Estimate the length of tubing to be passed by adding 8 to 10 cm to the distance from the nares to the xiphoid process (Fig. 10.1).

Prepare the child by explaining the procedure as fully as possible; sedation is rarely required. Older children who are alert can remain sitting. Infants and obtunded children require the supine position with their head turned to the side.

Straighten the curved tube out and check its patency with a syringe. If it is too pliable, stiffen it by immersion in ice water. Apply lubricant or lidocaine gel to facilitate atraumatic nasal passage. Grasp the tube 5 to 6 cm from the distal end and advance it posteriorly along the floor of the nose. If it is incorrectly directed up the nose, the tube may lacerate the inferior turbinate. Insert it with the natural curve of the tube pointing downward to pass the bend of the posterior pharynx. A cooperative child can be asked to flex his/her head slightly, as well as to swallow some water to assist in glottic closure and easy passage into the esophagus. An assistant should flex the infant's neck. If the child coughs and gags persistently or if the tube emerges from the mouth, temporarily discontinue the procedure and support the child until they recover from the episode.

When the tube is successfully passed to the measured length, check its position. Attach a syringe filled with air to the proximal end and, while depressing the plunger rapidly, listen

with a stethoscope for gurgling over the stomach. Other confirmatory tests in high risk patients should be considered prior to using include pH testing of gastric contents (pH should be less than 4) or a frontal single view of the chest and part of the upper abdomen to confirm location. Tape the tube securely to the nose, using tincture of benzoin on the skin in the uncooperative or diaphoretic child.

10.2. PERITONEAL TAP

Indications

1. To obtain peritoneal fluid for diagnostic purposes
2. Relief of respiratory distress secondary to a large peritoneal fluid collection

Contraindications

1. Second or third trimester pregnancy (ultrasound guidance recommended)

Complications

1. Perforation of abdominal viscera or vessels
2. Local bleeding or soft tissue infection
3. Peritonitis
4. Ascitic fluid leak

Procedure

The child undergoing a diagnostic peritoneal aspiration may require sedation to permit safe access to the peritoneal cavity. If a large amount of intraabdominal fluid has accumulated, it may elevate the diaphragm, causing respiratory compromise. This serves as a relative contraindication to the use of general anesthetic for sedation.

Before attempting this procedure, carefully evaluate the abdominal anatomy. Verify the presence of ascites by percussion, being certain to note shifting dullness after the child is turned. Place the patient in the position in which the procedure is to be done, either sitting (Fig. 10.2C) or lateral decubitus (Fig. 10.2A) with an adequate amount of restraint. If a large amount of fluid has collected, the child will have less respiratory embarrassment if allowed to be seated during the procedure. If concern remains regarding the location of viscera, adhesions, or a specific area to be entered for diagnostic studies, ultrasound can aid in localizing the best place to enter the abdominal cavity.

For a diagnostic tap, use an 18-, 20-, or 22-gauge metal needle or over-the-needle catheter. If a large amount of fluid must be evacuated, the plastic catheter, in contrast to a metal needle, allows repositioning of the patient and decreases the risk of bowel perforation during a prolonged procedure. There is a risk of kinking with a plastic catheter as well as a risk that the plastic catheter could be sheared off into the peritoneal cavity.

As shown in Figure 10.2B, a midline approach in either supraumbilical or infraumbilical location is probably the

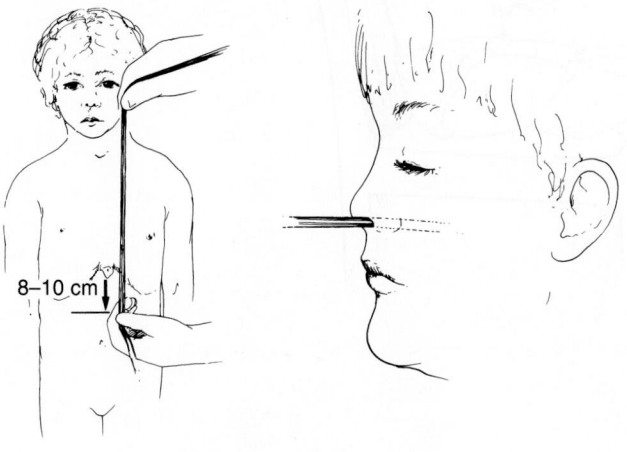

8–10 cm

10.1

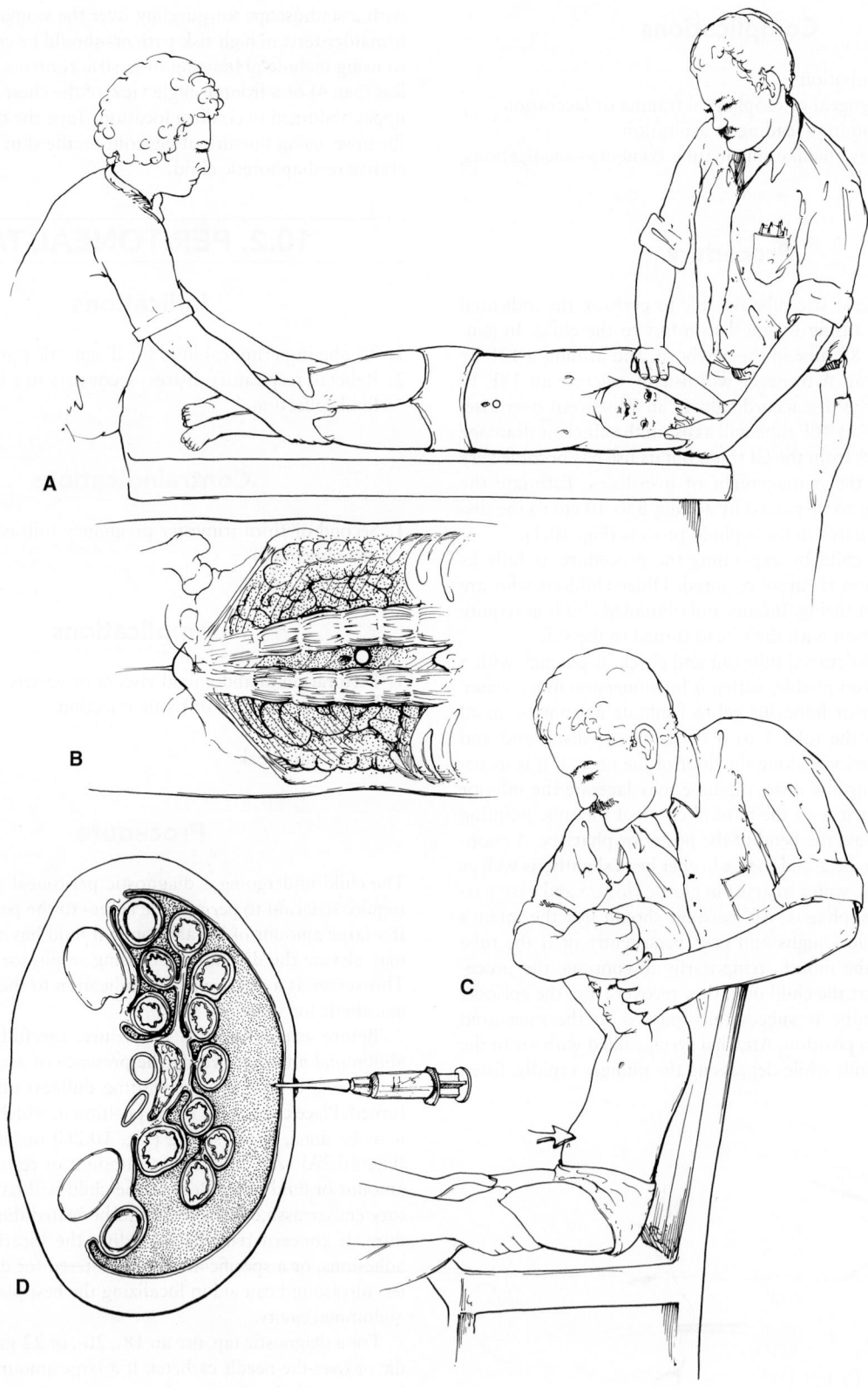

10.2

safest. Position the child in either the sitting or decubitus position. Cleanse a large area around the planned site with povidone–iodine solution. Then, if in the decubitus position, drape the patient with towels under and over the back; whereas if in the sitting position, drape towels on the lap. Wearing sterile gloves, inject the skin with 1% lidocaine.

After local anesthesia is achieved, take the needle and catheter in hand. Stabilize the tip of the needle with the thumb and index finger, placing the heel of this hand against the abdominal wall. With the other hand, direct the needle perpendicular to the abdominal wall. Puncture the skin, and then move the needle tip caudad and parallel to the midline for a short distance to make a Z-track. Advance the needle with support until a "popping sensation" or decreased resistance is appreciated. Immediately verify penetration through the peritoneum by drawing fluid into the syringe. As shown schematically in Figure 10.2D, the abdominal viscera lie slightly away from the peritoneum if a moderate amount of fluid has collected.

Slowly advance the needle several millimeters while continuing to aspirate fluid with the syringe. Then remove the needle and syringe from the catheter and cover the opening with the thumb. After attaching a larger syringe and T-connector, observe for a brisk flow of fluid. The catheter tip can be repositioned once the needle has been removed, and the patient safely turned to facilitate the collection of fluid. When the procedure is completed, quickly pull the catheter straight out, and firmly apply sterile gauze and then a pressure dressing to the puncture wound.

10.3. PERITONEAL LAVAGE

Indications

Evaluation of a patient with blunt multiple trauma, and/or penetrating thoracoabdominal trauma, with cardiovascular instability or coma, to determine the need for immediate laparotomy. It is not sensitive for retroperitoneal bleeding.

Complications

1. Iatrogenic injury to abdominal viscera or vessels (may be enhanced by prior abdominal adhesions)
2. Hemorrhage or bleeding from the procedure with potential to be false positive test.
3. Wound infection and/or peritonitis
4 Evisceration

Contraindications

1. Existing indication for celiotomy
2. Relative contraindications are recent abdominal surgery, preexisting coagulopathy, and/or morbid obesity

Equipment

1. Povidone–iodine solution; sterile drapes; gloves; gauze; 1% lidocaine with epinephrine; peritoneal dialysis/lavage catheter; Ringer's lactate and/or normal saline solution; IV catheter; collecting bag; sample tubes; sutures (reabsorbable and superficial); Steri-strips
2. Open technique—no. 15 scalpel blade and handle, and two hemostats
3. Closed technique—18-gauge needle, guidewire, no. 11 scalpel blade

Procedure

The child should receive an overall trauma assessment, an IV infusion of saline through at least one large-bore catheter, and the appropriate laboratory and radiographic evaluation. Correction of any cardiorespiratory disturbances is essential for the procedure to be safely performed.

Pass a nasogastric tube to decompress the stomach and a urinary catheter to empty the bladder. Select a site for the incision, either supraumbilical or infraumbilical, in the midline. A supraumbilical location is preferable in younger children in whom the bladder extends into the abdomen (Fig. 10.3A) and/or in pregnant patients (above the uterine fundus). Using aseptic technique, including sterile gown, gloves, and mask, prepare the anterior abdominal wall with povidone–iodine solution. Inject 1% lidocaine with epinephrine (to lessen bleeding) into the skin and subcutaneous tissue for local anesthesia.

Open Technique

When performing the open technique, make a 1.5- to 2-cm transverse incision in the skin with a no. 15 scalpel blade 1 to 2 cm above the umbilicus (Fig. 10.3A). The subcutaneous tissue should be divided and the linea alba exposed by blunt dissection. Make a transverse or vertical incision through the linea alba as shown in Figure 10.3B, with care not to penetrate deeper than this fascial plane.

Using two hemostats, grasp the peritoneum at the center of the fascial opening, as shown in Figure 10.3C. The field should be maintained free of blood to prevent a false-positive result. Between the hemostats, make a small incision through the peritoneum with the scalpel to provide access to the abdominal cavity. An immediate return of frankly bloody material constitutes a positive result.

If frankly bloody fluid is not obtained on opening the peritoneum, gently introduce a peritoneal dialysis catheter, without a trocar, through the peritoneal opening. Pass it caudally just inside the peritoneal lining into the pelvis to minimize the chance of perforating a viscus, as shown in cross-section in Figure 10.3D. If aspiration through the catheter yields frankly bloody fluid, significant intraabdominal bleeding has occurred.

Closed Technique

When performing the closed technique, insert an 18-gauge beveled needle attached to syringe through the skin, subcutaneous tissue, fascia, and into the peritoneum. (Light resistance may be noted when penetrating the fascia and the peritoneum.) Using Seldinger technique, pass a guidewire through the needle until resistance is met, or 3 cm of guidewire remains outside needle hub. Then remove the needle over the guidewire, with caution not to displace current guidewire location. Using an 11-blade scalpel, incise a small area of skin directly next to the guidewire (entrance site of the catheter).

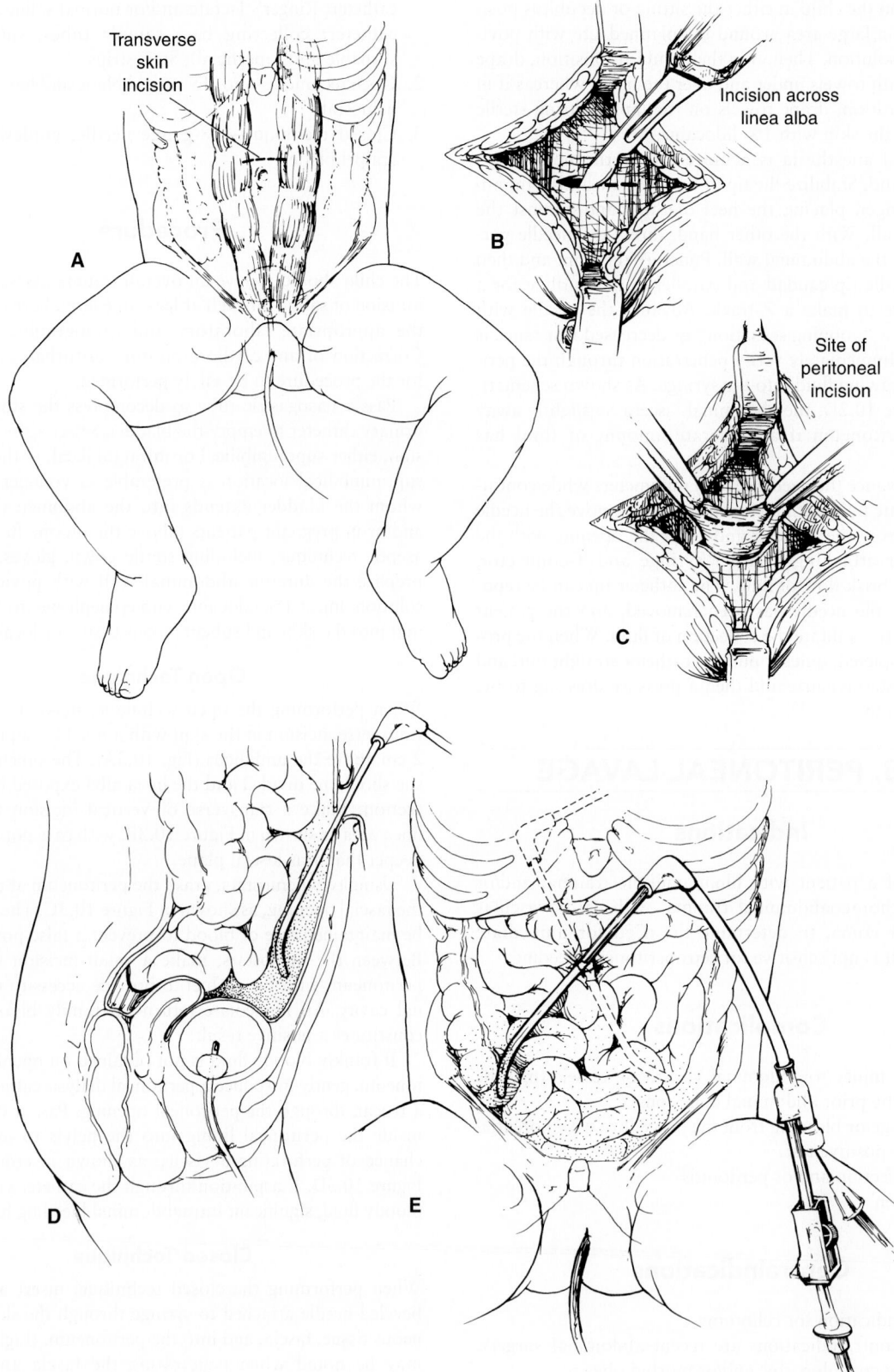

Transverse
skin
incision

A

Incision across
linea alba

B

Site of
peritoneal
incision

C

D

E

10.3

Next, pass peritoneal lavage catheter over the guidewire into the peritoneal cavity and withdraw the guidewire. Connect catheter to syringe and aspirate. If gross blood is obtained, significant intraabdominal bleeding has occurred.

Lavage (Open and Closed Techniques)

If no blood is obtained, quickly infuse 10 to 20 mL per kg of Ringer's lactate or normal saline solution into the abdominal cavity through the catheter, as shown in Figure 10.3E. After the fluid has been instilled, turn the patient from side to side to promote its distribution throughout the peritoneal cavity. Then, allow the fluid to run back out under gravity into a sterile collecting bag connected to IV tubing. Return of at least 200 ml of lavage represents adequate sample (at the rate 30% to 50% of fluid volume instilled). Effluent samples should be sent for determination of red blood cell (RBC) count, white blood cell (WBC) count, amylase level, Gram stain, and examination for stool or food particles. At the completion of the lavage, whether the result is positive or negative, carefully remove the catheter. Use chromic sutures to close the peritoneum, and 2-0 or 3-0 absorbable sutures for the fascia and subcutaneous tissue. Place Steri-strips across the skin.

Positive results include gross blood; more than 100,000 RBCs or 500 WBCs per high-power field in blunt trauma; greater than 10,000 RBCs in penetrating trauma; particulate matter or positive Gram stain for food fibers or bacteria; elevated lavage amylase or alkaline phosphatase. A negative diagnostic peritoneal lavage does not exclude retroperitoneal bleeding or diaphragmatic tears.

10.4. REPLACEMENT OF A GASTROSTOMY TUBE

Indications

Obstruction or dislodgment of a gastrostomy tube

Contraindications

1. Evidence of peritonitis
2. Freshly placed tube in first weeks after placement (relative)
3. Tubes out more than 4 to 6 hours (often require dilation)

Complications

1. Bleeding at the mucosal site
2. Separation of the stomach from the abdominal wall
3. Gastric outlet obstruction from an improperly positioned tube

Equipment

1. Replacement tube—Button, Bard, Mallincott, MIC KEY, PeeWee, or Foley catheter
2. Lubricant
3. Normal saline
4. Syringes (5 to 10 mL, 30 to 50 mL)
5. Absorbent dressing
6. Tape

Procedure

When a child with a gastrostomy appears in the ED after dislodgment of the tube, it should be replaced as soon as possible. The opening quickly narrows, making passage of a replacement difficult.

Perform a history and physical examination to rule out an intraabdominal obstruction, and examine the gastrostomy site for bleeding or tears. Pass a blunt-tipped stylet or lubricated cotton-tipped swab through the opening to assess the patency and direction of the tract.

Prepare the equipment. Fill the balloon with saline to ensure it works. When using "mushroom" or "ball" tubes, slide the tube over the stylet after lubricating the distal end, as in Figure 10.4A. When no replacement is available, an alternative is to use a Foley catheter of similar diameter. Hook the end of the tube and the handle of the stylet, and generously apply lubricant to the distal portion.

Restrain the child in the supine position. Holding the system perpendicular to the abdominal wall, as in Figure 10.4B, aim it in the direction of the stoma tract as determined by the previous probing. Grasp the distal end of the tube between the index finger and thumb of one hand and stabilize it by placing the heel of this hand against the abdominal wall to prevent slippage. When using a styletted tube, the other hand holds the handle of the stylet and the proximal portion of the tube.

Pass the tip of the catheter into the opening to the gastrostomy site and, with steady, firm pressure, push it down in the direction of the stomach, perpendicular to the abdominal wall. It may take 30 to 45 seconds of this steady pressure to stretch the site enough to permit entry. Avoid sudden jerking of the tip because this increases the chance of mucosal damage or separation.

When the stomach is entered, resistance suddenly lessons. As shown in Figure 10.4C, the tube must be inserted far enough so the entire tube or whole "mushroom" tip (balloon) is in the gastric cavity. For buttons, advance completely. Instill the saline to inflate the balloon. Remove the syringe. For a styletted tube, advance several centimeters if little resistance, detach the handle of the stylet from the catheter, and pass the catheter 4 to 5 cm farther. The balloon will spontaneously open on withdrawal of the stylet. Then fully withdraw the stylet and pull the tube gently out to appreciate the "clunk" on reaching the surface. If the tube is in the stomach, it will move freely and spontaneously drain gastric contents. If gastric contents do not spontaneously drain and the tube appears to be in, install 30 to 60 mL of normal saline and withdraw it to check for gastric contents. If still in doubt or with difficult placements, consider instilling barium or gastrograffin and obtaining a radiograph. Recent literature suggests that ultrasound with color Doppler can accurately define the location of the tube as can air insufflation as a contrast medium. Cover the distal end with clean gauze.

Occasionally, the catheter may not be advanced far enough, leaving the balloon in the wall of the stomach. If this is the case, remove the saline with the syringe or reinsert the stylet, stretch the tube, and with constant pressure, advance the catheter into the stomach. Similarly, if a child with a gastrostomy tube in place appears to be uncomfortable or have an obstructed tube,

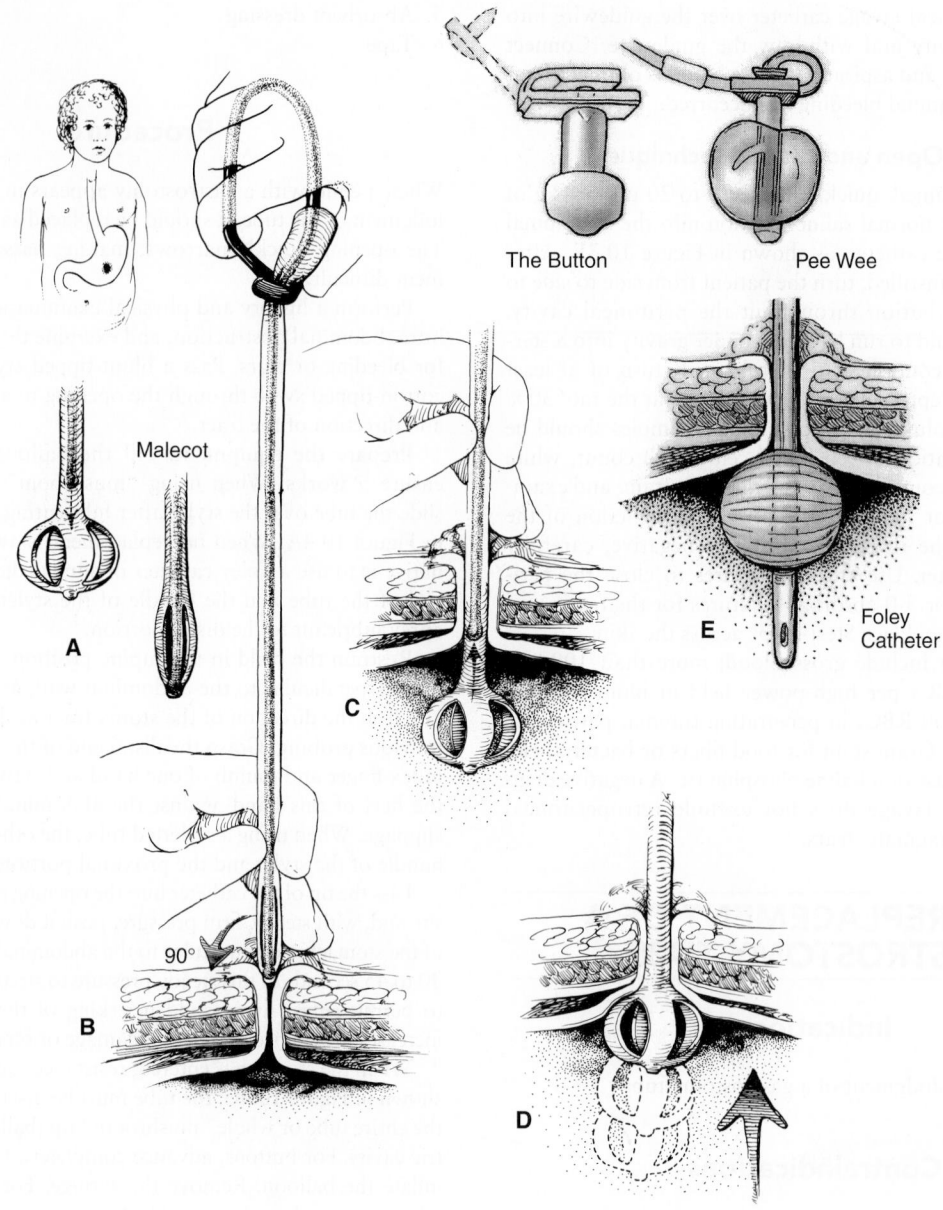

The Button

Pee Wee

Malecot

A

B

90°

C

D

E

Foley
Catheter

10.4

the tube may have been incorrectly placed or may have slipped out so the balloon is inflated in the gastric wall.

If the procedure causes mucosal trauma, the local application of lubricant gel or a neutralizing agent, such as an antacid, may decrease inflammation of the stoma.

10.5. REDUCTION OF AN INCARCERATED INGUINAL HERNIA

Indications

1. To prevent strangulation of incarcerated bowel, ovary, or other organs

2. To allow for edema to resolve, permitting a less hazardous, semi-elective repair of the hernia

Complications

1. Compression damage of the bowel or other incarcerated organ or tissue (may be related to the incarceration and not reduction).
2. Increased edema and pain

Procedure (Fig. 10.5)

Be careful to ascertain if the patient has a hernia and not the acute presentation of a hydrocele. Place the patient supine in a

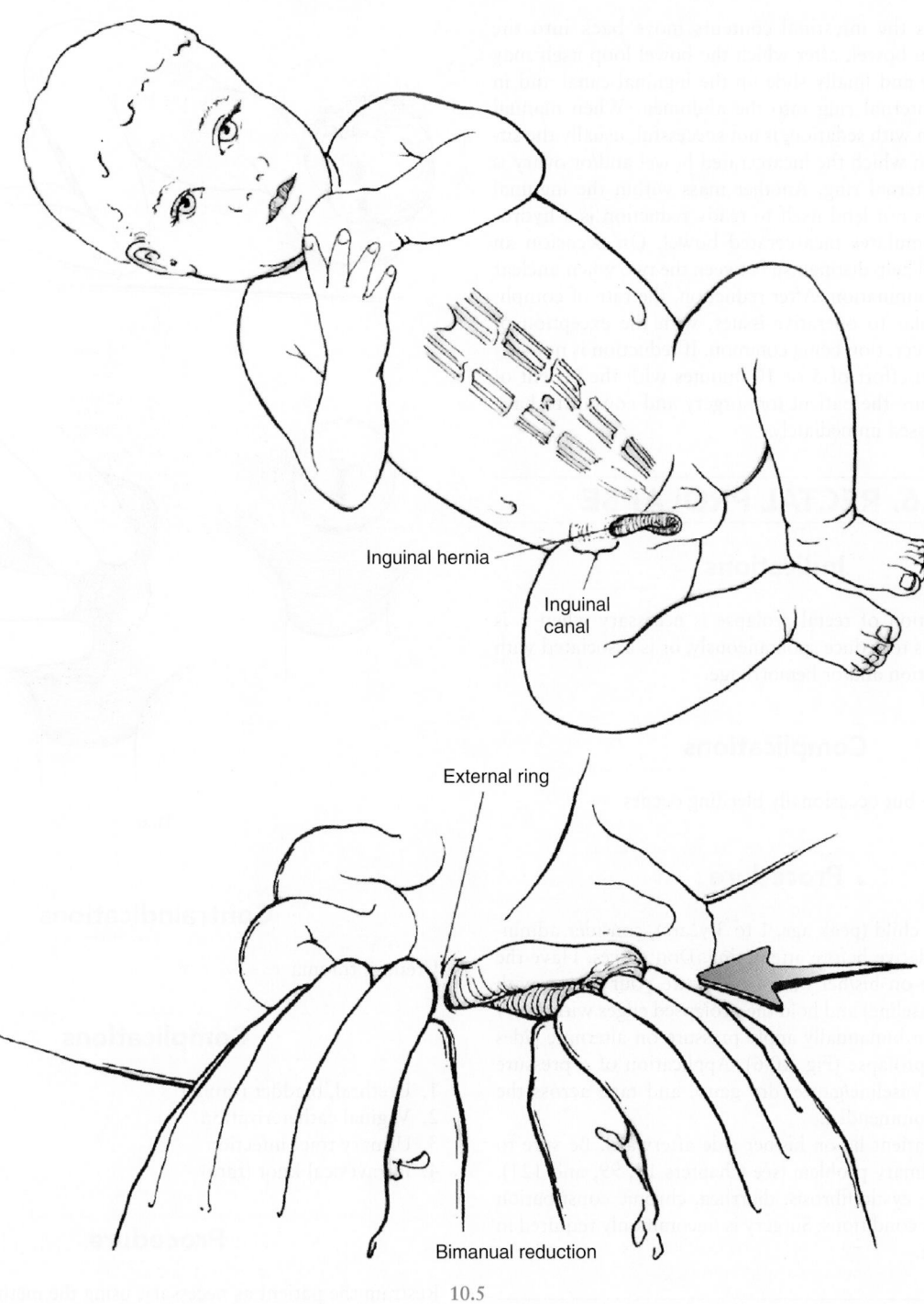

Inguinal hernia

Inguinal
canal

External ring

Bimanual reduction

10.5

mild Trendelenburg position to decrease edema in the incarcerated tissue. The primary principle of reduction is to reduce the contents of the bowel first, after which the edematous bowel itself may then be coaxed back into the abdominal cavity. Consider pharmacologic sedation and pain control to reduce discomfort and the infant's rising intraabdominal pressure. This is done by applying bimanual pressure along the entire inguinal canal so uniform pressure is placed on the incarcerated bowel. Begin to apply pressure gently with slightly increased pressure in the distal canal compared with the proximal canal to encourage reduction of intestinal contents into the bowel

within the abdomen. Apply a sustained, moderate pressure for up to 5 minutes or until reduction is achieved.

If reduction has not occurred at this point, it may be due to patient discomfort and tensing of the abdominal wall. Reassess the pain control or sedation used. When ready, reposition the patient gently in a Trendelenburg position and apply the same maneuver of sustained pressure along the inguinal canal. Use one of the ipsilateral hand having thumb and index finger compressing at the ring while the other hand is leading/pushing the hernia towards the ring will often be successful. If sustained pressure is successful, a gurgling sensation will first be felt as the intestinal contents move back into the intraabdominal bowel, after which the bowel loop itself may begin to move and finally slide up the inguinal canal and in through the internal ring into the abdomen. When manual reduction, even with sedation, is not successful, usually the situation is one in which the incarcerated bowel and/or ovary is outside the external ring. Another mass within the inguinal canal that does not lend itself to ready reduction is a hydrocele, which simulates incarcerated bowel. On occasion an ultrasound will help distinguish between the two when unclear on physical examination. After reduction, the rate of complications is similar to operative issues, with the exception of recurrent incarceration being common. If reduction is not successful after an effort of 5 or 10 minutes with the benefit of sedation, prepare the patient for surgery and consult to have the infant assessed immediately.

10.6. RECTAL PROLAPSE

Indications

Manual reduction of rectal prolapse is necessary when it is prolonged, fails to reduce spontaneously, or is associated with passive congestion and/or hemorrhage.

Complications

Extremely rare but occasionally bleeding occurs

Procedure

In the anxious child (peak age, 1 to 3 years), consider administration of sedative before attempting. Don gloves. Have the child lie prone on his/her knees. Lubricate your gloves with petrolatum (Vaseline) and hold the prolapsed edges with 4×4 in^2 gauze. Then bimanually apply pressure on alternate sides to reduce the prolapse (Fig. 10.6). Application of a pressure dressing with Vaseline/gauze, dry gauze and tape across the buttocks is recommended.

Have the patient lie on his/her side afterward. Be sure to address the primary problem (see Chapters 13, 99, and 121). Causes include cystic fibrosis, diarrhea, chronic constipation and neurologic conditions. Surgery is uncommonly required in young children.

11.1. CATHETERIZATION OF THE BLADDER

Indications

1. Multiple trauma, especially for evaluation of the urinary tract in the unconscious child
2. Monitoring of urine output in conditions such as shock or severe head injury
3. Relief of acute urinary retention
4. To obtain a urine specimen for diagnosis in a young child or other when they cannot give a clean catch specimen

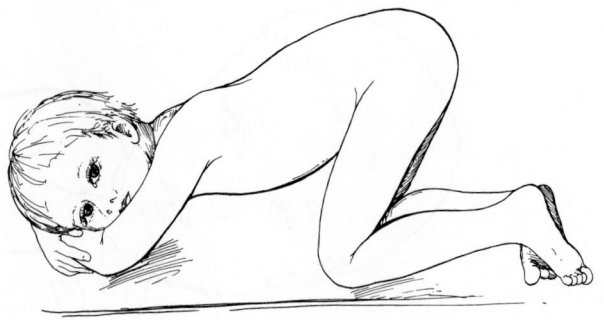

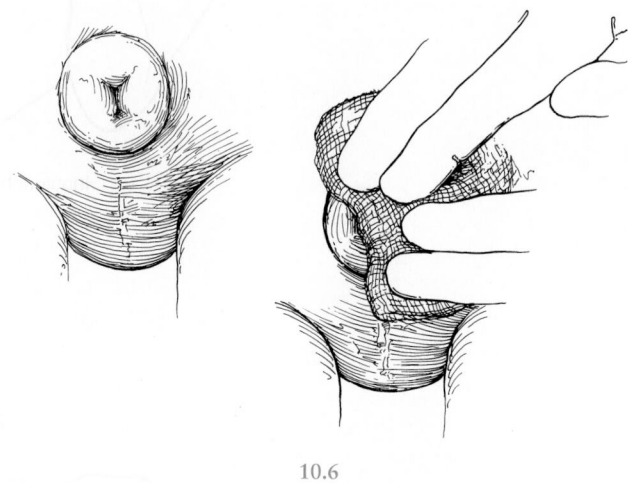

10.6

Contraindications

Urethral trauma

Complications

1. Urethral, bladder trauma
2. Vaginal catheterization
3. Urinary tract infection
4. Intravesical knot (rare)

Procedure

Restrain the patient as necessary, using the method shown for suprapubic bladder aspiration in infants (Fig. 11.1A). The older child may require additional restraint if he/she is uncooperative. Prepare the urethral meatus and penis or the perineal area thoroughly by scrubbing with a povidone–iodine solution; select a Foley catheter of the appropriate size (8F in newborns, 10F in most children, and 12F in older children). Inflate the balloon on the catheter with normal saline to test its competence. The catheter tip should be well lubricated with sterile lubricant to minimize local trauma.

Male

As shown in Figure 11.1A, gently grasp and extend the penile shaft to straighten out the urethral pathway. Hold the catheter

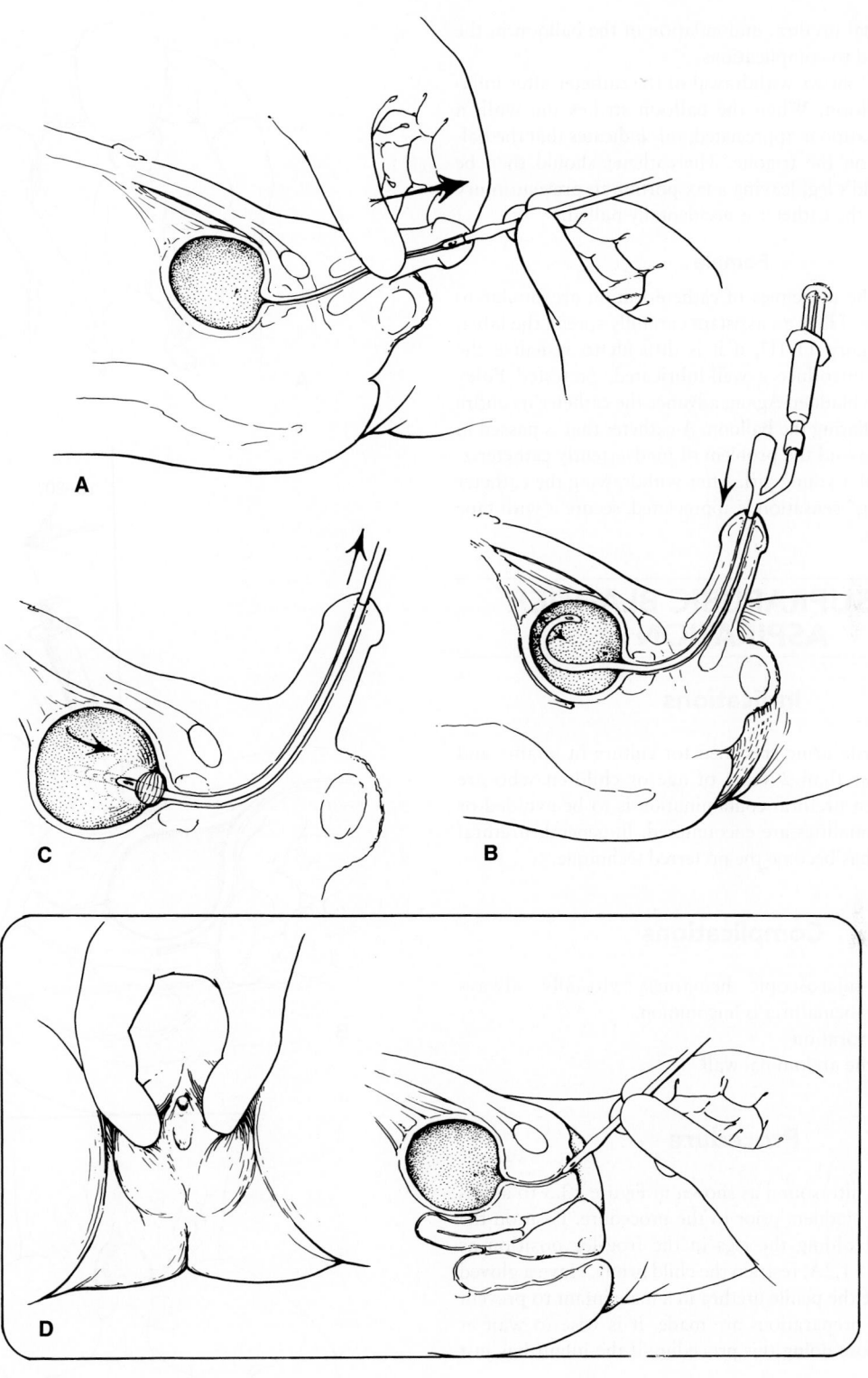

11.1

near the distal tip and advance it up the urethra unless resistance or an obstruction is encountered. If this occurs, select a smaller catheter. Generally, if an 8F is too large, a 5F, 15-cm length feeding tube is a satisfactory alternative, but it is more difficult to maintain in the bladder.

When the catheter reaches the junction of the penile shaft and the perineum, it may help to position the penis more vertically, as shown in Figure 11.1B. The catheter should be passed into the bladder all the way to the Y-connection; this is important because urine may begin to flow while the catheter is in the proximal urethra, and inflation of the balloon in the urethra may lead to complications.

Figure 11.1C shows withdrawal of the catheter after inflation of the balloon. When the balloon strikes the wall, a "clunking" sensation is appreciated; this indicates that the balloon is resting on the trigone. The catheter should then be taped to the child's leg, leaving a lax portion to prevent injury to the trigone if the catheter is accidentally pulled.

Female

In the female, the principles of catheterization are similar to those in the male. Have an assistant carefully spread the labia, as shown in Figure 11.1D, if it is difficult to visualize the urethra. Then, introduce a well-lubricated, pretested Foley catheter into the bladder. Again, advance the catheter its entire length before inflating the balloon. A catheter that is passed in its entirety will avoid the problem of inadvertently catheterizing the vagina of a young girl. After withdrawing the catheter until a "clunking" sensation is appreciated, secure it with tape to the child's leg.

11.2. SUPRAPUBIC BLADDER ASPIRATION

Indications

To obtain a sterile urine specimen for culture in infants and children younger than 2 years of age or children who are incontinent when urethral contamination is to be avoided or anatomic abnormalities are encountered. In general, urethral catheterization has become the preferred technique.

Complications

1. Hematuria—microscopic hematuria virtually always occurs. Gross hematuria is uncommon.
2. Intestinal perforation
3. Infection of the abdominal wall

Procedure

Consider use of ultrasound as shown in Figure 13.3 to assess for urine in the bladders prior to the procedure. Position the infant supine. Holding the legs in the frog-leg position as shown in Figure 11.2A, restrain the child firmly. Have a gloved assistant occlude the penile urethra in a male infant to prevent urination while preparations are made. It is wise to wait at least 1 hour before doing this procedure if the infant has just voided.

Select a puncture site in the midline of the abdomen, approximately 1 to 2 cm cephalad to the superior edge of the pubic bone (Figs. 11.2B and 11.2C). Prepare the skin by cleansing with povidone–iodine solution. After three applications of the antiseptic solution, wipe the dry area with 70% alcohol. Position a 1.5-in 22-gauge needle (with 3-mL syringe attached) at the planned puncture site perpendicular to the plane of the abdominal wall, which is generally 10 to 20 degrees from the true vertical (Fig. 11.2C). Pierce the skin and then, with a second quick stabbing

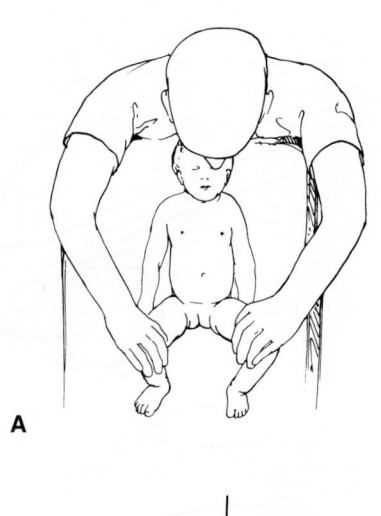

A

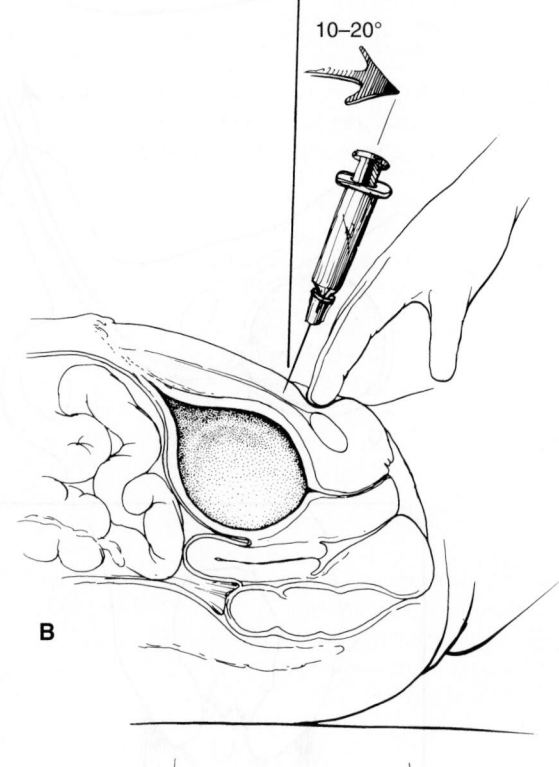

B

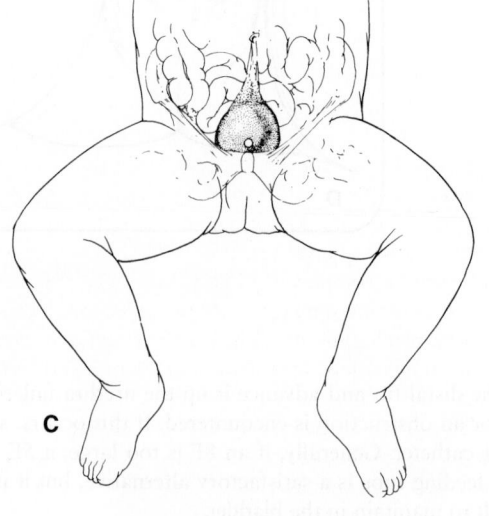

C

11.2

motion, enter the bladder. Withdraw the needle slowly while aspirating with the syringe. If urine is not obtained, do not remove the needle from below the surface of the abdomen. Instead, change the angle of the needle, and reinsert it as previously described. Attempt the procedure at two different angles; first, about 20 degrees caudad to the perpendicular, and second, above 20 degrees cephalad to the perpendicular. If urine is not obtained after the third attempt, further trials are unlikely to be successful. Either perform urethral catheterization or wait 1 to 2 hours and try the suprapubic bladder tap again. Alternatively, use simple ultrasound to know when the bladder is fuller to be able to better guarantee collection of urine specimen.

12.1. INCISION AND DRAINAGE OF AN ABSCESS

Indications

Diagnostic and therapeutic drainage of fluctuant adenitis or superficial soft tissue abscess. Community-acquired methicillin-resistant *Staphylococcus aureus* (MRSA) is commonly the etiologic agent.

Complications

1. Scar formation
2. Injury to local structures surrounding or underlying the abscess (arteries, veins, nerves, tendons)
3. Fistula formation—usually only with mycobacterial neck mass (scrofula)

Contraindications

1. Relative contraindications would include herpetic whitlow, which may increase spread of infection and atypical tubercular abscesses where fistula risk increases.
2. Consider surgical consultation with deep perianal or central facial abscesses.

Procedure

Preparation of the pediatric patient for abscess drainage is critical and includes pharmacologic anxiolysis and pain management in most instances. This may necessitate attention to the NPO status of the patient. Of less risk, is consideration of oral anxiolysis and amnesia with medication such as midazolam in dosing up to 0.5 mg per kg (maximum 20 mg). Parenteral use of ketamine for procedural sedation is much more satisfactory in children with a complex or large abscess. The application of EMLA® or other anesthetic cream may be of value anesthetizing the superficial epidermis when the procedure is not being performed immediately. Distraction techniques and the use of child life may also help to reduce anxiety and pain. Immediately prior to beginning the procedure, position the child to maximize the access to the abscess, and complete the preprocedural time out as required by your institution. For example, in case of a cervical neck mass, place the child supine

with head turned 90 degrees away from the midline to expose the neck. Have an assistant stabilize the patient at the site of the procedure, Figures 12.1A and 12.1B shows a neck abscess, and restrain as necessary. Local anesthetic (xylocaine 1%) injection in a field block 360 degrees surrounding the abscess will reduce pain. This should be followed by xylocaine injection linearly along the abscess where the incision is to be made. In very small ones, occasionally the topical anesthetic is sufficient if appropriate pain relief has been achieved with adjuvant medication.

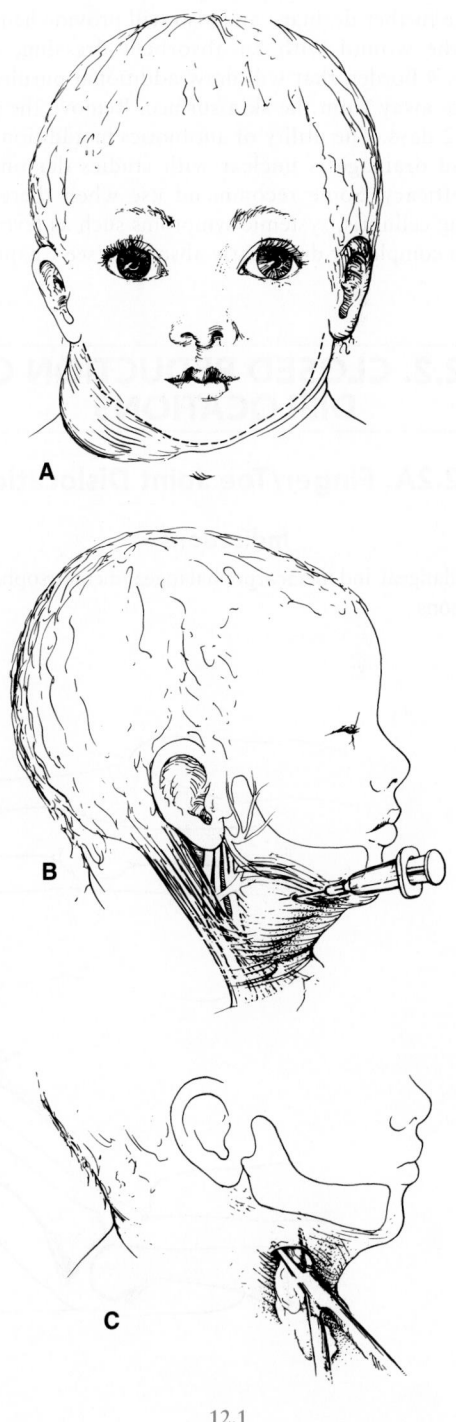

12.1

PROCEDURES

Incision and Drainage

Preparation of the site includes cleansing of the skin with povidone–iodine solution. With a no. 11 scalpel blade, incise the skin over the abscess parallel to the natural creases of the skin to the depth of the superficial fascia. Then, bluntly open the abscess with a hemostat for at least 1 cm, as shown in Figure 12.1C. Insert a gloved little finger into the abscess to break up any septae. The abscess cavity may be irrigated with normal saline to enhance removal of debris and purulence. Pack the wound lightly with a packing strip leaving 2 to 3 cm of the strip outside of the cavity. This will function to physically keep the wound open to promote further drainage and also will provide hemostasis. Dress the wound with an absorbent dressing, such as Mepilex® Border, that will draw additional purulence and drainage away from the skin surface. Remove the packing in 1 to 2 days. The utility of antibiotics in addition to incision and drainage is unclear with studies demonstrating equal efficacy. Some recommend use when there is surrounding cellulitis, systemic symptoms such as fever or difficult to completely drain early abscesses (see Chapter 92).

12.2. CLOSED REDUCTION OF DISLOCATIONS

12.2A. Finger/Toe Joint Dislocation

Indications

Interphalangeal and metacarpophalangeal/metatarsophalangeal dislocations

Complications

Fractures secondary to attempted reduction

Procedure

Check the neurovascular status in the affected phalanx. Splint the deformed phalanx for comfort if necessary. Radiographs of at least two views are usually taken to ascertain the presence of obvious fractures or interposition of the volar plate of the distal phalanx. It is important to note that closed reduction of a dislocation may not be possible when there is dorsal dislocation with interposition of the volar plate or entrapment of the metacarpal/metatarsal head (Fig. 12.2A).

Consider the use of procedural sedation, a digital block, or both. If necessary, have an assistant restrain the child. Grasp the extremity proximal to the dislocation to stabilize the joint. Grasp the tip of the distal phalanx and apply traction longitudinally. The joint will usually slide into proper position. If this method is unsuccessful, apply pressure distally to accentuate the deformity a few degrees, mild hyperextension, while applying traction to the phalanx longitudinally.

After reduction, obtain radiographs to ensure proper position of the joints and to evaluate for fractures. Immobilize the joint in slight flexion for 2 to 3 weeks in total, usually with a foam padded splint. Distal interphalangeal joints are immobilized in full extension and proximal interphalangeal joints with 20 to 30 degrees of flexion. If a small avulsion of the volar lip of the distal phalanx is evident, apply a dorsal splint to prevent hyperextension of the affected joint.

In cases in which the reduction is unsuccessful, the volar plate is interposed, or the second metacarpal bone is trapped, consult an orthopedic surgeon immediately to assess the need of open reduction. Volar dislocations are more complicated and often require open reduction.

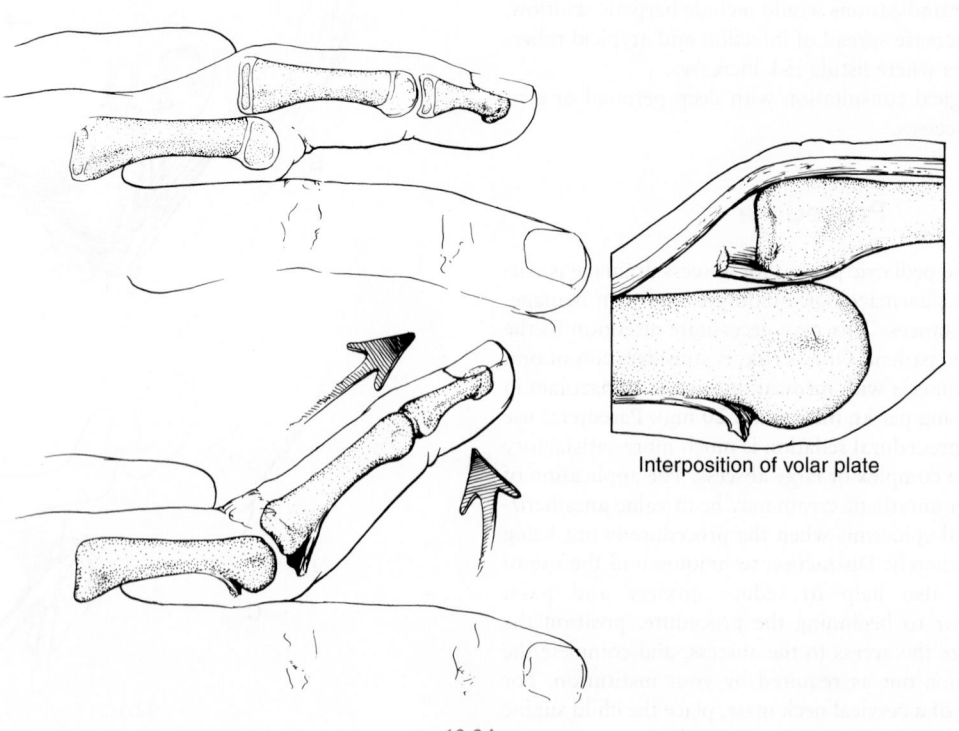

Interposition of volar plate

12.2A

12.2B. Shoulder (Glenohumeral) Joint Dislocation

Indications

Anterior shoulder dislocations in adolescents and young adults. For posterior shoulder dislocations, orthopedic consultation is recommended.

Complications

1. Nerve injury to the axillary nerve, brachial plexus, radial, ulnar, or distal nerves
2. Tear or detachment of the rotator cuff
3. Fractures of humeral head
4. Vascular injury
5. Recurrent dislocation

Procedure

There are multiple methods to reduce an anterior dislocation of the shoulder. Most pediatric emergency medicine physicians prefer techniques that require minimal force such as the external rotation techniques, the Stimson technique, or the scapular manipulation technique. The traditional traction–countertraction technique is still used in many circumstances but it requires more force and several assistants. Reduction of glenohumeral dislocation often requires administration of both intravenous narcotic analgesics and muscle relaxants (i.e., fentanyl and midazolam). However with some of the less forceful techniques, little to no medications are required.

1. The External Rotation Technique

    The patient is sitting upright or lying supine and has the elbow on the affected side adducted and flexed at 90 degrees. The clinician usually grasps the wrist and very slowly (over 5 to 10 minutes) externally rotates the shoulder while maintaining the arm adducted. The shoulder usually relocates when the arm is externally rotated between 70 to 110 degrees. A variation of this technique is called the Hennipen technique.

    Occasionally, the Milch technique is added to the external rotation technique to achieve reduction. After the arm is fully externally rotated, abduct the arm at the shoulder over the head while maintaining external rotation. Then apply traction in line with the humerus and apply posterior pressure over the humeral head—either with direct force over the anterior head of the axilla or pressure to the humeral head in the axilla using the clinician's thumb.

2. The Stimson Technique

    The patient lies prone with the affected arm hanging over the edge of the stretcher with 4–7 kg (10-15 lb) pounds of weight attached to the wrist. Muscular relaxation by use of benzodiazepine may facilitate reduction. Reduction usually takes approximately 20 to 30 minutes (Fig. 12.2B, part A)

3. Scapular Manipulation Technique

    The patient usually lies prone with the affected arm hanging off the edge of the stretcher. To facilitate reduction, apply downward traction using either an assistant or 10 to 15 pounds of weight attached to the wrist. The clinician will then pushes the inferior tip of the scapula medially while pulling the superior aspect laterally (Fig. 12.2B, part B). Muscular relaxation is a good adjunct for this procedure.

4. Traction and Countertraction

    Have an assistant apply countertraction with a folded sheet wrapped around the chest. Simultaneously, as the operator, exert traction to the arm as shown in Figure 12.2B, part C. After the linear traction frees the humeral head, apply slight lateral traction to reduce the proximal humerus.

Postreduction

Following successful reduction, splint the shoulder either using a sling and swath or shoulder immobilizer. Traditionally the shoulder has been immobilized in internal rotation and reduction, however some recent studies suggest that the incidence of redislocation is less with 10 degrees of external rotation. Most clinicians obtain a postreduction radiograph of the shoulder yet new findings are rarely found on postreduction films. The patient should be referred for orthopedic follow-up and rehabilitation.

12.2C. Patella Dislocation

Indications

Closed patellar dislocations, particularly laterally displaced

Complications

1. Intraarticular hematoma
2. Bony or ligamentous trauma

Procedure

Assess the joint and extremity for ligamentous stability and neurovascular integrity. Most practitioners will obtain a radiograph to evaluate for associated osteochondral fractures, which can be close to 25%. For an obvious patella dislocation that occurred without significant associated trauma, radiographs may not be necessary. The benefits of the radiograph must be weighed against the increased pain, swelling and resultant neurovascular compromise pain that occurs with delays by obtaining radiographs. Sedation/muscle relaxation and analgesia with administration of a benzodiazepine and narcotic may ease the reduction. In many instances, the reduction may be spontaneous after administration of benzodiazepine alone.

When laterally dislocated, the knee joint is usually held in mild flexion (20 to 30 degrees). Have an assistant stabilize the distal thigh, as shown in Figure 12.2C, part A. Then, while extending the knee joint, simultaneously apply gentle pressure on the lateral aspect of the patella to medially reposition it (Fig. 12.2C, part B). Knee mobility should be restored immediately on successful reduction. If radiographs were not initially obtained, they should be obtained after reduction. The use of an extended knee brace with crutches for a brief time provides appropriate restriction of activity with orthopedic follow-up in around a week. Some patients are at risk of recurrence and may benefit from evaluation.

12.2D. Hip Dislocation

Indications

For traumatic dislocations of the hip

Complications

1. Associated fractures
2. Avascular necrosis of the femoral head
3. Sciatic nerve injury (mainly with posterior dislocation)
4. Deep venous thrombosis

PROCEDURES

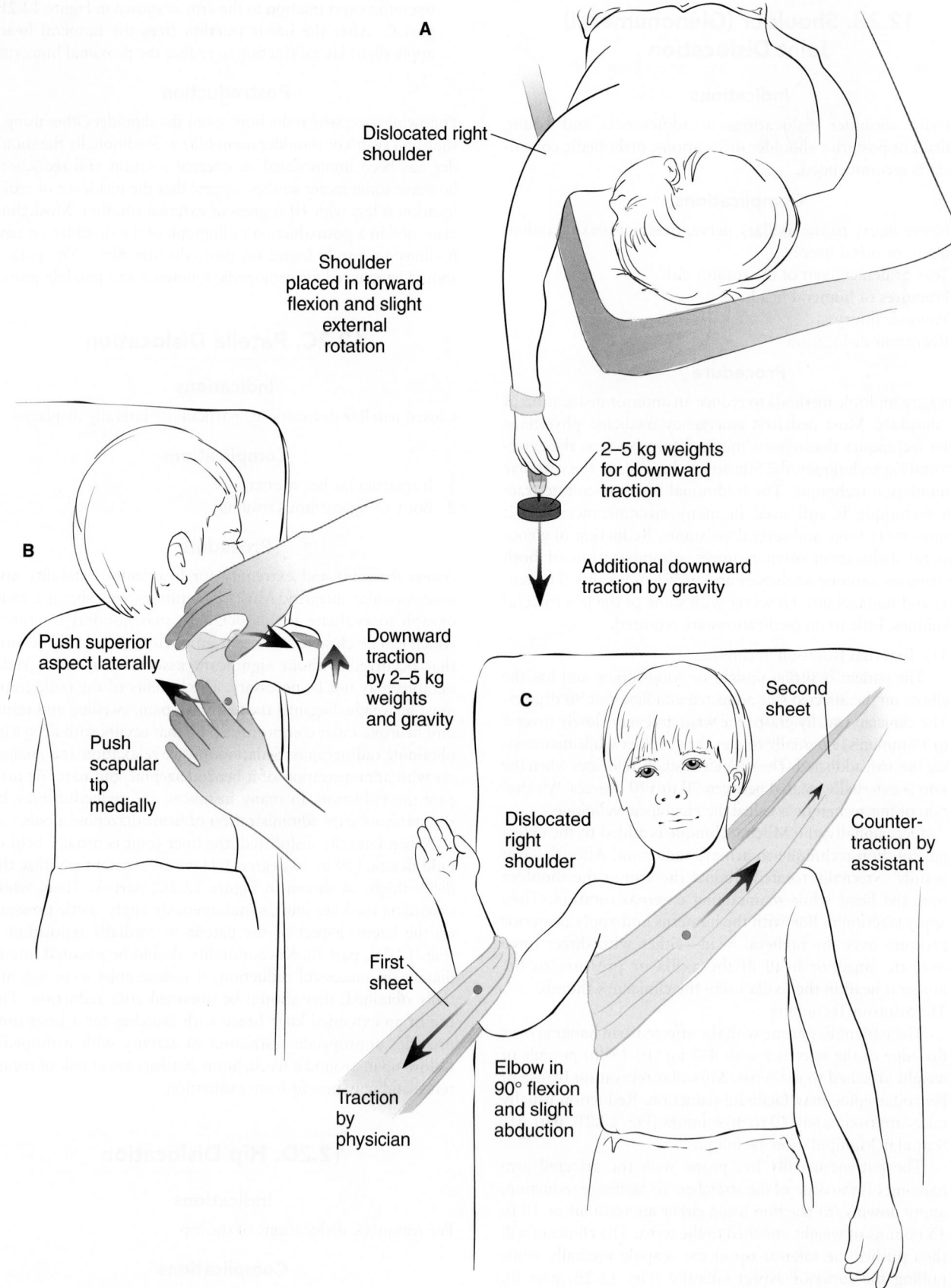

A

Dislocated right shoulder

Shoulder placed in forward flexion and slight external rotation

2–5 kg weights for downward traction

Additional downward traction by gravity

B

Push superior aspect laterally

Push scapular tip medially

Downward traction by 2–5 kg weights and gravity

C

Dislocated right shoulder

Second sheet

Counter-traction by assistant

First sheet

Elbow in 90° flexion and slight abduction

Traction by physician

12.2B

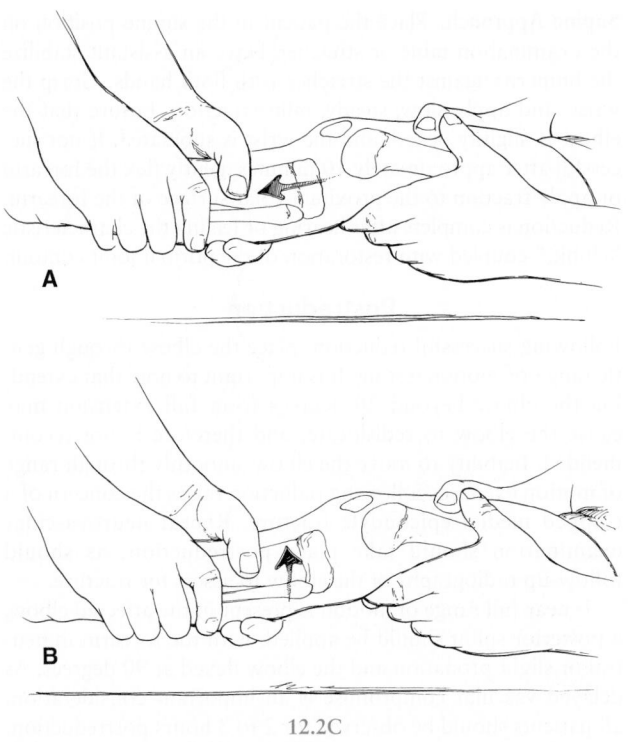

12.2C

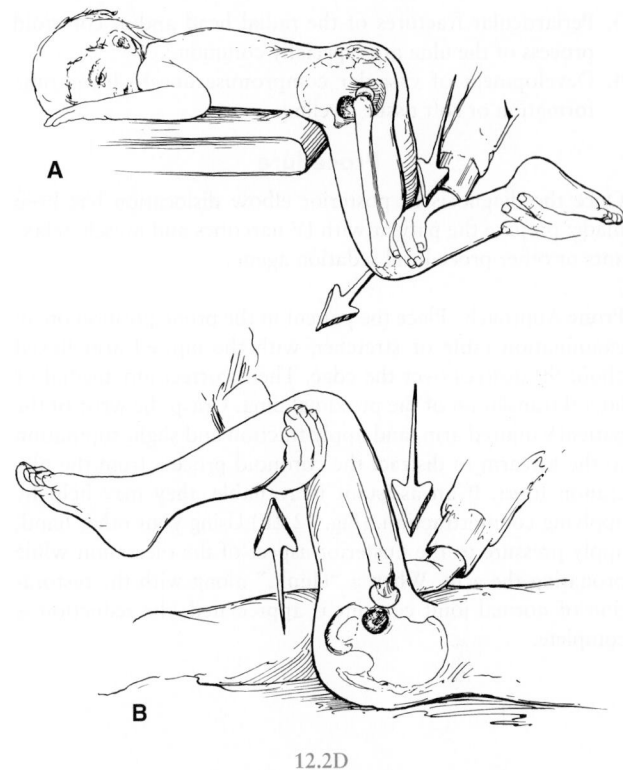

12.2D

Procedure

Assess the neurovascular status of the affected limb. Associated fractures are common due to the magnitude of force required to produce a hip injury, thus radiographs with at least two different views—anteroposterior and oblique should always be obtained. When the diagnosis is confirmed and there are no contraindications to proceed, attempt at reduction may be initiated in the ED. Given the high incidence of complications, as well as the need for traction, non—weight-bearing management, hospital admission and close follow-up, emergent orthopedic consultation prior to reduction with the goal to reduce the hip within 4 to 6 hours of injury. Failure to reduce after 2 to 3 attempts mandates open reduction.

Placement of an IV and administration of narcotic and/or benzodiazepine or other procedural sedation is usually necessary for optimal analgesia and relaxation to facilitate reduction. Sedation must be carefully monitored, especially if other injuries are present.

Posterior Dislocations. Posterior dislocations are more common. The mechanism of injury is often a flexed knee having a posterior-directed force applied (i.e., dashboard injury in motor vehicle accident). The femoral head in the dislocation lies posterior to the acetabulum (Fig. 12.2D, part A and B). Characteristically, the hip is flexed and the leg is adducted, internally rotated, and shortened. The preferred method of reduction is called the Stinson method (Fig. 12.2D, part A). Place the patient prone on the examination table. The affected extremity needs to be flexed 90 degrees at the hip. The physician must apply downward traction on the calf. Have an assistant press over the greater trochanter to slide the femoral head into position. Common practice is to place the patient in

Buck's traction following the procedure and after obtaining postreduction films.

Anterior Dislocations. Anterior dislocations are much less common but may occur with anterior-directed force in a motor vehicle crash or a fall associated with forced abduction. The femoral head may come to lie in the obturator canal or anterior to the symphysis pubis. On examination, the hip is extended and the leg is abducted and externally rotated with no obvious shortening.

Place the patient supine and apply strong downward pressure on both anterosuperior iliac crests to keep the trunk on the bed. Have an assistant grasp the affected limb flexing the hip and knee to 90 degrees (Fig. 12.2D, part B). Then, rotate the leg to a neutral position. This will make it a posterior slip. The assistant then must maintain steady forceful traction in the calf at 90 degrees to lift the femoral head into the acetabulum. While continuing the force, extend the knee and hip to bring the leg to the extended position. Obtain a radiograph before traction is applied.

12.2E. Elbow Joint Dislocation

Indications

Posterior elbow dislocations

Complications

1. Brachial artery injury (especially with open elbow dislocations)
2. Median and ulnar nerve injury as a result of stretching, entrapment, or severance.

PROCEDURES

3. Periarticular fractures of the radial head and/or coronoid process of the ulna are especially common.
4. Development of vascular compromise due to hematoma formation or soft tissue swelling.

Procedure

Once the diagnosis of posterior elbow dislocation has been made, prepare the patient with IV narcotics and muscle relaxants or other procedural sedation agents.

Prone Approach. Place the patient in the prone position on an examination table or stretcher, with the injured arm flexed about 90 degrees over the edge. Then, correct any medial or lateral translation of the proximal ulna. Grasp the wrist of the patient's injured arm, and apply traction and slight supination to the forearm to distract the coronoid process from the olecranon fossa. If an assistant is available, they may help by applying countertraction. (Fig. 12.2E) Using your other hand, apply pressure to the posterior aspect of the olecranon while pronating the arm. When a "clunk," along with the restoration of normal joint contour is appreciated, the reduction is complete.

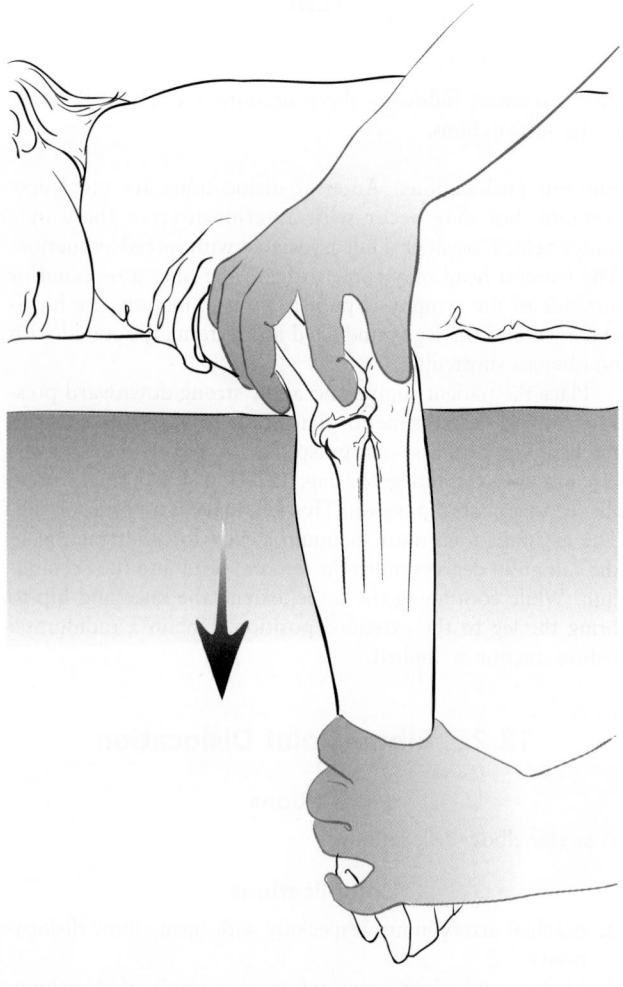

12.2E

Supine Approach. Place the patient in the supine position on the examination table or stretcher. Have an assistant stabilize the humerus against the stretcher with both hands. Grasp the wrist, and apply slow, steady, inline traction. Ensure that the elbow is slightly flexed, and the wrist is supinated. If not successful after approximately 10 minutes, gently flex the forearm or apply traction to the proximal volar surface of the forearm. Reduction is complete after hearing or feeling the characteristic "clunk," coupled with restoration of the normal joint contour.

Postreduction

Following successful reduction, place the elbow through gentle range-of-motion testing. It is important to note that extending the elbow beyond 20 degrees from full extension may cause the elbow to redislocate, and therefore is not recommended. Inability to move the elbow smoothly through range of motion exercises following reduction raises the concern of a trapped medial epicondyle fracture. Repeat neurovascular examination should take place postreduction, as should follow-up radiographs of the elbow to assess for fracture.

If near-full range of motion is present in the affected elbow, a posterior splint should be applied, with the forearm in neutral or slight pronation and the elbow flexed at 90 degrees. As delayed vascular compromise is an important consideration, all patients should be observed for 2 to 3 hours postreduction. If at the end of the observation period there is no evidence of vascular compromise, the patient may be discharged home with orthopedic referral for follow-up. Typically, after 5 to 10 days, range of motion exercises are initiated with interval splinting or with use of a sling for comfort and support. Immobilization for prolonged periods has been associated with a poorer ultimate range of motion of the elbow.

12.3. DRAINAGE OF A SUBUNGUAL HEMATOMA

Indications

Blood under pressure beneath a nail bed, either proximally or distally

Complications

1. Bleeding
2. Infection

Procedure

Subungual hematomas occur from trauma in the proximal or distal nail bed, as shown in Figure 12.3. Consider a radiograph to evaluate for a tuft fracture of the distal phalanx. Generally, the hematoma causes pain that is immediately relieved with drainage. A digital nerve block may be used for anesthesia but is useful in anxious children or those with an already painful injury.

A hematoma of the proximal nail bed is relieved by making a hole in the nail (trephination). Restrain the child and digit on a table. Soak the fingertip in povidone–iodine

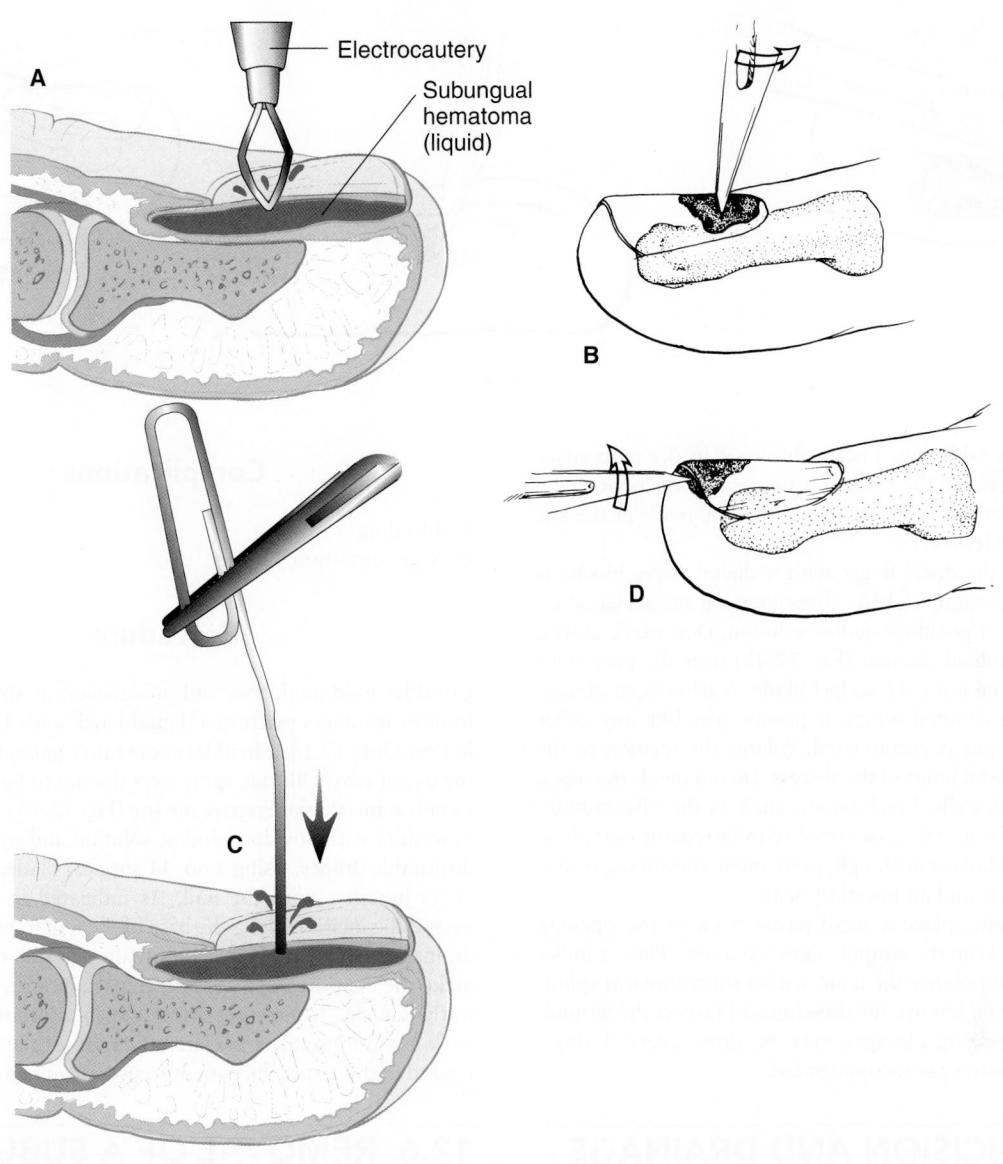

12.3A–D

solution for several minutes. A high temperature surgical one-use electrocautery pen can be used to puncture the nail and this technique is more rapid and less painful than making a hole with a scalpel (Fig. 12.3A). In the setting where electrocautery is not readily available, options include heating of a paper clip on a hemostat or the use of an 11 blade. Enter perpendicular to the nail in the center of the hematoma. Puncture the nail by simultaneously applying downward and rotary pressure, as shown in Figure 12.3B (blade) and Figure 12.3C (heated paper clip). Apply pressure sterile gauze to drain the blood for several minutes, and then cover with a sterile dressing.

A distal hematoma is shown in Figure 12.3D. Restrain the child and finger on a firm surface. Cleanse the nail with povidone–iodine solution. Take a scalpel with a no. 11 blade and lance the hematoma by inserting the blade directly under the nail parallel to its course. Keep the blade against the undersurface of the nail. Cover with a sterile gauze while blood is draining and apply a sterile dressing.

12.4. INCISION AND DRAINAGE OF A FELON

Indications

A felon, or digital pulp space abscess, requires drainage to relieve severe pain and to decrease the spread of infection.

Complications

1. Scar formation
2. Bleeding

Procedure

The use of procedural sedation may be a useful adjunct to digital block in an anxious child. Have an assistant hold the hand

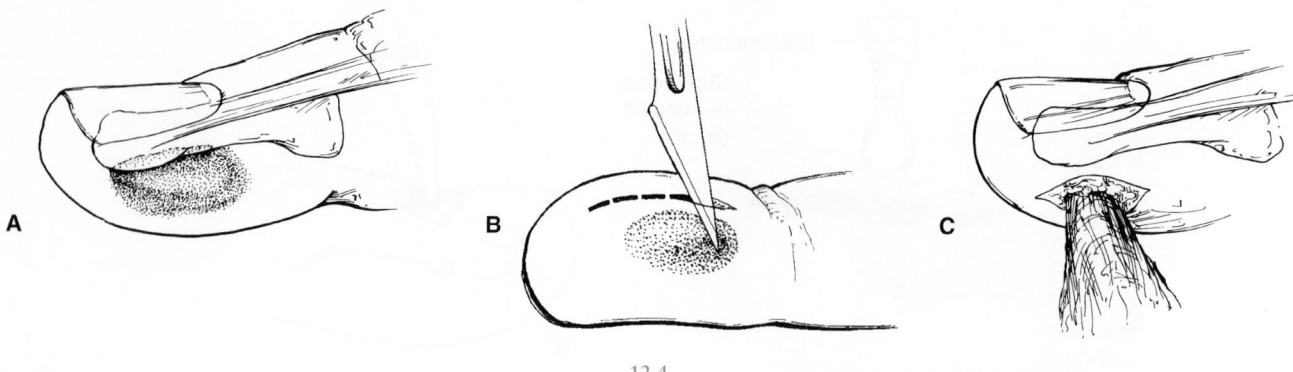

12.4

supinated on a table top. Locate the felon in the pulp space (Fig. 12.4A) between the volar soft tissues and the periosteum of the distal phalanx. The incision should be made at the site of maximal tenderness.

Anesthetize the distal finger with a digital nerve block, as described in Procedure 12.13A. After obtaining anesthesia, scrub the fingertip with povidone–iodine solution. Don sterile gloves. Make a longitudinal incision (Fig. 12.4B) over the previously selected site using a no. 11 scalpel blade. A felon is an abscess and should be drained where it points, just like any other abscess. When pus is encountered, enlarge the incision to the proximal and distal limits of the abscess. Do not divide the septa.

Previously described techniques, such as the "fishmouth" and lateral incisions, are associated with iatrogenic complications. These include skin slough, permanent anesthesia, unstable fat pad, pain, and an unsightly scar.

After drainage, place a small gauze wick in the opening (Fig. 12.4C) to keep the wound edges separated. Place a bulky dressing and immobilize the hand with a short forearm splint. In 24 to 48 hours, remove the dressing and inspect the wound. Subsequent dressing changes may be done every 3 days. Systemic antibiotics are recommended.

12.5. INCISION AND DRAINAGE OF A PARONYCHIA

Indications

Failure of a superficial infection of the soft tissue along the edges of the nail to respond to medical treatment or the development of pus beneath the surface.

Complications

1. Bleeding
2. Scar formation

Procedure

Consider mild anxiolysis with midazolam in anxious children. In most instances perform a digital block with 1% lidocaine as in Procedure 12.13A. In older cooperative patients, occasionally the use of ethyl chloride spray over the site to be lanced is sufficient for anesthesia. Prepare the site (Fig. 12.5A) for the surgical procedure with povidone–iodine solution and cover with sterile disposable drapes. Using a no. 11 surgical blade, incise the skin at its junction with the nail. As indicated in Figure 12.5B, extend the incision along the base of the nail to permit adequate drainage. If the paronychia is only on one side of the nail bed, make the incision along the lateral margin of the nail bed distal to the cuticle. To keep the wound open, placement of a gauze wick is often useful at the lateral margin of the nail. Dress the wound and instruct the patient to use warm compresses.

12.6. REMOVAL OF A SUBUNGUAL SPLINTER OR FOREIGN BODY

Indications

1. Painful subungual splinter
2. To prevent infection or a foreign-body reaction to a splinter in the nail bed

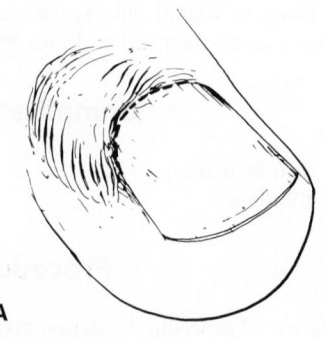

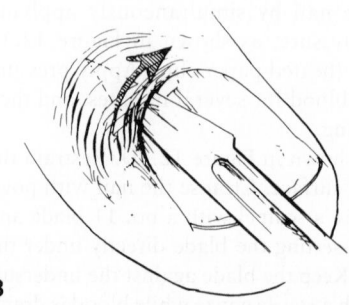

A   B

12.5

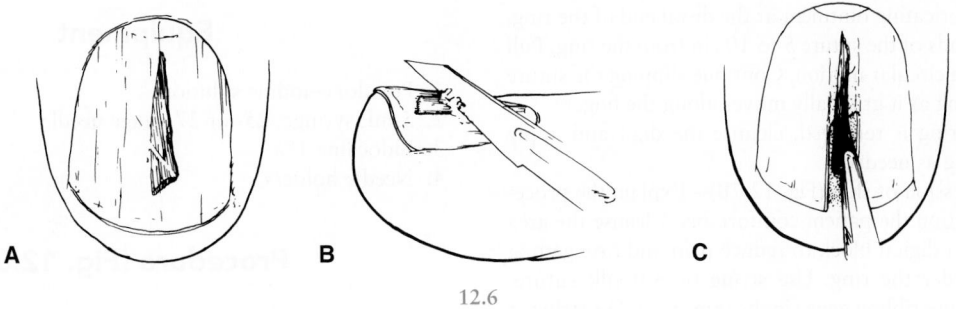

12.6

Complications

1. Bleeding
2. Infection

Procedure

Restrain the child's hand with the fingers extended (Fig. 12.6A). If the splinter end is visible, it may be possible to pull it out directly with tweezers or a hemostat. Consider use of a digital block if it is painful. An alternative is to use a no. 11 blade to scrape the nail down to the nail bed for the splinter to uncover enough splinter to remove it. Hold the blade perpendicular to the direction of the splinter and at 90 degrees from the horizontal, as in Figure 12.6B. Scrape the nail off in a proximal to distal fashion, applying pressure gently to minimize discomfort from squeezing the nail onto the splinter. The shape of the nail removed is similar to that of a "U." With a small tweezers or forceps, grasp the splinter once it is exposed and tug it gently to remove it from the nail bed (Fig. 12.6C). Soak the finger in a warm povidone–iodine and water solution several times per day to decrease the chance of infection.

Large splinters or those embedded deeply under the nail require prolonged scraping and are best removed by excision of a large portion of nail after a digital block.

12.7. REMOVAL OF RINGS

Indications

Strangulating ring on a digit

Complications

1. Vascular compromise
2. Trauma to digit

Procedure

1. String pull (Fig. 12.7A)—Explain the procedure and position the patient comfortably. Cleanse the area and consider a digital block. Use a string or heavy suture. Place one end of the string under the ring and pull it through. Place a small

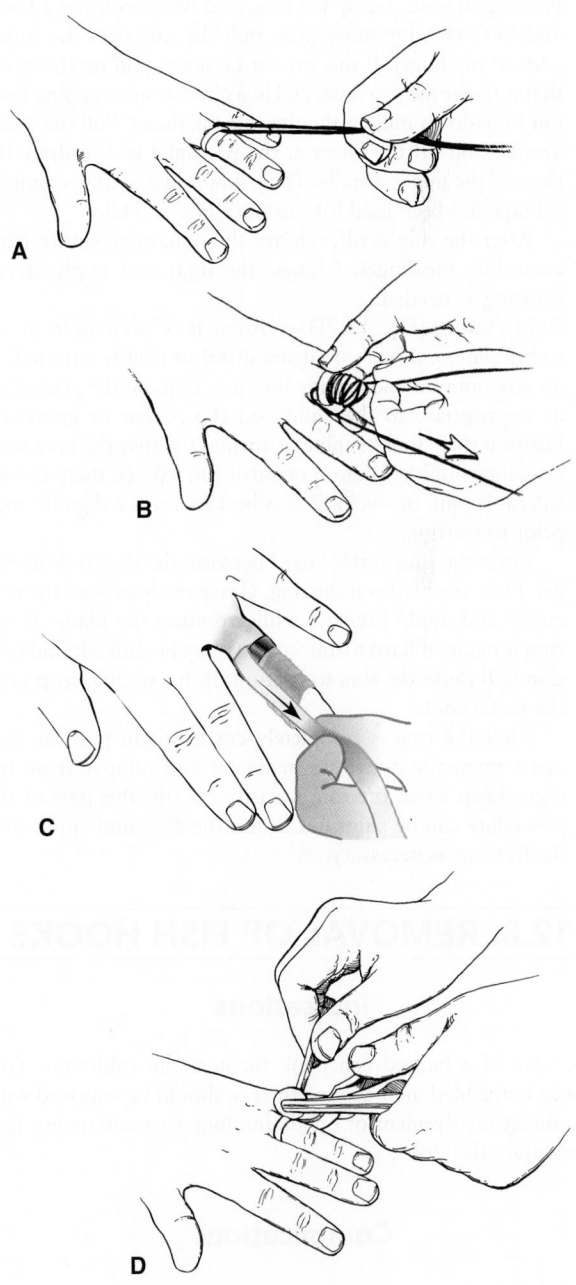

12.7

amount of lubricating ointment at the distal end of the ring. Grasp both ends of the suture 5 to 10 cm from the ring. Pull the suture in a circular motion. Continue slipping the suture around the ring as it gradually moves along the finger.

After the ring is removed, cleanse the digit and apply sterile dressing as needed.

2. String compression of skin (Fig. 12.7B)—Explain the procedure and position the patient comfortably. Cleanse the area and consider a digital block to reduce pain and ease getting the string under the ring. Use string or 3-0 silk suture. Alternatively, use ribbon gauze in the same way. The string at the proximal end should be placed under the ring. Then wrap the suture on the distal side around the finger. Continue to wrap the string tightly to compress the soft-tissue swelling on the finger until it covers the proximal interphalangeal joint. Grasp the ring, and while exerting a back-and-forth twisting movement, pull the ring over the suture and off the finger. If this cannot be done, pull on the string that is under the proximal end in a circular unwrapping fashion to assist in pulling the ring off the finger. Pull the string around and off the finger at the proximal end to draw the ring off the finger distally. Thin ribbon-like gauze or umbilical tape has been used for this also (Fig. 12.7C).

After the ring is off, remove the remaining suture from encircling the finger. Cleanse the digit and apply sterile dressing as needed.

3. Ring cutting (Fig. 12.7D)—Often, it is preferable to try technique no. 2 or 3, if edema distal to ring is minimal, in an attempt to avoid cutting the ring. Explain the procedure as appropriate to the child and the parent or guardian. Position the patient supine or sitting. Cleanse the area with povidone–iodine solution or substitute. When there is considerable pain or swelling, it is best to inject a digital block prior to starting.

Insert the ring-cutter guard between the ring and the finger. Place the blade on the ring. Grasp the handle of the ring cutter and apply pressure while rotating the blade. If the ring is made of hard metal, cutting may be difficult and friction will cause the ring to heat up. If this occurs, stop until the metal cools.

After the ring is completely cut through, pull the ring apart manually or with a hemostat and remove from the digit. Even when the ring is easily cut off, this part of the procedure can be painful. Cleanse the digit and apply sterile dressing as necessary.

12.8. REMOVAL OF FISH HOOKS

Indications

Presence of a barbed fish hook through the epidermis. Fish hooks embedded in or around the eye should be removed with the direct involvement of ophthalmology to avoid or not further injure the globe.

Complications

1. Infection
2. Direct damage to tissue

Equipment

1. Povidone–iodine solution
2. 5-mL syringe, 25- or 27-gauge needle
3. Lidocaine 1%
4. Needle holders

Procedure (Fig. 12.8)

1. Barb cut. Explain the procedure as appropriate to the child and the parent or guardian. Position and restrain the child to have easy access to the fish hook. Cleanse the area with povidone–iodine solution or substitute. Inject 1% lidocaine with a 25- or 27-gauge needle into the surrounding skin or when appropriate do a digital block.

   Wearing sterile gloves, grasp the fish hook with needle holders. Apply downward pressure along the curve of the fish hook (proximal to distal), forcing the barb end of the hook out through the skin (Fig. 12.8A, part 1). After the barb has been pushed through the skin, sever the barb with a wire cutter (Fig. 12.8A, part 2). The remainder of the hook can then be extracted by withdrawing it along its original path of entry (Fig. 12.8A, part 3).

2. String removal (Fig. 12.8B). When the fish hook lies too deep to force through a second wound, an alternate method can be used.

   Explain the procedure and restrain the child as necessary. Cleanse the area with povidone–iodine solution or

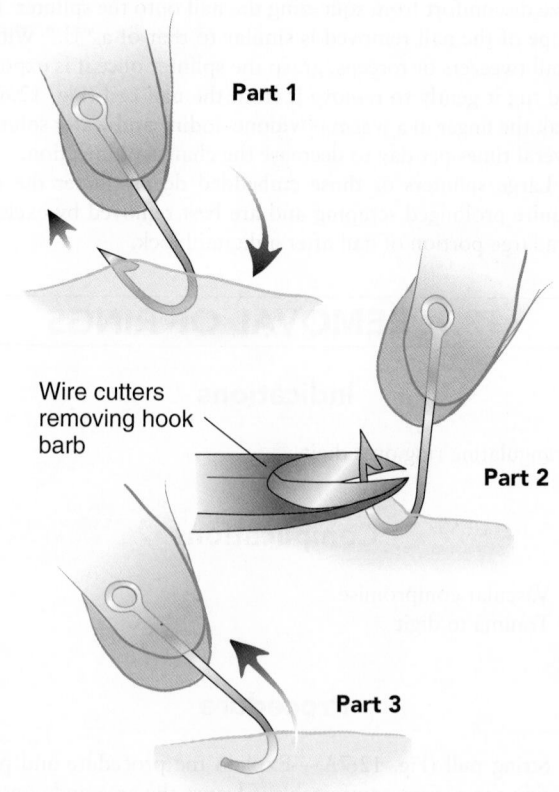

Part 1

Wire cutters removing hook barb

Part 2

Part 3

12.8A

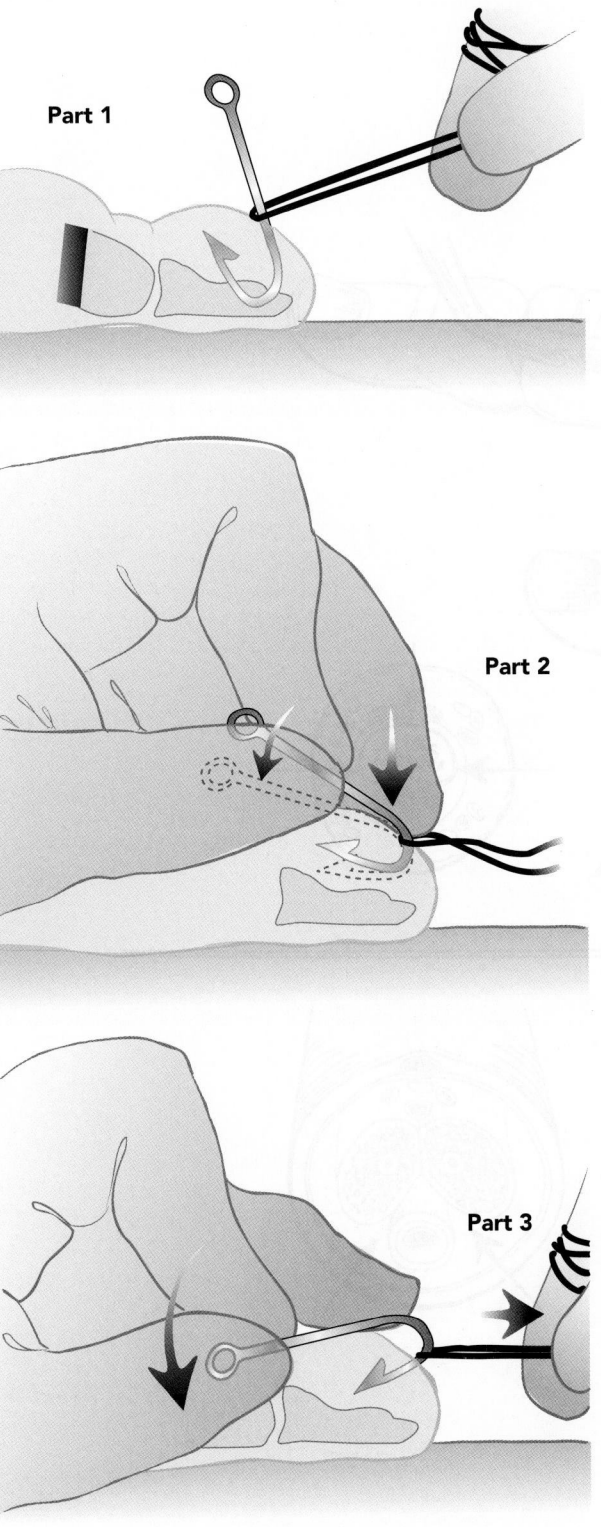

12.8B

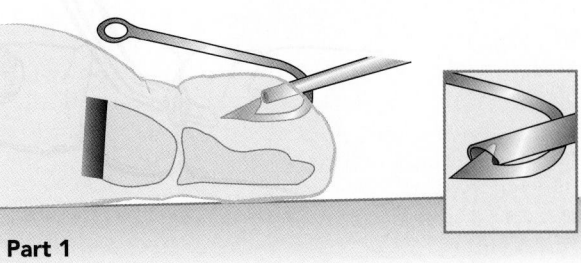

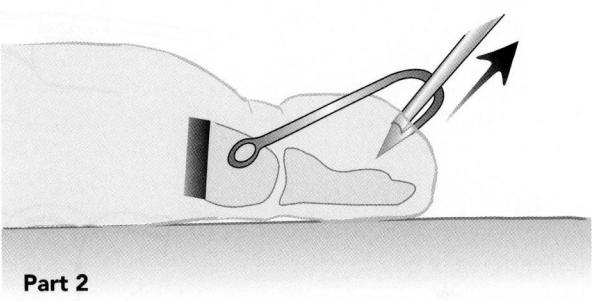

12.8C

the dominant hand and pull sharply (part 3). This action should disengage the barb, and the hook can be removed through the entry wound.

3. Needle technique (Fig. 12.8C). This uses the principle that a needle such as an 18 gauge may be large enough to cover the barb and allow the withdrawal of the fishhook without fear that the barb will continue to catch the hook. Prepare the site as before with the injection of 1% lidocaine. Enter the opening through the skin along the needle and then the needle can catch on the barb. It may be necessary to push the fishhook slightly in to more easily access the barb with the needle. Then pull the fishhook out the opening with the needle engaged.

Following removal, cleanse the area and apply sterile dressing. Give active or passive tetanus immunization as indicated. Consider antibiotic prophylaxis only in high risk patients with issues of immunity.

12.9. HAIR TOURNIQUET REMOVAL (FIG. 12.9)

Indications

To remove apparent constricting bands of hair or thread from finger, toe, penis, or clitoris

Complications

1. Damage to nerves or arterial supply (may be caused by prolonged ischemia from the tourniquet or incision)
2. Damage to tendons
3. Damage to corpus cavernosum, corpus spongiosum, clitoris or urethra

substitute. Inject 1% lidocaine with a 25- or 27-gauge needle into the surrounding skin.

Loop a piece of string around the hook (part 1). With the nondominant hand, depress the shaft of the hook against the skin (part 2). Grasp the end of the string with

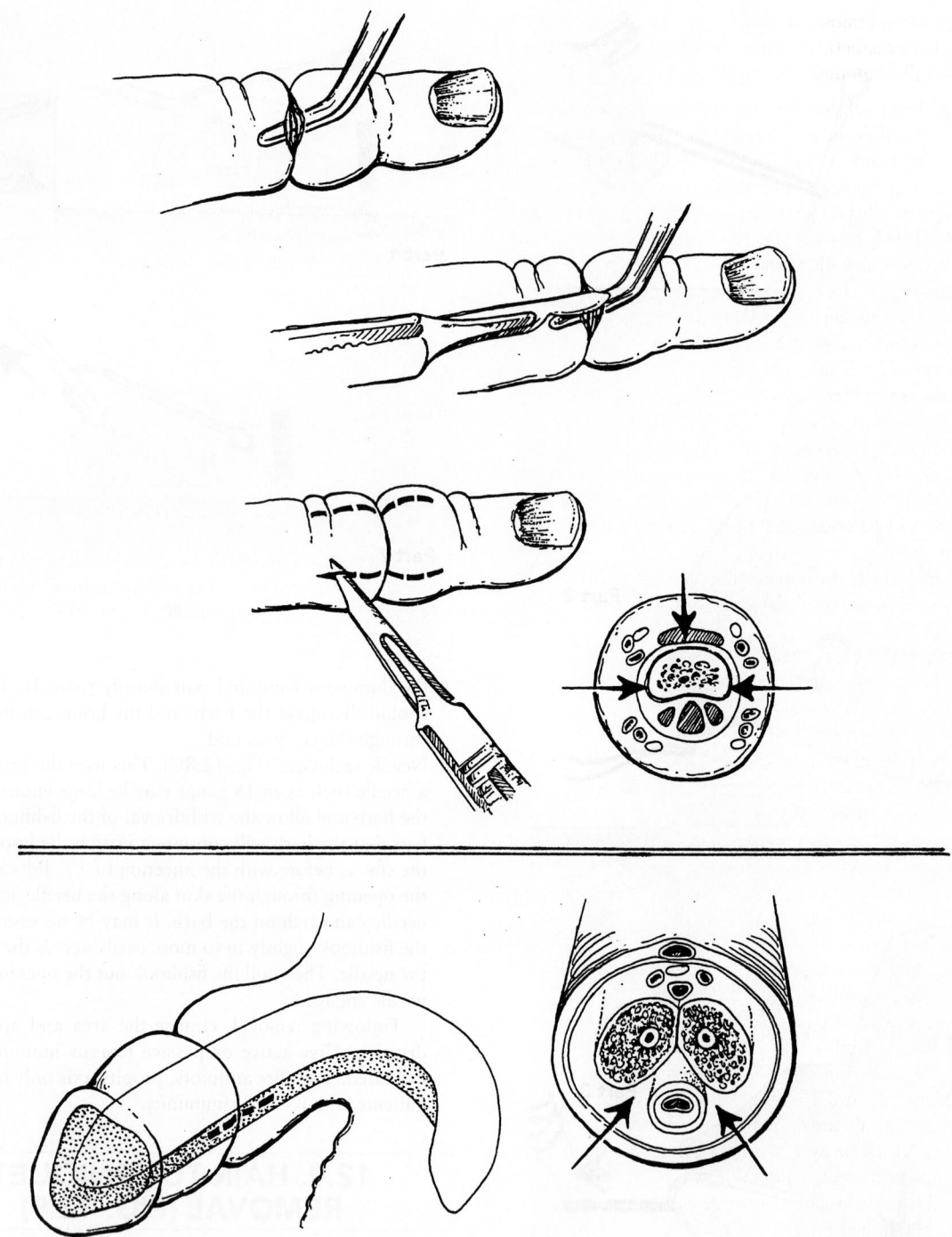

12.9

Equipment

1. Topical, local or regional anesthesia materials
2. Scalpel blade with handle—no. 11 blade
3. Povidone–iodine solution
4. Fine-tip forceps
5. Blunt probe
6. Fine-tip scissors

Procedure

Constriction by hair or thread of a digit or penis and occasionally the clitoris occurs most often in the first few months of life but can be seen in older children on occasion. On physical examination, a sharp circumferential demarcation is usually apparent. Hair tourniquets on digits have been confused with a felon or paronychia. Hair tourniquets on a penis have been confused with paraphimosis or balanitis. The application of EMLA® or other anesthetic cream to the site 45 minutes before the procedure will often make removal much less painful.

1. Isolating the band—If the hair or thread is not deeply embedded, a blunt metal probe may be used to isolate the constricting band. The band is best isolated by placing the probe under the hair or thread on the dorsal aspect of the finger or toe. Digital or penile block will assist in those where they can not be helped with topical anesthetic. Once the band is isolated, it may be cut with a fine-tip scissors or by placing a scalpel blade against the probe to protect the underlying skin. Improvement of the swelling and release of the constriction must be noted before discharging the patient.
2. Hair remover—Application of hair remover can dissolve a hair and provide relief. This method will not work with synthetic fibers. Hair remover should not be used if marked inflammation or swelling to the tissue is evident. This method is also not recommended for removing a constricting band from the penis. Improvement of the swelling and release of the constriction must be noted before discharging the patient.
3. Surgical removal—If the hair or fiber cannot be isolated by the aforementioned methods, then direct incision of the band is indicated.
   a. Digit—A digital block should be performed and the area should be cleansed and draped in a sterile fashion. To avoid the neurovascular bundles, an incision should be made at the 3-o'clock or the 9-o'clock position. The incision should be made longitudinally along the digit, perpendicular to the band. The incision should be extended to the bone to ensure removal. After improvement in the constriction is noted, a dressing may be applied.

   An incision on the dorsal aspect is an alternative, since the tourniquet may be less deeply embedded on the dorsal surface. This approach will probably result in a longitudinal incision into the extensor tendon. With splinting and general wound care, this incision should heal without complications.
   b. Penis—Urologic consultation is advisable before undertaking this procedure, unless ischemic damage might worsen because of a delay. A penile nerve block should be performed, and the area should be cleansed and draped in a sterile fashion. The incision should be made at the 4-o'clock or 8-o'clock position. This is the junction of the corpus cavernosum and corpus spongiosum. The goal is to release the constricting band without penetrating the lumen of the corpus. Reperfusion normally occurs within several minutes after relief of the constricting band; however, some swelling may persist for several days. A loose dressing should be applied.
   c. Clitoris—Although an uncommon occurrence, the procedure for such a situation has been described. Topical anesthetic such as EMLA® should be applied. If difficult to release the constricting band as previously described, immediate urologic or gynecologic consultation should be undertaken.

   Neurovascular status and tendon function should be documented after the procedure. Tetanus prophylaxis should be given as indicated, and reevaluation is suggested in 24 hours when the swelling should have mostly resolved.

12.10. ARTHROCENTESIS—GENERAL CONSIDERATIONS

Indications

1. Removal of a joint effusion causing severe pain and distension that limits function
2. Suspected septic arthritis
3. To obtain joint fluid for the diagnosis of systemic illness (i.e., collagen vascular disease)

Complications

1. Bleeding
2. Infection—joint space or bone

Contraindications (relative)

1. Bleeding diathesis—Patients with bleeding diatheses (i.e., hemophilia) as the cause of the joint effusion usually require only immobilization and replacement of coagulation factors.
2. Presence of a fracture around the joint space—Aspiration may increase the chance of infection when a fracture is present.

Equipment

1. Marking pen, povidone-iodine solution, gauze, bacteriostatic saline solution, adhesive bandage
2. Local anesthetic—1% lidocaine, topical anesthetic such as EMLA®
3. 23- or 25-gauge needles, 3-mL syringes, 18- or 20-gauge syringe, and 5- to 10-mL syringe, specimen collection tubes

12.10A. Knee Joint

Remember to use your institution's "hold point" procedure before starting.

Procedure

The knee is the joint that most commonly requires aspiration in children, primarily to evaluate possible bacterial infection or to drain large traumatic effusion. Radiographs should usually be obtained before tapping the joint. Ultrasound guided arthrocentesis has been tried but may not improve success rate in the knee joint.

Place the child supine on the examination table, with the knee actively extended as far as comfortable. A towel under the slightly flexed joint will usually be helpful for comfort and for positioning. Restrain the child as necessary. Have an assistant hold both the thigh and calf of the leg to be tapped. Consider pharmacologic sedation as necessary. When time allows, consider lidocaine-prilocaine paste (EMLA®) or other noninjectable anesthetic.

The lateral approach to the knee is preferred because it avoids passage through the vastus medialis muscle. Pick a

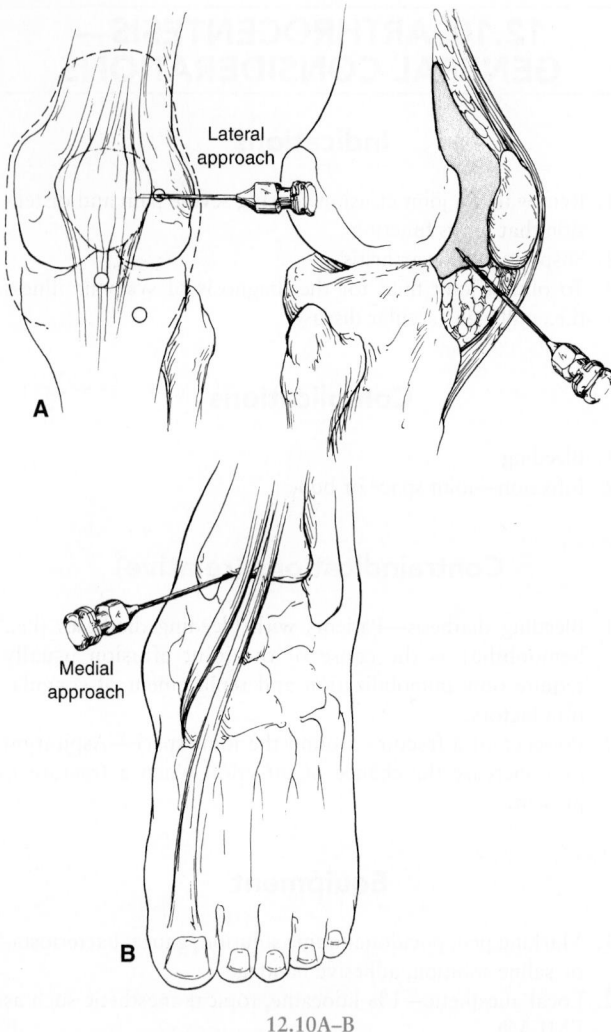

12.10A–B

12.10B. Ankle Joint

Procedure

Restrain the patient in the supine position on the examining table. Have an assistant hold the foot in slight plantar flexion (approximately 110 degrees). Place a soft brace under the plantar surface of the foot to provide further immobilization.

Identify two landmarks, the medial malleolus of the distal tibia and the thick halluces longus extensor tendon. The latter structure is found approximately 1 cm anterolateral to the medial malleolus, as shown in Figure 12.10B.

Pick a puncture site between these landmarks. Cleanse it circumferentially with povidone–iodine solution. Wear sterile gloves and inject 1% lidocaine locally to anesthetize the skin. Use either an 18- or 20-gauge plain or spinal needle attached to a 10-mL syringe.

Puncture the skin aiming the needle slightly inferiorly toward the tibial–talar articulation as shown. Apply suction to the syringe. Aspirate the fluid from the joint and remove the needle when satisfied that an adequate specimen has been obtained (often only a small amount). Apply sterile gauze to the puncture site and immobilize the joint.

12.10C. Elbow Joint

Procedure

Rest the child prone or seated, with his/her arm extended and elbow flexed 90 degrees to maximally open the joint space. Restrain the patient, maintaining the arm and forearm in this flexed position.

The needle puncture site should lie in the center of the triangle formed by the head of the radius, the lateral humeral epicondyle, and the olecranon, as demonstrated in Figure 12.10C. Sterilize the site with povidone–iodine solution. Wearing sterile gloves, inject the skin with 1% lidocaine or spray with ethyl chloride for anesthesia. Use a large-bore, 18- or 20-gauge needle on a 10-mL syringe.

Puncture the skin perpendicularly to the surface of the arm (Fig. 12.10C). Hold the syringe in one hand and guide the needle tip with the thumb and index finger of the other, leaning against the patient's arm. Advance the syringe while applying suction to the plunger, until the needle enters the elbow joint. If difficulty is encountered on entering the joint space, pull the needle back and reassess the location of the landmarks. Readvance it in a new line. Continue to stabilize the syringe while aspirating fluid. Remove the needle and press sterile gauze over the puncture site. Immobilize the joint.

12.10D. Interphalangeal Joint

Procedure

Have the child sit with the forearm extended over the examination table or place him/her prone with the arms extended over the head. Restrain, if necessary. Have an assistant immobilize the finger proximally and distally. Locate the joint to be aspirated, using the radiograph as necessary. Choose a puncture site on the dorsal surface because the skin of the palm is

puncture point at the midpatellar level in the anteroposterior view and at the posterior margin of the patella in the lateral view (Fig. 12.10A).

Cleanse the area to be punctured circumferentially with povidone–iodine solution. Use a 23- or 25-gauge needle attached to a 3-mL syringe to inject 1% lidocaine into the skin and subcutaneous tissues for anesthesia or, alternatively, spray ethyl chloride locally. Avoid injecting into the joint space prior to obtaining fluid for testing and culture.

Wearing sterile gloves, attach an 18-gauge needle to a 10-mL syringe. Hold the syringe in one hand while palpating the lateral margin of the patella with the other. Puncture the skin with syringe 10 to 20 degrees above the horizontal at the anesthetized site. Advance the needle, applying suction on the plunger of the syringe, until it passes into the joint space near the margin of the patella. When the joint space is entered, the syringe will fill the joint fluid. Stabilize the syringe against the patient's leg with the heel of the hand during the aspiration. Move the needle slightly in varied directions to effectively evacuate the joint and minimize the risk of injury to the synovium.

At completion, remove the syringe and apply a sterile gauze pad over the puncture site. Send the aspirate for appropriate studies. Immobilize the knee joint with a supportive dressing and avoid weight bearing during the treatment phase acutely.

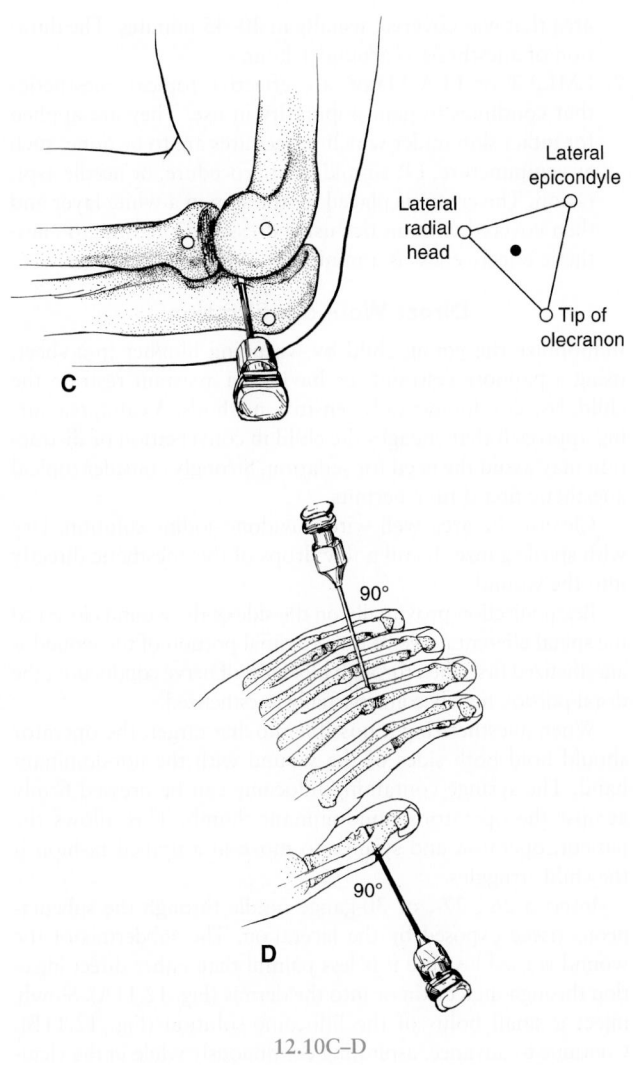

12.10C–D

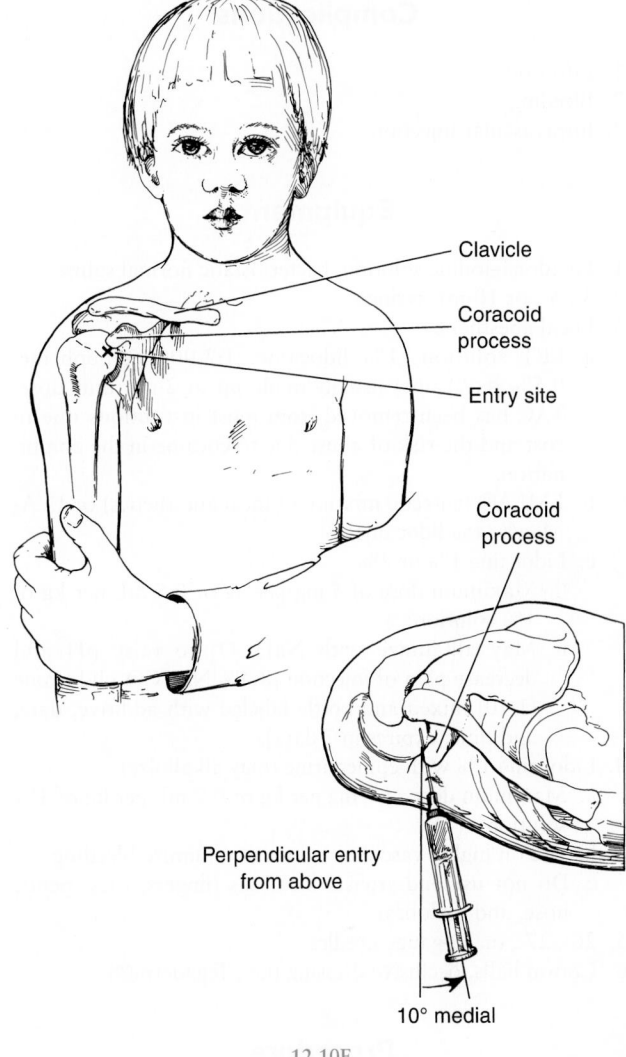

12.10E

tougher and because slight flexion opens the joint space, facilitating a dorsal approach (Fig. 12.10D).

Cleanse the surface with povidone–iodine solution and allow to dry. If using lidocaine, avoid preparations with epinephrine. A digital block may be considered. Using a 22-gauge needle attached to a 5-mL syringe, puncture the skin perpendicularly to the long axis of the finger and advance the needle to the joint space. Be sure to puncture the skin and joint in the middle of the finger to avoid the digital vessels, which run peripherally. Aspirate fluid with suction on the syringe. Remove the needle and press sterile gauze over the puncture. Immobilize the joint.

12.10E. Shoulder Joint

Procedure (Fig. 12.10E)

Rest the child supine or seated with his/her shoulder flexed (arm at the side). Restrain the patient as necessary. Have an assistant hold the arm next to the chest.

Use the anterior approach for joint aspiration. Identify the coracoid process found just below the distal end of the clavicle and immediately medial to the humeral head.

The puncture site is just below and immediately lateral to the tip of the coracoid process. Cleanse the area circumferentially with povidone–iodine solution. Wear sterile gloves and inject 1% lidocaine into the skin and subcutaneous tissue with a 25- to 27-gauge needle. For aspiration, use an 18- or 20-gauge needle attached to a 10-mL syringe.

Direct the needle perpendicular (neither caudal or cephalad) to the entry site, angling 10 degrees medially to enter the joint space. Apply suction to the syringe during entry. Aspirate the fluid and withdraw from the joint when adequate specimen has been obtained. Place sterile gauze over the puncture site and immobilize the joint in a sling or harness.

12.11. TOPICAL ANESTHESIA AND DIRECT WOUND INFILTRATION

Indications

Anesthesia for laceration repair, removal of foreign body, or other simple procedures of the skin

PROCEDURES

Complications

1. Infection
2. Bleeding
3. Intravascular injection

Equipment

1. Povidone–iodine solution, bacteriostatic normal saline
2. 3-, 5-, or 10-mL syringe
3. Local anesthetic
   a. LET solution (1% lidocaine, 1:2,000 epinephrine, 0.5% tetracaine) usually made up to 2-mL unit dose. TAC has been removed from most institutions due to cost and the risk of abuse due to cocaine in the combination.
   b. EMLA® (eutectic mixture of local anesthetics) or ELA-Max® (4% lidocaine)
   c. Lidocaine 1% or 2%
      i. Maximum dose of 5 mg per kg or 0.5 mL per kg of 1% solution
      ii. May alkalinize with $NaHCO_3$ to raise pH and decrease pain of injection [8.4% $NaHCO_3$: lidocaine (1:10) mixed and bottle labeled with additive, date, and time; expires in 7 days]
4. Lidocaine 1% with epinephrine (may alkalinize)
   a. Maximum dose of 7 mg per kg or 0.7 mL per kg of 1% solution
   b. Use on highly vascular regions to minimize bleeding
   c. Do not use end-arterial locations (fingers, toes, penis, nose, and earlobes)
5. 26-, 27-, or 30-gauge needles
6. Cotton balls, occlusive dressing (i.e., Tegaderm®)

Procedure

Check the region for blood supply, sensation, and motor nerve function before injecting the anesthetic. Prepare materials before the child enters the treatment room or out of view of the child. Have all equipment ready to use before beginning the procedure. Consider procedural sedation for complex or painful procedures even unless topical anesthetic is all required.

Topical Anesthetic

1. The placement of LET (less expensive and a noncontrolled substance) is particularly useful in locations with excellent vascularization and away from end arteries. Prepare the anesthetic wound with removal of debris and blood clots. Draw the solution into a 3-mL syringe. It is useful to place a few drops into the wound initially either directly or from a cotton swab. The remainder of the solution is then placed on a cotton ball and firmly pressed onto the wound for about 20 minutes. Where possible, covering with an occlusive clear dressing, such as Tegaderm®, can reduce the risk of the anesthetic contacting other nearby surfaces on the patient. Avoid placing the cotton ball near mucous membranes where systemic absorption of the cocaine can place the child at risk of seizure. The wound is ready for closure or other procedures when blanching of skin appears in the area that was covered, usually in 30–45 minutes. The duration of anesthesia is around 1 hour.
2. EMLA® or ELA-Max® are effective topical anesthetics that continues to gain popularity in use. They are applied for intact skin under which procedures are to be done, such as venipuncture, LP, simple local procedure, or needle aspiration. The cream is placed on the skin in a white layer and then covered with an occlusive dressing. The time to anesthetic effectiveness is a minimum of 45 to 60 minutes.

Direct Wound Infiltration

Immobilize the young child by wrapping him/her in a sheet, using a papoose restraint, or having an assistant restrain the child. Use developmentally sensitive methods. A calm, reassuring approach that engages the child in conversation or distraction may avoid the need for sedation. Strongly consider topical anesthetic first if time permits.

Cleanse the area well with povidone–iodine solution. Dry with sterile gauze. Instill a few drops of the anesthetic directly into the wound.

Begin injection proximally on the side of the wound closest to the spinal efferent nerve. If the proximal portion of the wound is anesthetized first, then through blockage of nerve conduction, the distal portion may become partially anesthetized.

When anesthetizing a possible moving target, the operator should hold both sides of the wound with the nondominant hand. The syringe containing lidocaine can be pressed firmly against the operator's nondominant thumb. This allows the patient, operator, and syringe to move in a unified fashion if the child struggles.

Insert a 26-, 27-, or 30-gauge needle through the subcutaneous tissue exposed by the laceration. The subdermis of the wound is used because it is less painful than either direct injection through intact skin or into the dermis (Fig. 12.11A). Slowly inject a small bolus of the lidocaine solution (Fig. 12.11B). Continue to advance, aspirating continuously while in the vicinity of large vessels. Otherwise, aspiration before injection is rarely necessary.

Remove the needle and reinsert subcutaneously into adjacent tissue that has already been anesthetized. Slowly inject another bolus of anesthetic and advance the needle while injecting (Fig. 12.11C).

Continue this process of injection, withdrawal, and reinsertion in a sequential fashion around the entire perimeter of the wound. Wait 5 minutes for anesthetic effect.

12.12. FIELD BLOCK

Indications

Local anesthesia for surgical procedures to be performed in areas of inflammation or infection (i.e., grossly contaminated lacerations, incision, and drainage of an abscess) or for local anesthesia with preservation of the wound architecture.

Complications

1. Infection
2. Bleeding

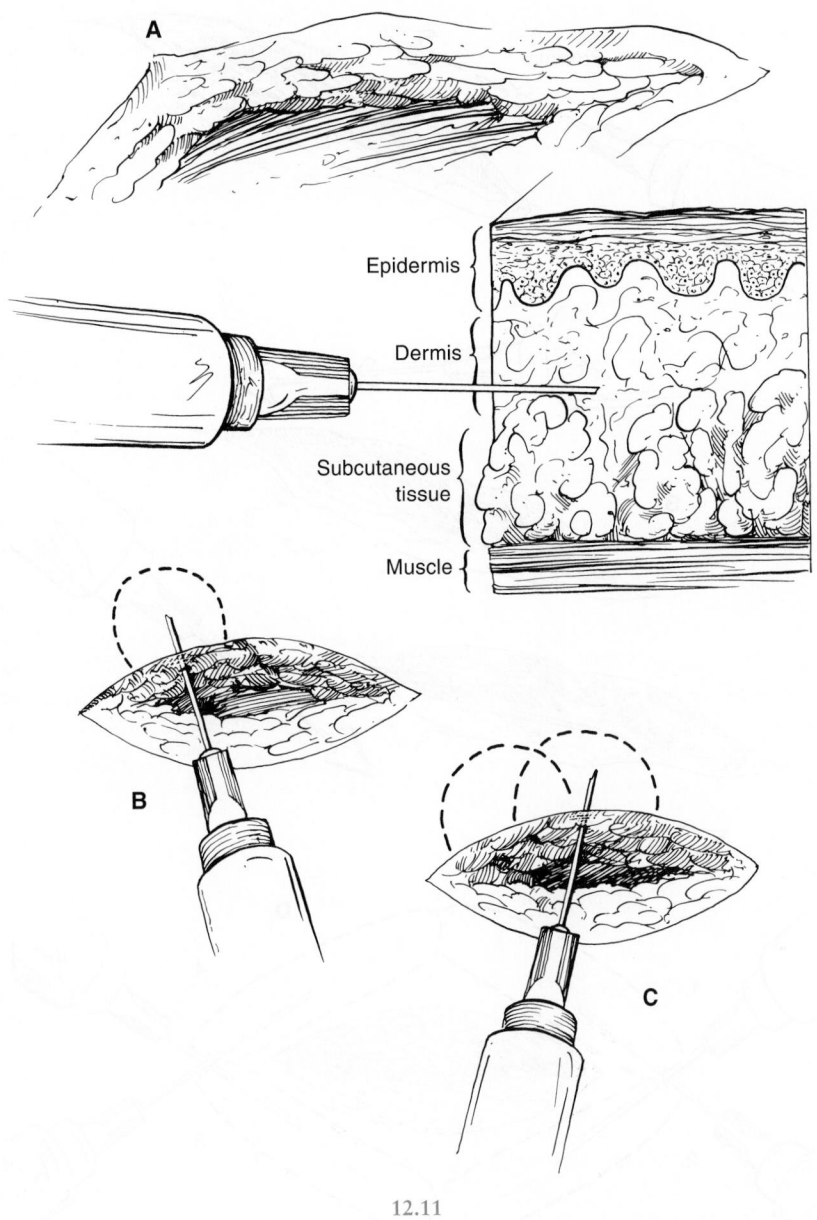

Epidermis

Dermis

Subcutaneous
tissue

Muscle

12.11

PROCEDURES

Equipment

1. Povidone–iodine solution
2. 3-, 5-, or 10-mL syringe
3. Local anesthetic
   a. Lidocaine 1% or 2% (may alkalinize with $NaHCO_3$)
   b. Lidocaine 1% with epinephrine (may alkalinize) (not for use on fingers, toes, penis, nose, and earlobes)
4. 25-, 27-, or 30-gauge needles

Procedure

Check the area for blood supply, sensation, and motor nerve function before injecting the anesthetic agent. Cleanse the area well with povidone–iodine solution. Dry with sterile gauze.

Field blocks use the same plane of injection as direct wound infiltration, but the subdermis is entered through intact skin to prevent carrying debris or bacteria into uncontaminated tissues.

Insert the needle through the skin into the superficial fascia at the proximal aspect of the laceration (Fig. 12.12A). Aspirate before injection in the vicinity of a large major vessel. Inject the lidocaine slowly in small amounts as the needle is advanced to approximately two-thirds the length of the needle. Continue to inject slowly as the needle is withdrawn from the insertion site. Reinsert the needle at the end of the first wheal, where the skin is becoming anesthetized. Repeat injections (Fig. 12.12B) in this fashion. Continue injections until complete infiltration of the circumference of the wound has been achieved (Fig. 12.12C). Allow 5 minutes for anesthesia.

If the field block is used to prevent distortion of the wound margins, then anesthetic is infiltrated in a diamond-shaped fashion around the wound. The needle is inserted at the

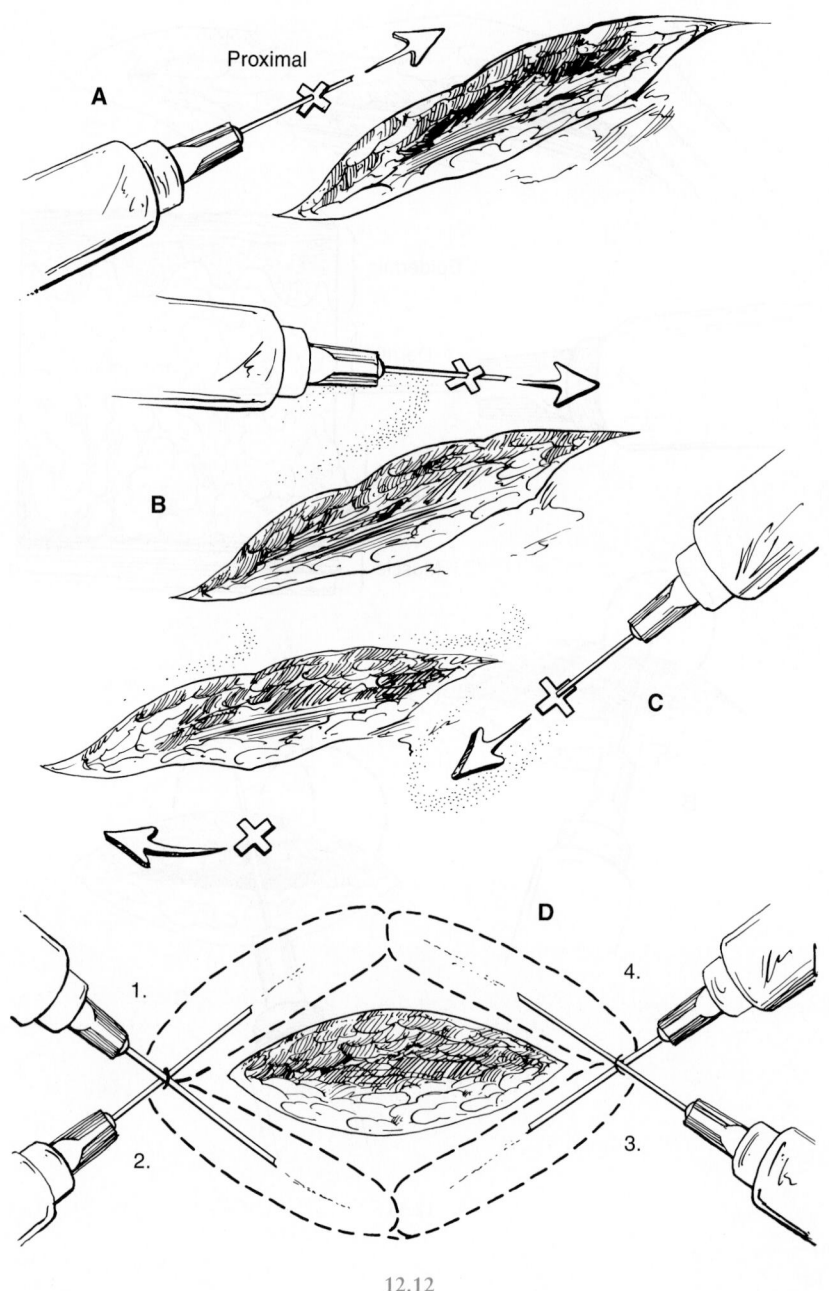

12.12

proximal end of the wound, and lidocaine is injected slowly as the needle is advanced. The needle is then withdrawn and redirected approximately 90 degrees, and infiltration is continued. The needle is then reinserted at the other end of the wound and the process repeated until the diamond-shaped ring of lidocaine is complete (Fig. 12.12D). This region should be anesthetized after 5 minutes.

12.13. PERIPHERAL NERVE BLOCKS—GENERAL PRINCIPLES

Following are the peripheral blocks, which are most commonly required in the emergency setting. As a summary, the lists of complications and equipment are as follows.

Complications

1. Infection
2. Bleeding
3. Intravascular, intraneural injections
4. Contracture if prolonged splint or not in position of function

Equipment

1. Povidone–iodine solution
2. 3- to 5-mL syringe
3. 1% lidocaine (may be alkalinized with 1 mL NaHCO$_3$ to 10 mL lidocaine)
4. 25- to 27-gauge 1- to 1.5-in needle

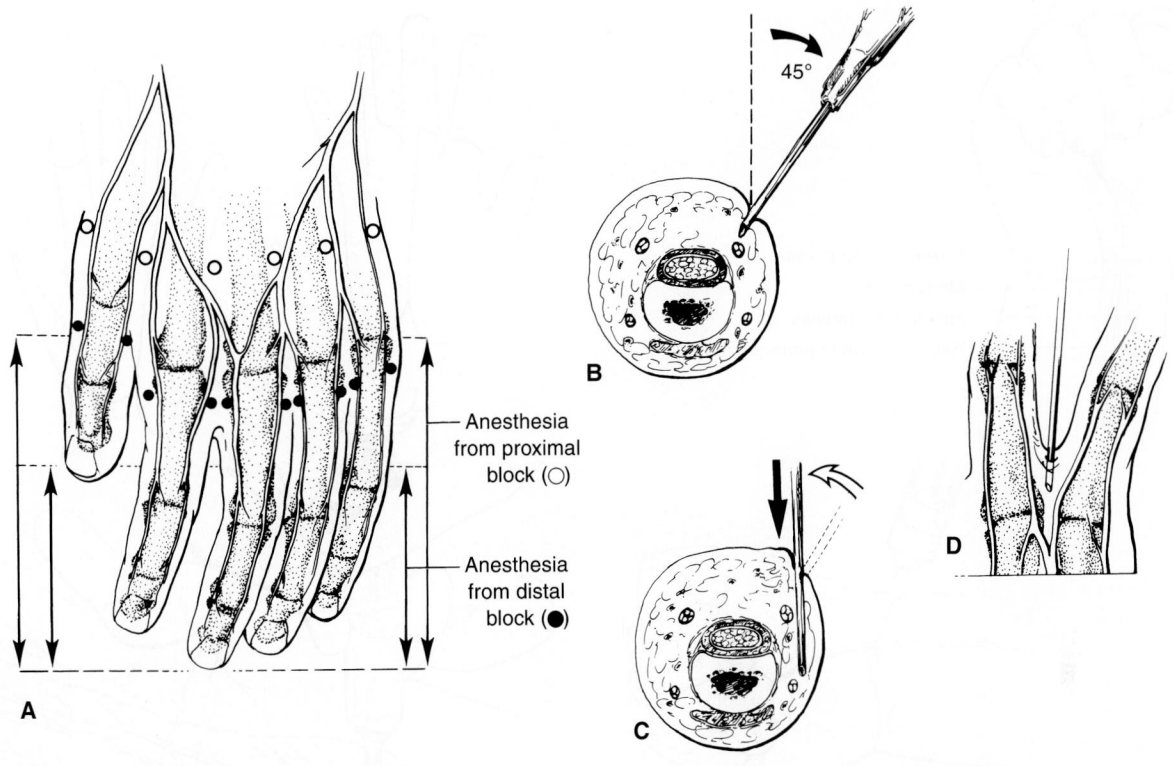

12.13A

12.13A. Digital and Metacarpal Nerve Block

Indications

Anesthesia of fingers and toes for surgical procedures (i.e., drainage of a felon or paronychia, removal of a foreign body, or laceration repair) including the proximal digit

Caution

Do not use a vasoconstrictor such as epinephrine with the anesthetic agent.

Procedure

Carefully identify the area that requires the anesthetic. If it includes more than the distal two-thirds to three-fourths of the fingers or toes, use the metacarpal nerve block. For more proximal procedures consider other options. Check the digit for blood supply, sensation, and motor nerve function before injecting the anesthetic agent. The site of puncture on the digits for each is shown in Figure 12.13A.

Consider procedural sedation, child life techniques, and restraint if required. Have an assistant grasp the extremity proximal to the digit to prevent movement.

The digital nerves, as shown in Figure 12.13A, part B, are both dorsal and volar in the body of the digit, and anesthesia must be injected at both levels (see closed circles, Fig. 12.13A).

Scrub the planned puncture sites on the medial and lateral aspect(s) of the finger thoroughly with povidone–iodine solution. Dry with sterile gauze and don gloves. Use a 22-gauge needle attached to a 5-mL syringe and 1% lidocaine (without epinephrine). Inject the site at a 45-degree angle from vertical until the needle hits the periosteum. Release the tension on the

needle and gently rotate the syringe to the vertical as shown in Figure 12.13A, part C. Then, advance the needle to the volar surface while injecting anesthetic until at least three-fourths through the digit. Remove the needle from the tissue, and then repeat the procedure on the other side of the digit in a similar manner. The digit should be anesthetized after several minutes.

An alternative approach to the digital nerve block is to block the nerve at the level of the metacarpophalangeal joint. This method may be less painful and may have fewer complications than a more distal block.

Achieve the block by inserting a 25-gauge, 5/8-in needle along each side of the finger at the intradigital fold in line with web space. Insert the needle into the web space until the tip is at the level of the metacarpal phalangeal joint (1 to 2 cm) and inject 1 to 2 mL of 1% lidocaine. For the index finger, place a half-ring wheal of lidocaine along the radial side of the proximal aspect of the finger. For the fifth digit, inject a similar wheal along the ulnar border to anesthetize the lateral aspect.

Proximal Digital Nerve Block. Figure 12.13A shows the location of more proximal block (see the open circles). Inject these areas when the entire finger, including the proximal phalanx, must be anesthetized. The nerve is closer to the palmar surface here, making it best to inject the anesthetic closer to the palmar surface.

12.13B. Median Nerve Block

Indications

1. Lacerations distal to the nerve's sensory distribution
2. Removal of a foreign body

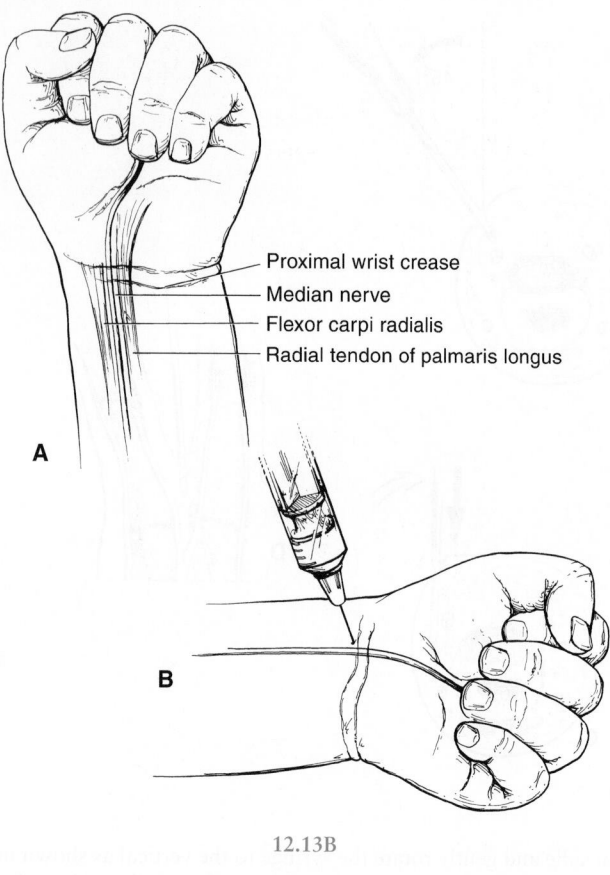

12.13B

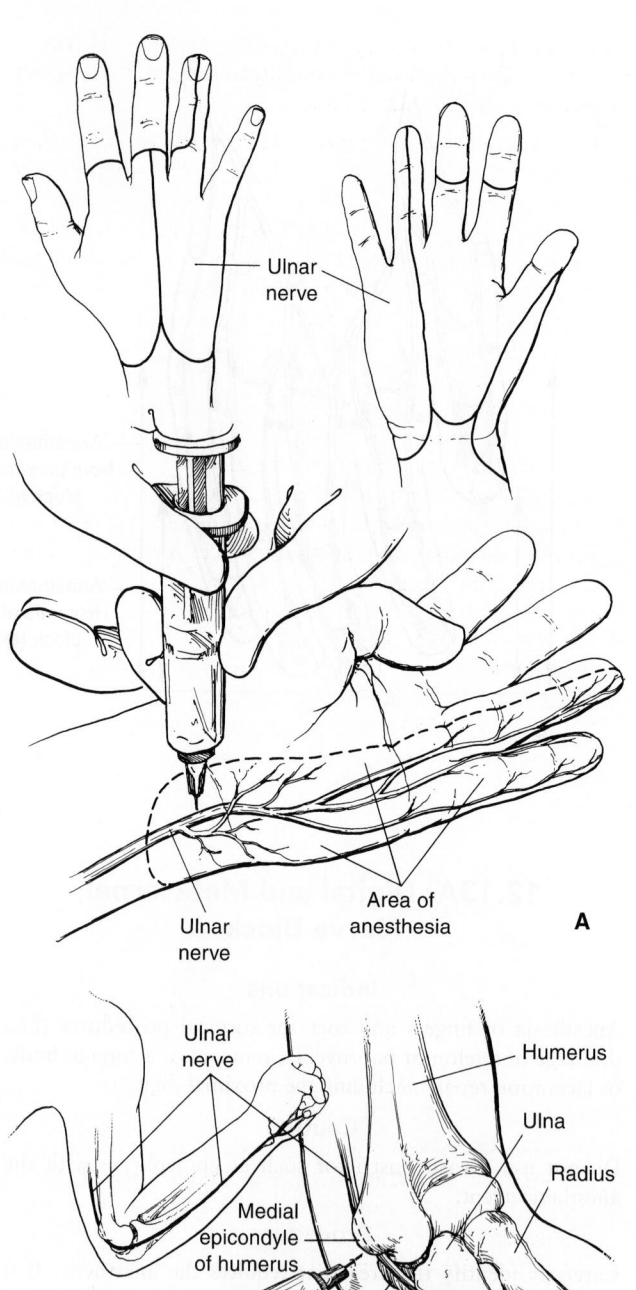

12.13C

Procedure (Fig. 12.13B)

The median nerve at the level of the proximal wrist crease courses superficially to lie between the more medial tendon of the flexor carpi radialis and the immediately radial tendon of the palmaris longus. Locate the two tendons by having the patient make a fist and flex the wrist. Cleanse the area with povidone–iodine solution. Insert a 25-gauge, 5/8-in needle at the level of the proximal skin crease on the distal forearm and at a right angle to the tendon. Depending on the size of the child, insert the needle 0.5 to 1 cm and inject 2 to 3 mL of 1% lidocaine. In the older child or adolescent, attempt to demonstrate paresthesia of the hand to ensure the nerve is touched by the needle point before injecting the lidocaine. If a paresthesia is elicited when entering the retinaculum, withdraw slightly prior to injection to avoid directly injecting the nerve. The effect will be best in 10 to 20 minutes.

12.13C. Ulnar Nerve Block

Indications

To provide anesthesia to the dorsal and palmar aspects of the hand, fifth finger, and ulnar side of the fourth finger to perform surgical procedures (i.e., laceration repair, debridement of hand burns or abrasions, reduction of hand fractures, or foreign-body removal)

Procedure

Carefully identify the area requiring anesthesia (Fig. 12.13C, part A). Check the hand and digits for blood supply, sensation, and motor nerve function before injecting lidocaine.

The ulnar nerve divides into two branches at the wrist. The palmar branch is located at the proximal wrist crease between the ulnar artery and the flexor carpi ulnaris tendon. The dorsal branch divides from the palmar branch 3 to 4 cm proximal to the wrist and courses under the flexor carpi ulnaris tendon.

The ulnar nerve can be blocked at the wrist or elbow. Ulnar nerve blocks at the wrist are not always successful because they require that both branches receive anesthetic. However, the risk of discomfort and of intraneural injection is slightly greater with blocks at the elbow.

1. Ulnar nerve block at the wrist—Cleanse the ventral surface of the wrist area well with povidone—iodine solution. Dry with sterile gauze.

   Using a 25-gauge needle, inject an intradermal skin wheal of lidocaine over the ulnar nerve at the proximal wrist crease at the level of the ulnar styloid. Insert the needle perpendicular to the skin on the ulnar side of the ulnar artery (Fig. 12.13C, Part A). At a depth of about 5 mm, paresthesia usually occurs. Aspirate to prevent intravascular injection, and then infuse 3 mL of lidocaine. If no paresthesia is elicited, inject an additional 2 mL of anesthetic. If the dorsal sensory branch of the ulnar nerve is not adequately anesthetized, inject approximately 3 mL of lidocaine subcutaneously on the dorsal surface of the wrist just distal to the ulnar styloid. Wait 10 to 15 minutes for anesthesia to take effect.

2. Ulnar nerve block at the elbow—Palpate the cordlike ulnar nerve between the medial epicondyle and olecranon by flexing the elbow. Cleanse the overlying skin with povidone–iodine solution. Dry with sterile gauze.

   With a 25-gauge needle, raise an intradermal skin wheal over the nerve. Through the skin wheal, inject 3 to 5 mL of 1% lidocaine on either side of the ulnar nerve (Fig. 12.19C, Part B). Do not inject directly into the nerve sheath. If paresthesias occur, remove the needle approximately 2 mm to avoid intraneural injection because this may result in postoperative paresthesias. Wait 15 minutes for anesthesia to take effect.

12.13D. Radial Nerve Block

Indications

1. Anesthesia of the dorsum of the thumb, index, and middle fingers, and radial portion of the dorsum of the hand for surgical procedures (i.e., laceration repair, debridement of hand burns or abrasions, or foreign-body removal)
2. A radial nerve block may be combined with median and ulnar nerve blocks for reduction of hand fractures

Procedure

Carefully identify the area requiring anesthesia (Fig. 12.13D). If it includes more than the dorsum and radial aspect of the hand, alternative methods must be performed to achieve adequate anesthesia.

Proximal to the wrist, a superficial cutaneous branch exits the main radial nerve. At the level of the wrist, this branch subdivides into several rami, which lie subcutaneously and provide sensory innervation to the dorsal–radial aspect of the wrist and hand.

Scrub the dorsal–radial aspect of the wrist thoroughly with povidone–iodine solution. Dry with sterile gauze. Identify the radial styloid. Insert a 25-gauge needle into the subcutaneous tissue 2 to 4 cm proximal to the prominence of the radial styloid. Slowly inject a small bolus of lidocaine (2 to 4 mL). To anesthetize the dorsal branches, lay down a continuous subcutaneous tract of lidocaine from the radial styloid to the lateral

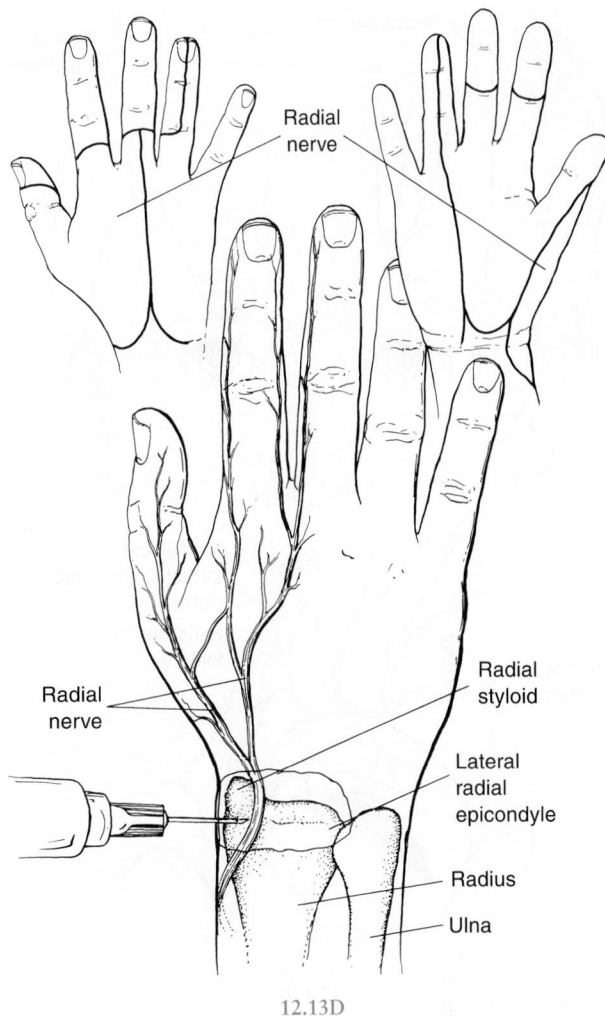

Radial nerve

Radial nerve

Radial styloid

Lateral radial epicondyle

Radius

Ulna

12.13D

radial epicondyle of up to 5 to 10 mL. Allow 10 to 15 minutes for a complete block.

12.13E. Supraorbital Nerve Block

Indications

1. Lacerations within sensory distribution of the nerve (Fig. 12.13E)
2. Removal of a foreign body

Procedure

The supraorbital nerve exits the skull at the foramen just above the supraorbital ridge. The supratrochlear nerve exits just medial to the supraorbital nerve. Locate the foramen by palpating over the medial aspect of the supraorbital ridge (Fig. 12.13E).

Cleanse the area with povidone–iodine solution. Insert a 25-gauge, 5/8-in needle just medial to the foramen, directed toward the foramen (Fig. 12.13E). Depending on the size of the child, insert the needle 0.5 to 1 cm and inject 1 to 3 mL of 1% lidocaine with epinephrine. In the older child or adolescent, attempt to demonstrate paresthesia of the forehead to ensure the nerve is touched by the needle point before injecting the lidocaine.

PROCEDURES

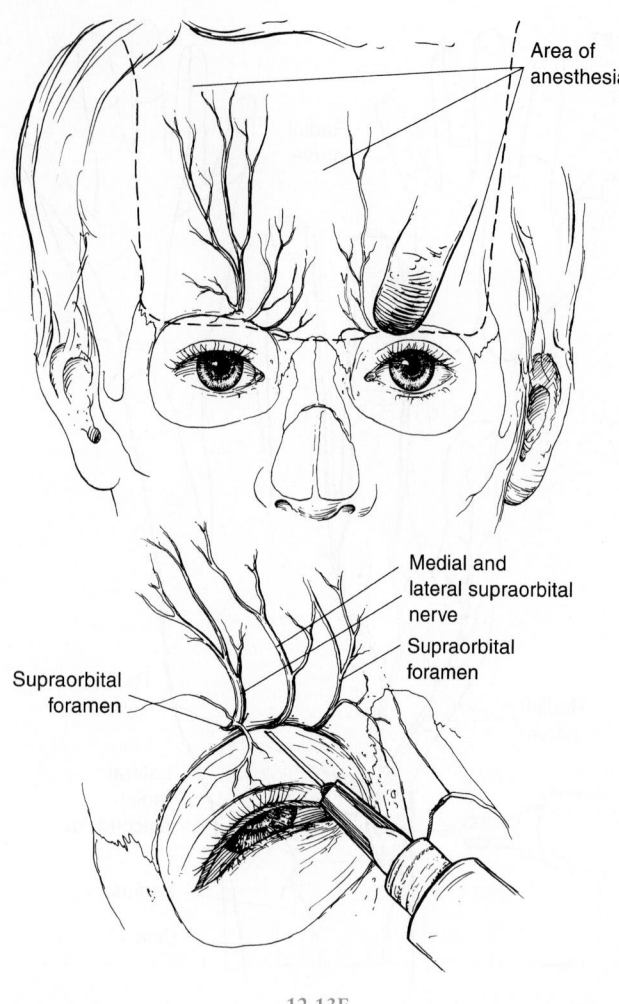

Area of
anesthesia

Medial and
lateral supraorbital
nerve

Supraorbital
foramen

Supraorbital
foramen

12.13E

12.13F. Infraorbital Nerve Block (Intraoral Approach)

Indications

1. Lacerations within sensory distribution of the nerve (Fig. 12.13F)—midface (skin of the upper lip, nose, and lower eyelid)
2. Removal of a foreign body

Procedure

The infraorbital nerve exits its foramen just below the infraorbital ridge. Locate the foramen by palpating over the cheek just below the infraorbital ridge.

Don gloves and place a finger over the infraorbital ridge while using the index finger to hold up the upper lip. Numb the upper gum near the second bicuspid with a topical anesthetic. Insert a 25-gauge, 1.5-in needle on a syringe with 1% lidocaine. Puncture the gum line along the long axis of the second upper bicuspid and advance until the needle is palpated at the foramen where the infraorbital nerve exits. The needle is inserted to about a depth of 2 cm in a full-grown teenager. Inject 1 to 2 mL of 1% lidocaine.

When tissue injury is sufficient to make palpation of the infraorbital ridge difficult, a field block may be used infiltrating 4 to 5 mL in a fanlike distribution along the upper buccal fold. Wait 5 minutes for anesthesia to occur.

12.13G. Mental (Infraoral) Nerve Block

Indications

1. Lacerations of the lower lip and chin
2. Removal of a foreign body

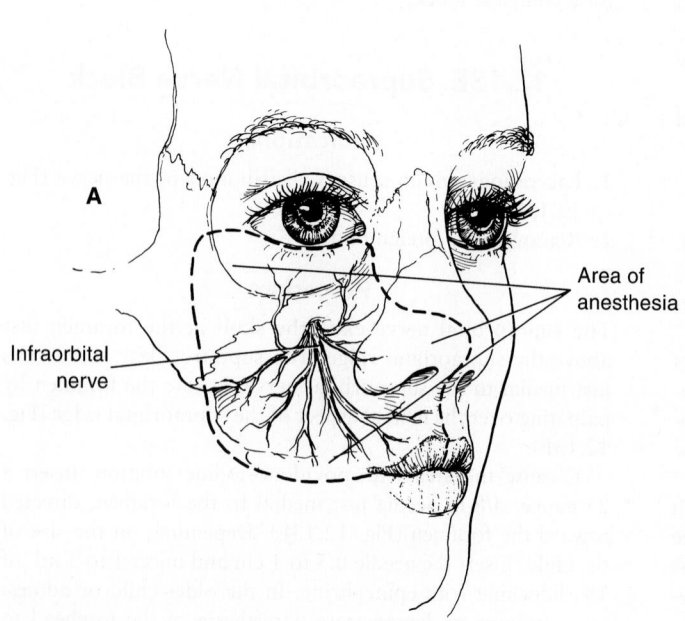

A

Area of
anesthesia

Infraorbital
nerve

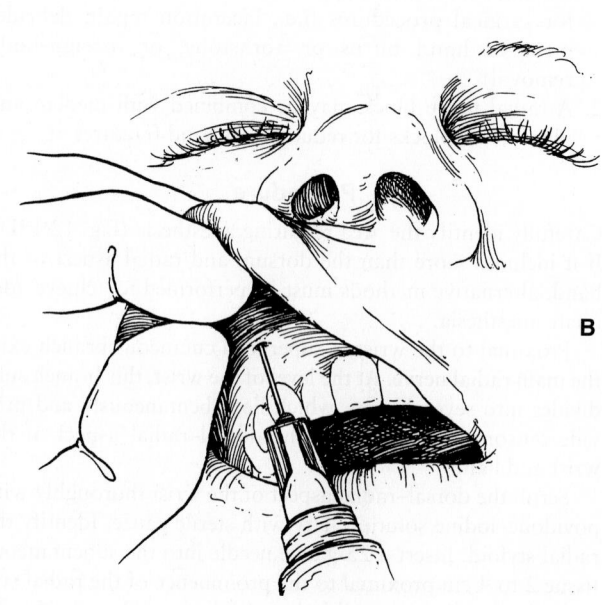

B

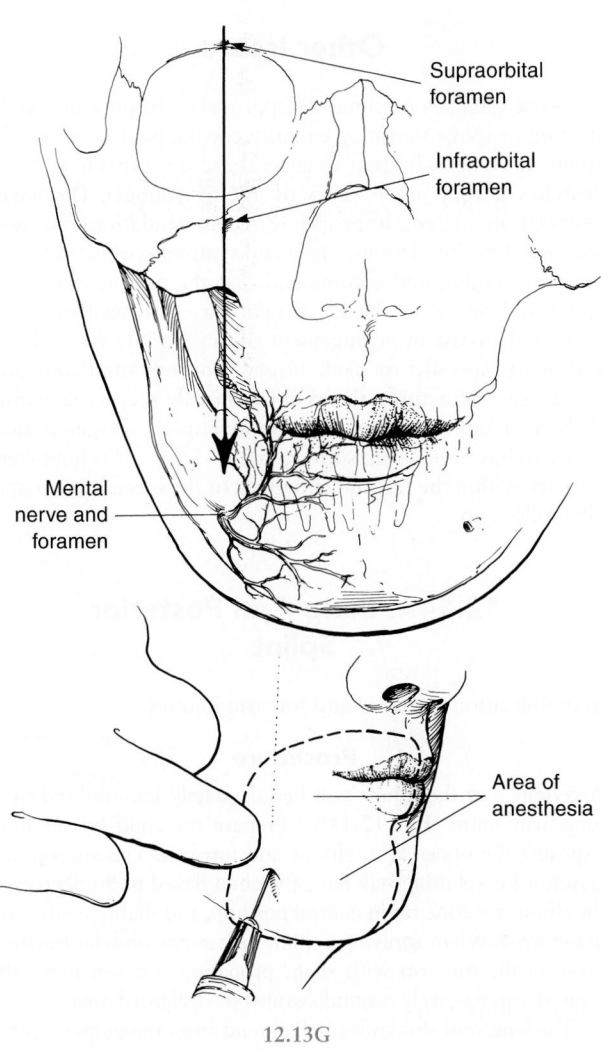

12.13G

Procedure

The mental nerve is a branch of the alveolar nerve with sensory distribution of the lower lip and chin (Fig. 12.13G). It exits its foramen in the mandible at the level of the premolar. Locate the foramen by palpating over the mandible in line with the supraorbital and infraorbital foramen (Fig. 12.13G).

Cleanse the area with topical anesthetic. Insert a 25-gauge, 5/8-in needle just medial to the foramen directed toward the foramen. Depending on the size of the child, insert the needle approximately 0.5 cm and inject 1 to 2 mL of 1% lidocaine with epinephrine. In the older child or adolescent, attempt to demonstrate paresthesia of the lower lip to ensure the nerve is touched by the needle point before injecting lidocaine.

12.14. SPLINTING OF MUSCULOSKELETAL INJURIES

General Splinting

Indications

To provide short-term stabilization and/or protection of musculoskeletal injuries (fractures, tendon injuries, lacerations, or tenosynovitis)

Complications

1. Neurovascular compromise
2. Pressure sores
3. Contact dermatitis

Equipment

1. Cotton bandage (Webril®)
2. Plaster slabs or rolls (2-, 3-, 4-, and 6-in widths) or prepadded material (OCL™ and Orthoglass®) of same widths
3. Room temperature tap water
4. Elastic (Ace™) bandage
5. Adhesive tape

Procedure

Determine the style of splint needed from the anatomic considerations of the injury. Remember that the injured extremity should be splinted in a position of function to minimize contractures. Skin lesions and wounds should be cleansed, repaired, and dressed in the usual manner before the application of plaster. Open fractures should be evaluated emergently by an orthopedic surgeon. Neurovascular status should be documented before and after the splint is applied.

Before applying the splint, it is important to completely expose the extremity to be splinted and anticipate the child's ability to remove his/her clothing once the splint is applied.

Plaster Splint

Measure and cut the appropriate length of plaster. It is better to cut the length slightly longer than necessary to account for any shrinkage of material. If the cut length is too long, the end can always be rolled on itself. The upper extremity requires 8 to 10 layers; the lower, 12 to 14 layers to withstand some weight bearing. In general, the slab should be wide enough to cover approximately one-half of the circumference of the extremity but should never be so wide that it overlaps itself.

Next, prepare the padding. If toes or fingers are to be incorporated within the splint, place padding between the digits to prevent maceration. Roll Webril® bandage around the injured extremity in a distal to proximal manner, making sure to overlap each turn by 50%. Extend the padding 2 to 3 cm distally and proximally beyond the area to be splinted. Wrinkles of the Webril can create pressure points and are best avoided by stretching and partially tearing the bandage during application. Bony prominences require additional padding with orthopedic felt or Webril to minimize pressure injury. Stockinette may be used under the Webril, if desired.

Immerse the plaster slab in room temperature water until bubbling stops. Because setting plaster elaborates heat, room temperature water is recommended to minimize risk of heat injury to the patient's skin. Remove the slab from the water and on an absorbent surface such as a towel; smooth the plaster to remove excess moisture and wrinkles and to laminate the layers. The setting time of the plaster is determined by the temperature of the water and the overall moisture content of the plaster, with warmer water and drier plaster shortening the set time. Properly position the splint onto the extremity. Using your palms, smooth and contour the splint to the extremity, taking care not to leave indentations. Indentations create pressure points that will be uncomfortable and cause skin breakdown. Fold the exposed Webril back over the ends of the splint.

PROCEDURES

Next, an optional layer of gauze or a single layer of Webril may be placed over the splint to prevent the Ace™ wrap from being incorporated into the plaster. Then, roll the Ace wrap over the splint in a distal to proximal manner and secure with tape. The extremity should be maintained in the desired position until the splint is sufficiently hard.

Fiberglass Splint

A good option is to use one of the commercially available splinting preparations (OCL™ or Orthoglass™), which incorporate the padding and a fiberglass splint material into a single preparation. These preparations are designed to provide a sufficient amount of padding by themselves and do not require the use of additional padding under the splint. However, some practitioners prefer to pad bony prominences, such as the malleoli, heel, or elbow, particularly when the splints may be kept on longer before follow-up. The advantages of these materials are their ease and neatness of application. The fiberglass products also appear to be more durable than the plaster splints. A relative disadvantage is that these commercially available products are not as moldable to the bends of an extremity as well as plaster seems to be.

It is important to follow the specific manufacturer's instructions when using these products to ensure appropriate application. In general, these products are cut to length; moistened with water; stretched, smoothed, and molded to the injured extremity; and then covered with an Ace bandage. Once the material is applied and secured, maintain the extremity in the proper position until the splint becomes sufficiently rigid. This takes place usually much quicker than plaster, as short as 10 minutes from application. It is helpful to cut the material slightly longer than necessary and to fold the excess length back on itself to make a smooth comfortable end to the splint. This technique is especially helpful at natural flexion areas, such as the palm or toes. *Remember* also that the cut ends of the fiberglass material become sharp when dry and require either taping of the exposed ends or a stretching of the padding material on its application to cover the exposed end and prevent skin laceration.

Other Issues

Dispense crutches or slings as appropriate to prevent weight bearing or usage that may enhance edema, pain, or cause the splint to break. Children in general are not capable of using crutches if they are 6 years of age or younger. Discharge instructions include appropriate recommendations for rest, ice, and elevation. Discuss signs and symptoms of neurovascular compromise, and recommend that the patient loosen the splint and return to the ED if neurovascular insufficiency is suspected. Assist in arrangement of appropriate referral and follow-up specific to each injury. For nonangulated and nondisplaced fractures, this visit is generally acceptable within 7 days of injury, although some orthopedic surgeons may desire to have follow-up sooner, in 2 to 3 days. It is important to work within the recommendations of the specialists for specific follow-up.

12.14A. Long Arm Posterior Splint

Immobilization of elbow and forearm injuries

Procedure

Ascertain that the injury will be adequately immobilized by a long arm splint (Fig. 12.14A). Prepare the child by carefully exposing the upper arm, elbow, and forearm. The appropriate position for splinting will have the child flexed to 90 degrees at the elbow, the forearm in neutral position, and slight dorsiflexion at the wrist. When applying a splint for a supracondylar fracture, position the forearm with slight pronation. Do not move the injured arm passively around swollen or disfigured areas.

The length of this splint will extend from the palmar crease of the hand to mid-arm being the length up the arm from the elbow. It will run along the ulnar side of the forearm and the posterior aspect of the humerus. Take care so the splint does not impinge on the axilla. The width should extend semicircularly

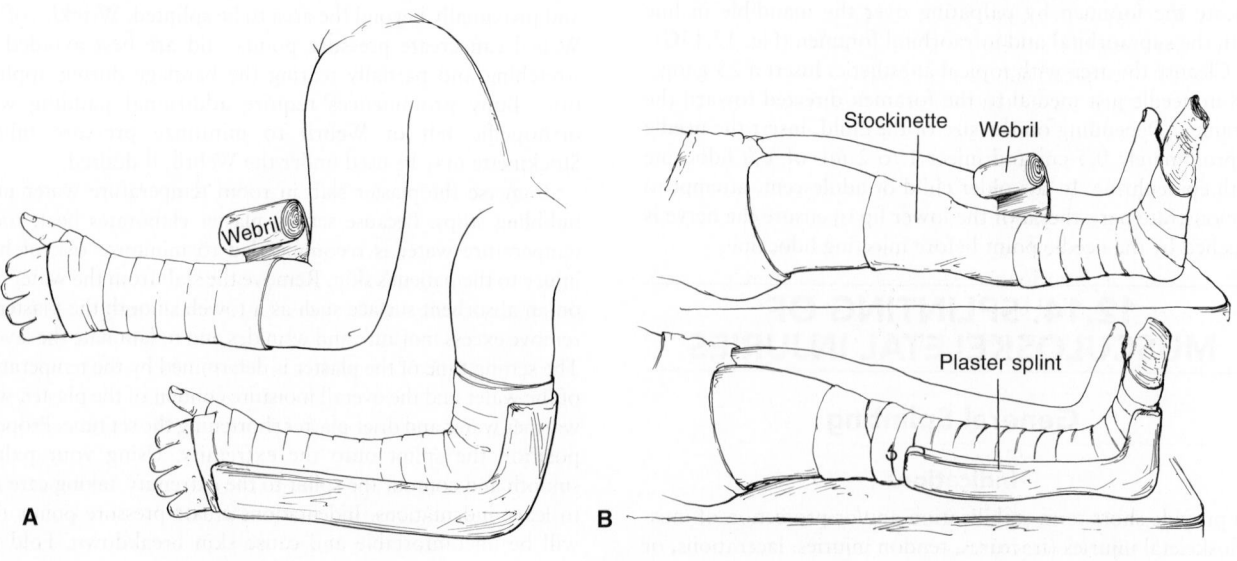

A   B

halfway around the arm. Prepare and apply the splint material as described in the "General Splinting" section. This splint requires the use of a sling.

Supracondylar fractures may require more urgent follow-up and should be discussed with an orthopedic surgeon.

12.14B. Posterior Ankle Splint

Indications

Immobilization of ankle sprains and fractures of the foot, ankle, and distal fibula

Procedure

This splint extends from the foot, including the ball of the foot, to proximal lower leg at the level of the fibular head. Ensure it does not impinge on the popliteal fossa when the leg is flexed. For metatarsal fractures, the splint is sometimes extended to include the toes. The material should be wide enough to support the entire width of the foot. The splint will maintain the foot at 90 degrees of flexion and is most easily applied with the child in the prone position with the leg flexed. Prepare and apply the splint materials as described in the "General Splinting" section. Consider additional padding at the malleoli and calcaneus. Once the splint is applied, it is often necessary to have someone maintain the foot at 90 degrees while the material hardens.

Discharge the patient with crutches and warn that this splint does not tolerate weight bearing well, particularly in school-age children or teens.

12.14C. Ankle Stirrup (Sugar Tong) Splint

Indications

Immobilization of injuries to the ankle, especially in adolescents

Procedure

This splint may be used alone or together with a posterior splint. It provides lateral and medial support to injured ankles. This splint extends in a U-shaped fashion from the fibular head around the ankle to just below the knee. The width of the material should be approximately one-half of the circumference of the narrowest portion of the lower leg. The material, however, should not overlap. Application occurs more easily with the patient in the prone position and the foot at 90 degrees. Consider padding the malleoli with felt or Webril™ to decrease the incidence of pressure sores. Prepare and apply the splint materials as described in the "General Splinting" section. When using the posterior and stirrup splint together, place the posterior splint on first closest to the leg.

Discharge the patient with crutches and discourage weight bearing.

12.14D. Long Leg Posterior Splint

Indications

Immobilization of knee injuries and fractures of the midshaft and proximal tibia and fibula

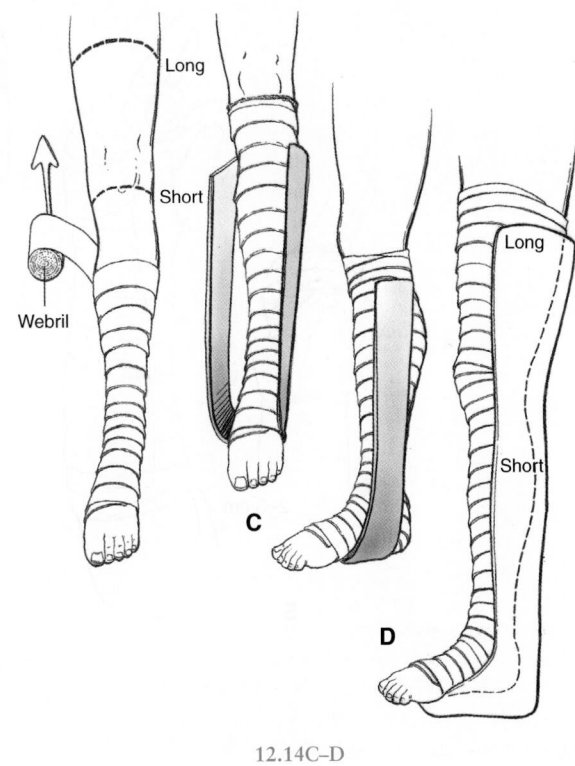

12.14C–D

Procedure

The injuries immobilized by this splint often require early orthopedic consultation. When used, the splint extends from just behind the toes to the area below the gluteal fold (Fig. 12.14C, D). The splint material must be sufficiently wide to support the proximal thigh and the knee. The final position will maintain the ankle at 90 degrees and the knee in slight flexion. The help of an assistant or two is necessary to support and elevate the leg during the procedure. Prepare and apply the splint materials as described in the "General Splinting" section. Discharge the patient with crutches and discourage weight bearing.

12.14E. Ulnar Gutter Splint

Indications

1. Boxer's fractures (up to 20 degrees angulation without rotation)
2. Uncomplicated fourth and fifth phalangeal fractures

Procedure (Fig. 12.14E)

This splint is U-shaped, incorporates the fourth and fifth phalanges, and extends along the ulnar side of the forearm. The final splint extends from the distal fingers to the proximal forearm. The proper splinting position maintains slight dorsiflexion of the wrist, 60 to 90 degrees of flexion of the metacarpophalangeal joint, and 20 degrees of flexion of the interphalangeal joints.

To determine the appropriate length of splint material, measure from the patient's fingertip to 2 to 3 cm shy of the volar crease at the elbow. The plaster material should be wide enough to enclose the fourth and fifth phalanges and overlie both the

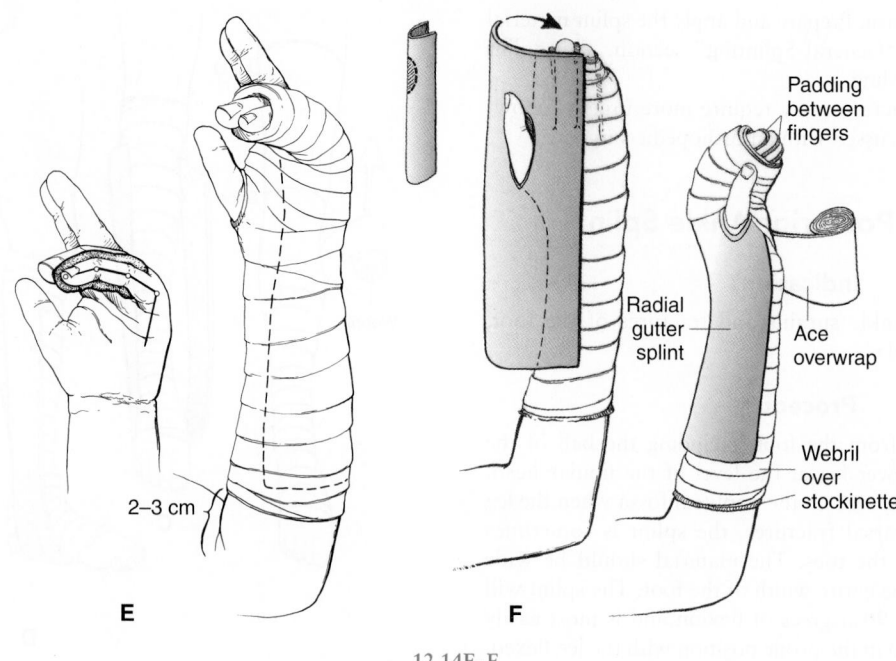

12.14E–F

volar and dorsal surfaces of the fourth and fifth metacarpals. Place the patient's elbow in a neutral position so no pronation or supination of the forearm is possible. Prepare and apply the splint materials as described in the "General Splinting" section. Remember to place padding between the digits. For metacarpal fractures, it is desirable to approach 90 degrees of flexion at the metacarpal phalangeal joint. This position tightens the collateral ligaments and helps maintain reduction.

Inform the patient that the knuckle contour at the fracture site may be less noticeable after this injury heals.

12.14F. Radial Gutter Splint

Indications

1. Second and third metacarpal fractures
2. Second and third phalangeal fractures

Procedure

This splint is U-shaped and lies along the radial side of the arm. It extends from the tips of the second and third phalanges to the proximal forearm a few inches shy of the flexural crease at the elbow. The width of the material will cover the second and third metacarpals on the volar and dorsal surfaces. The final position maintains the forearm in neutral position with the wrist in slight dorsiflexion, the metacarpal joint at 60 to 90 degrees of flexion, and up to slight flexion of the interphalangeal joints.

Prepare and apply the materials as described in the "General Splinting" section. A hole must be made in the splinting material to allow for the thumb. Accomplish this by locating the position of the thumb on the splint material, folding the material in half, and cutting a semicircle of material from the folded edge. If fiberglass is used, this cut edge is

sharp so the padding must be stretched well or additional padding placed around the thumb to keep fiberglass from direct contact with the skin. Remember also to place padding between the fingers.

A sling is not necessary but can be dispensed for comfort.

12.14G. Sugar Tong Splint—Forearm

Indications

Distal radius and wrist fractures in which pronation and supination are minimized and the elbow is immobilized.

Procedure

As shown in Figure 12.14G, the splint extends along the volar surface from the flexural crease of the palm, around the elbow, and dorsally to the metacarpal heads. The fingers and thumb remain free. As shown in the figure, the arm should be flexed 90 degrees at the elbow with no rotation of the forearm. The hand is dorsiflexed minimally (have the patient hold a small roll of tape or Webril™).

With the arm positioned as just described, measure from the midpalm around the elbow to the knuckles dorsally (add 1 to 2 in to allow for shrinkage). The splinting material should be wide enough to support the arm volarly and dorsally but not so wide as to overlap. Prepare and apply the materials as described in the "General Splinting" section. Ensure sufficient padding is placed over the elbow if simple plaster is used. A properly measured splint allows 90 degrees of flexion of the fingers and approaches, but does not cover, the knuckles dorsally. An assistant is helpful when applying this splint. Ensure the thumb is free to move in all directions.

Discharge the patient with a sling with the hand slightly above the level of the elbow.

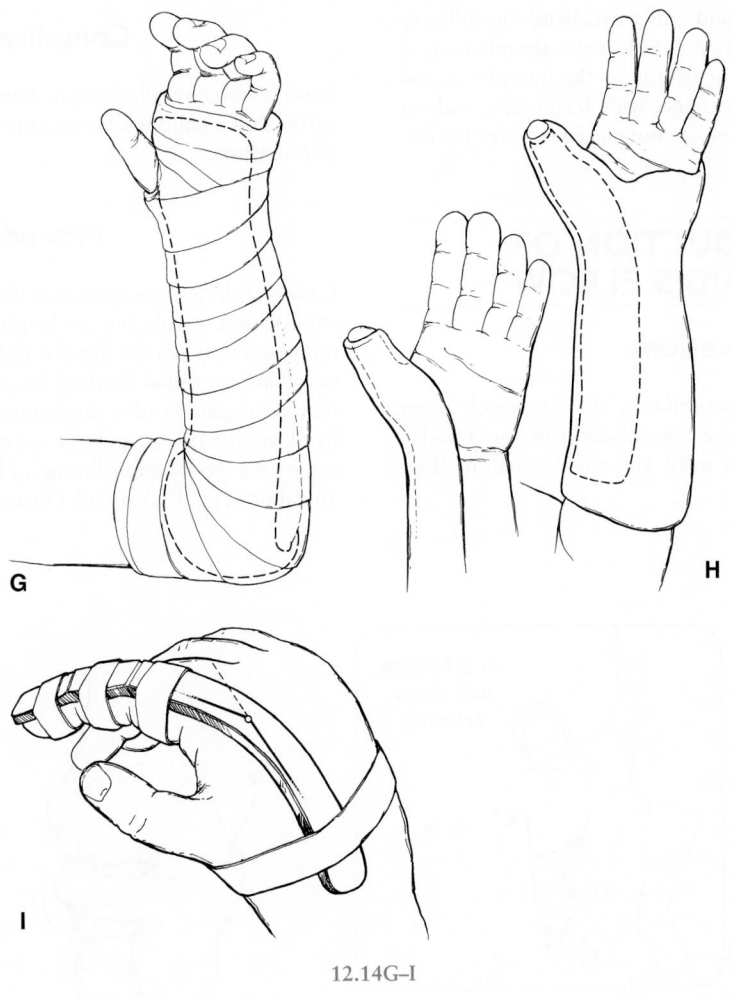

12.14G–I

12.14H. Thumb Spica Splint

Indications

1. Nonrotated, nonangulated, nonarticular fractures of the thumb metacarpal or phalanx
2. Ulnar collateral ligament injuries (gamekeeper's thumb)
3. Suspected or documented scaphoid (navicular) fracture

Procedure (Fig. 12.14H)

The splint extends in a U-shaped manner along the radial side of the thumb and forearm from the thumbnail to the midforearm. The proper splinting position maintains the wrist in slight dorsiflexion, the thumb in some flexion and abduction, and the interphalangeal joint in slight flexion. The final position is as though the patient were holding a glass or catching a ball, and will allow apposition of the index finger and thumb.

Determine the appropriate length of splint material by measuring from the patient's thumbnail to the midforearm. The splint should be wide enough to completely encircle the thumb. Prepare and apply the splint materials as described in the "General Splinting" section. The Webril should cover the thumb, hand, and forearm. Mold the splint so the thumb is maintained in the position previously described.

A sling is usually unnecessary.

12.14I. Dorsal Extension Block (Finger Splint)

Indications

1. Nonrotated, nonangulated fractures of the phalanges, not involving greater than 10% of the joint line
2. Immobilization after laceration or tendon repair
3. Sprains of the phalangeal ligaments
4. Note: Mallet and boutonniere fingers require an alternative splinting method

Equipment

1. Commercially available foam splints with aluminum backing
2. 1/2- and 1-in adhesive tape

Procedure

A dorsal splint is preferred to a volar splint because tactile sensation is maintained, it is more comfortable for the patient, and it is more protective of the injury as the splint lies between the patient and outside surfaces during ambulation.

The splint extends from the dorsum of the wrist to the end of the finger (Fig. 12.14I). The appropriate width will be equal to the diameter of the finger. Cut the splint to the proper length and place tape on the sharp edges. Tape the splint with 1-in tape to the dorsum of the hand and wrist. Bend the splint to obtain 50 to 90 degrees of flexion at the metacarpophalangeal joint and 15 to 20 degrees of flexion at the interphalangeal joints. Secure the splint of the finger with 1/2-in tape, making sure not to cover the joint lines. Do not place tape over the distal phalanx.

12.15. REDUCTION OF NURSEMAID'S ELBOW

Indications

Radial head subluxation (nursemaid's elbow), which is an injury that probably represents interposition of the annular ligament between the radial head and the capitellum (Fig. 12.15A).

Complications

Vascular or musculoskeletal damage if the maneuver is performed on a child with a fracture (i.e., supracondylar fracture of humerus).

Procedure

Radiographs are not necessary if the suspicion for radial head subluxation is high, but are helpful to be certain that no bony injury exists when the history and examination are equivocal. Suspicion for radial head subluxation is based on (i) A history that is suggestive of a mechanism that would lead to radial head subluxation, such as excessive axial traction placed across the elbow joint during a fall while holding hands with an adult (Fig. 12.15); (ii) Observation of the affected arm,

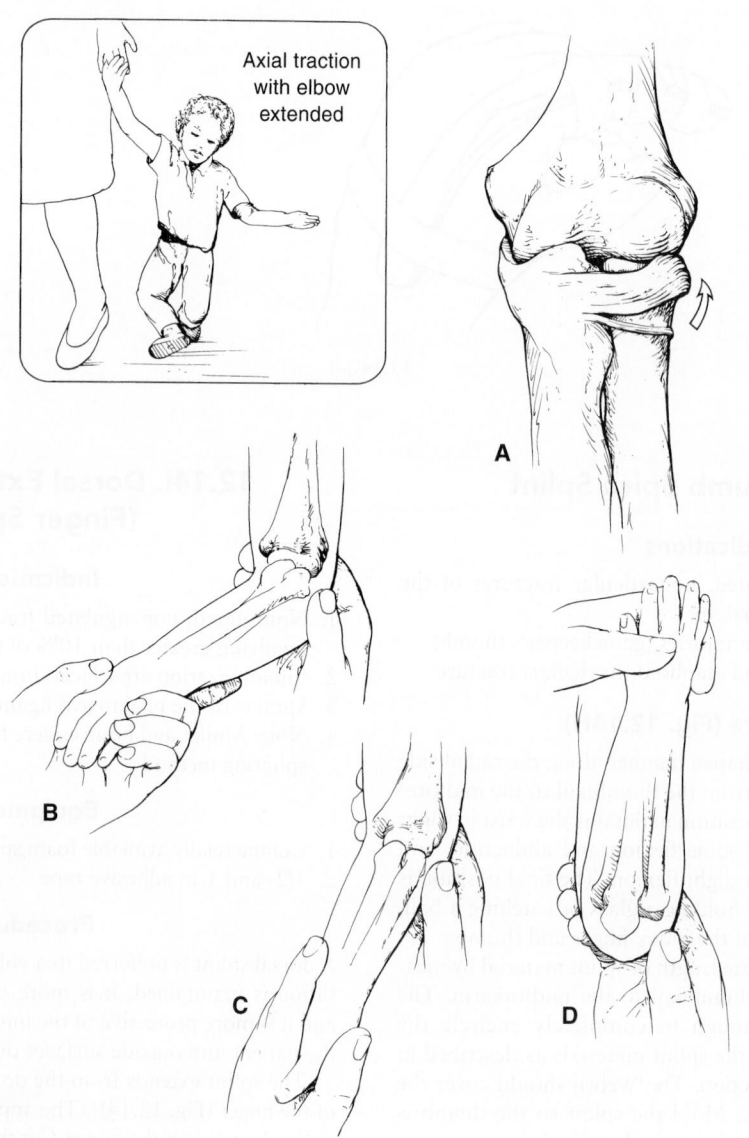

which is generally held at the child's side, slightly flexed at the elbow in pronation; and (iii) Absence of point tenderness along the length of the arm and shoulder during examination of the affected arm. An adequate examination requires that the child be comfortable and may entail some distraction. Oral analgesia with acetaminophen or ibuprofen may be useful.

Generally, it takes less than 10 to 15 minutes after the reduction before the child uses the arm normally. Rarely, when a prolonged period has elapsed before reduction, it will take somewhat longer for the child to regain normal function after the maneuver is performed. Repeat or try an alternative approach if unsatisfied with the child's use of the arm.

Supination and Flexion Approach

After explaining the procedure to the parent, have the parent or assistant gently restrain the child in the sitting position. As shown in Figure 12.15B, grasp the palm of the child's hand as if to shake it. Encircle the elbow with the other hand with the thumb over the annular ligament of the radius and position the elbow in some flexion. Gently distract the elbow joint and then supinate the palm of the hand (Fig. 12.15C), and in a continuous motion, flex the elbow to the shoulder (Fig. 12.15D). During the flexion maneuver, the physician feels a "pop" with the thumb that lies over the radial head.

Hyperpronation

In more recent years, an alternative approach utilizes hyperpronation with flexion to achieve reduction. Some clinicians use this method as their primary means of reduction, whereas others employ it after the supination-flexion technique fails. This approach may be less painful. As shown in Figure 12.15B, gently grasp the patient's hand on the affected side as if to shake it, stabilize the elbow joint in some flexion, and place pressure with a finger on the radial head. Gently distract the elbow joint and hyperpronate by rotating the hand on the affected side medially. As before, the physician will feel a "pop" with the hand placed over the radial head.

12.16. APPLICATION OF A FIGURE-OF-EIGHT HARNESS

Indications

An alternative to use of a sling for immobilizing of midshaft clavicle fractures

Complications

1. Pressure sores (tight application)
2. Pain (loose application)

Procedure

Obtain radiographs in two views to confirm the presence and location of the fracture. Then choose a figure-of-eight dressing by measuring the child's chest circumference and picking the closest available size (Table 12.16).

TABLE 12.16

FIGURE-OF-EIGHT HARNESS SIZES

Size	Chest circumference (cm)
Extra extra small	<20
Extra small	20–25
Small	25–30
Medium	30–35
Medium long	33–39

Stand the child up and loosely drape the harness over his/her shoulders to assess how much to tighten the straps. Remove the harness and manually adjust the straps by sliding the cloth through the metal clips. Make it slightly tighter than estimated during the fitting to pull the shoulders slightly back from their usual forward, rounded position.

Reapply the harness around the shoulders from the front to the back with the soft padding against the skin of the axillae. Approximate the buckles in the midline of the back and clip them. The harness should fit snugly, and the shoulders should be straight (Fig. 12.16). Tighten the straps as necessary.

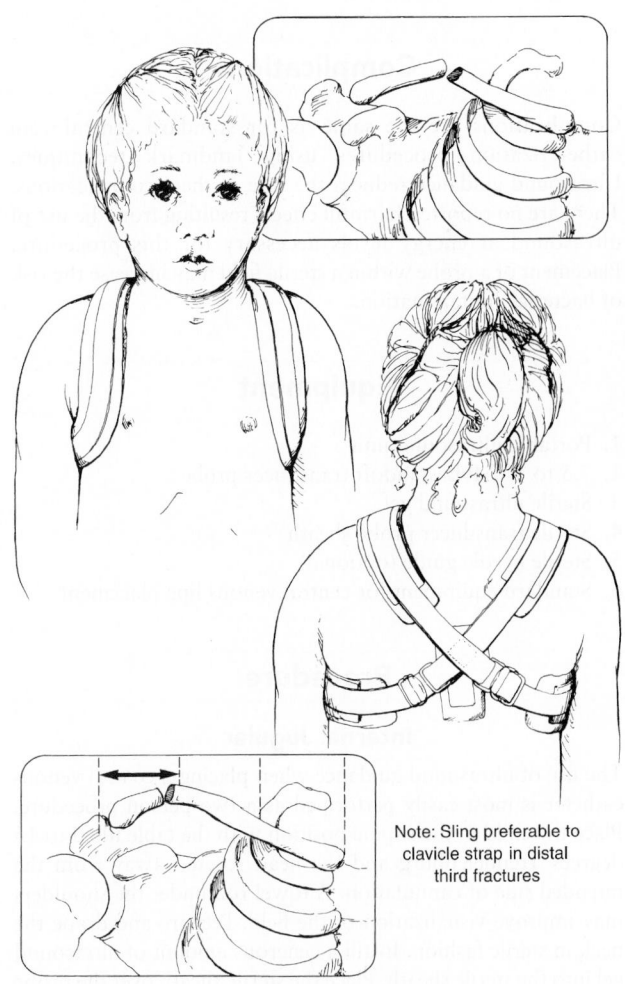

Note: Sling preferable to clavicle strap in distal third fractures

12.16

Have the patient wear the harness except during bathing for 3 weeks. The parent should demonstrate the successful reapplication of the harness before leaving the ED.

Alternative—Sling

The use of a figure of 8 harness versus a sling for conservative treatment of uncomplicated clavicle fracture has not clearly demonstrate strong evidence for better outcomes. Midshaft and greatly displaced fractures have been treated effectively with surgical intervention in older adolescents and adults. A number of experts have chosen the use of a sling for 3 weeks as equal therapy. An alternative to uncomplicated clavicle fractures is the use of an arm sling at close to 90 degrees.

13.1 ULTRASOUND GUIDANCE FOR CENTRAL VEIN CATHETERIZATION

Indications

In patients who require central venous access, ultrasound facilitates central vein catheterization by providing direct visualization and localization of vessels, as well as real-time guidance of the venipuncture needle.

Complications

Complications are the same as for standard central vein catheterization procedures using landmark techniques. Ultrasound guidance reduces the rate of these complications. There are no reported harmful effects resulting from the use of ultrasound at energy levels necessary for this procedure. Placement of a probe within a sterile field may increase the risk of bacterial contamination.

Equipment

1. Portable ultrasound unit
2. 7.5 to 10 MHz standoff transducer probe
3. Sterile ultrasound gel
4. Sterile transducer probe sheath
5. Sterile needle guide (optional)
6. Standard equipment for central venous line placement

Procedure

Internal Jugular

The use of ultrasound guidance when placing a central venous catheter is most easily performed as a two-person procedure. Place the child in the supine position with the table tilted to 15 degrees Trendelenburg and the head rotated away from the intended side of cannulation. A towel roll under the shoulders may improve visualization of the field. Prepare and drape the neck in sterile fashion. Instill a generous amount of ultrasound gel into the sterile sheath. Place the sterile sheath over the probe head and proximal length of cable. Ensure all air is removed

from between the probe head sheath. Apply an additional layer of sterile ultrasound gel to the sheath overlying the probe head. Attach the needle guide to the transducer probe. Position the probe on the skin surface above the clavicle and between the two heads of the sternocleidomastoid muscle. Hold the probe perpendicular to the path of the internal jugular vein with the needle guide facing the patient's head. Vessels appear as dark (anechoic) circular objects on the ultrasound screen. Maneuver the probe to produce a cross-sectional image of the jugular vein and carotid artery on the screen. An ultrasound unit with Doppler capabilities will facilitate identification of patent vessels. The jugular vein ordinarily lies superficial and lateral to the carotid artery. Pressure on the probe assists in distinguishing veins from arteries. The thinner-walled vein will collapse under pressure while the artery will not. A Valsalva maneuver in a cooperative patient will increase the diameter of the vein. Rotate the patient's head while transducing the vessels to find the optimal position in which the vessels lie side by side. Align the vein so it is centered beneath the probe and the electronic dot markers on the screen intersect it. Anesthetize the skin surface at the puncture site. Place the needle in the needle guide with the bevel facing the probe and advance through the skin. Observe the needle on the screen as it enters the vessel. The needle indents the vein as it comes in contact with the surface. The vein returns to its normal shape once it is punctured. Confirm placement through aspiration of blood into the syringe. Disengage the needle from the holder and remove the probe from the skin surface. Complete the placement of the central line as when using the landmark technique.

Femoral Vein

Position the child supine with the leg abducted and externally rotated. Prepare and drape the skin surface using sterile technique. Prepare the transducer probe as described previously. Place the probe on the skin surface just below the inguinal ligament at the point of the femoral artery pulsation (Fig. 13.1A). In the setting of a difficult-to-palpate pulse or cardiac arrest, place the probe midway between the anterior superior iliac crest and the pubic symphysis. Position the probe perpendicular to the direction of the femoral vein with the needle guide facing the feet. Identify the femoral vein and artery on the ultrasound screen (Fig. 13.1B). The vein lies medial to the artery. Use the previously mentioned techniques to distinguish the vein from the artery. Anesthetize the skin at the puncture site using sterile technique. Insert the needle through the needle guide with the bevel facing the probe (Fig. 13.1C), and advance through the skin surface until cannulation is visualized on the screen and confirmed through aspiration of blood into the syringe. Remove the needle from the guide and the probe from the skin surface. Complete femoral vein catheterization using standard Seldinger technique.

13.2. FOCUSED ABDOMINAL SONOGRAPHY FOR TRAUMA

Indications

Focused abdominal sonography for trauma (FAST) is a limited ultrasound examination performed in the setting of pediatric

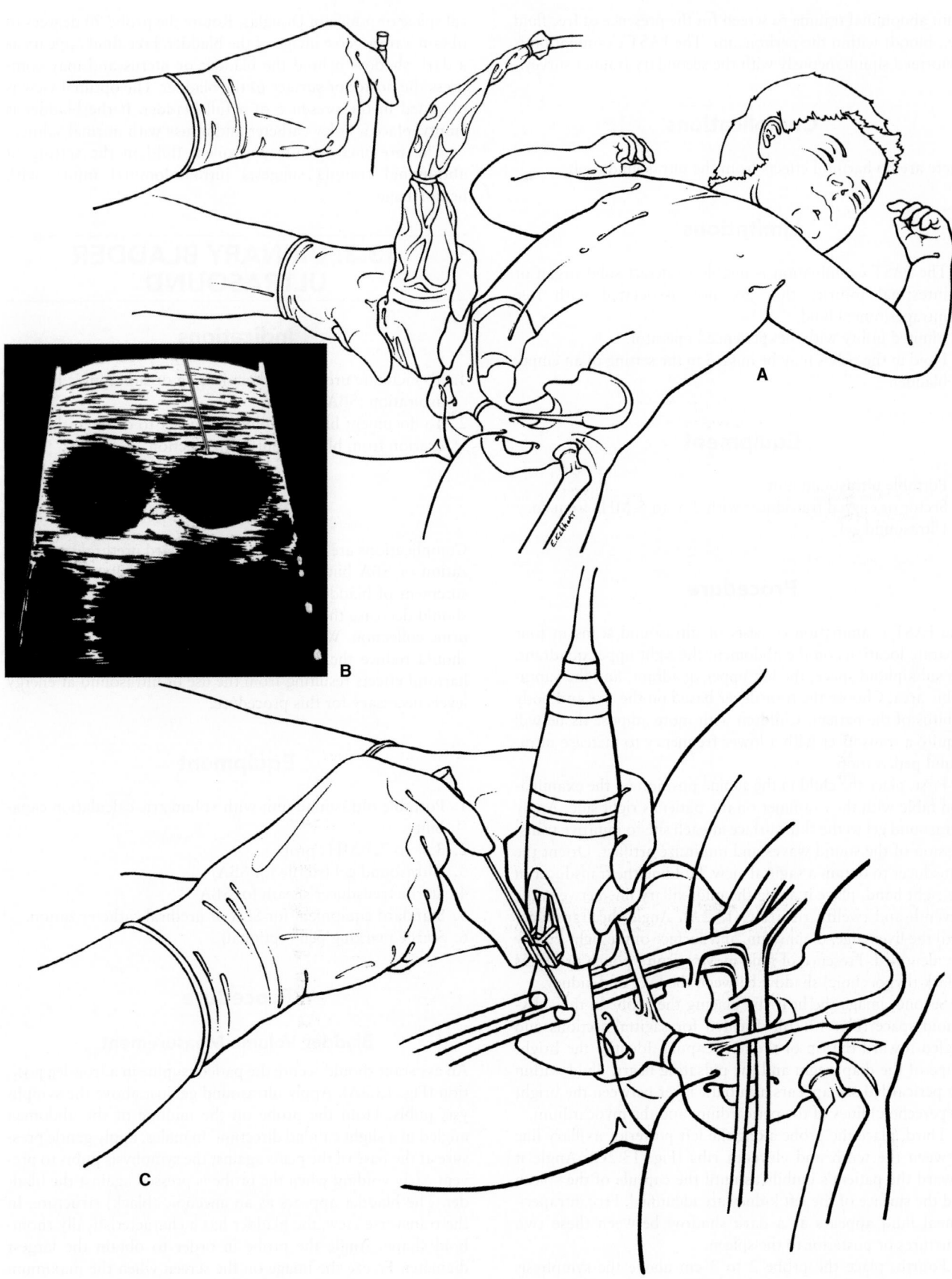

blunt abdominal trauma to screen for the presence of free fluid (i.e., blood) within the peritoneum. The FAST examination is performed simultaneously with the secondary trauma survey.

Complications

There are no harmful effects from the ultrasound itself.

Limitations

1. The FAST examination is unable to detect solid organ or intestinal injuries that are not associated with free intraperitoneal fluid.
2. Limited utility with inexperienced operator.
3. Fluid in the pelvis may be missed in the setting of an empty bladder.

Equipment

1. Portable ultrasound unit
2. Sector or curved transducer with 2.5- to 5-MHz frequency
3. Ultrasound gel

Procedure

The FAST examination consists of ultrasound scans in four separate locations on the abdomen: the right upper quadrant, the subxiphoid space, the left upper quadrant, and the suprapubic area. Choose the transducer based on the size and body habitus of the patient. Children with more adipose tissue will require a transducer with a lower frequency to increase ultrasound penetration.

First, place the child in the supine position on the examination table with the examiner on the patient's right side. Apply ultrasound gel to the skin surface at each site to improve transmission of the sound waves and minimize artifact. Orient the transducer to obtain a sagittal view. Holding the transducer in the right hand, place it along the midaxillary line between the eleventh and twelfth ribs (Fig. 13.2A). Angle the transducer until the liver edge, diaphragm, and surface of the right kidney are identified. Presence of fluid in Morrison's pouch produces a dark (hypoechoic) shadow between the liver and kidney.

Second, image the heart by placing the probe in the subxiphoid space (Fig. 13.2B), oriented for sagittal sections and angled toward the tip of the left scapula. Identify the bright stripe of the diaphragm and the pulsating heart. Fluid within the pericardial sac appears as a dark layer between the bright (hyperechoic) lines of the pericardium and the myocardium.

Third, place the probe along the left posterior axillary line between the tenth and eleventh ribs (Fig. 13.2C). Angle it toward the patient's umbilicus until the capsule of the spleen and the surface of the left kidney are identified. Free intraperitoneal fluid appears as a dark shadow between these two structures or posterior to the spleen.

Fourth, place the probe 2 to 3 cm above the symphysis pubis and direct the probe 30 degrees caudally (Fig. 13.2D). Orient the probe to obtain a sagittal view. Angle the transducer toward the patient's left and right to scan the retrovesi-

cal space or pouch of Douglas. Rotate the probe 90 degrees to obtain a transverse image of the bladder. Free fluid appears as a dark shadow behind the bladder or uterus and may compress the posterior surface of the bladder. The optimal view is obtained in the presence of a full bladder. If the bladder is empty, place a Foley catheter and infuse with normal saline.

The presence of intraperitoneal fluid in the setting of abdominal trauma suggests intraabdominal injury with hemorrhage.

13.3. URINARY BLADDER ULTRASOUND

Indications

1. To facilitate urethral catheterization or suprapubic bladder aspiration (SBA)
2. To document bladder volume in order to distinguish dehydration from bladder outlet obstruction

Complications

Complications are the same as for standard urethral catheterization or SBA but should be less frequent. Ultrasound measurement of bladder volume to confirm the presence of urine should decrease the number of attempts needed for successful urine collection. When used as an adjunct to SBA, ultrasound should reduce the complication rate. There are no reported harmful effects resulting from the use of ultrasound at energy levels necessary for this procedure.

Equipment

1. Portable ultrasound unit with volumetric calculation capability
2. 3.5- to 7.5-MHz probe
3. Ultrasound gel (sterile for SBA)
4. Sterile transducer sheath for SBA
5. Standard equipment for SBA or urethral catheterization.
6. Sterile marking pen (optional)

Procedure

Bladder Volume Measurement

An assistant should secure the patient supine in a frog-leg position (Fig. 13.3A). Apply ultrasound gel just above the symphysis pubis. Hold the probe on the midline of the abdomen angled in a slight caudad direction. In males, apply gentle pressure at the base of the penis against the symphysis pubis to prevent early voiding when the probe is pressed against the bladder. The bladder appears as an anechoic (black) structure. In the transverse view, the bladder has a characteristically rhomboid shape. Angle the probe in order to obtain the largest diameter. Freeze the image on the screen when the maximum bladder size is visualized. Measure the anterioposterior and transverse diameters. Turn the probe 90 degrees for a longitudinal view. Freeze the maximum diameter view and

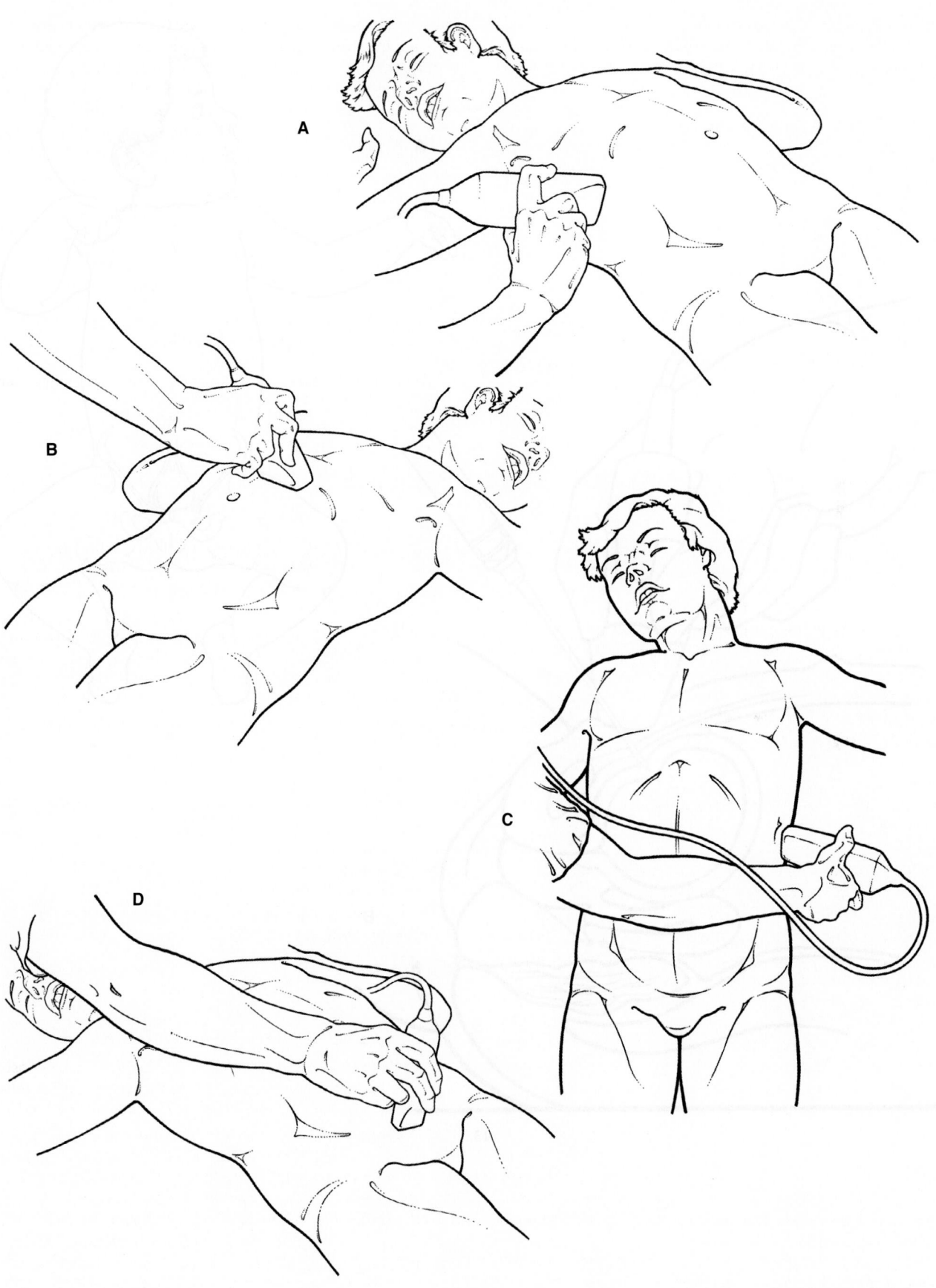

13.2

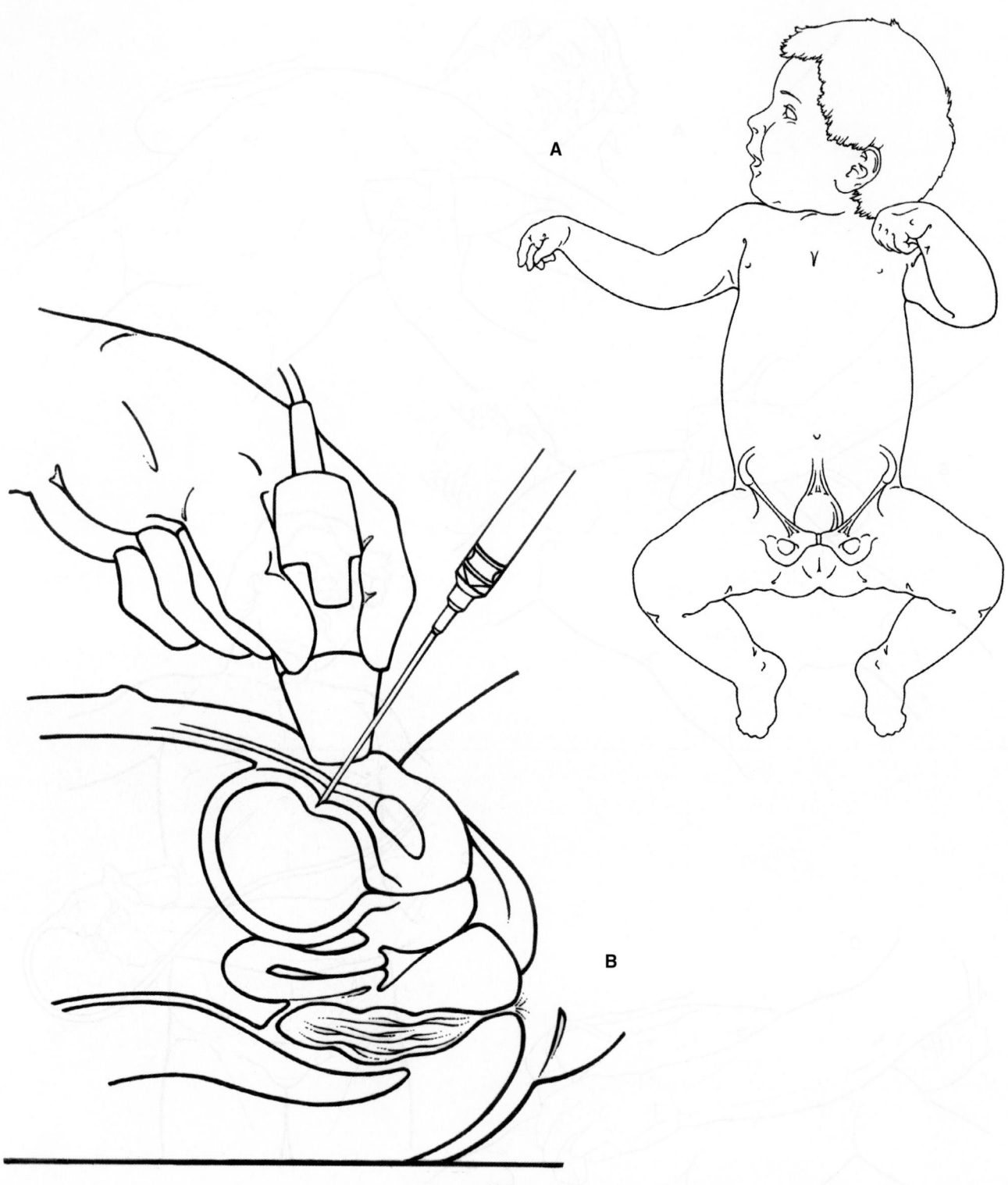

13.3

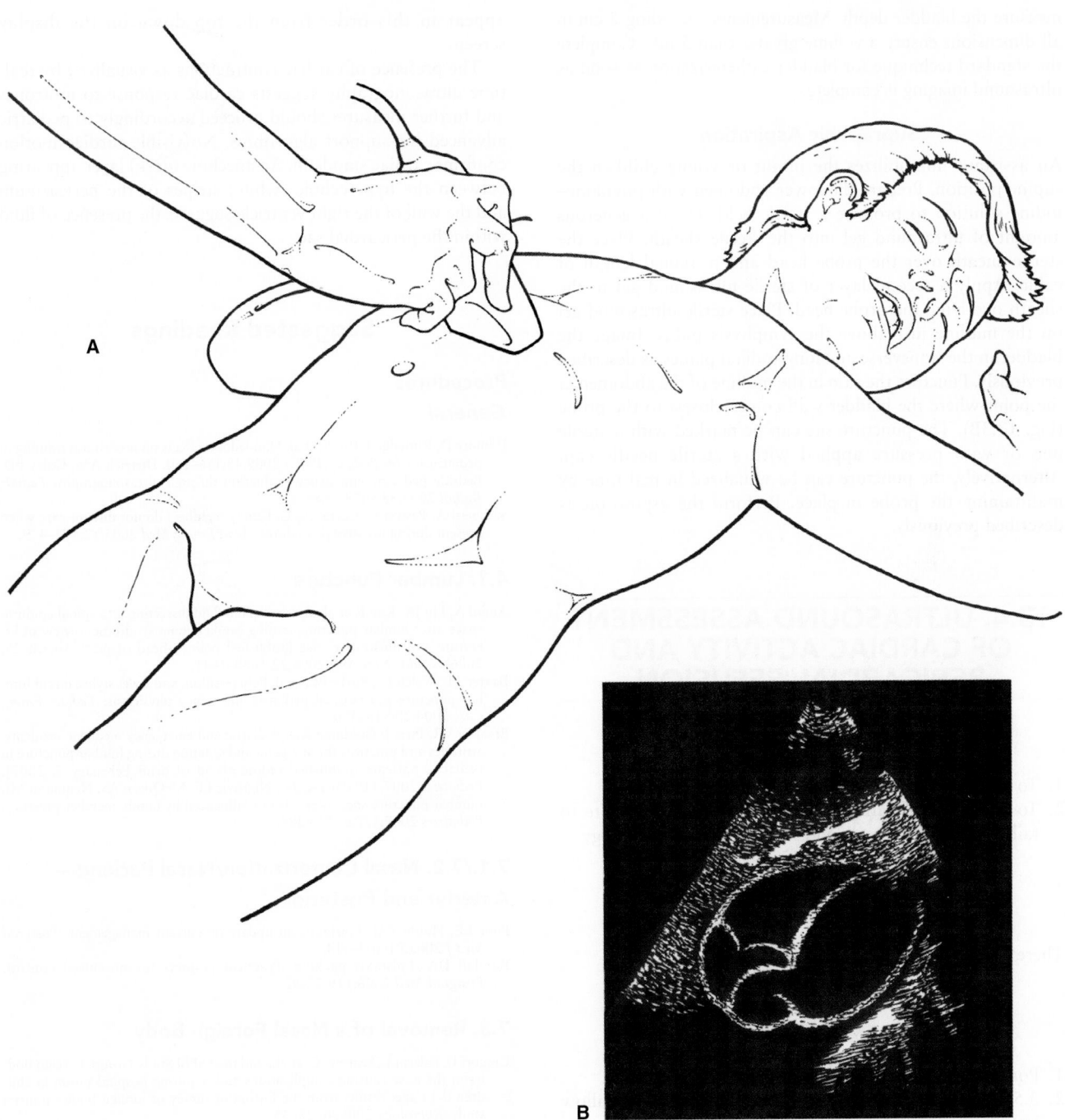

A

B

13.4

measure the bladder depth. Measurements exceeding 2 cm in all dimensions ensure a volume greater than 5 mL. Complete the standard technique for bladder catheterization as soon as ultrasound imaging is complete.

Suprapubic Aspiration

An assistant immobilizes the infant or young child in the supine position. Prepare the lower abdomen with povidone–iodine solution to produce a sterile field. Instill a generous amount of ultrasound gel into the sterile sheath. Place the sterile sheath over the probe head and proximal length of cable. Apply a second layer of sterile ultrasound gel to the sheath overlying the probe head. Place sterile ultrasound gel on the midline just above the symphysis pubis. Image the bladder in the transverse and longitudinal planes as described previously. Puncture the skin in the midline of the abdomen at the point where the bladder wall comes closest to the probe (Fig. 13.3B). The puncture site can be marked with a sterile pen or with pressure applied with a sterile needle cap. Alternatively, the puncture can be visualized in real time by maintaining the probe in place. Perform the aspiration as described previously.

13.4. ULTRASOUND ASSESSMENT OF CARDIAC ACTIVITY AND PERICARDIAL EFFUSION

Indications

1. To view cardiac activity during cardiac resuscitation
2. To diagnose pericardial effusion that may contribute to failed resuscitation or hypotension of unknown etiology

Complications

There are no complications of echocardiography.

Equipment

1. Portable ultrasound unit
2. 3.5 to 5 MHz transducer with a small footprint to allow imaging between the ribs
3. Ultrasound gel

Procedure

The subxiphoid view is the easiest to obtain and most commonly used. With the patient in the supine position, place ultrasound gel over the left costal margin at the xiphoid process. Place the probe in the transverse orientation on the ultrasound gel and pointing at the left shoulder (Fig. 13.4A). Adjust the angle and position of the probe until the bright (hyperechoic) stripe of the diaphragm, the dark (anechoic) pericardial space, and the hyperechoic wall of the right ventricle appear on one image (Fig. 13.4B). These structures

appear in this order from the top down on the display screen.

The presence of cardiac contractions as visualized by real-time ultrasonography suggests cardiac response to inotropes and further measures should proceed accordingly to pediatric advanced life-support algorithms. No visible cardiac motion confirms cardiac standstill. An anechoic (dark) layer appearing between the hyperechoic (white) stripes of the pericardium and the wall of the right ventricle suggests the presence of fluid within the pericardial sac.

Suggested Readings

Procedures

General

Damore D, Rutledge J, Pan S, et al. Handedness effects on procedural training in pediatrics. *Clin Pediatr (Phila)* 2009;48:156–160. Dietrich AM, Coley BD. Bedside pediatric emergency evaluation through ultrasonography. *Pediatr Radiol* 2008;38:S679–S684.

Sacchetti A, Paston C, Carraccio C. Family members do not disrupt care when present during invasive procedures. *Acad Emerg Med* 2005;12:477–479.

4.1. Lumbar Puncture

Amini A, Liu JK, Kan P, et al. Cerebrospinal fluid dissecting into spinal epidural space after lumbar puncture causing cauda equina syndrome: review of literature and illustrative case [published online ahead of print August 25, 2006]. *Childs Nerv Syst* 2006;22:1639–1641.

Baxter AL, Welch JC, Burke BL, et al. Pain position, and stylet styles: infant lumbar puncture practices of pediatric emergency physicians. *Pediatr Emerg Care* 2004;20:816–820.

Breakey VR, Pirie J, Goldman RD. Pediatric and emergency medicine residents' attitudes and practices for analgesia and sedation during lumbar puncture in pediatric patients [published online ahead of print February 5, 2007]. *Pediatrics* 2007;119:e361–e366. Nigrovic LE, McQueen AS, Neumann MI. Lumbar puncture success rate is not influenced by family-member presence. *Pediatrics* 2007;120:e377–e382.

7.1./7.2. Nasal Cauterization/Nasal Packing— Anterior and Posterior

Pope LE, Hobbs CG. Epistaxis: an update on current management. *Postgrad Med J* 2005;81:309–314.

Randall DA. Epistaxis packing. Practical pointers for nosebleed control. *Postgrad Med* 2006;119:77–82.

7.3. Removal of a Nasal Foreign Body

Gregori D, Salerni L, Scarinzi C, et al., and the ESFBI Study Group. Foreign bodies in the nose causing complications and requiring hospitalization in children 0-14 age: results from the European survey of foreign bodies injuries study. *Rhinology* 2008;46:28–33.

Kiger JR, Brenkert TE, Losek JD. Nasal foreign body removal in children. *Pediatr Emerg Care* 2008;24:785–792.

Purohit M, Ray S, Wilson T, et al. The 'parent's kiss': an effective way to remove paediatric nasal foreign bodies. *Ann R Coll Surg Engl* 2008;90:420–422.

7.5. Flexible Nasopharyngolarygoscopy

Hayes JT, Houston R. Flexible nasolaryngoscopy. A low-risk, high-yield procedure. *Postgrad Med* 1999;106:107–110, 114.

7.6. Endotracheal Intubation

American Heart Association. 2005 American Heart Association (AHA) guidelines for cardiopulmonary resuscitation (CPR) and emergency cardiovascular care (ECC) of pediatric and neonatal patients: pediatric basic life support. *Pediatrics* 2006;117:e989–e1004.

Duracher C, Schmautz E, Martinon C, et al. Evaluation of cuffed tracheal tube size predicted using the Khine formula in children. *Pediatr Anaesth* 2008;18:113–118.

7.7. Cricothyroidotomy/Percutaneous Tracheotomy

De Leyn P, Bedert L, Delcroix M, et al., and Belgian Association of Pneumology and Belgian Association of Cardiothoracic Surgery. Tracheotomy: clinical review and guidelines. *Eur J Cardiothorac Surg* 2007;32:412–421.

Helm M, Gries A, Mutzbauer T. Surgical approach in difficult airway management. *Best Pract Res Clin Anaesthesiol* 2005;19:623–640.

Patel KG, Zdanski CJ. Cricothyroidotomy vs. sternal tracheotomy for challenging airway anatomy. *Laryngoscope* 2008;118:1827–1829.

Scrase I, Woollard M. Needle vs surgical cricothyroidotomy: a short cut to effective ventilation. *Anaesthesia* 2006;61:962–974.

8.1. Insertion of a Chest Tube

Dev SP, Nascimiento B Jr, Simone C, et al. Videos in clinical medicine. Chest-tube insertion. *N Engl J Med* 2007;357:e15.

8.3. Resuscitative Thoracotomy

Hunt PA, Greaves I, Owens WA. Emergency thoracotomy in thoracic trauma—a review. *Injury* 2006;37:1–19.

Ladd AP, Gomez GA, Jacobson LE, et al. Emergency room thoracotomy: updated guidelines for a level I trauma center. *Am Surg* 2002;68:421–424.

9.2. Emergency Transvenous Pacing

Francis GS, Williams SV, Achord JL, et al. Clinical competence in insertion of a temporary transvenous ventricular pacemaker. A statement for physicians from the ACP/ACC/AHA Task Force on Clinical Privileges in Cardiology. *Circulation* 1994;89:1913–1916.

Wald DA. Therapeutic procedures in the emergency department patient with acute myocardial infarction. *Emerg Med Clin North Am* 2001;19:451–467.

Overbay D, Criddle L. Mastering temporary invasive cardiac pacing. *Crit Care Nurse* 2004;24:25–32.

10.3. Peritoneal Lavage

American College of Surgeons Committee on Trauma. *Advanced trauma life support for doctors; student manual*, 7th ed. Chicago: Second Impression, 2005.

Hodgson NF, Stewart TC, Girotti MJ. Open or closed diagnostic peritoneal lavage for abdominal trauma? A meta-analysis. *J Trauma* 2000;48:1091–1095.

Nagy KK, Roberts RR, Joseph KT, et al. Experience with over 2500 diagnostic peritoneal lavages. *Injury* 2000;31:479–482.

10.4. Replacement of a Gastrostomy Tube

Burke DR, El Shami A, Heinle E, et al. Comparision of gastrostomy tube replacement verification using air insufflation versus gastrograffin. *Arch Phys Med Rehabil* 2006;87:1530–1533.

Wu TS, Leech SJ, Rosenberg M, et al. Ultrasound can accurately guide gastrostomy tube replacement and confirm proper tube placement at the bedside. *J Emerg Med* 2009;36:280–284.

10.5. Reduction of an incarcerated Inguinal Hernia

Goldman RD, Balasubramanian S, Wales P, et al. Pediatric surgeons and pediatric emergency physicians' attitudes towards analgesia and sedation for incarcerated inguinal hernia reduction. *J Pain* 2005;6:650–655.

Niedzielski J, Kr I R, Gawlowska A. Could incarceration of inguinal hernia in children be prevented? *Med Sci Monit* 2003;9:CR16–CR18.

10.6. Rectal Prolapse

Antao B, Bradley V, Roberts JP, et al. Management of rectal prolapse in children. *Dis Colon Rectum* 2005;48:1620–1625.

Zempsky WT, Rosenstein BJ. The cause of rectal prolapse in children. *Am J Dis Child* 1988;142:338–339.

12.1. Incision and Drainage of an Abscess

Duong M, Markwell S, Peter J, et al. Randomized, controlled trial of antibiotics in the management of community-acquired skin abscesses in the pediatric patient [published online ahead of print April 29, 2009]. *Ann Emerg Med.* doi:10.1016/Jannnemergmed.2009.03.14

Hast MB, Klasner A, Kness S, et al. Cutaneous community-associated methicillin-resistant staphylococcal aureus among all skin and soft-tissue infections in two geographically distant pediatric emergency departments. *Acad Emerg Med* 2007;14:35–40.

Seal J, Glynn L, Statter M, et al. A high prevalence of methicillin-resistant *Staphylococcal aureus* among surgically drained soft-tissue infections in pediatric patients. *Pediatr Surg Int* 2006;22:683–687.

12.2B. Shoulder (Glenohumeral) Joint

Harvey RA, Trabulsy ME, Roe L. Are postreduction anteroposterior and scapular Y views useful in anterior dislocations? *Am J Emerg Med* 1992;10:149–151.

Itoi E, Hatakeyama Y, Kido T, et al. A new method of immobilization after traumatic anterior dislocation of the shoulder: a preliminary study. *J Shoulder Elbow Surg* 2003;12:413–415.

Miller BS, Sonnabend DH, Hatrick C, et al. Should acute anterior dislocations of the shoulder be immobilized in external rotation? A cadaveric study. *J Shoulder Elbow Surg* 2004;13:589–592.

Tannebaum RD, Kondabala RK, Stockmal PJ. Postreduction radiographs after anterior shoulder dislocation: a reappraisal. *Ann Emerge Med* 2001;37:418–419.

12.2C. Patella

Saunders TG, Paruchuri NB, Zlatkin MB. MRI of osteochondral defects of the lateral femoral condyle: incidence and pattern of injury after transient lateral dislocation of the patella. *AJR Am J Roentgenol* 2006;187:1332–1337.

Zaida A, Babyn P, Astori I, et al. MRI of traumatic dislocations in children. *Pediatr Radiol* 2006;36:1163–1170.

12.2D. Hip

Herrera-Soto JA, Price CT. Traumatic hip dislocations in children and adults: pitfalls and complications. *J Am Acad Orthop Surg* 2009;17:15–21.

Mehlman CT, Hubbard GW, Crawford AH, et al. Traumatic hip dislocation in children. Long-term follow up of 42 patients. *Clin Orthop Relat Res* 2000;376:68–79.

Vialle R, Odent T, Pannier S, et al. Traumatic hip dislocation in children. *J Pediatr Orthop* 2005;25:138–144.

Vontobel BJ, Hocevar Z, Jakob RP. Avascular necrosis following traumatic hip dislocation in an 8-year-old boy. *Arch Orthop Trauma Surg* 1994;113:83–85.

12.2E. Elbow

Cohen MS, Hastings H II. Acute elbow dislocation: evaluation and management. *J Am Acad Orthop Surg* 1998;6:15–23.

Kuhn MA, Ross G. Acute elbow dislocations. *Orthop Clin North Am* 2008;39:155–161.

Mehta JA, Bain GI. Elbow dislocations in adults and children. *Clin Sports Med* 2004;23:609–627.

Ross G. Acute elbow dislocation: on-site treatment. *Phys Sportsmed.* 1999;27:121–122.

Sheps DM, Hildebrand KA, Boorman RS. Simple dislocations of the elbow: evaluation and treatment. *Hand Clin* 2004;20:389–404.

Villarin LA Jr, Belk KE, Fried R. Emergency department evaluation and treatment of elbow and forearm injuries. *Emerg Med Clin North Am* 1999;17:843–858.

12.9. Hair Tourniquet Removal

Alverson B. A genital hair tourniquet in a 9-year old girl. *Pediatr Emerg Care* 2007;23:169–170.

Bacon JL, Burgis JT. Hair thread tourniquet syndrome in adolescents: a presentation and review of the literature. *J Pediatr Adolesc Gynecol* 2005;18:1555–1556.

Chegwissdden HJ, Poirier MP. Near strangulation as a result of hair tourniquet syndrome. *Clin Pediatr(Phila)* 2005;44:359–361.

12.10A. Knee Joint

Wiler JL, Costantino TG, Filippone L, et al. Comparison of ultrasound-guided and standard landmark techniques for knee arthrocentesis [published online ahead of print December 4, 2008]. *J Emerg Med.*

PROCEDURES

12.15. Reduction of Nursemaid's Elbow

Green DA, Linares MY, Garcia Pena BM, et al. Randomized comparison of pain perception during radial head subluxation reduction using supination-flexion or forced pronation. *Pediatr Emerg Care* 2006;22:235–238.

Macias CG, Bothner J, Wiebe R. A comparison of supination/flexion to hyperpronation in the reduction of radial head subluxations. *Pediatrics* 1998; 102:e10.

McDonald J, Whitelaw C, Goldsmith LJ. Radial head subluxation: comparing two methods of reduction. *Acad Emerg Med* 1999;6:715–718.

12.16. Application of a Figure-of-eight Harness

Chalidis B, Sachinis N, Samoladas E, et al. Acute management of clavicle fractures. A long term functional outcome study. *Acta Orthop Belg* 2008;74: 303–307.

Lenza M, Belloti JC, Andriolo RB, et al. Conservative interventions for treating middle third clavicle fractures in adolescents and adults. *Cochrane Database Syst Rev* 2009;15:CD007121.

Nordqvist A, Petersson CJ, Reflund-Johnell I. Mid-clavicle fractures in adults: end result study after conservative treatment. *J Orthop Trauma* 1998;12: 572–576.

APPENDIX A ■ PEDIATRIC EMERGENCY MEDICINE EQUIPMENT

STEPHEN LUDWIG, MD

A-1 EMERGENCY DEPARTMENT

1. Airway

1.1 Tongue depressors
1.2 Suction catheters, 6F, 8F, 10F (2 of each)
1.3 Yankauer suction tips (4)
1.4 Magill forceps (small, medium, large) (1 each)
1.5 Oxygen catheters for suction, 10F, 14F (2 of each)
1.6 Oropharyngeal airways, 4–10 (2 of each)
1.7 Nasopharyngeal airways, 12F, 14F, 16F, 18F, 20F, 22F, 24F, 26F, 28F, 30F (2 of each)
1.8 Tracheostomy Tubes, multiple sizes, types
1.9 Humidivent
1.10 Meconium aspirator

2. Breathing

2.1 Oxygen supply
2.2 Oxygen flow meter
2.3 Oxygen tubing
2.4 Cylinder key
2.5 Oxygen masks
2.6 Nasal cannula
2.7 Nonrebreather mask
2.8 Nebulizer and administration equipment
2.9 Self-inflating bags with oxygen reservoir (adult, infant)
2.10 Mapleson D bags with reservoir (0.5 L, 1 L, 5 L)
2.11 Laryngoscope handle with knurled finish (small, large)
2.12 Laryngoscope blades
    2.12.1 Miller 0, 1, 2, 3
    2.12.2 Wis-Hipple 1.5
    2.12.3 MacIntosh 2, 3, 4
2.13 Extra "C" batteries (2), "AA" batteries (2)
2.14 Extra laryngoscope bulbs
2.15 Endotracheal tubes
    2.15.1 Uncuffed sizes 2.5–8.5 (2 of each)
    2.15.2 Cuffed sizes 3.5, 4.0, 4.5, 5.0, 6.0, 7.0, 8.0 (2 of each)
2.16 Laryngeal mask airways
2.17 Stylets (1 adult, 1 infant)
2.18 Easycap (ETCO$_2$ analyzer), 2 sizes
2.19 Disposable Manometer, 15 mm, 22 mm

3. Circulation

3.1 Stat IV tray
3.2 Central venous pressure tray, 5, 10, 11 (2 of each)
3.3 Cutdown tray (2)
3.4 Umbilical catheterization tray
3.5 Intraosseous needles—16, 18 (2 of each); EZ-IO (3 sizes)
3.6 Radial artery tray (2.5F, 5 cm; 2.5F, 2.5 cm)
3.7 Drugs, prepackaged
    3.7.1 Epinephrine 1:1,000; 1:10,000
    3.7.2 Dextrose (D 25%) (D 10%)
    3.7.3 Atropine
    3.7.4 Sodium bicarbonate
    3.7.5 Calcium chloride
    3.7.6 Lidocaine 2%
3.8 Drugs
    3.8.1 Acyclovir
    3.8.2 Adenosine
    3.8.3 Afrin® nasal spray
    3.8.4 Amiodarone
    3.8.5 Ampicillin
    3.8.6 Benadryl®
    3.8.7 Bretylium
    3.8.8 Calcium gluconate
    3.8.9 Cefotaxime
    3.8.10 Ceftriaxone
    3.8.11 Charcoal
    3.8.12 Clindamycin
    3.8.13 Cyanide kit (Hydroxocobalamin)
    3.8.14 Dexamethasone
    3.8.15 Diazepam
    3.8.16 Diazoxide
    3.8.17 Digoxin
    3.8.18 Dilantin
    3.8.19 Diphenhydramine
    3.8.20 Dobutamine
    3.8.21 Dopamine
    3.8.22 Fentanyl
    3.8.23 Flumazenil
    3.8.24 Furosemide
    3.8.25 Gastrografin
    3.8.26 Gentamicin
    3.8.27 Glucagon
    3.8.28 Haloperidol
    3.8.29 Heparin vial

3.8.30 Hydralazine
3.8.31 Hydrocortisone
3.8.32 Insulin
3.8.33 Isoproterenol
3.8.34 Ketamine
3.8.35 Ketorolac
3.8.36 Lidocaine 1%
3.8.37 Lidocaine 2%
3.8.38 Magnesium sulfate
3.8.39 Mannitol
3.8.40 Midazolam
3.8.41 Milrinone
3.8.42 Morphine
3.8.43 Meperidine
3.8.44 Methylprednisolone
3.8.45 Naloxone (1 mg per mL)
3.8.46 Neostigmine
3.8.47 Nifedipine
3.8.48 Nitroprusside
3.8.49 Norepinephrine (Levophed®)
3.8.50 Oxacillin
3.8.51 Pentobarbital
3.8.52 Phenobarbital
3.8.53 Procainamide
3.8.54 Prostaglandin
3.8.55 Risperidone
3.8.56 Solu-Medrol®
3.8.57 Terbutaline
3.8.58 Thiopental
3.8.59 3% Saline
3.8.60 Vasopressin
3.8.61 Vancomycin
3.8.62 Vecuronium
3.8.63 Verapamil
3.9 IV fluids
  3.9.1 Tubing
  3.9.2 Stopcocks
  3.9.3 Normal saline solution, 1 L (10 bags)
  3.9.4 Lactated Ringer's solution, 1 L (10 bags)
  3.9.5 Albumin 5%, 25%
3.10 Syringes
3.11 Alcohol pads
3.12 Needles (all sizes)
3.13 Broselow Tape™ or dosage wall chart
3.14 Infusion pumps (3)
3.15 Cardiac board
3.16 Arm boards
3.17 Tape
3.18 Tincture of benzoin
3.19 Tegaderm

4. Monitoring

4.1 Sphygmomanometer Doppler and aneroid
4.2 Blood pressure cuffs (neonate, child, adult, large adult, thigh)
4.3 EKG/leads
4.4 Pulse oximeter
4.5 End-tidal CO_2 monitor
4.6 Doppler (handheld)
4.7 Defibrillator/defibrillator paste
4.8 Temperature probe
4.9 Hypothermia thermometer
4.10 Blood pressure-monitoring lines
4.11 Intracranial pressure-monitoring lines

5. Laboratory Testing

5.1 Syringes
5.2 Needles
5.3 Alcohol pads
5.4 Betadine
5.5 Tubes including culture media
5.6 Blood gas kit
5.7 Point-of-care testing (i-STAT)
5.8 Glucometer, test strips
5.9 Hemoccult cards
5.10 Sterile basins, bedpans, urinals
5.11 Evidence bags
5.12 Shroud, autopsy permits, related supplies

6. Trauma Care

6.1 Cervical collars: Stifneck® Baby no-neck or Pediatric no-neck, short, regular
6.2 Nasogastric tubes, 10, 16 (2 of each)
6.3 Feeding tubes, 3.5F–8F (2 of each)
6.4 Foley catheters, catheterization tray
6.5 Tracheostomy tray (2)
6.6 Thoracentesis tray
6.7 Chest tube insertion (2)
6.8 Chest tubes, 12F, 16F, 20F, 24F, 28F, 32F, 34F, 40F (2 of each)
6.9 Pleurovac
6.10 Thoracotomy tray
6.11 Minor procedure tray (3)
6.12 Peritoneal tray (11F dialysis set)
6.13 Obstetric pack
6.14 Blood administration sets
6.15 Blood warmer
6.16 Pressure bags
6.17 Garder-Walls tongs
6.18 Hare traction splint
6.19 Scalpels no. 10, 11, 15
6.20 Suture material (1 box of each):
  2.0 Silk ties
  3.0 Silk
  4.0 Vicryl
  Tevdek cardiovascular, 2.0, 4.0, 5.0
  TFE polymer pledgets (8677-01)
  TFE polymer pledgets (8675-01)

7. Other

7.1 Protective supplies
  7.1.1 Gloves, nonlatex (small, medium, large) (5 each)

7.1.2 Gowns
7.1.3 Masks
7.1.4 Shoe covers
7.1.5 Protective eye goggles/Fluidshield mask
7.1.6 Needle receptacles
7.1.7 Caps
7.2 Stat worksheet on clipboard
7.3 Key phone numbers
7.4 Drug formulary
7.5 Drug labels
7.6 Scissors, heavy gauge
7.7 Flashlight
7.8 Ophthalmoscope
7.9 Otoscope
7.10 Overbed warmers
7.11 Blankets
7.12 Bair hugger
7.13 Hand print kit

8. Transport Equipment

8.1 Portable suction
8.2 Portable monitors
8.3 Infusion pump
8.4 Airway box
8.5 Drug box

A-2 OFFICE OR CLINIC

1. Airway Equipment

1.1 Oxygen tank with flow meter
1.2 Face masks
1.3 Oxygen reservoir masks
1.4 Nasal cannula
1.5 Oxygen tubing
1.6 Oropharyngeal airways (all sizes)
1.7 Nasopharyngeal airways (all sizes)
1.8 Suction machine, portable
1.9 Suction catheters
1.10 Yankauer suction tips (4)
1.11 Magill forceps (small, medium, large)

2. Breathing Equipment

2.1 Bag-valve-mask with O_2 reservoir (adult, pediatric)
2.2 Masks (infant to adult sizes)
2.3 Pulse oximeter

3. Circulation Equipment

3.1 Cardiac board
3.2 IV catheter—25, 23, 21 (3 of each)
3.3 IV catheter—22, 20, 16 (3 of each)
3.4 Intraosseous needles (4)
3.5 Normal saline 5% dextrose, 500 mL (2)
3.6 Normal saline solution, 500 mL (2)
3.7 Solusets (2)
3.8 Sphygmomanometers—cuffs (4 sizes)
3.9 Drug box—prepackaged syringes
    3.9.1 Epinephrine 1:10,000
    3.9.2 Sodium bicarbonate, full strength
    3.9.3 Sodium bicarbonate, half strength
    3.9.4 Dextrose, 25%
    3.9.5 Atropine, 0.4 mg per 0.5 mL
    3.9.6 Naloxone
    3.9.7 Diazepam/lorazepam
    3.9.8 Phenobarbital
    3.9.9 Activated charcoal
    3.9.10 Tourniquets
    3.9.11 Betadine swabs
    3.9.12 Alcohol swabs
    3.9.13 Tape
    3.9.14 Syringes
    3.9.15 Arm boards

4. Other Equipment

4.1 Resuscitation cart checklist
4.2 Semirigid cervical collars (adult, pediatric)
4.3 Sandbags (3)
4.4 Splints, inflatable
4.5 Nasogastric tubes
4.6 Rubber gloves
4.7 Protective eyewear
4.8 Broselow Tape™ or wall chart

APPENDIX B ■ EMERGENCY DRUG COMPENDIUM

SHANNON F. MANZI, PHARMD

Appendix B provides an easily accessible resource for dosages and side effects of medications included in the main text. The dosages included here are based on literature available at the time the text was prepared. For medications that are relatively new to pediatrics (e.g., dexmedetomidine), further refinement in drug dosage recommendations will undoubtedly occur. Other frequently updated drug information resources, such as the online Lexi-Comp's Pediatric Dosing Handbook (updated continuously), American Hospital Formulary Service (updated quarterly), or Facts and Comparisons (updated monthly) may provide additional information. Finally, for added safety, prescribers should check the package insert and/or one or two additional resources for dosage information whenever prescribing an unfamiliar drug. Some medications only have the commonly used dosage forms listed.

A list of the abbreviations used and their definitions is presented at the end of this appendix. Please note that all drugs listed are to be given IV may also be given via an IO line.

RESUSCITATION DRUG LIST

Drug: ADENOSINE (ADENOCARD®)
Route of Administration: IV
Dose: *SVT; Initial:* 0.1 mg per kg per dose (max 6 mg per dose)
Subsequent: neonates: Increase by increments of 0.05 mg per kg to a maximum of 0.25 mg per kg per dose; *children:* Increase by increments of 0.1 mg per kg per dose (max 12 mg per dose) to a maximum of 0.3 mg per kg. Allow 2 minutes between incremental increases.
Precautions: Administer by rapid bolus IV injection over 1-2 seconds simultaneously with a rapid saline flush of 5-10 mL; use 3- or 4-way stopcock, if necessary. Continuous EKG and BP monitoring is mandatory. Theophylline and caffeine may antagonize the effect of adenosine; therefore, patients receiving these drugs may require higher dosages of adenosine.
Adverse Effects: Sinus bradycardia, ventricular ectopy
Availability: Injection: 3 mg per mL

Drug: ALPROSTADIL (PROSTIN VR Pediatric®)
Synonyms: Prostaglandin, PGE₁
Route of Administration: IV
Dose: *Initial: neonates and infants:* 0.05 to 0.1 mcg per kg per minute; *maintenance:* 0.01 to 0.4 mcg per kg per minute
Precautions: Dose should be titrated to lowest rate that produces desired side effects. Apnea occurs in approximately 10% of neonates with congenital heart defects within first hour of infusion.
Adverse Effects: Severe hypotension, apnea, bradycardia
Availability: Injection: 500 mcg per mL

Drug: AMIODARONE (CORDARONE®)
Use caution, sound-alike drugs include: Amrinone (Inocor®)
Route of Administration: IV
Dose: *VF/VT arrest:* 5 mg per kg IV rapid push (max 300 mg per dose)
Dysrhythmia (unstable): 5 mg per kg IV over 20 to 60 minutes (max 300 mg per dose)
Continuous infusion for tachyarrhythmias: 5 to 15 mcg per kg per minute
Precautions: Dilute with D5W only for continuous infusion. Up to 75% of patients will experience adverse effects. Many drug–drug interactions due to cytochrome P450 inhibition.
Adverse Effects: Arrhythmias, cardiogenic shock, hypotension, hepatotoxicity, headache, pulmonary fibrosis and interstitial pneumonitis, skin discoloration
Availability: Injection: 50 mg per mL

Drug: ATROPINE
Route of Administration: IV, ETT
Dose: *Initial:* 0.02 mg per kg (min single dose: 0.1 mg; max single dose: 1 mg adolescent, 2 mg adult). For ETT use, dose is 2 to 10 times the IV dose. Dilute with normal saline (NS) to a volume of 3 to 5 mL and follow with several positive-pressure breaths.
Subsequent: The initial dose may be repeated every 5 to 10 minutes to a maximum cumulative dose of 2 mg.
Note: Much higher doses are necessary in organophosphate/nerve agent toxicity.
Precautions: A minimum dose of 0.1 mg should be administered to avoid the paradoxical bradycardia that may occur with lower dosages.

1846

Adverse Effects: Tachycardia, excessive drying of secretions, mydriasis

Availability: Injection: many strengths available; most common concentrations are 0.4, 0.5, and 1 mg per mL

Drug: CALCIUM CHLORIDE

Use caution, sound-alike drugs include: Calcium gluconate

Route of Administration: IV

Dose: *Initial:* Calcium chloride: 20 mg per kg (max 1,000 mg per dose)

Subsequent: The initial dose may be repeated once, 10 minutes following initial dose. Total maximum dose 2,000 mg.

Precautions: Calcium chloride must be diluted and should be given through a central IV line whenever possible. Scalp, hand, and foot veins should not be used for administration unless in life-threatening situation. Calcium in any form should be infused slowly while monitoring the patient for bradycardia. Do not admix calcium with any solution containing sodium bicarbonate or phosphate salts (a fatal precipitation can occur). Calcium is contraindicated in digitalis toxicity. Calcium may antagonize the effects of verapamil.

Adverse Effects: Hypercalcemia, cardiac arrest, venous irritation.

Note: Extravasation may cause severe necrosis and sloughing.

Availability: Injection: 1 g in 10 mL (13.5 mEq calcium per g)

Drug: CALCIUM GLUCONATE

Use caution, sound-alike drugs include: Calcium chloride

Route of Administration: IV

Dose: *Initial:* Calcium gluconate: 100 mg per kg (max 3,000 mg per dose)

Subsequent: The initial dose may be repeated once, 10 minutes following initial dose. Total maximum dose 3,000 mg.

Precautions: Calcium gluconate should be diluted and ideally be given only through a central IV line; however, a large peripheral line may be used, if necessary. Calcium in any form should be infused slowly while monitoring the patient for bradycardia. Do not admix calcium with any solution containing sodium bicarbonate or phosphate salts (a fatal precipitation can occur). Calcium is contraindicated in digitalis toxicity. Calcium may antagonize the effects of verapamil.

Adverse Effects: Hypercalcemia, cardiac arrest, venous irritation.

Note: Extravasation may cause severe necrosis and sloughing.

Availability: Injection: 1 g in 10 mL (4.5 mEq of calcium per g)

Drug: DEXTROSE

Route of Administration: IV

Dose: *Initial:* 0.5 to 1 g per kg administered slowly (2 to 4 mL per kg of a 25% dextrose or 5 to 10 mL per kg of a 10% dextrose solution). If 25% dextrose is not available, dilute 50% dextrose 1:1 with sterile water or NS for injection to yield a 25% solution. Concentrations of continuous infusions greater than 12.5% should be infused via a central line when possible. For neonates with hypoglycemia, a dose of 0.25 to 0.5 g per kg (2.5 to 5 mL per kg) of a 10% dextrose solution should be used.

Subsequent: Subsequent doses and infusions should be based on the serum glucose concentration.

Adverse Effects: Hyperglycemia, hyperosmolarity

Availability: Injection: 0.1 g per mL (10% dextrose/water), 0.25 g per mL (25% dextrose/water), 0.5 g per mL (50% dextrose/water)

Drug: DOBUTAMINE (DOBUTREX®)

Use caution, sound-alike drugs include: Dopamine

Route of Administration: IV

Dose: 2 to 20 mcg per kg per minute (titrate to desired cardiovascular effect)

Precautions: Unstable in alkaline solutions. Solutions containing sodium bicarbonate should not be admixed with dobutamine. May begin administration via a peripheral line, changing to central access as soon as possible.

Adverse Effects: Tachycardia, exaggerated hypertensive response, ventricular ectopy

Availability: Injection: concentrate for IV infusion (must be further diluted): 12.5 mg per mL

Drug: DOPAMINE (INTROPIN®)

Use caution, sound-alike drugs include: Dobutamine

Route of Administration: IV

Dose: 2 to 20 mcg per kg per minute (titrate to desired renal or cardiovascular effect). If low perfusion state persists following adequate volume replacement, begin infusion at 10 mcg per kg per minute. Titrate as needed.

Precautions: Dopamine is unstable in alkaline solutions. Solutions containing sodium bicarbonate should not be admixed with dopamine (inactivation of dopamine may occur). May begin administration via a peripheral line, changing to central access as soon as possible.

Adverse Effects: Hypertension, tachycardia, and vasoconstriction may be seen with high infusion rates.

Availability: Injection (must be further diluted): 40 mg per mL

Drug: EPINEPHRINE

Route of Administration: IM, IV, ETT, SC

Dose: *Initial:* 10 mcg per kg (0.1 mL per kg of 1:10,000 solution) IV (max initial dose: 5 mL)

Subsequent: All subsequent doses should be the same as the initial dose. Beta-blocker overdose may require high dose (1:1,000) at 0.1 mL per kg if no response.

Intramuscular: 0.01 mL per kg (1:1,000 solution) max 0.5 mg per dose

Continuous infusion: 0.1 to 1 mcg per kg per minute.

Endotracheal: 0.1 mg per kg (0.1 mL of 1:1,000 solution) diluted in 3 to 5 mL of saline followed by several positive-pressure breaths.

Precautions: Epinephrine is inactivated in the presence of bicarbonate. Extravasations should be treated immediately with phentolamine.

Adverse Effects: Hypotension, hypertension, tachycardia, vasoconstriction

Availability: Injection: 100 mcg per mL (1:10,000); 1 mg per mL (1:1,000): Autoinjector: 0.15 mg, 0.3 mg

Drug: ETOMIDATE (AMIDATE®)

Route of Administration: IV

Dose: *RSI:* 0.3 mg per kg IV × 1 dose

Procedural Sedation: 0.15 mg per kg per dose IV PRN sedation × 2 doses

Precautions: May result in adrenal suppression if multiple doses or continuous infusion used. May cause pain on injection.

Adverse Effects: Injection site pain, involuntary skeletal muscle movement, nausea, and vomiting

Availability: Injection: 2 mg per mL

Drug: FLUMAZENIL (ROMAZICON®)

Route of Administration: IV

Dose: *Benzodiazepine reversal:* 0.01 mg per kg IV × 1 dose (max 0.2 mg per dose); may repeat as needed to a max of 0.05 mg per kg or 1 mg total, whichever is less.

Precautions: Use caution if patient is dependent on benzodiazepines. May result in abrupt withdrawal precipitating hypertension, myocardial infarction, and seizures.

Adverse Effects: Arrhythmias, hyper/hypotension, acute withdrawal symptoms

Availability: Injection: 0.1 mg per mL

Drug: KETAMINE (KETALAR®)

Use caution, sound-alike drugs include: Ketorolac (Toradol®)

Route of Administration: IV, IM

Dose: *Rapid sequence intubation:* 1 to 2 mg per kg IV or 3 to 7 mg per kg IM (1 dose)

See general medication section for procedural sedation dosing.

Precautions: Avoid use in patients with suspected head trauma or seizures of unknown origin, may increase ICP.

Adverse Effects: Laryngospasms, emergence reactions, tachycardia, hypertension

Availability: Injection: 10, 50, and 100 mg per mL

Drug: ISOPROTERENOL (ISUPREL®)

Route of Administration: IV infusion

Dose: 0.1 to 1 mcg per kg per minute

Precautions: Isoproterenol may aggravate arrhythmias associated with digitalis toxicity. In the dehydrated or hypovolemic patient, the vasodilatory properties of isoproterenol may produce exaggerated hypotension. Commercially available products contain sulfites and should be used with caution in patients known to be sensitive to sulfiting agents.

Adverse Effects: Tachyarrhythmias, myocardial ischemia, hypotension, hypertension, tremor, agitation

Availability: Injection: 0.02, 0.2 mg per mL

Drug: LIDOCAINE (XYLOCAINE®)

Route of Administration: IV, ETT

Dose: *Initial:* 1 mg per kg (max 100 mg per dose) IV over 2 to 4 minutes (maximum rate 0.7 mg per kg per minute or 50 mg per minute, whichever is less)

Note: If using via ETT, dose is two to four times the IV dose diluted in 3 to 5 mL of saline and followed by several positive-pressure breaths.

Subsequent: Initial dose may be repeated up to two to three times at 5- to 10-minute intervals (maximum dose during a 1-hour period: 200 to 300 mg). Once the initial bolus has been given, a continuous infusion of lidocaine at 20 to 50 mcg per kg per minute should be initiated. Lidocaine serum concentrations should be monitored.

Precautions: Dosage must be modified in children with CHF, shock, or liver disease.

Adverse Effects: *Early:* nausea, vomiting, altered CNS status, paresthesias

Later: seizures, cardiac toxicity (myocardial depression, arrhythmias)

Availability: Injection: various concentrations ranging from 10 to 200 mg per mL (dilute to a concentration of 10 to 20 mg per mL for IV push and 8 mg per mL for continuous infusion before use)

Drug: LORAZEPAM (ATIVAN®)

Route of Administration: IV, IM

Dose: *Status epilepticus:* 0.1 mg per kg per dose (max 4 mg per dose) IV/IM q5min × 2 to 3 doses

Continuous infusion: 0.05 to 0.1 mg per kg per hour

Precautions: Contains large amounts of propylene glycol, may result in metabolic acidosis, do NOT use in neonates as a continuous infusion. Precipitation may occur if final concentration is less than 1 mg per mL.

Adverse Effects: CNS depression, hypotension, bradycardia, respiratory depression

Availability: Injection: 2, 4 mg per mL

Drug: METHYLPREDNISOLONE SODIUM SUCCINATE (SOLU-MEDROL®)

Route of Administration: IV, IM

Dose: *Initial shock, acute SLE, multiple sclerosis, transverse myelitis:* 30 mg per kg by IV infusion over 15 to

30 minutes, max 1,500 mg per dose; *acute asthma and allergic reactions*: 1 to 2 mg per kg by slow IV push over 5 to 10 minutes (usual max 80 mg per dose).

Precautions: Use of high-dose methylprednisolone in treatment of shock and spinal cord injury remains controversial.

Adverse Effects: Hypotension and vasodilation may occur with rapid IV injection. Electrolyte abnormalities, mood disturbances, infection.

Availability: Injection: 40, 125, 500 mg; 1 or 2 g (powder for reconstitution).

Drug: NALOXONE (NARCAN®)
Route of Administration: IV, IM, SC, ETT
Dose: *Dose depends on degree of reversal needed.
Initial: age birth to 5 years (weight <20 kg): 0.1 mg per kg per dose; *age older than 5 years*: 2 mg per dose (max initial dose: 2 mg). Higher doses may be needed in refractory adults. If giving via ETT, dose is 2 to 10 times the IV dose diluted in 3 to 5 mL of saline followed by several positive-pressure breaths.
Subsequent: The initial dose may be repeated every 3 to 5 minutes up to a maximum of five doses.
*Graded reversal: 0.001 to 0.01 mg per kg (1 to 10 mcg per kg) IV q3–5min as needed for respiratory depression secondary to PCA/epidural or chronic opiate use.

Adverse Effects: May precipitate withdrawal symptoms in narcotic-dependent patients.

Availability: Injection: 0.4, 1 mg per mL

Drug: NICARDIPINE (CARDENE®)
Route of Administration: IV
Dose: *Hypertensive emergencies: initial:* 1 to 3 mcg per kg per minute as a continuous infusion, titrate as needed to maintain BP in desired range. Max of 5 mcg per kg per minute.

Note: Do not use in patients at risk for increased intracranial pressure.

Adverse Effects: Hypotension, reflex tachycardia, phlebitis, increased ICP

Availability: Injection: 2.5 mg per mL

Drug: NITROPRUSSIDE, SODIUM (NITROPRESS®, NIPRIDE®)
Route of Administration: IV
Dose: *Hypertensive emergencies: initial:* 0.5 to 1 mcg per kg per minute as a continuous infusion, titrate as needed to maintain BP in desired range. Average 3 mcg per kg per minute, max of 10 mcg per kg per minute. At doses higher than 4 mcg per kg per minute, thiocyanate levels need to be monitored.

Note: Sodium nitroprusside is only compatible with D5W and must be protected from light. Nitroprusside has an immediate onset of action. Careful hemodynamic monitoring is essential. Infusion should be adminis-

tered by infusion pump. Freshly prepared solutions may appear brownish; any solution discolored blue, green, orange, or red should be discarded. Other medications should not be admixed or run through the same line with nitroprusside.

Adverse Effects: Usually associated with excessive or rapid lowering of BP. Cyanide intoxication may occur in patients with renal dysfunction and prolonged duration of infusion. Cyanide and thiocyanate levels should be checked in patients receiving nitroprusside for more than 3 days or rates higher than 4 mcg per kg per minute. Other effects may include increased ICP, disorientation, nausea, and vomiting.

Availability: Injection: 10, 25 mg per mL

Drug: NOREPINEPHRINE (LEVOPHED®)
Route of Administration: IV
Dose: 0.05 to 1 mcg per kg per minute as a continuous infusion. Titrate as needed to maintain BP.

Precautions: May begin administration via a peripheral line, changing to central access as soon as possible. Must be further diluted for infusion.

Adverse Effects: Hypertension, organ ischemia, decreased peripheral perfusion

Availability: Injection: 1 mg per mL

Drug: ROCURONIUM (ZEMURON®)
Route of Administration: IV, IM
Dose: *RSI:* 0.6 to 1.2 mg per kg IV. For IM, use higher end of dosing range (up to 1.8 mg per kg per dose) if giving IM.

Precautions: Use only in the presence of personnel skilled in the management of an artificial airway.

Adverse Effects: Respiratory arrest, hyper/hypotension, arrhythmias (rare)

Availability: Injection: 10 mg per mL

Drug: SODIUM BICARBONATE
Route of Administration: IV
Dose: *Initial: age younger than 1 month or weight less than 5 kg:* 1 mEq per kg (2 mL per kg) of 0.5 mEq per mL (4.2%) solution. If only 7.5% or 8.4% solution (1 mEq per mL) is available, dilute 1:1 with D5W before administration; *age older than 1 month or >5 kg:* 1 mEq per kg (1 mL per kg) of 1 mEq per mL (8.4%) solution.
Subsequent: Corrective NaHCO dose (mEq) = 0.3 body weight (kg) × base deficit (mEq per L) OR 0.5 × body weight (kg) × (24 − serum HCO_3).

Note: Give one-half of this calculated estimate.
Continuous infusion: Up to 1 mEq per kg per hour
Tumor-lysis syndrome: D5W with sodium bicarbonate 75 mEq per L at 125 mL per m² per hour to maintain urine pH 7 to 8 and SG less than or equal to 1.010. Do not use bicarbonate hydration if also using rasburicase (Elitek®).

Precautions: Sodium bicarbonate should be given by direct IV administration slowly (max rate for infants 10 mEq per minute) and followed by NS flush to avoid precipitation in the IV line with other drugs such as calcium. Sodium bicarbonate should not be given via the ETT because it irritates the upper respiratory tract and lung parenchyma.

Adverse Effects: Hypernatremia (contains 11.9 mEq of sodium per 1 g), alkalosis, hyperosmolarity

Availability: Injection: most common concentrations are 0.5 mEq per mL (4.2%) and 1 mEq per mL (8.4%)

Drug: SUCCINYLCHOLINE (ANECTINE®)
Route of Administration: IV, IM
Dose: *Intubation:* 1 to 2 mg per kg IV or 2 to 4 mg per kg deep IM (max dose: 150 mg)
Use 2 mg per kg IV if younger than 2 years of age.
Precautions: Use only in the presence of personnel skilled in the management of an artificial airway. Avoid using in patients with personal or familial history of malignant hyperthermia, hyperkalemia, burns, renal failure, or myopathy associated with elevated CPK values.
Adverse Effects: Muscle fasciculations, respiratory depression, malignant hyperthermia, bradycardia, hypotension, cardiac arrhythmias (hyperkalemia)
Availability: Injection: 20, 50, 100 mg per mL

Drug: THIOPENTAL (PENTOTHAL®)
Route of Administration: IV
Dose: *RSI:* 3 to 6 mg per kg IV
Reduction of ICP: 1.5 to 5 mg per kg per dose IV
Precautions: Extravascular injection may cause pain, swelling, ulceration, and necrosis. Do not use in patients with hypotension.
Adverse Effects: Pronounced hypotension, respiratory depression, apnea, emergence delirium, nausea, vomiting, laryngospasm
Availability: Injection: 250 mg, 500 mg, 1 g, 2.5 g, 5 g

Drug: VASOPRESSIN (PITRESSIN®)
Route of Administration: IV
Dose: *VF or VT:* Adults: 40 units × 1 dose
GI hemorrhage: 0.002 to 0.005 units per kg per minute IV titrated up to a max of 0.01 unit per kg per minute
Diabetes Insipidus: 0.5 milliunits per kg per hour (0.005 units/kg/hr) IV to a max of 10 milliunits/kg/hr (0.01 units/kg/hr).
Precautions: Infiltration of the IV site can result in severe necrosis.
Adverse Effects: Pronounced hypertension, cardiac arrhythmias, vasoconstriction, abdominal cramping, nausea, vomiting, water intoxication
Availability: Injection: 20 units per mL

MEDICATIONS

Drug: ACETAMINOPHEN (FEVERALL®, LIQUIPRIN®, TEMPRA®, TYLENOL®)
Route of Administration: PO, PR
Dose: 10 to 15 mg per kg per dose in four to six divided doses (max daily dose: 90 mg per kg per day or 4 g, whichever is less); *loading dose:* 30 to 40 mg per kg PR × 1 dose
Precautions: Use cautiously in patients with liver disease and those who have not eaten in several days. Watch for duplicate therapy, especially with concurrent Percocet® or Vicodin® orders.
Availability (advise parents/patients that many strengths are available):
Chewable tablets: 80, 160 mg
Tablets: 325, 500 mg
Drops: 100 mg per mL
Oral suspension: 32 mg per mL
Capsules with powder for oral solution: 80, 160 mg (Feverall®)
Suppositories: 80, 120, 325, 650 mg

Drug: ACETAZOLAMIDE (DIAMOX®)
Route of Administration: IV, PO
Dose: 20 mg per kg per day IV/PO divided q6h, increase by 25 mg per kg per day (max 100 mg per kg per day)

Precautions: Do not use extended-release preparations for pseudotumor cerebri, diuresis, or epilepsy. Dosage adjustment required with renal dysfunction.
Adverse Effects: Electrolyte abnormalities, bone marrow suppression, headache, vertigo, GI upset
Availability: Injection: 500 mg
Tablets: 125 mg, 250 mg
Extended release capsule: 500 mg

Drug: ACETYLCYSTEINE (MUCOMYST®, ACETADOTE)
Route of Administration: PO, PR, IV
Dose: *Acetaminophen poisoning:* 150 mg per kg IV over 1 hour, then 50 mg per kg over 4 hours, then 100 mg per kg over 16 hours OR 140 mg per kg × 1 loading dose IV/PO, followed by 70 mg per kg per dose IV/PO q4h × 12 to 17 doses
Meconium ileus equivalent: 5 to 30 mL of 10% solution PO or PR three to six times per day
Prevention of contrast-induced nephrotoxicity: 10 mg per kg per dose PO BID (max 600 mg per dose) on day prior to and day of procedure
Precautions: Many regimens exist. Consult toxicologist. Higher rates of anaphylactoid reactions occur with IV administration. Consider late administration (more than 48 hours postingestion) as acetylcysteine

may provide benefit in acetaminophen toxicity. Acetylcysteine therapy may be discontinued prior to reaching 17 doses if acetaminophen levels are undetectable and LFTs return to baseline.

Adverse Effects: Nausea, vomiting, GI distress, anaphylactoid reactions, rash

Availability: Injection: 20% (200 mg per mL) solution
Oral: 20% (200 mg per mL) solution

Drug: ACYCLOVIR (ZOVIRAX®)

Route of Administration: IV, PO, topical

Dose: *Neonatal herpes simplex:* 30 to 60 mg per kg per day IV divided q8h. *Children and adults: mucocutaneous herpes simplex:* 750 mg per m^2 per day or 15 mg per kg per day IV divided q8h. *Varicella-zoster:* 1,500 mg per m^2 per day or 30 mg per kg per day IV divided q8h. *Herpes simplex encephalitis:* 60 mg per kg per day IV divided q8h. *Varicella (immunocompetent child only):* 80 mg per kg per day PO in four divided doses for 5 days (max 3,200 mg per day). *Genital herpes (initial treatment): adults:* 1 g per day PO in five divided doses or 1,200 mg per day PO in three divided doses for 7 to 10 days; *children:* 80 mg per kg per day PO in three to five divided doses (max 3,200 mg per day). *Topical:* Apply to cover each lesion six times daily for 7 days. A finger cot or glove should be used to apply ointment to prevent viral transmission.

Precautions: Patients should be adequately hydrated to prevent precipitation of acyclovir crystals in the renal tubules. Dosage adjustment required with renal dysfunction. Dose for obese patients should be based on ideal body weight.

Adverse Effects: Nephrotoxicity, headache, vertigo, GI upset, thrombophlebitis

Availability: Injection: 500 mg, 1 g
Capsules: 200 mg
Tablets: 400 mg, 800 mg
Oral suspension: 40 mg per mL
Topical ointment: 5%

Drug: ADENOSINE (see Resuscitation List)

Drug: ALBUTEROL (PROVENTIL®, VENTOLIN®)

Route of Administration: PO, inhalation

Dose: *Oral therapy generally not recommended. PO: children (age 2 to 6 years):* Initial dose 0.1 mg per kg per dose given TID (do not exceed 2 mg TID initially). May increase dose gradually to 0.2 mg per kg per dose given TID (not to exceed 12 mg per day); *children (6 to 14 years):* initial dose 2 mg given TID to QID. May cautiously increase to a maximum daily dose of 24 mg per day; *inhalation: MDI (90 mcg per puff): children younger than 12 years:* one to two inhalations four times per day; *children older than 12*

years: one to two inhalations given four to six times daily. *PO Rotahaler: older than 4 years:* 200 mcg every 4 to 6 hours; may increase to 400 mcg per dose. *Nebulizer:* 0.15 mg per kg (0.03 mL per kg of 0.5% solution) (maximum single dose: 5 mg or 1 mL of 0.5% solution) every 20 minutes for three doses (may use standard doses of 0.5 mL <30 kg and 1 mL for >30 kg), then q1–6h. Continuous nebulization 0.5 mg per kg per hour (suggested β_2-agonist total max 20 mg per hour). May be combined with ipratropium for nebulization.

Adverse Effects: Tachycardia, nervousness, tremor, palpitations, alterations in blood glucose, hypokalemia

Availability: Tablets: 2, 4 mg
Extended-release tablets: 4, 8 mg
Oral syrup: 0.4 mg per mL
Metered-dose aerosol: each actuation delivers 90 mcg of albuterol
Capsules containing powder for oral inhalation: 200 mcg
Solution for nebulization: 0.5% (5 mg per mL) concentrate, 0.083% (0.83 mg per mL) prediluted bullets

---

Drug: ALLOPURINOL (ZYLOPRIM®)

Route of Administration: IV. PO

Dose: *Tumor lysis syndrome:* 10 mg per kg per day divided BID (max 300 mg per dose)

Adverse Effects: Allergic reactions, hepatotoxicity, bone marrow suppression, rash

Availability: Injection: 100-mg vials. Tablets 100 mg, 300 mg

---

Drug: ALPROSTADIL (see Resuscitation List)

Drug: ALTEPLASE (tPA, ACTIVASE®)

Route of Administration: IV

Dose: *Catheter clearance:* Volume of catheter + 10%: max 2 mg in 2 mL in clogged port for 20 minutes to 2 hours, then withdraw

Catheter-directed thrombolysis: 0.01 to 0.2 mg per kg per hour at the site of the thrombus; Involvement of service managing the catheter recommended.

Systemic thrombotic therapy: 0.1 to 0.6 mg per kg per hour IV × 6 hours; Consider pediatric hematology consult.

Precautions: Recent major surgery, trauma, history of AVM or aneurysm, and uncontrolled hypertension are contraindications for use.

Adverse Effects: Hemorrhage, hypotension, fever, rash
Availability: Injection: 2-, 50-, 100-mg vials

Drug: AMINOCAPROIC ACID (AMICAR®)

Route of Administration: PO, IV

Dose: *Initial:* 50 to 100 mg per kg IV × 1 dose (infuse over 1 hour)

Subsequent: 30 mg per kg per hour IV as continuous infusion or 100 mg per kg per dose IV/PO q6h to achieve plasma concentration greater than or equal to 130 mg per L for inhibition of systemic hyperfibrinolysis (max 30 g per day)

Precautions: Rapid injection may result in arrhythmia and hypotension.

Availability: Injection: 250 mg per mL

Tablet: 500 mg

Oral syrup: 250 mg per mL

Drug: AMINOPHYLLINE (see THEOPHYLLINE®)

Drug: AMOXICILLIN (AMOXIL®, LAROTID®, POLYMOX®)

Route of Administration: PO

Dose: 20 to 120 mg per kg per day in two to three divided doses (max 3 g per day). If high-dose amoxicillin (80 mg per kg per day) is not required, may dose as follows: patients weighing less than 10 kg may receive 125 mg TID and patients weighing 10 to 50 kg may receive 250 mg TID, those greater than 50 kg may receive 500 mg TID.

Adverse Effects: Diarrhea, rash, hypersensitivity reactions

Availability: Capsules: 250, 500 mg

Tablets: 500, 875 mg

Chewable tablets: 125, 200, 250, 400 mg

Oral suspension: 125 mg per 5 mL, 200 mg per 5 mL, 250 mg per 5 mL, 400 mg per 5 mL

Drug: AMOXICILLIN/CLAVULANIC ACID (AUGMENTIN®)

Route of Administration: PO

Dose: 20 to 120 mg per kg per day of amoxicillin component in two to three divided doses (max 3 g per day of amoxicillin)

Precautions: PO suspension and chewable tablets contain a 4:1 ratio of amoxicillin to clavulanic acid. Film-coated tablets contain a 2:1 or 4:1 ratio of the drugs. Note that two 250-mg film-coated tablets should not be substituted for one 500-mg film-coated tablet to avoid GI side effects from excessive clavulanic acid. The BID formulation contains a 7:1 ratio of amoxicillin to clavulanic acid.

Adverse Effects: Similar to amoxicillin alone. Diarrhea or loose stools has been reported in 9% of patients, although is reportedly higher in practice. Limit dosage to 40 mg per kg per day of amoxicillin component and administer doses with food to minimize GI side effects. Nausea and vomiting appear related to the dose of clavulanic acid.

Availability: Powder for oral suspension:

200: Amoxicillin 200 mg and clavulanic acid 28.5 mg per 5 mL (100 mL)

400: Amoxicillin 400 mg and clavulanic acid 57 mg per 5 mL (100 mL)

125: Amoxicillin 125 mg and clavulanic acid 31.25 mg per 5 mL (75, 100, 150 mL)

250: Amoxicillin 250 mg and clavulanic acid 62.5 mg per 5 mL (75, 100, 150 mL)

ES-600: Amoxicillin 600 mg and clavulanic acid 42.9 mg per 5 mL (75, 125, 200 mL)

Tablet:

250: Amoxicillin 250 mg and clavulanic acid 125 mg

500: Amoxicillin 500 mg and clavulanic acid 125 mg

875: Amoxicillin 875 mg and clavulanic acid 125 mg

Tablet, chewable:

125: Amoxicillin 125 mg and clavulanic acid 31.25 mg

200: Amoxicillin 200 mg and clavulanic acid 28.5 mg

250: Amoxicillin 250 mg and clavulanic acid 62.5 mg

400: Amoxicillin 400 mg and clavulanic acid 57 mg

Tablet, extended release (Augmentin XR™):

Amoxicillin 1,000 mg and clavulanic acid 62.5 mg

Drug: AMPICILLIN (GENERIC)

Route of Administration: PO, IM, IV

Dose: *Injection: younger than 7 days of age:* 100 to 300 mg per kg per day divided every 12 hours; *older than 7 days of age:* 100 to 400 mg per kg per day in four to six divided doses. Use maximum doses for treatment of meningitis; *PO: older than 1 month of age:* 50 to 100 mg per kg per day in four divided doses (max 3 g per day).

Precautions: When given orally, ampicillin should be administered on an empty stomach.

Adverse Effects: See Amoxicillin. Diarrhea occurs with greater frequency as compared with amoxicillin.

Availability: Injection: 125-, 250-, 500-mg vials; 1-g vials

Oral suspension: 25, 50 mg per mL

Capsules: 250, 500 mg

Drug: AMPICILLIN/SULBACTAM (UNASYN®)

Route of Administration: IV

Dose: Dose based on ampicillin component: 200 mg per kg per day IV divided q6h

Precautions: Infuse over at least 30 minutes.

Adverse Effects: See Ampicillin.

Availability: Injection: 500-mg vials; 1-g vials (2-1 ration of amoxicillin to sulfbactam)

Drug: ASPIRIN (ACETYLSALICYLIC ACID, ASA)

Route of Administration: PO, PR

Dose: *Fever/analgesia:* 10 to 15 mg per kg per dose every 4 to 6 hours, max 4 g per day.

Rheumatoid arthritis: 60 to 90 mg per kg per day initial dose in four divided doses (max dose 4 g per day). Administer with food.

Kawasaki disease: 80 to 100 mg per kg per day divided every 6 hours until fever resolves, then 3 to 5 mg per kg per day.

Precautions: Avoid use in patients with varicella or influenza and during presumed outbreaks of influenza because of a possible associated risk of Reye's syndrome. Use with caution in bleeding disorders or when using concomitantly with other medications that carry a risk of bleeding. Serum concentrations should be monitored in patients receiving long-term therapy. Small changes in dose may result in disproportionate increases in serum concentration.

Adverse Effects: GI upset, GI bleeding, tinnitus, reduced platelet function, bronchospasm

Availability (many strengths are available):
Tablets: 75, 81, 165, 325, 500 mg
Suppositories: 300, 600 mg

Drug: ATENOLOL (TENORMIN®)
Route of Administration: PO
Dose: *Initial:* 0.8 to 1 mg per kg per day PO daily; *maintenance:* 0.8 to 2 mg per kg per day PO daily
Precautions: IV preparation not used in children.
Adverse Effects: Hypotension, heart block, headache, wheezing
Availability: Tablets: 25, 50, 100 mg
Injection: 0.5 mg per mL

Drug: ATROPINE (see Resuscitation Drug List)

Drug: AZATHIOPRINE (IMURAN®)
Route of Administration: PO, IV
Dose: *Initial:* 2 to 5 mg per kg per dose; *maintenance:* 1 to 3 mg per kg per day in one to two divided doses
Precautions: Reduce dosage to 25% to 30% of usual when allopurinol is also being administered. Concurrent use of ACE inhibitors may result in severe anemia.
Adverse Effects: Bone marrow suppression, nausea, vomiting, stomatitis
Availability: Injection: 5 mg per mL
Tablet: 50 mg

Drug: AZITHROMYCIN (ZITHROMAX®)
Route of Administration: PO, IV
Dose: *Otitis media (age older than 6 months):* 30 mg per kg PO as a single dose (max dose: 1,500 mg); alternatively, 10 mg per kg PO as a single dose (max dose: 500 mg) followed by 5 mg per kg per day PO (max daily dose: 250 mg) on days 2 to 5.
Streptococcal pharyngitis: 12 mg per kg PO single daily dose for 5 days (max dose: 500 mg per day); alternatively, 10 mg per kg PO as a single dose (max dose: 500 mg) followed by 5 mg per kg per day PO (max daily dose: 250 mg) on days 2 to 5.
Community-acquired pneumonia: 10 mg per kg PO/IV as a single dose (max dose: 500 mg) followed by 5 mg

per kg per day PO/IV (max daily dose: 250 mg) on days 2 to 5.
Uncomplicated chlamydial infections, chancroid (adolescents and adults): 1 g PO as a single dose.
Note: Although effective against gonorrhea, the 2-g oral dose is poorly tolerated and therefore not recommended as first-line therapy.
Adverse Effects: Nausea, vomiting, metallic taste, rash
Availability: Oral capsules: 250 mg
Tablets: 250, 500 mg
Oral suspension: 20, 40 mg per mL
Single-dose packets: 1 g per packet
Injection: 500 mg per vial

Drug: BARLEY MALT SOUP EXTRACT (MALTSUPEX®)
Route of Administration: PO
Dose: 5 to 30 mL per day or 4 to 32 g per day, usual 4 to 8 g per day; dilute per manufacturer instructions
Adverse Effects: diarrhea, allergic reactions
Availability: Liquid 16 g per 15 mL, powder 16 g per tbsp

Drug: BECLOMETHASONE (BECLOVENT®, VANCERIL®)
Route of Administration: Inhalation
Dose: *Asthma: age 6 to 12 years:* 1 to 2 puffs TID to QID by PO inhalation (max dose: 10 puffs per day). Each puff delivers 42 mcg.
Rhinitis (seasonal or perennial): age 6 to 12 years: spray (42 mcg) in each nostril BID to TID.
Precautions: Caution should be used in converting asthmatic patients from oral steroids to inhaled steroids. Monitor such patients for steroid withdrawal symptoms (muscle and joint pain, malaise, anorexia, nausea, hypotension, and other symptoms of acute adrenal insufficiency). Not recommended for "prn" use.
Adverse Effects: Hoarseness, oral candidiasis or aspergillosis, dry mouth, bronchospasm
Availability: Aerosol for oral inhalation: 42 mcg per metered spray
Aerosol for nasal insufflation: 42 mcg per metered spray

Drug: BENZTROPINE (COGENTIN®)
Route of Administration: PO, IM, IV
Dose: *Age older than 3 years:* 0.02 to 0.05 mg per kg per dose once or twice daily (max dose: 6 mg per day)
Precautions: Not for use in children younger than 3 years of age, unless life-threatening emergency. Use cautiously in older children.
Adverse Effects: Anticholinergic symptoms—dry mouth, tachyarrhythmias, nausea, vomiting, hallucinations, coma
Availability: Tablets: 0.5, 1, 2 mg
Injection: 1 mg per mL

Drug: BUPIVACAINE (MARCAINE, SENSORCAINE®)
Route of Administration: Infiltration
Dose: Depending on type of block, 5 to 50 mL is instilled
Precautions: Never inject intravenously. Intralipids should be immediately available in case of inadvertent intravenous or intra-arterial injection.
Adverse Effects: Respiratory arrest, seizures
Availability: Injection: 0.25%, 0.5%, 0.75%

Drug: C-1 INHIBITOR (CINRYZE®)
Route of Administration: IV
Dose: *Hereditary angioedema:* 10 to 20 units per kg acute; 1,000 units every 3 to 4 days for prophylaxis
Precautions: Should be given at room temperature at a rate of 1 mL per minute.
Adverse Effects: Severe hypersensitivity reactions, thrombosis, muscle pain
Availability: Injection 500 units

Drug: CALCIUM (see Resuscitation List)

Drug: CAPTOPRIL (CAPOTEN®)
Route of Administration: PO
Dose: *Hypertension: neonate:* 0.01 to 0.1 mg per kg per dose; *older infants and children:* 0.15 to 0.5 mg per kg per dose (max 12.5 mg initial dose). Twofold increments in the dosage can be made after an observation period of 1 to 2 hours if the initial doses are ineffective. Maintenance doses may be given every 8 to 12 hours.
CHF (or other patients who may be salt/volume depleted): An initial dose of 25% to 50% of the usual antihypertensive doses should be used. Max 6 mg per kg per day in two to three divided doses.
Precautions: Pronounced hypotension may be observed when captopril is administered in conjunction with diuretics or other antihypertensive drugs. Hyperkalemia may occur when used with potassium-sparing diuretics or potassium supplementation. Dosages should be reduced in patients with impaired renal function. Do not use in patients with bilateral renal artery stenosis or unilateral renal artery stenosis with a solitary kidney as renal blood flow may be severely impaired.
Adverse Effects: Excessive lowering of BP, cough, proteinuria, neutropenia, rash, altered taste perception, angioedema
Availability: Tablets: 12.5, 25, 50, 100 mg
Note: Several recipes for compounding captopril suspension have been published. Due to the relative instability in aqueous solutions, captopril suspensions have a relatively short stability of 7 to 10 days.

Drug: CARBAMAZEPINE (TEGRETOL®, CARBATROL®)
Route of Administration: PO

Dose: *Initial:* 5 to 10 mg per kg per day in three to four divided doses, increasing every 5 to 7 days as needed. *Usual maintenance:* 15 to 35 mg per kg per day in three to four divided doses for immediate-release products and in two divided doses for extended-release products (max 1,200 mg per day).
Adverse Effects: Transient leukopenia, aplastic anemia (rare), ataxia and other CNS disturbances, GI upset, constipation, rash, Stevens-Johnson syndrome, nystagmus, hepatotoxicity
Precautions: Major drug interactions may occur with other medications metabolized via the 3A3/4 and 2C19 enzyme pathways. Carbamazepine induces its own metabolism approximately 14 days after starting therapy; therefore, a dose increase may be required at this time. Serum trough concentrations of carbamazepine (therapeutic 4 to 12 mg per dL) and any other concomitant anticonvulsants should be monitored.
Availability: Tablets: 100 mg (chewable), 200-mg tablets, extended-release: 100, 200, 400 mg capsules, extended-release: 200, 300 mg
Oral suspension: 20 mg per mL
Note: May use suspension rectally as a temporary alternative to oral route.

Drug: CARNITINE (CARNITOR®)
Route of Administration: PO, IV
Dose: *Primary carnitine deficiency or prophylaxis of valproic acid-induced hepatotoxicity:* 50 to 100 mg per kg per day PO divided BID-TID, usual max 3 g per day; *severe cases:* 50 mg per kg IV load, then 50 to 300 mg per kg per day IV divided q4–6h
Adverse Effects: Nausea, vomiting, diarrhea, body odor
Availability: Oral solution: 100 mg per mL
Tablets: 330 mg
Injection: 200 mg per mL

Drug: CEFADROXIL (DURICEF®)
Route of Administration: PO
Dose: 30 mg per kg per day as a single dose or two equally divided doses, max 4 g per day
Adverse Effects: Rash, GI upset, transient leukopenia
Availability: Capsules: 500 mg
Tablets: 1 g
Oral suspension: 25, 50, 100 mg per mL

Drug: CEFAZOLIN (ANCEF®, KEFZOL®)
Route of Administration: IM, IV
Dose: 50 to 100 mg per kg per day in three divided doses, *osteomyelitis:* 150 mg per kg per day IV divided q8h (max 12 g per day)
Adverse Effects: Other than allergic reactions, adverse effects are rarely observed. Rare adverse effects include

elevations in serum transaminase values, positive Coombs' test, and hemolytic anemia.

Availability: Injection: 250-, 500-mg vials; 1-, 5-g vials

Drug: CEFDINIR (OMNICEF®)
Route of Administration: PO
Dose: *Age older than 6 months:* 14 mg per kg per day in two divided doses (max dose: 600 mg per day)
Adverse Effects: Nausea, vomiting, diarrhea
Availability: Oral suspension: mg per mL
Tablets: 300, 600 mg
Oral Suspension: 25 mg per mL

Drug: CEFIXIME (SUPRAX®)
Route of Administration: PO
Dose: *Age older than 6 months:* 8 mg per kg per day in one to two divided doses (max 400 mg per day); *gonorrhea:* 400 mg PO as a single dose
Adverse Effects: Nausea, vomiting, diarrhea
Availability: Oral suspension: 20 mg per mL
Tablets: 200, 400 mg

Drug: CEFOTAXIME (CLAFORAN®)
Route of Administration: IV, IM
Dose: *Age younger than 1 week:* 100 mg per kg per day in two divided doses; *age 1 to 4 weeks:* 150 mg per kg per day in three divided doses; *age 1 month to 12 years:* 50 to 200 mg per kg per day in four to six equally divided doses (max 12 g per day). *Penicillin intermediate or resistant pneumococcal meningitis:* 300 mg per kg per day in four divided doses.
Adverse Effects: See Cefazolin.
Availability: Injection: 1-, 2-g vials

Drug: CEFPROZIL (CEFZIL®)
Route of Administration: PO
Dose: 15 to 30 mg per kg per day in two divided doses (max 1 g per day)
Adverse Effects: Rash, diarrhea, nausea, vomiting
Availability: Tablets: 250, 500 mg
Oral suspension: 25, 50 mg per mL

Drug: CEFTAZIDIME (FORTAZ®, TAZIDIME®)
Route of Administration: IV, IM
Dose: *Age 0 to 4 weeks:* 100 to 150 mg per kg per day in two to three divided doses; *age 1 month to 12 years:* 100 to 150 mg per kg per day in three divided doses (max 6 g per day). *Cystic fibrosis:* 150 to 200 mg per kg per day IV divided q8h.
Adverse Effects: See Cefazolin. Transient neutropenia with positive Coombs.
Availability: Injection: 500-mg vials; 1-, 2-g vials

Drug: CEFTRIAXONE (ROCEPHIN®)
Route of Administration: IV, IM
Dose: *Usual dose:* 50 to 100 mg per kg per day in one or two divided doses. *Bacterial meningitis:* Initial dosage should be 100 mg per kg as a single dose followed by 100 mg per kg per day in two divided doses (max 2,000 mg per dose). *Uncomplicated gonorrhea:* 125 mg IM single dose; use 250 mg IM single dose if concomitant PID (max 4 g per day). *Chancroid:* 250 mg IM single dose.
Adverse Effects: See Cefazolin; also, biliary sludging/cholelithiasis; avoid use in neonates with hyperbilirubinemia because ceftriaxone has been shown to displace bilirubin from albumin-binding sites, possibly leading to kernicterus.
Availability: Injection: 250-, 500-mg vials; 1-, 2-g vials

Drug: CEFUROXIME (CEFTIN®, ZINACEF®)
Route of Administration: IV, PO
Dose: *Injection: Neonates:* 50 to 100 mg per kg per day divided q12h. *Age older than 3 months: usual dose:* 50 to 150 mg per kg per day in three or four divided doses. Because of limited penetration into cerebrospinal fluid, avoid use in patients with possible meningitis (max dose: 9 g per day).
Oral suspension: 20 to 30 mg per kg per day in two divided doses.
Oral tablets: 250 to 500 mg per day (total dose) in two divided doses.
Note: Tablets and oral suspension are NOT bioequivalent and are NOT substitutable on a mg-per-kg basis.
Adverse Effects: See Cefazolin. Rash, GI distress.
Availability: Injection: 750-, 1,500-mg vials per premixed infusions
Oral tablets: 125, 250, 500 mg
Oral suspension: 25 mg per mL

Drug: CEPHALEXIN (KEFLEX®)
Route of Administration: PO
Dose: 50 to 100 mg per kg per day given in four divided doses (max 4 g per day)
Adverse Effects: Nausea, vomiting, diarrhea; possible cross-hypersensitivity with penicillins
Availability: Capsules: 125, 250, 500 mg
Oral suspension: 25, 50 mg per mL

Drug: CETIRIZINE (ZYRTEC®)
Route of Administration: PO
Dose: *2 to 5 years:* 2 .5 to 5 mg per day in one to two divided doses. *Older than 5 years:* 5 to 10 mg per day in one to two divided doses.
Adverse Effects: Drowsiness, GI distress, paresthesias, cough, bronchospasm
Availability: Tablets: 5, 10 mg
Oral solution: 1 mg per mL

Drug: CHARCOAL, ACTIVATED (ACTA-CHAR®, ACTIDOSE®, LIQUI-CHAR®)

Route of Administration: PO

Dose: 1 g per kg (or approximately 5 to 10 times the amount of poison ingested), max 100 g per dose. Multiple doses should be considered for ingestions that are extended-release preparations, undergo enterohepatic recirculation, or form bezoars.

Precautions: Do not administer concurrently with syrup of ipecac or dairy products. Adequate airway protection is essential. Limited indications currently.

Adverse Effects: Use sorbitol-containing suspensions as initial dose with caution, generally not recommended in children. Sorbitol acts as a cathartic. Plain charcoal suspensions should be used for subsequent doses. Careful monitoring of fluid and electrolyte status is essential in patients receiving sorbitol. Vomiting, constipation, or diarrhea may occur. Stools will be black.

Availability: Loose powder for suspension, mix in 6 to 8 oz of water

Oral suspension in aqueous or sorbitol solution: many strengths such as 15 g in 75 mL or 120 mL, 30 g in 120 mL, or 50 g in 250 mL

Drug: CHLORAL HYDRATE (NOCTEC®)

Route of Administration: PO, PR

Dose: *Hypnosis:* 25 to 50 mg per kg per dose; may be repeated once at half the initial dose (max 1 g per dose). *Procedural sedation:* 50 to 100 mg per kg per dose; may be repeated once at 25 to 75 mg per kg per dose for inadequate sedation (total max 1g infants, 2 g children). Administer capsule with full glass of water or fruit juice. Dilute chloral hydrate syrup in water or fruit juice before administration.

Adverse Effects: CNS depression, vomiting (very common), abdominal pain, prolonged sedation, apnea

Availability: Capsule: 250, 500 mg

Oral syrup: 50, 100 mg per mL

Drug: CHLORAMPHENICOL (CHLOROMYCETIN®)

Route of Administration: IV

Dose: *Age younger than 7 days:* 20 mg per kg IV load, follow with maintenance dose 12 hours later of 25 mg per kg per day in two divided doses; *age 7 to 28 days:* 50 mg per kg per day in two divided doses; *age older than 1 month:* 50 to 100 mg per kg per day in four divided doses (max 6 g per day)

Precautions: Serum concentrations should be monitored.

Adverse Effects: Bone marrow depression, "gray baby syndrome" (failure to feed, abdominal distension, cyanosis, irregular respiration, cardiovascular collapse)

Availability: Injection: 1 g per vial

Drug: CHLOROQUINE

Route of Administration: IV, PO

Dose: *acute malaria:* Initial dose: 10 mg per kg of base (maximum 600 mg base per dose), followed by 5 mg base per kg at 6, 24, and 48 hours

Precautions: Adverse Effects: Cardiovascular collapse, GI distress, aplastic anemia, agranulocytosis, hepatic dysfunction

Availability: Injection: from CDC; Tablets: 500 mg (300 mg base)

Drug: CHLOROTHIAZIDE (DIURIL®)

Use caution, sound-alike drugs include: Hydrochlorothiazide (Hydrodiuril®)

Route of Administration: PO, IV

Dose: *PO:* 20 to 40 mg per kg per day in two divided doses (max dose: 2 g per day)

IV: 5 to 20 mg per kg per day in two divided doses

Precautions: Use with caution in patients with liver and severe renal disease.

Adverse Effects: Hypokalemia, metabolic alkalosis, hyperuricemia, hyperglycemia, rash

Availability: Tablets: 250, 500 mg

Oral suspension: 50 mg per mL (contains 9.5% alcohol)

Injection: 500-mg vial

Drug: CHLORPHENIRAMINE MALEATE (CHLOR-TRIMETON®)

Route of Administration: PO

Dose: *Age 2 to 5 years:* 1 mg every 4 to 6 hours (max 6 mg per day); *age 6 to 11 years:* 2 mg every 4 to 6 hours (max 12 mg per day); *age older than 12 years:* 4 mg every 4 to 6 hours (max 24 mg per day)

Precautions: May lower seizure threshold.

Adverse Effects: CNS stimulation or depression, anticholinergic effects

Availability: Syrup: 0.4 mg per mL (contains 7% alcohol)

Tablets: 2 mg (chewable), 4, 8, 12 mg

Sustained-released tablets and capsules: 8, 12 mg

Drug: CIMETIDINE (TAGAMET®)

Route of Administration: IV, PO

Dose: *Neonates:* 5 to 10 mg per kg per day every 8 to 12 hours; *older infants:* 10 to 20 mg per kg per day every 6 to 12 hours; *child:* 20 to 40 mg per kg per day in three to four divided doses (max 2,400 mg per day)

Precautions: Reduce dosage in patients with renal dysfunction. Extensive drug interactions because cimetidine inhibits the hepatic microsomal enzymes responsible for the metabolism of many drugs. Cimetidine may increase the plasma concentrations and pharmacologic activity of theophylline, phenytoin, propranolol, warfarin, lidocaine, and many more.

Availability: Tablets: 200, 300, 400, 800 mg

Oral solution: 60 mg per mL

Injection: 150 mg per mL

Drug: CIPROFLOXACIN (CIPRO®)
Route of Administration: PO, IV
Dose: 20 to 30 mg per kg per day in two divided doses (max 800 mg per day IV, 1,500 mg per day PO); *severe P. aeruginosa*: 30 mg IV per kg per day IV divided q12h (max 1,200 mg per day)
Precautions: Preliminary studies have shown cartilage damage in juvenile animals, currently not approved for use in children younger than 18 years of age EXCEPT for cases of suspected anthrax.
Adverse Effects: Headache, rash, photosensitivity, GI distress, interstitial nephritis, tendonitis
Availability: Oral suspension 50, 100 mg per mL
Tablets: 100, 250, 500, 750 mg
Injection: 200-, 400-mg premixed infusions per vials

Drug: CLARITHROMYCIN (BIAXIN®)
Route of Administration: PO
Dose: 15 mg per kg per day in two divided doses (max 1 g per day)
Precautions: Drug interactions with medications metabolized by the cytochrome P450 (hepatic) enzyme systems (see Erythromycin).
Adverse Effects: See Erythromycin. Incidence of side effects may be lower with clarithromycin.
Availability: Oral suspension 25, 50 mg per mL
Tablets: 250, 500 mg

Drug: CLINDAMYCIN (CLEOCIN®)
Route of Administration: IV, PO
Dose: *PO*: 10 to 30 mg per kg per day in three divided doses, max 1.8 g per day
IV: age younger than 1 month: 15 to 20 mg per kg per day in three divided doses; *age 1 month or older*: 25 to 40 mg per kg per day in three divided doses, max 4.8 g per day; *topical*: twice-daily application
Precautions: If diarrhea occurs during therapy, antibiotic-associated pseudomembranous colitis should be considered as a potential cause. IM use may result in formation of sterile abscesses, and this route of administration should not be used. The oral suspension has very poor palatability; compliance may be an issue.
Adverse Effects: GI disturbances (see Precautions), thrombophlebitis after IV administration, hypersensitivity reactions
Availability: Capsules: 75, 150, 300 mg
Granules for oral suspension: 15 mg per mL when reconstituted
Injection: 150 mg per mL
Topical solution: 1%

Drug: CLONAZEPAM (KLONOPIN®)
    Use caution, sound-alike drugs include: Clonidine (Catapres®)
Route of Administration: PO

Dose: *Initial*: 0.01 to 0.03 mg per kg per day in two to three divided doses, increase slowly
Maintenance: 0.1 to 0.2 mg per kg per day in two to three divided doses
Adverse Effects: Sedation, hypotension, nausea, vomiting, anorexia
Availability: Tablets: 0.5, 1, 2 mg
Note: Several recipes for suspensions have been published.

Drug: CLONIDINE (CATAPRES®)
    Use caution, sound-alike drugs include: Clonazepam (Klonopin®)
Route of Administration: PO, topical, epidural
Dose: *Hypertension: initial*: 0.005 to 0.01 mg per kg per day PO divided q8–12h; *maintenance*: 0.005 to 0.025 mg per kg per day PO divided q6h (max 0.9 mg per day); *ADHD: initial*: 0.05 mg per day, increase every 3 to 7 days to 0.003 to 0.008 mg per kg per day PO divided TID-QID (max 0.4 mg per day)
Transdermal patches may be used once a stable oral dose is achieved. Patches may be cut, if necessary. For hypertension, change patches once per week. For ADHD, it may be necessary to change the patch every 3 days.
Adverse Effects: Hypotension, sedation, rash, GI distress
Availability: Tablets: 0.1, 0.2 mg
Transdermal patches: 0.1, 0.2, 0.3 mg
Injection: 100 mcg per mL

Drug: CLOTRIMAZOLE (GYNE-LOTRIMIN®, MYCELEX-G®)
Route of Administration: Intravaginal
Dose: *Intravaginal tablet:* Two 100-mg vaginal tablets (total: 200 mg per dose) daily at bedtime for 3 consecutive days. Alternative treatment regimens include use of one 500-mg vaginal tablet for one dose or use of one 100-mg vaginal tablet daily for 7 days.
Intravaginal cream: Contents of one applicator at bedtime for 7 to 14 days, alternative 1- and 3-day preparations exist.
Adverse Effects: Rash, burning, or irritation at or near application site
Availability: Vaginal tablet: 100, 500 mg
Vaginal cream: 1%

Drug: COCAINE HYDROCHLORIDE
Route of Administration: Topical
Dose: Topical administration in each nostril for local anesthesia, refractory epistaxis (max single dose: 1 mg per kg)
Adverse Effects: CNS excitation or depression, euphoria, restlessness, hallucinations, increased BP, increase or decrease in heart rate, psychic dependence with repeated use
Availability: Topical solution: 4%

Drug: CODEINE
Route of Administration: PO
Dose: 0.5 to 1 mg per kg per dose PO q3–6h as needed (usual adult max 60 mg per dose)
Adverse Effects: Sedation, respiratory depression, GI distress, constipation
Availability: Tablet: 15, 30, 60 mg
Solution: 3 mg per mL

Drug: CROMOLYN SODIUM (INTAL®)
Route of Administration: Inhalation
Dose: *Asthma :* Usual dosage for adults and children 2 years of age and older is 20 mg QID via nebulizer or one to two puffs TID-QID via MDI; *allergic rhinitis:* 1 nasal spray in each nostril TID or QID
Precautions: Not for acute relief of bronchospasm. When used for exercise-induced bronchospasm, cromolyn should be administered 10 to 15 minutes before exercise (but no longer than 1 hour before exercise).
Adverse Effects: Oropharyngeal irritation, bronchospasm
Availability: MDI: 800 mcg per puff
Solution for nebulization: 10 mg per mL
Nasal solution: 40 mg per mL

Drug: CYCLOSPORINE (SANDIMMUNE®, NEORAL®, GENGRAF®)
Route of Administration: PO, IV
Dose: Dosage must be individualized based on blood or plasma concentration monitoring. For prevention of allograft rejection, the initial oral dose is 14 to 18 mg per kg preoperatively followed by 15 mg per kg per day divided in one to two doses for 1 to 2 weeks. Once patient is stabilized, the dosage is usually tapered over 6 to 8 weeks to a maintenance dosage of 5 to 9 mg per kg per day as a single daily dose. Oral preparations are not bioequivalent and are not interchangeable. The IV dose is *one-third* of the oral dose (initial 5 to 6 mg per kg IV preoperatively, then 2 to 10 mg per kg per day IV q8–24h).
Precautions: Blood or plasma concentrations should be monitored. Therapeutic plasma/blood concentration ranges differ according to assay method. Major adverse effects of cyclosporine include hypertension, hyperkalemia, renal dysfunction, hirsutism, gingival hyperplasia, tremor, seizures, hepatotoxicity, and abdominal discomfort. Anaphylaxis has occurred after IV administration and may be related to the polyoxyl castor oil component in the vehicle for the injectable product. The metabolism and toxicity of cyclosporine may be affected by many drugs, particularly those that are metabolized via cyp450 3A3/4 (antifungals, erythromycin, clarithromycin, calcium channel–blocking agents, corticosteroids, grapefruit juice, protease inhibitors, sirolimus, tacrolimus).
Note: Oral liquid doses may be mixed in a glass container with apple juice or orange juice to improve palatability. Do not mix the solution for emulsion (Neoral) in milk (may be unpalatable). Use mixture immediately to minimize adsorption to the secondary container. Rinse secondary container with diluting beverage to ensure complete administration of the dose. Solution for injection should be mixed in glass or hard plastic syringes only.
Availability: Oral solution (Sandimmune, Gengraf, Neoral): 100 mg per mL (may contain 12.5% alcohol)
Oral capsules: 25, 100 mg
Injection: 50 mg per mL

Drug: CYPROHEPTADINE (PERIACTIN®)
Route of Administration: PO
Dose: *Allergic conditions:* 0.25 to 0.5 mg per kg per day in three to four divided doses (max doses: age 2 to 6 years: 12 mg per day; age 7 to 14 years: 16 mg per day); *appetite stimulation:* older than 13 years: 2 mg PO QID, max 8 mg PO QID; *migraine headaches:* children 4 mg PO BID-TID, adolescents/adults 4 to 8 mg PO TID; *spasticity:* older than 12 years: 4 mg PO, max 36 mg per day
Adverse Effects: Anticholinergic effects, increased appetite
Availability: Tablets: 4 mg
Oral syrup: 0.4 mg per mL

Drug: DEFEROXAMINE (DESFERAL®)
Route of Administration: IM, IV, SC
Dose: *Chelation, iron acute:* 15 mg per kg per hour IV or 50 mg per kg IM q6h, max 360 mg per kg or 6 g per day, whichever is less
Adverse Effects: GI distress, hypotension, anaphylactoid reaction
Notes: Turns urine orange or pink when complex is excreted. Injection must be further diluted for IV infusion.
Availability: Injection 250 mg per mL

Drug: DESMOPRESSIN (DDAVP®)
Route of Administration: Intranasal, SC, IV
Dose: *Acute hemophilia, von Willebrands:* 0.3 mcg per kg IV over 30 minutes or HIGH-DOSE nasal spray. *Enuresis/diabetes insipidus:* LOW-DOSE nasal spray
Note: Do not use in patients younger than 2 years old.
Adverse Effects: Facial flushing, headache, hypertension, hypotension, water retention, hyponatremic seizures
Availability: Injection 4 mcg per mL; Intranasal 100 mcg per mL or 1.5 mg per mL; Tablet 0.1 mg, 0.2 mg; Tablet sublingual 60, 120, and 240 mcg

Drug: DEXAMETHASONE (DECADRON®, HEXADROL®)
Route of Administration: PO, IM, IV
Dose: *Dependent on disease:* usual range is 0.024 to 1 mg per kg per day. *Croup:* 0.6 mg per kg per dose (usual max 12 mg per dose); *inflammation:* 0.5 to 2 mg

per kg per day divided q6–8h; *bacterial meningitis:* 0.6 mg per kg per day IV in four divided doses beginning just previous to or with the first dose of antibiotics; *epidural abscess/cerebral edema:* 2 mg per kg IV load (max 100 mg) followed by 1 to 2 mg per kg per day in four divided doses for 24 hours.

Note: Equivalent dosing 5 mg methylprednisolone = 1 mg dexamethasone

Adverse Effects: Acute: sodium and water retention, hypokalemia, hyperglycemia, hypertension, leukocytosis, behavioral disturbances, peptic ulcer

Availability: Injection: 4, 8, 10, 16, 20, 24 mg per mL

Tablets: various strengths ranging from 0.25 to 6 mg per tablet

Oral liquid: 0.1 mg per mL, 1 mg per mL concentrate (oral liquid products contain 0% to 30% alcohol)

Drug: DEXTROAMPHETAMINE (DEXEDRINE®)

Route of Administration: PO

Dose: *3 to 5 years:* 2.5 to 5 mg daily, gradually increasing to a maximum of 40 mg per day

Precautions: Tolerance may develop and require adjustment of the dosage.

Adverse Effects: Insomnia, nervousness, loss of appetite, irritability, tachycardia

Availability: Tablets: 5, 10 mg

Sustained-release Spansules: 5, 10, 15 mg

Drug: DIAZEPAM (VALIUM®, DIASTAT®)

Route of Administration: PO, IV, PR

Dose: *Status epilepticus:* 0.05 to 0.3 mg per kg per dose IV over 3 to 5 minutes every 15 minutes to a cumulative maximum total dose of 0.75 mg per kg or 10 mg, whichever is less. Lower dose is used in neonates. *Epilepsy:* 0.1 to 0.8 mg per kg per day PO divided q6–8h; *sedation:* 1 to 2.5 mg per dose PO, TID-QID. Alternatively, initial dosages of 0.1 to 0.3 mg per kg per day PO in two to three divided doses may be used; *PR:* 0.5 mg per kg (max 20 mg per dose), then 0.25 mg per kg in 10 minutes if needed. Can also use injectable form of drug for PR administration.

Precautions: When given IV for status epilepticus, dose may be repeated at 15-minute intervals to a maximum total of 0.75 mg per kg or 10 mg, whichever is less. Lorazepam is usually the drug of choice in status epilepticus in children. Maintenance anticonvulsant therapy should also be initiated when status epilepticus has been controlled.

Adverse Effects: Sedation, cardiorespiratory depression, hypotension

Availability: Injection: 5 mg per mL

Tablets: 2, 5, 10 mg

Oral solution: 1, 5 mg per mL

Rectal gel: 2.5, 5, 10, 20 mg

Drug: DIAZOXIDE (HYPERSTAT®)

Route of Administration: IV, PO (for hypoglycemia only)

Dose: *For hypertensive crisis:* 1 to 3 mg per kg per dose (max: 150 mg) given by rapid IV injection: over 10 to 30 seconds. Dose may be repeated in 5 to 15 minutes, if necessary (max 10 to 15 mg per kg per day); *hyperinsulinemic hypoglycemia (PO): newborns/infants:* initial dosage of 10 mg per kg per day PO in two to three divided doses; *maintenance:* 8 to 15 mg per kg per day PO in two to three divided doses. *Children and adults:* initial dosage of 3 mg per kg per day PO in two to three divided doses; *maintenance:* 3 to 8 mg per kg per day PO in two to three divided doses

Precautions: Severe orthostatic hypotension may occur after IV administration. Hypersensitivity to thiazides or other sulfonamides.

Adverse Effects: Hyperglycemia, tachycardia, salt and water retention, nausea, vomiting, extrapyramidal reactions (after long-term oral use)

Availability: Injection: 15 mg per mL

Oral capsules: 50 mg

Oral suspension: 50 mg per mL

Drug: DICLOXACILLIN (DYNAPEN®, PATHOCIL®)

Route of Administration: PO

Dose: *Mild to moderate infections:* 25 to 100 mg per kg per day in four divided doses. *Osteomyelitis:* 50 to 100 mg per kg per day in four divided doses (max 2 g per day). Suspension unpalatable and is no longer made.

Precautions: See Oxacillin.

Adverse Effects: See Oxacillin.

Availability: Capsules: 125, 250, 500 mg

Drug: DIGOXIN (see Chapter 84)

Drug: DIGOXIN IMMUNE FAB (DigiFab®, Digibind®)

Route of Administration: IV

Dose: *Initial:* Determine the TBL (total body load) of digoxin:

$$\frac{\text{Serum level (ng/mL)} \times 5.6 \times \text{wt in kg}}{1{,}000} = \text{TBL}$$

Divide the TBL by 0.5 to get the initial number of vials to treat empirically. If the amount of digoxin ingested is known, multiply by 0.8 to determine TBL. Infuse over 5 minutes via a 1.2-micron filter.

Adverse Effects: Hives, anaphylaxis, hypotension, chills, wheezing, hypokalemia, ventricular dysfunction, atrial arrhythmias

Note: Fab fragments may persist in the body for days and interfere with subsequent digoxin assays. Infusion must be filtered.

Availability: Powder for injection: vial 38 mg

Drug: DIHYDROERGOTAMINE (DHE®)

Route of Administration: IV, IM, SC, intranasal

Dose: *Migraine headache:* 0.5 mg intranasal, may repeat in 15 minutes if necessary up to a total 4 mg. 1 mg if giving via IM/SC/IV injection, may repeat up to a total of 3 mg for IM/SC or 2 mg for IV. Maximum for all routes is 6 mg per week.

Adverse Effects: Nausea, vomiting, paresthesias, cramping, subarachnoid hemorrhage, ergot poisoning

Note: Prime nasal pump prior to using. Do not use in pregnancy, renal dysfunction, cardiac disease or if a triptan has been used in the past 24 hours. Many dangerous drug interactions, notably and inhibitors of cyp3A4.

Availability: Injection 1 mg per mL; nasal spray 4 mg per mL

Drug: DIMENHYDRINATE

Use caution, sound-alike drugs include: Diphenhydramine (Benadryl®)

Route of Administration: IV, IM, PO

Dose: *Antiemetic/antihistamine:* 2 to 5 years: 12.5 to 25 mg per dose every 6 to 8 hours (max 75 mg per day), 6 to 12 years: 25 to 50 mg per dose every 6 to 8 hours (max 150 mg per day), older than 12 years 50 to 100 mg per dose every 6 to 8 hours (max 400 mg per day)

Adverse Effects: Anticholinergic side effects: drowsiness, urinary retention, dry mouth, tachycardia

Availability: Tablet 50 mg

Drug: DIPHENHYDRAMINE (BENADRYL®)

Route of Administration: PO, IM, IV

Dose: 1 to 1.25 mg per kg per dose every 6 hours as needed (max 300 mg per day)

Adverse Effects: Anticholinergic effects, drowsiness, sedation, dry mouth, intramuscular injection can be very painful

Availability: Injection: 10, 50 mg per mL
Capsules/tablets: 25, 50 mg
Tablets, chewable: 12.5 mg
Elixir: 2.5 mg per mL (contains 14% alcohol)
Oral syrup: 1.25, 2.5 mg per mL (some products contain 5% alcohol)

Drug: DOBUTAMINE (see Resuscitation Drug List)

Drug: DOPAMINE (See Resuscitation Drug List)

Drug: DOXYCYCLINE (VIBRAMYCIN®)

Route of Administration: PO, IV

Dose: *For acute pelvic inflammatory disease/chlamydial infections:* 100 mg BID; *anthrax, other severe suscepti-ble infections:* 2 to 5 mg per kg per day in two divided doses (max 200 mg per day).

Precautions: Due to teeth staining, limit use to patients older than 8 years of age and weighing more than 45 kg. Rocky Mountain spotted fever and anthrax should be treated with doxycycline, regardless of age.

Adverse Effects: See Tetracycline.

Availability: Capsules: 50, 100 mg
Tablets: 100 mg
Powder for oral suspension: 5 mg per mL when reconstituted
Syrup, suspension: 10 mg per mL
Injection: 100 mg per vial

Drug: EDROPHONIUM (TENSILON®)

Route of Administration: IV, IM, SC

Dose: *myasthenia gravis diagnostic test:* 0.04 mg per kg over 1 minute followed by 0.16 mg per kg within 45 seconds if no response (max dose 10 mg total); IM/SC: <34 kg 2 mg, >34 kg 5 mg; adults 10 mg; *reversal of neuromuscular blocking agents (NMBA):* adult 10 mg over 30 to 45 seconds; may repeat every 5 to 10 minutes up to 40 mg.

Precautions: Atropine should be readily available during any use of edrophonium

Notes: IV route preferred for diagnostic testing. Always use atropine or glycopyrrolate in conjunction with edrophonium when reversing NMBAs to control secretions.

Adverse Effects: Hypotension, cardiac arrest, arrhythmias, seizures, GI distress, bronchoconstriction

Availability: Injection 10 mg per mL

Drug: ENOXAPARIN (LOVENOX®)

Route of Administration: SC

Dose: Adjust dose based on anti-Xa levels. Obese patients should receive adjusted body weight dosing. *Deep vein thrombosis (DVT) treatment: younger than 2 months:* 1.5 mg per kg per dose SC q12h; *older than 2 months:* 1 mg per kg per dose SC q12h
DVT prophylaxis: younger than 2 months: 0.75 mg per kg per dose SC q12h; *older than 2 months:* 0.5 mg per kg per dose SC q12h

Precautions: Do not use in patients with active hemorrhage or risk of GI bleeding.

Adverse Effects: Hemorrhage, edema, local irritation at injection site

Availability: Injection 100 mg per mL

Drug: EPINEPHRINE (see Resuscitation Drug List)

Drug: ERYTHROMYCIN (E-MYCIN®, E.E.S.®, PEDIAMYCIN®)

Route of Administration: PO, IV

Dose: *PO:* 30 to 50 mg per kg per day of erythromycin equivalent in three to four divided doses (max 4 g per day).

Note: Erythromycin base, erythromycin ethylsuccinate, and erythromycin estolate are available for oral use.

IV: 15 to 50 mg per kg per day of erythromycin equivalent in four divided doses (max 4 g per day).

Prokinetic: Initial 3 mg per kg IV over 60 minutes, then 20 mg per kg per day PO divided TID-QID before meals and at bedtime.

Precautions: Many significant drug interactions occur with erythromycin, particularly with medications metabolized via cyp3A3/4; use extreme caution when adding to a patient's existing drug regimen. Oral administration of the estolate salt has been associated with cholestatic jaundice. However, this reaction rarely occurs among children 12 years of age or younger. Erythromycin use in young infants is associated with pyloric stenosis. For IV use, the drug should be diluted to at least 5 mg per mL and infused over 30 to 60 minutes.

Adverse Effects: Rash, elevation of hepatic enzymes. IV administration of erythromycin may cause severe venous irritation and thrombophlebitis. PO administration may be associated with abdominal pain and cramping.

Availability: Injection: various concentrations

Estolate salt:

Capsules: 250 mg

Tablets: 500 mg

Oral suspension: 25, 50 mg per mL

Ethylsuccinate salt:

Chewable tablets: 200 mg

Tablets: 400 mg

Oral liquid: 40, 80 mg per mL

Lactobionate salt: 500-, 1,000-mg vials (for IV use)

Gluceptate salt: 250-, 500-, 1,000-mg vials (for IV use)

Drug: ERYTHROMYCIN ETHYLSUCCINATE AND SULFISOXAZOLE (PEDIAZOLE®)

Route of Administration: PO

Dose: Dose based on erythromycin component: 50 mg per kg per day in four divided doses (max 2 g per day erythromycin)

Adverse Effects: See Erythromycin and Sulfisoxazole.

Availability: Granules for oral suspension: erythromycin 40 mg per mL and sulfisoxazole 120 mg per mL when reconstituted.

Drug: ESMOLOL (BREVIBLOC®)

Route of Administration: IV

Dose: *Hypertensive crisis and supraventricular tachyarrhythmias:* Loading dose of 500 mcg per kg per minute over 1 minute, followed by 50 to 100 mcg per kg per minute for 4 minutes. If response is not adequate within 5 minutes, a second loading dose of 500 mcg per kg per minute for 1 minute, followed by an infusion of 100 mcg per

kg per minute for 4 minutes, may be administered. Again, if response is not adequate, additional loading doses of 500 mcg per kg per minute over 1 minute may be administered every 5 minutes, followed by maintenance infusions for 4 minutes that have been increased by 50 mcg per kg per minute to a maximum infusion rate of 200 mcg per kg per minute. *Other cardiology experts have advocated much lower initial loading doses of 50 mcg per kg in pediatric SVT, using extreme caution in infants.*

Precautions: May worsen inadequate cardiac function. Avoid use in patients with overt CHF or bronchospastic disease. May mask signs and symptoms of hypoglycemia. Do not use in sympathomimetic overdose.

Adverse Effects: Hypotension, bronchospasm, worsening of CHF

Availability: Injection: 10 mg per mL

Concentrate, for preparation of IV infusions: 250 mg per mL

Drug: ESTROGENS, CONJUGATED (PREMARIN®)

Route of Administration: PO, IM, IV

Dose: *Abnormal uterine bleeding, stable hematocrit:* 1.25 mg PO BID, may increase to 2.5 mg PO QID if bleeding persists

Abnormal uterine bleeding, unstable hematocrit: 20 to 40 mg IV q4h for up to 24 hours

Urethral prolapse: Use vaginal cream applied to area BID-TID

Precautions: For uterine bleeding, the IV route of administration is preferred for a more rapid response. Administer IV injection slowly to avoid flushing reaction.

Adverse Effects: Flushing (with IV administration), hypertension, nausea, vomiting

Availability: Injection: 25 mg

Tablets: 0.3, 0.625, 0.9, 1.25, 2.5 mg

Vaginal cream: 0.625 mg per g

Drug: ETHACRYNIC ACID (EDECRIN®)

Route of Administration: PO, IV

Dose: *PO:* 1 mg per kg daily or BID (usual adult starting dose: 25 mg daily, max 3 mg per kg per day)

IV: 0.5 to 1 mg per kg per dose given once (max dose: 50 to 100 mg)

Adverse Effects: Ototoxicity, electrolyte imbalance (see Furosemide)

Availability: Injection: 50-mg vial (as sodium ethacrynate)

Tablets: 25, 50 mg

Drug: ETOMIDATE (see Resuscitation Drug List)

Drug: FabAV (Crofab®)

Route of Administration: IV

Dose: *Initial:* 4 to 6 vials, repeated as needed based on response. Each vial is reconstituted with 10 mL of sterile water and then the total dose is mixed in 250 mL of NS. The infusion should be started slowly, at a rate of 25 to 50 mL per hour for 10 minutes, while observing for allergic reaction. The rate should then be increased so the 250 mL is given over 1 hour.

Adverse Effects: Hives, anaphylaxis, hypotension, chills, wheezing

Note: Intravenous diphenhydramine is recommended to be given in conjunction with infusion. Slowing the rate of infusion is generally necessary if side effects develop.

Availability: Injection: vial 10-mL serum

Drug: FENOLDOPAM (CORLOPAM®)

Route of Administration: IV

Dose: 0.2 mcg per kg per minute, titrating up by 0.3 to 0.5 mcg per kg per minute every 20 to 30 minutes. Maximum rate 0.8 mcg per kg per minute.

Adverse Effects: Hypotension, tachycardia, increased intracranial pressure, increased intraocular pressure

Availability: Injection: 10 mg per mL

Drug: FERROUS SULFATE (FER-IN-SOL®, VARIOUS GENERICS)

Route of Administration: PO

Dose: *Maintenance/prophylaxis:* 1 to 2 mg per kg per day elemental iron, max 15 mg elemental iron per day

Treatment: 4 to 6 mg per kg per day elemental iron given in three divided doses, max 195 mg elemental iron per day

Adverse Effects: GI irritation, constipation, dark stools, solution may stain teeth

Note: Always prescribe dose based on elemental iron content. Elemental iron 65 mg = ferrous sulfate 325 mg.

Availability: Various liquid products: 15, 18, 25, 45 mg per mL (content expressed as mg per mL of elemental iron)

Tablets: 325 mg ferrous sulfate (65 mg elemental iron per 325 mg ferrous sulfate)

Drug: FLUMAZENIL (see Resuscitation Drug List)

Drug: FLUTICASONE (FLOVENT®, FLONASE®)

Route of Administration: Oral inhalation, nasal spray

Dose: Oral inhalation (MDI) depends on disease severity and previous steroid requirements. Consult manufacturer package insert for more information.

Nasal spray: 1 squirt to each nostril daily

Adverse Effects: Dry, itchy mouth and throat, hoarseness, epistaxis (nasal spray)

Note: Use spacer device. Instruct patient to use bronchodilator prior to fluticasone dose. Nasal spray should be held in hand opposite of nostril to avoid direct force and subsequent bleeding of the septum.

Availability: Oral inhalation: 44, 110, 220 mcg per actuation

Nasal spray: 50 mcg per spray

Drug: FOLIC ACID (FOLVITE®)

Route of Administration: PO, IM, IV

Dose: *Deficiency:* *infants:* 15 mcg per kg per dose daily, max 50 mcg per day; *children:* 1 mg per day initial, decrease to 0.1 to 0.4 mg per day; *adolescents and adults:* 0.25 to 1 mg per day

Adverse Effects: Do not use in patients with undiagnosed anemia. Use in patients with pernicious anemia may alleviate the hematologic manifestations but allow the neurologic disorder to progress.

Availability: Injection: 5, 10 mg per mL

Tablets: 0.4, 0.8, 1 mg

Drug: FOMEPIZOLE (ANTIZOL®, 4-MP)

Route of Administration: IV

Dose: 15 mg per kg IV load, then 10 mg per kg per dose IV q12h; at 48 hours, increase dose to 15 mg per kg per dose IV q12h. If patient receiving hemodialysis, increase interval to q6h.

Adverse Effects: Nephrotoxicity, headache, tachycardia, hypotension, allergic reactions

Availability: Injection: 1.5-g vial

Drug: FOSPHENYTOIN (CEREBYX®)

Route of Administration: IV, IM

Dose: Fosphenytoin is dosed in Phenytoin equivalents (PE) to avoid error. Loading dose is 10 to 20 mg PE per kg, maintenance 5 to 8 mg PE per kg per day divided q8–12h. For status epilepticus, infuse at 3 mg PE per kg per minute, max 150 mg PE per minute. Monitor trough phenytoin levels.

Adverse Effects: Fosphenytoin is a prodrug of phenytoin and has similar adverse effects, with the notable exception of tissue necrosis and arrhythmia secondary to rapid infusion. Fosphenytoin may be given IM. Hypotension may occur with rapid infusion; slow rate if this occurs. Fosphenytoin may cause severe perineum itching due to deposition of phosphate.

Availability: Injection: 50 mg PE per mL

Drug: FUROSEMIDE (LASIX®)

Route of Administration: IV

Dose: *IV: Initial:* 1 mg per kg over 1 to 2 minutes (max initial dose: 40 mg); *subsequent:* if no response in 20 to 30 minutes, a repeat dose of 1 to 2 mg per kg may be given. *Continuous infusion:* 0.05 to 0.1 mg per kg per hour, usual max 6 mg per kg per day; *oral:* 1 to 2 mg per kg per dose every 6 hours

Precautions: Hypokalemia in a patient on digoxin may result in the development of life-threatening arrhythmias.

Adverse Effects: Hypokalemia, hypocalcemia, metabolic alkalosis, hypotension

Availability: Injection: 10 mg per mL

Tablet: 20, 40, 80 mg

Oral solution: 8, 10 mg per mL

Drug: GABAPENTIN (NEURONTIN®)

Route of Administration: PO

Dose: *Initial:* 5 mg per kg per day, increase to 5 to 35 mg per kg per day divided TID. Max 90 mg per kg per day or 3,600 mg per day, whichever is less

Adverse Effects: Dizziness and somnolence (especially with rapid titration), mood alterations, nausea, vomiting, weight gain, tremor

Availability: Capsule: 100, 300, 400 mg

Oral solution: 50 mg per mL

Drug: GENTAMICIN (GARAMYCIN®)

Route of Administration: IV, IM

Dose: Many protocols exist. *Age: younger than 30 days, gestational age less than 35 weeks:* 3 mg per kg every 24 hours; *age: younger than 30 days, gestational age more than 35 weeks:* 4 mg per kg IV q24h. *Age: older than 30 days to 10 years:* 7.5 mg per kg per IV q24h or 2.5 mg per kg per dose IV q8h. *Age: older than 10 years:* 6 mg per kg IV q24h or 2 mg per kg per dose IV q8h

Precautions: Reduce dosage in patients with renal insufficiency; monitor serum gentamicin concentrations; use adjusted dosing weight when dosing obese patients.

Adverse Effects: Ototoxicity, nephrotoxicity

Availability: Injection: 10, 40 mg per mL

Drug: GRISEOFULVIN (GRIFULVIN®, FULVICIN U/F®)

Route of Administration: PO

Dose: *Microsized:* 10 to 20 mg per kg per day in one or two divided doses (max 1,000 mg per day); *ultramicrosized:* 5 to 10 mg per kg per day in one or two divided doses (max 750 mg per day)

Precautions: Several drug interactions exist, including warfarin and phenobarbital.

Adverse Effects: Agranulocytosis, hepatic dysfunction

Availability: Microsized suspension: 25 mg per mL

Capsules: 250 mg

Tablets: 250, 500 mg

Ultramicrosized tablet: 125, 165, 250, 330 mg

Drug: HALOPERIDOL (HALDOL®)

Route of Administration: PO, IM

Dose: Note: Pediatric dosages are not well established. IV use reported but not routinely recommended. Never use deconoate preparation IV. *Age older than 3 years: initial dose:* 0.01 to 0.03 mg per kg per day in two to three divided doses. *Acute agitation:* 0.025 to 0.075 mg per kg per dose q6h. *Usual maintenance:* 0.05 to 0.15 mg per kg per day in two to three divided doses (max 6 mg per day)

Note: Injectable lactate salt is used for acute management; a long-acting decanoate salt is available but is generally used at monthly intervals for maintenance therapy.

Adverse Effects: Dystonic reactions, tardive dyskinesia, hypotension, rash

Availability: Injection (lactate salt): 5 mg per mL

Tablets: 0.5, 1, 2, 5, 10, 20 mg

Oral solution: 2 mg per mL

Drug: HEPARIN

Route of Administration: IV

Dose: *Acute treatment:* 50 to 100 units per kg IV bolus over 10 minutes followed by 20 to 28 units per kg per hour by continuous IV infusion

Catheter flushing: 30 to 50 units every 8 hours as needed

Implanted port access: 300 to 500 units (use 100 units per mL concentration)

Precautions: Titrate dose to achieve desired activated PTT (usually one and one-half to two times control value). Heparin levels may be a more sensitive measure in some institutions.

Adverse Effects: Hemorrhage, heparin-induced thrombocytopenia

Availability: Injection: various concentrations are available; most commonly used are 1,000, 5,000, 10,000, 20,000 units per mL.

Drug: HYDRALAZINE (APRESOLINE®)

Use caution, sound-alike drugs include: Hydroxyzine (Atarax®)

Route of Administration: PO, IM, IV

Dose: *PO:* 0.25 mg per kg per dose, up to four times a day (initial single dose should not exceed 25 mg), then increase gradually over 3 to 4 weeks as needed (max 7.5 mg per kg per day)

IV/IM: 0.1 to 0.2 mg per kg per dose every 4 to 6 hours as needed; initial dose should not exceed 20 mg IM/IV (max 1.5 to 3 mg per kg per day)

Precautions: When given IV, hydralazine should be infused over 15 to 20 minutes while BP is monitored.

Adverse Effects: Tachycardia, flushing, headache, vomiting, sodium and water retention

Availability: Injection: 20 mg per mL

Tablets: 10, 25, 50, 100 mg

Drug: HYDROCHLOROTHIAZIDE (ESIDRIX®, HYDRODIURIL®, ORETIC®)

Use caution, sound-alike drugs include: Chlorothiazide (Diuril®)

Route of Administration: PO
Dose: 2 to 3 mg per kg per day in two divided doses (max 200 mg per day)
Adverse Effects: See Chlorothiazide.
Availability: Tablets: 25, 50, 100 mg
Oral solution: 10 mg per mL

Drug: HYDROCORTISONE (SOLU-CORTEF®)
Route of Administration: PO, IM, IV
Dose: *Acute adrenal insufficiency:* 1 to 2 mg per kg IV initial dose, followed by 3 to 5 mg per kg per day in four divided doses
Status asthmaticus: 4 to 8 mg per kg IV initial dose followed by 2 to 4 mg per kg per day in four to six divided doses
Shock: 50 mg per kg IV initial dose followed by 50 to 75 mg per kg per day in four to six divided doses for 2 days (max 2 g per dose)
Adverse Effects: See Dexamethasone.
Availability: Injection: 100, 250, 500 mg, and 1 g per vial
Tablets: 20 mg (Cortef)
Oral suspension: 2 mg per mL (Cortef)

Drug: HYDROMORPHONE (DILAUDID®)
Route of Administration: PO, IV, SC
Dose: *Acute pain, moderate to severe: older than 6 months and weight less than 50 kg:* 0.015 mg per kg per dose IV/SC q3–6h (max 2 mg per dose) as needed OR 0.03 to 0.08 mg per kg per dose PO q3–4h as needed (max 4 mg per dose); *more than 50 kg:* 1 to 2 mg PO/IV/SC q3–4h as needed
Note: Patients with previous opiate exposure may require higher initial doses.
Adverse Effects: Respiratory depression, apnea, sedation, hypotension, allergic reaction
Availability: Injection: 1, 2, 3, 4, 10 mg per mL
Tablet: 2, 4, 8 mg

Drug: HYDROXOCOBALAMIN (CYANOKIT®)
Route of Administration: IV
Dose: *Cyanide toxicity:* 70 mg per kg IV over 15 minutes (max 5 g per dose), may repeat dose
Precautions: Will interfere with colorimetric tests, such as bilirubin, Scr, and co-oximetry.
Adverse Effects: Headache, hypertension, discoloration of skin
Availability: Injection: 5-g kit

Drug: HYDROXYCHLOROQUINE (PLAQUENIL®)
Route of Administration: PO
Dose: *Malaria prophylaxis:* 5 mg per kg (base) once per week; *malaria treatment:* 10 mg per kg (base) load, then 5 mg per kg (base) daily—consult CDC for recommendations; *rheumatoid arthritis:* 3 to 6 mg per kg

per day (sulfate) in a single daily dose (max 400 mg per day)
Precautions: This drug should be given with extreme caution to children and to any patients with potential G6PD deficiency; all patients should be followed with periodic complete blood cell counts and ophthalmologic examinations.
Adverse Effects: *Acute:* headache, drowsiness, visual disturbances, rash
Long-term: corneal deposits, retinopathy (may be irreversible), discoloration of skin and mucous membranes, alopecia, blood dyscrasias, behavioral changes
Availability: Tablets: 200-mg hydroxychloroquine sulfate (equivalent to 155 mg of hydroxychloroquine base)

Drug: HYDROXYZINE (ATARAX®, VISTARIL®)
Use caution, sound-alike drugs include: Hydralazine (Apresoline®)
Route of Administration: PO, IM, IV
Dose: *PO:* 2 mg per kg per day in three to four divided doses (max 100 mg per day); *IM/IV:* 0.5 to 1 mg per kg per dose given every 4 to 6 hours (max 100 mg)
Precautions: May potentiate effects of barbiturates or narcotics.
Adverse Effects: Drowsiness, dry mouth
Availability: Injection (HCl salt, Vistaril®): 25, 50 mg per mL
Tablets (HCl salt, Atarax®): 10, 25, 50, 100 mg
Capsules (pamoate salt, Vistaril®): 25, 50 mg
Oral syrup (Atarax®): 2 mg per mL
Oral suspension (Vistaril®): 5 mg per mL

Drug: IBUPROFEN (ADVIL®, MOTRIN®, NUPRIN®, PEDIAPROFEN®)
Route of Administration: PO
Dose: *Fever:* 10 mg per kg per dose every 6 to 8 hours (max 1,200 mg per day)
Inflammatory diseases: 30 to 50 mg per kg per day in three or four divided doses (max 3,200 mg per day)
Analgesia: 4 to 10 mg per kg per dose every 6 to 8 hours (max 1,200 mg per day)
Precautions: Avoid in patients with aspirin hypersensitivity, moderate to severe dehydration, bleeding disorders. Administer doses with food or milk.
Adverse Effects: GI upset, GI bleeding, headache, prolonged bleeding time, fluid retention, acute renal failure
Availability: Tablets: 200, 300, 400, 600 mg
Chewable tablets: 50, 100 mg
Oral suspension: 20 mg per mL
Oral drops: 40 mg per mL

Drug: IMIPENEM and CILASTATIN (PRIMAXIN®)
Route of Administration: IV
Dose: *Age: younger than 3 months:* 100 mg per kg per day divided q6h; *age: older than 3 months:* 60 to 100 mg per kg per day divided q6–8h (max 4 g per day)

Precautions: Administer drug diluted to 5 mg per mL over 20 to 60 minutes. Dosage must be adjusted in patients with renal dysfunction.

Adverse Effects: Hypotension, seizures, nausea, vomiting, neutropenia, transient elevation of liver enzymes

Availability: Injection: 500 mg, 1 g

Drug: INDOMETHACIN (INDOCIN®)

Route of Administration: PO, PR, IV

Dose: *Inflammatory diseases:* 1 to 4 mg per kg per day PO or PR in two to four divided doses (max 200 mg per day); *patent ductus arteriosus:* give the following doses IV at 12- to 24-hour intervals for three doses, interval determined by urine output:

Age at first dose	Dose (mg per kg)		
	1st	2nd	3rd
<48 h	0.2	0.1	0.1
2–7 day	0.2	0.2	0.2
>7 day	0.2	0.25	0.25

Precautions: Avoid in patients with a history of aspirin hypersensitivity. Indomethacin should be used with caution in patients with coagulation defects or impaired renal function. May inhibit naturetic effect of furosemide. May increase serum concentration of digoxin.

Adverse Effects: GI disturbances, GI bleeding, headache, visual changes, hypersensitivity reactions, renal dysfunction (reduced glomerular filtration rate, reduced urine output, fluid retention), inhibition of platelet aggregation

Availability: Capsules: 25, 50 mg
Oral suspension: 5 mg per mL
Rectal suppository: 50 mg
Injection: 1 mg per vial

Drug: INSULIN, HUMAN REGULAR (HUMULIN R®, NOVOLIN R®)

Route of Administration: IV, SC

Dose: *Acute management of DKA:* 0.1 units per kg SC/IV, followed by 0.1 units per kg per hour as a continuous infusion. *Emergent, symptomatic hyperkalemia:* 0.1 units per kg SC/IV × 1 dose along with 0.5 g per kg of dextrose. *Maintenance:* Highly variable; 0.5 to 1 units per kg per day divided two-thirds in the morning, one-third in the evening

Precautions: Tubing should be primed for 15 to 30 minutes prior to infusion, if possible, to ensure complete adsorption to binding sites. Do not consider all clear insulin preparations to be fast acting or appropriate for IV infusion. A diluent is provided by the manufacturer to dilute 100 units per mL to 10 units per mL for doses under 0.5 units.

Adverse Effects: Hypoglycemia, palpitations, tachycardia, confusion

Availability: Injection: 100 units per mL

Drug: IPRATROPIUM BROMIDE (ATROVENT®)

Route of Administration: Oral inhalation, nasal inhalation

Dose: *Nebulization: acute asthma: weight less than 10 kg:* 0.25 mg every 20 minutes for three doses, then q4–6h if needed; *weight more than 10 kg:* 0.5 mg every 20 minutes for three doses, then q4–6h if needed

MDI: 3 to 12 years: 1 to 2 puffs TID (max 6 puffs per 24 hours); *older than 12 years:* 2 puffs QID (max 12 puffs per 24 hours); *nasal spray:* 2 sprays each nostril two to four times per day.

Precautions: Do not use older MDI versions (non-HFA) in patients with peanut or soy allergy.

Adverse Effects: Exacerbation of respiratory symptoms, dyspnea, pharyngitis, blurred vision, nervousness, dizziness. Because of the drug's low lipid solubility, CNS side effects are uncommon.

Availability: Metered-dose aerosol: 18 mcg per spray
Solution for nebulization: 0.02% (0.5 mg per 2.5 mL)
Nasal spray: 0.03%, 0.06%

Drug: ISRADIPINE (DYNA-CIRC®)

Route of Administration: PO

Dose: *Severe hypertension and hypertensive emergencies:* 0.05 to 0.15 mg per kg per dose PO TID-QID, titrated up as needed, max 20 mg per day

Precautions: Use caution with concurrent use of CYP3A4 inhibitors as they can significantly increase the serum concentrations of isradipine. Should be used carefully in patients with CHF or hepatic dysfunction.

Adverse Effects: Nausea, excess hypotension, bradycardia, headache, dizziness

Availability: Tablets: 2.5, 5 mg
Tablets, controlled release: 5, 10 mg

Drug: KETAMINE (KETALAR®)

Use caution, sound-alike drugs include: Ketorolac (Toradol®)

Route of Administration: IV, IM, PO

Dose: *Procedural sedation:* 1 to 2 mg per kg per dose IV, may repeat 0.5 mg per kg per dose IV q2–5min as needed to maintain sedation (max 5 mg per kg or 500 mg, whichever is less) OR 4 to 5 mg per kg per dose IM, may repeat 2 mg per kg per dose IM × 1 if inadequate sedation in 10 minutes. Oral dose: 10 mg per kg × 1. *RSI:* see Resuscitation Drug List.

Precautions: Resources for managing laryngospasms must be immediately available. Do not use in emotionally labile children.

Adverse Effects: Emergence reactions, laryngospasm, possible increase in ICP
Availability: Injection: 10, 50, 100 mg per mL

Drug: KETOROLAC (TORADOL®)

Use caution, sound-alike drugs include: Ketamine (Ketalar®)
Route of Administration: IV, IM, PO
Dose: *IV, IM:* 0.5 mg per kg per dose every 6 hours to a maximum of 15 mg per dose for patients weighing less than 50 kg or a maximum of 30 mg per dose for patients weighing more than 50 kg.
PO: 16 years of age or older: 10 mg per dose every 6 hours. PO dosing recommendations are not available for children younger than 16 years of age.
Precautions: Treatment should be limited to a maximum of 5 days because of the increased risk of hemorrhage with long-term therapy.
Adverse Effects: GI bleed, edema, headache, dyspepsia, nausea, increased bleeding time, anaphylaxis, hypersensitivity reactions (contraindicated for use in patients with aspirin allergy)
Availability: Injection: 15, 30 mg per mL
Tablets: 10 mg

Drug: LABETALOL (NORMODYNE®, TRANDATE®)
Route of Administration: IV, PO
Dose: *Severe hypertension and hypertensive emergencies:* 0.25 to 1 mg per kg per dose IV q4–6h, max 20 mg per dose. Additional higher dosages may be administered at 10-minute intervals until control of supine BP or until a cumulative dose of 300 mg is achieved. Alternatively, continuous infusion rates of 0.25 to 1 mg per kg per hour have been used (max 3 mg per kg per hour). *Hypertension, oral:* Initial dose 3 mg per kg per day (max 100 mg PO BID); usual maintenance dosage is 5 to 20 mg per kg per day (max 1,200 mg per day).
Precautions: Due to extended half-life and duration of action, continuous infusions can be difficult to titrate. Additive hypotension occurs when administered with a diuretic. May worsen CHF; avoid use in patients with bronchial asthma, overt heart failure, or severe bradycardia. May mask signs and symptoms of hypoglycemia. Synergistic hypotension occurs with halothane anesthesia.
Adverse Effects: Nausea, excess hypotension, bradycardia, headache, bronchospasm
Availability: Tablets: 100, 200, 300 mg
Injection: 5 mg per mL

Drug: LACTULOSE (ENULOSE®)
Route of Administration: PO
Dose: *Portal systemic encephalopathy:* infants 2 to 10 mL per day, children 40 to 90 mL per day divided 3 to 4 times per day, titrate to 2 to 3 soft stools per day.
Constipation: children 7.5 mL per day, adults 15 to 30 mL per day

Adverse Effects: Nausea, vomiting
Availability: Syrup 667 mg per mL

Drug: LAMOTRIGINE (LAMICTAL®)
Route of Administration: PO
Dose: Note: Consult manufacturer's package insert for initial dosing regimens, weeks 1 to 4.
Patients receiving enzyme-inducing anti-epileptic drugs (AEDs) without valproic acid: 0.6 mg per kg per day in two divided doses, increasing gradually to a maximum of 15 mg per kg per day (max 400 mg per day).
Patients receiving enzyme-inducing AEDs with valproic acid: 0.2 mg per kg per day in one to two divided doses, increasing gradually to a maximum of 5 mg per kg per day (max 250 mg per day)
Adverse Effects: Life-threatening rash (especially in children), angioedema, Stevens-Johnson syndrome, photosensitivity, nausea, vomiting, diplopia, amblyopia, nystagmus, dizziness, ataxia
Availability: Chewable tablets: 5, 25 mg
Tablets: 25, 100, 150, 200 mg

Drug: LEVONORGESTEROL (PLAN B®)
Route of Administration: PO
Dose: 0.75 mg PO × 1 dose, then repeat in 12 hours OR 1.5 mg PO × 1 dose
Adverse Effects: Nausea, vomiting, headache
Availability: Tablets: 0.75 mg, 2 tablets per package

Drug: LEVOTHYROXINE (LEVOXYL®, SYNTHROID®)
Route of Administration: PO, IM, IV
Dose: Oral:
0 to 6 months: 8 to 10 mcg per kg daily or 25 to 50 mcg per day
6 to 12 months: 6 to 8 mcg per kg daily or 50 to 75 mcg per day
1 to 5 years: 5 to 6 mcg per kg daily or 75 to 100 mcg per day
6 to 12 years: 4 to 5 mcg per kg daily or 100 to 150 mcg per day
Older than 12 years: 2 to 3 mcg per kg daily or more than or equal to 150 mcg per day
Growth and puberty complete: 1.6 mcg per kg daily
Note: IV and IM doses are 50% to 75% of oral dose.
Adverse Effects: Hypertension, palpitations, tachycardia, insomnia, diarrhea, weight loss
Availability: Injection: 0.2, 0.5 mg per vial
Tablets: 25, 50, 75, 88, 100, 112, 125, 150, 175, 200, 300 mcg
Note: Many recipes for compounding oral suspensions have been published.

Drug: LIDOCAINE (see Resuscitation Drug List for IV/ETT)

Drug: LIDOCAINE (Xylocaine®, LMX-4)
Route of Administration: Oral, topical

Dose: *Minor procedures, IV insertion:* 1 g per site, applied in a thick layer and covered with an occlusive dressing for at least 20 minutes. *Oral mouthwash:* use in a 1:1:1 mixture with diphenhydramine and Maalox; do not exceed 3 mg per kg per dose or give within 3 hours of previous dose.

Precautions: Allergic reaction, toxic absorption.

Adverse Effects: Possible absorption of the lidocaine

Availability: Cream: 4%, viscous: 2%

Drug: LIDOCAINE and PRILOCAINE (emla®)

Route of Administration: Topical

Dose: *Minor procedures:* 2.5 g per site, applied in a thick layer and covered with an occlusive dressing for at least 60 minutes. *Painful procedures:* 2 g per 10 cm^2 of skin, covered and left in place for at least 2 hours.
Maximum doses: Less than 10 kg: 100 cm^2
10 to 20 kg: 600 cm^2
More than 20 kg: 2,000 cm^2

Neonates: Use smaller amount of cream. Methemoglobinemia is of theoretical concern in these patients; the manufacturer does not recommend its use in patients younger than 1 month of age or in patients younger than 12 months of age who are receiving treatment with methemoglobin-inducing agents.

Precautions: Avoid use near eyes or mouth, especially in children.

Adverse Effects: Possible absorption of the lidocaine and prilocaine

Availability: Cream: Lidocaine 2.5% and prilocaine 2.5%

Drug: LITHIUM CARBONATE (ESKALITH® AND OTHERS)

Route of Administration: PO

Dose: 15 to 60 mg per kg per day divided in three to four doses (max initial: 300 mg per day, max maintenance: 2,400 mg per day). Sustained-release preparations are given in two divided doses. Lithium serum concentrations should be maintained at 0.6 to 1.4 mEq per L.

Precautions: Serum lithium concentrations must be monitored because toxicity is related to serum concentration. Increased sodium intake may result in decreased lithium serum concentrations. The following factors may increase lithium serum concentrations: reduced sodium intake, vomiting, and concomitant therapy with nonsteroidal antiinflammatory agents or diuretics.

Adverse Effects: Mild thirst at initiation of therapy, transient and mild nausea during first few days of therapy, nephrogenic diabetes insipidus, goiter. Lithium toxicity is characterized by CNS disturbances (tremor, confusion, somnolence) and GI disturbances (anorexia, nausea, vomiting).

Availability: Capsules (immediate release): 150 mg (4.06 mEq), 300 mg (8.12 mEq), 600 mg (16.24 mEq)
Tablets: 300 mg

Oral solution: Lithium citrate 1.6 mEq of lithium per mL (equivalent to 60 mg of lithium carbonate per mL)
Tablets (sustained release): 300, 450 mg

Drug: LOPERAMIDE (IMODIUM®)

Route of Administration: PO

Dose: *Acute diarrhea:* First day of therapy (initial 24 hours): 2 to 5 years (13 to 20 kg), 1 mg TID; 5 to 8 years (20 to 30 kg), 2 mg BID; 8 to 12 years (more than 30 kg), 2 mg TID. On second and subsequent days, dosages of 0.1 mg per kg per dose (not to exceed dosage appropriate for age recommended for first day) may be given after each unformed stool. *Chronic diarrhea:* 0.08 to 0.24 mg per kg per day divided in two to three doses, max 2 mg per dose. *Traveler's diarrhea (max 2 days of therapy):* 6 to 8 years, 1 mg after each loose stool, max 4 mg per day; 9 to 11 years, 2 mg after first loose stool, followed by 1 mg after each loose stool, max 6 mg per day; older than 12 years, 4 mg after first loose stool, followed by 2 mg after each loose stool, max 8 mg per day.

Adverse Effects: Behavioral disturbances, sedation, abdominal cramping, constipation, dry mouth

Availability: Capsules, tablets: 2 mg
Oral solution: 0.2 mg per mL

Drug: LORACARBEF (LORABID®)

Route of Administration: PO

Dose: *Acute otitis media:* 30 mg per kg per day in two divided doses for 10 days using the suspension form of the drug because it yields higher plasma concentrations (max 800 mg per day). *Pharyngitis, tonsillitis:* 15 mg per kg per day in two divided doses (max 800 mg per day).

Adverse Effects: Possible cross-sensitivity with penicillin; diarrhea, nausea, vomiting, skin rashes

Availability: Capsules: 200 mg
Suspension: 100, 200 mg per 5 mL

Drug: LORAZEPAM (ATIVAN®)

Route of Administration: IV, PO

Dose: *Status epilepticus:* 0.1 mg per kg per dose IV every 5 to 15 minutes for two to three doses (max 4 mg per dose)
Anxiety: 0.05 to 0.1 mg per kg PO/IV q4–8h prn, max 4 mg per dose. Usual adult dose 2 mg
Antiemetic: 0.04 to 0.08 mg per kg per dose IV/PO (max 4 mg per dose)

Precautions: Avoid inadvertent intraarterial injection because it may induce arteriospasm leading to gangrene. Use caution with continuous infusions as propylene glycol may lead to toxicity and acute renal failure.

Adverse Effects: Excess sedation, respiratory depression, hypotension

Availability: Tablets: 0.5, 1, 2 mg

Injection: 2, 4 mg per mL
Oral solution: 2 mg per mL

Drug: MAGNESIUM SULFATE
Route of Administration: IV
Dose: *Acute asthma*: 40 mg per kg per dose IV over 20 minutes (max 2 g per dose)
Torsades de Pointes: 25 to 50 mg per kg per dose IV rapid infusion (max 2 g per dose)
Adverse Effects: Tachyarrhythmias, prolonged QRS, flushing, loss of deep tendon reflexes, change in mental status
Availability: Injection: 100, 125, 250, 500 mg per mL

Drug: MANNITOL (OSMITROL®)
Route of Administration: IV
Dose: Note: For patients with oliguria or suspected inadequate renal function, first establish adequate urine output with a test dose of 200 mg per kg (maximum 12.5 g) over 3 to 5 minutes (over 20 to 30 minutes for patients with cerebral edema/increased ICP) to produce at least 1 mL per kg per hour urine flow for 2 to 3 hours.
Initial dose: 0.5 to 1 g per kg, followed by 0.25 to 0.5 g per kg per dose every 4 to 6 hours as needed.
Precautions: Do not use in patients with hypotension, anuria, active intracranial bleeding, severe pulmonary edema or congestive heart disease. Mannitol must be filtered during administration. Never run as a continuous infusion.
Adverse Effects: Electrolyte imbalances, dehydration, CNS toxicity
Availability: Injection: 5%, 10%, 15%, 20%, 25%

Drug: MECLIZINE (ANTIVERT®)
Route of Administration: PO
Dose: *Motion sickness*: 12.5 to 25 mg 1 hour prior to travel, repeat every 12 to 14 hours. *Vertigo*: 25 to 100 mg per day in 2 to 3 divided doses
Precautions: Do not use in patients younger than 12 years old.
Adverse Effects: Sedation, weight gain
Availability: Tablets; 12.5, 25, 50 mg

Drug: MEDROXYPROGESTERONE ACETATE (PROVERA®)
Route of Administration: PO
Dose: *Amenorrhea, uterine bleeding:* 5 to 10 mg per day for 5 to 10 days
Precautions: Avoid during pregnancy and in patients with a history of thromboembolic disease, breast malignancy, migraine, undiagnosed vaginal bleeding, or depression.
Adverse Effects: Breast tenderness, weight loss or gain, edema, thrombophlebitis, menstrual abnormalities, cholestatic jaundice, mental depression
Availability: Tablets: 2.5, 5, 10 mg

Drug: MEPERIDINE (DEMEROL®)
Route of Administration: PO, IM, IV
Dose: Adult: 1 to 2 mg per kg per dose IM or PO every 3 to 4 hours; 1 to 1.5 mg per kg per dose IV every 4 hours, if needed (max 100 mg per dose).
Precautions: Not recommended in children. Neurotoxic metabolite may accumulate in patients with renal failure or after prolonged use. May potentiate other CNS depressants. May induce dependence. Never use in patients taking monamine oxidase inhibitors; use extreme caution with SSRIs and TCAs.
Adverse Effects: CNS depression, respiratory depression, orthostatic hypotension, nausea, vomiting, urinary retention, decreased GI motility
Availability: Injection: 25, 50, 75, 100 mg per mL
Tablets: 50, 100 mg
Oral solution: 10 mg per mL

Drug: MEROPENEM (MERREM®)
Route of Administration: IV
Dose: 60 to 120 mg per kg per day divided every 8 hours, use higher dose in meningitis (max 6 g per day)
Adverse Effects: See Imipenem.
Availability: Injection: 500 mg, 1 g

Drug: METAPROTERENOL (ALUPENT®, METAPREL®)
Route of Administration: PO, inhalation
Dose: *PO: age 6 to 9 years and weight less than 30 kg:* 10 mg TID or QID; *adults and children older than 9 years of age and weight more than 30 kg:* 20 mg TID or QID
There is less experience in children younger than 6 years of age but PO dosages of 1.3 to 2.6 mg per kg per day in divided doses have been well tolerated though infrequently indicated.
Inhalation : 2 puffs every 4 hours from metered-dose aerosol (max dose: six doses per day). Via intermittent positive-pressure breathing (for patients 12 years of age or older): 0.2 to 0.3 mL of 5% solution diluted in 2.5 mL of 0.45% or 0.9% NaCl. Alternatively, 2.5 mL of commercially available 0.6% solution may be used. Do not repeat these doses more often than every 4 hours.
Precautions: Patients should be carefully instructed in the proper use of the inhaler.
Adverse Effects: Nausea, headache, tremor, tachycardia, dizziness, flushing
Availability: Tablets: 10, 20 mg
Oral solution: 2 mg per mL
Aerosol: 0.65 mg per inhalation
Solution for nebulization: 0.4%, 0.6%, 5%

Drug: METHOTREXATE
Route of Administration: IM
Dose: *Ectopic pregnancy:* 50 mg per m^2 as a single IM dose. A repeat dose may be needed on an outpatient basis.

Adverse Effects: Nausea, vomiting, bone marrow suppression, esophagitis

Availability: Injection 10 mg per mL, 25 mg per mL

Drug: METHYLENE BLUE

Route of Administration: IV

Dose: *Methemoglobinemia:* 1 to 2 mg per kg per dose (infuse over 5 minutes); may repeat after 1 hour, if needed.

Adverse Effects: Hypertension, discoloration of urine and feces, nausea, vomiting, abdominal pain, excessive formation of methemoglobin, cyanosis

Availability: Injection: 10 mg per mL

Drug: METHYLPHENIDATE (CONCERTA®, RITALIN®)

Route of Administration: PO

Dose: *Initial dose (age older than 6 years):* 0.3 mg per kg per dose (max 5 mg per dose) at breakfast and lunch. Gradually titrate dosage by 0.1 mg per kg per dose every week to effect (max 2 mg per kg per day or 60 mg per day, whichever is less). Some patients may require TID dosing.

Precautions: Tolerance may develop and require dosage adjustment.

Adverse Effects: Insomnia, nervousness, loss of appetite, irritability, growth suppression, increased or decreased BP, tachycardia

Availability: Tablets: 5, 10, 20 mg

Sustained-released tablets: 18, 20, 27, 36, 54 mg

Drug: METHYLPREDNISOLONE (see Resuscitation Drug List)

Drug: METOCLOPRAMIDE (REGLAN®)

Route of Administration: PO, IV

Dose: 0.1 to 0.2 mg per kg per dose PO/IV every 6 hours, max 10 mg per dose. Higher doses of 1 mg per kg per dose (max 50 mg per dose) may be used for acetaminophen overdose or chemotherapy-induced nausea and vomiting. Prophylactic diphenhydramine may be beneficial in decreasing extrapyramidal side effects seen with higher doses.

Adverse Effects: Dystonic reactions, hypertension, bradycardia, agitation, hallucinations, constipation, diarrhea

Availability: Injection: 5 mg per mL

Solution: 1, 10 mg per mL

Tablets: 5, 10 mg

Drug: METRONIDAZOLE (FLAGYL®)

Route of Administration: PO, IV

Dose: *Antibiotic-associated pseudomembranous colitis:* 20 to 35 mg per kg per day in four divided doses.

Amebiasis: 35 to 50 mg per kg per day PO in three divided doses for 5 to 10 days (max 750 mg TID).

Giardiasis: 15 mg per kg per day PO in three divided doses for 5 days (max 250 mg TID).

Helicobacter pylori infection: 15 to 20 mg per kg per day in two divided doses for 4 weeks (max 1 to 1.5 g per day). Many combination regimens exist.

Trichomonas vaginalis: 15 mg per kg per day PO in three divided doses for 7 days (max 1 g per day); usual adult dose: 500 mg PO BID for 7 days or a single dose of 2 g.

IV (for treatment of anaerobic infections): 30 mg per kg per day divided every 6 hours; IV doses should be administered over 1 hour (max 4 g per day).

Precautions: Disulfiram-like reaction may occur with ingestion of alcohol. Palatability is poor and compliance may be an issue.

Adverse Effects: Metallic taste, GI distress, peripheral neuropathy

Availability: Tablets: 250, 500 mg

Injection: 5 mg per mL

Note: Several recipes for suspensions have been published.

Drug: MICONAZOLE (MONISTAT®)

Route of Administration: Topical

Dose: *Cream or lotion:* Twice-daily application for 2 to 4 weeks

Vaginal cream: One applicatorful daily for 3 to 7 days

Vaginal suppository: One 100-mg suppository intravaginally at bedtime for 7 days or one 200-mg suppository intravaginally at bedtime for 3 days

Availability: Cream, lotion, vaginal cream: 2%

Vaginal suppositories: 100, 200 mg

Drug: MIDAZOLAM (VERSED®)

Route of Administration: IV, IM, PO, intranasal

Dose: *IM/IV sedation for procedures:* 0.05 to 0.1 mg per kg IM/IV just before procedure (max 2 mg per dose*), may repeat every 3 minutes with a dose of 0.05 mg per kg as needed to maintain sedation (total max 0.3 mg per kg or 10 mg, whichever is less); *PO sedation:* 0.25 to 1 mg per kg PO 30 to 45 minutes before procedure (max dose: 15 mg); *intranasal:* 0.2 mg per kg using the 5 mg per mL injection administered with a needleless syringe into the nares; *maintainence of sedation (i.e., postintubation):* 0.05 to 0.1 mg per kg per dose IV/IM every 1 to 2 hours as needed (max 10 mg per dose); *continuous infusion:* 0.05 to 0.1 mg per kg per hour.

Note: *Adolescents and adults require smaller doses of midazolam than children.

Adverse Effects: Hypotension, bradycardia, paradoxical excitement, local pain at the injection site, laryngospasm, bronchospasm

Availability: Injection: 1, 5 mg per mL

Oral syrup: 2 mg per mL

Drug: MIDODRINE (PROAMANTINE®)
Route of Administration: PO
Dose: *Postural hypotension:* 10 mg TID while patient is awake and upright (max 40 mg per day); *vasovagal syncope:* 5 mg while patient is awake and upright (max 15 mg per day)
Precautions: Do not use in patients younger than 12 years old.
Adverse Effects: Bardycardia, hypertension, leg cramps, nausea, weight gain
Availability: Tablets: 2.5, 5 mg

Drug: MINERAL OIL
Route of Administration: PO
Dose: *Constipation:* 5 to 11 yr: 5 to 20 mL per day; >12 yr: 15 to 45 mL per day in divided doses
Note: Do not use in children less than 3 years of age or any patient who is at risk for aspiration
Adverse Effects: Aspiration pneumonitis, loss of fat soluble vitamins, abdominal cramping, diarrhea
Availability: Liquid 100%: 30 mL, 480 mL

Drug: MORPHINE SULFATE (GENERIC)
Route of Administration: PO, IM, IV, SC
Dose: *Oral:* 0.1 to 0.5 mg per kg per dose PO q4–6h as needed
Initial (SC, IM, IV): younger than 6 months: 0.05 mg per kg per dose IV every 2 to 4 hours as needed; *older than 6 months:* 0.1 mg per kg every 2 to 6 hours as needed (usual max 10 mg per dose).
Initial IV infusion: 0.01 to 0.04 mg per kg per hour (postoperative pain) or 0.04 to 0.07 mg per kg per hour (sickle cell or cancer pain). For neonates, use an initial rate of 0.01 mg per kg per hour. Maximum initial dose: 2 mg per hour; accumulation may occur—titrate as necessary.
Precautions: IV morphine should be administered slowly (over 4 to 5 minutes) while monitoring respiratory rate, BP, and heart rate. May potentiate other CNS depressants.
Adverse Effects: Respiratory depression, apnea, hypotension, bradycardia, rash, allergic reaction
Availability: Oral solution: 2, 4, 20 mg per mL
Tablets: 15, 30 mg
Sustained release tablets: 15, 30, 60 mg
Injection: Multiple concentrations ranging from 2 to 15 mg per mL

Drug: MUPIROCIN (BACTROBAN®)
Route of Administration: Topical
Dose: Application of a small amount to affected area TID for 1 to 2 weeks
Availability: Ointment 2% in polyethylene glycol base

Drug: NAFCILLIN
Route of Administration: IM, IV
Dose: *Age 0 to 4 weeks, weight less than 1,200 g:* 50 mg per kg per day in two divided doses

Age 7 days or younger, weight 1,200 to 2,000 g: 50 mg per kg per day in two divided doses
Age 7 days or younger, weight more than 2,000 g: 75 mg per kg per day in three divided doses
Age older than 7 days, weight 1,200 to 2,000 g: 75 mg per kg per day in three divided doses
Age older than 7 days, weight more than 2,000 g: 100 mg per kg per day in four divided doses
Older infants and children: 50 to 200 mg per kg per day in four to six divided doses (max 2 g per dose)
Precautions: See Oxacillin; each gram of nafcillin contains approximately 3 mEq sodium. Dose must be adjusted in renal dysfunction.
Adverse Effects: See Oxacillin.
Availability: Injection: 500 mg; 1, 2 g

Drug: NALOXONE (see Resuscitation List)

Drug: NAPROXEN (NAPROSYN®, ANAPROX®)
Route of Administration: PO
Dose: *Dysmenorrhea:* 500 mg initial dose followed by 250 mg every 6 to 8 hours
Juvenile rheumatoid arthritis: 10 to 15 mg per kg per day in two divided doses (max dose: 1 g per day)
Precautions: Use with extreme caution in patients with history of aspirin hypersensitivity.
Adverse Effects: See Ibuprofen.
Availability: Oral suspension: 25 mg per mL
Tablets: 250, 375, 500 mg
Tablets, naproxen sodium: 275 mg (equivalent to 250 mg Naprosyn®), 550 mg (equivalent to 500 mg Naprosyn®)

Drug: NIFEDIPINE (ADALAT®, PROCARDIA®)
Route of Administration: PO
Dose: *Hypertension (adult):* 30 to 60 mg per day PO of extended-release tablet. Titrate dosage at 7- to 14-day intervals (max 120 mg per day). Usual initial dose of liquid-filled capsules is 10 mg TID (max 180 mg per day).
Hypertensive emergencies (child): Clinical experience is limited but doses in the range of 0.25 to 0.5 mg per kg per dose have been used (max 10 mg per dose).
Note: Rapid reduction of BP occurs when administered sublingually or intrabuccally by puncturing or chewing the liquid-filled capsule and expressing the liquid into the mouth. Many clinicians prefer that capsules be bitten, then swallowed to achieve higher peak serum concentrations and less variation in response.
Precautions: May increase serum concentrations and pharmacologic activity of digoxin and phenytoin. Additive or synergistic hypotension occurs with β-adrenergic-blocking agents, fentanyl, hydralazine, and other antihypertensives. Patients receiving extended-release

tablets should not be alarmed if a tablet-like substance appears in the stool because drug is released from a nonabsorbable shell during passage through the GI tract.

Adverse Effects: Excessive lowering of BP, worsening of heart failure, dizziness, flushing, peripheral edema

Availability: Capsules: 10, 20 mg

Extended-release tablets: 30, 60, 90 mg

Note: The liquid-filled capsules may be pierced on each end and the contents withdrawn for doses lower than 10 mg. The volume of each capsule may be obtained from the manufacturer.

Drug: NITROFURANTOIN (MACRODANTIN®, MACROBID®)

Route of Administration: PO

Dose: *Acute urinary tract infection:* 5 to 7 mg per kg per day in four divided doses (max 400 mg per day)

Prophylaxis or long-term therapy: 1 to 2 mg per kg per dose as a single evening dose (max 100 mg per day)

Precautions: Medication should be administered with food to minimize GI distress. Dosage should be reduced in patients with impaired renal function.

Adverse Effects: GI distress, interstitial pneumonitis, pulmonary fibrosis, peripheral neuropathy

Availability: Capsules 25, 100 mg

Extended release capsules: 100 mg

Oral suspension: 5 mg per mL

Drug: NITROPRUSSIDE (see Resuscitation Drug List)

Drug: NORETHINDRONE (NORLUTIN®, NORLUTATE®)

Route of Administration: PO

Dose: *Amenorrhea, uterine bleeding:* 2.5 to 10 mg per day norethindrone acetate, 5 to 20 mg per day of norethindrone

Precautions: Contraindicated in patients with history of thrombotic or thromboembolic disorders.

Adverse Effects: Breakthrough bleeding, edema, weight loss or gain, mental depression

Availability: Tablets: 5 mg norethindrone, 5 mg norethindrone acetate

---

Drug: NYSTATIN (MYCOSTATIN®, NILSTAT®)

Route of Administration: PO, topical

Dose: *PO: age younger than 28 days:* 400,000 units per day in four divided doses; *age older than 28 days:* 400,000 to 2,000,000 units per day in four divided doses. Rub in oral doses well to affected areas in the mouth.

Adverse Effects: GI disturbances

Availability: Topical cream, ointment, and powder

Oral tablets: 500,000 units

Oral suspension: 100,000 units per mL

Drug: OCTREOTIDE (SANDOSTATIN®)

Route of Administration: IV, SC

Dose: *Diarrhea:* 1 to 10 mcg per kg per dose every 12 hours; *GI hemorrhage: initial:* 1 to 2 mcg per kg, max 50 mcg per dose, followed by a continuous infusion 1 to 2 mcg per kg per hour, max 50 mcg per hour; *sulfonylurea overdose:* 1 to 2 mcg per kg, max 50 mcg per dose

Adverse Effects: Hyper/hypotension, palpitations, anxiety, headache, fever, rash, hyper/hypoglycemia

Note: Depot injection for monthly administration in stable patients only. Do not use for IV administration.

Availability: Injection: 0.05, 0.1, 0.2, 0.5, 1 mg per mL

Depot injection: 10, 20, 30 mg

Drug: OLANZAPINE (ZYPREXA®)

Route of Administration: PO, IM

Dose: *Oral maintenance:* 2.5 to 20 mg per day, titrated slowly. *Acute agitation:* 5 to 10 mg IM

Adverse Effects: Hypersensitivity reactions, cardiac arrhythmias, blood dyscrasias, suicidal ideation, hyperglycemia, hyperlipidemia, seizures

Note: Should only be prescribed for maintenance therapy in conjunction with psychiatry consult.

Availability: Injection: 10 mg; Tablets: 2.5, 5, 7.5, 10, 15, 20 mg

---

Drug: OMEPRAZOLE (PRILOSEC®)

Route of Administration: PO

Dose: 0.6 to 1 mg per kg per dose daily, may increase to 3.3 mg per kg per day divided BID; *usual adult:* 20 mg per dose

Precautions: Possible drug interactions with other medications metabolized via the CYP3A3/4 enzyme pathway. Do not use in patients receiving high-dose methotrexate.

Adverse Effects: GI distress, tachycardia, bradycardia, insomnia, anxiety, rash, myalgias, tinnitus

Availability: Capsules, delayed release: 10, 20, 40 mg

Note: Several recipes for suspensions have been published.

Drug: ONDANSETRON (ZOFRAN®)

Route of Administration: PO, IV, IM

Dose: *Nononcology nausea and vomiting:* 0.15 mg per kg per dose PO/IV/IM every 8 hours as needed. Lower doses have been shown to be effective and better tolerated. *Age-based dosing: 6 months to 1 year:* 2 mg; *1 to 12 years:* 4 mg; *>12 years:* 8 mg per dose, *Chemotherapy-associated nausea and vomiting:* 0.45 mg per kg per day IV/PO divided every 8 to 24 hours

Adverse Effects: Headache, dizziness, seizures, tachycardia, bradycardia, rash, fever

Availability: Injection: 2 mg per mL

Solution: 0.8 mg per mL

Tablet: 4, 8 mg

Tablet, orally dissolving: 4, 8 mg

Drug: OXACILLIN
Route of Administration: IM, IV
Dose: *Younger than 1 week of age and weight less than 2,000 g:* 50 mg per kg per day given in two divided doses
Younger than 1 week of age and weight more than 2,000 g: 100 mg per kg per day in four divided doses
Children: 100 to 200 mg per kg per day given in four to six divided doses (max 12 g per day)
Precautions: Each gram of oxacillin contains approximately 3 mEq of sodium. Dose must be adjusted in renal dysfunction.
Adverse Effects: Hepatic dysfunction, hypersensitivity reactions, blood dyscrasias
Availability: Injection: Various size vials containing 250 mg to 10 g per vial
Capsules: 250, 500 mg
Oral solution: 500 mg per mL when reconstituted

Drug: OXCARBAZEPINE (TRILEPTAL®)
Route of Administration: PO
Dose: *Initial:* 8 to 10 mg per kg per day divided BID, titrate up slowly over 2 weeks to an average dose of 5 to 60 mg per kg per day (total 2,400 mg per day)
Precautions: Do not discontinue abruptly, do not use in pregnancy unless benefit outweighs risk.
Adverse Effects: Psychomotor slowing, cognitive dysfunction, Stevens-Johnson syndrome, hyponatremia, suicidal ideation
Availability: Tablet: 150, 300 mg
Liquid: 60 mg per mL

Drug: PANTOPRAZOLE (PROTONIX®)
Route of Administration: IV, PO
Dose: 0.5 to 1 mg per kg per day given IV/PO q12–24h, 0.1 mg per kg per hour for continuous infusion
Precautions: Vessel irritant: dilute to 4 mg per mL for intermittent infusion, 0.8 mg per mL for continuous infusion. Note current controversy about using a protein pump inhibitors while receiving clopidrogel for antiplatelet effect.
Adverse Effects: Phlebitis, GI distress, diarrhea, myalgia, arthralgia
Availability: Injection: 40 mg per vial
Tablets: 20,40 mg
Oral suspension (compounded): 2 mg per mL

Drug: PANCURONIUM (PAVULON®)
Route of Administration: IV
Dose: *Intubation in patients younger than 1 month of age:* 0.06 to 0.1 mg per kg; *children:* 0.15 mg per kg
Maintenance of paralysis: 0.1 mg per kg per hour via continuous infusion or 0.1 to 0.15 mg per kg per dose IV q1h prn
Precautions: Pancuronium is not generally used for RSI due to long onset time. Neonates are particularly sensitive

to the effects of neuromuscular-blocking agents and dosage must be individualized.
Adverse Effects: Tachycardia, respiratory depression, hypertension, excessive salivation
Availability: Injection: 1, 2 mg per mL

Drug: D-PENICILLAMINE (DEPEN®, CUPRIMINE®)
Route of Administration: PO
Dose: *Lead poisoning: initial:* 5 mg per kg per day in divided doses, titrate over several weeks to 20 to 30 mg per kg per day in three to four doses, max 1.5 g per day; *rheumatoid arthritis:* 3 to 10 mg per kg per day given as a single dose; start at a low dosage and titrate dosage upward over several months (max 1.5 g per day)
Precautions: Monitor CBC, urinalysis, renal and hepatic function. Give with food or flavored food substance to improve palatability.
Adverse Effects: Allergic reactions, rash, hematuria, proteinuria, anorexia, nausea, vomiting, diarrhea, bitter taste, stomatitis, blood dyscrasias, cross-sensitivity with penicillins, optic neuritis, obliterative bronchiolitis
Availability: Capsules: 125, 250 mg
Tablets: 250 mg

Drug: PENICILLIN G, BENZATHINE (BICILLIN®)
Route of Administration: IM only
Dose: *Staphylococcal and streptococcal infections: weight less than 27 kg:* single dose of 300,000 to 600,000 U; *weight more than 27 kg:* single dose of 900,000 U; *adult:* single dose of 1.2 million U; *syphilis:* single dose of 50,000 U per kg (max dose: 2.4 million U) only if neurosyphilis can be excluded; otherwise, penicillin G or penicillin G procaine are preferred
Precautions: Administer as deep IM injection; otherwise precautions are same as for penicillin G. Death has been reported after inadvertent IV administration.
Adverse Effects: See Penicillin G, Potassium.
Availability: Injection: 300,000, 600,000 U per mL

Drug: PENICILLIN G, POTASSIUM
Route of Administration: IM, IV
Dose: *Injection : age younger than 7 days:* 50,000 to 100,000 units per kg per day IV in two divided doses for most infections; *neonatal meningitis due to group B streptococcus:* 250,000 to 400,000 units per kg per day IV in four divided doses; *infants and children:* 100,000 to 400,000 units per kg per day IV in four to six divided doses (max 20,000,000 units per day)
Precautions: Each 1,000,000 units contains approximately 2 mEq of potassium.
Adverse Effects: Allergic reactions, interstitial nephritis, nausea, vomiting, diarrhea, seizures (with high doses)

Availability: Injection: many strengths ranging from 200,000 units per vial to 20,000,000 units per vial; sodium penicillin G is available in vials of 1,000,000 and 5,000,000 units.

Drug: PENICILLIN V, POTASSIUM (PEN VEE K®, V-CILLIN K®)

Route of Administration: PO

Dose: 25 to 50 mg per kg per day in three to four divided doses (max 2 g per day); *prophylaxis of pneumococcal infections or recurrent rheumatic fever: age younger than 5 years:* 125 mg BID; *age 5 years or older:* 250 mg BID

Precautions: Same as for penicillin G, potassium.

Adverse Effects: Same as for penicillin G, potassium

Availability: Tablets: 125, 250, 500 mg

Oral solution: 25, 50 mg per mL

Drug: PENTOBARBITAL (NEMBUTAL®)

Route of Administration: PO, IV

Dose: *Procedural sedation:* 1 to 2 mg per kg per dose IV every 5 minutes until adequately sedated, max 100 mg per dose; total max 300 mg or 6 mg per kg, whichever is less

Oral: 2 to 6 mg per kg PO × 1 dose

Adverse Effects: Prolonged sedation, respiratory depression, apnea, hypotension

Availability: Injection: 50 mg per mL

Capsule: 50, 100 mg

Oral solution: 3.64 mg per mL

Drug: PHENAZOPYRIDINE (PYRIDIUM®)

Route of Administration: PO

Dose: 12 mg per kg per day in three divided doses for 2 days (max 200 mg per dose)

Precautions: May mask signs of infection; therefore, do not use alone or for extended periods of time.

Adverse Effects: Headache, rash, discoloration of urine, methemoglobinemia

Availability: Tablets: 100, 200 mg

Drug: PHENOBARBITAL (LUMINAL®)

Route of Administration: PO, IM, IV

Dose: *Initial:* 10 to 20 mg per kg

Subsequent infants and children: 3 to 6 mg per kg per day in two divided doses

Adolescents: 1 to 2 mg per kg per day in one to two divided doses

Precautions: Administer by IV route at a rate no faster than 1 mg per kg per minute. Serum concentrations should be monitored. Be prepared to intubate if high doses are used in status epilepticus.

Adverse Effects: Sedation, ataxia, paradoxical excitation, hypotension, cardiorespiratory depression

Availability: Injection: 30, 60, 65, 130 mg per mL

Tablets: 8, 15, 30, 60, 100 mg

Oral elixir: 3, 4 mg per mL

Drug: PHENTOLAMINE (REGITINE®)

Route of Administration: IM, IV

Dose: *Hypertensive crisis:* 0.05 to 0.1 mg per kg per dose, do not exceed 5 mg per dose

Vasoconstrictor infiltration: Infants: 2.5 to 5 mg diluted in 10 mL of NS, administer as serial "pincushion" injections, do not exceed 0.1 mg per kg. Children and adolescents: 5 to 10 mg diluted in 10 mL of NS. Administer as above, do not exceed 5 mg.

Precautions: Must be on CV monitor for intravenous/intramuscular doses.

Adverse Effects: Hypotension, cardiac arrhythmias

Availability: Injection: 5 mg per mL

Drug: PHENYTOIN (DILANTIN®, VARIOUS GENERICS)

Route of Administration: PO, IV

Dose: *Initial loading dose:* 15 to 20 mg per kg (see Precautions)

Subsequent doses:

Age	Dosage
6 mo to 3 yr	8–10 mg per kg per day in two divided doses
4–6 yr	7.5–9 mg per kg per day in two divided doses
7–9 yr	7–8 mg per kg per day in two divided doses
10–16 yr	5–7 mg per kg per day in two divided doses

Precautions: IV phenytoin should be administered directly into a large vein or IV tubing at a rate no faster than 1 mg per kg per minute (25 to 50 mg per minute in an adult). Phenytoin should not be infused via small veins in the hand, foot, or scalp. Treat extravasations immediately. If dilution is necessary, NS should be used because other solutions cause precipitation of phenytoin. IM administration should be avoided because of erratic and incomplete absorption. Serum concentrations should be monitored.

Adverse Effects: Sedation, nystagmus, ataxia, gingival hyperplasia, rash, Stevens-Johnson syndrome. Drug interactions may occur when phenytoin is combined with phenobarbital, carbamazepine, chloramphenicol, isoniazid, salicylates, oral anticoagulants, and many others.

Availability: Injection: 50 mg per mL

Prompt-release oral capsules: 30, 100 mg

Extended-release oral capsules (Dilantin®): 30, 100 mg

Chewable tablets: 50 mg

Oral suspension: 6, 25 mg per mL

Drug: PHYTONADIONE (VITAMIN K, MEPHYTON®)

Route of Administration: Subcutaneous, IM, IV, PO

Dose: *Life-threatening bleeding:* Infants and children: 5 mg per dose IV, Adults: 2.5 to 10 mg per dose IV

Non-Life-threatening serious bleeding: Infants and children: 0.5 to 2.5 mg SC or IV

Precautions: Subcutaneous administration strongly preferred when possible due to serious infusion reactions occurring with IV administration. Dilute in 5 to 10 mL of NS for IV administration, give no faster than 1 mg per minute.

Adverse Effects: Anaphylactoid reactions, hypotension

Availability: Injection: 2, 10 mg per mL

Tablet: 5 mg

Drug: PIPERACILLIN/TAZOBACTAM (ZOSYN®)

Route of Administration: IV

Dose: Dose is based on piperacillin component. Usual 200 to 300 mg per kg per day divided every 6 hours. *Cystic fibrosis:* 300 to 500 mg per kg per day divided every 6 hours. Max 18 g per day as piperacillin

Adverse Effects: See Penicillin.

Availability: Injection: 2.25, 3.375, 4.5 g

Drug: POLYETHYLENE GLYCOL – PEG 3350 (MIRALAX®)

Route of Administration: PO

Dose: *Disimpaction:* 1 to 1.5 g per kg per day (max 100 g per day) PO daily × 3 days. *Constipation:* <10 kg: 4.25 g per day, 10 to 30 kg: 8.5 g per day, >30 kg: 17 g per day

Notes: 17 g = 1 tbsp = 1 capful or packet; mix every 17 g in 8 oz of fluid

Adverse Effects: Diarrhea, electrolyte imbalance with overdose

Availability: Powder for suspension

Drug: POLYETHYLENE GLYCOL with Electrolytes (GoLYTELY®)

Route of Administration: PO

Dose: *Disimpaction:*

Whole Bowel Irrigation (toxic exposure): Infants and young children: 500 mL per hour; Adolescents and adults: 2,000 mL per hour, max 4,000 mL

Adverse Effects: GI cramping, nausea, vomiting, electrolyte disturbances (rare with proper use)

Availability: Powder for solution

Drug: POLYSTYRENE SULFONATE, SODIUM (KAYEXALATE®)

Route of Administration: PO, PR

Dose: 1 g per kg per dose (max 60 g per dose); 1 g of resin binds approximately 1 mEq of potassium. Administer powder orally as a suspension in water. Dilute each 1 g of powder to at least 4 mL. If administering via NG tube, dilute suspension 1:1 with tap water to aid in delivery. If administered rectally, give as a retention enema. Dilute each 1 g of powder to at least 3 to 4 mL with 1% methylcellulose or 10% dextrose in water. PR administration is generally less effective than PO administration. Enema should be retained for at least 30 minutes.

Precautions: Monitor serum electrolytes. Each gram of resin contains approximately 4 mEq of sodium. Resin delivers 1 mEq of sodium for each 1 mEq of potassium removed. Resin may also bind other cations (e.g., calcium, magnesium).

Availability: Powder for suspension

Suspension: 0.25 g sodium polystyrene sulfonate per 1 mL (in approximately 30% sorbitol)

Drug: POTASSIUM CHLORIDE (MICROK, KLORCON®)

Route of Administration: PO, IV

Dose: *Oral, hypokalemia:* 1 to 2 mEq per kg per day; follow institutional guidelines for IV dosing and infusion restrictions – most use 0.5 mEq per kg per dose (max 40 mEq) infused over 2 hours at 0.1 mEq per mL for peripheral line, 0.2 mEq per mL for central line infusion

Precautions: Ensure adequate monitoring (laboratory, urine output, and cardiorespiratory), do not let patient break, chew, or crush extended release tablets or capsules. Use caution in patients with renal dysfunction.

Adverse Effects: Arrhythmias, GI erosion, rash

Availability: Capsules 8, 10 mEq

Liquid 20 mEq per 15 mL, 40 mEq per 15 mL

Capsules extended release 8, 10, 20 mEq

Powder for reconstitution 20, 25 mEq

Injection 2 mEq per mL concentrated; 10, 20, 30, and 40 mEq mixed in 100 mL NS

Drug: POTASSIUM IODIDE (IOST, THYROSHIELD, SSKI®)

Use caution, sound-alike drugs include: Potassium iodine (Lugol's solution®)

Route of Administration: PO

Dose: *Thyrotoxic crisis:* <1 year: 3 to 5 drops (150 to 250 mg) PO TID; >1 year: 6 to 10 drops (300 to 500 mg) PO TID; *Select radiation poisoning:* <1 month: 16.25 mg PO daily; 1 month to 3 year: 32.5 mg PO daily; 3 to 18 years: 65 mg PO daily; >68 kg: 130 mg PO daily until exposure is eliminated

Precautions: Dilute well prior to administration.

Adverse Effects: Gastritis, hypothyroidism, dermatitis, arrhythmias

Availability: Solution SSKI: 1 g per mL, ThyroShield 65 mg per mL

Tablets: 65, 130 mg

Drug: PREDNISOLONE (ORAPRED®, PRELONE®)

Route of Administration: PO

Dose: *Acute asthma*: 1-2 mg per kg × 1 dose, then 2 mg per kg per day in two divided doses; *antiinflammatory*: 0.5 to 2 mg per kg per day in divided doses. Max 80 mg per dose

Adverse Effects: See Methylprednisolone. Palatability may be an issue with compliance.

Availability: Oral solution: 3 mg per mL
Tablets: 5 mg
Oral disintegrating tablets: 15 mg, 30 mg

Drug: PREDNISONE (DELTASONE®)

Route of Administration: PO

Dose: *Physiologic replacement*: 0.1 to 0.15 mg per kg per day; *acute asthma*: 1-2 mg per kg × 1 dose then 1 to 2 mg per kg per day divided BID (max 80 mg per dose); *rheumatoid arthritis*: 1 to 2 mg per kg per day in one to four divided doses; *nephrotic syndrome*: 2 mg per kg per day

Precautions: Every-other-day therapy is advised once dosage is established to minimize adrenal suppression and growth retardation.

Adverse Effects: See Methylprednisolone.

Availability: Tablets: 1, 2.5, 5, 10, 20, 25, 50 mg
Oral solution: 1 mg per mL

Drug: PROCAINAMIDE (PRONESTYL®, PROCANBID®, PROCAN®)

Route of Administration: PO, IM, IV

Dose: *PO*: 15 to 50 mg per kg per day in four to eight divided doses (for prompt-release products); once stabilized, therapy can be changed to sustained-release product at same total daily dosage but administered in four divided doses (or two divided doses-Procanbid®).

IV: Initial loading dose of 3 to 7 mg per kg per dose (max 100 mg per dose) diluted and given slowly over 5 minutes, may be repeated after 10 to 30 minutes; *continuous IV infusion*: 20 to 80 mcg per kg per minute (0.02 to 0.08 mg per kg per minute); *maximum total daily dose*: 2 to 4 g PO or IM, or 1 to 2 g IV

Precautions: IV administration may cause hypotension if given too rapidly or in excessive doses. Dosage adjustment is recommended for patients with reduced renal function. Avoid using in patients with myasthenia gravis or second- or third-degree heart block.

Adverse Effects: Mental confusion, myocardial depression, cardiac arrhythmias (especially conduction block), lupus-like syndrome, nausea, vomiting

Availability: Injection: 100, 500 mg per mL
Capsules/tablets: 250, 375, 500 mg
Tablets, extended-release (Procan SR®): 250, 500, 750 mg; 1 g
Twice-daily extended-release (Procanbid®): 500 mg, 1 g

Drug: PROPRANOLOL (INDERAL®)

Route of Administration: PO, IV

Dose: *IV: acute antiarrhythmic*: 0.01 to 0.1 mg per kg per dose given slowly (max 1 mg per dose) every 6 to 8 hours as needed; *PO: hypertension*: usual starting dose 0.5 to 1 mg per kg per day in four divided doses; maintenance dose 1 to 5 mg per kg per day in two to four divided doses (max 240 mg per day); *migraine headache prophylaxis*: 0.6 to 1.5 mg per kg per day in three divided doses, max 4 mg per kg per day

Precautions: IV injection should be given slowly over 10 minutes. Use with extreme caution, if at all, in patients with asthma, diabetes, or CHF.

Adverse Effects: Myocardial depression, hypoglycemia, nausea, vomiting

Availability: Injection: 1 mg per mL
Tablets: 10, 20, 40, 60, 80 mg
Oral solution: 4, 8, 80 mg per mL

Drug: PSEUDOEPHEDRINE (SUDAFED®)

Route of Administration: PO

Dose: 4 mg per kg per day in four divided doses; or age 2 to 5 years: 15 mg every 4 to 6 hours (max 60 mg per day); age 6 to 11 years: 30 mg every 4 to 6 hours (max 120 mg per day); age 12 years or older: 60 mg every 4 to 6 hours (max 240 mg per day)

Precautions: Extended-release products containing 120 mg or greater should not be used in patients younger than 12 years of age.

Adverse Effects: CNS excitation or sedation, tachycardia, blurred vision, headache, hypertension

Availability: Tablets: 30, 60 mg
Capsules, timed-release: 120 mg
Liquid: 3, 6 mg per mL
Drops: 7.5 mg per 0.8 mL

Drug: PYRIDOSTIGMINE (MESTINON®)

Use caution, sound-alike drugs include: Physostigmine (Antilirium®)

Route of Administration: PO, IM, IV

Dose: *PO: myasthenia gravis*: usual starting dose 1 mg per kg per dose every four hours; IV/IM: 0.05 to 0.15 mg per kg per dose (max 10 mg per dose). *Reversal of NMBA*: 0.1 to 0.25 mg per kg per dose IV (max 20 mg per dose)

Precautions: Must use atropine or glycopyrrolate for secretion control when reversing NMBAs.

Adverse Effects: Nausea, vomiting, cramping, diarrhea, increased respiratory secretions

Availability: Tablets 60 mg
Injection: 5 mg per mL
Syrup: 12 mg per mL

Drug: QUINIDINE (VARIOUS)

Route of Administration: PO, IM, IV

Dose: *Test dose:* 2 mg per kg PO

Therapeutic: 15 to 60 mg per kg per day in four to six divided doses; *usual dose:* 30 mg per kg per day in five divided doses of quinidine sulfate PO or quinidine gluconate parenterally. Consult the CDC for dosing recommendations in the treatment of malaria.

Precautions: IV use of quinidine is recommended only when a cardiologist is in attendance. Absorption from IM injection sites is erratic and unreliable. Oral quinidine should be taken with food.

Adverse Effects: Adverse GI effects, hypotension, cardiac arrhythmias, blood dyscrasias, systemic lupus erythematosus-like syndrome. Cinchonism is a sign of quinidine toxicity, and is characterized by tinnitus, headache, vertigo, fever, nausea, and disturbed vision. Cinchonism may occur after single dose.

Availability: Sulfate injection: 200 mg per mL

Gluconate injection: 80 mg per mL

Quinidine sulfate tablets/capsules: 100, 200, 300 mg

Quinidine gluconate tablets (sustained release): 324 mg

Note: Sulfate salt contains 83% anhydrous quinidine; gluconate salt contains 62% anhydrous quinidine.

Drug: RABIES IMMUNE GLOBULIN (HYPERAB®)

Route of Administration: IM, infiltration around wound

Dose: 20 units per kg administered at the same time as rabies vaccine, but in a different site. Use one-half the dose to infiltrate the wound site unless the wound involves mucous membranes.

Adverse Effects: Local soreness, muscle stiffness at injection site, fever

Availability: Injection: 150 units per mL

Drug: RABIES VIRUS VACCINE (IMOVAX RABIES®, HDCV)

Route of Administration: IM

Dose: *Postexposure prophylaxis:* Five doses of 1 mL each administered on days 0, 3, 7, 14, and 28. Low risk patients do not require day 28 dose. The first dose should be administered at the same time as the immunoglobulin, but in a different muscle.

Adverse Effects: Local pain and erythema, fever, encephalomyelitis, peripheral neuropathy

Availability: Injection: 2.5 U per mL

Drug: RANITIDINE (ZANTAC®)

Route of Administration: IV, PO

Dose: *IV:* 1 mg per kg per dose IV every 8 hours (max 50 mg per dose); *continuous infusion:* 0.15 mg per kg per hour; *oral:* 2 mg per kg per dose PO every 12 hours (max 150 mg per dose). Higher dosages may be necessary in pathologic hypersecretory conditions.

Adverse Effects: Dizziness, headache, bradycardia, rash, thrombocytopenia

Availability: Injection: 25 mg per mL

Oral liquid: 15 mg per mL

Tablets: 75, 150, 300 mg

Drug: RASBURICASE (ELITEK®)

Route of Administration: IV

Dose: *IV:* 0.15 to 0.2 mg per kg per dose IV rounded to the nearest vial size

Note: All samples for uric acid levels must be sent on ice to avoid breakdown by the rasburicase in vitro. Do NOT use alkaline hydration prior to rasburicase (use hydration without sodium bicarbonate). Allopurinol should not be given simultaneously with rasburicase.

Adverse Effects: Dizziness, headache, nausea, severe hemolysis (G6PD)

Availability: Injection: 1.5, 7.5 mg

Drug: RIFAMPIN (RIFADIN®, RIMACTANE®)

Route of Administration: PO

Dose: *Prophylaxis against H. influenzae type b: age younger than 1 month:* 10 mg per kg per day as a single daily dose for 4 days; *age 1 month to 12 years:* 20 mg per kg per day as a single daily dose for 4 days (max 600 mg); *prophylaxis against Neisseria meningitidis: age younger than 1 month:* 10 mg per kg per day in two divided doses for 2 days; *age 1 month 12 years:* 20 mg per kg per day in two divided doses for 2 days (max 1,200 mg); *tuberculosis: age older than 1 week:* 10 to 20 mg per kg per day (maximum daily dose: 600 mg)

Precautions: When using rifampin in conjunction with isoniazid, limit rifampin dose to 15 mg per kg daily and isoniazid to 10 mg per kg daily to minimize risk of hepatotoxicity.

Adverse Effects: Hepatotoxicity, GI disturbances, flulike syndrome, red-orange discoloration of urine, feces, sweat, and tears. Discoloration of contact lenses may also occur.

Availability: Capsules: 150, 300 mg

Note: Several recipes for suspensions have been published usually reconstituted at 10 mg per mL.

Drug: RIMANTADINE (FLUMADINE®)

Route of Administration: PO

Dose: *Prophylaxis: children younger than 10 years of age:* 5 mg per kg daily (max 150 mg per day); *children older than 10 years of age:* 100 mg BID. Reduce dosage to 100 mg per day in patients with severe hepatic or renal dysfunction.

Precautions: Use with caution in patients with epilepsy.

Adverse Effects: Dizziness, headache, confusion, anxiety, restlessness, nausea, vomiting, urinary retention

Availability: Syrup: 10 mg per mL

Tablets: 100 mg

Drug: RISPERIDONE (CONSTA, RISPERDAL®)
Route of Administration: PO, IM
Dose: *Oral*: range is 0.5 mg per day titrated up to a max of 6 mg per day; IM 12.5 to 25 mg every two weeks
Adverse Effects: Prolonged QTc, arrhythmias, blood dyscrasias, neuroleptic malignant syndrome (NMS), dystonias, hyperglycemia, orthostatic hypotension, suicidal ideation
Note: IM is depot formulation, will not work acutely. Do NOT ever give intravenously. Orally-disintegrating tablets (ODTs) contain phenylalanine
Availability: Tablet: 0.25, 0.5, 1, 2, 3, 4 mg
Orally disintegrating tablet: 0.25, 0.5, 1, 2, 3, 4 mg
Oral solution: 1 mg per mL
Injection: 12.5, 25, 37.5, 50 mg with administration pack

Drug: ROCURONIUM (see Resuscitation Drug List)

Drug: SODIUM BICARBONATE (See Resuscitation Drug List)

Drug: SPIRONOLACTONE (ALDACTONE®)
Route of Administration: PO
Dose: 1 to 3.3 mg per kg per day in one or two divided doses (max 200 mg per day)
Adverse Effects: Hyperkalemia, hyponatremia, gynecomastia
Availability: Tablets: 25, 50, 100 mg
Note: Several recipes for suspensions have been published.

Drug: SUCCINYLCHOLINE (see Resuscitation Drug List)

Drug: SUCRALFATE (CARAFATE®)
Route of Administration: PO
Dose: 40 to 80 mg per kg per day divided q6h, max 1 g per dose
Precautions: Sucralfate binds many drugs, ensure adequate separation. Give on empty stomach. Aluminum toxicity may occur in patients with renal insufficiency.
Adverse Effects: Constipation, drug—drug interactions
Availability: Tablets: 1 g
Suspension: 100 mg per mL

Drug: SULFISOXAZOLE (GANTRISIN®)
Route of Administration: PO
Dose: *Initial*: 75 mg per kg as a single dose; *maintenance*: 120 to 150 mg per kg per day in four to six divided doses (max 4 to 8 g per day)

Precautions: Fluid intake should be encouraged to minimize risk of crystalluria.
Adverse Effects: GI distress, rash, fever, allergic reactions
Availability: Tablets: 500 mg
Pediatric solution/suspension: 100 mg per mL
Lipo-Gantrisin suspension (extended-release): 200 mg per mL

Drug: SUMATRIPTAN (IMITREX®)
Route of Administration: SC, PO, intranasal
Dose: Limited information suggests SC doses of 3 mg for children 6 years of age or older weighing 22 to 30 kg or 6 mg in children weighing more than 30 kg are safe and effective. Alternatively, a dose of 0.06 mg per kg SC has been used. Currently, only adult dosing is available for the oral and intranasal preparations.
Precautions: Use with caution in patients with preexisting coronary, hepatic, or renal disease or epilepsy.
Adverse Effects: Flushing, pain, and/ or edema at the injection site, chest tightness, and atypical nervous system effects such as tingling, numbness, feelings of warmth, heat, burning, cold or pressure, dizziness, or drowsiness
Availability: Injection: 12 mg per mL

Drug: TERBUTALINE (BRETHINE®, BRICANYL®)
Route of Administration: PO, IV, SC
Dose: *PO*: 0.05 mg per kg per dose three times per day, max 7.5 mg per day
SC: status asthmaticus load: 10 mcg per kg × 1 dose followed by continuous IV infusion (see below). Alternatively: 0.003 to 0.005 mg per kg per dose (3 to 5 mcg per kg per dose) to a maximum single dose of 0.25 mg; may repeat once after 15 to 20 minutes.
IV: status asthmaticus: load: 10 mcg per kg × 1 dose, followed by a continuous infusion of 0.4 mcg per kg per minute. Titrate as needed to maintain aeration and heart rate less than 200. Max dose 6 mcg per kg per minute. Suggested total β_2-agonist maximum: 20 mg per hour.
Precautions: Manufacturer does not recommend use in children younger than 12 years of age.
Adverse Effects: See Albuterol. Transient hypotension may occur at doses less than 2 mcg per kg per minute secondary to upregulation of the β_2-receptors in the vasculature.
Availability: Tablets: 2.5, 5 mg
Injection: 1 mg per mL

Drug: TETANUS IMMUNE GLOBULIN
Route of Administration: IM only (do NOT administer IV)
Dose: *Postexposure prophylaxis*: 250 units IM × 1 dose; *treatment*: therapeutic dose: 3,000 to 6,000 units IM × 1 dose.

Note: The need for TIG is dependent on previous immunization history. Consult the CDC website for further dosing recommendations.

Precautions: Allergic reactions are possible (epinephrine should be immediately available).

Adverse Effects: Pain at injection site, myalgias, fever, flulike symptoms, allergic reactions

Availability: Injection: 250 units per vial

Drug: TETANUS and DIPTHERIA TOXOID (Td, DT)
Route of Administration: IM
Dose: *Wound management: younger than 7 years:* 0.5 mL of the DT preparation IM × 1 dose; *older than 7 years:* 0.5 mL of the Td preparation IM × 1 dose.
Note: Number of postexposure doses and need for TIG is dependent on previous immunization history. Consult the CDC website for further dosing recommendations.
Adverse Effects: Fever, pain at injection site, allergic reaction
Availability: Injection: DT (pediatric), Td (adult)

Drug: TETANUS, reduced DIPTHERIA and PERTUSSIS (Tdap)
Route of Administration: IM
Dose: *Wound management:* 11 to 65 years: 0.5 mL IM × 1 dose
Note: At this time, only one booster of Tdap is recommended. Consult the CDC website for further dosing recommendations.
Adverse Effects: Fever, pain at injection site, allergic reaction
Availability: Injection

Drug: TETRACYCLINE (ACHROMYCIN®)
Route of Administration: PO
Dose: *PO:* >8 years: 25 to 50 mg per kg per day given in four divided doses (max 3 g per day)
Precautions: Avoid in children younger than 8 years of age because tetracycline may cause enamel hypoplasia and discoloration of permanent teeth. Tetracycline chelates divalent cations and should not be given with milk, iron, or antacids. Tetracycline should be given 1 hour before or 2 hours after meals or milk.
Adverse Effects: GI distress, photosensitivity, pseudotumor cerebri, and overgrowth of nonsusceptible organisms including fungi
Availability: Capsules: 100, 250, 500 mg
Oral suspension: 25 mg per mL

Drug: THEOPHYLLINE (SOMOPHYLLIN®, SLO-PHYLLIN®, THEOPHYL®, THEO-DUR®, MANY OTHERS)
Route of Administration: PO, IV form is aminophylline
Dose: *Acute asthma (age older than 1 year):* IV, initial dose of 6 mg per kg over 20 to 30 minutes followed by continuous infusion of 0.9 to 1.1 mg per kg per hour (adjust to maintain therapeutic serum concentra-

tion of 10 to 20 mg per L). Modify initial dose according to baseline serum concentration if patient is known to be on maintenance theophylline.
Chronic asthma: PO, 16 to 24 mg per kg per day in four divided doses. Sustained-release products may be given every 8 to 12 hours. Adjust dose to achieve serum concentration of 10 to 20 mg per L.
Apnea of prematurity: IV/PO: *initial:* 4 to 6 mg per kg (over 20 to 30 minutes if IV); *maintenance:* 3 to 5 mg per kg per day in two to three divided doses. Adjust to maintain therapeutic serum concentration (8 to 14 mg per L)
Adverse Effects: CNS irritability, tachycardia, nausea, vomiting, abdominal cramping, seizures (at toxic serum concentrations)
Availability: Many strengths and dosage forms (check local availability); most commonly used forms in children include oral liquid: 18 mg per mL; sustained-release capsules: 50, 60, 75, 100, 125, 200, 250, 300 mg
Injection as aminophylline: 25 mg per mL
Note: Aminophylline 0.8 mg = theophylline 1 mg. Alcohol- and dye-free liquid products are available.

Drug: THIAMINE (VITAMIN B1)
Route of Administration: IV, PO
Dose: *Neonatal seizures:* 100 mg IV × 1 dose; *mitochondrial defects:* 100 to 200 mg PO daily.
Adverse Effects: Cardiovascular collapse with rapid infusion of large doses, GI distress, discoloration of urine, rash
Availability: Injection: 100, 200 mg per mL
Tablets: 25, 50, 100, 250, 500 mg

Drug: TICARCILLIN (TICAR®)
Route of Administration: IV, IM
Dose: *Neonates: younger than 7 days, weight less than 2,000 g:* 150 mg per kg per day in two divided doses; *younger than 7 days, weight more than 2,000 g:* 225 mg per kg per day in three divided doses; *older than 7 days, weight more than 2,000 g:* 300 mg per kg per day in three to four divided doses; *age older than 1 month:* 200 to 300 mg per kg per day in four divided doses (max 24 g per day)
Precautions: Ticarcillin contains 5.2 to 6.5 mEq of sodium per gram.
Adverse Effects: Hypernatremia, hypokalemia, metabolic alkalosis, seizures, reduced platelet function
Availability: Injection: 1, 3, 6 g

Drug: TOBRAMYCIN (NEBCIN®)
Route of Administration: IV, IM
Dose: See Gentamicin
Precautions: See Gentamicin.

Adverse Effe cts: See Gentamicin.
Availability: Injection: 10, 40 mg per mL, also available as preservative free

---

Drug: TOPIRAMATE (TOPAMAX®)

Route of Administration: PO
Dose: *Initial:* 0.5 to 1 mg per kg, increasing by 1 mg per kg per day weekly until 6 to 15 mg per kg per day is reached. Dose is usually divided BID.
Precautions: Sulfa allergy cross-reactivity
Adverse Effects: Drowsiness, ataxia, cognitive word finding difficulties, parasthesias, kidney stones, suicidal ideation
Availability: Tablet 25, 50, 100, 200 mg
Sprinkle capsules: 15, 25 mg

Drug: TRIMETHOPRIM -SULFAMETHOXAZOLE (BACTRIM®, SEPTRA®)

Route of Administration: PO, IV
Dose: Note: Dosage is expressed in terms of the trimethoprim component. Dosage forms contain a ratio of 5 mg of sulfamethoxazole (SMX) to 1 mg of trimethoprim (TMP).
Minor infections: 8 mg per kg per day TMP in two divided doses (max 320 mg per day TMP); *Pneumocystis carinii pneumonia (treatment dose):* 20 mg per kg per day TMP (PO) or 15 to 20 mg per kg per day TMP (IV) in four divided doses every 6 hours.
Precautions: Dilute IV doses and infuse over no less than 60 to 90 minutes. Dosage modification required in patients with renal impairment.
Adverse Effects: Most common are rashes and GI upset. Most serious are severe hypersensitivity reactions (e.g., Stevens-Johnson syndrome, erythema multiforme), blood dyscrasias, and hepatocellular necrosis.
Availability: Oral suspension: TMP 8 mg per mL and SMX 40 mg per mL
Tablets: TMP 80 mg and SMX 400 mg
Double-strength tablets: TMP 160 mg and SMX 800 mg
Injection: TMP 16 mg per mL and SMX 80 mg per mL

Drug: TROPICAMIDE (Mydracil®)

Route of Administration: Opthalamic
Dose: 1 to 2 drops within 30 minutes of eye exam
Precautions: Use with caution in young children.
Adverse Effects: Psychotic disturbances, blurred vision, increased intraocular pressure
Availability: Opthalamic solution 0.5, 1%

Drug: TYPHOID VACCINE (TYPHIM®)

Route of Administration: IM, PO
Dose: IM vaccination: 0.5 mL × 1 dose; Oral vaccine: 1 capsule PO every other day for 4 doses

Note: The injectable vaccine provides immunity for approximately 2 to 3 years. The live oral vaccine provides immunity for up to 5 years.
Precautions: ORAL typhoid vaccine can cause stomach upset, and is recommended to be taken in the evening prior to bedtime. Antibiotics should not be given concurrently with ORAL typhoid vaccine.
Adverse Effects: Nausea, vomiting
Availability: Capsules, Injection

Drug: VALPROIC ACID (DEPACON®, DEPAKENE®, DEPAKOTE®)

Route of Administration: IV, PO, PR
Dose: *Status epilepticus:* Load 20 mg per kg IV over 5 minutes; *epilepsy:* 15 to 60 mg per kg per day in two to three divided doses. If taking other enzyme-inducing AEDs, may require 100 mg per kg per day. Supplemental carnitine is recommended by some experts if using high doses.
Precautions: Valproic acid may interact with the following drugs: clonazepam, phenobarbital, phenytoin, salicylates, and warfarin. Serum drug concentrations should be carefully monitored in patients taking multiple drug products. Monitor liver function tests before and at frequent intervals during therapy (see Adverse Effects). IV doses may need to be divided q6h to maintain adequate levels. Infusion rate is 60 minutes, unless in status epilepticus.
Adverse Effects: Nausea, vomiting, sedation, hyperammonemia (with or without coma), thrombocytopenia, inhibition of platelet aggregation, pancreatitis, severe and potentially fatal hepatotoxicity
Availability: Capsules: 250 mg (valproic acid)
Capsules (containing coated particles or "sprinkles"): 125 mg
Delayed-release tablets: 125, 250, 500 mg (as divalproex sodium)
Injection: 100 mg per mL
Syrup: 50 mg per mL (sodium valproate)
Note: The syrup has been successfully administered by the PR route after dilution with water. Depakote ER has only been approved for migraine prophylaxis and should not be used for epilepsy at this time.

Drug: VANCOMYCIN (VANCOCIN®)

Route of Administration: IV, PO
Dose: *IV: age 1 to 2 months:* 10 mg per kg per dose every 12 hours; *age older than 2 months:* 40 to 60 mg per kg per day in three to four divided doses. Use higher doses for CNS infections.
PO, for treatment of antibiotic-associated pseudomembranous colitis only: 10 mg per kg per dose every 6 hours (max 2 g per day). Usual adult dose is 125 mg PO QID.
Precautions: Administer IV over 60 minutes to minimize risk of "red-man's syndrome" (hypotension and rash). PO route should not be used for treatment of systemic infections. Monitor trough levels. Poor palatability of oral solutions may influence compliance.

Adverse Effects: Ototoxicity and nephrotoxicity (especially when used in conjunction with other ototoxic and/or nephrotoxic drugs), thrombophlebitis, hypotension, rash
Availability: Capsules: 125, 250 mg
Injection: 500 mg, 1, 2 g per vial
Powder for oral solution: 1, 10 g

Drug: VARICELLA-ZOSTER IMMUNE GLOBULIN (VariZIG®)
Route of Administration: IM, IV
Dose: 125 units for every 10 kg of weight (min dose 125 units, max 625 units)
Notes: Give within 96 hours of exposure. May diminish efficacy of live vaccines, ensure administration of varicella vaccine if needed prior to or at the same time as the administration of VariZIG.
Precautions: Use only the supplied diluent. Watch for signs of varicella for 28 days post administration.
Adverse Effects: Site reaction, fever, anaphylaxis, pulmonary edema, renal dysfunction
Availability: Injection 125 units per vial

Drug: VECURONIUM (NORCURON®)
Route of Administration: IV
Dose: *Maintanence of paralysis postintubation:* 0.1 mg per kg per dose every 1 hour or more frequently as needed to maintain paralysis; *continuous infusion:* 0.05 to 0.07 mg per kg per hour. *RSI:* 0.3 mg per kg IV × 1 dose
Precautions: A higher dose is needed to obtain rapid onset needed for RSI; therefore, paralysis may persist for more than 2 hours postdose.
Adverse Effects: See Rocuronium.
Availability: Injection: 10-mg vial

Drug: VERAPAMIL (CALAN®, ISOPTIN®)
Route of Administration: IV
Dose: *Supraventricular tachycardia: age 1 to 16 years:* 0.1 to 0.3 mg per kg over 2 minutes (max dose: 5 mg). May repeat dose once after 30 minutes if adequate response is not achieved. Repeat dose in children 2 to 15 years of age should not exceed 10 mg.
Note: Although oral dosage forms are available, oral dosage requirements in children have not been established.

Precautions: Because of the risk of severe hypotensive responses, use with extreme caution, if at all, in neonates and children younger than 1 year of age. Use with continuous EKG monitoring in all children.
Adverse Effects: Hypotension, bradycardia, tachycardia, dizziness, headache, nausea. Hypotension or bradycardia caused by verapamil may be reversed by administration of calcium salts or β-adrenergic agents. IV fluids should also be used to treat hypotension. Atropine sulfate may counteract the bradycardia.
Availability: Injection: 2.5 mg per mL

Drug: WARFARIN (COUMADIN®)
Route of Administration: PO
Dose: *Load on day 1:* 0.2 mg per kg × 1 dose (max 10 mg per dose)
Maintenance: Dosing is based on INR. Usual maintenance is 0.1 mg per kg per day but is highly variable.
Precautions: Food and drug interactions should be thoroughly discussed with the patient. The potential for many serious drug interactions exist.
Adverse Effects: Hemorrhage, fever, skin lesions, anorexia
Availability: Tablet: 1, 2, 2.5, 4, 5, 7.5, 10 mg

Drug: ZINC SULFATE
Route of Administration: PO
Dose: 0.5 to 1 mg elemental zinc per kg per day in 1 to 3 divided doses, normal adult dose 25 to 50 mg elemental zinc (110 to 220 mg zinc sulfate) PO daily-TID
Precautions: Clinical response often takes several weeks, up to two months.
Adverse Effects: GI distress
Availability: Capsule 220 mg (50 mg elemental zinc); liquid can be compounded

---

Drug: ZIPRASIDONE (GEODON®)
Route of Administration: PO, IM
Dose: 20 to 100 mg per day depending on disease state and titration. *Acute agitation:* 10 mg IM every 2 hours or 20 mg every 4 hours, max 40 mg per day
Adverse Effects: Prolonged QTc, extrapyramidal side effects, nausea, chest pain, weight gain
Note: Change to oral therapy as soon as possible.
Availability: Injection: 20 mg
Capsule: 20, 40, 60, 80 mg

ABBREVIATIONS

AED, antiepileptic drug; BID, twice daily; BP, blood pressure; CBC, complete blood count; CDC, Centers for Disease Control and Prevention; CHF, congestive heart failure; CNS, central nervous system; CPK, creatine phosphokinase; D5W, dextrose 5% in water; EKG, electrocardiogram; ETT, endotracheal tube; G6PD, glucose-6-phosphate dehydrogenase deficiency; GI, gastrointestinal; ICP, intracranial pressure; IM, intramuscular(ly); INR, international normalized ratio; IO, intraosseous; IV, intravenous(ly); MAOi, Monoamine oxidase inhibitor; MDI, metered-dose inhaler; NMS, neuroleptic malignant syndrome; ODT, orally disintegrating tablets; PCA, patient-controlled analgesia; PE, phenytoin equivalents; PO, oral(ly); PPI, proton pump inhibitor; PR, rectal(ly); PRN, as needed; PTT, partial thromboplastin time; QHS (at bedtime); QID, four times daily; QTc, QT corrected; RSI, rapid sequence intubation; SC, subcutaneous(ly); TID, three times daily.

APPENDIX C ■ PRACTICAL INFORMATION

JOSHUA NAGLER, MD

VITAL SIGNS

Blood Pressure

Values:
Neonatal blood pressures vary significantly with age: systolic 40 to 80 mm Hg and diastolic 20 to 55 mm Hg.

| Age (yr) | Percentile (systolic/diastolic) | |
	50%	95%
2	96/60	108/66
6	106/68	112/72
9	112/72	116/76
12	118/76	122/82

Lower extremity pressures usually measure 10 to 40 mm Hg higher.

Complete blood pressure tables for children and adolescents are available from the National Heart Lung and Blood Institute at http://www.nhlbi.nih.gov/guidelines/hypertension/child_tbl.htm.

Pulsus Paradoxicus

Pulsus paradoxicus is defined as a drop in systolic blood pressure of greater than 10 mm Hg when first taken during inspiration and then taken during expiration.

Resting Respiratory Rate

Age	Breaths/min
Neonate	30–50
2–12 mo	30–40
12 mo—2 yr	22–30
2–12 yr	16–24
Adolescent	12–20

Resting Heart Rate

Age	Beats/min
Newborn	92–180
1 wk–1 mo	100–180
3 mo–2 yr	100–150
2–10 yr	65–120
10 yr–adult	55–110

Temperature

Conversion:
Fahrenheit versus centigrade

$$°C = (°F - 32) \times 5/9$$

Example: $°C = (98.6 - 32)$ (or 66.6) $\times 5 (=333)/9 = 37$
$°F = (°C \times 9/5) + 32$
Example: $°F = (39 \times 9 = 351) (/5 = 70.2) + 32 = 102.2$
Extrapolating points: 38°C = 100.4°F
39°C = 102.2°F
40°C = 104.0°F
41°C = 105.8°F

End-tidal Carbon Dioxide

End-tidal carbon dioxide level: normal 35 to 45 mm Hg. See Fig. C.1 for normal capnogram.

Weight

Conversion: Wt (lb)/2.2 = Wt (kg)

$$Wt (kg) \times 2.2 = Wt (lb)$$

Rapid weight estimation for children 10 years or younger: Wt (kg) = [2 × age (yr)] + 8

| Age | Percentile (using kg) | | |
	5%	50%	95%
Neonate, wk			
32	1.3	1.8	2.8
40	2.7	3.5	4.2
6 mo			
Female	5.9	7.2	8.6
Male	6.3	7.7	9.5
1 yr			
Female	7.8	9.5	11.4
Male	8.4	10.1	12.0
2 yr			
Female	9.8	11.8	14.0
Male	10.5	12.7	14.7
5 yr			
Female	14.1	17.9	22.2
Male	15.2	19.0	22.8
7 yr			
Female	15.5	19.5	29.0
Male	16.6	21.0	29.8
9 yr			
Female	21.7	28.0	40.6
Male	22.6	28.0	40.2

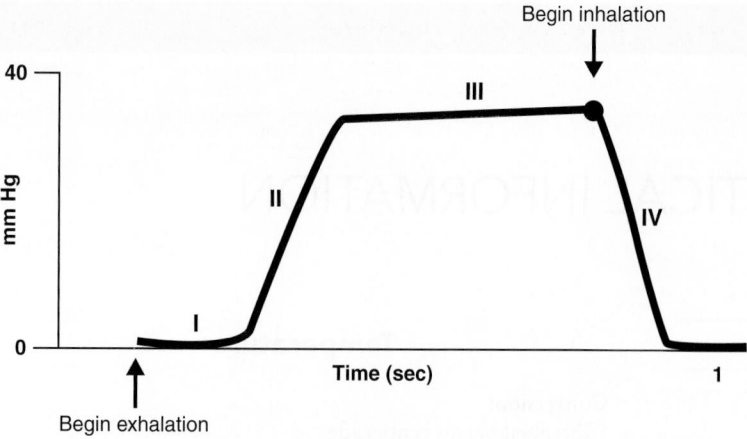

Phase I: Beginning of exhalation. Dead space is cleared from the upper airway.

Phase II: Rapid rise in CO_2 concentration as alveolar CO_2 reaches the upper airway.

Phase III: Plateau. Entire exhaled breath stream is alveolar gas. Maximum value for that tidal breath is the end-tidal CO_2.

Phase IV: Beginning of inhalation. Atmospheric air replaces alveolar CO_2.

FIGURE C.1 Normal capnogram.

Body Surface Area

Nomogram Method:
Body surface area (BSA) can be determined by connecting the height and weight numbers with a straight line. The point at which the line intersects the surface area abscissa is the reading for surface area in meters squared (Fig. C.2). To determine the approximate body surface area for normally proportioned children, use either the second line from the left in Fig. C.2 or the following formula:

Formulaic Method:

Mosteller's Formula: BSA (m^2) = Square root of: [Ht (cm) $\times$ Wt (kg)] $\div$ 3600

Dubois Formula: BSA = $(W^{0.425} \times H^{0.725}) \times 0.007184$

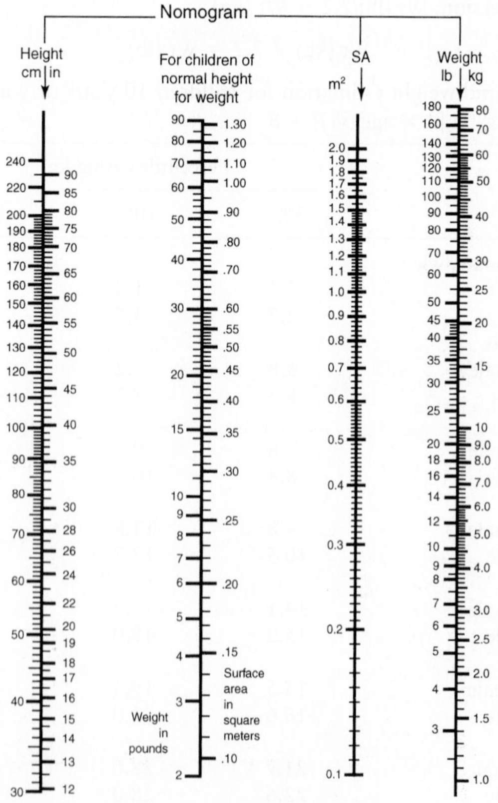

Body Mass Index

Body Mass Index (BMI) = weight (kg)/[height (m)]^2

Body Mass Index Calculator is available at the Centers for Disease Control and Prevention Web site at: http://apps.nccd.cdc.gov/dnpabmi/Calculator.aspx.

For children 2 years and older:

BMI < 5th percentile: Underweight
BMI > 85th percentile: Overweight
BMI > 95th percentile: Obese

IMMUNIZATIONS

HIV and other severely immunodeficient or immunosuppressed patients should be immunized in consultation with their primary caregivers and probably should not receive measles, mumps, or rubella (MMR) or varicella vaccine.

Recommendations for management upon exposure to tetanus; rabies; meningococcemia; *Haemophilus influenzae* type b; rubeola; rubella; hepatitis A, B, and C; pertussis; and varicella are defined in the "Prophylaxis After Exposure to Serious Disease" section, later in this appendix.

BEDSIDE LABORATORY TESTING

Rapid Screening Test for Cold Agglutinins

Collect a few drops of blood in a purple-top tube (small test tube with about 0.2 mL of 3.8 NaEDTA). Place in ice water bath for about 60 seconds. Tilt tube and look for flocculation

FIGURE C.2 Surface area. (Adapted from *Harriet Lane handbook*. 18th ed. St. Louis, MO: Mosby, 2008.)

Recommended Immunization Schedule for Persons Aged 0 Through 6 Years—United States • 2009

For those who fall behind or start late, see the catch-up schedule

Vaccine ▼ Age ►	Birth	1 month	2 months	4 months	6 months	12 months	15 months	18 months	19–23 months	2–3 years	4–6 years
Hepatitis B	HepB	HepB			HepB						
Rotavirus			RV	RV	*RV*						
Diphtheria, tetanus, pertussis			DTaP	DTaP	DTaP		DTaP				DTaP
***Haemophilus influenzae* type b**			Hib	Hib	*Hib*	Hib					
Pneumococcal			PCV	PCV	PCV	PCV				PPSV	
Inactivated poliovirus			IPV	IPV	IPV						IPV
Influenza						Influenza (Yearly)					
Measles, mumps, rubella						MMR					MMR
Varicella						Varicella					Varicella
Hepatitis A						HepA (2 doses)				HepA Series	
Meningococcal										MCV	

Range of recommended ages

Certain high-risk groups

This schedule indicates the recommended ages for routine administration of currently licensed vaccines, as of December 1, 2008, for children aged 0 through 6 years. Any dose not administered at the recommended age should be administered at a subsequent visit, when indicated and feasible. Licensed combination vaccines may be used whenever any component of the combination is indicated and other components are not contraindicated and if approved by the Food and Drug Administration for that dose of the series. Providers should consult the relevant Advisory Committee on Immunization Practices statement for detailed recommendations, including high-risk conditions: http://www.cdc.gov/vaccines/pubs/acip-list.htm. Clinically significant adverse events that follow immunization should be reported to the Vaccine Adverse Event Reporting System (VAERS). Guidance about how to obtain and complete a VAERS form is available at http://www.vaers.hhs.gov or by telephone, 800-822-7967.

FIGURE C.3 Immunization schedule for persons aged 0 through 6 years. (Adapted from Centers for Disease Control and Prevention. Recommended immunization schedules for persons aged 0 through 18 Years, United States, 2009. *MMWR 2008*; 57(51/52).) Also available at http://www.cdc.gov/vaccines/recs/schedules/child-schedule.htm.

Recommended Immunization Schedule for Persons Aged 7 Through 18 Years—United States • 2009

For those who fall behind or start late, see the schedule below and the catch-up schedule

Vaccine ▼ Age ►	7–10 years	11–12 years	13–18 years
Tetanus, diphtheria, pertussis		Tdap	Tdap
Human papillomavirus		HPV (3 doses)	HPV Series
Meningococcal	MCV	MCV	MCV
Influenza		Influenza (yearly)	
Pneumococcal		PPSV	
Hepatitis A		HepA series	
Hepatitis B		HepB series	
Inactivated poliovirus		IPV series	
Measles, mumps, rubella		MMR series	
Varicella		Varicella series	

Range of recommended ages

Catch-up immunization

Certain high-risk groups

This schedule indicates the recommended ages for routine administration of currently licensed vaccines, as of December 1, 2008, for children aged 7 through 18 years. Any dose not administered at the recommended age should be administered at a subsequent visit, when indicated and feasible. Licensed combination vaccines may be used whenever any component of the combination is indicated and other components are not contraindicated and if approved by the Food and Drug Administration for that dose of the series. Providers should consult the relevant Advisory Committee on Immunization Practices statement for detailed recommendations, including high-risk conditions: http://www.cdc.gov/vaccines/pubs/acip-list.htm. Clinically significant adverse events that follow immunization should be reported to the Vaccine Adverse Event Reporting System (VAERS). Guidance about how to obtain and complete a VAERS form is available at http://www.vaers.hhs.gov or by telephone, 800-822-7967.

FIGURE C.4 Immunization schedule for persons aged 7 through 18 years. (Adapted from Centers for Disease Control and Prevention. Recommended immunization schedules for persons aged 0 through 18 years, United States, 2009. *MMWR 2008*; 57(51/52).) Also available at http://www.cdc.gov/vaccines/recs/schedules/child-schedule.htm.

in the blood as it starts up the side of the tube. Warm the tube to room temperature and see if the flocculation disappears. Presence of flocculation when observed by the naked eye with subsequent disappearance on warming is a positive test for cold agglutinins and equates with about a 1:64 or greater cold agglutinin titer. There are widely varying reported sensitivities and specificities for positive cold agglutination tests for Mycoplasma or other diseases, and caution should be used in decision making based on this test alone.

Apt Test for Fetal Blood

If a stool specimen passed by a neonate is grossly bloody, mix a small sample of the specimen in a test tube with an equal quantity of tap water. Centrifuge briefly or filter out the solid material. The supernate should have a pink color due to the suspended blood. Add 1 part of 1.0% NaOH to 5 parts of the supernate. Wait for 2 minutes. A persistent pink color indicates presence of fetal hemoglobin because fetal hemoglobin is resistant to alkali denaturation; if the supernate turns yellow or brown, the hemoglobin is from an adult, suggesting swallowed maternal blood.

Stool Examination for Leukocytes

Smear a small specimen of stool on a glass slide. Mix with 1 to 2 drops of methylene blue stain. Cover with thin cover slip. Wait for 3 minutes before microscopic examination. Presence of more than 5 white blood cells per high-power field may increase the probability of a specific bacterial cause of diarrhea; however, widely varied sensitivities and specificities of this test have been reported.

Gram Stain

Make a thin smear of blood, spinal fluid, or vaginal or urethral secretion on a glass slide. Allow to air dry. Apply gentian violet; allow to sit for 1 minute; and then wash with water. Next, apply iodine solution for 1 minute and wash. Decolorize by applying acetone/alcohol for a few seconds and wash. Stain with safranin for 15 seconds and wash. Examine under high-power microscope.

Tzanck Preparation

Unroof a vesicular or bullous lesion, blot it, and scrape the base with the edge of a glass slide or scalpel. Spread the scraped material onto a glass slide and fix with methyl alcohol. Stain for 30 seconds with Wright stain and wash. Microscopic examination showing multinucleated giant cells is indicative of herpetic or zoster lesions.

Pinworm Evaluation

1. Place a piece of cellophane or tape over the end of a tongue depressor with sticky side out. Place over the perianal mucosa, applying moderate pressure for 1 minute. Spread the sticky side of the tape over a glass slide. Look through the microscope for ova.

   or

2. Instruct the parents to turn over the child who has been asleep for about an hour and look carefully at the perianal area. Live, threadlike worms, about 1 cm in length can be seen wiggling out of the anus to lay their ova.

Methemoglobin Screening Test

To evaluate for methemoglobinemia in the cyanotic patient who has no cardiac or respiratory impairment and does not respond to oxygen, place a drop of blood on white filter paper. Wave it in the air for 60 seconds. Dark red or violet blood without methemoglobin (i.e., deoxyhemoglobin) will brighten after exposure to atmospheric oxygen, whereas the dark (often chocolate brown) blood with methemoglobin will not change color. This differential response can be accelerated by gently blowing on the sample.

ELECTROCARDIOGRAPHIC CAVEATS

In young children, the right ventricle normally extends to the right of the sternum, as can be seen graphically on an anteroposterior chest radiograph. Because of this, an electrocardiogram in children younger than 5 years should include a chest lead taken on the right side of the chest, at a point analogous to the left-sided V4 lead (midclavicular line). This lead is called V4R. Rarely, if a heart is grossly enlarged and extends well to the right of the sternum, a V6R and even a V7R lead must be taken to complete a tracing that properly displays right ventricular potentials.

The right ventricle is normally the dominant ventricle in young children. Right axis is normal, and aVR usually has a dominant R wave in its QRS complex. The QRS progression across the chest leads usually goes from dominant R wave in V4R through the transitional zone to dominant R wave again in the left-sided chest leads. This may be true until as late as 4 years of age.

On the right-sided chest leads and in extremity lead III, T waves are normally inverted in infants and young children.

Determining whether a QT interval is prolonged is of particular importance in evaluating the patient with syncope and fainting. The following formula is used:

$$\text{Corrected QT (QTc)} = \text{Measured QT (in fractions of a second)} \div \sqrt{R - R} \text{ interval in fractions of a second)}$$

QTc should not exceed: 0.45 in young infants
0.44 in older infants and children
0.43 in adolescents and adults

FLUID AND ELECTROLYTE AIDES

A *millimole* is the atomic weight expressed in milligrams.
Equivalents are the number of electric charges per liter or the atomic weight divided by valence.
A *milliequivalent* is the equivalent weight expressed in milligrams.
Serum osmolality is calculated with the formula:

$$\text{Calculated osm} = 2(\text{Na}) + \text{Glucose (mg/dL)} \div 18 + \text{BUN (mg/dL)} \div 2.8$$

Normal range is about 285 to 295 mOsm per L.

$$\text{Osmolar gap} = \text{Measured (osm)} - \text{calculated (osm)}.$$

A gap of more than 10 units is considered abnormal, most commonly seen with ingestion of various types of alcohol.

Anion gap is the difference between measured cations and measured anions in the serum. In practice, the formula most commonly used is:

$$\text{Anion gap} = (\text{Na}) - (\text{Cl} + \text{bicarb})$$

An anion gap of more than 15 mEq per L is considered elevated.

Maintenance fluid requirements for children:

For 24-hour calculations:

For the first 10 kg: 100 mL per kg
For the second 10 kg: additional 50 mL per kg
For each kg beyond 20 kg: additional 20 mL per kg

For per-hour calculations:

For the first 10 kg: 4 mL per kg
For the second 10 kg: additional 2 mL per kg
For each kg beyond 20 kg: additional 1 mL per kg

Maintenance electrolytes:

Sodium: 2–3 mEq per kg per day
Potassium: 1–2 mEq per kg per day
Chloride: 2 mEq per kg per day

Total body water (as percentage of body weight):

80% at birth
70% at 6 months
60% at 1 year
Two-thirds is intracellular fluid and one-third is extracellular.

Fluids Used for Enteral Rehydration and Maintenance

Ideally, oral fluids should have a carbohydrate concentration of 2% to 2.5%, sodium concentration of at least 70 mEq/L for rehydration and 40 to 45 mEq/L for maintenance, and potassium concentration of 20 to 25 mEq/L.

	CHO (g/dL)	Na⁺ mEq/L	K⁺ mEq/L	mOsm/kg H₂O Osmolarity
Pedialyte®	2.5	45	20	250
Naturalyte®	2.5	45	20	260
Rehydralyte®	2.5	75	20	310
WHO rehydration solution	2	90	20	310
Gatorade®[a]	5.9	21	2.5	377
Cow's milk[a]	4.9	22	36	260

[a]Not recommended as first-line therapies for rehydration; less effective for maintenance hydration.

SENSORY NERVE DERMATOMES

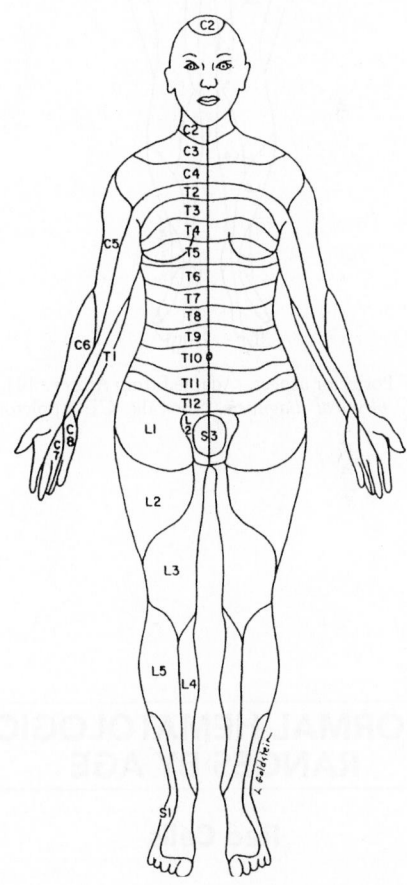

FIGURE C.5 Anterior aspect. (Adapted from Athreya BH, Silverman BK. *Pediatric physical diagnosis.* Norwalk, CT: Appleton-Century-Croft, 1985.)

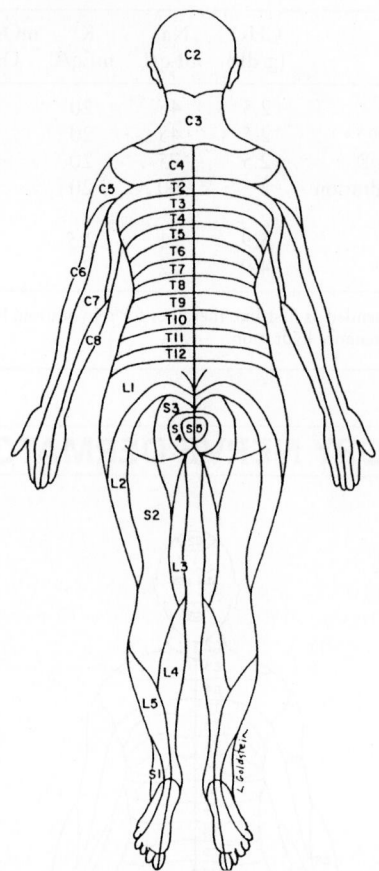

FIGURE C.6 Posterior aspect. (Adapted from Athreya BH, Silverman BK. *Pediatric physical diagnosis*. Norwalk, CT: Appleton-Century-Croft, 1985.)

NORMAL HEMATOLOGIC RANGES BY AGE

Red Cells

Age	Hemoglobin (g/dL) Mean	Hemoglobin (g/dL) Range	Hematocrit (%) Mean	Hematocrit (%) Range	Reticulocytes (%) Mean	MCV (fl) Mean
Cord blood	16.8	13.7–20.1	55	45–65	5.0	110
1–2 wk	16.5	13.0–20.0	50	42–66	1.0	
1 mo	12.0	9.5–14.5	36	31–41	1.0	
6 mo–6 yr	12.0	10.5–14.0	37	33–42	1.0	74
7–12 yr	13.0	11.0–16.0	38	34–40	1.0	78
Adult						
Female	14	12.0–16.0	42	37–47	1.6	80
Male	16	14.0–18.0	47	42–52		80

MCV, mean corpuscular volume.

White Cells

Age	Leukocytes (WBC/mm³) Mean	Leukocytes (WBC/mm³) Range	Neutrophils (%) Mean	Neutrophils (%) Range	Lymphocytes (%) Mean	Eosinophils (%) Mean
Cord blood	18,000	9,000–30,000	61	40–80	31	2
1–2 wk	12,000	5,000–21,000	40		63	3
1 mo	12,000	6,000–18,000	30		48	2
6 mo–6 yr	10,000	6,000–15,000	45		48	2
7–12 yr	8,000	4,500–13,500	55		38	2
Adult	7,500	5,000–10,000	55	35–70	35	3

WBC, white blood cell.

PROPHYLAXIS AFTER EXPOSURE TO SERIOUS DISEASE

Tetanus Exposure

Exposure to *Clostridium tetani*, the causative organism for tetanus (lockjaw), occurs primarily through wounds incurred at a site contaminated by human or animal excreta. The first step in prevention involves thorough cleaning, irrigation, and possibly debridement of potentially contaminated wounds. A decision about the need for and extent of immunoprophylaxis should be based on the nature and severity of the wound and on the tetanus immunization status of the patient. The following table serves as a guide:

Prior tetanus toxoid immunization (doses)	Clean, minor wound	All other wounds
Infants <6 weeks old, no prior tetanus immunization	None	TIG only
Uncertain or did not complete primary series	DTaP (if <7 yr), Td (if 7–9 yr, or prior Tdap) Tdap (> 10 yr)	DTaP, Td, or Tdap *and* TIG
Primary series complete (most recent within past 5 yr)	None	None
Primary series complete (most recent between 5 and 10 yr ago)	None	Td (if 7–9 yr, or prior Tdap) or Tdap
Primary series complete (most recent more than 10 yr ago)	Td	Td (if prior Tdap) or Tdap

Primary series = minimum of 3 doses of tetanus and diphtheria containing vaccine (DTap, DTP, Tdap, DT, Td). DTaP; diphtheria, tetanus, acellular pertussis; Td, adult formulation of diphtheria, tetanus toxoid; TIG, tetanus immunoglobulin [dose: 250 U IM (intramuscularly) for all ages]. All immunocompromised patients with non clean, minor wounds should receive TIG.

Rabies Exposure

A bite or very close contact with the saliva of an animal carrying the rabies virus is considered a potential rabies exposure.

The most common animal reservoirs include bats, skunks, raccoons, foxes, and woodchucks. Dogs and cats that have been bitten by rabid animals will carry the virus in their saliva before becoming symptomatic and may transmit it to humans by bite or abrasion during this time. In the United States, the majority of rabies deaths have been associated with bat variants of the rabies virus, in most cases with no clear history of a bite. Worldwide, however, most cases result from dog bites.

The decision about when to institute prophylaxis after an exposure must be guided by the location and severity of the wound, the status of the offending animal if known, and knowledge of the local epidemiology. In the northeastern United States, for instance, rabies is prevalent in the raccoon population, with resultant fear of infection in the dog and cat population. Incarceration and observation of a biting animal for 10 days is advisable, if the offending animal is known. If a patient has closed-space exposure to bats in the home or workplace, whether or not there is history of a bite, prophylaxis with human diploid cell vaccine (HDCV) is recommended.

Active Immunization (Postexposure)

Prophylaxis should begin with thorough cleaning and irrigation of the wound.

Five doses of HDCV, 1 mL each, should be given in the deltoid muscle in adults, or in the anterior thigh in children, on days 0, 3, 7, 14, and 28* after exposure. Alternatively, purified chick embryo cell vaccine (PCECV) may be used on the same dosage schedule. Dosages are not decreased for children. Occasional allergic reactions have been reported with HDCV, particularly with booster doses.

Passive Immunization

In addition to HDCV, human rabies immunoglobulin (HRIG) should be given to patients who have had no prior immunization, in a dose of 20 IU per kg on day 0 of exposure. Most of the dose should be infiltrated around the wound and the remainder given IM, remote from the side of the HDCV administration.

Preexposure prophylaxis for those at high risk of exposure because of travel to or work in endemic areas consists of three injections of HDCV or PCECV, given IM on days 0, 7, and 21 or 28.

Meningococcal Infection Exposure

Any person who has had close contact with an index patient during the 14 days prior to onset of invasive disease should receive antibiotic prophylaxis. Chemoprophylaxis is most effective when given within 24 hours of exposure. Close contacts include household, day care center, and nursery school contacts, as well as medical personnel with exposure to oral secretions (i.e., anyone involved with intubation, suctioning, or mouth-to-mouth resuscitation).

Chemoprophylaxis

Rifampin—10 mg per kg per dose (maximum 600 mg/dose), twice a day for 2 days (infants younger than 1

month, 5 mg/kg/dose); not for pregnant women; urine and contact lenses may turn red. Consider alternative therapy in young women, using oral contraceptives.

Ceftriaxone—single IM dose of 125 mg for ages 15 years and younger and 250 mg for those older than 15 years.

Ciprofloxacin—single oral dose of 500 mg for nonpregnant contacts 18 years and older or for younger children if no acceptable alternative therapy is available.

Immunoprophylaxis

Meningococcal quadrivalent polysaccharide vaccine (groups A, C, Y, and W-135)—Current recommendations are for children 11 to 18 years of age to be vaccinated at routine 11 to 12 year health-care visits or at their earliest convenience. In addition, immunization should occur for those at increased risk of meningococcal disease including college students living in dormitories, military recruits, persons with complement deficiencies, and persons with anatomic or functional asplenia. Vaccination can be used as an adjunct to chemoprophylaxis following exposure, although serotype B is not included in current vaccines. Type-specific vaccine C is available for infants and children in Canada and Europe.

Varicella Exposure

Varicella-zoster virus (VZV) is highly contagious. Administration of the varicella vaccine is essentially free of risk, although effectiveness in preventing clinical illness if given within 3 days of exposure is not uniform.

The only assured protection for the contact is provided by varicella-zoster immunoglobulin (VZIG). Its use should be confined to those who have been exposed and who are at high risk of developing complications of varicella. In emergency medicine, this will be largely limited to those who are immunosuppressed or immunodeficient (including HIV patients). Other patients who may require treatment with VZIG include varicella exposures in the following groups: premature infants weighing less than 1,000 g and neonates born to mothers who develop the disease within 5 days before or 2 days after delivery.

The dosage of VZIG is 125 U [1.25 mL (1 vial) IM] per each 10 kg or less, up to a maximum of 625 U [6.25 mL (5 vials)].

With the advent of acyclovir as an effective modifier for varicella, it is not necessary to give VZIG to the healthy susceptible adolescents or adult patients who are exposed to the disease. Treatment of varicella and zoster infection is discussed in Chapter 92.

Pertussis Exposure

Older siblings, adolescents, and adults, often with only mild and atypical disease, can be a significant source of exposure of pertussis for infants and young children.

Maintaining high vaccination rates is the most effective means of prevention. Current immunization schedules include acellular pertussis vaccinations at 2, 4, 6, and 15 to 18 months and 4 to 6 years. Tdap booster at 11 to 18 years has recently been added. Exposed children younger than 7 years who are

---

*The 28-day dose is not necessary in healthy nonimmunocompromised patients except in high-risk areas.

not immunized or who are partially immunized should have immunization initiated or brought to completion.

Chemoprophylaxis for close contacts for asymptomatic household contacts within 21 days of onset of cough in the index patient can prevent symptomatic infection. Potential regimens include the following:

■ Azithromycin:
  ■ First line in most children given equivalent efficacy, better tolerated, and no effect on liver metabolism.
  ■ Infants younger than 6 months: 10 mg per kg per day for 5 days.
  ■ Infants and children 6 months or older: 10 mg per kg (max 500 mg) on day 1, followed by 5 mg per kg per day (max 250 mg) on days 2 to 5.
  ■ Adults: 500 mg on day 1, followed by 250 mg per day on days 2 to 5.
■ Erythromycin:
  ■ Cheaper, generics available
  ■ Infants younger than 1 month: increased risk for pyloric stenosis.
  ■ Dose: 40 to 50 mg per kg per day in four divided doses (max 2 g/day) for 14 days.
■ Clarithromycin:
  ■ Infants younger than 1 month: not recommended.
  ■ Infants and children 1 month or older: 15 mg per kg per day (max 1 g/day) in two divided doses for 7 days.
  ■ Adults: 1 g per day in two divided doses for 7 days.
■ Trimethoprim-sulfamethoxazole:
  ■ Infants younger than 2 months: not recommended.
  ■ Infants 2 months or older and children: trimethoprim 8 mg per kg per day, sulfamethoxazole 40 mg per kg per day in two divided doses for 14 days.
  ■ Adults: trimethoprim 320 mg per day, sulfamethoxazole 1,600 mg per day in two divided doses for 14 days.

Hepatitis A Exposure

Hepatitis A virus is food- and waterborne. It is also transmitted by close person-to-person contact with infected individuals, who may or may not be symptomatic, and less commonly by needle sharing and sexual contact. The hygienic measure of careful handwashing for all medical, day care center, and restaurant personnel should be followed at all times. Potentially contaminated food and water should be avoided.

Immunoprophylaxis

Routine Hepatitis A vaccination is now recommended for all children at 1 year of age, and any child 2 to 18 years of age who lives in a community with a high incidence of disease. Therefore, the number of patients requiring postexposure prophylaxis is likely to decrease in coming years.

Unimmunized household and close personal contacts and children and staff at day care centers (particularly those with diapered children) who are exposed to an index case should receive immunoprophylaxis. Household contacts of children exposed at day care center should also be treated. Exposure in schools, offices, and hospital settings do not require prophylaxis unless there has been a spread within the institution.

Prophylaxis for children older than 1 year is single-antigen hepatitis A vaccine. For children younger than 12 months or

those with immunocompromised or chronic liver disease, low-dose immunoglobulin (IG) (0.02 mL/kg IM) should be given. Prophylaxis should be initiated as soon as possible, up to 14 days of exposure.

Hepatitis B Exposure

Hepatitis B virus (HBV) is transmitted by exposure to contaminated blood, semen, cervical secretions, or saliva through open wounds, needle exposure, medical management, improperly prepared transfusion, sexual activity, and maternal–child transmission.

Universal administration of HBV vaccine is begun in infancy. Medical and institutional personnel and others at high risk of exposure should also be vaccinated with HBV vaccine. There are two approved vaccines, both without thimerosal, and doses will vary for each. Higher doses should be considered for immunodeficient patients.

Postexposure prophylaxis guidelines depend on whether the source is known to be hepatitis B positive, on the immunization status of the exposed, and on whether the exposure is occupational or not. For nonoccupational exposure, anyone who is unimmunized or partially immunized and is exposed to a known hepatitis B-positive source should receive vaccination as well as Hepatitis B immunoglobulin (HBIG) at 0.06 mL per kg (minimum dose: 0.5 mL). Anyone who has completed the hepatitis B series but has not had a documented postvaccination response should receive a hepatitis B vaccine booster. For exposure to a source with an unknown hepatitis B status, immunizations series should be initiated/completed but HBIG is not required. In the occupational setting, providers are more likely to know (or can rapidly determine) their postvaccination status, and guidelines for vaccination and HBIG can be made accordingly. See *MMWR Recomm Rep* 2001;50(RR-11) and *MMWR Recomm Rep* 2008;57(RR08), the latter also available at http://www.cdc.gov/mmwr/preview/mmwrhtml/rr5708a1.htm, for details on prophylaxis following occupational exposure. Where warranted, prophylaxis should be given as soon as possible, preferably within 24 hours.

Neonates born to hepatitis B surface antigen–positive mothers should receive HBV vaccine within 12 hours of birth. HBIG (0.5 mL) should be given simultaneously but at a different site.

Hepatitis C Exposure

Hepatitis C is parenterally transmitted through contaminated blood or blood products and through maternal–infant transmission. Transmission through breast-feeding has not been reported. IG prophylaxis is not recommended. No vaccine is available.

For additional information, refer to Pickering LK, ed. *Red book: 2006 report of the Committee on Infectious Diseases*, 27th ed. Elk Grove Village, IL: American Academy of Pediatrics, 2006.

HIV Health-care Occupational Exposure

Medical and dental personnel (MDP), particularly those working in emergency departments and in the various surgical and laboratory areas, are susceptible to inadvertent exposure to

HIV. This may occur (i) percutaneously (needle stick or scalpel wound); (ii) by contact of MDP skin or mucous membranes with potentially contaminated body fluid such as blood, semen, or vaginal secretions; or (iii) by direct MDP skin or mucous membrane contact with laboratory specimens. If MDP skin is previously irritated or abraded, the risks under (ii) and (iii) are increased. Actual incidents of infection under such circumstances is minimal (less than 0.3% to 0.1%).

The first step in prophylaxis is always, when possible, prevention of exposure. This is best accomplished by MDP carefully following the guidelines of appropriate handwashing, use of gloves, proper cleaning and draping for any procedure that may involve exposure, careful disposal of all needles and other disposable instruments and syringes, and effective sterilization of all reusable equipment and devices.

When exposure does occur to MDP, careful cleaning of the wound area is essential. Relevant details of the exposure should be documented in a confidential record, including date and time, job duty being performed, full details of the circumstances and nature of the exposure, and description of the source of the exposure material. An ongoing record should include details of counseling, postexposure management, and follow-up of the MDP and the individual who was the source of the exposure material.

With permission, HIV testing should be performed on the source individual and, if found negative, testing should be repeated periodically for 6 months. The exposed MDP should undergo baseline HIV testing at the time of exposure. If the source individual for the exposure material is HIV positive, becomes HIV positive, or refuses to be tested, the MDP should be retested at 4- to 6-week intervals for up to 6 months. Seroconversion usually occurs within 3 months of exposure.

Consideration should be given to early initiation of postexposure prophylaxis for the MDP when the source individual is known to be, or is at high risk for being, HIV positive. A 4-week course of two drugs should be prescribed (zidovudine plus lamivudine, stavudine plus lamivudine, or stavudine plus didanosine). A third antiretroviral drug should also be added for highest-risk exposures. The potential toxicity of the drug regimens should be balanced against the degree of risk imposed by the exposure to the MDP. A decision must be made by the MDP and personal physician after adequate and appropriate counseling and after consideration of all factors involved in weighing benefit versus risk and toxicity. Hepatitis B prophylaxis should be considered as described previously.

Further details are available at: Centers for Disease Control and Prevention. Updated guidelines for management of occupational exposures to HBV, HCV, and HIV. *MMWR Recomm Rep* 2001;50(RR-11):1–42. Also see *MMWR Recomm Rep* 2006;55(RR-16), available at http://www.cdc.gov/mmwr/preview/mmwrhtml/rr5516a2.htm..

Postexposure prophylaxis for nonoccupational exposures is discussed in Chapter 93, with additional information available at CDC: Centers for Disease Control and Prevention. Antiretroviral postexposure prophylaxis after sexual, injection-drug use, or other nonoccupational exposure to HIV in the United States: recommendations from the U.S. Department of Health and Human Services. *MMWR* 2005;54 (No. RR-2).

SCORES

Glasgow Coma Scale

Older children	Infants	Points
Eye Opening		
Spontaneous	Spontaneous	4
To verbal command	To verbal stimuli	3
To pain	To pain	2
None	None	1
Best Motor Response		
To verbal command		
Obeys	Moves spontaneously and purposefully	6
To painful stimulus		
Localizes	Withdraws to touch	5
Flexion withdrawal	Withdraws to pain	4
Flexion decorticate	Flexion decorticate	3
Extension decerebrate	Extension decerebrate	2
No response	No response	1
Best Verbal Response		
Oriented and interactive	Smiles, babbles, or coos	5
Disoriented	Cries but consolable	4
Inappropriate words	Persistent inappropriate crying or screaming	3
Incomprehensible	Moans or grunts	2
No response	No response	1

AVPU

A—alert
V—responds to vocal stimuli
P—responds to painful stimuli
U—unresponsive

Note: The following two trauma scores have some limited value in determining whether to triage a pediatric trauma patient to a level I trauma center. Higher scores are generally associated with more favorable outcomes. Refer to Furnival RA, Schunk JE. ABCs of scoring systems for pediatric trauma. *Pediatr Emerg Care* 1999;15:215–223; and Narci A, Solak O, Turhan-Haktanir N, et al. The prognostic importance of trauma scoring systems in pediatric patients. *Pediatr Surg Int* 2009;25:25–30.

Revised Trauma Score

Attribute	Coded value
Respiratory Rate	
10–29	4
>29	3
6–9	2
1–5	1
0	0
Systolic Blood Pressure	
>89	4
76–89	3
50–75	2
1–49	1
0	0

Glasgow Coma Scale	
13–15	4
9–12	3
6–8	2
4–5	1
3	0

Unweighted Revised Trauma Score

Pediatric Trauma Score

Component	+2	+1	−1
Size	>20 kg (40#)	10–20 kg	>10 kg
Airway	Normal	Maintainable	Unmaintainable
Systolic blood pressure	>90 mm Hg	50–90 mm Hg	<50 mm Hg
Central nervous system	Awake	Obtunded/ loss of consciousness	Coma/ decerebrate
Skeletal	None	Closed fracture	Open/multiple fractures
Cutaneous	None	Minor	Major/ penetrating

Assign a value to each component. A score of 8 or less may suggest that care should be provided in a pediatric trauma center.

APGAR Score

Sign	0	1	2
Heart rate	Absent	<100 beats/min	>100 beats/min
Respiratory effort	Absent	Slow, irregular	Good, crying
Muscle tone	Limp	Some flexion of extremities	Active motion
Response to catheter in nostril (tested after oropharynx is clear)	No response	Grimace	Cough or sneeze
Color	Blue, pale	Body pink, extremities blue	Completely pink

To be checked on each newborn at 1 minute and again at 5 minutes after completion of birth.

Trauma Protocol

To be done simultaneously under direction of a team leader and including a recorder if sufficient personnel are available in unstable patients or those with significant risk of morbidity/mortality.

Primary Survey and Resuscitation

"A" AIRWAY—Evaluate for: adequacy of air movement, positioning, foreign material (blood or emesis), speech, midline trachea, subcutaneous air

Interventions: oral or nasopharyngeal airway, bag-mask ventilation, or intubation as needed; maintain C-spine immobilization

"B" BREATHING—Evaluate for: breath sounds, open pneumothorax, tension pneumothorax, hemothorax, flail chest, gastric distension, hypoxia

Interventions: supplemental oxygen; positive pressure ventilation as indicated

"C" CIRCULATION—Evaluate for: hemorrhage, peripheral pulses, heart sounds, capillary refill, jugular vein distension

Interventions: vascular access (venous, intraosseous), bloods for laboratory tests, including type and cross-match

"D" DISABILITY—Evaluate for: pupils, level of consciousness, AVPU, Glasgow Coma Scale and/or Revised Trauma Score, other cranial nerves, if possible

"E" EXPOSURE—Evaluate for: open wounds, penetrating trauma, front and back

Interventions: Avoid prolonged exposure, hypothermia

"F" FOLLOW—monitors, rhythm strip, catheter, nasogastric tube

"G"—blood gases if indicated

"H" HISTORY—preliminary

Secondary Survey

■ Complete physical examination, ventral and dorsal, including cranial nerve check, fundoscopic examination, careful neurologic screening, abdominal examination, check for blood from penis, rectal examination, and evaluation of all open wounds

■ Complete history of the current episode and medical history, if possible

■ C-spine film, chest radiograph, abdominal and pelvic films; consideration of emergency ultrasound and/or computed tomography scan

■ Careful splinting and wound dressing as indicated

■ Continuous reevaluation and ongoing monitoring.

APPENDIX D ■ PARENTAL INSTRUCTION SHEETS

NANETTE C. DUDLEY, MD

ABSCESS/MRSA

Your child has an abscess. An abscess is a skin infection that has a collection of pus. Larger abscesses are drained and the pus removed. Most abscesses are treated with antibiotics. The *Staphylococcus aureus* causes most abscesses and the term MRSA (methicillin-resistant *S. aureus*) is used if the bacteria is resistant to many antibiotics. This bacteria can spread to family members and close contacts. Your child will need close follow-up until he/she is better.

Your antibiotic is _____
Your follow-up is _____

Home Treatment

1. Keep any draining wound covered with a clean, dry bandage. If a drain was placed, do not remove it and follow-up with your child's doctor as recommended to remove it or have the abscess checked.
2. Wash your hands and your child's hands with soap and water or hand sanitizer after touching the infected area or any item with drainage from the wound.
3. Wash and dry thoroughly any towels, clothes, bedding that touches the skin, and do not share bar soap or razors.
4. Do not allow your child to play sports, return to day care, or be part of any activity with skin-to-skin contact until the wound is healed.

Call your Doctor or Return to the Emergency Department If:

1. Your child has fever, looks sick or is extremely irritable or lethargic.
2. The wound seems more painful, has spreading redness, looks more swollen.
3. You think your child is not improving or is getting worse after 2 to 3 days of antibiotics.

To Prevent Spreading the Bacteria to Others in Your Family

1. Do not share anything that comes in contact with the infected skin (bath products, athletic equipment, sheets/towels, etc.).
2. Clean surfaces and equipment (doorknobs, light switches, counters) touched by bare skin with a disinfectant (Lysol® or Pine-Sol® or similar product) that says it works for *S. aureus* on the label.
3. Discard all old razors and toothbrushes.

4. Your doctor may want to try using medicine or a cleansing routine to get rid of the staphylococci in your household. These treatments do not always work, but to have the best result **all household** members need to be treated at the same time. Your doctor recommends:

_____
_____

ANIMAL BITES

Your child was bitten by an animal. This can be frightening to some children, and your child may need some extra comfort to feel better. Your doctor suggests the following if needed for comfort.

The examining doctor cleaned the bite wound. The doctor may have given you instructions to clean the wound at home. They are:

_____
_____

[ ] Your child was given a **tetanus** shot in the emergency department (ED). Show this to your child's doctor to update his/her records.

_____

[ ] Your doctor has decided that **antirabies** treatment is needed. Your child was given the first injection (shot) today. He/she will need to return to the ED for the rest of the shots. The 28th day injection is only necessary under certain circumstances.

3rd day_____ 7th day_____ 14th day_____
28th day*_____

If your child gets a fever or the needle site is red or swollen, call your doctor. All the shots must be given to protect your child.

[ ] Your doctor has given your child a prescription for **antibiotics.** Not all bites need antibiotic treatment. Your child must take all the medicine as directed. Your dose is:

_____

Signs of Infection

Call your doctor or return to the ED if any of these signs develop after your visit:

1. Increased redness around the bite
2. Pain
3. Discharge or pus from the bite
4. Increased swelling
5. Bad smell
6. Fever

ASTHMA

Children with asthma have a reactive airway. The tubes that carry air to the lungs and the small passages in the lungs are sensitive to many things. When triggered, the airways react by getting smaller, swelling, and forming mucous plugs. This reaction can occur with colds and viruses; with exposure to pets, dust, odors, or allergens; or with exercise and emotional stress. The treatment your child received in the ED helps open the airways and reduce the swelling.

Asthma is a condition that can affect your child for many years. Identifying something that triggers wheezing in your child may help avoid future episodes. **No smoking** should be allowed in the house because smoke irritates the airways of all children with asthma or respiratory illness. Your child can return to school if he/she is feeling better. If medicine needs to be taken at school, talk with your doctor and the school nurse. If an older child uses an inhaler, get permission for him/her to carry it. Your child can participate in gym class but may need to be excused during a cold if coughing or mild wheezing is present. If your child has multiple episodes of asthma, he/she should wear a medical alert bracelet.

Home Treatment

1. If your child starts wheezing, keep him/her calm or playing quietly. Excitement and physical activity can make the wheezing worse.
2. Give the medicine as prescribed. Talk with your doctor about an **asthma action plan** giving you instructions on how to manage your child's asthma to prevent future episodes.
3. Home treatment can be a combination of both quick relief medicine and medicine for long-term control of asthma.
4. Do not run out of the medicine. Make sure you always have refills.
5. Over-the-counter medicines often do not work in asthma. Call your doctor before giving your child a nonprescription medicine.

Your doctor has prescribed the medicine below:

Quick Relief Medicine _____ *(works fast)*
   Inhaler
   [ ] Use _____ puffs_____ inhaler _____.
   [ ] Use a spacer with the inhaler to help your child get all the medicine.

   Nebulized Medicine (Aerosol)
   [ ] Give _____ by aerosol _____.

   Steroids (used to decrease airway swelling)
   [ ] _____

Long-term Control Medicine (used regularly, helps keep asthma "under control")
   [ ] _____
_____

Call Your Doctor or Return to the Emergency Department If:

1. Your child has increasing shortness of breath or trouble breathing.
2. Your child is breathing hard or fast.

3. Your child looks blue or passes out (**call an ambulance immediately, do not drive yourself**).
4. Your child looks sick or anxious.
5. You have any questions or concerns.

BRONCHIOLITIS

Children with bronchiolitis have an infection with a virus that produces wheezing and trouble breathing. The tubes that carry air to the lungs and the small passages in the lungs themselves are infected by the virus. The symptoms can last a few weeks. This condition causes the most problems in young babies (younger than 3 months), children with heart or lung problems, and babies who were premature or have other medical problems. Breathing cigarette smoke can make your baby worse. The most common virus causing bronchiolitis is the respiratory syncytial virus (RSV) but other viruses lead to similar illness. Because it is a virus, antibiotics do not help. We do try to make children more comfortable and help them breathe easier. Your doctor has decided that your child can be treated at home, but we know that this infection can sometimes worsen. If you think your child is getting worse, you need to return to the ED.

Home Treatment

1. If your child starts wheezing, keep him/her calm or playing quietly. Excitement and physical activity can make the wheezing worse.
2. Run a vaporizer in your child's room. (We prefer a cool mist vaporizer to avoid the risk of burns.)
3. If your child's nose is stuffy you may use a bulb syringe and salt water drops to suction the mucus.
4. Encourage fluids.
5. Over-the-counter medicines often do not work in bronchiolitis. Check with your doctor before giving your child a nonprescription medicine.

Sometimes breathing treatments with asthma medications that open the airways help children breathe easier. Sometimes these treatments do not help. If your doctor prescribes breathing treatments, he/she believes these will help. Use them as instructed. However, if you do not think the treatments are helping and your child has trouble breathing, please return to the ED.

Your doctor has prescribed the medicine below:

   Inhaler
   [ ] Use _____ puffs _____ inhaler _____.

Use a spacer with the inhaler to help your child get all the medicine.

   Nebulized Medicine (Aerosol)
   [ ] Give _____ by aerosol _____.

   Other Medicines
   [ ] _____
_____

Call Your Doctor or Return to the Emergency Department If:

1. Your child has increasing shortness of breath or trouble breathing.

2. Your child is breathing fast (faster than 60 times per minute).
3. Your child stops breathing (even without turning blue) or seems tired or lethargic.
4. Your child is unable to drink (often a sign of trouble breathing).
5. Your child looks blue or passes out (**call an ambulance immediately, do not drive yourself**).
6. Your child looks sick or anxious.
7. You have any questions or concerns.

BURNS

Your child was treated for a burn. Burns occur when the skin is injured by contact with heat, fire, chemicals, or electricity. Your child has a clean dressing on the burn to protect it and prevent infection. For some burns, it is important to schedule a recheck in 24 to 48 hours to reassess the depth of the burn injury. Other burns can be cared for at home. Your doctor's instructions are:

Your child may have received a tetanus booster in the ED. If so, notify your child's doctor to update his/her records.

How to Change the Dressing at Home

1. Wash your hands thoroughly with soap and water.
2. Remove the old bandage. If it sticks, you can soak it for a few minutes in warm (not hot) water.
3. Wash the burn with warm, soapy water.
4. Rinse and pat dry with a clean towel.
5. With a sterile tongue depressor, apply the antibiotic _____ to the burned area in a thin layer. Do not reuse a dirty tongue depressor.
6. Carefully rewrap the burn with a sterile bandage as directed by your doctor.

Signs of Infection

1. Increasing redness or red streaks around the burn
2. Swelling
3. Pain
4. Yellow pus or discharge
5. Fever

If you notice any signs of infection, call your doctor immediately or return to the ED.

Pain

Acetaminophen (e.g., Tylenol®) or ibuprofen (e.g., Advil®, Motrin®) can be used for pain. Table D.1, Table D.2. If your child was given a prescription for a different pain medication, you should use that medication as prescribed. Speak with your doctor about timing the dose with the dressing changes to relieve pain. Your medication is: _____

Exercise/Physical Therapy

Your doctor may have directed your child to perform certain exercises or physical therapy to help maintain or regain use of the burned area. Please ask your doctor if you have questions about the exercises or if you think your child is becoming stiff or tight around a burned area.

Long-term Care

Once the skin has healed, apply a lubricating cream or lotion to the burned area. This treatment will keep it soft and decrease itching. Avoid extremes of heat or cold for 1 year after the burn. Avoid direct sunlight for 1 year after the burn and apply a sunscreen to any burned areas to protect the new skin.

CAST OR SPLINT CARE

Your child has a serious injury or fracture that the doctors want to keep quiet and immobile in a cast or splint. A cast completely covers the injured body part with solid fiberglass or plaster. A splint has a hard frame, but some areas are not covered by a hard surface and are wrapped with padding or an ace wrap only. A splint is often put on right after an injury to allow for swelling and rechecking the injury site.

What to Do in the First 48 Hours

1. Keep the injured area with the cast elevated as much as possible to prevent swelling.
2. If your child has a splint and there is a lot of pain or the fingers or toes are cold and pale, unwrap the bandage wrap to relieve the pressure from swelling. If this helps, rewrap it a little looser. If this does not help, rewrap the splint, call your child's doctor or return to the ED.
3. Give ibuprofen (e.g., Motrin®, Advil®) every 6 hours as needed for pain. Your child's dose is:

[ ] Your child may need additional pain medicine. Your doctor has written a prescription for:

General Cast or Splint Care

1. Do not allow your child to walk or put weight on the cast unless your doctor specifically tells you to do this.
2. Keep long arm casts in a sling at all times, except when sleeping.
3. Do not get the cast wet unless you are told this is okay.
4. Do not allow your child to place objects inside the cast.
5. Do not use devices such as knitting needles, coat hangers, and so forth to scratch underneath the cast.
6. Your child can take a bath if the cast is covered with a plastic bag and kept above the water.
7. Keep the skin around the cast edges clean and dry. You can put rubbing alcohol on the skin near the cast edge to prevent irritation.

8. If the cast edge feels rough, you can put adhesive tape around it or "petal" around the edge with moleskin. Ask your doctor or nurse how to do this.

9. If your child is unable to go to school, have his/her teacher provide homework assignments and ask for a tutor, if necessary.

Return to the Emergency Department or See Your Orthopedic Doctor If:

1. Your child's fingers or toes feel numb or cold, look blue or pale, and unwrapping the splint does not help.

2. Your child complains of tingling, tightness, or worsening pain in the injured arm or leg.

3. There is pain under the cast in one spot, or pain anywhere for no apparent reason.

4. It hurts your child to move the fingers or toes.

5. Your child has a fever.

6. You smell a bad odor coming from the cast.

7. The skin around the cast edge is red or irritated.

8. The cast gets soft or cracked.

9. The pain medication does not make your child feel better.

[ ] *Use of Crutches*

1. Help your child walk with crutches as demonstrated. Do not allow him/her to put weight on the cast unless told to do so.

2. Help your child go up and down stairs until you are comfortable he/she can do it well.

3. Do not have your child rest his/her underarms on the crutches. Putting weight on the underarms can cause nerve damage.

4. Always use crutches with rubber tips, and wipe the tips dry if they get wet so they are not slippery.

COMMON COLD (UPPER RESPIRATORY INFECTION)

The common cold is an infection of the nose and throat that is usually caused by a virus. It can make your child have sneezing, coughing, fever, and not feel well. Cold symptoms can last as long as 7 to 10 days. Colds spread from person to person by coughing or direct breathing and when people do not wash their hands well after blowing their nose or sneezing. Over-the-counter cold medicines do not "cure" a cold and do not help cold symptoms for children. They can have dangerous side effects and are not recommended at all for children younger than 2 years. Your child can return to school or day care when he/she feels well and does not have a fever. During cold season, send your child to school with a pack of tissues and hand sanitizer to help prevent spreading infection.

Home Treatment

1. Home treatment is aimed at keeping your child comfortable. If your child is uncomfortable or looks sick, he/she may need to see a doctor for a reexamination.

2. Encourage your child to drink plenty of fluids such as juice, soda, or Kool-Aid®. Do not force him/her to eat because it may cause vomiting. Your child may not feel like eating, but it is important that he/she drinks to prevent dehydra-

tion. If your child is interested in his/her regular diet, that should be encouraged.

3. Warm liquids sometimes ease a sore throat and help open a clogged nose. Grandmother's chicken soup may be the perfect meal for a child with a cold!

4. For nasal congestion (runny nose), you can use salt water drops to loosen the mucus. These drops should be used before feeding your child and at bedtime, but they can also be used in between if you think your child's nose is clogged and he/she has trouble breathing. You can buy saline (salt water) drops at the grocery or drug store or make your own.

To make salt water drops:

Mix ¼ tsp salt with ½ cup warm water. If you have a clean medicine bottle, you can store this solution for 24 hours (label it salt water). If you do not have a clean bottle, throw away the salt water after each use.

Using a medicine dropper, put two drops of the salt water in one nostril. Have your child lying flat when you do this. You may want to support his/her neck or shoulders with a rolled-up towel. Wait 30 to 60 seconds before suctioning the mucus with a rubber bulb syringe. Squeeze the air out of the bulb, put the tip of the bulb into the nostril. Let the air come back into the bulb, and the suction will pull the mucus out of the nose. Squeeze the mucus out of the bulb onto a tissue.

Repeat this process with the other nostril. Do not do this more often than six times per day. In young infants, the best time to do this is often before meals or a bottle. Wash the bulb syringe in warm soapy water after each use. Squeeze it in the water to clean the inside.

5. Do not use over-the-counter cold medicines without discussing this with your doctor first. **Do not use an adult cold medicine for a child!**

6. Use a cool mist vaporizer in your child's room. This will moisten the air and help loosen your child's nasal secretions. We prefer a cool mist vaporizer to avoid the risk of burns. Do not add medicine to the vaporizer; use plain water. Wash the vaporizer as instructed after each use.

7. Give acetaminophen (e.g., Tylenol®) or ibuprofen (e.g., Advil®, Motrin®) if your child has a fever. Your dose is:

Call Your Doctor or Return to the Emergency Department If:

1. Your child has trouble breathing or starts wheezing.

2. Your child gets a new fever higher than 102° F (38.5° C) [or higher than 100.5° F (38.0° C) if your baby is younger than 6 months].

3. Your child has trouble swallowing.

4. Your child is not drinking well or you think he/she is dehydrated (dry).

5. Your child complains of ear pain or you have concern of an ear infection.

6. Your child is sleepy or lethargic.

7. Your child looks sick.

8. You have any questions or concerns.

CONCUSSION

Your child was diagnosed with a concussion. A concussion is a head injury that causes symptoms of neurologic (brain) dysfunction. Usually with a concussion, images of the brain (CT or MRI) are normal and often not necessary. Your child's symptoms may include confusion, headache, amnesia, dizziness, unsteadiness or incoordination, nausea and vomiting, problems concentrating or focusing, problems sleeping, mood or behavior changes, and problems with speech. Rest is an important part of treatment. Children who are reinjured in the week or so after a concussion can occasionally have more serious problems if the return to full activity after the first injury was premature. Having more than one concussion may put your child at risk for life-long problems, so it is important to wear helmets and other athletic equipment to prevent future head injuries.

Home Treatment

1. Quiet activities and rest from both physical and mental exertion (including videogames or school) is recommended after a concussion.
2. Acetaminophen (e.g., Tylenol®) or ibuprofen (e.g., Motrin®, Advil®) may be given for headache.
3. Clear liquids should be given if your child is nauseous or vomiting.
4. Ice can be applied to any areas of swelling or bruising on the scalp.

Return to Play

When your child returns to sports, physical activity, or school, depends on his/her symptoms and whether this is a first concussion or if your child has had other concussions. A doctor should examine your child before allowing him/her to participate in contact or competitive sports. At minimum, your child should be completely symptom free (both at rest and when active) for at least 1 week before being allowed to participate in competitive sports. A slow return to full activity is recommended before returning to a specific sport. Your doctor has written specific instructions for your child's concussion and return to play:

Call Your Doctor or Return to the Emergency Department If:

1. You are unable to awaken your child or he/she seems more sleepy or confused.
2. Your child has severe or worsening headache.
3. Your child has a seizure.
4. Your child has continued or worsening vomiting, fever, or neck stiffness.
5. Your child loses control of urine or stool.
6. Your child has weakness or numbness of the face or an arm or leg.
7. Your child has trouble walking, seems more unsteady.

CONJUNCTIVITIS (PINK EYE)

Conjunctivitis is an infection or irritation of the outer part of the eye. It makes the "white" of the eye appear pink or red and is commonly called pink eye. It can be caused by allergies or infections from viruses (most common) or bacteria. Most pink

eye is contagious. All members of your household should wash their hands carefully, and other children should not touch your child's eye. Your child should have his/her own washcloth and towel. Whenever you touch his/her eye, you must wash your hands.

Treatment

1. Clean any pus or drainage with a warm, wet washcloth or cotton ball.
2. Your doctor may have prescribed antibiotic drops or ointment. Place this medicine in your child's eyes as directed by the doctor. Do not use the same medicine for other people in the house. Have them examined by a doctor and given their own medicine. Your medicine is:

3. Try not to get the medicine in the other eye if it is not affected.
4. Do not use the medicine longer than directed. If the infection persists, see your doctor.

Call Your Doctor If:

1. The eyelids get red or swollen.
2. Your child has trouble seeing or blurry vision.
3. Your child gets a fever or looks sick.
4. The infection is not better in 2 to 3 days.
5. You have any other questions or concerns.

CONSTIPATION

Constipation is the delayed or difficult passage of hard, dry stools. They usually hurt or cause pain when they are passed. There are no rules about the number of stools a child needs to have in a day or week. As long as your child has soft stools, he/she probably is not constipated. It can be normal for babies or small children to grunt, strain, and even cry while they are having a bowel movement. It can also be normal for a baby to go a few days without a bowel movement. Each child develops a pattern of his/her own.

The doctor who examined your child decided that he/she is constipated. Most constipation can be treated by some **dietary changes.**

1. If your baby is younger than 4 months, add 1 to 2 oz of apple, prune, or pear juice to your baby's diet each day until stools are soft and regular. Constipation is very rare in breast-fed babies; talk with your doctor if you breast-feed. Do not continue the juice for more than 1 week without checking with your doctor. You can also move your baby's legs in gentle bicycle motions if you think he/she is having trouble passing a hard stool.
2. If your baby is older than 4 months, give him/her one 4-oz bottle of apple, prune, or pear juice per day, and encourage fruits and vegetables if he/she has begun taking baby food.
3. If your child is eating table food:
   a. Increase the amount of fruits and vegetables he/she eats. Adding raw ones provides increased "roughage."
   b. Increase the bran content of his/her foods. Feed your child bran cereal, bran muffins, oatmeal, and whole wheat bread if possible.

c. Make sure your child drinks enough fluids, encourage 4 to 6 oz apple, prune, or pear juice each day.

4. Some children have severe constipation or a long-term problem that needs additional help with medication. Your doctor has written any additional instructions below.

_____

_____

Additional Tips

If your child complains of pain with a bowel movement, he/she may have a small tear or fissure in the rectal area. You can put Vaseline® or a protective diaper cream in this area to allow it to heal.

Give older constipated children protected time at least twice each day for toilet sitting. Your child should be able to sit on the toilet for about 15 uninterrupted minutes two times per day. After meals is the best time for your child to sit on the toilet.

Exercise also helps improve constipation, and you and your child may want to participate in activities together.

Call Your Doctor If:

1. The constipation does not improve in 2 weeks.
2. Your child has severe abdominal pain or vomiting.
3. You see more than a few drops of blood in the stool.
4. Your child begins losing control of bowel movements or soiling his/her underwear.

Final Note: Although you may reward your child for a successful bowel movement, never punish your child for not having a bowel movement or for soiling his/her underwear.

CORNEAL ABRASION

Your child has a scratch on the cornea, which is the outer surface of the eye. The doctor who examined your child put some drops in the eye. These drops ease the pain and prevent the scratch from getting infected. Some doctors will place a patch over your child's eye. This helps protect the eye from further injury and allows it to rest while it heals. We understand that some children try to remove the patch. If this occurs, the scratch should still heal without a problem. Pain medication (Tylenol®, Motrin®, or Advil®) may help your child. Most corneal abrasions will heal overnight.

It is **very important** to be checked within a day or two to see if the scratch is healed. An infected scratch or one that does not heal well can cause a permanent scar on the surface of the eye. Your doctor has arranged the following follow-up: _____

Call us if you have any questions or concerns.

CROUP

Croup is a swelling of the upper airway in the area commonly called the windpipe and voice box, or more technically, the trachea and larynx. Most children with croup have a virus, and some children are likely to get croup more than once. Croup is worse at night and during sleep in infants and better during the day. It usually lasts about 5 days.

Children with croup may have a fever and cold symptoms. The cough is harsh like a barking dog or seal. The noisy breathing is called stridor and is caused by the narrowing of the airway from the swelling.

Treatment

[ ] A steroid medicine dexamethasone (Decadron®) can help with the airway swelling in croup. Your doctor has decided to use this medicine for your child. Your dose is: _____

Home Treatment

1. Stay calm and keep your child calm. It can be frightening when your child has trouble breathing, but if he/she is anxious or crying, it will make things worse.
2. Use a cool mist vaporizer in your child's room to humidify the air. Do not use a hot steam vaporizer because it could burn your child if he/she gets too close.
3. Prop your child's head up with a few pillows, or sit up with him/her. Your child may find his/her own position that makes breathing easier, but sitting up often helps.
4. Give acetaminophen (e.g., Tylenol®) for fever. Use a suppository if your child has trouble breathing or is throwing up.
5. Encourage your child to drink clear liquids. Do not force your child to eat if he/she does not want to eat or has difficulty in breathing.
6. If your child's breathing sounds worse or the noisy stridor is louder, turn on the hot water in the bathroom shower or sink. Close the door and let the room steam up. Take your child in the bathroom with you and sit down for about 15 minutes. Keep your child occupied by reading to him/her or playing with toys. **Stay calm!**
7. Sometimes cool air will also help your child. If the steamy bathroom does not help, you can dress your child for the outdoors and then take him/her outside for 10 minutes.

Return to the Emergency Department Immediately If:

1. Your child has trouble breathing, is using his neck or abdominal muscles to breathe, is pulling in his chest to breathe.
2. Your child looks pale or has blue areas around the mouth/lips, fingernails, or toenails.
3. Your child passes out.
4. Coughing is continuous, or there is no improvement after mist or cool air is tried.
5. Your child is uncomfortable or unable to sleep.
6. Your child is drooling or has trouble swallowing.
7. Your child has a high fever [greater than 102° F (38.5° C)].
8. Your child seems to be getting tired of breathing.
9. You have any concerns or the child is rapidly getting worse.

Transport your child yourself if you have your own car, the drive is less than 15 minutes, and your child seems comfortable and stable. When driving with a sick child, have two people in the car, one in the back with the child and one in front driving. Keep the child in his/her car seat. Open the windows and allow some cool air inside. **Call an ambulance if your child has trouble breathing, is passed out, looks blue, or is getting worse.**

DIAPER RASH

A diaper rash is usually caused by irritation of the baby's skin from contact with urine or bowel movements. Sometimes the skin can also be infected with yeast or bacteria, and your doctor will let you know if your baby has an infection.

Treatment of Diaper Rash

1. Keep the baby's bottom as clean and dry as possible. Change the diapers often. Wash the diaper area gently with soap and water at each change and pat dry. Avoid premoistened wipes while the rash is present because they may irritate and sting.
2. Leave the diaper off, if you can, to allow the air to dry and heal the rash. This can best be done at naptime with your baby lying on his/her back on an open diaper.
3. If your doctor ordered a protective ointment, you should apply this with each diaper change. Medicated ointments or creams should be used as prescribed.

_____

4. Do not use talcum powder or baby powder because it can injure your baby's lungs if inhaled.
5. Avoid plastic pants if possible. They trap in moisture and make the rash worse. If you use cloth diapers, consider changing to disposable while your child has a rash.

Call Your Doctor or Return to the Emergency Department If:

1. Your baby develops a fever.
2. The rash does not appear to be improving after 5 to 7 days.
3. The rash is getting worse or pimples or blisters develop in the diaper area.
4. You are concerned about your baby.

EAR INFECTIONS

Your child has an ear infection, which is an infection of the middle ear, the space behind the eardrum. Ear infections can be caused by viruses or bacteria and are more common in the winter months. An ear infection is not contagious, but it can start as a cold. The germs in the throat or nose migrate into the middle ear. Fluid also can build up in the middle ear and swelling from a cold prevents it from draining into the throat. The combination of germs and fluid becomes an infection and pus is produced, putting pressure on the eardrum and causing pain. If your child has drainage from the ear, this may mean the eardrum has torn. The small tear in the eardrum will heal itself if the infection is treated. However, if fluid stays behind the eardrum for long periods, your child may have hearing problems. Any child with hearing problems or problems with speech/language should follow up with his/her doctor to make sure the fluid is gone. Your child can return to school or day care as soon as he/she is feeling better.

Treatment

1. **Pain and Fever:** Your child may have a fever or some ear pain. Acetaminophen (e.g., Tylenol®) or ibuprofen (e.g., Motrin®, Advil®) will treat this pain. Your child's dose is:

_____

Your doctor may also give you drops to numb the eardrum and help the pain. These drops should not be used if there is fluid draining out of the ear. Your instructions are:

_____

2. **Observation:** Ear infections caused by viruses may get better without antibiotics. If you and your doctor decided to watch your child without antibiotics, then you can still use

medicine for pain and fever to help your child. Your child should get better in 2 to 3 days, and if not getting better you need to follow up with your doctor.

3. **Antibiotics:** Ear infections are often treated with antibiotics. The fever and pain may continue for 2 to 3 days after starting the antibiotic. Some antibiotics cause diarrhea. If the diarrhea is severe or you think your child is getting dehydrated (not urinating well, not drinking well, no tears when crying), see your doctor. If your child gets a rash, he/she may be allergic to the antibiotic. See your doctor. Your dose of medicine is:

_____

Give your child the antibiotic prescribed, even if your child feels better. The full course is needed to kill the infection. Keep all medicines out of reach of small children.

4. **Ear Drops:** Your doctor may give you ear drops to treat an infection in the ear canal or external ear. Have your child lie on your lap with the infected ear up. Put drops in the ear canal and massage in front of the ear to help the drops fall into the canal. Do not put anything else in the ear canal. Ear drops: _____. Use the drops _____ times per day for _____ days.

5. **Follow-up:** Follow-up with your regular doctor in 2 to 3 days if your child is not feeling better (still has pain, fever, or ear drainage).

Call Your Doctor or Return to the Emergency Department If:

1. Your child looks sick or fever continues for more than 2 days after starting antibiotics.
2. Your child has a new drainage from the ear.
3. Your child gets a rash.
4. Diarrhea becomes severe or you think your child is dehydrated (dry).
5. Your child is sleepy or lethargic, or if you have any questions or concerns.

ECZEMA (ATOPIC DERMATITIS)

Eczema is common. Children with eczema may have a family history of allergies, hay fever, or asthma. All children with eczema have dry skin. Keeping your child's skin moist, and avoiding skin irritants will help control the eczema. Eczema usually improves as your child gets older.

Avoiding Skin Irritation

1. Avoid wool or synthetic clothing because it can be irritating. Dress your child in cotton when possible, and try to keep his/her arms and legs covered (tights or long pants, long-sleeve shirts).
2. Keep your child's room free of dust, and keep the air moist with a cool mist vaporizer or humidifier.
3. Wash your child's clothes in a mild detergent and avoid fabric softeners that can be irritating.

Skin Care

1. Do not overdo bathing. A **short** daily bath is fine, but your doctor may recommend changing to every other day baths.

Use a mild soap with moisturizer. Avoid deodorant soaps or those with scents. Avoid vigorous scrubbing, and bathe in warm, not hot, water. Do not use bubble baths. After bathing, pat dry and apply any medicated creams or moisturizing creams immediately (within 3 minutes) to seal in the moisture.

2. Your doctor may have prescribed a cream for specific areas. Apply this medicated cream as directed to those areas. Apply _____

3. After applying the medicated cream, apply a general moisturizing cream or ointment to your child's entire body. Apply this moisturizer two times per day, *everyday*.

_____

4. If itching is a problem, your doctor may prescribe a medicine to be used for a short period.

_____

These medicines can make your child sleepy and teenagers should not drive a car while taking this medicine. Keep your child's fingernails cut short if scratching is a problem. Some children need to wear socks on their hands when they go to sleep to keep them from scratching.

Call Your Doctor If:

1. The eczema is red or irritated looking, your child develops sores or scabs or painful lumps, or your child gets a fever.
2. You think the eczema is not under good control.
3. You have any questions or concerns.

FEBRILE SEIZURE

A febrile seizure is a "fit" or "convulsion" that occurs with a fever. Most children who have febrile seizures outgrow them by 4 to 5 years of age. Having a febrile seizure does not mean that your child has brain damage or will be delayed. They are fairly common, often happening in the first day of a fever and are not related to development of a seizure disorder or epilepsy. There is a chance, however, that your child may have another seizure when he/she has a fever.

When your child becomes sick, the suggestions below will help you control the fever and prevent a seizure:

1. Give acetaminophen (e.g., Tylenol®) or ibuprofen (e.g., Advil®, Motrin®) in the correct dose for your child's age. Table D.1, Table D.2 Acetaminophen can be given every 4 hours, ibuprofen every 6 hours while your child's temperature is 101° F (38.0° C) or higher.
2. Do not bundle or overdress your child. The body loses heat through the skin, and if you bundle him/her, the excess heat cannot escape.
3. Sponge your child with lukewarm water or put him/her in a shallow tub containing 2 to 3 in of water and drip water over his/her body. **Do not** use alcohol or cold water to bring your child's fever down. If your child begins shivering or shaking, stop sponging and remove him/her from the bath water.
4. While your child has a fever, give plenty of fluids to prevent dehydration.
5. Give any medications prescribed by your doctor.
   Your child may have another febrile seizure because they can occur before you realize your child is ill.

If Your Child Has Another Seizure:

1. Stay calm.
2. Do not put anything in your child's mouth.
3. Place your child on his/her side to help drain secretions.
4. Loosen clothing.
5. Do not try to hold your child still. Move objects away from your child so he/she does not get hurt.
6. Support your child's head with a pillow or soft object.

Call an ambulance if the seizure is lasting longer than 5 minutes or if your child has difficulty breathing or looks blue. Otherwise, once the seizure stops, call your doctor for further instructions or bring your child to the office or ED for a physical examination. Your child may be sleepy after the seizure and need to be checked by a doctor for the cause of the fever.

FEVER

Your child has a fever. This means the body temperature is above normal. In the mouth, normal temperature is 98.6° F (37° C); under the arm, normal is 98° F (36.6° C); and by rectum, normal is 100° F (37.7° C). A fever is the body's way of fighting an infection and is not always a bad thing. You only need to treat the fever if it is high [greater than 102° F (38.5° C)] or if your child is uncomfortable. The height of the temperature does not indicate how severe the illness is that causes the fever. Your child should see a doctor if you have any concerns.

What to Do to Keep Your Child Comfortable

1. Dress your child lightly to be comfortable in your home's temperature. Do not overbundle or use heavy blankets because this will raise your child's temperature further. A T-shirt and underwear or diaper with a light sheet or blanket is fine for sleeping.
2. Encourage plenty of liquids. Your child may not be hungry but it is important that he/she continues to drink and does not get dehydrated.
3. Keep the room around 70° F if possible. In the winter, do not overheat, and in the summer, use a fan or air conditioner if available.
4. Acetaminophen (e.g., Tylenol®) lowers fever. Your pharmacy may sell acetaminophen as a generic fever product. This is just as effective and may cost less. Check your child's temperature before giving the medicine. The dose can be repeated every 4 hours. Table D.1
   If your child is vomiting or does not like to take medicine, you can buy acetaminophen suppositories at your pharmacy without a prescription. Ask your doctor or nurse about how to use a suppository.
5. Ibuprofen (e.g., Advil®, Motrin®) may also be used for fever control in children 6 months and older. The dose can be repeated every 6 hours. Table D.2
6. Do not use aspirin for fever control in children.
7. Sponging your child with lukewarm water will also lower his/her temperature but is not as helpful as fever medicine. Do not use alcohol or add alcohol to a bath. Never leave your child alone in a bath. If your child starts shivering,

TABLE D.1

ACETAMINOPHEN DOSAGE BY AGE AND WEIGHT

Age	Weight (lb)	Drops[a] (80 mg/0.8 mL)	Liquid (160 mg/5 mL)	Chewable (80 mg)	Junior Caplet, Junior Chew (160 mg)
0–2 mo	Consult your doctor right away				
2–3 mo	6–11	½ dropper			
4–11 mo	12–17	1 dropper	½ tsp		
12–23 mo	18–23	1½ droppers	¾ tsp		
2–3 yr	24–35	2 droppers	1 tsp	2 tablets	1 tablet
4–5 yr	36–47	3 droppers	1½ tsp	3 tablets	1½ tablets
5–8 yr	48–59	4 droppers	2 tsp	4 tablets	2 tablets
9–10 yr	60–71		2½ tsp	5 tablets	2½ tablets
11–12 yr	72–95		3 tsp	6 tablets	3 tablets

[a]Use the dropper that comes with the acetaminophen bottle. Other droppers may be of a different size.

take him/her out of the bath and dry off. Shivering can raise the body temperature.

Call Your Doctor or Return to the Emergency Department If:

1. Your child is younger than 6 months and has a fever greater than 101° F (38.2° C).
2. The fever continues for more than 2 additional days without other symptoms.
3. Your child has the fever with other symptoms—rash, trouble breathing, ear pain, headache, stiff neck, vomiting, diarrhea, joint swelling, or pain.
4. Your child acts sick, is irritable, sleeps a lot, stops playing, or does not eat or drink.
5. You have any questions or concerns.

FEVER LESS THAN 2 MONTHS

Your baby has a fever. This means the body temperature is above normal. We worry about young babies with fever because they can have more trouble fighting a serious infection, and it is harder for parents and doctors to tell when they are getting sick. Your baby was evaluated in the ED and the doctor decided he/she could be cared for at home. You should follow-up as instructed.

What to Do to Keep Your Baby Comfortable

1. Dress your child lightly to be comfortable in your home's temperature. Do not overbundle or use heavy blankets because this will raise your child's temperature further. A T-shirt and diaper with a light sheet or blanket is fine for sleeping.
2. Encourage plenty of liquids. It is important that he/she continues to drink and does not get dehydrated.
3. Keep the room around 70°F if possible. In the winter, do not overheat, and in the summer, use a fan or air conditioner if available.
4. Acetaminophen (e.g., Tylenol®) lowers fever. Your pharmacy may sell a generic fever product with acetaminophen. These are just as effective and may cost less. Check your baby's temperature before giving the medicine. The dose can be repeated every 4 hours.

   Your baby's dose is: _____

   Use the dropper that comes with the acetaminophen bottle. Other droppers may be of a different size.

TABLE D.2

IBUPROFEN DOSAGE BY AGE AND WEIGHT

Age	Weight (lb)	Drops[a] (50 mg/1.25 mL)	Liquid (100 mg/5 mL)	Chewable (50 mg)	Junior Caplet (100 mg)
0–6 mo	Consult your doctor before using				
7–11 mo	15–17	1½ droppers	¾ tsp		
12–23 mo	18–23	2 droppers	1 tsp		
2–3 yr	24–35	3 droppers	1½ tsp	3 tablets	
4–5 yr	36–47	4 droppers	2 tsp	4 tablets	
6–8 yr	48–59		2½ tsp	5 tablets	2½ tablets
9–10 yr	60–71		3 tsp	6 tablets	3 tablets
11–12 yr	72–95		4 tsp	8 tablets	4 tablets

[a]Use the dropper that comes with the Ibuprofen (Advil®, Motrin®) bottle. Other droppers may be of a different size.

5. Follow-up is usually arranged with your physician or the ED within 24 hours of this visit. **Your follow-up is:** _____

Return to the Emergency Department If:

1. The fever continues for more than 2 additional days without other symptoms.
2. Your baby has other symptoms—rash, grunting or trouble breathing, stiff neck, vomiting, diarrhea, or pain.
3. Your child acts sick, is irritable, sleeps a lot, or does not drink.
4. You have any questions or concerns.

HEAD INJURY

The doctor who examined your child determined that he/she can safely be observed at home. You will need to watch your child for the next 24 to 72 hours and bring him/her back to the ED, if necessary. Please tell your nurse or doctor before leaving the ED if you do not think you can do this. If you were told your child has a concussion, he/she should not play sports until symptom free at least 1 week and cleared by a doctor.

Normal Behaviors in the First 8 Hours After a Head Injury

1. Your child may be **sleepy.** It is okay to let him/her sleep. Your child should be able to wake up and behave normally, recognize people and things, and speak clearly.
2. **Vomiting,** or throwing up, is also normal in the first few hours following a head injury.
3. Your child may complain of a **headache.** You can give acetaminophen (e.g., Tylenol®).

What to Do

1. Have your child rest or play quietly for the first 24 to 72 hours.
2. Feed your child a lighter than normal diet.
3. Give acetaminophen for a headache.

Return to the Emergency Department Immediately If:

1. **Vomiting** continues after the first 8 hours or begins later than the first few hours after the injury.
2. Your child is **difficult to wake up** or is **not acting normally** when awakened.
3. Your child's **headache worsens,** changes your child's behavior, or is not relieved by acetaminophen.
4. Your child has **trouble seeing** or **walking** or **acts clumsy** or uncoordinated.
5. Your child has **bleeding** or **clear drainage** from his/her **nose** or **ears.**
6. Your child has a **convulsion** or **seizure.**
7. Your child is unusually **sleepy** or has any **unusual behavior** or **change in behavior.**

HIVES

Urticaria, or hives, are red blotches on the skin due to a substance called histamine. They can be of many different sizes and are very itchy. Most hives are an allergic reaction to something your child touched, ate, or put on his/her skin. Hives can also be a reaction to cold, heat, emotional stress, or a viral infection. Some common substances that cause hives are milk, eggs, peanuts, strawberries, shellfish, plants, perfumes, medicines, pets, insect bites, soaps, and detergents. Hives can last only a few hours or several weeks. Often, the cause is unknown, but if you think you know what caused the hives, you should try to avoid reexposing your child to this substance.

Treatment

1. Sometimes no treatment is necessary, and the hives go away on their own.
2. Warmth makes the itching worse, so use a cool washcloth or cool bath to make your child more comfortable.
3. Your doctor may prescribe a medicine (usually an antihistamine) for itching. These medicines can make your child sleepy. Teenagers should not drive while using this medicine. Your medicine is _____
4. The best treatment is to avoid whatever caused the hives, so try to determine what caused them.

Call the Doctor If:

1. Your child has **trouble breathing** or feels a **tightness in his/her throat or chest or has lip or tongue swelling. Call an ambulance immediately and get to the nearest ED.**
2. The itching is not relieved by the medicine prescribed.
3. The hives do not go away after a few weeks.

IMPETIGO

Impetigo is a skin infection caused by bacteria. You can get impetigo by scratching and infecting insect bites or dry skin or by touching sores on other people. It is easily spread to other parts of the body and to other people, so your child should not return to day care or school until the crusts are gone.

Things to Do If Your Child Has Impetigo

1. Wash your hands before and after caring for your child or use a hand sanitizer to kill bacteria.
2. Gently wash the crusty areas three times each day with soap and water. You may need to soak the area in warm water to remove all the crusts.
3. Blot the areas dry.
4. If your doctor prescribed an ointment, apply this to the sore and the area around it. Rub it in well. _____
5. If your doctor prescribed a medication by mouth, give it to your child as directed until it is all gone. Your dose is: _____
6. Carefully wash the bathtub or bathroom sink your child used with soap and water. Do not use the kitchen sink if possible. Wash your child's towel, washcloth, and bed linens separately. Do not allow your child to share these.
7. Keep your child's fingernails cut short and try to keep him/her from scratching.

Call Your Doctor or Return to the Emergency Department If:

1. Your child gets a fever.
2. The infection is not improving in 3 to 4 days.
3. The sores appear to be spreading, the skin is red, painful, swollen, or draining pus.
4. The sores are not cleared up after 10 days.

LICE

Head lice are small, gray insects that live on humans. They can be spread by direct contact and by shared combs, hats, and clothes. They live in the hair and lay tiny white eggs called nits that stick to each hair shaft. Lice can cause itching.

Treatment

Your child was given a prescription for either cream rinse or shampoo (permethrin or pyrethrin) to treat the lice. **To use the shampoo:**

1. Apply to dry hair until thoroughly coated. (Wear rubber gloves when applying the shampoo.)
2. Leave the shampoo on the hair for 10 minutes and not longer.
3. Add a small amount of water to get lather and shampoo the hair.
4. Do not get shampoo in the eyes or mouth. If you do, rinse immediately with water.
5. Rinse the hair with water and towel dry. Use a fine-tooth comb to remove all nits. They may stick to the hair shaft and be difficult to remove. If so, rinse hair with a dilute vinegar and water solution (dilute vinegar with an equal amount water). This will make nits easier to remove.

To Use the Cream Rinse

1. Wash the hair with your regular shampoo and towel dry.
2. Apply the cream rinse to coat the hair thoroughly.
3. Leave the cream rinse on the hair for 10 minutes.
4. Rinse the hair with water and towel dry. Remove nits as previously described.

Re-treat with the shampoo or cream rinse in 7 days. Two treatments are recommended to kill all lice. Itching may continue for a few weeks even though the lice are gone.

To Eliminate Lice From Your Home

1. Vacuum all surfaces thoroughly.
2. Clean combs and brushes in hot water with some antilice shampoo or cream rinse.
3. Wash all pieces of clothing worn in the last 2 days and any sheets, blankets, and pillow cases your child used in hot water (more than 130° F) and dry in a hot dryer for at least 20 minutes.
4. Any items not washable—stuffed toys, coats, hats—must be set aside in airtight plastic bags for 2 weeks.

NOSEBLEEDS

Nosebleeds are common in children. They are usually caused by dryness inside the nose plus some irritation from rubbing, picking, or cold symptoms. They can begin suddenly and sometimes occur during sleep.

How to Stop a Nosebleed

1. Have your child sit up and lean forward. You may need a container so that your child can spit out any blood that has drained into his/her throat.
2. Firmly pinch the soft part of the nostrils (not the tip or the bone) together for a **full** 5 minutes. Use a clock to time this, and do not let go sooner. Tell your child to breathe through his/her mouth.
3. When you release the pressure, if the bleeding begins again, repeat step 2 one time.
4. If the bleeding continues, call your doctor or take your child to the ED. If possible, have someone hold pressure on the nose while traveling to the ED.
5. Do not place anything inside the nose while it is bleeding (e.g., gauze, tissue).
6. Cold washcloths or ice to the face will not help stop the bleeding.
7. Swallowed blood can irritate the stomach, causing your child to vomit up bloody material.

How to Prevent Nosebleeds

1. Using your finger, gently place a small amount of Vaseline® on the inside of the nose. This will help ease the dryness and irritation.
2. Use a cool mist vaporizer or humidifier in your child's room.
3. Discourage your child from picking his/her nose, and keep fingernails cut short.
4. If your child has a stuffy nose, you can use saline nose drops to make the mucus easier to clear. Avoid vigorous nose blowing.
5. Do not give your child aspirin unless directed by your doctor. If your child has many nosebleeds and is on aspirin, tell your doctor.

Call Your Doctor If:

1. You cannot stop the bleeding or your child has many nosebleeds in one day.
2. You think a lot of blood was lost, or your child faints, or looks dizzy or pale.
3. You see blood elsewhere—in urine, stool—or your child has bruises or a rash.
4. Your child looks sick.

RINGWORM

Ringworm is a fungal infection that can cause a skin rash or infect the scalp and cause hair loss, scaling or pimples, and pus. Your doctor can usually diagnose this condition by looking at it. Sometimes he/she will scrape the rash and take a culture. Ringworm is spread from person to person; from animals; or from shared combs, towels, or hats.

Treatment

Skin Infection: Your doctor prescribed a cream. Put this cream on the rash as directed. The rash should improve in 7 to 10 days, but you should continue the cream for a full 2-week course. If it is not gone after 2 weeks, call your doctor.

Scalp Infection: Your doctor prescribed a medicine (griseofulvin) to be taken orally. Your child's dose is _____. This medicine should be taken for the full course and is best taken with milk or a fatty meal. If your child begins vomiting or experiences diarrhea, abdominal pain, or a rash, or if he/she looks ill while taking this medicine, call your doctor. Your doctor also prescribed a special shampoo (selenium sulfide 2.5%) to decrease the time that your child is contagious. This shampoo can be used twice a week or as directed by your doctor. If your child wears braids or ponytails, they should be undone so the shampoo can penetrate to the scalp. Your child's combs, brushes, and clothing should be cleaned with ordinary soap and water. Ask your doctor or school nurse about when your child can return to school.

Call Your Doctor If:

1. The rash is not gone after a full course of the medicine.
2. Your child gets ill while taking griseofulvin.
3. You have any questions or concerns.

SCABIES

Scabies are little bugs that burrow in the skin and cause severe itching and a rash. These bugs are best seen with a microscope. They can spread easily from person to person by direct contact or by wearing clothes that have the scabies bug living in them. The itching and rash may last for 2 to 4 weeks after treatment. Your doctor may be able to give your child some medicine that helps the itching. If it continues longer than this, return to your doctor. Everyone in your household should be treated at the same time because scabies spread easily from person to person. Even people without symptoms should be treated; ask your doctor about this.

Treatment

[ ] Your doctor has prescribed a special cream containing 5% permethrin (Elimite®). Massage the cream into the skin from the head to the soles of the feet, including the scalp for an infant. Try to avoid the eyes because the cream can irritate them. If any of the cream gets in the eyes, wash them with cool water. Scabies like to live between the fingers and toes, under arms, and around the waist and genitals. Make sure to include all these areas. Leave the cream on for at least 8 hours, and then give your child a bath to wash off the cream.

[ ] Older children (more than 33 lb) can also be treated with a medicine (ivermectin), one dose now and one in 2 weeks. Your dose is: _____

The itching and rash may last for 2 to 4 weeks after treatment. Your doctor may be able to give your child some medi-

cine that helps the itching. If it continues longer than this, return to your doctor. Everyone in your household should be treated at the same time because scabies spread easily from person to person. Even people without symptoms should be treated; ask your doctor about this.

Medication for itching: _____

Cleaning Your House

1. Scabies can live on clothing or bed linens for up to 1 week.
2. Using hot water (more than 120°F), wash all clothing, bed linens, towels, and washcloths used in the past week, and dry them with high heat for 20 minutes to kill the scabies.
3. Items that cannot be washed (e.g., toys, blankets) should be placed in a plastic bag and stored for 1 week.
4. Clean clothes and clean sheets should be used after applying the cream.

Your child can return to school after treatment with the cream. Remember to keep the cream stored out of reach of your child because it can be poisonous if swallowed.

Call Your Doctor If:

1. The itching persists longer than 4 weeks after using the cream.
2. You think the skin has become infected or looks red with blistering or crusting.

SEDATION

Your child was given sedation in the ED. The sedation medicine was _____.

After sedation, your child may still be sleepy and may be unsteady when walking. Keep your child safe and avoid climbing, riding a bike, operating motorized equipment, or other activities where your child could get hurt for at least 6 hours after sedation. Vomiting may also occur. If your child vomits, allow him/her to rest and offer small sips of clear liquids.

What to Do

1. It is okay to let your child sleep, but he/she should be able to wake up and behave normally, recognize people and things, and speak clearly.
2. Plan quiet activities for the rest of the day.
3. Feed your child a lighter than normal diet. Some sedation medicines lead to nausea or some vomiting.
4. If your child has pain, offer pain medications as instructed.

Call or Return to the Emergency Department If:

1. Your child is not acting normally 6 hours after sedation.
2. Your child is difficult to arouse or unable to recognize you.
3. Your child is vomiting frequently and unable to keep down small sips of fluids.
4. Your child has trouble breathing, coughing, or fast breathing.
5. Your child has fever greater than 101°F (38.5° C).
6. Your child's pain is not eased by the pain medication.
7. You have any questions or concerns.

SEIZURE

Your child has had a seizure. A seizure occurs when the brain cells send electrical discharges that cause the arms and legs to jerk or twitch and the eyes to stare or blink. Usually, a child is sleepy or confused after having a seizure.

What to Do If Your Child Has a Seizure

1. Stay calm.
2. Do not put anything in your child's mouth.
3. Place your child on his/her side to help drain secretions.
4. Loosen clothing.
5. Do not try to hold your child still. Move objects away from your child so that he/she does not get hurt.
6. Support your child's head with a pillow or soft object.
7. Do not try to give your child any medicine by mouth during a seizure. It may cause him/her to choke.
8. Try to observe what your child looks like during the seizure and how long the seizure lasts. This information may help your doctor decide how to treat the seizure.

[ ] Rescue Medicine

Your doctor wants your child to use a "rescue" medicine if the seizure lasts more than 5 minutes. This medicine is _____. Your instructions are: _____
_____

Keep this medicine out of reach of children.

Call for Help If:

1. Your child has trouble breathing or looks blue.
2. The seizure is lasting longer than 5 minutes (even if you used a rescue medicine).
3. You cannot wake your child 30 minutes after the seizure.

After the Seizure

Your child may be sleepy and should be allowed to rest. Continue to give any medications prescribed for the seizure disorder. Do not give extra medicine or change the dosage without calling your doctor. Make sure you do not run out of the medication. Give all medicine as scheduled.

Follow-up with your regular doctor when a seizure occurs. This can be a good time to review your child's medical care and make changes if necessary. Your child may want to participate in sports or activities such as bicycle riding, swimming, or driving a car or motorcycle. Discuss this with your doctor before you allow your child to participate.

SORE THROAT

A sore throat occurs when the tonsils or back of the mouth become infected by a virus or bacteria. The infection usually spreads from person to person by coughing or sneezing but can also spread by sharing drinking cups or eating utensils.

Your doctor may have sent a swab of your child's throat for a culture. The culture will diagnose a strep throat caused by the streptococci. The culture may take up to 2 days for a result, and so a quicker test called rapid strep is used. The quick test misses some of the streptococci that may show on the culture.

[ ] **The rapid strep test was negative or not available at this time.** If the rapid test was negative, this does not absolutely mean your child does not have strep throat. Call _____ for the culture results on _____ from _____. Have your pharmacy phone number ready in case the doctor needs to phone in a prescription for your child.

[ ] **The rapid strep test was positive.** Your child has strep throat and needs antibiotic treatment. Your doctor may give you a prescription for an antibiotic, or your child can get a shot of long-acting penicillin in the ED. Both medicines will treat the infection. If you choose the antibiotic at home, you need to give your child all the medicine.

Your dose is:_____

Home Treatment

1. The antibiotic will not make your child feel better right away. It may take 2 to 3 days to see improvement. Watch for a rash; trouble breathing; or swelling of the face, hands, or feet as signs of an allergic reaction to the antibiotic.
2. Encourage your child to drink plenty of fluids such as juice, soda, and fruit drinks. Soft foods such as applesauce, pudding, and mashed potatoes may be less irritating to the throat.
3. Give acetaminophen (e.g., Tylenol®) or ibuprofen (e.g., Motrin®, Advil®) for fever. Your child's dose is: _____
_____
4. Salt water gargles (½ tsp salt in 1 cup warm water) may make an older child's sore throat feel better. Do not let your child swallow the salt water. Have him/her spit it out. Use over-the-counter medicine that soothes the throat in school-age children as recommended.
5. Your child may go back to school 24 hours after starting the antibiotic as long as he/she feels well and does not have a fever.

Call Your Doctor or Return to the Emergency Department If:

1. Your child has drooling or difficulty in swallowing.
2. Your child has a stiff neck.
3. Your child has trouble breathing.
4. Your child has a rash or swelling of the hands or feet.
5. Your child still has a fever 2 to 3 days after starting antibiotics.
6. You are unable to give your child the antibiotic.
7. Your child looks sick or you have any questions or concerns.

SPRAINS AND STRAINS

A *sprain* is an injury to the ligaments that hold your bones together. A *strain* is an injury to the muscle or muscle tendon from stretching or pulling.

Treatment

1. Keep the injured area quiet. If your doctor gave you a splint or crutches, have your child use these as instructed. If you

were given an elastic bandage, keep it on as much as possible to help with swelling.

2. Keep the injured area elevated as much as possible. Prop up an arm or leg with pillows.

3. Use an ice pack for the first 48 hours. Do not put the ice directly against the skin; wrap it in a towel first. Keep the ice on the area for 15 minutes every 3 hours while awake.

4. You may give your child ibuprofen (e.g., Motrin®, Advil®) for pain. Your dose is: _____

5. Follow-up with your doctor or with an orthopedic surgeon in _____ days.

Exercise

Follow your doctor's instructions for exercise. Sprains often improve faster when exercises are begun early. Moving the injured area in all directions without putting weight or stress on the area is a good start. (For an ankle sprain, your child can write the alphabet with his/her foot.) Do not advance your activity if you are having a lot of pain. Do not stop using crutches until you can walk normally without pain. Your instructions are: _____

Call Your Doctor or Return to the Emergency Department If:

1. Your child has increased redness or swelling at the injury site or worsening pain.

2. Your child gets a fever.

3. Your child has no feeling in the injured arm or leg or it feels cold.

4. Your child is not feeling better in 3 to 5 days or is not making steady progress in 3 to 5 days.

5. You have any questions or concerns.

STOMATITIS

Stomatitis is a viral infection that can cause sores or blisters on the gums, tongue, and other areas inside the mouth. Your child may have a fever, and the ulcers are painful. He/she may not want to eat or drink. Because this is a viral infection, it will usually clear up by itself within 5 days. However, some children may have sores in the mouth for 1 to 2 weeks.

To Keep Your Child Comfortable and Prevent Dehydration

1. Give acetaminophen (e.g., Tylenol®) or ibuprofen (e.g., Advil®, Motrin®) at the correct dosage for your child's age. This medicine will help with the pain and fever. Acetaminophen suppositories are available at your pharmacy without a prescription. Your dose is: _____.

2. Encourage cold or cool liquids. These may be soothing to the mouth and help numb the pain. Avoid citrus and carbonated drinks (e.g., orange and grapefruit juices, lemonade, soda). Soft foods such as applesauce, yogurt, or pudding may be less irritating to the mouth.

3. Avoid salty or spicy foods.

4. If your doctor has given you a mouthwash or other medication, use as directed.

_____

To Prevent Spread of This Infection

1. Wash your hands and your child's hands frequently and before eating.

2. Do not share your child's eating utensils or drinking cups while sick; wash after each use.

3. Wash any toys your child places in his/her mouth before and after your child plays with them.

Call Your Doctor or Return to the Emergency Department If:

1. Your child is repeatedly refusing to drink or cannot swallow.

2. Your child appears dehydrated (no urine output in the last 8 hours, no tears when crying, lips are dry or cracked).

3. You think your child looks worse than when you were initially seen in the ED.

4. Your child is not getting better after 1 week.

URINARY TRACT INFECTION

Your child has been diagnosed with a urinary tract infection. This is an infection of the bladder or kidneys. It can cause symptoms of fever, abdominal or back pain, vomiting, or burning with urination, or it may have no symptoms in small babies. The diagnosis is made by looking at a clean sample of urine under a microscope and then growing bacteria with a urine culture.

Treatment

1. Antibiotics are used to treat the infection. Your child's medicine is _____.
   Make sure to give all doses for the full course to completely get rid of the infection. Diarrhea can be a side effect of antibiotics, so do not stop them if this occurs. If your child does get a rash or severe diarrhea, call your doctor.

2. Encourage extra fluids by mouth to help clear the infection.

3. Allow your child to urinate as often as he/she desires, and encourage him/her not to "hold" the urine.

4. Follow-up is important to ensure the infection is cured.

Long-term Follow-up

Urinary tract infections can sometimes come back. Your doctor may want to follow your child more frequently and look at urine samples. Most children with a first time infection need to have their kidneys and bladder evaluated to ensure there is not a problem that led to the infection. Your doctor may schedule tests to look for this.

Tips for Prevention

1. Teach your child to wipe from front to back and then throw away the toilet paper.

2. Have girls wear cotton underwear. Synthetics can irritate the genital area and lead to infection.
3. Bubble baths, creams, or powders in the genital area may be irritating and lead to holding urine, causing an infection.
4. Encourage your child to drink plenty of fluids each day.
5. Encourage him/her to empty the bladder completely every 3 to 4 hours during the day and to urinate before bedtime.

Call Your Doctor or Return to the Emergency Department If:

1. Fever lasts longer than 2 days with antibiotic treatment or your child develops a fever while taking the antibiotic.
2. Your child stops urinating or the urine becomes bloody.
3. Your child gets worse.
4. Your child refuses to take the antibiotic.
5. Your child gets a rash or has severe diarrhea while taking the antibiotic.

VIRAL INFECTION

Your child is sick with a viral infection. This does not mean that there is nothing wrong with your child. Viruses are microbes that survive on living cells and cause many types of illnesses. There are many viruses, and we do not always know which one is causing your child's illness. We do know that antibiotics do not help treat viral infections and that overuse of antibiotics can make some harmful bacteria more difficult to treat. We do not give children with viral infections antibiotics because they will usually get better without them, and we want to keep levels of resistant bacteria low. Children with viral infections often have fever and body aches. You can help your child feel better by treating his/her symptoms. **Ask your doctor or nurse for fever instructions to take home.**

Treatment

Pain and Fever: Use acetaminophen (e.g., Tylenol®) or ibuprofen (e.g., Motrin®, Advil®) to ease body aches and treat fever. Your child's dose is:_____.

Fluids: Offer your child liquids to drink to keep him/her from getting dehydrated (dry). Children should urinate at least two to three times per day.

Other Instructions: _____

_____

_____

Follow-up: A typical viral infection may last 5 to 7 days. If your child is getting worse or not improving, particularly if vomiting persistently, you need to see a doctor.

Call Your Doctor or Return to the Emergency Department If:

1. Your child is irritable, and it is difficult to calm him/her down.
2. Your child is unable to take fluids or is weak, sleepy, or lethargic.
3. You think your child looks dry (eyes look sunken, soft spot is depressed, no tears when crying, mouth looks dry).
4. Your child has other symptoms—rash, trouble breathing, ear pain, headache, stiff neck, vomiting, diarrhea, joint swelling, or pain.
5. You think your child looks sick or is getting worse.
6. You have any questions or concerns.

VOMITING AND/OR DIARRHEA

Vomiting or diarrhea occurs when the lining of the stomach or intestines is irritated by an infection. Usually, the infection is a virus and needs to run its course, which may vary from 1 day to 1 week. The doctor who examined your child decided that you could treat this illness at home. To make your child feel better, he/she needs to rest the stomach and intestines and help prevent more vomiting and diarrhea. This can be done by giving your child clear liquids and foods that are easily digested and by avoiding spicy or greasy foods that can further irritate the gastrointestinal tract. The goal is to keep your child from becoming dehydrated (dry). Your child can return to school or day care when the diarrhea or vomiting have resolved and he/she is feeling better.

Follow the Instructions Below

For Babies 2 Months to 1 Year

1. Feed your baby an oral electrolyte solution (e.g., Pedialyte®, Infalyte®) until he/she has not vomited for 2 hours. If your baby vomits the electrolyte solution, then give small amounts at frequent intervals (e.g., ½ to 1 oz every 15 minutes for babies 5 to 10 kg or 11 to 22 lb).
2. **Do not give plain water.**
3. If your child is not vomiting, continue his/her regular diet. You may give extra oral electrolyte solution (e.g., Pedialyte®, Infalyte®) to keep your child from getting dehydrated. You can give your child food even if he/she has diarrhea.
4. If you are breast-feeding, continue breast-feeding on demand.
5. If you are formula feeding, restart formula when your child has not vomited for 2 hours. Continue formula even if your child has diarrhea. If the diarrhea is worse with formula, your baby may have trouble absorbing the formula. Call or see your child's doctor.
6. See your doctor or return to the ED if the vomiting and diarrhea continue. **Do not give your baby only Pedialyte® or Infalyte® for more than 24 hours.**

For Children Older Than 1 Year

1. Give your child clear liquids (ones you can see through) until the vomiting improves and allow the stomach to rest. Oral electrolyte solutions (e.g., Pedialyte®, Infalyte®) are best for your child with the right amount of sugar and salt. Use of these alone for more than 24 hours is NOT RECOMMENDED. Other clear liquids may have high amounts of sugar and can worsen diarrhea. Some children do not like the taste of the electrolyte solution. If your child will not drink the oral electrolyte solutions, other clear liquids may keep him/her from getting dry. Examples are flat soda (shake out the fizz), Kool-Aid®, Gatorade® diluted with an equal amount of water, Hawaiian Punch®, juices (not apple, orange, grapefruit), tea with sugar, Jell-O®, popsicles, water ice, sherbet, clear soups, or broth. DO NOT GIVE MILK. If your child vomits the clear liquids, try giving only small sips. Giving your child a straw may keep him/her from drinking large amounts.

2. If the vomiting improves, you may continue your child's regular diet. Soft, bland foods such as oatmeal, rice cereal, bananas, applesauce, dry toast, crackers, vanilla wafers, dry mashed potatoes, noodles, lean meats, vegetables, and fruits may be better. STAY AWAY FROM FRIED OR SPICY FOODS. You can give your child food even if he/she has diarrhea.

3. Resume milk if your child's stomach feels better and if vomiting and diarrhea are improving.

4. See your doctor if the vomiting and diarrhea continue. Do not give your child only clear liquids for more than 48 hours without calling your doctor.

Call Your Doctor or Return to the Emergency Department If:

1. The vomiting and diarrhea do not improve.
2. Your child is unable to take fluids or is weak, sleepy, or lethargic.
3. You think your child looks dry (eyes look sunken, soft spot is depressed, no tears when crying, mouth looks dry).
4. Your child has not urinated in 8 hours.
5. There is blood in the vomit or stool, brown flecks like coffee grounds in the vomit, or green vomiting.
6. Your child has abdominal pain.
7. Your child has a fever higher than 102°F (39°C).
8. You think your child looks sick or is getting worse.
9. You have any questions or concerns.

WOUND CARE

Your child has an injury in which the skin was broken. These injuries can be fixed in different ways, depending on the age of your child and the size and location of the injury. However, all such wounds heal with a scar. This scar will remodel itself within 12 months.

Stitches (Sutures) or Staples

[ ] Your child had _____ stitches or staples placed for an injury to his/her _____. These must be removed in _____ days. Call your doctor for an appointment to remove the stitches or return to the ED for removal.

[ ] The stitches do not need to be removed. They will come out by themselves. Follow-up with your regular doctor in _____ days.

[ ] Your child's wound should be rechecked in _____ days. Call your doctor for an appointment or return to the ED.

Washing with a washcloth or a quick shower is okay. Do not take a bath, soak the stitches/staples, or allow your child to swim with them. If the stitches should loosen or if the wound pops open, bring your child back to the ED. If the wound starts bleeding, apply direct pressure for 15 minutes. If it continues to bleed, call your doctor or return to the ED.

Apply an antibiotic ointment to the stitches _____ times per day.

Keep the area covered with a clean bandage.

No cover is necessary after the first 48 hours.

Apply sunscreen to wound area when outdoors to protect new skin.

[ ] Wound Adhesive

Your child had a special glue (Dermabond®) used to fix your child's wound. Keep clean and dry. Do not soak in water or allow your child to swim for the next 7 days. Allow the glue to peel off by itself (usually in 7 days).

[ ] Your child received a tetanus shot in the ED. Show this to your child's doctor to update their records.

[ ] Your doctor has given your child a prescription for antibiotics. Not all wounds need antibiotic treatment. Your child must take all the medicine as directed. Your dose is:

Signs of Infection

Call your doctor or return to the ED if any of these signs develop:

1. Increased redness around the wound
2. Pain
3. Discharge or pus from the wound
4. Increased swelling
5. Bad smell
6. Fever

APPENDIX E ■ CLINICAL PATHWAYS IN EMERGENCY MEDICINE

JANE M. LAVELLE, MD, AND CYNTHIA R. JACOBSTEIN, MD, MSE

The ability to provide effective, safe, and reliable bedside care for a wide range of presenting complaints in the emergency department (ED) is of the utmost importance. This task has become increasingly complex and challenging with the explosion of knowledge and technology. Incorporating education to physicians in training in a setting that demands efficient (reduction of unnecessary testing) and timely practice is an additional challenge. The ED clinical pathways were created to meet these competing goals. The availability of the intranet browser, the electronic medical record, and physician order entry were the catalysts needed to make the clinical pathways and order sets that are immediately available to bedside clinicians a reality. We believe that use of these pathways reduces variability of bedside care, error, unnecessary testing and treatment, as well as reducing length of stay and cost. We and others believe that use of these pathways/guidelines helps us standardize the care for the large majority of patients with common and important conditions and leaves the ED team more effective time to provide medical decision making for complex and higher risk patients. To date, the Children's Hospital of Philadelphia Emergency Department has developed 22 clinical pathways for a variety of common and uncommon chief complaints. We have provided five of these in this chapter: asthma, bronchiolitis, dehydration, diabetic ketoacidosis, and suspected appendicitis.

The clinical decision-making algorithms are based on current evidence in the medical literature as well as expert consensus from providers within our institution. Multidisciplinary teams work together to review literature and create the algorithm for critical clinical decision making as well as for the necessary processes to execute the care. For example, the appendicitis pathway was created by physicians and nurses from radiology, general surgery, and the emergency department. Each pathway contains certain standard elements. These include triage parameters, a clinical decision-making algorithm, key components of physician and nursing assessment, nursing bedside procedure, educational PowerPoint presentations for nurses and physicians, and links to key articles and useful websites. Each pathway is also accompanied by computerized order sets specific to each complaint, which can assist in decision support to follow the pathway/guideline. When a patient presents with a complaint for which a pathway exists, a brief discussion between the bedside nurse and physician allows care, including IV placement, lab draws, and other initial care to begin as early in the ED visit as possible.

We have made these pathways available on our intranet site, so they are readily accessible to all bedside providers. We have reproduced the clinical algorithm here. The underlined text represents a hyperlink on our internet website, which is represented in table form here.

We intend to link each pathway to a quality metrics allowing the bedside team of providers to receive feedback to improve clinical decision making as well as to identify system issues that need to be addressed. These pathways are currently being used for nursing and physician education. We eventually hope to include these as part of the resident curriculum during their ED rotations.

ED Guidelines for Evaluation/Treatment of Children with Asthma

JOSEPH ZORC, M.D., JANE LAVELLE, M.D.

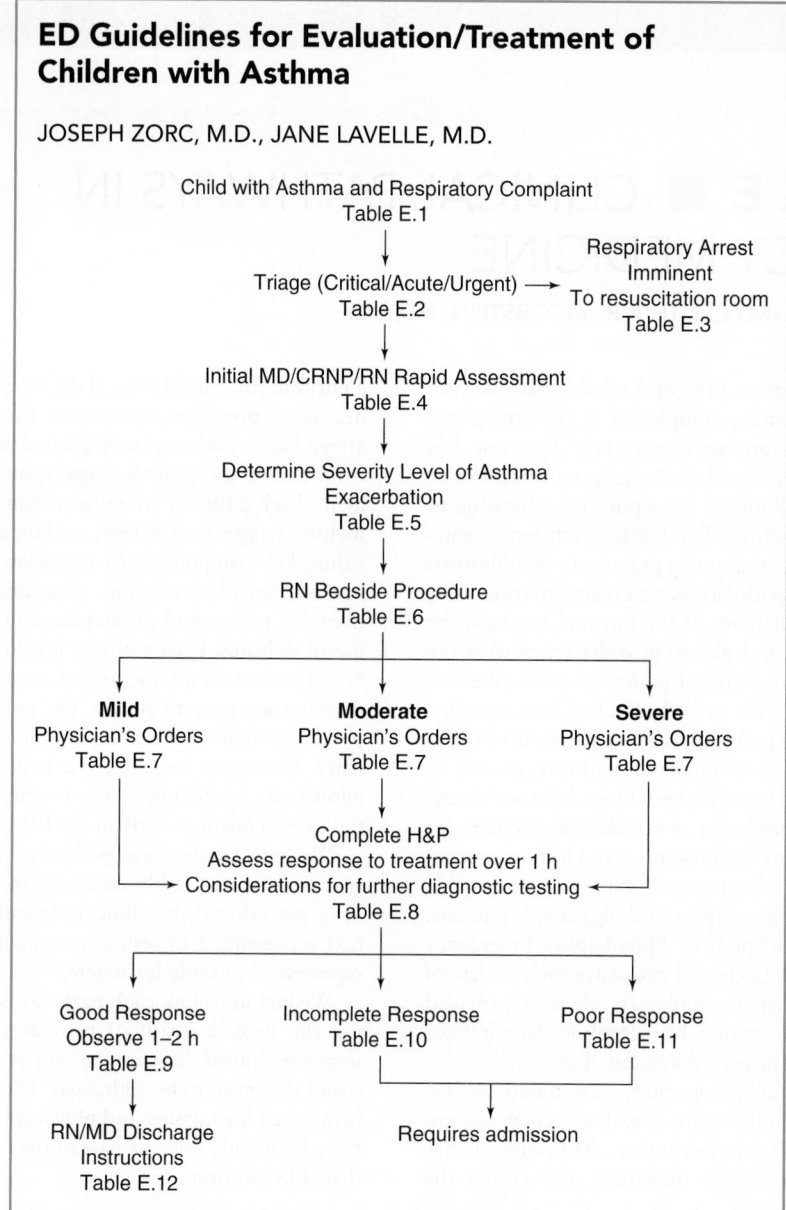

Child with Asthma and Respiratory Complaint
Table E.1

↓

Triage (Critical/Acute/Urgent) ⟶ Respiratory Arrest Imminent
Table E.2   To resuscitation room
                                       Table E.3

↓

Initial MD/CRNP/RN Rapid Assessment
Table E.4

↓

Determine Severity Level of Asthma
Exacerbation
Table E.5

↓

RN Bedside Procedure
Table E.6

Mild   **Moderate**   **Severe**
Physician's Orders   Physician's Orders   Physician's Orders
Table E.7   Table E.7   Table E.7

Complete H&P
Assess response to treatment over 1 h
Considerations for further diagnostic testing
Table E.8

Good Response   Incomplete Response   Poor Response
Observe 1–2 h   Table E.10   Table E.11
Table E.9

RN/MD Discharge
Instructions   Requires admission
Table E.12

TABLE E.1

CHILD WITH ASTHMA AND RESPIRATORY COMPLAINT

Asthma definition for pathway:
- Acute trouble breathing/wheezing
- Age >12 mo, and
- Prior diagnosis of asthma or history of two significant wheezing episodes

TABLE E.2

TRIAGE (CRITICAL/ACUTE/URGENT)

Respiratory distress		
Critical	**Acute**	**Urgent**

■ Severe wheezing with:
  Severe tachypnea
  Bradypnea/apnea
  Severe retractions
  Nasal flaring
  Grunting respirations
  Decreased muscle tone
  Lethargy
■ Absent breath sounds
■ Agonal respirations
■ Pulse oximetry <92%
	■ Wheezing with moderate:
	  Increased work of breathing
	  (WOB)
	  Tachypnea
	  Retractions
	  Intermittent grunt
	■ Decreased aeration with
	  moderate tachypnea and
	  WOB
	■ Pulse oximetry <95%
		■ Wheezing with mild:
		  Increased WOB
		  Tachypnea
		  Mild retractions
		■ Pulse oximetry ≥95%

Guide to rates of breathing in awake children	
Age	**Normal rate (in min)**
<2 mo	<60
2–12 mo	<50
1–5 yr	<40
6–8 yr	<30

TABLE E.3

RESPIRATORY ARREST IMMINENT

■ Drowsy, confused
■ Paradoxical breathing, absence of wheeze
■ Bradycardia

Impending Respiratory Failure
■ ABCs
■ Consider IM epinephrine (1:1,000) 0.01 mL/kg (maximum 0.5 mL)
■ Methylprednisolone (Solumedrol®) 2 mg/kg IV (maximum 60 mg)
■ Albuterol nebs × 3 plus Ipratropium

Albuterol weight-based dosing		
Weight (kg)	**Unit dose (0.5%)**	**Continuous**
<5	1.25 mg (0.25 mL)	5 mg/h (1 mL/h)
5–10	2.5 mg (0.5 mL)	10 mg/h (2 mL/h)
10–20	3.75 mg (0.75 mL)	15 mg/h (3 mL/h)
>20	5 mg (1.0 mL)	20 mg/h (4 mL/h)

Ipratroprium weight-based dosing	
5–10	250 μg q20min × 3
>10	500 μg q20min × 3

■ IV magnesium sulfate 50 mg/kg, maximum 2 g
■ IV terbutaline
  Bolus: 2–10 μg/kg
  Infusion: 0.08–0.4 μg/kg/min (maximum 6 μg/kg/min)
■ Heliox (consult critical care medicine)
■ Rapid sequence intubation
  Atropine 0.01 mg/kg IV, maximum 1 mg
  Midazolam 0.05 mg/kg IV, maximum 2 mg
  Ketamine 1–3 mg/kg IV
  Vecuronium 0.2 mg/kg IV

TABLE E.4

INITIAL MD/CRNP/RN RAPID ASSESSMENT

General
■ Reassess VS, pulse and perfusion
■ General appearance
■ Respiratory status—rate, work of breathing (WOB), and air entry

Brief History
■ Onset of symptoms
■ Use of bronchodilators
■ Chronic asthma medications
■ Symptoms of infectious disease

TABLE E.6

RN BEDSIDE PROCEDURE

■ Obtain and administer PO prednisone/prednisolone as soon as ordered
■ Identify if:
   Family has an asthma care plan for flares
   Child uses a controller medication
   Child has a source for follow-up care

TABLE E.5

DETERMINE SEVERITY LEVEL OF ASTHMA EXACERBATION

Mild	Moderate	Severe
Pulse oximetry >95%	Pulse oximetry 90–95%	Pulse oximetry <90%
Mild tachypnea	Moderate tachypnea	Severe tachypnea
Normal mental status	Mildly anxious	Anxious
Minimal ↑ WOB	Moderate ↑ WOB	Severe ↑ WOB
Good aeration	Fair–good aeration	Poor aeration
End expiratory wheeze	Loud expiratory wheeze	Inspiratory, expiratory wheezing, or no wheezing
PEF ≥70%	PEF 40–69%	PEF <40%

Guide to rates of breathing in awake children

Age	Normal rate (min)
<2 mo	<60
2–12 mo	<50
1–5 yr	<40
6–8 yr	<30

TABLE E.7

PHYSICIAN'S ORDERS FOR MILD/MODERATE/SEVERE ASTHMA

Options:
■ Albuterol puffs × 3 with MDI spacer are the preferred treatment for patients with mild wheezing
■ Albuterol nebs × 3 (plus Ipratropium)
   Consider IM epinephrine (1:1000) 0.01 mL/kg (maximum 0.5 mL)
   See Table E.3 for further therapy for severe asthma

Albuterol weight-based dosing

Weight (kg)	Unit dose (0.5%)	MDI puffs	Continuous
<5	1.25 mg (0.25 mL)	2	5 mg/h (1 mL/h)
5–10	2.5 mg (0.5 mL)	4	10 mg/h (2 mL/h)
10–20	3.75 mg (0.75 mL)	6	15 mg/h (3 mL/h)
>20	5 mg (1.0 mL)	8	20 mg/h (4 mL/h)

Ipratroprium weight-based dosing

5–10	250 μg q20min × 3
>10	500 μg q20min × 3

Prednisone/Prednisolone—Administer 2 mg/kg PO (maximum of 60 mg) for moderate/severe or mild with incomplete response

TABLE E.8

COMPLETE HISTORY AND PHYSICAL

History
- Duration of symptoms
- Presence of infectious disease or allergic symptoms
- Home therapy
- Most recent oral steroid use
- Prior ED visits/hospitalizations, particularly in the last year
- Prior ICU admissions, intubations
- Chronic lung or heart disease, immunodeficiency
- Asthma management doctor

Physical Exam
- Vital signs, mental status, pulse oximetry
- Consider peak expiratory flow (PEF) in children ≥6 yr following initial β-agonist therapy
- WOB, wheezing, aeration

Further Diagnostic Testing
Consider chest x-ray:
- Persistent asymmetry
- Persistent pulse oximetry <90%
- Prolonged fever
- ICU admission

TABLE E.9

GOOD RESPONSE

Patient has **mild** symptoms:
  Pulse oximetry >95%
  Mild tachypnea
  Normal mental status
  Minimal ↑ WOB
  Good aeration
  End expiratory wheeze
  PEF >80%

- Observe minimum of 30 min if only single nebulization given
- Observe 1–2 h following albuterol nebulization ×3

TABLE E.10

INCOMPLETE RESPONSE

Patient continues with **moderate** symptoms:
  Pulse oximetry 90–94%
  Moderate tachypnea
  Mildly anxious
  Moderate ↑ WOB
  Fair–good aeration
  Loud expiratory wheeze
  PEF 40–70%

- Continue q2h albuterol nebulizations (weight-based)
- Consider continuous albuterol nebulization
- Assess need for additional therapies (see poor response)

TABLE E.11

POOR RESPONSE

Patient continues with severe symptoms:
  Pulse oximetry <90%
  Severe tachypnea
  Anxious
  Severe ↑ WOB
  Poor aeration
  Inspiratory, expiratory wheezing

- Place IV, send basic metabolic panel
- Continuous albuterol nebulization
- IV magnesium sulfate 50 mg/kg, maximum of 2 g
- IV terbutaline
  Bolus infusion 2–10 μg/kg
  Infusion 0.08–0.4 μg/kg/min (maximum 6 μg/kg/min)

TABLE E.12

RN/MD DISCHARGE INSTRUCTIONS

At Discharge from ED
1. ED discharge instructions, review asthma recovery plan
2. Prescribe oral steroids for 4 days if indicated
3. Review dosing of medications at discharge
4. Review home medications
5. Review need for follow-up with a primary care provider within 3–5 days
6. Review signs that would require a return to the ED

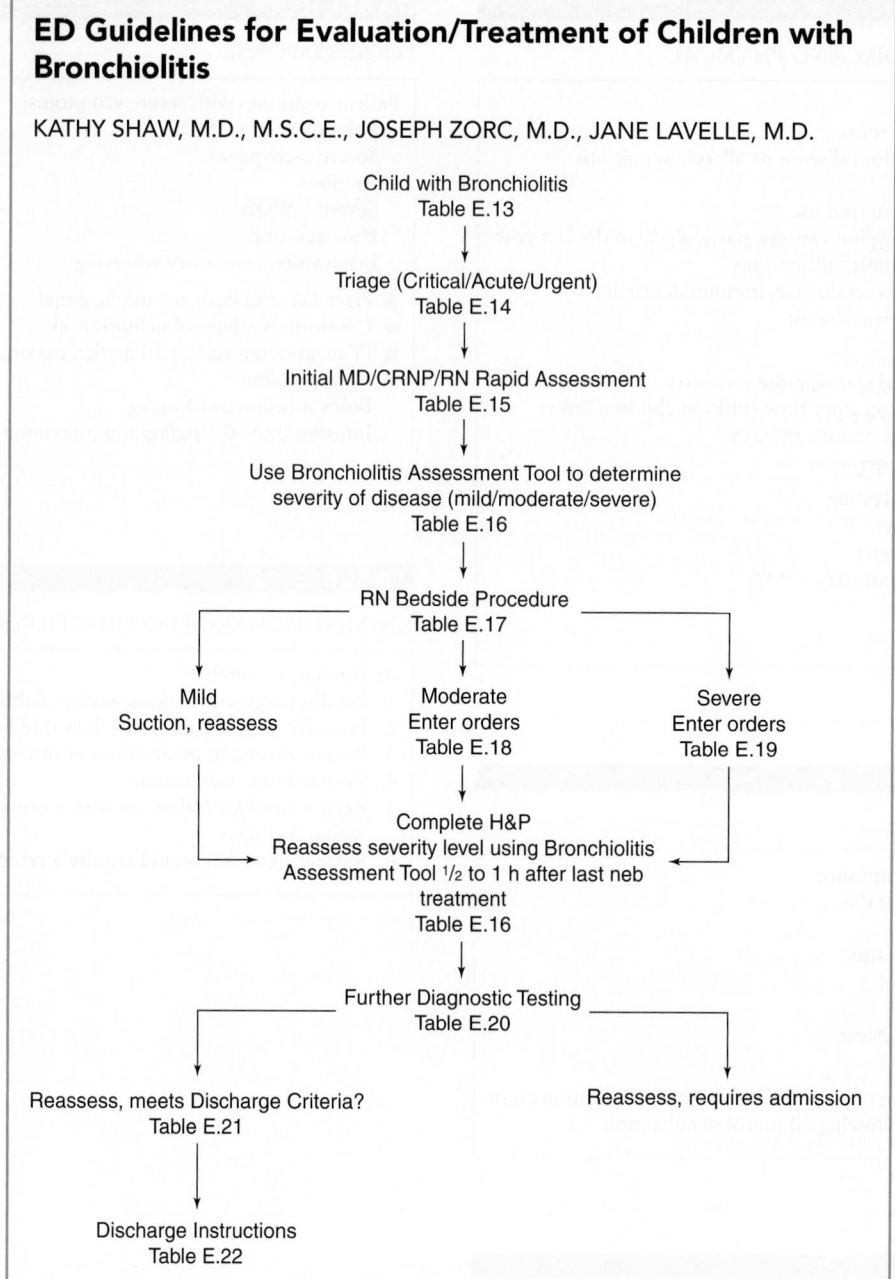

ED Guidelines for Evaluation/Treatment of Children with Bronchiolitis

KATHY SHAW, M.D., M.S.C.E., JOSEPH ZORC, M.D., JANE LAVELLE, M.D.

Child with Bronchiolitis
Table E.13

Triage (Critical/Acute/Urgent)
Table E.14

Initial MD/CRNP/RN Rapid Assessment
Table E.15

Use Bronchiolitis Assessment Tool to determine
severity of disease (mild/moderate/severe)
Table E.16

RN Bedside Procedure
Table E.17

Mild
Suction, reassess

Moderate
Enter orders
Table E.18

Severe
Enter orders
Table E.19

Complete H&P
Reassess severity level using Bronchiolitis
Assessment Tool ½ to 1 h after last neb
treatment
Table E.16

Further Diagnostic Testing
Table E.20

Reassess, meets Discharge Criteria?
Table E.21

Reassess, requires admission

Discharge Instructions
Table E.22

TABLE E.13

CHILD WITH BRONCHIOLITIS

Bronchiolitis definition for pathway
  Previous healthy infant
  <12 mo of age with URI symptoms and wheezing

TABLE E.14

TRIAGE (CRITICAL/ACUTE/URGENT)

Respiratory distress		
Critical	Acute	Urgent

■ Agonal respirations
  Severe wheezing with:
  Severe tachypnea (RR ≥80)
  Bradypnea/apnea
  Severe retractions
  Nasal flaring
  Grunting respirations
  Absent breath sounds
■ Decreased muscle tone or
  Lethargy
■ Pulse oximetry <90%
	■ Wheezing with moderate:
	  Increased work of breathing
	  (WOB)
	  Tachypnea (RR ≥70)
	  Retractions
	  Intermittent grunting
	■ Decreased aeration with
	  moderate tachypnea and
	  WOB
	■ Pulse oximetry <95%
		■ Wheezing with mild:
		  Increased WOB
		  Tachypnea
		  Mild retractions
		■ Pulse oximetry >95%

Guide to rates of breathing in awake children	
Age	Normal rate (per min)
Newborn	<65
<2 mo	<60
2–6 mo	<55
7–12 mo	<50

TABLE E.15

MD/CRNP/RN RAPID ASSESSMENT

History of Illness
■ Preceding upper respiratory illness and/or rhinorrhea
■ Symptoms, when they began, presence of fever
■ History of apnea?
■ Ability to maintain hydration
■ Infectious exposures
■ Medications received
■ Identify high risk factors:
  History of prematurity, gestational age <34 wk
  Receiving Synagis™ treatments
  Heart disease
  Lung disease
  Immunodeficiency
■ Allergies

Physical Exam
■ Overall appearance
■ Vital signs, pulse oximetry reading
■ Mental status
■ Respiratory status
  Work of breathing
  Flaring
  Grunting
  Breath sounds
  Wheezing
  Crackles

TABLE E.16

BRONCHIOLITIS ASSESSMENT TOOL

Respiratory assessment	Mild	Moderate	Severe
Pulse ox in room air	≥95%	91–94%	≤90%
Respiratory rate	<60	60–70	>70
Mental status	Normal	Irritable but active	Lethargic
Feeding	Normal	Less but adequate	Poor
Increased WOB			
Retractions	Minimal/None	Intercostal	Substernal
Accessory muscles			Neck or abdominal muscles
Wheeze	Minimal/none	Moderate expiratory	Severe inspiratory/expiratory
Air exchange	Good, equal BS	Localized decreased BS	Multiple areas decreased

Classification of severity by using assessment tool	
Single Severity	
Mild	≥5 factors in the mild category
Moderate	≥5 factors in the moderate category
Severe	≥5 factors in the severe category
Mixed Severity	
Mild/moderate	Majority of factors are in mild and moderate categories
Moderate/severe	Majority of factors are in moderate and severe categories

Measuring response to albuterol/racemic epi using the assessment tool
Improvement noted in at least 3 of 7 categories

TABLE E.17

RN BEDSIDE PROCEDURE

1. Suction nasopharynx/oropharynx
2. Obtain pulse oximetry reading
3. Administer oxygen for SaO_2 < 90% and consider for consistently 91–94%
4. Babies in the severe category should have continuous pulse oximetry and CR monitoring
5. Obtain physician's respiratory orders for treatment, as needed
6. Assess hydration:
   a. Infants with mild/moderate distress, offer Pedialyte™
   b. Infants with severe distress, assess need for IV fluids, maintain NPO status
7. Obtain order for IV, laboratory studies for infants <2 mo with a temperature >38.2°C
8. Document vital signs, pulse oximetry every hour in moderate and severe categories

TABLE E.18

IMMEDIATE PHYSICIAN'S ORDERS FOR MODERATE BRONCHIOLITIS

Albuterol trial × 1 treatment, MDI with spacer is the preferred method of delivery
Pulse oximetry prior to each nebulization treatment
Administer steroids if 2 prior episodes of wheezing
Consider racemic epinephrine treatment for moderate/severe patients

Albuterol weight-based dosing

Weight (kg)	Unit dose (0.5%)[a]	MDI puffs (90 µg)	Continuous
<5	1.25 mg (0.25 mL)	2	5 mg/h
5–10	2.5 mg (0.5 mL)	2	10 mg/h

Single dose: 0.083%—1.5 mL <5 kg, 3 mL >5 kg
Racemic Epi (1% solution) with NS to volume of 2.5 mL

<5 kg	0.25 mL	
5–10 kg	0.5 mL	

OR

L-epinephrine (1:1,000)

<5 kg	1.25 mL	
5–10 kg	2.5 mL	

[a]Dilute with 2 mL NS.

TABLE E.19

IMMEDIATE PHYSICIAN'S ORDERS FOR SEVERE BRONCHIOLITIS

Continuous pulse oximetry and CR monitor
Albuterol trial × 2
Consider racemic epinephrine treatment
Administer steroids if any prior episode of wheezing

Albuterol weight-based dosing

Weight (kg)	Unit dose (0.5%)[a]	MDI puffs (90 µg)	Continuous
<5	1.25 mg (0.25 mL)	2	5 mg/h
5–10	2.5 mg (0.5 mL)	2	10 mg/h

Single dose: 0.083%–1.5 mL <5 kg, 3 mL >5 kg
Racemic Epi (1% solution) in 2 mL NS

<5 kg	0.25 mL	
5–10 kg	0.5 mL	

OR

L-epinephrine (1:1,000)

<5 kg	1.25 mL	
5–10 kg	2.5 mL	

[a]Dilute with 2 mL NS

TABLE E.20

FURTHER DIAGNOSTIC TESTING

Chest x-ray
Obtain chest x-ray on infants with:
  Age <2–3 mo
  Persistent fever beyond third day of illness
  Severe disease
  Signs, symptoms concerning for another diagnosis
  High risk factors
  – Heart disease
  – Lung disease
  – Immunodeficiency
Routine radiographs are not indicated in babies with mild/moderate disease

Viral Antigen Testing
RSV or other viral antigen testing **ONLY** for patients requiring admission for cohorting for infection control.

Other Laboratory Studies
Consider work up for serious bacterial illness in infants <2 mo presenting with fever >38.2°C or who appear ill out of proportion to bronchiolitis.
Electrolytes, bedside glucose testing in patients with significant dehydration

TABLE E.21

DISCHARGE CRITERIA (MUST MEET ALL CRITERIA)

1. Patient severity score
   ■ Mild severity score
   ■ Mild to moderate severity score
     i. Not in first 1–2 days of illness
     ii. Absence of high-risk factors
       – History of prematurity, gestational age <34 wk
       – Receiving Synagis™ treatments
       – History of apnea
       – Heart disease
       – Lung disease
       – Immunodeficiency
2. Patient is able to maintain hydration at home
3. Caregivers able to assess infant and understand care and follow-up instructions
4. MD follow-up is recommended within 24 h for:
   ■ All infants presenting in the first 2 days of illness
   ■ All infants with moderate severity of illness

TABLE E.22

RN/MD DISCHARGE INSTRUCTIONS

1. If patient had a good response to β-agonists, discharge home with:
   ■ MDI and spacer: requires practice with patient, family in ED.
   ■ Respiratory therapist should review use of the above with the family
2. Use bronchiolitis discharge instructions
3. Focus instructions on:
   ■ Use of saline nose drops, humidifier
   ■ Tylenol for analgesia and fever
   ■ Signs of inadequate hydration
   ■ Signs of respiratory distress
   ■ When to return to the ED
   ■ When follow-up is required

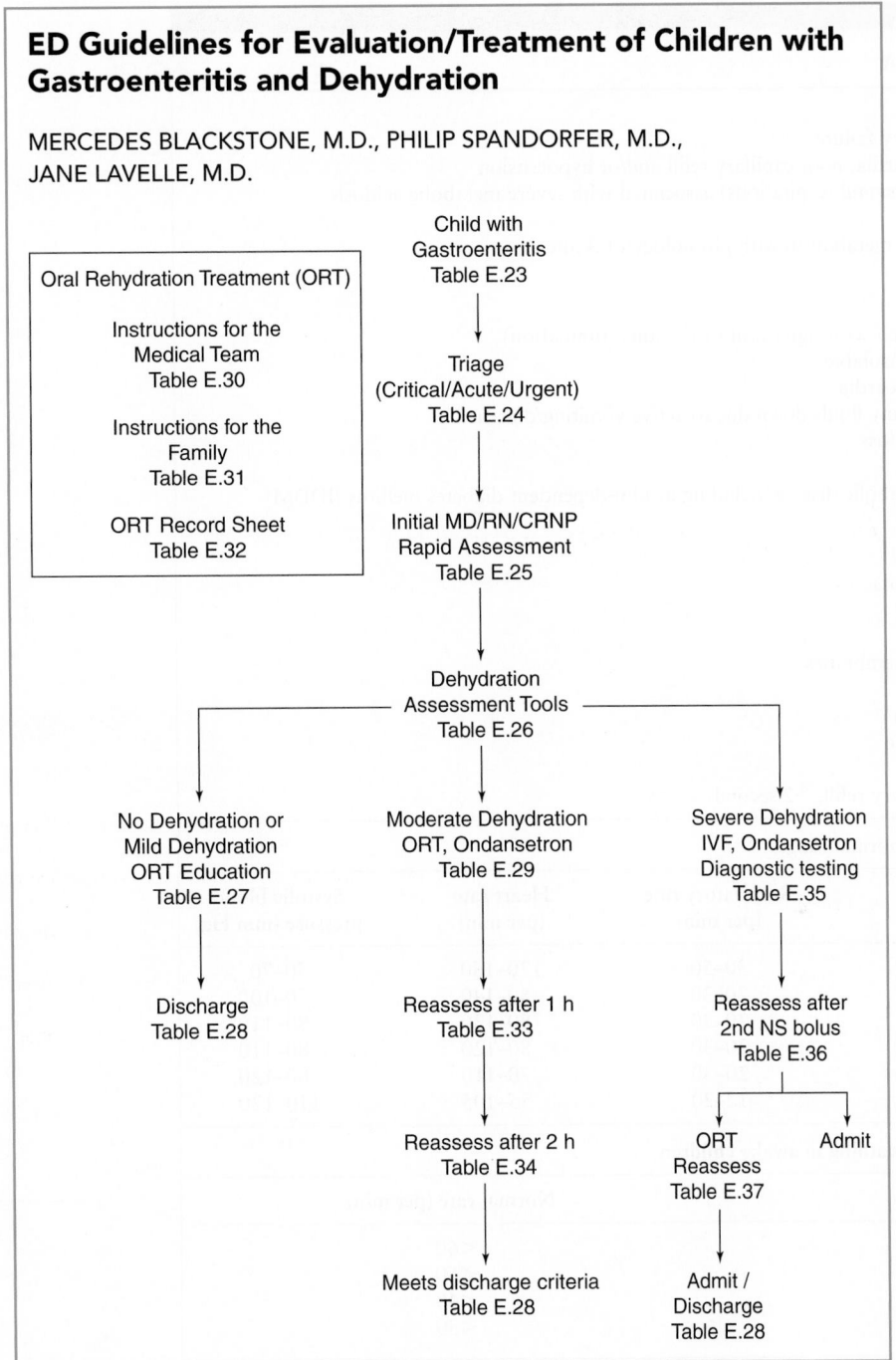

ED Guidelines for Evaluation/Treatment of Children with Gastroenteritis and Dehydration

MERCEDES BLACKSTONE, M.D., PHILIP SPANDORFER, M.D., JANE LAVELLE, M.D.

Child with
Gastroenteritis
Table E.23

Oral Rehydration Treatment (ORT)

Instructions for the
Medical Team
Table E.30

Instructions for the
Family
Table E.31

ORT Record Sheet
Table E.32

Triage
(Critical/Acute/Urgent)
Table E.24

Initial MD/RN/CRNP
Rapid Assessment
Table E.25

Dehydration
Assessment Tools
Table E.26

No Dehydration or
Mild Dehydration
ORT Education
Table E.27

Moderate Dehydration
ORT, Ondansetron
Table E.29

Severe Dehydration
IVF, Ondansetron
Diagnostic testing
Table E.35

Discharge
Table E.28

Reassess after 1 h
Table E.33

Reassess after
2nd NS bolus
Table E.36

Reassess after 2 h
Table E.34

ORT
Reassess
Table E.37

Admit

Meets discharge criteria
Table E.28

Admit /
Discharge
Table E.28

TABLE E.23

CHILD WITH GASTROENTERITIS

This pathway is to be used for the treatment of children with gastroenteritis and associated dehydration. It is important to assess the child for surgical, neurologic, and metabolic conditions before using this treatment pathway. Oral rehydration therapy (ORT) may also be used for other causes of dehydration, e.g., fever, pharyngitis, stomatitis.

Children who have vomiting or diarrhea but who are not dehydrated or have only mild dehydration, do not need to be rehydrated in the ED. These patients and families will benefit from education about use of ORT at home.

TABLE E.24

TRIAGE CRITERIA

Critical
- Cardiopulmonary failure
- Extreme tachycardia, poor capillary refill and/or hypotension
- Hyperpnea (Kussmaul respirations) associated with severe metabolic acidosis
- Unresponsive
- Inborn errors of metabolism with physiology of **Acute**

Acute
- Ill-appearing
- Lethargic (awaken with significant or noxious stimulation)
- Irritable or inconsolable
- Significant tachycardia
- Unable to keep any fluids down due to active vomiting/diarrhea
- 10–15% weight loss
- Abdominal pain
- Pre-existing metabolic disease including insulin-dependent diabetes mellitus (IDDM)

Urgent
- Listless
- 5–10% weight loss
- Any two:
  Oliguria
  Tacky mucous membranes
  Absent tears`
  Mild tachycardia
  Sunken fontanelle
  Sunken eyes
  Prolonged capillary refill, >2 second

Pediatric vital sign normal ranges

Age group	Respiratory rate (per min)	Heart rate (per min)	Systolic blood pressure (mm Hg)
Newborn	30–50	120–160	50–70
Infant (1–12 mo)	20–30	80–140	70–100
Toddler (1–3 yr)	20–30	80–130	80–110
Preschooler (3–5 yr)	20–30	80–120	80–110
School Age (6–12 yr)	20–30	70–110	80–120
Adolescent (13+ yr)	12–20	55–105	110–120

Guide to rates of breathing in awake children

Age	Normal rate (per min)
<2 mo	<60
2–12 mo	<50
1–5 yr	<40
6–8 yr	<30

TABLE E.25

INITIAL MD/RN/CRNP RAPID ASSESSMENT

Goal
- Rapidly assess degree of dehydration
- Identify patients who have other underlying cause for their symptoms (surgical, metabolic or CNS Disease)

History

Onset of symptoms, presence of fever	
Emesis	How many, last time, bilious/bloody, worse in the AM
Diarrhea	How many, last time, blood/mucous
Intake	Type and amount of fluid given
Urination	How many times, last time, color/odor
Exposure	Ill-contacts, new foods, farm animals, foreign travel
Pain	Location, quality, radiation, duration
Preillness weight	Compare current weight with recent previous weight, weight loss is a sensitive indicator of dehydration
Identify high-risk factors:	Underlying medical problem, such as cardiac, GI, renal, metabolic, endocrine (diabetes), immunodeficiency, history of abdominal surgery

Physical Exam
- General appearance, VS, Weight
- Mental status (lethargic, listless, decreased activity)
- Respiratory status: tachypnea, hyperpnea (Kussmaul respirations)
- Abdominal tenderness, rebound, or guarding; sunken or distended?
- Concerns for increased ICP (focal neurologic exam, papilledema)

Signs of Dehydration
- Tachycardia, tachypnea, capillary refill >2 seconds
- Absence of tears
- Sunken fontanelle, sunken eyes, tenting, sunken abdomen
- Dry mucous membranes
- Poor skin turgor

Gorelick MH, Shaw KN, Murphy KO. Validity and reliability of clinical signs in the diagnosis of dehydration in children. *Pediatrics* 1997;99(5):e6.

TABLE E.26

DEHYDRATION ASSESSMENT TOOLS

10 Point Dehydration Assessment Tool
- Ill-appearance
- Tachycardia (HR >150/min)
- Abnormal respirations
- Sunken eyes
- Absent tears
- Dry mucous membranes
- Abnormal radial pulse
- Capillary refill >2 seconds
- Decreased skin elasticity
- Decreased urine output

4 Point Dehydration Assessment Tool
- Ill-appearance
- Dry mucous membranes
- Absent tears
- Capillary refill >2 seconds

10 Point score			4 Point score		
# Features present	Degree of dehydration	% Fluid deficit	# Features present	Degree of dehydration	% Fluid deficit
<3	Mild	<5	1	Mild	<5
≥3 and <7	Moderate	5–10	2	Moderate	5–10
≥7	Severe	>10	3–4	Severe	>10

Gorelick MH, Shaw KN, Murphy KO. Validity and reliability of clinical signs in the diagnosis of dehydration in children. *Pediatrics* 1997;99(5):e6.

TABLE E.27

NO DEHYDRATION OR MILD DEHYDRATION

RN Bedside Care
■ Initial weight, VS
■ Antipyretics as appropriate
■ Education:
 a. Give specific written and verbal instructions on use of ORT
 b. Provide oral syringes and/or medicine cup for home use
 c. Give clear instructions for follow-up should condition change

TABLE E.28

DISCHARGE

Discharge Criteria
■ Clinical signs of dehydration are absent, mild or have resolved
■ Caregivers understand how to give ORT and can continue to do so at home
■ Caregivers understand discharge instructions and know what to look for

Discharge Instructions
Print out gastroenteritis/dehydration instructions with emphasis on the facts that:
■ Oral rehydration solution alone replaces fluid but won't stop the diarrhea
■ Breastfeeding should be continued through the illness
■ Start appropriate diet once the patient is rehydrated (and preferably early)
 ■ Complex carbohydrates, fresh fruits, vegetables, lean meats, yogurt
 ■ Full-strength formula
■ Avoid antidiarrheal medications
■ Antipyretics as usual

TABLE E.29

MODERATE DEHYDRATION (5–10% DEHYDRATION)

RN Bedside Care
■ Initial weight, VS
■ Antipyretics as appropriate
■ Monitor and document I/O's, urine-specific gravity, and dip with first void
■ Initiate ORT, refer to:
 ■ Instructions for the Medical Team
 ■ Instructions for the Family
 ■ ORT Record Sheet—to print instructions, open link, then right click and select print
 ■ Teach the family to document on the I/O Worksheet
 ■ Enter I/O in EHR

Ondansetron (Oral)
Consider using for patients with:
■ Persistent emesis
■ Severe nausea

Patient weight (kg)	Oral dose of ondansetron (mg)
8–15	2
>15–30	4
>30	8
Less than 6 mo or 8 kg, off label use, review with pharmacy/attending staff	

TABLE E.30

ORT INSTRUCTIONS FOR THE MEDICAL TEAM

ORT works via the sodium glucose cotransport mechanism, which optimizes intestinal absorption of water. Utilizing the correct electrolyte solution is critical for its success. Adding juice to the solutions alters the sodium to glucose concentration and diminishes the efficacy of ORT.

Appropriate Solutions
- Pedialyte
- Gatorade ½ strength with saltine crackers in older patients

Total Volume to be Given over 3–4 h

Mild/moderate dehydration	5–10% dehydration	50 mL/kg
Moderate/severe dehydration	>10% dehydration	100 mL/kg

Ongoing Losses

- 5–10 mL/kg for each diarrheal stool
- 2 mL/kg for each emesis

Aliquot Volume to be given every 5 min

Mild/moderate dehydration	1 mL/kg
Moderate/severe dehydration	2 mL/kg

Double the aliquot volume as tolerated after the first 30 min
Maximum aliquot volume is 30 mL

TABLE E.31

ORAL REHYDRATION THERAPY INSTRUCTIONS FOR FAMILIES

- ORT is a treatment we use for dehydrated patients.
- A small amount of liquid (1–2 mL/kg of the child's body weight is administered every 5 min with a syringe or small cup over 3–4 h. To treat your child today, we will start with _____mL every 5 min.
- Pedialyte is the best fluid choice for young children. Older children may refuse this, so ½ strength Gatorade with saltine crackers is substituted. These fluids have the most favorable ratio of glucose and sodium, which helps the intestines to reabsorb water.
- Although your child may want more, it is important to give the fluid slowly. This allows the stomach to absorb the liquid and helps prevent vomiting. Please watch the clock and give only the recommended amount every 5 min.
- Your child may refuse the fluid initially, but with a few feeds it often gets much easier and the child begins to take the fluids.
- If your child vomits, let your nurse know. If it is only a small amount, we will continue ORT. If it is a large amount, we may need to stop and place an IV.
- If your child repeatedly refuses the feeds or is passing frequent, large-volume stools, we may need to place an IV.

TABLE E.32

HOME ORAL REHYDRATION THERAPY RECORD SHEET

Pre-weight:_____
Post-weight:_____

Time	Amount of fluid taken (mL)	Emesis (# times)	Diarrhea (# times)

TABLE E.33

REASSESS AFTER 1 HOUR

RN Bedside Care
■ Repeat VS
■ Antipyretics as appropriate
■ Assess I/O's and Urine Specific Gravity (USG)
■ Repeat Dehydration Assessment Tools

ORT Success
■ After 30–60 min, double aliquot volume if patient is doing well

ORT Failure
■ Patient has received less than half of hourly requirement
■ Patient repeatedly refusing ORT
■ Persistent emesis, significant ongoing losses from diarrhea (see "Severe Dehydration" for IVF recommendations)

TABLE E.34

REASSESS AFTER 2 HOURS

RN Bedside Care
■ Repeat VS
■ Antipyretics as appropriate
■ Assess I/O's and USG
■ Repeat Dehydration Assessment Tools

ORT Success
■ Prepare patient and family for discharge

ORT Failure
■ Patient has received less than half of hourly requirement
■ Patient repeatedly refusing ORT
■ Persistent emesis, significant ongoing losses from diarrhea (see "Severe Dehydration" for IVF recommendations)

TABLE E.35

SEVERE DEHYDRATION

MD/RN Bedside Care
General
Initial weight, VS
Antipyretics as appropriate
Monitor and document I/O's, urine-specific gravity, and dip
  with first void

Place IV
Bedside glucose, alert MD immediately if result <70 mg/dL
D_{10} bolus when indicated, repeat glucose in 30 min
Dextrose 10%—0.25–0.5 g/kg OR 2.5–5 mL/kg
Serum electrolytes for all patients
Consider other labs as indicated for individual patients

IVF
NS 20 mL/kg over 15–30 min
Reassess with Dehydration Assessment Tool
Repeat NS 20 mL/kg as needed

Ondansetron (Oral or IV)
Consider using for patients with:
Persistent emesis
Severe nausea

Patient weight (kg)	Oral dose of ondansetron (mg)
8-15	2
>15–30	4
>30	8
(Less than 6 mo or 8 kg consultation regarding usage)	

Recommended IV dose for Ondansetron is 0.15 mg/kg,
maximum dose 8 mg
Further Diagnostic Testing
■ Consider need for urinalysis, urine culture
■ Stool for bacterial culture and *Clostridium difficile*
Bloody, mucous stools
Diarrhea >7–10 days

ORT
■ Initiate when patient is able
  Refer to ORT Box
  To print instructions, open link, then right click and select
  print
  Teach the family to document on the I/O Worksheet
  Enter I/O in EHR

TABLE E.36

REASSESS AFTER 2ND NS BOLUS

RN Bedside Care
■ Repeat VS
■ Antipyretics as appropriate
■ Assess I/O's, and USG
■ Repeat Dehydration Assessment Tools

Criteria for ORT
■ Significant improvement in Dehydration Assessment Score
■ Emesis resolving
■ Diarrheal output not excessive
■ Laboratory studies not concerning
■ Initiate ORT
  ■ Refer to ORT box
  ■ To print instructions, open link, then right click and
    select print
  ■ Teach the family to document on the I/O Worksheet
  ■ Enter I/O in EHR

Criteria for Continued IV Therapy/Admission
■ Little to no improvement in Dehydration Assessment Score
■ Persistent significant losses
■ Hypoglycemia, significant electrolyte abnormalities

IVF

Consider need for third NS bolus

Moderate dehydration	1.5 × maintenance
Severe dehydration	2 × maintenance

To calculate maintenance mL/h, use patient's weight in kg:
4 mL/kg for the first 10 kg
+ 2 mL/kg for the next 10 kg
+ 1 mL/kg for each kg over 20 kg

Example: 25 kg
4 × 10 = 40
+ 2 × 10 = 20
+ 1 × 5 = 5

Maintenance rate is 65 mL/h
1½ Maintenance is 98 mL/h

TABLE E.37

ORT/REASSESS

RN Bedside Care
■ Repeat VS
■ Antipyretics as appropriate
■ Assess I/O's and USG
■ Repeat Dehydration Assessment Tools

ORT Success
■ Prepare patients and family for discharge

ORT Failure/Admission
■ Patient has received less than half of hourly requirement
■ Patient repeatedly refusing ORT
■ Persistent emesis, significant ongoing losses from diarrhea
■ Reinstitute IVF, admit

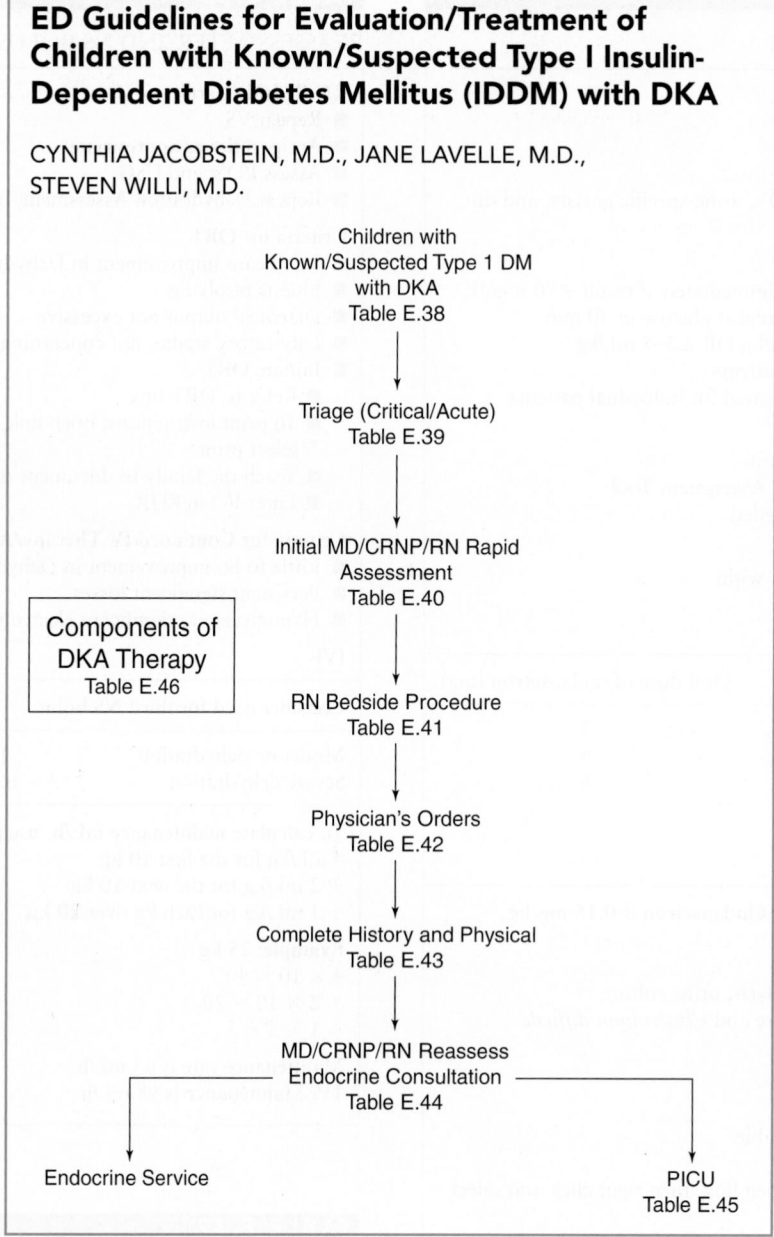

ED Guidelines for Evaluation/Treatment of Children with Known/Suspected Type I Insulin-Dependent Diabetes Mellitus (IDDM) with DKA

CYNTHIA JACOBSTEIN, M.D., JANE LAVELLE, M.D., STEVEN WILLI, M.D.

Children with Known/Suspected Type 1 DM with DKA
Table E.38

↓

Triage (Critical/Acute)
Table E.39

↓

Initial MD/CRNP/RN Rapid Assessment
Table E.40

Components of DKA Therapy
Table E.46

↓

RN Bedside Procedure
Table E.41

↓

Physician's Orders
Table E.42

↓

Complete History and Physical
Table E.43

↓

MD/CRNP/RN Reassess
Endocrine Consultation
Table E.44

Endocrine Service   PICU
Table E.45

TABLE E.38

CHILDREN WITH KNOWN/SUSPECTED TYPE 1 DM WITH DKA

Definition:	
■ Hyperglycemia	Blood sugar >200 mg/dL
■ Acidosis	pH <7.3
■ Ketonuria/Ketonemia	HCO_3 <15 mEq/L

TABLE E.39

TRIAGE (CRITICAL/ACUTE)

Critical	Acute
Hypotension	IDDM with illness:
Abnormal Mental Status	Vomiting
Severe tachycardia, hyperpnea	Fever
(Kussmaul respirations)	H/O hyperglycemia
	H/O ketonuria

TABLE E.40

INITIAL MD/CRNP/RN RAPID ASSESSMENT

History
- Serum glucose levels (home, office, EMS provider)
- Home urine ketones
- Insulin use, most recent dose?
- Insulin pump?
- Other symptoms—fever, vomiting, other

Physical Exam
- Vital signs
- Brief neurologic assessment
  Level of alertness/AVPU/GCS
  Pupils—size and responsiveness
- Respiratory status—distress, hyperpnea, other?
- Perfusion
  Capillary refill
  Pulses

TABLE E.41

RN BEDSIDE PROCEDURE

General
- Place patient on CR monitor
- Begin documentation on DKA flowsheet
- Document vital signs every 15 min

IV Placement
- Discuss the need for IV placement with patient/family, obtain the following specimens:
  Bedside glucose
  Venous blood gas (VBG) or bedside I-stat/other
  Serum electrolytes, glucose, Mg, PO_4
  CBC with differential

Urine Specimens
- Obtain urine for ketones, glucose
- Pregnancy tests in postpubertal girls

IVF Fluids
- Begin normal saline (NS) bolus 10 mL/kg over 30 min

TABLE E.42

PHYSICIAN'S ORDERS

Use the DKA Order Set that includes the following:
Laboratory
  Venous blood gas
  Serum electrolytes with glucose, Mg, PO_4
  CBC with differential
  UA dip
  Bedside glucose
  Urine for HCG (as needed)

IV Fluids
  NS bolus (complete 20 mL/kg bolus)
  Confer with ED physician/provider for subsequent boluses
  Two bag IVF system:
    D_0 NS with 20 mEq KCl/L and 13.6 mmoles KPO_4/L[a]
    D_{10} NS with 20 mEq KCl/L and 13.6 mmoles KPO_4/L

Insulin Infusion
Administer 0.1 units/kg/h of regular insulin (based on standard concentrations of continuous infusion at your institution)
Discontinue the patient's personal insulin pump when the insulin infusion is ready

[a]13.6 mmoles KPO_4 provides 20 mEq of potassium.

TABLE E.43

COMPLETE HISTORY AND PHYSICAL—IDENTIFY POSSIBLE CAUSES FOR DKA

History
- Onset of symptoms
  - If first onset, obtain history of polyuria, polydipsia, amount of weight loss, etc.
- Other systemic symptoms:
  Fever
  Respiratory
  GI/GU
- Recent blood glucose levels, urine ketones, insulin use
- Age at diagnosis of IDDM
- Past history of DKA
- Other PMH
- Medications, allergies

Physical Examination
- Review vital signs
- Complete exam with focus on:
  Airway
  Breathing
  Circulation (perfusion, capillary refill)
  Neurologic system
  Other systems related to complaints

TABLE E.44

MD/CRNP/RN REASSESS

MD/CRNP Reassess
- Mental status, vital signs, I/O
- Review venous blood gas or I-stat, glucose, urine ketones
- Consider 12 lead ECG for patients who have K > 6

Characteristics of High-Risk Patients
Age <5 yr, especially <2 yr
Obtunded or decline in mental status in the ED
pH <7.1
Glucose >1,000 mg/dL
Na (measured) >155 mEq/L or falling calculated Na
K <3.5 mEq/L
- Endocrine consultation
- Evaluate the need for CNS imaging if mental status not good, improving in first few hours of RX.

RN Reassess/Documentation on DKA Flowsheet
- Frequent vital signs (q15min)
- Mental status check (q30min)
- Hourly (time from start of IV)
  Blood glucose
  I/O
- One hour after insulin infusion begins:
  Repeat VBG (or bedside I-stat), serum electrolytes with Mg, PO$_4$
  Repeat these every 2 h as needed, discuss with the MD

TABLE E.45

CRITERIA FOR PICU ADMISSION

- Obtundation, coma, or decline in mental status during therapy
- Uncompensated shock; labile compensated shock
- Respiratory—failure of ability to compensate for metabolic acidosis
- Significant metabolic acidosis

Consider also:
- Age <2 yr
- Glucose >1,000 mg/dL
- Falling corrected serum Na[a] see Table E.46
- Significant hypokalemia (K persistently <3.5 mEq/L)

TABLE E.46

THREE KEY COMPONENTS OF DKA THERAPY

1. **Fluid Therapy**
   NS Resuscitation
   NS bolus 20 mL/kg
   Repeat NS boluses only with EM staff review
   Two Bag System (IVF following the initial saline bolus)
   Bag #1: NS, KCl, KPO$_4$
   Bag #2: Same as bag#1 plus D$_{10}$

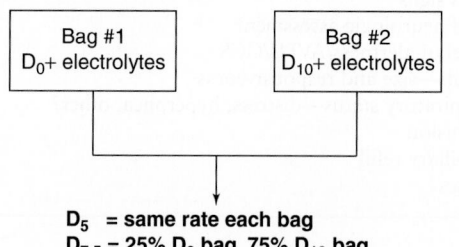

D_5 = same rate each bag
$D_{7.5}$ = 25% D_0 bag, 75% D_{10} bag

Electrolytes

Patient's K mEq/L	mEq KCL/L	mEq KPO$_4$/L	mmol KPO$_4$/L[a]
<3.5	30	30	20.4
3.5–5	20	20	13.6
5–6	10	10	6.8
>6	0	0	0

Dextrose
Start dextrose when the patient's glucose is <300 mg/dL
Change dextrose delivered by changing flow rates of the two bags

Rate
Run IVF at 1½ maintenance rate based on patient weight
To calculate maintenance cc/h, use patient's weight in kg:
4 mL/kg for the first 10 kg
+ 2 mL/kg for the next 10 kg
+ 1 mL/kg for each kg over 20 kg

Example: 25 kg
4 × 10 = 40
+ 2 × 10 = 20
+ 1 × 5 = 5
Maintenance rate is 65 mL/h
1½ Maintenance is 98 mL/h
2. **Insulin Infusion**
   Regular insulin at rate of 0.1 unit/kg/h
   No insulin boluses
   Goal—Drop glucose by 50–100 mg/dL every hour
3. **Reassessment**
   Frequent vital signs (q15min)
   Mental status check (q30min)

Hourly:
Blood glucose
I/O

One hour after insulin infusion begins:
Repeat VBG or I-stat as needed, serum electrolytes with Mg, PO$_4$
http://www.guidelines.gov/summary/summary.aspx?doc_id=6826&nbr=004193&string=dka

[a]Formula for correction of serum Na: Na$_{corrected}$ = Na$_{measured}$ + 1.6 × [Serum glucose − 100]/100

ED Evaluation of Children with Suspected Appendicitis without Known GI Disease

JANE LAVELLE, M.D., MICHAEL NANCE, M.D., KASSA DARGE, M.D., MARK JOFFE, M.D.

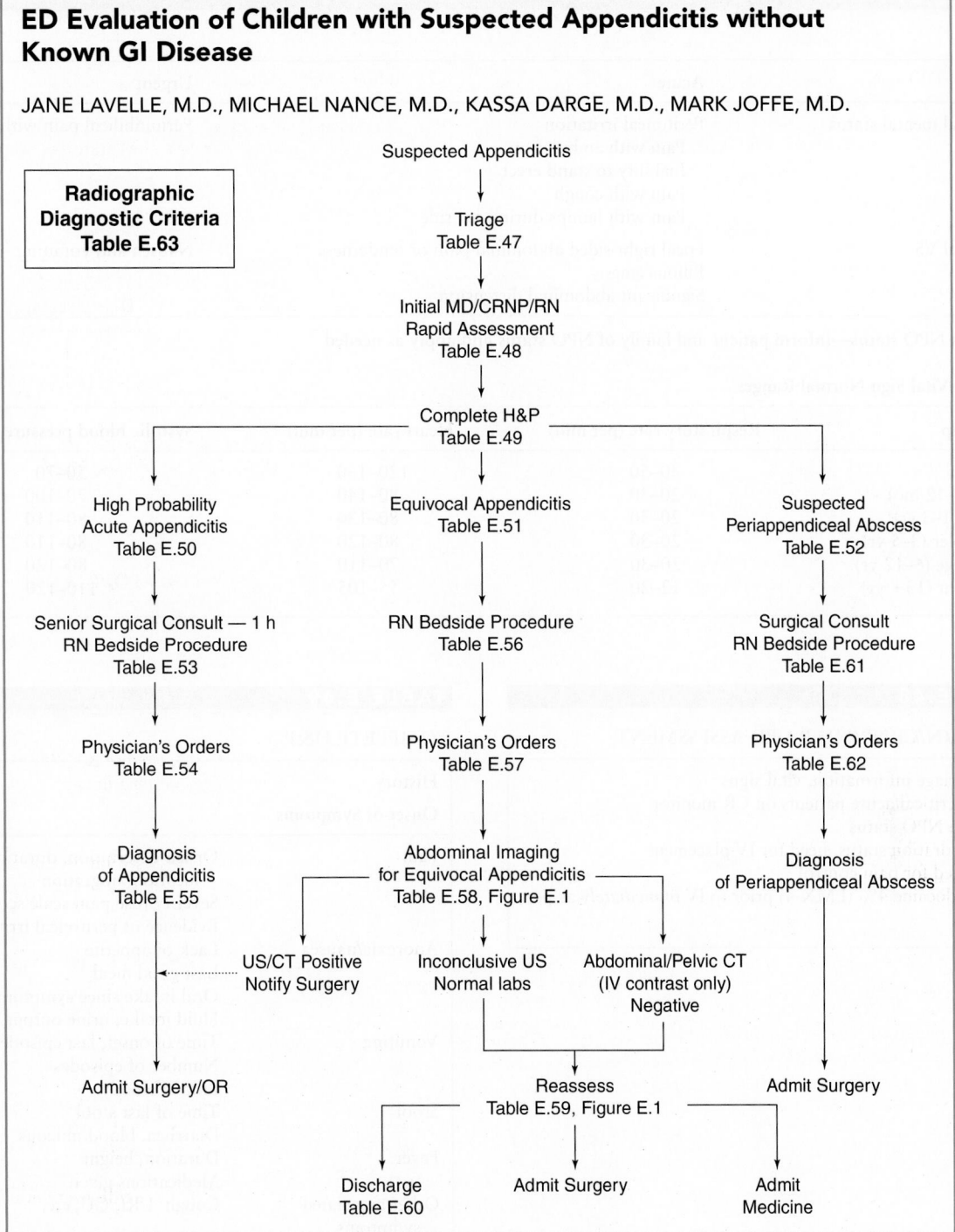

TABLE E.47

TRIAGE

Critical	Acute	Urgent
Abnormal mental status	Peritoneal irritation 　Pain with ambulation 　Inability to stand erect 　Pain with cough 　Pain with bumps during car ride	Periumbilical pain with anorexia
Abnormal VS	Focal right-sided abdominal pain or tenderness Bilious emesis Significant abdominal distension	Nausea and vomiting

Maintain NPO status—Inform patient and family of NPO status and apply as needed

Pediatric Vital Sign Normal Ranges

Age group	Respiratory rate (per min)	Heart rate (per min)	Systolic blood pressure (mm Hg)
Newborn	30–50	120–160	50–70
Infant (1–12 mo)	20–30	80–140	70–100
Toddler (1–3 yr)	20–30	80–130	80–110
Preschooler (3–5 yr)	20–30	80–120	80–110
School Age (6–12 yr)	20–30	70–110	80–120
Adolescent (13+ yr)	12–20	55–105	110–120

TABLE E.48

INITIAL RN/CRNP/MD RAPID ASSESSMENT

Review triage information, vital signs
Place all critical/acute patients on CR monitor
Reinforce NPO status
Assess hydration status, need for IV placement
Assess need for pain control
Apply Lidocaine 4% (LMX-4) prior to IV *immediately* as per protocol

TABLE E.49

COMPLETE H&P

History **Onset of Symptoms**	
Pain	Onset, description, duration, location, migration Severity (use pain scale score) Evidence of peritoneal irritation
Anorexia/nausea	Lack of appetite Last good meal Oral intake since symptom onset Fluid intake, urine output
Vomiting	Time of onset, last episode Number of episodes Bilious/bloody
Stool	Time of last stool Diarrhea, blood/mucous
Fever	Duration, height Medications given
Other associated symptoms	Cough, URI, GU, etc.
Past medical history	Prior abdominal pain episodes
Physical Examination **General Appearance,** **Vital Signs**	
Abdomen	Focal tenderness, guarding/rebound, distension Psoas, obturator, Rovsing's signs CVA tenderness
Genital	Tanner stage Inguinal canal abnormality Scrotum/testicles abnormalities Bimanual exam, as indicated Rectal exam, as indicated

TABLE E.50

HIGH-PROBABILITY ACUTE APPENDICITIS

RLQ tenderness with or without rebound
Pain with movement (cough, car ride, jumping on right foot)
Symptoms less than 24–48 h
Anorexia, followed by vomiting
Pain **preceding** vomiting
Migration of pain from periumbilical region to RLQ

TABLE E.51

EQUIVOCAL ACUTE APPENDICITIS

Presenting with focal abdominal tenderness (usually right-sided) with variable number of the features of high-probability acute appendicitis

TABLE E.52

SUSPECTED PERIAPPENDICEAL ABSCESS

Systemic toxicity
Fever
Symptoms >48–72 h
Diffuse abdominal tenderness and guarding
Urinary and/or rectal urgency
Palpable RLQ mass
WBC, ANC, CRP consistent with marked inflammation

TABLE E.53

SENIOR SURGICAL CONSULT/RN BEDSIDE PROCEDURE

Senior Surgical Consultation
- Goal—Surgery fellow/attending to evaluate patient **within 30–60 min**

RN Bedside Procedure
General
- Place critical/acute patients on CR monitor
- Document VS q1h
- Document IVF, voids, urine concentration specific gravity

IV Placement
Discuss the need for IV placement with patient/family, obtain the following specimens:
- CBC, C-reactive protein, serum electrolytes and glucose, other as indicated.
- Consider need for bedside glucose testing
- Blood culture for toxic patients

Urine Specimens
- Urinalysis (i.e., urine dip or laboratory)
- Urine HCG (for girls ≥12 yr of age).

IVF Fluids
Begin NS bolus 20 mL/kg over 60 min

TABLE E.54

USE PHYSICIAN'S ORDERS FOR SUSPECTED APPENDICITIS

Laboratory
CBC with differential, C-reactive protein, electrolytes and glucose
Urinalysis or UA dip, Urine HCG

IV Fluids
NS bolus 20 mL/kg; repeat as needed
Continued fluids:
Use D_5 ½ NS with 20mEq KCl/L (add KCl after patient urinates)
Rate 1½ maintenance

To calculate maintenance mL/h, use patient's weight in kg:
4 mL/kg for the first 10 kg
+ 2 mL/kg for the next 10 kg
+ 1 mL/kg for each kg over 20 kg

Example: 25 kg
4 × 10 = 40
+ 2 × 10 = 20
+ 1 × 5 = 5
Maintenance rate is 65 mL/h
1½ Maintenance is 98 mL/h

Analgesia
Assess pain and treat with parenteral medication

Antibiotics with high-risk appendicitis preoperatively or with abscess to be admitted.

Administer:
Unasyn® (ampicillin/sulbactam) Dose—50 mg/kg ampicillin component up to 2 g IV
Clindamycin (in PCN allergic patients)—10–15 mg/kg (maximum 600 mg) IV

TABLE E.55

DIAGNOSIS OF APPENDICITIS

Other Criteria Supporting High Probability
- ANC > 6,750
- CRP > 2
- WBC > normal for age
- Negative UA
- Fecalith

Further Radiographic Testing
The need for further imaging should be discussed between responsible ED staff and surgical consult. Ultrasound is the study of choice for nonobese patients. Its advantages include lack of patient exposure to ionizing radiation, as well as evaluation of ovarian anatomy and flow.

Optimal study in nonobese patients	Ultrasound
Alternative choice	Abdominal/pelvic CT with IV contrast only
	Use pediatric CT settings to minimize radiation exposure

TABLE E.56

RN BEDSIDE PROCEDURE

General
Place critical/acute patients on CR monitor
Document vital signs as per protocol
Document IVF, urine output and urinalysis with specific gravity

IV Placement
Discuss the need for IV placement with patient/family, obtain the following specimens:
  CBC, C-reactive protein, electrolytes, and glucose
  Consider need for bedside glucose
  Blood culture for toxic patients

Urine Specimens
Urine dip
If urine dip is positive, send for formal lab UA
Send urine culture if formal lab UA suggests UTI

For postpubertal girls add:
Urine pregnancy test
Consider urine screen for GC/Chlamydia

IVF Fluids
Begin NS bolus 20 mL/kg
Prepare for bladder catheterization as per US-Foley protocol

TABLE E.57

PHYSICIAN'S ORDERS

Use ED Physician's Orders for Suspected Appendicitis

Laboratory
CBC, C-reactive protein, electrolytes and glucose.
UA dip
Urine for HCG, culture and screen for GC/Chlamydia as needed

Radiology
Consider obstruction series
See Abdominal Imaging for radiographic study indicated (Figure E.1)

IV Fluids
NS bolus 20 mL/kg; repeat as needed
Continued fluids:
Use D_5 ½ NS with 20mEq KCl/L (add KCl after patient urinates)
Rate 1½ maintenance

To calculate maintenance mL/h, use patient's weight in kg:
4 mL/kg for the first 10 kg
+ 2 mL/kg for the next 10 kg
+ 1 mL/kg for each kg over 20 kg

Example: 25 kg
$4 \times 10 = 40$
$+ 2 \times 10 = 20$
$+ 1 \times 5 = 5$
Maintenance rate is 65 mL/h
1½ Maintenance is 98 mL/h

Analgesia
Assess pain and treat

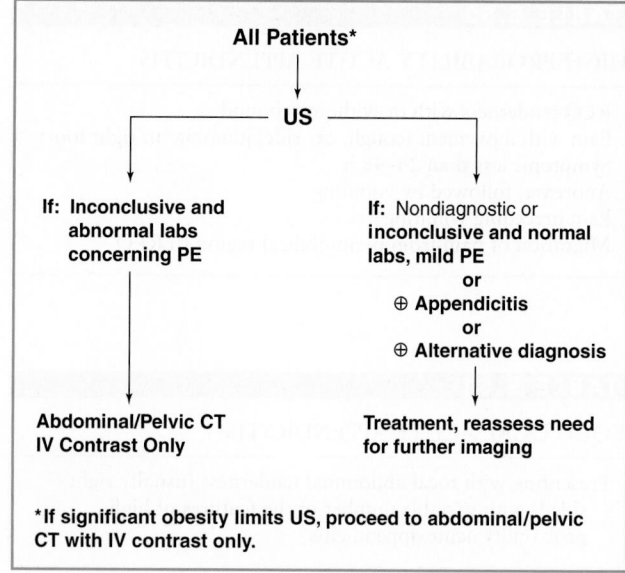

FIGURE E.1 Abdominal Imaging for Equivocal Appendicitis.

TABLE E.58

ORDERS FOR ABDOMINAL IMAGING

US	Male	Limited abdomen, focus on RLQ
	Female	Limited abdomen, focus on RLQ
		Pelvic with Doppler study

Abdominal/pelvic CT IV Contrast Only

TABLE E.59

REASSESS

- VS, pain, abdominal exam
- Review all laboratory and radiology studies
- Reassess need for further imaging with abdominal/pelvic CT with IV contrast only
- Consider other diagnoses vs. very early appendicitis
- Complete surgical consultation, as needed
- Consider po challenge as clinically indicated

Negative Predictors for Appendicitis
- WBC <10,000/μL
- ANC <6,750/μL
- No percussion tenderness on physical examination
- No guarding on physical examination
- No nausea, emesis

Patients with symptoms >24 h, CRP <2, and ANC < 6,750 are highly unlikely to have acute appendicitis

TABLE E.60

DISCHARGE

Anticipatory Guidance
Return to MD for persistent/worsening symptoms
Monitor hydration
Analgesia instructions
Treatment for disease identified
Use discharge instructions for abdominal pain

TABLE E.61

SURGICAL CONSULT/RN BEDSIDE PROCEDURE

Surgical Consult
Consult surgery resident/fellow/attending for suspected acute
    abdomen, especially with potential periappendiceal abscess

RN Bedside Procedure
General
Place critical/acute patients on CR monitor
Document vital signs as per protocol
Document IVF, urine output, urine specific gravity

IV Placement
Discuss the need for IV placement with patient/family, obtain
    the following specimens:
    CBC, C-reactive protein, serum electrolytes, with glucose
    Consider need for bedside glucose
    Blood culture for toxic patients

Urine Specimens
    Urine dip
    Urine HCG

IVF Fluids
Begin NS bolus 20 mL/kg over 30–60 min

TABLE E.62

PHYSICIAN'S ORDERS WITH SUSPECTED ABSCESS

Use Physician's Orders for Suspected Periappendiceal Abscess
Laboratory
CBC, CRP, electrolytes and glucose
UA dip, Urine HCG

Radiology
Order abdominal/pelvic CT with oral and PO contrast at 0 h
    and 2 h, and IV contrast

IV Fluids
NS bolus 20 mL/kg; repeat as needed
Continued fluids:
Use D_5 ½ NS with 20 mEq KCl/L (add KCl after patient uri-
    nates)
Rate 1½ maintenance

To calculate maintenance mL/h, use patient's weight in kg:
4 mL/kg for the first 10 kg
+ 2 mL/kg for the next 10 kg
+ 1 mL/kg for each kg over 20 kg

Example: 25 kg
$4 \times 10 = 40$
$+ 2 \times 10 = 20$
$+ 1 \times 5 = 5$
Maintenance rate is 65 mL/h
1½ Maintenance is 98 mL/h

Analgesia
Assess pain and treat

Antibiotics
Administer:
    Unasyn (dosing noted) + Gentamycin (2–2.5 mg/kg, max
        120 mg)
    Clindamycin + Gentamycin (PCN allergic patients)

TABLE E.63

RADIOGRAPHIC DIAGNOSTIC CRITERIA

Ultrasound
Positive for Appendicitis
Noncompressible fluid-filled distended tubular structure with
    diameter ≥ 6 mm
With or without an appendicolith
No peristaltic activity
Constant shape and position
Anterior to the psoas muscle or in the retrocecal position
Suggestive for Appendicitis
Pericecal inflammatory changes in the absence of visualizing
    an abnormal appendix

CT
Positive for Appendicitis
Enlarged appendix >6 mm
Nonopacified appendiceal lumen
Significant wall enhancement with IV contrast material
Periappendiceal fat stranding
Appendicolith
Free fluid or abscess in RLQ/pelvis
Focal cecal wall thickening

References

Asthma

National Asthma Education and Prevention Program. Expert Panel Report 3: Guidelines for the Diagnosis and Management of Asthma. Full Report 2007. U.S. Department of Health and Human Services, National Institute of Health, National Heart, Lung, and Blood Institute. http://www.nhlbi.nih. gov/guidelines/asthma/asthgdln.htm.

Scarfone RJ, Fuchs SM, Nager AL, et al. Controlled trial of oral prednisone in the emergency department treatment of children with acute asthma. *Pediatrics* 1993;92(4):513–518.

Zorc JJ, Scarfone RJ, Li Y, et al. Scheduled follow-up after a pediatric emergency department visit for asthma: a randomized trial. *Pediatrics* 2003;111:495.

Bronchiolitis

Bordley WC, Viswanathan M, King VJ, et al. Diagnosis and testing in bronchiolitis. *Arch Pediatr Adolesc Med* 2004;158:119.

Corneli MC, Zorc JJ, Mahajan P, et al. A mulicenter, randomized, controlled trial of dexamethasone for bronchiolitis. *N Engl J Med* 2008;359:1972.

Diagnosis and Management of Bronchiolitis, Clinical Practice Guideline, Subcommittee on the Diagnosis and Management of Bronchiolitis, 2003–2006. American Academy of Pediatrics. http://www.pediatrics.org/cgi/dai/10.1542/peds.2006–2223.

Schuh S, Lalani A, Allen U, et al. Evaluation of the utility of radiography in acute bronchiolitis. *J Pediatr* 2007;150:429.

Dehydration

Freedman SB, Adler M, Seshadri R, et al. Oral ondansetron for gastroenteritis in a pediatric emergency department. *N Engl J Med* 2006;354:1698–1705.

King CK, Glass R, Bresee JS, et al. Managing acute gastroenteritis among children: oral rehydration, maintenance, and nutritional therapy. *MMWR Recomm Rep* 2003;52(RR-16):1–16.

Spandorfer PR, Alessandrini EA, Joffe MD, et al. Oral versus intravenous rehydration of moderately dehydrated children: a randomized, controlled trial. *Pediatrics* 2005;115(2):295–301. doi:10.1542/peds.2004–0245.

Stork CM, Brown KM, Reilly TH, et al. Emergency department treatment of viral gastritis using intravenous ondansetron or dexamethasone in children. *Acad Emerg Med* 2006;13(10):1027–1033.

Diabetic Ketoacidosis

Agus MS, Wolfsdorf JI. Diabetic ketoacidosis in children. *Pediatr Clin North Am* 2005;52(4):1147–1163.

Dunger DB, Sperling MA, Acerini CL, et al. European society for paediatric endocrinology/lawson wilkins pediatric endocrine society consensus statement on diabetic ketoacidosis in children and adolescents. *Pediatrics* 2004;113(2):e133–e140.

Glaser N, Barnet P, McCaslin I, et al. Risk factors for cerebral edema in children with diabetic ketoacidosis. The Pediatric Emergency Medicine Collaborative Research Committee of the American Academy of Pediatrics. *N Engl J Med* 2001;344:264–269.

Wolfsdorf J, Craig ME, Daneman D, et al. Diabetic ketoacidosis in children and adolescents with diabetes. *Pediatr Diabetes* 2009;10(Suppl 12): 118–133.

Appendicitis

Bundy DG, Byerley JS, et al. Does this child have appendicitis? *JAMA* 2007;298(4):438.

Kharbanda AB, Taylor GA, Bachur RG. Suspected appendicitis in children: rectal and intravenous contrast-enhanced versus intravenous contrast-enhanced CT. *Radiology* 2007;243(2):520.

Kharbanda AB, Taylor GA, Fishman SJ, et al. A clinical decision rule to identify children at low risk for appendicitis. *Pediatrics* 2005;116(3):709–716.

Kwok MY, Kim MK, Gorelick MH. Evidence-based approach to the diagnosis of appendicitis in children. *Pediatr Emerg Care* 2004;20(10):690.

Rothrock SG, Pagnane J. Acute appendicitis in children: emergency department diagnosis and management. *Ann Emerg Med* 2000:36:39–51.

Pages followed by *f* indicate figures; pages followed by *t* indicate tables.